Antiparasitic Drugs in Small Animal Practice: Spectrum of Activity

Etienne Côté, DVM, DACVIM
Dwight D. Bowman, PhD

Disclaimer: These data are based on reported efficacies and personal experience. Several products and/or indications are not approved for use in small animals by the Food and Drug Administration. Any drug may be listed as efficacious but pose a risk of toxicosis in certain individuals of a species or all individuals of other species. Several drugs carry risks of adverse effects. The clinician using or advocating the use of any product bears the responsibility for becoming fully informed regarding possible limitations, adverse effects, warnings, or contraindications, and acting accordingly. It is the responsibility of the veterinarian using or advocating the use of these drugs to properly and completely research all the relevant characteristics of any of these drugs and to act in the patient's best interest.

	Ectoparasites							Endoparasites: heartworm			Endoparasites: gastrointestinal								Endoparasites: respiratory					
Drug **Commercial name (generic name)**	Flea adulticide	Flea preventative	Ticks	Sarcoptes	Demodex	Cheyletiella	Ear mites	Heartworm preventative	Heartworm microfilaricide	Heartworm adulticide	Roundworms	Hookworms	Tapeworms	Whipworms	Giardia	Cryptosporidium	Paragonimus	Tritrichomonas	Capillaria	Crenosoma	Oslerus	Filaroides	Nasal mite	Aelurostrongylus
Acarexx (ivermectin topical)							•																	
Advantage (imidacloprid)	•	•																						
Advocate/Advantage Multi (imidacloprid + moxidectin)	•	•		•	•		•	•			•	•		•										
Capstar (nitenpyram)	•																							
Droncit (praziquantel)													•											
Drontal (praziquantel + pyrantel)											•	•	•											
Drontal Plus (praziquantel + pyrantel + febantel)											•	•	•	•	•									
Filaribits (diethylcarbamazine)								•																
Flagyl (metronidazole)															•									
Frontline (fipronil)	•	•	•	•		•																		
HeartGard (ivermectin 0.006 mg/kg)								•	•															
HeartGard Plus (ivermectin + pyrantel)								•	•		•	•												
Immiticide (melarsomine)										•														
Interceptor (milbemycin)				•	•	•		•	•		•	•		•									•	
Ivomec (ivermectin 0.2 mg/kg PO or IM)				•	•	•	•	•	•		±	•							•	•	•		•	
Levamisole (several brand names)									•										•	•		•		•
Milbemite (milbemycin topical)							•																	
Panacur (fenbendazole)											•	•		•	•		•		•	•		•		•
Program (lufenuron)		•																						
ProHeart (moxidectin) (1)					•			•																
Pyrantel (several brand names)											•	•												
Pyrethrin/pyrethroids (several brand names)	•		±			•	•																	
Revolution (selamectin)	•	•	±	•		•	•	•	•		•	•												•
Sentinel (milbemycin + lufenuron)		•		•	•	•		•	•		•	•		•						•			•	
Valbazen (albendazole)															•		•		•			•		

(1) Extensive reports of life threatening or fatal adverse reaction with sustained-release (6-month duration) injection
±: documented efficacy against some species or types but not others

Glossary: parasites
Fleas: *Ctenocephalides felis*; Sarcoptes: scabies (*Sarcoptes scabei*); Ear mites: *Otodectes cynotis*; Heartworm: *Dirofilaria immitis*; Hookworms: *Ancylostoma caninum, Uncinaria* spp.; Roundworms: *Toxocara canis, Toxocara felis, Toxascaris leonina*; Tapeworms: *Dipylidium caninum, Taenia* spp.; Whipworms: *Trichuris vulpis*; Nasal mite: *Pneumonyssoides caninum*

Vicki Ambrose
ambrose35@gmail.com

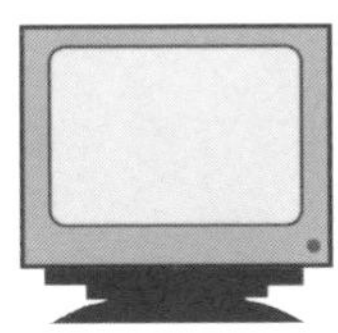

To access **Côté's *Clinical Veterinary Advisor: Dogs and Cats Online***, please scratch off the area below for your unique password.
Then log in at: http://www.cote.clinicalvetadvisor.com/

Please enter the following serial number when prompted:
SCRATCH OFF BELOW

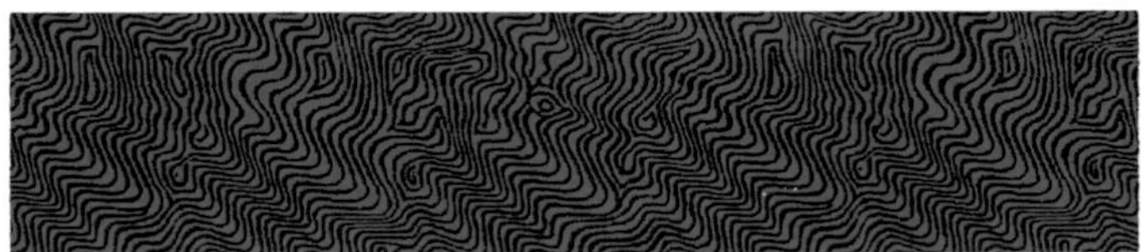

THIS SERIAL NUMBER IS FOR ONE-TIME USE ONLY.

When you have accessed the site, you will be prompted to set up your user name and password. You will also need to provide your e-mail address. Once you have followed these steps, you will be able to access the website.

Important note: Purchase of this book includes access to the online version of this edition for use exclusively by the individual purchaser from the launch of the site. This license and access to the online version operates strictly on the basis of a single user per PIN number. The sharing of passwords is strictly prohibited, and any attempt to do so will invalidate the password. Access to this site is available until the next edition publishes.

Technical Support
Technical support for this product is available between 7:30 a.m. and 7 p.m. CST, Monday through Friday. Inside the United States, call 1-800-692-9010. Outside the United States, call 314-872-8370. You may also fax your questions to +1-314-997-5080 or e-mail Technical Support at: technical.support@elsevier.com.

Part Number: 9996046826

CLINICAL VETERINARY ADVISOR

Dogs and Cats

Editor-in-Chief

Etienne Côté
Assistant Professor
Department of Companion Animals
Atlantic Veterinary College
University of Prince Edward Island
Charlottetown, Prince Edward Island, Canada

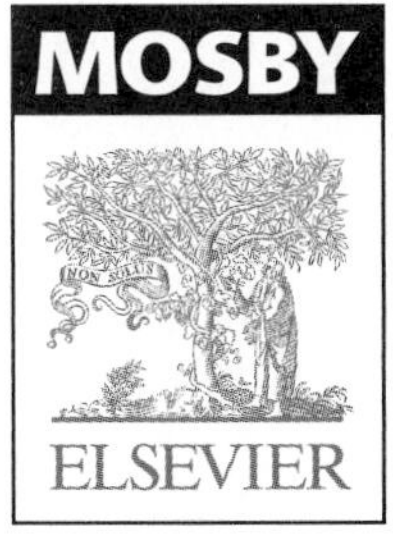

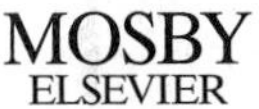

11830 Westline Industrial Drive
St. Louis, Missouri 63146

CLINICAL VETERINARY ADVISOR: DOGS AND CATS

ISBN-13: 978-0-323-03698-6
ISBN-10: 0-323-03698-8

Notice

Knowledge and best practice in this field are constantly changing. As new research and experience broaden our knowledge, changes in practice, treatment and drug therapy may become necessary or appropriate. Readers are advised to check the most current information provided (i) on procedures featured or (ii) by the manufacturer of each product to be administered, to verify the recommended dose or formula, the method and duration of administration, and contraindications. It is the responsibility of the practitioner, relying on their own experience and knowledge of the patient, to make diagnoses, to determine dosages and the best treatment for each individual patient, and to take all appropriate safety precautions. To the fullest extent of the law, neither the Publisher nor the Editors assumes any liability for any injury and/or damage to persons or property arising out or related to any use of the material contained in this book.

The Publisher

ISBN-13: 978-0-323-03698-6
ISBN-10: 0-323-03698-8

Publishing Director: Linda Duncan
Veterinary Publisher: Penny Rudolph
Managing Editor: Jolynn Gower
Publishing Services Manager: Melissa Lastarria
Senior Project Manager: Joy Moore
Design Direction: Mark Oberkrom

Printed in the United States of America

Last digit is the print number: 9 8 7 6 5 4 3 2 1

Editor-in-Chief

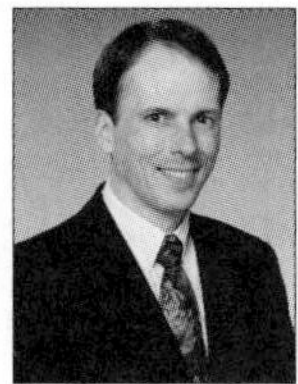

Etienne Côté, DVM, DACVIM (Cardiology, SAIM)
Cardiology, Chief Complaints, Procedures and Techniques, Differential Diagnosis
Assistant Professor
Department of Companion Animals
Atlantic Veterinary College
University of Prince Edward Island
Charlottetown, Prince Edward Island, Canada

Editors

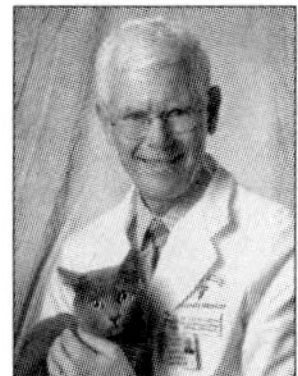

C. A. Tony Buffington, DVM, PhD, DACVN
Nutrition
Professor of Veterinary Clinical Sciences
Veterinary Teaching Hospital
The Ohio State University
Columbus, Ohio

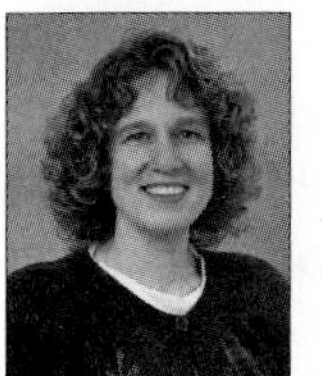

Leah A. Cohn, DVM, PhD, DACVIM (SAIM)
Urology
Associate Professor
Department of Veterinary Medicine and Surgery
College of Veterinary Medicine
University of Missouri
Columbia, Missouri

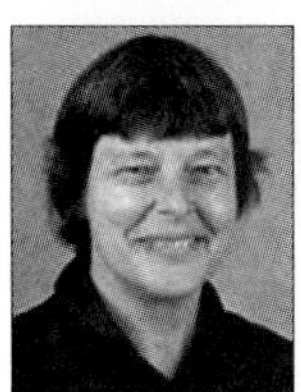

Susan M. Cotter, DVM, DACVIM (SAIM, Oncology)
Hematologic/Immunologic
Distinguished Professor
Department of Clinical Sciences
Cummings School of Veterinary Medicine
Tufts University
North Grafton, Massachusetts

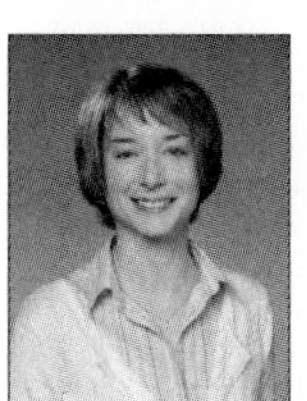

Cheryl L. Cullen, DVM, MVetSc, DACVO
Ophthalmology
Clinical Associate Professor, Comparative Ophthalmology
Department of Companion Animals
Atlantic Veterinary College
University of Prince Edward Island
Charlottetown, Prince Edward Island, Canada

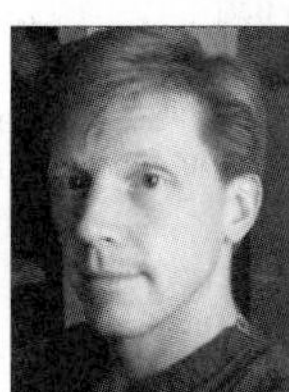

Curtis W. Dewey, DVM, MS, DACVIM (Neurology), DACVS
Neurology
Associate Professor, Neurology/Neurosurgery
Department of Clinical Sciences
Hospital for Animals
Cornell University
Ithaca, New York

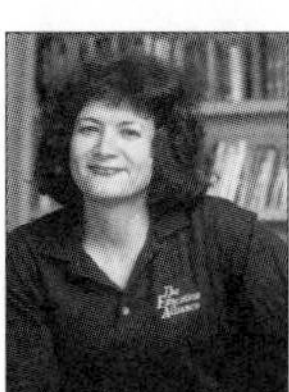

Jan A. Hall, BVM&S, MS, MRCVS, DACVD
Dermatology
Assistant Professor
Department of Clinical Studies
Ontario Veterinary College
Guelph, Ontario, Canada

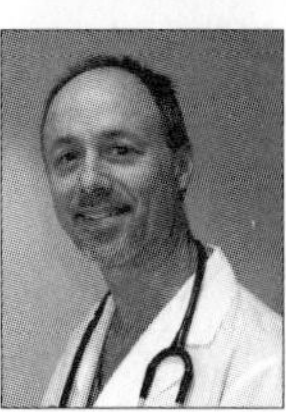

Joseph Harari, DVM, MS, DACVS
Orthopedics
Veterinary Surgical Specialists
Spokane, Washington

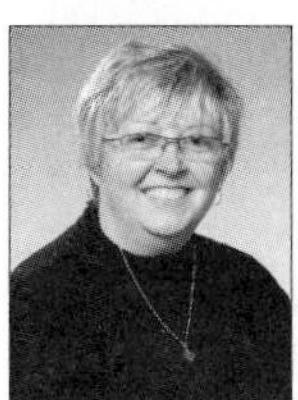

Sherri Ihle, DVM, MSc, DACVIM (SAIM)
Endocrinology
Associate Professor of Small Animal Medicine
Department of Companion Animals
Atlantic Veterinary College
University of Prince Edward Island
Charlottetown, Prince Edward Island, Canada

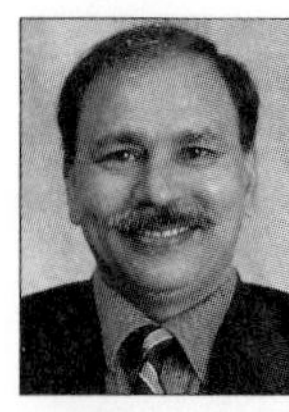

Safdar A. Khan, DVM, MS, PhD, DABVT
Toxicology
Director of Toxicology Research
ASPCA Animal Poison Control Center
Urbana, Illinois

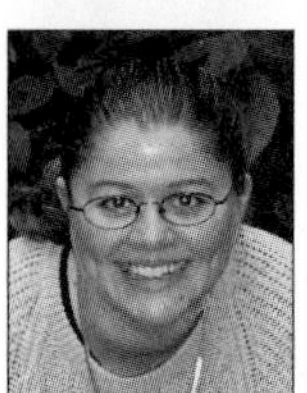

Michelle A. Kutzler, DVM, PhD, DACT
Theriogenology
Assistant Professor
Clinical Sciences
Oregon State University
College of Veterinary Medicine
Corvallis, Oregon

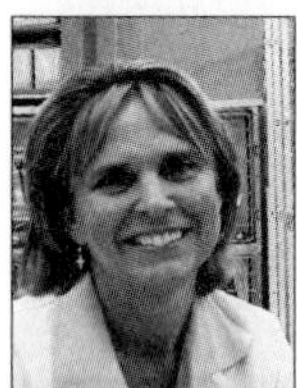

Douglass K. Macintire, DVM, MS, DACVIM (SAIM), DACVECC
Infectious Diseases
Professor of Acute Medicine and Critical Care
Department of Clinical Sciences
College of Veterinary Medicine
Auburn University
Auburn, Alabama

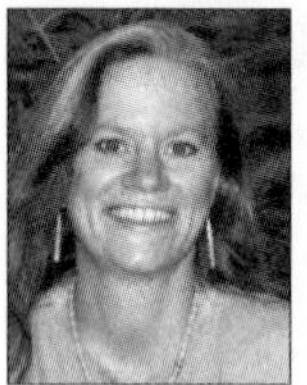

Karen L. Overall, MA, VMD, PhD, DACVB
Behavior
Center for Neurobiology and Behavior
Psychiatry Department
School of Medicine
University of Pennsylvania
Philadelphia, Pennsylvania

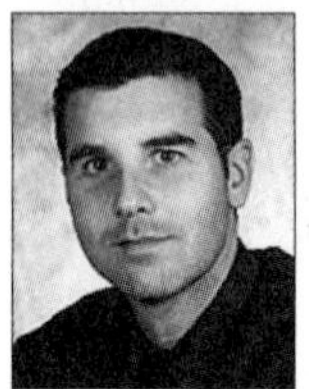

Kenneth M. Rassnick, DVM, DACVIM (Oncology)
Oncology
Assistant Professor of Oncology
College of Veterinary Medicine
Cornell University
Ithaca, New York

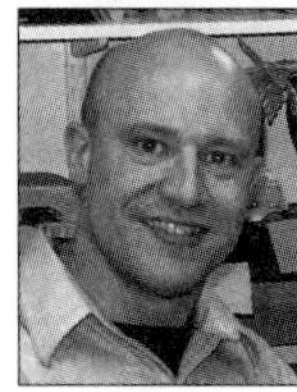

Alexander M. Reiter, DMV, Dipl-Tzt, DAVDC, DEVDC
Dentistry
Assistant Professor of Dentistry and Oral Surgery
School of Veterinary Medicine
University of Pennsylvania
Philadelphia, Pennsylvania

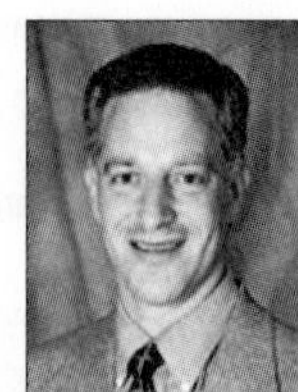

Keith P. Richter, DVM, DACVIM (SAIM)
Hepatic-Pancreatic
Veterinary Specialty Hospital of San Diego
San Diego, California

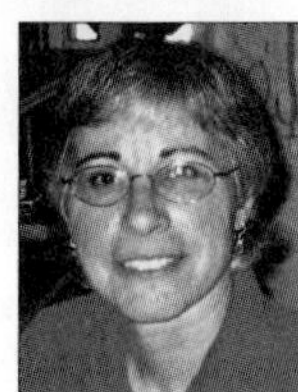

Lois Roth-Johnson, DVM, PhD, DACVP
Laboratory Tests
Pathologist
IDEXX Laboratories
North Grafton, Massachusetts

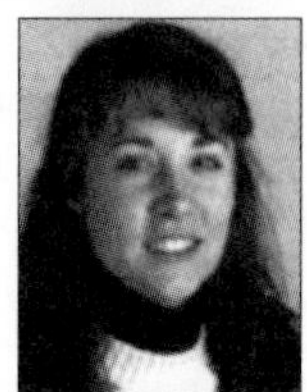

Elizabeth Rozanski, DVM, DACVECC, DACVIM (SAIM)
Emergency and Critical Care
Assistant Professor
Cummings School of Veterinary Medicine
Tufts University
North Grafton, Massachusetts

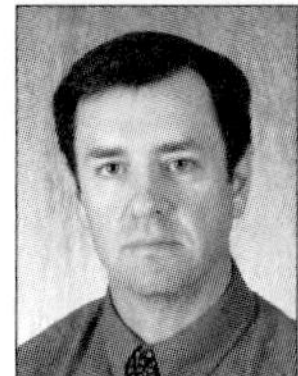

Rance K. Sellon, DVM, PhD, DACVIM (SAIM)
Respiratory Disorders
Associate Professor
Department of Veterinary Clinical Sciences
Washington State University
Pullman, Washington

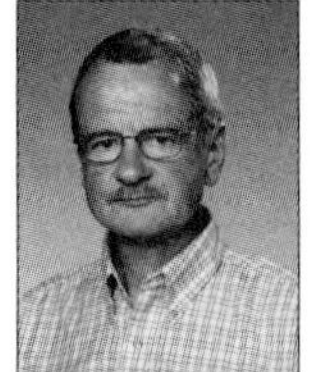

Richard Walshaw, BVMS, DACVS
Soft Tissue Surgery
Professor, Companion Animal Surgery
Department of Companion Animals
Atlantic Veterinary College
University of Prince Edward Island
Charlottetown, Prince Edward Island, Canada

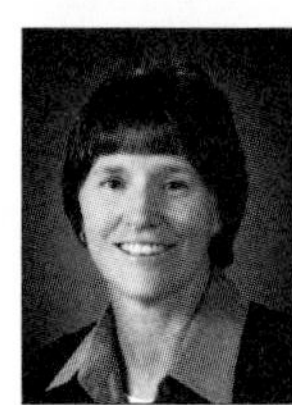

Debra L. Zoran, DVM, MS, PhD, DACVIM (SAIM)
Gastroenterology
Clinical Associate Professor
Texas A&M University
College Station, Texas

Contributors

Kirsten Aarbo, DVM
Woodstock Veterinary Hospital
Woodstock, Vermont

Jonathan A. Abbott, DVM, DACVIM
Associate Professor
Department of Small Animal Clinical Sciences
Virginia-Maryland Regional College of Veterinary Medicine
Virginia Polytechnic Institute and State University
Blacksburg, Virginia

Lisa M. Abbott, DVM
Resident, Emergency and Critical Care
Southern Oregon Veterinary Specialty Center
Medford, Oregon

Sarah K. Abood, DVM, PhD
Coordinator, Student Programs
Assistant Professor
Small Animal Clinical Sciences
College of Veterinary Medicine
Michigan State University
East Lansing, Michigan

Christopher A. Adin, DVM, DACVS
Assistant Professor of Surgery
Department of Clinical Sciences
College of Veterinary Medicine
University of Florida
Gainesville, Florida

Darcy B. Adin, DVM, DACVIM (Cardiology)
Veterinary Specialists of Rochester
Rochester, New York

Sarah Allen, DVM
Angell Animal Medical Center
Boston, Massachusetts

Robin W. Allison, DVM, PhD, DACVP
Assistant Professor
Department of Veterinary Pathobiology
Oklahoma State University
Stillwater, Oklahoma

Amanda P. Amaratunga, DVM
Associate Veterinarian
Boyne Veterinary Clinic
Alliston, Ontario, Canada

Jamie G. Anderson, RDH, DVM, MS, DAVDC, DACVIM (SAIM)
Co-Owner, San Francisco Veterinary Specialists
San Francisco, California

Elizabeth A. Armitage, VetMB, MA, MRCVS
Anesthesia Resident
Department of Clinical Sciences
Cummings School of Veterinary Medicine
Tufts University
North Grafton, Massachusetts

Clarke E. Atkins, DVM, DACVIM (SAIM, Cardiology)
Professor of Medicine and Cardiology
Department of Clinical Sciences
College of Veterinary Medicine
North Carolina State University
Raleigh, North Carolina

Todd W. Axlund, DVM, MS, DACVIM (Neurology)
Associate Professor, Neurology and Neurosurgery
Department of Clinical Sciences
College of Veterinary Medicine
Auburn University
Auburn, Alabama

Jonathan Bach, DVM
Department of Clinical Sciences
Cummings School of Veterinary Medicine
Tufts University
North Grafton, Massachusetts

Dennis B. Bailey, DVM, DACVIM (Oncology)
Long Island Veterinary Specialists
Plainview, New York

Raviv J. Balfour, DVM, DACVS
Animal Surgical Emergency Center
Los Angeles, California

Carsten Bandt, DVM
Resident, Emergency Critical Care Department
Cummings School of Veterinary Medicine
Tufts University
North Grafton, Massachusetts

Lisa G. Barber, DVM, DACVIM (Oncology)
Assistant Professor
Department of Clinical Sciences
Cummings School of Veterinary Medicine
Tufts University
North Grafton, Massachusetts

Georgina Barone, DVM, DACVIM (Neurology)
Staff Neurologist
Long Island Veterinary Specialists
Plainview, New York

Kirstie A. Barrett, DVM, DACVIM (Cardiology)
California Animal Hospital
Los Angeles, California

Cary L. M. Bassett, DVM, PhD, DACVIM (SAIM)
Small Animal Internist
Carolina Veterinary Specialists
Greensboro, North Carolina

Jeff D. Bay, DVM, DACVIM (SAIM)
Wisconsin Veterinary Referral Center
Waukesha, Wisconsin

Daniela Bedenice, DMV, DACVIM (SAIM)
Assistant Professor
Department of Clinical Sciences
Cummings School of Veterinary Medicine
Tufts University
North Grafton, Massachusetts

Marie-Claude Bélanger, DVM, MS, DACVIM (SAIM)
Assistant Professor
Department of Clinical Sciences
Faculty of Veterinary Medicine
University of Montreal
St-Hyacinthe, Québec, Canada

Ellison Bentley, DVM, DACVO
Clinical Assistant Professor, Comparative Ophthalmology
School of Veterinary Medicine
University of Wisconsin-Madison
Madison, Wisconsin

Michael Bernstein, DVM, DACVIM (SAIM)
Medical Director
VCA South Shore Animal Hospital
South Weymouth, Massachusetts

Adam Birkenheuer, DVM, PhD, DACVIM (SAIM)
Assistant Professor of Internal Medicine
Department of Clinical Sciences
College of Veterinary Medicine
North Carolina State University
Raleigh, North Carolina

Mark W. Bohling, DVM
Assistant Professor of Surgery
Department of Small Animal Clinical Sciences
College of Veterinary Medicine
University of Tennessee
Knoxville, Tennessee

Bernard D. Boisvert, BSc (Hons), DVM
Mission Ridge Animal Hospital
St. Albert, Alberta, Canada

John D. Bonagura, DVM, MS, DACVIM (Cardiology, SAIM)
Professor
Department of Veterinary Clinical Sciences
Member, Davis Heart & Lung Research Institute
Veterinary Teaching Hospital
The Ohio State University
Columbus, Ohio

Betsy R. Bond, DVM, DACVIM (Cardiology)
Staff Cardiologist
The Animal Medical Center
New York, New York

James P. Boulay, DVM, MS, DACVS
Surgeon
Veterinary Specialty Center of Tucson
Tucson, Arizona

Søren R. Boysen, DVM, DACVECC
Assistant Professor
Emergency and Critical Care
Faculty of Veterinary Medicine
University of Montreal
St-Hyacinthe, Québec, Canada

Marjory B. Brooks, DVM, DACVIM (SAIM)
Associate Director
Comparative Coagulation Section, Animal Health Diagnostic Laboratory
College of Veterinary Medicine
Cornell University
Ithaca, New York

Michael R. Broome, DVM, MS, DABVP
Advanced Veterinary Medical Imaging
Tustin, California

Andrew J. Brown, MA, VetMB, MRCVS
Assistant Professor, Emergency and Critical Care Medicine
College of Veterinary Medicine
Michigan State University
East Lansing, Michigan

M. Raquel Brown, DVM, DACVIM (Internal Medicine)
Veterinary Clinical Associate
Department of Veterinary Clinical Sciences
Texas A&M University
College Station, Texas

Lisa Brownlee, DVM, DACVIM (SAIM)
Assistant Professor
Department of Veterinary Medicine
College of Veterinary Medicine
Oregon State University
Corvallis, Oregon

Stephanie R. Bruner, DVM, DACVD
Staff Dermatologist
Greater Cincinnati Veterinary Specialists
Wilder, Kentucky

Jeffrey N. Bryan, DVM, MS
Research Assistant Professor
Department of Veterinary Medicine and Surgery
University of Missouri
Columbia, Missouri

James W. Buchanan, DVM, MMS, DACVIM (Cardiology)
Emeritus Professor of Cardiology
Department of Clinical Studies
School of Veterinary Medicine
University of Pennsylvania
Philadelphia, Pennsylvania

Barret J. Bulmer, DVM, MS, DACVIM (Cardiology)
Assistant Professor
Department of Clinical Sciences
College of Veterinary Medicine
Kansas State University
Manhattan, Kansas

Lisa Carioto, DVM, DVSc, DACVIM (SAIM)
Mobile Veterinary Internal Medicine Referral Service
Montreal, Québec, Canada

Khristen J. Carlson, DVM
Resident, Small Animal Internal Medicine
College of Veterinary Medicine
Auburn University
Auburn, Alabama

Maureen Carroll, DVM, DACVIM (SAIM)
Angell Animal Medical Center
Boston, Massachusetts

Tara Chapman, DVM, DACVIM (SAIM)
Alta Vista Animal Hospital
Ottawa, Ontario, Canada

Dennis J. Chew, DVM, DACVIM (SAIM)
Professor
Department of Veterinary Clinical Sciences
The Ohio State University
Columbus, Ohio

Jane O. Cho, DVM, DACVO
Veterinary Eye Specialists, PLLC
Ardsley, New York

Ruthanne Chun, DVM, DACVIM (Oncology)
Associate Professor
Department of Clinical Sciences
Kansas State University
Manhattan, Kansas

Cécile Clercx, DVM, PhD, DECVIM-CA (Internal Medicine)
Professor
Department of Veterinary Clinical Sciences
Faculty of Veterinary Medicine
University of Liège
Belgium

Joan R. Coates, DVM, MS, DACVIM (Neurology)
Associate Professor, Veterinary Neurology/Neurosurgery
Department of Veterinary Medicine and Surgery
College of Veterinary Medicine
University of Missouri
Columbia, Missouri

Cynthia S. Cook, DVM, PhD, DACVO
Veterinary Vision, Inc.
San Mateo, California

Lilian Cornejo, DVM
Clinical Assistant Professor of Internal Medicine
Department of Clinical Sciences
Cummings School of Veterinary Medicine
Tufts University
North Grafton, Massachusetts

Yonaira Cortés, DVM
Resident, Emergency and Critical Care
Angell Animal Medical Center
Boston, Massachusetts

Nancy B. Cottrill, DVM, MS, DACVO
Staff Ophthalmologist
Angell Animal Medical Center
Springfield, Massachusetts

Kate E. Creevy, DVM
Resident, Small Animal Medicine
College of Veterinary Medicine
University of Georgia
Athens, Georgia

Andrew Cruikshank, DVM
Resident, Emergency and Critical Care
Animal Surgical and Emergency Center
Los Angeles, California

Anne M. Dalby, DVM
Veterinary Referral Clinic
Bedford Heights, Ohio

Sylvie Daminet, DVM, PhD, DACVIM, DECVIM-CA (Internal Medicine)
Associate Professor
Department of Medicine and Clinical Biology of Small Animals
Faculty of Veterinary Medicine
Ghent University
Merelbeke, Belgium

Autumn P. Davidson, DVM, MS, DACVIM (SAIM)
Clinical Professor
Department of Medicine and Epidemiology
School of Veterinary Medicine
University of California
Davis, California

Benjamin Davidson, BVSc (Hons), MACVSc
New York City Veterinary Specialists
New York, New York

Ellen B. Davidson Domnick, DVM, DACVS
Associate Professor, Small Animal Surgery
Department of Veterinary Clinical Sciences
Boren Veterinary Medical Teaching Hospital
College of Veterinary Medicine
Oklahoma State University
Stillwater, Oklahoma

Deborah G. Davis, DVM, DACVP
Clinical Pathologist
IDEXX Laboratories
North Grafton, Massachusetts

Amy E. DeClue, DVM
Resident, Small Animal Internal Medicine
Veterinary Medicine and Surgery
Veterinary Teaching Hospital
University of Missouri
Columbia, Missouri

Vincent E. Defalque, DMV
Dermatology Resident
Department of Small Animal Clinical Sciences
Michigan State University
East Lansing, Michigan

Teresa DeFrancesco, DVM, DACVIM (Cardiology), DACVECC
Associate Professor of Cardiology and Critical Care
Department of Clinical Sciences
College of Veterinary Medicine
North Carolina State University
Raleigh, North Carolina

Caroline de Jaham, DMV, MSc, DACVD
Veterinary Dermatologist
DMV Veterinary Centre
Montreal (Lachine), Québec, Canada

Alexander deLahunta, DVM, PhD
James Law Professor of Veterinary Anatomy, Emeritus
College of Veterinary Medicine
Cornell University
Ithaca, New York

Eric de Madron, DVM, DACVIM (Cardiology), DECVIM (Internal Medicine)
Partner, Head of Referral Services, Director of Internal Medicine
Alta Vista Animal Hospital
Ottawa, Ontario, Canada

Helio Autran de Morais, DVM, PhD, DACVIM (SAIM, Cardiology)
Department of Medical Sciences
University of Wisconsin
Madison, Wisconsin

Erika de Papp, DVM, DACVIM (SAIM)
Director
Department of Internal Medicine
Angell Animal Medical Center
Boston, Massachusetts

Ravinder S. Dhaliwal, DVM, MS, DACVIM (Oncology), DABVP (Canine and Feline)
Staff Oncologist
South Bay Veterinary Specialists
San Jose, California

Ursula M. Dietrich, DMV, MRCVS, DACVO, DECVO
Assistant Professor
Department of Small Animal Surgery and Medicine
College of Veterinary Medicine
University of Georgia
Athens, Georgia

Caroline W. Donaldson, DVM
Consulting Veterinarian in Clinical Toxicology
ASPCA Animal Poison Control Center
Urbana, Illinois

Sharon Drellich, DVM, DACVECC
Staff Veterinarian, Emergency and Critical Care Medicine
Angell Animal Medical Center
Boston, Massachusetts

Kenneth Drobatz, DVM, MSCE
Professor, Section of Critical Care
Director, Emergency Service
Department of Clinical Studies
Matthew J. Ryan Veterinary Hospital
University of Pennsylvania
Philadelphia, Pennsylvania

Yvan Dumais, DMV, DAVDC
Montreal, Québec, Canada

Eric K. Dunayer, MS, VMD
Consulting Veterinarian in Clinical Toxicology
ASPCA Animal Poison Control Center
Urbana, Illinois

Marilyn Dunn, DMV, IPSAV, MVSc, DACVIM (SAIM)
Associate Professor
Department of Clinical Sciences
Faculty of Veterinary Medicine
University of Montreal
St-Hyacinthe, Québec, Canada

Samuel Durkan, DVM
Resident, Emergency and Critical Care Medicine
Cummings School of Veterinary Medicine
Tufts University
North Grafton, Massachusetts

N. Joel Edwards, DVM, DACVIM (Cardiology)
Upstate Veterinary Specialties, PLLC
Latham, New York

Bruce E. Eilts, DVM, MS, DACT
Professor of Theriogenology
Department of Veterinary Clinical Sciences
School of Veterinary Medicine
Louisiana State University
Baton Rouge, Louisisana

Stephen J. Ettinger, DVM, DACVIM (Cardiology, SAIM), FACC, FAHA
California Animal Hospital
Los Angeles, California

Susan N. Ettinger, DVM, DACVIM (Oncology)
Staff Oncologist
Department of Oncology
South Bay Veterinary Specialists
San Jose, California

Paul A. Eubig, DVM
Consulting Veterinarian in Clinical Toxicology
ASPCA Animal Poison Control Center
Urbana, Illinois

James F. Evermann, MS, PhD
Professor
Department of Veterinary Clinical Sciences
College of Veterinary Medicine
Washington State University
Pullman, Washington

Patty J. Ewing, DVM, MS, DACVP
Senior Pathologist
Department of Pathology
Genzyme Corporation
Framingham, Massachusetts

John Farrelly, DVM, DACVIM (Oncology), DACVR (Radiation Oncology)
Head of Radiation Therapy
The Animal Medical Center
New York, New York

Wenche Farstad, DVM, PhD, DECAR
Department of Production Animal Clinical Sciences
Norwegian School of Veterinary Science
Oslo, Norway

Karen K. Faunt, DVM, MS, DACVIM (SAIM)
Director of Medical Support
Banfield The Pet Hospital
Portland, Oregon

Edward C. Feldman, DVM, DACVIM (SAIM)
Professor
Department of Medicine and Epidemiology
School of Veterinary Medicine
University of California
Davis, California

Nathaniel Fenollosa, DVM, DACVIM (Cardiology)
Staff Cardiologist
Angell Animal Medical Center
Springfield, Massachusetts

Fidelia R. Fernandez, DVM, MS, DACVP (Clinical Pathology)
Clinical Pathologist
Antech Diagnostics
Cary, North Carolina

Janean L. Fidel, DVM, MS, DACVIM (Oncology), DACVR (Radiation Oncology)
Assistant Professor
Department of Veterinary Clinical Sciences
Washington State University
Pullman, Washington

Wendy D. Fife, DVM, MS, DACVR
Radiologist
Diagnostic Imaging
Denver, Colorado

Deborah M. Fine, DVM, MS, DACVIM (Cardiology)
Assistant Professor
Department of Veterinary Medicine and Surgery
University of Missouri
Columbia, Missouri

Linda S. Fineman, DVM, DACVIM (Oncology)
Clinical Oncologist
Pacific Veterinary Specialists and Emergency Service
Capitola, California
Veterinary Tumor Institute
Santa Cruz, California

James M. Fingeroth, DVM, DACVS
Chief of Surgery
Veterinary Specialists of Rochester
Rochester, New York

James A. Flanders, DVM, DACVS
Associate Professor
Department of Clinical Sciences
College of Veterinary Medicine
Cornell University
Ithaca, New York

Polly A. Fleckenstein, DVM, MS, CVA
Chief of Staff
Emergency and Intensive Care Service
Veterinary Medical Center of Central New York
Veterinary Medical Officer
Safety Officer, Veterinary Medical Assistance Team—National Disaster Medical System
Federal Emergency Management Agency
Department of Homeland Security, USA
Syracuse, New York

Andrea B. Flory, DVM
Resident, Medical Oncology
Cornell University Hospital for Animals
Ithaca, New York

Peter Foley, MSc, DVM, DACVIM (SAIM)
Assistant Professor of Companion Animal Medicine
Department of Companion Animals
Atlantic Veterinary College
University of Prince Edward Island
Charlottetown, Prince Edward Island, Canada

Thierry Francey, DVM
Lecturer
Department of Medicine and Epidemiology
School of Veterinary Medicine
University of California
Davis, California

Boel A. Fransson, DVM, PhD, DACVS
Clinical Instructor
Department of Veterinary Clinical Sciences
Washington State University
Pullman, Washington

Lisa M. Freeman, DVM, PhD, DACVN
Associate Professor
Department of Clinical Sciences
Cummings School of Veterinary Medicine
Tufts University
North Grafton, Massachusetts

Kristi M. Gannon, DVM, DACVECC
Oradell Animal Hospital, Inc.
Paramus, New Jersey

Laura D. Garrett, DVM, DACVIM (Oncology)
Assistant Professor
Veterinary Clinical Medicine
University of Illinois
Urbana, Illinois

Cynthia Gaskill, DVM, PhD
Assistant Professor
Department of Biomedical Sciences
Atlantic Veterinary College
University of Prince Edward Island
Charlottetown, Prince Edward Island, Canada

Stephen D. Gaunt, DVM, PhD, DACVP
Professor of Veterinary Clinical Pathology
Department of Pathobiological Sciences
School of Veterinary Medicine
Louisiana State University
Baton Rouge, Louisiana

Kirk N. Gelatt, VMD, DACVO
Distinguished Professor of Comparative Ophthalmology
Department of Small Animal Clinical Sciences
College of Veterinary Medicine
University of Florida
Gainesville, Florida

Hans Gelens, DVM, MSc, DACVIM (SAIM)
Assistant Professor
Department of Companion Animals
Atlantic Veterinary College
Charlottetown, Prince Edward Island, Canada

Anna R. M. Gelzer, DMV, DACVIM, DECVIM (Cardiology)
Assistant Professor
Department of Clinical Sciences
College of Veterinary Medicine
Cornell University
Ithaca, New York

Anne J. Gemensky-Metzler, DVM, MS, DACVO
Associate Professor—Clinical Comparative Ophthalmology
Department of Veterinary Clinical Sciences
The Ohio State University College of Veterinary Medicine
Columbus, Ohio

Tracy Gieger, DVM, DACVIM (SAIM, Oncology)
Assistant Professor
Department of Small Animal Medicine and Surgery
University of Georgia
Athens, Georgia

Tony M. Glaus, PD, DMV, DACVIM (SAIM), DECVIM (Internal Medicine, Cardiology)
Head, Division of Cardiology
Clinic for Small Animal Internal Medicine
Vetsuisse Faculty
University of Zurich
Zurich, Switzerland

Joseph C. Glennon, VMD, DACVS
Surgeon
Veterinary Specialties Referral Center
Pattersonville, New York

Cristina Gobello, DVM
Institute of Theriogenology
Small Animal Area
Faculty of Veterinary Sciences
National University of La Plata
Argentina

Kristine L. Gonzales, DVM
Staff Veterinarian
Guide Dogs for the Blind, Inc.
San Rafael, California

Lillian I. Good, DVM, DACVECC
Criticalist
Pacific Veterinary Specialists and Emergency Service
Capitola, California

Barbara R. Gores, DVM, DACVS
Surgeon
Veterinary Specialty Center of Tucson
Tucson, Arizona

Cecilia Gorrel, BSc, MA, Vet MB, DDS, Hon FAVD, DEVDC, MRCVS
Veterinary Dentistry and Oral Surgery Referrals
Veterinary Oral Health Consultancy
Hampshire, United Kingdom

Kinga Gortel, DVM, MS, DACVD
Animal Dermatology Specialty Clinic
Marina del Rey, California

Ruanna Gossett, DVM, PhD, DACVP
Clinical Pathologist
IDEXX, Inc.
West Sacramento, California

Margherita Gracis, DVM, DAVDC, DEVDC
Clinica Veterinaria Città di Monza
Italy

Carlos Gradil, DVM, PhD, DACT
University of Massachusetts
Veterinary and Animal Sciences
Amherst, Massachusetts

Kristi L. Graham, DVM, MS, DACVIM (SAIM)
Veterinary Specialty Center, LLC
Indianapolis, Indiana
Visiting Instructor
Veterinary Technology Program
Purdue University
West Lafayette, Indiana
Carmel, Indiana

Bradley A. Green, DVM
Internal Medicine Resident
Department of Medical Sciences
University of Wisconsin—Madison
Madison, Wisconsin

Pascale Griessmayr, DMV
Resident, Medical Oncology
Cummings School of Veterinary Medicine
Tufts University
North Grafton, Massachusetts

Sophie A. Grundy, BVSc (Hons), MACVSc, DACVIM (SAIM)
Dayton, Indiana

Sharon M. Gwaltney-Brant, DVM, PhD, DABVT, DABT
Medical Director
ASPCA Animal Poison Control Center
Urbana, Illinois

John J. Haburjak, DVM, DACVS
Head, Department of Surgery
Berkeley Center for Special Veterinary Services
Berkeley, California

Jens Häggström, DVM, PhD, DECVIM-CA (Cardiology)
Professor of Internal Medicine
Department of Clinical Sciences, Uppsala
Faculty of Veterinary Medicine and Animal Science
Swedish University of Agricultural Sciences
Sweden

Edward J. Hall, MA, VetMB, PhD, DECVIM-CA
Professor of Small Animal Internal Medicine
Head of the Division of Companion Animal Studies
Department of Clinical Veterinary Science
University of Bristol
Bristol, United Kingdom

Michael Hannigan, BVMS, CertSAD, MRCVS
Senior Veterinarian
Properties Animal Clinic
Calgary, Alberta, Canada

Kenneth R. Harkin, DVM, DACVIM (SAIM)
Associate Professor
Small Animal Internal Medicine
Kansas State University
Manhattan, Kansas

John R. Hart, Jr., DVM, DACVIM (SAIM)
Staff Internist
Veterinary Specialty Hospital of San Diego
San Diego, California

Colin E. Harvey, BVSc, FRCVS, DACVS, DAVDC
Professor of Surgery and Dentistry
Department of Clinical Studies
School of Veterinary Medicine
University of Pennsylvania
Philadelphia, Pennsylvania

Timothy V. Hatt, DVM, CCRP
Department Head and Associate Veterinarian
Physical Rehabilitation
Oradell Animal Hospital
Paramus, New Jersey

Herman A. W. Hazewinkel, DVM, PhD, DECVS, DECVCN
Professor in Companion Animal Orthopaedics
Department of Clinical Sciences of Companion Animals
Utrecht University
The Netherlands

Timothy M. Hazzard, PhD, DVM
Research Associate
Department of Clinical Sciences
College of Veterinary Medicine
Oregon State University
Corvallis, Oregon

Geoff Heffner, DVM
Resident, Emergency and Critical Care Medicine
Department of Clinical Sciences
Cummings School of Veterinary Medicine
Tufts University
North Grafton, Massachusetts

Alicia K. Henderson, DVM
Resident, Small Animal Internal Medicine
Department of Clinical Sciences
Cummings School of Veterinary Medicine
Tufts University
North Grafton, Massachusetts

Kate Hill, BVSc, DACVIM (SAIM)
Assistant Professor of Medicine
Department of Small Animal Clinical Sciences
University of Tennessee
Knoxville, Tennessee

Steve Hill, DVM, MS, DACVIM (SAIM)
Veterinary Specialty Hospital of San Diego
San Diego, California

Andrew Hillier, BVSc, MACVSc, DACVD
Associate Professor
Veterinary Clinical Sciences
The Ohio State University
Columbus, Ohio

Mark E. Hitt, DVM, DACVIM (SAIM)
Atlantic Veterinary Internal Medicine
Annapolis, Maryland

Daniel F. Hogan, DVM, DACVIM (Cardiology)
Assistant Professor
Veterinary Clinical Sciences
Purdue University
West Lafayette, Indiana

Steven R. Hollingsworth, DVM, DACVO
Lecturer, Department of Surgical and Radiological Sciences
School of Veterinary Medicine
University of California
Davis, California

Cheryl A. Holloway, RVT
Animal Health Technician
College of Veterinary Medicine
The Ohio State University
Columbus, Ohio

Jennifer L. Holm, DVM, DACVECC
Staff Veterinarian—Critical Care Unit
Angell Animal Medical Center
Boston, Massachusetts

David Holt, BVSc, DACVS
Associate Professor of Surgery
University of Pennsylvania School of Veterinary Medicine
Philadelphia, Pennsylvania

Heidi Hottinger, DVM, DACVS
Gulf Coast Veterinary Specialists
Houston, Texas

Katherine Albro Houpt, VMD, PhD, DACVB
Professor of Physiology
Deparment of Biomedical Sciences
College of Veterinary Medicine
Cornell University
Ithaca, New York

Andrew Isaacs, DVM
Resident, Neurology and Neurosurgery
Department of Clinical Sciences
Auburn University College of Veterinary Medicine
Auburn, Alabama

Joli M. Jarboe, DVM, DACVIM (Neurology)
Veterinary Neurological Center
Las Vegas, Nevada

Edward Jazic, DVM
Resident in Dermatology
Dermatology Clinic for Animals, Arizona Vet Specialists
Gilbert, Arizona

Albert E. Jergens, DVM, MS, DACVIM (SAIM)
Associate Professor
Department of Veterinary Clinical Sciences
Iowa State University
Ames, Iowa

Cheri A. Johnson, DVM, MS, DACVIM (SAIM)
Professor and Chief of Staff
Department of Small Animal Clinical Sciences
College of Veterinary Medicine
Michigan State University
East Lansing, Michigan

Susan E. Johnson, DVM, MS, DACVIM (SAIM)
Associate Professor
Department of Veterinary Clinical Sciences
College of Veterinary Medicine
The Ohio State University
Coliumbus, Ohio

Christopher J. Jones, DVM, DACVIM (SAIM)
Associate Internist
Gulf Coast Veterinary Internists
Houston, Texas

Soraya V. Juarbe-Diaz, DVM, DACVB
ABS Applied Animal Behaviorist
Florida Veterinary Specialists
Tampa, Florida
North Florida Veterinary Specialists
Jacksonville, Florida
Palm Beach Veterinary Referral and Critical Care Center
West Palm Beach, Florida
Coral Springs Animal Hospital
Coral Springs, Florida

Brett Kantrowitz, DVM, DACVR
Ojai, California

Bruce W. Keene, DVM, MSc, DACVIM (Cardiology)
Professor
Department of Clinical Sciences
North Carolina State University
College of Veterinary Medicine
Raleigh, North Carolina

Ninette Keller, BVSc (Hons), MMedVet (Med)
Lecturer, Department of Companion Animal Clinical Studies
Small Animal Medicine
Faculty of Veterinary Science
Onderstepoort, Pretoria, South Africa

Marc Kent, DVM, DACVIM (Neurology, SAIM)
Assistant Professor
Department of Small Animal Medicine and Surgery
University of Georgia
Athens, Georgia

Marie E. Kerl, DVM, DACVIM (SAIM), DACVECC
Assistant Professor
Department of Veterinary Medicine and Surgery
University of Missouri
Columbia, Missouri

Frank Kettner, BSc (Hons), BVSc (Hons)
Lecturer
Section of Small Animal Medicine
Department of Companion Animal Clinical Studies
Faculty of Veterinary Science
University of Pretoria
Onderstepoort, South Africa

Moazzam A. Khan, DVM, MSc, MS, PhD
Biologist (Toxicology Evaluator)
Existing Substances Division
Ottawa, Canada

Greg Kilburn, DVM
Resident, Neurology/Neurosurgery
Veterinary Neurological Center
Las Vegas, Nevada

Lesley G. King, MVB, MRCVS, DACVECC, DACVIM (SAIM), DECVIM-CA
Emergency and Critical Care Section
Department of Clinical Sciences
University of Pennsylvania School of Veterinary Medicine
Philadelphia, Pennsylvania

Barbara E. Kitchell, DVM, PhD, DACVIM (SAIM, Oncology)
Professor and Director
Center for Comparative Oncology
Michigan State University
College of Veterinary Medicine
East Lansing, Michigan

Karen L. Kline, DVM, MS, DACVIM (Neurology)
Associate Professor of Neurology and Neurosurgery
Veterinary Clinical Sciences
Iowa State University
College of Veterinary Medicine
Ames, Iowa

Michael W. Knight, DVM
Senior Consulting Veterinary Toxicologist
ASPCA Animal Poison Control Center
Urbana, Illinois

Amie Koenig, DVM, DACVIM (SAIM), DACVECC
Assistant Professor
Department of Small Animal Medicine and Surgery
College of Veterinary Medicine
University of Georgia
Athens, Georgia

Kara A. Kolster, DVM
Resident in Theriogenology
Department of Large Animal Clinical Sciences
Virginia-Maryland Regional College of Veterinary Medicine
Virginia Polytechnic Institute and State University
Blacksburg, Virginia

Bruce G. Kornreich, DVM, PhD, DACVIM (Cardiology)
Biomedical Sciences
Cornell University
Ithaca, New York

Janet Kovak, DVM, DACVS
Staff Surgeon
The Animal Medical Center
New York, New York

Marc S. Kraus, DVM, DACVIM (SAIM, Cardiology)
Department of Clinical Sciences
College of Veterinary Medicine
Cornell University
Ithaca, New York

Donald R. Krawiec, DVM, MS, PhD, DACVIM (SAIM)
President
California Veterinary Specialists, Inc.
San Marcos and Murrieta, California

Natali Krekeler, DMV, DACT
Clinical Instructor
Department of Clinical Sciences
Cornell University
Ithaca, New York

Tracy A. LaDue, DVM, DACVIM (SAIM), DACVR
Medical and Radiation Oncologist
Southeast Veterinary Oncology
Jacksonville, Florida

Elizabeth J. Laing, DVM, DVSc, DACVS
Surgical Referral Service
Fort Atkinson, Wisconsin

Leigh A. Lamont, DVM, MS, DACVA
Assistant Professor of Anesthesiology
Department of Companion Animals
Atlantic Veterinary College
University of Prince Edward Island
Charlottetown, Prince Edward Island, Canada

Cathy Langston, DVM, DACVIM (Internal Medicine)
Staff Veterinarian
Nephrology, Urology
Hemodialysis and Renal Transplantation Unit
Animal Medical Center
New York, New York

Nancy J. Laste, DVM, DACVIM (Cardiology)
Section Head, Cardiology
Department of Internal Medicine
Angell Animal Medical Center
Boston, Massachusetts

Susanne K. Lauer, DMV
Assistant Professor
Veterinary Clinical Sciences
School of Veterinary Medicine
Louisiana State University
Baton Rouge, Louisiana

Andrew Leisewitz, BVSc, MMedVet, PhD, DECVIM
Companion Animal Clinical Sciences
Faculty of Veterinary Science
University of Pretoria
Onderstepoort, South Africa

Bruce E. LeRoy, DVM, PhD, DACVP (Clinical Pathology)
Assistant Professor
Comparative Oncology Program
Department of Pathology
College of Veterinary Medicine
University of Georgia
Athens, Georgia

John R. Lewis, VMD, FAVD
Lecturer in Dentistry
School of Veterinary Medicine
University of Pennsylvania
Philadelphia, Pennsylvania

James D. Lincoln, DVM, MS
Associate Professor in Small Animal Surgery
Department of Veterinary Clinical Sciences
College of Veterinary Medicine
Washington State University
Pullman, Washington

David S. Lindsay, PhD
Professor
Department of Biomedical Sciences and Pathobiology
Virginia-Maryland Regional College of Veterinary Medicine
Virginia Polytechnic Institute and State University
Blacksburg, Virginia

Remo Lobetti, BVSc, MMedVet (Med), DECVIM (Internal Medicine)
Internist
Bryanston Veterinary Hospital
Bryanston, South Africa

Jennifer E. Locke, DVM, DACVIM (Oncology)
Assistant Professor, Oncology
Veterinary Clinical Sciences
Iowa State University
Ames, Iowa

Andrea L. Looney, DVM, DACVA
Lecturer, Section of Anesthesiology
College of Veterinary Medicine
Cornell University
Ithaca, New York

Cheryl Lopate, MS, DVM, DACVT
Private Practice
Reproductive Revolutions, Inc.
Newberg, Oregon

Andrew Lowe, DVM
Dermatology Resident
Veterinary Clinical Medicine
Department of Veterinary Clinical Medicine
Small Animal Clinic
University of Illinois
Urbana, Illinois

Lori Ludwig, VMD, MS, DACVS
Associate Surgeon
Veterinary Surgical Care
Mount Pleasant, South Carolina

Virginia Luis Fuentes, MA, VetMB, PhD, CertVR, DVC, MRCVS, DACVIM (Cardiology), DECVIM-CA (Cardiology)
Senior Lecturer
Department of Veterinary Clinical Sciences
Royal Veterinary College
North Mymms
Hatfield, Hertfordshire, United Kingdom

Jody P. Lulich, DVM, PhD, DACVIM (SAIM)
Minnesota Urolith Centre
Department of Veterinary Clinical Sciences
University of Minnesota
St. Paul, Minnesota

Bertrand Lussier, DMV, MSc, DACVS
Assistant Professor
Department of Clinical Sciences
Faculty of Veterinary Medicine
University of Montreal
St-Hyacinthe, Québec, Canada

Kristin MacDonald, DVM, PhD, DACVIM (Cardiology)
Staff Veterinary Cardiologist
Department of Veterinary Medicine and Epidemiology
University of California
Davis, California
Veterinary Cardiologist
The Animal Care Center of Sonoma
Rohnert Park, California

David J. Maggs, BVSc, DACVO
Assistant Professor
Department of Surgical and Radiological Sciences
School of Veterinary Medicine
University of California
Davis, California

Orla Mahony, MVB, DACVIM (Oncology), DECVIM
Clinical Assistant Professor
Department of Small Animal Clinical Sciences
Cummings School of Veterinary Medicine
Tufts University
North Grafton, Massachusetts

Rebecca L. Malakoff, DVM, DACVIM (Cardiology)
Staff Veterinarian
Cardiology Department
Angell Animal Medical Center
Boston, Massachusetts

Ann Marie Manning, DVM, DACVECC
Chief Medical Officer
Angell Animal Medical Center
Boston, Massachusetts

Steven L. Marks, BVSc, MS, MRCVS, DACVIM (SAIM)
Clinical Associate Professor of Critical Care and Internal Medicine
Department of Clinical Sciences
North Carolina State University
Raleigh, North Carolina

Melissa Marshall, DVM
Director, Emergency and Critical Care
Red Bank Veterinary Hospital
Tinton Falls, New Jersey

Charles L. Martin, DVM, MS, DACVO
Professor Emeritus
Department of Small Animal Medicine
University of Georgia
Athens, Georgia

Kyle G. Mathews, DVM, MS, DACVS
Associate Professor
Department of Clinical Sciences
College of Veterinary Medicine
North Carolina State University
Raleigh, North Carolina

Glenna E. Mauldin, DVM, MS, DACVIM (Oncology), DACVN
Associate Professor of Veterinary Oncology
Department of Veterinary Clinical Sciences
Louisiana State University School of Veterinary Medicine
Baton Rouge, Louisiana

Carol A. McClure, DVM, MS, PhD, DACT
Research Scientist
University of Prince Edward Island
Charlottetown, Prince Edward Island, Canada

Brendan C. McKiernan, DVM, DACVIM
Wheat Ridge Veterinary Specialists
Wheat Ridge Animal Hospital
Wheat Ridge, Colorado

Elizabeth A. McNiel, DVM, PhD, DACVIM (Oncology), DACVR (Radiation Oncology)
Assistant Professor
Department of Veterinary Clinical Sciences
University of Minnesota
St. Paul, Minnesota

Charlotte Means, DVM, MLIS
Consulting Veterinarian in Clinical Toxicology
ASPCA Animal Poison Control Center
Urbana, Illinois

James H. Meinkoth, DVM, PhD, DACVP
Professor
Department of Pathobiology
College of Veterinary Medicine
Oklahoma State University
Stillwater, Oklahoma

Mushtaq A. Memon, BVSc, PhD, DACT
Theriogenologist, Veterinary Teaching Hospital
Associate Professor
Department of Veterinary Clinical Sciences
Washington State University
Pullman, Washington

Michèle Menard, DVM, MS, PhD, DACVP
President
Veterinary Cytopathology
Clackamas, Oregon

Kathryn M. Meurs, DVM, PhD, DACVIM (Cardiology)
Professor
Veterinary Clinical Sciences
College of Veterinary Medicine
Washington State University
Pullman, Washington

Kathryn E. Michel, DVM, MS, DACVN
Assistant Professor of Nutrition
Chief, Section of Medicine
Department of Clinical Studies
School of Veterinary Medicine
University of Pennsylvania
Philadelphia, Pennsylvania

David Miller, BVSc (Hons), MMedVet (Med)
Senior Physician
Ridgemall Veterinary Referral Hospital
Johannesburg, South Africa

James B. Miller, DVM, MS, DACVIM (SAIM)
Professor, Department of Companion Animals
Atlantic Veterinary College
University of Prince Edward Island
Charlottetown, Prince Edward Island, Canada

Sarah J. Miller, DVM, DACVIM (Cardiology)
Staff Cardiologist
Advanced Veterinary Care Center
Lawndale, California

Michael B. Mison, DVM, DACVS
Staff Surgeon
Veterinary Specialty Center of Seattle
Lynnwood, Washington

Elise Mittleman, DVM, DACVECC
Emergency and Critical Care
Animal Critical Care and Specialty Group at Veterinary Referral Center
Malvern, Pennsylvania

Peter Moak, DVM
Assistant Professor
Department of Companion Animals
Atlantic Veterinary College
University of Prince Edward Island
Charlottetown, Prince Edward Island, Canada

Lisa E. Moore, DVM, DACVIM (SAIM)
Clinical Associate Professor
Veterinary Medical Teaching Hospital
College of Veterinary Medicine
Kansas State University
Manhattan, Kansas

Phillip A. Moore, DVM, DACVO
Assistant Professor
Department of Small Animal Medicine and Surgery
College of Veterinary Medicine
University of Georgia
Athens, Georgia

Adam Mordecai, DVM
Resident, Small Animal Internal Medicine
Department of Veterinary Clinical Sciences
Washington State University
Pullman, Washington

Sherry J. Morgan, DVM, PhD, DACVP, ABT, ABVT
Scientific Director, Preclinical Safety
Abbott Laboratories
Abbott Park, Illinois

Helen Munro, BVMS, MRCVS
Honorary Fellow
Veterinary Pathology
Royal (Dick) School of Veterinary Studies
University of Edinburgh
Edinburgh, Scotland

Michelle Murray Scibelli, DVM, MS, DACVIM (Neurology)
Tustin, California

Sarah L. Naidoo, DVM, MSc, DACVIM (SAIM)
Dove-Lewis Emergency Animal Hospital
Portland, Oregon

Jill Narak, DVM
Intern, Small Animal Medicine and Surgery
Department of Clinical Sciences
Auburn University College of Veterinary Medicine
Auburn, Alabama

Mirinda Nel (van Schoor), BVSc
Clinical Instructor in Small Animal Medicine
Department of Companion Animal Clinical Sciences
Faculty of Veterinary Science
University of Pretoria
Onderstepoort, South Africa

O. Lynne Nelson, DVM, MS, DACVIM (SAIM, Cardiology)
Assistant Professor
Department of Veterinary Clinical Sciences
Washington State University
Pullman, Washington

Richard W. Nelson, DVM, DACVIM (SAIM)
Professor, Internal Medicine
Department of Medicine and Epidemiology
School of Veterinary Medicine
University of California
Davis, California

Andrea Nicastro, DVM, DACVIM (SAIM)
Staff Internist
Veterinary Medical Care, L.L.C.
Mount Pleasant, South Carolina

E. Kelly Nitsche, BVSc, DVM, DABVP (Canine/Feline), DACVIM (SAIM)
Chief of Medicine
Veterinary Specialists of North Texas
Dallas, Texas

Nicole C. Northrup, DVM, DACVIM (Oncology)
Assistant Professor
Comparative Oncology Program
Department of Small Animal Medicine and Surgery
College of Veterinary Medicine
University of Georgia
Athens, Georgia

Dennis P. O'Brien, DVM, PhD, DACVIM
Professor of Neurology
Department of Veterinary Medicine and Surgery
Veterinary Medical Teaching Hospital
University of Missouri
Columbia, Missouri

Karine M. Onclin, DVM, MSc, PhD, DECAR
Lecturer
Small Animal Theriogenology
Large Animal Clinical Sciences
College of Veterinary Medicine
University of Florida
Gainesville, Florida

Joao S. Orvalho, DVM
Cardiology Resident
Veterinary Medical Teaching Hospital
University of California
Davis, California

Carl A. Osborne, DVM, PhD, DACVIM (SAIM)
Minnesota Urolith Centre
Department of Veterinary Clinical Sciences
University of Minnesota
St. Paul, Minnesota

M. Lynne O'Sullivan, DVM, DVSc, DACVIM (Cardiology)
Assistant Professor
Department of Clinical Studies
Ontario Veterinary College
University of Guelph
Guelph, Ontario, Canada

Elizabeth O'Toole, BSc, DVM, DVSc, DACVECC
Assistant Professor
Veterinary Clinical Sciences
College of Veterinary Medicine
The Ohio State University
Columbus, Ohio

Therese E. O'Toole, DVM, DACVIM (SAIM)
Assistant Clinical Faculty
Department of Clinical Sciences
Cummings School of Veterinary Medicine
Tufts University
North Grafton, Massachusetts

Nicole Pacifico, DVM
Ross University
St. Kitts, West Indies

LeeAnn Pack, DVM
Staff Radiologist
Atlantic Veterinary College
University of Prince Edward Island
Charlottetown, Prince Edward Island, Canada

Rebecca A. Packer, DVM, MS
Resident, Neurology/Neurosurgery
Department of Veterinary Medicine and Surgery
University of Missouri
Columbia, Missouri

Philip Padrid, DVM
Midwest Regional Medical Director
Veterinary Centers of America Hospitals
Associate Professor of Medicine
Section of Pulmonary/Critical Care Medicine
University of Chicago
Chicago, Illinois

Nadia Pagé, DMV, MSc, DACVD
Veterinary Dermatologist
DMV Veterinary Center
Montreal (Lachine) (QC), Canada

Marc Papageorges, DVM, MS, PhD, DACVR
President
Veterinary Diagnostic Imaging, P.C.
Clackamas, Oregon

Manon Paradis, DMV, MVSc, DACVD
Professor
Department of Clinical Sciences
Faculty of Veterinary Medicine
University of Montreal
St-Hyacinthe, Québec, Canada

Rosa María Páramo Ramirez, MVZ, PhD
Full Time Lecturer
Reproduction Department
Facultad de Medicina Veterinaria y Zootecnia
Universidad Nacional Autónoma de México
Ciudad Universitaria
Tlalpan, Mexico D.F.

Adam P. Patterson, DVM, DACVD
Chesapeake Veterinary Dermatology Associates
Towson, Maryland

April Paul, DVM
Resident, Emergency and Critical Care Medicine
Department of Clinical Sciences
Cummings School of Veterinary Medicine
Tufts University
North Grafton, Massachusetts

Michael Pavletic, DVM, DACVS
Head, Department of Surgery
Angell Animal Medical Center
Boston, Massachusetts

Michael E. Peterson, DVM, MS
Associate Veterinarian
Reid Veterinary Hospital
Albany, Oregon

Polly B. Peterson, DVM, DACVIM (SAIM)
Associate Veterinarian
Veterinary Specialty Center of Seattle
Lynnwood, Washington

Elisa A. Petrollini, CVT, VTS (ECC)
Assistant Nursing Supervisor, Nursing Services
Ryan Veterinary Hospital of the University of Pennsylvania
Philadelphia, Pennsylvania

Fred S. Pike, DVM, DACVS
Staff Surgeon
Veterinary Specialty Hospital of San Diego
San Diego, California

Chantale L. Pinard, DVM, MSc, DACVO
Clinical Instructor
Faculty of Veterinary Medicine
University of Montreal
St-Hyacinthe, Québec, Canada

Dan Polidoro, DVM
Animal Surgical & Emergency Center
Los Angeles, California

Eric R. Pope, DVM, MS, DACVS
Associate Professor
Department of Veterinary Medicine and Surgery
University of Missouri
Columbia, Missouri

Brandy Porterpan, DVM
Lecturer
Small Animal Teaching Hospital
Texas A&M College of Veterinary Medicine
College Station, Texas

Barrak M. Pressler, DVM, DACVIM (SAIM)
Graduate Student, Immunology Graduate Group
Department of Clinical Sciences
College of Veterinary Medicine
North Carolina State University
Raleigh, North Carolina
Postdoctoral Fellow
Division of Nephrology and Hypertension
Department of Medicine
School of Medicine
University of North Carolina
Chapel Hill, North Carolina

Robert Prošek, DVM, MS, DACVIM (Cardiology)
Director
Heart & Eye Center for Animals
Homestead, Florida
Director
Cardiology Service at Miami Veterinary Specialists
Coral Gables, Florida
Adjunct Professor
University of Florida
Gainesville, Florida

David R. Proulx, MSpVM, DACVIM (Oncology), DACVR (Radiation Oncology)
California Veterinary Specialists
San Marcos, California

David A. Puerto, DVM, DACVS
Chief of Surgery
Center for Animal Referral and Emergency Services
Langhorne, Pennsylvania

Beverly J. Purswell, DVM, PhD, DACT
Professor and Interim Head
Department of Large Animal Clinical Sciences
Virginia-Maryland Regional College of Veterinary Medicine
Virginia Polytechnic Institute and State University
Blacksburg, Virginia

Fonzie Quance-Fitch, DVM, DACVP
Chief, Pathobiology
59th Clinical Research Squadron
Wilford Hall Medical Center
Lackland AFB, Texas

Richard F. Quinn, DVM, DVSc, DACVO
Veterinary Ophthalmologist
Veterinary Eye Specialists
London, Ontario, Canada
Adjunct Professor
Department of Ophthalmology
University of Western Ontario
London, Ontario, Canada
Veterinary Eye Specialists
Denfield, Ontario, Canada

MaryAnn G. Radlinsky, DVM, MS, DACVS
Associate Professor
Department of Small Animal Medicine and Surgery
University of Georgia
Athens, Georgia

Gregg Rapoport, DVM, DACVIM (Cardiology)
Staff Cardiologist
Cardiology Service
Angell Animal Medical Center
Boston, Massachusetts

Jennifer E. Rawlinson, DVM
Dental Resident
School of Veterinary Medicine
University of Pennsylvania
Philadelphia, Pennsylvania

Carol Reinero, DVM, DACVIM (SAIM), PhD
Assistant Professor
Department of Veterinary Medicine and Surgery
University of Missouri
Columbia, Missouri

Adam J. Reiss, DVM, DACVECC
Chief of Emergency Medicine
Southern Oregon Veterinary Specialty Center
Medford, Oregon

Valeria Rickard, DVM
North Oatlands Animal Hospital, PC
Senior Veterinarian/Owner
Leesburg, Virginia

Laura G. Ridge, DVM
Internal Medicine Resident
Department of Small Animal Medicine
University of Georgia
Athens, Georgia

Carlos O. Rodriguez, Jr., DVM, PhD, DACVIM (Oncology)
Lecturer
Department of Surgical and Radiological Sciences
University of California
Davis, California
Staff Oncologist
San Francisco Veterinary Specialists
San Francisco, California

Margaret V. Root Kustritz, DVM, PhD, DACT
Department of Veterinary Clinical Sciences
University of Minnesota
College of Veterinary Medicine
St. Paul, Minnesota

Patricia L. Rose, DVM, MS, DACVS, DACVR
Atlantic Veterinary College
University of Prince Edward Island
Charlottetown, Prince Edward Island, Canada

Tracey A. Rossi, DVM
Resident, Small Animal Internal Medicine
Department of Clinical Sciences
Cummings School of Veterinary Medicine
Tufts University
North Grafton, Massachusetts

Philip Roudebush, DVM, DACVIM
Scientific Spokesperson
Technical Information Services
Hill's Pet Nutrition, Inc.
Topeka, Kansas
Adjunct Professor
Department of Clinical Sciences
College of Veterinary Medicine
Kansas State University
Manhattan, Kansas

Véronique Sammut, DMV, MS, DACVIM (Neurology)
Associate
California Animal Hospital
Los Angeles, California

Lynne Sandmeyer, DVM, DVSc, DACVO
Associate Professor
Department of Small Animal Clinical Sciences
Western College of Veterinary Medicine
University of Saskatchewan
Saskatoon, Saskatchewan

John S. Sapienza, DVM, DACVO
Long Island Veterinary Specialists
Plainview, New York

Frédéric Sauvé, DVM, MSc, DES, DACVD
Clinical Instructor
Centre Hospitalier Universitaire Vétérinaire
Faculty of Veterinary Medicine
University of Montreal
St-Hyacinthe, Québec, Canada

Michael Schaer, DVM, DACVIM (SAIM), DACVECC
Professor and Associate Chief of Staff
Small Animal Clinical Sciences
College of Veterinary Medicine
University of Florida
Gainesville, Florida

Mary M. Schell, DVM, DABT
Consultant in Veterinary Clinical Toxicology
ASPCA—Animal Poison Control Center
Urbana, Illinois

Patricia A. Schenck, DVM, MS, PhD
Assistant Professor
Diagnostic Center for Population and Animal Health
Endocrine Diagnostic Section
Michigan State University
Lansing, Michigan

Johan P. Schoeman, BVSc, DSAM (RCVS-London), MMedVet (Pretoria), DECVIM-CA (Internal Medicine), MRCVS
Associate Professor and Head
Section of Small Animal Medicine
Department of Companion Animal Clinical Studies
Faculty of Veterinary Sciences
University of Pretoria
Onderstepoort, South Africa

Diana M. Schropp, DVM
Southern Oregon Veterinary Specialty Center
Medford, Oregon

Wayne S. Schwark, DVM, MSc, PhD
Professor of Pharmacology
Department of Molecular Medicine
College of Veterinary Medicine
Cornell University
Ithaca, New York

Kersti Seksel, BVSc (Hons), MRCVS, MA (Hons), FACVSc (Animal Behavior), DACVB
Sydney Animal Behavior Service
Managing Director and Principal Consultant
Seaforth, New South Wales, Australia

Kim A. Selting, DVM, MS, DACVIM (Oncology)
Assistant Professor
Department of Veterinary Medicine and Surgery
University of Missouri—Columbia
Columbia, Missouri

Jonathan Shani, BSc (Mechanical Engineering), DVM, DECVS
Surgeon
Mobile Surgical Services
Tel-Aviv, Israel

Darcy H. Shaw, DVM, MSc, DACVIM (SAIM)
Department of Companion Animals
Atlantic Veterinary College
University of Prince Edward Island
Charlottetown, Prince Edward Island, Canada

Scott P. Shaw, DVM, DACVECC
Assistant Professor
Department of Clinical Sciences
Cummings School of Veterinary Medicine
Tufts University
North Grafton, Massachusetts

Jenifer G. Sheehy, DVM
Staff Veterinarian
Veterinary Emergency Referral Group, Inc.
Houston, Texas

G. Diane Shelton, DVM, PhD, DACVIM (SAIM)
Professor
Department of Pathology
University of California
San Diego, California

Sharon L. Shields, DVM, DACVS
Animal Surgical Emergency Center
Los Angeles, California

Jeffery Simmons, DVM
Resident, Veterinary Emergency and Critical Care
Auburn University
Department of Clinical Sciences
Auburn University
Auburn, Alabama

Daniela Simon, DMV, DECVIM-CA (Oncology)
Small Animal Hospital
School of Veterinary Medicine Hannover
Hannover, Germany

D. David Sisson, DVM, DACVIM (Cardiology)
Professor and Head
Department of Clinical Sciences
College of Veterinary Medicine
Oregon State University
Corvallis, Oregon

Meg Sleeper, VMD, DACVIM (Cardiology)
Assistant Professor of Cardiology
Cardiology Section Chief
Department of Clinical Studies—Philadelphia
University of Pennsylvania School of Veterinary Medicine
Philadelphia, Pennsylvania

Laura J. Smallwood, DVM, DACVIM (SAIM)
Northlake Veterinary Specialists
Clarkston, Georgia

Frances O. Smith, DVM, PhD, DACT
Owner
Smith Veterinary Hospital, Inc.
Burnsville, Minnesota
Adjunct Professor
University of Minnesota
School of Veterinary Medicine
St. Paul, Minnesota
President
Orthopedic Foundation for Animals
Columbia, Missouri

Jodi D. Smith, DVM
Department of Clinical Sciences
College of Veterinary Medicine
Auburn University
Auburn, Alabama

Kerry Smith Bailey, DVM
Long Island Veterinary Specialists
Plainview, New York

Mark M. Smith, VMD, DACVS, DAVDC
Dentistry and Oral Surgery
Red Bank Veterinary Hospital
Red Bank, New Jersey

Saralyn Smith-Carr, DVM, PhD, DACVIM (SAIM)
Associate Professor
Department of Clinical Sciences
College of Veterinary Medicine
Auburn University
Auburn, Alabama

Elisabeth Snead, BSc, DVM, DACVIM (SAIM)
Assistant Professor
Small Animal Clinical Sciences
Western College of Veterinary Medicine
University of Saskatchewan
Saskatoon, Saskatchewan, Canada

Mary E. Somerville, DVM, DACVS
Animal Surgical and Emergency Center
Los Angeles, California

Dennis Spann, DVM, DACVIM (SAIM)
Staff Internist
Loomis Basin Veterinary Clinic
Loomis, California

Jonathan Spears, BSc, DVM
Theriogenology Resident
Atlantic Veterinary College
University of Prince Edward Island
Charlottetown, Prince Edward Island, Canada

Alan W. Spier, DVM, PhD, DACVIM (Cardiology)
Florida Veterinary Specialists
Tampa, Florida

Jörg M. Steiner, DMV, PhD, DACVIM (SAIM), DECVIM-CA
Clinical Associate Professor and Co-Director
Gastrointestinal Laboratory
Department of Small Animal Clinical Sciences
College of Veterinary Medicine and Biomedical Sciences
Texas A&M University
College Station, Texas

Rebecca L. Stepien, DVM, MS, DACVIM (Cardiology)
Clinical Associate Professor—Cardiology
Department of Medical Sciences
University of Wisconsin School of Veterinary Medicine
Madison, Wisconsin

Michael Stone, DVM, DACVIM (SAIM)
Clinical Assistant Professor
Cummings School of Veterinary Medicine
Tufts University
North Grafton, Massachusetts
Consultant
Veterinary Internal Medicine Mobile Specialists
Woodstock, Connecticut

Elizabeth M. Streeter, DVM, DACVECC
Clinician
Veterinary Clinical Sciences
Iowa State University
College of Veterinary Medicine
Veterinary Teaching Hospital
Ames, Iowa

Keith Nelson Strickland, BSc (Zoology), DVM, DACVIM (Cardiology)
Associate Professor of Cardiology
Department of Veterinary Clinical Sciences
School of Veterinary Medicine
Louisiana State University
Baton Rouge, Louisiana

Shannon T. Stroup, DVM
Resident, Internal Medicine
Department of Clinical Sciences
Auburn University College of Veterinary Medicine
Auburn, Alabama

Vivien Surman, DVM, MRCVS
Ameriland Animal Hospital
Ovid, New York

Graham Swinney, BVSc, FACVSc, DVLS
Clinical Assistant Professor
Department of Veterinary Clinical Sciences
Washington State University
Pullman, Washington

Jane Sykes, BVSc (Hons), PhD, DACVIM (SAIM)
Assistant Professor
Department of Medicine and Epidemiology
University of California
Davis, California

Joseph Taboada, DVM, DACVIM (SAIM)
School of Veterinary Medicine
Louisiana State University
Baton Rouge, Louisiana

Kathryn Taylor, DVM
Resident
Department of Clinical Sciences
Auburn University
Auburn, Alabama

William B. Thomas, DVM, MS, DACVIM (Neurology)
Associate Professor, Neurology & Neurosurgery
Department of Small Animal Clinical Sciences
University of Tennessee
Knoxville, Tennessee

Juliene L. Throop, VMD, DACVIM (SAIM)
Internal Medicine Consultant
IDEXX Laboratories
Westbrook, Maine

Michael Thrusfield, MSc, BVMS, DTVM, CBiol, FIBiol, DECVPH, MRCVS
Senior Lecturer
Royal (Dick) School of Veterinary Studies
University of Edinburgh, Scotland
Veterinary Clinical Studies
Easter Bush Veterinary Centre
Roslin, Midlothian, United Kingdom

Lisa M. Tieber Nielson, DVM, MS
Neurology Resident
Department of Clinical Sciences
College of Veterinary Medicine
Small Animal Teaching Hospital
Auburn University
Auburn, Alabama

D. Michael Tillson, DVM, MS, DACVS
Associate Professor
Small Animal Surgery
Department of Clinical Sciences
College of Veterinary Medicine
Auburn University
Auburn, Alabama

Karen M. Tobias, DVM, MS, DACVS
Professor
Department of Small Animal Clinical Sciences
University of Tennessee
College of Veterinary Medicine
Knoxville, Tennessee

Danna M. Torre, DVM
Resident, Emergency and Critical Care Medicine
Cummings School of Veterinary Medicine
Tufts University
North Grafton, Massachusetts

Nicholas J. Trout, MA, VetMB, MRCVS, DACVS, DECVS
Staff Surgeon
Angell Animal Medical Center
Boston, Massachusetts

Mark T. Troxel, DVM, DACVIM (Neurology)
Staff Neurologist/ Neurosurgeon
Neurology and Neurosurgery Department
Massachusetts Referral Hospital
Woburn, Massachusetts

David C. Twedt, DVM, DACVIM (SAIM)
Professor
Department of Clinical Sciences
College of Veterinary Medicine and Biomedical Sciences
Colorado State University
Fort Collins, Colorado

Shelly Vaden, DVM, PhD, DACVIM (SAIM)
Professor of Internal Medicine
North Carolina State University
College of Veterinary Medicine
Raleigh, North Carolina

Beth A. Valentine, DVM, PhD, DACVP
Associate Professor
Department of Biomedical Sciences
College of Veterinary Medicine
Oregon State University
Corvallis, Oregon

Liesel van der Merwe, BVSc (Hons) Pret, MRCVS
Senior Lecturer
Department of Companion Animal Clinical Studies
Faculty of Veterinary Science
University of Pretoria
Onderstepoort, South Africa

Leen Verhaert, DVM, DEVDC
Associate
TRIVET Veterinary Private Practice
Hove, Belgium
Scientific Co-Worker
Department of Medicine and Clinical Biology of Small Animals
Ghent University
Ghent, Belgium

John Verstegen, DVM, MSc, PhD, DECAR
Associate Professor
Small Animal Theriogenology
Large Animal Clinical Sciences
College of Veterinary Medicine
University of Florida
Gainesville, Florida

Erin D. Vicari, VMD
Emergency Clinician
Veterinary Specialty Center of Delaware
Wilmington, Delaware

Dietrich Volkmann, BVSc, MMedVet (Gynecology), DACT
Staff Veterinarian
Section of Reproductive Studies
New Bolton Center
University of Pennsylvania
Kennett Square, Pennsylvania

Lori S. Waddell, DVM, DACVECC
Adjunct Assistant Professor
Intensive Care Unit
Section of Critical Care
Matthew J. Ryan Veterinary Hospital of the University of Pennsylvania
Philadelphia, Pennsylvania

Stephen Waisglass, BSc, DVM, MRCVS, CertSAD
Dermatology Consultant
Doncaster Animal Clinic
Thornhill
Ontario, Canada
ACVD Resident
Ontario Veterinary College
Guelph, Ontario, Canada

Thomas J. Walker, DVM
Resident
Emergency and Critical Care Medicine
Department of Small Animal Clinical Sciences
Cummings School of Veterinary Medicine
Tufts University
North Grafton, Massachusetts

Aubrey A. Webb, DVM, PhD
Department of Biomedical Sciences
Atlantic Veterinary College
University of Prince Edward Island
Charlottetown, Prince Edward Island, Canada

Craig B. Webb, PhD, DVM, DACVIM (SAIM)
Assistant Professor
Clinical Sciences Department
Colorado State University
Veterinary Teaching Hospital
Fort Collins, Colorado

Cynthia R. L. Webster, DVM, DACVIM (SAIM)
Associate Professor
Department of Clinical Sciences
Cummings School of Veterinary Medicine
Tufts University
North Grafton, Massachusetts

Claire Weigand, DVM, DACVIM (SAIM)
Angell Animal Medical Center—Western New England
Springfield, Massachusetts

Sharon L. Welch, DVM
Consulting Veterinarian in Clinical Toxicology
ASPCA Animal Poison Control Center
Urbana, Illinois

Elizabeth G. Welles, DVM, PhD
Associate Professor
Department of Pathobiology
Auburn University
Auburn, Alabama

Jocelyn Wellington, DVM, DACVD
Animal Dermatology Services
London, Ontario, Canada

Aaron Wey, DVM, DACVIM (Cardiology)
Upstate Veterinary Specialties
Latham, New York

Richard Wheeler, DVM, DACT
Poudre River Veterinary Clinic
Fort Collins, Colorado
Associate Faculty
Small Animal Medicine
Colorado State University
Fort Collins, Colorado

Megan Whelan, DVM
Resident
Emergency and Critical Care Medicine
Cummings School of Veterinary Medicine
Tufts University
North Grafton, Massachusetts

Christine L. Wilford, DVM
Associate Veterinarian
Cats Exclusive Veterinary Center
Seattle, Washington

David A. Wilkie, DVM, MS, DACVO
Associate Professor
Head, Comparative Ophthalmology
Department of Clinical Sciences
The Ohio State University
Veterinary Hospital
Columbus, Ohio

Michael Willard, DVM, MS, DACVIM (SAIM)
Professor
Department of Small Animal Medicine and Surgery
Texas A&M University
College Station, Texas

Laurel E. Williams, DVM, DACVIM (Oncology)
Assistant Professor (Oncology)
Department of Clinical Sciences
College of Veterinary Medicine
North Carolina State University
Raleigh, North Carolina

Kimberly B. Winters, DVM
Resident, Small Animal Internal Medicine
Department of Clinical Sciences
Cummings School of Veterinary Medicine
Tufts University
North Grafton, Massachusetts

Tina Wismer, DVM, DABVT, DABT
Senior Toxicologist
ASPCA Animal Poison Control Center
Urbana, Illinois

Christina Wolf, DVM
Intern, Veterinary Clinical Sciences
College of Veterinary Medicine
University of Tennessee
Knoxville, Tennessee

Michael W. Wood, DVM
Clinical Investigator
Department of Clinical Sciences
College of Veterinary Medicine
North Carolina State University
Raleigh, North Carolina

Deanna R. Worley, DVM
Department of Clinical Studies
University of Pennsylvania
School of Veterinary Medicine
Matthew J. Ryan Veterinary Hospital
Philadelphia, Pennsylvania

Kathy Wright, DVM, DACVIM (Cardiology, SAIM)
Cardiologist
The Cincinnati Animal Referral and Emergency Center
Cincinnati, Ohio

Anthony Yu, DVM, MS, DACVD
Associate Professor
Department of Clinical Studies
Ontario Veterinary College
University of Guelph
Guelph, Ontario, Canada

For guidance past and present
For generosity, both professional and personal
For embodying the saying that
"In matters of teaching, example is not the most important thing, it is the only thing"
For friendship
This book is dedicated with gratitude to my mentor
Stephen J. Ettinger

Foreword

When Dr. Côté completed his medicine and cardiology studies at the California Animal Hospital, he left our group much as most newly trained residents do. He had a heart full of desire to change the practice of Veterinary Medicine. In doing so, his ideals were wonderfully broad and challenging. He knew that there were many who could benefit from his "new ways" of thinking and teaching. During the training years, one of the things that was very apparent was his desire to teach the younger staff members and to present points to them in ways that were unique and that approached problems in a way that could be understood readily and remembered. This book is an extension of that thought process. Certainly, one would say initially that his goal was to present the more exotic, but as time passed, Dr. Côté saw that the basics represented challenges every bit as exciting and pressing to the veterinarian and to the client.

Dr. Côté's career at our teaching hospital began with helping the younger staff to understand the use of over-the-counter human medications. These enlightened him to the importance of basic and clear instructions that could readily and effectively be passed on to the staff or the client. I believe that Dr. Côté has established in this book a similar point of reference in that the disease conditions and problems are covered quickly but in enough detail to readily distinguish each problem from complicating or easily mistaken conditions. The approach used in this textbook involves covering the major areas within small animal veterinary practice: diseases and disorders, procedures and techniques, differential diagnoses, decision making based on an algorithmic tree-like methodology, and laboratory testing and medications, identified by functional category and clinical efficacy in disease.

In order to make this an effective mechanism of teaching, he has chosen a template-based approach that allows for a quick and thorough review of the varying processes. These templates thus permit the reader easy access to the basic testing necessary to identify a problem, the usual approach to a reliable physical examination and history as well as to the possibilities that develop regarding the mechanism, and the approach to the differential diagnosis. Minimum database testing comes first as well it should. The authors of the sections have incorporated only reasonable diagnostic testing limited to those tests that are routinely performed in most general practices. With either a secure diagnosis in hand or a reasonable differential diagnosis considered, the clinician may take the opportunity to confirm the diagnosis with additional appropriate testing or be able to ford the treatment process effectively.

This approach allows the reader to have ready access to information on a scale that is handy and sufficiently brief so as not to inundate a busy time period. Selected references are available to allow further research or study into each process described and to guide the reader to sources that describe the condition in greater detail. While the editor of this book is keenly aware that medicine may be far more complex than that which is presented, the obvious and the requisite information provided identify to the reader a clear and distinct pathway to each process. Ultimately this is directed at a successful conclusion by utilizing this easy-to-read and readily discernible method of approach.

Treatment portions of the text cover therapeutic goals, acute and chronic treatments, drug interactions, likely and possible complications, and recommended monitoring. A modified up-to-date drug summary is provided also, and the reader is encouraged to utilize this easy-to-use format that describes the various drugs we utilize daily in small animal practice. Therapeutic products are identified as being designed for human beings, dogs, cats, or a combination so that the reader may select the appropriate products to use. When these are available as human drug products, the veterinarian also has the option to offer written prescriptions for immediate filling at local human pharmacies or through the World Wide Web, as many people opt for prescription agents through that source. This makes it easier for the reader to determine the availability of the product so that written prescriptions can be provided for many of the ailments.

The end of each topic includes a section referred to as clinical pearls, which are most useful nuggets regarding the subject. This pearl is one that often is something one learns only in the process of treating real disease. It does, however, transcend from lecturer to student easily and, if utilized properly, the reader will find an abundance of information from these quotes. I suggest that the reader does not gloss over them but rather realizes the value that such short, succinct statements permit in allowing one to recognize a disease that otherwise might be quickly overlooked or simply missed. Enjoy reading this book, keep it handy, and utilize it as a daily reference source to make certain that today's medicine becomes tomorrow's cures.

Stephen J. Ettinger, DVM, DACVIM (Cardiology, SAIM), FACC, FAHA

California Animal Hospital
Los Angeles, California

Preface

"Everything should be made as simple as possible, but no simpler."

Albert Einstein

Keeping pace with current knowledge in any aspect of veterinary medicine is an enormous challenge, let alone staying up to date in all of them. For a busy practitioner, specialty textbooks, reviews, and original articles may be too detailed to be immediately useful. Simplified information often is more accessible, but the appeal can be misleading if the information is not peer-reviewed or even scientifically defensible. The *Clinical Veterinary Advisor* provides an entry point between these two extremes using a template-based format, illustrations, and a multi-faceted approach. It is designed to present the most current information in a concise and useful manner. Accordingly, the *Advisor* is organized to cover six major components of small animal practice: diseases and disorders, procedures and techniques, differential diagnoses, algorithm-based decision making, laboratory tests, and medications.

The first section of this book is Diseases and Disorders. It describes the most important elements of commonly encountered illnesses and initial problems of dogs and cats. The material is presented following the natural progression of a case: background information is first, including the definition of the topic, synonyms, and epidemiologic facts. Next come the reason underlying the veterinary visit (chief complaint) and important or typical elements of the history as it pertains to the particular disorder. After physical examination findings, diagnostic testing is presented in two consequent parts: the initial database includes diagnostic tests that are routinely performed first in most general practices. Immediately after come advanced or confirmatory tests, which encompass the more specific evaluations that either can be done in some general practices or require referral to a university hospital or specialty center. This staged approach reflects the process that we so commonly use with our patients. Treatment is similarly described as initial, acute treatment, and then separately, chronic or long-term treatment for disorders requiring ongoing care. Drug dosages and routes of administration are included directly, to avoid forcing the reader to leaf through the drug formulary for every medication. The end of each topic in Diseases and Disorders includes a section for clinical pearls, which are the nuggets of information that are most valuable based on the experience of the author and editor—a counterintuitive point, an easily made mistake to avoid, a concern about the nature of the disease or process, or other facts to provide medical hints that often escape the written word.

Procedures and Techniques, the second section, describes over 80 diagnostic and therapeutic procedures specific to small animal practice. The breadth of this material is wide, ranging from the simple, such as cystocentesis or rectal palpation, to the advanced, such as temporary cardiac pacing or hemodialysis. The material is presented in a streamlined and formatted way by specialists who have either pioneered these procedures or are considered experts in their application. The intent is to allow a reader to feel prepared for performing the procedures if the reader's training and skills are adequate, or else to understand what is involved in a procedure when referring a patient to another institution for having it performed.

The third section, Differential Diagnosis, regroups tables that list the causes of some 250 of the most common abnormalities encountered in small animal practice. This section is perhaps most useful for students and young veterinarians, or for any veterinarian reviewing the breadth of potential etiologies for a particular disorder.

The fourth section, Laboratory Tests, has been designed to combine the clinical pathologist's expertise with the needs of the small animal practitioner. This section presents some 140 concise summaries of commonly—and uncommonly—used small animal laboratory tests. As in other parts of the book, the information for each topic is arranged in an intuitive and user-friendly manner: basic information comes first (definition, normal range of results, underlying physiology), followed by causes of abnormal levels, the next test or diagnostic step to consider, and finally, a listing of artifacts, specimen handling instructions, and clinical pearls.

Section five, the Clinical Algorithms section, approaches the management of some of the most common or challenging disorders in small animal practice using the "decision tree" format. Younger veterinarians or those veterinarians looking for information in an unfamiliar part of small animal practice may find this section most helpful, since it represents a starting point of information stripped of nuances and caveats. This basic, streamlined approach simply provides an initial framework for addressing a particular disorder, from which individual variations can then radiate.

Finally, the sixth section is the Drug Formulary. This section is the result of combining the practitioner's need for coverage of relevant medications with the pharmacologist's information base. Described and summarized in tabular format are 450 medications that are in common use or that are emerging in practice. Space constraints preclude a very detailed description, so an emphasis is placed on the most immediately useful elements of individual drugs.

Throughout this textbook, information is included based on its clinical importance. Some topics are discussed in greater detail than others, or even as separate stand-alone topics if their occurrence in practice justifies it. For example, chronic renal failure is a common disease and it occurs in two very different contexts: some animals are overtly ill, whereas in others the disorder is discovered incidentally on routine lab tests. Since both situations occur often in practice, and both are managed very differently, there are two separate whole topics in the *Advisor* to address this situation: "Chronic renal failure, occult ('asymptomatic')," and "Chronic renal failure, overt ('symptomatic')." The same is true for lymphoma, hyperadrenocorticism, and other diseases with variable presentations or subtypes.

Given a fixed allotment of photographs and images, topics most suitable for illustrations have been identified, and images included accordingly. Photographs and illustrations occupy a premium in terms of space, and therefore a determined effort has been made to include only photographs with immediate clinical relevance. Histopathologic images, necropsy images, images that are unclear or ambiguous, and the like, with little in-clinic impact, have been excluded in favor of single-frame images that clearly illustrate a condition, series of photographs that illustrate a process, or paired images (1 normal, 1 abnormal) that help demonstrate a lesion by comparison. It is not enough for a picture to be worth a thousand words—the "words" must be clear and useful.

Simplicity can be deceptive. Teaching students, interns, and residents reminds us of our own first exposure to master clinicians. Some of them made clinical reasoning and medical procedures seem so easy. Unbeknownst to us then (and to our own students and trainees now, perhaps), the ease and polish was not necessarily spontaneous. It often was the result of incalculable hours of practice, refinement, awareness, patience, understanding, and persistence. The same can be said of this book. The highly formatted presentation and compact nature of the information aim to be user-friendly. However, this apparent simplicity conceals an enormous amount of painstaking work. "What is written without effort is in general read without pleasure," said the lexicographer Samuel Johnson. By that measure, the *Advisor* should be a joy to read. One topic at a time, and then as a whole, the material that makes up the *Advisor* has been conceived, written out, reworked, amended, compromised on, refined, and ultimately accepted. As a result, it is my intent and my hope that this book will stand out as cohesive and immediately useful.

It would be a pleasure to say that the *Advisor* will answer every question that comes up in small animal practice. We all know that an honest assessment of any book says otherwise. A truer goal for this textbook is for it to provide its readers with a solid summary of the information needed to properly handle most of what one encounters in practice, from the old to the new, from the routine to the exceptional. The governing principles have been to make the material accurate, practical, current, and rapidly accessible. Now the book is ready to enter the information stream and let its content speak for itself.

Acknowledgments

We—all of us—are keenly aware in these times of the value of our own time. To many of us it is our most precious commodity. In this manner, the authors and editors of the *Advisor* have been most generous: the more time authors and editors have spent on streamlining a manuscript, the easier it is for reader-practitioners to grasp the information quickly. In addition to medical knowledge, the act of taking a chapter from start to finish requires patience and dedication. For having accepted to contribute the material that makes up the totality of the *Advisor*, and lived up to these commitments, I offer each individual author and editor my heartfelt, sincere thanks. Their tireless efforts were the backbone and the flesh of this project. These are the colleagues who provided great material, answered my many questions, and rolled with the punches. Authors wrote and submitted manuscripts under an enormous array of circumstances including tremendous hardships such as the manuscripts from Gulf Coast authors that arrived, within deadline, despite the Hurricane Katrina disaster. Editors contended with the unpredictable and inevitable changes and snags that occur with any undertaking of this size, and did so with a smile. My heart is filled with deep gratitude and pride when I think of what we have accomplished, and the way we have done so.

The team at Elsevier, including Penny Rudolph, Jolynn Gower, Stacy Beane, Melissa Lastarria, Joy Moore, Jennifer Hong, Liz Fathman, and John Dedeke, as well as Amanda Hellenthal and the SPi group, provided positive support and all the essentials that transformed our 7000 pages of raw information in MS Word into this attractive book. I thank each of you. The illustrations of Glenda Clements-Smith and Don O'Connor added substantially to the clarity and the impact of the information and their work is gratefully acknowledged.

I wish to thank my colleagues and friends, without whom this book would be different or nonexistent. Steve Ettinger, my mentor in the truest sense, helped with his insights on countless crucial occasions. An editor could not possibly hope for a better source of advice and feedback. I am grateful to my students and trainees past and present for the courage, curiosity, or both, that led them to ask questions that needed asking, and thus to keep the wheel of learning in motion. In a similar respect, I thank any and all readers in advance for sending comments, corrections, or modifications that help improve future versions of the *Advisor*. I wish to thank my university colleagues and particularly Peter Foley for their informal comments, opinions, and unwavering support. In addition to multiple Atlantic Veterinary College editors and authors, I thank Hans Gelens, Darcy Shaw, Pat Rose, and Lee Ann Pack for their additional contributions and support of the project. I am grateful to the Radiology staff at AVC, particularly Wayne McKenna and Nancy Hogan, for continuing to accept my requests for images and for their unfailingly quick turnaround. Karen Roche and Ruth Bigney provided invaluable administrative and secretarial help, and I thank them sincerely. From the very beginning, Navin Khanna, Michel Racicot, and Nicole Cloutier offered me their expertise with incredible generosity, and I am indebted to them for their kindness. Finally, I particularly wish to thank the Yeh family and the Formosa Tea House for providing a haven that allowed me to work in a peaceful and welcoming setting for many, many hours on this book.

Etienne Côté
Charlottetown, Canada

Contents

ALPHABETICAL LISTING

CES: Client Education Sheet, found on the companion website at **www.coteclinicalvetadvisor.com.**

SECTION II PROCEDURES AND TECHNIQUES

SECTION III DIFFERENTIAL DIAGNOSIS

(web): indicates an entry that is available only on the companion website at **www.coteclinicalvetadvisor.com.**

SECTION V CLINICAL ALGORITHMS

CLIENT EDUCATION SHEETS

The following client education sheets can be found on the companion website at **www.coteclinicalvetadvisor.com.**

SECTION I

Diseases and Disorders

EDITORS

C. A. Tony Buffington, DVM, PhD, DACVN
Nutrition

Leah A. Cohn, DVM, PhD, DACVIM (SAIM)
Urology

Etienne Côté, DVM, DACVIM (Cardiology, SAIM) Cardiology; Chief Complaints; Other Topics

Susan M. Cotter, DVM, DACVIM (SAIM, Oncology) Hematologic and Immune-Mediated Diseases

Cheryl L. Cullen, DVM, MVetSc, DACVO
Ophthalmology

Curtis W. Dewey, DVM, MS, DACVIM (Neurology), DACVS Neurology

Jan A. Hall, BVM&S, MS, MRCVS, DACVD
Dermatology

Joseph Harari, DVM, MS, DACVS
Orthopedics

Sherri Ihle, DVM, MSc, DACVIM (SAIM)
Endocrinology

Safdar A. Khan, DVM, MS, PhD, DABVT
Toxicology

Michelle A. Kutzler, DVM, PhD, DACT
Theriogenology

Douglass K. Macintire, DVM, MS, DACVIM (SAIM), DACVECC Infectious Diseases

Karen L. Overall, MA, VMD, PhD, DACVB
Behavior

Kenneth M. Rassnick, DVM, DACVIM (Oncology) Oncology

Alexander M. Reiter, DMV, Dipl-Tzt, DAVDC, DEVDC Dentistry

Keith P. Richter, DVM, DACVIM (SAIM)
Hepatobiliary and Pancreatic Diseases

Elizabeth Rozanski, DVM, DACVECC, DACVIM (SAIM) Emergency and Critical Care

Rance K. Sellon, DVM, PhD, DACVIM (SAIM)
Respiratory Diseases

Richard Walshaw, BVMS, DACVS Soft Tissue Surgery

Debra L. Zoran, DVM, MS, PhD, DACVIM (SAIM) Gastroenterology

Abdominal Compartment Syndrome

BASIC INFORMATION

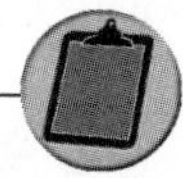

DEFINITION

Impaired organ function resulting from increased intra-abdominal pressure (IAP)

SYNONYM(S)

ACS
Increased IAP
Intra-abdominal hypertension (IAH)

EPIDEMIOLOGY

- An underlying disease leading to either gas or fluid buildup in the abdominal compartment, or interference with the abdominal wall's ability to expand and compensate for increased abdominal contents, is the initiating factor. There is no breed, sex, or species predilection.
- Partial list of predisposing conditions:
  - Abdominal effusions (any type)
  - Abdominal wraps/bandages
  - Pancreatitis
  - Hepatic abscess
  - Peritonitis
  - Abdominal trauma
  - Sepsis of any origin
  - Abdominal neoplasia
  - Antishock trousers

CLINICAL PRESENTATION

PHYSICAL EXAM FINDINGS

- Any patient with abdominal disease or accumulations of fluid, gas, or tissue (neoplastic, inflammatory, etc.) in the abdominal cavity can develop intra-abdominal hypertension and abdominal compartment syndrome.
- Indications to check IAP are (usually in combination):
  - Progressive abdominal distention or tympany
  - Azotemia, reduced urine output
  - Elevated central venous, mean arterial, right and left atrial pressures
  - Distended jugular veins may be evident
  - Rising intracranial pressure and altered mentation
  - Vomiting and diarrhea new to the patient
  - Rising blood lactate
  - Tachypnea and tachycardia

ETIOLOGY AND PATHOPHYSIOLOGY

- Increased pressure in the abdomen leads to impaired blood flow to abdominal organs and, when severe, direct compression of blood vessels. This leads to alterations in renal, hepatic, and gastrointestinal functions.
- Reduced ability for the diaphragm to contract against the tense abdomen impairs tidal volume and therefore compromises ventilation. Mechanical/positive pressure ventilation is similarly affected.
- An increase in central venous pressure (CVP) and drop in cardiac output (from increased systemic vascular resistance) lead to the previously noted changes in cardiovascular function.
- Hormonal changes occur in response to the altered cardiovascular status in the body's attempt to compensate, including elevations in renin-angiotensin activity, antidiuretic hormone, and catecholamine levels.

DIAGNOSIS

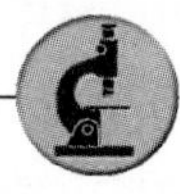

DIFFERENTIAL DIAGNOSIS

IAP must be measured to make the diagnosis of abdominal compartment syndrome.

INITIAL DATABASE

- IAP is measured using a water manometer attached to a stopcock in the evacuation line from a urethral catheter, the tip of which must reach the lumen of the bladder.
- The urinary bladder is emptied, and a few milliliters of saline are placed in the bladder (3–10 ml, depending on patient size).
- The setup is zeroed, the three-way stopcock is closed (to interrupt flow between the urethral catheter and the manometer), and the zero mark on the column is held at the same approximate horizontal level as the atria of the heart:
  - The level of the point of the shoulder in the standing animal
  - The level of the umbilicus in the laterally recumbent animal
- The manometer is filled to the top of the column and then reopened to the bladder.
- The reading is taken when the column of saline stops falling. The meniscus may move slightly up and down with ventilation.
- Alternatively, a venous catheter in the caudal vena cava gives similar information but can be more cumbersome to place and to maintain.
- An abdominal drain already in place can be used to monitor IAP. A three-way stopcock and manometer can be set into the system at an appropriate evacuation point.
- As with central venous pressure measurements, trends in pressure parameters may be more important than any single number, especially in the lower ranges. The patient should be in the same position each time a measurement is taken.

ADVANCED OR CONFIRMATORY TESTING

- Repeated measurements.
- Supplementing the data with lactate levels, liver enzyme changes, urine output, blood urea nitrogen, and creatinine levels can assist in identifying the primary cause and secondary changes.
- Measurements of cardiac output and other cardiovascular parameters and monitoring of mentation and intracranial pressure give a more extensive assessment of cardiovascular function and perfusion.

TREATMENT

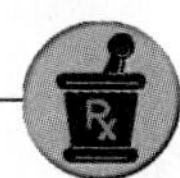

THERAPEUTIC GOAL(S)

Normal IAP is 0–5 cm H_2O, or <10 cm H_2O after abdominal surgery.

ACUTE, GENERAL TREATMENT

- Acute management of abdominal compartment syndrome requires immediate reduction of IAP by paracentesis or exploratory surgery and direct removal of the fluid or tissue causing the problem.
- Maintain appropriate vascular volume with fluid and blood product administration.
- IAP of 10–20 cm H_2O is a mild elevation.
  - Ensure adequate vascular volume (IV fluids as necessary) and monitor for changes in IAP.
- IAP 20–35 cm H_2O is a moderate to severe elevation.
  - Ensure adequate vascular volume (IV fluids as necessary).
  - Use diagnostics to identify underlying cause if not known.
  - Monitor for progression using repeated measurements.
  - Consider active decompression if pressure continues to rise or if other parameters continue to deteriorate. Decompression may involve abdominocentesis to remove fluid or surgical reduction of the problem.
- IAP >35 cm H_2O is a severe elevation.
  - Abdominal compartment syndrome is extremely likely.
  - Decompression of the abdomen is required.

- If a correctible source is not identified, exploratory laparotomy is indicated.

CHRONIC TREATMENT

- Placement of abdominal drains or repeated drainages/centeses in chronic conditions to maintain reduced pressure may be necessary. Treatment of the underlying disease is essential.
- Maintain appropriate vascular volume with IV fluid and blood product administration.

RECOMMENDED MONITORING

IAP, central venous pressure, blood pressure, blood chemistry, lactate, urine output

PROGNOSIS AND OUTCOME

Prognosis depends on underlying cause and associated abnormalities, organ dysfunction, and disease. If end-organ function is deteriorating, prognosis worsens.

PEARLS & CONSIDERATIONS

Most critically ill patients should have urethral catheters in place to monitor urine output. Addition of a three-way stopcock for manometer placement (using aseptic technique) is simple and makes collection of IAP data simple.

COMMENTS

It is advised that monitoring and management of patients this ill take place in an adequately staffed 24-hour facility.

PREVENTION

Careful monitoring with preventive action taken if IAP rises

SUGGESTED READING

Drellich S: Intraabdominal pressure and abdominal compartment syndrome. *Compend Contin Educ Prac Vet* 22:764–769, 2000.

Cheatham ML: Intra-abdominal hypertension and abdominal compartment syndrome. *New Horizons* 7:96–115, 1999.

AUTHOR: **SHARON DRELLICH**

EDITOR: **ELIZABETH ROZANSKI**

Abdominal Distention

BASIC INFORMATION

DEFINITION

Enlargement of the abdominal cavity

EPIDEMIOLOGY

SPECIES, AGE, SEX: Dependent on underlying cause.

CLINICAL PRESENTATION

HISTORY, CHIEF COMPLAINT

- Abdominal enlargement (rate of distention is extremely variable, varies from acute to chronic and insidious).
- Perceived weight gain.
- Decreased activity.
- Anorexia.
- Tachypnea.
- Abdominal discomfort/pain.
- When ascites is present and the fluid accumulation is rapid, clinical signs of weakness and dyspnea are more likely to be apparent.
- History may include clinical signs associated with the primary disease (e.g., repeated, unproductive attempts at vomiting if gastric dilatation and volvulus; dyspnea, cough if cardiac disease; icterus if liver disease).

PHYSICAL EXAM FINDINGS

- Visible abdominal enlargement (Figs. I-1 and I-2)
- Abdominal palpation:
  - Fluid wave may be present (ballottement) with ascites.
  - An abdominal mass or organomegaly (liver, spleen, kidney, etc.) may be palpable.
- Physical abnormalities associated with primary disease may be present:
  - Cardiovascular abnormalities (heart murmur, arrhythmia, gallop sound, jugular distention) should warrant further investigation into the possibility of right heart failure.
  - Marked generalized lymphadenopathy may suggest lymphoma.
  - Muffled heart sounds are consistent with pericardial effusion and tamponade if ascites is present.

ETIOLOGY AND PATHOPHYSIOLOGY

- Ascites: all causes
- Hyperadrenocorticism/Cushing's disease
- Cyst (renal, hepatic)
- Gastrointestinal dilation (food, air, water, foreign material)
- Lipoma
- Lymphadenopathy
- Mass—non-neoplastic (hematoma, granuloma, abscess)
- Neoplasia
- Pancreatitis
- Parasitic (*Mesocestoides*)
- Peritonitis
- Pneumoperitoneum (peritonitis or postsurgical)
- Pyometra/hydrometra
- Obstipation
- Organomegaly (hepatomegaly, splenomegaly, renomegaly)
- Torsion (splenic, gastric dilation/volvulus, etc.)
- Urinary obstruction/bladder distention

DIAGNOSIS

DIFFERENTIAL DIAGNOSIS

- Normal variation
- Obesity
- Pregnancy

INITIAL DATABASE

- Abdominal radiographs
  - Loss of serosal detail (focal or generalized) is common if ascites is present
  - May have "ground-glass" appearance (carcinomatosis, peritonitis)
  - Mass lesions, fat, or organomegaly may be apparent or suggested by displacement of gas-filled organs
  - Free air may be present with peritonitis (ruptured viscus)
- Thoracic radiographs
  - Enlarged cardiac silhouette and/or caudal vena cava if congestive heart failure or pericardial effusion (rule out as cause of ascites)
  - Metastatic pulmonary disease
  - Pleural effusion
- Complete blood count, biochemistry panel, and urinalysis are indicated for any animal with ascites or abnormal abdominal distention. Abnormalities depend on underlying cause and extent of organ damage
- Abdominal ultrasonography
  - Confirms presence of fluid if present and differentiates fluid from soft tissue or fat
  - Identification of mass lesions, organomegaly, cyst, etc.
- Echocardiography
  - Confirms diagnosis of right heart enlargement or pericardial effusion (rule out as cause of ascites)
- Abdominal paracentesis if ascites; obtain fluid for cytology and biochemical evaluation
- Characterize fluid based on protein concentration, specific gravity, and total cell count
  - Transudate (pure)

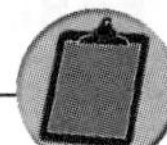

        - Clear and colorless
        - Protein <2.5 g/dl
        - Specific gravity <1.018
        - Cells <1000/mm³: neutrophils and mesothelial cells
    - Modified transudate
        - Red or pink; may be slightly cloudy
        - Protein 2.5–5.0 g/dl
        - Specific gravity >1.018
        - Cells <5000/mm³: neutrophils, mesothelial cells, erythrocytes, and lymphocytes
    - Exudate (nonseptic)
        - Pink or white; cloudy
        - Protein 2.5–5.0 g/dl
        - Specific gravity >1.018
        - Cells 5000–50,000/mm³: neutrophils, mesothelial cells, macrophages, erythrocytes, and lymphocytes
    - Exudate (septic)
        - Red, white, or yellow; cloudy
        - Protein >4.0 g/dl
        - Specific gravity >1.018
        - Cells 5000–100,000/mm³: neutrophils, mesothelial cells, macrophages, erythrocytes, lymphocytes, and bacteria
    - Hemorrhage
        - Red
        - Protein >5.5 g/dl
        - Specific gravity 1.007–1.027
        - Cells consistent with peripheral blood; usually does not clot
    - Chyle
        - Pink, straw, or white
        - Protein 2.5–7.0 g/dl
        - Specific gravity 1.007–1.040

ADVANCED OR CONFIRMATORY TESTING

- Fine-needle aspirate or needle biopsy (mass, enlarged organs, etc.). Biopsy not recommended if area is infected (abscess, pyometra) or likely to hemorrhage (e.g., suspected hemangiosarcoma)
- Prothrombin time if anticoagulant intoxication is suspected as cause of ascites (paracentesis contraindicated if coagulopathy is suspected)
- Computed tomography, magnetic resonance imaging
- Abdominal exploratory may be indicated

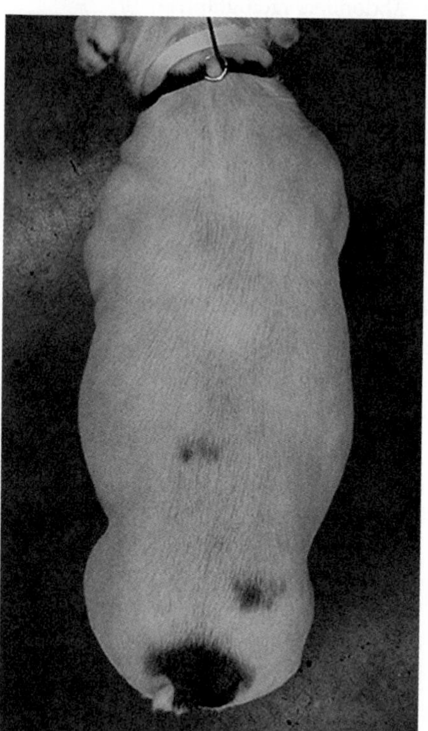

FIGURE I-1 Dorsal view of a young English bulldog with marked ascites caused by right-sided congestive heart failure due to severe pulmonic stenosis. The fluid abdominal distention hides the dog's weight loss and may be mistaken by the owner as an increase in lean body mass. This degree of abdominal distention was associated with poor appetite, lethargy, and dyspnea in this dog.

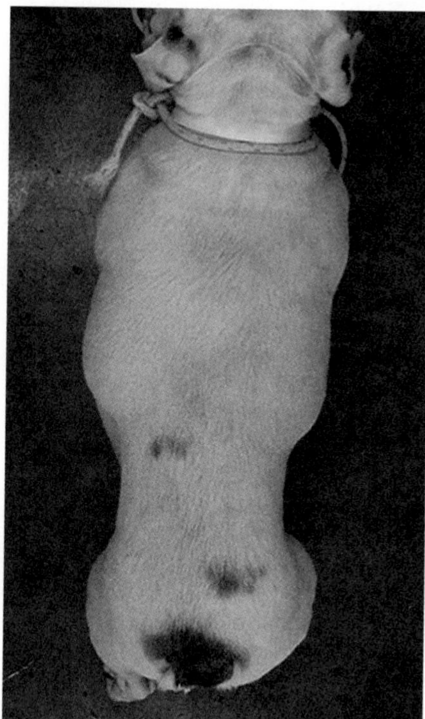

FIGURE I-2 Same dog as in Fig. I-1, 2 hours later when large-volume abdominal drainage was complete. The dog was breathing normally, was more active, and appeared markedly more comfortable. The extent of cardiac cachexia is revealed.

TREATMENT

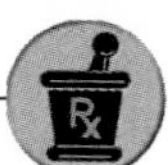

THERAPEUTIC GOAL(S)

Treatment of underlying disease

ACUTE GENERAL TREATMENT

- Treatment of underlying disease:
    - Chemotherapy if lymphoma
    - Pericardiocentesis if pericardial effusion is present
    - Drug therapy for congestive heart failure
- Removal of fluid if discomfort or respiratory difficulty is present (see Abdominal Drainage, p 1176).
- Surgery may be indicated for neoplasia, pyometra, peritonitis, and some causes of hemorrhage (e.g., ruptured splenic or hepatic hemangiosarcoma).

PROGNOSIS AND OUTCOME

Dependent on underlying cause

PEARLS & CONSIDERATIONS

COMMENTS

- Approach to patient with abdominal distention is to determine the nature of the primary problem.
- Thoracic radiographs should be part of the routine evaluation for a patient with ascites so as not to overlook the possibility of cardiac, pericardial, or metastatic disease—or pleural effusion.
- The cause of abdominal distention may be benign (obesity, intra-abdominal lipoma, cyst).

SUGGESTED READING

Ettinger SJ, Barrett KA: Ascites, peritonitis, and other causes of abdominal distention. In Ettinger SJ, Feldman EC, eds: *Textbook of Veterinary Internal Medicine*, ed 4. Philadelphia, WB Saunders, 1995, pp 66–71.

AUTHOR: **KIRSTIE A. BARRETT**
EDITOR: **ETIENNE CÔTÉ**

Aberrant Adrenocortical Disease (Increased Adrenal Sex Hormone Production)

BASIC INFORMATION

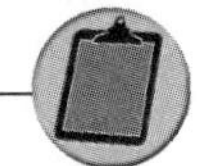

DEFINITION

Clinical signs of hyperadrenocorticism are present, but cortisol test results are normal and one or more of the adrenal sex hormones are increased

SYNONYM(S)

Atypical hyperadrenocorticism
Sex hormone abnormality

EPIDEMIOLOGY

SPECIES, AGE, SEX

- Uncommon
- Middle-aged/old dogs and cats

ASSOCIATED CONDITIONS AND DISORDERS: Hyperadrenocorticism.

CLINICAL PRESENTATION

DISEASE FORMS/SUBTYPES

- Pituitary dependent
- Adrenal dependent: adrenal carcinoma has mainly been reported (two cats and six dogs with hyperprogesteronism reported)

HISTORY, CHIEF COMPLAINT: Identical to Hyperadrenocorticism, p 537.

PHYSICAL EXAM FINDINGS: Identical to Hyperadrenocorticism, p 537.

ETIOLOGY AND PATHOPHYSIOLOGY

- The adrenal gland(s) secretes an excessive amount of one or more adrenal sex hormones.
- Adrenal tumors (particularly adenocarcinomas) may secrete adrenal sex hormones due to disruption of adrenal tissue.
- Progestagens can act as glucocorticoid agonists.
- Cortisol concentrations may be normal to subnormal with sex-hormone secreting adrenal tumors, as high progestagen concentrations can suppress cortisol secretion.

DIAGNOSIS

DIFFERENTIAL DIAGNOSIS

- See Polyuria/Polydipsia, p 878
- See Polyphagia, p 877
- See Alopecia, p 52

INITIAL DATABASE

See Hyperadrenocorticism, p 537

ADVANCED OR CONFIRMATORY TESTING

- Adrenocorticotropic hormone (ACTH) stimulation test with sex hormone panel (progesterone, 17-hydroxyprogesterone, estradiol, androstenedione, testosterone):
  - Dogs with nonadrenal illness may have mildly increased adrenal sex hormones.
  - Approximately 71% sensitivity and specificity for 17-hydroxyprogesterone concentrations if a cutoff greater than 8.5 ng/ml is used for diagnosing atypical hyperadrenocorticism.
- Low-dose dexamethasone suppression test to rule out typical hyperadrenocorticism ± endogenous ACTH concentrations, computer tomography, magnetic resonance imaging (see Hyperadrenocorticism, p 537)

TREATMENT

THERAPEUTIC GOAL(S)

Resolution of clinical signs

ACUTE GENERAL TREATMENT

- See Adrenal Neoplasia (Adenoma/Carcinoma), p 43
- Pituitary-dependent (see Hyperadrenocorticism, p 537)

CHRONIC TREATMENT

See Acute General Treatment above

DRUG INTERACTIONS

See Hyperadrenocorticism, p 537; Adrenal Neoplasia (Adenoma/Carcinoma), p 43

POSSIBLE COMPLICATIONS

See Hyperadrenocorticism, p 537; Adrenal Neoplasia (Adenoma/Carcinoma), p 43

RECOMMENDED MONITORING

Medical therapy: Perform an ACTH stimulation test every 3 months.

- Mitotane therapy: sex hormone concentrations (and cortisol, if also increased) should decrease to normal.
- Trilostane therapy: Progesterone and 17-hydroxyprogesterone concentrations may increase despite resolution of clinical signs and a decrease in cortisol concentrations.

PROGNOSIS AND OUTCOME

- Adrenal tumor: good if surgically resectable
- Pituitary dependent: good with treatment

PEARLS & CONSIDERATIONS

COMMENTS

- Limited information is available regarding this disease and the sensitivity and specificity of adrenal sex hormones in nonadrenal illness. Further research in this area is required.
- Adrenal sex hormones are increased in dogs with typical hyperadrenocorticism (i.e., hypercortisolemia).

SUGGESTED READING

Chapman PS, et al: Evaluation of the basal and post adrenocortical serum concentrations of 17-hydroxyprogesterone in the diagnosis of hyperadrenocorticism in dogs. *Vet Rec* 153:771-775, 2003.

Ristic JM, et al: Plasma 17-hydroxyprogesterone concentrations in the diagnosis of canine hyperadrenocorticism. *J Vet Intern Med* 16:433-439, 2002.

Syme HM, et al: Hyperadrenocorticism associated with excessive sex hormone production by an adrenocortical tumor in two dogs. *J Am Vet Med Assoc* 219:1725-1728, 2001.

AUTHOR: **KATE HILL**
EDITOR: **SHERRI IHLE**

Abortion (Canine)

BASIC INFORMATION

DEFINITION

The expulsion of one or more fetuses before full term pregnancy (i.e., before the conceptus is capable of independent life)

SYNONYM(S)

Fetal loss
Pregnancy wastage

EPIDEMIOLOGY

SPECIES, AGE, SEX: Female dog; no specific age.

RISK FACTORS

- Inbreeding (inbreeding coefficient >0.25): early embryonic death, conceptus resorption
- Malnutrition (pregnancy ketosis)
- Endocrinopathies (hypothyroidism, hypoluteoidism)
- Infection (*Brucella canis, Listeria monocytogenes, Escherichia coli, Campylobacter* spp, *Salmonella* spp, canine herpesvirus 1, minute virus of canines, bluetongue virus, *Neospora caninum*, *Toxoplasma gondii*)

CONTAGION AND ZOONOSIS

- *B. canis* is zoonotic.
- Canine herpesvirus 1, minute virus of canines: transmission through direct contact via nasal secretions, air particles, contact with aborted fetuses/placentae.
- Male-to-female venereal contact is *not* a significant means of viral transmission.

GEOGRAPHY AND SEASONALITY: Canine brucellosis: endemic in parts of North and South America, not Europe since 1996. Canine herpesvirus: worldwide prevalence.

CLINICAL PRESENTATION

HISTORY, CHIEF COMPLAINT

- Pregnant bitch whelps prematurely with nonviable pups, or has no pups at term.
- Abnormal vulvar discharge during pregnancy, fever, or signs of abdominal pain may be noted by owner.
- Usually abortion in the bitch goes unnoticed by the owner, because she may eat the fetuses.

PHYSICAL EXAM FINDINGS

- Often unremarkable.
- Vaginal discharge occurs normally in pregnant bitches and is clear to mucoid or pink-tinged and odorless; purulent, hemorrhagic, greenish, blackish, or malodorous vaginal discharge may indicate pregnancy complications that could lead to abortion.

ETIOLOGY AND PATHOPHYSIOLOGY

- Canine pregnancy requires normal luteal function throughout its duration. Any toxic or hormonal substance that may induce endogenous release of prostaglandins and subsequent luteolysis may result in abortion.
  - Bacterial toxins (*E. coli*, staphylococcal)
  - Adrenergic agonists (e.g., phenylepinephrine)
- Fetal survival requires normal placental function and placental relaxin production. Pathogens that influence placental function (i.e., herpesvirus placentitis) may cause abortion.

DIAGNOSIS

DIFFERENTIAL DIAGNOSIS

- Pseudocyesis (false pregnancy)
- Vaginal discharge due to vaginitis or metritis

INITIAL DATABASE

- Serology of affected dam (*B. canis,* herpesvirus)
- Virus or bacterial isolation from fetuses, placenta, and/or birth canal (infectious agents as listed previously)
- Fetal necropsy (e.g., renal subcapsular hemorrhages typical of herpesvirus)
- Serum progesterone level of dam:
  - Needs to be >2 ng/ml (>6 nmol/L) to sustain pregnancy.
  - Lower level at any time, from ovulation to day 55 of canine pregnancy, suggests hypoluteoidism (luteal dysfunction/failure).
  - Since low serum progesterone levels may occur secondary to fetal death rather than vice versa, the diagnosis of hypoluteoidism is based on a low serum progesterone level, positive effect of progesterone supplementation in a bitch that once aborted, and absence of other risk factors.
- Thyroid hormone analyses:
  - May reveal subclinical hypothyroidism aggravated to a clinically significant disease during periods of stress, such as pregnancy (see Hypothyroidism, p 575).
- Hematology:
  - Normal hematocrit values: 45–55% (nonpregnant) 30–35% (pregnant).
  - Immune-mediated hemolytic anemia may cause abortion.

ADVANCED OR CONFIRMATORY TESTING

- Ultrasonography may reveal fetal death before onset of abortion
- Contact diagnostic laboratory for further recommendations for specific pathogens

TREATMENT

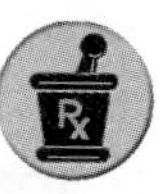

THERAPEUTIC GOAL(S)

Usually it is not possible to save the aborting pregnancy. However, in cases of hypoluteoidism (see Serum progesterone, above), progesterone supplementation may be attempted.

ACUTE GENERAL TREATMENT

Supportive:

- Intravenous fluids (e.g., lactated Ringer's solution) and antibiotics if fever
- Antibiotics: empiric for first few days
  - Amoxicillin (22 mg/kg PO q 8h), cephalexin or cefadroxil (20 mg PO q 8–12h), or pivampicillin (30 mg/kg PO q 12h).
  - Enrofloxacin (5 mg/kg SC, IM, or PO q 24h) or trimethoprim/sulfadiazine (15 mg/kg PO q 12h) is a lesser consideration, as cartilaginous (fluoroquinolone) and teratogenic (trimethoprim-sulfa) adverse effects are possible.
  - Longer-term based on culture and sensitivity results and clinical state.

CHRONIC TREATMENT

If hypoluteoidism is confirmed, treatment may include intramuscular injections of progesterone in oil 2 mg/kg every second day until 10 days before term. Cessation is necessary for parturition to occur.

DRUG INTERACTIONS

Glucocorticoids are unpredictable abortefacient drugs in dogs.

POSSIBLE COMPLICATIONS

- Supplementation with progesterone analogs (i.e., altrenogest) before fetal sexual differentiation: not recommended if whelping date is not known.
- Poor timing may result in masculinization of female fetuses, and failure to discontinue supplementation can cause prolonged gestation, fetal death, and lactation failure.

RECOMMENDED MONITORING

If suspicious of possible abortion, weekly monitoring of progesterone concentrations and fetal viability with abdominal ultrasound examinations should be performed.

PROGNOSIS AND OUTCOME

- Poor for saving an ongoing pregnancy. Usually there is no problem in subsequent pregnancies, except in cases of *Brucella* infections and occasionally in herpesvirus-infected bitches with recrudescent infection.
- Bitches with hypoluteoidism may experience recurrent abortion.

PEARLS & CONSIDERATIONS

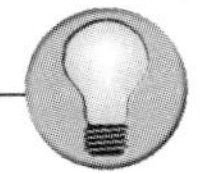

COMMENTS

- Abortion is uncommon in the bitch; fetal resorption or mummification is more common.
- Usually abortion in the bitch goes unnoticed by the owner, as the bitch may eat the fetuses.
- The diagnosis of abortion should prompt a search for an underlying cause (see Risk Factors above).

PREVENTION

- Limit contact with external dogs at breeding and during pregnancy
- Isolate pregnant bitches from showing or performing dogs during pregnancy, especially if herpesvirus is endemic
- Apply an adequate vaccination and deworming program

CLIENT EDUCATION

- Accurate pregnancy diagnosis should be done in bitches on days 25 to 30 (ultrasonography or relaxin test)
- Regular medical evaluation of breeding dogs

SUGGESTED READING

Concannon PW, McCann JP, Temple M: Biology and endocrinology of ovulation, pregnancy and parturition in the dog. *J Reprod Fertil* 39(Suppl):2–25, 1989.

Farstad W: Infectious causes of pregnancy loss in the dog. In Günzel-Apel A-R (ed): *Pathology of Canine and Feline Reproduction, Physiology and Pathology of the Neonate.* The 2nd Course in Reproduction in Companion, Exotic and Laboratory Animals of The European School of Advanced Veterinary Studies, Hannover, Germany, 2003, Volume 2, pp 15.1–15.8.

Gunzel-Apel A-R: Noninfectious causes of pregnancy loss/abnormal pregnancy in the bitch. In Günzel-Apel A-R (ed): *Pathology of Canine and Feline Reproduction, Physiology and Pathology of the Neonate.* The 2nd Course in Reproduction in Companion, Exotic and Laboratory Animals of The European School of Advanced Veterinary Studies, Hannover, Germany, 2003, Volume 2, pp 17.1–17.11.

Ronsse V, et al: Seroprevalence of canine herpesvirus 1 in the Belgian dog population in 2000. *Reprod Domest Anim* 37:299–304, 2002.

England GW, Gary CW: Pregnancy diagnosis, abnormalities of pregnancy and pregnancy termination. In Simpson G, England GW, Harvey M (eds): *Manual of Small Animal Reproduction and Neonatology.* United Kingdom, British Small Animal Veterinary Association, 1998, pp 113–125.

AUTHOR: **WENCHE FARSTAD**
EDITOR: **MICHELLE A. KUTZLER**

Abscess, Apical (Tooth Root)

BASIC INFORMATION

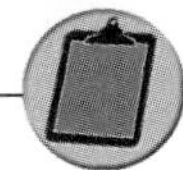

DEFINITION

An apical abscess is a suppurative process of the periapical region of a tooth.

SYNONYM(S)

Periapical abscess
Periradicular abscess
Tooth root abscess

EPIDEMIOLOGY

RISK FACTORS

- Dental trauma (infective, mechanical, thermal, chemical)
- Pulp and periapical disease (Fig. I-3)

ASSOCIATED CONDITIONS AND DISORDERS: Pulp and periapical disease (see Fig. I-3).

CLINICAL PRESENTATION

DISEASE FORMS/SUBTYPES

- Acute
- Chronic (more common)

HISTORY, CHIEF COMPLAINT

- The acute apical abscess presents features of an acute inflammation of the apical periodontium. The affected tooth is extremely painful and slightly extruded from its socket. Localized swelling or cellulitis may be present (e.g., maxillary/facial swelling with or without draining tract), as well as regional lymphadenitis and fever. Rapid extension to adjacent tissues may occur.
- The chronic apical abscess generally presents with no clinical signs, because it is essentially a mild, well-circumscribed area of suppuration. It may undergo rapid exacerbation to become an acute abscess.

PHYSICAL EXAM FINDINGS

- Variable, depending on whether the abscess is acute or chronic
- Fractured and/or discolored tooth crowns
- Severe periodontal disease
- Drainage tracts (oral cavity or skin of face/maxilla)

ETIOLOGY AND PATHOPHYSIOLOGY

- The primary cause is tooth trauma (infective, mechanical, thermal, chemical), resulting in irreversible pulpitis and necrosis.
- If untreated, the inflammatory reaction spreads to involve the periapical region.
- A number of different tissue reactions (including abscessation) may occur, as illustrated in Fig. I-3.
- Periapical lesions do not represent individual, distinct entities. In most cases there is a subtle transformation from one type of lesion into another.
- The apical abscess may develop directly as a result of pulp necrosis, but more commonly originates from an apical granuloma or cyst.

DIAGNOSIS

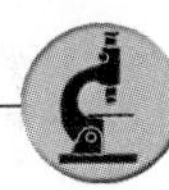

DIFFERENTIAL DIAGNOSIS

- Periapical (apical) granuloma: periapical bone lysis; accumulation of mononuclear inflammatory cells, fibroblasts, and collagen
- Periapical (radicular) cyst: periapical bone lysis; bone walls covered by cystic epithelium
- Osteomyelitis: diffuse regional bony lysis

INITIAL DATABASE

- General physical examination (fever, regional lymphadenitis, facial swelling, oral or facial draining tract[s])
- Meticulous oral examination under general anesthesia to identify tooth (teeth) with pulpal pathology (fractured teeth with pulpal exposure, discolored teeth, caries, drainage tracts)
- Dental radiography to assess periapical status of affected tooth (teeth)
- Variable radiographic appearance depending on whether acute or chronic process
- Acute abscess (arising directly from a necrotic pulp) may show only widening of apical periodontal space
- Chronic abscess is associated with bone destruction (periapical lucency) around the apex of the tooth

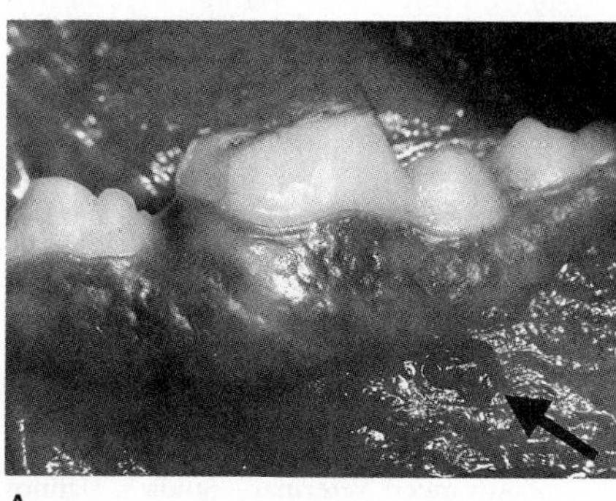
A

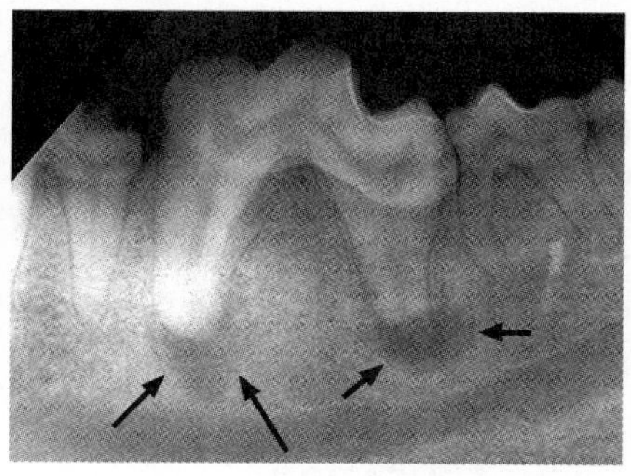
B

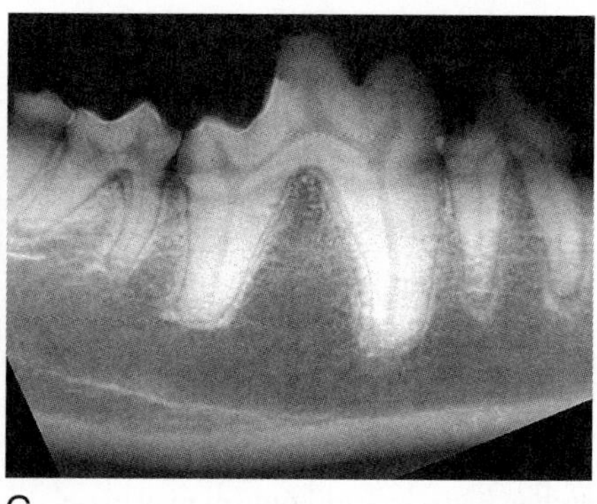
C

FIGURE I-3 **A**, Left M1 fistula: clinical picture of the left lower first molar; the cusps of the tooth are fractured or worn with pulp exposure; a fistula is visible at the mucogingival junction near the distal root of this tooth (*arrow*). **B**, Left M1 fistula, same patient: radiograph of the left lower first molar; the cusps of the tooth are fractured or worn with pulp exposure; radiolucencies are apparent around the apices of both roots. **C**, Right M1 normal, for comparison: normal appearance of periodontal and periapical tissues. Although the cusps of this tooth also are fractured or worn (uncomplicated crown fractures [i.e., without pulp involvement], there is no evidence of pockets of lucency (which would suggest abscessation) at the root tips. Courtesy of Dr. Alexander M. Reiter, University of Pennsylvania.

ADVANCED OR CONFIRMATORY TESTING

An intraoral dental radiographic technique is required to assess the periapical region.

TREATMENT

THERAPEUTIC GOAL(S)

- Achieve drainage
- Remove cause of inflammatory reaction

ACUTE GENERAL TREATMENT

- Extraction or endodontic therapy (total pulpectomy and root canal filling) (see Dental Extraction, p 1220).
- Endodontic therapy may need to be staged (i.e., performed in several sessions).
- Concurrent systemic antibiotic treatment is indicated if systemic signs (fever, regional lymphadenopathy) are present, the associated swelling is diffuse, or cellulitis occurs.
- The use of systemic antibiotics alone is not appropriate treatment.
- Analgesic treatment with nonsteroidal anti-inflammatory drugs (e.g., in dogs: meloxicam 0.1 mg/kg PO q 24h or carprofen 2 mg/kg PO q 12h).

CHRONIC TREATMENT

- Extraction or endodontic therapy
- Monitor teeth at risk of pulpal disease (e.g., uncomplicated crown fracture)

DRUG INTERACTIONS

Adverse reactions to systemic antibiotics and/or analgesics

POSSIBLE COMPLICATIONS

- Incomplete extraction
- Endodontic: incomplete drainage, incomplete removal of pulp, substandard obturation and restoration

RECOMMENDED MONITORING

- Physical examination
- Radiographic evaluation to confirm healing

PROGNOSIS AND OUTCOME

Excellent if therapeutic goals (drainage and removal of cause of inflammation) are achieved

PEARLS & CONSIDERATIONS

COMMENTS

- Chronic abscess is more common than acute.
- An abscess associated with a drainage tract usually causes less discomfort.
- Drainage tracts commonly occur on the buccal aspect of the tooth in the oral cavity.
- An acute apical abscess with systemic signs and diffuse swelling (cellulitis) is a true emergency.

PREVENTION

- Minimize risk of dental trauma
- Monitor (clinically and radiographically) teeth that have been subjected to trauma and may develop periapical pathology (e.g., uncomplicated crown fracture)
- Prompt treatment (extraction or endodontic therapy) of teeth that have pulpal disease (e.g., complicated crown fracture)

CLIENT EDUCATION

- Explain the pathophysiology of pulpal and periapical disease (see Fig. I-3)
- Train owners to examine the oral cavity and look for "abnormal" teeth

SUGGESTED READING

Cohen AS, Brown DC: Orofacial dental pain emergencies: Endodontic diagnoses and management. In Cohen S, Burns RC (eds): *Pathways of the Pulp*. St. Louis, Mosby, 2002, pp 31–75.

Gorrel C: Common oral conditions. In Gorrel C (ed): *Veterinary Dentistry for the General Practitioner*. Philadelphia, WB Saunders, 2004, pp 79–81.

Gorrel C, Robinson J: Endodontics in small carnivores. In Crossley DA, Penman S (eds): *Manual of Small Animal Dentistry*. Cheltenham, British Small Animal Veterinary Association, 1995, pp 168–181.

AUTHOR: **CECILIA GORREL**

EDITOR: **ALEXANDER M. REITER**

Abscess, Cat Bite

BASIC INFORMATION

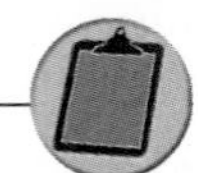

DEFINITION

Subcutaneous abscess in a cat secondary to a bite wound from another cat

EPIDEMIOLOGY

SPECIES, AGE, SEX

- Cat, any age, either sex
- Potentially more common in males

RISK FACTORS

- Intact male
- Outdoor existence

CONTAGION AND ZOONOSIS

- Bacteria flora of oral cavity and skin:
  - *Pasteurella multocida*: major causative organism
  - *Staphylococcus* sp.
  - *Streptococcus* sp.
- Humans can develop severe cellulitis and abscess formation from these bacteria secondary to a cat bite.
- Feline immunodeficiency virus (FIV) infection: main source of transmission in cats is bite wounds.

GEOGRAPHY AND SEASONALITY: Possibly greater occurrence in warmer months when cats are outdoors more frequently.

ASSOCIATED CONDITIONS AND DISORDERS

- Cellulitis
- Skin necrosis
- Osteomyelitis of underlying bone

CLINICAL PRESENTATION

HISTORY, CHIEF COMPLAINT

- Nonspecific complaints:
  - Lethargy
  - Anorexia
- Subcutaneous mass/swelling:
  - Soft/turgid
  - Painful
  - Warm to touch
- Open wound with purulent drainage or with crusted, dried discharge interpreted as matted hair

PHYSICAL EXAM FINDINGS: Abscess may be well circumscribed and easily delineated, or broad-based and difficult to identify.

- Nonspecific findings:
  - Fever
  - Dehydration
  - Lethargy
- Subcutaneous mass/swelling:
  - Soft/turgid
  - Painful on palpation
  - ± Draining tract
- Possibly:
  - Evidence of necrosis of overlying skin
  - Inflammation/induration of surrounding skin
    - Developing cellulitis

ETIOLOGY AND PATHOPHYSIOLOGY

- Bite results in puncture or laceration of skin and underlying tissues
- Potential for "iceberg" effect
  - Damage to underlying tissue greater than skin puncture wound
- Bacteria from oral cavity, hair, skin, and surrounding environment are injected into the subcutaneous tissues
  - *Pasteurella multocida*
  - *Staphylococcus* and *Streptococcus* spp.
  - Anaerobes
- Devitalized tissue, dead space, and tissue fluid accumulation provide excellent medium for bacterial growth and abscess formation
- Associated problems that can develop include:
  - Cellulitis
  - Draining tract
  - Necrosis of overlying skin
  - Osteomyelitis of underlying bone
  - Fistula formation due to perforation of a hollow organ
    - Rectum

DIAGNOSIS

DIFFERENTIAL DIAGNOSIS

Dependent on site of abscess but may include:

- Foreign body abscess
- Blunt or other penetrating trauma with abscess formation
- Neoplasia
- Anal sac abscess
- Salivary mucocele
  - Extremely rare in cats

INITIAL DATABASE

- Complete blood count
  - Neutrophilia ± toxic changes
    - Inflammation, infection
  - Neutropenia with toxic changes (degenerative left shift)
    - Severe inflammation (cellulitis)/infection
    - Sepsis
- Radiographs of affected area
  - Underlying osteomyelitis
    - Ilium, sacrum, or coccygeal vertebrae in particular
- Fine-needle aspiration of mass
  - Cytology to confirm abscess
  - Bacterial culture and sensitivity testing
    - Aerobic and anaerobic
    - Generally not performed in routine cases without systemic signs of illness
    - Indicated in cases where systemic illness, osteomyelitis, or concurrent immunosuppression or other diseases are present
- Serologic testing for FIV
  - Indicated in all cats with bite wounds, because this is the main route of transmission for FIV

TREATMENT

Most abscesses will resolve with lancing, establishment of drainage, and wound debridement if necessary, with or without systemic antibiotic therapy. Failure to resolve or presence of systemic signs warrants further evaluation and treatment.

THERAPEUTIC GOAL(S)

- Resolve abscess and prevent early recurrence
- Prevent development of sepsis

ACUTE GENERAL TREATMENT

- Surgical exploration, debridement and lavage of abscess pocket(s)
  - See Suggested Reading below.
  - Wounds should be closed *only* if all devitalized, necrotic tissue has been removed and infection has been controlled.
- Provide postoperative drainage
- Antibiotic therapy for bacterial infection
  - Long-term therapy based on results of microbiologic culture and sensitivity tests.
  - Empiric therapy until results available:
    - Cefazolin, 22 mg/kg, IV q 6h, or
    - Amoxicillin, 10–20 mg/kg, orally, q 12h

CHRONIC TREATMENT

- Open wound and drain management until wounds have healed
  - Appropriate bandaging techniques to provide suitable environment for wound healing and to protect drains
- Antibiotic therapy (see above) until resolution of infection
- Castration/ovariohysterectomy to decrease roaming and fighting

POSSIBLE COMPLICATIONS

- Progressing cellulitis and necrosis of tissues due to inadequate surgical debridement and wound management

- Failure to resolve abscess
  - Inadequate surgical exploration, debridement, and drainage
  - Primary wound closure in the face of infection
- Dehiscence of surgically closed wound
  - Primary wound closure in the face of infection
  - Inadequate debridement of devitalized tissue
- Development of nonhealing open wound (pocket wound)
  - Axillary and inguinal regions in particular
  - Significant problem in cats
  - Can be difficult to resolve; consider referral

RECOMMENDED MONITORING

- Repeat visits to veterinarian as necessary for bandage changes and drain removal until abscess has resolved and wounds have healed
- Observe for recurrence of abscess
- Observe for development of new abscesses

PROGNOSIS AND OUTCOME

- Excellent provided appropriate surgical and postoperative care instituted
- Guarded if:
  - Cellulitis and tissue necrosis develops
    - May require repeated surgical debridement and prolonged open wound management
    - May require reconstructive surgery
  - Nonhealing/pocket wound develops
    - Requires complex reconstructive surgery

PEARLS & CONSIDERATIONS

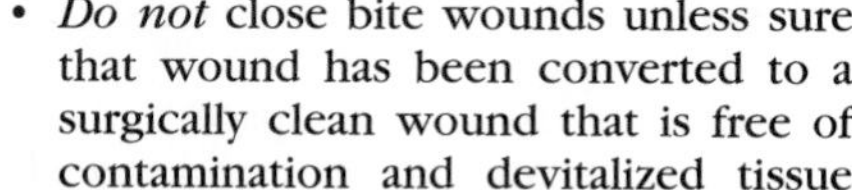

COMMENTS

- *Do not* close bite wounds unless sure that wound has been converted to a surgically clean wound that is free of contamination and devitalized tissue and that adequate postoperative drainage can be provided.
- If in doubt, leave the wound open to heal by contraction and epithelialization.

PREVENTION

- Have cat castrated/spayed
- Keep cat indoors

CLIENT EDUCATION

- Keep cats indoors to prevent problem
- Neuter cats to decrease fighting
- Seek early veterinary care if suspect abscess developing

SUGGESTED READING

Swaim SF, Henderson RA: Wounds on the limbs. In *Small Animal Wound Management*. Philadelphia, Lea & Febiger, 1990, pp 69–72.

Bowling MW, et al: Cutaneous wound healing in the cat: A macroscopic description and comparison with cutaneous wound healing in the dog. *Vet Surg* 33:579–587, 2004.

AUTHOR & EDITOR: **RICHARD WALSHAW**

Abscess, Lung

BASIC INFORMATION

DEFINITION

Localized collection of exudate due to suppuration of lung tissue, resulting in pulmonary cavitation

SYNONYM(S)

Pulmonary abscess

EPIDEMIOLOGY

SPECIES, AGE, SEX: Dog and cat, any age, either sex.

RISK FACTORS: Foreign body inhalation.

GEOGRAPHY AND SEASONALITY: Inhalation of plant foreign body (e.g., grass awn) in endemic areas.

ASSOCIATED CONDITIONS AND DISORDERS: Hypertrophic osteopathy.

- Reported in dogs with chronic pulmonary abscessation
- Results in slowly progressive lameness in affected patients

CLINICAL PRESENTATION

HISTORY, CHIEF COMPLAINT

- Chronic, progressive respiratory signs
  - Cough, increased respiratory effort, respiratory distress
- Acute dyspnea/respiratory decompensation
  - Due to rupture of the abscess, resulting in pneumothorax
- Nonspecific signs of illness (inappetence, weight loss) associated with fever

PHYSICAL EXAM FINDINGS

- Poor body condition
- Fever may be present, but absence of fever does not rule out the diagnosis
- Increased lung sounds (moist rales) on auscultation
- If an associated pyothorax/pneumothorax is/are present:
  - Tachypnea/dyspnea
  - Decreased heart and lung sounds on auscultation

ETIOLOGY AND PATHOPHYSIOLOGY

Possible etiologies for pulmonary abscess include:

- Foreign body migration
- Pneumonia (primary bacterial, aspiration)
- Fungal infection (blastomycosis, histoplasmosis, coccidioidomycosis)
- Parasitic infestation (*Paragonimus*)
- Primary pulmonary neoplasia

DIAGNOSIS

DIFFERENTIAL DIAGNOSIS

Other possible mass(es) in the pulmonary parenchyma:

- Neoplasia
- Cyst
- Granuloma
- Parasitic nodules

INITIAL DATABASE

- Complete blood count:
  - Possible neutrophilic leukocytosis with or without a left shift.
  - Anemia (generally mild, nonregenerative) may result if chronic abscessation is present.
- Survey thoracic radiographs (Figs. I-4 and I-5):
  - Mass within pulmonary parenchyma.
    - Cavitation/gas present in lesion is pathognomonic
  - Pneumothorax.
  - Pleural effusion (if pyothorax).
- Analysis of pleural effusion:
  - Cytology.
  - Bacterial culture and sensitivity testing: both aerobic and anaerobic.

ADVANCED OR CONFIRMATORY TESTING

Computed tomography scan:

- Assess involvement of other intrathoracic structures—superior visualization, especially when pleural effusion is present
  - Additional pulmonary involvement
  - Mediastinal abscess
  - Pleural involvement

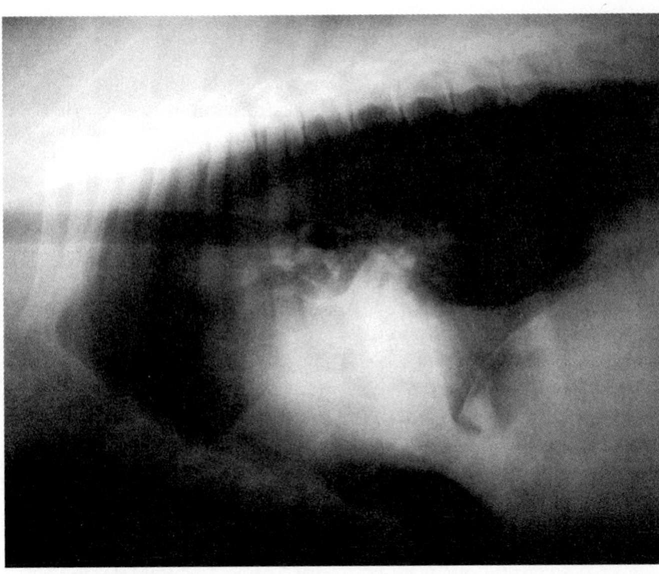

FIGURE I-4 Lateral radiograph of the thorax of a dog with a lung abscess. The abscessed lobe is the right middle lung lobe, which overlies the cardiac silhouette in this projection. Courtesy of Dr. Richard Walshaw.

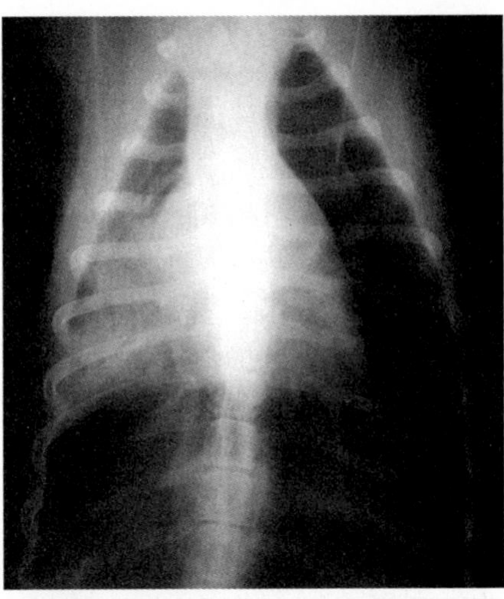

FIGURE I-5 Dorsoventral thoracic radiograph of the same dog. Opacities of the right middle lung lobe suggest extensive consolidation, consistent with lung abscess. Courtesy of Dr. Richard Walshaw.

- Assess if lesion amenable to surgical resection
- Possibly identify cause of abscess
- Rule out other causes of pulmonary mass

TREATMENT

THERAPEUTIC GOAL(S)

- Medically stabilize patient in preparation for anesthesia and surgery
- Surgical removal of affected lung lobe (remove source of infection)
- Long-term antimicrobial therapy based on culture and sensitivity test results
    - Prevent other lung lobes from being affected
    - Treatment of associated pyothorax

ACUTE GENERAL TREATMENT

- Correction of fluid and electrolyte deficits
- Respiratory system support if needed:
    - Oxygen supplementation
    - Thoracocentesis may be required if associated pneumothorax or pyothorax
- Antimicrobial therapy:
    - Initially, empiric therapy active against aerobic and anaerobic bacteria
        - Second-generation cephalosporin
            - Cefoxitin: 22 mg/kg IV, q 6h
        - Amoxicillin (± clavulanic acid): 10–20 mg/kg PO, q 12h
    - Definitive antimicrobial therapy should be based on results of aerobic and anaerobic microbiologic culture and sensitivity testing
        - Continued for 4 to 6 weeks
- Thoracotomy:
    - Removal of affected lung lobe
    - Treatment of pyothorax, if present
        - See Pyothorax, p 935

CHRONIC TREATMENT

Long-term antibiotic therapy based on microbiologic culture and sensitivity result:

- 4 to 6 weeks

POSSIBLE COMPLICATIONS

Depending on etiology:

- Development of chronic pneumonia
- Development of abscess(es) in other lung lobes
- Failure to resolve associated pyothorax (e.g., failure to entirely remove inciting cause, such as foreign body having migrated outside the removed lung lobe/resected tissue)

RECOMMENDED MONITORING

Survey thoracic radiographs:

- At completion of antibiotic therapy
- Periodically (every 3 months)

PROGNOSIS AND OUTCOME

Prognosis depends on the underlying cause:

- Pulmonary abscessation can be associated with sepsis and severe systemic illness, in which case the prognosis is guarded to poor, or may be an incidental finding in an otherwise stable patient, in which case the prognosis is fair provided complete excision is possible.
- Non-neoplastic abscessation is associated with a fair to good prognosis.

PEARLS & CONSIDERATIONS

COMMENTS

- Important to determine underlying cause of pulmonary abscess
- Medical treatment to stabilize the patient
    - Ideally, antimicrobial choice is based on culture and susceptibility testing as early in the course of treatment as possible
- Surgical removal of affected lobe required
    - Obtain definitive diagnosis
    - Remove source of chronic infection

SUGGESTED READING

Fossum TW: Surgery of the lower respiratory system: lungs and thoracic wall. In Fossum TW: *Small Animal Surgery*. St. Louis, Mosby, 2002, pp 760–787.

Hesselink JW, et al: Hypertrophic osteopathy in a dog with a chronic lung abscess. *J Am Vet Med Assoc* 196:760, 1990.

Nelson AW, et al: Lungs. In Slatter D (ed): *Textbook of Small Animal Surgery*. Philadelphia, WB Saunders, 2003, pp 880–889.

AUTHOR: **MARYANN G. RADLINSKY**

EDITOR: **RICHARD WALSHAW**

Abscess, Prostatic

BASIC INFORMATION

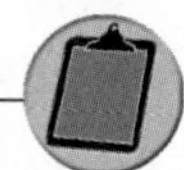

DEFINITION

Severe disorder involving infection of the prostate gland resulting in the production of pocket(s) of suppurative material and destruction of glandular tissue

EPIDEMIOLOGY

SPECIES, AGE, SEX: Intact male dogs of any age can be affected, but dogs are usually over 5 years old.

GENETICS AND BREED PREDISPOSITIONS: Doberman pinschers have been reported to have a high incidence of prostatic disease in general.

RISK FACTORS: Sexually intact males are at greatest risk; advancing age also increases risk.

ASSOCIATED CONDITIONS AND DISORDERS: Benign prostatic hypertrophy (BPH), squamous metaplasia of the ducts, and prostatic neoplasia predispose to infection, and therefore may also increase chances of abscess formation.

CLINICAL PRESENTATION

HISTORY, CHIEF COMPLAINT (SOME OR ALL MAY BE PRESENT)

- May be without clinical signs (incidental finding)
- Clinical signs arise from compression of adjacent structures, or from systemic illness (sepsis):
  - Dysuria
  - Urethral discharge
  - Tenesmus
  - Ribbon-like stool
  - Anorexia
  - Depression
  - Pyrexia
  - Shock

PHYSICAL EXAM FINDINGS

- Urethral/preputial discharge (may be bloody).
- Prostatomegaly on rectal exam (asymmetric).
- Prostate may be felt as an abdominal mass if severely enlarged.
- Prostatic and/or abdominal pain may be present.
- Systemic signs of illness may be present such as fever, depression, or even signs of septic shock.

ETIOLOGY AND PATHOPHYSIOLOGY

- Bacterial infection arises from elsewhere in the urinary tract, hematogenously, or from a prostatic cyst that has become infected.
- Associated conditions that predispose to infection can alter normal defenses (abnormalities in urine flow during micturition, the urethral high pressure zone, bactericidal effects of prostatic fluid, and/or local IgA production).
- Most common bacterial organisms cultured: *Escherichia coli*, *Staphylococcus* sp., *Streptococcus* sp., *Proteus* sp., *Pseudomonas* sp.

DIAGNOSIS

DIFFERENTIAL DIAGNOSIS

- Other prostatic disease: prostatic/paraprostatic cyst, prostatitis, prostatic neoplasia, benign prostatic hypertrophy
- Other lower urinary tract disease: neoplasia (transitional cell carcinoma, others), urethral calculi, cystitis
- Colonic disease: colitis, neoplasia
- Mass of other tissue origin (e.g., fibrosarcoma)

INITIAL DATABASE

- Complete blood count: may have an inflammatory leukogram
- Chemistry profile: generally unremarkable
- Urinalysis:
  - May have inflammatory sediment
  - Caution if obtaining urine by cystocentesis: do not enter/lacerate a large prostatic abscess
- Urine culture and sensitivity:
  - Often positive for bacteria
  - Essential for the most accurate antibiotic selection
- Abdominal radiographs: prostatomegaly
- Prostatic ultrasound: mixed echogenicity (focal hypoechoic/anechoic area[s] with focal hyperechoic areas)

ADVANCED OR CONFIRMATORY TESTING

- Prostatic wash/ejaculate: cytologic evidence of inflammation, bacteria (depends on whether abscess is walled off) (see Prostatic Massage, p 1303)
- Prostatic fine-needle aspirate (see Prostatic Diagnostic Sampling: Biopsy, Fine-Needle Aspiration, p 1302)
  - Cytology of abscess contents reveals septic suppurative inflammation
  - Caution: may risk spread of infection, causing peritonitis
- Culture of prostatic fluid/abscess contents
  - Generally a single bacterial species isolated

TREATMENT

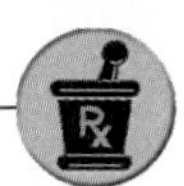

THERAPEUTIC GOAL(S)

Drain abscess and resolve infection without allowing peritonitis to develop

ACUTE GENERAL TREATMENT

- Surgical drainage of cavities greater than 1 cm on ultrasound is the standard of care.
  - Current recommendations involve debridement and intracapsular omentalization.
- Castration (or drug therapy [e.g., finasteride 5 mg/dog PO q 24h assuming 10–40 kg body weight]) causes atrophy of prostatic tissue and is an important component of therapy.
- Institute antibiotic therapy appropriate for the prostate gland and ideally based on culture and sensitivity testing.
- Antibiotics that readily cross the prostate barrier:
  - Chloramphenicol 30–50 mg/kg PO q 8h (bacteriostatic).
  - Trimethoprim-sulfamethoxazole 15 mg/kg PO q 12h (bactericidal).
  - Fluoroquinolones:
    - Enrofloxacin 5 mg/kg PO q 12–24h (bactericidal).
    - Ciprofloxacin has poorer penetration to the prostate than does enrofloxacin.
- Antibiotic penetration into an abscess may be inadequate and therefore must be combined with surgical or percutaneous drainage.

CHRONIC TREATMENT

Postdrainage antibiotic therapy:

- At least 4 to 6 weeks in duration
- Based on bacterial culture and sensitivity

POSSIBLE COMPLICATIONS

- Morbidity can be high with surgical intervention, but incidence of complications is decreased with prostatic omentalization technique versus older techniques (e.g., placement of Penrose drains and marsupialization).
- Possible complications include urinary incontinence; chronic draining tracts; and with uncontrolled abscesses that rupture and/or produce sepsis, peritonitis, septic shock, and death are possible.

RECOMMENDED MONITORING

- Repeat examination including rectal palpation
- Repeat ultrasound of the prostate 2 to 3 weeks following initial treatment and

as needed thereafter to ensure resolution of the abscess
- Urine and/or prostatic fluid should be cultured 1 to 2 weeks following cessation of antibiotic therapy. If positive for bacteria, antibiotic therapy reinstituted
- Follow up complete blood count, chemistry panel, urinalysis recommended 2 to 3 weeks after initial treatment, and thereafter until abnormalities resolved

PROGNOSIS AND OUTCOME

- Guarded to poor
- Historically, reported mortality rates of 24–51% within the first year following therapy, but prognosis appears to be better if prostatic omentalizaion technique is used

PEARLS & CONSIDERATIONS

- Report of ultrasound-guided percutaneous prostate drainage offers promise for a less invasive treatment option.
- Owners need to be aware that percutaneous drainage may need to be performed more than one time.

PREVENTION

Castration will decrease incidence dramatically, although rarely the disease may occur in neutered males

CLIENT EDUCATION

Owner needs to be made aware of the guarded prognosis, long-term problems of possible urinary incontinence, and possible need for subsequent surgery

SUGGESTED READING

Boland LE, et al: Ultrasound-guided percutaneous drainage as the primary treatment for prostatic abscesses and cysts in dogs. *J Am Anim Hosp Assoc* 39:151, 2003.

White RA, et al: Intracapsular prostatic omentalization: A new technique for management of prostatic abscesses in dogs. *Vet Surg* 24:390, 1995.

AUTHOR: **LISA BROWNLEE**

EDITOR: **LEAH A. COHN**

Abscess, Retropharyngeal

BASIC INFORMATION

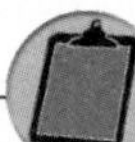

DEFINITION

Abscess that develops in the soft tissues dorsocaudal to the pharynx and dorsal and/or lateral to the esophagus

SYNONYM(S)

Retropharyngeal foreign body abscess

EPIDEMIOLOGY

SPECIES, AGE, SEX: Dogs: tend to be younger.

RISK FACTORS

- Playing catch with, or chewing on, objects such as sticks that could penetrate the pharynx
- Interacting with a porcupine

CONTAGION AND ZOONOSIS: Any possibility of a bite by a wild animal carries the possibility of rabies in endemic regions (see Rabies, p 939).

GEOGRAPHY AND SEASONALITY: Possibly more common in warmer months when dogs play outside.

CLINICAL PRESENTATION

HISTORY, CHIEF COMPLAINT

- History of:
  - Playing catch with a stick
  - Chewing on a stick
  - Interacting with a porcupine
- Nonspecific complaints:
  - Lethargy
  - Decreased appetite
- Dysphagia, particularly with solid food
- Drooling
- Respiratory stridor
- Reluctance to move head and neck

PHYSICAL EXAM FINDINGS

- Nonspecific findings:
  - Depression, lethargy
  - Fever
- Ptyalism:
  - Hemorrhagic discharge.
- Dyspnea (upper airway), stridor:
  - Laryngotracheal compression due to expanding mass in the neck
- Reluctance to move head and neck
- Reluctance to have mouth opened
- Palpation of cranial cervical area:
  - Pain
  - Mass/thickening cranial dorsal cervical region that may extend lateral to esophagus and trachea and toward the thoracic inlet
- Possible cervical draining tract

ETIOLOGY AND PATHOPHYSIOLOGY

- Generally caused by penetrating trauma to dorsocaudal wall of pharynx
  - Catching/landing on a stick
  - Attacking a porcupine, with resultant quills in the oropharynx
- Infection, and possibly also foreign body, enters soft tissues caudodorsal to pharynx
- Pharyngeal wound heals rapidly
- Walled-off abscess develops in soft tissues of neck
- Abscess extends down fascial planes of neck to thoracic inlet

DIAGNOSIS

DIFFERENTIAL DIAGNOSIS

- Retropharyngeal lymphadenopathy
  - Inflammation
  - Neoplasia
    - Primary
    - Metastatic
- Retropharyngeal neoplasia
  - Lymphoma
  - Carotid body tumor
  - Metastatic neoplasia

INITIAL DATABASE

- Complete blood count
  - Neutrophilia associated with inflammation/infection (toxic changes, left shift)
- Survey cervical radiographs (lateral projection)
  - Soft tissue mass dorsal/dorsolateral to larynx
  - Ventral/lateral deviation of trachea/esophagus
  - Rarely identify foreign body
    - Radiolucent
- Survey thoracic radiographs
  - Rule out thoracic involvement
- Ultrasound examination of retropharyngeal area
  - Differentiate abscess/cellulitis from mass
  - Identify enlarged lymph nodes
- Fine-needle aspiration (ultrasound guided)
  - Cytology to determine etiology
  - Bacterial culture and sensitivity testing
    - Aerobic and anaerobic
      - *Actinomyces* spp and *Nocardia* spp can be associated with penetrating foreign body/wild animal bite abscesses

ADVANCED OR CONFIRMATORY TESTING

- Contrast radiography, if draining tract present
  - Identify extent of abscess

- Identify contained foreign body
- Computed tomography
  - Presurgical identification of extent of abscess/tracts in complex cases

TREATMENT

THERAPEUTIC GOAL(S)

- Remove foreign body, if present
- Resolve abscess and prevent early recurrence

ACUTE GENERAL TREATMENT

- Oropharyngeal examination under general anesthesia:
  - Identify site of penetration, if pharyngeal wound still present.
  - Endoscopic examination of abscess cavity through pharyngeal wound.
    - Foreign body removal.
    - Lavage abscess cavity.
  - Rule out other potential causes of retropharyngeal mass (e.g., metastatic tonsillar carcinoma).
- Surgical exploration, debridement, and lavage of abscess pocket(s):
  - Rarely can the abscess be totally excised, because its walls are usually intimately involved with the fascial planes and other vital structures of the neck.
- Provide postoperative drainage until abscess has resolved:
  - Abscess usually cannot be totally excised; treatment is most easily accomplished by leaving wound open and allowing it to heal by contraction and epithelialization.
    - Open wound management aims to prevent formation of new abscess pockets.
- Antibiotic therapy for bacterial infection:
  - Long-term therapy based on results of microbiologic culture and sensitivity tests.
    - If *Actinomyces* spp. or *Nocardia* spp. present, antibiotic therapy for 2 to 3 months is often recommended.
  - Empiric therapy until results available.
    - Cefazolin, 22 mg/kg, IV q 6h, if animal is receiving IV fluids and is unable to take oral medications.
    - Amoxicillin, 10–20 mg/kg, orally, q 12h.

CHRONIC TREATMENT

- Open wound management until wounds have healed
  - Appropriate bandaging techniques to provide suitable environment for wound healing
- Antibiotic therapy (see above) until resolution of infection
- If open wound is present in pharynx, will need to provide alternate route for nutrition, and antibiotic administration, to allow wound to heal and prevent further contamination of abscess cavity
  - PEG tube to bypass pharynx and esophagus (see Feeding Tube Placement: Percutaneous Endoscopic Gastrostomy [PEG], p 1247)
  - Reexamine pharynx in 10 to 14 days
    - If pharynx healed, patient can return to oral feeding, and tube can be removed

POSSIBLE COMPLICATIONS

- Failure to resolve abscess/development of a chronic draining tract
  - Inadequate surgical exploration and drainage
  - Failure to remove all foreign material
  - Primary wound closure in the face of infection
- Extension of the abscess into the thorax
  - Mediastinal abscess
  - Pyothorax

RECOMMENDED MONITORING

- Repeat visits to veterinarian as necessary for open wound management and bandage changes until abscess has resolved and wounds have healed
- Observe for recurrence of abscess, development of draining tract
- If open wound in pharynx and feeding tube placed
  - Reexamination of pharynx in 10 to 14 days
    - Evaluation of wound healing
  - Feeding tube removal

PROGNOSIS AND OUTCOME

- Usually good with appropriate surgical procedures
- Recurrence likely, or chronic draining tract will develop, if:
  - Inadequate surgical exploration and drainage
  - Failure to remove all foreign material
  - Primary wound closure is performed in the face of infection

PEARLS & CONSIDERATIONS

COMMENTS

It is always better to leave this type of wound open, and allow it to heal by second intention, rather than to close it and have recurrence of the abscess.

PREVENTION

Avoid situations that would lead to a possible penetrating pharyngeal injury (see below)

CLIENT EDUCATION

- Do not let dogs play with or chew on objects such as sticks that could cause penetrating pharyngeal injuries
- Do not let dogs interact with porcupines

SUGGESTED READING

Lamb CR, et al: Sinography in the investigation of draining tracts in small animals: Retrospective review of 25 cases. *Vet Surg* 23:129–134, 1994.

White RAS, Lane JG: Pharyngeal stick penetration injuries in the dog. *J Small Anim Pract* 29:13–35, 1988.

Harvey CE: In *Veterinary Dentistry*, Philadelphia, WB Saunders, 1985, pp 185–186.

AUTHOR & EDITOR: **RICHARD WALSHAW**

Abuse

BASIC INFORMATION

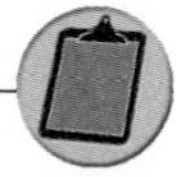

DEFINITION

- Physical abuse: physical actions such as kicking, punching, beating, burning, microwaving, drowning, asphyxiation, and administration of drugs or poisons
- Sexual abuse: any use of an animal for sexual gratification
- Emotional abuse: threatening behavior
- Neglect: failure to provide the basic physical and/or emotional necessities of life (e.g., food, shelter, veterinary attention)

SYNONYM(S)

Physical abuse:
- Battered pet syndrome
- Nonaccidental injury

EPIDEMIOLOGY

SPECIES, AGE, SEX: Young male dogs and young cats particularly at risk.

GENETICS AND BREED PREDISPOSITIONS, RISK FACTORS: Crossbred dogs, Staffordshire bull terriers, and domestic short-haired cats at increased risk in the United Kingdom, but this may represent favoring of particular breeds by owners of low socioeconomic status.

CONTAGION AND ZOONOSIS: There is an association between animal abuse, domestic violence, and child abuse. Links within the community (e.g., social workers, police, child protection teams, animal welfare organizations) are highly advantageous for addressing the public health aspects of abuse. Interagency collaboration is effective and helps to reduce stress on the veterinarian.

CLINICAL PRESENTATION

DISEASE FORMS/SUBTYPES: Variant of abuse: fabricated or induced illness. Synonyms:

- Factitious illness by proxy
- Munchausen syndrome by proxy
  - Uncommon
  - Involves invention or falsification of illness in animal by owner, motivation being attention seeking by owner
  - May involve repetitive injury

HISTORY, CHIEF COMPLAINT: Crucial to note that none of the following features alone is diagnostic. A combination raises suspicion, and this combination varies.

- History supplied is inconsistent with the injury. Usually the injury is too severe to "fit" the history. Owner's "explanation" to account for the pet's injuries merits attention by its lack of plausibility (e.g., it might be reported that an animal with severe burns "sat too close to the radiator" or "lay too close to the fire," or that an animal with fractures "fell down the stairs," "fell off the sofa," "fell from child's arms," "fell off the bed," or "fell off the steps").
- Discrepant history (e.g., the person presenting the animal may change his/her story, or the history may differ from person to person).
- Particular person implicated (e.g., partner, child, or even self-admission).
- Repetitive injury (i.e., animal presented more than once with injuries, and/or different ages of injury are present). All body systems may be involved, but fractures are important.
- Previous injury/death of another animal in the same home, particularly when unexplained.
- Lack of history of motor vehicle accident, or any possible accident.
- The behavior of the *owner* causes concern (e.g., implausible, aggressive, embarrassed, obviously discomforted, or shows a lack of concern for the animal).
- The behavior of the *animal* causes concern (e.g., shows fear of owner, or happier when hospitalized away from owner).
- Family violence known or suspected.

When obtaining the history of a case where abuse is on the differential diagnosis, some points are essential:

- It is important to be objective and avoid jumping to conclusions.
- Likewise, it is necessary to remain polite and calm, and to avoid being confrontational.
- If the decision is made to discuss concerns with the client, it can be helpful to present those concerns nonconfrontationally, along the lines of the following: "It's difficult for me to match Spot's injuries with what you are saying. Is there anything else you'd like to tell me?"
- It is important to ensure that clinical notes are comprehensive and thorough, and that they are retained because of potential legal ramifications. Relying on memory can be problematic, because it may be some time before the case goes to court.

PHYSICAL EXAM FINDINGS

- Wide spectrum of possible injuries.
- Superficial injuries are common: bruising of head, thorax, abdomen, and limbs; scleral/conjunctival hemorrhages. Shaving of the hair can reveal bruising, even in animals with very dark coats. Bruising is likely to be present over bony structures like ribs or vertebrae but may be absent in the (soft) abdominal wall. Necropsy examination of suspected fatal cases must include thorough examination of all subcutaneous areas for bruising.
- Fractures and locomotor injuries: The most common fractures involve the skull, ribs, and femurs, although other bones may also be involved.
- Physical signs of internal thoracoabdominal injuries: rupture of major organs (liver, kidney, spleen, urinary bladder); intrapulmonary hemorrhage; rupture of bowel uncommon.
- Sexual abuse injuries involve the genitalia and/or the anal/rectal area. Both sexes may be abused.

ETIOLOGY AND PATHOPHYSIOLOGY

- Owner-associated risk factors for the animal include domestic abuse, alcoholism, substance abuse, and mental illness.
- Some authors suggest that animal abuse is more common in areas of social deprivation, but this is largely anecdotal, and abuse does occur in affluent groups.

DIAGNOSIS

DIFFERENTIAL DIAGNOSIS

- Naturally occurring conditions, such as skeletal disorders (e.g., metabolic bone disease) and blood dyscrasias.
- Motor vehicle accidents/hit by car. History helps to differentiate (e.g., is the animal ever allowed out, or is always kept in house?), as does physical exam (animals hit by cars often have tattered nails, skin abrasions, and dirt in the haircoat).

INITIAL DATABASE

- Much of the diagnostic information in cases of abuse is obtained from the history and physical exam as previously described.
- Ancillary diagnostic tests depend on the specific details of each case.
  - Radiographic examination, particularly for fractures. Fractures of differing ages may be present.
  - Necropsy of fatal cases. Radiographic examination can also be helpful in fatal cases before necropsy.

TREATMENT

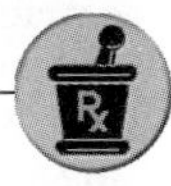

ACUTE GENERAL TREATMENT

As dictated by nature and extent of injuries

PROGNOSIS AND OUTCOME

- Dependent on the severity of the abuse. Fatal cases occur.
- Can be poor with fabricated or induced illness (Munchausen's syndrome by proxy) if the pet remains with the owner.

PEARLS & CONSIDERATIONS

COMMENTS

- No single injury or group of injuries, when divorced from the circumstances surrounding a suspect case, can currently be considered to conclusively indicate physical abuse.
- Considerable knowledge is available on injuries specifically associated with child abuse. Further research on equivalent animal abuse injuries is needed. The medical experience of child abuse injuries provides a useful starting point for researchers.
- It is highly desirable that an experienced veterinary pathologist perform necropsy of fatal suspected abuse cases, preferably one with forensic experience.
- Injury from sexual abuse may be absent. Common sense dictates that injury depends on animal size and the actual type of sex act, which can be variable.
- It is not the veterinarian's remit to *prove* abuse. That is the responsibility of law courts. The veterinarian's responsibility is limited to provision of veterinary evidence to the court.
- In so doing, it may be reassuring to be aware that investigation of an abuse case is multidisciplinary (e.g., animal welfare organizations, police) and that there may be lay witnesses of the abuse.
- The veterinarian may feel that in some cases there are extenuating circumstances with regard to the person per-

petrating the abuse (e.g., emotional problems or other personal difficulties) (see Etiology and Pathophysiology above). These feelings may influence the veterinarian's decision to report a case. *These circumstances are not the veterinarian's responsibility*, nor does he or she have the relevant expertise to judge them. In the UK, for example, the law courts consider such circumstances.

- Each veterinary practice needs to consider its own procedures in relation to this difficult area. It is advisable to have a practice policy available for guidance.
- The law varies from country to country and within countries. Currently, reporting systems for dealing with child abuse cases are in place in many countries, but in general have not been developed for animal abuse cases. Advice may be available from an animal welfare organization or veterinary association.
- In some circumstances the veterinarian may feel that the welfare of the animal is so severely compromised that client confidentiality should be breached. In the UK, for example, this is fully recognized in the Royal College of Veterinary Surgeons *Guide to Professional Conduct*. The veterinarian is advised "in the first instance to attempt to discuss concerns with the client. In cases where this would not be appropriate, or the client's reaction increases rather than allays concerns, the veterinarian should contact the relevant authorities." Appropriate contact details are listed in this guide. Advice, with contact details, is also given on the reporting of concerns about child abuse or domestic violence to appropriate authorities (regardless of whether animal abuse is present).

SUGGESTED READING

Arkow P: Child abuse, animal abuse and the veterinarian. *J Am Vet Med Assoc* 204:1004, 1994.
Beirne P: Rethinking bestiality: Towards a concept of interspecies sexual assault. *Theor Criminol* 1:317, 1997.
Feldman MD: Canine variant of factitious disorder by proxy. *Am J Psychiatry* 154:1316, 1997.
Hobbs CJ, Wynne JM: *Physical Signs of Child Abuse*, ed 2. London, WB Saunders, 2001.
Kempe CH, et al: The battered-child syndrome, *JAMA* 181:17–24, 1962.
Lockwood R, Ascione FR (eds): *Cruelty to Animals and Interpersonal Violence: Readings in Research and Application*. West Lafayette, Purdue University Press, 1998.
Munro HMC, Thrusfield MV: "Battered pets": Features that raise suspicion of Non-accidental injury. *J Small Anim Pract* 42:218, 2001.
Munro HMC, Thrusfield MV: "Battered pets": Non-accidental physical injuries found in dogs and cats. *J Small Anim Pract* 42:279, 2001.
Munro HMC, Thrusfield MV: "Battered pets": sexual abuse. *J Small Anim Pract* 42:333, 2001.
Munro HMC, Thrusfield MV: "Battered Pets": Munchausen syndrome by proxy (factitious illness by proxy). *J Small Anim Pract* 42: 385, 2001.
Munro HMC, Thrusfield MV: The battered-pet syndrome. *Veterinary Times* 32:13, 2002.
Royal College of Veterinary Surgeons (2004). Guide to Professional Conduct. Part 3. Annexes. *Animal Abuse, Child Abuse and Domestic Violence:* www.rcvs.org.uk.

AUTHORS: **MICHAEL THRUSFIELD, HELEN MUNRO**
EDITOR: **ETIENNE CÔTÉ**

Acetaminophen Intoxication

BASIC INFORMATION

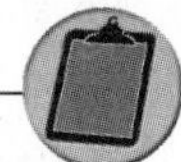

DEFINITION

An oral intoxication resulting from acetaminophen-containing medications (usually human over-the-counter products), which is characterized by methemoglobinemia, acute hepatic damage, or both

SYNONYM(S)

Acetominofen (Mexican)
N-acetyl-p-aminophenol (APAP)
Nonaspirin pain reliever
Paracetamol
Common brand names include Feverall, Liquiprin, Panadol, Tempra, Tylenol, Pamprin, Excedrin, Midol

EPIDEMIOLOGY

SPECIES, AGE, SEX

- Dogs and cats. Cats are much more susceptible to toxic effects (develop toxicity at lower doses than do dogs and have signs that are more severe for equivalent doses).
- Immature animals may be more resistant to the adverse liver effects, because the P-450 pathways are not fully functional (toxic metabolite not formed readily).

RISK FACTORS: Age, species, underlying liver disease, preexisting anemia.

ASSOCIATED CONDITIONS AND DISORDERS

- Hemolytic anemia
- Acute liver failure

CLINICAL PRESENTATION

HISTORY, CHIEF COMPLAINT

- History of ingestion
- Lethargy, inappetence, weakness, depression
- Facial and paw edema (especially cats)
- Dyspnea
- Vomiting

PHYSICAL EXAM FINDINGS

- Lethargy, depression.
- Mucous membranes may be pale due to anemia, or muddy, cyanotic, or brownish due to methemoglobinemia.
- Facial and paw edema (cats).
- Dyspnea.
- Coma (late).

ETIOLOGY AND PATHOPHYSIOLOGY

Source

- Acetaminophen is available as tablets, liquids, liquigels, chewables, and rectal suppositories.
- Available as 325-mg tablets (regular strength), 500 mg (extra strength), 80 mg (children's chewable), 160 mg (junior strength), 160 mg/5 ml (children's elixir), 100 mg/ml or 120 mg/2.5 ml (infant drops).
- Found in many combination products (antihistamines, decongestants, cough suppressants, opiates), including most "aspirin-free" products.

Pathophysiology

- When acetaminophen undergoes hepatic metabolism, P-450 enzymes produce oxidative metabolite (*N*-acetyl-para-benzoquinoneimine or NAPQI).
- NAPQI is conjugated via hepatic glucuronidation or sulfation, rendering it nontoxic. However, nonconjugated fraction can bind to lipid bilayer of hepatocytes, resulting in acute hepatic damage.
- Cats, deficient in glucuronyl transferase, are therefore extremely susceptible to toxic effects.
- NAPQI also causes oxidative damage to red blood cells (RBCs) leading to methemoglobinemia and Heinz body formation within 2 to 4 hours of ingestion, with subsequent lysis of the defective RBCs, causing anemia.
- Dogs may have decreased tear production with doses >30 mg/kg and hepatotoxicity at doses >75–100 mg/kg.
- Cats have increasing methemoglobin levels with doses >30–40 mg/kg.

DIAGNOSIS

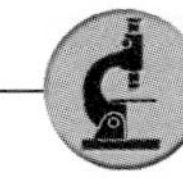

DIFFERENTIAL DIAGNOSIS

- Rule out other causes of methemoglobinemia, generally toxicities: resorcinol in cats; naphthalene, local anesthetics, oxidative drugs (pyridium, phenazopyridine), nitrite, chlorates, garlic or onions in dogs, cats, and other pets
- Rule out other causes of acute hepatic damage, commonly toxic in origin: iron, aflatoxins mycotoxins, cycas palm, castor beans, blue-green algae, metaldehyde, and amanita mushrooms

INITIAL DATABASE

- Complete blood count, serum chemistry profile
- Estimate methemoglobin (metHb). Drop of blood on white filter paper is brownish if metHb >15% (normal <1%). 20–40% metHb generally causes dyspnea; 40–55% metHb generally causes neurologic depression; 70% metHb is acutely life threatening. Higher metHb warrants more intense therapy
- Urinalysis: brown color with methemoglobinuria
- Schirmer tear test (acetaminophen idiosyncratic reaction causing keratoconjuntivitis sicca)

ADVANCED OR CONFIRMATORY TESTING

Acetaminophen serum levels can be measured by many human hospital laboratories.

- Helpful in confirming exposure if history is questionable

TREATMENT

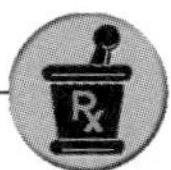

THERAPEUTIC GOAL(S)

- Protect RBC integrity
- Prevent liver damage
- Replenish glutathione stores in liver to enhance glucuronidation/inactivation of NAPQI
- Convert methemoglobin back to hemoglobin
- Supportive care (fluids, ensure adequate tissue oxygen levels)

ACUTE GENERAL TREATMENT

- Gastrointestinal decontamination (emesis and/or activated charcoal) if known ingestion less than 4 hours before presentation (see Vomiting, Induction of, p 1328; Gastric Intubation, Gavage, Lavage, p 1258)
- *N*-acetylcysteine provides sulfhydryl source to bind NAPQI, protecting hepatocytes and RBCs. Initial dose 140 mg/kg, repeat at 70 mg/kg/dose, q 6h, for total of eight doses. Can be given orally, or diluted in IV fluids if bacteriostatic filter is available for administration
- S-adenosyl methionine: as recommended on package (e.g., 90 mg PO per small dog or cat q 24h, up to 225 mg PO per large dog q 24h)
- Cimetidine at 5–10 mg/kg IV, q 6–8h, inhibits P-450 enzyme activity and may reduce metabolism of acetaminophen to NAPQI. Used as an adjunct to *N*-acetylcysteine
- Ascorbic acid (ascorbate, vitamin C), at 30 mg/kg PO q 8h, may help stabilize RBC membranes and reverse some methemoglobinemia
- IV fluids (e.g., if dehydrated: isotonic crystalloid fluids at 40–60 ml/kg/day plus volume to correct dehydration) to improve tissue perfusion

CHRONIC TREATMENT

- S-adenosylmethionine: continue treatment until liver enzymes are within normal range; may require weeks to months
- Artificial tears until normal production resumes

DRUG INTERACTIONS

Treatment with medications that induce P-450 enzyme system activation (e.g., phenobarbital) increases NAPQI production capacity (may produce greater toxicity)

POSSIBLE COMPLICATIONS

Keratoconjunctivitis sicca (dry eye) is sometimes seen in dogs at doses below those causing other adverse effects; toy breeds may be more susceptible

RECOMMENDED MONITORING

- Hematocrit
- Liver enzymes
- Schirmer tear test, baseline and at 48 hours

PROGNOSIS AND OUTCOME

- Early decontamination (induction of vomiting, administration of activated charcoal) before the onset of clinical signs is associated with a fair to good prognosis.
    - If <14 hours between ingestion and treatment, most patients can survive even a high dose
- Once clinical signs are noted, the prognosis is guarded because of the possibility of life-threatening methemoglobinemia and hemolysis (hemolysis mostly in cats), hepatopathy (primarily in dogs), and pigment-induced nephropathy in any animal with hemolysis.

PEARLS & CONSIDERATIONS

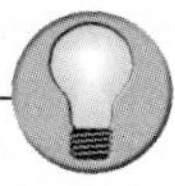

COMMENTS

Availability of s-adenosylmethionine provides a clinically useful alternative to treatment of acetaminophen toxicosis

PREVENTION

Keep all medication in closed cabinets or drawers, not on countertops.

CLIENT EDUCATION

Animals are very sensitive to many medications that humans take with relative safety.

SUGGESTED READING

Mariani CL, Fulton RB Jr: Atypical reaction to acetaminophen intoxication in a dog. *JVECCS* 11:123–126, 2001.

Osweiler GD: Acetaminophen. In *Toxicology*. Philadelphia, Williams & Wilkins, 1996, pp 303–304.

Roder J: Analgesics. In Plumlee KA (ed): *Clinical Veterinary Toxicology*. St. Louis, Mosby, 2004, p 284.

AUTHOR: **MARY M. SCHELL**

EDITOR: **SAFDAR A. KHAN**

Achilles Tendon Injury

BASIC INFORMATION

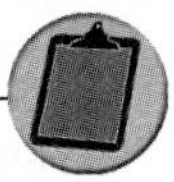

DEFINITION

- The Achilles tendon is composed of three tendons inserting on the calcaneus: the gastrocnemius tendon; the common tendon of biceps femoris, semitendinosus, and gracilis; and the superficial digital flexor tendon.
- Injuries described include insertional avulsion (most common), avulsion of gastrocnemius origin from the femur, musculotendinous ruptures, midsubstance tendon laceration(s), and chronic inflammatory disease.

SYNONYM(S)

Achilles mechanism failure
Common calcaneal tendon rupture
Dropped hock

EPIDEMIOLOGY

SPECIES, AGE, SEX: Mature dogs; working or racing breeds.

CLINICAL PRESENTATION

HISTORY, CHIEF COMPLAINT: Hind limb trauma, excessive athletic activity.
PHYSICAL EXAM FINDINGS: Variable lameness, palpable gap or excessive swelling along tendons, plantigrade stance, dropped hock (excessive tarsal flexion during stand), excessive toe flexion (intact superficial digital flexor tendon).

ETIOLOGY AND PATHOPHYSIOLOGY

- Most lesions are caused by trauma, excessive overload; repetitive stresses can lead to chronic degenerative changes.
- Injuries can be classified based on location of lesion.
- Chronic lesions contain gaps and fibrous connective tissue between tendon ends.

DIAGNOSIS

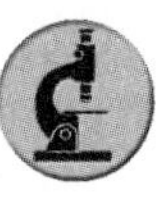

DIFFERENTIAL DIAGNOSIS

- Fracture of the calcaneus
- Tarsal hyperextension injury
- Distal tibia/fibula fractures

INITIAL DATABASE

- Lameness examination, palpation of Achilles tendon, flexion/extension maneuvers of stifle and hock joints
- Mediolateral and caudocranial radiographic projections of stifle and hock
- Ultrasound of Achilles complex
- Complete blood count and chemistry panel based on signalment and nature of injury; generally unremarkable with tendon injury alone

ADVANCED OR CONFIRMATORY TESTING

Magnetic resonance imaging provides superior detail, but not often performed (yet) in animals

TREATMENT

THERAPEUTIC GOAL(S)

Restoration of Achilles tendon length and strength

ACUTE GENERAL TREATMENT

- Avulsed head(s) of gastrocnemius muscle is(are) repaired with wire around fabella and into distal femur.
- Acute mid tendon cuts of each tendon are anastomosed (three-loop pulley, Bunnell, or locking-loop pattern).
- Avulsed tendon(s) from tuber calcani is(are) reattached by Krakow suture passed through bone tunnels.
- Avulsion of tuber calcanei bone fragment is stabilized with small pins and tension band wiring.
- All repairs are externally supported by an external fixator, internal bone screw, splint, or cast with the hock in extension.

CHRONIC TREATMENT

In chronic injuries, devitalized and fibrous tissues are resected and tendon ends reapposed; fascial grafts, tendon transposition, and muscle lengthening procedures have been used to stabilize tendon gaps or defects. Adjunctive support with the hock in extension is also required.

POSSIBLE COMPLICATIONS

- Repair failure
- Infection
- Morbidity with cast, splint, or fixator

RECOMMENDED MONITORING

- Weekly examination of limb to reduce problems associated with cast, splint, or fixator
- Removal of external support or screw 6 to 8 weeks after surgery
- Controlled exercise and rehabilitation for 6 months to avoid reinjury

PROGNOSIS AND OUTCOME

- Good to excellent with appropriate early treatment and postoperative care
- Fair for chronic or repeat injuries
- Poor with nonsurgical treatments

PEARLS & CONSIDERATIONS

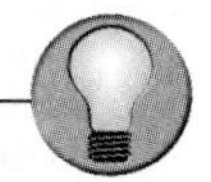

COMMENTS

- Postoperative support is critical in protecting the tendon during the first 2 months of healing.
- Controlled exercise and rehabilitation will enhance recovery of tendon strength and gliding functions, and possibly reduce fibrous adhesions.

SUGGESTED READING

King M, Jerram R: Achilles tendon rupture in dogs. *Comp Contin Educ Pract Vet* 25:613, 2003.

Piermattei DL, Flo GL: Avulsion of the gastrocnemius muscle. In Piermattei DL, Flo GL (eds): *Handbook of Small Animal Orthopedics and Fracture Repair*, ed 3. Philadelphia, WB Saunders, 1997, pp 620–922.

AUTHOR: **JONATHAN SHANI**
EDITOR: **JOSEPH HARARI**

Acid or Alkali (Corrosives) Toxicosis

BASIC INFORMATION

DEFINITION

Exposure, usually by ingestion, to any of a number of household or commercial products containing acids (e.g., hydrochloric, sulfuric, nitric, phosphoric acid) or alkalies (e.g., sodium or potassium carbonate, ammonium hydroxide, potassium permanganate) or free halogens (e.g., chlorine, iodine, or bromine) in quantities sufficient to cause corrosive damage to superficial tissue or produce systemic toxicity in animals

SYNONYM(S)

Toxicosis due to caustic agents

EPIDEMIOLOGY

SPECIES, AGE, SEX

- Dogs and cats of all ages and breeds are vulnerable.
- Dogs are more likely to be involved.
- Cats can ingest clinically significant amounts due to their grooming habits.

RISK FACTORS: Easy access to household or commercial products including alkaline batteries, antirust compounds, toilet bowl cleaners, drain openers, and bleaches.

CLINICAL PRESENTATION

DISEASE FORMS/SUBTYPES

- Acids cause localized coagulative necrosis and superficial burns (perforation less likely).
- Alkalies can cause deep penetrating (liquefactive) lesions by solubilizing the mucous membranes of tissues (perforation more likely compared to acids).

HISTORY, CHIEF COMPLAINT

- Exposure is usually via accidental ingestion, skin or eye contact, or inhalation (rare).
- History typically is specific: exposure to a household cleaning product.
- Salivation, protrusion of tongue (common in cats), vomiting (few minutes to hours) may be noted by owners.

PHYSICAL EXAM FINDINGS

- Oral ulcers (lips, gingiva, tongue)
  - Initially, corrosive burns appear milky white or gray, then turn black.
- Dysphagia
- Hyersalivation/ptyalism/excessive licking
- Protrusion of tongue, tongue swelling
- Corrosive burns on the skin
- Signs of pain (abdominal or generalized)
- Vomiting, diarrhea
- Lethargy
- Anorexia
- Signs indicating esophageal perforation (rare), such as discomfort when swallowing, or signs of mediastinitis or of sepsis
- Corneal ulcer, blepharitis (ocular exposures)

ETIOLOGY AND PATHOPHYSIOLOGY

Source

- Common household products that contain acids include antirust compounds, gun barrel cleaning fluids, automobile batteries, and swimming pool cleaning agents.
- Alkali-containing products in the household include drain cleaner, washing products, liquid cleaner, toilet bowl cleaner, alkaline batteries, and radiator cleaning agents.

Pathophysiology

- Acids and similar corrosive agents cause rapid coagulative necrosis and pain. Mucosal penetration or perforation is rare.
- Concentrated alkali solutions can rapidly penetrate the mucous membranes by dissolving the lipoprotein matrix of cell membranes. They induce deep, penetrating lesions, including liquefactive necrosis and vascular hemolysis. Perforation is more likely compared to acids.

DIAGNOSIS

DIFFERENTIAL DIAGNOSIS

- Oral ulcers from uremia
- Foreign body obstruction (intractable vomiting)
- Viral or bacterial gastroenteritis
- Garbage toxicosis

INITIAL DATABASE

- Complete blood count (may see leukocytosis due to inflammation/stress)
- Serum biochemisty profile: electrolyte changes due to vomiting, dehydration are possible
- Urinalysis: generally unremarkable
- Thoracic radiographs: indicated if coughing, dyspnea, or fever of unknown origin. May show evidence of pleural effusion (rare due to esophageal rupture) and/or aspiration pneumonia
- Abdominal radiographs: may show evidence of peritonitis if perforation has occurred

ADVANCED OR CONFIRMATORY TESTING

- Abdominal ultrasound if peritonitis is suspected on physical exam or radiographically
- Upper gastrointestinal endoscopy to evaluate mucosal damage or to assess for esophageal or gastric perforation

TREATMENT

THERAPEUTIC GOAL(S)

- Decontamination of patient
- Protect gastrointestinal (GI) mucosa if oral exposure
- Supportive therapy

ACUTE GENERAL TREATMENT

- Decontamination:
  - Dermal: wash exposed area with water for 20 to 30 minutes. If severe burns, surgical debridement may be necessary.
  - Ocular: Flush eyes with tepid tap water (or isotonic saline) for 20 to 30 minutes. Stain the cornea with fluorescein to assess for corneal ulcers (see Corneal Ulceration, p 246).
  - Oral exposure: immediately dilute with milk or water. Chemical neutralization with weak acid or alkali is contraindicated. This can cause an exothermic reaction and more thermal injuries.
  - Emesis: contraindicated (can cause more damage).
  - Activated charcoal: do not use because it is ineffective against caustic agents.
  - Gastric lavage: contraindicated (risk of perforation).
  - Inhalation (rare): in case of inhalation exposure, remove animal to fresh air.
  - If esophageal perforation is suspected, do not allow food or water until the extent of injury is evaluated.
- Protect GI mucosa:
  - H_2 receptor antagonists:
    - Famotidine: dogs/cats: 0.5 mg/kg PO, SC, IM, IV q 12-24h
    - Cimetidine: dogs/cats: 10 mg/kg PO q 6h
  - Sucralfate. Dogs: 0.5-1 g PO q 8-12h; cats: 0.25-0.5 g PO q 8-12h
- Supportive care:
  - IV fluids for rehydration (e.g., lactated Ringer's solution) or maintenance.
  - Broad-spectrum antibiotics (e.g., ampicillin 22 mg/kg IV q 8h plus enrofloxacin 5 mg/kg IM or diluted 1:1 with sterile saline and given slowly IV q 12h [q 24h in cats]) if GI mucosal integrity is compromised and/or if secondary infection is identified.
  - Corticosteroids (dexamethasone 0.5-1.0 mg/kg IV or IM for 3 to 5 days or prednisolone 0.25-1.0 mg/kg PO). Use is controversial; can help

prevent esophageal stricture secondary to esophagitis, but delay healing and predispose to infection; concurrent broad-spectrum antibiotic use of unproven benefit.
  - Manage pain: opiates (e.g., fentanyl patch or butorphanol 0.1-1.0 mg/kg IM, IV, or SC).

RECOMMENDED MONITORING

- Acutely: blood pressure, respiratory effort, exam: monitor for shock
- Chronically: body temperature; thoracic radiographs; complete blood count: evidence of esophageal rupture and mediastinitis, or of aspiration pneumonia possibly due to esophageal stricture

POSSIBLE COMPLICATIONS

- Aspiration pneumonitis/pneumonia
- Esophageal perforation and mediastinitis; gastroenteric perforation and peritonitis
- Esophageal stricture

PROGNOSIS AND OUTCOME

- Good to excellent if animal is treated immediately after exposure
- Poor in patients in hypovolemic shock or if esophageal or stomach perforation occurs

PEARLS & CONSIDERATIONS

COMMENTS

- Alkaline products with a pH of 12.5 can cause esophageal ulcers; products with a pH of 14 can cause esophageal perforation and stricture formation.
- Most household cleansing agents are complex mixtures of chemicals. The clinician must carefully determine the most toxic ingredient and hazard resulting from exposure; consultation with a poison control center is advised.

PREVENTION

Keep household cleaning products out of reach of pets

SUGGESTED READING

Anderson KD: Alkali injury. In Haddad LM, Winchester JF (eds): *Clinical Management of Poisoning and Drug Overdose*. Philadelphia, WB Saunders, 1990, pp 1056-1061.

Coppock RW, et al: The toxicology of detergents, bleaches, antiseptics and disinfectants in small Animals. *Vet Hum Toxicol* 30(5):463-472, 1988.

Winchester JF: Acids and antacids. In Haddad LM, Winchester, JF (eds): *Clinical Management of Poisoning and Drug Overdose*. 1990, pp 1065-1069.

AUTHOR: **MOAZZAM A. KHAN**
EDITOR: **SAFDAR A. KHAN**

Acidosis

BASIC INFORMATION

DEFINITION

Acidosis is a condition in which there is a net increase in the $[H^+]$ in the body (and hence a lower pH). Acidosis may be metabolic (reflected in decreased $[HCO_3^-]$ due to the accumulation of a nonvolatile fixed acid) or respiratory (reflected in increased pCO_2).

EPIDEMIOLOGY

RISK FACTORS: Numerous diseases result in body pH abnormalities. Serious illness is almost always associated with acid-base disturbance.

ASSOCIATED CONDITIONS AND DISORDERS

- Numerous.
- Metabolic acidosis is most commonly associated with conditions of reduced circulation, leading to excessive acid generation or reduced H^+ loss or increased H^+ retention.
- Respiratory acidosis is caused by reduced alveolar ventilation.
- Each primary abnormality will be accompanied by a secondary compensatory response.
  - The exception is with cats; as a species, they less commonly show respiratory compensation for metabolic acidosis.
- Respiratory compensation for metabolic acidosis results in a 0.7 mmHg drop in pCO_2 for every 1 mEq/L drop in $[HCO_3^-]$.
- Metabolic compensation for respiratory acidosis results in an increase in $[HCO_3^-]$ by 0.15 (acute) to 0.35 mEq/L (chronic) for every 1 mmHg increase in arterial pCO_2.

CLINICAL PRESENTATION

DISEASE FORMS/SUBTYPES: Metabolic acidosis may be associated with an increased anion gap (normochloremic metabolic acidosis) or normal anion gap (hyperchloremic metabolic acidosis). Respiratory acidosis has no subclassifications.

HISTORY, CHIEF COMPLAINT: Dependent on the underlying disease process.

PHYSICAL EXAM FINDINGS

- Dependent on the underlying disease process.
- Severe acidosis causes reduced cardiac output, arterial vasodilation, and central nervous system depression.
- Respiratory compensation may be associated with deep rhythmic breathing.
- Primary respiratory acidosis may be associated with clinically observable abnormalities in breathing (such as dyspnea or reduced respiratory effort in cases of muscular paralysis or exhaustion). Mucous membranes may be cyanotic.

ETIOLOGY AND PATHOPHYSIOLOGY

- Metabolic acidosis is characterized by a primary decrease in plasma $[HCO_3^-]$, increased $[H^+]$, decreased pH, and a secondary or adaptive decrease in pCO_2.
- Metabolic acidosis is caused by:
  - Loss of HCO_3^- rich fluid from the body (usually from the gut, but also through the kidney).
  - Failure of excretion of fixed acid (e.g., tissue hypoperfusion, renal insufficiency).
  - Addition of fixed acids to the body (like ethylene glycol or salicylates). Fixed acids may also be produced in excess by the body (like lactate or ketones), leading or contributing to metabolic acidosis.
- Metabolic acidosis may be associated with an increase in anion gap (suggesting accumulation of organic acids such as lactate; the corrected serum $[Cl^-]$ is normal) or a normal anion gap (suggesting HCO_3^- loss; the corrected serum Cl^- is elevated).
  - Corrected Cl^- is defined as patient $Cl^- \times$ normal Na^+/patient Na^+.
  - Anion gap can be calculated by the formula: $(Na^+ + K^+) - (Cl^- + HCO_3^-)$, and normal values for dogs are between 12 and 24 mEq/L.

- The anion gap represents the ions in a blood sample that are not measured in the anion gap formula.
- Increased anion gap acidosis is normally associated with an accumulation of organic acids such as lactate or ketones, and [Cl^-] remains unchanged.
- The only important cause of a low anion gap is hypoalbuminemia, and this should be borne in mind as a potential confounder of high anion gap acidosis, because hypoalbuminemia occurs commonly in critical illness that itself is a common cause of high anion gap acidosis.
- Normal anion gap metabolic acidosis is associated with an increased corrected [Cl^-].

- Respiratory acidosis is associated with reduced alveolar ventilation, generally from an abnormally low respiratory rate or decreased tidal volume (e.g., large volume pleural effusion, excessively tight chest wrap bandage, altered lung compliance as seen in lung edema, neuromuscular junction disruption as seen with neurotoxins and some peripheral neuropathies). The result is an increase in pCO_2 leading to a reduced pH with a secondary or compensatory partial increase in [HCO_3^-] or reduction in blood [Cl^-].
- Simple respiratory acidosis will not alter anion gap, but the metabolic compensatory response can be expected to drop [Cl^-].
- The presence of severe acidosis may be masked by an equally severe alkalosis from retention of HCO_3^- or low pCO_2 (i.e., mixed acid-base disorder). Therefore acidosis cannot be said to be absent only on the basis of normal blood pH (absence of acidemia); pCO_2 and [HCO_3^-] also must be normal.

DIAGNOSIS

DIFFERENTIAL DIAGNOSIS

- Acidosis is never a primary diagnosis. It is always the consequence of another disease and, as such, each disease that causes acidosis will have its own differential diagnosis list.
- More than one primary acid-base imbalance may occur concurrently, and these combinations are then termed *mixed acid-base disorders*. For example, metabolic and respiratory acidosis may occur concurrently.
- Causes of increased anion gap metabolic acidosis:
  - Ethylene glycol toxicity
  - Diabetic ketoacidosis
  - Uremic acidosis
  - Lactic acidosis (e.g., due to cardiovascular collapse during shock)
- Causes of normal anion gap acidosis:
  - Diarrhea
  - Renal tubular acidosis
  - Dilutional acidosis (rapid saline administration)
  - Hypoadrenocorticism

INITIAL DATABASE: Complete blood count, serum biochemistry panel, urinalysis.

- Bicarbonate (HCO_3^-): low, unless mixed acid-base disorder (opposing/offsetting disorders).
- Total protein, albumin: hypoalbuminemia explains a low anion gap; a normal anion gap metabolic acidosis with concurrent hypoalbuminemia should raise the suspicion that a high anion gap metabolic acidosis is present but that the high anion gap is concealed by the effect of hypoalbuminemia.
- Electrolyte abnormalities: as described previously.
- Overall, these routine laboratory tests are an essential part of basic evaluation of all systemic disorders that could cause acidosis.

ADVANCED OR CONFIRMATORY TESTING

- Diagnosis and characterization of acidosis requires a blood gas analysis in addition to determination of serum electrolytes and albumin concentrations.
  - A venous blood sample is generally adequate for pCO_2, HCO_3^-, and electrolytes, but an arterial sample is preferable because PaO_2 may then be assessed as a measure of lung function.
- Special diagnostic evaluations should be tailored to the specific diagnosis of disease processes suspected on the initial database.
- Thoracic imaging (radiographs ± other modalities based on findings) should be performed in cases of respiratory acidosis.

TREATMENT

THERAPEUTIC GOAL(S)

The primary aim is to correct the underlying cause of the acid-base derangement. Treating the inciting cause should return the blood pH to normal/close normal. As a general rule, one should correct the most life-threatening, most treatable condition first. For example, if one decompresses the stomach of a gastric dilation-volvulus (GDV) patient and aggressively supports vascular volume, direct intervention to manage acid-base abnormalities will not be necessary. The acid-base parameters are a good indication of the success of the interventions used for dealing with the GDV but should not require direct management.

ACUTE GENERAL TREATMENT

- Specific adjustment of blood pH by the administration of HCO_3^- is almost never required and should only be considered if blood pH ≤7.1. The aim of treatment is to raise pH to 7.2. Treatment is more important in dogs with (HCO_3^-) ≤5 mmol/L, because very small decreases in (HCO_3^-) at this level result in large decreases in pH. An *approximate* dose of HCO_3^- can be calculated from the formula:

$$\text{mEq } HCO_3^- \text{ required} = 0.5 \times \text{body weight (kg)} \times (\text{base deficit} - \text{patient } HCO_3^-).$$

- Administer half of this dose intravenously over 3 to 4 hours and recheck acid-base status with a blood gas measurement. The balance of the dose may be administered if the pH remains <7.2 at that time.
- HCO_3^- is not indicated in the treatment of respiratory acidosis. If arterial pO_2 ≤60 mmHg in respiratory acidosis, oxygen should be administered to raise it to approximately 60 mmHg (but no higher). Cl^- rich fluids (e.g., 0.9% NaCl) assist compensation in chronic respiratory acidosis by preventing the development of rebound metabolic alkalosis once the respiratory problem has been dealt with and pO_2 has normalized.

CHRONIC TREATMENT

Oral supplementation of $NaHCO_3$ (0.5-1 mEq/kg/day) may be helpful in chronic metabolic acidosis (as in cases of chronic renal failure). Dietary chloride supplementation (e.g., KCl) assists metabolic compensation in cases of chronic respiratory acidosis.

DRUG INTERACTIONS

Intravenous $NaHCO_3$ should not be given in dextrose- or alcohol-containing fluids, and it is best administered as a separate infusion.

POSSIBLE COMPLICATIONS

Rapid administration of $NaHCO_3$ can be dangerous, and treatment of mixed metabolic and respiratory acidosis with $NaHCO_3$ can compound the respiratory acidosis, because the CO_2 generated by the $NaHCO_3$ cannot be blown off.

RECOMMENDED MONITORING

Blood gas and serum electrolyte and protein evaluation

PROGNOSIS AND OUTCOME

Dependent on the reversibility of the underlying disease disorder and the trend of the acid-base variables over time

PEARLS & CONSIDERATIONS

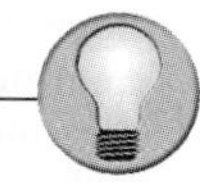

COMMENTS

- Almost all critically ill patients will have an acid-base abnormality, but few require treatment beyond correction/management of the underlying cause.
- Venous or arterial blood samples are adequate for measuring pH, pCO_2, HCO_3^-, and electrolytes, but only arterial samples can be used for pO_2 (PaO_2) measurement.
- Animals can have serious acid-base abnormalities with normal blood pH ("mixed acid-base disorders"). A common pitfall is to fail to notice a severe, mixed acid-base disturbance because a patient has a normal blood pH; HCO_3^-, pCO_2, and electrolytes must also be evaluated.
- Mixed acid-base disorders should be suspected if:
    - pCO_2 and HCO_3^- change in opposite directions
    - pH is normal with an abnormal pCO_2 and/or HCO_3^-
    - pH changes in a direction opposite to what is expected for the underlying disease
- One type of mixed acid-base disorder, the combination of metabolic acidosis with respiratory alkalosis (neutralizing pH abnormalities) commonly occurs in conditions like septic shock, GDV; liver disease and cardiopulmonary resuscitation.
- Another type of mixed acid-base disorder, the combination of respiratory acidosis together with metabolic alkalosis, may occur in cases of GDV, and of pulmonary edema treated with diuretics.
- The combination of respiratory acidosis together with metabolic acidosis usually occurs in patients with acute severe respiratory disease that also have lactic acidosis due to hypoxemia, shock, or low cardiac output.
- Hyperchloremic and high anion gap acidosis together are usually seen in renal failure, resolving ketoacidosis or in patients with high anion gap acidosis that develop diarrhea or receive fluid therapy.
- Unlike dogs, cats with metabolic acidosis do not commonly generate compensatory respiratory alkalosis.

PREVENTION

Treat precipitating causes aggressively

SUGGESTED READING

DiBartola SP, de Morais HA: Acid-base disorders. In DiBartola SP (ed): *Fluid Therapy in Small Animal Practice*, 2nd ed. Philadelphia, WB Saunders, 2000, pp 189-264.

AUTHOR: **ANDREW LEISEWITZ**
EDITOR: **ELIZABETH ROZANSKI**

Acne

BASIC INFORMATION

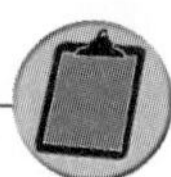

DEFINITION

- Canine acne is a chronic inflammatory disorder of the chin and lips of young dogs, characterized by deep folliculitis and furunculosis.
- Feline acne is an idiopathic disorder of follicular keratinization.

SYNONYM(S)

Canine acne:

- Chin pyoderma
- Muzzle folliculitis and furunculosis

EPIDEMIOLOGY

SPECIES, AGE, SEX

- Canine acne is common, particularly in young, short-coated breeds.
- Feline acne is not confined to adolescence.
- There is no reported gender predisposition.

GENETICS AND BREED PREDISPOSITION

- Large short-coated dog breeds appear predisposed: boxers, Doberman pinschers, English bulldogs, Great Danes, weimaraners, mastiffs, rottweilers, and German short-haired pointers.
- No documented breed predilection in cats.

CLINICAL PRESENTATION

HISTORY, CHIEF COMPLAINT

- Skin lesions restricted to the chin area, sometimes involving the lips, noted by the owner (see below)
- Lesions may be an incidental finding during routine examination

PHYSICAL EXAM FINDINGS

- Canine acne: Early lesions consist of erythematous papules. Lesions can progress to pustules, bullae, or occasional ulcerated draining tracts with serosanguineous discharge on the chin or muzzle (Fig. I-6).
- Feline acne: incidentally discovered comedones on the chin, and occasionally the lips, that do not seem to bother the cat. These lesions can evolve to papules, pustules, and even furunculosis and cellulitis when secondarily infected.

ETIOLOGY AND PATHOPHYSIOLOGY

- Unknown cause.
- Bacterial involvement is secondary.
- Canine acne can be triggered by local trauma, and genetic predisposition has been suggested.
- Feline acne could be aggravated by poor grooming habits, underlying predisposition to seborrhea, the production of abnormal sebum, hair cycle influences, stress, viruses, and immunosuppression.

DIAGNOSIS

DIFFERENTIAL DIAGNOSIS

- Demodicosis
- Dermatophytosis
- *Malassezia* dermatitis
- Eosinophilic granuloma (feline)
- Early juvenile cellulitis (canine)
- Contact dermatitis
- Sebaceous gland or other localized skin tumors

INITIAL DATABASE

- Diagnosis is usually based on history, clinical findings, and ruling out other differentials
- Cytology (pustules or exudates): suppurative inflammation and phagocytosed bacteria when secondarily infected
- Skin scrapings are routinely performed to rule out demodicosis

ADVANCED OR CONFIRMATORY TESTING

- Dermatohistopathology: follicular hyperkeratosis, folliculitis and/or furunculosis, and even cellulitis
- Bacterial culture and sensitivity test may be needed if nonresponsive to appropriate empiric antibiotic therapy
- Dermatophyte testing medium if dermatophytosis is suspected

TREATMENT

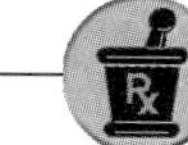

THERAPEUTIC GOAL(S)

Eliminate secondary bacterial infection if present, and control recurrences

ACUTE GENERAL TREATMENT

- Choice of treatment will depend on the severity of the disease.
- Minimize trauma to the chin (dogs).
- Clipping the affected area can increase the efficacy of topical treatment (cats).

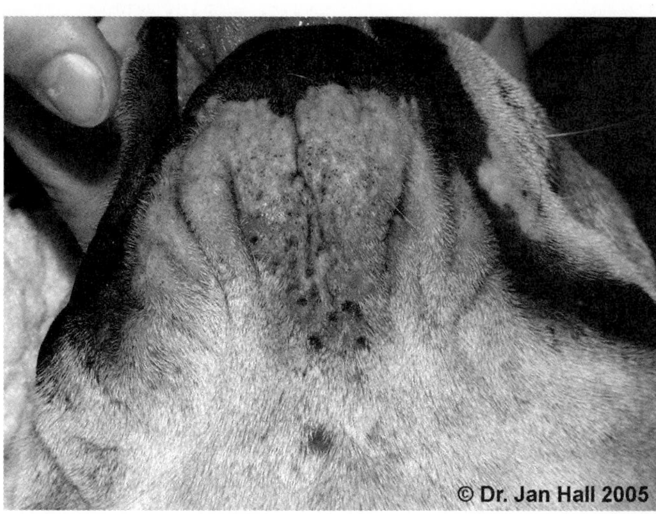

FIGURE I-6 Comedones and pustules on the chin of a 2-year-old English bulldog with chin acne secondary to canine atopy. Courtesy of Dr. Jan A. Hall.

Topical treatment:
- Mild lesions can be controlled with application of benzoyl peroxide shampoo or gel (maximum of 5% concentration) q 24h until resolution, then 1 to 2 times per week as needed.
- Mupirocin or fusidic acid ointments or creams may be applied. These medications may be considered initially or if there is a lack of response to treatment with benzoyl peroxide.
- Tretinoin 0.01-0.05% cream or lotion may be used in refractory cases. May be drying or irritating.
- Glucocorticoid creams may be needed to reduce inflammation, once secondary bacterial infection has been eliminated.
- Others: sulphur-salicylic acid shampoos, 0.75% metronidazole gel, other topical medications containing clindamycin, erythromycin, or tetracycline (cats).

Systemic treatment:
- Treat secondary bacterial infection with appropriate systemic antibiotics for 4 to 8 weeks. Culture and sensitivity may be warranted if empirical treatment (e.g., cephalexin 22 mg/kg PO q 8h or 30 mg/kg q 12h [dogs], clavulanic acid potentiated amoxicillin 62.5 mg PO q 12h [cats]) is ineffective after 1 to 2 weeks.
- Refractory feline cases may benefit from systemic isotretinoin administration: 2 mg/kg PO q 24h until resolution (approximately one month), then every 2 to 3 days as needed.

CHRONIC TREATMENT

For recurring lesions, topical medication can be used as needed for long-term therapy.

POSSIBLE COMPLICATIONS

- Localized irritation with topical preparations containing benzoyl peroxide or tretinoin.
- Chronic topical steroids can cause adrenal suppression and local skin atrophy.
- Oral isotretinoin can induce side effects: diarrhea, anorexia, vomiting, conjunctivitis, increased liver enzyme levels. It is teratogenic. With chronic use, skeletal abnormalities are a concern. In addition, it can possibly be harmful in case of accidental human ingestion.

RECOMMENDED MONITORING

With oral isotretinoin therapy: pretreatment measurement of tear production, complete blood count, chemistry profile, and urinalysis. Repeat in 1 to 2 months, if normal, then repeat as needed

PROGNOSIS AND OUTCOME

- Canine acne carries a good prognosis, with many dogs achieving a permanent cure. Some dogs require lifelong topical therapy.
- Feline acne also has a good prognosis, but lifelong intermittent or continuous therapy is often needed.
- In severe cases, active lesions can resolve with scarring.

PEARLS & CONSIDERATIONS

COMMENTS

- Owners should avoid expressing the lesions, because of possible internal rupture of the hair follicles, inducing local inflammation.
- Benzoyl peroxide-containing medications can bleach carpets and fabrics.
- When it is not secondarily infected, feline acne is a cosmetic disease that does not affect the cat's quality of life. It could be left untreated if not visually objectionable.

SUGGESTED READING

Medleau L, et al: Bacterial diseases (chapter 3) and Keratinization and seborrheic disorders (chapter 12). In *Small Animal Dermatology: A Color Atlas and Therapeutic Guide*. Philadelphia, WB Saunders, 2001, pp 38-39, 323-324.

Scott DW, et al: Bacterial skin diseases (chapter 3) and keratinization defects (chapter 14). In *Muller & Kirk's Small Animal Dermatology*, ed 6. Philadelphia, WB Saunders, 2001, pp 303-306, 1042-1043.

AUTHOR: **NADIA PAGÉ**
EDITOR: **JAN A. HALL**

Acral Lick Dermatitis

Client Education Sheet on Website

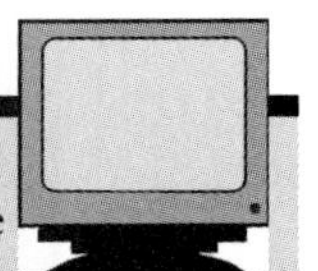

BASIC INFORMATION

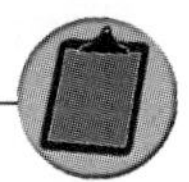

DEFINITION

Development of a firm, alopecic plaque lesion on the skin secondary to excessive licking

SYNONYM(S)

Lick granuloma

EPIDEMIOLOGY

SPECIES, AGE, SEX

- Dogs
- Most >5 years old
- May occur more frequently in males

GENETICS AND BREED PREDISPOSITION

- Seen primarily in large-breed dogs
- Predisposed breeds include the Doberman pinscher, Labrador retriever, Great Dane, Irish setter, golden retriever, German shepherd

RISK FACTORS: Underlying conditions include allergic disease and bacterial infections.

ASSOCIATED CONDITIONS AND DISORDERS: Hyperadrenocorticism (occasional finding).

CLINICAL PRESENTATION

HISTORY, CHIEF COMPLAINT

- Patient usually presents with a unilateral firm, alopecic plaque lesion on the distal limb
- History of pruritus or constant licking is an important feature of the condition
- Occasional history of trauma or joint disease in the affected area

PHYSICAL EXAM FINDINGS

- Generally only a single lesion is noted. Most common sites include dorsal carpus, metacarpus, or metatarsus.
- A firm, erythematous, alopecic, eroded, or ulcerated lesion is typical. Saliva staining of the surrounding hair, purulent oozing tracts, and dependent edema may also be noted. Frequently a hard fibrous nodule develops. The presence of multiple lesions is usually associated with an underlying skin disorder (e.g., atopy, food hypersensitivity, pyoderma).

ETIOLOGY AND PATHOPHYSIOLOGY

- Acral lick lesions have a multifactorial etiology. Most cases have an organic cause (hypersensitivity skin disease, joint disease, neoplasia, etc.) with secondary behavioral involvement.
- Lesion development is normally secondary to localized or generalized pruritus and associated with chronic licking of the affected area. Chronic licking elicits a deep inflammatory response leading to the development of an erosive plaque, secondary bacterial folliculitis, and furunculosis.
- After initiation of the lesion, constant licking maintains the problem.
- In some cases, no organic cause can be identified. In these individuals obsessive-compulsive behavior associated with boredom and separation anxiety is important.

DIAGNOSIS

DIFFERENTIAL DIAGNOSIS

For underlying cause:

- Demodicosis (affected individuals normally have more widespread skin lesions)
- Dermatophytosis
- Hypersensitivity disorders; food, flea, environmental (affected dogs have more widespread skin lesions)
- Pyoderma (affected dogs have more widespread skin lesions, including pustules and crusts)
- Spontaneous hyperadrenocorticism (acral lick dermatitis is noted occasionally)
- Foreign body granuloma (historic information)
- Previous trauma (historic information of injury)
- Degenerative joint disease
- Neoplasia (histiocytoma, mastocytoma)
- Pressure point granuloma
- Calcinosis circumscripta
- Behavioral; boredom, separation anxiety (rule out organic skin disease)

INITIAL DATABASE

Tentative diagnosis is based on history and clinical presentation:

- Skin cytology (exfoliative cytology, to rule out neoplasia). Mixed inflammatory infiltrate with fibroblasts noted
- Skin scrapings (to rule out demodicosis)
- Fungal culture (to rule out dermatophytosis)
- Skin biopsy (to rule out neoplasia). Histopathologic evaluation of acral lick lesions reveals ulceration and irregular epidermal hyperplasia that may be pronounced. Dermal infiltrate may vary from mild perivascular dermatitis to severe folliculitis and furunculosis.
- Routine hematologic evaluation, chemistry profile, and urinalysis (to look for evidence to suggest underlying spontaneous hyperadrenocorticism)

ADVANCED OR CONFIRMATORY TESTING

- Radiographic study of chronic lesions may reveal a secondary periosteal reaction. Underlying joint disease may be noted
- Behavioral consultation

TREATMENT

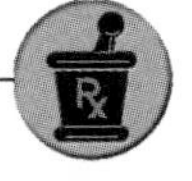

THERAPEUTIC GOAL(S)

- Eliminate secondary infection and inflammation.
- Control behavioral factors. Behavioral modification is more effective once inflammation and secondary infection are controlled.
- It is critical that the patient is not allowed to lick the affected area once treatment commences.

ACUTE AND CHRONIC TREATMENT

Choice of treatment will depend on the severity of the condition:

- Topical therapy: apply until lesion resolves before gradually weaning off.
  - 8.0 ml of flucinolone with DMSO (SynOtic) mixed with 3.0 ml of flunixin meglumine (Banamine): apply directly to the affected area q 12h while wearing gloves. Numbs nerve endings in the lesion.
  - Capsaicin (Zostrix): Apply 2 to 3 times daily.
- Intralesional therapy:
  - Triamcinolone acetonide (Vetalog) or methylprednisolone acetate (Depo-Medrol) injected directly into the lesion. Volume is generally less than recommended injectable dose due to limitations of injection volume into the mass.
- Systemic therapy:
  - Antibiotic therapy.
    - Aggressive antibiotic therapy (cephalexin 30 mg/kg q PO 12h) for up to 12 weeks may dramatically improve long-standing lesions, even decreasing pruritus.
  - Anti-inflammatory therapy.
    - The addition of systemic steroid therapy after 4 weeks of antibiotic therapy may be beneficial.
    - Prednisone (inflammation): 1–2 mg/kg PO q 24h initially, before weaning down to lowest effective dose.
  - Antihistamines:
    - Hydroxyzine 2.2 mg/kg PO q 8–12h; or
    - Chlorpheniramine 4–8 mg/dog PO q 8–12h.

- Narcotic analgesics:
  - Naltrexone 2.2 mg/kg PO q 12-24h.
- Behavior-modifying drugs:
  - Clomipramine 1-3 mg/kg PO q 24h; or
  - Fluoxetine HCl 1 mg/kg PO q 24h; or
  - Doxepin 3-5 mg/kg PO q 12h; maximum 150 mg q 12h; or
  - Amitriptyline 1.1-2.2 mg/kg PO q 12h.
- Physical restraint (Elizabethan collar, bandaging) is often essential.
- Surgical excision should generally not be attempted because of difficulties with closure and a high incidence of wound breakdown.
- Laser therapy may be less likely to lead to wound breakdown and postoperative pain.
- Cryosurgery may be considered to destroy nerve endings, breaking the itch-scratch cycle.

DRUG INTERACTIONS

- Do not use drugs with central nervous system depressant activity (e.g., antihistamines, clomipramine, amitriptyline, doxepin, fluoxetine) concurrently.
- Avoid use of tricyclic antidepressants with monoamine oxidase inhibitors or antihistamines.
- Cimetidine may inhibit tricyclic antidepressant metabolism.

POSSIBLE COMPLICATIONS

Wound breakdown may require postsurgical intervention.

RECOMMENDED MONITORING

Tricyclic antidepressant drugs may affect liver and heart function. Perform routine hematology, chemistry profile, and ECG every 6 to 8 weeks.

PROGNOSIS AND OUTCOME

Guarded prognosis. Therapy must focus on organic dermatologic nature of the condition, as well as behavioral factors involved

PEARLS & CONSIDERATIONS

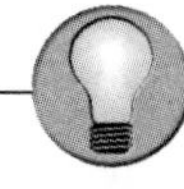

COMMENTS

- Behavioral component is often secondary. Investigate potential for underlying skin disease and treat accordingly.
- Development of a new lesion close to where a lesion was covered is strongly indicative of a significant behavioral component to the disorder.

CLIENT EDUCATION

Behavioral modification

SUGGESTED READING

Scott DW, Miller WH, Griffin CE: Skin immune system and allergic diseases. In *Muller and Kirk's Small Animal Dermatology*, 6th ed. Philadelphia, WB Saunders, 2001, pp 1058-1064.

Virga V: Behavioral dermatology. *Vet Clin North Am Small Anim Pract* 33(2):231-251, v-vi, 2003.

AUTHOR & EDITOR: **JAN A. HALL**

Acromegaly

BASIC INFORMATION

DEFINITION

A rare disorder of cats and dogs caused by chronic increased serum growth hormone concentrations. Acromegaly causes overgrowth of connective tissue, bone, and viscera

SYNONYM(S)

Hypersomatotropism

EPIDEMIOLOGY

SPECIES, AGE, SEX

- Cats: middle-aged/old (mean, 10 years; range, 4 to 17 years). Male predominance
- Dogs: older unspayed females overrepresented

RISK FACTORS: Progestin administration (dogs).

ASSOCIATED CONDITIONS AND DISORDERS: Insulin-resistant diabetes mellitus.

CLINICAL PRESENTATION

DISEASE FORMS/SUBTYPES

- Cats: growth hormone-secreting pituitary adenoma
- Dogs:
  - Usually secondary to increased exogenous (drugs administered to prevent estrus) or endogenous (diestrus) progesterone concentrations. Progesterone stimulates growth hormone production by mammary tissue
  - One report of acromegaly due to pituitary adenoma

HISTORY, CHIEF COMPLAINT: Polyuria; polydipsia; polyphagia; progestin drug administration (e.g., megesterol acetate); insulin-resistant diabetes mellitus (i.e., poor glycemic control despite insulin doses > 1.5-2.0 U/kg/dose [dogs] or 7-10 U/dose [cats]), especially in cats.

PHYSICAL EXAM FINDINGS

- Cats: large cat with a prominent head (most common), gallop sound ("gallop rhythm") on cardiac auscultation, signs of congestive heart failure (tachypnea, crackles, muffled heart sounds), lameness. Neurologic signs (e.g., stupor, adipsia, altered thermoregulation, seizures, behavior change) may be seen with a pituitary macroadenoma.
- Dogs: thick, puffy skin with excessive folds around the head, neck, and extremities.
- Dogs and cats: diffuse thickening of oropharyngeal soft tissues, stridor/snoring, protrusion of the mandible, widening of the interdental space, hepatomegaly, and renomegaly.

ETIOLOGY AND PATHOPHYSIOLOGY

- Chronic growth hormone excess has both catabolic and anabolic effects.
- Anabolic effects: increased insulin-like growth factor-1 (IGF-1) causes proliferation of bone, cartilage, soft tissues, and viscera.
- Catabolic effects: anti-insulin effect on tissues causes decreased carbohydrate utilization and ultimately leads to insulin-resistant diabetes mellitus.

DIAGNOSIS

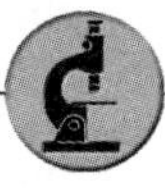

DIFFERENTIAL DIAGNOSIS

Differentials for insulin antagonism/resistance: hyperadrenocorticism; infection; drugs (e.g., glucocorticoids, progestins); hyperthyroidism (cats); chronic pancreatitis; renal insufficiency; obesity; or problems with insulin type, storage, or administration

INITIAL DATABASE

- Complete blood count, serum biochemical profile, urinalysis:
  - Hyperglycemia, glycosuria, hypercholesterolemia, and mild elevations in alanine aminotransferase and alkaline phosphatase (secondary to poorly controlled diabetes mellitus) are common in cats. Overt diabetes mellitus is less common in dogs.

  - Mild polycythemia, hyperphosphatemia without concurrent azotemia, and hyperglobulinemia also possible in some cats.
- Tests for hyperadrenocorticism (see Hyperadrenocorticism, p 537; Hyperadrenocorticism Suspect/Conflicting Results, p 540) should be performed, because both acromegaly and hyperadrenocorticism can cause insulin resistance, bilateral adrenomegaly, and a pituitary mass.
- Radiographs:
  - Hallmark findings: diffuse oropharyngeal soft tissue hypertrophy; degenerative arthropathy of multiple joints (cats); spinal spondylosis deformans (cats); manibular enlargement; hyperostosis of the bony calvarium.
  - Also possible with acromegaly, but in cats in general, these findings are far more commonly due to disorders other than acromegaly: mild to severe cardiomegaly, pulmonary edema and/or pleural fluid (cats); hepatomegaly, renomegaly.
- Abdominal ultrasound: normal or possible hepatomegaly, renomegaly, and adrenomegaly.
- Echocardiography: possible left ventricular thickening.

ADVANCED OR CONFIRMATORY TESTING

- Cats:
  - Brain computed tomography or magnetic resonance imaging: contrast-enhancing pituitary mass is usually visible; failure to identify a mass does not rule out acromegaly.
  - Increased serum growth hormone concentration is diagnostic for feline acromegaly but because of extremely limited availability of this test, diagnosis is often based on appropriate clinical findings, increased serum IGF-1 concentration, and documentation of a pituitary mass. Growth hormone and IGF-1 values should be interpreted in consultation with the laboratory performing the assay(s).
- Dogs:
  - Presumptive diagnosis is based on appropriate history, clinical signs, and physical examination findings. Increased serum growth hormone and IGF-1 concentrations are required to establish a definitive diagnosis, which is rarely possible due to the extremely limited availability of the growth hormone assay.

TREATMENT

THERAPEUTIC GOAL(S)

- Cats: Decrease the size of the pituitary mass and return serum growth hormone concentrations to normal.
- Dogs: Decrease serum progesterone concentrations so serum growth hormone concentrations normalize.

ACUTE GENERAL TREATMENT

- Cats: if diabetic, insulin dosage should be adjusted to try to attain/maintain glycemic control (see Diabetes Mellitus, p 289)
- Dogs:
  - Progesterone-induced: The dog should be spayed and/or exogenous progestin therapy discontinued. Anabolic effects of growth hormone will resolve, but diabetes mellitus, if present, may not resolve
  - Pituitary growth hormone-secreting adenoma: treat as in cats

CHRONIC TREATMENT

Cats: There is no consistently effective treatment.

- Radiation therapy (pituitary): considered the best option, but response is variable and is usually transient. Limited availability, expense, the need for repeated anesthesia, prolonged hospitalization, and unpredictable response are disadvantages.
- Surgery (transsphenoidal hypophysectomy): has been used for treating some cats with pituitary-dependent hyperadrenocorticism but has not yet been used with acromegaly.
- Medical treatment: octreotide, a somatostatin analog, has not been effective in cats.

POSSIBLE COMPLICATIONS

- Radiation therapy: post-treatment hypopituitarism, hypoglycemia as tissue response to insulin improves.
- Cats: Severe hypoglycemia from an insulin overdose can occur with treatment or due to unpredictable fluctuations in the severity of insulin resistance. The risk of hypoglycemia increases with higher insulin doses, so caution and careful monitoring are necessary if insulin doses must exceed 12 to 15 U/dose.

RECOMMENDED MONITORING

- Physical exam
- Blood and urine glucose if diabetic

PROGNOSIS AND OUTCOME

- Cats: guarded to poor. Survival times range from 4 to 60 months. Most cats are euthanized because of failure to control diabetes mellitus, or because of acromegalic complications (congestive heart failure, respiratory distress, renal failure, neurologic signs).
- Dogs (progestin-induced acromegaly): good.

SUGGESTED READING

Feldman EC, Nelson RW: Disorders of growth hormone. In Feldman EC, Nelson RW (eds): *Canine and Feline Endocrinology and Reproduction*. Philadelphia, WB Saunders, 2004, pp 45–84.

Goossens MMC, et al: Cobalt 60 irradiation of pituitary gland tumors in three cats with acromegaly. *J Am Vet Med Assoc* 213:374, 1998.

Hurty CA, Flatland B: Feline acromegaly: a review of the syndrome. *J Am Anim Hosp Assoc* 41:292–297, 2005.

Peterson ME, et al: Acromegaly in 14 cats. *J Vet Intern Med* 4:192, 1990.

Rijnberk A: Acromegaly. In Ettinger SJ, Feldman EC (eds): *Textbook of Veterinary Internal Medicine*, ed 5. Philadelphia, WB Saunders, 2000, pp 1370–1373.

AUTHOR: **ELISABETH SNEAD**

EDITOR: **SHERRI IHLE**

Actinomycosis and Nocardiosis

BASIC INFORMATION

DEFINITION

- Actinomycosis: chronic, pyogranulomatous disease due to infection by anaerobic, gram-positive, non-acid–fast, pleomorphic, branching, rod-shaped bacteria that are members of the genus *Actinomyces* (dogs: *Actinomyces viscosus* and *A. bordeovulneris;* cats: *A. viscosus* and *A. meyeri*)
- Nocardiosis: chronic, pyogranulomatous disease due to infection by aerobic, gram-positive, partially acid-fast, branching, rod-shaped bacteria that are members of the genus *Nocardia* (dogs and cats: *N. asteroides* and *N. brasiliensis*; dogs only: *N. otitidiscaviarum*; cats only: *N. caviae*)

EPIDEMIOLOGY

SPECIES, AGE, SEX

- Actinomycosis: canine, adult to middle-aged, males more commonly infected
- Nocardiosis: canine, young (<2 years), males more commonly infected

RISK FACTORS

- Actinomycosis: housing and/or use in outdoor environment (primarily hunting dogs). Coinfection with other bacteria predisposes to development of the pyogranulomatous disease form
- Nocardiosis: immunosuppressive drug therapy or concurrent diseases

GEOGRAPHY AND SEASONALITY: Environmental presence of grass awns (foxtails), which may be inhaled or ingested: associated with higher incidence, especially of actinomycosis.

CONTAGION AND ZOONOSIS: Actinomycosis and nocardiosis: not significant zoonotic agents, except for severely immunocompromised individuals.

ASSOCIATED CONDITIONS AND DISORDERS: Actinomycosis and nocardiosis: associated with bite wounds in cats often resulting in chronic draining tracts.

CLINICAL PRESENTATION

DISEASE FORMS/SUBTYPES

- Pyothorax/body cavity effusion
- Chronic cutaneous draining tracts/nonhealing wounds (actinomycosis) or subcutaneous abscesses (nocardiosis)
- Systemic/disseminated infection

HISTORY AND CHIEF COMPLAINT

- Nonspecific systemic signs (e.g., lethargy, inappetence) due to sepsis
- Respiratory abnormalities (cough, dyspnea)
- Visible skin lesions (e.g., soft subcutaneous masses, draining tracts)

PHYSICAL EXAM FINDINGS

- **Actinomycosis:**
  - Pyothorax/body cavity effusion:
    - Thorax:
      - Cough
      - Tachypnea
      - Dyspnea
      - Decreased lung sounds
      - Subcutaneous masses on lateral thorax:
        - Often develop draining sinus
      - Chronic and progressive weight loss and fever
      - Involvement of associated tissues (mediastinum, heart, pleura, and chest wall) can produce additional physical signs (e.g., arrhythmia)
    - Retroperitoneal space:
      - Back pain
      - Rear leg paresis or paralysis
      - Subcutaneous masses on caudal thorax or flank
    - Abdomen:
      - Palpable masses
      - Abdominal distention
      - Subcutaneous masses on lateral abdomen (not as common as with thoracic disease):
        - Often develop draining sinus
  - Chronic subcutaneous soft tissue masses, cutaneous draining tracts, and nonhealing wounds:
    - Cervicofacial region and subcutaneous tissue:
      - Mandible, submandibular region, and ventral or lateral cervical areas most frequently affected
      - Acute to chronic subcutaneous soft tissue swelling of the neck or head region
      - Lesions are fluctuant to firm with ulcerations or draining sinuses
      - Adjacent bone can have periosteal new bone formation or osteomyelitis with chronic infections
      - Fluid discharged or aspirated from masses:
        - Serosanguineous to purulent
        - Yellow-tan granules ("sulfur granules"), which are colonies of *Actinomyces*
  - Systemic/disseminated infection:
    - Any of the preceding forms may become systemic
- **Nocardiosis:**
  - Pyothorax/body cavity effusion:
    - Thorax:
      - Distemper-like signs:
        - Mucopurulent oculonasal discharge
        - Anorexia
        - Weight loss
        - Cough
        - Dyspnea
        - Diarrhea
        - Hyperthermia
    - Coinfection with canine distemper virus is commonly seen
  - Subcutaneous:
    - Firm to fluctuant swellings
    - May ulcerate or develop fistulous tracts
    - Reddish-brown exudate
  - Disseminated:
    - Skin, subcutaneous tissue, kidney, liver, spleen, lymph nodes, central nervous system, bone, and joints

ETIOLOGY AND PATHOPHYSIOLOGY

- **Actinomycosis:**
  - *Actinomyces* spp. are dependent on disruption of the normal protective mucosal barriers.
  - Typically, the disease spreads by direct extension through, not along, normal tissue planes:
    - Often initiated by a migrating grass awn that penetrated the skin or oral, pharyngeal, or other mucosa.
  - Rarely, hematogenous dissemination occurs.
  - The pathogenicity of *Actinomyces* spp. is dramatically increased in mixed infections:
    - Pure culture inoculation typically does not result in infection.
    - *Actinomyces* fimbriae bind to cell surface receptors on other bacteria or neutrophils:
      - Inhibits neutrophil phagocytosis and bactericidal activity on bacteria complex
  - *Actinomyces* spp. induce neutrophil chemotaxis, activate macrophages, and stimulate B-lymphocyte hyperplasia:
    - The preceding characteristics lead to the typical finding of a dense mat of *Actinomyces* spp. and mixed infection surrounded by neutrophils, macrophages, and plasma cells.
  - Extension of the disease through normal tissue planes is facilitated by release of proteolytic enzymes from macrophages and degranulated neutrophils.
  - Cervicofacial region infections:
    - Bite wounds.
    - Foreign body perforation.
    - Chronic gingivitis-peridontitis.
  - Thorax:
    - Direct extension.
    - Migration of foreign body (grass awn).

        - Aspiration of organisms.
        - Esophageal perforation.
    - Abdominal:
        - Direct extension.
        - Migration of foreign body (grass awn).
        - Penetrated gastrointestinal (GI) tract mucosa by ingested foreign body.
        - Abdominal trauma (gunshot).
    - Retroperitoneal space:
        - Direct extension.
        - Migration of foreign body (grass awn):
            - Migration through lung to the dorsal attachment of the diaphragm
            - Migration through the intestines by the attachment of the root of the mesentery
    - Limbs:
        - Bite wounds.
        - Foreign body.
        - Lacerations contaminated by licking.
    - Subcutaneous:
        - Extension for other forms.
        - Bite wounds (primarily in cats).
- **Nocardiosis:**
    - Virulent strains of *Nocardia* spp. are facultative intracellular pathogens:
        - Inhibit/alter neutrophil and macrophage neutralizing ability.
    - Thorax:
        - Direct extension.
        - Aspiration of organisms.
        - Systemic disease may result from erosion into blood vessels from alveoli.
    - Subcutaneous:
        - Extension for other forms.
        - Bite wounds (primarily in cats).

DIAGNOSIS

DIFFERENTIAL DIAGNOSIS

- Pyothorax:
    - Bacterial pyothorax
    - Thoracic neoplasia
    - Chronic diaphragmatic hernia
- Cutaneous:
    - Bite wound abscess
    - Draining tracts from foreign bodies
- Disseminated:
    - Feline infectious peritonitis
    - Anaerobic bacterial infections
    - Systemic mycoses
    - Canine distemper (nocardiosis)

INITIAL DATABASE

- **Actinomycosis:**
    - Thoracic radiographs:
        - Alveolar and interstitial infiltrates with consolidation
        - Pleural thickening
        - Pleural effusion (often localized to one side)
        - Pericardial effusion
        - Widening of the mediastinum
        - Mass lesions
        - Periosteal new bone formation or osteomyelitis of adjacent ribs, vertebral bodies, or sternebrae
    - Abdominal radiographs/abdominal ultrasound:
        - Peritoneal effusion
        - Mass lesions
    - Vertebral radiographs:
        - Periosteal new bone formation on the ventral aspects of two to three adjacent vertebrae:
            - T13–L3 most common sites
            - Intervertebral disk space is not commonly affected
        - Osteomyelitis and compression fractures with chronic infections
    - Cytology of aspirates (pleural effusions, bronchial lavages, abscesses):
        - Slightly viscous, translucent/opaque fluid, possibly containing yellow macroscopic particles several millimeters in diameter ("sulfur granules") that, when present, represent pure cultures of *Actinomyces* (Fig. I-7)
- **Nocardiosis:**
    - Thoracic radiographs:
        - Variable:
            - Multiple, diffuse pulmonary nodules
            - Intrapulmonary or extrapulmonary solitary masses
            - Focal or diffuse bronchointerstitial to alveolar infiltrates
            - Lobar consolidations
            - Pleural effusions
            - Significant hilar lymphadenopathy
    - Other radiographic findings:
        - Soft tissue swelling
        - Bone lysis
        - Periosteal new bone growth
    - Cytology of aspirates (pleural effusions, bronchial lavages, abscesses):
        - Suppurative to pyogranulomatous inflammation, with evidence of gram-positive, branching, filamentous rod bacteria

ADVANCED OR CONFIRMATORY TESTING

- **Actinomycosis:**
    - Histopathologic examination may demonstrate filamentous bacteria with or without sulfur granules
    - Culture provides definitive diagnosis
    - Gram-positive, acid-fast staining negative
- **Nocardiosis:**
    - Gram-positive, acid-fast staining positive (partial or weak)
    - Uncommonly see sulfur granules
    - Usually not a mixed culture

TREATMENT

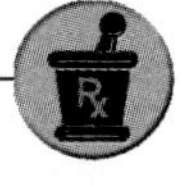

ACUTE GENERAL TREATMENT

Actinomycosis and nocardiosis:

- Pyothorax (see Pyothorax, p 935):
    - Drainage of thoracic cavity via single or bilateral chest drains
    - Lavage q 8–12h with warm sterile saline:
        - Add heparin 1500 IU/100 ml lavage fluid to prevent formation of adhesions
    - Continue for 5 to 7 days or until the retrieved fluid is clear and no bacteria are seen on cytology
- Open and drain abscesses:
    - May require Penrose drain or closed suction drain
- Bony lesions may require debridement.

CHRONIC TREATMENT

- **Actinomycosis:**
    - Penicillin G: 100,000 U/kg IV, IM, SC q 6–8h or 40 mg/kg PO q 8h
        - Minimum of 3 to 4 months treatment after resolution of clinical signs
    - Surgery may be warranted to remove diseased tissue after initial course of antibiotics
- **Nocardiosis:**
    - Sulfonamides

TABLE I-1 Actinomycosis versus Nocardiosis

Actinomyces	Nocardia
Culture	
Facultative or obligate anaerobe	Aerobe
Often not cultured	Usually cultured
Mixed bacterial culture	Sole isolate (unless from contaminated sample)
Staining Characteristics	
Gram-positive, nonacid fast (negative)	Gram-positive, partially acid fast (positive)
Clinical Disease	
Adult outdoor dogs	Dogs <2 years old
Fight wounds and pyothorax in cats	Fight wounds in cats
Treatment	
Penicillins	Sulfonamides

Table modified from Edwards DF: Actinomycosis and nocardiosis. In Greene CE (ed): *Infectious Diseases of the Dog and Cat*. Philadelphia, WB Saunders, 1998, pp 303–313.

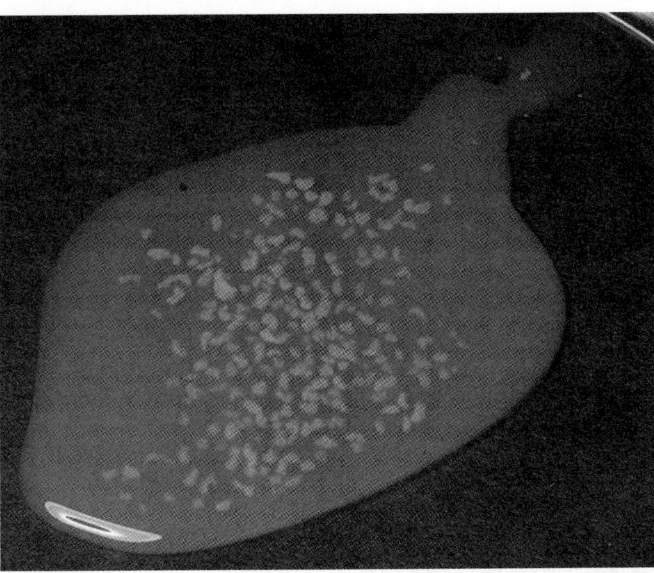

FIGURE I-7 Thoracic exudate in Petri dish, demonstrating numerous macroscopic "sulfur granules." These soft, yellow granules are colonies of *Actinomyces*. Reprinted from Edwards DF: Actinomycosis and nocardiosis. In Greene CE: *Infectious Diseases of the Dog and Cat*, ed 3. Philadelphia, WB Saunders, 1998, p 452 (with permission).

- Trimethoprim-sulfadiazine: 15–30 mg/kg PO q 12h
  - Susceptibility results warranted:
    - Not all isolates sensitive to sulfonamides
    - Amikacin and/or imipenem may be required

DRUG INTERACTIONS

Actinomycosis:

- Oxacillin, dicloxacillin, cephalexin, metronidazole, and aminoglycosides have poor in vitro activity against *Actinomyces* spp.

POSSIBLE COMPLICATIONS

Actinomycosis:

- *A. hordeovulneris* does not respond well to penicillin:
  - Clindamycin, chloramphenicol, or erythromycin warranted

RECOMMENDED MONITORING

Actinomycosis and nocardiosis:

- Cytologic and radiologic studies and repeated cultures can be used to determine the duration of therapy.

PROGNOSIS AND OUTCOME

- **Actinomycosis:**
  - In almost half the cases, the infection recurs. Therefore, identification and removal of any foreign material (e.g., grass awn) and careful monitoring for recurrence are important.
  - Due to the high reinfection rate, the prognosis is poor.
- **Nocardiosis:**
  - Due to predisposing conditions and delayed diagnosis, the prognosis is poor.

PEARLS & CONSIDERATIONS

COMMENTS

See Table I-1

SUGGESTED READING

Edwards DF: Actinomycosis and nocardiosis. In Greene CE (ed): *Infectious Diseases of the Dog and Cat*. Philadelphia, WB Saunders, 2006, pp 451–461.

AUTHOR: **ANDREW ISAACS**
EDITOR: **DOUGLASS K. MACINTIRE**

Acute Abdomen

BASIC INFORMATION

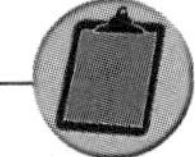

DEFINITION

A sudden onset of abdominal discomfort or pain

EPIDEMIOLOGY

SPECIES, AGE, SEX

- Dogs more commonly affected
- Specific causes vary with age, breed, and sex

GENETICS AND BREED PREDISPOSITION: Large-breed, deep-chested dogs are more prone to developing gastric dilation-volvulus (GDV) and splenic torsion.

RISK FACTORS: Prior intestinal surgery.

CONTAGION AND ZOONOSIS: Parvovirus is highly contagious to dogs but not other species.

ASSOCIATED CONDITIONS AND DISORDERS: Sepsis, hemorrhage, hypoalbuminemia, hypovolemia/hypovolemic shock (depending on cause).

CLINICAL PRESENTATION

HISTORY, CHIEF COMPLAINT

- Apparent abdominal pain
- Collapse
- Vomiting: projectile and acute onset are suggestive of obstruction
- Diarrhea: small bowel, large bowel, or dark feces (gastrointestinal bleeding)
  - Melena: upper gastrointestinal bleeding
  - Hematochezia: colonic or rectal bleeding
- Weight loss
- Anorexia
- Dietary indiscretion
- Intoxication

PHYSICAL EXAM FINDINGS

- Signs of abdominal pain (by definition)
  - The stoic nature of some patients may mask the manifestations of pain.
- Collapse
- Tachycardia (e.g., >140 bpm in a medium-sized dog)
- Poor peripheral pulses
- Dehydration may coexist with hypovolemia

ETIOLOGY AND PATHOPHYSIOLOGY

- Abdominal pain is due to the stretching of the nerve fibers located in the abdominal organs and body wall.
- The nerve endings can be stimulated with stretching or inflammation from generalized peritonitis.

- Generalized peritonitis can result from inflammatory, infectious, neoplastic, or obstructive disease processes.
- See Differential Diagnosis below.

DIAGNOSIS

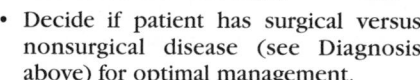

Acute abdomen is approached either surgically or medically, and this important decision depends fundamentally on an accurate diagnosis of the underlying cause.

DIFFERENTIAL DIAGNOSIS

The differential diagnosis can be divided into specific organ systems:

- Gastrointestinal (GI): infectious (parvovirus [dogs], panleukopenia [cats], or parasites), hemorrhagic, obstructive (neoplasia, foreign material, intussusception, or incarceration), gastric dilation with or without volvulus, ulceration, or perforation
- Liver: infectious (leptospirosis, ascending portal infection, other), toxic, neoplasia hemangiosarcoma, carcinoma, others, abscess, cholangiohepatitis, obstruction/rupture of the biliary system
- Pancreas: pancreatitis, neoplasia, or abscess
- Spleen: torsion, neoplasia (hemangiosarcoma, hemangioma, others), and trauma-induced injury
- Urogenital: trauma (urinary bladder rupture, ureteral avulsion), urolithiasis (ureteral, cystic, urethral), pyelonephritis, ureteral or urethral obstruction, neoplasia (renal carcinoma, hemangiosarcoma, other; transitional cell carcinoma), prostatic infection, abscessation, or neoplasia, pyometra, metritis, or uterine or testicular torsion
- Adrenal: carcinoma, pheochromocytoma (± caval thromboembolism)
- Generalized peritoneal disease: chemical peritonitis (bile or urine), infectious peritonitis (ruptured viscus or penetrating trauma), neoplasia (carcinomatosis, mesothelioma)
- Systemic disorders that may manifest with an acute abdomen include hemorrhage (peritoneal, retroperitoneal), thromboembolism (GI tract, liver, kidney), congestive heart failure (uncommon; generally chronic), hypoalbuminemia, and vasculitis

INITIAL DATABASE

- Complete blood count: evidence of sepsis or blood loss.
- Serum chemistry panel (including lipase): azotemia ± hyperkalemia with uroabdomen; elevated liver values with hepatobiliary disease; electrolyte changes secondary to vomiting or diarrhea of any cause.
- Urinalysis:
  - Avoid cystocentesis when pyometra is suspected.
- Abdominal radiographs: evaluate for foreign bodies, obstructive patterns, organ enlargement or displacements ("double bubble" sign with GDV), loss of detail seen with effusive disease (pancreatitis, peritonitis of any cause), or with free gas (ruptured viscus, penetrating trauma).
  - A minimum of two views should be taken, and horizontal-beam views may also be helpful when looking for pneumoperitoneum.
- Abdominal ultrasound should be considered to evaluate for effusions, obstructions, masses, or abscesses in abdominal organs; foreign material; evaluation of the biliary tree, pancreas, and urogenital system.
- Abdominocentesis is warranted to evaluate cytologic characteristics of abdominal effusions.

ADVANCED OR CONFIRMATORY TESTING

- Fine-needle aspirates or biopsies using ultrasound guidance can be obtained of the liver, spleen, pancreas, lymph nodes, prostate, and some abdominal masses depending on vascularity
- Additionally, measurement of abdominal effusion glucose concentration is useful to detect intra-abdominal sepsis
- Abdominal effusion lipase levels are increased with pancreatitis
- Increased effusion blood urea nitrogen, creatinine, and potassium are found in uroabdomen
- Blood coagulation panel to evaluate for coagulopathies

TREATMENT

THERAPEUTIC GOAL(S)

- Decide if patient has surgical versus nonsurgical disease (see Diagnosis above) for optimal management.
- Specific treatment is based on the underlying cause.
- The main goals of supportive care are to optimize cardiac output and tissue perfusion, and to ameliorate any signs of shock as early as possible.

ACUTE GENERAL TREATMENT

- Cardiovascular support is accomplished through the use of crystalloids, colloids, blood products, and pressors or inotropes to maintain blood pressure and vital organ perfusion (see Hypotension, Systemic, p 572; Transfusion Therapy and Collection Techniques for Blood Banking, p 1312).
- Pain management is warranted (relief of discomfort and to decrease sympathetic stimulation on heart rate from uncontrolled pain).
- Intravenous fluids:
  - Type and rate tailored based on heart rate, pulse quality, maintaining normal blood pressure, urinary output, mucous membrane color, and capillary refill time
- Abdominal exploration:
  - Removal of obstruction
  - Resection/removal of nonviable tissue
  - Correction of GDV
  - Resection/removal of masses
  - Repair or removal of source of hemorrhage if focal
  - Resection of abscesses, abdominal lavage

DRUG INTERACTIONS

Aminoglycosides should be withheld in cases of renal dysfunction or dehydration.

POSSIBLE COMPLICATIONS

- Severe complications can ensue if a surgical disease is not detected before intestinal perforation.
- Death can result from inadequate treatment or progression of underlying disease.
- Dehiscence of surgical sites, especially with low plasma albumin.
- Overwhelming infection from septic processes.
- Multiple organ dysfunction and failure.
- Disseminated intravascular coagulation from activation of coagulation cascade.

RECOMMENDED MONITORING

Heart rate, respiratory rate, temperature, urine output, PCV/TS, blood pressure, lactate, and electrolyte levels

PROGNOSIS AND OUTCOME

Prognosis depends highly on the underlying cause. If shock is present, earlier resolution is associated with a better outcome.

PEARLS & CONSIDERATIONS

COMMENTS

- It is essential to rapidly and accurately determine if a surgical condition is present. This is best accomplished with a complete history and physical exam and using the minimum database and advanced testing.
- Occasionally, dogs with back pain will appear to have abdominal pain.

SUGGESTED READING

Heeren V, et al: Acute abdomen: diagnosis. *Compend Contin Educ Pract Vet* 26(5): 350–363, 2004.

Heeren V, et al: Acute abdomen: treatment. *Compend Contin Educ Pract Vet* 26(5): 366–373, 2004.

AUTHOR: **SAMUEL DURKAN**

EDITOR: **ELIZABETH ROZANSKI**

Acute Moist Dermatitis

Client Education Sheet on Website

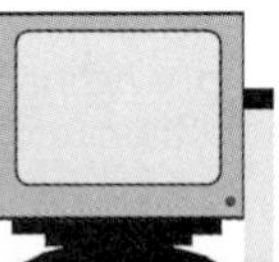

BASIC INFORMATION

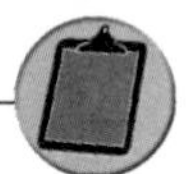

DEFINITION

An acute and rapidly progressive surface bacterial skin infection secondary to trauma that is self-inflicted in an attempt to relieve pain or pruritus

SYNONYM(S)

"Hot spot"
Moist eczema
Pyotraumatic dermatitis

EPIDEMIOLOGY

SPECIES, AGE, SEX: Acute moist dermatitis is most common in dogs less than 4 years old.

GENETICS AND BREED PREDISPOSITION: It can develop in any breed, but golden retrievers, rottweilers, Saint Bernards, and German shepherds appear over-represented.

RISK FACTORS: The prevalence is greater in hot, humid weather and more likely to occur in dense-coated, long-haired breeds. Other factors associated with acute moist dermatitis include allergy (flea, atopy, adverse food reaction, contact), ectoparasites (flea, scabies, ticks, cheyletiellosis), otitis externa, anal sac disease, excess moisture (e.g., swimming), unkempt coat, and painful musculoskeletal disease.

CLINICAL PRESENTATION

HISTORY, CHIEF COMPLAINT

- Acute onset of well-demarcated alopecic area that exudes serum and becomes matted with hair at the periphery
- Lesion(s) is(are) pruritic and often very painful

PHYSICAL EXAM FINDINGS

- Variably sized erosive to ulcerative lesion exuding serum (Fig. I-8)
- Erythematous margins sharply demarcate lesion from surrounding normal skin
- Erythematous papules at periphery of lesion suggest deep pyoderma
- Lesions most frequently found on face, neck, and dorsal lumbosacral area of lateral thigh
- Single lesion in one body region is more common than multiple lesions

ETIOLOGY AND PATHOPHYSIOLOGY

- Unknown
- Any factor that initiates an "itch-scratch" cycle may predispose to acute moist dermatitis

DIAGNOSIS

DIFFERENTIAL DIAGNOSIS

- Demodicosis
- Dermatophytosis
- Staphylococcal pyoderma
- Calcinosis cutis

INITIAL DATABASE

- Skin scrapes: negative for mites
- Impression cytologic evaluation: suppurative inflammation

ADVANCED OR CONFIRMATORY TESTING

Skin biopsy: only indicated in resistant cases. On histologic examination, an acute exudative reaction affecting only the epidermis is noted.

TREATMENT

THERAPEUTIC GOAL(S)

- Control inflammation and pruritus
- Identify and control or resolve underlying cause(s)
- Clip and cleanse lesion(s)

ACUTE GENERAL TREATMENT

- Sedation or general anesthesia warranted in some cases due to intense pain.
- Clip hair from lesion(s) to allow cleaning and easier topical treatment.
- Flush area with 2% or 4% chlorhexidine solution (diluted at least 20:1 [tap water: chlorhexidine]) to remove crusts and exudation.
  - Affected area is exquisitely sensitive to temperature (of greatest concern if no sedation/anesthesia). Ensure that diluted chlorhexidine, surface of clipper blades, and anything else coming in contact with the lesion is approximately at body temperature.
- Topical therapy: often sole therapy warranted with small lesions; apply astringent (aluminum acetate) topically q 8–12 h for 3 to 7 days; more extensive or painful lesions benefit from topical glucocorticoid cream or combination steroid/antibiotic topical cream applied q 12h for 3 to 7 days.
- Systemic glucocorticoids: recommended for extensive or very painful lesion; prednisone 0.5–1.0 mg/kg PO q 24h; length of treatment depends on severity of lesion but typically is 5 to 10 days.
- Nonsteroidal anti-inflammatory (e.g., meloxicam 0.1 mg/kg PO q 24h for 3 to 5 days): for pain management; do not administer in conjunction with systemic glucocorticoids.
- Systemic antibiotics: not indicated unless erythematous papules noted at periphery of lesion. Cephalexin at 30 mg/kg q 12h for 30 days would be a good choice for antibiotic therapy.

RECOMMENDED MONITORING

Reevaluation in 5 to 7 days recommended for extensive lesion or if lesion is not responding to appropriate therapy

PROGNOSIS AND OUTCOME

- Most lesions respond rapidly and completely to topical and/or systemic therapy.

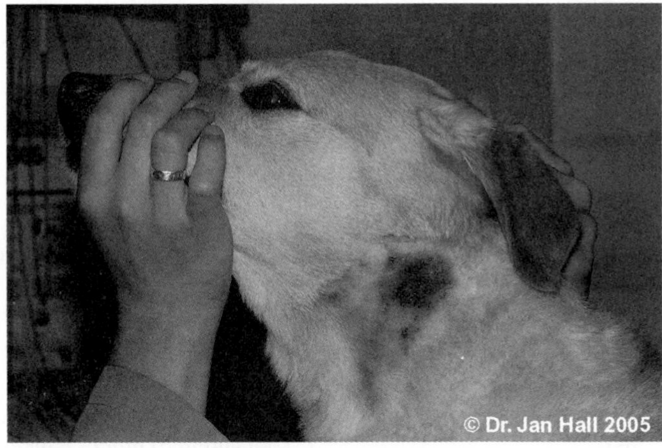

FIGURE I-8 Hot spot (area of acute moist dermatitis) on the neck of a 5-year-old mixed-breed dog associated with a minor bite wound. Courtesy of Dr. Jan A. Hall.

- Acute moist dermatitis will recur when predisposing causes have not been eliminated or controlled.

PEARLS & CONSIDERATIONS

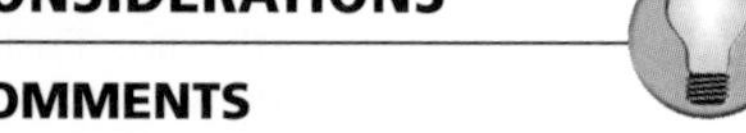

COMMENTS

- Whenever an acute moist dermatitis lesion responds poorly to appropriate therapy or relapses quickly, an alternative diagnosis should be considered. Routine dermatologic diagnostics including skin biopsy may be indicated.
- Papules and pustules surrounding an acute moist dermatitis lesion (satellite lesions) may indicate a primary follicular condition (bacterial folliculitis, superficial pyoderma), with the acute dermatitis as a secondary, self-traumatic complication.
- Systemic antibiotics for a minimum of 30 days are recommended in the treatment of all acute moist dermatitis lesions.

CLIENT EDUCATION

Owners often underestimate the extent of the lesion and may be shocked when the lesion is exposed after hair clipping. For this reason, barring the pet's extreme discomfort, initial clipping of the hair of a suspected acute moist dermatitis lesion should often be done in front of the owner to avoid the perception that part of the wound was inflicted iatrogenically.

SUGGESTED READING

Holm BR, et al: A prospective study of clinical findings, treatment and histopathology of 44 cases of pyotraumatic dermatitis. *Vet Dermatol* 15(6):369, 2004.

Scott DW, Miller WH JR, Griffin CE (eds): *Mueller & Kirk's Small Animal Dermatology.* Philadelphia, WB Saunders, 2001, pp 1163-1167.

AUTHOR: **JOCELYN WELLINGTON**

EDITOR: **JAN A. HALL**

Acute Renal Failure

BASIC INFORMATION

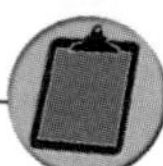

DEFINITION

- Abrupt decline of glomerular filtration rate resulting in an accumulation of nitrogenous waste products and inability to maintain normal fluid balance
- Azotemia: biochemical abnormality (elevation in blood urea nitrogen, creatinine)
- Uremia: overt clinical signs caused by renal failure
- Oliguria: urine production <0.25 ml/kg/hr
- Normal urine production: 1-2 ml/kg/hr
- Polyuria: urine production >2 ml/kg/hr

SYNONYM(S)

Acute kidney failure
Anuric/oliguric renal failure
ARF

EPIDEMIOLOGY

SPECIES, AGE, SEX: Both dogs and cats susceptible. Often, animals with acute renal failure are younger than those with chronic renal failure.

GENETICS AND BREED PREDISPOSITION: Dogs: large-breed, free-roaming. Cats: free-roaming.

RISK FACTORS: Dogs and cats:

- Nephrotoxins:
  - Ethylene glycol
  - Plants (e.g., Easter lily, raisins, grapes)
  - Phosphate enemas
  - Heavy metals
  - Hypervitaminosis D (e.g., cholecalciferol-containing rodenticides, pharmaceuticals)
  - Drugs (e.g., aminoglycosides, amphotericin B, cisplatin, sulfonamides, tetracyclines, nonsteroidal anti-inflammatory drugs, radiocontrast agents)
- Ischemia: hypotension, trauma, shock, hypoadrenocorticism, congestive heart failure, temperature extremes, prolonged anesthesia, anaphylaxis
- Infection:
  - Dogs: leptospirosis, pyelonephritis, Rocky mountain spotted fever, borreliosis
  - Cats: pyelonephritis, feline infectious peritonitis
- Other: thromboembolic disease, hypercalcemia, transfusion reaction, myoglobin/hemoglobinuria, vasculitis, envenomation, trauma, urinary tract obstruction, renal lymphoma (cats > dogs)

CONTAGION AND ZOONOSIS: Dogs: leptospirosis.

CLINICAL PRESENTATION

DISEASE FORMS/SUBTYPES

- Oliguric/anuric ARF
- Polyuric ARF

HISTORY, CHIEF COMPLAINT (SOME OR ALL MAY BE PRESENT)

- Lethargy, depression
- Vomiting, anorexia
- Collapse
- Abdominal/general discomfort
- Renomegaly
- Recent onset polydipsia, polyuria
- No urination (no urine production and no attempts to urinate)

PHYSICAL EXAM FINDINGS

- Dehydration
- Small bladder
- Abdominal/renal pain
- Normal size/enlarged kidneys
- Oral (uremic) mucosal ulcerations
- Oral cavity debris/secretions (vomitus, saliva)
- Halitosis
- Tachycardia, tachypnea

ETIOLOGY AND PATHOPHYSIOLOGY

- Renal injury initiated by various causes (e.g., ischemia, toxicant, infection)
- Renal response causes extension of insult through four mechanisms:
  - Impaired glomerular filtration via reduced ultrafiltration coefficient
  - Tubular obstruction (cellular casts, protein, hemoglobin, crystals)
  - Tubular back leak of ultrafiltrate
  - Intrarenal vasoconstriction
- Injury leads to failure of renal excretory, regulatory, and endocrine functions with resultant uremia

DIAGNOSIS

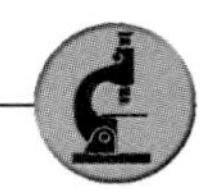

DIFFERENTIAL DIAGNOSIS

Specific causes: see Etiology and Pathophysiology above

- Azotemia differential diagnosis:
  - Prerenal azotemia* (dehydration, gastrointestinal bleeding)
  - Renal failure (acute or chronic)
  - Postrenal azotemia (urinary tract obstruction, rupture)

*Note: conditions that impair urine concentration but result in profound dehydration and prerenal azotemia difficult to differentiate from ARF (e.g., hypoadrenocorticism)

INITIAL DATABASE

- Complete blood count: Anemia (which often characterizes chronic renal failure) typically is absent.

- Serum biochemical profile: azotemia (elevated blood urea nitrogen, creatinine, phosphorus), hyperkalemia, hypocalcemia or hypercalcemia, metabolic acidosis.
- Urinalysis: isosthenuria, tubular casts, calcium oxalate monohydrate crystalluria (ethylene glycol toxicity), pyuria (pyelonephritis), hematuria, bacteriuria.
- Abdominal radiographs: renomegaly (unlike most cases of chronic renal failure).
- Abdominal ultrasound: renomegaly; renal pelvic dilation; alterations in renal parynchemal echogenicity; loss of corticomedullary distinction; hyperechoic cortices (ethylene glycol toxicity, but also common in normal, healthy cats).
- Electrocardiogram (ECG): altered by pronounced hyperkalemia (bradycardia [more common in dogs than cats], absent P waves, wide QRS complexes).
- Measurement of urine output:Assess following complete rehydration. Although polyuric ARF can be seen, the classic presentation is oliguria (urine production <0.25 ml/kg/hr) or anuria (absent urine production). By way of contrast, chronic renal failure is associated with normal or excessive (>2 ml/kg/hr) volumes of urine.

ADVANCED OR CONFIRMATORY TESTING

- Ethylene glycol testing (positive within 24 hours of toxin ingestion in dogs, false positive after propylene glycol administration) (see Ethylene Glycol Intoxication, p 367)
- Comparison of measured to calculated osmolality (osmole gap; measured osmolality >10 mOsm/L above calculated osmolality suggests ethylene glycol toxicity)
- Serology or polymerase chain reaction: leptospirosis (acute and convalescent titers), Lyme borreliosis, others
- Adrenocorticotropic hormone stimulation test: hypoadrenocorticism
- Renal biopsy: etiologic as well as prognostic information
- Glomerular filtration rate: seldom required

TREATMENT

THERAPEUTIC GOAL(S)

- Resolve life-threatening electrolyte/acid-base disorders
- Restore urine production
- Resolve azotemia
- Address specific causation

ACUTE GENERAL TREATMENT

- Isotonic crystalloid fluid therapy:
  - Resolve dehydration within the first 6 to 12 hours.
    - Percent dehydration (expressed as a decimal [i.e., 10% = 0.1]) × body weight (kg) = deficit (liters).
  - Compensate for estimated ongoing losses (e.g., vomiting, panting).
  - Provide maintenance fluids (60 ml/kg/day).
    - Promote diuresis by increasing fluid rate above maintenance. Practically, two to three times maintenance rates are appropriate assuming adequate urine production.
    - In oliguric/anuric animals, maintenance fluid rates may be excessive, so monitor (see later).
  - Avoid overhydration.
    - Body weight q 6-12h.
      - Weight loss represents fluid loss or muscle wasting.
      - Weight gain in hydrated animal implies fluid retention (i.e., overhydration).
    - Central venous pressure (CVP) q 2-12h. (See Central Venous Pressure Monitoring, p 1206.)
      - CVP 6-8 cm H_2O represents maximum safe intravascular volume.
      - CVP >10 cm H_2O associated with risk of pulmonary edema.
    - Closed-system indwelling urinary catheter facilitates early recognition of polyuria (>2 ml/kg/hr), oliguria (<0.25 ml/kg/hr), or anuria in the hydrated animal.
      - If oliguria/anuria documented, discontinue maintenance fluid therapy and institute "ins and outs" fluid therapy to maintain appropriate hydration.
        - Even if anuric, provide 20 ml/kg/day crystalloid fluid (i.e., insensible losses).
        - Measure and record urine volume q 1-4h. Add that volume of intravenous crystalloid to insensible loss for the next 1 to 4 hours.
        - Continue until oliguria/anuria resolves.
  - Promote urine production with drugs if urine production <0.25 ml/kg/hr.
    - Furosemide 2-6 mg/kg IV bolus. If oliguria persists, repeat bolus. If urine production >1 ml/kg/hr after bolus therapy, institute constant rate infusion (0.25-1.0 mg/kg/hr).
    - Mannitol 250-500 mg/kg IV once.
      - Caution: increased vascular volume may result in pulmonary edema if overhydrated.
    - Dopamine: not recommended.
  - If oliguria or anuria persist despite therapy, institute hemodialysis or peritoneal dialysis, or euthanize.
- Address acid-base and electrolyte disorders:
  - If potassium >7 mEq/L, consider one or more of the following:
    - Regular insulin (1/4 unit/kg IV bolus) with intravenous dextrose (2 g/unit insulin over 6 hours). 2 g dextrose/unit insulin is 4 ml 50% dextrose (needs to be diluted at least 1:5 with sterile water)/unit insulin.
    - Sodium bicarbonate 1 mEq/kg IV bolus.
    - Calcium gluconate 1 ml/kg *slow* IV bolus (cardioprotective) with ECG monitoring and discontinuation of the infusion if heart rate slows, or sudden QT interval shortening or ST segment elevation or depression occurs.
  - If pH <7.1, institute sodium bicarbonate therapy.
    - Calculate bicarbonate deficit ([0.3] × [BW kg] × [Base deficit]).
    - Administer 1/2 of the deficit in intravenous fluids over 6 hours.
- Monitor blood pressure.
  - Maintain mean arterial pressure >60 mmHg, systolic >80 mmHg.
  - Systemic hypertension (systolic pressure >170 mmHg) can accompany ARF. Persistent hypertension should be addressed medically (amlodipine 0.025 mg/kg q 24h). (See Systemic Hypertension, p 1058.)
- Medical therapy to decrease gastric acidity.
  - Famotidine 0.5-1.0 mg/kg PO, IM, IV q 12-24h.
  - Omeprazole 0.5-1.0 mg/kg PO q 24h.
- Antiemetic therapy as necessary.
  - Metoclopramide 0.1-0.5 mg/kg PO, IM, SQ q 6-8h, or 0.01-0.02 mg/kg/hr constant rate infusion.
  - Dolasetron 0.5 mg/kg PO, IV, SQ q 24h.
- Specific therapy for underlying disorders.
  - Leptospirosis: Ampicillin 22 mg/kg IV q 6h for 2 weeks followed by a 2-week course of doxycycline 2.5-5 mg/kg PO q 24h to address urinary shedding.
  - Ethylene glycol: see also Ethylene Glycol Intoxication, p 367.
    - Ethanol (20%) 5.5 ml/kg IV q 4h × 5 treatments, then 5.5 ml/kg IV q 6h for 4 treatments (dogs and cats).
    - 4-methylpyrrazole 20 mg/kg IV first treatment, then 15 mg/kg @ 12 and 24 hours, then 5 mg/kg @ 36 hours (dogs only).
- Discontinue nephrotoxic drugs.

CHRONIC TREATMENT

- Manage underlying cause of renal failure
- Maintain fluid balance throughout recovery period (6 to 8 weeks):
  - Intravenous fluids continued until the animal is producing urine, drinking, maintaining hydration.
  - Wean intravenous fluids gradually (2 to 3 days).
  - Duration of hospitalization expected to take days to weeks.

- For owners considering peritoneal dialysis or hemodialysis (Hemodialysis, see p 1263) for persistently oliguric animals, facilitate early referral
- Provide nutritional support:
  - Protein and phosphorus restriction are ideal, but not at the expense of appetite/palatability.
  - Anorexia is common in ARF.
    - If vomiting is rare/absent and anorexia is chronic, consider enteral tube feeding.
    - If vomiting is intractable, consider total parenteral nutrition.
- Treat chronic renal failure if necessary (see Chronic Renal Failure, Occult ["Asymptomatic"], p 204; Chronic Renal Failure, Overt ["Symptomatic"], p 205)

POSSIBLE COMPLICATIONS

- Failure to produce urine
- Overhydration
- Hyperkalemia and cardiac dysrhythmia
- Severe metabolic acidosis
- Chronic renal failure
- Uremic pneumonitis/encephalitis

RECOMMENDED MONITORING

- Until azotemia is resolving, urine output is >1 mg/kg/hr, and animal is drinking voluntarily
  - Body weight q 6-12h
  - CVP q 2-12h
  - Serum blood urea nitrogen/creatinine q 24-48h
  - Electrolytes (Na^+, K^+, Cl^-) acid-base status and blood pressure q 6-24h
  - Packed cell volume and total protein q 24h
  - Measure urine output
    - Indwelling urinary catheters predispose to urinary infection and should not be left in place longer than necessary.
    - Maintain good aseptic technique with catheters.
    - Closed, sterile urine collection systems and catheters should be replaced daily.
    - Remove catheter once urine output has been appropriate for >24 hours.
- Convalescent serologic evaluation as appropriate (e.g., leptospirosis, *Rickettsia rickettsii*)
- As uremic signs abate, reduce monitoring frequency
- Body weight, serum chemistry, and packed cell volume monitored at least weekly until azotemia resolves or plateaus
- With residual azotemia, long-term monitoring should proceed as for chronic renal failure

PROGNOSIS AND OUTCOME

- Short term: poor (60% mortality rate all causes of ARF; >90% mortality for ethylene glycol intoxication).
- If animal survives short term (6 to 8 weeks), long-term prognosis can be good.
- Renal failure may become chronic or may resolve. Animals with resolved ARF may develop chronic renal failure later in life.

PEARLS & CONSIDERATIONS

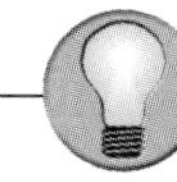

COMMENTS

- Differentiating acute from chronic renal failure is essential for treatment and prognostication.
- Because of the zoonotic importance of leptospirosis, handle urine carefully with all dogs in ARF unless a specific cause has been defined.
- Renal biopsy should be performed for all animals before dialysis. Histopathology can provide a more accurate prognosis before beginning a costly and complicated treatment.
- Hypoadrenocorticism and diabetes insipidus are possible explanations for the combination of azotemia and isosthenuria without renal failure.

PREVENTION

- If considering drugs with nephrotoxic potential, ensure hydration first and monitor renal function
- Educate owners regarding nephrotoxins
- Formulate vaccination programs considering regional prevalence of infectious causes of ARF

CLIENT EDUCATION

- Educate clients regarding nephrotoxins.
- Treatment of ARF may be costly, and recovery may require at least 6 to 8 weeks.
- Lifelong therapy of chronic renal failure may be required for surviving animals.

SUGGESTED READING

Stokes JE, Forrester SD: New and unusual causes of acute renal failure in dogs and cats. *Vet Clin North Am Small Anim Pract* 34:909, 2004.

Labato MA: Strategies for management of acute renal failure. *Vet Clin North Am Small Anim Pract* 31:1265, 2001.

Vaden SL, et al: A retrospective case-control of acute renal failure in 99 dogs. *J Vet Intern Med* 11:58, 1997.

AUTHOR: **MARIE E. KERL**
EDITOR: **LEAH A. COHN**

Acute Respiratory Distress Syndrome

BASIC INFORMATION

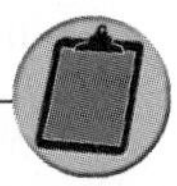

DEFINITION

Broadly, any pathologic condition that results in the development of respiratory difficulty. However, usually acute respiratory distress syndrome (ARDS) refers to the development of noncardiogenic pulmonary edema as an inflammatory response to any severe illness.

SYNONYM(S)

Adult respiratory distress syndrome
ARDS
Shock lung

EPIDEMIOLOGY

SPECIES, AGE, SEX: Any critically ill dog may be affected; it is unclear at this time if cats are affected with ARDS.

RISK FACTORS: Severe critical illness or injury.

ASSOCIATED CONDITIONS AND DISORDERS

- Sepsis and septic shock
- Polytrauma
- Neoplasia

CLINICAL PRESENTATION

DISEASE FORMS/SUBTYPES

- Acute lung injury (ALI) is a less severe form of pulmonary dysfunction. ALI may progress to ARDS or it may regress with supportive care.
- Pulmonary ARDS may develop as a result of a direct pulmonary insult such as pneumonia or pulmonary contusion.
- Extrapulmonary ARDS may develop in a critically ill or injured dog as part of the multiple organ dysfunction syndrome, when the initial insult was outside the lung (e.g., septic abdomen).

HISTORY, CHIEF COMPLAINT

- Reflects the initial presenting complaint
- ARDS is a hospitalized dog diagnosis

PHYSICAL EXAM FINDINGS

- Increased respiratory rate and effort

- Orthopnea
- Cyanosis in advanced cases

ETIOLOGY AND PATHOPHYSIOLOGY

- A pulmonary or extrapulmonary insult results in the formation of severe systemic inflammation.
- Cytokines and other proinflammatory products cause vasculitis and, when diffuse alveolar damage occurs, a protein-rich pulmonary edema is the result.
- Pulmonary edema results in ventilation-perfusion (V-Q) mismatch and severe hypoxemia.
- Three stages of ARDS have been described: exudative, proliferative, and fibrotic. Surviving patients will proceed through each stage. The actual time course for each stage in dogs is not known. However, the clinician should anticipate that recovery from ARDS requires weeks.
- ARDS in humans is considered a clinical diagnosis. The criteria for diagnosis include:
  - Underlying event (severe trauma/sepsis, etc.)
  - Diffuse bilateral pulmonary infiltrates on thoracic radiographs
  - Hypoxemia (PaO_2:F_iO_2 ratio of <200)
  - Decreased pulmonary compliance ("stiff lungs")
  - Absence of heart failure (normal pulmonary capillary wedge pressure)
- Equivalent criteria have not been validated for veterinary patients.

DIAGNOSIS

DIFFERENTIAL DIAGNOSIS

- Pneumonia
- Volume overload or congestive heart failure/cardiogenic pulmonary edema
- Pulmonary thromboembolism

INITIAL DATABASE

- Thoracic radiographs to exclude other causes of respiratory distress.
- Arterial blood gas analysis: In a severely dyspneic dog, the risks accompanying collection of an arterial blood sample may outweigh the benefits.
  - Calculation of the ratio of PaO_2:F_iO_2 can be used to distinguish ARDS and ALI. PaO_2 is measured on an arterial blood gas sample; F_iO_2 is the fraction of inspired oxygen (room air = 0.21; 40% oxygen = 0.4; 100% oxygen = 1).
    - Normal patient ratio >475.
    - Acute lung injury <300.
    - Acute respiratory distress <200.
- If available, the protein content of expectorated pulmonary edema fluid/foam may be evaluated on a refractometer.
  - Pulmonary edema from noncardiac sources like ARDS has a protein content at least 75% that of the serum, whereas cardiogenic pulmonary edema has a protein content 30% that of the serum.
- Other tests as indicated by primary disease process.

ADVANCED OR CONFIRMATORY TESTING

- Computed tomography of lungs; advantage of superior resolution, drawbacks of general anesthesia and lesser availability
- Echocardiography to exclude cardiac dysfunction or pulmonary thromboembolism
- Transtracheal wash or bronchoalveolar lavage with cytologic evaluation and culture to exclude infection or neoplasia

TREATMENT

Intubation and ventilation should be aggressively pursued if respiratory effort is elevated for longer than 1 hour or is increasing, or if SPO_2 <89% despite supplemental oxygen

THERAPEUTIC GOAL(S)

- Treatment of the underlying systemic disease and, if necessary, positive-pressure ventilation are the cornerstones of management of ARDS.
- No specific therapy for ARDS.
- Provide support for the damaged lung parenchyma to permit healing.

ACUTE GENERAL TREATMENT

- Oxygenation with mechanical ventilation with positive end-expiratory pressure:
  - Low tidal volumes with an attempt to limit barotrauma are recommended
  - May result in increased P_aCO_2 ("permissive hypercarbia")
  - See Ventilation, Positive Pressure, p 1325
- Other supportive measures:
  - Antibiotics (e.g., ampicillin 22 mg/kg IV q 8h, with or without enrofloxacin 5 mg/kg IV diluted in sterile saline and given slowly IV q 12h [q 24h in cats])
  - Heparin 75 IU/kg SQ q 8h if disseminated intravascular coagulation is suspected
  - Surgery if indicated for primary disease
- Diuretics are not directly indicated, although every effort should be made to prevent volume overload. If clinically it is unclear if volume overload may be present, 1 to 2 mg/kg furosemide IV may be administered q 6h.
- Colloids are not indicated for acute lung injury or ARDS. Due to the altered permeability of the capillary-alveolar membrane, synthetic colloids may cross into the pulmonary parenchyma and worsen gas exchange.

CHRONIC TREATMENT

Prednisone 0.5-1 mg/kg PO q 24h during recovery phase to delay/prevent pulmonary fibrosis; empiric and unsupported by objective evidence to date

POSSIBLE COMPLICATIONS

- Failure of other organ systems
- Chronic pulmonary insufficiency

RECOMMENDED MONITORING

Affected patients need *intense* nursing care.

- Ventilation parameters
- Oxygen saturation and arterial blood gas analysis
- Direct blood pressure
- Continuous electrocardiographic monitoring
- Urine output

PROGNOSIS AND OUTCOME

Guarded to grave. Survival after ARDS is possible but rare. Multiple organ failure, progressive hypoxemia, circulatory collapse, and ongoing costs associated with intensive care have limited survival in affected dogs.

PEARLS & CONSIDERATIONS

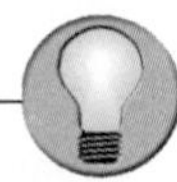

COMMENTS

Accuracy in diagnosis: identify and treat causes of hospital-acquired respiratory distress that are more commonly responsive (better prognosis):

- Pneumonia
- Pulmonary thromboembolism
- Volume overload/congestive heart failure

PREVENTION

Early identification of patients at risk, and implementation of intensive supportive care:

- Prevent sepsis from progressing to septic shock
- Adequately treat severely injured patients

CLIENT EDUCATION

ARDS is a severe disease associated with critical illness. Committed clients with adequate emotional and financial resources or pet insurance are necessary for successful treatment.

SUGGESTED READING

Parent C, et al: Clinical and clinicopathologic findings in dogs with acute respiratory distress syndrome: 19 cases (1985-1993). *J Am Vet Med Assoc* 208:1419-1427, 1996.

Parent C, et al: Respiratory function and treatment in dogs with acute respiratory distress syndrome: 19 cases (1985-1993). *J Am Vet Med Assoc* 208:1428-1433, 1996.

AUTHOR & EDITOR: **ELIZABETH ROZANSKI**

Acute Tumor Lysis Syndrome

BASIC INFORMATION

DEFINITION

Acute tumor lysis syndrome (ATLS) is a rare disorder consisting of a group of metabolic disturbances caused by massive death of neoplastic cells and subsequent release of intracellular contents. Veterinary ATLS is characterized by hyperphosphatemia, hyperkalemia, hypocalcemia, with or without azotemia. ATLS rarely occurs spontaneously; it occurs in patients after antineoplastic therapy.

SYNONYM(S)

Tumor lysis syndrome

EPIDEMIOLOGY

SPECIES, AGE, SEX: ATLS can occur in any dog or cat with a large tumor burden following rapid cytoreduction (neoplastic cell death) after treatment.

RISK FACTORS

- Patients at highest risk are dogs and cats with large tumor burdens and with some degree of volume contraction that rapidly responds to cytolytic therapy.
- Clinically, it is most common in patients with advanced-stage lymphoma or leukemia, as these are highly chemosensitive tumors.
- Associated risk factors include:
  - Large tumor burden
  - Preexisting renal disease
  - Hypercalcemia
  - High tumor growth fraction
  - High serum lactate dehydrogenase activity
- It is rare in patients with solid tumors.

CLINICAL PRESENTATION

HISTORY, CHIEF COMPLAINT: Clinical signs include anorexia, vomiting, diarrhea, lethargy, and collapse. Typically, signs occur within 48 hours after chemotherapy or radiation therapy; rarely, ATLS has been reported to occur up to 8 days after treatment.

PHYSICAL EXAM FINDINGS: Patients can present in shock with signs such as mental depression, dehydration, tachypnea, pale mucous membranes, decreased capillary refill time, and cardiac arrhythmias.

ETIOLOGY AND PATHOPHYSIOLOGY

- With treatment of very sensitive tumors, rapid tumor lysis liberates large quantities of intracellular contents into the circulation.
- Acute release of intracellular phosphates (adenosine triphosphate, nucleic acids) causes hyperphosphatemia, usually within 48 to 96 hours.
- Elevated serum phosphate precipitates with serum calcium, forming $CaPO_4$ salts and causing secondary hypocalcemia.
- Acute release of intracellular potassium leads to hyperkalemia within 12 hours, which can cause bradycardia and arrhythmias. Hyperkalmia may be accentuated by renal impairment.
- Hyperuricemia is seen in humans with ATLS due to release of intracellular urate from nucleic acids. Hyperuricemia and resulting obstructive nephropathy seem to occur less clinically in animals. Dogs at increased risk include dogs that are azotemic, have a large tumor burden, dalmatians, or dogs with severe liver disease.
- Renal failure is related to precipitation of $CaPO_4$ in renal tubules and to cardiovascular collapse. In humans, serum urate precipitation contributes to acute renal failure.
- Metabolic acidosis is typically a high anion gap lactic acidosis.

DIAGNOSIS

DIFFERENTIAL DIAGNOSIS

- Disorders associated with chemotoxicity, such as severe gastrointestinal toxicity and dehydration, neutropenia and/or sepsis after chemotherapy
- Disorders secondary to primary neoplasia, such as coagulopathies and organ failure

INITIAL DATABASE

- Minimum database (complete blood count, biochemical profile, urinalysis).
- Blood gas analysis.
- In dogs, the most consistent abnormality is hyperphosphatemia, with or without azotemia and metabolic acidosis. Hypocalcemia and hyperkalemia are not prominent in ATLS, and patients are not typically clinical for these metabolic abnormalities.

TREATMENT

THERAPEUTIC GOAL(S)

- Treat shock, correct dehydration and fluid deficits, and correct electrolyte abnormalities
- Increase elimination of excess electrolytes with fluid diuresis

ACUTE GENERAL TREATMENT

- Aggressive crystalloid fluid therapy; consider non-lactate-, non-potassium-containing fluids, such as 0.9% NaCl, to address hyperphosphatemia or hyperkalemia. Administer fluids at rates appropriate for patients in shock.
- Monitor the patient closely. Rate of fluid administration should be adjusted based on patient's hydration, cardiovascular, renal, and electrolyte status.
- Delay further treatment for neoplasia until patient has been stabilized.
- Urine alkalinization is used in humans to increase the solubility of uric acid. It is not recommended in veterinary patients, because urate nephropathy is less significant, and alkalinization increases urine phosphate deposition.
- Allopurinol, which inhibits xanthine oxidase, is used in humans to prevent uric acid formation. In dogs, it is only recommended in those with urate metabolism problems (i.e., dalmatians) at a dose of 10 mg/kg PO q 8-24h.
- Monitor for acute renal failure and treat appropriately. Hemodialysis, if available, can be performed until renal function resumes.

PROGNOSIS AND OUTCOME

Prompt diagnosis and aggressive treatment to correct fluid deficits and electrolytes and acid-bases disturbances are essential to prevent renal damage and further decompensation.

PEARLS & CONSIDERATIONS

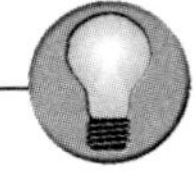

PREVENTION

Prevention is key to avoid ATLS in patients undergoing therapy:

- Recognition of risk factors is essential (see Risk Factors above).
- In patients at risk, initiate fluid therapy 24 to 48 hours before treatment, and continue for 24 to 96 hours after chemotherapy.
- Monitor these patients for early biochemical abnormalities and adjust treatment accordingly.

SUGGESTED READING

Brooks DG: Acute tumor lysis syndrome in dogs. *Compend Contin Educ Pract Vet* 17:1103-1106, 1995.

Ogilvie GK, Moore AS: Acute tumor lysis syndrome. In Ogilvie GK, Moore AS (eds): *Feline Oncology: A Comprehensive to Compassionate Care.* Trenton, NJ, Veterinary Learning Systems, 2001, pp 144-145.

AUTHOR: **SUSAN N. ETTINGER**
EDITOR: **KENNETH M. RASSNICK**

Adenocarcinoma, Anal Sac

BASIC INFORMATION

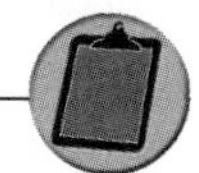

DEFINITION

Malignant neoplasm that develops from the apocrine glands of the anal sac

SYNONYM(S)

Apocrine adenocarcinoma

EPIDEMIOLOGY

SPECIES, AGE, SEX

- Male and female dogs appear to be equally affected, in contrast to initial reports suggesting a female predominance.
- Older age, with a median of 10 years.
- Cats are rarely affected.

GENETICS AND BREED PREDISPOSITION: Certain breeds appear to be at risk, suggesting a possible genetic predisposition:

- Cocker spaniel
- English springer spaniel
- German shepherd

ASSOCIATED CONDITIONS AND DISORDERS: Hypercalcemia occurs in 25-50% of dogs with anal sac adenocarcinoma.

CLINICAL PRESENTATION

HISTORY, CHIEF COMPLAINT

- Signs associated with mass effect:
  - Perineal swelling
  - Tenesmus
  - Biting/licking perineum
  - Scooting
- Signs associated with hypercalcemia:
  - Polyuria/polydipsia
  - Depression
  - Weakness
  - Vomiting
- As many as 30% of anal sac adenocarcinomas are detected incidentally on a routine physical examination. This underscores the importance of complete rectal examination on routine exams.

PHYSICAL EXAM FINDINGS: Evidence of an anal sac mass and/or evidence of sublumbar lymphadenopathy; the latter may be detectable by either abdominal or rectal palpation.

ETIOLOGY AND PATHOPHYSIOLOGY

- Anal sacs are paired scent glands in carnivores that are located between the internal and external anal sphincter. The sacs empty through a single duct that opens at the lateral margins of the anus.
- Malignant tumors may develop from the apocrine glands that line the sacs or, rarely, from the sac epithelium (squamous cell carcinoma).
- Anal sac adenocarcinomas tend to metastasize early in the course of the disease, and more than 50% of dogs have metastasis at the time of initial diagnosis.
  - Metastasis to regional (iliac) lymph nodes is common.
  - Other sites of metastasis include lung, liver, and spleen.
- Hypercalcemia occurs in 25-50% of dogs with anal sac adenocarcinoma and is secondary to the production of parathormone-related peptide (PTHrp) by tumor cells.
  - PTHrp binds to parathormone (PTH) receptors, but, unlike PTH, its production is not inhibited by elevated serum calcium.
  - PTHrp increases calcium mobilization from bone and absorption from the intestine while decreasing renal excretion of calcium.

DIAGNOSIS

An initial suspicion is based on physical exam (visualization or palpation). Cytologic evaluation may be sufficiently suggestive of the diagnosis to prompt an appropriately wide surgical excision. Confirmation of the diagnosis requires histopathologic assessment of tissue.

DIFFERENTIAL DIAGNOSIS

- Perianal adenoma or adenocarcinoma
- Perineal hernia
- Anal sac abscess
- Other cutaneous neoplasia

INITIAL DATABASE

- Complete blood count, serum chemistry profile, urinalysis, ± ionized calcium
- Clinical staging for anal sac tumors involves:
  - Measurement of primary tumor diameter
  - Evaluation of regional (iliac) lymph nodes
  - Evaluation for distant metastases to lungs, liver, or spleen
- Thoracic and abdominal radiographs and abdominal ultrasonography are indicated for clinical staging

ADVANCED OR CONFIRMATORY TESTING

- Although definitive diagnosis is based on histopathologic evaluation, cytologic evaluation may be helpful in determining the optimum biopsy approach.
- In some cases, the clinical and cytologic data may be sufficient to plan a wide surgical excision without a prior surgical biopsy.
- It is particularly important, however, that a definitive plan be formulated before excision.
- Given the perianal location, there are restrictions on the margin of excision.
  - Roughly half of the anal sphincter can be removed without the development of fecal incontinence.
  - Poorly planned excisions and biopsies could disseminate tumor cells locally and severely compromise the success of treatment.
- Computed tomography or magnetic resonance imaging of the perineal region (local extent of disease) and caudal abdomen can be useful in the clinical staging of anal sac adenocarcinoma, as well as in planning surgical approach or radiation therapy.

TREATMENT

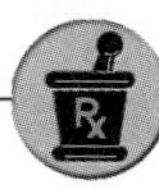

THERAPEUTIC GOAL(S)

Control the tumor both locally and systemically to palliate signs of disease

ACUTE GENERAL TREATMENT

- Surgery is the most effective treatment modality for anal sac adenocarcinomas that can be excised with clean histologic margins and have not metastasized.
- Radiation therapy may be useful in cases where surgery alone is unlikely to achieve tumor control.
- In cases where there is evidence of regional lymph node involvement, surgery and/or radiation therapy should still be considered.
- Chemotherapy with cisplatin (50-70 mg/m^2 IV plus saline diuresis), carboplatin (250-350 mg/m^2 IV), doxorubicin (30 mg/m^2 IV), or a combination of these agents might be effective in reducing or delaying systemic metastasis. Special handling requirements and potentially severe or life-threatening adverse effects exist with these chemotherapeutic drugs; these concerns, and rapid evolution of protocols, warrant consultation with/referral to an oncologist.
- Hypercalcemia should resolve upon treating the primary tumor. Additional therapy for hypercalcemia may be indicated in the interval between diagnosis and treatment or in cases in which

tumor control cannot be achieved (see Hypercalcemia, p 543).
- In dogs with advanced disease, palliative use of chemotherapy or radiation therapy may be indicated.

POSSIBLE COMPLICATIONS

- Surgical complications include wound infection, fecal incontinence, and anal stricture.
- Acute, self-limiting reactions in the perineal skin and the mucosa of the rectum and colon are expected side effects of radiation.
- Late radiation effects, which could include chronic diarrhea and even rupture of the bowel, may rarely occur.

PROGNOSIS AND OUTCOME

- Overall median survival is 18 months.
- The presence of hypercalcemia appears to have a negative impact on the survival of dogs with anal sac adenocarcinoma. Reported median survival for dogs with hypercalcemia is 6 to 9 months compared to 11 to 19 months for normocalcemic dogs.
- Dogs with large tumors (>10 cm^2) and dogs with pulmonary metastases have shorter survival times.
- The presence of iliac lymphadenopathy has not been a consistently negative predictor of survival.

PEARLS & CONSIDERATIONS

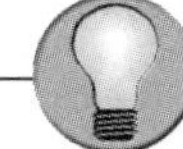

COMMENTS

As many as 30% of anal sac adenocarcinomas are detected incidentally on a routine physical examination. This underscores the importance of complete rectal examination on routine exams.

SUGGESTED READING

Bennett PF, et al: Canine anal sac adenocarcinomas: Clinical presentation and response to therapy. *J Vet Intern Med* 16:100–104, 2002.

Goldschmidt MH, Hendrick MJ: Tumors of the skin and soft tissues: Anal sac gland carcinoma. In Meuten DJ (ed): *Tumors in Domestic Animals*. Ames, IA, Iowa State Press, 2002, pp 74–76.

Williams LE, et al: Carcinoma of the apocrine glands of the anal sac in dogs: 113 cases (1985–1995). *J Am Vet Med Assoc* 223:825–831, 2003.

AUTHOR: **ELIZABETH A. McNIEL**

EDITOR: **KENNETH M. RASSNICK**

Adenocarcinoma, Intestinal/Colonic

BASIC INFORMATION

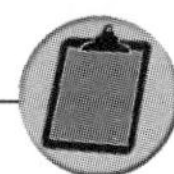

DEFINITION

Malignant tumor that rises from gastrointestinal (GI) tract epithelium

EPIDEMIOLOGY

SPECIES, AGE, SEX: Intestinal carcinoma is rare in dogs and cats, accounting for 1% of tumors in necropsied cats and 0.1% of tumors in dogs. Colorectal adenocarcinoma is slightly more common.

- Mean age of cats with small intestinal adenocarcinoma is 11 years; colorectal tumors in cats occur at a mean age of 16 years
- Mean age of dogs with intestinal and colorectal adenocarcinomas is 9 years

GENETICS AND BREED PREDISPOSITION

- Intestinal adenocarcinoma is most common in boxers, collies, poodles, West Highland white terriers, German shepherds, and Doberman pinschers, as well as Siamese cats (70% of adenocarcinomas of the small intestine of cats are seen in the Siamese breed).
- Shar-pei dogs may have increased incidence of intestinal adenocarcinoma.
- In dogs, colorectal tumors are most common in collies and German shepherds.

ASSOCIATED CONDITIONS AND DISORDERS

- Intestinal obstruction
- Melena
- Hematochezia

CLINICAL PRESENTATION

HISTORY, CHIEF COMPLAINT

- Intestinal adenocarcinoma signs depend on lesion location and include intermittent vomiting, hematemesis, anorexia, dehydration, melena, hematochezia, diarrhea, signs associated with intestinal obstruction or peritonitis, abdominal distention from peritoneal effusion due to carcinomatosis.
- Colorectal adenocarcinomas cause hematochezia, tenesmus, and dyschezia.
- Slowly progressive, nonobstructive tumors may cause anorexia, weight loss, and nonregenerative iron deficiency anemia.

PHYSICAL EXAM FINDINGS: Depending on lesion location:

- Palpable abdominal mass
- Palpable mass and/or rectal bleeding on rectal examination
- Abdominal effusion from carcinomatosis or peritonitis
- Signs of anemia in chronic lesions, poor body condition (body condition score 1–2/9)

ETIOLOGY AND PATHOPHYSIOLOGY

Etiology is unknown, but genetic predisposition is probable

DIAGNOSIS

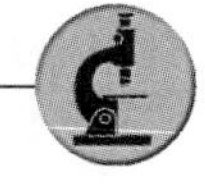

DIFFERENTIAL DIAGNOSIS

Depending on lesion location and signs:

- Foreign body
- Infectious enteropathy, chronic parasitism
- Inflammatory bowel disease
- Alimentary lymphoma
- Alimentary mast cell tumor in cats
- Colorectal polyps, adenomas
- Smooth muscle tumors (leiomyoma, leiomyosarcoma, GIST)

INITIAL DATABASE

- Complete blood count results often are nonspecific (neutrophilia, regenerative or nonregenerative anemia secondary to acute or chronic blood loss).
- Serum biochemistry panel: elevation in alkaline phosphatase may be seen.
- Urinalysis: generally unremarkable.
- Thoracic radiographs for metastasis staging.
- Abdominal radiographs may demonstrate signs of intestinal obstruction, mass effect, or may be noncontributory.
- Positive contrast gastrointestinal study or barium enema may reveal mass or annular constrictive lesion.
- Ultrasonography can define primary mass as well as intra-abdominal lymph node or organ metastasis, and may guide fine-needle aspiration cytologic evaluation.

ADVANCED OR CONFIRMATORY TESTING

Endoscopic or surgical biopsy is required for definitive diagnosis: choice of approach depends on the location of the lesion, because colonoscopy is the procedure of choice for colonic neoplasia diagnosis, but endoscopy will often be nondiagnostic if the lesion is in the jejunum (unable to reach the lesion)

TREATMENT

THERAPEUTIC GOAL(S)

Surgical resection is the treatment of choice for intestinal and colonic adenocarcinoma.

ACUTE GENERAL TREATMENT

General supportive care includes:

- Rehydration and restoring electrolyte homeostasis
- Managing anemia with transfusions and hematinics as indicated by clinical condition
- Antibiotic and emergency management for peritonitis (see Peritonitis, Septic, p 840)
- Analgesic management as indicated for pain in obstructive lesions or peritonitis
- Pro-motility agents are contraindicated in obstructive disease

CHRONIC TREATMENT

- Curative therapy for nonmetastatic intestinal and colonic adenocarcinoma is complete surgical excision.
- Radiation therapy may be palliative or curative for nonresectable colonic lesions.
- Chemotherapy is generally unsuccessful, but therapy with nonsteroidal anti-inflammatory drugs, doxorubicin, platinum agents, antimetabolites (gemcitabine, fluorouracil), or taxanes may be attempted in cases with nonresectable, metastatic, or carcinomatosis disease.

POSSIBLE COMPLICATIONS

- Surgical wound dehiscence with secondary peritonitis, pneumoperitoneum
- Chemotherapy-induced leukopenia might predispose to infection
- Chemotherapy-induced thrombocytopenia might increase tumor hemorrhage
- Chemotherapy might result in perforation of transmural lesions

RECOMMENDED MONITORING

If primary lesion can be successfully resected, ultrasonography for metastasis or recurrence, as well as thoracic radiographs, are indicated.

PROGNOSIS AND OUTCOME

Prognosis is dependent on:

- Histologic type and grade of the primary lesion: low-grade lesions or carcinoma in situ may be completely resected with curative intent.
- Annular constrictive lesions are particularly aggressive.
- Potential for curative resection depends on tumor size and location.
- Metastatic disease and carcinomatosis are incurable and are associated with a poor prognosis.

PEARLS & CONSIDERATIONS

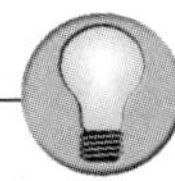

COMMENTS

- The small intestine contains more than 90% of the epithelial cells in the gut, but it is associated with only 10% of all GI malignancies.
- Etiology is unknown for GI cancer, but animals may have multicentric primary lesions due to field carcinogenesis.

SUGGESTED READING

Crawshaw J, Berg J, Sardinas JC, et al: Prognosis for dogs with nonlymphomatous, small intestinal tumors treated by surgical excision. *J Am Anim Hosp Assoc* 34:451, 1998.

Church EM, Mehlhaff CJ, Patnaik AK: Colorectal adenocarinoma in dogs: 78 cases (1973-1984). *J Am Vet Med Assoc* 191:727, 1987.

Slawienski MJ, Mauldin GE, Mauldin GN, et al: Malignant colonic neoplasia in cats: 46 cases (1990-1996). *J Am Vet Med Assoc* 211:878, 1997.

Morrison WB: Nonlymphomatous cancers of the esophagus, stomach and intestines. In Morrison WB (ed): *Cancer in Dogs and Cats: Medical and Surgical Management*, ed 2. Jackson, WY, Teton NewMedia, 2002, pp 527-533.

AUTHOR: **BARBARA E. KITCHELL**
EDITOR: **DEBRA L. ZORAN**

Adenoma/Adenocarcinoma, Perianal

BASIC INFORMATION

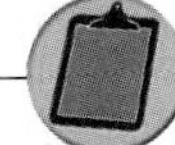

DEFINITION

Neoplastic proliferation of the perianal sebaceous glands. These glands are widely distributed over the skin of the caudal half of the body.

SYNONYM(S)

Hepatoid tumor

EPIDEMIOLOGY

SPECIES, AGE, SEX

- Tumors of perianal glands develop almost exclusively in mature, adult, male dogs that are sexually intact or were neutered late in life.
- Females diagnosed with perianal adenoma are invariably spayed and may be affected by hypertestosteronism occurring with hyperadrenocorticism.
- Perianal adenomas occur very commonly in adult male dogs; perianal adenocarcinomas in dogs are uncommon.

GENETICS AND BREED PREDISPOSITION

- Perianal adenomas:
  - Alaskan malamute
  - Beagle
  - Cocker spaniel
  - Siberian husky
  - Samoyed
  - Shih tzu
- Perianal adenocarcinomas:
  - German shepherds
  - Arctic breeds (samoyed, Alaskan malamute, Siberian husky)

RISK FACTORS

- Perianal adenoma:
  - Sexually intact males
  - Dogs with hyperadrenocorticism (Cushing's disease) and secondary hypertestosteronism
- Perianal adenocarcinoma:
  - Both neutered and intact males

CLINICAL PRESENTATION

HISTORY, CHIEF COMPLAINT

- Dogs with perianal gland tumors are typically presented for the evaluation of one or more masses, usually in the perineal region.
- Because of the wide distribution of perianal glands in the skin of the caudal body, masses may occur at other locations.

PHYSICAL EXAM FINDINGS

- Cutaneous mass in the perineal region. The masses tend to be well circumscribed, superficial, and may be finely lobulated or cauliflower-like in appearance.
- ± Ulceration.
- ± Diffuse skin thickening.
- Differentiation from anal sac disorders and perineal hernia:

  - Visual inspection, as described previously
  - Rectal palpation: perianal adenomas are palpably superficial (cutaneous) and not associated with the anal sacs; the pelvic diaphragm is intact and without herniation

ETIOLOGY AND PATHOPHYSIOLOGY

- Perianal glands are modified sebaceous glands.
- Development of the perianal glands occurs under the influence of testosterone.
- Similarly, tumorigenesis appears to be influenced by hormones, particularly testosterone.
  - Sexually intact males.
  - Hyperadrenocorticism if there is hyperfunction of the zona reticularis. This results in elevated testosterone levels regardless of neuter status.

DIAGNOSIS

Perianal adenomas are often suspected based on physical appearance and palpation in an intact male dog and should resolve with neutering.

DIFFERENTIAL DIAGNOSIS

- Anal sac adenocarcinoma
- Perineal hernia
- Anal sac abscess
- Other cutaneous neoplasia

INITIAL DATABASE

- Complete blood count, serum chemistry, and urinalysis can be helpful in assessing the possibility of hyperadrenocorticism in neutered dogs with perianal adenomas.
- Cytologic evaluation is helpful in the assessment of perianal gland tumors.
  - Cytologically, the perianal glands and their tumors are composed of hepatoid cells, which resemble hepatocytes. The cells are round and arranged in clusters reminiscent of hepatic lobules. There is abundant cytoplasm and a round, centrally located nucleus usually exhibiting a single large nucleolus. The degree of cellular pleomorphism is variable and is not consistently associated with malignancy.
- A definitive diagnosis of benign vs. malignant perianal gland tumor must be made based on histologic examination. Invasion of tissue is the strongest characteristic of malignancy.

TREATMENT

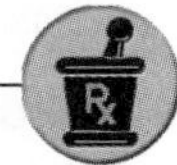

THERAPEUTIC GOAL(S)

The goals of treatment are to control the tumor and to eliminate the source of testosterone.

ACUTE GENERAL TREATMENT

- Perianal adenoma:
  - For most dogs, eliminating testosterone will result in full or partial tumor regression. Thus neutering is recommended and often curative.
- Tumors that persist after neutering should be removed surgically. Tumors can also be resected marginally at the time of the neuter. Marginal resection will provide sufficient biopsy material to ensure a diagnosis of adenoma. Cryosurgery combined with marginal resection may decrease the chance of tumor recurrence.
- For histologically confirmed adenocarcinomas, wide surgical resection is indicated. Wide resection may also be helpful in cases of persistent or recurrent tumors that have not demonstrated malignancy on previous biopsies.
- Anatomic limitations may preclude wide resection in the anal area.
  - At least half of the anal sphincter must be intact to provide fecal continence.
  - For large tumors that do not regress after neutering, radiation therapy may be considered. Radiation may be used after marginal resection or can be used presurgically. Presurgical use of radiation may allow for smaller resections later.
- Although perianal tumors may regress under their influence, administration of estrogens is not recommended due to the potential for toxicity when given at doses required for tumor response.
- In dogs with hyperadrenocorticism, control of that disease may be essential for tumor control (see Hyperadrenocorticism, p 537).

CHRONIC TREATMENT

Perianal tumors may recur after treatment or in dogs with a persistent stimulus for tumorigenesis (hyperadrenocorticism, or breeding animals that are not neutered). Treatment options remain the same.

PROGNOSIS AND OUTCOME

- For benign perianal adenomas, prognosis is excellent.
- Adenocarcinomas can recur locally (16% metastasis rate). Tumors >5 cm in diameter are more likely to recur, and these dogs are more likely to die of their disease.
  - Prognosis worsens with lymph node or distant metastasis
- For dogs with adenocarcinomas <5 cm and >5 cm in diameter without evidence of metastasis, median survival = 24 and 12 months, respectively.
- For dogs with adenocarcinomas that exhibit evidence of local or distant metastasis, median survival = 7 months.

PEARLS & CONSIDERATIONS

COMMENTS

- Perianal adenocarcinomas are not commonly associated with paraneoplastic hypercalcemia, unlike anal sac adenocarcinoma.
- Neutering of male dogs early in life can prevent the development of perianal gland tumors.
- Neutering at the time of diagnosis may allow for full or partial tumor regression.
- Tumors that do not regress after neutering or are recurrent may be exhibiting malignant transformation and more aggressive resection, and/or radiation therapy may be indicated.

SUGGESTED READING

Goldschmidt MH, Hendrick MJ: Tumors of the skin and soft tissue: Hepatoid gland adenoma and hepatoid gland epithelioma. In Meuten DJ (ed): *Tumors in Domestic Animals*. Ames, IA, Iowa State Press, 2002, pp 68-70.

Vail DM, et al: Perianal adenocarcinoma in the canine male: A retrospective study of 41 cases. *J Am Anim Hosp Assoc* 26:329-334, 1990.

AUTHOR: **ELIZABETH A. McNIEL**
EDITOR: **KENNETH M. RASSNICK**

Adhesives and Glues Toxicosis

BASIC INFORMATION

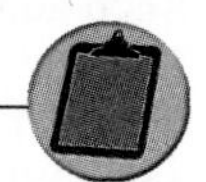

DEFINITION

Adverse physical effects caused by oral, ocular, aural, or dermal exposure to common household adhesives including super glue, expandable polyurethane glue, and white glue

EPIDEMIOLOGY

SPECIES, AGE, SEX

- All animals of all ages and sexes susceptible; exposure is more common in dogs.
- Dermal exposure in cats can result in clinically significant oral exposure (grooming).

RISK FACTORS: Availability of common household adhesives in pet's environment.

CLINICAL PRESENTATION

HISTORY, CHIEF COMPLAINT

- Accidental, acute exposure to adhesives
- Salivation, retching, vomiting, anorexia, lethargy after oral exposure (super glue, polyurethane, white glue)

PHYSICAL EXAM FINDINGS

- Tissue adhesions after ocular or dermal exposure to super glues
- Presence of dried adhesive on the animal (skin, paws, fur, teeth, eye, ear)
- Abdominal distention/discomfort (polyurethane glue ingestion)
- Blepharospasm, epiphora, conjunctivitis, or keratitis with ocular exposure
- Salivation, lethargy, anorexia with oral exposure (all adhesives)

ETIOLOGY AND PATHOPHYSIOLOGY

- Super glues:
  - Contain ethyl-2-cyanoacrylate 60-100% and poly (methylmethacrylate) 2-30%.
  - Super glues (cyanoacrylates) cause rapid adhesion of body structures on contact. These glues are generally mildly irritating to the mucous membranes.
- Expandable polyurethane glue, industrial strength wood glue:
  - Contain diphenylmethane diisocyanate and polymethylene polyphenyl isocyanate in various concentrations.
  - Ingestion of expandable polyurethane glues (isocyanates) is detrimental due to space-occupying properties; can form an expanding gastric foreign body. This is more likely to occur in dogs that chew the bottle of glue. These glues are generally mildly irritating.
- White glues: contain polyvinyl acetate in various concentrations. They are mildly irritating to the mucous membranes.

DIAGNOSIS

DIFFERENTIAL DIAGNOSIS

- Other foreign body injury or ingestions (plastic, woods, metals)
- Garbage toxicosis
- Exposure to corrosives, detergents, bleaches, irritants
- Viral or bacterial gastroenteritis

INITIAL DATABASE

- Abdominal radiographs 12 to 24 hours after ingesting polyurethane glue typically indicate a large, mottled density resembling kibble in the stomach.
- Complete blood count (inflammatory leukogram), chemistry profile, urinalysis.
- Fluorescein staining to identify corneal ulcers.

ADVANCED OR CONFIRMATORY TESTING

Endoscopy may help determine the size of foreign body (polyurethane glue) and also evaluate esophageal and gastric mucosal damage (irritation, ulcers, perforation); rarely useful for removing foreign material (too friable or too large)

TREATMENT

THERAPEUTIC GOAL(S)

- Assess tissue damage
- Separate adhered tissues if needed
- Gastrostomy to remove gastric foreign body if present (polyurethane glue)

ACUTE GENERAL TREATMENT

Super Glue:

- Oral: Adhered tissues typically will separate in 1 to 4 days. If necessary, separate tissues under general anesthesia. Apply margarine, mineral oil, or petroleum jelly, wait 15 to 30 minutes; gently peel or roll adherent tissues apart. Do not pull adherent planes of tissue directly apart due to high tensile strength of the bond. Expand-able foreign body is not expected from ingestion of super glue (cyanoacrylates).
- Aural: Glue may bond to tympanum. Repeatedly applying 3% H_2O_2 (preferred) or acetone on cotton balls may loosen the bond to allow slow extraction of the glue cast. Lavage external ear canal with sterile water afterwards.
- Ocular: rinse eye with 0.9% saline or water for 15 minutes. If the cornea is adhered to lids or lashes, may need to separate under general anesthesia as for oral exposure. If the lids or lashes are adhered to themselves, forced separation is often *not* needed. Assess the cornea for damage and treat abrasions with ophthalmic antibiotics and mydriatics (see Corneal Ulceration, p 246).
- Dermal: as for Oral.

Polyurethane Adhesives:

- Oral: do not induce emesis.
- Do not administer activated charcoal, because it can significantly increase chances of aspiration due to retching and vomiting.
- Perform gastrostomy if concretion (gastric foreign body) is present. Routine premedication (atropine 0.02 mg/kg IV) and general anesthesia (e.g., propofol induction [up to 4 mg/kg IV to effect] and isoflurane maintenance).
- Sucralfate and H_2 antagonist advised if GI signs present or if foreign body is removed.
  - H_2 receptor antagonists:
    - Famotidine: dogs/cats: 0.5 mg/kg PO, SC, IM, IV q 12-24h; or
    - Cimetidine: dogs/cats: 5-10 mg/kg PO q 6h.
  - Sucralfate: dogs: 0.5-1 g PO q 8-12h; cats: 0.25-0.5 g PO q 8-12h.
- Postoperative:
  - Administer broad-spectrum antibiotics after gastrostomy if evidence of contamination or infection (e.g., enrofloxacin 5 mg/kg PO q 12h for 10 days, ampicillin 22 mg/kg IV q 6h for 2 days).
  - Metoclopramide 0.4 mg/kg SC q 8h for 1 to 2 days. Contraindication: gastrointestinal obstruction.
  - Restrict food and water intake for first 12 to 24 hours after surgery.
  - Postoperative pain control (e.g., oxymorphone 0.08 mg/kg IM q 6h or hydromorphone 0.1-0.2 mg/kg IM, IV, or SC q 2-6h).
  - IV fluids as needed.
- Dermal, ocular, aural: treat as for super glues.

White Glue or Other Glues:

- Most exposures do not need aggressive treatment because signs are usually mild and self-limiting. Treat mild to moderate gastrointestinal irritation supportively. Gastric foreign body is not expected.

POSSIBLE COMPLICATIONS

Stomach rupture and peritonitis

RECOMMENDED MONITORING

- Complete blood count
- Chemistry profile

PROGNOSIS AND OUTCOME

- Very good in all situations unless extensive corneal or tympanic membrane damage occurs
- Very good in uncomplicated cases for gastric foreign body removal
- Guarded to poor if stomach rupture, torsion, or peritonitis has occurred

PEARLS & CONSIDERATIONS

COMMENTS

- General negative effects are as follows: super glues, binding of tissues; polyurethane glues, expansion to form gastrointestinal foreign body; white glues, minimal.
- After the ingestion of expandable polyurethane glue (isocyanates), it is vital to verify the presence of a foreign body before performing a gastrostomy.
- Ingestion of dried, already polymerized polyurethane glue (isocyanates) will not expand further in the stomach.
- Expandable gastric foreign body is not expected from super glue and white glue ingestion.
- Complete recovery may take several days after surgical removal of gastric foreign body.

PREVENTION

Keep adhesives out of reach of pets

SUGGESTED READING

Abadir WF, et al: Removal of superglue from the external ear using acetone: Case report and literature review. *J Laryngol Otolaryngol* 109(12):1219–1221, 1995.

Horstman CL, et al: Gastric outflow obstruction after ingestion of wood glue in a dog. *J Am Anim Hosp Assoc* 39(1): 47–51, 2003.

McLean CJ: Ocular superglue injury. *J Accid Emerg Med* 14(1):40–41, 1997.

AUTHOR: **PAUL A. EUBIG**

EDITOR: **SAFDAR A. KHAN**

Adrenal Mass, Incidental

BASIC INFORMATION

DEFINITION

An adrenal mass discovered incidentally with abdominal imaging (radiography, ultrasonography, computed tomography [CT] or magnetic resonance imaging [MRI]) (see also Adrenal Neoplasia [Adenoma/Carcinoma], p 43)

SYNONYM(S)

Adrenal incidentaloma
Adrenaloma
Inapparent adrenal mass

EPIDEMIOLOGY

SPECIES, AGE, SEX

- Usually middle-aged/old dogs and cats
- True incidence is not known

ASSOCIATED CONDITIONS AND DISORDERS

- Nonfunctional: none
- Functional: see Hyperadrenocorticism, p 537; Aberrant Adrenocortical Disease (Increased Adrenal Sex Hormone Production), p 5; Hyperaldosteronism, Primary, p 541; Pheochromocytoma, p 846

CLINICAL PRESENTATION

DISEASE FORMS/SUBTYPES

- Functional:
  - Cortisol-secreting
  - Aldosterone-secreting
  - Sex-hormone-secreting
  - Pheochromocytoma
- Nonfunctional
- Benign
- Malignant

HISTORY, CHIEF COMPLAINT

- By definition, these are incidental findings.
- Nonfunctional: usually none.
- Functional: further questioning may reveal historical clinical signs.
  - See Hyperadrenocorticism, p 537
  - See Hyperaldosteronism, Primary, p 541
  - See Aberrant Adrenocortical Disease (Increased Adrenal Sex Hormone Production), p 5
  - See Pheochromocytoma, p 846

PHYSICAL EXAM FINDINGS

- Usually absent or not suggestive of adrenal disease, because these are incidental findings
- Nonfunctional: usually none
- Functional: subtle signs may be apparent if these were overlooked initially (or may become apparent with progression over time)
  - See Hyperadrenocorticism, p 537
  - See Hyperaldosteronism, Primary, p 541
  - See Aberrant Adrenocortical Disease (Increased Adrenal Sex Hormone Production), p 5
  - See Pheochromocytoma, p 846

ETIOLOGY AND PATHOPHYSIOLOGY

See Hyperadrenocorticism, p 537; Adrenal Neoplasia (Adenoma/Carcinoma), p 43; Hyperaldosteronism, Primary, p 541; Aberrant Adrenocortical Disease (Increased Adrenal Sex Hormone Production), p 5; Pheochromocytoma, p 846

DIAGNOSIS

Although surgical removal and histopathologic examination can provide a definitive diagnosis, a more conservative approach should be considered in patients with incidentally discovered adrenal masses with no invasion of surrounding structures, no evidence of metastasis, and no clinical or biochemical evidence of adrenal disease.

DIFFERENTIAL DIAGNOSIS

- Adrenal carcinoma
- Adrenal adenoma:
  - Androgen-secreting tumor
  - Cortisol-secreting tumor
  - Aldosterone-secreting tumor
- Pheochromocytoma
- Granuloma
- Metastatic disease:
  - Mammary tumor
  - Lymphoma
  - Other carcinomas
- Adrenal nodular hyperplasia
- Adrenal cyst
- Adrenal myelolipoma
- Adrenal teratoma
- Adrenal hematoma

INITIAL DATABASE

- Revisit a detailed history and physical examination to identify any previously missed signs or abnormalities that could be attributed to one of the functional tumor types.
- See Hyperadrenocorticism, p 537; Aberrant Adrenocortical Disease (Increased Adrenal Sex Hormone

Production), p 5, Hyperaldosteronism, Primary, p 541; and Pheochromocytoma, p 846 for compatible results on the following tests:
  - Complete blood count, serum biochemical profile, urinalysis
  - Blood pressure
  - Fundic examination
  - Thoracic radiographs (three views)
  - Electrocardiogram
- In addition to finding the mass, abdominal radiographs and ultrasonography can help in assessing the size of the mass, local invasion of adjacent structures, and potential intra-abdominal metastasis.
- Cytologic examination of a fine-needle aspirate (if feasible based on the location and appearance of the mass) may help assess malignancy.

ADVANCED OR CONFIRMATORY TESTING

- Possible tests to identify a functional mass:
  - Adrenocorticotropic hormone stimulation test with adrenal sex hormone panel and aldosterone concentrations
  - Low-dose dexamethasone suppression test
  - Urine cortisol: creatinine ratio (urine collected at home by owner)
  - Serial blood pressure measurements.
  - Urine catecholamines (limited availability; see Pheochromocytoma, p 846)
- CT or MRI of abdomen can help assess size of the mass, local invasion of adjacent structures, and intra-abdominal metastasis

TREATMENT

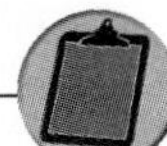

THERAPEUTIC GOAL(S)

- Nonfunctional benign tumors: no treatment needed/monitoring only
- Functional or malignant tumors: surgical excision

ACUTE GENERAL TREATMENT

- Surgery to remove a malignant tumor or functional benign tissue. If functional, see the appropriate chapter for perioperative management recommendations.
- If the neoplastic status of the mass is unknown, surgical removal is controversial if no clinical signs are observed by the owner, the mass is small (<3 cm), hormonal tests are normal, and there are no clinical signs of pheochromocytoma.

CHRONIC TREATMENT

Functional tumor: see the specific topic

POSSIBLE COMPLICATIONS

- Wound dehiscence, hemorrhage, thromboembolism
- For functional tumors, also see the specific topic

RECOMMENDED MONITORING

- Benign, nonfunctional mass: reassess size at 2, 4, and 6 months, then q 4-6 months. If there is no change in size, then adrenalectomy may be avoided.
- Client to monitor for clinical signs of hyperadrenocorticism, such as polyuria and polydipsia or signs of pheochromocytoma, such as collapse, weakness, tachycardia, etc.

PROGNOSIS AND OUTCOME

- Benign tumor: excellent to good
- Malignant tumor with no metastasis: fair to good with surgical excision
- Functional tumors: also see the specific topic
- Some dogs with incidentally discovered adrenal masses on ultrasound and no sign of local invasion nor overt clinical signs of adrenal disease have been monitored medically until they died. Necropsy results in 30 dogs indicate:
  - Nonsecreting/clinically unimportant adrenal tumors or granulomas: 40%
  - No abnormalities ("mass" was normal variation in adrenal tissue): 30%
  - Pheochromocytoma: 30%

PEARLS & CONSIDERATIONS

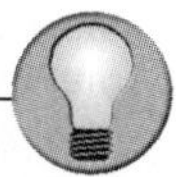

COMMENTS

The seeming absence of clinical signs may in fact be a presence of subtle signs that are only apparent retrospectively after treatment. In humans with incidentally discovered adrenal masses and subtle or subclinical hyperadrenocorticism (defined as hypercortisolemia in two standard tests for hyperadrenocorticism in the absence of clinical signs), surgical removal of the masses led to the animals showing an improved demeanor despite no previous recognition of clinical signs. Resolution of hypercortisolemia was also seen.

SUGGESTED READING

Feldman EC, Nelson RW: Canine hyperadrenocorticism. In Feldman EC, Nelson RW (eds): *Canine and Feline Endocrinology and Reproduction*, ed 2. Philadelphia, WB Saunders, 2004, pp 252-357.

Mansmann G, et al: The clinically inapparent adrenal mass: update in diagnosis and management. *Endocrine Rev* 25(2):309-340, 2004.

Melian C, Peterson ME: The incidentally discovered adrenal mass. In Bonagura JD (ed): *Kirk's Current Veterinary Therapy XIII*. Philadelphia, WB Saunders, 2000, pp 368-372.

AUTHOR: **KATE HILL**

EDITOR: **SHERRI IHLE**

Adrenal Neoplasia (Adenoma/Carcinoma)

BASIC INFORMATION

DEFINITION

A benign or malignant tumor of the adrenal gland that can be functional (secreting adrenal hormones) or nonfunctional (nonsecretory). Cortisol-secreting and nonsecretory tumors are discussed here (also see Aberrant Adrenocortical Disease (Increased Adrenal Sex Hormone Production), p 5; Hyperaldosteronism, Primary, p 541; Pheochromocytoma, p 846).

SYNONYM(S)

Adrenal tumor

Adrenal dependent hyperadrenocorticism

Canine Cushing's syndrome (more general term)

EPIDEMIOLOGY

SPECIES, AGE, SEX

- Dogs: median age 11.3 years; more common in females (60-70%) and large breeds (46% > 20 kg)
- Cats: mean age 12 years; no sex predilection

GENETICS AND BREED PREDISPOSITION

- Dogs: dachshunds, German shepherds, Labrador retrievers, poodles
- Cats: none

ASSOCIATED CONDITIONS AND DISORDERS: Functional tumors are one cause of hyperadrenocorticism.

CLINICAL PRESENTATION

DISEASE FORMS/SUBTYPES

- Functional
- Nonfunctional (nonsecretory)

HISTORY, CHIEF COMPLAINT

- Functional: see Hyperadrenocorticism, p 537
- Nonfunctional: often none

PHYSICAL EXAM FINDINGS

- Functional: see Hyperadrenocorticism, p 537
- Nonfunctional: usually normal

ETIOLOGY AND PATHOPHYSIOLOGY

- Most adrenal tumors secrete cortisol, but oversecretion of other hormones (see Aberrant Adrenocortical Disease (Increased Adrenal Sex Hormone Production), p 5; Hyperaldosteronism, Primary, p 541; Pheochromocytoma, p 846) or lack of function is also possible.
- The excess cortisol causes a decrease in pituitary adrenocorticotropic hormone (ACTH) secretion, but the tumor continues to function autonomously. The contralateral adrenal often decreases in size due to lack of stimulation.
- Adrenal adenomas and adenocarcinomas are equally represented.
- In the dog, the right and left adrenal glands are affected with equal frequency. Rarely, bilateral masses occur. Data are limited for the cat.

DIAGNOSIS

DIFFERENTIAL DIAGNOSIS

- Granuloma
- Metastatic disease
- Pheochromocytoma
- Aldosterone-secreting tumor
- Sex-hormone–secreting tumor (aberrant adrenocortical disease)
- Adrenal nodular hyperplasia

INITIAL DATABASE

- Complete blood count, serum biochemical profile, urinalysis:
  - Functional tumor: see Hyperadrenocorticism, p 537
  - Nonfunctional tumor: usually normal
- Thoracic radiographs (three views):
  - Functional tumor: see Hyperadrenocorticism, p 537
  - Nonfunctional tumor: possible metastasis
- Abdominal radiographs: hepatomegaly (if functional), possible mineralized adrenal gland
- Abdominal ultrasonography: unilateral adrenal enlargement with small contralateral adrenal, possible tumor invasion of adjacent tissues
- Blood pressure: may be elevated with functional tumors

ADVANCED OR CONFIRMATORY TESTING

- To determine if the tumor is cortisol-secreting, see tests for Hyperadrenocorticism (p 537).
- Measurement of adrenal sex hormones and aldosterone, in addition to cortisol, before and after stimulation with synthetic ACTH may also be useful. (See Aberrant Adrenocortical Disease [Increased Adrenal Sex Hormone Production], p 5; Hyperaldosteronism, Primary, p 541).
- Endogenous ACTH concentration will be low.
- Abdominal computed tomography or magnetic resonance imaging: can demonstrate local tissue invasion.
- Histopathologic examination and immunohistochemistry of the excised tumor is confirmatory, but histopathologic determination of malignancy can be challenging. Gross evidence of metastasis provides conclusive evidence of malignancy.

TREATMENT

THERAPEUTIC GOAL(S)

Removal or destruction of malignant tissue:

- Control of clinical signs

ACUTE GENERAL TREATMENT

- Dogs: Stabilization before surgery may include medical management with ketoconazole (e.g., 10–15 mg/kg/day; see Hyperadrenocorticism, p 537) before surgery, and control of hypertension if present (e.g., amlodipine 0.0625–0.25 mg/kg PO q 24h; see Systemic Hypertension, p 1058)
- Cats: Trilostane, metyrapone, and aminoglutethimide have been used for stabilization before surgery (see Hyperadrenocorticism, p 537)
- Assess thromboembolic risk with coagulation profile including antithrombin III and D-dimers

CHRONIC TREATMENT

- Surgical excision is preferred if obvious metastatic disease is not present.
- Intraoperative support should include 0.9% saline IV and dexamethasone IV (0.1 mg/kg in IV fluids over 6 hours (intraoperatively ± overlapping into postoperative period).
- Postoperatively, dexamethasone should be continued (0.1 mg/kg SQ q 6–12h) for 2 to 3 days or until the dog is eating and oral prednisone therapy (0.1 mg/kg PO q 12h initially, tapered over several months) can be started.
- If postoperative hyperkalemia occurs (rare with unilateral adrenalectomy), treat as for Hypoadrenocorticism (p 561).
- Hypercortisolism due to residual disease after surgery can be managed with mitotane in dogs (see below).
- Primary medical management of cortisol-secreting tumors can be difficult, because higher doses are required. Relapses occur in approximately 50% of dogs.
  - Mitotane (o'p-DDD):
    - Induction therapy: 25–37.5 mg/kg/day (after a meal PO q 12h). Perform an ACTH stimulation test every 10 to 14 days. Increase dose in 10 mg/kg PO q 12h increments up to 45 mg/kg q 12h if no response.
    - Maintenance therapy: 50–100 mg/kg/week divided in two to four treatments.
    - Monitor therapy with an ACTH stimulation test q 3 months. Also see Hyperadrenocorticism, p 537, for other induction guidelines.

DRUG INTERACTIONS

See Hyperadrenocorticism, p 537

POSSIBLE COMPLICATIONS

- Hemorrhage
- Thromboembolism
- Wound dehiscence
- Infection

RECOMMENDED MONITORING

Thoracic radiographs and abdominal ultrasonography every 2 to 3 months to check for metastasis

PROGNOSIS AND OUTCOME

- Prognosis is poor with metastatic disease or local invasion
- Surgery with excision of tumor (if no metastasis): dogs: median survival 17.5 to 36 months (range 1 day to 53 months); cats: range 14 days to 30 months
- Medical management with mitotane: Dogs without metastasis respond better. Mean survival of dogs with adrenal tumors is 16.4 months (median 11.5 months, range 20 days to 5.1 years)

PEARLS & CONSIDERATIONS

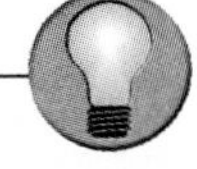

COMMENTS

- Surgical therapy is preferred if metastatic disease is not evident.
- Medical therapy and long-term management can be as expensive as surgical therapy.
- Because the surgery and perioperative management can be complex, consideration should be given to referral.

SUGGESTED READING

Anderson CR, Birchard SJ, et al: Surgical treatment of adrenocortical tumors: 21 cases (1990–1996). *JAAHA* 37:93–97, 2001.

Hill KE, Scott-Moncrieff JC: Tumors of the adrenal cortex causing hyperadrenocorticism. *Vet Med* 96(9): 686–706, 2001.

AUTHOR: **KATE HILL**

EDITOR: **SHERRI IHLE**

Aggression, Cat

Client Education Sheet on Website

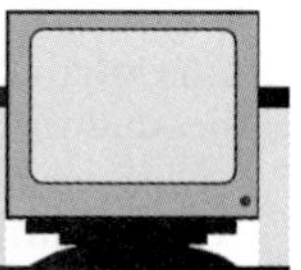

BASIC INFORMATION

DEFINITION

A threat, challenge, or attack directed toward one or more individuals. Feline aggression can be intraspecific (between cats) or interspecific (between different species).

EPIDEMIOLOGY

SPECIES, AGE, SEX: All feline breeds, sexes, and age groups. Onset commonly at social maturity (2 to 4 years).

RISK FACTORS

- Anxiety
- Hand-rearing (failure to learn social rules from cats): intraspecific aggression
- Lack of exposure to humans between 2 and 9 weeks old: aggression to humans
- Severe in utero malnutrition

CONTAGION AND ZOONOSIS

- Contagion: bite wounds
- Zoonosis: cat-scratch fever/bartonellosis, bite wounds

GEOGRAPHY AND SEASONALITY: Redirected aggression, and aggression involving the visitation of other cats and/or urine marking may be more common as the seasons change (e.g., during spring and fall) and the odor environment and access to that environment changes.

ASSOCIATED CONDITIONS AND DISORDERS

- Medical conditions such as intracranial disease, lead poisoning, arthritis, sensory deficits, hyperthyroidism, feline lower urinary tract disease, feline immunodeficiency virus, and rabies have been associated with feline aggression.
- Feline elimination complaints that don't resolve with basic treatment (see Inappropriate Elimination, Cat, p 583) are almost always associated with unrecognized aggression.

CLINICAL PRESENTATION

HISTORY, CHIEF COMPLAINT

- Passive (covert) or active (overt) aggression can be noted.
- May involve a threat, challenge, or actual attack.
- Typical elements of the history include aggression between two cats in the household, or directed toward the clients when the cat is handled or when the clients move. The cat may bite when the client attempts to approach or handle the cat (overt aggression). The cat may also block access to areas (e.g., by sitting in doorways and staring [covert aggression]).
- Signs may be:
  - Visual (changes in body posture, piloerection)
  - Auditory (hissing, spitting)
  - Olfactory (spraying, scratching, or rubbing areas rich in sebaceous glands [chin, head, cheeks, base of tail], whisker area)
  - May involve use of teeth and/or claws

PHYSICAL EXAM FINDINGS: Unremarkable, unless aggression is associated with a medical condition.

ETIOLOGY AND PATHOPHYSIOLOGY

- The hypothalamus and amygdala are involved in defense and aggression.
- Monoamines and androgenic steroids act as modulators of established offensive and defensive aggressive behaviors.

DIAGNOSIS

DIFFERENTIAL DIAGNOSIS

Aggression as part of a medical illness (see Associated Conditions and Disorders above)

INITIAL DATABASE

- Behavioral Assessment, see p 1188
- Complete blood count, serum biochemistry panel, thyroid panel, urinalysis ± urine culture, neurologic examination: to help rule out medical disorders that trigger aggression

TREATMENT

THERAPEUTIC GOAL(S)

- Intercat aggression: intercat tolerance through reduction of anxiety
- Aggression directed toward clients: management of the cat's behavior by helping clients address underlying causes

ACUTE GENERAL TREATMENT

- Any highly aroused cat should not be approached, especially to try to calm or reassure it. The cat should be left alone until it is calmer. Arousal can last 24 to 48 hours due to hypothalamic stimulation. If necessary, heavy blankets or cardboard can be used to herd the cat into an unused room for sequestration until calmer. Water, food, and a litterbox can be slipped through the door if the cat's behavior permits.
- If another cat is involved, then the cats should initially be separated. They should be placed in separate rooms so that they can hear and smell each other, but no visual contact occurs.
- If the aggression is directed toward humans, all situations that provoke aggression (e.g., patting) should be avoided.

CHRONIC TREATMENT: AGGRESSION BETWEEN CATS

- For aggression between cats within the same household, each cat should be placed separately in each room of the house for a few days until its scent is present in all the rooms.
- While the cats are separated, a regular routine should be established with each cat so that feeding and playing occur at a set time each day. Ideally, the cats are fed five to six small meals each day. This may need to be done while the cat is in a cat cage.
- Treatment then involves slowly reintroducing the cats to each other. This is the same way a new cat is introduced into the household. The aim is for them to have a positive association with each other. This essentially means that "good" things, such as play or feeding, only happen in the presence of the other cat.
  - As the cats are slowly reintroduced, they initially are only in the same room during mealtimes. This can be accomplished using leads and harnesses or cages/crates. Caution should be urged to avoid overzealous use of cages/crates. Clients often attempt to use cages in the hope of "flooding" the cats. The idea behind successful flooding is that the cats stop caring about the presence of each other; however, flooding can be viewed as entrapment and may be traumatic, resulting in permanently phobic cats who panic or are depressed.
  - Cats—in or out of cages—are placed at opposite ends of the room and are fed at this time. This should create a positive association with food and the presence of the other cat.
  - If no hissing or spitting occurs and each cat eats the food, the cats are gradually brought closer and closer to each other over a period of days and meals. This may take several weeks or even months.
  - Then one cat at a time is allowed to freely explore, and if no aggression occurs, then both are allowed to interact under supervision.
  - The reintroduction needs to be very slow.

- Anxiolytic medication may also be needed to treat one or both cats.
  - Tricyclic antidepressants (TCAs) such as amitriptyline (0.5-1 mg/kg PO q 12-24h, average 5-10 mg/cat PO q 24h) or clomipramine (0.5 mg/kg PO q 24h).
  - Selective serotonin reuptake inhibitors (SSRIs) such as fluoxetine (0.5 mg/kg PO q 24h) may be useful for the aggressor cat.
  - Benzodiazepines, such as diazepam (0.2-0.4 mg/kg PO q 12h; average 1-2 mg/cat PO q 12h), has been helpful for some timid cats who become victims.
  - The cats may require medication for a prolonged period. This may be up to 6 to 12 months, and then the cats should be slowly weaned off medication.
- Synthetic pheromone analog Feliway may be beneficial in simple cases of the introduction of unfamiliar cats.

CHRONIC TREATMENT: AGGRESSION TO HUMANS

- For cases involving aggression toward the client, it is important to identify and then avoid all situations that may be provocative (e.g., approaching, stroking, handling).
- Then the client needs to instigate a behavior modification program in which the cat is taught to earn all attention or rewards by deferring to the client:
  - It has to come or sit at the client's request, before any interaction with the client.
  - It is not allowed to initiate any interaction. If the cat does solicit attention, the client should completely ignore the cat or walk away.
  - No reward/attention is given until the cat defers and responds to the command (e.g., sit or come).
- Desensitization and counterconditioning to handling and moving are indicated and the cat rewarded for appropriate acceptable behavior.
- No physical punishment should be used, because that will exacerbate the problem.
- Anxiolytic medication may also be needed to treat the cat to alter the neurochemical environment.
  - TCAs such as amitriptyline (0.5-1 mg/kg PO q 24h, average of 5-10 mg/cat PO q 24h) or clomipramine (0.5 mg/kg PO q 24h) have proved useful in some cases.
  - SSRIs such as fluoxetine (0.5 mg/kg PO q 24h) have also proved useful because they are available in a liquid formulation.
  - Benzodiazepines are generally not recommended, because they may disinhibit aggression associated with inhibited fear. If this is not an issue, benzodiazepines can be used and may facilitate food-reward-based behavior modification programs because they make cats hungry.
- In some cases these cats require lifelong medication or for prolonged periods of time with a minimum period usually of 6 to 12 months. Attempts to slowly wean off medication may be made.

DRUG INTERACTIONS

TCAs and SSRIs should not be used with monoamine oxidase inhibitors such as selegiline (Anipryl), amitraz, and some tick collars.

POSSIBLE COMPLICATIONS

Long-term use of diazepam is occasionally associated with hepatotoxicity; preference of other drugs, or regular monitoring if inevitable, is recommended.

RECOMMENDED MONITORING

All animals being treated with medication should have full physical and laboratory evaluations before medication initiation to determine a baseline, especially for liver and kidney parameters. These evaluations should be checked every 6 to 12 months or more frequently as indicated by results, overt signs or behaviors, client concerns, and the age and general health status of the cat.

PROGNOSIS AND OUTCOME

The behavior can usually be managed, not cured, with client education and compliance.

PEARLS & CONSIDERATIONS

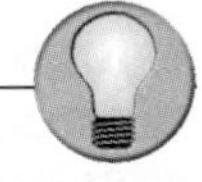

COMMENTS

- Punishment of aggression should be avoided because it tends to aggravate the aggression.
- With intercat aggression, an excellent way of demonstrating cats' behaviors, and having clients understand intercat processes, is to have clients videotape the cats. Reviewing videotapes helps clients understand their cats' behaviors.

PREVENTION AND CLIENT EDUCATION

Attendance at Kitten Kindy classes

SUGGESTED READING

Beaver BV: Fractious cats and feline aggression. *J Feline Med Surg* 6:13-18, 2004.

Crowell-Davis SL, Curtis TM, Knowles RJ: The social organization of the cat: A modern synthesis. *J Feline Med Surg* 6:19-28, 2004.

Overall KL: *Clinical Behavioral Medicine for Small Animals*. St. Louis, Mosby, 1997.

Overall KL, Rodan I, Beaver BV, et al: Feline behavior guidelines from the American Association of Feline Practitioners. *J Am Vet Med Assoc* 227:70-84, 2005.

Seksel K: *Training Your Cat*. Melbourne, Australia, Hyland House, 2001.

AUTHOR: **KERSTI SEKSEL**

EDITOR: **KAREN L. OVERALL**

Aggression, Dog

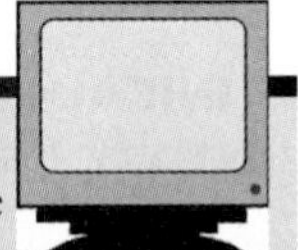

Client Education Sheet on Website

BASIC INFORMATION

DEFINITION

An appropriate or inappropriate threat or challenge that is ultimately resolved by combat or deference

SYNONYM(S)

Impulse-control aggression: dominance aggression

EPIDEMIOLOGY

SPECIES, AGE, SEX

- Any age and either gender
- May be manifest at the end of sexual maturity (6 to 9 months) and become refined during social maturity (12 to 36 months)
- Impulse-control aggression: 90% male. In females, often very young (8 weeks old)

GENETICS AND BREED PREDISPOSITION

- Impulse control aggression. United States: English springer spaniels (bench), dalmatians. United Kingdom: English cocker spaniels, golden retrievers, and others
- Fear aggression. United States: border collies, German shepherds, other breeds

RISK FACTORS

- Largest risk factor for pathologic aggression likely is genetic liability.

- Dogs that are chained are overrepresented in dog-bite statistics.
- Dog parks (dogs unknown to each other; clients may see interaction as a form of treatment for fearful or aggressive dogs, which it is not).
- Misconceptions may worsen the problem. Clients are often mistakenly advised to "dominate" the dog or to be "alpha." These terms and their usage are based in profound misunderstandings of canine behavior, and this approach must not be used.

CONTAGION AND ZOONOSIS

- Risk of physical trauma and of zoonosis (rabies, others) with bite wounds.
  - Boys aged 5 to 9 years at highest risk for bites; dog is usually known to them
- Physical punishment (by humans) in response to canine aggression will almost always increase the risk to humans and worsen the condition.

ASSOCIATED CONDITIONS AND DISORDERS

- Coexistence of more than one form of aggression, or other behavioral disorders, is common.
- Obtaining an accurate diagnosis of type of aggression is essential to help identify triggers.

CLINICAL PRESENTATION

DISEASE FORMS/SUBTYPES: Five commonly encountered types of aggression:

- Impulse-control ("dominance") aggression. Can involve growling, baring teeth, staring, and/or biting, especially in response to certain human behaviors (staring at dog, reaching towards or over dog, punishment)
- Fear aggression. Characterized by trembling; growling, barking, or snapping while backing up; cowering; possibly biting from behind and running away
- Interdog aggression. Characterized by threats, staring, and challenges. Interactions with other dogs change with social maturity. Usually male-male or female-female. May be neuter-responsive, particularly in males that fight with non-household members
- Protective/territorial aggression. Characterized by barking, growling, snarling, biting to protect stationary (e.g., house) or mobile (e.g., car) property. Worse with discrete boundaries (e.g., fence). Not aggressive away from territory
- Food-related aggression. Characterized by growling when eating if approached (even from far away), biting if food/treat is threatened. Possible correlation to future impulse-control aggression

HISTORY, CHIEF COMPLAINT

- Early signs are often not noticed by clients and must be inquired about by veterinarians.
- Biting, growling, snarling, lip-lifting, snapping, staring, and body posturing (e.g., blocking of access) are common early signs of aggression.
- Abuse, neglect, or "lack of socialization" seldom factor into histories of pathological aggression.

PHYSICAL EXAM FINDINGS: Exam is almost always unremarkable, barring dog bite wounds in interdog aggression.

ETIOLOGY AND PATHOPHYSIOLOGY

- Dogs with impulse-control aggression may have abnormal levels of cerebrospinal neurochemical metabolites and may excrete metabolites of excitatory neurotransmitters in their urine.
- Amygdala and caudate nuclei proposed as anatomic diagnosis.

DIAGNOSIS

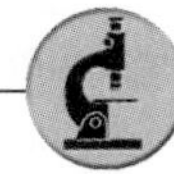

DIFFERENTIAL DIAGNOSIS

Primary neurologic disease (encephalitis, adverse medication reaction, etc.). Brain mass/neoplasm is an uncommon cause for aggression.

INITIAL DATABASE

Complete blood count, serum biochemistry profile, and urinalysis to rule out underlying medical conditions and contraindications for psychotropic medication. Generally unremarkable

ADVANCED OR CONFIRMATORY TESTING

A video of the dog will provide the needed subjective and objective data to distinguish among all forms of aggression.

TREATMENT

THERAPEUTIC GOAL(S)

- Abort the exhibition of the aggressive behaviors to render the dog safer and to prevent the dog from learning to be more aggressive.
- Enhance public and familial safety and the emotional bonds with the dog.
- Alleviate or prevent the anxiety underlying the aggression.
- Render the dog happier by meeting its needs; this may mean that there are certain circumstances in which these patients should never be placed.
- Aggression is a set of rules that allows the dog to cope with what it perceives to be an uncertain world, and so it is ideally suited to treatment by substituting a more humane set of rules that helps to make the world more predictable to the dog.

ACUTE GENERAL TREATMENT

- The key to keeping clients and dogs safe is to avoid known provocative circumstances, which applies to all forms of aggression.
- Physical punishment or threats are strictly contraindicated, because they will intensify pathologic aggression.
- The trigger in impulse control aggression is about the dog's perception of, or response to, humans who exhibit any type of action associated with control or access to control of the dog's behavior such as reaching for the dog. Instead of reaching for the dog, the clients can learn to call the dog to them and teach the dog, with positive reinforcement, to offer behaviors that are appropriate (e.g., lifting up the head and neck for a collar to be slipped on).
- For fear aggression, protect the dog. Do not continue to expose the dog thinking the dog will "get used to it"; the dog will only suffer and become worse.
- For interdog aggression, separate the dogs when not supervised, regardless of who is perceived as the aggressor. A video of the dogs when they are not fighting reveals body postures and signals, indicating which dog is the aggressor. The aggressor must be prevented from actively or passively threatening other dogs, even if this means walking dogs separately or banishing the aggressor.
- For food-related aggression, if the food over which the dog is aggressive is a food toy (e.g., treat cube, rawhide, vegetable bone), remove these from the dog's repertoire. If the dog is aggressive over meals, feed the dog separately behind a locked door, and do not take the food dish until the dog is out of the room and otherwise focused.
- Do not kennel, crate, tie, chain, or put aggressive dogs in a run if they can be approached and harassed, or if it makes them more reactive.
- If the client is thinking of euthanizing the dog or afraid of living with the dog, consider boarding the dog for a week so that they can make an informed, nonimpulsive decision. The vast majority of these dogs improve dramatically, and because clients understand triggers for biting, these dogs may be less at risk for future bites than is the average dog.

CHRONIC TREATMENT

- Dogs should be taught to relax while making eye contact with the clients as a preferred default/substitute behavior when the dog encounters a situation about which it is anxious or unsure.
- Systematic desensitization can be used if the triggers can be identified and manipulated.
- Head collars can be used indoors and outdoors, and allow a dog's mouth to be humanely closed, while redirecting their behavior in a way that mimics normal dog signaling.

- More specific behavior modification designed to teach the dog to trust the client and to take cues about the appropriateness of their behavior from the client should be coupled with medications.
  - Amitriptyline: 1–2 mg/kg PO q 12h × 30 days to start, or
  - Fluoxetine: 1 mg/kg PO q 24h × 60 days to start, or
  - Clomipramine: up to 3 mg/kg PO q 12h × 60 days
  - Combinations of lower doses of amitriptyline and fluoxetine (synergistic)

DRUG INTERACTIONS

These drugs should not be used with monoamine oxidase inhibitors (e.g., some parasiticide collars and dips, and some medications of cognitive dysfunction).

POSSIBLE COMPLICATIONS

Failure to improve can be due to overly rapid behavior modifications; discordant approaches in the household; or history of choke chain, or pinch collar "corrections" (dog perceives clients as a threat)

RECOMMENDED MONITORING

- Frequent (weekly) contact with clients.
- All instructions, including warnings, must be in writing and understood by the clients.

PROGNOSIS AND OUTCOME

- The best prognosticators for canine aggression are the client's determination to help the dog and his/her ability to provide a predictable environment in which the dog can improve.
- Clients who are afraid of the dog often have trouble with treatment (behavior modification).
- Clients with chaotic households have trouble protecting the dog, and preventing the dog from being a risk to others.
- Clients who commit to treating the dog because treatment will relieve the dog's anxiety and suffering see the dog improve dramatically, regardless of the diagnosis or level of aggression.
- With appropriate treatment, the vast majority of these dogs improve to the extent that it is hard to tell they had a behavior problem, but many dogs would benefit from lifetime restricted access in certain physical or social situations.
- Medication may be lifelong for these dogs, but studies indicate no untoward events.

PEARLS & CONSIDERATIONS

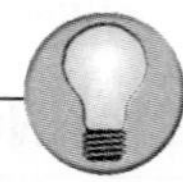

COMMENTS

- Shock collars have *no* place in the treatment of any behavioral condition. They will *always* exacerbate anxiety, even if they may suppress some parts of the behavioral signs. Their determined use by clients should prompt the suspicion of physical abuse (animal or human) in the household.
- The widely held belief that pathologic aggression in dogs stems from abusive handling in the past is entirely unsubstantiated.

PREVENTION

- Humane training methods teach clients to read and understand dog signaling, a skill that leads to early detection of problematic behavior.
- Head collars and harnesses now make it possible to raise even the most rambunctious dog to be relatively calm. All puppies should be fitted with these at their first appointment.

CLIENT EDUCATION

- Consistency is key because it makes the world a more predictable place. Predictability lessens anxiety in a dog.
- Forceful training, training by compulsion, and training that involves physical restraint has no place in modern treatments of aggression. Clients are often told differently. The Association of Pet Dog Trainers (www.apdt.com) certifies pet dog trainers (CPDT) who are trained and skilled in using only positive methods that enhance learning.
- With respect to impulse-control aggression, clients must understand that struggling with the dog will make the dog more dangerous. Treating these dogs is not about being their "master"; it's about treating their anxiety.
- With respect to interdog aggression, clients must understand that the dog that they see being overtly aggressive may not have been the instigator. This is a complicated diagnosis. Quick fixes that are implied by simplistic recommendations ("reinforce the alpha dog") almost always make this condition worse.

SUGGESTED READING

de Keuster T, Lamoureux J, Kahn A: Epidemiology of dog bites: A Belgian experience of canine behaviour and public health concerns. *Vet J* 2005, in press.

Love M, Overall KL: Dogs and children: how anticipating relationships can help avoid disasters. *J Am Vet Med Assoc* 219:446–453, 2001.

Overall KL: Canine behavioral disorders. In Morgan RV (ed): *Handbook of Veterinary Internal Medicine,* ed 4. Philadelphia, Churchill Livingstone, 2003, pp 1149–1162.

Overall KL: Pharmacological treatment in behavioral medicine: the importance of neurochemistry, molecular biology, and mechanistic hypotheses. *Vet J* 62:9–23, 2001.

Overall KL, Love M: Dog bites to humans: demography, epidemiology, and risk. *J Am Vet Med Assoc* 218:1–12, 2001.

Schilder MBH, van der Borg JAM: Training dogs with help of the shock collar: short and long term behavioural effects. *Appl Anim Behav Sci* 85:319–334, 2004.

AUTHOR & EDITOR: **KAREN L. OVERALL**

Alcohol Intoxication (Ethanol, Isopropyl Alcohol, and Methanol)

BASIC INFORMATION

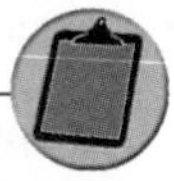

DEFINITION

Acute toxicosis associated with accidental ingestion of alcoholic beverages, alcohol-containing household products such as windshield wiper fluid, or uncooked bread dough and characterized by vomiting, lethargy, ataxia, weakness, coma, and acidosis. Improper dosing or rate of administration of ethanol for ethylene glycol toxicosis can also result in ethanol toxicosis.

SYNONYM(S)

Ethanol: aethanolum grain alcohol, alcohol etílico, alkohol, ethanolum, ethyl alcohol, spiritus

Isopropyl alcohol: isopropol alcohol, alcojel, isohol, rubbing alcohol (70% isopropanol)

Methanol: wood alcohol, Manhattan spirit, colonial spirit

EPIDEMIOLOGY

SPECIES, AGE, SEX

- Dogs more likely to ingest alcoholic beverages or alcohol-containing household products.
- Dogs and cats of both sexes and all breeds and ages are susceptible.

GEOGRAPHY AND SEASONALITY: Toxicosis more likely to occur in winter months (windshield washer fluid) and during holiday season (alcoholic beverages).

CLINICAL PRESENTATION

HISTORY, CHIEF COMPLAINT

- History of exposure to alcohol-containing beverage or household products, or circumstances favoring exposure (e.g., recent social gathering without supervision of the pet).
- Acute vomiting, lethargy, central nervous system (CNS) depression, ataxia, disorientation, vocalization, or excitability.
- In severe cases dyspnea, tremors, seizures, and coma are possible.

PHYSICAL EXAM FINDINGS

- Vomiting, abdominal pain
- Hypotension
- Tachycardia
- CNS depression, ataxia, vocalization, disorientation, or coma
- Dehydration
- Hypothermia

ETIOLOGY AND PATHOPHYSIOLOGY

Source

- Alcohols are transparent, colorless, mobile, volatile liquids composed of a hydrocarbon chain and a hydroxyl group miscible with water, ether, and chloroform.

Pathophysiology

- The basic mechanism of action of alcohols is thought to be due to dissolution of lipid biomembranes affecting ion channels and their proteins, causing a depressant effects on the CNS.
- Ethanol can also augment γ-aminobutyric acid-mediated synaptic inhibition, as well as changes in chloride ions.

DIAGNOSIS

DIFFERENTIAL DIAGNOSIS

- Ethylene glycol intoxication
- Marijuana intoxication
- Uremia
- Diabetic ketoacidosis
- Hepatic encephalopathy
- Primary CNS disease (inflammation, neoplasia, other)

INITIAL DATABASE

- Complete blood count: generally within normal range
- Serum chemistry profile: some electrolyte abnormalities and azotemia possible due to vomiting and dehydration
- Urinalysis: generally unremarkable
- Blood gas analysis may be consistent with metabolic acidosis, often with a high anion gap (>25 mEq/L)
- Serum osmolality: may be increased (osmole gap >20 mOsm/kg); major differential diagnosis is ethylene glycol intoxication
- Electrocardiogram (ECG) may reveal cardiac arrhythmias
- Arterial blood pressure: rule out hypotension

ADVANCED OR CONFIRMATORY TESTING

Serum or blood alcohol levels can be requested from a human hospital to confirm exposure.

TREATMENT

THERAPEUTIC GOAL(S)

- Decontamination
- Supportive care
- Monitor and correct acid-base abnormalities

ACUTE GENERAL TREATMENT

- Decontamination:
  - Emesis: indicated in patients within 30 minutes of exposure if not showing clinical signs of toxicosis. Apomor-phine (0.03-0.04 mg/kg IV or IM, or crush tablet portion with water and instill into conjunctival sac, rinse following emesis) or hydrogen peroxide 3% (2 ml/kg, max 45 ml PO, repeat in 10 to 15 minutes if no vomiting).
  - Activated charcoal (1-3 g/kg mixed with water; give as a slurry). Give if patient is showing no clinical signs or if ingestion is large. If the patient is unconscious, may be administered via gastric tube (see Gastric Intubation, Gavage, Lavage, p 1258). In such cases, use a cuffed endotracheal tube to prevent aspiration, and ensure that a mouth speculum is in place to avoid the patient's chewing and inhaling the endotracheal tube.
- Supportive care:
  - Fluid diuresis. Isotonic fluids if normoglycemia. If hypoglycemia is present, use dextrose containing fluids (e.g., 2.5% dextrose: add 50 ml of 50% dextrose per liter of fluids) and add B vitamins.
  - Mechanical ventilation may be necessary in comatose patients (see Ventilation, Positive Pressure, p 1325).
  - Thermoregulation (judicious rewarming, as with heating pads, for hypothermia).
  - Cardiovascular support: monitor ECG and perfusion. If ventricular arrhythmias are present, check serum potassium and other possible triggers (see Ventricular Arrhythmias [Premature Ventricular Complexes, Ventricular Tachycardia], p 1148; Sinus Bradycardia, p 1005).
  - Yohimbine (0.1 mg/kg IV) or naloxone (0.02-0.04 mg/kg IV) may help to reverse alcohol-induced coma although their efficacy to reverse alcohol-induced coma has not been determined.
- Correct acid-base abnormalities.
  - Correct acidosis if severe (HCO_3^- <12) and persistent despite rehydration and good perfusion. Sodium bicarbonate (1-3 mEq/kg IV as needed).

POSSIBLE COMPLICATIONS

- Aspiration pneumonia
- Renal failure due to myoglobinuria (rare)

RECOMMENDED MONITORING

- Acid-base status
- ECG
- Blood pressure
- Heart rate
- Temperature
- Blood glucose

PROGNOSIS AND OUTCOME

Fair short-term prognosis (risk of complications), good long-term prognosis: recovery expected within 12 to 24 hours with treatment

PEARLS & CONSIDERATIONS

COMMENTS

- Ethanol: minimum lethal dose in humans: adult: 5-6 g/kg in nontolerant adults; pediatric: 3 g/kg (1 ml = 0.789 g).
- Methanol causes blindness and neuronal necrosis in primates. This is not an issue in nonprimates due to differences in methanol metabolism.
- Alcohols are rapidly and completely absorbed from the GI tract (within 30 minutes to 2 hours).
- Isopropanol and methanol persist in circulation longer than ethanol. Methanol and isopropanol generally produce greater CNS depression than ethanol.
- Uncooked bread dough, when ingested by dogs, ferments in the GI tract and produces ethanol, causing signs of drunkenness, and potentially causes foreign body obstruction.

- Windshield washer fluids contain 20–100% ethanol.
- Windshield washer fluid is generally translucent blue, and nonviscous (like water); antifreeze (ethylene glycol, not methanol) is generally fluorescent green and viscous (like light syrup).

PREVENTION

Keep alcoholic beverages and alcohol-containing household products out of the reach of pets

SUGGESTED READING

Valentine WM: Short chain alcohols. In Beasley VR (ed): *Vet Clin North Am Small Anim Pract* 20(2):515–523, 1990.

Hardman JG, Limbird LE: Ethanol. In *Goodman & Gilman's The Pharmacological Basis of Therapeutics,* ed 9. 1996, pp 386–396, 1682.

Poisindex Editorial Staff. Alcohol (Toxicologic Managements). Rumack BH, Hess AJ, Gelman CR. Micromedex, Engelwood, CO.

Spyker DA: Oxygenated compounds: Alcohols, glycols, ketones and esters. In Sullivan JB, Krieger GR (eds): *Hazardous Materials Toxicology.* Philadelphia, Williams & Wilkins, 1992, pp 1105–1108.

AUTHOR: **SHARON L. WELCH**

EDITOR: **SAFDAR A. KHAN**

Alkalosis

BASIC INFORMATION

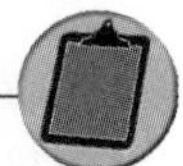

DEFINITION

Metabolic alkalosis is characterized by a primary increase in plasma (HCO_3^-), decreased (H^+), increased pH, and a secondary adaptive partial increase in pCO_2. Respiratory alkalosis results from a primary decrease in pCO_2 in blood (hypocapnia), and this results in a raised pH and a compensatory increase in blood (HCO_3^-).

EPIDEMIOLOGY

RISK FACTORS: Alkalosis is never a primary diagnosis, and many diseases may result in this acid-base abnormality.

ASSOCIATED CONDITIONS AND DISORDERS

- Metabolic alkalosis:
  - Chloride responsive:
    - Vomiting of stomach contents
    - Diuretic drugs
  - Chloride nonresponsive (rare):
    - Hyperadrenocorticism
    - Hyperaldosteronism
  - Alkali administration (oral $NaHCO_3$)
  - Refeeding after fasting
  - High-dose penicillin
  - Severe K^+ or Mg^+ deficiency
- Respiratory alkalosis:
  - Hypoxemia and all its many causes, such as congestive heart failure, severe anemia, hypotension, ventilation-perfusion mismatching (which itself has many causes such as pneumonia, pulmonary embolic disease, and pulmonary edema)
  - Pulmonary disease (such as pneumonia, embolism, edema, acute respiratory distress syndrome)
  - CNS-mediated hyperventilation (liver disease, sepsis, postmetabolic acidosis, primary CNS disease)
  - Heat stroke
  - Eclampsia (alkalosis also worsens the availability of Ca^{++})
  - Mechanical ventilation with inappropriate settings
  - Pain and/or panting

CLINICAL PRESENTATION

DISEASE FORMS/SUBTYPES: Metabolic lkalosis may be chloride responsive (common) or chloride unresponsive. Respiratory alkalosis has no subclassification.

HISTORY, CHIEF COMPLAINT: Variable, depending on the nature of the disease leading to this acid-base disturbance (see the list of possible causes under Associated Conditions and Disorders above).

PHYSICAL EXAM FINDINGS: This is dependent on the nature of the disease leading to this acid-base disturbance (see the list of possible causes under Associated Conditions and Disorders above). The clinical signs of metabolic alkalosis (e.g., weakness, cardiac arrhythmias, altered renal function, ileus) may be attributed to hypokalemia if it is present. Severe alkalosis may result in lowered (Ca^{++}), and this may cause muscle twitching and irritability.

ETIOLOGY AND PATHOPHYSIOLOGY

- Chloride-responsive metabolic alkalosis results from the loss of chloride-rich fluid from the body (such as in gastric vomiting, which results in the loss of Cl^- rich gastric fluid and a loss of extracellular fluid volume). This is followed by vigorous renal reabsorption of Na^+ and Cl^- from the glomerular filtrate. All chloride administered to the chloride-unresponsive group is lost in renal filtrate, and this group of patients has adequate extracellular fluid volume. The chloride-responsive type is more common. For each 1 mEq/L increase in HCO_3^-, an increase of 0.7 mmHg in pCO_2 can be expected in compensation in both dogs and cats.
- Persistent metabolic alkalosis will result in hypokalemia, because in most cases of metabolic alkalosis, there is renal sodium retention, and hypokalemia develops as the kidneys increase Na^+-K^+ exchange. Therefore K^+ loss is not the cause of alkalosis; it is the result of it. K^+ supplementation alone will not correct an alkalosis, KCl supplementation will correct the disturbance because of the Cl^- supplementation.
- Respiratory alkalosis develops when the degree of alveolar ventilation exceeds that required to eliminate the metabolic load of CO_2 produced. Compensation is biphasic. Acute respiratory alkalosis will result in a 2.5 mEq/L drop in HCO_3^- for each 10 mmHg drop in pCO_2. This is true for both dogs and cats. Chronic respiratory alkalosis results in a 5.5 mEq/L drop in HCO_3^- for each 10 mmHg drop in pCO_2. Compensation for respiratory alkalosis usually results in a normal or very near normal blood pH.

DIAGNOSIS

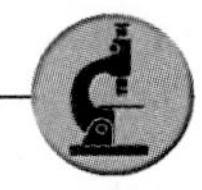

DIFFERENTIAL DIAGNOSIS

Each possible cause of alkalosis as previously listed will have its own differential diagnosis list.

INITIAL DATABASE

- Complete blood count, serum biochemistry panel, urinalysis:
  - Overall, these routine laboratory tests are an essential part of basic evaluation of all systemic disorders that could cause alkalosis.
  - Bicarbonate (HCO_3^-): high (by definition) in alkalosis, unless mixed acid-base disorder (opposing/offsetting disorders) is present.

- ◦ Potassium, chloride, and calcium abnormalities possible, as described previously.

ADVANCED OR CONFIRMATORY TESTING

Alkalosis may be defined on a routine serum biochemistry panel (elevated [TCO_2]). Arterial blood gas analysis is necessary to define an alkalosis as metabolic or respiratory. Also, it is necessary to measure serum electrolytes for complete evaluation of this acid-base disturbance. Because respiratory alkalosis is frequently associated with respiratory disease, investigations should focus on pulmonary disease (possibly including such techniques as thoracic imaging and airway endoscopy and sample collection).

TREATMENT

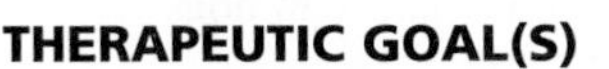

THERAPEUTIC GOAL(S)

- The goal of treatment in chloride-responsive metabolic alkalosis is to provide sufficient Cl^- to replace the deficit, while supplementing K^+ and Na^+. K^+ supplementation without correcting Cl^- deficits will not resolve the alkalosis. The permanent solution to the problem will involve resolution of the precipitating cause (e.g., resolving the cause of gastric vomiting). Chloride-resistant alkalosis is rare in veterinary medicine and requires resolution of the underlying disease process for correction of the acid-base abnormality.
- A point to remember: giving oxygen to patients that are hypoxemic with metabolic alkalosis may aggravate hypercapnia, because the increased pO_2 lessens the drive on ventilation.

ACUTE GENERAL TREATMENT

The intravenous fluid of choice in the treatment of patients with chloride responsive metabolic alkalosis is 0.9% NaCl (normal saline) with added KCl. It is important to supplement K^+, because most patients with metabolic alkalosis will have been sick long enough to be K^+-depleted, and a K^+ deficit will not correct on its own even if the acid-base balance corrects. In fact, saline-induced diuresis may worsen K^+ deficiency. Some have recommended the use of rebreathing bags (such as a paper bag over the patient's muzzle) to encourage the rise of pCO_2 in acute cases of respiratory alkalosis such as that seen with eclampsia; however, one should beware of hyperthermia in this setting.

CHRONIC TREATMENT

- Fluid therapy may be required for several days to correct all deficits. In cases in which the loss of gastric fluid has induced metabolic alkalosis, gastric acid secretion may be reduced by treatment with a proton pump inhibitor or H_2-blocker drug. Patients with congestive heart failure receiving loop diuretics to control pulmonary edema may require oral KCl supplementation to lessen or prevent metabolic alkalosis.
- Treatment of respiratory alkalosis requires correction of the underlying causes of hypocapnia.

POSSIBLE COMPLICATIONS

Patients with chronic pulmonary disease and chronic hypercapnea are at greater risk of metabolic alkalosis than others because superimposition of metabolic alkalosis on the chronic lung disorder can further reduce ventilation and lead to worsened hypoxemia. The clinician should avoid giving oxygen to animals with metabolic alkalosis if possible, because this may reduce alveolar ventilation and aggravate hypoxemia.

PROGNOSIS AND OUTCOME

Dependent on the underlying disease process

PEARLS & CONSIDERATIONS

COMMENTS

- Almost all critically ill patients will have an acid-base abnormality, but few require intervention beyond treatment of the inciting cause.
- Venous or arterial blood samples are adequate for measuring pH, pCO_2, and HCO_3^-, but only arterial samples can be used for pO_2 (PaO_2) measurement.
- Patients with chronic pulmonary disease that have hypoxemia and hypercapnia are at risk for developing metabolic alkalosis (usually because of diuretic use) and, if metabolic alkalosis develops, this may can further reduce ventilation and worsen hypoxemia. Therefore, metabolic alkalosis should not be overlooked if the patient has a chronic lung disease.
- Chronic respiratory alkalosis may present with a normal pH, because compensation may be complete.
- Animals can have serious acid-base abnormalities with normal blood pH ("mixed acid-base disorders").
- Mixed disorders should be suspected if:
  - ◦ pCO_2 and HCO_3^- change in opposite directions
  - ◦ pH is normal with an abnormal pCO_2 and/or HCO_3^-
  - ◦ pH changes in a direction opposite to what is expected for the primary disorder
- One type of mixed acid-base disorder, respiratory alkalosis with metabolic acidosis, (neutralizing pH abnormalities) may occur in conditions such as septic shock, gastric dilation-volvulus (GDV), liver disease, and cardiopulmonary resuscitation.
- The development of respiratory alkalosis in an animal with metabolic acidosis may indicate the development of septicemia.
- Respiratory acidosis may occur together with metabolic alkalosis in cases of pulmonary edema treated with diuretics, and in cases of GDV.
- Mixed metabolic alkalosis with metabolic acidosis is usually seen in animals with long-standing high anion gap acidosis (such as with renal failure) that begin vomiting and develop hypochloremia as a result. Alternatively, this mixed disturbance may begin as a metabolic alkalosis followed by the development of severe volume depletion and lactic acidosis. Recognition of this mixture of disorders is important because treatment of the one imbalance allows the other to emerge unopposed.
- Respiratory alkalosis may occur together with metabolic alkalosis and may develop in dogs with chronic respiratory disease that are receiving diuretics. Sudden ventilation of dogs with established respiratory acidosis may acutely drop pCO_2 in a dog that has established compensatory increased (HCO_3^-), and this can lead to severe alkalemia.

PREVENTION

Clinicians should be aware of the conditions that may lead to alkalosis and the treatments that may precipitate metabolic alkalosis particularly. The timely supplementation of chloride may prevent this.

SUGGESTED READING

DiBartola SP, de Morais HA: Acid-base disorders. In DiBartola SP (ed): *Fluid Therapy in Small Animal Practice*, ed 2. Philadelphia, WB Saunders, 2000, pp 189–264.

AUTHOR: **ANDREW LEISEWITZ**
EDITOR: **ELIZABETH ROZANSKI**

Alopecia

BASIC INFORMATION

DEFINITION

- Complete or partial loss of hair in areas where it is normally present
- May be localized, multifocal, or generalized

SYNONYM(S)

Excessive shedding
Hair loss
Hypotrichosis

EPIDEMIOLOGY

SPECIES, AGE, SEX: Depends on underlying cause.

GENETICS AND BREED PREDISPOSITION
Breed predisposition for several causes of alopecia:
- Color dilution alopecia: Doberman pinscher, many other breeds
- Recurrent seasonal flank alopecia: boxer, bulldog, Airedale terrier
- Alopecia X/adrenal reproductive hormone imbalance: Pomeranian, chow chow, keeshond and other plush-coated breeds, Arctic breeds (e.g., Samoyed, Alaskan malamute, Siberian husky), as well as miniature poodles

CONTAGION AND ZOONOSIS: Dermatophytosis should be considered when patchy or focal alopecia is present.

GEOGRAPHY AND SEASONALITY: Recurrent seasonal flank alopecia may be present for several months each year.

ASSOCIATED CONDITIONS AND DISORDERS
- Hypothyroidism: other clinical signs associated with thyroid hormone deficiency
- Hyperadrenocorticism: other clinical signs associated with cortisol excess
- Sertoli cell tumor: male feminization
- Bacterial pyoderma or *Malassezia* dermatitis, often associated with underlying hypersensitivity dermatitis (atopy, dermatologic adverse food reaction)

CLINICAL PRESENTATION

HISTORY, CHIEF COMPLAINT
- Progressive loss of hair from one or more areas of the body
- May be associated with pruritus
- Onset and progression are variable
- Clinical signs other than hair loss may be present (e.g., polyuria/polydipsia, lethargy)

PHYSICAL EXAM FINDINGS
- Is alopecia diffuse or localized/multifocal?
- Is the hair absent or broken off near the skin surface (e.g., feline symmetric alopecia)?
- Does hair epilate easily?
- Is there evidence of skin inflammation (e.g., erythema or crusting)?
- Is there any evidence to support endocrine disease (e.g., muscle atrophy, pendulous abdomen, obesity)?

ETIOLOGY AND PATHOPHYSIOLOGY

Loss of hair may be due to different processes, depending on the underlying cause:
- New hair failing to grow when old hairs are lost (often endocrine disease)
- Inflammation in hair follicles leading to hair loss (infectious folliculitis: bacteria, dermatophyte, *Demodex*)
- Breakage of hair due to trauma (e.g., feline symmetric alopecia associated with excessive grooming)
- Other causes include structural defects (e.g., color dilution alopecia), ischemia (e.g., postvaccinal vasculitis), or hair loss secondary to sebaceous adenitis

DIAGNOSIS

DIFFERENTIAL DIAGNOSIS

- Symmetric/diffuse with minimal inflammation:
  - Hyperadrenocorticism (including iatrogenic form caused by systemic or topical corticosteroids)
  - Hypothyroidism
  - Alopecia X/adrenal reproductive hormone imbalance
  - Seasonal flank alopecia
  - Feline symmetric alopecia (usually self-induced due to pruritus)
  - Postclipping alopecia
  - Pattern baldness
  - Follicular dysplasia (including black hair follicular dysplasia)
  - Alopecia secondary to testicular neoplasia
  - Other sex hormone dermatoses
  - Feline paraneoplastic alopecia
- Symmetric/diffuse with inflammation:
  - Sebaceous adenitis
  - Color dilution alopecia
- Localized or multifocal:
  - Bacterial (staphylococcal folliculitis): most common cause in dogs
  - Demodicosis
  - Dermatophytosis
  - *Malassezia* dermatitis
  - Immune-mediated diseases (including hypersensitivity dermatitis)
  - Less common: cutaneous lymphoma, alopecia areata, vaccine-induced ischemia

INITIAL DATABASE

- Symmetric/diffuse alopecia with minimal inflammation:
  - Minimum database: complete blood count, chemistry profile, urinalysis
  - Thyroid analysis
  - Trichography (microscopic examination of hair follicles) (e.g., "barbered" hairs in cats grooming excessively)
- Localized, multifocal, or inflammatory alopecia:
  - Skin scrapings

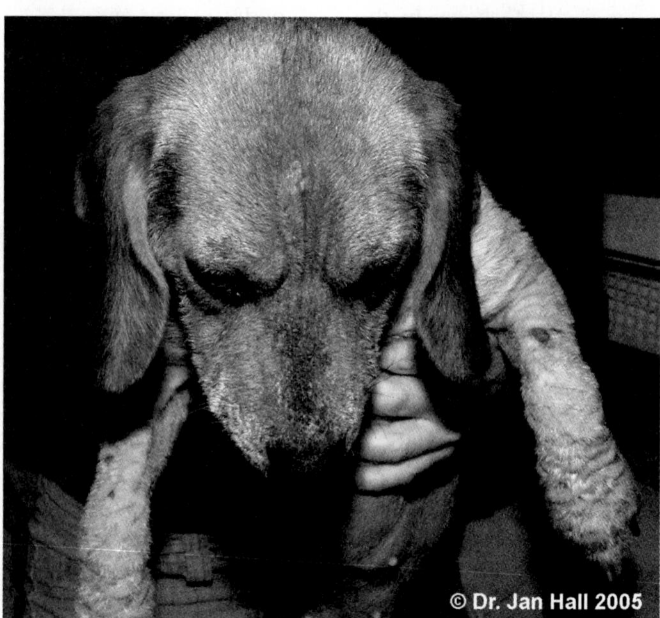

FIGURE I-9 Alopecia associated with demodicosis in a puppy. Courtesy of Dr. Jan A. Hall.

- Wood's light examination and fungal culture for dermatophytes
- Skin cytologic examination for bacteria and *Malassezia*
- Trichography

ADVANCED OR CONFIRMATORY TESTING

- Symmetric/diffuse alopecia with minimal inflammation:
  - Skin biopsy
  - ACTH stimulation or low-dose dexamethasone suppression test
  - Adrenal reproductive hormone panel
  - Abdominal radiography/ultrasonography
- Localized, multifocal, or inflammatory alopecia:
  - Skin biopsy
  - Response to therapy in dogs if bacterial folliculitis is suspected (e.g., minimum 3 weeks of cephalexin 22 mg/kg PO q 12h, with the exact duration depending on response)

TREATMENT

THERAPEUTIC GOAL(S)

Correct underlying cause of alopecia

CHRONIC TREATMENT

Variable, depending on cause

RECOMMENDED MONITORING

Variable, depending on underlying cause

PROGNOSIS AND OUTCOME

- The prognosis for alopecia in most cases is good if the underlying cause of hair loss is identified and treated.
- Extensive scarring limits hair regrowth.

PEARLS & CONSIDERATIONS

COMMENTS

- Cats with feline symmetric alopecia often lose hair due to excessive grooming associated with pruritus. Owners do not always observe excessive grooming.
- In dogs, multifocal alopecia with variable or intermittent pruritus and inflammation is most commonly caused by bacterial folliculitis. Treat appropriately for bacterial folliculitis then reevaluate.
- Dermatophytosis is a common cause of alopecia in cats. Always consider and test for dermatophytosis when multifocal or localized alopecia is noted.
- Alopecia X/adrenal reproductive hormone imbalance should always be considered in healthy plush-coated or Arctic breed dogs exhibiting truncal alopecia.
- Melatonin 3-6 mg PO q 12h for 3 to 4 months is a safe and variably effective supplement to stimulate hair regrowth in the treatment of recurrent seasonal flank alopecia and alopecia X (see Alopecia X, p 53).

SUGGESTED READING

Frank LA, et al: Retrospective evaluation of sex hormones and steroid hormone intermediates in dogs with alopecia. *Vet Dermatol* 14:91-97, 2003.

Paradis M: Melatonin therapy in canine alopecia. In Bonagura J (ed): *Current Veterinary Therapy XIII*. Philadelphia, WB Saunders, 2000, pp 546-549.

AUTHOR: **KINGA GORTEL**

EDITOR: **JAN A. HALL**

Alopecia X

BASIC INFORMATION

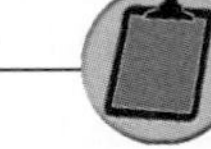

DEFINITION

Acquired, progressive, noninflammatory alopecia of unknown etiology seen typically in plush-coated type dogs and in miniature poodles. A myriad of names—etiopathogeneses, diagnostic procedures, and therapeutic modalities—has been proposed with varied validity and outcome.

SYNONYM(S)

Adrenal sex hormone imbalance
Black skin disease of Pomeranians
Castration-responsive dermatosis
Coat funk in Alaskan malamutes
Congenital adrenal hyperplasia-like-syndrome
Follicular dysplasia of Nordic breeds
Follicular growth dysfunction of plush-coated breeds
Growth hormone-responsive alopecia
Hyposomatotropism of the adult dog
Lysodren-responsive dermatosis
Pseudo-Cushing's

EPIDEMIOLOGY

SPECIES, AGE, SEX

- Male and female adult dogs
- Regardless of neuter status
- Typically 2 to 5 years old
- Breeds at greater risk include Pomeranian, chow chow, keeshond, Samoyed, Alaskan malamute, Siberian husky, and miniature poodle

CLINICAL PRESENTATION

HISTORY, CHIEF COMPLAINT

- Partial to complete alopecia of the ventrum, perineum, caudal aspect of thighs, tail and tail base, around the neck, and ultimately the trunk, sparing the head and forelimbs.
- Marked hyperpigmentation is common.
- Occasionally, seborrhea and superficial pyoderma are noted.

PHYSICAL EXAM FINDINGS: No systemic signs of illness.

ETIOLOGY AND PATHOPHYSIOLOGY

- Etiopathogenesis of this condition is not known.
- Previous hypotheses such as growth hormone deficiency or hydroxylase-21 abnormality have been abandoned.
- Current popular hypotheses include:
  - Genetic predisposition to a nonidentified hormonal imbalance and/or a change in receptor sensitivity at the hair follicle level
  - Primary disorder of hair growth cycle
  - Mild but prolonged increase of basal cortisolemia

DIAGNOSIS

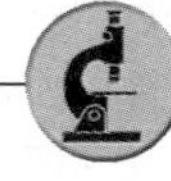

DIFFERENTIAL DIAGNOSIS

- Hypothyroidism
- Hyperadrenocorticism
- Functional gonadal neoplasm
- Sebaceous adenitis
- Telogen defluxion
- Other follicular dysplasias

INITIAL DATABASE

- History and physical examination findings
- Ruling out other differentials

ADVANCED OR CONFIRMATORY TESTING

- Dermatohistopathology: reveals nonspecific changes of endocrinopathy.
- Excessive trichilemmal keratinization (flame follicles), seen in many but not all cases, is suggestive of this disorder.
- Sex hormone panels (baseline and post-adrenocorticotropic hormone stimulation) have been recommended but usefulness has recently been questioned.

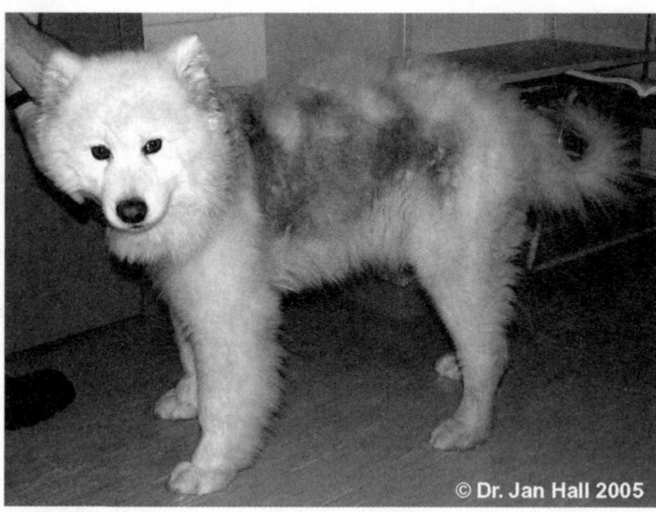

FIGURE I-10 Alopecia X in a Samoyed dog. Courtesy of Dr. Jan A. Hall.

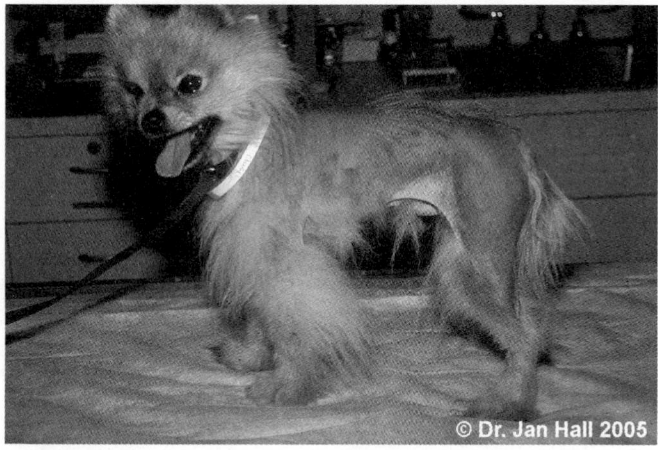

FIGURE I-11 Alopecia X in a 4-year-old, male castrate, Pomeranian. Note that characteristically, the head and all four legs are not affected. Courtesy of Dr. Jan A. Hall

TREATMENT

THERAPEUTIC GOAL(S)

- The therapeutic approach is highly empiric.
- Castration or ovariohysterectomy in an intact animal. A normal haircoat may regrow in 50–75% of cases. Many affected dogs were sterilized long before the first clinical signs were noted.
- Currently recommended therapeutic modalities include:
  - Melatonin (3–6 mg PO q 8–12h for 3 to 4 months) is effective in 30–60% of the cases.
  - Mitotane (25 mg/kg q 24h or 25–50 mg/kg two to three times weekly has been suggested) is effective in ~50% of cases. However, the risk of side effects (e.g., hypoadrenocorticism) should be carefully considered, and close monitoring is essential.
  - Trilostane, given at a mean daily dose of ~11 mg/kg (range ~6–23 mg/kg/day) was recently reported to promote hair regrowth in 90% of treated Pomeranians and miniature poodles.

PROGNOSIS AND OUTCOME

- Alopecia X is a purely cosmetic disorder. Benign neglect without any treatment is therefore a valid option.
- The progression of hair loss is variable. Some dogs will retain hair (puppy coat appearance) on the trunk for years; others become completely alopecic over the trunk within months.
- Hair regrowth is not predictable with any of the current therapies and may not last lifelong.

PEARLS & CONSIDERATIONS

COMMENTS

Affected dogs may regrow hair at the site of skin biopsy or other external traumatic stimuli (skin scraping, sunburn, etc.)

SUGGESTED READING

Cerundolo R, et al: Treatment of canine alopecia X with trilostane. *Vet Dermatol* 15:285–293, 2004.

Frank LA: Growth hormone-responsive alopecia in dogs. *J Am Vet Med Assoc* 226:1494–1497, 2005.

Frank LA, Hnilica KA, Rohrbach BW, Oliver JW: Retrospective evaluation of sex hormones and steroid hormone intermediates in dogs with alopecia. *Vet Dermatol* 4:91–97, 2003.

Frank LA, et al: Adrenal steroid hormone concentrations in dogs with hair cycle arrest (alopecia X) before and during treatment with melatonin and mitotane. *Vet Dermatol* 15:278, 2004.

AUTHOR: **MANON PARADIS**
EDITOR: **JAN A. HALL**

Amitraz Toxicosis

BASIC INFORMATION

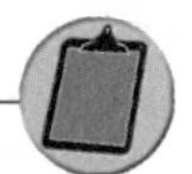

DEFINITION

- Amitraz, a formamidine pesticide, is used as an orchard spray to control many pests. As a potent acaracide, it is used in dogs for the treatment of demodicosis; use for treating demodicosis may be decreasing due to the availability of alternatives with fewer potential side effects. Amitraz-containing collars for control of ticks remain popular, because they have been shown to prevent transmission of tick-borne Lyme disease.
- Toxicosis occurs mostly in dogs from dermal or oral exposure of amitraz-containing products and is characterized by

depression, ataxia, bradycardia or tachycardia, hypotension, hypothermia, gastrointestinal (GI) stasis, and mydriasis.

SYNONYM(S)

Some amitraz-containing products are:

- Mitaban 19.9% topical solution for dilution in 10.6 ml bottle (each ml Mitaban contains 199 mg/ml of amitraz)
- Preventic Tick collar (9% amitraz) weighs approximately 27.5 g and is 25 inches (65 cm) long (99 mg of amitraz/inch of collar)
- Taktic 12.5% concentrated solution for dilution and topical application to swine, dairy or beef cattle in 760 ml cans (extralabel use by some small-animal veterinarians)

EPIDEMIOLOGY

SPECIES, AGE, SEX

- Cats are extremely sensitive.
- Toy or small breeds, debilitated or geriatric animals are more prone to adverse neurologic effects (sedation, ataxia); dosage adjustment or use of other treatments instead of amitraz is advised for these animals when treating demodicosis.
- Safety not determined in dogs <4 months old.
- Safety in pregnant animals not tested. Use as a last resort only when benefits outweigh risks.

RISK FACTORS

- Amitraz has α-2 adrenergic properties; concurrent use of other medications possessing α-2 adrenergic properties (xylazine) may worsen hypotension.
- Amitraz is a minor monoamine oxidase inhibitor (MAOI); concurrent use of other MAOI (selegiline) or tricyclic antidepressants (clomipramine, amitriptyline) not recommended.
- Amitraz can cause a marked increase in plasma glucose level by inhibiting insulin release. Use with caution in diabetic patients.
- Do not use if animal has deep pyodermas with draining tracts; damaged skin may allow enhanced amitraz absorption.

CLINICAL PRESENTATION

HISTORY, CHIEF COMPLAINT

- Use of amitraz-containing dips
- Pieces or whole amitraz-containing tick collar missing
- Transient, mild depression lasting 24 to 72 hours after topical use of amitraz is common. Conversely, toxicosis involves progression of signs such as marked depression with bradycardia, slowed peristalsis
- Ataxia

PHYSICAL EXAM FINDINGS

- Heart rate: bradycardia common (often less than 50 bpm)
- Ataxia
- Vomiting
- Body temperature (below normal)
- GI motility (absent or stasis)
- Signs of hypotension

ETIOLOGY AND PATHOPHYSIOLOGY

- Exact mechanism in mammals unknown. Amitraz possesses α-2 adrenergic properties, which results in stimulation of presynaptic and postsynaptic α-2 adrenergic receptors leading to hypotension, depression, and ataxia.
- Amitraz is also a weak inhibitor of MAO activity.
- Amitraz can cause hyperglycemia by inhibiting insulin release.
- Rapidly absorbed orally and dermally; peak blood levels in dogs in 3 hours.
- Quickly metabolized in liver; excreted through urine (78%) and feces (9%).

DIAGNOSIS

DIFFERENTIAL DIAGNOSIS

- Ivermectin toxicosis
- Macadamia nuts toxicosis
- Marijuana toxicosis

INITIAL DATABASE

- Arterial blood pressure: hypotension common
- Blood glucose: hyperglycemia common
- Serum chemistry profile: hyperglycemia common
- Abdominal radiographs: pieces of collar, evidence of ileus
- CBC: generally without significant changes
- Urinalysis: generally without significant changes

ADVANCED OR CONFIRMATORY TESTING

- If amitraz is the suspected agent, can evaluate response to therapeutic dose of yohimbine or atipamezole (doses: see below)
- Amitraz is detectable in stomach contents, urine, and feces; generally only for preventive, academic, or legal concerns (turnaround time likely too long to affect immediate management)

TREATMENT

THERAPEUTIC GOAL(S)

- Decontamination
- Use specific α-2 antagonist
- Supportive care

ACUTE GENERAL TREATMENT

- Use specific α-2 antagonists:
  - Yohimbine 0.1–0.2 mg/kg IV in dogs. Repeat in 1 to 3 hours as needed; or
  - Atipamezole (Antisedan) 50 μg/kg (0.05 mg/kg) IM in dogs (effect is gradual [up to 20 minutes]).
- Decontamination of patient:
  - All cases:
    - Dermal exposure: bathe, using diluted dishwashing liquid; dry off and keep warm.
  - If known inappropriate exposure (e.g., ate amitraz collar) but not showing clinical signs:
    - Emesis: apomorphine (0.03–0.04 mg/kg IV or IM, or crush tablet portion with water and instill into conjunctival sac, rinse out after emesis) or hydrogen peroxide 3% (2 ml/kg, max 45 ml PO, repeat in 10 to 15 minutes if no vomiting). Successful emesis is more likely if food is present in the stomach.
    - Whole wheat bread to add bulk to diet, accelerating passage of collar through GI system.
    - Activated charcoal: not very effective in binding amitraz; several sources recommend it. 1–3 g/kg PO; give labeled dose for commercial preparations.
  - If known inappropriate exposure (e.g., ate amitraz collar) and moderate or severe clinical signs:
    - Gastric lavage or endoscopy may help remove pieces of collars from the stomach.
    - If clinical signs are controlled by α-2 antagonist drug, consider emesis induction.
    - Warm water enema may accelerate elimination of pieces of collar.
    - Surgery; last resort to remove pieces of collars.
- Supportive care:
  - IV fluids as necessary based on hydration, perfusion, and electrolyte status.
  - Thermoregulation (e.g., heating pads).
  - Diazepam 0.5–2 mg/kg IV for seizures.

POSSIBLE COMPLICATIONS

Paralytic ileus

RECOMMENDED MONITORING

- Heart rate
- Blood pressure
- Body temperature
- Blood glucose
- Central nervous system status

PROGNOSIS AND OUTCOME

- Good with prompt treatment
- Poor if comatose, seizures, moribund, or complete ileus

PEARLS & CONSIDERATIONS

COMMENTS

- Avoid atropine, glycopyrrolate, or any other drug with anticholinergic effects when treating bradycardia. Use an α-2 receptor antagonist like yohimbine or atipamezole (see Acute General Treatment above).
- Clinical signs of toxicosis can continue, because pieces of collars are still in the GI tract.
- Collars are not generally radiopaque, but may be suspected on abdominal radiographs if ingested with metal buckle.

PREVENTION

- Make amitraz dilutions according to label directions
- Use well-fitted collars to avoid being pulled off and ingested
- Monitor condition of tick collars, especially in multi-dog households; do not use collars on dogs who are likely to chew on each other

SUGGESTED READING

Gwaltney-Brant S: Amitraz. In Plumlee KA (ed): *Clinical Veterinary Toxicology*. St. Louis, Mosby, 2003, pp 177–178.

Extension Toxicology Network: http://extoxnet.orst.edu.

AUTHOR: **MARY M. SCHELL**

EDITOR: **SAFDAR A. KHAN**

Amphetamine Toxicosis

BASIC INFORMATION

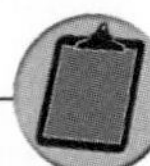

DEFINITION

Intoxication due to ingestion of human stimulant drugs in the amphetamine class (prescribed, or obtained illicitly)

SYNONYM(S)

Commonly encountered amphetamines or related drugs are benzphetamine, dextroamphetamine (Dexedrine), methamphetamine, dextroamphetamine, pemoline, methylphenidate (Ritalin), phentermine, diethylpropion, phendimetrazine, and phenmetrazine.

Street names: speed, bennies, uppers. Commonly used adulterants are caffeine, ephedrine, or phenylpropanolamine, and these substances may enhance the effects of amphetamines.

EPIDEMIOLOGY

SPECIES, AGE, SEX

- Any species; dogs more likely due to indiscriminate eating habits
- Geriatric patients and animals with preexisting seizure disorders or cardiovascular disease: higher risk for life-threatening intoxication

RISK FACTORS: Availability of amphetamines (prescription or illicit) in the pet's environment.

CLINICAL PRESENTATION

HISTORY, CHIEF COMPLAINT

- History of exposure to amphetamines.
- Acute onset of restlessness, hyperactivity, panting, tremors, shaking, or seizures. Onset generally 2 to 4 hours postingestion, slightly longer if sustained-release preparation.
- Ataxia, weakness, circling, and collapse possible.
- Sudden death is possible.
- Signs generally last >12 hours and up to 48 hours with sustained-release pharmaceutical formulations.

PHYSICAL EXAM FINDINGS

- Restlessness, hyperactivity
- Tachypnea
- Mydriasis (bilateral)
- Hyperthemia (104–106°F)
- Cardiac arrhythmias, tachycardia, systemic hypertension
- Tremors, shaking, circling, seizures
- Collapse

ETIOLOGY AND PATHOPHYSIOLOGY

- Amphetamines are sympathomimetic amines that cause central nervous system (CNS) and cardiovascular stimulation.
  - Commonly used in humans for suppression of appetite, narcolepsy, attention deficit disorder, Parkinsonism, and some behavior disorders
- Mechanism of action.
  - Medullary respiratory center and reticular activating system stimulation
  - Stimulation of release of norepinephrine from stores in adrenergic nerve terminals, and direct stimulation of α- and β-adrenergic receptors. Increase in amount of catecholamine at nerve endings is via increased release and inhibition of reuptake and metabolism
  - Amphetamines also increase presynaptic release of serotonin
- Rapid oral absorption (peak plasma levels 1 to 5 hours postingestion).

DIAGNOSIS

DIFFERENTIAL DIAGNOSIS

- Other forms of toxicosis: methylxanthines (e.g., chocolate), pseudoephedrine, zinc phosphide, nicotine, metaldehyde, other illicit drugs (e.g., cocaine)
- Other seizure disorders (see Seizures, p 990)

INITIAL DATABASE

- Electrocardiogram (ECG): sinus tachycardia, ventricular arrhythmias
- Serum electrolytes: hypokalemia may be present
- Blood gas analysis: metabolic acidosis.
- Blood pressure: hypertension
- Urinalysis: myoglobinuria due to rhabdomyolysis

ADVANCED OR CONFIRMATORY TESTING

- Amphetamines can be detected readily in the urine or stomach contents (difficult in plasma unless large exposure) by human hospital laboratories. Call for instructions before submitting samples.
- Several over-the-counter illicit drug kits (available in pharmacies) are available for screening illicit drugs, including amphetamines. These kits are quick, fairly reliable, and relatively inexpensive.
- Necropsy samples: gastric contents, urine, plasma.

TREATMENT

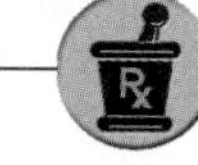

THERAPEUTIC GOAL(S)

- Treat life-threatening CNS and cardiovascular signs
- Decontamination of patient
- Enhance excretion of amphetamines
- Supportive care

ACUTE GENERAL TREATMENT

- Treat life-threatening CNS and cardiovascular signs:
  - For severe agitation: Acepromazine 0.05–1 mg/kg IV or IM, beginning at 0.05 mg/kg and repeating as needed; doses as high as 1 mg/kg are sometimes needed with extreme agitation; chlorpromazine 0.5–4.4 mg/kg IV q 6–24h.
  - For seizures: diazepam (0.5–2 mg/kg IV) or barbiturates (pentobarbital

3-20 mg/kg IV to effect) with caution. Use inhalant anesthesia such as isoflurane if other methods ineffective.
  - Cyproheptadine (1.1 mg/kg PO or can mix with saline and give per rectum) for serotonin syndrome (hyperthermia, CNS signs).
  - For tachycardia and serotonin syndrome: propranolol (0.02-0.06 mg/kg IV; start low and titrate up as needed).
- Decontamination of patient:
  - Emesis: effective within a couple of hours after exposure; use only in patients not showing clinical signs; 3% hydrogen peroxide (1 tsp/5 kg of body weight); repeat once if needed. Apomorphine, dogs 0.03 mg/kg IV or 0.04 mg/kg IM; the use of apomorphine is controversial in cats; dose for cats is 0.04 mg/kg IV or 0.08 mg/kg IM or SC). Alternatively, crush a portion of an apomorphine tablet, mix with sterile water, and place a few drops in the conjunctival sac. Rinse eye after successful emesis. Xylazine can be used as an emetic in cats at 0.44 mg/kg IM (reverse with yohimbine 0.1 mg/kg IV).
  - Gastric lavage only if a very large dose has been ingested and emesis cannot be induced (e.g., comatose animal).
  - Activated charcoal 1-4 g/kg PO. Protect airway with cuffed endotracheal tube if patient is unconscious.
  - Enhance excretion of amphetamines:
    - Acidify urine to 4.5-5.5 pH with ammonium chloride 25-50 mg/kg PO q 6h, or ascorbic acid 20-30 mg/kg PO, SC, or IM to hasten elimination. Note: Monitor acid-base status while acidifying urine.
    - Fluid diuresis.
  - Supportive care:
    - Thermoregulation (fans, cool-water bath).
    - Minimize sensory stimuli.

DRUG INTERACTIONS

Other CNS stimulants (e.g., phenylpropanolamine)

POSSIBLE COMPLICATIONS

- Hemodynamic complications such as disseminated intravascular coagulation secondary to severe hyperthermia
- Rhabdomyolysis, secondary renal damage

RECOMMENDED MONITORING

- Heart rate, ECG
- Blood pressure
- Central nervous system
- Temperature
- Electrolytes
- Acid-base status
- Urinalysis

PROGNOSIS AND OUTCOME

- Presence of severe hyperthermia (> 106°F), tachycardia, or seizures: guarded to poor prognosis
- Good prognosis with mild CNS and cardiovascular signs

PEARLS & CONSIDERATIONS

COMMENTS

- LD50 in dogs: methamphetamine 11 mg/kg PO; amphetamine sulfate 20-27 mg/kg PO
- Clinical signs of toxicosis can be seen with methylphenidate (Ritalin) at about 1 mg/kg
- Minimum lethal dose for most amphetamines: 10-23 mg/kg

SUGGESTED READING

Beasley VR: *Amphetamines. A Systemic Approach to Toxicology*. 1997, pp 133-134.
Gilman AG, Goodman LS, Gilman A (eds): *The Pharmacological Basis of Therapeutics*, ed 6. New York, Macmillan, pp 159-163.
Hautekeete LA: A retrospective study of pemoline toxicosis in dogs: 101 cases. *J Vet Emerg Crit Care* 203-207, 1999.
Khan S: Amphetamines and related drugs. In *Merck Veterinary Manual,* ed 9. Whitehouse Station, NJ, Merck & Co., 2005, pp 2539-2540.
Plumb DC: *Veterinary Drug Handbook*, ed 5. Ames, IA, Iowa State University Press, 2005.

AUTHOR: **SHARON L. WELCH**
EDITOR: **SAFDAR A. KHAN**

Amyloidosis

BASIC INFORMATION

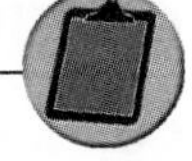

DEFINITION

- Pathologic deposition of polymerized proteins in a β-pleated sheet conformation in various organs, particularly the kidneys
- *Reactive* or *secondary* amyloidosis: associated with/secondary to chronic systemic inflammation

SYNONYM(S)

Amyloidosis in shar-peis (see Shar-Pei Fever, p 998):
- Familial Mediterranean fever
- Swollen hock syndrome

EPIDEMIOLOGY

SPECIES, AGE, SEX: Uncommon in dogs; rare in cats. Usually middle-aged to older dogs and cats, but shar-pei dogs may present at a younger age.

GENETICS AND BREED PREDISPOSITION
- Dogs: shar-pei (renal and hepatic amyloidosis); any breed may be affected by reactive form
- Cats: Abyssinians (renal amyloidosis), Siamese/Oriental cats (systemic amyloidosis)

RISK FACTORS: Chronic inflammatory and infectious disease may predispose to reactive amyloidosis.

ASSOCIATED CONDITIONS AND DISORDERS
- Protein-losing nephropathy (PLN)
- Nephrotic syndrome
- Chronic renal failure
- Thromboembolic disease
- Other organ dysfunction depends on sites of amyloid deposition

CLINICAL PRESENTATION

DISEASE FORMS/SUBTYPES
- Dogs: glomerular deposition with progressive protein-losing nephropathy (PLN) and renal failure
  - Non-shar-pei dogs: Reactive amyloidosis usually causes PLN before azotemic renal failure.
  - Shar-peis: Glomerular and/or medullary deposition with variable proteinuria; renal failure may precede PLN. History may include intermittent fever and inflammatory nonerosive polyarthritis. Hepatic amyloidosis with or without renal amyloidosis may also occur.
- Cats: amyloid deposition without clinical signs most common, but still rare
  - Abyssinians: Glomerular and/or medullary deposition with variable degrees of proteinuria; renal failure may develop without PLN.

- Siamese/Oriental cats: systemic amyloid deposition with clinical signs dependent on organs affected.

HISTORY, CHIEF COMPLAINT

- Early stages of disease: no clinical signs.
  - Exception: with reactive amyloidosis, a chronic infection/inflammatory process may cause overt signs, while amyloid deposition occurs concurrently but "silently."
- As amyloidosis progresses, complications of nephrotic syndrome (e.g., edema/ascites), hypercoagulability (e.g., pulmonary thromboembolism), or renal failure (e.g., polyuria/polydipsia, uremia) develop.
- Shar-peis may be intermittently febrile or lame.
- Siamese or Oriental cats may present with life-threatening intra-abdominal hemorrhage due to liver lobe fracture.

PHYSICAL EXAM FINDINGS

- Often unremarkable
- Ascites or peripheral edema (see Nephrotic Syndrome, p 749)
- Mild enlargement of involved organs may be present
- Shar-peis may be febrile and have joint effusion and/or arthralgia; distal joints most commonly affected

ETIOLOGY AND PATHOPHYSIOLOGY

- Proteins with β-pleated sheet conformation accumulate within extracellular spaces, leading to organ dysfunction.
  - Accumulation within glomeruli common in dogs, leading to proteinuria followed by renal failure.
  - Renal medulla, liver, or systemic deposition may occur.
  - Evidence suggests a dysregulated inflammatory respose leads to amyloid deposition.
- *Reactive amyloidosis* is most common.
  - Deposited protein is amyloid protein A, a fragment of serum amyloid A (SAA).
  - SAA increases secondary to inflammatory diseases.
- *Immunoglobulin light chain-associated amyloidosis* is much rarer.
  - Associated with monoclonal gammopathy (e.g., multiple myeloma, some lymphomas).

DIAGNOSIS

DIFFERENTIAL DIAGNOSIS

See Protein-Losing Nephropathy, p 900; Proteinuria, p 1400

INITIAL DATABASE

- Complete blood count: usually unremarkable
- Chemistry profile: changes of Nephrotic Syndrome, p 749 and/or Chronic Renal Failure, Occult ["Asymptomatic"], p 204; Chronic Renal Failure, Overt ["Symptomatic"], p 205. Azotemia often mild or absent at presentation except in shar-pei dogs and cats
- Urinalysis: proteinuria if glomerular amyloid deposition. Minimally concentrated to isosthenuric urine is seen as renal damage progresses
- Arterial blood pressure with Doppler: to assess for systemic hypertension
- Urine protein/creatinine (UPC) ratio: often dramatically increased (except shar-pei dogs, cats)
  - Normal: <0.5 (dogs), <0.4 (cats). Amyloidosis often elevates UPC >10.
  - Concurrent lower urinary tract disease should be ruled out; bacterial cystitis, uroliths, or neoplasia may increase the UPC ratio.
- Imaging: often unremarkable; kidneys and liver may be mildly enlarged and hyperechoic on ultrasound examination

ADVANCED OR CONFIRMATORY TESTING

Biopsy required for definitive diagnosis:

- A renal core biopsy must always be performed parallel to the long axis of the kidney (i.e., cortex only); biopsy instruments directed toward the renal medulla or hilus may lacerate a renal arcuate artery (arterial hemorrhage).
- Histologic findings:
  - Hematoxylin and eosin stain: homogenous eosinophilic material within affected organs
  - Congo red stain: apple-green birefringence when viewed under polarized light
- Shar-peis and Abyssinians preferentially deposit amyloid in the renal medulla, so renal biopsy may not be diagnostic. Hepatic biopsy may be preferred in patients with clinicopathologic evidence of liver dysfunction.

TREATMENT

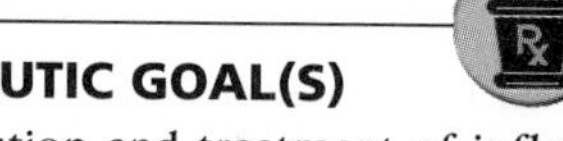

THERAPEUTIC GOAL(S)

- Identification and treatment of inflammatory disease, if present
- Reduction of proteinuria
- Treatment of renal failure
- Treatment of hypertension

ACUTE GENERAL TREATMENT

- Stabilization and treatment of uremic crisis if renal failure present
- Specific therapy for PLN: see Glomerulonephritis, p 442; Protein-Losing Nephropathy, p 900
- Treatment of complications if they occur: see Acute Renal Failure, p 32; Chronic Renal Failure, Occult ["Asymptomatic"], p 204; Chronic Renal Failure, Overt ["Symptomatic"], p 205; Nephrotic Syndrome, p 749; Pulmonary Thromboembolism, p 920; Systemic Hypertension, p 1058

CHRONIC TREATMENT

- Management/resolution of concurrent inflammatory disease.
- Continued management of PLN.
- Dimethyl sulfoxide may slow or prevent progression of amyloidosis in dogs. 300 mg/kg PO q 24h, or dilute 90% solution 1:4 in sterile water and administer 20–80 mg/kg SQ three times/week. Owners should wear gloves when administering. SQ injections may cause local irritation.
- Colchicine should be used in shar-peis at earliest diagnosis, regardless of disease severity or presence of proteinuria. 0.01–0.03 mg/kg PO q 24h. If vomiting/diarrhea develop, decrease dose.

RECOMMENDED MONITORING

Urine protein:creatinine ratio, urinalysis, serum albumin and creatinine, blood pressure, body weight, and condition score should be monitored weekly to monthly initially. Once stable, every 3 to 6 months unless therapy or condition changes

PROGNOSIS AND OUTCOME

- Overall, guarded to poor (months to 1 to 2 years). Worse if concurrent azotemia: often rapidly progress to uremic crisis once azotemia develops
- Prognosis improved (occasional resolution) if inflammatory diseases are identified and eliminated
- Early colchicine therapy (before renal failure) for shar-pei dogs may greatly improve prognosis

PEARLS & CONSIDERATIONS

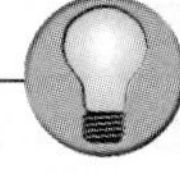

COMMENTS

- Differentiation of amyloidosis from other causes of protein-losing nephropathy requires biopsy. Histologic diagnosis allows tailored therapy and prognosis.
- Renal amyloidosis is primarily a renal cortical disease in dogs other than shar-peis.
- It is reasonable to assume a shar-pei with consistent clinical signs (recurrent lameness, fever, and pathologic proteinuria) is affected even without biopsy.
- Substantial renal amyloidosis may be present despite normal blood urea nitrogen, creatinine, and urine specific gravity values.

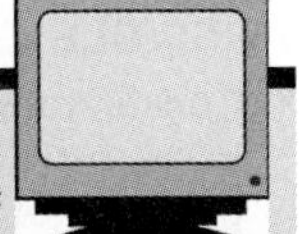

PREVENTION

Affected shar-pei dogs and Abyssinian, Oriental, and Siamese cats should not be bred.

SUGGESTED READING

DiBartola SP, et al: Familial renal amyloidosis in Chinese shar pei dogs. *J Am Vet Med Assoc* 197:483, 1990.

Pressler B, Vaden SL: Managing renal amyloidosis in dogs and cats. *Vet Med* 98:320, 2003.

AUTHOR: **BARRAK M. PRESSLER**
EDITOR: **LEAH A. COHN**

Anal Sac Diseases

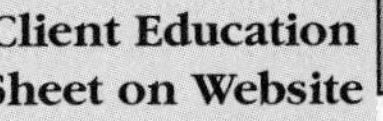

BASIC INFORMATION

DEFINITION

Anal sac diseases include anal sac impaction, anal sacculitis, anal sac abscess, and anal sac neoplasia (anal sac adenocarcinoma of the apocrine glands, squamous cell carcinoma).

SYNONYM(S)

Anal glands (a misnomer)

EPIDEMIOLOGY

SPECIES, AGE, SEX

- Dogs and cats have anal sacs. Dogs are much more commonly affected than cats.
- Older, female dogs are predisposed to anal sac tumors.

RISK FACTORS: Abnormal anal tone, diarrhea, obesity, increased secretions due to seborrhea, and obstruction of the anal sac ducts may predispose to impaction and possibly infection.

ASSOCIATED CONDITIONS AND DISORDERS: Some dogs may have associated atopy, food allergy, or seborrhea.

CLINICAL PRESENTATION

HISTORY, CHIEF COMPLAINT: Mild cases will likely involve the dog or cat's licking or biting at the perineal area, as well as "scooting" (rubbing the perineum on the floor) or reluctance to sit. The owner may notice a foul odor. With more severe disease, dyschezia, tenesmus, or bloody discharge from the area may be seen.

PHYSICAL EXAM FINDINGS: Visual and digital rectal examination are essential; pain may require sedation or anesthesia of the patient.

- A swelling in the area of the sacs (i.e., immediately lateral and ventral to the anus) may be seen, suggesting distention with secretions or a mass.
- If an anal sac has ruptured, an ulcerated, draining tract may be seen.
- Upon digital palpation, a firm, painful anal sac may be noted, suggesting inflammation (impaction, infection).
- With anal sac impaction, the contents may be very difficult to express. With anal sacculitis or abscess, the secretions may be bloody, purulent, and thicker than normal.
- A mass rather than a fluid-filled structure may be palpated and extend beyond the margins of the anal sac if neoplasia is present.

ETIOLOGY AND PATHOPHYSIOLOGY

Anal sacs are paired structures located on either side of the anus between the internal and external anal sphincter muscles. Each sac opens onto the margin of the anus via a single duct. The sacs function as reservoirs for apocrine and sebaceous gland secretions. Normal anal sac secretions are a viscous, foul-smelling liquid or paste with a yellow, gray, or brown color that are usually expressed during defecation. The secretions may be granular or contain solid material.

DIAGNOSIS

DIFFERENTIAL DIAGNOSIS

- Anal sac impaction: firm enlargement of sac(s), often painful. Expression possible under general anesthesia with or without cannulation
- Anal sacculitis: inflammation and pain with/without excessive accumulation of secretions
- Anal sac abscess: infected, enclosed anal sac secretions and pus. Often discovered after abscess ruptures through perianal skin
- Anal sac neoplasia: see Adenocarcinoma, Anal Sac, p 37
- Perianal fistula: anal sacs are normal
- Perineal hernia: rectal examination reveals rent in pelvic diaphragm
- Trauma: history and physical examination
- Perineal dermatitis: often affects dorsal lumbosacral/tailhead area and medial thighs

INITIAL DATABASE

- Complete blood count/serum chemistry panel/urinalysis: usually within normal limits; hypercalcemia possible with adenocarcinoma of anal sacs
- Thoracic and pelvic radiographs, and abdominal ultrasound exam: rule out metastatic lesions
- Cytologic examination of anal sac contents: may reveal neutrophils, bacteria, or yeast
- Culture of anal sac contents: may be difficult to interpret due to normal flora; pure culture of single bacterial species suggests infection
- Cytologic examination of mass aspirate: used for aiding in diagnosis of neoplasia

ADVANCED OR CONFIRMATORY TESTING

- Parathyroid hormone-related protein levels may be elevated in dogs with an anal sac mass and hypercalcemia.
- Abdominal ultrasound to rule out metastasis to lymph nodes.

TREATMENT

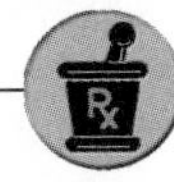

THERAPEUTIC GOAL(S)

- Empty the anal sacs
- Control infection
- Definitive therapy for neoplasia: see Adenocarcinoma, Anal Sac, p 37

ACUTE GENERAL TREATMENT

- Anal sac impaction: gently, manually express the sacs. Frequent recurrence or refractory impaction may lead to need for anal sacculectomy.
- Anal sacculitis: manually express the sacs followed by flushing with sterile saline. An antibiotic or antibiotic/corticosteroid combination ointment or solution can then be instilled into the sacs. Sedation and analgesia are usually needed for the procedure.
- Anal sac abscess/rupture: sedation and analgesia. Expression of material (if possible) followed by copious flushing of the area with sterile saline. If the sac is not ruptured, topical warm packing for several days may bring the abscess to a point where it can be lanced. Antibiotic ointment or solution may be instilled, but systemic antibiotics (e.g., enrofloxacin 5 mg/kg PO q 24h) are recommended.

CHRONIC TREATMENT

- Weight loss if the patient is obese
- Dietary fiber to increase stool bulk: may help prevent recurrence
- Therapy of associated conditions (e.g., seborrhea, food allergy)

POSSIBLE COMPLICATIONS

- Constipation if defecation is painful
- Fecal incontinence: uncommon complication of anal sacculectomy
- Fistulous tracts may form if the entire anal sac is not removed during anal sacculectomy

RECOMMENDED MONITORING

Monitor the area of anal sacculitis, abscesses q 2-3 days to ensure adequate resolution. Abscess drainage may need to be repeated if the initial opening seals.

PROGNOSIS AND OUTCOME

- Prognosis for non-neoplastic diseases of the anal sacs is generally good. Most animals will respond to medical management.
- Prognosis for animals that require surgical removal of the anal sacs is good to guarded.
- Prognosis for neoplastic diseases of the anal sacs is fair to guarded.

PEARLS & CONSIDERATIONS

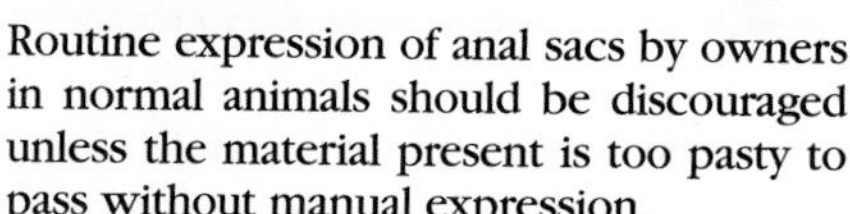

COMMENTS

Routine expression of anal sacs by owners in normal animals should be discouraged unless the material present is too pasty to pass without manual expression.

PREVENTION

- Adequate dietary fiber
- Avoid obesity

CLIENT EDUCATION

- Early intervention and treatment may help prevent the need for anal sacculectomy.
- If anal sac disease makes expression of anal sacs at home by the owners necessary, they should be taught an appropriate technique, to prevent excessive irritation or inflammation from the procedure.

SUGGESTED READING

Down MO, Stampley AR: Use of a Foley catheter to facilitate anal sac removal in the dog. *J Am Anim Hosp Assoc* 34:395-397, 1998.

Esplin DG, Wilson SR, Hullinger GA: Squamous cell carcinoma of the anal sac in five dogs. *Vet Pathol* 40:332-334, 2003.

Hill LN, Smeak DD: Open versus closed bilateral anal sacculectomy for treatment of non-neoplastic anal sac disease in dogs: 95 cases (1969-1994). *J Am Anim Hosp Assoc* 221:662-665, 2002.

Pappalardo E, Martine PA, Noli C: Macroscopic, cytological, and bacteriological evaluation of anal sac content in normal dogs and dogs with selected dermatologic diseases. *Vet Dermatol* 13:315-322, 2002.

van Duijkeren E: Disease conditions of canine anal sacs. *J Small Anim Pract* 36:12-16, 1995.

AUTHOR: **LISA E. MOORE**

EDITOR: **DEBRA L. ZORAN**

Anaphylaxis

BASIC INFORMATION

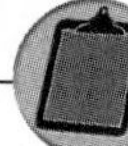

DEFINITION

An acute, hypersensitive immune reaction that results in the massive, generalized release of inflammatory mediators from basophils and mast cells. This life-threatening systemic allergic reaction can result in rapid cardiovascular collapse, respiratory distress, and death.

- *Urticaria:* a cutaneous manifestation of anaphylaxis consisting of pruritic wheals
- *Angioedema:* nonpainful cutaneous and visceral swelling (regional or generalized) that is one of the hallmarks of anaphylaxis

SYNONYM(S)

Allergic reaction
Anaphylactic reaction
Anaphylactic shock
Type I immune hypersensitivity

EPIDEMIOLOGY

SPECIES, AGE, SEX: Has been reported in most species; no age or sex predilection.

GENETICS AND BREED PREDISPOSITION: Boxers and pit bulls are most often affected with urticaria.

RISK FACTORS

- Previous exposure to an antigen or hapten suspected to cause anaphylaxis increases risk, but previous exposure is not always recognized
- Can be triggered by a number of medications including hormones, antibiotics, chemotherapy agents, parasiticides, vaccines

GEOGRAPHY AND SEASONALITY: Summer or warm weather for insect-related anaphylaxis.

CLINICAL PRESENTATION

DISEASE FORMS/SUBTYPES

- *Anaphylactic reactions* occur as a result of the interaction of an antigen or hapten with an antibody molecule, IgE, that has been formed from a previous exposure.
- *Anaphylactoid reactions* occur without an antibody and do not require previous exposure.
- Both reactions result in the rapid, systemic release of inflammatory mediators from mast cells and have identical clinical presentation and treatment.

HISTORY, CHIEF COMPLAINT

- Recent exposure to an inciting antigen or hapten (vaccine, topical paraciticide, ophthalmic antibiotics, parenteral antibiotic, snake bite, food ingredient)
- Excitation
- Severe pruritis with urticaria
- Vomiting/diarrhea
- Respiratory distress
- Hypersalivation
- Collapse

PHYSICAL EXAM FINDINGS

- Generalized wheals, facial angioedema
- Weakness
- Mentation changes: depression or excitation
- Pale mucous membranes
- Prolonged capillary refill time
- Poor pulse quality
- Tachycardia
- Dyspnea (cats)
- Rarely, an insect stinger is found in the skin, confirming insect bite
- Coma

ETIOLOGY AND PATHOPHYSIOLOGY

- Anaphylactic reactions:

   - Initial exposure to an antigen results in the production of specific IgE (antibody).
   - Subsequent reexposure to the antigen results in the binding of the antigen to IgE on the surface of basophils in circulation and mast cells in tissues.
   - Activated basophils and mast cells release granules containing primary mediators of anaphylaxis: histamine, heparin, proteases, and chemotactic factors.
   - Activation of the arachadonic acid cascade results in the release of secondary mediators including leukotrienes, prostaglandins, thromboxanes, and platelet-activating factor.
   - Cytokine synthesis also occurs within 2 to 24 hours, contributing to the inflammatory process.
- Anaphylactoid reactions:
   - Exposure to the antigen or hapten results in the activation of the complement cascade, leading to the production of anaphylatoxins (C3a and C5a), which causes the activation of mast cells and basophils and the release of primary mediators not involving an antibody response.
- The activation, synthesis, and release of the inflammatory mediators result in peripheral vasodilation, increased vascular permeability, hypotension, bronchospasm, laryngeal edema, increased airway secretion production, intestinal hypermotility, cardiac arrhythmias, stimulation of pain receptors, and pruritus.

DIAGNOSIS

The diagnosis is based on history and physical exam findings alone. It is *essential* that treatment for anaphylaxis be instituted before diagnostic testing, because the onset of treatment is the primary determinant of survival.

DIFFERENTIAL DIAGNOSIS

- Shock (hypovolemic, cardiogenic, septic)
- Pulmonary edema
- Heart disease: arrhythmias
- Feline asthma
- Acute gastrointestinal disease

INITIAL DATABASE

- Blood pressure: monitor for hypotension
- Complete blood count, serum chemistry, urinalysis: generally unremarkable
- Survey radiographs: to rule out pulmonary disease if dyspnea is present

TREATMENT

THERAPEUTIC GOAL(S)

- Cardiovascular and respiratory support
- Antagonize inflammatory mediators
- Block further release of inflammatory mediators
- Remove causative agent

ACUTE GENERAL TREATMENT

Instituted in severe cases (those patients with dyspnea, hemodynamic instability, or depression/coma):

- IV catheter placement first
- IV fluids for volume resuscitation
   - Crystalloids:
      - Dog: 90 ml/kg/hr
      - Cat: 40–60 ml/kg/hr
   - Synthetic colloids:
      - Dog: 10–20 ml/kg slow bolus
      - Cat: 5–10 ml/kg slow bolus
   - Fluid therapy should be guided by the patient's monitoring parameters.
- If severe clinical signs: epinephrine to treat hypotension, bronchoconstriction, and block the release of inflammatory mediators
   - 0.01–0.2 mg/kg IV (IM or SQ for less severe cases), or
   - 0.02–0.4 mg/kg intratracheal administration
- Establish an airway in patients with upper airway dyspnea or apnea caused by severe laryngeal edema
   - Endotracheal intubation
   - Tracheostomy
- Oxygen therapy if evidence of hypoxemia
- Bronchodilation if bronchospasm persists after epinephrine administration
   - Aminophylline:
      - Dog: 5–10 mg/kg IV, IM
      - Cat: 5 mg/kg IV, IM
   - Inhaled albuterol
- Vasopressor therapy if hypotension persists despite fluid therapy and epinephrine
   - Dopamine:
      - 5–15 µg/kg/min

CHRONIC TREATMENT

May be instituted instead of acute general treatment if a patient is showing only mild clinical signs and is hemodynamically stable. In general, treatment of anaphylaxis is complete within 24 to 72 hours of presentation.

- Glucocorticoid therapy to block the release of secondary mediators:
   - Dexamethasone sodium phosphate: 0.1–0.2 mg/kg IV once
- Antihistamine therapy:
   - H_1 blockers
      - Diphenhydramine: 0.5–1 mg/kg IM once
   - H_2 blockers
      - Famotidine 0.5–1 mg/kg IV, IM, SQ q 12h

DRUG INTERACTIONS

Epinephrine, aminophylline: arrhythmogenic. Use caution when both used together. Aminophylline: use only after fluid resuscitation has been accomplished

POSSIBLE COMPLICATIONS

- Cardiac arrhythmias
- Organ dysfunction

RECOMMENDED MONITORING

- Frequent monitoring should be continued for 24 to 48 hours after reaction
- Heart rate, respiratory rate, respiratory effort, pulse rate, pulse quality, mentation, mucous membrane color, capillary refill time, temperature
- Blood pressure
- Central venous pressure
- Electrocardiogram
- Pulse oximetry or arterial blood gases
- Packed cell volume and total solids
- Serum chemistry
- Coagulation profile

PROGNOSIS AND OUTCOME

- Immediate recognition and prompt intervention are the keys for a successful outcome.
- Anaphylaxis can result in death within 1 hour of exposure to the inciting agent.

PEARLS & CONSIDERATIONS

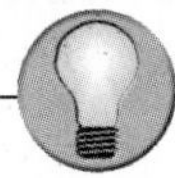

COMMENT

- Anaphylactic shock does not always involve a previous exposure and sensitization.
- Anaphylaxis should be suspected in patients with unexplained, acute cardiovascular and respiratory collapse.
- Aggressive fluid therapy and epinephrine are the first line of treatment in severe anaphylaxis.

PREVENTION

- Minimize the chance of an anaphylactic reaction by administering IV medications slowly.
- Be aware of, and use caution with, medications that are known to be associated with anaphylaxis.
- Pretreatment of patients with a history of previous anaphylaxis with antihistamines and glucocorticoids may be useful in blunting the inflammatory response.

CLIENT EDUCATION

- Be familiar with your pet's medical history and alert your veterinarian of all medications your pet has received, previous blood product transfusions, and previous allergic reactions.
- A pediatric Epi-pen may be prescribed for animals with prior life-threatening reactions.

SUGGESTED READING

Cohen RD: Systemic anaphylaxis. In Bonagura JD, Kirk RW (eds): *Kirk's Current Veterinary Therapy XII Small Animal Practice*. Philadelphia, WB Saunders, 1995, pp 150–152.

Plunkett SJ: Anaphylaxis to ophthalmic medication in a cat. *J Vet Emerg Crit Care* 10 (3):169–171.

Waddell LS: Systemic anaphylaxis. In Ettinger SJ, Feldman EC (eds): *Textbook of Veterinary Internal Medicine Diseases of the Dog and Cat*. St. Louis, Elsevier, 2005, pp 458–460.

AUTHOR: **KRISTI M. GANNON**

EDITOR: **ELIZABETH ROZANSKI**

Anemia, Aplastic

BASIC INFORMATION

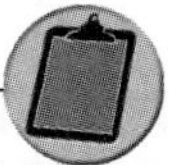

DEFINITION

Pancytopenia (decrease in erythrocytes, leukocytes, and platelets in peripheral blood) due to failure of the bone marrow to produce all hematopoietic cell lines. Erythrocytes only: see Anemia: Nonregenerative, and Pure Red Cell Aplasia, p 69

SYNONYM(S)

Aplastic pancytopenia
Hypoplastic anemia

EPIDEMIOLOGY

SPECIES, AGE, SEX: Dogs and cats of any age and all breeds may be affected.

CLINICAL PRESENTATION

DISEASE FORMS/SUBTYPES

- Acute form occurs within 2 weeks of bone marrow injury; proliferating and progenitor cells affected within the bone marrow
- Chronic form results from injury to hematopoietic stem cells

HISTORY, CHIEF COMPLAINT

- Acute form: lethargy, inappetence, fever
- Chronic form: as above with weakness, tachypnea, collapse

PHYSICAL EXAM FINDINGS

- Acute form: fever, possible mucosal bleeding
- Chronic form: as above with pallor, tachypnea, tachycardia, and soft systolic heart murmur (anemia-related)

ETIOLOGY AND PATHOPHYSIOLOGY

- Infectious: *Ehrlichia* spp., parvovirus, feline leukemia virus (FeLV)
- Drugs: chemotherapy, sulfa drugs, phenylbutazone, estrogen (dogs), thiacetarsemide, griseofulvin (cats)
- Toxins
- Radiation
- Immune-mediated
- Idiopathic: most common
- Neutropenia develops 5 to 6 days and thrombocytopenia develops 8 to 10 days after marrow insult
- Fever usually secondary to opportunistic infection due to invasion of bacteria from gastrointestinal or respiratory tracts

DIAGNOSIS

DIFFERENTIAL DIAGNOSIS

- Infiltration of the bone marrow with malignant cells
- Myelodysplasia, see p 725
- Myelofibrosis

INITIAL DATABASE

- Complete blood count (CBC): granulocytopenia (neutropenia, eosinopenia), and thrombocytopenia occur first, followed by moderate to severe nonregenerative anemia
  - Reticulocyte count: corrected count < 1%; absolute count < 60,000/µl
- Blood smear evaluation: for red blood cell morphology and to identify abnormal circulating cells present in small numbers
- Bone marrow aspirate: panhypoplasia (variable severity), necrosis, and increased macrophages may be seen
- Serum biochemistry profile and urinalysis usually unremarkable or reflect underlying disease
- FeLV testing (cats)
- *Ehrlichia canis* testing (dogs)

ADVANCED OR CONFIRMATORY TESTING

Bone marrow aspiration and core biopsy:

- Marked decrease in all hematopoietic cell lines; typically in aplastic anemia patients, hematopoietic cells constitute <25% of the marrow (normal marrow contains 50% hematopoietic cells and 50% fat).
- Core biopsy required to confirm hypoplastic marrow.
- Dysplastic changes may be expected during the recovery phase.

TREATMENT

THERAPEUTIC GOAL(S)

Provide supportive care while awaiting marrow regeneration

ACUTE GENERAL TREATMENT

- Discontinue medications potentially associated with aplastic anemia.
- Transfusion (usually packed red blood cells) to increase in oxygen-carrying capacity if hematocrit < 15% or if significant clinical signs of anemia are present (see Transfusion Therapy and Collection Techniques for Blood Banking, p 1312).
- Broad-spectrum antibiotics (if signs of infection, or prophylactically if neutrophils < 500–1000 µl). For prophylaxis, antibiotics with good gram-negative spectrum, but sparing of anaerobic flora; specifically, enrofloxacin 5 mg/kg PO q 24h or trimethoprim sulfa 15 mg/kg PO q 12h. Caution: trimethoprim sulfa has caused aplastic anemia.
- Platelet transfusions if platelet count is <50,000/µl in patients requiring surgery.

CHRONIC TREATMENT

- Immunosuppressive drugs may be tried for idiopathic aplastic anemia, including:
  - Prednisone: 1–2 mg/kg PO q 12h
  - Azathioprine (dogs): 2 mg/kg PO q 24h to every other day
  - Cyclophosphamide: 50 mg/m^2 PO × 4 days, repeat weekly
  - Cyclosporine A: 5–10 mg/kg PO q 12h (target blood levels of 200–300 mg/ml)
  - Intravenous immune globulin
- Bone marrow transplantation with matched full sibling donor when spontaneous recovery is absent: investigational therapy
- The role of hematopoietic growth factors, such as erythropoietin and granulocyte-colony stimulating factor in dogs and cats with aplastic anemia is unknown. Concern about cross-reactive neutralizing antibody formation with human recombinant products

DRUG INTERACTIONS

Immunosuppressive and especially myelosuppressive drugs (cyclophosphamide, azathioprine) may increase risk of sepsis

POSSIBLE COMPLICATIONS

Sepsis and bleeding

RECOMMENDED MONITORING

- Repeat CBC weekly until full recovery
  - Usually 3 weeks for acute aplastic anemia
  - May spread out to every 2 weeks in chronic form
- Upon recovery, continue to monitor CBC monthly for additional 3 months

PROGNOSIS AND OUTCOME

- Dependent on underlying cause.
- Acute aplastic anemias often are reversible within 2 to 3 weeks after withdrawal of inciting agents.
- Idiopathic and chronic aplastic anemias tend to be less responsive, with recovery times up to months. Many dogs are euthanized shortly after diagnosis.
- Young dogs (<3 years old) may be more likely to respond to immunosuppressive drugs or recover spontaneously.

PEARLS & CONSIDERATIONS

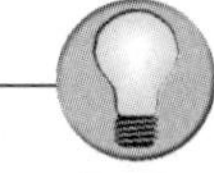

COMMENTS

- In acute aplastic anemia, granulocytopenia and thrombocytopenia occur before the hematocrit and drop due to longer circulating half-life of erythrocytes.
- Anemia is often moderate to severe in chronic aplastic anemia.
- Early recognition of aplastic anemia may improve the chance of recovery.

PREVENTION

CBCs should be monitored in animals receiving medications associated with aplastic anemia.

SUGGESTED READING

Bacigalupo A: Bone marrow transplantation for severe aplastic anemia from HLA identical siblings. *Haematologica* 84:2-4, 1999.

Dornsife RE, et al: Induction of aplastic anemia by intra-bone marrow inoculation of a molecularly cloned feline retrovirus. *Leukemia Res* 13:745-755, 1989.

Weiss DJ, Klausner JS: Drug-associated aplastic anemia in dogs: eight cases (1984-1988). *J Am Vet Med Assoc* 196:472-479, 1990.

Weiss DJ: Aplastic anemia. In Feldman BF, Zinkl JG, Jain NC (eds): *Schalm's Veterinary Hematology,* ed 5. Philadelphia, Lippincott, Williams & Wilkins, 2000, pp 212-215.

AUTHOR: **LISA G. BARBER**
EDITOR: **SUSAN M. COTTER**

Anemia Due to Blood Loss

BASIC INFORMATION

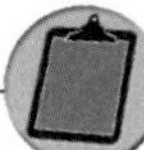

DEFINITION

A decrease in total red blood cell (RBC) mass secondary to loss of RBCs from the vascular space

SYNONYM(S)

Hemorrhagic anemia
Iron deficiency anemia

EPIDEMIOLOGY

SPECIES, AGE, SEX: Variable depending on underlying cause.

RISK FACTORS: Neoplasia, gastrointestinal ulcers, coagulopathy, heavy parasite load (e.g., fleas, hookworms).

CLINICAL PRESENTATION

HISTORY, CHIEF COMPLAINT

- Weakness, lethargy, collapse, anorexia, exercise intolerance
- Acute blood loss
  - Trauma
  - Abdominal distention
- Chronic blood loss
  - Melena, epistaxis, hematuria
  - Pica

PHYSICAL EXAM FINDINGS: Varies with severity and duration:

- Pale mucous membranes/pallor
- Weakness, exercise intolerance; collapse or syncope possible
- Tachycardia, tachypnea, bounding pulses
- Heart murmur: systolic, left-sided, and generally soft (< III/VI)
- Hemorrhage from surgery, trauma, or underlying cause
- Hemoabdomen
- Petechiation, ecchymoses: suggestive of generalized bleeding disorder as underlying cause

ETIOLOGY AND PATHOPHYSIOLOGY

- Acute blood loss:
  - Trauma
  - Surgical bleeding
  - Bleeding neoplasm (hemangiosarcoma)
  - Gastrointestinal ulcer
  - Bleeding disorder (thrombocytopenia, anticoagulant rodenticide toxicity, hemophilia)
- Chronic blood loss/iron deficiency anemia:
  - Gastrointestinal bleeding most common: neoplasia, hookworms, ulcerations
  - Less common: heavy flea infestation, urinary tract hemorrhage
  - Overuse of blood donors or frequent phlebotomy
  - Iron deficiency anemia can develop with chronic external blood loss:
    - Iron depletion leads to decreased synthesis of hemoglobin and delayed cell maturation. RBCs are less deformable with accelerated lysis.
    - Young animals at increased risk due to decreased iron storage.

DIAGNOSIS

DIFFERENTIAL DIAGNOSIS

Differentiate from Anemia, Hemolytic, p 64. Blood loss characterized by decreased plasma total protein (TP) without autoagglutination, spherocytes, hyperbilirubinemia/uria, or hemoglobinemia/uria

INITIAL DATABASE

- Acute blood loss
  - Packed cell volume (PCV)/plasma TP: initially little change in PCV because of concurrent loss of plasma with RBCs. Over hours, redistribution of fluid occurs, resulting in lowered PCV and plasma protein
  - Complete blood count (CBC):
    - Normocytic, normochromic RBCs initially
    - Reticulocytosis 3 to 5 days after acute loss: hypochromic macrocytosis and polychromasia
    - Platelet count usually normal
    - Schistocytes associated with hemangiosarcoma or other splenic mass
  - Serum biochemistry panel:
    - Panhypoproteinemia if external blood loss
  - Abdominocentesis: hemoabdomen secondary to trauma, splenic disease, hemangiosarcoma, bleeding disorder
  - Coagulation panel and buccal mucosal bleeding time to rule out hemostatic defect
- Chronic blood loss/iron deficiency anemia
  - CBC:
    - Regenerative or nonregenerative
    - Microcytosis, increased red cell distribution width, hypochromasia
    - Thrombocytosis
  - Serum biochemistry panel: panhypoproteinemia
  - Fecal flotation/fecal occult blood
  - Abdominal radiographs, ultrasound, endoscopy: neoplasia, gastrointestinal ulceration

ADVANCED OR CONFIRMATORY TESTING

- Iron deficiency anemia
  - Low serum iron concentration (<60 μg/dl), low serum ferritin concentra-

 tion (<70 μg/dl), and low transferrin saturation (<20%)
 - Bone marrow: erythroid hyperplasia. Prussian blue stain: absence of iron particles (hemosiderin) in dogs
- Nuclear scintigraphy scan may confirm occult gastrointestinal blood loss

TREATMENT

THERAPEUTIC GOAL(S)

- Acute blood loss:
  - Control hemorrhage
  - Restore circulating volume and tissue oxygenation
- Chronic blood loss/iron deficiency anemia:
  - Identify and correct underlying cause
  - Iron deficiency resolves 6 to 8 weeks after eliminating cause
    - Ensure adequate diet
    - Administer iron until hematologic abnormalities resolve

ACUTE GENERAL TREATMENT

- Acute blood loss:
  - IV fluid therapy with crystalloids ± colloids to correct hypovolemia
  - If signs of hypoxia (weakness, tachycardia, tachypnea) consider transfusion: packed RBCs (6-10 ml/kg) best if available; whole blood (10-20 ml/kg), oxyglobin (10-30 ml/kg). See Transfusion Therapy and Collection Techniques for Blood Banking, p 1312
  - Autotransfusion if hemorrhage in a body cavity and no blood contamination with bacteria or neoplastic cells
  - If coagulopathy, correct with vitamin K1, 1-5 mg/kg/day SC, fresh frozen plasma (6-10 ml/kg), cryoprecipitate (1 unit/10 kg IV) depending on cause
- Chronic blood loss:
  - Transfusion if severe
  - Treatment of underlying cause (may involve gastrointestinal protectants, dewormer, surgery for intestinal tumor, etc.). See specific disorders

CHRONIC TREATMENT

Chronic blood loss/iron deficiency anemia (see characteristic CBC and iron changes, above):

- Replace iron with iron dextran 10-20 mg/kg IM or ferrous sulfate 100-300 mg/dog/day or 50-100 mg/cat/day PO

POSSIBLE COMPLICATIONS

- Massive blood loss: hypovolemic shock, hypoxia, possible death
- See Transfusion Reactions, p 1098
  - Dogs: blood typing should be performed before transfusion. If recipient is not typed, donor should be negative for DEA-1.1. Additionally, previously transfused dogs should be crossmatched before any transfusions.
  - Cats: possess naturally occurring antibodies against the blood type antigen they lack (alloantibodies). Cats must be typed or crossmatched before any transfusions.
- Adverse drug reactions: iron dextran: injection site pain, anaphylactic reaction; ferrous sulfate: vomiting, diarrhea, dark stools

RECOMMENDED MONITORING

- Acute blood loss:
  - Monitor PCV/TP once to twice daily initially; monitor heart rate, respiratory rate, blood pressure, mucous membrane color, and capillary refill time.
  - Polymerized bovine hemoglobin (Oxyglobin) increases oxygen carrying capacity without increasing PCV; need to monitor hemoglobin concentration.
- Chronic blood loss:
  - Monitor CBC every 1 to 4 weeks.
  - Reticulocytosis may be the first sign of response.

PROGNOSIS AND OUTCOME

- Good with blood loss secondary to trauma or surgery once hemorrhage is controlled and cardiovascular status is stabilized
- Excellent with parasites and appropriate treatment
- Fair with various coagulopathies, depending on severity of blood loss on presentation and ability to control blood loss
- Fair with gastrointestinal ulcers once underlying disease treated
- Guarded to grave with neoplasia. Short-term response with surgery with or without additional chemotherapy, depending on tumor type and extent

PEARLS & CONSIDERATIONS

COMMENTS

- In acute blood loss, PCV is not a good indicator of patient status. Indicators of perfusion (pulse strength, capillary refill time, blood pressure, and blood lactate concentration) are more important in acute situations.
- Decision to transfuse a patient should be based on clinical signs rather than PCV. However, at a PCV <12%, patients generally decompensate and require a transfusion.
- Do not treat iron deficiency anemia without searching for an underlying cause of blood loss.

CLIENT EDUCATION

Counsel clients on importance of follow-up with chronic/iron deficiency anemia

SUGGESTED READING

Giger U: Regenerative anemias caused by blood loss or hemolysis. In Ettinger SJ, Feldman EC (eds): *Textbook of Veterinary Internal Medicine*. St. Louis, Elsevier, 2005, pp 1886-1890.

AUTHOR: **ALICIA K. HENDERSON**
EDITOR: **SUSAN M. COTTER**

Anemia, Hemolytic

BASIC INFORMATION

DEFINITION

Decrease in red blood cell (RBC) mass due to destruction or shortened lifespan of RBCs. Immune-mediated hemolytic anemia is discussed as a separate topic (see Anemia, Immune-Mediated Hemolytic, p 66).

EPIDEMIOLOGY

SPECIES, AGE, SEX: Variable depending on underlying cause.

GENETICS AND BREED PREDISPOSITION

- Inherited RBC defects:
  - Phosphofructokinase (PFK) deficiency: English springer spaniels, rarely cocker spaniels
  - Pyruvate kinase (PK) deficiency: basenjis, beagles, West Highland white terriers, Cairn terriers, miniature poodles, toy Eskimos, dachshunds, Abyssinian and Somali cats
  - Feline porphyria: Siamese, domestic shorthairs
- Infectious:
  - Babesiosis: greyhounds and pit bulls at increased risk

RISK FACTORS

- Oxidative damage: propofol, lidocaine, onions, garlic, chives, vitamin K_3, naphthalene, acetaminophen, zinc, propylene glycol. Cats at increased risk
- Microangiopathic: hemangiosarcoma, disseminated intravascular coagulopathy (DIC), hepatic/splenic disease, heartworm, vasculitis
- Hypophosphatemia: complication of diabetes mellitus/diabetic ketoacidosis, hepatic lipidosis, refeeding syndrome, phosphate-binding antacids

GEOGRAPHY AND SEASONALITY

- Cytauxzoonosis: southeast United States
- Babesiosis: southern United States, California

CLINICAL PRESENTATION

DISEASE FORMS/SUBTYPES

- Intravascular: direct RBC lysis within vasculature. Results in hemoglobinemia/uria, icterus
- Extravascular: RBCs phagocytosed by mononuclear phagocytic system. Results in splenomegaly, hepatomegaly icterus
- Both intravascular and extravascular may occur simultaneously

HISTORY, CHIEF COMPLAINT

- Anorexia, weakness, exercise intolerance, collapse
- Exposure to oxidant drug, food, chemical

PHYSICAL EXAM FINDINGS: Depends on degree of anemia and rapidity of onset.

- Pallor, weakness, lethargy, depression, tachycardia, tachypnea
- Icterus
- Hepatosplenomegaly
- Fever, lymphadenopathy
- Murmur: systolic, soft (grade II/VI or less), left-sided
- Cyanosis if methemoglobinemia

ETIOLOGY AND PATHOPHYSIOLOGY

- Immune-mediated, see p 66
- Oxidant toxicity: Oxidant damage causes Heinz body formation or methemoglobinemia, with decreased RBC lifespan and decreased delivery of oxygen to tissues, respectively
  - Heinz bodies make RBCs prone to intravascular lysis or phagocytosis. Heinz bodies are considered an absolute marker of oxidative RBC injury in dogs, less so in cats (present in 10–50% of healthy cats).
  - Methemoglobinemia, suspected with cyanosis or brown-colored blood, does not affect RBC lifespan nor induce hemolysis; it decreases the oxygen-carrying capacity of RBC.
  - Oxidant RBC toxicity can cause Heinz bodies, methemoglobinemia, or both; Heinz bodies are more routinely identified first (blood smear).
- Infectious organisms: can infect RBCs directly and cause hemolysis. Other infectious agents may trigger secondary RBC destruction
  - Mycoplasmosis (*M. haemofelis, M. haemominutum*): formerly hemobartonellosis; feline; transmitted primarily via fleas/ticks, but also by transfusion or transplacentally; feline leukemia virus exaggerates severity; loss of RBC deformability and antibody response leads to phagocytosis; secondary immune destruction.
  - Babesiosis (*B. canis, B. gibsoni*): canine; tick-borne; transplacental and transfusion transmission reported.
  - Cytauxzoonosis (*C. felis*): feline; high mortality.
- Microangiopathic: hemangiosarcoma, DIC. Fragmentation of RBCs by abnormal vascular structures or narrowing of vessels
- Hypophosphatemia: most common with phosphorus < 1.5 mg/dl; depletion of erythrocyte adenosine triphosphate (ATP), diphosphoglycerate (DPG), and reduced glutathione; decreased RBC deformability, increased osmotic fragility, and susceptibility to oxidative injury
- Hereditary erythrocyte defects:
  - PK deficiency: glycolytic enzyme deficiency causing decreased ATP leading to osmotic fragility.
  - PFK deficiency: glycolytic enzyme deficiency causing decreased 2,3-DPG; results in increased intracellular pH and RBC fragility in alkaline conditions such as hyperventilation during exercise.
  - Feline porphyria: deficiency of uroporphyrinogen II cosynthetase; inability to produce normal amounts of hemoglobin.
- Feline neonatal isoerythrolysis: Maternal anti-A alloantibodies in colostrum destroy RBCs in kittens with type A blood

DIAGNOSIS

DIFFERENTIAL DIAGNOSIS

- Blood loss anemia
- Immune-mediated hemolytic anemia

INITIAL DATABASE

- CBC:
  - Decreased hematocrit, RBC count, and hemoglobin
  - Evidence of regeneration:
    - Absolute reticulocytes > 60,000/μl, corrected reticulocyte count > 1%
    - Macrocytosis, hypochromasia
    - Regeneration may not be evident for 3 to 5 days (until bone marrow responds)
  - Morphology: anisocytosis, polychromasia, Heinz bodies, schistocytes (microangiopathy), parasites
- Serum biochemistry panel and urinalysis: hyperbilirubinemia/uria if marked hemolysis. Total protein normal
- Hemoglobinemia/uria with intravascular hemolysis
- Slide agglutination and Coombs' test to rule out immune-mediated hemolytic anemia
- Coagulation panel to assess for DIC
- Bone marrow: not indicated if regenerative; erythroid hyperplasia
- Radiographs to rule out metallic foreign body. Ultrasound for neoplasia or splenic abnormalities (e.g., torsion)

ADVANCED OR CONFIRMATORY TESTING

- Polymerase chain reaction for *Mycoplasma;* immunofluorescent antibody and enzyme-linked immunosorbent assay for *Babesia*
- DNA tests for PK/PFK deficiency; porphyrins in urine and RBCs for porphyria

TREATMENT

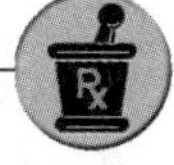

THERAPEUTIC GOAL(S)

- Identify and remove cause
- Supportive therapy
- ± Corticosteroids to suppress mononuclear phagocytic system while etiologic agent is eliminated

ACUTE GENERAL TREATMENT

- If severe, may require transfusion: packed RBCs (6–10 ml/kg IV), whole blood (10–20 ml/kg IV), or polymerized bovine hemoglobin (Oxyglobin) (10–30 ml/kg IV). See Transfusion Therapy and Collection Techniques for Blood Banking, p 1312
- Toxicity:
  - Zinc foreign body: remove via endoscopy/surgery
  - Acetaminophen: N-acetylcysteine at 140 mg/kg IV, then 70 mg/kg q 6h × six doses. See Acetaminophen Intoxication, p 16
- Hypophosphatemia: potassium phosphate at 0.01 to 0.03 mmol/kg/hr IV until normal
- Parasites:
  - *Mycoplasma haemofelis*: doxycycline 5 mg/kg PO q12h × 3 weeks. See Hemobartonellosis, Feline, p 479
  - Babesiosis: Imidocarb dipropionate 3.5 mg/lb IM

CHRONIC TREATMENT

- Avoid excitement/exercise with PFK deficiency
- Prednisone and splenectomy in feline PK deficiency

POSSIBLE COMPLICATIONS

- Hypercoagulation/pulmonary thromboembolism
- See Transfusion Reactions, p 1098
  - Dogs: blood typing should be performed prior to transfusion. If recipient is not typed, donor should be negative for DEA-1.1. Previously

transfused dogs should be cross-matched.
  - Cats: have naturally occurring alloantibodies. Fatal transfusion reactions can occur; cats must be typed or cross-matched before any transfusions.

RECOMMENDED MONITORING

Monitor PCV every 12 to 24 hours initially, then every 3 to 5 days. Heart rate, respiratory rate, mucous membrane color, and capillary refill time

PROGNOSIS AND OUTCOME

- Good once cause is removed and hemolytic crisis is over
- Poor for cytauxzoonosis (although a less virulent, nonfatal form has been reported), isoerythrolysis, canine PK deficiency, hemangiosarcoma, DIC

PEARLS & CONSIDERATIONS

COMMENTS

- Decision to transfuse should be based on clinical signs rather than PCV. However, when PCV <12%, patients generally decompensate and require transfusion.
- Although immune-mediated hemolytic anemia is the most common cause of hemolysis in dogs, other causes of hemolysis should be considered, especially in young or old dogs.

CLIENT EDUCATION

- Clinician should counsel clients on causes of oxidative damage and that acetaminophen use should especially be avoided
- Clinician should counsel owners and breeders on heritable defects to avoid breeding of affected dogs

SUGGESTED READING

Giger U: Regenerative anemias caused by blood loss or hemolysis. In Ettinger SJ, Feldman EC (eds): *Textbook of Veterinary Internal Medicine*. St. Louis, Elsevier, 2005, pp 1890–1907.

AUTHOR: **ALICIA K. HENDERSON**
EDITOR: **SUSAN M. COTTER**

Anemia, Immune-Mediated Hemolytic

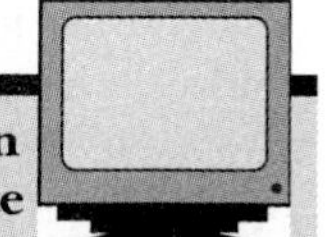

BASIC INFORMATION

DEFINITION

A common hemolytic disease in dogs resulting from increased destruction or phagocytosis of red blood cells (RBC) that have been coated with immunoglobulin, complement, or both. Immune-mediated hemolytic anemia (IMHA) occurs less commonly in cats.

SYNONYM(S)

Autoimmune hemolytic anemia
Idiopathic nonregenerative immune-mediated hemolytic anemia
IMHA
Pure red cell aplasia (PRCA) can be considered as a variant of IMHA in which destruction is directed at RBC precursors in the bone marrow.
Evans syndrome (if coexists with immune-mediated thrombocytopenia)

EPIDEMIOLOGY

SPECIES, AGE, SEX
- Dogs: both sexes, 1 to 13 years old. Many studies report an overrepresentation of middle-aged, spayed female dogs.
- Feline IMHA occurs more frequently in young cats.

GENETICS AND BREED PREDISPOSITION
- Canine breeds most commonly represented include the cocker spaniel, English springer spaniel, miniature poodle, Irish setter, collie, miniature schnauzer, Doberman pinscher, miniature pinscher, bichon frise, old English sheepdog, and Finnish spitz.
- No breed predisposition has been reported in cats.

RISK FACTORS: Recent vaccination has been reported as a risk factor in dogs with primary IMHA. However, this association has inconsistent support in a number of other studies.

GEOGRAPHY AND SEASONALITY: An increased incidence in dogs has been reported in the spring, with as many as 40% of cases seen in May and June.

ASSOCIATED CONDITIONS AND DISORDERS
- Thromboembolism
- Disseminated intravascular coagulopathy (DIC)
- Severe thrombocytopenia (< 50,000 platelets/µl) has been reported in 20–30% of dogs with IMHA and has been associated with both development of thromboembolism and increased mortality (see Thrombocytopenia, Immune-Mediated, p 1079)

CLINICAL PRESENTATION

DISEASE FORMS/SUBTYPES
- *Primary* (idiopathic): hemolysis results from antibody targeting red blood cell (RBC) membrane antigen
- *Secondary:* hemolysis results from antibody targeting novel membrane antigen, exposed during membrane alteration by underlying disease (neoplasia, infection, or microangiopathy), or by reaction to drugs, toxins, blood transfusion, or bee envenomation
- *Intravascular* hemolysis: red blood cells are destroyed in the vasculature in a process mediated by complement
- *Extravascular* hemolysis: RBCs are selected and destroyed by macrophages in the spleen and/or liver

HISTORY, CHIEF COMPLAINT
- Signs of anemia including lethargy, progressive weakness
- Inappetence to anorexia
- Vomiting
- Icterus
- Discolored urine (bilirubinuria or hemoglobinuria)
- Less common are signs of acute hemolysis including cardiovascular collapse, dyspnea, or central nervous system signs

PHYSICAL EXAM FINDINGS
- Weakness
- Pale mucous membranes
- Icterus
- Tachycardia
- Tachypnea, dyspnea
- Bounding pulses
- Heart murmur
- Splenomegaly and hepatomegaly
- Discolored urine

ETIOLOGY AND PATHOPHYSIOLOGY

- Targeting of RBCs by the immune system initiates a series of events that results in hemolysis.
- Immunoglobulin may target RBC membrane antigens directly (*primary* or idiopathic IMHA), or the membrane may be altered by a variety of conditions, exposing novel antigens that are then targeted by immunoglobulin (*secondary* IMHA).
- In dogs, 75% of cases are estimated to be *primary*. *Primary* IMHA is uncommon in cats.
- Neoplasia has been estimated to be the most common cause of *secondary* IMHA in dogs. In cats, IMHA has been associated with drug reaction, feline leukemia (FeLV), lymphoma, and RBC

parasitism (*Mycoplasma hemofelis*, formerly *Haemobartonella*).

- *Extravascular hemolysis* occurs when RBCs coated with immunoglobulin (mostly IgG), complement, or both, circulate through the spleen and liver and are destroyed.
- Splenomegaly reflects active erythrophagocytosis by macrophages within the spleen, in addition to extramedullary hematopoiesis.
- Partial erythrophagocytosis by macrophages within the spleen produces spherocytes, a hallmark of IMHA.
- *Intravascular hemolysis* occurs in the vasculature when RBCs coated with immunoglobulin directly activate complement and are destroyed. *Intravascular hemolysis* can rarely occur by direct membrane attack mediated by complement without immunoglobulin involvement.
- IgM or IgG plus complement can also agglutinate RBCs, another hallmark of IMHA.
- Some erythrophagocytosis occurs in the liver in the presence of both excessive amounts of IgG, and some IgM; and hepatomegaly results from both erythrophagocytosis, and extramedullary hematopoeisis.
- Rapid decreases in hematocrit can cause ischemic injury to the liver, resulting in elevated serum alkaline phosphatase and severe leukocytosis. These changes have been associated with decreased survival.
- Leukocytosis may also result from increased red cell fragments in circulation and increased bone marrow activity.
- A regenerative response to anemia requires 3 to 5 days. Reticulocytosis, another hallmark of IMHA, has been reported in more than 80% of dogs.
- Elevated total bilirubin resulting from hemolysis and liver disease has been associated with decreased survival.
- A nonregenerative response (lack of reticulocytosis) may reflect inadequate time for the bone marrow to mount a response, or immune-mediated destruction of RBCs before their release, or as they are being released from the bone marrow (PRCA). See Anemia: Nonregenerative, and Pure Red Cell Aplasia, p 69.

DIAGNOSIS

DIFFERENTIAL DIAGNOSIS

- Anemia:
  - Blood loss (see Anemia Due to Blood Loss, p 63) and other hemolytic anemia (see Anemia, Hemolytic, p 64)
  - Abdominal hemorrhage
  - Bleeding disorder
  - Bone marrow failure (see Anemia [Aplastic], p 1336)
  - Anemia of chronic disease
- Nonimmune hemolytic anemia:
  - Heinz body anemia
  - Blood cell parasites (*Babesia* [dog], *Mycoplasma* [cat])
  - Genetic disorders such as phosphofructokinase deficiency, pyruvate kinase deficiency
- Icterus:
  - Hepatitis
  - Cirrhotic/fibrosing liver disease (see p 210)
  - Biliary obstruction
  - Pancreatitis
  - Cholangitis

INITIAL DATABASE

- Complete blood count with RBC morphology and reticulocyte count:
  - Hallmarks of IMHA include spherocytosis, autoagglutination, polychromasia, anisocytosis, and reticulocytosis. Autoagglutination has been reported in 42-66% of dogs; spherocytosis in 79% of dogs; polychromasia in 90% of dogs, and some combination of these in 96% of dogs with IMHA.
  - RBC parasites may be identified on a smear (e.g., *Babesia* spp [dogs], *Mycoplasma hemofelis* (formerly *Haemobartonella*) [cats]).
- Serum chemistry profile documents baseline total bilirubin, and serum liver and renal values. Hypoalbuminemia has been associated with increased risk of thromboembolism and possibly increased mortality.
- Urinalysis can provide a baseline measure of renal function in conjunction with serum chemistry profile. Pyuria or bacteriuria should prompt culture and antibiotic therapy.
- FeLV and feline immunodeficiency virus serologic testing in cats.
- In saline agglutination (slide autoagglutination test): see Cross-Match and Blood Typing, p 1212.
- Direct antibody test (DAT) (Coombs') or flow cytometry: flow cytometry has reported greater sensitivity and specificity than the DAT.
- Coagulation panel (activated partial thromboplastin time, prothrombin time, fibrinogen, fibrin degradation products, platelet count): dogs with IMHA are in a hypercoagulable state and are at risk of developing pulmonary thromboembolism and DIC. Dogs with IMHA may have elevations in prothrombin time (PT), activated partial thromboplastin time (aPTT), or have increased D-dimers, as a result of DIC. Note that decreases in PT or aPTT do *not* indicate a hypercoagulable state, nor do normal results in these parameters indicate absence of hypercoagulability.
- Survey thoracic radiography (three views) to exclude metastatic disease.
- Abdominal ultrasonography or survey abdominal radiography to assess for neoplasia.

ADVANCED OR CONFIRMATORY TESTING

- Serology. Dogs: heartworm, *Ehrlichia*, *Anaplasma*, rickettsial diseases, *Babesia*, *Bartonella*, antinuclear antibody titer; cats: FeLV, FIV, *Mycoplasma*
- Polymerase chain reaction test for *M. haemofelis* if suspected

TREATMENT

THERAPEUTIC GOAL(S)

- Maintain adequate oxygen-carrying capacity
- Immunosuppression
- Maintain perfusion of tissues
- Prophylactic anticoagulant therapy

ACUTE GENERAL TREATMENT

- Packed red blood cell (pRBC) transfusion is indicated if tachycardia, tachypnea, bounding pulses, and weakness accompany anemia (see Transfusion Reactions, p 1098)
- Immunosuppressive therapy: prednisone (1-2 mg/kg PO, SC, or IM q 12h), or dexamethasone sodium phosphate (0.15-0.25 mg/kg IV q 12h)
- Anticoagulant therapy: low molecular weight heparin (Fragmin 100-150

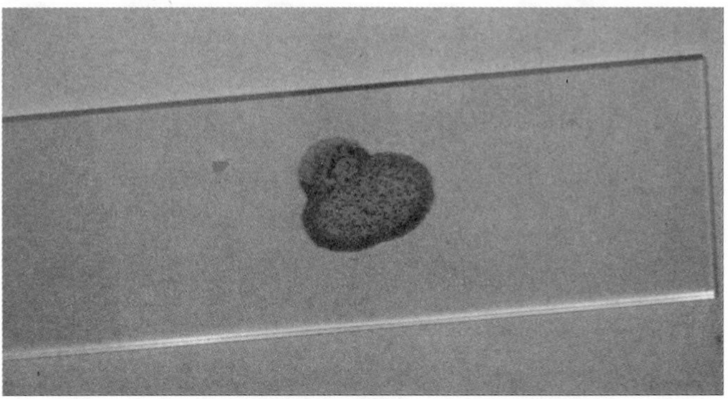

FIGURE I-12 Positive slide autoagglutination test from a dog with IMHA. Note clumping of red cells on a slide in a drop of anticoagulated blood mixed with a drop of saline. The plasma was also icteric.

IU/kg SC q 12–24h), or unfractionated ("regular") heparin (250–300 IU/kg SC q 6–8h)
- Gastric protectants: H_2 blockers (e.g., famotidine 0.5 mg/kg IV or PO q 12–24h)
- Intravenous crystalloids to support renal perfusion
- Antibiotic therapy if underlying infectious disease identified
- Anticancer therapy if underlying neoplastic disease identified

CHRONIC TREATMENT

- Continue immunosuppression with prednisone 1 mg/kg q 12h for 3 to 6 months, with tapering doses of 25% recommended every 3 to 4 weeks if hematocrit remains stable.
- An effective immunosuppressant treatment protocol beyond glucocorticoids has not been accepted in veterinary medicine. Additional therapies that have been used include:
  - Azathioprine (2 mg/kg PO q 24h for 10 days, then once every other day).
  - Cyclosporine (10 mg/kg PO q 24h; monitor blood levels).
  - Intravenous immunoglobulin (0.5 g/kg IV q 24h for 3 days) is costly.
  - Cyclophosphamide has been associated with decreased survival, and hence its use is not recommended.

POSSIBLE COMPLICATIONS

- Hospital-acquired infection: bacteremia, aspiration pneumonia, urinary tract infection
- Due to increased risk of pulmonary thromboembolism, use of jugular IV catheters is discouraged
- Adverse drug side effects:
  - Prednisone: gastrointestinal signs, pancreatitis, iatrogenic hyperadrenocorticism
  - Azathioprine: pancreatitis, hepatopathy, bone marrow suppression
  - Anticoagulants: bleeding

RECOMMENDED MONITORING

- During acute crisis, packed cell volume (PCV) should be assessed q 8–12h
- Once stabilized, PCV should be evaluated q 12–24h daily in hospital
- After discharge, PCV should be monitored weekly for first month, and then at each time of deciding on tapering medication to ensure remission

PROGNOSIS AND OUTCOME

- Mortality for dogs with IMHA has been estimated at 40–60%.
- Negative prognostic indicators include:
  - Severe serum bilirubin elevation
  - Severe thrombocytopenia
  - Thromboembolism
  - Severe leukocytosis
- A large number of dogs may relapse within a year, necessitating reinstitution of immunosuppressive therapy.
- Cats with underlying disease tend to respond poorly.

PEARLS & CONSIDERATIONS

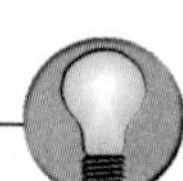

COMMENTS

- Because spherocytosis may result after transfusion, complete blood count and/or a fresh blood smear should be evaluated before transfusion therapy.
- Dogs with IMHA die of one of two causes: anemia or thromboembolism. Therefore, in addition to immunosuppression, the cornerstones of treatment include pRBC transfusion and adequate anticoagulation,
- The thought that transfusions "add fuel to the fire" has not been shown to be true.

CLIENT EDUCATION

After treatment is complete, clients should watch for early signs of relapse.

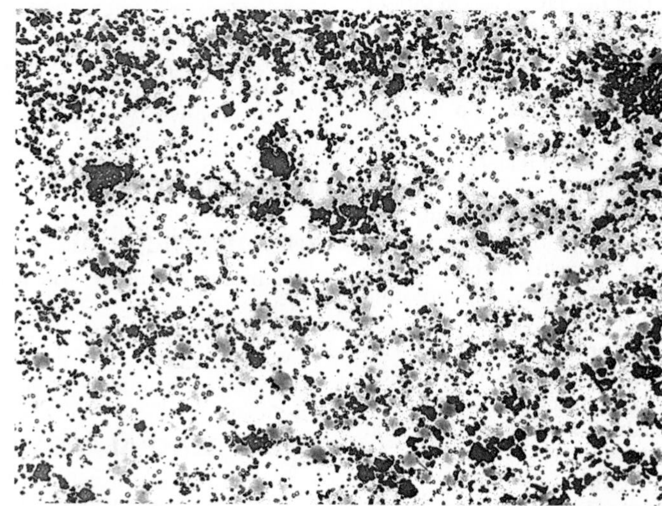

FIGURE I-13 Microscopic evidence of autoagglutination: clustering/clumping of red blood cells. This finding could be seen either on an unstained blood smear or one stained with Wright's or DiffQuick stains. Figs. I-13 and I-14 copyright Department of Clinical Pathology, Atlantic Veterinary College, and reproduced with permission.

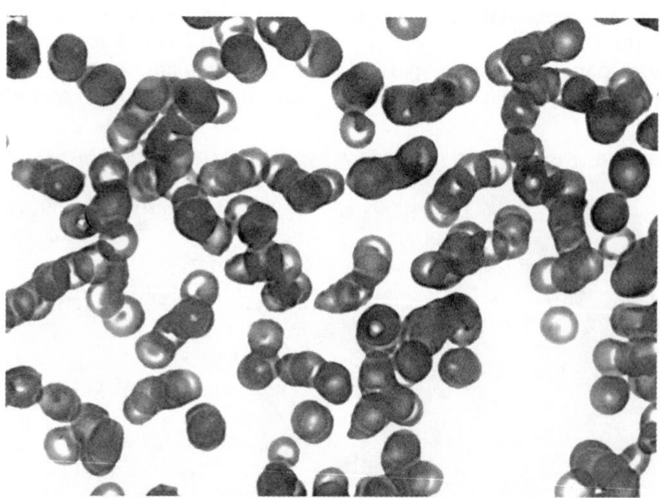

FIGURE I-14 NOT autoagglutination. This roll-of-coins appearance of red blood cells is characteristic of rouleaux formation, which may occur with hyperglobulinemias, or have no pathologic significance.

SUGGESTED READING

Carr AP, et al: Prognostic factors for mortality and thromboembolism in canine immune-mediated hemolytic anemia: a retrospective study of 72 dogs. *J Vet Intern Med* 16(5):501, 2002.

McCullough S: Immune-mediated hemolytic anemia: understanding the nemesis. *Vet Clin North Am Small Anim Pract* 33(6):1295, 2003.

AUTHOR: **THERESE E. O'TOOLE**
EDITOR: **SUSAN M. COTTER**

DISEASES AND DISORDERS

Anemia: Nonregenerative, and Pure Red Cell Aplasia

BASIC INFORMATION

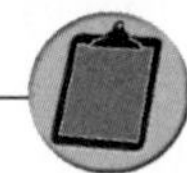

DEFINITION

- Decrease in hemoglobin and red blood cell (RBC) mass without a regenerative response, specifically reticulocytosis.
- Pure red cell aplasia (PRCA) is a specific form of severe nonregenerative anemia in which erythroid precursors are absent in the bone marrow. Myeloid lines are normal in numbers and maturation.

SYNONYM(S)

Erythrocyte aplasia

EPIDEMIOLOGY

SPECIES, AGE, SEX

- Dependent on underlying cause of nonregenerative anemia
- PRCA:
  - Middle-aged, female dogs
  - In feline leukemia virus-(FeLV-) and feline immunodeficiency virus-(FIV-) negative cats, most <2 years old

RISK FACTORS: Nonregenerative anemia: chronic renal failure, chronic systemic illness, FeLV- or FIV-positive status (cats).

CLINICAL PRESENTATION

HISTORY, CHIEF COMPLAINT: Lethargy, weakness, exercise intolerance, collapse, tachypnea.

PHYSICAL EXAM FINDINGS: Pale mucous membranes, tachycardia, tachypnea, soft systolic heart murmur, intolerance to handling (particularly cats).

ETIOLOGY AND PATHOPHYSIOLOGY

- Etiologies of nonregenerative anemia:
  - Defective hemogloblin synthesis: iron deficiency/chronic blood loss, copper deficiency, lead toxicity
  - Defective erythrocyte maturation: folate or cobalamin (cyanocobalamin, vitamin B_{12}) deficiency
  - Primary failure of erythropoiesis: inherited, acquired (immune-mediated)
  - Secondary failure of erythropoiesis: chronic renal failure or anemia of inflammatory disease (e.g., inflammatory or chronic diseases, neoplasia)
  - See Anemia (Aplastic), p 1336: drugs, toxins, radiation, infections (FeLV, FIV, ehrlichiosis)
  - Bone marrow infiltration: neoplasia, myelofibrosis
- PRCA is believed to be immune-mediated based on responsiveness to immunosuppressive therapy.
- Nonregenerative anemia may occur when the immune system destroys reticulocytes or earlier erythroid precursors.

DIAGNOSIS

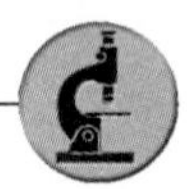

DIFFERENTIAL DIAGNOSIS

Acute blood loss or destruction with insufficient time for reticulocytosis (3 to 4 days)

INITIAL DATABASE

- Complete blood count: anemia, erythrocyte morphology dependent on cause. In immune-mediated forms, erythrocytes are often normocytic, normochromic
  - PRCA in dogs: median hematocrit 10% (range 5-18%), reticulocyte count 0.1%
  - PRCA in cats: median hematocrit 7% (range 6-15%)
- Reticulocyte count: <1% corrected, absolute count <60,000/μl
- Blood smear: basophilic stippling in lead poisoning, spherocytosis in early IMHA, or abnormal cells
- Total protein: decreases with hemorrhage, normal to slightly increased with hemolysis or marrow failure
- Serum biochemistry profile and urinalysis reflect underlying disorders (e.g., renal failure). Liver enzymes may be elevated in immune-mediated anemia
- Cats: FeLV and FIV testing

ADVANCED OR CONFIRMATORY TESTING

- Bone marrow aspirate or core biopsy: evaluates cellularity, myeloid: erythroid ratio, completeness and orderliness of maturation, presence of abnormal cells
  - M/E ratio often >75:1 in PRCA (normal: 1:1 to 2:1)
  - Mature lymphocytosis common in cats with PRCA; lymphocytosis and plasmacytosis sometimes seen in dogs
- Coombs' test
  - Dogs: usually negative with PRCA, but may be positive with autoimmune-associated nonregenerative immune-mediated anemia
  - Cats: positive in approximately 50%
- Testing for underlying disorders
  - For example, consider thoracic radiographs and abdominal ultrasound if neoplasia suspected

TREATMENT

THERAPEUTIC GOAL(S)

- Increase oxygen-carrying capacity through correction of anemia
- Identify and correct underlying disorders
- Anemia of inflammatory disease does not require treatment; often improves with treatment of underlying cause

ACUTE GENERAL TREATMENT

Transfusion with packed RBCs if hematocrit <15% or with significant clinical signs

CHRONIC TREATMENT

- Treat underlying disorders
- For PRCA and nonregenerative immune-mediated anemia, immunosuppressive therapy
  - Prednisone: 1-2 mg/kg PO q 12h, then taper once response seen
  - If inadequate response, consider other immunosuppressive drugs:
    - Cyclophosphamide: 50 mg/m^2 PO q 24h × 4 days; repeat weekly
    - Azathioprine (dogs): 2 mg/kg PO q 24h × 5 days, then every other day
    - Cyclosporine microemulsion [Atopica, Neoral] 2-5 mg/kg PO q 12h, adjusted to achieve trough serum concentrations of 200-500 ng/ml; concurrent ketoconazole 10 mg/kg PO q 24h allows cyclosporine dosage of 2-5 mg/kg PO q 24h
  - Pure red cell aplasia may require > 1 month (sometimes several months) before hematocrit rises by 5%

RECOMMENDED MONITORING

Repeat hematocrit periodically:

- In PRCA, recheck every 3 to 4 days until RBC count begins to rise, then weekly until normal for 1 month, monthly thereafter until stable

PROGNOSIS AND OUTCOME

Depends on underlying disorder and severity of anemia:

- Good for PRCA and other correctable disorders that respond to treatment
- Guarded to poor for nonregenerative anemia secondary to retroviruses, ehrlichiosis, or chronic renal failure

PEARLS & CONSIDERATIONS

COMMENTS

- With acute anemia, sufficient time may not have elapsed (3 to 4 days) to detect reticulocytosis.
- Anemia in PRCA is usually severe at presentation, because the onset generally is gradual.
- Anemia of inflammatory disease usually is mild, except in end-stage renal failure.

- Bone marrow evaluation is needed to distinguish PRCA from other nonregenerative anemias.
- Canine PRCA usually is immune-mediated
- Feline nonregenerative anemia commonly is secondary to renal failure or retroviruses.

SUGGESTED READING

Cotter SM: Non-regenerative anemia. In Ettinger SJ, Feldman EC (eds): *Textbook of Veterinary Internal Medicine*, ed 5. Philadelphia, WB Saunders, 2000, pp 1804-1816.

Stokol T, Blue JT: Pure red cell aplasia in cats: 9 cases (1989-1997). *J Am Vet Med Assoc* 214:75-79, 1999.

Stokol T, et al: Idiopathic pure red cell aplasia and nonregnerative immune-mediated anemia in dogs: 43 cases (1988-1999). *J Am Vet Med Assoc* 216:1429-1436, 2000.

Weiss DJ: Primary pure red cell aplasia in dogs: 13 cases (1996-2000). *J Am Vet Med Assoc* 221:93-95, 2002.

AUTHOR: **LISA G. BARBER**
EDITOR: **SUSAN M. COTTER**

Anesthetic-Related Complications

BASIC INFORMATION

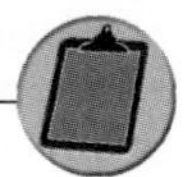

DEFINITION

Anesthetic-related complications include overdosage of anesthetic agents, idiosyncratic reactions to anesthetic agents, anesthetic equipment failure, and pathologic complications attributed to anesthesia.

SYNONYM(S)

Anesthesia equipment malfunction
Anesthetic accidents
Drug reaction

EPIDEMIOLOGY

SPECIES, AGE, SEX: Dogs or cats of any age and either sex can be affected.

RISK FACTORS: Increased risk:

- Very young animals, very old animals, animals with comorbidities. Specifically, cardiac disease and cardiovascular instability are associated with higher risk of mortality
- Failure to adequately monitor anesthetized patients impairs the detection of anesthetic equipment malfunction and anesthetic-related complications

ASSOCIATED CONDITIONS AND DISORDERS: Respiratory arrest, cardiac arrest.

CLINICAL PRESENTATION

DISEASE FORMS/SUBTYPES

- Equipment failure
- Cardiovascular, respiratory, or neurologic complications
- Anaphylactic reactions
- Anesthesia-related hyperthermia or hypothermia
- Prolonged anesthetic recovery

HISTORY, CHIEF COMPLAINT

- During general anesthesia: onset of:
  - Apnea
  - Dyspnea
  - Acute pallor and/or cyanosis
  - Bradycardia
  - Tachycardia/tachyarrhythmia
  - Hypotension
  - Hypothermia
- During anesthetic recovery: neurologic dysfunction

PHYSICAL EXAM: See History, Chief Complaint above.

ETIOLOGY AND PATHOPHYSIOLOGY

- Primary respiratory system effects, potentially leading to hypotension, bradycardia, and cardiac arrest if left unchecked:
  - Equipment malfunction causing hypercapnia and/or hypoxemia
  - Accidental closure of the pressure release valve ("pop-off valve") causing pulmonary barotrauma and bradycardia
  - Tracheal tears from overinflated endotracheal cuffs, causing pneumomediastinum, subcutaneous emphysema, possibly pneumothorax
  - Endotracheal tube occlusion (overinsertion beyond the carina, or occlusion with secretions [especially if internal tube diameter <4.0 mm])
  - Opioid overdosage
- Primary cardiovascular effects, potentially leading to cardiac arrhythmias or congestive heart failure:
  - Exacerbation of undetected cardiac disease if excessive doses of drugs that stress the cardiovascular system (atropine, glycopyrrolate, isoproterenol, dopamine, dobutamine, epinephrine) are used
- Neurologic signs during recovery: most commonly due to hypoxia-induced cerebral edema
- Potential causes of any signs of adverse reactions:
  - Administration of particular anesthetic agents to which the patient has an idiosyncratic reaction (rare) or in dosages that the patient fails to appropriately metabolize (common)
  - Underestimation of patient's ability to tolerate cardiovascular or respiratory suppressive effects of anesthetic agents

DIAGNOSIS

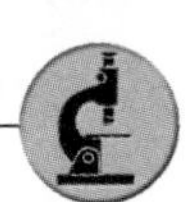

DIFFERENTIAL DIAGNOSIS

- Respiratory system decompensation from development of surgically induced pneumothorax
- Cardiovascular and respiratory dysfunction from primary disease (e.g., sepsis, traumatic brain injury)
- Cardiovascular decompensation from surgical complication (e.g., surgical bleeding, excessive sympathetic discharge, vagal-mediated reflexes)
- Monitoring equipment malfunction (e.g., disconnected electrocardiogram [ECG] leads, malpositioned pulse oximeter probe)
- Anesthesia machine malfunction (e.g., disconnected oxygen supply/tubing or breathing circuits; malfunctioning one-way inspiratory and expiratory valves; failure of non-rebreathing circuits)

INITIAL DATABASE

- Assessment of endotracheal tube position for dislodgement (too shallow/extubated, or too deep/obstructing mainstem bronchus)
- Assessment of pulse quality: systolic pulse < 60 mmHg may not be palpable
- Heart rate assessed via an esophageal stethoscope or direct palpation on the chest
- Monitoring of blood pressure, pulse oximetry, end-tidal CO_2
- Check anesthetic circuit for leaks, malfunction, inadvertently closed pressure valves
- Arterial blood gas analysis, packed cell volume/total solids: elucidate causes of cyanosis, pallor
- Review drugs and doses administered

TREATMENT

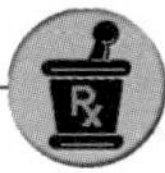

THERAPEUTIC GOAL(S)

- Restore cardiovascular stability
- Reverse respiratory depression

- Manage secondary (e.g., neurologic) effects
- Remove malfunctioning equipment

ACUTE GENERAL TREATMENT

- Apnea, cyanosis, acute pallor:
  - Assess anesthetic depth; reduce/stop anesthetic administration if too deep
  - Assess pupillary light response and if negative, assess for cardiac arrest (see Cardiopulmonary Cerebral Resuscitation, p 1202)
  - Ensure airway, oxygen supply, and breathing circuit are open
  - Opioid antagonists (e.g., naloxone 0.01–0.04 mg/kg IV to effect) if opioid overdosage
- Tachypnea/dyspnea:
  - Assess anesthetic depth; increase anesthetic administration if too shallow
  - Rule out pneumothorax (ensure valves are open; percussion and auscultation; radiograph)
  - Rule out severe hyperthermia (idiosyncratic)
- Bradycardia:
  - Assess airway, oxygen supply, breathing circuit for patency
  - May treat with glycopyrrolate (0.11 mg/kg IV)
  - If instantaneous change from severe tachycardia to severe bradycardia, prepare for cardiac arrest
- Tachycardia/tachyarrhythmia: see Sinus Tachycardia, p 1007; Ventricular Arrhythmias (Premature Ventricular Complexes, Ventricular Tachycardia), p 1148
- Hypotension:
  - Lighten anesthetic level if too deep
  - Administer intravenous fluids if hypovolemic
  - Administer inotropic agents if necessary
- Hypothermia: common. Rewarm carefully (unconscious patient cannot avoid iatrogenic overheating and burns). Target: T >98° F (36.7° C), then stop and monitor
- Neurologic complications postanesthesia: treat as for Head Trauma, p 454

POSSIBLE COMPLICATIONS

- Severe hypoxemia or hypercarbia: neurologic dysfunction
- Prolonged anesthetic recovery, hypothermia, hypotension may require intensive supportive measures such as external heating, inotropes, and mechanical ventilation

RECOMMENDED MONITORING

- Continuous ECG
- Respiration rate, effort
- Blood gas analysis to assess oxygenation and ventilation
- Blood pressure monitoring
- Temperature monitoring

PROGNOSIS AND OUTCOME

- With prompt recognition and immediate intervention, most anesthesia-related complications have a fair to good prognosis for full recovery.
- Improvement in patient monitoring, allowing early detection of complications, have resulted in the reduction of anesthetic-associated mortality to 0.1–0.4%.

PEARLS & CONSIDERATIONS

COMMENTS

- Vigilant monitoring, rapid detection of abnormalities, and prompt treatment prevent serious consequences and decrease anesthetic-associated mortality.
- Selection of cardiovascular or respiratory-sparing anesthetic agents or those that are readily reversible may be preferable in high-risk populations.

PREVENTION

- Thorough patient evaluation before anesthesia
- Reversible anesthetic agents
- Thorough monitoring, including audible monitoring devices
- Complete maintenance of anesthetic equipment

SUGGESTED READING

Cooper JB, et al: Preventable anesthesia mishaps: A study of human factors. *Qual Saf Health Care* 11:277–283, 2002.

Dyson DH, et al: Morbidity and mortality associated with anesthetic management in small animal veterinary practice in Ontario. *J Am Anim Hosp Assoc* 34:325–335, 1998.

Gaynor JS, et al: Complications and mortality associated with anesthesia in dogs and cats. *J Am Anim Hosp Assoc* 35:13–17, 1999.

AUTHOR: **ELIZABETH A. ARMITAGE**

EDITOR: **ELIZABETH ROZANSKI**

Angular Limb Deformities

BASIC INFORMATION

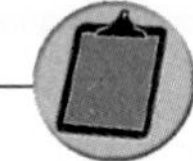

DEFINITION

An abnormal growth of the limb due to premature closure of a physis (growth plate)

- Most commonly occurs in the forelimb with radial or ulnar physeal closure(s)
- Rarely, affects the hind limb with premature closure of the tibial physis

SYNONYM(S)

Premature closure of radial, ulnar, or tibial physis

Radius curvus

EPIDEMIOLOGY

SPECIES, AGE, SEX: Primarily young dogs.

RISK FACTORS: Trauma to limb and physis.

CLINICAL PRESENTATION

HISTORY, CHIEF COMPLAINT

- Trauma to the limb 3 to 4 weeks before deformity
- Often, dog is presented when the leg begins to appear deformed

PHYSICAL EXAM FINDINGS

- Lameness of affected limb with pain on palpation of carpus or elbow.
- The limb may appear shortened or have an angular deviation.

ETIOLOGY AND PATHOPHYSIOLOGY

- Premature closure of the distal ulnar physis is the most common physeal injury, likely due to the conical shape of this physis in dogs.
  - Because of the paired bone system, cessation of growth in the ulna causes cranial bowing, external rotation, and valgus deformity of the radius. Elbow and carpal incongruities can also occur.
- Asymmetric closure of the distal radial physis can cause an angular deformity similar to closure of the ulnar physis.
- Symmetric closure of the distal radial physis will often lead to radial shortening and elbow incongruity, but no angular deformity.

DIAGNOSIS

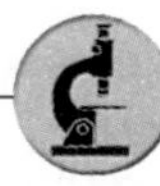

DIFFERENTIAL DIAGNOSIS

- Malunion of a fracture
- Ligamentous or tendinous damage at the elbow or antebrachiocarpal joint
- Retained cartilaginous cores of the ulna

INITIAL DATABASE

- Complete blood count and serum chemistry panel: no abnormal findings expected with this disorder
- Mediolateral and craniocaudal elbow to carpus radiographs of the affected and contralateral limb to assess degree of deformation

TREATMENT

THERAPEUTIC GOAL(S)

- Immature dogs:
  - Restore unrestricted growth
  - Maximize limb length
  - Correct angular deformities and joint incongruencies
- Mature dogs:
  - Correct angular, rotational deformities, and joint incongruency
  - Preserve limb length

ACUTE GENERAL TREATMENT

- An ulnar ostectomy is used in an immature dog with premature closure of the ulnar physis to restore growth potential.
  - A fat graft placed in the ostectomy prevents premature bone union.
- Premature closure of the distal radius is treated with distraction osteogenesis using circular external fixation.
  - This allows for limb lengthening and correction of angular deformities.
- A corrective closing radial wedge osteotomy, stabilized with a tplate or external fixation, is performed in mature dogs for acute correction of angular and rotational deformities.
- With severe elbow incongruity, a dynamic proximal ulnar osteotomy permits realignment.

CHRONIC TREATMENT

- In the postoperative period, a soft padded bandage or metasplint may be placed to protect the limb. Physical rehabilitation (see Physical Rehabilitation, p 1300) to reduce risk of complications
- Exercise restriction for at least 6 weeks until radiographs confirm bone healing

POSSIBLE COMPLICATIONS

- External fixation may have premature loosening of the fixation pins or pin tract infection
- Inappropriate amount of surgical correction may result in persistent valgus
- Distal radial plating may result in decreased antebrachiocarpal joint range of motion
- Distraction osteogenesis may lead to flexor tendon contracture.

RECOMMENDED MONITORING

- Suture removal and recheck 2 weeks after surgery
- Radiographs at 4 to 6 weeks to evaluate bone healing

PROGNOSIS AND OUTCOME

- Guarded after ulnar ostectomy alone. Often, an additional surgical procedure is necessary at skeletal maturity to correct the angular deformity.
- Good after definitive corrective osteotomy if the amount of correction is adequate.

PEARLS & CONSIDERATIONS

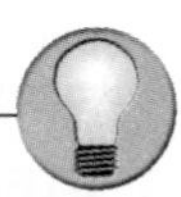

COMMENTS

- Corrective osteotomy is performed at the point of maximum deformity to provide optimal realignment of the articular surfaces and appropriate limb alignment.
- If there is minimal radial shortening but radial head subluxation, a proximal ulnar ostectomy will shorten the ulna and restore elbow congruity.
- During ulnar ostectomy, the periosteum must be removed completely to prevent premature healing of the ostectomy site.
- Pes varus is a rare condition associated with distal tibial physeal closure in dachshunds.

SUGGESTED READING

Johnson AL, Hulse DA: Radial and ulnar growth deformities. In Fossum TW (ed): *Small Animal Surgery*, ed 2. St. Louis, Mosby, 2002, pp 955–963.

Piermattei DL, Flo GL: Correction of abnormal bone growth and healing. In *Brinker, Piermattei, and Flo's Handbook of Small Animal Orthopedics and Fracture Repair*, ed 3. Philadelphia, WB Saunders, 1997, pp 686–712.

Boudrieau RJ: Deformities caused by premature closure of radial and ulnar physes. In Slatter D (ed): *Textbook of Small Animal Surgery*, ed 3. Philadelphia, WB Saunders, 2002, pp 1964–1973.

AUTHOR: **RAVIV J. BALFOUR**
EDITOR: **JOSEPH HARARI**

Anorexia

BASIC INFORMATION

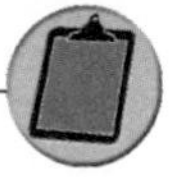

DEFINITION

The loss of appetite for food

SYNONYM(S)

Decreased appetite
Inappetence
Loss of appetite

EPIDEMIOLOGY

GENETICS AND BREED PREDISPOSITION: Toy breeds of dogs are inclined to have a capricious, finicky appetite.

CLINICAL PRESENTATION

HISTORY, CHIEF COMPLAINT: History is important:

- Differentiate between a pet that wants to eat but is unable to (pseudoanorexia) and a pet that shows no inclination to eat.
- Food palatability: smell, taste, texture, and temperature all affect acceptability.
- Pain, vomiting, or nausea associated with eating may cause the development of food aversion, which may result in complete anorexia in cats and a capricious appetite in dogs.

PHYSICAL EXAM FINDINGS

- Extended anorexia will be associated with weight loss and muscle atrophy.
- Patients with anorexia due to systemic disease will usually present with additional clinical signs of the underlying disorder.
- Oropharyngeal examination in patients may show relevant abnormalities (e.g., marked periodontal disease).
- Neurologic examination in patients with dysphagia or esophageal disease.
- Patients with psychological eating disorders will appear clinically normal.

ETIOLOGY AND PATHOPHYSIOLOGY

- Mechanisms triggering the onset of true anorexia are complex due to the interplay of numerous factors controlling satiety and hunger.
- Central nervous system:
  - Hypothalamus and solitary nucleus associated with satiety and hunger

- Serotonin inhibits appetite, whereas γ-aminobutyric acid (GABA) stimulates appetite
- Gastrointestinal factors:
  - Gastric and duodenal distention
  - Gastric "satiety hormones": cholecystokinin, somatostatin, glucagon, leptin
  - Plasma concentration of nutrients
- Environmental, sensory and psychological factors:
  - Learned behavior
  - Palatability of diet or altered diet
  - Environment
  - Pain/stress
  - Food aversion
- Systemic disease.
- Organic disease and neoplasia can cause the release of cachectin and interleukin-1, which have inhibitory effects on appetite.

DIAGNOSIS

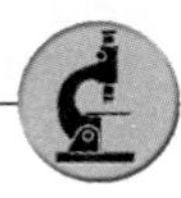

DIFFERENTIAL DIAGNOSIS

- Disinterested in food altogether (true anorexia):
  - Systemic disease
  - Infection/inflammation
  - Neoplasia
  - Food aversion
- Reluctance to eat (pseudoanorexia):
  - Associated with pain/discomfort:
    - Painful prehension or mastication, odynophagia (repeated, painful attempts at swallowing)
      - Retrobulbar (apical/tooth root) abscesses
      - Intraoral masses/foreign bodies
      - Mandibular fractures/temporomandibular joint disease
      - Masticatory muscle myositis
      - Periodontal disease
      - Salivary gland disorders
    - Oropharyngeal dysphagia
    - Esophageal disease (masses, foreign bodies)
  - Associated with nausea:
    - Gastrointestinal inflammatory disease
    - Ileus
    - Delayed gastric emptying
    - Vestibular disease

INITIAL DATABASE

- Pseudo-anorexia:
  - Neurologic examination
  - Oral, dental, and cranial examination (sedation or general anesthesia)
  - Radiographs of the teeth, mandible, or nasal cavity may be required
  - Thoracic radiographs and/or endoscopy to evaluate the esophagus for any obstruction (e.g., masses, foreign bodies)
- True anorexia

For the truly anorexic patient, the causes may be legion. Anorexia is one of the *least specific* clinical signs and will not, in itself, direct the clinical evaluation. Anorexia is purely an indicator of underlying systemic disease.

ADVANCED OR CONFIRMATORY TESTING

Will be dictated by clinical findings:

- Pseudo-anorexia: imaging, radiographs, esophageal endoscopy
- True anorexia: laboratory tests and imaging as suggested by history, physical exam findings, and the initial database

TREATMENT

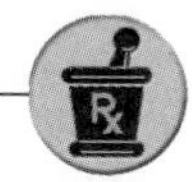

THERAPEUTIC GOAL(S)

- Management of anorexia is a vital basic supportive therapy in the ill patient and will decrease both morbidity and mortality. Protein energy malnutrition has adverse effects on the immune system and causes delayed healing, muscle weakness, insulin resistance, and increased metabolic rate due to activation of the sympathetic nervous system. Anorexia will also result in breakdown of the intestinal mucosal barrier.
- Nutritional support should be initiated early in the management of a patient to prevent malnutrition.

ACUTE GENERAL TREATMENT

- Proper identification and treatment of the underlying cause.
- General supportive therapy:
  - Maintain fluid and electrolyte balances.
- Nutritional supportive therapy:
  - Dietary manipulation:
    - Ensure the availability of highly palatable food (taste, odor, and texture).
    - Avoid oral medication in anorexic patients.
  - Anorexia that persists for 3 to 5 days requires a form of nutritional support:
    - *If the gut works, use it*: enterocytes rely on luminal nutrition. Enteral feeding via nasoesophageal, esophagostomy, or gastrostomy tubes. Esophagostomy tubes are easily placed and maintained (see Feeding Tube Placement: Esophagostomy Tube, p 1243).
    - Parenteral feeding.
  - Control of nausea:
    - Metoclopramide: 0.2-0.4 mg/kg IV q 8h (IV constant rate infusion that administers 1-2 mg/kg/day is effective). Improves gastrointestinal motility, gastric emptying, decreases ileus, and has central antidopaminonergic effects.
- Appetite stimulation: This is a short-term *adjunctive* treatment to be used while an effort is made to ascertain the underlying cause. It is rarely of long-term benefit, and the drugs can have side effects.
  - Diazepam: 0.2 mg/kg IV every 2 hours (facilitates GABA activity).
  - Cyproheptadine: 1-2 mg/kg PO q 8-24h (serotonin antagonist).

CHRONIC TREATMENT

Long-term/permanent esophagostomy or gastrostomy tubes may be required (see Feeding Tube Placement: Percutaneous Endoscopic Gastrostomy [PEG], p 1247)

POSSIBLE COMPLICATIONS

- Avoid antiemetics if gastrointestinal obstruction is suspected
- Benzodiazepines are contraindicated in cats with hepatic disease

RECOMMENDED MONITORING

Monitor body weight, serum albumin levels, electrolyte levels

PROGNOSIS AND OUTCOME

Anorexia is a clinical manifestation only. The outcome is dependent on the cause.

PEARLS & CONSIDERATIONS

COMMENTS

- The most important consideration when presented with an "anorexic" patient is to determine whether it wants to eat. This is a vital decision-making piece of information and is based on a good history, physical examination, and observation of the animals.
- Patients may be choosy in what they eat, and anorexic animals should be tempted with a variety of food before establishing a diagnosis of anorexia.
- Oral medications can cause anorexia.
- Anorexia is an early sign of nausea.
- Animals, especially cats, develop learned aversions to foods with negative associations.
- *If the gut works, use it.*

SUGGESTED READING

Sanderson S, Bartges JW: Management of anorexia. In Bonagura JD (ed): *Kirk's Current Veterinary Therapy XIII: Small Animal Practice*. Philadelphia, WB Saunders, 2000, pp 69–74.

Bowlin CL: Anorexia and weight loss. In Lappin MR (ed): *Feline Internal Medicine Secrets*. Philadelphia, Hanley & Belfus, 2001.

AUTHOR: **LIESEL VAN DER MERWE**

EDITOR: **ETIENNE CÔTÉ**

Antibiotic-Responsive Diarrhea

BASIC INFORMATION

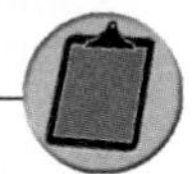

DEFINITION

Strictly defined as any diarrhea (including diarrhea associated with *Clostridium* spp., *Campylobacter* spp., *Salmonella* spp.) demonstrating responsiveness to and resolution with antibiotic therapy; however, it is conventionally defined as increased numbers of aerobic and/or anaerobic bacteria appropriately cultured from the small intestine in patients with associated clinical signs. There is considerable controversy regarding the definition of antibiotic-responsive diarrhea (ARD)/antibiotic-responsive enteropathy (ARE) versus small intestinal bacterial overgrowth (SIBO), which are often used interchangeably; the current trend is to refer to this condition as *antibiotic-responsive diarrhea* until the pathogenesis is more clearly defined (see below).

SYNONYM(S)

ARD
ARE
SIBO
Small bowel bacterial overgrowth

EPIDEMIOLOGY

SPECIES, AGE, SEX: Young animals predominate; no gender bias.
GENETICS AND BREED PREDISPOSITION: German shepherd dogs, beagles (IgA dysregulation/deficiency).
RISK FACTORS: Underlying immunologic gastrointestinal (GI) disease, pancreatic insufficiency, achlorhydria, intestinal motility disorders, GI obstructive disease, GI bypass surgery (secondary ARD).
CONTAGION AND ZOONOSIS: None other than zoonotic potential of enteric (e.g., *Salmonella* spp., *Campylobacter* spp.) infections.

CLINICAL PRESENTATION

DISEASE FORMS/SUBTYPES

- Primary: idiopathic ARD in which no underlying functional abnormality or disease is identified (rarely seen)
- Secondary: ARD as a complication of other underlying primary GI/pancreatic disease (common)

HISTORY, CHIEF COMPLAINT: Small bowel diarrhea (variable severity); variable weight loss, poor body condition, borborygmus, flatulence, vomiting (occasional).
PHYSICAL EXAM FINDINGS: No physical findings are diagnostic of ARD other than nonspecific small bowel diarrhea and occasionally weight loss. Steatorrhea may occur.

ETIOLOGY AND PATHOPHYSIOLOGY

- At this time, until investigators are better able to define the normal ranges for duodenal flora in dogs and cats, the term *SIBO* is difficult to apply and impossible to distinguish from ARD that is not due to bacterial overgrowth. Thus, ARD is used for describing patients with clinical signs of GI disease responsive only to antibiotic therapy.
- Normal host protective mechanisms prevent overgrowth of normal flora or pathogens through gastric acid secretion, intestinal motility (peristalsis and interdigestive migrating complexes), pancreatic and bile antimicrobial secretions (enzymes, immunoglobulins), and local enteric immunoglobulin production.
- Normal dogs: aerobic bacteria predominate (*E. coli, Staphylococcus* spp., *Streptococcus* spp., *Proteus* spp., *Corynebacterium* spp); anaerobes are rare (*Bacteroides* spp., *Propionibacterium* spp., *Peptostreptococcus* spp.); proximal small bowel bacterial numbers in healthy dogs reported to range from 10^2–10^5 colony-forming units (CFU)/ml.
- Cats: much higher bacterial counts are found (10^5–10^8 CFU/ml): aerobic *Pasteurella* sp. predominate; anaerobes are common (*Bacteroides* spp., *Fusobac-terium* spp., *Eubacterium* spp.); SIBO is not reported in the cat (based on the normal higher bacterial counts).
- Current research suggests these numbers (derived from human values and initial reports in dogs) represent an inappropriately low adopted cut-off value; healthy dogs may have much higher bacterial counts.
- The pathophysiology of ARD is thought to involve intraluminal effects of proliferating bacteria, damage to the mucosal enterocytes, injury to brush border enzymes and carrier proteins, secretion of enterotoxins, deconjugation of bile acids, hydroxylation of fatty acids, decreased mucin production, bacterial competition for nutrients, and increased mucosal permeability.
- Mucosal morphologic changes on biopsy are usually minimal: mild, patchy lymphoplasmacytic infiltrates, villous blunting (may be more pronounced with anaerobic infections).
- Increased lamina propria CD4$^+$ lymphocytes and increased cytokine production (TNFα, TGFβ) have been demonstrated in affected dogs.
- The net result is intermittent small bowel diarrhea with or without weight loss, variable vomiting, anorexia and anemia due to cobalamin deficiency, and malnutrition due to malabsorption of fats, carbohydrates, proteins, and fat-soluble vitamins.

DIAGNOSIS

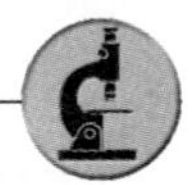

DIFFERENTIAL DIAGNOSIS

- Intestinal parasitism (helminth, giardiasis)
- Dietary intolerance/hypersensitivity
- Inflammatory bowel disease
- Intestinal lymphosarcoma
- Exocrine pancreatic insufficiency (EPI)
- Intestinal obstruction: stricture, intussusception, neoplasia, foreign body
- Motility disorders
- Surgical causes: bypass procedures, ileocolic valve resection

INITIAL DATABASE

- Fecal flotation and rectal scraping cytologic study to rule out other causes of diarrhea
- Complete blood count: may demonstrate mild anemia due to malnutrition (decreased B_{12} absorption; anemia not specifically macrocytic, in contrast to human pernicious anemia) or anemia of chronic disease (typically mild and nonregenerative)
- Biochemistry panel and urinalysis: usually nonspecific; hypoproteinemia may suggest protein-losing enteropathy or nephropathy
- Abdominal radiography and/or ultrasonography for obstructive disease or neoplasia

ADVANCED OR CONFIRMATORY TESTING

- Most cases of ARD are diagnosed retrospectively, based on response to a brief course of oral antibiotics implemented when other common causes of diarrhea have been ruled out.
- Increased serum folate levels, decreased serum cobalamin levels (or both): lacking in sensitivity and specificity.
- Serum trypsin-like immunoreactivity to rule out EPI.
- Increased serum unconjugated bile acids have been reported in dogs with

SIBO; however, elevated levels in control dogs limit specificity.
- Endoscopic mucosal biopsies demonstrate minimal inflammatory infiltrates/changes in primary ARD; in secondary ARD, GI biopsies may demonstrate the underlying, primary disease.
- Fecal culture: rarely helpful except for the isolated case of *Salmonella* or *Campylobacter* infection.
- Duodenal juice culture (handled anaerobically) is the gold standard for SIBO with total bacterial counts $>10^5$ CFU/ml or anaerobes $>10^4$ CFU/ml considered diagnostic of bacterial overgrowth (dogs only). The validity of simple quantification is currently under intense debate and is impractical for general practice.
- More sophisticated and specific DNA testing for bacterial species and numbers is being investigated and may improve our ability to determine true bacterial overgrowth versus antibiotic-responsive enteropathies.

TREATMENT

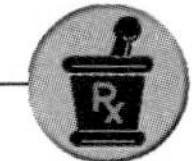

THERAPEUTIC GOAL(S)

Resolution of diarrhea with appropriate antibiotic therapy

ACUTE GENERAL TREATMENT

- Identify and treat underlying contributory disorders
- Fenbendazole 50 mg/kg daily for 3 to 5 days should be considered for occult parasitism before antibiotic therapy
- Unless specifically directed by fecal culture, antibiotic choices for 10 to 14 days include:
  - Metronidazole: 10-15 mg/kg PO q 12h (anaerobes, only)
  - Tylosin: 10-40 mg/kg PO q 12h
  - Oxytetracycline: 10 mg/kg PO q 8h
  - Enrofloxacin: 5-10 mg/kg PO q 24h
  - Amoxicillin: 20 mg/kg PO q 12h
- Parenteral B_{12} supplementation (250-500 µg/week IM or SC) may be required to normalize serum levels
- Low-fat, highly digestible diet (many available)
- Prebiotic therapy: fructo-oligosaccharides feed normal flora ("beneficial bacteria")
- Dietary fiber: increase, decrease, or change in type (soluble versus insoluble) to alter flora

CHRONIC TREATMENT

- Some animals have recurrent signs when antibiotic treatment ends; long-term, low-dose antibiotic therapy may be required, but only when underlying causes have definitively been addressed.
- Recognize underlying contributory disorders that may be associated with ARD/SIBO and require other treatment.

DRUG INTERACTIONS

- History of sensitivity to any of the antibiotics listed.
- Metronidazole is a radiation sensitizer in animals undergoing concurrent radiation therapy.

POSSIBLE COMPLICATIONS

Central nervous system signs with high-dose metronidazole (do not exceed 30 mg/kg/day, and do not exceed 2 weeks of treatment at this dose)

RECOMMENDED MONITORING

Monitor for recurrence of diarrhea after therapy

PROGNOSIS AND OUTCOME

Usually excellent; may require chronic treatment, especially if underlying GI disease is present and ARD is secondary

PEARLS & CONSIDERATIONS

COMMENTS

- Primary (idiopathic) ARD is rare; always evaluate for underlying GI tract disease.
- Decreased intestinal motility is probably the most important cause of ARD; in addition to GI tract disease, consider endocrine (hypothyroidism, diabetes mellitus, hypoadrenocorticism) and neurologic causes.
- Chronic use of potent H_2 blockers (cimetidine, ranitidine, famotidine, nizatidine) or proton pump inhibitors (omeprazole, lansoprazole) may predispose to ARD due to hypochlorhydria.
- German shepherd dogs are likely predisposed to ARD due to IgA deficiency and exocrine pancreatic insufficiency.
- Enzyme replacement for exocrine pancreatic insufficiency may not be efficacious until antibiotic therapy is instituted.
- The ideal antibiotic would be concentrated in bile and delivered at effective levels directly to the upper small intestine.
- Histiocytic ulcerative colitis (large bowel disease) has recently been reported as an antibiotic-responsive diarrhea in dogs.

CLIENT EDUCATION

Long-term diet control (low-fat, highly digestible) in addition to antibiotic therapy may be required.

SUGGESTED READING

German AJ, Hall EJ, Day MJ: Chronic intestinal inflammation and intestinal disease in dogs. *J Vet Intern Med* 17(1):8-20, 2003.

German AJ, et al: Comparison of direct and indirect tests for small intestinal bacterial overgrowth and antibiotic-responsive diarrhea in dogs. *J Vet Intern Med* 17(1):33-43, 2003.

Hall EJ, Simpson KW: Diseases of the small intestine. *In* Ettinger SJ, Feldman EC (eds): *Textbook of Veterinary Internal Medicine,* ed 5. Philadelphia, WB Saunders, 2000, pp 1182-1238.

Hostutler RA, et al: Antibiotic-responsive histiocytic ulcerative colitis in 9 dogs. *J Vet Intern Med* 18(4):499-504, 2004.

Ludlow CL, Davenport DJ: Small intestinal bacterial overgrowth. In Bonagura JD (ed): *Kirk's Current Veterinary Therapy XIII.* Philadelphia, WB Saunders, 2000, pp 637-641.

Marks SL: Editorial: Small intestinal bacterial overgrowth in dogs-less common than you think? *J Vet Intern Med* 17(1):5-7, 2003.

Willard MD: Chronic small bowel diarrhea-part II. In *ACVIM Proceedings 22nd Annual Veterinary Medical Forum.* Minneapolis, 2004, pp 505-507.

Williams DA: Small intestinal bacterial overgrowth. In *ACVIM Proceedings 19th Annual Veterinary Medical Forum.* Denver, 2001, pp 544-546.

AUTHOR: **E. KELLY NITSCHE**

EDITOR: **DEBRA L. ZORAN**

Anticoagulant Rodenticide Toxicosis

Client Education Sheet on Website

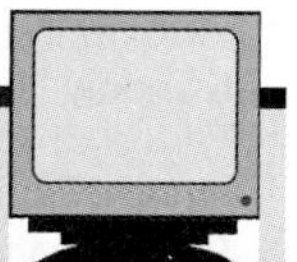

BASIC INFORMATION

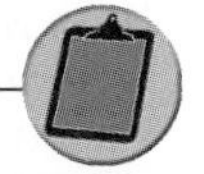

DEFINITION

Anticoagulant rodenticides are designed to kill rats, mice, and other rodents by internal bleeding. Toxicosis in small animals generally occurs 3 to 5 days after consuming the bait and is characterized by generalized hemorrhages, pale mucous membranes, presence of external hematomas, anorexia, lethargy, swollen joints, bloody feces, dyspnea, weakness, and sudden death.

SYNONYM(S)

Agent name	Examples of trade names
Warfarin	Anchor Rat and Mouse Bait, Cat-in-a-Bag
Pindone	Purina Rat Kill Soluble, Eaton's AC formula 50
Diphacinone	Assassin Rodenticide Bait, Exterminator's Choice
Difethialone	D-Cease, Generations, D-Con Rat and Mouse Bait
Brodifacoum	D-Con Mouse Prufe II, Havoc, Jaguar, Final Blox
Bromadiolone	Boot Hill, Hawk, Just One Bite

EPIDEMIOLOGY

SPECIES, AGE, SEX: Potentially all are susceptible. Young and elderly animals more sensitive.

RISK FACTORS

- Underlying hepatic disease can enhance toxicity.
- A high-fat diet can enhance anticoagulant absorption.
- Prolonged treatment with sulfaquinoxalin can enhance toxicity by reducing the synthesis of vitamin K_1.

GEOGRAPHY AND SEASONALITY: Poisoning more common in fall and winter months; possible any time of the year.

CLINICAL PRESENTATION

HISTORY, CHIEF COMPLAINT

- History or evidence of exposure several days prior.
  - Many times there is no history of exposure.
- Typically, vague initial clinical signs occur as the first manifestation.
  - Lethargy, exercise intolerance, anorexia.
- Dyspnea, coughing.
- Lameness, swollen joints.
- Sudden death with no reported clinical signs is possible.

PHYSICAL EXAM FINDINGS

- Pale mucous membranes
- Tachycardia, dyspnea, harsh lung sounds.
  - Pulmonary hemorrhage
  - Hemorrhagic pleural effusion
  - Airway hematoma
  - Hypovolemic shock
- Weakness, exercise intolerance
- Subcutaneous masses (external hematomas)
- Oozing or bleeding at venipuncture sites or wounds
- Lameness, swollen joints
- Exophthalmos (retrobulbar hemorrhage)
- Petechiae, ecchymoses
- Frank bleeding from the mouth, rectum (rare)

ETIOLOGY AND PATHOPHYSIOLOGY

Source

- Mainly two types of anticoagulant rodenticides: first generation and second generation.
  - First generation: warfarin and indanediones:
    - Warfarin products list "4-hydroxycoumarin" in active ingredients.
    - Indanedione products list "1,3 indanedione" in active ingredients.
    - Indanedione examples include pindone, chlorphacinone, and difethialone.
  - Second-generation anticoagulants:
    - Brodifacoum, bromadiolone, diphacinone, others.
    - Longer acting and more toxic.
- Many generics and trade names (see table under Synonyms, above).
  - Some companies have multiple products with the same trade name but different active ingredients.
  - Older products, such as warfarin and pindone, are not actively marketed but may still be available.
- Indanedione and second-generation anticoagulants frequently have concentrations of 0.005%, while warfarin-containing baits often have concentrations of 0.025%, and difethialone products usually have a concentration of 0.0025%.

Pathophysiology

- Anticoagulants block activation of vitamin K–dependent clotting factors.
  - Affected clotting factors include II, VII, IX, and X, affecting the extrinsic, intrinsic, and common pathways.
    - Factor VII has the shortest half-life; therefore the extrinsic pathway is affected first in anticoagulant rodenticide toxicity, and thus prothrombin time (PT) is elevated before activated partial thromboplastin time (aPTT).
  - Vitamin K_1 epoxide reductase is the specific enzyme that is inhibited.
    - Without this enzyme's function, vitamin K_1 cannot be recycled from its inactive form, vitamin K_1 epoxide, to vitamin K_1.
    - The resulting vitamin K_1 deficiency is responsible for clinical signs of bleeding and is also the basis for treatment with vitamin K_1.
  - Coagulation factors already present degrade naturally and are used up slowly. Therefore, clinical signs are not expected for 3 to 5 days postingestion. Second-generation anticoagulants are generally more toxic and longer-acting than first-generation anticoagulants, resulting in more persistent effects.

DIAGNOSIS

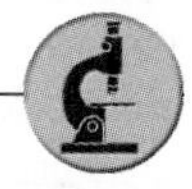

DIFFERENTIAL DIAGNOSIS

Bleeding disorders due to liver disease, hemophilia, von Willebrand disease, thrombocytopenia, disseminated intravascular coagulopathy. Differentiation is often straightforward on the basis of signalment, history, physical examination, and routine laboratory tests.

INITIAL DATABASE

- Complete blood count:
  - Regenerative anemia may be present.
  - Mild to moderate thrombocytopenia may occur (50,000–150,000/µl).
- Serum chemistry panel.
- Hematocrit (may be low if bleeding occurring).
- Coagulation panel:
  - One-stage PT and aPTT or PTT will elevate before hemorrhage occurs, and elevation persists during clinical signs.
    - PT is the more sensitive of the two for anticoagulant rodenticide toxicosis.
  - PIVKA (proteins induced by vitamin K_1 absence or antagonism) will be prolonged.
    - More sensitive than PT/aPTT.
    - Not as widely available.
  - A threefold increase in PT or PIVKA is supportive of anticoagulant rodenticide toxicosis.
  - Prior administration of vitamin K_1 can interfere with the PT.
- Radiographs may reveal thoracic or abdominal effusions. Tracheal narrowing or soft tissue opacity may be present.

ADVANCED OR CONFIRMATORY TESTING

- Stomach contents, blood, and serum may be analyzed for anticoagulants. Results are generally not received in time to make a difference in treatment, but can be important in legal cases.
- Necropsy samples include serum, liver, and kidney. Most veterinary diagnostic labs have an anticoagulant screen that can detect most of the anticoagulants available on the market.

TREATMENT

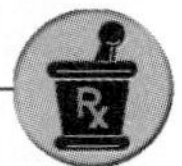

THERAPEUTIC GOAL(S)

- Decontamination of patient and monitoring (animals not showing clinical signs) to determine if vitamin K_1 is necessary
- Stop bleeding (animals with overt clinical signs)
- Supportive care

ACUTE GENERAL TREATMENT

- Decontamination and monitoring for animals without overt clinical signs:
  - Induction of emesis (hydrogen peroxide 3%: 0.25–0.5 ml/kg PO once, or syrup of ipecac: 2 to 6 ml total dose PO once) useful within 4 hr of ingestion, followed by administration of activated charcoal (dose according to packaging label of product [e.g., 10 ml of activated charcoal suspension PO made from 2 g activated charcoal suspended in 10 ml tap water]) and a cathartic (use labeled doses for commercial products).
  - Monitor PT, aPTT, or PIVKA at baseline, 48 and 72 hours. If the 72-hour PT/PIVKA is normal, no additional treatment needed.
  - Confine animals and limit exercise while monitoring PT or PIVKA.
  - If PT or PIVKA elevates, start oral vitamin K_1 therapy at 1.5–2.5 mg/kg q 12h or 3–5 mg/kg once daily.
    - Continue treatment for 14 to 30 days, depending on the specific anticoagulant.
    - PT or PIVKA should be checked 48 hours after the last dose of vitamin K_1.
      - If PT or PIVKA is still elevated 48 hours after last dose (16 to 32 days postexposure), resume vitamin K_1 treatment for 1 week, and then remeasure PT or PIVKA 48 hours after last dose. Some animals will require prolonged treatment.
    - Once the PT or PIVKA is normal at 48 hours, vitamin K_1 therapy can be discontinued.
- Treatment of hemorrhaging animals:
  - Decontamination (emesis, activated charcoal administration) is unnecessary, since ingestion will have occurred >24 hours before clinical signs.
  - Blood or plasma transfusions to provide clotting factors immediately. See Transfusion Reactions, p 1098.
  - Vitamin K_1 therapy at 5 mg/kg PO divided q 8–12h.
  - In cases of hemorrhagic pleural effusion causing severe dyspnea, chest tubes may be necessary.
- Supportive care (as needed):
  - Intravenous fluids.
  - Oxygen supplementation.
  - Thermoregulation.
  - Nutritional support (high-fat diet with vitamin K_1 can enhance its absorption).
  - Broad-spectrum antibiotics if concurrent infection is identified.
  - Cage rest.

DRUG INTERACTIONS

Anticoagulants are highly protein bound. Concurrent use of highly protein-bound drugs such as corticosteroids or nonsteroidal anti-inflammatory drugs can increase anticoagulant toxicity.

POSSIBLE COMPLICATIONS

- Retrobulbar hemorrhage: temporary blindness.
- Permanent paresis may develop if bleeding occurs in the spinal cord.

RECOMMENDED MONITORING

- Clinical signs
- PT
- Hematocrit

PROGNOSIS AND OUTCOME

- Excellent if animal presented before clinical signs develop. Most animals respond very well to vitamin K_1 therapy.
- Prognosis guarded to poor if animal bleeds in the chest or in the central nervous system.

PEARLS & CONSIDERATIONS

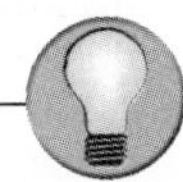

COMMENTS

- Brodifacoum is among the most toxic and most commonly involved anticoagulants; LD50 for dogs is 0.2–4 mg/kg.
  - Animals can develop toxicosis between the LD50 and 1/10 of the LD50.
  - Therefore, animals ingesting a dose >0.02 mg/kg should be decontaminated and monitored.
  - For example, decontamination is recommended if a 20-lb (9-kg) dog eats approximately 5 g (1 tsp) of 0.005% brodifacoum.
  - Most brodifacoum-containing commercial baits are available as either 1.5-oz or 3-oz packages.
- Animals can ingest subtoxic doses over several days, eventually developing toxicosis.
- Relay toxicosis (ingestion of prey that has consumed the toxin) is possible but rare.
  - Barn cats ingesting large numbers of rodents are at risk.
- Anticoagulants can cause fetal loss at doses that are not toxic to the dam.
- Vitamin K_1 injection (even when given SC) can cause anaphylaxis in some animals.
- Injectable vitamin K_1 has no advantage over oral vitamin K_1 therapy (both have similar bioavailability).
- Vitamin K_1 comes as injection, 5-mg tablets (human) or 25-mg capsules (veterinary).
- Vitamin K_1 should be given with fatty food (such as canned dog food, peanut butter, cheese, etc.). Nonfat milk and some meats are very lean.
- The color and form (bar, pellet, tracking powder, etc.) do not differentiate between brands or active ingredients. The packaging will contain the active ingredient and the EPA registration number that can be used to determine the class of rodenticide and the specific treatment required.

PREVENTION

- Keep all baits out of the reach of pets. Rodents may drag packages within reach of pets.
- Baits are attractive to pets. Remove the bait from the animal's environment.

SUGGESTED READING

Means C: Anticoagulant rodenticides. In Plumlee KH (ed): *Clinical Veterinary Toxicology*. St. Louis, Mosby, 2004, pp 444–446.

Merola V: Anticoagulant rodenticides: deadly for pests, dangerous for pets. *Vet Med* 97:716–722, 2002.

ASPCA Animal Poison Control Center hotline and website:

- 1-800-548-2423
- 1-888-426-4435
- www.apcc.aspca.org

AUTHOR: **CHARLOTTE MEANS**

EDITOR: **SAFDAR A. KHAN**

Aortic Thromboembolism, Feline

BASIC INFORMATION

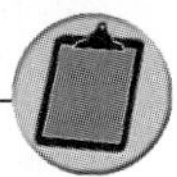

DEFINITION

- Occlusion of a systemic artery (typically the aortic trifurcation) by an embolus that has dislodged from the site of thrombus formation (typically the left side of the heart) and the associated clinical sequelae.
- *Thrombus* refers to a concretion of cells and blood constituents (clot) in a discrete location in the circulation.
- *Embolus* refers to a thrombus or thrombus fragment that has traveled through the circulation and obstructs a vessel in an organ or tissue.
- Thrombi (and subsequent emboli) are most commonly a sterile matrix of fibrin, platelets, and associated red and white blood cells, but tumor or septic emboli are occasionally the cause of thromboembolic disease.

SYNONYM(S)

Aortic thromboembolism (ATE)
Feline aortic thromboembolism (FATE)
Saddle embolus
Saddle thrombus

EPIDEMIOLOGY

SPECIES, AGE, SEX: Feline, all age adults reported, male predisposition.

GENETICS AND BREED PREDISPOSITION: No genetic or breed predisposition beyond the male predisposition for hypertrophic cardiomyopathy, the leading cause of feline aortic thromboembolism (FATE).

RISK FACTORS

- Heart disease (hypertrophic cardiomyopathy, restrictive cardiomyopathy, dilated cardiomyopathy, congenital cardiac disorders)
- Spontaneous contrast in the left atrium or left ventricle on the echocardiographic study
- Pulmonary neoplasia
- Other neoplasia

CLINICAL PRESENTATION

DISEASE FORMS/SUBTYPES

- Saddle thrombus: total or partial occlusion of the distal aortic trifurcation
- Brachial artery embolus (single forelimb affected)
- Visceral artery thromboembolism (renal artery, mesenteric artery): less common; may accompany saddle thrombus

HISTORY, CHIEF COMPLAINT

- Patients may have a prior history of heart disease or reported physical findings of cardiac disease (murmur, arrhythmia).
  - A preexisting heart murmur is less commonly noted in the history of cats with restrictive cardiomyopathy.
- Saddle thrombus: peracute onset of pain and paresis/paralysis of hindlimbs.
- Brachial artery thrombus: sudden onset of lameness or disuse of a forelimb.
- Visceral thomboemboli: acute onset abdominal pain, vomiting, lethargy.

PHYSICAL EXAM FINDINGS

- Saddle thrombus:
  - Pain and varying degrees of paralysis of the hind limbs
  - Typically absence of femoral pulses
    - Incomplete forms may have unilateral loss of femoral pulse or a differential in the femoral pulse strength
  - Firm, painful quadriceps and gastrocnemius musculature
  - Hypothermia is common
  - Foot pads are cyanotic and cool to the touch; nail beds are cyanotic
  - Dyspnea is common; diagnostic testing must distinguish between pain and congestive heart failure (CHF) as the cause
- Brachial artery embolus: varying degree of forelimb paralysis (typically paw knuckled under). Absence of brachial pulse, foot pad cyanotic and cool to the touch

ETIOLOGY AND PATHOPHYSIOLOGY

- Thromboembolism is positively correlated with increasing left atrial size.
- Less common causes include primary tumor emboli and sterile emboli related to pulmonary neoplasia.

DIAGNOSIS

DIFFERENTIAL DIAGNOSIS

- Trauma (pelvic fractures, femoral fractures, spinal injury)
- Primary neurologic disease (spinal infarction, intervertebral disk disease, spinal neoplasia, trauma)

INITIAL DATABASE

- Complete blood count, biochemical profile, urinalysis: commonly noted abnormalities include hyperglycemia, elevations in ALT and AST, hypocalcemia, and varying degrees of azotemia (suggests concomitant renal infarction)
- Thyroid hormone analysis (if ≥6 years old)
- Feline leukemia, feline immunodeficiency serology (if at risk for these diseases)
- Full coagulation profile (prothrombin time [PT], activated partial thromboplastin time [aPTT], fibrinogen, fibrin/fibrinogen degradation product [FDPs], platelet count)
  - With FATE, FDP levels may be elevated and fibrinogen levels may be decreased, but these findings are not sensitive or specific.
  - Decreased PT and/or aPTT: no correlation to whether a cat is in a procoagulant state.
- Full-body radiographs
  - Thorax: signs of congestive heart failure (pulmonary edema, pleural effusion), signs of cardiac disease (cardiac chamber enlargement).
  - Spine: fractures, neoplasia (differential diagnosis).
- Echocardiography (once stable)
- Electrocardiography (once stable)
- Blood pressure determinations

ADVANCED OR CONFIRMATORY TESTING

- Nonselective angiography: can confirm extent of vessel occlusion and associated visceral artery occlusion
- Abdominal ultrasound: may be helpful in identifying extent of vessel occlusion and coexisting abdominal organ infarction
- Computed tomography/magnetic resonance imaging: can establish detailed information about the extent of the vascular occlusions but requires general anesthesia, which is problematic in these unstable patients

TREATMENT

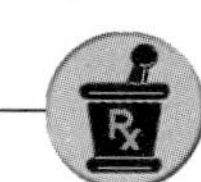

THERAPEUTIC GOAL(S)

- Pain control
- Supportive care (maintain hydration, treat associated CHF, maintain electrolyte balance and renal perfusion)
- Clot dissolution: the goal *if* thrombolytic therapy is attempted
- Preventing extension of the thromboembolus: anticoagulant and antiplatelet therapy

ACUTE GENERAL TREATMENT

- Pain management (oxymorphone 0.05–0.1 mg/kg SQ or IV q 4–8h, hydromorphone 0.1–0.2 mg/kg SQ or IV q 4–8h, morphine 0.05–0.2 mg/kg SQ q 6–8h, buprenorphine 0.01–0.015 mg/kg SQ or IV q 6–12h, or butorphanol 0.1–0.4 mg/kg SQ or IV q 2–4h)
- Diuretics, if CHF present (furosemide 1.0–4.0 mg/kg SQ or IV q 4–12h)
- Vasodilators: if blood pressure is adequate, may help collateral circulation in the hind legs (hydralazine 0.5–1.0

mg/kg PO q 12h, acepromazine 0.025-0.05 mg/kg SQ q 12-24h), angiotensin-converting enzyme inhibitors (enalapril, benazepril) usually avoided in the acute setting due to potential coexisting renal infarctions
- Oxygen therapy: if CHF, dyspnea
- Fluid therapy: Conservative crystalloid therapy is typically administered in patients in the absence of fulminant CHF

CHRONIC TREATMENT

- Aimed at treatment for the underlying condition (treatment of heart disease, removal of primary lung tumor)
- Anticoagulant therapy:
  - Warfarin (0.25 ml of 1 mg/ml suspension initially administered per cat q 24h, dose titrated q 5-7 days to maintain a PT or international normalized ratio 1.5 to 2.0 times upper limit of normal. Ideally patients are initially anticoagulated with heparin 150 IU/kg SQ q 8h and have a 48-hour heparin-warfarin overlap), or
  - Low molecular-weight heparin (e.g., dalteparin 100 IU/kg SQ q 12-24h)
- Antiplatelet therapy:
  - Aspirin (doses range from 5 mg PO per cat every 72 hours to 81 mg per cat every 48 hours), or
  - Clopidogrel (dose recently reported at 18.75 mg PO per cat per day)

DRUG INTERACTIONS

Multiple drug interactions reported for warfarin, including amiodarone, barbiturates, cimetidine, corticosteroids, erythromycin, estrogens, griseofulvin, ibuprofen, indomethacin, ketoprofen, metronidazole, neomycin, pentoxifylline, phenylbutazone, quinidine, salicylates, spironolactone, vitamin K, and others (see drug formularies for detailed list)

POSSIBLE COMPLICATIONS

- Disease complications: gangrenous necrosis of a hind limb; self-mutilation of the limb; visceral occlusions leading to organ infarction, organ failure, and death; cardiac arrhythmias
- Thrombolytic therapy: hemorrhagic complications, acute reperfusion syndromes (hyperkalemia, acidosis, death)
- Anticoagulant therapy: bleeding complications
- Diuretic therapy: volume contraction, azotemia
- Vasodilator therapy: hypovolemia, decompensation of renal function
- Fluid therapy: volume overload, CHF

RECOMMENDED MONITORING

- Frequent physical examination
- Daily renal, electrolyte, and coagulation profile monitoring during hospitalization
- Continuous ECG (arrhythmias common)

PROGNOSIS AND OUTCOME

- Guarded prognosis: 33-50% chance of discharge from the hospital, high chance of rethrombosis
- Prognosis more favorable for partial or forelimb emboli (75% chance of discharge from the hospital)
- Grave prognosis with visceral artery occlusions
- Body temperature at admission appears to be positively correlated with prognosis: more favorable if T > 98.9°F (37.2°C)

PEARLS & CONSIDERATIONS

COMMENTS

- Although much anecdotal discussion exists, to date there have been no studies proving that any preventative measures decrease the chance of suffering a saddle thrombus or recurrent embolic event.
- Intermittent claudication (lameness) may signal a patient to be at high risk for FATE and should prompt a discussion about preventive therapy.

PREVENTION

- Treatment of associated cardiac disease
- Use of antiplatelet agents in patients at lower risk and the use of anticoagulant therapy in patients at high risk (severe left atrial enlargement, patients who have had a previous embolic event, patients with spontaneous contrast on the echocardiogram)

CLIENT EDUCATION

- All cats with cardiac disease are presumed to be at risk for thromboembolic complications.
- Cats with increasing amounts of left atrial enlargement and with spontaneous contrast are at high risk for thromboembolism.
- Risk/benefit discussion of preventative measures.

SUGGESTED READING

Hogan DF, et al: Antiplatelet effects and pharmacodynamics of clopidogrel in cats. *J Am Vet Med Assoc* 225(9):1406-1411, 2004.

Laste NJ, Harpster NK: A retrospective study of 100 cases of feline distal aortic thromboembolism: 1977-1993. *J Am Anim Hosp Assoc* 31(6):492-500, 1995.

Smith CE, et al: Use of low molecular weight heparin in cats: 57 cases (1999-2003). *J Am Vet Med Assoc* 225(8):1237-1241, 2004.

Smith SA, et al: Arterial thromboembolism in cats: acute crisis in 127 cases (1992-2001) and long-term management with low-dose aspirin in 24 cases. *J Vet Intern Med* 17(1):73-83, 2003.

AUTHOR: **NANCY J. LASTE**
EDITOR: **ETIENNE CÔTÉ**

Arrhythmogenic Right Ventricular Cardiomyopathy

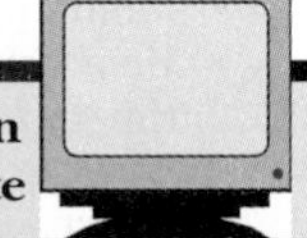

Client Education Sheet on Website

BASIC INFORMATION

DEFINITION

Primary myocardial disease involving fatty and/or fibrous replacement of atrophic myocardium predominantly, but not exclusively, of the right ventricle

SYNONYM(S)

Arrhythmic right ventricular dysplasia
Arrhythmogenic cardiomyopathy
ARVC

Similar terms (boxers): boxer cardiomyopathy, boxer myocarditis.

The form of this disease that affects boxer dogs is discussed in greater detail under Boxer Cardiomyopathy (see p 145).

EPIDEMIOLOGY

SPECIES, AGE, SEX: Dogs: none. Cats: trend toward more males.

GENETICS AND BREED PREDISPOSITION: Dogs: boxers, either autosomal dominant or variable penetrance. Cats: unknown.

ASSOCIATED CONDITIONS AND DISORDERS: Dilated Cardiomyopathy, see p 302.

CLINICAL PRESENTATION

DISEASE FORMS/SUBTYPES

- **Boxers:**
  - Latent ("asymptomatic") ventricular arrhythmias
  - Ventricular arrhythmias with syncope

- **Cats:** none

HISTORY, CHIEF COMPLAINT
- **Boxers:** syncope
- **Cats:**
  - Dyspnea
  - Abdominal distention
  - Syncope
  - Anorexia
  - Lethargy

PHYSICAL EXAM FINDINGS
- **Boxers:**
  - Arrhythmias
  - Tachycardia
- **Cats:**
  - Muffled heart/lung sounds
  - Arrhythmias
  - Ascites
  - Heart murmur

ETIOLOGY AND PATHOPHYSIOLOGY

Possible genetic cause
- Amount of pleural/abdominal effusion determines clinical signs (cats)
- Rate of ventricular tachycardia determines presence of syncope; syncope more likely in sustained and faster heart rates (dogs and cats)

DIAGNOSIS

DIFFERENTIAL DIAGNOSIS

- **Dogs:**
  - Electrocardiography: ventricular arrhythmias
    - Idiopathic: uncommon in boxers
    - Neoplasia, metabolic derangements
  - Syncope
    - Seizures
- **Cats:**
  - Radiographic (pleural or abdominal effusion)
    - Neoplasia (lymphoma, thymoma, mesothelioma)
    - Idiopathic chylous effusion (thorax)
    - Infectious (feline infectious peritonitis, pyothorax)
    - Hemorrhagic (primary coagulopathy [rare], trauma, neoplasia)
  - Electrocardiographic
    - Other cardiomyopathies (hypertrophic, restrictive, dilated, or unclassified)
  - Echocardiographic
    - Congenital tricuspid dysplasia (rare in cats)
  - Syncope
    - Seizures

INITIAL DATABASE

- **Dogs:**
  - Thoracic radiographs: usually normal
  - Electrocardiogram: right-sided ventricular premature complexes (upright in lead II, wide, bizarre, no associated P wave), usually of one shape (monomorphic) but may be polymorphic, may be singles, or sustained/nonsustained ventricular tachycardia. Single electrocardiogram may not reveal presence or extent of ventricular arrhythmias
  - Echocardiogram: usually normal left ventricle and atrium with variably dilated right ventricle and atrium that may only be appreciated on the left apical or left parasternal long-axis views
  - Complete blood count, biochemistry profile, urinalysis are usually normal
- **Cats:**
  - Thoracic radiographs: pleural effusion and right atrial/ventricular cardiac enlargement. May need to perform thoracocentesis before cardiac silhouette can be appreciated
  - Electrocardiogram: atrial and/or ventricular arrhythmias; may be normal
  - Echocardiogram: dilated right atrium and ventricle with normal velocity tricuspid regurgitation
  - Complete blood count, biochemistry profile, urinalysis, T4 (in cats >7 years old), FeLV and FIV, usually unremarkable in arrhythmogenic right ventricular cardiomyopathy (ARVC) unless there are secondary metabolic changes
  - Thoracic/abdominal fluid analysis

ADVANCED OR CONFIRMATORY TESTING

- **Dogs:** 24-hour Holter monitor
- **Dogs and cats:** percutaneous right ventricular myocardial biopsy (not recommended)

TREATMENT

THERAPEUTIC GOAL(S)

- **Dogs:**
  - Prevent syncope
  - Prevent sudden death (may not be achievable despite treatment)
- **Cats:**
  - Relieve clinical signs of heart failure, if present
  - Prevent syncope
  - Prevent sudden death (may not be achievable despite treatment)

ACUTE GENERAL TREATMENT

- **Dogs:**
  - If sustained, rapid ventricular tachycardia:
    - Lidocaine, initial bolus of 2-4 mg/kg IV slowly followed by constant rate infusion of 40-80 μg/kg/min; or procainamide, 20-50 μg/kg/min IV or 6-15 mg/kg q 4-6h IM
- **Cats:**
  - If congestive heart failure is present:
    - Thoracocentesis and/or abdominocentesis
    - Oxygen therapy
    - Furosemide: 1-2 mg/kg IV q 6-24h
    - *No stress!*
  - If life-threatening ventricular arrhythmias are present:
    - Lidocaine, 0.05 mg/kg IV slowly, or sotalol, 1/8 to 1/4 of an 80 mg tab PO q 12h

CHRONIC TREATMENT

- **Dogs:**
  - For ventricular arrhythmias:
    - Sotalol: 1-3 mg/kg PO q 12h; titrate up as needed, or
    - Mexiletine: 4-8 mg/kg PO q 8h plus atenolol: 0.5 mg/kg PO q 12-24h
    - L-carnitine: 50 mg/kg q 8-12h (rare positive response)
- **Cats:**
  - For congestive heart failure:
    - Lasix: 1-2 mg/kg PO q 12h
    - Enalapril: 0.5 mg/kg PO q 12-24h
    - Digoxin: 1/4 of a 0.125 mg tab PO q 2-3 days
  - For ventricular arrhythmias:
    - Sotalol: 10-20 mg per cat PO q 12h

POSSIBLE COMPLICATIONS

Sudden death in both species, even with treatment

RECOMMENDED MONITORING

- **Cats:**
  - Electrocardiograms
  - Thoracic radiographs
  - Serum biochemistry profiles
- **Dogs:**
  - Holter monitor 1 to 2 weeks after diagnosis
  - Electrocardiograms every 3 to 4 months

PROGNOSIS AND OUTCOME

- Variable
- Dogs tend to do better than cats
- Sudden death common in both

PEARLS & CONSIDERATIONS

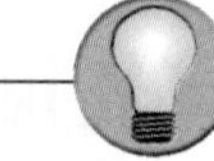

COMMENTS

- Arrhythmogenic right ventricular cardiomyopathy is a disease that has been described in both dogs and cats.
- It is much worse in cats; cats generally live only weeks to months after diagnosis.
- Dogs with no clinical signs generally do well unless there is concomitant myocardial failure.
- Antiarrhythmic drugs may not prevent sudden death.

CLIENT EDUCATION

- Cats: monitor for signs of heart failure; sudden death is possible
- Dogs: monitor for syncope; sudden death is possible

SUGGESTED READING

Fox PR, et al: Spontaneously occurring arrhythmogenic right ventricular cardiomyopathy in the domestic cat. A new animal model similar to the human disease. *Circulation* 102:1863-1870, 2000.

Basso C, et al: Arrhythmogenic right ventricular cardiomyopathy causing sudden cardiac death in boxer dogs. A new animal model of human disease. *Circulation* 109:1180-1185, 2004.

AUTHOR: **BETSY R. BOND**
EDITOR: **ETIENNE CÔTÉ**

Arsenic Toxicosis

BASIC INFORMATION

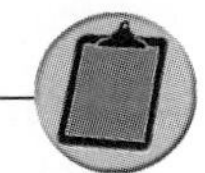

DEFINITION

Condition resulting from exposure to injurious levels of arsenic

EPIDEMIOLOGY

SPECIES, AGE, SEX

- Cats more sensitive
- Young animals more susceptible

RISK FACTORS: Sources: contaminated ground water, pesticides (ant baits, termite baits), herbicides (crabgrass killers), wood preservatives, mining and manufacturing, iatrogenic (heartworm adulticides), animal feeds (phenylarsonics-swine, poultry).

CLINICAL PRESENTATION

DISEASE FORMS/SUBTYPES

- Peracute or acute toxicosis: single toxic dose
- Subacute toxicosis: lower dosages over several days

HISTORY, CHIEF COMPLAINT

- Exposure to arsenic-containing product
- Peracute death (no premonitory signs)
- Acute: severe gastrointestinal (GI) signs, weakness, recumbency, shock, and death
- Subacute: persistent, watery diarrhea; signs of renal failure within 3 days

PHYSICAL EXAM FINDINGS

- Acute toxicosis:
  - Vomiting
  - Abdominal pain
  - Watery diarrhea
  - Weakness
  - Rapid, weak pulses
  - Dehydration
  - Hypothermia
- Subacute toxicosis:
  - Persistent GI signs, especially watery diarrhea
  - Oliguria, polyuria, or anuria
  - Anorexia
  - Weakness
  - Hypothermia

ETIOLOGY AND PATHOPHYSIOLOGY

- Arsenic binds sulfhydryl groups on enzymes and other cellular proteins, impairing cellular respiration and depleting energy stores.
- Tissues most affected are those rich in oxidative enzymes (GI tract, endothelium, lung, kidney, liver, and epidermis).
  - GI inflammation and necrosis causes hemorrhagic gastroenteritis.
  - Endothelial damage results in fluid loss into interstitium, hypovolemia, hypotension, and noncardiogenic pulmonary edema.
  - Hepatic and renal damage from direct effect of arsenic or secondary to hypovolemia and organ hypoperfusion.
- Toxicity varies with physical form, solubility, and valence.
  - Inorganic arsenic (e.g., arsenic trioxide) more toxic than organic forms (e.g., melarsomine, arsanilic acid).
  - Trivalent arsenic (arsenite) more toxic than pentavalent forms (arsenate).
  - Highly soluble forms (e.g., arsenious acid, arsenic acid) more toxic than insoluble forms.
- Single lethal dose of sodium arsenite = 1-25 mg/kg of body weight.
- Arsenic trioxide 3 to 10 times less toxic than sodium arsenite.

DIAGNOSIS

DIFFERENTIAL DIAGNOSIS

- Enteritis (e.g., parvoviral enteritis)
- Hemorrhagic gastroenteritis
- Pancreatitis
- Zinc phosphide toxicosis
- Garbage toxicosis

INITIAL DATABASE

- Arterial blood pressure measurement: hypotension is common and may require treatment (e.g., IV fluids)
- Complete blood count
  - Evidence of hemoconcentration initially; may normalize or progress to mild anemia once rehydrated
- Serum chemistry profile
  - Azotemia, acidosis in subacute cases (surviving >3 days)
- Urinalysis
  - Proteinuria
  - Cellular casts
  - Urine specific gravity (USG) of 1.008-1.012 with concurrent azotemia signifies chronic renal failure (see Chronic Renal Failure, pp 204-207). Acute renal failure (see Acute Renal Failure, p 32) may produce oliguria/anuria before affecting the urine specific gravity

ADVANCED OR CONFIRMATORY TESTING

- Urine arsenic levels useful in first 48 hours
  - Background levels generally <1 ppm
- Arsenic analysis in vomitus, feces, GI contents
- Tissue levels in kidney or liver
  - Level >10 ppm wet weight confirms arsenic toxicosis
- Hair: not useful diagnostically: chronic toxicosis not reported in domestic animals
- Blood: *not* reliable specimen for confirming arsenic exposures

TREATMENT

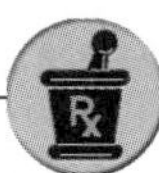

THERAPEUTIC GOAL(S)

- Control life-threatening signs
- Prevent systemic absorption
- Chelation therapy
- Manage GI effects

ACUTE GENERAL TREATMENT

- Control life-threatening signs:
  - Aggressive fluid therapy if hypovolemia/dehydration
  - Manage hypovolemic shock (see Shock, Hypovolemic, p 999)
  - Blood replacement therapy if required due to GI blood loss (see Transfusion Reactions, p 1098)
  - Correct acid/base or electrolyte imbalances (see Acidosis, p 20)
  - Manage cardiac arrhythmias if present (see Ventricular Arrhythmias [Premature Ventricular Complexes, Ventricular Tachycardia], p 1148)
  - Thermoregulation (e.g., heating blankets if hypothermia)
- Prevent systemic absorption:
  - Only if subclinically affected (no clinical signs)
  - Emesis:
    - Useful <30 minutes of exposure
    - Apomorphine (0.03-0.04 mg/kg IV or IM, or crush tablet portion with water and instil into conjunctival sac, rinse following emesis)

- Hydrogen peroxide 3% (2 ml/kg PO, maximum 45 ml)
  - Gastric lavage:
    - Consider if large ingestion
    - Contraindicated in vomiting animals, due to potential for gastric wall rupture
  - Activated charcoal:
    - Adsorbs arsenic poorly; most sources recommend its use, but efficacy is limited
    - Contraindicated with vomiting or GI hemorrhage
- Chelation therapy:
  - Recommended if progressive signs or very high exposure
  - Succimer is preferable over British Anti-Lewisite (fewer adverse effects, administration more convenient)
  - Use with caution in patients with prior renal insufficiency:
    - Maintain adequate hydration
  - Succimer:
    - Dimercaptosuccinic acid, DMSA, *Chemet*
    - 10 mg/kg PO q 8h for 10 days
    - Can be given rectally in vomiting animals
  - British Anti-Lewisite:
    - Generally replaced by succimer for this application
- Manage GI effects:
  - Antiemetics
    - Chlorpromazine 0.2–0.5 mg/kg IM or SC q 6–8h
    - Metoclopramide: do not use in patients with GI hemorrhage
  - Sucralfate:
    - 0.5–1 g q 8h PO
  - Antibiotics effective against gram-negative organisms and anaerobes (e.g., combination of enrofloxacin 2.5 mg/kg diluted 1:1 with sterile water and given slowly IV q 12h and ampicillin 10–20 mg/kg IV q 8h) if signs of sepsis due to translocation of GI bacteria
  - Parenteral nutrition, vitamin supplementation as needed (see Parenteral Nutrition, p 1296)
- General supportive care:
  - Manage renal insufficiency as needed

CHRONIC TREATMENT

Hepatoprotectants as needed:

- SAM-E (*Denosyl*) 18 mg/kg PO for 1 to 3 months

POSSIBLE COMPLICATIONS

Permanent renal insufficiency

RECOMMENDED MONITORING

- Blood pressure
- Hydration
- Hematocrit, total solids
- Acid-base status
- Renal values

PROGNOSIS AND OUTCOME

- Good with prompt treatment or if only mild GI signs are present
- Guarded to poor with severe clinical signs

PEARLS & CONSIDERATIONS

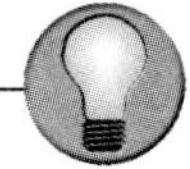

COMMENTS

- Toxicosis less common due to decreased use of arsenic-containing pesticides.
- Sources accessible to pets include ant baits, termite baits, crabgrass killers, and ashes from arsenic-treated lumber (unburned lumber is unlikely to be associated with acute arsenic toxicosis).

PREVENTION

- Avoid arsenic-containing products in areas to which pets have access
- Avoid burning copper-chromium-arsenic treated wood; dispose of ashes from such wood to prevent exposure to pets

SUGGESTED READING

Ensley S: Arsenic. In Plumlee KH (ed): *Clinical Veterinary Toxicology*. St. Louis, Mosby, 2004, pp 193–195.

Neiger RD: Arsenic. In Peterson ME, Talcott PA (eds): *Small Animal Toxicology*. Philadelphia, WB Saunders, 2001, pp 420–430.

AUTHOR: **SHARON M. GWALTNEY-BRANT**

EDITOR: **SAFDAR A. KHAN**

Arteriovenous Fistula

BASIC INFORMATION

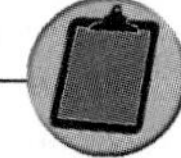

DEFINITION

Arteriovenous (AV) fistulas are abnormal communications between an artery and a vein resulting in the bypass of the capillary network. If located in the liver, the communication usually is between the hepatic artery and portal vein; hepatic artery to hepatic vein communications may occur.

SYNONYM(S)

Congenital hepatic AV fistula:

- Hamartoma
- Hemangioma

EPIDEMIOLOGY

SPECIES, AGE, SEX

- Variable; congenital—younger than 1.5 years. Secondary to neoplasia in older animals
- Genetics and breed predispositions: uncommon in dogs and rare in cats

ASSOCIATED CONDITIONS AND DISORDERS

- Portal hypertension
- Ascites
- Multiple acquired portosystemic shunts (PSS)
- Neoplasia

CLINICAL PRESENTATION

DISEASE FORMS/SUBTYPES

- Peripheral:
  - Swelling, SQ edema, especially over a limb, often after trauma or surgery
- Hepatic:
  - Acute onset of gastrointestinal clinical signs/ascites
- High output heart failure
- Other reported:
  - Renal; hepatic microvascular; subsequent to hemorrhagic gastroenteritis

HISTORY, CHIEF COMPLAINT

- Depends on location, size, duration, and etiopathology
- Peripheral:
  - Swollen leg, with or without pain, with or without inflammation
  - Soft swelling over the trunk
- Hepatic:
  - Depression
  - Lethargy
  - Ascites
  - Vomiting
  - Diarrhea
  - Absence of overt signs possible
- High output heart failure:
  - Dyspnea
  - Exercise intolerance
  - Cough

PHYSICAL EXAM FINDINGS

- Peripheral:
  - Painless, easily compressible, warm mass, usually over a limb. Mass is a

result of grossly distended blood vessels and edema
  - Auscultable continuous murmur (bruit) over the mass/fistula
  - Increased pulse and heart rate (large fistulas)
  - Distal to the fistula: swelling, warmer or colder than proximal area, possibly painful if secondary inflammatory edema
  - Pressure proximal to the fistula may cause the heart rate to drop
- Hepatic:
  - Continuous murmur (bruit) through the abdominal wall at level of liver (cranial abdomen, ventrally or laterally)
  - Ascites
  - Abdominal pain

ETIOLOGY AND PATHOPHYSIOLOGY

- Etiology:
  - Trauma, neoplasia, iatrogenic (venipuncture, surgery, perivascular injection of irritating substances), idiopathic
- Pathophysiology:
  - Reduced peripheral resistance, venous hypertension, increased cardiac preload, and potentially high-output heart failure
  - Shunted blood can cause local edema and ischemia, followed by tissue necrosis, ulceration, or organ dysfunction

DIAGNOSIS

DIFFERENTIAL DIAGNOSIS

- Hepatic:
  - Congenital PSS (will rarely have ascites) (see Portosystemic Shunt, p 880)
  - Congenital defects causing right-sided heart failure
  - Idiopathic hepatic fibrosis
  - Portal vein hypoplasia
  - Lobular dissecting hepatitis
  - Noncirrhotic portal hypertension
- Peripheral: very few differential diagnoses; local continuous murmur virtually pathognomonic:
  - Vasculitis

INITIAL DATABASE

- Hepatic:
  - Complete blood cell count: mild anemia
  - Serum biochemical profile: hypoproteinemia, increased liver enzymes, and bile acids
  - Thoracic radiographs: usually unremarkable
  - Abdominal sonography: large, tortuous, pulsating vessels; pulsatile blood flow on Doppler evaluation. Multiple PSS often occur secondarily, seen as enlarged tortuous vessels caudal to the liver
- Peripheral:
  - Thoracic radiographs: cardiomegaly if high-output heart failure
  - Radiograph the affected area to look for neoplasia
  - Ultrasound of affected area: direct visualization of fistula (tortuous vessels); turbulent flow seen with color flow Doppler

ADVANCED OR CONFIRMATORY TESTING

- Selective or nonselective angiography
- Exploratory surgery

TREATMENT

THERAPEUTIC GOAL(S)

- Removal of the swelling
- Restore normal hepatic, pulmonary function
- Prevent high-output heart failure

ACUTE GENERAL TREATMENT

- Hepatic:
  - Ligation of multiple PSS is contraindicated
  - Partial hepatectomy if fistula is in one lobe
  - Treatment for ascites and hepatic encephalopathy, if needed
- Peripheral:
  - Surgical removal (ligation of all vessels often a challenging, complex surgical procedure)
  - Transcatheter embolization

CHRONIC TREATMENT

- None with successful surgical removal of peripheral AV fistula
- For hepatic AV fistula: treat for ascites, hepatic encephalopathy, if needed; treat for hypoproteinemia, if needed

POSSIBLE COMPLICATIONS

- Surgical ligation of multiple PSS: fatal portal hypertension
- Hepatic function may not return to normal after lobectomy
- Complex and long duration of peripheral AV fistula ligation surgery (hours)

PROGNOSIS AND OUTCOME

Depends on cause and complications:
- Peripheral generally better prognosis than hepatic unless the cause is neoplasia or the heart is adversely affected
- Prognosis of hepatic depends on degree/presence of liver failure and portal hypertension

PEARLS & CONSIDERATIONS

COMMENTS

- AV fistulas produce focal continuous murmurs at the fistula site; therefore, auscultation of enlarged limbs or of the hepatic region of patients with clinical signs suggesting hepatic AV fistulas is an essential part of the initial diagnostic evaluation.
- In general, peripheral AV fistulas and hepatic AV fistulas are rare findings.
- Peripheral AV fistulas will only involve one limb; other diagnoses should be pursued if multiple limbs are involved.
- Pulmonary AV fistulas have not been reported in veterinary medicine.
- "Hamartomas" are also defined as normal structures that have formed abnormally and are not isolated to describing hepatic AV fistulas.

SUGGESTED READING

Whiting PG, et al: Partial hepatectomy with temporary hepatic vascular occlusion in dogs with hepatic arteriovenous fistulas. *Vet Surg* 15:171, 1986.

AUTHOR: **BETSY R. BOND**
EDITOR: **ETIENNE CÔTÉ**

Ascites

BASIC INFORMATION

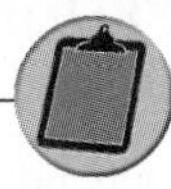

DEFINITION

Pathologic accumulation of fluid (transudate, modified transudate, exudate, or chyle; or more specifically, serum, pus, urine, bile, blood, or neoplastic cells) in the abdominal cavity

SYNONYM(S)

Abdominal fluid accumulation/effusion
Peritoneal fluid accumulation/effusion

EPIDEMIOLOGY

SPECIES, AGE, SEX: Dependent on underlying cause. Ascites is a sign of disease rather than a primary cause.

CLINICAL PRESENTATION

HISTORY, CHIEF COMPLAINT

- Abdominal enlargement (rate of distention is extremely variable, varying according to inciting cause)
- Perceived "weight gain" (abdominal distention)
- Decreased activity
- Anorexia
- Tachypnea
- Abdominal discomfort/pain
- When fluid accumulation is rapid, clinical signs of weakness and dyspnea more likely to be apparent
- History may include clinical signs associated with the primary disease (dyspnea/cough if cardiac disease, icterus if liver disease)

PHYSICAL EXAM FINDINGS

- Abdominal distention.
- Abdominal palpation:
    - Fluid wave may be present.
    - An abdominal mass or organomegaly (liver, spleen, kidney, etc.) may be palpable.
- Physical abnormalities associated with primary disease may be present. For example, cardiovascular abnormalities such as a murmur, arrhythmia, gallop rhythm, or jugular distention should warrant further investigation into the possibility of right heart failure. Generalized lymphadenopathy could suggest lymphoma. Muffled heart sounds with tachycardia and a weak pulse are consistent with pericardial effusion/tamponade if ascites is present.

ETIOLOGY AND PATHOPHYSIOLOGY

- Chylous effusion (obstructive, traumatic)
- Congestive heart failure (right-sided, pericardial effusion, and tamponade)
- Diaphragmatic hernia
- Hemorrhage (warfarin poisoning, trauma, neoplasia)
- Hypoalbuminemia
- Infectious (bacterial, viral [feline infectious peritonitis], parasitic [*Mesocestoides*])
- Liver disease/portal hypertension
- Neoplasia
- Pancreatitis
- Urinary tract rupture

DIAGNOSIS

DIFFERENTIAL DIAGNOSIS

Rule out causes of abdominal distention without ascites:

- Abscess (intact)
- Bladder distention
- Cyst
- Cushing's disease
- Gastrointestinal dilation (gastric torsion, ileus, aerophagia, overeating, parasitism)
- Lipoma (intra-abdominal)
- Lymphadenopathy
- Neoplasia
- Obesity
- Obstipation
- Organomegaly
- Pyometra/hydrometra

INITIAL DATABASE

- Abdominal radiographs:
    - Loss of serosal detail (focal or generalized)
    - Abdomen may have a diffuse, "ground-glass" appearance (carcinomatosis, peritonitis)
    - Mass lesions, fat, or organomegaly may be apparent or suggested by displacement of gas-filled organs
    - Free air may be present with peritonitis (ruptured viscus)
- Complete blood count, biochemistry panel, urinalysis: indicated for any animal with ascites. Abnormalities depend on underlying cause and extent of organ damage
- Thoracic radiographs:
    - Enlarged cardiac silhouette/caudal vena cava if cardiac disease or pericardial effusion
    - Metastatic pulmonary disease
    - Pleural effusion (with ascites: "bicavitary effusion")
- Abdominal ultrasonography:
    - Confirms presence of fluid and differentiates fluid from soft tissue or fat
    - Identification of mass lesions or organomegaly
    - Localizes small amounts of fluid for centesis
- Echocardiography:
    - Confirms diagnosis of right heart abnormalities or pericardial effusion

ADVANCED OR CONFIRMATORY TESTING

- Abdominal paracentesis:
    - Obtain fluid for cytologic and biochemical evaluation
    - Contraindicated if anticoagulant rodenticide toxicity (or other coagulopathy) suspected
- Fluid characteristics:
    - Transudate (typical causes: hypoalbuminemia, preportal hypertension, cyst rupture):
        - Clear and colorless, waterlike
        - Protein <2.5 g/dl
        - Specific gravity <1.018
        - Cell <1000/mm^3: neutrophils and mesothelial cells
    - Modified transudate (typical causes: congestive heart failure, neoplasia, hepatopathy):
        - Red or pink; may be slightly cloudy, slightly viscous/gummy
        - Protein 2.5-5.0 g/dl
        - Specific gravity >1.018
        - Cells <5000/mm^3: neutrophils, mesothelial cells, erythrocytes, and lymphocytes
    - Exudate, nonseptic (typical causes: pancreatitis, bile peritonitis, uroabdomen, neoplasia):
        - Pink or white; cloudy
        - Protein 2.5-5.0 g/dl
        - Specific gravity >1.018
        - Cells 5000-50,000/mm^3: neutrophils, mesothelial cells, macrophages, erythrocytes, and lymphocytes
    - Exudate, septic (typical causes: penetrating injury, gastrointestinal rupture, ruptured pyometra, ruptured abscess, pancreatitis):
        - Red, white, or yellow; cloudy
        - Foul odor common (suggests anaerobic infection)
        - Protein >4.0 g/dl
        - Specific gravity >1.018
        - Cells 5000-100,000/mm^3: neutrophils, mesothelial cells, macrophages, erythrocytes, lymphocytes, and bacteria
    - Hemorrhage (typical causes: ruptured neoplasm [benign or malignant], anticoagulant toxicity, trauma [splenic/hepatic fracture]):
        - Red
        - Protein >5.5 g/dl
        - Specific gravity 1.007-1.027
        - Cells consistent with peripheral blood; does not clot

- Chyle (typical cause: lymphatic disease):
  - Pink, straw, or white
  - Protein 2.5-7.0 g/dl
  - Specific gravity 1.007-1.040
- Prothrombin time if suspect anticoagulant intoxication
- Computed tomography, magnetic resonance imaging
- Consider abdominal exploratory to determine cause of ascites if all noninvasive diagnostics have been unremarkable

TREATMENT

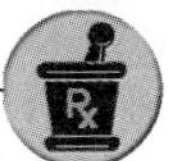

THERAPEUTIC GOAL(S)

Treatment of underlying disease:
- Delaying or eliminating recurrent effusion is long-term goal with chronic etiologies

ACUTE GENERAL TREATMENT

- Treatment of underlying disease, for example:
  - Chemotherapy if lymphoma
  - Pericardiocentesis if pericardial effusion is present
  - Drug therapy for congestive heart failure
- Removal of fluid if discomfort or respiratory difficulty is present: abdominal drainage (see Abdominal Drainage, p 1176).
- Urgent surgery may be indicated for septic peritonitis, ruptured masses, and briskly hemorrhagic hemoabdomen cases.

CHRONIC TREATMENT

- Abdominal drainage (see Abdominal Drainage, p 1176) if recurrent ascites causing discomfort/dyspnea
- Diuretics (furosemide 1-3 mg/kg PO, SC, IM, or IV q 8-24h; or spironolactone 0.5-1.5 mg/kg PO q 12-24h) are less effective at mobilizing transudates than centesis/drainage, but may help reduce the rate of reaccumulation medium to long term

POSSIBLE COMPLICATIONS

- Systemic effects of disorder that produced ascites (hypovolemia and anemia if hemoabdomen, sepsis with septic ascites, hemodynamic compromise if congestive heart failure, etc.).
- "Tense ascites" (marked ascites that stretches the abdominal wall and increases intra-abdominal pressure) can cause discomfort and inappetence, can cause dyspnea through cranial displacement of the diaphragm, and can reduce the arterial perfusion of vital intra-abdominal organs. This situation is referred to as the abdominal compartment syndrome (see Abdominal Compartment Syndrome, p 2).

RECOMMENDED MONITORING

- Girth measurement
- Body weight
- Respiratory ease/comfort

PROGNOSIS AND OUTCOME

Dependent on underlying cause

PEARLS & CONSIDERATIONS

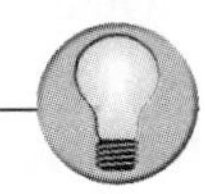

COMMENTS

- The approach to a patient with ascites is to determine the nature of the primary problem.
- Abdominocentesis is a safe and effective procedure that can be repeated in chronic conditions as periodic large-volume abdominal drainage.
- Thoracic radiographs should be part of the routine evaluation for a patient with ascites so as not to overlook the possibility of cardiac, pericardial, or metastatic disease.

SUGGESTED READING

Ettinger SJ, Barrett KA: Ascites, peritonitis, and other causes of abdominal distention. In Ettinger SJ, Feldman EC (eds): *Textbook of Veterinary Internal Medicine*, ed 4. Philadelphia, WB Saunders, 1995, pp 66-71.

AUTHOR: **KIRSTIE A. BARRETT**
EDITOR: **ETIENNE CÔTÉ**

Aseptic Necrosis of the Femoral Head

BASIC INFORMATION

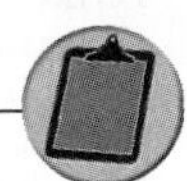

DEFINITION

A painful hip condition caused by interruption of blood supply to the proximal femoral epiphysis, producing bone necrosis and collapse of the articular cartilage. This process results in malformation of the coxofemoral joint and subsequent degenerative joint disease.

SYNONYM(S)

Legg-Calvé-Perthes disease
Legg-Perthes disease
Perthes disease

EPIDEMIOLOGY

SPECIES, AGE, SEX
- Small-breed dogs 5 to 10 months old
- Uncommon in cats

GENETICS AND BREED PREDISPOSITIONS
- Terrier breeds at increased risk
- Affected breeds include Yorkshire terrier, Manchester terrier, miniature pincher, poodle (toy and miniature), Lakeland terrier, West Highland white terrier, Cairn terrier, Australian shepherd, Chihuahua, dachshund, Lhasa apso, pug

CLINICAL PRESENTATION

HISTORY, CHIEF COMPLAINT: Rear leg lameness: unilateral or bilateral.

PHYSICAL EXAM FINDINGS
- Pain on extension and flexion of the affected coxofemoral joint(s)
- Crepitus is unusual in early stages but may be a residual finding in untreated dogs
- Muscle atrophy of the affected leg(s)

ETIOLOGY AND PATHOPHYSIOLOGY

- Aseptic necrosis of the femoral head is considered to be a primary degenerative arthropathy.
- Its etiology and pathogenesis are still unknown.
- The primary lesion appears to be ischemic injury and subsequent necrosis of the subchondral bone of the proximal femoral physis (capital physis).
- Once the subchondral bone is dead, it is replaced by granulation tissue and fibrous tissue.
- There is a loss of the structural integrity, and subsequent weight-bearing causes articular cartilage fibrillation and collapse.
- Bone death, inflammatory mediators, and the seepage of synovial fluids through the damaged cartilage produce a painful condition.

DIAGNOSIS

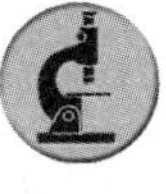

Based on signalment, physical examination, and radiographic study

DIFFERENTIAL DIAGNOSIS

- Traumatic injury (fractures) to the femoral head or neck
- Hip dysplasia
- Coxofemoral luxation
- Septic arthritis of the coxofemoral joint
- Other causes of rear limb lameness (patellar luxation, stifle injury, etc.)

INITIAL DATABASE

- Routine clinical pathologic tests (complete blood count, serum chemistry panel, urinalyisis) based on signalment
- Physical examination of hip joint
- Pelvic or coxofemoral radiographs (lateral and ventrodorsal projections) (see Fig. I-15)

ADVANCED OR CONFIRMATORY TESTING

Advanced imaging techniques (computed tomography, magnetic resonance imaging, or nuclear scintigraphy) are not routinely required.

TREATMENT

- Femoral head and neck excision
- Total hip replacement (an option in large dogs)
- Use of a non-weight-bearing sling/bandage (controversial)
- Medical management to relieve pain (will not prevent progressive joint degeneration)

THERAPEUTIC GOAL(S)

Return animal to normal, pain-free activity

ACUTE GENERAL TREATMENT

- A femoral head and neck ostectomy (FHO) is recommended for most cases.
  - Postoperative radiographs are taken to assess the surgical site.
- Non-weight-bearing sling.
  - Long-term application of an Ehmer sling reportedly allowed one dog to remodel the damaged proximal femur and maintain a pain-free coxofemoral joint.

CHRONIC TREATMENT

In some cases, chronic changes in the coxofemoral joint may necessitate intermittent or chronic nonsteroidal anti-inflammatory drug (NSAID) administration.

- Optimally, NSAIDs are given on an intermittent basis; however, in more advanced cases, long-term daily use might be indicated.
- Buffered aspirin 22 mg/kg PO q 12h; or
- Carprofen 2.2 mg/kg PO q 12h; or
- Etodolac 10-15 mg/kg PO q 24h; or
- Deracoxib 1-2 mg/kg PO q 24h; or
- Meloxicam 0.1 mg/kg PO q 24h.

DRUG INTERACTIONS

- Codosing glucocorticosteroids and NSAIDs can result in severe gastrointestinal irritation, ulceration, and perforation.
- Use of NSAIDs should be closely monitored in dogs with a history or biochemical findings of liver or renal dysfunction.

POSSIBLE COMPLICATIONS

- Hip joint pain secondary to inadequate bone removal
- Limb dysfunction secondary to disuse atrophy

RECOMMENDED MONITORING

- Postoperative radiographic testing to evaluate bone excision
- Monthly physical examinations to evaluate limb function until "normal"

PROGNOSIS AND OUTCOME

Good to excellent for return of functional leg use after FHO if rehabilitation and physical activity are performed. A pseudoarthrosis composed of fibrous tissue is formed.

PEARLS & CONSIDERATIONS

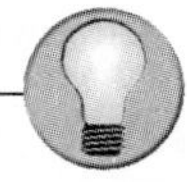

COMMENTS

Physical rehabilitation is important for obtaining the best results after FHO. Range of motion exercises, swimming, and limited weight-bearing exercises will help create a good pseudoarthrosis.

CLIENT EDUCATION

- Breeders of dogs at risk should be questioned regarding incidence of this condition in their animals.
- Affected animals should be removed from the breeding pool.

SUGGESTED READING

Johnson AL, Hulse DA: Diseases of joints. In Fossum TW (ed): *Small Animal Surgery*, ed 2. St. Louis, Mosby, 2002, pp 1109-1110.

Cook WT, Smith MM: Perthes disease. In Slatter D (ed): *Textbook of Small Animal Surgery*, ed 3. Philadelphia, WB Saunders, 2002, pp 2260-2264.

Roperto F, Papparella S, Crovace A: Legg-Calve-Perthes disease in dogs: Histological and ultrastructural investigations. *J Am Anim Hosp Assoc* 28:156-162, 1992.

LaFond E, Breur GJ, Austin CC: Breed susceptibility for developmental orthopedic diseases in dogs. *J Am Anim Hosp Assoc* 38:467-477, 2002.

AUTHOR: **D. MICHAEL TILLSON**
EDITOR: **JOSEPH HARARI**

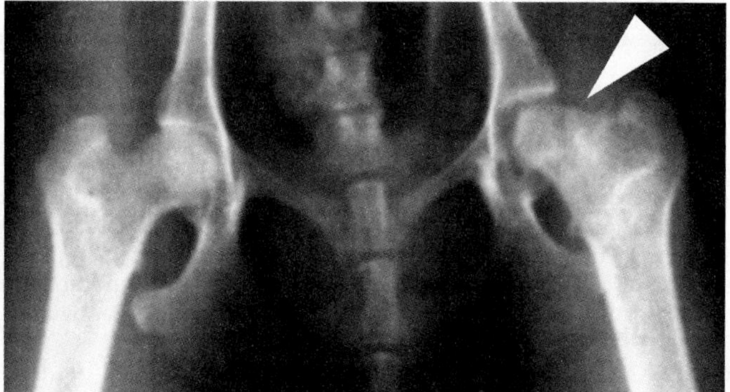

FIGURE I-15 Asceptic necrosis of the femoral head. Ventrodorsal view of the coxofemoral joints of a 10-month-old pug with left hind limb lameness and hip joint pain. Note the bone deformation of the left femoral head (*arrowhead*) compared to the normal right joint.

Aspergillosis

BASIC INFORMATION

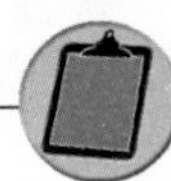

DEFINITION

Regional or disseminated infection with the opportunistic fungus, *Aspergillus* spp.

EPIDEMIOLOGY

SPECIES, AGE, SEX: Dogs more commonly affected than cats.

GENETICS AND BREED PREDISPOSITION

- Middle-aged German shepherd dogs are overrepresented in cases of systemic aspergillosis.
- Medium- to large-breed, dolichocephalic dogs are overrepresented in cases of nasal aspergillosis.

RISK FACTORS

- Systemic/disseminated: immunosuppression (excessive glucocorticoids, neutropenia, diabetes mellitus) or primary immune deficiencies
- Nasal: other primary nasal disease; immunoglobulin A deficiency; prolonged antibiotic use; nasal conformation

CONTAGION AND ZOONOSIS: Aspergillosis is an opportunistic infection; not zoonotic or contagious.

ASSOCIATED CONDITIONS AND DISORDERS

- Systemic: diskospondylitis
- Nasal: chronic rhinitis; fungal sinusitis

CLINICAL PRESENTATION

DISEASE FORMS/SUBTYPES

- Systemic
- Nasal

HISTORY, CHIEF COMPLAINT

- Systemic:
  - Nonspecific signs predominate (lethargy, inappetence, decreased activity, etc.).
  - Retrospectively, signs may have been present and slowly progressive for weeks to months.
  - Acute signs related to diskospondylitis (e.g., acute paresis/paralysis) occur in some cases.
- Nasal: chronic nasal discharge, sneezing, epistaxis, depigmentation of nares

PHYSICAL EXAM FINDINGS

- Systemic:
  - Signs of ill thrift (lethargy, weight loss, poor haircoat, dehydration).
  - Spinal pain during deep palpation.
  - Firm/hard limb swelling with adjacent cutaneous draining tracts may be present.
  - Signs of uveitis (e.g., conjunctival redness, photophobia) are possible and may occur sooner than other signs.
- Nasal:
  - Nasal discharge is common, generally mucopurulent.
  - Evidence of nasal pain.
  - Depigmentation/ulceration of the ventral nares (the path of nasal discharge) is common.
  - Epistaxis (unilateral or bilateral).
  - Nasal air flow often sounds congested/obstructed due to nasal discharge, but may be clearer sounding than normal if no discharge is present and extensive turbinate destruction has occurred.

ETIOLOGY AND PATHOPHYSIOLOGY

- Nasal: *Aspergillus fumigatus* most common.
- Systemic: *Aspergillus terreus* most common.
- *Aspergillus* spp. fungi are normal environmental organisms that often are found incidentally on the skin and mucosa of dogs. Their presence alone does not indicate infection.
- *Aspergillus* fungi are routinely inhaled, ingested, and inoculated during normal activities and are eradicated by the host, especially via cell-mediated immune mechanisms.
- With systemic aspergillosis, multiplication and proliferation of *Aspergillus* spp. occurs when the patient fails to eradicate the organism, typically after routine exposure via inhalation.
  - Therefore, systemic aspergillosis requires both management of the mycosis and identification and management of any underlying immunodeficient trigger.
- With nasal aspergillosis, the role of immunocompromise is unclear.
  - Affected dogs generally do not have any evidence of systemic illness or immunocompromise.
  - Lymphocyte function is low both pretreatment and post-treatment for nasal aspergillosis in dogs.
  - A dominant Th1-regulated cell-mediated immune response has been identified.
- Mutual exclusion: nasal aspergillosis is not suspected to lead to disseminated aspergillosis, and disseminated aspergillosis essentially never causes signs of nasal disease.

DIAGNOSIS

DIFFERENTIAL DIAGNOSIS

- Systemic: other opportunistic mycoses, bacterial diskospondylitis, vertebral or other bone neoplasm
- Nasal: neoplasia, bacterial rhinitis, foreign body, bleeding disorder (if epistaxis)

INITIAL DATABASE

- Complete blood count, serum biochemistry panel: mature neutrophilia/stress leukogram common and nonspecific
- Systemic:
  - Urinalysis may show fungal hyphae
  - Radiographs of the spine may reveal evidence of diskospondylitis (vertebral end-plate lysis)
  - Radiographs of bony swellings can reveal lytic-productive lesions
  - Abdominal ultrasound is indicated to identify visceral fungal granulomas
- Nasal:
  - Swabs of nasal exudates are not useful; generally identify secondary bacterial infection only, and when *Aspergillus* is present, it may only be a contaminant

ADVANCED OR CONFIRMATORY TESTING

- Systemic:
  - Fine-needle aspirates of enlarged lymph nodes, affected intervertebral disks, or bone lesions may show hyphae.
  - Serology variable. Poor immune function, predisposing to systemic aspergillosis, may translate to poor titers despite infection. Also, different species of *Aspergillus* have individual seroreactivities.
  - Histologic evaluation of biopsied tissue is diagnostic—fungal granulomas. If a clinical suspicion of aspergillosis exists at the time of biopsy, a portion of the specimen should also be submitted for fungal culture.
- Nasal: diagnosis is confirmed when fungal hyphae can be demonstrated histologically within nasal tissue and/or when at least two of the following three criteria are fulfilled: positive serum titer for *Aspergillus fumigatus*, positive *Aspergillus* fungal culture, and supportive imaging (radiographic/computed tomographic) findings.
  - Imaging: computed tomography is the modality of choice (greater resolution than radiographs, good bone detail unlike magnetic resonance imaging). Typical findings are nasal turbinate loss, intranasal fluid opacity (exudates), and possibly fluid opacity in the frontal sinus(es).
  - Nasal radiographs show regional or diffuse, asymmetric turbinate loss, and either increase (due to intranasal exudate) or decrease (if scant exudate, and loss of turbinate and overlying mucosa) soft tissue/fluid opacity. A drawback is the difficulty in determining whether soft tissue/fluid opacity in the nasal passages is due

to discharge (fluid) or mass (e.g., neoplasm).
  - Rhinoscopy is the preferred method for direct observation and sampling. An abnormally vast, cavernous nasal cavity is common (turbinate loss). Fungal plaques or granulomas may be observed directly (Fig. I-18). Microscopic identification of *Aspergillus* from a macroscopically visible intranasal or intrasinus colony is considered pathognomonic. Both left and right nasal cavities are examined, as findings often are asymmetric.
  - Rhinotomy is highly invasive, and surgical exploration offers little or no advantage over rhinoscopy in patients with nasal aspergillosis.
  - *Aspergillus* serology results are variable, and titers may not be used as a sole diagnostic test for nasal aspergillosis.
  - Fungal culture results that demonstrate *Aspergillus* from samples not involving a macroscopic fungal colony are equivocal and must be supported by additional tests to make the diagnosis.

TREATMENT

THERAPEUTIC GOAL(S)

Elimination of the organism and return to normal function

ACUTE AND CHRONIC TREATMENT

- Systemic
  - Amphotericin B 0.25 IV infusion q 48h until nephrotoxicity develops or a cumulative dose is reached (8-12 mg/kg, dogs). Risks include nephrotoxicity, anaphylaxis, perivascular irritation/sloughing if extravasation, and lack of efficacy.
  - Amphotericin B lipid-based formula 3-5 mg/kg IV infusion q 48h until nephrotoxicity develops or a cumulative dose is reached (12 mg/kg, dogs and cats). Same risks as previous, but less nephrotoxicity.
  - Itraconazole 2.5-5 mg/kg PO q 12h indefinitely and often lifelong. Monitor for liver adverse effects. Absorption enhanced substantially by administering with food.
- Nasal
  - Endoscopic/nonsurgical intranasal clotrimazole infusion is the treatment of choice. See Nasal Infusion of Clotrimazole, p 1284.
  - Repeating treatment is warranted if nasal discharge has not resolved at 2 weeks post-treatment.
  - In a minority of patients, it is necessary to repeat the clotrimazole

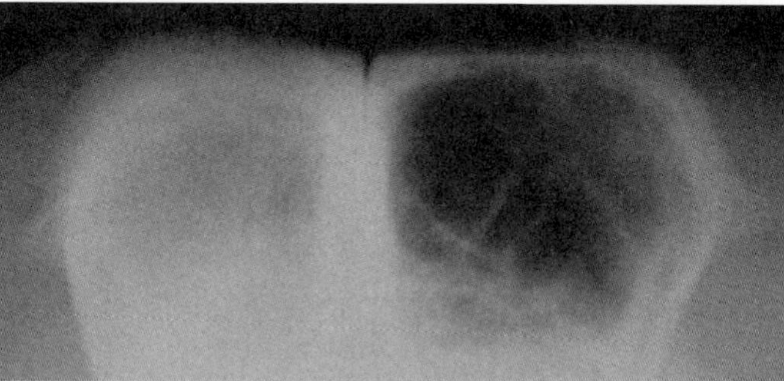

FIGURE I-16 Radiograph of the frontal sinuses of a dog. Marked opacification of the right frontal sinus and thickening of the frontal bone are present. These findings are suggestive of sinonasal aspergillosis but other inflammation, a primary tumor of the sinuses, or extension of a nasal tumor into the sinuses cannot be ruled out. Courtesy of Drs. Jimmy H. Saunders and Cécile Clercx, University of Liège.

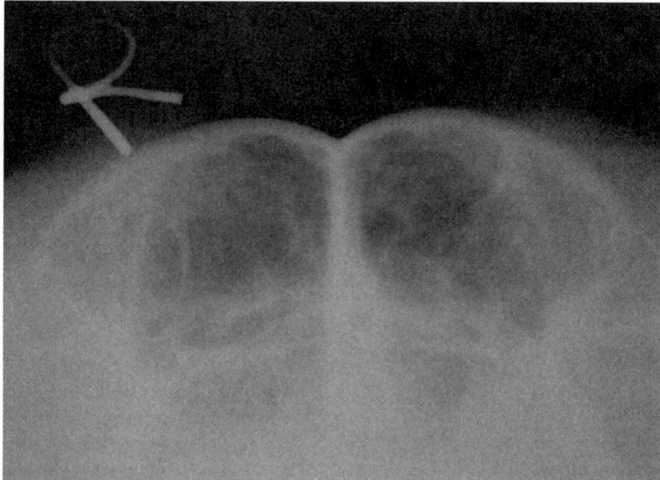

FIGURE I-17 Radiograph of the frontal sinuses of a normal dog for comparison. Courtesy of Drs. Jimmy H. Saunders and Cécile Clercx, University of Liège.

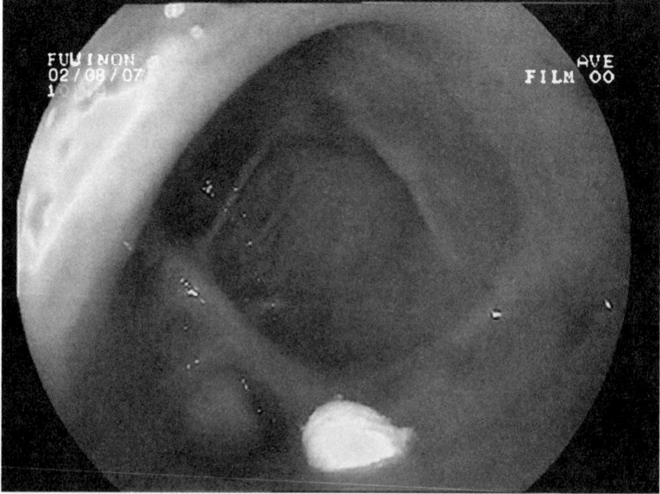

FIGURE I-18 Endoscopic view of the frontal sinus of a patient with sinonasal aspergillosis. Diffuse inflammation and a fungal accumulation, or aspergilloma (fluffy white nodule at bottom of image), are present. Courtesy of Dr. Cécile Clercx, University of Liège.

DISEASES AND DISORDERS

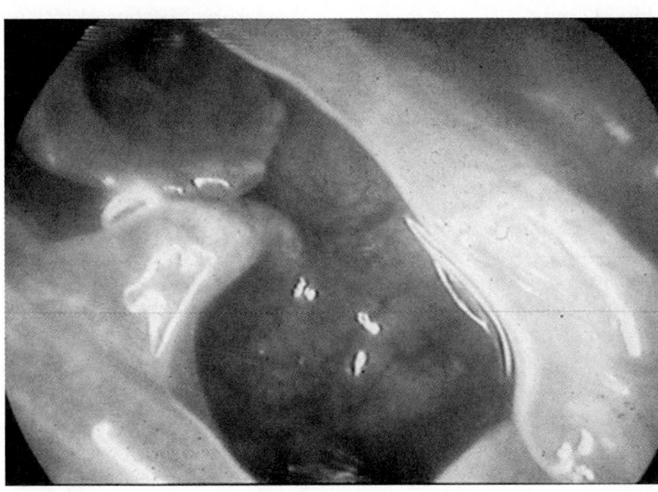

FIGURE I-19 Endoscopic view of the frontal sinus of a patient with a history of sinonasal aspergillosis and successful treatment. Courtesy of Dr. Cécile Clercx, University of Liège.

intranasal infusion once or, rarely, more than once.

POSSIBLE COMPLICATIONS

Intractable infection

RECOMMENDED MONITORING

- Evolution/resolution of clinical signs.
- Serial titers are not useful.

PROGNOSIS AND OUTCOME

- Systemic:
  - The prognosis is almost universally poor, although some dogs may obtain palliation with itraconazole (lifelong therapy; 3-year survival reported in one non-German shepherd case).
  - Many affected dogs are euthanized at the time of conclusive diagnosis due to the extent of lesions and underlying deficiencies in immunity.
- Nasal: fair to good
  - Clinical signs resolve with a single treatment in 65% of dogs, and 87% of dogs with a total of one or more treatments.
  - A lesser extent of radiographic lesions is associated with a better prognosis.

PEARLS & CONSIDERATIONS

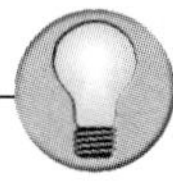

COMMENTS

- For nasal aspergillosis, nasal discharge ceases (permanently) in most dogs within 2 weeks of treatment.
- The frontal sinuses should also be imaged in any patient suspected of having nasal aspergillosis.

CLIENT EDUCATION

Diagnosis of aspergillosis is complex but is important, because diagnostic tests help to determine the likelihood of success

SUGGESTED READING

Day MJ: Canine disseminated aspergillosis. In Greene CE (ed): *Infectious Diseases of the Dog and Cat*. Philadelphia, WB Saunders, 1998, pp 409–413.

Mathews KG, et al: Comparison of topical administration of clotrimazole through surgically placed versus nonsurgically placed catheters for treatment of nasal aspergillosis in dogs: 60 cases (1990–1996). *J Am Vet Med Assoc* 213:501–506, 1998.

Peeters D, et al: An immunohistochemical study of canine nasal aspergillosis. *J Comp Pathol* 132:283–288, 2005.

Saunders JH, et al: Radiographic, magnetic resonance imaging, computed tomographic, and rhinoscopic features of nasal aspergillosis in dogs. *J Am Vet Med Assoc* 225:1703–1712, 2004.

Sharp NJH: Canine nasal aspergillosis-penicilliosis. In Greene CE (ed): *Infectious Diseases of the Dog and Cat*. Philadelphia, WB Saunders, 1998, pp 404–409.

AUTHOR: **ETIENNE CÔTÉ**

EDITOR: **DOUGLASS K. MACINTIRE**

Asthma, Cat

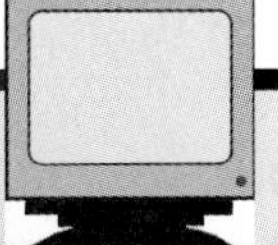

Client Education Sheet on Website

BASIC INFORMATION

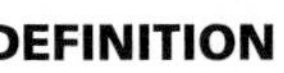

DEFINITION

A syndrome triggered by allergen-specific activation of immune cells leading to clinical signs of cough, wheeze and/or respiratory distress, eosinophilic inflammation of the airways, bronchoconstriction, and structural changes in the lung

SYNONYM(S)

Feline allergic asthma
Feline allergic bronchitis
Feline eosinophilic bronchitis
Feline lower airway disease

EPIDEMIOLOGY

SPECIES, AGE, SEX: Affected cats are usually young to middle-aged at onset; either gender can be affected.

GENETICS AND BREED PREDISPOSITION: There is a possible breed predisposition for Siamese cats.

GEOGRAPHY AND SEASONALITY: Seasonality of clinical signs depends on the allergen. Indoor allergens tend to be present year-round, while outdoor allergens are more seasonal.

CLINICAL PRESENTATION

DISEASE FORMS/SUBTYPES

- May be an acute, life-threatening disease ("status asthmaticus")
- May have chronic persistent signs
- May have waxing and waning signs

HISTORY, CHIEF COMPLAINT

- Cough (often confused with "hacking up a hairball")
- Wheeze
- Tachypnea
- Respiratory distress

PHYSICAL EXAM FINDINGS

- Cough, which may be inducible with tracheal palpation.
- Wheezes may be audible with or without a stethoscope.
- Respiratory distress tends to have a prominent expiratory component ("expiratory push").
- Tachypnea is common.

ETIOLOGY AND PATHOPHYSIOLOGY

- Sensitization to allergens activates T-helper 2 lymphocytes, leading to production of cytokines.
- Cytokines are responsible for allergen-specific IgE production, inflammatory cell influx (the hallmark cell is the eosinophil), airway hyper-reactivity, and remodeling changes in the lung.
- Airway inflammation and hyper-reactivity provoke bronchoconstriction, leading to clinical signs of cough and respiratory difficulty; remodelling changes can further reduce luminal diameter of small airways contributing to respiratory difficulty.
- Reduction in diameter of small airways impairs expiration more than inspiration, leading to the expiratory push observed during physical examination and the phenomenon of "air-trapping" on thoracic radiographs.

DIAGNOSIS

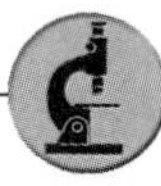

DIFFERENTIAL DIAGNOSIS

- Physical examination findings (cough, dyspnea, wheeze):
  - Pleural effusion
  - Cardiogenic or noncardiogenic pulmonary edema
  - Pneumonia (infectious, aspiration, foreign body)
  - Neoplasia
  - Interstitial lung disease
  - Laryngeal disease
    - Should be easily distinguished from asthma, because musical noises will be loudest when auscultation is performed over the larynx
- Radiographic findings:
  - Chronic bronchitis
  - Lung worms
  - Heartworm disease

INITIAL DATABASE

- Thoracic radiographs:
  - Bronchial or bronchointerstitial pattern.
  - Hyperinflation of lungs ("air trapping").
    - Expanded lung fields
    - Increased radiolucency of lung fields (especially caudodorsal lung regions)
    - Flattened diaphragm
    - Increased distance between the caudal aspect of the cardiac silhouette and the diaphragm on the lateral view
  - Collapse of lung lobe (most commonly the right middle lung lobe), thought to be associated with overproduction of mucoid respiratory secretions and mucus plugging of bronchus.
  - May be normal.
- Complete blood count:
  - Eosinophilia is compatible with either allergic or parasitic disease.
  - Absence of eosinophilia does not rule out feline asthma.
- Fecal Baermann:
  - Should be done multiple times on different stool samples since respiratory parasites are intermittently shed in the feces.
  - Alternatively, a trial with an antiparasitic like fenbendazole (25–50 mg/kg PO q 12h for 10 to 14 days) can be administered to help rule out parasites.
- Heartworm antibody/antigen test:
  - Helps rule out a cause of cough and peripheral eosinophilia in cats.
  - Refer to other sources on the interpretation of these tests (see Heartworm Disease, Cat, p 462).

ADVANCED OR CONFIRMATORY TESTING

- Echocardiogram to help rule out heartworm disease
- Respiratory wash cytology:
  - Collected by blind bronchoalveolar lavage through an endotracheal tube or via bronchoscopy.
  - Submission of a portion of the wash sample for culture to exclude secondary bacterial infection is encouraged.
  - Cytologic examination of lavage fluid will show increased numbers of eosinophils with asthma and increased numbers of neutrophils with chronic bronchitis.
    - The concurrent presence of both can indicate either *chronic asthmatic bronchitis* (the presence of long-standing inflammation associated with asthma can lead to the development of superimposed chronic bronchitis, the hallmark cell of which is the neutrophil) or secondary bacterial infection.
- Pulmonary function testing with bronchoprovocation:
  - Only available at a few referral centers.

TREATMENT

THERAPEUTIC GOAL(S)

- In an acute crisis, stabilize respiratory function.
- For chronic therapy:
  - Minimize exposure to environmental allergens and irritants
  - Decrease inflammation
  - Alleviate bronchoconstriction
- Future therapeutics will likely focus on upstream modulation of the immune response to either induce tolerance to allergen, or alter the T-helper 2 cell-driven immune response so that it is less damaging, instead of palliative measures to control inflammation and bronchoconstriction after they have already been triggered.

ACUTE GENERAL TREATMENT

- Minimize handling and stress to reduce oxygen requirements
- Administer oxygen
- Bronchodilators:
  - Delivered by nebulization or metered dose inhalers:
    - Albuterol 0.5% solution for nebulization: give 0.1–0.25 ml diluted in 2 ml of sterile saline through a nebulizer every 4 hours.
    - Metered dose inhalants are delivered by using a "spacer" with a face mask designed for cats (see Medication Administration by Inhalation, p 1278).
      - Albuterol 17 g inhalant: 1–2 actuations ("puffs") into the spacer while the cat takes about 10 breaths; can be repeated every 30 minutes if necessary for 1 to 4 hours.
  - Parenteral routes:
    - Terbutaline 0.01 mg/kg SC or IM q 4–8h.
    - In severe cases, epinephrine 0.1 mg/cat SC, IM, or IV may be beneficial.
      - Hypoxia can cause epinephrine to be arrhythmogenic, so oxygen should be administered concurrently, and this treatment should not be used in cats with preexisting heart disease or systemic hypertension.
- Glucocorticoids: administer via parenteral route:
  - Prednisolone sodium succinate 1–2 mg/kg slowly IV or dexamethasone 0.2–0.5 mg/kg IV or IM
  - Inhalant glucocorticoids do not work fast enough to be of benefit in acute treatment

CHRONIC TREATMENT

- Environmental modulation:
  - Ideally, remove the allergen causing clinical signs.
    - In practice, this is difficult or impossible to do.
  - Minimize exposure to dusts (e.g., cat litter), smoke, aerosols.
  - Hepa-type air filters.
- Bronchodilators:
  - Oral route best for chronic therapy while aerosolized route best for "rescue" therapy intermittently given for acute clinical signs.
    - Sustained release theophylline (Theo-Dur) 25 mg/kg PO q 24h.
    - Aminophylline 4–5 mg/kg PO q 8h.
    - Terbutaline 0.625 mg/cat PO q 12h.
  - In severe cases where cats develop status asthmaticus at home, owners

can be taught to give a subcutaneous injection of terbutaline 0.01 mg/kg.

- Glucocorticoids:
  - Oral glucocorticoids preferred initially to control inflammation with a transition to a metered dose inhalant form.
    - Prednisone or prednisolone 1-2 mg/kg/day.
  - Reposital ("depo") glucocorticoids often appear to lose their efficacy over time and must be given more and more frequently.
- If a secondary bacterial infection is documented based on culture and sensitivity (this is uncommon), administer an appropriate antibiotic. Alternatively, if the response to glucocorticoids is less than expected, a short course of a broad-spectrum antibiotic that penetrates into the bronchial secretions and bronchial epithelium (e.g., doxycycline [5 mg/kg PO q 12h]), may also be tried.
- Cyclosporine (5 mg/kg q 12h to start) is not routinely recommended for feline asthma but may be considered in severe cases refractory to other medications.
  - Should be considered a "last resort" and not standard practice.
  - Therapeutic blood monitoring is required.
- Cyproheptadine (2 mg PO q 12h; higher doses may be required in some cats) may be beneficial in alleviating airway hyper-reactivity in a subpopulation of asthmatic cats.

DRUG INTERACTIONS

Do not give propranolol or other nonspecific β-adrenergic blockers to asthmatics, because these drugs can exacerbate bronchoconstriction.

POSSIBLE COMPLICATIONS

Theophyllines have a low therapeutic index, and dosages should be based on lean body weight. They are relatively contraindicated in patients with hypertension, hyperthyroidism, and cardiac disease. In particular, the sustained-release oral formulations of theophylline are not designed for absorption by the gastrointestinal tracts of small animals, and variable assimilation of the drug (underabsorption or overabsorption) is possible. Manifestations of toxicity include tachycardia and behavior changes such as agitation and anxiety (similar to theobromine toxicosis).

RECOMMENDED MONITORING

- Clinical signs at home
- Physical examination
- Thoracic radiographs

PROGNOSIS AND OUTCOME

- If respiratory distress is a manifestation of disease, sudden death could occur before veterinary intervention.
- Prognosis can range from grave to good and depends on the number and severity of status asthmaticus episodes and their response to acute and chronic management.
- If respiratory distress is not a manifestation of the disease, and inflammation can be controlled with corticosteroids and environmental modulation, prognosis is good to excellent.
- If inflammation is not well controlled, damage to the lungs can occur and lead to airflow limitation, in which case the prognosis is guarded to fair.

PEARLS & CONSIDERATIONS

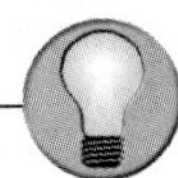

COMMENTS

- Bronchodilators should not be given as monotherapy, because they do not adequately suppress airway inflammation; chronic airway inflammation leads to permanent damage and structural changes.
- Unlike in humans, leukotrienes do not appear to play an important role in the pathogenesis of feline asthma; therefore, there is no indication to administer leukotriene receptor antagonists like zafirlukast to cats.
- Allergen-specific immunotherapy may one day prove to be a useful therapeutic strategy; however, development of safe and effective protocols is still in the early stages of research.

CLIENT EDUCATION

Keeping a record of when clinical signs occur can help establish the seasonality to allergen exposure.

SUGGESTED READING

Dye J, et al: Bronchopulmonary disease in the cat: historical, physical, radiographic, clinicopathologic, and pulmonary functional evaluation of 24 affected and 15 healthy cats. *J Vet Intern Med* 10:385, 1996.

Moise N, et al: Clinical, radiographic, and bronchial cytologic features of cats with bronchial disease: 65 cases (1980–1986). *J Am Vet Med Assoc* 194:1467, 1989.

Reinero CR, et al: Effect of drug therapy on airway inflammation and hyperreactivity, and immune parameters in a feline model of asthma. *Am J Vet Res* 66:1121-1127, 2005.

AUTHOR: **CAROL REINERO**
EDITOR: **RANCE K. SELLON**

Ataxia

BASIC INFORMATION

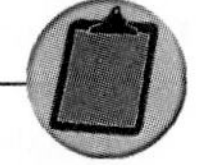

DEFINITION

Failure of muscular coordination; a sign of sensory dysfunction within the nervous system

SYNONYM(S)

Incoordination

EPIDEMIOLOGY

SPECIES, AGE, SEX: Dependent on underlying cause.

GENETICS AND BREED PREDISPOSITION: Dependent on underlying cause.

CLINICAL PRESENTATION

DISEASE FORMS/SUBTYPES

- *Proprioceptive (sensory) ataxia*: due to dysfunction of the proprioceptive pathways in any or all of the spinal cord, brainstem, or cerebrum. The appearance is that of a patient's failure to perceive where its limbs are in space.
- *Vestibular ataxia* (see also Vestibular Disease, p 1152): due to dysfunction of the peripheral vestibular system within the inner ear or the central vestibular system within the brainstem. The appearance is that of a patient with loss of balance/disequilibrium.
- *Cerebellar ataxia*: results from diseases affecting the cerebellum. The appearance is that of loss of fine motor control despite normal initiation of movements.

HISTORY, CHIEF COMPLAINT

- Onset: peracute to chronic/insidious, depending on cause.
- Signs of pain may be associated with proprioceptive ataxia.
- "Walking as if intoxicated" may be reported for cerebellar or vestibular ataxia.
- Owners of animals with acute onset of vestibular ataxia often think their animal is seizuring.
- History of otitis externa (vestibular ataxia).
- Recent therapy with metronidazole or aminoglycosides (vestibular ataxia).

PHYSICAL AND NEUROLOGIC EXAM FINDINGS (SOME OR ALL MAY BE PRESENT)

Proprioceptive ataxia:
- Generally accompanied by paresis
- Basewide stance
- Circumduction, abduction, and crossing over of the limbs
- Delayed limb protraction with an elongated stride
- Mild hypermetria
- Standing on the dorsum of the paw; "knuckling over"
  - Ulceration of the dorsal aspect of the paw and wear of the nails

Vestibular ataxia:
- The hallmark of vestibular ataxia is a head tilt with the ventral ear indicating the side of the lesion.
  - Very rarely, the head tilt may be directed away from the lesion in the paradoxic vestibular syndrome.
- The trunk may lean, fall, or curve toward the side of the lesion, causing patients to press against a wall.
- Ipsilateral limb flexion and contralateral limb extension may be noted.
- Paresis is not a component of peripheral vestibular disease but may be seen with central vestibular disease.
- Tight circling toward the side of the lesion (as opposed to wide circles with forebrain disease).
- With peripheral vestibular disease, nystagmus is horizontal or rotary with the fast phase away from the lesion and does not change with different head positions.
- In central vestibular disease, nystagmus may be horizontal, rotary, vertical, or may change direction with different head positions.
- Abnormal eye position (strabismus).
- Mental status is normal with peripheral vestibular disease and may be depressed with central vestibular disease.
- Postural reactions are normal with peripheral vestibular disease and delayed with central vestibular disease.
  - Note: in acute peripheral disease, postural reactions may appear delayed; careful examination is necessary.
- Bilateral peripheral vestibular disease (rare) causes a crouched posture with wide head excursions bilaterally, absent physiologic nystagmus without the presence of head tilt, resting nystagmus, or postural deficits.

Cerebellar ataxia:
- Broad-based stance
- Dysmetria, hypermetria, spasticity (abnormal, excessive, stiff movement of the limbs, respectively)
- Intention tremor (i.e., tremor precipitated by the onset of voluntary movement, such as responding to a command)
- Preservation of strength and postural reactions
- Absent menace response possible with cerebellar disease
- Head tilt away from the lesion in the rare case of paradoxical vestibular syndrome
- Opisthotonos with thoracic ± pelvic limb extensor rigidity with acute severe lesions

ETIOLOGY AND PATHOPHYSIOLOGY
- Proprioceptive ataxia:
  - Intervertebral disk disease
  - Caudal cervical spondylomyelopathy/"wobbler syndrome"
  - Degenerative myelopathy
  - Congenital malformations (spina bifida)
  - Fibrocartilaginous emboli
  - Neoplasia
  - Myelitis
  - Trauma
- Vestibular ataxia:
  - Idiopathic peripheral vestibular disease (old dog, any age cat)
  - Otitis media/interna
  - Vascular
  - Neoplasia
  - Inflammatory polyp (cat, middle ear)
  - Hypothyroidism (older dog)
  - Polyneuropathy
  - Toxic (e.g., aminoglycosides, metronidazole) (especially topical [ear medication] with disrupted tympanum)
  - Thiamine deficiency (cats)
- Cerebellar ataxia:
  - Abiotrophy
  - Atrophy/hypoplasia (in utero panleukopenia infection in cats, herpes virus in dogs, others)
  - Infectious (feline infectious peritonitis, distemper)
  - Inflammatory (meningoencephalitis: granulomatous, steroid-responsive, necrotizing)
  - Neoplasia
  - Caudal occipital malformation syndrome (chiari-like malformation)
  - Vascular

DIAGNOSIS

DIFFERENTIAL DIAGNOSIS
- Orthopedic disease (e.g., ruptured cranial cruciate ligament, hip dysplasia)
- Weakness (metabolic, neuromuscular)

INITIAL DATABASE
- Complete physical and neurologic examination, including fundic and otoscopic exam
- Complete blood count, serum chemistry, urinalysis, thyroid profile to evaluate systemic causes of ataxia

ADVANCED OR CONFIRMATORY TESTING
- Imaging modalities (radiography, myelography, computed tomography, magnetic resonance imaging)
- Cerebrospinal fluid analysis
- Electrodiagnostics (e.g., brainstem auditory evoked response)
- Serum and cerebrospinal fluid titers for infectious diseases

TREATMENT

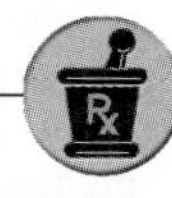

THERAPEUTIC GOAL(S)
Identify and eliminate the underlying cause

ACUTE GENERAL TREATMENT
See specific disease descriptions

CHRONIC TREATMENT
See specific disease descriptions

POSSIBLE COMPLICATIONS
- Trauma resulting from falls associated with ataxia/incoordination
- Anorexia and dehydration due to incapacitation or nausea
- Respiratory dysfunction with severe cervical spinal cord lesions

RECOMMENDED MONITORING
Follow-up exam and serial diagnostic studies as directed by the patient's clinical progression

PROGNOSIS AND OUTCOME

- Dependent on the underlying cause.
- In general, diseases with an acute onset have a more favorable prognosis than those with a chronic course.

PEARLS & CONSIDERATIONS

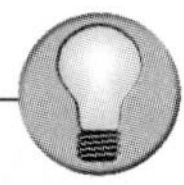

COMMENTS
- Accurate identification and characterization of ataxia are the most important aspects of neurologic localization.
- Diffuse lower motor neuron disease causes weakness but not ataxia; affected animals are short-strided, but careful examination reveals that although they may not have the strength to appropriately place their limbs, they are aware of the position of the limbs in space.

SUGGESTED READING

De Lahunta A: *Veterinary Neuroanatomy and Clinical Neurology*, ed 2. Philadelphia, WB Saunders, 1983.

Lorenz MD, Kornegay JN: Ataxia of the Head and the Limbs. In Lorenz MD, Kornegay JN: *Handbook of Veterinary Neurology*, ed 4. St. Louis, WB Saunders, 2004, pp 219–244.

AUTHORS: **GREG KILBURN, JOLI M. JARBOE**

EDITOR: **ETIENNE CÔTÉ**

Atlantoaxial Subluxation

BASIC INFORMATION

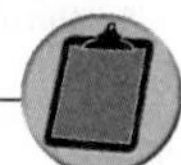

DEFINITION

An instability of the articulation between the first (atlas) and second (axis) cervical vertebra, often resulting from a congenital malformation, trauma, or a combination of both. The instability causes compression of the associated spinal cord, varying degrees of neurologic impairment, and neck pain (cervical hyperesthesia).

SYNONYM(S)

AAS
Atlantoaxial instability
Atlantoaxial luxation
Atlantoaxial malformation

EPIDEMIOLOGY

SPECIES, AGE, SEX: Dogs and cats. Most cases are diagnosed in dogs <2 years old.
GENETICS AND BREED PREDISPOSITION: Small/toy breeds (toy poodle, Pomeranian, Yorkshire terrier, Japanese Chin, Pekingese).
RISK FACTORS: Trauma-induced atlantoaxial subluxation (AAS) usually results from excessive ventroflexion of the cranial cervical spine.
ASSOCIATED CONDITIONS AND DISORDERS: Other conditions common to toy breeds (portosystemic shunt, hydrocephalus, patellar luxation) may coexist and should be considered before definitive treatment of AAS.

CLINICAL PRESENTATION

DISEASE FORMS/SUBTYPES

- Congenital
- Traumatic

HISTORY, CHIEF COMPLAINT: Congenital: history of cervical pain, abnormal head carriage, ataxia, or tetraparesis is typical. Commonly, mild/moderate slowly progressive gait dysfunction exists, and an incident of cervical pain possibly associated with an incident of hyperflexion (trauma) of the neck prompts evaluation.
PHYSICAL EXAM FINDINGS

- Neurologic deficits suggesting a cervical spinal cord (C1-C5) lesion: tetraparesis and rarely tetraplegia, with normal or increased thoracic and pelvic limb reflexes.
- Rarely, severe spinal cord compression can cause respiratory paralysis and death (disruption of descending fibers of the brainstem respiratory centers).

ETIOLOGY AND PATHOPHYSIOLOGY

- Instability of the atlantoaxial joint arises from agenesis or hypoplasia of the dens (odontoid process); dorsal deviation of the dens; absence or laxity of the atlantoaxial (transverse, apical, and alar) ligaments; traumatic fracture of the dens, atlas, or axis; or traumatic rupture of the atlantoaxial ligaments.
- With interruption of the normal anatomy of the C1-C2 junction, excessive flexion can occur at the atlantoaxial joint, allowing the cranial aspect of C2 (axis) to deviate dorsally into the vertebral canal and impinge on the cervical spinal cord.

DIAGNOSIS

DIFFERENTIAL DIAGNOSIS

- Intervertebral disk disease
- Trauma of other spinal column components (C1-C5) such as a vertebral body fracture or luxation
- Meningomyelitis (infectious or idiopathic inflammatory)
- Diskospondylitis
- Neoplasia

INITIAL DATABASE

Definitive diagnosis of AAS is made by survey radiography:

- Static instability can be noted on plain films by the increased space between the dorsal spine of the axis and the dorsal arch of the atlas, as well as by dorsal displacement of the body of the axis.
- Occasionally, a diagnosis cannot be made using a static, nonstressed radiographic technique. If the index of suspicion for AAS is high, a dynamic lateral spinal radiograph may be performed by placing the dog or cat in lateral recumbency and gently ventroflexing the neck. A dramatic widening of the C1-C2 space is noted dorsally in dogs with AAS. It is important to use extreme caution when ventroflexing the neck because of increased spinal cord compression and damage that can occur with this type of positioning.

ADVANCED OR CONFIRMATORY TESTING

Computed tomography or magnetic resonance imaging:

- Not usually necessary to confirm AAS
- Provide greater anatomic detail, which may be useful for preoperative decision making

TREATMENT

THERAPEUTIC GOAL(S)

- Stabilization of the atlantoaxial joint
- Preservation or improvement of neurologic status
- Relief of cervical pain

ACUTE GENERAL TREATMENT

- Ventilation management must be instituted immediately in animals with respiratory compromise.
- Stabilization of the cervical spine:
    - Cage restriction; avoidance of collar/neck leads; soft padded neck wrap or fiberglass-type orthotic.
- Medical management of spinal cord trauma:
    - Varying opinions, without consensus. Dexamethasone or methylprednisolone sodium succinate has been recommended at an anti-inflammatory dose in acute spinal cord injury (<8 hours in duration). (See Spinal Cord Trauma, p 1023.)

CHRONIC TREATMENT

- Stabilization of the atlantoaxial joint is best achieved through surgical intervention
    - Connection of the dorsal spinous processes of atlas and axis using wire or endogenous ligaments
    - Ventral cervical approach to fuse atlas and axis. More technically demanding procedure, but it allows removal of the dens
- Nonsurgical stabilization of the atlantoaxial joint: neck braces (orthotics) and severely restricted activity
    - Palliative, and therefore reserved for mild cases or cases in which clients decline surgical correction
    - Side effects include atrophy of neck muscles, which increases risk of injury when the brace is removed

POSSIBLE COMPLICATIONS

- Fracture of the fixation device, requiring reoperation
- Nonsurgical management: permanent dependency on brace, no correction of lesion, risk of acute worsening if brace is removed

PROGNOSIS AND OUTCOME

- Medical treatment will not provide a definitive solution. Initial improvement in clinical signs may be apparent, but signs eventually recur.
- Surgical success depends on age at onset of clinical signs, duration of signs before surgery, and the preoperative neurologic status.

- Indicators for a more positive prognosis: onset of signs at <24 months old, duration of signs <10 months, and normal or mildly ataxic gait preoperatively (versus paresis/plegia).
- Not prognostically significant: type of surgery performed, grade of AAS, radiographic appearance of the dens, or need for a second surgery.

PEARLS & CONSIDERATIONS

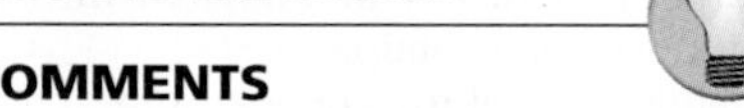

COMMENTS

Patients with AAS can be most effectively treated with surgical intervention, which carries a 70–75% success rate.

PREVENTION

Breeding affected animals should be avoided

CLIENT EDUCATION

- Clinical signs may not present until a minor traumatic episode occurs. Therefore, activity restriction of affected animals and supervision of playtime is advisable.
- Surgical success has been shown to be most effective when this condition is addressed before the onset of severe neurologic deficits.

SUGGESTED READING

Beal MW, et al: Ventilatory failure, ventilator management, and outcome in dogs with cervical spinal disorders: 14 cases (1991–1999). *J Am Vet Med Assoc* 218(10):1598–1602, 2001.

Braund, KG: Developmental disorders. In Braund (ed): *Clinical Neurology in Small Animals-Localization, Diagnosis, and Treatment*. Ithaca, IVIS, 2003. www.ivis.org/special_books/Braund/braund16.

Beaver DR, et al: Risk factors affecting the outcome of surgery for atlantoaxial subluxation in dogs: 46 cases (1978–1998). *J Am Vet Med Assoc* 216(7):1104–1109, 2000.

LeCouteur RA, Grandy JL: Diseases of the spinal cord. In Ettinger, SJ, Feldman, EC (eds): *Textbook of Veterinary Internal Medicine*. Philadelphia, WB Saunders, 2000, pp 615–616.

Platt SR, et al: A modified ventral fixation for surgical management of atlantoaxial subluxation in 19 dogs. *Vet Surg* 33:349–354, 2004.

Thomas WB, et al: Surgical management of atlantoaxial subluxation in 23 dogs. *Vet Surg* 20(6):409–412, 1991.

AUTHORS: **TODD W. AXLUND, CHRISTINA WOLF**

EDITOR: **CURTIS W. DEWEY**

Atonic or Hypotonic Urinary Bladder

BASIC INFORMATION

DEFINITION

Absent or incomplete detrusor muscle (bladder wall) contraction

SYNONYM(S)

Bladder atony
Bladder overdistention
Lower motor neuron (LMN) bladder

EPIDEMIOLOGY

RISK FACTORS: Spinal cord injury/disease, peripheral nervous system disorders (including dysautonomia), urine retention.

GEOGRAPHY AND SEASONALITY: See Dysautonomia, p 323.

ASSOCIATED CONDITIONS AND DISORDERS: See Cystitis, Bacterial, p 270; Incontinence, Urinary, p 589.

CLINICAL PRESENTATION

DISEASE FORMS/SUBTYPES

- Detrusor atony/hypotonia with sphincter atonia/hypotonia (LMN bladder)
- Detrusor atony/hypotonia with normal or hypertonic sphincter tone
  - Neurogenic: upper motor neuron (UMN) bladder
  - Non-neurogenic: as a result of bladder overdistention from any cause

HISTORY, CHIEF COMPLAINT

- Absent/weak attempts to void
- Leakage or dribbling of urine
- Associated signs of neurologic dysfunction unrelated to micturition (e.g., paresis)

PHYSICAL EXAM FINDINGS

- Distended bladder
- Large volume of residual urine
- Bladder expression may be easy or difficult (depending on sphincter tone, obstruction)
  - LMN (sacral lesion or peripheral nervous system): flaccid bladder, flaccid anus and tail
  - UMN (suprasacral lesion): turgid bladder, perineal tone intact

ETIOLOGY AND PATHOPHYSIOLOGY

- LMN dysfunction disrupts parasympathetic control of detrusor muscle.
  - Intramural bladder weakness causing inability to contract and empty normally and completely.
  - Lesions in sacral spinal cord, sacral nerves, or pelvic plexus.
  - Internal urethral sphincter tone may be retained because sympathetic innervation (hypogastric nerve) is not affected by LMN lesions.
- Severe UMN lesions (L7 to pons) may lead to loss of voluntary micturition and resultant overdistension.
  - Disinhibition of sympathetic innervation may increase urethral sphincter tone.
- Non-neurogenic bladder atonia results from urethral outflow obstruction or pelvic disease (i.e., pain, fractures).
  - Bladder overdistention results in disruption of tight junctions between detrusor smooth muscle fibers.
  - Disruption inhibits the wave of excitation between myofibers, resulting in a flaccid bladder.

DIAGNOSIS

DIFFERENTIAL DIAGNOSIS

- Hypotonia from LMN disease
  - Sacral spinal cord, vertebrae, caudal equina area, or nerve roots lesions:
    - Degenerative: intervertebral disk disease, degenerative lumbosacral stenosis
    - Anomalous: vertebral malformation
    - Neoplasia, including extradural (primary bone, metastatic tumors [prostatic carcinoma, lymphoma]), intradural extramedullary (meningioma, nerve sheath tumor), and intramedullary (oligodendroglioma, astrocytoma, ependymoma, metastatic [lymphoma, hemangiosarcoma])
    - Infectious: diskospondylitis
    - Traumatic: fracture/luxation, traction spinal cord injury (tail pull/avulsion)
    - Vascular: thromboembolic disease, fibrocartilaginous emboli
  - Peripheral nervous system disease:
    - Neuropathy
    - Dysautonomia
    - Myopathy
    - Neuromuscular junction
      - Myasthenia gravis

- Hypotonia from overdistention
  - Neurogenic:
    - UMN lesions (suprasacral: L7 to pons)
  - Non-neurogenic:
    - Inability to ambulate or posture for urination leading to urine retention (e.g., pain, pelvic fracture, inflammation, confinement/ behavior)
    - Urethral obstruction (e.g., calculi, intraluminal or extraluminal mass compression)

INITIAL DATABASE

- Residual urine volume increased (normal, <0.2-0.4 ml/kg in dogs). Urinary catheterization may allow detection of urethral obstruction
- Rectal examination
  - Anal tone
    - LMN disease: decreased or absent
    - UMN or non-neurogenic disease: present
  - Urethra/prostate: possible obstruction, mass effect
- Neurologic examination and neuroanatomic localization
  - Complete neurologic examination, including perineal and bulbocavernosus reflex, tail tone
    - UMN lesion (usually T3 to L3): sacral reflexes intact
    - LMN lesion (L7 to coccygeal region; peripheral nerves): decreased or absent reflexes (may lack sensation)
- Clinical pathology
  - Complete blood count: unremarkable
  - Serum biochemistry: unremarkable (with urethral obstruction, may reflect postrenal azotemia, hyperkalemia)
  - Urinalysis, urine culture and sensitivity: secondary urinary tract infection common
- Abdominal radiography: distended bladder; possible evidence of vertebral, pelvic, prostatic disease, or urethral calculi

ADVANCED OR CONFIRMATORY TESTING

- Neurodiagnostic testing:
  - Myelography
  - Epidurography
  - Electromyography
  - Nerve conduction studies
  - Somatosensory-evoked response testing
  - Advanced imaging:
    - Magnetic resonance imaging
    - Computed tomography
- Contrast radiography:
  - Retrograde urethrography
- Abdominal ultrasonography
- Urodynamic testing:
  - Cystometry: determine bladder contractile function
  - Urethral pressure profile: evaluate urethral tone
  - Leak point pressure measurement: evaluate urethral resistance

TREATMENT

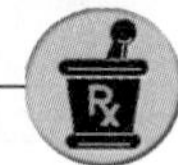

THERAPEUTIC GOAL(S)

- Maintain empty bladder
- Restoration of bladder wall function
- Treat underlying condition and secondary urinary infection

ACUTE GENERAL TREATMENT

- Indwelling urinary catheter (closed-system)
- Urethral sphincter relaxation:
  - Smooth muscle relaxation (α-antagonists)
    - Phenoxybenzamine. Dogs: 5-15 mg/dog PO q 12-24h; cats: 1.25-5 mg/cat PO q 12h. Onset of action is delayed up to 4 days. Side effects: hypotension, tachycardia, increased intraocular pressure. Contraindications: cardiovascular disease, glaucoma, renal failure
    - Prazosin. Dogs: 1 mg/15 kg PO q 8-12h; cats 0.25-0.5 mg/cat PO q 12-24h. Side effects: hypotension, mild sedation. Contraindications: see phenoxybenzamine
  - Striated muscle relaxation (skeletal muscle relaxants)
    - Diazepam. Dogs: 2-10 mg/dog PO q 8h; cats: 2-5 mg/cat PO q 8h or 0.2-0.5 mg/kg IV as needed. Side effects: sedation, excitation, idiosyncratic hepatic necrosis in cats
    - Methocarbamol. Dogs: 15-20 mg/ kg PO q 8h; cats: 61-132 mg/kg/ day PO divided q 8-12h. Side effects: weakness, sedation, vomiting
- Detrusor muscle contraction:
  - Bethanechol (parasympathomimetic). Dogs: 5-25 mg/dog PO q 8h; cats: 1.25-5 mg/cat PO q 8h. Side effects include ptyalism, vomiting, diarrhea, bronchoconstriction. Contraindications: urinary or gastrointestinal obstruction
  - Cisapride (prokinetic; enhances acetylcholine release). Dogs: 0.5 mg/kg PO q 8h; cats: 1.25-5 mg/cat PO q 8-12h. Side effects: diarrhea, abdominal pain

CHRONIC TREATMENT

- Resolution of underlying disorder
- Long-term supportive drug therapy
- Maintain a small or empty bladder (intermittent catheterization may be required)

DRUG INTERACTIONS

- Bethanechol minimally effective if tight junctions completely disrupted or when nerves have been avulsed or transected
- Bethanechol may enhance urethral sphincter tone, so it is important to treat with α-antagonist (e.g., phenoxybenzamine) before starting bethanechol

POSSIBLE COMPLICATIONS

- Bladder wall fibrosis and permanent bladder hypotonia
- Recurrent urinary tract infection

RECOMMENDED MONITORING

- Frequently monitor voiding activity (provide opportunity to urinate)
- Monitor residual urine volume during catheterization procedures. If residual volume normalizes, catheterization no longer required
- Periodic urinalysis ± urine culture; initially every several weeks

PROGNOSIS AND OUTCOME

- Good if cause is non-neurogenic
- Guarded for sacral spinal cord lesions
- Poor for dysautonomia, nerve avulsion, or severe sacral spinal cord injury

PEARLS & CONSIDERATIONS

COMMENTS

Expedient and early management of overdistended bladder is crucial for resolution and prevention of bladder wall fibrosis

PREVENTION

- Successful management depends on identification and treatment of underlying disorder.
- Monitoring voiding is important for postoperative neurosurgical and orthopedic patients.

CLIENT EDUCATION

- If signs persist, the client will need instructions for intermittent bladder catheterization.
- The client should be educated to differentiate urine overflow from voluntary micturition.

SUGGESTED READING

Dewey CW: Neurology and neuropharmacology of normal and abnormal urination. In Dewey CW (ed): *A Practical Guide to Canine and Feline Neurology*. Ames, IA, Iowa State Press, 2003, pp 357-366.

Fischer JR, Lane IF: Medical treatment of voiding dysfunction in dogs and cats. *Vet Med* 98:67, 2003.

Lane IF: A diagnostic approach to micturition disorders. *Vet Med* 98: 49, 2003.

Lorenz MD, Kornegay JN: Disorders of micturition. In Lorenz MD, Kornegay JN (eds): *Handbook of Veterinary Neurology,* ed 4. Philadelphia, Elsevier Science, 2004, pp 75-90.

AUTHOR: **JOAN R. COATES**

EDITOR: **LEAH A. COHN**

Atopy

Client Education Sheet on Website

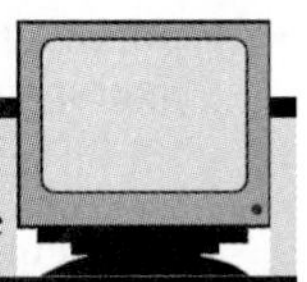

BASIC INFORMATION

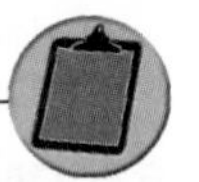

DEFINITION

A genetically programmed disease of dogs and cats characterized by chronic pruritus, in which the patient develops a hypersensitivity to one or more allergens in the environment that are inhaled or absorbed through the skin

SYNONYM(S)

Allergic inhalant dermatitis
Atopic disease
Atopic eczema

EPIDEMIOLOGY

SPECIES, AGE, SEX

- There is no clear sex predisposition, although atopy may be slightly more common in females.
- Age of onset: from 6 months to 7 years (70% of cases start within 1 to 3 years of age).

GENETICS AND BREED PREDISPOSITION

- Dogs: Chinese shar-peis, Cairn terriers, West Highland white terriers, Scottish terriers, Lhasa apsos, shih tzus, wire-haired fox terriers, dalmatians, Irish setters, English setters, golden retrievers, Labrador retrievers, miniature schnauzers
- Cats: No breed predispositions have been demonstrated

RISK FACTORS

- Certain breeds (familial involvement)
- Age (most cases start between 1 and 3 years old)
- Concurrent parasitic disease, viral diseases, and vaccines may augment IgE production

GEOGRAPHY AND SEASONALITY

- There is marked geographic variation in specific allergen exposure
- An animal may be seasonally or nonseasonally atopic, depending on exposure to sensitizing allergens
- 80% of dogs with seasonal atopy will progress to nonseasonal disease

ASSOCIATED CONDITIONS AND DISORDERS

- 20–30% of cases have concurrent dermatologic adverse food reactions or flea allergy dermatitis.
- Secondary infections with bacteria and yeast are common.
- Seborrheic skin disease.
- Otitis externa.
- Feline eosinophilic granuloma complex.
- Anal sacculitis.
- Atopic conjunctivitis.
- Atopic rhinitis.

CLINICAL PRESENTATION

HISTORY, CHIEF COMPLAINT

- Pruritus is a dominant chief complaint.
- Other clinical signs may be similar to those of dermatologic adverse reactions to food/food allergy and other pruritic skin conditions.

PHYSICAL EXAM FINDINGS

- Pruritus (itching, scratching, licking, rubbing), usually affecting the face, feet, and ventrum.
- Areas most commonly affected include muzzle, periocular region, ear canals/pinnae, interdigital spaces, axillae, and groin.
- Self-trauma, redness, and secondary skin changes may be noted, particularly in chronic cases.
- Saliva staining of hair may be noted.
- Secondary bacterial and yeast infections, ear infections, and acute moist dermatitis ("hot spots") may also be noted.

ETIOLOGY AND PATHOPHYSIOLOGY

- Atopy is a genetically programmed type-1 hypersensitivity in which the patient becomes sensitized to environmental allergens that do not cause problems in nonatopic animals.
- Predisposed dogs inhale, or more likely percutaneously absorb, allergens that provoke the production of allergen-specific IgE (and possibly, IgG). Late-phase (delayed 8–12h) reactions may also be involved.
- The antibody molecules circulate through the body before attaching to tissue mast cells, especially those in the skin, where they cross-link, leading to degranulation and production of inflammatory mediators, as well as chemotactic factors for other inflammatory cells.
- Parasitic diseases, viral infections, and vaccination with modified live vaccines have all been shown to augment production of IgE specific for environmental allergens.

DIAGNOSIS

DIFFERENTIAL DIAGNOSIS

The first step when dealing with any dog that is suspected of being atopic is to make sure that other causes of pruritus have been ruled out:

- Ectoparasites (*Sarcoptes, Demodex* [uncommon], *Cheyletiella, Notoedres, Otodectes,* fleas, lice)
- Bacterial infections (*Staphylococcus intermedius*)
- Fungal infections (*Malassezia*, ringworm [dermatophytes])
- Seborrhea
- Other allergies/hypersensitivities (flea bite hypersensitivity, other ectoparasite hypersensitivities, adverse food reaction/food allergy, contact hypersensitivity, drug hypersensitivity)
- Behavioral disorders (feline psychogenic alopecia, flank sucking, tail-biting, self-nursing)
- Neoplasia (mast cell tumor, epitheliotropic lymphoma)

INITIAL DATABASE

- The minimum database for a pruritic patient should include a complete history and physical examination and a thorough dermatologic examination for ectoparasites, bacteria, and yeast.
- An initial dermatologic database:
  - Deep skin scrapings
  - Trichography (microscopic examination of plucked hairs)
  - Skin and ear cytologic examination
  - Fungal culture

ADVANCED OR CONFIRMATORY TESTING

- Specific diagnostic testing for environmental allergens should be carried out only after elimination of ectoparasites, especially *Sarcoptes*, and elimination and/or control of bacterial and yeast infections.
- In nonseasonal cases, evaluation for dermatologic adverse food reactions/food allergy is often performed in advance of testing for environmental hypersensitivities.
- Allergy testing is available as an intradermal test performed by specialist practitioners or as a blood test. Regardless of method, test results must be reviewed in light of allergen exposure.
  - **Intradermal testing**
    - Intradermal testing is regarded as the gold standard for diagnosis, because it identifies mast-cell-bound IgE within the skin.
    - Usually performed at the start or just after the allergy season in seasonal patients.
    - Because drug therapy may suppress test results, oral corticosteroids (prednisone, dexamethasone) should be withdrawn for a minimum 4 weeks (1 week per month of long-term therapy), and long-acting injectable depo steroids for up to 12 weeks. Antihistamines

and fatty acid supplements are generally withdrawn for 2 weeks.

- **Serum testing**
  - Radioallergosorbent and enzyme-linked immunosorbent assays tests detect relative levels of IgE in serum, *not* within the skin.
  - Serum tests have less risk, are much more convenient, and appear to be less affected by drug therapy.
  - Serum testing is best performed at the height of the allergy season.
  - Currently serum testing is recommended for animals that are strongly suspected to be atopic but have negative intradermal tests, or where intradermal testing is unavailable.

TREATMENT

THERAPEUTIC GOAL(S)

- Atopy is often a lifelong problem, so the goal is to eliminate or minimize allergen exposure while maintaining the pet's comfort and homeostasis of the skin.
- Appropriate clinical protocol depends on the seasonality of the problem, distribution, severity of lesions, client compliance, and cost of therapy.
- Although allergen-specific therapy is the ideal, additional antipruritic therapy is often required.
- Secondary yeast and bacterial infections should be controlled by appropriate therapy before any attempt is made to further control pruritus.

ACUTE GENERAL TREATMENT

- Antihistamines
  - Antihistamines, in combination with omega-3 essential fatty acids, may alleviate pruritus in up to 30% of cases. Antihistamines shown to be of benefit for dogs include:
    - Hydroxyzine 2.2 mg/kg q 8-12h.
    - Diphenhydramine 2.2 mg/kg q 8-12h.
    - Chlorpheniramine 0.4 mg/kg q 8-12h.
    - Amitriptyline 1 mg/kg q 12h.
  - Chlorpheniramine and amitriptyline have also been useful in cats.
  - Side effects, such as drowsiness, lethargy, or nervousness, are sometimes noted. Reducing the frequency of administration and dose may minimize these effects.
  - Nonsedating antihistamines have not generally been found to be effective.
- Essential fatty acids (EFA)
  - Omega-3 EFA in capsule form as a supplement (eicasopentanoic acid, 30 mg/kg/day) or in food may help manage pruritus by decreasing the production of pro-inflammatory mediators.
  - The optimum ratio of supplementation within the diet appears to lie between 10:1 and 5:1, omega-6/omega-3.
- Corticosteroids
  - Corticosteroids are effective for controlling pruritus associated with environmental allergies.
  - Prednisone at an initial daily dose of 0.5-1.0 mg/kg for dogs (1-2 mg/kg for cats) before weaning to an alternate day schedule is regarded as the first choice when using glucocorticoids for atopy.
  - A corticosteroid-antihistamine combination containing prednisolone 2 mg and trimeprazine 5 mg (Temaril-P) has been shown to control pruritus better than antihistamines alone and equivalent to a much higher dose of corticosteroid, reducing the risk of steroid side effects.
    - Recommended frequency is twice daily for 4 days then once a day until pruritus is controlled before weaning down to the lowest possible alternate day dosage (starting dose q 12h as follows: <5 kg = 0.5 tab; 5-10 kg = 1 tab; 10-20 kg = 2 tab; >20 kg = 3 tab).
- Cyclosporine
  - Cyclosporine (microemulsion type [e.g., Neoral, Atopica]) at a dose of 5 mg/kg q 24h.
  - Treatment may be expensive, especially in medium- or large-breed dogs.
  - Vomiting appears to be the most common side effect, although an increase in hair growth and gingival hyperplasia have been noted.
- Topical antipruritic therapy
  - Topical antipruritic therapy can be a useful way to decrease pruritus.
  - A tepid bath will have an antipruritic effect related to the cooling effect of evaporation and general rehydrating of the skin.
  - Mild cleansing or colloidal oatmeal shampoos may also be beneficial.
- Physical restraint
  - Elizabethan collars, foot bandages, or T-shirts may be helpful in preventing self-trauma and secondary infections.

CHRONIC TREATMENT

Immunotherapy:

- Subcutaneous administration of a gradually increasing dose of allergens that produced positive reactions on allergy testing and are present in the patient's environment.
- May be beneficial in approximately 70% of cases.
- Immunotherapy is usually considered for patients diagnosed with atopy with a long allergy season (e.g., nonseasonal cases) or where antipruritic therapy does not provide sufficient relief.
- Response to therapy is very individualized, and may be seen as early as 1 month or may take up to a year.
- Maintenance injections are given as often as needed to maintain the response (usually every 1 to 3 weeks), and usually therapy is lifelong.

DRUG INTERACTIONS

Drugs that inhibit cytochrome P-450 enzymes (imidazoles, macrolides, anticonvulsants, corticosteroids) will increase cyclosporine blood levels.

PROGNOSIS AND OUTCOME

- With environmental allergy, it is imperative that clients understand that the allergy problems are likely to affect the pet for the rest of its life.

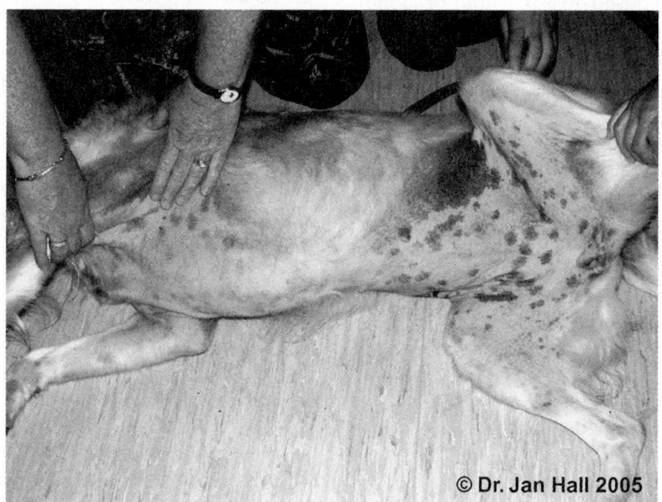

FIGURE I-20 Erythema of the ventral inguinal region (right of image) and axillary region (left of image) in this dog with atopy. Courtesy of Dr. Jan A. Hall.

- Studies have shown that with good client compliance and individualized therapy, greater than 90% of cases can be satisfactorily managed.

PEARLS & CONSIDERATIONS

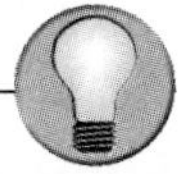

COMMENTS

- Client counselling is very important before starting treatment, as unrealistic expectations are a great cause of client dissatisfaction.
- Client compliance is markedly increased if immunotherapy is included as part of an individualized management protocol that, at least initially, includes topical and/or systemic antipruritic therapy.
- Secondary yeast and bacterial infections are common and should be controlled first by appropriate therapy before any attempt is made to further control pruritus.
- Routine follow-up evaluations, including physical exam, hematology, chemistry profile, and urinalysis are recommended every 6 to 12 months for dogs on long-term corticosteroid therapy.

SUGGESTED READING

DeBoer DJ, Hillier A: The ACVD task force on canine atopic dermatitis (XV): fundamental concepts in clinical diagnosis. *Vet Immunol Immunopathol* 81:271-276, 2001.

Griffin CE, DeBoer DJ: The ACVD task force on canine atopic dermatitis (XIV): Clinical manifestations of canine atopic dermatitis. *Vet Immunol Immunopathol* 81:255-269, 2001.

AUTHORS: **JAN A. HALL, AMANDA P. AMARATUNGA**
EDITOR: **JAN A. HALL**

Atrial Fibrillation

BASIC INFORMATION

DEFINITION

A cardiac arrhythmia characterized by multiple ectopic atrial electrical discharges. Only an occasional, random atrial depolarization reaches the atrioventricular (AV) node and is conducted to the ventricles, resulting in an irregular (usually rapid) ventricular rhythm.

EPIDEMIOLOGY

SPECIES, AGE, SEX

- After ventricular arrhythmias, atrial fibrillation (AF) is the most common clinically significant arrhythmia in dogs.
- AF is rare in cats.

GENETICS AND BREED PREDISPOSITION

- The incidence of AF is higher in large-breed dogs than small-breed dogs.
- Giant-breed dogs (e.g., Irish wolfhounds) are predisposed to idiopathic or "lone" AF, which occurs in the absence of underlying heart disease.

RISK FACTORS

- Most commonly associated with cardiac disease, especially those causing severe atrial enlargement:
  - Chronic AV valvular heart disease (endocardiosis)
  - Dilated, hypertrophic, or restrictive cardiomyopathy
  - Congenital heart disease
  - Cardiac trauma
- Other causes/associations include:
  - Severe systemic or metabolic diseases:
    - Addison's disease
    - Gastric dilation-volvulus
  - Drugs:
    - Digoxin toxicity
    - Anesthetic agents (especially opiates)
  - Lone atrial fibrillation in giant-breed dogs

CLINICAL PRESENTATION

HISTORY, CHIEF COMPLAINT

- May be an incidental finding
- Exercise intolerance, weakness
- Syncope
- Patient may present with signs of congestive heart failure: coughing, dyspnea

PHYSICAL EXAM FINDINGS

- Irregularly irregular heart rhythm (classically described as sounding like "sneakers in a dryer")
- Irregular pulses with deficits
- Patient may have dyspnea, pulmonary crackles, ascites with concurrent congestive heart failure
- Physical examination alone is poor for assessing the ventricular rate of dogs with AF (25% accuracy)

ETIOLOGY AND PATHOPHYSIOLOGY

- The rapid cascade of impulses from multiple atrial foci tends to cancel each other out, such that no single impulse depolarizes the atria completely. Hence, there is no P wave on the electrocardiogram (ECG), but instead rapid tiny undulations or f waves.
- An occasional, random impulse reaches the AV node, finds it ready to be depolarized, and sends the signal for ventricular contraction. Thus, atrial fibrillation results in a ventricular rhythm that is *always* irregular (irregularly irregular R-R interval).
  - Because the impulses are conducted normally through the AV node and ventricles, the shape of the QRS complexes is normal (narrow and positive in lead II).
- The loss of the atrial contraction or "atrial kick" to ventricular filling typically decreases stroke volume by 20%.
  - This loss may not be important to an otherwise healthy animal, especially if the ventricular rate is not rapid (no clinical signs; AF is an incidental finding).
  - However, if primary heart disease exists, AF combined with rapid ventricular response rates can lead to significant decreases in cardiac output and congestive heart failure.

DIAGNOSIS

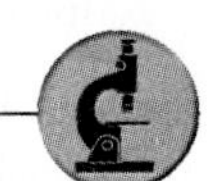

DIFFERENTIAL DIAGNOSIS

Exam:

- AF cannot be distinguished from polymorphic (multifocal) ventricular tachycardia on physical exam

ECG:

- Atrial flutter: a more organized arrhythmia with a saw toothed pattern of rapid atrial depolarizations (F waves). Atrial flutter can degenerate into AF, or the ECG pattern can alternate between the two. Uncommon in dogs and cats
- Atrial tachycardia: characterized by P' waves, which may be hidden in previous T waves or not apparent in all leads
- Ventricular tachycardia (VT):
  - Rarely, AF can be combined with bundle branch block or aberrant conduction, resulting in wide QRS complexes that may appear very similar to VT.
  - Look for subtle irregularity of rhythm (more common with AF than VT).
  - Perform a vagal maneuver (ventricular rate slows if AF, not if VT).
- Baseline noise or artifact (e.g., shivering, purring) on the ECG may mimic F waves:

   - However, the actual rhythm (R-R intervals) is regular, unlike AF.

INITIAL DATABASE

- ECG is the gold standard for diagnosis. ECG features of AF:
   - An irregularly irregular rhythm (irregular R-R intervals)
   - No P waves (in any leads)
   - f waves (fine oscillations) typically visible along the baseline
   - Narrow QRS complexes (rarely, may appear wide with coexistant bundle branch block or aberrant conduction)
   - The ventricular rate is typically fast, but may be normal
- Vagal maneuver (see Vagal Maneuver, p 1323): may lead to a decrease in ventricular rate, and aid in the diagnosis of AF by revealing the irregular rhythm and lack of P waves (which may not be as obvious at faster rates). Calipers may also be useful in demonstrating irregularity.
- Thoracic radiography and echocardiography may be used in diagnosing underlying cardiac disease or concurrent congestive heart failure.

TREATMENT

THERAPEUTIC GOAL(S)

- Correct underlying disease if possible
- Medical conversion to sustained normal sinus rhythm is rarely possible with chronic atrial fibrillation in small animals
- Control of ventricular response rate becomes the achievable goal in most cases. The desired rate will vary with size of the patient and underlying cardiac disease (i.e., target of <140-160 bpm in a dog not actively in congestive heart failure)

ACUTE GENERAL TREATMENT

- Above all, eliminate or manage factors that may be increasing the ventricular rate.
   - Treat congestive heart failure (especially pulmonary edema or pleural effusion).
   - Minimize stress.
- Consider aggressive treatment for AF cases in which ventricular rates remain markedly elevated (e.g., >230 bpm in a medium-sized dog) despite these measures (uncommon situation).
- Goal in first few hours is a modest (10-15%) decrease in heart rate; target heart rate (see Therapeutic Goal[s] above) is often achieved over weeks of titration.
- If impaired systolic function is suspected (i.e., with dilated cardiomyopathy), caution is advised with use of calcium channel blockers or β-blockers due to their negative inotropic effects (choose lowest dose and titrate upward based on response).
- Patients with markedly rapid AF (e.g., ventricular rate >230 bpm in a medium-sized dog) should have an intravenous (IV) catheter and be on continuous ECG monitoring during drug administration.
   - Digoxin: traditionally considered the first-choice therapy with AF. Benefits include decreasing ventricular rate without decreasing systolic function. However, the acute benefit of IV administration is limited due to slow onset of action and toxic side effects, causing this administration to lose favor.
      - May start oral use with 0.005-0.01 mg/kg q 12h, not to exceed 0.25 mg q 12h (or use elixir at 0.00425 mg/kg q 12h).
   - Calcium channel blockers: commonly used as first-choice IV agents when AF is associated with a persistently elevated ventricular rate despite identification and treatment of coexisting factors such as pulmonary edema.
      - Diltiazem: slow IV bolus of 0.05-0.15 mg/kg.
      - Verapamil: slow IV bolus of 0.05-0.3 mg/kg.
   - β-blockers:
      - Esmolol: slow IV bolus of 0.05 to 0.5 mg/kg, constant rate infusion (CRI) of 0.05-0.2 mg/kg/min.
      - Propranolol: slow IV bolus of 0.01-0.1 mg/kg, every 2 minutes until ventricular rate is controlled.
- With concurrent heart failure, higher mean heart rates of 170 to 220 bpm in a large-breed dog are common and may be necessary to maintain adequate cardiac output. Appropriate treatment to relieve the congestion will decrease the heart rate accordingly. Aggressive treatment to lower the heart rate before stabilization of the heart failure should be avoided, because it may cause worsening of congestion.

CHRONIC TREATMENT

- Digoxin, β-blockers, and calcium channel blockers are classically used alone, or in combination to control heart rate. The exact drug chosen reflects the underlying heart disease if present (e.g., digoxin is appropriate if AF is associated with dilated cardiomyopathy but not hypertrophic cardiomyopathy).
   - Digoxin: traditional first-choice oral agent:
      - Dog: 0.005-0.1 mg/kg PO q 12h, not to exceed 0.25 mg q 12h (or 0.00425 mg/kg q 12h for elixir)
      - Cat: 0.03125 mg (one quarter of 0.125 mg tablet) PO q 48-72h
- Calcium channel blockers:
   - Diltiazem (Cardizem):
      - Dog: 0.5-1.5 mg/kg PO q 8h
      - Cat: 7.5 mg PO q 8-12h
   - Diltiazem sustained-release (Dilacor, Cardizem-CD):
      - Dog: 1.5-6 mg/kg PO q 12-24h
      - Cat: 30-60 mg PO q 12-24h
   - Verapamil:
      - Dog: 1-3 mg/kg PO q 8h
- β-Blockers:
   - Atenolol:
      - Dog: 0.5-1 mg/kg PO q 12-24h, or start at 6.25-12.5 mg q 12-24h and titrate to effect
      - Cat: 6.25 mg PO q 12-24h

DRUG INTERACTIONS

- Simultaneous administration of digoxin with verapamil, amiodarone, or quinidine can increase digoxin serum concentrations and potentially cause digoxin toxicity.
- It is generally not recommended to use calcium channel blockers in conjunction with β-blockers due to combined effects on blood pressure and contractility.

POSSIBLE COMPLICATIONS

- Digoxin:
   - Gastrointestinal (GI) signs (anorexia, vomiting, diarrhea) related to toxicity
   - AV block, other arrhythmias
- Calcium channel blockers, β-blockers: much more likely to see complications with IV use.
   - Negative inotropism (especially verapamil): use with caution with left ventricular dysfunction
   - Hypotension (lesser risk with β-blockers compared to calcium channel blockers
   - Severe bradycardia or asystole
   - GI upset with oral calcium channel blockers
- Chronic use of β-blocker therapy should not be abruptly discontinued (sudden stopping can lead to excessive catecholamine-mediated tachycardia related to upregulation of β-receptors).

RECOMMENDED MONITORING

- Digoxin: measure trough digoxin serum level 7 to 10 days after starting therapy (8 to 10 hours postdose)
- All three classes of drugs: regular monitoring of heart rate and blood pressure is advised

PROGNOSIS AND OUTCOME

- Dependent on underlying cardiac disease:
   - Large-breed dogs with idiopathic/lone AF may do well for years with appropriate treatment, but progressive atrial enlargement and cardiac disease may develop.

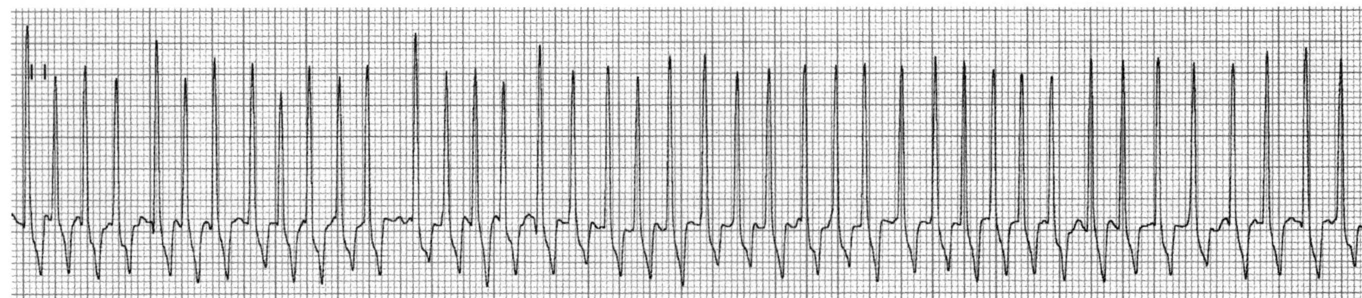

A

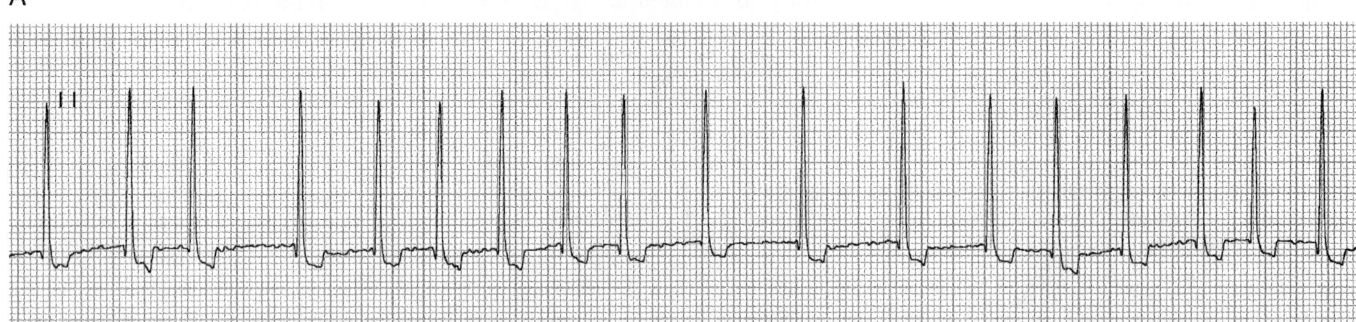

B

FIGURE I-21 **A,** Lead II ECG showing atrial fibrillation with a rapid ventricular response rate (290–300 bpm) in a dog with congestive heart failure. Note that the QRS complexes are narrow in appearance and the R-R intervals are irregular (less apparent at rapid ventricular rates). 25 mm/sec. **B,** Lead II ECG showing atrial fibrillation in the same dog 2 weeks after appropriate treatment for the congestive heart failure and initiation of treatment with digoxin. The ventricular response rate has decreased to 120–130 bpm, and the irregularity to the R-R intervals and lack of P waves is now more apparent. 25 mm/sec.

    - Prognosis with severe cardiac disease is guarded (atrial fibrillation has been found to be a negative prognostic indicator when present in diagnoses of dilated cardiomyopathy).
- Cats with AF have a prognosis that is not appreciably different from that of cats with the same underlying heart disease and sinus rhythm.

PEARLS & CONSIDERATIONS

COMMENTS

- ECG monitors often are poor at detecting QRS complexes when heart rate is rapid (may count T waves also, or miss QRS complexes). Heart rate on an ECG monitor is determined by counting QRS complexes for 15 seconds and multiplying by 4.
- If AF and congestive heart failure (especially pulmonary edema) are present simultaneously, treatment of the congestive heart failure (e.g., diuretics) must be instituted at the same time as, or before, treatment to reduce the ventricular rate.

PREVENTION

The high prevalence of AF in certain breeds (e.g., Irish wolfhound) supports the hypothesis that a genetic predisposition may be a risk factor for developing lone AF. It may be advisable not to use affected dogs for breeding.

SUGGESTED READING

Cote E, et al: Atrial fibrillation in cats: 50 cases (1979–2002). *JAVMA* 225(2): 256–260, 2004.

Gelzer ARM, Kraus MS: Management of atrial fibrillation. *Vet Clin Small Anim* 34: 1127–1144, 2004.

Tilley LP: Analysis of common canine cardiac arrhythmias. In Tilley LP (ed): *Essentials of Canine and Feline Electrocardiography*. Philadelphia, Lippincott, Williams & Wilkins, 1992, pp 127–207.

AUTHOR: **REBECCA L. MALAKOFF**
EDITOR: **ETIENNE CÔTÉ**

Atrial Premature Complexes and Atrial/Supraventricular Tachycardia

BASIC INFORMATION

DEFINITION

- Atrial premature complex (APC): a premature beat originating from ectopic focus in the atria
- Atrial tachycardia (AT): a rapid, regular rhythm originating from a focus in the atria other than the sinus node (three or more consecutive APCs are considered atrial tachycardia)
- Supraventricular tachycardia (SVT): originates from the atria or the AV junction (includes atrial tachycardia and AV junctional tachycardia)
    - This definition may also be considered to include atrial fibrillation and atrial flutter, which are discussed in a separate section and will not be specifically addressed here.

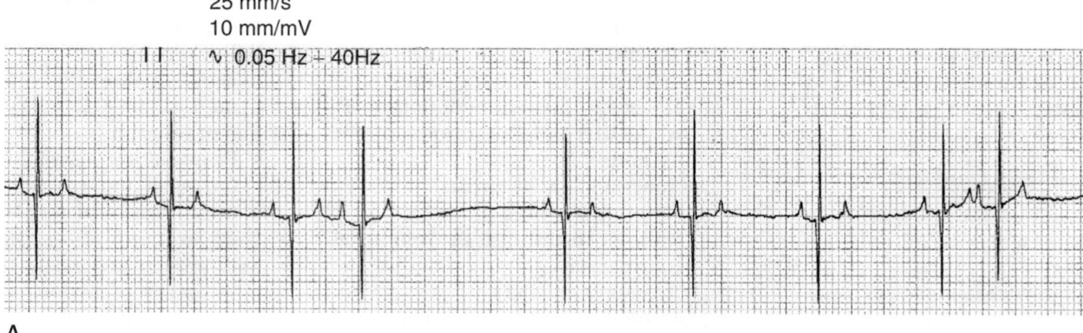

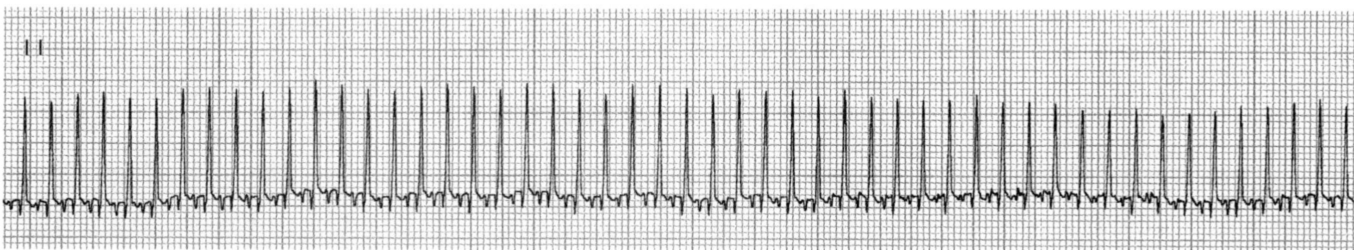

FIGURE I-22 **A,** Lead II ECG showing APCs (the fourth and last beats). A premature P′ wave is followed by a narrow complex QRS and a noncompensatory pause. 25 mm/sec. **B,** Atrial/supraventricular tachycardia lead II ECG showing a rapid, narrow-complex, monomorphic (QRS complexes all of the same shape) tachycardia. The heart rate is 330 bpm. A supraventricular tachycardia is diagnosed on the basis of the narrow, upright QRS complexes in this lead II tracing. 25 mm/sec.

SYNONYM(S)

APCs: premature atrial or supraventricular complexes
Atrial or supraventricular extrasystoles
Atrial or supraventricular premature contractions
Atrial or supraventricular premature impulses

EPIDEMIOLOGY

SPECIES, AGE, SEX: APCs can be a normal occurrence in very old dogs.

GENETICS AND BREED PREDISPOSITION: An orthodromic (conduction through the AV node and retrograde back to the atria via a bypass tract) reciprocating tachycardia has been identified in Labrador retrievers (see Wolff-Parkinson-White Syndrome, p 1166).

RISK FACTORS

- Cardiac disease, especially those causing atrial enlargement:
  - Chronic valvular heart disease (endocardiosis): common cause of APCs
  - Dilated, hypertrophic, or restrictive cardiomyopathy: common cause of APCs
  - Congenital heart disease
  - Atrial tumors such as hemangiosarcoma
- Noncardiac disease:
  - Increased sympathetic tone
  - Hyperthyroidism
  - Sepsis
  - Electrolyte and acid-base abnormalities (i.e., hypokalemia)
  - Hypoxia
  - Anemia
- Drugs:
  - Digoxin toxicity (often produces atrial tachycardia with AV block)
  - Sympathomimetics
  - Anesthetic agents
- Ventricular preexcitation:
  - Wolff-Parkinson-White Syndrome (see Wolff-Parkinson-White Syndrome, p 1166)

CLINICAL PRESENTATION

DISEASE FORMS/SUBTYPES

- Isolated APCs (by definition, no more than three in a row)
- AT, SVT: paroxysmal (intermittent bursts) or sustained (continuous)

HISTORY, CHIEF COMPLAINT

- May be an incidental finding in a patient without clinical signs
- Syncope, weakness with rapid tachycardias are possible
- Patient may have dyspnea related to congestive heart failure
- SVTs may rarely precipitate sudden death if resultant myocardial ischemia leads to ventricular tachycardia or fibrillation, or if antiarrhythmic medications used in treatment have a proarrhythmic effect

PHYSICAL EXAM FINDINGS

- An irregular heart rhythm is ausculted with APCs.
  - Premature beats are heard; pulse deficits are also noted when beats are very premature.
  - It is not possible to determine the nature of a premature beat (i.e., whether it is an APC or a ventricular premature complex [VPC]) on physical examination alone.
- One or more bursts of a rapid rhythm can be ausculted with paroxysmal AT/SVT.
- A sustained, rapid, regular rhythm is ausculted with continuous AT/SVT.

ETIOLOGY AND PATHOPHYSIOLOGY

- Several electrophysiologic mechanisms, including enhanced automaticity, reentry, and bypass tracts can cause AT/SVT. It can be difficult to determine the underlying mechanism from surface electrocardiograms (ECGs). Clinical implications of determining such mechanisms are minimal but important for some cases: eligibility for catheter-based ablation (cure) of SVT if caused by a bypass tract (see Wolff-Parkinson-White Syndrome, p 1166).
- Hemodynamic effects of atrial tachyarrhythmias depend on the underlying disease, ventricular rate, and whether the patient is at rest or exercising.
  - Excessively rapid ventricular rates will reduce cardiac output, systemic blood pressure, and coronary artery perfusion due to shortened diastolic interval.
- Sustained or frequently recurrent atrial tachycardias may lead to tachycardia induced cardiomyopathy, which may be reversible with appropriate treatment.

DIAGNOSIS

Initial suspicion is usually based on auscultation of premature beats or a rapid heart rate. Definitive diagnosis requires an ECG

DIFFERENTIAL DIAGNOSIS

- APCs and AT: indistinguishable from VPCs and ventricular tachycardia on physical exam.
- AT must be differentiated from sinus tachycardia, because sinus tachycardia is usually an appropriate physiologic rhythm responding to a systemic disturbance.
- Uncommonly, atrial arrhythmias may coexist with aberrant conduction/bundle branch block, producing wide QRS complexes and causing APCs and AT to appear similar to VPCs and ventricular tachycardia.
    - With APCs and AT/SVT, a P wave precedes each QRS complex at a repeatable interval; conversely, with VPCs, P waves are present but are not associated with the QRS complexes.

INITIAL DATABASE

- ECG:
    - APCs:
        - P'-QRS-T complexes occur earlier than next expected sinus complex.
        - Have a P' wave that is different in appearance from normal sinus P waves.
            - Occasionally P' waves may not be visible if the rate is so high that they are "buried" in the preceding T wave (consider performing a vagal maneuver [see p 1323]), or if they are isoelectric in that lead (examine other ECG leads for P' waves).
        - Narrow QRS complexes (rarely, can be wide with coexisting bundle branch block or aberrant conduction).
        - APCs are usually followed by a noncompensatory pause (i.e., the R-R interval of two normal sinus complexes enclosing the APC is less than the R-R intervals of three consecutive sinus complexes, caused by resetting of the sinus node by the ectopic atrial impulse).
    - Atrial tachycardia:
        - Three or more APCs in a row.
            - Therefore, rapid rate (e.g., >160/min [large dog], >200/min [small dog], >260/min [cat]).
        - May be paroxysmal or continuous.
        - Regular or slightly irregular rhythm.
        - P' waves are present, but again may be hidden or superimposed on previous T waves.
        - The P'-R interval is usually constant.
        - Narrow QRS complexes (rarely, can be wide with coexisting bundle branch block or aberrant conduction).
        - At extremely rapid atrial rates, there may be varying degrees of AV block (i.e., nonconducted P' waves due to refractoriness of the AV node).
    - AV junctional tachycardia:
        - Negative P' waves in lead II.
        - Difficult to distinguish from atrial tachycardia.
- Vagal maneuver, p 1323:
    - May suddenly terminate atrial and junctional tachycardias, or slow rate to aid in diagnosis.
    - Should have no effect on ventricular tachycardia.

ADVANCED OR CONFIRMATORY TESTING

Electrophysiologic studies: may be used for determining the underlying mechanism of arrhythmia. Not widely available

TREATMENT

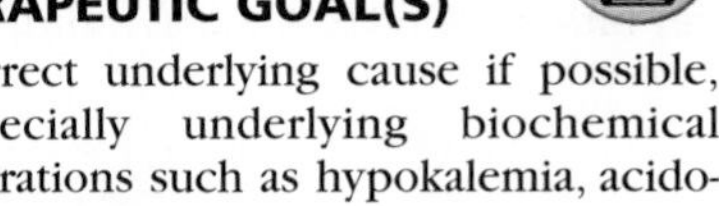

THERAPEUTIC GOAL(S)

- Correct underlying cause if possible, especially underlying biochemical alterations such as hypokalemia, acidosis, hypoxia.
- Return hemodynamic stability: isolated, infrequent APCs do not cause hemodynamic instability, and no specific treatment is required.
- Conversion of the arrhythmia to sinus rhythm: not always possible.
- Control the ventricular response rate.
    - This is the goal in many cases when AT/SVT is rapid, especially when structural atrial disease (e.g., enlargement) signifies that the atrial arrhythmia is likely to persist.
    - The desired or target rate will be achieved with drugs that slow transmission of the atrial impulses to the ventricles (i.e., induce AV nodal slowing or even AV block) to optimize the ventricular rate.
    - The desired or target rate will vary with the size of the patient and the underlying cardiac disease.

ACUTE GENERAL TREATMENT

AT/SVT producing ventricular rates >250 bpm should be considered critical and usually require aggressive IV therapy (with goal of decreasing ventricular rate). Patients should have an IV catheter and be on continuous ECG monitoring during drug administration.

- Perform vagal maneuver first. Some ATs/SVTs will terminate. If not, use drugs
- Calcium channel blockers: commonly used as first-choice agents:
    - Diltiazem: slow IV bolus of 0.05-0.15 mg/kg
    - Verapamil: slow IV bolus of 0.05-0.3 mg/kg
- β-Blockers:
    - Esmolol: slow IV bolus of 0.05-0.5 mg/kg, 0.05-0.2 mg/kg/min constant rate infusion
    - Propranolol: slow IV bolus of 0.01-0.1 mg/kg, every 2 minutes until ventricular rate is controlled
- Digoxin: used historically IV to treat SVT, but limited acute benefit due to slow onset of action, and toxic side effects have caused this administration to lose favor

CHRONIC TREATMENT

- Calcium channel blockers:
    - Diltiazem (Cardizem):
        - Dog: 0.5-1.5 mg/kg PO q 8h
        - Cat: 7.5 mg PO q 8-12h
    - Diltiazem-sustained release (Dilacor, Cardizem-CD):
        - Dog: 1.5-6 mg/kg PO q 12-24h
        - Cat: 30-60 mg PO q 12-24h
    - Verapamil:
        - Dog: 1-3 mg/kg PO q 8h
- β-Blockers:
    - Atenolol:
        - Dog: 0.5-1 mg/kg PO q 12-24h, or start at 6.25-12.5 mg q 12-24h and titrate to effect
        - Cat: 6.25-12.5 mg PO q 12-24h (start low, titrate to effect)
- Digoxin:
    - Dog: 0.005-0.01 mg/kg PO q 12h, not to exceed 0.25 mg PO q 12h (or 0.00425 mg/kg q 12h for elixir)
    - Cat: 0.03125 mg (one quarter of 0.125 mg tablet) PO q 48-72h
- Combination therapy is sometimes necessary (see Drug Interactions).

DRUG INTERACTIONS

- Simultaneous administration of digoxin with verapamil, amiodarone, or quinidine can increase digoxin serum concentrations and potentially cause digoxin toxicity.
- It is generally not recommended to use calcium channel blockers in conjunction with β-blockers due to combined effects on blood pressure and contractility.

POSSIBLE COMPLICATIONS

- Calcium channel blockers, β-blockers: much more likely to see complications with IV use. Use repeated small doses with monitoring, instead of single large dose.
    - Negative inotropism (especially verapamil): contractility-reducing effects mean that these drugs should be used with caution with left ventricular dysfunction (dilated cardiomyopathy, virtually any advanced heart disease) or congestive heart failure
    - Hypotension (lesser risk with β-blockers compared to calcium channel blockers)

  - Severe bradycardia or asystole
  - Gastrointestinal (GI) signs with oral calcium channel blockers
- Chronic use of β-blocker therapy should not be abruptly discontinued (sudden stopping can lead to excessive catecholamine-mediated tachycardia related to upregulation of β-receptors).
- Digoxin:
  - GI signs related to toxicity (anorexia, vomiting, diarrhea)
  - AV block, other arrhythmias

RECOMMENDED MONITORING

Digoxin: measure trough digoxin serum level 7 to 10 days after starting therapy or adjusting dose (8 to 10 hours postdose)

PROGNOSIS AND OUTCOME

Dependent on underlying cause and cardiac disease

SUGGESTED READING

Tilley LP: Analysis of common canine cardiac arrhythmias. In Tilley LP (ed): *Essentials of Canine and Feline Electrocardiography*. Philadelphia, Lippincott, Williams & Wilkins, 1992, pp 127–207.

Tilley LP: Analysis of common feline cardiac arrhythmias. In Tilley LP (ed): *Essentials of Canine and Feline Electrocardiography*. Philadelphia, Lippincott, Williams & Wilkins, 1992, pp 208–252.

AUTHOR: **REBECCA L. MALAKOFF**
EDITOR: **ETIENNE CÔTÉ**

Atrial Rupture (Left)

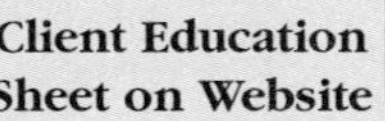

Client Education Sheet on Website

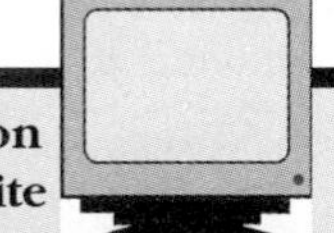

BASIC INFORMATION

DEFINITION

Spontaneous endomyocardial splitting leads to left atrial rupture in dogs with marked left atrial enlargement and elevated left atrial pressure

SYNONYM(S)

Endomyocardial split of the left atrium
Left atrial tear
Left atrial split

EPIDEMIOLOGY

SPECIES, AGE, SEX

- Most often seen in older dogs
- More common in males

GENETICS AND BREED PREDISPOSITION: More common in Cavalier King Charles spaniels and other chondrodystrophoid breeds such as cocker spaniels, dachshunds, and miniature poodles.

RISK FACTORS

- Left atrial enlargement due to long-standing mitral regurgitation
- Ruptured chordae tendineae
- Chronic mitral valve endocardiosis (mitral regurgitation due to myxomatous valve disease)

ASSOCIATED CONDITIONS AND DISORDERS

- Congestive heart failure
- Hemopericardium

CLINICAL PRESENTATION

DISEASE FORMS/SUBTYPES

- Nonperforating endocardial splits are only found at necropsy.
- Perforating endomyocardial splits cause hemopericardium or atrial septal defects.

HISTORY, CHIEF COMPLAINT

- Long-standing mitral insufficiency
- Dyspnea
- Acute collapse

PHYSICAL EXAM FINDINGS

- Nonspecific acute collapse
- Tachycardia
- Weak pulse
- Pale mucous membranes
- Loud systolic murmur at left apex

ETIOLOGY AND PATHOPHYSIOLOGY

- Left atrial rupture is caused by increased wall tension associated with marked left atrial enlargement and elevated left atrial pressure.
- These changes usually are due to chronic mitral valve disease with valve incompetence and coexisting endocardial degeneration, but endocardial splitting also may occur in young dogs with patent ductus arteriosus and marked left atrial enlargement.
- Multiple splits are usually present, and a deep, endomyocardial split may perforate the left atrial wall, resulting in hemopericardium or an acquired atrial septal defect depending on its location.
- Healed, endothelialized splits are often present in dogs with fresh thrombus-covered splits.
- Dogs with acquired atrial septal defects always have had otherwise healed splits.

DIAGNOSIS

DIFFERENTIAL DIAGNOSIS

- Other myocardial disease
- Atrial neoplasm
- Neoplastic pericardial effusion
- Idiopathic pericardial effusion
- Congenital atrial septal defect

INITIAL DATABASE

- Radiographs to detect large globoid cardiac silhouette plus left atrial enlargement
- Electrocardiogram to identify arrhythmias such as atrial premature beats or atrial fibrillation and conduction abnormalities such as wide, notched P waves

ADVANCED OR CONFIRMATORY TESTING

Echocardiogram to detect pericardial effusion and a laminar blood clot usually near the left atrium in the long axis view

TREATMENT

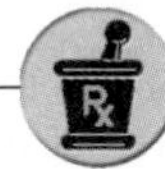

THERAPEUTIC GOAL(S)

- Relieve signs of congestive heart failure
- Relieve cardiac tamponade
- Stop atrial hemorrhage

ACUTE GENERAL TREATMENT

- Oxygen supplementation
- Vasodilator to reduce systemic afterload, promote forward flow, and reduce mitral regurgitant flow:
  - Nitroprusside 1 μg/kg/min IV constant rate infusion, titrating up to a maximum of 5 μg/kg/min
  - Requires constant blood pressure monitoring and stabilization or reduction of infusion rate if systemic blood pressure decreases
  - Not recommended if systemic hypotension is already present
- Partial pericardiocentesis to reduce cardiac tamponade if causing clinical signs
- Thoracotomy and suture closure of epicardial perforation
- Circumferential suture of the mitral annulus

CHRONIC TREATMENT

- Vasodilator
- Create atrial septal defect to decompress the left atrium

DRUG INTERACTIONS

Nonspecific

POSSIBLE COMPLICATIONS

- Additional atrial hemorrhage
- Death

RECOMMENDED MONITORING

Periodic radiographs or echocardiogram to monitor atrial size

PROGNOSIS AND OUTCOME

- Poor, but some dogs have survived with aggressive vasodilator therapy.
- Survival has been observed for several months if an atrial septal defect develops.

PEARLS & CONSIDERATIONS

COMMENTS

- The chief radiographic signs are pericardial effusion and a large left atrium.
- The chief echocardiographic signs are pericardial effusion and a blood clot near the left atrium. Hemopericardium due to other causes typically is chronic in nature, larger in volume, and does not develop blood clots.
- If the animal is hemodynamically stable and a blood clot is on the left atrium, there is merit in not removing the hemopericardium so that counterpressure is maintained on the left atrium until vasodilator therapy can be initiated and/or preparations can be made for surgery.

PREVENTION

- No preventive treatment is known
- Aggressive vasodilator therapy may help

CLIENT EDUCATION

Avoid stress and hyperactivity

SUGGESTED READING

Buchanan JW: Spontaneous left atrial rupture in dogs. *Adv Exp Med Biol* 22:315-324, 1972.

Buchanan JW: Left atrial rupture. 2003, http://www.vin.com/library/general/JWBCardio2.htm.

Buchanan JW, Kelly AM: Endocardial splitting of the left atrium in dogs with hemorrhage and hemopericardium. *J Am Vet Radiol Soc* 5:28-39, 1964.

Buchanan JW, Sammarco CD: Circumferential suture of the mitral annulus for correction of mitral regurgitation in dogs. *Vet Surg* 27:182-193, 1998.

Sadanaga KK, MacDonald MJ, Buchanan JW: Echocardiography and surgery in a dog with left atrial rupture and hemopericardium. *JVIM* 4:216-221, 1990.

AUTHOR: **JAMES W. BUCHANAN**

EDITOR: **ETIENNE CÔTÉ**

Atrial Septal Defect

BASIC INFORMATION

DEFINITION

One of a number of congenital cardiac defects characterized by incomplete formation of the interatrial septum and communication between the left and right atrium

SYNONYM(S)

ASD

Atrial septum: interatrial septum

Ostium primum defect

Ostium secundum defect

Patent foramen ovale (incorrect)

Persistent atrioventricular canal/atrioventricular septal defect/endocardial cushion defect (together with ventricular septal defect)

Sinus venosus defect

EPIDEMIOLOGY

SPECIES: All mammalian species.

AGE: Usually early in life. Small defects may go undetected or be incidental findings.

SEX: Unknown.

GENETICS AND BREED PREDISPOSITION: Dogs: boxer, Doberman pinscher, and Samoyed.

CLINICAL PRESENTATION

DISEASE FORMS/SUBTYPES

- Incidental murmur
- Incidental finding of thoracic radiographic abnormalities
- Incidental echocardiographic identification
- Clinical signs of pulmonary hypertension and right-to-left or bidirectional shunting (large defects), such as collapse, cyanosis

HISTORY/CHIEF COMPLAINT

- With mild defects, there may be no overt signs, and signs of the defect are encountered incidentally.
- With larger defects, signs of congestive heart failure, pulmonary hypertension, hypoxemia, or polycythemia may be evident.

PHYSICAL FINDINGS

- Patient may have no physical findings with mild defects.
- Heart murmur present due to increased transvalvular flow in right heart:
  - Murmur of relative pulmonic stenosis (soft, systolic murmur loudest at left heart base/cranially on left hemithorax).
  - Murmur of relative tricuspid stenosis (soft, diastolic right-sided murmur; rare).
  - With endocardial cushion defects, murmurs of mitral or tricuspid regurgitation may be present.
- Split second heart sound.
- If congestive heart failure (CHF) is present:
  - Ascites, peripheral edema, dyspnea due to pleural effusion.
- With right-to-left or bidirectional shunting, murmur will be absent and cyanosis is possible.

ETIOLOGY AND PATHOPHYSIOLOGY

- Presumed genetic etiology, although specific mutations have not been identified.
- Direction of blood flow depends on the caliber of the defect and the relative resistance to flow into the left and right ventricle.
- Small (restrictive) defects maintain left atrial pressures higher than right atrial, resulting in left-to-right flow and subsequent right heart volume overload and pulmonary overcirculation. Right heart failure may develop.
- Large defects may result in increased pulmonary vascular resistance, right ventricular hypertrophy, and bidirectional/balanced or right-to-left shunting lesion with signs of pulmonary hypertension (Eisenmenger physiology), arterial hypoxemia.

DIAGNOSIS

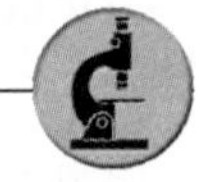

DIFFERENTIAL DIAGNOSIS

- Physical/radiographic: pulmonic stenosis, tricuspid dysplasia, tetralogy of Fallot
- Echocardiographic: normal echo "dropout," patent foramen ovale, mild pulmonic stenosis

INITIAL DATABASE

- Echocardiogram: defect noted in atrial septum with two-dimensional imaging.

Unlike normal echo "drop-out," an ASD has sharp, not tapered, edges, is generally observable in more than one echo view, and may be located at the very base of the atrial septum (septum primum defect). Color/spectral Doppler assists in characterizing increased pulmonic/tricuspid velocities, flow across defect. Quantitative Doppler can estimate the pulmonary/systemic shunt flow ratio.

- Thoracic radiographs: variable, ranging from normal to right-sided cardiomegaly, pulmonary artery enlargement, pulmonary overcirculation. Pulmonary arterial tortuosity/enlargement or pulmonary undercirculation are possible with pulmonary hypertension.
- Electrocardiogram: normal or may have evidence of right heart enlargement (S-waves I, II, III, aVL, aVF; right axis deviation; tall P waves).
- Complete blood count, serum chemistry panel, urinalysis usually unremarkable. Polycythemia may be present with bidirectional shunting.
- Arterial blood gas analysis may indicate hypoxemia in cases of bidirectional or right-to-left shunting.

ADVANCED OR CONFIRMATORY TESTING

Rarely needed or used:

- Transesophageal echocardiography
- Cardiac catheterization may yield quantitative information, confirm defect, and identify concurrent defects

TREATMENT

THERAPEUTIC GOAL(S)

Prevent/delay increases in pulmonary vascular resistance and CHF

ACUTE GENERAL TREATMENT

See Heart Failure, Acute/Decompensated, p 458; Hyperviscosity Syndrome, p 558.

- In cases of CHF, therapy should reduce venous congestion (diuretics), inhibit sodium/water retention, and counteract vasoconstriction (ACE inhibitors, vasodilators).
- Digoxin may be indicated with atrial tachyarrhythmias, myocardial failure, or baroreceptor dysfunction.
- Abdominocentesis/thoracocentesis may be needed for body cavity effusions.
- Phlebotomy as indicated for hyperviscosity syndrome associated with polycythemia.

CHRONIC TREATMENT

See Heart Failure, Chronic, p 459; Hyperviscosity Syndrome, p 558

- Recurrent centeses as necessary.
- Recheck evaluations are essential for CHF management (monitor renal function, albumin/total protein, blood pressure, heart rate/rhythm).
- Definitive surgical repair has been reported and is available at selected academic institutions. Catheter closure has also been reported. These advanced techniques are not always indicated and are rarely used.
- Phlebotomy as indicated for hyperviscosity syndrome associated with polycythemia.

POSSIBLE COMPLICATIONS

- Recurrent CHF
- Syncope (from pulmonary hypertension, right-to-left shunting)
- Polycythemia

RECOMMENDED MONITORING

- Serum chemistry panel, complete blood count, urinalysis, and blood pressure prior to initiation of therapy for CHF
- Recheck serum blood urea nitrogen, creatinine, and electrolytes 1 week after initiating oral therapy
- Hematocrit in patients with evidence of bidirectional shunting (polycythemia and/or hypoxemia)
- Serial echocardiography and thoracic radiographs as dictated by rate of progression

PROGNOSIS AND OUTCOME

- Excellent with mild (small) defects
- Guarded with large defects, pulmonary hypertension, right-to-left shunting, or animals with CHF

PEARLS & CONSIDERATIONS

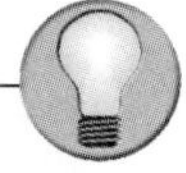

CLIENT EDUCATION

- Although a definitive genetic basis is not established, affected animals should not be used for breeding.
- Recheck evaluations are a necessary part of management of polycythemia or CHF.
- A common error of inexperienced echocardiographers is the misdiagnosis of normal, mid-atrial septal echo dropout (the normal fossa ovalis) as an ASD.

RECOMMENDED READING

Bonagura JD, Lehmkuhl LB: Congenital heart disease. In Fox PR, Sisson DD, Moïse NS (eds): *Textbook of Canine and Feline Cardiology: Principles and Practice*, ed 2. Philadelphia, WB Saunders, 1999, pp 471-535.

Kittleson MD, Kienle RD: Septal defects. In Kittleson MD, Kienle RD (eds): *Small Animal Cardiovascular Medicine*. New York, Mosby, 1998, pp 231-239.

Monnet E, et al: Diagnosis and surgical repair of partial atrioventricular septal defects in two dogs. *J Am Vet Med Assoc* 211(5):569-572, 1997.

AUTHOR: **AARON WEY**
EDITOR: **ETIENNE CÔTÉ**

Atrial Standstill

BASIC INFORMATION

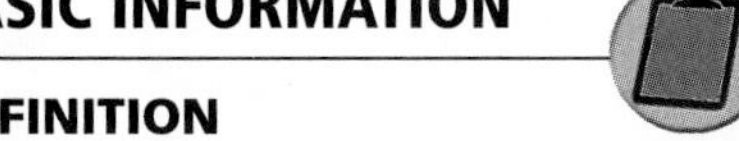

DEFINITION

Cardiac arrhythmia in which the atria do not depolarize. The two main causes are hyperkalemia and atrial myopathy.

SYNONYM(S)

Atrial paralysis
Silent atria

EPIDEMIOLOGY

SPECIES, AGE, SEX: Dogs and cats: any age, either sex.

RISK FACTORS: Diseases that can cause hyperkalemia, and in turn, atrial standstill, include:

- Hypoadrenocorticism
- Urethral obstruction
- Urinary bladder rupture
- Acute renal failure
- Iatrogenic (improper addition of KCl to IV fluids; direct IV administration of undiluted KCl or potassium penicillin)
- Muscle necrosis (reperfusion injury, massive trauma)

CLINICAL PRESENTATION

DISEASE FORMS/SUBTYPES

- Hyperkalemia-induced
- Atrial myopathy-induced

HISTORY, CHIEF COMPLAINT

- Hyperkalemia-induced: generally reflective of underlying disorder (e.g., lethargy, inappetence, vomiting in dogs with hyperkalemia due to hypoadrenocorticism), dysuria, stranguria, and malaise in dogs or cats with urethral obstruction, etc.
- Atrial myopathy-induced: exercise intolerance, lethargy, weakness, possibly syncope
- May be an incidental finding on electrocardiogram (ECG)

PHYSICAL EXAM FINDINGS

- Hyperkalemia or atrial myopathy-induced: Bradycardia is a highly suggestive finding.
    - Typical ventricular rates range from 40–100 bpm in dogs with atrial standstill.
    - In cats, bradycardia may be present, and cats with severe, life-threatening hyperkalemia and atrial standstill may still have heart rates >200 bpm.
- Other signs depend on the inciting cause (e.g., markedly enlarged urinary bladder with urethral obstruction).

ETIOLOGY AND PATHOPHYSIOLOGY

- Atrial myopathy-associated atrial standstill:
    - Atrial stretch and replacement of atrial myocytes with fibrous tissue.
    - Physical disruption of myocyte-to-myocyte conduction of electrical impulses through atria.
    - The heartbeat originates from the atrioventricular junction ("junctional escape rhythm").
    - Most commonly occurs in cats with marked atrial enlargement due to cardiomyopathy, but sporadic cases in dogs and cats with normal atria (and normokalemia) are seen.
    - Atrial standstill is permanent.
- Hyperkalemia causes atrial standstill:
    - Rising serum potassium concentrations decrease the transmembrane concentration gradient of cardiomyocytes, slowing repolarization (phases 1-4 of depolarization).
    - High serum potassium concentrations slow, or may totally inhibit, the sodium channel, and attendant phase 0 depolarization.
    - Atrial myocardium is exquisitely sensitive to the paralytic effects of hyperkalemia, much more so than ventricular myocardium. Sinoatrial nodal tissue is most resistant.
    - The heartbeat originates from the sinoatrial node, travels through the atria normally along the internodal pathways, and reaches the atrioventricular node normally, but fails to depolarize the surrounding atrial tissue along the way ("sinoventricular rhythm"). Thus, no P wave is seen on the ECG.
    - Atrial standstill caused by hyperkalemia is reversible with normalization of serum potassium.

DIAGNOSIS

DIFFERENTIAL DIAGNOSIS

Bradycardia on physical examination:

- Second-degree atrioventricular block
- Third-degree atrioventricular block
- Sinus bradycardia
- Sick sinus syndrome

INITIAL DATABASE

- ECG. Gold standard of clinical diagnosis:
    - Absence of P waves in all leads.
    - Regular rhythm (constant R-R interval).
    - Heart rate: bradycardia (dogs: typically <100 bpm) or any heart rate (cats: 120–260 bpm in most cases, but possibly <80 bpm if terminally ill).
    - ECG *must* display multiple leads (e.g., not just lead II) to make a diagnosis of atrial standstill. Otherwise, P waves may be isoelectric in one lead, which may give the impression of atrial standstill on single-lead ECGs of patients in normal sinus rhythm.
- Serum electrolyte panel:
    - Serum potassium concentration is an essential test in every patient with atrial standstill. Hyperkalemia severe enough to produce atrial standstill is a medical emergency.
    - Absence of hyperkalemia in a patient with atrial standstill provides the diagnosis of atrial myopathy (by exclusion).

ADVANCED OR CONFIRMATORY TESTING

- Thoracic radiographs and echocardiography: if atrial standstill coexists with normokalemia, to assess atrial structure
- Serum ionized calcium level: in cats with atrial standstill caused by urethral obstruction-related hyperkalemia. Hypocalcemia commonly present and may be arrhythmogenic

TREATMENT

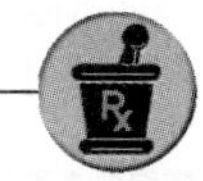

THERAPEUTIC GOAL(S)

Identify cause and reverse it if possible

ACUTE AND CHRONIC TREATMENT

Depends on cause:

- Treatment for hyperkalemia if present (see Hyperkalemia, p 546).

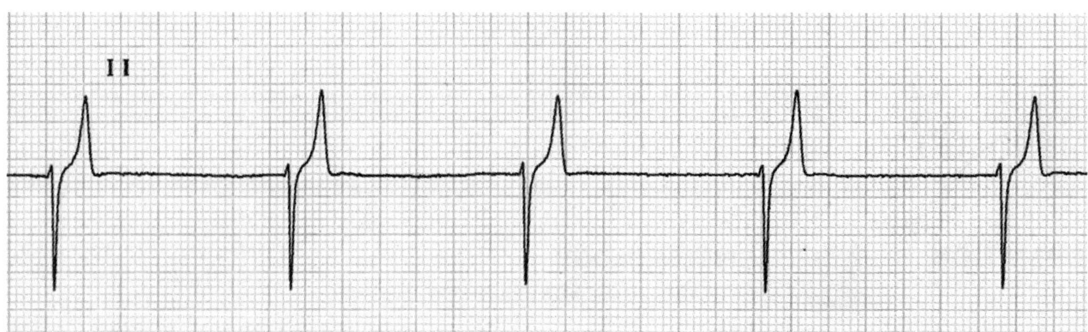

FIGURE I-23 Electrocardiogram of a golden retriever with atrial standstill. The cause is atrial myopathy, based on a normal serum potassium level. The rhythm is regular, and no P waves are seen in this lead II tracing, nor were they present in any other lead. The negative QRS complexes suggest a concurrent intraventricular conduction disturbance. 25 mm/sec, 1 cm/mV.

- Treatment for atrial myopathy-associated atrial standstill involves treatment of the underlying cardiac disorder, as indicated, regardless of atrial standstill. If overt clinical signs (e.g., exercise intolerance, syncope) occur despite treatment for the underlying heart problem, pacemaker implantation may be necessary.

RECOMMENDED MONITORING

For hyperkalemia-associated atrial standstill: continuous ECG monitoring until P waves reappear

PROGNOSIS AND OUTCOME

- Hyperkalemia-associated atrial standstill: immediate prognosis is guarded. Successful management of hyperkalemia and its inciting cause often results in a good long-term prognosis.
- Atrial myopathy-associated atrial standstill: guarded prognosis, specifically dependent on degree of atrial enlargement and severity of clinical signs.

PEARLS & CONSIDERATIONS

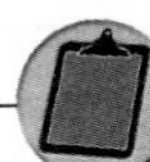

COMMENTS

- Atrial standstill in hyperkalemic patients is a harbinger of life-threatening arrhythmias. Failure to note atrial standstill (loss of P waves on ECG) in patients with hyperkalemia may allow hyperkalemia to worsen, leading to cardiac arrest.
- Artifactual hyperkalemia is common in dogs and cats: platelets release potassium in vitro when activated (e.g., blood clotting in a red top tube). Artifact is ruled out by measuring potassium on blood from a green top tube.
- In cats, tachycardia (or normal heart rate) does not rule out atrial standstill, but in dogs, atrial standstill almost always causes bradycardia.

SUGGESTED READING

Tilley LP: *Essentials of Canine and Feline Electrocardiography*, ed 3. Philadelphia, Lea & Febiger, 1993, pp 182–183.

Gavaghan BJ, et al: Persistent atrial standstill in a cat. *Aust Vet J* 77:574–579, 1999.

AUTHOR & EDITOR: **ETIENNE CÔTÉ**

Atrioventricular Block, First-Degree

BASIC INFORMATION

DEFINITION

Delayed conduction of an electrical impulse from the sinoatrial (SA) node or atria through the atrioventricular (AV) junction (AV node and bundle of His). The hallmark manifestation on an electrocardiogram is a prolonged PR interval.

SYNONYM(S)

First-degree AV block
First-degree heart block

EPIDEMIOLOGY

SPECIES, AGE, SEX

- Most common in older dogs, but can occur in dogs and cats of any age
- No reported gender predisposition

GENETICS AND BREED PREDISPOSITION: Dogs: cocker spaniels, dachshunds, brachycephalic breeds.

CLINICAL PRESENTATION

HISTORY, CHIEF COMPLAINT

- First-degree AV block produces no clinical signs: as a sole entity, it is detected only as an incidental finding on electrocardiogram (ECG)
- Historic problems relate to underlying condition, if any

PHYSICAL EXAM FINDINGS: Undetectable on physical examination as sole entity:

- First-degree AV block produces no audible disturbance in cardiac rhythm

ETIOLOGY AND PATHOPHYSIOLOGY

The PR interval (or PQ interval) encompasses the duration of atrial depolarization—the P wave—and duration of conduction through the AV node—the PR segment—and its duration is normally ≤0.13 seconds in dogs, or ≤0.09 seconds in cats.

ETIOLOGY

- Physiologic first-degree AV block: may occur as normal variant, often concurrently with respiratory sinus arrhythmia (both are manifestations of prevailing vagal tone)
- Iatrogenic first-degree AV block: medications that decrease the rate of conduction through the AV node. Common: digoxin, opioids (morphine, hydromorphone, oxymorphone, fentanyl, etc.), quinidine. Also possible: β-adrenergic antagonists/β-blockers, calcium channel antagonists/blockers, procainamide)
- Pathologic conditions resulting in increased vagal tone (e.g., respiratory, gastrointestinal, and intracranial central nervous system disorders)
- "Primary" cardiomyopathies (e.g., hypertrophic cardiomyopathy)
- Idiopathic fibrosis of the AV node
- Infiltrative myocardial disease
- Myocardial infarction

PATHOPHYSIOLOGY: All of the above pathological, physiologic, and iatrogenic etiologies may result in decreased velocity of electrical conduction through the specialized cardiac myocytes of the AV junction to the ventricles.

DIAGNOSIS

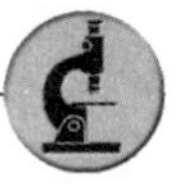

The diagnosis is by ECG only

DIFFERENTIAL DIAGNOSIS

Artifact (e.g., abnormal/changing ECG paper speed)

INITIAL DATABASE

- Electrocardiogram: PR interval >0.13 sec (dog); PR >0.09 sec (cat)

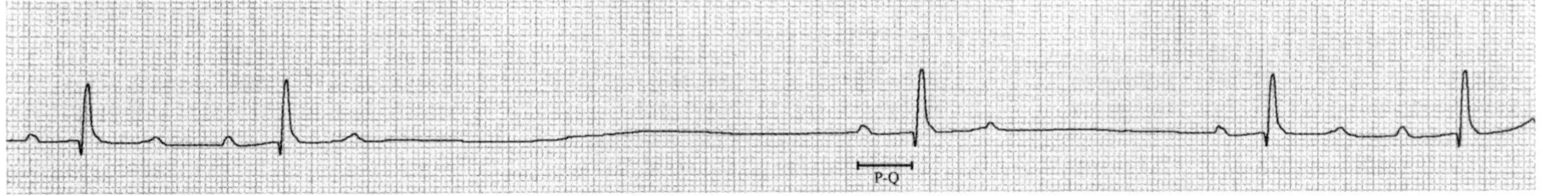

FIGURE I-24 First-degree AV block in a 5-year-old German shepherd with severe inflammatory bowel disease. PR interval (PQ interval) is prolonged at 0.20 seconds; upper limit of normal = 0.13 seconds. 50 mm/sec.

- Additional testing as pertains to underlying/concurrent condition, if any

ADVANCED OR CONFIRMATORY TESTING

Not applicable nor required

TREATMENT

THERAPEUTIC GOAL(S)

None unless an underlying condition exists

ACUTE GENERAL TREATMENT

As discussed previously

CHRONIC TREATMENT

As discussed previously

RECOMMENDED MONITORING

No specific monitoring necessary

PROGNOSIS AND OUTCOME

Excellent: no negative implications as sole entity

PEARLS & CONSIDERATIONS

COMMENTS

- First-degree AV block does not cause clinical signs; it is simply an indicator of delayed AV nodal conduction and as such, it is a clue that an underlying cardiac or systemic problem may be present.
- The onset of first-degree AV block in a patient may be an indicator of drug toxicity (e.g., digoxin) if the patient is receiving a drug that delays AV nodal conduction and if a previous ECG indicates absence of first-degree AV block.

SUGGESTED READING

Miller MS, et al: Electrocardiography. In Fox PR, Sisson D, Moïse NS (eds): *Textbook of Canine and Feline Cardiology*. Philadelphia, WB Saunders, 1999, pp 67–105.

Tilley LP: Interpretation of common cardiac arrhythmias. In Tilley LP (ed): *Essentials of Canine and Feline Electrocardiography*. Philadelphia, Lea & Febiger, 1992, pp 127–252.

AUTHOR: **GREGG RAPOPORT**

EDITOR: **ETIENNE CÔTÉ**

Atrioventricular Block, Second-Degree

BASIC INFORMATION

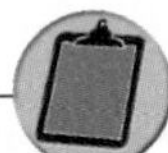

DEFINITION

A cardiac arrhythmia (bradycardia) characterized by intermittent failure of transmission of atrial electrical impulses to the ventricles. Electrocardiographically, some proportion of P waves not followed by QRS complexes

SYNONYM(S)

Second-degree AV block
Second-degree heart block
Mobitz type I: Wenckebach phenomenon

EPIDEMIOLOGY

SPECIES, AGE, SEX

- Dogs affected more often than cats
- No gender predisposition

GENETICS AND BREED PREDISPOSITION

- Older cocker spaniels and dachshunds
- Hereditary: pugs with His bundle stenosis

CLINICAL PRESENTATION

DISEASE FORMS/SUBTYPES

- Mobitz type I (Wenckebach): progressive lengthening of PR interval from heartbeat to heartbeat until a nonconducted/blocked P wave (P wave not followed by QRS complex) occurs
- Mobitz type II: PR interval is constant, but some P waves are intermittently blocked
  - "High-grade"/"advanced" second-degree atrioventricular (AV) block: three or more consecutive nonconducted P waves
  - Mobitz type II second-degree AV block: further described with the ratio of P waves to QRS complexes (e.g., 5:4)

HISTORY, CHIEF COMPLAINT

- Mobitz type I: no clinical signs; patient is normal, or historic complaints relate to underlying condition
- Mobitz type II: may include episodic or persistent signs of low-output heart failure (e.g., lethargy, weakness, syncope) or congestive heart failure (e.g., cough, tachypnea, dyspnea, abdominal distention) if overall heart rate (ventricular rate) is low

PHYSICAL EXAM FINDINGS

- Heart rate typically normal or decreased.
- Cardiac rhythm typically "regularly irregular" with occasional "skipped beats" (no ventricular activity after the blocked atrial impulse). Atrial impulse (blocked at AV node) generally is not auscultable
- Femoral pulse strength typically normal, or stronger for beats following pauses; no pulse deficit
- High-grade Mobitz type II only: signs of low-output or congestive heart failure possible

ETIOLOGY AND PATHOPHYSIOLOGY

- For first-degree AV block, see Atrioventricular Block, First-Degree, p 107
- Also may occur transiently seconds to a few minutes after intravenous atropine administration

DIAGNOSIS

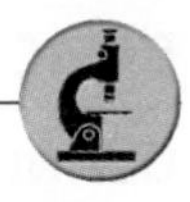

DIFFERENTIAL DIAGNOSIS

- Auscultatory:
  - Pronounced respiratory sinus arrhythmia (common)
  - Sinoatrial arrest or block (uncommon)
- Electrocardiogram (ECG):
  - Third-degree AV block (see Atrioventricular Block, Third-Degree, p 110)
  - Rhythmic motion artifact (purring, shivering)

INITIAL DATABASE

- ECG:
  - Confirm diagnosis and rule out other arrhythmias
  - Second-degree AV block: some proportion of P waves not followed by QRS complexes. Therefore atrial rate is faster than ventricular rate
- Echocardiogram: rule out structural intracardiac causes
- Thoracic radiographs: rule out congestive heart failure
- Complete blood count, serum biochemistry profile, and urinalysis: unremarkable unless concurrent conditions

ADVANCED OR CONFIRMATORY TESTING

- See Atropine response test (see Sick Sinus Syndrome, p 1003). Differentiation between physiologic (atropine abolishes block) and pathologic (atropine has incomplete or no effect)

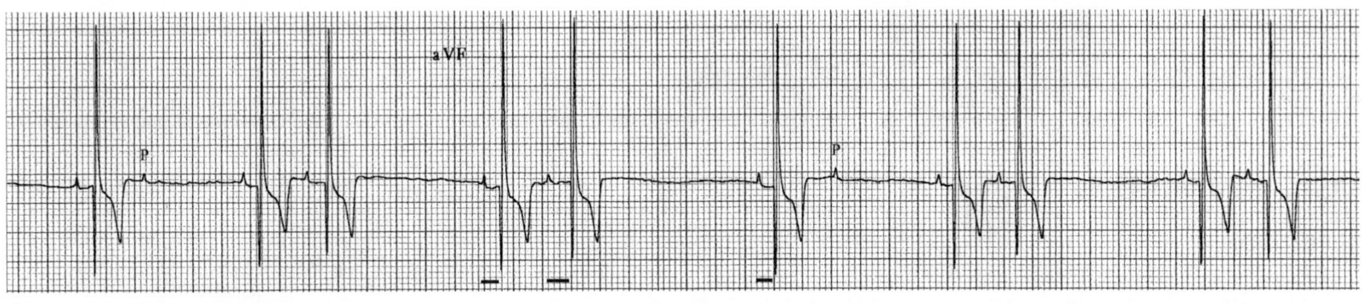

A

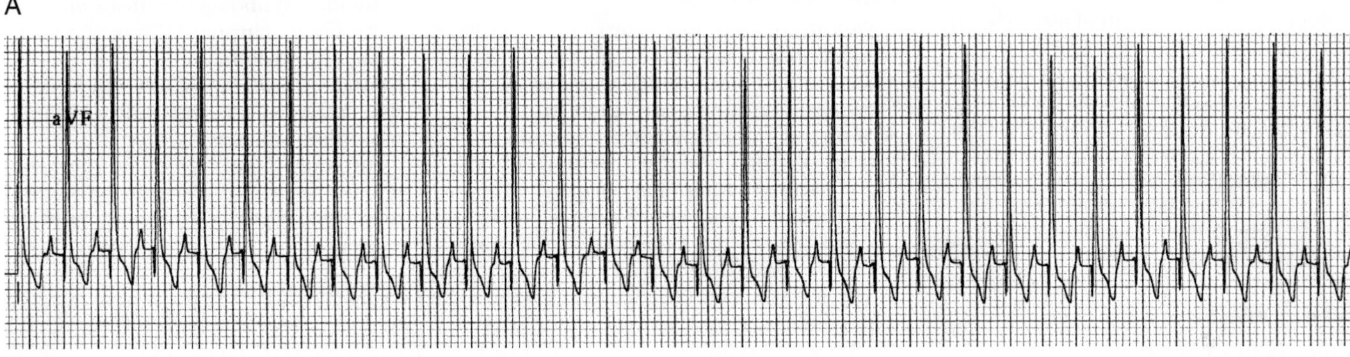

B

FIGURE I-25 **A**, Second-degree AV block Mobitz type I in an 11-year-old cocker spaniel evaluated for lethargy. Mobitz type I classification (note 2 nonconducted P waves and solid lines marking variable PQ intervals). **B**, ECG obtained 30 minutes following intramuscular atropine injection (0.04 mg/kg) shows positive response: HR has increased from 70/min to 230/min and AV block has resolved; suggests AV block is physiologic and not responsible for reported clinical signs.

- For Mobitz type II (or Mobitz type I if accompanied by sinus bradycardia and vague clinical signs)
- Complete positive response: heart rate increase ≥50% and total resolution of AV block
- Consider use of ambulatory ECG (24-hour Holter monitor, event monitor) if relationship of arrhythmia to clinical signs remains unclear

TREATMENT

THERAPEUTIC GOAL(S)

- Restore normal cardiac output
  - The ventricular rate is a major determinant of clinical impact and need for treatment.
- Resolve congestive heart failure if present

ACUTE GENERAL TREATMENT

Generally needed only with high-grade Mobitz II block causing clinical signs:

- Standard therapy for congestive heart failure if applicable (see Heart Failure, Chronic, p 459)
- Temporary pacemaker implantation
- Intravenous isoproterenol (0.4 mg in 250 ml saline, IV infusion titrated to increase atrial rate) can be administered prior to pacemaker implantation. Response is variable and often unrewarding

CHRONIC TREATMENT

Generally needed only with high-grade Mobitz II block causing clinical signs:

- Permanent pacemaker implantation
- Oral positive chronotropic medications (e.g., propantheline 0.5-1 mg/kg PO q 8h) can be used; response is variable and generally inadequate

POSSIBLE COMPLICATIONS

- Mobitz type II second-degree AV block may progress to third-degree AV block (see Atrioventricular Block, Third-Degree, p 110).
- Patients with high-grade Mobitz II second-degree AV block and clinical signs are at risk for sudden death.

RECOMMENDED MONITORING

- Mobitz type I: consider periodic ECGs to ensure no progression
- Mobitz type II: without therapy, periodic ECGs (every few months or as dictated by clinical signs)

PROGNOSIS AND OUTCOME

- Mobitz type I: excellent
- Mobitz type II:
  - If no clinical signs, fair to good
  - If clinical signs, or if high grade, guarded without treatment, but generally fair to good with permanent pacemaker

PEARLS & CONSIDERATIONS

COMMENTS

- Mobitz type I second-degree AV block rarely causes clinical signs and does not predict degeneration to Mobitz type II or third-degree AV block.
- Therapy for congestive heart failure can often be tapered or discontinued after successful pacemaker implantation.

SUGGESTED READING

Miller MS, et al: Electrocardiography. In Fox PR, Sisson D, Moïse NS (eds): *Textbook of Canine and Feline Cardiology*. Philadelphia, WB Saunders, 1999, pp 67-105.

Tilley LP: Interpretation of common cardiac arrhythmias. In Tilley LP (ed): *Essentials of Canine and Feline Electrocardiography*. Philadelphia, Lea & Febiger, 1992, pp 127-252.

AUTHOR: **GREGG RAPOPORT**
EDITOR: **ETIENNE CÔTÉ**

Atrioventricular Block, Third-Degree

BASIC INFORMATION

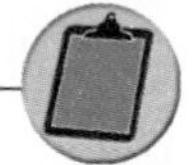

DEFINITION

- A cardiac arrhythmia (bradycardia) characterized by persistent, complete blockage of conduction of atrial electrical impulses to the ventricles.
- Electrocardiographically, P waves occur regularly and at a normal or elevated rate but are not followed by QRS complexes. Ventricular activity consists of QRS complexes that occur regularly but at a very slow rate (ventricular escape rhythm) and are often wide and bizarre in morphology.

SYNONYM(S)

Complete heart block
Third-degree AV block
Third-degree heart block

EPIDEMIOLOGY

SPECIES, AGE, SEX

- Occurs in dogs and cats
- More common in older animals but can occur at any age

GENETICS AND BREED PREDISPOSITION

- Reported as hereditary in pugs with His bundle stenosis
- Doberman pinschers overrepresented in one study

ASSOCIATED CONDITIONS AND DISORDERS

- Reported association between borreliosis (Lyme disease) in dogs and people
- Concurrent myasthenia gravis has been reported in a small number of dogs

CLINICAL PRESENTATION

HISTORY, CHIEF COMPLAINT

- Syncope
- Episodic or persistent lethargy and weakness
- If concurrent congestive heart failure: tachypnea, dyspnea, abdominal distention

PHYSICAL EXAM FINDINGS

- Bradycardia: heart rate typically <50/min in dogs, <120/min in cats
- Variable intensity of first heart sound due to beat-to-beat variation in end-diastolic ventricular volume
- Intermittent, prominent jugular pulsations: "cannon *a* waves" caused by intermittent right atrial contraction against closed tricuspid valve
- Intermittently noted third and fourth heart sounds (subtle, variable)
- Other findings referable to low-output or congestive heart failure in some animals

ETIOLOGY AND PATHOPHYSIOLOGY

- Failure of the atrioventricular (AV) junction (AV node and bundle of His) to conduct supraventricular electrical impulses distal to a site of interruption.
- Ventricular depolarization (and contraction) occurs due to the development of an "escape rhythm" that emanates from pacemaker cells either in the more distal part of the AV junction (the His bundle) or in the ventricles.
- The result is a faster atrial rate (P waves per minute) and slower ventricular rate (QRS complexes per minute) that occur independently of one another.

Causes:

- Idiopathic fibrosis of the AV node
- "Primary" cardiomyopathies (e.g., hypertrophic cardiomyopathy)
- Infiltrative myocardial disease
- Certain congenital heart defects (e.g., ventricular septal defect)
- Bacterial endocarditis
- Myocardial infarction
- Severe hyperkalemia
- Iatrogenic: toxicity secondary to specific cardiac medications (e.g., β-adrenergic antagonists, calcium channel antagonists, digitalis glycosides)
- All of the above may lead to failure of the specialized cardiac myocytes of the AV junction to transmit supraventricular electrical impulses

DIAGNOSIS

DIFFERENTIAL DIAGNOSIS

- Historic:
  - Other causes of syncope (e.g., tachyarrhythmias, structural heart disease, pulmonary hypertension, intracranial disease, metabolic disease)
- Auscultatory:
  - Other bradyarrhythmias (e.g., sinus bradycardia, persistent atrial standstill, high-grade second-degree AV block)

INITIAL DATABASE

- Electrocardiogram: confirm diagnosis and rule out other arrhythmias
  - Escape rhythm: QRS complexes may appear wide and bizarre, or normal (presumably arising from ventricles or from lower AV junction, respectively). Rate: 30–70 bpm (dogs), 70–140 bpm (cats)
- Echocardiogram: rule out structural intracardiac causes (see Etiology and Pathophysiology above)
  - Incidental finding of other abnormalities (e.g., chronic AV valve endocardiosis) is common
- Thoracic radiographs: rule out congestive heart failure and other intrathoracic abnormalities
- Complete blood count, serum biochemistry profile, and urinalysis: unremarkable unless concurrent conditions present

TREATMENT

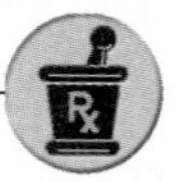

THERAPEUTIC GOAL(S)

- Restore normal cardiac output
- Resolve congestive heart failure if present

ACUTE GENERAL TREATMENT

- Standard therapy for acute heart failure if applicable (see Heart Failure, Acute, p 459)
- Temporary and/or permanent artificial pacemaker implantation (see Pacemaker: Transthoracic Cardiac Pacing, p 1294)
- Intravenous positive chronotropic medications (e.g., isoproterenol 0.4 mg in 250 ml saline, IV infusion titrated to increase atrial rate) can be administered; response is variable and almost always unrewarding with third-degree AV block

CHRONIC TREATMENT

- Permanent artificial pacemaker implantation
- Therapy for congestive heart failure can often be tapered or discontinued after successful pacemaker implantation

POSSIBLE COMPLICATIONS

Sudden death may occur without artificial pacemaker implantation

RECOMMENDED MONITORING

Postoperative monitoring referable to pacemaker implantation

PROGNOSIS AND OUTCOME

Variable but generally fair to good after successful implantation of permanent pacemaker (better if congestive heart failure has not been present)

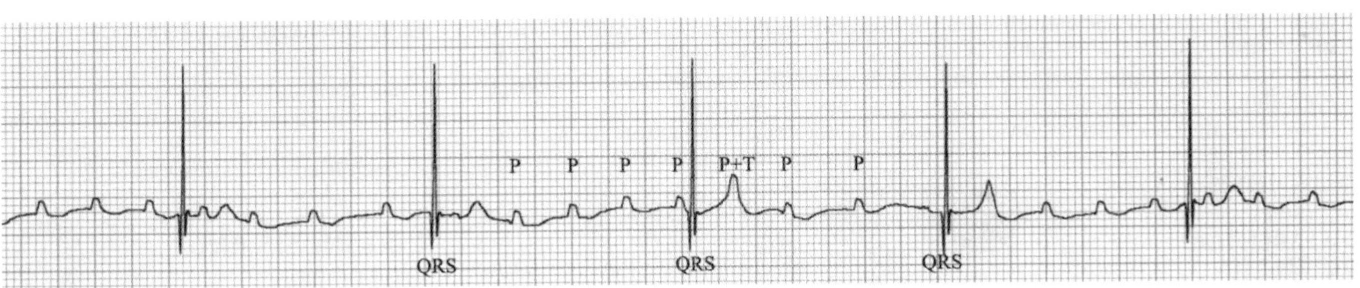

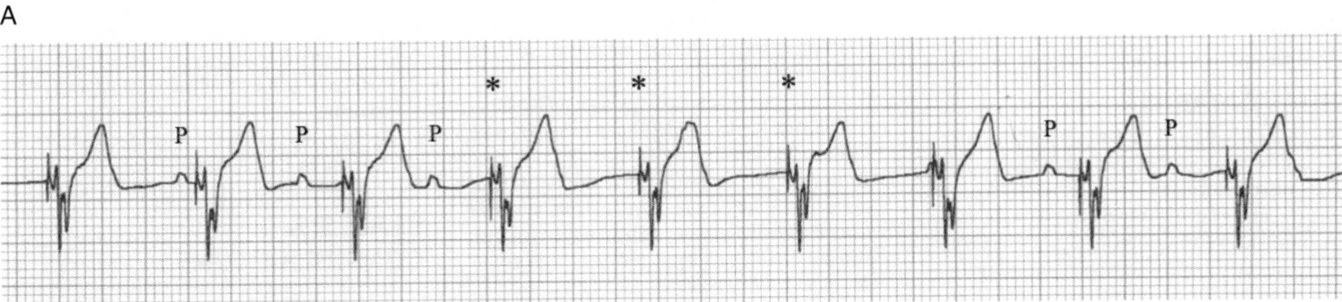

FIGURE I-26 Third-degree AV block in a 2-year-old Irish spaniel with syncope, before and after permanent jugular transvenous pacemaker implantation. **A**, (Admission): note atrial rhythm (P waves, 190/min) and unrelated ventricular rhythm (QRS complexes, 40/min). One P wave is superimposed on a T wave ("P+T"). **B**, (After pacemaker implantation): ventricular-paced rhythm at a rate of 90/min. Unrelated P waves can still be seen. Pacemaker spikes (*asterisk*) precede each QRS complex.

PEARLS & CONSIDERATIONS

COMMENTS

- Ventricular antiarrhythmic agents are contraindicated until artificial pacing has been established, due to potential for suppression of ventricular escape foci.
- Therapy for congestive heart failure can often be tapered or discontinued after successful pacemaker implantation.
- Clinical signs may be subtle (e.g., progressive lethargy) and most apparent retrospectively after pacemaker implantation.

SUGGESTED READING

Miller MS, et al: Electrocardiography. In Fox PR, Sisson D, Moïse NS (eds): *Textbook of Canine and Feline Cardiology*. Philadelphia, WB Saunders, 1999, pp 67–105.

Tilley LP: Interpretation of common cardiac arrhythmias. In Tilley LP (ed): *Essentials of Canine and Feline Electrocardiography*. Philadelphia, Lea & Febiger, 1992, pp 127–252.

AUTHOR: **GREGG RAPOPORT**

EDITOR: **ETIENNE CÔTÉ**

Aural Hematoma

BASIC INFORMATION

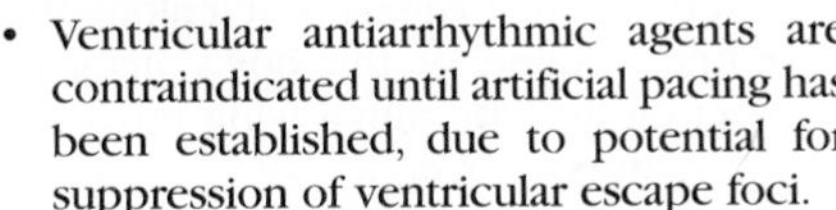

DEFINITION

- A collection of blood within the cartilage plate of the ear
- A fluctuant, fluid-filled swelling on the concave surface of the ear pinna

EPIDEMIOLOGY

SPECIES, AGE, SEX: Dogs and cats. It is the seventh most commonly treated surgical condition in small animal practice.

GENETICS AND BREED PREDISPOSITION: Dogs with pendulous pinnae may be at increased risk to rupture capillaries during self-trauma.

RISK FACTORS: Dogs and cats with otitis externa are at increased risk.

CONTAGION AND ZOONOSIS: Parasitic infestation (*Otodectes* spp.).

GEOGRAPHY AND SEASONALITY

- Geographic distribution of parasitic causes of otitis externa
- Associated with seasonal incidence of otitis externa
  - Warmer weather (humidity, swimming)
  - Atopic disease

CLINICAL PRESENTATION

HISTORY, CHIEF COMPLAINT

- Head shaking or scratching ears
- History of otitis externa: acute or chronic
- History of generalized dermatologic problems

PHYSICAL EXAM FINDINGS

- Soft, fluid-filled, or fluctuant swelling on concave surface of pinna:
  - Swelling may become firm and "cauliflower-like" as fibrosis develops
- Otitis externa:
  - Evidence of parasitic infestation
  - Evidence of other causes (excessively hairy ear canals, structural anomaly)
- Evidence of a generalized dermatologic problem

ETIOLOGY AND PATHOPHYSIOLOGY

- Aural hematomas are most often caused by self-trauma (head shaking or scratching) to the pinna secondary to otitis externa.
- Sinusoidal wave motions of the ear fracture the auricular cartilage.
- Because of the inflammation and fragility of the superficial blood vessels,

rupture of epithelial and intrachondral blood vessels occurs with subsequent entrapment of blood between the epithelium and auricular cartilage, resulting in hematoma formation.

DIAGNOSIS

DIFFERENTIAL DIAGNOSIS

- Abscess
- Seroma
- Soft tissue neoplasia

INITIAL DATABASE

- Complete blood count, serum biochemistry profile, and urinalysis: generally unremarkable
- Otic examination under anesthesia
    - Samples of exudate are collected for:
        - Microscopic examination to look for evidence of inflammation, bacterial, and/or yeast proliferation, parasitic infestation
        - Microbiologic culture and sensitivity testing if significant bacterial involvement
    - Thorough examination for foreign bodies (e.g., grass awn) and integrity of tympana

ADVANCED OR CONFIRMATORY TESTING

- Work-up to determine cause of generalized dermatologic problem:
    - Thyroid profile
    - Skin testing for atopic disease
    - Food trial for possible food allergy
    - Examination for parasite infestations (fleas)
- Computed tomography scan (preferred) or skull radiographs of bulla to detect and diagnose concurrent otitis media

TREATMENT

THERAPEUTIC GOAL(S)

- Complete evacuation of the hematoma
- Establishment of continued drainage until adhesion occurs within the layers of the pinna
- Providing means for epithelium-cartilage tissue contact so that adhesion occurs
- Prevention of deformity by reducing scarring

ACUTE GENERAL TREATMENT

- Treatment is surgical:
    - Incisional method, using longitudinal, S-shaped, or elliptical incision. The incision is made full-thickness through the inner concave skin layer only, *not* including the cartilage plate or outer convex skin layer. More aggressive skin incisions potentially cause necrosis. Closure: mattress sutures to prevent deformation and "cauliflower ear," then healing by second intention
    - Fine-needle aspiration (FNA) of the hematoma: invariably ineffective long term
    - Temporary insertion of a self-retaining teat cannula. Effective in resolving hematoma and allowing controlled scar formation. More effective in preventing recurrence than FNA. Ineffective if much scar tissue has formed
    - Oral corticosteroids (prednisone, 0.5 mg/kg PO q 24h) and indwelling Penrose drains
- Pinna needs to be appropriately bandaged to head to prevent further trauma and to allow tissue adhesion to occur during the healing process (2 to 3 weeks)

CHRONIC TREATMENT

- Control/treatment of underlying dermatologic problem is imperative to limit recurrence.
- Affected patients should have regular otic examinations with cleaning, if necessary. General anesthesia (or heavy sedation) is usually necessary to allow thorough examination and cleaning, because the procedure can be uncomfortable (even painful) and to avoid iatrogenic damage to the ear canal.

POSSIBLE COMPLICATIONS

- Recurrence of the hematoma due to inadequate/ineffective treatment and failure to identify or control underlying cause
- Associated with surgical treatment:
    - Incisional technique:
        - Insufficient size of incision may cause premature closure, hematoma recurrence
        - Incorrect orientation of incision and inadvertent ligation of an auricular artery may cause loss of blood supply to sections of the pinna, resulting in necrosis
    - Teat cannula technique:
        - Premature removal of cannula by patient
    - Fine-needle aspiration technique:
        - Inability to remove all fluid, preventing tissue adhesion
    - Passive drainage and corticosteroids:
        - Side effects from systemic corticosteroids
        - Premature removal of passive drains
    - With any of the above techniques, failure to adequately immobilize pinna to allow tissue adhesion and healing to occur results in recurrence.

RECOMMENDED MONITORING

- Appropriate regular otic examination and cleaning
- Reevaluation to ensure that underlying cause of otitis externa is being adequately controlled/treated

PROGNOSIS AND OUTCOME

- Prognosis is good to excellent with appropriate treatment of the hematoma and management of the underlying otitis externa.
- Recurrence is likely if underlying otitis externa is not managed appropriately.

PEARLS & CONSIDERATIONS

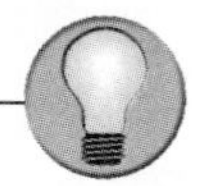

COMMENTS

- Evacuation of the contents of the hematoma, establishment of drainage, and prevention of pinna deformation are necessary for successful surgical treatment of aural hematomas.
- Aural hematomas are caused by trauma to the pinna, most often due to head shaking or vigorous scratching by the animal.
- Always examine the complete external canals of both ears.
- To remove the bandage, cut it along the ventral midline of the dog's neck to avoid cutting the pinna lying reflected on the dorsal head.

PREVENTION

Determination of the underlying cause of the head shaking or scratching is essential to prevent recurrence.

CLIENT EDUCATION

- Evacuation of the contents of the hematoma, establishment of drainage, and prevention of pinna deformation are necessary for successful surgical treatment of aural hematomas.
- Aural hematomas are caused by underlying trauma to the ear pinna, most often due to head shaking or vigorous scratching by the animal.

SUGGESTED READING

Henderson RA, Horne R: Aural hematomas. In Slatter D (ed): *Textbook of Small Animal Surgery*, ed 3. Philadelphia, WB Saunders, 2003, pp 1737–1741.

Joyce JA: Treatment of canine aural hematoma using an indwelling drain and corticosteroids. *J Small Anim Pract* 35:341–344, 1994.

AUTHOR: **ELLEN B. DAVIDSON DOMNICK**

EDITOR: **RICHARD WALSHAW**

Babesiosis

BASIC INFORMATION

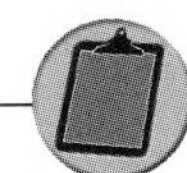

DEFINITION

Canine babesiosis is a tick-borne disease caused by a hemoprotozoan parasite that infects red blood cells of dogs causing hemolytic anemia and thrombocytopenia. Two species have been identified: *Babesia canis* (large babesia) and *Babesia gibsoni* (small babesia).

SYNONYM(S)

A third small babesia has been identified in dogs living in Spain.

Babesia canis has three subspecies (*B. canis vogeli, B. canis canis, B. canis rossi*).

B. gibsoni is present in Asia and has recently been found in American pit bull terriers. A second small piroplasm found in California dogs was initially thought to be *B. gibsoni* but has now been tentatively named *Theileria annae*.

EPIDEMIOLOGY

GENETICS AND BREED PREDISPOSITION

- American pit bull terriers at risk for *B. gibsoni*
- Greyhounds at risk for *B. canis vogeli*

RISK FACTORS

- Tick infestation
- Blood transfusion
- Shared needles or surgical instruments
- Dog fights
- Vertical transmission in affected breeds

CONTAGION AND ZOONOSIS

- Transmission is through blood contamination or arthropod infestation (*Rhipicephalus, Haemaphysalis*, or *Dermacentor* spp.).
- Canine babesiosis is not a zoonotic disease; *B. microti* is a small babesia infecting human red blood cells. Canine species of *Babesia* have not been reported in humans.

GEOGRAPHY AND SEASONALITY

- *B. gibsoni* is an emerging pathogen in North America, reported most often in pit bull terriers. It is endemic in Asia. *Babesia gibsoni* has been reported in American pit bull terriers as far north as Wisconsin and Michigan and as far south as Texas and Florida.
- *Babesia canis rossi* causes severe disease in South African dogs.

ASSOCIATED CONDITIONS AND DISORDERS: Clinical signs of babesiosis can be indistinguishable from hemolytic anemia associated with immune-mediated hemolytic anemia or thrombocytopenia seen with immune-mediated or other tick-borne diseases.

CLINICAL PRESENTATION

DISEASE FORMS/SUBTYPES: Babesiosis can cause severe, life-threatening disease in some dogs; others show few or no outward clinical signs.

HISTORY, CHIEF COMPLAINT: Owners may observe weakness, lethargy, anorexia, pallor, icterus, and port-wine colored urine. Other historic findings may include tick exposure, recent blood transfusion, or recent dog fight (especially with a pit bull terrier).

PHYSICAL EXAM FINDINGS: Icterus, pallor, splenomegaly, lymphadenopathy, fever.

ETIOLOGY AND PATHOPHYSIOLOGY

- Sporozoites in tick salivary glands transmitted to dog during feeding (requires 2 to 3 days).
- Sporozoites enter red blood cells (RBCs).
- Parasites induce fibrin-like proteases (FLPs) that cause RBCs to become sticky and clump.
- Intravascular and extravascular hemolysis occur.
- Secondary immune-mediated destruction of RBCs may occur.

DIAGNOSIS

DIFFERENTIAL DIAGNOSIS

- Immune-mediated hemolytic anemia
- Immune-mediated thrombocytopenia
- Zinc toxicity
- Splenic torsion
- Ehrlichiosis
- Leptospirosis
- Dirofilariasis with caval syndrome

INITIAL DATABASE

- Hematocrit: decreased
- Platelet count: decreased
- Blood smear: identification of babesia organisms
  - Small babesiosis: 1-3 μm signet ring forms
  - Large babesiosis: 3-6 μm paired tear drop forms
- Serum bilirubin: increased
- Urinalysis: bilirubinuria or hemoglobinuria
- Coombs' test: positive in up to 85% of cases

ADVANCED OR CONFIRMATORY TESTING

- PCR test: only way to determine species or subspecies. More sensitive than blood smear
- IFA test >1:64 is considered positive
  - Cannot differentiate species
  - False-negative results can occur with acute or peracute disease or severe immunosuppression

TREATMENT

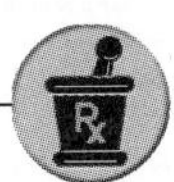

THERAPEUTIC GOAL(S)

It may not be possible to completely eradicate the parasite, but clinical signs usually improve with supportive care and antiparasitic therapy.

ACUTE GENERAL TREATMENT

Supportive treatment may require blood transfusion or hemoglobin polymer (e.g., Oxyglobin) for animals that are anemic:

- IV fluids may be required in animals that are febrile and dehydrated.
- Imidocarb diproprionate (6.6 mg/kg IM once, repeat in 7 to 14 days). Pretreatment with atropine (0.04 mg/kg IM or SC 30 minutes before imidocarb injection) may reduce cholinergic side effects.
- Atovaquone (13.5 mg/kg PO q 8h with fatty meal for 10 days) plus azithromycin (10 mg/kg PO q 24h for 10 days). Best chance for cure but very expensive.
- If anemia/thrombocytopenia does not improve, immunosuppressive therapy may be needed (prednisone 1 mg/kg q 12h), tapered gradually after anemia resolves.

CHRONIC TREATMENT

- Vector control: topical acaricide (e.g., fipronil) plus flea/tick collar
- Dogs with positive *Babesia* titer should not be used as blood donors

POSSIBLE COMPLICATIONS

Prolonged immunosuppressive therapy before specific antibabesial treatment can worsen outcome and should not be used in sick, hospitalized dogs

RECOMMENDED MONITORING

- Monitor hematocrit and platelet count daily until improvement is seen and then every 1 to 3 weeks until anemia and thrombocytopenia resolve.

- PCR should be negative 60 days posttreatment if the parasite has been successfully eradicated.

PROGNOSIS AND OUTCOME

- Good prognosis with early diagnosis and treatment
- Animals may remain subclinically infected for life
- Severely anemic or thrombocytopenic animals may die

PEARLS & CONSIDERATIONS

COMMENTS

B. gibsoni is an emerging infectious disease in North America. New species are being identified through molecular techniques.

PREVENTION

Effective tick control

CLIENT EDUCATION

- In endemic areas, use both a topical acaricide and a repellent flea/tick collar. Avoid blood transmission (shared needles, vaccines, etc.).
- Babesiosis can be transmitted vertically and should be considered in puppies with weakness and pallor.

SUGGESTED READING

Birkenhauer AJ, Levy MG, Breitschwerdt EB: Double-blind placebo controlled trial evaluating the efficacy of an atovaquone azithromycin combination therapy for chronic *Babesia gibsoni* infections. *J Vet Intern Med* 18:494–498, 2004.

Boozer AL, Macintire DK: Canine babesiosis. *Vet Clin North Am Small Anim Pract* 33:885–904, 2003.

AUTHOR & EDITOR: **DOUGLASS K. MACINTIRE**

Back Pain

BASIC INFORMATION

DEFINITION

Pain localized to the thoracolumbar spinal column

SYNONYM(S)

Spinal hyperesthesia
Spinal hyperpathia

EPIDEMIOLOGY

SPECIES, AGE, SEX

- Dependent on the underlying cause
- Dogs: middle-aged (type I intervertebral disk disease), older adults (type II intervertebral disk disease, neoplasia)
- Cats: older adults (neoplasia), males more commonly represented (aortic thromboembolism)

GENETICS AND BREED PREDISPOSITION: Dogs: chondrodystrophic breeds (type I intervertebral disk disease).

RISK FACTORS: Cats: thromboembolism associated with cardiomyopathy.

CLINICAL PRESENTATION

HISTORY, CHIEF COMPLAINT: Vocalization, reluctance to movement or activity, pain elicited if patient touched or moved.

PHYSICAL EXAM FINDINGS

- Hunched posture (kyphosis), pain elicited on epaxial palpation; ataxia, paresis, or paralysis; heat or swelling in epaxial region; splinting and pain on abdominal palpation
- Fever, if back pain is associated with infection (e.g., diskospondylitis)
- Heart murmur, diminished femoral pulses, cyanosis of toenails if back pain is associated with aortic thromboembolism

ETIOLOGY AND PATHOPHYSIOLOGY

- Neurogenic: compression, inflammation, or traumatic disruption of spinal cord, spinal roots, spinal nerves, dorsal root ganglia, or meninges
- Vertebral column: trauma, inflammation, or lysis of vertebral bone, intervertebral disks, or articular facets
- Epaxial muscle: inflammation, abscessation, ischemia, or trauma

DIAGNOSIS

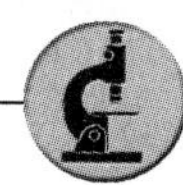

DIFFERENTIAL DIAGNOSIS

- Intervertebral disk disease (IVDD)
- Vertebral fracture or luxation
- Meningitis or meningomyelitis (granulomatous)
- Polyarthritis (immune mediated or infectious)
- Diskospondylitis
- Vertebral osteomyelitis
- Spondylosis deformans/degenerative joint disease of articular facets
- Neoplasia (primary or metastatic)
- Polymyopathy (traumatic or inflammatory myositis)
- Fibrocartilaginous embolism (FCE; acute but transient pain, resolving within hours)
- Pain not localized to the spinal column: aortic thromboembolism, abdominal pain

INITIAL DATABASE

- Neurologic examination
- Complete blood count, serum biochemistry, urinalysis: often unremarkable unless systemic disease or infection present
- Radiographs: bone lysis or proliferation (neoplasia, osteomyelitis), vertebral fracture or luxation (trauma), intervertebral disk mineralization, disk space narrowing, wedging or displacement (IVDD), vertebral endplate lysis or proliferation (diskospondylitis), articular facet sclerosis and malformation, spondylosis

ADVANCED OR CONFIRMATORY TESTING

Selection based on history, clinical signs, and results of initial database:

- Cerebrospinal fluid tap: cytologic evaluation, culture, serologic testing for IgA or infectious agents
- Myelogram: identify and discern between extradural compression (IVDD), intradural/extramedullary lesion (meningioma), or intramedullary lesion (other neoplasia or cord swelling [e.g., due to FCE])
- Urine culture (diskospondylitis)
- Blood culture and sensitivity (diskospondylitis, osteomyelitis, bacterial meningitis)

- Needle aspirate of intervertebral disk (diskospondylitis)
- Serology: *Brucella canis* (diskospondylitis), rickettsial diseases (polyarthritis, meningitis)
- Arthrocentesis: cytology (polyarthritis), culture (septic polyarthritis or meningitis)
- Advanced imaging: computed tomography or magnetic resonance imaging, if lesion is suspected but not identified on myelogram
- Biopsy of vertebral bone (neoplasia, osteomyelitis)

TREATMENT

THERAPEUTIC GOAL(S)

- Elimination of infectious or noninfectious paraspinal inflammatory causes
- Elimination of any compressive lesion on spinal cord or nerve roots
- Stabilization of vertebral column

ACUTE GENERAL TREATMENT

Address the underlying cause

CHRONIC TREATMENT

- Degenerative joint disease may require persistent or recurrent nonsteroidal anti-inflammatory drug (NSAID) administration.
- Chronic intervertebral disk disease or immune-mediated disease may require intermittent or persistent corticosteroid treatment.
- Antibiotic therapy for diskospondylitis (see Diskospondylitis, p 310) or vertebral osteomyelitis continued for 6 weeks beyond resolution of clinical signs.

DRUG INTERACTIONS

Corticosteroids and NSAIDs must not be administered concurrently due to the risk of severe gastrointestinal ulceration.

POSSIBLE COMPLICATIONS

- Worsening or recurrence of signs
- Progression of spinal cord lesions
- Myelomalacia
- Valvular endocarditis, for infectious conditions

RECOMMENDED MONITORING

- Repeat physical and neurologic examination within 12 to 24 hours of treatment
- Follow-up examination and radiographs as needed

PROGNOSIS AND OUTCOME

Variable, depending on underlying cause

PEARLS & CONSIDERATIONS

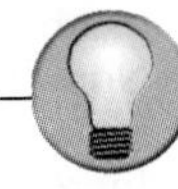

COMMENTS

- Localization of pain requires thorough physical and neurologic examination.
- Acute back pain with neurologic deficits may represent a surgical emergency and should be evaluated immediately.

CLIENT EDUCATION

- Owner should monitor for recurrence of signs
- Acute worsening of signs warrants emergency evaluation and treatment

SUGGESTED READING

Lorenz MD, Kornegay JN: *Handbook of Veterinary Neurology*. St. Louis, WB Saunders, 2004, pp 345–353.

Webb AA: Potential sources of neck and back pain in clinical conditions of dogs and cats: a review. *Vet J* 165:193–213, 2003.

AUTHOR: **PETER MOAK**

EDITOR: **ETIENNE CÔTÉ**

Barbiturates Toxicosis

BASIC INFORMATION

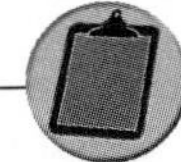

DEFINITION

Barbiturates are substituted pyrimidine derivatives with hypnotic, sedative, and anticonvulsant properties. Barbiturate toxicosis refers to the onset of clinical signs caused by an acute, excessive exposure (generally by ingestion) to this class of substances. The chronic effects of therapeutic phenobarbital use are discussed in greater detail in Phenobarbital: Adverse Effects/Toxicoses (p 844).

SYNONYM(S)

Based on their half-lives, barbiturates are divided into ultra-short-acting, short-acting, and long-acting drugs:

- Ultra-short-acting: methohexital (Brevital), thiamylal (Surital), thiopental (Pentothal)
- Short-acting: butabarbital (Buticaps, Butisol, Barbased, Butolan), hexobarbital (Evipal), pentobarbital (Nembutal), secobarbital (Seconal)
- Long-acting: phenobarbital, primidone (metabolized to phenobarbital), metharbital (not available in United States)

EPIDEMIOLOGY

SPECIES, AGE, SEX: All species, breeds, and sexes of companion animals susceptible; dogs more likely to be involved.

GENETICS AND BREED PREDISPOSITION

- Underlying liver disease can result in prolonged blood levels of any barbiturates
- Patients with renal insufficiency may accumulate unmetabolized drug (may require dose adjustment)

RISK FACTORS

- Change in diet, body weight, body composition, and age of animal may alter pharmacokinetics
- Low body fat (greyhounds and other sight hounds): metabolize more slowly
- Available sources include prescription medications, euthanized animals not properly disposed of (e.g., carcass not buried to a sufficient depth)

CLINICAL PRESENTATION

HISTORY, CHIEF COMPLAINT

- History/evidence of exposure
- Rapid onset of somnolence, lack of response to stimulation, ataxia, hyporeflexia

PHYSICAL EXAM FINDINGS

- Slow, shallow respiration
- Hypothermia
- Decreased response to stimuli
- Hypotension
    - Poor pulse quality
    - Prolonged capillary refill time

ETIOLOGY AND PATHOPHYSIOLOGY

- Toxicosis occurs when animals accidentally eat large amounts (phenobarbital) or from an overdose of injectable barbiturate (pentobarbital, euthanasia solution given to the wrong patient) or due to eating flesh from an animal that had been euthanized with a barbiturate-containing product.
- Toxicosis is characterized by hyporeflexia, ataxia, hypothermia, hypotension,

coma, slow shallow respiration, and death.
- Nonselective depression of both presynaptic and postsynaptic excitability.
- Increased threshold for electrical stimulation in motor cortex.

DIAGNOSIS

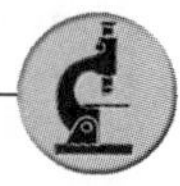

DIFFERENTIAL DIAGNOSIS

- Other intoxications:
  - Nonbarbiturate sedatives (benzodiazepines)
  - Ethanol, ethylene glycol
  - Muscle relaxants (baclofen)
  - Marijuana
  - Opioids
  - Ivermectin
- Nontoxicologic disorders:
  - Hepatic encephalopathy
  - Hypoglycemia
  - Hypocalcemia
  - Primary intracranial disorder (encephalitis, neoplasia, etc.)

INITIAL DATABASE

- Complete blood count, serum chemistry profile: expected to be within normal range
- Increased liver enzymes with chronic phenobarbital use in dogs are not necessarily due to liver dysfunction (see Phenobarbital: Adverse Effects/ Toxicoses, p 844)
- Arterial blood pressure: establish baseline and continue to monitor for hypotension

ADVANCED OR CONFIRMATORY TESTING

- Abdominal radiography. Intact phenobarbital tablets may be radiopaque.
- Semiquantitative and qualitative immunoassays available for secobarbital, amobarbital, butabarbital, pentobarbital, phenobarbital, and talbutal: use urine, serum, or plasma.

TREATMENT

THERAPEUTIC GOAL(S)

- Decontamination of patient
- Supportive care

ACUTE GENERAL TREATMENT

- Supportive care:
  - Intravenous administration of isotonic crystalloid fluids (warmed if animal in hypothermic as well), rate titrated to support blood pressure
  - If hypothermia: external warmth (see Hypothermia, p 573)
  - If hypoventilation or apnea:
    - Positive-pressure ventilation
    - Cuffed endotracheal tube to protect airway (always with mouth gag/speculum in place to avoid tube chewing). Monitoring and airway care essential (hourly [or more] tube cleaning, avoiding pressure injury from overinflated cuff, etc.)
- Decontamination of patient:
  - Emesis: useful within 2 to 4 hours only in animals not showing clinical signs (3% hydrogen peroxide 2 ml/kg PO once, to maximum 45 ml)
  - Activated charcoal (1-2 g/kg PO once, with sorbital or other cathartic); repeating charcoal (half of the original dose) two to three times every 6 to 8 hours will help decrease severity and duration of signs. May be ingested by patient if conscious and stable, or given by stomach tube (see Gastric Intubation, Gavage, Lavage, p 1258)
  - Gastric lavage: consider where emesis is contraindicated (coma) or where large toxic doses have been ingested (see Gastric Intubation, Gavage, Lavage, p 1258)
  - Enema may help promote gastrointestinal evacuation; administer additional activated charcoal (as an enema; same as PO dose, but diluted to make more watery)
  - Peritoneal or hemodialysis may be considered if hemodynamic compromise occurs, but likely not any more helpful than fluids and repeated doses of activated charcoal

DRUG INTERACTIONS

- Benzodiazepines: additive central nervous system and respiratory depressive effects
- Preexisting liver disease may prolong duration of signs

POSSIBLE COMPLICATIONS

- Aspiration pneumonia
- Renal impairment secondary to hypotension

RECOMMENDED MONITORING

- Respiration rate, blood pressure, body temperature, level of alertness
- Monitor electrolytes if using repeat doses of cathartic in the activated charcoal

PROGNOSIS AND OUTCOME

- With coma, prognosis guarded until signs of improved consciousness are seen
- Respiratory arrest is a primary risk

PEARLS & CONSIDERATIONS

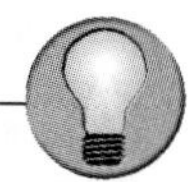

COMMENTS

- At-home decontamination (induction of vomiting) should be considered only if no clinical signs are present, if an observed ingestion took place, or if the pet was found with the container.
- Boiling or freezing of meat does not destroy barbiturates. Barbiturate-contaminated meat is a true risk for relay (secondary) poisoning.
- Acute signs of toxicosis (depending on the dose and the type of agent involved) can last several days.
- Orally administered activated charcoal acts as a "sink" that draws in barbiturates such as phenobarbital. Therefore, administration of repeated doses of activated charcoal is useful in all instances of acute barbiturate toxicosis, even when overdose occurs from barbiturate injection.

PREVENTION

- Keep medications out of animal's reach.
- Awareness of where pets roam when unsupervised.
- To prevent secondary acute poisoning, animals euthanized with barbiturates should not be used for animal (or human) consumption.

CLIENT EDUCATION

- Need to control or monitor pet's environment
- Location of nearest veterinary hospital at any time of day or night

SUGGESTED READING

Plumb DC: Pentobarbital sodium. In *Plumb's Veterinary Drug Handbook*. Ames, IA, Blackwell, 2005, pp 811-813.

Plumb DC: Phenobarbital sodium. In *Plumb's Veterinary Drug Handbook*. Ames, IA, Blackwell, 2005, pp 820-823.

Rader JD: Anticonvulsants. In Plumlee K (ed): *Clinical Veterinary Toxicology*. St. Louis, Mosby, 2003, pp 284-285.

AUTHOR: **MARY M. SCHELL**

EDITOR: **SAFDAR A. KHAN**

Barking, Excessive

BASIC INFORMATION

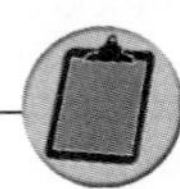

DEFINITION

One of a number of canine vocalizations. Excessive barking usually involves either a normal amount of barking that is unacceptable in the human context, or a pathologic amount of barking as part of an anxiety disorder or other behavioral disorder.

SYNONYM(S)

The predominant vocalization for some breeds may be a bay or howl (e.g., hounds and northern breeds such as the Siberian husky) or a whine/yodel (e.g., basenji).

EPIDEMIOLOGY

SPECIES, AGE, SEX: Dogs of any age or gender can bark, although puppy vocalizations may more often be associated with care-seeking behaviors, and adult vocalizations may more often be associated with care-giving behaviors and those associated with social interaction and cohesion.

GENETICS AND BREED PREDISPOSITION: Normal barking quality and quantity have been greatly influenced by human-selection for specific behaviors. Pathologic barking (defined by its excessiveness and quality, given the context of the situation eliciting the barking) is devoid of breed or gender preference, although a dog's body size may affect the pitch.

RISK FACTORS

- Dogs in multidog households may experience social facilitation in which the behaviors of one individual in a group encourage similar behaviors in others.
- In breeds that have been selected for specific vocalization behaviors, such vocalizations may become more annoying to the clients and/or their neighbors and still be normal.
- Dogs that are naturally vocal may have excessive barking as a salient sign that is part of a true behavioral disorder (see Associated Conditions and Disorders below).

CONTAGION AND ZOONOSIS: In the case of undesirable or abnormal behaviors, naïve and newly added puppies or adults may learn barking and other vocalization behaviors by observation. This will reinforce the patient's barking and may compound any anxiety-related problem.

GEOGRAPHY AND SEASONALITY: Dogs kept outdoors are more likely to use barking as a routine form of communication with other dogs in the vicinity. This may be especially true if the dogs are confined and not leash-walked, and so unable to obtain as much environmental information through olfaction.

ASSOCIATED CONDITIONS AND DISORDERS: Barking may be a nonspecific sign in any anxiety-based disorder, including separation anxiety, aggression, obsessive-compulsive disorder, and noise and storm phobias.

CLINICAL PRESENTATION

HISTORY, CHIEF COMPLAINT

- Excessive barking is noted by client at home. In some cases, however, clients may not know about the barking unless neighbors complain, unless they can listen at home, or unless they record the dogs in their absence.
- Barking can appear indiscriminate or as a response to external stimuli. For example, barking that is associated with an anxiety disorder may also be characterized by hypervigilant behavior (continuous monitoring of the social and physical environments). In these cases, dogs may scan at windows, along fences, and at doors. Clients may also describe the patient as unable to rest or settle down for any considerable amount of time.
- Important elements of the history that should be elicited include whether it occurs in the owner's absence (e.g., associated with separation anxiety), whether it ends with the owner's inadvertently rewarding the behavior, as with a treat to "silence" the dog (i.e., learned behavior), etc.

PHYSICAL EXAM FINDINGS

- Generally unremarkable
- If barking represents a change in behavior, vocal cords and surrounding tissue may become edematous
- Rarely, a source of pain or other physical abnormality can be identified as a trigger for barking or whining

ETIOLOGY AND PATHOPHYSIOLOGY

- A simplistic interpretation is to believe that barking is only used agonistically (e.g., to increase the distance between two or more interacting individuals.) However, depending on the pitch, tone, frequency, and pattern, barking may be used for making contact with other individuals (including when reuniting after being apart), to signal alarm, to signal concern or distress, and to solicit information from other dogs. Barking can also be a sign of an anxiety disorder, including obsessive-compulsive disorder (also see Separation Anxiety, p 993).
- As with other animal species, slight variations in vocalization/barking are likely capable of conveying subtle shades of meaning that may be overlooked by clients; however, if queried carefully and without prejudice, clients can describe these nuances even if their interpretation of the meaning is inexact.

DIAGNOSIS

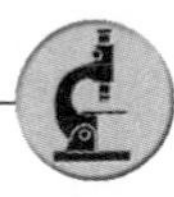

DIFFERENTIAL DIAGNOSIS

Excessive barking

- Normal barking, especially alarm barking by watch and guard dogs selected to alert by barking, reactive barking in terrier and hound breeds, and working barking in some herding breeds. These barking behaviors can be modified with humane training and are typically context-appropriate, although inconvenient or undesirable for some clients.
- Learned behavior. Barking that elicits a response/reward from the client (e.g., the client lets the dog out when it barks, or pets it to "calm it down").
- Separation anxiety.
- Thunderstorm phobia.
- Noise phobia.
- Obsessive-compulsive disorder.

Change in vocalization

- Laryngeal paralysis, laryngeal masses, and thyroid neoplasia can result in changes in bark quality (see Voice Change, p 1157), which must be differentiated from barking-induced hoarseness and for owner-induced trauma to the cervical region through leash, choke chain, or pinch collar "corrections."

INITIAL DATABASE

Minimum database: complete blood count, serum chemistry profile, and urinalysis to rule out any underlying contraindications for psychotropic medication, if their use is warranted. Other laboratory or imaging procedures should address any other concurrent physical exam findings.

ADVANCED OR CONFIRMATORY TESTING

Learned behaviors are ruled out if they are extinguished by complete removal of the reward. The longer the behavior has been ongoing, reinforced, or rewarded, the longer eradication of the learned behavior will take.

TREATMENT

THERAPEUTIC GOAL(S)

To treat the disorder based on accurate identification of cause

ACUTE GENERAL TREATMENT

- If barking is within the normal behavioral repertoire, given triggers and context, the dog can be taught when and when not to bark. This can be done by rewarding "good barking" and not "bad barking," and coupling both to words used only in those situations.
- If barking is pathologic, the anxiety state that leads to the abnormal vocalization must be treated.
  - Identify triggers and limit exposure to them whenever possible.
  - When barking occurs, redirect the dog's attention and activity to alternative behaviors (play, relaxation), and reward for compliance. It may be necessary to use a leash to remove the dog from the situation before asking for the alternative behavior. Reward any and all decreases in barking in response to triggers. A head collar can be used to gently close the dog's mouth and interrupt the cycle of barking, but this strategy must be accompanied by others that indicate to the dog which behaviors will be rewarded.
  - A neutral stimulus (noise, citronella spray burst) may be used for interrupting the behavior followed by positive engagement in a different, non-barking-related behavior that can be rewarded.
  - Treatment with psychotropic medication is only appropriate if barking is abnormal (i.e., one manifestation of a behavioral disorder) (e.g., anxiety). Under such circumstances, an accurate diagnosis is essential, and treatment may include such medications as amitriptyline, fluoxetine, or clomipramine.
  - Punishment, yelling, and shock should be avoided. Aversive responses serve only to increase, rather than decrease, arousal and may exacerbate the barking behavior.

CHRONIC TREATMENT

- Dogs should be taught to relax while making eye contact with the clients as a preferred default/substitute behavior when the dog encounters a situation about which it is anxious or unsure.
- Systematic desensitization can be used if the triggers can be identified and manipulated.
- Alternative ways of alerting (sitting in a designated spot or in front of the clients) should be taught, so that the dog is still allowed to signal information.

DRUG INTERACTIONS

Amitriptyline, fluoxetine, and clomipramine should not be used with monoamine oxidase inhibitors (e.g., some tick collars, and flea, tick, and mite dips, and some medications used for treating cognitive dysfunction).

POSSIBLE COMPLICATIONS

- Clients who try to work with behavior modification too quickly (e.g., rewarding sitting even if the dog is distressed, instead or working to teach the dog to relax) may experience slow or no progress. In some cases, forcefulness of working with the dog can make the dog worse. Lack of consensus in application of treatment modification within a multiple-person household can have the same effect.
- Clients who have used leash, choke chain, or pinch collar "corrections" may have damaged the dog's esophagus, trachea, larynx, thyroid, and recurrent laryngeal nerves, resulting in changes in the quality of vocalization, with or without changes in swallowing and respiratory functions.

RECOMMENDED MONITORING

Follow-up in each case is individualized. Frequent follow-up with the clients—at least weekly—is helpful. Medications should be monitored for any cardiac, renal, or hepatic side effects (uncommon) or sedation (more common).

PROGNOSIS AND OUTCOME

- For species-appropriate but inconvenient barking, prognosis is very good to excellent
- For pathologic barking, prognosis ranges from fair to very good depending on severity and chronicity of disorder
- Both are influenced by client compliance, environmental circumstances, and response to psychotropic medication in the case of pathologic barking

PEARLS & CONSIDERATIONS

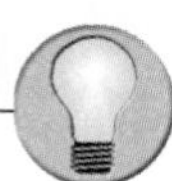

COMMENTS

Shock collars have *no* place in the treatment of any behavioral condition. They will *always* exacerbate anxiety, even if they may suppress some aspects of behavioral signs. In normal dogs, the likelihood for intended or unintended abuse or misuse greatly outweighs any potential benefit. Because the desire to use such methods may be associated with client anger, assessment for the potential risk of abuse directed at pets, spouses, and children should be made in any case in which such techniques have been used or the clients wish to use them (see Abuse, p 14). Animals learn from shock, but they are not learning what the clients think they are: rather, they are learning fear and avoidance. This is far below the level of teaching to which we should all aspire, and may in turn lead to other behavioral disorders.

PREVENTION

Early intervention. When dogs are added to the home, education of the dog as to what level of barking is acceptable to the client should be instituted on the first episode of unwanted barking.

CLIENT EDUCATION

Yelling at a dog to be quiet will increase arousal and is therefore counterproductive. Clients can teach their dog the level of alarm barking they will tolerate by calmly taking the barking dog away from the trigger (using a leash if necessary), asking for an alternative behavior (sitting while looking at the client in a relaxed fashion), and then rewarding the quiet response.

SUGGESTED READING

Ascione FR, Arkow P (eds): *Child Abuse, Domestic Violence, and Animal Abuse: Linking the Circles of Compassion for Prevention and Intervention*. West Lafayette, IN, Purdue University Press, 1999.

Juarbe-Diaz SV: Assessment and treatment of excessive barking in the domestic dog. *Vet Clin North Am Small Anim Pract* 27:515-532, 1997.

Schilder MBH, van der Borg JAM: Training dogs with help of the shock collar: Short and long term behavioral effects. *Appl Anim Behav Sci* 85:319-334, 2004.

AUTHOR: **SORAYA V. JUARBE-DIAZ**

EDITOR: **KAREN L. OVERALL**

Bartonellosis

BASIC INFORMATION

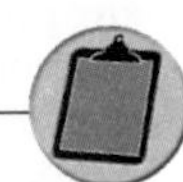

DEFINITION

Bartonellosis is an emerging vector-transmitted disease of humans and domestic and wild mammals caused by bacteria of the genus *Bartonella*. These organisms are fastidious, pleomorphic, aerobic, gram-negative rods. In vivo *Bartonella* spp. can cause intracellular infections and are known to infect erythrocytes and endothelial cells.

EPIDEMIOLOGY

SPECIES, AGE, SEX
- Dogs: any age and sex
- Cats: any age and sex

GENETICS AND BREED PREDISPOSITION
- Dogs: herding dogs may be at increased risk, while toy breeds may have a decreased risk for infection (these correlations may be environmentally related rather than true breed predilections)
- Cats: no reported breed predispositions

RISK FACTORS: The risk of infection increases with exposure to vectors such as sand flies, lice, fleas, and ticks. Hence dogs that live in rural environments, have free access to roam the outdoors, and contact other animals regularly have higher rates of infection. Immunocompromised individuals may also be at increased risk of infection.

CONTAGION AND ZOONOSIS: Eight *Bartonella* spp. or subspecies are known to infect humans:
- *B. henselae*: cat scratch disease, endocarditis, bacillary angiomatosis
- *B. vinsonii* subsp. *berkhoffi*: endocarditis
- *B. vinsonii* subsp. *arupensis*: endocarditis
- *B. clarridgeiae*: cat scratch disease
- *B. elizabethae*: endocarditis
- *B. washoensis*: endocarditis
- *B. quintana*: trench fever, endocarditis, bacillary angiomatosis
- *B. bacilliformis*: Carrion's disease, Oroya fever, verruca peruana

GEOGRAPHY AND SEASONALITY: Seroprevalence is increased in warm humid climates, although *Bartonella* spp. are being identified worldwide. Seasonal occurrence of disease may be seen in association with vector exposure.

ASSOCIATED CONDITIONS AND DISORDERS
- Dogs:
  - Endocarditis
  - Myocarditis and arrhythmias
  - Peliosis hepatis
  - Granulomatous and lymphocytic hepatitis.
  - Granulomatous lymphadenitis
  - Epistaxis
  - Granulomatous rhinitis
  - Polyarthritis
- Evidence of *Bartonella* exposure has been identified in patients with the following disorders; however, a cause/effect relationship has not been established:
  - Immune-mediated hemolytic anemia
  - Cutaneous vasculitis
  - Anterior uveitis and choroiditis
  - Meningoencephalitis
- Cats:
  - Endocarditis (rare)
  - The high prevalence of *Bartonella* infections in cats makes clinical associations with diseases difficult to make. A correlation with some conditions such as stomatitis and uveitis has been suggested.

CLINICAL PRESENTATION

DISEASE FORMS/SUBTYPES
- Dogs: naturally infected with *B. vinsonii* subspecies *berkhoffi*, *B. henselae*, *B. clarridgeiae*, *B. elizabethae*, *B. washoensis*.
- Cats: naturally infected with *B. henselae*, *B. clarridgeiae*, *B. koehlerae*, and *B. bovis*. Cats may be bacteremic for several weeks to more than a year.

HISTORY, CHIEF COMPLAINT: Dogs: affected individuals may have one or more of the following presentations:
- Weakness
- Lethargy
- Anorexia
- Nasal discharge and/or epistaxis
- Lameness
- Other reported signs include vomiting, diarrhea, cough, and seizures
- Subclinical and nonspecific signs are also possible

Cats: affected individuals may have one or more of the following presentations:
- Lethargy
- Anorexia
- Reproductive difficulty
- Subclinical infections are very common

PHYSICAL EXAM FINDINGS
- Dogs: affected individuals may have one or more of the following findings:
  - Fever
  - Splenomegaly
  - Lameness
  - Evidence of vasculitis
  - Heart murmur
  - Lymphadenopathy
  - Hepatomegaly
  - Neurologic dysfunction
  - Uveitis
  - Nasal discharge/epistaxis
  - Some affected dogs have no abnormal findings detected during physical examination
- Cats: affected individuals may have one or more of the following findings:
  - Many cats have no abnormal findings
  - Fever
  - Lymphadenitis
  - *Bartonella*-associated stomatitis, uveitis, and neurologic dysfunction have also been reported
  - Coinfection with feline immunodeficiency virus (FIV) may be associated with stomatitis and lymphadenopathy

ETIOLOGY AND PATHOPHYSIOLOGY

- Dogs: Data support that a tick vector (*Rhipicephalus sanguineus*, *Dermacentor* spp., or *Ixodes* spp.) is the likely source of *Bartonella vinsonii* subspecies *berkhoffi* and possibly other *Bartonella* infections.
  - *Bartonella* infections are associated with a cyclical CD8+ cell lymphopenia, modulation of adhesion molecules on CD8+ T-cells, defective monocytic phagocytosis, and impaired B-cell antigen presentation within lymph nodes.
- Cats: *Bartonella henselae* is believed to be transmitted via the inoculation of infected flea (*Ctenocephalides felis*) feces rather than flea bites. Direct and vertical transmission from cat to cat has not been identified. The sources of other feline *Bartonella* infections are unknown.
- Ultimately, clinical disease appears to be dependent on the status and response of the host immune system, resulting in focal suppurative/granulomatous reactions, endovascular *Bartonella* multiplication, or a multifocal angioproliferative response.

DIAGNOSIS

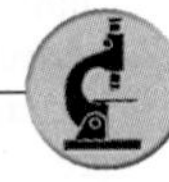

DIFFERENTIAL DIAGNOSIS

- Bacterial endocarditis
- Other vector-borne diseases, including *Rickettsia*, *Ehrlichia*, *Babesia*, and *Borrelia* infections
- Systemic fungal infections, including histoplasmosis, blastomycosis, and coccidioidomycosis
- Neoplasia
- Immune-mediated disease
- Feline leukemia virus and feline immunodeficiency virus (cats)

- Endocarditis, infective
- Polyarthritis

INITIAL DATABASE

- Complete blood count
  - Dogs: Thrombocytopenia, anemia, neutrophilic leukocytosis, monocytosis, and eosinophilia are the most commonly reported abnormalities detected in patients infected with *B. vinsonii* subspecies *berkhoffi*.
  - Cats: No consistent abnormalities have been identified, although a transient anemia and persistent eosinophilia have been reported.
- Serum biochemistry panel
  - Dogs: Increased liver enzymes and hypoalbuminemia are the most commonly reported abnormalities. Other changes may be detected secondary to end-organ damage rather than a direct effect of *Bartonella* infection.
  - Cats: No consistent abnormalities have been identified.
- Urinalysis
  - Dogs: No consistent abnormalities have been identified.
  - Cats: No consistent abnormalities have been identified.
- Arthrocentesis
  - Dogs: neutrophilic, lymphocytic, or mononuclear polyarthritis.
- Cerebral spinal fluid
  - Dogs: No consistent abnormalities have been identified.

ADVANCED OR CONFIRMATORY TESTING

- Dogs:
  - Immunofluorescence assays (IFA) for IgG antibodies are widely used for confirming exposure to *Bartonella*. Cross reactivity and non-reactivity are potential pitfalls. Sensitivity and specificity have not been clearly established. In most laboratories, titers ≥1:64 are considered seroreactive.
  - Amplification of *Bartonella* DNA by polymerase chain reaction (PCR) from blood and tissue samples can be used to establish a diagnosis of infection. Cross-priming and sample contamination may result in false-positive results. Low number of circulating organisms can result in false-negative results.
  - Routine microbiologic techniques are often not adequate for the growth of *Bartonella* spp. Isolation via culture on blood agar plates has poor diagnostic sensitivity in dogs and may take as long as 30 to 60 days to result in detectable growth of *Bartonella* organisms. A recently described liquid media preparation (*Bartonella-Alphaproteobacteria* growth medium) has resulted in faster, more sensitive detection of *Bartonella*, but it is not yet routinely available for diagnostic use.
- Cats: Definitive identification of *Bartonella* as a causative agent of disease is difficult given the large number of chronically infected healthy cats.
  - Antibody testing is recommended on adopting new cats, especially kittens that immunocompromised individuals wish to adopt. Seronegative antibody tests have a strong correlation with the lack of bacteremia.
  - Serology is of otherwise limited utility in cats.
  - Both IFA and Western blot testing for anti-*B. henselae* antibodies are widely available.
  - PCR can accurately identify *Bartonella* infections in cats but does not necessarily indicate that bartonellosis is the cause of disease.
  - Definitive isolation via culture on agar plates is still considered the gold standard for confirming bacteremia, although multiple cultures may be necessary because of intermittent bacteremia.

TREATMENT

THERAPEUTIC GOAL(S)

At the current time there is not a treatment consensus. Treatment should be considered in bacteremic individuals, particularly if clinical signs are apparent. A lack of resolution of disease after treatment should prompt clinicians to consider alternative diagnoses. Seroreactive patients (titers >1:64) should be treated only after first considering the *Bartonella* species identified and the antibody prevalence within the population before instituting therapy.

GENERAL TREATMENT

- A well-established antibiotic protocol does not yet exist for the treatment of *Bartonella* in dogs or cats, and current protocols are extrapolated from experimental studies or human medicine. In human medicine, prolonged use of tetracyclines, erythromycin, rifampin, azithromycin, doxycycline, or a combination of these antibiotics has been used effectively.
- Dogs: Azithromycin (e.g., small dogs: 10 mg/kg, medium dogs: 7 mg/kg, large dogs: 5 mg/kg. Give PO q 24h × 7 days, then q 48h × 5 weeks) and other macrolides have been used given their ability to obtain high intracellular concentrations. Alternatively, other antibiotics that can obtain high intracellular concentrations (doxycycline [10 mg/kg PO q 24h], enrofloxacin) could possibly be beneficial, but efficacy has not been proven for any of these drugs in clinical veterinary medicine. In principle, prolonged treatment for 4 to 6 weeks is recommended. However, the high rate of incidentally discovered infections in otherwise normal animals indicates that initiation of treatment should be considered only if compatible clinical signs are present and other possible causes have been ruled out.
- Cats: Azithromycin (10 mg/kg PO q 24h × 7 days, then q 48h × 5 weeks) has been used; however, there is no antibiotic protocol that has been shown to clear cats of infection. At the present time, there are no definitive recommendations for treatment.

CHRONIC TREATMENT

- There are no clear recommendations for chronic relapsing disease in dogs and cats. Alternative diagnoses should be strongly considered in patients that "fail" treatment.
- In human medicine, a course of antibiotics for 4 to 6 months is recommended for patients who experience a relapse of bacteremia.

POSSIBLE COMPLICATIONS

Recurrent/persistent infection

RECOMMENDED MONITORING

- Resolution of clinical signs after therapy.
- Antibody titers can be followed during treatment (at 1 month) and post-treatment (at 6 months) to follow antibody trends. A resolution of detectable antibodies is generally considered a positive outcome. The significance of persistent antibody titers after treatment is unknown.

PROGNOSIS AND OUTCOME

Depending on the clinical presentation, the prognosis can vary tremendously.

PEARLS & CONSIDERATIONS

COMMENTS

- Coinfection with multiple *Bar-tonella* spp. and subtypes, as well as with other vector transmitted infections, is possible and should be considered in some cases.
- Defining bartonellosis as a clinical entity is still in its infancy.
- It remains unknown in many circumstances whether *Bartonella* is a primary pathogen, opportunistic invader, or incidental finding.
- It is well established that *Bartonella vinsonii* subspecies *berkhoffi* is an important infective agent in dogs, while the clinical implications of *Bartonella henselae* bacteremia in both dogs and cats remains to be elucidated.

PREVENTION

Consistent use of flea and tick preventatives is recommended.

CLIENT EDUCATION

- Monitor for recurrence of presenting signs.
- Since the current understanding of the pathology and treatment of bartonellosis is far from complete, clients should be cautioned that treatment may not result in resolution of clinical disease. Some reasons for treatment failure may include failure to eradicate the infection or other disease conditions besides *Bartonella* causing the clinical signs.
- Zoonosis is possible, and immunocompromised individuals should be particularly cautious when adopting new pets.

SUGGESTED READING

Boulouis H, et al: Factors associated with the rapid emergence of zoonotic *Bartonella* infections. *Vet Res* 36:383–410, 2005.

Breitschwerdt E, et al: Clinicopathological abnormalities and treatment response in 24 dogs seroreactive to *Bartonella vinsonii (berkhoffi)* antigens. *J Am Anim Hosp Assoc* 40:92–101, 2004.

Chomel B, et al: Cat scratch disease and other zoonotic *Bartonella* infections. *J Am Vet Med Assoc* 224:1270–1279, 2004.

Glaus T, et al: Seroprevalence of *Bartonella henselae* infection and correlation with disease status in cats in Switzerland. *J Clin Mircobiol* 35:2883–2885, 1997.

Guptill L. Bartonellosis. *Vet Clin Small Anim* 33:809–825, 2003.

Guptill L, et al: Prevalence, risk factors, and genetic diversity of *Bartonella henselae* infections in pet cats in four regions of the United States. *J Clin Mircobiol* 42:652–659, 2004.

Henn J, et al: Seroprevalence of antibodies against *Bartonella* species and evaluation of risk factors and clinical signs associated with seropositivity in dogs. *Am J Vet Res* 66:688–694, 2005.

Maggi R, et al: Novel chemically modified liquid growth medium that will support the growth of seven *Bartonella* species. *J Clin Mircobiol* 43:2651–2655, 2005.

AUTHORS: **MICHAEL W. WOOD, ADAM BIRKENHEUER**
EDITOR: **DOUGLASS K. MACINTIRE**

Baylisascaris Infection

BASIC INFORMATION

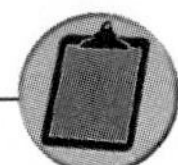

DEFINITION

A rare but potentially devastating zoonosis involving parasitic infection with the raccoon roundworm *Baylisascaris procyonis*

SYNONYM(S)

Ocular or neural larval migrans
Raccoon roundworm, visceral

EPIDEMIOLOGY

SPECIES, AGE, SEX

- Raccoons are the natural host for the mature enteric parasite. However, larvae can infect more than 90 species of birds and mammals, including dogs.
- Cats appear to be only marginally susceptible, or even resistant, to disease due to *Baylisascaris* larva migrans.

RISK FACTORS

- Zoonosis occurs when humans acquire the parasite by the fecal-oral route. Therefore, exposure to raccoon feces is a major risk factor (e.g., in uncovered outdoor sandboxes or similar "latrines," which are areas where raccoons specifically choose to defecate).
- Dog feces have also been shown to contain *Baylisascaris* eggs when the dog is infected with intestinal, adult *B. procyonis*.
- Ingestion of intermediate hosts such as small rodents by raccoons or other mammals (e.g., dogs) may also cause infection if the intermediate host's tissues contain *Baylisascaris* larvae.

CONTAGION AND ZOONOSIS: Infective eggs within the environment can cause an often fatal meningoencephalitis in humans with children less than 2 years old at highest risk.

GEOGRAPHY AND SEASONALITY: More common in the midwestern and northeastern United States and California. Infected raccoons have also been reported in Georgia.

CLINICAL PRESENTATION

DISEASE FORMS/SUBTYPES

- Clinical illness due to *B. procyonis* is extremely uncommon in small animal medicine; neurologic and ocular signs are theoretically possible.
- Rather, the greatest concern is regarding the zoonotic potential of *B. procyonis* eggs passed in raccoon, or rarely, canine, feces.
- In humans, visceral larval migrans (VLM), ocular larval migrans (OLM), and neural larval migrans (NLM) may be observed.

HISTORY, CHIEF COMPLAINT

- Dogs infected with *B. procyonis* generally show no clinical signs, and harbor the parasite without outward evidence of infection. Rarely, dogs may sustain larva migrans that causes overt clinical signs as early as 9 to 10 days after ingestion of raccoon feces.
- Signs often progress rapidly over several days.

PHYSICAL EXAM FINDINGS

- NLM: Depression, ataxia, head tilt, circling, nystagmus, opisthotonos, recumbency, coma
- OLM: Blindness, signs of uveitis (red eye, photophobia, etc.), observable larvae within the eye/retina
- VLM: Usually an incidental finding without clinical signs

ETIOLOGY AND PATHOPHYSIOLOGY

- All animals (including dogs and humans) are infected by ingesting the eggs of *Baylisascaris* shed in the feces of raccoons. Raccoons originally become infected in the same manner, or by ingesting intermediate hosts (see Risk Factors).
- Once ingested, the larvae hatch within the intestine and begin to migrate (*larva migrans*) through the liver, lungs, brain, and eyes as early as 3 days postinfection.
- Migration of only one or two larvae through the brain can cause destruction of the white matter (leukomalacia) and severe inflammation and necrosis.
- Eggs become infective 24 to 48 hours after being passed by the raccoon. Infective eggs are highly stable and may remain viable within the environment for years.
- Eggs are most susceptible to heat.

DIAGNOSIS

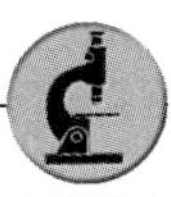

DIFFERENTIAL DIAGNOSIS

In dogs and raccoons, signs of central nervous system dysfunction are *very uncommonly* due to *Baylisascaris* infection. Causes that are much more common include:

- Other infectious causes of encephalitis: toxoplasmosis, tick-borne diseases, neospora, canine distemper virus
- Granulomatous meningoencephalitis
- Toxin exposure

- Neoplasia
- Metabolic disease (e.g., hepatic encephalopathy, hypoglycemia)

INITIAL DATABASE

- Complete blood count: possible eosinophilia
- Serum biochemistry profile, urinalysis: may rule out toxic or metabolic diseases
- Complete neurologic and ocular examination: asymmetry of deficits is expected if any deficits are present
- Fecal flotation and examination: More than 20 dogs in the Midwest have been shown to have a mature intestinal infection of *Baylisascaris* with infective eggs shed in their feces
- Cerebrospinal fluid tap with cytology: meningoencephalitis with increased eosinophils

ADVANCED OR CONFIRMATORY TESTING

Virtually never performed in small animal medicine given the rarity of clinical disease in dogs and cats

- Magnetic resonance imaging (brain): preferential destruction of white matter.
- Serologic testing is available for humans but is not commercially available for veterinary patients.
- Definitive diagnosis may not be possible until postmortem.

TREATMENT

THERAPEUTIC GOAL(S)

Rapid identification and treatment to prevent progression of leukomalacia and neurologic signs

ACUTE GENERAL TREATMENT

- Neurologic larva migrans (rare in dogs and cats): Corticosteroids (e.g., dexamethasone 0.1-0.2 mg/kg IV q 8-24h) are essential to stabilize the inflammatory component of the encephalitis.
- Anthelmintics: when *Baylisascaris* eggs are found incidentally on a fecal flotation.
  - Albendazole (50 mg/kg PO q 24h × 10 days or more): traditionally the antihelmintic of choice. Administration for >3 days may risk myelosuppression.
  - Milbemycin oxime (0.5-1 mg/kg PO): newer treatment. About 75% effective at eliminating *Baylisacaris* infection in dogs with one dose.
- Ocular larvae within the retina may be killed using laser photocoagulation or removed via enucleation.

CHRONIC TREATMENT

- Patients surviving the initial neurologic disease may be permanently handicapped and require supportive and nursing care.
- A long course of corticosteroids may be necessary to control the necrosis and inflammation associated with larval migration and death.

PROGNOSIS AND OUTCOME

- Severity of signs and speed of progression are related to the egg burden ingested
- Prognosis is poor if clinical signs are advanced at time of diagnosis or treatment. Fair to good if signs are mild and treated quickly

PEARLS & CONSIDERATIONS

COMMENTS

- Consider larval migrans in an animal with acute onset of neurologic disease consistent with encephalitis, especially if recent contact with raccoon environments is possible.
- *Baylisascaris* does not usually cause any outwardly observable clinical signs in raccoons.

PREVENTION

- Prevention is the most effective therapy.
- Preventing exposure to raccoons and their feces is paramount. Covering sandboxes when unused and avoiding raccoon latrines are essential.

CLIENT EDUCATION

- People and pets should avoid raccoon latrines (bases of trees, fallen logs or large rocks, forks of trees, and also attics, haylofts), which may contain raccoon feces with millions of infective eggs.
- Raccoons are attracted to sources of food. People should not attempt to feed them.
- Young children should be closely observed when outside to avoid ingestion of infective eggs.

SUGGESTED READING

Kazacos KR: Raccoon roundworms as a cause of animal and human disease. In *Proceedings,* Tufts Animal Expo, 2002.

Kazacos KR: *Baylisascaris procyonis* and related species. In Samuel WM, Pybus MJ, Kocan AA (eds): *Parasitic Diseases of Wild Mammals.* Ames, IA, Iowa State University Press, 2001, pp 301-340.

AUTHOR: **KATHRYN TAYLOR**

EDITOR: **DOUGLASS K. MACINTIRE**

Bee and Other Insect Stings

BASIC INFORMATION

DEFINITION

Stings from insects such as bees, wasps, and hornets, as well as bites from members of the class *Arachnida* such as spiders and scorpions, can result in clinical signs.

SYNONYM(S)

Insect bites

EPIDEMIOLOGY

SPECIES, AGE, SEX: Bites and stings are more likely to occur in young, inquisitive animals. Cats may be more tolerant than dogs to many insect toxins.

GENETICS AND BREED PREDISPOSITION: Boxers seem especially prone to insect reactions.

GEOGRAPHY AND SEASONALITY: Bee stings are more common during warm weather when the insects are active. Spiders and scorpions are more commonly encountered in the fall and winter when they move indoors in response to cooler temperatures outdoors.

CLINICAL PRESENTATION

DISEASE FORMS/SUBTYPES

- Bees, wasps, hornets
- Spiders and scorpions

HISTORY, CHIEF COMPLAINT

- **Bees, wasps, hornets** (order Hymenoptera):

- Animals frequently present with no known history of an insect sting. Instead, they present for clinical signs associated with an allergic reaction. Severity of signs will depend on the type of venom, location of the sting, number of stings, and sensitivity of the animal receiving the sting.
- **Spiders and scorpions:**
  - Animals may have a history of a bite from a spider or scorpion. If possible, the owner should be asked to present the insect for examination (taking care not to be stung during handling).
  - *Black widow spider* (*Latrodectus* spp.): characterized by the typical hourglass-shaped marking on the spider's abdomen.
- **Spiders:**
  - *Brown recluse spider* (*Loxosceles* spp.): Most are brown with a violin-shaped marking in the dorsal surface of the cephalothorax.
  - *Scorpion* (family Scorpaenidae): typically brown in color with a flat body and eight legs. They have two pincers and a segmented tail.
  - In many cases, there is no known exposure, and a diagnosis is made based on clinical signs.

PHYSICAL EXAM FINDINGS

- **Bees, wasps, hornets:**
  - Local reaction associated with an immunologic response is the most common finding. This may include a swollen head/face or diffuse urticaria. Cases with severe facial swelling can develop respiratory distress from upper airway obstruction and occlusion.
  - Less commonly, an animal may develop anaphylaxis. Signs of anaphylaxis may develop within 15 minutes of a sting. Anaphylaxis in dogs can manifest as vomiting, defecation, urination, muscular weakness, respiratory depression, and convulsions. Cats most often show signs of pruritis, dyspnea, salivation, incoordination, and collapse. Animals with massive envenomation may show signs of acute respiratory distress syndrome or disseminated intravascular coagulation.
- **Spiders and scorpions:**
  - *Black widow spider*: Clinical signs may develop within minutes of the bite. Clinical signs vary and include pain at the site of the bite and abdominal pain. The most severe signs can include hypersalivation, arrhythmia, diarrhea, seizures, flaccid paralysis, and death.
  - *Brown recluse spider*: Bites from the brown recluse spider are noted for the dermonecrotic effects. These effects result in a slow-healing ulcerative lesion. Initially, the bite is characterized by ecchymosis surrounded by blanching and edema. Systemic signs are less common.
  - *Scorpion*: The bites of most scorpions found in North America cause only mild discomfort and rarely require treatment. *C. sculturatus* has a neurotoxin that produces signs of parasympathetic involvement including miosis, hypotension, bronchial constriction, salivation, lacrimation, urination, and defecation.

ETIOLOGY AND PATHOPHYSIOLOGY

- Most systemic signs result from an IgE-mediated allergic reaction.
- A small number of dogs and cats may develop anaphylaxis.
- Black widow spider bites are more often associated with clinical signs than those from the brown recluse spider or the scorpion.

DIAGNOSIS

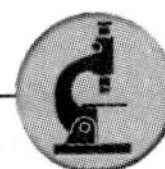

DIFFERENTIAL DIAGNOSIS

- Cellulitis
- Peripheral edema
- Acute abdomen (black widow spider)
- Nonhealing wound (brown recluse spider)

INITIAL DATABASE

- Packed cell volume
- Serum total protein
- Blood glucose
- Azo stick

TREATMENT

THERAPEUTIC GOAL(S)

- Relief of discomfort
- Prevent further edema/urticaria formation

ACUTE GENERAL TREATMENT

- Facial edema/urticaria:
  - Remove stinger, if present. Use fine forceps/tweezers or a flat object (e.g., dull side of a scalpel blade), taking care not to press on the stinger's sac (if present) to avoid injecting the remaining contents of the stinger into the patient
  - Diphenhydramine 1-2 mg/kg IM
  - Dexamethasone sodium phosphate SP 0.2 mg/kg IV slowly
- Anaphylaxis (see p 60):
  - Epinephrine 0.01 mg/kg IV
  - Intravenous fluid support
  - Diphenhydramine 1-2 mg/kg IM
  - Dexamethasone SP 0.2 mg/kg IV slowly
- Black widow spider:
  - Wound care
  - IV fluid support
- Brown recluse spider:
  - Wound excision

RECOMMENDED MONITORING

Animals with facial swelling or urticaria should be monitored for 20 to 30 minutes after therapy to ensure clinical signs are not progressing.

PROGNOSIS AND OUTCOME

Most animals with insect bites and stings have an excellent prognosis. Animals with severe systemic signs have a more guarded short-term prognosis as dictated by the severity of signs.

PEARLS & CONSIDERATIONS

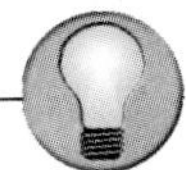

COMMENTS

Animals with facial edema of unknown origin should have their face and lips closely examined for the presence of a stinger.

PREVENTION

Avoid insects and spiders

SUGGESTED READING

Cowell AK, Cowell RL: Management of bee and other Hymenoptera stings. In Bonagura JD (ed): *Current Veterinary Therapy XII*. Philadelphia, WB Saunders, 1995, pp 226–228.

AUTHOR: **SCOTT P. SHAW**
EDITOR: **ELIZABETH ROZANSKI**

Behavioral Problem Prevention: Kittens

BASIC INFORMATION

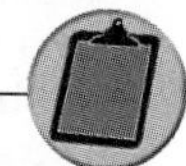

DEFINITION

The first few kitten visits set the stage for future veterinary visits because they help the new kitten owner understand normal feline behavior and help with preventing problems with litter training, scratching, biting, and chewing.

SYNONYM(S)

Kitten kindergarten
Kitten kindy
Kitten socialization
Kitten training

EPIDEMIOLOGY

SPECIES, AGE, SEX: Cats <4 months old; both sexes.
CONTAGION AND ZOONOSIS: Cat scratch fever is most commonly transmitted by kittens with fleas. Unless cats are exposed to humans when the kittens are between 2 and 9 weeks old, they are unlikely to fully adjust to people and are more at risk for such transmissions.
GEOGRAPHY AND SEASONALITY: There is seasonality to kittens in some regions of the world. Veterinary practices should remember this when structuring kitten and neutering programs.
ASSOCIATED CONDITIONS AND DISORDERS

- Increased risk of abandonment and euthanasia if owners do not understand normal feline behavior. Behavior problems are the most common reason for relinquishment of cats.
- The single biggest cause of euthanasia in pet cats in the United States is nonuse of litter boxes.

CLINICAL PRESENTATION

HISTORY, CHIEF COMPLAINT: The owner may not report any difficulties or may report difficulties with litter training, scratching, biting, or chewing.
PHYSICAL EXAM FINDINGS: Unremarkable.

ETIOLOGY AND PATHOPHYSIOLOGY

- Multifactorial.
- People keep cats ~2 years after they exhibit any problem, which often occurs at the onset or in the midst of social maturity (2 to 4 years), explaining the demographics of the relinquished cats.

DIAGNOSIS

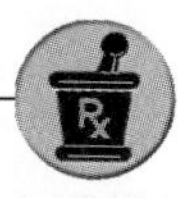

DIFFERENTIAL DIAGNOSIS

Based on the presenting signs and complaints of the owner

INITIAL DATABASE

History and physical exam are generally sufficient

TREATMENT

THERAPEUTIC GOAL(S)

- Educate owners about normal feline behavior
- Reduce the risk of surrender in the future
- Make veterinary visits as stress-free as possible for the owner and the cat

ACUTE GENERAL TREATMENT

- Rewards (e.g., treats, pats) should be given for appropriate behaviors.
- Inappropriate behaviors should be redirected and more appropriate behaviors substituted.
- Cats should not be verbally or physically punished for inappropriate behaviors.
- Cat basket training so that the cat associates the cat basket with pleasant experiences.
- Feline synthetic pheromone analog may help to decrease anxiety in some cases associated with introductions to new homes or environments, although conclusive data are lacking.

CHRONIC TREATMENT

- Appropriate behaviors must be reinforced long-term for them to be maintained.
- All future veterinary visits should use minimal restraint.
- Appropriate physical and mental stimulation is necessary, especially for indoor cats. These can include:
  - Scratching posts. These can be commercially bought or built at home from pieces of wood nailed together and covered with carpet. The posts need to be stable (so they do not fall over) and generally the larger the better (so the cat can stretch out). Some cats prefer to scratch on horizontal surfaces, others on vertical, so the posts should allow for both preferences. Cover in a material that the cat wants to use. Attaching toys on strings can also make these posts more interesting.
  - Indoor garden box. Grow grass, catnip, or catmint for cats to nibble; can provide enjoyment for many cats.
  - Tunnels, paper bags, and cardboard boxes provide good hiding places, especially if placed up high.
  - Commercially available toys such as the Bizzy Kitty, Cat Track, Kitty Kong, and Cat Dancer can provide hours of mental and physical enrichment.
  - Two kittens keep each other company and play together while the owners are at work.
  - Hide dry cat food in lots of places around the house and let the cat "hunt" for its dinner. Commercially available devices can be filled with food and left in locations for cats to find and play with to encourage cats to get more physical and mental exercise.
  - Train behaviors on cue: cats can be trained to come on cue, sit, roll over, etc.
  - Agility training. Cats are taught similar techniques to dogs (i.e., negotiating various stimuli).

PROGNOSIS AND OUTCOME

Because many new kitten owners are very open to learning, prognosis should be favorable

PEARLS & CONSIDERATIONS

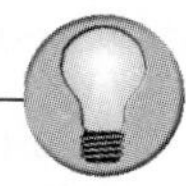

COMMENTS

- Educate owners that rewarding appropriate behaviors and ignoring or redirecting inappropriate behaviors are the best ways to manage behavioral problems and avoid kitten behavioral disorders in the future.
- If behavior problems persist, referral to a veterinary behaviorist early in the process is preferable to waiting to see if the cat "will grow out of it," because the problems may become more firmly ingrained.

PREVENTION

Attendance at kitten socialization and training classes can help owners to have realistic expectations of their cat's behavior.

CLIENT EDUCATION

It is just as important to socialize and train kittens as puppies for them to grow up into well-behaved and accepted members of society.

SUGGESTED READING

Hunthausen W, Seksel K: Preventative behavioural medicine. In Horwitz D, Mills D, Heath S (eds): *BSAVA Manual of Canine and Feline Behavioural Medicine*. Gloucester, UK, British Small Animal Association, 2002, 49–60.

Landsberg G, Hunthausen W, Ackerman L: *Handbook of Behaviour Problems of the Dog and Cat*. Oxford, Butterworth-Heineman, 2003.

Overall KL: *Clinical Behavioral Medicine for Small Animals*. St. Louis, Mosby, 1997.

Overall KL, et al: *Feline Behavior Guidelines from the American Association of Feline Practitioners*. AAFP, 2004.

Seksel K: *Training Your Cat*. Melbourne Australia, Hyland House, 2001.

AUTHOR: **KERSTI SEKSEL**
EDITOR: **KAREN L. OVERALL**

Behavioral Problem Prevention: Puppies

BASIC INFORMATION

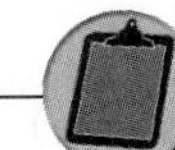

DEFINITION

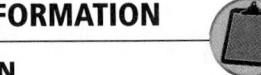

The first few puppy visits set the stage for future veterinary visits. They help the new puppy client understand normal canine behavior and help prevent problems with toilet training, digging, jumping up, barking, mouthing, and chewing.

SYNONYM(S)

Puppy socialization/training/preschool

EPIDEMIOLOGY

SPECIES, AGE, SEX

- Dogs <4–6 months old.
- Problematic behavior in puppies becomes more pronounced at social maturity (about 18 to 24 months old), when pathologic behaviors usually develop.

GENETICS AND BREED DISPOSITION Variability in normal, playful behavior is breed and line-dependent.

CONTAGION AND ZOONOSIS: Dog bites are a public health risk.

GEOGRAPHY AND SEASONALITY: Dog bites are more prevalent in warmer months.

ASSOCIATED CONDITIONS AND DISORDERS

- Dogs not adequately exposed to varied stimuli may be more at risk for developing neophobia, fear of other dogs, and fear of humans.
- Increased risk of abandonment and euthanasia if clients do not understand normal canine behavior. The average client with a problem dog keeps the dog 3 months before relinquishment.
- Inherited disorders (e.g., lissencephaly present with abnormal behavior).

CLINICAL PRESENTATION

HISTORY, CHIEF COMPLAINT

- May be unremarkable (routine evaluation).
- Alternatively, common chief complaints include toilet training problems, digging, jumping up, barking, mouthing, or chewing.
- Every veterinary visit should review a puppy's behavior, thus educating the client about age-specific normal behavior, and allowing early intervention, when behavioral problems are easiest to fix. Sample questions could include: (1) Does your dog urinate in the house? (2) Is your dog afraid of other dogs or strangers? (3) Does your dog vocalize when you wish it to be quiet? (4) Does your dog destroy anything when left alone? (5) Does your dog have any mouthing, biting, or other behaviors that concern you?

PHYSICAL EXAM FINDINGS: Unremarkable.

DIAGNOSIS

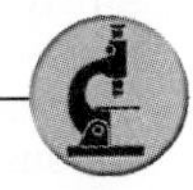

DIFFERENTIAL DIAGNOSIS

Based on complaints of the client

INITIAL DATABASE

Diagnostic testing only as indicated by abnormalities in history or physical exam

TREATMENT

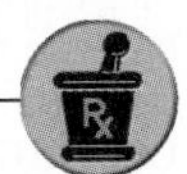

THERAPEUTIC GOAL(S)

- Educate clients about normal canine behaviors
- Reduce risk of surrender by addressing these factors

ACUTE GENERAL TREATMENT

- Rewards (e.g., treats) should be given for appropriate behaviors.
- Inappropriate behaviors should be redirected and more appropriate behaviors substituted.
- Dogs should not be verbally or physically punished for inappropriate behaviors.
- Dogs should be taught to sit on cue; sitting is a natural "stop" signal in dogs.
- Head collars (e.g., Gentle Leaders, Haltis) and harnesses (e.g., Easy Walker Harness, No-pull Harness) should be used for all puppies because they appropriately direct dogs towards good behavior, preempting the need for "corrections." These devices also prevent problem behaviors and allow the clients to succeed in getting the dog to behave calmly.
- Choke chains, prong collars, and electronic collars have no place in changing or preventing inappropriate behaviors; these methods are outdated and not recommended.

CHRONIC TREATMENT

- Appropriate behaviors must be reinforced long-term.
- Most behaviors such as jumping up, digging, or mouthing are not true behavior problems but normal behaviors that are a problem to the clients.
- Many may be best resolved by ignoring the behavior and teaching the dog an alternative response instead (response substitution).
- Jumping up:
  - The client must *not* pay attention (look, touch, or speak) to the dog when it jumps up. Instead, the client should stand still or turn his/her back on the dog and wait until all of the dog's four feet are firmly on the ground.
  - Interactions occur only when the dog is relatively calm.
- Chewing objects:
  - Dogs need suitable toys to chew as alternatives to household objects. These toys need to be changed regularly (daily) to maintain the dog's interest.
  - Avoid old shoes or other belongings (dog does not know the difference between unwanted objects and valuable ones).
  - May need to apply bittering agent to off-limits objects.
- Digging:

  - A digging pit the size of a child's size sandpit filled with loose sand or soil encourages digging in this area.
  - Burying bones, toys, and other treats in this area rewards the dog for digging there.
- Mouthing:
  - It is important for clients to reinforce the rules of play (i.e., not too rough).
  - If a puppy mouths or bites, the client should stop play and just walk away. If the puppy persists in play biting, then the client needs to entirely discontinue any interaction or play and temporarily remove the puppy from the environment.
  - Clients should not use hands to hit the puppy or push him away because this will encourage mouthing or biting. Puppies may think this is a game and will persist in biting.
- Barking: see Barking, Excessive, p 117.

DRUG INTERACTIONS

- Very young puppies generally should not need medication for anxiety-related conditions.
- The synthetic analog of dog appeasement pheromone may help decrease anxiety; objective data are lacking.

RECOMMENDED MONITORING

See History, Chief Complaint above

PROGNOSIS AND OUTCOME

Because new puppy clients often are very open to learning, it should be favorable

PEARLS & CONSIDERATIONS

COMMENTS

- Educate clients that rewarding appropriate behaviors and ignoring or redirecting the inappropriate behaviors is the best basis for their puppy.
- If behavior problems persist, referral to a veterinary behaviorist early in the process is preferable to waiting to see if the dog "will grow out of it."

PREVENTION

- Offer pre-pet selection advice.
- Attendance at puppy socialization and training classes educates the puppies to behave politely in society. The classes also help clients to understand their dog's behavior and have realistic expectations of their dog.

CLIENT EDUCATION

The Humane Society of the United States has free brochures for a variety of early training approaches and management-related behavior problems (www.hsus.org).

SUGGESTED READING

Hunthausen W, Seksel K: Preventative behavioural medicine. In Horwitz D, Mills D, Heath S (eds): *BSAVA Manual of Canine and Feline Behavioural Medicine.* Gloucester, UK, British Small Animal Association, 2002, 49-60.

Love M, Overall KL: Dogs and children: how anticipating relationships can help avoid disasters. *J Am Vet Med Assoc* 219:446-453, 2001.

Miller P: The power of positive dog training, available at www.dogwise.com

Overall KL: *Clinical Behavioral Medicine for Small Animals*. St. Louis, Mosby, 1997.

AUTHOR: **KERSTI SEKSEL**

EDITOR: **KAREN L. OVERALL**

Behavior Problems, Miscellaneous

BASIC INFORMATION

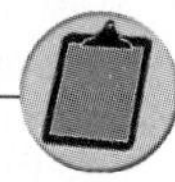

DEFINITION

Species-typical and normal behaviors that may inconvenience clients

- Dogs:
  - Coprophagy
  - Chewing
  - Digging
  - Mounting/humping
  - Roaming
  - Fence-running/scratching
- Cats:
  - Scratching of furnishings
  - Late night activity, climbing on counters

EPIDEMIOLOGY

SPECIES, AGE, SEX: Younger animals of both sexes and species are more likely to exhibit exploratory and play behaviors that may irritate clients. Intact males may roam more frequently and greater distances.

GENETICS AND BREED PREDISPOSITION

- Hounds and northern dog breeds (e.g., husky, malamute, Samoyed) are anecdotally reported to look more readily for opportunities to roam.
- Highly active breeds or individuals with inadequate stimulation and exercise to satisfy their behavioral and cognitive needs may look for alternatives for behavioral expression, and these actions may be intolerable to owners.

RISK FACTORS: Management practices that decrease enrichment (both mental and physical) or that fail to establish a humane rule structure that meet a pet's physical, social, developmental, behavioral, and cognitive needs. Examples are lengthy confinement within a day for dogs (e.g., 8 of 24 hours), lack of interactive toys, lack of basic training, inadequate aerobic exercise, and inadequate social exposure.

CONTAGION AND ZOONOSIS: Multiple-dog and multiple-cat households may experience social facilitation that fosters many of these behaviors. In social facilitation, the behaviors of one individual in a group stimulate others to do the same or similar behaviors.

GEOGRAPHY AND SEASONALITY: Access (e.g., digging in soil) and the level of provocative stimuli (e.g., other cats outside) may vary seasonally.

ASSOCIATED CONDITIONS AND DISORDERS: Obsessive-compulsive disorders.

CLINICAL PRESENTATION

DISEASE FORMS/SUBTYPES: Bouts of behaviors that can be interrupted and that seem only to occur opportunistically may be normal but annoying behaviors or management-related behavior problems. If the behaviors cannot be easily interrupted, or the animal is constantly seeking ways to get access to do them, a more serious disorder should be suspected (e.g., obsessive-compulsive disorder).

HISTORY, CHIEF COMPLAINT

- Clients complain that the dog or cat behaves in a way that is annoying (e.g., cat walking on counters) or disgusting (e.g., dog rolling in feces) to the client, but not threatening or dangerous.
- The first step in eliciting relevant information is to get a good and complete description of the behaviors and the context in which they occur. Context is critical for assessment of whether the behaviors are "normal" or species-typical ones that can be redirected or managed, while still meeting the animal's needs. For example, a cat's scratching at an inanimate object (e.g., furniture) is part of normal behavior and can be redirected, but scratching at humans or other cats may represent aggression.

PHYSICAL EXAM FINDINGS: Usually unremarkable, although history or evidence of minor self-trauma acquired during exploratory or escape behaviors may be present.

ETIOLOGY AND PATHOPHYSIOLOGY

- Clients must understand that animals do not undertake these behaviors to "spite" them or out of "jealousy"; attention-seeking is commonly involved, but the key to managing these disorders is having clients understand the significance of these behaviors in terms of normal dog and cat behavior.
- Most of these behaviors are normal behaviors in context, intensity, and frequency, at least at first.
- With time, if the behaviors are becoming increasingly abnormal, the context, intensity, and frequency with which they are exhibited will change, as will the animal's focus, interactions with humans and other animals, and daily time budget.
- Behavior modification is based on the concept that positive behaviors should be encouraged and repeated if they result in a pleasurable outcome. This repetition leads to learning at the neurochemical level where new proteins at synapses are made. These more efficient neuronal connections make it more likely that the dog or cat will continue with the behavior. This is why it is so important to routinely screen for behaviors clients consider annoying and why we must encourage them to seek us out with their questions. Intervention before too many neurochemical changes have occurred will make it easier to stop and redirect the behaviors.

DIAGNOSIS

DIFFERENTIAL DIAGNOSIS

If any of the signs are excessive, repetitive, and performed to the exclusion of other comfort, social, and maintenance behaviors, an anxiety disorder such as obsessive-compulsive disorder must be considered.

INITIAL DATABASE

- Complete blood count, serum biochemistry profile, urinalysis: generally unremarkable
- Feces or other ingestions: fecal flotation; abdominal radiographs if obstruction is suspected

TREATMENT

THERAPEUTIC GOAL(S)

Provide an acceptable outlet for the unmet behavioral, cognitive, and species-typical needs that lead the pet to engage in the behavior that the client finds objectionable.

ACUTE GENERAL TREATMENT

- Increase aerobic activity through exercise and interactive play with humans or fellow dogs/cats. Dogs playing with other dogs, in particular, usually provides more effective exercise with greater aerobic scope than does play with humans.
- Environmental modification should be used for preventing access to or limiting the repetition of the undesirable behavior, and fostering alternative, acceptable behaviors.

CHRONIC TREATMENT

- Behavior modification can provide outlets or encourage substitute behaviors that allow acceptable expression of the individual's mental and social needs. Depending on the problem, this may consist of continued aerobic exercise, goal-oriented activities (obedience, agility, tracking, coursing training in dogs, interactive predatory play in cats). Rewards—verbal, physical, food—should be given for all spontaneous and calm behaviors (e.g., chewing on chew-toys, clawing on provided surfaces, digging in a sandbox provided for this purpose).
- Attention-seeking behaviors, such as jumping, "playful" whining or biting, etc., need to be ignored completely. Elimination of the reward will extinguish the behavior if, and only if, the client is consistent in not responding. Clients must be made aware that unlearning takes longer than learning because of the neurochemical changes involved.
- In mild cases, devices that interrupt the behavior with an aversive stimulus can be useful early in the course of the problem, only if the animal is not afraid of the stimulus, and only if appropriate outlets to which the behavior can be redirected are also provided.
- Examples of aversive, but not harmful or fear-inducing, disruptive stimuli include inverted plastic carpet runners (spike side up) or static electricity mats for surfaces that the client wants to be off-limits to the pet, and pressurized air blasts triggered by motion detector sensors. Note that some animals will be afraid of these stimuli. If this is the case, the devices should not be used. The purpose of a disruptive stimulus is *only* to stop the behavior in a way that encourages the animal to seek more information. If the animal is afraid, it cannot do this.

POSSIBLE COMPLICATIONS

- Poor client compliance will lead to continued self-reinforcement and worsening of the problem, which, in turn, will lead to a worsening of the relationship between the pet and client. Therefore a cornerstone of treatment is owner understanding of the basis for the behavior and the intention of the proposed treatment.
- Abandonment and death are frequent sequelae to behaviors clients find undesirable, whether or not the behaviors were the dog's or cat's "fault." The impact of this pattern on veterinary economics is huge. The impact on veterinary ethics should also be huge.

RECOMMENDED MONITORING

- Frequent follow-up will help many clients comply more reliably.
- Demonstrations that show clients new ways to interact with their pet are essential.
- By dedicating these tasks to one staff member, continuity and consistency in advice and follow-up are maintained. Clients also feel that their veterinarians care more about them under these conditions.

PROGNOSIS AND OUTCOME

- Excellent if the clients understand the pets' needs and are willing and able to meet them
- Poor if clients had unrealistic expectations, consider pets recyclable, feel guilty about discussing the issue with their vet, or are unwilling or unable to meet their pets' needs

PEARLS & CONSIDERATIONS

COMMENTS

- In extreme forms that interfere with normal physical and social functioning, most of these "annoyance" behaviors are also characteristic of obsessive-compulsive disorder and other anxiety-related conditions. This does not mean that exhibition of these miscellaneous concerns will lead to obsessive-compulsive disorder. It does mean that the nonspecific signs and complaints can be similar, and clients should be aware of this and not dismiss unusual behaviors out of hand as just bratty behaviors without having them evaluated first.
- Behavior problems are among the top reasons otherwise healthy pets are relinquished to shelters, which substantially impacts a population of fundamentally healthy animals, as well as having effects on veterinary economics, veterinary staff morale, etc.

PREVENTION

Puppy and kitten classes; basic obedience and agility training; and understanding of basic behavioral, physical, and social needs of dogs and cats will help clients to intervene before behaviors become problems.

CLIENT EDUCATION

Veterinarians are encouraged to keep a loaning library of books, newsletters, videos covering basic behaviors of dog and cats, and a list of trainers and facilities that a staff member has verified use humane training techniques. This will provide the atmosphere of caring that will make it easier for clients to seek and get the help they need.

SUGGESTED READING

Donaldson J: *The Culture Clash*. Berkeley, Calif., James and Kenneth Publishers, 1996.

Miller P: *The Power of Positive Dog Training*. Dog Wise, 2003.

Seksel K: *Training Your Cat*. Melbourne, Australia, Hyland House, 2001.

AUTHOR: **SORAYA V. JUARBE-DIAZ**
EDITOR: **KAREN L. OVERALL**

Benign Prostatic Hyperplasia

BASIC INFORMATION

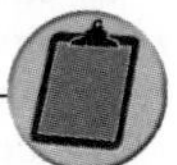

DEFINITION

A disorder that causes symmetric enlargement of the prostate gland due to an androgen-dependent, age-related increase in the number of cells in both the stromal and glandular elements of the prostate. It is the most common cause of prostatomegaly in dogs.

SYNONYM(S)

Benign prostatic hypertrophy
BPH

EPIDEMIOLOGY

SPECIES, AGE, SEX: Sexually intact, adult male dogs.

RISK FACTORS

- The condition is androgen-dependent; therefore, it is essentially exclusive to intact males.
- Age dependency: 50% prevalence at age 5 years; 95% prevalence by age 9 years.

ASSOCIATED CONDITIONS AND DISORDERS: Some dogs with benign prostatic hyperplasia (BPH) also have small cystic changes within the prostate. These may be prone to bacterial infection, but often they are merely an incidental finding during prostate ultrasonography.

CLINICAL PRESENTATION

HISTORY, CHIEF COMPLAINT

- BPH often causes no clinical signs.
- When it does, sanguineous urethral discharge that is not associated with urination, and tenesmus, are the two most common signs.
- Less commonly there may be a history of hematuria or of subfertility.

Note: Unlike the situation in men, BPH rarely causes stranguria or urine retention in dogs.

PHYSICAL EXAM FINDINGS

- Sexually intact, adult male dog
- Careful rectal and abdominal palpation of the prostate:
  - Symmetric, nonpainful enlargement of the prostate.
  - Prostatomegaly in a castrated dog should prompt a search for neoplasia, not a diagnosis of BPH.
- ± Sanguineous urethral (preputial) discharge
- Otherwise healthy

ETIOLOGY AND PATHOPHYSIOLOGY

- Androgen-dependent
- Progresses with age. The mean age of onset of clinical signs is 8 year
- Normal reflux of prostatic fluid into the urinary tract results in sanguineous urethral (preputial) discharge
- Prostatomegaly may cause mechanical interference with defecation

DIAGNOSIS

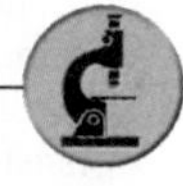

DIFFERENTIAL DIAGNOSIS

- Cystic prostatic disease (retention cysts; paraprostatic cysts)
- Prostatic neoplasia
- Squamous metaplasia of the prostate
- Bacterial prostatitis

INITIAL DATABASE

- Ultrasound:
  - Prostatomegaly with homogeneous parenchyma, ± a few small (<10 mm) cysts. The urethra is normal.
- Abdominal radiographs, indicated if tenesmus is present:
  - Prostatomegaly, ± dorsal displacement of colon.
- Urinalysis and urine culture, indicated if urinary signs are present:
  - Macroscopic or microscopic hematuria may be found.
  - Culture results negative with BPH. Positive culture results indicate concomitant urinary tract infection and/or bacterial prostatitis.

ADVANCED OR CONFIRMATORY TESTING

- Complete blood count and serum biochemical profile:
  - Dogs with BPH are usually otherwise healthy, and results should be normal. If they are not, or if the dog is ill, a diagnosis other than, or in addition to, BPH should be pursued.
- Other causes of prostatomegaly are excluded by the following:
  - Prostatic fluid culture and cytology (see Prostatic Massage, p 1303):
    - Prostatic samples can be obtained by fine-needle aspiration under ultrasound guidance, by prostatic wash, or by collecting the third fraction of the ejaculate.
    - Culture results are negative with BPH. Positive culture results indicate concomitant bacterial prostatitis, and/or urinary tract infection, and/or contamination of the ejaculate with preputial organisms.
    - Hematospermia is often present, ± the occasional macrophage and nondegenerative neutrophil.
  - Retrograde cystourethrogram (see Cystogram, p 1214):
    - Urethra is normal with BPH. Reflux of contrast into prostatic parenchyma is absent or minimal (relative to the measurement of maximal urethral diameter)
  - Biopsy, histopathologic evaluation:
    - Although the definitive diagnosis is established histopathologically, it is rarely necessary or indicated when all the testing described above is consistent with BPH, and only BPH.

TREATMENT

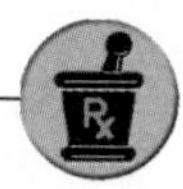

THERAPEUTIC GOAL(S)

- Resolution of clinical signs.
- Animals showing no clinical signs do not necessarily require treatment, only watchful waiting. Treatment can be delayed until clinical signs occur. BPH may predispose the prostate gland to ascending infection by urethral flora.

TREATMENT

SURGICAL: Castration is the treatment of choice for dogs with clinical signs

because it is curative and more effective than pharmacologic management.
- Prostatic involution is detectable within days of castration.
- Prostatic size is expected to decrease by 50% within 3 weeks and by 70% within 9 weeks.
- Clinical signs typically are completely resolved within 4 weeks after castration.

PHARMACOLOGIC
- Response to pharmacologic therapy is temporary
- 5α-reductase inhibitor: Finasteride (Proscar, Merck) 0.1-0.2 mg/kg PO q 24h; or 5 mg/dog/day PO
- Progestins (e.g., medroxyprogesterone 3 mg/kg, SQ once)

POSSIBLE COMPLICATIONS OF PHARMACOLOGIC THERAPY
- Decreased fertility (semen quality, libido, and testicular size)
- Increased appetite and diabetes mellitus with progestins

RECOMMENDED MONITORING
If castration is not performed, watchful waiting

PROGNOSIS AND OUTCOME

- Excellent:
  - Dogs not showing clinical signs may remain so for months to years
  - Castration is curative of clinical signs
- Pharmacologic therapy will temporarily improve clinical signs, but signs eventually (usually many months) recur after treatment ends.

PEARLS & CONSIDERATIONS

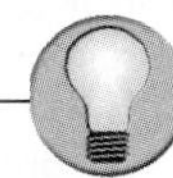

COMMENTS
- Unlike the situation in men, BPH in dogs rarely causes stranguria or urine retention. When canine prostatic disease causes those signs, or urethral involvement, it is more likely due to neoplasia than to BPH.
- Prostatomegaly in a castrated dog should prompt a search for neoplasia, not BPH.
- Dogs with BPH are usually otherwise healthy. If the dog is ill, a diagnosis other than, or in addition to, BPH should be pursued.
- The herbal remedy from the saw palmetto plant (*Serenoa repens*) does not significantly affect the prostate gland of dogs with BPH.

PREVENTION
Castration of juvenile dogs prevents BPH.

SUGGESTED READING

Barsanti JA, et al: Effects of an extract of *Serenoa repens* on dogs with hyperplasia of the prostate gland. *Am J Vet Res* 61:880, 2000.

Disorders of the canine prostate. In Johnston SD, Root Kustritz MV, Olson PN (eds): *Canine and Feline Theriogenology*. Philadelphia, WB Saunders, 2001, pp 337-355.

Johnson CA: Disorders of the prostate gland. In Nelson RW, Couto CG (eds): *Small Animal Internal Medicine*, ed 3. St. Louis, Mosby, 2003, pp 927-933.

Kutzler MA, et al: Prostatic diseases. In Ettinger SJ, Feldman EC (eds): *Textbook of Veterinary Internal Medicine*, ed 6. St. Louis, Elsevier-Saunders, 2005, pp 1809-1819.

AUTHOR: **CHERI A. JOHNSON**

EDITOR: **MICHELLE A. KUTZLER**

Bicipital Tenosynovitis

BASIC INFORMATION

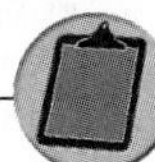

DEFINITION
Inflammation of the biceps brachii tendon and surrounding synovial sheath

SYNONYM(S)
Bicipital bursitis (inaccurate)

EPIDEMIOLOGY
SPECIES, AGE, SEX
- Dogs
- Medium and large breeds
- Middle-aged to older

RISK FACTORS: Trauma, overuse of muscle, shoulder joint osteoarthritis.

ASSOCIATED CONDITIONS AND DISORDERS: Osteoarthritis or osteochondrosis of shoulder joint, supraspinatus tendonitis.

CLINICAL PRESENTATION
HISTORY, CHIEF COMPLAINT: Forelimb lameness exacerbated by exercise and unresponsive to nonsteroidal anti-inflammatory drugs (NSAIDs); caused by trauma to shoulder or insidious in onset.

PHYSICAL EXAM FINDINGS
- Shortened forelimb stride with head lifted as affected forelimb is advanced
- Pain on palpation of the bicipital tendon in the intertubercular groove
- Pain on flexion of shoulder and extension of the elbow while placing tendon and muscle under tension

ETIOLOGY AND PATHOPHYSIOLOGY
- Can be caused by blow to cranial aspect of shoulder during flexion
- Tendon may be strained or stretched with disruption of fibers
- In chronic conditions, dystrophic mineralization occurs in tendon
- Secondary to shoulder joint osteoarthritis or osteochondrosis if cartilage fragments collect within the communicating tendon sheath and cause inflammation
- Adhesions between tendon sheath and tendon can occur secondary to trauma
- Tendon can also be avulsed from supraglenoid tubercle

DIAGNOSIS

DIFFERENTIAL DIAGNOSIS
- Supraspinatus tendonitis
- Supraglenoid tubercle fracture
- Shoulder joint collateral ligament injury
- Shoulder joint osteoarthritis
- Cervical nerve root compression

INITIAL DATABASE
- Patient database as indicated by stability and American Society of Anesthesiologists classification (p 1134)
- Medial to lateral radiograph of the scapulohumeral joint
- Skyline radiographic view of the intertubercular groove

ADVANCED OR CONFIRMATORY TESTING
- Contrast arthrography may reveal irregularity of tendon surface or sheath.
- Arthrocentesis may be consistent with osteoarthritis (increase nucleated cell counts 1500-4800 cells/μl, primarily mononuclear; aseptic).
- Ultrasonography of the biceps tendon will identify irregular fiber arrangement and increased synovial sheath fluid content.
- Magnetic resonance imaging (MRI) may be considered to identify tendon and sheath lesions.
- Arthroscopy for direct visualization of tendon and sheath.

TREATMENT

THERAPEUTIC GOAL(S)

Relieve pain due to tenosynovitis

ACUTE GENERAL TREATMENT

- Local injection with methylprednisolone acetate (10–40 mg) followed by 2 weeks of rest. Repeat at 2-week intervals for three treatments; if no improvement, surgery is considered
- Surgical treatment:
  - Tenotomy via arthrotomy or arthroscopy
  - Tenodesis to the proximal humerus by screw/washer or passing tendon through a bone tunnel and suturing to the periosteum

CHRONIC TREATMENT

Exercise restriction for 6 to 8 weeks

POSSIBLE COMPLICATIONS

- Poor response to steroid treatment
- Chondromalacia in shoulder joint or biceps tendon rupture secondary to steroid injection
- Persistent lameness due to inadequate tenodesis

RECOMMENDED MONITORING

- Short-term postoperatively for seroma
- Long-term for restoration of limb function

PROGNOSIS AND OUTCOME

- Fair to good after steroid injection and rest
- Good after tenodesis or tenotomy (arthroscopic)

PEARLS & CONSIDERATIONS

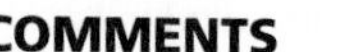

COMMENTS

- Establishing a diagnosis of bicipital tenosynovitis can be difficult.
- Disease of the supraspinatus tendon can be a conflicting cause of shoulder joint pain. This condition is best evaluated by MRI or arthroscopy to identify tendon impingement into the groove; splitting this tendon resolves pain and lameness.
- The synovial sheath of the biceps tendon is continuous with the shoulder joint capsule.

SUGGESTED READING

Stobie D, et al: Chronic bicipital tenosynovitis in dogs: 29 cases (1985–1992). *J Am Vet Med Assoc* 207:201, 1995.

Montgomery R, Fitch R: Muscle and tendon disorders. In Slatter D (ed): *Textbook of Small Animal Surgery*, ed 3. Philadelphia, WB Saunders, 2003, p 2217.

AUTHOR: **JAMES D. LINCOLN**

EDITOR: **JOSEPH HARARI**

Bile Duct Obstruction, Extrahepatic

BASIC INFORMATION

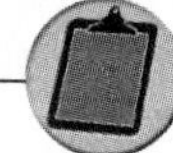

DEFINITION

Pathologic obstruction of the extrahepatic bile duct system

EPIDEMIOLOGY

SPECIES, AGE, SEX: Dependent on the underlying cause.

- Dogs:
  - Middle-aged to older adults:
    - Pancreatitis; less commonly, neoplasia
- Cats:
  - Middle-aged to older adults:
    - Neoplasia

RISK FACTORS

- Dogs:
  - Pancreatitis
- Cats:
  - Pancreatitis
  - Cholangitis/cholangiohepatitis
  - Inflammatory bowel disease
  - Neoplasia

ASSOCIATED CONDITIONS AND DISORDERS

- Dogs:
  - Cholecystitis
  - Gall bladder mucocele
- Dogs and cats:
  - Coagulopathy possible due to lack of absorption of fat-soluble vitamin K
  - Cholelithiasis
  - Bile peritonitis
  - Neoplasia

CLINICAL PRESENTATION

HISTORY, CHIEF COMPLAINT

- Dogs:
  - Anorexia
  - Lethargy
  - Vomiting
  - Diarrhea
- Cats:
  - Anorexia
  - Lethargy
  - Weight loss
  - Vomiting

PHYSICAL EXAM FINDINGS

- Dogs:
  - Icterus
  - Fever
  - Tachycardia
- Cats:
  - Icterus
  - Dehydration
  - Fever or hypothermia

ETIOLOGY AND PATHOPHYSIOLOGY

- Dogs:
  - See Pancreatitis, Dog, p 796
  - Cholelithiasis:
    - Etiology poorly understood
- Cats:
  - Extrahepatic biliary obstruction often associated with a "triad" of diseases:
    - Cholangitis
    - Pancreatitis (see Pancreatitis, Cat, p 794)
    - Inflammatory bowel disease
      - Common opening of the pancreatic and common bile ducts into the duodenum and the increased duodenal bacterial content may predispose cats to ascending cholangitis and pancreatitis after vomiting associated with inflammatory bowel disease (Fig. I-27)
- Both species: lack of bile entering intestinal tract:
  - Decreases absorption of fat and fat soluble vitamins, notably vitamin K:
    - Potential coagulopathy
  - May result in increased absorption of endotoxin from the gut

DIAGNOSIS

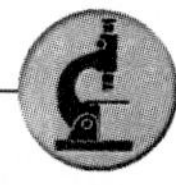

DIFFERENTIAL DIAGNOSIS

- Hyperbilirubinemia:
  - Rule out hemolysis:
    - Immune-mediated hemolytic anemia, toxicity (zinc, onions, etc.) and other diseases causing hemolytic anemia

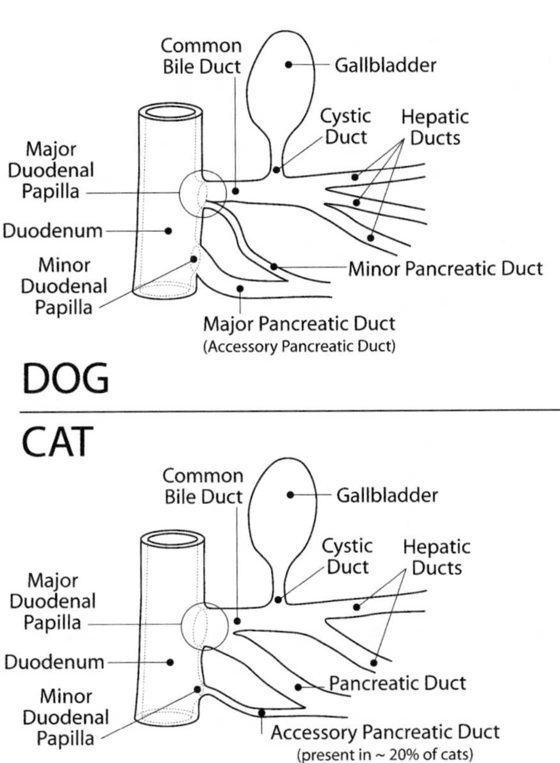

FIGURE I-27 Comparative anatomy of the canine and feline biliary systems. Courtesy of Glenda Clements-Smith.

- Rule out hepatic disease:
  - Hepatitis: acute, chronic
  - Cirrhotic/fibrosing liver disease
  - Neoplasia
  - Copper and other toxins in dogs, acetaminophen toxicosis in cats
- Extrahepatic biliary obstruction:
  - Pancreatitis
  - Cholelithiasis
  - Cholangitis
  - Neoplasia
  - Stricture in biliary system
  - Foreign body duodenal obstruction
  - Diaphragmatic hernia
  - Parasitic infection

INITIAL DATABASE

- Complete blood count:
  - Possible anemia; generally very mild if any (unless concurrent gastrointestinal ulceration). By contrast, hyperbilirubinemia/icterus caused by hemolysis generally produces moderate to marked anemia
  - Inflammatory leukogram
- Serum biochemistry profile:
  - Elevated bilirubin concentration
  - Elevated liver enzyme concentrations
  - Possible elevated amylase and lipase concentrations
  - Hypokalemia
- Urinalysis: bilirubinuria is common in both species (but mild bilirubinuria also is normal in the dog)
- Survey abdominal radiographs:
  - May delineate radiopaque choleliths
- Survey thoracic radiographs:
  - Rule out metastatic disease if neoplasia is suspected

ADVANCED OR CONFIRMATORY TESTING

- Abdominal ultrasound examination:
  - Common bile duct dilation
    - >5 mm diameter: diagnostic of bile duct obstruction in the cat
  - Visible contraction of the gallbladder is not expected in either healthy or diseased states
- Peritoneal fluid analysis (obtained during abdominal ultrasound examination):
  - Elevated bilirubin concentration
    - Bile peritonitis
  - Cytology and microbiologic (aerobic and anaerobic) culture and sensitivity testing
    - Septic peritonitis
- Coagulation profile

TREATMENT

THERAPEUTIC GOAL(S)

- Correction of fluid deficits
- Normalization of serum electrolyte concentrations
- Normalization of coagulation status before surgery:
  - Vitamin K administration
  - Fresh frozen plasma
- Relief of extrahepatic biliary obstruction
- Nutritional support if indicated

ACUTE GENERAL TREATMENT

- Rehydration by intravenous administration of balanced electrolyte solution
- Parenteral antibiotics effective against gram-negative bacteria and anaerobes:
  - Empiric therapy:
    - Cefoxitin, 22 mg/kg, IV, q 2h perioperatively, then q 6h
    - Metronidazole, 7.5-15 mg/kg, IV, q 12h
    - Enrofloxacin, 2.5-5 mg/kg, IV, q 12h (q 24h in cats, due to risk of retinal toxicity)
  - Specific, long-term therapy based on culture and sensitivity test results
- Possible administration of fresh frozen plasma:
  - Hypoproteinemia
  - Possible coagulopathy
- Vitamin K administration: 2.5 mg/kg SQ q 12h × 3-5 days, then once weekly
- Relief of extrahepatic biliary obstruction: surgical intervention:
  - Retrograde and antegrade flushing of biliary system: all cases
  - Common bile duct stenting: if dynamic obstruction
  - Cholecystoduodenostomy/jejunostomy: if advanced or permanent obstruction
  - Tube cholecystostomy
  - Cholecystectomy: if gallbladder wall is devitalized
- Nutritional support:
  - Provide access for enteral feeding (e.g., gastrostomy tube) if patient is anorexic

CHRONIC TREATMENT

Maintenance of bile flow:

- Ursodeoxycholic acid, 10-15 mg/kg PO q 24h. Contraindicated if biliary obstruction is still present

POSSIBLE COMPLICATIONS

- Ongoing pancreatitis
- Bile leakage
- Peritonitis
- Endotoxemia
- Sepsis
- Death

RECOMMENDED MONITORING

- Clinical and laboratory parameters assessing perfusion, including capillary refill time, pulse rate and quality, blood pressure, urine output, arterial pH, and lactate concentrations
- Respiratory function
- Serum liver enzyme and bilirubin concentrations
- Coagulation profile

PROGNOSIS AND OUTCOME

- Poor if biliary obstruction associated with neoplasia: 100% mortality in cats
- Guarded if biliary obstruction associated with non-neoplastic causes in cats
- Guarded to fair if biliary obstruction associated with non-neoplastic causes in dogs

PEARLS & CONSIDERATIONS

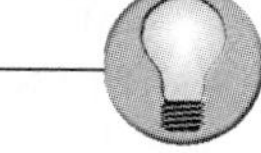

COMMENTS

- Given the association of biliary obstructive disease in cats with cholangitis/cholangiohepatitis and inflammatory bowel disease, a liver biopsy and culture, bile culture, and small intestinal biopsies must be obtained at the time of surgery in this species. A convenient site for duodenal biopsy is the edge of the duodenotomy performed to cannulate the duodenal papilla(e) or to perform a cholecystoduodenostomy.
- In assessing hyperbilirubinemia, total bilirubin concentration is important. Conjugated versus unconjugated bilirubin is not linked to the source of hyperbilirubinemia in dogs and cats as it is in humans.

SUGGESTED READING

Mayhew PD, et al: Pathogenesis and outcome of extrahepatic biliary obstruction in cats. *J Small Anim Pract.* 43:247, 2002.

Mehler SJ, et al: Variables associated with outcome in dogs undergoing extrahepatic biliary surgery: 60 cases (1988–2002). *Vet Surg* 33:644, 2004.

AUTHOR: **DAVID HOLT**
EDITOR: **RICHARD WALSHAW**

Bilious Vomiting Syndrome

BASIC INFORMATION

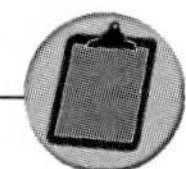

DEFINITION

A disorder resulting in vomiting of a bile-stained fluid, most likely due to gastric hypomotility or gastroduodenal reflux

SYNONYM(S)

Gastroduodenal reflux
Idiopathic gastric hypomotility

EPIDEMIOLOGY

SPECIES, AGE, SEX: No predisposition. Only reported in dogs, but likely occurs in cats.
RISK FACTORS: Concurrent gastric or intestinal disease (i.e., outflow obstruction) possible but usually affects otherwise normal dogs.

CLINICAL PRESENTATION

DISEASE FORMS/SUBTYPES

- Gastric hypomotility causing vomiting when stomach empty, otherwise healthy
- Gastric hypomotility causing chronic vomiting and weight loss

HISTORY, CHIEF COMPLAINT (SOME OR ALL MAY BE PRESENT)

- Vomiting, typically in the morning (especially in animals fed once daily)
- Abdominal discomfort or increased stomach "noises" (borborygmi)
- Nausea
- Anorexia
- Weight loss

PHYSICAL EXAM FINDINGS

- Typically normal; abdominal palpation is unremarkable
- Dehydration and lethargy (chronic vomiting)

ETIOLOGY AND PATHOPHYSIOLOGY

- Presumed to be caused by gastroduodenal reflux that occurs when the dog's stomach is empty for long periods or due to abnormal gastroduodenal motility.
- Classically, the pet vomits bile-stained fluid, usually late at night or in the morning, just before eating, but otherwise feels well.
- Anatomic abnormalities or pyloric obstruction are not present, and there are no inflammatory changes in the gastrointestinal mucosa.

DIAGNOSIS

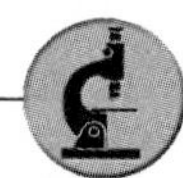

DIFFERENTIAL DIAGNOSIS

- Outflow obstruction (i.e., congenital stenosis, foreign bodies, polyps, neoplasia)
- Dietary intolerance or hypersensitivity
- Defective propulsion
- Gastric disorders (gastritis, gastroenteritis)
- Metabolic (hypokalemia, hypocalcemia, hypoadrenocorticism)
- Nervous inhibition (trauma, stress)
- Drugs (anticholinergics, others)

INITIAL DATABASE

- Complete blood count, serum biochemistry profile, urinalysis usually unremarkable. Hypokalemia, hypochloremia, and metabolic alkalosis possible with voluminous or chronic vomiting
- Abdominal radiographs:
  - Normal
- Retention of food or fluid in the stomach longer than 8 hours, and often 12 to 16 hours after a meal, is suggestive of outflow obstruction or a motility disturbance

ADVANCED OR CONFIRMATORY TESTING

- Motility studies are frequently difficult to perform, are not routinely available outside of referral centers, and the repeatability and sensitivity of these studies are often questioned.
- Positive contrast radiography (see Upper Gastrointestinal Radiographic Contrast Series, p 1316):
  - Typically normal
  - Incomplete gastric emptying following 4 hours (wide variability)
- Fluoroscopy:
  - Often normal
  - Decreased frequency of gastric contractions and incoordination of antropyloric movement (objective criteria are lacking)
- Abdominal ultrasound:
  - Normal
  - Abnormal contractile activity (subjective)
- Scintigraphy:
  - Handling of radioisotopes limits the availability of scintigraphy to referral institutions
- Gastroduodenoscopy is suggested to help rule out inflammatory, infectious, or structural causes of vomiting.

TREATMENT

THERAPEUTIC GOAL(S)

- Increase gastric peristalsis
- Promote gastric emptying

ACUTE GENERAL TREATMENT

Management/resolution of systemic disorder if present, including fluid and electrolyte disturbances or acid-base abnormalities

CHRONIC TREATMENT

- Dietary management:
  - Feeding small, frequent meals (especially late at night) to prevent the stomach from being empty for long periods and to increase normal gastric motility.
  - Diets low in fat and fiber promote gastric emptying and may be helpful to reduce gastric retention.
  - Canned or liquefied diets (solids are retained in the stomach longer) are also beneficial in animals with abnormal gastric retention of foods.
- Medical management: Structural disease first must be ruled out
  - Metoclopramide (0.2-0.4 mg/kg PO or SQ q 8h); increases gastric peristalsis in some but not all affected dogs.
  - Cisapride (0.5-1 mg/kg PO q 24h); accelerates gastric emptying in dogs by stimulating pyloric motor activity.
  - Erythromycin (1 mg/kg PO q 8-12h); accelerates gastric emptying by inducing antral contractions.
  - Ranitidine (1-2 mg/kg PO or SQ q 12h) and nizatidine (2-5 mg/kg PO q 12h); stimulate gastric antral contractions.

POSSIBLE COMPLICATIONS

- Acid/base or electrolyte disorders may occur secondary to chronic vomiting.
- Weight loss.

PROGNOSIS AND OUTCOME

Prognosis is typically excellent; most dogs respond well to dietary and/or prokinetic therapy

PEARLS & CONSIDERATIONS

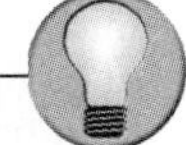

COMMENTS

- Differential diagnoses for bilious vomiting syndrome include a number of primary or secondary disorders of gastric emptying.
- Primary disorders of gastric emptying may arise from mechanical obstruction or defective propulsion.
- Secondary disorders of gastric emptying include metabolic and electrolyte disturbances.
- Nutrition, and medical management using prokinetic therapy, are important components of therapy.
- Weight loss should prompt a complete diagnostic evaluation, because it is not a common feature of uncomplicated bilious vomiting syndrome.

RECOMMENDED READING

Hall JA, et al: Diagnosis and treatment of gastric motility disorders. *Vet Clin North Am Small Anim Pract* 29:377-395, 1999.

Washabau RJ, et al: Diagnosis and management of gastrointestinal motility disorders in dogs and cats. *Compend Contin Educ Pract Vet* 19(6):721-737, 1997.

AUTHOR: **BRANDY PORTERPAN**
EDITOR: **DEBRA L. ZORAN**

Blastomycosis

BASIC INFORMATION

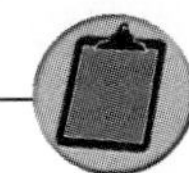

DEFINITION

Systemic mycotic infection affecting many mammalian species, with a predilection for the lungs, skin, eyes, and bone

SYNONYM(S)

Chicago disease (humans)
Gilchrist's disease

EPIDEMIOLOGY

SPECIES, AGE, SEX

- Most often reported in humans and dogs. Has been reported in cats, sea lions, lions, wolves, ferrets, and polar bears
- Usually seen in large-breed, male, young dogs (1 to 5 years old)

GENETICS AND BREED PREDISPOSITION: Doberman pinschers may be at increased risk.

RISK FACTORS

- Outdoor, hunting dogs in endemic areas. Living near a waterway is a risk factor for infection.
- Exposure to disrupted soil (construction involving earth moving or excavation), especially of the sandy, acidic types, is associated with infection.
- Proximity of the face to soil is highly correlated with inhalation and infection, which may help explain the higher risk in dogs compared to humans.

CONTAGION AND ZOONOSIS

- Penetrating wounds (surgical instruments, bite wounds) contaminated by organisms can cause infection in humans.
- Organisms can be transmitted when cultured (aerosol).
- Direct airborne animal-human or human-animal transmission does not occur because the yeast phase (in the infected patient) is not transmissible by aerosol.
- Dogs and humans may acquire blastomycosis from the same environmental source, but illness often is noted in the dog first; thus dogs serve as sentinels for the human disease.

GEOGRAPHY AND SEASONALITY

- *Blastomyces dermatitidis* is present in North America, Africa, and Central America. Endemic areas include the Mississippi, Missouri, and Ohio River valleys; mid-Atlantic states; and the Canadian provinces of Alberta, Quebec, Manitoba, and Ontario (Fig. I-28).
- No seasonal distribution in the southeastern United States.
- May be seasonally distributed in the U.S. Midwest, with more cases seen during late spring through late fall in Wisconsin.
- The specific location of the fungus in soil is unknown; the fungal colonies are not grossly visible and are exceedingly difficult to isolate from the environment.
- A "microfocus" model of ecology for *B. dermatitidis* suggests that environmental pockets of fungal growth and spore release occur when a suitable combination of soil type, moisture, and soil disruption is present.

CLINICAL PRESENTATION

DISEASE FORMS/SUBTYPES: Cutaneous, pulmonary, and osseous forms.

HISTORY, CHIEF COMPLAINT: Anorexia, weight loss, cough, dyspnea, exercise intolerance, ocular changes, lameness, skin lesions, and neurologic signs.

PHYSICAL EXAM FINDINGS

- Highly variable. Fever, depression, emaciation, lymphadenomegaly common
- Pulmonary involvement:
  - Harsh, dry lung sounds; cough; dyspnea at rest
  - Cyanosis, respiratory arrest possible in very advanced stages
- Ocular changes: signs of uveitis, endophthalmitis
- Skin lesions (nasal planum, face, nail beds): subcutaneous abscesses, ulcerated draining lesions, or granulomatous proliferative lesions
- Bone involvement: lameness due to fungal osteomyelitis

ETIOLOGY AND PATHOPHYSIOLOGY

- *Blastomyces dermatitidis* is a dimorphic fungus.
  - The mycelial form grows in soil, mulch, or decaying organic matter (saprophyte) that produces infective spores, which are released into the air most readily when a combination of moisture and soil disruption occurs.
  - The yeast phase grows at body temperature and is not easily airborne; aerosol transmission of the organism from an infected dog is not a recognized risk.
- The route of infection is by inhalation. Mycelial spores are inhaled from the environment (soil or other organic matter) and enter the terminal airways.
- At body temperature the organism transforms into the yeast form, which establishes within the lungs and then disseminates throughout the body via the blood and lymphatics.
- Organism causes a pyogranulomatous inflammation with a predilection for the skin, eyes, bones, lymph nodes, subcutaneous tissues, nares, brain, and testes.
- Direct inoculation into a wound from soil is uncommon.

DIAGNOSIS

The diagnosis depends on demonstration of the organism or serologic evidence of active infection in a patient with compatible clinical signs.

DIFFERENTIAL DIAGNOSIS

- Pulmonary form: bacterial or viral pneumonia (canine distemper or adenovirus), metastatic neoplasia
- Bone form: bacterial osteomyelitis, primary or metastatic bone tumors
- Cutaneous form: bacterial, fungal, parasitic, autoimmune dermatitides
- Other systemic mycoses

INITIAL DATABASE

- Complete blood cell count:
  - Mild normocytic normochromic anemia
  - Moderate leukocytosis (17,000 to 30,000 white blood cell/μl), left shift, lymphopenia
- Serum chemistry panel:
  - Hyperglobulinemia
  - Hypoalbuminemia
  - Hypercalcemia possible (10% of cases)
- Thoracic radiographs:
  - Diffuse, nodular interstitial and bronchointerstitial lung patterns
  - Solitary to multiple nodules may be seen
  - Tracheobronchial lymphadenomegaly
  - Less commonly: pleural effusion, pneumomediastinum
- Radiographs of bones: osteolytic or periosteal proliferation with soft tissue swelling

ADVANCED OR CONFIRMATORY TESTING

- Cytologic examination of lymph node aspirates, draining exudates, skin impression smears, or vitreous aspirates may reveal the organism in more than half the cases.
  - Identification of the thick-walled, broad-based budding yeast is diagnostic.
- Less commonly, the organism may be found in transtracheal wash and lung aspirates.
- Agar-gel immunodiffusion test: positive serum antibody titer is a presumptive diagnosis combined with clinical signs and history:
  - False-negative results occur with early infection or inadequate immune responses.
  - False-positive results may occur with exposure (subclinical cases).

TREATMENT

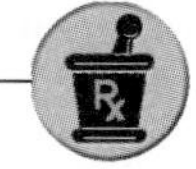

THERAPEUTIC GOAL(S)

Long-term therapy is necessary to eradicate the infection.

ACUTE AND CHRONIC TREATMENT

- General supportive care to include intravenous fluid therapy, oxygen therapy, and other treatments as indicated by the patient's status.
- Antifungal drugs:
  - Itraconazole is considered the drug of choice; however, oral formulation and fungistatic mechanism may be insufficient for critically ill patients.
  - Amphotericin B is used for more severe cases because of its intravenous administration and fungicidal properties; however, its toxicity profile (mainly renal) may be limiting.
- Itraconazole:
  - Dogs: 5 mg/kg q 12h PO for 5 days, then 5 mg/kg/day for at least 30 days after all signs of disease have resolved.
  - Cats: 5 mg/kg PO q 12h.

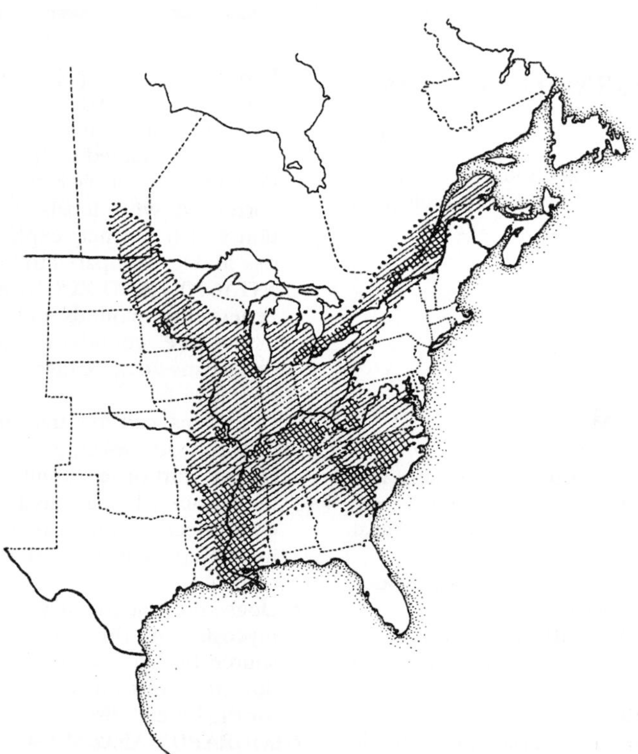

FIGURE I-28 Geographic area in which blastomycosis is endemic. Areas of highest prevalence are cross-hatched. From Rippon JW: *Medical Mycology*, ed 3. Philadelphia, Saunders, 1988, pp 474–505. Reprinted with permission.

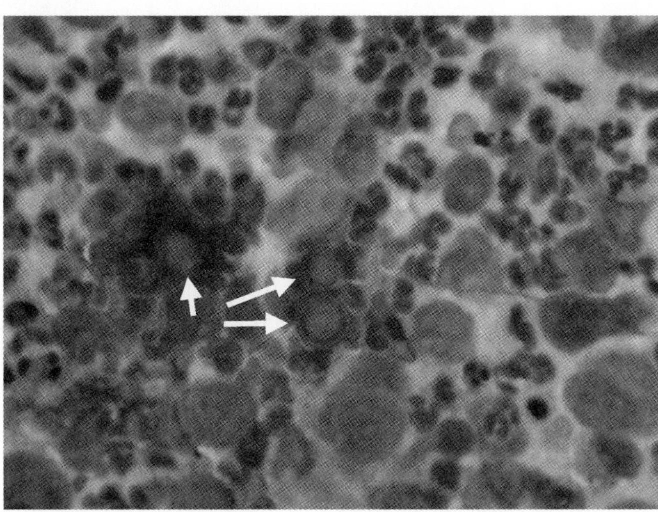

FIGURE I-29 Cytologic evaluation of a fine-needle aspiration from a patient with blastomycosis. The cytologic diagnosis is made based on the thick-walled, basophilic, spherical *B. dermatitidis*. The intense inflammatory infiltrate surrounding the yeasts (*arrows*) is typical.

- Formulation may make dosage challenging (100-mg capsules)
- Oral liquid formulation available (10 mg/ml)
  - Administer with food to maximize absorption.
- Amphotericin B (IV):
  - Dogs: 0.5 mg/kg IV three times weekly × 60 days or until signs of toxicity.
  - Cats: 0.25 mg/kg IV three times weekly or less if signs of toxicity.
- Amphotericin B (SC):
  - Dogs, cats: 0.5-0.8 mg/kg SC diluted with 400-500 ml 0.45% saline/2.5% dextrose and given two to three times weekly to a cumulative dose of 8-26 mg/kg or until signs of toxicity.
- Lipid-soluble amphotericin B:
  - Dogs, cats: 1 mg/kg IV three times weekly × 60 days or less if signs of toxicity.
- Animals must be adequately hydrated and undergoing fluid diuresis before administration of amphotericin B formulas.
- Duration of treatment should continue for 1 month beyond the resolution of clinical signs.
- Combination therapy of amphotericin B with an imidazole (itraconazole or fluconazole, which has superior penetration characteristics) is advised for central nervous system (CNS) and ocular infections. Amphotericin B does not readily cross the blood-brain barrier.

DRUG INTERACTIONS

- Itraconazole and ketoconazole should not be administered with other hepatically metabolized drugs.
- Itraconazole and ketoconazole should always be administered with food to optimize absorption.
- Amphotericin B formulas should not be administered with other renally excreted drugs.

POSSIBLE COMPLICATIONS

- Itraconazole may result in hepatotoxicity and anorexia but has fewer side effects than amphotericin B.
- Ketoconazole may cause gastrointestinal signs and elevated serum liver enzymes. Increased risk of hepatotoxicity in cats. Use in cats is controversial.
- Amphotericin B is potentially nephrotoxic, hepatotoxic, and can cause phlebitis.
  - Lipid-soluble amphotericin B may be less nephrotoxic.
- Lung disease often worsens initially with treatment due to inflammation secondary to organism death.

RECOMMENDED MONITORING

- Liver enzymes should be monitored in animals treated with itraconazole.
- Blood urea nitrogen (BUN), creatinine, γ-glutamyltransferase, and urine sediment should be monitored in animals treated with amphotericin B formulas. A rising BUN and/or casts in the urine sediment may necessitate discontinuing or lowering the dose of amphotericin B.
- Thoracic radiographs on a regular basis if lung disease.

PROGNOSIS AND OUTCOME

- Animals with significant lung involvement or CNS involvement have a poor prognosis.
- Can be cured if treated aggressively, but recurrence or reinfection are possible.
- Recurrence rate: 20%. If recurrence occurs, it usually does so within 1 year of completion of treatment. Common causes of recurrence include severe disease (especially when the central nervous system is affected) and inadequate duration of treatment.
- Severe ocular lesions may result in permanent vision loss.

PEARLS & CONSIDERATIONS

COMMENTS

- Early aggressive treatment is essential
- Recurrence is possible

PREVENTION

- No vaccine
- Restrict activity in endemic areas, particularly lakes, creeks, and heavily shaded areas with moist soil

CLIENT EDUCATION

- Long-term treatment is necessary
- Can be fatal
- Yeast form found in animal tissues is not directly transmissible
- Can be transmitted via penetrating wounds

SUGGESTED READING

Arceneaux KA, Taboada J, Hosgood G: Blastomycosis in dogs: 115 cases (1980-1995). *JAVMA* 213(5) 658-664, 1998.

Boothe DM: *Small Animal Clinical Pharmacology and Therapeutics*. Philadelphia, WB Saunders, 2001, pp 222-236.

Legendre AM: Blastomycosis. In Greene CE (ed): *Infectious Diseases of The Dog and Cat*. Philadelphia, WB Saunders, 2006, pp 569-576.

AUTHOR: **LISA M. TIEBER NIELSON**
EDITOR: **DOUGLASS K. MACINTIRE**

Blindness

BASIC INFORMATION

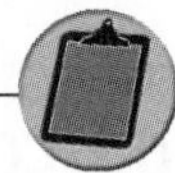

DEFINITION

Loss of vision

SYNONYM(S)

Amaurosis, central blindness: loss of vision due to a lesion in the central nervous system

EPIDEMIOLOGY

SPECIES, AGE, SEX: Dogs and cats; any age and sex may be affected, depending on etiology.

GENETICS AND BREED PREDISPOSITION

- Primary glaucoma: beagle, bassett hound, Bouvier des Flandres, chow chow, cocker spaniel, dachshund, dalmatian, Great Dane, poodle, shar-pei, arctic breeds, spaniel breeds (see Glaucoma, p 440)
- Lens luxation: terrier breeds, spaniel breeds, German shepherd, miniature and toy poodle, Chihuahua (see Lens Luxation, p 628)
- Retinal detachment: shih tzu (see Retinal Detachment, p 965)

RISK FACTORS

- Age: older animals may be predisposed to diseases associated with blindness, including neoplasia (intracranial, intraocular, optic chiasmal) and retinal detachment (see Retinal Detachment, p 965)
- Outdoor access may predispose to infectious diseases associated with blindness (see Uveitis, p 1134, and Optic Neuritis, p 768)

CLINICAL PRESENTATION

DISEASE FORMS/SUBTYPES

- Unilateral or bilateral
- Sudden or progressive
- "Red eye" blindness: associated with visible conjunctival redness on physical examination:
  - Glaucoma (see Glaucoma, p 440)
  - Severe uveitis (see Uveitis, p 1134)
  - Cataracts (see Cataracts, p 182)
  - Lens luxation (see Lens Luxation, p 628)
  - Complex corneal ulceration (see Corneal Ulceration, p 246)
  - Orbital disease (see Orbital Disease, p 773)
- Nonred, noninflamed eye ("quiet eye") blindness: no conjunctival redness is observed in the blind eye(s):
  - Prechiasmal/chiasmal blindness
    - Lesion affecting retina, optic nerve, optic chiasm (Fig. I-30)
    - Associated with dilated pupils and pupillary light reflex (PLR) abnormalities
  - Postchiasmal/cortical blindness
    - Lesion affecting optic tract, lateral geniculate nucleus, optic radiations, or visual cortex of the cerebrum
    - Pupil size and PLRs usually normal unless optic tracts affected along portions common to PLR and vision pathways (see Fig. I-30) and/or unrelated, concurrent iris condition (see Pupil Abnormalities, p 924)

HISTORY, CHIEF COMPLAINT

- Variable depending on the underlying cause, whether the blindness is unilateral or bilateral, and sudden or progressive in onset
- In cases of sudden blindness, all or some of the following may be reported:
  - Disorientation (see Disorientation/Confusion, p 312)
  - Suddenly starts bumping into objects
  - Inability to find food bowl, toys, etc.
  - Lethargy
  - Anxiety
- In cases of progressive blindness, all or some of the following may be reported:
  - Occasionally bumping into objects in own environment
  - Frequently bumping into objects in unfamiliar or suddenly altered environment
  - Vision deficits in dim light and/or darkness (loss of night vision) (e.g., progressive retinal degeneration/atrophy; see Retinal Degeneration, p 963)
  - Patients may be lethargic and/or anxious but generally adjust better and compensate well with progressive vision loss, especially if slowly progressive

PHYSICAL EXAM FINDINGS

- "Red eye" blindness (see Glaucoma, p 440; Uveitis, p 1134; Orbital Disease, p 773)
- Nonred, quiet eye blindness
  - Prechiasmal/chiasmal blindness:
    - Menace response absent
    - Dazzle reflex (bright light perception) absent
    - Pupil(s) dilated or fixed and dilated
    - PLR(s) decreased (i.e., sluggish and incomplete) or absent
    - ± Anisocoria (asymmetry between the size of the pupils), especially seen in unilateral lesions where only the affected pupil is more dilated)
  - Postchiasmal/cortical blindness:
    - Menace response variable depending on localization and severity of lesion
    - Menace response may be absent in contralateral eye if a unilateral lesion present
    - Small percentage of nasal/medial visual field may be preserved due to undecussated (those not crossed-over) optic nerve fibers
    - Menace response absent in both eyes in bilateral/diffuse optic tract, lateral geniculate nucleus, optic radiation, or visual cortical lesions
    - Dazzle reflex(es) normal
    - Pupil size and PLRs normal unless certain portions of optic tract(s) affected that are common to both the PLR and visual pathways (see Fig. I-30) and/or unrelated, concurrent iris condition (see Pupil Abnormalities, p 924)

ETIOLOGY AND PATHOPHYSIOLOGY

- "Red eye" blindness: the lesion is ocular or intraocular:
  - Opacity of the ocular media (e.g., cornea, aqueous humor, lens, vitreous) in cases of corneal ulceration, uveitis, and glaucoma
  - Retinal degeneration with or without detachment and optic nerve atrophy in glaucoma (see Glaucoma, p 440)
- Nonred, quiet eye blindness:
  - Prechiasmal/chiasmal: the lesion lies along the retina–optic nerve–optic chiasm pathway
    - Retinal diseases (see Retinal Detachment, p 965; see Retinal Degeneration, p 963)
    - Optic nerve lesions (e.g., congenital optic nerve hypoplasia, inflammation [see Optic Neuritis, p 768]), neoplasia (e.g., meningioma), or atrophy (e.g., glaucoma, trauma)
    - Optic chiasmal lesions (e.g., neoplasia, abscess)
  - Postchiasmal/cortical: the lesion affects the optic radiation to and including the visual (occipital) cerebral cortex
    - Cerebral edema
    - Cerebral infectious, inflammatory, or neoplastic disease

DIAGNOSIS

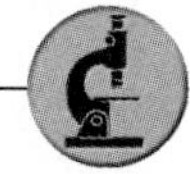

DIFFERENTIAL DIAGNOSIS

- "Red eye" blindness:
  - May be confused with disorientation due to causes other than blindness (see Disorientation/Confusion, p 312) and concurrent non-vision-threatening cause(s) of "red eye" including:

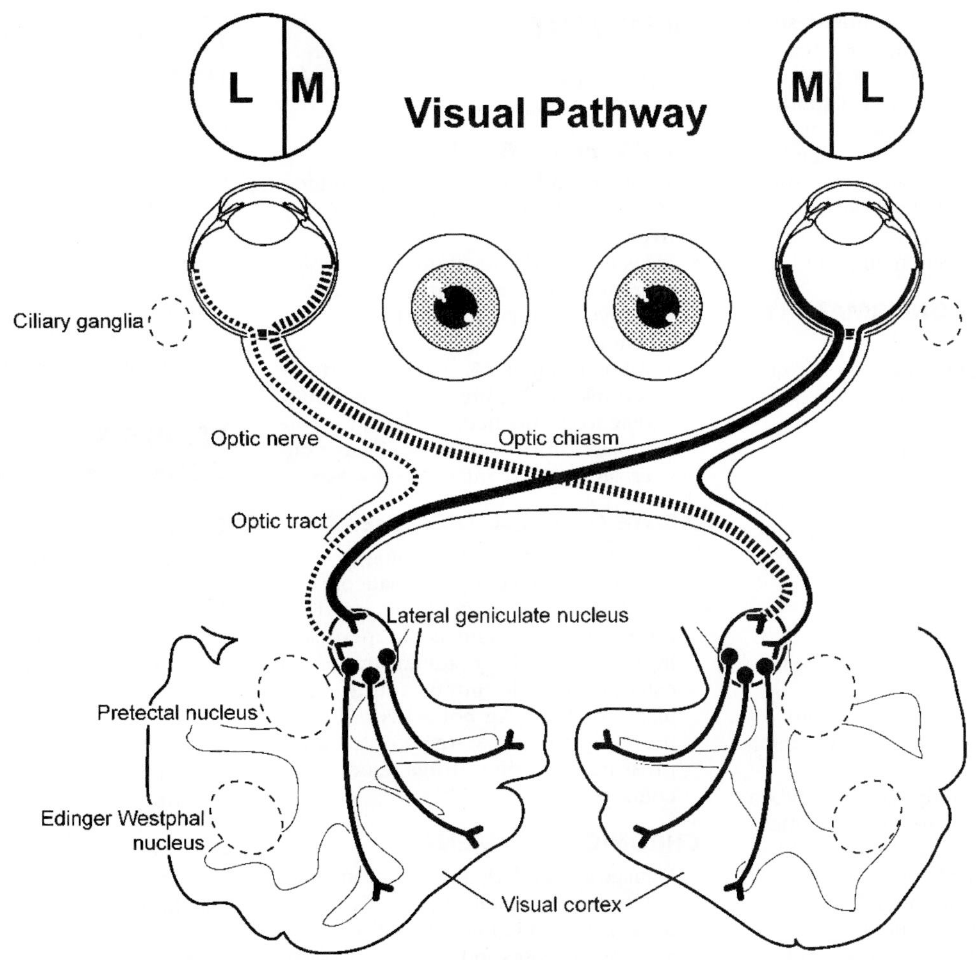

FIGURE I-30 Anatomy of visual pathway from the eye to the visual cortex of the cerebrum. The circles adjacent to "Visual Pathway" title indicate visual fields. M = medial; L = lateral.

    - Conjunctivitis (see Conjunctivitis: Dogs, p 233; Conjunctivitis: Cats, p 231)
    - Episcleritis (see Episcleritis/Scleritis, p 353)
    - Simple or indolent corneal ulcer (see Corneal Ulceration, p 246)
- Nonred, noninflamed eye ("quiet eye") blindness:
  - May be confused with disorientation due to causes other than blindness (see Disorientation/Confusion, p 312)
- Blindness may also be characterized as unilateral or bilateral. Note: unilateral processes by definition more commonly affect only one eye, but if they are very extensive, they can affect both eyes in some cases; disorders that affect one or both eyes with equal frequency are listed in both categories.
  - Unilateral: corneal trauma, complex corneal ulceration, lens luxation, retinal detachment, retinal hemorrhage, glaucoma, cerebral lesions (optic radiation/visual occipital cortex)
  - Bilateral: cataracts, retinal detachment, retinal hemorrhage, severe uveitis, glaucoma, optic neuritis, optic chiasm lesions, sudden acquired retinal degeneration progressive retinal degeneration/atrophy

INITIAL DATABASE

- Cranial nerve examination is imperative to localize the lesion causing blindness:
  - Menace response, assessment of pupil symmetry and size, direct and consensual PLRs, dazzle, palpebral and corneal reflexes, assessment of physiologic nystagmus (i.e., vestibulo-ocular reflex), evaluation of facial sensation and motor function
    - Normal PLRs: lesion usually postchiasmal/cortical (with "nonred, noninflamed eye" ["quiet eye"] blindness) or opacity of ocular media
    - Sluggish, incomplete/absent PLR and dilated pupil: lesion involves retina, optic nerve, optic chiasm (causes bilateral blindness), or optic tract; or a separate, primary lesion of the pupil is present
- General neurologic examination
- Complete ophthalmic examination including:
  - Fluorescein stain and intraocular pressure assessments
  - Examination of anterior segments
    - Evaluate for opacity of the cornea, aqueous humor, lens, or vitreous
  - Posterior segment/fundic examination after pharmacologic pupil dilation (1% tropicamide)
    - Pharmacologic pupil dilation is contraindicated with glaucoma
    - Evaluate optic nerve (size, shape, color; see Glaucoma, p 440 and Optic Neuritis, p 768)
    - Evaluate tapetum (dorsal reflective mirror) for brightness and/or color changes (e.g., hyperreflective/bright with retinal degeneration and/or certain forms of retinal detachment; hyporeflective/dull grey to pigmented with inflammation and/or certain forms of retinal detachment)
    - Evaluate nontapetal fundus (typically pigmented and located ventrally) for whitish/grey discoloration (e.g., depigmentation from past or active inflammation; retinal detachments) or hemorrhages
    - Evaluate vasculature of retina (should see small arteries and larger veins coming from the optic disk and coursing peripherally)

and look for inflammatory lesions (hyporeflective/dull grey to pigmented lesions in the tapetal fundus and in the nontapetal fundus), hemorrhages, or detachment
- Complete blood count, serum chemistry profile, urinalysis to assess systemic status
- Blood pressure (see Retinal Detachment, p 965; Systemic Hypertension, p 1058; Blood Pressure Measurement, p 1191)

ADVANCED OR CONFIRMATORY TESTING

- Thoracic radiographs (screen for neoplasia or systemic infectious disease)
- Serologic titers for infectious diseases unique to geographic area:
  - Rickettsial diseases
  - Systemic mycoses (blastomycosis, cryptococcosis, histoplasmosis, coccidioidomycosis)
  - Lyme disease
  - Bartonellosis
  - Toxoplasmosis
- Aspiration of enlarged lymph nodes for cytologic evaluation
- Ocular ultrasonography if opacity of ocular media precludes fundic examination
- Histopathologic study in cases when eye is blind and painful and enucleation is advised
- Referral is advisable for all cases of blindness of undetermined cause for additional work-up including:
  - Electroretinography to assess retinal function
  - Visual-evoked potentials
  - Cerebrospinal fluid tap
  - Magnetic resonance imaging or computed tomography
  - Vitreous centesis with cytologic study, culture, titers
- Rectal scrape, cytologic study for protothecosis

TREATMENT

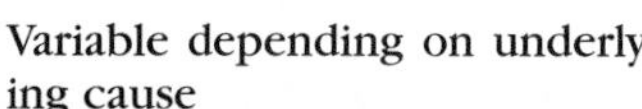

Variable depending on underlying cause

THERAPEUTIC GOAL(S)

- Treat any underlying cause of blindness such as hypertensive retinopathy, uveitis, etc.
- In general, administration of empiric therapy is not recommended until a tentative or final diagnosis has been reached.
  - Administration of systemic corticosteroids prematurely may preclude diagnosis of neoplasia and some inflammatory disorders and may exacerbate systemic infectious diseases

ACUTE GENERAL TREATMENT

- Depends on underlying etiology
- Example: acute congestive glaucoma. Administration of systemic corticosteroids to reduce effects of reperfusion injury followed by administration of osmotic diuretic intravenously (e.g., mannitol 1-2 g/kg bolus over 20 minutes), topical and systemic intraocular pressure-lowering drugs (see Glaucoma, p 440)

CHRONIC TREATMENT

- Manage any underlying conditions such as chronic renal failure, systemic hypertension, systemic infectious disease
- Systemic mycoses and immune-mediated disorders require long-term therapy
- Treat primary cause of blindness when possible (e.g., refer for cataract surgery in cases with mature cataracts)

RECOMMENDED MONITORING

- Monitor for return of vision, PLR, dazzle reflex after commencing therapy
- Serial fundic examinations

PROGNOSIS AND OUTCOME

- Variable depending on underlying cause.
- Restoration of vision after acute vision loss may be possible after rapid diagnosis of underlying condition and aggressive appropriate therapy.
- In many cases, however, blindness is irreversible, and long-term management aims to provide comfort if pain is likely (e.g., glaucoma).

PEARLS & CONSIDERATIONS

COMMENTS

- Assessment of the direct and consensual PLRs and dazzle reflexes is imperative in evaluation of blindness.
  - Absence of the PLR and/or dazzle reflex is a poor prognostic indicator because minimal retinal function is required to retain these reflexes
- The PLR and dazzle reflexes are subcortical pathways (do not involve the cerebral cortex) and therefore are normal with blindness caused by cortical lesions.
- A PLR is dependent only on quantity of light; vision is dependent on quality of light; therefore, the PLR should remain intact despite opacity of the ocular media if there is no concurrent retinal or optic nerve damage.

SUGGESTED READING

Martin CL: Evaluation of patients with decreased vision or blindness. *Clin Tech Small Anim Pract* 16(1):62-70, 2001.

AUTHOR: **ANNE J. GEMENSKY-METZLER**
EDITOR: **CHERYL L. CULLEN**

Blue-Green Algae Toxicosis

BASIC INFORMATION

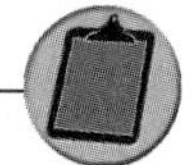

DEFINITION

Sudden-onset neurologic signs or acute liver failure in dogs, caused by ingestion of blue-green algae

SYNONYM(S)

BGA toxicosis
Cyanobacteria toxicosis

EPIDEMIOLOGY

SPECIES, AGE, SEX

- Dogs: all breeds, ages, and sexes susceptible
- Cats: none reported

RISK FACTORS: BGA blooms are favored by stagnant water; warm water temperatures; ample sunlight; and high nutrients from fertilizer, animal waste, and sewage runoff.

GEOGRAPHY AND SEASONALITY: Blooms occur mostly in summer or fall.

CLINICAL PRESENTATION

DISEASE FORMS/SUBTYPES

- Acute hepatotoxic syndrome
- Subacute neurotoxic syndrome

HISTORY, CHIEF COMPLAINT

- History of swimming or drinking water from a pond, lake, or river
- Vomiting, diarrhea, weakness, and collapse (>6 hrs after exposure): hepatotoxic syndrome
- Salivation, vomiting, diarrhea, dyspnea, tremors, muscle fasciculations, ataxia, weakness, seizures, and death (>15 min after exposure): neurotoxic syndrome

PHYSICAL EXAM FINDINGS

- Presence of algae on the muzzle or on the fur elsewhere on the body is common. Bluish-green and slimy, or may be dried if later presentation
- Hepatotoxic syndrome: see History, Chief Complaint above; plus pale mucous membranes, poor capillary refill time, tachycardia or bradycardia,

signs of abdominal pain, rapid weak pulse, hypothermia, and shock
- Neurotoxic syndrome: see History, Chief Complaint above

ETIOLOGY AND PATHOPHYSIOLOGY

- BGA are microscopic organisms that form colonies visible to the naked eye, rely on photosynthesis for energy, and have a cell wall similar to gram-negative bacteria.
- Accumulations of large amounts of BGA in lakes, ponds, or rivers are known as *waterblooms*. BGA blooms can be found throughout the world and are light to dark green or sometimes reddish-brown. Wind propels toxic algae to the shoreline where animals are exposed to the organism by ingestion when they drink BGA-contaminated water.
- Common toxin-producing genera of fresh and brackish water BGA include *Microcystis, Anabaena, Oscillatoria, Aphanizomenon, Nodularia,* and *Nostoc* spp.
- Acute hepatotoxic syndrome:
  - Most commonly described poisoning by BGA caused by low-molecular-weight cyclic heptapeptides and pentapeptides known as *microcystins* and *nodularins*. Microcystin-LR (MCLR) is the most toxic and the most frequently encountered of approximately 50 similar peptides.
  - After ingestion, BGA toxins are released from the cells and preferentially absorbed from the ileum.
  - Once inside hepatocytes, toxins inhibit protein phosphatases (PP) types 1 and 2A (PP1 and 2A), causing hyperphosphorylation of cytosolic and cytoskeletal proteins, leading to cytoskeletal disruption, damage, and necrosis.
  - Death occurs due to massive intrahepatic hemorrhage, hypovolemia, and liver failure.
- Subacute neurotoxic syndrome: Responsible toxins are:
  - Anatoxin-a: an alkaloid and a potent postsynaptic depolarizing neuromuscular blocking agent that affects nicotinic and muscarinic acetylcholine receptors.
  - Anatoxin-a(s): inhibits peripheral (but not central) cholinesterase irreversibly and is the only known naturally occurring organophosphorus cholinesterase inhibitor (similar to organophosphate pesticides).

DIAGNOSIS

DIFFERENTIAL DIAGNOSIS

- Differentiate from other hepatotoxic agents: amanita mushroom, sago palm, acetaminophen
- Primary hepatic diseases (see Hepatic Injury, Acute, p 491)

INITIAL DATABASE

- Hepatotoxic syndrome:
  - Complete blood count (CBC): leukocytosis and thrombocytopenia.
  - Serum biochemistry panel: increased alanine aminotransferase (ALT), aspartate aminotransferase (AST), alkaline phosphatase, γ-glutamyltransferase (GGT), glucose, and possibly creatine phosphokinase, lactate dehydrogenase. Hypoglycemia is possible after hyperglycemia.
  - Serum bile acids: increase commonly occurs early.
  - Coagulation profile: Whole blood clotting time may be normal; prothrombin time and activated thromboplastin times increase twofold to fourfold.
- Neurotoxic syndrome:
  - Due to rapid effect of the toxins, no significant serum biochemical changes are expected.

ADVANCED OR CONFIRMATORY TESTING

- Postmortem (hepatotoxicosis): rounding of hepatocytes, disruption of hepatic cords, loss of sinusoidal integrity, intrahepatic hemorrhage, and centrilobular necrosis.
- Blood cholinesterase analysis may help (see Organophosphate and Carbamate Insecticide Toxicosis, p 775).
- Microscopic identification of toxigenic algae. Obtain large specimen (1-2 L) of the algae by straining the cells out of the water with cheesecloth. Specimens can be sent for identification, purification, and quantification of algal toxins; mouse bioassay; or for enzyme-linked immunosorbent assay to Dr. Wayne Carmichael's laboratories; call before shipping the specimens: http://www. wright.edu/biology/faculty/carmichael/ labhome/labhome.htm.

TREATMENT

THERAPEUTIC GOAL(S)

- Decontamination of patient
- Control muscarinic and neurologic signs
- Supportive care

ACUTE GENERAL TREATMENT

- Decontamination:
  - Emesis: only in animals not showing any clinical signs (see Vomiting, Induction of, p 1328).
  - Activated charcoal 2-4 g/kg PO.
  - Cholestyramine (200-300 mg/kg PO) may be more effective than charcoal (it is more expensive and must be obtained from a pharmacy).
  - The noncompetitive, bile-acid transport inhibitors, rifampicin, and bile salts, such as cholate and deoxycholate, can inhibit uptake of microcystins. Their utility, however, in clinical algal toxicoses needs to be determined.
- Control muscarinic and neurologic signs:
  - Atropine sulfate for muscarinic signs (0.04-0.1 mg/kg IV prn).
  - Diazepam for seizures 0.5-2 mg/kg IV prn; other antiseizure medications such as barbiturates can be used if diazepam is ineffective.
- Supportive care:
  - Control severe vomiting with metoclopramide (0.1-0.4 mg/kg PO, SC, or IM q 6h), only if intestinal obstruction has been ruled out (if present, usually unrelated to BGA).
  - Treat signs of acute hepatic failure (see Hepatic Encephalopathy, p 489; Hemorrhage, p 485; Hepatic Injury, Acute, p 491). Typical therapeutics may include:
    - Lactulose
    - S-adenosyl methionine
    - Dietary management
    - Vitamin K_1
    - Plasma and/or whole blood transfusions as needed
    - IV fluids (possibly including 5% dextrose)
    - Broad-spectrum antibiotics for secondary infection

POSSIBLE COMPLICATIONS

Permanent hepatic insufficiency

RECOMMENDED MONITORING

- Serum chemistry profile, especially liver-specific enzymes (ALT, AST, GGT, alkaline phosphatase)
- Serum bile acids
- CBC
- Hematocrit
- Body temperature
- Blood glucose

PROGNOSIS AND OUTCOME

Poor prognosis with systemic signs of acute hepatic damage or severe neurologic dysfunction

PEARLS & CONSIDERATIONS

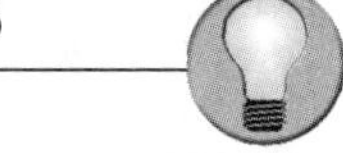

COMMENTS

- In dogs, BGA poisoning is a sporadic but recurrent cause of acute illness and death.

- Lethal doses of purified MCLR: rat, 160 μg/kg IP; mouse, 100 μg/kg IP; LD50 of purified anatoxin-a in mouse = 200 μg/kg IP and anatoxin-a(s) = 30 μg/kg IP.

SUGGESTED READING

Beasley VR, et al: Diagnostic and clinically important aspects of cyanobacterial (blue-green algae) toxicoses. *J Vet Diag Invest,* 1:359–365, 1989.

Khan SA, et al: Comparative pathology of microcystin-LR in cultured hepatocytes, fibroblasts, and renal epithelial cells. *Natural Toxins* 3:119–128, 1995.

AUTHOR & EDITOR: **SAFDAR A. KHAN**

Bordetellosis

BASIC INFORMATION

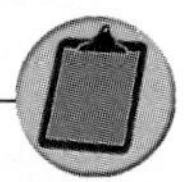

DEFINITION

Highly contagious infection caused by *Bordetella bronchoseptica* that is implicated in respiratory diseases, including tracheitis, bronchitis, and possibly pneumonia

SYNONYM(S)

Canine respiratory disease complex
Infectious tracheobronchitis
Kennel cough

EPIDEMIOLOGY

SPECIES, AGE, SEX

- Young dogs more commonly affected than adults
- Cats are also potentially affected with clinical disease

RISK FACTORS: An increased risk is seen in dogs and cats housed in close proximity, as seen in shelters and breeding facilities.

CONTAGION AND ZOONOSIS: The disease is transmitted either directly via animal-to-animal contact, or contact with aerosolized microdroplets from infected animals. Bordetellosis is a known zoonotic disease, especially in immunocompromised people.

GEOGRAPHY AND SEASONALITY: Probably worldwide distribution, with no significant seasonality.

ASSOCIATED CONDITIONS AND DISORDERS

- Bordetellosis is often part of a disease complex, not a solitary disease. As such, in dogs it often is associated with canine parainfluenza; canine adenovirus-2; canine distemper; and infections with *Mycoplasma* spp., *Streptococcus* sp., *Pasteurella* sp., *Pseudomonas* sp., and others. In cats, *Bordetella bronchiseptica* has been linked with feline respiratory disease complex organisms such as feline rhinotracheitis (feline herpesvirus), feline calicivirus, and other bacterial organisms.
- Bordetellosis is generally limited to the upper respiratory tract; in some cases pneumonia can occur.

CLINICAL PRESENTATION

HISTORY, CHIEF COMPLAINT

- History usually includes exposure to a multi-housing environment (kennel, dog show, other) several days before onset of coughing
- The chief complaint depends on severity
  - Mild tracheitis may present with a dry cough that is worse with excitement, and nasal discharge is possible.
  - Severe tracheobronchitis presents with dyspnea, coughing, anorexia, mucopurulent discharge, and lethargy.

PHYSICAL EXAM FINDINGS

- Spontaneous cough and/or cough inducible with palpation of trachea in dogs
- Sneezing is more common in cats
- ± Mild to moderate fever in severe cases
- ± Possibly increased lung sounds
- ± Nasal or ocular discharge

ETIOLOGY AND PATHOPHYSIOLOGY

- *B. bronchiseptica* is shed from oropharyngeal secretions for up to 3 months in infected animals.
- When secretions reach the oropharynx, the organism attaches to the cilia of the respiratory epithelium and causes stasis of the mucociliary apparatus.
- Due to impairment of immune function, infection facilitates colonization of the respiratory tract by other organisms.

DIAGNOSIS

DIFFERENTIAL DIAGNOSIS

- In dogs:
  - Canine distemper
  - Canine parainfluenza
  - Canine adenovirus infection
  - Mycoplasmosis
  - Chronic sterile tracheobronchitis of older dogs
  - Other causes of pneumonia (aspiration, etc.)
  - Collapsing trachea
  - Airway foreign body
- In cats:
  - Feline rhinotracheitis (feline herpesvirus-1)
  - Feline calicivirus infection
  - *Chlamydophila felis* infection
  - Other bacterial causes of pneumonia

INITIAL DATABASE

- Complete blood count: often unremarkable; neutrophilia with left shift or toxic neutrophil changes may be seen with pneumonia
- Thoracic radiographs: often unremarkable (mild cases); evidence of pneumonia possible (severe/complicated cases)

ADVANCED OR CONFIRMATORY TESTING

- Transtracheal wash or bronchoalveolar lavage if pneumonia or lower airway disease suspected
- Bacterial culture and sensitivity (positive cultures noted in healthy patients as well)
- Swabs of the oropharynx can be performed but should be placed on a special medium to decrease other respiratory flora

TREATMENT

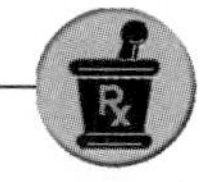

THERAPEUTIC GOAL(S)

- Appropriate antibiotic therapy
- Supportive care

ACUTE GENERAL TREATMENT

- Antimicrobials:
  - Ideally based on culture and sensitivity.
  - Initial choices include:
    - Amoxicillin-clavulanate (12.5–25 mg/kg PO q 12h)
    - Trimethoprim-sulfonamide (15 mg/kg PO q 12h)
    - Doxycycline (5 mg/kg PO q 12h).
  - In severe cases, other choices may include gentamicin, enrofloxacin, and cefazolin.
- Antitussives:
  - Reduce clearance of organisms and may allow for further colonization.
  - Not recommended in cases of pneumonia.
  - For suppression of dry, nonproductive coughs only (mild cases, in

which animal is otherwise well). Dose is titrated to reduce cough without causing sedation.
  - Butorphanol 0.05–1 mg/kg PO q 8–12h
  - Hydrocodone 0.22 mg/kg PO q 8–12h
- Bronchodilators:
  - May be indicated in cases of severe pneumonia.
- Aerosol therapy:
  - May help with clearance of tracheal or bronchial secretions.
  - May also be used for nebulizing antibiotics, especially gentamicin, kanamycin, and polymyxin B although variable or inadequate tissue concentrations of some of these drugs administered via this route have been reported.
- Glucocorticoids:
  - Anti-inflammatory doses orally may help cough.
  - Prednisolone 0.25–0.5 mg/kg PO q 12h for 2 to 3 days only.
- Adequate hydration is very important to facilitate clearance of mucoid secretions

RECOMMENDED MONITORING

Repeat thoracic radiographs should be done in cases of pneumonia.

PROGNOSIS AND OUTCOME

- Often self-limiting infection, especially in adults.
- Severe (potentially fatal) pneumonia may be seen in the young or debilitated.

PEARLS & CONSIDERATIONS

COMMENTS

Once clinical signs have resolved, shedding of organisms may nevertheless last for up to 3 months. Therefore, infection of other animals and immunocompromised people may continue during that time, and suitable precautions (avoidance of direct or indirect contact) should be taken.

PREVENTION

- Quarantine of new animals and infected animals may decrease spread in multi-animal housing.
- Decreasing stress with adequate hygiene and care are strongly recommended. Cages can be disinfected with diluted bleach (1:32 solution).
- Vaccination:
  - Parenteral and nasal vaccinations are available, although effectiveness is questionable.
  - One recent study suggests that intranasal and parenteral vaccines used sequentially may be superior.
  - Depending on vaccine, intranasal vaccines may be used as soon as 2 weeks of age.
  - Intranasal vaccines may induce cough and/or nasal discharge.
- Natural immunity may last up to 6 months after infection.

SUGGESTED READING

Edinboro CH, et al: A placebo-controlled trial of two intranasal vaccines to prevent kennel cough in dogs entering a humane shelter. *Prev Vet Med* 62:89–99, 2004.

Ellis JA, et al: Effect of vaccination on experimental infection with *Bordetella bronchiseptica* in dogs. *J Am Vet Med Assoc* 218: 267–275, 2001.

Ford RB, et al: Canine infectious tracheobronchitis. In Greene CE (ed): *Infectious Disease of the Dog and Cat*. Philadelphia, WB Saunders, 1998, pp 33–38.

Gaskell R, et al: Feline respiratory disease. In Greene CE (ed): *Infectious Disease of the Dog and Cat*. Philadelphia, WB Saunders, 1998, pp 97–105.

AUTHOR: **JEFFERY SIMMONS**

EDITOR: **DOUGLASS K. MACINTIRE**

Boric Acid Toxicosis

BASIC INFORMATION

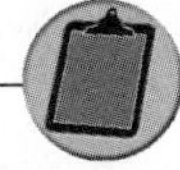

DEFINITION

Toxicosis resulting from ingestion of inorganic compound of boron used in ant or roach baits, flea products for dogs and cats, cleaning compounds, buffering agent, eye wash, and anticaking agent. Toxicosis is uncommon because of the relatively large amount of product that needs to be ingested, but when this occurs, it is characterized by vomiting, diarrhea, anorexia, lethargy, and rarely renal damage.

SYNONYM(S)

Borax
Orthoboric acid
Sodium biborate
Sodium borate
Sodium perborate
Sodium pyroborate
Sodium tetraborate

EPIDEMIOLOGY

SPECIES, AGE, SEX

- All breeds of cats and dogs are susceptible.
- Cats can be exposed after walking through the agent (e.g., gels [generally 5.4% concentration] that are put out on small pieces of cardboard or in small cups or powder forms [5–99% concentration] that can be placed in cupboards or in closets) or when flea powders containing boric acid are used topically.

RISK FACTORS: Preexisting renal disease may increase the risk of nephrotoxicity from large ingestions.

CLINICAL PRESENTATION

HISTORY, CHIEF COMPLAINT

- History of using a boric acid-containing product on the animal or in the house (for fleas or control of other insects)
- Vomiting
- Hypersalivation
- Anorexia
- Lethargy

PHYSICAL EXAM FINDINGS

- Findings tend to be nonspecific
- Common:
  - Hypersalivation
  - Lethargy
  - Vomiting, diarrhea
- Possible:
  - Oliguria/anuria
  - Anorexia
  - Ataxia (rare)
  - Seizures (rare)

ETIOLOGY AND PATHOPHYSIOLOGY

Source:

- Some ant baits may contain less than 1% boric acid, whereas some roach products can contain 100% boric acid.
- Boric acid-containing formulations are available as powder, liquid, or gels.
- Borates have been used in pharmaceutical preparations (mouthwash, toothpastes, cosmetics), as toiletries, in cleaning compounds, and as insecticides.

Pathophysiology:

- The exact mechanism is unknown. Boric acid is considered cytotoxic to all cells.
- Rapidly absorbed after oral ingestion through mucous membranes, as well as through abraded skin.
- Concentrated in the kidneys before excretion, excreted unchanged in the urine.

- Half-life in dogs is 12 hours, but total elimination may take up to 7 days.
- No death or serious systemic toxicity reported in dogs when given 1.54–6.51 g/kg of borax or 1–3 g/kg of boric acid. Examples:
  - 20 ounces of a 5.4% boric acid ant bait would have to be ingested by a 20-kg dog to reach a dose of 1.5 g/kg.
  - Similarly, 1.1 ounces of a 99% boric acid agent would need to be ingested by a 20-kg dog to reach a dose of 1.5 g/kg.
  - In either case, systemic signs are not likely except for possibly vomiting and diarrhea.

DIAGNOSIS

DIFFERENTIAL DIAGNOSIS

- Garbage toxicosis
- Dietary indiscretion
- Infectious enteritis (parvoviral, coronaviral, bacterial, etc.)
- Foreign body
- Nephrotoxic agents (ethylene glycol, pharmaceuticals, lilies [cats], grapes and raisins [dogs])

INITIAL DATABASE

- Complete blood count: microcytic hypochromic anemia
- Serum biochemistry panel: azotemia, hyperchloremia, hypernatremia, hyperkalemia, and metabolic acidosis may be noted in severe cases. Rarely, elevated liver enzymes
- Urinalysis: in severe cases causing oliguria or anuria with tubular necrosis, albuminuria, hematuria, proteinuria, and epithelial casts (acute renal failure), or isosthenuria concurrently with azotemia (chronic renal failure) may be noted

ADVANCED OR CONFIRMATORY TESTING

Boric acid may be detected in the urine, cerebrospinal fluid, blood, and plasma.

TREATMENT

THERAPEUTIC GOAL(S)

- Decontamination of patient
- Supportive care

ACUTE GENERAL TREATMENT

- Decontamination of patient:
  - Emesis: induce emesis in cases involving large ingestions. Approximately 3% hydrogen peroxide at 1–2 ml/kg PO, maximum dose 45 ml. Repeat in 10 minutes if vomiting does not occur the first time, or use apomorphine 0.04 mg/kg IM or IV or instill part of a crushed tablet dissolved in water into conjunctival sac and rinse out when vomiting begins
  - Activated charcoal not useful in binding boric acid
  - Bathe the animal for dermal exposures, using diluted, liquid dishwashing detergent
- Supportive care:
  - Control excessive vomiting with metoclopramide at 0.022–0.044 mg/kg PO, SQ, or IM, barring gastrointestinal obstruction
  - Gastrointestinal protectants: sucralfate 0.5–1 g q 8h, PO and famotidine 0.5 mg/kg PO, SQ, or IM q 12–24h for 5 to 7 days
  - IV fluid diuresis for 24 to 48 hours with large ingestion
  - Treat renal failure as needed (see Acute Renal Failure, p 32)
  - Control seizures with diazepam 0.5–2 mg/kg IV unless underlying metabolic (e.g., hypoglycemia, hypocalcemia) or hepatic (see Hepatic Encephalopathy, p 489) cause

CHRONIC TREATMENT

- Chronic problems not expected
- Renal damage generally responds to fluid therapy and supportive care

POSSIBLE COMPLICATIONS

May exacerbate preexisting renal disease

RECOMMENDED MONITORING

- Recheck renal parameters (blood urea nitrogen, creatinine, urinalysis) at 24 and 48 hours postexposure
- If renal parameters are within normal limits at that time, further problems not expected

PROGNOSIS AND OUTCOME

Excellent in animals with signs limited to vomiting/diarrhea after a low-dose exposure

PEARLS & CONSIDERATIONS

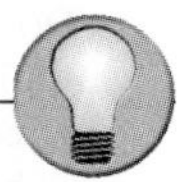

COMMENTS

- Activated charcoal adsorbs boric acid poorly (boron compounds do not adhere well to charcoal). A 30:1 ratio of activated charcoal to boric acid was needed to absorb 38% of boric acid in an in vitro study; 5 to 10 times the normal activated charcoal dose would be required to be effective, and therefore activated charcoal is not recommended as a routine part of treatment of boric acid toxicosis.
- In general, boron compounds have a wide margin of safety and in most cases of toxicity, only vomiting and diarrhea are noted.
- Ant baits containing 1–5% boric acid are not expected to cause a serious problem in dogs or cats.
- Concentrated boric acid product greater than 50% should be avoided, but products containing less than 5.4% concentration are considered relatively safe.
- In general, boron compounds have a wide margin of safety, and in most cases of toxicity, only vomiting and diarrhea are noted.

PREVENTION

Avoid using highly concentrated boric-acid products directly on animals or in the house (on the carpet especially if cats are around) where direct exposure to pets is likely.

SUGGESTED READING

Kiesch-Nesselrodt A, Hooser SB: Boric acid. In Beasley VR (eds): Toxicology of selected pesticides, drugs, and chemicals. *Vet Clin North Am Small Anim Pract* 369–373, 1990.

Welch S: Boric acid. In Plumlee KH (ed): *Clinical Veterinary Toxicology*. St. Louis, Mosby, 2004, pp 143–145.

AUTHOR: **CAROLINE W. DONALDSON**
EDITOR: **SAFDAR A. KHAN**

Borreliosis

BASIC INFORMATION

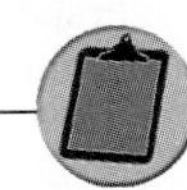

DEFINITION

Borreliosis is a bacterial disease that affects humans and other mammals. It is caused by a unicellular, spiral-shaped, gram-negative bacteria that is transmitted primarily by *Ixodes* ticks.

SYNONYM(S)

Lyme disease
Lyme borreliosis
Ixodes tick: deer tick

EPIDEMIOLOGY

SPECIES, AGE, SEX

- Susceptibility: humans > dogs > cats
- Dogs more commonly affected at younger age

GENETICS AND BREED PREDISPOSITION

- Breeds associated with outdoor activities
- Labradors, golden retrievers, and Shetland sheepdogs may be predisposed to renal effects ("Lyme nephritis/nephropathy")

RISK FACTORS: Higher risk of infection when greater opportunity for tick bite (e.g., proximity of animal to undisturbed dense vegetation in endemic area).

CONTAGION AND ZOONOSIS

- Direct horizontal spread of the tick from dogs to humans is unlikely.
- Dogs and cats act as sentinel carriers.

GEOGRAPHY AND SEASONALITY

- The *Ixodes* ticks inhabit mostly temperate latitudes. Most cases of borreliosis are found in the northeastern and mid-Atlantic United States (accounting for 83% of human cases in 2002) and the upper midwest and coastal Pacific northwest.
- Most cases are reported between May and November.

ASSOCIATED CONDITIONS AND DISORDERS: Lyme nephritis/nephropathy can develop in chronic cases in predisposed animals.

CLINICAL PRESENTATION

HISTORY, CHIEF COMPLAINT

- Exposure to ticks is commonly known to have occurred.
- Animals may show anorexia, lethargy, fever, swelling of one or more joints (often carpi/hocks).
    - Clinical signs usually occur 1 to 5 months after exposure.
- Animals with Lyme nephropathy usually present in early spring to late fall for evaluation of vomiting and anorexia.

PHYSICAL EXAM FINDINGS

- Absence of any clinical signs is most common
    - Most dogs with a positive *Borrelia* titer have no overt manifestations of illness.
    - Fewer than 5% exhibit clinical signs of disease.
- Lymphadenopathy
- Warm, swollen, painful joints
- Fever (103–106°F, [40–41°C])

ETIOLOGY AND PATHOPHYSIOLOGY

- *Borrelia burgdorferi* is a small microaerophilic spirochete.
- The form of Lyme borreliae in North America is *B. burgdorferi sensu stricto.*
- The organism multiplies in the tick and enters the host at the end of the tick's bloodmeal (when it regurgitates) after 48 to 72 hours of attachment.
- Replication occurs in skin at the site of tick bite, followed by migration throughout the tissues.
- A persistent carrier state is likely, both in infected animals with overt clinical signs and in latent infections.
- Vectors are the small (<3 mm) *Ixodes* spp. ticks. The white-footed deer mouse is the main reservoir and preferred host of larval and nymphal ticks.

DIAGNOSIS

DIFFERENTIAL DIAGNOSIS

- Septic arthritis
- Other tick-borne arthritides (ehrlichiosis, Rocky Mountain spotted fever [RMSF], bartonellosis)
- Immune-mediated polyarthritits (systemic lupus erythematosus, rheumatoid arthritis)
- Polymyositis
- Panosteitis
- Neoplasia
- Degenerative joint disease
- Trauma
- Osteomyelitis

INITIAL DATABASE

Initial database is usually directed at ruling out other causes of fever of unknown origin (see Fever of Unknown Origin, p 386) and includes:

- Complete blood count and serum biochemistry profile: no specific findings expected
- Urinalysis: pathologic proteinuria in cases of Lyme nephritis/nephropathy
- Arhtrocentesis: leukocyte counts range from 2000 to 100,000 nucleated cells per microliter
- Serologic tests: RMSF, *Ehrlichia* spp., *Anaplasma*, *Babesia*, *Leptospira interrogans* (multiple serovars)
- Abdominal ultrasound
- Antinuclear antibody test

ADVANCED OR CONFIRMATORY TESTING

- Serologic test:
    - Detects serum antibody against C6 peptide of VlsE antigen (not found in the vaccine)
    - It can be detected at 3 to 5 weeks postexposure
    - It is found in the SNAP-3 test by IDEXX labs
    - Use titer information with caution, because a positive titer indicates exposure rather than active infection
- Renal biopsy: glomerulonephritis, tubular necrosis, interstitial lymphoplasmacytic inflammation
- Culture of spirochetes is the most definitive diagnosis. Skin of the infected patient is the best to culture
- Polymerase chain reaction (PCR) of skin: very sensitive. PCR of urine is less sensitive

TREATMENT

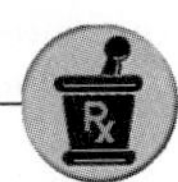

THERAPEUTIC GOAL(S)

- Resolution of lameness and fever if present
- Palliative and supportive care for complications associated with glomerulonephritis caused by Lyme nephropathy

ACUTE GENERAL TREATMENT

Doxycycline (10 mg/kg PO 24h) or amoxicillin (11 mg/kg PO q 12h). Usually treatment is continued for 4 weeks in an effort to eliminate the carrier state.

CHRONIC TREATMENT

- Because no studies have proven the length of time antibiotics need to be administerd to clear the carrier state, prolonged antibiotic therapy may be necessary in cases of Lyme nephropathy.
- Treatment for Lyme nephropathy may include a combination of doxycyline with angiotensin-converting enzyme inhibitor (e.g., enalapril, 0.5 mg/kg PO q 12–24h), low-dose aspirin (0.5 mg/kg PO q 12h), and omega-3-fatty acids.
- Supportive care of renal disease may be warranted and can include antiemetics, phosphate binders, intravenous fluids, and antihypertensives.
- Some dogs with Lyme arthritis do not improve with antibiotics alone.

Corticosteroids can be added for suspected immune-mediated polyarthritis (e.g., prednisone 2.2 mg/kg PO q 24h, tapering to 0.5 mg/kg PO 24h), noting that high doses and prolonged treatment should be avoided whenever possible (immunosuppression).

RECOMMENDED MONITORING

For dogs with Lyme nephropathy: Monthly monitoring of hematocrit, serum creatinine, serum albumin, urine protein:creatinine ratio, and blood pressure can be decreased to every 3 to 6 months if the animal becomes stable clinically.

PROGNOSIS AND OUTCOME

- Prognosis is good for acute presentation with arthritis and fever. Most dogs respond well to antibiotic treatment, although titer remains positive
- Prognosis is guarded to poor for Lyme nephropathy, especially when hypoalbuminemia, dehydration, and azotemia are present, with a life expectancy in some cases of days to weeks

PEARLS & CONSIDERATIONS

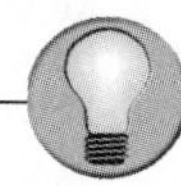

COMMENTS

In humans, the *Borrelia* vaccine was removed from the market because of concern that it might increase the risk of immune-mediated polyarthritis in genetically predisposed individuals.

PREVENTION

- Vector control is the primary means of prevention:
  - Keep lawns mowed
  - Preventic collars (amitraz) or other flea/tick preventative (e.g., fipronil)
  - Check for ticks daily
- Lyme disease vaccine: use is controversial because it may promote immune complex glomerulonephritis in predisposed individuals

CLIENT EDUCATION

Clients should be educated on proper tick removal and tick control.

SUGGESTED READING

Fritz CL, et al: Lyme borreliosis. *JAVMA* 223:9, 2003.

Littman MP: Canine borreliosis. *Vet Clin North Am Small Anim Pract* 33, 2003.

AUTHOR: **KHRISTEN J. CARLSON**

EDITOR: **DOUGLASS K. MACINTIRE**

Botulism

BASIC INFORMATION

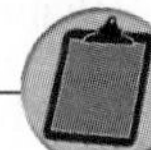

DEFINITION

An acute, rapidly progressive generalized lower motor neuron (LMN) paralytic disorder caused by ingestion of an exotoxin produced by the bacterium *Clostridium botulinum*

EPIDEMIOLOGY

SPECIES, AGE, SEX: Any breed, either sex. Cats appear highly resistant to botulism (no natural cases reported).

GENETICS AND BREED PREDISPOSITION: No breed predilection.

RISK FACTORS: Ingestion of contaminated food or carrion.

CONTAGION AND ZOONOSIS: There are seven antigenically identified types of botulinum neurotoxins (A–G). Dogs: type C. Large animals: type B. Humans: types A, B, F.

GEOGRAPHY AND SEASONALITY: Worldwide distribution, all seasons.

ASSOCIATED CONDITIONS AND DISORDERS: Aspiration pneumonia, ventilatory failure (respiratory arrest).

CLINICAL PRESENTATION

HISTORY, CHIEF COMPLAINT

- Lower motor neuron paresis/paralysis that is often ascending
  - Begins as weakness in the pelvic limbs and can progress to quadriplegia.
- History of ingestion of carrion or other source of anaerobic bacterial contamination
  - The incubation period after ingestion ranges from hours to 6 days.
  - Botulism is especially likely if multiple animals are affected.

PHYSICAL EXAM FINDINGS

- Decreased LMN reflexes (patellar, others) and muscle tone in all limbs.
- Cranial nerve abnormalities (decreased/absent palpebral and menace, decreased jaw tone and gag, mydriasis, voice change).
- Level of consciousness maintained, pain perception preserved.
- In severely affected animals, decreased abdominal and intercostal muscle tone is observed, which can require ventilation or lead to death from ventilatory failure.
- Tail wag is maintained.
- Parasympathetic dysfunction can also be observed (heart rate changes, megaesophagus).

ETIOLOGY AND PATHOPHYSIOLOGY

- *C. botulinum* is a gram-positive, saprophytic, spore-forming bacterial rod in soil.
- Clinical signs develop after ingestion of the preformed toxin; it is absorbed from the stomach and small intestine and enters the lymphatics where it is transported by an unknown mechanism to the neuromuscular junction of cholinergic nerves.
- A metalloproteinase (botulinal toxin) prevents the presynaptic release of acetylcholine at the neuromuscular junction. Toxin binding is quick, irreversible, and independent of temperature and neural activity. Cell membrane receptors have a high affinity for the toxin (species and individual variation in sensitivity to toxin).
- The severity of the signs varies with the amount of toxin ingested and individual susceptibility.
- The blockage of release of acetylcholine from the presynaptic membrane results in progressive, symmetric, ascending lower motor neuron paresis/paralysis.
- Duration of illness in the dog: 14 to 24 days.

DIAGNOSIS

The diagnosis is based on a history suggestive of toxin ingestion and the resultant clinical signs.

DIFFERENTIAL DIAGNOSIS

- Early tick paralysis
- Early polyradiculoneuritis

INITIAL DATABASE

- Complete blood cell count, serum biochemical analysis, and urinalysis: usually normal
- Neurologic examination consistent with diffuse lower motor neuron dysfunction
- Thoracic and abdominal radiographs may reveal megaesophagus (with or without signs of aspiration pneumonia)

and carrion skeletal remains in the gastrointestinal tract, respectively

ADVANCED OR CONFIRMATORY TESTING

- Confirmatory diagnosis is based on finding the toxin in serum, feces, vomitus, or food samples.
- Preferred method of toxin identification is the mouse neutralization test.
- Other in vitro tests (radioimmunoassay, passive hemagglutination, enzyme-linked immunosorbent assay and polymerase chain reaction) exist but have not replaced the mouse test to date.
- Electrophysiology:
  - Marked reduction in muscle action potential amplitude evoked by electrical stimulation of the motor nerve
  - Normal or only mildly reduced nerve conduction velocities
  - Normal electromyography

TREATMENT

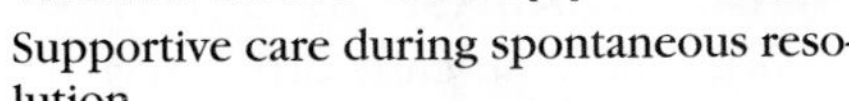

THERAPEUTIC GOAL(S)

Supportive care during spontaneous resolution

ACUTE GENERAL TREATMENT

- Antitoxin (type specific) must be administered before the botulinal toxin binds to receptors at the myoneural junction.
  - Type C polyvalent antitoxin (dog): 10,000-15,000 IU/dog IV or IM, two doses given 4 hours apart.
  - Anaphylaxis is a potential risk; intradermal skin testing is recommended prior to administration.
  - Antitoxin may be effective to prevent further toxin binding if ongoing intestinal absorption/circulation.
- Antibiotic use is debated; penicillin and metronidazole have been given to dogs and humans to reduce potential intestinal growth of *C. botulinum,* but use is controversial (disease occurs due to ingestion of preformed toxin, and these drugs could alter gastrointestinal flora).
- Antibiotics if secondary infection (i.e., aspiration pneumonia; based on culture and sensitivity testing).

CHRONIC TREATMENT

Long-term physical therapy, frequent turning, and soft bedding are essential.

DRUG INTERACTIONS

Avoid aminoglycosides (associated with neuromuscular blockade)

POSSIBLE COMPLICATIONS

- Aspiration pneumonia
- Decubital ulcers
- Muscle atrophy and fibrosis
- Ventilatory failure

RECOMMENDED MONITORING

- Respiratory rate and character; temperature and pulse
- Chest radiographs
- Serial neurologic examinations

PROGNOSIS AND OUTCOME

- Good to guarded.
- Recovery usually occurs 2 to 3 weeks after regrowth of terminal motor branches; dependent on severity of signs and complications.
- Complete recovery can occur spontaneously in moderately affected animals.

PEARLS & CONSIDERATIONS

COMMENTS

- The index of suspicion for botulism increases markedly if more than one animal is affected simultaneously.
- Referral may be necessary if long-term supportive care and ventilatory support are needed.

PREVENTION

- Prevention of access to carrion and spoiled food.
- Thorough cooking of any foods fed to dogs and cats.
- Botulinal toxin is destroyed by heating to 80°C for 30 minutes or 100°C for 10 minutes.

CLIENT EDUCATION

See Prevention above

SUGGESTED READING

Barsanti JA: Botulism. In Greene CE (ed): *Infectious Diseases of the Dog and Cat.* Philadelphia, Elsevier, 2001, pp 263-267.

Hartman K, Greene CE: Diseases caused by systemic bacterial infections. In Ettinger SJ, Feldman EC (eds): *Textbook of Veterinary Internal Medicine.* ed 6. Philadelphia, Elsevier, 2005, pp 629-631.

Shelton GD: Myasthenia gravis and disorders of neuromuscular transmission. In Shelton GD (ed): *Vet Clin North Am Small Anim Pract* 32:189-206, 2002.

AUTHOR: **KAREN L. KLINE**

EDITOR: **CURTIS W. DEWEY**

Boxer Cardiomyopathy

Client Education Sheet on Website

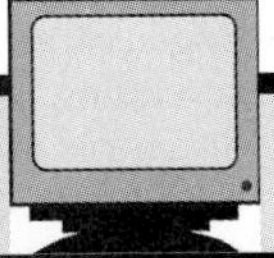

BASIC INFORMATION

DEFINITION

An inherited myocardial abnormality of boxer dogs characterized by the presence of ventricular arrhythmias. Affected dogs are predisposed to the development of syncope, sudden death, and, rarely, congestive heart failure. The disease exhibits many clinical, pathologic, and genetic features of arrhythmogenic right ventricular cardiomyopathy (ARVC) in humans, and this term may be a more appropriate name for the disease in boxers.

SYNONYM(S)

Arrhythmogenic cardiomyopathy

Arrhythmogenic right ventricular cardiomyopathy (ARVC)

Arrhythmogenic right ventricular dysplasia

Familial ventricular arrhythmia (FVA) of boxers

EPIDEMIOLOGY

SPECIES, AGE, SEX

- Species/breed: boxer dogs
- Age incidence: ARVC is mostly an adult onset disease, increasing in frequency and severity with age. Dogs as young as 6 months old have been reported, but the median age is 9.1 ± 2.3 years
- Sex incidence: none reported

GENETICS AND BREED PREDISPOSITION: The disorder is believed to be inherited as an autosomal dominant trait with variable penetrance, meaning it may be transmitted by the sire or the dam, and the extent to which offspring are affected is individually variable.

RISK FACTORS: The single most important predisposing factor is a family history of disease. Not all animals with this disorder are overtly affected, which precludes readily identifying affected animals that should be excluded from breeding.

GEOGRAPHY AND SEASONALITY: Geographic distribution reflects the gene pool. Boxer cardiomyopathy/ARVC is seen in North America, Europe, and elsewhere; geographic differences based on variation in gene pools are described both within and among countries.

CLINICAL PRESENTATION

DISEASE FORMS/SUBTYPES

Boxer cardiomyopathy is categorized into three types:

- Type I—dogs with latent ventricular arrhythmias.The arrhythmias are apparent on an electrocardiogram (ECG), but overt clinical manifestations such as syncope are not seen.
- Type II—dogs that show clinical signs associated with the arrhythmias. Generally, syncope or sudden death occurs in association with ventricular tachyarrhythmias (ventricular tachycardia/ventricular fibrillation).
- Type III—uncommon form of boxer cardiomyopathy involving cardiac chamber enlargement and mechanical (systolic) dysfunction; this form of the disease more closely resembles dilated cardiomyopathy (DCM) than an arrhythmogenic cardiomyopathy. Many of these dogs also manifest atrial arrhythmias, especially atrial fibrillation, in addition to the more typical ventricular arrhythmias. Dogs with type III disease are more likely to develop signs of congestive heart failure (CHF) than dogs with types I and II disease, in whom mechanical cardiac function and normal cardiac dimensions are preserved as long as rapid ventricular arrhythmias are not occurring.

HISTORY, CHIEF COMPLAINT

- The manner of presentation will depend on which type of boxer cardiomyopathy/ARVC a particular dog has.
- Type I: no overt clinical signs. These dogs often present specifically for screening exams for the disease, or the disease is identified incidentally during evaluation of an unrelated disease or purpose (e.g., ventricular arrhythmia noted during annual wellness exam or preanesthetic monitoring).
- Type II: chief complaint is the occurrence of signs referrable to the arrhythmia. These signs typically include weakness, exercise intolerance, syncope, or collapse. In some cases, sudden death is the initial (and only) evidence of this disease.
- Type III: dogs may present for signs related to their arrhythmia (ventricular or atrial) or subsequent to myocardial failure. This most commonly manifests as signs of CHF, including coughing, dyspnea or other respiratory difficulty; abdominal distention (ascites); exercise intolerance; and weakness.

PHYSICAL EXAM FINDINGS

- Type I and type II dogs are almost always normal on physical examination. The only evidence of disease is the identification of ventricular arrhythmias, which, due to their intermittence and varying degrees of prematurity, may not be evident on routine physical examination.
- Type III: Physical findings reflect the presence of CHF (dyspnea, pulmonary crackles, jugular distention, ascites). A murmur of mitral regurgitation (left apical systolic) may also be heard. Arrhythmias may also be detected, especially tachycardias such as sinus tachycardia (from CHF), ventricular arrhythmias, and atrial fibrillation.

ETIOLOGY AND PATHOPHYSIOLOGY

- The specific genetic defect is unknown; research to identify specific genes is ongoing.
- The cause of the arrhythmia is unknown but may be related to ventricular fibrofatty infiltration and possibly to altered cellular calcium dynamics.
- On histologic examination, affected dogs have a fibrofatty myocardial infiltration that appears to originate in the right ventricle and interventricular septum; left ventricular involvement occurs later in the course of disease.
- This pattern is consistent with the clinical manifestation of disease, in that ventricular arrhythmias are most commonly of right ventricular origin. Abnormal left ventricular morphology and impaired function seen less commonly and only in more severe cases (type III dogs).

DIAGNOSIS

DIFFERENTIAL DIAGNOSIS

- Differentials for type I dogs (ventricular arrhythmias with no overt manifestations such as syncope) include any cause for premature ventricular complexes/ventricular arrhythmias:
  - Underlying cardiac disease
  - Systemic abnormalities (endocrinopathy, metabolic or acid/base disturbance, immune-mediated/inflammatory disease, neoplasia)
  - Autonomic imbalance (stress, sympathetic activation)
  - Drug-induced arrhythmias (digoxin, catecholamines, methylxanthines, chemotherapy)
  - Splenic disease
  - Traumatic injury (e.g., hit by car)
  - Gastric dilatation/volvulus
- Differentials for type II dogs (syncope; see also Syncope, p 1053):
  - Reduced cardiac output:
    - Outflow tract obstruction (e.g., subaortic stenosis, pulmonic stenosis)
    - CHF
    - Inappropriate bradycardia (e.g., due to advanced second-degree or third-degree atrioventricular block or reflex sinus bradycardia due to pulmonary hypertension or other causes)
    - Impaired ventricular filling (hypovolemia, pericardial disease, diastolic dysfunction, obstruction to venous return)
  - Neurocardiogenic syncope
  - Hypoxemia/hypoglycemia
  - Seizure disorders (or other primary neurologic disease)
- Differentials for type III disease:
  - DCM (or other cardiomyopathy)
  - Valve degeneration (endocardiosis): advanced state, with ventricular hypocontractility
  - Other causes of CHF

INITIAL DATABASE

- Document ventricular arrhythmia by in-hospital ECG and/or 24-hour ambulatory ECG (Holter monitor).
  - Identification of an arrhythmia in the absence of other causes for ventricular premature complex (VPCs) (see above) can make for a straightforward diagnosis.
  - There is no clear consensus on the "normal" number of VPCs in healthy boxers, and there is wide variation in the degree of arrhythmia required for a patient to be considered "abnormal." Some believe that 100 VPCs/24 hr is consistent with a diagnosis of boxer cardiomyopathy/ARVC; others consider any boxer with >50 VPCs/24 hr as affected.
- Results of comprehensive diagnostic testing (complete blood count, serum biochemistry profile, urinalysis, thoracic radiographs, abdominal ultrasound exam, echocardiogram) are normal with boxer cardiomyopathy/ARVC types I and II. Since ventricular arrhythmias can be caused by such a large variety of disorders, both cardiac and noncardiac, boxer cardiomyopathy/ARVC is considered a diagnosis of exclusion.

ADVANCED OR CONFIRMATORY TESTING

- Histopathologic evaluation:
  - Infiltration of a fibrofatty material in the right ventricle (± left ventricle) is commonly seen. Areas of inflammation and/or necrosis may also be seen. Dogs with more advanced disease may be more likely to demon-

strate myocyte degeneration and replacement fibrosis.
- Magnetic resonance imaging is being used investigationally to identify fibrosis/fibrofatty infiltration in the right ventricular/left ventricular walls.

TREATMENT

THERAPEUTIC GOAL(S)

- Reduce arrhythmia frequency and severity
- Reduce clinical signs (syncope) in patients with type II disease
- Reduce risk of sudden death—very controversial (antiarrhythmic therapy has never been shown to reduce risk of death)
- Control clinical signs and improve survival in dogs with CHF (type III)

ACUTE GENERAL TREATMENT

- Life-threatening ventricular tachycardia requires intravenous antiarrhythmic therapy (ideally lidocaine; procainamide as an alternative). See Ventricular Arrhythmias (Premature Ventricular Complexes, Ventricular Tachycardia), p 1148.
- Acute CHF (type III) therapy includes diuretics (furosemide) and oxygen support; nitrates and inotropes (dobutamine) may also be considered. Thoracocentesis and abdominocentesis for pleural effusion and ascites, respectively. See Heart Failure, Acute/Decompensated, p 458.

CHRONIC TREATMENT

- Chronic treatment for dogs without clinical signs (type I) is very controversial and not definitively indicated. Antiarrhythmic therapy has not been shown to reduce the risk of sudden death. Reduction of arrhythmia frequency does not always translate to a favorable clinical outcome.
- Treatment of dogs may be warranted even if no overt signs such as syncope are present; such treatment decisions should be guided by the results of Holter monitoring. Generally, treatment is considered when the arrhythmia is severe, especially if runs of ventricular tachycardia are seen.
- Treatment of dogs that have experienced syncope is generally more widely accepted, since antiarrhythmic therapy can reduce the occurrence of syncope, regardless of its limited (if any) long-term effect on sudden death.
- Common drugs used as oral antiarrhythmics include sotalol (1-6.6 mg/kg PO q 12h); mexiletine (4-8 mg/kg PO q 8-12h; with or without atenolol 0.35-0.6 mg/kg PO q 12h); or procainamide (10-12 mg/kg PO q 8h). Amiodarone is routinely used in humans, but not in veterinary medicine.
- Type III: Angiotensin-converting enzyme inhibitors (enalapril) and diuretics (furosemide and spironolactone) for CHF; positive inotropes (digoxin or pimobendan). See Heart Failure, Chronic, p 459.
- Carnitine deficiency has been described in one family of boxers with type III disease; supplementation of carnitine may be indicated in type III dogs.

DRUG INTERACTIONS

Proarrhythmic effects of antiarrhythmics can be additive. The use of multiple antiarrhythmics should be undertaken cautiously, especially with drugs that prolong QT interval (sotalol, amiodarone, procainamide).

POSSIBLE COMPLICATIONS

- Proarrhythmia is always a concern with antiarrhythmic therapy. Reevaluation once therapy is underway is essential to verify that the arrhythmias have not worsened subsequent to therapy.
- Positive inotropes (digoxin, dobutamine, pimobendan) should be used cautiously in patients with ventricular arrhythmias, because they may exacerbate arrhythmia.
- β-Blockers are useful antiarrhythmics but must be used with caution in patients with a history of CHF and should not be initiated during acute CHF.

RECOMMENDED MONITORING

- Arrhythmia monitoring by in-hospital ECG for acute cases, or by Holter for chronic management.
- Monitoring the patient with type III disease and CHF includes evaluation of respiratory rate and effort, blood pressure, serum chemistries (renal function), and thoracic radiography to monitor pulmonary edema and/or pleural effusion.
- Periodic blood pressure evaluation is important if β-blockers (atenolol or sotalol) are used, or if CHF is present.

PROGNOSIS AND OUTCOME

- The prognosis for dogs with types I and II disease is extremely variable. Some dogs will experience sudden death or continued syncope. Other dogs will live the rest of their lives without clinical signs and succumb to an unrelated disease process.
- Dogs with type III disease have a poor prognosis, similar to that of DCM. Life expectancies of weeks to months are typical.

PEARLS & CONSIDERATIONS

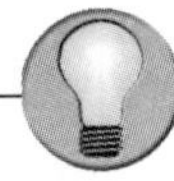

COMMENTS

- There is some debate regarding the relationship between types I and II disease relative to type III disease. Some speculate that there is a spectrum of disease, with progression to chamber enlargement and systolic failure as the most extreme form of ARVC. Others contend that type III disease is identical to dilated cardiomyopathy seen in other breeds (e.g. Doberman pinschers) and is unrelated to ARVC. The precise relationship between these forms of disease remains to be fully elucidated.
- Dogs with types I and II disease have structurally normal hearts, and the presence of a murmur in these dogs must be considered different from a murmur in a type III dog. Murmurs in types I and II disease often reflect mild congenital disease (subaortic stenosis) or a functional murmur, which is completely unrelated to boxer cardiomyopathy/ARVC.
- The controversy regarding the ability of antiarrhythmics to reduce risk of death should be acknowledged when deciding to treat dogs showing no clinical signs.

PREVENTION

At this time, the only way to prevent the disease is to avoid breeding affected dogs.

CLIENT EDUCATION

Identification of affected dogs is complicated by the lack of universally accepted criteria for disease; the presence of affected but externally normal-appearing dogs further complicates disease diagnosis. As a rule, a 24-hour Holter monitor recording should be obtained before making any breeding decisions.

SUGGESTED READING

Basso C, et al: Arrhythmogenic right ventricular cardiomyopathy causing sudden cardiac death in boxer dogs: A new animal model of human disease. *Circulation* 109:1180, 2004.

Harpster NK: Boxer cardiomyopathy. In Kirk RW (ed): *Current Veterinary Therapy: Small Animal Practice*. Philadelphia, WB Saunders, 1983, pp 329-337.

Meurs KM, et al: Comparison of the effects of four antiarrhythmic treatments for familial ventricular arrhythmias in boxers. *J Am Vet Med Assoc* 221:522, 2002.

Meurs KM, et al: Familial ventricular dysrhythmias in boxer dogs. *J Vet Intern Med* 13:437, 1999.

AUTHOR: **ALAN W. SPIER**

EDITOR: **ETIENNE CÔTÉ**

DISEASES AND DISORDERS

Brachial Plexus Abnormalities

BASIC INFORMATION

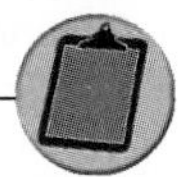

DEFINITION

Dysfunction of the peripheral nerves or nerve roots of the brachial plexus (C6-T2 spinal segments)

SYNONYM(S)

Brachial plexus neuropathy

EPIDEMIOLOGY

RISK FACTORS

Dependent on disease subtype:

- Trauma
- Antigenic stimulation

ASSOCIATED CONDITIONS AND DISORDERS

None directly; concurrent traumatic injuries:

- Shock, hypotension, head trauma, pneumothorax

CLINICAL PRESENTATION

DISEASE FORMS/SUBTYPES

- Traumatic brachial plexus injury:
  - Complete brachial plexus avulsion
    - Neurotmesis (avulsion) of all brachial plexus nerves
    - Unilateral or bilateral
  - Partial brachial plexus avulsion
    - Neurotmesis of some, but not all, nerves in the brachial plexus
    - Typically cranial or caudal portion of plexus
  - Stretching (neurapraxia) and damage to nerve(s), without avulsion
- Brachial plexus neuritis:
  - Idiopathic inflammatory neuropathy of the brachial plexus
- Nerve sheath tumors (see p 751)

HISTORY, CHIEF COMPLAINT

- Thoracic limb lameness, paresis, or paralysis
- History of trauma or antigenic stimulation (e.g., vaccination, allergic hypersensitivity [see Anaphylaxis, p 60], food allergy [see p 396–400])

PHYSICAL EXAM FINDINGS

- Varies with respect to nerve root(s) affected (see Suggested Reading below).
- Abnormalities *may* include:
  - Focal muscle atrophy
    - Evident 5 to 10 days postinjury
  - Neurologic deficits in thoracic limb(s): normal pelvic limbs
    - Thoracic limb monoparesis/monoplegia, or bilateral thoracic limb paresis/plegia
    - Proprioceptive deficits
    - Hyporeflexia/areflexia
    - Loss of nociception (superficial or deep pain sensation) to various autonomous zones of thoracic limb(s): evaluate *all* autonomous zones and *all digits* for sensory loss (see Nerves of the Forelimb, p 1389)
  - Ipsilateral loss of cutaneous trunci reflex
    - May occur with lateral thoracic nerve injury (C8-T1 spinal nerve roots)
  - Ipsilateral Horner's syndrome
    - May occur with injury of the sympathetic pathway (T1-T3 spinal nerve roots)

ETIOLOGY AND PATHOPHYSIOLOGY

- Brachial plexus avulsion: trauma to the thoracic limb(s) that results in abduction, caudal displacement, or extreme flexion/extension of the shoulder joint; results in traction injury to the nerve roots of the brachial plexus as they attach to the spinal cord.
- Brachial plexus neuritis: idiopathic inflammatory response; theories include antigenic stimulation by vaccination, allergic reactions, or diet hypersensitivities (particularly diets containing horse meat).

DIAGNOSIS

DIFFERENTIAL DIAGNOSIS

- Neoplasia
- Musculoskeletal injury:
  - Fractures
  - Dislocations
  - Muscle avulsions
- Central cord syndrome:
  - Injury or dysfunction of the central spinal cord parenchyma (grey matter)
  - Very rare; reported sporadically with spinal trauma, disk herniation, or intramedullary neoplasia
- Other focal neuropathies (e.g., early stages of rabies encephalomyelitis or acute canine polyradiculoneuropathy/Coonhound paralysis)

INITIAL DATABASE

- Neurologic examination
- Cutaneous sensory evaluation (autonomous zones) and deep pain assessment (see Nerves of the Forelimb, p 1389)

ADVANCED OR CONFIRMATORY TESTING

- Electrophysiologic studies
- Myelography, computed tomography, and magnetic resonance imaging: often not effective in diagnosing brachial plexus injury; may rule out other compressive myelopathies or neuropathies

TREATMENT

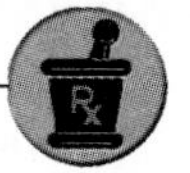

THERAPEUTIC GOAL(S)

- Regain neurologic function, ability to ambulate
- Maintain joint mobility, prevent muscle contractures
- Prevent self-mutilation of affected limb(s)

ACUTE GENERAL TREATMENT

- Supportive care/trauma resuscitation.
- Prevent self-mutilation and external trauma to affected limb(s):
  - Booties to protect paw from abrasions and scuffing
  - E-collar to prevent licking, chewing, or other self-mutilation
- Corticosteroids may be beneficial in brachial plexus neuritis; however, insufficient information exists to confirm their efficacy.

CHRONIC TREATMENT

- Prevent self-mutilation.
- Physical therapy (see Physical Rehabilitation, p 1300): prevent muscle contracture and maintain range of motion/extensor ability should neurologic function return:
  - Target all joints, including carpus and digits.
  - Perform range of motion (ROM) exercises for 10 to 15 minutes three to five times daily.
- Limb amputation: treatment of choice for permanent unilateral brachial plexus avulsion.
- Euthanasia is warranted in permanent bilateral avulsions.
- Limb-sparing treatments for brachial plexus avulsion have been attempted, including nerve root transplantation, transposition, neurotization, and muscle transposition. Treatment results are generally unsatisfactory. Transposition and neurotization of the intact contralateral C8 ventral root in dogs shows some promise; however, at this time recovery of neurologic function remains limited.

POSSIBLE COMPLICATIONS

- Paresthesias/sensory nerve injuries promote self-mutilation.
- Abrasions may occur on the dorsum of the paw from scuffing/dragging the affected limb during ambulation, creating a potential portal for infection.

RECOMMENDED MONITORING

Serial assessment of cutaneous sensation and motor function every 2 to 4 weeks

PROGNOSIS AND OUTCOME

- Loss of deep pain sensation suggests avulsion and warrants a grave prognosis for return of function.
- Preservation of deep pain sensation warrants a guarded to good prognosis for return of function over weeks to months.
- Lack of any neurologic improvement over a 4-week period suggests permanent deficit.
- Brachial plexus neuritis has a guarded prognosis; recovery is possible.

PEARLS & CONSIDERATIONS

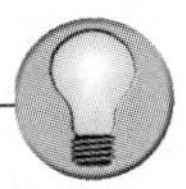

COMMENTS

- Physical therapy is *imperative* in cases with potential for recovery.
  - Splints or bandages are generally *not* recommended because they impair mobility.
- Evaluate all digits for deep pain sensation; peripheral nerve deficits may be localized and identified in only one digit.

PREVENTION

Minimize risk of motor vehicle trauma (e.g., riding in open truck beds where pets could jump or be thrown from the vehicle)

CLIENT EDUCATION

- If recovery is possible/attempted, train clients to perform effective physical therapy
- If amputation is necessary, discuss benefits of amputation and how well pets adapt
- Discuss importance of maintaining pet at a lean body weight and the negative impact of concurrent osteoarthritis or hip dysplasia on their pet's ability to ambulate

SUGGESTED READING

Bailey CS: Patterns of cutaneous anesthesia associated with brachial plexus avulsions in the dog. *J Am Vet Med Assoc* 185:889–899, 1984.

Cummings JF, et al: Canine brachial plexus neuritis: A syndrome resembling serum neuritis in man. *Cornell Vet* 63:589–617, 1973.

AUTHOR: **REBECCA A. PACKER**

EDITOR: **CURTIS W. DEWEY**

Brachycephalic Airway Syndrome

Client Education Sheet on Website

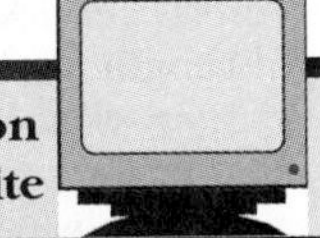

BASIC INFORMATION

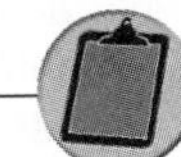

DEFINITION

A syndrome of anatomic and functional abnormalities of the upper airway found in brachycephalic (short-nosed) dogs that result in variable degrees of upper airway distress

SYNONYM(S)

Brachycephalic syndrome
Brachycephalic upper airway syndrome
Upper airway syndrome

EPIDEMIOLOGY

SPECIES, AGE, SEX

- Brachycephalic airway syndrome occurs only in dogs.
- Mean age at time of presentation: 3 to 4 years.
- Presentation with clinical problems in one of two age groups:
  - Young dogs (3 to 12 months old) already having respiratory difficulty
  - Middle-aged dogs with increasingly severe respiratory problems over several years

GENETICS AND BREED PREDISPOSITION: Breeds predisposed: English and French bulldogs, Boston terrier, pug, boxer, pekingese, shih tzu.

RISK FACTORS: Deterioration/decompensation producing severe dyspnea:

- Hot, humid weather
- Hot ambient temperature (e.g., in car with inadequate ventilation)
- Exertion

GEOGRAPHY AND SEASONALITY: More likely to trigger owner concern during summer, when increased ambient temperatures and activity can lead to episodes of severe dyspnea.

ASSOCIATED CONDITIONS AND DISORDERS

- Three primary anatomic components of the brachycephalic airway syndrome:
  - Stenotic nares
  - Elongated soft palate
  - Hypoplastic trachea
- Any or all may be present in any given brachycephalic dog
- Secondary airway changes that can develop due to increased airway resistance include:
  - Laryngeal saccule eversion
  - Laryngeal collapse
    - More commonly seen in young dogs, particularly Boston terriers and pugs (laryngeal cartilages very pliable)
- Obesity: aggravating factor
- Noncardiogenic pulmonary edema/acute respiratory distress syndrome:
  - Occurs if patient inspires forcefully and excessively against severe upper airway obstruction
  - Can cause persistence of cyanosis/hypoxemia despite relief of upper airway obstruction

CLINICAL PRESENTATION

HISTORY, CHIEF COMPLAINT

- History of exercise intolerance, cyanosis, or collapse
- Gagging or coughing
- Stertor, stridor

PHYSICAL EXAM FINDINGS

- Stenotic or narrowed nares
- Stridor or stertor; increased inspiratory sounds
- Increased expiratory sounds on auscultation if concurrent pneumonia, bronchitis, or noncardiogenic pulmonary edema
- If in severe respiratory distress: cyanosis, stridor or apnea, hyperthermia

ETIOLOGY AND PATHOPHYSIOLOGY

- Breeding selection has led to dorsoventral flattening, and rostrocaudal shortening, of the skull and nasal passages of these dogs. The result is an increased negative pressure in the nasal passages and pharynx during inspiration.
- These anatomic characteristics coupled with redundant and edematous nasopharyngeal and oropharyngeal soft tissues contribute to increased airway resistance and obstruction.
- If untreated, stenotic nares and an elongated soft palate increasingly interfere with breathing.
- Excessive negative nasopharyngeal pressure results in laryngeal saccule eversion and laryngeal collapse (inward folding of the epiglottis and arytenoid cartilages).

- As the nasopharyngeal mucosa becomes edematous and inflamed, it contributes to upper airway obstruction.

DIAGNOSIS

The characteristic inspiratory stridor in brachycephalic breeds is suggestive of the diagnosis on physical examination alone. Confirmation requires a sedated oropharyngeal examination and cervical and thoracic radiographs.

DIFFERENTIAL DIAGNOSIS

- Upper airway mass: neoplasia, polyp, granuloma, foreign body, abscess
- Laryngeal paralysis
- Cervical or laryngeal trauma
- Coagulopathy resulting in laryngeal hematoma
- Collapsing trachea

INITIAL DATABASE

- Complete blood count, serum biochemistry profile, urinalysis: generally unremarkable
- Lateral cervical radiographs:
  - Length of soft palate
  - Hypoplastic trachea
- Inspiratory and expiratory thoracic radiographs (complications; differential diagnosis):
  - Tracheal collapse
  - Chronic small airway disease
  - Pneumonia
  - Noncardiogenic pulmonary edema

ADVANCED OR CONFIRMATORY TESTING

Rapid-acting anesthetic induction and oropharyngeal/laryngeal examination (e.g., propofol 4-6 mg given slow IV to effect): be prepared to intubate and ventilate if necessary, given propofol's apnea-inducing qualities:

- Determine if soft palate excessively long
- Presence of laryngeal saccule eversion
- Presence of laryngeal collapse

TREATMENT

THERAPEUTIC GOAL(S)

- Immediately, if severe dyspnea:
  - Relieve upper airway obstruction via sedation with or without endotracheal intubation or tracheostomy
  - Minimize patient's anxiety and thus reduce the risk of noncardiogenic pulmonary edema, hyperthermia, and worsening dyspnea
- Long-term:
  - Relieve upper airway obstruction via surgical correction

ACUTE GENERAL TREATMENT

- Stenotic nares:
  - Remove excessive cartilaginous tissue of alae (wings) of nostrils
  - Vertical, lateral, or horizontal wedge resection of the alar tissue using scalpel or CO_2 laser
- Elongated soft palate:
  - Shorten soft palate by removing excessive or redundant palatal tissue to improve glottal airflow, eliminate excessive negative pressure, and improve functional glottal size
  - Soft palate resection using sharp transection or CO_2 laser
- Everted laryngeal saccules:
  - Excise everted mucosal tissue
  - Traction and amputation of everted mucosa with scissors, scalpel, or CO_2 laser
- Laryngeal collapse:
  - Cannot be surgically corrected
  - If causing clinically significant airway obstruction, bilateral ventriculocordectomy and unilateral partial arytenoidectomy or permanent tracheostomy may be necessary
- Hypoplastic trachea:
  - No surgical treatment
- Complications

CHRONIC TREATMENT

- Avoid exposure to high ambient temperatures and humidity and other sources of stress
- Maintain optimal body weight

POSSIBLE COMPLICATIONS

- Hyperthermia, see p 1371
- Noncardiogenic pulmonary edema (see Pulmonary Edema, Noncardiogenic, p 913). Sedate early to reduce the risk of this complication
- Aspiration pneumonia: see Pneumonia, Aspiration, p 862
- Excessive shortening of soft palate will result in nasal reflux of food or water or, more rarely, aspiration pneumonia
- Laryngeal saccule eversion and collapse may develop if upper airway obstruction persists

RECOMMENDED MONITORING

Owner should be aware of any recurrent signs of upper airway obstruction (exercise intolerance, coughing, gagging, stridor, or stertor), which might indicate progressive degenerative changes in upper airway (laryngeal collapse)

PROGNOSIS AND OUTCOME

- Guarded prognosis if acute, severe dyspnea: a life-threatening state may exist, but with a good response to treatment, full resolution of signs is possible
- Good to excellent long-term prognosis after correction of stenotic nares and resection of elongated soft palate provided dog does not have a hypoplastic trachea and secondary changes have not developed
- Variable (poor to good) prognosis if laryngeal collapse has developed or if dog has a hypoplastic trachea, depending on degree of airway obstruction

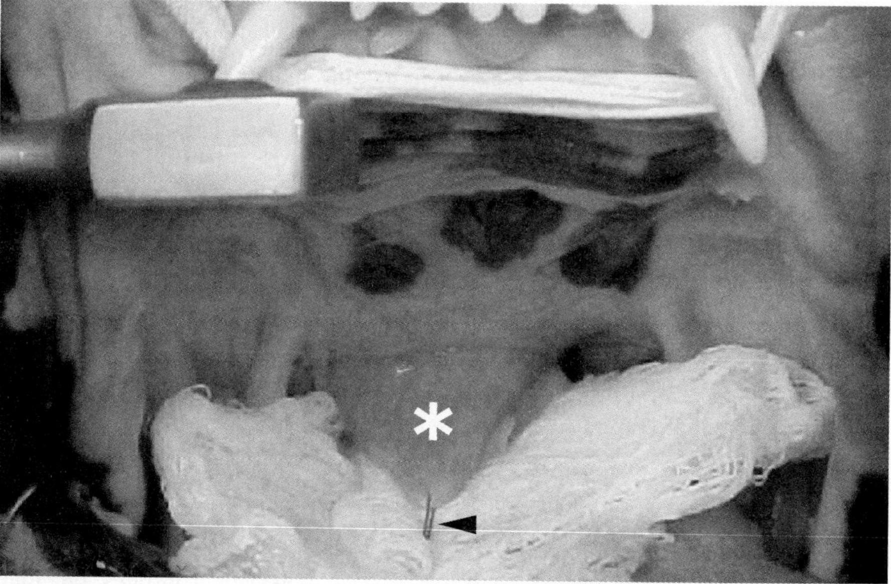

FIGURE I-31 Preoperative open-mouth view of the elongated soft palate (*asterisk*) of a French bulldog with brachycephalic airway syndrome. A stay suture (*arrowhead at bottom*) is placed through the caudal tip of the soft palate in preparation for resection. Courtesy of Dr. Richard Walshaw.

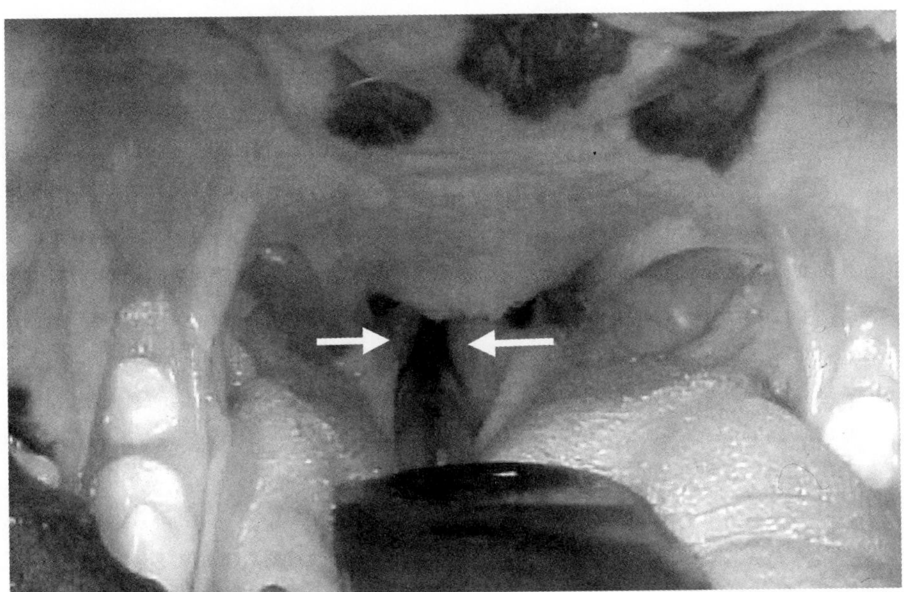

FIGURE I-32 Postoperative view of the same dog. Resection of the elongated soft palate is complete, creating a pharynx with a more normal conformation. Consequently, the larynx (*arrows*) is more easily seen illustrating the improvement brought by the soft palate resection. Courtesy of Dr. Richard Walshaw.

PEARLS & CONSIDERATIONS

COMMENTS

- Early detection and surgical treatment are recommended for best outcome and avoidance of secondary changes/complications
- Lifestyle modifications are often necessary to minimize episodes of airway distress:
  - Maintain ideal body weight
  - Avoid stressful situations
- Hypoplastic trachea may affect long-term prognosis and outcome after surgery

PREVENTION

- Because brachycephalic syndrome is breed-associated and heritable, it is not preventable.
- Episodes of respiratory distress may be minimized by avoiding stress, moderating exercise, preventing obesity, avoiding exposure to high ambient temperatures, and early surgical treatment for elongated soft palate and stenotic nares.

CLIENT EDUCATION

- Discuss breed association and heritability in brachycephalic dogs
- Syndrome is progressive and exacerbated by stress, obesity, and exposure to high ambient temperatures
- Early surgical intervention is important for most successful outcome

SUGGESTED READING

Davidson EB, et al: Evaluation of carbon dioxide laser and conventional incisional techniques for resection of soft palates in brachycephalic dogs. *J Am Vet Med Assoc* 219:776–781, 2001.

Monnet E: Brachycephalic airway syndrome. In Slatter D (ed): *Textbook of Small Animal Surgery*. ed 3. Philadelphia, WB Saunders, 2002, pp 808–813.

Orsher RJ: Brachycephalic airway disease. In Bojrab MJ (ed): *Disease Mechanisms in Small Animal Surgery*, ed 2. Philadelphia, Lea & Febiger, 1993, pp 369–370.

Rozanski EA, et al: Measurement of upper airway resistance in awake untrained dolichocephalic and mesaticephalic dogs. *Am J Vet Res* 55:1055–1059, 1994.

AUTHOR: **ELLEN B. DAVIDSON DOMNICK**
EDITOR: **RICHARD WALSHAW**

Brain Neoplasia

BASIC INFORMATION

DEFINITION

- Primary brain tumors include meningioma (discussed separately; see Meningioma, p 696), glioma (astrocytoma, oligodendroglioma), choroid plexus tumor, ependymoma, medulloblastoma, olfactory neuroblastoma, and primitive neuroectodermal tumor.
- Secondary brain tumors include pituitary tumors, tumors that invade by direct extension into the brain (e.g., nasal tumors), and metastatic tumors to the brain (e.g., hemangiosarcoma, lymphoma [latter is discussed separately; see Lymphoma, Central Nervous System, p 652]).

SYNONYM(S)

Brain tumor

EPIDEMIOLOGY

SPECIES, AGE, SEX

- Occurs in both dogs and cats.
- Incidence reported as high as 2.6% in dogs and 2.8% in cats.
- Brain tumors typically occur in older dogs and cats. Most dogs are older than 5 years. The median age for dogs and cats to develop brain tumors is approximately 9 and 11 years, respectively.
- Both males and females are affected.

GENETICS AND BREED PREDISPOSITION

- Canine: Brachycephalic breeds (e.g., boxer, Boston terrier) appear prone to developing gliomas.
- Feline: no breed predisposition.

GEOGRAPHY AND SEASONALITY: Reported worldwide. No seasonality.

CLINICAL PRESENTATION

DISEASE FORMS/SUBTYPES

- Meningioma: tumor of the arachnoid membrane
- Glioma: tumor of the cells that form the interstitial tissue of the central nervous system (CNS)
- Choroid plexus papilloma: tumor of the cells of the choroid plexus, the intracranial vascular structure responsible for the formation of cerebrospinal fluid
- Ependymoma: tumor of the ependymal cells that line the ventricular system

HISTORY, CHIEF COMPLAINT

- A brain tumor should be suspected in any older patient with an insidious onset of slowly progressive neurologic signs, and in any patient older than 5 years with an acute onset of seizures.
- Historic findings depend on lesion location. Clinical signs are often insidious and progressive; however, recent onset of clinical signs is possible.
- The most common chief complaints include seizures, circling, behavior change (aggression), altered consciousness, and nonspecific signs such as inappetence and lethargy.

PHYSICAL EXAM FINDINGS

- Neurologic exam findings vary depending on lesion location (see Neurologic Examination, p 1286).
- Findings generally reflect a focal lesion with asymmetric clinical signs.
- Cerebral brain tumors: seizures, contralateral menace and postural reaction deficits, behavior change, contralateral hemiparesis, altered mental status.
- Brainstem brain tumors: ipsilateral cranial nerve deficits, hemiparesis or tetraparesis or tetraplegia, altered mental status, central vestibular dysfunction.
- Cerebellar brain tumors: hypermetria, intention tremors, truncal sway, broad-based stance, paradoxical vestibular dysfunction.

ETIOLOGY AND PATHOPHYSIOLOGY

- Etiology is unknown.
- Usually occur as solitary masses. Multiple tumors may be seen with metastatic disease.
- Most commonly reported in the supratentorial compartment (rostral to the tentorium cerebelli, including the cerebrum and diencephalon).
- Biologic behavior (benign vs. malignant) is generally irrelevant, because neoplasia of the brain is detrimental via space-occupying effects.

DIAGNOSIS

Neoplasia of the brain is suspected based on signalment, history, and neurologic examination results. Confirmation requires intracranial imaging (computed tomography [CT] or magnetic resonance imaging [MRI]).

DIFFERENTIAL DIAGNOSIS

- Infectious diseases (bacterial, viral, fungal, protozoal)
- Inflammatory diseases (e.g., granulomatous meningoencephalomyelitis)
- Cerebrovascular infarction if clinical signs are acute, nonprogressive, and asymmetric
- Toxin and metabolic diseases if clinical signs are acute, nonprogressive, and symmetric

INITIAL DATABASE

- Complete blood count/biochemical analysis/urinalysis: usually normal
- Thoracic and abdominal radiographs: usually normal, but performed to rule out extracranial neoplasia

ADVANCED OR CONFIRMATORY TESTING

- CT or MRI:
  - MRI is markedly superior for soft tissue detail (brain, spinal cord) and has higher resolution than CT. As a result, this is the current gold standard for brain imaging.
  - CT is an adequate imaging modality, is superior for bone lesions (e.g., skull tumors), and may be cheaper than MRI.
  - Focal mass identified for most brain tumors; however, multiple tumors may be identified with metastatic neoplasia.
  - CT and MRI features are variable between tumor types.
- Cerebrospinal fluid (CSF) analysis:
  - Used as an adjunct to advanced imaging, primarily to assess encephalitis.
  - With brain neoplasia, results are generally nonspecific and reveal normal to mildly elevated protein.
  - Albuminocytologic dissociation (elevated CSF protein with normal white blood cell count) can be seen but is not pathognomonic.
  - Neoplastic cells are rarely identified within the CSF; however, the presence of lymphoblasts within the CSF supports a diagnosis of CNS lymphoma.
- Histopathologic analysis of tissue is required for definitive diagnosis. Tissue samples can be obtained via surgical excision or stereotactic brain biopsy.

TREATMENT

THERAPEUTIC GOAL(S)

Definitive treatment involving surgical excision and/or radiation therapy

ACUTE GENERAL TREATMENT

- Surgical excision: used for removing or debulking the tumor, if accessible, and for providing a definitive histologic diagnosis.
- Radiation therapy: used as an adjunctive treatment to surgery or as a primary treatment.
- Chemotherapy: generally not effective because the blood-brain barrier (BBB) prevents chemotherapeutic agents from entering the brain and spinal cord.
  - Nitrosourea agents such as lomustine (CCNU; 60-90 mg/m^2 PO q 6 weeks) or carmustine (BCNU 50 mg/m^2 IV q 6 weeks), which can cross the BBB, appear to have some effect in canine gliomas and canine CNS lymphoma.
  - The most serious potential adverse effects are bone marrow suppression (anemia, thrombocytopenia, leukopenia) and hepatotoxicity.
- Cluster seizures or status epilepticus: Diazepam 0.5 mg/kg IV (can be repeated at 5-minute intervals for a maximum of three doses). If diazepam is initially effective, but seizures recur, consider diazepam IV constant rate infusion (0.25–0.50 mg/kg/hr) or loading dose of phenobarbital IV (to effect, up to 16–20 mg/kg total dose). See Seizures, p 990.
- Cerebral edema/brain herniation: Mannitol 0.5 g/kg IV slowly over 10 to 15 minutes; furosemide (2 mg/kg IV) has synergistic effects with mannitol and can be given if needed.

CHRONIC TREATMENT

- Seizures: Anticonvulsants should be used if there is more than one seizure every 6 to 8 weeks.
  - Phenobarbital: 2–4 mg/kg PO or IV q 12h.
  - Potassium bromide: 20–50 mg/kg PO SID; dose can be divided BID to reduce nausea and vomiting. Use with caution in cats; frequently causes reversible clinical signs consistent with bronchial asthma, but in rare cases has been fatal.
- Cerebral edema: Prednisone 0.5 mg/kg PO q 12h initially then taper to lowest dose that will control clinical signs.

DRUG INTERACTIONS

- Drug interactions or altered metabolism of medications have been reported between corticosteroids and amphotericin B, furosemide, thiazide diuretics, digitalis glycosides, cyclosporine, phenytoin, phenobarbital, and mitotane.
- Corticosteroids should not be given concurrently with nonsteroidal anti-inflammatory drugs or other potentially ulcerogenic medications.
- Phenobarbital may cause excessive sedation in dogs with intracranial mass lesions, even at low doses.

POSSIBLE COMPLICATIONS

Progression of clinical signs, including status epilepticus, brain herniation, and sudden death

RECOMMENDED MONITORING

- Serial neurologic exam every 4 to 6 weeks
- Serum phenobarbital blood level 2 weks after starting medication or any change in dosage, or immediately after loading dose
- Serum bromide blood level 3 to 4 months after starting medication or any change in dosage in dogs and 2 months in cats, or immediately after loading dose

PROGNOSIS AND OUTCOME

- In general, the prognosis is fair to guarded in both dogs and cats.
- In dogs, several small-scale reports have shown a median survival time of approximately 2 to 4 months with supportive care and nonspecific treatment only, 6 to 12 months with surgery alone, 7 to 24 months with radiation therapy alone, 6 to 18 months with surgery and radiation, and 7 months with chemotherapy alone.
- There are no large-scale reports of survival times in cats with the exception of meningiomas (see Meningioma, p 696). However, the long-term prognosis for cats with other brain tumors is likely similar to that for dogs.

PEARLS & CONSIDERATIONS

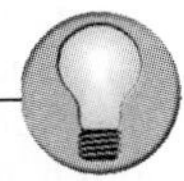

COMMENTS

With neoplasia of the brain, asymmetric neurologic deficits are much more common than symmetric deficits. Symmetric neurologic deficits make other diagnoses more likely.

PREVENTION

No known method to prevent disease

CLIENT EDUCATION

- Warn owner of corticosteroid side effects (e.g., polyuria, polydipsia, polyphagia, weight gain, gastrointestinal ulceration, iatrogenic hyperadrenocorticism).
- Phenobarbital and KBr: Short-term side effects include sedation/lethargy and pelvic limb weakness and ataxia. Long-term side effects include polyuria, polydipsia, polyphagia, weight gain. Less common adverse effects include hepatotoxicity and blood dyscrasias for phenobarbital and pancreatitis for KBr.
- See other sources for additional information.

SUGGESTED READING

Bagley RS, et al: Clinical signs associated with brain tumors in dogs: 97 cases (1992–1997). *J Am Vet Med Assoc* 214:818, 1999.

Dewey CW, et al: How I treat primary brain tumors in dogs and cats. *Comp Cont Educ Pract Vet* 22:756, 2000.

LeCouteur RA: Current concepts in the diagnosis and treatment of brain tumors in dogs and cats. *J Small Anim Pract* 40:411,1999.

Troxel MT, et al: Feline intracranial neoplasia: Retrospective review of 160 cases (1985–2001). *J Vet Intern Med* 17:850, 2003.

AUTHOR: **MARK T. TROXEL**

EDITOR: **CURTIS W. DEWEY**

Breeding Management

BASIC INFORMATION

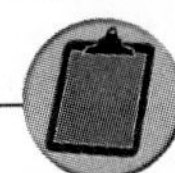

DEFINITION

Diagnostic and treatment approaches that optimize a bitch's reproductive performance

SYNONYM(S)

Breeding timing
Estrus monitoring

EPIDEMIOLOGY

SPECIES, AGE, SEX: Dogs, postpubertal, female.

GENETICS AND BREED PREDISPOSITION

- Breeding animals should be tested for heritable disorders, because more than 400 genetic diseases have been identified in dogs.
- Breeding management is indicated in any breed that cannot breed or deliver offspring naturally. Bitches requiring elective caesarean section (e.g., brachycephalics) require intense monitoring to establish the time of their luteinizing hormone (LH) surge during estrus.

RISK FACTORS

- Advanced age of dam and/or sire
- Use of cooled or frozen semen
- Dam's or sire's history of unsatisfactory fertility
- Degenerative and/or infectious conditions within the reproductive tract

CONTAGION AND ZOONOSIS: *Brucella canis.*

GEOGRAPHY AND SEASONALITY: Bitches cycle at any time of the year (except Basenji—late summer/early fall).

ASSOCIATED CONDITIONS AND DISORDERS: Estrus induction, artificial insemination (AI), pregnancy diagnosis.

CLINICAL PRESENTATION

HISTORY, CHIEF COMPLAINT: Owner desires litter from dam and wants to maximize fertility and fecundity.

PHYSICAL EXAM FINDINGS: Physical exam should be unremarkable. Overt signs of estrus should be evident:

- Swollen, edematous vulva
- Serosanguineous vaginal discharge
- Perineal stimulation results in lateral deviation of the tail ("flagging"), elevation of the vulva and lordosis

DIAGNOSIS

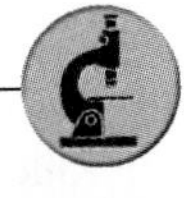

DIFFERENTIAL DIAGNOSIS

- Persistence of estrous behavior: granulosa cell tumor, cystic ovarian disease
- Discharge from an open pyometra
- Vaginal or uterine trauma resulting in bleeding

INITIAL DATABASE

- Vaginoscopy:
  - Start 0 to 5 days after onset of vaginal bleeding; continue q 48h to monitor estrogenization of the vaginal mucosa.
  - Tubular Plexiglas speculum, 10–20 mm inner diameter, 15–25 cm length.
  - Maximal development of the squamous epithelium (evident as paleness) and edema (evident as swollen, rounded folds) of the vaginal mucosa coincides with peak estrogen concentrations, just before LH surge.
- Vaginal cytology:
  - Start 0 to 5 days after the onset of vaginal bleeding and continue q 48h to monitor estrogenization of the vaginal mucosa.
  - Use a cotton swab, moistened with saline, and extended with hemostat or AI pipette to reach through a vaginal speculum for collection of cells from cranial vagina.
  - The vaginal cytology will contain 100% superficial cells (large, angular, often with folded edges), many of which still have nuclear remnants or pyknotic nuclei.
- Serum progesterone concentration:
  - Start determining serum progesterone concentration once there is maximal development of the squamous epithelium and/or the vaginal cytology contains 100% superficial cells.
  - Refrigeration of whole blood during the first 2 hours after sample collection significantly decreases measured serum progesterone concentrations in dogs. When whole, clotted blood is not centrifuged immediately after

collection, it must not be refrigerated for at least 2 hours because this will affect serum progesterone concentrations.
  - The day of LH surge (d0) is the day preceding the first day on which serum progesterone concentration exceeds 2 ng/ml.
- *Brucella* testing is essential.

TREATMENT

THERAPEUTIC GOAL(S)

Under most circumstances, no treatment is indicated.

- When no breeding management is used, bitches are bred naturally every other day as long as they are receptive (in behavioral estrus):
  - When the male is not freely available or when AI is intended, breeding management is needed to optimize fertility, while reducing the number of breedings to one or two per cycle.
  - A single, well-timed breeding with an adequate sperm number can yield better results than multiple, ill-timed breedings.

ACUTE GENERAL TREATMENT

BREEDING STRATEGIES: Natural service, fresh or shipped (cooled) semen AI:

- Breed on days 4 and 6 after LH surge.
- Inseminate vaginally, using a 5 mm thick plastic pipette that is advanced to the caudal end of the cervix (confirm placement by abdominal palpation).
- Once the pipette is placed, the semen is injected slowly through a syringe attached to the pipette, the pipette is withdrawn, and a finger is placed into the vestibulum and used to massage the floor of the cranial vestibulum ("feathering") for 1 to 10 minutes (vaginal contractions result and facilitate movement of semen through the cervix).
- Elevation of the bitch's hindquarters is often practiced but does not improve fertility.

AI with frozen or poor quality fresh/cooled semen:

- Breed on day 5 after LH surge:
  - Perform laparotomy and inject semen through uterine wall.
  - Perform transcervical AI, using endoscopically guided transcervical catheterization (dedicated equipment) or Norwegian catheter guided through the cervix by abdominal palpation (advanced skill and experience needed).
  - The latter two techniques allow for repeat inseminations on multiple days (usually days 5 to 7 after LH surge). With frozen semen, more than one insemination at daily intervals and a lower sperm dose produces better results than a single, well-timed insemination with a high sperm dose.
  - Two to four daily vaginal inseminations with frozen-thawed semen extended with prostatic fluid have yielded excellent results as well.

RECOMMENDED MONITORING

Rarely, persistent estrus results from failure of ovulation, cystic ovarian degeneration, or a granulosa cell tumor

PEARLS & CONSIDERATIONS

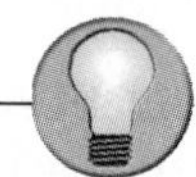

COMMENTS

- Animals should be tested for brucellosis and heritable disorders before breeding.
- Semen quality should be assessed in advance.
- Test kits for semiquantitative determination of serum progesterone and luteinizing hormone concentrations of bitches are available for use when laboratory services are not available.
- The day of LH surge (d0) is the day preceding the first day on which serum progesterone concentration exceeds 2 ng/ml.

CLIENT EDUCATION

- Fourth to sixth days after the LH surge are most fertile in bitches, but pregnancies can result from breeding up to 3 days earlier or 2 days later using fresh semen.
- Estrus monitoring is also used to predict the most likely whelping date: 65 (±1) days after the LH surge or 57 (±1) days after D1 of cytologic diestrus.

SUGGESTED READING

Goodman M: Ovulation timing. *Vet Clin North Am Sm Anim Pract* 31:219, 2001.

Lindsay FEF, Concannon PW: Normal canine vaginoscopy. In Burke TJ (ed): *Small Animal Reproduction and Infertility*. Philadelphia, Lea & Febiger, 1986, pp 112–120.

Nothling JO, Gerstenberg C, Volkmann DH: Success with intravaginal insemination of frozen-thawed dog semen: A retrospective study. *J So Afr Vet Assoc* 66:49, 1995.

Volkmann DH: The effects of storage time and temperature and anticoagulant on laboratory measurements of canine blood progesterone concentrations. *Theriogenology* 2006 Feb 7 (Epub ahead of print).

Wilson MS: Transcervical insemination techniques in the bitch. *Vet Clin North Am Small Anim Pract* 31:291, 2001.

AUTHOR: **DIETRICH VOLKMANN**

EDITOR: **MICHELLE A. KUTZLER**

Bromethalin Toxicosis

BASIC INFORMATION

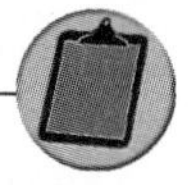

DEFINITION

A neurotoxic syndrome resulting from ingestion of bromethalin rodenticide.

Commercial products contain 0.01% bromethalin or 2.84 mg bromethalin per 1 oz of bait.

SYNONYM(S)

- (2,4-dinitro-*N*-methyl-*N*-[2,4,6-tribromophenyl]-6-[trifluoromethyl] benzenamine)
- Sold under numerous trade names, including:
  - Assault mouse/rat Place Pack
  - Fastrac Mouse Seed Place Pacs
  - Green thumb mouse killer
  - Hot Shot Sudden Death Brand Mouse Killer$_1$
  - Purina Assault Meal
  - Rampage Rodenticide Place Pacs
  - Real-Kill Mouse Killer Placepacs
  - Real-Kill Rat And Mouse Killer All Weather Bars
  - Real-Kill Rat And Mouse Killer Pellets
  - Real-Kill Rat Killer Placepack
  - Top gun Pellet Rodenticide Place Pack
  - Vengence

EPIDEMIOLOGY

SPECIES, AGE, SEX

- Cats much more sensitive than dogs
- Ingestion more common in dogs than cats
- All breeds, sexes susceptible; young animals may be more sensitive

GEOGRAPHY AND SEASONALITY: Toxicity is more prevalent during fall or winter months.

CLINICAL PRESENTATION

DISEASE FORMS/SUBTYPES

- Dogs ingesting doses close to or greater than the LD_{50} (approximately 3.65 mg/kg) may develop a convulsant syndrome with onset of seizures within 24 hours.
- Dogs consuming less than the LD_{50} manifest a paralytic syndrome in 1 to 7 days.

- Cats typically develop a paralytic syndrome regardless of the ingested dose.

HISTORY, CHIEF COMPLAINT
- History or evidence of exposure
- Central nervous system (CNS) depression, hind limb weakness, or ataxia without evidence of pain
- Twitching, seizures

PHYSICAL EXAM FINDINGS
- Convulsant syndrome:
  - Focal or generalized seizures (possibly triggered by environmental stimuli)
- Tremors:
  - Hyperthermia
- Paralytic form:
  - Hind limb weakness, ataxia
  - Depression, tremors, areflexive hind limb paralysis, seizures
  - Cats may also show nystagmus, anisocoria, opisthotonos, and occasionally abdominal distention from paralytic ileus

ETIOLOGY AND PATHOPHYSIOLOGY
- Bromethalin and its major metabolite desmobromethalin are potent uncouplers of oxidative phosphorylation.
- Cerebral and spinal edema secondary to decreased ATP production and failure of Na-K ATPase pumps.
- Elevated CSF pressure causes neurologic dysfunction.

DIAGNOSIS

DIFFERENTIAL DIAGNOSIS
- Convulsant form:
  - Primary CNS disease
  - Metaldehyde toxicosis
  - Strychnine toxicosis
  - Zinc phosphide toxicosis
  - Ethylene glycol toxicosis
- Paralytic form:
  - Neuromuscular disease (polyradiculoneuritis, tick paralysis, botulism, myasthenia gravis)
  - Spinal cord/CNS trauma
  - Intervertebral disk disease

INITIAL DATABASE
- The diagnosis is generally presumptive, based on clinical presentation, physical examination, and history if available.
- Complete blood count, serum biochemistry panel, radiology: no significant changes.

ADVANCED OR CONFIRMATORY TESTING
Rarely performed.
- Cerebrospinal fluid (CSF) tap: increased CSF pressure; no inflammatory changes.
- CNS edema, demyelination, and vacuolization on histopathologic exam.
- Bromethalin can be detected in tissues post mortem (liver, kidney, brain, and fat).

TREATMENT

THERAPEUTIC GOAL(S)
- Decontamination of patient
- Supportive care

ACUTE GENERAL TREATMENT
Emesis and/or activated charcoal (A/C) treatment recommendations:

Recommendation for Dogs

Time since Exposure (hrs)	Dose Ingested (mg/kg)	Treatment
<4	0.1-0.49	Emesis or 1 dose of A/C
>4	0.1-0.49	One dose of A/C
<4	0.5-0.75	Emesis and 3 doses of A/C over 24 hours
>4	0.5-0.75	3 doses of A/C over 24 hours
<4	>0.75	Emesis and 3 doses of A/C a day for 48 hours
>4	>0.75	3 doses of A/C a day for 48 hours

A/C, activated charcoal.

Recommendations for Cats

Time since Exposure (hrs)	Dose Ingested (mg/kg)	Treatment
< 4	0.05-0.1	Emesis or 1 dose of A/C
>4	0.05-0.1	1 dose of A/C
<4	0.1-0.3	Emesis and 3 doses of A/C over 24 hours
>4	0.1-0.3	3 doses of A/C over 24 hours
<4	>0.3	Emesis and 3 doses of A/C a day for 48 hours
>4	>0.3	3 doses of A/C a day for 48 hours

A/C, activated charcoal.

CHRONIC TREATMENT
- Supportive care for clinically ill patients (fluids, nutritional support, seizure control, etc.)
- Cerebral edema may not respond well to furosemide, mannitol, or corticosteroids
- Diazepam, barbiturates, and other anticonvulsants for CNS signs

POSSIBLE COMPLICATIONS
Permanent CNS damage/dysfunction due to demyelination and vacuolization

RECOMMENDED MONITORING
Animals with a suspected or confirmed exposure to bromethalin but without overt clinical signs need to be monitored for an onset of hind limb weakness or other CNS signs for 7 days postexposure.

PROGNOSIS AND OUTCOME

- Good with decontamination of patient prior to the onset of signs
- Guarded if signs develop; recovery may take days to weeks
- Poor if paralysis or seizures develop

PEARLS & CONSIDERATIONS

COMMENTS
- Commercial products contain 0.01% bromethalin or 2.84 mg/oz bromethalin.
- Doses of 0.95-1.05 mg/kg in dogs and 0.24 mg/kg in cats can be lethal.
- The various rodenticides (see Anticoagulant Rodenticide Toxicosis, p 76), bromethalin, and cholecalciferol (see Cholecalciferol Toxicosis, p 198) cannot be identified by appearance alone.
- Vitamin K_1 therapy, used for anticoagulant rodenticides, is not indicated for bromethalin ingestion.
- Potential for relay toxicosis (intoxication through consumption of prey that has itself ingested the toxin) appears low except for cats whose diet consists largely of rodents.

PREVENTION
Placement of baits in areas not accessible to dogs and cats

SUGGESTED READING

Dorman D: Bromethalin. In Plumlee KH (ed): *Clinical Veterinary Toxicology*. St. Louis, Mosby, 2004, pp 446–448.

Dunayer, EK: Bromethalin: The other rodenticide. *Veterinary Medicine* 98:732, 2003.

AUTHOR: **ERIC K. DUNAYER**
EDITOR: **SAFDAR A. KHAN**

Bronchiectasis

BASIC INFORMATION

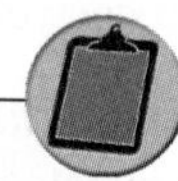

DEFINITION

Irreversible, pathologic dilation of airways due to destruction of the elastic and muscular components of the airway walls

EPIDEMIOLOGY

SPECIES, AGE, SEX

- Dogs are affected more commonly than cats.
- Young animals are affected if associated with a congenital abnormality (rare); animals are older if associated with chronic inflammation, infection, or neoplasia.
- Either gender can be affected.

GENETICS AND BREED PREDISPOSITION: American cocker spaniels, West Highland white terriers, miniature poodles, Siberian huskies, and English springer spaniels may have an increased risk.

RISK FACTORS

- Congenital defects (e.g., primary ciliary dyskinesia)
- Chronic infection or inflammation
- Neoplasia

ASSOCIATED CONDITIONS AND DISORDERS

- Congenital defects in mucociliary function, such as primary ciliary dyskinesia
- Immunodeficiency diseases
- Acquired diseases, such as:
  - Chronic bronchitis
  - Eosinophilic bronchitis
  - Bronchopneumonia
  - Neoplasia

CLINICAL PRESENTATION

DISEASE FORMS/SUBTYPES

- Focal, multifocal, diffuse distribution
- Cylindrical, saccular, and cystic forms

HISTORY, CHIEF COMPLAINT

- Incidental radiographic finding in the absence of clinical signs (especially in cats)
- Cough
- Tachypnea
- Respiratory distress
- Other signs that reflect underlying disease (e.g., nasal discharge with ciliary dyskinesia)

PHYSICAL EXAM FINDINGS

- Cough may be inducible on tracheal palpation; however, several other diseases, including nonairway disorders, may also produce an inducible cough
- Other findings may be referable to underlying disease (e.g., fever with bacterial pneumonia)

ETIOLOGY AND PATHOPHYSIOLOGY

- Congenital or acquired conditions lead to a cycle of damage to the bronchial epithelium and/or their cilia, inflammation, impairment of mucociliary function, and secondary infection.
- Cellular damage, inflammation, and infection perpetuate the cycle of airway wall destruction, leading to bronchiectasis.

DIAGNOSIS

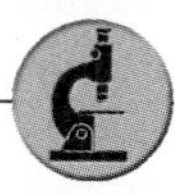

DIFFERENTIAL DIAGNOSIS

Physical exam (cough or respiratory distress):

- Other airway diseases (e.g., chronic sterile bronchitis, eosinophilic bronchitis)
- Pneumonia (infectious, aspiration, eosinophilic, foreign body)
- Neoplasia
- Pulmonary thromboembolism
- Cardiogenic or noncardiogenic pulmonary edema
- Pleural effusion
- Pneumothorax
- Interstitial lung disease

INITIAL DATABASE

- Complete blood count: may provide evidence of underlying infection or eosinophilic inflammation
- Thoracic radiographs:
  - Bronchiectasis has a pathognomonic radiographic appearance.
    - Cylindrical form: dilated bronchi with nontapering ends
    - Saccular form: "cluster of grapes" appearance to airways
    - Cystic form: rounded ends of the very small bronchi
  - Evidence of concurrent/underlying pulmonary disease is frequently present.
  - Radiographs may be unremarkable in the early stages of disease.

ADVANCED OR CONFIRMATORY TESTING

- Computed tomography may help detect subtle lesions.
- Bronchoscopy and bronchoalveolar lavage or fine-needle aspiration (cytology and culture) are useful in identification of underlying/concurrent diseases.
- Specialized functional and immunologic studies such as mucociliary scintigraphy, IgA levels, and others may be needed to evaluate patients for suspected congenital disease.
- Lung biopsy is sometimes needed to identify underlying/concurrent disease.

TREATMENT

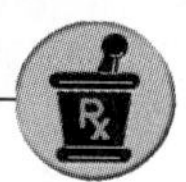

THERAPEUTIC GOAL(S)

- Dampen inflammation
- Enhance mucociliary clearance
- Address secondary infections if present

ACUTE GENERAL TREATMENT

Address underlying illness and secondary complications (e.g., bacterial bronchopneumonia)

CHRONIC TREATMENT

- Environmental modulation:
  - Minimize exposure to irritants such as dust, smoke, and aerosols.
  - Hepa-type air filters.
- Humidification or nebulization enhances mucociliary function by increasing water content of the mucociliary blanket.
- Bronchodilators are unlikely to be helpful.
- Glucocorticoids:
  - Oral (e.g., prednisone 0.25–0.5 mg/kg/day) preferred initially to control inflammation.
  - Continuation of glucocorticoids is based clinically on the underlying disease contributing to bronchiectasis.
    - If bronchiectasis is due to resolved pneumonia or obstructive disease, then short courses leading to discontinuation may be considered.
    - If bronchiectasis is secondary to noninfectious inflammatory disease (e.g., chronic bronchitis), inflammation often will need to be controlled with long-term, low-dose glucocorticoids.
  - The metered dose inhalant glucocorticoids (e.g., flunisolide: can start at 110 µg/actuation, one puff using a spacer q 12h; decrease to 44 µg/actuation, one puff using a spacer q 12h thereafter) may minimize systemic effects in the long term. See Medication Administration by Inhalation, p 1278.
- Treat recurrent secondary bacterial infections if present, ideally based on culture and sensitivity.
- In cases in which bronchiectasis is confined to a single lung lobe (e.g., due to a prior bacterial pneumonia), lobectomy may be curative.

POSSIBLE COMPLICATIONS

Attempting to control inflammation with glucocorticoids may impair immunologic clearance of secondary infection; additionally, bronchiectasis is itself associated with impaired mucociliary function, which also predisposes to bacterial infections. Frequent use of antibiotics may lead to development of bacterial resistance.

RECOMMENDED MONITORING

- Clinical signs at home
- Physical examination
- Thoracic radiography
- Repeated airway cultures as indicated

PROGNOSIS AND OUTCOME

- If disease is focal and the lobe removed (e.g., bronchiectasis secondary to chronic obstruction from neoplasia or a foreign body) and the underlying disease is cured, prognosis is excellent.
- Otherwise, the disease cannot be cured and must be treated chronically by balancing antibiotics for secondary infections and anti-inflammatory doses of corticosteroids; in the absence of life-threatening infection or serious underlying disease (e.g., neoplasia), long-term survival is possible.

PEARLS & CONSIDERATIONS

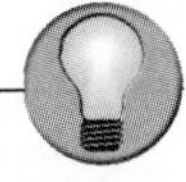

COMMENTS

- Bronchiectasis is always secondary to an underlying condition, although the primary disease may have resolved by the time of evaluation (e.g., bacterial pneumonia).
- Management of secondary bacterial infections should be done on the basis of culture and sensitivity whenever possible to prevent development of antibiotic resistance.

CLIENT EDUCATION

Owners must understand that aside from focal disease treated with lobectomy, this is not a curable disease; in multifocal and diffuse cases, recurrent secondary bacterial infections are common and can potentially be life-threatening.

SUGGESTED READING

Hawkins EC, et al: Demographic, clinical, and radiographic features of bronchiectasis in dogs: 316 cases (1988–2000). *J Am Vet Med Assoc* 223:1628, 2003.

Norris CR, et al: Clinical, radiographic, and pathologic features of bronchiectasis in cats: 12 cases (1987–1999). *J Am Vet Med Assoc* 216:530, 2000.

AUTHOR: **CAROL REINERO**
EDITOR: **RANCE K. SELLON**

Bronchiolar and Pulmonary Neoplasia

BASIC INFORMATION

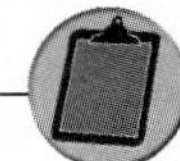

DEFINITION

Neoplastic growth originating in the bronchi or lower airways

SYNONYM(S)

Lung cancer
Primary lung tumors
Primary pulmonary tumors

EPIDEMIOLOGY

SPECIES, AGE, SEX

- Rare in dogs (1.24% of dogs at necropsy) and cats (0.38% at necropsy)
- Older animals:
  - 9.3 to 10.9 years in dogs
  - 11 to 12.5 years in cats
- No sex predilection

GENETICS AND BREED PREDISPOSITION: No breed predisposition known but increased incidence in boxer dogs and tricolor cats found in single studies.

RISK FACTORS: Weak links to urban environment, secondhand smoke, brachycephalic confirmation.

ASSOCIATED CONDITIONS AND DISORDERS

- Hypertrophic osteopathy.
- Digital, ocular, or muscular signs secondary to metastasis are common in cats.

CLINICAL PRESENTATION

DISEASE FORMS/SUBTYPES: Malignant:

- Adenocarcinomas are the most common in dogs and cats and can be of different subtypes:
  - Bronchial
  - Alveolar
  - Bronchoalveolar
- Squamous cell carcinoma
- Variety of sarcomas also possible, but rare

Benign:

- Papillary and bronchial adenoma
- Hemangioma
- Fibroma
- Myxochondroma
- Blastoma

HISTORY, CHIEF COMPLAINT

- Nonproductive cough most common complaint
- Dyspnea, lethargy, tachypnea less common
- Occasionally spontaneous pneumothorax or hemothorax
- Occasionally, chief complaint involves problems secondary to hypertrophic osteopathy or metastatic disease (e.g., swollen painful limbs or digital pain)

PHYSICAL EXAM FINDINGS

- Can be normal.
- Increased respiratory rate and/or effort possible.
- Easily elicited cough with tracheal palpation. However, this finding is nonspecific, because many other disorders (including many pulmonary parenchymal disorders) may cause an easily elicited cough.
- Lung auscultation is often normal, although silent areas may be noted over large masses.

ETIOLOGY AND PATHOPHYSIOLOGY

Exact etiology is unknown, but inhalation of carcinogens provoking malignant transformation is suspected.

- Dogs trained to smoke cigarettes (through a tracheostomy) or that inhaled radioactive substances developed lung tumors at a dramatically increased rate.

DIAGNOSIS

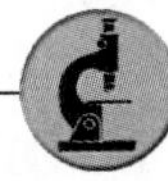

DIFFERENTIAL DIAGNOSIS

- Metastatic disease (usually multiple nodules of similar size)
- Malignant histiocytosis (usually also includes disease at other locations)
- Tumors of pleura, mediastinum, or heart base
- Abscess, fungal or bacterial disease
- Lymphoid granulomatosis
- Eosinophilic granulomatosis
- Foreign body granuloma
- Hematoma or infarct
- Lung lobe torsion
- Bronchial foreign body (causes lung lobe collapse/atelectasis)
- Mediastinal masses

INITIAL DATABASE

- Complete blood count, serum biochemistry profile, and urinalysis are often normal.
- Thoracic radiographs:
  - Primary lung tumors usually appear as single nodules or one large nodule/mass and several smaller nodules.
  - Cats can have more diffuse infiltrative patterns within a lung lobe.

ADVANCED OR CONFIRMATORY TESTING

- Thoracic computed tomography is the best modality to identify the full extent of disease and assess possibility of surgical removal.
- Bronchoscopy and brush biopsy of bronchial lesions or transthoracic needle aspiration of peripheral lesions may yield sufficient cells for cytologic diagnosis.
  - Nonspecific inflammation is a common cytologic feature of respiratory samples obtained from patients with pulmonary neoplasia and thus does not rule out neoplasia.
  - Transthoracic needle biopsy carries acute risks of pneumothorax and hemothorax, and a long-term risk of tumor seeding.

TREATMENT

THERAPEUTIC GOAL(S)

Removal of tumor

ACUTE GENERAL TREATMENT

- If dyspneic, give oxygen.
- Fluid or air in the thorax should be evacuated if respiration is impaired by pleural effusion or pneumothorax, respectively.

CHRONIC TREATMENT

- Single nodule/mass:
  - The appropriate therapy for a single isolated nodule is surgical resection.
- If metastatic disease is identified (within lung parenchyma, pleura, hilar nodes, or distant sites), or the tumor is not removable due to size or other factors, surgery should not be attempted.
  - Incomplete removal of lung tumors will not increase quality of life or lifespan.
  - Chemotherapy can be considered for malignant tumors.
    - Vinblastine and platinum-containing drugs are most often recommended for carcinomas, but pulmonary carcinomas are generally poorly responsive to chemotherapy.
    - Doxorubicin-based protocols may be helpful for patients with sarcomas.
- Radiation therapy for palliation of clinical signs can be considered if tumor is confined to one area.

POSSIBLE COMPLICATIONS

- Pneumothorax
- Hemothorax
- Pleural effusion

RECOMMENDED MONITORING

Thoracic radiographs for tumor progression, return (postoperatively), or response to therapy

PROGNOSIS AND OUTCOME

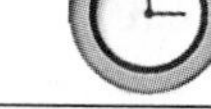

- Small tumors carry better prognosis.
  - Median survival after resection of tumors <5 cm diameter is 20 months; >5 cm diameter is 8 to 9 months
- Adenocarcinoma has a better prognosis than squamous cell carcinoma or undifferentiated carcinomas (median survival 251 days versus 160 days).
- Hilar lymph node enlargement is associated with a poor prognosis (median survival 60 days versus 12 months if no lymph node enlargement).

PEARLS & CONSIDERATIONS

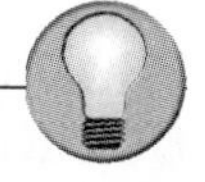

COMMENTS

Patients with lung tumors should always be evaluated fully before attempting surgical resection.

- If the tumors are small, peripherally located, and there is no obvious lymph node enlargement, surgery should be recommended, and survival after resection could be greater than 1 year.

SUGGESTED READING

Fox LE, King RR: Cancers of the respiratory system. In Morrison WB (ed): *Cancer in Dogs and Cats*. Baltimore, Williams & Wilkins, 2002, pp 497–512.

Withrow SJ: Lung cancer. In Withrow SJ, MacEwen (eds): *Small Animal Clinical Oncology*. Philadelphia, WB Saunders, 2001, pp 361–370.

AUTHOR: **JANEAN L. FIDEL**
EDITOR: **RANCE K. SELLON**

Bronchitis: Chronic, Sterile

Client Education Sheet on Website

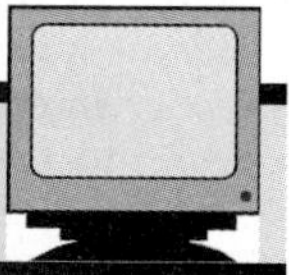

BASIC INFORMATION

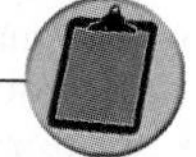

DEFINITION

A common noninfectious airway disease of older adult dogs. The hallmark is a chronic cough lasting longer than 2 months and not attributable to a known cause.

SYNONYM(S)

Chronic bronchial disease
Chronic bronchitis
Chronic obstructive pulmonary disease (COPD)
Noninfectious sterile bronchitis
Old dog sterile bronchitis

EPIDEMIOLOGY

SPECIES, AGE, SEX

- Most common in dogs; rarely reported in cats
- Mainly middle-aged to older dogs of either sex

GENETICS AND BREED PREDISPOSITION: Primarily a disease of small-breed dogs but should not be overlooked in large-breed dogs.

RISK FACTORS: Inhaled environmental irritants such as cigarette smoke, room deodorizers or carpet cleaners, and wood-burning stoves or fireplaces can exacerbate chronic sterile bronchitis.

GEOGRAPHY AND SEASONALITY: There may be seasonal exacerbations in individual pets, although no specific seasonality is described for all dogs.

ASSOCIATED CONDITIONS AND DISORDERS

- Pneumonia
- Collapsing trachea
- Bronchiectasis
- Pulmonary hypertension and cor pulmonale

CLINICAL PRESENTATION

HISTORY, CHIEF COMPLAINT: The primary clinical sign is a dry, hacking cough.

- Cough can be moderately productive (expectoration of mucus):
  - Not specifically diurnal or nocturnal
  - May have loud, "goose-honk" character
  - Often triggered by physical exertion, especially if it involves the dog's pulling on a leash (tracheal pressure from collar)
- Owners may note post-tussive retching or gagging and mistakenly describe this as "vomiting."

In severe cases, signs may include:
- Exercise intolerance
- Syncope
  - Tachypnea
  - Cyanosis

PHYSICAL EXAM FINDINGS

- Cough:
  - The characteristic finding of this disorder.
  - Commonly with sterile chronic bronchitis, the cough occurs less frequently or not at all when the dog is in a veterinary facility (sympathetically mediated bronchodilation due to anxiety?).
- Tracheal sensitivity:
  - Applying light to moderate external pressure on the trachea using the fingers may elicit a cough.
  - In affected dogs, it may be possible to elicit a cough with tracheal pressure. However, many other respiratory disorders also have this feature, even if the airway is *not* the source of the problem (e.g., dogs with cardiogenic pulmonary edema virtually always cough in response to tracheal pressure). Therefore, the finding of tracheal sensitivity is nonspecific.
- Auscultatory abnormalities (increased bronchovesicular sounds, crackles, wheezes):
  - Crackles can often be heard on auscultation of the lungs in patients with sterile chronic bronchitis. They can be erroneously attributed to congestive heart failure; therefore, both conditions should be investigated when crackles are heard, especially in a dog in which no heart murmur is ausculted.
- Tachypnea

ETIOLOGY AND PATHOPHYSIOLOGY

Airway inflammation, characterized by cellular infiltrates, glandular hyperplasia, smooth muscle hypertrophy, and loss of ciliated epithelial cells provokes cough:
- Although inhaled irritants and environmental pollutants could be partially responsible, definitive underlying causes have not been identified.

DIAGNOSIS

DIFFERENTIAL DIAGNOSIS

- Pneumonia
- Collapsing trachea
- Congestive heart failure
- Respiratory neoplasia
- Heartworm disease
- Canine infectious tracheobronchitis

INITIAL DATABASE

- Thoracic radiograph abnormalities can include:
  - Mild to moderate diffuse interstitial pattern
  - Hyperinflation of lung field ("air trapping"). See Asthma, Cat, p 89
  - Bronchial markings ("doughnuts," "tram lines")
  - If pulmonary hypertension present, possible findings include:
    - Right-sided cardiomegaly
    - ± Enlarged, tortuous pulmonary arteries
- Normal thoracic radiographs do not exclude the possibility of sterile chronic bronchitis:
  - Lateral cervical radiographs should be obtained in suspected cases to avoid misdiagnosis of sterile chronic bronchitis as a result of overlooking cervical collapsing trachea

ADVANCED OR CONFIRMATORY TESTING

- Cytologic examination of samples collected by bronchoalveolar lavage or transtracheal wash often demonstrates a predominance of nondegenerate neutrophils:
  - Occasionally, a predominance of eosinophils is seen.
  - Although bacterial infection is uncommon with this disease, quantitative culture of airway samples is recommended to exclude secondary infection or colonization exacerbating the disease.
- Bronchoscopy often reveals inflammation, hyperemia, and edema of the mucosa and accumulation of secretions in the tracheobronchial tree.
  - Collapse or hypoplasia of the trachea or bronchi may also be appreciated in cases in which sterile chronic bronchitis coexists with collapsing trachea.
- Arterial blood gas measurement: consider if severe dyspnea/respiratory distress (uncommon). May reveal:
  - Hypoxemia.
  - Hypocarbia.
    - Hypercarbia from respiratory failure may be seen in advanced cases and usually signals a grave prognosis.

TREATMENT

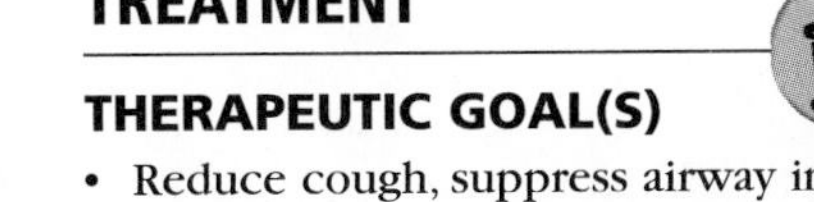

THERAPEUTIC GOAL(S)

- Reduce cough, suppress airway inflammation, reduce airway obstructions, and minimize the potential for secondary infections
- Complete resolution of cough is virtually never possible. The therapeutic goal is reduction of frequency and severity of cough so that the animal is more comfortable

ACUTE GENERAL TREATMENT

- Bronchodilators, anti-inflammatory medications, and cough suppressants are indicated in acute exacerbations.
  - Cough suppressants:
    - Cough suppressants are indicated to decrease coughing frequency and severity. Cough suppressants should not be used if the cough is moderately productive or if there is suspicion of an underlying infection.
    - Hydrocodone 0.22 mg/kg PO q 6–12h.
    - Butorphanol 0.25–1 mg/kg PO q 6–12h; the higher dosage may cause sedation. The oral dosage is many times greater than the injectable dose and should **not** be used for calculating injectable doses of butorphanol.
  - Anti-inflammatory medications:
    - Prednisone 0.5–1.0 mg/kg q 12h for 5 to 7 days to induce remission of cough.
    - Decrease prednisone dose by half every 7 days and, when possible, move to alternate-day dosing to achieve minimum dose necessary to control clinical signs.
  - Bronchodilators:
    - β_2 agonists:
      - Terbutaline (total amount per dose): small dogs 0.625–1.25 mg PO q 12h, medium dogs 1.25–2.5 mg PO q 12h, large dogs 2.5–5 mg PO q 12h.
      - Albuterol: 0.05 mg/kg PO q 8h.
    - Methylxanthines:
      - Not all long-acting theophylline products have equivalent bioavailability in dogs. Implica-tions are that failure to respond to a certain product should prompt the consideration of switching bronchodilators (to a different brand of theophylline or a different class of bronchodilator altogether [e.g., a $\beta 2$ agonist]), and that certain individuals may develop signs of toxicosis when receiving doses that are well tolerated by others.
        - Theocap ER or Theochron ER (Inwood Laboratories) are recommended at 10 mg/kg PO q 12h.
        - Aminophylline or theophylline 10 mg/kg PO q 8h.
- Oxygen therapy is indicated if hypoxemia is present (usually in patients with respiratory distress, which is uncommon).

CHRONIC TREATMENT

- Eliminate sources of airway irritation (see Risk Factors above).
- Weight loss:
  - Obesity is a common exacerbating factor, potentially leading to the Pickwickian syndrome (respiratory compromise due to obesity).
  - Weight loss helps increase lung volume and compliance.
- Bronchodilators, either oral or inhaled, are often used for decreasing airway resistance.
  - Doses for oral management are listed under Acute General Treatment above.
  - Metered dose inhaler of salmeterol (β_2-agonist): one puff (21 μg) by inhalation q 12h. See Medication Administration by Inhalation, p 1278.
- Cough suppressants decrease cough frequency and severity:
  - Antitussives should not be used if cough is moderately productive or if there is suspicion of underlying infection. Doses are listed under Acute General Treatment above.
  - For long-term use, dose is typically titrated to reduce or eliminate cough, without reaching levels that produce drowsiness.
  - Cough suppressants may be administered daily at first (days to weeks) to obtain palliation of cough, and then reduced or dosed intermittently on an as-needed basis to manage flare-ups of coughing.
- Anti-inflammatory medications, either oral or inhaled corticosteroids, are often required:
  - Dose for oral management is listed under Acute General Treatment above.
  - Metered dose inhaler of fluticasone: one puff (220 μg) by inhalation q 12h. See Medication Administration by Inhalation, p 1278.
- The decision to incorporate antibiotic therapy should be based on cytologic evaluation and culture of airway samples.

DRUG INTERACTIONS

Fluoroquinolone antibiotics inhibit the metabolism of methylxanthine bronchodilators such as theophylline and aminophylline; their concurrent use can result in toxic plasma levels of the bronchodilator.

POSSIBLE COMPLICATIONS

- Bronchiectasis
- Pulmonary hypertension and right-sided congestive heart failure

RECOMMENDED MONITORING

Clinical signs

PROGNOSIS AND OUTCOME

- Guarded:
  - Complete resolution of the disorder (and its associated cough) is essentially never possible, because sterile chronic bronchitis is a progressive disease.
  - However, it is rarely life-threatening. Properly managed and treated, many or most patients with sterile chronic bronchitis can enjoy an excellent quality of life and normal life expectancy.
- Long-term complications of bronchitis can include bronchiectasis and pulmonary hypertension.

PEARLS & CONSIDERATIONS

COMMENTS

- Diagnosis of sterile chronic bronchitis is by exclusion of other causes of chronic cough.
- Middle-aged to older small-breed dogs often have mitral or tricuspid endocardiosis. The combination of cough, heart murmur, and pulmonary crackles on auscultation, and some degree of cardiomegaly from valvular insufficiency radiographically, can lead to the erroneous diagnosis of a cardiogenic cause for the cough, when in fact the cause is sterile chronic bronchitis and concurrent (but compensated, clinically insignificant) mitral or tricuspid endocardiosis.
  - Dogs with sterile chronic bronchitis, in contrast to dogs with congestive heart failure, often have normal or lower than normal heart rates.
  - Similarly, dogs with sterile chronic bronchitis often have respiratory sinus arrhythmia, whereas dogs with acute pulmonary edema virtually never do (sinus tachycardia instead).
  - If pulmonary crackles are ausculted yet there is no heart murmur, extra care should be taken to differentiate sterile chronic bronchitis from congestive heart failure (pulmonary edema) through radiographs, because the two diseases often present with very similar clinical features.
  - The diagnosis of sterile chronic bronchitis should be exclusive of any signs of pulmonary edema on thoracic radiographs. In the absence of thoracic radiographs, the diagnosis of congestive heart failure/pulmonary edema in a coughing dog cannot be made, and long-term treatment with diuretics is not supported.
- Medications delivered by metered dose inhaler are gaining attention for treatment of sterile chronic bronchitis. See Medication Administration by Inhalation, p 1278.
  - The proposed advantage is minimization of the adverse effects of oral treatment.
- Obesity is a common complicating factor. For this reason (and many others related to various adverse effects of long-term use), corticosteroid administration of more than a few days' duration should be avoided as much as possible.

CLIENT EDUCATION

The clinical signs of sterile chronic bronchitis can be controlled in many dogs, but cure is unlikely

SUGGESTED READING

Bach JF, Kukanich B, Papich MG, McKiernan BC: Evaluation of the bioavailability and pharmacokinetics of two extended-release theophylline formulations in dogs. *J Am Vet Med Assoc* 224:1113, 2004.

Johnson L: CVT update: Canine chronic bronchitis. In Bonagura JD (ed): *Kirk's Current Veterinary Therapy XIII Small Animal Practice*. Philadelphia, WB Saunders, 2000, pp 801-804.

McKiernan BC: Diagnosis and treatment of canine chronic bronchitis: Twenty years of experience. *Vet Clin North Am Small Anim Pract* 30:1267, 2000.

AUTHOR: **LAURA G. RIDGE**

EDITOR: **RANCE K. SELLON**

Bronchoesophageal Fistula

BASIC INFORMATION

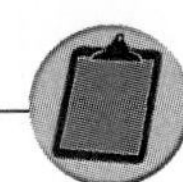

DEFINITION

A communicating tract between the esophagus and a bronchus

SYNONYM(S)

Esophageal fistula

EPIDEMIOLOGY

SPECIES, AGE, SEX

- An uncommon disease that occurs primarily in dogs; occasional cases in cats have been reported.
- Most reported cases have been described in young dogs (<7 years old) of either sex.

GENETICS AND BREED PREDISPOSITION

- Most cases of bronchoesophageal fistula have been seen in small-breed dogs; this predisposition also reflects the increased prevalence of esophageal foreign bodies in small-breed dogs. Conceivably, however, any breed could be affected in the presence of appropriate risk factors.
- Congenital bronchoesophageal fistula has also been described in dogs and cats, although the genetic basis for the disease has not been established.

RISK FACTORS: An esophageal foreign body is the single biggest risk factor for the subsequent development of a bronchoesophageal fistula.

ASSOCIATED CONDITIONS AND DISORDERS

- Focal pneumonia/aspiration pneumonia
- Esophageal diverticulum

CLINICAL PRESENTATION

DISEASE FORMS/SUBTYPES

- Congenital
- Acquired

HISTORY, CHIEF COMPLAINT

- Chronic cough is the most common clinical sign; coughing after drinking water is seen in some, but not all, cases. The cough is often responsive to therapy with antimicrobials but typically recurs at some point after cessation of antimicrobial therapy
- Regurgitation
- Anorexia, lethargy, depression
- Tachypnea, increased respiratory effort
- Weight loss

PHYSICAL EXAM FINDINGS

- Cough
- Fever
- Tachypnea, increased respiratory effort
- Increased bronchovesicular sounds, or diminished breath sounds from pleural effusion, may be appreciated during thoracic auscultation; thoracic auscultation may also be normal

ETIOLOGY AND PATHOPHYSIOLOGY

- Congenital:
  - Failure of tracheobronchial tree to completely separate from gastrointestinal tract during embryologic development
- Acquired (more common form of bronchoesophageal fistula):
  - Esophageal perforation from an esophageal foreign body is the usual cause. The foreign body can perforate the esophagus itself, or perforation may result from pressure necrosis of the esophagus
  - Esophageal diverticulum formation that predisposes to entrapment of an esophageal foreign body and subsequent perforation of the esophagus can also lead to a bronchoesophageal fistula

DIAGNOSIS

DIFFERENTIAL DIAGNOSIS

Other causes of chronic cough include:

- Aspiration pneumonia secondary to other esophageal diseases
- Other causes of recurring pneumonia such as seen with immune deficiencies (e.g., IgA deficiency) or abnormalities in pulmonary defense mechanisms (e.g., ciliary dyskinesia/immotile cilia syndrome)
- Respiratory foreign bodies
- Respiratory neoplasia
- Inflammatory respiratory diseases (e.g., chronic bronchitis, eosinophilic bronchopneumopathy)

INITIAL DATABASE

- Completed blood count: inflammatory leukogram; mild nonregenerative anemia possible (anemia of chronic inflammatory disease)
- Thoracic radiographs can have several abnormalities:
  - Localized alveolar, interstitial, or bronchial changes; the right caudal and right intermediate lung lobes are most commonly affected
  - Esophageal foreign body
  - Esophageal diverticulum
  - Pleural fluid

ADVANCED OR CONFIRMATORY TESTING

- Contrast esophagrams will demonstrate the fistula in most cases. Performing a contrast esophagram with fluoroscopy is considered more sensitive for the detection of small fistulas and for differentiating a fistula from aspirated contrast agent.
- Esophagoscopy/bronchoscopy are considered less sensitive than contrast esophagrams but will be helpful in some cases; bronchoscopy can help rule out other causes of focal pneumonia such as respiratory foreign bodies or bronchial neoplasia.
- Respiratory washes (transtracheal wash, bronchoalveolar lavage) will be important in some cases, particularly those with a history of having received multiple antimicrobials, to guide appropriate antimicrobial selections.

TREATMENT

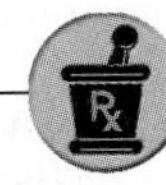

THERAPEUTIC GOAL(S)

- Remove communication between esophagus and airway
- Control pulmonary infection

ACUTE GENERAL TREATMENT

Surgical resection of the fistula with primary closure of the esophageal defect; remove esophageal foreign body if present

CHRONIC TREATMENT

Antimicrobials for pneumonia with selection best guided by culture and sensitivity testing of respiratory washes

POSSIBLE COMPLICATIONS

- Complications of treatment or the primary disease have not been described for those animals that survive.
- Complications of untreated bronchoesophageal fistula include persistent or recurring pneumonia, pleuritis, and pulmonary parenchymal abscessation.

RECOMMENDED MONITORING

- Clinical signs
- Thoracic radiographs for radiographic resolution of pneumonia

PROGNOSIS AND OUTCOME

A good prognosis is expected if respiratory complications are not serious. For patients with severe respiratory complications, the prognosis is guarded.

PEARLS & CONSIDERATIONS

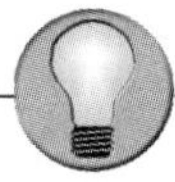

COMMENTS

Administration of a dilute concentration of barium sulfate (20–30% weight/volume) for an esophagram can facilitate demonstration of a bronchoesophageal fistula. The use of oral iodinated contrast agents for the documentation of bronchoesophageal fistulae has been discouraged because of the potential for more local adverse effects (cough, pulmonary edema) and the lower degree of radiographic contrast achieved with these substances (see Barium Esophagram, Dynamic, p 1187; Upper Gastrointestinal Radiographic Contrast Series, p 1316).

SUGGESTED READING

Kyles AE: Esophagus. In Slatter D: *Textbook of Small Animal Surgery*, ed 3. Philadelphia, Elsevier Science, 2003, pp 573–592.

Park RD: Bronchoesophageal fistula in the dog: Literature survey, case presentations, and radiographic manifestations. *Comp Cont Educ Pract Vet* 6:669, 1984.

Spielman BL, et al: Esophageal foreign body in dogs: A retrospective study of 23 cases. *J Am Anim Hosp Assoc* 28:570, 1992.

AUTHOR & EDITOR: **RANCE K. SELLON**

Brucellosis, Dog

BASIC INFORMATION

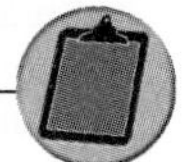

DEFINITION

Infection with *Brucella canis*

EPIDEMIOLOGY

SPECIES, AGE, SEX

- No age or gender predisposition reported
- Cats rarely affected

RISK FACTORS: Housing or breeding with infected animals.

CONTAGION AND ZOONOSIS: Highly contagious among dogs. Primary mode of transmission is oral; exposure is via infected body fluids, including vulvar discharge of estrus, parturition, or abortion; semen; and urine. Slight zoonotic potential exists. Canine brucellosis is a reportable disease in the United States (report to local health department, state department of health, state veterinarian's office, and/or veterinary public health program, depending on the state).

CLINICAL PRESENTATION

HISTORY, CHIEF COMPLAINT: Classic presentation in bitches is abortion at 45 to 55 days of gestation. Other signs include prolonged exudation of mucopurulent vulvar discharge and birth of stillborn or weak pups. Classic presentation in male dogs is epididymitis. Other signs include scrotal dermatitis, testicular atrophy, and poor semen quality. Either gender may present for infertility.

PHYSICAL EXAM FINDINGS: Bitches may abort partially autolyzed puppies and have persistent mucopurulent vulvar discharge. Males may present with painful scrotal enlargement and scrotal dermatitis (acute infection) or with testicular atrophy (chronic infection). Either gender may present for lymphadenopathy or signs of diskospondylitis.

ETIOLOGY AND PATHOPHYSIOLOGY

- After exposure by ingestion, or less commonly by venereal transfer, transient lymphadenopathy is followed by colonization of bacteria in genital tissues.
- Bacteremia develops 1 to 4 weeks after infection, persists for at least 6 months, and is intermittent thereafter.
- Clinical signs of reproductive tract disease in bitches are due to placentitis and metritis and, in male dogs, are due to epididymal inflammation and subsequent autoimmune destruction of testicular tissue.

DIAGNOSIS

DIFFERENTIAL DIAGNOSIS

- Abortion: canine herpesvirus infection, hypoluteoidism, other bacterial infections
- Infertility/poor semen quality/azoospermia: improper timing of breeding, subclinical uterine infection, testicular or prostatic disease
- Scrotal enlargement: torsion of spermatic cord, hernia, testicular neoplasia

INITIAL DATABASE

Rapid slide agglutination test with 2-mercaptoethanol (RSAT with 2-ME; D-Tec, Synbiotics, San Diego CA); identifies infection from 8 to 12 weeks postinfection. Negative results reliable unless dog only recently exposed. False-positive results common; all animals testing positive should be reevaluated (see Advanced or Confirmatory Testing below)

ADVANCED OR CONFIRMATORY TESTING

- Agar gel immunodiffusion test using cytoplasmic antigens (AGID; Cornell University): very specific, identifies infected animals from 12 weeks postinfection until 3 years after abacteremic
- Bacterial culture of blood, disease-related tissue or fluid; definitive, but false-negative results are common

TREATMENT

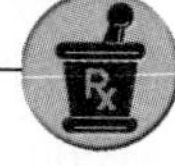

THERAPEUTIC GOAL(S)

Minimize spread to other animals and humans, stop progression of disease in affected animals

ACUTE GENERAL TREATMENT

- Euthanasia should be considered in kennel situations.
- Ovariohysterectomy or castration decreases shedding of organisms.
- Antibiotic therapy: No regimen is 100% effective; animals should never be considered cleared of the organism. Regimens described include tetracycline (30 mg/kg PO q 12h for 28 days) and streptomycin (20 mg/kg IV q 24h for 14 days); and enrofloxacin (5 mg/kg PO q 24h for 4 weeks). However, the latter regimen (enrofloxacin) has not been rigorously evaluated in a clinical setting.

CHRONIC TREATMENT

- Animals should not be housed with persons susceptible to infection. Periodic antibiotic therapy as described previously may be beneficial.
- In kennel situation: close kennel: no animals in or out; test all animals and euthanize or remove all that test positive; repeat test-and-removal monthly until all animals test negative for 3 consecutive months; quarantine all incoming animals for 8 to 12 weeks and test before introduction into kennel population.

RECOMMENDED MONITORING

Animals diagnosed with canine brucellosis should be considered positive for life and perhaps treated with antibiotics periodically to decrease risk of bacteremia and subsequent shedding

PROGNOSIS AND OUTCOME

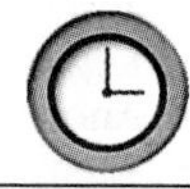

Dogs infected with *B. canis* should be considered positive for life. No dog infected with *Brucella* should be used for breeding, even if treated with antibiotics.

PEARLS & CONSIDERATIONS

RSAT is a good screening test. Dogs testing negative with an

RSAT, especially those that show no overt clinical signs, are considered *not* to be infected with *B. canis* unless testing is within 12 weeks postinfection. Likewise, dogs testing positive with an RSAT that are immediately tested with AGID and have a negative AGID result are considered *not* to be infected with *B. canis* unless testing is within 12 weeks postinfection or more than 3 years abacteremic.

PREVENTION

All intact male and female dogs should be screened for *B. canis* every 3 to 6 months, not just before breeding.

CLIENT EDUCATION

- Incurable, zoonotic disease
- Regular testing greatly decreases risk of introduction of *B. canis* into kennel and loss of breeding stock

SUGGESTED READING

Johnston SD, Root Kustritz MV, Olson PN: Canine brucellosis. In *Canine and Feline Theriogenology*. Philadelphia, WB Saunders, 2001, pp 88-91, 319-321.

Wanke MM: Canine brucellosis. *Anim Repro Sci* 82:195, 2004.

AUTHOR: **MARGARET V. ROOT KUSTRITZ**
EDITOR: **MICHELLE A. KUTZLER**

Budd-Chiari-Like Syndrome and Cor Triatriatum Dexter

BASIC INFORMATION

DEFINITION

Uncommon cardiovascular defects that partially obstruct the flow of blood into, or through, the right atrium

- Cor triatriatum dexter:
  - Congenital cardiac defect resulting from persistence of the embryologic right sinus venosus valve.
  - The result is a membranous division of the right atrium, which obstructs hepatic venous return to the heart.
  - Cranial vena caval flow is unaffected.
- Budd-Chiari syndrome:
  - Originally described as hepatic postsinusoidal hypertension secondary to inflammation and thrombosis of small hepatic veins.
    - Result: obstruction of venous return to the heart, resulting in ascites, hepatomegaly, and abdominal pain.
  - Currently, it is often used loosely to describe obstruction of venous return to the right heart caused by such diverse entities as cor triatriatum dexter, right atrial neoplasia, and caudal vena cava obstruction secondary to masses or traumatic kinking/fibrosis.
    - These disorders are more appropriately referred to as Budd-Chiari-like syndromes.

SYNONYM(S)

BCLS
CTD

EPIDEMIOLOGY

SPECIES, AGE, SEX

- Canine: most often in patients <2 years old; males more commonly affected than females
- Feline: no cases reported (see Cor Triatriatum Sinister and Supravalvular Mitral Stenosis, p 238)

CLINICAL PRESENTATION

DISEASE FORMS/SUBTYPES

- CTD: membrane can cause partial or complete division of right atrium. If the membrane is complete, then blood flowing into the caudal chamber must pass to the cranial chamber via a vascular connection with the azygous vein.
- Budd-Chiari-like syndrome: obstruction to venous flow may be acquired (e.g., caudal vena cava trauma and subsequent fibrosis) or congenital.

HISTORY, CHIEF COMPLAINT

- Lethargy
- Inappetence
- Severe abdominal distention

PHYSICAL EXAM FINDINGS

- Hepatomegaly
- Ascites
- Abdominal discomfort
- Distention of superficial abdominal vasculature
- Muscle wasting (cardiac cachexia)

ETIOLOGY AND PATHOPHYSIOLOGY

- Obstruction of venous return elevates intrahepatic pressure
- Increased pressure causes leakage of protein and fluid from the hepatic sinusoids, resulting in high protein ascites (modified transudate)

DIAGNOSIS

DIFFERENTIAL DIAGNOSIS

- Pericardial effusion
- Right atrial tumor
- Tricuspid dysplasia
- Cor pulmonale (pulmonary hypertension)
- Dilated cardiomyopathy (biventricular)
- Arrhythmogenic right ventricular cardiomyopathy

INITIAL DATABASE

- Ascites without jugular distention supports the diagnosis of CTD or BCLS over other causes of right heart failure signs.
  - Primary intra-abdominal causes of ascites (e.g., hemoabdomen, portal hypertension) are important differential diagnoses.
- Fluid analysis of the ascites indicates a modified transudate: high protein (>2.5 g/dl), relatively low nucleated cell count (usually <5000 cells/μl).
- Thoracic radiographs most often show normal cardiac silhouette and lung fields; enlargement of the caudal vena cava is expected if CTD or BCLS is causing ascites.
- Serum biochemistry panel will often show mild elevation in hepatic enzymes; complete blood count may show a stress leukogram; urinalysis is unremarkable.
- Electrocardiogram may show tall P waves consistent with right atrial enlargement.

ADVANCED OR CONFIRMATORY TESTING

- CTD: two-dimensional echocardiography will display a membrane dividing the right atrium. Doppler echocardiography will demonstrate blood flow through an opening in the membrane if the membrane is perforate.
- BCLS: two-dimensional echocardiography may reveal evidence of an obstruction or may be normal, necessitating other modalities.
- Abdominal ultrasound demonstrates ascites, hepatomegaly, distended hepatic veins, and the absence of a primary intra-abdominal cause for the ascites (e.g., mass).
- Angiography is an alternate imaging technique to define blood flow and to diagnose causes of BCLS other than CTD.

- Pressure measurements of the hepatic veins, caudal vena cava, and right atrium normally should be approximately equal (normal: 0-5 mmHg). A drop in elevated pressure measured from the liver to the right heart indicates an obstruction is present.

TREATMENT

THERAPEUTIC GOAL(S)

Alleviate clinical signs of right heart failure

ACUTE GENERAL TREATMENT

- Abdominocentesis will improve patient's comfort level (see Abdominocentesis, p 1178; Abdominal Drainage, p 1176).
- CTD has been successfully corrected with both surgery and balloon dilation.
- Budd-Chiari-like syndromes: surgery may be indicated, depending on the underlying cause.

CHRONIC TREATMENT

If definitive treatment is not possible, furosemide (1-4 mg/kg PO q 12h) and an angiotensin-converting enzyme inhibitor (e.g., enalapril 0.5 mg PO q 12-24h) should be administered along with periodic abdominocenteses to control fluid accumulation.

DRUG INTERACTIONS

Electrolyte depletion and dehydration may result from overzealous diuretic administration.

POSSIBLE COMPLICATIONS

- Surgery is highly invasive, and therefore the risk of mortality is increased with an inexperienced surgeon.
- Balloon dilation of CTS may not create a sufficient opening in the membrane to alleviate clinical signs.

RECOMMENDED MONITORING

- Ascites should resolve with successful reduction/removal of obstruction.
- Renal and hepatic function should be periodically monitored if medical therapy is chosen.

PROGNOSIS AND OUTCOME

- Excellent with successful reduction/removal of the obstruction.
- Medical management alone is unlikely to be satisfactory on a long-term basis if clinical signs (e.g., marked abdominal distention from ascites) are already present.

PEARLS & CONSIDERATIONS

COMMENTS

- Jugular distention is *not* present with CTS and other BCLS, unlike other cardiovascular diseases that cause signs of right heart failure.
- Diseases that result in signs of right heart failure are the most common causes of a modified transudate in the abdomen of dogs. Therefore, a modified transudate ascites should always prompt a cardiac work-up.

CLIENT EDUCATION

- Advise that surgery or balloon dilation offers the best chance for cure.
- Medical therapy is palliative but is unlikely to be satisfactory on a long-term basis.

SUGGESTED READING

Grooters AM, Smeak DD: Budd-Chiari-like syndromes in dogs. In Bonagura JD (ed): *Current Veterinary Therapy XII*. Philadelphia, WB Saunders, 1995, pp 876-879.

Johnson MS, et al: Management of cor triatriatum dexter by balloon dilatation in three dogs. *J Small Anim Pract* 45:16, 2004.

Mitten RW, et al: Diagnosis and management of cor triatriatum dexter in a Pyrenean mountain dog and an Akita Inu. *Aust Vet J* 79:177, 2001.

AUTHOR: **DEBORAH M. FINE**

EDITOR: **ETIENNE CÔTÉ**

Burns

BASIC INFORMATION

DEFINITION

- Burns are the injuries that result from exposure to flame, extreme heat, scalding, inhalation, or chemical or electrical trauma. Burns produce clinical syndromes ranging from self-limiting injury to devastating long-term incapacitation and potentially death.
- Eschar: a thick, coagulated crust or slough that develops as a result of a burn.
- Compartmentalization: a condition associated with third- and fourth-degree burns in which swelling within tissue compartments creates strictures that can decrease thoracic wall motion and ventilation, or ischemic injury to limbs.

EPIDEMIOLOGY

SPECIES, AGE, SEX

- Animals of any signalment are susceptible to burn injury.
- Debilitating conditions such as chronic renal disease or immunoincompetence carry increased risks for fatal complications.

CLINICAL PRESENTATION

DISEASE FORMS/SUBTYPES

- First-degree burns:
  - Superficial layers of dermis.
  - Typically red.
  - Typically dry and painful.
- Second-degree burns:
  - Superficial layers of dermis.
  - Typically red.
  - Typically wet and very painful.
- Third- and fourth-degree burns:
  - Superficial layers of dermis (third-degree) and subcutaneous layers, tendon, and bone (fourth-degree).
  - Typically waxy and leathery in appearance.
  - Typically less painful than first- or second-degree.
  - Third- and fourth-degree burns carry a greater risk of wound sepsis, coagulation disorders, limb ischemia, or compression severe enough to cause ventilatory compromise or abdominal problems.
- Electrical burns (see Electrocution, p 340):
  - High-voltage: associated with compartmental syndromes and ischemia.
  - Low-voltage: seldom associated with complication.
- Chemical or tar burns usually involve the superficial dermis layers.

HISTORY, CHIEF COMPLAINT

- History and chief complaint reflect acute trauma
- Recent anesthetic procedures should prompt suspicion of heating blanket or heating lamp burn
- With acts of malicious intent, history may be unknown

PHYSICAL EXAM FINDINGS

- Physical examination findings depend on the location and extent of the burn.
- Thermal burn resulting from a heating blanket or lamp will present as a defined injury reflective of the size of the blanket and the positioning of the animal during recumbency.
- Hypothermia may be present with serious burns.
- Animals with extensive burns may present in shock.
- The presence of singed whiskers or burn debris in the mouth is strongly suggestive of inhalation (see Smoke Inhalation, p 1011).
- Dyspnea or respiratory distress can occur rapidly from pharyngeal and laryngeal edema, progressive upper airway obstruction, pulmonary edema, inhalation of burn debris, or carbon monoxide toxicity.
- Corneal trauma.

ETIOLOGY AND PATHOPHYSIOLOGY

- Localized wound inflammation results in release of inflammatory mediators and capillary leakage, causing extravasation of fluid.
- If the syndrome of leaky capillaries occurs systemically, fluid losses may be severe and result in hypotension or cardiac collapse necessitating aggressive intravenous fluid resuscitation.
- Inhalation injury can result in upper airway obstruction secondary to pharyngeal and laryngeal mucosal injury, swelling, and increasing amounts sedation and exudative debris.
- Inhalation or aspiration of burn debris can result in direct lung injury.
- Inhalation traumatizes the clearance ability of the large airways, predisposing to aspiration pneumonia. Colonization of the respiratory system is initially by normal flora. Nosocomial infection may occur within 2 to 3 days of hospitalization.
- Extravasation of fluid into alveoli may result in noncardiogenic pulmonary edema, further as exacerbating inhalation lung injury.
- Carbon monoxide toxicity results in carboxyhemoglobinemia and hypoxemia.
- Large area burns are at high risk for infection.
- Third- and fourth-degree burns may result in compartmentalization (see Definition above).
- Generalized sepsis may result from wound infection, or nosocomial infection due to the presence of multiple invasive catheters or the development of pneumonia.
- Systemic inflammation may result in coagulopathy, including disseminated intravascular coagulopathy.

DIAGNOSIS

DIFFERENTIAL DIAGNOSIS

- Severe bacterial pyoderma
- Immune-mediated disease
- Fungal infection
- Abscess
- Aspiration pneumonia
- Sepsis

INITIAL DATABASE

- Complete blood count, including manual platelet count
- Serum biochemistry profile
- Urinalysis
- Coagulation panel, including prothrombin and partial thromboplastin times
- Survey radiographs, including thorax and limbs for fractures if lameness is present
- Appropriate cultures if evidence of pneumonia

ADVANCED OR CONFIRMATORY TESTING

- Wound culture if infected
- Brain computed tomography or magnetic resonance imaging if unexplained mental alteration

TREATMENT

THERAPEUTIC GOAL(S)

- Maintenance of mean arterial blood pressure and adequate urine production
- Maintenance of patent airway and oxygen saturation
- Maintenance of plasma oncotic pressure
- Wound management
- Prevention or limitation of complications, including pneumonia, sepsis, and coagulopathy

ACUTE GENERAL TREATMENT

- Intensive intravenous fluid resuscitation with crystalloids (e.g., 0.9% NaCl, lactated Ringer's solution, others—dictated by specifics of case) during the initial 8 to 12 hours of injury to maintain adequate mean arterial blood pressure and urine production at 1–2 ml/kg/h.
- Maintenance of airway patency in presence of pharyngeal or laryngeal edema, with early elective intubation if necessary.
- Early wound care: before surgical assessment, apply dry dressings to wounds. First- and second-degree burns may be self-limiting.
- Greasy or oil-based dressings (e.g., Vaseline-impregnated gauze) should be avoided.
- Third- and fourth-degree burns may require early escharotomy (debridement/burn excision) or fasciotomy to limit wound sepsis, stricture, or limb ischemia.
- In cases with concurrent smoke inhalation, supplemental oxygen provided within the first 12 hours of injury will help treat carboxyhemoglobinemia.
- Mechanical ventilation may be required to maintain oxygen saturation.
- Broad-spectrum antimicrobial coverage if evidence of pneumonia until culture results are available (e.g., ampicillin 22 mg/kg IV q 8h plus enrofloxacin 3 to 5 mg/kg IM or off-label use [diluted 1:1 in 0.9% sterile saline and given slowly IV] q 12–24h; maximum 5 mg/kg q 24h in cats).

CHRONIC TREATMENT

- First- and second-degree burn wounds may require little debridement. Application of antimicrobial topical creams such as silver sulfadiazine or 0.5% silver nitrate is recommended.
- Small eschars should be debrided for primary closure early in the course of wound care.
- Large eschars not amenable to primary closure should be debrided and treated with grafts. Open wound management presents a high potential for wound sepsis and is thus not advised if avoidable.
- Serious burns involving the limbs should be debrided to avoid limb ischemia and treated with variations of splinting to avoid contracture.
- Intravenous fluid therapy should be titrated to replace losses/correct dehydration, maintain arterial blood pressure, and sustain appropriate urine production.
- Systemic inflammation and leaky vessels may result in protein loss and severe hypoalbuminemia. Judicious use of synthetic colloids (Hetastarch at 20 ml/kg/24h) or concentrated human albumin infusion may be required to maintain colloid oncotic pressure and mean arterial blood pressure. Transfusion with fresh frozen plasma is recommended in cases of coagulopathy (see Transfusion Reactions, p 1098).
- Serum electrolytes should be monitored, especially with usage of topical medications that can cause excessive loss of water or sodium.
- In cases of severe inhalation injury, maintenance of long-term intubation or tracheostomy may be required until resolution of burn trauma and associated pharyngeal laryngeal, and airway edema.
- Lavage of the airway to help clear burn (carbon) debris and excessive secretions.
- Mechanical ventilation for management of direct lung injury from inhalation of carbon debris, aspiration pneumonia, or pulmonary edema.
- Nutrition.
- Physical therapy.

POSSIBLE COMPLICATIONS

- Wound infection
- Aspiration pneumonia
- Nosocomial infection
- Sepsis
- Limb ischemia from wound contracture
- Coagulopathy

RECOMMENDED MONITORING

- Mean arterial blood pressure
- Central venous pressure
- Quantification of urine production
- Oxygen saturation
- Complete blood count, serum biochemistry profile, coagulation tests

PROGNOSIS AND OUTCOME

- Outcome is generally good with first- and second-degree burns and more guarded with third- and fourth-degree burns
- Prognosis guarded to poor with inhalation injury
- Prognosis relies on response to fluid resuscitation in severe burn injury
- Prognosis improves with appropriate and successful wound management
- Prognosis worsens with development of complications, including nosocomial infection and sepsis

PEARLS & CONSIDERATIONS

COMMENTS

- The severity of burn injury is determined by depth of the burn, extension or size of the injury, and presence of inhalation injury.
- Third- and fourth-degree burns, and/or inhalation, are best treated in a tertiary care facility with 24-hour intensive care management and surgeons skilled in surgical burn management.
- Severe eschars causing constriction of ventilatory muscles or limb ischemia require early debridement, with primary would closure or grafting, to limit wound infection and reduce the risk of compartmentalization.
- Large burns resulting in marked protein loss may be best treated with fresh frozen plasma transfusion to replenish proteins for tissue repair, oncotic support, coagulation factors, and acute phase proteins.
- Respiratory distress in a patient with evidence of inhalation (e.g., burned whiskers) may be due to pharyngeal or laryngeal edema and warrants intubation to obtain and maintain airway patency.
- Iatrogenic thermal burns as a complication from heating pads or lamps during anesthetic procedures may be the most common type of burn injury not resulting in death.
- Burn injury resulting in death occurs most commonly from house fires or malicious acts.

SUGGESTED READING

Sheridan RL: Burns. *Crit Care Med* 30[Suppl]: S500–S514, 2002.

AUTHOR: **THERESE E. O'TOOLE**
EDITOR: **ELIZABETH ROZANSKI**

Cachexia, Cancer-Associated

BASIC INFORMATION

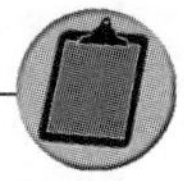

DEFINITION

The term *cancer cachexia* refers to weight loss in an animal or person with underlying neoplastic disease. Classic defining features of the syndrome include severe involuntary weight loss, fatigue, anemia, and progressive depletion of both lean body mass and adipose stores.

SYNONYM(S)

Cancer-associated weight loss

EPIDEMIOLOGY

SPECIES, AGE, SEX: Cancer cachexia has been reported in association with neoplastic disease in many species including people, cats, and dogs with naturally occurring malignancies, as well as laboratory rodents bearing implanted tumors. Animals of any age and either sex may be affected.

RISK FACTORS

- Advanced clinical stage of neoplastic disease.
- Tumors of the upper gastrointestinal tract (esophagus, stomach, and pancreas) in humans.
- Lower risk in people with treatment-responsive lymphomas, soft tissue sarcomas, and breast cancer.
- Cancer cachexia appears to be less common in cats and dogs than in people.

ASSOCIATED CONDITIONS AND DISORDERS: Cancer cachexia is a form of protein-energy malnutrition. Protein-energy malnutrition is the most common form of malnutrition found in critically ill animals and people and occurs when protein and energy intake is insufficient to meet requirements. Protein-energy malnutrition is associated with hypoproteinemia; delayed wound healing; immunosuppression; and compromised gastrointestinal, pulmonary, and cardiovascular function. Multiorgan failure and death will be the eventual outcome unless nutritional support is provided and the primary underlying disease process is resolved.

CLINICAL PRESENTATION

HISTORY, CHIEF COMPLAINT: Although weight loss is the primary abnormality in all cats and dogs with cancer cachexia, specific historic findings differ substantially from animal to animal. Weight loss may be mild to profound in severity, and ranges from acute to chronic in duration. Weight loss is also superimposed on any clinical signs associated with the underlying neoplastic disease, which vary with the specific diagnosis.

PHYSICAL EXAM FINDINGS: Physical exam findings in animals with cancer cachexia can be divided into two groups: abnormalities related to cancer cachexia, and abnormalities caused by the animal's underlying cancer. The clinical signs associated with cancer cachexia are nonspecific, initially may be subtle, and can easily be overlooked. Findings may include muscle wasting, pallor, weakness, poor haircoat, hepatomegaly, splenomegaly, evidence of chronic infections, and lymphadenopathy. Peripheral edema could be present in severe cases. Physical exam findings related to the underlying malignancy are highly variable and depend on the animal's specific histopathologic diagnosis and stage of disease. No two animals with cancer cachexia have exactly the same presentation.

ETIOLOGY AND PATHOPHYSIOLOGY

- The etiology of cancer cachexia is highly variable and multifactorial.
- There are two major categories of cancer cachexia: primary and secondary.
- Primary cancer cachexia is an incompletely understood paraneoplastic syndrome in which tumor-related changes in host metabolism lead to inefficient use of consumed calories, in turn leading to gradual depletion of lean body mass and adipose stores. No matter how

many calories are fed or by what route, host requirements cannot be met.

- Recent studies suggest that primary cancer cachexia may be an inflammatory disorder caused by alterations in proinflammatory mediators such as interleukin-1α (IL-1α), IL-1β, IL-6, tumor necrosis factor-α (TNF-α), and various eicosanoids.
- Secondary cancer cachexia is caused by one or more of a variety of functional abnormalities that decrease nutrient intake, digestion, or absorption. Examples include the physical presence of tumor within the digestive tract causing gastrointestinal dysfunction, or side effects of radiotherapy or chemotherapy such as stomatitis, vomiting, and gastroenteritis.

DIAGNOSIS

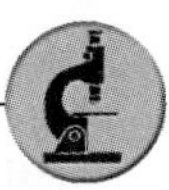

DIFFERENTIAL DIAGNOSIS

Differential diagnoses for weight loss in a cat or dog with cancer:

- Primary cancer cachexia (paraneoplastic abnormalities in energy metabolism)
- Secondary cancer cachexia:
  - Tumor involving the intestinal tract
  - Paraneoplastic syndromes other than cancer cachexia:
    - Hypercalcemia
    - Pyrexia
  - Treatment-related toxicity:
    - Altered taste and smell perception
    - Learned food aversions
    - Stomatitis/mucositis
    - Gastroenteritis
    - Centrally mediated nausea and vomiting
- Concurrent disease:
  - Infection:
    - Bacterial, viral, fungal, oomycotic, or rickettsial
  - Organ dysfunction/failure (i.e., liver, kidney, lung)
  - Diabetes mellitus
  - Hyperthyroidism (cats)
- Inappropriate nutritional management (unsuitable diet, inadequate caloric intake)

INITIAL DATABASE

- Diet history (specific ration fed and quantity consumed, plus all treats, supplements, and medications)
- Body weight and body condition score
- Complete blood count
- Serum biochemical profile
- Urinalysis
- Chest and abdominal radiographs
- Retroviral screening (cats)
- Serum thyroxine concentration (cats)

ADVANCED OR CONFIRMATORY TESTING

- Thoracic and abdominal ultrasonography
- Cross-sectional imaging (computed tomography, magnetic resonance imaging)
- Endoscopy
- Urine culture and sensitivity
- Fine-needle aspiration cytology, impression smears, or tissue biopsy to confirm the presence or absence of neoplastic cells, organisms, or other abnormalities in suspected lesions

TREATMENT

THERAPEUTIC GOAL(S)

The basic goals of therapy in the cat or dog suffering from cancer cachexia are twofold:

- Return the animal to ideal body condition
- Maintain the animal in ideal body condition long term

ACUTE GENERAL TREATMENT

- Cancer cachexia is a paraneoplastic syndrome, so eradication of the underlying neoplastic disease is the best treatment. This goal can be met by:
  - Obtaining a rapid and accurate definitive diagnosis of neoplasia, including neoplasm type and clinical stage.
  - Initiating timely and effective antineoplastic therapy.
- An individualized feeding protocol is instituted concurrently and is based on the animal's nutritional assessment, as defined by the minimum database outlined previously. Components of this feeding protocol must include:
  - Fluid requirement in milliliters per day.
  - Energy requirement in kilocalories per day.
  - A choice of commercial ration that meets the animal's needs:
    - Calories appropriately distributed among protein, fat, and carbohydrate
    - All necessary nutrients (i.e., vitamins and minerals) present in correct quantities and ratios
  - A method of feeding that will be tolerated by the animal.
- No single diet is appropriate for every animal with cancer cachexia, because underlying disease, nutritional status, and nutrient requirements are highly variable from case to case.
  - Rations with ample protein and fat are often recommended for weight-losing cats and dogs with cancer.
  - Individual restriction of protein, fat, or carbohydrate intake may be indicated depending on preexisting or concurrent conditions such as renal or hepatic insufficiency, pancreatitis, or diabetes mellitus.
- Voluntary intake is the most practical feeding technique, but quantities of food and water consumed must be measured to ensure that requirements are actually met.
- Assisted feeding should be instituted without delay in animals unable to meet their own nutrient requirements.
- Assisted enteral feeding using some type of feeding tube is usually preferred, because it allows nutrients to be metabolized through normal pathways and is more effective in maintaining gut health.
- Fluid deficits and electrolyte or acid-base imbalances should be corrected before any type of assisted feeding is attempted.

CHRONIC TREATMENT

Nutritional recommendations are adjusted as necessary based on repeat nutritional assessment, with the goal of maintaining ideal body condition:

- Food intake is increased or decreased as needed in response to changes in body weight and condition.
- Assisted feeding can be used intermittently to maintain nutrient intake.
- The specific ration recommended for an individual animal may change depending on the progression of the underlying neoplastic disease and concurrent conditions.

POSSIBLE COMPLICATIONS

- Gastrointestinal intolerance
- Refeeding Syndrome, see p 948

RECOMMENDED MONITORING

- Nutritional assessment, including diet history, body weight, and body condition score, needs to be repeated at regular intervals.
- Diagnostics are repeated as indicated based on underlying neoplastic disease and nutritional status; this commonly includes complete blood count, serum biochemical profile, urinalysis, and imaging studies.

PROGNOSIS AND OUTCOME

- Cancer cachexia has a well-documented negative effect on quality of life and prognosis in people, and its impact is highly likely to be the same in cats and dogs.
- Increased incidence and severity of treatment-related toxicities, lower treatment response rates, shorter remission durations, and shorter survival times should be expected in weight-losing animals when compared to weight-stable animals with the same tumor.

PEARLS & CONSIDERATIONS

COMMENTS

Recent work suggests that many dogs with cancer are actually obese. Indiscriminate use of high-fat diets in these animals will simply promote additional weight gain and its associated health problems. The primary goal of nutritional therapy in any cat or dog with cancer is always to maintain ideal body weight and condition.

SUGGESTED READING

Mauldin GE, Davidson JR: Nutritional support of hospitalized cats and dogs. In Slatter D (ed): *Textbook of Small Animal Surgery,* ed 3. Philadelphia, WB Saunders, 2003, pp 87–113.

Michel KE, Sorenmo K, Shofer FS: Evaluation of body condition and weight loss in dogs presented to a veterinary oncology service. *J Vet Intern Med* 18:692, 2004.

Ogilvie GK, et al: Effect of fish oil, arginine, and doxorubicin chemotherapy on remission and survival time for dogs with lymphoma: A double-blind, randomized placebo-controlled study. *Cancer* 88:1916, 2000.

Strasser F, Bruera ED: Update on anorexia and cachexia. *Hematol Oncol Clin North Am* 16:589, 2002.

AUTHOR: **GLENNA E. MAULDIN**

EDITOR: **KENNETH M. RASSNICK**

Cachexia, Cardiac

BASIC INFORMATION

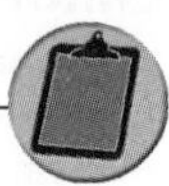

DEFINITION

Weight and lean tissue loss associated with congestive heart failure (CHF)

EPIDEMIOLOGY

SPECIES, AGE, SEX: More common in dogs than in cats.

RISK FACTORS: More common in right-sided or biventricular than in isolated left-sided CHF but can occur regardless of underlying cause.

ASSOCIATED CONDITIONS AND DISORDERS: Occurs secondary to CHF.

CLINICAL PRESENTATION

DISEASE FORMS/SUBTYPES: Variable severity, not necessarily restricted to emaciated, end-stage patients.

HISTORY, CHIEF COMPLAINT: Heart failure (see Heart Failure, Acute/Decompensated, p 458; Heart Failure, Chronic, p 459).

PHYSICAL EXAM FINDINGS

- Loss of lean body mass first noted in epaxial, gluteal, scapular, or temporal muscles; may be subtle initially
- Palpate obese animals and animals with ascites or subcutaneous edema carefully to determine whether muscle loss is present

ETIOLOGY AND PATHOPHYSIOLOGY

- Cardiac cachexia reduces strength, immune function, and survival.
- Decreased food intake, increased energy requirements, and production of the inflammatory cytokines tumor necrosis factor (TNF) and interleukin-1 (IL-1).
  - TNF and IL-1 cause anorexia, increased energy requirements, catabolism of lean body mass, myocardial fibrosis, and decreased cardiac contractility (negative inotropy).

DIAGNOSIS

DIFFERENTIAL DIAGNOSIS

Cachexia from other diseases (e.g., cancer, renal failure)

INITIAL DATABASE

- Diet history, including specific types and amounts of food eaten, dietary supplements, treats, and foods used for administering medications
- Evaluation for potential causes of anorexia (e.g., worsening CHF; medication side effects such as azotemia, hyperkalemia, or hypotension; unpalatable diet)

TREATMENT

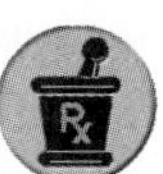

THERAPEUTIC GOAL(S)

- Optimally manage CHF
- Minimize anorexia (see Chronic Treatment below)
- Reduce energy requirements
- Ensure adequate protein intake
- Modulate cytokine production

ACUTE GENERAL TREATMENT

- In acute CHF episodes, avoid diet changes until the patient is home and stabilized on medications.
- Introduce new diet gradually when patient is stabilized, to avoid food aversions.

CHRONIC TREATMENT

- Ensure optimal therapy for CHF (See Heart Failure, Chronic, p 459)
- Minimize anorexia:
  - Reduced sodium diet palatable to individual patient may require diet changes (e.g., dry to canned, or different brand or flavor).
  - Balanced homemade diet formulated by veterinary nutritionist.
  - Smaller, more frequent meals.
  - Palatability enhancers (cooked meat, low-sodium broth).
  - Fish oil supplementation (see "Modulate cytokine production" below).
- Reduce energy requirements:
  - Optimal management of CHF.
  - Exercise restriction.
- Ensure adequate protein intake:
  - Avoid protein-restricted diets (e.g., "renal" diets).
- Modulate cytokine production:
  - Administer one 1-gram fish oil capsule (containing 180 mg eicosapentaenoic acid and 120 mg dehydroepiandrosterone) per 10 pounds body weight per day.
  - Fish oil should contain vitamin E as an antioxidant, but no other nutrients.
  - Cod liver oil and flax seed oil should not be used.

DRUG INTERACTIONS

Medication side effects can contribute to cachexia by causing anorexia (e.g., digoxin toxicity, azotemia secondary to angiotensin-converting enzyme inhibitor, or overzealous diuretic use).

RECOMMENDED MONITORING

- Body weight (be sure to adjust for ascites) and assessment of muscle loss
- Appetite and food intake

PROGNOSIS AND OUTCOME

Prognosis depends on the underlying cardiac disease. However, anorexia is a common contributing factor to an owner's decision for euthanasia.

PEARLS & CONSIDERATIONS

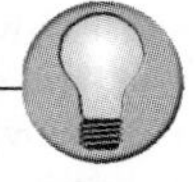

COMMENTS

- Animals with CHF often have variable and cyclical appetites. Reassure owners that this is common and that they can offer favorite foods when this occurs. However, anorexia longer than 24 to 48 hours should trigger reevaluation of CHF and medications.

- Centesis should be performed on anorectic animals with a significant ascites or pleural effusion to reduce fluid accumulation (for comfort).
- Animals with CHF may prefer foods at a particular temperature (e.g., room temperature, warmed, refrigerated).
- Dogs with CHF often prefer sweet tastes, particularly as the disease progresses. Adding items such as maple syrup, fruit-flavored yogurt, or applesauce to the dog's food may improve food intake.

PREVENTION

- None known
- Early detection in more subtle stages
- Minimize by ensuring adequate food intake and optimal therapy for CHF

CLIENT EDUCATION

- Sodium intake:
  - Provide owner specific instructions regarding foods high in sodium, appropriate dog foods, acceptable low-salt treats, and methods for administering medications
- Appetite:
  - Provide the owner with suggestions for improving the animal's appetite (see Chronic Treatment above)

SUGGESTED READING

Freeman L, Roubenoff R: Nutrition implications of cardiac cachexia. *Nutr Rev* 52:340–347, 1994.

Freeman LM, et al: Nutritional alterations and the effect of fish oil supplementation in dogs with heart failure. *J Vet Intern Med* 12:440–448, 1998.

Freeman LM, et al: Evaluation of dietary patterns in dogs with cardiac disease. *J Am Vet Med Assoc* 223:1301–1305, 2003.

Freeman LM, Rush JE, Farabaugh AE, Must A: Assessment of health-related quality of life in dogs with cardiac disease. *J Am Vet Med Assoc* 226:1864–1868, 2005.

Freeman LM, Rush JE: Nutritional management of cardiac disease. In Ettinger SJ, Feldman EC (eds): *Textbook of Veterinary Internal Medicine*, ed 6. St. Louis, Elsevier, 2005, pp 579–563.

Mallery KF, Freeman LM, Harpster NK, Rush JE: Factors contributing to the decision for euthanasia of dogs with congestive heart failure. *J Am Vet Med Assoc* 214:1201–1204, 1999.

AUTHOR: **LISA M. FREEMAN**

EDITOR: **C. A. TONY BUFFINGTON**

Calcinosis Cutis and Calcinosis Circumscripta

BASIC INFORMATION

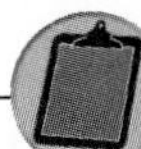

DEFINITION

- Calcinosis cutis is uncommon and characterized by inappropriate deposition of calcium within the skin. Calcinosis cutis typically denotes a specific form of dystrophic calcification associated with spontaneous or iatrogenic hyperadrenocorticism.
- Calcinosis circumscripta is a localized nodular deposition of calcium in subcutaneous tissue or in other areas such as the tongue, tendons, and ligaments.

SYNONYM(S)

Calcium gout
Tumoral calcinosis

EPIDEMIOLOGY

SPECIES, AGE, SEX

- Calcinosis cutis develops as a result of another underlying disorder in dogs, most commonly spontaneous or iatrogenic hyperadrenocorticism.
- Calcinosis circumscripta is an uncommon disorder found in dogs less than 2 years old. It is rare in cats.

GENETICS AND BREED PREDISPOSITION: Calcinosis circumscripta is typically found in large-breed dogs, with German shepherds being predisposed.

RISK FACTORS

- Increased risk of calcinosis cutis with chronic administration of exogenous corticosteroids.
- Calcinosis circumscripta lesions develop at sites of repetitive trauma.

ASSOCIATED CONDITIONS AND DISORDERS

- Calcinosis cutis: hypertrophic osteodystrophy and idiopathic polyarthritis
- Calcinosis circumscripta: hypervitaminosis D, primary hyperparathyroidism, nutritional hypercalcemia

CLINICAL PRESENTATION

DISEASE FORMS/SUBTYPES

- Calcinosis cutis is classified as dystrophic, metastatic, or iatrogenic.
- *Dystrophic calcification* is either localized or generalized. Localized dystrophic calcification occurs as a result of tissue abnormalities or injury. Generalized dystrophic calcification in dogs most commonly occurs with spontaneous or iatrogenic hyperadrenocorticism.
- *Metastatic calcification* is the result of an underlying defect in calcium or phosphorus metabolism (e.g., hypercalcemia of malignancy, of primary hyperparathyroidism, or of vitamin D rodenticide toxicosis). Canine metastatic calcification restricted to the footpads is associated with chronic renal failure.
- *Iatrogenic calcinosis cutis* occurs secondary to percutaneous absorption or penetration of calcium-containing products (e.g., calcium chloride).

HISTORY, CHIEF COMPLAINT

- Dogs affected with calcinosis cutis may present for evaluation of erythematous papules or plaques with gritty surfaces with or without concurrent pruritus. Alternatively, in many cases, the dominant clinical signs relate to the underlying disorder (e.g., hyperadrenocorticism).
- In calcinosis circumscripta, dogs present with a solitary mass over bony prominences or in the oral cavity, particularly the tongue.

PHYSICAL EXAM FINDINGS

- Calcinosis cutis lesions may be found anywhere on the body but typically develop along the dorsum of the trunk, inguinal region, and axillae. Early lesions are erythematous papules that coalesce to form firm, gritty plaques. A chalky white to pink material can be seen through intact epidermis of early nonulcerated lesions. Ulceration and crusting occur during transepidermal elimination of mineralized debris. Lesions can be quite pruritic, leading to extreme self-trauma.
- Calcinosis circumscripta is usually a solitary lesion but multiple masses are possible. The lesion is a firm, haired to alopecic, well-circumscribed, subcutaneous or deep dermal mass that may ulcerate and discharge a chalky or gritty substance. Nodules vary tremendously in size.

ETIOLOGY AND PATHOPHYSIOLOGY

- The exact mechanism of mineral deposition in calcinosis cutis and calcinosis circumscripta is unknown. The pathogenesis probably involves abnormally high mitochondrial calcium phosphate

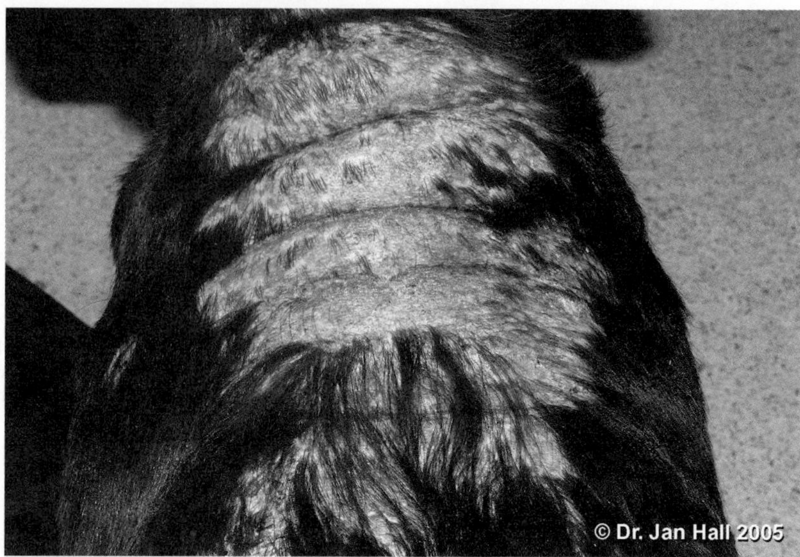

FIGURE I-33 Calcinosis cutis affecting the dorsal neck of a 2-year-old female spayed Labrador retriever with iatrogenic hyperadrenocorticism secondary to antipruritic therapy for canine atopy. Courtesy of Dr. Jan A. Hall.

levels, resulting in crystal formation and cell death.
- Calcium salts are deposited along collagen and elastin fibers.

DIAGNOSIS

DIFFERENTIAL DIAGNOSIS

- Calcinosis cutis: bacterial pyoderma, deep fungal infection, demodicosis, neoplasia
- Calcinosis circumscripta: neoplasia, foreign body

INITIAL DATABASE

- Cytologic evaluation of exudates: amorphorous gritty material.
- Skin scrapings: a gritty consistency will be noted when smearing the sample on a microscope slide.
- Routine hematologic and biochemical profile: Changes associated with hypercortisolism are usually noted in spontaneous and iatrogenic hyperadrenocorticism cases. Calcium and phosphorus levels are usually normal, except in cases of metastatic calcification.

ADVANCED OR CONFIRMATORY TESTING

- Histopathologic study: multifocal accumulations of finely or coarsely granular amorphous basophilic debris in deep dermal or subcutaneous tissue encompassed by granulomatous inflammation
- Radiographs:
  - Calcinosis cutis: occasionally, may be noted as small, sheetlike regions of mineralization in the subcutis or skin
  - Calcinosis circumscripta: conglomerated calcified mass in skin or subcutis

TREATMENT

THERAPEUTIC GOAL(S)

- Control or eliminate underlying disease process if present
- Surgical excision curative for solitary lesion of calcinosis circumscripta

ACUTE GENERAL TREATMENT

Pruritus control: Because corticosteroid use should be limited or avoided in patients with hyperadrenocorticism, antihistamines such as hydroxyzine 2.2 mg/kg PO q 8-12h or diphenhydramine 2.2 mg/kg PO q 8-12h in combination with oral omega-3 essential fatty acids may be used for managing pruritus.

CHRONIC TREATMENT

- Topical dimethyl sulfoxide may be useful to dissolve the calcium. Apply to no more than one third of the body at one time. If lesions are extensive, serum calcium levels should be monitored at the same time.
- Antibiotics to control secondary pyoderma associated with widespread calcinosis cutis (e.g., cephalexin 22-30 mg/kg PO q 8-12h for 21 to 30 days or amoxicillin-clavulanate 12.5 mg/kg PO q 12h for 21 to 30 days).
- Hydrotherapy and frequent bathing with antibacterial shampoo.

DRUG INTERACTIONS

Avoid systemic or topical corticosteroid use in patients with calcinosis cutis associated with spontaneous or iatrogenic hyperadrenocorticism

PROGNOSIS AND OUTCOME

- Subclinical lesions of calcinosis cutis may slowly regress spontaneously without treatment over weeks to months, providing that the underlying hyperadrenocorticism is handled.
- Recurrence of calcinosis circumscripta lesions postsurgical excision does not occur.

PEARLS & CONSIDERATIONS

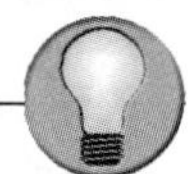

COMMENTS

In patients with iatrogenic calcinosis cutis associated with excessive glucocorticoid administration, lesions may progress and increase in size for approximately 30 to 90 days after discontinuing the glucocorticoid use.

SUGGESTED READING

Scott DW, Miller WH Jr, Griffin CE (eds): *Mueller & Kirk's Small Animal Dermatology*. Philadelphia, WB Saunders, 2001, pp 1398-1401.

AUTHOR: **JOCELYN WELLINGTON**
EDITOR: **JAN A. HALL**

Calicivirus, Cat

BASIC INFORMATION

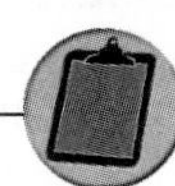

DEFINITION

Common viral disease in domestic and some exotic cats characterized by upper respiratory signs, oral ulceration, and less commonly arthritis

SYNONYM(S)

Upper respiratory infection (calicivirus is one possible etiology)
Limping kitten syndrome
Older literature: classification as picornavirus
Virulent systemic feline calicivirus (FCV) is also known as *hemorrhagic fever-like FCV*.

EPIDEMIOLOGY

SPECIES, AGE, SEX

- All domestic cats, and some exotic feline species, are susceptible.
- All ages affected, but susceptibility for typical infection is highest in kittens.
  - However, adults are more likely to experience the virulent systemic form of infection.
- No gender predilection.

RISK FACTORS

- Multiple-cat environments
- Crowding
- Stress
- Poor husbandry
- Coinfection with other respiratory pathogens worsens disease

CONTAGION AND ZOONOSIS: FCV is a highly contagious disease of cats. No zoonotic implications are known.

GEOGRAPHY AND SEASONALITY: Worldwide with no seasonality.

ASSOCIATED CONDITIONS AND DISORDERS

- Lymphocytic-plasmacytic stomatitis and gingivitis linked to chronic carriers
- Frequent coinfection with other upper respiratory pathogens

CLINICAL PRESENTATION

DISEASE FORMS/SUBTYPES

- Pneumotropic isolates affect primarily the upper, and uncommonly the lower, respiratory tract.
- Rheumatic isolates cause joint pain and lameness in naturally infected kittens.
  - Also reported after administration of modified-live calicivirus vaccine.
- Virulent systemic form recently identified that causes more severe clinical signs in adults.
  - Vaccinated cats can be affected.

HISTORY, CHIEF COMPLAINT

- Malaise: lethargy, listlessness
- Inappetence/anorexia
- Ocular signs (see Physical Exam Findings below)
- Sneezing
- Nasal discharge (serous or purulent)
- Drooling
- Reluctance to walk, lameness

PHYSICAL EXAM FINDINGS

- Conjunctivitis: diffuse, bilateral
- Epiphora
- Blepharospasm
- Chemosis: may be dramatic; entire globe may become hidden behind swollen conjunctiva
- Oculonasal discharge (serous or purulent)
- Fever
- Vesicles or erosions on tongue, palate, nasal planum:
  - Visible during routine examination of mouth
  - Characteristic of calicivirus, in contrast to other upper respiratory tract-related etiologies (e.g., chlamydiosis or feline viral rhinotracheitis/herpesvirus infection)
  - May cause drooling
- Dehydration
- Cough is uncommon
- Rheumatic form:
  - Fever; temperature often >104° F (>40° C)
  - Joint swelling
  - Pain
  - Myalgia
  - Oral ulcers possible
  - Kitten/cat may eat well but be reluctant to walk
- Virulent systemic form:
  - Fever
  - Facial and limb edema that may progress to necrosis
  - Upper respiratory signs
  - Pancreatitis with icterus
  - Dyspnea
  - Epistaxis and/or hematochezia
  - Ulcerations in mouth, face, muzzle, pinna, and extremities
  - Pneumonia
  - Pericarditis
  - Death

ETIOLOGY AND PATHOPHYSIOLOGY

- Infection with FCV, an RNA virus with multiple subtypes of varying degrees of virulence and cross-reactivity, is acquired predominantly via ingestion.
  - Spread by aerosol route less likely
- Replication occurs in oropharyngeal tissues with spread primarily to epithelium of conjunctiva, nose, and oral cavity, including the tongue and palate.
  - Rapid cytolysis of infected cells ensues
  - In the virulent systemic form, signs result from vasculitis and development of disseminated intravascular coagulation/systemic inflammatory response syndrome

DIAGNOSIS

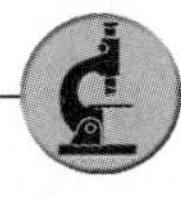

DIFFERENTIAL DIAGNOSIS

- Feline herpesvirus 1:
  - Cough and keratitis more likely with feline herpesvirus infection
  - Oral ulceration less likely with feline herpesvirus infection
- Chlamydiosis
- Mycoplasmosis
- Bordetellosis
- Corneal injury/trauma

INITIAL DATABASE

- Fluorescein staining of corneas to rule out corneal ulcers/injury
- Feline leukemia/feline immunodeficiency virus tests to rule out underlying immune compromise
- No characteristic findings on complete blood count, biochemical profiles, or urinalysis

ADVANCED OR CONFIRMATORY TESTING

- Viral culture
- Viral identification usually not warranted except in cases of virulent systemic calicivirus infection

TREATMENT

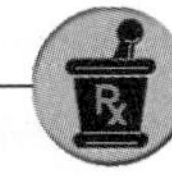

THERAPEUTIC GOAL(S)

- Maintain hydration and nutrition
- Pain relief for ulcers, joint/muscle pain
- Control secondary bacterial infection

ACUTE GENERAL TREATMENT

- Fluids to maintain hydration.
- Syringe feeding if anorexic.
- Erythromycin ophthalmic ointment to combat potential secondary *Chlamydia* or *Mycoplasma* infections.
- Buprenorphine (0.01-0.03 mg/kg q 8-12h IM, IV, PO) may be considered for analgesia.
- α-Interferon may inhibit replication.

CHRONIC TREATMENT

- Recrudescence of clinical disease is uncommon.
- Cats may be susceptible to infection with new subtypes.

POSSIBLE COMPLICATIONS

- Interstitial viral pneumonia and/or secondary bacterial pneumonia can be life-threatening complications.
- Oral ulcers and arthritis usually resolve without complication.
- Sudden dyspnea may occur if pneumonia develops.

RECOMMENDED MONITORING

Clinical signs

PROGNOSIS AND OUTCOME

- Prognosis is good for recovery from typical calicivirus infection with supportive care.
- By contrast, a mortality rate of 40% is reported for the virulent systemic form.

PEARLS & CONSIDERATIONS

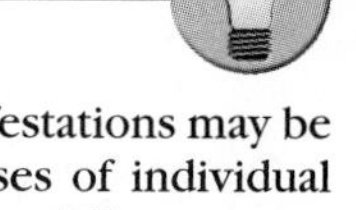

COMMENTS

- Different disease manifestations may be due to unique responses of individual cats to virus rather than different virus subtypes.
- Recovered cats remain lifelong carriers. Virus is shed continuously from oral cavity regardless of health status or stress.
- Properly vaccinated cats may become infected with different subtypes.

PREVENTION

- Proper husbandry to prevent cat-to-cat contact and cross-contamination during cleaning and feeding procedures.
- FCV is stable and resistant to many disinfectants, except bleach (sodium hypochlorite) diluted 1 part bleach:32 parts tap water.
- Proper vaccination at 8 to 10 weeks, after 12 weeks of age, 1 year later, and every 3 years afterward.

CLIENT EDUCATION

- Emphasize proper vaccination
- In catteries, consider immunizing kittens from carrier queen as early as 6 weeks of age

SUGGESTED READING

Hurley KF, et al: An outbreak of virulent systemic calicivirus disease. *J Am Vet Med Assoc* 224:241, 2004.

Pesavento PA, et al: Pathologic, immunohistochemical, and electron microscopic findings in naturally occurring virulent systemic feline calicivirus infection in cats. *Vet Pathol* 41:257, 2004.

AUTHOR: **CHRISTINE L. WILFORD**
EDITOR: **RANCE K. SELLON**

Callus/Hygroma/Pressure Sores

BASIC INFORMATION

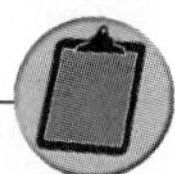

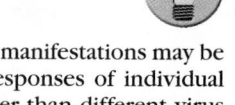

DEFINITION

- Callus: a thickened alopecic area of skin over a pressure point
- Hygroma: a subcutaneous bursa that develops over a pressure point
- Pressure sore: an area of tissue damage or necrosis concentrated over a bony prominence resulting from prolonged application of pressure

SYNONYM(S)

Decubital ulcer (pressure sores)

EPIDEMIOLOGY

SPECIES, AGE, SEX: Any patient can develop a callus, hygroma, or pressure sores.
GENETICS AND BREED PREDISPOSITION: Large- or giant-breed dogs because of their size and weight are disproportionately more commonly affected.
RISK FACTORS

- Immunosuppressed individuals may be more prone to secondary focal pyoderma of pressure point lesions.
- Animals that are weak or emaciated, as well as those that are recumbent for long periods on hard surfaces, are at a high risk for developing pressure sores.

CLINICAL PRESENTATION

HISTORY, CHIEF COMPLAINT

- Often have a history of prolonged recumbency, or sleeping on hard surfaces such as wood, cement, or brick
- Owner may notice progressive lesions over bony prominences. Some owners may not notice sores until they break open, or see the patient further aggravating the lesions by licking them

PHYSICAL EXAM FINDINGS

- A callus initially appears as a thickened, hyperkeratotic, lichenified, and alopecic area of skin over a bony prominence, commonly affecting the elbows, hocks, and sternum.
- A hygroma produces a subcutaneous fluid sac over the pressure point (e.g., elbows).
- The severity of pressure sores is variable:
    - They can be erythematous to purple in color, with a serous, sanguineous, or purulent discharge.
    - Ulcers and fistulae may be noted, depending on severity and progression of the lesion.

ETIOLOGY AND PATHOPHYSIOLOGY

- A callus is caused by trauma over bony prominences.
- A hygroma may develop as an acquired bursa over a pressure point as a reaction to pressure.
- Pathogenic bacteria may invade a fissure in a callus leading to secondary infection.
- Prolonged pressure compresses capillary circulation, causing tissue damage or necrosis, producing a pressure sore:
    - Grade I lesions affect the epidermis and superficial epidermis.
    - Grade II lesions extend to the subcutis. Within 24 to 48 hours, the ulcer edges become undermined.
    - Grade III lesions extend to the deep fascia.
    - Grade IV lesions involve the underlying bone.

DIAGNOSIS

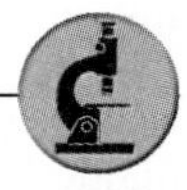

DIFFERENTIAL DIAGNOSIS

- Ulcerated soft tissue tumor
- Infected/necrotic wound as a result of trauma

INITIAL DATABASE

- A thorough history and physical exam are most important.
    - Diagnosis is generally based on physical location of the lesion(s) over pressure points, typical appearance (see Clinical Presentation above), and owner's description of the environment and surfaces on which the dog lies
- Radiographs of the affected area may help to ascertain bony involvement (uncommon).

ADVANCED OR CONFIRMATORY TESTING

Histopathologic evaluation of biopsies can be used for distinguishing a pressure sore from an ulcerated/necrotic tumor

TREATMENT

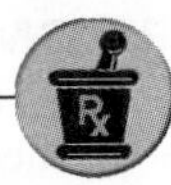

THERAPEUTIC GOAL(S)

- Providing a soft, padded environment may be all that is required to decrease the size of callus lesions and prevent progression.
- Resolving pressure sores and preventing new lesions depend on providing an optimum environment for healing by treating infection and encouraging blood supply to the area.

ACUTE GENERAL TREATMENT

- Pressure sores should be cleaned daily with an antiseptic solution such as chlorhexidene diluted to 0.05%.
  - With standard 4% chlorhexidine solution, dilute 1 part chlorhexidine to 80 parts water to obtain 0.05% concentration.
  - For example, 12 ml 4% chlorhexidine solution (approximately 1/3 to 1/2 fluid oz) in 1 L water.
- Various treatments have been suggested to accelerate healing of pressure sores, including wound-healing creams, raw honey, or a topical antibiotic, mupirocin.
- Although systemic antibiotics are not said to penetrate well due to the area of capillary and venous congestion at the base and tissue margins of the pressure sore, coverage is prudent.
  - Cephalexin 30 mg/kg PO q 12h for 30 days may be beneficial.
- Grade II-IV pressure sores often require surgical debridement and closure, but not until the patient is ambulatory. Otherwise, the wound may dehisce.
- Physical barriers such as Elizabethan collars may help to deter self-trauma to pressure point lesions.

POSSIBLE COMPLICATIONS

- Wound dehiscence after surgery
- Slow healing

PROGNOSIS AND OUTCOME

- Callus lesions can be controlled by attention to home environment and bedding.
- Since the severity of pressure sores varies, severe lesions are accordingly more difficult to manage.
- If the patient recovers from the underlying disease/reason for recumbency quickly, the pressure sore should heal spontaneously, but often slowly.

PEARLS & CONSIDERATIONS

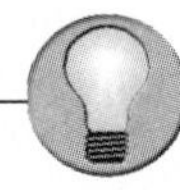

COMMENTS

Prevention of pressure sores is of utmost importance, because they can be difficult to manage, prone to infection, and slow to heal.

PREVENTION

- All recumbent patients should be turned frequently and given massage, physiotherapy, and/or hydrotherapy to stimulate blood flow.
- Recumbent animals should be kept on a well-padded surface such as a waterbed, soft egg crate, foam rubber pad, or airbed.

SUGGESTED READING

Kanj LF, et al: Pressure ulcers. *J Am Acad Dermatol* 38:517, 1998.

Swaim SF, et al: Pressure wounds in animals. *Comp Contin Educ Pract Vet* 18:203, 1996.

AUTHORS: **AMANDA P. AMARATUNGA, JAN A. HALL**

EDITOR: **JAN A. HALL**

Campylobacter Enteritis

BASIC INFORMATION

DEFINITION

Diarrheal disease resulting from invasive and toxigenic effects of *Campylobacter* spp. infection

EPIDEMIOLOGY

SPECIES, AGE, SEX

- Most commonly occurs in young animals <6 months old
- Pathogen of dogs, cats, humans, and various wild and domestic animals

GENETICS AND BREED PREDISPOSITION: None.

RISK FACTORS

- Young age
- Crowded conditions such as kennels or catteries and animal shelters
- Conditions with poor hygiene and sanitation
- Immunocompetence/immunodeficiency of individual patient
- Concomitant gastrointestinal infections
- Antibiotic therapy may predispose

CONTAGION AND ZOONOSIS

- Contagious between animals and species.
- Commonly spread between animals by fecal-oral route through contaminated food and water sources.
- Humans appear to be more susceptible than dogs or cats to clinical disease.
  - Dogs and cats are a major source of *Campylobacter jejuni* infection in people.
  - Other sources of infection to humans include eating raw or undercooked meat, especially poultry.
  - Owners of pets should be warned of the risks and practice good hygiene to minimize risk of zoonosis.

GEOGRAPHY AND SEASONALITY: Appears to be more common in the summer and fall months.

ASSOCIATED CONDITIONS AND DISORDERS: May be associated with other gastrointestinal infections or parasites:

- Parvovirus
- Coronavirus
- *Giardia*
- *Salmonella*

CLINICAL PRESENTATION

DISEASE FORMS/SUBTYPES

- Most cases of *Campylobacter* infection show no clinical signs.
- Clinical disease usually in young dogs and cats.

HISTORY, CHIEF COMPLAINT

- Most affected dogs and cats show no signs of the infection.
- Acute diarrhea ranging from watery to mucoid diarrhea with or without blood:
  - Tenesmus
  - Vomiting possible
- Chronic diarrhea that may be intermittent.
- Cholecystitis has been reported in two dogs associated with *C. jejuni*.

PHYSICAL EXAM FINDINGS: Acute cases may have fever and/or signs of dehydration.

ETIOLOGY AND PATHOPHYSIOLOGY

- Gram-negative, curved, motile, microaerophilic bacterial rods
- Component of the normal intestinal flora
- Clinical disease depends on number of organisms ingested as well as degree of development of protective antibody
- Disease localizes in jejunum, ileum, cecum, and colon, and histologic changes occur primarily in colon

- Virulence factors, including cytotoxin production, allow organism to invade epithelium
- Enterotoxin results in secretory diarrhea

DIAGNOSIS

DIFFERENTIAL DIAGNOSIS

- Viral diarrhea: parvovirus, coronavirus, rotavirus
- Bacterial diarrhea: *Salmonella, Clostridium*
- Parasites
- Dietary indiscretion

INITIAL DATABASE

Complete blood count, serum chemistry profile, and urinalysis results usually normal or nonspecific

- Mild hemoconcentration may be seen with dehydration
- Leukocytosis may be seen with invasion of mucosa
- Serum chemistry profile may show elevated total proteins and prerenal azotemia with dehydration

ADVANCED OR CONFIRMATORY TESTING

- Microscopic examination of feces:
    - Evaluation of stained smears of fresh feces for presence of characteristic organisms.
    - Increased numbers of fecal white blood cells also may be present.
    - *Campylobacter* may be difficult to distinguish from other similar species, including *Helicobacter*, on cytologic evaluation alone.
    - *Campylobacter* enteritis is difficult to diagnose cytologically, because many dogs have this organism as part of normal flora.
    - Dark field or phase contrast microscopy if available.
- Fecal culture:
    - Requires special *Campylobacter* plates and microaerophilic conditions.
    - Samples of fresh feces should be collected and placed in anaerobic transport medium.
    - Organisms remain viable for 3 days at room temperature and 1 week if refrigerated, but viability is improved with shorter delays.
- Serology:
    - Polymerase chain reaction is most reliable method of definitive identification of *Campylobacter* species, but tests are expensive and not available in all labs, and the presence of the organism does not prove that it is the cause of clinical signs.

TREATMENT

THERAPEUTIC GOAL(S)

- Elimination of organism from environment to minimize risk to humans
- Resolution of clinical signs

ACUTE GENERAL TREATMENT

- Efficacy of antibiotic therapy in altering course of disease is unknown.
- Erythromycin 10 to 20 mg/kg PO q 8h (or drugs from this family, including azithromycin 5-10 mg/kg PO q 24h) are the drugs of choice.
- Tetracyclines also have activity against *Campylobacter* (doxycycline 5 mg/kg PO q 12-24h).
- Chloramphenicol has questionable efficacy.
- Quinolones (e.g., enrofloxacin 5 mg/kg PO q 24h [4 mg/kg PO q 24h in cats]) thought to be effective, but a high rate of resistance exists.
    - Deleterious effects on joint cartilage is a concern, because many patients are young, growing animals.
- Duration of treatment with any of these antibiotics is typically several weeks.

CHRONIC TREATMENT

May be indicated in carrier animals (treatment for 4 to 6 months has been reportedly necessary to completely clear the organism)

RECOMMENDED MONITORING

- Monitor clinical signs
- Recheck fecal culture to assess fecal shedding and potential exposure to humans

PROGNOSIS AND OUTCOME

- Prognosis for recovery is good in the absence of other serious, concomitant disease
- Worse prognosis if underlying immunodeficiency or complicating disease

PEARLS & CONSIDERATIONS

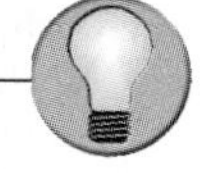

COMMENTS

- May be difficult to attribute *Campylobacter* as cause of diarrhea in dogs and cats since also part of normal flora
- However, infected animals should be treated due to potential exposure and transmission to humans

PREVENTION

- Good sanitation and avoidance of overcrowding
- Avoid undercooked meats

CLIENT EDUCATION

- Owners should be informed that this is a zoonotic disease and that humans are very susceptible.
- Good hygiene is essential, especially with a puppy or kitten with diarrhea.

SUGGESTED READING

Fox JG: Campylobacter infections. In Greene CE (ed): *Infectious Diseases of the Dog and Cat.* Philadelphia, WB Saunders, 1998, pp 226-229.

Marks SL, Kather EJ: Bacterial-associated diarrhea in the dog: A critical appraisal. *Vet Clin Small Anim* 33:5, 2000.

AUTHOR: **CHRISTOPHER J. JONES**

EDITOR: **DEBRA L. ZORAN**

Cardiac Glycosides-Containing Plant Toxicosis

BASIC INFORMATION

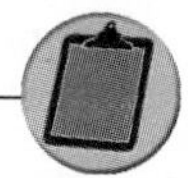

DEFINITION

Toxicosis occuring as a result of ingestion of plants that produce cardiovascular effects. For specific details concerning pharmacologic (digoxin) toxicosis, see Digoxin Toxicity, p 301.

SYNONYM(S)

Some cardiac glycoside-containing plants:

- *Asclepias* sp. (some): milkweed
- *Convallaria majalis*: lily of the valley
- *Digitalis purpurea*: foxglove (Fig. I-34)
- Hellebore sp.
- Kalanchoes sp.
- *Nerium oleander*: oleander
- *Thevitia nerifolia*: yellow oleander
- *Thevetia peruviana*: yellow oleander

Some grayanotoxins-containing plants:

- *Rhododendron* sp.: rhododendron, azalea, rosebay
- *Kalmia* sp.: laurels
- *Pieris* sp.: Japanese pieris, Mountain pieris

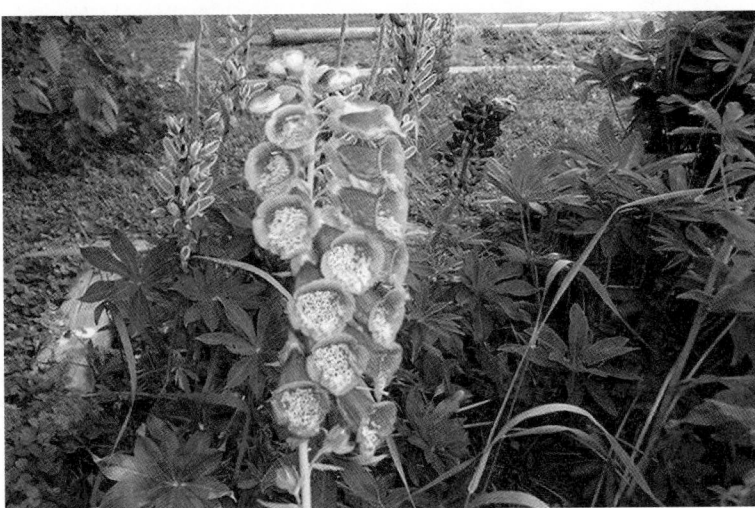

FIGURE I-34 Foxglove plant (*Digitalis purpurea*) is a source of cardiac glycosides such as digitalis.

EPIDEMIOLOGY

SPECIES, AGE, SEX: All ages and breeds are susceptible; dogs are more likely to be involved.

RISK FACTORS: Plants or flower bouquets present in pet's environment.

GEOGRAPHY AND SEASONALITY: Toxicosis occurs throughout the year but more likely to occur in spring and summer months (outdoor exposures).

CLINICAL PRESENTATION

HISTORY, CHIEF COMPLAINT

- History or evidence of exposure (witnessed ingestion, or chewed plant, or plant material present in the vomitus).
- Cardiac glycosides: onset of clinical signs within 2 to 8 hours of ingestion.
- Most common signs include salivation, vomiting, lethargy, depression, and ataxia. With severe intoxications, convulsions and death are possible.
- Grayanotoxins: signs occur within 6 hours of ingestion: lethargy, salivation, vomiting, signs of abdominal pain, ataxia, lateral recumbency, and seizures are possible.

PHYSICAL EXAM FINDINGS

- Cardiac glycoside-containing plants: pale mucous membranes, weak pulses, tachypnea, bradycardia or paroxysmal tachycardias.
- Extracardiac findings may include: vomiting, lethargy, diarrhea, tremors, seizures, and collapse.
- Grayanotoxins-containing plants: tachycardia, tachypnea, hyperthermia, vomiting, lethargy, diarrhea, hypotension, and bradycardia.

ETIOLOGY AND PATHOPHYSIOLOGY

- Cardiac glycosides:
    - Inhibition of Na-K-ATPase pump in the myocardial cell.
    - Result: decreased intracellular potassium, increased intracellular sodium. Intracellular sodium is exchanged for calcium, raising intracellular calcium levels.
        - Effects noted include: Heart block due to progressive interference with electrical conduction and increased vagal tone. Decrease in normal resting membrane potential. Decreased myocardial cell pacemaker activity, leading (in severe toxicoses) to malignant cardiac arrhythmias (ventricular) or asystole.
- Grayanotoxins: structurally distinct from cardiac glycosides but with a similar mechanism of action. Like cardiac glycosides, they bind to sodium channels, slowing their opening and closing, and decreasing their ion selectivity, and therefore produce similar clinical signs. Many cells are affected, especially excitable cells (neurologic, cardiac, muscle cells).

DIAGNOSIS

DIFFERENTIAL DIAGNOSIS

- Bufo toad ingestion
- Primary cardiac disease
- Systemic illness causing ventricular arrhythmias

INITIAL DATABASE

- Complete blood count (no significant changes expected)
- Serum chemistry panel: hyperkalemia possible; *hypo*kalemia markedly worsens the toxic effects (including making the heart refractory to antiarrhythmics such as lidocaine and procainamide) and needs to be treated (see Hypokalemia, p 566)
- Serum digoxin levels if needed (cardiac glycoside containing plants). Test can be performed at a local human hospital
- Electrocardiogram (ECG) to assess cardiovascular status
    - A combination of first- or second-degree AV block together with possibility of exposure to incriminating plant and compatible clinical signs is highly suggestive of the clinical diagnosis of glycoside plant cardiotoxicity.
    - Ventricular or atrial arrhythmias of virtually any type are possible.
    - The most common electrocardiogram (ECG) changes include first-, second-, or even third-degree atrioventricular (AV) block, ventricular arrhythmias, and ST segment changes.
- Blood pressure (may see hypotension)

ADVANCED OR CONFIRMATORY TESTING

- Serum digoxin levels (cardiac glycoside containing plants). Any detectable amount in a patient not receiving digoxin pharmaceutically confirms the diagnosis.
- Presence of oleandrin in gastrointestinal (GI) contents and body fluids can confirm exposure (available in some veterinary diagnostic laboratories)

TREATMENT

THERAPEUTIC GOAL(S)

See Oleander Poisoning, p 765 for more information on treatment or other aspects of cardiac glycosides-containing plant toxicosis.

- Decontamination of patient
- Supportive care (most cases; signs are mild or moderate)
- Severe cardiac arrhythmias/systemic signs: hospitalization and intensive care

ACUTE GENERAL TREATMENT

- Decontamination of patient:
    - Emesis: If no clinical signs apparent; apomorphine (0.03-0.04 mg/kg IV or IM, or crush tablet portion with water and instill into conjunctival sac; rinse following emesis).

- Hydrogen peroxide 3% (2 ml/kg, max 45 ml) PO; repeat in 10 to 15 minutes if no vomiting.
- Activated charcoal; after emesis or if few hours have elapsed after exposure; (1-4 g/kg) with a cathartic such as 70% sorbitol (3 ml/kg) PO.

- Treat cardiac arrhythmias:
  - Bradyarrhythmias in a normotensive patient: atropine 0.02-0.04 mg/kg IV, repeat as needed.
  - See Ventricular Arrhythmias, p 1148.
  - Digoxin immune Fab (Digibind) may be used for treating cardiac glycoside toxicosis (see Digoxin Toxicity, p 301).
- Supportive care:
  - IV fluids as needed; avoid calcium-containing fluids.
  - Correct acid-base status and electrolytes as needed.
  - Control central nervous system signs with benzodiazipine if needed (e.g., diazepam 0.5-1.0 mg/kg IV).
  - Control severe vomiting with metoclopramide (0.1-0.4 mg/kg PO, SC or IM q 6h), provided GI obstruction is ruled out.

POSSIBLE COMPLICATIONS

Permanent cardiac damage

RECOMMENDED MONITORING

- ECG
- Electrolytes
- Blood pressure
- Heart rate and pulse

PROGNOSIS AND OUTCOME

- Cardiac glycosides: Animals with moderate to severe cardiovascular signs have a guarded prognosis; even with intensive supportive care, serious intoxications may require several hours to several days of in-hospital treatment.
- Animals with only GI signs but no subsequent cardiovascular signs have a good prognosis.
- Grayanotoxins: prognosis is generally good with grayanotoxin-containing plants.

PEARLS & CONSIDERATIONS

COMMENTS

- Most ingestions of plants containing grayanotoxins in small amounts cause only vomiting and diarrhea.
- Cardiotoxicity of these plants is exclusively arrhythmogenic; structural heart disease (e.g., valve disease) is not caused by these plants.

SUGGESTED READING

Borrows GE: Toxic plants of North America. Ames, IA, Iowa State Press, 2001, pp 430-444, 1092-1096.

Galey FD: Cardiac Glycosides. In Plumlee KH (ed): *Clinical Veterinary Toxicology*. St. Louis, Mosby, 2004, pp 386-388.

Puschner B: Grananotoxins. In Plumlee KH (ed): *Clinical Veterinary Toxicology*. St. Louis, Mosby, 2004, pp 412-414.

AUTHOR: **CAROLINE W. DONALDSON**

EDITOR: **SAFDAR A. KHAN**

Cardiomegaly (Radiographic)

BASIC INFORMATION

DEFINITION

Enlargement of the cardiac silhouette relative to the thorax

- Radiographic assessment:
  - Subjective
    - Empiric: based on clinical experience
    - Compare to previous radiographs of same patient or other patient of same breed/conformation
  - Objective
    - Vertebral heart score: sum of long and short axes of cardiac silhouette on lateral view compared to length of thoracic vertebrae, beginning at T4 and continuing caudally
      - Canine normal = 9.7 ± 0.5
      - Feline normal = 7.5 ± 0.3
      - Has not proven to be more accurate than subjective assessment

EPIDEMIOLOGY

GENETICS AND BREED PREDISPOSITION

Dog Breeds Predisposed to Heart Disease

Disease	Some commonly affected breeds
Congenital	
Patent ductus arteriosus	Maltese, poodle, keeshond, bichon frise, Pomeranian
Subaortic stenosis	Newfoundland, bloodhound, boxer, golden retriever, rottweiler
Tricuspid dysplasia	Labrador retriever
Pulmonic stenosis	English bulldog, Scottish terrier, wirehaired fox terrier
Ventricular septal defect	Lakeland terrier, West Highland white terrier
Acquired	
Valvular endocardiosis	Cavalier King Charles spaniel, small breeds
Dilated cardiomyopathy	Doberman pinscher, Irish wolfhound, Great Dane, boxer, Saint Bernard, Afghan hound, Newfoundland, Old English sheepdog
Pericardial effusion	Retrievers, German shepherds, other large breeds (hemangiosarcoma, idiopathic sterile pericarditis); brachycephalic dogs (chemodectomas)

CLINICAL PRESENTATION

HISTORY, CHIEF COMPLAINT

- Dyspnea, tachypnea, cough, exercise intolerance, syncope
- May be incidental finding

PHYSICAL EXAM FINDINGS: Cardiac murmur, arrhythmia, tachycardia, muffled heart sounds, increased lung sounds, pulse alterations, ascites, jugular venous distention.

ETIOLOGY AND PATHOPHYSIOLOGY

- Pressure overload: outflow obstruction, hypertension
- Volume overload: valvular insufficiency, cardiomyopathy, shunt
- Pericardial effusion: neoplasia, inflammation, hemorrhage; rarely, infection

DIAGNOSIS

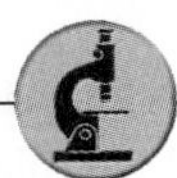

DIFFERENTIAL DIAGNOSIS

Enlarged chamber	Appearance on lateral view	Appearance on VD/DV view
Left atrium	Dorsal deviation of left mainstem bronchus	Increase in soft tissue opacity causing splaying of the mainstem bronchi
Left ventricle	Dorsal deviation of trachea	Enlargement of apex at 3 to 5 o'clock
Right atrium	Bulge at cranial aspect of cardiac silhouette	Bulge at 9:30 to 11:30 o'clock
Right ventricle	Widening of the cardiac silhouette, increased cardiosternal contact	Rounding and enlargement at 5 to 8 o'clock "Reverse D" appearance

- Left-sided cardiomegaly:
  - Valvular disease: mitral insufficiency
  - Cardiomyopathy
    - Dilated (dilated cardiomyopathy, DCM): canine
    - Hypertrophic (hypertrophic cardiomyopathy, HCM), restrictive: feline
  - Congenital
    - Left-to-right shunts: pulmonary overcirculation
      - Patent ductus arteriosus: ± main pulmonary artery, descending aorta, left auricular bulge
      - Ventricular or atrial septal defect
    - Subaortic stenosis: aortic arch dilation
    - Mitral dysplasia
- Left-sided congestive heart failure:
  - Enlarged left atrium
  - Interstitial to alveolar pulmonary infiltrates; perihilar, caudal distribution
  - In dogs with DCM and in cats, cardiogenic edema may have patchy, diffuse distribution
  - ± Enlarged pulmonary veins
- Right-sided cardiomegaly:
  - Valvular disease: tricuspid insufficiency
  - Congenital
    - Pulmonic stenosis: main pulmonary artery dilation
    - Tetralogy of Fallot: no main pulmonary artery enlargement, ± pulmonary underperfusion
    - Tricuspid dysplasia: can resemble generalized cardiomegaly, pericardial effusion on radiographs
    - Right-to-left patent ductus arteriosus or ventricular septal defect: heart may be of normal size, ± pulmonary underperfusion, main pulmonary artery, and lobar artery dilation
  - Cor pulmonale
    - Secondary to pulmonary hypertension: main pulmonary artery and lobar artery dilation
    - Example: heartworm disease, pulmonary thromboembolism, chronic pulmonary disease
- Right-sided congestive heart failure:
  - Pleural effusion
  - Enlarged caudal vena cava
  - Hepatomegaly
- Generalized cardiomegaly:
  - Pericardial effusion: globoid appearance; loss of normal heart shape. No enlarged left atrium
    - Idiopathic
    - Heart base, right atrial/auricular mass
    - Mesothelioma
    - Congestive heart failure
    - Left atrial rupture
    - Peritoneal-pericardial diaphragmatic hernia
  - Dilated cardiomyopathy
  - Mitral and tricuspid insufficiency
    - Individual chamber enlargement, including left atrial enlargement
- Great vessels:
  - Pulmonary trunk dilation: 1 to 2 o'clock on ventrodorsal/dorsoventral (VD/DV) view
    - Pulmonic stenosis, pulmonary hypertension
  - Aortic arch dilation: 11 to 1 o'clock on VD/DV view
    - Aortic stenosis, patent ductus arteriosus. May be normal in geriatric cats
  - Caudal vena cava enlargement
    - Right-sided congestive heart failure, cardiac tamponade, right atrial obstruction
- Pulmonary vasculature: corresponding pulmonary arteries and veins should be of equal size:
  - Large pulmonary arteries
    - Pulmonary hypertention: heartworm disease, pulmonary thromboembolism, chronic pulmonary disease
  - Large pulmonary veins
    - Venous congestion associated with left atrial enlargement
  - Large pulmonary arteries and veins
    - Left-to-right shunts
  - Small pulmonary arteries and veins
    - Right-to-left shunts, low cardiac output

INITIAL DATABASE

- Right or left lateral and VD or DV thoracic radiographs made during full inspiration
- Electrocardiogram, blood pressure, serum biochemistry profile

ADVANCED TESTING

- Echocardiography
- Nonselective or selective angiography

TREATMENT

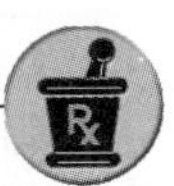

THERAPEUTIC GOAL(S)

- Reduce preload and afterload
- Improve diastolic and systolic function

ACUTE AND CHRONIC TREATMENT

As required based on underlying cause

PROGNOSIS AND OUTCOME

Variable depending on underlying disease

PEARLS & CONSIDERATIONS

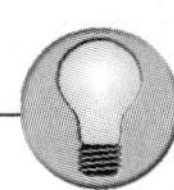

COMMENTS

- Things that mimic cardiomegaly:
  - Chondrodystrophic, shallow-chested patient
  - Films made during expiration
  - Excess pericardial fat
  - Patient obliquity
- Things that mimic pulmonary disease:
  - Films made during expiration
  - Underexposure
  - Excess intrathoracic and/or extrathoracic fat
- Positional differences:
  - Cardiac apex is normally rounded and dorsally displaced on left lateral view
  - Cardiac silhouette is normally more elongated on VD view and more oval in shape on DV view
  - With pleural effusion, cardiac silhouette is better outlined on VD view
- Breed/conformation differences:
  - Deep-chested patients: cardiac silhouette more narrow and vertically oriented on lateral projection compared to patients with other chest conformations

- Chondrodystrophic, shallow-chested patients: cardiac silhouette appears large relative to thorax. Trachea deviated dorsally on lateral projection (normal)
- Normal geriatric felines:
  - Horizontal orientation of heart
  - Tortuous, prominent aorta
- Cardiomegaly is present in 80% of dogs with hemodynamically significant pericardial effusion (cardiac tamponade); for the remaining 20%, diagnosis depends on physical exam (tachycardia + weak pulse + muffled heart sounds) and echocardiography.

SUGGESTED READING

Berry CR, Love NE, Thrall DE: Interpretation paradigms for the small animal thorax. In Thrall DE (ed): *Textbook of Veterinary Diagnostic Radiology*. Philadelphia, WB Saunders, 2002, pp 307–322.

Lord PF, Suter PF: Radiology. In Fox PR, Sisson D, Moise NS (eds): *Textbook of Canine and Feline Cardiology*. Philadelphia, WB Saunders, 1999, pp 107–129.

Root CR, Bahr RJ: The heart and great vessels. In Thrall DE (ed): *Textbook of Veterinary Diagnostic Radiology*. Philadelphia, WB Saunders, 2002, pp 402–419.

AUTHOR: **WENDY D. FIFE**
EDITOR: **ETIENNE CÔTÉ**

Carnitine Deficiency

BASIC INFORMATION

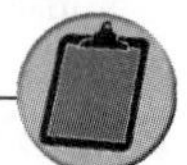

DEFINITION

Inadequate synthesis, intake or availability of dietary L-carnitine (only the L isomer can be used by the body)

SYNONYM(S)

Since L-carnitine is the biologically active isomer, the terms *carnitine* and *L-carnitine* are used interchangeably in the clinical setting.

EPIDEMIOLOGY

SPECIES, AGE, SEX: L-carnitine (β-hydroxy-γ-trimethylaminobutyric acid) appears to be a conditionally essential nutrient for dogs and cats. Although not essential under normal circumstances, deficiency can occur under some circumstances in some animals.

GENETICS AND BREED PREDISPOSITION
- Cats: none reported.
- Dogs: Members of isolated families of various breeds may have carnitine deficiency or insufficiency. For example, some boxers with dilated cardiomyopathy (DCM) appear to respond to oral L-carnitine supplementation, and similarly, some American cocker spaniels with DCM respond to oral supplementation with taurine (500 mg) and L-carnitine (1g) PO q 8h.

RISK FACTORS: Cats: rapid weight loss in obese cats, idiopathic hepatic lipidosis.

CLINICAL PRESENTATION

DISEASE FORMS/SUBTYPES
- Cats: idiopathic hepatic lipidosis. No cardiac effects of carnitine deficiency have been identified.
- Dogs: DCM.

HISTORY, CHIEF COMPLAINT
- Cats: compatible with idiopathic hepatic lipidosis (see p 493)
- Dogs: compatible with congestive heart failure (exercise intolerance and weight loss progressing to cough, respiratory distress, and eventually, ascites)

PHYSICAL EXAM FINDINGS
- Cats: obesity (?); signs of idiopathic hepatic lipidosis: icterus, hepatomegaly, ± dehydration
- Dogs: variable combinations of tachypnea, dyspnea, tachycardia, tachyarrhythmia, and lethargy. Soft systolic murmur at the apex on the left side, gallop rhythm in severe cases

ETIOLOGY AND PATHOPHYSIOLOGY

- L-carnitine is synthesized from lysine and methionine in the liver. Some prepared pet foods may have less available L-carnitine than unprocessed meat, which could unmask inadequate endogenous synthesis in predisposed animals, or in unusual circumstances. L-carnitine participates in cellular metabolism through free fatty acid transport into the mitochondria for catabolism, and apparently also by modulating glucose metabolism.
- Dogs: DCM associated with carnitine deficiency appears to result from inadequate L-carnitine-mediated fatty acid transport for mitochondrial energy production.
- Cats: association between L-carnitine and idiopathic hepatic lipidosis is less clear but may be related to inadequate synthesis or tissue availability.

DIAGNOSIS

DIFFERENTIAL DIAGNOSIS

- Cats: other hepatopathies, other influences on hepatic lipidosis
- Dogs: idiopathic DCM and other causes of myocardial failure

INITIAL DATABASE

Low plasma L-carnitine concentration suggests carnitine deficiency and need for supplementation of dogs, but the test is not sensitive. That is, myocardial carnitine deficiency may occur with normal plasma carnitine concentrations. Collect samples for plasma L-carnitine determination in heparinized syringes; one's clinical laboratory should be contacted for detailed instructions on collection, preparation, and shipping of samples. Reported normal plasma concentrations (μmol/L) are:

	Total	Free	Esterified
Dogs	12-38	8-36	0-7
Cats: male (9)	5-22	4-18	0-6
Cats: female (4)	5-44	5-34	0-12

ADVANCED OR CONFIRMATORY TESTING

Dogs: fluoroscopic-guided endomyocardial biopsy may be used for determining muscle L-carnitine concentrations, but this currently is unavailable to most practices. One may supplement for 3 to 4 months and monitor for regression of cardiac dysfunction while providing routine treatment for DCM and congestive heart failure as indicated. (Treatments are *not* expected to reverse the cardiomegaly and congestive heart failure as medications are tapered or stopped.)

TREATMENT

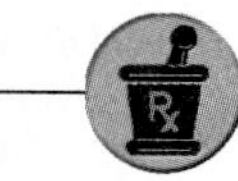

THERAPEUTIC GOAL(S)

Restore carnitine homeostasis:
- Cats: improve liver function
- Dogs: improve cardiac function

ACUTE GENERAL TREATMENT

- Cats: supportive care for Idiopathic Hepatic Lipidosis, p 493

- Dogs: supportive care for congestive heart failure and cardiac arrhythmias (see Atrial Fibrillation, p 98; Ventricular Arrhythmias, p 1148)
- L-carnitine supplementation pending confirmation of diagnosis (?)

CHRONIC TREATMENT

- Cats: L-carnitine 200 to 500 mg PO per day during enteral nutritional support for idiopathic hepatic lipidosis has been recommended.
- Dogs:L-carnitine 200 mg/kg PO q 8h has been suggested. Validate potency of L-carnitine preparation used, because significant variation exists in commercially available L-carnitine, or use pharmaceutic grade. Advise clients that L-carnitine could be a significant expense in addition to usual care for a large dog. Supplementation for as long as 4 months may be needed to identify echocardiographic improvement (if it occurs).

RECOMMENDED MONITORING

- Cats: clinical condition, return to food intake
- Dogs: clinical condition, thoracic radiography

PROGNOSIS AND OUTCOME

- Cats: poor to good (± L-carnitine supplementation) depending on severity of idiopathic hepatic lipidosis and rapidity with which adequate nutritional support occurs
- Dogs: guarded to poor; few dogs with DCM respond to L-carnitine

PEARLS & CONSIDERATIONS

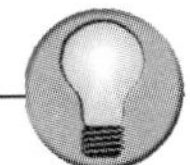

COMMENTS

- Recently estimated that ~5% of cases of DCM are carnitine-deficient
- In cats, recovery of function and appetite occurs within days to weeks of provision of L-carnitine
- In dogs, months may be required to determine efficacy

PREVENTION

Feed a properly formulated diet

CLIENT EDUCATION

Explain the importance of feeding a properly formulated diet

SUGGESTED READING

Carroll MC, Côté E: Carnitine: A review. *Compend Contin Educ Pract Vet* 23:45, 2001.

Center SA: Feline hepatic lipidosis. *Vet Clin North Am* 35:225, 2005.

Pion PD: Traditional and non-traditional effective and noneffective therapies for cardiac disease in dogs and cats. *Vet Clin North Am* 34:187, 2004.

AUTHOR & EDITOR: **C. A. TONY BUFFINGTON**

Carpal Trauma

BASIC INFORMATION

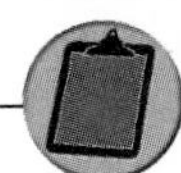

DEFINITION

Carpal trauma includes ligamentous (sprain), fibrocartilagenous (hyperextension), fracture, or shearing injuries

SYNONYM(S)

Carpal breakdown

EPIDEMIOLOGY

GENETICS AND BREED PREDISPOSITION: Racing greyhounds: accessory carpal bone fractures.

RISK FACTORS: Racing or agility activities; distal forelimb trauma.

CLINICAL PRESENTATION

DISEASE FORMS/SUBTYPES

- Sprains (hyperextension)
- Fractures
- Shearing/degloving wounds
- Coaptation-related injuries, including pressure sores from casts or splints; dermatitis from soiled bandages; and wound infection or dehiscence from old, dirty dressings

HISTORY, CHIEF COMPLAINT

- Forelimb trauma
- Lameness after competition; slowing or drifting wide on racetrack turns

PHYSICAL EXAM FINDINGS

- Lameness
- Carpal swelling
- Open wounds around the carpus
- Pain or crepitation during palpation of the carpus
- Gross instability characterized by palmigrade stance (Fig. I-35)

ETIOLOGY AND PATHOPHYSIOLOGY

- Track animals racing counterclockwise are predisposed to right-sided injuries (80%).
- In pets, carpal fractures (usually radial carpal bone) are less common than ligament injury.
- In racing animals, fractures usually involve the accessory carpal bone

DIAGNOSIS

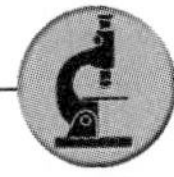

DIFFERENTIAL DIAGNOSIS

- Autoimmune polyarthropathy (systemic lupus erythematosus, rheumatoid arthritis)
- Infectious (Lyme borreliosis, rickettsial diseases)

INITIAL DATABASE

- Mediolateral and dorsopalmar radiographic projections of the distal limb (pes and carpus)
- Complete blood count and chemistry panel based on American Society of Anesthesiologists (ASA) (see American Society of Anesthesiologists: Classification System, p 1334) patient classification
- Electrocardiography and thoracic radiography (if part of massive trauma)

ADVANCED OR CONFIRMATORY TESTING

- Oblique radiographic views to outline nondisplaced fractures
- Stress radiography (mediolateral radiograph with carpus manually forced into hyperextension) for localizing joint instability

TREATMENT

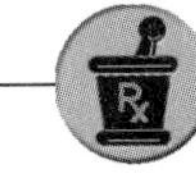

THERAPEUTIC GOAL(S)

- Fractures: stabilization and anatomic reduction
- Ligamentous injuries: reestablishment of carpal support with ligament repair or arthrodesis
- Shearing injuries: wound management

ACUTE GENERAL TREATMENT

- Minimally displaced, nonarticular fractures, grade I, and most grade II ligament sprains are externally splinted for 6 to 8 weeks.
- Luxated joints, intra-articular fractures, and grade III sprains are initially supported in a modified Robert-Jones bandage until definitive surgery.
- Shearing injuries, after initial wound management protocols, are covered

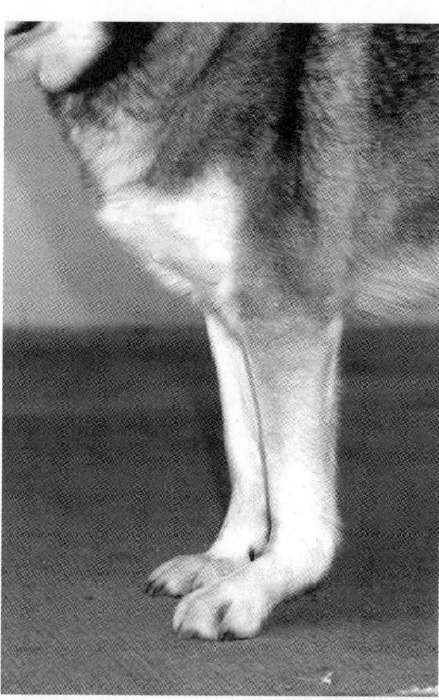

FIGURE I-35 Lateral view of a mature malamute with a left forelimb lameness due to palmar carpal breakdown following a jump from a deck.

and supported until definitive treatment is performed.

- Gentle lavage using warm saline, lactated Ringer's solution, dilute chlorhexidine solutions of open wounds to reduce gross contamination (patients are sedated and given analgesics).
- Coverage of tissues with moistened (above solutions) gauze sponges useful in debridement (wet-to-dry-bandages) since they are changed daily.
- Alternatively, direct application of sugar or honey has been used to reduce infection and promote healing in highly contaminated, traumatic open wounds, but the role of such treatment in the joint space is unclear.
- Final surgical debridement and joint lavage can be performed during orthopedic stabilization surgery.
- Wounds with healthy granulation tissue, reduced contamination, and early epithelialization can be closed with sutures or covered with a nonadherent dressing and allowed to heal via second intention.

CHRONIC TREATMENT

- Surgical repairs require 6 to 12 weeks of external coaptation (e.g., splint, cast, or external fixator), and exercise restriction.
- Radial carpal bone luxation is treated with open joint tissues repair.
- Large radial carpal and accessory carpal bone fractures are treated with lag-screw fixation.
- Small radial carpal and accessory carpal bone fractures are excised and have good outcomes.
- Avulsion fractures are treated with tension band techniques.
- Hyperextension injuries are managed with partial carpal arthrodesis (middle and distal carpal joints) or pancarpal arthrodesis (injuries involving the antebrachial carpal joint).
- Collateral ligament injuries are primarily repaired or replaced with synthetic suture.

POSSIBLE COMPLICATIONS

- Reduction/implant failure
- Delayed or failed arthrodesis
- Wound infection
- Coaptation-related morbidity
- Degenerative joint disease

RECOMMENDED MONITORING

- Lameness evaluation 1 to 3 months after injury and treatment
- Serial radiographic studies to evaluate fracture healing or progression of arthrodesis

PROGNOSIS AND OUTCOME

- Good to excellent for noncompeting dogs.
- Variable for athletic dogs needing to return to preinjury competition levels.
- Severe shearing injuries with neurovascular compromise may necessitate limb amputation.

PEARLS & CONSIDERATIONS

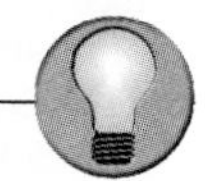

COMMENTS

- Complete palmar carpal breakdown (grade III sprain) requires pancarpal arthrodesis.
- Intra-articular fractures, when treated conservatively, rarely heal with osseous bridging, thus leading to degenerative joint disease.
- Partial carpal arthrodesis can promote a return to most preinjury activities.
- In racing greyhounds, treatment of radial carpal or accessory carpal bone fractures with lag-screw fixation (preferred) or fragment excision provides a return to competitive performance.

SUGGESTED READING

Johnson KA: Carpal Injuries. In Bloomberg MS, Dee JF, Taylor RA (eds): *Canine Sports Medicine and Surgery*. Philadelphia, WB Saunders, 1998, pp 100–119.

Piermattei DL, Flo GL: Orthopedic conditions of the carpus. In *Brinker, Piermattei, and Flo's Handbook of Small Animal Orthopedics and Fracture Repair*, ed 3. Philadelphia, WB Saunders, 1997, pp 344–394.

AUTHOR: **JOHN J. HABURJAK**
EDITOR: **JOSEPH HARARI**

Castor Bean Toxicosis

BASIC INFORMATION

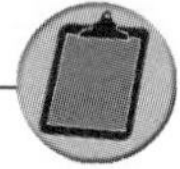

DEFINITION

Acute clinical signs, commonly including vomiting and diarrhea, initially and frequently progressing to coma and death, that occur in dogs as a result of eating castor beans

SYNONYM(S)

African coffee tree
Mexico weed
Mole bean
Palma Christi
Wonder tree
Ricinus communis

EPIDEMIOLOGY

SPECIES, AGE, SEX: All breeds, ages, and sexes susceptible; dogs involved more often than cats.

RISK FACTORS: Presence of castor beans in pet's environment.

GEOGRAPHY AND SEASONALITY

- Year round; more cases in October and November, when castor beans mature and are released from their spiny pods.
- Castor beans for jewelry and other ornamental purposes are available throughout the year.

CLINICAL PRESENTATION

HISTORY, CHIEF COMPLAINT

- History of exposure to castor bean plant or ornamentals (e.g., jewelry)

- A lag period of 6 to 12 hours or up to 48 hours before signs appear
- Vomiting and diarrhea (with or without blood), anorexia, lethargy

PHYSICAL EXAM FINDINGS

- No remarkable physical exam findings if recent exposure (<6 hours).
- Within 6 to 48 hours of exposure, anorexia, depression, lethargy, mild to severe vomiting, diarrhea, and abdominal tenderness may begin.
- In severe cases, dehydration, weakness, tremors, or seizures can ensue.
- Tachycardia, hypotension, and shock may be present (potentially fatal).
- Presence of castor beans or leaves in the vomitus.

ETIOLOGY AND PATHOPHYSIOLOGY

- Castor bean is a large decorative, ornamental, Caribbean plant now present throughout the warmer parts of the United States. The beans are commercially grown for castor oil or may be used for ornamental purposes (e.g., jewelry). The plant produces spiny pods that burst open after drying, releasing seeds. The seeds have color markings resembling some ticks or beetles.
- All parts of the castor bean plant contain ricin and therefore are considered toxic if ingested; the highest concentration of ricin is in the bean. Ricin, a heterodimeric glycoprotein, is a cellular toxin (toxalbumin) that inhibits protein synthesis. When protein synthesis cannot occur, the cell dies. Cell death in the gastrointestinal (GI) tract results in vomiting, diarrhea, abdominal pain, and hemorrhages.

DIAGNOSIS

DIFFERENTIAL DIAGNOSIS

- Dietary intolerance/garbage toxicosis
- Sago palm toxicosis
- Pancreatitis
- Viral and bacterial gastroenteritis
- GI tract obstruction

INITIAL DATABASE

- Complete blood count (CBC), serum biochemistry profile, or other changes may be seen 12 to 24 hours after ingestion
- CBC:
    - Leukocytosis
- Serum biochemistry panel:
    - Elevated alanine aminotransferase, aspartate aminotransferase, and lactate dehydrogenase, indicative of liver damage
    - Increased blood urea nitrogen and serum creatinine: may be renal or prerenal
    - Increased serum albumin and globulin possible, suggesting dehydration

ADVANCED OR CONFIRMATORY TESTING

Postmortem findings may include necrosis and hemorrhages in the heart, stomach, GI tract, lungs, liver, kidney, and pancreas.

TREATMENT

THERAPEUTIC GOAL(S)

- Decontamination of patient
- Protect GI mucosa
- Supportive care

ACUTE GENERAL TREATMENT

- Decontamination of patient:
    - Emesis: only animals not showing any clinical signs (see Vomiting, Induction of, p 1328). May be effective within several hours after exposure, especially if seeds have been ingested, since seeds are hard to digest
    - Gastric lavage: only if a potentially lethal dose has been ingested (see Pearls & Considerations below) and emesis cannot be induced (comatose animal)
    - Activated charcoal 2-4 g/kg PO; may be effective even several hours after exposure if seeds have been ingested. Protect airway with cuffed endotracheal tube if patient is unconscious
- Protect GI mucosa:
    - Administer GI protectants such as sucralfate (0.5-1 g/dog, or 125-250 mg/cat) PO q 8-12h and H_2 blockers (e.g., famotidine 0.5 mg/kg PO, SC, IM, or IV q 12-24h or ranitidine 0.5-2 mg/kg PO, IM, or IV q 8-12h
    - Control severe vomiting with metoclopramide (0.1-0.4 mg/kg PO, SC or IM q 6h), provided no evidence of GI obstruction is present
- Supportive care:
    - IV fluids for 2 to 3 days or as long as needed, typically at 1.5 to 2 times maintenance rates
    - Diazepam for seizures (0.5-2 mg/kg IV prn)
    - Lactulose (15-30 ml PO every 6 to 8 hours in dogs, and 0.25-1 ml PO every 8 to 12 hours in cats) may reduce the risk of hepatic encephalopathy if liver damage has occurred
    - SAM-e (s-adenosylmethionine) (18 mg/kg PO in dogs and cats q 24-72h for 1 to 3 months) for liver damage
    - Dietary management: soft bland diet in small amounts for 1 to 5 days

CHRONIC TREATMENT

SAM-e for chronic hepatopathy

POSSIBLE COMPLICATIONS

Possible liver or renal compromise

RECOMMENDED MONITORING

- CBC
- Liver enzymes on presentation: 24, 48 hours, or until resolution of signs
- Kidney profile on presentation: 24, 48 hours, or until resolution of signs
- Electrolytes
- Blood pressure and heart rate

PROGNOSIS AND OUTCOME

- Prognosis depends on the amount ingested and whether the beans were chewed or broken (prognosis worse) and if spontaneous vomiting occurred after the ingestion. Spontaneous vomiting after ingestion in dogs may prevent serious toxicosis due to self-decontamination.
- Most dogs respond well to supportive treatment.
- Poor prognosis if multiple organ damage, shock, or seizures occur.
- Mortality rate in dogs ingesting castor beans is approximately 9%.

PEARLS & CONSIDERATIONS

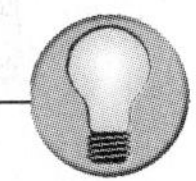

COMMENTS

- Severity of signs increases if the seed is chewed open. Ricin is not likely to be released from the seed unless the coat is masticated, broken, or damaged.
- All known or potential ingestions should be considered serious and treated aggressively to avoid serious consequences.
- In humans, ingestion of one to eight seeds can be lethal; the same may be true for dogs or cats.
- The toxalbumin is one of the most deadly substances known. Lethal dose in mice is 0.025 µg/kg IP and 1 mg/kg PO in humans.
- Latin name *(Ricinus)* means "insect," since beans resemble some ticks or beetles.

PREVENTION

Keep castor beans out of reach of pets

SUGGESTED READING

Albretsen JC, et al: Evaluation of castor bean toxicosis in dogs: 98 cases. *J Am Anim Hosp Assoc* 36:229-233, 2000.

Fodstad O, et al: Toxicity of abrin and ricin in mice and dogs. *J Toxicol Environ Health* 5:1073-1084, 1979.

Knight MW, et al: Selected poisonous plant concerns in small animals. *Vet Med* 92:260-272, 1997.

AUTHOR & EDITOR: **SAFDAR A. KHAN**

Cataracts

Client Education Sheet on Website

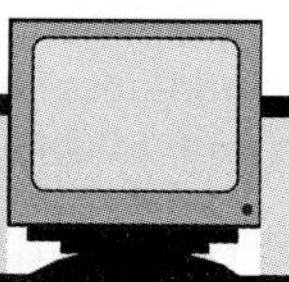

BASIC INFORMATION

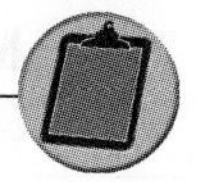

DEFINITION

Any opacity, regardless of size, of the lens or its capsule is termed a *cataract*. A cataract results from a change in the lens protein composition or lens fiber arrangement.

EPIDEMIOLOGY

SPECIES, AGE, SEX

- Dogs and cats
- Variable age of onset depending on breed affected and cause
- Cataracts reported to affect 16.8% of mixed-breed dogs ages 7–15+ years
- No sex predisposition

GENETICS AND BREED PREDISPOSITION

- In dogs, most cataracts have an inherited or genetic component; most common mode of inheritance is autosomal recessive.
- Breeds of dogs with the highest prevalence of cataracts include: smooth fox terrier, Havanese, bichon frise, Boston terrier, poodles (toy, miniature, standard), silky terrier, American cocker spaniel, and miniature schnauzer.
- Canine cataracts can also occur secondary to diabetes mellitus, which has a genetic predisposition in some breeds (see Diabetes Mellitus, p 289).
- Presumed congenital feline cataracts reported in Persian, Birman, Himalayan, and domestic shorthair.

RISK FACTORS

- Diabetes mellitus
- Hypocalcemia
- Anterior uveitis
- Retinal degeneration
- Retinal detachment
- Lens luxation

CLINICAL PRESENTATION

DISEASE FORMS/SUBTYPES: Cataracts are classified by age at onset, location, and severity, in addition to etiology.

- Age at onset:
  - Congenital: present at birth
  - Juvenile: few months to 6 years
  - Senile: >6 years
- Location:
  - Capsule: anterior, posterior
  - Cortex: anterior, posterior, equatorial
  - Nucleus
- Severity:
  - Incipient: <10% of retinal examination obstructed
  - Immature:
    - Early: 10–50% of retinal examination obstructed
    - Late: 50–99% of retinal examination obstructed
  - Mature: 100% of retinal examination obstructed
  - Hypermature: liquefaction/resorption with associated lens-induced uveitis (see Uveitis, p 1134)
  - Morgagnian: nucleus falls ventrally in the capsule

HISTORY, CHIEF COMPLAINT

- Vision disturbance
- Cloudy, white pupil
- The chief complaint may reflect a systemic cause of cataracts (e.g., polyuria-polydipsia with diabetes mellitus)

PHYSICAL EXAM FINDINGS

- Opacity of the lens (unilateral or bilateral) with any or all of the following:
  - Anterior uveitis (see Uveitis, p 1134)
  - Glaucoma, p 440
  - Lens subluxation/luxation (see Lens Luxation, p 628)
  - Retinal Degeneration, p 963; Retinal Detachment, p 965
- Systemic abnormalities may be present when cataracts are caused by a generalized disorder (e.g., weight loss with diabetes mellitus).

ETIOLOGY AND PATHOPHYSIOLOGY

- Regardless of etiology, all cataracts occur through a change in the lens protein composition or lens fiber arrangement:
  - Inherited: numerous breeds of dogs, some cats
  - Diabetes mellitus: increased blood glucose results in diffusion of increased glucose into the lens, overwhelming standard metabolism of the lens, causing excess glucose to be shunted to the sorbitol pathway, which forms polyols and subsequently osmotically draws water into the lens, causing opacification (dogs)
  - Secondary to intraocular disease:
    - Uveitis
    - Glaucoma
    - Retinal degeneration/detachment
    - Lens luxation
  - Trauma to lens: blunt or penetrating
  - Age-related
  - Nutritional: in puppies and kittens fed milk replacer. Proposed mechanism: amino acid deficiency(ies), such as arginine, at crucial stage during lens development
  - Hypocalcemia, p 564
  - Radiation therapy/injury (see Radiation Therapy: Adverse Reactions, p 940), when primary beam near or on globe
  - Medications (e.g., long-term oral ketoconazole; mostly in young, large-breed dogs given higher doses [6–13.9 mg/kg/day])
  - Toxins (e.g., dinitrophenol; diazoxide)
  - Electric shock
- Not all cataracts are progressive.
- Cataracts can progress to become hypermature and result in lens-induced uveitis.

DIAGNOSIS

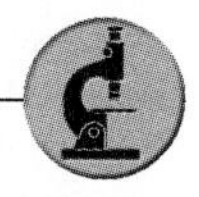

DIFFERENTIAL DIAGNOSIS

- Nuclear/lenticular sclerosis: normal aging change; usually seen in animals ≥7 years old; does not cause vision loss; center of lens becomes opalescent to hazy, but tapetal reflection in pupil (usually greenish) is still visible, versus cataracts, which obstruct this reflection
- Diseases causing diffuse corneal edema (bluish-white opacity on *cornea*, not in pupil; may obstruct ability to see the pupil) including:
  - Glaucoma
  - Anterior uveitis
  - Corneal endothelial degeneration or dystrophy
- Diseases causing secondary cataracts:
  - Retinal degeneration, or detachment
  - Anterior uveitis (cataracts typically incomplete if due to inflammation; uveitis may also occur secondary to cataracts; if cataracts occupying large extent of lens in predisposed breed, assume lens-induced uveitis)
  - Lens luxation

INITIAL DATABASE

- Complete ophthalmic examination including:
  - Menace response
  - Evaluation of pupil size, symmetry, and pupillary light reflexes
  - Intraocular pressure (IOP): rule out glaucoma (>30 mmHg)
  - After IOP assessment (assuming normal result), dilate pupil with 1% tropicamide
  - Penlight or transilluminator to characterize the cataract, evaluate for concurrent uveitis
  - Fundic (posterior segment) examination using indirect or direct ophthalmoscopy
- Blood and urine glucose determination (dogs primarily)

ADVANCED OR CONFIRMATORY TESTING

- Complete blood count, chemistry profile, and urinalysis to rule out systemic metabolic disease (e.g., diabetes mellitus, hypocalcemia) as cause of cataracts and/or to assess patient before considering referral for possible cataract surgery
- Ocular ultrasound if the cataract is immature or worse in severity and precludes accurate evaluation of the posterior segment of the eye
- Electroretinogram (ERG) to assess retinal function (routinely conducted by veterinary ophthalmologists before cataract surgery)

TREATMENT

THERAPEUTIC GOAL(S)

- Incipient and nonprogressive early immature cataracts do not require treatment.
- Progressive immature, mature, and hypermature cataracts are treated to:
  - Restore vision (i.e., cataract surgery)
  - Prevent secondary sequelae of cataracts: uveitis, glaucoma, and retinal detachment

ACUTE GENERAL TREATMENT

- Treat associated uveitis with topical mydriatics and anti-inflammatories (see Uveitis, p 1134)
- Treat secondary glaucoma accordingly (see Glaucoma, p 440)
- Referral for cataract surgery if cataract is vision-threatening and animal systemically stable (e.g., concurrent diabetes mellitus is controlled):
  - Cataract surgery requires preliminary ocular ultrasound and ERG that indicate that the posterior segment of the eye is normal
  - Phacoemulsification (ultrasonic lens fragmentation) to remove the cataract:
    - Followed by implantation of an artificial intraocular lens to restore emmetropia (normal vision, neither far-nor near-sighted) (Fig. I-36).
    - Without an intraocular lens implant, animals are 14 diopters hyperopic (far-sighted) with little useful vision.

CHRONIC TREATMENT

- After cataract surgery, treat as directed by the veterinary ophthalmologist:
  - Topical antibiotics and anti-inflammatories.
  - Exercise restriction/Elizabethan collar: 2 weeks.
  - Anti-inflammatory therapy may be continued in a decreasing fashion for months or, in some cases, indefinitely.
  - Frequent reevaluation of intraocular lens position, IOP, retinal examination, and inflammation control.
- If cataract surgery is not an option:
  - Monitor cataracts for progression and treat associated uveitis with topical anti-inflammatory(ies) (see Uveitis, p 1134) long-term.
  - Use IOP-lowering drugs in combination with anti-inflammatories if secondary glaucoma develops (see Glaucoma, p 440).
  - Enucleation or evisceration and intrascleral prosthesis of end-stage, blind, painful globes.

DRUG INTERACTIONS

Corticosteroids (topical ophthalmic or oral) may interfere with management of diabetes mellitus.

POSSIBLE COMPLICATIONS

- Without cataract surgery, the following can occur:
  - Uveitis
  - Glaucoma
  - Blindness, p 136
- After cataract surgery, the following can occur:
  - Uveitis
  - Glaucoma
  - Corneal Ulceration, p 246
  - Surgical wound/incisional dehiscence
  - Intraocular infection (see Hypopyon, p 571)
  - Retinal detachment
  - Intraocular lens displacement
  - Lens capsule fibrosis
  - Corneal endothelial degeneration and secondary corneal edema
  - Keratoconjunctivitis Sicca, p 614

RECOMMENDED MONITORING

- Without cataract surgery, monitor for cataract progression and secondary complications (see Possible Complications above) every 2 to 4 months, or more or less frequently, depending on the extent of cataract, rate of cataract development, and presence or absence of associated ocular complications.
- After cataract surgery, monitor according to veterinary ophthalmologist's recommendations; generally involves:
  - Reevaluations at postoperative weeks 2, 8, and 20.
  - Long-term follow-up every 6 to 12 months for life.
  - In addition to routine ophthalmic examinations, Schirmer tear test, IOP, menace response, and pupillary light reflexes should be evaluated each time the animal is presented to the veterinarian.

PROGNOSIS AND OUTCOME

- Rate of cataract progression variable depending on cause and location of the cataract and age of the animal.
- Success of cataract surgery (i.e., phacoemulsification), as determined by a positive visual outcome, is 90–95%.
- Success is increased with early referral (i.e., before animal is blind) and sur-

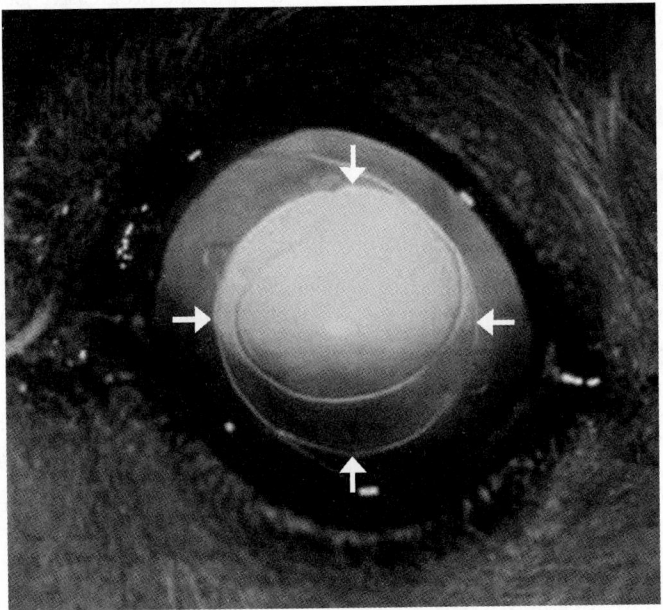

FIGURE I-36 Canine eye 24 hours after cataract surgery and intraocular lens implantation. Note the dilated pupil and intraocular lens implant centered within the pupil (*arrows*).

gery, and with diligent postoperative monitoring and treatment.

PEARLS & CONSIDERATIONS

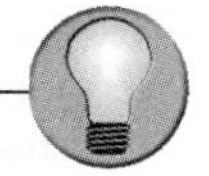

COMMENTS

- Early referral and prompt surgical intervention before the onset of hypermaturity and lens-induced uveitis will result in a more successful outcome.
- Animals affected with cataracts, regardless of the severity, should not be used for breeding unless it is known specifically that the cataract is of nongenetic origin.

PREVENTION

- Ophthalmic screening of animals used for breeding by a board-certified veterinary ophthalmologist and registration through the Canine Eye Registration Foundation will help to remove affected animals from the breeding population.
- Prompt treatment of intraocular inflammation will decrease the likelihood of secondary cataracts.
- Early diagnosis and proper management of diabetes mellitus will help prevent cataract formation, but even the most well-managed diabetics may still develop cataracts. Once present, cataracts caused by diabetes mellitus are irreversible and will not resorb, even with good diabetic control.
- In the future, use of aldose reductase inhibitors and antioxidants may have a role in the delay and prevention of cataracts.

CLIENT EDUCATION

- It is essential that clients understand that not all cataracts are progressive.
- If a cataract is progressive, the client must make a decision with regard to surgery.
- Although surgery is associated with some risks, not opting for surgery is also associated with risks of lens-induced uveitis, secondary glaucoma, retinal detachment, and ocular pain.
- Animals undergoing cataract removal surgery that do not receive an intraocular lens implant have vision that, in human equivalence, is worse than 20/400, and corresponds to being "legally blind."

SUGGESTED READING

Colitz CMH: Diseases of the lens and vitreous. In Morgan RV, Bright RM, Swartout MS (eds): *Handbook of Small Animal Practice*. Philadelphia, WB Saunders, 2003, pp 995–1003.

Davidson MG, Nelms SR: Diseases of the lens and cataract formation. In Gelatt KN (ed): *Veterinary Ophthalmology*. Philadelphia, Lippincott, Williams & Wilkins, 1999, pp 797–925.

Gelatt KN, MacKay EO: Prevalence of primary breed-related cataracts in the dog in North America. *Vet Ophthalmol* 8:101–111, 2005.

Wilkie DA, Gilmour M: Diseases of the lens. In Birchard SJ, Sherding RG (eds): *Saunders Manual of Small Animal Practice*. Philadelphia, WB Saunders, 2000, pp 1342–1346.

AUTHOR: **DAVID A. WILKIE**
EDITOR: **CHERYL L. CULLEN**

Caudal Cervical Spondylomyelopathy

Client Education Sheet on Website

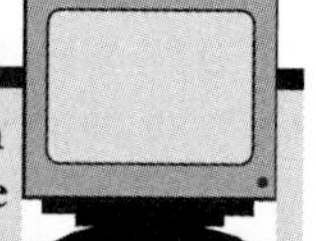

BASIC INFORMATION

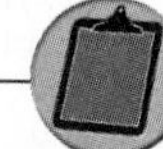

DEFINITION

A combination of vertebral malformation and malarticulation that affects caudal cervical vertebrae and associated ligamentous structures

SYNONYM(S)

CCSM
Cervical malformation/malarticulation syndrome
Cervical spondylopathy
Cervical vertebral instability
Spondylolisthesis
"Wobbler syndrome"

EPIDEMIOLOGY

SPECIES, AGE, SEX: Most commonly encountered in middle-aged to older, large-breed dogs of either sex. Some reports describe a predilection in males (2:1–4:1) over females.

GENETICS AND BREED PREDISPOSITION: Doberman pinschers appear to be most prone to developing caudal cervical spondylomyelopathy (CCSM). Other commonly affected breeds include rottweilers, German shepherds, and dalmatians.

CLINICAL PRESENTATION

HISTORY, CHIEF COMPLAINT

- The majority of cases have histories that include progressive gait abnormalities noted for months to years.
- Occasionally, CCSM patients experience acute-onset and rapid development of neurologic dysfunction.
- With CCSM, abnormalities of thoracic limb gait are usually present but can be subtle and may be overlooked. When apparent, these abnormalities manifest as a stiff, stilted thoracic limb gait.
- Other less common historic/clinical complaints include nonambulatory tetraparesis/tetraplegia, neck pain, and thoracic limb lameness.

PHYSICAL EXAM FINDINGS

- Neurologic examination findings are consistent with a C6-T2 spinal cord lesion/myelopathy.
  - In ambulatory dogs, a characteristic "choppy," short-strided forelimb gait with a wide-based, ataxic hind limb gait is common.
  - Patellar reflexes may be increased, and there may be delayed postural reactions in the pelvic limbs (including when the patient's weight is supported—delayed hopping response from proprioceptive deficits).
  - The remainder of the neurologic examination is unremarkable.
- Classic lower motor neuron signs to the thoracic limbs are not frequently encountered in ambulatory patients (more common in nonambulatory tetraparetic or tetraplegic dogs).
- Careful palpation of the ventral processes of the cervical vertebrae, as well as side-to-side movements of the head and neck, usually reveal some evidence of pain/cervical hyperesthesia.

ETIOLOGY AND PATHOPHYSIOLOGY

- Affected dogs are believed to have a malformation/malarticulation of caudal cervical vertebrae. The resultant instability of these abnormal vertebral segments leads to hypertrophy of supportive soft tissue structures, including the intervertebral disk. Such hypertrophy and movement lead to spinal cord impingement.
- Genetic (affected breeds), nutritional (overfeeding during growth), and conformational (long neck with large head) influences have been suggested as causative or contributory.

- Vertebral malalignment ("tipping") as seen radiographically can be part of the malformation but is not necessarily indicative of a spinal cord lesion.

DIAGNOSIS

The diagnosis is suspected based on signalment, history, characteristic gait abnormalities, and evidence of cervical pain on physical examination and is confirmed with imaging.

DIFFERENTIAL DIAGNOSIS

- Type I disk extrusion
- Type II disk protrusion
- Neoplasia
- Spinal arachnoid cyst

INITIAL DATABASE

- Complete blood count, serum chemistry profile, urinalysis: generally unremarkable
- Thoracic and cervical radiographs: if other diagnoses (e.g., vertebral neoplasia) are being considered
- Imaging of the cervical spine:
  - Myelography or magnetic resonance imaging (MRI) are both acceptable.
  - MRI is preferable, because it provides superior detail and images within the spinal cord parenchyma and is better tolerated by the patient.
  - With either modality, static, as well as dynamic, views of the spine should be obtained.

TREATMENT

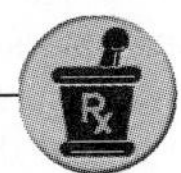

THERAPEUTIC GOAL(S)

- Return to normal or near-normal gait
- Elimination of neck pain

ACUTE GENERAL TREATMENT

- Exercise restriction
- Low-dose oral prednisone therapy (e.g., 0.5 mg/kg, PO q 12h)

CHRONIC TREATMENT

Most patients respond transiently, if at all, to medical therapy. Surgical distraction/stabilization is recommended in most cases. Some cases may require dorsal decompression.

PROGNOSIS AND OUTCOME

The majority of dogs (>80%) will respond favorably to surgical distraction/stabilization. Dogs that require dorsal decompression typically have a prolonged convalescent period (i.e., they may be nonambulatory for several months postoperatively).

PEARLS & CONSIDERATIONS

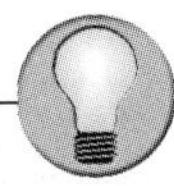

COMMENTS

- Poor responses to surgical correction tend to be dramatic and are usually due to either failure of surgical implants or compression at a site cranial or caudal to the operative site.
- The radiographic appearance alone does not correlate to the clinical impact of the lesion; imaging and examination are complementary.

SUGGESTED READING

DeRisio L, et al: Dorsal laminectomy for caudal cervical spondylomyelopathy: Postoperative recovery and long term follow-up in 20 dogs. *Vet Surg* 31:418, 2002.

Dewey CW: Myelopathies: Disorders of the spinal cord. In Dewey CW (ed): *A Practical Guide to Canine and Feline Neurology*. Ames, IA, Iowa State Press, 2003, pp 277–336.

Bruecker KA, et al: Caudal cervical spondylomyelopathy: Decompression by linear traction and stabilization with Steinman pins and polymethyl methacrylate. *J Am Anim Hosp Assoc* 25:677, 1989.

Dixon BC, et al: Modified distraction-stabilization technique using an interbody polymethyl methacrylate plug in dogs with caudal cervical spondylomyelopathy. *J Am Vet Med Assoc* 208:61, 1996.

AUTHOR & EDITOR: **CURTIS W. DEWEY**

Caudal Occipital Malformation Syndrome

BASIC INFORMATION

DEFINITION

Caudal occipital malformation syndrome (COMS) is a congenital malformation of the caudal occipital bone region that results in overcrowding of the caudal fossa and compression of the cervicomedullary junction at the level of the foramen magnum. It is commonly associated with syringohydromyelia, usually involving the cervical spinal cord.

SYNONYM(S)

Chiari type I malformation
COMS
Occipital bone hypoplasia

EPIDEMIOLOGY

SPECIES, AGE, SEX

- This is a disorder of small-breed dogs, with the Cavalier King Charles spaniel being the most overrepresented.
- The age at onset of disease is variable, with mean age at diagnosis of 4 to 6 years.
- There is no apparent sex predilection.

GENETICS AND BREED PREDISPOSITION

- Cavalier King Charles spaniel
  - Most common
  - Evidence of heritability, but mode of inheritance has not been determined
- Yorkshire terriers
- Miniature/toy poodles

ASSOCIATED CONDITIONS AND DISORDERS

- The vast majority of dogs with COMS have associated syringohydromyelia, usually affecting the cervical spinal cord.
- Occasionally, COMS patients also have hydrocephalus, intracranial intraarachnoid cysts (quadrigeminal cysts), and malformation of the C1 and/or C2 vertebrae (basilar invagination).

CLINICAL PRESENTATION

HISTORY, CHIEF COMPLAINT

- Dogs present for a wide variety of clinical manifestations, the most common of which are cerebellovestibular dysfunction and cervical myelopathy.
- A unique presentation of dogs with COMS that have concurrent cervical syringohydromyelia is incessant scratching at the shoulder region and head/neck region (suspected paresthesia).
- In a small percentage of COMS cases, seizure activity is the chief complaint.
- Clinical signs are often intermittent, often worsening in periods of stress or excitement.

PHYSICAL EXAM FINDINGS

- General examination is usually normal.
- Neurologic examination is usually indicative of cervical myelopathy (e.g., upper motor neuron signs to all four limbs), cerebellovestibular dysfunction (head tilt, resting nystagmus, circling, loss of balance, cerebellar ataxia, intention tremor, loss of menace response despite normal vision), or both.
- Neck and/or head pain on palpation is often present.

ETIOLOGY AND PATHOPHYSIOLOGY

- The underlying problem is a malformed caudal occipital bone region, which is probably an inherited trait.

- The malformed occiput leads to cerebellar compression and constriction of the cervicomedullary junction at the level of the foramen magnum.
- Over time, the meninges at the constricted cervicomedullary junction become progressively hypertrophied.
- Pressure in intracranial and spinal cerebrospinal fluid (CSF) spaces builds over time; CSF is preferentially diverted into the central canal region of the cervical spinal cord (with resultant syringohydromyelia).

DIAGNOSIS

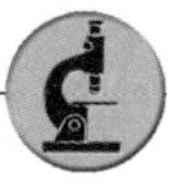

DIFFERENTIAL DIAGNOSIS

Differential diagnosis depends on the nature of the neurologic dysfunction in an individual patient:

- For example, in a dog with COMS that has multifocal central nervous system dysfunction, a likely differential diagnosis would be granulomatous meningoencephalomyelitis.
- In a dog with COMS manifesting with neck pain alone, a likely differential diagnosis would be intervertebral disk extrusion/protrusion.

INITIAL DATABASE

- The diagnosis of COMS is dependent on magnetic resonance imaging (MRI), especially the mid-sagittal T2-weighted view.
- CSF analysis is often performed to rule out concurrent inflammatory brain/spinal cord disease.

TREATMENT

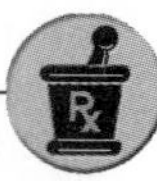

THERAPEUTIC GOAL(S)

The therapeutic goal is to halt disease progression and achieve either improvement or resolution of clinical signs of neurologic dysfunction.

ACUTE GENERAL TREATMENT

- Most dogs respond favorably to oral prednisone therapy (e.g., 0.5 mg/kg PO q 12h, tapering if chronic use).
- Excessive scratching activity is usually ameliorated with oral gabapentin (10 mg/kg, PO, q 8h).

CHRONIC TREATMENT

In most cases, surgical decompression of the foramen magnum (FMD) is indicated to achieve long-term therapeutic success.

POSSIBLE COMPLICATIONS

- Long-term corticosteroid administration can lead to side effects. These can vary from mild (e.g., weight gain, polyuria and polydipsia) to severe (e.g., life-threatening gastrointestinal disturbance).
- Potential surgical complications include intraoperative/early postoperative death (rare), postoperative worsening of neurologic status (uncommon and usually temporary), and need for future reoperation (typically due to excessive scar formation at FMD site).

PROGNOSIS AND OUTCOME

- There is little information regarding prognosis for COMS.
- Most dogs respond favorably to medical therapy; however, the disease tends to progress over time. In one study, 5 of 10 dogs with COMS that were treated medically were euthanized within 2 years due to disease progression.
- Surgical therapy (FMD) is associated with an 81% success rate. The reoperative rate is 25%.

PEARLS & CONSIDERATIONS

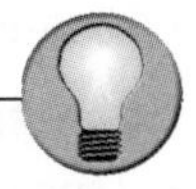

COMMENTS

- Success of surgery appears to be inversely related to duration of clinical signs before surgical intervention.
- Anecdotally, the author has seen fewer postoperative recurrences in cases that underwent cranioplasty performed in conjunction with FMD.

SUGGESTED READING

Dewey CW, et al: Caudal occipital malformation syndrome in dogs. *Compend Contin Educ Pract Vet* 26:886, 2004.

Dewey CW, et al: Foramen magnum decompression for treatment of caudal occipital malformation syndrome in dogs. *J Am Vet Med Assoc* 227:1270, 2005.

Dewey CW, et al: Foramen magnum decompression with cranioplasty for treatment of caudal occipital malformation syndrome in dogs. *J Vet Intern Med* (abstract) in press, 2006.

Rusbridge C, et al: Inheritance of occipital bone hypoplasia (Chiari type I malformation) in cavalier King Charles spaniels. *J Vet Intern Med* 18:673, 2004.

AUTHOR & EDITOR: **CURTIS W. DEWEY**

Cerebellar Abiotrophy

BASIC INFORMATION

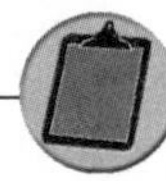

DEFINITION

The spontaneous, premature, progressive degeneration of fully developed cerebellar tissue. Specifically, it involves the loss and degeneration of Purkinje cells (most commonly) within the cerebellar cortex. In contrast, cerebellar hypoplasia is the incomplete development of the cerebellum as a result of an in utero or perinatal insult or genetic abnormality.

SYNONYM(S)

Cerebellar cortical degeneration

EPIDEMIOLOGY

SPECIES, AGE, SEX

- Cerebellar abiotrophy has been reported in dogs and, less commonly, cats.
- The age of onset varies by breed and species:
  - Early onset of clinical signs (birth to 3 to 4 weeks of age) is seen in the beagle, miniature poodle, rough-coated collie, Irish setter, Airedale terrier, coton de tulear, Finnish harrier, Jack Russell terrier, Rhodesian ridgeback, and Samoyed.
  - Dogs that show clinical signs from 6 weeks to 6 months of age include the Australian kelpie, Bernese mountain dog, border collie, bull mastiff, coton de tulear, Gordon setter, Kerry blue terrier, and Labrador retriever.
  - Mixed-breed cats also show clinical signs between the ages of 6 to 16 weeks.
  - Late-onset cerebellar abiotrophy is reported in the English sheepdog, American Staffordshire terrier, Brittany spaniel, and the Siamese and domestic short-haired cat.
- There is no apparent sex predisposition.

GENETICS AND BREED PREDISPOSITION: The genetic basis, where established, is an autosomal recessive pattern, affecting both sexes equally. See Species, Age, Sex above for specific breed predispositions.

CLINICAL PRESENTATION

HISTORY, CHIEF COMPLAINT: Typically, animals are normal at birth and present for progressive cerebellar ataxia or other cerebellar clinical signs beginning at the age appropriate for the particular breed.

There is no known trauma history or toxin exposure, and the animals are usually otherwise healthy.

PHYSICAL EXAM FINDINGS

- Clinical signs reflect cerebellar dysfunction and may include:
  - Cerebellar ataxia
  - Base wide stance
  - Truncal swaying
  - Intention tremors
  - Nystagmus
  - Poor menace response with normal vision
  - Hypermetric gait
  - Opisthotonos
- Postural responses and spinal reflexes are within normal limits
  - Care must be taken to support the animal's weight when performing postural responses, because the animal's balance is often abnormal.

ETIOLOGY AND PATHOPHYSIOLOGY

The cause of cerebellar abiotrophy is unknown. However, it is believed to be an intrinsic metabolic defect such as a defect in glutamate metabolism, causing excitotoxic injury to the cerebellar Purkinje cells.

DIAGNOSIS

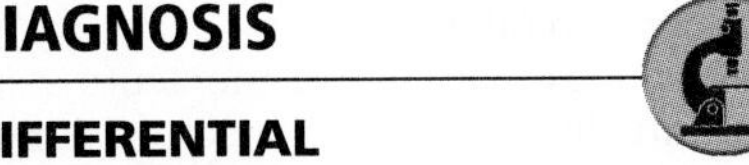

DIFFERENTIAL DIAGNOSIS

- Cerebellar hypoplasia should not be confused with this disorder, because hypoplasia is a nonprogressive disorder, and clinical signs are present at the onset of ambulation.
- Differential diagnoses include inherited lysosomal storage diseases (gangliosidosis, mannosidosis, hereditary neuroaxonal dystrophy, others), inflammatory causes such as granulomatous meningoencephalitis, and other congenital causes such as quadrigeminal cisternal cysts and caudal occipital malformation syndrome. Diseases less likely are infectious causes secondary to *Cryptococcus neoformans*, canine distemper virus, feline infectious peritonitis, *Toxoplasma gondii*, and tick-borne agents.

INITIAL DATABASE

- The diagnosis is based on signalment, history, and physical and neurologic clinical exams.
- Typically, initial diagnostics and neurodiagnostics are normal and not useful in the antemortem diagnosis of this disorder.

ADVANCED OR CONFIRMATORY TESTING

Definitive diagnosis of cerebellar abiotrophy is gained histologically at the time of necropsy. The only gross abnormality noted is a decreased cerebellar mass (<10% of the total brain weight). Unique to the Kerry blue terrier is a pallor gelatinous change, and cavitation of the caudate nuclei. Histologically, lesions are confined to the cortex and include symmetric degeneration and loss of Purkinje cells with subsequent proliferation of astroglia (Bergmann astrocytes). Secondary to Purkinje cell loss, Wallerian degeneration of the white matter of the folia may occur. The molecular layer is reduced in size because of a decreased number of cell processes due to Purkinje cell loss. The granular layer is also reduced in thickness with a diminished granular cell population, which is related to the severity of the loss of Purkinje cells.

TREATMENT

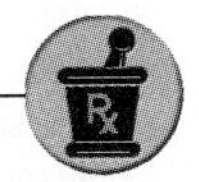

THERAPEUTIC GOAL(S)

Because there are no effective treatments for this progressive disorder, therapeutic goals are palliative only.

PROGNOSIS AND OUTCOME

Prognosis is grave because this disease is progressive (both slowly in certain breeds and rapidly in others). Rarely, the clinical signs may stabilize, as seen in the rough-coated collie.

PEARLS & CONSIDERATIONS

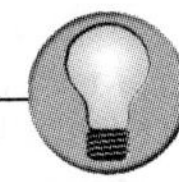

COMMENTS

- Cerebellar abiotrophy must be differentiated from cerebellar hypoplasia, which is a nonprogressive disease that results from the abnormal development of the cerebellum with some differentiation of tissue.
- Unlike abiotrophy, which involves an intrinsic metabolic defect, hypoplasia results from an extrinsic cause, most notably a parvovirus. For example, kittens infected with the feline panleukopenia virus either in utero or in the perinatal period may develop cerebellar dysfunction secondary to cerebellar hypoplasia. The virus causes inflammation and destruction of cells in the external germinal layer of the cerebellum, which results in failure to reach normal size.
- Another difference between hypoplasia and abiotrophy is that with hypoplasia, clinical signs are first noted at the onset of ambulation. Due to the disease's nonprogressive nature, most cats will compensate for the dysfunction, or the clinical signs may lessen. Therefore, this disease carries a more favorable prognosis than cerebellar abiotrophy.

SUGGESTED READING

Inada S, et al: Study of hereditary cerebellar degeneration in cats. *Am J Vet Res* 57(3):296-301, 1996.

Sanders SG, Bagley RS: Cerebellar diseases and tremor syndromes. In Dewey CW (ed): *A Practical Guide to Canine and Feline Neurology*. Ames, IA, Iowa State Press, 2003, pp 252-256.

Summers BA, Cummings JF, de Lahunta A: Degenerative diseases of the central nervous system. In Summers BA, Cummings JF, de Lahunta A: *Veterinary Neuropathology*. St. Louis, Mosby, 1995, pp 300-305.

AUTHOR: **KERRY SMITH BAILEY**

EDITOR: **CURTIS W. DEWEY**

Chagas' Disease

BASIC INFORMATION

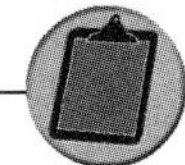

DEFINITION

Chagas' disease is a rare condition caused by infection with the hemoflagellate protozoa, *Trypanosoma cruzi (T.cruzi)*, resulting primarily in cardiomyopathy.

SYNONYM(S)

American Trypanosomiasis

EPIDEMIOLOGY

SPECIES, AGE, SEX

- Hunting dogs have been shown to be at risk for increased exposure. One study in 1995 found the disease to be endemic in a population of Walker hounds in Virginia. Animals that present with acute disease usually are younger than one year of age.
- Limited information on infection in cats.

RISK FACTOR: Exposure to the vector is the primary risk factor.

CONTAGION AND ZOONOSIS

- *T. cruzi* infects dogs and humans via vector arthropods ("kissing bugs," family Reduviidae). Reservoir mammals include armadillos, opossums, raccoons, dogs, and cats.
- The disease can be transmitted from the blood of infected dogs to human beings

via the same vector. Blood transfusions and organ transplantation have been implicated in infection in humans.

GEOGRAPHY AND SEASONALITY: *T. cruzi* infection is a major human health problem in South America, Mexico and Central America. Cases of canine infections are on the rise in the Southern United States, primarily in Texas, close to the Mexican border.

CLINICAL PRESENTATION

DISEASE FORMS/SUBTYPES: The disease occurs in three stages:
- Acute stage
- An extended latent period if the patient survives the acute stage
- Chronic stage

HISTORY, CHIEF COMPLAINT: Most commonly related to cardiac dysfunction (dilated cardiomyopathy) which occurs in the chronic stage. Animals usually present with acute signs including exercise intolerance, weakness, collapse or sudden death of a healthy dog. Generalized lymphadenopathy may be seen prior to acute disease.

PHYSICAL EXAM FINDINGS
- Acute stage: lethargy, pale mucous membranes, weak pulse, tachycardia, hepatomegaly, splenomegaly. Anorexia, diarrhea possible.
- Latent stage: Clinical signs appear to regress.
- Chronic stage: Animals that survive the acute form of the disease may have signs of progressive right sided heart disease including hepatomegaly with ascites, pleural effusion, and jugular vein distention.

ETIOLOGY AND PATHOPHYSIOLOGY

- Three life stages of the organism:
  - Trypomastigotes (flagellated form found in blood)
  - Amastigotes (nonflagellated intracellular form)
  - Epimastigotes (flagellated form found in vector)
- Arthropod vector, which contains epimastigote form of the organism, defecates during feeding.
  - The bite of reduviid bugs is usually nocturnal and nonpainful (unnoticed by the victim)
- Epimastigotes enter vertebrate hosts and then enter macrophages/monocytes, forming amastigotes.
- After binary fission of amastigotes into trypomastigotes, host cell ruptures.
- Trypomastigotes enter circulation, causing damage primarily in cardiomyocytes.
- Organism/infection may also be transmitted via blood transfusions, transplacentally, or by ingestion of infected tissue or milk.

DIAGNOSIS

DIFFERENTIAL DIAGNOSIS

- Idiopathic dilated cardiomyopathy
- Myocarditis of other cause (see Myocarditis, p 728)
- Other causes of right heart failure (heartworm disease—caval syndrome; pericardial effusion; others)

INITIAL DATABASE

- Complete blood count: lymphocytosis common
- Blood smear stained with Giemsa or Wright's stain: may provide definitive diagnosis if organism is seen (trypomastigotes; flagellate organisms, two to three times as long as the diameter of erythrocytes)
- Serum biochemstry profile: liver enzymes commonly elevated
- Thoracic radiographs: cardiomegaly, with or without evidence of congestive heart failure (e.g., pleural effusion), in chronic stage
- Cytology of lymph nodes, buffy coat or ascitic fluid: may reveal trypomastigotes before or during acute disease
- Electrocardiography (ECG): a variety of arrhythmias and ECG changes can occur with Chagas' disease:
  - Supraventricular arrhythmias
  - Ventricular arrhythmias
  - ST segment elevation or depression
  - Low amplitude QRS complexes
  - First-, second-, or third-degree AV block, or right bundle branch block

ADVANCED OR CONFIRMATORY TESTING

- Serologic testing: titer usually positive at 3 weeks postinfection
  - Indirect fluorescent antibody
  - Direct hemagglutination
  - Complement fixation
- PCR
- Blood culture: may reveal trypomastigotes
- Histopathologic evaluation of cardiac tissue: may reveal amastigotes

TREATMENT

THERAPEUTIC GOAL(S)

- Control of the organism (elimination of infection often is not possible)
- Management of clinical signs caused by congestive heart failure and/or arrhythmias

ACUTE GENERAL TREATMENT

- See Heart Failure, Acute/Decompensated, p 458
- Nifurtimox: 2–7 mg/kg PO q 6h for 3 to 5 months
  - May be difficult to obtain
  - Should be implemented during acute stage; helps to blunt severity of acute stage, but ineffective if administered only in chronic stage
  - Toxicity common (e.g., vomiting, anorexia, neurologic signs) but few alternatives available
- Glucocorticoids: anti-inflammatory dose (prednisone 0.5–1.0 mg/kg PO q 12–24h)

CHRONIC TREATMENT

Treatment for chronic management of congestive heart failure (see Heart Failure, Chronic, p 459) if needed

POSSIBLE COMPLICATIONS

Dilated cardiomyopathy usually occurs 8 to 36 months after the acute stage.

PROGNOSIS AND OUTCOME

- Prognosis is guarded, with survival time in animals surviving the acute stage being 0 to 60 months.
- Most dogs that survive the acute stage eventually develop dilated cardiomyopathy.

PEARLS & CONSIDERATIONS

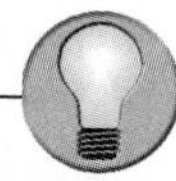

PREVENTION

- Blood products from animals with known infection should be handled with caution by all laboratory staff.
- Vector control is the primary form of prevention.
- Limit the contact with infected reservoir hosts such as opossums, raccoons, and armadillos.
- Screen all blood donors closely that are from endemic areas.

SUGGESTED READING

Bradley KK, et al: Prevalence of American trypanosomiasis (Chagas' disease) among dogs in Oklahoma. *JAVMA* 217:12, 2000.

Busch MP, et al: Current and emerging infectious risks of blood transfusions. *JAMA* 289:8, 2003.

AUTHOR: **KHRISTEN J. CARLSON**

EDITOR: **DOUGLASS K. MACINTIRE**

Chemotherapy: Adverse Reactions

BASIC INFORMATION

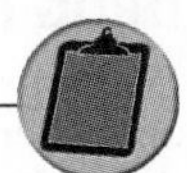

DEFINITION

Chemotherapy targets rapidly dividing cells. However, normal proliferating cells (gastrointestinal [GI] epithelial, bone marrow, others) may be affected, resulting in adverse reactions. In addition, some chemotherapy agents cause unique toxicities.

EPIDEMIOLOGY

SPECIES, AGE, SEX

- Drugs that should not be administered to cats:
  - Cisplatin: fatal pulmonary edema
  - 5-Fluorouracil: fatal neurologic signs
- Toxicities not generally observed clinically in cats:
  - Cyclophosphamide: hemorrhagic cystitis
  - Doxorubicin: documented histopathologic changes, but cardiotoxicity not seen clinically

GENETICS AND BREED PREDISPOSITION: Collies, shelties, border collies, and sight hounds have been reported to have mutations in the MDR1 gene, which may result in decreased expression of P glycoprotein and increased risk of toxicity with drugs that are substrates for this protein.

RISK FACTORS

- Significant infiltration of the bone marrow by neoplastic cells: myelosuppression.
- Neoplastic GI involvement: GI toxicity.
- Clinically ill patients may be more likely to develop adverse effects and should receive concurrent supportive care.
- Preexisting cardiomyopathy: increased risk of doxorubicin cardiotoxicity.
- Preexisting renal dysfunction: increased risk of toxicity with renally excreted drugs; increased risk of cisplatin nephrotoxicity.
- Preexisting hepatic dysfunction: increased risk of toxicity with drugs eliminated by the liver and possible increased risk of hepatotoxicity.

CLINICAL PRESENTATION

HISTORY, CHIEF COMPLAINT: Administration of associated chemotherapeutic agent.

PHYSICAL EXAM FINDINGS

- Adverse reactions occurring during administration:
  - Allergic reactions (L-asparaginase, doxorubicin, taxanes [rarely used])
    - Facial swelling, erythema, urticaria, panting, agitation, vomiting, diarrhea, dyspnea, tachypnea, collapse, hypotension
  - Extravasation injury (vincristine/vinblastine, doxorubicin, actinomycin D, dacarbazine, mechlorethamine, cisplatin)
    - No immediate signs
    - Erythema, inflammation, licking site 7 to 14 days post-treatment
    - Can progress to slough of skin and subcutis
  - Acute vomiting (common: cisplatin, dacarbazine, streptozotocin. Less common: doxorubicin, cyclophosphamide, mechlorethamine, procarbazine)
    - Vomiting during/within 24 hours of chemotherapy
- Delayed adverse reactions:
  - GI toxicity (common: doxorubicin, MOPP (mechlorethamine, vincristine, procarbazine, prednisone) protocol, cisplatin, dacarbazine. Less common: vincristine, vinblastine, cyclophosphamide, mitoxantrone, carboplatin, actinomycin, methotrexate)
    - Vomiting, diarrhea, lethargy, anorexia 2 to 5 days after chemotherapy
    - Vincristine: may cause paralytic ileus and associated GI signs
    - Doxorubicin: may cause life-threatening hemorrhagic colitis
  - Myelosuppression/sepsis (most common: CCNU (lomustine; 1-[2-chlorethyl]-3-cyclohexyl-nitrosourea), carboplatin. Also common: doxorubicin, mitoxantrone, cyclophosphamide [especially combined with vincristine])
    - Usually no overt manifestations
    - Possible: lethargy, loss of appetite, fever with sepsis generally around 7 days postadministration
    - Neutrophil count lowest (nadir) generally 7 days after administration
    - Onset of signs with cisplatin, carboplatin, and CCNU (in cats) is more variable (7 days or later)
- Unique adverse reactions:
  - Cardiac toxicity (doxorubicin)
    - Arrhythmia, exercise intolerance, weakness, collapse, tachypnea, tachycardia
  - Hemorrhagic cystitis (cyclophosphamide, ifosfamide)
    - Stranguria, pollakiuria, hematuria
  - Nepthrotoxicity (cisplatin, streptozotocin. Rare: doxorubicin, CCNU. Extremely rare: carboplatin)
    - Often no clinical signs
    - With progression, polyuria, polydipsia, lethargy, decreased appetite
  - Hepatotoxicity (CCNU, streptozotocin)
    - Often no clinical signs
    - If progresses, icterus, lethargy, loss of appetite, GI signs, and abdominal effusion

ETIOLOGY AND PATHOPHYSIOLOGY

- Allergic reactions: L-asparaginase: type I hypersensitivity reaction. Doxorubicin: stimulates mast cell degranulation.
- Extravasation injury: vesicant injury to local tissue.
- Acute vomiting: irritation of chemoreceptor trigger zone.
- Gastrointestinal toxicity: injury to GI crypt epithelium.
- Myelosuppression/sepsis: Injury to proliferating bone marrow cells causes neutropenia and possibly thrombocytopenia. Severe neutropenia allows opportunistic infection, usually by GI bacteria (usually gram-negative, but gram-positive and anaerobic infections possible).
- Cardiac toxicity: cumulative toxicity (doses ≥180–240 mg/m^2). Myocardium has less catalase; damaged by free radicals produced by doxorubicin. Causes arrhythmias and decreased contractility, progressing to dilated cardiomyopathy weeks to months after treatment.
- Hemorrhagic cystitis: metabolite (acrolein) directly toxic to the bladder urothelium.
- Nephrotoxicity: cisplatin, streptozotocin: tubular injury and decreased glomerular filtration (cisplatin).

DIAGNOSIS

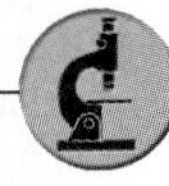

INITIAL DATABASE

- Complete blood count (CBC), serum biochemistry profile, urinalysis:
  - Neutropenia, possibly thrombocytopenia (myelosuppression)
  - Azotemia, low urine specific gravity (USG) (nephrotoxicity)
  - Hematuria (hemorrhagic cystitis)
  - Elevated liver enzymes (hepatotoxicity)
- Additional tests (e.g., diagnostic imaging) as determined by history, exam, and lab test results

TREATMENT

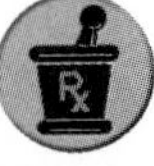

THERAPEUTIC GOAL(S)

Control of toxic effects and prevention of secondary complications

ACUTE GENERAL TREATMENT

- Adverse reactions occurring during administration:
  - Allergic reactions
    - Depends on severity.
    - Dexamethasone SP 0.5–2 mg/kg IV.
    - Diphenhydramine 1–2 mg/kg IM.
    - Intravenous fluids 90 ml/kg/hr (dog), 50 ml/kg/hr (cat).
    - Epinephrine if severe (dilute 1 ml of 1:1000 solution in 9 ml of 0.9% NaCl. Give 0.1 ml/kg of 1:10,000 solution IV).
  - Extravasation injury
    - Aspirate drug back before removing catheter.
    - Vincristine/vinblastine: infuse 1 ml 1% hyaluronidase for each milliliter extravasated.
    - Apply compresses (cold for doxorubicin; warm for vincristine/vinblastine) for 10 minutes q 6h for 72 hours after extravasation.
    - Doxorubicin: administer dexrazoxane (anecdotal dose: 400–600 mg/m^2 IV within 3 hours of administration, repeat at 24 and 48 hours). Topical DMSO (dimethyl sulfoxide) gel may also be helpful.
    - Wound management: E collar, clip/clean, topical or systemic antibiotic, ± topical or systemic anti-inflammatory.
    - Surgical debridement/grafting if severe.
  - Acute vomiting
    - Stop administration.
    - Nothing by mouth.
    - Antiemetic therapy (see section on delayed vomiting for drugs and dosages below).
    - IV fluid support if indicated.
- Delayed adverse reactions:
  - Gastrointestinal toxicity
    - Nothing by mouth.
    - Patient acting normally, self-limiting vomiting: water trial then bland diet trial.
    - Patient acting normally, diarrhea not bloody or watery: bland diet, consider metronidazole 15 mg/kg PO q 12h for colitis.
    - Patient lethargic, vomiting/diarrhea continuing, or watery or bloody diarrhea: admit to hospital for supportive care.
      - Intravenous fluids
      - Antiemetics
        - Metoclopramide: 0.2–0.5 mg/kg SC q 8h or IV as a CRI at 1.1–2.2 mg/kg/day. Also for vincristine-induced ileus
        - If refractory:
          - Dolasetron (dogs/cats): 0.6–1 mg/kg IV slowly q 12–24h
          - Ondansetron (dogs): 0.1–1 mg/kg IV slowly q 8–24h; (cats) 0.1–0.15 mg/kg IV slowly q 6–12h
      - H_2 receptor antagonist
        - Ranitidine 1–2 mg/kg slow IV q 12h
      - Antibiotic therapy if bloody vomit/diarrhea, neutropenic, or febrile
      - Enteral feeding tube if prolonged anorexia (rare)
      - Usually resolves in 2 to 3 days
  - Myelosuppression/sepsis
    - Usually no treatment required. Counts generally normalize within 2 to 3 days (except carboplatin-prolonged nadirs).
    - If neutrophil count <1000 cells/μl, consider prophylactic antibiotics. For dogs that are not Doberman pinschers and do not have decreased tear production, a common choice is sufadiazine-trimethoprim 15 mg/kg PO q 12h for 5 to 7 days. Cats do not usually need prophylactic antibiotics.
    - If febrile or ill, admit to hospital for intravenous fluids and intravenous antibiotics:
      - Base on culture and sensitivity if available (urine, blood, wound swab)
      - Empiric option while culture results pending: ampicillin 22 mg/kg IV q 8h with either amikacin 20 mg/kg IV q 24h (caution: risk of renal injury) or enrofloxacin 5 mg/kg dilute and given slowly IV q 12h (dogs) or q 24h (cats)
- Unique adverse reactions:
  - Cardiac toxicity (doxorubicin)
    - No treatment beyond management of cardiac disease.
    - Avoid additional doxorubicin.
  - Hemorrhagic cystitis (HC)
    - Treat bacterial cystitis if present.
    - Self-limiting, but may take weeks to months to resolve.
    - Anti-inflammatory: nonsteroidal anti-inflammatory drug or prednisone.
    - Oxybutynin hydrochloride (0.2 mg/kg PO q 8–12h) for straining, pollakiuria.
    - Instillation of diluted dimethyl sulfoxide into the bladder may be helpful if refractory.
    - After HC, cyclophosphamide should not be administered again. Often chlorambucil is substituted.
  - Nephrotoxicity
    - Discontinue drug.
    - Treatment usually not necessary, but if clinical or acute renal failure, hospitalize for therapy.
  - Hepatotoxicity
    - Discontinue drug.
    - Treat hepatic dysfunction if indicated.

CHRONIC TREATMENT

Cardiac toxicity, chronic bone marrow toxicity, nephrotoxicity, and hepatotoxicity may require chronic management.

DRUG INTERACTIONS

Many possible interactions of chemotherapy agents with each other and other drugs. It is the responsibility of veterinarians treating patients with chemotherapy to review possible interactions associated with each agent before administration.

RECOMMENDED MONITORING

For all patients undergoing chemotherapy:

- CBC at the expected time of the neutrophil nadir the first time they receive each drug. CBC rechecked as indicated, especially before administration of potentially myelosuppressive chemotherapy.
- A serum chemistry profile should be performed every 2 to 3 months or more frequently if indicated.
- A urinalysis should be performed every 3 to 6 months or more often if indicated.

PROGNOSIS AND OUTCOME

With appropriate treatment and supportive care, most patients will recover from delayed adverse reactions and those that occur during administration. Cardiac toxicity, chronic bone marrow toxicity, nephrotoxicity, and hepatoxicity generally do not resolve but may improve or stabilize.

PEARLS & CONSIDERATIONS

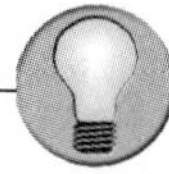

COMMENTS

- It is essential that clinicians treating veterinary cancer patients review possible complications associated with chemotherapy agents so that they are able to take axppropriate preventive measures and manage adverse effects.
- It is also important to review metabolism and excretion of chemotherapy agents when treating patients with organ dysfunction, because dose reductions or avoidance of certain drugs may be necessary.

PREVENTION

Double check all dose calculations, route of administration, and patient's history, exam, and lab test results, prior to administration.

- Allergic reactions
  - Premedicate (20 minutes pretreatment): diphenhydramine 2 mg/kg IM ± dexamethasone SP 0.5 mg/kg SQ),

then monitor patient 30 minutes post-treatment.
  - Administer doxorubicin slowly (1 mg/min).
- Extravasation injury
  - Administer chemotherapy through intravenous catheter placed on first attempt in vein not punctured within 24 hours.
  - Comfortably restrain patient; sedate if fractious.
  - Flush catheter with 3 to 5 ml of 0.9% NaCl before and after administration.
  - Monitor site during treatment.
- Acute vomiting
  - Administer chemotherapy slowly.
  - Pretreatment antiemetic agents are given prior to cisplatin, streptozotocin, or dacarbazine administration. Options include:
    - Butorphanol (dog): 0.2–0.4 mg/kg IM 20 minutes before chemotherapy.
    - Dolasetron (dog/cat): 0.6–1 mg/kg slow IV immediately before chemotherapy.
    - Ondansetron (dog): 0.1–1 mg/kg PO or IV slowly 30 minutes prior and 90 minutes after starting cisplatin; (cat) 0.1–0.3 mg/kg IV slowly 15 minutes before and 12 hours after chemotherapy.
  - For less emetogenic agents:
  - Metoclopramide (dog/cat): 0.2- 0.5 mg/kg PO or SC q 8h starting at least 30 minutes before treatment.
- Gastrointestinal toxicity
  - Double check chemotherapy doses.
  - If patient hospitalized with gastrointestinal toxicity, reduce subsequent doses of that drug by 25%.
  - Prophylactic antiemetic if history of gastrointestinal toxicity (metoclopramide 0.2–0.5 mg/kg PO q 8h).
- Myelosuppression/sepsis
  - CBC before myelosuppressive chemotherapy. Do not treat if <3000 neutrophils/µl or <100,000 platelets/µl.
  - Due to the potential for cumulative thrombocytopenia, CCNU chemotherapy may need to be discontinued if a pretreatment CBC reveals a platelet count that has decreased below the reference range.
  - Double check chemotherapy doses.
  - CBC at expected neutrophil nadir the first time patient receives each agent.
  - If neutrophil count at nadir is <1000 cells/µl, reduce subsequent doses of that drug by 25%.
  - If overdose, treatment with recombinant human granulocyte colony stimulating factor (rhG-CSF) 5 µg/kg q 24h SQ for 3 to 5 days starting 24 hours after treatment.
- Cardiac toxicity. Do not treat dogs with myocardial dysfunction.
  - Cardiac evaluation for breeds at risk for dilated cardiomyopathy and dogs with cardiac abnormalities (heart murmur, arrhythmia, cardiomegaly) before doxorubicin.
  - Limit total lifetime cumulative doxorubicin dose to <180–240 mg/m^2; substitute noncardiac toxic agents (mitoxantrone, actinomycin-D) after 150 mg/m^2.
  - Dexrazoxane: 10 mg for every 1 mg of doxorubicin given IV within 30 minutes of each dose. Not helpful once cardiac injury present. Not used routinely in veterinary oncology.
- Hemorrhagic cystitis
  - Administer in morning.
  - Give furosemide (2 mg/kg PO, IV, or SC) with cyclophosphamide.
  - Ad lib access to water.
  - Encourage frequent urination.
  - After HC, cyclophosphamide should not be administered again. Often chlorambucil is substituted.
- Nephrotoxicity
  - Urine specific gravity and serum creatinine before every dose of cisplatin, streptozotocin.
  - Serum biochemistry profiles and urinalyses for all patients at least every 3 months, more frequently if indicated
  - Fluid diuresis protocol required with cisplatin, streptozotocin.
- Hepatotoxicity
  - Check liver enzymes with every other dose or more frequently if indicated; discontinue drug if an increase in liver enzymes is noted.

CLIENT EDUCATION

Provide information that allows clients to recognize adverse effects of chemotherapy and encourage them to seek veterinary care promptly.

SUGGESTED READING

Chun R, et al: Cancer chemotherapy. In Withrow SJ, MacEwen EG (eds): *Small Animal Clinical Oncology*, ed 3. Philadelphia, Elsevier, 2001, pp 92–118.

Kisseberth WC, MacEwen EG: Complications of cancer and its treatment: Adverse effects. In Withrow SJ, MacEwen EG (eds): *Small Animal Clinical Oncology*, ed 3. Philadelphia, Elsevier, 2001, pp 198–215.

Moore AS, Ogilvie GK: Treatment of nausea and vomiting. In Ogilvie GK, Moore AS (eds): *Feline Oncology: A Comprehensive Guide to Compassionate Care*. Trenton, NJ, Veterinary Learning Systems, 2001, pp 109–112.

Rassnick KM: Toxicology of antineoplastic treatments. In Wingfield WE, Raffe MR (eds): *The Veterinary ICU Book*. Jackson, WY, Teton NewMedia, 2002, pp 1137–1146.

AUTHOR: **NICOLE C. NORTHRUP**
EDITOR: **KENNETH M. RASSNICK**

Cheyletiellosis

BASIC INFORMATION

DEFINITION

Cheyletiellosis is a highly contagious, zoonotic skin mite infestation of dogs and cats caused by *Cheyletiella* spp.

SYNONYM(S)

Walking dandruff

EPIDEMIOLOGY

SPECIES, AGE, SEX

- *Cheyletiella blakei*: cats.
- *C. yasguri*: dogs.
- *C. parasitivorax*: rabbits (cross-infections to other species, including humans, are common).
- In general, young animals are more frequently affected.

GENETICS AND BREED PREDISPOSITION: Cocker spaniels and long-haired cats appear predisposed.

RISK FACTORS: Contact with an infected animal (may or may not be showing clinical signs; infections may not necessarily produce overt manifestations of pruritus or other signs).

CONTAGION AND ZOONOSIS

- Since cheyletiellosis is a zoonotic disease, humans are at risk if exposed to an infected individual pet (whether or not overt clinical signs are present), and likewise a pet may acquire the parasite from an infected human.
- *Cheyletiella* spp. are not host-specific and may transfer readily between dogs, cats, and rabbits.
- The mites are very contagious, so animals in shelter and breeding establishments and those that visit groomers can be at a higher risk.

CLINICAL PRESENTATION

HISTORY, CHIEF COMPLAINT

- Scale ("dandruff") is common, may be copious, and is usually noted dorsally.
- The patient may or may not be pruritic.
- Cats may present for overgrooming.
- Apparently normal individual pets may be presented for evaluation because of suspect human lesions.

PHYSICAL EXAM FINDINGS

- The scale is most frequently noted over the dorsum. It may consist of just flakes of dried skin, or a combination of scale and *Cheyletiella* mites.
- This scale is often referred to as "walking dandruff" because it can be seen to move on the examination room table (i.e., some of the scales are mites).
- Pruritus varies from none to severe.
- Erythema of the skin may or may not be noted.

ETIOLOGY AND PATHOPHYSIOLOGY

- *Cheyletiella* is a relatively large mite (visible to the naked eye), with prominent hooklike mouth parts, that lives on the skin surface and feeds on surface debris and exudates. These mites form pseudotunnels in the surface keratin.
- The entire life cycle is completed on the host within 21 days.
- The mite is an obligate parasite, since the larvae, nymphs, and adult males die soon after leaving the host.
- The mite eggs, smaller than lice eggs, are loosely attached to the hairs.
- Eggs are shed into the environment with the pet's hair and may be an important source of reinfestation.

DIAGNOSIS

DIFFERENTIAL DIAGNOSIS

- In dogs, differential diagnosis depends on the clinical presentation.
- If only scaling is present, differential diagnoses include:
  - Primary seborrhea
  - Ectoparasites (*Demodex, Otodectes*, fleas, lice)
  - Ill thrift or nutritional imbalance (intestinal parasitism, poor nutrition, etc.)
- If intense pruritus is present, differentials include:
  - Sarcoptic mange
  - Allergies/hypersensitivities (atopy, flea bite hypersensitivity, other ectoparasite hypersensitivities, food allergy/adverse food reaction, contact hypersensitivity, drug hypersensitivity)
  - Bacterial infections (*Staphylococcus intermedius*)
  - Fungal infections (*Malassezia*, ringworm [dermatophytes])
- In cats, military dermatitis due to other causes such as flea allergy or other hypersensitivity should be considered as well as other causes of generalized seborrhea and pruritus.

INITIAL DATABASE

Diagnosis is based on the collection and identification of the mites. This can be difficult, especially in cats, because of grooming habits. The mites are relatively easy to kill since they live on the surface of the skin.

- The most reliable method involves picking up scale and debris from the coat or table with acetate tape (e.g., transparent-type Scotch tape) for microscopic examination.
- A flea comb can be useful for helping to collect the sample.

ADVANCED OR CONFIRMATORY TESTING

Cheyletiella eggs and mites can sometimes be identified in a fecal flotation.

TREATMENT

THERAPEUTIC GOAL(S)

- All in-contact animals should be treated (i.e., including animals in the same household, even if not showing clinical signs).
- Environmental treatment may be required in severe cases.

ACUTE GENERAL TREATMENT

- Weekly application for 3 to 4 weeks of insecticidal shampoos or sprays containing pyrethrins, 2% lime sulfur (e.g., Lym Dyp; DVM) or 0.025% amitraz (Mitaban; Pfizer) dips appears to be very effective.
- Two to four treatments of ivermectin (Ivomec Bovine Injection, 10 mg/ml, Merial) at 0.2-0.4 mg/kg PO or SQ (typical dose for 20 kg [44 lb] dog = 0.4-0.8 ml) at 7- to 14-day intervals are also effective but should not be used in collies and other sensitive individuals given possible neurologic side effects.
- The topical products selamectin (Revolution; Pfizer), imidacloprid (Advantage; Bayer), and fipronil (Frontline; Merial) are also claimed to be effective.

POSSIBLE COMPLICATIONS

- In collie breeds and other sensitive individuals, clinical signs of a reaction to ivermectin include hypersalivation, disorientation, ataxia, mydriasis (dilated pupils), coma, and possibly death if supportive care is not instituted. A different treatment should be used for such animals.
- Although amitraz is an effective therapy for cheyletiellosis, side effects and the risk to the operator are of concern, gloves must be worn, and treatment must be done in a well-ventilated area.
- Side effects of amitraz can include transient sedation, depression, lethargy, pruritus, gastrointestinal signs, and hyperglycemia (diabetics). Yohimbine (Yobine; Vet-A-Mix) can be used as an antidote when side effects are of concern. See Amitraz Toxicosis, p 54.

PROGNOSIS AND OUTCOME

Prognosis is good

PEARLS & CONSIDERATIONS

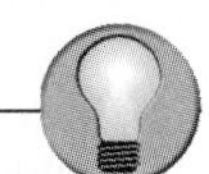

COMMENTS

Infected animals do not always show clinical signs of pruritus, erythema, or alopecia.

CLIENT EDUCATION

Humans transiently infected with *Cheyletiella* spp. may develop an uncomfortable, pruritic dermatosis characterized by papular lesions that typically affect the arms, legs, trunk, and buttocks. Any suspicion of human dermatopathy should prompt the individual to consult with a physician.

SUGGESTED READING

Chailleux N, Paradis M: Efficacy of selamectin in the treatment of naturally acquired cheyletiellosis in cats. *Can Vet J* 43(10):767-770, 2002.

Scott DW, Miller WH Jr, Griffin CE: In *Muller & Kirk's Small Animal Dermatology*, ed 6. Philadelphia, WB Saunders, 2001, pp 423-516.

AUTHORS: **JAN A. HALL, AMANDA P. AMARATUNGA**

EDITOR: **JAN A. HALL**

Chlamydiosis, Cat

BASIC INFORMATION

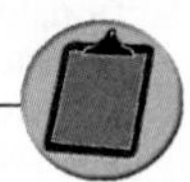

DEFINITION

A bacterial infection associated mainly with acute and chronic conjunctivitis in cats

SYNONYM(S)

Chlamydia psittaci infection (outdated; current name is *Chlamydophila felis*)
Chlamydophila felis infection
Feline pneumonitis (outdated term: the organism is primarily a conjunctival pathogen)

EPIDEMIOLOGY

SPECIES, AGE, SEX: The prevalence of *C. felis* in cats with upper respiratory tract disease has ranged from 10–31%. Cats <5 years old, and especially <1 year old, are predisposed. There is no strong sex predilection.
RISK FACTORS: Young age is the most significant risk factor.
CONTAGION AND ZOONOSIS: There are isolated reports of *C. felis*-associated conjunctivitis in humans, and possibly community-acquired pneumonia. Maintenance of hygienic conditions and prompt treatment of cats should help prevent human disease.
GEOGRAPHY AND SEASONALITY: Worldwide distribution; may be more common in summer.
ASSOCIATED CONDITIONS AND DISORDERS: May be associated with concurrent feline herpesvirus 1 or feline calicivirus infection.

CLINICAL PRESENTATION

HISTORY, CHIEF COMPLAINT
- Ocular discharge and redness
- Occasionally decreased appetite
- Nasal discharge
- Sneezing

PHYSICAL EXAM FINDINGS
- Blepharospasm
- Chemosis
- Conjunctivitis
- Serous to mucopurulent ocular discharge
- Serous to mucopurulent nasal discharge (always accompanied by conjunctivitis)
- Possible fever
- Possible vaginal discharge

ETIOLOGY AND PATHOPHYSIOLOGY

- *Chlamydophila felis* is an obligately intracellular bacterium related to gram-negative bacteria.
- The life cycle alternates between an extracellular, infectious elementary body and an intracellular reticulate body.
- Reticulate bodies divide within a cytoplasmic vacuole called an *inclusion*, and are released from the host cell as elementary bodies.
- Natural transmission probably occurs by close contact with other cats and their aerosols, and via fomites.
- The incubation period is 3 to 5 days, and infection may persist for months.
- Feline chlamydiosis is a systemic disease, and organisms are shed from the conjunctiva, vagina, and rectum.
- Recently, another chlamydial species has been identified in cats, *Neochlamydia hartmannellae*; the clinical significance of this organism is yet to be determined.

DIAGNOSIS

Diagnosis may be suspected based on clinical signs (i.e., marked persistent conjunctivitis) and response to appropriate antimicrobials

DIFFERENTIAL DIAGNOSIS

- Infectious causes:
  - Feline herpesvirus 1
  - Feline calicivirus
  - *Bordetella bronchiseptica*
  - *Mycoplasma* spp.
  - *Cryptococcus neoformans*
  - *Aspergillus* spp.
- Noninfective causes:
  - Eyelid and nasal neoplasia (including nasopharygeal polyps)
  - Dental disease
  - Congenital eyelid malformations
  - Palate defects
  - Chemical irritants
  - Foreign bodies
  - Trauma
  - Immune-mediated/inflammatory (e.g., eosinophilic keratoconjunctivitis)

INITIAL DATABASE

Conjunctival scrapings: may reveal inclusion bodies within epithelial cells when stained with Giemsa; notoriously unreliable

ADVANCED OR CONFIRMATORY TESTING

- Human enzyme-linked immunosorbent assay antigen kits for *Chlamydia trachomatis*: performed on conjunctival swabs, have variable sensitivity and specificity
- Cell culture: available in specialized laboratories, requires special transport media, and sensitivity varies depending on equipment and technical expertise
- Polymerase chain reaction (PCR): performed on conjunctival swabs, sensitivity and specificity varies with the laboratory; quality control may be problematic in some laboratories; ensure positive and negative extraction controls are included with each run
- Positive serology: correlates well with infection in unvaccinated cats, but reliable assays are not readily available

TREATMENT

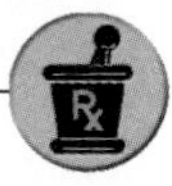

THERAPEUTIC GOAL(S)

Relieve clinical signs and eliminate infection.

ACUTE GENERAL TREATMENT

- Doxycycline, 10 mg/kg PO q 24h for at least 4 weeks.
- Treat all cats in the household simultaneously.
- Because infection is systemic, use of topical treatment alone is not likely to be effective.
- Doxycycline is superior to azithromycin.
- A 4-week course of amoxicillin-clavulanic acid (2.5 mg/kg PO q 12h) may also eliminate *C. felis*.

POSSIBLE COMPLICATIONS

- Risk of teeth discoloration in kittens if tetracyclines are used in the last 2 to 3 weeks of pregnancy or kittens in the first few months of life.
- Little evidence that this occurs with doxycycline; amoxicillin-clavulanic acid is an acceptable alternative in this situation.
- Administration of doxycycline liquid oral suspension minimizes the risk of doxycycline-induced esophagitis associated with tablets (or follow tablet administration with a water bolus by syringe).

RECOMMENDED MONITORING

Consider retesting with PCR or cell culture in problem cattery situations after treatment to ensure infection has been eliminated

PROGNOSIS AND OUTCOME

- Excellent in households with low numbers of cats.
- Fair in cattery situations; recurrent cases involve large numbers of cats and poor compliance. All cats in the household must be treated with the full course of antimicrobials and proper hygiene and quarantine maintained. Concurrent infections with feline calicivirus and feline herpesvirus 1 are a common problem.

PEARLS & CONSIDERATIONS

COMMENTS

- There is some evidence that *C. felis* may infect the reproductive tract and cause vaginal discharge. Abortion and infertility have been documented in some cats infected with *C. felis*, but in general it appears that *C. felis* does not cause feline reproductive disease.
- There is experimental evidence that *C. felis* may be associated with lameness in cats.

PREVENTION

- Maintenance of environmental hygiene in catteries and disinfection of fomites with a 1:32 solution of bleach in tap water, to which detergent may be added.
- Modified live and inactivated cell culture vaccines are available, which do not prevent infection or clinical signs, although the latter are reduced in severity.
  - Associated with atypical reactions in a small percentage of cats, including fever, anorexia, and lameness 7 to 21 days after vaccination
  - May be useful as part of a control program in catteries with endemic chlamydiosis

SUGGESTED READING

Dean R, et al: Use of quantitative real-time PCR to monitor the response of *Chlamydophila felis* infection to doxycycline treatment. *J Clin Microbiol* 43(4):1858-1864, 2005.

McDonald M, et al: A comparison of DNA amplification, isolation and serology for the detection of *Chlamydia psittaci* infection in cats. *Vet Rec* 143:97-101, 1998.

Sykes JE: Feline chlamydiosis. *Clin Tech Small Anim Pract* 20:129-134, 2005.

Von Bomhard W, et al: Detection of novel chlamydiae in cats with ocular disease. *Am J Vet Res* 64:1421-1428, 2003.

AUTHOR: **JANE SYKES**
EDITOR: **DOUGLASS K. MACINTIRE**

Chocolate Toxicosis

BASIC INFORMATION

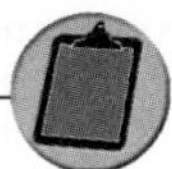

DEFINITION

Acute toxicosis from ingestion of chocolate products and byproducts

SYNONYM(S)

Methylxanthine toxicosis

EPIDEMIOLOGY

SPECIES, AGE, SEX: Dogs are most commonly affected; all breeds, ages, sexes susceptible.

RISK FACTORS: Animals with cardiac or seizure disorders may be at increased risk for signs.

GEOGRAPHY AND SEASONALITY: Toxicosis can occur year-round; most prevalent during holiday seasons, such as Easter, Christmas, and Valentine's Day.

CLINICAL PRESENTATION

DISEASE FORMS/SUBTYPES

- Severity and onset of signs depend on amount and type of chocolate ingested
- Chocolate and its byproducts contain methylxanthines; theobromine (primary) and caffeine (secondary), sugars, and fat
- See Table I-2 for methylxanthine content of products
- Variable individual sensitivity to methylxanthines
- Methylxanthine dosages:
  - 20-40 mg/kg: mild to moderate clinical signs
  - 40-50 mg/kg: cardiac arrhythmias; potentially life-threatening
  - >60 mg/kg: seizures

HISTORY, CHIEF COMPLAINT

- Known ingestion of chocolate most common
- Onset of signs 6 to 12 hours postingestion possible
- Initially: bloating, vomiting, diarrhea; polydipsia; restlessness
- Can progress to polyuria, agitation, tremors, rigidity, ataxia, seizures, collapse, coma

PHYSICAL EXAM FINDINGS

- Agitation, nervousness
- Tachycardia
- Tachypnea
- Hypertension
- Hyperthermia
- Cardiac arrhythmias (premature ventricular contractions, sinus tachycardia, sinus bradycardia, others)
- Ataxia, tremors, seizures

ETIOLOGY AND PATHOPHYSIOLOGY

- Behavior changes, central nervous system stimulation, and cardiovascular abnormalities: competitive inhibition of cellular adenosine receptors
- Enhanced cardiac and skeletal muscle contractility: increase in free intracellular calcium concentrations from inhibition of sarcoplasmic calcium reuptake and increased calcium entry into cells
- Death likely due to cardiac arrhythmias, respiratory failure, or hyperthermia-induced disseminated intravascular coagulation (DIC)
- High sugar contents and fat in chocolate: gastrointestinal signs, possibly pancreatitis

DIAGNOSIS

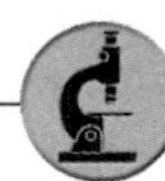

DIFFERENTIAL DIAGNOSIS

- Other toxicoses that can cause central nervous system (CNS) excitation: amphetamines, pseudoephedrine, phenylpropanolamine, metaldehyde, cocaine, antidepressants, antihistamines
- Causes of cardiac arrhythmias (see Ventricular Arrhythmias, p 1148; Sinus Tachycardia, p 1007; Sinus Bradycardia, p 1005)
- Causes of dyspnea/tachypnea (see Dyspnea, p 326)
- Causes of hyperthermia (see Heat Stroke/Hyperthermia, p 467)
- Causes of Systemic Hypertension, p 1058

INITIAL DATABASE

- Temperature
- Heart rate, rhythm
- ECG
- Blood pressure
- Serum biochemistry panel:
  - Renal values in animals with severe clinical signs
  - Serum electrolyte levels in animals with overt clinical signs
- Evaluation of pancreas (serum assays, ultrasound) in animals with severe clinical signs

TREATMENT

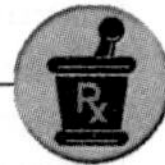

THERAPEUTIC GOAL(S)

- Manage severe clinical signs
- Decrease systemic absorption
- Enhance methylxanthine elimination

ACUTE GENERAL TREATMENT

- Manage clinical signs:
  - CNS signs/neuromuscular
    - Diazepam (0.5-2 mg/kg IV) for seizures
    - Barbiturates, gas anesthetics if diazepam ineffective
    - Methocarbamol (50-200 mg/kg slow IV, do not exceed 330 mg/kg/24 hr) for tremors, rigidity

TABLE I-2 Approximate methylxanthine content of various products*

Product	Theobromine	Caffeine
Cocoa powder	737 mg/oz	42 mg/oz
Baker's chocolate	393 mg/oz	118 mg/oz
Semisweet chocolate	138 mg/oz	22 mg/oz
Sweet dark chocolate		
Instant cocoa mix powder	136 mg/oz	15 mg/oz
Milk chocolate	56 mg/oz	6 mg/oz
White chocolate	0.25 mg/oz	0.85 mg/oz
Cocoa bean shell mulch	225 mg/oz	

*Exact methylxanthine content varies with growing conditions for cocoa beans as well as individual commercial formulations of products. Approximate methylxanthine dose ingested (in mg/kg) is: 1. Add product's theobromine concentration, in mg/oz (above) + product's caffeine concentration, in mg/oz (above). 2. Multiply this number by number of ounces of chocolate product ingested. 3. Divide by dog's body weight in kg.

- Cardiac arrhythmias:
  - IV fluid therapy as needed
  - β-Blockers for supraventricular tachyarrhythmias
    - Metoprolol (0.2-0.4 mg/kg PO q 8h)
    - Propranolol (0.04-0.06 mg/kg slow IV over 2 to 3 minutes; max 0.2 mg/kg)
  - Lidocaine for rapid sustained ventricular arrhythmias
    - Dogs: 1-4 mg/kg IV, then 30 to 50 µg/kg/min if necessary (if β-blockers ineffective). Cats (use with caution): 0.5-2 mg/kg IV
  - Atropine (0.01-0.02 mg/kg IV) for bradyarrhythmias
- Control hyperthermia:
  - Fluids, fans, etc.
- Decontaminate patient after life-threatening issues addressed:
  - Subclinical (or stabilized clinical) patient only
    - Emesis (effective up to 8 to 12 hours postingestion): see Vomiting, Induction of, p 1328
- Gastric Intubation, Gavage, Lavage, p 1258:
  - Consider when emesis is contraindicated (comatose, anesthetized)
- Activated charcoal:
  - 1-4 g/kg (or labelled dosage) after emesis/lavage; repeat q 8h during clinical signs of toxicosis
- Animals without clinical signs/preclinical cases: monitor 8 to 12 hours for development of signs:
  - Maintain urine output (IV fluid diuresis) ± potassium supplementation
- Urinary catheter placement:
  - Caffeine is resorbed from the urine; urinary catheter helps increase caffeine excretion

DRUG INTERACTIONS

Erythromycin, cimetidine, corticosteroids may delay methylxanthine clearance

POSSIBLE COMPLICATIONS

- DIC from hyperthermia
- Myoglobinuria from seizure-induced rhabdomyolysis
- Renal failure
- Pancreatitis

RECOMMENDED MONITORING

- ECG, blood pressure, body temperature
- Serum electrolytes
- Fluid ins/outs
- Urinalysis
- Pancreatic ultrasound ± enzymes

PROGNOSIS AND OUTCOME

- Prognosis is generally good with prompt and aggressive care.
- If severe clinical signs are not controlled, prognosis is guarded to poor.
- Signs generally resolve in 12 to 72 hours, depending on methylxanthine dose, severity of signs, and aggressiveness of treatment.

PEARLS & CONSIDERATIONS

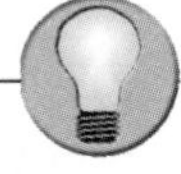

COMMENTS

- The darker the chocolate, the more dangerous it is.
- To estimate amount of methylxanthine ingested, add amount of caffeine and theobromine together (see Table I-2), multiply by number of ounces ingested, and divide by body weight in kilograms.
- Half-life in dogs: theobromine = 17.5 hours; caffeine = 4.5 hours.

PREVENTION

- Keep chocolate-containing products away from pets
- Avoid leaving chocolate-containing gifts unsupervised (e.g., under the Christmas tree)

CLIENT EDUCATION

Pets fed small amounts of chocolate may develop a taste for it and actively seek out chocolate, leading to intoxication.

SUGGESTED READING

Albretsen JC: Methylxanthines. In Plumlee KH (ed): *Clinical Veterinary Toxicology*. St. Louis, Mosby, 2004, pp 322-325.

Gwaltney-Brant SM: Chocolate intoxication. *Vet Med* 96:108-110, 2001. Available in PDF form online at: http://www.aspca.org/site/DocServer/toxbrief_0201.pdf?docID=111.

AUTHOR: **SHARON M. GWALTNEY-BRANT**

EDITOR: **SAFDAR A. KHAN**

Cholangitis/Cholangiohepatitis Complex of Cats

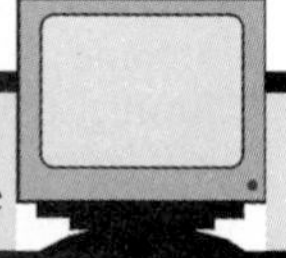

Client Education Sheet on Website

BASIC INFORMATION

DEFINITION

- Inflammation of the biliary tree and surrounding hepatocellular parenchyma. May occur as a primary process, a coexisting condition, or secondary to a variety of other feline diseases.
- Cholangitis: inflammation is centered around the bile ducts.
- Cholangiohepatitis: extension of cholangitis into the surrounding hepatic parenchyma.
- Cholangitis/cholangiohepatitis (CCH) has been referred to as both a "complex" (CCHC) and a "syndrome" (CCHS).
  - In either case, this designation emphasizes the fact that a variety of distinct forms of disease are included within a single umbrella term (see disease forms/subtype, below).

SYNONYM(S)

Acute neutrophilic CCH: suppurative CCH

Chronic, lymphoplasmacytic CCH: nonsuppurative, lymphoplasmacytic, or lymphoproliferative CCH

EPIDEMIOLOGY

SPECIES, AGE, SEX

- The CCHC of cats is one of the most common feline hepatobiliary disorders.
- Patients with this disease range in age from <1 to >16 years old, but most are middle-aged.
- Cats presenting for acute (suppurative) disease are several years younger than those with chronic (nonsuppurative) disease.
- Male cats appear to be overrepresented.

GENETICS AND BREED PREDISPOSITION: Himalayan, Persian, and Siamese cats may be predisposed.

RISK FACTORS: Extrahepatic biliary obstruction, inflammatory bowel disease (IBD), pancreatitis, cholestatic disease, cholelithiasis, bacterial infection or splenic abscess, feline infectious peritonitis (FIP), toxoplasmosis, immunodeficiencies, drugs (diazepam, tetracyclines).

CONTAGION AND ZOONOSIS: Not considered either a contagious or zoonotic disease.

ASSOCIATED CONDITIONS AND DISORDERS: *Triaditis* is the term used for describing the combination of CCH with IBD and pancreatitis: IBD or pancreatitis is seen in 50–85% of the cases of CCHC, with both present in up to 40% of CCHC patients. Cholangitis/cholangiohepatitis can also be associated with hepatic lipidosis, or secondary to a variety of other diseases/conditions (see Risk Factors above).

CLINICAL PRESENTATION

DISEASE FORMS/SUBTYPES

- Three distinct entities exist within the CCHC, as defined by the World Small Animal Veterinary Association Liver Diseases and Pathology Standardization Research Group on the basis of histopathologic findings:
  - Acute neutrophilic (suppurative).
  - Chronic (lymphoplasmacytic or mixed).
  - Lymphocytic (nonsuppurative).
- The forms can be quite different clinically (history, initial presentation, chief complaint, etiology, progression, and outcome).
- Chronic lymphocytic cholangitis is a form seen predominantly in Europe and is progressive:
  - Some pathologists classify this as low grade (well-differentiated) lymphoma.
- Lymphocytic portal hepatitis is a separate entity confined to portal triads and is often an incidental finding in older cats.

HISTORY, CHIEF COMPLAINT

- Patients with the suppurative form of CCH usually present for an acute onset of illness: anorexia, fever, and vomiting in a jaundiced cat with abdominal discomfort.
- Patients with the nonsuppurative form of CCH usually present for a more chronic condition with subtle nonspecific signs and less commonly present with acute signs.
- Patients with either form are usually jaundiced, and a few may have ascites.
- Patients with the chronic condition may be polyphagic, although rarely they will be presented for lethargy, anorexia, vomiting, and weight loss.

PHYSICAL EXAM FINDINGS

- Suppurative CCH: The patient is usually febrile, dehydrated, and jaundiced and may have abdominal discomfort with palpation.
- Patients with the nonsuppurative form of CCH may have minimal physical exam abnormalities or may present jaundiced.
  - Hepatomegaly may be appreciated with abdominal palpation

ETIOLOGY AND PATHOPHYSIOLOGY

- Bacterial infection (*Escherichia coli, Streptococcus*, other enteric organisms, anaerobes); ascending infection of the biliary tract (acute suppurative/neutrophilic cholangitis)
- In association with other infectious agents (i.e., toxoplasmosis, FIP)
- Immune-mediated disorder (chronic nonsuppurative/lymphocytic cholangitis)
- Extrahepatic biliary obstruction
- Secondary or concurrent pancreatitis (especially with suppurative form; pancreatic and bile ducts enter duodenum through a common opening in the cat). See Bile Duct Obstruction, Extrahepatic, p 130
- IBD

DIAGNOSIS

DIFFERENTIAL DIAGNOSIS

- Hepatic lipidosis
- Hepatic neoplasia (especially lymphoma)
- Extrahepatic biliary duct obstruction
- Pancreatitis
- Inflammatory bowel disease
- FIP
- Sepsis

INITIAL DATABASE

- Complete blood count:
  - Leukocytosis; neutrophilia with a left shift and/or toxic neutrophils
  - Lymphocytosis (nonsuppurative CCH)
  - Mild nonregenerative anemia with poikilocytes and/or Heinz bodies
- Serum biochemistry panel:
  - Elevated liver enzyme activities (alanine aminotransferase, ALP, aspartate aminotransferase, γ-glutamyltransferase)
  - Possibly elevated total bilirubin
  - Increased bile acids (fasting and postprandial)
  - Hyperglobulinemia (nonsuppurative CCH)
- Other:
  - High trypsin-like immunoreactivity or feline pancreatic lipase immunoreactivity (fPLI) possible with pancreatitis
  - Low cobalamin with severe IBD
  - Possible clotting time abnormalities (prothrombin time, activated partial thromboplastin time, activated clotting time [ACT], proteins induced by vitamin K absence [PIVKA])
  - Hepatomegaly (radiographs or laparoscopy)

ADVANCED OR CONFIRMATORY TESTING

- Abdominal ultrasound:
  - Hepatic parenchyma: mixed echogenicity, multifocal hyperechogenicity, diffuse hypoechogenicity, or a coarse or nodular appearance:
  - Prominent portal vasculature.
  - Biliary tree abnormalities.
  - Gallbladder distention, cholelithiasis, biliary sludge, thickened gallbladder wall.
  - Abdominal lymphadenopathy.
  - Evidence of pancreatic or intestinal inflammation.
  - Ascites (nonsuppurative CCH; high protein, low cellularity).
- Fine-needle aspiration (FNA) of the liver:
  - Hepatocellular vacuolation (concurrent lipidosis is possible).
  - Cellular infiltration: neutrophils, lymphocytes, mixed, intraluminal biliary inflammation.
  - Bacterial culture and sensitivity.
  - In general, fine-needle aspirations result in a greater number of false-negative and false-positive diagnoses compared to core or wedge biopsies.
- Liver biopsy (wedge [laparotomy, laparoscopy] or ultrasound-guided core: as above for FNA, plus:
  - Periportal hepatocellular necrosis, bile duct dilation and proliferation (suppurative).
  - Periductal fibrosis, diminished bile duct number and sclerosing cholangitis (nonsuppurative).
- Laparoscopy:
  - Abdominal lymphadenopathy.
  - Ability to obtain wedge biopsy sample.
- Laparotomy: as above for laparoscopy:
  - Assess biliary system for extrahepatic biliary obstruction.
  - Feeding tube placement possible.

TREATMENT

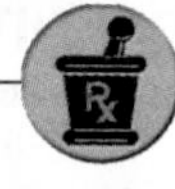

THERAPEUTIC GOAL(S)

- Provide supportive, nonspecific care necessary for patient comfort/stabilization (e.g., fluids)

- Remove or treat underlying etiology if identified (e.g., obstruction, infection)
- Treat underlying condition if cholangiohepatitis is secondary (e.g., toxoplasmosis)
- Treat concurrent conditions (e.g., pancreatitis, IBD)
- Provide/maintain appropriate plane of nutrition

ACUTE GENERAL TREATMENT

- Treatment should be tailored to the individual patient.
- Fluids (Normosol, lactated Ringer's solution) with potassium supplementation.
- Antibiotics (based on culture and sensitivity when possible):
  - Amoxicillin-clavulanate 62.5-125 mg PO q 12h; or
  - Amoxicillin 10-20 mg/kg PO q 12h, or
  - Cephalexin or cefadroxil 22 mg/kg PO q 8h; or
  - Enrofloxacin 5 mg/kg PO q 24h combined with metronidazole 7.5 mg/kg PO q 12h.
- Ursodeoxycholic acid (10-15 mg/kg PO q 24h) for choleresis, unless physical obstruction to gallbladder outflow exists.
- Vitamin K_1 (5 mg PO q 24h) in cases of coagulation abnormalities.
- Nutritional support:
  - Route determined by clinical condition.
  - Protein restriction in cats is problematic because they are strict carnivores; protein restriction should be avoided unless there is clear evidence of hepatic encephalopathy (rare).
  - Consider supplementation with L-carnitine (250 mg/cat PO q 24h), taurine (250-500 mg/cat PO q 24h), thiamine (B_1) 50-100 mg PO q 24h for 3 days, and vitamin B_{12} (1 mg SC repeated weekly).
- Cannulation for removal of inspissated bile, surgery for extrahepatic biliary obstruction, and necessary treatments for associated conditions (especially pancreatitis, IBD, hepatic lipidosis).

CHRONIC TREATMENT

- Long-term management is highly dependent on an accurate diagnosis and requires histopathologic analysis of a liver biopsy.
- Continued antibiotics and ursodeoxycholic acid (see Acute General Treatment above) 3 to 6 months if suppurative CCH.
- Prednisolone (for chronic or nonsuppurative CCH; 4 mg/kg/day initially, gradual taper over 2 to 4 months) combined with metronidazole (see Acute General Treatment above).
- Refractory cases of nonsuppurative CCH may require chemotherapeutics (e.g., methotrexate [0.13 mg PO q 8h for 3 doses at 7-day intervals, if tolerated], cyclosporine [3-5 mg/kg PO q 12h], or chlorambucil [4 mg/m2 PO q 48h]). Given the potential for severely detrimental side effects with these drugs and the need for close monitoring, their use is recommended only in consultation with an internist.
- Vitamin E (α-tocopherol acetate, 10-30 IU/kg) for all forms of CCHS.
- S-adenosylmethionine (20 mg/kg PO q 24h [enteric coated tablet]) for all forms of CCHS.
- Ursodeoxycholic acid, carnitine (see Acute General Treatment above)
- Continued treatment of concurrent conditions such as pancreatitis and/or IBD.
- Treatment for ascites if present (furosemide [1-3 mg/kg PO q 12h and/or spironolactone [1 mg/kg PO q 12h], ACE-inhibitors [enalapril, 0.5 mg/kg PO q 12-24 h], salt restriction).
- For biliary cirrhosis (sclerosing CCHC), consider the addition of pulsatile therapy with methotrexate (0.13 mg q 8h for 3 doses, at 7 day intervals, if tolerated), being cognizant of potentially adverse side-effects (GI, hepatic toxicity and renal toxicity, bone marrow suppression).

DRUG INTERACTIONS

- Drug availability may be affected by cholestasis.
- Pharmacokinetics may be affected by altered liver function.

POSSIBLE COMPLICATIONS

- Hepatic lipidosis with prolonged anorexia or inadequate nutritional support
- Diabetes mellitus with steroid treatment of nonsuppurative disease or IBD
- Hepatic sclerosis
- Progression of acute to chronic disease
- Necrotizing cholecystitis, choleliths

RECOMMENDED MONITORING

- Hepatic enzyme activity and total bilirubin levels (at 2-week intervals until stable, then monthly)
- PIVKA and/or clotting times if abnormalities are present or to monitor vitamin K_1 therapy
- Consider repeat bile acids to monitor liver function

PROGNOSIS AND OUTCOME

- Acute suppurative cholangiohepatitis may be a single curable event, or it may recur (especially if antibiotic therapy is curtailed), but the prognosis is generally good with timely diagnosis and appropriate treatment.
- Nonsuppurative cholangiohepatitis is a chronic condition but carries a fair to good prognosis with lifelong therapy.
- Concurrent pancreatitis and/or IBD may also affect the prognosis negatively.

PEARLS & CONSIDERATIONS

COMMENTS

- The cholangitis/cholangiohepatitis complex of cats is a complex or constellation of distinct clinical signs, biochemical abnormalities, and histopatholologic derangements. The underlying etiology may be distinct as well, and determining whether an infectious process is a contributing factor has a critical bearing on treatment decisions. Following the appropriate and sufficient diagnostic steps in the work-up of a cat with inflammatory liver disease is critical for therapeutic success.
- Suppurative CCH is often infectious in nature (and therefore treated initially with antibiotics), whereas nonsuppurative CCH may have an immune-mediated basis (and is therefore treated with immunosuppressive drugs).

PREVENTION

Avoid and/or treat contributing or concurrent conditions such as chronic pancreatitis or IBD

CLIENT EDUCATION

- Vigilant monitoring is important for early detection of anorexia, lethargy, vomiting, or abdominal discomfort, because suppurative cholangiohepatitis may recur.
- Compliance with medication administration may be a lifelong commitment.
- Proper nutritional support (optimal high-protein diet) is important.

SUGGESTED READING

Center SA: Cholangitis/cholangiohepatitis in the cat. *Proc Annual Meeting ACVIM,* pp 409-412, 1997.

Gagne JM, et al: Clinical features of inflammatory liver disease in cats: 41 cases (1983-1993). *JAVMA* 214:513-516, 1999.

AUTHOR: **CRAIG B. WEBB**
EDITOR: **KEITH P. RICHTER**

Cholecalciferol Toxicosis

BASIC INFORMATION

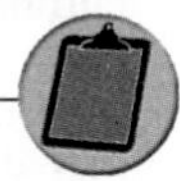

DEFINITION

Cholecalciferol (vitamin D_3) is used as a dietary supplement and as a rodenticide. Toxicity is characterized by clinical manifestations of hypercalcemia and hyperphosphatemia, anorexia and lethargy due to renal failure, cardiac arrhythmias, seizures, and tissue mineralization.

SYNONYM(S)

Vitamin D_3

Common trade names are: Mouse-B-Gon, Rat-B-Gon, Quintox, Rampage, and True Grit. Most baits contain 0.075% cholecalciferol (0.75 mg cholecalciferol/gram bait).

One IU of cholecalciferol (e.g., in dietary supplements) is equivalent to 0.025 µg of cholecalciferol.

Practitioners should be aware that products with the same name may contain various active ingredients. For example, Rampage may contain bromethalin or cholecalciferol. It is imperative that active ingredients be verified on the package.

EPIDEMIOLOGY

SPECIES, AGE, SEX

- All animals susceptible
- Dogs more likely to be involved
- Young animals may be more sensitive

RISK FACTORS: Preexisting disease such as chronic renal failure can increase susceptibility.

CONTAGION AND ZOONOSIS: Relay toxicosis (intoxication via consumption of prey that has itself consumed cholecalciferol) has not been reported.

GEOGRAPHY AND SEASONALITY: More cases in the fall and the winter months when more rodenticides are used.

CLINICAL PRESENTATION

HISTORY, CHIEF COMPLAINT

- History or evidence of consuming bait
- Lethargy, anorexia, vomiting ± diarrhea, polyuria and polydipsia 12 to 72 hours postingestion
- Renal failure 24 to 72 hours postingestion

PHYSICAL EXAM FINDINGS

- Anorexia, lethargy
- Dehydration
- Signs of abdominal pain
- Hematemesis, melena
- Dyspnea, cardiac arrhythmias (especially bradycardia)
- Seizures (uncommon)

ETIOLOGY AND PATHOPHYSIOLOGY

- Cholecalciferol is metabolized to calcitriol (1,25 dihydroxyvitamin D).
  - Calcitriol increases intestinal absorption of calcium, stimulates bone resorption of calcium, and increases renal tubular resorption of calcium.
- Toxicologic effects are due to hypercalcemia and hyperphosphatemia.
- Parathyroid hormone synthesis is suppressed.

DIAGNOSIS

DIFFERENTIAL DIAGNOSIS

Hypercalcemia:

- Synthetic vitamin D_3 ointments (Dovonex, Tacalitol) used for treating psoriasis in humans
- Hypercalcemia of malignancy (lymphoma, perianal adenocarcinoma, multiple myeloma, others)
- Primary renal failure
- Primary hyperparathyroidism
- Addison's disease (hypoadrenocorticism)
- Granulomatous diseases (e.g., blastomycosis, schistosomiasis)
- Chronic overdose of vitamin D_3 supplements

INITIAL DATABASE

- Complete blood count, serum chemistry profile:
  - Baseline if possible (<8 hour postexposure)
  - Calcium, phosphorus, blood urea nitrogen (BUN), creatinine should be included
  - Monitor daily for 4 days
- Ca (mg/dl) X P (mg/dl) product. If > 60, increased risk of soft tissue calcification
- Urinalysis:
  - Isosthenuria (specific gravity 1.008 to 1.012) or hyposthenuria (specific gravity of 1.002 to 1.006) are common; indicate renal failure if concurrent azotemia
- Radiographs for soft tissue calcification
- Ultrasound may suggest soft tissue mineralization (generally, radiography is superior)

ADVANCED OR CONFIRMATORY TESTING

- Serum 25-hydroxycholecalciferol level; can be used for differentiating between cholecalciferol rodenticides and vitamin D_3 ointments. The test cannot detect calcipotriene found in ointments; of limited clinical benefit.
- Necropsy: fresh or frozen kidney. Total wet weight kidney calcium will be elevated (300 to 1000 ppm; normal ranges 100 to 150 ppm).
- Histopathologic evaluation of lungs, kidney, aorta, myocardium, and gastric mucosa can reveal soft tissue mineralization and necrosis.

TREATMENT

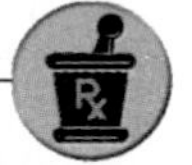

THERAPEUTIC GOAL(S)

- Prevent or lower elevations in serum calcium and phosphorus
- Treat acute renal failure
- Supportive care

ACUTE GENERAL TREATMENT

- Decontamination of patient: induction of vomiting within 4 hours of ingestion (apomorphine: 0.04 mg/kg, either sprinkled in the conjunctival sac and rinsed after emesis, or IV. Alternatively, hydrogen peroxide 3% may be given PO: 0.45 ml/kg to a maximum of 45 ml. Can be repeated once if the animal does not vomit in 15 minutes.
- Repeated doses of activated charcoal (dose according to packaging label of product; e.g., 10 ml of activated charcoal suspension PO made from 2 g activated charcoal suspended in 10 ml tap water) and a cathartic, given q 8h × 24 hours.
- Cholecalciferol doses > 0.1 mg/kg require decontamination and monitoring.
- Treat hypercalcemia in animals showing overt clinical signs:
  - Saline diuresis 0.9% saline at 130 ml/kg/day.
    - Avoid calcium-containing fluids.
    - Adjust dose if cardiac disease or other vascular volume-compromising condition.
  - Furosemide 2.5–4.5 mg/kg PO, SC, IM, or IV q 6–8h.
    - Do not use thiazide diuretics (calcium-retaining).
  - Prednisolone 1–3 mg/kg PO q 8–12h.
  - High doses of dexamethasone at 1–2 mg/kg IV or SQ q 24h have been recommended. Because dexamethasone has 10 times the glucocorticoid potency of prednisone, these high doses can cause substantial gastrointestinal ulceration and hemorrhage and should only be used as a last resort.
  - Phosphate binders: aluminium hydroxide 10–30 mg/kg PO q 8h.
  - Low-calcium diet.
  - Avoid sunlight.

- Specific antagonists (must choose one or the other; do not combine):
  - Pamidronate (preferred) 1.3-2.0 mg/kg as a slow IV infusion. Repeat in 5 to 7 days if needed. May see a transient increase in BUN or creatinine.
  - Calcitonin: Use if supportive treatments are not effective. 4-6 IU/kg SQ q 8-12h. Some animals become refractory to salmon calcitonin.
- Continue treatment until serum calcium stabilized, or Ca X P < than 60 (days to weeks of treatment).
- Treat other signs (renal failure, seizures, arrhythmias).
- Gradually wean off prednisolone/dexamethasone and furosemide.
- Stop phosphate binders when phosphorus level stabilizes.

POSSIBLE COMPLICATIONS

- Soft tissue mineralization (irreversible)
- Pulmonary edema (mineralization and leakage of pulmonary vessels), hemorrhage, or aspiration pneumonia
- Sudden death associated with myocardial or aortic mineralization
- Gastric ulceration, hematemesis, shock, and collapse
- Hypocalcemia if animals are not weaned from treatment after calcium levels are normalized

RECOMMENDED MONITORING

Monitor serum calcium and phosphorus for 5 to 7 days after values are normalized, then two to three times a week for 2 weeks, and then once at 1 month postexposure

PROGNOSIS AND OUTCOME

- Prognosis good if animal receives prompt treatment, and if soft tissue mineralization has not occurred
- Prognosis poor to guarded with prolonged elevations in calcium and phosphorus, causing soft tissue mineralization

PEARLS & CONSIDERATIONS

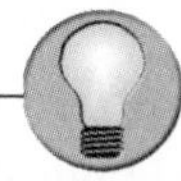

COMMENTS

- Total wet kidney calcium concentrations can be used for differentiating between ethylene glycol toxicosis (3000 to 12,000 ppm) and cholecalciferol toxicosis (300 to 1000 ppm).
- Dietary supplements generally list cholecalciferol, or vitamin D, in IU.
  - One IU of cholecalciferol is equivalent to 0.025 μg of cholecalciferol.

PREVENTION

Keep rodenticides out of the reach of pets

CLIENT EDUCATION

- Provide information about pet proofing homes
- Remind clients that rodenticides may be appealing to pets

SUGGESTED READING

Rumbeiha WK: Cholecalciferol. In Peterson ME, Talcott PA (eds): *Small Animal Toxicology*. Philadelphia, WB Saunders, 2001, pp 452-465.

AUTHOR: **CHARLOTTE MEANS**
EDITOR: **SAFDAR A. KHAN**

Cholecystitis

BASIC INFORMATION

DEFINITION

Inflammation of the gallbladder wall. Can be acute, chronic, necrotizing and/or emphysematous

EPIDEMIOLOGY

SPECIES, AGE, SEX

- Necrotizing and emphysematous cholecystitis occur infrequently in dogs and are extremely rare in cats.
- Acute cholecystitis may occur in cats secondary to bacterial cholangitis/cholangiohepatitis.
- Mean age: 9.5 years.
- Male dogs are at increased risk.
- Breed predisposition has not been reported.

GENETICS AND BREED PREDISPOSITION: Older, female, small-breed dogs appear to be at increased risk for cholelithiasis.

RISK FACTORS: Age (increased risk with age), history of previous cholecystitis, and concurrent systemic disease are associated with increased risk of cholecystitis.

ASSOCIATED CONDITIONS AND DISORDERS

- Cholangitis (inflammation of the bile ducts), choledochitis (inflammation of the common bile duct), and cholangiohepatitis (inflammation of the biliary tree and periportal hepatic parenchyma)
- Cholelithiasis, gallbladder rupture/perforation, and subsequent bile peritonitis (septic or sterile) can be sequelae to cholecystitis
- Can occur as the result of gallbladder mucocele
- Diabetes mellitus and cystic duct obstruction: emphysematous cholecystitis (weak association)

CLINICAL PRESENTATION

DISEASE FORMS/SUBTYPES

- Chronic and emphysematous forms may be incidental findings noted on abdominal ultrasound or abdominal radiographs (emphysematous—gas within gallbladder)
- Acute and necrotizing forms generally result in systemic illness

HISTORY, CHIEF COMPLAINT

- Presenting complaints are generally vague. May include vomiting, diarrhea, depression, lethargy, weight loss.
- Profound weakness or collapse can occur with gallbladder perforation and peritonitis.

PHYSICAL EXAM FINDINGS

- Nonspecific findings may include tachycardia, tachypnea, pyrexia, dehydration, and cranial abdominal pain.
- Icterus often is present when there is concurrent extrahepatic biliary obstruction.

ETIOLOGY AND PATHOPHYSIOLOGY

- Necrotizing cholecystitis (type I):
  - Secondary to infection with subsequent loss of viability of the gallbladder wall.
  - Gallbladder perforation does not occur despite wall necrosis.
- Acute (type II) and chronic (type III) cholecystitis:
  - Etiology is poorly defined.
  - Bacterial infection (ascending from the common bile duct or via hematogenous spread) suspected.
  - Type II cholecystitis results in gallbladder perforation and peritonitis.
  - Type III cholecystitis results in cholecystic adhesions (omental and hepatic adhesions) and/or fistulation.

- Emphysematous cholecystitis:
  - Invasion of the wall with gas-forming bacteria.
  - Tympanic cholecystitis is the result of gas distention of the lumen of the gallbladder by gas-forming bacteria.
  - Severe tympanic cholecystitis can be associated with emphysematous cholecystitis (gas dissection into the gallbladder wall).

DIAGNOSIS

DIFFERENTIAL DIAGNOSIS

- Other hepatobiliary disease
- Pancreatitis
- Proximal small bowel disease

INITIAL DATABASE

- Complete blood count results are variable depending upon severity and suddenness in onset of cholecystitis.
- Increased serum liver enzyme and bilirubin levels are possible.
- Hypoglycemia possible in cases involving septic peritonitis.
- Hyperglycemia may be seen in cases with concurrent diabetes mellitus and emphysematous cholecystitis.
- Abdominal radiographs may show air or calculi in gallbladder. Loss of cranial abdominal detail may be apparent (peritonitis).
- Abdominal ultrasound highly reliable for the identification of gallbladder rupture (86% sensitivity).
  - Loss of gallbladder wall continuity, hyperechoic fat in the cranial portion of the abdomen, and free abdominal fluid are possible findings. Choleliths may be seen.

ADVANCED OR CONFIRMATORY TESTING

- Definitive diagnosis requires surgical biopsy and histopathologic evaluation of a specimen of the gallbladder wall.
  - Cultures of bile and/or gallbladder mucosa should be performed (*Escherichia coli* and *Klebsiella* spp. most common, but aerobic and anaerobic culture and sensitivity are warranted).
- Laparoscopic evaluation and liver biopsy may prove useful. Conversion to an open procedure and cholecystectomy should be anticipated.
- Ultrasonographic-guided, percutaneous cholecystocentesis: bile cytology and bacterial culture and sensitivity.
- Cholangiography: radiographic imaging of the biliary system; very uncommonly performed.
- Abdominal paracentesis (p 1176) or diagnostic peritoneal lavage (p 1225) are secondary choices if ultrasound not available.
- Scintigraphy is an accurate indicator of canine extrahepatic biliary obstruction (EHBO).

TREATMENT

THERAPEUTIC GOAL(S)

- Relief of EHBO (if present)
- Surgical removal of severely compromised gallbladder, if present
- Appropriate treatment of infectious etiologies

ACUTE GENERAL TREATMENT

- Immediate surgical intervention in cases with gallbladder wall rupture and/or concurrent bile peritonitis
- Patients that are systemically ill must be aggressively supported before surgical management (fluids, antibiotics, colloids)

CHRONIC TREATMENT

Select cases of cholecystitis can be managed without surgical intervention, provided there are no signs of systemic illness such as severe lethargy, vomiting, or anorexia; there is no evidence of EHBO or compromise of the gallbladder's integrity; and serum biochemical values (liver enzymes and bilirubin) are decreasing over time or have normalized. Treatments that may be used in conservative (nonsurgical) management of these select cases include long-term antibiotic therapy (e.g., ampicillin 10–20 mg/kg IV q 8h or amoxicillin-clavulanic acid 10–20 mg/kg PO q 12h until culture and sensitivity results are available), choleretics (ursodiol, 15 mg/kg PO q 24h), and treatment of any underlying disease (e.g., pancreatitis, diabetes mellitus)

POSSIBLE COMPLICATIONS

- Gallbladder rupture and bile peritonitis (septic versus nonseptic)
- Recurrence of cholecystitis with inappropriate treatment
- EHBO

RECOMMENDED MONITORING

- Intensive monitoring in a critical care setting is indicated in markedly compromised patients (e.g., necrotizing cholecystitis, bile peritonitis).
- Serial serum biochemistry profiles and serial abdominal ultrasounds as indicated.
- Monitoring coagulation profiles and vitamin K supplementation (0.5 mg/kg IM q 12h until relief of obstruction) is indicated in patients with complete EHBO.

PROGNOSIS AND OUTCOME

- Mortality rates of 39% with canine-necrotizing cholecystitis
- Overall mortality rates of 50% with canine bile peritonitis (0% with nonseptic effusions and 73% with septic effusions)

PEARLS & CONSIDERATIONS

COMMENTS

- Select cases can be managed medically.
- Surgical management is indicated in all cases involving gallbladder compromise, bile peritonitis, or EHBO (excluding select cases of pancreatitis).

CLIENT EDUCATION

- Recurrence is possible if cholecystectomy is not performed
- Early intervention likely improves outcome

SUGGESTED READING

Church EM, Matthiesen DT: Surgical treatment of 23 dogs with necrotizing cholecystitis. *J Am Anim Hosp Assoc* 24:305, 1988.

Ludwig LL, et al: Surgical treatment of bile peritonitis in 24 dogs and 2 cats: A retrospective study (1987–1994). *Vet Surg* 26:90, 1997.

Pike FS, et al: Gallbladder mucoceles in dogs: 30 cases (2000–2002). *J Am Vet Med Assoc* 224(10):1615, 2004.

AUTHOR: **FRED S. PIKE**
EDITOR: **KEITH P. RICHTER**

Chole(cysto)lithiasis

BASIC INFORMATION

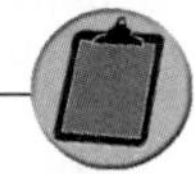

DEFINITION

Formation of stones in the extrahepatic bile duct system (choleliths) and/or specifically in the gallbladder (cholecytoliths)

SYNONYM(S)

Gallstones

EPIDEMIOLOGY

SPECIES, AGE, SEX

- Dogs:
  - Older, small-breed, spayed females appear to be predisposed.
- Cats:
  - Middle-aged to older adults.

ASSOCIATED CONDITIONS AND DISORDERS

- Cats:
  - In some cats, possible association with:
    - Cholangitis
    - Pancreatitis
    - Inflammatory bowel disease
- Dogs:
  - Cholecystitis
  - Gallbladder perforation
  - Bile peritonitis due to gallbladder rupture
  - Rarely biliary adenocarcinoma

CLINICAL PRESENTATION

DISEASE FORMS/SUBTYPES

- Cholelithiasis without specific clinical signs:
  - Incidental finding on abdominal radiographs or ultrasound performed for another reason
- Cholelithiasis associated with clinical signs of:
  - Gastrointestinal disease
  - Biliary obstruction
  - Peritonitis when cholelithiasis is associated with biliary disruption/rupture

HISTORY, CHIEF COMPLAINT

- Generally nonspecific: malaise and gastrointestinal signs predominate.
- Dogs:
  - Vomiting, anorexia, lethargy, weakness, polydipsia, polyuria, weight loss.
- Cats:
  - Vomiting, dehydration, anorexia, lethargy.
- **Note:**
  - Choleliths may be an incidental finding in both dogs and cats and may not be associated with any clinical signs.

PHYSICAL EXAM FINDINGS

- Icterus is commonly noted when cholelithiasis is associated with cholangitis, cholecystitis, and/or gallbladder obstruction.
- Fever may be noted in dogs, in association with infection and/or bile peritonitis.
- Signs of abdominal pain are not consistently noted, even when biliary obstruction is present.

ETIOLOGY AND PATHOPHYSIOLOGY

- Etiology unknown.
- In dogs and cats, most choleliths contain mainly calcium rather than cholesterol as seen in humans.
- Choleliths may obstruct the extrahepatic biliary system (see Bile Duct Obstruction, Extrahepatic, p 130):
  - Decreased absorption of fat and fat-soluble vitamins, notably vitamin K, and subsequent coagulopathy
  - Decreased bile secretion into the intestine may result in decreased binding of endotoxin predisposing to endotoxemia
- Cholelithiasis has been associated with concurrent cholecystitis and gallbladder rupture, resulting in bile peritonitis.

DIAGNOSIS

DIFFERENTIAL DIAGNOSIS

- Cholelithiasis with extrahepatic biliary obstruction and jaundice:
  - Hyperbilirubinemia due to hemolysis:
    - Immune-mediated hemolytic anemia
    - Other diseases causing severe intravascular hemolysis
  - Hepatic disease:
    - Cholangiohepatitis, feline
    - Idiopathic chronic hepatitis (dogs)
    - Cirrhosis
    - Neoplasia
    - Copper and other toxins in dogs
    - Acetaminophen toxicosis in cats
  - Extrahepatic biliary obstruction:
    - Pancreatitis
    - Cholangitis
    - Neoplasia
    - Stricture
    - Foreign body obstruction
    - Diaphragmatic hernia
- Cholelithiasis without biliary obstruction:
  - Other causes of vomiting and anorexia, because choleliths are an incidental finding:
    - Viral enteritis
    - Foreign body obstruction
    - Gastric, intestinal, or pancreatic neoplasia
    - Inflammatory bowel disease
    - Ingested toxins
    - Hepatic and renal diseases

INITIAL DATABASE

- Complete blood count:
  - Possible anemia, though usually mild
  - Inflammatory leukogram
- Serum biochemistry profile:
  - Elevated bilirubin concentration
  - Elevated liver enzyme concentration
  - Possible elevations of amylase and lipase concentrations
  - Hypokalemia
- Survey abdominal radiographs:
  - May delineate radiopaque choleliths
- Survey thoracic radiographs:
  - Rule out metastatic disease if neoplasia is suspected

ADVANCED OR CONFIRMATORY TESTING

- Abdominal ultrasound examination:
  - Common bile duct dilation:
    - Further delineate choleliths
    - >5 mm diameter is diagnostic of bile duct obstruction in the cat
  - Evaluate gallbladder in dogs with concurrent cholecystitis:
    - Wall thickness
    - Contents:
      - Choleliths
      - Mucocele
    - Presence of attached omentum
    - Surrounding fluid
- Peritoneal fluid analysis (obtained during abdominal ultrasound examination):
  - Bilirubin concentration
    - Bile peritonitis
  - Cytology and microbiologic culture and sensitivity testing
    - Septic peritonitis
- Coagulation profile

TREATMENT

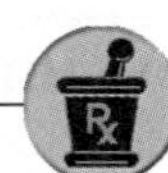

THERAPEUTIC GOAL(S)

- No hepatobiliary-specific clinical signs (choleliths are an incidental finding):
  - No treatment is required
  - Monitor for development of clinical signs associated with cholelithiasis
- Signs of biliary stasis, disruption, or obstruction:
  - Correction of fluid deficits
  - Normalization of serum electrolyte concentrations
  - Normalization of coagulation status prior to surgery
  - Removal of choleliths/relief of biliary obstruction
  - Treatment of bile peritonitis if biliary disruption has occurred
  - Nutritional support if indicated (see Feeding Tube Placement: Esopha-

gostomy Tube, p 1243; Feeding Tube Placement: Percutaneous Endoscopic Gastrostomy [PEG], p 1247; Parenteral Nutrition, p 1296)

ACUTE GENERAL TREATMENT

- Rehydation by intravenous administration of balanced electrolyte solution
- Parenteral antibiotics effective against gram-negative bacteria and anaerobes:
  - Empiric therapy:
    - Cefoxitin, 22 mg/kg, IV, q 2h perioperatively, then q 6h
    - Metronidazole, 7.5–15 mg/kg, IV, q 12h
    - Enrofloxacin, 5–15 mg/kg q 24h for dogs, 5 mg/kg q 24h for cats
  - Specific, long-term therapy based on culture and sensitivity test results
- Possible administration of fresh frozen plasma:
  - Hypoproteinemia
  - Possible coagulopathy
- Vitamin K administration
- Removal of choleliths/relief of extrahepatic biliary obstruction:
  - Cholecystectomy:
    - Results in the best long-term prognosis if all stones are removed and biliary system is patent
  - Retrograde and antegrade flushing of biliary system
  - Common bile duct stenting
  - Cholecystoduodenostomy/jejunostomy
  - Tube cholecystostomy
- Nutritional support:
  - Provide access for enteral feeding if patient is anorexic

CHRONIC TREATMENT

Maintenance of bile flow: Urseodeoxycholic acid 10–15 mg/kg PO q 24h

POSSIBLE COMPLICATIONS

- Recurrence of cholelithiasis
- Bile leakage
- Pancreatitis
- Peritonitis
- Endotoxemia
- Sepsis
- Death

RECOMMENDED MONITORING

- If clinical signs were/are present:
  - Clinical and laboratory parameters assessing perfusion including capillary refill time, pulse rate and quality, blood pressure, urine output, arterial pH, and lactate concentrations
  - Respiratory function
  - Serum liver enzymes and bilirubin concentrations
  - Coagulation profile
- If incidental finding:
  - Physical exam and serum biochemistry profile every 6 months

PROGNOSIS AND OUTCOME

- Fair in clinically ill animals if all choleliths removed and a cholecystectomy is performed
- Guarded if cholelithiasis is associated with biliary leakage and aseptic bile peritonitis
- Poor in patients with septic bile peritonitis
- Open prognosis in patients without clinical signs (incidental finding)

PEARLS & CONSIDERATIONS

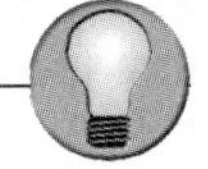

COMMENTS

Given the association of biliary obstructive disease (cholelithiasis) in cats with cholangitis/cholangiohepatitis and inflammatory bowel disease, a liver biopsy and culture, bile culture, and small intestinal biopsies should be obtained at the time of surgery in this species.

SUGGESTED READING

Eich CS, et al: The surgical treatment of cholelithiasis in cats: A study of nine cases. *J Am Anim Hosp Assoc* 38:290, 2002.

Kirpensteijn J, et al: Cholelithiasis in dogs: 29 cases (1980–1990). *J Am Vet Med Assoc* 202:1137, 1993.

AUTHOR: **DAVID HOLT**

EDITOR: **RICHARD WALSHAW**

Chondrosarcoma

BASIC INFORMATION

DEFINITION

Chondrosarcoma (CSA) is a malignant mesenchymal tumor that produces chondroid and fibrillar matrix, but never osteoid.

EPIDEMIOLOGY

SPECIES, AGE, SEX

- In dogs, CSA is the second most common primary bone tumor, accounting for 10% of all primary bone tumors:
  - Median age is around 8 years, but CSA has been reported at ages ranging from 1 to 15 years.
  - There is no gender predilection.
- In cats, CSA and other primary bone tumors are uncommon. CSA may rarely occur in the soft tissues at sites of previous vaccinations (see Vaccine-Site Sarcoma, p 1136).

GENETICS AND BREED PREDISPOSITION

- Large-breed dogs. Approximately 75% of dogs with CSA weigh >20 kg.
- Mixed-breed dogs, golden retrievers, boxers, and German shepherds are overrepresented.

ASSOCIATED CONDITIONS AND DISORDERS: Osteochondromatosis (multiple cartilaginous exostoses) lesions may undergo malignant transformation, resulting in CSA or, less commonly, osteosarcoma.

CLINICAL PRESENTATION

DISEASE FORMS/SUBTYPES

- The majority of CSAs arise from flat bones. Approximately 30% occur in the nasal cavity, accounting for 15% of all nasal tumors; 20% of CSAs arise from the ribs, accounting for 30–40% of all primary rib tumors.
- A total of 20% of CSAs arise from the appendicular skeleton, often but not always at sites where osteosarcoma typically occurs. CSA accounts for only 3–5% of all primary bone tumors in the appendicular skeleton.
- Other reported sites include facial bones, vertebrae, pelvis, digits, and os penis.

HISTORY, CHIEF COMPLAINT

- Patients often present with a visible mass at the affected site. Additional clinical signs vary with the site of skeletal involvement.
- Nasal CSA is usually associated with unilateral or bilateral epistaxis. Other clinical signs include sneezing, dyspnea, and swelling over the nasal cavity.
- Appendicular CSA is usually associated with lameness.

PHYSICAL EXAM FINDINGS

- Findings for CSA will depend on the anatomic location. Often, but not always, a firm to hard mass will be palpable.

- Patients with nasal CSA often have reduced airflow through the nares, and hemorrhagic discharge may be present. More advanced tumors may be associated with a visible mass effect (externally or orally). The ipsilateral eye may not retropulse or may be exophthalmic.
- Rib CSA most commonly arises near the costochondral junction. Any rib may be affected.
- Patients with appendicular and digital CSA are variably lame, ranging from minimal to non-weight-bearing.

ETIOLOGY AND PATHOPHYSIOLOGY

Etiology is unknown

DIAGNOSIS

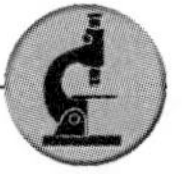

DIFFERENTIAL DIAGNOSIS

- General differential diagnoses for aggressive bone lesions:
  - Other primary bone tumors (osteosarcoma, fibrosarcoma, hemangiosarcoma).
  - Metastatic bone tumors (transitional cell, prostatic, mammary, thyroid, anal sac apocrine gland carcinomas).
  - Tumors that locally invade adjacent bone (nasal carcinoma; oral squamous cell carcinoma, melanoma, fibrosarcoma, epulides; digital squamous cell carcinoma, melanoma; synovial cell sarcoma; histiocytic sarcoma).
  - Hematopoietic tumors (myeloma, lymphoma). Radiographic lesions typically are purely lytic.
  - Bacterial or fungal osteomyelitis.
- Additional differentials for epistaxis:
  - Thrombocytopenia or coagulopathy.
  - Fungal rhinitis (usually *Aspergillus*).
  - Systemic hypertension.
  - Foreign body.

INITIAL DATABASE

- Radiographic imaging of the primary tumor:
  - The bony changes associated with CSA are the same as those seen with osteosarcoma (see Osteosarcoma, p 783).
  - Nasal neoplasia is most often associated with soft-tissue opacity in the nasal cavity and/or frontal sinuses, as well as destruction of the turbinates, nasal septum, vomer, or surrounding palatine, maxillary, and/or frontal bones.
  - Primary rib tumors often can be distinguished from tumors originating from the lung by the presence of an extrapleural sign.
    - An extrapleural sign is characterized by a smoothly marginated indentation of the lung that tapers gradually at the junction with the thoracic wall.
- After a radiographic or histologic diagnosis, patients should be completely staged with a CBC, chemistry panel, urinalysis, and three-view thoracic radiographs

ADVANCED OR CONFIRMATORY TESTING

- For axial tumors, computed tomography (CT) imaging is recommended to more accurately stage local disease and help with planning surgery and/or radiation therapy. CT imaging can be done in place of radiographic studies.
  - For nasal tumors, CT is superior to radiographs for detecting soft tissue opacity within the nasal cavity and surrounding sinuses, bony destruction, and extension through the cribriform plate into the brain.
- Histopathologic evaluation is required to confirm the diagnosis of CSA.
  - For nasal tumors and large, nonresectable tumors, an incisional biopsy is recommended. For resectable tumors, an incisional biopsy is not contraindicated, but it is reasonable to surgically remove the local disease, with biopsy submission after surgery.

TREATMENT

THERAPEUTIC GOAL(S)

- Relieve pain and other clinical signs associated with the primary tumor
- Prolong disease-free interval and prolong survival

ACUTE GENERAL TREATMENT

- Treatment of nasal CSA (see also Nasal Tumors):
  - Radiation therapy is the treatment of choice. Definitive treatment schemes typically use total doses of 48 to 57 Gy administered in 16 to 19 fractions or 3.0 Gy each.
  - Surgery is not an effective treatment modality for nasal tumors. It has been used before orthovoltage radiation therapy, but it is no longer routinely recommended because most radiation treatment facilities currently use megavoltage units (cobalt-60 or linear accelerator).
- The treatment of choice for rib CSA is wide surgical resection. Multiple ribs and/or underlying lung may need to be removed. Polypropylene mesh may be needed to obtain thoracic wall closure, and diaphragmatic advancement techniques may be necessary for caudal thoracic tumors.
  - Adjuvant radiation therapy is recommended if excision is incomplete, but there is little information regarding efficacy.
- The treatment of choice for appendicular CSA is amputation. Limb salvage techniques may be considered for tumors arising from the distal radius or ulna.
- For CSA arising from other sites, wide surgical excision is recommended whenever possible. When excision is incomplete, adjuvant radiation therapy may help improve local control, but there is limited information regarding efficacy.
- There is no information regarding the efficacy of chemotherapy for the treatment of CSA in veterinary patients.
  - In humans with CSA, adjuvant chemotherapy is recommended for patients with high-grade (dedifferentiated) tumors. Protocols typically include doxorubicin, ifosfamide, cisplatin, and/or methotrexate, but it remains uncertain whether adjuvant chemotherapy improves disease-free interval or survival.
- Palliative care is indicated for patients with advanced local disease or visible metastasis, and when owners decline definitive therapy.
  - Oral analgesics such as nonsteroidal anti-inflammatory drugs (NSAIDs, including aspirin 10-25 mg/kg PO q 8-24h, carprofen 2 mg/kg PO q 12h, etodolac 10-15 mg/kg PO q 24h, deracoxib 1-2 mg/kg PO q 24h [may use 3-4 mg/kg PO q 24h for first 7 days only], or meloxicam 0.1 mg/kg PO q 24h; or acetaminophen with codeine), are recommended, but are rarely sufficient to completely control pain.
  - Palliative radiation therapy very effectively controls the pain associated with bony tumors. Most information regarding efficacy is from the treatment of osteosarcoma (see Osteosarcoma, p 783), but similar benefits are seen in patients with chondrosarcoma.
  - Patients with pulmonary metastasis often benefit from oral corticosteroids (do not combine corticosteroids with NSAIDs).

RECOMMENDED MONITORING

Patients should be evaluated every 2 to 3 months for evidence of local recurrence and metastatic disease. At a minimum, this includes a thorough physical examination and three-view thoracic radiographs. Imaging of the site of the primary tumor may be indicated as well, depending on location, completeness of excision, and clinical signs.

PROGNOSIS AND OUTCOME

- Overall, 30-40% of patients with CSA die due to local disease.
- Fewer than 10% of patients present with gross metastatic disease, and overall metastatic rates range from 20-50%.

Nasal CSA may have a lower metastatic potential.

- In dogs with nasal CSA treated with definitive radiation therapy (megavoltage), 1-year progression-free survival rate is around 50%, and 2-year progression-free survival rate is around 30%.
  - Patients with nasal CSA are three times less likely to have local recurrence than are patients with nasal adenocarcinoma.
  - For patients with nasal tumors in general, extension into the frontal sinuses and/or erosion through the bones of the nasal passage is associated with a threefold increase in risk of local recurrence. Unilateral versus bilateral involvement is not a significant prognostic factor.
- For dogs with rib CSA treated with surgical resection, reported median survival times range from 1 to 3 years. Clean surgical margins are associated with lower rates of local recurrence and metastasis.
- For dogs with appendicular CSA treated with amputation, median survival is around 18 months.
- When treated with supportive care alone, survival times typically are 1 to 2 months. For some animals, though, progression of local and/or metastatic disease may be relatively slow, allowing them to continue enjoying good quality of life for extended periods of time.

SUGGESTED READING

Pirkey-Ehrhart N, et al: Primary rib tumors in 54 dogs. *J Am Anim Hosp Assoc* 31:65, 1995.

Popovitch CA, et al: Chondrosarcoma: A retrospective study of 97 dogs (1987–1990). *J Am Anim Hosp Assoc* 30:81, 1994.

Théon AP, et al: Megavoltage irradiation of neoplasms of the nasal and paranasal cavities in 77 dogs. *J Am Vet Med Assoc* 202:1469, 1993.

AUTHOR: **DENNIS B. BAILEY**
EDITOR: **KENNETH M. RASSNICK**

Chronic Renal Failure, Occult ("Asymptomatic")

Client Education Sheet on Website

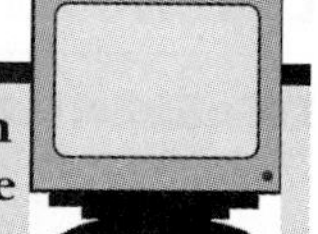

BASIC INFORMATION

DEFINITION

- Chronic renal failure (CRF): azotemia with inadequately concentrated urine (specific gravity < 1.035 in cats; < 1.030 in dogs).
- Occult CRF: CRF in which no clinical signs are present. Renal disease causing inadequately concentrated urine without azotemia is termed *renal insufficiency.*
- For information on CRF causing overt clinical signs, see Chronic Renal Failure, Overt ("Symptomatic"), p 205.

SYNONYM(S)

Latent CRF
Preclinical CRF
Asymptomatic CRF
Compensated CRF
CRF: chronic kidney disease
Incidentally discovered CRF

EPIDEMIOLOGY

SPECIES, AGE, SEX:

- More common in cats than dogs
- Any age but more common in older animals

GENETICS AND BREED PREDISPOSITIONS: Familial nephropathies are reported in a number of dog and cat breeds (see Chronic Renal Failure, Overt ["Symptomatic"], p 205). These nephropathies may lead to an early onset of renal failure.

RISK FACTORS: Advanced age, prior episode of acute renal failure, prior nephrotoxic exposure, pyelonephritis, nephrolith/ureterolith.

CLINICAL PRESENTATION

DISEASE FORMS/SUBTYPES: Incidental CRF is usually detected via routine geriatric or preanesthetic screening, or during investigation of unrelated illness.

PHYSICAL EXAM FINDINGS: Frequently no abnormal physical exam findings. The patient may have small or irregular kidneys.

ETIOLOGY AND PATHOPHYSIOLOGY

- CRF can be the end result of a variety of insults to the kidney, which may start as tubular, glomerular, or interstitial, because each nephron works as a unit. If the glomerulus is irreversibly damaged, the associated tubule will degenerate and vice versa.
- As nephrons are lost, the remaining nephrons hypertrophy. Although initially adaptive, glomerular hypertension damages the nephron, leading to further nephron loss. After a certain amount of damage has been sustained (generally when creatinine >3.5 mg/dl), renal failure may be progressive despite resolution of initiating cause.
- The specific etiology of CRF is frequently undetermined:
  - Tubulointerstitial nephritis most common cause (70% of cats, 60% of dogs)
  - Glomerulonephritis also a common cause (30% of dogs, 15% of cats)
  - Other demonstrable causes: amyloidosis, renal dysplasia, polycystic kidney disease, tubulonephrosis, lymphoma, chronic pyelonephritis, nephroliths or ureteroliths resulting in partial obstruction, vasculitis, infarction, and sequelae to acute renal failure with incomplete resolution

DIAGNOSIS

DIFFERENTIAL DIAGNOSIS

Azotemia:

- Prerenal azotemia (e.g., dehydration, high-protein diet, gastrointestinal bleeding) typically characterized by concentrated urine specific gravity.
- Azotemia with inadequately concentrated urine may be due either to renal failure or to dehydration (i.e., prerenal azotemia) combined with extrarenal impairment of urine concentration:
  - Drug therapy (e.g., diuretics, glucocorticoids)
  - Osmotic diuresis (e.g., diabetes mellitus)
  - Impaired medullary concentration gradient (e.g., hypoadrenocorticism, portosystemic shunting)
  - Central diabetes insipidus
  - Nephrogenic diabetes insipidus (e.g., hypercalcemia, pyometra, pyelonephritis)
- Postrenal azotemia (urinary obstruction, rupture) is generally easily differentiated from renal failure by dysuria.

INITIAL DATABASE

- Complete blood count (CBC): usually unremarkable; occasionally mild anemia.
- Serum biochemistry profile: azotemia; sometimes hyperphosphatemia, hypokalemia.
- Urinalysis: isosthenuric or minimally concentrated specific gravity (dogs <1.030; cats <1.035). Active sediment may indicate urinary tract infection.
- Urine culture.
- Abdominal radiographs or ultrasound: kidneys may be small and irregular.
- Blood pressure.

ADVANCED OR CONFIRMATORY TESTING

- Glomerular filtration rate (GFR) measurement: can confirm inadequate GFR, particularly when azotemia is mild and cause of impaired urine concentration unclear. All methods are

somewhat cumbersome, but iohexol clearance, creatinine clearance, and nuclear scintigraphy are most commonly used.
- Urine protein: creatinine ratio. An increased ratio when urine sediment exam is inactive suggests glomerular disease.

TREATMENT

THERAPEUTIC GOAL(S)

Slow the progression of disease

ACUTE GENERAL TREATMENT

Restricted quantity (but high quality) protein and restricted phosphorus diet ("renal diet") slows progression in dogs with CRF:
- Although cats are obligate carnivores and diet recommendations cannot be generalized, renal diets are typically recommended.
- There are many different brands of renal diet, and palatability varies with individual patient.
- Homemade diets may also be used.
- It is important to maintain adequate caloric intake.

CHRONIC TREATMENT

- For dogs and cats with protein-losing nephropathy, angiotensin-converting enzyme inhibition (ACEi) may slow progression of renal failure (enalapril or benazepril, 0.25–0.5 mg/kg PO q 12–24h).
- While ACEi is not proven to slow progression of renal disease in cats with UPC <0.43, it is widely used for this purpose in the UK.
- As renal failure progresses, animals may decompensate (show overt signs caused by CRF). See Chronic Renal Failure, Overt ("Symptomatic"), p 205, for specific therapeutic recommendations.

RECOMMENDED MONITORING

- Stable patients with incidental CRF should be monitored every 6 months.
- Recheck should include body weight, CBC (or minimally packed cell volume), biochemical profile with electrolytes, and blood pressure measurement.
- Clinical signs of hypokalemia, hyperphosphatemia, anemia, and hypertension may not occur until devastating; therefore early interventions can be based on detection by routine screening
- Urinalysis and urine culture twice a year due to increased risk of clinically silent urinary tract infection.

PROGNOSIS AND OUTCOME

- Some animals with incidental CRF may remain stable and free of clinical signs for years, while others progress more rapidly.
- The rate of progression to overt CRF is unpredictable.

PEARLS & CONSIDERATIONS

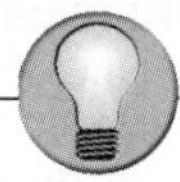

COMMENTS

Avoid nephrotoxic drugs (e.g., aminoglycosides) or drug combinations (e.g., nonsteroidal anti-inflammatory drugs with ACEi). If use of these drugs is necessary, ensure adequate hydration and monitor carefully for deterioration in renal function.

CLIENT EDUCATION

Animals should be presented for care promptly for signs of clinical illness. Progression of renal failure may lead to decompensation, and patients with CRF are less able to cope with extrarenal illness. Vomiting from any cause may lead to dehydration, which may worsen renal function, leading to exacerbation of vomiting, anorexia, and dehydration. Prompt fluid therapy (either IV or SQ, depending on severity and underlying illness) may be needed to stop the cycle.

SUGGESTED READING

Brown SA: Evaluation of chronic renal disease: A staged approach. *Compend Contin Educ Pract Vet* 21:752, 1999.

AUTHOR: **CATHY LANGSTON**
EDITOR: **LEAH A. COHN**

Chronic Renal Failure, Overt ("Symptomatic")

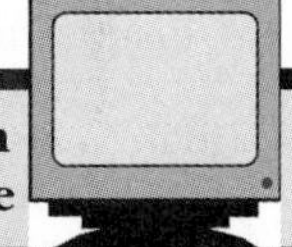

Client Education Sheet on Website

BASIC INFORMATION

DEFINITION

- Chronic renal failure (CRF): azotemia (elevated blood urea nitrogen and/or creatinine) with inadequately concentrated urine (specific gravity <1.035 for cats, <1.030 for dogs) present long term (usually months to years).
- Overt CRF: CRF that is responsible for clinical signs in a patient.
- Uremia is the constellation of clinical signs associated with renal failure (i.e., not all animals with renal failure are uremic).
- For information on incidentally discovered CRF (not producing overt signs), see Chronic Renal Failure, Occult ("Asymptomatic"), p 204.

SYNONYM(S)

Clinical CRF
Decompensated CRF
Symptomatic CRF
CRF: chronic interstitial nephritis, tubulointerstitial nephritis, nephrosclerosis chronic kidney disease, kidney failure

EPIDEMIOLOGY

SPECIES, AGE, SEX
- More common in cats than in dogs
- Common in older animals but can occur in animals of any age

GENETICS AND BREED PREDISPOSITIONS
- Increased frequency in Maine coon, Abyssinian, Siamese, Russian blue, and Burmese cats
- Familial nephropathies may lead to early-onset CRF. Familial nephropathies reported in:
  - Abyssinian cats
  - Persian cats
  - Basenjis
  - Beagles
  - Bedlington terriers
  - Bernese mountain dogs
  - Bull terriers
  - Cairn terriers
  - Chow chows
  - Cocker spaniels
  - Doberman pinschers
  - Golden retrievers
  - Keeshonds
  - Lhasa apsos
  - Newfoundlands
  - Norwegian elkhounds
  - Pembroke Welsh corgis
  - Rottweilers
  - Samoyeds
  - Shar-peis
  - Shih tzus
  - Soft-coated Wheaten terriers
  - Standard poodles

RISK FACTORS: Advanced age, prior episode of acute renal failure, prior nephrotoxic exposure, pyelonephritis, nephrolith/ureterolith, glomerulonephritis, amyloidosis.

ASSOCIATED CONDITIONS AND DISORDERS: Anemia, dehydration, urinary tract infection, renal secondary hyperparathyroidism, systemic hypertension, hypokalemia, metabolic acidosis, ulcers (gastric or oral), vomiting, weight loss.

CLINICAL PRESENTATION

DISEASE FORMS/SUBTYPES

- Incidentally diagnosed in apparently healthy animals (see occult/asymptomatic CRF, p 204)
- Overtly ill ("symptomatic") but stable patients (managed as outpatients)
- Decompensated patients (require hospitalization until stabilized)

HISTORY, CHIEF COMPLAINT (SOME OR ALL MAY BE PRESENT)

- Polyuria/polydipsia
- Anorexia
- Weight loss
- Vomiting
- Lethargy
- Halitosis
- Altered consciousness
- Seizures
- Bleeding problems

PHYSICAL EXAM FINDINGS (SOME OR ALL MAY BE PRESENT)

- Dehydration
- Frequently small, irregular kidneys, rarely large kidneys
- Signs of renal pain unusual
- Uremic halitosis
- Oral ulceration
- Poor haircoat
- Poor body condition
- Mild pallor

ETIOLOGY AND PATHOPHYSIOLOGY

- CRF can be the end result of a variety of insults to the kidney, which may start as tubular, glomerular, or interstitial.
- Even if an inciting cause can be cured, after a certain amount of damage has been sustained, renal failure may be progressive (generally when creatinine >3.5 mg/dl).
- The specific etiology of CRF is frequently undetermined:
  - Tubulointerstitial nephritis most common cause (70% of cats, 60% of dogs)
  - Glomerulonephritis also a common cause (30% of dogs, 15% of cats)
  - Other demonstrable causes: amyloidosis, renal dysplasia, polycystic kidney disease, tubulonephrosis, lymphoma, chronic pyelonephritis, nephroliths or ureteroliths resulting in partial obstruction, vasculitis, infarction, and sequelae to acute renal failure with incomplete resolution

DIAGNOSIS

DIFFERENTIAL DIAGNOSIS

Differential diagnosis of azotemia:

- Prerenal azotemia (dehydration, hypoadrenocorticism, gastrointestinal bleeding)
  - Urine specific gravity is usually >1.030 (dogs) or >1.035 (cats)
- Renal azotemia (acute renal failure, chronic renal failure)
- Postrenal azotemia (urinary tract obstruction, rupture)
  - Dysuria and/or additional clinical pathologic abnormalities (e.g., hyperkalemia)

INITIAL DATABASE

- Assess hydration: azotemia may be caused or worsened by dehydration.
- Serum biochemical profile: azotemia, variable hyperphosphatemia, hypokalemia, hypercalcemia or hypocalcemia, metabolic acidosis.
- Complete blood count (CBC): anemia due to lack of erythropoietin (EPO), gastrointestinal (GI) bleeding, anemia of chronic disease common. EPO deficiency results in nonregenerative anemia with normal to increased total protein, while GI blood loss results in low total protein.
- Urinalysis: isosthenuric urine specific gravity. Active sediment may suggest urinary tract infection (UTI).
- Urine culture: incidental, clinically silent UTI may occur with CRF; UTI may be cause of CRF.
- Thyroid level (elderly cats): rule out hyperthyroidism as concurrent disorder.
  - Correction of hyperthyroidism can worsen renal function in cats with CRF.
  - In cats that have both hyperthyroidism and CRF concurrently, treatment emphasis is placed on the disease that is most responsible for clinical signs.
- Blood pressure (BP): hypertension (systolic BP >160–180 mmHg, diastolic BP >95 mmHg) present in 20–60% of cats with CRF, may cause end-organ damage (especially heart, eyes, central nervous system, kidneys).
- Abdominal imaging: abdominal radiography or ultrasonography may further elucidate cause of CRF (i.e., obstructing or partially obstructing nephroliths or ureteroliths, renal neoplasia, cystic disease, perinephric pseudocysts). Alterations of shape, size, and echogenicity of kidneys are common.

ADVANCED OR CONFIRMATORY TESTING

- Urine protein:creatinine ratio. In dogs and cats with CRF, pathologic proteinuria (urine protein:creatinine [UPC] ratio >0.5 in dogs, >0.4 in cats; urinary sediment is inactive and culture is negative) may indicate a benefit from angiotensin-converting enzyme inhibition.
- Glomerular filtration rate (GFR) measurement: rarely used when azotemia is present.
- Renal biopsy: indicated primarily with renomegaly (rule out lymphoma, feline infectious peritonitis, amyloidosis).

TREATMENT

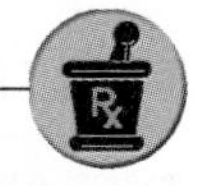

THERAPEUTIC GOAL(S)

- Alleviate uremic signs
- Delay progression of renal failure

ACUTE GENERAL TREATMENT

- Compensated state: see Chronic Treatment below.
- Decompensated state (e.g., dehydrated, anorexic, vomiting):
  - Hospitalization is ideal since oral therapies often are poorly tolerated.
  - Rehydration over 24 to 36 hours usually appropriate.
    - Intravenous crystalloid fluid therapy (i.e., lactated Ringer's solution, Plasmalyte, 0.9% saline).
    - Fluid rate: maintenance (66 ml/kg/day) plus replacement of dehydration (percent dehydration [as a decimal, e.g., 10% = 0.1] × kg body weight = liters deficit) plus ongoing losses (estimated volume of polyuria, vomiting).
  - Maintenance:
    - Maintenance rate plus 5–6% body weight per 24 hours to promote diuresis.
    - Practically, twice the calculated maintenance rate is sufficient for most.
    - Potassium supplementation of fluids based on potassium measurement (not to exceed 0.5 mEq/kg/hr; see Hypokalemia, p 566).
  - Other treatments described for chronic therapy may be applicable (e.g., H_2 blockers, antiemetics; see chronic treatment below), but injectable forms are used until oral medications are tolerated.

CHRONIC TREATMENT

- Delay of progression: see Chronic Renal Failure, Occult ("Asymptomatic"), p 204.
- Appropriate high-quality restricted protein and restricted phosphorus diets ("renal diet") slow progression and decrease clinical uremia.
  - Acceptance of diet changes can be problematic, particularly in severely affected patients.
  - Maintaining adequate caloric intake to avoid weight loss takes precedence over nutrient composition of the diet.
  - Renal diets should be introduced when uremia (illness) is minimized.
  - Nutritional support occasionally requires appetite stimulation (cats:

cyproheptadine 1 to 2 mg PO q 12h) or tube feeding.

- Additional therapies may be used depending on presence of particular uremic signs.
  - Anorexia or vomiting: decrease gastric acidity. Histamine blockers (famotidine, 0.5 mg/kg IV, SC, PO q 24h; ranitidine, 0.5-2.5 mg/kg SC, PO q 24h [avoid rapid IV administration, which may cause nausea] q 12-24h; cimetidine) or proton pump inhibitors (e.g., omeprazole 0.7 mg/kg PO q 24h).
  - Persistent vomiting: antiemetics (metoclopramide 0.2-0.4 mg/kg SC q 6h or 0.01-0.02 mg/kg/hr as constant rate infusion; phenothiazines); 5HT serotonin antagonists for intractable vomiting (ondansetron 0.22 mg/kg IV q 8-12h or dolasetron).
  - GI ulceration (e.g., hematemesis, melena, anemia, elevated blood urea nitrogen:creatinine ratio): sucralfate 0.25-1 g PO q 8h until signs resolve.
  - Hyperphosphatemia: diet ± medications.
    - Phosphate binders to prevent absorption of phosphorus from ingested food.
    - Aluminum hydroxide or aluminum carbonate 30-90 mg/kg/day divided and administered with meals. Dose is titrated based on serum phosphorus concentration.
    - Calcium acetate 60-90 mg/kg/day. Hypercalcemia possible side effect.
    - Selavemer hydrochloride is a newer, expensive phosphorus binder. Limited veterinary experience.
  - Hypokalemia (more likely in cats than dogs): potassium gluconate (2 mEq per 4.5 kg per day) or potassium citrate (75 mg/kg PO q 12h).
  - Acidosis (more likely in cats than dogs): consider treatment if total CO_2 <16 mEq/L or pH <7.2. Potassium citrate 75 mg/kg PO q 12h (also addresses hypokalemia), sodium bicarbonate 10 mg/kg PO q 12h.
  - Anemia: transfusion based on clinical need. Human recombinant EPO (Epogen 100 IU SQ q 48-72h until hematocrit rises; then q 7 days to maintain low-normal hematocrit) plus iron supplementation can be used for stimulating red blood cell production. Up to 25% of animals treated with Epogen (EPO) develop cross-reactive antibodies and must discontinue therapy.
  - Hypertension: Calcium channel blockers recommended. If proteinuria is present or calcium channel blocker is insufficient, use or add ACE inhibitor. See Systemic Hypertension, p 1058.
  - Chronic dehydration, or persistent signs of uremia: subcutaneous fluid administration. Dose is empiric, based on subjective assessment of the patient's well-being, hydration status, and presence of other disorders (e.g., heart disease).Typically for cats without heart problems, 100 to 150 ml daily to every other day.
  - Renal secondary hyperparathyroidism (see Renal Secondary Hyperparathyroidism, p 956).
- Renal transplantation may be appropriate for some animals/owners. May be preceded by hemodialysis (see Hemodialysis, p 1263). Greatest chance of success in mildly to moderately azotemic cats without concurrent illness or infection.

DRUG INTERACTIONS

- Phosphate binders can interfere with absorption of orally administered medications, especially antibiotics.
- Sucralfate works best in an acid environment and should be given at least 30 minutes before antacid therapy.

POSSIBLE COMPLICATIONS

- Anorexia, vomiting, GI ulceration, hyperphosphatemia, hypokalemia, acidosis, anemia, and hypertension are common sequelae of CRF.
- Volume overload (pleural effusion, pulmonary edema, dyspnea, or peripheral fluid accumulation) is a concern at high rates of fluid administration, particularly in anemic animals or those with concurrent heart disease.
- Platelet dysfunction in CRF increases risks of bleeding (gingival, GI, bruising, bleeding after invasive procedures).

RECOMMENDED MONITORING

- Routine recheck including physical exam, weight, chemistry panel, CBC, or packed cell volume. Frequency depends on disease severity.
  - Low-grade azotemia (i.e., creatinine >3.5 mg/dl, relatively asymptomatic), recheck every 6 months
  - Moderate azotemia (i.e., creatinine 3.5-5 mg/dl, stable on therapy), recheck every 2 months
  - Severe azotemia (i.e., creatinine >5 mg/dl, SQ fluids on a daily basis), recheck monthly
- Urinalysis and urine culture should be performed at least twice a year.
- Blood pressure measurement should be performed at least every 3 months, or 1 week after antihypertensive drug dose adjustments.
- Changes in clinical signs warrant recheck as well.

PROGNOSIS AND OUTCOME

- Longevity is difficult to predict in an individual patient, with a range of days to years.
- There are no known predictors of impending decompensation.
- Most patients with overt ("symptomatic") CRF will die of CRF or related complications, although some maintain stable renal function and die of unrelated disease (such as neoplasia).

PEARLS & CONSIDERATIONS

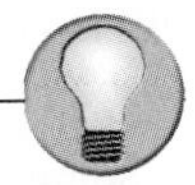

COMMENTS

- At an early stage of decompensation, renal transplant can be considered for otherwise healthy cats.
- Renal biopsy is rarely informative in cats with chronic renal failure and small kidneys (the inciting cause is virtually never identified).
- Urine culture and sensitivity in patients with CRF is essential at the time of diagnosis, and periodically thereafter.
  - UTIs commonly occur without an active urine sediment on urinalysis in CRF patients.
  - Correction of the UTI may improve renal function if subclinical pyelonephritis is present.
  - Few other complicating factors can be treated so easily and effectively.

CLIENT EDUCATION

- CRF is in incurable condition in which treatments are aimed primarily at improving the quality of life
- Renal transplantation is limited in availability and expensive. With successful renal transplant, intensive lifelong medication and frequent rechecks are required.

SUGGESTED READING

Brown SA: Evaluation of chronic renal disease: A staged approach. *Compend Contin Educ Pract Vet* 21:752, 1999.

Elliott J, Barber PJ: Feline chronic renal failure: Clinical findings in 80 cases diagnosed between 1992 and 1995. *J Small Anim Pract* 39:78, 1998.

Lulich JP, Osborne CA, O'Brien, TD, Polzin DJ: Feline renal failure: Questions, answers, questions. *Compend Contin Educ Pract Vet* 14:127, 1992.

AUTHOR: **CATHY LANGSTON**

EDITOR: **LEAH A. COHN**

Chylothorax

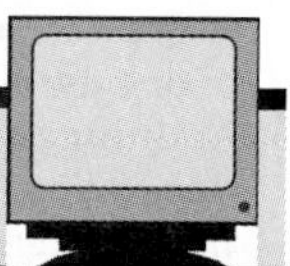
Client Education Sheet on Website

BASIC INFORMATION

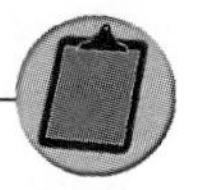

DEFINITION

Accumulation of fluid with a high triglyceride concentration (chyle) within the pleural space

EPIDEMIOLOGY

SPECIES, AGE, SEX

- Cats and dogs of any age can develop chylothorax.
- Some diseases associated with chylothorax are more common in middle-aged to older patients.

GENETICS AND BREED PREDISPOSITION: Possible breed predispositions include Afghan hounds and Shiba Inu dogs, and purebred cats, especially Oriental type cats.

RISK FACTORS

- Trauma
- Intestinal lymphangiectasia
- Congestive heart failure (CHF; cats more commonly develop chylothorax as part of CHF than dogs do)
- Thoracic neoplasia

ASSOCIATED CONDITIONS AND DISORDERS: Fibrosing pleuritis.

CLINICAL PRESENTATION

HISTORY, CHIEF COMPLAINT

- Typical clinical signs include:
  - Tachypnea
  - Increased inspiratory effort
  - Shallow respiration
  - Restrictive breathing pattern
  - Open-mouth breathing
  - Lethargy or exercise intolerance
  - Coughing
  - Possibly cyanosis
- Some animals, especially cats, may show minimal clinical signs until effusion volume is quite large

PHYSICAL EXAM FINDINGS

- Respiratory distress.
- Thoracic auscultation:
  - Muffled heart and lung sounds ventrally.
    - Careful auscultation for cardiac murmurs or arrhythmias is warranted, or for displacement of heart sounds to one side or caudally that may suggest a mass effect.
  - Increased bronchovesicular lung sounds dorsally.
  - Abnormalities of thoracic auscultation can be very subtle in cats.
- Thoracic percussion: hyporesonance ventrally.
- Jugular vein distention or pulsation may be present in animals with heart failure or pericardial disease.
  - Large-volume pleural effusions can contribute to increased central venous pressure and possibly jugular venous distention (i.e., appearance is identical to that seen when the jugular vein is raised manually for blood sampling) or jugular pulsation.
  - Radiation of a normal carotid pulse to the overlying jugular vein should not be misinterpreted as jugular pulsation.
- Peripheral lymphadenomegaly.
- Peritoneal effusion.
- Decreased cranial thoracic compressibility (cats) if associated with mediastinal mass.

ETIOLOGY AND PATHOPHYSIOLOGY

- Chyle is the fluid formed from lymphatic drainage of the gastrointestinal tract, which is collected in a small abdominal reservoir, the cisterna chyli. The sole outflow of the cisterna chyli is the thoracic duct, a single or paired structure that courses dorsally though the thorax and empties into the cranial vena cava.
- Impaired or disrupted lymphatic drainage:
  - Trauma and subsequent rupture of the thoracic duct
  - Neoplasia, including mediastinal, thoracic wall, or affecting thoracic duct.
  - Thoracic lymphangiectasia
    - May be associated with intestinal lymphangiectasia
  - Infectious causes such as fungal granulomas
- Increased central venous hydrostatic pressure (thoracic duct empties into cranial vena cava):
  - CHF (right-sided in dogs, left or right-sided in cats)
  - Pericardial disease:
    - Pericardial effusion
    - Restrictive pericardial disease
  - Pulmonary thromboembolism
  - Heartworm disease
- In many cases the cause of chylothorax cannot be determined (classification as idiopathic).
- Pleural effusion causes hypoxemia through a combination of hypoventilation and ventilation:perfusion mismatching.

DIAGNOSIS

DIFFERENTIAL DIAGNOSIS

- Other causes of pleural effusion:
  - Hypoalbuminemia
  - CHF
  - Intrathoracic neoplasia
  - Lung lobe torsion
  - Pyothorax
  - Pseudochylothorax
  - Hemothorax
- Pneumothorax
- Pulmonary parenchymal disease

INITIAL DATABASE

- Thoracic radiographs:
  - Interlobar fissure lines.
  - Reduced visualization of the heart, especially on dorsoventral views.
  - Retraction of lung margins from the thoracic wall, with an interposed fluid opacity.
  - Blunting of the lung margins at the costophrenic angles.
  - Increased opacity dorsal to the sternum on lateral views, with rounding of the lung margins ventrally.
  - The diaphragm is often obscured.
  - Widened mediastinum.
- Thoracocentesis: chyle is often grossly white or pink and opaque and remains so after centrifugation.
  - Chyle may be classified as a modified transudate (<3000–5000 nucleated cells/μl) or a nonseptic exudate (>5000 nucleated cells/μl).
    - Early chylothorax usually has a predominance of lymphocytes.
    - With chronicity, increased numbers of nondegenerate neutrophils, and some macrophages, may appear.
- Postdrainage thoracic films are advised to check for radiographic signs of pulmonary parenchymal, mediastinal, or cardiac disease.
  - Atelectatic lung lobes may give a false impression of lung masses.
  - Fibrosing/constrictive pleuritis secondary to chronic chylothorax may prevent complete reexpansion postdrainage.
- Thoracic ultrasonography can detect pulmonary or mediastinal masses/lesions, lymphadenomegaly, pulmonary consolidation, lung lobe torsion.
  - If the patient is stable, ultrasound is ideally performed before effusion is completely drained to provide an acoustic window.
  - Thoracic ultrasound can detect small volume effusions, guide thoracocentesis if fluid is compartmentalized, or guide fine-needle aspiration of masses or other pathology.

ADVANCED OR CONFIRMATORY TESTING

- Complete blood count:
  - Lymphopenia is possible.

- Leukogram changes are rarely specific.
- Serum biochemical profile:
  - Hypocalcemia and hypoalbuminemia are possible if chylothorax is secondary to intestinal lymphangiectasia.
- Urinalysis: generally unremarkable.
- Echocardiography can help rule in or rule out myocardial, valvular, or pericardial disease as the cause.
- Biochemical analysis of pleural fluid:
  - Compared to serum concentrations, increased pleural fluid triglyceride, and decreased pleural fluid cholesterol levels are consistent with chylous effusion.
- Pseudochylous effusions (rare) have a pleural fluid cholesterol concentration greater than the serum cholesterol concentration, and pleural fluid triglyceride concentration lower than the serum triglyceride concentration.
- Occasionally in fasted or anorexic animals, pleural fluid is not milky and can have a reduced triglyceride concentration; consider checking the pleural fluid and serum triglyceride levels postprandially.
- Computed tomography or magnetic resonance imaging may aid assessment of structural abnormalities in the thoracic cavity.

TREATMENT

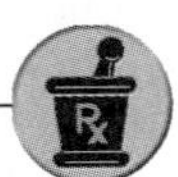

THERAPEUTIC GOAL(S)

- Improve respiratory function
- Identify and treat (when possible) the underlying cause

ACUTE GENERAL TREATMENT

- Oxygen if respiratory distress.
- Thoracocentesis is the initial therapy of choice.
  - Complete drainage is not necessary to relieve clinical signs and may be hazardous if fibrosing pleuritis is present, limiting the degree of lung expansion.

CHRONIC TREATMENT

- Specific treatment of the underlying disease, when identified, may be enough to resolve chylothorax.
- Intermittent thoracocentesis during the treatment period may be needed as respiratory signs dictate.
  - If regular thoracocentesis is performed, monitor electrolytes as hyponatremia (secondary to loss in pleural fluid) and hyperkalemia (secondary to reduced renal excretion) can develop.
- If fluid accumulation is rapid, thoracostomy tubes may be required.
- If the underlying disease cannot be determined, medical therapy may be attempted initially.
  - A low-fat diet, either commercial or homemade, helps reduce the flow of chyle.
  - Rutin (50 mg/kg PO q 8h) has been used for treating lymphedema in humans and has been used in chylothorax with some apparent success and no documented adverse effects.
- If medical therapy is unsuccessful, surgical intervention is indicated.
  - Some clinicans advocate surgical intervention as the initial treatment of choice to reduce the risk of fibrosing pleuritis.
  - The optimal timing for surgery in chylothorax is controversial and remains undetermined. Delaying surgery increases the risk of development of fibrosing/restrictive pleuritis.
  - The most common procedure is ligation of the thoracic duct and its branches, often in combination with lymphangiography.
    - Thoracic duct rupture is rarely detected by lymphangiography.
    - Ligation is accomplished via an intercostal or trans-diaphragmatic approach.
    - Lymphangiography is often repeated after ligation to ensure all branches have been ligated.
    - Success rates reported for cats vary from 20–53% (complete resolution).
    - For dogs resolution rate is reported at 53%.
    - En bloc ligation of the thoracic duct has been described in dogs without lymphangiography, with similar success rates (50%).
  - After ligation, abdominal lymphaticovenous anastomoses form to transport chyle to the venous system, bypassing the thoracic duct.
  - Thoracoscopic thoracic duct ligation combined with mesenteric lymphangiography has been described.
- A number of other techniques have been suggested in combination with thoracic duct ligation.
  - Pleurodesis promotes development of diffuse adhesions between the parietal and visceral pleura but is not recommended.
  - Passive pleuroperitoneal drainage techniques have been described, but success rates are low due to drain obstruction.
  - Active pleuroperitoneal or pleurovenous drainage techniques have been used, but disadvantages include cost, thrombosis, catheter obstruction, air embolism, venous occlusion, sepsis, abdominal distention (if pleuroperitoneal), and potential lack of owner compliance.
  - Omentalization of the pleural space exploits the large surface area and lymph-draining capability of the omentum.
  - Thoracic duct ligation with pericardectomy has been recently reported.
    - A thickened pericardium may increase right-sided venous pressures, impeding drainage of chyle after thoracic duct ligation.
    - Success rates reported are 100% for dogs and 80% for cats.

POSSIBLE COMPLICATIONS

- Incomplete resolution of chylothorax can occur with any treatment technique.
- Surgical and anesthetic risks for invasive procedures.
- Fibrosing pleuritis, pleural thickening by fibrous tissue that restricts normal lung expansion, is a consequence of chronic chylothorax.

RECOMMENDED MONITORING

- Thoracic radiographs to assess pleural fluid accumulation/resolution.
- Postoperative patients should also be monitored for re-accumulation of fluid.

PROGNOSIS AND OUTCOME

- Some patients will have resolution of chylothorax if the underlying disease can be corrected.
- For patients with idiopathic chylothorax or thoracic lymphangiectasia, the newly described approach of combining pericardectomy with thoracic duct ligation is showing some promising results.
- If the underlying disease cannot be managed successfully, the prognosis is poorer.

PEARLS & CONSIDERATIONS

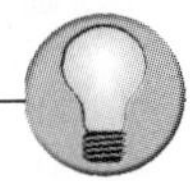

COMMENTS

- Cats with pleural effusion can be clinically fragile and must be handled carefully if dyspneic (e.g., during restraint).
- Long-standing chylous pleural effusion can lead to fibrotic pleural disease, an irreversible cause of respiratory impairment.

PREVENTION

Not available

CLIENT EDUCATION

Chylothorax can be a frustrating disease and requires diagnostic assessment to identify treatable underlying causes.

SUGGESTED READING

Birchard SJ, Smeak DD, Fossum TW: Results of thoracic duct ligation in dogs with chylothorax. *J Am Vet Med Assoc* 193:68, 1988.

Enwiller TM, et al: Popliteal and mesenteric lymph node injection with methylene blue

for coloration of the thoracic duct in dogs. *Vet Surg* 32:359, 2003.
Fossum TW, et al: Thoracic duct ligation and pericardectomy for treatment of idiopathic chylothorax. *J Vet Intern Med* 18: 307, 2004.
Fossum TW, et al: Severe bilateral fibrosing pleuritis associated with chronic chylothorax in five dogs and two cats. *J Am Vet Med Assoc* 201:317, 1992.
Radlinsky MG, et al: Thoracoscopic visualization and ligation of the thoracic duct in dogs. *Vet Surg* 31:138, 2002.
Thompson MS, Cohn LA, Jordan RC: Use of rutin for medical management of idiopathic chylothorax in 4 cats. *J Am Vet Med Assoc* 215:345, 1999.

AUTHOR: **GRAHAM SWINNEY**
EDITOR: **RANCE K. SELLON**

Cirrhotic/Fibrosing Liver Disease

BASIC INFORMATION

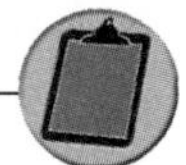

DEFINITION

- Fibrosis: replacement of hepatic parenchyma with extracellular matrix (ECM), collagen, and connective tissue
- Cirrhosis: diffuse hepatic fibrosis with concurrent formation of regenerative nodules that results in irreversible loss of normal hepatic architecture

EPIDEMIOLOGY

SPECIES, AGE, SEX

- Incidence is highest in middle-aged to older dogs (>7 years) with chronic liver disease.
- Middle-age cats with cholangiohepatitis may suffer from biliary cirrhosis.
- Copper storage hepatopathy (~1-5 years) and idiopathic fibrosis are seen in younger dogs (<2 years).
- Male cocker spaniels, female doberman pinschers, and Labrador retrievers appear more prone to disease than the opposite gender.

GENETICS AND BREED PREDISPOSITION

- Doberman pinschers, cocker spaniels, Scottish terriers, and Labrador retrievers have a familial predisposition for chronic active (idiopathic) hepatitis. See Hepatitis (Chronic) of Doberman Pinscher Dogs, p 500; Hepatitis (Chronic) of Cocker Spaniel Dogs, p 499.
- Copper storage disease is inherited in Bedlington terriers, West Highland white terriers, Skye terriers, and dalmatians.
- German shepherds and standard poodles develop juvenile idiopathic hepatic fibrosis.

RISK FACTORS: Idiopathic chronic hepatitis (chronic active hepatitis) in dogs, excess hepatic copper or iron storage, extrahepatic biliary obstruction.

ASSOCIATED CONDITIONS AND DISORDERS

- Portal hypertension, ascites, hepatic encephalopathy, coagulopathies, urolithiasis, acquired portosystemic shunts, gastric ulceration, fat malabsorption and steatorrhea, hypoglycemia, and hypoalbuminemia may result from fibrosing liver disease.
- Rare occurrence of pulmonary edema (hypoalbuminemia) or renal failure (hepatorenal syndrome).

CLINICAL PRESENTATION

HISTORY, CHIEF COMPLAINT

- Chronic condition of variable intensity that usually includes lethargy, anorexia, and weight loss.
- Vomiting, diarrhea, melena, and polyuria/polydipsia also frequently are part of the history.
- Jaundice or signs of coagulopathy uncommonly are reported by owners.
- Owners may report abdominal distention from ascites as "weight gain," even as the patient loses muscle mass.

PHYSICAL EXAM FINDINGS

- May be unremarkable except for weight loss and muscle wasting.
- Jaundice occurs commonly.
- Ascites and evidence of coagulopathies in advanced cases.
- Halitosis.
- Microhepatica may be present (dogs), although cats with biliary cirrhosis may have large livers.
- Manifestations of cerebral dysfunction (depression, stupor, others) due to hepatic encephalopathy. See Hepatic Encephalopathy, p 489.

ETIOLOGY AND PATHOPHYSIOLOGY

- ECM deposition (fibrosis) is stimulated by inflammatory mediators.
- ECM deposition may also be an idiopathic or congenital defect.
- Chronic fibrosis and regenerative nodule formation results in cirrhosis.
- Chronic progressive collagen deposition irreversibly destroys normal hepatic architecture.
- Normal hepatic blood flow and bile flow are disrupted, perpetuating hepatocellular injury.
- Any chronic inflammatory hepatic condition may be responsible, although a specific cause is not often identified (i.e., idiopathic).
- Possible underlying etiologies include cholangitis/cholangiohepatitis (cats), copper storage disease (dogs), drugs and/or toxins (anticonvulsants, azole antifungals, trimethoprim-sulfa), immune-mediated, leptospirosis, canine infectious hepatitis, hypoxia, extrahepatic biliary obstruction, or a single episode of massive hepatic necrosis (i.e., postnecrotic cirrhosis).
- Hepatic vascular resistance may increase, resulting in portal hypertension, ascites, acquired shunts, and encephalopathy.

DIAGNOSIS

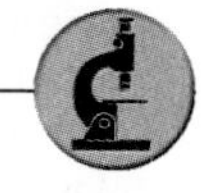

DIFFERENTIAL DIAGNOSIS

- Chronic active/idiopathic hepatitis (dogs)
- Cholangitis/cholangiohepatitis (cats)
- Noncirrhotic portal hypertension
- Biliary obstruction
- Pancreatitis
- Hepatic neoplasia (primary or metastatic)
- Feline infectious peritonitis, toxoplasmosis
- Chronic fibrosing pancreatitis
- Congenital portosystemic shunt
- Hepatic lipidosis (cats)
- Hemolytic anemia
- Right-sided heart failure

INITIAL DATABASE

- Complete blood count:
  - Nonregenerative anemia (normocytic, normochromic, or microcytic)
  - Acanthocytes (cats)
- Serum biochemistry panel:
  - Elevated hepatic enzyme activities (alkaline phosphatase, alanine aminotransferase, aspartate aminotransferase, γ-glutamyl transferase)
  - Hyperbilirubinemia
  - Low blood urea nitrogen (BUN) (variable)
  - Hypoalbuminemia and hyperglobulinemia (variable)
  - Hypocholesterolemia (variable)
  - Hypoglycemia (variable)
  - Electrolyte abnormalities (hypokalemia, hyponatremia)
- Urinalysis:
  - Isosthenuria
  - Ammonium biurate crystalluria (variable)

ADVANCED OR CONFIRMATORY TESTING

- Abdominocentesis and fluid analysis of ascites: pure transudate (hypoalbuminemia) or modified transudate (portal hypertension).
- Coagulation studies: prolonged activated clotting time, partial thromboplastin time (PT), activated partial thromboplastin time (aPTT), proteins induced by vitamin K antagonism or absence (PIVKA), buccal mucosal bleeding time. Of these, the PIVKA test is most sensitive, although PT and aPTT are acceptable and more readily available. It has not been shown that any of these studies will help predict bleeding following hepatic biopsy.
- Serum bile acids: elevated (fasting and postprandial).
- Radiographs: small liver (dogs), large liver (cats), loss of abdominal detail.
- Abdominal ultrasound:
  - Nodular hyperechoic/mixed echogenicity of hepatic parenchyma with abdominal effusion.
  - Acquired portosystemic shunt(s).
- Laparoscopy or laparotomy:
  - Small, firm, irregular liver.
- Liver biopsy for histopathologic analysis: confirmatory.
  - Fibrosis: inflammatory (bridging), or noninflammatory (sinusoidal, triads).
  - Cirrhosis, nodular regeneration, loss of normal hepatic architecture.
  - Note: suspicion of cirrhotic/fibrosing liver disease should prompt the consideration of wedge biopsy of the liver rather than ultrasound-guided core biopsy, because a firm, severely fibrotic liver may be difficult to penetrate safely with core biopsy instruments, especially if ascites is present. Additionally, needle core biopsies are often inaccurate in cirrhotic livers.

TREATMENT

THERAPEUTIC GOAL(S)

- Nonspecific supportive care
- Restoration of biochemical imbalances secondary to decreased liver function
- Specific treatment if underlying etiology is identified (e.g., excess copper, infection)

ACUTE GENERAL TREATMENT

- Intravenous fluids (balanced electrolyte solution) as needed:
  - Avoid 0.9% NaCl with ascites and hypoalbuminemia.
  - Avoid lactate with hepatic failure.
  - Potassium (20–40 mEq/L or more, based on serum potassium level) and dextrose (2.5–5%) supplementation may be necessary.
  - Dextrans or plasma transfusion for oncotic pressure support.
    - Plasma advantages include presence of albumin (contributes positively to protein balance), presence of clotting factors, and persistence in circulation (versus protein-losing enteropathy or nephropathy, in which the transfused proteins may be lost quickly); drawbacks include cost and short shelf life (fresh) or need to freeze (fresh frozen).
- Therapeutic abdominocentesis when necessary (i.e., respiratory compromise, significant abdominal discomfort)

CHRONIC TREATMENT

See also Hepatic Encephalopathy, p 489.

- Nutrition:
  - Most commercial geriatric, liver, or renal diets are appropriate.
  - Adjust protein consumption in the face of hepatic encephalopathy (decreased/optimal quantity, replace meat proteins with dairy and/or vegetable protein).
  - Fermentable fiber in cases of hepatic encephalopathy.
  - Water-soluble vitamin supplementation.
  - Avoid mineral supplements containing copper.
- Antibiotics:
  - Specific to infectious agent if identified as underlying etiology (rarely in dogs).
  - For signs of hepatic encephalopathy consider:
    - Metronidazole (7.5 mg/kg PO q 12h), or
    - Amoxicillin-clavulanate (15 mg/kg PO q 12h), or
    - Ampicillin (20 mg/kg PO q 8h), or
    - Neomycin (20 mg/kg PO q 8h)
- Anti-inflammatory: with histopathologic confirmation of chronic noninfectious inflammation, consider prednisone or prednisolone (1–4 mg/kg PO q 24–48h, taper if possible), and/or azathioprine (1 mg/kg PO q 24–48h).
- Antifibrotic: Colchicine (0.03 mg/kg PO q 24h), although no published data support its use or clearly demonstrate a beneficial effect. Prednisone (anti-inflammatory) and d-penicillamine (copper chelator; 10–15 mg/kg PO q 12h) also have antifibrotic properties.
- Lactulose (0.25–0.5 ml/kg PO q 8h, titrated to achieve loose fecal consistency) with cleansing and/or retention enemas (povidone-iodine diluted 1:10 with tap water or lactulose diluted 1:3 with tap water) to decrease ammonia production/absorption in cases of hepatic encephalopathy.
- Ursodiol (10–15 mg/kg PO q 24h) as a choleretic in cases of cholestasis.
- d-α-tocopherol (200–600 IU q 24h), S-adenosylmethionine (20 mg/kg q 24h), and milk thistle/silymarin (exact dose unknown) may act as hepatoprotective antioxidants.
- Spironolactone (1–2 mg/kg PO q 12h) or furosemide (1–2 mg/kg PO q 12h) in cases of ascites.
- Vitamin K_1 (5–20 mg SQ or IM) if overt clinical bleeding is identified or if PT or aPTT is prolonged greater than twice normal.
- Sucralfate (1 g/25 kg PO q 8–12h) and/or famotidine (Pepcid 0.5 mg/kg q 24h) as gastrointestinal ulcer therapy.

DRUG INTERACTIONS

- Animals with hepatic failure are anesthetic risks. Barbiturates should be avoided, and benzodiazepines should be used with care. Isoflurane or sevoflurane are the gas anesthetics of choice. Propofol, although hepatically metabolized, may be administered to effect (usually requiring a small fraction of normal doses) for controlling seizures due to hepatic encephalopathy.
- Lidocaine, theophylline, propranolol, captopril, and tetracyclines should be avoided.
- Diuretics may worsen hepatic encephalopathy, promote dehydration or metabolic alkalosis, and should be used only in otherwise stable patients for the long-term delay of return of ascites.
- Corticosteroids should be avoided in animals with active infection, may precipitate hepatic failure and/or gastric ulceration, and cause sodium retention (may use dexamethasone [no mineralocorticoid activity] as an alternative to prednisone).
- Nonsteroidal anti-inflammatory drugs may exacerbate gastrointestinal ulceration.
- Avoid medications that rely solely or predominantly on hepatic metabolism for effectiveness or clearance.

POSSIBLE COMPLICATIONS

Hepatic encephalopathy, septicemia, hemorrhage/coagulopathy, disseminated intravascular coagulation

RECOMMENDED MONITORING

Body weight, abdominal girth, liver enzymes, albumin, BUN, and bile acids should be monitored on a monthly basis.

PROGNOSIS AND OUTCOME

- In one recent report, 94% of dogs with hepatic fibrosis/cirrhosis were dead within 1 week of diagnosis.
- Dogs with idiopathic hepatic fibrosis/cirrhosis have been reported to survive for up to 6 years, and aggressive therapy may extend the survival of cirrhotic patients, although the prognosis is usually very poor with advanced disease.
- Histopathologic findings may be helpful as a prognostic indicator.

- Patients with hepatic fibrosis/cirrhosis causing clinical signs of hepatic encephalopathy or of coagulopathy, or with histologically severe changes (cirrhosis, advanced fibrosis), usually have a poor prognosis.

PEARLS & CONSIDERATIONS

COMMENTS

- Hepatic fibrosis and cirrhotic changes indicate a progressive, terminal condition that is, unfortunately, not often recognized or appreciated until the patient is in an advanced state of the disease. An underlying etiology is not often identified, making specific therapy impossible. A histopathologic diagnosis is essential in cases of suspected hepatic fibrosis/cirrhosis.
- Even with severe cirrhotic/fibrosing liver disease, patients may have little active liver inflammation and therefore can have normal or near-normal liver enzyme values.
  - Bile acids (especially postprandial) are much more sensitive for detection.
- Treatment of hepatic encephalopathy-induced seizures with diazepam may induce a profoundly depressed or obtunded state that should be avoided. If such a state occurs, it may respond to flumazenil (0.1 mg/kg IV). Generally, induction and maintenance of anesthesia with either propofol constant rate infusion or isoflurane inhalation may be a better choice in such cases. See Hepatic Encephalopathy, p 489.

PREVENTION

- Being aware of breed predispositions and early testing of appropriate animals (i.e., Bedlington terriers) may lead to early intervention.
- Avoid oversupplementation with copper-containing products.

CLIENT EDUCATION

Encephalopathic patients that can be clinically stabilized need attention to nutrition: even extremely small amounts of meat protein (e.g., one small meat-based treat) may precipitate severe signs of hepatic encephalopathy.

SUGGESTED READING

Rutgers HC, et al: Idiopathic hepatic fibrosis in 15 dogs. *Vet Rec* 133:115, 1993.

Sevelius E: Diagnosis and prognosis of chronic hepatitis and cirrhosis in dogs. *J Small Anim Pract* 36:521, 1995.

AUTHOR: **CRAIG B. WEBB**
EDITOR: **KEITH P. RICHTER**

Citrus Oil Extract Toxicosis

BASIC INFORMATION

DEFINITION

Adverse effects typically caused by excessive dermal exposure of D-limonene. Toxicity is characterized by excessive salivation, weakness, ataxia, hypothermia, tremors, and erythema. Clinical signs are usually temporary, and an affected animal generally recovers fully within a few hours to a couple of days. Toxicosis usually occurs when concentrated products are not diluted properly.

EPIDEMIOLOGY

SPECIES, AGE, SEX

- Dogs and cats of all ages, sexes, and breeds are vulnerable.
- Cats are more sensitive than dogs.

RISK FACTORS

- Inappropriate dilution or excessive use (i.e., more than 5 to 10 times the manufacturer's recommended use)
- Risk of D-limonene or linalool toxicity increases when formulated with other solvents or essential oils

GEOGRAPHY AND SEASONALITY: Toxicosis more prevalent in summer months during flea season.

CLINICAL PRESENTATION

HISTORY, CHIEF COMPLAINT

- History of exposure (use of spray, shampoo, or dip containing citrus oil extracts)
- Hypersalivation, hypothermia, muscle weakness
- Ataxia and tremors

PHYSICAL EXAM FINDINGS

- A distinct citrus smell virtually always is present on the animal and is an important diagnostic finding.
- Hypersalivation.
- Muscle weakness.
- Tremors, shivering, or ataxia.
- Body temperature: mild to severe hypothermia.
- Irritation of eyes and skin. Cutaneous erythema, especially in the scrotal and perineal areas, is a common finding.

ETIOLOGY AND PATHOPHYSIOLOGY

- Crude citrus oil extracts including D-limonene and linalool have some insecticidal properties and are used in shampoos, sprays, or dips for control of fleas on dogs and cats.
- Concentration of D-limonene and linalool in most sprays is less than 1%. Shampoos usually contain D-limonene 5%. Some dips contain 78.2% D-limonene and need to be diluted before use on animals.
- Limonene (occurs in D or L form) is a monoterpene that occurs naturally in some fruits (citrus), trees, and bushes. It is commonly used as a flavoring agent, fragrance, feed additive, and in many household cleaning products.
- Linalool is found in nature as a monoterpene in volatile oils, various herbs, leaves, flowers, wood, and citrus products. It is used as a fragrance in soaps, detergents, and perfumes and as a flavoring agent in beverages, chewing gum, and candy.
- The exact mechanism of action of these products in mammals is not clear. Linalool has been ruled out to be a cholinesterase inhibitor.
- It has been suggested that these products cause centrally and peripherally acting vasodilation, resulting in hypothermia and muscle weakness.

DIAGNOSIS

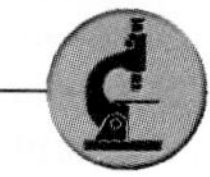

DIFFERENTIAL DIAGNOSIS

- Head trauma
- Toxicosis from pyrethrins/pyrethroids
- Portosystemic shunt

INITIAL DATABASE

- The diagnosis is generally established based on history and physical exam. Additional diagnostic testing may be used for ruling out other disorders with similar presenting signs.
- Complete blood count, serum biochemistry profile, urinalysis: typically unremarkable.

TREATMENT

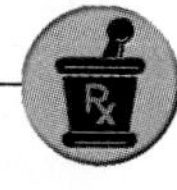

THERAPEUTIC GOAL(S)

- Dermal decontamination
- Thermoregulation
- Supportive care

ACUTE GENERAL TREATMENT

- Dermal decontamination:

- In case of dermal exposure, it is recommended to bathe the affected animal with an unmedicated detergent or soap and warm water. Drying the animal thoroughly, keeping the animal warm, and monitoring the body temperature frequently are essential to minimize hypothermia while not overcompensating and causing hyperthermia. Bathing can be repeated until the citrus smell is gone.
- Thermoregulation:
  - Monitoring of body temperature for hypothermia and keeping the animal warm and dry are essential.
  - Use of heating pads as needed, and warm water enema if hypothermia is severe, should be considered; however, warm water enema usage will eliminate rectal temperature as a reliable way of measuring core body temperature.
  - Avoidance of overcompensation (risk of iatrogenic hyperthermia); active rewarming of the patient should be terminated, and switched to passive warmth retention with ongoing monitoring, once the body temperature >98°F (36.7°C).
- Supportive care:
  - Administer intravenous fluids if necessary (e.g., dehydration, hypotension, electrolyte deficits).

PROGNOSIS AND OUTCOME

- Usually good to excellent; recovery within hours to a couple of days.
- Deaths have been reported in cats.

PEARLS & CONSIDERATIONS

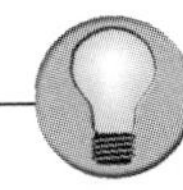

COMMENTS

- Animals treated with citrus oil extracts have a distinct smell.
- Hypersalivation is an immediate sign of d-limonene toxicosis in cats; it may last from 15 minutes to 1 hour. Severely affected cats show hypothermia and tremors.
- Linalool exposure produces more severe signs and for longer duration than d-limonene.
- d-limonene and linalool are well absorbed orally.
- When dips are used in higher concentration than recommended, limonene may be absorbed in significant quantities through the skin, causing systemic effects.

PREVENTION

Follow manufacturer's instructions for dilutions

SUGGESTED READING

Hooser SB: D-limonene, linalool, and crude citrus oil extracts. *Toxicol Select Pesticides Drugs Chem* 20(2):383–385, 1990.
http://www.getipm.com/sitemap.htm.
http://www.peteducation.com.

AUTHOR: **MOAZZAM A. KHAN**
EDITOR: **SAFDAR A. KHAN**

Cleaning Products Toxicosis

BASIC INFORMATION

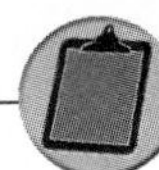

DEFINITION

Accidental exposure (dermal, oral, or ocular) of pets to household cleaning products, including soaps, detergents, bleaches, and disinfectants. Bleaches are discussed in greater detail in Acid or Alkali (Corrosives) Toxicosis, p 19.

EPIDEMIOLOGY

SPECIES, AGE, SEX

- Dogs more commonly involved than cats
- Cats more sensitive to cationic detergents, phenol, and pine oil-containing products

CLINICAL PRESENTATION

HISTORY, CHIEF COMPLAINT

- History of known exposure to a household cleaning product
- Rapid onset of clinical signs (minutes to a few hours)

PHYSICAL EXAM FINDINGS

- Hypersalivation, vomiting, diarrhea, lethargy (soaps, anionic, nonionic, and Zwitter detergents)
- Oral ulcers (phenol, cationic detergents)
- Corneal ulcer, conjunctivitis/blepharitis (phenol, cationic detergents)
- Central nervous system depression, aspiration (pine oil)
- Distinct smells: bleach, pine oil
- Salivation, vomiting (bleach, pine oil)

ETIOLOGY AND PATHOPHYSIOLOGY

- Sources:
  - Soaps are salts of fatty acids made by the reaction of alkali with fatty acids.
  - Detergents are nonsoap surfactants in combination with inorganic ingredients such as phosphates, silicates, or carbonates.
  - Detergents are classified into nonionic, anionic, cationic, or Zwitter agents according to charge present in solution. The classification depends on the active substance in the product (listed on label on product container).
    - Nonionic detergents: most heavy-duty laundry liquids, nonphosphate granular products, and many low-sudsing laundry products; alkyl ethoxylate, alkyl phenoxy polyethoxy ethanol, polyethylene glycol stearates
    - Anionic detergents: soap, emulsifiers for ointments and creams, dish wash liquids, solvent/detergent degreasers; alkyl sodium sulfonates, alkyl sodium sulfates, dioctyl sodium sulfosuccinates, sodium lauryl sulfates, tetrapropylene benzene sulfonate
    - Cationic detergents (quaternary ammonium compounds): benzethonium chloride, benzalkonium chloride, alkyl dimethyl 3, 4-dichlorobenzene, cetyl pyridinium chloride
    - Zwitter detergents: most shampoos, bath products, and nonirritant toiletries
  - Disinfectants: chemicals applied on inanimate objects to inhibit or kill micro-organisms (e.g., quaternary ammonium compounds [cationic detergents], phenols, pine oils, bleaches).
  - Most household bleach products contain sodium hypochlorite 3–6%. Nonchlorine/colorfast bleaches contain sodium peroxide, or sodium perborates.
- Pathophysiology:
  - Depending on dose and concentration, soaps, anionic, nonionic, and Zwitter detergents, and chlorine bleaches are mildly irritating to the mucous membranes. Oral or skin burns are rare.
  - Inhalation of chlorine fumes can cause pulmonary irritation, coughing, and if severe, dyspnea and noncardiogenic pulmonary edema.
  - Quaternary ammonium compounds are structurally similar to dexamethonium (neuromuscular blocking

agent) and hexamethonium (ganglionic blocking agent). Therefore, systemic effects may resemble organophosphate insecticide toxicosis (see p 775). They also cause corrosive damage to skin and oral mucosa.
    - Phenol (1-5%) can cause oral or dermal burns. Phenol (or other phenolic derivatives) can also cause respiratory stimulation and alkalosis followed by metabolic acidosis.
    - Pine oil disinfectants are irritating to the mucous membranes.

DIAGNOSIS

DIFFERENTIAL DIAGNOSIS

- Corrosives toxicosis (alkali, acids)
- Uremia (oral ulcers)
- Acute vomiting: foreign body obstruction, viral or bacterial gastroenteritis, garbage toxicosis, pancreatitis

INITIAL DATABASE

- Complete blood count (leukocytosis with cationic detergents, phenol; within normal limits for others)
- Serum chemistry profile: electrolyte changes (from severe vomiting or dehydration; cationic detergents, phenols) may be present
- Urinalysis: results should be unremarkable
- Fluorescein staining for corneal ulcers (cationic detergents, phenol)

ADVANCED OR CONFIRMATORY TESTING

- Thoracic radiographs: indicated if coughing, dyspnea, or fever of unknown origin. May show evidence of aspiration pneumonia and/or noncardiogenic pulmonary edema
- Abdominal imaging (radiographs, ultrasound): to rule out other causes of acute severe vomiting
- Endoscopic examination of esophagus to rule out perforation within 12 to 24 hours (cationic detergents, phenol)

TREATMENT

THERAPEUTIC GOAL(S)

- Decontamination of patient
- Protect gastrointestinal (GI) mucosa
- Supportive therapy

ACUTE GENERAL TREATMENT

- Decontamination:
    - Oral dilution: *Best option*. Immediately administer milk or water (approximately, 0.25 to 0.5 cups for a 30-lb [14-kg] dog and 1 to 2 tablespoons for a 10-lb [4.5-kg] cat). Follow with milk of magnesia (0.2-0.3 ml/kg PO).
    - Emesis induction in cases of toxicosis with soaps, detergents (other than cationic); *rarely needed*. Use within 2 to 4 hours only if very large amounts have been ingested. *Do not induce vomiting: cationic detergents, phenol, or pine oils.*
        - Apomorphine 0.03-0.04 mg/kg IV, IM, or dissolved and instilled into conjunctival sac
        - Hydrogen peroxide 3%: 2 ml/kg PO (max 45 ml)
    - Activated charcoal: rarely needed; 1-3 g/kg PO with a cathartic such as 70% sorbitol (3 ml/kg). Not needed for cationic detergents, phenol, or pine oils.
    - Dermal: wash exposed area (cationic detergents, phenol) with water for 20 to 30 minutes.
    - Ocular: flush eyes with tepid tap water (or saline) for 20 to 30 minutes. Repeat fluorescein stain to assess for corneal ulcers.
- Protect GI mucosa (cationic detergents, phenol):
    - H_2 receptor antagonists:
        - Famotidine: dogs/cats: 0.5 mg/kg PO, SC, IM, IV q 12-24h, or
        - Cimetidine: dogs/cats: 5-10 mg/kg PO q 6h)
    - Sucralfate: dog: 0.5-1 g PO q 8-12h; cat: 0.25-0.5 g PO q 8-12h.
- Supportive care:
    - Intravenous fluids for rehydration (e.g., lactated Ringer's solution) or maintenance.
    - Broad-spectrum antibiotics (e.g., ampicillin 22 mg/kg IV q 8h plus enrofloxacin 5 mg/kg IM or diluted 1:1 with sterile saline and given slowly IV q 12h [q 24h in cats]) if caustic burns and/or secondary infection.
    - Manage pain (caustic burns): opiates (e.g., fentanyl patch or butorphanol 0.1-1.0 mg/kg IM, IV, or SC).
- Nutrition: feed watery slurry or soft mashed food while visible mucosal erosions are present

RECOMMENDED MONITORING

- Complete blood count, serum chemistry profile: electrolyte changes and other effects of vomiting
- Monitor oral cavity, perioral skin for caustic burns (cationic detergents, phenol) to determine when to introduce solid food
- Pulse oximetry, thoracic radiography if aspiration (pine oils)

PROGNOSIS AND OUTCOME

- Excellent with soaps, detergents (other than cationic), and household bleaches
- Good to guarded if pulmonary edema develops (bleaches) or if caustic burns are present (cationic detergents, phenols in cats)

PEARLS & CONSIDERATIONS

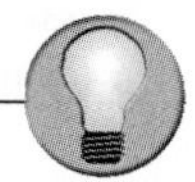

COMMENTS

Soaps, detergents (other than cationic), and household bleaches have a low order of toxicity and can be treated by immediate dilution (oral administration of milk or water).

PREVENTION

Keep household cleaning products out of reach of pets

SUGGESTED READING

Coppock RW, et al: The toxicology of detergents, bleaches, antiseptics and disinfectants in small animals. *Vet Hum Toxicol* 30(5):463-472, 1988.

Kore AM, et al: Toxicology of household cleaning products and disinfectants. *Vet Clin North Am Small Anim Pract* 20(2):525-536, 1990.

AUTHOR: **MOAZZAM A. KHAN**
EDITOR: **SAFDAR A. KHAN**

Cleft Palate

BASIC INFORMATION

DEFINITION

A congenital, physical defect of the lips, hard, and/or soft palate

SYNONYM(S)

Primary cleft palate: "harelip," "cleft lip"

EPIDEMIOLOGY

SPECIES, AGE, SEX

- Dogs and cats of either sex
- Incidence higher in brachycephalic dog breeds and Siamese cats
- Problem noted in puppies and kittens soon after birth: nursing problems

GENETICS AND BREED PREDISPOSITION

- Inherited as either autosomal recessive or irregularly dominant genes
- Mating of parents with cleft palate results in 41% incidence in offspring

ASSOCIATED CONDITIONS AND DISORDERS

- Aspiration pneumonia
- Chronic rhinitis

CLINICAL PRESENTATION

DISEASE FORMS/SUBTYPES

Two types of cleft palate:

- Primary. Upper lip and/or rostralmost hard palate. Unilateral defects are more commonly on the left side.
- Secondary. Involves hard and/or soft palate:
  - Midline cleft of soft ± hard palate
  - Unilateral or bilateral absence of soft palate

HISTORY, CHIEF COMPLAINT

- Primary cleft palate: mild nasal congestion and discharge
- Secondary cleft palate: inability to suckle (failure to create negative pressure for nursing); chronic nasal discharge of milk, mucus, or pus; coughing, gagging, and/or sneezing; poor weight gain; unthriftiness

PHYSICAL EXAM FINDINGS

- Small stature
- Nasal discharge (milk reflux into nasal cavity)
- Auscultation: increased lung sounds, wheezing, or crackles (aspiration pneumonia); dyspnea
- Oral examination:
  - Primary cleft: "harelip" often obvious. Primary cleft palate can present as unilateral or bilateral lip defect only; as defect of the rostral hard palate only; or as defects both of the lip and rostralmost hard palate. Can also be associated with abnormalities of the secondary palate
  - Secondary cleft: midline defect can usually be visualized, but soft palate may be difficult to evaluate

ETIOLOGY AND PATHOPHYSIOLOGY

- Etiology:
  - Hormonal: gestational corticosteroid administration.
  - Infectious-viral-induced.
  - Mechanical.
  - Metabolic.
  - Nutritional.
  - Toxic: secondary to drug, viral toxins.
  - Hereditary:
    - Autosomal recessive or irregularly dominant genes.
    - Growth of palatine bones in the fetus may compete with the growth of skull, especially in broad-skulled (brachycephalic) dogs, to achieve normal closure of the palatine plates.
- Pathophysiology:
  - The *primary palate* is formed by the lips and most rostral hard palate. The rest of the hard palate and the soft palate constitute the *secondary palate*.
  - In cleft palate, any of several bones may be affected, including the incisive, maxillary, and palatine bones.
  - Defects of the primary and secondary palate result from a *failure of fusion* of paired (and one unpaired) structures during development.

DIAGNOSIS

DIFFERENTIAL DIAGNOSIS

Acquired oronasal fistula

INITIAL DATABASE

- Complete blood count, thoracic radiographs:
  - Possible aspiration pneumonia
- Serum biochemistry panel, urinalysis:
  - Routine to assess unthrifty patients

ADVANCED OR CONFIRMATORY TESTING

Oral examination under general anesthesia:

- Define extent of secondary cleft palate defects

TREATMENT

THERAPEUTIC GOAL(S)

- Treat and resolve aspiration pneumonia prior to surgery
- Nutritional support (tube feeding) until patient of adequate age and health for surgery
- Complete closure of palatine defects

ACUTE GENERAL TREATMENT

- Treat aspiration pneumonia (see p 862)
- Tube feeding (orogastric) with milk replacer or other suitable diet (e.g., Hills' a/d) until surgical candidate (>2-4 months old):
  - Supplies nutritional needs
  - Minimizes rhinitis
  - Allows patient to mature: anesthetic purposes, greater strength of palatal tissue, more working room in the oropharynx to effect repair

CHRONIC TREATMENT

- Surgical repair of primary cleft requires accurate reconstruction of the columella (rostral margin of nasal septum) and philtrum (natural groove ventral to nasal septum)
- Surgical repair of secondary cleft palate:
  - Hard palate repair involves utilization of mucoperiosteal flaps supplied by major palatine arteries; exposed bone is left to granulate and epithelialize (Fig. I-37). Overlapping double flaps, medially positioned double flaps, or unilateral rotation (single pedicle) flaps may be used.
  - Soft palate repair involves either an overlapping flap or medially positioned technique with a two- or three-layer closure.

POSTOPERATIVE MANAGEMENT

- Pain control: opioids (e.g., hydromorphone 0.1-0.2 mg/kg IV or IM as needed up to q 2-4h) and nonsteroidal anti-inflammatory drugs (e.g., carprofen 2 mg/kg PO q 12h)
- Antibiotics: usually not required unless aspiration
- Nutritional support: soft food; no chewing toys/treats for 4 weeks; esophagostomy and gastrostomy tubes are rarely needed
- Wound management: oral application of dilute chlorhexidine solution or gel for 4 weeks; Elizabethan collar to prevent pawing at surgical site; reexamination in 2 weeks for removal of skin sutures at lips

POSSIBLE COMPLICATIONS

- Dehiscence:
  - Excess tension if inadequate mobilization of tissue for closure
  - Tongue movements, prehension, chewing (consider postoperative tube feeding)

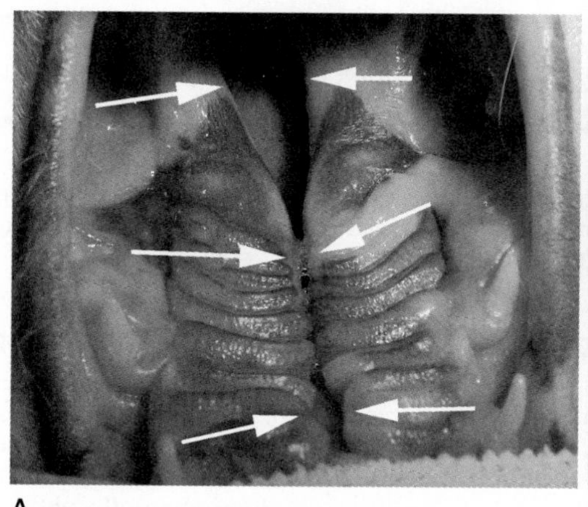

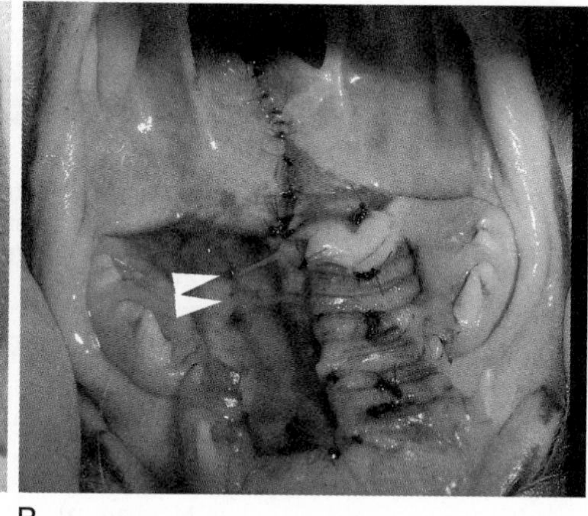

FIGURE I-37 **A**, Congenital cleft palate. This 14-week-old dog is under general anesthesia and in dorsal recumbency; rostral is towards the bottom of the image. A congenital defect of the secondary palate (midline cleft of the hard and soft palate) is seen (*arrows*). **B**, Congenital cleft palate, repaired: the hard palate defect was repaired utilizing the overlapping double flap technique (note the exposed major and accessory palatine arteries—*arrowheads*); the donor area is left to granulate and epithelialize. The soft palate defect was repaired utilizing the medially positioned double flap technique. Courtesy of Dr. Alexander M. Reiter, University of Pennsylvania.

- Palatal flap necrosis if major palatine artery is compromised during surgery

RECOMMENDED MONITORING

Owner should watch for recurrence of clinical signs that could indicate dehiscence

PROGNOSIS AND OUTCOME

- Multiple procedures may be required to close a cleft. Follow-up surgeries should not be attempted before healing of all tissues involved (6 weeks)
- Poor prognosis for congenital soft palate absence
- Guarded prognosis for secondary cleft palate without surgical repair (risk of aspiration)

PEARLS & CONSIDERATIONS

COMMENTS

The best chance of success is with the first surgical procedure; avoid electrocoagulation for hemostasis, handle flaps as carefully as possible, and avoid creating closure that is under tension.

PREVENTION

- Avoid breeding parents that have cleft palate
- Avoid giving corticosteroids or other potential teratogens during pregnancy

CLIENT EDUCATION

Management of patients with cleft palate requires intensive nursing care for 2 to 4 months until surgery can be performed

SUGGESTED READING

Nelson AW: Cleft palate. In Slatter D (ed): *Textbook of Small Animal Surgery*, ed 3. Philadelphia, WB Saunders, 2003, pp 814–823.

Robertson JJ: The palate. In Bojrab MJ (ed): *Disease Mechanisms in Small Animal Surgery*, ed 2. Philadephia, Lea & Febiger, 1993, pp 191–194.

AUTHORS: **ELLEN B. DAVIDSON DOMNICK, ALEXANDER M. REITER**
EDITORS: **ALEXANDER M. REITER, RICHARD WALSHAW**

Clostridial Enterocolitis

BASIC INFORMATION

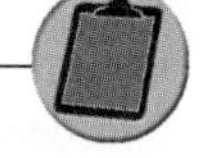

DEFINITION

Clostridial enterocolitis is a form of intestinal disease that causes diarrhea in dogs and cats and is suspected to be caused by *Clostridium perfringens*. It typically causes large intestinal diarrhea that may be acute and self-limiting, or may be chronic in nature.

SYNONYM(S)

Acute nosocomial colitis
Canine nosocomial diarrhea
Clostidial enterotoxicosis

EPIDEMIOLOGY

SPECIES, AGE, SEX: Dogs are more commonly affected than cats. No apparent age or sex predilection. Acute disease can occur in any age animal, whereas chronic disease can occur in middle-aged to older animals.

CLINICAL PRESENTATION

HISTORY, CHIEF COMPLAINT (SOME OR ALL MAY BE PRESENT)

- Large intestinal diarrhea. Small volumes of feces, increased frequency of defecation, and straining are common, and mucus and/or fresh blood may been visualized in the feces. Vomiting and flatulence may also be present in some patients. Many patients show no clinical signs other than the diarrhea.
- A small number of patients may also have small bowel diarrhea marked by large volumes of feces.

PHYSICAL EXAM FINDINGS

- Findings are nonspecific and relate to large intestinal diarrhea. There may be abdominal discomfort during palpation. There may also be signs of pain during digital rectal examination.
- Acute nosocomial diarrhea associated with *C. perfringens* is often seen 1 to

5 days after boarding or kenneling. This syndrome appears to be self-limiting and responds well to supportive care.

ETIOLOGY AND PATHOPHYSIOLOGY

- *C. perfringens* is an anaerobic, spore-forming, gram-positive bacillus that is also found in normal dogs and cats.
- Sporulation of toxigenic strains causes release of enterotoxin A. This enterotoxin can cause mucosal damage and fluid secretion in the colon.
- Other factors must also be involved. Enterotoxin-related damage cannot be the sole explanation for this disorder, because enterotoxin has been identified in the feces of normal animals.

DIAGNOSIS

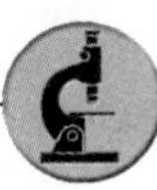

DIFFERENTIAL DIAGNOSIS

- All causes of large intestinal diarrhea, both primary gastrointestinal and systemic/nonprimary gastrointestinal, need to be considered.
- Primary gastrointestinal disease includes parasites, inflammatory bowel disease, neoplasia, fungal disease, and histiocytic ulcerative colitis.
- Systemic/extraintestinal causes of acute diarrhea include anxiety/nervousness, other intra-abdominal disorders, and intoxications (e.g., organophosphates).

INITIAL DATABASE

- Complete blood count, biochemical profile, urinalysis, fecal flotation: generally unremarkable.
- Fecal enzyme-linked immunosorbent assay (ELISA) for *Giardia* or other pathogens.
- Fecal smear with Gram stain.
- Rectal scraping for cytologic study (to rule out histoplasmosis, lymphoma) using a vaginal or bone marrow harvesting-type curette.
- Fecal analysis is very important in all cases of large bowel diarrhea, because this test is noninvasive and may yield important clues to the problem, even if the diagnosis is elusive.

ADVANCED OR CONFIRMATORY TESTING

- Advanced diagnostic evaluation may include fecal culture, and evaluation for the presence of enterotoxin in feces.
- Abdominal imaging with radiographs or ultrasound is often normal but can be warranted to rule out extra gastrointestinal diseases.
- Colonoscopy is rarely indicated to diagnose this condition, but in severe cases may be necessary to rule out other causes of colitis:
  - Mucosal hyperemia or ulceration are typical.
  - Histopathologic analysis of biopsies may indicate neutrophilic colitis, the presence of other inflammatory bowel disease, or may be normal.
- Fecal cytologic study may indicate the presence of sporulating clostridial organisms, which have the appearance of safety pins. However, the presence of these organisms does not confirm that a clostridium is the cause of the clinical disease.
- Anaerobic fecal cultures will typically identify high concentrations of *C. perfringens* (>3-5 organisms/field on oil immersion).
- Other diagnostic tests that are available include ELISA enterotoxin assays and polymerase chain reaction enterotoxin genotyping.

TREATMENT

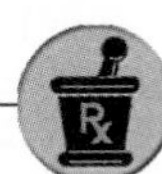

THERAPEUTIC GOAL(S)

Therapeutic goals are to provide supportive care and eliminate large bowel diarrhea. These patients may be dehydrated, anorexic, and lethargic. Supportive care should be directed toward correcting volume deficits and reducing intestinal discomfort so that the patient will eat and be more comfortable.

ACUTE GENERAL TREATMENT

- Treatment with intravenous crystalloids to correct volume deficits is very important.
- The use of antimicrobials, including amoxicillin (20 mg/kg PO q 8h), erythromycin (10-20 mg/kg PO q 8h), tylosin (5-10 mg/kg PO q 12h), or metronidazole (15-20 mg/kg PO q 12h × 7 days maximum) is generally beneficial. Parenteral antibiotics with anaerobic bactericidal activity (e.g., ampicillin 20 mg/kg IV q 6-8h) are indicated if the patient is systemically ill.
- Dietary management with high-fiber diets has also been shown to reduce clinical signs and speed recovery.

CHRONIC TREATMENT

- Long-term antimicrobial therapy may be required along with dietary management.
- In some cases, the antibiotic therapy may be discontinued as long as the high-fiber diet is maintained.

RECOMMENDED MONITORING

Based on the presence or absence of diarrhea

PROGNOSIS AND OUTCOME

The prognosis is dependent on the presenting condition of the patient. In most cases the prognosis is excellent.

PEARLS & CONSIDERATIONS

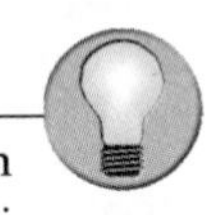

- There is no gold standard on how to treat this disease; treatment is adapted based on specific abnormalities identified on physical exam and diagnostic testing.
- There is still some question as to whether Koch's postulates have been fulfilled regarding causality of *C. perfringens* and this form of enteritis.

CLIENT EDUCATION

In most cases the signs associated with this disease subside with supportive care, but some patients may be chronically affected.

SUGGESTED READING

Kruth SA, et al: Nosocomial diarrhea associated with enterotoxigenic *Clostridium perfringens* infection in dogs. *J Am Vet Med Assoc* 195:331-334, 1989.

Twedt DC: *Clostridium perfringens*-associated enterotoxicosis in dogs. In Kirk RW, Bonagura JD (eds): *Current Veterinary Therapy XI: Small Animal Practice*. Philadelphia, WB Saunders, 1992, 602-604.

Weese JS, et al: The roles of *Clostridium difficile* and enterotoxigenic *Clostridium perfringens* in diarrhea in dogs. *J Vet Intern Med* 15:374-378, 2001.

AUTHOR: **STEVEN L. MARKS**

EDITOR: **DEBRA L. ZORAN**

Coccidioidomycosis

BASIC INFORMATION

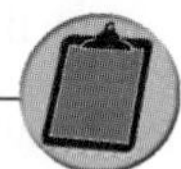

DEFINITION

A respiratory and systemic fungal infection caused by the fungus *Coccidioides immitis*

SYNONYM(S)

San Joaquin Valley fever
Valley fever

EPIDEMIOLOGY

SPECIES, AGE, SEX: Young, male, medium- to large-breed dogs that are housed outside are more commonly infected. Cats are more resistant to infection but can develop clinical illness.

GENETICS AND BREED PREDISPOSITION: Illness has been reported in a large number of breeds and is more commonly reported in the boxer, pointer, Australian shepherd, beagle, Scottish terrier, Doberman pinscher, and cocker spaniel breeds.

RISK FACTORS

- When in endemic area, increased risk with:
  - Daytime spent predominantly outdoors
  - Amount of roaming space > 1 acre
  - Walking in the desert
  - ± Immunosuppression
- When in endemic area, decreased risk with walking preferentially on sidewalks

CONTAGION AND ZOONOSIS

- Coccidioidomycosis occurs in humans, who may become infected at the same environmental source as dogs and other animals.
- Direct transmission from animals to humans is extremely unlikely, because the yeast phase (present at body temperature) is not transmitted by aerosol.
- Conversion of the yeast phase to the mycelial phase, which produces infectious spores (arthroconidia) that may be inhaled, could occur on bandages, tissue samples, or instruments; such material should be dealt with safely and immediately (e.g., disinfected or autoclaved).
- The mycelial/hyphal form of *C. immitis*, which grows in vitro and in nature, is a serious zoonotic risk. Any tissue or fluid that may contain *C. immitis* should never be cultured unless this is done with high-level biosafety containment (by a specialized laboratory with appropriate notification).

GEOGRAPHY AND SEASONALITY

- Coccidioidomycosis is most common in the southwestern United States, including California, Arizona, and Texas (the lower Sonoran life zone). A few endemic areas are found in Central and South America.
- Having lived in or traveled through these regions is an essential component of the history of patients with coccidioidomycosis.
- Because the disease is acquired through inhalation of airborne spores, the incidence of disease increases when rainy seasons are followed by drought and dust storms.

CLINICAL PRESENTATION

HISTORY, CHIEF COMPLAINT

- Typically, the earliest sign of infection is a mild chronic cough. The cough may be dry and harsh, or moist and productive.
- Other presenting complaints may include inappetence, weight loss, lethargy, lameness, signs of head or neck pain, signs of vision loss, or cutaneous draining tracts.
- Cats are more likely to present with skin lesions than dogs.
- See Geography and seasonality above.

PHYSICAL EXAM FINDINGS: Respiratory findings may be limited to mild signs of coughing or include harsh lung sounds, dyspnea, and tachypnea. Systemic signs may include fever, depression, weakness, lameness, peripheral lymphadenopathy, firm/ hard swelling over long bones, draining skin lesions, and signs of keratitis or uveitis.

ETIOLOGY AND PATHOPHYSIOLOGY

- *Coccidioides immitis* is a dimorphic fungus; it has both yeast and mycelial (hyphal) forms:
  - The mycelial form exists in the environment and produces arthroconidia that are easily inhaled and highly infectious.
  - The yeast form grows in tissue and results in clinical illness.
  - Inhalation of 10 or fewer arthroconidia is sufficient to cause infection that produces clinical signs.
- After inhalation, arthroconidia enter the pulmonary alveoli and cause subpleural lesions:
  - In this location, the fungus changes morphology to the yeast form, producing endospores that can disseminate to other tissues.
  - The incubation period from the time of inhalation to the appearance of respiratory signs is 1 to 3 weeks.
- Similar to most fungi, the response to infection results in the development of pyogranulomatous inflammation.
- The most common form of infection is a lower respiratory tract infection, which may progress to systemic illness affecting the lymph nodes, bones, eyes, and skin most commonly.
  - Dissemination can happen within 10 days of inhalation, but overt clinical signs of disseminated coccidioidomycosis are usually only noted ≥4 months after the onset of respiratory signs.
- The course of illness may be protracted over several months to years.
- Many animals that inhale *C. immitis* have subclinical, self-resolving infections or recover from the respiratory phase without therapy.
  - Approximately 28% of dogs living in an endemic region develop antibodies to *C. immitis* by age 2 years, and approximately 6% develop clinical infection.

DIAGNOSIS

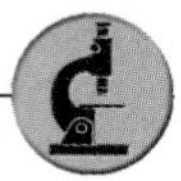

DIFFERENTIAL DIAGNOSIS

- Cough:
  - Initially, a dry hacking cough may be mistaken for tracheobronchitis.
  - A productive cough may also be due to bacterial pneumonia, other systemic fungal infection, or neoplasia.
  - Other important differential diagnoses include chronic sterile bronchitis, collapsing trachea, and congestive heart failure.
- Considerations for bone lesions should include bacterial osteomyelitis, other fungal infections, or neoplasia.
- Skin lesions: differential diagnoses include draining tracts due to other systemic mycoses, bony lesions such as infected sequestra, or abscesses due to bite wounds or other penetrating injuries.
- Causes of ocular lesions could include other systemic infectious illnesses and immune-mediated diseases.

INITIAL DATABASE

- Complete blood count may reveal an inflammatory leukogram and a mild nonregenerative anemia.
- Hypoalbuminemia (virtually all cases) and hyperglobulinemia (approximately 50% of cases) are common. Hypercalcemia has not been described with this form of fungal infection.
- Urinalysis is not expected to show specific abnormalities.
- Thoracic radiographs are frequently abnormal and are indicated in any patient suspected of having coccidioidomycosis:

- Common findings include a diffuse interstitial pulmonary pattern and hilar lymphadenopathy, which may be profound.
- Alveolar infiltrates and nodules with or without pleural effusion or evidence of pericardial effusion may also be seen.
- Radiographs of long bones may reveal proliferative and lytic lesions, typically distally in the bone (distal diaphysis, metaphysis, and epiphysis).

ADVANCED OR CONFIRMATORY TESTING

- Coccidioidomycosis can be definitively diagnosed via cytologic examination of exudates, sputum, or aspirates, or histopathologic examination of tissue:
  - The organism is a large (1 to 10 times the diameter of a red blood cell), round structure typically surrounded by neutrophils and macrophages.
  - Transtracheal washes and lymph node aspirates are often falsely negative. Cytologic evaluation of fluid from draining tracts and of pleural effusion are more likely to yield organisms.
  - Organisms can be difficult to find histopathologically on bone biopsies but are readily identified within bony microabscesses.
- Serologic testing is available for dogs and cats. Several serologic tests are available for both IgM and IgG:
  - As with other forms of serology, IgM reflects acute response. A positive titer can be noted within 2 weeks of exposure (i.e., during or just after the incubation period) and may last 4 to 6 weeks.
  - IgG indicates exposure or infection. The magnitude of titer is considered important, with higher titers (≥1:64), suggesting disseminated or severe pulmonary infections.
  - IgG titer is expected to decrease slowly, but may not reach zero, with successful treatment.
  - Positive IgG titers from dogs living in endemic areas are more likely due to exposure than from active infection.

TREATMENT

THERAPEUTIC GOAL(S)

- Prevention of further systemic dissemination of the organism.
- Eradication of the organism in the patient.
- Mild respiratory cases will often resolve without antifungal therapy.

ACUTE GENERAL TREATMENT

- Supportive care for systemic illness and respiratory distress as warranted:
  - See Oxygen Supplementation, p 1292.
  - See Hypotension, Systemic, p 572.
- Rapid diagnosis should be followed by antifungal therapy. Broad-spectrum antibiotics should be avoided.
- Antifungal oral drugs (azoles) should be given with food to enhance bioavailability.
  - Ketoconazole (5 to 10 mg/kg PO q 12h). Effective, least costly; may produce adverse hepatic effects or vomiting/inappetence.
  - Itraconazole (5 mg/kg PO q 12h). More effective than ketoconazole in some cases, less so in others (not predictable). Costly. May have fewer adverse effects.
  - Fluconazole (5 mg/kg PO q 12h). Highly lipid soluble, best penetration of eye, central nervous system. Costly.
- Cats generally receive 25 to 50 mg total of the antifungal azole agent every 12 to 24 hours.
- Amphotericin B (0.4–0.5 mg/kg IV q 48–72h; caution regarding perivascular irritation/sloughing; monitor renal parameters); can be used in patients that do not tolerate azole drugs (e.g., anorexia, vomiting, hepatic dysfunction) or who are critically ill, because amphotericin B is fungicidal, whereas the azole drugs are fungistatic.
- Lufenuron 5 mg/kg PO q 24h for 4 months has shown promising results.

CHRONIC TREATMENT

Therapy must persist at least 2 months beyond the resolution of clinical signs, which may be as long as 12 months with disseminated disease.

DRUG INTERACTIONS

- Care should be taken in prescribing antifungal therapy for long-term use. Some patients receiving azole drugs can develop liver dysfunction, intestinal upset, thrombocytopenia, and skin reactions.
- Compatibility of other medications with antifungal agents should be investigated before use. Antifungal agents should not be used in conjunction with H_2 blockers or cisapride.
- Caution should be taken in patients receiving op'DDD, warfarin, digoxin, phenytoin, methylprednisolone, cyclosporine, and oral antidiabetic agents.

POSSIBLE COMPLICATIONS

If clinically significant respiratory signs are left untreated, systemic spread of illness is likely

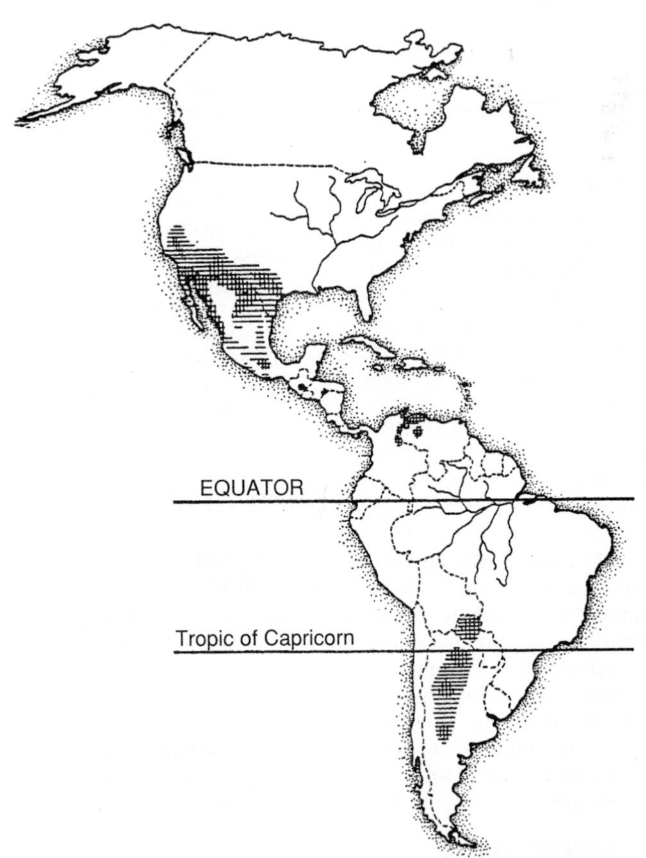

FIGURE I-38 Geographic area in which coccidioidomycosis is endemic. Areas of highest prevalence are cross-hatched. From Rippon JW: *Medical Mycology*, ed 3. Philadelphia, Saunders, 1988, p 436. Reprinted with permission.

PROGNOSIS AND OUTCOME

- Prognosis for patients with only respiratory signs is fair to good.
- Patients with disseminated disease have a guarded to poor prognosis for full recovery.

PEARLS & CONSIDERATIONS

COMMENTS

- Diagnosis based on serology alone is not recommended but occasionally necessary. Due to the prognosis, expense of therapy and length of therapy, all efforts should be made to obtain a cytologic or histologic diagnosis.
- Fungal culture of *Coccidioides* should not be attempted in a veterinary practice, because the hyphae are the infectious form of the fungus and are highly infectious to humans as well as domestic animals.
- Bandages used for covering cutaneous draining tracts may be highly infectious to humans if the lesion is due to coccidioidomycosis; therefore, bandages should be avoided in such situations, or if indispensable, should be disinfected or destroyed (autoclaved) immediately when removed.

SUGGESTED READING

Butkiewicz CD, et al: Risk factors associated with *Coccidioides* infection in dogs. *J Am Vet Med Assoc* 226(11):1851-1854, 2005.

Greene RT: Coccidioidomycosis. In Greene CE (ed): *Infectious Diseases of the Dog and Cat.* Philadelphia, WB Saunders, 1998, pp 391-398.

Johnson LR, et al. Clinical, clinicopathologic, and radiographic findings in dogs with coccidioidomycosis: 24 cases (1995-2000). *J Am Vet Med Assoc* 222(4):461-466, 2003.

Shubitz LE: Incidence of coccidioides infection among dogs residing in a region in which the organism is endemic. *J Am Vet Med Assoc* 226(11):1846-1850, 2005.

Taboada J: Systemic mycoses. In Ettinger SJ, Feldman EC (eds): *Textbook of Veterinary Internal Medicine*. Philadelphia, WB Saunders, 2000, pp 453-476.

AUTHOR: **KATHRYN TAYLOR**

EDITOR: **DOUGLASS K. MACINTIRE**

Coccidiosis, Intestinal

BASIC INFORMATION

DEFINITION

A diarrheal disease caused by infection of the intestinal tract with Apicomplexan parasites in the Genus *Cystoisospora*

SYNONYM(S)

Isospora

EPIDEMIOLOGY

SPECIES, AGE, SEX: Intestinal coccidiois occurs both in dogs and cats. Males and females are equally susceptible. Young animals are more likely to have clinical signs than are older animals. Animals that are stressed are also more likely to develop clinical coccidiosis than are nonstressed animals.

GENETICS AND BREED PREDISPOSITION: None.

RISK FACTORS: Recent weaning or overcrowded conditions. Animals less than 1 year old.

CONTAGION AND ZOONOSIS: Oocysts of *Cystoisospora* species can infect and cause asymptomatic infections in a number of paratenic hosts. Infections in humans have been reported in immunocompromised hosts, but usually with coccidian species not found in dogs and cats.

GEOGRAPHY AND SEASONALITY: *Cystoisospora* species have a worldwide distribution and are present year round.

CLINICAL PRESENTATION

HISTORY, CHIEF COMPLAINT: Diarrhea or diarrhea and vomiting are the main complaints. Diarrhea is nonbloody, often foul smelling, pasty, and semiformed to liquid.

PHYSICAL EXAM FINDINGS: Weight loss (or poor growth), dull haircoat, dehydration, and slightly elevated temperature may be present.

ETIOLOGY AND PATHOPHYSIOLOGY

- Intestinal coccidiosis in cats is caused by *Cystoisospora felis* and *Cystoisospora rivolta*. Intestinal coccidiosis in dogs is caused by *Cystoisospora canis* and *Cystoisospora ohioensis* complex (*C. ohioensis; C. neorivolta; C. burrowsi*).
- Intestinal damage is caused by rupture of host cells lining the intestinal villi of the small intestines. Villous atrophy and villous erosions occur due to parasite multiplication.

DIAGNOSIS

DIFFERENTIAL DIAGNOSIS

Giardiasis or other protozoal enteric infections, viral or bacterial induced diarrhea, dietary indiscretion, other parasitic (helminths) diseases of the intestines

INITIAL DATABASE

- Fecal examination and demonstration of characteristic oocysts.
- Parvovirus enzyme-linked immunosorbent assay may be indicated in affected puppies with severe diarrhea, to rule out concurrent parvoviral enteritis.
- Kittens should be tested for feline leukemia virus or feline immunodeficiency virus (older than 4 months).

ADVANCED OR CONFIRMATORY TESTING

None needed

TREATMENT

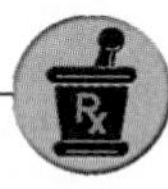

THERAPEUTIC GOAL(S)

Remission of diarrhea and cessation of oocyst production

ACUTE GENERAL TREATMENT

- Sulfadimethoxine (Albon oral suspension 5%):
  - 55 mg/kg PO once, followed 24h later by 27.5 mg/kg PO q 24h in dogs.
  - Treatment is continued until clinical signs have resolved for 48 hours.
  - Adequate water intake must be maintained during treatment to prevent dehydration.
  - Supportive care includes fluids; providing a warm, dry environment; and an appropriate diet.
- Off-label:
  - Toltrazuril (Baycox) 30 mg/kg PO as a single treatment.
  - Ponazuril (Marquis) 30 mg/kg PO as a single treatment.
  - A combination of sulfadimethoxine with ormetoprim (Primor) 55 mg/kg PO q 24h (for up to 21 days) is also effective.
  - Amprolium (Corid) 300-400 mg/kg PO q 24h for 5 days or 110-220

mg/kg for 7 to 12 days. Amprolium is bitter, and care should be taken that the appropriate dose is ingested and not spit out by the treated dogs.

CHRONIC TREATMENT

Same as for acute

DRUG INTERACTIONS

See sulfonamides

RECOMMENDED MONITORING

Adult animals with documented coccidiosis should be evaluated for other causes of intestinal disease (e.g., inflammatory bowel disease, lymphoma) or immunocompromise (e.g., Cushing's disease).

PROGNOSIS AND OUTCOME

Good; most animals will respond readily to anticoccidial treatment.

PEARLS & CONSIDERATIONS

COMMENTS

- It is virtually impossible to prevent exposure to coccidia in dogs and cats. Clinical disease often develops around weaning or after other stressful events like shipping or moving locations.
- The use of newer anticoccidials (Ponazuril or Toltrazuril) strategically, at times when animals are likely to develop coccidiosis, may become common practice in the future. An example of a strategic treatment would be administration of ponazuril a few days prior to or at weaning to prevent development of coccidiosis in recently weaned puppies.

PREVENTION

Reduce environmental contamination as much as possible (control populations, keep the environment clean, and remove fecal contamination of all litter boxes and living areas)

CLIENT EDUCATION

Coccidian parasites can be zoonotic to immunocompromised humans.

SUGGESTED READING

Daugschies A, et al: Toltrazuril treatment of cystoisosporosis in dogs under experimental and field conditions. *Parasitol Res* 86:797–799, 2000.

Lindsay DS, et al: Biology of *Isospora* spp. from humans, nonhuman primates, and domestic animals. *Clin Microbiol Rev* 10:19–34, 1997.

AUTHOR: **DAVID S. LINDSAY**

EDITOR: **DEBRA L. ZORAN**

Cognitive Dysfunction

BASIC INFORMATION

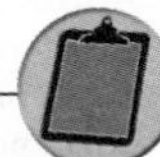

DEFINITION

The decline in behavioral condition with advanced age, in the absence of causative physical or medical conditions

SYNONYM(S)

Senility

EPIDEMIOLOG3Y

SPECIES, AGE, SEX

- Cats: typically >10 years old.
- Dogs: typically >6 years old (large breeds), >12 years (small breeds).

GENETICS AND BREED PREDISPOSITION: Dogs and cats, like humans, may have "susceptibility genes" for the development of lesions associated with clinical cognitive syndromes.

ASSOCIATED CONDITIONS AND DISORDERS: Concurrent anxiety-related conditions are common.

CLINICAL PRESENTATION

HISTORY, CHIEF COMPLAINT: Disorientation, changes in social and interactive behavior (becoming "needier," or, conversely, more aloof), changes in locomotor and sleep cycle behaviors, and loss of "housetraining."

In early-onset cognitive dysfunction, animals may have only slightly altered sleep cycles and appear more anxious.

PHYSICAL EXAM FINDINGS

- May be unremarkable.
- Possible abnormalities include worn claws or scraped nose if "trapped" in corners or if exhibiting ritualistic locomotor behavior.
- Weight loss (from excessive locomotion and/or inappetence due to anxiety).
- When examined on video, the behaviors exhibited by an animal with cognitive dysfunction often seem without purpose.

ETIOLOGY AND PATHOPHYSIOLOGY

- Dogs, like humans, develop lesions of amyloid plaques, the density of which appears to roughly correlate with the level of impairment in some patients.
- Unlike humans, dogs do not appear to develop neurofibrillary tangles that are associated with the tauopathy, Alzheimer's disease.
- Both cats and dogs experience a decrease in brain cortical mass and a relative increase in ventricular volume with aging. These changes may be more extreme in patients with cognitive dysfunction.

DIAGNOSIS

DIFFERENTIAL DIAGNOSIS

- Generalized anxiety disorder
- Anxiety: usually transient; associated with changes in physical capabilities (e.g., diminished or changing sensory or locomotor capabilities)
- Separation anxiety: old age onset
- Panic disorder
- Attention-seeking behavior

INITIAL DATABASE

- Complete blood count, serum biochemistry profile, and urinalysis: generally unremarkable
- Neurologic examination: generally unremarkable
- Thyroid profile: rule out hyperthyroidism or hypothyroidism

ADVANCED OR CONFIRMATORY TESTING

If neurologic signs are present or develop, a full neurologic evaluation, including spinal fluid analysis and brain computed tomography or magnetic resonance imaging, may be indicated.

TREATMENT

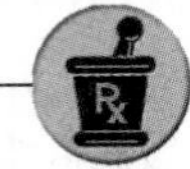

THERAPEUTIC GOAL(S)

Decrease in the rate at which the animal appears to mentally fail, while relieving pain and distress associated with changes in physical and mental status

ACUTE GENERAL TREATMENT

- Avoid exposure stimuli known to distress the animal.

- Early rewarding of any normal, preferred, or good interactive or elimination behaviors and encourage normal locomotion.
- There should be absolutely no punishment—physical, verbal, deprivational, or mental—for any undesirable behavior that occurs as a result of this condition. Such actions will render the patient more anxious.
- Protect the patient from attendant wanderings or odd behaviors while keeping it comfortable. The latter may involve containing it in an area with an absorbent surface when left alone.
- Mental stimulation in the early stages is essential and may delay clinical progression. Treat balls, food toys, games involving puzzle solving, safe exercise, interactive tasks ("get the mouse," "bring the ball," etc.), and olfactory stimulation are useful.

CHRONIC TREATMENT

- As stated, plus physically and mentally stimulating exercises: swimming, massage, range of motion exercises, etc.
- Encourage relaxation.
- If "loss of housetraining" occurs, ensure that the animal is taken out frequently to minimize the cost of "mistakes."
- Encourage reestablishment of daily cycles by feeding at regular hours and at least a few hours before bedtime, and using a benzodiazepine before bed, if needed.
- Protect the pet from accidents (e.g., falling into the swimming pool, falling down stairs).
- Specialized diets rich in antioxidants decrease the rate of cognitive dysfunction progression, improve behavioral function, and may have a protective effect (e.g., Hill's B/D [Brain Diet]).
- In the United Kingdom, nutraceutical food additives are available and have been shown to improve function in dogs with cognitive changes (e.g., Aktivait).
- The monoamine oxidase inhibitor (MAOI), selegiline (Anipryl) (0.5 mg/kg PO q 24h; may double dose after 1 month if ineffective) is the drug of choice and licensed for use for the treatment of canine cognitive dysfunction in the United States.

POSSIBLE COMPLICATIONS

Any concurrent, untreated, anxiety-related, or behavioral conditions generally worsen with age and will render the signs of cognitive dysfunction worse.

RECOMMENDED MONITORING

Examination, complete blood count, serum chemistry profile, urinalysis, ± thyroid profile as needed, and at least q 6–12 months if medications

PROGNOSIS AND OUTCOME

- The course is inexorable, but with diet, exercise, and with stimulation, patients in early stages can have years of quality life.
- Prognosis is improved by early diagnosis, comprehensive treatment, and client compliance.

PEARLS & CONSIDERATIONS

COMMENTS

- If the clients videotape the animal early in the development of the condition, they will be better able to monitor changes, assess treatment, and make quality-of-life decisions.
- Clients often are made the saddest by the feeling that they are losing their emotional and intellectual connection with their pet. Treatment must acknowledge this concern and address it when possible.
- Other cats or dogs in the household can often help calm these patients and help them with activities that they may now find challenging.

PREVENTION

- Diets rich in antioxidants may decrease risk
- Mental and physical activity

CLIENT EDUCATION

- Clients must understand that problematic behaviors attendant with cognitive dysfunction are not willful acts of disobedience by a vengeful pet.
- Treatment of this condition is an ongoing process and will continue for the life of the pet. Relapses may occur with treatment discontinuation or with added stressors.

SUGGESTED READING

Colle M-A, et al: Vascular and parenchymal beta amyloid deposition in the aging dog: Correlation with behavior. *Neurobiol Aging* 21(5):695–704, 2000.

Heath SE: Behaviour problems in the geriatric pet. In Horwitz D, Mills, DS, Heath SE (eds): *British Small Animal Veterinary Association Manual of Canine and Feline Behavioural Medicine*. Gloucester, UK, BSAVA, Lookers, Pool and Dorset, 2002, pp 109–118.

Milgram NW, et al: Dietary enrichment counteracts age-associated cognitive dysfunction in canines. *Neurobiol Aging* 23(5):737–745, 2002.

Neilson JC, et al: Prevalence of behavioral changes associated with age-related cognitive impairment in dogs. *J Am Vet Med Assoc* 218:1787–1791, 2001.

AUTHOR & EDITOR: **KAREN L. OVERALL**

Colitis, Acute

Client Education Sheet on Website

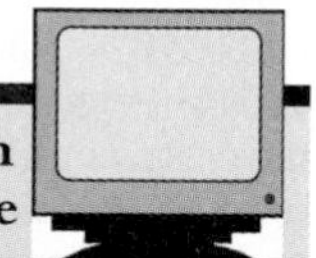

BASIC INFORMATION

DEFINITION

Sudden onset (<72 hours) of colonic inflammation (large bowel diarrhea and straining to defecate), which is generally not associated with systemic signs of illness. Diarrhea is usually characterized as mild, of small volume, and containing mucus and/or fresh blood. Also see Diarrhea, Acute, p 294.

SYNONYM(S)

"Stress" colitis

EPIDEMIOLOGY

SPECIES, AGE, SEX: Predominantly seen in young dogs and cats (<1 year old) as a consequence of parasitism, bacterial enteropathogens, or dietary indiscretion.

GENETICS AND BREED PREDISPOSITION: None.

RISK FACTORS: Age (predominantly young animals), recently kenneled animals, dietary factors, free-roaming pets, gastrointestinal tract parasitism.

CONTAGION AND ZOONOSIS: Helminth parasites (*Trichuris* spp.), protozoa (*Giardia* spp., *Tritrichomonas* spp.), and bacteria (*Campylobacter* spp., *Clostridium* spp., enterotoxigenic *Escherichia coli*, *Salmonella* spp.) have potential for contagion and zoonosis.

CLINICAL PRESENTATION

HISTORY, CHIEF COMPLAINT: Large bowel diarrhea, which is characterized by tenesmus (straining to defecate), increased frequency of defecation, mucoid feces, and fresh (red) blood.

PHYSICAL EXAM FINDINGS: Generally well fleshed without systemic signs (e.g., unthriftiness or weight loss) of illness.

Rectal examination fails to reveal significant abnormalities except to the character of the feces.

ETIOLOGY AND PATHOPHYSIOLOGY

- Parasites: both helminth and protozoa.
- Dietary causes: gluttony, spoiled food, dietary indiscretion with ingestion of foreign or abrasive materials (e.g., cat litter, rocks, nondigestible materials such as hair in long-haired cats).
- Specific bacterial pathogens may cause colonic inflammation via invasion or enterotoxin production.

DIAGNOSIS

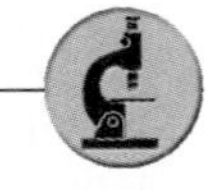

DIFFERENTIAL DIAGNOSIS

Specific causes: see Etiology and Pathophysiology above.

INITIAL DATABASE

- Physical examination: perform abdominal palpation and digital rectal examination with collection of feces.
- Fecal examination for nematode and protozoal parasites. Both fecal flotations and direct fecal smears should be performed. Note that multiple (three) zinc sulfate flotation tests using fresh feces may be required for identification of *Giardia* spp. trophozoites. See Giardiasis, p 439.
- Commercial enzyme-linked immunosorbent assay kits are also sensitive for the detection of *Giardia* antigen.
- Rectal cytologic evaluation may indicate evidence of bacterial pathogens (e.g., vegetative spores of *Clostridia* or increased numbers of fecal leukocytes indicative of acute mucosal inflammation).

ADVANCED OR CONFIRMATORY TESTING

Generally not indicated. Animals that fail to respond to empiric therapy (see below) will require confirmatory testing (e.g., fecal cultures, polymerase chain reaction, or other assays) for suspect bacterial pathogens.

TREATMENT

THERAPEUTIC GOAL(S)

Initial management of animals with acute colitis is nonspecific and supportive. In most instances, signs are self-limiting and/or respond readily to empiric therapy.

ACUTE GENERAL TREATMENT

- Treat for suspect nematode and protozoan parasites using appropriate broad-spectrum anthelmintics or antiprotozoal medications (e.g., fenbendazole 50 mg/kg PO q 24 h for 3 days).
- Feed a bland or mixed fiber diet (either commercial or homemade), giving small volumes at increasingly frequent interval for 3 to 5 days.
- Avoid all treats and dietary supplements during the dietary trial period.
- If using a bland diet, add fiber (small amounts of soluble fiber, such as psyllium mucilloid 1 teaspoon/10 kg at each feeding) to the diet to reduce tenesmus and facilitate colonic epithelial repair.
- Avoid the use of antibiotics in animals, except those with confirmed bacterial causes for their signs.

RECOMMENDED MONITORING

Have clients communicate their pet's progress after 72 hours of therapy

PROGNOSIS AND OUTCOME

Generally excellent for full recovery

PEARLS & CONSIDERATIONS

COMMENTS

- Acute colitis is a common complaint in general practice that is very responsive to supportive therapy.
- The elimination of infectious and parasitic causes is the key to treating acute colitis.

PREVENTION

- Prophylactic deworming.
- Avoid dietary indiscretion.
- Avoid free-roaming pets.
- In cats with recurrent colitis due to hair, frequent brushing, administration of hairball laxatives, or removing excess hair (shaving) may be indicated to control signs.

CLIENT EDUCATION

Monitor for failure to respond to empiric treatments

SUGGESTED READING

Marks SL, et al: Bacterial-associated diarrhea in the dog: A critical appraisal. *Vet Clin North Am Small Anim Pract* 33:1029, 2003.

AUTHOR: **ALBERT E. JERGENS**
EDITOR: **DEBRA L. ZORAN**

Colitis, Chronic

BASIC INFORMATION

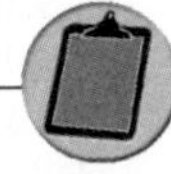

DEFINITION

Denotes persistent (>3 weeks' duration) signs of colonic inflammation, characterized by large bowel diarrhea with tenesmus/dyschezia, urgency, and increased frequency of defecation. Feces often contain mucus and/or fresh blood. Systemic signs attributable to nutrient malabsorption (e.g., anorexia, weight loss) are uncommon.

EPIDEMIOLOGY

SPECIES, AGE, SEX: More common in middle-aged and older dogs and cats as a consequence of infiltrative mucosal disorders (e.g., inflammatory bowel disease [IBD] and neoplasia). Infectious disorders (e.g., *Trichuris vulpis*, gastrointestinal [GI] histoplasmosis) may be seen in younger dogs and less commonly in cats.

GENETICS AND BREED PREDISPOSITION: Boxers are predisposed to histiocytic ulcerative colitis (HUC). German shepherds and purebred cats are at increased risk for lymphocytic-plasmacytic IBD.

CONTAGION AND ZOONOSIS: Some bacterial enteropathogens (e.g., *Clostridium perfringens*, potentially contagious) may cause chronic colitis if not detected early. Also, some helminth parasites (*Trichuris* spp., potentially contagious) and protozoa (*Giardia* spp., potentially zoootic; *Tritrichomonas* spp., potentially contagious and zoonotic) may cause persistent signs of colitis in pets.

GEOGRAPHY AND SEASONALITY: Midwestern United States for GI histoplasmosis.

ASSOCIATED CONDITIONS AND DISORDERS: Colonic motility disorders (e.g., irritable bowel syndrome in dogs and colonic constipation/obstipation in cats) may mimic mucosal inflammation and cause signs of large bowel diarrhea with tenesmus. Note that these diseases are due to functional defects in colonic motility and have no mucosal/structural disease.

CLINICAL PRESENTATION

DISEASE FORMS/SUBTYPES

- Dietary responsive disorders: includes both food intolerance (nonimmunologically mediated) and dietary sensitivity (immunologically mediated; see Food Allergy, Gastrointestinal, p 398)
- Infectious disorders: includes select nematode/protozoal parasites, bacteria, and fungal organisms (especially GI histoplasmosis)
- Infiltrative mucosal diseases: includes fungal, benign (e.g., IBD), and malignant (e.g., mucosal neoplasia) diseases

HISTORY, CHIEF COMPLAINT: Persistent large bowel diarrhea, which is characterized by tenesmus (straining to defecate), increased frequency of defecation, mucoid feces, and fresh (red) blood. Note that some disorders (e.g., IBD, GI histoplasmosis, GI lymphoma) may affect the small intestines as well as causing mixed large-small bowel signs.

PHYSICAL EXAM FINDINGS

- The animal is often well fleshed without systemic signs (e.g., unthriftiness, weight loss) of illness. Fungal disease, IBD, and neoplasia may selectively cause fever, alterations in appetite, and peripheral/mesenteric lymphadenopathy.
- Rectal examination: evaluate the character of the feces, obtain fecal samples for parasitic examination, procure exfoliative cytologic specimens, and evaluate the rectum for possible mass lesions.

ETIOLOGY AND PATHOPHYSIOLOGY

- Large bowel diarrhea is characterized by increased amounts of mucus due to the large numbers of mucus-secreting goblet cells in the colon.
- Hematochezia indicates severe mucosal disruption of the distal colon and rectum.
- Parasites: both helminth and protozoa. *Trichuris vulpis* (dogs), *Tritrichomonas foetus* (cats), *Giardia lamblia* (dogs, cats).
- Dietary causes: incriminating antigens or dietary ingredients (nonimmunologic).
- Specific bacterial pathogens: cause colonic inflammation via invasion or enterotoxin production.
- Infiltrative mucosal disorders: either benign, malignant, or infectious (e.g., fungal).

DIAGNOSIS

DIFFERENTIAL DIAGNOSIS

- Specific causes: see Etiology and Pathophysiology above.
- Occasionally patients with rectal diseases (e.g., perineal hernia, perineal fistula, diverticuli, or rectal polyps or masses) will present with signs of large bowel disease. These are generally distinguished by digital examination and careful inspection; normal pelvic and rectal structure on examination more strongly suggests large bowel disease in such cases.

INITIAL DATABASE

- Physical examination: perform abdominal palpation and digital examination with collection of feces.
- Fecal examination for nematode and protozoal parasites. Both fecal flotations and fecal smears should be performed. Note that multiple (three) zinc sulfate flotation tests using fresh feces may be required for identification of *Giardia* spp. trophozoites.
    - Commercial enzyme-linked immunosorbent assay kits are also sensitive for the detection of *Giardia* antigen.
- Rectal cytology may indicate evidence of bacterial pathogens (e.g., vegetative spores of *Clostridia* or increased numbers of fecal leukocytes indicative of acute mucosal inflammation). Exfoliative cytology (e.g., rectal scrape using a uterine curette or a curette of the same type used for bone graft harvesting) is also a useful tool for confirming the presence of *Histoplasma* organisms contained within colonic macrophages.
- Abdominal imaging (survey radiographs, pneumocolonography, and/or ultrasonography) may identify fecal impaction, mass lesions, or evidence of significant mesenteric lymphadenopathy. Generally, ultrasonography is a poor screening tool for colonic disease due to the obstructive effect of air in the colonic lumen on the ultrasound beam and because intestinal wall thickness is difficult to standardize.

ADVANCED OR CONFIRMATORY TESTING

- Colonoscopy with procurement of multiple mucosal biopsy specimens is required to diagnose most infiltrative diseases. Exfoliative cytology at the time of GI endoscopy is a useful adjunct to mucosal biopsy.
- Proctoscopy can also be used to examine and obtain biopsy specimens of the distal colon and rectum when the disease is confined to distal aspects or when colonoscopy is unavailable.
- Colonic biopsies should not be obtained routinely by laparotomy, since the bacterial content of the colon and attendant risk of bacterial peritonitis after biopsy of a diseased colon is markedly greater than in the small intestine.

TREATMENT

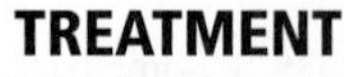

THERAPEUTIC GOAL(S)

- Treatment of chronic colitis generally requires a specific definitive diagnosis because empiric therapies are often inadequate or deleterious (e.g., use of corticosteroids in animals with GI histoplasmosis).
- Appropriate dietary management is important, regardless of the cause for colonic inflammation and may include elimination, fiber-supplemented, or low-residue diets.
- Fiber supplementation is an important component of therapy because these dietary additives bind colonic irritants, normalize dysmotility, and promote colonic epithelial repair and renewal.

CHRONIC TREATMENT

- Treat for suspect nematode and protozoan parasites (even if fecal exams are negative for parasites) using appropriate broad-spectrum anthelmintics or antiprotozoal (fenbendazole 50 mg/kg PO q 24h for 3 to 5 days) medications. Confirm efficacy of therapy with repeat follow-up fecal examinations.
- Feed a hypoallergenic diet to animals with dietary-responsive disorders and IBD. Reduction in the quantity of dietary antigens will assist in reducing mucosal inflammation with these disorders. Other animals with colitis but not requiring a specific antigen-restricted diet will benefit from being fed a low-fat, fiber-enriched, and highly digestible commercial ration.
- Choose diets (or supplement the diet) with increased n-3:n-6 fatty acids to reduce mucosal inflammation.
- Avoid all treats and supplements containing protein or flavors during the dietary trial period.
- Use diets with added soluble or mixed fiber or add small to moderate amounts of soluble fiber to the diet to reduce tenesmus and to facilitate colonic epithelial repair.
- Only use antibiotics in animals with confirmed bacterial causes (e.g., colonization with enteropathogenic bacteria) for their signs. Antimicrobials used in this fashion are best chosen based on susceptibility testing to the incriminating pathogen. Obvious exceptions to this caveat are animals with HUC (which may respond to oral fluoroquinolone therapy, enrofloxacin 10 mg/kg PO q 24h) and lymphocytic-plasmacytic colitis (IBD), which may respond to metronidazole (10 mg/kg PO q 12h, used as an immunomodulator) alone or in combination with other immunosuppressive drugs.
- Sulfasalazine (20–30 mg/kg PO q 8h typically for 3 to 6 weeks in dogs), or newer mesalamine drugs, and glucocorticoids (e.g., prednisone or prednisolone 1 mg/kg PO q 12h for dogs, 1–2 mg/kg PO q 12h for cats) are first-choice immunosuppressive drugs for therapy of colonic IBD.
- Drugs effective against GI histoplasmosis include itraconazole (10 mg/kg/day PO

for 6 to 9 months), and/or amphotericin B (used most often in dogs with systemic histoplasmosis, but must ensure normal renal function before administration, and is often used in combination with itraconazole). See Histoplasmosis, p 525.

- Treatment for colonic neoplasia varies as to the type of neoplasm. Focal lesions (e.g., adenocarcinoma, leiomyoma/sarcoma) respond best to surgical excision followed by chemotherapy. Diffuse mucosal tumors (e.g., lymphosarcoma) will require multidrug chemotherapy regimens. Selective cyclooxygenase II inhibitors may be useful in the treatment of some colonic tumors.

POSSIBLE COMPLICATIONS

- Cure is not possible with colonic IBD, but the prognosis for control of signs is good with effective therapy.
- Animals treated with amphotericin B for GI histoplasmosis are at risk for drug-induced renal disease.

RECOMMENDED MONITORING

- Rechecks initially are required at 2- to 4-week intervals in animals with IBD.
- Monitor renal function in animals treated with amphotericin B.
- Assess for leukopenia in patients receiving chemotherapy for malignant colonic neoplasia.
- Ideally, animals responsive to elimination diets (e.g., those having dietary responsive causes for chronic colitis) should be returned to their normal (incriminating) diet to see if large bowel signs recrudesce. This is impractical in most instances.

PROGNOSIS AND OUTCOME

- The prognosis for dietary-responsive disorders is excellent.
- The prognosis for infiltrative disorders varies depending on the cause.
- Most forms of IBD respond readily to a combination of dietary and pharmacologic therapies, but relapses should be expected. HUC requires a more guarded prognosis, although recent therapy with fluoroquinolones has improved success.
- GI histoplasmosis carries a guarded prognosis because long-term therapy (months to years) may be required; however, most animals respond favorably to antifungal therapy in spite of disease burden.
- Colonic neoplasia carries a guarded prognosis with the exception of benign colonic polyps, in which the prognosis is excellent.

PEARLS & CONSIDERATIONS

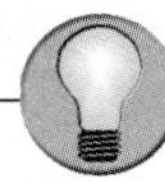

COMMENTS

- Major causes for chronic colitis include dietary, infectious, and infiltrative disorders.
- Most animals with chronic signs of large intestinal disease will require a thorough diagnostic evaluation to rule out the varied causes for colonic inflammation.
- Colonoscopy with mucosal biopsy is imperative for diagnosis of most forms of chronic colitis.

PREVENTION

- Prophylactic deworming
- Avoid dietary indiscretion

CLIENT EDUCATION

Dietary modification to a diet suitable for colonic disease may be required for the life of the pet.

SUGGESTED READING

Sherding RG, Johnson SE: Diseases of the intestines. In Birchard SJ, Sherding RG (eds): *Saunder's Manual of Small Animal Practice*, ed 2. Philadelphia, WB Saunders, 2000, pp 787–815.

Zoran D: Pathophysiology and management of canine colonic diseases. *Comp Contin Educ Pract Vet* 21:824, 1999.

AUTHOR: **ALBERT E. JERGENS**

EDITOR: **DEBRA L. ZORAN**

Collapse

BASIC INFORMATION

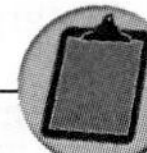

DEFINITION

Loss of the ability to support weight and ambulate without assistance and may include the loss of consciousness

EPIDEMIOLOGY

SPECIES, AGE, SEX

- Dogs, cats
- Age and sex depend on underlying disease

GENETICS AND BREED PREDISPOSITION: Exercise-induced collapse in Labrador retrievers. Intervertebral disk extrusion in chondrodystrophic breeds.

RISK FACTORS: Increased ambient temperature, obesity.

CONTAGION AND ZOONOSIS

- Agents causing polyarthritis such as *Borrelia burgdorferi*
- Agents affecting the neuromuscular junction such as *Clostridium botulinum*

GEOGRAPHY AND SEASONALITY: Areas with a high incidence of infectious agents that can cause collapse.

RISK FACTORS: Diabetes mellitus, cardiomyopathies, hypoadrenocorticism, immune-mediated hemolytic anemia, hemangiosarcoma, caudal cervical spondylomyelopathy (wobbler's syndrome).

CLINICAL PRESENTATION

DISEASE FORMS/SUBTYPES

- Neuromuscular: paresis/paralysis but mentation normal
- Neurologic: alterations in intracranial (mentation, cranial nerves) and/or spinal (reflexes, reactions) function, without an underlying systemic cause
- Orthopedic: signs of joint or bone pain, reduced range of motion, or fracture
- Metabolic/endocrine: characteristic systemic signs
- Cardiovascular: characteristic signs or heart disease and/or vascular disturbances
- Respiratory: overt respiratory signs (usually dyspnea) in the absence of systemic, neuromuscular, or cardiovascular causes

HISTORY, CHIEF COMPLAINT: Dependent on underlying cause. Often includes one or more of the following: weakness, inability to rise, incontinence (urine or feces), anxiety/distress, abdominal distention, vomiting, diarrhea, respiratory distress, unconsciousness.

PHYSICAL EXAM FINDINGS

- Dependent on underlying cause:
  - Nonspecific signs commonly include recumbency, alterations in mentation (disorientation, unconsciousness), vomiting, variable heart rate (normal, bradycardic or tachycardic), variable pulse quality (absent, weak to hyperdynamic), and pale to hyperemic membranes.
- Some underlying causes may be more likely in the presence of certain physical findings:

- Asynchronous pulse quality (cardiac arrhythmias), muffled heart sounds (pericardial effusion/cardiac tamponade, pleural effusion if muffled lung sounds also), stertorous upper airway noises (upper airway obstruction), abdominal fluid wave (hemoabdomen, right-sided congestive heart failure, or pyoabdomen/sepsis), moist lung sounds (respiratory, cardiovascular, or pulmonary hemorrhage), flaccid to fasciculating muscles (neuromuscular), decreased to increased spinal reflexes (neuromuscular or neurologic), neck or back pain (orthopedic, neurologic), joint effusion (orthopedic).

ETIOLOGY AND PATHOPHYSIOLOGY

Collapse is caused by loss of normal, coordinated function of muscles that support the body.

- Neuromuscular: reduced nerve conduction, disturbance of neuromuscular junction, or primary myopathy (rare)
- Neurologic: intracranial or spinal failure to generate or communicate impulses for normal mentation and/or limb function
- Orthopedic: failure of the skeleton and/or joints to support weight
- Metabolic/endocrine: limitation of metabolic fuel for muscles, nerves, or the cental nervous system (e.g., hypoglycemia, hypocalcemia, hypokalemia)
- Cardiovascular: inadequate perfusion of muscles and/or the central nervous system
- Respiratory: inadequate oxygenation of blood, and therefore, of tissues

DIAGNOSIS

DIFFERENTIAL DIAGNOSIS

- Neuromuscular: myasthenia gravis, polyradiculoneuritis, tick paralysis, botulism, polyarthritis
- Neurologic: intervertebral disk extrusion, fibrocartilaginous emboli, spinal fracture, spinal tumor, meningitis, intracranial neoplasia, narcolepsy (rare)
- Metabolic/endocrine: anemia, shock/sepsis, insulin overdose, insulinoma, eclampsia, hypoparathyroidism, renal disease, hepatic dysfunction, hypoadrenocortism, toxins that affect oxygen binding to hemoglobin such as carbon monoxide and acetaminophen toxicity, shock (hemorrhagic, anaphylactic)
- Cardiovascular: arrhythmias, arterial thromboembolism, cardiac tamponade
- Respiratory: laryngeal paralysis, brachycephalic upper airway syndrome, laryngeal masses, pharyngeal swelling/foreign body, tracheal collapse, tracheal foreign body, nasopharyngeal polyp

INITIAL DATABASE

Complete blood count, biochemical profile, electrolytes. Electrocardiogram (ECG), blood pressure (multiple limbs if thromboembolism suspected), thoracic and abdominal radiographs, remove any ectoparasites (ticks)

- Results variable depending on underlying cause

ADVANCED OR CONFIRMATORY TESTING

As dictated by history, physical findings, and initial test results

- Arterial blood gas, saline agglutination testing, tick-borne disease titers, arthrocentesis, adrenocorticotropic hormone stimulation, abdominal ultrasound, echocardiography, magnetic resonance imaging or myelogram, cerebrospinal fluid analysis, pharyngeal examination, laryngeal function assessment, abdomino/thoraco/pericardiocentesis, acetylcholine receptor antibody titers, Holter monitor/event recorder, insulin: glucose ratio, parathormone and ionized calcium, edrophonium (Tensilon) response test.

TREATMENT

THERAPEUTIC GOAL(S)

- Correct acute/life-threatening disturbances (severe biochemical or electrolyte abnormalities, severe anemia, hypotension, body temperature abnormalities)
- Address underlying problem

ACUTE GENERAL TREATMENT

- Intravenous fluids, oxygen supplementation, and/or intubation if needed, blood transfusion, dextrose supplementation (hypoglycemia), electrolyte supplementation, insulin (combined with dextrose) for hyperkalemia, analgesia/sedation if indicated.
- Antibiotics, anti-inflammatories, diuretics, and antiarrhythmic medications may be indicated depending on underlying problem.
- Dexamethasone (0.2–1 mg/kg IV) may be given if a hypoadrenocortical crisis is suspected; it will not interfere with diagnostic testing.

CHRONIC TREATMENT

Dependent on underlying disease process

DRUG INTERACTIONS

Edrophonium's cardiac effects may be potentiated by digoxin.

POSSIBLE COMPLICATIONS

Edrophonium can cause acute cholinergic crisis

RECOMMENDED MONITORING

Blood glucose, electrolytes, ECG, blood pressure

PROGNOSIS AND OUTCOME

In general prognosis is guarded but varies from good to poor depending on underlying disease process

PEARLS & CONSIDERATIONS

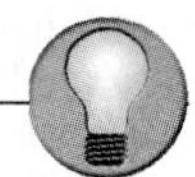

COMMENTS

- Many of the pathologic processes that cause collapse are not common, and establishing the diagnosis can be difficult.
- Common diseases, such as intervertebral disk disease, should be considered first, and the diagnostic evaluation can proceed to less common etiologies afterwards.
- The two diseases leading to collapse that are most commonly overlooked in general practice are pericardial effusion and hypoadrenocorticism.

SUGGESTED READING

Platt SR, Garosi LS: Neuromuscular weakness and collapse. *Vet Clin North Am Small Anim Pract* 34(6):1281–1230, 2004.

Smith SA, et al: Arterial thromboembolism in cats: Acute crisis in 127 cases (1992–2001) and long-term management with low-dose aspirin in 24 cases. *J Vet Intern Med* 17(1):73–83, 2003.

Stafford Johnson M, et al: A retrospective study of clinical findings, treatment and outcome in 143 dogs with pericardial effusion. *J Small Anim Pract* 45(11):546–552, 2004.

AUTHOR: **ADAM J. REISS**
EDITOR: **ETIENNE CÔTÉ**

Collapsing Trachea

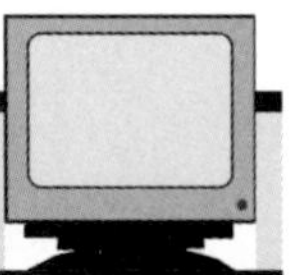

Client Education Sheet on Website

BASIC INFORMATION

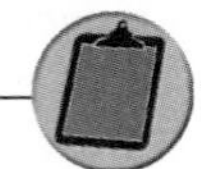

DEFINITION

Weakening of tracheal cartilage support for large airways resulting in cough and impaired conduction of air

SYNONYM(S)

Collapsed trachea
Tracheal collapse

EPIDEMIOLOGY

SPECIES, AGE, SEX

- Primarily a disease of middle-aged, small-breed dogs; rarely reported in large-breed dogs
- No known sex predilection

GENETICS AND BREED PREDISPOSITION: Breeds commonly affected include the Yorkshire terrier, toy and miniature poodle, and Pomeranian.

RISK FACTORS: Obesity may exacerbate frequency and severity of signs.

ASSOCIATED CONDITIONS AND DISORDERS: Small-breed dogs with collapsing trachea often have concurrent noninfectious chronic tracheitis and bronchitis.

CLINICAL PRESENTATION

DISEASE FORMS/SUBTYPES

Grades of tracheal collapse:

- I: Minor protrusion of dorsal membrane into airway lumen, <25% reduction in diameter. Generally not associated with clinical signs
- II: 50% reduction in airway lumen, tracheal rings elongated and mildly flattened
- III: 75% reduction in airway lumen, tracheal rings markedly flattened
- IV: >90% reduction in airway lumen, severely flattened tracheal rings, possibly with dorsal deviation of ventral tracheal surface. Generally associated with frequent or constant advanced clinical signs

HISTORY, CHIEF COMPLAINT

- Owners often complain of a recurrent, loud, honking cough with gagging or retching commonly observed at the end of a series of coughs.
  - Signs may worsen with excitement, heat, eating or drinking, or exercise.
- Milder clinical signs may have been present since early in life.
- Severely affected animals may exhibit cyanosis or syncope in addition to severe coughing.

PHYSICAL EXAM FINDINGS

- Dry cough elicited with tracheal palpation.
  - This finding is nonspecific, however, since many other respiratory disorders, including pulmonary parenchymal disorders (e.g., pulmonary edema), may cause a cough to be elicited easily with tracheal palpation.
- With cervical collapsing trachea, wheezes may be ausculted over the cervical tracheal region.
- With thoracic collapsing trachea, loud snapping noises may be ausculted due to the dynamic opening and collapse of large airways (sound is due to airway opening during inspiration).
- Increased expiratory effort may be seen.

ETIOLOGY AND PATHOPHYSIOLOGY

- Decreased rigidity of tracheal cartilage rings results in dynamic collapse during inspiration with cervical involvement and during expiration with thoracic involvement.
- The etiology is unknown, but suggested mechanisms include:
  - Failure of chondrogenesis
  - Acquired secondary to chronic small airway disease
  - Cartilage degeneration
  - Trauma
  - Loss of innervation of the trachealis dorsalis muscle

DIAGNOSIS

DIFFERENTIAL DIAGNOSIS

- Sterile chronic bronchitis
- Congestive heart failure
- Infectious tracheobronchitis
- Bronchial compression due to left atrial enlargement or lymphadenopathy
- Pneumonia
- Tracheal or laryngeal obstruction

INITIAL DATABASE

- Routine laboratory testing is usually unremarkable.
- Thoracic and lateral cervical radiographs may reveal collapse.
  - Ideally, obtain images during inspiration for cervical collapse and expiration for thoracic collapse.

ADVANCED OR CONFIRMATORY TESTING

- Fluoroscopy is usually helpful in identifying dynamic collapse with an elicited cough.
- Bronchoscopy can identify severity, characterize the collapse location, and facilitate collection of airway wash samples to rule out concurrent infectious and inflammatory conditions.

TREATMENT

THERAPEUTIC GOAL(S)

- Decrease the severity and frequency of cough and associated clinical signs
- Treat any secondary conditions exacerbating the collapsing trachea

ACUTE GENERAL TREATMENT

- Oxygen and judicious use of sedatives and cough suppressants may be necessary in an acute crisis.
- Butorphanol (0.02–0.1 mg/kg SC q 4–6h) can lessen acute severe cough and respiratory distress.
- Low-dose acepromazine (0.05–0.1 mg/kg IM) can provide sedation that breaks the cycle of airway irritation and coughing when a bout of extremely severe, collapsing trachea-related coughing occurs.

CHRONIC TREATMENT

- Obesity leads to decreased lung expansion and increased breathing effort. Therefore, weight loss is important in any obese dog diagnosed with collapsing trachea.
- Antitussives help reduce irritation or damage to the tracheal epithelium from chronic cough:
  - Hydrocodone 0.22 mg/kg PO q 6–12h; or
  - Butorphanol 0.55–1.1 mg/kg PO q 8–12h.
- Anti-inflammatory therapy may be needed to decrease laryngeal or tracheal inflammation:
  - Prednisone 0.5–1 mg/kg PO q 12h tapered and discontinued after 5 to 7 days of use.
  - Only short-term use is recommended.
- Bronchodilators may benefit dogs with intrathoracic collapse or expiratory effort that do not improve with initial therapy:
  - β-2 agonists.
    - Terbutaline (total amount per dose): small dogs 0.625–1.25 mg PO q 12h, medium dogs 1.25–2.5 mg PO q 12h, large dogs 2.5–5 mg PO q 12h.
    - Albuterol: 0.05 mg/kg PO q 8h.
  - Methylxanthines.
    - Not all long-acting theophylline products are equivalent in bioavailability in dogs. Implications are that failure to respond to a certain product should prompt the consideration of switching bronchodilators (to a different brand of theophylline or a different class of bronchodilator altogether [e.g.,

a β-2 agonist]), and that certain animals may develop signs of toxicosis when receiving doses that are well tolerated by others.
    - TheocapER or Theochron ER (Inwood Laboratories) are recommended at 10 mg/kg PO q 12h.
    - Aminophylline or theophylline 10 mg/kg PO q 8h.
- Surgical implantation of external prosthetic rings can be considered in patients with grade II-IV collapse that fail medical management.
    - Implants are more practical for cervical collapse but can be attempted for thoracic collapse through cranial retraction of the trachea. Several potential drawbacks exist, including implant failure and extension of the collapsing process beyond the length of the implant over time.

POSSIBLE COMPLICATIONS

Cough suppressants: somnolence, sluggishness at higher doses

RECOMMENDED MONITORING

Clinical signs

PROGNOSIS AND OUTCOME

- The prognosis for survival is good. Most dogs show improvement, but varying degrees of persistent clinical signs, with appropriate treatment. The prognosis for cure is poor, because collapsing trachea is irreversible and progressive.
- Dogs with severe clinical signs (cyanosis, syncope) have a guarded prognosis for comfortable survival if not effectively treated with medical therapy.

PEARLS & CONSIDERATIONS

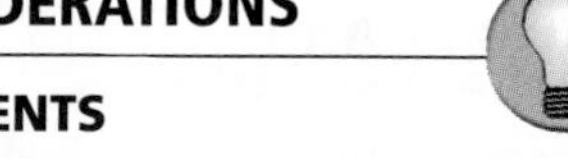

COMMENTS

- Techniques involving intratracheal stents are being investigated and have shown some potential in the treatment of thoracic tracheal collapse.
- By reducing bronchial smooth muscle contraction during cough (lessens dynamic component of cough), and slowing the velocity of air flow during coughing (by increasing bronchial diameter), bronchodilators may help patients with collapsing trachea even though the drugs do not act directly at the site of the lesion.

PREVENTION

Affected dogs should probably not be bred.

CLIENT EDUCATION

For most dogs, the tracheal collapse is managed with weight control, antitussives, and periodic administration of anti-inflammatory drugs.

SUGGESTED READING

Johnson L: Tracheal collapse. *Vet Clin North Am Small Anim Pract* 30:1253–1266, 2000.

AUTHOR: **LAURA G. RIDGE**
EDITOR: **RANCE K. SELLON**

Color Disorders of the Skin and Haircoat

BASIC INFORMATION

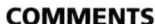

DEFINITION

Innate or acquired pigmentary abnormality of the skin or hair

SYNONYM(S)

Hyperpigmentation: melanoderma, melanotrichia
Hypopigmentation: leukoderma, leukotrichia, poliosis, graying

EPIDEMIOLOGY

SPECIES, AGE, SEX

- Some conditions present at birth (e.g., albinism)
- Most are acquired at any age in dogs and cats

GENETICS AND BREED PREDISPOSITION

- Hyperpigmentation:
    - Acanthosis nigricans: dachshund
    - Recurrent seasonal flank alopecia: boxer, English bulldog, Airedale terrier
    - Papillomavirus-associated plaques: pug, miniature schnauzer, shar-pei
- Hypopigmentation:
    - Vitiligo: Belgian tervuren, Siamese cat, rottweiler, Doberman pinscher, German shepherd, others
    - Waardenburg-Klein syndrome: dalmatian, bull terrier, Sealyham terrier, collie
    - Premature greying: golden retriever, Labrador retriever, Irish setter
    - Dermatomyositis: collie, Shetland sheepdog
    - Canine cyclic hematopoiesis: collie
    - Chédiak-Higashi syndrome: Persian cat

RISK FACTORS: Depends on underlying cause.

CONTAGION AND ZOONOSIS: Dermatophytosis and *Sarcoptes scabei* (hyperpigmentation).

GEOGRAPHY AND SEASONALITY

- "Snow nose": decreased nasal pigmentation during winter months
- Seasonal flank alopecia: marked localized alopecia and hyperpigmentation, often in spring or fall

ASSOCIATED CONDITIONS AND DISORDERS

- Waardenburg-Klein syndrome: deafness
- Uveodermatologic syndrome: uveitis
- Dermatomyositis: may exhibit myositis
- Chédiak-Higashi syndrome: immunologic deficiency
- Canine cyclic hematopoiesis: usually lethal before age 6 months

CLINICAL PRESENTATION

HISTORY, CHIEF COMPLAINT

- Acquired change in skin or coat color tends to be gradual
- Question owners about sun exposure, general changes, any evidence of inflammation (e.g., pruritus)

PHYSICAL EXAM FINDINGS

- Examine skin for evidence of inflammation (e.g., erythema, lichenification).
- Certain physical abnormalities are associated with specific pigmentation disorders (e.g., uveitis, myositis, deafness, obesity).

ETIOLOGY AND PATHOPHYSIOLOGY

Normal pigmentation of the skin and hair is a highly complex process susceptible to influence of numerous genetic and acquired factors

DIAGNOSIS

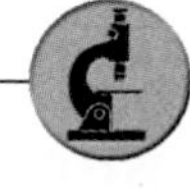

DIFFERENTIAL DIAGNOSIS

- Acquired hyperpigmentation:
    - Postinflammatory: common in dogs, can occur with any chronic inflammatory process but particularly common with hypersensitivity disorders, demodicosis, pyoderma. May affect hair in dogs; frequently affects hair in Siamese and Himalayan cats.
    - Endocrinopathy: hyperadrenocorticism, hypothyroidism, alopecia X, sex hormone dermatoses.
    - Neoplasia: feline Bowen's disease, other pigmented tumors.
    - Acanthosis nigricans in dachshunds: localized to axillae. Usually a reaction

pattern with multiple causes (friction, infection, hypersensitivity), but a primary genetic form also exists.
  - Lentigenes: macular melanosis (orange cats).
  - Other: recurrent seasonal flank alopecia, sun exposure, drug therapy-induced, papillomavirus-associated plaques.
- Acquired hypopigmentation:
  - Postinflammatory: common. On the nasal planum, consider discoid lupus erythematosus, as well as pemphigus erythematosus, pemphigus foliaceus, uveodermatologic syndrome, other immune-mediated diseases. Pyoderma, dermatomyositis, and other inflammatory conditions also may cause depigmentation in affected areas.
  - Neoplasia: particularly epitheliotropic lymphoma.
  - Other: drug-induced, periocular leukotrichia/depigmentation in Siamese cats.
  - Vitiligo: multifactorial genetic cause likely. Symmetric patchy loss of pigment from hair and skin, most often on the face (including nose and lips).
  - Mucocutaneous hypopigmentation: common congenital finding in some breeds.
  - Others: albinism, Waardenburg-Klein syndrome, canine cyclic hematopoiesis, Chédiak-Higashi syndrome.
  - Nasal hypopigmentation: includes Dudley nose, a gradual loss of pigment from a normally black nasal planum, and "snow nose," in which depigmentation is less complete (usually occurs in winter).
  - Red coat syndrome: black hair lightens to reddish-brown, may be due to dietary factors (inadequate levels of tyrosine and phenylalanine).
  - Lightening of the coat can occur with excessive exposure to chlorinated water, sunlight, or if hair growth is very slow.

INITIAL DATABASE

May include:
- Skin scrapings
- Cytologic examination
- Skin biopsy
- Trichograms (microscopic examination of plucked hairs)
- Complete blood count, serum biochemistry profile, urinalysis

ADVANCED OR CONFIRMATORY TESTING

For specific diseases, additional testing may include:
- Screening tests for endocrinopathy (hyperadrenocorticism, hypothyroidism)
- Ocular examination (uveodermatologic syndrome)
- Muscle evaluation (dermatomyositis)
- Auditory evaluation (Waardenburg-Klein syndrome)

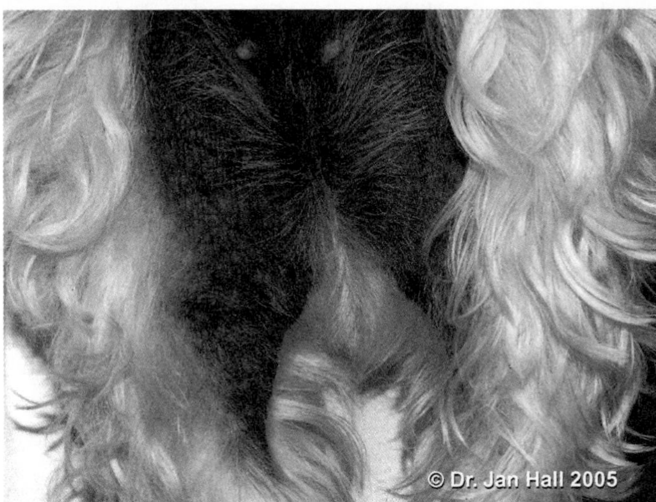

FIGURE I-39 Hyperpigmentation of the ventral abdomen of a 3-year-old West Highland white terrier with canine atopy. Hyperpigmentation of the skin in this case is secondary to chronic skin irritation. Courtesy of Dr. Jan A. Hall.

TREATMENT

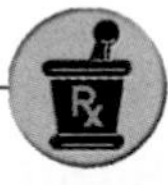

THERAPEUTIC GOAL(S)

Restore normal pigmentation to skin and hair

ACUTE GENERAL TREATMENT

Depends on underlying cause:
- Many conditions do not require or respond to treatment.
- Inflammation, endocrinopathy, or neoplasia may be treatable.
- Reduce sun exposure in alopecic dogs.

PROGNOSIS AND OUTCOME

- Good prognosis for acquired hyperpigmentation providing the underlying condition can be controlled; variable for other conditions.
- Improvement may be very slow for all conditions.

PEARLS & CONSIDERATIONS

COMMENTS

- When examining a nasal planum exhibiting hypopigmentation or depigmentation, inflammatory or infiltrative processes typically exhibit loss of the normal cobblestone architecture, while processes with minimal or no inflammation (e.g., vitiligo) spare the normal surface pattern.
- The best place to biopsy a nasal planum (or other mucocutaneous junction) exhibiting depigmentation is in an area that is gray, rather than completely depigmented, because it is likely most actively losing pigment.

SUGGESTED READING

Alhaidari Z, Olivry T, Ortonne J: Melanocytogenesis and melanogenesis: Genetic regulation and comparative clinical diseases. *Vet Dermatol* 10:3-16, 1999.

AUTHOR: **KINGA GORTEL**
EDITOR: **JAN A. HALL**

Coma

BASIC INFORMATION

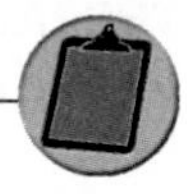

DEFINITION

A state of unconsciousness unresponsive to all stimuli; a neurologic emergency

EPIDEMIOLOGY

RISK FACTORS

- Any condition that increases intracranial pressure
- Older animals: neoplasia
- Younger animals: trauma and toxins

CONTAGION AND ZOONOSIS: Consider rabies.

CLINICAL PRESENTATION

DISEASE FORMS/SUBTYPES

- Obtunded: conscious state with mild to moderate reduction in alertness
- Stupor: unconscious state that requires strong stimuli (usually noxious; toe pinch) to evoke a response (often reduced)

HISTORY, CHIEF COMPLAINT

- Acute onset or rapid deterioration: consider toxin, trauma, rapidly bleeding tumor, or embolism/infarction
- Chronic slow progression: consider tumor, metabolic disease, or encephalitis

PHYSICAL EXAM FINDINGS

- Recumbent with minimal to no response
- Patient may present in shock
- Neurologic exam: focus on level of consciousness (response to toe pinch and loud noise), pupillary size and light reflexes, ability to elicit physiologic nystagmus, limb rigidity, and respiratory patterns to determine prognosis

ETIOLOGY AND PATHOPHYSIOLOGY

- There are two general causes of unconsciousness:
  - Diffuse cortical injury.
  - Interruption of the ascending reticular activating system located in the brainstem.
- Diffuse cortical injury generally carries a better prognosis than brainstem injury.
- Brainstem (midbrain, medulla) injury may be suspected based on:
  - Deficits in pupillary light response or pupil size: midbrain (assuming exam reveals no evidence of ocular or optic nerve lesion).
  - Inability to elicit normal physiologic nystagmus: medulla (assuming no evidence of middle/inner ear abnormality on exam).
  - Limb rigidity: medulla (assuming no spinal cord or neuromuscular signs).
  - Respiration abnormalities: medulla or midbrain (barring primary airway/lung lesion).
    - Kussmaul (rapid, deep, labored breathing, associated with diabetic coma).
    - Cheyne-Stokes (abnormal breathing pattern with alternating periods of apnea and deep, rapid breathing; the cycle begins with slow, shallow breaths that gradually increase in depth and rate and is then followed by a period of apnea).

DIAGNOSIS

DIFFERENTIAL DIAGNOSIS

- Intracranial:
  - Trauma, tumor, hemorrhage, status epilepticus, embolism/ischemic encephalopathy, granuloma, abscess, developmental disorders (hydrocephalus, storage diseases), and infections (rabies, feline infectious peritonitis, canine distemper, fungal, parasitic).
- Systemic:
  - Toxins: lead, barbiturates, antidepressants, tranquilizers, alcohol, ethylene glycol.
  - Metabolic: hypoglycemia, diabetic ketoacidosis, hepatic encephalopathy, uremic encephalopathy, hypoadrenocorticism, myxedema coma.
  - Hyperosmolar syndromes: hyperosmolar nonketotic diabetes mellitus, ethylene glycol, hypernatremia.
  - Hyperviscosity: polycythemia, hyperglobulinemia.
  - Miscellaneous: severe hypovolemia/shock, post arrest, heat stroke, hyponatremia.

INITIAL DATABASE

LABORATORY TESTS

- Complete blood count (infection or thrombocytopenia)
- Serum biochemistry panel (metabolic disorders)
- Urinalysis:
  - Glucose, ketones (diabetes mellitus/ketoacidosis)
  - Calcium oxalate monohydrate crystals (ethylene glycol intoxication)
  - Ammonium biurate crystals (portosystemic shunt)
  - Low urine specific gravity (USG)/casts (renal disease [consider other causes of low USG])
- Prothrombin time/partial thromboplastin time or activated clotting time (coagulopathies)
- Serum bile acids (liver failure)

IMAGING

- Thoracic radiographs (metastatic lesions, trauma, or infections)
- Skull radiographs (trauma/skull fractures)

ADVANCED OR CONFIRMATORY TESTING

Magnetic resonance imaging or computed tomography followed by cerebrospinal fluid analysis after systemic disease is eliminated.

TREATMENT

THERAPEUTIC GOAL(S)

- Stabilize and provide supportive care
- Specific therapy when diagnosis confirmed

ACUTE GENERAL TREATMENT

AIRWAY AND BREATHING

- Endotracheal intubation assists ventilation and protects the airways (comatose patients cannot swallow; salivary secretions, regurgitation, and vomiting may cause airway obstruction and aspiration pneumonia).
- Provide supplemental oxygen (maintain PaO_2>60 mmHg, SaO_2>90%).
- Caution: nasal oxygen lines can induce sneezing, which increases intracranial pressure (ICP).
- Ensure ventilation (maintain pCO_2 between 35-45 mmHg).

CIRCULATION

- Place intravenous catheter (avoid jugular veins if ICP elevated).
- Correct hypovolemia.
  - Fluid choice is controversial.
    - Crystalloids usually sufficient. Administer 1/4 shock dose (15 ml/kg dogs, 10 ml/kg cats) repeatedly in rapid IV increments until cardiovascularly stable.
  - Avoid overhydration.
- Provide maintenance and ongoing fluid losses.
- With cardiac disease or hyperosmolar syndromes, administer fluids cautiously.

DECREASE ICP

- In comatose patient, assume ICP elevated until proven otherwise.
- Elevate head 20 to 30 degrees.
- Avoid pressure on jugular veins.
- Give mannitol (0.5-2 mg/kg IV over 20 to 30 minutes) if diagnosis is unconfirmed or patient shows neurologic deterioration.
- Avoid mannitol in dehydrated, hypovolemic patients and when underlying cardiac disease or hyperosmolar states are present.

SUPPORTIVE CARE

- Control seizures:
  - Diazepam (0.5–1 mg/kg IV; can repeat twice in 15 minutes. If ineffective, then use constant rate infusion or different drug); or
  - Phenobarbital (2–15 mg/kg slow IV bolus [monitor respiration]); or
  - Propofol (if severe hepatopathy/hepatic coma) (1–6 mg/kg IV bolus; can repeat or switch to constant rate infusion [monitor respiration]).
- Treat hypoglycemia with intravenous dextrose:
  - Dose: 0.5 g/kg slow IV. Dilute 50% dextrose 1 ml/kg into 0.9% NaCl 3 ml/kg and administer IV slowly.
  - Avoid hyperglycemia.
- Glucocorticoids (e.g., methylprednisolone sodium succinate 30 mg/kg IV initial dose, then according to standard protocols) may be beneficial (neoplasia) or harmful (trauma).
- Confirm diagnosis before giving glucocorticoids.
- If life-threatening deterioration occurs before the diagnosis is confirmed, rapid-acting intravenous glucocorticoids can be administered for suspected neoplasia or encephalitis.
- Physical therapy, turning, lubrication of the eyes, and moistening the mouth every 4 hours.
- A urinary catheter assists with monitoring urine output and preventing urine scald.

SPECIFIC THERAPY: See specific diseases

POSSIBLE COMPLICATIONS

- Hypotension
- Hypothermia
- Brain herniation
- Cardiac arrhythmias
- Hypoventilation
- Aspiration pneumonia
- Seizures

RECOMMENDED MONITORING

- Rapid deterioration possible: monitor until stable and deterioration unlikely.
- Neurologic examination every 30 to 60 minutes.
- Continuous electrocardiogram.
- Blood pressure every 30 to 60 minutes (systolic: >90 mmHg but <180 mmHg; mean: >60 mmHg but <140 mmHg).
- Blood gases ($PaCO_2$ and PaO_2) every 60 minutes or capnography and pulse oximetry continuously.
- Blood glucose and electrolytes as needed.

PROGNOSIS AND OUTCOME

- Varies with underlying disease.
- Generally guarded until diagnosis confirmed.
- Declines as level of consciousness decreases.
- Worse with systemic complications.
- Unresponsive pupils, decerebrate rigidity, abnormal respiratory patterns, and loss of physiologic nystagmus carry a grave prognosis.
- Miotic responsive pupils suggest cortical lesions and a better prognosis.
- Can use modified Glasgow Coma Scale for prognosis in dogs with head trauma (see p 454).
- Failure to improve over 5 to 7 days warrants poor prognosis.

PEARLS & CONSIDERATIONS

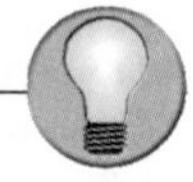

COMMENTS

- Animals that display decerebrate rigidity are also comatose.
- Bradycardia with concurrent hypertension suggests elevated ICP.
- Can use caloric test to evaluate nystagmus (infusion of warm or cold water into the ear canal normally results in nystagmus).
- Administration of lidocaine during intubation (0.75 mg/kg IV) may suppress gag and cough reflexes, which would otherwise increase ICP.

CLIENT EDUCATION

- Full neurologic recovery can take weeks to months.
- Long-term neurologic deficits and seizures can occur.

SUGGESTED READING

Dayrell-Hart B, Klide AM: Intracranial dysfunction: Stupor and coma. *Vet Clin North Am Sm Anim Pract* 19(6):1209–1222, 1989.

AUTHOR: **SØREN R. BOYSEN**
EDITOR: **ETIENNE CÔTÉ**

Conjunctivitis: Cats

BASIC INFORMATION

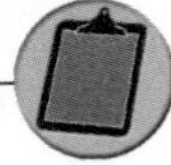

DEFINITION

Conjunctivitis is an inflammation of the conjunctiva, a thin mucous membrane lining the inner surface of the upper and lower eyelids, and both sides of the third eyelid (palpebral conjunctiva). In the conjunctival fornix ("cul-de-sac"), the conjunctiva reflects onto the globe (bulbar conjunctiva) and becomes continuous with the corneal epithelium. Conjunctivitis is one of the most common feline ocular diseases.

SYNONYM(S)

Red eye

Chalmydophila felis: formerly *Chlamydia psittaci*

Feline herpesvirus (FHV-1): feline viral rhinotracheitis

EPIDEMIOLOGY

SPECIES, AGE, SEX

- Younger cats: FHV-1, *C. felis*, *Mycoplasma* spp., eosinophilic conjunctivitis
- Older cats: lipogranulomatous conjunctivitis; neoplasia
- No sex predisposition

GENETICS AND BREED PREDISPOSITION: Lightly colored (white cats) predisposed to actinic-related conjunctivitis, lipogranulomatous conjunctivitis, squamous cell carcinoma.

RISK FACTORS

- Multicat household, catteries, boarding kennels, veterinary hospitals, cat shows, free-roaming cats (infectious conjunctivitis)
- Underlying systemic viral infection (feline leukemia virus [FeLV], feline immunodeficiency virus [FIV]) may predispose to FHV-1 infection

CONTAGION AND ZOONOSIS

- FHV-1, *C. felis*, *Mycoplasma* spp.: contagious cat-to-cat
- *C. felis*: identified in humans with conjunctivitis

ASSOCIATED CONDITIONS AND DISORDERS: Most cats with upper respiratory syndrome (see Upper Respiratory Infection, Feline, p 1115) present with conjunctivitis.

CLINICAL PRESENTATION

DISEASE FORMS/SUBTYPES

- Unilateral (e.g., trauma, topical irritants, intraocular neoplasm, uveitis) versus bilateral (e.g., systemic illness, infectious conjunctivitis)
- Primary:
  - Infectious causes common in cats (see above).
- Secondary:

- Underlying ocular and/or systemic disease (e.g., uveitis, lymphosarcoma).

HISTORY, CHIEF COMPLAINT

- Painful, red eye (unilateral or bilateral)
- Ocular discharge
- Signs of upper respiratory tract infection (FHV-1) including sneezing, nasal discharge, inappetence
- Recurrent signs of red, painful eye and/or ocular discharge (FHV-1)

PHYSICAL EXAM FINDINGS

- Conjunctival hyperemia
- Conjunctival edema (chemosis)
- Lymphoid follicles on conjunctiva
- Smooth, cream or white conjunctival nodules (lipogranulomatous)
- Ocular discharge (see Ocular Discharge, p 762; sometimes dark-brown to black, waxy discharge in Persian, Himalayan, Siamese cats)
- Blepharospasm
- Protrusion of the third eyelid

ETIOLOGY AND PATHOPHYSIOLOGY

- Primary:
  - Viral:
    - FHV-1 is considered one of the most important causative agents of feline conjunctivitis; has high affinity for conjunctival and respiratory epithelia and causes epithelial necrosis.
    - Other viruses involved in feline upper respiratory syndrome, but less likely to cause conjunctivitis, include calicivirus and reovirus.
  - Bacterial:
    - *C. felis*.
    - *Mycoplasma* spp.
    - Other bacterial infections (e.g. *Staphylococcus* spp., *Bacillus* spp., *Corynebacterium* spp.); uncommon in cats.
  - Immune-mediated:
    - Eosinophilic conjunctivitis
    - Allergic conjunctivitis; rare in cats
- Secondary:
  - Other ocular causes of red eye (see Red Eye, p 946) including:
    - Mechanical ocular irritation (e.g., entropion, trichiasis, distichiasis, exophthalmos (cranial displacement of the globe), lagophthalmos (incomplete closure of the eyelids), foreign body.
    - Corneal Ulceration, p 246.
    - Anterior Uveitis (see Uveitis, p 1134).
    - Ocular trauma.
    - Glaucoma, p 440.
    - Blepharitis.
  - Obliteration of lacrimal puncta/ducts due to symblepharon (adhesions of conjunctiva to surrounding tissues).
  - Actinic-related conjunctivitis.
  - Lipogranulomatous conjunctivitis:
    - Likely a reaction to sebaceous secretions from damaged meibomian glands.
    - May be a form of chalazion (see Eyelid Defects: Trauma, Masses, p 371).
    - Possible role of actinic radiation.
  - Systemic infectious diseases:
    - Viral (FeLV, FIV).
    - Systemic mycoses.
  - Neoplasia (e.g., squamous cell carcinoma, lymphosarcoma).

DIAGNOSIS

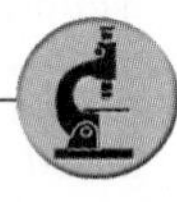

DIFFERENTIAL DIAGNOSIS

Primary conjunctivitis must be differentiated from secondary conjunctivitis (i.e., other causes of red eye; see Etiology and Pathophysiology above).

INITIAL DATABASE

Complete ophthalmic examination including:

- Examination of all conjunctival surfaces, including lacrimal puncta, with diffuse light and magnification.
- Conjunctival swabs for bacterial ± fungal culture(s) and sensitivity (done before other diagnostic tests).
- Conjunctival scrapings for cytology; diagnosis of bacterial or fungal infection, *C. felis* and *Mycoplasma* spp. inclusions; eosinophils (eosinophilic conjunctivitis).
- Schirmer tear test (normal >15 mm/min but can be variable in cats).
- Fluorescein dye application (monitor nares for exit of dye to determine if nasolacrimal system patent).
- Intraocular pressures (normal >15 mmHg and <25 mmHg).

ADVANCED OR CONFIRMATORY TESTING

- Conjunctival samples may be submitted for polymerase chain reaction testing for infectious diseases (FHV-1, *C. felis*, *Mycoplasma* spp., FeLV).
- Conjunctival samples for indirect fluorescent antibody staining (FHV-1).
- Flush nasolacrimal system if suspect occlusion (see Dacryocystitis, p 275).
- Conjunctival biopsy and histopathology (neoplasia).

TREATMENT

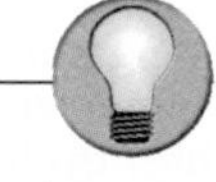

THERAPEUTIC GOAL(S)

- Treat underlying cause
- Eliminate infection, if possible
- Eliminate ocular pain

ACUTE GENERAL TREATMENT

- Primary:
  - FHV-1 or bacterial:
    - Topical broad-spectrum antibiotics (e.g., tobramycin or bacitracin-neomycin-polymyxin B ointment) q 6-8 hours for 7 to 10 days (to prevent secondary bacterial conjunctivitis if FHV-1-induced).
  - *C. felis* and/or *Mycoplasma* spp.:
    - Topical tetracycline ointment q 6–8h; continued for 10 to 14 days after clinical signs have resolved.
  - Eosinophilic:
    - Topical corticosteroids (e.g., prednisolone acetate 1% suspension or 0.1% dexamethasone solution or ointment) q 6–8h, tapered to indefinite maintenance dose.
    - Topical cyclosporine A (CsA; 0.2–2%) q 8–12h as indefinite treatment.
- Secondary: treat underlying cause:
  - Lipogranulomatous:
    - Surgical excision typically curative

CHRONIC TREATMENT

- FHV-1: see Herpesviral Keratitis in Cats, p 513.
- *C. felis* and/or *Mycoplasma* spp.:
  - Prolonged topical tetracycline if concurrent infection with FIV is confirmed.
  - Oral antibiotics (e.g., doxycycline-5 mg/kg PO q 12h for 3 to 4 weeks for difficult cases).

POSSIBLE COMPLICATIONS

FHV-1 may cause:

- Corneal Sequestration: Cats, p 245
- Symblepharon
- Keratoconjunctivitis sicca, p 614

PROGNOSIS AND OUTCOME

- Variable depending on cause.
- Usually good.
- Conjunctivitis caused by *C. felis* may become chronic.
- Recurrent conjunctivitis is observed with FHV-1 infection.

PEARLS & CONSIDERATIONS

COMMENTS

- FHV-1 infection may not only cause conjunctivitis, but may also cause keratitis in cats (see Herpesviral Keratitis in Cats, p 513).
- Topical corticosteroids should be avoided in cats with conjunctivitis, unless eosinophilic or lipogranulomatous conjunctivitis is confirmed cytologically and/or histologically.

PREVENTION

Reduction of known stresses is useful (FHV-1).

CLIENT EDUCATION

- Monitor for recurrent signs of conjunctivitis (FHV-1).
- Stress factors (e.g., concurrent systemic disease (FeLV, FIV), systemic or topical corticosteroids, general anesthesia, multicat household, moving) can trigger flare-up of FHV-1-induced conjunctivitis.

SUGGESTED READING

Allgoewer I, Schaffer E, Stockhaus C, Voegtlin A: Feline eosinophilic conjunctivitis. *Vet Ophthalmol* 4:69-74, 2001.

Read RA, Lucas J: Lipogranulomatous conjunctivitis: Clinical findings from 21 eyes in 13 cats. *Vet Ophthalmol* 4:93-98, 2001.

Stiles J, Townsend WM, Rogers QR, Krohne SG: Effect of oral administration of L-lysine on conjunctivitis caused by feline herpesvirus in cats. *Am J Vet Res* 63:99-103, 2002.

AUTHOR: **URSULA M. DIETRICH**
EDITOR: **CHERYL L. CULLEN**

Conjunctivitis: Dogs

BASIC INFORMATION

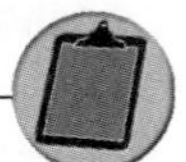

DEFINITION

Conjunctivitis is an inflammation of the conjunctiva, a thin mucous membrane lining the inner surface of the upper and lower eyelids, and both sides of the third eyelid (palpebral conjunctiva). In the conjunctival fornix ("cul-de-sac"), the conjunctiva reflects onto the globe (bulbar conjunctiva) and becomes continuous with the corneal epithelium. Conjunctivitis is one of the most commonly diagnosed ocular disorders in dogs.

SYNONYM(S)

Red eye

Canine adenovirus 1: infectious canine hepatitis

EPIDEMIOLOGY

SPECIES, AGE, SEX

- Typically no age predisposition, although allergic conjunctivitis and follicular conjunctivitis typically occur in younger dogs
- No sex predisposition

GENETICS AND BREED PREDISPOSITION: Breeds predisposed to:

- Pannus (Chronic Superficial Keratitis), p 802
- Plasmacellular conjunctivitis: German shepherd, collie
- Keratoconjunctivitis Sicca, p 614
- Abnormal eyelid conformation (e.g., Entropion/Ectropion, p 345)
- Deep orbits, narrow skull conformation, and inadequate tear drainage (i.e., medial canthal pocket syndrome): dolichocephalic breeds including Afghan hound, Doberman pinscher, standard poodle
- Ligneous conjunctivitis (rare): Doberman pinscher

RISK FACTORS

- Outdoor activities (e.g., hunting) (allergic conjunctivitis)
- Nonvaccinated animals, dog shelters, dog shows (Distemper, Canine, p 315); canine adenovirus (CAV-1, CAV-2) conjunctivitis)

CONTAGION AND ZOONOSIS: Canine distemper virus and CAV-1, CAV-2: contagious dog-to-dog.

ASSOCIATED CONDITIONS AND DISORDERS: Skin allergies, otitis externa (allergic conjunctivitis).

CLINICAL PRESENTATION

DISEASE FORMS/SUBTYPES

Unilateral or bilateral:

- Primary: allergic, infectious
- Secondary: underlying ocular and/or systemic disease (e.g., pannus/CSK, keratoconjunctivitis sicca, uveitis, canine distemper, histiocytosis)

HISTORY, CHIEF COMPLAINT

- Painful, red eye (unilateral or bilateral)
- Ocular discharge

PHYSICAL EXAM FINDINGS

- Conjunctival hyperemia
- Conjunctival edema (chemosis)
- Lymphoid follicles on conjunctiva
- Thick, opaque palpebral conjunctival membrane formation (ligneous conjunctivitis)
- Ocular Discharge, p 762
- Blepharospasm
- Protrusion of the third eyelid

ETIOLOGY AND PATHOPHYSIOLOGY

- Primary:
  - Allergic conjunctivitis
  - Follicular conjunctivitis (chronic antigenic stimulation)
  - Immune-mediated conjunctivitis (clinical signs together with plasmacellular infiltration on cytologic/histologic evaluation, suggestive of immune-mediated condition)
  - Bacterial conjunctivitis (*Staphylococcus* spp., other gram-positive organisms; uncommon)
- Secondary:
  - Other ocular causes of red eye (see Red Eye, p 946) including:
    - Keratoconjunctivitis Sicca, p 614
    - Mechanical ocular irritation (e.g., entropion, ectropion, trichiasis, distichiasis, ectopic cilia, eyelid mass, exophthalmos [cranial displacement of the globe], lagophthalmos [incomplete closure of the eyelids], foreign body)
    - Corneal Ulceration, p 246
    - Anterior uveitis (see Uveitis, p 1134)
    - Ocular trauma
    - Glaucoma, p 440
    - Blepharitis
    - Dacryocystitis, p 275
    - Scrolled cartilage of the third eyelid and/or prolapsed gland of the third eyelid (see Third Eyelid Abnormalities/Protrusion, p 1077)
    - Periocular skin disease (e.g., pemphigus foliaceus, demodicosis)
  - Environmental:
    - Irritation from dust, smoke, or chemicals
    - Actinic-related/solar conjunctivitis in dogs lacking pigment along margin of third eyelid
  - Systemic infectious diseases:
    - Viral (canine distemper, CAV-1 and CAV-2)
    - Systemic mycoses (see Blastomycosis, p 133; Coccidioidomycosis, p 218; Cryptococcosis, p 259; Histoplasmosis, p 525)
    - Leishmaniasis, p 627
  - Systemic noninfectious diseases (e.g., systemic histiocytosis, polycythemia vera)
  - Neoplasia (e.g., lymphosarcoma, multiple myeloma, mast cell tumor, squamous cell carcinoma)
  - Idiopathic:
    - Ligneous conjunctivitis
      - Conjunctival injury and exaggerated, inflammatory immune response implicated in human form of disease
      - May be associated with membrane formation involving the oral mucosa, upper respiratory tract, or urinary tract

DIAGNOSIS

DIFFERENTIAL DIAGNOSIS

Primary conjunctivitis must be differentiated from secondary conjunctivitis (i.e..

other causes of red eye; see Etiology and Pathophysiology).

INITIAL DATABASE

Complete ophthalmic examination including:

- Examination of all conjunctival surfaces, including lacrimal puncta, with diffuse light and magnification
- Conjunctival swabs for bacterial ± fungal culture(s) and sensitivity (done before other diagnostic tests)
- Conjunctival scrapings for cytologic evaluation; diagnosis of bacterial or fungal infection, intracytoplasmic inclusions in conjunctival epithelial cells in distemper infection
- Schirmer tear test (normal >15 mm/min)
- Fluorescein dye application (monitor nares for exit of dye to determine if nasolacrimal system patent)
- Intraocular pressures (normal >15 mmHg and <30 mmHg)

ADVANCED OR CONFIRMATORY TESTING

- Conjunctival samples may be submitted for polymerase chain reaction testing for infectious diseases (e.g., distemper virus).
- Conjunctival samples for indirect fluorescent antibody staining (distemper virus, adenovirus).
- Flush nasolacrimal system if suspect occlusion (see Dacryocystitis, p 275).
- Conjunctival biopsy and histopathology (neoplasia; ligneous conjunctivitis).

TREATMENT

THERAPEUTIC GOAL(S)

- Treat underlying cause.
- Eliminate infection, if possible.
- Eliminate ocular pain.

ACUTE GENERAL TREATMENT

- Primary:
  - Bacterial:
    - Topical broad-spectrum antibiotics (e.g., bacitracin/neomycin/polymyxin B; or based on culture and sensitivity results) q 6-8h for 7 to 10 days.
  - Allergic or follicular or plasmacellular:
    - Topical corticosteroid or corticosteroid/antibiotic combination (e.g., 0.1% dexamethasone ± neomycin/ polymyxin B solution or ointment) q 6-8h, tapered slowly based on response to treatment; may recur; address contributing factors (e.g., atopy, food allergy).
    - Topical cyclosporine A (CsA; 0.2-2%) q 12h (plasmacellular); usually required long-term.
- Secondary: treat underlying cause:
  - Ligneous:
    - Topical CsA (0.2-2%) q 12h.
    - Azathioprine orally 1.5-2 mg/kg PO q 24h until clinical improvement; then gradually tapered to as low a dose as possible (e.g., 1 mg/kg PO q 24h, then every other day, then weekly for maintenance).
    - ± Prednisone orally 1-2 mg/kg PO q 24h until clinical improvement; then gradually tapered over 3 to 4 weeks until maintenance dose reached.

CHRONIC TREATMENT

Indefinite maintenance therapy usually required for immune-mediated causes of conjunctivitis (i.e., plasmacellular conjunctivitis [see Pannus (Chronic Superficial Keratitis), p 802]), and ligneous conjunctivitis; see Acute General Treatment above.

PROGNOSIS AND OUTCOME

- Variable depending on cause.
- Usually good if underlying cause addressed.
- Some breeds with medial canthal pocket syndrome develop chronic conjunctivitis and may need indefinite topical treatment.
- Immune-mediated causes of conjunctivitis typically require lifelong treatment.

PEARLS & CONSIDERATIONS

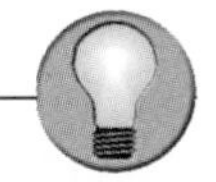

COMMENTS

Do not use topical corticosteroids if corneal ulceration is noted.

PREVENTION

Conjunctivitis due to breed predisposition: avoid breeding affected or closely related dogs

SUGGESTED READING

Gerding PA, McLaughlin SA, Troop MW: Pathogenic bacteria and fungi associated with external ocular diseases in dogs: 131 cases (1981-1986). *J Am Vet Med Assoc* 193:242-244, 1988.

Ramsey DT, Ketring KL, Glaze MB, et al: Ligneous conjunctivitis in four Doberman pinschers. *J Am Anim Hosp Assoc* 32:439-447, 1996.

Stone A, Schrock J: Bacterial conjunctivitis in the dog: Preliminary findings. *J Am Anim Hosp Assoc* 8:10-12, 1972.

AUTHOR: **URSULA M. DIETRICH**

EDITOR: **CHERYL L. CULLEN**

Constipation/Obstipation and Megacolon

BASIC INFORMATION

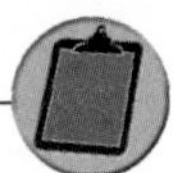

DEFINITION

- Constipation: infrequent or difficult evacuation of feces, but does not imply loss of function.
- Obstipation: intractable constipation that is refractory to control.
- Megacolon: persistent dilation of the large intestine associated with chronic constipation or obstipation, or occurring secondary to idiopathic loss of colon function. Dilated megacolon implies permanent loss of colonic structure and function.

EPIDEMIOLOGY

SPECIES, AGE, SEX: Constipation can occur in both dogs and cats. Megacolon is rarely reported in dogs and only secondary to uncorrected pelvic fractures or colonic/rectal obstruction. Obstipation/megacolon is reported to be more common in middle-aged, male cats of the domestic shorthair, domestic long hair, or Siamese breeds.

GENETICS AND BREED PREDISPOSITION: Manx cats may be predisposed to neurogenic megacolon.

RISK FACTORS

- Functional obstruction preventing passage of feces: neurologic disease or trauma, dysautonomia
- Mechanical obstruction preventing passage of feces: pelvic fracture, colonic stricture or neoplasia, extraluminal mass compressing colon, anal stricture, colonic foreign body

ASSOCIATED CONDITIONS AND DISORDERS: Perineal hernia may be cause of, or result of, megacolon.

CLINICAL PRESENTATION

DISEASE FORMS/SUBTYPES

- Hypertrophic megacolon: develops as a consequence of obstructive lesions, and thus may be reversible with early therapy
- Dilated megacolon: end stage of colonic dysfunction (both idio-

pathic or untreated hypertrophic megacolon)

HISTORY, CHIEF COMPLAINT

- Reduced, absent, or painful defecation is typical presentation.
- Fecal balls are often very hard if passed, and occasionally watery diarrhea may be passed around fecal concretion.
- Prolonged constipation will result in anorexia, lethargy, weight loss, or vomiting (may be projectile).

PHYSICAL EXAM FINDINGS

- Poor body condition.
- Dehydration.
- Colon distended with hard feces on abdominal palpation. Signs of abdominal pain may be present.
- Perineal irritation/ulceration.
- Rectal exam (dogs): hard feces, possible pelvic narrowing or mass palpated, perineal hernia (usually must be performed under sedation).

ETIOLOGY AND PATHOPHYSIOLOGY

- Prolonged retention of feces in colon due to functional (neurogenic) or mechanical obstruction (e.g., pelvic fractures, intraluminal or extraluminal masses).
- Inflammation can also be associated with constipation (perianal fistula, proctitis, anal sac abscess, or perianal bite wounds).
- Water absorption from feces in colon results in concretion that is difficult or impossible to pass (common in cats with chronic progressive renal disease or diabetes mellitus).
- Neurogenic dysfunction from dysautonomia (autonomic system failure), trauma to pelvic or hypogastric nerves (pelvic fracture), neoplasia of spinal cord, or caudal spinal cord diseases (e.g., lumbosacral disease, cauda equina syndrome, Manx cat sacral deformities).
- Prolonged distention of colon causes irreversible changes in colonic smooth muscles and nerves.
- Retained bacterial toxins may be absorbed, resulting in endotoxemia and signs of illness (anorexia, lethargy, vomiting).

DIAGNOSIS

DIFFERENTIAL DIAGNOSIS

- Reversible causes of constipation:
  - Dehydration, electrolyte disorders, inflammatory diseases of the anorectum
  - Drug administration (opioids, anticholinergics)
  - Environmental changes (inactivity, litter box changes)
- Any of the risk factors causing mechanical obstruction

INITIAL DATABASE

- Complete blood cell count: leukocytosis (mature neutrophilia/stress leukogram), occasionally anemia.
- Serum biochemistry profile: azotemia (associated with dehydration or concurrent chronic renal failure); hypokalemia; hypercalcemia.
- Urinalysis: no specific changes. Isosthenuria in azotemic patients if chronic renal failure.
- Abdominal radiographs: feces distended colon. Underlying cause of initial colonic distention/fecal retention may be evident: pelvic fractures, evidence of spinal trauma (vertebral fracture/luxation), extraluminal compressive masses, foreign material in colon.

ADVANCED OR CONFIRMATORY TESTING

- Ultrasonography: identifies suspected extraluminal masses. Poor utility for intraluminal visualization because even minute amounts of colonic gas block ultrasound waves.
- Barium enema: defines strictures or intraluminal masses (see Barium Enema, p 1185).
- Endoscopy: identifies colorectal neoplasia, stricture, inflammatory lesions, sacculations and diverticula, etc.
- Evaluation of animals with suspected neurologic impairment may include cerebrospinal fluid analysis, computed tomography/magnetic resonance imaging scanning of distal spinal cord and cauda equina region, myelogram, and electrophysiologic studies (electromyography).
- Diagnosis of dysautonomia is based on finding other systemic evidence of the disease (megaesophagus, mydriasis, decreased lacrimation, prolapsed nictitans, and bradycardia) but is considered a rare cause of megacolon. See Dysautonomia, p 323.

TREATMENT

THERAPEUTIC GOAL(S)

- Correct dehydration and electrolyte abnormalities.
- Evacuate colon.
- Control recurrent constipation.
- Correct underlying cause of constipation prior to onset of irreversible changes in colonic smooth muscle and nerves.
- For end-stage megacolon, focus may be oriented mainly toward surgical methods of relieving recurrent obstruction.

ACUTE GENERAL TREATMENT

- Fluid therapy for dehydration with supplementation to correct hypokalemia if present. Intravenous fluid therapy (60-90 ml/kg/day) is often needed for most severely affected cats. Correction of dehydration assists in constipation relief through rehydration of the colonic mucosa.
- Enemas and careful manual extraction of feces if obstipated. In most cats, sedation or anesthesia will be required. Multiple procedures over a day or two may be needed in the most severely obstipated/impacted cats to prevent additional injury or rupture of the diseased colon.
- Warm water enemas (30-50 ml water/dose) using a 12-14 Fr, well-lubricated, red rubber catheter for insertion are well tolerated. Higher volumes of water must be used with caution, because they may cause vomiting (and aspiration). If multiple enemas are administered in a short period of time, saline is preferred instead of tap water to avoid an excessive osmotic shift of sodium and other electrolytes into the colon and resultant hyponatremia.
- Enemas should not contain soaps or other irritants; lactulose or mineral oil can be used.
- Enemas containing sodium phosphate (e.g., Fleet) are contraindicated in cats and small dogs due to the severe hyperphosphatemia and subsequent hypocalcemia they can cause.
- Broad-spectrum antibiotics (e.g., ampicillin 22 mg/kg IV q 8h and enrofloxacin 5 mg/kg diluted 1:1 in saline and given slowly IV q 12h [q 24h in cats]) are indicated if signs of endotoxemia or fever are noted.

CHRONIC TREATMENT

- Control recurrent constipation with high-fiber or low-residue diet. High-fiber diets are useful in management of constipation when the cat still has a functional colon and if the cat is well hydrated. However, cats that are prone to dehydration will be even more prone to it with high-fiber diets. Low-residue diets are often best in cats with chronic recurrent episodes of obstipation or true megacolon because they reduce the amount of material reaching the colon and make it easier to keep a soft stool.
- Medical therapy includes stool softeners or laxatives (e.g., lactulose 0.25-0.5 ml/kg PO q 8-12h; or docusate sodium/dioctyl sulfosuccinate 50 mg/cat PO q 12-24h; or mineral oil) and prokinetics (cisapride, 1 mg/kg PO q 24h). Lactulose is the most effective stool softener and is given to effect daily to maintain a soft to semi-formed stool (usual dose after titration: 1-4 ml/cat PO q 8-12h).
- Bulk-forming laxatives (cellulose, psyllium) will not be effective in cats prone to dehydration or in cats with poor colonic muscle function, because their mechanism of action is similar to high-fiber diets.

- Stimulant laxatives (e.g., bisacodyl, castor oil, cascara) should not be used for relieving constipation but are best used as a preventative in cats that still have normal colonic function.
- Prokinetic therapy may assist smooth muscle function in cats with recurrent constipation or obstipation. The most effective drugs are the serotonergic agonists (cisapride, prucalamide), and histamine H_2 receptor antagonists (ranitidine 1–2 mg/kg PO q 8–12h, or nizatidine [dogs only] 5 mg/kg PO q 24h; famotidine does not have this effect).
- Correct underlying cause: remove masses causing obstruction to outflow or correct pelvic fractures obstructing outflow with pelvic osteotomy.
- Perform subtotal colectomy (with or without preservation of the ileocolic valve) if lack of response to medical treatment or pelvic fracture malunion >6 months from onset of obstipation.

POSSIBLE COMPLICATIONS

- Medical treatment: perforation due to trauma from enemas and evacuation of feces; gentle manipulation and being patient (don't be in a hurry to remove the concretion) are essential.
- Subtotal colectomy: leakage, dehiscence, and peritonitis; chronic diarrhea (may be associated with bacterial overgrowth from loss of ileocolic sphincter); recurrent constipation; stricture.

RECOMMENDED MONITORING

- For cats undergoing medical management, close observation of fecal passage by the owner is essential for prevention of severe recurrent constipation.
- After subtotal colectomy, monitor:
  - Hydration
  - Appetite
  - Temperature, blood glucose, abdominal pain (signs of leakage or dehiscence of anastomosis)

PROGNOSIS AND OUTCOME

- Fair prognosis with medical management. Recurrent constipation requiring repeated enemas and manual evacuation is common.
- Good to excellent prognosis with subtotal colectomy. Owner needs to be aware that stools are usually soft, and the frequency of defecation is increased, for 2 to 3 months after surgery. Occasionally diarrhea is a persistent long-term problem.
- Guarded prognosis with pelvic osteotomy for pelvic fracture malunion. Correction of obstruction may not resolve megacolon and constipation.

PEARLS & CONSIDERATIONS

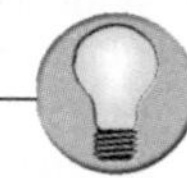

COMMENTS

- Do not attempt correction of pelvic malunion by pelvic osteotomy if >6 months from onset of signs of obstipation. Perform subtotal colectomy instead.
- Do not perform enema immediately before surgery for megacolon. It is more difficult to control contamination of the abdomen with liquid feces during surgery.

PREVENTION

Repair pelvic fractures that cause obstruction of pelvic canal early

CLIENT EDUCATION

Warn owners that diarrhea can be severe after subtotal colectomy but that it usually resolves within 8 weeks. If the cecum is removed during surgery, consider treatment for bacterial overgrowth if diarrhea persists >8 weeks.

SUGGESTED READING

Hasler AH, et al: Cisapride stimulates contraction of idiopathic megacolonic smooth muscle in cats. *J Vet Intern Med* 11:313, 1997.

Matthiesen DT, et al: Subtotal colectomy for the treatment of obstipation secondary to pelvic fracture malunion in cats. *Vet Surg* 20:113, 1991.

Rosin E, et al: Subtotal colectomy for treatment of chronic constipation associated with idiopathic megacolon in cats: 38 cases (1979–1985). *J Am Vet Med Assoc* 193:850, 1988.

Schrader SC, et al: Pelvic osteotomy as a treatment for obstipation in cats with acquired stenosis of the pelvic canal: Six cases (1978–1989). *J Am Vet Med Assoc* 200:208, 1992.

Washabau RJ, Holt DE: Diseases of the large intestine. In Ettinger SJ, Feldman EC (eds): *Textbook of Veterinary Internal Medicine,* ed 6. St. Louis, Elsevier, 2005, pp 1378–1408.

AUTHOR: **LORI LUDWIG**

EDITOR: **RICHARD WALSHAW**

Contact Dermatitis

BASIC INFORMATION

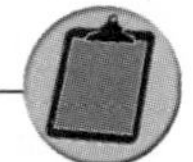

DEFINITION

Cutaneous inflammation that occurs after contact with an irritant or antigenic substance

SYNONYM(S)

Allergic contact dermatitis
Contact hypersensitivity
Irritant contact dermatitis

EPIDEMIOLOGY

SPECIES, AGE, SEX

- An uncommon disorder in dogs comprising only 1–10% of referral dermatology cases; rare in cats.
- Allergic contact dermatitis typically occurs in animals older than 1 year; irritant contact dermatitis may occur at any age.
- No sex predisposition.

GENETICS AND BREED PREDISPOSITION: Terrier breeds, French poodles, and golden retrievers may be at increased risk.

RISK FACTORS: Concurrent inflammatory dermatoses.

ASSOCIATED CONDITIONS AND DISORDERS

- Atopy.
- Secondary bacterial or *Malassezia* dermatitis is common.

CLINICAL PRESENTATION

DISEASE FORMS/SUBTYPES

- Allergic contact dermatitis
- Irritant contact dermatitis

HISTORY, CHIEF COMPLAINT

- Allergic contact dermatitis:
  - The chief complaint is typically chronic pruritus that may be seasonal or nonseasonal depending on the allergen.
  - A recent change in environment or housing is typically not noted, because signs may take longer than 2 years to develop from the time of initial exposure.
  - The animal is typically the only one in the household affected.
- Irritant contact dermatitis:
  - The chief complaint may be acute cutaneous pain rather than pruritus.
  - Onset of the condition often correlates with the introduction of a new substance.
  - There may be more than one individual affected (including the owner).

PHYSICAL EXAM FINDINGS: Lesion distribution reflects the area of the body in contact with the offending substance.

- Sparsely haired areas and those areas in contact with the environment are more frequently affected (ventral sufaces of the feet, chest, and abdomen, perineum, scrotum).
- Regional dermatitis of the muzzle and chin may occur with reactions to substances such as plastic food dishes or rubber chew toys.
- A generalized distribution may be present with contact reactions to shampoos.
- The ears may be the only area affected if topical otic medications have been administered.
- The primary lesion is an erythematous papular and macular eruption.
- Vesicles are occasionally present.
- With chronic exposure, alopecia, lichenification, and hyperpigmentation develop.

ETIOLOGY AND PATHOPHYSIOLOGY

- Allergic contact dermatitis is a type IV hypersensitivity disorder. The development of clinical disease requires two stages: induction and elicitation. The induction phase is the time from allergen exposure until the time lymphocytes become programmed to recognize the allergen. This phase may take months to years, during which time there is no evidence of clinical disease. Elicitation is the time from reexposure to the allergen to the development of cutaneous inflammation. This phase may take several days.
- Reported causes include shampoos, insecticides, topical/otic medications, plastic, detergents, wool, synthetic rugs, fertilizers, cement, perfumed cat litter, and several species of plants.
- Irritant contact dermatitis is an antigen-independent process that is the result of direct keratinocyte damage by the offending compound. No induction phase is necessary. Acids, alkalis, surfactants, solvents, enzymes, and oxidants may cause irritant contact dermatitis.

DIAGNOSIS

DIFFERENTIAL DIAGNOSIS

- Atopy
- Adverse food reaction/food allergy
- Flea allergy dermatitis
- Bacterial pyoderma
- Demodicosis
- Sarcoptes
- *Malassezia* dermatitis
- Demodicosis
- Dermatophytosis
- Pelodera dermatitis
- Hookworm dermatitis
- Erythema multiforme
- Drug eruptions
- Lupus erythematosus

INITIAL DATABASE

Contact dermatitis is an uncommon disorder in veterinary medicine. More common causes of the apparent clinical signs should be ruled out first.

- Skin scrapings and cytologic study should be performed to detect microbial or parasitic infections.
- A fungal culture should be considered, especially in cats, to detect dermatophytosis.
- An elimination food trial may be performed to rule out dermatologic adverse food reactions/food allergy.
- Intradermal skin testing or in vitro serum allergy testing may be performed to investigate atopy.

ADVANCED OR CONFIRMATORY TESTING

- Histopathologic evaluation may provide supportive evidence and help differentiate between allergic and irritant contact dermatitis if the biopsies are taken early in the disease process. Biopsies of chronically diseased skin are usually nonspecific.
- Patch testing is a specific test for investigating contact dermatitis. A series of compounds is applied to the skin for 48 hours, and the degree of erythema, induration, and papular eruptions caused by each agent is evaluated. Standardized kits for veterinary medicine are not available, but human standardized kits have been used successfully in dogs.
- Restriction and provocative exposure is the most reliable test. Ideally the animal should be bathed to remove all possible allergens and removed completely from the home environment for 2 to 4 weeks. After resolution the animal is reintroduced to the environment. A return of clinical signs will typically occur within 24 to 72 hours in cases of contact dermatitis.

TREATMENT

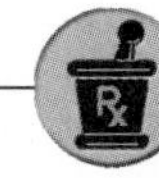

THERAPEUTIC GOAL(S)

Resolution of the skin lesions and pruritus or pain

ACUTE GENERAL TREATMENT

- Treat any secondary microbial infections.
- Identify and remove the offending substance.
- Palliative therapy with glucocorticoids (prednisone 0.5-1.0 mg/kg PO q 24h initially, before weaning down based on response), pentoxifylline (20 mg/kg PO q 12h) or topical tacrolimus (0.1% ointment) may provide relief in cases of allergic contact dermatitis.

PROGNOSIS AND OUTCOME

Excellent if the offending substance is identified and removed

PEARLS & CONSIDERATIONS

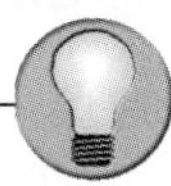

COMMENTS

Substances may cause both irritation and allergic contact dermatitis.

SUGGESTED READING

Marsella R: Contact hypersensitivity. In Campbell KL (ed): *Small Animal Dermatology Secrets*. Philadelphia, Hanley and Belfus, 2004, pp 202-208.

Olivry T: Allergic contact dermatitis in the dog: Principles and diagnosis. *Vet Clin North Am Small Anim Pract* 20:6, 1990.

White PD: Contact dermatitis in the dog and cat. *Semin Vet Med Surg Small Anim* 6:4, 1991.

AUTHOR: **ANDREW LOWE**
EDITOR: **JAN A. HALL**

Cor Triatriatum Sinister and Supravalvular Mitral Stenosis

BASIC INFORMATION

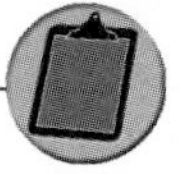

DEFINITION

- Congenital cardiac malformations involving membranous division of the left atrium into a proximal high pressure chamber and a distal low pressure chamber.
- Cor triatriatum sinister (CTS) can be distinguished from supravalvular mitral stenosis (SVMS) by the location of the membrane relative to the left auricle. Cor triatriatum ("three atria") sinister ("left"): the auricle is distal to the dividing membrane and connected with the distal low-pressure left atrial chamber.
- Supravalvular mitral stenosis: the left auricle is proximal to the dividing membrane and is connected with the proximal high-pressure left atrial chamber.

SYNONYM(S)

CTS
SVMS

EPIDEMIOLOGY

SPECIES, AGE, SEX

- Feline; most often diagnosed in cats less than 1 year of age but has been reported in older cats; males reported more frequently.
- Canine: no cases reported (see cor triatriatum dexter).

GENETICS AND BREED PREDISPOSITION: Uncommon. No known breed predisposition or genetic defect defined.
RISK FACTORS: None known.

CLINICAL PRESENTATION

HISTORY, CHIEF COMPLAINT

- Respiratory distress
- Anorexia
- Lethargy

PHYSICAL EXAM FINDINGS: Not all signs will be present in every patient:

- Tachypnea
- Dyspnea
- Tachycardia
- Gallop
- Diastolic murmur
- Arrhythmias with pulse deficits
- Crackles and/or wheezes
- Muffled lung sounds (pleural effusion)

ETIOLOGY AND PATHOPHYSIOLOGY

- CTS results from incomplete incorporation of the embryologic pulmonary venous chamber into the developing left atrium.
- SVMS results from embryologic malformation of the mitral valve apparatus.
- Both CTS and SVMS cause left atrial inflow obstruction, which may result in signs of left-sided congestive heart failure, including pulmonary edema, pleural effusion, and pericardial effusion. Therefore, clinical signs of CTS and SVMS are identical.

DIAGNOSIS

DIFFERENTIAL DIAGNOSIS

- Mitral valve stenosis
- Hypertrophic cardiomyopathy
- Dilated cardiomyopathy
- Thyrotoxic heart disease
- Left atrial tumor

INITIAL DATABASE

- Thoracic radiographs demonstrate marked left atrial enlargement, ± left ventricular enlargement. Signs of congestive heart failure may also be present: pulmonary venous distention, interstitial to alveolar infiltrate, and/or pleural effusion.
- Electrocardiogram may show wide P waves consistent with left atrial enlargement, and tall R waves consistent with left ventricular enlargement.
- Complete blood count may show a stress leukogram. Biochemistry panel and urinalysis are likely to be unremarkable.

ADVANCED OR CONFIRMATORY TESTING

- Echocardiography:
  - Two-dimensional echocardiography will display a membrane dividing the atrium and indicating the position of the membrane relative to the auricle.
  - Doppler echocardiography can be used for determining the degree of obstruction by measuring the velocity of blood flow across orifice.
    - The modified Bernoulli equation can be used for calculating the pressure gradient across the membrane (Pressure change = $4 \times \text{velocity}^2$).
- Angiography is an alternate imaging technique to define the location of the obstruction and determine if other concurrent cardiac defects are present, but invasiveness of angiography makes echocardiography a superior first choice.

TREATMENT

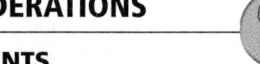

THERAPEUTIC GOAL(S)

Alleviate clinical signs of left heart failure.

ACUTE GENERAL TREATMENT

If patient is in acute heart failure, then treat with furosemide, oxygen, and nitroglycerin. See Heart Failure, Acute/Decompensated, p 458.

CHRONIC TREATMENT

- Furosemide and an angiotensin-converting enzyme inhibitor to control fluid accumulation. See Heart Failure, Chronic, p 459.
- Periodic thoracocenteses may be necessary to treat pleural effusion.
- Successful surgical correction of CTS has been reported.

DRUG INTERACTIONS

Electrolyte depletion and dehydration may result from overzealous diuretic administration.

POSSIBLE COMPLICATIONS

Surgery is highly invasive and therefore the risk of mortality is increased with an inexperienced surgeon.

RECOMMENDED MONITORING

- Pulmonary edema/pleural effusion should resolve with successful reduction/removal of the membranous obstruction.
- Renal function should be periodically monitored if medical therapy chosen.

PROGNOSIS AND OUTCOME

- Excellent with successful reduction/removal of the obstruction.
- Medical management alone is unlikely to be satisfactory on a long-term basis if signs of congestive heart failure have already occurred, but the small number of recorded veterinary cases of CTS/SVMS limits the extent of this conclusion.

PEARLS & CONSIDERATIONS

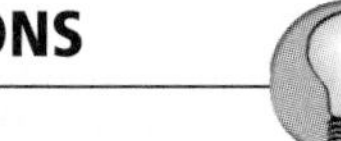

COMMENTS

These defects are rare but represent potentially curable abnormalities. Any cat presenting with signs of heart failure should have an echocardiogram performed to rule out CTS or SVMS.

CLIENT EDUCATION

Owner should monitor for recurrence of heart failure: increased respiratory rate or effort, lethargy, or anorexia. Owner should monitor patient's resting respiratory rate and call clinician if rate exceeds 40 breaths/minute when the patient is asleep.

SUGGESTED READING

Fine DM, et al: Supravalvular mitral stenosis in a cat. *J Am Anim Hosp Assoc* 38:403, 2002.

Heaney AM, et al: Cor triatriatum sinister and persistent left cranial vena cava in a kitten. *J Vet Intern Med* 18(6):895–898, 2004.

Wander KW, et al: Surgical correction of cor triatriatum sinister in a kitten. *J Am Anim Hosp Assoc* 34:383, 1998.

AUTHOR: **DEBORAH M. FINE**
EDITOR: **ETIENNE CÔTÉ**

Corneal Discoloration

BASIC INFORMATION

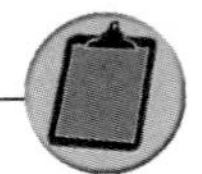

DEFINITION

Corneal discoloration is any alteration of corneal clarity.

SYNONYM(S)

Corneal opacification
Corneal opacity

EPIDEMIOLOGY

SPECIES, AGE, SEX: Varies depending on the underlying cause.

CLINICAL PRESENTATION

HISTORY, CHIEF COMPLAINT

- Brown, white, white/yellow, white/pink, blue/grey, or red spot(s) on or within the cornea.
- Vision may be reduced depending on the location and size of discoloration.
- Discomfort and ocular discharge may be present depending on the cause.

PHYSICAL EXAM FINDINGS

- Focal to diffuse brown, white, white/yellow, white/pink, blue/grey, or red discoloration of the corneal surface, stroma, or endothelium
- Reduced or absent menace response if lesion covers significant portion of axial cornea

ETIOLOGY AND PATHOPHYSIOLOGY

- Brown discolorations:
  - Epithelial and stromal pigmentation occurs secondary to chronic irritation or inflammation:
    - Melanin is produced by melanocytes in the epithelium and superficial stroma in response to chronic corneal irritation from desiccation or mechanical trauma.
    - Proliferation and migration of limbal melanocytes into the stroma may also occur secondary to chronic inflammation in response to ulceration, degeneration, or an immune response to corneal antigen.
  - Endothelial pigmentation:
    - Adherence of melanin or melanin-containing cells, usually arising from the anterior uvea, to the endothelium.
  - Stromal infiltration at the limbus as extension of a melanin-containing neoplasm.
  - Protrusion of pigmented tissue through a corneal defect (i.e., iris prolapse).
  - Corneal sequestrum (cats):
    - Associated with chronic irritation: the central/paracentral stroma becomes necrotic, stained, and overlying epithelium is usually disrupted.
    - Cause of stromal discoloration is unresolved.
    - See Corneal Sequestration: Cats, p 245.
- White discolorations:
  - Fibrosis/scarring:
    - During the healing of stromal injury, such as ulceration, trauma, or inflammation, fibroplasia occurs, and newly produced collagen is laid down in a disorganized fashion.
  - Lipid (see Corneal Lipid Infiltrates, p 241):
    - Lipid deposition is associated with a primary defect of corneal lipid metabolism in inherited corneal dystrophy in some breeds.
    - Lipid deposition may be associated with secondary defect of corneal metabolism such as in corneal degeneration caused by trauma, ulceration, chronic irritation, uveitis, or glaucoma.
    - Lipid infiltration in the cornea may occur in systemic disorders of lipid metabolism due to leakage of lipid-laden serum at the limbus (arc-shaped) or in association with corneal vascularization.
  - Calcium:
    - Calcium deposition may be associated with secondary defect of corneal metabolism such as in corneal degeneration caused by trauma, ulceration, chronic irritation, uveitis, or glaucoma.
    - Calcium deposition in the cornea may occur due to derangements in systemic calcium and phosphorus metabolism.
- White/yellow or white/pink discolorations:
  - Epithelial or stromal infiltration of inflammatory cells occurs in association with sterile inflammation or secondary to infection.
  - Endothelial deposition of inflammatory cells occurs in association with chronic uveitis (keratic precipitates).
  - Epithelial inclusion cysts usually form when mitotically active basal epithelial cells become displaced into the corneal stroma, due to trauma or surgery, and continue to grow.
- Grey/blue discolorations:
  - Corneal edema:
    - Fluid from the tear film may enter the corneal stroma secondary to loss of corneal epithelium (i.e., corneal erosion, ulcer, or other trauma).
    - Aqueous humor may enter corneal stroma due to loss or damage of corneal endothelium or endothelial pump function.
    - Fluid from vascular leakage secondary to newly formed blood vessels may enter the cornea.
  - Florida spots:
    - Slowly to nonprogressive corneal disease that does not cause other overt clinical signs.
    - Typically characterized by bilateral multifocal, grey-white opacities within the cornea.
    - Recognized in dogs and cats in the southeastern United States.
    - Etiology is unknown, possibly mycobacterial organism.
- Red discolorations:
  - Corneal vascularization:
    - Vascularization occurs as a response to injury of the corneal epithelium or stroma as a normal component of healing.
    - Vascularization may occur as part of an immune-mediated inflammatory response.
    - Vascularization may occur secondary to disease of adjacent ocular

tissues including uveitis, episcleritis, and glaucoma.
- Hemorrhage into the cornea may occur due to trauma to blood vessels invading the cornea or as an extension of conjunctival hemorrhage.

DIAGNOSIS

DIFFERENTIAL DIAGNOSIS

- Brown discolorations:
  - Corneal Pigmentation, p 242:
    - Chronic irritation/inflammation:
      - Pigmentary keratitis (in brachycephalic dogs primarily).
        - Large palpebral fissure.
        - Lagophthalmos (incomplete closure of the eyelids).
        - Ectopic cilia.
        - Trichiasis: entropion, nasal folds, aberrant dermis at medial canthus.
      - Exposure keratitis.
        - Buphthalmos (chronic glaucoma).
        - Neuroparalytic keratitis (cranial nerve VII lesion).
      - Keratoconjunctivitis sicca (KCS).
      - Chronic superficial keratitis (CSK/pannus) (dogs).
    - Protrusion of iris tissue through corneal defect.
    - Persistent pupillary membrane (iris to cornea).
    - Anterior synechia.
    - Rupture of pigmented uveal cyst.
    - Neoplasia.
      - Limbal melanocytoma.
      - Invasive anterior uveal melanoma (see Intraocular Neoplasia, p 603).
  - Corneal sequestrum, cats.
  - Brown foreign material.
- White discolorations:
  - Corneal fibrosis/scarring (hazy grey-white) (see Corneal/Scleral Trauma, p 244).
  - Corneal lipid infiltrate or deposition (bright white, crystalline; see Corneal Lipid Infiltrates, p 241):
    - Corneal dystrophy.
    - Corneal degeneration (Fig. I-40)
    - Lipid keratopathy: systemic lipid abnormalities.
      - Diabetes mellitus
      - Pancreatitis
      - Hypothyroidism
      - Hyperadrenocorticisim
      - Thyroid carcinoma
      - Hepatic disease
      - Primary hyperlipoproteinemia
      - Postprandial hyperlipoproteinemia
  - Corneal calcium deposition (dense, chalky-white).
    - Corneal degeneration.
    - Systemic disease.
      - Hypercalcemia
      - Hyperphosphatemia
      - Hyperadrenocorticism
      - Renal disease
      - Hyperparathyroidism
      - Hypervitaminosis D
- White/yellow or white/pink discolorations:
  - Inflammatory cell infiltration:
    - Infected corneal ulcer.
    - Corneal abscess.
      - Infectious
      - Sterile
  - Feline proliferative keratoconjunctivitis (plaques and infiltrates).
  - Corneal epithelial inclusion cyst.
- Grey-blue discolorations:
  - Corneal edema:
    - Corneal endothelial loss or damage.
      - Endothelial dystrophy
      - Uveitis
      - Glaucoma
      - Trauma
        - Anterior lens luxation with endothelial contact.
        - Intraocular surgery.
    - Corneal epithelial loss.
      - Corneal ulceration
    - Associated with corneal vascularization.
  - Florida spots (see Etiology and Pathophysiology above).
- Red/pink discolorations:
  - Corneal vascularization
    - Corneal injury or inflammation:
      - Corneal ulceration
      - Chemical irritation
      - Mechanical irritation:
        - Trichiasis
        - Ectopic cilia
        - Entropion
      - Exposure:
        - Large palpebral fissure
        - Lagophthalmos (incomplete closure of the eyelids)
        - Ectropion
        - Buphthalmos (chronic glaucoma)
        - Exophthalmos
        - Neuroparalytic keratitis (cranial nerve VII lesion)
      - Neurotrophic keratitis (cranial nerve V lesion)
      - Keratoconjunctivitis sicca
      - Qualitative tear film abnormalities
      - Chronic superficial keratitis/"pannus" (dogs)
      - Feline proliferative keratoconjunctivitis (cats)
      - Corneal degeneration (see Fig. I-40)
    - Adjacent ocular disease:
      - Uveitis
      - Episcleritis
      - Scleritis
      - Orbital disease
      - Glaucoma

INITIAL DATABASE

Complete ophthalmic examination is essential, including the following:

- Schirmer tear test: values <10 mm/min are consistent with KCS; values of 10 to 15 mm/min suggestive of KCS and should be interpreted in light of other clinical signs
- Tear film break-up time: values <10 seconds are suggestive of a qualitative tear film abnormality
- Fluorescein staining: positive in corneal ulceration
- Tonometry: elevated intraocular pressure (>30 mmHg) in glaucoma, and reduced (<10 mmHg) in cases of uveitis

ADVANCED OR CONFIRMATORY TESTING

- Complete blood cell count, serum biochemistry, urinalysis, serum lipid profile (total serum lipids, cholesterol, triglycerides, lipoprotein electrophoresis, ± cholesterol esters and phospholipids), thyroid, ± adrenal gland testing are recommended if lipid or calcium

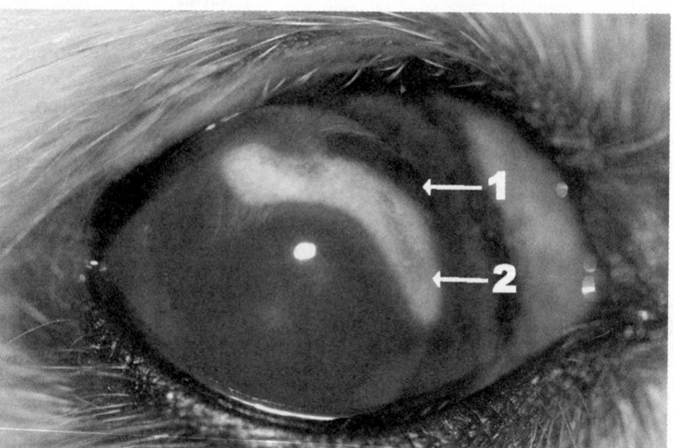

FIGURE I-40 Corneal degeneration in a dog. There is a horizontally ovoid area of corneal pigmentation *(1)* and a white arc of corneal lipid deposit *(2)*.

infiltration is suspected in association with systemic disease.
- Cytologic evaluation of conjunctival scraping or conjunctival biopsy is useful in diseases associated with conjunctival inflammation or proliferation.
- Cytologic evaluation of corneal scrapings is useful in proliferative disease of the cornea, or inflammatory cell infiltration of a corneal ulcer.

TREATMENT

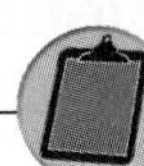

THERAPEUTIC GOAL(S)

- Halting progression of the lesion
- Treat underlying cause
- Reduce ocular discomfort

ACUTE GENERAL TREATMENT

Treatment will vary depending on the underlying cause.

PROGNOSIS AND OUTCOME

Prognosis and outcome will vary depending on the underlying cause.

PEARLS & CONSIDERATIONS

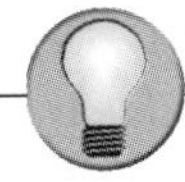

COMMENTS

In determining the underlying cause, documenting the location, color, shape, and pattern of corneal discoloration, as well determining the presence of other concurrent ocular disease, are extremely helpful.

SUGGESTED READING

Bellhorn R, et al: Superficial pigmentary keratitis in the dog. *J Am Vet Med Assoc* 149:173, 1966.

Chavkin MJ, et al: Risk factors for development of chronic superficial keratitis in dogs. *J Am Vet Med Assoc* 204:1630–1634, 1994.

Crispin SM, et al: Dystrophy, degeneration and infiltration of the canine cornea. *J Small Anim Pract* 24:63–83, 1983.

Featherstone HJ, et al: Feline corneal sequestra: A review of 64 cases (80 eyes) from 1993 to 2000. *Vet Ophthalmol* 7:213, 2004.

Morgan RV, et al: Feline eosinophilic keratitis: A retrospective study of 54 cases: (1989–1994). *Vet Comp Ophthalmol* 6:131, 1996.

Morreale RJ: Corneal diagnostic procedures. *Clin Tech Small Anim Pract* 18:145–151, 2003.

AUTHOR: **LYNNE SANDMEYER**

EDITOR: **CHERYL L. CULLEN**

Corneal Lipid Infiltrates

BASIC INFORMATION

DEFINITION

- *Corneal dystrophy* is a hereditary, noninflammatory, often bilateral infiltration of lipid not associated with systemic disease.
- *Corneal degeneration* is stromal lipid and/or mineral deposition secondary to previous or concurrent corneal disease.
- *Lipid keratopathy* is a typically bilateral, predominantly peripheral corneal stromal lipid infiltrate, secondary to dyslipoproteinemias of systemic disease origin.

SYNONYM(S)

Arcus lipoides corneae; corneal arcus; corneal limbal lipid infiltrates

Calcareous (calcium) degeneration; lipid (fatty) degeneration

Corneal epithelial dystrophy; corneal stromal dystrophy

EPIDEMIOLOGY

SPECIES, AGE, SEX

- Dogs; rare in cats
- Corneal dystrophy: usually develops between 2 and 4 years of age

GENETICS AND BREED PREDISPOSITION: Corneal dystrophy: any breed of dog, rare in cats; most commonly diagnosed breeds include the beagle, Cavalier King Charles spaniel, Siberian husky, Alaskan malamute, Samoyed, American cocker spaniel, and Labrador retriever.

ASSOCIATED CONDITIONS AND DISORDERS

- Corneal degeneration: ulcerative and nonulcerative keratitides including:
  - Chronic superficial keratitis (see Pannus [Chronic Superficial Keratitis], p 802)
  - Limbal melanocytoma
  - Nodular granulomatous episclerokeratitis (see Episcleritis/Scleritis, p 353)
  - Keratoconjunctivitis Sicca, p 614
  - Ocular trauma (see Corneal/Scleral Trauma, p 244)
- Lipid keratopathy: hyperlipoproteinemias/systemic diseases including:
  - Hypothyroidism, p 575
  - Hyperadrenocorticism, p 537
  - Diabetes Mellitus, p 289
  - Pancreatitis Dog, p 796; Pancreatitis, Cat, p 794
  - Primary hyperlipidemia (see Hyperlipidemia, p 547)

CLINICAL PRESENTATION

DISEASE FORMS/SUBTYPES

- Corneal dystrophy: well demarcated, oval to round grey-white or silver opacities in the central or paracentral cornea, often ringlike with a clear central zone
- Corneal degeneration: highly variable appearance, dense white to greyish stromal scars, irregular shape and distribution, often with ulceration and stromal vascularization
- Lipid keratopathy: dense, often arc-shaped, white-to-yellow crystalline opacities in the peripheral cornea, often separated from the limbus by a clear zone; additional opacity centrally if the cornea is vascularized

HISTORY, CHIEF COMPLAINT

- Corneal opacity
- Visual behavior change (uncommon in corneal dystrophy)
- Blepharospasm, serous ocular discharge/tearing (with ulceration in corneal degeneration)

PHYSICAL EXAM FINDINGS

- See Disease Forms/Subtypes above
- Corneal abnormalities (corneal dystrophy, corneal degeneration)
- Variable, dependent on systemic disorder involved (lipid keratopathy)

ETIOLOGY AND PATHOPHYSIOLOGY

- Heritable genetic mutation (corneal dystrophy)
- Secondary pathologic changes including altered lipid metabolism and dystrophic calcification (corneal degeneration)
- Deposition of lipid-laden serum across the limbus from systemic hyperlipidemia (lipid keratopathy)

DIAGNOSIS

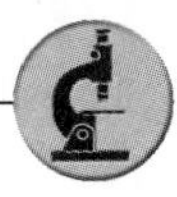

DIFFERENTIAL DIAGNOSIS

Other types of grey to white corneal opacities (see Corneal Discoloration, p 239) including:

- Scar: dull grey to white; does not retain fluorescein stain
- Edema: bluish to grey; indistinct borders
- Ulcer: retains fluorescein stain (see Corneal Ulceration, p 246)
- Inflammatory cell infiltrate: grey to yellow; indistinct borders and varying degrees of uveitis (see Uveitis, p 1134)

INITIAL DATABASE

- Complete ophthalmic examination including:
  - Assessing corneal appearance (see Disease Forms/Subtypes above).
  - Schirmer tear test (may be low in cases of corneal degeneration, which can occur as a result of Keratoconjunctivitis sicca [see p 614]). Normal >15 mm in 1 minute in dogs, variable in cats.
  - Fluorescein dye application (positive staining of cornea most common with corneal degeneration).
- Complete blood count, serum biochemistry panel (including fasting cholesterol, triglycerides, blood glucose, calcium, phosphorus) to screen for underlying disorders, and urinalysis (typically unremarkable except for systemic disorders).

ADVANCED OR CONFIRMATORY TESTING

- Referral to a veterinary ophthalmologist to confirm/document crystalline nature and depth/distribution (often breed-specific) of presumed lipid infiltrate via slit-lamp biomicroscopic examination (corneal dystrophy)
- Evaluation of thyroid and adrenal function (see Hypothyroidism, p 575 and Hyperadrenocorticism, p 537); serum lipid electrophoresis (lipid keratopathy)

TREATMENT

THERAPEUTIC GOAL(S)

- Minimize further deposition of lipid infiltrate if possible
- Surgically remove infiltrate if significant visual impairment and/or chronic corneal ulceration (referral to veterinary ophthalmologist)
- Manage any underlying systemic disease

ACUTE GENERAL TREATMENT

- Corneal dystrophy:
  - Treatment typically not required.
  - Poor response to medical management.
  - If advanced epithelial or stromal disease with vision impairment and/or corneal ulceration, may require surgical removal (lamellar keratectomy); may or may not recur.
- Corneal degeneration:
  - Therapy aimed at underlying corneal disease.
  - If progressive and interfering with functional vision or creates ocular discomfort (chronic ulceration), lamellar keratectomy.
  - Topical application of disodium ethylenediaminetetraacetic acid in an ophthalmic preparation (0.4–1.38% q 6–8h) if calcium component suspected.
  - Anecdotal evidence of improvement subsequent to dietary restriction of lipid/cholesterol, or following use of dietary additives to reduce cholesterol (flaxseed oil, oat bran, niacin).
- Lipid keratopathy:
  - Therapy aimed at underlying systemic disease (dogs); treat anterior segment inflammation/uveitis (often seen concurrently in cats; see Uveitis, p 1134).

CHRONIC TREATMENT

Management/resolution of systemic disorder if present

RECOMMENDED MONITORING

Dictated by concurrent corneal disease management (corneal degeneration) or systemic disease management (lipid keratopathy)

PROGNOSIS AND OUTCOME

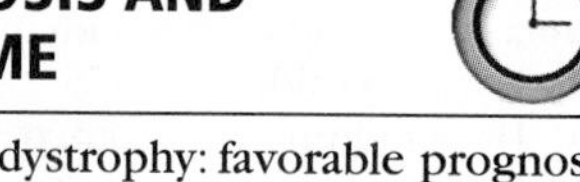

- Corneal dystrophy: favorable prognosis because the opacities are focal, and the lesion is typically nonprogressive; may resolve spontaneously.
- Corneal degeneration: prognosis dependent on underlying corneal disease; may progress with chronic inflammatory or neoplastic disease; typically static after trauma.
- Lipid keratopathy: may improve post-resolution or control of underlying systemic abnormality.

PEARLS & CONSIDERATIONS

COMMENTS

- The most common cause of corneal lipid infiltrate is corneal dystrophy; it is often discovered as an incidental finding and rarely causes appreciable vision impairment.
- At this time, there are serious questions about the safety and efficacy of systemically administered "lipid-lowering" medications for small-animal ocular disease.

CLIENT EDUCATION

Corneal dystrophy: suspected cases should be evaluated by a veterinary ophthalmologist, because the disease has genetic implications.

SUGGESTED READING

Crispin SM: Ocular manifestations of hyperlipoproteinemia. *J Small Anim Pract* 34:500, 1993.

Crispin SM, et al: Dystrophy, degeneration, and infiltration of the canine cornea. *J Small Anim Pract* 24:63, 1983.

Cooley PL, et al: Corneal dystrophy in the dog and cat. *Vet Clin North Am* 20:681, 1990.

AUTHOR: **RICHARD F. QUINN**

EDITOR: **CHERYL L. CULLEN**

Corneal Pigmentation

BASIC INFORMATION

DEFINITION

Brown to black discoloration of the cornea, usually due to the presence of melanin

EPIDEMIOLOGY

SPECIES, AGE, SEX

- Dogs: pigmentary keratitis: brachycephalic breeds; no age or sex predilection; chronic superficial keratitis (CSK; see Pannus [Chronic Superficial Keratitis], p 802)
- Cats: corneal sequestrum (see Corneal Sequestration: Cats, p 245)

CLINICAL PRESENTATION

HISTORY, CHIEF COMPLAINT

- Brown discoloration of cornea
- Concurrently:
  - Redness of the conjunctiva
  - Ocular discharge
  - Ocular pain
  - Reduced vision

PHYSICAL EXAM FINDINGS

- Brown or black discoloration of the corneal epithelium, stroma, or endothelium.
- Extensive pigmentation may cause reduced or absent menace response.
- Other findings will vary depending on underlying cause.

ETIOLOGY AND PATHOPHYSIOLOGY

- Epithelial and stromal pigmentation:
  - Melanin is produced by melanocytes in the epithelium and superficial

stroma in response to chronic corneal irritation from desiccation or mechanical trauma.
  - Proliferation and migration of limbal melanocytes into the stroma may also occur secondary to chronic inflammation in response to corneal ulceration, degeneration, or an immune response to corneal antigen.
- Endothelial pigmentation:
  - Adherence of melanin or melanin-containing cells, usually arising from the anterior uvea, to the endothelium.
- Stromal infiltration at the limbus as extension of a melanin-containing neoplasm.
- Protrusion of pigmented tissue through a corneal defect (see Corneal/Scleral Trauma, p 244).
- Corneal sequestrum (cats; see Corneal Sequestration: Cats, p 245):
  - Associated with chronic irritation.
  - The central/paracentral corneal stroma becomes necrotic, stained, and the overlying epithelium is usually disrupted.
  - Cause of stromal discoloration is unresolved.

DIAGNOSIS

DIFFERENTIAL DIAGNOSIS

- Epithelial and stromal pigmentation:
  - Pigmentary keratitis (Fig. I-41):
    - Large palpebral fissure
    - Lagophthalmos (incomplete closure of the eyelids)
    - Distichiasis/ectopic cilia
    - Trichiasis: entropion, nasal folds, aberrant dermis at medial canthus
  - Exposure keratitis:
    - Buphthalmos (chronic glaucoma)
    - Neuroparalytic keratitis (cranial nerve VII lesion)
  - Keratoconjunctivitis sicca
  - Chronic superficial keratitis (dogs)
  - Limbal melanocytoma (note: melanomas of the limbus in dogs and cats are almost always benign and therefore are appropriately called *melanocytomas* benign tumor of melanocyte origin)
  - Invasive anterior uveal melanoma/melanocytoma
  - Protrusion of iris tissue through corneal defect (i.e., iris prolapse)
  - Corneal sequestrum (cats)
- Endothelial pigmentation:
  - Persistant pupillary membrane (iris-to-cornea)
  - Anterior synechia
  - Uveal melanoma/melanocytoma
  - Rupture of pigmented uveal cyst

INITIAL DATABASE

- Neuro-ophthalmic examination: evaluate palpebral reflexes and completeness of eyelid closure
- Schirmer tear test (STT): values <10 mm/min and clinical signs consistent with keratoconjunctivitis = KCS
- Fluorescein staining: positive if corneal ulceration is present. Fluorescein uptake usually occurs only around the edge of a corneal sequestrum
- Ophthalmic examination: evaluate for abnormalities of eyelids and aberrant cilia

TREATMENT

THERAPEUTIC GOAL(S)

- Treat underlying cause
- Halt progression
- Reduce pigmentation
- Reduce discomfort

ACUTE GENERAL TREATMENT

Treatment will vary depending on underlying cause

RECOMMENDED MONITORING

- Recheck at regular intervals (every 4 to 6 months or more frequently depending on the cause)
- Photographs help monitor progression of lesions

PROGNOSIS AND OUTCOME

Prognosis and outcome will vary depending on the underlying cause

PEARLS & CONSIDERATIONS

COMMENTS

Ocular examination is an essential part of the routine physical examination, because corneal pigmentation may go unnoticed by owners until it is severe enough to affect vision.

SUGGESTED READING

Bellhorn R, et al: Superficial pigmentary keratitis in the dog. *J Am Vet Med Assoc* 149:173, 1966.

Carter R, et al: The causes, diagnosis, and treatment of canine keratoconjunctivitis sicca. *Vet Med* 97:683–694, 2002.

Chavkin MJ, et al: Risk factors for development of chronic superficial keratitis in dogs. *J Am Vet Med Assoc* 204:1630–1634, 1994.

Clerc B: Chronic superficial keratitis in German shepherd dogs and other breeds. *Canine Pract* 21(6):6–12, 1996.

Featherstone HJ, et al: Feline corneal sequestra: A review of 64 cases (80 eyes) from 1993 to 2000. *Vet Ophthalmol* 7:213, 2004.

AUTHOR: **LYNNE SANDMEYER**

EDITOR: **CHERYL L. CULLEN**

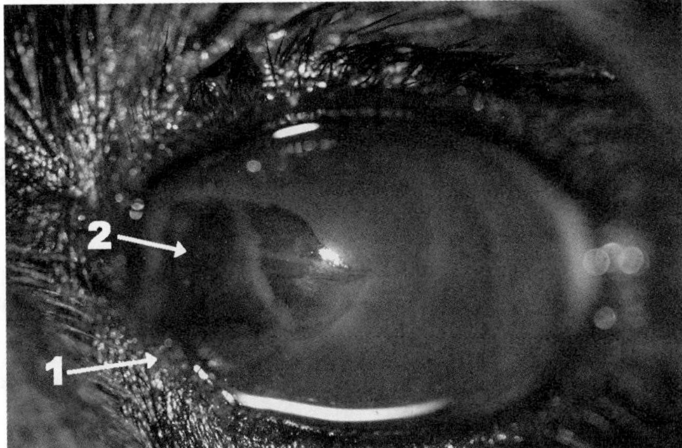

FIGURE I-41 Pigmentary keratitis of the left eye in a brachycephalic dog. There is medial entropion *(1)* and a triangular area of corneal pigmentation *(2)* overlying the medial cornea secondary, in part, to the entropion. Courtesy of Dr. Bruce Grahn.

Corneal/Scleral Trauma

BASIC INFORMATION

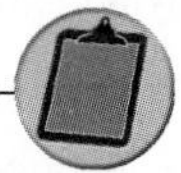

DEFINITION

Occurs secondary to blunt or sharp trauma. Penetrating infers partial-thickness injury; perforating infers full-thickness injury. Simple wounds involve only cornea or sclera; complicated wounds involve multiple ocular structures.

SYNONYM(S)

Corneoscleral laceration

EPIDEMIOLOGY

SPECIES, AGE, SEX: Any species, age, or sex.

RISK FACTORS

- Young active animals
- Hunting animals
- Interanimal fighting
- Dog's head out the window while car is in motion

ASSOCIATED CONDITIONS AND DISORDERS: Existing visual impairment may predispose.

CLINICAL PRESENTATION

HISTORY, CHIEF COMPLAINT

- Running through dense or dry vegetation just before onset of clinical signs
- Owner may or may not observe trauma or causal event
- Acute onset of any or all of the following:
  - Blepharospasm
  - Ocular discharge
  - Blood or fluid coming from eye
  - Cloudy eye

PHYSICAL EXAM FINDINGS

- Signs of pain on ophthalmic examination manifested by blepharospasm and resistance to ophthalmic examination.
- Linear, V-shaped, or stellate corneal lesion of acute onset accompanied by any or all of the following:
  - Hyphema (see Hyphema, p 560) and/or subconjunctival hemorrhage
  - Corneal edema with or without cellular infiltrate
  - Uveal prolapse: appears as pigmented structure in damaged cornea or sclera; associated with:
    - Dyscoric/misshapen pupil
    - Hyphema (see Hyphema, p 560)
  - Foreign body embedded in cornea or perforating cornea
  - Signs of uveitis, particularly with perforating trauma (see Uveitis, p 1134)
  - Fibrin in cornea may fill perforation; light brown in color, may be associated with blood
  - Yellowish lens material in anterior chamber and cataract (see Cataracts, p 182) if lens involved
  - Shallow anterior chamber if wound actively leaking
- A thorough examination of the entire conjunctival sac is necessary to identify any retained foreign material; sedation, general anesthesia, or referral may be required in difficult cases or if this procedure is unfamiliar to the practitioner.
- Subconjunctival hemorrhage and hyphema should alert clinician to possibility of posterior scleral rupture if no anterior segment lesions are present, particularly if accompanied by very low intraocular pressure (i.e., < 10 mmHg).

ETIOLOGY AND PATHOPHYSIOLOGY

- Variable; usually traumatic (sharp or blunt) in origin
- Foreign body may be retained in laceration

DIAGNOSIS

DIFFERENTIAL DIAGNOSIS

If traumatic event not evident, consider other causes:

- Corneal ulceration
- Uveitis
- Hyphema

INITIAL DATABASE

- Assess vision: menace response, dazzle reflex, direct and consensual pupillary light reflexes (if deficient, see Blindness, p 136)
- Cytologic study and aerobic culture and sensitivity of wound
- Complete blood count, serum chemistry, urinalysis for preanesthetic purposes if surgery necessary

ADVANCED OR CONFIRMATORY TESTING

- Consider ocular ultrasound to determine extent of intraocular involvement, presence of intraocular foreign body, or posterior globe rupture.
- Orbital radiographs or computed tomography to determine presence or path of foreign body.
- Seidel test to determine if cornea or scleral wound is sealed: apply dry fluorescein strip carefully to surface of wound to cover surface with stain; leaking aqueous will appear as a green rivulet.

TREATMENT

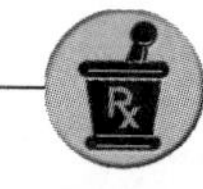

THERAPEUTIC GOAL(S)

- Remove foreign bodies if present
- Repair lacerations that penetrate greater than 50% of the stroma or perforate the cornea or sclera
- Eliminate infection
- Control intraocular inflammation

ACUTE GENERAL TREATMENT

- Do not put pressure on the globe until the possibility of rupture is eliminated.
- Elizabethan collar placement to prevent self-trauma.
- Small, nonperforating or very small sealed perforating wounds without uveal prolapse: consider conservative therapy:
  - Topical antibiotic solution (e.g., neomycin/polymyxin/gramicidin, gentamicin, ciprofloxacin) q 6h.
  - Add broad-spectrum systemic antibiotics if perforating (e.g., amoxicillin-clavulanate 13.75 mg/kg PO q 12h; base long-term choice on culture and sensitivity).
  - Systemic anti-inflammatory therapy with either nonsteroidal anti-inflammatories (e.g., meloxicam 0.1 mg/kg PO q 24h or carprofen 2 mg/kg PO q 12h) or anti-inflammatory doses of prednisone (e.g., 0.5-1 mg/kg PO q 24h).
  - Topical atropine 1% solution q 6-24h if significant uveitis present (see Uveitis, p 1134).
- Perforating or deep, large, or gaping penetrating wounds, and wounds with uveal prolapse require primary surgical repair (referrable procedure) involving:
  - Replacement of viable uveal tissue or resection of nonviable uveal tissue.
  - Irrigation and reinflation of anterior chamber.
  - Repair of cornea with appropriate-size suture material (8-0 to 10-0).
  - Careful inspection of lens; if lens rupture noted, lens should be removed by phacoemulsification.

CHRONIC TREATMENT

- Monitor and treat for uveitis and wound dehiscence
- Consider changing antibiotics if indicated by culture and sensitivity results

DRUG INTERACTIONS

Do not use topical ophthalmic ointments if globe rupture is suspected.

POSSIBLE COMPLICATIONS

- Retinal Detachment, p 965
- Cataracts, p 182
- Chronic Uveitis, p 1134

- Glaucoma, p 440
- Endophthalmitis (inflammation of the uveal tract and anterior and posterior compartments of the eye)
- Loss of vision and eye
- Cats may develop post-traumatic ocular sarcomas years after original injury (see Intraocular Neoplasia, p 603)

RECOMMENDED MONITORING

- Reevaluate in 24 to 48 hours to ensure that wounds are sealed, inflammation is improving, and that there are no signs of infection.
- Frequency of examination then depends on response to therapy.

PROGNOSIS AND OUTCOME

- Intuitively, small, shallow penetrating wounds of the cornea or lacerations involving only the cornea have a good prognosis, whereas complicated, perforating wounds with uveal and/or lens involvement have a poorer prognosis.
- Posterior wounds involving sclera or sclera and uvea have a grave prognosis.
- Blunt trauma usually has a grave prognosis, particularly if extensive hyphema is present.
- Negative menace response, and negative dazzle and pupillary light reflexes at initial examination of a patient with corneal or scleral trauma indicate grave prognosis for vision.

PEARLS & CONSIDERATIONS

COMMENTS

- Consider sedation to keep animal calm and to prevent self-trauma.
- Use an Elizabethan collar to prevent self-trauma.

PREVENTION

Animals should be monitored when introduced to new environment with other animals

CLIENT EDUCATION

Discuss the possibility of long-term complications that could lead to loss of vision and loss of an eye.

SUGGESTED READING

Slatter D: Ocular emergencies. In Slatter D (ed): *Fundamentals of Veterinary Ophthalmology*. Philadelphia, WB Saunders, 2001, pp 562–570.

AUTHOR: **ELLISON BENTLEY**
EDITOR: **CHERYL L. CULLEN**

Corneal Sequestration: Cats

BASIC INFORMATION

DEFINITION

Corneal sequestration is a disease unique to cats characterized by an area of necrotic cornea that is variably pigmented.

SYNONYM(S)

Corneal mummification
Corneal necrosis
Corneal sequestrum
Corneal nigrum
Necrotizing keratitis

EPIDEMIOLOGY

SPECIES, AGE, SEX

- Cats
- Any age; average age of 5 years in retrospective studies
- No sex predilection

GENETICS AND BREED PREDISPOSITION: All breeds, but Persian, Himalayan, Burmese appear predisposed.

RISK FACTORS

- Feline herpesvirus type-1 (FHV-1), particularly in domestic shorthairs and longhairs.
- Any corneal insult, particularly chronic.
- Brachycephalic cats are predisposed.
- Grid keratotomy performed for nonhealing/indolent corneal ulcers (see Corneal Ulceration, p 246) in cats may predispose to sequestrum formation.

CLINICAL PRESENTATION

HISTORY, CHIEF COMPLAINT

- "Black spot on eye"
- Blepharospasm
- Ocular discharge
- "Red" eye

PHYSICAL EXAM FINDINGS

- Circular to oval, pigmented lesion in central to paracentral cornea is pathognomonic (Fig. I-42).
- Pigmentation varies from subtle, tan discoloration of cornea to a dense black, opaque lesion (see Fig. I-42).
- Lesion may form a slightly raised, irregular corneal plaque.
- Corneal neovascularization with chronicity.
- Variable corneal edema and inflammation surrounding sequestrum.
- A rim of loose, edematous corneal epithelium may develop around the sequestrum.
- Depth of corneal involvement (i.e., extent of lesion) difficult to ascertain because sequestrum often opaque.

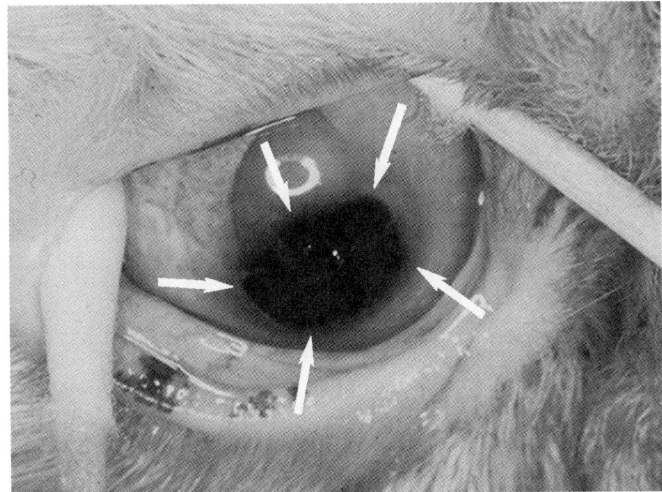

FIGURE I-42 Corneal sequestrum in a cat (*arrows*). Note its dark appearance and paracentral location.

ETIOLOGY AND PATHOPHYSIOLOGY

- The fundamental problems generated by corneal sequestration are (1) pain, (2) obstruction of vision, and (3) cosmetic appearance.
- Chronic corneal irritation, such as that found in brachycephalic cats with entropion (see Entropion/Ectropion, p 345) and/or lagophthalmos (incomplete closure of the eyelids), is a common feature.
- FHV-1 is linked to sequestrum formation, particularly in nonbrachycephalic cats (see Herpesviral Keratitis in Cats, p 513).
- Tear film deficiencies (e.g., Keratoconjunctivitis Sicca, p 614; qualitative tear film abnormality [e.g., mucin deficiency]) have been reported in cats with sequestra.
- Source of pigment unknown; cats with sequestra noted to have pigmented tears and contact lenses placed in cats with sequestra (see Acute General Treatment below) often become discolored.

DIAGNOSIS

The diagnosis is generally based on the signalment (species) and the physical appearance of the lesion.

DIFFERENTIAL DIAGNOSIS

Corneal rupture with iris prolapse (should have dyscoric/misshapen pupil and uveitis if this has occurred; see Corneal/Scleral Trauma, p 244)

INITIAL DATABASE

Complete ophthalmic examination to assess for underlying causes of corneal irritation:

- Schirmer tear test (if < 5 mm/min, see Keratoconjunctivitis Sicca, p 614)
- Fluorescein dye application (sequestrum itself often does not retain fluorescein dye; there may be positive fluorescein dye retention around sequestrum)

ADVANCED OR CONFIRMATORY TESTING

- Consider testing for FHV-1 (see Herpesviral Keratitis in Cats, p 513)
- Tear film break-up time (see Corneal Ulceration, p 246)

TREATMENT

THERAPEUTIC GOAL(S)

- Completely remove the sequestrum and prevent recurrence.
- Eliminate ocular pain.
- Minimize corneal scarring.

ACUTE GENERAL TREATMENT

- Prophylactic topical antibiotic therapy (can be ointment or solution formulation) such as ciprofloxacin or neomycin/polymyxin/gramicidin q 6-8h, particularly if fluorescein positive.
- If sequestrum appears small and superficial, and the affected eye is comfortable, observation is a treatment option:
  - Sequestrum may spontaneously slough, resulting in minimal scarring; however, sequestra can take months to years to slough.
- If sequestrum is long-standing, large, or eye is painful, surgical removal is indicated through:
  - Keratectomy (sequestrum excision using a corneal dissector; generally a referrable procedure).
  - No postoperative pigmented corneal tissue should remain; a contact lens may be placed for protection for 2 weeks.
  - Very large sequestra may require conjunctival or frozen donor corneal grafting.

CHRONIC TREATMENT

Treat underlying contributing factors/causes such as entropion or lagophthalmos (see Entropion/Ectropion, p 345) and FHV-1 (see Herpesviral Keratitis in Cats, p 513).

POSSIBLE COMPLICATIONS

- Recurrence of the sequestrum in the surgical site.
- If the sequestrum is allowed to slough, descemetocele (see Corneal Ulceration, p 246) formation or corneal rupture is a possibility.

RECOMMENDED MONITORING

- If the lesion is not treated surgically, owners should monitor carefully for sequestrum sloughing and return to the veterinarian immediately after the sequestrum sloughs to avoid complications from deep corneal defects. At the time of sequestrum sloughing, initiation of prophylactic topical antibiotics (e.g., neomycin/polymyxin/gramicidin, or ciprofloxacin) q 6-8h is indicated, and referral for further evaluation (with or without surgical treatment) should again be considered.
- Surgical treatment: usually several rechecks at 1- to 2-week intervals until defect is epithelialized.

PROGNOSIS AND OUTCOME

Good, but recurrence is possible

PEARLS & CONSIDERATIONS

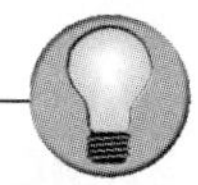

COMMENTS

Avoid topical corticosteroid use, because this may induce herpetic stromal keratitis if FHV-1 is an underlying cause.

CLIENT EDUCATION

Recurrence possible, as is involvement of contralateral eye

SUGGESTED READING

Featherstone HM, Sansom J: Feline corneal sequestra: A review of 64 cases (80 eyes) from 1993 to 2000. *Vet Ophthalmol* 7:213-227, 2004.

Morgan RV: Feline corneal sequestration: A retrospective study of 42 cases (1987-1991). *J Am Anim Hosp Assoc* 30:24-30, 1994.

AUTHOR: **ELLISON BENTLEY**

EDITOR: **CHERYL L. CULLEN**

Corneal Ulceration

Client Education Sheet on Website

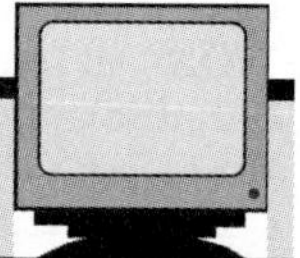

BASIC INFORMATION

DEFINITION

A loss of superficial corneal epithelium with or without loss of varying amounts of the underlying corneal stroma. Three main categories of corneal ulceration:

- *Simple* corneal ulcer: an acute loss of epithelial layers of the cornea due to trauma; usually noninfected.
- *Complex* corneal ulcer: an acute or chronic loss of epithelial and stromal layers of the cornea due to trauma and/or infection.
- *Indolent/refractory* corneal ulcer: a superficial ulcer resulting from failure of epithelial adhesion to the corneal basement membrane and stroma.

SYNONYM(S)

Corneal abrasion

Corneal erosion

Keratomalacia
Ulcerative keratitis

EPIDEMIOLOGY

SPECIES, AGE, SEX

- Simple/complex ulcers: dogs and cats of any age or sex
- Indolent ulcers: middle-aged to older dogs; cats may also be affected

GENETICS AND BREED PREDISPOSITION

- Simple/complex ulcers: brachycephalic breeds (dogs and cats) predisposed, but any breed may be affected
- Indolent ulcers: dogs: Boxers predisposed, but any breed may be affected; cats: breeds predisposed to corneal sequestration (see Corneal Sequestration: Cats, p 245) including Persians and Himalayans

RISK FACTORS

- Keratoconjunctivitis sicca (dry eye; see Keratoconjunctivitis Sicca, p 614)
- Brachycephalic conformation
- Eyelid conformational abnormalities (see Entropion/Ectropion, p 345; Distichiasis/Ectopic Cilia/Trichiasis, p 317)
- Feline herpesvirus-1 (FHV-1, feline viral rhinotracheitis) infection (see Herpesviral Keratitis in Cats, p 513)

CONTAGION AND ZOONOSIS: FHV-1 keratoconjunctivitis is contagious among cats.

CLINICAL PRESENTATION

DISEASE FORMS/SUBTYPES: Three main categories of corneal ulceration:

- Simple corneal ulcer
- Complex corneal ulcer:
  - Stromal ulcer (ulcer with loss of varying amounts of the corneal stroma)
  - Keratomalacia/melting ulcer (softening and necrosis of the cornea, often associated with infection)
  - Descemetocele (a loss of all stromal layers down to Descemet's membrane [basement membrane of the corneal endothelium] and the endothelium)
  - Ruptured ulcer (perforation of the cornea)
- Indolent/refractory corneal ulcer

HISTORY, CHIEF COMPLAINT

- Variable onset from acute to insidious or chronic
- Occasional history of trauma
- Ocular pain (squinting and/or rubbing at eye)
- Cloudiness to surface of eye
- "Red" eye
- Ocular discharge
- Occasionally upper respiratory signs in cats (see Herpesviral Keratitis in Cats, p 513)

PHYSICAL EXAM FINDINGS

- Simple and indolent corneal ulcers; any or all of the following may be present:
  - Blepharospasm (squinting)
  - Conjunctival injection
  - Third eyelid prolapse
  - Ocular discharge: often serous
  - Corneal edema
  - Obvious defect in corneal epithelium
  - Fluorescein dye retention
  - Miotic (small) pupil (reflex uveitis; see Uveitis, p 1134)
  - Aqueous flare (see Uveitis, p 1134)
- Complex corneal ulcer; any or all of the above *and* one or more of the following:
  - Mucopurulent ocular discharge
  - Corneal blood vessels (see Corneal Vascularization, p 249)
  - Corneal white-yellow cellular infiltrate
  - Corneal stromal defect (i.e., crater appearance to affected cornea)
  - Keratomalacia/melting (softening and necrosis of the cornea as evidenced by a gelatinous appearance to the affected tissues)
  - Hypopyon (see Hypopyon, p 571)
- Descemetocele; any or all of the above *and* the following:
  - Fluorescein-negative clear center of a stromal ulcer (Descemet's membrane is hydrophobic and does not retain fluid or fluorescein stain)
- Ruptured corneal ulcer; any or all of the above *and* one or more of the following:
  - Copious ocular discharge with fibrin and/or blood (see Hyphema, p 560) in the anterior chamber
  - Visible tan-brown iris prolapse (iris filling the corneal defect) and/or fibrin clot within ulcer
  - Shallow anterior chamber
  - Dyscoria (abnormal pupil shape)
  - Visible anterior synechia (iris adhesion) to the ulcerated area
- Indolent ulcer; any or all of the findings of a *simple ulcer and* the following:
  - Rim of loose epithelium
  - Minimal to moderate pain
  - Corneal vascularization, variable
  - Slow to vascularize
  - Noninfected

ETIOLOGY AND PATHOPHYSIOLOGY

- Trauma.
- Ocular foreign body.
- Tear film abnormalities:
  - Keratoconjunctivitis Sicca, p 614 (i.e., quantitative tear film deficiency)
  - Mucin and/or lipid deficiency (i.e., qualitative tear film deficiency)
- Eyelid conformational abnormalities:
  - Entropion
  - Trichiasis
  - Distichiasis
  - Ectopic cilia
  - Lagophthalmos (incomplete closure of the eyelids, usually in brachycephalics)
  - Neurologic disorders (e.g., facial nerve paralysis, neuroparalytic keratitis [cranial nerve VII lesion]; corneal denervation, neurotrophic keratitis [cranial nerve V lesion])
- FHV-1 infection.
- Corneal sequestration (cats).
- Simple corneal ulcers may progress to complex or ruptured corneal ulcers secondary to infection or sterile inflammation.
- Indolent ulcers result from a primary defect of corneal epithelial adhesion to the underlying corneal basement membrane and stroma:
  - Look for and address any other underlying cause(s) (as listed previously) to promote healing of these refractory corneal ulcers

DIAGNOSIS

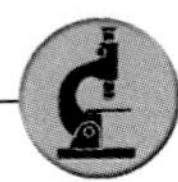

DIFFERENTIAL DIAGNOSIS

- Corneal dystrophy or degeneration
- Proliferative/eosinophilic keratoconjunctivitis (cats)
- Anterior uveitis
- Glaucoma
- Horner's syndrome

INITIAL DATABASE

- Neuro-ophthalmic (cranial nerve) examination: menace response, pupillary light reflexes, palpebral and corneal reflexes.
- Schirmer tear test. Normal >15 mm/min in dogs, variable in cats.
- Fluorescein dye application.
- Tear film break-up time (TFBUT):
  - Test that subjectively evaluates the rate at which the tear film evaporates.
  - Mean TFBUTs = 19.7 seconds (dog) and 16.7 seconds (cat).
  - If too rapid (i.e., <5–10 seconds), suspect qualitative tear film deficiency such as mucin and/or lipid.
- Corneal cytologic study to assess for microbial agents (i.e., bacteria, fungi) to help direct initial treatments.
- Corneal culture and sensitivity.
- Intraocular pressure to rule out glaucoma.

ADVANCED OR CONFIRMATORY TESTING

- Keratectomy sample for corneal histopathologic evaluation
- Corneal swab and/or keratectomy sample for polymerase chain reaction (FHV-1, bacterial, fungal)

TREATMENT

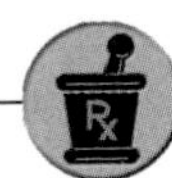

THERAPEUTIC GOAL(S)

- Prevent progressive loss of corneal stroma and corneal rupture.
- Eliminate ocular pain.
- Prevent or eliminate corneal infection.

- Promote corneal epithelialization.
- Minimize corneal scarring.

ACUTE GENERAL TREATMENT

- Simple corneal ulcer:
  - Broad-spectrum topical antibiotic solution or ointment (e.g., triple antibiotic or oxytetracycline) q 4-6h.
    - Gentamicin is a *poor* first choice due to its narrow spectrum for only gram-negative bacteria (ocular flora is primarily gram-positive bacteria).
  - Topical atropine 1% ophthalmic solution or ointment q 12-48h.
  - ± Systemic nonsteroidal anti-inflammatory drug.
- Complex corneal ulcer: Any or all of the above *and* the following:
  - Autogenous serum (prepared by obtaining a sample of the patient's own blood, anticoagulating and centrifuging, and using the supernatant [serum] topically for its antiprotease, anticollagenase properties [to slow or halt corneal melting]) and/or oxytetracycline (5 mg/g) ointment topically q 4-6h, or more frequently if keratomalacia/melting ulcer.
  - Topical fluoroquinolone antibiotic (e.g., ciprofloxacin or ofloxacin) for improved corneal penetration and spectrum of activity at increased frequency if keratomalacia/melting ulcer (q 2-4h).
  - Topical antifungal agent q 4-6h (e.g., natamycin; those derived from systemically administered agents such as itraconazole or miconazole) if fungal keratitis suspected based on corneal cytology and/or culture.
  - Hospitalization of animals with deep or rapidly progressive ulcers for frequent medical treatments and monitoring.
  - Structural surgical repair (i.e., keratectomy to remove the diseased cornea with placement of a graft: conjunctival, corneal); referable procedure is advisable if:
    - Stromal loss continues despite aggressive appropriate medical management.
    - If ulcer exceeds 50% stromal depth or is ruptured.
  - Indolent ulcer:
    - Application of topical ophthalmic anesthetic (e.g., proparacaine 0.5% solution) with or without sedation or general anesthesia (depending on the animal).
    - Debridement of all loose corneal epithelium with dry, sterile, cotton-tipped applicators (Figs. I-43, I-44).
    - Perform multiple grid keratotomy (may predispose to sequestrum formation in cats [see Corneal Sequestration: Cats, p 245]) with the bevelled edge of a 25-gauge needle held at a 45-degree angle to the cornea (Fig. I-44, *C*):
      - Gentle vertical and horizontal scratches every 0.5 mm over ulcerated area just through basement membrane into superficial stroma (grid lines should be barely visible).
  - Broad-spectrum topical antibiotic (as for simple corneal ulcer above) q 6-8h.

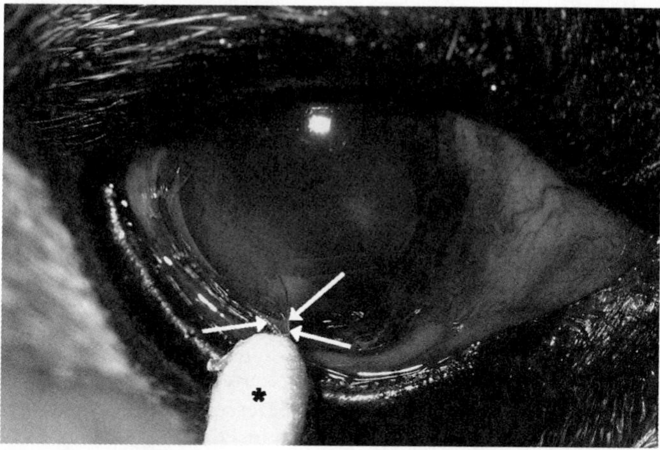

FIGURE I-43 Debridement of an indolent corneal ulcer of the right eye in a dog. Note the lip of nonadherent corneal epithelium (*arrows*) attached to the sterile cotton-tipped applicator (*asterisk*).

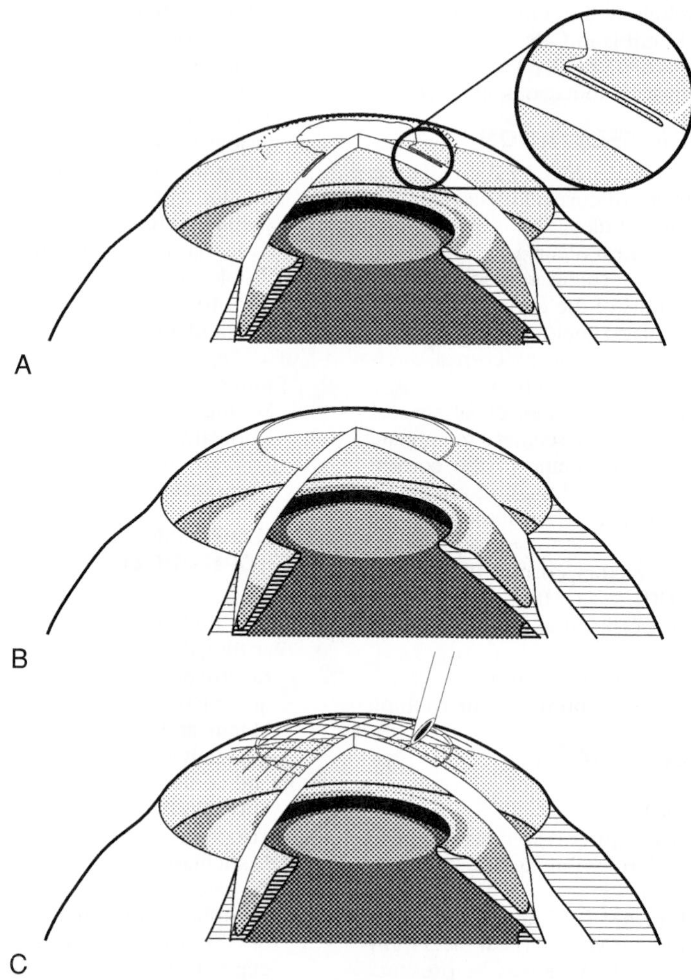

FIGURE I-44 Grid keratotomy. **A,** Indolent ulcer with corneal epithelial flaps (e.g., at time of presentation). **B,** After topical anesthesia and debridement (as in Fig. I-43); **C,** Performing the grid keratotomy.

- Atropine 1% ophthalmic solution or ointment q 24–72h.
- ± Tear supplement.
- ± Application of a bandage soft contact lens to improve comfort and minimize mechanical forces of eyelids on migrating corneal epithelium.

CHRONIC TREATMENT

- Antimicrobial therapy as directed by culture and susceptibility results.
- Topical antibiotic with expanded spectrum and/or improved corneal penetration (e.g., fluoroquinolones).
- FHV-1 ulcer:
  - Topical antiviral solution or ointment (idoxuridine, trifluridine, vidarabine) q 4–6h.
  - See Herpesviral Keratitis in Cats, p 513, for details.

DRUG INTERACTIONS

Must separate application of a bacteriostatic (oxytetracycline) from a bactericidal antibiotic by at least 1 to 2 hours

POSSIBLE COMPLICATIONS

- Corneal perforation
- Corneal scarring
- Corneal pigmentation
- Corneal stromal permanent defect (i.e., facet)
- Corneal sequestration (cats)
- Vision impairment/loss

RECOMMENDED MONITORING

- Schirmer tear tests
- Evaluate for progressive loss of corneal stromal layers
- Repeat corneal cytology and/or culture to monitor response to antimicrobial therapy, especially if noting progressive stromal loss despite current therapies

PROGNOSIS AND OUTCOME

- Simple/indolent: most heal with minimal scarring within 5 to 10 days with appropriate treatment.
- Complex: healing may take 2 to 8 weeks, and substantial corneal scarring is expected.

PEARLS & CONSIDERATIONS

COMMENTS

- Topical corticosteroids are contraindicated with corneal ulceration; they delay healing and promote keratomalacia/melting.
- Referral to a veterinary ophthalmologist is recommended if ulcer progresses despite aggressive appropriate medical management and/or if ulcer exceeds 50% stromal depth or is ruptured, because structural surgical repair is usually required.
- Any simple corneal ulcer that does not heal within 5 to 10 days should be considered a complex ulcer, and underlying causes such as infection, foreign body, ectopic cilia, distichia, etc. must be ruled out.
- Gentamicin is a poor first choice for the treatment of simple corneal ulcers due to its limited spectrum of activity (gram-negative only).

PREVENTION

Avoid or treat underlying cause(s)

CLIENT EDUCATION

- Simple corneal ulcers may become complex; therefore, topical antibiotic treatment and regular follow-up to assess ulcer healing are crucial.
- Indolent corneal ulcers may recur in the same eye or occur in the opposite eye.
- The patient's eye is frequently more uncomfortable for 24 to 48 hours after epithelial debridement and multiple grid keratotomy have been performed to treat an indolent corneal ulcer.

SUGGESTED READING

Gelatt KN: Diseases and surgery of the canine cornea and sclera. In Gelatt KN (ed): *Essentials of Veterinary Ophthalmology*. Baltimore, Lippincott Williams & Wilkins, 2000, pp 125–145.

Gelatt KN: Feline ophthalmology. In Gelatt KN (ed): *Essentials of Veterinary Ophthalmology*. Baltimore, Lippincott Williams & Wilkins, 2000, pp 308–315.

AUTHOR: **ANNE J. GEMENSKY-METZLER**
EDITOR: **CHERYL L. CULLEN**

Corneal Vascularization

BASIC INFORMATION

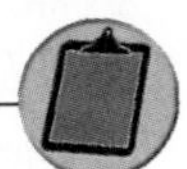

DEFINITION

The presence of blood vessels in or on the cornea

SYNONYM(S)

Corneal neovascularization
Vascularized keratitis

EPIDEMIOLOGY

SPECIES, AGE, SEX: Varies depending on underlying cause.
ASSOCIATED CONDITIONS AND DISORDERS: Corneal ulceration, irritation, desiccation, uveitis, episcleritis, or scleritis.

CLINICAL PRESENTATION

HISTORY, CHIEF COMPLAINT (SOME OR ALL MAY BE PRESENT)

- History:
  - Ocular trauma
  - Chronic ophthalmic disorder (e.g., keratoconjunctivitis sicca, indolent corneal ulcer, others)
- Chief complaint:
  - Red discoloration of the eye
  - Ocular discharge
  - Signs of ocular pain, manifesting as behavior change, blepharospasm

PHYSICAL EXAM FINDINGS

- Focal to diffuse red discoloration of the corneal surface or stroma.
- New corneal vessels enter stroma at the limbus and may be small:
  - May give the affected cornea a reddish haze
  - Are leaky and cause surrounding corneal edema (bluish haze)
  - May be missed altogether due to a cursory exam
- Other findings will vary depending on the cause.

ETIOLOGY AND PATHOPHYSIOLOGY

Blood vessel ingrowth occurs:

- As a response to injury of the corneal epithelium or stroma as a normal component of healing
  - Neutrophils, which enter the cornea from the tear film and the limbus, are important sources for angioblast and fibroblast growth factors.
  - There is a 3- to 4-day delay before the ingrowth of corneal blood vessels.
  - Ingrowth then occurs at a rate of approximately 1 mm/day.
- As part of an immune-mediated inflammatory response
- Secondary to disease of adjacent ocular tissues including uveitis, episcleritis, scleritis, glaucoma, and orbital disease

DIAGNOSIS

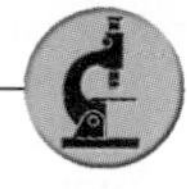

DIFFERENTIAL DIAGNOSIS

- Corneal injury or inflammation:
  - Corneal ulceration
  - Chemical irritation
  - Mechanical irritation:
    - Distichiasis/ectopic cilia/trichiasis
    - Entropion
  - Exposure:
    - Large palpebral fissure
    - Lagophthalmos (incomplete closure of the eyelids)
    - Ectropion
    - Buphthalmos (chronic glaucoma)
    - Exophthalmos
  - Neuroparalytic keratitis (cranial nerve VII lesion)
  - Neurotrophic keratitis (cranial nerve V lesion)
  - Keratoconjunctivitis sicca
  - Qualitative tear film abnormalities
  - Chronic superficial keratitis (pannus; dogs)
  - Proliferative keratoconjunctivitis (cats)
  - Corneal degeneration
- Adjacent ocular disease:
  - Uveitis
  - Episcleritis/scleritis
  - Orbital disease
  - Glaucoma

INITIAL DATABASE

- Neuro-ophthalmic examination: evaluate palpebral reflexes (cranial nerves V and VII) and completeness of eyelid closure.
- Schirmer tear test: values <10 mm/min and clinical signs consistent with keratoconjunctivitis = KCS.
- Tear film break-up time: values <10 seconds are suggestive of qualitative tear film abnormalities.
- Fluorescein staining: positive in corneal ulceration.
- Tonometry: elevated intraocular pressure (>30 mmHg) in glaucoma, or reduced (< 10 mmHg) in cases of uveitis.
- Ophthalmic examination: evaluate for abnormalities of eyelids and aberrant cilia, sclera, and intraocular structures.

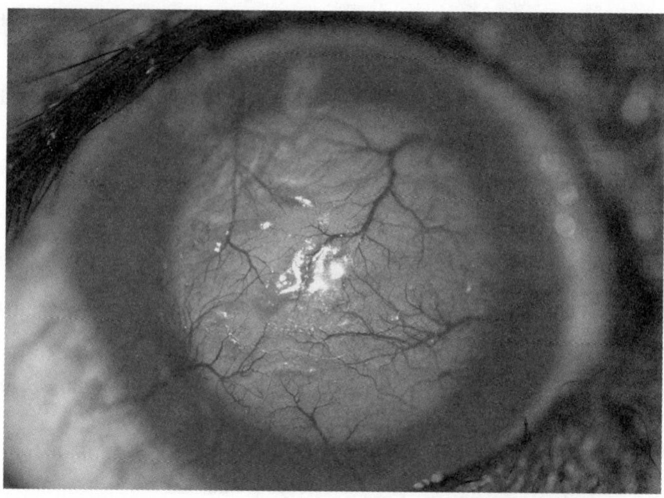

FIGURE I-45 Superficial corneal vascularization in a dog secondary to keratoconjunctivitis sicca. Note the numerous branching blood vessels located diffusely throughout the cornea. Courtesy of Dr. Bruce Grahn.

TREATMENT

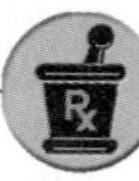

THERAPEUTIC GOAL(S)

- Treat underlzying cause
- Prevent progression
- Reduce discomfort

ACUTE GENERAL TREATMENT

Treatment will vary depending on underlying cause

POSSIBLE COMPLICATIONS

- Corneal vascularization may lead to pigmentation and scarring.
- Vascularization is often part of normal healing and should not be inappropriately suppressed.

PROGNOSIS AND OUTCOME

- Prognosis and outcome will vary depending on the underlying cause.
- In corneal injury, corneal vascularization denotes progression toward healing and is therefore a positive sign, provided the underlying problem can be controlled or eliminated.

PEARLS & CONSIDERATIONS

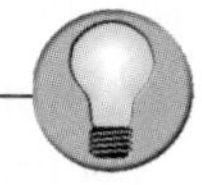

COMMENTS

It may be useful to distinguish between superficial and deep vascularization:

- Superficial vascularization occurs in response to superficial corneal or external ocular disease.
  - Superficial blood vessels arise from the conjunctiva, cross the limbus, are bright red, and branch frequently (Fig. I-45).
- Deep vascularization occurs in response to deep corneal or intraocular disease.
  - Deep blood vessels arise from the ciliary circulation, disappear at the limbus, and appear darker red and straight.

SUGGESTED READING

Chavkin MJ, et al: Risk factors for development of chronic superficial keratitis in dogs. *J Am Vet Med Assoc* 204:1630–1634, 1994.

Morgan RV, et al: Feline eosinophilic keratitis: A retrospective study of 54 cases: (1989–1994). *Vet Comp Ophthalmol* 6:131, 1996.

AUTHOR: **LYNNE SANDMEYER**
EDITOR: **CHERYL L. CULLEN**

Coronaviral Enteritis

BASIC INFORMATION

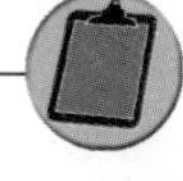

DEFINITION

Infectious intestinal disease that causes a generally mild diarrhea in dogs and cats

SYNONYM(S)

CCV (canine coronavirus)
FECV (feline enteric coronavirus)

EPIDEMIOLOGY

SPECIES, AGE, SEX: Dogs: neonatal puppies are more severely affected. Cats: virus virtually ubiquitous in the cat population; however, clinical disease is more common in young kittens in catteries and shelters.

RISK FACTORS: Dogs: Infection is prevalent in animal shelters and breeding farms (dense populations and concurrent infections). Cats: Multi-cat households (more than five cats) or catteries.

CONTAGION AND ZOONOSIS: Dogs: CCV is highly contagious and spreads rapidly through groups of susceptible dogs (dog to dog). Cats: FECV is highly contagious and spreads rapidly through multi-cat households (cat to cat). Transmission is by the fecal-oral route. CCV and FECV are not known to infect people.

CLINICAL PRESENTATION

DISEASE FORMS/SUBTYPES

- Dogs:
  - Subclinical in adult dogs
  - Diarrhea and vomiting (neonatal puppies)
- Cats:
  - Subclinical in adult cats
  - Mild to moderately severe diarrhea in kittens
  - Mutation to feline infectious peritonitis virus resulting in multisystemic disease (see Feline Infectious Peritonitis, p 378)

HISTORY, CHIEF COMPLAINT (SOME OR ALL MAY BE PRESENT)

- Mild to moderately severe diarrhea.
- Blood in feces (infrequent).
- Vomiting is more common in dogs.
- Lethargy and inappetance.
- Weight loss.

PHYSICAL EXAM FINDINGS

- Dehydration. The degree depends on the severity of the diarrhea.
- Occasionally concurrent ocular and nasal discharge, or weight loss in chronically infected kittens.

ETIOLOGY AND PATHOPHYSIOLOGY

- Member of the virus family Coronaviridae.
- Single-stranded RNA virus.
- Dogs and cats: virus infects epithelial cells in the tips of small intestine villi, causing a malabsorptive diarrhea. The virus remains infective for 2 to 3 days at room temperature (several days longer at temperatures just above freezing), and may be transmitted to other animals via infected litter boxes or fomites.
- Cats only: RNA mutations of FECV result in the formation of a new virus (feline infectious peritonitis [FIP] variant) that is able to enter and replicate within feline macrophages. Cats infected with this variant of FECV virus that do not mount an appropriate immune response may develop severe systemic illness (see Feline Infectious Peritonitis, p 378).

DIAGNOSIS

DIFFERENTIAL DIAGNOSIS

- Intestinal disease caused by enteric bacteria (*Campylobacter*, salmonellosis), protozoa (coccidiosis), or other viruses (i.e., canine parvoviral enteritis, feline panleukopenia-associated enteritis)
- Dietary indiscretion (dogs)
- Parasites (both dogs and cats)
- Dietary intolerance (cats)

INITIAL DATABASE

- Complete blood count, biochemistry panel, urinalysis: nonspecific changes
  - Severe diarrhea can result in marked dehydration and electrolyte abnormalities.
- Fecal testing for parasites and protozoa

ADVANCED OR CONFIRMATORY TESTING

Generally not performed, since coronaviral enteritis is usually self-limiting (exception: FIP) and, even in severe cases, responsive to supportive care.

- Dogs:
  - Detection of CCV in fresh feces by electron microscopy (false-negative findings are possible).
  - Virus isolation. However, CCV does not grow well.
  - Reverse transcriptase polymerase chain reaction (PCR) has been developed to detect CCV in fecal specimens (not commercially available).
  - Serologic evaluation (positive titers only confirm exposure to CCV, not necessarily active infection).
- Cats:
  - Serologic evaluation (indirect immunofluorescent antibody; enzyme-linked immunosorbent assay.
  - Does not differentiate FECV that causes isolated enteritis from FECV that causes FIP.
  - Does not correlate with severity of disease.
  - Positive titers only confirm exposure to FECV, not necessarily active infection.
  - In multi-cat (more than six cats) households, virtually all cats are seropositive.
  - Reverse transcriptase PCR has been developed to detect FECV in fecal specimens.
  - Does not reliably differentiate FECV that causes isolated enteritis from FECV that causes FIP.

TREATMENT

THERAPEUTIC GOAL(S)

Treatment is primarily supportive during the time needed for the disease to run its natural course.

ACUTE GENERAL TREATMENT

- Parenteral fluids to maintain fluid and electrolyte balance.
- Broad-spectrum antimicrobial agents to treat secondary bacterial infections are rarely indicated.
- Good nursing care and hygiene.

POSSIBLE COMPLICATIONS

- Dogs:
  - Clinical course (typically 7 to 10 days) may be longer and more severe in dogs that develop secondary complications or infection.
  - Dehydration, acidosis, shock.
  - Concurrent canine parvovirus or parasitic infections.
- Cats:
  - In immunocompromised kittens or cats, the virus may persist, resulting in chronic diarrhea or vomiting (months).
  - Enteric coronavirus can mutate into feline infectious peritonitis virus. Monitoring the affected cat and others in contact with it for signs of FIP (e.g., abdominal distention, fever, weight loss, neurologic signs, and icterus). However, the occurrence of coronaviral enteritis in an individual cat is not predictive of FIP.

RECOMMENDED MONITORING

Response to therapy

PROGNOSIS AND OUTCOME

- Dogs:
  - Good; neonatal puppies with concurrent parvovirus and coronavirus infections have a more guarded prognosis.
- Cats:
  - Generally good; guarded to poor in cats in whom FECV mutates and causes FIP.

PEARLS & CONSIDERATIONS

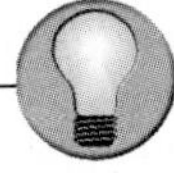

COMMENTS

- Clinical disease is considered infrequent compared with other viral enteropathies.
- Dogs:
  - CCV vaccines are not considered core vaccines but should be reserved for animals in which the risk of exposure may be higher (dense, stressful environments).
- Cats:
  - Inapparent infection is common in normal cats.
  - FECV-associated enteritis does not predispose a cat to development of FIP.

CLIENT EDUCATION

Reducing the number of cats per household (especially kittens less than 12 months old) and keeping potentially FECV-contaminated surfaces clean (e.g., litterboxes) can reduce population loads of FECV, and thus also reduce the risk of FIP.

RECOMMENDED READING

Pederson NC, et al: Common virus infection in cats, before and after being placed in shelters, with emphasis on feline enteric coronavirus. *J Feline Med Surg* 6(2):83–88, 2004.

Sanchez-Morgado JM, et al: Molecular characterization of a virulent canine coronavirus BG strain. *Virus Res* 104(1):27–31, 2004.

AUTHOR: **BRANDY PORTERPAN**
EDITOR: **DEBRA L. ZORAN**

Cough

BASIC INFORMATION

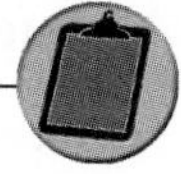

DEFINITION

A reflexive, forceful expulsion of air from the lungs and airways

EPIDEMIOLOGY

SPECIES, AGE, SEX: Dogs and cats of any age and either sex.

RISK FACTORS

- Exposure to airborne irritants or allergens
- Contact with other animals (infectious causes)

CONTAGION AND ZOONOSIS

- Dogs:
  - Infectious tracheobronchitis ("kennel cough")
  - Canine distemper
- Cats:
  - Viral rhinotracheitis

ASSOCIATED CONDITIONS AND DISORDERS: Vomiting: the "terminal retch" that occurs at the end of a paroxysm of coughing may be misinterpreted as vomiting by clients.

CLINICAL PRESENTATION

DISEASE FORMS/SUBTYPES: A useful way to consider the causes of cough, and the way to manage a coughing patient, involves the following categories:

- Purposeful cough. The cough is beneficial in expelling foreign material (e.g., inhaled foreign body) or substances (e.g., pus in pneumonia patients).
- Warning cough. The cough is a respiratory manifestation of a systemic disturbance that may become life-threatening (e.g., pulmonary edema from congestive heart failure, pulmonary hemorrhage from anticoagulant rodenticide toxicosis).
- Nuisance cough. The cough is disturbing or distressing to the patient and/or the owner but is not immediately life-threatening (e.g., infectious tracheobronchitis/"kennel cough," chronic sterile bronchitis).

HISTORY, CHIEF COMPLAINT

- Character (moist versus dry, soft versus hacking, nocturnal versus diurnal): may offer some insight regarding cause, but much overlap exists between different diseases.
- Dyspnea concurrently: generally indicates a more pressing need for diagnosis and treatment (purposeful and warning categories).
- Exposure to detrimental environment: contagion, inhalation of irritant substances.
- Duration of the cough: coughs that have maintained an equal intensity for months or more are commonly associated with disorders in the "nuisance cough" category.

PHYSICAL EXAM FINDINGS

- Dyspnea. See History, Chief Complaint above.
- Inducible cough. A cough that is elicited with application of tracheal pressure may occur with tracheobronchial diseases, with pulmonary parenchymal disease, or in unaffected animals. It does not indicate an anatomic source of the underlying problem. Tracheal pressure may be useful for confirmatory purposes if the owner is unsure whether the clinical sign observed at home is a cough.
- Pulmonary auscultation. Possible abnormalities include crackles/rales (interstitial fibrosing lung disease, pulmonary edema, others), loud bronchovesicular sounds (pulmonary edema, airway disease, others), wheezes (airway disease), and decreased lung sounds (pleural effusion, pneumothorax, intrathoracic mass).
- Cardiac auscultation. The presence of a heart murmur in a coughing dog raises the possibility of pulmonary edema (see Heart Failure, Acute/Decompensated, p 458). However, unrelated cardiac and respiratory diseases often coexist.
- A complete physical examination is indicated, because many disorders produce cough as only one manifestation of the underlying disease.

ETIOLOGY AND PATHOPHYSIOLOGY

- Abnormal presence of gases, substances, or material on the respiratory epithelium triggers afferent vagal impulses to the brainstem.
- Efferent impulses cause a sequence of glottis closure, abdominal and thoracic muscle contraction, and sudden glottis opening, causing the burst of air flow that is the cough.

DIAGNOSIS

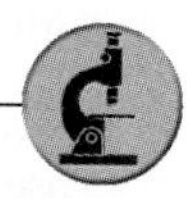

DIFFERENTIAL DIAGNOSIS

Causes of cough:

- Tracheobronchitis
- Collapsing trachea (dogs only)
- Chronic sterile bronchitis
- Asthma/allergic airway disease (cats)
- Bronchiectasis
- Allergic bronchitis
- Tracheal neoplasia
- Tracheal/bronchial foreign body
- Pneumonia (aspiration, bacterial, fungal, protozoal)
- Cardiogenic pulmonary edema (dogs only)
- Noncardiogenic pulmonary edema/acute respiratory distress syndrome
- Eosinophilic bronchopneumopathy
- Pulmonary hemorrhage
- Heartworm disease
- Pulmonary thromboembolism
- Pulmonary neoplasia
- Lungworms
- Tracheobronchial lymphadenopathy
- Left atrial enlargement
- Mediastinal mass

INITIAL DATABASE

- Thoracic radiographs and lateral cervical radiograph:
  - Radiographs are the initial diagnostic test of choice for coughing patients.
  - Indicated in any patient with signs of systemic illness, any patient with a cough of >10 days' duration, and any patient whose owner is concerned and wishes more than an exam-room evaluation.
- Fecal analysis (Baermann) if lungworms are locally endemic.
- Heartworm serology in endemic areas.
- Routine medical evaluation, including complete blood count, serum biochemistry profile, and urinalysis if patient shows systemic signs.

- Prothrombin time, partial thromboplastin time, platelet count if the patient roams outdoors or could otherwise have been exposed to anticoagulant rodenticide.

ADVANCED OR CONFIRMATORY TESTING

Based on specifics of case as assessed with history, presenting signs, physical exam findings, and initial database results

TREATMENT

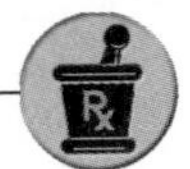

THERAPEUTIC GOAL(S)

- Correction/cure of inciting disorder, when possible
- Palliation of cough if underlying cause cannot be eliminated

ACUTE AND CHRONIC TREATMENT

- Dependent on underlying cause:
  - Purposeful cough: primary respiratory lesion requires correction (e.g., pneumonia treatment, foreign body removal, lung lobectomy) and treatments that increase the efficacy of the cough (e.g., nebulization and coupage). Cough suppression is contraindicated.
  - Warning cough: systemic disorder must be identified and addressed promptly (cardiogenic pulmonary edema: diuretics. Pulmonary hemorrhage from anticoagulant toxicity: plasma transfusion, vitamin K_1 replacement). Treatments to increase the efficacy of the cough, such as nebulization and coupage, or treatments aimed at decreasing the cough (cough suppressants), are contraindicated.
  - Nuisance cough: avoidance of triggers (e.g., allergens, dusts) and cough suppression. Treatment of complicating factors if they occur (e.g., infection).
- Cough suppressants (e.g., butorphanol 0.25–1 mg/kg PO q 8–24h as needed, or hydrocodone 0.25 mg/kg PO q 6–24h as needed, or codeine 0.5–2 mg/kg PO q 6–12h as needed):
  - Only used when a sterile, uncomplicated process is responsible for the cough, and the patient is systemically well. Examples: collapsing trachea, chronic sterile bronchitis, uncomplicated allergic airway disease.
- Empiric antibiotics or corticosteroids are not recommended in the absence of a diagnosis for the cause of the cough (minimum: completion of the initial database).

RECOMMENDED MONITORING

- Respiratory effort.
- Resolution of cough is expected in 7 to 10 days, with no worsening or new clinical signs of illness, in cases of benign, self-contained processes such as infectious tracheobronchitis. Failure to self-resolve may indicate a more complex cause and warrants further evaluation.

PROGNOSIS AND OUTCOME

Based on cause:

- Purposeful cough: prognosis fair to good if underlying cause can be controlled (eradication of pneumonia, removal of foreign body).
- Warning cough: short-term prognosis guarded. Long-term prognosis variable, based on response to acute treatment and underlying cause.
- Nuisance cough: short-term prognosis generally good, long-term prognosis fair (e.g., with collapsing trachea patients responding well to treatment) to good (e.g., patients with infectious tracheobronchitis).

PEARLS & CONSIDERATIONS

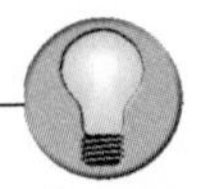

COMMENTS

- Cough is a clinical sign, not a disease. Optimal management must involve an accurate diagnosis of the underlying cause.
- Cigarette smoke inhalation and obesity are common but reversible complicating factors in patients with chronic cough.

SUGGESTED READING

Côté E: Diagnosis and management of cough: A new clinical approach. Proceedings, 24th Annual ACVIM Forum, Louisville, KY, 2006.

Rozanski EA, Rush JE: Acute and chronic cough. In King LG (ed): *Textbook of Respiratory Diseases in Dogs and Cats*. St. Louis, WB Saunders, 2004, pp 42–46.

AUTHOR & EDITOR: **ETIENNE CÔTÉ**

Cranial Cruciate Ligament Injury

Client Education Sheet on Website

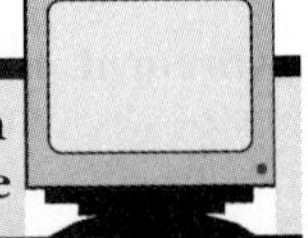

BASIC INFORMATION

DEFINITION

Partial or complete tearing of the cranial cruciate ligament (CrCL) causing stifle instability

SYNONYM(S)

Anterior cruciate ligament (ACL) rupture

EPIDEMIOLOGY

SPECIES, AGE, SEX: Seen in dogs, and less frequently in cats, of all ages.

RISK FACTORS

- Hereditary or developmental factors causing limb conformation or stifle joint deformation/malalignment
- Athletic injury
- Underlying systemic disease weakening the stifle (rare)

ASSOCIATED CONDITIONS AND DISORDERS

- Patellar instability
- Hip dysplasia
- Meniscal injury
- Osteochondritis dissecans
- Osteoarthritis
- Intracondylar notch stenosis
- Immune-mediated arthritis

CLINICAL PRESENTATION

DISEASE FORMS/SUBTYPES

- Partial CrCL rupture
- Complete CrCL rupture

HISTORY, CHIEF COMPLAINT

- Variable lameness of one or both hind limbs
- Lameness worsening with exercise and improving with rest
- Morning stiffness and "warming out" of lameness
- Weakness in, or reluctance to, jump/rise
- "Sloppy" (tilted) sitting position in which limb or stifle is splayed to the side
- Active, athletic ambulation (hunting, retrieving etc.) and sudden lameness

PHYSICAL EXAM FINDINGS

- Slanted sitting position
- Unilateral or bilateral, variably weight-bearing lameness
- Stifle instability:
  - Stifle joint effusion
  - Medial fibrosis of proximal tibial tissues (buttress formation)
  - Overall thickening of joint capsule

- Pain on manual hyperextension and/or hyperflexion of stifle
- Meniscal clicking during joint manipulation
- Limb muscle atrophy
- Arched spine due to forward weight shifting in bilaterally affected dogs

ETIOLOGY AND PATHOPHYSIOLOGY

- Biomechanical instability of the stifle joint resulting from an imbalance of muscular and weight-bearing forces necessary to control cranial tibial thrust, excessive internal rotation, and hyperextension of the stifle.
  - All lead to degeneration and rupture of the CrCL.
- Direct trauma is an infrequent cause of ligament rupture.

DIAGNOSIS

DIFFERENTIAL DIAGNOSIS

- Muscle strain
- Joint sprain
- Patella luxation
- Caudal cruciate ligament injury
- Long digital extensor tendon avulsion
- Immune-mediated arthritis
- Osteochondrosis of the stifle
- Lumbosacral disease
- Hip dysplasia or osteoarthritis
- Rickettsial and fungal disease
- Bone/joint neoplasia

INITIAL DATABASE

- Complete blood count, biochemical profile, urinalysis based on patient stability/American Society of Anesthesiologists classification (see American Society of Anesthesiologists Classification System, p 1334).
- Rickettsial and/or fungal titers (based on geography).
- Palpation of stifle joints for instability; this may require sedation:
  - Patients with partial ligament rupture may have instability only with stifle in flexion.
  - Cranial drawer sign (static).
    - Cranial displacement (manual) of tibia relative to femur (Fig. I-46).
  - Cranial tibial translation or thrust (dynamic) (Fig. I-47).
    - Cranial movement of tibial tuberosity as hock is flexed and gastrocnemius muscle contracts.
    - Increased internal rotation of proximal tibia.
- Lateral and craniocaudal stifle radiographs.
  - In cases of limb malalignment, radiographs should include the femur, tibia, hip, and tarsal joints to characterize limb conformation and joint conditions.
  - Calculation of tibial plateau slope angle to assist in choice of stabilization technique (Figs. I-48 and I-49).

ADVANCED OR CONFIRMATORY TESTING

- Arthrocentesis (to eliminate other possible causes)
- Arthroscopy (to eliminate other possible causes)
- Magnetic resonance imaging:
  - Possibly most useful for partial ruptures

TREATMENT

THERAPEUTIC GOAL(S)

- To relieve pain, improve function, and minimize progression of degenerative changes by stabilizing the stifle joint
- To treat meniscal injury

ACUTE GENERAL TREATMENT

- Medical management:
  - Nonsteroidal anti-inflammatory drugs (NSAIDs):
    - Aspirin 10–25 mg/kg PO q 8–24h; or
    - Carprofen 2 mg/kg PO q 12h; or
    - Etodolac 10–15 mg/kg PO q 24h; or

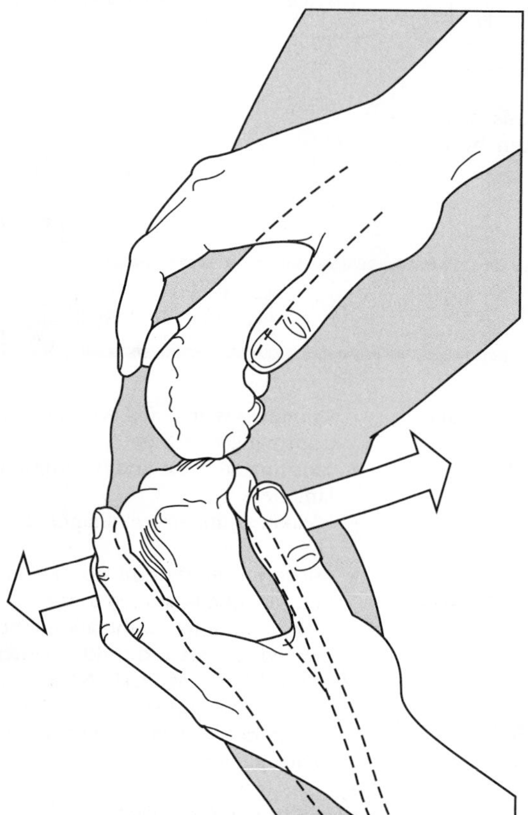

FIGURE I-46 Palpation of the stifle joint for cranial drawer motion of the tibia relative to the femur with cranial cruciate ligament insufficiency.

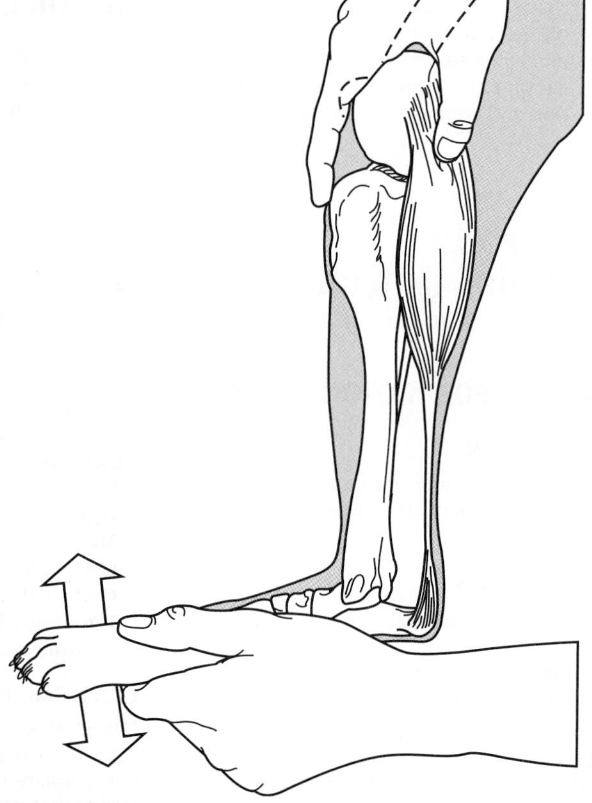

FIGURE I-47 Palpation of the stifle joint using tibial compression test for cranial cruciate ligament injury. Flexion of the hock will cause cranial displacement of the tibia.

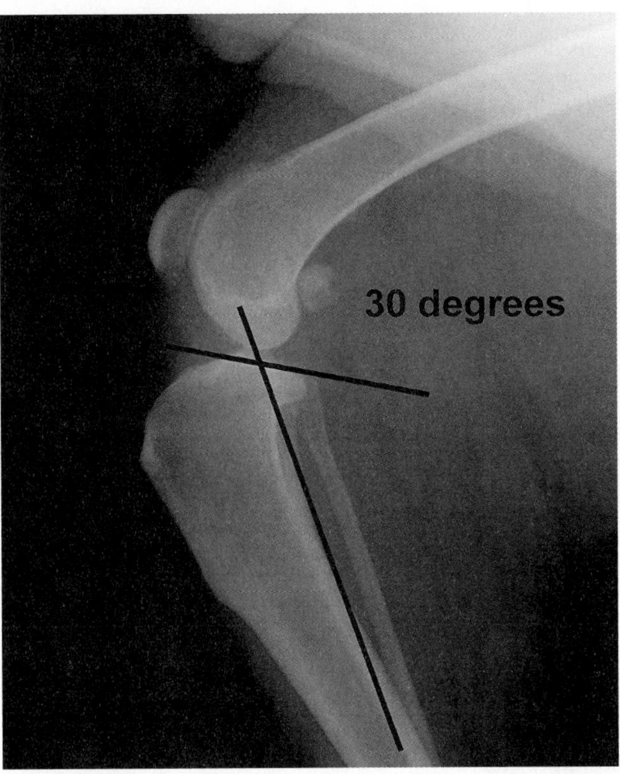

FIGURE I-48 Preoperative radiograph of the stifle of a dog with cranial cruciate ligament rupture. The tibial plateau angle is 30°.

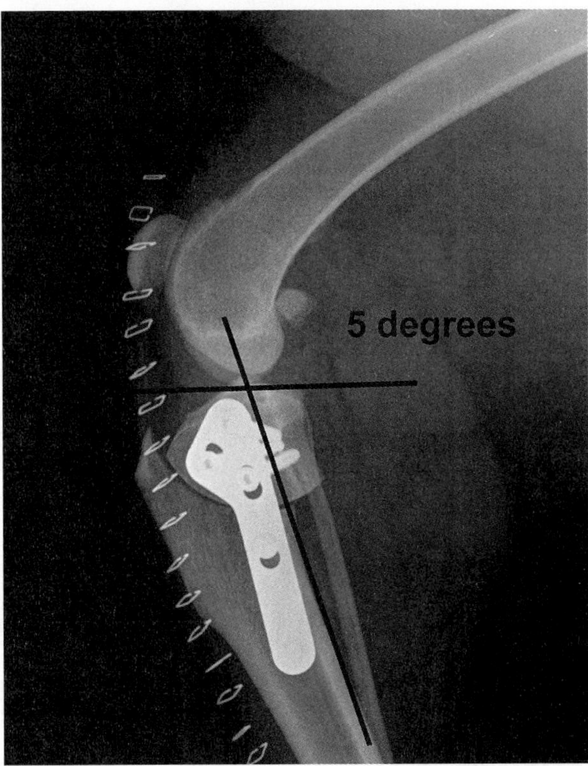

FIGURE I-49 Photograph of the same stifle after tibial plateau leveling osteotomy (TPLO). The tibial plateau angle is satisfactory at 5°.

        - Deracoxib 1-2 mg/kg PO q 24h (may use 3-4 mg/kg PO q 24h for first 7 days only); or
        - Meloxicam 0.1 mg/kg PO q 24h; or
        - Meclofenamic acid 1.1 mg/kg, PO q 24h after eating, for 5 days maximum; or
        - Tepoxalin 10 mg/kg PO q 24h (new product, objective data pending); or
        - Others.
- Conservative treatment (rest and NSAIDs)
    - Best tolerated in patients weighing <10-15 kg.
    - Generally unsuccessful in larger dogs.
    - Lameness usually resolves within 2 to 4 months:
        - Instability persists, and secondary degenerative joint disease develops despite "normal" function.
        - Increased risk of meniscal damage due to joint instability.
        - Body weight often is shifted to the contralateral limb.
- Surgical stabilization of the stifle:
    - Intra-articular fascia lata or patella tendon autogenous graft: limits cranial motion and internal rotation of the tibia.
    - Extracapsular suture stabilization (fabella to tibial tubercle): limits drawer motion and rotation.
    - Fibular head transposition: uses the lateral collateral ligament to reduce drawer motion and internal rotation.

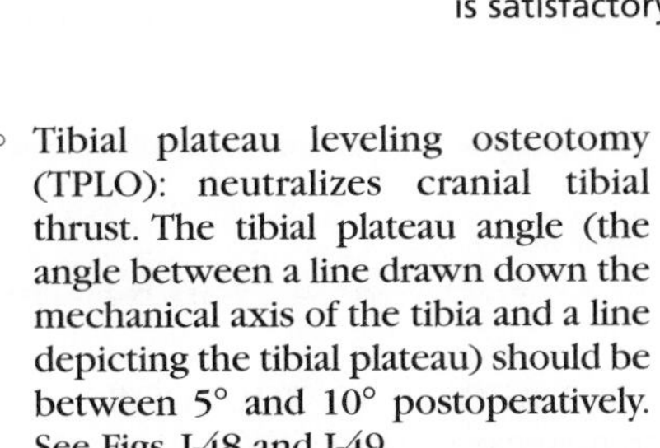

    - Tibial plateau leveling osteotomy (TPLO): neutralizes cranial tibial thrust. The tibial plateau angle (the angle between a line drawn down the mechanical axis of the tibia and a line depicting the tibial plateau) should be between 5° and 10° postoperatively. See Figs. I-48 and I-49.
    - Tibial tubercle advancement (TTA): a new technique to neutralize cranial tibial thrust.
    - Arthroscopic-assisted reconstruction: for debridement of ligament and meniscus.
    - Pinning or wiring of avulsion injuries: to reattach ligament origin or insertion.
- Meniscal treatment:
    - Medial meniscal release.
    - Medial meniscectomy (partial or complete).

CHRONIC TREATMENT

- Management includes the same treatments as in acute cases but may require more long-term medical management for the treatment of osteoarthritis.
    - NSAIDs as listed previously.
    - A chondroprotective agent:
        - Polysulfated glycosaminoglycan 5 mg/kg IM once weekly × 4-6 weeks; or
        - Pentosan polysulfate (from beechwood hemicellulose) 3 mg/kg, SC once weekly; or
        - Oral formulations (glucosamine, chondroitin sulphate, hyaluronan): according to formulation/labeled instructions).
- Nutrition (energy-restricted diet, as appropriate).
- Weight control.
- Exercise moderation.
- Physical therapy (see also Physical Rehabilitation, p 1300):
    - Controlled leash walks for 5 to 10 minutes two to three times a day, slowly on inclines/declines.
    - Passive flexion/extension exercises of the limb can be performed for 5 to 10 minutes, two to three times a day; this regimen can be increased in frequency and duration during the second and third postoperative month.
    - Gentle swimming three times a week for 10 to 15 minutes can also be incorporated during the third and fourth month.
    - A gradual return to normal activity is encouraged during month 5.
- In chronic cases with degenerative joint disease and minimal instability, some surgeons believe surgical stabilization should be limited to techniques (TPLO, TTA) that neutralize cranial tibial thrust.

POSSIBLE COMPLICATIONS

- Medical management:

- Gastrointestinal, hepatic, renal, or other systemic reactions from NSAID therapy
- Continued progression of degenerative joint disease
- Failure of medical management to control pain
- Surgical management:
  - Failure to stabilize the stifle joint
  - Progression of degenerative joint disease
  - Postoperative meniscal injury:
    - Damage not recognized at surgery
    - Shear forces not neutralized
  - Implant failure
  - Infection (soft tissue or bone)

RECOMMENDED MONITORING

- Basic laboratory monitoring of patients on NSAID therapy
- Weight loss, exercise levels (rehabilitation), and clinical signs as dictated by the patient
- Radiographic monitoring if clinical signs worsen

PROGNOSIS AND OUTCOME

- Long-term function for patients that have undergone a reconstructive procedure is good. Published assessments of most techniques in the past 25 years describe improvement in 80–90% of dogs after surgery, regardless of the methodology.
- Postoperative rehabilitation is critical for clinical recovery.
- Techniques that neutralize cranial tibial thrust are successful in:
  - Returning dogs to normal function and activity
  - Minimizing or stopping the progression of osteoarthritis

PEARLS & CONSIDERATIONS

COMMENTS

- Bilateral lameness may be difficult to recognize and is often confused with neurologic disease.
  - A careful orthopedic examination is essential.
- Injury of the contralateral cranial cruciate ligament occurs in 40% of patients.
  - A 60% incidence if radiographic changes are visible in the uninjured joint.
- Some surgeons recommend surgery for patients of any size to ensure optimum function.
- In partial CrCL ruptures with minimal or no cranial drawer, some surgeons prefer to use only stabilization techniques that neutralize cranial tibial thrust.
- In one arthroscopic study of partial CrCL injury, TPLO stopped the progression of further ligament rupture in six of seven dogs.
- *Editor's note:* Practitioners should consider consultation and referral with an orthopedic surgeon; selection of the "best" procedure continues to be controversial among specialists.

SUGGESTED READING

Dejardin LM: Tibial plateau leveling osteotomy. In Slatter D (ed): *Textbook of Small Animal Surgery*, ed 3. Philadelphia, 2002, pp 2090–2133.

Hayashi K, Manley PA, Muir P: Cranial cruciate ligament pathophysiology in dogs with cruciate disease: A review. *J Am Anim Hosp Assoc* 40:385, 2004.

Johnson AL, Hulse DA: Cranial cruciate ligament rupture. In Fossum TW (ed): *Small Animal Surgery*, ed 2. St. Louis, Mosby, 2002, pp 1110–1122.

Vasseur PB: Stifle joint. In Slatter D (ed): *Textbook of Small Animal Surgery*, ed 3. Philadelphia, WB Saunders, 2002, pp 2090–2133.

AUTHORS: **JAMES P. BOULAY, BARBARA R. GORES**

EDITOR: **JOSEPH HARARI**

Cranial Vena Cava Syndrome

BASIC INFORMATION

DEFINITION

Cranial vena cava syndrome is an uncommon sequela to extraluminal compression, invasion, or intraluminal obstruction of the cranial vena cava (CrVC). Obstruction of the CrVC results in pitting edema of the head, neck, and forelimbs.

SYNONYM(S)

Caval syndrome
Precaval syndrome
Superior vena caval syndrome

EPIDEMIOLOGY

SPECIES, AGE, SEX: Depends on underlying cause.

RISK FACTORS

- Jugular catheters
- Cranial mediastinal neoplasia (e.g., thymoma, lymphoma, carcinoma, aortic body tumors)
- Hypercoagulable conditions (e.g., sepsis, immune-mediated hemolytic anemia, protein-losing nephropathies, corticosteroid excess, neoplasia, pancreatitis)
- Mycoses leading to the formation of granulomas (e.g., blastomycosis, cryptococcosis)

CONTAGION AND ZOONOSIS: Fungal granulomas causing CrVC syndrome may be caused by organisms that can also infect humans (*Blastomyces dermatitidis, Cryptococcus neoformans*), but these would be common-source infections, not zoonoses.

GEOGRAPHY AND SEASONALITY: Infectious causes (e.g., blastomycosis) are more prevalent in certain geographic areas.

CLINICAL PRESENTATION

HISTORY, CHIEF COMPLAINT

- Head, neck, and forelimb swelling
- Additional clinical signs depend on underlying cause

PHYSICAL EXAM FINDINGS

- Symmetric, nonpainful pitting edema of head, neck, and forelimbs
- Dyspnea, tachypnea, muffled heart/lung sounds (if pleural effusion present)
- Weakness, tachycardia, arrhythmias, muffled heart sounds (if pericardial effusion present)
- ± Jugular venous distention
- ± Engorgement of conjunctival and scleral vessels
- Additional physical exam findings depend on underlying cause

ETIOLOGY AND PATHOPHYSIOLOGY

- Extraluminal compression, invasion, or intraluminal obstruction of the CrVC causes impaired venous return from the cranial portion of the body. This leads to interstitial fluid accumulation, resulting in edema of the head, neck, and forelimbs.
- The most common causes include mediastinal neoplasia, fungal granulomas, and cranial vena caval thrombosis (e.g., secondary to hypercoagulable states, tumor emboli, jugular catheters).

DIAGNOSIS

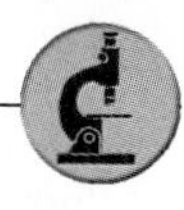

DIFFERENTIAL DIAGNOSIS

For head and neck swelling:

- Angioedema (e.g., vaccine reaction, insect bite hypersensitivity)
- Generalized peripheral edema (e.g., secondary to hypoalbuminemia, vasculitis, right-sided congestive heart failure)
- Acute blunt trauma to head/neck
- Subcutaneous emphysema
- Lymphangiosarcoma of the head and neck

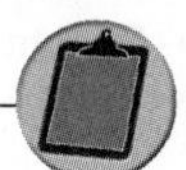

- Myxedema (e.g., secondary to hypothyroidism)
- Foreign body around neck (e.g., elastic band)
- Salivary mucocele (cervical)
- Jugular vein thrombosis or mass
- Abscessation or cellulitis
- Rattlesnake bite

INITIAL DATABASE

To help determine underlying cause:
- Complete blood count
- Serum biochemistry profile
- Urinalysis
- Feline leukemia and feline immunodeficiency tests (to help evaluate for the presence of lymphoma in cats)
- Thoracic radiographs (to identify cranial mediastinal masses, pleural and/or pericardial effusion)

ADVANCED OR CONFIRMATORY TESTING

- Thoracic ultrasonography (to visualize emboli or tumor compression/invasion of cranial vena cava)
- Nonselective angiography (to identify CrVC filling defects, localize site of obstruction, highlight collateral circulation)
- Computed tomography or magnetic resonance imaging
- Echocardiography (to identify pericardial effusion or masses at the level of the terminal CrVC)
- Fine-needle aspiration or biopsy of thoracic masses

TREATMENT

THERAPEUTIC GOAL(S)

- Remove obstructive lesion from CrVC
- Treat predisposing cause

ACUTE GENERAL TREATMENT

- Mediastinal masses: depending on tumor type, treatment may include surgery, chemotherapy, or radiation (alone or in combination)
- Fungal granulomas: systemic antifungal drugs (e.g., itraconazole, fluconazole, depending on extent and type of mycosis)
- CrVC thrombosis:
  - Treat underlying cause
  - Remove jugular catheters if present
  - ± Anticoagulants (e.g., heparin): efficacy unproven
  - ± Thrombolytic agents (e.g., streptokinase): efficacy unproven; may result in life-threatening hemorrhage
- ± Diuretics (to minimize edema formation): efficacy limited

CHRONIC TREATMENT

Depends on underlying disease

POSSIBLE COMPLICATIONS

Thrombolytic agents may result in life-threatening hemorrhage

PROGNOSIS AND OUTCOME

- Prognosis depends on severity of underlying illness; presence of CrVC syndrome does not appear to confer a worse prognosis than that of the underlying disorder alone.
- Head, neck, and forelimb edema may abate if CrVC obstruction removed and/or if adequate collateral circulation develops.

PEARLS & CONSIDERATIONS

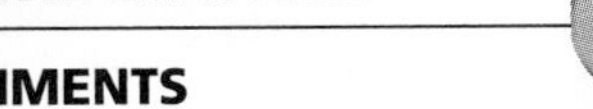

COMMENTS

- Although the name is similar, heartworm caval syndrome is a totally different clinical entity involving right-sided heart failure, hemolysis, and hemoglobinuria as a consequence of advanced heartworm disease.
- Human medicine offers promising alternatives to the current therapies available in veterinary medicine:
  - Surgical bypass of the CrVC obstruction.
  - Endovascular therapy: a combination of:
    - Thrombolytic agents
    - Angioplasty (balloon dilation of obstructed vessel)
    - Stent placement at the level of vascular obstruction
    - ± Anticoagulants

PREVENTION

- Avoid jugular catheters in hypercoagulable patients.
- Consider prophylactic anticoagulant therapy in patients with hypercoagulable disorders.

SUGGESTED READING

Howard J, Arceneaux KA, Paugh-Partington B, Oliver J: Blastomycosis granuloma involving the cranial vena cava associated with chylothorax and cranial vena caval syndrome in a dog. *J Am Anim Hosp Assoc* 36:159–161, 2000.

Nicastro A, Côté E: Cranial vena cava syndrome. *Compend Contin Educ Pract Vet* 24(9):701–710, 2002.

Peaston AE, Church DB, Allen GS, Haigh S: Combined chylothorax, chylopericardium, and cranial vena cava syndrome in a dog with thymoma. *J Am Vet Med Assoc* 197:1354–1356, 1990.

AUTHOR: **ANDREA NICASTRO**
EDITOR: **ETIENNE CÔTÉ**

Cricopharyngeal Achalasia/Dysphagia

BASIC INFORMATION

DEFINITION

Failure of upper esophageal sphincter (cricopharyngeal muscle) relaxation and lack of synchrony with pharyngeal muscle activity

SYNONYM(S)

Cricopharyngeal asynchrony
Cricopharyngeal dysphagia

EPIDEMIOLOGY

SPECIES, AGE, SEX
Dog:
- Problem noted at time of weaning
  - Eating solid food

GENETICS AND BREED PREDISPOSITION: Purebred dogs:
- Congenital anomaly
- Smaller breeds
  - Spaniels overrepresented

RISK FACTORS: Smaller, purebred dog.

ASSOCIATED CONDITIONS AND DISORDERS: Potentially other congenital swallowing disorders:
- Pharyngeal paresis
- Megaesophagus

CLINICAL PRESENTATION

HISTORY, CHIEF COMPLAINT: Onset of clinical signs at time of weaning/introduction of solid food:
- Gagging, retching

- Dysphagia with repeated attempts to swallow food
- Coughing, nasal reflux
- Poor body condition, failure to grow and gain weight
- Weight loss

PHYSICAL EXAM FINDINGS

- Poor body condition:
  - Smaller when compared to littermates
- Possible clinical signs of aspiration pneumonia:
  - Coughing
  - Fever
  - Increased lung sounds on auscultation
- Observation of animal attempting to eat:
  - Dysphagia
  - Repeated attempts to swallow

ETIOLOGY AND PATHOPHYSIOLOGY

- Result of asynchronous/failure of relaxation of the cricopharyngeal muscle in response to pharyngeal contraction
- Normal physiology:
  - Food bolus formed by pharyngeal muscular activity is pushed caudally by the base of the tongue
  - Cricopharyngeal muscle relaxes, allowing passage of the bolus into the upper esophagus
- Cricopharyngeal achalasia:
  - Asynchronous cricopharyngeal relaxation results in repeated caudal movement of a bolus against persistent cricopharyngeal contraction
  - Causes dysphagia with possible aspiration into the trachea

DIAGNOSIS

DIFFERENTIAL DIAGNOSIS

See Dysphagia, p 325

- Neurologic dysfunction associated with ability to prehend food
- Neurologic dysfunction of tongue
- Pharyngeal paresis
- Megaesophagus
- Pharyngeal or esophageal foreign body or mass

INITIAL DATABASE

- Complete blood count:
  - Neutrophilia with left shift, toxic changes: associated with inflammation/ infection if aspiration pneumonia. Stress leukogram alone neither supports nor rules out aspiration pneumonia. Normal complete blood count results do not rule out aspiration pneumonia.
- Serum biochemistry profile:
  - Hypoproteinemia:
    - Evidence of malnutrition.
- Diagnostic imaging:
  - Survey thoracic radiographs:
    - Rule out aspiration pneumonia.
    - Rule out megaesophagus.
  - Dynamic swallowing study (canned food mixed with barium):.
    - Failure of relaxation of upper esophageal sphincter to allow bolus into esophagus.
    - Rule out other causes of dysphagia/ regurgitation:
      - Pharyngeal paresis
      - Esophageal hypomotility (megaesophagus)
        - Contraindication to surgical correction
      - Pharyngeal or esophageal foreign body
    - See Barium Esophagram, Dynamic, p 1187.

TREATMENT

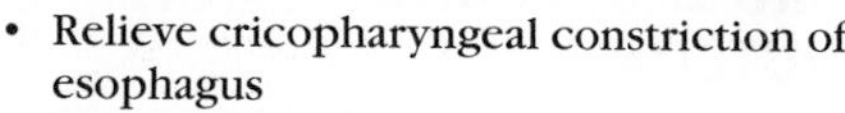

THERAPEUTIC GOAL(S)

- Relieve cricopharyngeal constriction of esophagus
- Treat associated aspiration pneumonia
- Provide nutritional support until oral intake has returned to normal

ACUTE GENERAL TREATMENT

- Before surgical correction:
  - Correction of fluid and electrolyte deficits, if present
  - Aggressive treatment of aspiration pneumonia, if present (see Pneumonia, Aspiration, p 862):
    - Antibiotic therapy
    - Oxygen therapy
    - Physical therapy:
      - Coupage
  - Nutritional support:
    - Feeding tube
- Surgical correction:
  - Cricopharyngeal myotomy/myectomy:
    - ± Thyropharyngeal myotomy/myectomy
- Postoperative feeding regimen:
  - Small, frequent feedings
  - Canned food diet:
    - Chopped up so that there are no large pieces
  - Feed in an elevated position

CHRONIC TREATMENT

- Gradual return to normal feeding regimen as swallowing function improves
- Continued treatment of aspiration pneumonia until resolved

POSSIBLE COMPLICATIONS

- Recurrence of problem due to:
  - Inadequate separation/excision of cricopharyngeal (± thyropharyngeal) muscle
  - Fibrosis of surgical site with stricture development
- Failure to recognize associated esophageal hypomotility:
  - Persistent reflux of esophageal contents
  - Increased risk of developing aspiration pneumonia

RECOMMENDED MONITORING

Repeat dynamic swallowing study 4 to 6 weeks after surgery.

- Demonstrate resolution of failure of upper esophageal sphincter to relax

PROGNOSIS AND OUTCOME

Good provided:

- No associated pharyngeal or esophageal dysfunction
- Aspiration pneumonia resolves

PEARLS & CONSIDERATIONS

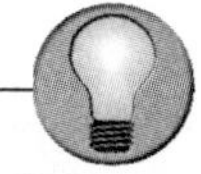

COMMENTS

- Aggressively treat severe malnutrition and/or aspiration pneumonia before surgical intervention to decrease morbidity and mortality associated with anesthesia and surgery.
- Rule out esophageal motility problems before surgery.
  - Significantly increases risk of aspiration pneumonia.
- Consider re-operation if clinical signs recur and diagnosis is accurate.

CLIENT EDUCATION

Recognize problem as soon as possible to:

- Minimize risk of development of aspiration pneumonia
- Prevent malnutrition

SUGGESTED READING

Ladlow J, Hardie RJ: Cricopharyngeal achalasia in dogs. *Compend Contin Ed Pract Vet* 22:750–755, 2000.

Nile JD, et al: Resolution of dysphagia following cricopharyngeal myectomy in six young dogs. *J Small Anim Pract* 42:32–35, 2001.

Warnock JJ, et al: Surgical management of cricopharyngeal achalasia in dogs: 14 cases (1989–2001). *J Am Vet Med Assoc* 223:1462–1468, 2003.

AUTHORS: **MARYANN G. RADLINSKY, RICHARD WALSHAW**

EDITOR: **RICHARD WALSHAW**

Cryptococcosis

BASIC INFORMATION

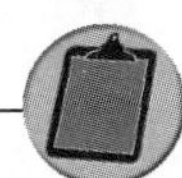

DEFINITION

A systemic mycosis caused by a dimorphic fungus with the yeast phase being infective unlike other mycoses. Clinically, there is a predilection for the upper respiratory tract, central nervous system (CNS), skin, and eyes.

EPIDEMIOLOGY

SPECIES, AGE, SEX

- Both domestic and wild animals may be infected as well as humans.
- Cats may be more susceptible than dogs.
- No age or sex predilection in cats.
- Young adult dogs more commonly affected.

RISK FACTORS

- Exposure to pigeon droppings and soil in warm, humid climates.
- Immunosuppressed states (glucocorticoids) and diseases (feline immunodeficiency virus [FIV] or feline leukemia virus [FeLV] infections in cats, ehrlichiosis in dogs) may be a risk factor.

CONTAGION AND ZOONOSIS: Zoonosis is unlikely, but caution is warranted. The yeast form is infective, and this does not aerosolize from infected tissues or body fluid.

GEOGRAPHY AND SEASONALITY: Worldwide distribution.

CLINICAL PRESENTATION

DISEASE FORMS/SUBTYPES: Respiratory, cutaneous, CNS, and ocular forms.

HISTORY, CHIEF COMPLAINT

- Cats typically present with upper respiratory tract signs (sneezing, nasal discharge), swelling of the nose, skin lesions. Neurologic or ophthalmic signs may also be present.
- Dogs may present with weight loss, anorexia, lethargy, and neurologic or ophthalmic signs.

PHYSICAL EXAM FINDINGS

- Cats: unilateral or bilateral nasal discharge, sneezing, firm swelling over bridge of nose. Submandibular lymphadenomegaly.
- Dogs and cats: Multifocal neurologic signs with cranial nerve involvement. Ocular abnormalities including retinal detachment, chorioretinitis, panophthalmitis, optic neuritis. Cutaneous lesions including papules, nodules, or ulcerated draining lesions. Fever possible.

ETIOLOGY AND PATHOPHYSIOLOGY

- *Cryptococcus neoformans* is a saprophytic, round, yeastlike dimorphic fungus with a large heteropolysaccharide capsule (Fig. I-50).
- Inhalation of yeastlike nonencapsulated airborne organisms is the most likely route of infection.
- The organism may then establish itself in the upper respiratory tract or in the alveoli, forming granulomas.
- In tissues, the organism forms a capsule that interferes with the immune response, preventing clearance of the organism.
- Hematogenous dissemination and invasion into the CNS and eyes may follow.
- Establishment of the organism in tissues and dissemination will occur if there is a poor cell-mediated immune response.

DIAGNOSIS

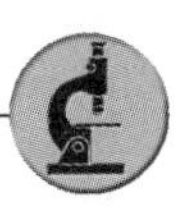

DIFFERENTIAL DIAGNOSIS

- Other systemic fungal disease
- Lymphosarcoma
- Respiratory: chronic rhinitis (bacterial or viral), nasal tumors, other systemic fungal diseases, toxoplasmosis
- CNS:
  - Feline infectious diseases (FeLV, FIV, feline coronavirus/feline infectious peritonitis, toxoplasmosis, rabies)
  - Canine infectious diseases (canine distemper, rabies, ehrlichiosis, Rocky Mountain spotted fever, toxoplasmosis)
  - Noninfectious CNS diseases such as granulomatous meningoencephalitis or neoplasia
- Cutaneous: bacterial pyoderma, abscesses, autoimmune skin disease

INITIAL DATABASE

- Complete blood cell count, serum chemistry panel, and urinalysis can be within normal limits.
- May find cryptococcus in urine sediment.
  - Stain to help differentiate organisms from fat droplets
- Thoracic radiographs may show pulmonary nodules.
- Nasal radiographs may show lysis or proliferative lesions.

ADVANCED OR CONFIRMATORY TESTING

- Cytology of nasal exudates, skin exudates, lymph node aspirate, cerebrospinal fluid (CSF), ocular fluid, tissue biopsy may reveal organisms (see Fig. I-50)
- Latex agglutination test for capsular antigen in serum, urine, or CSF:
  - Diagnostic test of choice
  - False-negative results possible with localized infection
- Fungal culture from exudates, CSF, urine, ocular or joint fluid, and tissue samples
  - Represent a possible zoonotic hazard (aerosol) and should be performed in a specialized laboratory only

TREATMENT

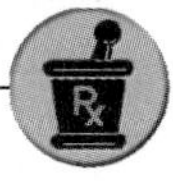

THERAPEUTIC GOAL(S)

Long-term therapy is necessary to eradicate the infection.

ACUTE AND CHRONIC TREATMENT

- Treatment of dogs and cats with any antifungal should continue at least 1 month past resolution of clinical signs.
- Monitoring of serial titers may help assess response to therapy:
  - A decrease in serum antigen titer implies a favorable prognosis. Specifically, a favorable prognosis is associated with a progressive decrease in serum antigen titer of at least 10-fold by the end of 2 months.
  - Use of antigen titers to guide duration of treatment: treatment should be continued for 1 month after complete resolution of clinical signs and a decrease in titer by at least two orders of magnitude (e.g., if 1:512 at diagnosis, then 1:128, 1:64, or lower) but ideally when there is an undetectable titer.
  - Although titers often decrease with treatment, in some cats it may take 3 to 5 years to reach a negative titer.
- In cats, fluconazole and itraconazole have been successful and associated with less severe side effects than amphotericin B and ketoconazole.
- Amphotericin B and ketoconazole are not useful in treatment of CNS cryptococcosis (fail to cross the blood-brain barrier).
- Animals must be adequately hydrated and should be undergoing fluid diuresis before administration of amphotericin B formulas.

- Many treatment options exist. In cats, the treatment of first choice is generally fluconazole, whereas in dogs, the cost may make other medication options more attractive.
  - Fluconazole: 5–15 mg/kg PO q 12–24h (dogs and cats).
  - Amphotericin B SC: 0.5–0.8 mg/kg diluted with 400–500 ml 0.45% saline/2.5% dextrose and given two to three times weekly to a cumulative dose of 8–26 mg/kg (dogs and cats).
  - Amphotericin B IV:
    - 0.5 mg/kg IV q 48–72h (dogs).
    - 0.25 mg/kg IV q 48–72h (cats).
    - Maintenance dose recommendations vary.
    - Total cumulative dose of 4–10 mg/kg and 4–8 mg/kg for dogs and cats, respectively.
  - Lipid-soluble amphotericin B: 1 mg/kg IV q 48–72h for 60 days (dogs, cats).
  - Itraconazole: 5 mg/kg PO with food q 12h (cats).
    - Formulation may make dosage challenging (100-mg capsules).
    - Oral liquid formulation available (10 mg/ml).
  - Ketoconazole 5–15 mg/kg PO q 12h (dogs).

DRUG INTERACTIONS

- Itraconazole and ketoconazole should not be administered with other hepatically metabolized drugs.
- Amphotericin B should not be administered with other renally excreted drugs.
- Fluconazole is renally eliminated, and dose must be decreased in patients with renal failure.

POSSIBLE COMPLICATIONS

- Itraconazole may result in gastrointestinal signs and hepatotoxicity (initially manifested with elevated serum alanine aminotransferase). Rare side effects include vasculitis and cutaneous ulcerations.
- Ketoconazole may cause gastrointestinal signs and elevated serum liver enzymes. Cats have an increased risk for hepatotoxicity, and use of this drug is controversial in this species.
- Amphotericin B is potentially nephrotoxic and can cause phlebitis.
  - Lipid-soluble amphotericin B may be less nephrotoxic.

RECOMMENDED MONITORING

- Liver enzymes and renal values should be routinely monitored while animal is treated with antifungals.
- Animals treated with amphotericin B should have blood urea nitrogen (BUN), creatinine, renal γ-glutamyltransferase, and urine sediment examinations performed routinely. A rising BUN and/or casts in the urine sediment may necessitate discontinuing or lowering the dose of amphotericin B.

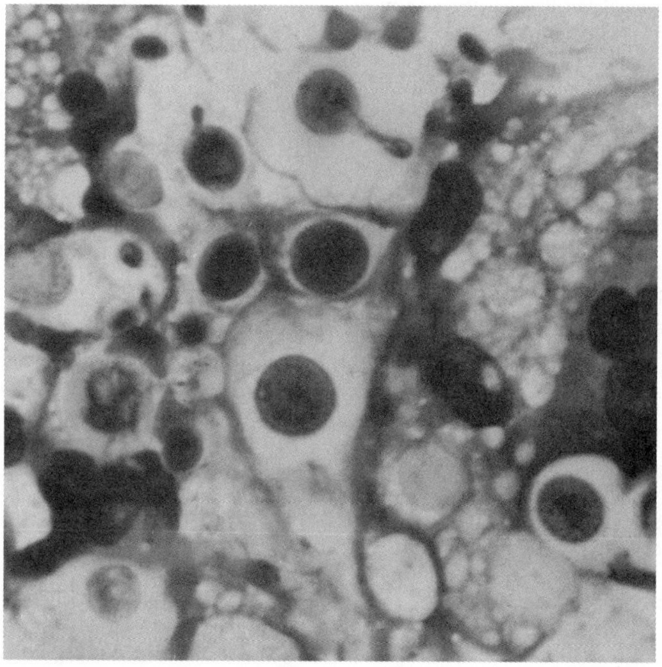

FIGURE I-50 Cytology shows capsulate yeasts, with narrow-neck budding in a DiffQuik-stained smear. Courtesy of R. Malik, University of Sydney, Sydney, Australia. (In Greene CE: *Infectious Diseases of the Dog and Cat*, ed 3. St. Louis, WB Saunders, 2006, p 587, with permission.)

PROGNOSIS AND OUTCOME

- Infection may be cleared in cats; however, maintenance antifungal therapy may be necessary in FeLV/FIV-positive cats.
- FeLV/FIV seronegative status is significantly associated with treatment success (using itraconazole) in cats with nasal cryptococcosis. FeLV/FIV-positive cases are associated with severe signs involving the CNS and eyes.
- CNS infections and disseminated infections are more likely to exist in cats with FeLV or FIV and may be more difficult to clear.
- Magnitude of pretreatment antigen titers has no significant effect on treatment outcome using itraconazole.
- More cats with the cutaneous forms of cryptococcosis (82%) were treated successfully than cats with intranasal (53%) cryptococcosis or cryptococcal infection of other sites (43%).
- Guarded prognosis in dogs.

PEARLS & CONSIDERATIONS

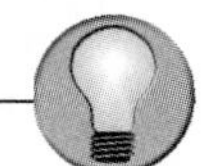

PREVENTION

- No vaccine available
- Avoid pigeon droppings and damp, shaded soil

SUGGESTED READING

Boothe DM: *Small Animal Clinical Pharmacology and Therapeutics*. Philadelphia, WB Saunders, 2001, pp 222–236.

Flatland B, Greene RT, Lappin MR: Clinical and serologic evaluation of cats with cryptococcosis. *J AM Vet Med Assoc* 209:1110–1113, 1996.

Gerds-Grogan S, Dyrell-Hart B: Feline cryptococcosis: A retrospective evaluation. *J Am Anim Hosp Assoc* 33:118–122, 1997.

Jacobs GH, Medleau L, Calvert CC, Brown J: Cryptococcal infection in cats: Factors influencing treatment outcome and results of sequential serum antigen titers in 35 cats. *J Vet Intern Med* 11:1–4, 1997.

Jacobs GJ, Medleau L: Cryptococcosis. In Greene CE (ed): *Infectious Diseases of The Dog and Cat*. Philadelphia, WB Saunders, 1998, pp 383–390.

O'Toole TE, Sato AF, Rozanski EA: Cryptococcosis of the central nervous system in a dog. *J Am Vet Med Assoc* 222(12):1722–1725, 2003.

AUTHOR: **LISA M. TIEBER NIELSON**
EDITOR: **DOUGLASS K. MACINTIRE**

Cryptorchidism

BASIC INFORMATION

DEFINITION

Failure of one or both testicles to descend into the scrotum. Literally, "hidden testicle"

SYNONYM(S)

Monorchid or anorchid (a misnomer, because it technically designates testicular aplasia—complete failure of testicle to develop)
Retained testicle(s)

EPIDEMIOLOGY

SPECIES, AGE, SEX: Intact males, canine and feline. A presumptive diagnosis can be made at 8 weeks, and a definitive diagnosis can be made by 6 months.

GENETICS AND BREED PREDISPOSITION: Considered to be a simple, autosomal recessive trait. Incomplete penetrance and failure of Mendelian probability suggest a multifactoral or polygenic mode of inhertitance.

INCIDENCE
- Mixed-breed dogs ~3.9%
- Purebred dogs ~8.7% (toy and miniature breeds show a significantly higher rate of occurrence)
- Cats (mixed and purebred) ~1.3%

RISK FACTORS
- Familial
- Drugs used during pregnancy with antiandrogen effects: diethylstilbesterol, estradiol cypionate, progestagens, cimetidine, flutamide, finasteride

ASSOCIATED CONDITIONS AND DISORDERS
- Testicular neoplasia: a retained testicle has a 10-fold greater risk of tumorgenesis
- Intersex: male pseudo-hermaphrodite, Klinefelter's syndrome
- Infertility: only if bilaterally cryptorchid

CLINICAL PRESENTATION

DISEASE FORMS/SUBTYPES
- Unilateral: one testicle retained (the right testicle is twice as likely to be retained as the left)
- Bilateral: both testicles retained (less common than unilateral cryptorchidism)
- Abdominal: testicle(s) retained within the abdomen (usually near the internal inguinal ring; rarely at the caudal pole of the kidney)
- Inguinal: testicle(s) retained within the inguinal canal (most common presentation)

HISTORY, CHIEF COMPLAINT
- Absence of one or both testicles in scrotum
- Male breeding behavior in a "neutered" animal

PHYSICAL EXAM FINDINGS: Only one or no testes are palpable within the scrotum. Testes should be easily palpable and normally descended by 8 weeks of age.

ETIOLOGY AND PATHOPHYSIOLOGY

- Testosterone is responsible for testicular descent in three stages of migration—abdominal, inguinal, and scrotal—through the dissolution of the cranial suspensory ligament and contraction of the gubernaculum.
- Testicular descent in cats is complete at birth, but the testicles can move freely into the inguinal canal for up to 6 months.
- Testicular descent in dogs is not completed until approximately 40 days after birth.

DIAGNOSIS

DIFFERENTIAL DIAGNOSIS

- Monorchidism (unilateral testicular aplasia)
- Anorchidism (bilateral testicular aplasia)
- Intersex: male pseudo-hermaphrodite, Klinefelter's syndrome

INITIAL DATABASE

- Palpation. In tense or nervous animals, the testicle(s) may be drawn proximally toward the inguinal canal and may be palpable under sedation or general anesthesia.
- Penile examination. In cats, presence of penile spines indicates circulating androgens most likely of testicular origin.
- Ultrasonography may be useful in evaluating testicles retained in the abdomen.

ADVANCED OR CONFIRMATORY TESTING

In animals where cryptorchidism is suspected but castration history is unknown:
- Exploratory surgery.
- Human chorionic gonadotropin (hCG) stimulation test: measure blood testosterone concentrations before and 24 hours after 750 IU hCG given IV to dogs or cats regardless of body weight. Presence of testicular tissue should yield a twofold increase in testosterone concentration.

TREATMENT

THERAPEUTIC GOAL(S)

- Prevent development of testicular tumors
- Render the animal sterile to prevent propagation of heritable abnormalities
- Remove testosterone-producing tissues to eliminate undesirable male behavior

TREATMENT

Castration:
- Parainguinal approach for inguinally retained testicle(s)
- Abdominal approach for abdominally retained testicle(s)

PROGNOSIS AND OUTCOME

Prognosis for life is excellent. Castration will also eliminate risks of testicular cancer and greatly reduce the risk of prostatic disease.

PEARLS & CONSIDERATIONS

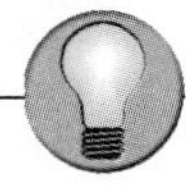

COMMENTS

Surgical correction or medical treatment (using gonadotropin-releasing hormone [GnRH] or hCG) to induce the descent of the aberrant testicle into the scrotum have been reported in dogs (GnRH: two injections 50-100 μg given SC or IV with a 7-day interval; hCG: four injections of 100-1000 IU given IM with a 3- to 4-day interval between injections), but efficacy and ethics of such protocols are suspect. In addition, artificially corrected, cryptorchid testicles have the same 10-fold increased potential for neoplasia as retained testicles.

PREVENTION

- Removal of affected animals from the breeding population results in reduced incidence within the breed.
- The dam and female siblings of affected males may be homozygous or heterozygous carriers.
- The sire and some male siblings will be heterozygous carriers not showing any manifestations of cryptorchidism.

CLIENT EDUCATION

Do not breed animals that are cryptorchid or have sired cryptorchid offspring.

SUGGESTED READING

Johnson S, Root Kustritz M, Olson P: *Canine and Feline Theriogenology*. Philadelphia, WB Saunders, 2001, pp 313-317, 530-532.

Klonisch T, et al: molecular and genetic regulation of testis descent and external genitalia development. *Develop Biol* 270:1-18, 2004.

AUTHOR: **RICHARD WHEELER**
EDITOR: **MICHELLE A. KUTZLER**

Cryptosporidiosis, Gastrointestinal

BASIC INFORMATION

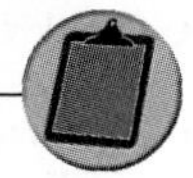

DEFINITION

A primary gastroenterocolitis caused by the ubiquitous coccidian parasite *Cryptosporidia parvum*

EPIDEMIOLOGY

SPECIES, AGE, SEX: Cats of any age and gender can be affected. Canine cryptosporidiosis is almost entirely seen in puppies less than 6 months old.

RISK FACTORS

- Immunosuppression primarily caused by feline leukemia virus (FeLV) and/or feline immunodeficiency virus (FIV): particularly in multicat environments (humane shelters, catteries, etc.)
- Overcrowding raises prevalence of infection since oocysts shed in feces are highly infective
- Adult cats with severe intestinal disease (e.g., inflammatory bowel disease, lymphoma)

CONTAGION AND ZOONOSIS: Exposure and transmission are from fecally contaminated water or food sources. Mammalian species affected with clinical disease are primarily feline, bovine, and human (one canine case only). In immunocompromised humans, cryptosporidiosis is a significant cause of morbidity. Therefore, pets living with these individuals should be screened to ensure that they are not shedding the oocysts.

CLINICAL PRESENTATION

HISTORY, CHIEF COMPLAINT: Chronic diarrhea (see p 297) that is small bowel in character is the main clinical sign in early infection. Vomiting may occur but is less likely. Tenesmus, hematochezia, and weight loss may occur in long-standing infections.

PHYSICAL EXAM FINDINGS: Many cats with cryptosporidiosis have subclinical infection. In cats with overt clinical signs, gas- and fluid-filled intestinal loops can be identified on abdominal palpation; cats may appear thin, unthrifty, and malnourished with chronic disease. Fever usually does not occur.

ETIOLOGY AND PATHOPHYSIOLOGY

- *Cryptosporidium parvum* oocysts are found in feces. They may be shed at any time—during diarrhea, or in the absence of clinical signs—but the incidence of shedding from carriers (not showing signs) is not high.
- Transmission is by fecal-oral route.
- Infection occurs without invasion into intestinal epithelium.
- The mechanism of clinical disease is postulated to be an interruption of normal flora by the parasite and later influx of inflammatory cells into the intestinal epithelium, leading to villous atrophy, secretory diarrhea, and malabsorption.
- The terminal ileum usually has the highest parasite load.

DIAGNOSIS

Routine screening specifically for *Cryptosporidium* is a low-yield procedure given current techniques and the low prevalence of shedding, but testing should be considered in animals with compatible clinical signs and/or immunocompromised pets or owners.

DIFFERENTIAL DIAGNOSIS

- Causes of gastroenterocolitis that prevail in overcrowded conditions: *Giardia* spp., *Cystoisospora* spp., *Tritrichomonas foetus, Toxoplasma gondii, Entamoeba histolytica.*
- Other causes of diarrhea and weight loss: inflammatory bowel disease, gastrointestinal lymphoma, hyperthyroidism.

INITIAL DATABASE

- Complete fecal examination consisting of direct smear, Sheather's solution flotation, and $ZnSO_4$ analysis should always be performed on cats with diarrhea:
  - *Cryptosporidium* oocysts (4 μm; about half the diameter of an erythrocyte) may be identified by light microscopy in direct smear of feces stained with crystal violet.
  - Phase microscopy is usually required on unstained preparations from a Sheather's fecal float.
  - In general, microscopic identification of oocysts requires expertise, is challenging, even with staining or immunofluorescence, and is inferior to enzyme-linked immunosorbent assay (ELISA).
- Complete blood count, serum chemistry, urinalysis, total T_4 analysis, abdominal imaging: if diarrhea and weight loss are present (rule out other disorders).
- FeLV and FIV ELISA.

ADVANCED OR CONFIRMATORY TESTING

- Specimens shipped to commercial laboratories should be sent in a 38% formaldehyde (100% formalin) solution added to feces in a 1:10 dilution to kill oocysts but still allow detection.
- Feline serum cryptosporidial IgG ELISA: highly correlates with exposure to parasite but not necessarily active infection.
- ELISA tests for cryptosporidial antigen in feces of humans and rodents are available. Diagnostic efficacy is unproven in cats and dogs.
- Intestinal biopsy can differentiate from other intestinal disease but is costly, time consuming, and less effective than fecal examination.
- If necropsy is used for primary diagnosis, intestinal samples should be taken within hours after death; otherwise postmortem autolysis will prevent confirmation.

TREATMENT

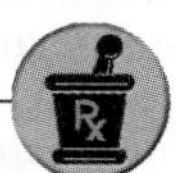

THERAPEUTIC GOAL(S)

- Complete resolution of infection
- Prevention of further oocyst shedding

ACUTE GENERAL TREATMENT

- Initial treatment consists of parenteral fluid therapy to correct hypovolemia, electrolyte imbalances, and acid-base disturbances if present.
- Antiprotozoal and antibiotic agents have been shown to be effective:
  - Azithromycin 7-15 mg/kg PO q 12h for 5 to 7 days. Current drug of choice for treatment of human cryptosporidiosis. Studies in cats have not been performed, but efficacy would be expected.
  - Paromomycin 125-165 mg/kg PO q 12h for 5 days was the traditional drug of choice, but because of side effects, it has fallen from favor.
  - Tylosin 11 mg/kg PO q 12h for 28 days.

CHRONIC TREATMENT

Treatment of concurrent antibiotic-responsive enteritis/small intestinal bacterial overgrowth (metronidazole 10-15 mg/kg PO q 12-24h for 5 to 7 days) may be beneficial in addition to treatment for *Cryptosporidium*.

POSSIBLE COMPLICATIONS

Chronic infection: intestinal intussusception or lymphangiectasia are possible

RECOMMENDED MONITORING

- Fecal analysis after treatment to determine if fecal shedding is still occurring.
- Another fecal analysis may be required if diarrhea persists and/or recurs after treatment.
- Animals with chronic infection should be reevaluated at frequent intervals to assess progress.

PROGNOSIS AND OUTCOME

Prognosis is good with treatment in cats that do not have FeLV/FIV infection

PEARLS & CONSIDERATIONS

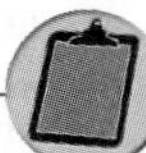

COMMENTS

- This disease occurs in immunocompromised cats.
- Glucocorticoids and other immunosuppressive agents should be avoided until the infection is resolved.

PREVENTION

- This is a disease that is prevalent in overcrowded and unsanitary conditions.
- Reducing environmental contamination with improved sanitation is an important aspect of prevention.
- Although 5% ammonia will kill parasites, it requires 18 hours of contact for effect. Therefore, higher concentrations of ammonia are required if contact time is shortened. Dilute sodium hypochlorite (bleach diluted 1 part bleach:32 parts water) kills *Cryptosporidium*.

CLIENT EDUCATION

- Potential for zoonosis
- Caution with immunosuppressed individuals and young children (greatest potential for infection)

SUGGESTED READING

Barr SC: Cryptosporidiosis and cyclosporiasis. In Greene CE (ed): *Infectious Diseases of the Dog and Cat*. Philadelphia, WB Saunders, 1998, pp 518-524.

Lappin MR: Enteric protozoal diseases. *Vet Clin North Am Small Anim Pract* 35(1):81-88, 2005.

AUTHOR: **SARALYN SMITH-CARR**
EDITOR: **DEBRA L. ZORAN**

Cutaneous Cysts

BASIC INFORMATION

DEFINITION

Variable-sized non-neoplastic masses within the skin, forming saclike structures with an epithelial lining. Identification of cyst origin depends on epithelial lining or the structure from which the cyst developed. Most common are follicular cysts. Dermoid cysts are congenital and hereditary.

SYNONYM(S)

Infundibular cyst (epidermal inclusion cyst, epidermoid cyst, sebaceous cyst)

EPIDEMIOLOGY

SPECIES, AGE, SEX

- Common in dogs, rare in cats.
- Multiple follicular cysts may be noted in young dogs (congenital).
- Solitary follicular cysts may occur at any age.

GENETICS AND BREED PREDISPOSITION

- Follicular cysts: commonly noted in boxers, Doberman pinschers, shih tzus, and miniature schnauzers
- Dermoid cysts: common in boxers, Kerry blue terriers, Rhodesian ridgebacks

ASSOCIATED CONDITIONS AND DISORDERS: Dermoid sinus (Rhodesian ridgebacks). See Pilonidal Cyst, p 851.

CLINICAL PRESENTATION

DISEASE FORMS/SUBTYPES

- Follicular cysts
- Infundibular cysts
- Dermoid cysts

HISTORY, CHIEF COMPLAINT

- Patients often presented for evaluation of a fluctuant to solid, nonpainful, freely movable mass anywhere within the skin.
- Cysts may drain a yellow to brown liquid with caseous material. May refill over time.

PHYSICAL EXAM FINDINGS

- Majority of dogs do not show clinical signs.
- Multiple follicular cysts may be noted over the dorsal midline or pressure points (associated with trauma).
- Solitary follicular cysts are firm to fluctuant dermal or subcutaneous masses; 0.5-5 cm in diameter; often found on the head, neck, sacral area, and proximal limbs.
- Dermoid cysts are solitary or multiple and are found on the dorsal midline.
- Ruptured cysts may be painful and pruritic with evidence of inflammation, infection, and self-trauma.

ETIOLOGY AND PATHOPHYSIOLOGY

- Majority of cysts are follicular and classified as either infundibular, metrical, or of hybrid type, based on whether the cyst develops from the infundibulum of the hair follicle, hair follicle matrix, or a combination of the two, respectively.
- Multiple follicular cysts are thought to be congenital, as are dermoid cysts.
- Solitary follicular cysts may develop because of dermal fibrosis, microtrauma, or blockage of follicular ostia.

DIAGNOSIS

DIFFERENTIAL DIAGNOSIS

- Keratoacanthoma: benign skin tumors, thought to be of follicular origin, that superficially appear very similar to follicular cysts. Usually have a pore with a keratinous plug. May be multiple and generalized
- Papilloma
- Trichofolliculoma
- Cutaneous horn
- Caseous abscess

INITIAL DATABASE AND ADVANCED OR CONFIRMATORY TESTING

- Excisional biopsy and histopathologic examination to determine specific cyst origin and rule out skin neoplasia
- Fine-needle aspirate with impression smears demonstrates sebaceous or keratinous debris

TREATMENT

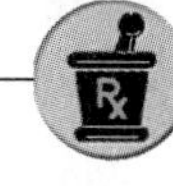

THERAPEUTIC GOAL(S)

Nonrecurrence

ACUTE GENERAL TREATMENT

- Surgical excision
- Observation without treatment

CHRONIC TREATMENT

Retinoids such as isotretinoin (Accutane) 1-2 mg/kg q 12h PO or acitretin (Soriatane) 0.5-1.0 mg/kg PO q 12h may be helpful as prophylactic therapy for multiple follicular cysts.

POSSIBLE COMPLICATIONS

- Cysts may rupture, leading to inflammation, secondary infection, and a foreign body reaction.
- Retinoid therapy: keratoconjunctivitis sicca, conjunctivitis, pruritus, hyperactivity, stiffness, mucocutaneous junction, erythema, vomiting, diarrhea, teratogenicity, elevated liver enzymes.

RECOMMENDED MONITORING

Retinoids: monitor liver enzymes, tear production

PROGNOSIS AND OUTCOME

Good

PEARLS & CONSIDERATIONS

COMMENTS

- Never squeeze a cyst firmly to evacuate it, because this will increase the risk of inward cyst rupture, leading to a foreign body reaction and secondary infection.
- If the client is concerned enough to present the patient for examination of a skin mass, benign neglect should not be encouraged.

SUGGESTED READING

Scott DW, Miller WH, Griffin CE: In Scott DW, Miller WH, Griffen GE (eds): *Muller and Kirk's Small Animal Dermatology*, ed 6. Philadelphia, WB Saunders, 2001, pp 1375–1379.

AUTHORS: **BERNARD D. BOISVERT, JAN A. HALL**
EDITOR: **JAN A. HALL**

Cutaneous Neoplasia

BASIC INFORMATION

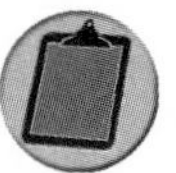

DEFINITION

Neoplasia arising from cells within the skin and adnexa. Skin tumors may be benign or malignant. Most common cutaneous neoplasms in dogs are, in descending order of frequency, lipoma, sebaceous gland hyperplasia, mast cell tumor, histiocytoma, and papilloma. In cats, basal cell tumors are the most common, followed by squamous cell carcinoma and fibrosarcoma. Squamous cell carcinoma is discussed separately (Oral, p 1034; Cutaneous, p 1032).

SYNONYM(S)

Basal cell tumor: basal cell epithelioma
Keratoacanthoma: intracutaneous cornifying epithelioma, infundibular keratinizing acanthoma

EPIDEMIOLOGY

SPECIES, AGE, SEX

- Dog: 30% of all tumors arise within the skin
- Cat: 20% of all tumors arise within the skin
- Median age for cutaneous neoplasia is 10.5 years for dogs and 12 years for cats
- Predilection for histiocytoma in young dogs
- Canine: males predisposed to keratoacanthoma
- Feline: males predisposed to mast cell tumor and hemangioma

GENETICS AND BREED PREDISPOSITION

- Canine breeds with highest incidence of skin tumors include the boxer, Scottish terrier, bullmastiff, basset hound, Kerry blue terrier, and Norwegian elkhound.
- Shar-peis tend to develop mast cell tumors at a younger age (mean 4 years).
- Feline breeds with highest incidence are the Siamese and Persian.
- Keratoacanthoma: The generalized form may have a hereditary basis in Norwegian elkhound and keeshond.

RISK FACTORS

- Basal cell carcinoma: A strong correlation in humans exists with exposure to ultraviolet light and development. This association has not been established in dogs and cats.
- Cutaneous hemangioma/hemangiosarcoma: Short-coated dogs with nonpigmented skin in sun-exposed areas such as the glabrous skin of the ventral abdomen and white cats are at higher risk.

CLINICAL PRESENTATION

DISEASE FORMS/SUBTYPES

- Basal cell tumors: benign or malignant (basal cell carcinoma) tumors arising from the pluripotential basal epithelial cells in the epidermis and adnexa.
- Hemangioma/Hemangiosarcoma: benign or malignant neoplasms arising from endothelial cells of blood vessels.
- Histiocytoma: benign neoplasm that arises from epidermal Langerhans cells.
- Keratoacanthoma: benign neoplasms of hair follicle origin.
- Mast cell tumors: common neoplasms of dogs and cats that arise from mast cells. All mast cell tumors should be considered malignant, because each tumor has metastatic potential.
- Trichoepithelioma: benign neoplasms that arise from keratinocytes that differentiate toward all three segments of the hair follicle.
- Sebaceous gland hyperplasia: epithelial growths arising from sebocytes.

HISTORY, CHIEF COMPLAINT: Solitary to multiple cutaneous masses.

PHYSICAL EXAM FINDINGS

- Basal cell tumor: Solitary, well-circumscribed, firm to cystic, alopecic, commonly ulcerated, often pigmented; mass typically located on the head, neck, shoulders, or thorax. In cats, malignant lesions also can occur on the nasal planum and eyelids.
- Cutaneous hemangioma/hemangiosarcoma: Dermal or subcutaneous, solitary or multiple, oval masses, or red to dark red plaques, usually located along the limbs and ventral abdomen. Feline masses are bluish to reddish-black nodules to plaques.
- Histiocytoma: Solitary, well-circumscribed, firm, erythematous, intradermal nodule found most frequently on the head, limbs, and thorax. Fast growing but benign. Occasionally observed as multiple cutaneous nodules or plaques.
- Keratoacanthoma: Most commonly found on the back, neck, thorax, and limbs. Well-circumscribed dermal or subcutaneous masses with a pore opening to the skin surface; pore usually consists of a keratin plug. Not metastatic.
- Mast cell tumor (Fig. I-51): Highly variable in appearance: most commonly a small, raised, firm, well-circumscribed mass that may be erythematous, alopecic, or ulcerated. However, can appear as any other skin or subcutaneous tumor. Regional distribution: 50% trunk, 40% extremities, 10% head. Darier's sign (local edema and inflammation) can occur on palpation of some lesions. Regional lymphadenopathy may occur; most patients have no systemic signs; splenomegaly and hepatomegaly are features of disseminated mastocytosis. Feline: Variable appearance: solitary to multiple; nodular or papular or plaquelike lesions (see Fig. I-51) in the dermis or subcutis. There may be a positive association between cutaneous mast cell tumors and feline immunodeficiency virus. Variable metastatic potential to lymph nodes and viscera.
- Trichoepithelioma: Usually solitary, solid or cystic, elevated, round, and well-circumscribed; frequently become ulcerated and alopecic.
- Sebaceous gland tumors: Solitary or multiple raised, wartlike to smooth,

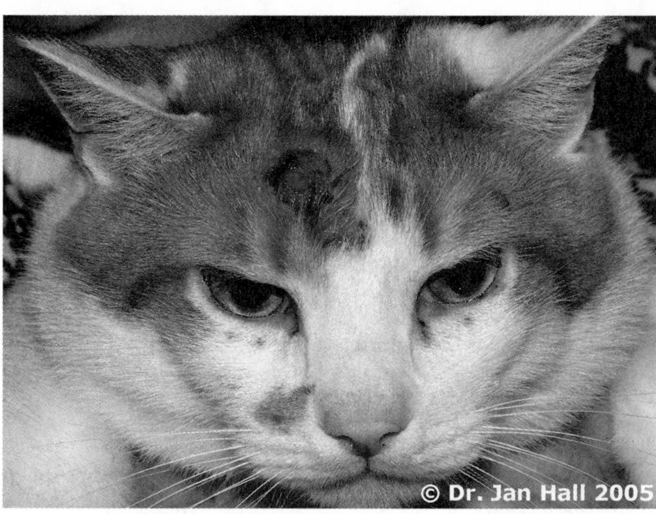

FIGURE I-51 Mast cell tumor on the head of an 8-year-old male, castrated, domestic short-haired cat. Courtesy of Dr. Jan A. Hall.

may ulcerate; most commonly found on limbs, trunk, eyelids, head.

ETIOLOGY AND PATHOPHYSIOLOGY

- Neoplastic transformation relies on changes within specific growth-regulating genes
- Principal growth-regulating genes include:
  - Oncogenes that code for proteins that increase growth
  - Tumor-suppressor genes that decrease proliferation and differentiation

DIAGNOSIS

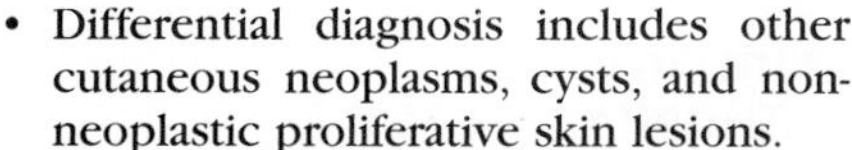

DIFFERENTIAL DIAGNOSIS

- Differential diagnosis includes other cutaneous neoplasms, cysts, and non-neoplastic proliferative skin lesions.
- The only way to distinguish between benign neoplasms from malignant neoplasms and non-neoplastic proliferative skin disease is histopathologic examination of tissue. Malignant lesions show rapid, invasive growth, infiltration, and metastasis.

INITIAL DATABASE

- Complete blood count, serum biochemistry profile, urinalysis: assess systemic abnormalities, if any
- Cytologic exam (fine-needle aspirate):
  - Basal cell tumor: small, round to cuboidal epithelial cells arranged in groups or ribbons. Basal cell carcinomas are difficult to differentiate cytologically from benign lesions.
  - Histiocytoma: sheets of round cells with a pale blue cytoplasm and variable size and shape to the nuclei; variable numbers of neutrophils and lymphocytes depending on stage of growth and involution.
  - Mast cell tumor: round cells with blue to purple granules.
  - Sebaceous gland hyperplasia: clusters of lipid sebocytes.
- Histopathologic exam (biopsy):
  - Basal cell tumor: well-circumscribed, symmetric proliferation of basal epithelial cells that has a broad zone of connection to the overlying epidermis.
  - Basal cell carcinoma: circumscribed, irregular dermal mass comprising multiple epithelial cell aggregates embedded in a fibrous stroma that may extend into the underlying subcutis.
  - Hemangioma: proliferation of blood-filled vascular spaces lined by single layers of well-differentiated endothelial cells.
  - Hemangiosarcoma: invasive proliferation of atypical endothelial cells with areas of vascular space formation.
  - Histiocytoma: uniform sheets and cords of histiocytes infiltrating the dermis and subcutis; characteristic high mitotic index.
  - Keratoacanthoma: keratin-filled crypt in the dermis that has an opening to the skin surface.
  - Mast cell tumor: characterized by a diffuse to multinodular proliferation of mast cells. Histopathologic grading system for dogs (not cats): Grade I-III (III represents most aggressive lesions). Feline cutaneous mast cell tumors can be confused with other round cell tumors and eosinophilic plaques.

ADVANCED OR CONFIRMATORY TESTING

- Abdominal and cardiac ultrasonography to determine if hemangiosarcoma lesions are primary or metastatic.
- See Mast Cell Tumors, Cat, p 683; Mast Cell Tumors, Dog, p 685 regarding diagnostic testing for staging.

TREATMENT

THERAPEUTIC GOAL(S)

Goals of therapy include surgery, chemotherapy, cryotherapy, laser therapy, immunotherapy, and radiotherapy

ACUTE GENERAL TREATMENT

- Basal cell tumor: surgical excision is curative.
- Hemangioma: surgical excision, cryotherapy, or electrosurgery usually curative.
- Hemangiosarcoma: Aggressive surgical excision is treatment of choice; complete excision of subcutaneous tumor is difficult.
- Histiocytoma: Spontaneous remission may occur within 3 months. Surgical excision is curative for lesions that do not regress.
- Keratoacanthoma: May resolve spontaneously. Surgical excision, cryosurgery, or observation without treatment are also options.
- Mast cell tumor (see Mast Cell Tumors, Cat, p 683; Mast Cell Tumors, Dog, p 685): treatment of choice is aggressive surgical excision:
  - Wide surgical excision is necessary. Surgical margins of 3 cm laterally and one fascial plane deep to the tumor are recommended. All surgical margins should be carefully examined to determine if clear margins have been obtained. If the tumor is microscopically present in the surgical margins, then reexcision (3-cm margins) and/or radiation therapy should be performed.
  - For neoplasms located in inoperable regions, radiation therapy is a good palliative choice. When possible, surgery before radiation therapy to reduce tumor volume is advisable.
  - If lymph nodes are affected but no systemic metastasis has occurred, surgical excision of the lymph node followed by chemotherapy is recommended.
  - The presence of abnormal numbers of mast cells in fine-needle aspirate cytologic evaluation of the spleen, liver, or bone marrow, or within buffy coat smears or peripheral blood smears (less reliable), may be indicative of dissemination and the need for systemic chemotherapy.
- Trichoepithelioma: Surgical excision, cryosurgery, electrosurgery, or observation without treatment.
- Sebaceous gland hyperplasia: Surgical excision, cryotherapy, or observation without treatment. May recur after sur-

gery. Sebaceous gland carcinomas rarely metastasize.

CHRONIC TREATMENT

- Hemangiosarcoma: Chemotherapy can be used before surgery to reduce tumor size; median postsurgical survival of 425 days with the use of a regimen including doxorubicin, cyclophosphamide, and vincristine (study of six dogs).
- Mast cell tumor: Prednisone, when used alone, can provide short-term remission. By adding chemotherapeutic agents such as vinblastine and cyclophosphamide, remission to prednisone-sensitive mass cell tumors can be increased. See Mast Cell Tumors, Cat, p 683, Dog, p 685.

POSSIBLE COMPLICATIONS

- Hemangiosarcoma: Local recurrence and metastasis are common in dogs; metastasis is rare in cats.
- Mast cell tumor: gastrointestinal bleeding, bleeding at surgical site, delayed wound healing.

PROGNOSIS AND OUTCOME

- Prognoses for excised basal cell tumor, and trichoepithelioma are generally very good.
- Prognosis for strictly intradermal hemangiosarcoma is excellent, but the prognosis for subcutaneous hemangiosarcoma is poor.
- Prognosis for excised histiocytoma is excellent. However, the generalized form is likely to recur.
- Mast cell tumor: Metastasis occurs in 30% of canine cases; tumors that arise from the prepuce, perineum, scrotum, digits, and mucocutaneous sites are more commonly aggressive and malignant; prognosis is based on tumor growth rate, tumor site, local tumor recurrence, systemic signs, tumor staging, previous chemotherapy, and histologic grading. Solitary feline tumors have excellent prognosis because the majority are benign; < 20% of affected cats experience dissemination, and then the prognosis is poor.

PEARLS & CONSIDERATIONS

COMMENTS

- The most effective way to separate benign neoplasms from malignant neoplasms and non-neoplastic proliferative skin disease is histopathologic examination of tissue.
- The key to successful management is an accurate diagnosis.
- Skin cytology may provide valuable information about the cell type.
- Immunohistochemistry has markedly improved our ability to determine progenitor cells for many skin neoplasms.

CLIENT EDUCATION

Mast cell tumor: Animals that have more than one cutaneous tumor are likely to develop more.

SUGGESTED READING

Morrison W: *Cancer in Dogs and Cats: Medical and Surgical Management.* Baltimore, Williams & Wilkins, 1998, pp 489–511.

Scott D, et al: *Muller and Kirk's Small Animal Dermatology*, ed 6. Philadelphia, WB Saunders, 2001, pp 1236–1414.

AUTHOR: **EDWARD JAZIC**
EDITOR: **JAN A. HALL**

Cyanosis

BASIC INFORMATION

DEFINITION

A bluish or grayish discoloration of the mucous membranes or skin due to hypoxemia

SYNONYM(S)

Oxidized hemoglobin: oxygenated hemoglobin

Reduced hemoglobin: deoxygenated hemoglobin

EPIDEMIOLOGY

SPECIES, AGE, SEX: Dog or cat of any age and either sex.

GENETICS AND BREED PREDISPOSITION: Predispositions for underlying causes.

CLINICAL PRESENTATION

DISEASE FORMS/SUBTYPES

- Generalized cyanosis: all mucous membranes have a bluish tinge
- Regional cyanosis: due to localized hypoxia. Not discussed further

HISTORY, CHIEF COMPLAINT

- Dyspnea
- Exercise intolerance
- Collapse; hind limb collapse (described by owners as unexplained periods of sitting during walks) in cases of cyanosis affecting only the caudal half of the body (differential cyanosis)
- Syncope
- Visible cyanosis noted by owner

PHYSICAL EXAM FINDINGS

- Dyspnea may range in severity from mild to severe, in positive correlation to the severity of the underlying problem.
    - An exception is right-to-left shunting heart disease, which may cause pronounced cyanosis even in a patient with minimal dyspnea.
- Heart murmur possible with some right-to-left shunts (e.g., tetralogy of Fallot).
- Stunted growth if congenital right-to-left cardiac shunts.

ETIOLOGY AND PATHOPHYSIOLOGY

ETIOLOGY

- Severe pulmonary disease (e.g., pneumonia, pulmonary edema, hemorrhage):
    - Ventilation/perfusion (V/Q) mismatch
    - Pulmonary diffusion disorder
- Severe bronchial disease (e.g., asthma)
- Airway obstruction (laryngeal paralysis, elongated soft palate/brachycephalic airway syndrome, foreign body, mass)
- Hypoventilation
- Pulmonary arterial disease (pulmonary hypertension, pulmonary thromboembolism)
- Diminished lung capacity (severe pleural effusion, pneumothorax, intrathoracic mass, obesity)
- Right-to-left shunting heart disease:
    - Cyanosis is usually generalized (tetralogy of Fallot, Eisenmenger's complex, others).
    - Differential cyanosis, with pink oral and conjunctival mucous membranes

and cyanotic vulvar/preputial mucosa, is characteristic of right-to-left shunting patent ductus arteriosus.

PATHOPHYSIOLOGY

- Reduced (deoxygenated) hemoglobin is blue, whereas oxidized (oxygenated) hemoglobin is red.
- Cyanosis appears when there is a substantial quantity of reduced hemoglobin in the blood:
    - The deep blue color of a reduced hemoglobin molecule overwhelms the red color of an oxidized hemoglobin molecule.
    - Therefore, when cyanosis first appears, there is less reduced hemoglobin than oxidized hemoglobin.
    - Typically, in a patient with a normal hematocrit, the presence of cyanosis indicates a blood concentration of reduced hemoglobin of >5 g/dl (normal total blood hemoglobin concentration: 12.4-19.1 g/dl [dog], 8.5-14.4 g/dl [cat]).
- When cyanosis is observed, severe hypoxemia is present. In a patient with a normal hematocrit, cyanosis begins to appear when PaO_2 <50 mmHg, which corresponds to SaO_2 <80%, (normal PaO_2 = 90-100 mmHg when breathing room air; normal SaO_2 >95%).
- It is the *absolute* amount of reduced hemoglobin that determines the presence of cyanosis, not the proportion of total hemoglobin that is reduced. Therefore, anemic animals are cyanotic only when they have a very severe degree of hypoxemia, whereas polycythemic animals can be cyanotic with proportionally less oxidized hemoglobin, or even under normal conditions.
- Carboxyhemoglobin, which is elevated in carbon monoxide poisoning, confers a "cherry-colored flush" to the skin and mucous membranes, and this may mask cyanosis in a severely hypoxemic, carbon monoxide-intoxicated patient.

DIAGNOSIS

DIFFERENTIAL DIAGNOSIS

- Methemoglobinemia, from oxidative injury to red blood cells (e.g., acetaminophen toxicosis in cats):
    - Methemoglobin gives a "muddy" color to the mucous membranes, which may be indistinguishable from cyanosis.
    - Differentiation is possible based on the gross appearance of the blood. A drop of blood is applied to a white paper towel. With cyanosis, the blood is dark blue, whereas with methemoglobinemia, it is chocolate-brown.
- Normal pigmentation/melanin. Differentiation involves evaluation of other, nonpigmented mucous membranes or measurement of an arterial blood gas sample for oxygen content.
- Normal pink mucous membranes observed in certain lighting conditions (e.g., fluorescent lights) may falsely appear cyanotic.

INITIAL DATABASE

- Thoracic and lateral cervical radiographs: identify airway or lung structural lesions
- Complete blood count: identify clues indicating cause (e.g., polycythemia with right-to-left shunts or chronic lung disease)
- Arterial blood gas: confirm hypoxemia
- Echocardiography: identify cardiac shunts
- Oral and pharyngeal exam if upper airway dyspnea or apnea: identify and correct obstruction

TREATMENT

THERAPEUTIC GOAL(S)

Correct critical hypoxemia

ACUTE GENERAL TREATMENT

Oxygen supplementation. Beneficial effect expected in most cases, although right-to-left shunts are minimally to poorly responsive to oxygen supplementation.

CHRONIC TREATMENT

Management or correction of the underlying cause

POSSIBLE COMPLICATIONS

Worsening hypoxemia leading to respiratory arrest

RECOMMENDED MONITORING

- Observation of respiratory effort
- Mucous membrane color
- Pulse oximetry and/or arterial blood gas measurements help to quantify response to treatment but are not a replacement for careful observation of respiratory effort and monitoring of underlying cause

PROGNOSIS AND OUTCOME

- Short term: always guarded, because severe hypoxemia is present.
- Long term: varies widely, depending on underlying cause. Ranges from excellent (e.g., with good response to treatment for lung disease) to poor (e.g., with end-stage heart disease).

PEARLS & CONSIDERATIONS

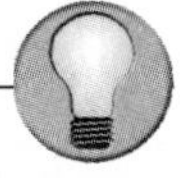

COMMENTS

- Cyanosis depends on the absolute amount of reduced, or deoxygenated, hemoglobin in the circulation. Therefore, anemic animals or animals with hypoperfusion (e.g., shock) are less cyanotic despite severe hypoxemia, whereas polycythemic animals may show cyanosis with minimal hypoxemia.
- A patient with marked cyanosis and minimal dyspnea should be suspected of having right-to-left shunting or a hematologic problem (e.g., methemoglobinemia from oxidative red blood cell injury).

SUGGESTED READING

Guyton AC, Hall JE: Respiratory insufficiency-pathophysiology, diagnosis, oxygen therapy. In Guyton AC, Hall JE (eds): *Textbook of Medical Physiology*, ed 9. Philadelphia, WB Saunders, 1996, pp 543-544.

Lee JA, Drobatz KJ: Respiratory distress and cyanosis in dogs. In King LG (ed): *Textbook of Respiratory Diseases in Dogs and Cats*. St. Louis, WB Saunders, 2004, pp 1-12.

Petrie J-P: Cyanosis. In Ettinger SJ, Feldman EC (eds): *Textbook of Veterinary Internal Medicine*, ed 6. St. Louis, Elsevier, 2005, pp 219-222.

AUTHOR & EDITOR: **ETIENNE CÔTÉ**

Cyclic Thrombocytopenia

BASIC INFORMATION

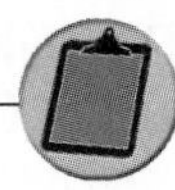

DEFINITION

A tick-borne disease characterized by periodic parasitemia of platelets, leading to intermittent episodes of thrombocytopenia

SYNONYM(S)

Anaplasma platys infection. Formerly canine thrombocytic ehrlichiosis or *Ehrlichia platys* infection.

EPIDEMIOLOGY

SPECIES, AGE, SEX: Dogs. No sex or age predilection.

RISK FACTORS: Dogs at risk for increased tick exposure, especially sporting dogs.

CONTAGION AND ZOONOSIS: Transmitted by tick vectors, such as *Rhipicephalus sanguineus* (brown dog tick); possible transmission via other arthropods. Has not been reported to affect humans.

GEOGRAPHY AND SEASONALITY

- Geographic distribution reflects that of the tick vector.
- Reported worldwide. United States strains considered less pathogenic.

ASSOCIATED CONDITIONS AND DISORDERS: Coinfection with other tick-borne diseases (e.g., *Babesia*, *Borrelia,* other *Ehrlichia* spp.) is common and likely potentiates severity of both diseases.

CLINICAL PRESENTATION

For less pathogenic strains, history and physical exam are often unremarkable. Thrombocytopenia may be an incidental finding on work-up for other disease.

DISEASE FORMS/SUBTYPES: Note that the organism found in the United States rarely causes any clinical signs or hematologic abnormalities other than thrombocytopenia itself. A more virulent strain exists outside the U.S., especially in the Middle East, where affected dogs often present with overt clinical signs.

HISTORY, CHIEF COMPLAINT

- Commonly none (see above)
- When present, may include:
  - Lethargy
  - Anorexia
  - Ocular changes
  - Epistaxis
  - Petechia and ecchymoses
  - Excessive hemorrhage after trauma or surgery (rare)

PHYSICAL EXAM FINDINGS

- Commonly none (e.g., organism may be incidental hematologic finding)
- When present, may include:
  - Pale mucous membranes
  - Mild to severe fever
  - Petechiae/ecchymoses of skin, gums, sclera, mucous membranes
  - Excessive hemorrhage after trauma or surgery
  - Signs of uveitis
  - Hyphema
  - Lymphadenopathy
  - Mucopurulent nasal discharge

ETIOLOGY AND PATHOPHYSIOLOGY

- Ribosomal RNA genetic sequencing has led to reclassification of causative organism. Formerly *Ehrlichia platys* (family Rickettsiaceae). Renamed *Anaplasma platys* (family Anaplasmataceae).
- Two mechanisms of platelet destruction:
  - Direct injury due to replicating organisms.
  - Immune-mediated destruction and clearance.
- Organisms parasitize platelets after incubation period of 8 to 15 days after tick bite.
- Within days, there is rapid decline in platelet numbers, followed by rapid recovery.
- Cycles occur every 1 to 2 weeks, lessening in severity with each recurrence.

DIAGNOSIS

DIFFERENTIAL DIAGNOSIS

- Other tick-borne diseases:
  - *Ehrlichia canis*
  - *Rickettsia rickettsii* (Rocky Mountain spotted fever)
  - *Ehrlichia equi*
- Immune-mediated thrombocytopenia.
- Toxin- or drug-induced thrombocytopenia (cisplatin, cyclophosphamide, chlorambucil, doxorubicin, hydroxyurea).
- Bone marrow suppression/pancytopenia.
- Disseminated intravascular coagulation (DIC).
- Platelet consumption due to internal or external hemorrhage or vasculitis.
- Vaccination with modified live canine distemper vaccine can rarely cause a transient, nonclinical thrombocytopenia.
- Cyclical congenital thrombocytopenia of grey collie dogs (canine cyclic hematopoiesis; see Color Disorders of the Skin and Haircoat, p 228).

INITIAL DATABASE

- Complete blood count (CBC):
  - Thrombocytopenia. Severity can vary, with platelet counts ranging from less than 10,000 to more than 100,000 platelets/fl.
  - Giant platelets often noted.
  - ± Regenerative anemia if extensive hemorrhage.
  - Mild nonregenerative anemia with repeated disease cycles.
  - Mild leukopenia (occasional).
- Serum biochemistry profile: often unremarkable.
- Activated clotting time and buccal mucosal bleeding time will be prolonged with severe thrombocytopenia. Other coagulation test results are within normal limits.
- Bone marrow exam: megakaryocytes normal or increased in number.
- Radiographic imaging of thorax and abdomen: typically unremarkable. Diagnostic imaging is typically indicated in these cases for ruling out other causes of thrombocytopenia such as internal hemorrhage or neoplasia.

ADVANCED OR CONFIRMATORY TESTING

- Giemsa-stained blood smear may demonstrate organisms within platelets, which appear as dark-staining morulae. Organism may be identified in fewer than 10% of affected animals, indicating a high rate of false-negative results.
- Immunocytochemical staining with avidin-biotin can help identify morulae in platelets.
- Serology: indirect immunofluorescent antibody test is available. Does not cross-react with *Ehrlichia canis* antibody test. Monitor convalescent antibody titers every 2 to 3 weeks.

TREATMENT

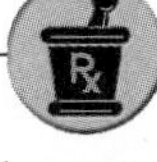

THERAPEUTIC GOAL(S)

- Removal of organisms should be curative
- Focus on supportive care for complications of thrombocytopenia

ACUTE GENERAL TREATMENT

- Drugs of choice: doxycycline (5-10 mg/kg PO or IV q 12h) or tetracycline (20-30 mg/kg PO q 8h).
- Blood transfusion, transfusion of oxygen-carrying solutions, intravenous crystalloid/colloid administration as indicated for acute hemorrhage.
- Platelet-rich-plasma may be administered for severe thrombocytopenia. Expensive, poorly available (refrigerated shelf life = 2 to 3 days), and is often unsuccessful.
- Vincristine: induces thrombocytosis via an unknown mechanism. Give 0.02 mg/kg IV once, maximum once weekly.

CHRONIC TREATMENT

Tick control imperative to prevent reinfection.

DRUG INTERACTIONS

- Common side effects of doxycycline/tetracycline are anorexia, vomiting, and diarrhea.
- Many oral drugs and foods may decrease absorption of oral tetracyclines: aluminum- or calcium-containing antacids, iron products, kaolin-pectin, bismuth salicylate, or milk products. Coadministration of theophylline may enhance adverse gastrointestinal side effects.
- Doxycycline has fewer issues with the listed drug interactions than tetracycline.
- Vincristine can cause sloughing of soft tissues if extravasation occurs during intravenous injection.

RECOMMENDED MONITORING

Serial CBCs q 1-2 weeks post-treatment to monitor recurrence.

PROGNOSIS AND OUTCOME

- Good with effective treatment and less pathogenic strains in most cases.
- Guarded if severe hemorrhage, DIC.

PEARLS & CONSIDERATIONS

COMMENTS

Since coinfection with other tick-borne diseases is common, diagnostics should include work-up for multiple causative agents.

PREVENTION

Tick control is most important.

CLIENT EDUCATION

Has not been reported to affect humans.

SUGGESTED READING

Bradfield JF, Vore SJ, Pryor WHJ: *Ehrlichia platys* infection in dogs. *Lab Anim Sci* 46:5, 1996.

Cohn LA: Ehrlichiosis and related infections. In Macintire DK, Breitschwerdt EB (eds): *The Veterinary Clinics of North America: Small Animal Practice. Emerging and Re-emerging Infectious Diseases.* Philadelphia, WB Saunders, 2003, pp 863-884.

Harvey JW: Thrombocytotropic anaplasmosis. In Greene CE (ed): *Infectious Diseases of the Dog and Cat.* Philadelphia, WB Saunders, 2006, pp 229-231.

AUTHOR: **SHANNON T. STROUP**
EDITOR: **DOUGLASS K. MACINTIRE**

Cystadenoma, Hepatobiliary

BASIC INFORMATION

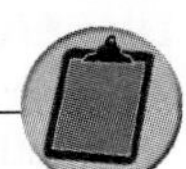

DEFINITION

Benign hepatic tumor primarily seen in older cats that may occur as focal or multifocal cystic lesions of the liver. The cysts are lined by cuboidal, occasionally vacuolated, epithelium. Histogenesis remains uncertain

SYNONYM(S)

Bile duct adenoma
Bile duct cystadenoma
Biliary cystadenoma
Cystadenoma

EPIDEMIOLOGY

SPECIES, AGE, SEX: Primarily cats older than 10 years. No sex predisposition. Rare in dogs.

GENETICS AND BREED PREDISPOSITION: Domestic short-haired cats.

CLINICAL PRESENTATION

DISEASE FORMS/SUBTYPES

- Focal or multifocal hepatic lesions most common.
- Unilocular masses are far less common.

HISTORY, CHIEF COMPLAINT: Abdominal enlargement, lethargy, vomiting, and polydipsia. Patients may show no overt clinical signs, with cystadenomas identified as incidental findings on abdominal palpation, radiographs, or abdominal ultrasound.

PHYSICAL EXAM FINDINGS: Generally unremarkable. Cranial abdominal organomegaly may be noted with very large cystadenomas.

ETIOLOGY AND PATHOPHYSIOLOGY

Etiopathogenesis remains unknown

DIAGNOSIS

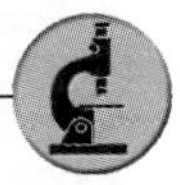

DIFFERENTIAL DIAGNOSIS

Congenital or acquired hepatic cysts, hepatic abscessation, malignant hepatobiliary tumors (e.g., cystadenocarcinoma), metastatic hepatic neoplasia

INITIAL DATABASE

- Serum biochemical profile, complete blood count, and urinalysis are generally unremarkable.
- Abdominal radiographs may prove useful with large cysts that displace surrounding structures.
- Ultrasonography is the diagnostic test of choice. It reveals fluid-filled mass(es) with internal septae, with a variable tissue component. The mass can appear hypoechoic or anechoic due to the cystic nature of the lesion.
- Aspiration of the cystic fluid yields an acellular fluid with a low total protein concentration (<2.0 g/dl).

ADVANCED OR CONFIRMATORY TESTING

- Advanced imaging is generally not indicated.
- Histopathologic evaluation is required for a definitive diagnosis; a presumptive diagnosis may be made by a skilled ultrasonographer.

TREATMENT

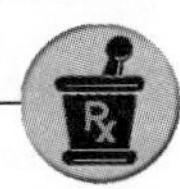

THERAPEUTIC GOAL(S)

Surgical excision if indicated

TREATMENT

- Surgical removal to prevent progressive enlargement and associated clinical signs.
  - The decision to excise the mass must be weighed against the condition of the patient (e.g., patients with comorbid conditions in which cystadenoma is an incidental finding).
- Enteral feeding should be considered postoperatively in patients that are anorectic (esophagostomy or gastrostomy tubes).

POSSIBLE COMPLICATIONS

Hemorrhage and bile leakage and resultant bile peritonitis are potential postoperative complications.

RECOMMENDED MONITORING

Follow-up hepatic ultrasound may be considered to monitor for recurrence in cases with incomplete excision.

PROGNOSIS AND OUTCOME

- Complete tumor excision warrants an excellent prognosis.
- Given the slow-growing nature of the tumor, surgical debulking of nonresectable lesions may provide long-term palliation.

- Hepatobiliary cystadenomas are not known to have malignant potential in veterinary medicine.

PEARLS & CONSIDERATIONS

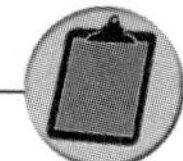

COMMENTS

- Given the potential for malignancy, histopathologic study should be advised for all cystic hepatic lesions.
- Malignant transformation has been reported in humans with hepatobiliary cystadenoma.

PREVENTION

Not applicable given unknown etiology

CLIENT EDUCATION

Percutaneous cyst drainage may be palliative in select cases; however, given the excellent prognosis associated with complete excision, surgical intervention is advised.

SUGGESTED READING

Nyland TG, et al: Ultrasonographic evaluation of biliary cystadenomas in cats. *Vet Radiol Ultrasound* 40:300, 1999.

Trout NJ, et al: Surgical treatment of hepatobiliary cystadenoma in cats: Five cases (1988–1993). *J Am Vet Med Assoc* 206:505, 1995.

AUTHOR: **FRED S. PIKE**

EDITOR: **KEITH P. RICHTER**

Cystitis, Bacterial

BASIC INFORMATION

DEFINITION

Bacterial infection of the urinary bladder

SYNONYM(S)

Bladder infection

Lower urinary tract infection

EPIDEMIOLOGY

SPECIES, AGE, SEX

- Dogs affected more often than cats.
- Females affected more often than males.

RISK FACTORS

- Bladder disease, including cystic calculi and neoplasia
- Congenital or acquired structural defects of the lower urinary tract
- Conditions causing formation of dilute urine, including diabetes mellitus and hyperadrenocorticism
- Immunosuppressive drug therapy, including glucocorticoids
- Disorders of micturition, including urine retention, urinary incontinence, and vulvar (or, rarely, preputial) conformational abnormalities
- Bacteremia
- Urinary catheterization
- Perineal urethrostomy

ASSOCIATED CONDITIONS AND DISORDERS: Diabetes mellitus, hyperadrenocorticism, urinary retention disorders, struvite urolithiasis, nonstruvite urolithiasis, transitional cell carcinoma, glucocorticoid therapy, ectopic ureter, urachal diverticulum, urethral stenosis, vaginitis, prostatitis, pyelonephritis, neurogenic urine retention.

CLINICAL PRESENTATION

DISEASE FORMS/SUBTYPES

- Uncomplicated: infection in the absence of structural or functional host defects.
- Complicated: infection in a host with structural or functional defects (see Risk Factors)
- Recurrent: repeated infections with the same or different species of bacteria.
- Persistent: continued infection with the same bacteria despite antibiotic treatment.

HISTORY, CHIEF COMPLAINT

- Clinical signs may be absent.
- When present:
  - Pollakiuria
  - Stranguria/dysuria
  - Hematuria
  - Inappropriate elimination
  - Malodorous urine
  - Perivulvar dermatitis

PHYSICAL EXAM FINDINGS

- Usually unremarkable
- Occasionally:
  - Painful bladder
  - Palpably thickened urethra on rectal exam (if concurrent urethritis)
  - Findings related to predisposing illness or condition (e.g., findings suggestive of endocrine disorder, urolithiasis, prostatitis)

ETIOLOGY AND PATHOPHYSIOLOGY

- Infecting bacteria usually ascend through the urethra to the bladder, but hematogenous infection or infection from pyelonephritis is possible.
- Bacterial virulence factors and numbers influence likelihood of infection. Flora adapted for preputial and vaginal environments are protective from uropathogenic infection.
- Multiple physical (e.g., intact uroepithelium, voiding action of urination, urethral pressure and length), chemical (e.g., urine osmolality, urea content, pH), and immunologic host defenses protect from infection. Disruption or defects in these defenses predispose to infection.
- The most common pathogens are *Escherichia coli*, *Staphylococcus*, *Proteus*, *Enterococcus*, *Klebsiella*, *Streptococcus*, *Enterobacter*, and *Pseudomonas*. Only ~20% of infections involve more than one species.
- Bacterial resistance to antibiotics can be problematic. Resistance may be inherent or may result from genetic transfer of resistance factors or from mutation and selection pressures.

DIAGNOSIS

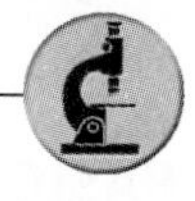

DIFFERENTIAL DIAGNOSIS

- Urolithiasis
- Prostatitis
- Lower urinary tract neoplasia
- Feline lower urinary tract signs/disease/interstitial cystitis
- Obstructive uropathy

INITIAL DATABASE

- Complete blood count: may reflect predisposing illness or condition.
- Serum biochemistry profile: may reflect predisposing illness or condition.
- Urinalysis: bacteriuria, pyuria, hematuria, proteinuria. Sample should be obtained via midstream catch, clean catheterization, or cystocentesis (ideal):
  - May reflect predisposing illness or condition (e.g., crystals, glucosuria).
  - Sediment exam may be inactive despite infection, especially with diabetes mellitus, hyperadrenocorticism, or other conditions producing dilute urine.
  - "Leukocyte" squares on urine dipstick are notoriously inaccurate.
- Gram stain of urine sediment.
- Urine culture/sensitivity:
  - Samples should be collected via clean catheterization or cystocentesis (ideal). If urine is collected via catheter, bacterial number should be quantified to distinguish contamination ($<10^3$ bacteria/ml) from infection.
  - Although preferred, culture is not necessary for first occurrence of uncomplicated infection.
  - Culture/sensitivity should always be obtained from complicated, recurrent, or persistent infection.

- An inactive sediment does not eliminate the need for culture and sensitivity, because many concurrent disorders produce dilute urine, limit leukocyte responses in the urine, or both, producing a negative microscopic sediment exam despite active cystitis.

ADVANCED OR CONFIRMATORY TESTING

- Reserved for complicated, recurrent, or resistant infection
- Abdominal radiographs: radiopaque uroliths, prostatomegaly, rarely emphysematous cystitis
- Abdominal ultrasound: identify radiolucent uroliths, thickened bladder wall or mass, evidence of pyelonephritis or prostatic disease
- Urinary contrast studies: identify radiolucent uroliths, bladder mass, evidence of pyelonephritis, urethral abnormalities

TREATMENT

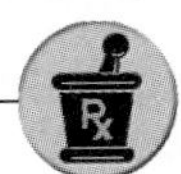

THERAPEUTIC GOAL(S)

- Eliminate infection
- Address predisposing illnesses or conditions

ACUTE GENERAL TREATMENT

Several antibiotic choices are appropriate for empiric treatment of uncomplicated infection, or pending culture/sensitivity results in complicated infection:

- Gram-positive infections: amoxicillin (15-20 mg/kg PO q 8-12h) or amoxicillin-clavulanic acid (10 mg/kg PO q 12h).
- Gram-negative infections: trimethoprim/sulfadiazine ([TMS]; 15-30 mg/kg q 12h) or enrofloxacin (5-10 mg/kg q 12h).
  - In cats, a maximum enrofloxacin dosage of 5 mg/kg/day is recommended to reduce the risk of ocular toxicity (permanent retinal degeneration).

CHRONIC TREATMENT

- Predisposing illnesses or conditions should be addressed.
- Duration of antibiotic therapy:
  - Uncomplicated: 7 to 14 days.
  - Complicated: 4 weeks or more.
- Antibiotic therapy is adjusted based on in vitro susceptibility results while considering cost effectiveness, potential adverse reactions, and the likelihood of developing resistance.
- Multidrug resistant *E. coli* infections may be encountered in complicated or persistent infections. Susceptibility may be limited to expensive, potentially toxic, or parenterally administered antibiotics:
  - Amikacin (5-10 mg/kg SQ [or IV, IM] q 24h) or gentamicin (2-6 mg/kg SQ [or IV, IM] q 24h):
    - Nephrotoxic.
    - Avoid use in dehydrated animals or those with compromised renal function.
  - Imipenem-cilastatin (2-5 mg/kg SQ [or IV,IM] q 8h):
    - Although not an approved route of administration, the 250- or 500-mg powder for injection may be diluted in 10 ml of saline and the appropriate dose of the resultant solution given SQ.
  - The vial may be kept refrigerated for up to 24 hours.
  - Expensive.

POSSIBLE COMPLICATIONS

- Emphysematous cystitis: uncommon complication resulting in gas formation in bladder wall; most often identified in diabetic animals.
- Pyelonephritis: vesicoureteral junction usually prevents bacterial ascension to kidneys.
- Urolithiasis: especially struvite.
- Adverse reactions to antibiotics are possible (e.g., TMS may cause keratoconjunctivitis sicca, gentamicin is nephrotoxic, enrofloxacin is detrimental to cartilage in growing dogs and, in high doses, may irreversibly damage the feline retina).

RECOMMENDED MONITORING

- For uncomplicated infection, urinalysis should be repeated just before discontinuing antibiotic. If sediment is inactive, antibiotic may be stopped, and analysis should again be evaluated 2 to 3 weeks later.
- For recurrent or relapsing infection, urine culture is repeated 3 to 5 days after initiation of appropriate antibiotic and again 2 to 3 weeks after completion of course. Urine sediment should be inactive just before discontinuing antibiotic. If it is not, culture is repeated.
- For animals with continuing predisposing illness or conditions, periodic urine culture may be warranted even without signs of lower urinary tract disease. Inactive sediment exam cannot be substituted for urine culture in animals with diabetes mellitus, hyperadrenocorticism, or dilute urine from any cause.

PROGNOSIS AND OUTCOME

- Prognosis of uncomplicated infection is excellent
- Prognosis of complicated infection depends on ability to correct predisposing illness or condition

PEARLS & CONSIDERATIONS

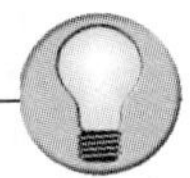

COMMENTS

- Any bacterial cystitis in a male dog should be viewed as a complicated infection.
- Struvite crystalluria in dogs is most commonly due to bacterial urinary tract infection or delayed microscopic examination of the sediment, and virtually never is related to diet.
- Lower urinary tract signs in cats are seldom caused by bacterial cystitis (<5% of cats age 10 years or younger with lower urinary tract signs have bacterial cystitis), making empiric antibiotic therapy inappropriate in cats. Therefore, urine from such cats should first be cultured to rule out an infectious contribution.
- Concurrent pyelonephritis commonly occurs in the absence of "classic" signs such as signs of lumbar pain, intermittent fever, or neutrophilia. The absence of these signs in a patient with recurrent bacterial cystitis should not defer an evaluation for pyelonephritis (e.g., abdominal ultrasound).
- Many antibiotics are present in high concentration in the urine as a result of renal excretion:
  - Disk diffusion assays of sensitivity evaluate expected serum drug concentration, so sensitivity of a uropathogen in vivo may be greater than that predicted in vitro.
  - If expected urine concentration of antibiotic exceeds minimum inhibitory concentration by four times, the antibiotic should be effective.
- Persistent bacterial cystitis usually results from either inappropriate choice of antibiotic or inadequate dose/duration of administration, emergence of bacterial resistance to the chosen antibiotic, or failure to correct underlying illness or condition allowing infection to occur.

PREVENTION

- Correction of predisposing illness or conditions is the most effective strategy to prevent infection.
- For animals in which predisposing factors cannot be corrected and recurrent infections are problematic, prophylactic antibiotic use or urinary antiseptics may be warranted:
  - Antibiotics: one third to one half of usual daily dose amoxicillin, TMS, or fluoroquinolone administered once daily before bed.
  - Antiseptics (dogs):
    - Methenamine mandelate (10 mg/kg PO q 6-8h) or methenamine hippurate (500 mg PO q 12h).
    - Both effective in acidic urine; may require addition of ammonium

chloride as acidifying agent (60–100 mg/kg q 12h). Caution: urinary acidification may precipitate formation of certain uroliths.

CLIENT EDUCATION

Antibiotics should be given as prescribed to completion even if clinical signs resolve quickly.

SUGGESTED READING

Bartges JW: Diagnosis of urinary tract infections. *Vet Clin North Am Small Anim Pract* 34:923, 2004.

Cohn LA, et al: Trends in fluoroquinolone resistance of bacteria isolated from canine urinary tracts. *J Vet Diag Invest* 15:338, 2003.

Forrester SD, et al: Retrospective evaluation of urinary tract infection in 42 dogs with hyperadrenocorticism or diabetes mellitus or both. *J Vet Intern Med* 13:557, 1999.

Seguin MA, et al: Persistent urinary tract infections and reinfections in 100 dogs (1989–1999). *J Vet Intern Med* 17:622, 2003.

AUTHOR & EDITOR: **LEAH A. COHN**

Cystitis, Fungal/Algal

BASIC INFORMATION

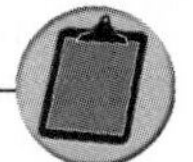

DEFINITION

Infection of the urinary tract by fungal or algal organisms (most commonly *Candida* sp.). Infections can be primary (confined to the urinary tract) or secondary (systemic or disseminated infection).

SYNONYM(S)

Candiduria
Fungal urinary tract infection
Funguria

EPIDEMIOLOGY

SPECIES, AGE, SEX: Reported in dogs and cats. Secondary algal infections only reported in dogs. No age predilection, but associated risk factors more common in older animals. Females possibly at increased risk.

RISK FACTORS: Diabetes mellitus; urinary tract stoma formation (e.g., perineal urethrostomy); urinary tract catheterization; concurrent lower urinary tract disease (e.g., neoplasia, recurrent bacterial cystitis); prolonged antibiotic administration; immunosuppressive drug administration (e.g., glucocorticoids, chemotherapeutics).

CONTAGION AND ZOONOSIS: No zoonotic risk because organisms are ubiquitous in the environment.

ASSOCIATED CONDITIONS AND DISORDERS: Fungal pyelonephritis; fungal septicemia; disseminated/systemic fungal or algal infection.

CLINICAL PRESENTATION

DISEASE FORMS/SUBTYPES

- Primary fungal cystitis: infection confined to bladder/lower urinary tract.
- Fungal pyelonephritis: infection of renal pelvis and parenchyma. Usually due to ascending lower urinary tract infection.
- Secondary fungal/algal cystitis: Urinary shedding of fungal or algal organisms due to systemic/disseminated infection with renal involvement.

HISTORY, CHIEF COMPLAINT

- Primary fungal cystitis often produces no overt clinical signs.
- Lower urinary tract disease signs (dysuria, pollakiuria, stranguria) possible.
- Clinical signs associated with renal failure (see Chronic Renal Failure, Occult ["Asymptomatic"], p 204; Chronic Renal Failure, Overt ["Symptomatic"], p 205) may accompany fungal pyelonephritis or secondary infection.
- Signs of other organ system disease may occur with secondary fungal/algal cystitis.

PHYSICAL EXAM FINDINGS

- Primary fungal cystitis or pyelonephritis: usually unremarkable
- Secondary fungal/algal cystitis: depends on organism and distribution (See Aspergillosis, p 87; Cryptococcosis, p 259; Protothecosis, p 903)

ETIOLOGY AND PATHOPHYSIOLOGY

- Primary fungal cystitis: Disruption of urinary tract defense mechanisms allows ascending infection from genital mucosa and environment:
  - Pyelonephritis results when organisms ascend from the bladder to renal pelvis.
  - Reported primary fungal infections include those caused by *Candida* sp.; *Cryptococcus neoformans; Trichosporon* sp., *Rhodotorula* sp.
- Secondary fungal/algal cystitis: disseminated/systemic infection that includes colonization of the kidneys results in urinary shedding of organisms.
  - Fungal organisms isolated from urine in dogs or cats with disseminated infections: *Acremonium* sp.; *Aspergillus* sp.; *Blastomyces dermatiditis*; *Candida* sp.; *Cryptococcus neoformans; Paecilomyces* sp.; *Penicillium* sp.; *Phialemonium obovatum*; *Trichosporon* sp.
  - Algal organisms isolated from urine in dogs with disseminated infections: *Prototheca wickerhamii; Prototheca zopfii*.

DIAGNOSIS

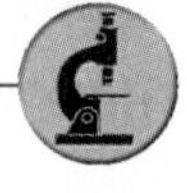

DIFFERENTIAL DIAGNOSIS

Differentials for fungal elements in urine: contamination from genital mucosa, contamination from skin, primary or secondary infection

INITIAL DATABASE

- Complete blood count and chemistry profile:
  - Unremarkable with primary fungal cystitis.
  - Changes associated with renal failure may occur with pyelonephritis or disseminated infection.
- Urinalysis:
  - Organisms may be seen on urine sediment examination or urine cystospin preparations.

ADVANCED OR CONFIRMATORY TESTING

- Urine culture:
  - Identification of fungal or algal organisms in urine sediment should be followed by urine culture (cystocentesis).
  - Most fungal and algal organisms grow readily on standard culture media.
    - *Candida* sp. (most commonly isolated agent) grows on blood agar within 2 to 3 days.
    - Other fungal organisms may require culture for longer periods.
  - Speciation requires culture on specific media (e.g., Sabouraud's).
- Antifungal drug susceptibility testing.
  - Recommended for *Candida albicans* infections that do not respond to standard therapy

- Recommended for all non-*C. albicans* fungal infections (including non-*C. albicans* candidal infections) because of likelihood of resistance.
- Recommended for *Prototheca zopfii* infections, because reported cases have had widely varying susceptibility patterns.

TREATMENT

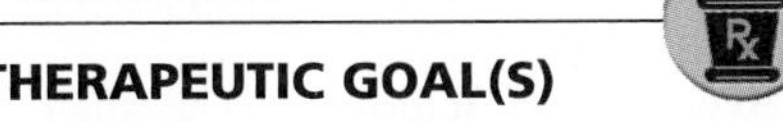

THERAPEUTIC GOAL(S)

- Resolution or control of predisposing conditions
- Elimination of infection using antifungal drugs

ACUTE GENERAL TREATMENT

- Primary *C. albicans* infections: Fluconazole 5 mg/kg PO q 12h.
- Primary non-*C. albicans* candidal infections, other fungal agents, and secondary/systemic fungal and algal infections: drug therapy based on susceptibility testing.
  - Primary infections: start fluconazole while waiting for susceptibility results.
  - Secondary/systemic infections: start itraconazole while waiting for susceptibility.

CHRONIC TREATMENT

- Primary fungal infections treated as "complicated" infections:
  - Reculture urine 1 to 2 weeks after starting therapy to assess efficacy.
  - Continue treatment until two successive negative urine cultures, 2 weeks apart.
- If infection does not respond or recurs, repeat susceptibility testing.
- Intravesicular clotrimazole infusion recently described:
  - Comparative trials are lacking.
  - Suggested protocol:
    - Place Foley catheter, empty bladder.
    - Infuse 5-10 ml/kg 1% clotrimazole solution.
    - Solution should be retained for a minimum of 30 minutes if possible.
    - Repeat q 1 wk for 3 to 4 weeks.
    - Maintain patient on oral antifungal therapy between infusions.

POSSIBLE COMPLICATIONS

Primary infections may progress to pyelonephritis or disseminated/systemic infection.

RECOMMENDED MONITORING

Culture urine regularly (q 2-4 months) after resolution to monitor for recurrence

PROGNOSIS AND OUTCOME

- Primary fungal infections are very difficult to treat; prognosis is fair.
  - Intravesicular clotrimazole infusion protocol may improve treatment success in the future.
- Prognosis for secondary nonbacterial cystitis due to disseminated/systemic infections is poor.

PEARLS & CONSIDERATIONS

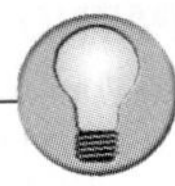

COMMENTS

- Control or elimination of predisposing factors is critical for resolution of fungal infections.
- Patients with nonbacterial cystitis should be screened for diabetes mellitus and concurrent lower urinary tract diseases.
- Urine culture in animals suspected of having disseminated or systemic fungal or algal disease is a noninvasive method of organism identification.

SUGGESTED READING

Jin Y, et al. Fungal urinary tract infections in the dog and cat: A retrospective study (2001-2004). *J Am Anim Hosp Assoc* 41:373, 2005.

Pressler BM, et al: *Candida* spp. urinary tract infections in 13 dogs and 7 cats: Predisposing factors, treatment, and outcome. *J Am Anim Hosp Assoc* 39:263, 2003.

Pressler BM, et al: Urinary tract manifestations of protothecosis in dogs. *J Vet Intern Med* 19:115-119, 2005.

Toll J, et al: Intravesicular administration of clotrimazole for treatment of candiduria in a cat with diabetes mellitus. *J Am Vet Med Assoc* 223:1156, 2003.

Watt PR, et al: Disseminated opportunistic fungal disease in dogs: 10 cases (1982-1990). *J Am Vet Med Assoc* 207:67, 1995.

AUTHOR: **BARRAK M. PRESSLER**

EDITOR: **LEAH A. COHN**

Cytauxzoonosis

BASIC INFORMATION

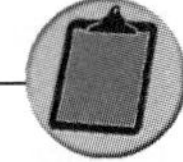

DEFINITION

Cytauxzoon felis is a protozoal organism transmitted by ticks that causes fatal illness in domestic cats.

- Piroplasm: the form of the organism that is found in red blood cells.
- Merozoite: the free organisms that are released when the macrophage ruptures. These become piroplasms when they enter circulating red blood cells.
- Schizont: the asexual reproductive phase of the organism that occurs (via binary fission) within macrophages that have phagocytized infective organisms transmitted by the tick vector.

EPIDEMIOLOGY

SPECIES, AGE, SEX: *C. felis* infects only felidae (both domestic and wild cats). There is no age or sex predilection.

RISK FACTORS: Outdoor cats with tick exposure in endemic areas are at risk.

CONTAGION AND ZOONOSIS: Extensive investigation of *C. felis* has shown that nonfelidae species, including humans, cannot be infected.

GEOGRAPHY AND SEASONALITY: *C. felis* infection has been reported in the south-central and southeastern United States.

CLINICAL PRESENTATION

DISEASE FORMS/SUBTYPES: Until recently, almost all reported cases of *C. felis* in domestic cats were fatal. The existence of a less virulent strain is now suspected, because erythroparasitemia has been detected in cats in Oklahoma with no history of clinical illness.

HISTORY, CHIEF COMPLAINT: Clinical signs are acute and nonspecific and include anorexia, lethargy, dyspnea, icterus, and pallor.

PHYSICAL EXAM FINDINGS: Affected cats are usually febrile (103-107°F [39.4-41.7°C]), but hypothermia is seen in moribund, terminally ill cats. Abdominal palpation reveals splenomegaly and hepatomegaly. Tachypnea, tachycardia, altered mentation, vocalization, seizures, and coma can be seen in the later stages of disease. Most cats exhibit a rapid course, with death occurring within 1 week of onset of signs.

ETIOLOGY AND PATHOPHYSIOLOGY

- The natural host is thought to be the eastern bobcat (*Lynx rufus rufus*), which develops a mild or subclinical infection compared to the rapidly progressive and usually fatal disease seen in domestic cats.
- The organism is transmitted by the *Dermacentor variabilis* tick during feeding.
- Organisms are phagocytized by macrophages and carried to various tissues (liver, spleen, lung, and lymph nodes).
- Asexual reproduction occurs within the host macrophage during the schizont phase. Schizonts occlude venules, causing organ failure and clinical illness.
- When the schizonts rupture, merozoites are released to infect erythrocytes.
- Organisms must be ingested by a tick to produce the virulent schizont form that is infective to cats.

DIAGNOSIS

DIFFERENTIAL DIAGNOSIS

- Immune-mediated hemolytic anemia
- *Mycoplasma hemofelis* infection (formerly hemobartonellosis)
- Feline leukemia virus infection
- Feline immunodeficiency virus
- Feline infectious peritonitis
- Feline cholangiohepatitis
- Toxoplasmosis

INITIAL DATABASE

- Blood smear: Piroplasms usually appear as 1-1.5-μm signet rings, "safety pins," or chains of cocci in red blood cells. Infected macrophages may also be seen on the feathered edge.
- Complete blood count: normocytic, normochromic, nonregenerative anemia ± leukopenia and thrombocytopenia.
- Serum chemistry profile: elevated liver enzymes, hyperbilirubinemia, azotemia, hyperglycemia, and electrolyte or acid-base disturbances are common.
- Abdominal radiographs or ultrasound reveal splenomegaly and hepatomegaly but do not contribute directly to the diagnosis.
- Urinalysis reveals bilirubinuria.
- Coagulation testing may be consistent with disseminated intravascular coagulation (DIC).

ADVANCED OR CONFIRMATORY TESTING

- Bone marrow aspiration and cytologic study reveal macrophages laden with schizonts.
- Fine-needle aspirates of lymph nodes, liver, or spleen may reveal *C. felis* organisms.

TREATMENT

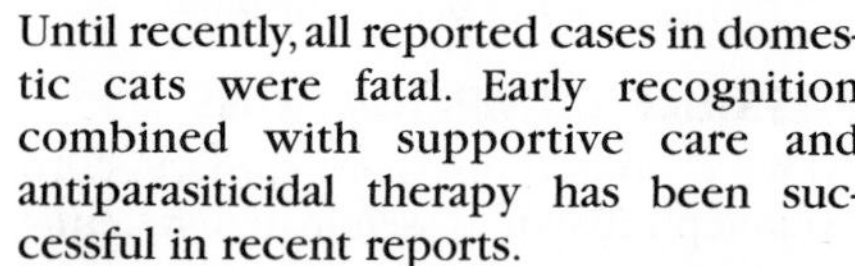

THERAPEUTIC GOAL(S)

Until recently, all reported cases in domestic cats were fatal. Early recognition combined with supportive care and antiparasiticidal therapy has been successful in recent reports.

ACUTE GENERAL TREATMENT

- Crystalloid fluids are given to correct dehydration, restore intravascular volume, and maintain perfusion.
- In anemic animals, oxygen delivery to tissues must be restored with a transfusion of whole blood, packed red blood cells, or polymerized hemoglobin (e.g., Oxyglobin), 20 ml/kg IV administered over 4 hours.
- Some clinicians treat DIC with heparin (150-250 IU/kg SC q 8h or 18 IU/kg/h IV CRI [constant rate infusion]).
- Antiprotozoal therapy:
  - Imidocarb dipropionate (Imizol, Schering-Plough, Kenilworth, N.J.): 5 mg/kg IM repeated in 7 to 14 days after pretreatment with atropine (0.04 mg/kg SC) to minimize cholinergic side effects. (Efficacy not proven.)
  - Diminazene aceturate (Ganaseg, ER Squibb, Princeton, N.J.).
  - Doxycycline (5 mg/kg PO q 12-24h × 14 days) is recommended as treatment for coinfection with other tick-borne pathogens.

CHRONIC TREATMENT

- There is currently no treatment recommended to reduce the carrier state, because this is usually not seen in domestic cats.
- A recent report of 18 parasitemic cats that survived may indicate a less virulent strain in Oklahoma.

PROGNOSIS AND OUTCOME

- Death usually occurs within 1 to 3 weeks after infection or within 1 week of developing clinical signs.
- Circulating parasitemia is often a terminal finding.
- Hypothermia, icterus, severe anemia, and collapse warrant a poor prognosis.

PEARLS & CONSIDERATIONS

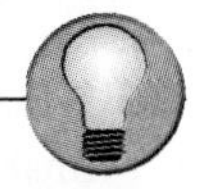

COMMENTS

Clinical suspicion and early diagnosis through tissue aspiration and cytology have resulted in successful response to treatment.

PREVENTION

In endemic areas, an effective acaricide and tick repellent should be used to prevent exposure to ticks.

CLIENT EDUCATION

Outdoor cats in areas where bobcats roam are at risk for this deadly disease.

SUGGESTED READING

Greene CE, et al: Administration of diminazene aceturate or imidocarb diproprionate for treatment of cytauxzoonosis in cats. *J Am Vet Med Assoc* 215 (4):497-500, 1999.

Kier AB, Greene CE: Cytauxzoonosis. In Greene CE (ed): *Infectious Diseases of the Dog and Cat*. St. Louis, WB Saunders, pp 470-473, 1998.

Meinkoth J, et al: Cats surviving natural infection with *Cytauxzoon felis*: 18 cases (1997-1998). *J Vet Intern Med* 14 (5):521-525, 2000.

AUTHOR & EDITOR: **DOUGLASS K. MACINTIRE**

Dacryocystitis

BASIC INFORMATION

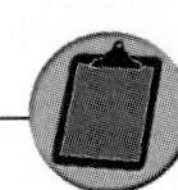

DEFINITION

Although dacryocystitis is technically inflammation of the lacrimal sac, the term is commonly used for describing inflammation anywhere along the tear drainage (i.e., nasolacrimal) system, including the lacrimal puncta, canaliculi, lacrimal sac, and nasolacrimal duct. Dacryocystitis is an acquired condition resulting in ocular discharge (see Ocular Discharge, p 762).

EPIDEMIOLOGY

SPECIES, AGE, SEX

- Dogs and cats
- No age or sex predisposition

GENETICS AND BREED PREDISPOSITION

- Brachycephalic breeds (lacrimal stasis): most common conformation associated with dacryocystitis
- Some extremely dolichocephalic breeds (Doberman pinschers, collies, etc.) also have poor tear drainage and stasis due to a small, deeply set eye and loss of eye to lid contact in the medial canthal area

RISK FACTORS

- The most common causes of dacryocystitis in dogs and cats are foreign bodies, such as plant awns, that become lodged in the nasolacrimal system, and descending infections due to poor conformation and subsequent lacrimal stasis.
- Animals that spend time outdoors are at increased risk.

GEOGRAPHY AND SEASONALITY

- Areas with an abundance of plants
- Increased incidence in spring and summer

CLINICAL PRESENTATION

HISTORY, CHIEF COMPLAINT

- Ocular discharge (serous, mucoid, purulent, or a combination)
- Owner may report swelling and/or draining tract in skin ventral to medial canthus

PHYSICAL EXAM FINDINGS: Ocular discharge in the form of tears, mucus, or pus with any or all of the following:

- Conjunctivitis.
- Lacrimal punctal foreign body.
- Swelling and signs of pain in the medial canthal area.
- If sufficiently chronic, fistulous tracts may be present in the medial canthal area.

ETIOLOGY AND PATHOPHYSIOLOGY

- Most common cause of dacryocystitis is migration of foreign bodies, most frequently plant material, into the nasolacrimal system.
- Descending infections from ocular surface flora, often associated with poor tear drainage and lacrimal stasis, also incriminated with initiating inflammation.

DIAGNOSIS

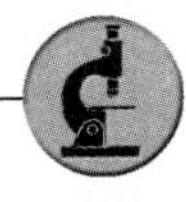

DIFFERENTIAL DIAGNOSIS

- Other causes of blockage of the nasolacrimal system:
  - Congenital disorders including micropunctum or imperforate lacrimal punctum
  - Acquired disorders including traumatic lacerations, or neoplastic invasion or compression of the nasolacrimal drainage apparatus
- Other causes of ocular discharge (see Ocular Discharge, p 762)

INITIAL DATABASE

- Complete ophthalmic examination including:
  - Schirmer tear test (rule out keratoconjunctivitis sicca [KCS; see p 614] as cause for ocular discharge). Normal >15 mm after 1 minute in dogs, variable in cats.
  - Fluorescein dye application.
    - Rule out corneal ulceration as cause for ocular discharge.
    - Fluorescein dye application also tests for nasolacrimal system patency.
      - Dye normally traverses the nasolacrimal apparatus to exit the nares within 5 minutes (dogs and cats).
      - Visualization of the dye in the nares can be assisted with a Wood's lamp (dye fluoresces).
      - False-negative results may occur if animal licks dye from nares before dye is visualized or dye may drain caudally into nasopharynx (mainly brachycephalic breeds).
- Nasolacrimal flushing if suspect complete or partial nasolacrimal duct blockage:
  - May be done under firm restraint with topical ocular anesthesia (e.g., proparacaine 0.5%) (dogs).
  - Resistant animals or signs of discomfort warrant routine preanesthetic evaluation and subsequent sedation or general anesthesia (cats have small lacrimal puncta).
  - Lacrimal puncta can be cannulated, not distal nasal puncta (dogs and cats), which are difficult to identify in many or most individuals irrespective of dacryocystitis.
  - Identify dorsal and ventral lacrimal puncta (oval in dog and round in cat, with or without circumferential pigment), 1 to 2 mm from eyelid margin in palpebral conjunctiva near medial canthus.
  - Gently insert cannula or intravenous catheter (stylet removed; 22 to 24 gauge, dogs; 24 to 26 gauge, cats), with 3-ml syringe filled with sterile saline or eyewash attached, approximately 3 mm into the dorsal lacrimal punctum.
  - Slowly inject the saline/eyewash until it flows from the ventral lacrimal punctum (confirms puncta, canaliculi, and lacrimal sac are patent).
  - Next occlude ventral lacrimal punctum with digital pressure and flush 3 to 12 ml saline/eyewash through the nasolacrimal duct.
  - Collect fluid/discharge at naris in sterile basin.
- Culture and sensitivity testing of purulent discharge, if present.
- Consider referral to a veterinary ophthalmologist if unable to establish patency of nasolacrimal system.

ADVANCED OR CONFIRMATORY TESTING

- Dacryocystorhinography (contrast study of nasolacrimal system) with standard radiography can identify an obstruction site.
- Recently, computed tomography-dacryocystorhinography has been demonstrated to allow highly accurate characterization of lesions obstructing the nasolacrimal duct.

TREATMENT

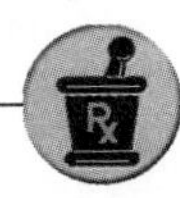

THERAPEUTIC GOAL(S)

Determine nature and location of obstruction and relieve it

ACUTE GENERAL TREATMENT

- If foreign body lodged in canaliculi or lacrimal sac, it may be manually removed by flushing fellow lacrimal punctum.

- If a foreign body is present in nasolacrimal duct, removal may be accomplished by dacryocystotomy (surgical incision of nasolacrimal duct; referable procedure).

CHRONIC TREATMENT

- Care after any of the preceding surgeries would include topical antibiotic-steroid combination medication (neomycin/polymyxin/dexamethasone suspension or ointment q 4-6h) for the first 2 to 4 postoperative weeks.
- Dacryocystotomy requires the placement and maintenance of a Silastic cannula and oral antibiotics for 3 to 4 weeks after surgery.

POSSIBLE COMPLICATIONS

If foreign bodies are left in the nasolacrimal drainage system, scarring, permanent occlusion, and chronic epiphora may result.

PROGNOSIS AND OUTCOME

- Depends on underlying cause
- Good prognosis with successful removal of foreign body

PEARLS & CONSIDERATIONS

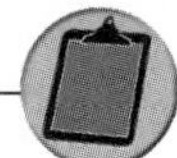

COMMENTS

- Prompt retrieval of foreign bodies from the proximal portions of the nasolacrimal system is essential as surgical removal from the nasolacrimal duct is technically difficult and has many potential complications.
- False-negative results can occur when attempting nasolacrimal fluorescein dye passage in brachycephalic breeds because fluorescein may drain into the back of the oral cavity due to the characteristic shape of a brachycephalic dog or cat's maxilla.

PREVENTION

Keep pets away from areas with tall grass, especially in the late summer

SUGGESTED READING

Grahn BH: Diseases and surgery of the canine nasolacrimal system. In Gelatt KN (ed): *Veterinary Ophthalmology*, ed 3. Philadelphia, Lippincott Williams & Wilkins, 1999, pp 569–581.

Ocular Disorders Presumed to be Inherited in Purebred Dogs, ed 3. Genetics Committee of the American College of Veterinary Ophthalmologists, 1999.

Nykamp SG, et al: Computed tomography dacryocystography evaluation of the nasolacrimal apparatus. *Vet Radiol Ultrasound* 45:23, 2004.

AUTHOR: **STEVEN R. HOLLINGSWORTH**
EDITOR: **CHERYL L. CULLEN**

Deafness

BASIC INFORMATION

DEFINITION

- Deafness is the inability to hear.
- *Sensorineural deafness* results from an abnormality in the inner ear and/or vestibulocochlear nerve and/or the auditory pathways in the brain.
- *Conduction deafness* results from a lesion in the outer ear and/or tympanum and/or middle ear.

SYNONYM(S)

Hearing loss

EPIDEMIOLOGY

SPECIES, AGE, SEX

- Dogs and cats
- Any age or gender

GENETICS AND BREED PREDISPOSITION

- Congenital, inherited, sensorineural deafness is associated with coat and iris color.
  - Cats with white haircoats and blue irides are commonly affected by congenital deafness.
  - Dog breeds with white, spotted, merle, or dapple haircoats are predisposed to congenital deafness.
- Inherited sensorineural deafness is also seen in breeds not related to white, spotted, merle, or dapple coat colors (e.g., Doberman pinscher).

RISK FACTORS

- Genotype: white, piebald, extreme piebald, or merle genes.
- Old age.
- Repeated exposure to loud noises.
- Breeds of dogs susceptible to otitis externa and/or otitis media.
- Exposure to high dosages of systemic ototoxic drugs, such as aminoglycosides, erythromycin, loop diuretics, cisplatin, nitrogen mustard, or topical chlorhexidine antiseptic. Topical drugs are potentially more ototoxic if the tympanum is not intact.

ASSOCIATED CONDITIONS AND DISORDERS

- Otitis externa and/or media
- External or middle ear canal neoplasia
- Nasopharyngeal polyps (cats)

CLINICAL PRESENTATION

DISEASE FORMS/SUBTYPE: Described as:

- Congenital or adult-onset
- Inherited or noninherited
- Sensorineural or conduction deafness

HISTORY, CHIEF COMPLAINT

- Animals with bilateral congenital or adult-onset deafness:
  - Overly aggressive with other puppies in a litter (congenital deafness)
  - Nonresponsive to auditory stimuli (particular frequencies and/or magnitudes)
  - Difficult to obedience train
  - Tendency to startle when approached from a position out of visual field
  - Increased tendency to sleep
  - Not aroused from sleep with auditory stimuli
- Diagnosis of unilateral deafness is not possible with behavioral markers alone; electrodiagnostic evaluation to establish a diagnosis of unilateral deafness.

PHYSICAL EXAM FINDINGS

- Animals with normal hearing may not respond to loud sounds in the clinical setting—behavioral response to auditory stimuli is unreliable for evaluating deafness.
- Animals with peripheral sensorineural deafness typically have no abnormal physical examination findings.
- Animals with acquired conduction deafness may have one or all of the following clinical signs:
  - Abnormal aural examination
  - Head tilt
  - Facial droop
  - Horner's syndrome
  - Head shaking
  - Signs of pain upon manipulation of the ears
- Animals with deafness resulting from diseases affecting the vestibulocochlear nerve or central components of the auditory pathways will typically demonstrate other concurrent abnormal neurologic signs.

ETIOLOGY AND PATHOPHYSIOLOGY

- Acquired conduction deafness resulting from otitis externa/media.
  - Impaired conduction of sound waves to the tympanic membrane from hyperplasia and exuberant sebum

production or the presence of pus in the external ear canal.
  - Impaired transduction of sound waves to the otic ossicles because of stiffened, fibrotic, or ruptured tympanic membrane.
  - Impaired mechanoelectrical transduction due to sclerosis of otic ossicles.
- Acquired conduction deafness from external or middle ear masses.
  - Obstruction of sound waves to the tympanic membrane.
  - Destruction of middle ear structures.
- Presbycusis (senile deafness).
  - Degeneration of the neural components of the inner ear.
  - ± Stiffening of the tympanic membrane.
  - ± Ankylosis of the otic ossicles.
- Loud noise exposure.
  - Damage to inner ear hair cells and/or ossicles and/or tympanic membrane.
- Congenital hereditary deafness associated with coat color.
  - Associated with coat color genes.
  - Abnormal migration of neural crest cells (precursor to melanocytes) to the inner ear (thought to provide nourishment to inner ear) associated with sacculocochlear type degeneration.

DIAGNOSIS

DIFFERENTIAL DIAGNOSIS

- Primary behavioral disorder
- Canine cognitive dysfunction syndrome (geriatric dogs)

INITIAL DATABASE

- Distant and proximal physical examinations
- Neurologic examination
- Thorough aural examination

ADVANCED OR CONFIRMATORY TESTING

Brainstem auditory evoked response/potential (BAER or BAEP) testing using air or bone-conducting stimuli (see Brainstem Auditory Evoked Response, p 1197).

TREATMENT

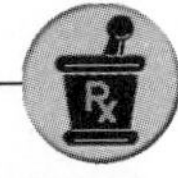

THERAPEUTIC GOAL(S)

- Prevent deafness from developing
- Improve hearing ability

ACUTE GENERAL TREATMENT

- No treatment for congenital inherited deafness; careful selection of breeding animals by only using nondeaf animals for breeding (perform BAER tests on nontested adults and all puppies).
- No practical treatments for animals with sensorineural deafness. Custom-fit hearing aids are offered by some specialty practices (consult with neurologist or audiologist).
- For acquired conduction deafness, treat the underlying cause of the disease.
- Use ototoxic drugs with caution or not at all (topically) if the tympanum is not known to be intact.

RECOMMENDED MONITORING

Repeated BAER testing to monitor response to therapy in animals with incomplete deafness

PROGNOSIS AND OUTCOME

- Inherited sensorineural deafness and deafness resulting from degeneration of inner ear is permanent
- Variable prognosis for animals with conduction deafness (depends on chronicity and/or severity of the disease)

PEARLS & CONSIDERATIONS

COMMENTS

- Unilaterally deaf animals are as likely to produce deaf offspring as bilaterally deaf animals.
- Animals with bilateral deafness require special care including:
  - Keeping animals on leash, especially when near traffic.
  - Obedience training using hand signals.
  - Prevent children from startling the animal to minimize the risk of bite injury.
- Animals with presbycusis may have concurrent cognitive decline accounting for behavioral changes.

PREVENTION

- Use nondeaf animals for breeding.
- For breeds predisposed to congenital deafness, use animals with nonblue irides for breeding.

CLIENT EDUCATION

- For dog breeders:
  - Inherited sensorineural deafness is a multifactorial genetic condition and is not easily eliminated from particular breeds.
  - Breeding unilaterally or bilaterally deaf animals together increases the incidence of deafness in the offspring; conversely, the incidence of deafness decreases when two hearing dogs are bred together.
  - Breeding two hearing dogs together can still result in producing unilaterally or bilaterally deaf puppies (for inherited deafness).
- For owners:
  - Inform owners that the dog has special training needs.
  - Recommend the following book:

Becker SC: *Living with a Deaf Dog: A Book of Advice, Facts and Experiences about Canine Deafness.* Cincinnati, Susan Cope Becker, 1997.

SUGGESTED READING

Deafness in dogs and cats: Information on deafness prevalence, causes and management for owners, breeders and researchers © George M. Strain: http://www.lsu.edu/deafness/deaf.htm.

Listing of worldwide BAER test sites © George M. Strain: http://www.lsu.edu/deafness/baersite.htm.

AUTHOR: **AUBREY A. WEBB**

EDITOR: **ETIENNE CÔTÉ**

Deciduous Teeth, Persistent ("Retained")

BASIC INFORMATION

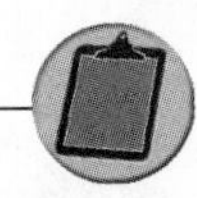

DEFINITION

Deciduous teeth that failed to exfoliate

SYNONYM(S)

Retained deciduous teeth: "retained" refers to failure to erupt; the term *persistent* meaning failure to exfoliate is more accurate.

EPIDEMIOLOGY

SPECIES, AGE, SEX: Dogs and cats. Permanent dentition eruption schedules dictate when a deciduous tooth is considered persistent (Table I-3). One tooth in one place at one time is the general rule of thumb. If deciduous and permanent teeth of the same type are occupying the same space, the deciduous tooth is persistent.

GENETICS AND BREED PREDISPOSITION: High prevalence in toy breeds (Yorkshire terriers, miniature poodles, and Pomeranians) suggests inheritance, but unproven.

ASSOCIATED CONDITIONS AND DISORDERS: As a result of persistence of deciduous teeth:
- Periodontal disease
- Malocclusion
- Malposition, retarded eruption, impaction of permanent teeth
- Palatal/labial trauma

CLINICAL PRESENTATION

HISTORY, CHIEF COMPLAINT: Teeth appear too numerous or are angled abnormally. A large percentage of persistent deciduous teeth are found on physical examination of adolescent cats and dogs presented for neutering.

PHYSICAL EXAM FINDINGS

The deciduous canine and incisor teeth are most commonly affected, though persistent deciduous premolars do occur (there are no deciduous molars or first premolars).

ETIOLOGY AND PATHOPHYSIOLOGY

- Persistent deciduous teeth may result in malpositioned permanent teeth.
- Permanent mandibular incisors, canines, and premolars erupt lingual (i.e., toward the tongue) relative to persistent deciduous teeth (Fig. I-52); lingually deviated permanent mandibular canine teeth may cause palatal trauma.
- Maxillary permanent incisors and premolars erupt palatal (i.e., toward the palate) relative to persistent deciduous teeth.
- Permanent maxillary fourth premolars erupt buccal (i.e., labial) and distal (i.e., away from the midline of the dental arch) relative to persistent deciduous teeth.
- Permanent maxillary canine teeth erupt mesial (i.e., toward the midline of the dental arch) relative to persistent deciduous teeth.
- Food debris, plaque, and calculus accumulating on and between deciduous and permanent teeth may cause periodontal disease even in young animals.

The exact mechanism is not fully understood, but there are four commonly reported causes:
- Lack of permanent successors
- Dentoalveolar ankylosis of persistent deciduous teeth
- Failure of the erupting permanent crown to contact and apply pressure to the deciduous tooth root
- Hormonal abnormalities affecting growth or metabolism

TABLE I-3 Permanent Dentition Eruption Times in the Dog and Cat

	Dog	Cat
Incisors	3-5 months	3-4 months
Canines	4-6 months	4-5 months
Premolars	4-6 months	4-6 months
Molars	5-7 months	4-5 months

DIAGNOSIS

DIFFERENTIAL DIAGNOSIS

- Missing, malformed, malpositioned, or unerupted permanent tooth
- Supernumerary permanent tooth
- Malocclusion

INITIAL DATABASE

- Complete blood count, serum chemistry panel, urinalysis: preoperative, and generally unremarkable
- Full-mouth dental radiographs: evaluate root structures, confirm and document presence of healthy permanent teeth

ADVANCED OR CONFIRMATORY TESTING

Hormone levels if metabolic/endocrine disease is suspected

TREATMENT

THERAPEUTIC GOAL(S)

- To alleviate dental crowding, soft tissue trauma, and/or dental interlock
- To prevent periodontal disease
- To prevent malpositioning of permanent dentition and malocclusion
- To correct existing malposition of dentition

ACUTE GENERAL TREATMENT

- No treatment is needed for uncrowded, healthy persistent deciduous teeth that have no permanent counterpart.
- Extraction of all other persistent deciduous teeth is advised.
- Closed and open extraction techniques are acceptable depending on tooth to be extracted and degree of root resorption.
  - Closed extraction for mobile teeth.
  - Open extraction via creation of a mucoperiosteal flap and alveolar bone removal for solid teeth with complete root structures.
  - Slow, steady pressure with a dental elevator is key for periodontal ligament fatigue.
  - Be sure to keep all instrumentation away from the erupting permanent tooth.
- Extraction sites should be closed, using absorbable synthetic suture material while avoiding placing sutures directly over an erupting tooth.
- Postoperative dental radiographs are recommended to ensure complete extraction, to evaluate surrounding structures for damage, and to provide documentation.
- Antibiotics are not usually necessary postextraction.

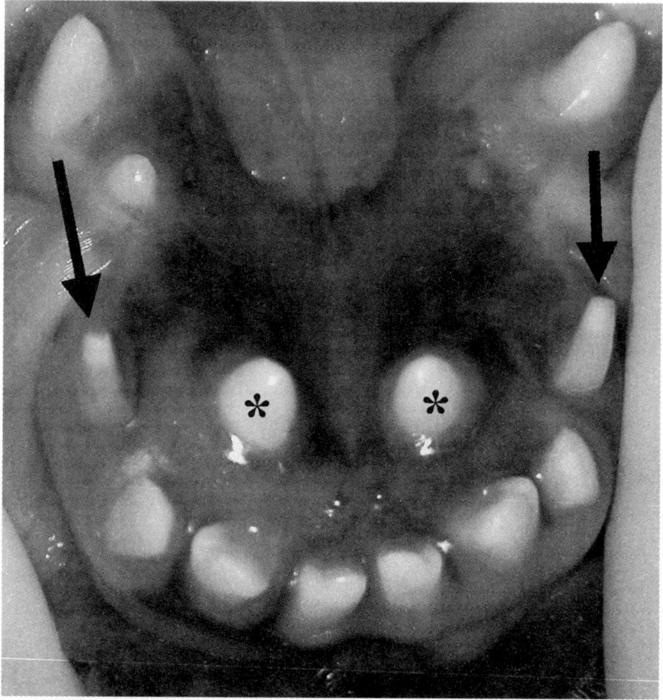

FIGURE I-52 Bilateral persistent deciduous lower canine teeth in a dog (*arrows*), causing the permanent canines (*asterisks*) to be displaced lingually. Courtesy of Dr. Alexander M. Reiter, University of Pennsylvania.

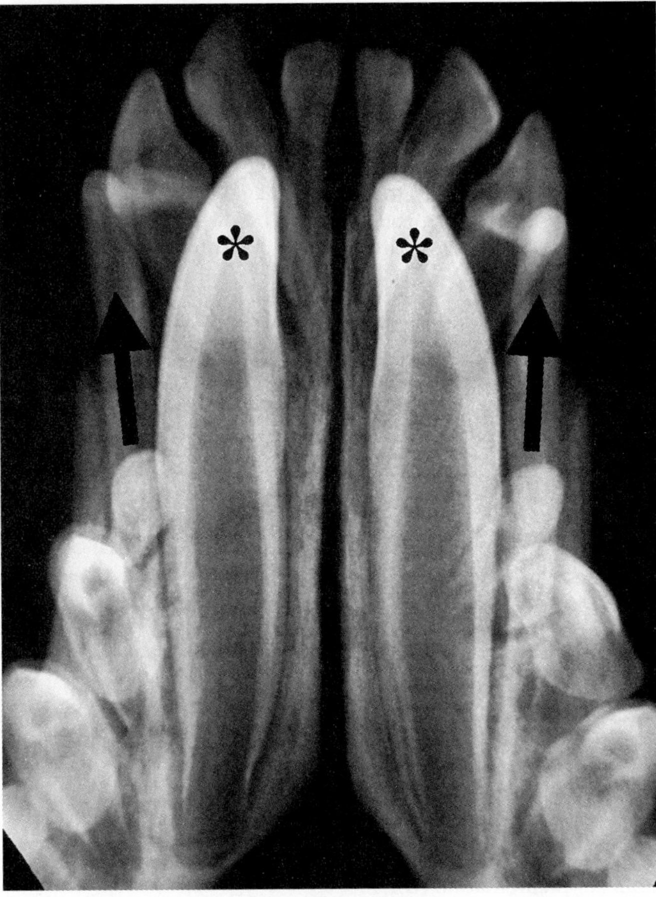

FIGURE I-53 Radiograph of the lower jaw of the same dog; persistent deciduous canine teeth (*arrows*) block the normal eruption pathway of the permanent successors (*asterisks*). Radiograph is arranged in labial mounting; rostral is toward the top of the image, and the patient's left is on the right of the image. Courtesy of Dr. Alexander M. Reiter, University of Pennsylvania.

- Pain management: intraoperative local nerve block (0.5% bupivacaine hydrochloride; 0.3 to 0.5 ml near mental, inferior alveolar, or infraorbital nerve), followed by oral nonsteroidal anti-inflammatory (e.g., deracoxib 2 mg/kg PO q 24h) ± opioid medications (e.g., butorphanol 0.2-0.4 mg/kg PO q 8h) for 2 to 3 days postoperatively.

POSSIBLE COMPLICATIONS

- Root fracture and retained root tips leading to infection of the permanent tooth
- Retarded eruption, malpositioning, and/or mechanical damage to the permanent tooth (Figs. I-52 and I-53)
- Accidental extraction of permanent tooth

RECOMMENDED MONITORING

- Examination 1 to 2 weeks to evaluate extraction sites
- Examination 4 to 6 weeks to evaluate occlusion if necessary; if abnormalities persist, therapeutic recommendations are offered

PROGNOSIS AND OUTCOME

Excellent for regional healing and reduction of risk of periodontal disease

PEARLS & CONSIDERATIONS

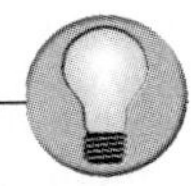

COMMENTS

- Early extraction of persistent deciduous teeth is key to success.
- Deciduous teeth have a thin dentinal layer and long, spindly roots. They are difficult to extract and break easily. The first rule is to *go slow*!

PREVENTION

Selective breeding

CLIENT EDUCATION

Genetic counseling

SUGGESTED READING

Harvey CE, Emily PP: *Small Animal Dentistry*. St. Louis, Mosby, 1993, pp 276-281.

Holstrom SE, et al: *Veterinary Dental Techniques*, ed 3. Philadelphia, WB Saunders, 2004, pp 291-339.

Mulligan TW, et al: *Atlas of Canine and Feline Dental Radiography*. Trenton, N.J., Veterinary Learning Systems, 1998, 91-103.

Wiggs RB, Lobprise HB: *Veterinary Dentistry: Principles and Practice*. Philadelphia, Lippincott-Raven, 1997, pp 167-179.

AUTHOR: **JENNIFER E. RAWLINSON**
EDITOR: **ALEXANDER M. REITER**

Degenerative Myelopathy

BASIC INFORMATION

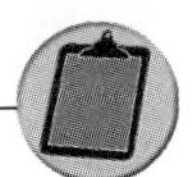

DEFINITION

Canine degenerative myelopathy is a degenerative disease of unknown etiology most severely affecting the thoracolumbar spinal cord.

SYNONYM(S)

Canine degenerative radiculomyelopathy
German shepherd dog myelopathy

EPIDEMIOLOGY

SPECIES, AGE, SEX: Canine, age: usually 5 years or older; younger dogs rarely can be affected; mean age 9 years.

GENETICS AND BREED PREDISPOSITION

- Unknown
- Breed predisposition: purebred dogs: German shepherd, Pembroke and Cardigan Welsh corgi, standard poodle, Rhodesian Ridgeback, collie, boxer, Chesapeake Bay retriever, Irish setter

CLINICAL PRESENTATION

HISTORY, CHIEF COMPLAINT

- Progressive weakness of pelvic limbs
- Initially affected dogs will drag nails and show pelvic limb ataxia
- Difficulty jumping
- The disease is progressive over 4 to 6 months from time of suspected diagnosis

PHYSICAL EXAM FINDINGS

- Pelvic limb tremors
- Asymmetric truncal ataxia to severe paraparesis and paraplegia

- Long spastic stride in gait
- Proprioceptive loss (toe dragging, absent conscious proprioception)
- Spinal reflexes present or exaggerated
- Patellar reflex may be decreased to absent
- Variable presence of crossed extensor reflex
- Disuse muscle atrophy of pelvic limbs
- Absence of paraspinal hyperesthesia
- Urinary and fecal incontinence in later disease stage
- Thoracic limb function may be affected late in the disease course

ETIOLOGY AND PATHOPHYSIOLOGY

- The etiology of degenerative myelopathy remains unknown.
- Hypotheses include toxic, immune-mediated, vitamin deficiencies, oxidative stress, and genetic.
- Neuropathologic lesion distribution involves axons and myelin in all funiculi of the spinal cord; most severe in the thoracolumbar spinal cord and have been described as discontinuous, bilateral, and asymmetric.
- Recent studies have shown degenerative changes in some neurons of the brainstem.

DIAGNOSIS

DIFFERENTIAL DIAGNOSIS

Other spinal cord disorders mimic signs of degenerative myelopathy:

- Intervertebral disk disease: Hansen type II
- Inflammatory disease of the spinal cord: myelitis
- Spinal cord neoplasia
- Degenerative lumbosacral stenosis
- Hip dysplasia
- Other coexisting orthopedic diseases

INITIAL DATABASE

- Neurologic examination.
  - See Physical Exam Findings above for clinical findings.
    - Nonpainful progressive myelopathy
  - Neuroanatomic localization: T3 to L3 spinal cord.
- Clinical pathology: generally unremarkable.
  - Complete blood count.
  - Serum biochemistry.
  - Urinalysis.
- Thoracic radiography.
  - Screening for metastatic neoplasia (central nervous system neoplasia differential diagnosis).

ADVANCED OR CONFIRMATORY TESTING

- Clinical working diagnosis is based on ruling out other diseases that cause progressive myelopathy.
- Cerebrospinal fluid analysis: may show increased protein concentration.
- Electrophysiologic testing.
  - Electromyography and nerve conduction studies (see p 1231).
  - Used for ruling out other neuropathic disorders.
  - Some dogs with degenerative myelopathy will show evidence of axonopathy, but these may just be age-related changes.
- Survey spinal radiography.
- Myelography: no evidence of a compressive myelopathy.
- Advanced imaging: no evidence of a compressive myelopathy.
  - Computed tomography combined with myelography.
  - Magnetic resonance imaging.
- Definitive diagnosis is only ever determined postmortem by histopathologic examination of the spinal cord.

TREATMENT

THERAPEUTIC GOAL(S)

There are no proven effective therapies for degenerative myelopathy.

ACUTE AND CHRONIC TREATMENT

Exercise, vitamin supplementation (B_{12}, E, and C), and protease inhibitors (aminocaproic acid) have been advocated as potential therapies. Disclaimer: Although the following drugs have been recommended as supplements in dogs with degenerative myelopathy, efficacy still remains to be proven.

- Aminocaproic acid (500 mg/dog; 15 mg/kg PO q 8h)
- Vitamin E (1000-2000 IU/dog PO q 24h)
- Vitamin B_{12} (100-200 μg/dog PO q 24h)
- Encourage exercise and physical therapy to slow onset of disuse muscle atrophy
- Monitor for urinary and fecal incontinence
  - Basic nursing care and hygiene if incontinence occurs, to prevent the onset of urine scald, infected decubital ulcers, or similar skin lesions
- When patient becomes nonambulatory, keep on a well-padded surface

POSSIBLE COMPLICATIONS

- Urinary tract infections
- Decubital ulcer formation (see Callus/Hygroma/Pressure Sores, p 172)

RECOMMENDED MONITORING

- Monitor for secondary urinary tract infection
- Monitor for proper nursing care

PROGNOSIS AND OUTCOME

- Long-term prognosis is considered poor.
- Dogs often lose their ability to ambulate within 4 to 6 months from time of diagnosis.
- The disease eventually will progress to affect the thoracic limbs.

PEARLS & CONSIDERATIONS

COMMENTS

- Lack of paraspinal hyperesthesia is a key clinical feature of degenerative myelopathy.
- A suspected diagnosis is based on exclusion of other spinal cord disorders.
- Histopathologic evaluation is the only definitive method by which to confirm a diagnosis of degenerative myelopathy.

CLIENT EDUCATION

- The disease eventually will progress to paraplegia and will affect the thoracic limbs.
- Meticulous nursing care is essential in the recumbent patient.
  - Keep patient clean and dry to prevent urine scald
  - Keep patient on a protective surface (optimize padding, traction, and ease of cleaning)
- A sling with wheels or a cart may assist with patient mobility.
- Physical therapy using range-of motion and isometric exercises will help maintain joint flexibility and muscle strength (see Physical Rehabilitation, p 1300).

SUGGESTED READING

Braund KG, Vandevelde M: German shepherd dog myelopathy: a morphologic and morphometric study. *Am J Vet Res* 39:1309, 1978.

Griffiths IR, Duncan ID: Chronic degenerative radiculomyelopathy in the dog. *J Sm Anim Pract* 16:461, 1975.

Johnston PE, et al: Central nervous system pathology in 25 dogs with chronic degenerative radiculomyelopathy. *Vet Rec* 146:629, 2000.

Johnston PE, Knox K, Gettinby G, Griffiths IR: Serum alpha-tocopherol concentrations in German shepherd dogs with chronic degenerative radiculomyelopathy. *Vet Rec* 148:403, 2001.

AUTHOR: **JOAN R. COATES**
EDITOR: **CURTIS W. DEWEY**

Dehydration

BASIC INFORMATION

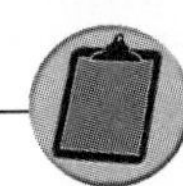

DEFINITION

Dehydration occurs when fluid losses (sensible loss [renal]; and insensible loss [gastrointesinal, respiratory]) exceed fluid intake.

SYNONYM(S)

Decreased circulating blood volume
Negative fluid balance

EPIDEMIOLOGY

SPECIES, AGE, SEX: All animals are susceptible to dehydration, depending on the underlying disease process. Due to a high body surface area to volume ratio, smaller animals (<10 kg) are more prone to dehydration.

RISK FACTORS: Diseases and toxins that affect appetite, decreased water ingestion, decreased renal and intestinal conservation of water, and poor vascular integrity predispose to dehydration.

Infectious diseases such as parvoviral enteritis and coccidiosis; metabolic disturbances resulting from diseases, such as renal failure or hypoadrenocorticism; endocrinopathies such as diabetes mellitus or insipidus; intoxications with substances such as ethylene glycol; and any cause of decreased water and food intake can all result in dehydration.

CONTAGION AND ZOONOSIS: Dehydration is not contagious; however, some of the diseases that cause dehydration (such as parvoviral enteritis and leptospirosis) can be contagious to other pets and/or have zoonotic potential.

GEOGRAPHY AND SEASONALITY

- Hotter weather in the summer may make a sick animal become dehydrated more rapidly.
- Frozen water bowls in the winter may cause pets to become dehydrated.

CLINICAL PRESENTATION

DISEASE FORMS/SUBTYPES: Hypertonic dehydration, isotonic dehydration, hypotonic dehydration.

HISTORY, CHIEF COMPLAINT: Anorexia, vomiting, diarrhea, lethargy, weakness, panting.

PHYSICAL EXAM FINDINGS: Lethargy, dry/tacky mucous membranes, tachycardia, poor pulse quality, skin tenting, sunken eyes/enophthalmos, and weight loss. The approximate level of dehydration is estimated based on the following physical exam findings: 5% = dry/tacky mucous membranes; 6–8% = dry mucous membranes and delayed skin tent test, 10–12% = the patient is in shock, and signs include all of the above plus bilaterally symmetric enophthalmos, tachycardia (dogs), weakness, slow capillary refill time, poor pulse, and lethargy or obtundation.

ETIOLOGY AND PATHOPHYSIOLOGY

- Gastroenteritis (clostridial, parvoviral, parasitic, foreign body-induced, obstruction-induced)
- Renal failure (acute, chronic)
- Endocrine disease (hypoadrenocortism, diabetes mellitus or insipidus)
- Intoxication (ethylene glycol, or any other toxin that causes vomiting, diarrhea, or renal failure)

PATHOPHYSIOLOGY: Regardless of cause, dehydration results in a decrease in circulating blood volume, which directly affects perfusion and oxygen delivery to essential tissues/organs. Mild cases may be clinically insignificant, but in moderate or severe dehydration, the metabolic processes in hypoperfused tissues must then rely on anaerobic pathways to produce adenosine triphosphate, which is a less efficient process. Furthermore, a byproduct of anaerobic metabolic pathways is lactic acid, which accumulates in states of decreased perfusion and results in metabolic acidosis.

DIAGNOSIS

DIFFERENTIAL DIAGNOSIS

- Skin tent: old age, thin/emaciated body condition (false increase), obesity (false decrease)
- Tacky mucous membranes: may occur in healthy individuals

INITIAL DATABASE

Complete blood count, serum biochemical profile, urinalysis, fecal exam

ADVANCED OR CONFIRMATORY TESTING

Urine/fecal culture, parvoviral fecal antigen testing, gastrointestinal barium series, thoracic and abdominal radiographs, abdominal ultrasound, adrenocorticotropic hormone stimulation testing, ethylene glycol testing—all as dictated by initial diagnostic information and case evolution.

TREATMENT

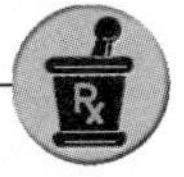

THERAPEUTIC GOAL(S)

- Fluid replacement
- Correction of electrolyte abnormalities
- Treatment of underlying disease

ACUTE GENERAL TREATMENT

- Fluid replacement should be performed with an isotonic crystalloid such as lactated Ringer's solution, Normosol R, or 0.9% sodium chloride.
- Maintenance rate and dehydration replacement must be calculated.
- Dehydration volume is delivered over 24 to 48 hours and is added to maintenance rates.
- Maintenance rate = 40 ml/kg/24 hr for large dogs (>10 kg), 60 ml/kg/24 hr for cats and small dogs (<10 kg).
- Dehydration replacement volume (ml) = % dehydration as a decimal (e.g., 10% is 0.1) × body weight in kg × 1000.
- Adjustment of fluid rate and frequent, close monitoring of respiratory rate and comfort if heart disease, renal disease, or systemic hypertension is present.
- Electrolyte replacement:
  - Do not supplement potassium at a rate of greater than 0.5 mEq/kg/hr.
  - Do not raise or lower serum sodium at a rate of greater than 1 mEq/L/hr.

CHRONIC TREATMENT

Depends on underlying disease process

DRUG INTERACTIONS

Do not add sodium bicarbonate to calcium-containing fluids (precipitation reaction)

POSSIBLE COMPLICATIONS

Overhydration: pulmonary edema, pleural or peritoneal effusion, hemodilution, cerebral edema, peripheral edema. Monitor more closely if heart or renal disease; consider colloid therapy if hypoalbuminemia.

RECOMMENDED MONITORING

Body weight, urine output, heart rate, pulse quality capillary refill time, skin turgor, blood pressure, packed cell volume/total solids, blood urea nitrogen, creatinine

PROGNOSIS AND OUTCOME

Prognosis is good if the underlying disease process is identified and can be corrected

PEARLS & CONSIDERATIONS

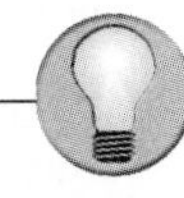

COMMENTS

Recheck electrolytes (sodium, potassium, chloride, and phosphorus) imbalances and acid base status frequently (every 4 to 8 hours) during the first 24 hours of therapy to ensure that treatment goals are being achieved. Body weight and urine output are among the easiest and most accurate ways to gauge the level of hydration.

PREVENTION

See specific disease information

CLIENT EDUCATION

Anorexic animals, or those vomiting and having diarrhea (especially very young or very old), can become dehydrated quickly and should be examined by a veterinarian as soon as possible.

SUGGESTED READING

DiBartola SB: *Fluid Therapy in Small Animal Practice*. Philadelphia, WB Saunders Company, 2000.

AUTHOR: **ADAM J. REISS**
EDITOR: **ETIENNE CÔTÉ**

Demodicosis

Client Education Sheet on Website

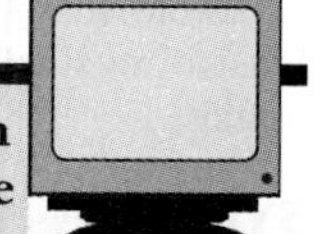

BASIC INFORMATION

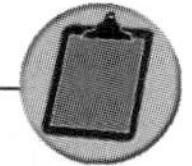

DEFINITION

Demodicosis is an inflammatory disease associated with a local or generalized increase in the number of *Demodex* mites found on the skin. *Demodex*, a commensal organism, is normally found in very small numbers in hair follicles and sebaceous glands of healthy animals.

SYNONYM(S)

Demodectic mange

EPIDEMIOLOGY

SPECIES, AGE, SEX

- *Demodex canis* is a normal resident of dog skin and is present in small numbers on the skin of most healthy dogs. Transmission occurs from bitch to pups in the first 2 to 3 days of life.
- Juvenile demodicosis is normally first noted in young dogs, often by 3 to 6 months of age.
- Adult-onset demodicosis often occurs in middle-aged to old dogs associated with internal disease and immunosuppression.
- Feline demodicosis is uncommon, is poorly understood, and is usually associated with underlying immunosuppressive disorders. Mites have been identified on the skin and in the otic canal of cats without internal disease signs.

GENETICS AND BREED PREDISPOSITION

- Affected individuals should not be bred.
- Dog breeds commonly affected by juvenile demodicosis are: Afghan hounds, American Staffordshire terrier, American pit bull terrier, Boston terrier, boxer, Chihuahua, collie, dalmatian, Doberman pinscher, English bulldog, German shepherd dog, Great Dane, Old English sheepdog, pug, and Shar-Pei.
- Burmese and Siamese cats may be at increased risk.

RISK FACTORS: Whether a dog develops demodicosis depends on immunologic factors that are affected by genetic influences.

CONTAGION AND ZOONOSIS: Not considered to be contagious.

GEOGRAPHY AND SEASONALITY: Although no geographic distribution has been identified for *D. canis*, anecdotal reports suggest that *Demodex gatoi* may be more common in the southeastern United States (see Etiology and Pathophysiology below).

CLINICAL PRESENTATION

DISEASE FORMS/SUBTYPES

- Juvenile demodicosis
- Adult-onset demodicosis

HISTORY, CHIEF COMPLAINT

- Lesions and history may vary from localized alopecia to generalized alopecia, with scaling, crusting, and in severe cases, systemic disease.
- Pruritus may be noted, especially in generalized cases that present with erythema.
- Adult-onset demodicosis usually accompanies internal disease or immunosuppression.

PHYSICAL EXAM FINDINGS

- Classic demodicosis (juvenile) starting in puppyhood may be localized (focal), multifocal, or generalized, depending on severity.
  - Localized demodicosis typically presents as one to three small areas of patchy alopecia, mild erythema, and scaling on the face or forelimbs.
  - Multifocal demodicosis cases have small areas affected, but they are generalized over the body rather than just on the face and forelimbs. They represent an intermediate stage in the disease progression, although they typically require aggressive treatment.
  - Generalized demodicosis cases have much more extensive alopecia, scaling, and plugging of hair follicles. Pododermatitis is also common. Generalized demodicosis may be associated with the development of a severe secondary deep pyoderma that may further suppress the immune system, allowing further mite proliferation.
- Adult-onset demodicosis often presents as multifocal or generalized and is unique because in many cases no obvious internal disease can be found at the time of diagnosis, despite extensive investigation. However, within 1 to 2 years, signs of severe internal disease become apparent.

ETIOLOGY AND PATHOPHYSIOLOGY

- In dogs, short-bodied and long-bodied versions of the mite have been noted. It is not clear whether these represent mutant forms or different species.
- Large-bodied *Demodex* mites have also been reported in adult-onset demodicosis cases associated with immunosuppressive illness as well as anecdotally in seborrheic disorders.
- In cats, a short-bodied, "stubby," surface-living species, *D. gatoi*, has also been found. This mite has been associated with alopecia and pruritus, whether associated with scaling or excessive grooming.
- The exact mechanism that allows *Demodex* mites to proliferate is not known. Genetic factors are believed to predispose dogs to demodicosis.
- In adult dogs, changes in the immune system relating to internal systemic disease appear to allow the mites to proliferate.
- Estrus, vaccination and heartworm infection, and inappropriate treatment (corticosteroids) can all potentially aggravate *Demodex* infections.

DIAGNOSIS

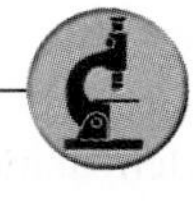

DIFFERENTIAL DIAGNOSIS

Because skin scrapings reveal the mites easily, demodicosis should not be confused with other disorders.

- Dogs:
  - Bacterial folliculitis/furunculosis
  - Deep pyoderma
  - Dermatophytosis
  - Dermatomyositis (facial lesions)
  - Pemphigus foliaceus
  - Erythema multiforme
  - Systemic lupus erythematosus
  - Sebaceous adenitis
  - Epitheliotropic lymphoma

- Cats (*D. gatoi*—pruritus):
  - Scabies
  - Cheyletiellosis
  - Hypersensitivity disorders
  - Psychogenic alopecia

INITIAL DATABASE

- The initial database should include history, physical examination, trichograms (microscopic examination of hair plucks from the edge of the lesion), and deep skin scrapings from four to five sites on the body.
- Skin should be squeezed to express mites from the hair follicles immediately before scraping, and should ooze a small amount of blood after an appropriately taken skin scraping.

ADVANCED OR CONFIRMATORY TESTING

- Skin biopsy, rather than scrapings, may be used for making a diagnosis in cases affecting the feet (pododermatitis) and in shar-peis where, because of thick skin and deeply extending follicles, it is more challenging to detect mites on skin scrapings.
- Adult-onset demodicosis cases require a full diagnostic work-up for internal disease, including routine hematology, chemistry profile, urinalysis, imaging, screening tests for endocrinopathies, retroviral feline immunovirus/feline leukemia virus serologic evaluation in cats, etc.

TREATMENT

THERAPEUTIC GOAL(S)

- Demodicosis can be a challenging condition to treat. The key to a successful outcome is early recognition.
- Most cases of localized demodicosis will resolve spontaneously as the immune system of the puppy matures. Self-cure is believed to occur because, as the immune system matures, it is finally able to suppress mite growth.
- Resistance issues or the risk of relapse is minimized by an intensive treatment program, for all of the treatments listed in this section.

ACUTE GENERAL TREATMENT

- Therapy for generalized demodicosis normally depends on the use of daily oral ivermectin or milbemycin, or periodic amitraz dips, and takes place over several months.
- Response to therapy is monitored by monthly skin scrapings and/or trichograms.
  - Ivermectin (10 mg/ml bovine injection solution, given orally):
    - Currently the treatment of choice, at a dose of 0.3-0.6 mg/kg PO until resolution.
    - After clinical cure is achieved, the dog is gradually weaned off the ivermectin over 2 or 3 months.
    - This treatment is contraindicated in certain individuals and breeds (see Possible Complications below).
  - Milbemycin:
    - Acceptable alternative.
    - 1 mg/kg daily PO initially, increasing to 2 mg/kg if there is a lack of response.
    - Daily treatment should be continued until clinical cure, followed by gradual weaning.
  - Moxidectin (Cydectin Injection solution 10 mg/ml; Wyeth):
    - Has also been recommended.
    - 0.4 mg/kg PO q 24h.
    - There is only a limited amount of information on its use in the veterinary literature.
  - Amitraz:
    - Monoamine oxidase inhibitor and α-2 agonist.
    - An approved therapy for demodicosis, but side effects and the risk to the operator are of concern.
      - Gloves must be worn.
      - Treatment should be performed in a well-ventilated area.
      - Other specifications as required by EPA.
    - Treat small (<5 kg) and medium dogs (5-15 kg) at the labeled recommendation of 250 ppm or 0.025%.
    - In very small dogs, treat only half the body at a time to minimize the risk of side effects.
    - Large dogs (>15 kg) are treated at twice label strength (500 ppm or 0.05%).
    - Perform eight weekly dips, followed by two every other week dips, then two monthly dips.
      - The total treatment period is 12 dips in 20 weeks.
    - Before the use of amitraz, a benzoyl peroxide shampoo should be used because of its follicular flushing ability.
    - Localized demodicosis or pododemodectic mange can be treated with a 1:10 solution of amitraz in mineral oil or propylene glycol.
  - The use of vitamin E 200 IU PO (up to five times daily) and nonspecific immunomodulators remains critically unproven, but can be used as an adjunct to standard therapy.
- Pyoderma may be a significant secondary problem; antibiotic therapy should be continued for 4 to 12 weeks depending on response.
- Although localized demodicosis lesions should resolve on their own with maturity of the immune system, focal use of a benzoyl peroxide gel, or amitraz dips may be beneficial.

POSSIBLE COMPLICATIONS

- The challenge with ivermectin is to monitor carefully for neurotoxicity and to make sure that clients are briefed about the signs to watch for (mydriasis, ataxia, weakness, hypersalivation, etc.) and risks (coma and death) before therapy.
- Although toxicity can occur in any breed, collies and collie crosses are most at risk. The problem is due to a mutation in the multidrug resistance gene (MDR-1). Dogs with the mutant gene have a defect in the pump that clears ivermectin from the central nervous system, resulting in the accumulation of the drug and the neurologic signs described.
- Side effects of amitraz can include transient sedation depression, lethargy, pruritus, vomiting/diarrhea, and hyperglycemia (diabetics). Yohimbine can be used as an antidote when side effects are of concern.

RECOMMENDED MONITORING

Scrapings and/or hair plucks are normally performed periodically during therapy.

PROGNOSIS AND OUTCOME

- Prognosis assessment is normally based on the ratios of eggs and larval forms to adults, as well as the number of live to dead mites. Generally, the larger the number of juvenile forms the worse the prognosis. Approximately 10% of cases cannot be cured and may require long-term management.
- As treatment progresses, increased numbers of dead mites and decreased numbers of juvenile stages would be regarded as pointing toward a favorable prognosis.
- For most cases of localized juvenile demodicosis, the prognosis is good.
- In all cases of adult-onset demodicosis, the prognosis is guarded.

PEARLS & CONSIDERATIONS

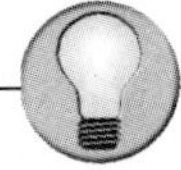

COMMENTS

- As pruritus may be noted in some demodicosis cases, likely associated with a hypersensitivity reaction to the presence of the mite, it is very important to use a good diagnostic approach. Electing to use glucocorticoids in a suspected pruritic pet without ruling out *Demodex* may have a significant impact on the progression of the condition.
- Ivermectin sensitivity testing (for the presence of the MDR-1 mutant gene) is available from the Washington State University College of Veterinary Medicine Clinical Pharmacology Laboratory (Phone/

FAX 509-335 3745). A cheek brush sample is sent for analysis. According to the laboratory, dogs at risk for ivermectin toxicity are homozygous or heterozygous for the presence of the mutant gene.

SUGGESTED READING

Holm BR: Efficacy of milbemycin oxime in the treatment of canine generalized demodicosis: A retrospective study of 99 dogs (1995–2000). *Vet Dermatol* 14(4):189–195, 2003.

Hugnet C, Bentjen SA, Mealey KL: Frequency of the mutant MDR1 allele associated with multidrug sensitivity in a sample of collies from France. *J Vet Pharmacol Ther* 27(4): 227–229, 2004.

Mealey KL, Bentjen SA, Gay JM, Cantor GH: Ivermectin sensitivity in collies is associated with a deletion mutation of the MDR-1 gene. *Pharmacogenetics* 11(8):727–733, 2001.

Muller RS: Treatment protocols for demodicosis: An evidence-based review. *Vet Dermatol* 15(2):75–89, 2004.

Wagner R, Wendlberger U: Field efficacy of moxidectin in dogs and rabbits naturally infested with *Sarcoptes* spp., *Demodex* spp. and *Psoroptes* spp. mites. *Vet Parasitol* 93(2):149–158, 2000.

AUTHORS: **JAN A. HALL, AMANDA P. AMARATUNGA**
EDITOR: **JAN A. HALL**

Dermatomyositis

BASIC INFORMATION

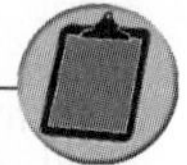

DEFINITION

Familial canine dermatomyositis is a hereditary, idiopathic inflammatory skin disease producing alopecia, erosions, and crusting, predominantly over bony prominences in collies and Shetland sheepdogs. Myositis and vasculitis may be noted as the disease progresses. Acquired dermatomyositis may be noted in other breeds.

EPIDEMIOLOGY

SPECIES, AGE, SEX

- Dogs: primarily young dogs (<6 months old). Full extent of the disease is usually noted by 1 year. Number of lesions and severity usually decreases from then on
- Cats: do not appear to get dermatomyositis
- No sex predilection

GENETICS AND BREED PREDISPOSITION

- Dermatomyositis is classically overrepresented in collies and Shetland sheepdogs, Beauceron shepherds, and their crossbreeds.
- Acquired dermatomyositis has been reported in Welsh corgis, Lakeland terriers, chow chows, German shepherds, and Kuvasz and Australian cattle dogs but has an unproven familial basis.

RISK FACTORS: Mechanical trauma and sunlight (UV) and reproductive stress (estrus, parturition, lactation) may worsen the lesions.

GEOGRAPHY AND SEASONALITY: Populations of familial dermatomyositis occur in collies and Shetland sheepdogs where the autosomal dominant trait is strongly expressed.

ASSOCIATED CONDITIONS AND DISORDERS

- Myositis may lead to dysphagia; megaesophagus with subsequent aspiration pneumonia; and lameness.
- Idiopathic ulcerative dermatosis of collies and Shetland sheepdogs may represent an adult-onset version of the condition characterized by well-demarcated ulcers within the axillary and inguinal area.

CLINICAL PRESENTATION

DISEASE FORMS/SUBTYPES: Familial versus acquired (see Genetics and Breed Disposition above).

HISTORY, CHIEF COMPLAINT: Owner generally presents a young collie or Shetland sheepdog puppy with skin lesions over bony prominences.

- Puppies may be painful or inappetent.
- Inappetence is directly related to the degree of myositis affecting pharyngeal muscles.
- Stunted growth, lameness, and muscle wasting may occur as the disease progresses.

PHYSICAL EXAM FINDINGS

- Clinical signs wax and wane and vary from minor skin lesions (papules/rarely vesicles) to severe ulceration of the skin with a generalized debilitating myositis affecting the head and distal limbs.
- Skin lesions generally present as erosive and crusting lesions around the eyes, on the bridge of the nose, lips, ear, and prominences of elbows, hocks, digits, and the tail tip. Vesicles are occasionally noted.
- Pruritus is not normally feature unless complicated by another condition.
- Pyoderma may or may not be noted.
- Some dogs present with onychodystrophy. Ulcers of the footpads are rarely noted.
- Healing may lead to scarring alopecia.
- Megaesophagus and aspiration pneumonia are occasionally noted.
- Littermates may be affected to different degrees.

ETIOLOGY AND PATHOPHYSIOLOGY

- Etiology and exact pathogenesis are unknown.
- The condition is thought to be associated with a hereditary autosomal dominant trait of variable expression in affected collies and Shetland sheepdogs.
- Most researchers believe that the condition has an immune-mediated or autoimmune basis, although others have suggested that a viral or environmental trigger could be important.

DIAGNOSIS

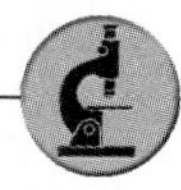

DIFFERENTIAL DIAGNOSIS

- Demodicosis
- Dermatophytosis
- Bacterial folliculitis (superficial pyoderma)
- *Malassezia* dermatitis
- Discoid lupus erythematosus
- Vasculitis
- Epidermolysis bullosa simplex (presence of vesicles)

INITIAL DATABASE

- Skin cytology: negative.
- Skin biopsy for histopathologic evaluation (may be nondiagnostic in mild cases). Characteristic hydropic degeneration in the basal cell layer with a mild perivascular to interstitial dermatitis. Follicular atrophy may be noted in chronic lesions. Vasculitis is occasionally noted.
- Complete blood count, serum biochemistry profile, urinalysis: usually within normal limits.

ADVANCED OR CONFIRMATORY TESTING

- Electromyograms are abnormal in cases with subclinical or clinical myositis
- Muscle biopsy reveals myofibrillar degeneration and atrophy with accumulations of mixed inflammatory cells
- Neurologic examination is usually normal

TREATMENT

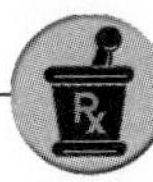

THERAPEUTIC GOAL(S)

Minimize scarring of facial skin and subsequent debilitating myositis

ACUTE AND CHRONIC GENERAL TREATMENT

Therapeutic options include:

- Pentoxifylline 20 mg/kg q 12h PO.
- Tetracycline and niacinamide (*adult dogs only*): given for minimum 3 months, weaning down based on a favorable response.
  - >10 kg: 500 mg of each drug PO q 8h
  - <10 kg: 250 mg of each drug PO q 8h
- Prednisone 1–2 mg/kg PO q 12–24h, weaning down to an alternate day regimen based on a favorable response.
- Vitamin E 400–800 IU per day PO for minimum 1 to 2 months.
- Omega-3 EFA (Derm Caps).
- Cyclosporine emulsion form (Atopica, Neoral): 5 mg/kg q 12–24h PO.
- These drugs may be used alone or in combination, depending on the severity of the disease.
- Supportive care includes controlling secondary infection with appropriate therapy and avoiding mechanical trauma to the face (avoid "gentle leaders" type muzzle collars), aggressive bathing, or harsh shampoos.
- Soften dry foods and raise bowls to minimize dysphagia.
- Avoid intense sunlight.

POSSIBLE COMPLICATIONS

- Chronic prednisone use can cause iatrogence hyperadrenocorticism and immune suppression.
- Pentoxifylline can cause gastric irritation, elevated clotting times, and nervous irritability.
- Cyclosporine: diarrhea, vomiting, anorexia, gingival hyperplasia, and gingivitis. Monitor for tumors.

RECOMMENDED MONITORING

Cyclosporine: Check trough cyclosporine levels if adverse reactions are noted or there is a poor clinical response. A level of 500–700 ng/ml has been associated with efficacy.

PROGNOSIS AND OUTCOME

Prognosis is variable depending on severity. Mild cases may resolve without further problems, although scarring may be noted. Dogs with more severe skin lesions may be prone to recurrent skin problems Cases with severe myositis have a poor prognosis for long-term survival

PEARLS & CONSIDERATIONS

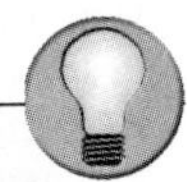

PREVENTION

- Do not breed affected individuals
- Minimize exposure to UV light for affected individuals

CLIENT EDUCATION

Affected individuals will likely require a higher level of skin care than nonaffected dogs.

SUGGESTED READING

Rees CA, Boothe DM: Therapeutic response to pentoxifylline and its active metabolites in dogs with familial canine dermatomyositis. *The Vet.* 4(3):234–241, 2003.

Scott DW, Miller WH, Griffin CE: Dermatomyositis. In Scott DW, Miller WH, Griffin CE (eds): *Muller and Kirk's Small Animal Dermatology*, ed 6. Philadelphia, WB Saunders, 2001, pp 940–946.

AUTHORS: **BERNARD D. BOISVERT, JAN A. HALL**

EDITOR: **JAN A. HALL**

Dermatophytosis

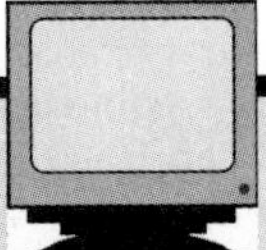

Client Education Sheet on Website

BASIC INFORMATION

DEFINITION

- *Dermatophytosis* is a fungal disease affecting the keratinized tissues of the body (hair, nail, and stratum corneum) caused by a parasitic species of fungus.
- The term *dermatomycosis* is used to denote a fungal infection of skin, hair, or nail caused by a nonparasitic (saprophytic) species of fungus.

SYNONYM(S)

Ringworm

Microsporum canis (zoophilic [cat and dog are normal hosts])

Microsporum gypseum (geophilic [soil species])

Trichophyton mentagrophytes (zoophilic [rodents are the normal host])

EPIDEMIOLOGY

SPECIES, AGE, SEX

- Overall incidence of canine dermatophytosis is very low; there is a tendency toward overdiagnosis.
- Incidence of feline dermatophytosis is higher and it tends to be underdiagnosed.
- Young animals appear predisposed because of the delay in the development of adequate cell-mediated immunity.

GENETICS AND BREED PREDISPOSITION: Some individuals are resistant to infection and remain as carriers that show no overt clinical signs.

RISK FACTORS

- Dermatophytosis is a zoonotic disease that tends to occur in immunocompromised individuals.
- In veterinary medicine, specific predisposing factors include: high population density (shelters or catteries), immunodeficiency syndromes (feline immunodeficiency virus [FIV], feline leukemia virus [FeLV]), cancer, immunosuppressive therapy, poor nutrition, and stress associated with pregnancy and lactation.
- Ectoparasites may be important factors in the development of cattery infections as they encourage self-trauma.
- Carriers showing no clinical signs may be an important source of the disease for stressed individuals.

CONTAGION AND ZOONOSIS

- Since dermatophytosis is a zoonotic disease, humans are at risk if exposed to an infected individual or asymptomatic carrier pet, and vice versa.
- Transmission is also by contact with infected fomites or soil.
- Fungal spores may be viable for years under ideal conditions.

GEOGRAPHY AND SEASONALITY

- In the Northern Hemisphere, *M. canis* has an increased incidence in the winter months, whereas *M. gypseum* has an increased incidence in the summer and fall.
- The incidence of *M. canis* infection and isolation is consistently higher in hot and humid locales.

CLINICAL PRESENTATION

HISTORY, CHIEF COMPLAINT

- Often a young patient, sometimes from a multianimal environment presenting

with one or more areas of alopecia, or a poor haircoat.
- The patient may be pruritic.

PHYSICAL EXAM FINDINGS

- Dermatophytosis can present as circular patches of alopecia (annular lesions), with variable degrees of inflammation, scaling, and crusting.
- Occasionally, ruptured hair follicles may produce abscess or cellulitis (mycetoma).
- Kerions (local areas of folliculitis and furunculosis) and pseudomycetomas (cutaneous or subcutaneous areas of granulomatous folliculitis and furunculosis) may also be seen.
- In cats, dermatophytosis is a common cause of miliary dermatitis, chin acne, and generalized seborrhea, as well as classic annular lesions.
- *Trichophyton* dermatophytosis may produce facial alopecia, erythema, and hyperpigmentation that clinically and histologically resemble pemphigus erythematosus.

ETIOLOGY AND PATHOPHYSIOLOGY

- Dermatophytes live in nonviable, keratinized tissue (skin, hair, nails).
- Mechanical disruption of the stratum corneum provides a portal of entry for organisms.
- As the upper third of the hair follicle is keratinized, dermatophytosis is a common cause of folliculitis due to the plugging of the follicle with keratin and debris.
- Dermatophytes grow only in actively growing (*anagen*) hairs, weakening the hair shafts and causing them to break.
- Spontaneous resolution occurs as infected hairs go into the resting phase, *telogen*. As hair growth ceases, the fungus must move to another follicle in the growth phase, typically creating a circular lesion.

DIAGNOSIS

DIFFERENTIAL DIAGNOSIS

- Dermatophytosis will be greatly overdiagnosed if clinicians depend on clinical signs alone.
- In dogs, top differentials include bacterial folliculitis and demodicosis, which mimic a classic ringworm lesion.
- In the dog, if the lesion looks like ringworm, it is likely a staphylococcal infection instead.
- In cats military dermatitis due to other causes such as flea allergy or other hypersensitivity should be considered, as well as other causes of generalized seborrhea and pruritus.

INITIAL DATABASE

Diagnosis is based on the history and clinical presentation and the results of diagnostic testing.

- Trichogram
  - Hairs can be plucked from the edge of a lesion and placed in oil or potassium hydroxide with Indian ink (50:50) to look for evidence of fungal spores.
- Wood's lamp
  - The lamp contains a UV light of 253.7 nm wavelength and needs to be warmed up for 5 to 10 minutes before use to ensure that the correct wavelength of light is emitted.
  - Approximately 50% of strains of *M. canis* will fluoresce with an apple-green color. Many other materials, including keratin scale, soaps, dyes, and medications, may fluoresce, giving false-positive results.
- Fungal culture
  - In-clinic fungal cultures can be carried out using Dermatophyte Test Media (DTM).
  - Two types of in-clinic DTM are available: Fungassay (turns red for positive within 7 days) or Derm Duet (contains two different media, a DTM and a rapidly sporulating Sabouraud's medium that will turn royal blue with the growth of a dermatophyte).
  - Hair and scale are removed from the edge of new or expanding lesions using hemostats or needle holders, and pressed into the DTM with a sterile needle.
  - Sampling lesions that appear to fluoresce with the Wood's lamp may be especially helpful.
  - Specimens can be collected from suspected carrier individuals, using a sterile toothbrush, and be inoculated directly into fungal media.
  - All positive cultures should be examined for typical colony characteristics (dermatophyte cultures are usually white or lightly colored, whereas saprophytes/contaminants will usually be pigmented).

ADVANCED OR CONFIRMATORY TESTING

Histopathology: Dermatophytes may be visible on histopathologic study. However, a negative result should not be used as clear evidence that a dermatophyte was not present. Special stains can be used to look for evidence of fungal infection.

TREATMENT

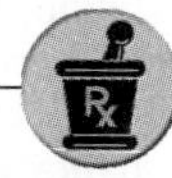

THERAPEUTIC GOAL(S)

- Treatment protocols for dermatophytosis normally rely on topical therapy, systemic therapy, or a combination of both.
- Any approach to dermatophytosis in a multicat situation should focus as much on environmental factors and management practices as it does on the diagnosis and treatment of affected individuals. Nonaffected animals should either be separated from infected animals or treated prophylactically with a whole body topical therapy.

ACUTE GENERAL TREATMENT

- Animals with individual lesions should have the hair carefully clipped out.
- A total body hair clipping may be indicated in severe cases, and long-haired animals.
- Single lesions may be spot-treated with an antifungal cream to an area 6 cm beyond the margin of the lesion. However, full body therapy is often preferable.
- Twice weekly topical therapy with a chlorhexidine 2% shampoo, followed by a 0.2% enilconazole rinse, has proved effective.
- Systemic treatment options for dermatophytosis include:
  - Griseofulvin
    - Fungistatic antifungal agent that inhibits cell division.
    - 25-60 mg/kg PO q 12h for a minimum of 6 weeks.
    - Teratogenic; should not be administered to pregnant animals.
    - Vomiting, diarrhea, and idiosyncratic bone marrow suppression may also occur (especially in cats that are FIV positive).
  - Itraconazole
    - Fungistatic (and at higher doses fungicidal) triazole derivative that alters the fungal cell membrane permeability by inhibiting ergosterol synthesis.
    - 5-10 mg/kg PO q 24h for 30 to 60 days has been recommended.
    - Administered with food for optimal absorption.
    - Adverse effects include elevated liver enzymes, anorexia, and gastrointestinal upset.
  - Ketoconazole
    - 10 mg/kg PO q 24h or divided twice daily.
    - Administered with food for optimal absorption.
    - Side effects are more common and may be more severe than with itraconazole and include elevated liver enzymes, anorexia, and gastrointestinal upset.
  - Terbinafine
    - Fungistatic allylamine antifungal agent that also suppresses biosynthesis of ergosterol.
    - Has been recommended for the treatment of dermatophytosis at a

dose of 30-40 mg/kg PO q 24h for 30 to 60 days.
  - Drug has been shown to be well tolerated, with vomiting as the main side effect reported.
- Lufenuron
  - Chitin inhibitor
  - 60-100 mg/kg PO q 2-4 weeks has been suggested, but contradictory results exist.
  - Until clear evidence shows that lufenuron is effective as a sole therapy, it should be used only as an adjunctive treatment.
- Environmental management is also necessary: Any item that is not needed should be destroyed. The environment should be thoroughly vacuumed and steam-cleaned before disinfection with a 0.5% sodium hypochlorite solution (bleach), which can also be used for cleaning any washable items.
- Vaccination against *M. canis* has not been shown to be very effective except as an adjunctive therapy during severe outbreaks.

POSSIBLE COMPLICATIONS

False-negative fungal cultures may delay therapy. False-positive cultures may lead to unnecessary and potentially erroneous treatment, especially in dogs.

RECOMMENDED MONITORING

- Successful therapy is normally confirmed by two negative fungal cultures.
- Routine hematologic evaluation should be performed biweekly during feline therapy with griseofulvin (neutropenia/bone marrow suppression).
- Liver function should be assessed before considering therapy with itraconazole or ketoconazole.
- Clients should be briefed about potential side effects to therapy.

PROGNOSIS AND OUTCOME

- The prognosis in most cases is generally good except in immunocompromised animals.
- In some long-haired cats dermatophytosis may take several years to resolve completely, and require more aggressive treatment.

PEARLS & CONSIDERATIONS

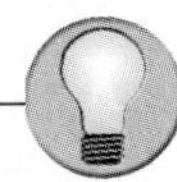

COMMENTS

- It is important to discuss this zoonotic disease with clients, particularly if they have young children or elderly humans in the household.
- In the dog, if the lesion looks like ringworm, it is likely a staphylococcal infection instead.
- It is recommended that any feline being adopted from a cattery or shelter be tested for FIV/FeLV if being introduced into a household with another cat. Persistent infection with dermatophytosis, or even infection in an adult cat, is another good reason to test.
- Side effects from antifungal drugs can be severe, especially in cats. It is important to become familiar with side effects and make sure clients are aware of associated clinical signs.

SUGGESTED READING

DeBoer DJ, Moriello KA, Blum JL, Volk LM: Effects of lufenuron treatment in cats on the establishment and course of *Microsporum canis* infection following exposure to infected cats. *J Am Vet Med Assoc* 222(9):1216-1220, 2003.

Kotnik T, et al: Terbinafine hydrochloride treatment of *Microsporum canis* experimentally-induced ringworm in cats. *Vet Microbiol* 83:161-168, 2001.

Moriello KA: Treatment of dermatophytosis in dogs and cats: review of published studies. *Vet Dermatol* 15(2):99-107, 2004.

Moriello KA, DeBoer DJ: Feline dermatophytosis. Recent advances and recommendations for therapy. *Vet Clin North Am Small Anim Pract* 25(4):901-921, 1995.

Moriello KA: Management of dermatophyte infections in catteries and multiple-cat households. *Vet Clin North Am Small Anim Pract* 20(6):1457-1474, 1990.

AUTHORS: **JAN A. HALL, AMANDA P. AMARATUNGA**

EDITOR: **JAN A. HALL**

Diabetes Insipidus

BASIC INFORMATION

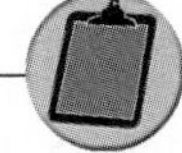

DEFINITION

Insufficient antidiuretic hormone (ADH) secretion (central diabetes insipidus) or action (nephrogenic diabetes insipidus) resulting in inadequate urine concentrating ability

EPIDEMIOLOGY

SPECIES, AGE, SEX

- Affects both dogs and cats
- No breed, gender, or age predilection

CLINICAL PRESENTATION

DISEASE FORMS/SUBTYPES

- Central diabetes insipidus
- Nephrogenic diabetes insipidus

HISTORY, CHIEF COMPLAINT

- Polyuria, polydipsia, loss of house-training, perceived urinary incontinence.
- Stupor, disorientation, ataxia, and seizures may be reported if an underlying neurologic disorder is present.

PHYSICAL EXAM FINDINGS

- Usually normal.
- Dehydration may be noted if the animal has not had free access to water.
- Neurologic abnormalities (e.g., stupor, disorientation, ataxia) may be seen in cases with underlying neurologic disease.

ETIOLOGY AND PATHOPHYSIOLOGY

- Normal daily water consumption: <70 ml/kg/day (dogs; higher in dogs <4 kg), <250 ml/day (average-size cat).
- ADH is released by the neurohypophysis in response to increased plasma osmolality, and to a lesser degree to reduced blood volume.
- ADH binds to receptors at the renal distal tubules and collecting ducts and allows water to be resorbed from the lumen of the duct into the renal interstitium, resulting in concentrated urine. Water resorption is also dependent on the osmotic gradient of the renal intersitium.
- Central diabetes insipidus (CDI) results from a lack of hypothalamic production of ADH secondary to cerebral trauma, cranial neoplasia (primary or metastatic), or hypothalamic/pituitary cysts. Those animals without a discernable underlying cause are classified as having idiopathic CDI.
- Nephrogenic diabetes insipidus (NDI) results from a reduced capacity of ADH to bind to its renal receptors and exert its renal actions. Interference with the binding capacity of ADH can be secondary to *Escherichia coli* endotoxins (pyometra, pyelonephritis), hypercalcemia, hypokalemia, hyperaldosteronism, and hyperadrenocorticism.

- Congenital NDI and congenital CDI are very rare.

DIAGNOSIS

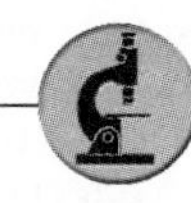

DIFFERENTIAL DIAGNOSIS

Polyuria/polydipsia (see also Polyuria/Polydipsia, p 878):
- Chronic renal insufficiency
- Hyperadrenocorticism
- Psychogenic polydipsia
- Pyelonephritis
- Pyometra
- Hypoadrenocorticism
- Liver disease
- Hyperthyroidism
- Diabetes mellitus
- Hypercalcemia
- Hypokalemia
- Primary hyperaldosteronism
- Primary renal glycosuria

INITIAL DATABASE

- Complete blood count: usually normal; mild hemoconcentration may be present if the animal is dehydrated.
- Serum biochemical profile:
  - Urea may be decreased due to increased renal loss or mildly increased in dehydrated patients
  - Mild hyponatremia or hypokalemia occasionally seen
- Urinalysis: Usually hyposthenuria (urine specific gravity <1.008) but can concentrate up to 1.015 in cases with partial ADH deficiency.
- Other tests to rule out causes of of secondary NDI usually include urine culture, abdominal ultrasound, and a test(s) for hyperadrenocorticism (see Hyperadrenocorticism, p 537).

ADVANCED OR CONFIRMATORY TESTING

- Endogenous creatinine clearance testing or nuclear scintigraphy to estimate glomerular filtration rate: considered if persistent isosthenuria is present.
- Random plasma osmolality:
  - A large overlap can occur between results from patients with a primary polyuric disorder (e.g., CDI or NDI) and a primary polydipsic disorder (i.e., psychogenic polydipsia).
  - Plasma osmolality of <280 mOsm/kg is suggestive of psychogenic polydipsia.
  - Plasma osmolality of >280 mOsm/kg can be seen with CDI, NDI, or psychogenic polydipsia.
- Modified water deprivation test:
  - Used for differentiating between diabetes insipidus and psychogenic polydipsia.
  - Causes of secondary NDI should be ruled out before performing this test.
  - Should not be performed if renal disease or dehydration is present.
  - The patient must be monitored throughout the test.
  - Procedure:
    - Slowly decrease the patient's water intake to 70–100 ml/kg/day over 3 to 5 days before starting the test to help correct any secondary renal medullary solute washout.
    - Fast the patient for 12 hours before the test.
    - At the start of the water deprivation, empty the patient's bladder, and determine the patient's weight, blood urea nitrogen (BUN) (via an Azostick is sufficient), urine specific gravity (USG), and urine osmolality (if readily available).
    - Withhold water and monitor clinical demeanor, weight (after emptying bladder), and USG (± urine osmolality) q 1h. Assess the BUN every few hours.
    - This portion of the test is stopped when 3% of the body weight has been lost, USG increases to >1.030, azotemia occurs, or the pet becomes clinically dehydrated or depressed.
    - If 3% of the body weight has been lost, urine concentration is <1.030, and the pet is still clinically normal, administer ADH (aqueous vasopressin: 0.55 U/kg IM to a maximum of 5 U) and reassess USG at 30, 60, and 120 minutes.
    - Slowly reintroduce water when the test is completed.
  - Interpretation:
    - Patients with psychogenic polydipsia will slowly increase their USG to >1.030 with water deprivation alone.
    - Patients with complete CDI will show little or no increase in urine concentration (still <1.015–1.020) by the time they have lost 3–5% of their body weight, but will show a 50+% increase in USG after ADH administration.
    - Patients with partial CDI will show little increase in urine concentration by the time they have lost 3–5% of their body weight, but will show an increase in USG of >15% but <50% after ADH administration.
    - Patients with NDI will show little increase in USG even with ADH administration.
  - Possible complications of the test: hypernatremia/hypertonic dehydration (irritability, weakness, ataxia, stupor, coma).
- Computed tomography or magnetic resonance imaging of the brain can be used to image a potential underlying cranial mass in older patients with CDI.

TREATMENT

THERAPEUTIC GOAL(S)

- Reduce or resolve the polyuria/polydipsia
- Address the underlying cause

ACUTE GENERAL TREATMENT

None generally required

CHRONIC TREATMENT

- Exogenous ADH administration (desmopressin acetate [DDAVP]: either as tablets (0.1 mg/dog PO q 8h; increase dose if no response within 1 week) or intranasal drops administered into the conjunctival sac [1–4 drops/patient q 12h]) is the treatment of choice for CDI. Patients with NDI are unresponsive to DDAVP therapy.
- Thiazide diuretics can be used in cases of primary NDI or partial CDI to reduce total body sodium concentrations, thereby increasing renal sodium and water resorption and reducing urine volume. Chlorothiazide (20–40 mg/kg PO q 12h) or hydrochlorothiazide (1–4 mg/kg PO q 12h) should be used in conjunction with a low-sodium diet.
- Chlorpropamide is an oral hypoglycemic agent that potentiates renal ADH action and may be useful in cases of partial CDI. Doses of 10–40 mg/kg PO q 24h have been suggested, but clinical responses in cats and dogs have been variable.
- A sodium-restricted diet alone may be useful at reducing urine volume in patients with CDI and NDI.
- If the polyuria/polydipsia is not disruptive to the owners, and the animal has free access to water, therapy for CDI or NDI may not be required.

DRUG INTERACTIONS

Chlorpropamide may enhance the antidiuretic effects of desmopressin, and displaces nonsteroidal anti-inflammatory drugs, warfarin, and many others from circulating protein binding sites, elevating serum levels.

POSSIBLE COMPLICATIONS

- Cellular overhydration can theoretically occur in patients that consume large volumes of water shortly after receiving DDAVP, due to a decreased ability to excrete the free water once DDAVP reaches therapeutic effect. Neurologic signs (ataxia, depression, tremors) can occur as a consequence of cerebral edema. It is recommended that pets do not have free access to water immediately after each dose.
- Conjunctival irritation is occasionally seen with conjunctival administration of DDAVP but is usually mild.

- Thiazide diuretics may cause hypokalemia and, if given to a patient with primary polydipsia, could lead to cellular overhydration due to decreased free water excretion.
- Hypoglycemia is the most common complication of chlorpropamide therapy.

RECOMMENDED MONITORING

- Clinical response should be monitored in those patients receiving DDAVP therapy.
- Serum electrolytes should be periodically monitored if thiazide diuretics are used, as should blood glucose levels if chlorpropamide is used.

PROGNOSIS AND OUTCOME

- In patients with congenital or idiopathic CDI, clinical signs generally resolve completely with DDAVP therapy, and they can have a normal life expectancy. The expense of DDAVP therapy, however, can make lifelong treatment not feasible for some pet owners.
- CDI secondary to an underlying cranial tumor has a very guarded prognosis, as progressive neurologic signs often develop in the ensuing months.
- The polyuria/polydipsia of primary NDI is often difficult to manage medically and therefore is associated with a guarded prognosis.

PEARLS & CONSIDERATIONS

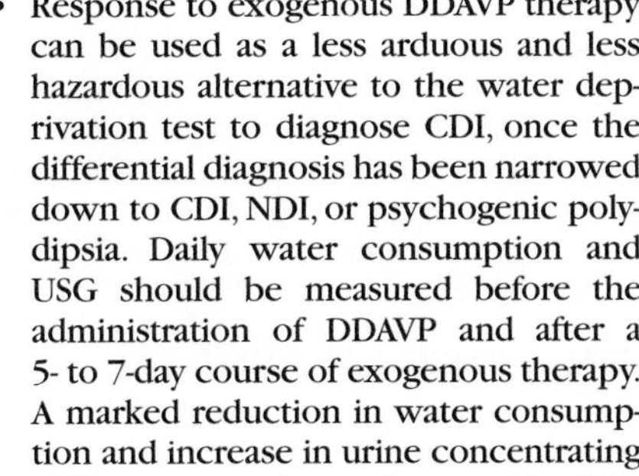

COMMENTS

- Response to exogenous DDAVP therapy can be used as a less arduous and less hazardous alternative to the water deprivation test to diagnose CDI, once the differential diagnosis has been narrowed down to CDI, NDI, or psychogenic polydipsia. Daily water consumption and USG should be measured before the administration of DDAVP and after a 5- to 7-day course of exogenous therapy. A marked reduction in water consumption and increase in urine concentrating ability occurs in patients with CDI. Patients with NDI or psychogenic polydipsia do not have a clinical response to DDAVP.
- Hyperadrenocorticism is a likely differential in a patient that initially responds to exogenous DDAVP therapy but later has recurrence of polyuria and polydipsia.
- The water deprivation test requires extremely diligent *hourly* monitoring for the entire duration of the test, without which there is a risk of rapidly progressive life-threatening dehydration in these patients.

CLIENT EDUCATION

Patients with diabetes insipidus must always have free access to water.

SUGGESTED READING

Feldman EC, Nelson RW: Water metabolism and diabetes insipidus. In Feldman EC, Nelson RW (eds): *Canine and Feline Endocrinology and Reproduction,* ed 3. St. Louis, Saunders, 2004, pp 2–41.

AUTHOR: **SARAH L. NAIDOO**
EDITOR: **SHERRI IHLE**

Diabetes Mellitus

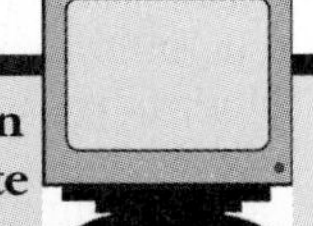

Client Education Sheet on Website

BASIC INFORMATION

DEFINITION

Diabetes mellitus is a complex metabolic disorder caused by deficiency of insulin, usually after destruction of pancreatic islet β-cells

SYNONYM(S)

Diabetes
Insulin-dependent diabetes
Non-insulin-dependent diabetes

EPIDEMIOLOGY

SPECIES/AGE/SEX

- Diabetes mellitus typically occurs in older dogs and cats.
- Peak prevalence: 7 to 9 years (dogs), 9 to 11 years (cats).
- Juvenile-onset diabetes occurs in dogs and cats less than 1 year of age and is uncommon.
- In dogs, females are affected twice as frequently as males. In cats, diabetes occurs predominately in neutered males.

GENETICS AND BREED PREDISPOSITION

- The role of genetics remains to be determined. Genetic predispositions for diabetes have been suggested by familial associations in dogs and by pedigree analysis of Keeshonden.
- Dog breeds at increased risk:
  - Australian terrier
  - Bichon frise
  - Cairn terrier
  - Fox terrier
  - Keeshond
  - Poodle (miniature)
  - Poodle (standard)
  - Samoyed
  - Schnauzer (miniature)
  - Schnauzer (standard)
  - Spitz
- There is no apparent breed predisposition in cats, although Burmese cats are overrepresented in Australia.

RISK FACTORS

- Obesity
- Recurring pancreatitis
- Diestrus in the older intact female dog
- Diseases causing insulin resistance, most notably hyperadrenocorticism and acromegaly
- Insulin antagonistic drugs, most notably glucocorticoids and progestagens

ASSOCIATED CONDITIONS AND DISORDERS

- Renal insufficiency
- Hyperlipidemia
- Systemic hypertension
- Bacterial infections
- Cataracts and blindness (dogs)
- Peripheral neuropathy causing weakness and plantigrade stance (cats)

CLINICAL PRESENTATION

DISEASE FORMS/SUBTYPES: Subtypes:

- Insulin-dependent diabetes mellitus (type 1) is identified in 99% of dogs and 50–70% of cats at the time diabetes is diagnosed. It is characterized by an absolute deficiency of insulin and mandatory need for insulin injections to control clinical signs of the disease.
- Non-insulin-dependent diabetes mellitus (type 2) is identified in approximately 30% of cats at the time diabetes is diagnosed and it is characterized by reduced population of β-cells and potential for clinical response to weight loss, diet, oral hypoglycemic drugs, and correction of concurrent insulin antagonistic disease or drugs.
- Transient or subclinical diabetes is identified in approximately 20% of cats and is characterized by resolution of the clinical diabetic state weeks to months after initiating insulin treatment. Clinical diabetes may or may not recur in the future.

HISTORY/CHIEF COMPLAINT

- Polydipsia, polyuria, polyphagia, and weight loss in virtually all diabetics
- Additional clinical signs can include:
  - Lethargy
  - Poor body condition
  - Blindness from cataracts (dogs)

- Lack of grooming behavior, poor haircoat (cats)
- Decreased jumping ability, rear limb weakness, or development of a plantigrade posture (cats)

PHYSICAL EXAMINATION: There are no classic physical examination findings. Body weight ranges from obese to thin. Lethargy; a dry, lusterless haircoat and scales from hyperkeratosis; hepatomegaly from hepatic lipidosis; lenticular changes consistent with cataract formation (dogs); and impaired ability to jump, weakness in the rear limbs, ataxia, or a plantigrade posture from peripheral neuropathy (cats) may be identified.

ETIOLOGY AND PATHOPHYSIOLOGY

- The etiology of diabetes is multifactorial and involves a combination of genetic predisposition, environmental factors, insulin resistance, and decreased numbers of β-cells.
- Decreased numbers of β-cells typically result from destruction secondary to vacuolar degeneration, islet amyloidosis (cats), immune destruction (dogs), pancreatitis, or congenital islet hypoplasia.
- Insulin deficiency causes decreased tissue utilization of glucose, amino acids, and fatty acids; accelerated hepatic glycogenolysis and gluconeogenesis; and accumulation of glucose in the circulation, causing hyperglycemia.
- Progressively worsening hyperglycemia leads to glycosuria, which creates an osmotic diuresis causing polyuria. Compensatory polydipsia prevents dehydration.
- The diminished peripheral tissue utilization of ingested glucose results in weight loss.
- Insulin deficiency results in failure of the satiety center to inhibit the feeding center in the hypothalamus, causing polyphagia.

DIAGNOSIS

The diagnosis is based on the presence of appropriate clinical signs (i.e., polyuria, polydipsia, polyphagia, weight loss) and documentation of persistent fasting hyperglycemia (blood glucose greater than 200 mg/dl (11 mmol/L)) and persistent glycosuria.

INITIAL DATABASE

- A thorough diagnostic evaluation is indicated to identify any disease that might be causing or contributing to the diabetic state, that may result from the diabetic state or that may force modification of therapy.
- Complete blood count: typically normal.
- Common serum biochemical profile findings: hyperglycemia, hypercholesterolemia, and increased serum alanine transaminase and alkaline phosphatase activities.
- Common urinalysis findings: specific gravity >1.025, glycosuria, findings consistent with concurrent bacterial urinary tract infection (see Urinary Tract Infections, Recurrent and Persistent, p 1416). Ketonuria establishes a diagnosis of diabetic ketosis or ketoacidosis.
- Findings on abdominal ultrasound include hepatomegaly, changes suggesting pancreatitis, and bilateral adrenomegaly or an adrenal mass if concurrent hyperadrenocorticism is present.
- Additional diagnostic tests to consider include serum thyroxine concentration in an older diabetic cat, serum pancreatic lipase immunoreactivity for pancreatitis, serum progesterone concentration in an intact female diabetic dog, and bacterial culture of urine.

DIFFERENTIAL DIAGNOSES

See Polyphagia, p 877; Polyuria/Polydipsia, p 878; Weight Loss, p 1162

TREATMENT

THERAPEUTIC GOAL(S)

- The primary goal is elimination of owner-observed clinical signs and maintenance of a healthy, active pet.
- Normal findings on physical examination.
- Stable body weight once obesity is corrected.
- Avoidance of clinical signs of hypoglycemia.
- Avoidance of chronic complications of diabetes mellitus, most notably recurring ketosis, clinical signs of poor control of glycemia (e.g., lethargy, weight loss, poor body condition), cataracts (dogs), and clinical signs of peripheral neuropathy (cats).

TREATMENT

- For dogs, recombinant human or pork-source NPH or lente insulin at an initial dosage of 0.25 U/kg SC q 12h.
- For cats, recombinant human or pork-source lente or beef/pork-source PZI insulin at an initial dose of 1 unit per cat SC q 12h.
- Adjust dietary caloric intake to correct or prevent obesity.
- Divide total daily caloric intake in half and offer at the time of each insulin injection. Consumption may be immediate or intermittent throughout the 12-hour period, depending on eating habits of the dog or cat.
- In dogs, increase fiber content of the diet unless concurrent disease or adverse effects dictate otherwise. Amount of fiber depends on fiber type: insoluble fiber should be greater than 10%, soluble fiber should be 4–8%, and mixtures of soluble and insoluble fiber should be greater than 8% of diet on dry matter basis.
- In cats, restrict carbohydrate content of diet, ideally to 15% or less of metabolizable energy. Fiber content of the diet can also be increased as described for dogs.
- Initiate daily exercise routine for dogs.
- Identify and treat concurrent disorders that interfere with insulin effectiveness.
- Treatment with the oral sulfonylurea glipizide may be considered in diabetic cats when the owner refuses to administer insulin; ketonuria and peripheral neuropathy are not identified; and the cat is relatively healthy.
- Treatment of DKA: see Diabetic Ketoacidosis, p 291.

POSSIBLE COMPLICATIONS

Insulin-induced hypoglycemia

RECOMMENDED MONITORING

- Initially, monitor clinical response and blood glucose concentrations weekly until diabetic control is attained, defined as resolution of clinical signs and blood glucose concentrations ranging between 100 and 300 mg/dl (5.5 and 16.7 mmol/L) during the 12 hours after insulin administration.
- Monitor history, physical examination, body weight, and serum fructosamine concentration every 3 to 6 months once diabetes is controlled.
- Evaluate multiple blood glucose concentrations during the 12 hours after insulin administration if diabetic control is lost (i.e., return of clinical signs, abnormalities identified on physical examination, or progressive loss of body weight). Adjust insulin therapy accordingly.

PROGNOSIS AND OUTCOME

- The prognosis depends on owner commitment to treating the disorder, ease of glycemic regulation, presence and reversibility of concurrent disorders, and avoidance of chronic complications associated with the diabetic state.
- Mean survival time for diabetic dogs and cats is approximately 3 years from time of diagnosis, although diabetic dogs and cats that survive the first 6 months can easily maintain a good quality of life for longer than 5 years with proper care.

SUGGESTED READING

Briggs C, et al: Reliability of history and physical examination findings for assessing control of glycemia in dogs with diabetes mellitus: 53 cases (1995–1998). *J Am Vet Med Assoc* 217: 48, 2000.

Cohn LA, et al: Assessment of five portable blood glucose meters, a point-of-care analyzer, and color test strips for measuring blood glucose concentration in dogs. *J Am Vet Med Assoc* 216:198, 2000.
Feldman EC, Nelson RW: Canine diabetes mellitus. In Feldman EC, Nelson RW (eds): *Canine and Feline Endocrinology and Reproduction*, ed 3. St. Louis, Saunders, 2004, pp 486-538.
Feldman EC, Nelson RW: Feline diabetes mellitus. In Feldman EC, Nelson RW (eds): *Canine and Feline Endocrinology and Reproduction*, ed 3. St. Louis, Saunders, 2004, pp 539-579.
Goossens M, et al: Response to insulin treatment and survival in diabetic cats: 104 cases (1985-1995). *J Vet Intern Med* 12:1, 1998.
Hess RS, Ward CR: Effect of insulin dosage on glycemic response in dogs with diabetes mellitus: 221 cases (1993-1998). *J Am Vet Med Assoc* 216:217, 2000.
Nelson RW, et al: Transient clinical diabetes mellitus in cats: 10 cases (1989-1991). *J Vet Intern Med* 13:28, 1998.
Nelson RW, et al: Efficacy of protamine zinc insulin for treatment of diabetes mellitus in cats. *J Am Vet Med Assoc* 218:38, 2001.
Wess G, Reusch C: Capillary blood sampling from the ear of dogs and cats and use of portable meters to measure glucose concentration. *J Small Anim Pract* 41:60, 2000.

AUTHOR: **RICHARD W. NELSON**
EDITOR: **SHERRI IHLE**

DISEASES AND DISORDERS

Diabetic Ketoacidosis

BASIC INFORMATION

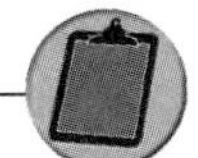

DEFINITION

Diabetic ketoacidosis (DKA) is a life-threatening metabolic disorder caused by insulin deficiency and insulin resistance that leads to excess hepatic production of ketoacids and progressively worsening metabolic acidosis, hyperosmolality, serum electrolyte derangements, and systemic signs of illness.

EPIDEMIOLOGY

See Diabetes Mellitus, p 289

CLINICAL PRESENTATION

HISTORY/CHIEF COMPLAINT: The history and physical examination findings are variable because of the progressive nature of DKA and the variable time between the onset of DKA and owner recognition of a problem. The classic clinical signs of diabetes (i.e., polyuria, polydipsia, polyphagia, weight loss) develop initially, followed by systemic signs of illness (lethargy, anorexia, vomiting) as ketonemia and metabolic acidosis develop and worsen. Underlying illness that precipitates DKA (e.g., pancreatitis, infection) also contributes to the clinical picture. The time interval from onset of diabetes to onset of DKA is unpredictable but once ketoacidosis develops, severe illness usually becomes evident within days.

PHYSICAL EXAMINATION: Findings are variable for reasons discussed above. Common physical examination findings in addition to those found in nonketotic diabetic dogs and cats include dehydration, depression, weakness, tachypnea, and sometimes a strong odor of acetone on the breath. Slow, deep breathing (i.e., Kussmaul's respiration) may be observed in animals with severe metabolic acidosis. Such signs as vomiting and abdominal pain are common because of the common concurrent occurrence of pancreatitis.

ETIOLOGY AND PATHOPHYSIOLOGY

- Synthesis of ketone bodies (i.e., acetoacetic acid, β-hydroxybutyric acid, and acetone) requires mobilization of free fatty acids (FFAs) from triglycerides stored in adipose tissue and a shift in hepatic metabolism from fat synthesis to fat oxidation and ketogenesis.
- Accelerated production of ketones requires insulin deficiency, insulin resistance, and increased production of diabetogenic hormones, most notably glucagon.
- Insulin deficiency "allows" lipolysis to increase, thus increasing the availability of FFAs to the liver and in turn promoting ketogenesis.
- Insulin deficiency may be absolute or relative; that is, DKA may develop in some diabetic dogs and cats despite daily injections of insulin.
- Increased concentrations of diabetogenic hormones (glucagon, epinephrine, cortisol, growth hormone) combined with concurrent illness and an altered metabolic milieu (e.g., increased concentrations of plasma FFAs and amino acids, metabolic acidosis) causes insulin resistance and stimulates lipolysis, ketogenesis, and gluconeogenesis, which worsens hyperglycemia and promotes ketonemia.
- Progressive accumulation of ketones in the blood overwhelms the body's buffering system, causing metabolic acidosis and surpasses the renal tubular threshold for complete resorption causing ketonuria.
- Ketonuria contributes to the osmotic diuresis caused by glycosuria and enhances excretion of solutes (e.g., sodium, potassium, magnesium).
- Excessive renal loss of water and electrolytes combined with fluid loss secondary to vomiting leads to volume contraction, an underperfusion of tissues, and development of prerenal azotemia.
- Progressively worsening hyperglycemia combined with urinary losses of water leads to hyperosmolality, a shift of water out of cells and cellular dehydration.
- The severe metabolic consequences of DKA, which include severe metabolic acidosis, hyperosmolality, obligatory osmotic diuresis, dehydration, and electrolyte derangements, quickly become life-threatening.

DIAGNOSIS

- Diagnosis of diabetes mellitus requires appropriate clinical signs and documentation of persistent fasting hyperglycemia and glycosuria. The concurrent documentation of ketonuria establishes the diagnosis of diabetic ketosis (DK) and documentation of metabolic acidosis establishes the diagnosis of DKA.
- Commonly used urine reagent strips do not detect β-hydroxybutyrate. If ketonuria is not present but DKA is suspected, blood can be tested for acetoacetic acid and acetone using Acetest tablets (Ames Division, Miles Laboratories, Elkhart, Ind.) or for β-hydroxybutyrate using a benchtop chemistry analyzer.

INITIAL DATABASE

- The laboratory evaluation of healthy dogs and cats with ketonuria is similar to the nonketotic diabetic.
- The laboratory evaluation of sick dogs and cats with DKA should include a complete blood count, serum biochemical profile, serum electrolytes, arterial acid-base evaluation, and urinalysis with culture.
- Additional data such as radiographs, abdominal ultrasound, or further clinical pathologic studies may be needed depending on results of the history, physical examination, and nature of concurrent illnesses.

- Typical findings in DKA include severe hyperglycemia, metabolic acidosis, hyperosmolality, hyponatremia, hypokalemia, hypochloremia, prerenal azotemia, increased liver enzyme activities, hypercholesterolemia, and urinary tract infection. Alterations associated with concurrent pancreatitis are also common.

TREATMENT

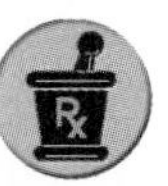

THERAPEUTIC GOAL(S)

- Provide adequate amounts of insulin to maintain the blood glucose concentration between 100 and 300 mg/dl (5.5–16.7 mmol/L).
- Restore water and electrolyte losses and maintain hydration and normal serum electrolyte concentrations.
- Correct metabolic acidosis.
- Identify and treat concurrent illness.
- Provide dextrose or food as needed to avoid hypoglycemia.
- Avoid overly aggressive therapy; slowly correct abnormalities over 24 to 48 hours.

TREATMENT

- For "healthy" dogs and cats with DK, short-acting Regular insulin can be administered SC q 8h until ketonuria resolves. The patient should be fed a third of its daily caloric intake at the time of each insulin injection. The insulin dose should be adjusted based on blood glucose concentrations. Longer-acting insulin preparations can be administered once DK has resolved.
- Treatment for systemically ill dogs and cats with DKA includes intravenous fluids with appropriate supplements, Regular (crystalline) insulin, bicarbonate, dextrose, and ancillary therapy depending on concurrent illness.
  1. Initial type of fluid depends on serum electrolyte concentrations. If not known, use 0.9% saline solution at a rate of 60–100 ml/kg/24 hr initially; adjust based on hydration status, urine output, and persistence of fluid losses.
  2. Potassium supplementation in fluids depends on serum potassium concentration; if unknown, initially add 40 mEq KCl to each liter of fluids.
  3. Phosphate supplementation in fluids is indicated if serum phosphorus concentration <1.5 mg/dl (0.48 mmol/L) or hemolytic anemia develops; initial IV infusion rate is 0.01 to 0.03 mmol/kg/hr in calcium-free fluids (e.g., 0.9% saline).
  4. Dextrose supplementation in fluids is indicated when blood glucose approaches 250 mg/dl (13.9 mmol/L); initially add dextrose to make 5% solution.
  5. Magnesium supplementation is not indicated unless persistent lethargy, anorexia, weakness, or refractory hypokalemia or hypocalcemia are encountered after 24 to 48 hours of fluid and insulin therapy and hypomagnesemia is documented.
  6. Bicarbonate supplementation is indicated if plasma bicarbonate <12 mEq/L (total venous CO_2 <12 mmol/L); if not known, do not administer unless animal is severely ill and then only once. Amount of supplement is based on formula: mEq HCO_3^- = body weight (kg) × 0.4 × (12 − animal's HCO_3^-) × 0.5; if animal's HCO_3^- or total CO_2 concentration is unknown, use 10 in place of (12 − animal's HCO_3^-). Add to IV fluids and give over 6 hours; do not give as bolus infusion. Re-treat if plasma bicarbonate concentration remains less than 12 mEq/L after 6 hours of therapy.
  7. Begin insulin therapy 2 to 4 hours after initiating fluid therapy. If serum potassium is normal, begin insulin treatment as described below. If hypokalemia is present, decrease insulin dose by 50% during initial 2 to 3 hours.
     - Regular insulin is administered using one of two techniques:
     - For the intermittent IM technique, the initial insulin dosage is 0.2 U/kg IM, then 0.1 U/kg IM hourly; switch to Regular insulin SC every 6 to 8 hours once blood glucose approaches 250 mg/dl (13.9 mmol/L) and add dextrose to IV fluids.
     - For the low-dose IV infusion technique, the initial insulin infusion rate is 0.05 U/kg/hr (cat) or 0.1 U/kg/hr (dog), diluted in 0.9% saline and administered via infusion or syringe pump in a line separate from that used for fluid therapy. Adjust infusion rate based on hourly blood glucose measurements; as blood glucose level decreases, switch to Regular insulin SC every 6 to 8 hours once blood glucose approaches 250 mg/dl (13.9 mmol/L) and add dextrose to IV fluids.
     - The goal of insulin treatment is a gradual decline in blood glucose concentration, preferably 50–75 mg/dl/hr (2.8–4.2 mmol/L/hr).

POSSIBLE COMPLICATIONS

- Complications result from overly aggressive treatment, inadequate patient monitoring, inadequate fluid replacement, and failure to reevaluate biochemical parameters in a timely manner.
- Common complications include hypokalemia, hypoglycemia, hypernatremia, hemolytic anemia induced by hypophosphatemia, and neurologic signs secondary to cerebral edema.
- Slow correction of abnormalities over 24 to 48 hours will minimize complications.

RECOMMENDED MONITORING

- Blood glucose measurement every 1 to 2 hours initially; as blood glucose level decreases in response to treatment, adjust insulin therapy and begin dextrose infusion when approaches 250 mg/dl (13.9 mmol/L).
- Hydration status, respiration, pulse every 2 to 4 hours; adjust fluids accordingly.
- Serum electrolyte and total venous CO_2 concentrations every 6 to 12 hours; adjust fluid and bicarbonate therapy accordingly.
- Urine output, glycosuria, ketonuria every 2 to 4 hours; adjust fluid therapy accordingly.
- Body weight, packed cell volume, temperature, blood pressure: daily.
- Additional monitoring, depending on concurrent disease.

PROGNOSIS AND OUTCOME

The prognosis for successful treatment of DKA is dependent, in part, on the severity of the metabolic derangements at the time DKA is diagnosed, underlying illnesses that precipitated DKA, and complications that develop during treatment. Close supervision and monitoring are imperative for a successful outcome.

SUGGESTED READING

Bruskiewicz KA, et al: Diabetic ketosis and ketoacidosis in cats: 42 cases (1980–1995). *J Am Vet Med Assoc* 211:188, 1997.

Duarte R, et al: Accuracy of serum β-hydroxybutyrate measurements for the diagnosis of diabetic ketoacidosis in 116 dogs. *J Vet Intern Med* 16:411, 2002.

Feldman EC, Nelson RW: Diabetic ketoacidosis. In Feldman EC, Nelson RW (eds): *Canine and Feline Endocrinology and Reproduction*, ed 3. St. Louis, Saunders, 2004, pp 580–615.

Macintire DK: Treatment of diabetic ketoacidosis in dogs by continuous low-dose intravenous infusion of insulin. *J Am Vet Med Assoc* 202:1266, 1993.

AUTHOR: **RICHARD W. NELSON**

EDITOR: **SHERRI IHLE**

Diaphragmatic Hernia

BASIC INFORMATION

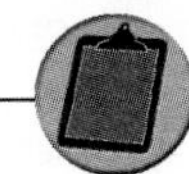

DEFINITION

Disruption of the continuity of the diaphragm such that abdominal organs can shift into the thoracic cavity

SYNONYM(S)

Pleuroperitoneal hernia

Note: peritoneopericardial diaphragmatic hernias are covered separately (see Peritoneopericardial Diaphragmatic Hernia, p 836)

EPIDEMIOLOGY

SPECIES, AGE, SEX

- Both dogs and cats.
- Congenital pleuroperitoneal hernias are rarely reported since many affected animals die soon after birth.
- Traumatic: commonly in male dogs 1 to 3 years old.

RISK FACTORS: Trauma is the most common cause of diaphragmatic hernia.

ASSOCIATED CONDITIONS AND DISORDERS

- Incarceration, obstruction, and strangulation of abdominal viscera
- Hepatic venous stasis, biliary tract obstruction, icterus, and ascites secondary to liver herniation
- Pleural effusion, hemothorax, chylothorax, bile pleuritis, and pneumothorax can complicate hernias
- Musculoskeletal or neurologic abnormalities secondary to trauma

CLINICAL PRESENTATION

DISEASE FORMS/SUBTYPES

- Congenital pleuroperitoneal hernia
  - Animals are dead at birth or die soon after with severe respiratory deficiency
- Traumatic diaphragmatic hernia
  - Clinical course can be acute or chronic

HISTORY, CHIEF COMPLAINT

- Acute:
  - History of trauma
  - Shock
  - Respiratory distress
  - Pale or cyanotic mucous membranes
- Chronic:
  - Dyspnea or tachypnea
  - Exercise intolerance
  - Anorexia
  - Depression
  - Vomiting
  - Dysphagia
  - Diarrhea
  - Constipation
  - Weight loss
  - Difficulty in lying down
  - Abdominal distention
- Some animals can be clinically normal, and the hernia is an incidental (typically radiographic) finding.

PHYSICAL EXAM FINDINGS

- Signs of hypovolemic shock
- Dyspnea and/or tachypnea
- Pale or cyanotic mucous membranes
- Tachycardia
- Cardiac arrhythmias
- Muffled heart and lung sounds on thoracic auscultation
- Borborygmi on thoracic auscultation
- Hyporesonance on chest wall percussion (pleural effusion)
- Hyperresonance on chest wall percussion (gastric tympany)
- Tucked-up or empty appearance of the abdomen
- Abdominal distention with fluid wave if ascites

ETIOLOGY AND PATHOPHYSIOLOGY

- Congenital:
  - Defect in the dorsolateral part of the diaphragm.
  - The intermediate part of the left lumbar muscle of the crus may be absent, or the defect may be more extensive with both crura and parts of the central tendon missing.
- Traumatic:
  - Direct:
    - Thoracoabdominal stab and gunshot wounds.
    - Iatrogenic injury during thoracocentesis.
  - Indirect:
    - Primarily motor vehicle accidents, but other blunt abdominal trauma can cause diaphragmatic hernia.
    - An abrupt increase in intra-abdominal pressure with the glottis open results in a large pleuroperitoneal pressure gradient.
      - This pressure gradient causes the diaphragm to tear at its weakest points, which are usually the muscular portions.
      - The location and size of the tear are dependent on the position of the animal on impact and the location of the viscera.
      - Viscera malpositioned in the thoracic cavity can suffer ischemic injury from alterations in blood flow.
      - Venous congestion of entrapped liver lobes can lead to pleural or abdominal effusion.
    - Clinical signs reflect respiratory dysfunction secondary to loss of diaphragmatic integrity, pleural effusion, or displacement of pulmonary parenchyma.
    - Clinical signs may also reflect dysfunction of displaced abdominal viscera.

DIAGNOSIS

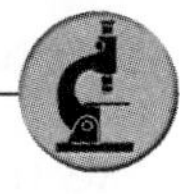

DIFFERENTIAL DIAGNOSIS

- Peritoneal-pericardial diaphragmatic hernia (see p 836)
- Other causes of pleural effusion
- Pneumothorax
- Pneumonia
- Other causes of abdominal distention or ascites

INITIAL DATABASE

- Complete blood count, biochemistry panel, urinalysis: variable results depending on time of presentation, severity of clinical signs, and organs displaced into the thorax.
- Thoracic radiographs may show:
  - Loss of the diaphragmatic line
  - Loss of cardiac silhouette
  - Dorsal displacement of lung fields
  - Pleural effusion
  - Presence of gas (stomach or intestines) in the thoracic cavity
- Thoracocentesis may be necessary for diagnostic thoracic radiographs (if large volume pleural effusion).
- Abdominal radiographs may show absence or cranial displacement of normal abdominal viscera.

ADVANCED OR CONFIRMATORY TESTING

- Ultrasonography may demonstrate a rent in the diaphragm, the organs herniating through it, or viscera in abnormal positions.
- Positive contrast celiography may demonstrate contrast medium in the pleural cavity, absence of a normal liver lobe outline, and incomplete visualization of the abdominal surface of the diaphragm.
- Contrast radiography of the intestinal tract may show barium-filled stomach or intestine in the thoracic cavity.
- In some animals, the diagnosis is confirmed during exploratory surgery.

TREATMENT

THERAPEUTIC GOAL(S)

- Stabilize patient
- Resolve respiratory distress
- Replace the abdominal organs in the abdominal cavity
- Repair the diaphragmatic defect

ACUTE GENERAL TREATMENT

- Oxygen administered via face mask, nasal cannula, or oxygen cage
- Fluid therapy as needed to stabilize cardiovascular status (particularly for acute trauma patients)
- Thoracocentesis if needed (see p 1308)
- Position the patient in sternal recumbency with the head elevated above the rear limbs (forelimbs elevated) if tolerated

CHRONIC TREATMENT

Surgical treatment:

- Replace the abdominal organs in the abdominal cavity
  - The diaphragmatic defect can be enlarged if necessary to reposition organs that have become swollen/ congested or that have developed adhesions.
- Close the diaphragmatic defect via standard herniorraphy, abdominal flaps, porcine small intestinal submucosal patches (Vet BioSIS), or synthetic material (Silastic sheeting)
- Remove air and fluid from the pleural cavity after closing the diaphragmatic defect
- Explore the entire abdominal cavity for associated injuries if traumatic etiology

POSSIBLE COMPLICATIONS

- Reexpansion pulmonary edema can follow rapid lung reexpansion
- Hypoventilation or hypoxia due to pain, pneumothorax, hemothorax, or tight bandages

RECOMMENDED MONITORING

- Vital signs
- Respiratory patterns
- Pain

PROGNOSIS AND OUTCOME

Prognosis is good if the animal survives the early postoperative period (12 to 24 hours)

PEARLS & CONSIDERATIONS

COMMENTS

- Findings on physical examination may be normal in some animals.
  - Diaphragmatic hernias are occasionally discovered as incidental findings in patients evaluated for other reasons.
- The radiographic diagnosis of diaphragmatic hernia can be surprisingly difficult in some cases.
  - Ultrasonography may be more useful in making the diagnosis especially if moderate to severe pleural effusion is present.
- Surgery should be delayed until the patient's condition has stabilized.
- Perform surgery as soon as possible if the stomach has herniated into the thoracic cavity.

PREVENTION

Routine use of leashes to avoid hit-by-car injuries

CLIENT EDUCATION

Patients with diaphragmatic hernia usually have a history of trauma, but failure to perform radiographic examination of the thorax often results in delayed diagnosis

SUGGESTED READING

Boudrieau SJ, Muir WW: Pathophysiology of traumatic diaphragmatic hernia in dogs. *Compend Contin Educ Pract Vet* 9:379, 1987.

Downs MC, Bjorling DE: Traumatic diaphragmatic hernias: A review of 1674 cases. *Vet Surg* 16:87, 1987.

Hyun C: Radiographic diagnosis of diaphragmatic hernia: review of 60 cases in dogs and cats. *J Vet Sci* 5:157, 2004.

Spattini G, et al.: Use of ultrasound to diagnose diaphragmatic rupture in dogs and cats. *Vet Radiol Ultrasound* 44:226, 2003.

AUTHOR: **MICHAEL B. MISON**
EDITOR: **RANCE K. SELLON**

Diarrhea, Acute

BASIC INFORMATION

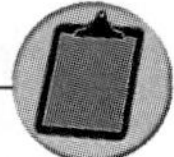

DEFINITION

- Increase in:
  - Frequency of defecation, and/or
  - Stool fluidity or loose consistency, and/or
  - Fecal volume (increased water content or fecal solids)
- Sudden onset
- Short duration (<2 weeks)

EPIDEMIOLOGY

RISK FACTORS

- Environment: overcrowding, poor sanitation, immune-compromised (infectious).
- Puppies, kittens: intestinal parasites, certain viral infections.
- Habitation: farm, free-roaming, left unsupervised (dietary indiscretion).
- Dog/cat shows: stress, close contact, animals from large geographic areas.
- Raw diets: Salmonellosis, *Escherichia coli* infection (young children, immune-compromised).
- Stress: increased shedding of organisms.

CONTAGION AND ZOONOSIS

- Potential zoonoses:
  - *Salmonella* spp.
  - *E. coli*
  - *Campylobacter* spp.
  - *Clostridium difficile*
  - *Yersinia enterocolitica*
  - *Shigella* spp.
  - *Giardia*
  - *Cryptosporidium parvum*
  - *Toxoplasma gondii*
  - *Balantidium coli*
  - *Entamoeba histolytica*
  - *Pentatrichomonas hominis*
  - *Echinococcus* spp.
  - *Ancylostoma caninum* (cutaneous larval migrans)
  - *Toxocara* spp. (visceral and ocular larval migrans)
- Species-specific viral infections: feline leukemia virus (FeLV)/feline immunovirus (FIV)/feline infectious peritonitis/ feline panleukopenia (cat to cat); canine parvovirus (dog to dog).

GEOGRAPHY AND SEASONALITY

- Warmer, humid conditions: optimize conditions for proliferation.
- Cooler conditions: inactivate organism/ prevent further contagion.

CLINICAL PRESENTATION

DISEASE FORMS/SUBTYPES: Small or large intestine, or combination.

HISTORY, CHIEF COMPLAINT

- Duration of clinical signs/course.
- Age.
- When/where pet acquired.
- Vaccination history.
- Assess dietary history:
  - Abrupt diet change
  - Well-balanced commercial diet
  - Raw diet
- Environment:

- Potential for dietary indiscretion (food, foreign body, garbage, compost, manure)
- Exposure to infectious agents, parasites (recent hospitalization, boarding, grooming, travel)

- Recent medications.
- Stressful episode: recent move, changes in family routine, renovations, police/working dog
- Depression/lethargy.
- Differentiate small intestinal diarrhea from large (see Table I-4, p 298).

PHYSICAL EXAM FINDINGS

- Mentation: depression and dehydration in acute diarrhea patient: infectious or toxicity most likely.
- Mucous membrane color.
  - Brick red/injected: sepsis.
  - Pale: hypoperfusion/shock/pain.
- Hydration (nauseated/vomiting animal may have moist mucous membranes).
- Signs of shock, sepsis.
  - Pyrexia/subnormal temperature.
  - Tachycardia.
  - Tachypnea.
  - Cool extremities.
- Posture: "dog-praying" position/arched back (abdominal pain).
- Body weight.
- Body condition score.
- Abdominal palpation:
  - Lymphadenopathy (neoplasia, inflammation, infection).
  - Thickened bowel (inflammatory, neoplastic infiltration).
  - Fluid- or gas-filled bowel.
  - Intussusception (sausage shape), especially puppies with viral gastroenteritis or parasitism.
  - Pain: splinting/groans/turns toward examiner.
  - Assess fullness of urinary bladder (urine production with respect to hydration status and renal function).
  - Abdominal mass.
- Perineal area:
  - Perianal fistulas.
  - Perineal hernia may cause signs of large bowel disease.
  - Anal gland disease.
- Rectal palpation:
  - Pain/increased mucosal sensitivity.
  - Narrowing of rectum (infiltrative disease, stricture).
  - Foreign body.
  - Mass (polyp[s], neoplasia).
- Cats: Palpate for thyroid nodule (hyperthyroidism).
- Observe animal defecating (tenesmus, signs of pain, character of feces).

ETIOLOGY AND PATHOPHYSIOLOGY

- Abnormality of transmucosal movement of water and solute:
  - Osmotic (decreased solute absorption)
  - Secretory (hypersecretion of ions)
  - Exudative (increased permeability)
  - Abnormal motility
- More than one mechanism possible, depending on underlying cause

ETIOLOGY

- **Diet**
  - Food intolerance/allergy
  - Poor quality food
  - Abrupt diet change
  - Dietary indiscretion/toxin ingestion (mycotoxins, spoiled foods)
  - Overeating
- **Parasites**
  - Helminths
    - Hookworms: *Ancylostoma/Uncinaria* spp.
    - Whipworms: *Trichuris vulpis*
    - Ascarids/roundworms: *Toxocara* spp.
    - *Strongyloides*
  - Cestodes
  - Trematodes
  - *Trichinella*
  - Protozoa
    - *Isospora* spp. (coccidiosis)
    - *Giardia* spp.
    - *Cryptosporidium spp.*
    - *Pentatrichomonas*
    - *Balantidium coli*
    - *Entamoeba*
  - *Neorickettsial* spp. (rickettsia): salmon poisoning
  - *Histoplasma capsulatum*
  - Pythiosis
  - *Prototheca* (algae)
- **Bacteria**
  - *Campylobacter jejuni*
  - *Clostridium* spp. (*perfringens, difficile, upsaliensis*)
  - *E. coli*
  - *Salmonella* spp.
  - *Y. enterocolitica*
  - *Shigella* spp.
  - Small intestinal bacterial overgrowth (*Enterobacteraciae*)/antibiotic-responsive diarrhea
  - *Bacillus piliformis*
- **Viral**
  - Astrovirus
  - Coronaviruses
  - Canine distemper
  - Canine parvovirus
  - FeLV (secondary infections)
  - FIV (secondary infections)
  - Feline panleukopenia
  - Rotavirus
- **Chemicals**
  - Heavy metals/organophosphates
- **Drugs**
  - Various antibiotics
  - Antineoplastics
  - Anthelmintics
  - Anti-inflammatory nonsteroidals
  - Cardiac glycosides (digoxin)
  - Lactulose
- Hemorrhagic gastroenteritis (HGE)
- Intestinal foreign body
- Intussusception (especially puppies with viral gastroenteritis)
- Intestinal volvulus
- Irritable bowel syndrome
- Lymphangiectasia
- Neoplasia
  - Malignant lymphoma (most common)
  - Adenocarcinoma
- **Extragastrointestinal causes**
- Acute pancreatitis
- Hypoadrenocorticism
- Hepatic disease, cholangiohepatitis
- Renal disease
- Diabetes mellitus
- Exocrine pancreatic insufficiency (EPI)
- Hyperthyroidism (cats)

DIAGNOSIS

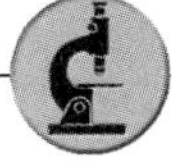

DIFFERENTIAL DIAGNOSIS

See Etology and Pathophysiology above

INITIAL DATABASE

- Fecal examinations:
  - Cytology (fresh saline smears): ova, larvae, motile protozoa, certain bacteria.
  - Flotation.
  - Zinc sulfate centrifugal flotation (*Giardia* cysts).
  - Enzyme-linked immunosorbent assay: *Giardia*-specific antigen.
  - Iodine stain: enhances visualization of *Giardia* trophozoites, stops motion of organism and cysts (stain light brown).
- Complete blood count (CBC) (if depressed, dehydrated, pyrexic):
  - Leukocytosis, leukopenia.
  - Presence/absence of left shift.
  - Elevated packed cell volume (PCV)/total solids (TS) (dehydration).
  - Elevated PCV without concomitant elevation in TS: hemorrhagic gastroenteritis.
  - Absence of stress leukogram suggestive of hypoadrenocorticism (CBC: lymphocytosis, eosinophilia, mild anemia, normal neutrophil count suggestive of hypoadrenocortiscism [i.e., absence of stress leukogram]).
- Serum biochemical profile:
  - Decreased electrolytes: gastrointestinal (GI) tract loss.
  - Hypoglycemia: sepsis, anorexia (young).
  - Elevated liver enzyme activities: hepatic disease, pancreatitis, or primary GI tract disease with portal bacterial translocation.
- Urinalysis: specific gravity (renal function/degree of dehydration).
- Serum thyroxine concentration (older cats).
- Parvoviral fecal antigen test (enzyme-linked immunosorbent assay).
- Abdominal radiographs, contrast radiography and/or ultrasonography.

ADVANCED OR CONFIRMATORY TESTS

- Adrenocorticotropic hormone stimulation test.
- Fecal cultures (*E. coli*, *Salmonella* spp., *C. jejuni*, *Clostridium* spp., *Y. enterocolitica*). However, efficacy in determining true infection is controversial; many of these bacteria are commensal organisms, and their presence in feces does not necessarily correlate with disease.
- *C. perfringens* fecal endospore enumeration (unreliable).
- *C. perfringens* enterotoxin: caution, discordant results amongst detection methods.
- Molecular techniques (polymerase chain reaction): increasing commercial availability.

TREATMENT

THERAPEUTIC GOAL(S)

- Correct volume deficits
- Prevent further dehydration
- Identify (if possible) and eliminate underlying cause
- Prevent contagion (other hospitalized patients)

ACUTE GENERAL TREATMENT

- Dietary restriction (24 to 48 hours, depending on severity of diarrhea and systemic status of patient).
- Gradual reintroduction of a bland, easily digestible, low-fat diet (small, frequent meals) for 3 to 5 days, with gradual reintroduction of the regular diet or new maintenance diet.
- Nonspecific or mild acute diarrhea: often self-limiting (1 to 2 days).
- Empiric or supportive treatments if indicated.
  - Fluid therapy:
    - Parenteral fluids if dehydration.
    - Mild diarrhea: over-the-counter oral glucose and electrolyte solutions, and/or subcutaneous fluids.
    - Severe cases: colloids and/or plasma transfusions.
  - Deworming medications.
  - Antimicrobials:
    - Reserved for cases associated with severe mucosal damage and high risk of secondary sepsis/endotoxemia (e.g., parvovirus, HGE).
    - Metronidazole (*Clostridium* spp.) 10-20 mg/kg IV as a constant rate infusion (CRI) over 1 hour, or PO q 12h.
    - Alternative: Ampicillin 22 mg/kg IV q 8h.
    - Erythromycin (*C. jejuni*) 10 mg/kg PO q 8h.
    - Enrofloxacin (*Salmonella* spp.) 2.5-5 mg/kg PO q 24h.
    - Trimethoprim/sulfadiazine 7-15 mg/kg PO q 12h.
  - Motility-modifying drugs (use with caution or not at all if GI obstruction or infectious diarrhea is suspected).
    - Short-term use (5 days or less).
    - Narcotic analgesics (contraindicated in infectious diarrhea).
      - Diphenoxylate (Lomotil): 0.1-0.2 mg/kg PO q 8-12h.
      - Loperamide (Imodium): 0.1-0.2 mg/kg PO q 8-12h.
    - Anticholinergics/antispasmodics.
      - Aminopentamide (Centrine): 0.01-0.03 mg/kg PO q 8-12h.
      - Hyoscyamine (Levsin): 0.003-0.006 mg/kg PO q 8-12h.
    - Combination central nervous system depressants and anticholinergics.
      - Prochlorperazine and isopropamide (Darbazine):
        - <10 kg: No. 1 capsule PO q 8h.
        - >10 kg: No. 3 capsule PO q 8h.
      - Chlordiazepoxide and clinidium (Librax): 0.1-0.25 mg/kg (dose based on clinidium) PO q 8-12h.
  - Antisecretory/protectant:
    - Bismuth subsalicylate (Pepto-Bismol): 0.1-1.0 mg/kg PO, tapering dose q 8-12h (caution in cats due to salicylates; may cause melenic-appearing stools; avoid chewable tablets [not well absorbed]).
  - Analgesics (butorphanol, fentanyl).
  - Nutritional support, if prolonged fasting required.
  - Antiemetics if severe nausea/vomiting (dogs and cats unless stated otherwise):
    - *Prochlorperazine: 0.1-0.5 mg/kg IM, SC, IV (slowly) q 6-8h; 1 mg/kg PO q 12h.
    - *Chlorpromazine: 0.2-0.5 mg/kg IM, SC q 6-8h; 0.05 mg/kg IV (slowly) q 4h; 1 mg/kg rectally q 8h (dog).
    - *†Metoclopramide: 0.2-0.5 mg/kg SC q 8h; 1-2 mg/kg/day IV as a CRI.
    - Ondansetron: 0.05-0.15 mg/kg IV q 8-24h; 0.5-1.0 mg/kg PO q 8-12h.
    - Dolasetron: 0.5 mg/kg IV, SC, PO q 24h.
    - Butorphanol: 0.2 mg/kg SC, IM, IV q 4-6h; 0.1 mg/kg IV as CRI.
    - Cyproheptadine: 1-2 mg per CAT PO q 8-12h.
    - Ranitidine: 0.5 mg/kg IV (slowly), SC, PO q 12h.

POSSIBLE COMPLICATIONS

- Further/ongoing dehydration.
- Severe mucosal damage: pyrexia, secondary sepsis/endotoxemia.
- Development of intussusception/other intestinal accident.

RECOMMENDED MONITORING

- Patient can deteriorate rapidly
- Frequent or constant monitoring:
  - Body weight (minimum q 24h)
  - Temperature
  - PCV/TS
  - Blood glucose
  - Electrolytes

PROGNOSIS AND OUTCOME

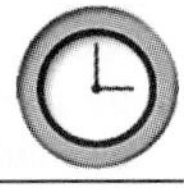

- Dependent on underlying cause.
- Infectious causes, intoxications, mechanical/functional obstruction, HGE, acute pancreatitis, hepatitis, renal disease, hypoadrenocorticism: potentially life-threatening.
- Dietary indiscretion, parasitic diseases: often not as serious.
- Appropriate monitoring and subsequent treatment influence outcome.

PEARLS & CONSIDERATIONS

COMMENTS

- Advanced diagnostic evaluation may not be necessary in a patient with first-time acute diarrhea when that patient is otherwise stable and well; however, failure of diarrhea to respond to treatment in 24 to 48 hours, or deterioration at any time, warrants further diagnostic testing and treatment.
- Establish a hospital infectious protocol: prevent contagion.
  - Follow protocol on admission (any patient with a suspicion of contagion).
  - Parasite control, good sanitation habits, impervious flooring in kennels/dog runs: paramount importance.
- Routine deworming of bitches and puppies (every 2 weeks) decreases transmission.
- Routine antibiotic use (uncomplicated diarrhea) is discouraged.
  - Adverse effects on normal GI flora.
  - Promotes resistant strains of bacteria.

CLIENT EDUCATION

- Pets are occasionally reservoirs for human infection.
  - Proper hygiene:
    - Frequent hand washing (one's own and childrens').
    - Regular cleaning of pet's bedding and litterbox (cats).
- Feeding of raw diets is discouraged.
  - Risk of transmission of zoonotic pathogens (*E. coli.*, *Salmonella* spp.).

---

*May precipitate seizures in animals with a history of seizure activity.

†Do not use if obstruction is suspected.

- Strict (yet basic) hygiene protocols required (if feeding of raw diets cannot be prevented).
  - Wash pet's food bowls (hot water/soap) after *each* meal, one's hands, utensils, kitchen counters.

SUGGESTED READING

German AJ, et al: Comparison of direct and indirect tests for small intestinal bacterial overgrowth and antibiotic-responsive diarrhea in dogs. *J Vet Intern Med* 17:33–43, 2004.

Guilford WG: Approach to clinical problems in gastroenterology. In Guilford WG, et al (eds): *Strombeck's Small Animal Gastroenterology*, ed 2. Philadelphia, WB Saunders, 1996, pp 50–76.

Guilford WG, Strombeck DR: Classification, pathophysiology, and symptomatic treatment of diarrheal diseases. In Guilford WG, et al (eds): *Strombeck's Small Animal Gastroenterology*, ed 2. Philadelphia, WB Saunders, 1996, pp 351–366.

Marks SL: Editorial. Small intestinal bacterial overgrowth in dogs: Less common than you think. *J Vet Intern Med* 17:5–7, 2004.

Marks SL, Kather EJ: Bacterial-associated diarrhea in the dog: A critical appraisal. *Vet Clin Small Anim* 33:1029–1060, 2003.

Tams TR: Diarrhea. In Ettinger SJ, Feldman EC (eds): *Textbook of Veterinary Internal Medicine* Vol. I, ed 5. Philadelphia, WB Saunders, 2000, pp 121–126.

Tams TR: Gastrointestinal symptoms. In Tams TR (ed): *Small Animal Gastroenterology*, ed 2. St. Louis, Saunders (Elsevier Science), 2003, pp 1–50.

Washabau RJ, Elie MS: Anti-emetic therapy. In Bonagura JD (ed): *Kirk's Current Veterinary Therapy XII Small Animal Practice*. Philadelphia, WB Saunders, 1995, pp 679–684.

Willard M: Clinical manifestations of gastrointestinal disorders. In Nelson RW, Couto CG (eds): *Essentials of Small Animal Internal Medicine*, ed 2. St. Louis: Mosby, 1998, pp 346–369.

AUTHOR: **LISA CARIOTO**
EDITOR: **ETIENNE CÔTÉ**

Diarrhea, Chronic

BASIC INFORMATION

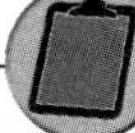

DEFINITION

- Increase in:
  - Frequency of defecation, and/or
  - Stool fluidity or loose consistency, and/or
  - Fecal volume (increased water content or fecal solids)
- Persistent clinical signs (more than 2 to 3 weeks) or episodic occurrence

EPIDEMIOLOGY

CONTAGION AND ZOONOSIS: Potentially zoonotic organisms. See Diarrhea, Acute, p 294.

GEOGRAPHY AND SEASONALITY: See Diarrhea, Acute, p 294

CLINICAL PRESENTATION

DISEASE FORMS/SUBTYPES: Small versus large bowel, or both (Table I-4).
- Further segregated into diseases caused by maldigestion or malabsorption
- Malabsorption:
  - Nonprotein versus protein-losing disease

HISTORY, CHIEF COMPLAINT
- Duration of clinical signs/course
- Age
- When/where pet acquired
- Vaccination history
- Assess dietary history
  - Abrupt diet change
  - Well-balanced commercial diet
  - Raw diet
- Recent medications
- Stressful episode: recent move, changes in family routine, renovations, police/working dog
- Depression/lethargy
- Differentiate small intestinal diarrhea from large (Table I-4)

PHYSICAL EXAM FINDINGS
- Hydration status
- Depression/weakness/lethargy
- Emaciation: malnutrition, chronic malabsorption, protein-losing enteropathy
- Dull haircoat: malabsorption (fatty acids, protein, vitamins)
- Fever: inflammation, infection, neoplasia
- Edema, ascites, decreased lung/heart sounds: protein-losing enteropathy
- Pale mucous membranes: chronic GI blood loss, anemia of chronic illness/inflammation
- Abdominal palpation:
  - Mass(es): foreign body, neoplasm, granuloma
  - Thickened bowel loops: inflammation, neoplastic infiltration
  - "Aggregated" bowel loops: mass, peritoneal adhesions
  - "Sausage"-shaped loop: intussusception
  - Pain: inflammation, obstruction, ischemia
  - Gas/fluid distention: diarrhea, obstruction (mass), ileus
  - Mesenteric lymphadenopathy: neoplasia, inflammation
- Rectal palpation:
  - Mass(es): polyp, neoplasm, granuloma
  - Circumferential narrowing: stricture, spasm, neoplasm
  - Irregular mucosal texture: colitis, neoplasm

ETIOLOGY AND PATHOPHYSIOLOGY

- Small intestine:
  - Decreased fluid and electrolytes absorption
  - Incomplete nutrient absorption (fats, carbohydrates)
  - Increased fluid and electrolytes secretion
- Large intestine:
  - Decreased fluid and electrolytes absorption
  - Secretion of fluid and electrolytes
  - Failure of reservoir function

CAUSES OF CHRONIC SMALL (S) AND LARGE (L) INTESTINAL DIARRHEA
- Parasites:
  - *Giardia*—s/l
  - Hookworms—s
  - Roundworms—s
  - Whipworms (*Trichuris*)—l
  - Amoebiasis—l
  - Balantidium coli—l
- Dietary intolerance—s/l.
- Dietary allergy—s/l.
- Inflammatory bowel disease (IBD):
  - Lymphocytic-plasmacytic—s/l
  - Eosinophilic—s/l
  - Granulomatous enteritis—s/l
  - Hypereosinophilic syndrome (cats primarily)—s
  - Neutrophilic (suppurative/purulent) enteritis—s
  - Breed-specific (shar-pei, basenji, soft-coated wheaten terrier)—s
  - Chronic ulcerative colitis—l
  - Histiocytic ulcerative colitis (primarily boxers)—l
- Neoplasia—s/l:
  - Lymphoma
  - Adenocarcinoma
  - Leiomyoma/leiomyosarcoma
  - Mast cell tumor
- Infectious:
  - Salmonellosis—l
  - Campylobacteriosis—s/l
  - Clostridial infection—s/l
  - Histoplasmosis—s/l
  - Yersiniosis—l
  - *Bacillus piliformis*—l
  - Pythiosis—l
  - Protothecosis—l
  - Tritrichomoniasis (cats)—s/l

TABLE I-4 **Clinical Signs of Small Intestinal vs. Large Intestinal Diarrhea**

Characteristic	Small Intestine	Large Intestine
Feces		
Mucus	Uncommon	Common
Hematochezia (fresh blood in/on feces)	Absent	Often present
Melena (digested blood in feces)	± Present	Absent
Volume	Often increased	Normal to decreased (due to increased frequency)
Quality	Nearly formed to watery ("cowpile"); ± undigested food/fat; possibly malodorous	Loose to semi-solid
Shape	Variable (dependent upon amount of water present)	Normal or narrowed
Steatorrhea (undigested fat in feces)	Present with maldigestive or malabsorptive disorders	Absent
Defecation		
Frequency	Normal to mildly increased (2 to 4 times/day)	Greatly increased (4 to 10 times/day)
Dyschezia (inability to defecate without straining or signs of pain)	Absent	Dogs: frequent; cats: less common
Tenesmus (straining)	Absent	Common (dog). Cats: less common, rule out stranguria
Urgency	Less common, unless severe acute enteritis	Frequent
Associated Signs		
Weight loss	Common	Uncommon. Possible with severe chronic colitis, diffuse neoplasia, histoplasmosis, pythiosis
Vomiting	Possible	May be seen, especially with acute colitis (30%). Possible before onset of abnormal stools
Appetite	Usually normal; may be ↑ or ↓ in bowel infiltration/inflammation depending on severity of lesion	Normal to decreased if severe disease (neoplasia, histoplasmosis)
Halitosis	± Present (maldigestion/malabsorption)	Absent
Borborygmus	Possible	Absent
Flatulence	Possible	Common
Fecal incontinence	Rare	Possible
"Scooting" or chewing of perianal area	Absent	Possible with proctitis

 - Feline leukemia virua (FeLV)—s/l
 - Feline immunodeficiency virus (FIV)—s/l
 - Feline infectious peritonitis (FIP)—s/l
- Chronic small intestinal bacterial overgrowth (SIBO) in dogs secondary to:
 - Immunoglobulin A deficiency—s
 - Partial obstruction (chronic intussusception) or blind loops—s
 - Exocrine pancreatic insufficiency (EPI)—s
 - Abnormal motility with underlying gastrointestinal (GI) disease—s
 - Gastric acid deficiency—s
 - Antibiotic-responsive enteritis/diarrhea (considered equivalent to SIBO by some)—s
 - Idiopathic—s
- Villous atrophy—s:
 - Idiopathic
 - Gastrinoma
 - Gluten-responsive
- Hyperthyroidism (cats)
- Hypoadrenocorticism
- Protein-losing enteropathy:
 - Intestinal lymphangiectasia
 - *Any of the preceding disorders can cause protein-losing enteropathy (disease progression and severity)*
- Maldigestive diseases—s:
 - EPI
 - Lactase deficiency (especially cats)
- Functional disorder:
 - Irritable bowel syndrome (IBS)—l

DIAGNOSIS

DIFFERENTIAL DIAGNOSIS

See Etiology and Pathophysiology above

INITIAL DATABASE

- Fecal tests
 - Flotation (including zinc sulfate flotation)
 - Direct smear: *Giardia, Entamoeba, Balantidium coli*
 - Enzyme-linked immunosorbent assay (ELISA): *Giardia*-specific antigen
 - Cytologic evaluation (rectal scraping)
 - Culture and sensitivity
 - *Clostridium perfringens* enterotoxin assay
 - *Cryptosporidium* fecal ELISA test
 - Occult blood neoplasia; meat-based diet may cause false positives with some kits
- Complete blood count (CBC)
 - Hydration status (PCV/TS)
 - Leukocytosis: inflammation, infection, stress
 - Eosinophilia: eosinophilic IBD, endoparasitism
 - Lymphopenia: lymphangiectasia
 - Anemia: chronic GI blood loss, anemia of chronic illness/inflammation, nutrient malabsorption
 - Absence of a stress leukogram: hypoadrenocorticism
- Serum biochemistry profile
 - Hypoalbuminemia, hypoproteinemia
 - Azotemia
 - Abnormal liver enzyme levels
 - Hypocholesterolemia: lymphangiectasia, hepatopathy
- Urinalysis
 - Specific gravity: renal function, hydration
 - Proteinuria
- Serum T4 (cats)
- FeLV/FIV

ADVANCED OR CONFIRMATORY TESTING

- Urine protein: creatinine ratio if proteinuric
- Serum bile acids

- Adrenocorticotropic hormone stimulation test
- Trypsin-like immunoreactivity test: EPI (species-specific test)
- Serum cobalamin (vitamin B_{12}), folate
  - Folate: depends on jejunum's absorptive function (proximal small intestine)
  - Cobalamin: depends on pancreatic intrinsic factor secretion and absorption in ileum (distal small intestine)
  - ↓ Folate and ↓ cobalamin: diffuse malabsorptive disease
  - ↓ Cobalamin, ↑ folate: antibiotic-responsive enteritis/SIBO
- Gastrin levels
- Serology (histoplasmosis)
- Radiography:
  - Survey
  - Contrast
- Abdominal ultrasonography: mass lesion, thickened bowel loops, loss of detail of GI wall architecture/wall layering
  - Exception: mass lesion
- Endoscopy: upper and lower (determine extent of disease)
- Exploratory laparotomy: full-thickness biopsies *(biopsy even if no gross lesions)*
- Empiric therapy (may be elected due to client's financial constraints):
  - Anthelmintics
  - Antimicrobials
  - Anti-inflammatories
  - Dietary trials
- Molecular techniques (polymerase chain reaction): increasing commercial availability

TREATMENT

THERAPEUTIC GOAL(S)

Treat underlying cause

ACUTE GENERAL TREATMENT

- Low-fat, highly digestible low-fiber diets (low-fat cottage cheese/tofu and rice or potatoes)
- Small, frequent meals (3–6/day)
- High-fiber diets (colitis)
- Empiric treatment: anthelmintics (fenbendazole) or metronidazole, even with negative tests

CHRONIC TREATMENT

- Dependent on underlying cause; see specific disorders for details
- Dietary modifications (general):
  - Novel protein source
  - Trial period: minimum 3 to 4 weeks
  - Eliminate all other foods (antigen sources [treats, toys, flavored medications])

PROGNOSIS AND OUTCOME

- Dependent on underlying cause, response to treatment, owner compliance, and interindividual variation.
- Guarded:
  - Histoplasmosis.
  - Protothecosis.
  - Pythiosis.
  - Yersiniosis.
  - Regional granulomatous enterocolitis.
- Poor to guarded:
  - Basenji, shar-pei, soft-coated Wheaten terrier-associated IBD.
  - FIP.
  - Villous atrophy (clinical signs often persist despite treatment).
  - Feline hypereosinophilic syndrome.
- Fair:
  - Histiocytic-ulcerative colitis (lifetime therapy needed, difficult to control).
- Fair to good:
  - Antibiotic-responsive enteritis/SIBO: depending on underlying cause. Some require frequent or continuous treatment; others have prolonged remission with one course of antibiotics.
  - FeLV/FIV (when secondary infections controlled).
- Fair to excellent:
  - IBD (realistic expectation: maintenance of remission/control of relapses, rather than cure).
- Good:
  - Dietary intolerance/food allergy.
  - Giardiasis.
  - *Salmonella* (although mortality rate can be high [hospitalized, young, immune-compromised]).
  - *Campylobacter*
  - *Clostridium* spp. (although fatalities reported)
- Good to excellent:
  - EPI (continual treatment)
  - Hyperthyroidism
  - Hypoadrenocorticism (lifelong treatment)
  - Hookworms/roundworms/whipworms
- Lymphangiectasia: unpredictable. Remission in some (months to years), cachexia, cavity effusions, intractable diarrhea in others.
- Neoplasia: dependent on tumor type.

POSSIBLE COMPLICATIONS

- Immunosuppressive therapy (azathioprine, chlorambucil): myelosuppression
- 5-aminosalicylates: keratoconjunctivitis sicca
- Iatrogenic hyperadrenocorticism with chronic glucocorticoid use
- Excessive protein loss: edema/cavity effusions
- Buccal mucosal irritation: pancreatic enzyme supplementation (EPI)

RECOMMENDED MONITORING

- Body weight
- Serum protein concentration
- Frequent CBCs (immunosuppressive agents)
- Schirmer tear test (sulfasalazine)
- Steroids: use minimum effective dose

PEARLS & CONSIDERATIONS

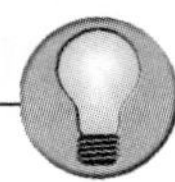

COMMENTS

- SIBO: difficult to diagnose (antibiotic-responsive diarrhea considered separate disease by some).
- Culture and sensitivity: efficacy in determining true infection controversial; many of the bacteria are commensal organisms and their presence in the feces does not necessarily correlate with disease.
- *C. perfringens* enterotoxin assay: significance of positive result not truly understood (nondiarrheic dogs can be positive).
- Intestinal biopsies strongly recommended.
- During laparotomy or endoscopy, always obtain biopsies, even if tissues appear grossly normal.
- Corticosteroids: use minimum effective dose.

CLIENT EDUCATION

Some of the preceding diseases can be frustrating to treat (waxing and waning nature). Inform owner at time of diagnosis: avoids unrealistic expectations/disappointment).

SUGGESTED READING

Guilford WG: Approach to clinical problems in gastroenterology. In Guilford WG, et al (eds): *Strombeck's Small Animal Gastroenterology*, ed 2. Philadelphia, WB Saunders, 1996, pp 50–76.

Guilford WG, Strombeck DR: Classification, pathophysiology, and symptomatic treatment of diarrheal diseases. In Guilford WG, et al (eds): *Strombeck's Small Animal Gastroenterology*, ed 2. Philadelphia, WB Saunders, 1996, pp 351–366.

Marks SL, Kather EJ: Bacterial-associated diarrhea in the dog: A critical appraisal. *Vet Clin Small Anim* 33:1029–1060, 2003.

Tams TR: Diarrhea. In Ettinger SJ, Feldman EC (eds): *Textbook of Veterinary Internal Medicine*, Vol. I, ed 5. Philadelphia, WB Saunders, 2000, pp 121–126.

Tams TR: Gastrointestinal symptoms. In Tams TR (ed): *Small Animal Gastroenterology*, ed 2. St. Louis, WB Saunders (Elsevier Science), 2003, pp 1–50.

Willard M: Clinical manifestations of gastrointestinal disorders. In Nelson RW, Couto CG (eds): *Essentials of Small Animal Internal Medicine*, ed 2. St. Louis, Mosby, 1998, pp 346–369.

AUTHOR: **LISA CARIOTO**
EDITOR: **ETIENNE CÔTÉ**

Dietary Intolerance

BASIC INFORMATION

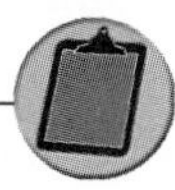

DEFINITION

Adverse reactions to an ingested food or food additive due to nonimmunologic mechanisms

SYNONYM(S)

Adverse reaction to food
Food intolerance
Lactose intolerance

EPIDEMIOLOGY

SPECIES, AGE, SEX: Dogs and cats: no age or gender predilection.

RISK FACTORS

- Food contaminated with microorganisms or their toxic metabolites
- Specific foods (onions, chocolate)
- Toxic food preservatives (e.g., propylene glycol in cats)
- Preformed vasoactive amines (e.g., histamine) in food, such as fish
- Dairy products
- Dietary indiscretion (gluttony, pica, ingestion of indigestible materials)

ASSOCIATED CONDITIONS AND DISORDERS

- Dietary hypersensitivity
- Inflammatory bowel disease

CLINICAL PRESENTATION

HISTORY, CHIEF COMPLAINT: Vomiting, diarrhea, intermittent abdominal pain, abdominal distention, soft feces, flatulence, increased frequency of defecation.

PHYSICAL EXAM FINDINGS: Diarrhea (small or large bowel), vomiting, abdominal distention, urticaria, angioedema.

ETIOLOGY AND PATHOPHYSIOLOGY

- Food poisoning:
  - Eating foods (e.g., through scavenging, improperly cooked homemade foods, raw diets, contaminated canned or dry commercial foods [e.g., aflatoxin]) that are contaminated with bacteria, fungal toxins, or other toxins that cause an immediate gastrointestinal (GI) response. (See Garbage Toxicosis, p 425.)
- Idiosyncratic adverse reactions to food additives:
  - The more common examples are reactions to food colorings (red or green dyes) or to certain preservatives.
  - Occur infrequently and unpredictably in individuals, and are not apparently dose related.
  - Histaminergic reactions mediated by type 1 (mast cell mediated) or 2 (receptors for gastric acid release in the stomach) histamine receptors.
- Pharmacologic reactions to vasoactive amines (e.g., histamine) found in food
- Carbohydrate intolerance (lactase deficiency):
  - Mediated by lack of carbohydrate digestion due to mucosal disease, lack of enzyme activity—either congenital or acquired—or due to a true allergic reaction to proteins in milk (lactose intolerance). Which of these types of reactions are causing the problem is rarely defined and not clinically relevant.
- Dietary indiscretion:
  - Typically defined as the consumption of unusual or rotten foods (as can occur with scavenging or raiding the garbage can), the consumption of too much food (gluttony), or pica (eating nonfood substances such as hair, rocks, bones, etc.).
  - The insult occurring in the GI tract varies with the type of indiscretion that is observed, and thus, no consistent clinical presentation is recognized.

DIAGNOSIS

Food intolerance is suspected on the basis of acute vomiting and/or diarrhea, often but not always occurring as a result of acute dietary alterations; confirmatory diagnosis is often retrospective, with resolution of clinical signs as a result of proper diet. In contrast to dietary hypersensitivity (food allergy), the response to the change in food is more rapid (1 to 2 weeks) with dietary intolerance. Therefore, if no response occurs during this time frame, the diagnosis of intolerance should be questioned.

DIFFERENTIAL DIAGNOSIS

- Any chronic disorder affecting the GIT (e.g., hypoadrenocorticism, protein-losing enteropathy, infiltrative disease)
- Inflammatory bowel disease
- GI neoplasia
- Chronic parasitism
- Food hypersensitivity

INITIAL DATABASE

- Complete blood count: nonspecific and usually normal
- Serum biochemistry profile: nonspecific and usually normal
- Urinalysis: nonspecific
- Fecal flotations to rule out parasitic causes of vomiting/diarrhea

ADVANCED OR CONFIRMATORY TESTING

- Proper nutrition/elimination food trial.
- Further testing generally unnecessary for the primary diagnosis; used for identifying other disorders with similar signs or for identifying inciting causes (differential diagnosis).
- Abdominal radiography and ultrasonography: used for ruling out the other causes of vomiting and diarrhea for which imaging modalities are diagnostic (e.g., intestinal obstruction, intestinal mass).
- Endoscopy with biopsy and histopathologic evaluation of GI mucosa: Mucosa may be normal, or may show increases in lamina propria lymphocytes or plasma cells; however, the inflammatory changes seen in dogs or cats with food intolerance are generally less profound than found in those with IBD or other diseases of the mucosa.

TREATMENT

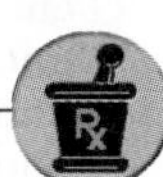

THERAPEUTIC GOAL(S)

- Avoid exposure to food toxins, dairy products, certain (or excess) carbohydrates, and dietary sources of vasoactive amines (e.g., certain types of fish)
- Control episodes of dietary indiscretion

ACUTE GENERAL TREATMENT

- Nonspecific supportive care based on clinical signs (e.g., parenteral fluid administration for dehydration).
- Perform an elimination food trial (in general, a shorter trial of 7 to 10 days is all that is required to result in the resolution of the signs of dietary intolerance).
- Clinical signs of GI disease usually resolve within a few days on the new diet that does not contain the offending substance.

CHRONIC TREATMENT

- Maintain strict avoidance of offending foods or ingredients (e.g., dairy products)
- Find an acceptable commercial or homemade food for long-term maintenance
- Control episodes of gluttony, pica, or ingestion of indigestible materials

POSSIBLE COMPLICATIONS

Certain types of food poisoning can cause serious and life-threatening disease.

PROGNOSIS AND OUTCOME

Good prognosis if offending foods or ingredients are eliminated from the diet

PEARLS & CONSIDERATIONS

COMMENTS

In instances of recurrent food intolerance (versus one-time events), use of a food diary by the animal owner is important to monitor clinical response and compliance.

CLIENT EDUCATION

Human food sources, snacks, treats and food for other animals in the household (e.g., dog having access to cat food) can be a problem.

SUGGESTED READING

Roudebush P, Guilford WG, Shanley KV: Adverse reactions to food. In Hand MS, Thatcher CD, Remillard RL, Roudebush P (eds): *Small Animal Clinical Nutrition,* ed 4. Topeka, Mark Morris Institute, 2000, pp 431–453.

AUTHOR: **PHILIP ROUDEBUSH**
EDITOR: **DEBRA L. ZORAN**

Digoxin Toxicity

BASIC INFORMATION

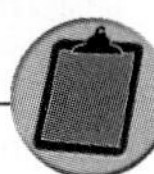

DEFINITION

Clinical signs caused by excessive administration of, or individual intolerance to normal doses of, digoxin

SYNONYM(S)

Digitalis poisoning
Digoxin intoxication
Digoxin and *digitalis* are used interchangeably: other digitalis derivatives, such as digitoxin, are no longer used clinically.

EPIDEMIOLOGY

SPECIES, AGE, SEX: Dogs and cats
GENETICS AND BREED PREDISPOSITION: Doberman pinschers appear predisposed.
RISK FACTORS
- Renal failure
- Hypovolemia, dehydration
- Hypokalemia
- Concurrent administration of drugs that increase serum digoxin levels: diazepam, erythromycin, quinidine, tetracycline, verapamil
- Obesity (if digoxin is dosed on total body weight, rather than lean body weight)
- Intravenous digoxin
- MDR-1 gene mutant

ASSOCIATED CONDITIONS AND DISORDERS: Underlying heart disease prompting digoxin treatment.

CLINICAL PRESENTATION

DISEASE FORMS/SUBTYPES
- Systemic signs
- Cardiac arrhythmias

HISTORY, CHIEF COMPLAINT
- Hallmarks of digoxin toxicity: lethargy, anorexia, vomiting, and diarrhea, together or individually.
- May be intermittent in mild cases.
- Severe toxicity: refractory vomiting, tenesmus, collapse, death.
- Except for massive overdoses, digoxin treatment needs to have been underway for >24 hours (and usually weeks) to produce signs of toxicity.
- Most commonly, patients are receiving digoxin as part of long-term cardiac treatment. Much less commonly, digoxin toxicity occurs from a pet's consuming plants or human medication.

PHYSICAL EXAM FINDINGS
- Lethargy, dehydration
- Physical findings attributable to underlying heart disease
- Digoxin toxicity can also produce virtually any cardiac arrhythmia
  - Bradycardia or tachycardia on examination

ETIOLOGY AND PATHOPHYSIOLOGY

- Digoxin is a cardiac glycoside drug derived from the foxglove plant.
  - It is absorbed slowly (6 to 8 hours to peak serum concentration with oral tablets in dogs; faster with elixir) and is mainly excreted renally (>60%).
- The half-life is long: 14 to 56 hours (dogs), 30 to 173 hours (cats).
- Therefore, when intoxication occurs, it more often is a cumulative process (chronic treatment).
- Acute overdoses are amenable to activated charcoal administration for several hours after ingestion.
- All cardiac glycosides (therapeutic, e.g., digoxin, digitoxin [historic]; or botanical, e.g., foxglove, oleander) act on the sodium-potassium-adenosine triphosphate pump of mammalian cells to increase intracellular Na^+ and Ca^{2+} concentrations.
- Cardiovascular, neurologic, and gastrointestinal effects are responsible for clinical signs.
- With digoxin toxicity, systemic clinical signs precede, or occur concurrently with, cardiac arrhythmias.

DIAGNOSIS

The diagnosis is strongly suspected on the basis of medication history and clinical signs. Initial testing offers supportive evidence, but the diagnosis is often established based on resolution of clinical signs when the drug is stopped.

DIFFERENTIAL DIAGNOSIS

- Primary gastrointestinal disease
- Uremia/renal failure
- Cardiac arrhythmias of primary cardiac, or systemic, origin

INITIAL DATABASE

- Serum biochemistry profile, urinalysis:
  - Evidence of chronic renal failure or hypokalemia increases likelihood of intoxication.
  - Concurrent treatment with diuretics may cause azotemia and isosthenuria.
  - Generally if azotemia is severe (blood urea nitrogen >80 mg/dl and creatinine >3 mg/dl), some degree of reduced renal function is expected and digoxin elimination is likely reduced, predisposing to toxicity.
- Electrocardiogram (ECG):
  - First-degree atrioventricular (AV) block (see Atrioventricular Block, First-Degree, p 107): early ECG manifestation of digoxin toxicity.
  - Higher degrees of AV block, premature atrial or ventricular complexes common.

ADVANCED OR CONFIRMATORY TESTING

- Serum digoxin concentration: confirmation (retrospective)
  - Therapeutic level: 0.8–2.0 ng/ml
  - >2–3 ng/ml with clinical signs: digoxin toxicity
  - Turnaround time of test limits immediate usefulness but some local human hospitals may provide stat service

- Evaluations of renal/central nervous/gastrointestinal systems: as dictated by clinical signs

TREATMENT

THERAPEUTIC GOAL(S)

- Acute overdoses: prevent digoxin assimilation
- All cases: reduce serum digoxin concentration

ACUTE GENERAL TREATMENT

- Acute overdoses (uncommon): activated charcoal and supportive care (see Etiology and Pathophysiology above).
- Toxicity in dogs receiving normal digoxin doses chronically: the cornerstone of treatment is discontinuation of the drug.
    - Treatment may be restarted 48 hours later at half the dose after signs of toxicity have resolved.
- Intravenous fluid therapy: judicious, if patient has cardiac disease.
- Potassium supplementation in hypokalemic patients: essential, since hypokalemia may potentiate arrhythmias.
- Ventricular antiarrhythmics if rapid ventricular arrhythmias (see Ventricular Arrhythmias [Premature Ventricular Complexes, Ventricular Tachycardia], p 1149).
- Treatment for supraventricular arrythmias if very rapid (see Atrial Premature Complexes and Atrial/Supraventricular Tachycardia, p 100).
- Soluble antidigoxin antibodies may be administered in severely ill patients.
    - Number of vials (38 mg each) given slowly IV = serum digoxin level [ng/ml] × body weight (kg)/100.
    - For example, 2 vials slow IV single dose for a 35 lb (16 kg) dog with serum digoxin level 12 ng/ml.
    - Very costly ($500 per vial).

RECOMMENDED MONITORING

Monitoring serum concentrations is secondary to monitoring of clinical signs alone.

PROGNOSIS AND OUTCOME

- Dependent on dose, elimination (renal function, hydration), extent of signs, and response to treatment.
- Severe digoxin intoxication can be fatal.

PEARLS & CONSIDERATIONS

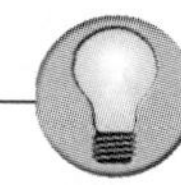

COMMENTS

- Differentiation between digoxin toxicity and an unrelated problem (e.g., primary GI disturbance, renal failure, other) may be challenging.
- It is virtually always preferable to assume that digoxin toxicity exists and discontinue the drug and use other cardiac drugs (e.g., beta blockers, inotropes) as replacements if necessary, while evaluation of the other differential diagnoses takes place; response to discontinuation helps to confirm toxicity retrospectively.

PREVENTION

Early detection of clinical signs of toxicity by owners, and if signs occur, discontinuation of the drug, monitoring, and supportive care.

SUGGESTED READING

Knight DH: Efficacy of inotropic support of the failing heart. *Vet Clin North Am* 21:879-904, 1991.

Ward DM, Forrester SD, DeFrancesco TC, Troy GC: Treatment of severe chronic digoxin toxicosis in a dog with cardiac disease, using ovine digoxin-specific immunoglobulin G Fab fragments. *J Am Vet Med Assoc* 215:1808–1812, 1999.

AUTHOR & EDITOR: **ETIENNE CÔTÉ**

Dilated Cardiomyopathy

Client Education Sheet on Website

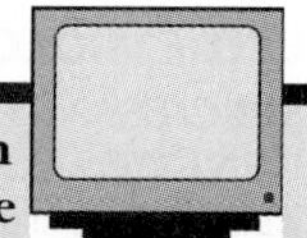

BASIC INFORMATION

DEFINITION

A primary myocardial disease characterized by impaired systolic function (pump failure) of one or both ventricles leading to cardiac enlargement and potential congestive heart failure, arrhythmias, or both. Diastolic dysfunction may also be observed.

SYNONYM(S)

Congestive cardiomyopathy
DCM

EPIDEMIOLOGY

SPECIES, AGE, SEX

- Dogs:
    - Adult-onset disease (4 to 10 years) except in Portuguese water dogs (juvenile; weeks to months of age)
    - Male > female
- Cats:
    - 2 to 20 years (mean, 9.8 ± 4.4 years)
    - Male > female

GENETICS AND BREED PREDISPOSITION

- Dogs
    - Large/giant-breed dogs overrepresented (Doberman pinscher, Irish wolfhound, Great Dane, Scottish deerhound, boxer,Afghan hound, Old English sheepdog, Dalmatian).
    - Variety of spaniel breeds (English, American cocker spaniels; others).
    - Young Portuguese waterdogs.
    - Irish wolfhounds, Newfoundlands, Doberman pinschers, boxers: autosomal dominant trait. Portuguese water-dogs: autosomal recessive trait (suspected).
- Cats: Abyssinian, Burmese, and Siamese overrepresented.

RISK FACTORS

- Taurine deficiency in cats (common cause of DCM in cats, mainly before 1987)
- Dalmatians fed a low-protein diet
- Cocker spaniels, golden retrievers (taurine deficiency)

GEOGRAPHY AND SEASONALITY: Chagas' disease–associated DCM (southern United States): clinical presentation is indistinguishable from idiopathic dilated cardiomyopathy.

CLINICAL PRESENTATION

DISEASE FORMS/SUBTYPES

- Occult DCM: earliest level. Overtly healthy dog with evidence of systolic dysfunction by echocardiography.
- Congestive heart failure (CHF).
- Cardiac arrhythmias: atrial fibrillation [especially giant breeds], ventricular arrhythmias [boxers, Doberman pinschers].
- Sudden cardiac death.

HISTORY, CHIEF COMPLAINT

- Occult DCM: by definition, without clinical signs (screening exam or incidental finding).
- CHF (left-sided): tachypnea, coughing, abdominal distention, lethargy, inappetence, respiratory distress, nasal discharge.

- CHF (right-sided): ascites, hepatomegaly, abdominal distention, lethargy, inappetence, jugular distention/pulses, respiratory distress.
- Cardiac arrhythmias: syncope, collapse, lethargy, precipitation of CHF.

PHYSICAL EXAM FINDINGS

- Weakness, depression, weight loss/cachexia, cardiogenic shock due to decreased arterial blood pressure, soft grade 1-3/6 systolic left and/or right apical murmur, S3 or summation gallops, arrhythmia.
- Right-sided CHF: jugular pulse/distention, muffled heart and ventral lung sounds with pleural effusion, hepatomegaly due to congestion (± ascites).
- Left-sided CHF: pulmonary crackles/rales, muffled lung sounds with pleural effusion [cats].
- Hypokinetic femoral pulses, pulse deficits with ventricular premature beats or atrial fibrillation.
- Subcutaneous edema is rare.

ETIOLOGY AND PATHOPHYSIOLOGY

- Proposed etiologies for idiopathic DCM include viral infection, nutritional deficiency, immune-mediated, microvascular hyperreactivity, and a variety of genetic disorders.
- Many believe that majority of cases represent genetic familial abnormalities of structural and/or contractile myocardial proteins.
- Before clinical signs, onset of myocardial failure leads to reduced cardiac output followed by activation of various neurohormones and cytokines to support blood pressure. This leads to short-term stability but long-term further myocardial damage.
- Very rare cases due to infection (parvoviral, protozoal) or toxicity (doxorubicin, radiation).

DIAGNOSIS

DIFFERENTIAL DIAGNOSIS

- Clinical:
  - Primary respiratory disease, noncardiogenic pulmonary edema, pleural space disorders (pneumothorax, noncardiogenic effusions), heartworm disease, endocardiosis, infectious endocarditis or myocarditis, cardiac tumors and pericardial effusion, diaphragmatic hernia, pulmonary hemorrhage, airway obstruction (laryngeal paralysis, tumor, foreign body, collapsing trachea), congenital heart disease, toxic cardiomyopathy (doxorubicin).
- Radiographic:
  - Pericardial effusion, peritoneopericardial diaphragmatic hernia, endocardiosis and other causes of chronic cardiac volume overload (arteriovenous fistula), congenital heart disease, other pleural effusions.
- Echocardiographic:
  - Myocardial failure due to advanced or end-stage valvular disease (endocardiosis) or shunts (patent ductus arteriosus, fistulas, septal defects). Subnormal fractional shortening (FS) % may be normal in many healthy individuals; check left ventricle (LV) diameter, E-point to septal separation, or even premature ventricular contractions on ECG/Holter for support of DCM, as well as myocarditis, ischemic cardiomyopathy, acute systemic hypertension.

INITIAL DATABASE

- Thoracic radiography: generalized cardiomegaly and signs of CHF (left-sided: interstitial or alveolar pulmonary edema [dogs, cats] and/or pleural effusion [cats]), (right-sided: pleural effusion, enlarged caudal vena cava, hepatomegaly, ascites [much more common in dogs]). Preclinical often unremarkable although left atrial and/or left ventricular enlargement may be noted.
- ECG: Sinus tachycardia possibly with atrial or ventricular premature beats; atrial fibrillation; ventricular tachycardia especially in boxers and Doberman pinschers; prolonged and/or increased voltage QRS complexes suggestive of LV enlargement; low voltage QRS complexes with pleural or pericardial effusion.
- Routine hematologic tests and urinalysis: usually normal. Exceptions:
  - Severe DCM
    - Prerenal azotemia
    - High alanine aminotransferase
    - Hyponatremia and hypochloremia, if noted with CHF, confer a poorer prognosis as they indicate free water retention
  - Concurrent disease
  - Result of therapy for heart failure (hypokalemia, metabolic alkalosis, prerenal azotemia)
- Effusion analysis: usually modified transudate (nucleated cell count <2500/ml, total protein <4.0 g/dl); chylous effusion possible in cats.

ADVANCED OR CONFIRMATORY TESTING

- Echocardiography: ventricular and atrial dilation, reduced myocardial systolic function (reduced left ventricular FS% and ejection fraction), increased E-point septal separation. Doppler studies confirm mitral and tricuspid regurgitation, low velocity transaortic flow, diastolic ventricular dysfunction and possibly pulmonary hypertension (if severe left-sided heart failure).
- Taurine concentrations: Deficiency if <40-50 nmoles/ml (plasma) or <250 nmoles/ml (whole blood). Taurine assays require special handling (green top tube or myocardium only; frozen)
- Histopathologic study: lesions include absence of inflammation, myocyte loss, attenuated wavy fibers, and increased myocardial fibrosis.

TREATMENT

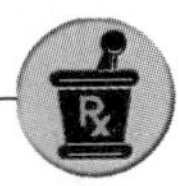

THERAPEUTIC GOAL(S)

- Resolution of congestive heart failure
- Control of detrimental or life-threatening arrhythmias
- Improved quality of life (e.g., appetite, exercise capacity)

ACUTE GENERAL TREATMENT

In cases of severe cardiogenic pulmonary edema: See Heart Failure, Acute.

- Minimize stress (e.g., keep cats separated from canine patients).
- Absolute rest.
- Oxygen supplementation.
- Furosemide (dogs: 2–6 mg/kg IV or IM initial dose, then 1–2 mg/kg q 2–3h as needed for resolution of pulmonary edema then q 8–12h for the first 3 days) (cats: 1–4 mg/kg parenterally q 4–12h as needed; duration of effect around 1 to 2 hours).
- Pleurocentesis if large-volume pleural effusion (therapeutic, diagnostic).

Additionally, as needed (based on severity of presenting signs, and response to above):

- 2% nitroglycerin paste applied topically: 1" q 8h [dog], 0.25" q8 h [cat].
- Life-threatening arrhythmias (see Ventricular Arrhythmias [Premature Ventricular Complexes, Ventricular Tachycardia], p 1149; Atrial Premature Complexes and Atrial/ Supraventricular Tachycardia, p 100).
- Sodium nitroprusside [dogs]: effective for treating critical cardiogenic pulmonary edema, but requires constant-rate infusion, protection from light, and careful monitoring. Start at 2 μg/kg/min IV and titrate upward. Mean blood pressure must remain >70 mmHg. Maximum = 10 μg/kg/min.
- Dobutamine (if severe heart failure or cardiogenic shock; ECG monitoring needed):
  - Dogs: start at 2.5–5 μg/kg/min, titrate upwards q 30–60 min in 2.5 μg/kg/min IV increments until heart rate increases by >10% or PVCs develop/become more frequent. Maximum infusion rate 15 μg/kg/min IV.
  - Cats: >2.5 μg/kg/min not recommended.

CHRONIC TREATMENT

- Pleurocentesis and abdominocentesis as needed.
- Diuretics (as needed to control edema):
  - Furosemide [dog] 1–4 mg/kg PO q 8–24h, [cat] 1–2 mg/kg PO q 8–24h.

- For chronic treatment of CHF where fluid retention is refractory to furosemide alone, add:
  - Spironolactone [dog, cat] 1–2 mg/kg q 12–24h PO; and/or
  - Hydrochlorothiazide [dog, cat] 2–4 mg/kg q 12h PO.
- ACE inhibitors:
  - Enalapril [dog] 0.5 mg/kg q 12–24h PO, [cat] 0.5mg/kg q 24h PO; or
  - Benazepril [dog] 0.5 mg/kg q 12–24h PO, [cat] 0.25–0.5 mg/kg q 24h PO; or
  - Lisinopril [dog] 0.5 mg/kg q 24h PO.
- Digoxin. Dogs: 0.003 mg/kg q 12h PO. Cats: 0.01 mg/kg or 1/4 of a 0.125 mg tablet PO q 48h.
- Pimobendan [dogs] 0.25 mg/kg q 12h PO for CHF caused by DCM in Doberman pinschers; unproven in other breeds or other heart diseases.
  - Novel Therapy (use after careful consideration of benefits and risks).
- β-Blockers blunt cardiotoxic effects of sympathetic nervous system; however, heart failure must be well controlled first, and dose begun low and up-titrated slowly (days to weeks) with careful monitoring. Options include:
  - Carvedilol [dogs] up to 0.5 mg/kg q 12h PO (start with 1/4 dose initially).
  - Metoprolol [dogs, cats] up to 1 mg/kg q 8h PO (start with 1/4 dose initially).
  - Atenolol [dogs, cats] up to 1 mg/kg q 12h PO (start with 1/4 to 1/2 dose initially).

ARRHYTHMIAS

- In *atrial fibrillation*, slowing of ventricular response rate in dogs is achieved with digoxin combined with atenolol or carvedilol (above) if necessary, or diltiazem (1–1.5 mg/kg PO q 8h). If CHF is present, diuretic treatment must be initiated first or simultaneously.
- Serious *ventricular arrhythmias* are managed with identification and treatment of underlying causes (e.g., hypoxemia from pulmonary edema) and, if rapid or causing clinical signs, can be treated with mexiletine (5–8 mg/kg PO q 8h), sotalol (2 mg/kg PO q 12h), tocainide (10–20 mg/kg PO q 8h) or procainamide (8–20 mg/kg PO q 6–8h). Often mexiletine is combined with a low dose β-blocker (atenolol, sotalol). See Ventricular Arrhythmias [Premature Ventricular Complexes, Ventricular Tachycardia], p 1149.
- Diet
  - Keep patient eating with adequate level of protein intake.
  - Elimination of high salt containing snacks.
  - Sodium-restricted commercial diets such as Purina CV or Hills H/D (not at the expense of good appetite).
- Taurine: recommended in all cats (250 mg PO q 12h) with DCM until demonstrated that patient is unresponsive to taurine; dose in dogs 500 mg PO q 12h.
- Omega-3 fatty acids may improve appetite and reduce cachexia (EPA 30–40 mg/kg q 24h; DHA 20–25 mg/kg PO q 24h).
- Consider L-carnitine (110 mg/kg PO q 12h) in boxers and American cocker spaniels not responding to taurine.

DRUG INTERACTIONS

- Quinidine, verapamil: will increase serum digoxin level (risk of toxicity)
- Hypokalemia, hypercalcemia, renal dysfunction, and hypothyroidism predispose to digitalis intoxication (therefore, decrease dose of digoxin)

POSSIBLE COMPLICATIONS

- Sudden death due to arrhythmias (especially uncontrolled ventricular tachycardia)
- Renal insufficiency (due to low cardiac output, medical treatment); however, mild to moderate azotemia (without associated clinical signs) is expected with diuretic treatment
- Iatrogenic complications due to medical treatment (hypokalemia, azotemia, other electrolyte abnormalities)

RECOMMENDED MONITORING

- Monitor 7 to 10 days after discharge, then as needed (e.g., q 1–4 months barring decompensation): Physical examination, thoracic radiographs, ECG, serum renal, and electrolyte profile.
- Holter/event monitors, echocardiography, other: if significant or unexpected change in patient's condition.
- Serum digoxin levels 1 week [dogs] or 2 weeks [cats] after start of therapy (therapeutic range = 0.8–1.8 ng/ml) taken 6 to 8 hours postpill.
- Renal/electrolyte panel 5 to 7 days after starting angiotensin-converting enzyme inhibitors.
- Repeat echocardiogram in 3 to 6 months after initiating taurine supplementation to determine response to therapy.

PROGNOSIS AND OUTCOME

- Overall, death usually occurs 3 to 24 months after diagnosis.
- Paroxysmal ventricular tachycardia and atrial fibrillation are probable markers of shorter survival.
- Plasma cardiac Tn-I >0.20 ng/ml is suggestive of shorter survival time.
- Prognosis is influenced by treatment, time of diagnosis, and client compliance.
- Prognosis generally worse in Portuguese water dogs and Doberman pinschers than in other breeds, but some Dobermans live months to years after diagnosis.
- Prognosis in Irish wolfhounds with DCM is fair; lifespan virtually unaffected.
- In cats with DCM not due to taurine deficiency, the prognosis is usually grave.

PEARLS & CONSIDERATIONS

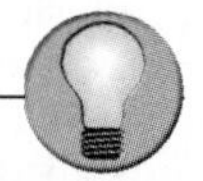

COMMENTS

- Most dogs should have left atrial enlargement, pulmonary venous enlargement and perihilar/caudodorsal pulmonary edema if pulmonary infiltrates are cardiogenic, whereas cats usually have atrial enlargement with variable edema location and pulmonary vein enlargement.
- Low echocardiographic LV fractional shortening (FS%) is not pathognomonic for DCM; many normal hearts contract more in apical to basilar direction and this motion is not accounted for by the FS%.
- Most small-breed dogs more likely to have chronic mitral valve endocardiosis > collapsing trachea > primary respiratory disease > DCM causing similar clinical presentation.
- DCM in cats is rare, hypertrophic cardiomyopathy is common; the opposite is true in dogs.

CLIENT EDUCATION

Monitor for signs associated with progression of disease (coughing [dogs], open mouth breathing [cats], respiratory changes, lethargy, collapse) and adverse side effects of medications (vomiting, diarrhea, anorexia)

SUGGESTED READING

Sisson DD, Thomas WP, Keene BW: Primary myocardial disease in the dog. In Ettinger SJ, Feldman EC (eds): *Textbook of Veterinary Internal Medicine*, ed 5. Philadelphia, WB Saunders, 2000, pp 874–895.

Website: Proposed Guidelines for the Diagnosis of Canine Idiopathic Dilated Cardiomyopathy: www.esvc.net/guidelines/cidc/index.htm.

AUTHOR: **ROBERT PROŠEK**
EDITOR: **ETIENNE CÔTÉ**

Disaster Working Dog Management and Health

BASIC INFORMATION

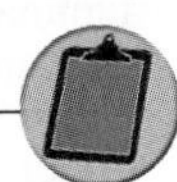

DEFINITION

Working dogs are highly trained for a specific task or tasks by an individual or organization for the purpose of assistance in a disaster, emergency, or disaster prevention.The nature of their work exposes them to environmental risks less commonly encountered by pet dogs.

SYNONYM(S)

Accelerant detection dog
Bomb sniffer
Drug detection dog; search and rescue dog
Dual purpose dog: does patrol and some type of detection work
Explosives detection dog
Military working dog
Patrol dog

EPIDEMIOLOGY

SPECIES, AGE, SEX: Primarily young adult male dogs (2 to 8 years old).

GENETICS AND BREED PREDISPOSITION: German shepherd, Labrador retriever, Belgian malinois, other breeds or crossbreeds.

RISK FACTORS

- Physical safety of working and training environment, risk of exposure, environmental conditions.
- Specific risk factors include long hours; stressful environment; oral, dermal, and respiratory exposure to toxins; hazardous footing; work low to the ground and in inaccessible areas, risking exposure to pockets of toxins/gases not apparent to handlers.

CONTAGION AND ZOONOSIS

- Agents of bioterrorism, foreign animal diseases, biologic weapons of mass destruction
- Infectious agents: *Leptospira*, rabies, other endemic infectious agents, ectoparasites and endoparasites

GEOGRAPHY AND SEASONALITY: Consider effects of weather conditions, especially temperature extremes, on working dogs.

ASSOCIATED CONDITIONS AND DISORDERS: Nutritional (dehydration, diet change, or anorexia when working), stress-related (GDV, anorexia/adipsia, "burnout").

CLINICAL PRESENTATION

DISEASE FORMS/SUBTYPES

- Environmental concerns
- Foot problems
- Trauma
- Explosives
- Toxins
- Lacrimators
- Pharmaceuticals and illicit drugs
- Weapons of mass destruction (biologic, chemical, radiologic)

HISTORY, CHIEF COMPLAINT

- Known exposure.
- Inability to work or perform task.
- General signs of illness that may include vocalizing, hypersalivation, lameness, ocular signs, nasal discharge, sneezing, diarrhea, vomit, poor or no appetite, manifestations of anaphylaxis, ataxia, depression, hyperactivity, cough, weakness, petechiae, hemorrhage, collapse, central nervous system depression, collapse, muscle tremors, polyuria/polydipsia, seizure, coma.

PHYSICAL EXAM FINDINGS

- Variable, based on exact disorder.
- Most commonly, abnormalities include dehydration, heat or cold stress, exhaustion, foot disorders.
- May be none initially (chronic, organ involvement, carcinogenic).

ETIOLOGY AND PATHOPHYSIOLOGY

- Environmental: dehydration, heat stroke, hypothermia, inadequate nutrition, inadequate conditioning, drowning, choking, plant toxins, moldy food (tremorgenic mycotoxins), zootoxins.
- Foot problems: laceration, abrasion, torn nail(s), contact dermatitis.
- Trauma: fracture, laceration, abrasion, projectiles, blunt trauma, crushing injury, sprain, strain.
- Explosives: cyclonite (c-4); 2,4,6-trinitrotoluene (TNT); pentaerthritol tetranitrate, dynamite (nitroglycerin + stabilizing agent), nitrates, smokeless powders, chlorates, nitromethane, triacetone triperoxide.
- Toxins: ethylene glycol; rodenticides; herbicides; insecticides; toxic agents released at disaster site (gas, smoke, particulates, liquids, solids) such as hydrocarbons, polychlorinated biphenyls, hazardous metals, asbestos, gases (hydrogen cyanide, hydrogen sulfide, freon, halogenated gases, carbon monoxide), soaps/detergents/acids/alkalis, propylene glycol, phenol, alcohols.
- Lacrimators: oleoresin capsicum (pepper spray), o-chlorobenzylidene malonitrile, 1-chloroacetophenone (mace), dibenzoxazepine.
- Illicit/legal drugs/supplements: marijuana, cocaine, amphetamines, opiates, phencyclidine, prescription medications, over-the-counter medications; herbal prepartaions and supplements.
- Routes of exposure: dermal, inhalation, ocular or ingestion. Swallowing of inhaled large particulate (2 to 5 µg) material moved to the oropharynx by mucociliary apparatus.

DIAGNOSIS

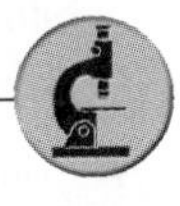

DIFFERENTIAL DIAGNOSIS

Varies with presentation, history, and physical exam findings

INITIAL DATABASE

- Complete blood count (CBC), serum biochemistry profile, urinalysis: common abnormalities include evidence of renal failure (azotemia + isosthenuria) from toxins, evidence of hepatopathy from trauma, thrombocytopenia and coagulopathy from heat stroke, calcium oxalate monohydrate crystalluria with ethylene glycol toxicosis, cylindruria (urinary casts) with renal trauma/toxin/heat stroke.
- Arterial blood gas and/or pulse oximetry.
  - Oxygen saturation (SpO_2) low with near drowning, noncardiogenic pulmonary edema (shock, seizure, trauma).
  - Note for carbon monoxide poisoning (combustion of gasoline): pulse oximetry cannot evaluate the true severity of hypoxemia because of its inability to differentiate between oxygenated hemoglobin and carboxyhemoglobin.
- Arterial blood pressure: for diagnosis and monitoring of hypotension in hypovolemic shock, or identification of hypertension with some intoxications.
- Electrocardiogram: sinus tachycardia with some intoxications; ventricular arrhythmias with hypoxemia, myocarditis, ischemic events, heat stroke.
- Radiographs as appropriate for trauma, respiratory signs, neurologic signs.

ADVANCED OR CONFIRMATORY TESTING

- Ethylene glycol test.
- Specific diagnostic tests exist but availability varies. Tests available include heavy metals, cholinesterase, polychlorinated biphenyl (PCBs), carboxyhemoglobin (CO poisoning), anticoagulants, pharmaceutical and illicit drugs.
- Obtain and store preexposure blood.
- Necropsy for unexplained death, and consider for any working dog.

TREATMENT

THERAPEUTIC GOAL(S)

- Stabilize the patient
- Decrease ongoing exposure and absorption
- Supportive care

ACUTE GENERAL TREATMENT

- Stabilize the patient:
  - General emergency medicine and stabilization of vital signs and specific derangements with appropriate cardiovascular and respiratory support.
  - Control hemorrhage, shock.
  - Control dyspnea, oxygen therapy, move to fresh air.
  - Control seizures, tremors.
  - Control pain.
- Decrease ongoing exposure and absorption:
  - Induce vomiting, gastric lavage (exceptions include corrosive agents, hydrocarbons, PCBs, soaps and detergents [cationic agents], acids and alkalis, phenol).
  - Administer water or milk orally for dilution (useful for corrosive agents, soaps, detergents, acids and alkalis, explosives [C-4, nitrates, nitromethane]).
  - Activated charcoal ± saline cathartic or sorbitol for noncorrosive agents (minimally effective for some heavy metals or short-chain solvents, hydrocarbons, soaps and detergents, acids and alkalis, ethylene glycol).
  - Gastrointestinal protectants.
  - Dermal decontamination using copious amounts of water and liquid dish detergent; ocular and nasal flushing using water or saline; washing or clipping hair in feet if buildup of debris or concrete dust. Clip affected haired areas to facilitate removal. Body temperature of the patient must be monitored to avoid hypothermia.
- Supportive care:
  - Fluid therapy: diuresis to help promote removal of agents that are primarily excreted renally and to address shock, dehydration and metabolic derangements.
  - Treat dehydration, hypothermia/hyperthermia, stress colitis, hemorrhagic gastroenteritis, and hemorrhagic cystitis.

CHRONIC TREATMENT

As indicated for specific case

DRUG INTERACTIONS

As indicated for individual treatments

POSSIBLE COMPLICATIONS

As indicated for individual case

RECOMMENDED MONITORING

- As indicated:
  - Monitoring may improve mentation and demeanor.
  - Temperature: during decontamination procedures and/or shock, to help prevent hypothermia.
  - Hydration, electrolytes, hematocrit/total solids, blood glucose, blood urea nitrogen, urine production and serial urinalyses.
  - Pain.
- May be lifelong if injury or exposure leads to permanent lesions.
- Baseline (yearly or biannually) bloodwork including CBC, serum biochemistry profile, heartworm antigen test, urinalysis and thyroid profile. Consider infectious disease screening as appropriate for location: Lyme disease, ehrlichiosis, bartonellosis, leishmaniasis, etc.

PROGNOSIS AND OUTCOME

Prognosis depends on source, speed of identification of inciting cause, and speed of appropriate decontamination, emergency, and supportive care. Prognosis improves with proper prevention, awareness, and monitoring work site for potential concerns.

PEARLS & CONSIDERATIONS

COMMENTS

- Important resources:
  - Center for Disease Control: www.cdc.gov.
  - American Veterinary Medical Association: www.avma.org.
  - Veterinary Medical Assistance Team: www.VMAT.org.
  - American Society for the Prevention of Cruelty to Animals, Animal Poison Control Center, www.ASPCA.org; 1-888-426-4435.
- Most common problems are hydration, exhaustion, foot/pad disorders.
- Health problems should be treated with the highest standards of veterinary care. Chronic diseases (e.g. allergies, degenerative joint disease, epilepsy, cardiopulmonary disease, gastrointestinal diseases) may benefit from treatment by a specialist and/or by complementary therapies such as acupuncture, massage, physical therapy, and nutrition.
- Proper nutrition and adequate exercise are important for working dogs as these can affect behavior, scent detecting ability, and ability to work long hours.
- Handler physical and mental health must be appropriate to complement the team work needed.
- Handling and training should include obedience, crate training, restraint, and muzzling to aid in situations where working dog is injured, contaminated, or needs veterinary care.
- Person(s) providing treatment should utilize proper personal protective equipment including gloves, eye protection, mask, apron, etc. Disasters with mass casualties may include human contamination as potential risk (human immunodeficiency virus, hepatitis, etc.).
- Knowledge of chronic medications' effects on work (i.e., prednisone may affect odor detection) and interactions with toxicants (i.e., hydrocarbons and certain medications) is important.

PREVENTION

- Heat Index guidelines are not established but should be considered. Rest and hydration at least every 30 to 60 minutes. Fluids (subcutaneous by site veterinarian) before work in stressful environments may be beneficial.
- Working dogs should be in top health to work at their best ability and without distraction.
- Ample time for play and rest and recovery from stressful work situations is essential.
- Routine veterinary preventive health care is paramount.
- Acclimation of dogs to personal protective devices such as goggles and foot protection before field work is important. Masks may not be appropriate due to panting and need for olfactory sense.
- Decontamination procedures including bathing, ocular, and nasal flushing are particularly important in disaster situations. Dogs should be accustomed to bathing and mass-decontamination procedures (may include muzzle for procedures and to prevent drinking of decontamination effluent; crate or kennel for decontamination protocol).
- Regular cleaning during work of nose, muzzle, and body to prevent licking (including licking the nose, where material may collect on the nasal planum) and ingestion.
- Knowledge of the type of agent(s) at the scene.
- Prevent drinking unknown sources by keeping well hydrated.
- Prevent ingestion by using "basket" type muzzle.
- Reflective safety vest.
- Canine floatation device.
- Appropriate holding/travelling area environment: fans/air-conditioning or heat, water, crate, good footing/bedding while travelling or at staging area. Consider vehicle alarm for excessive vehicle temperatures.

CLIENT EDUCATION

- Search out veterinary and disaster assistance in advance; Veterinary Medical Assistance Teams (VMAT) (federal resource, Department of Homeland Security); local Veterinary Medical Association and veterinary emergency

hospital, Society for the Prevention of Cruelty to Animals (SPCA); Office of Emergency Preparedness, State and County Emergency Management Resources.
- Employer should have access for handlers to ASPCA—Animal Poison Control Center (1-888-426-4435) with credit card on file or account established. Handlers should have phone number at all times.
- Personal protective equipment for handler and dog.
- Training in first aid procedures and kits: include bandaging and splint materials, sterile saline for flushing eyes and wounds, apomorphine and/or hydrogen peroxide for inducing vomiting, activated charcoal with a cathartic, resuscitator bag, stethoscope, thermometer, ophthalmic ointment, booties, liquid dish soap for decontamination of skin and coat, towels for drying.
- Knowledge of normal vital signs and physical exam findings.
- Canine field cardiopulmonary cerebral resuscitation.
- Obtain or locate ample source of safe water for hydration and decontamination.
- Knowledge of possible risks in animal's line of work: define ahead of time or search out site Safety Officer or VMAT veterinarian.
- Save vomitus, urine, and/or feces if dog is not acting normally: may be diagnostic. Save sample of material or liquid that the animal ingested or drank. (Keep sample bags or sterile plastic sample containers in vehicle or jump-pack.)

SUGGESTED READING

Altom EK, et al: Effect of dietary fat source and exercise on odorant-detecting ability of canine athletes. *Res Vet Sci* 75:149, 2003.
DeClementi C: Emergency management of lacrimator exposure for canine and equine handlers, ASPCA Animal Poison Control Center, 2004.
DeClementi C: Issues of concern for drug and explosive detection dogs, ASPCA Animal Poison Control Center, 2004.
DeClementi, et al: VMAT decontamination standard operating procedure, presented at the National Disaster Medical System Conference. Dallas, 2004.
Gwaltney-Brant SM, et al: General toxicologic hazards and risks for search and rescue dogs responding to urban disasters. *J Am Vet Med Assoc* 222:292, 2003.
Morris A: Using the 9/11 VMAT experience to improve on-site medical care of search and rescue dogs, presented at the National Disaster Medical System Conference. Dallas, 2004.
Murphy LA, et al:Toxicologic agents of concern for search-and-rescue dogs responding to urban disasters. *J Am Vet Med Assoc* 222:296, 2003.
Otto CM, et al: Field treatment of search dogs: lessons learned from the World Trade Center disaster. *J Vet Emerg Crit Care* 12:33, 2002.
Otto CM: Medical and behavioural surveillance of dogs deployed to the World Trade Center and the Pentagon 10/01–06/02, presented at The National Disaster Medical System Conference. Dallas, 2004.
Wismer TA, et al: Management and prevention of toxicoses in search-and-rescue dogs responding to urban disasters. *J Am Vet Med Assoc* 222:305, 2003.

AUTHOR: **POLLY A. FLECKENSTEIN**
EDITOR: **ETIENNE CÔTÉ**

Discoid Lupus Erythematosus

BASIC INFORMATION

DEFINITION

A relatively benign cutaneous disease with no systemic involvement

SYNONYM(S)

Collie nose
Cutaneous lupus erythematosus
DLE
Nasal solar dermatitis

EPIDEMIOLOGY

SPECIES, AGE, SEX
- Canine; very rare in cats
- No age or clear sex predilection

GENETICS AND BREED PREDISPOSITION: Breed predispositions include Rough collie, German shepherd, Shetland sheepdog, Siberian husky, Brittany spaniel, German short-haired pointer, and Australian herding breeds.

RISK FACTORS
- Breed
- Exposure to ultraviolet light

GEOGRAPHY AND SEASONALITY: More common in summer months and sunny climates.

CLINICAL PRESENTATION

DISEASE FORMS/SUBTYPES: Usually localized to the planum nasale (nasal planum: the unhaired, dorsal, rostral most surface of the nose). Less commonly, lesions affect other sites including lip folds, oral cavity, periocular area, pinnae, genitalia and, rarely, distal limbs.

HISTORY, CHIEF COMPLAINT
- Owners typically present dogs for evaluation of changes in the appearance of the nasal planum.
- Mild to severe erythema, depigmentation, scaling and crusting of the planum nasale with ulceration and erosions are commonly noted by owners. Pruritus and pain are variable. When other sites are affected, crusting, erosions, and ulceration may be noted.

PHYSICAL EXAM FINDINGS
- Erythema, depigmentation, and scaling of the nose.
  - Early depigmentation manifests itself as a change in color from normal black to gray/white.
  - Early depigmentation manifests itself as a change in surface texture of the nasal planum from the normal rough "cobblestone"-like appearance to a smooth, shiny surface (Fig. I-54).
  - Scaling and crusting may be present at the junction between nasal planum and haired skin.
- When other sites are affected; crusting, erosions, and ulceration may be noted.
- Dogs with discoid lupus erythematosus are otherwise healthy.

ETIOLOGY AND PATHOPHYSIOLOGY

- The pathogenesis is thought to involve autoreactive T cells that stimulate B cells to produce antibodies to a number of different nuclear proteins. Ultraviolet light may initiate the process of expression in photosensitive individuals (50% of cases).
- Antibodies are deposited in the basement membrane, and subsequently, epidermal basal layer cells are damaged. This results in subepidermal vesicle formation and immune complex deposition in the basement membrane zone.

DIAGNOSIS

A strong suspicion exists on physical examination alone; characteristic nasal depigmentation with erythema and/or erosions/ulcerations in the absence of nasal discharge or any other sign of systemic illness is generally considered diagnostic.

DIFFERENTIAL DIAGNOSIS

- Bacterial infection: mucocutaneous pyoderma (may mimic discoid lupus

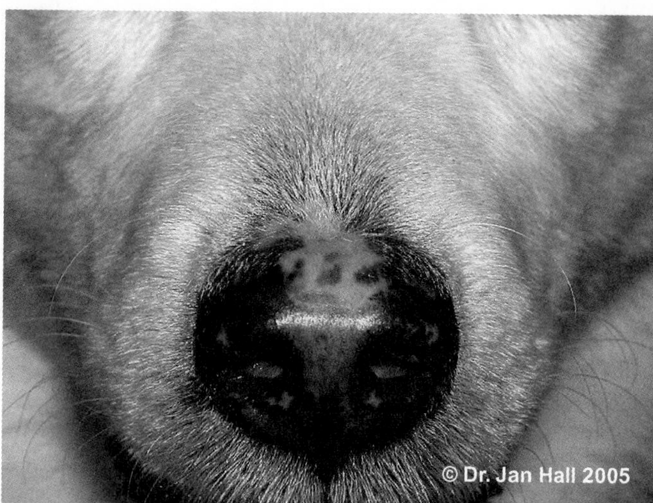

FIGURE I-54 Discoid lupus erythematosus affecting the nasal planum of a Siberian husky mixed-breed dog. Note the depigmentation, erosion along the dorsal edge, and general loss of the normal "cobblestone" appearance of the nasal planum. Courtesy of Dr. Jan A. Hall.

erythematosus [DLE]), staphylococcal folliculitis
- Immune-mediated diseases: systemic lupus erythematosus (SLE), pemphigus foliaceus/pemphigus erythematosus, drug reaction, uveodermatologic syndrome
- Vitiligo
- Neoplasia: squamous cell carcinoma, epitheliotropic lymphoma
- Trauma
- Dermatophytosis
- Dermatomyositis (collie breeds)

INITIAL DATABASE

- Deep skin scrapings
- Skin cytology (impression smear)
- Dermatophyte culture
- Routine hematology, chemistry profile and urinalysis: generally unremarkable
- Serum antinuclear antibody test: usually negative with DLE (helps to rule out SLE)

ADVANCED OR CONFIRMATORY TESTING

- Biopsy (under general anesthesia) for histopathologic evaluation, which is the gold standard for diagnosis. Biopsy reveals an interface dermatitis, with mononuclear lichenoid pattern, pigmentary incontinence, hydropic degeneration, Civatte bodies (dyskeratotic cells in the epidermis) and increased amounts of dermal mucin. By contrast, mucocutaneous pyoderma reveals a mononuclear licnenoid infiltrate but no evidence of interface dermatitis.
- Immunohistochemistry is rarely required.
- Biopsy for fungal and bacterial culture.

TREATMENT

THERAPEUTIC GOAL(S)

Control and resolution of existing lesions

ACUTE GENERAL TREATMENT

PRIMARY: Some or all may be necessary:
- Routine antibiotic therapy: cephalexin 30 mg/kg PO q 12h for 30 days to rule out mucocutaneous pyoderma.
- Topical corticosteroids: potent glucocorticoids including betamethasone, 0.1% amcinonide or flucinolone in dimethyl sulfoxide (Synotic). Switch to a low potency product such as 1.0% hydrocortisone cream once a favorable response is noted.
- Topical tacrolimus 0.1% ointment (ProTopic): q 12h initially, wean based on a favorable response.
- Vitamin E 400-800 IU/day PO.
- Essential fatty acids (n3 EFA, eicasopentanoic acid) 30 mg/kg PO q 24h.
- Tetracycline and niacinamide: >10 kg, 500 mg PO q 12h (< 10 kg, 250 mg) of each drug PO q 8h. May take 6 to 8 weeks to produce improvement. If good response, wean gradually (several weeks). Doxycycline, as an alternative to tetracycline: 10 mg/kg PO q 24h.

IN REFRACTORY CASES
- Systemic corticosteroids: prednisone, 2.2-4.4 mg/kg/day PO initially, then weaning based on a favorable response.
- Azathioprine 2.2 mg/kg PO q 24-48h while administering prednisone. Monitor for adverse bone marrow effects (or rarely, adverse hepatic effects or pancreatitis).

CHRONIC TREATMENT

- Avoid intense sunlight (e.g., 0800 to 1700 hr)
- Topical sunscreens if sunlight exposure is unavoidable
- Bilateral rotational nasal flaps for refractory cases

POSSIBLE COMPLICATIONS

- Nasal cartilage erosion and arteriole hemorrhage
- Squamous cell carcinoma

RECOMMENDED MONITORING

- Routine hematology and chemistry profiles if using azathioprine. Initially, q 14 days reducing to q 3 months.
- High-dose corticosteroids are rarely required; however, appropriate serum chemistries and urinalysis should be used in such cases.
- With chronic use of intermediate or long-acting topical corticosteroid application, adrenal function should be monitored.

PROGNOSIS AND OUTCOME

Good, but may require chronic therapy

PEARLS & CONSIDERATIONS

COMMENTS

- Dogs with DLE typically feel and act well; the disorder is usually confined to the hairless skin of the nose.
- Depigmentation on the inner surfaces of the nostrils accompanied by nasal discharge suggests an intranasal problem (e.g., nasal aspergillosis) rather than DLE.

CLIENT EDUCATION

- Avoid intense ultraviolet light
- Sunscreen use

SUGGESTED READING

Scott DW, Miller WH, Griffin CE: Immune mediated disorders. In *Muller and Kirk's Small Animal Dermatology*, ed 6. Philadelphia, WB Saunders, 2001, pp 712-717.

AUTHOR: **MICHAEL HANNIGAN**
EDITOR: **JAN A. HALL**

Discolored Urine

BASIC INFORMATION

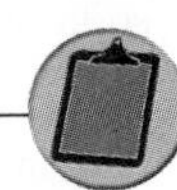

DEFINITION

Urine that is any other color besides yellow or amber; most often caused by the presence of blood, hemoglobin, myoglobin, or bilirubin

EPIDEMIOLOGY

SPECIES, AGE, SEX: Dependent on underlying cause.

CLINICAL PRESENTATION

HISTORY, CHIEF COMPLAINT

- Owner may note discolored urine with no other clinical signs.
- Signs may relate to primary cause. For example:
  - Pollakiuria, dysuria, stranguria associated with lower urinary tract disease.
  - Weakness, collapse, pallor associated with severe hemolysis.
  - Weakness or pain associated with severe muscle damage.

PHYSICAL EXAM FINDINGS

- Lower urinary tract disease:
  - Vaginal disease (infection, inflammation, mass)
    - Vaginal discharge
    - Vaginal mass
    - Vulvar abnormalities
  - Prostatomegaly
  - Thickenened, abnormal urethra
  - Distended bladder
- Hemolysis:
  - Pallor
  - Tachycardia
  - Weakness, collapse
  - Splenomegaly
- Muscle damage:
  - Weakness
  - Signs of pain
  - Signs of blunt trauma or of prolonged recumbency
- Icterus:
  - Yellow mucous membranes, sclera, skin

ETIOLOGY AND PATHOPHYSIOLOGY

- Yellow, dark yellow
  - Normal
- Red, pink, red/brown, orange
  - Hematuria
  - Hemoglobinuria
  - Myoglobinuria,
- Orange/yellow
  - Very concentrated normal urine
  - Excess urobilin
  - Bilirubin
- Yellow/brown, green/brown
  - Bile pigments
- Brown to black
  - Methemoglobin
  - Myoglobin
  - Bile pigments
- Colorless
  - Very dilute urine

DIAGNOSIS

DIFFERENTIAL DIAGNOSIS

- Dark yellow/orange
  - Normal
  - Prehepatic icterus (extravascular hemolytic anemia)
  - Hepatic icterus:
    - Dogs/cats: hepatic neoplasia, toxin-induced hepatopathy.
    - Dogs: idiopathic or breed-associated hepatitis.
    - Cats: hepatic lipidosis, cholangitis/cholangiohepatitis.
  - Posthepatic icterus (biliary disease, pancreatic disease, duodenal disease)
- Red, pink, red/brown, orange
  - Urinary tract infection
  - Idiopathic cystitis/feline lower urinary tract signs (FLUTS) (cats)
  - Urolithiasis
  - Urethritis
  - Prostatitis, prostatic neoplasia
  - Vaginitis
  - Intravascular hemolytic anemia
  - Hemoglobin transfusion
  - Neoplasia (e.g., transitional cell carcinoma, renal carcinoma, others)
  - Coagulopathy
  - Trauma
  - Estrus
- Brown to black
  - Trauma
  - Heinz body hemolysis-inducing toxins:
    - Zinc
    - Copper
    - Onions, garlic, broccoli
    - Drugs (acetaminophen, methylene blue)
- Colorless
  - Normal
  - Fluid therapy/overhydration
  - See Polyuria/Polydipsia, p 878:
    - Diabetes mellitus
    - Diabetes insipidus
    - Diuretics
    - Hepatic diseases
    - Hyperthyroidism
    - Hypoadrenocorticism
    - Hypokalemia
    - Pyometra
    - Renal failure
    - Glucocorticoid excess (hyperadrenocorticism, iatrogenic)
    - Psychogenic polydipsia

INITIAL DATABASE

- Complete blood count (CBC)
  - Anemia
- Serum biochemistry profile
  - Metabolic diseases (see Polyuria/Polydipsia above)
  - Evaluate color of serum:
    - Clear: consider myoglobin.
    - Pink: hemolysis.
    - Yellow: icterus.
- Urinalysis
  - Comparing free-catch to cystocentesis sample often aids in localization:
    - Discoloration of urine in both samples suggests a systemic, renal, ureteral, or urinary bladder disorder.
    - Discoloration of free-catch urine but normal-color cystocentesis urine suggests a urethral, uterine, prostatic, testicular, preputial, vulvar, or vaginal problem.
    - Discoloration of cystocentesis urine with a normal color free-catch sample suggests erroneous switching of the samples or other error.
  - Hematuria:
    - Cystitis.
    - Urolithiasis.
    - Urethritis.
    - Neoplasia.
    - Prostatitis/prostatic abscess.
    - Prostatic neoplasia.
    - Bladder neoplasia.
    - Trauma.
    - Estrus.
    - Idiopathic renal hematuria.
  - Pyuria:
    - Cystitis, pyelonephritis.
    - Inflammation, sterile (idiopathic cystitis/FLUTS).
    - Neoplasia.
  - Hemoglobinuria: hemolysis
  - Myoglobinuria: muscle damage
- Urine culture and sensitivity
- Abdominal radiographs
  - Calculi
  - Mass effect
  - Prostatomegaly
  - Metal in gastrointestinal tract (e.g., zinc)
  - Enlargement/mineralization of sublumbar lymph nodes, suggesting prostatic or urinary bladder neoplasia
- Abdominal ultrasound
  - Renal disease (pyelonephritis, mass, diffuse infiltration, other)
  - Bladder wall tumor (transitional cell carcinoma, other)
  - Prostatic disease
  - Urolithiasis
  - Sublumbar lymphadenopathy

- Other neoplasia/abnormality contributing to hemolysis
- Sedated vaginal examination
  - Mass
  - Inflammation/infection
  - Conformational abnormality

ADVANCED OR CONFIRMATORY TESTING

As dictated by findings for the individual case:

- Laboratory testing
  - Vaginal smear
  - Urine protein/creatinine ratio
  - Ejaculate examination
  - Fine-needle aspirate
- Imaging
  - Excretory urogram
  - Double contrast cystogram
  - Contrast vaginogram
- Biopsy
  - Cystoscopy
  - Exploratory laparotomy (virtually always replaced by lesser-invasive means, unless laparotomy is also therapeutic [e.g., urolith removal])

TREATMENT

THERAPEUTIC GOAL(S)

- Correct underlying cause based on accurate diagnosis
- Most life-threatening situations evaluated/addressed first

PROGNOSIS AND OUTCOME

Varies based on underlying cause

PEARLS & CONSIDERATIONS

- Physical examination and minimum laboratory work (CBC, serum biochemistry profile, urinalysis) to help quickly narrow the differential list.
- Comparison of urine color to plasma color and of free catch versus cystocentesis urine samples are simple but vital steps for narrowing the differential diagnosis list.
- Basic imaging (abdominal radiographs and ultrasound) can rule in or rule out many common causes of discolored urine.
- Dark yellow urine is not necessarily of that color because of adequate concentration; urinalysis with specific gravity is indicated for differentiation from pathologic conditions.
- Bilirubin conjugation and excretion is normal in the dog but not the cat; therefore trace or mild bilirubinuria in dogs may be normal and is not necessarily indicative of hepatobiliary or hemolytic disease.

SUGGESTED READING

Bartges JW: Diagnosis of urinary tract infections. *Vet Clin North Am Small Anim Pract* 34(4):923–933, 2004.

Cahill-Morasco R, DePasquale MA: Zinc toxicosis in small animals. *Compend Contin Educ Pract Vet* 24(9):712–720, 2002.

Forrester SD: Diagnostic approach to hematuria in dogs and cats. *Vet Clin North Am Small Anim Pract* 34(4):849–866, 2004.

Grundy SA, Barton C: Influence of drug treatment on survival of dogs with immune-mediated hemolytic anemia: 88 cases (1989–1999). *J Am Vet Med Assoc* 218(4):543–546, 2001.

Labato MA: Managing urolithiasis in cats. *Vet Med* 96(9):708–717, 2001.

Lulich JP, Osborne CA: Urine culture as a test for cure: why, when, and how? *Vet Clin North Am Small Anim Pract* 34(4):1027–1041, 2004.

AUTHOR: **CLAIRE WEIGAND**
EDITOR: **ETIENNE CÔTÉ**

Diskospondylitis

BASIC INFORMATION

DEFINITION

An inflammation/infection of the intervertebral disk and the adjacent end plates and vertebral bodies. Bacterial (usually *Staphylococcus*) is most common; occasionally, it is due to the fungal organism *Aspergillus*.

EPIDEMIOLOGY

SPECIES, AGE, SEX

- Most commonly seen in medium- to giant-breed male dogs (males outnumber females 2:1).
- Typically, young to middle-aged dogs are affected (median age 9 years).
- Has also been seen in small breed dogs as well as in cats.

GENETICS AND BREED PREDISPOSITION: German shepherds are overrepresented for fungal diskospondylitis.

CONTAGION AND ZOONOSIS: Diskospondylitis caused by *Brucella canis* carries the possibility of zoonosis.

CLINICAL PRESENTATION

HISTORY, CHIEF COMPLAINT

- Variable clinical presentation.
- Most dogs show progressive clinical signs over several weeks; however, some dogs develop clinical signs acutely.
- Clinical signs are often nonspecific (pyrexia, anorexia, weight loss, lethargy, depression), but usually include hyperesthesia associated with the spinal lesion.

PHYSICAL EXAM FINDINGS

- General physical and neurologic examinations vary depending on the location, severity, and secondary effects of the infection.
- Patients examined early in the course of the disease often only show signs of spinal hyperpathia, without paraparesis.
- Later, patients may have more severe spinal hyperpathia with varying degrees of paraparesis.
- Occasionally, patients present with an acute onset of back pain with associated ambulatory or nonambulatory paraparesis/paraplegia.

ETIOLOGY AND PATHOPHYSIOLOGY

- Some dogs that develop diskospondylitis may have underlying immune compromise.
- Infectious organisms may gain access to the disk space and vertebrae via several mechanisms.
  - Hematogenous spread of bacteria or fungi: the most common mechanism, although the primary source of infection, is not always found.
    - The urinary tract is the most likely source of infection.
    - Other sources, although rare, are bacterial endocarditis and dental disease.
  - Foreign body migration: most commonly a grass awn.
    - The plant materials have barbed ends that allow them to migrate through tissues.
    - The awns may carry bacteria with them to the disk space and/or serve as a nidus for bacterial localization once they arrive at the disk space.

TABLE I-5 Organisms that Cause Diskospondylitis and Recommended Antibiotics (Pending Culture and Sensitivity)

Organism	Antibiotic	Dosage
Staphylococcus species	Cephalexin	22 mg/kg PO q 8h
	Amoxicillin-clavulanate	13.75 mg/kg PO q 12h
Streptococcus species	Amoxicillin	22 mg/kg PO q 12h
Brucella canis	Enrofloxacin	5 mg/kg PO q 12h
	Doxycycline	25 mg/kg PO q 12h
Escherichia coli	Enrofloxacin	5 mg/kg PO q 12h
	Cephalexin	22 mg/kg PO q 12h
	Amoxicillin-clavulanate	13.75 mg/kg PO q 12h
Actinomyces species	Penicillin G	100,000 U/kg IV, IM, SC q 6h
Aspergillus species	Itraconazole	5 mg/kg PO q 12h

   - Proposed mechanisms for the site of entry include inhalation with migration through the lungs or diaphragm, ingestion and subsequent penetration through the bowel wall, and entrance through overlying skin.
- Iatrogenic: infection may develop after spinal surgery or paravertebral injection.
- Bacterial organisms that are involved are usually coagulase-positive *Staphylococcus* organisms (*S. intermedius, S. aureus*.) Other bacterial pathogens include *Streptococcus* species, *Brucella canis*, and *Escherichia coli*. Less frequently isolated bacteria are *Pasteurella*, *Proteus*, *Corynebacterium*, *Actinomyces*, *Nocardia*, *Bacteroides*, and *Mycobacterium* species.
- Fungal organisms include *Aspergillus* and *Paecilomyces* species.

DIAGNOSIS

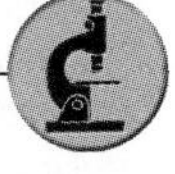

DIFFERENTIAL DIAGNOSIS

Diskospondylitis must be distinguished from spondylosis deformans and spinal neoplasia:

- Spondylosis and sclerosis are common both in spondylosis deformans and diskospondylitis; however, vertebral end-plate lysis is seen only in diskospondylitis.
- Typically in spinal neoplasia, the lytic lesion is confined to a single vertebra, whereas in diskospondylitis, the lysis is associated with adjacent vertebrae.

INITIAL DATABASE

- Complete blood count, serum biochemistry panel: typically unremarkable.
  - Leukocytosis may be seen if there are concurrent systemic abnormalities (e.g., pyometra, prostatic abscess, endocarditis).
- Urinalysis reveals bacterial cystitis in up to 40% of cases.
  - The same organism is occasionally identified in both the urine and blood cultures.
- Blood cultures should be obtained whenever possible.
- Cerebrospinal fluid is typically normal.
- *Brucella* titers may be positive. Because of the zoonotic potential, this titer should be performed in all sexually intact patients suspected of having diskospondylitis.
- Radiographs are the most useful diagnostic tool. Changes first appear 2 to 4 weeks after the onset of clinical signs.
  - Collapse of the disk space.
  - Proliferative bony changes adjacent to the intervertebral disk space.
  - Sclerosis at the bony margins.
  - The first radiographic signs are usually a collapsed intervertebral disk space with or without subtle vertebral end plate erosion.
  - With more chronic infections, the bone becomes more sclerotic and ventral spur formation occurs. This is often accompanied by marked osteolysis and inflammatory new bone formation.

ADVANCED OR CONFIRMATORY TESTING

- The most sensitive procedure for identifying infectious organisms associated with diskospondylitis is culture of surgically obtained tissue. Samples can be taken at the time of surgery, if indicated for decompression, but otherwise it is an invasive diagnostic tool.
- Fluoroscopically guided percutaneous disk aspiration has been shown to be useful in obtaining a positive culture in approximately 75% of cases.
- Myelography and MRI are useful tools to identify spinal cord compression. The vertebral endplates often demonstrate strong contrast enhancement with MRI.

TREATMENT

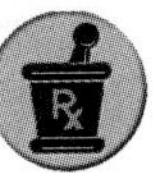

ACUTE AND CHRONIC TREATMENT

- When a specific causative agent is not identified, empiric treatment with antibiotics is warranted. The most common causative bacteria are coagulase-positive *Staphylococcus* species, which are generally sensitive to first generation cephalosporins or β-lactamase-resistant penicillins (Table I-5).
- Antibiotic treatment usually results in improvement of spinal hyperesthesia within 4 to 5 days. If there is no improvement within 7 to 10 days of starting antibiotics, the case should be reevaluated (if not already done, consider blood or urine culture, fungal titers, aspiration of the lesion, etc.).
- Antibiotic therapy should be continued for at least 6 weeks after clinical and radiographic improvement is seen. Specifically, antibiotic therapy should be continued until there is no additional or persistent bony lysis, which is considered a radiographic sign of progression of the disease.
- With *Brucella* positive dogs, a combination of tetracyclines and aminoglycosides or fluoroquinolones is useful. There is a high rate of recurrence of brucellosis after treatment, likely because *Brucella* is an intracellular organism. *Brucella*-positive dogs should be castrated, both to decrease the risk of spread to dogs and humans, as well as to cause the regression of gonadal steroid-dependent tissues that act as reservoirs for the organism. (See Brucellosis, Dog, p 162.)
- Limited success is seen using itraconazole in fungal diskospondylitis.
- Surgical treatment: Based on imaging studies and clinical signs (e.g., vertebral instability or spinal cord compression associated with neurologic deficits) spinal cord decompression via a dorsal or hemilaminectomy may be indicated.

RECOMMENDED MONITORING

- In addition to clinical signs, radiographs should be monitored during the healing phase.
  - The radiographic signs of healing diskospondylitis lesions are disappearance of the lytic focus and its replacement by bridging or fusion of involved vertebrae.
- In young dogs (<1 year) radiographic improvement parallels clinical improvement and includes minimal additional bony lysis along with increased sclerosis and bridging.
- In older dogs, there is a lag of 3 to 9 weeks between the time of clinical improvement and the appearance of radiographic characteristics of recovery.

- During the lag period, radiographic findings are consistent with progression of disease, showing increased bony lysis without additional sclerosis or bridging. The bony lysis is likely secondary to bone being resorbed at the site of the lesion before new bone formation can occur.

PROGNOSIS AND OUTCOME

- The prognosis is variable and depends mainly on the severity of neurologic deficits and the causative agent.
  - Patients with only spinal hyperpathia and no neurologic deficits have an excellent prognosis.
  - As the severity of the neurologic signs worsens, so does the prognosis.
- Prognosis is also based on response to treatment and is less favorable when the animal does not respond to medical management. In such cases, a different antibiotic may be considered or a disk/bone culture can be performed to rule out fungal disease and identify an organism.
- Fungal diskospondylitis carries a grave prognosis.
- Patients who require surgery carry a guarded prognosis that worsens with the degree of spinal instability.

PEARLS & CONSIDERATIONS

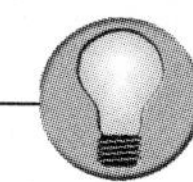

COMMENTS

Approximately 56% of dogs with diskospondylitis have associated spinal cord compression. In the majority of these dogs (76%), the compression is cause by soft tissue (i.e., proliferation of the annulus secondary to instability, steatitis) rather than subluxation (20%).

SUGGESTED READING

Dewey CW: Disorders of the cauda equina. In Dewey CW (ed): *A Practical Guide to Canine and Feline Neurology*. Ames, IA, Iowa State Press, 2003, pp 348–351.

Jaffe MH, et al: Canine diskospondylitis. *The Comp Cont Ed Pract Vet* 19:551–555, 1997.

Shamir MH, et al: Radiographic findings during recovery from discospondylitis. *Vet Radiol Ultrasound* 42:496–503, 2001.

AUTHOR: **KERRY SMITH BAILEY**

EDITOR: **CURTIS W. DEWEY**

Disorientation/Confusion

BASIC INFORMATION

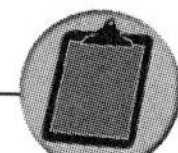

DEFINITION

An inappropriate state of confusion with respect to time and/or place and/or identity

EPIDEMIOLOGY

SPECIES, AGE, SEX

- Dogs and cats
- Any age or gender

GENETICS AND BREED PREDISPOSITION: Cats and dogs are predisposed (brachycephalic and dome-headed breeds) to congenital hydrocephalus.

RISK FACTORS

- Old age: canine cognitive dysfunction syndrome (similar condition probably exists in cats)
- Access to psychoactive drugs or potentially neurotoxic substances
- Preexisting liver or kidney disease, diabetes mellitus, hypothyroidism, or other diseases causing osmotic, electrolyte, and/or acid-base disturbances

CLINICAL PRESENTATION

HISTORY, CHIEF COMPLAINT

- External trauma
- Ingestion of toxic substance with central nervous system effects
- Barring observed trauma or intoxication, owners may describe any combination of the following signs:
  - Not responding to being called by name
  - Wandering aimlessly
  - Behaving unaware or "forgetful" of surroundings or of owner/family members
  - Urinating or defecating in inappropriate places
  - Not behaving in anticipatory manner with regard to daily routines (e.g., not being excited to being fed at usual time)
- Clear concise description of primary complaint and ask questions pertaining to:
  - Vision or hearing changes
  - Potential access to toxins or psychotropic drugs
  - Signs associated with metabolic disturbances (e.g., thirst and appetite; gastrointestinal and urological behaviors)
  - History of recent trauma
  - History of seizures (animals can be disoriented during the postictal period)

PHYSICAL EXAM FINDINGS

- Physical examination findings depend on the etiology (see specific diseases).
- For accurate treatment and prognosis, it is important to identify whether the cause of the disorientation is of:
  - Primary brain origin (e.g., canine cognitive dysfunction syndrome, congenital hydrocephalus, brain neoplasia)
  - Secondary to some other cause (e.g., trauma, various metabolic encephalopathies, various toxicities)
  - Resulting from visual impairment: may note mydriasis in normal ambient lighting (see Blindness)
  - Resulting from hearing impairment
  - Benign behavioral origin

ETIOLOGY AND PATHOPHYSIOLOGY

- Disorientation can result when a disease affects the cerebrum.
- Exact pathophysiologic explanation of altered frontal and temporal lobe function varies with each disease but may include:
  - Alterations in neuronal metabolism (e.g., hypoglycemia, hypothyroidism, hypocalcemia).
  - Accumulation of neurotoxic substances (e.g., hepatic encephalopathy).
  - Chronic oxidative stress in the brain leading to neurodegeneration (e.g., canine cognitive dysfunction syndrome).
  - Alterations in brain neurotransmitters (e.g., hepatic encephalopathy, epilepsy).
  - Alterations in neuronal excitability (e.g., electrolyte disturbances).
  - Direct mechanical damage (head trauma).
- Animals can become disoriented despite normal cerebral function when they are blind and/or deaf (see Deafness, p 276 and Blindness, p 136).

DIAGNOSIS

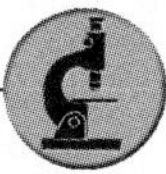

DIFFERENTIAL DIAGNOSIS

- See Etiology and Pathophysiology above for differentiation of specific inciting causes
- Differential diagnosis for disorientation:
  - Stereotypic behavior
  - Complex partial seizure

INITIAL DATABASE

- Age of onset.

- Complete neurologic examination (see p 1286).
- Complete ophthalmic examination (see p 1288).
- Complete blood count, serum biochemistry, urinalysis to (1) determine any underlying systemic condition and (2) preanesthetic work-up (if needed).
- NOTE: Diagnosis of age-related cognitive dysfunction is a diagnosis of exclusion in elderly patients; therefore, one should first consider other diseases resulting in disorientation.

ADVANCED OR CONFIRMATORY TESTING

- Brainstem auditory evoked response testing; rule out deafness.
- Scotopic and photopic maze testing/obstacle course: vision.
- Electroretinogram: retinal function.
- Computed tomography or magnetic resonance imaging of brain.
- Cerebrospinal fluid cytologic with biochemical ± serologic assessment.
- Clinical laboratory diagnostic tests for various endocrinopathies, for liver function, toxicology screen, etc.

TREATMENT

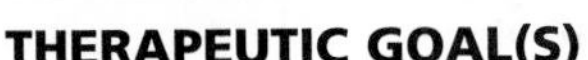

THERAPEUTIC GOAL(S)

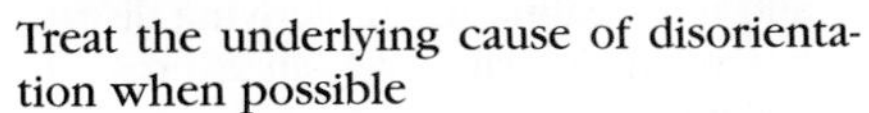

Treat the underlying cause of disorientation when possible

ACUTE GENERAL TREATMENT

Acute treatment varies according to the etiology (see specific etiology)

CHRONIC TREATMENT

Animals with incurable disorientation (e.g., age-related cognitive dysfunction) may need special care including:

- Being confined within a yard or home (e.g., to prevent wandering away and getting lost)
- Taking animal outside to urinate/defecate more frequently (dogs) (if dog is inappropriately urinating/defecating in the house)

PROGNOSIS AND OUTCOME

Prognosis depends on the etiology

PEARLS & CONSIDERATIONS

COMMENTS

- Up to 75% of dogs, 7 years or older, will demonstrate at least one clinical sign consistent with canine cognitive dysfunction syndrome.
- Animals with clinical signs of disorientation, related to vision or hearing loss, will commonly adapt to their surroundings and will have a good quality of life provided they are not used for tasks requiring these senses.

SUGGESTED READING

ASPCA Poison Control Center: http://www.aspca.org/site/PageServer?pagename=apcc (useful for information and links pertaining to toxicologic information on various plants and drugs).

Cuddon PA: Metabolic encephalopathies. *Vet Clin N Am Small Anim Pract* 26:893–923, 1996.

Head E, Zicker SC: Nutraceuticals, aging, and cognitive dysfunction. *Vet Clin North Am Small Anim Pract* 34:217–228, 2004.

Richardson JA, et al: Clinical syndrome associated with zolpidem *(Ambien® -ed.)* ingestion in dogs: 33 cases (January 1998–July 2000). *J Vet Intern Med* 16:208–210, 2002.

Wismer TA: Accidental ingestion of alprazolam *(Xanax® -ed.)* in 415 dogs. *Vet Hum Toxicol* 44:22–23, 2002.

AUTHOR: **AUBREY A. WEBB**
EDITOR: **ETIENNE CÔTÉ**

DISEASES AND DISORDERS

Disseminated Intravascular Coagulation

BASIC INFORMATION

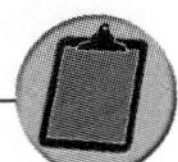

DEFINITION

An acquired syndrome of coagulation system dysregulation in which coagulation is abnormally and inappropriately activated, resulting in widespread deposition of fibrin in the microvasculature. Depletion of platelets and coagulation factors causes bleeding in a subset of patients with disseminated intravascular coagulation (DIC).

SYNONYM(S)

DIC
Dysfibrinogen syndrome

EPIDEMIOLOGY

SPECIES, AGE, SEX: Dogs of any age or sex. Rarely identified in cats.

RISK FACTORS: Primary disorders that initiate DIC: Neoplasia, sepsis, polytrauma, shock, multiple organ dysfunction syndrome, gastric dilation-volvulus, severe inflammatory and immune reactions (pancreatitis, immune hemolysis, envenomation), liver failure.

ASSOCIATED CONDITIONS AND DISORDERS: DIC always develops secondary to an underlying or primary disease process (see Risk Factors above).

CLINICAL PRESENTATION

DISEASE FORMS/SUBTYPES

- Acute DIC: associated with fulminant diseases (e.g., sepsis, anaphylaxis, heatstroke, pancreatitis, envenomation)
- Chronic DIC: develops secondary to solid tumors and hematopoietic neoplasia; common in dogs with hemangiosarcoma

HISTORY, CHIEF COMPLAINT: Typically reflects the primary disease, e.g., gastric dilation-volvulus, heatstroke, neoplasia. Signs of organ failure and dyspnea (due to tissue thrombosis and pulmonary thromboembolism) and hemorrhage may complicate disease presentation.

PHYSICAL EXAM FINDINGS: Variable, depending on primary disease and extent of thrombosis/factor depletion:

- Collapse
- Pale mucous membranes
- Tachycardia
- Tachypnea
- Diffuse bruising (ecchymoses)
- Melena
- Icterus

ETIOLOGY AND PATHOPHYSIOLOGY

- Two major pathways initiate DIC:
  - Systemic inflammatory response accompanied by cytokine activation and coagulation cascade activation (e.g.,. sepsis, polytrauma).
  - Release or exposure of procoagulant stimuli into the vascular space initiates widespread activation of coagulation (e.g., hemangiosarcoma, mammary carcinoma).
- Systemic fibrin deposition is insufficiently balanced by opposing anticoagulant mechanisms.
  - Antithrombin depletion from consumption, degradation, and suppressed synthesis.

   - Protein C system: downregulated by proinflammatory cytokines.
- Fibrinolysis is concomitantly suppressed.
   - High plasminogen activator inhibitor levels impair fibrinolysis.
- Subsequent depletion of coagulation factors, including consumption of platelets develops in some patients.
- Local thrombosis contributes to acidosis, ischemia, and necrosis, which can perpetuate the syndrome.

DIAGNOSIS

DIFFERENTIAL DIAGNOSIS

- Hemorrhagic DIC:
   - Anticoagulant rodenticide exposure
   - Severe thrombocytopenia
   - Inherited or acquired platelet dysfunction
   - Dextran or hetastarch administration (prolonged clotting times)
   - Liver failure
- Thrombotic DIC:
   - Organ failure or pulmonary thrombosis/thromboemboli (PTE) due to:
      - Cardiac disease
      - Heartworm disease
      - Tumor emboli
      - "Hypercoagulability" associated with antithrombin loss

INITIAL DATABASE

- Complete blood count, platelet count, blood smear evaluation.
   - Thrombocytopenia.
   - Schistocytosis (fragmented red blood cells) from shredding effect of intravascular fibrin strands.
- Serum chemistry profile.
- Urinalysis.
- Chest and abdominal radiographs.
- Coagulation testing (prothrombin time [PT], activated partial thromboplastin times [aPTT], fibrinogen).
- D-dimer or fibrin/fibrinogen degradation product (FDP) concentration: typically increased in DIC.
- Antithrombin III activity: typically decreased in DIC.

ADVANCED OR CONFIRMATORY TESTING

- No single laboratory test is diagnostic for DIC.
- The presence of a primary disease capable of initiating DIC and combined laboratory abnormalities of hemostatic pathways support the diagnosis.
   - Elevated aPTT or activated clotting time (ACT)
   - Elevated PT
   - Thrombocytopenia or falling platelet count
   - Elevated FDPs or D-dimers
   - Schistocytosis
   - Hypofibrinogenemia

TREATMENT

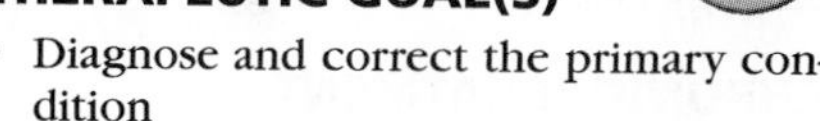

THERAPEUTIC GOAL(S)

- Diagnose and correct the primary condition
- Control active hemorrhage
- Prevent organ failure due to thrombosis

ACUTE GENERAL TREATMENT

- Always treat the primary condition.
- Support adequate perfusion with intravenous fluids.
- Supplemental oxygen therapy if indicated.
- Red blood cell transfusion or polymerized hemoglobin solution: considered in anemia cases. See Transfusion Reactions, p 1098.
- Fresh-frozen plasma (FFP) transfusion if fibrinogen and clotting factor depletion cause overt signs of hemorrhage, or if fibrinogen deficient patients require surgery. High volume and repeated doses of FFP may be needed (10–15 ml/kg IV q 8–12h).
- Heparin (either unfractionated or low-molecular weight heparin) should be considered in cases with signs of dyspnea due to PTE or organ failure due to thrombosis.
   - "Regular," unfractionated heparin (UFH) 100–200 U/kg SQ q 8h, or 15–25 U/kg/hr IV continuous rate infusion.
   - Low-molecular-weight heparin: dalteparin (Fragmin) 100 IU/kg SQ q 12h; enoxaparin (Lovenox) 1–1.5 mg/kg SQ q 12h.

CHRONIC TREATMENT

DIC is always a sequela and chronic treatment should be directed toward the primary condition.

DRUG INTERACTIONS

Avoid heparin, hetastarch, and dextrans when prolonged clotting times due to severe factor and fibrinogen depletion, or severe thrombocytopenia, are present.

POSSIBLE COMPLICATIONS

- Pulmonary thromboembolism
- Thromboembolism to other organs (e.g., renal, neurologic, aortic thromboembolism, hepatoportal)
- Hemorrhage into other organs leading to organ dysfunction

RECOMMENDED MONITORING

- Serial platelet counts and coagulation times.
- Monitor organ function and tissue oxygenation.
- If heparin treatment: closely monitor to detect signs of hemorrhage, falling platelet count, or excessive prolongation of in vitro clotting time (UFH therapy).
- A target prolongation of aPTT to 1.5 to 2 times patient baseline is considered evidence of UFH high-dose anticoagulant effect.
- UFH and low-molecular-weight heparins can be monitored based on their inhibition of Factor Xa. In human studies, the target range of anti-Xa activity for UFH = 0.3 to 0.7 U/ml (UFH) and for low-molecular-weight heparin = 0.5 to 1.0 U/ml .

PROGNOSIS AND OUTCOME

- Guarded
- Prognosis depends primarily on the underlying condition

PEARLS & CONSIDERATIONS

COMMENTS

- The development of DIC contributes to the morbidity and mortality of the primary disease process.
- Treating DIC late in the disease process is difficult.
- Having an early suspicion that DIC may develop is important for selecting appropriate tests to document and monitor the syndrome.
- Treating DIC alone (e.g., with heparin) and not treating the underlying disease has been described as "an exercise in futility."

PREVENTION

The critical factors in preventing or ameliorating DIC are specific and aggressive correction of the primary disease process.

CLIENT EDUCATION

The development of DIC represents a severe complication of many different systemic diseases.

SUGGESTED READING

Feldman B, Kirby R, Caldin M: Recognition and treatment of disseminated intravascular coagulation. In Bonagura JD: *Current Veterinary Therapy XIII*. Philadelphia, WB Saunders, 2000, pp 190–194.

Bateman SW, et al: Disseminated intravascular coagulation in dogs: review of the literature. *J Vet Emerg Crit Care* 8(1):29–45, 1998.

Boudreaux M, et al: Evaluation of antithrombin-III activity as a coindicator of disseminated intravascular coagulation in cats with induced feline infectious peritonitis virus infection. *Am J Vet Res* 50(11):1910–1913, 1989.

Levi M: Current understanding of disseminated intravascular coagulation. *Br J Haematol* 124:567–576, 2003.

AUTHORS: **JONATHAN BACH, MARJORY B. BROOKS**

EDITORS: **ELIZABETH ROZANSKI, SUSAN M. COTTER**

Distemper, Canine

BASIC INFORMATION

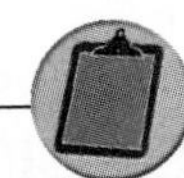

DEFINITION

Canine distemper is a viral disease primarily of young dogs caused by canine distemper virus, a *Morbillivirus* of the family Paramyxoviridae. Clinical disease can range from subclinical or mild signs to severe systemic illness with high morbidity and variable mortality. Mortality is largely dependent on the development of central nervous system (CNS) signs.

SYNONYM(S)

Distemper
Hardpad disease

EPIDEMIOLOGY

SPECIES, AGE, SEX

- Disease can occur in members of the family Canidae (dog, coyote, fox, etc.), Mustelidae (ferret, skunk, etc.), Procyonidae (raccoon, etc.), and Felidae (cat, lion, etc.).
- Young dogs (3 to 6 months old) are most commonly affected.

GENETICS AND BREED PREDISPOSITION: Breed predisposition with regard to disease susceptibility has been suspected, but not proven. Dolichocephalic breeds reportedly have higher disease prevalence and mortality rates versus brachycephalic breeds.

RISK FACTORS

- Lack of vaccination.
- Exposure of a naïve dog to an animal with subclinical or clinical disease.
- Puppies born to a bitch with mild or inapparent disease (transplacental infection).
- Protection in an immunocompetent dog may be compromised during periods of stress or immunosuppression.

CONTAGION AND ZOONOSIS

- During periods of viral shedding, canine distemper virus is abundant in respiratory secretions, and is most commonly transmitted by aerosol exposure. Direct contact with contaminated urine, feces, or skin may also result in infection.
- Canine distemper is not considered a zoonotic disease.

ASSOCIATED CONDITIONS AND DISORDERS

- Mild disease in dogs may be difficult to clinically distinguish from canine infectious tracheobronchitis ("kennel cough"). Canine distemper typically manifests initially as rhinitis accompanied by fever. Later, signs of bronchitis and pneumonia, gastroenteritis, and neurologic dysfunction may develop.
- Hyperkeratosis of the footpads and ocular signs (anterior uveitis, optic neuritis, retinal degeneration) may accompany canine distemper.
- Keratoconjunctivitis sicca may develop as a sequela to systemic disease.
- Potential dental abnormalities (enamel hypoplasia, impacted teeth, oligodontia) in dogs that survive neonatal infection.

CLINICAL PRESENTATION

DISEASE FORMS/SUBTYPES: Subclinical to mild disease is probably the most common result of CDV infection, but generalized distemper is the most commonly recognized form. Generalized distemper manifests initially as respiratory disease. Gastrointestinal disease usually follows, and the potential exists for signs of neurologic dysfunction to develop concomitant with or after the resolution of systemic illness.

HISTORY, CHIEF COMPLAINT: Variable; depends on the stage of disease recognized by the client. The history may include complaints of lethargy, inappetence, signs of respiratory disease (ocular and/or nasal discharge, coughing, dyspnea), vomiting, diarrhea, and/or varying neurologic abnormalities depending on which portion of the CNS may be affected.

PHYSICAL EXAM FINDINGS

- Systemic disease (epithelial stage): serous to mucopurulent oculonasal discharge and conjunctivitis are very commonly observed; coughing, dyspnea, increased lung sounds are nonpecific but also occur commonly; diarrhea, vomiting, dehydration, cachexia, and fever can occur.
- Neurologic disease: signs indicative of encephalitis (seizures, vestibular disease, cerebellar signs, paraparesis or tetraparesis accompanied by proprioceptive ataxia) are more common than signs of meningitis (hyperesthesia). Myoclonus (involuntary twitching of the head and neck, or of the limbs) is very suggestive of canine distemper.
- Note: Because of the pathogenesis of canine distemper, signs of systemic disease and signs of neurologic disease are not observed at the same time. Therefore, if such signs are present simultaneously, it is unlikely that both are due to canine distemper.

ETIOLOGY AND PATHOPHYSIOLOGY

- Once exposure to canine distemper virus has occurred, the virus replicates within tissue macrophages of the respiratory epithelium, and virus-infected mononuclear cells spread to various lymphoid organs. Viral proliferation in multiple lymphoid organs is related to the initial, but often unnoticed, febrile response and occasionally observed lymphopenia (secondary to viral damage of lymphocytes).
- Viremia ensues, and depending on the dog's level of immunity, canine distemper virus may infect multiple epithelial tissues (skin, epithelium of the gastrointestinal [GI], respiratory, and urogenital tracts), invade the CNS, or both. Clinical signs due to epithelial/mucosal effects usually begin approximately 2 weeks after infection and last for 1 to 2 weeks. Neurologic signs begin at the earliest 1 to 3 weeks *after resolution* of oculonasal discharge, coughing, and other epithelial/mucosal signs.
- Shedding of canine distemper virus occurs once epithelial cells are affected, typically about 2 weeks after infection. Shedding may persist for up to 60 to 90 days postinfection.
- If canine distemper virus is able to colonize CNS tissues, acute and/or chronic encephalitis may be observed secondary to neuronal death and demyelination.
- Dogs with adequate immunity against canine distemper virus tend to develop inapparent disease and clear the virus by day 14 postinfection.

DIAGNOSIS

Canine distemper is suspected when young, especially unvaccinated dogs present for evaluation of mucosal signs (oculonasal discharge, cough, vomiting/diarrhea) or neurologic signs possibly with a history of mucosal signs having resolved at least 1 week earlier. Confirmation requires demonstration of the organism directly (uncommon), or via fluorescent antibody testing or similar analysis.

DIFFERENTIAL DIAGNOSIS

- Canine infectious tracheobronchitis
- Canine parvoviral enteritis
- Other causes of CNS disease in young dogs (congenital structural abnormalities, infectious/inflammatory disease)

INITIAL DATABASE

- Complete blood count may reveal an absolute lymphopenia secondary to lymphoid depletion. Distemper inclusions may rarely be identified within lymphocytes, monocytes, neutrophils, or erythrocytes on peripheral blood smears.

- Serum chemistry profile and urinalysis abnormalities are variable and nonspecific.
- Thoracic radiographs may reveal an interstitial pattern in early stages of canine distemper. Signs of pneumonia (increased soft tissue opacity, alveolar pattern) may be apparent later (usually due to secondary bacterial infection).

ADVANCED OR CONFIRMATORY TESTING

- Serum canine distemper virus antibody titers may or may not be helpful. IgM is uncommonly measured, and IgG levels do not discern recent infection from vaccination or from past infection.
- Cerebrospinal fluid (CSF)
    - Increased protein concentration and total nucleated cell count, predominantly consisting of lymphocytes, characterize canine distemper viral encephalitis. Dogs with noninflammatory demyelinating lesions may have normal CSF results, however.
    - An elevated anticanine distemper CSF antibody titer is diagnostic for canine distemper encephalitis. Contamination of CSF with peripheral blood could mistakenly introduce canine distemper antibodies into CSF, however, giving a false-positive diagnosis. Therefore, in instances where it is possible that the CSF sample was contaminated by peripheral blood, it is recommended that both canine distemper virus and canine parvovirus titers be assessed on both CSF and serum; presence of a positive canine parvovirus titer in both CSF and serum indicates blood contamination and invalidates the significance of a positive CSF canine distemper titer.
- Fluorescent antibody testing provides the best result for antemortem diagnosis.
    - May be performed on cytologic smears prepared from buffy coat (most common), respiratory or tonsillar epithelium, CSF, bone marrow, or urine sediment.
    - May be rewarding when performed on conjunctival scrapings early in the disease (e.g., when conjunctivitis and ocular discharge are present), but becomes negative as the disease progresses and these signs subside.
- Some laboratories offer a polymerase chain reaction test for canine distemper virus in whole blood, serum, and CSF.
- Definitive postmortem diagnosis of canine distemper can be made via immunofluorescent techniques on frozen tissue sections obtained at necropsy. Sections of tonsil, lymph nodes, lung, stomach, duodenum, spleen, urinary bladder, and brain should be collected for testing.

TREATMENT

THERAPEUTIC GOAL(S)

- No specific antiviral agents are currently available for canine distemper virus.
- Treatment of generalized canine distemper is supportive and aimed at managing clinical signs.
- Supportive care of patients with neurologic disease is less rewarding, as signs frequently progress or may initially be incompatible with life.

ACUTE GENERAL TREATMENT

- Broad-spectrum antibiotic therapy and expectorants or nebulization and coupage if secondary bacterial pneumonia is present (see Pneumonia, Bacterial, p 863)
- Intravenous fluids as needed for dehydration
- Diazepam or midazolam (0.5 mg/kg IV or 1.0 mg/kg per rectum) for acute seizure control

CHRONIC TREATMENT

- Nutritional support for cachectic dogs.
- Maintenance antiepileptic drugs may be required in some neurologic cases. (See Seizures, p 990.)
- Anti-inflammatory doses of corticosteroids (e.g., prednisone 0.5-1 mg/kg PO q 24-48h, tapering to lowest effective dose) may be beneficial in controlling signs of optic neuritis or chronic inflammatory encephalitis. Such treatment is contraindicated during the systemic (epithelial/mucosal) stage of canine distemper.

POSSIBLE COMPLICATIONS

Clients should be cautioned that even if a dog recovers from generalized illness without evidence of neurologic disease, it is possible for neurologic signs to develop at a later time.

PROGNOSIS AND OUTCOME

- Neurologic complications are the most important factor that influences prognosis.
- Recovery from canine distemper is largely dependent on the effectiveness of the host's immune response.
- Dogs with adequate immunity tend to show no clinical signs of illness and clear the virus within 2 weeks postinfection. The incidence of later-onset CNS signs in these animals is low.
- Dogs with inadequate immunity (poor to no antibody response) tend to develop mild to severe systemic illness, and have a greater likelihood of eventually developing neurologic signs.

PEARLS & CONSIDERATIONS

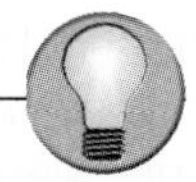

COMMENTS

Puppies and young adult dogs with "kennel cough" may in fact have canine distemper. The likelihood is greater if vaccine history is deficient, and if other mucosal signs (particularly conjunctivitis) and/or signs of pneumonia are present.

PREVENTION

- Routine vaccination with a modified live canine distemper virus (ML-CDV) vaccine in puppies (every 3 to 4 weeks between 6 and 16 weeks old with a booster vaccination 1 year later) followed by periodic boosters (every 3 years).
- Vaccination generally confers adequate immunity in dogs, but disease may still occur if a dog is stressed or immunocompromised, or exposed to a highly virulent strain or a large quantity of canine distemper virus.
- A recombinant canine distemper vaccine (canarypox virus-vectored; Recombitek® Distemper, Merial) is currently available, and initial studies indicate comparable efficacy to ML-CDV vaccines in dogs.

CLIENT EDUCATION

- Dogs with distemper should be isolated from other healthy dogs (especially puppies) at least 2 weeks beyond resolution of clinical signs.
- Dogs typically shed virus for 1 to 2 weeks after recovery from acute systemic illness; however, some dogs may shed virus in body secretions for up to 2 months (especially those that developed severe systemic disease and/or neurologic signs).
- Canine distemper virus is sensitive to ultraviolet light, heat, and drying. In warm climates, canine distemper virus does not usually persist in kennels after the removal of infected dogs. Colder climates allow a longer persistence of virus in the environment.

SUGGESTED READING

Greene CE, Appel MJ: Canine distemper. In Greene CE (ed): *Infectious Diseases of the Dog and Cat,* ed 2. Philadephia, WB Saunders, 1998, pp 9-22.

AUTHOR: **JODI D. SMITH**
EDITOR: **DOUGLASS K. MACINTIRE**

Distichiasis/Ectopic Cilia/Trichiasis

BASIC INFORMATION

DEFINITION

- *Distichiasis*: the presence of an additional row of adventitious lashes on the eyelid margin arising from the meibomian glands (Fig. I-55), in addition to the normal eyelashes emerging from the usual peripheral eyelid margin
- *Ectopic cilia*: aberrant individual eyelashes that arise from the meibomian glands and grow through the palpebral conjunctiva toward the globe
- *Trichiasis*: a normal eyelid/facial hair that is directed toward and contacts the conjunctiva or cornea

SYNONYM(S)

Aberrant cilia
"Abnormal eyelashes"
Distichia

EPIDEMIOLOGY

SPECIES, AGE, SEX

- Common in dogs; rare in cats
- Most often in young dogs, but can occur at any age
- No sex predisposition

GENETICS AND BREED PREDISPOSITION

- *Distichiasis*: any breed, but common in American and English cocker spaniels, miniature long-haired dachshund, English bulldog, golden retriever, Cavalier King Charles spaniel, Pekingese, toy and miniature poodles, Yorkshire terrier, and Shetland sheepdog.
- *Ectopic cilia*: any breed, but common in boxers.
- *Trichiasis*:
  - Congenital trichiasis: English cocker spaniel and small breed dogs such as brachycephalic breeds with prominent facial folds (e.g., Pekingese, pug).
  - Acquired trichiasis: breeds with redundant dorsal skin folds (English bulldog, shar-pei, chow chow, bloodhound, St. Bernard).

ASSOCIATED CONDITIONS AND DISORDERS

- Conjunctivitis (see Conjunctivitis: Dogs, p 233)
- Ulcerative keratitis (see Corneal Ulceration, p 246)
- Nonulcerative keratitis (see Corneal Pigmentation, p 242; Corneal Vascularization, p 249)

CLINICAL PRESENTATION

HISTORY, CHIEF COMPLAINT

- *Distichiasis*:
  - Generally does not produce clinical signs; most cases are clinically silent.
  - Epiphora and blepharospasm may be seen if ocular irritation is present.
- *Ectopic cilia*:
  - Acute onset of signs of ocular pain such as severe blepharospasm and epiphora.
- *Trichiasis*:
  - Signs of ocular irritation such as blepharospasm and epiphora.

PHYSICAL EXAM FINDINGS

- *Distichiasis*:
  - Single to multiple cilia along eyelid margin (see Fig. I-55).
  - Usually not causing overt clinical signs.
  - Epiphora, mild conjunctivitis, and nonulcerative keratitis are seen if cilia are causing ocular irritation.
  - Blepharospasm and ulcerative keratitis are seen if causing severe corneal irritation.
  - Entropion (secondary/spastic) may be seen if blepharospasm is severe.
- *Ectopic cilia*:
  - Most common at the 12-o'clock position (center of upper eyelid).
  - Emerge through the palpebral conjunctiva 4 to 6 mm posterior (caudal) to the eyelid margin.
  - Magnification is needed to identify the cilia.
  - Acute blepharospasm and epiphora are typical.
  - Focal signs of nonulcerative and ulcerative keratitis often are seen.
  - Keratitis, whether ulcerative or nonulcerative, often presents in a vertical pattern that follows the path of eyelid movement.
- *Trichiasis*:
  - Congenital trichiasis: The cilia occur on the lateral two thirds of the upper eyelid.
  - Medial canthal trichiasis: The hairs arise along the medial eyelid margin and in the area of the caruncle (aberrant dermis at the medial canthus and present on the conjunctiva).
  - Trichiasis is often associated with eyelid agenesis of the lateral two thirds of the upper eyelid in cats.
  - Signs of ocular irritation, such as epiphora, if mild.
  - Keratitis (ulcerative and nonulcerative), if severe.

ETIOLOGY AND PATHOPHYSIOLOGY

- Meibomian glands without cilia may spontaneously develop distichiasis or ectopic cilia if the glands become metaplastic.
- *Distichiasis*:
  - Cilia originate from the meibomian glands.

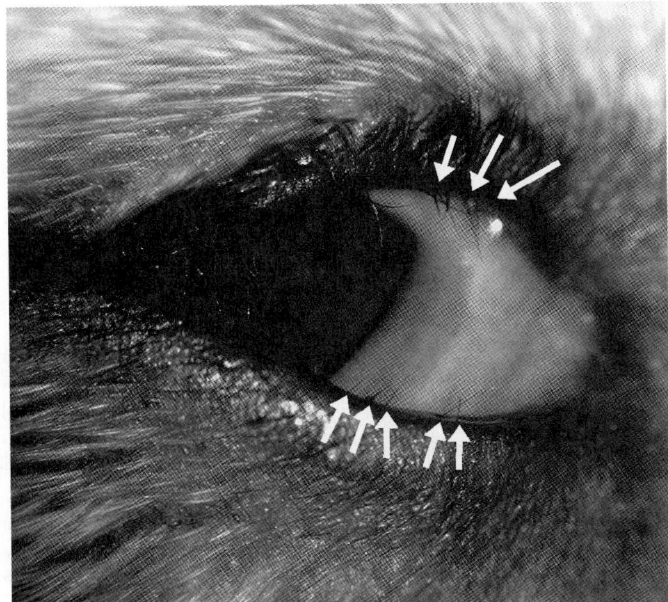

FIGURE I-55 Distichiasis in a dog. Note the numerous, long aberrant hairs along the upper and lower eyelid margins and arising from the meibomian gland ducts (*arrows*). These hairs were an incidental finding and caused no clinical signs; therefore no treatment was warranted.

  - Develop from metaplastic meibomian glands.
  - Arise secondary to chronic inflammation (meibomianitis), i.e., acquired condition.
  - May or may not contact cornea.
- *Ectopic cilia*:
  - Cilia originate from the meibomian glands and emerge through the palpebral conjunctiva.
  - Always contact cornea.
  - Can occur at any time in the animal's life.
- *Trichiasis*:
  - Normal hairs that are abnormally directed toward the eye.
  - Congenital trichiasis of the upper eyelid can be bilateral or unilateral.
  - Acquired trichiasis develops secondary to ptosis associated with redundant dorsal skin folds (see Genetics and Breed Predisposition).
  - Acquired trichiasis develops secondary to loss of muscle tone in older dogs.
  - Associated with entropion, prominent nasal folds, and medial canthal hairs (eyelids and caruncle).

DIAGNOSIS

DIFFERENTIAL DIAGNOSIS

- Trichomegaly (excessively long eyelashes)
- Other causes of blepharospasm including:
  - Corneal ulceration
  - Conjunctivitis
  - Uveitis
- Other causes of epiphora
- Entropion

INITIAL DATABASE

Complete ophthalmic examination including:

- Schirmer tear test (normal >15 mm after 1 minute in dogs, variable in cats)
- Fluorescein dye application
- Intraocular pressure (normal: 10-25 mmHg)
- Examination of the eyelid margin and palpebral conjunctiva with magnification and a good light source
- Examination of the cornea

ADVANCED OR CONFIRMATORY TESTING

5 to 10 × magnification is often needed to visualize ectopic cilia

TREATMENT

THERAPEUTIC GOAL(S)

- Eliminate ocular irritation
- Determine if distichiasis and/or trichiasis are responsible for clinical signs of ocular disease
- Remove the offending cilia or direct the cilia away from the globe

ACUTE GENERAL TREATMENT

- *Distichiasis*:
  - Usually does not produce clinical signs; no treatment required.
  - Hairs regrow within 4 to 5 weeks with mechanical epilation/plucking.
  - If producing clinical signs, may treat surgically:
    - Before removal, expression of the meibomian glands pushes hidden hairs from the glands.
    - Cryotherapy along the palpebral surface of the meibomian glands using a double freeze-thaw cycle is effective treatment for a large number of distichia in a patient.
    - Electrolysis is useful for single or a low number of cilia; procedure is tedious and excessive current may cause tissue damage.
    - Carbon dioxide laser removal is tedious and can predispose to excessive tissue damage.
    - Resection from the conjunctival surface effective for single or multiple cilia.
    - Eyelid splitting techniques are not recommended due to the potential for postoperative eyelid deformities and regrowth of the hairs.
- *Ectopic cilia*:
  - Typically produce clinical signs; therefore treated surgically.
  - En-bloc resection of aberrant cilia including associated conjunctiva and underlying meibomian gland.
  - Surgical removal usually successful, but regrowth can occur.
- *Trichiasis*:
  - If minor ocular irritation, conservative management may be effective:
    - Clipping hairs short to prevent ocular contact.
  - Variable surgical therapies depending on location of trichiasis:
    - Many procedures complex; consider referral to veterinary ophthalmologist.
    - Medial canthal trichiasis may be corrected by permanent medial canthoplasty (pocket technique or Wyman technique) or cryotherapy.
    - Nasal fold trichiasis may require resection of prominent nasal skin folds
    - Trichiasis associated with ptosis (drooping of the upper eyelid) may be corrected by a Stades procedure.
    - Trichiasis associated with redundant dorsal skin folds may be corrected by extensive removal of tissue or by the use of anchoring sutures to the periosteum.
    - Trichiasis associated with eyelid agenesis in cats may be corrected by cryotherapy until kitten is old enough for permanent surgery (e.g., rotational flap).

CHRONIC TREATMENT

If recurrence, repeat treatment may be required

POSSIBLE COMPLICATIONS

- The most common complication to correction of distichiasis, ectopic cilia, and trichiasis is recurrence
- Postoperative eyelid scarring ± entropion

RECOMMENDED MONITORING

Have owner monitor animal for signs of recurrent ocular irritation postoperatively; may indicate regrowth of offending hair(s)

PROGNOSIS AND OUTCOME

Generally good prognosis, but recurrence is possible regardless of treatment

PEARLS & CONSIDERATIONS

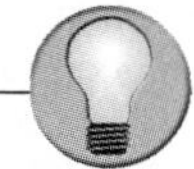

COMMENTS

- Distichiasis and trichiasis are among the most common eyelid abnormalities.
- Goal is not simply to diagnose distichiasis or trichiasis, but to determine if the abnormal hair(s) is/are causing ocular irritation, as this determination will help decide whether treatment is necessary.
- Keratitis that presents in a vertical pattern that follows the path of eyelid movement should raise the suspicion of an ectopic cilium in the upper eyelid.
- Magnification commonly is needed to identify ectopic cilia, and the diagnosis should not be ruled out based on absence of visualization without a magnifying glass or loupe.
- Ectopic cilia and hairs causing distichiasis will regrow within 4 to 5 weeks with mechanical epilation/plucking.
- No single treatment guarantees permanent resolution of distichia, ectopic cilia, or trichiasis.

PREVENTION

Avoid breeding affected or closely related dogs

CLIENT EDUCATION

- Presence of distichiasis or trichiasis does not indicate disease.

- Animals with distichiasis, ectopic cilia, or trichiasis are monitored for signs of ocular irritation.
- Recurrence is possible regardless of treatment.

SUGGESTED READING

Bedford PGC: Diseases and surgery of the canine eyelid. In Gelatt KN (ed): *Veterinary Ophthalmology*. Philadelphia, Lippincott Williams & Wilkins, 1999, pp 535-568.

Lackner PA: Techniques for surgical correction of adnexal disease. *Clin Tech Small Anim Pract* 16 (1):40, 2001.

Martin CL: Eyelids. In Martin CL (ed): *Ophthalmic Disease in Veterinary Medicine*. London, Manson Publishing, Ltd, 2005, pp 145-182.

AUTHOR: **PHILLIP A. MOORE**
EDITOR: **CHERYL L. CULLEN**

Draining Tracts, Cutaneous

BASIC INFORMATION

DEFINITION

A tract that connects an area of subcutaneous or deeper soft tissue inflammation to the skin surface

SYNONYM(S)

Fistulous tract

EPIDEMIOLOGY

SPECIES, AGE, SEX: Variable depending on etiology.

RISK FACTORS: Penetrating injuries, chronic exposure of the skin to trauma or moisture, wound contamination, contact with infected individuals, immunodeficiency syndromes.

CONTAGION AND ZOONOSIS: Pathogens with zoonotic potential include: *Nocardia*, *Blastomyces*, *Sporothrix*, and *Leishmania* among others.

GEOGRAPHY AND SEASONALITY: In warm, dry climates: grass awns as penetrating foreign bodies.

ASSOCIATED CONDITIONS AND DISORDERS

- Frequently associated with cutaneous nodular disease.
- May be associated with underlying immunosuppressive disorders.

CLINICAL PRESENTATION

DISEASE FORMS/SUBTYPES: Infectious, noninfectious, neoplastic

HISTORY, CHIEF COMPLAINT: There may be a history of a previous penetrating injury, typically associated with infectious causes. For all three forms/subtypes, a common complaint is of a nonhealing cutaneous wound that may fail to respond to topical antimicrobial therapy.

PHYSICAL EXAM FINDINGS

- Lesions may be solitary or multiple.
- Draining tracts are often associated with cutaneous nodules (fungal or bacterial granuloma, idiopathic sterile pyogranuloma/granuloma; sterile nodular panniculitis) scattered over the trunk.
- Lesions may or may not be painful.
- Exudate from the tracts may be serous, serosanguineous, or purulent. Tissue granules may be found within the exudate (e.g., actinomycosis, actinobacillosis, nocardiosis, and bacterial pseudomycetoma).

ETIOLOGY AND PATHOPHYSIOLOGY

- Infectious causes are often the result of direct inoculation of the organism into the subcutaneous tissue by way of a penetrating injury. A major exception is the systemic mycoses (histoplasmosis, blastomycosis, coccidioidomycosis, cryptococcosis), which are acquired mainly through inhalation and only very rarely through direct inoculation.
- Immunosuppressive diseases may increase the risk of infection or colonization with opportunistic pathogens.

DIAGNOSIS

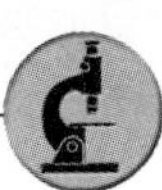

DIFFERENTIAL DIAGNOSIS

Differential diagnosis includes many infectious and noninfectious conditions.

- Infectious:
  - Bacterial (including feline subcutaneous abscesses, actinomycotic infections [*Actinomyces, Nocardia*], *Streptomyces griseus, Dermatophilus congolensis*, actinobacillosis, mycobacteria, bacterial pseudomycetoma)
  - Fungal (including blastomycosis, histoplasmosis, cryptococcosis, coccidioidomycosis, zygomycosis, pythiosis, sporotrichosis, and dermatophytic pseudomycetoma)
  - Parasitic (including leishmaniasis, neosporosis, dracunculiasis, cutaneous dirofilariasis, and cutaneous habronemiasis)
- Noninfectious:
  - Foreign bodies (although secondary bacterial infection is virtually inevitable)
  - Immune-mediated (sterile nodular panniculitis [Fig. I-55], systemic lupus erythematosus, drug eruption)
  - Xanthomatosis
  - Neoplasia

INITIAL DATABASE

A thorough diagnostic approach is indicated with draining tracts: all of the following diagnostic tests are indicated for a complete evaluation.

- Culture and sensitivity: Bacterial (aerobic and anaerobic), fungal, and mycobacterial cultures should be considered in cases of persistent draining tracts and are required. Culture of the superficial exudate will likely not reflect the true, deeper disease process. Samples of deep tissue should be obtained by biopsy for culture. Many of the potential pathogens are difficult to successfully culture, which could result in false-negative results. Notify the lab as to which differentials are being considered so that appropriate sampling, transport, and culture procedures are performed (many fungal organisms are highly infectious to humans under laboratory conditions).
- Cytologic evaluation: As well as the exudate, any tissue granules present should be crushed between two slides and examined. Fine needle aspirates of nodules or impression smears of biopsy samples may also prove useful (Diff-Quik, followed by acid-fast and period acid-Schiff staining). If samples are submitted to an outside laboratory, be sure to send unstained slides and notify the lab as to which differentials are being considered.
- Histopathologic evaluation: Obtain multiple specimens from both open and closed lesions. Wedge or elliptical biopsies provide a better yield for deep subcutaneous lesions than punch biopsies. Special stains may be required to positively identify some pathogens, and the pathologist should be provided with a complete list of differentials.
- A lack of organisms on cytologic study, histopathologic study, and culture, if performed correctly, may indicate a noninfectious etiology.
- Routine hematology, chemistry profile, urinalysis.

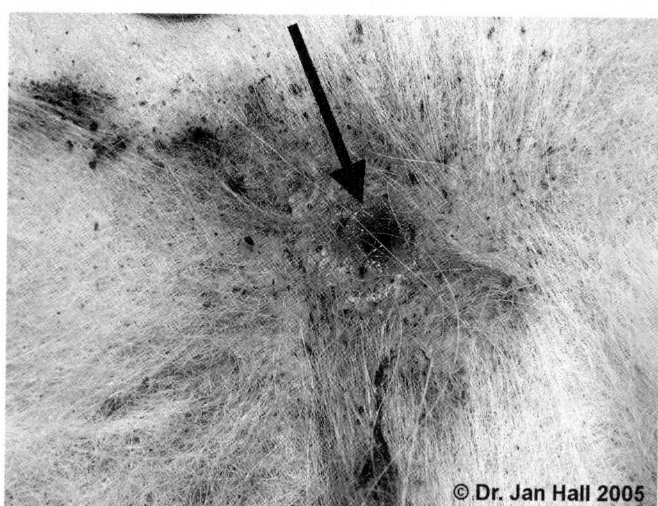

FIGURE I-56 Draining tract (*arrow*) on the ventral thorax of a Shetland sheepdog with sterile nodular panniculitis. Courtesy of Dr. Jan A. Hall.

ADVANCED OR CONFIRMATORY TESTING

- Radiographs: may help to identify foreign bodies or diseases with systemic manifestations, such as pulmonary involvement with blastomycosis.
- Serology: A fourfold rise in titer from two samples taken 3 weeks apart may help confirm the diagnosis with some pathogens, especially the mycotic pathogens (e.g. cryptococcosis, blastomycosis, *Pythium*).
- Fundic examination.
- Antinuclear antibody.

TREATMENT

THERAPEUTIC GOAL(S)

Resolution of the draining tracts

ACUTE GENERAL TREATMENT

- Treatment varies depending on the etiology.
- In general, an inciting cause (e.g., foreign body, neoplasm) should always be sought and, if present, needs to be removed for an optimal outcome/potential for cure.
- Lavage and debridement of the lesions in combination with appropriate antimicrobial therapy based on culture and sensitivity are indicated for infectious etiologies.
- Noninfectious etiologies (e.g., sterile nodular panniculitis) may respond to immunosuppressive doses of glucocorticoids and other immunosuppressive therapies.

PROGNOSIS AND OUTCOME

Variable depending on etiology

PEARLS & CONSIDERATIONS

COMMENTS

- Patients with chronic or recurrent infectious draining tracts should be evaluated for underlying immunosuppressive diseases or persistent local/focal abnormalities (foreign body, neoplasm, etc.).
- Only after infectious agents have been completely ruled out, and a definitive diagnosis reached, should treatment be considered for noninfectious diseases that respond to glucocorticoid therapy.

SUGGESTED READING

Beale KM: Nodules and draining tracts. *Vet Clin North Am Small Anim Pract* 25:4, 1995.

Daigle JC, et al: Draining tracts and nodules in dogs and cats. *Clin Techn Small Anim Pract* 16:4, 2001.

AUTHOR: **ANDREW LOWE**

EDITOR: **JAN A. HALL**

Drowning

BASIC INFORMATION

DEFINITION

Death by asphyxia due to submersion in a liquid medium

EPIDEMIOLOGY

SPECIES, AGE, SEX: Dogs and cats of either sex and any age.

RISK FACTORS: Preexisting disorder (orthopedic injury, neurologic dysfunction, visual deficits, respiratory abnormality) can predispose an incapacitated patient to fall into water or become submerged during aquatic activity.

CLINICAL PRESENTATION

DISEASE FORMS/SUBTYPES: Fresh water versus salt water aspiration.

HISTORY, CHIEF COMPLAINT: There is almost always a known submersion incident. If possible, it is helpful to obtain information regarding factors that have been reported to influence prognosis in human medicine.

- Circumstances surrounding submersion (severe internal injuries worsen prognosis)
- Duration of submersion (prognosis worsens with increased time)
- Tonicity and temperature of the water (prognosis better with fresh/ice water)
- Apnea after rescue (spontaneous breathing improves prognosis)
- Immediate neurologic condition after rescue (poor condition worsens prognosis)

PHYSICAL EXAM FINDINGS: Variable depending on severity. May include collapse, dyspnea, tachypnea, tachycardia, bradycardia, cyanosis, hypoperfusion, hypothermia, increased bronchovesicular sounds, or cardiac or respiratory arrest.

ETIOLOGY AND PATHOPHYSIOLOGY

- Pulmonary: fresh water. Affects the surface tension properties of pulmonary surfactant (surfactant washout), leading to alveolar instability, the possibility of noncardiogenic pulmonary edema, and alterations in the ventilation-perfusion ratio. Due to the relative hypotonicity of fresh water, aspirated fluid is generally quickly absorbed into the circulation. If enough fluid is absorbed, hyponatremia causes hemolysis (with hemoglobinemia, hyperkalemia).
- Pulmonary: sea water. Results in a net influx of fluid into the pulmonary parenchyma (osmotic gradient) and alveolar flooding. The net flux of fluid from the circulation to the lungs may be so great as to cause hypovolemia.
- Cardiovascular. Elevated systemic and pulmonary vascular resistance, cardiac

arrhythmias and cardiac arrest are primarily due to hypoxia; they are positively related to the length of anoxic insult, and negatively to the effects of hypothermia and effectiveness of resuscitation.
- Neurologic pathophysiology. Ischemia leads to an elevation in extracellular central nervous tissue glutamate concentration, which is thought to be directly related to neuronal damage. Both cerebral ischemia and hypoxia can lead to irreversible neurologic dysfunction.
- In all, 90% of drowning victims aspirate fluid into the lungs; in 10%, drowning is associated with laryngospasm and inhalation against a closed glottis, causing noncardiogenic pulmonary edema without aspiration of water.

DIAGNOSIS

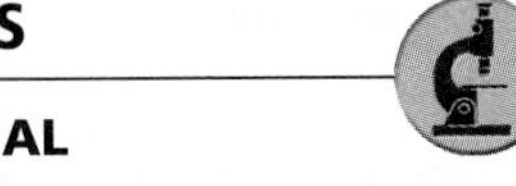

DIFFERENTIAL DIAGNOSIS

Known history of recent submersion is generally sufficient to make the diagnosis

INITIAL DATABASE

- Arterial blood gas analysis (hypoxemia variable with degree of aspiration/noncardiogenic pulmonary edema; metabolic acidosis possible and appears detrimental to prognosis)
- Pulse oximetry. Low SpO_2 with hypoxemia
- Electrocardiogram: ventricular arrhythmias
- Complete blood count (usually unremarkable)
- Serum chemistry (increased liver enzymes, possibly hypoproteinemia)
- Urinalysis (usually unremarkable)
- Thoracic radiographs (pulmonary infiltrates of varying location and type)
- Blood pressure (usually unremarkable)

ADVANCED OR CONFIRMATORY TESTING

Bronchoalveolar lavage or transtracheal wash is indicated if warranted by clinical suspicion of pulmonary infection

TREATMENT

THERAPEUTIC GOAL(S)

- Improve ventilation
- Maintain appropriate intravascular volume and tissue perfusion (*mean* arterial blood pressure >60–80 mmHg, central venous pressure = 2–5 cm H_2O, urine production >1–2 ml/kg/hr)
- Ensure adequate blood oxygen saturation (SpO_2 >92%, PaO_2 >80 mmHg [room air])
- Correct electrolyte imbalances or severe acidosis (e.g., if pH <7.1)

ACUTE GENERAL TREATMENT

- Regain spontaneous ventilation and circulation (see Cardiopulmonary Cerebral Resuscitation, p 1202).
- Oxygen supplementation (see p 1292).
- IV fluid administration as indicated.
- Mechanical ventilation with positive end-expiratory pressure where indicated (see p 1325).
- Abdominal thrust or gravitational drainage offers *no* advantage and may increase complications such as regurgitation and aspiration and delaying adequate treatment.
- Antibiotic therapy is not indicated unless clinical and radiographic evidence of pulmonary infection. Antibiotic use should be based on culture and sensitivity results.
- Corticosteroid therapy was once suggested but has failed to demonstrate any therapeautic advantage in large studies and may predispose patients to infection.

POSSIBLE COMPLICATIONS

- In addition to being predisposing factors, preexisting problems such as respiratory disease, heart disease, or seizure disorders should be identified because they may complicate resuscitation.
- Infrequently, grossly contaminated water can cause lower airway obstruction by particulate matter or cause pulmonary infection.
- Uncommonly, renal function can become compromised due to decreased renal perfusion, hypoxemia, or severe hemoglobinuria.
- Cerebral hypoxia, cerebral hypoperfusion or carbon dioxide narcosis can cause varying degrees of neurologic impairment that may be permanent.

RECOMMENDED MONITORING

- Thoracic auscultation
- Respiratory rate and effort
- Arterial blood gas analysis
- Urine output
- Neurologic status
- Hematocrit, electrolyte and pH imbalances
- Electrocardiogram

PROGNOSIS AND OUTCOME

- Most near-drowning animals are markedly improved within 24 hours. Failure to rapidly improve is associated with a grave prognosis, as is persistent hypoxemia.
- By extrapolation from human medicine, the need for CPR on presentation, pH <7.0, and apnea or coma, are poor prognostic indicators.
- Similarly in human beings, submersion for >25 minutes, resuscitation for >25 minutes, cardiac arrest at time of presentation, and lack of return of purposeful movements within 24 hours of the incident are associated with severe neurologic deficits or death.

PEARLS & CONSIDERATIONS

COMMENTS

Abdominal thrust and gravitational pull (suspended upside-down) offer no benefits and may increase complications such as regurgitation, aspiration, and delayed resuscitation.

PREVENTION

- Outdoor supervision
- Avoidance of swimming by dogs with disorders causing episodic lack of control (seizures, syncope)
- Precautionary pool-side safety measures such as pool covers and gated pool areas
- Boating safety measures: flotation devices; keeping animals in boat cabin, on boat floor, or away from railings
- Avoid semi-frozen lakes, ponds, or rivers

SUGGESTED READING

Powell LL: Accidental drowning and submersion injury. In King LG (ed): *Textbook of Respiratory Disease in Dogs and Cats.* St. Louis, Saunders, 2004, pp 484–486.

Modell JH: Current concepts: drowning. *N Engl J Med* 328(4):253–256, 1993.

AUTHOR: **GEOFF HEFFNER**

EDITOR: **ELIZABETH ROZANSKI**

Drug Eruption

BASIC INFORMATION

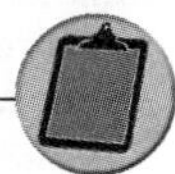

DEFINITION

Development of cutaneous or mucocutaneous lesions following drug administration (topical, oral, or injectable). These uncommon reactions can be either predictable (pharmacologic) or unpredictable (idiosyncratic). It is likely that many drug reactions, by their subtlety, go unreported.

SYNONYM(S)

Adverse drug reaction
Cutaneous drug reaction

EPIDEMIOLOGY

SPECIES, AGE, SEX: The incidence of drug eruptions in dogs and cats has been reported as 2% and 1.6%, respectively.

GENETICS AND BREED PREDISPOSITION: No clear breed predisposition. Shetland sheepdog, dalmatian, Yorkshire terrier, miniature poodle, miniature schnauzer, Australian shepherd, Old English sheepdog, Scottish terrier, wirehaired fox terrier, and greyhound breeds may be overrepresented.

CLINICAL PRESENTATION

HISTORY, CHIEF COMPLAINT

- History of drug administration.
- The chief complaint may be variable because of the wide spectrum of clinical signs.
- Depending if the reaction is predictable or not, the reaction can occur following the first treatment or as the result of several days to years of drug administration (see below).

PHYSICAL EXAM FINDINGS: Several clinical presentations have been described:

- Erythroderma/exfoliative dermatitis: localized or diffuse erythema that can lead to scales, crusts, and alopecia.
- Urticaria/angioedema: edematous papules and wheals; variable erythema and pruritus.
- Autoimmune diseases (pemphigus [Fig. I-57], bullous pemphigoid, systemic lupus erythematosus): clinical presentation varies from pustules and crusts to vesicles, bullae, and ulcers depending the autoimmune dermatosis mimicked.
- Erythema multiforme (EM)/toxic epidermal necrolysis (TEN): group of diseases manifested by an acute reaction pattern of skin and mucous membranes characterized by erythematous maculopapules and flat or raised annular or polycyclic lesions with minimal epidermal detachment in EM; and widespread erythema, blistering, and severe epidermal detachment in TEN.
- Fixed reactions: well-demarcated erythematous lesions sometimes associated with blistering and necrosis.
- Macules and papules: usually erythematous; pruritic or not.
- Pruritus: localized or widespread, can lead to self-induced lesions.
- Injection site reactions: local reaction characterized by alopecia, inflammation, necrosis, or ulceration.
- Vasculitis: purpura, necrosis and punctate ulcers especially localized over extremities, pressure points and oral mucosa.

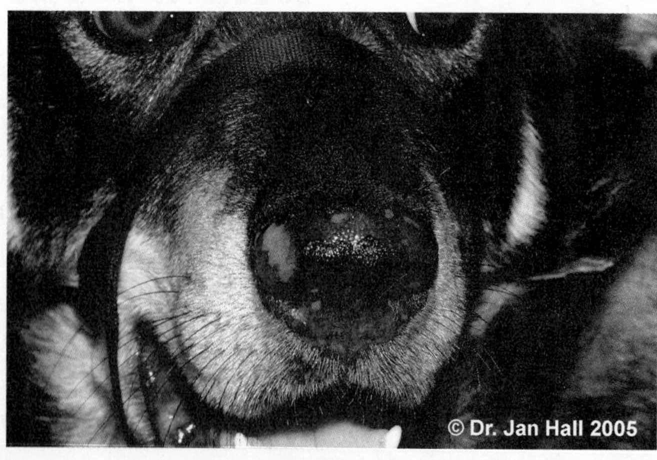

FIGURE I-57 Drug-induced pemphigus vulgaris affecting the nasal planum of a 5-year-old, male, castrated, mixed breed dog. The normal, black epithelium of the nasal planum has sloughed entirely over a period of hours, exposing a mostly denuded dermis. Courtesy of Dr. Jan A. Hall.

ETIOLOGY AND PATHOPHYSIOLOGY

- Although some drugs are more frequently associated with drug reactions, all kind of drugs are at risk to cause a cutaneous drug eruption.
- Reactions may be immediate after first administration or after weeks to months of administration without prior apparent reaction.
- The predictable (pharmacologic) reactions are related to the pharmacologic actions of the drugs and thus more common. They are dose-dependent and reversed when the drugs are discontinued.
- The unpredictable (idiosyncratic) reactions are usually considered immunologically mediated. They can also be associated to genetic individual differences in the metabolism of drugs leading to inappropriate generation or accumulation of toxic metabolites. These reactions are often serious and potentially fatal.

DIAGNOSIS

The key elements necessary for identifying a cutaneous drug eruption are: a thorough history including drug administration and appropriate timing for the development of skin eruptions, a lack of alternative explanations for the lesions, and dechallenge, with resolution of skin lesions within 1 to 2 weeks. Rechallenging with the suspected drug confirms the diagnosis but is not recommended.

DIFFERENTIAL DIAGNOSIS

- Erythroderma/exfoliative dermatitis: epitheliotropic lymphoma.
- Urticaria/angioedema; macules/papules; pruritus: hypersensitivity disorders, ectoparasitosis, superficial bacterial or fungal infection, and mast cell tumor.
- Autoimmune diseases: spontaneous autoimmune disease not related to drugs, which is more common.
- EM/TEN: superficial and deep infection (bacterial and fungal), urticaria, autoimmune diseases, burns, ulcerative stomatitis, and epitheliotropic lymphoma.
- Fixed reactions: contact dermatitis, hypersensitivity disorders, pyoderma, and fungal infection.
- Injection site reactions: traction alopecia, hypersensitivity disorders, pyoderma, dermatophytosis, alopecia areata, and neoplasia.

- Vasculitis: urticaria, autoimmune diseases, EM/TEN, disseminated intravascular coagulation, coagulopathy, frostbite, and neoplasia.

INITIAL DATABASE

- History of drug administration before onset of skin lesions.
- No specific laboratory findings.
- Routine dermatologic diagnostics should be performed as appropriate (skin scrapings, skin cytology, skin biopsy, fungal culture) based on differential diagnosis.

ADVANCED OR CONFIRMATORY TESTING

- Suspected vasculitis: rickettsial titers, if other clinical signs suggestive of rickettsial diseases are present
- Suspected systemic lupus erythematosus: antinuclear antibody test
- Cats: feline immunodeficiency virus (FIV)/feline leukemia virus (FeLV) serology, if considered appropriate based on clinical signs

TREATMENT

THERAPEUTIC GOAL(S)

- Stop the pharmacologic or immunologic reactions causing the drug eruption.
- Prevent secondary skin infection if the cutaneous barrier is ruptured.
- Supportive care is important when the animal is debilitated.

ACUTE AND CHRONIC GENERAL TREATMENT

- Discontinue use of the offending medication.
- Supportive care as needed, including fluid therapy, nutritional support, analgesics, antipruritic therapy, or wound care. Depending on the clinical presentation, corticosteroids may be used (controversial).

PROGNOSIS AND OUTCOME

Good, except if internal organs are affected or if there is extensive epidermal necrosis

PEARLS & CONSIDERATIONS

COMMENTS

- Lesions can persist for days to weeks after discontinuing the medication.
- Hospitalization may be indicated.
- Consider short-term glucocorticoid or immunosuppressive therapy if severe pruritus or immune-mediated dermatosis exists and concurrent infection is absent.
- Immunomodulatory therapy can be beneficial in EM/TEN, injection site reactions, or vasculitis.
- Avoid future use of the offending medication or chemically related drugs.

SUGGESTED READING

Scott DW, Miller WH: Idiosyncratic cutaneous adverse drug reactions in the cat: literature review and report of 14 cases (1990–1996). *Feline Pract* 26:10, 1998.

Scott DW, Miller WH: Idiosyncratic cutaneous adverse drug reactions in the dog: literature review and report of 101 cases (1990–1996). *Canine Pract* 24:16, 1999.

Scott DW, Miller WH, Griffin CE: In *Muller and Kirk's Small Animal Dermatology*, ed 6. Philadelphia, WB Saunders, 2001, pp 720–729.

AUTHOR: **FRÉDÉRIC SAUVÉ**

EDITOR: **JAN A. HALL**

Dysautonomia

BASIC INFORMATION

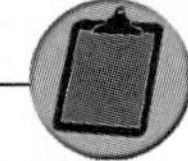

DEFINITION

Syndrome characterized by degeneration of the autonomic ganglia, producing failure of parasympathetic and sympathetic function in multiple organs

SYNONYM(S)

Autonomic neuropathy
Key-Gaskell syndrome
Pure autonomic failure
Pandysautonomia

EPIDEMIOLOGY

SPECIES, AGE, SEX

- In the United States, dogs are most commonly affected, with occasional feline cases. In the United Kingdom, horses are most commonly affected.
- Any age animal may be affected, but dysautonomia most commonly affects young adult dogs (median age 18 months).
- No sex predilection.

RISK FACTORS: Free-roaming, rural dogs are at higher risk.

CONTAGION AND ZOONOSIS

- Except for rare reports of multiple dogs in a household affected, no evidence of contagion
- No evidence of zoonosis

GEOGRAPHY AND SEASONALITY

- In the United States, the greatest concentration of dysautonomia centers around the borders between Missouri, Kansas, and Oklahoma. Cases are also seen in the northern Colorado and southern Wyoming front range, with occasional cases elsewhere in the country.
- The disease is most common in the late winter–early spring, with the incidence decreasing during the summer months.

ASSOCIATED CONDITIONS AND DISORDER: Autonomic failure can be a part of a more diffuse peripheral neuropathy or neuromuscular junction disorder.

CLINICAL PRESENTATION

DISEASE FORMS/SUBTYPES: Different combinations of organ failure may be seen.

HISTORY, CHIEF COMPLAINT

- Acute disease: most cases less than 5 to 14 days' duration
- Most common complaint is gastrointestinal (GI) disturbances: vomiting/regurgitation and diarrhea, although some animals will be constipated
- Dysuria
- Photophobia, dilated pupils, or third eyelid elevation
- Coughing
- Nasal discharge
- Weight loss

PHYSICAL EXAM FINDINGS

- Diminished anal sphincter tone
- Dry eyes and mucous membranes with normal hydration; crusty nose
- Midrange or dilated pupils with no pupillary light reflex, but normal vision
- Elevated third eyelid, enophthalmos, and ptosis
- Distended, easily expressed bladder

- Abdominal discomfort
- Heart rate and blood pressure are usually at the low end of normal range
- Nasal discharge or crackles on lung auscultation if secondary rhinitis or aspiration pneumonia
- Cachexia can be dramatic even in relatively short duration disease

ETIOLOGY AND PATHOPHYSIOLOGY

- Histologically, there is loss of neurons in the autonomic ganglia with little inflammation
- Cause is unknown, but toxic and immune-mediated hypotheses are being investigated

DIAGNOSIS

It is necessary to document autonomic failure in multiple organs without significant deficits in sensory or motor function before being confident in the diagnosis.

DIFFERENTIAL DIAGNOSIS

- The most dramatic signs reflect parasympathetic loss, so anticholinergic toxicity (organophosphate, carbamate) needs to be ruled out.
- Other differentials would be determined by the specific organ that is most prominently affected:
  - GI: gastroenteritis, GI foreign body, metabolic causes, idiopathic megaesophagus, focal myasthenia gravis.
  - Dry mucous membranes: dehydration.
  - Dilated pupils: intraocular or retrobulbar disease.
  - Photophobia: corneal ulcer or anterior uveitis.
  - Elevated third eyelid, enophthalmos and ptosis: any cause of Horner's syndrome especially retrobulbar, mediastinal, or middle ear disease.
  - Dysuria: urinary tract infection, disease affecting sacral spinal cord, cauda equina, or pelvic nerves.
  - Loss of anal sphincter tone: disease affecting sacral spinal cord, cauda equina, or pudendal nerves.
  - Respiratory: any cause of pneumonia or rhinitis.

INITIAL DATABASE

- Complete blood count, serum biochemistry panel, urinalysis: unremarkable.
- Radiographs may reveal signs of ileus, distended bladder, megaesophagus, and/or aspiration pneumonia.
- Abdominal ultrasound or barium series may show lack of intestinal motility.
- Ocular pilocarpine test will rule out anticholinergic toxicity in animals with dilated pupils.
  - Place 2 to 3 drops of 0.05% pilocarpine (1% diluted 1:20 with saline or eye flush) in one eye.
  - Compare pupil size every 15 minutes for up to 1 hour.
  - Pupil should constrict in dysautonomia; anticholinergic toxicity or normal pupil does not respond.
- Atropine test: does not rule out anticholinergic toxicity, but documents cardiac involvement.
  - Measure heart rate before and 15 minutes after IV atropine 0.04 mg/kg.
  - Rate should increase in normal animal. Does not change in dysautonomia.

ADVANCED OR CONFIRMATORY TESTING

Diagnosis can be confirmed on histopathologic study by cell loss and gliosis in autonomic ganglia. The celiacomesenteric ganglia can be found surrounding the origin of the cranial mesenteric artery from the aorta, and there are usually autonomic ganglia in the periadrenal tissues.

TREATMENT

THERAPEUTIC GOAL(S)

Since the cause is unknown, treatment is supportive and nonspecific.

ACUTE GENERAL TREATMENT

- Support nutrition and hydration:
  - Intravenous fluids.
  - Percutaneous endoscopic gastrostomy tube may be of value, but if complete GI atony exists parenteral nutrition may be necessary.
  - Prokinetic drugs (e.g., metoclopramide 0.2-0.5 mg/kg IM or SC, q 6-8h, or cisapride 0.1-0.5 mg/kg PO q 8h).
- Eye lubrication.
- Humidification of air.
- Manually express the bladder. Low dose bethanechol (5-25 mg total dose PO per dog q 8h) may help bladder contraction but may cause increased vomiting.
- Antibiotics for secondary infections (based on culture and sensitivity).

DRUG INTERACTIONS

Animals with dysautonomia develop supersensitivity to direct acting cholinergic or adrenergic drugs as evidenced by the ocular pilocarpine test. Therefore all of these drugs need to be used cautiously beginning at about 10% of the normally used dose and escalating the dose as needed.

POSSIBLE COMPLICATIONS

Aspiration pneumonia can occur at any time in animals that are vomiting or regurgitating.

PROGNOSIS AND OUTCOME

- Prognosis is grave with 70-90% fatality.
- Animals either die of aspiration pneumonia or are euthanized because of poor quality of life.
- Occasional animal will recover but may have permanent dysfunction of one or more organs.

PEARLS & CONSIDERATIONS

COMMENTS

Because the cause is unknown, it is difficult to provide clients with firm recommendations for preventing future occurrences. Dogs in the same household do not appear to be at greater risk.

SUGGESTED READING

Berghaus RD, et al. Risk factors for development of dysautonomia in dogs. *J Am Vet Med Assoc* 218:1285-1292, 2001.

Harkin KR, et al: Dysautonomia in dogs: 65 cases (1993-2000). *J Am Vet Med Assoc* 220 (5):633-639, 2001.

O'Brien DP, Johnson GC: Autonomic neuropathies and dysautonomia. *Vet Clin North Am Small Anim Pract* 32:251-265, 2002.

AUTHOR: **DENNIS P. O'BRIEN**

EDITOR: **CURTIS W. DEWEY**

Dysphagia

BASIC INFORMATION

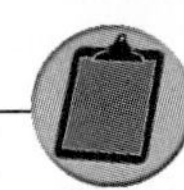

DEFINITION

Difficulty in swallowing resulting from the inability to prehend, form, and/or move a bolus of food from the mouth into the esophagus

EPIDEMIOLOGY

SPECIES, AGE, SEX: Dependent on underlying cause:

- Young dogs: congenital, foreign objects, facial trauma
- Young cats: congenital, inflammatory polyps
- Older animals: neoplasia

GENETICS AND BREED PREDISPOSITIONS: Cricopharyngeal achalasia (toy breeds), myasthenia gravis (Jack Russell and fox terriers, English spaniel, Samoyed, Siamese).

RISK FACTORS: Neuromuscular conditions may have breed predispositions.

CONTAGION AND ZOONOSIS: Rabies, especially if the animal's rabies vaccination status is unknown or if it has been exposed to a potentially rabid animal.

CLINICAL PRESENTATION

DISEASE FORMS/SUBTYPES

- Oral dysphagia
  - Modified eating behavior (eating with head tilted to one side and throwing head back while eating) common.
  - Mandibular/tongue paralysis, dental disease, masticatory muscle swelling or atrophy, inability to open the mouth, and food packed in the buccal folds without retention of saliva.
- Pharyngeal dysphagia
  - Normal prehension.
  - Repeated attempts at swallowing while repeatedly flexing and extending the head and neck, excessive chewing, and gagging.
  - Saliva-coated food retained in the buccal folds, diminished gag reflex, and nasal discharge from aspiration may exist.
- Cricopharyngeal dysphagia
  - Repeated, nonproductive efforts to swallow and gag associated with regurgitation immediately after swallowing.
  - Normal gag reflex and prehension.

HISTORY, CHIEF COMPLAINT (SOME OR ALL MAY BE PRESENT)

- Ptyalism/hypersalivation, gagging, weight loss, ravenous appetite, repeated attempts at swallowing, swallowing with the head in an abnormal position, coughing, regurgitation, painful swallowing, and occasionally anorexia.
- Foreign bodies cause acute-onset dysphagia.
- Pharyngeal dysphagia may be chronic and intermittent.

ETIOLOGY AND PATHOPHYSIOLOGY

- Anatomic or mechanical lesions:
  - Pharyngeal inflammation (trauma, abscess, eosinophilic granuloma)
  - Retropharyngeal lymphadenopathy/neoplasia
  - Pharyngeal/retropharyngeal foreign body
  - Salivary mucocele
  - Temporomandibular joint disorders (luxation, fracture, craniomandibular osteopathy)
  - Mandibular fracture
  - Cleft palate
- Pain because of dental disease, trauma, stomatitis, glossitis, and pharyngeal inflammation.
- Neuromuscular disorders (idiopathic trigeminal neuropathy, lingual paralysis).
- Masticatory muscle myositis.
- Pharyngeal weakness/paresis/paralysis:
  - Infectious polymyositis (toxoplasmosis, neosporosis)
  - Immune-mediated polymyositis
  - Muscular dystrophy
  - Polyneuropathies
  - Myoneural junction disorders (myasthenia gravis, tick paralysis, botulism)
- Rabies can cause dysphagia by affecting both the brainstem and peripheral nerves.
- Other brainstem disorders.

DIAGNOSIS

DIFFERENTIAL DIAGNOSIS

- Vomiting
- Regurgitation

INITIAL DATABASE

- Complete blood count: Inflammatory conditions can cause leukocytosis, sometimes with a left shift.
- Urinalysis:
  - Usually normal.
  - Isosthenuria can be associated with renal failure.
- Biochemistry: elevated serum creatine phosphokinase activity with muscular disorders.

ADVANCED OR CONFIRMATORY TESTING

- Other laboratory tests:
  - Type 2M-muscle antibody serology (masticatory muscle myositis).
  - Acetylcholinesterase receptor antibody test (acquired myasthenia gravis).
  - Antinuclear antibody test (immune-mediated diseases).
- Imaging:
  - Survey radiographs of the skull and neck, with attention to the mandibles, temporomandibular joint, teeth, pharyngeal and retropharyngeal area, and position of the hyoid apparatus.
  - Ultrasonography of the pharynx may be useful with mass lesions and for obtaining ultrasound-guided biopsy specimens.
  - Fluoroscopy to evaluate pharyngeal movement in patients with suspected pharyngeal or cricopharyngeal dysphagia.
  - Computed tomography or magnetic resonance imaging for suspected intracranial mass.
- Other diagnostic procedures:
  - Biopsy of a mass lesion.
  - Pharyngoscopy.
  - Electromyography of the pharyngeal musculature to confirm the presence of a neuromuscular disorder.
  - Repetitive nerve stimulation and edrophonium chloride test for suspected myasthenia gravis (suboptimal).
  - Cerebrospinal fluid analysis.

TREATMENT

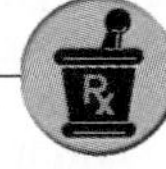

THERAPEUTIC GOAL(S)

- Determine underlying cause.
- Direct primary treatment at the underlying cause.
- Nutritional support:
  - Care taken to avoid aspiration when feeding orally.
  - Animals with oral dysphagia may be able to swallow if a bolus of food is placed in the caudal pharynx; other animals may find a gruel that can be lapped easier to swallow.
  - Elevating the head and neck may make swallowing easier for animals with pharyngeal or cricopharyngeal dysphagia and help prevent aspiration of food.
- If nutritional requirements cannot be met orally an esophagostomy or gastrostomy tube may be necessary.
- Surgical excision of a mass lesion.
- Foreign body removal.
- Cricopharyngeal myotomy may benefit patients with cricopharyngeal dysphagia; however a correct diagnosis is essential as cricopharyngeal myotomy will exacerbate dysphagia with oropharyngeal dysphagia.

POSSIBLE COMPLICATIONS

Aspiration pneumonia is a common complication.

RECOMMENDED MONITORING

- Daily for signs of aspiration pneumonia
- Body condition and hydration status daily
- If oral nutrition does not meet requirements, use esophagostomy/gastrostomy tube feeding

PROGNOSIS AND OUTCOME

Dependent on the cause, and on the associated complication of aspiration pneumonia

PEARLS & CONSIDERATIONS

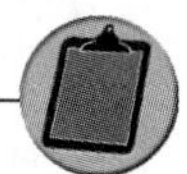

COMMENTS

- Uncommon problem
- Dysphagia not a diagnosis but a clinical sign

CLIENT EDUCATION

Monitor for aspiration pneumonia

RECOMMENDED READING

Hitt ME: Pharyngeal and swallowing disorders. In Morgan RV, Bright RN, Swartout MS (eds): *Handbook of Small Animal Practice,* ed 4. Philadelphia, WB Saunders, 2003, pp 305-306.

Jenkins CC: Dysphagia and regurgitation. In Ettinger SJ, Feldman EC: *Textbook of Veterinary Internal Medicine,* ed 5. Philadelphia, WB Saunders, 2000, pp 114-115.

AUTHOR: **REMO LOBETTI**
EDITOR: **ETIENNE CÔTÉ**

Dyspnea

BASIC INFORMATION

DEFINITION

Abnormal breathing. In clinical practice, "dyspnea" specifically refers to difficulty breathing.

SYNONYM(S)

Labored breathing
Respiratory difficulty
Severe dyspnea: respiratory distress

EPIDEMIOLOGY

SPECIES, AGE, SEX: Dogs and cats of any breed and either sex.

CONTAGION AND ZOONOSIS

- Animal-to-animal contagion with certain infectious etiologies
- Public health concern: severly dyspneic dog or cat may bite if distressed/disoriented

GEOGRAPHY AND SEASONALITY: Dependent on etiology.

ASSOCIATED CONDITIONS AND DISORDERS: Respiratory stridor, hypoxemia, syncope.

CLINICAL PRESENTATION

DISEASE FORMS/SUBTYPES

- Inspiratory dyspnea: generally caused by upper airway obstruction
- Inspiratory-expiratory dyspnea, or expiratory dyspnea: generally caused by lower airway, pulmonary circulatory, pleural, mediastinal, or metabolic problems

HISTORY, CHIEF COMPLAINT

- Dyspnea may be the presenting complaint if severe and/or the owner is observant.
- Nonspecific systemic complaints (anorexia, lethargy; hiding [cats]) may be reported in pets that are more mildly dyspneic or with owners who are less observant.
- Owners may describe excessive abdominal wall excursions ("belly breathing") as the first manifestation of dyspnea, especially in cats.
- Concurrent complaints, including exercise intolerance, lethargy, and inappetence are common but nonspecific.
- Medical history may be very informative (previous respiratory or systemic problems, current medications, etc.).
- Inciting cause (observed foreign body inhalation, anticoagulant ingestion few days earlier, etc) occasionally is reported by the owner.

PHYSICAL EXAM FINDINGS

- Increased respiratory effort: should be assessed immediately at the beginning of the consultation (e.g., exam room), before the hands-on physical examination increases the respiratory rate in nervous patients.
- Animals with moderate or severe dyspnea often manifest an anxious facial expression, reluctance to lie down, and other signs of discomfort.
- Inspiratory dyspnea.
  - Severity varies from mild inspiratory wheeze to extreme gasping actions.
  - The sound of turbulent air at the level of the obstruction may suggest the site of obstruction (e.g., nasal versus tracheal).
  - If nasal obstruction, dyspnea disappears when the animal breathes with the mouth open.
  - Other than potentially severe respiratory distress, animals with upper airway dyspnea are otherwise generally well: no weight loss, no other physical abnormalities.
- Expiratory or expiratory-inspiratory dyspnea.
  - With lower airway disease, dyspnea is often accompanied by cough, with or without other general systemic signs (lethargy, anorexia, etc.) or signs more closely related to respiratory disease (e.g., cyanosis).
  - If lower airway dyspnea is severe, the animal's posture can include abducted elbows, an extended neck, and the canthi of the lips drawn caudally.
  - Cough inducible with tracheal pressure does not indicate whether the problem originates from the upper or lower airway.
- Auscultation
  - Decreased intensity or absence of lung sounds suggests pneumothorax, pleural effusion, intrathoracic mass, or diaphragmatic hernia.
  - Presence of crackles and wheezes is nonspecific.

ETIOLOGY AND PATHOPHYSIOLOGY

- Respiratory center in medulla oblongata and pons is stimulated by $\uparrow CO_2$, $\uparrow H^+$, but not $\downarrow O_2$.
- Chemoreceptors (carotid bodies, aortic bodies) are stimulated by $\uparrow CO_2$, $\uparrow H^+$, and $\downarrow O_2$, feeding back to the respiratory center.
- Impulses from the respiratory center activate the intercostal muscles (intercostal nerves, which are branches of thoracic spinal nerves) and diaphragm (phrenic nerves).
- Disturbances in this process can occur at many levels, causing dyspnea.
  - Hypercapnea
  - Acidosis
  - Hypoxemia
  - Physical reduction of lung volume (obesity, diaphragmatic hernia, severe ascites)

- ◦ Respiratory paralysis
- ◦ Airway obstruction
- Causes of dyspnea: pulmonary edema, pleural effusion, upper airway obstruction (laryngeal paralysis, foreign body, brachycephalic syndrome), pneumonia, chronic sterile bronchitis, pulmonary hypertension, pulmonary thromboembolism, pulmonary hemorrhage, marked ascites, hyperthermia, neuromuscular weakness/paralysis, compensation for metabolic acidosis, anxiety.

DIAGNOSIS

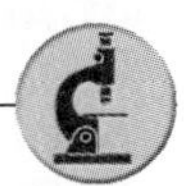

DIFFERENTIAL DIAGNOSIS

- Panting. Unlike dogs that are panting, dogs with dyspnea are likely to show wide chest excursions, an anxious facial expression, and unwillingness to lie down or rest.
- Reverse sneezing. Loud, inspiratory noises that are sudden in onset and in termination can be terminated by opening the mouth.

INITIAL DATABASE

- Thoracic radiographs. Diagnostic test of choice for expiratory or expiratory-inspiratory dyspnea.
- Oral/pharyngeal exam (may require sedation) and lateral cervical radiograph. If upper airway dyspnea is suspected.
- Complete blood count/serum biochemistry profile/urinalysis: no specific changes; results depend on etiology.

ADVANCED OR CONFIRMATORY TESTING

- Arterial blood gas. Degree of hypoxemia helps determine intensity of acute treatment.
- Pulse oximetry. Results may fluctuate; less invasive than arterial blood sampling.
- Coagulation profile. If rodenticide/pulmonary hemorrhage is suspected.
- Transtracheal wash. For evaluation of mild dyspnea associated with chronic cough.
- Bronchoscopy. For tracheal and bronchial visualization, and retrieval of secretions, tissue samples, foreign bodies.
- Rhinoscopy. If nasal obstruction, discharge, or other physical nasal signs are present.
- Echocardiography. If a cardiac cause is suspected (e.g., cardiomegaly; heart murmur).
- Computed tomography (thorax, nose). Especially to identify/characterize mass lesions.

TREATMENT

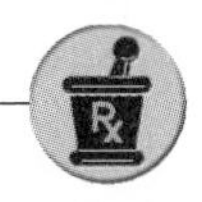

THERAPEUTIC GOAL(S)

- Control dyspnea immediately if life-threatening
- Address/eliminate underlying cause

ACUTE GENERAL TREATMENT

- Oxygen supplementation.
- Specific treatment is highly dependent on underlying cause and is initially based on history, physical findings, and thoracic radiographs. Acute general treatment may include removal of upper airway foreign body; thoracocentesis; diuretic; tracheostomy; or many others, depending on etiology.

CHRONIC TREATMENT

Depends on underlying cause

POSSIBLE COMPLICATIONS

Uncontrolled dyspnea, producing hypoxemia, cyanosis

RECOMMENDED MONITORING

- Respiratory effort
- Thoracic radiographs
- Arterial blood gases

PROGNOSIS AND OUTCOME

Highly variable, based mainly on severity of dyspnea at presentation, and ability to control underlying cause

PEARLS & CONSIDERATIONS

COMMENTS

- Dyspneic patients may be fragile. Simple procedures such as thoracic radiography or thoracocentesis need to be accomplished with the lowest effective degree of restraint in severely dyspneic patients, or else postponed.
- A simple way of establishing whether nasal obstruction is present and if so, which side(s) is/are affected involves simply occluding the nostrils, one at a time, and watching to see if airflow flutters a tuft of a few hairs plucked from the patient's coat and held in front of the nonoccluded nostril.

CLIENT EDUCATION

- At the time of diagnosis, patients are usually in serious or critical condition even if they do not appear to have been very ill.
- The long-term outlook depends on the cause of the labored breathing, and tests are necessary to find what the most likely cause is.

SUGGESTED READING

Mawby DI: Dyspnea and tachypnea. In Ettinger SJ, Feldman EC (eds): *Textbook of Veterinary Internal Medicine*, ed 6. St. Louis: Elsevier Saunders, 2005, pp 192–195.

AUTHOR & EDITOR: **ETIENNE CÔTÉ**

Dystocia

BASIC INFORMATION

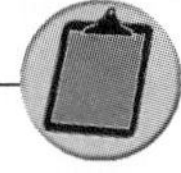

DEFINITION

Difficulty in the normal vaginal delivery of a neonate from the uterus

SYNONYM(S)

Ineffective labor

EPIDEMIOLOGY

SPECIES, AGE, SEX

- Dystocia occurs more commonly in the bitch than the queen.
- Older dams reportedly have a higher incidence of dystocia than younger ones.

GENETICS AND BREED PREDISPOSITION

- Brachycephalic breeds (bulldog, French bulldog, pug, Boston terrier, etc.) have a higher incidence of dystocia due to mismatch between the size of the maternal birth canal and the fetal head and shoulders, and a steep angle of the entrance of the maternal pelvic canal from the abdomen.
- Certain giant breeds (mastiffs) are believed to have a higher incidence of dystocia; this has not been confirmed by a controlled study.
- Some purebred colonies (assistance dog colonies) have a higher than breed average incidence of dystocia, suggesting heritability.
- Breed, parity (number of previous litters), and litter size can influence gestational length by 1 to 2 days.

RISK FACTORS

- Large litters.
- Poor condition of the dam.
- Small litters with oversized fetuses or prolonged gestation.

- Breed conformation, obesity, preeclampsia, malnutrition, vaginal canal abnormalities (strictures), pelvic abnormalities (healed fractures with reduction in pelvic canal), and abdominal wall defects (hernias) can predispose a dam to dystocia.
- A previous normal cesarean section does not predispose a bitch to dystocia.

CLINICAL PRESENTATION

DISEASE FORMS/SUBTYPE: Dystocia can be categorized as resulting from maternal causes, fetal causes, or a combination of maternal and fetal causes.

HISTORY, CHIEF COMPLAINT

- A client's perception that labor is not initiated or progressing as expected, most commonly due to:
  - Time between stages of labor.
  - Time between sequential deliveries of neonates.
- Alternatively, the presence of stillbirths can prompt presentation for dystocia.
- The clinician must quickly obtain a careful reproductive history detailing.
  - Breeding dates.
  - Any ovulation timing performed.
  - Historic and recent labor.
  - General medical history.

PHYSICAL EXAM FINDINGS

- Physical examination may be unremarkable; normal physical exam findings do not rule out dystocia.
- Typically dams in stage I (uterine contractions) or II (uterine and abdominal contractions) are euthermic, mildly agitated, trembling, mildly hyperpneic, and nesting.
- Variable abnormal physical findings include atypical vulvar discharge (green, malodorous, frankly hemorrhagic), a fetus in the birth canal (i.e., presence of a fetus caudal to the cervix, which may be palpable over the brim of the pelvis, or may be partially protruding out of the vulva), muscle tremors, fatigue, persistent vomiting, and protracted tenesmus.
  - Uteroverdin (green vaginal discharge) indicates placental separation and indicates the need for intervention if fetal delivery is not prompt.
  - Malodorous discharge suggests fetal death and necrosis or metritis.
  - Inappropriately voluminous hemorrhage should prompt evaluation for uterine trauma (surgical exploration) or abnormal placental site coagulation (medical ± surgical evaluation).
- Persistence of a fetus in the birth canal beyond 5 to 10 minutes warrants assisted delivery.
  - Placental separation and the potential for fetal hypoxemia are likely.
  - Caution: Traction applied to a fetus retained in the birth canal must be very gentle to avoid trauma to the fetus.
  - Traction is advised only if the veterinarian can position his/her fingers around the fetus's shoulders or hips for gentle traction.
  - Lubrication delivered via a red rubber catheter and KY jelly can be helpful.
- Protracted muscle tremors, vomiting, or marked fatigue suggest metabolic abnormalities (hypoglycemia, hypocalcemia) or exhaustion.
- Protracted tenesmus suggests obstruction or uterine inertia.

ETIOLOGY AND PATHOPHYSIOLOGY

- Normal labor proceeds through three stages.
  - Stage I labor is characterized by a progressive increase in the frequency and strength of uterine contractions. The dam may be restless or agitated. No external contractions are visible.
  - Stage II labor begins when abdominal efforts (tenesmus) coincide with uterine contractions, resulting in the delivery of a neonate through the birth canal.
  - Stage III labor consists of the delivery of the placenta.
  - Dams typically progress through stage I labor in 12 to 24 hours, and alternate between stages II and III until all neonates and placentae are delivered. Placentae normally may be delivered with the neonate, or separately.
- Etiology of dystocia: maternal/fetal causes
  - Maternal dystocia: primary or secondary uterine inertia, birth canal or abdominal wall defects (strictures, hernias), lack of lubrication in the birth canal, uterine torsion or tear, metabolic derangements.
  - Fetal dystocia: oversized, malformed (anasarca), malpositioned, malpostured fetus.
  - Combined maternal/fetal dystocia: mismatch of birth canal size versus fetal size.
  - "Breech" (caudal) presentations in dogs and cats are normal.

DIAGNOSIS

A correct diagnosis of dystocia is dependent on taking an accurate history and performing a thorough physical examination in a timely manner.

DIFFERENTIAL DIAGNOSIS

- Normal labor.
- Misinformation about gestational length, in which case lack of labor is then normal.
  - In the bitch, gestation is normally terminated 64 to 66 days from the initial rise in progesterone corresponding to the LH surge, or 56 to 58 days from the first day of diestrus.
  - Gestational length from the first breeding date can vary from 58 to 72 days.
  - In the queen, the mean gestation is 65 to 66 days from breeding.
- Completion of labor, misinformation about litter size.

INITIAL DATABASE

- Minimally, hematocrit and total protein, blood glucose, serum electrolytes, and ionized calcium should be evaluated.
  - Evidence of dehydration (elevated total protein/albumin, possibly normal or elevated hematocrit due to hemoconcentration) possible.
  - Mild dilutional anemia of pregnancy is expected. Marked anemia (packed cell volume <32) suggests blood loss or malcondition.
  - Electrolyte derangements (e.g., hypokalemia, hypochloremia) secondary to vomiting, diarrhea (not uncommon with labor), and fasting are possible.
  - Hypoglycemia and hypocalcemia can result from prolonged labor.
  - Ketosis (ketones in the serum or urine) with or without hypoglycemia indicates malnutrition.
- Abdominal ultrasound or fetal Doppler evaluation to assess fetal viability.
- Abdominal radiograph to evaluate litter size, relative fetal size and position.

ADVANCED OR CONFIRMATORY TESTING

Uterine monitoring to assess strength and frequency of contractions.

- Currently, canine and feline uterine monitors are available for short- or long-term lease through Veterinary Perinatal Services Inc. (www.whelpwise.com).

TREATMENT

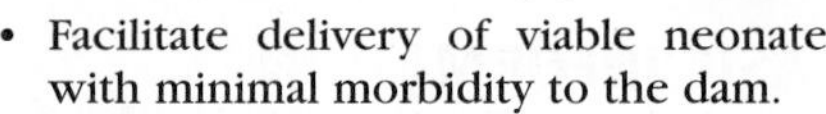

THERAPEUTIC GOAL(S)

- Facilitate delivery of viable neonates with minimal morbidity to the dam.
- Avoid unnecessary surgical intervention via timely diagnosis and medical intervention.
- Differentiate cases requiring surgical versus medical intervention: surgery is warranted if:
  - Refractory (unresponsive) uterine inertia.
  - Fetal distress and suboptimal response to medical management.
  - Intractable pain in bitch or queen.

- Obvious mismatch of fetal-maternal birth canal size.
- Birth canal abnormalities such as strictures or pelvic stenosis that cannot be remedied.
- Minimize fetal stress as neonatal death during the first week of life is related to stress during labor and the immediate postpartum period.
- Avoid fetal or maternal mortality.
- Preserve the reproductive capacity of a valuable dam.

ACUTE GENERAL TREATMENT

- Supportive: Intravenous balanced electrolyte containing fluids with 5% dextrose if appropriate (dam is hypovolemic, dehydrated, or hypoglycemic).
- Calcium: Calcium gluconate 10% solution (= 10 g/100 ml solution, or 0.465 mEq Ca^{++}/ml) (Fujisawa Inc., USA).
  - Given subcutaneously at 1 ml/4.5 kg (10 lb) body weight as indicated by the strength of uterine contractions—generally no more frequently than every 4 to 6 hours during the second stage of labor.
  - Large volumes of calcium gluconate given subcutaneously may cause local irritation; doses >4 ml should be divided.
  - Intravenous use: generally unnecessary unless systemic signs of severe hypocalcemia are present (see Hypocalcemia, p 564, for signs and intravenous doses).
  - While most dams are eucalcemic, the benefit of calcium administration is still seen, suggesting a cellular or subcellular effect.
- Oxytocin:
  - The administration of oxytocin increases the frequency of uterine contractions, while the administration of calcium increases their strength.
  - Oxytocin, 10 USP units/ml (American Pharmaceutical Partners Inc., Los Angeles) is most effective at mini doses, starting with 0.25 units SC or IM to a maximum dose of 4 units per bitch or queen.
  - The frequency of oxytocin administration is dictated by the labor pattern, and it is generally not given more frequently than hourly.
  - Absolute contraindications to oxytocin therapy: fetal obstruction in any part of the uterus or birth canal, uterine torsion, uterine laceration or rupture.
- Persistence of a fetus in the birth canal beyond 5 to 10 minutes warrants assisted delivery.
  - Placental separation and the potential for fetal hypoxemia are likely.
  - Caution: Traction applied to a fetus retained in the birth canal must be very gentle to avoid trauma to the fetus.
  - Traction is only advised if the veterinarian can position his/her fingers around the fetus's shoulders or hips for gentle traction.
  - Lubrication delivered via a red rubber catheter and water-soluble lubricant jelly can be helpful.

CHRONIC TREATMENT

Medical therapy for dystocia, based on the administration of calcium gluconate and oxytocin, can be directed and tailored based on the results of monitoring.

DRUG INTERACTIONS

Calcium is given before oxytocin in most cases, improving contractile strength before increasing frequency of contractions. The action of oxytocin is improved when given 15 minutes subsequent to calcium.

POSSIBLE COMPLICATIONS

- Hypercalcemia-induced arrhythmias if calcium solution is given intravenously at too rapid of a rate.
- Fetal hypoxia secondary to placental compression during uterine contractions induced by parenteral oxytocin administration, particularly if given inappropriately (too early in labor, when fetal obstruction is present, if uterine torsion is present, too frequently, too rapidly), or at excessive doses.
- Uterine rupture with fetal and maternal morbidity and mortality if ecbolic agents (oxytocin) are given excessively, inappropriately (too early in labor, when fetal obstruction is present, if uterine torsion is present, too frequently, too rapidly) or when the uterine wall is compromised, or torn.

RECOMMENDED MONITORING

- Progression of labor with viable neonates delivered.
- Using real-time transabdominal ultrasonography, fetal heart rates should be >180 bpm. Sustained fetal heart rates <180 bpm are associated with fetal distress.
- Continued uterine monitoring using tocodynamometry showing continuation and progression of appropriate contractile strength and frequency.

PROGNOSIS AND OUTCOME

Fair to good with timely intervention and appropriate monitoring

PEARLS & CONSIDERATIONS

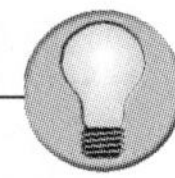

COMMENTS

- Obstruction of the uterus or birth canal (regardless of cause-fetal malposition, fetal-dam size mismatch, or anatomic defects of dam) must be ruled out by vaginal palpation, as it is an indication for cesarean section and an absolute contraindication for treatment with oxytocin.
- If appropriate monitoring is not available and obstruction of the uterus and birth canal have been ruled out, giving calcium gluconate subcutaneously is less hazardous than giving oxytocin.

PREVENTION

- Complete prebreeding evaluation of the bitch, including a vaginal examination
- Prepartum abdominal radiography to estimate fetal number and relative size in comparison to the dam

CLIENT EDUCATION

Client education about proper prenatal husbandry, accurate gestational length interpretation based on ovulation timing, client recognition of dystocia.

SUGGESTED READING

Davidson AP: Approaches to reducing perinatal mortality in dogs. In Concannon P (ed): *International Veterinary Information Service* (www.Ivis.org). Ithaca, NY, March 2003.

Davidson AP: Dystocia management. In Bonagura JD (ed): *Kirk's Veterinary Therapy XIV*. Philadelphia, WB Saunders, in press.

Davidson AP: Obstetrical monitoring in dogs. *Vet Med* 6:508, 2003.

Davidson AP: Uterine and fetal monitoring in the bitch. In Davidson AP (ed): *Vet Clin North Am* 31(2), Philadelphia, WB Saunders, March, 2001.

Eilts BE, et al: Factors influencing gestational length in the bitch. *Proc Third European Vet Soc for Sm An Reprod; European Congress on Companion, Exotic and Laboratory Animals,* May 2002.

Newman RB, et al: Objective tocodynamometry identifies labor onset earlier than subjective maternal perception. *Obstet Gynecol* 76:1089, 1998.

Stabenfeldt GH, et al: Pregnancy and parturition. In Cunningham JG (ed): *Textbook of Veterinary Physiology*, ed 3. Philadelphia, WB Saunders, 2002.

Wallace MS, et al: Abnormalities in pregnancy, parturition and the periparturient period. In Ettinger SJ, Feldman EC (eds): *Textbook of Veterinary Internal Medicine*. Philadelphia, WB Saunders, 1995.

AUTHOR: **AUTUMN P. DAVIDSON**
EDITOR: **MICHELLE A. KUTZLER**

Echinococcosis

BASIC INFORMATION

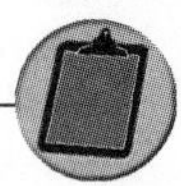

DEFINITION

- Cestode (tapeworm) infestation with larval stages that causes disease primarily in humans:
  - Cystic echinococcosis is caused by *Echinococcus granulosus*.
  - Alveolar echinococcosis is caused by *E. multilocularis*.
  - Polycystic echinococcosis is caused by *E. vogelii* or *E. oligarthrus*.
- Hydatid cyst disease refers to the clinical condition in which intermediate hosts have multiple, often large intraparenchymal cysts containing serous fluid and echinococcal segments.

SYNONYM(S)

Hydatid disease
Hydatidosis

EPIDEMIOLOGY

SPECIES, AGE, SEX

- *E. granulosus* definitive hosts are dogs and other canids; intermediate hosts are sheep, goats, swine, cattle, horses, camels, and humans.
- *E. multilocularis* definitive hosts are foxes and, less frequently, dogs, cats, coyotes, and wolves. Intermediate hosts are small rodents.
- *E. vogelii* definitive hosts are bush dogs and dogs; intermediate hosts are rodents.
- *E. oligarthrus* definitive hosts are wild felids; rodents are intermediate hosts.

RISK FACTORS: Exposure and ingestion of intermediate hosts (rodents, cattle, sheep).

CONTAGION AND ZOONOSIS

- Highly zoonotic.
- Humans become infected by ingestion of eggs from the feces of definitive hosts or in uncooked tissue/meat from other intermediate hosts such as cattle or sheep.
- Once ingested, organism spreads and cysts may develop in various organs.

GEOGRAPHY AND SEASONALITY

- *E. granulosus* occurs worldwide. More frequent in rural, grazing areas.
- *E. multilocularis*: northern hemisphere.
- *E. vogelii* and *E. oligarthrus*: Central and South America.

CLINICAL PRESENTATION

DISEASE FORMS/SUBTYPES

- Absence of clinical signs (definitive hosts, e.g., dogs and cats).
- Diarrhea (occasionally, dogs and cats).
- Hydatid cyst disease (intermediate hosts, e.g., humans, sheep, cattle).

HISTORY, CHIEF COMPLAINT

- Clinical signs in domesticated animals are uncommon; humans are most commonly affected by disease.
- Intermediate host's signs relate to location and size of cyst.
- Definitive hosts with adult tapeworms may have enteritis.

PHYSICAL EXAM FINDINGS

- Generally unremarkable (dogs, cats).
- Proglottids may be present in feces or around anus.
- Respiratory signs, abdominal distention, and other signs of hydatid cyst disease are not expected in dogs or cats, because they are definitive hosts, not intermediate hosts.

ETIOLOGY AND PATHOPHYSIOLOGY

- *E. granulosus* adults reside in the small intestine of the definitive host (dogs, coyotes, wolves).
- Eggs are passed into the feces where they are ingested by an intermediate host (e.g., cattle, sheep, horses).
- In the intermediate host, the organism invades the small intestine and spreads through the circulatory system, entering organs of predilection. The organism develops into a cyst that gradually enlarges.
  - Typically, liver, lungs, and other organs (central nervous system, bone, heart) are affected.
- Definitive host becomes infected by ingestion of raw, cyst-containing organs of intermediate hosts.
- *E. multilocularis* larval growth remains in the proliferative stage, resulting in invasion of surrounding tissues. The liver is primarily affected, with occasional metastasis to the brain and lungs.
- *E. vogelii* larvae have a predilection for the liver.

DIAGNOSIS

DIFFERENTIAL DIAGNOSIS

Other taenioids

INITIAL DATABASE

Fecal examination may reveal eggs, which are identical to other taenioids

ADVANCED OR CONFIRMATORY TESTING

- Diagnosis in definitive hosts is by coproantigen or DNA detection
- Hydatid cysts at necropsy

TREATMENT

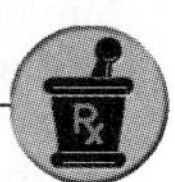

THERAPEUTIC GOAL(S)

Elimination of shedding

TREATMENT

- Adults may be treated with praziquantel 2.5-7.5 mg/kg PO or SC once.
- Hydatids require surgical removal.
- Epsiprantel (Cestex): dogs 5.5 mg/kg PO once; cats 2.75 mg/kg PO once. Single dosages eliminate *E. multilocularis* in over 99% of animals, but there may be residual worm burdens in some animals.

POSSIBLE COMPLICATIONS

Gastrointestinal signs may be seen with antiparasitics

RECOMMENDED MONITORING

Regular fecal flotation

PROGNOSIS AND OUTCOME

- Definitive hosts may have enteritis.
- Prognosis for intermediate hosts including humans depends on location of cysts.

PEARLS & CONSIDERATIONS

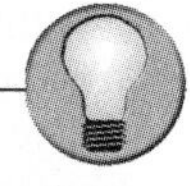

COMMENTS

Echinococcosis does not cause hydatid cyst disease in definitive hosts such as dogs and cats. Therefore, its interest in small animal medicine mainly revolves around the risk of zoonosis.

PREVENTION

- Vaccine available for intermediate hosts (sheep and cattle)
- Hygiene, to avoid human acquisition of the infection through fecal-oral contamination from dogs and cats
- Avoid consumption of raw or undercooked meat or viscera by humans, dogs, or cats

CLIENT EDUCATION

Eggs can infect humans by contamination via poor hygiene (dog licking face) and transfer to the mouth.

SUGGESTED READING

Eckert J, Thompson RC, Bucklar H, Bilger B, Deplazes P: Efficacy evaluation of epsiprantel (Cestex) against *Echinococcus multilocularis* in dogs and cats. *Berl Munc Tierarztl Wochenchr* 114(3-4):121-126, 2001.

Jenkins DJ, Romig T: Milbemycin oxime in a new formulation, combined with praziquantel, does not reduce the efficacy of praziquantel against *E. multilocularis* in cats. *J Helminthol* 77(4):367-370, 2003.

AUTHOR: **LISA M. TIEBER NIELSON**
EDITOR: **DOUGLASS K. MACINTIRE**

Eclampsia

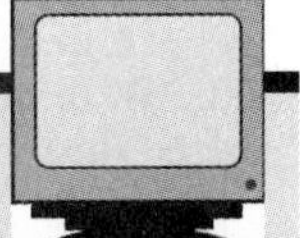

Client Education Sheet on Website

BASIC INFORMATION

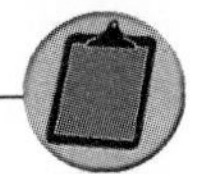

DEFINITION

Moderate to severe hypocalcemia of the lactating female, most commonly occurring in the first four weeks postpartum

SYNONYM(S)

Lactation tetany
Periparturient hypocalcemia
Puerperal tetany

EPIDEMIOLOGY

SPECIES, AGE, SEX

- Dogs: younger, postparturient bitches
- Cats: rare in queens

GENETICS AND BREED PREDISPOSITION: More common in small-breed dogs, although any lactating bitch may be affected.

RISK FACTORS

- Primiparous bitches may be at greater risk
- Decreased nutrition in the periparturient period as a result of stress or underlying illness
- Excess dietary calcium during gestation
- Large litter size is thought to be a risk factor

ASSOCIATED CONDITIONS AND DISORDERS: Hypoglycemia can arise secondarily due to energy demands of tetany.

CLINICAL PRESENTATION

HISTORY, CHIEF COMPLAINT: Lactating bitch with signs of aberrant behavior, ataxia, muscle tremors, seizures, and/or tetany.

PHYSICAL EXAM FINDINGS: Some or all of the following may be present:

- Nervousness, restlessness, pacing, whining, disinterest in pups
- Pruritus and biting at feet
- Ataxia, staggering, and muscle stiffness
- Muscle tremors, collapse, clonic spasms (tetany), and seizures (musculoskeletal signs are often exaggerated with tactile stimulus)
- Hyperthermia secondary to tetanic muscle contractions
- Panting; respiration eventually becomes labored as the condition progresses
- Tachycardia or bradycardia
- Arrhythmias: premature ventricular complexes
- Mydriasis and diminished pupillary light reflexes

ETIOLOGY AND PATHOPHYSIOLOGY

- Circulating ionized calcium is depleted due to lactation and fetal development, possibly in conjunction with underlying nutritional imbalance.
- Decreased circulating ionized calcium alters cellular membrane potentials and allows for spontaneous discharge of nerve fibers to induce contraction of skeletal muscles and alteration of central nervous system function.

DIAGNOSIS

DIFFERENTIAL DIAGNOSIS

- Hypocalcemia of alternate origin
- Hypoglycemia (may be concurrent)
- Cerebral edema (possibly secondary in eclampsia ± hypoglycemia)
- Toxin ingestion

INITIAL DATABASE

- Therapy should be initiated based on history, clinical signs, and physical exam if further diagnostic testing is not immediately available.
- Response to therapy is the most reliable diagnostic aid.
- Total serum calcium <6-7 mg/dl (<1.5-1.74 mmol/L) is the characteristic biochemical finding of eclampsia.
    - Calculated ionized calcium <3.5-4 mg/dl (<0.87-1 mmol/L).

ADVANCED OR CONFIRMATORY TESTING

Blood glucose should be evaluated to rule out hypoglycemia as a primary or secondary contributor to clinical signs, particularly for refractory cases.

TREATMENT

THERAPEUTIC GOAL(S)

- Return serum calcium concentration to normal by parenteral calcium therapy
- Control hyperthermia if present

ACUTE GENERAL TREATMENT

- Intravenous administration of a 10% calcium gluconate or calcium borogluconate solution *slowly*, at a rate of 1-1.5 ml/kg over 10 to 30 minutes or until resolution of clinical signs.
    - Calcium chloride solutions are not recommended due to perivascular corrosive effects if the solution extravasates.
    - Electrocardiographic (ECG) monitoring is warranted during administration (see Recommended Monitoring below).
- Intravenous (IV) calcium gluconate administration may be repeated in the event of a relapse; refractory cases should be reevaluated for hypoglycemia.
- The intravenous dose of calcium gluconate required to resolve clinical signs can be diluted 1:1 in saline for subcutaneous administration in three equal doses over 24 to 48 hours to prevent immediate relapse.
- Severe hyperthermia >104°F should be controlled with ice packs or alcohol baths (see Hyperthermia, p 1371).

CHRONIC TREATMENT

- Remove puppies for 24 to 36 hours to reduce maternal calcium loss through lactation; in the event of recurrence, remove puppies permanently.
- Puppies can be fed milk replacer every other day to decrease lactation demand on the bitch until weaning at age 3 weeks.
- Oral calcium replacement therapy for the bitch is recommended until weaning.
    - 20 mg/kg calcium carbonate PO q 8h.
    - Calcium carbonate antacid tablets available over the counter, such as Titralac or Tums, typically contain 500-750 mg calcium carbonate per tablet. See label for exact content.

POSSIBLE COMPLICATIONS

Overly rapid or unmonitored intravenous calcium administration can lead to severe bradycardia, ventricular arrhythmias, hypotension, and death.

RECOMMENDED MONITORING

- Cardiac monitoring by auscultation and/or ECG is required during intravenous calcium therapy. If severe bradycardia and/or arrhythmias develop, discontinue IV calcium until heart rate and rhythm normalize and then readminister at a decreased rate.
- Rectal temperature should be monitored until hyperthermia has resolved.

PROGNOSIS AND OUTCOME

Prognosis is good to excellent with immediate treatment and subsequent management

PEARLS & CONSIDERATIONS

COMMENTS

- Treatment should be initiated immediately based on signalment, history, and physical examination.
- Recurrence is possible up to the end of lactation.
- Preventive *prepartum* calcium supplementation is *not* recommended, as it may promote the development of eclampsia.
- Preventative *postpartum* calcium supplementation is recommended, as it may prevent recurrence during a subsequent lactation.
- Hypoglycemia is a common concurrent disorder, and blood/serum glucose should be measured in addition to blood/serum calcium in patients suspected of having eclampsia.

PREVENTION

Bitches should be maintained on a high-quality food during pregnancy.

CLIENT EDUCATION

Owners are to be cautioned that affected bitches may develop eclampsia in subsequent litters, and nutritional management and careful attention to early clinical signs are required.

SUGGESTED READING

Drobatz KJ, Casey KK: Eclampsia in dogs: 31 cases (1995-1998). *J Am Vet Med Assoc* 217(2):216-219, 2000.

Feldman EC, Nelson RW: *Canine and Feline Endocrinology and Reproduction*, ed 3. Philadelphia, WB Saunders, 2004, pp 829-831.

Johnston SD, Root-Kustritz MV, Olson PNS: Periparturient disorders in the bitch. In *Canine and Feline Theriogenology*. Philadelphia, WB Saunders, 2001, pp 141-143.

AUTHOR: **JONATHAN SPEARS**
EDITOR: **MICHELLE A. KUTZLER**

Ehrlichiosis, Canine Granulocytic

BASIC INFORMATION

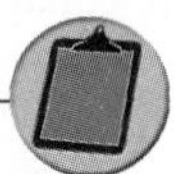

DEFINITION

Disease associated with infection by *Ehrlichia ewingii* and *Anaplasma phagocytophila* (formerly *E. equi*) in dogs.

These organisms predominantly infect circulating granulocytes (mainly neutrophils) and cause clinical illness that manifests with nonspecific signs (fever, lethargy, inappetence) and cytopenias. Clinically, granulocytic ehrlichiosis is similar to monocytic ehrlichiosis, with notable exceptions including the absence of a chronic phase in granulocytic ehrlichiosis, as well as a greater prevalence of lameness/polyarthritis.

SYNONYM(S)

Canine granulocytic ehrlichiosis (*E. ewingii*)
Equine ehrlichiosis (*A. phagocytophila*)
Human granulocytic ehrlichiosis (*A. phagocytophila*)
Tick fever (*A. phagocytophila*)

EPIDEMIOLOGY

SPECIES, AGE, SEX

- The dog is the predominantly affected species; one cat with granulocytic ehrlichiosis has been reported.
- As with other tick-borne infections, there is no clear age or sex predilection, but young adult males are overrepresented, likely due to increased exposure to the vector.
- One study found females overrepresented with *A. phagocytophila* infection.

RISK FACTORS: Due to the obligate tick vector, an increased incidence is noted in dogs near wooded areas with inadequate tick control.

CONTAGION AND ZOONOSIS: Most *Ehrlichia* spp. may be infectious to humans, but dogs appear to be minimally implicated in the human acquisition of ehrlichial infection. There is no direct dog-to-dog or dog-to-human transmission.

GEOGRAPHY AND SEASONALITY: Granulocytic ehrlichiosis due to *E. ewingii* is more commonly associated with the spring and summer months, correlating with the tick life cycle. *E. ewingii* is transmitted in part by the lone star tick (*Amblyomma americanum*) and therefore is found most often in the southeastern and southcentral United States.

Disease associated with *A. phagocytophila* is noted more predominantly in the autumn. *A. phagoctyophila* is transmitted by *Ixodes* spp. ticks and is found in the northwestern, north central, and northeastern United States.

ASSOCIATED CONDITIONS AND DISORDERS: Other tick-borne organisms such as those that cause Rocky Mountain spotted fever, cyclic thrombocytopenia, hepatozoonosis, monocytic ehrlichiosis, and babesiosis may be transmitted simultaneously, and these diseases can occur concurrently with granulocytic ehrlichiosis.

CLINICAL PRESENTATION

HISTORY, CHIEF COMPLAINT

- History usually includes tick exposure.
- Common clinical signs include lameness (due to polyarthropathy, especially with *E. ewingii*), depression, oculonasal discharge, and anorexia.
- Additional signs possible if coinfection with other tick-borne organisms.

PHYSICAL EXAM FINDINGS

- Fever
- Joint effusion, signs of joint pain
- Abdominal pain
- Lymphadenopathy
- Splenomegaly
- Ataxia

ETIOLOGY AND PATHOPHYSIOLOGY

- Ticks acquire the organism by feeding as either larvae or nymphs on infected animals. No transovarial transmission occurs in the tick.
- When an infected tick ingests a blood meal, the organism is transmitted via saliva to the vertebrate host.

- Infection leads to multiplication in granulocytic cells (predominantly neutrophils) and tissues (spleen, liver, and lymph nodes), producing cytopenias and overt physical signs.
- Infected dogs may clear the infection without therapy or clinical signs and thus not be presented for veterinary care.

DIAGNOSIS

DIFFERENTIAL DIAGNOSIS

- Rocky Mountain spotted fever (vs. acute phase of ehrlichiosis)
- Monocytic ehrlichiosis
- Hepatozoonosis
- Babesiosis
- Immune-mediated diseases (systemic lupus erythematosus, immune-mediated thrombocytopenia, immune-mediated arthropathies)
- Myeloma, lymphoma, and other diseases potentially characterized by hyperglobulinemia
- Leukemia
- Malignant histiocytosis

INITIAL DATABASE

- Complete blood count, serum biochemistry profile, urinalysis.
    - Thrombocytopenia (mild to severe) is the typical finding, but absence does not rule out ehrlichiosis.
    - Neutropenia, nonregenerative anemia, lymphocytosis, monocytosis, and eosinophilia may be observed.
    - Hyperglobulinemia is common; polyclonal is more frequent than monoclonal.
    - Pathologic proteinuria (e.g., elevated urine protein:creatinine ratio in the absence of urinary tract infection) may occur due to glomerulonephritis and other renal lesions.
- Fundic examination: retinal hemorrhages/detachment may be seen.
- Abdominal imaging if splenomegaly/signs of abdominal pain.
- Lymph node aspirates if lymphadenopathy (rule out other diagnoses).
- Arthrocentesis and limb radiography if signs of polyarthritis. Sterile, nonerosive polyarthritis with predominance of nondegenerate neutrophils is expected with ehrlichiosis.
- Bone marrow aspirate if thrombocytopenia is present and nonregenerative (low to normal MPV).
- Cerebrospinal fluid tap if neurologic signs.
- Antinuclear antibody and Coombs' tests: to help identify primary immune-mediated disease.

ADVANCED OR CONFIRMATORY TESTING

- Buffy coat and blood smear evaluation may identify morulae in granulocytes. Uncommon (many false-negative results).
- Serology: IFA or ELISA (antibody tests).
    - Positive results suggest infection, not exposure. Most infected dogs become seronegative within 6 to 9 months.
    - Confirmation with a convalescent titer (2 to 4 weeks later; should be higher) is recommended.
    - Cross-reactivity with *E. chaffeensis* and *E. canis* is noted with *E. ewingii* cases but cross-reactivity is not as likely with *A. phagoctyophila*.
- Polymerase chain reaction amplification: may be applied to tissue or whole blood. Can differentiate between *E. canis, E. chaffeensis,* and *E. ewingii* or can identify *A. phagoctyophila*.

TREATMENT

THERAPEUTIC GOAL(S)

- Supportive therapy
- Clear organism

ACUTE GENERAL TREATMENT

- Clear organism:
    - Tetracycline 22 mg/kg PO q 8h for 14 days; or
    - Doxycycline 5-10 mg/kg PO or IV q 12h for 21 days.
- Supportive care depends on clinical manifestation (i.e., transfusions for anemia, analgesics for polyarthritis pain).
- Glucocorticoids at immunosuppressive doses (e.g., prednisone 2-4 mg/kg PO q 24h): controversial, but may be considered during first 2 to 7 days of treatment.

CHRONIC TREATMENT

Chronic infections are rare with granulocytic ehrlichiosis, and response to doxycycline is typical.

POSSIBLE COMPLICATIONS

- Hemorrhage from severe thrombocytopenia or disseminated intravascular coagulation (DIC), especially if multiple concurrent infections.
- Protein-losing glomerular disease is not as common with granulocytic ehrlichiosis, due to lack of chronic disease.

RECOMMENDED MONITORING

Reevaluation of titers in 4 weeks; rise is confirmatory

PROGNOSIS AND OUTCOME

Good prognosis when rapid resolution of signs is seen (typical)

PEARLS & CONSIDERATIONS

COMMENTS

- Serologic cross-reactivity: *A. phagocytophila* may not be identified with titers for *E. canis. E. ewingii* may be identified with *E. canis* titers, although the amount may be reduced.
- The degree of hyperglobulinemia does *not* correlate with the efficacy of immune response.
- In some regions, *E. ewingii*, rather than *E. canis,* may be the more prevalent cause of ehrlichiosis.
- In a review by the University of Missouri, lameness was present in all affected dogs.

PREVENTION

Adequate tick control is the best prevention for ehrlichiosis.

SUGGESTED READING

Breitschwerdt EB: The rickettsioses. In Ettinger SJ, Feldman EC (eds): *Textbook of Veterinary Internal Medicine*. Philadelphia, WB Saunders, 2000, pp 402-404.

Cohn LA: Ehrlichiosis and related infections. *Vet Clin Small Anim* 33:863-884, 2003.

Liddell AM, et al: Predominance of *Ehrlichia ewingii* in Missouri dogs. *J Clin Microbiol* 41(10):4617-4622, 2003.

Neer TM: Ehrlichiosis. In Greene CE (ed): *Infectious Disease of the Dog and Cat*. Philadelphia, WB Saunders, 1998, pp 131-154.

Neer TM, et al: Consensus statement on ehrlichial disease of small animals from the Infectious Disease Study Group of the ACVIM. *J Vet Intern Med* 16:309-315, 2002.

AUTHOR: **JEFFERY SIMMONS**
EDITOR: **DOUGLASS K. MACINTIRE**

Ehrlichiosis, Canine Monocytic

BASIC INFORMATION

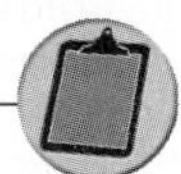

DEFINITION

Disease associated with infection by *Ehrlichia canis* and *E. chaffeensis*. These organisms predominantly infect circulating monocytes, macrophages, and lymphocytes and cause clinical illness that manifests with nonspecific signs (fever, lethargy, inappetence) and cytopenias.

SYNONYM(S)

Canine monocytic ehrlichiosis (*E. canis*)
Human monocytic ehrlichiosis (*E. chaffeensis*)
Tropical pancytopenia

EPIDEMIOLOGY

SPECIES, AGE, SEX: Ehrlichiosis is most commonly seen in dogs; rare in cats.
GENETICS AND BREED PREDISPOSITION: German shepherd dogs are thought to have a more fulminant illness.
RISK FACTORS: Because of the obligate tick vector, an increased incidence is noted in animals near wooded areas with inadequate tick control.
CONTAGION AND ZOONOSIS: Most *Ehrlichia* spp. may be infectious to humans, but dogs appear to be minimally implicated in the human acquisition of ehrlichial infection.There is no direct dog-to-dog or dog-to-human transmission.
GEOGRAPHY AND SEASONALITY: Monocytic ehrlichiosis has been found in most tropical and subtropical regions in the world based on the distribution of the vector, *Rhipicephalus sanguineus*, the brown dog tick. Because of different disease forms (acute, subacute, and chronic), there is no true seasonality. However, inoculation most commonly occurs in the warmer months.
ASSOCIATED CONDITIONS AND DISORDERS: Other tick-borne diseases such as Rocky Mountain spotted fever, cyclic thrombocytopenia, and hepatozoonosis may occur concurrently with ehrlichiosis.

CLINICAL PRESENTATION

DISEASE FORMS/SUBTYPES

- Acute phase: onset 8 to 20 days postinoculation; signs last 2 to 4 weeks, usually resolve spontaneously.
- Subclinical phase: onset 6 to 9 weeks postinoculation; clinically inapparent cytopenias.
- The infection may be cleared spontaneously at this time, but if not, the chronic phase ensues.
- Chronic phase: onset is weeks to months after inoculation; signs are variable in severity, ranging from mild illness to life-threatening cytopenic complications.

HISTORY, CHIEF COMPLAINT

- History usually includes tick exposure.
- Clinical signs associated with acute disease include depression, anorexia, weight loss, ocular and nasal discharges, lameness, and peripheral edema.
- Clinical signs of the chronic phase may include overt bleeding, cachexia, abdominal pain, lameness, and neurologic abnormalities.

PHYSICAL EXAM FINDINGS

- As described above (History, Chief Complaint).
- Fever is commonly present, as are signs of joint pain.
- Abdominal pain, signs of uveitis, epistaxis, cutaneous or mucous membrane petechiation, peripheral lymphadenopathy, pitting subcutaneous edema, splenomegaly, ataxia, seizures, vestibular signs, and blindness are variably present.

ETIOLOGY AND PATHOPHYSIOLOGY

- Ticks acquire the organism by feeding as either larvae or nymphs on infected animals. No transovarial transmission occurs in the tick.
- When an infected tick ingests a blood meal, the organism is transmitted via saliva to the vertebrate host.
- Infection leads to multiplication in mononuclear cells and tissues (spleen, liver, and lymph nodes).
- Infected cells attach to vascular endothelium in other organs such as lungs, kidneys, joints, and meninges, leading to vasculitis and subendothelial tissue infection and the acute phase of disease initially.
- Platelet consumption also occurs, with varying degrees of thrombosis, red cell destruction, and systemic inflammation.
- Subclinical phase is a result of ongoing bone marrow effects.
- Those unable to clear the infection in the subclinical phase develop chronic disease with hyperglobulinemia and immune complex formation, as well as bone marrow suppression, possibly leading to pancytopenia.

DIAGNOSIS

DIFFERENTIAL DIAGNOSIS

- Acute phase is similar to Rocky Mountain spotted fever (see p 975).
- Chronic disease differentials include immune-mediated diseases, myeloma, lymphoma, hepatozoonosis, malignant histiocytosis, leukemia, myelodysplasia, leptospirosis, and babesiosis.

INITIAL DATABASE

- Complete blood count, serum biochemistry profile, urinalysis
  - Thrombocytopenia (mild to severe) is the typical finding in all stages of illness, but absence does not rule out ehrlichiosis.
  - Neutropenia, nonregenerative anemia, lymphocytosis (sometimes marked), monocytosis, and eosinophilia may be observed.
  - Hyperglobulinemia is common; polyclonal > monoclonal.
  - Pathologic proteinuria (e.g., elevated urine protein:creatinine ratio in the absence of urinary tract infection) may occur due to glomerulonephritis.
- Fundic examination: retinal hemorrhages/detachment may be seen.
- Abdominal imaging if splenomegaly/signs of abdominal pain.
- Lymph node aspirates if lymphadenopathy.
- Arthrocentesis and limb radiography if signs of polyarthritis. Sterile, nonerosive polyarthritis with predominance of nondegenerate neutrophils is expected.
- Bone marrow aspirate if thrombocytopenia or pancytopenia is present.
- Cerebrospinal fluid tap if neurologic signs are present.
- Antinuclear antibody and Coombs' tests: to help identify primary immune-mediated disease.
- Protein electrophoresis to identify monoclonal gammopathy (e.g., myeloma) versus polyclonal gammopathy more commonly seen in ehrlichiosis.

ADVANCED OR CONFIRMATORY TESTING

- Buffy coat, blood smear evaluation: rarely identify morulae in mononuclear cells.
- Serology: IFA or ELISA (antibody tests):
  - Positive results suggest infection, not exposure. Most infected dogs become seronegative within 6 to 9 months.
  - Confirmation with a convalescent titer (2 to 4 weeks later; should be higher) is recommended.
  - Cross-reactivity exits with *E. chaffensis* and *E. ewingii*.
- Polymerase chain reaction amplification: may be applied to tissue or whole blood. May differentiate among *E. canis, E. chafeensis,* and *E. ewingii*.

TREATMENT

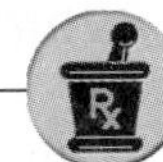

THERAPEUTIC GOAL(S)

- Supportive therapy
- Clear organism

ACUTE GENERAL TREATMENT

- Clear organism:
    - Tetracycline 22 mg/kg PO q 8h for 14 days; or
    - Doxycycline 5-10 mg/kg PO or IV q 12h for 21 days.
- Supportive care depends on clinical manifestation (i.e., transfusions for anemia, analgesics for polyarthritis pain).
- Glucocorticoids at immunosuppressive doses (e.g., prednisone 2-4 mg/kg PO q 24h): controversial, but generally recommended during first 2 to 7 days of acute stage.

CHRONIC TREATMENT

Some clinicians suggest resistant infections exist that may be treated with imidocarb dipropionate (5 mg/kg IM once, and repeat 14 to 21 days later; transient cholinergic side effects possible), long-term tetracycline (6.6 mg/kg PO q 24h), or repositol oxytetracycline (20 mg/kg up to 200 mg per dose IM twice weekly).

POSSIBLE COMPLICATIONS

- Hemorrhage from severe thrombocytopenia or disseminated intravascular coagulation (DIC)
- Protein-losing glomerular disease
- Blindness associated with retinal hemorrhages and detachment
- Immune-mediated diseases
- Long-term tetracycline therapy may prolong hematologic complications

PROGNOSIS AND OUTCOME

- Good prognosis with quick improvement in acute and mild chronic cases. Expect dramatic positive response to doxycycline or tetracycline within 48 hours.
- Severely pancytopenic patients with hemorrhagic complications or concurrent infections have a guarded to poor prognosis.

PEARLS & CONSIDERATIONS

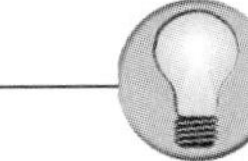

COMMENTS

- *E. canis* occurs in some cats, with clinical signs resembling acute canine monocytic ehrlichiosis.
- *E. canis* has been found in at least one human.
- *E. chaffeensis* may produce similar but less severe signs in dogs as *E. canis*, although as a result of cross-reactivity, the true incidence of *E. chaffeensis* in dogs is poorly defined.

PREVENTION

Adequate tick control is the best prevention.

SUGGESTED READING

Breitschwerdt EB: The rickettsioses. In Ettinger SJ, Feldman EC (eds): *Textbook of Veterinary Internal Medicine*. Philadelphia, WB Saunders, 2000, pp 402-404.

Breitschwerdt EB, et al: Molecular evidence supporting *Ehrlichia canis*-like infection in cats. *J Vet Intern Med* 16(6):642-649, 2002.

Cohn LA: Ehrlichiosis and related infections. *Vet Clin Small Anim* 33:863-884, 2003.

Neer TM: Ehrlichiosis. In Greene CE (ed): *Infectious Disease of the Dog and Cat*. Philadelphia, WB Saunders, 1998, pp 131-154.

Neer TM, et al: Consensus statement on ehrlichial disease of small animals from the Infectious Disease Study Group of the ACVIM. *J Vet Intern Med* 16:309-315, 2002.

AUTHOR: **JEFFERY SIMMONS**

EDITOR: **DOUGLASS K. MACINTIRE**

Eisenmenger's Syndrome

BASIC INFORMATION

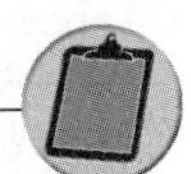

DEFINITION

Any large communication between the left and right sides of the heart, in association with severe pulmonary hypertension, which results in right to left shunting of blood

SYNONYM(S)

Eisenmenger's physiology

Eisenmenger's reaction

Eisenmenger's complex (large, nonrestrictive ventricular septal defect [VSD] plus pulmonary hypertension causing right-to-left shunting with or without dextroaorta)

The term "cyanotic congenital heart disease" includes Eisenmenger's syndrome, as well as right-to-left cardiac shunts without pulmonary hypertension (e.g., VSD with concurrent pulmonic stenosis).

EPIDEMIOLOGY

SPECIES, AGE, SEX

- Dogs and cats
- Young animals
- Female dogs more predisposed to patent ductus arteriosus (PDA); 15% of dogs with PDA have pulmonary hypertension

GENETICS AND BREED PREDISPOSITION: Dependent on the underlying cause:

- PDA: quasi-continuous or threshold trait with high degree of heritability. Miniature and toy poodles, collie, Pomeranian, Shetland sheepdog, American cocker spaniel, German shepherd, Maltese, keeshond, Yorkshire terrier.
- VSD: autosomal-dominant trait with incomplete penetrance or a polygenic trait. English springer spaniel, English bulldog.

RISK FACTORS: Living at high altitude.

ASSOCIATED CONDITIONS AND DISORDERS: Eisenmenger's syndrome can originate from an isolated cardiac defect (i.e., PDA) or from a combination of VSD and PDA.

CLINICAL PRESENTATION

HISTORY, CHIEF COMPLAINT

- Dyspnea (most common sign in cats)
- Exercise intolerance
- Syncope
- Lethargy
- Cough
- Cyanosis
- Hind limb collapse

PHYSICAL EXAM FINDINGS

- Soft (II-III/VI) left basilar systolic murmur (inconsistent)
- Right or left apical systolic murmurs (inconsistent)
- Tachycardia
- Tachypnea
- Generalized or regional cyanosis depending on underlying cause
- Loud second heart sound
- Split second heart sound

ETIOLOGY AND PATHOPHYSIOLOGY

- Size of the defect and severity of pulmonary hypertension determine the degree of shunting and thus the occurrence and extent of clinical signs.
    - Hypoxemia from shunting of venous blood into the arterial circulation leads to erythropoietin production and polycythemia.

- Polycythemia, if severe, can produce hyperviscosity and pulmonary embolism, central neurologic signs, and/or coagulopathies.

- Congenital:
  - High pulmonary vascular resistance is maintained after birth.
  - Abnormal maturation of the pulmonary vasculature.
- Acquired:
  - Large systemic-pulmonary communication (left-to-right shunt) offers minimal resistance to systolic flow.
  - Relative flows are determined by systemic and pulmonary vascular resistance.
  - Prolonged pulmonary hypertension leads to pulmonary vascular disease, an abnormal maturation of the pulmonary vasculature, and right ventricular hypertrophy.
  - Pulmonary arterial histologic features: medial muscular hypertrophy, laminar intimal fibrosis, necrotizing arteritis, plexiform lesions.
  - With progression, pulmonary vascular resistance may increase to a value greater than the systemic vascular resistance, causing right-to-left or bidirectional shunting (mixing of venous and arterial blood).

DIAGNOSIS

DIFFERENTIAL DIAGNOSIS

- Radiographic/electrocardiographic:
  - Right heart enlargement: other types of cardiac disease (pulmonic stenosis, tetralogy of Fallot, heartworm disease, tricuspid valve dysplasia), cor pulmonale
- Echocardiographic:
  - Pulmonic stenosis
  - Tetralogy of Fallot
  - Heartworm disease

INITIAL DATABASE

- Complete blood count (CBC): polycythemia (usually progressive with age)
- Heartworm test: antigen, antibody (cats), and microfilaria tests
- Thoracic radiographs: right heart enlargement, enlarged main pulmonary artery, normal to mildly enlarged pulmonary vasculature
- Systemic arterial blood pressure measurement: hypotension contraindicates performing phlebotomy without fluid replacement
- Electrocardiogram: tall P waves in lead II, deep S waves in lead II, right axis deviation; arrhythmias are uncommon
- Echocardiogram:
  - 2D: right ventricular hypertrophy, enlarged main pulmonary artery, identification of structural defects.
  - M mode: right ventricular free wall and septal hypertrophy, septal flattening, paradoxical septal motion.
  - Color flow Doppler: aliased or laminar flow across the congenital defect, tricuspid regurgitation (uncommon).
  - Spectral Doppler: tricuspid regurgitant velocity >3.5 m/s, pulmonic insufficiency velocity >3 m/s, reversed E/A ratio of mitral valve inflow profile, midsystolic notching of the pulmonary flow profile (severe cases).
  - Contrast echo: contrast appears in the left heart (intracardiac shunt) or in the abdominal aorta (extracardiac shunt).

ADVANCED OR CONFIRMATORY TESTING

- Cardiac catheterization: used for confirming diagnosis and to assess degree of shunting
- Angiogram: outlines the congenital defect(s) (PDA, VSD, or aorticopulmonary communication)
- Pressure measurements: increased pulmonary artery pressures. With large defects, right and left ventricular pressures have a tendency to equalize
- Oximetry: decreased aortic PO_2
- Transesophageal echocardiography: better identification of the congenital defect

TREATMENT

THERAPEUTIC GOAL(S)

- Control polycythemia and signs of hyperviscosity
- Reduce severity of pulmonary hypertension
- Control congestive heart failure
- Management of arrhythmias

ACUTE GENERAL TREATMENT

- Phlebotomy: if PVC >60%. Withdrawal of 10-20% of circulating blood volume (= 1-2 ml/kg) with or without intravenous fluid replacement. Repeated as needed (typically every several weeks) based on recurrence of clinical signs.
- Calcium channel blocker, phosphodiasterase V inhibitors: reduce pulmonary hypertension. See Pulmonary Hypertension (Arterial), p 914.

CHRONIC TREATMENT

Medical therapy:

- Hydroxyurea 20-25 mg/kg PO q 12-24h until hematocrit is lower; then 25-50 mg/kg PO q 48h as needed to maintain stable hematocrit. Recommended when patient requires frequent phlebotomies.
- Diuretics, ACE inhibitors, and antiarrhythmics following the treatment guidelines. See Heart Failure, Acute/Decompensated, p 458; Heart Failure, Chronic, p 459; Ventricular Arrhythmias (Premature Ventricular Complexes, Ventricular Tachycardia), p 1148.

DRUG INTERACTIONS

Hydroxyurea: reversible bone marrow suppression (pancytopenia), anorexia, vomiting and diarrhea, sloughing of nails are possible

RECOMMENDED MONITORING

Recheck examinations should include: CBC, serum renal profile, and systolic blood pressure measurement.

PROGNOSIS AND OUTCOME

Long-term prognosis is guarded to poor depending on the severity of the pulmonary hypertension

PEARLS & CONSIDERATIONS

COMMENTS

- Large systemic-pulmonary communications are uncommon in dogs and cats.
- Surgery is contraindicated due to severe pulmonary hypertension.

PREVENTION

Do not breed affected animals.

CLIENT EDUCATION

- Monitor respiratory rate at rest, exercise tolerance, and appetite
- Advise client not to breed affected animals

SUGGESTED READING

Feldman EC, et al: Eisenmenger's syndrome in the dog: Case reports. *J Am Anim Hosp Assoc* 17:477-483, 1981.

AUTHOR: **JOAO S. ORVALHO**
EDITOR: **ETIENNE CÔTÉ**

Elbow Dysplasia

Client Education Sheet on Website

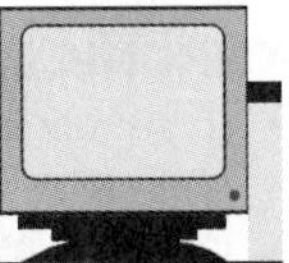

BASIC INFORMATION

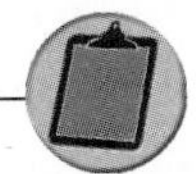

DEFINITION

- A group of diseases including fragmented medial coronoid process (FCP), ununited anconeal process (UAP), osteochondritis dissecans (OCD), and elbow incongruity (uneven radial head and medial coronoid surfaces) causing degenerative joint disease in the elbow.
- FCP is a separation of the medial aspect of the coronoid process from the ulna.
- UAP is a failure of the anconeal process to fuse to the ulna.
- Osteochondrosis is an abnormality of endochondral ossification, whereas OCD implies separation of the diseased cartilage from the subchondral bone.

EPIDEMIOLOGY

SPECIES, AGE, SEX

- Primarily in dogs between 6 and 9 months old.
- FCP may be present in older dogs with degenerative joint disease.

GENETICS AND BREED PREDISPOSITION: Elbow dysplasia is hereditary but also is associated with rapid growth and high-energy diet.

- UAP is found primarily in German shepherds, basset hounds, and Saint Bernards.
- FCP and OCD affect primarily retriever breeds, Bernese mountain dogs, and rottweilers.

Other large breed dogs may be affected by elbow dysplasia including the Newfoundland, mastiff, and Australian shepherd.

CLINICAL PRESENTATION

HISTORY, CHIEF COMPLAINT

- History of lameness on one or both front legs, often worse after exercise
- Reluctance to play or take long walks

PHYSICAL EXAM FINDINGS

- Lameness on one or both forelimbs.
- Pain on manipulation of the elbow, especially on extension.
- If osteoarthrosis is advanced, crepitation or effusion may be palpable along with a decreased amount of flexion to the joint (reduced range of motion).

ETIOLOGY AND PATHOPHYSIOLOGY

- OCD occurs when there is osteochondrosis (a failure of endochondral ossification), which leads to cartilage thickening and fissure formation.
    - Factors such as diet, rapid growth, hormonal imbalance, trauma, and genetics may lead to the development of OCD, as well as FCP and UAP.
- Joint incongruity, leading to increased pressure on the anconeus, has been implicated as a cause for UAP.
    - UAP may also be a form of osteochondrosis with abnormal, thickened cartilage, leading to failure of unification.
- The underlying pathophysiology of FCP is unknown but is believed to be secondary to elbow incongruity or a form of osteochondrosis.
    - Incongruity of the joint, especially an increase in length of the ulna in relation to the radius, can lead to increased weight-bearing load on the medial aspect of the coronoid process, leading to fissuring and fragmentation.
    - Osteochondrosis may lead to a delay in ossification of the coronoid region and subject to fragmentation when weight-bearing.

DIAGNOSIS

DIFFERENTIAL DIAGNOSIS

- Panosteitis
- OCD of the shoulder
- Elbow luxation

INITIAL DATABASE

- Complete blood count and serum chemistry panel based on signalment:
    - Consider before treatment or sedation/anesthesia.
    - Generally unremarkable for elbow dysplasia alone.
- Mediolateral, craniocaudal, and flexed lateral radiographs of both elbows (Fig. I-58):
    - An oblique craniocaudal view with the elbow flexed 30 degrees and rotated medially 15 degrees may help to assess the medial coronoid process.
    - The flexed lateral is the best radiographic view to identify a UAP (Fig. I-59).
    - OCD is seen on the medial condyle of the humerus, primarily on the craniocaudal view.
    - Elbow congruity is best assessed on the mediolateral view, and the beam should be centered on the elbow joint.

ADVANCED OR CONFIRMATORY TESTING

- A bone scan can be used for localizing the lameness if a complete orthopedic examination and radiographs are inconclusive.
- Computed tomography (CT) or magnetic resonance imaging (MRI) can be used for characterizing and delineating the elbow lesion.
- Arthrocentesis may be performed to rule out other causes of joint effusion.

TREATMENT

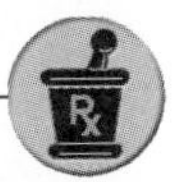

THERAPEUTIC GOAL(S)

- In persistently lame dogs, removal of the FCP, OCD, or UAP fragment will result in an improvement in limb function. However, degenerative joint disease is still expected to progress.
- In dogs with elbow incongruity, surgery will improve congruity and minimize ongoing degenerative changes to the joint.

ACUTE GENERAL TREATMENT

- Elbow arthroscopy, via a medial portal, is used for treatment of FCP and OCD and to assess elbow incongruity.
    - The FCP is identified and removed with grasping forceps.
    - OCD lesion is identified and the cartilage flap removed. A motorized shaver is used for removing fragments and to treat the underlying subchondral bone.
- In skeletally mature dogs, a UAP is often surgically removed via a lateral approach.
    - Various other surgical procedures have been described, such as lag screw fixation. However, these approaches result in no better success and have a higher complication rate related to the implants.
- In skeletally immature dogs, a dynamic ulnar osteotomy may be used for removing the pressure on the anconeal process and allowing bone or fibrous union of the fragment.
    - This may be used simultaneously with lag screw fixation of the anconeal process. Lag screw fixation causes compression of the anconeal process to the ulna and leads to bone fusion.
- If elbow incongruity exists, a dynamic ulnar osteotomy is performed to allow proximal movement (triceps muscles pull) of the ulna to improve joint congruency.
    - An intramedullary pin is placed, by some surgeons, in the ulna to provide stabilization and reduce callus formation.

CHRONIC TREATMENT

- If an ulnar osteotomy is performed, postoperative placement of a soft padded bandage for 2 to 4 weeks is used for support.
- Exercise should be restricted to short leash walks for 4 to 6 weeks after surgery.
- Medical therapy may be necessary after surgery if a significant amount of degenerative joint disease is present.
  - Nonsteroidal anti-inflammatory drugs (NSAIDs):
    - Aspirin 10–25 mg/kg PO q 8–24h; or
    - Carprofen 2 mg/kg PO q 12h; or
    - Etodolac 10–15 mg/kg PO q 24h; or
    - Deracoxib 1–2 mg/kg PO q 24h (may use 3–4 mg/kg PO q 24h for first 7 days only); or
    - Meloxicam 0.1 mg/kg PO q 24h; or
    - Meclofenamic acid 1.1 mg/kg PO q 24h after eating, for 5 days maximum; or
    - Tepoxalin 10 mg/kg PO q 24h (new product, objective data pending); or
    - Others
  - Chondroprotective agents:
    - Polysulfated glycosaminoglycan 5 mg/kg IM once weekly × 4–6 weeks; or
    - Pentosan polysulfate (from beechwood hemicellulose) 3 mg/kg SC once weekly; or
    - Oral formulations (glucosamine, chondroitin sulfate, hyaluronan): according to formulation/labeled instructions

POSSIBLE COMPLICATIONS

- Infection
- Implant failure if performing lag screw fixation

RECOMMENDED MONITORING

- Suture removal and recheck 2 postoperative weeks.
- Recheck 6 postoperative weeks to assess bone healing of the lag screw fixation (of 2 bone pieces) or the ulnar osteotomy (bone incision). Also helps evaluate progression of degenerative joint disease (DJD).
- Repeat radiographs 6 postoperative weeks if an ulnar osteotomy or lag screw fixation of the anconeal process was performed.

PROGNOSIS AND OUTCOME

- Surgery will help to alleviate lameness for OCD, FCP, and UAP. However, most affected dogs will continue to have progressive DJD and need medical therapy.
- Prognosis for return to full function depends on the degree of preexisting DJD.
- Medical treatment consisting of weight control, exercise restriction, NSAIDs, and polysulfated glycosaminoglycan therapy is reported to have a similar outcome to surgical treatment of OCD and FCP.

PEARLS & CONSIDERATIONS

COMMENTS

- Clinical signs of a FCP may not correlate with radiographic evidence of disease.
  - The initial radiographic change will be mild osteophytosis on the anconeal process.
  - Some dogs may show mild or no radiographic changes, yet be profoundly lame; such a patient needs MRI, CT, or arthroscopy.
  - Conversely, some dogs are not lame, yet have radiographic evidence of DJD.
  - Hence, treatment is directed toward the patient and not the radiograph.
- Unilateral forelimb lameness may not be detectable if bilateral forelimb disease is present.
- Because of the prevalence of bilateral disease, both elbows may undergo arthroscopy with one anesthetic episode, if clinically indicated.

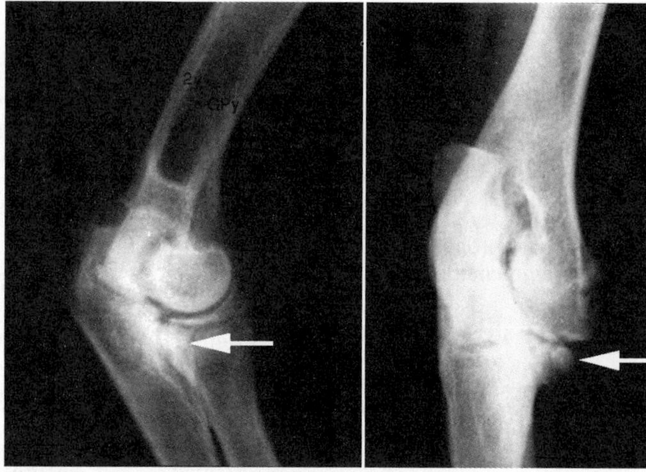

FIGURE I-58 Mediolateral (*left panel*) and craniocaudal (*right panel*) projections of a canine elbow with fragmented medial coronoid process (*arrows*). Courtesy of Dr. J. Harari; reproduced with permission.

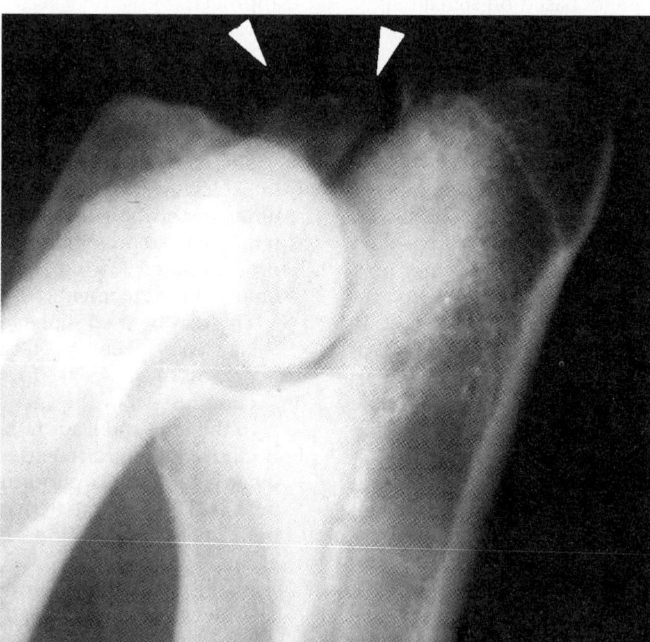

FIGURE I-59 Mediolateral projection of a flexed canine elbow joint with an ununited anconeal process (*arrowheads*). Courtesy of Dr. J. Harari; reproduced with permission.

- The anconeal process does not fuse until 4 to 5 months of age and cannot be diagnosed radiographically as ununited before that time.
- When manipulating the elbow to check for pain, avoid movement of the shoulder, which may obscure localization of the discomfort.

CLIENT EDUCATION

Because of the hereditary component of elbow dysplasia, affected dogs should not be used for breeding.

SUGGESTED READING

Bouck GR, et al: A comparison of surgical and medical treatment of fragmented coronoid process and osteochondritis dissecans of the canine elbow. *Vet Comp Orthop Traumatol* 8:177–183, 1995.

Johnson AL, et al: Canine elbow dysplasia. In Fossum TW (ed): *Small Animal Surgery*, ed 2, St. Louis, Mosby, Inc., 2002, pp 1066–1078.

Schulz KS, Krotscheck U: Canine elbow dysplasia. In Slatter D (ed): *Textbook of Small Animal Surgery*, ed 3. Philadelphia, WB Saunders, 2002, pp 1927–1952.

Turner BM, et al: Dynamic proximal ulnar osteotomy for the treatment of ununited anconeal process in 17 dogs. *Vet Comp Orthop Traumatol* 11:76–79, 1998.

AUTHOR: **RAVIV J. BALFOUR**
EDITOR: **JOSEPH HARARI**

Elbow Luxation

BASIC INFORMATION

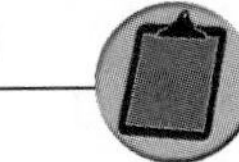

DEFINITION

Dislocation between brachium (humerus) and antebrachium (radius and ulna)

SYNONYM(S)

Elbow dislocation

EPIDEMIOLOGY

- Any breed, age, or sex for traumatic luxations
- Juvenile dogs for congenital luxations

GENETIC AND BREED PREDISPOSITION

- Congenital luxations generally more common in small breeds of dogs, but radial head luxation specifically occurs more frequently in larger breeds
- Suspected hereditary predisposition

RISK FACTORS: Forelimb trauma.

ASSOCIATED CONDITIONS AND DISORDERS: Some forms of congenital luxation may be associated with more generalized joint laxity syndromes or ectrodactyly.

CLINICAL PRESENTATION

DISEASE FORMS/SUBTYPES

- Traumatic
- Congenital, complete
- Congenital, partial (radial head luxation only)

HISTORY, CHIEF COMPLAINT

- Forelimb trauma secondary to motor vehicle accident, fall, or rough play/fighting
- Spontaneous lameness/deformity in young dog

PHYSICAL EXAM FINDINGS

- Traumatic: non-weight-bearing lameness with antebrachium and paw abducted, elbow flexed, and severe elbow swelling and pain.
- Congenital: partial weight-bearing lameness and joint thickening; discomfort during range of motion maneuvers.

ETIOLOGY AND PATHOPHYSIOLOGY

- Majority of traumatic luxations are lateral (proximal radius/ulna are lateral to distal humerus).
- Medial luxations are associated with severe soft tissue derangements.
- Traumatic injuries may have avulsion fracture(s) of collateral ligament(s).
- Congenital/developmental luxations and subluxations may be associated with asynchronous growth of the radius and ulna.

DIAGNOSIS

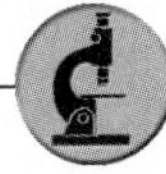

DIFFERENTIAL DIAGNOSIS

- Distal humeral fracture
- Monteggia lesion (cranial displacement of radial head and proximal ulna fracture)
- Elbow neoplasia

INITIAL DATABASE

- Orthogonal view (cranial-caudal and medial-lateral) radiographs of the elbow.
- Patient survey for other traumatic injuries, especially thoracic.
- Appropriate preanesthetic assessments as warranted for patient signalment.
- Radiographs of the contralateral elbow with congenital or developmental luxations.

TREATMENT

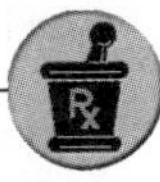

THERAPEUTIC GOAL(S)

- Anatomic reduction of joint surfaces
- Restoration of normal joint mobility
- Return to full weight bearing
- Elimination of discomfort

ACUTE GENERAL TREATMENT

- Traumatic elbow luxations are best managed via early closed reduction before muscle contraction makes manipulations difficult (see Luxation Reduction (Closed): Shoulder, Elbow, or Hip, p 1277).
- Patient must be anesthetized for reduction.
- If closed reduction is not achieved, open reduction and reconstruction of the collateral ligaments are indicated.
- If open reduction is needed, the limb should be bandaged to reduce patient discomfort and tissue swelling before surgery.
- Appropriate analgesics should be administered.
- Congenital/developmental luxations do not require "acute" treatment, but intervention is preferred to help slow progression of secondary osteoarthritis.
- Congenital luxations are less amenable to closed reduction.
- Congenital luxations may require osteotomies or ostectomies for treatment.

CHRONIC TREATMENT

- Immobilization with elbow bandaged in extension for 1 to 2 weeks.
- Initially, a heavy padded bandage (or more rigid splint for open reductions and those with severe collateral ligament damage), with gradual reduction in bandage thickness/stiffness as swelling subsides and stability increases.
- Gentle, passive range of motion (flexion/extension) physiotherapy instituted after bandage removal.
- Continued use of analgesics/anti-inflammatory agents, as needed, for patient comfort.

POSSIBLE COMPLICATIONS

- Recurrent luxation/instability
- Articular cartilage damage and secondary osteoarthritis
- Ligament damage
- Reduced range of motion from pericapsular fibrosis
- Chronic lameness

RECOMMENDED MONITORING

- Postreduction radiographs to confirm restoration of joint congruency
- Periodic lameness evaluations/elbow palpation until fully recovered

PROGNOSIS AND OUTCOME

- Good if mild articular cartilage or ligamentous lesions.
- Chronic fibrosis will result in a permanently thickened elbow.
- Most dogs with properly treated traumatic luxations will return to normal or near-normal function.
- More guarded prognosis for congenital/ developmental luxations.
- Severe complications/failures might necessitate salvage surgery (arthrodesis, total joint arthroplasty, or amputation).

PEARLS & CONSIDERATIONS

COMMENTS

- Early diagnosis is critical for promoting successful closed reduction.
- Closed reduction achieved by flexing elbow (moves anconeal process caudally), followed by abduction of the antebrachium with the paw flexed (moves anconeal process medially, attempting to "hook" anconeal process medial to lateral epicondylar crest of the humerus), followed by adduction and pronation of the antebrachium (attempting to "snap" the radial head medially to its proper location under the capitalum of the humerus, as the anconeal process acts as a fulcrum).
- Can consider paralyzing patient pharmacologically (requires ventilation of patient for gas exchange) to achieve greater muscle relaxation to facilitate reduction maneuvers.

CLIENT EDUCATION

- Bandage/splint care
- Controlled activity (kennel/leash)
- Passive range of motion physiotherapy after after removal
- Neuter dogs with congenital luxations due to potential heritability

SUGGESTED READING

Dassler C, Vasseur PB: Elbow luxation. In Slatter DH (ed): *Textbook of Small Animal Surgery*, ed 3. Philadelphia, WB Saunders, 2003, pp 1919–1927.

O'Brien MG, et al: Traumatic luxation of the cubital joint (elbow) in dogs: 44 cases (1978–1988). *J Am Vet Med Assoc* 201:1760, 1992.

Piermattei DL, Flo GL: The elbow joint. In *Brinker, Piermattei, and Flo's Handbook of Small Animal Orthopedics and Fracture Repair*, ed 3. Philadelphia, WB Saunders, 1997, pp 288–300.

AUTHOR: **JAMES M. FINGEROTH**
EDITOR: **JOSEPH HARARI**

Electrocution

BASIC INFORMATION

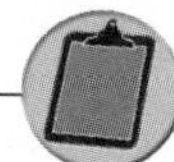

DEFINITION

The passage of electricity through tissue resulting in electrophysiologic disruption of the tissue

SYNONYM(S)

Electrical injury

EPIDEMIOLOGY

SPECIES, AGE, SEX: Most common in young cats and dogs (5 weeks to 1.5 years of age), with no sex predilection.
RISK FACTORS: Young age and environmental access.
GEOGRAPHY AND SEASONALITY: Tend to occur seasonally, perhaps most often from March until August, when owners are likely to operate electrical devices (e.g., fans).
ASSOCIATED CONDITIONS AND DISORDERS: Noncardiogenic pulmonary edema, oral burns.

CLINICAL PRESENTATION

DISEASE FORMS/SUBTYPES: High-voltage injury versus low-voltage injury based on the nature and intensity of the current. The most severe injuries result from a high current and high voltage situation and thus produce a worst clinical outcome. Electrical sources can produce energy levels that range from relatively low (e.g., 9-volt battery) to intermediate (e.g., household outlets), to very high (e.g., electrical metal utility cover). Household current is the most common.
HISTORY, CHIEF COMPLAINT: Sometimes witnessed; other times the owner reports sudden onset of dyspnea, collapse, or dysphagia.
PHYSICAL EXAM FINDINGS

- Oral burns: to the tongue, palate, and commissures of the lips
- Respiratory problems: dyspnea, cyanosis, coughing
- Cardiac problems: arrhythmias

ETIOLOGY AND PATHOPHYSIOLOGY

- Electricity (usually 60 Hz of alternating current or 120 volts is found in most households in the United States; in Europe it is usually 50 Hz of alternating current or 220 volts) disrupts the electrophysiologic activity of tissue causing muscle spasms, ventricular fibrillation, and vasomotor changes in the central nervous system, resulting in acute pulmonary edema. The electrical energy is also transformed into heat, which can cause coagulation of tissue proteins. Sudden death may result from these processes.
- Electrocution is almost always accidental, typically with a young pet chewing on an electric cord.

DIAGNOSIS

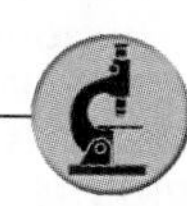

DIFFERENTIAL DIAGNOSIS

Chemical or thermal burns, exposure to fire, and smoke inhalation

INITIAL DATABASE

Initial database is dependent on the severity of injury. In some cases, if the animal has no physical exam abnormalities, no testing is required. In others cases, if the pet is dyspneic or pulmonary crackles are auscultated, chest radiographs are warranted. In severely affected animals, complete blood count, serum biochemistry profile, coagulation profile, and urinalysis are warranted.

ADVANCED OR CONFIRMATORY TESTING

Arterial blood gas analysis may be useful to document hypoxemia. However, in young or small animals, the stress of the sample collection should be weighed against the potential benefits.

TREATMENT

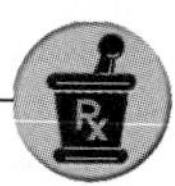

THERAPEUTIC GOAL(S)

- Treatment of pulmonary edema
- Treatment of burns

ACUTE GENERAL TREATMENT

Noncardiogenic pulmonary edema is treated with rest and supplemental oxygen. Bronchodilators (such as albuterol 0.05 mg/kg PO q 8h, or by aerosol; aminophylline 20 mg/kg PO q 12h or 6-11 mg/kg PO, IM, or slow IV q 8h) may help in clearing edema fluid. Intravenous fluid support may be required. Diuretics and glucocorticoids are usually not warranted. Positive pressure ventilation with positive end-expiratory pressure in theory should help maximally distend the alveoli that are available and keep the smaller airways open during the expiratory phase of respiration. However, if mechanical ventilation is deemed necessary, a poor outcome is likely.

CHRONIC TREATMENT

Treat burns with antibiotics, wound cleaning, soft food/feeding tube if burns are in the mouth, surgical debridement and closure. Puppies in particular will commonly eat despite severe oral injury.

POSSIBLE COMPLICATIONS

Infection of nonhealing burns, acute lung injury, acute respiratory distress syndrome

RECOMMENDED MONITORING

Respiratory rate and effort, as well as the healing of any burns, should be monitored.

PROGNOSIS AND OUTCOME

Depends on the degree of noncardiogenic pulmonary edema. Cats appear to do better than dogs in overall survival. Critical period is the first 24 to 48 hours after electrical shock; if the animal survives this period, he/she will likely survive.

PEARLS & CONSIDERATIONS

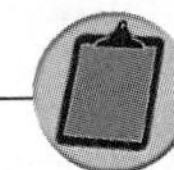

COMMENTS

Noncardiogenic pulmonary edema can be difficult to treat. There are no known specific treatment recommendations.

PREVENTION

Remove access to wires that are plugged into outlets

CLIENT EDUCATION

Education about reexposure, and removal of damaged or faulty electrical cords

SUGGESTED READING

Drobatz KJ, et al: Noncardiogenic pulmonary edema in dogs and cats: 26 cases (1987-1993). *J Am Vet Med Assoc* 206:1732-1736, 1995.

Morgan RV, Mawby D: Environmental injuries. In Hoskins JD (ed): *Veterinary Pediatrics*. Philadelphia, WB Saunders, 1995, pp 545-547.

AUTHOR: **MEGAN WHELAN**

EDITOR: **ELIZABETH ROZANSKI**

Emphysema and Pulmonary Bullae

BASIC INFORMATION

DEFINITION

- *Emphysema*: pathologic accumulation of air within an organ or tissue
- *Bulla*: an air-filled space within the pulmonary parenchyma that arises from alveolar distention or destruction of alveolar walls
- *Bleb*: an accumulation of air within the mesothelial covering and layers of elastic fibers and connective tissue cells that comprise the visceral pleura

SYNONYM(S)

Bullous emphysema

EPIDEMIOLOGY

SPECIES, AGE, SEX: Reported most commonly in dogs of middle age, although dogs of any age can be affected. Cats are rarely affected.

GENETICS AND BREED PREDISPOSITION

- A familial or genetic predisposition has not been demonstrated
- Large, deep-chested dog breeds are considered at greater risk of pulmonary blebs and bullae

RISK FACTORS

- Congenital bronchial hypoplasia (uncommon) reported in both dogs and cats.
- Chronic obstructive pulmonary diseases are a recognized risk factor in people and could be so in dogs (e.g., chronic sterile bronchitis).

ASSOCIATED CONDITIONS AND DISORDERS

- Congenital bronchial hypoplasia
- Spontaneous pneumothorax
- Pneumomediastinum (uncommon)
- Subcutaneous emphysema (uncommon)

CLINICAL PRESENTATION

DISEASE FORMS/SUBTYPES: Congenital forms of bullous lung disease have been described, usually secondary to bronchial hypoplasia.

HISTORY, CHIEF COMPLAINT: Animals may be clinically normal:

- A pulmonary bleb or bulla may be found incidentally during thoracotomy or thoracoscopy

Clinical signs, when present, can be acute, intermittent, or slowly progressive:

- Anorexia
- Lethargy
- Respiratory distress
- Cough
- Exercise intolerance

The rupture of a bleb or bulla, causing spontaneous pneumothorax, is typically associated with acute dyspnea.

PHYSICAL EXAM FINDINGS

- Respiratory distress
- Increased inspiratory effort (pneumothorax from ruptured bleb or bulla)
- Increased expiratory effort (pulmonary emphysema without pneumothorax)
- Tachypnea
- Tachycardia
- Diminished heart and lung sounds on one or both sides if pneumothorax
- Subcutaneous emphysema in occasional patients

ETIOLOGY AND PATHOPHYSIOLOGY

- Histopathologic assessment of resected tissues classifies lesions as blebs or bullae.
- Exact mechanisms leading to bulla or bleb formation are not defined:
  - Suspected to reflect the effects of distensile or traction forces on the lung surface, or the effects of inflammation or degradative enzymes in the alveoli to break down alveolar walls.
  - Increased alveolar pressure relative to transpleural pressure may also contribute.

DIAGNOSIS

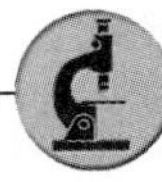

DIFFERENTIAL DIAGNOSIS

Other causes of pneumothorax:

- Trauma, either blunt or penetrating, to the thoracic wall, trachea, esophagus, or pulmonary parenchyma
- Inflammatory lung disease
- Neoplastic lung disease
- Parasitic lung disease, especially *Paragonimus kellicotti* and *Dirofilaria immitis*

INITIAL DATABASE

- Thoracic radiographs:
  - May demonstrate the features of pneumothorax (see Pneumothorax, p 866).
  - Often unremarkable; observation of a bleb or bulla is uncommon.
  - Animals with paragonimiasis may have thick-walled bullae evident, even with pneumothorax.
  - Thoracic radiographs may in some cases show air-filled dilations within the parenchyma.
  - Occasional animals may have pneumomediastinum and subcutaneous emphysema evident.
- Results of a complete blood count, biochemical profile, and urinalysis are typically unaffected by the disease.
- Hypoxemia will be the most consistently present abnormality on arterial blood gas analysis.
- Fecal examinations (flotation and sedimentation techniques) to rule out respiratory parasites.

ADVANCED OR CONFIRMATORY TESTING

- Definitive diagnosis is usually made by detection of bullae, blebs, or air leaking from the lung surface during thoracotomy or thoracoscopy and confirmed with histopathologic examination of resected tissue.
  - Median sternotomy is the preferred approach in patients with spontaneous pneumothorax.
  - Cranial lung lobes are most commonly affected, although other lung lobes can also have lesions.
- Tracheoscopy, bronchoscopy, and esophagoscopy are usually normal in patients with bullous lung disease unless airway hypoplasia is present.
- The role of computed tomographic scans in the diagnosis of bullous lung disease has not been evaluated, but would be expected to be more sensitive than plain radiography for the detection of bullous lesions.

TREATMENT

THERAPEUTIC GOAL(S)

- Improve respiratory function and oxygenation in patients with respiratory distress
- Remove bullae or blebs

ACUTE GENERAL TREATMENT

- Thoracocentesis if pneumothorax is present (see Thoracocentesis, p 1308):
  - Thoracostomy tubes with continuous suction may be needed in some patients for management of persistent air accumulation
- Oxygen provided by mask, nasal catheter, oxygen cage
- Cage rest

CHRONIC TREATMENT

- Long-term resolution of spontaneous pneumothorax from rupture of blebs or bullous lung lesions, if not from parasitic diseases, is most reliably achieved with surgical resection of the affected lung tissue by either partial or complete lung lobectomy.
  - Persistence or recurrence of clinical signs is more likely if the patient is managed nonsurgically.
  - Partial or complete lung lobectomy may be accomplished via thoracotomy or thoracoscopy.

POSSIBLE COMPLICATIONS

- Pneumothorax from leakage at suture or staple site
- Postoperative complications of infection, wound dehiscence

RECOMMENDED MONITORING

- Clinical signs
- Thoracic radiographs

PROGNOSIS AND OUTCOME

Prognosis is good with surgical resection of bullous lung lesions

PEARLS & CONSIDERATIONS

COMMENTS

- Often, in patients with spontaneous pneumothorax of uncertain origin and no history of trauma, bleb or bulla rupture ultimately is found to be the underlying cause.
- Some animals can be successfully managed with nonsurgical methods (thoracocentesis, thoracostomy tubes), but the literature supports early lung lobectomy for the best long-term outcomes.
- Affected animals can have multiple lesions scattered over different lung lobes, and lung lobes on both sides of the thoracic cavity can be affected. It is thus imperative to examine the entirety of both lungs during thoracotomy or thoracoscopy.

PREVENTION

There is no means of preventing the disease. Animals with congenital bronchial hypoplasia should probably not be bred.

CLIENT EDUCATION

Nonsurgical treatment approaches are more likely to be associated with persistence or recurrence of clinical signs. Postsurgical outcomes are usually excellent.

SUGGESTED READING

Brissot HN, et al: Thoracoscopic treatment of bullous emphysema in 3 dogs. *Vet Surg* 32:524, 2003.

Lipscomb VJ, et al: Spontaneous pneumothorax caused by pulmonary blebs and bullae in 12 dogs. *J Am Anim Hosp Assoc* 39:435, 2003.

Puerto DA, et al: Surgical and nonsurgical management of and selected risk factors for spontaneous pneumothorax in dogs: 64 cases (1986–1999). *J Am Vet Med Assoc* 220:1670, 2002.

AUTHOR & EDITOR: **RANCE K. SELLON**

Encephalopathy, Vascular

BASIC INFORMATION

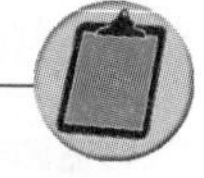

DEFINITION

Brain dysfunction caused by ischemia, or lack of oxygen delivery. These are most commonly focal events (i.e., infarcts or strokes), but occasionally manifest as widespread brain ischemia (i.e., global ischemia).

SYNONYM(S)

Infarct
Ischemic encephalopathy
Stroke

EPIDEMIOLOGY

SPECIES, AGE, SEX: There are no signalment restrictions for focal or global brain ischemia in dogs and cats.

GENETICS AND BREED PREDISPOSITION: Cavalier King Charles spaniels may be predisposed to cerebellar infarcts; this may be related to local pressure abnormalities due to caudal occipital malformation syndrome in this breed.

Brachycephalic breeds may be predisposed to developing global brain ischemia.

RISK FACTORS

- Focal ischemic events (strokes): hypertension, hypercoagulability, and hyperviscosity. The most prevalent of these diseases that cause these disturbances in patients with vascular encephalopathy are chronic renal failure and hyperadrenocorticism. Other conditions include diabetes mellitus, hypothyroidism, hyperthyroidism, hepatic failure, pheochromocytoma, and infectious diseases. Feline ischemic encephalopathy has been linked to intracranial migration of *Cuterebra* larvae. Other parasites have been occasionally implicated in dogs and cats.
- Risk factors for global brain ischemia include inadequate anesthetic monitoring, cardiac arrest, severe hypoxemia, and the use of ketamine in anesthetic protocols (especially in brachycephalic breeds).

CLINICAL PRESENTATION

DISEASE FORMS/SUBTYPES: Focal brain ischemic events (strokes, infarcts) can be small (lacunar) or large (territorial), and either hemorrhagic or nonhemorrhagic (the latter are more common). Global brain ischemia usually involves some degree of diffuse oxygen deprivation in the brain and is much less common than focal brain ischemia.

HISTORY, CHIEF COMPLAINT

- The characteristic historic feature of both focal and global ischemic encephalopathy is acute to peracute onset of brain dysfunction, which is nonprogressive after the first 24 hours.
- Typical chief complaints include sudden onset disorientation, mentation change, vocalizing/crying, or seizures.

PHYSICAL EXAM FINDINGS

- Physical and neurologic examination findings depend primarily on the underlying disorder leading to the ischemic event (physical examination findings) and the region of the brain affected by the ischemic event.
- Strokes affecting the cerebrum (e.g., propulsive pacing, disorientation, seizures), diencephalon/midbrain (e.g., depression, obtundation/coma), or cerebellum (hypermetria, intention tremor) are seen with some frequency in affected dogs.

ETIOLOGY AND PATHOPHYSIOLOGY

- Interruption of oxygen delivery to brain tissue
- Disruption of cellular energy metabolism (i.e., ATP production)
- Brain necrosis and edema
- Generation of cytotoxic mediators of secondary brain injury

DIAGNOSIS

DIFFERENTIAL DIAGNOSIS

- Brain neoplasm
- Inflammatory brain disease: sterile or infectious encephalitides
- Trauma (suggested at outset if history unknown, or supportive of trauma)

INITIAL DATABASE

- Complete blood count, serum biochemistry profile: abnormalities depend on underlying cause (e.g., polycythemia or hyperglobulinemia with hyperviscosity syndrome); changes consistent with renal disease if hypertension; hypoalbuminemia with hypercoagulability due to loss of antithrombin III (protein-losing nephropathy or enteropathy).
- Neurologic examination: deficits according to site of ischemia. Symmetric deficits with global ischemia, asymmetric with focal ischemia.
- Serial blood pressure measurement: rule out systemic hypertension.
- Urinalysis: pathologic proteinuria in cases of protein-losing nephropathy.

ADVANCED OR CONFIRMATORY TESTING

- Magnetic resonance imaging of brain: diagnostic test of choice
  - Helps to differentiate focal from global ischemia, but this distinction should be apparent from the history and neurologic exam alone
- Cerebrospinal fluid examination: may be unremarkable, or show nonspecific changes

TREATMENT

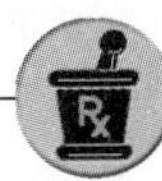

THERAPEUTIC GOAL(S)

- Minimize secondary brain swelling and tissue damage
- Treat underlying cause of brain ischemia
- Physical rehabilitation

ACUTE GENERAL TREATMENT

- Mannitol 0.5-1.0 g/kg body weight slowly IV over 10 to 15 minutes
- Oxygen supplementation

CHRONIC TREATMENT

- Treat underlying condition (e.g., antihypertensive drugs if hypertension is documented)
- Physical therapy

POSSIBLE COMPLICATIONS

- Recumbency-associated pneumonia
- Pressure sores
- Recurrent stroke
- Exacerbation of underlying condition leading to ischemic event

RECOMMENDED MONITORING

- Serial neurologic examinations
- Blood pressure (if hypertension documented)
- Progression or regression of underlying condition (e.g., diabetes control, control of hyperadrenocorticism)

PROGNOSIS AND OUTCOME

- Most patients recover fully from focal ischemic events.
- Prognosis for stroke is more closely associated with the underlying cause than the stroke event itself.
- Global brain ischemia is associated with a more guarded prognosis than focal brain ischemia.

PEARLS & CONSIDERATIONS

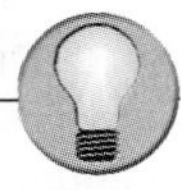

COMMENTS

- Recovery from vascular encephalopathy may take several weeks to several months.
- Aggressive physical therapy and nursing care are essential to a positive outcome.
- History and symmetry versus asymmetry of neurologic deficits are the main elements that allow the differentiation of global versus focal ischemia, respectively.
- Although dogs and cats can develop vascular encephalopathy (a true stroke) as described previously, overall this disorder occurs much less commonly than acute vestibular syndrome, which is an acute disorder that does not involve the brain (peripheral vestibular disease), does not involve infarction, and yet is often referred to inaccurately as a "stroke."

SUGGESTED READING

Cook LB, et al: Vascular encephalopathy associated with bacterial endocarditis in four dogs. *J Am Anim Hosp Assoc* 41: 252, 2005.

Glass EN, et al. Clinical and clinicopathologic features in 11 cats with *Cuterebra* larvae myiasis of the central nervous system. *J Vet Intern Med* 12:365, 1998.

Hillock, et al: Vascular encephalopathies in dogs. *Compend Contin Educ Pract Vet*. In press, 2005.

McConnell JF, et al: Magnetic resonance imaging findings of presumed cerebellar cerebrovascular accident in twelve dogs. *Vet Rad Ultrasound* 46:1, 2005.

Panarello G, et al: Magnetic resonance imaging of two suspected cases of global brain ischemia. *J Vet Emerg Crit Care* 14: 269, 2004.

AUTHOR & EDITOR: **CURTIS W. DEWEY**

Endocarditis, Infective

BASIC INFORMATION

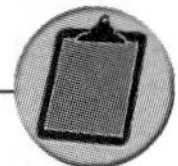

DEFINITION

Endocarditis is inflammation of the endocardial surface of the heart (endocardium).

- Infective endocarditis is microbial infection of the endocardium.
- Vegetative endocarditis is a specific form of endocarditis where structures (vegetations) composed of platelets, fibrin, microorganisms, and inflammatory cells adhere to heart valves or cling to septal defects, chordae tendineae, or the mural endocardium.

Endocarditis (both the term and the disease) is pathophysiologically and epidemiologically unrelated to the most common form of chronic valvular heart disease in dogs, known as endocardiosis.

EPIDEMIOLOGY

SPECIES, AGE, SEX

- Endocarditis is uncommon in dogs and very rare in cats.
- Male dogs are more commonly affected than females, and large breeds are affected more commonly than small.
- In the dog, the left-sided heart valves (aortic and mitral) are by far the most frequently affected.

RISK FACTORS

- Congenital aortic valve disease (e.g., subaortic stenosis) and other congenital heart diseases that cause disturbances of blood flow and subsequent changes in the endocardium.
- Glucocorticoid use predisposes to endocarditis, and many cases appear to have a nosocomial origin. Infected intravenous catheters, prosthetic heart valves, heart surgery, and interventional cardiac catheterization all enhance the risk.
- Infection with potentially immunosuppressive organisms (e.g., *Bartonella* spp., *Ehrlichia* spp.) enhances the risk of endocarditis.
- Predisposing factors for endocarditis in dogs include sources of chronic bacteremia (e.g., urinary tract infection, diskospondylitis) and systemic illnesses that facilitate bacterial infection (e.g., diabetes mellitus, hyperadrenocorticism/Cushing's disease).

GEOGRAPHY AND SEASONALITY: Infective endocarditis is recognized more in warmer climates (e.g., southern and western United States).

CLINICAL PRESENTATION

DISEASE FORMS/SUBTYPES: Endocarditis is classified as acute or subacute-chronic, based on the duration, rate of progression, and severity of clinical signs.

HISTORY, CHIEF COMPLAINT

- Extracardiac manifestations of systemic infection and inflammation are the source of most of the historic complaints.
- Manifestations of fever (e.g., lethargy, anorexia) are the most common sign, although they may be intermittent, minimal, or even absent in patients with less virulent organisms (e.g., *Bartonella* spp., some gram-positive organisms) or severe debilitation.
- Weight loss.
- Reluctance to move (back pain, polyarthritis).
- Intermittent lameness (muscle embolization, polyarthritis).

PHYSICAL EXAM FINDINGS: Most patients diagnosed with endocarditis have a heart murmur.

- The murmur may be newly recognized, or may have changed in intensity, quality, timing, or duration. Many animals with endocarditis have a preexisting heart murmur (e.g., from subaortic stenosis).
- The presence of a diastolic murmur in a systemically ill animal dramatically raises the index of suspicion for infective endocarditis.
- Aortic insufficiency often causes a soft, blowing murmur with a distant quality that is difficult to hear.

ETIOLOGY AND PATHOPHYSIOLOGY

- *Staphylococcus* spp., *Streptococcus* spp., *Erysipelothrix* spp., *Corynebacterium* spp., and *Escherichia coli* have been the most common bacterial isolates in canine infective endocarditis.
- *Bartonella* spp. is being isolated with increasing frequency.
- A wide variety of other organisms has been cultured from individual cases, with many nosocomial cases involving *Pseudomonas* spp., *Proteus* spp., or other antibiotic-resistant isolates. Anaerobic bacteria (e.g., *Bacteroides* spp.) are occasionally found.

DIAGNOSIS

Endocarditis is suspected based on clinical signs and the presence of a heart murmur on physical exam. The index of suspicion may increase substantially based on echocardiographic findings, but a positive bacterial blood culture is required to establish the clinical diagnosis.

DIFFERENTIAL DIAGNOSIS

- Presenting complaints of animals with infective endocarditis tend to be vague and associated with some aspect of systemic illness (e.g., fever, lameness).
- Endocarditis should be included in the differential diagnosis of any persistent fever of unknown origin, especially in the presence of a heart murmur.

INITIAL DATABASE

- Definitive diagnosis requires the synthesis of clinical, laboratory (microbiologic), and echocardiographic data.
- Complete blood count or serum biochemical changes are not specific.
- Echocardiography reveals an oscillating mass at a site of endocardial injury (i.e., a mass near but separate from the valve, whose movements are distinct from those of the valve; it is important to note that this excludes valves that are merely thickened, as in endocardiosis).
- Two separate blood cultures must be positive for a typical organism and obtained by separate venipunctures an hour apart (three cultures are recommended if time, money, and patient size permits; at least two must be positive).
- In acutely ill patients with apparent sepsis syndrome, three blood cultures 5 to 10 minutes apart should be obtained if the patient's size permits, followed by empiric antibiotic therapy.

ADVANCED OR CONFIRMATORY TESTING

- Patients with suspected or definite endocarditis should have electrocardiograms recorded (and repeated regularly during their clinical course), because the onset of AV or bundle-branch block suggests perivalvular extension of the infection.
- When blood cultures from suspected infective endocarditis patients remain sterile after 72 hours of incubation, the laboratory should intensify efforts to grow fastidious organisms such as *Bartonella* spp., and the clinician should initiate alternative (e.g., serologic, polymerase chain reaction) assessment.

TREATMENT

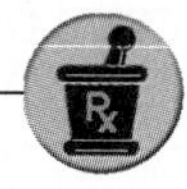

THERAPEUTIC GOAL(S)

- Provide effective anti-infective therapy to minimize valve damage
- Manage complications (e.g., heart failure)

ACUTE GENERAL TREATMENT

- Treatment is usually begun with parenteral antibiotic combinations in hospitalized dogs, but once the fever has resolved and clinical improvement (e.g., return of appetite) is evident (generally not more than 3 to 5 days), treatment is completed on an outpatient basis with oral antibiotics.
- Treatment is based on blood culture and sensitivity results; these results are not available for the first critical hours or days of therapy.
- Empiric antibiotic therapy for dogs with a clinical history and echocardiographic findings compatible with endocarditis is started with a combination of fluoroquinolone and penicillin-based antibiotics. Parenteral enrofloxacin (5 mg/kg IV q 12h) and amoxicillin (20 mg/kg IV q 8h) are most often chosen.
- Although discussed by some veterinary authors, anticoagulation does not appear to diminish the risk of bacterial embolization in humans, and is not generally recommended.

CHRONIC TREATMENT

- Therapy is generally continued for 12 weeks, and blood cultures are ideally obtained after 10 to 14 days (on antibiotics), and then again 1 week after stopping antibiotics.
- If *Bartonella* spp. is identified by culture or serology, azithromycin, 5-10 mg/kg PO q 24h is recommended for the first 7 days, then every other day for 6 to 12 weeks.

POSSIBLE COMPLICATIONS

Congestive heart failure, renal failure, or neurologic events are the complications that appear to have the greatest influence on prognosis.

PROGNOSIS AND OUTCOME

- Prognosis at the time of diagnosis is guarded due to the future possibilities of embolic complications and/or congestive heart failure.
- Long-term prognosis depends primarily on the valve damage that has been done at the time of diagnosis, as well as the response to antibiotic therapy.
- Recurrence or treatment failure is likely with inadequate duration of therapy, inappropriate antibiotic selection, or owner noncompliance.
- Despite optimal therapy and therapeutic monitoring, cure rates for endocarditis do not appear to be especially promising in dogs, and heart failure or deteriorations due to recurrent embolic events is often the long-term result.

PEARLS & CONSIDERATIONS

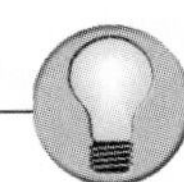

COMMENTS

- Although both can cause valve thickening and heart murmurs, taking a broader perspective of the case can more clearly demonstrate the differences between acute bacterial endocarditis (typically medium- to large-breed dogs of any age; overt clinical signs of recurrent infection/sepsis; new onset heart murmur; overall, occurs fairly rarely) and endocardiosis (medium to small breed dog, generally older adult; no link to overt signs of infection; murmur may be new in onset or long-standing; very common).
- The murmur of aortic insufficiency is often heard best by placing the diaphragm of the stethoscope in the animal's left armpit with the animal lying on its left side (on top of the stethoscope).
- A high index of suspicion for endocarditis is warranted in cases of diskospondylitis, and in any animal with fever and a diastolic murmur.
- With appropriate therapy, prognosis appears to be better for animals with less aggressive organisms such as *Bartonella* spp. if valve damage is not too severe at time of diagnosis.

PREVENTION

Animals with subaortic stenosis, animals with cardiac implants (e.g., transvenous pacemakers), and animals that have undergone balloon valvuloplasty should receive routine antibiotic prophylaxis for all procedures that are likely to induce transient bacteremia.

CLIENT EDUCATION

Owner compliance is perhaps an even bigger issue in the treatment of endocarditis than it is with other heart diseases, and effective explanation of the rationale for extended (often expensive) antibiotic treatment and a guarded prognosis is therefore critical.

SUGGESTED READING

Breitschwerdt EB, et al: Clinicopathological abnormalities and treatment response in 24 dogs seroreactive to *Bartonella vinsonii* (berkhoffii) antigens. *J Am Anim Hosp Assoc* 40(2):92, 2004.

MacDonald KA, et al: A prospective study of canine infective endocarditis in northern California (1999–2001): Emergence of *Bartonella* as a prevalent etiologic agent. *J Vet Intern Med* 1:56, 2004.

Wall M, Calvert C, Greene CE: Infective endocarditis in dogs. *Compend Cont Ed Pract Vet* 10(8):614–625, 2002.

AUTHOR: **BRUCE W. KEENE**

EDITOR: **ETIENNE CÔTÉ**

Entropion/Ectropion

BASIC INFORMATION

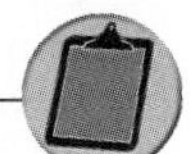

DEFINITION

- *Entropion* is the inversion of part or the entire eyelid margin toward the eye (Fig. I-60); may be developmental or acquired.
- *Ectropion* is the eversion of part or the entire eyelid margin away from the eye; may be developmental or acquired.

SYNONYM(S)

Inrolled eyelid (entropion)
Everted eyelid (ectropion)

EPIDEMIOLOGY

SPECIES, AGE, SEX

Entropion:

- Dogs common; cats less common
- Can occur at any age; developmental entropion usually develops in dogs <1 year of age
- No sex predisposition

Ectropion:

- Dogs
- Age variable, depends on cause
- No sex predisposition

GENETICS AND BREED PREDISPOSITION

Developmental entropion:

- Lateral entropion: English bulldog, chow chow, shar-pei, Saint Bernard, boxer, rottweiler, pointers, spaniels, and all retrievers.
- Medial canthal entropion: miniature and toy poodles, English bulldog, Cavalier King Charles spaniel, Maltese, and brachycephalic breeds including Pekingese, pug, and shih tzu; brachycephalic cats.
- Genetic basis not fully understood; considered inherited as a simple dominant trait, with complete penetrance in some breeds of dogs.

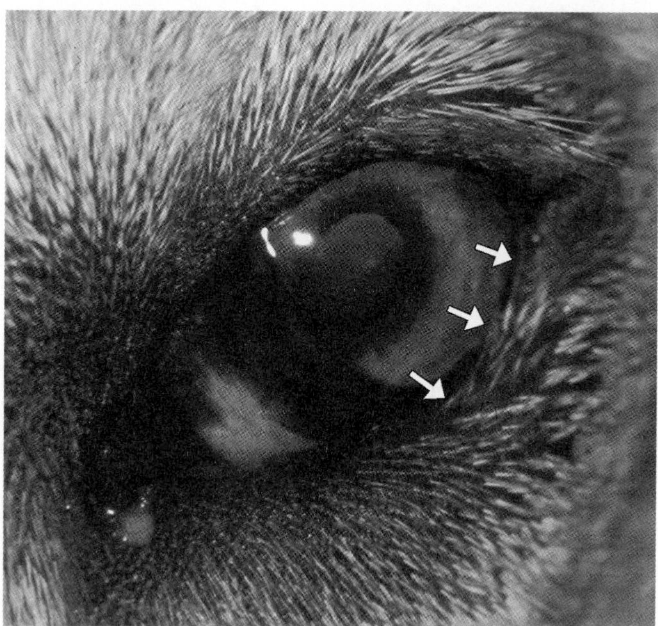

FIGURE I-60 Entropion of the ventrolateral eyelid in a dog (*arrows*). Note the prolapse of the third eyelid and mild mucoid ocular discharge at the medial canthus, which are common concurrent findings.

Developmental ectropion: bloodhound, St. Bernard, Great Dane, bullmastiff, Newfoundland, and some spaniel breeds.

Combination entropion-ectropion affecting the same lid: bloodhound, Saint Bernard, and English bulldog.

RISK FACTORS

Developmental entropion and ectropion:

- Breed predisposition

Acquired entropion:

- Ocular conditions that stimulate blepharospasm (e.g., see Conjunctivitis: Dogs, p 233, Cats, p 231; Corneal Ulceration, p 246)
- Eyelid trauma (see Eyelid Defects: Trauma, Masses, p 371)
- Blepharitis
- Old age and associated loss of orbicularis oculi muscle tone
- Phthisis bulbi (see Ocular Size Abnormalities, p 763)
- Enophthalmos (see Orbital Disease, p 773)

Acquired ectropion:

- Eyelid trauma (see Eyelid Defects: Trauma, Masses, p 371)
- Blepharitis
- Old age and associated loss of orbicularis oculi muscle tone
- Facial nerve paralysis

ASSOCIATED CONDITIONS AND DISORDERS

- Conjunctivitis
- Keratitis (ulcerative and nonulcerative)
- See Risk Factors above

CLINICAL PRESENTATION

DISEASE FORMS/SUBTYPES: Developmental and acquired forms.

HISTORY, CHIEF COMPLAINT

Entropion:

- Ocular discharge
- Blepharospasm
- "Red" eye
- Visible inrolling of eyelid
- ± Vision impairment in severe cases

Ectropion:

- Ocular discharge
- "Red" eye
- "Droopy"/"long" lower eyelid

PHYSICAL EXAM FINDINGS

- *Entropion*:
  - Inversion of the eyelid (see Fig. I-60) and some or all of the following:
    - Conjunctivitis (Cats, see p 231; Dogs, see p 233)
    - Epiphora or mucoid to mucopurulent ocular discharge
    - Blepharospasm
    - Protrusion of the third eyelid (see Fig. I-60)
    - Nonulcerative keratitis (see Corneal Pigmentation, p 242; Corneal Vascularization, p 249)
    - Ulcerative keratitis (see Corneal Ulceration, p 246)
- *Ectropion*:
  - Eversion of the lower eyelid and some or all of the following:
    - Conjunctivitis (Dogs, see p 233)
    - Lagophthalmos (incomplete closure of the eyelids)

ETIOLOGY AND PATHOPHYSIOLOGY

Dogs:

- *Developmental entropion*:
  - Related to abnormal skull and palpebral fissure (eyelid opening) conformation.
  - Associated with misdirection of the lateral canthal ligament in mesaticephalic breeds.
  - Upper eyelid entropion can be associated with ptosis and weight from excessive dorsal skinfolds.
  - Associated with microblepharon (small eyelids).
- *Acquired entropion*:
  - Decreased orbital support (decreased orbital mass, phthisis bulbi, or retractor bulbi muscle contraction) predisposes to loss of lid support (see Orbital Disease, p 773).
  - Secondary to blepharospasm.
  - Secondary to scarring and contraction of the eyelid from a previous eyelid injury and/or inflammation.
- *Developmental ectropion*:
  - Mild ectropion is a desired feature in some breeds (i.e., hounds).
  - Related to abnormal skull and palpebral fissure conformation.
  - Associated with laxity of the palpebral fissure related to macroblepharon.
- *Acquired ectropion*:
  - Transient ectropion results from laxity of the eyelid from relaxation or following excessive exercise in breeds with long lower eyelids.
  - Scarring and contraction of the eyelid from a previous eyelid injury and/or inflammation.
  - Facial nerve paralysis.

Cats:

- *Developmental entropion*:
  - Medial canthal entropion in brachycephalic breeds.
- *Acquired entropion*:
  - Decreased orbital support associated with loss of orbital and periorbital fat predisposes to loss of eyelid support.
  - Secondary to blepharospasm.
  - Associated with scarring and contraction from chronic conjunctival and/or eyelid inflammation.

DIAGNOSIS

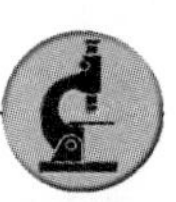

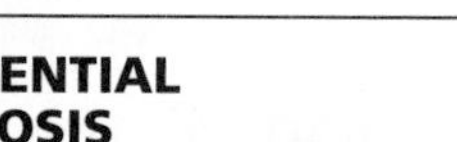

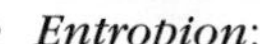

DIFFERENTIAL DIAGNOSIS

- *Entropion*:
  - Usually readily diagnosed on clinical examination; must be differentiated from:
    - Distichiasis (see Distichiasis/Ectopic Cilia/Trichiasis, p 317): one or more cilia emerge from the meibomian glands instead of the normal peripheral lid margin.
    - Trichiasis (see Distichiasis/Ectopic Cilia/Trichiasis, p 317): normal eyelid or facial hair directed toward, and contacting, the conjunctiva or cornea.
- *Ectropion*:
  - Usually readily diagnosed on clinical examination: apparent even before handling the patient.

INITIAL DATABASE

Complete ophthalmic examination including:

- Schirmer tear test (normal >15 mm after 1 minute in dogs, variable in cats)
- Fluorescein dye application
- Intraocular pressures
- Careful examination of conformation of eyelid margins, conjunctiva, and cornea

ADVANCED OR CONFIRMATORY TESTING

- Variable depending on underlying cause of acquired entropion and/or ectropion.
- With entropion, apply topical anesthetic (e.g., proparacaine 0.5%) to eye to evaluate degree of spastic entropion (i.e., entropion secondary to ocular pain versus developmental entropion or entropion from primary ocular disease such as ulcerative or nonulcerative keratitis). Spastic entropion temporarily resolves or decreases in severity within a few minutes of proparacaine application.
- Examine animal in a relaxed state to determine extent of entropion and/or ectropion and to select most appropriate corrective surgical technique; restraining the animal or manipulation of the head at examination can increase the severity of blepharospasm and exaggerate the degree of entropion.

TREATMENT

THERAPEUTIC GOAL(S)

- Resolve any underlying painful ocular disease (e.g., conjunctivitis, keratitis)
- Correct entropion (temporary versus permanent repair; see Acute General Treatment)
- Correct ectropion (if severe and predisposing to chronic ocular irritation)

ACUTE GENERAL TREATMENT

Entropion:

- Treat underlying condition(s) (see Corneal Ulceration, p 246; Conjunctivitis: Cats, p 231; Conjunctivitis: Dogs, p 233)
- Temporary correction until adult conformation reached (i.e., in puppies), or until underlying condition resolved:
    - Roll eyelids away from eye by placing temporary tacking or temporary tarsorrhaphy sutures to prevent chronic ocular pain and blepharospasm, and to prevent corneal pigmentation, vascularization, ulceration, and scarring
    - If successful, may not require permanent repair
- Permanent correction once adult conformation reached (increases success) and no other underlying condition (see Chronic Treatment)

CHRONIC TREATMENT

- Chronic *entropion* in mature animal:
    - Requires some form of surgery to evert the eyelid margin including:
    - Cases of mild entropion:
        - Consider Hotz-Celsus procedure (surgical procedure involving excision of an elliptic section of skin adjacent to the lid margin)
    - Lateral canthal entropion:
        - Creation or cutting of the lateral canthal ligament (modified Wyman's lateral canthoplasty or lateral canthal tenotomy, respectively)
        - Hotz-Celsus procedure and eyelid shortening procedure may be needed
    - Medial canthal entropion:
        - Medial canthoplasty procedure (e.g., pocket flap or Wyman technique)
        - Localized Hotz-Celsus procedure
    - Ptosis and upper eyelid entropion:
        - Stades' procedure to evert upper eyelid margin
- *Ectropion*:
    - Surgery rarely needed unless severe or if concurrent with entropion elsewhere on the lid
    - Cases of severe ectropion:
        - Consider modified Khunt-Szymanowski technique (lid-shortening procedure)
    - Cicatricial ectropion
        - V-Y blepharoplasty may be used

POSSIBLE COMPLICATIONS

- Temporary tacking sutures may pull through skin, necessitating repeat procedure(s) until animal is mature or until underlying condition is resolved
- Undercorrection or overcorrection of entropion
- Correction of subclinical ectropion predisposing to entropion

RECOMMENDED MONITORING

- Leave the temporary tacking sutures or temporary tarsorrhaphy in place until adult conformation reached, or for 2 to 3 weeks until concurrent ocular disease resolves.
- Permanent entropion and/or ectropion repairs require suture removal approximately 10 to 14 days after surgery.

PROGNOSIS AND OUTCOME

- Prognosis for restoring normal eyelid conformation is good
- Recurrence of entropion is possible depending on underlying cause and surgical treatment

PEARLS & CONSIDERATIONS

COMMENTS

- Treat any concurrent ocular disease before surgically correcting entropion.
- No single surgical procedure is effective for correction of all forms of entropion and/or ectropion (see Chronic Treatment above for some options).
- Shy on the side of undercorrection when performing entropion surgery; further future correction is much easier to manage than the other extreme (overcorrection causing ectropion).
- Correction of naturally occurring ectropion is rarely needed unless severe or occurs in conjunction with entropion on the same eyelid.

PREVENTION

Avoid breeding affected or closely related dogs with developmental entropion or clinically significant developmental ectropion.

CLIENT EDUCATION

If the initial repair is ineffective, additional surgical procedures may be needed.

SUGGESTED READING

Bedford PGC: Diseases and surgery of the canine eyelid. In Gelatt KN (ed): *Veterinary Ophthalmology*. Philadelphia, Lippincott Williams & Wilkins, 1999, pp 535-568.

Lackner PA: Techniques for surgical correction of adnexal disease. *Clin Tech Small Anim Pract* 16(1):40, 2001.

Martin CL: Eyelids. In Martin CL (ed): *Ophthalmic Disease in Veterinary Medicine*. London, Manson Publishing, Ltd, 2005, pp 145-182.

AUTHOR: **PHILLIP A. MOORE**

EDITOR: **CHERYL L. CULLEN**

Eosinophilic Granuloma Complex, Dermatologic

Client Education Sheet on Website

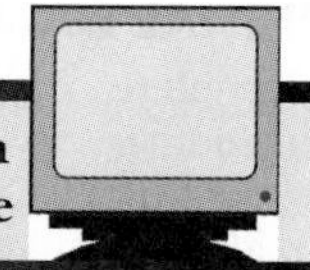

BASIC INFORMATION

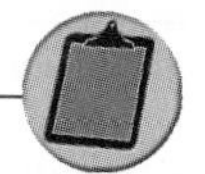

DEFINITION

A group of conditions likely erroneously grouped together based on typical clinical presentation and a possible eosinophilic dermatitis on histopathology

SYNONYM(S)

Eosinophilic granuloma: collagenolytic granuloma, linear granuloma

Eosinophilic ulcer: indolent ulcer, rodent ulcer

Feline eosinophilic skin diseases (dermatoses)

EPIDEMIOLOGY

SPECIES, AGE, SEX: Cats. No age or gender predisposition. However, eosinophilic plaques and granulomas may be more common in younger cats.

GENETICS AND BREED PREDISPOSITION: A genetic predisposition has been hypothesized because of lesion development in a colony of related pathogen-free cats. No breed or coat color predisposition.

GEOGRAPHY AND SEASONALITY: Warm weather seasonality may be observed.

ASSOCIATED CONDITIONS AND DISORDERS: Miliary dermatitis or feline symmetric alopecia may also be noted.

CLINICAL PRESENTATION

DISEASE FORMS/SUBTYPES: Three major forms:

- Eosinophilic plaque.
- Eosinophilic granuloma: A distinct form of eosinophilic granuloma is seen in cases of mosquito-bite hypersensitivity.
- Eosinophilic ulcer.

HISTORY, CHIEF COMPLAINT: Affected individuals usually present for pain or pruritus associated with lesion development. Lesions may be insidious in onset.

PHYSICAL EXAM FINDINGS

- Eosinophilic plaque: erythematous papules and raised plaquelike lesions, commonly on the ventral abdomen and medial thighs.
- Eosinophilic granuloma: erythematous, raised, alopecic lesions.
- Three distinct forms:
  - Nodules found in oral cavity (see Eosinophilic Granuloma Complex, Oral, p 349).
  - Linear lesions may be found on the lateral thorax, lateral shoulder, or caudal aspect of thighs in young cats, usually without pruritus.
  - Mosquito bite hypersensitivity: papules and crusts affecting bridge of nose, preauricular region, or pinnae.
- Eosinophilic ulcer: well-demarcated ulcer with a raised edge surrounding a pink-yellow ulcerated surface, developing in the midline of the upper lip, or adjacent to the upper canine tooth; may also affect the philtrum (Fig. I-61).
- All three forms may be observed in an individual cat. These lesions may also be seen in cats presenting with miliary dermatitis and/or feline symmetric alopecia.

ETIOLOGY AND PATHOPHYSIOLOGY

- Different forms may be regarded as different reaction patterns to the same underlying etiology, most commonly thought to be a hypersensitivity disorder to arthropods (flea, mosquito), food, or environmental allergens.
- Other suggested causes include viral and bacterial infections, chronic trauma, and autoimmune reactions.

DIAGNOSIS

DIFFERENTIAL DIAGNOSIS

- Allergic causes: contact dermatitis
- Infectious causes: viral (poxvirus, herpesvirus, calicivirus), fungal (dermatophytosis)
- Ectoparasites: *Otodectes*, *Notoedres*, *Cheyletiella*, trombiculosis, pediculosis, demodicosis
- Neoplasia: squamous cell carcinoma, mast cell tumor, fibrosarcoma, cutaneous lymphoma
- Autoimmune/immune-mediated causes: pemphigus foliaceus, drug reaction
- Actinic dermatitis

INITIAL DATABASE

- Trichogram: microscopic examination of plucked hairs may reveal broken hair tips indicating self-trauma.
- Ectoparasite examination: Skin scrapings are negative; flea combing may confirm the presence of a flea infestation.
- Cytology: large numbers of eosinophils with neutrophils, extracellular bacteria may be noted.
- Routine hematology: Mild to moderate eosinophilia may be noted.
- Retroviral testing (feline leukemia virus/feline immunodeficiency virus).

ADVANCED OR CONFIRMATORY TESTING

- Bacterial, fungal, mycobacterial cultures: negative
- Skin biopsy: a predominantly eosinophilic dermal infiltrate with possible flame figures (collagen fibers surrounded by eosinophilic material)
- Elimination diet trial: 8 to 10 weeks. If skin lesions resolve, rechallenge with original diet to confirm (reappearance of lesions)
- Intradermal and/or serologic allergy testing: positive reaction to fleas and other environmental allergens

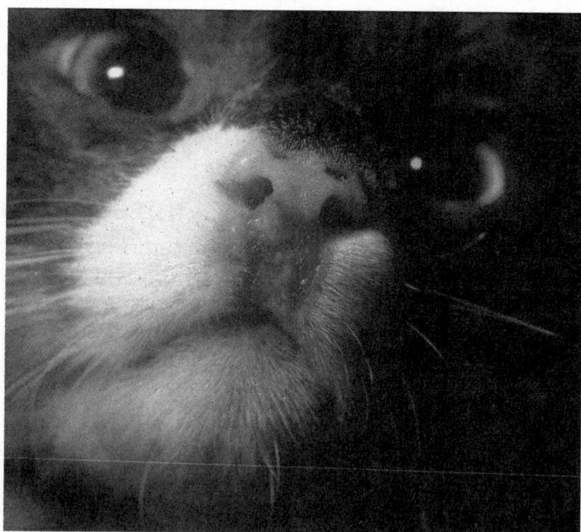

FIGURE I-61 Eosinophilic ulcer of the upper lip midline and the philtrum in a cat. Courtesy of Dr. Edmund J. Rosser, Michigan State University.

- Empiric ectoparasiticidal therapy: topical selamectin (Revolution) q 2 weeks for three doses or topical lime sulfur (LymDip; DVM) q 7 days for three treatments for all cats in the household

TREATMENT

THERAPEUTIC GOAL(S)

- Benign neglect in young cats with single linear eosinophilic granuloma lesions and no overt signs of pruritus
- Treat the underlying cause where appropriate
- Supportive nonspecific therapy, especially if the cat is extremely pruritic

ACUTE AND CHRONIC TREATMENT

Etiologic therapy:

- Flea control: treat all cats in the household and, where appropriate, the environment
- Hypoallergenic diet
- Allergen specific immunotherapy (desensitization)

Supportive nonspecific therapy—classical:

- Oral glucocortioids: 1 to 2 mg/kg prednisone (or prednisolone) PO q 12h initially, then weaning down to lowest effective dose.
- Injectable glucocorticoids: 4 mg/kg methylprednisolone (maximum 20 mg) IM (Depo-Medrol).
- Risks include induction of diabetes mellitus, iatrogenic Cushing's disease, and delayed tissue healing.

Supportive nonspecific therapy—alternative options for cats that respond poorly to glucocorticoid therapy may include:

- Oral antibiotics: clavulanic acid potentiated amoxicillin (Clavamox) 12.5 mg/kg PO q 12h for 3 weeks.
- Oral antihistamines: chlorpheniramine maleate (2-4 mg/cat PO q 12h), or amitriptyline (5 mg/cat PO q 12h) for 3 weeks. Use in combination with essential fatty acids PO.
- Oral cyclosporine: 5-10 mg/kg PO q 24h initially, then 5-10 mg/kg PO q 48h. Potential side effects include vomiting, diarrhea, and possible fatal acute toxoplasmosis.
- Oral chlorambucil: 2 mg/cat PO q 48h (in addition to prednisone). Monitor for adverse bone marrow effects. Use chemotherapy precautions.
- Injectable sodium aurothiomalate: 1 mg/kg IM q 7d.
- Megestrol acetate: 2.5-5 mg q 2-7d. Risk of severe side effects.
- Oral interferon alpha: 30-60 units/cat PO q 24h for 30 days.

Others: surgical excision, cryosurgery, laser and radiation therapies for single lesions.

PROGNOSIS AND OUTCOME

Prognosis is good

PEARLS & CONSIDERATIONS

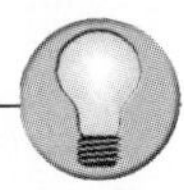

COMMENTS

Feline eosinophilic granuloma complex is not a specific diagnosis. A primary underlying cause is likely to be present, and should be investigated and treated.

SUGGESTED READING

Fondati A: Histopathologic study of feline eosinophilic dermatoses. *Vet Dermatol* 12:333, 2001.

Power HT, et al: Selected feline eosinophilic skin diseases. *Vet Clin North Am Small Anim Pract* 25:833, 1995.

AUTHOR: **VINCENT E. DEFALQUE**

EDITOR: **JAN A. HALL**

Eosinophilic Granuloma Complex, Oral

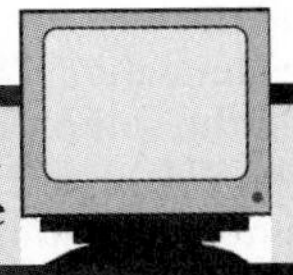

Client Education Sheet on Website

BASIC INFORMATION

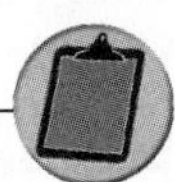

DEFINITION

- In cats, eosinophilic granuloma is one manifestation of an idiopathic complex of frequently encountered chronic, progressive lesions involving the oral cavity, lips, skin of the trunk, and extremities.
- In dogs, eosinophilic granuloma is a rare disease process characterized by single or multiple ulcerated lesions in the oral cavity.

SYNONYM(S)

The eosinophilic granuloma complex of cats can be divided into three separate lesions: eosinophilic ulcer ("rodent ulcer"), eosinophilic plaque, and linear granuloma.

EPIDEMIOLOGY

SPECIES, AGE, SEX

- Eosinophilic ulcer is seen in cats with a 3:1 female predisposition.
- Eosinophilic plaque is seen in cats from 2 to 6 years of age, and without a sex predilection.
- Linear granuloma is seen in 6-month-old to 5-year-old cats, and in females over males, 2:1.
- Canine oral eosinophilic granulomas are rare, and epidemiologic data are limited. Reported cases have been less than 4 years of age, with an 80% male predisposition.

GENETICS AND BREED PREDISPOSITION

- There is no known breed predilection in cats. A high incidence was reported in a group of interrelated specific pathogen-free cats in a closed breeding colony, suggesting a heritable predisposition.
- Siberian huskies and Cavalier King Charles spaniels have an increased frequency of oral eosinophilic granulomas. The hereditary basis in dogs is unknown.

RISK FACTORS: In one publication, 90% of cats with eosinophilic ulcers were feline leukemia virus positive.

CONTAGION AND ZOONOSIS: Multiple cases in a multicat household, and experimental transmission from one area on a cat to another, suggest an infectious etiology.

GEOGRAPHY AND SEASONALITY: Seasonal recurrence has been noted in Cavalier King Charles spaniels.

ASSOCIATED CONDITIONS AND DISORDERS: Eosinophilic plaques are occasionally seen with flea and food allergies.

CLINICAL PRESENTATION

DISEASE FORMS/SUBTYPES

- Feline:
  - Eosinophilic ulcers and plaques: 20% occur in the oral cavity and present as well-circumscribed, raised, ulcerated, and erythematous lesions of variable size.
  - Linear granulomas: symmetric, well-circumscribed, raised, firm, yellow or white, and gritty in appearance.
- Canine:
  - Cavalier King Charles spaniels: single or multiple ulcerated lesions on the lateral or ventral surface of the tongue and soft palate; do not appear as granulomas.
  - Siberian huskies: raised, firm, yellowish (ulcerated) masses with well demarcated edges appearing on the

lateral or ventral surface of the tongue or frenulum.

HISTORY, CHIEF COMPLAINTS: Dysphagia, hypersalivation, halitosis, difficulty eating, reduced appetite, and occasionally coughing.

PHYSICAL EXAM FINDINGS

- Abnormalities are, in general, confined to the oral cavity as described above.
- Skin lesions associated with feline eosinophilic ulcers and plaques are confined to the dermis and epidermis, are alopecic, and are intensely pruritic (see Eosinophilic Granuloma Complex, Dermatologic, p 348).
- Linear granulomas are linear, confined to the dermis, and otherwise associated with no other specific clinical signs.

ETIOLOGY AND PATHOPHYSIOLOGY

Unknown etiology, but associations have been made with:

- Hypersensitivity reactions (flea and food allergies)
- Self-inflicted trauma due to grooming
- Poor oral hygiene
- Genetic factors

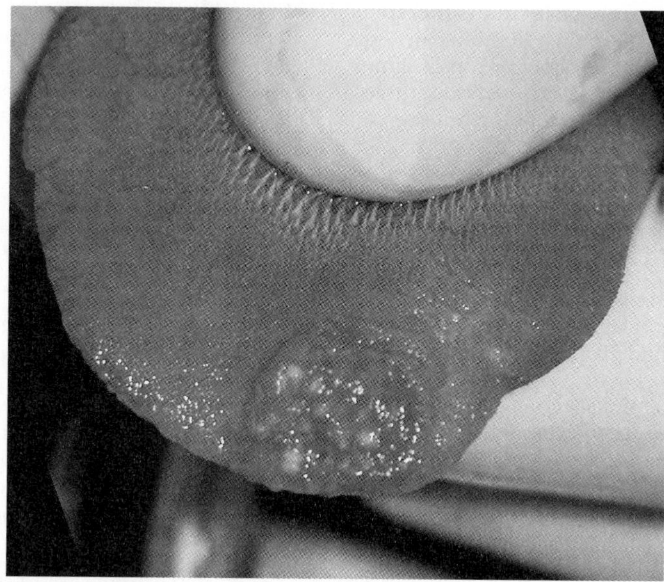

FIGURE I-62 Eosinophilic lesion near the tip of the tongue in a cat. Courtesy of Dr. Alexander M. Reiter, University of Pennsylvania.

DIAGNOSIS

Veterinarians familiar with this disease may be able to recognize an eosinophilic ulcer on the upper lip in cats by means of physical (oral) examination. The same is true for lesions on the soft palate in Cavalier King Charles spaniels. For any tongue lesions, biopsy and histopathologic evaluation of tissue are essential, to rule out squamous cell carcinoma; both conditions can be very similar in appearance. Soft palate fibrosarcomas in young dogs may often start as slightly raised and ulcerated lesions. To be certain and avoid misdiagnosis, biopsy is recommended in all suspected cases regardless of location.

DIFFERENTIAL DIAGNOSIS

- Neoplasia
- Focal inflammation due to a foreign body, trauma, or an infectious agent

INITIAL DATABASE

- History and physical exam are central to the diagnosis.
- Complete blood count.
  - Peripheral eosinophilia:
    - Reported with a 33-60% frequency
    - Occurs with feline eosinophilic plaques
- Lesion cytology cannot be used for confirming the diagnosis.

ADVANCED OR CONFIRMATORY TESTING

- Histopathologic evaluation of lesions details ulceration of the epidermis and infiltration of the dermis with eosinophils, lymphocytes, plasma cells, histiocytes, and mast cells; collagen necrosis.
- Recent ultrastructural studies show massive eosinophil degranulation and no alteration in collagen fibrils.

TREATMENT

THERAPEUTIC GOAL(S)

Complete regression of the lesion

ACUTE GENERAL TREATMENT

- Prednisone 1-2 mg/kg PO q 12-24h × 7 days, then tapered to the lowest effective dosage q 48h over several weeks to months. Transdermal application of prednisone ointment onto the pinnae may be an alternative to oral administration; or
- Methylprednisolone 20 mg SQ every 3 weeks for 2-3 doses; if chronic case, maintenance therapy at 20 mg SQ prn unless adverse effects are noted (history, exam, lab tests).
- Surgical excision in selected cases (e.g., certain lesions in sublingual tissue).

CHRONIC TREATMENT

- Radiation therapy is effective in cats.
- Levamisole will induce complete remission in 75% of feline cases.

POSSIBLE COMPLICATIONS

- Inadequate initial therapy may result in refractory lesions.
- Adverse effects to medications (glucocorticoids: polyuria, polydipsia, polyphagia, iatrogenic hyperadrenocorticism; levamisole: vomiting, neurologic abnormalities).

RECOMMENDED MONITORING

Until complete lesion regression

PROGNOSIS AND OUTCOME

Good if complete remission with initial course of therapy

PEARLS & CONSIDERATIONS

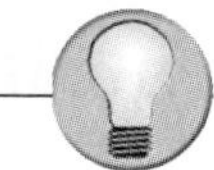

COMMENTS

Treat early and aggressively with glucocorticoids

SUGGESTED READING

Bardagi M, et al: Ultrastructural study of cutaneous lesions in feline eosinophilic granuloma complex. *Vet Dermatol* 14:297, 2003.

Bredal WP, et al: Oral eosinophilic granuloma in three Cavalier King Charles spaniels. *J Small Anim Pract* 37(10):499, 1996.

Madewell BR, et al: Oral eosinophilic granuloma in Siberian husky dogs. *J Am Vet Med Assoc* 177(8):323, 1983.

Pedersen NC: Inflammatory oral cavity diseases of the cat. *Vet Clin North Am Small Anim Pract* 22(6):1323, 1992.

Power HT, Ihrke PJ: Selected feline eosinophilic skin diseases. *Vet Clin North Am* 25(4):833, 1995.

Russell RG, et al: Filamentous bacteria in oral eosinophilic granulomas of a cat. *Vet Pathol* 25(3):249, 1988.

AUTHOR: **JAMIE G. ANDERSON**

EDITOR: **ALEXANDER M. REITER**

Epilepsy, Idiopathic

BASIC INFORMATION

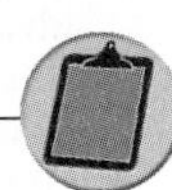

DEFINITION

A syndrome characterized by chronic recurrent seizures for which there is no identifiable cause.

Other terms:

- Status epilepticus: a seizure lasting more than 5 minutes, or two or more seizures in which there is incomplete recovery of consciousness.
- Cluster seizures (also called serial or acute repetitive seizures): three or more isolated seizures occuring within a short period of time.

SYNONYM(S)

Primary epilepsy

EPIDEMIOLOGY

SPECIES, AGE, SEX

- Dogs: commonly affected, 1 to 5 years old, slightly more common in males
- Cats: uncommonly affected

GENETICS AND BREED PREDISPOSITION

- More common in large-breed dogs but any breed can be affected
- Inherited in beagle, Belgian Tervuren, keeshond, dachshund, British Alsatian, labrador retriever, golden retriever, collie, and probably others

ASSOCIATED CONDITIONS AND DISORDERS: Hyperthermia can occur during status epilepticus due to muscle activity.

CLINICAL PRESENTATION

HISTORY, CHIEF COMPLAINT

- One or more seizures.
- Most common are generalized tonic-clonic seizures, characterized by loss of consciousness and sustained contraction of all muscles followed by paddling motions of the limbs or rhythmic muscle contractions, especially of the limbs and masticatory muscles.
- Also possible are milder generalized tonic-clonic seizures, in which consciousness is maintained, and focal seizures in which only part of the body is involved (e.g., fly-biting movements).
- With idiopathic epilepsy, the interictal period (period between seizures, after recovery) is normal and owners do not report evidence of ongoing neurologic deficits.
- An effort should be made to clarify any possible sources of intoxication (e.g., lead, ethylene glycol, organophosphate, carbamate, metaldehyde).

PHYSICAL EXAM FINDINGS

- Normal unless examined immediately after a seizure when temporary postictal deficits are possible, including generalized ataxia, abnormal behavior, and blindness that proceed to resolve over minutes to hours.
- Persistent neurologic deficits, such as hemiparesis, abnormal behavior, or visual deficits, are inconsistent with idiopathic epilepsy and suggest an underlying structural neurologic lesion.
- Persistent fontanelle may or may not be associated with hydrocephalus; however, it offers an acoustic window for ultrasonography to pursue this diagnosis.
- A fundic examination is essential. Uveal, retinal, or optic disk diseases that may correlate with causes of seizures and are inconsistent with idiopathic epilepsy include optic neuritis, feline infectious peritonitis, toxoplasmosis/neosporosis, systemic mycoses, rickettsial diseases, systemic hypertension, lymphoma, and metastatic neoplasia.

ETIOLOGY AND PATHOPHYSIOLOGY

Theories include inborn abnormalities in neuronal excitability, neurotransmitter, or receptor function

DIAGNOSIS

Idiopathic epilepsy is a clinical diagnosis based on the typical age of onset, lack of persistent neurologic deficits, and exclusion of other potential causes based on laboratory testing. A presumptive diagnosis of idiopathic epilepsy may be made without comprehensive diagnostic testing, when the patient's signalment and history are consistent with epilepsy, and physical and neurologic examination findings and initial database results are normal. In such cases, further testing may be pursued if deterioration or failure to respond to medication is noted. By declining a comprehensive evaluation, the patient's owner must assume the responsibility that an underlying, progressive lesion, rather than epilepsy, may be present.

DIFFERENTIAL DIAGNOSIS

- Metabolic disorders: hepatic encephalopathy including portosystemic shunt, hypoglycemia, polycythemia, hypocalcemia.
- Toxins: lead, ethylene glycol, organophosphate, carbamate, metaldehyde.
- Brain malformations: hydrocephalus, lissencephaly.
- Inherited degenerative diseases such as lysosomal storage diseases.
- Encephalitis: granulomatous meningoencephalitis, necrotizing encephalitis, distemper, tick-borne infections, fungal encephalitis, *Neospora caninum*, *Toxoplasma gondii*, feline infectious peritonitis.
- Neoplasia: primary and metastatic brain tumor.
- Vascular lesions: infarct, hemorrhage.
- Head injury.
- Also consider nonepileptic episodes such as syncope, narcolepsy, exercise-induced weakness, vestibular dysfunction, and episodes of pain.

INITIAL DATABASE

- Complete blood count: generally unremarkable. Nucleated red blood cells and/or basophilic stippling suggest lead toxicity rather than epilepsy; acanthocytes nonspecifically suggest hepatic disease.
- Serum chemistry profile, urinalysis: help to identify hypoglycemia, hepatic encephalopathy, and renal failure (uremic encephalopathy) as possible causes of seizures instead of idiopathic epilepsy. Fasting hypercholesterolemia may suggest hypothyroidism and attendant central nervous system effects if hyperlipidemia is severe. Hypocalcemia can produce intense muscle tremors that may be misinterpreted as seizures. Hyperglobulinemia in cats raises the possibility of feline infectious peritonitis-based encephalitis as the cause of seizures rather than epilepsy.
- Serum bile acids (preprandial and postprandial):
  - Elevation of either or both suggests hepatic encephalopathy (portosystemic shunt, cirrhotic/fibrosing liver disease, other) rather than idiopathic epilepsy.
  - However, moderate elevations in bile acids routinely may occur soon after a seizure of any cause. In these cases, it is warranted to recheck bile acids 2 to 4 weeks later to see if the abnormality persists.
- Blood lead concentration if potential exposure.

ADVANCED OR CONFIRMATORY TESTING

- Brain computed tomography (CT)/magnetic resonance imaging (MRI) and cerebrospinal fluid (CSF) analysis are

indicated in the following patients presenting with seizures and no identifiable systemic cause: dogs younger than 1 year or older than 5 years, dogs with persistent neurologic deficits, and cats. Results of these imaging procedures and CSF analysis are normal with idiopathic epilepsy (diagnosis of exclusion).
- EEG may show abnormalities that confirm seizure activity but do not definitively diagnose idiopathic epilepsy as the cause.

TREATMENT

Status epilepticus and cluster seizures require emergency treatment because they can lead to life-threatening complications such as hyperthermia and brain damage. Also, prolonged seizures become progressively refractory to treatment.

THERAPEUTIC GOAL(S)

- Reduce the frequency and severity of seizures to a level that does not substantially compromise the patient's and family's quality of life, while avoiding severe side effects.
- Daily medication is not indicated in patients with a single seizure, seizures caused by a transient condition (e.g., acute intoxication), or isolated seizures separated by a long period of time.
- Daily medication is indicated in patients with more than one isolated seizure per month, clusters of multiple seizures per day, or a clear pattern of increasing frequency or severity of seizures.

ACUTE GENERAL TREATMENT

- To stop an active seizure: diazepam 0.5-1 mg/kg IV to effect.
- If the seizure does not stop with three doses of diazepam, administer:
  - Pentobarbital 3-15 mg/kg, slow IV; or
  - Propofol 1-8 mg/kg IV to effect followed by continuous infusion at 0.1 mg/kg/min titrated to effect.
- If the seizure stops with the above therapy but recurs soon after, there are several options:
  - Load with phenobarbital: 12-24 mg/kg slow IV or IM, single dose, followed by maintenance doses of 2-3 mg/kg slow IV, IM, or PO, q 12h; or
  - Diazepam continuous rate infusion: 0.5-1 mg/kg/hr in 2.5% dextrose + 0.45% saline. Titrate based on seizure control and sedation.

CHRONIC TREATMENT

- Initial therapy with either phenobarbital or bromide.
- Phenobarbital:
  - Initial dose: 2-3 mg/kg PO q 12h (dog, cat) subsequently adjusted based on clinical effects and therapeutic monitoring.
  - Steady-state serum concentrations are reached about 10 days after starting therapy or changing the dose.
  - Common side effects: polyuria/polyphagia, sedation, ataxia.
- Potassium bromide:
  - Initial dose: 20-30 mg/kg PO q 24h (dog), subsequently changed based on clinical effects and therapeutic monitoring.
  - Cats: substantial risk of pneumonitis.
  - Steady-state serum concentrations are reached 2 to 3 months after starting therapy or changing the dose.
  - For more rapid control of seizures in dogs with frequent, severe seizures, administer a loading dose: 400 mg/kg total, divided into 6 to 8 doses over 48 hours.
  - Common side effects: polyuria/polyphagia, sedation, ataxia.
- If seizures are not adequately controlled despite target serum concentrations of the first drug, add a second drug while continuing the first drug. If the seizures become well controlled, it may be possible to gradually wean the first drug.
- Second-line drugs:
  - Zonisamide (10 mg/kg PO q 12h; dog).
  - Levetiracetam (20 mg/kg PO q 8h; dog, cat).
  - Gabapentin (100-300 mg PO total, q 8h; dog, cat).
  - Clorazepate (0.5-1 mg/kg PO q 8h; dog, cat).
  - Felbamate (15-45 mg/kg PO q 8h, dog).
- For dogs that suffer clusters of multiple seizures despite daily medication, at-home administration of diazepam per rectum can decrease the need for emergency veterinary care. The client administers 2 mg/kg of parenteral diazepam solution per rectum using a syringe and urinary catheter or teat cannula, repeated for a maximum total of three doses within 24 hours.

DRUG INTERACTIONS

- Phenobarbital may decrease the effect of chloramphenicol, corticosteroids, doxycycline, propanolol, and metronidazole. Other depressants and chloramphenicol may increase the effect of phenobarbital.
- Bromide: higher chloride intake increases bromide elimination, which increases the dose requirement; lower chloride decreases bromide elimination.

POSSIBLE COMPLICATIONS

- Phenobarbital-induced hepatotoxicity (see Phenobarbital: Adverse Effects/Toxicoses, p 844):
  - Minimized by avoiding serum concentrations >35 μg/ml.
  - Evidence of hepatotoxicity: increases in bile acid concentrations; proportionally larger increases of ALT compared to alkaline phosphatase; icterus, weight loss, ascites if very severe and advanced.
  - Potentially reversible if phenobarbital is stopped early enough.
- Phenobarbital rarely causes hematologic abnormalities, including neutropenia, anemia, and thrombocytopenia and the drug must be stopped if these abnormalities occur.
- Bromide increases the risk of pancreatitis and may be associated with megaesophagus.

RECOMMENDED MONITORING

- Phenobarbital:
  - Measure serum concentrations 14 days after starting therapy or changing dose, when seizures are not adequately controlled, when signs of dose-related toxicity occur, and every 6 to 12 months.
  - Blood sample is obtained immediately before the next dose is due (trough serum level), namely 8 to 12 hours after preceding dose was given.
  - Blood should *not* be drawn into serum separator tubes, as the separator material may artifactually reduce phenobarbital concentrations in vitro.
  - Target range: 20-35 μg/ml (85-150 μmol/L).
  - Measure bile acids every 6 to 12 months to screen for hepatotoxicity.
- Bromide:
  - Measure serum concentrations 1 month and 3 to 4 months after starting therapy or changing dose, when seizures are not adequately controlled, when signs of dose-related toxicity occur, and every 6 to 12 months.
  - Blood sample need not be drawn a certain number of hours after dosing, because of the drug's extremely long elimination half-life.
  - Target range: 1-2 mg/ml (100-200 mg/dl; 1000-2000 μg/ml) when used concurrently with phenobarbital and 2-3 mg/ml (200-300 mg/dl; 2000-3000 μg/ml) when used as monotherapy.

PROGNOSIS AND OUTCOME

- About 70% of dogs with idiopathic epilepsy can be adequately treated with phenobarbital and/or bromide and enjoy a good quality of life.
- In general, dogs with idiopathic epilepsy have a normal lifespan. However, some dogs with recurrent episodes of status epilepticus requiring emergency treatment have a decreased expected lifespan (about 8 years, compared to about 11 years).

PEARLS & CONSIDERATIONS

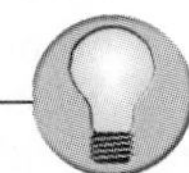

COMMENTS

- A common cause of poor seizure control is failure to reach target serum concentrations before switching to a second drug.
- Referral to a neurologist is considered if the diagnosis is uncertain or if the seizures are not adequately controlled within 3 months.

PREVENTION

- Animals with idiopathic epilepsy should not be bred because of potential genetic factors.
- Females should be spayed because estrus tends to increase seizures.

CLIENT EDUCATION

Client education is vital; the client must understand the goal of treatment, potential side effects, and need for periodic monitoring and dose adjustment. The client must agree that the benefits of treatment outweigh the side effects and must not alter treatment without consulting the attending veterinarian.

SUGGESTED READING

Podell M: The use of diazepam per rectum at home for the acute management of cluster seizures in dogs. *J Vet Int Med* 9:68, 1995.
Thomas WB: Seizures and narcolepsy. In Dewey CW (ed): *A Practical Guide to Canine and Feline Neurology*. Ames, Iowa State Press, 2003, pp 193–212.

AUTHOR: **WILLIAM B. THOMAS**
EDITOR: **CURTIS W. DEWEY**

DISEASES AND DISORDERS

Episcleritis/Scleritis

BASIC INFORMATION

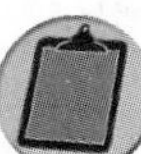

DEFINITION

Episcleritis: focal or diffuse inflammation of the episclera, a thin collagenous and vascular membrane that makes up the superficial layer of the sclera.
Scleritis: inflammation and thickening of the anterior and posterior sclera, involving cornea, uvea, and retina in advanced cases.

SYNONYM(S)

Collie granuloma
Fibrous histiocytoma
Necrotizing scleritis
Nodular fasciitis
Nodular granulomatous episcleritis/episclerokeratitis (NGE)
Non-necrotizing deep scleritis
Non-necrotizing superficial scleritis

EPIDEMIOLOGY

SPECIES, AGE, SEX
- Dogs
- No age or sex predisposition

GENETICS AND BREED PREDISPOSITION: Spaniel breeds, especially American cocker spaniel (episcleritis, scleritis), collie, Shetland sheepdog (NGE).

CLINICAL PRESENTATION

DISEASE FORMS/SUBTYPES
- Episcleritis:
  - Primary:
    - Simple
    - Nodular
  - Secondary
- Scleritis:
  - Non-necrotizing granulomatous
  - Necrotizing granulomatous

HISTORY, CHIEF COMPLAINT
- Episcleritis:
  - Pinkish-red growth on eye (nodular)
  - "Red" eye (diffuse)
  - Typically painless
- Scleritis:
  - Signs of ocular pain noted by owner:
    - Photophobia
    - Blepharospasm
    - Excessive tearing

PHYSICAL EXAM FINDINGS
Episcleritis:
- Conjunctival hyperemia
- Engorgement of episcleral vessels
- Thickening of episclera (partial or diffuse)
- With nodular forms, multiple or single, raised, pinkish-red mass(es) may be apparent at limbus; typically bilateral
- ± Perilimbal keratitis with corneal vascularization and edema (e.g., nodular granulomatous episclerokeratitis)

Scleritis:
- Conjunctival hyperemia
- Engorgement of episcleral vessels
- Typically bilateral, mildly elevated, red lesions in the anterior sclera
- Peripheral corneal vascularization and edema
- Nongranulomatous anterior uveitis, (see Uveitis, p 1134)

Advanced scleritis: presence of signs of scleritis and any or all of the following:
- Stromal keratitis (see Corneal Discoloration, p 239)
- Inflammation of the vitreous
- Secondary glaucoma (see Glaucoma, p 440)
- Retinochoroidal degeneration (see Retinal Degeneration, p 963)
- Cystic retinal detachment (see Retinal Detachment, p 965)
- Scleral thinning, which may cause subconjunctival iris prolapse

ETIOLOGY AND PATHOPHYSIOLOGY

- *Episcleritis/scleritis*:
  - Often idiopathic; immune-mediated disease
  - Association with positive *Toxoplasma* titers has been found
- *Episcleritis*:
  - Primary:
    - Simple (uncommon):
      - Not associated with systemic disease
      - Usually responsive to therapy; often self-limiting
    - Nodular (common):
      - Proposed pathogenesis of nodular granulomatous episcleritis involves production of inflammatory mediators by T lymphocytes and subsequent chemotaxis of histiocytes
  - Secondary:
    - Develops as a result of inflammation extending to episclera from severe intraocular diseases including:
      - Panophthalmitis/endophthalmitis (see Hypopyon, p 571)
      - Chronic glaucoma
      - Ocular trauma
- *Scleritis*:
  - Non-necrotizing granulomatous:
    - Characterized by infiltration of lymphocytes, plasma cells, and macrophages
    - Granulomatous response seen in cornea with corneal extension
    - ± Secondary uveitis
    - Damaged sclera replaced by fibrous tissue and/or cystic spaces causing scleral thinning after several episodes
  - Necrotizing granulomatous (rare):
    - Aggressive disease causing necrosis of scleral collagen
    - Typically affects both anterior and posterior segments of the eye
    - Commonly associated with secondary uveitis, glaucoma, and retinal detachment (e.g., see Uveitis, p 1134)
    - *Ehrlichia canis* reported in certain cases

DIAGNOSIS

DIFFERENTIAL DIAGNOSIS

Nodular episcleritis; other pinkish, raised lesions:
- Neoplasia:
  - Conjunctival neoplasia (e.g., mast cell tumor; hemangiosarcoma; histiocytoma)
  - Extension of intraocular tumor
- Granuloma (e.g., foreign body; parasitic—*Onchocerca* spp.)
- Granulation tissue

Diffuse episcleritis/scleritis; other causes of red eye:
- Conjunctivitis
- Glaucoma
- Uveitis

INITIAL DATABASE

- Complete ophthalmic examination including:
  - Schirmer tear test (normal >15 mm in one minute in dogs)
  - Fluorescein dye application
  - Intraocular pressures (normal >15 mmHg and <25 mmHg)
  - Examination of the anterior and posterior segments of the eye
- Cytologic examination of nodular lesion; may help differentiate neoplasia from inflammation (see Differential Diagnosis)

ADVANCED OR CONFIRMATORY TESTING

- Episcleral biopsy and histopathologic evaluation (nodular granulomatous episcleritis characterized by histiocytes, plasma cells, lymphocytes, and fibroblasts)
- Serologic titers for infectious diseases (e.g., *E. canis*; *T. gondii*)
- Laboratory testing: canine rheumatoid factor; antinuclear antibody; lupus erythematosus cell identification; negative in most cases
- Ocular ultrasound if ocular media opaque, compromising evaluation of deeper ocular structures; useful for ruling out concurrent ocular abnormalities (i.e., retinal detachment)

TREATMENT

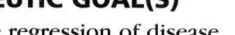

THERAPEUTIC GOAL(S)

- Promote regression of disease
- Eliminate ocular pain
- Keep disease in remission with maintenance therapy

ACUTE GENERAL TREATMENT

To be implemented only if fluorescein staining has ruled out corneal ulceration:
- Topical corticosteroids (e.g., 0.1% dexamethasone solution or ointment; or prednisolone acetate 1%) q 6-8h for 2 to 3 weeks, then gradually tapered.
- ±Topical cyclosporine (0.2-2%) q 12h. Used in addition to corticosteroids in refractory cases.

CHRONIC TREATMENT

NGE and scleritis often require topical (see Acute General Treatment) and systemic therapy(ies) including:
- Prednisone 1-2 mg/kg PO q 24h until clinical improvement, then gradually tapered over 3 to 4 weeks until maintenance dose reached.
- ± Azathioprine 1.5-2 mg/kg PO q 24h until clinical improvement; then gradually tapered to as low a dose as possible (e.g., 1 mg/kg PO q 24h, then q 48h, then once weekly for maintenance).
- Options if medical management ineffective:
  - Cryosurgery
  - Surgical excision

Alternative medical treatment includes:
- Tetracycline combined with niacinamide (PO q 8h); 250 mg of each for dogs ≤10 kg; 500 mg of each for dogs >10 kg; clinical response may take 1 to 2 months; occasional gastrointestinal side effects from niacinamide.

POSSIBLE COMPLICATIONS

- Chronic ocular pain
- Uveitis
- Secondary glaucoma
- Blindness
- Azathioprine may cause severe, life-threatening, myelosuppression; potentially hepatotoxic

RECOMMENDED MONITORING

- Monitor for regression of disease every 2 to 3 weeks until clinical signs resolve, then as needed depending on response to therapy.
- Complete blood count and liver enzymes should be assessed every 1 to 2 weeks for the first 2 months, then regularly (e.g., monthly) once clinically stable, in animals receiving azathioprine therapy.

PROGNOSIS AND OUTCOME

- Variable depending on underlying condition and cause
- Episcleritis—prognosis usually good.
- Recurrence possible

PEARLS & CONSIDERATIONS

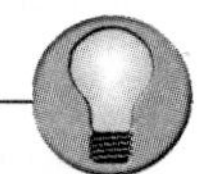

COMMENTS

Lifelong treatment is typically required

SUGGESTED READING

Paulsen M, et al: Nodular granulomatous episclerokeratitis in dogs: 19 cases (1973-1985). *J Am Vet Med Assoc* 190:1581-1587, 1987.

Rothstein E, Scott DW, Riis RC: Tetracycline and niacinamide for the treatment of sterile pyogranuloma/granuloma syndrome in a dog. *J Am Anim Hosp Assoc* 33:540-543, 1997.

Schadler H: Azathioprine in treatment for ocular nodular episcleritis. *Vet Med* 80:64-67, 1985.

AUTHOR: **URSULA M. DIETRICH**
EDITOR: **CHERYL L. CULLEN**

Epistaxis

BASIC INFORMATION

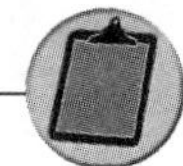

DEFINITION

Bleeding from the nasal cavity

SYNONYM(S)

Hemorrhagic nasal discharge
Nosebleed

EPIDEMIOLOGY

SPECIES, AGE, SEX

Dependent on underlying cause:
- Young purebred animals: coagulopathies
- Young to middle-aged animals: infectious diseases, trauma
- Middle-aged animals: acquired immune-mediated diseases
- Older animals: neoplasia

GENETICS, BREED PREDISPOSITION, AND RISK FACTORS

- Immune-mediated thrombocytopenia: young to middle-aged, small to medium female dogs
- Rickettsial disease: dogs living or traveling to endemic areas
- Thrombasthenia: otter hounds

- Thrombopathia: basset hounds
- von Willebrand disease: Doberman pinscher, Airedale, German shepherd, Scottish terrier, Chesapeake Bay retriever, and many other breeds; cats: Himalayan
- Hemophilia A: German shepherd and many other breeds; cats
- Hemophilia B: Cairn terrier, coonhounds, Saint Bernard, and other breeds; cats
- Nasal lesions:
  - Aspergillosis: German shepherd, dolichocephalic breeds
  - Neoplasia: dolichocephalic breeds

CONTAGION AND ZOONOSIS: Fungal infections (transmission potential appears low).

CLINICAL PRESENTATION

HISTORY, CHIEF COMPLAINT (SOME OR ALL MAY BE PRESENT)
- Nasal hemorrhage
- Sneezing
- Pawing at mouth/nose
- With coagulopathy: hematochezia, melena, hematuria, or hemorrhages
- Blindness, central nervous system (CNS) deficits possible with systemic hypertension

PHYSICAL EXAM FINDINGS
- Melena: from swallowing blood
- Nasal hemorrhage
- With coagulopathy: petechia, ecchymosis, hematomas, hematochezia, melena, and hematuria
- With coagulopathy or hypertension: retinal hemorrhages or detachment, CNS deficits

ETIOLOGY AND PATHOPHYSIOLOGY

Coagulopathy:
- Thrombocytopenia:
  - Immune-mediated disease: idiopathic disease, systemic lupus erythematosus (SLE), drug reaction
  - Rickettsial disease: ehrlichiosis, Rocky Mountain spotted fever
  - Bone marrow disease: neoplasia, aplastic anemia, infectious (fungal, rickettsial, or viral)
  - Disseminated intravascular coagulopathy (DIC)
- Thrombopathia:
  - Congenital: von Willebrand disease, thrombasthenia, thrombopathia
  - Acquired: nonsteroidal anti-inflammatory drugs (NSAIDs), hyperglobulinemia (*Ehrlichia,* multiple myeloma), uremia, DIC
- Coagulation factor defect:
  - Congenital: hemophilia A (factor VIIIc deficiency) and hemophilia B (factor IX deficiency)
  - Acquired: anticoagulant rodenticide (warfarin) intoxication, liver disease, DIC

Nasal disease:
- Foreign body
- Trauma
- Infection: fungal (*Aspergillus, Cryptococcus, Rhinosporidium*), viral, or bacterial
- Inflammation: lymphoplasmacytic rhinitis
- Neoplasia
- Vascular malformations

Systemic disease:
- Hypertension: renal disease; hyperthyroidism; hyperadrenocorticism; idiopathic
- Hyperviscosity: multiple myeloma; *Ehrlichia;* polycythemia
- Vasculitis: immune-mediated and rickettsial diseases

DIAGNOSIS

DIFFERENTIAL DIAGNOSIS

See Etiology and Pathophysiology above

INITIAL DATABASE

- Complete blood count:
  - Anemia if enough hemorrhage has occurred
  - Thrombocytopenia or thrombocytosis
  - Neutrophilia: infection; neoplasia
  - Pancytopenia: bone marrow disease
- Urinalysis:
  - Usually normal
  - Hematuria (coagulopathy), isosthenuria with renal failure, proteinuria
- Serum biochemistry profile:
  - Hypoproteinemia if enough hemorrhage has occurred
  - Elevated urea with normal creatinine: gastrointestinal blood
  - Hyperglobulinemia: ehrlichiosis, multiple myeloma
  - Azotemia (with isosthenuria): renal failure–induced systemic hypertension
  - Elevated liver enzymes and total bilirubin: severe hepatic disease causing coagulopathy

ADVANCED OR CONFIRMATORY TESTING

- Other laboratory tests:
  - Coagulation profile: prolonged times with coagulation factor defects; normal with thrombocytopenia and thrombopathia
  - Antinuclear antibody test: SLE
  - Platelet function testing (bleeding time, von Willebrand factor analysis)
  - *Ehrlichia* and Rocky Mountain spotted fever titers/polymerase chain reaction
  - Thyroid hormone assay: old cats
- Diagnostic imaging:
  - Thoracic radiograph: metastatic neoplasia
  - Nasal series: open mouth and frontal sinus views
  - CT scan: more sensitive than radiographs for many nasal diseases
- Other diagnostic procedures:
  - Rhinoscopy, nasal flush, nasal biopsy: indicated for suspected space-occupying disease; aimed at removing foreign bodies and sampling nasal tissue
  - Cytologic and histopathologic examination
  - Bacterial and fungal culture and sensitivity testing
  - Bone marrow aspiration and cytology (± core biopsy) with pancytopenia
  - Blood pressure evaluation

TREATMENT

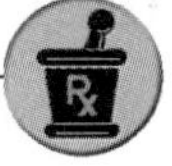

THERAPEUTIC GOAL(S)

- Stop epistaxis
- Treat primary cause

ACUTE GENERAL TREATMENT

- Minimize activity or stimuli that precipitate hemorrhage episodes.
  - Environment
  - Consider tranquilization (e.g., opiate)
- Whole blood or packed red blood cell (RBC) transfusion; may be needed with severe anemia.
- In life-threatening cases of refractory, exuberant arterial epistaxis, both carotid arteries may be ligated without adversely affecting perfusion of the head (vertebral artery collaterals).

SPECIFIC TREATMENT

Coagulopathy:
- von Willebrand disease: plasma or cryoprecipitate for acute bleeding
- Hemophilia: plasma or cryoprecipitate for acute bleeding; no long-term treatment
- Anticoagulant rodenticide intoxication: plasma for acute bleeding and vitamin K supplementation
- Liver disease and DIC; treat underlying cause; plasma may be beneficial
- Discontinue all NSAIDs
- Hyperglobulinemia: plasmapheresis

Nasal disease:
- Radiotherapy: nasal tumors
- Topical clotrimazole therapy for fungal disease
- Surgery: if foreign body unremovable by rhinoscopy; fungal rhinitis (*Aspergillus* and *Rhinosporidium*), neoplasia

Systemic disease:
- Hyperviscosity: treat underlying disease (e.g., ehrlichiosis and multiple myeloma); plasmapheresis
- Vasculitis: doxycycline for rickettsial disease; prednisone for immune-mediated disease
- Hypertension: treat underlying disease (e.g., renal disease, hyperthy-

roidism, and hyperadrenocorticism); reduce weight if obesity is present; restrict sodium; antihypertensive medication

POSSIBLE COMPLICATIONS

Anemia and collapsed state

RECOMMENDED MONITORING

- Platelet count with thrombocytopenia
- Coagulation profile with coagulation factor defects
- Blood pressure with hypertension
- Monitor clinical signs

PROGNOSIS AND OUTCOME

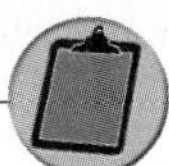

Dependent on cause

PEARLS & CONSIDERATIONS

COMMENTS

- Remember that epistaxis may indicate a systemic coagulopathy; use care when deciding which vein to use for blood sampling (prefer limb to jugular, for compression), whether to perform centeses, etc.
- Epistaxis is not a diagnosis but a clinical sign.
- Coagulopathy may present as unilateral epistaxis.
- Rule out systemic diseases and coagulopathy before focusing on nasal disease.

CLIENT EDUCATION

Monitor for recurrence of presenting signs

RECOMMENDED READING

Madden SN: Diseases of the nasal cavity and paranasal sinuses. In Morgan RV, Bright RN, Swartout MS (eds): *Handbook of Small Animal Practice*, ed 4. Philadelphia, WB Saunders, 2003, pp 136-143.

Mahony O: Bleeding disorders: Epistaxis and hemoptysis. In Ettinger SJ, Feldman EC (eds): *Textbook of Veterinary Internal Medicine*, ed 5. Philadelphia, WB Saunders, 2000, pp 213-217.

AUTHOR: **REMO LOBETTI**

EDITOR: **ETIENNE CÔTÉ**

Epulides and Odontogenic Tumors

BASIC INFORMATION

DEFINITION

- Epulis means "on the gums." Epulides (plural) consist of benign, gingival proliferations of tissue in the oral cavity arising from the periodontal ligament.
- In dogs, these are classified by the presence of bone *(ossifying epulis)* or by the lack of bone *(fibrous epulis)*. A third class of epulis, *acanthomatous epulis* (ACE), is characterized by a locally aggressive biologic behavior and typically involves bony invasion.
- Epulides do not metastasize.
- Feline epulides are rare.
- In cats, odontogenic tumors arise from the components of teeth, and these are benign and minimally invasive.
- Feline odontogenic tumors are often described as inductive or noninductive, which refers to the ability or inability of the tumor to induce reactive proliferation of connective tissue, respectively.
- Metastasis has not been reported in cats.

SYNONYM(S)

ACE previously termed as adamantinoma and ameloblastoma, although ameloblastoma may be a distinct tumor in young dogs

Dental tumor

Fibrous epulides are also called fibromatous epulides

EPIDEMIOLOGY

SPECIES, AGE, SEX

- Collectively, oral tumors account for 6% of canine cancer. Of canine oral tumors, 5% are dental tumors. Dental tumors can affect dogs of all ages, but they occur typically in middle-aged dogs. Ameloblastomas are seen in young dogs.
- Sex predilection information is conflicting. Female dogs have been reported to be affected more than males; however, equal incidence rates have also been documented.
- Epulides are much less common in cats, and all have been classified as ossifying or fibrous. ACE has not been reported. Cats of all ages can be affected. Multiple epulides have been reported in cats. Inductive fibroameloblastoma is a rare odontogenic tumor that affects young cats 6 months to 2 years old. The most common noninductive tumor is calcifying epithelial odontogenic tumor (CEOT). CEOT is typically reported in middle-aged and older cats.

GENETICS AND BREED PREDISPOSITION: Despite the increased incidence of gingival hyperplasia in boxers, this breed does not appear to be at increased risk for developing epulis.

CLINICAL PRESENTATION

HISTORY, CHIEF COMPLAINT

- Most commonly, the owner notices an oral mass.
- Presenting complaints include weight loss, dysphagia, increased salivation, bloody oral discharge, and halitosis.

PHYSICAL EXAM FINDINGS: Fibrous and ossifying epulides are typically firm gingival masses that measure 1 to 4 cm in diameter. They are discrete, located near teeth, and variably fixed to the gum line. They are covered by oral epithelium, and ulceration is not common. Similarly, ACE is covered by an intact epithelium, is firm, but is more rapidly growing. ACE is most commonly located in the rostral mandible and is more locally invasive with bone infiltration.

Inductive fibroameloblastoma in young cats has a predilection for the region of the maxillary canine teeth. The maxilla and teeth are commonly deformed. CEOTs can appear grossly similar to squamous cell carcinoma and are often ulcerated and friable. Some CEOTs appear pigmented and can be confused grossly with oral melanoma.

ETIOLOGY AND PATHOPHYSIOLOGY

- All canine epulides arise from the periodontal ligament.
- Canine ameloblastomas also arise from odontogenic tissue, but they are considered a distinct group that develop from the dental lamina.
- Feline fibroameloblastomas are inductive tumors that histologically resemble the embryonic connective tissue of the dental pulp. These tumors grow by expansion, rather than invasion.
- CEOT contains amyloid deposits within its stroma.

DIAGNOSIS

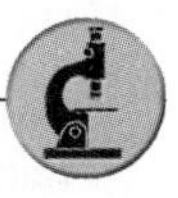

DIFFERENTIAL DIAGNOSIS

- In dogs, the most common malignant oral cancers are malignant melanoma, squamous cell carcinoma, and fibrosar-

coma. Non-neoplastic lesions include viral papillomatosis and eosinophilic granulomas.
- In the cat, squamous cell carcinoma is the most common malignant oral tumor. Oral fibrosarcomas are the second most common neoplasm. Benign differentials include eosinophilic granulomas and inflammatory polyps.

INITIAL DATABASE

- Most patients require a short general anesthetic. This will allow a good examination of the oral cavity with palpation, regional radiographs, and biopsy.
- Biopsy is the only definitive test to confirm the diagnosis.
  - For small lesions, curative intent excisional biopsy can be performed during the initial oral exam under anesthesia.
  - For larger lesions, a large incisional biopsy should be performed to rule out other forms of malignant oral neoplasia. Confirmation of the tumor type will allow the clinician to properly plan for an appropriate first surgery.
- Of the epulides, fibrous and ossifying epulides are not invasive, and radiographic changes to bone are unlikely. In contrast, radiographs are necessary for ACE, keeping in mind that normal skull films do not rule out bony invasion. (Greater than 40-50% cortical destruction is required for radiographically detectable bony lysis.) Radiographs may not delineate tumor margins, and caution should used in relying on skull films for surgical planning.
- Skull radiographs should also be taken for cats to evaluate for bony destruction. Ameloblastomas cause variable degrees of bone expansion, lysis, and production. Teeth may be missing, and the nasal cavity can be invaded. For CEOT, there is typically marked osteolysis.
- In general, computed tomography (CT) is considerably superior to radiography for imaging patients with epulides or ontogenic tumors.

ADVANCED OR CONFIRMATORY TESTING

Preoperative CT can be valuable to determine local disease extension and bony invasion. CT may assist in achieving wide surgical margins for ACE and is used for radiation planning.

TREATMENT

THERAPEUTIC GOAL(S)

The primary goal of managing patients with dental tumors is adequate local tumor control.

ACUTE GENERAL TREATMENT

- Surgery:
  - In dogs with epulides, local gingival excision is rarely curative, as these tumors arise from the periodontal ligament. Recurrence from the subgingival tissue in the tooth socket is likely, but ossifying and fibromatous epulides may be slow to recur. To prevent regrowth, the affected tooth root should be included in the excision.
  - For ACE, wide margins with bone resection are necessary to achieve local control. With aggressive resection (maxillectomy/mandibulectomy), recurrence rates are low, typically less than 5%. Postoperative radiation therapy (RT) may be necessary for local control.
  - Surgery is the treatment of choice for feline ameloblastoma and CEOT but is difficult for large tumors. Premaxillectomy may be required for local control of ameloblastoma.
- Radiation therapy:
  - RT can be considered for nonresectable masses, for incomplete resections, and for recurrent tumors.
  - RT is effective for ACE. Tumor control is achieved in about 90% of dogs, especially for smaller tumors. In contrast, larger tumors (>4 cm) are more likely to recur (30% control rates).
  - Feline ameloblastomas and CEOT that are too large for surgery generally will respond to RT.
- Cryosurgery:
  - Cryosurgery causes cellular death after controlled freezing and thawing of the tumor. It is best for low-grade tumors that are less than 2 cm in diameter and adherent or minimally invasive into one cortex. The tumor should be debulked and biopsied. Cryosurgery is applied to the underlying bone. Despite maintenance of the bony framework and preservation of oral function, recurrence is more common than with wide excision.
  - Tumors with extensive fixation to bone or invasion, such as ACE, should be removed surgically. Full-thickness freezing of the maxilla or mandible can lead to oronasal fistula or fracture, respectively.

PROGNOSIS AND OUTCOME

- Prognosis is excellent for canine epulides if treated aggressively.
- Wide surgical excision and RT have high cure rates. An exception is feline multiple epulides, which have a higher recurrence rate (72%).
- For canine ACE, median survival times of 2 to 3 years are reported.
- As with malignant oral tumors, smaller tumors and rostral location are positive prognostic factors. These masses are typically detected earlier, easier to operate, and more likely to have complete surgical margins.
- Similarly, tumor stage (size) is prognostic for local control when treated with RT.

PEARLS & CONSIDERATIONS

COMMENTS

- Because canine epulides arise from the periodontal ligament, excision limited to the gingiva will be inadequate, resulting in regrowth.
- Aggressive surgical excision may be curative in dogs and cats with these benign oral tumors.
- RT is an excellent alternative to surgery and an excellent adjuvant therapy in the postoperative setting.

SUGGESTED READING

Moore AS, Ogilvie GK: Tumors of the alimentary tract. In Ogilvie GK, Moore AS (eds): *Feline Oncology: A Comprehensive Guide to Compassionate Care*. Trenton, NJ, Veterinary Learning Systems, 2001, pp 271-294.

Théon AP, et al: Analysis of prognostic factor and patterns of failure in dogs with periodontal tumors treated with megavoltage irradiation. *J Am Vet Med Assoc* 210:785-788, 1997.

Withrow SJ: Cancer of the oral cavity. In Withrow SJ, MacEwen EG (eds): *Small Animal Clinical Oncology*, ed 3. Philadelphia, WB Saunders, 2001, pp 305-318.

AUTHOR: **SUSAN N. ETTINGER**

EDITOR: **KENNETH M. RASSNICK**

Erythema Multiforme and Toxic Epidermal Necrolysis

BASIC INFORMATION

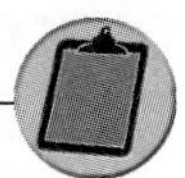

DEFINITION

Spectrum of acute, potentially severe epidermal and/or mucosal diseases defined by distinctive clinical and histopathologic findings. This diagnosis is considered if dermatologic findings include annular ("target") lesions (Fig. I-63), erythematous eruptions, and epidermal detachment with secondary ulcerations.

EPIDEMIOLOGY

SPECIES, AGE, SEX: Dogs and cats of any age and both sexes.

CLINICAL PRESENTATION

DISEASE FORMS/SUBTYPES: Based on clinical and histopathologic features, the erythema multiforme (EM)–toxic epidermal necrolysis (TEN) spectrum is divided into five different categories adapted from the human international consensus clinical classification: EM minor, EM major, Stevens-Johnson syndrome (SJS), overlap syndrome (OS), and TEN. However, this classification should be considered as a general guideline. Indeed, some cases can overlap these categories or present only a few clinical signs.

HISTORY, CHIEF COMPLAINT: A dermatosis with an acute onset and rapid deterioration. Systemic signs of illness and severe skin lesions are usually the main complaints. Drug administration can be an important element of the history.

PHYSICAL EXAM FINDINGS

- See Definition above.
- This classification is a broad description of the diseases and does not encompass all possible situations.
- The animal can be debilitated, especially with TEN. Fever precedes virtually all cases of TEN in humans.

ETIOLOGY AND PATHOPHYSIOLOGY

- In dogs and cats, EM is usually associated with either drug therapy, infections (herpesvirus, parvovirus), or is idiopathic.
- TEN is usually associated with drug therapy but can be idiopathic.
- The pathophysiology of EM: TEN spectrum diseases seems to be the result of an immune-mediated disorder. A cell-mediated immune response directed toward various antigens is suspected in EM, while a defective epidermal detoxification of drug byproducts, in addition to the cellular immune reaction, is proposed to explain TEN. Both processes lead to keratinocyte apoptosis (programmed cell death).

DIAGNOSIS

DIFFERENTIAL DIAGNOSIS

- Superficial and deep infection (bacterial and fungal)
- Urticaria
- Systemic and cutaneous lupus erythematosus
- Cutaneous drug eruption
- Pemphigus vulgaris
- Vasculitis
- Bullous pemphigoid
- Epidermolysis bullosa
- Burns
- Ulcerative stomatitis
- Epitheliotropic lymphoma

INITIAL DATABASE

- No specific laboratory findings.
- Routine dermatologic diagnostics should be performed as appropriate (skin scrapings, skin cytology, skin biopsy, fungal culture) based on differential diagnosis (see Dermatologic Diagnostic Procedures, p 1223)

Dermatologic examination	EM minor	EM major	SJS	OS	TEN
Flat or raised, focal or multifocal, target (concentric rings around a clear or crusty center) or polycyclic lesions	Yes	Yes	No	No	No
Number of mucosal surfaces involved	1 or fewer	>1	>1	>1	>1
Erythematous or purpuric, macular or patchy eruption (% of body surface affected)	<50	<50	>50	>50	>50
Epidermal detachment (vesicles, bullae, erosions, and ulcers) (% of body surface affected)	<10	<10	<10	10–30	>30

EM, erythema multiforme; SJS, Stevens-Johnson syndrome; OS, overlap syndrome; TEN, toxic epidermal necrolysis.

ADVANCED OR CONFIRMATORY TESTING

- Definitive diagnosis is based on the histopathologic findings (hydropic degeneration, single-cell apoptosis to full-thickness necrosis of the epidermis, dermal lymphohistiocytic cells infiltration, and subepidermal vesicles; hair follicles may be similarly affected).
- Some authors distinguish EM from TEN based on the histopathologic findings, but others argue that there is an overlap between these entities and thus, the disease should be defined based on the clinical classification.

TREATMENT

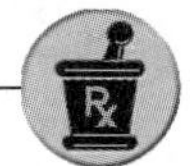

THERAPEUTIC GOAL(S)

- Stop the immunologic reactions causing the epidermal necrosis
- Prevent skin infection if the cutaneous barrier is ruptured
- Supportive care when the animal is debilitated

ACUTE GENERAL TREATMENT

- Try to find and correct the underlying cause. If a drug is being administered at the time of initial presentation, the first rule is to discontinue its use.
- May resolve spontaneously (EM).
- Severe cases of EM and TEN should receive supportive care, if needed:
    - Fluid therapy if fluid deficits/electrolyte imbalances/acid base disturbances
    - Nutritional support
    - Wound care (gentle washes with saline or chlorhexidine gluconate 0.05% solution, dermal protection to prevent complication such as infection or dessication, and topical antibiotics)
- Necrotic epidermis, rich in cytokines, can help reepithelialization. Therefore some authors recommend not to debride skin lesions.
- Systemic antibiotic therapy is warranted if evidence of bacteremia or sepsis is present and may be considered if ulcerations are present.
- Use of glucocorticoids is controversial and usually not beneficial.
- Pentoxifylline (10 mg/kg PO q 8h) has been useful in some cases.
- Intravenous immunoglobulin (Ig) therapy using human Ig (1 g/kg infused slowly over 4 to 6 hours) has been

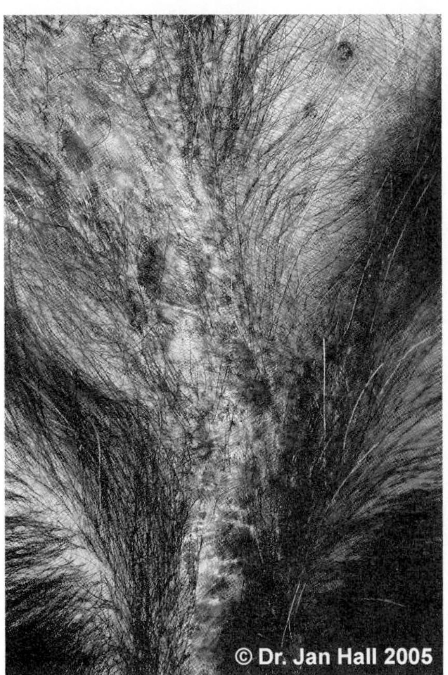

FIGURE I-63 Erythema multiforme annular (target) lesions on the caudal ventral abdomen of a dog. Courtesy of Dr. Jan A. Hall.

shown beneficial in a few cases. A similar equine product is also available, but there are anecdotal reports of serious side effects.
- Severe oral ulcerations may require oral rinses with chlorhexidine 0.1-0.2% solution or gel, or viscous lidocaine 2% application to the oral ulcers for comfort.

PROGNOSIS AND OUTCOME

- The prognosis is usually good in EM (except if the lesions are severe and extensive) and poor in TEN.
- The condition should improve within 3 weeks when the underlying cause is identified and eliminated.

PEARLS & CONSIDERATIONS

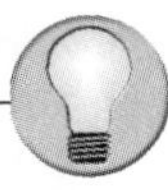

COMMENTS

- Hospitalization may be indicated, especially for TEN.
- Some cases have been related to diet. Thus, animals with an idiopathic case should receive a hypoallergenic diet.

SUGGESTED READING

Scott DW, Miller WH, Griffin CE: In *Muller and Kirk's Small Animal Dermatology*, ed 6. Philadelphia, WB Saunders, 2001, pp 729-742.

AUTHOR: **FRÉDÉRIC SAUVÉ**
EDITOR: **JAN A. HALL**

Esophageal Diverticulum

BASIC INFORMATION

DEFINITION

A rare disorder characterized by a pouch-like sacculation of the esophageal wall resulting in an area in which material can accumulate and remain

SYNONYM(S)

Pulsion: also called "true" diverticula
Traction: also called "false" diverticula

EPIDEMIOLOGY

SPECIES, AGE, SEX: Can happen in any age or sex, dog or cat.
ASSOCIATED CONDITIONS AND DISORDERS: Traction diverticula can be caused by tumors or infections.

CLINICAL PRESENTATION

DISEASE FORMS/SUBTYPES
- Congenital versus acquired
- Pulsion versus traction

HISTORY, CHIEF COMPLAINT
- Regurgitation may be seen, particularly with large diverticula
- Prior thoracic inflammatory disease may be suggestive (opportunity for adhesion formation and therefore traction diverticulum), although diverticulum perforation or rupture with secondary pyothorax can occur with any type of diverticulum

PHYSICAL EXAM FINDINGS
- Regurgitation may be noted in the exam room
- No other findings are considered specific

ETIOLOGY AND PATHOPHYSIOLOGY

- Pulsion diverticula are caused by herniation of the mucosa through the muscular wall of the esophagus, resulting in food retention within the diverticulum. This can be an acquired problem due to increased esophageal luminal pressure secondary to obstruction, esophagitis, stricture, foreign body, etc.; or it can be congenital, resulting from an inherent weakness in the esophageal wall or an abnormality of embryonic separation during development.
- Traction diverticuli are caused by an extraesophageal lesion such as maturing fibrous connective tissue (typically an adhesion between the esophagus and another intrathoracic structure such as tracheal or hilar lymph nodes). This adhesion pulls a portion of the esophageal wall out of position as the connective tissue matures and contracts, creating a pouch. In dogs, it is suspected that the most likely cause of traction diverticula is a penetrating esophageal foreign body that results in adhesion formation outside the esophagus. See Foreign Body, Esophageal, p 402; Foreign Body Removal, Esophageal (Endoscopic), p 1256.
- The main clinical utility of differentiating between these types is that surgery may correct a traction diverticulum (release adhesion), but pulsion diverticula are often due to an esophageal problem that may or may not be surgical (e.g., vascular ring anomaly versus esophageal stricture, respectively).

DIAGNOSIS

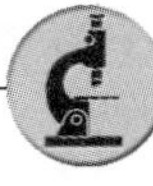

DIFFERENTIAL DIAGNOSIS

Regurgitation:
- Esophagitis.
- Megaesophagus (idiopathic; secondary to systemic disease; or pediatric: transient and congenital). Diverticula cause focal esophageal enlargement, whereas generalized esophageal enlargement should prompt the consideration of causes of megaesophagus (see Megaesophagus, p 691).
- Esophageal mass.
- Esophageal stricture.
- Vascular ring anomaly.

INITIAL DATABASE

- Complete blood count, serum chemistry profile, and urinalysis results are often normal unless there is systemic inflammatory disease
- Plain thoracic radiographs:
  - Look for a localized density
  - Distinguish focal from generalized esophageal disease (e.g., see Megaesophagus, p 691)
  - Assess for evidence of aspiration pneumonia
  - Assess for evidence of mediastinitis or pleuritis (e.g., mediastinal widening, pleural effusion), as can occur with esophageal perforation
- Contrast esophagram (see Barium Esophagram, Dynamic, p 1187):
  - Look for localized collection of contrast in a pouch outside the expected plane of the esophageal lumen
  - Distinguish esophageal disease from pleural or pulmonary disease
  - Distinguish from normal redundant esophagus seen in bulldogs and shar-peis

ADVANCED OR CONFIRMATORY TESTING

- Esophagoscopy: find the outpouching and distinguish traction from pulsion types
- Histopathology of resected pouch to look for cause of traction diverticulum

TREATMENT

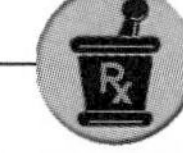

THERAPEUTIC GOAL(S)

- Try to resect pouch in animals that show clinical signs but do not have generalized esophageal weakness; however, there is substantial risk of dehiscence.
- Clinically silent diverticula should generally be left alone unless there appears to be substantial risk of perforation.

ACUTE GENERAL TREATMENT

- Treat aspiration pneumonia, if present (see Pneumonia, Aspiration, p 862)
- Treat septic pleuritis/mediastinitis, if present (see Pyothorax, p 935)
- Treat esophagitis or esophageal stricture as appropriate (see Esophagitis, p 366)
- Remove diverticulum surgically, if appropriate

CHRONIC TREATMENT

None, unless esophageal stricture or esophageal hypomotility is present after diverticulectomy

POSSIBLE COMPLICATIONS

- Perforation of diverticulum leading to pleural or mediastinal sepsis
- Aspiration pneumonia

PROGNOSIS AND OUTCOME

Guarded: Too few such cases have been identified and treated to produce objective prognostic information. No instances of self-resolution have been documented, however.

PEARLS & CONSIDERATIONS

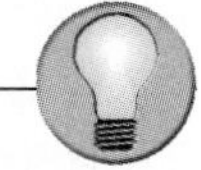

COMMENTS

- A very rare condition in dogs and cats.
- Must distinguish from the clinically insignificant redundant esophagus often seen in bulldogs and shar-peis.
- Can be difficult to recognize at esophagoscopy. If food is retained within them, diverticula can be seen easily during esophagoscopy. However, if the diverticulum is empty, it is just a fold of tissue that can be overlooked, especially if there is inadequate insufflation of the esophagus during the endoscopic examination. Adequate insufflation may require closing off the esophagus manually to hold in the air to facilitate evaluation of the esophagus.

SUGGESTED READING

Jergens AE: Diseases of the esophagus. In Ettinger SJ, Feldman EC (eds): *Textbook of Veterinary Internal Medicine*, ed 6. St. Louis, Elsevier Saunders, 2005, pp 1298–1310.

Woods CB, et al: Esophageal deviation in four English bulldogs. *J Am Vet Med Assoc* 172:934, 1978.

AUTHOR: **MICHAEL WILLARD**

EDITOR: **DEBRA L. ZORAN**

Esophageal Neoplasia

BASIC INFORMATION

DEFINITION

Benign or malignant tumor of the esophagus

EPIDEMIOLOGY

SPECIES, AGE, SEX

- Rare in dogs and cats
- Older animals predisposed
- No sex predilection, although squamous cell carcinoma is more common in female cats

GENETICS AND BREED PREDISPOSITION: No breed predilection.

RISK FACTORS: *S. lupi* infection, resulting in secondary sarcoma formation.

GEOGRAPHY AND SEASONALITY: Areas where *Spirocerca lupi* is endemic, including the Middle East, Africa, and the southeastern United States.

ASSOCIATED CONDITIONS AND DISORDERS: Hypertrophic osteopathy has been reported, especially in *Spirocerca lupi*-induced sarcomas.

CLINICAL PRESENTATION

DISEASE FORMS/SUBTYPES

- The most common primary esophageal tumors are squamous cell carcinoma (cats), leiomyosarcoma (dogs), osteosarcoma and fibrosarcoma; rarely benign tumors such as leiomyoma or plasmacytomas may occur.
- Primary thyroid gland or mammary gland tumors may metastasize to the esophagus.
- Lymphoma may involve the esophagus and generally when it does, multicentric lymphoma is present.
- Primary tumors arising from the thymus, heart base, or thyroid gland may extend directly into the esophagus.

HISTORY, CHIEF COMPLAINT

- Weight loss
- Discomfort with swallowing
- Dysphagia
- Regurgitation
- Lethargy, inappetence, dyspnea, cough (aspiration pneumonia)
- Less commonly lameness or pain of the extremities associated with hypertrophic osteopathy

PHYSICAL EXAM FINDINGS

- Rarely, a palpable mass may be found in the ventral cervical region. Most often,

however, no significant physical abnormalities are found.
- Thin body condition.
- Melena.
- Back pain from spondylitis of the caudal thoracic vertebrae caused by spirocercosis.

ETIOLOGY AND PATHOPHYSIOLOGY

- Sarcoma formation has been correlated to infection with *S. lupi*.
- *S. lupi* causes persistent tissue irritation, resulting in aortic scarring and nodular esophageal granulomas, which can undergo neoplastic transformation.
- Metastasis to the esophagus from primary thyroid gland or mammary gland tumors is more common than primary esophageal neoplasia.
- Primary esophageal malignancies may metastasize to regional lymph nodes or lungs, less commonly to other organs.

DIAGNOSIS

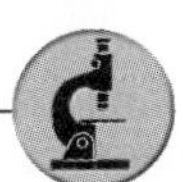

DIFFERENTIAL DIAGNOSIS

Any disease causing signs of partial esophageal obstruction (see Foreign Body, Esophageal, p 402) or megaesophagus (see Megaesophagus, p 691)

INITIAL DATABASE

- Plain radiographs of the thorax (three views) and neck may show repeatable, excessive gas in the esophagus, presence of a mass, or megaesophagus, all proximal (orad) to the obstruction. Lung fields should be evaluated for metastases.
- Barium swallow to show an esophageal stricture or mass.
- Esophagoscopy to visualize mass(es); often ulcerated, but leiomyomas are usually submucosal, well circumscribed, and not attached to overlying mucosa.
- Biopsy and histopathology, with samples usually obtained at the time of esophagoscopy.
- Complete blood count, serum biochemical profile, and urinalysis are usually normal, although some patients may be anemic due to chronic blood loss from friable esophageal tumors.
- Fecal flotation may show *S. lupi* ova, although a negative test does not rule out infection, as esophageal neoplasia may form long after initial exposure.
- Cytology of enlarged lymph nodes to differentiate reactive lymphadenopathy from metastasis.

ADVANCED OR CONFIRMATORY TESTING

- Computed tomography or magnetic resonance imaging to better delineate mass when radiographs are equivocal
- Exploratory surgery for histopathology when samples obtained during esophagoscopy are nondiagnostic

TREATMENT

THERAPEUTIC GOAL(S)

Goal is relief of signs of partial esophageal obstruction and delay or prevention of disease progression

ACUTE GENERAL TREATMENT

- Surgery, when feasible; in general, difficult due to length of resection required in advanced cases and inability to obtain good exposure of the esophagus
- Placement of esophagostomy or gastrostomy tubes for feeding (see Feeding Tube Placement: PEG, pp 1243–1249)

CHRONIC TREATMENT

- Nutritional palliation with placement of feeding tubes
- Palliative radiation therapy for cervical esophageal masses
- Photodynamic therapy may be considered for superficial mucosal tumors, but efficacy currently unknown

POSSIBLE COMPLICATIONS

- Risk of short-term dehiscence or long-term stricture formation after esophageal surgery
- Risks associated with thoracotomy
- Risk of infection at site of feeding tube
- Palliative radiation usually not attempted for intrathoracic lesions due to relative intolerance of adjacent normal tissues such as the heart, lungs, and trachea

RECOMMENDED MONITORING

- Monitor body weight, as ability to obtain adequate nutrition orally is often compromised
- Thoracic radiographs and regional lymph nodes, looking for metastasis

PROGNOSIS AND OUTCOME

Long-term prognosis is usually very poor due to low likelihood of relieving clinical signs or preventing metastasis

PEARLS & CONSIDERATIONS

COMMENTS

Little information is available about treating dogs with esophageal neoplasia, primarily due to the rarity of these tumors.

PREVENTION

Sarcoma formation may be prevented by avoiding *S. lupi* infection.

CLIENT EDUCATION

Quality of life is often very poor unless the tumor is benign and can be surgically excised

SUGGESTED READING

Jacobs TM, Rosen GM: Photodynamic therapy as a treatment for esophageal squamous cell carcinoma in a dog. *J Am Anim Hosp Assoc* 36:257, 2000.

Ranen E, et al: Partial esophagectomy with single layer closure for treatment of esophageal sarcomas in 6 dogs. *Vet Surg* 33:428, 2004.

AUTHOR: **LINDA S. FINEMAN**
EDITOR: **KENNETH M. RASSNICK**

Esophageal Perforation

BASIC INFORMATION

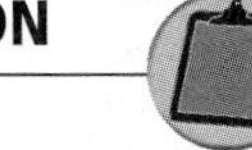

DEFINITION

Full-thickness defect in the esophagus with leakage of esophageal contents into the mediastinum and potentially the pleural space; see Foreign Body, Esophageal, p 402; Esophagitis, p 366 for related information

EPIDEMIOLOGY

SPECIES, AGE, SEX

- No age or sex predilection
- Perforation has been reported in more dogs than cats:
  - Attributed to the less discriminate feeding behavior of dogs

GENETICS AND BREED PREDISPOSITION: Eighty-six percent of esophageal foreign bodies are reported in dogs weighing <12 kg (26 lb).

RISK FACTORS: Foreign body ingestion. See Foreign Body, Esophageal, p 402.

ASSOCIATED CONDITIONS AND DISORDERS
- Mediastinal abscess
- Pneumothorax
- Pyothorax
- Bronchoesophageal fistula

CLINICAL PRESENTATION

HISTORY, CHIEF COMPLAINT
Historic findings associated with esophageal perforation include:
- Retching, regurgitation, vomiting, ptyalism, anorexia
- Coughing, dyspnea
- Restlessness
- Cervical swelling, subcutaneous emphysema

PHYSICAL EXAM FINDINGS
- Physical findings may include:
  - Fever
  - Subcutaneous emphysema
  - Rapid shallow respiration consistent with pneumothorax or pyothorax
  - Moist rales on auscultation if aspiration pneumonia is present
  - Dehydration
- The duration of clinical signs associated with esophageal perforation is reported to be longer than with esophageal foreign body alone. See Foreign Body, Esophageal, p 402.

ETIOLOGY AND PATHOPHYSIOLOGY
- Sharp edges of a foreign body may lacerate the esophagus and more rarely the great vessels.
- Large foreign bodies can result in pressure necrosis of the esophageal wall; the greatest damage is usually associated with pressure points of the foreign body against the esophageal wall.
- The most common site of foreign body lodgement is the distal esophagus just cranial to the gastroesophageal junction; other sites include the thoracic inlet, heart base, and less often the cervical esophagus. See Foreign Body, Esophageal, p 402.
- Esophageal perforation can also be associated with esophageal trauma or balloon dilation of esophageal strictures.

DIAGNOSIS

DIFFERENTIAL DIAGNOSIS
- Megaesophagus
- Hiatal hernia or gastroesophageal intussusception
- Intrinsic or extrinsic esophageal masses
- Neoplasia
- Parasite infestation
- Esophagitis
- Esophageal diverticulum
- Vascular ring anomaly
- Abnormal pharyngeal or esophageal motility

INITIAL DATABASE
- Complete blood count:
  - Neutrophilic leukocytosis.
  - More immature neutrophils are present with a perforated esophagus than with esophageal foreign body alone.
- Diagnostic imaging:
  - Survey cervical and thoracic radiographs.
    - Esophageal foreign body.
    - Pneumothorax.
    - Pleural effusion/pyothorax.
    - Increased lung density with concurrent aspiration pneumonia.
  - Contrast esophagram (see Barium Esophagram, Dynamic, p 1187).
    - Should be performed with water-soluble contrast if perforation is suspected.
    - Has a false-negative rate of 14.5%.
- Esophagoscopy:
  - Performed with care.
    - Do not create or worsen pneumothorax.
  - Evaluate integrity and viability of esophagus.
    - Identify site of perforation.
  - Possible foreign body removal.
- Analysis of pleural effusion, if present:
  - Cytology.
  - Bacterial culture and sensitivity testing (both aerobic and anaerobic).

TREATMENT

THERAPEUTIC GOAL(S)
- Repair of esophageal perforation
- Treatment of associated problems:
  - Mediastinal abscess
  - Pyothorax
- Nutritional support until esophageal injury has healed and function has returned
- Treatment/prevention of esophagitis:
  - Prevention of esophageal stricture formation

ACUTE GENERAL TREATMENT
- Correction of fluid and electrolyte deficits
- Antimicrobial therapy:
  - Empiric therapy using an antibiotic with a broad spectrum of aerobic activity.
    - Cefazolin: 22 mg/kg IV, q 6h.
  - Definitive antimicrobial therapy should be based on results of microbiologic culture and sensitivity testing.
    - Pleural fluid.
    - Mediastinal abscess.
- Surgical intervention:
  - Removal of foreign body if underlying cause.
  - Repair of perforation.
    - Primary closure.
    - Resection and anastomosis.
  - Debridement and lavage.
    - Mediastinal abscess.
    - Pyothorax.
- Treatment of esophagitis:
  - H_2 antagonists (e.g., famotidine 0.5 mg/kg IV q 12-24h)/antisecretory agents (e.g., omeprazole 0.7 mg/kg via feeding tube q 24h) to decrease gastric acid production.
  - Motility agents (metoclopramide 0.2-0.5 mg/kg SQ or PO q 6-12h, or cisapride 0.1-1 mg/kg PO q 8-12h) to promote normal gastroesophageal sphincter tone (reduce gastroesophageal reflux and esophagitis) and gastric emptying.
- Nutritional support until esophagus has healed and normal function has returned:
  - Feeding tube (PEG) to bypass esophagus.
    - 10 to 14 days.

CHRONIC TREATMENT
Treatment of pyothorax (see Pyothorax, p 935):
- Long-term antibiotic therapy:
  - Based on accurate identification of organism(s) involved
  - Up to 3 months of therapy may be required

POSSIBLE COMPLICATIONS
- Dehiscence of esophageal repair:
  - Recurrent leakage
- Esophageal diverticulum formation:
  - Secondary to the presence of a foreign body
- Esophageal stricture formation:
  - Secondary to damage caused by foreign body, surgical technique, or esophagitis

RECOMMENDED MONITORING
- If PEG tube has been placed:
  - Removal in 10 to 14 days.
- Ensure that normal esophageal function returns:
  - Esophageal stricture, if it occurs, usually becomes clinically apparent 3 to 4 weeks postinjury.
    - Increasing problem of regurgitation

PROGNOSIS AND OUTCOME

Prognosis associated with esophageal perforation is guarded due to multiple possible complications and is specifically influenced by the presence or absence of:
- Mediastinitis/mediastinal abscess formation
- Development of pyothorax
- Development of esophageal stricture

PEARLS & CONSIDERATIONS

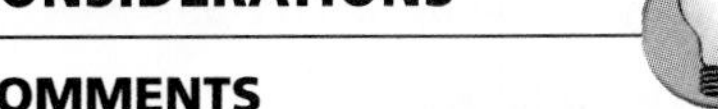

COMMENTS

Endoscopic evaluation and removal of esophageal foreign bodies must be done carefully, with special attention paid to the patient's ventilatory pattern, oxygen saturation, heart rate, and blood pressure. Insufflation with air in the presence of an esophageal perforation can lead to tension pneumothorax and acute cardiopulmonary compromise of anesthetized patients.

PREVENTION

Do not let dogs and cats eat foreign objects that have the potential to become lodged in the esophagus.

SUGGESTED READING

Houlton JF, et al: Thoracic oesophageal foreign bodies in the dog: A review of ninety cases. *J Small Anim Pract* 26:521, 1985.

Parker NR, et al: Diagnosis and surgical management of esophageal perforation. *J Am Anim Hosp Assoc* 25:587, 1989.

Spielman BL, et al: Esophageal foreign body in dogs: A retrospective study of 23 cases. *J Am Anim Hosp Assoc* 28:570, 1992.

AUTHOR: **MARYANN G. RADLINSKY**
EDITOR: **RICHARD WALSHAW**

Esophageal Stricture

BASIC INFORMATION

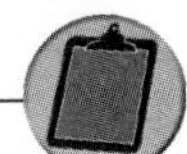

DEFINITION

A circular band of scar tissue that forms after deep esophageal injury (foreign body or esophagitis resulting in inflammation that extends into the submucosal and muscular layers) and compromises food passage through the esophageal lumen; see Foreign Body, Esophageal, p 402; Esophagitis, p 366 for related information

EPIDEMIOLOGY

SPECIES, AGE, SEX: No age, sex, or species predisposition, although strictures due to foreign bodies (bones, fish hooks) are more common in dogs, and those due to chemical esophagitis (pills, caustic agents) are more common in cats.

RISK FACTORS

- Dogs: ingestion of bones, rocks, other foreign objects
- Cats: administration of medications that are not followed with water or food (capsules or uncoated tablets are the most common medications that lodge and cause esophagitis or stricture)
- Dogs or cats: gastroesophageal reflux due to anesthesia, persistent vomiting

ASSOCIATED CONDITIONS AND DISORDERS

- Esophagitis (common)
- Esophageal foreign bodies (common)
- Esophageal neoplasia (rare)

CLINICAL PRESENTATION

HISTORY, CHIEF COMPLAINT

- Regurgitation is the classic presenting sign (distinguish from vomiting: regurgitation involves no prodromal signs or active retching)
- Difficulty swallowing or pain associated with swallowing (repeated swallowing efforts)
- Ptyalism/hypersalivation
- Inappetence
- Lethargy
- Weight loss (if the condition is longstanding)
- Cough, increased respiratory rate or effort may be seen if the patient has concurrent aspiration pneumonia

PHYSICAL EXAM FINDINGS

- May be normal
- Weight loss
- Ptyalism or gagging
- Coughing, fever, or increased bronchovesicular sounds if aspiration pneumonia has occurred

ETIOLOGY AND PATHOPHYSIOLOGY

- Some of the more frequently reported causes of stricture formation are esophagitis secondary to chronic, persistent vomiting, foreign bodies that lodge in the esophagus, and ingestion of caustic substances (including medications that lodge in the esophagus).
- A commonly reported cause of esophagitis in dogs and cats is reflux esophagitis due to general anesthesia; however, the incidence of stricture secondary to this cause of esophagitis is much less frequent.
- Infrequently reported causes of stricture formation in dogs and cats are hiatal hernias, esophageal *Pythium* spp. infection, esophageal neoplasia (the most common cause of stricture formation in humans), and esophageal surgery (to remove foreign bodies, masses).
- Esophageal stricture formation requires substantial esophageal injury (usually chemical or mechanical) resulting in penetration or inflammation that extends to the submucosa or muscular layers. The normal repair process that follows this injury results in formation of fibrous connective tissue, and many times this occurs in a circular band of scar tissue that closes the esophageal lumen.

DIAGNOSIS

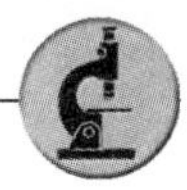

DIFFERENTIAL DIAGNOSIS

Regurgitation:

- Esophagitis
- Esophageal foreign body
- Esophageal mass (granuloma, parasites, neoplasia)
- Esophageal motility disorders (megaesophagus, congenital or acquired)
- Esophageal diverticulum
- Persistent right aortic arch
- Gastroesophageal reflux during anesthesia (history of anesthesia is important)
- Gagging/dysphagia
- Oropharyngeal, nasopharyngeal disease

INITIAL DATABASE

- Complete blood count, serum chemistry panel, urinalysis likely normal; changes are nonspecific.
  - Inflammatory leukogram present if aspiration pneumonia.
  - Evidence of dehydration possible if patient is unable to eat or drink.
- Thoracic/abdominal radiographs are indicated in all regurgitating patients.
  - Plain thoracic films may be normal, may show evidence of megaesophagus (or air/food in esophagus cranial to the stricture), or may reveal signs of aspiration pneumonia.
  - Plain abdominal films are usually unremarkable, unless there is a gastric outflow obstruction that is obvious and causing persistent vomiting/gastroesophageal reflux.

ADVANCED OR CONFIRMATORY TESTING

- Endoscopy is the preferred diagnostic imaging tool of choice for definitive identification of esophagitis, other esophageal anomalies, and esophageal strictures. In addition, endoscopy can be used for facilitating balloon dilation of the stricture site—the best approach for long-term stricture management (Fig. I-65).

- Contrast films may reveal stricture site or esophageal motility defect if food or paste is used, but liquid barium or iodinated contrast agents may pass through the stricture undetected. Contrast studies are helpful if multiple strictures are suspected, as visualization with the endoscope will be limited to the first stricture site in many animals. Caution is advised when administration of contrast is contemplated, as regurgitation of barium may result in aspiration.
- Fluoroscopy is often needed to identify a hiatal hernia or distal lower esophageal sphincter defect leading to reflux.
- Abdominal ultrasound is indicated to rule out abdominal causes of persistent vomiting that may lead to reflux esophagitis.

TREATMENT

THERAPEUTIC GOAL(S)

- Protecting the esophageal mucosa from additional injury
- Elimination of the underlying cause of the injury (if possible)
- Adequate resolution of regurgitaton, to allow the patient to maintain nutrition and hydration by oral feeding

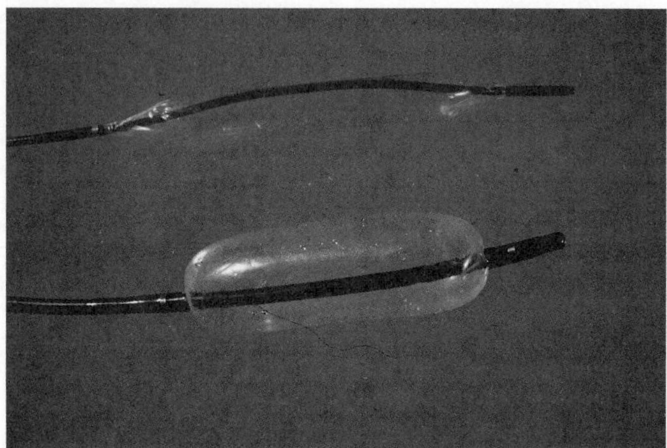

FIGURE I-64 Photo illustration of a 180-cm, 15-mm OD esophageal/pyloric balloon (CRE Wireguided balloon, Boston Scientific, Natick, MA). The upper balloon in the figure is undilated for comparison.

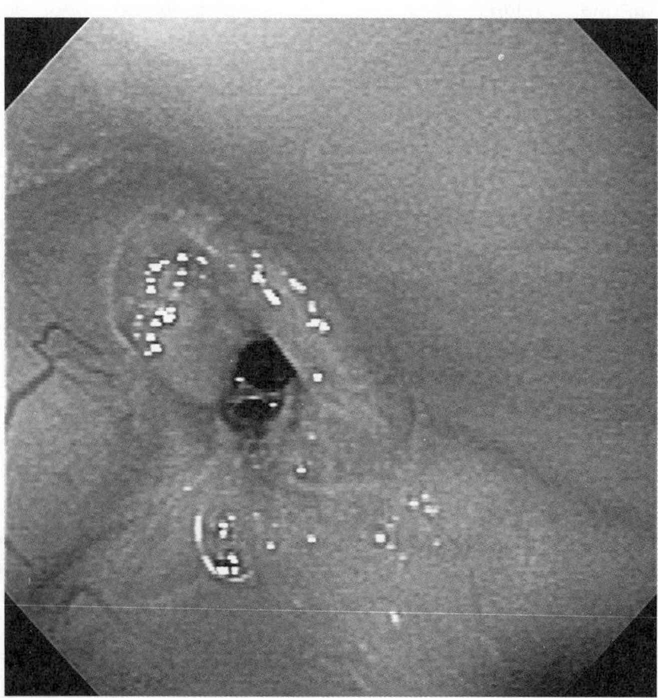

FIGURE I-65 Digital image obtained during esophagoscopy. A stricture site is apparent at the center of the image. Note that very little material (except small amounts of liquids) could pass through this opening.

ACUTE GENERAL TREATMENT

- Treatment of esophagitis if present (see Esophagitis, p 366) or other underlying causes of the stricture (control vomiting, remove foreign body, etc.).
- If the stricture is mild (liquid or canned foods can pass through the stricture site with few or no clinical signs, and no weight loss is evident), management may be accomplished by dietary modifications (feeding liquid, gruel, or canned foods in frequent, small meals).
- In severe strictures refractory to such conservative management, the stricture must be dilated (stretched) to allow liquids or gruels to pass. If this is not possible, a gastric feeding tube must be placed to allow maintenance of hydration and nutrition.
- Dilation can be accomplished by balloon or by esophageal bougienage. Balloon dilation is the preferred means of dilation and entails passage of an inflatable balloon catheter into the stricture site, inflating the balloon to allow the pressure to tear/break down the scar tissue, and thus increase the diameter of the esophageal lumen (Figs. I-64, I-66, I-67). Alternatively, bougienage involves the passage of rigid dilators of gradually increasing size through the stricture site. Both of these procedures are facilitated by concurrent use of endoscopic (or fluoroscopic) guidance to monitor the procedural success and to identify complications (e.g., esophageal tear) early.
- Corticosteroids (e.g., prednisone 0.5-1 mg/kg PO q 24h × 5-10 days) may be considered in an attempt to delay fibrosis of recently dilated strictures. Delayed healing and the risk of immunosuppression are drawbacks that contraindicate higher dose or longer term treatment.
- Lifelong dietary management is usually necessary, as complete resolution of the stricture and normalization of esophageal function are unlikely.

CHRONIC TREATMENT

- Many animals require several dilation procedures to achieve an esophageal opening that is sufficiently large to accommodate liquid or gruel diets.
- As for animals with esophagitis (see Esophagitis, p 366), long-term therapy may be needed. A cornerstone of treatment is the avoidance of hard foods.

POSSIBLE COMPLICATIONS

- The most important complication of esophageal stricture therapy is rupture or perforation of the esophagus during the ballooning or bougienage procedure.
- Complete recurrence of the stricture can occur if the dilation procedure is

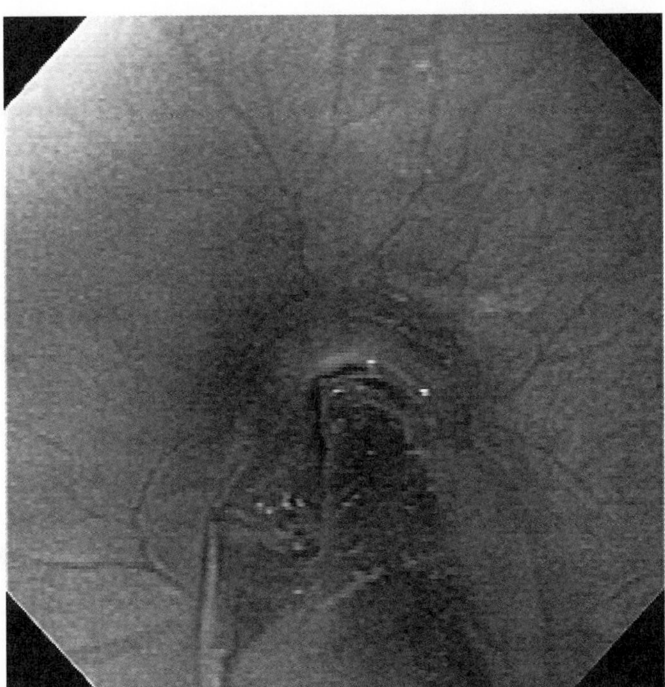

FIGURE I-66 Digital image obtained during esophagoscopy of the same patient as in Fig. I-65. This figure illustrates placement of the balloon in the stricture site. The balloon is partially inflated and momentarily will be fully inflated for stretching of the fibrous stricture, or cicatrix.

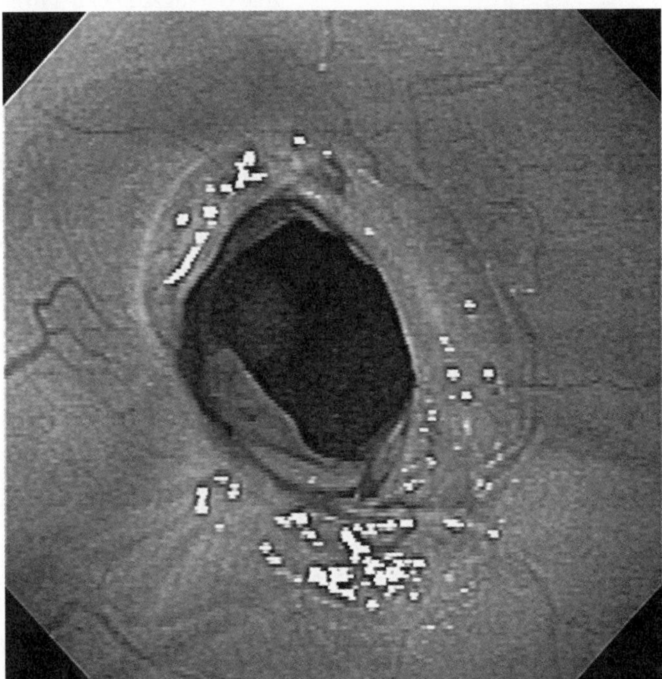

FIGURE I-67 Digital image obtained during esophagoscopy after balloon dilation of the stricture in the same dog as in the two preceding figures. Note that there is a degree of inflammation and bleeding at the site, but the lumen is markedly enlarged in diameter. The goal is to minimize the degree of inflammation created to avoid stricture redevelopment postballooning.

too aggressive, resulting in excessive inflammation.

- Aspiration pneumonia remains a possible complication if the stricture remains and the patient has episodes of regurgitation or does not have well-controlled dietary management (e.g., the dog gets into the garbage or is allowed to eat foods that will not pass).

PROGNOSIS AND OUTCOME

- The prognosis for mild strictures is generally good.
- The prognosis for severe strictures requiring multiple balloon dilation procedures is guarded.
- If the patient is able to be managed on liquid or gruel diets, with minimal to no regurgitation, the treatment is considered to be successful. Most animals with severe strictures must consume a softened, semi-liquid to liquid diet, as complete resolution of the stricture is not possible.

PEARLS & CONSIDERATIONS

COMMENTS

- Esophageal strictures are easy to diagnose (with endoscopy), but the difficult part is that there is a degree of clinical suspicion necessary to put the pieces together from the historic and physical exam findings.
- Esophageal strictures should be viewed as a clinical problem with a favorable outcome as long as appropriate dilation procedures are implemented and appropriate client expectations are achieved.

PREVENTION

- Prevent all dogs from eating bones, rocks, fish hooks, and other foreign objects.
- Oral medications should not be administered alone. They should either be given with food, followed with food, or, if the medication must be given on an empty stomach, it should be followed with water to prevent capsules or tablets from lodging in the esophagus.
- Do not tip surgical tables to a degree that will allow gastroesophageal reflux and esophagitis (a risk factor for strictures).

CLIENT EDUCATION

- The importance of using water after administration of medications cannot be overstressed.
- The long-term successful management of dogs or cats with strictures requires strict, lifelong dietary management.

SUGGESTED READING

Adamama-Moraitou KK, et al: Benign esophageal stricture in the dog and cat: A retrospective study of 20 cases. *Can J Vet Res* 66:55–59, 2002.

Leib MS, et al: Endoscopic balloon dilation of benign esophageal strictures in dogs and cats. *J Vet Intern Med* 15:547–552, 2001.

Westfall DS, et al: Evaluation of esophageal transit of tablets and capsules in 30 cats. *J Vet Intern Med* 15:467–470, 2001.

Willard MD, et al: Iatrogenic tears associated with ballooning of esophageal strictures. *J Am Anim Hosp Assoc* 30:431–435, 1994.

AUTHOR & EDITOR: **DEBRA L. ZORAN**

Esophagitis

BASIC INFORMATION

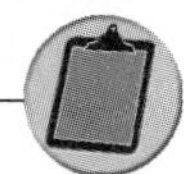

DEFINITION

Acute or chronic inflammation of the esophagus, most often secondary to reflux of gastric and/or duodenal contents

SYNONYM(S)

Gastroesophageal reflux
Reflux esophagitis

EPIDEMIOLOGY

SPECIES, AGE, SEX

- Dog and cat
- Any age, either sex can be affected; females may be overrepresented

RISK FACTORS

- General anesthesia, even of short duration:
  - Most common cause of reflux esophagitis in the dog and cat
- Congenital hiatal hernia
- Esophageal foreign body
- Oral medications (e.g., tetracyclines in cats) given without being followed by food or water administration
- Persistent vomiting

CLINICAL PRESENTATION

HISTORY, CHIEF COMPLAINT

- Mild esophagitis may be subclinical.
- Features noted by some owners include:
  - Increased swallowing motions, ptyalism (Fig. I-68).
  - Inappetence or anorexia, regurgitation, odynophagia (painful swallowing).
  - Reluctance to move or lie down.
  - Cats may vocalize after eating as an indication of esophageal pain.
- Affected patients may have a history that reveals risk factors (above).

PHYSICAL EXAM FINDINGS: May be normal.

When present, abnormalities can include:

- Thin body condition
- Dehydration
- Ptyalism (Fig. I-68)
- Pharyngitis
- Cranial abdominal/thoracic discomfort:
  - Hunched-up appearance
  - Guarding or pain on palpation

ETIOLOGY AND PATHOPHYSIOLOGY

- Etiology:
  - Premedicant drugs (atropine, benzodiazepines, phenothiazines, opioids) and anesthetic induction agents decrease lower esophageal sphincter tone, which may allow gastroesophageal reflux.
  - Anatomic abnormalities (e.g., hiatal hernia) of the distal esophageal region increase the risk of reflux esophagitis.
  - Ingestion of medications or chemicals can damage the esophagus mainly based on their pH and hyperosmolarity.
- Pathophysiology:
  - Esophageal mucosal contact with low pH gastric fluid, pepsin, trypsin, bile salts, and alkaline fluid results in damage and inflammation, which may remain mucosal or can involve all layers of the esophagus.
  - The volume, frequency, and duration of contact of material with the esophagus affect the severity of esophageal damage.

DIAGNOSIS

DIFFERENTIAL DIAGNOSIS

- Caustic agent ingestion (e.g., detergents, alkalis, acids)
- Thermal damage (e.g., gavage/tube feeding with excessively hot liquids)
- Esophageal foreign body
- Megaesophagus
- Vomiting
- Neoplasia or mass lesions (intrinsic or extrinsic)
- Vascular ring anomaly
- Hiatal hernia
- Gastroesophageal intussusception

INITIAL DATABASE

- Complete blood count, serum biochemistry profile, urinalysis: often within normal limits.
- Diagnostic imaging:
  - Survey thoracic radiographs:
    - Often no significant abnormal findings
    - Possible esophageal dilation
  - Contrast esophagram:
    - May demonstrate mucosal ulceration, mucosal hyperplasia, or decreased esophageal motility

ADVANCED OR CONFIRMATORY TESTING

- Esophagoscopy:
  - Definitive diagnosis:
    - Gross evaluation of the mucosa (Fig. I-69):
      - Extent of disease
      - Possible stricture formation
    - Evaluation of gastroesophageal junction:
      - Function
      - Evidence of reflux
    - Collection of samples for histopathologic examination

TREATMENT

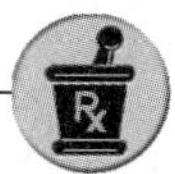

THERAPEUTIC GOAL(S)

- Decrease the amount and frequency of reflux
- Alter the composition of the reflux
- Protect the esophageal mucosa from further damage:
  - Allow healing
  - Prevent stricture formation

ACUTE GENERAL TREATMENT

- Feed a high-protein, low-fat diet:
  - Increases lower esophageal tone and encourages gastric emptying
- H_2 blockers (e.g., ranitidine 1-2 mg/kg PO or slow IV q 8-12h, or famotidine 0.5-1 mg/kg PO or IV q 12-24h):
  - Decrease the acidity of reflux
- Proton pump inhibitors (e.g., omeprazole 0.7 mg/kg PO q 24h):
  - May be more effective in decreasing the acidity of reflux
  - May result in faster healing of esophageal mucosal damage
- Prokinetic drugs (e.g., metoclopramide 0.2-0.5 mg/kg PO or SQ q 8h, or cisapride 0.1-1 mg/kg PO q 8-12h):
  - Increase lower esophageal tone
  - Promote aborad gastric contractions
  - Relax the pyloric region
- Sucralfate slurry (0.25-1 g/patient PO q 8h):
  - Protects the esophageal mucosa from further damage

CHRONIC TREATMENT

Continuation of treatments listed previously to prevent continuation/recurrence of problem until underlying cause identified and corrected:

- Decrease risk of stricture formation

POSSIBLE COMPLICATIONS

Esophageal stricture formation due to severe or unrecognized esophagitis

RECOMMENDED MONITORING

Ensure that normal esophageal function returns:

- Esophageal stricture usually becomes clinically apparent 3 to 4 weeks postinjury.
  - Increasing problem of regurgitation

PROGNOSIS AND OUTCOME

- Prognosis is good if esophagitis is recognized early and treated aggressively.

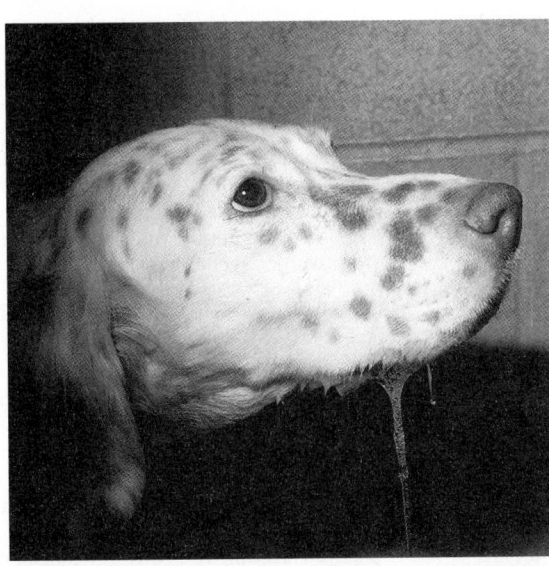

FIGURE I-68 Ptyalism in a dog with dysphagia caused by esophagitis. The underlying cause was gastroesophageal reflux. Courtesy of Dr. Richard Walshaw.

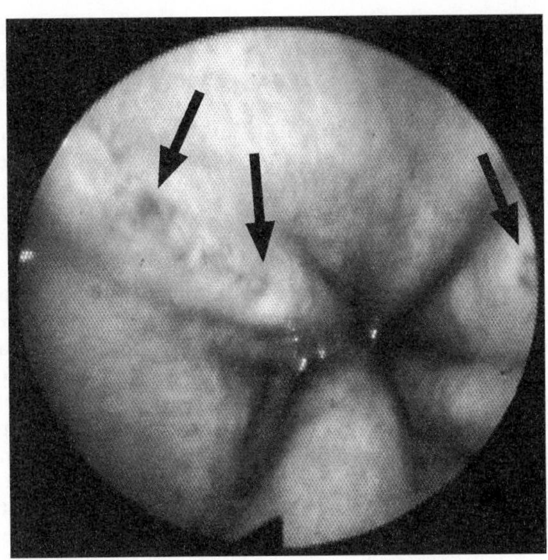

FIGURE I-69 Endoscopic view of the dog shown in Fig. I-68. Characteristic lesions are pinpoint mucosal petechiae or hemorrhages (*arrows*). Courtesy of Dr. Richard Walshaw.

- Prognosis is guarded for patients that develop long esophageal strictures.

PEARLS & CONSIDERATIONS

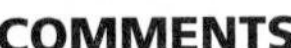

COMMENTS

Administer water (e.g., 5-10 ml by syringe) following any dry oral medication (tablet or capsule) given without food, to decrease the risk of prolonged contact of the tablet or capsule with the esophageal mucosa.

PREVENTION

Lavage and suction the esophagus after general anesthesia

- May decrease the acidity and volume of esophageal contents after anesthesia
- Has not been proven to decrease the incidence of reflux esophagitis

CLIENT EDUCATION

Administer water (e.g., 5-10 ml by syringe trickled in the cheek pouch) following any dry oral medication (tablet or capsule) given without food, to decrease the risk of prolonged contact of the tablet or capsule with the esophageal mucosa.

SUGGESTED READING

Han E: Diagnosis and management of reflux esophagitis. *Clin Tech Small Anim Pract* 18:231, 2003.

Han E, et al: Feline esophagitis secondary to gastroesophageal reflux disease: Clinical signs and radiographic, endoscopic, and histopathological findings. *J Am Anim Hosp Assoc* 39:161, 2003.

Sellon RK, et al: Esophagitis and esophageal strictures. *Vet Clin North Am Small Anim Pract* 33:945, 2003.

Tams TR: Diseases of the esophagus. In Tams TR (ed): *Handbook of Small Animal Gastroenterology*. St. Louis, Saunders, 2003, pp 118-157.

Westfall DS, et al: Evaluation of esophageal transit of tablets and capsules in 30 cats. *J Vet Intern Med* 15:467-470, 2001.

Wilson DV, et al: Postanesthetic esophageal dysfunction in 13 dogs. *J Am Anim Hosp Assoc* 40:455, 2004.

AUTHOR: **MARYANN G. RADLINSKY**
EDITOR: **RICHARD WALSHAW**

Ethylene Glycol Intoxication

BASIC INFORMATION

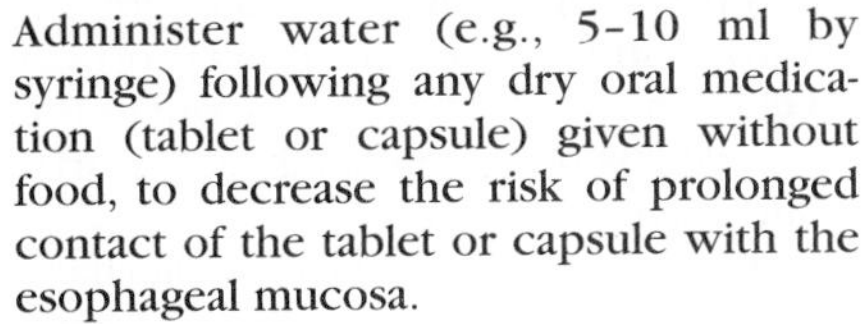

DEFINITION

Ethylene glycol (EG) intoxication manifests as the peracute onset of marked central nervous system (CNS) depression and progressive, dose-related systemic metabolic acidosis and renal failure secondary to ingestion of ethylene glycol. Sources of EG are commonly found in automobile radiator fluid, aircraft and runway deicing products, home solar units, and portable basketball goal post bases, among others.

SYNONYM(S)

Ethylene alcohol poisoning
Radiator antifreeze poisoning
CAS 107-21-1 poisoning
1,2-Ethanediolmonoethylene glycol poisoning

EPIDEMIOLOGY

SPECIES, AGE, SEX

- Animals of all ages, breeds, and sexes are equally susceptible to EG poisoning.
- Cats are most sensitive to EG intoxication.
- Dogs are intermediate in sensitivity among the species.
- Dogs are more commonly exposed than cats. Intact male dogs may be more likely to be involved.

RISK FACTORS

- Pets living outdoors or having free-range access to EG sources (e.g., garages).
- Northern climates or freezing temperatures provide increased opportunity, especially when water sources are limited (frozen) and antifreeze remains in the liquid state due to low freezing point.

- Engine leak is the most common source of exposure in pets.
- In the home, the garage is one of the most common exposure locations.

GEOGRAPHY AND SEASONALITY

- EG poisoning cases can occur throughout the year; it is no longer considered a seasonal problem.
- Northern and colder climates, but anywhere radiator fluid flushing is common. Summer automobile radiator flushing procedure is considered routine maintenance.

CLINICAL PRESENTATION

HISTORY, CHIEF COMPLAINT

- Evidence of exposure:
  - Pet being near an automobile garage or work area.
  - Roaming free in areas suspected or known to have EG sources.
- Classic "drunken sailor" behavior (stupor, narcosis, stumbling, ataxia, falling, nausea) is noted within 1 to 2 hours.
- Stupor phase gradually subsides over several hours.
  - Stupor phase may go unnoticed altogether in outdoor pets.
  - Owner may note the pet "getting better."
  - Patient is quiet, depressed, polydipsic, and polyuric.
- Patient gradually and steadily shows more weakness, depression, anorexia, and tachypnea/dyspnea as acute renal failure occurs (12 to 72 hours after ingestion).

PHYSICAL EXAM FINDINGS

- CNS depression, generalized weakness, hyporeflexia, knuckling, hypothermia, hypotension, tachycardia, vomiting, and polyuria.
- Urinary bladder may be empty on palpation.
- Patient may have already progressed beyond the initial "drunk" phase, and may not present as "classic," thus potentially confusing the picture.
  - Overt signs of acute renal failure (oliguria/anuria, anorexia, vomiting, renomegaly with signs of renal pain) begin 24 to 72 hours postingestion.
- In severe intoxications, seizures, nystagmus, and tremors may occur in the first few hours postingestion (grave prognosis).

ETIOLOGY AND PATHOPHYSIOLOGY

- Lethal dose of 95% ethylene glycol: 4.4 ml/kg (dog), 1.4 ml/kg (cat).
- Rapid oral absorption of EG.
  - Blood levels detectable in <30 minutes.
  - Initial CNS depression and narcosis, vasodilation, and hypotension with reflex tachycardia, diuretic effect.
- Metabolism involves hepatic alcohol dehydrogenase oxidation of EG to the aldehyde (glycoaldehyde).
  - This oxidation is a saturable process.
  - Therefore, it is the rate-limiting step.
  - The metabolic progression can be interrupted at this point with fomepizole or ethanol.
- Glycoaldehyde is very toxic but quickly converts to glycolic acid.
- Glycolic acid (30–45% of metabolite load) is fairly stable, further oxidizes to glyoxylic acid, then further metabolism occurs along several paths to oxalic acid, glycine, formate, hippurate, CO_2, etc. Aldehyde and acid load create a high anion gap metabolic acidosis.
- Metabolites inhibit the citric acid cycle and substrate-level phosphorylation, depress serotonin and pyruvate metabolism, and alter CNS amine levels.
- Secondary lactate accumulation, hypoperfusion, calcium oxalate formation, and precipitation in microvasculature and renal tubules occur.

DIAGNOSIS

DIFFERENTIAL DIAGNOSIS

Rule out other causes of acute CNS depression, ataxia, acidosis, or acute renal failure such as encephalitis, cranial trauma, intracranial neoplasia, diabetic ketoacidosis, or intoxication with barbiturates, aspirin, methanol, ethanol, isopropanol, propylene glycol, glycol ethers, vitamin D3, *Lilium* and *Hemerocallis* spp. (cats), nonsteroidal anti-inflammatory drugs, grapes, or raisins.

INITIAL DATABASE

- Ethylene Glycol Test Kit screening tool (Allelic Biosystems: PRN Pharmacal, Inc., Pensacola, FL, 800-874-9764). Recommended for use in dogs. Test can produce false-positive results with propylene glycol, glycerol, diethylene glycol (or other *cis* 1,2 diols), metaldehyde, and formaldehyde.
- Serum chemistry panel including serum electrolytes (especially Ca^{++}, Mg^{++}, K^{+}, and P).
- Acid-base: blood pH, pCO_2, pO_2, serum bicarbonate.
- Urinalysis: specific gravity, crystals, glucose, cellular debris.
  - As in any cause of acute anuric renal failure, specific gravity will not necessarily be low.
  - Calcium oxalate monohydrate crystals ("picket fence boards," flattened hexagon shapes: ⬡) can be observed 3 to 18 hours after EG ingestion, and are much more specific to ethylene glycol intoxication than calcium oxalate dihydrate crystals ("Maltese cross" or "square envelope" appearance: ☒), which can occur from nutritional or laboratory artifactual causes, as well as EG intoxication.
- Fluids: measure total input and output; body weight.
- Optional Wood's lamp detection of fluorescein dye added to the antifreeze; scan of muzzle, paws, vomitus, urine (excretes <3-6 hours in humans) for fluorescence that subjectively supports exposure.

ADVANCED OR CONFIRMATORY TESTING

- EG and glycolic acid levels (serum, urine). Requires STAT turnaround time to benefit early diagnosis in determining treatment approach.
- Serum osmolality:
  - Normal osmole gap: 5–10 mOsm/kg water (dogs and cats).
  - >20 mOsm/kg is strongly suggestive of EG intoxication.
  - Parallels EG blood level.
  - Significant increase <1-2 hours of exposure.
  - Osmole gap = measured osmolality − calculated osmolality.
- Anion gap
  - Normal anion gap: 10–25 mEq/L (dogs and cats).
  - >25 mEq/L is significant for diagnostic purposes.
  - May note change by 3 hours, but may require 6 hours. Therefore, less preferred as an early diagnostic tool.
- Ultrasound: Increased renal cortical echogenicity at 4 to 6 hours; late in the course, "halo sign" indicative of anuria, and grave prognosis.
  - Note: many normal, healthy cats have diffuse hyperechogenicity of renal cortices (avoid overinterpretation).
- Renal calcium level in postmortem tissue sample.

TREATMENT

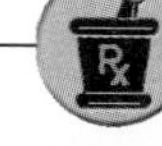

THERAPEUTIC GOAL(S)

- Interrupt conversion of EG to toxic metabolites early postexposure (window of opportunity: dogs, <8-12 hours; cats <2 hours)
- Prevent oliguria and rapidly progressive acute renal failure
- Acid base management

ACUTE GENERAL TREATMENT

- Induction of vomiting (hydrogen peroxide 3%: 0.25–0.5 ml/kg PO once, or syrup of ipecac: 2–6 ml total dose PO once) and administration of activated charcoal (dose according to packaging label of product; e.g., 10 ml of activated charcoal suspension PO made from 2 g activated charcoal suspended in 10 ml tap water) can reduce absorption within 30 to 60 minutes and are indicated if patient is a good risk.

- Interrupt conversion to toxic metabolites with fomepizole (4-MP, 4-methylpyrazole, Antizol-Vet, Orphan Medical).
  - Loading dose: 20 mg/kg slow IV infusion.
  - Then 15 mg/kg slow IV q 12h × 3 treatments in the dog.
  - Not effective in cats at labeled dose.
- Extralabel fomepizole: use in cats <3 hours after ingestion, at 125 mg/kg slow IV infusion, then 31.25 mg/kg q 12h × 3 treatments, has shown significant success.
- 7% ethanol solution.
  - Loading dose: 8.6 ml/kg slow IV.
  - Maintenance dose: 1.43–2.86 ml/kg/hr constant rate infusion (CRI) to effect.
    - Achieve serum ethanol concentrations of 100 mg/dl, or lethargic/comatose state.
    - Duration: approximately 48 hours.
  - Dogs treated with ethanol starting at 3 hours postingestion of EG excrete 80% of EG intact.
- Hemodialysis greater than peritoneal dialysis while on ethanol or fomepizole. Immediate dialysis on any patient showing clinical signs of toxicity will tend to increase the survival rate.
- Acid base and perfusion management is critical to survival. Sodium bicarbonate CRI as needed for metabolic acidosis.
- Crystalloids: high infusion rate required to correct severe dehydration and hypoperfusion.
- Provide cofactors for metabolism of toxic compounds.
  - Pyridoxine 1–2 mg/kg IV q 6h.
  - Thiamine 50 mg slow IV q 6h.

CHRONIC TREATMENT

Dialysis to allow regeneration of damaged tubular basement membrane

POSSIBLE COMPLICATIONS

Renal compromise. May be salvageable, depending on degree of insult and response to aggressive treatment

RECOMMENDED MONITORING

Renal function (urinalysis, serum chemistry, biopsy, etc.) should be monitored as needed in surviving patients.

PROGNOSIS AND OUTCOME

- Dogs: fair to good if proper, aggressive intervention within 8 to 12 hours; prognosis worsens by the hour if clinical signs are apparent and/or if a large dose was ingested.
- Cats: guarded to poor at best in any case showing clinical signs. Aggressive intervention (interruption of metabolism with high doses of fomepizole, dialysis, acid-base management) within 3 hours may prove successful.

PEARLS & CONSIDERATIONS

COMMENTS

- Progression of irreversible, potentially life-threatening effects in patients that have ingested EG is rapid (hours); therefore, evaluation and treatment are urgent, even in animals without overt clinical signs.
- "Safe antifreeze" contains propylene glycol, which is less toxic compared to EG; much less risk of renal injury. Dogs would generally need to ingest three to four times more propylene glycol to develop clinical signs as compared to ethylene glycol.
- Use of injectable valium, phenobarbital or pentobarbital, or some commercial oral preparations of activated charcoal before using EG test kit can give a false-positive result due to presence of propylene glycol in them.
- Calcium oxalate monohydrate urinary crystals (⬡) are strongly suggestive of ethylene glycol intoxication, whereas calcium oxalate dihydrate crystals (☒) may also be caused by nutrition, or refrigeration of the urine sample).
- EG test kit detects EG blood concentration >50 mg/dl. Shelf life of EG test kit is about 2 years.
  - Since cats are more sensitive to EG than dogs, a negative result (below the kit's detection limit) could possibly be misleading.
- Many human hospital laboratories have the capability of detecting and quantifying EG quickly in different body fluids and can be helpful if an EG test kit is not available on site.
- Antifreeze (ethylene glycol) is generally fluorescent green, viscous (like light syrup), and does not have a volatile odor; windshield washer fluid (not ethylene glycol) is generally translucent blue, pungent (volatile odor), and nonviscous (like water).

PREVENTION

Keep animals indoors, especially in freezing temperatures (frozen water sources, antifreeze remain in liquid state, thus are more attractive).

CLIENT EDUCATION

Lock antifreeze plastic containers away from chewing dogs. Use cat litter to clean up any spills, leaks. About 1 tsp (5 ml) of radiator antifreeze is lethal to an adult cat.

SUGGESTED READING

Connally HE, Thrall MA: Safety and efficacy of high dose fomepizole as therapy for EG intoxication in cats (Abstract). Proceedings, 8th IVECCS, San Antonio, TX, September, 2002.

Khan SA, et al: Ethylene glycol exposures managed by the ASPCA National Animal Poison Control Center from July 1995 to December 1997. *Vet Human Tox* 41(6):403–406, 1999.

Thrall MA, Grauer GF, Dial SM: Antifreeze poisoning. In Bonagura JD, Kirk RW (eds): *Kirk's Current Veterinary Therapy XII Small Animal Practice*. Philadelphia, WB Saunders, 1995, pp 232–237.

AUTHOR: **MICHAEL W. KNIGHT**
EDITOR: **SAFDAR A. KHAN**

Exocrine Pancreatic Insufficiency

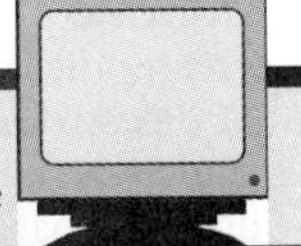

BASIC INFORMATION

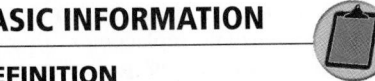

DEFINITION

A syndrome caused by insufficient secretion of pancreatic digestive enzymes by the exocrine pancreas

SYNONYM(S)

EPI

EPIDEMIOLOGY

SPECIES, AGE, SEX: Occurs more commonly in dogs than in cats. No known sex predilection. Patients of any age can be affected, but in dogs exocrine pancreatic insufficiency (EPI) is most commonly diagnosed in young adults. Cats with EPI can be of any age.

GENETICS AND BREED PREDISPOSITION: In dogs, EPI most commonly occurs in the German shepherd, for which an autosomal recessive inheritance has been proposed. A breed predilection has also been reported for rough coated collies. There is no known breed predilection in cats.

RISK FACTORS

- Chronic pancreatitis can lead to destruction of exocrine pancreatic tissue and lead to EPI.
- Pancreatic adenocarcinoma could lead to obstruction of the pancreatic duct, leading to lack of pancreatic enzyme secretion in the small intestine.

ASSOCIATED CONDITIONS AND DISORDERS Many canine and feline patients with EPI have other gastrointestinal disorders. Dogs with EPI commonly have secondary small intestinal bacterial overgrowth (also termed Antibiotic-Responsive Diarrhea, see p 74) while cats often have concurrent inflammatory bowel disease (see Inflammatory Bowel Disease, p 594).

CLINICAL PRESENTATION

HISTORY, CHIEF COMPLAINT

- Weight loss.
- Ravenous appetite.
- Loose stools and/or diarrhea.
- Poor haircoat.
- Uncommonly, diabetic cats and dogs with signs due to poor glycemic control are found to have EPI, and successful management of EPI is associated with an improvement in the diabetic state.

PHYSICAL EXAM FINDINGS

- Poor body condition
- Poor haircoat

ETIOLOGY AND PATHOPHYSIOLOGY

- The most common cause of EPI in the dog is pancreatic acinar atrophy.
- The most common cause of EPI in the cat and the second most common cause of EPI in the dog is chronic pancreatitis.
- Potential causes of EPI are obstruction of the pancreatic duct by a pancreatic adenocarcinoma and pancreatic aplasia or hypoplasia, but these have not yet been reported in dogs or cats.
- Decreased secretion of exocrine pancreatic digestive enzymes leads to lack of digestive enzymes in the small intestine, which will lead to maldigestion and associated clinical signs.
- Secondary cobalamin deficiency and in dogs small intestinal bacterial overgrowth (termed antibiotic-responsive diarrhea by some) are common.
- Diabetes mellitus may be due to chronic pancreatitis, which may also lead to EPI.

DIAGNOSIS

DIFFERENTIAL DIAGNOSIS

- Primary small intestinal disease
- Other secondary causes of chronic diarrhea and weight loss (i.e., hepatic failure, renal failure, hypoadrenocorticism, inflammatory or infiltrative bowel diseases, hyperthyroidism [cats])

INITIAL DATABASE

- Complete blood count, serum chemistry profile, and urinalysis are usually within normal limits.
- Imaging studies are usually within normal limits.

ADVANCED OR CONFIRMATORY TESTING

- Serum trypsin-like immunoreactivity (TLI) is the diagnostic test of choice for the diagnosis of EPI.
  - Serum TLI is species-specific.
  - A severely decreased serum TLI concentration is diagnostic of EPI.
    - In affected dogs: ≤2.5 μg/L (canine TLI).
    - In affected cats: ≤8.0 μg/L (feline TLI).
  - Some patients with EPI may have a serum TLI concentration in the questionable range (>2.5 but <5.0 μg/L [dog]; >8.0 but <12.0 μg/L [cat]).
    - These patients most likely have chronic small intestinal disease and should be evaluated for such, then retested 4 to 6 weeks later.
- Other diagnostic tests are much less reliable and should *not* be used for the diagnosis of EPI:
  - Fecal proteolytic activity.
  - Fecal elastase concentration.
  - Bentiromide absorption test.

TREATMENT

THERAPEUTIC GOAL(S)

- Pancreatic enzyme replacement
- Replenishment of body's vitamin stores
- Treatment of concurrent conditions if present:
  - Antibiotic-responsive enteritis/small intestinal bacterial overgrowth
  - Diabetes mellitus
  - Inflammatory bowel disease

ACUTE GENERAL TREATMENT

- Oral enzyme replacement therapy.
  - Starting dose: 1 tsp per 10 kg body weight with each meal.
  - Tablets and capsules are not as effective as powder.
  - Premixing the pancreatic enzymes with the diet is not necessary.
- Parenteral cobalamin supplementation if the patient is cobalamin-deficient (approximately 50% of dogs with EPI and virtually all cats with EPI are cobalamin-deficient).
  - Dose: 150–250 μg pure cobalamin (cats) or 250–1000 μg pure cobalamin (for small and large dogs, respectively), given once weekly × 6 weeks, then every other week for 6 weeks, followed by one additional dose 1 month later, and a recheck of serum cobalamin concentration 1 month after the last dose.

CHRONIC TREATMENT

- Oral enzyme replacement therapy:
  - Once patients have fully responded and gained back their original body weight, the amount of enzyme can be decreased to the lowest effective dose, titrated based on stool consistency and body weight
- Oral antibiotic therapy (i.e., tylosin 25 mg/kg PO q 12h for 6 weeks) if canine patient does not respond to enzyme replacement therapy and has antibiotic-responsive enteritis
- Insulin therapy if patient has concurrent diabetes mellitus

POSSIBLE COMPLICATIONS

Enzyme supplementation can lead to oral bleeding in approximately 10% of patients:

- Most of these patients will normalize after reduction of the dose

RECOMMENDED MONITORING

Body weight and fecal quality

PROGNOSIS AND OUTCOME

Most patients with EPI respond to therapy and have a normal life.

PEARLS & CONSIDERATIONS

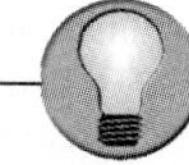

COMMENTS

- Some patients may not respond to enzyme replacement therapy and cobalamin supplementation alone.
  - Many of these patients have concurrent small intestinal disease (i.e., small intestinal bacterial overgrowth/antibiotic-responsive enteritis, and/or inflammatory bowel disease).
  - If concurrent disease cannot be identified, gastric acid inhibition can be tried (traditionally cimetidine has been used, but recently omeprazole 0.7 mg/kg PO q 24h has been used successfully).
- Fresh-frozen raw pancreas can also be used for enzyme replacement therapy (1–2 oz of ground raw pancreas equals about 1 tsp of powdered pancreatic extract).

SUGGESTED READING

Steiner JM, Williams DA: Serum feline trypsin-like immunoreactivity in cats with exocrine pancreatic insufficiency. *J Vet Intern Med* 14:627, 2000.

Westermarck E, Wiberg M, Steiner JM, Williams DA: Exocrine pancreatic insufficiency in dogs and cats. In Ettinger SJ, Feldman EC (eds): *Textbook of Veterinary Internal Medicine*, ed 6. St. Louis, Elsevier Saunders, 2005, pp 1492–1495.

AUTHOR: **JÖRG M. STEINER**
EDITOR: **KEITH P. RICHTER**

Eyelid Defects: Trauma, Masses

BASIC INFORMATION

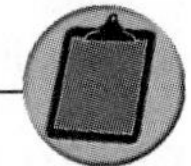

DEFINITION

Eyelid trauma is associated with any external injury to the eyelid, predisposing to inflammation or laceration.

Eyelid masses are associated with neoplasic or inflammatory conditions.

SYNONYM(S)

Chalazion: hordeolum, meibomian gland cyst

Meibomian glands: tarsal glands, palpebral glands

EPIDEMIOLOGY

SPECIES, AGE, SEX

- Dogs and cats.
- No sex predisposition.
- *Eyelid trauma* may occur at any age.
- *Eyelid mass*: average age 9 to 10 years (eyelid neoplasia; dogs), but depends on type of mass.

GENETICS AND BREED PREDISPOSITION

- *Eyelid trauma*: more common in young animals, outdoor animals, and sporting breeds of dogs.
- *Eyelid mass* (dogs): more common in the American cocker spaniel, boxer, poodle, golden retriever, Labrador retriever, English springer spaniel, beagle, collie, Siberian husky, and English setter.

RISK FACTORS

- Prevalence of eyelid neoplasia in cats increases with age
- White hair in the periocular region predisposes to squamous cell carcinoma (SCC), the most common eyelid neoplasm in cats
- Excessive sunlight predisposes to the development of SCC

ASSOCIATED CONDITIONS AND DISORDERS

Eyelid trauma:

- Corneal/scleral trauma (see Corneal/Scleral Trauma, p 244)
- Uveitis (see Uveitis, p 1134)

Eyelid mass:

- Blepharitis (eyelid inflammation)
- Conjunctivitis (see Conjunctivitis: Dogs, p 233; Cats, p 231)
- Corneal ulceration (see Corneal Ulceration, p 246)

CLINICAL PRESENTATION

HISTORY, CHIEF COMPLAINT

Eyelid trauma:

- Witnessed traumatic event
- Swollen eyelid(s) (blepharoedema)
- ± Eyelid laceration

Eyelid mass:

- Growth on eyelid and/or eyelid margin
- Persistent or intermittant bleeding of eyelid
- Signs of ocular pain if mass large and causing conjunctival and/or corneal irritation
- Ocular discharge

PHYSICAL EXAM FINDINGS

- *Eyelid trauma* (some or all of the following):
  - Blepharoedema
  - Eyelid laceration (partial or full-thickness)
  - Blepharospasm
  - Ocular discharge
  - Conjunctival hyperemia/edema (chemosis)
  - Keratitis (ulcerative or nonulcerative)
- *Eyelid mass* (some or all of the following):
  - Mass located along eyelid margin or adjacent to margin of eyelid
  - Size, location, and appearance vary with type of mass:
    - Neoplasm associated with the meibomian gland appears as an irregular, raised, variably sized mass ± pigment.
    - SCC appears as an erosive, ulcerated mass along the eyelid, often near the medial canthus.
    - Chalazion (meibomian gland cyst) presents as smooth, raised, yellow to white mass associated with the meibomian gland.
  - Ocular discharge, blepharospasm, conjunctivitis, keratitis if mass irritating the eye
  - Eyelid hemorrhage
  - Lagophthalmos (incomplete closure of the eyelids)

ETIOLOGY AND PATHOPHYSIOLOGY

- *Eyelid trauma* is generally associated with blunt trauma, penetration by sharp objects, or self-mutilation (pawing at eye).
- *Eyelid mass*:
  - Eyelid neoplasia:
    - Common in dogs; most are benign.
    - Rare in cats; most are SCC (malignant).
    - Similar to those of the skin; arise from epithelial, mesenchymal, and melanogenic cells.
    - Eighty-two percent of eyelid neoplasms in dogs are sebaceous adenomas, papillomas, or melanomas.
    - Sebaceous gland tumors (sebaceous adenoma, sebaceous epithelioma, and sebaceous adenocarcinoma) arise from the meibomian glands.
  - Focal eyelid inflammation:
    - A chalazion is a pyogranuloma associated with retained meibomian gland secretions.

DIAGNOSIS

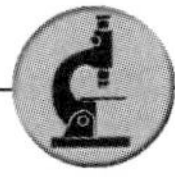

DIFFERENTIAL DIAGNOSIS

Eyelid swelling:

- Anaphylaxis
- Conjunctival/subpalpebral foreign body

INITIAL DATABASE

Complete ophthalmic examination including:

- Schirmer tear test (Normal >15 mm after 1 minute in dogs, variable in cats)
- Fluorescein dye application
- Intraocular pressures (Normal 20 ± 5 mmHg by applanation tonometry)
- Examination of periocular (e.g., conjunctiva) and intraocular structures, especially if trauma suspected
- Examination of eyelid margin for extent of laceration or extent and point of origin of mass

ADVANCED OR CONFIRMATORY TESTING

- Fine-needle aspiration and cytology of eyelid masses

- Histopathologic evaluation of all surgically removed eyelid masses

TREATMENT

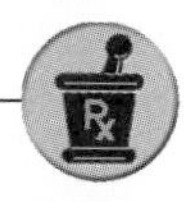

THERAPEUTIC GOAL(S)

- Restore normal eyelid conformation
- Eliminate ocular irritation
- Prevent recurrence of eyelid mass

ACUTE GENERAL TREATMENT

- *Eyelid trauma*:
  - Laceration requires primary/surgical closure of wound.
  - If full-thickness, close in two layers (conjunctiva followed by skin), starting at eyelid margin, to ensure accurate apposition of eyelid margin.
- *Eyelid mass*:
  - Neoplasia:
    - Surgical removal:
      - If involves eyelid margin and ≤1/3 length of eyelid, remove by a full-thickness "V"- or "house"-shaped excision.
      - Close in two layers (see *Eyelid Trauma* under Acute General Treatment above).
      - Eyelid margin mass >$\frac{1}{3}$ eyelid length requires a plasty procedure to ensure proper eyelid length (e.g., H-plasty). Consider referral to ophthalmologist or surgeon.
    - Cryosurgery:
      - Useful in treating benign eyelid mass in older animals.
      - May be performed under sedation.
      - Recurrence rate higher with cryotherapy than with full-thickness excision.
- Chalazion:
  - Surgical treatment:
    - Scalpel incision of overlying palpebral conjunctiva with curettage; heals by second intention.
  - Topical antibiotic-corticosteroid (e.g., neomycin-polymyxin-dexamethasone suspension) q 8h for 7 days after surgery.

POSSIBLE COMPLICATIONS

- Poor apposition of eyelid margin results in cicatrix (scar) formation predisposing to entropion or ectropion, or "step" to eyelid margin, resulting in corneal irritation and ulceration
- Improperly placed sutures at the eyelid margin can predispose to corneal ulceration
- Local regrowth of eyelid mass, if mass not completely removed

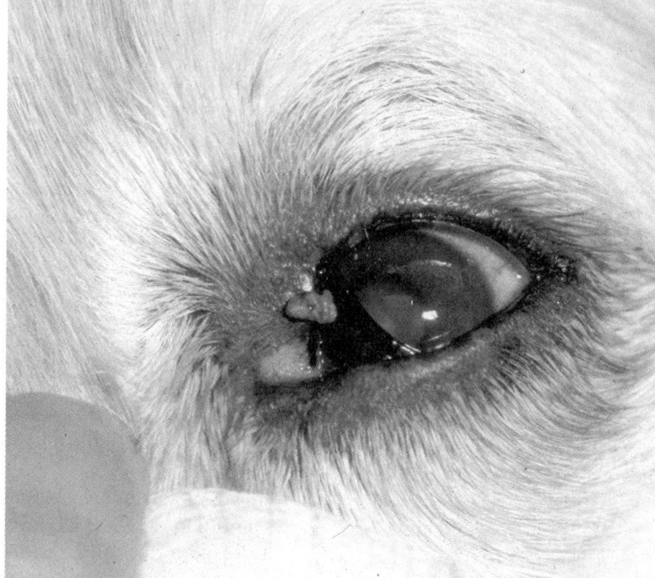

FIGURE I-70 Eyelid mass. Courtesy of Dr. Phillip A. Moore.

RECOMMENDED MONITORING

Reevaluate apposition of eyelid margin and remove skin sutures 10 days after surgery

PROGNOSIS AND OUTCOME

- Eyelid laceration: prognosis good if apposition of eyelid margin is achieved.
- Removal of eyelid neoplasm—dogs: prognosis good, majority are benign; cats: prognosis guarded, majority are malignant.
- Local recurrence is possible if an eyelid mass is not completely excised.

PEARLS & CONSIDERATIONS

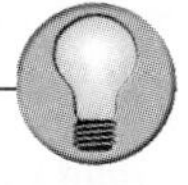

COMMENTS

- Eyelid lacerations are treated surgically, not as open wounds, to prevent eyelid scarring, contraction, and distortion of the eyelid margin.
- Eyelid masses should be removed early to prevent the need for plasty procedures.

PREVENTION

Limit actinic radiation (sunlight) exposure in white cats to decrease the potential for SCC

CLIENT EDUCATION

Recurrence is possible after the removal of any eyelid mass

SUGGESTED READING

Bedford PGC: Diseases and surgery of the canine eyelid. In Gelatt KN (ed): *Veterinary Ophthalmology*. Philadelphia, Lippincott Williams & Wilkins, 1999, pp 535–568.

Martin CL: Eyelids. In Martin CL (ed): *Ophthalmic Disease in Veterinary Medicine*. London, Manson Publishing, Ltd, 2005, pp 145–182.

AUTHOR: **PHILLIP A. MOORE**
EDITOR: **CHERYL L. CULLEN**

Facial Muscle Wasting

BASIC INFORMATION

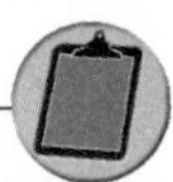

DEFINITION

Atrophy of the muscles of mastication, mainly the temporal and masseter muscles

SYNONYM(S)

Masticatory muscle atrophy

EPIDEMIOLOGY

SPECIES, AGE, SEX: Dogs (most commonly) and cats (rarely), any age, any sex; with muscular dystrophy (MD), only males affected; with hereditary Labrador retriever myopathy (HLRM), males and females affected.

GENETICS AND BREED PREDISPOSITION

- German shepherd, retrievers, Doberman pinscher, spaniels: masticatory muscle myositis (MMM)
- Shetland sheepdogs, rough and smooth-coated collies: dermatomyositis
- German shepherds, other large breeds: idiopathic polymyositis (IP)
- Large-breed dogs: glucocorticoid induced muscle atrophy
- Young male golden retriever: muscular dystrophy
- Labrador retriever: HLRM
- Bassett hounds: temporomandibular joint (TMJ) dysplasia

ASSOCIATED CONDITIONS AND DISORDERS

- Submandibular and prescapular lymphadenopathy (see Lymphadenopathy, p 644)
- Generalized muscle atrophy

CLINICAL PRESENTATION

HISTORY, CHIEF COMPLAINT

- Detailed history to include inquiries regarding previous bouts of painful mastication or chronic corticosteroid use.
- History may reflect abnormalities isolated to facial musculature or reflective of generalized myopathy.
  - Facial:
    - Prominence of external occipital protuberance noticed by owner.
    - Difficulty or inability to prehend food (less common).
    - Reflects either weakness (decreased jaw tone) or masticatory muscle fibrosis (increased jaw tone or trismus [inability to open the mouth]).
    - Prior episode(s) of painful mastication and crying while chewing: MMM.
  - Generalized:
    - Concomitant mild to severe weakness, exacerbated by exercise; generalized muscle atrophy: IP.
    - Bunny hopping gait, progressing to a more stilted gait with a plantigrade stance: MD.

PHYSICAL EXAM FINDINGS

- Full physical examination, paying particular attention to the head, the condition of other muscle groups, and the skin.
- Bilateral atrophy of the temporal and masseter muscles; skull-like appearance of the head.
  - Dogs with MMM can show salivation, dysphagia, and difficulty in opening their mouths, progressing to trismus.
  - Dogs with dermatomyositis can show generalized muscle atrophy, decreased jaw tone, facial nerve paralysis, stiff gait, dysphagia, regurgitation, and skin lesions.
- Enophthalmos, with third eyelid protrusion and small palpebral fissure due to dramatic loss of retrobulbar muscular support.
- Unilateral temporal muscle atrophy: ipsilateral denervation of the mandibular branch of the trigeminal nerve.

ETIOLOGY AND PATHOPHYSIOLOGY

- Developmental
  - MD
  - HLRM
  - Dermatomyositis
- Idiopathic
  - Trigeminal neuropathy
- Infectious
  - Toxoplasmosis (rare)
  - Neosporosis (rare)
- Immune-mediated
  - Systemic lupus erythematosus
  - Idiopathic polymyositis
  - MMM
- Iatrogenic
  - Glucocorticoid administration
- Metabolic
  - Hyperadrenocorticism
  - Cardiac cachexia
- Neoplastic
  - Cachexia and protein energy malnutrition resulting in muscle atrophy are features of many chronic neoplastic and inflammatory conditions
- Disuse atrophy
  - TMJ dysplasia
  - Traumatic luxation of the TMJ (cats)
  - TMJ ankylosis (cats)

DIAGNOSIS

DIFFERENTIAL DIAGNOSIS

- Masticatory muscle myositis
- Chronic idiopathic polymyositis
- Trigeminal neuropathy
- Protozoal myositis
- MD
- HLRM
- Dermatomyositis

INITIAL DATABASE

- Complete blood count usually normal by the time the muscles are atrophied
- Serum biochemistry profile
  - Elevated muscle enzyme levels (creatine kinase and aspartate aminotransferase): IP, MMM, DM, MD, HLRM
  - Hyperglobulinemia: IP

ADVANCED OR CONFIRMATORY TESTING

- Muscle biopsies and histopathology (see Muscle and Nerve Biopsy, p 1279):
  - Immunohistochemistry shows lack of dystrophin (MD).
  - Paucity of type 2 myofibers (HLRM).
  - Antibodies against type 2 myofibers on frozen sections of muscle (MMM).
  - Myofiber necrosis with mononuclear cell infiltrates, atrophy, and fibrosis (dermatomyositis).
  - Multifocal necrosis and phagocytosis of type 1 and type 2 myofibers (IP).
- Circulating serum antibodies against type 2 myofiber muscle fibers: MMM.
- Serology for *Toxoplasma* and *Neospora*: protozoal myositis.
- Electromyography more useful in determining neurologic, rather than muscular, etiology of the atrophy.

TREATMENT

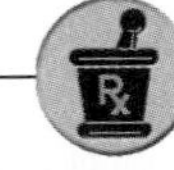

THERAPEUTIC GOAL(S)

Halt process of muscle inflammation and atrophy

CHRONIC TREATMENT

- Glucocorticoid therapy
  - Masticatory muscle myositis (prednisone 1 mg/kg q 12h, must continue for at least 21 days, then taper according to need and avoidance of side effects).
  - Idiopathic polymyositis (prednisone 1–2 mg/kg q 12h for 14 days, then tapering over at least 4 weeks to 12 months or longer).
  - Dermatomyositis (variable response).
- Upright feeding of dogs with concomitant megaesophagus.
- Clindamycin (12–25 mg/kg PO q 12h): protozoal myositis.

POSSIBLE COMPLICATIONS

Corticosteroid side effects

RECOMMENDED MONITORING

Monitor for corticosteroid side effects and taper the dose depending on muscle condition and function

PROGNOSIS AND OUTCOME

Variable, depending on the underlying etiology. Process is reversible, provided the muscles have not yet undergone extensive fibrosis

PEARLS & CONSIDERATIONS

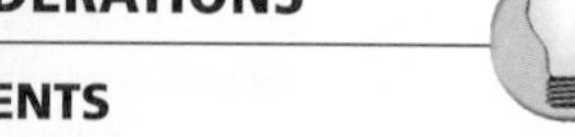

COMMENTS

- Facial muscle atrophy is a common feature of many emaciating conditions in which there is also accompanying generalized loss of lean body mass.
- Generalized muscle atrophy is often first noticed in the facial muscles, especially in long-haired breeds.
- Of all the differentials discussed in this section, only trigeminal nerve abnormalities, MMM, and anomalies of the TMJs are strictly confined to facial muscle atrophy.

CLIENT EDUCATION

Encourage clients to present patients early in the disease process

SUGGESTED READING

Gilmour MA, et al: Masticatory myopathy in the dog: A retrospective study of 18 cases. *J Am Anim Hosp Assoc* 28:300, 1992.

Taylor SM: Disorders of muscle. In Nelson RW, Couto CG (eds): *Small Animal Internal Medicine*. St. Louis, Mosby, 2003, pp 1062–1070.

AUTHOR: **JOHAN P. SCHOEMAN**

EDITOR: **ETIENNE CÔTÉ**

Facial Paralysis, Idiopathic

BASIC INFORMATION

DEFINITION

An acute neuropathy of unknown etiology affecting one or both facial nerves

EPIDEMIOLOGY

SPECIES, AGE, SEX

- Mature (>5 years) dogs and cats may be affected
- No known gender predisposition

GENETICS AND BREED PREDISPOSITION: Cocker spaniels, golden retrievers, and domestic long-haired cats are overrepresented.

CLINICAL PRESENTATION

HISTORY, CHIEF COMPLAINT

- Rapid onset of drooling from one side of the mouth.
- Inability to blink:
  - This deficit may be somewhat inapparent to owners since dogs and cats with facial paralysis retain the ability to periodically retract the globe (oculomotor nerve), which may give the appearance of a blink due to passive motion of the third eyelid.
- Dogs usually have an apparent ear droop and occasionally will have deviation of the nose away from the affected side. Food may collect in the affected commissure, and there may be associated halitosis.
- Occasionally clinical signs are bilateral, but may begin on one side and take several days or weeks to affect the contralateral side.

PHYSICAL EXAM FINDINGS

- The menace response and palpebral reflex on the affected side are absent.
- Facial drooping, ptyalism, and ptosis may be evident.
- When a noxious stimulus is applied to the upper lip, the muscles of facial expression will fail to contract (trigeminofacial reflex); sensation of the face remains unaffected.
- In chronic cases, there may be permanent lip contracture.
- Corneal ulceration may be evident due to damage to the parasympathetic fibers responsible for tear production and/or exposure keratitis from the inability to blink.

ETIOLOGY AND PATHOPHYSIOLOGY

- The pathogenesis in domestic animals is unknown, but in humans, a similar condition (Bell's palsy) is associated with herpes simplex virus infection.
- Histopathologic studies reveal active degeneration of large- and small-caliber myelinated fibers. Inflammation is absent.

DIAGNOSIS

DIFFERENTIAL DIAGNOSIS

- Idiopathic facial paralysis must be differentiated from other conditions involving the peripheral aspect of the facial nerve (e.g., otitis media-interna, hypothyroidism, ear polyps, and polyneuropathies).
- When they cause facial paralysis, disorders of the central nervous system such as neoplasia, encephalitis, congenital malformations, and trauma are usually accompanied by additional neurologic deficits.

INITIAL DATABASE

- Complete neurologic and otoscopic examination
- Serum chemistry panel and complete blood count; unremarkable with idiopathic facial paralysis
- Thyroid panel
- Schirmer tear test

ADVANCED OR CONFIRMATORY TESTING

Advanced imaging (e.g., magnetic resonance imaging, computed tomography scan) may be indicated for evaluation of the tympanic bullae and brainstem.

TREATMENT

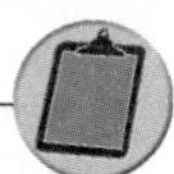

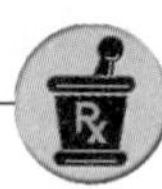

THERAPEUTIC GOAL(S)

Prevention of corneal ulceration. No specific therapy is indicated for the remaining manifestations of facial paralysis

ACUTE GENERAL TREATMENT

- Treatment is primarily supportive. Sterile lubricant ophthalmic ointment should be applied to the affected eye(s) at least 3 to 4 times/daily to prevent exposure keratitis and corneal ulceration.
- The use of corticosteroids is controversial and unlikely to be of benefit, given the paucity of inflammation. However, in people with Bell's palsy, such drugs may be efficacious in hastening recovery.

CHRONIC TREATMENT

Some animals require lifelong eye lubrication. Others will eventually begin to reflexively use the third eyelid to moisten the cornea and will no longer need topical medication.

PROGNOSIS AND OUTCOME

Prognosis for complete recovery is guarded. Some animals will regain variable levels of function to the facial nerve, but the majority have some degree of residual deficit.

HISTORY, CHIEF COMPLAINT

- Nonspecific clinical signs are most common, including lethargy, inappetence, and weight loss.
- Cats with FIP may have a history of failure to grow and usually have received multiple antibiotic therapies with no success.
- In cats with ascites due to effusive FIP, owners uncommonly notice the abdominal distention.
- Diarrhea is noted only occasionally in cases of FIP; gastrointestinal signs suggesting intestinal obstruction are sometimes noted when the FIP lesion is confined to the intestine (rare).

PHYSICAL EXAM FINDINGS

- Effusive form: abdominal distention with palpable fluid wave; dyspnea, muffled heart sounds, and muffled lung sounds due to pleural effusion.
- Noneffusive form:
  - Signs of central nervous system dysfunction, including ataxia, personality changes, nystagmus, seizures.
  - Ocular abnormalities, including change in iris color due to iritis/uveitis; hyphema; aqueous flare; vitreous clouding; and vascular cuffing, manifesting as gray lines parallel to retinal vessels.
  - Icterus.
  - Palpable abdominal mass(es), usually due to organomegaly (e.g., enlarged mesenteric lymph nodes, nodules in other organs, intestinal thickening).

ETIOLOGY AND PATHOPHYSIOLOGY

- FCoV related to transmissible gastroenteritis virus in pigs, canine and human coronaviruses.
- Largest known RNA genome; therefore, highly susceptible to mutation.
- FIP virus is a mutation of the ubiquitous and otherwise benign FCoV.
  - Factors that allow or trigger mutation are not known, although breed susceptibility appears to play a role.
  - Once mutated, the virus replicates within macrophages, and travels to the regional lymph nodes for further replication.
- The FIP virus can then undergo one of the following, depending on virus pathogenicity and the cat's immune response:
  - Elimination.
  - Complement mediated pyogranulomatous vasculitis. Result is effusive FIP.
  - Partial cell-mediated response, causing the formation of "classic granulomas." Result is noneffusive FIP.
  - Antibody-antigen complex formation and deposition in vascular endothelium, causing vasculitis.

DIAGNOSIS

- The most reliable diagnostic test for FIP is biopsy of affected tissue (e.g., intestine) with or without immunohistochemical staining. Noninvasive clinical tests all have limitations, and an initial diagnosis of FIP generally relies on a combination of information:
  - Compatible signalment and history.
  - Nonspecific (e.g., fever) and more specific (e.g., nonseptic exudative body cavity effusion, neurologic abnormalities, or characteristic ocular changes) on physical exam findings.
  - Suggestive results on laboratory tests (e.g., with effusion: positive polymerase chain reaction [PCR] result, presence of antibody titer, or immunofluorescent staining of antigen in macrophages).

DIFFERENTIAL DIAGNOSIS

- Neoplasia (lymphoma)
- Lymphocytic/nonsuppurative cholangitis
- Pyothorax/chylothorax
- Congestive heart failure

INITIAL DATABASE

- Complete blood count: lymphopenia, nonregenerative anemia, neutrophilic leukocytosis.
- Serum biochemistry profile.
  - Hyperglobulinemia (and secondary low albumin:globulin ratio) are hallmarks of both the effusive and noneffusive forms of FIP.
  - Elevated liver enzymes: common.
  - Elevated bilirubin: common, especially with noneffusive FIP.
- Thoracic and abdominal radiographs: pleural effusion and ascites (effusive FIP).
- Ocular and neurologic examination.
- Fluid analysis (asictes, pleural/pericardial effusion).
  - Clear, viscous (may contain clumped/precipitated protein), straw colored.
  - Exudate: protein >3.5 mg/dl and often much higher.
  - Nonseptic: total cell count low (e.g., 20×10^6 ml); lymphocytes, nondegenerate neutrophils, macrophages predominate.
  - High globulin concentration (>32%) strongly suggests FIP. Effusion albumin:globulin ratio <0.9 is 74% sensitive and 86% specific for FIP.
- Feline coronavirus serologic study.
  - Positive titer only represents exposure to FCoV, not specifically FIP.
  - Therefore titer result must be interpreted jointly with remaining clinical and laboratory information.
  - Most cats with positive titers for feline coronavirus never develop FIP.
  - Titers >1:16,000 are suggestive of FIP in cats showing signs of clinical disease.
  - Rarely, cats with FIP can have negative titers, especially in the terminal stages of disease.

ADVANCED OR CONFIRMATORY TESTING

- Serum protein electrophoresis in hyperglobulinemic patients:
  - To differentiate from neoplastic causes, which typically produce a monoclonal gammopathy
  - Polyclonal gammopathy with FIP (effusive and noneffusive forms), elevated globulins (usually α-2 and γ globulins)
- Cerebrospinal fluid (CSF) analysis:
  - High protein content (>20 mg/dl, often markedly higher) and cell count (>5 cells/μl, often much higher. Mononuclear pleocytosis with some neutrophils)
  - Caution: patient may be at increased risk of cerebellar/medullary herniation after CSF tap
- PCR:
  - Must involve reverse transcription, because test amplifies DNA but coronavirus is an RNA virus
  - Blood test: interpret results with caution. Cannot differentiate between enteric coronavirus and FIP
  - Effusion test: sensitive and specific, as are conventional means (fluid analysis, serology)
  - Note: Handle all PCR samples carefully, keep frozen and analyze as soon as possible after collection
- Definitive diagnosis only by histopathologic examination of suspected affected tissues: pyogranulommatous inflammation with vasculitis and perivascular cuffing. Immunohistochemical staining of tissues can confirm FIP

TREATMENT

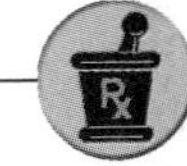

THERAPEUTIC GOAL(S)

Incurable disease; therefore goal is to provide comfort and supportive/palliative care

ACUTE GENERAL TREATMENT

- See Thoracocentesis, p 1308
- Oxygen therapy (see Oxygen Supplementation, p 1292)
- Fluid therapy

CHRONIC TREATMENT

Various drugs have been used. None has been shown effective, and the possibility of adverse effects often contraindicates use.

- Antiviral drugs: Ribavirin (shown to have severe toxicity in cats)
- Immunomodulating drugs:

- α-Interferon (human): 30 U PO q 24h on alternating weeks. Few to no adverse effects
  - Recombinant feline interferon
  - Acemannan
- Immune suppression: prednisone (4 mg/kg PO q 24h) ± cyclophosphamide (2-4 mg/kg PO q 24h for 4 days a week)
- Supportive therapy as indicated by clinical condition:
  - Environmental management: reduction of stress, including providing place to nest/hide, reducing conflicting cat-cat interactions
  - Nutritional support, including warming of food, offering multiple types of dry and moist food, and hand-feeding if ill cats are unwilling to eat
  - Intravenous fluids
  - Broad spectrum antibiotics for secondary bacterial infections (uncommon)

PROGNOSIS AND OUTCOME

Poor irrespective of treatment:
- Cats with the effusive form generally die within 2 months of onset of clinical signs.
- Cats with the noneffusive form tend to have a more chronic disease course that is also generally fatal.

PEARLS & CONSIDERATIONS

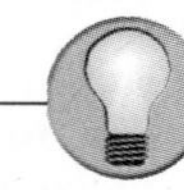

COMMENTS

A "feline infectious peritonitis titer" does not exist. A positive FCoV titer indicates only exposure to a feline coronavirus, which may be pathogenic (e.g., FIP) or benign.

PREVENTION

- Intranasal FIP vaccination:
  - Replicates only in respiratory epithelium. Does not cause systemic infection.
  - Protects 50-75% of cats from exposure to virulent FIP virus.
  - Not recommended for routine use in low-risk cats.
- Optimize husbandry practices:
  - A minority of cats are seronegative to FCoV. In catteries, these cats should be kept apart from other cats, as they can be used for breeding and raising litters with a low risk of any coronavirus.
  - In catteries, remove kittens from positive queens at 5 to 6 weeks old to reduce risk of acquisition of coronavirus.
  - When possible, only seronegative cats should be added to the cattery. Otherwise, seropositive cats may be kept with other seropositive cats.

CLIENT EDUCATION

- Select new cats from reputable breeder with low numbers of cats
- See Cornell Feline Health Center brochure on FIP: www.vet.cornell.edu/fhc/resources/brochure/fip.html

SUGGESTED READING

American Association of Feline Practitioners. 2000 Report of the American Association of Feline Practitioners and Academy of Feline Medicine Advisory Panel on Feline Vaccines: www.aafponline.org/resources/practice_guidelines.htm.

Hartmann K: Feline infectious peritonitis. *Vet Clin North Am Small Animal Pract* 35:39-79, 2005.

Hartmann K, et al: Comparison of different tests to diagnose feline infectious peritonitis. *J Vet Internal Med* 17:781-790, 2003.

Ishida T, et al: Use of recombinant feline interferon and glucocorticoids in treatment of feline infectious peritonitis. *J Fel Med Surg* 6:107-109, 2004.

Rohrbach BW, et al: Epidemiology of feline infectious peritonitis among cats examined at veterinary medical teaching hospitals. *J Am Vet Med Assoc* 218:1111-1118, 2001.

Sparks A: Feline coronavirus infection. In *Feline Medicine and Therapeutics*. Rapid City, IA, Blackwell Publishing, 2004, pp 623-636.

AUTHOR: **KHRISTEN J. CARLSON**
EDITOR: **DOUGLASS K. MACINTIRE**

Feline Leukemia Virus Infection

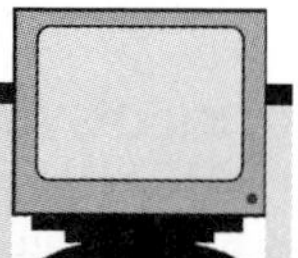

BASIC INFORMATION

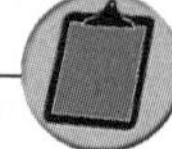

DEFINITION

Viral infection of cats that can result in immunosuppression and malignant neoplasia

SYNONYM(S)

FeLV

EPIDEMIOLOGY

SPECIES, AGE, SEX: Only cats are known to develop FeLV. Kittens less than 4 months old are more likely to become infected. There is no sex predilection.

RISK FACTORS: Multicat households or catteries, chronic exposure to free-roaming infected cats.

CONTAGION AND ZOONOSIS
- Most commonly transmitted through saliva during grooming and playing. FeLV is shed continually from saliva of infected cats.
- Can be transmitted through blood (e.g., transfusion).
- Transplacental transmission is possible. However, kittens are exposed to larger quantities of virus when an infected queen cleans and grooms them.
- Environmental contamination is of lesser concern because the virus is highly sensitive to desiccation, disinfectants, and heat.
- FeLV is not zoonotic.

ASSOCIATED CONDITIONS AND DISORDERS
- FeLV causes immunosuppression, which in turn is associated with opportunistic emergence of infectious diseases such as upper respiratory infections, stomatitis, toxoplasmosis, *Mycoplasma haemofelis*, feline infectious peritonitis (FIP), and feline panleukopenia.
- FeLV has been associated with feline sarcoma virus infection.

CLINICAL PRESENTATION

DISEASE FORMS/SUBTYPES
- FeLV has three subgroups: A, B, and C. Subgroup A is associated with all cases of clinical illness and viremia. Subgroup B occurs in combination with subgroup A in 50% of cats with viral-induced neoplasia. Subgroup C occurs rarely and always in combination with subgroup A to cause nonregenerative anemia.
- Infection with FeLV may result in the development of multiple hematologic abnormalities or syndromes including lymphoma, acute lymphoblastic or myeloblastic leukemia, myelodysplasia, and anemia.

HISTORY, CHIEF COMPLAINT
- Acute viremia in young cats causes fever, inappetence, and lethargy as potential chief complaints.
- Persistent viremia may cause owners to notice signs due to recurrent infections (e.g., weight loss, diarrhea, nasal or ocular discharge), or nonspecific signs attributable to anemia or malignancy, such as weakness, lethargy, or inappetence.
- FeLV may cause abortion and infertility.
- Specific clinical signs may be associated with individual syndromes.

PHYSICAL EXAM FINDINGS

- Findings are often nonspecific, including poor body condition, depression, or weakness. Signs may be attributable to immunosuppression, chronic or recurrent infections, or neoplasia (lymphoma).
- Newborn kittens may have "fading kitten syndrome" and die within the first 2 weeks of life.
- Acutely viremic cats may develop peripheral lymphadenopathy.
- Clinical signs of hematologic abnormalities may include pale mucous membranes resulting from anemia, or signs of sepsis or hemorrhage resulting from neutropenia or thrombocytopenia, respectively.
- The most common sign attributable to FeLV-associated lymphoma is dyspnea resulting from a mediastinal mass and pleural effusion. The initial examination of any dyspneic cat should include palpation with compression of the cranial thorax; in cats with large mediastinal masses, the cranial thorax is noticeably firm and noncompliant.
- Less commonly, signs arising from immune-mediated hemolytic anemia (see Anemia, Immune-Mediated Hemolytic, p 66), glomerulonephritis (see Glomerulonephritis, p 442), or polyarthritis (see Polyarthritis, p 871) may be noted, as these syndromes have been reported in cats with FeLV.
- The occurrence of FeLV-associated osteochondromas (multiple cartilaginous exostoses) may produce orthopedic abonormalities (palpable bony enlargements) or neurologic deficits, depending on site of involvement.

ETIOLOGY AND PATHOPHYSIOLOGY

- FeLV is an oncornavirus of the family *Retroviridae*.
- Infection occurs most commonly through exposure to saliva or blood through the oral or nasal cavity. The virus replicates in the oropharyngeal lymphoid tissues.
- Cats can mount a full immune response and eliminate the infection, or mount an ineffective immune response resulting in viremia.
- Once the patient is viremic, the virus replicates within disseminated lymphoid tissues and the bone marrow. An effective immune response at this stage can result in elimination of the virus, but more commonly results in the development of a latent carrier. If an ineffective immune response occurs during the viremic stage, the cat may become persistently viremic and is more likely to develop a hematologic abnormality, malignancy, chronic infection, or other clinical signs.
- Latent carriers of FeLV may become transiently viremic during times of stress or illness.

DIAGNOSIS

DIFFERENTIAL DIAGNOSIS

- Feline immunodeficiency virus, FIP, or neoplasia.
- Nonregenerative anemia may be associated with any chronic, infectious, or inflammatory disease.
- Lymphoma in cats is now more commonly *not* associated with FeLV.
- Viral upper respiratory infections, *M. haemofelis*, toxoplasmosis or fungal infections often accompany FeLV, and the presence of any of these infections in any cat should prompt evaluation for FeLV.

INITIAL DATABASE

- Complete blood count: may reveal mild to marked abnormalities with bone marrow infection, including nonregenerative anemia, neutropenia, thrombocytopenia, leukemia, or aplastic anemia.
- Serum chemistry profile: normal or changes may be nonspecific.
- Urinalysis: generally unremarkable. Opportunistic infections may include those of the urinary tract; glomerulonephritis or urinary tract infection may cause proteinuria.
- Chest radiographs: mediastinal mass and pleural effusion possible in patients with FeLV-associated lymphoma.
- Enzyme-linked immunosorbent assay (ELISA) of blood and immunofluorescent antibody (IFA) testing of blood and bone marrow are available to detect viral antigen.
    - ELISA is more sensitive (more likely to identify all true positives, but also produces some false-positive results) compared to IFA. Therefore ELISA is the diagnostic test of choice for general screening.
    - IFA is more specific (more effective at identifying true negative results) and therefore it is the confirmatory test of choice whenever an ELISA test is positive.
    - Positive results for both tests indicate that a cat is viremic and will be infected for life.
    - Positive ELISA and negative IFA usually indicate transient infection (will become negative for both) or early permanent infection (will become positive for both). Therefore cats with positive ELISA and negative IFA results should be retested in 3 to 4 months.
    - Latent carriers should be negative for both ELISA and IFA testing. Rarely, some cases of latent infection have been IFA-positive.
    - In some cats, FeLV is confined to the bone marrow. Therefore, any cat with signs prompting bone marrow aspiration for cytology (e.g., nonregenerative anemia) should be tested with FeLV IFA performed on the bone marrow, irrespective of prior negative FeLV blood test results.
- Saliva- or tear-based tests are not recommended (poor sensitivity; intermittent shedding).

ADVANCED OR CONFIRMATORY TESTING

Polymerase chain reaction (PCR) testing is available for use in cats with discordant ELISA and IFA test results. PCR may also be used for detecting minute viral particles in fixed tumor tissues.

TREATMENT

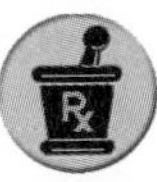

THERAPEUTIC GOAL(S)

There is no effective therapy to eliminate FeLV infection. The goals of therapy are to control clinical signs caused by secondary infection and hematologic abnormalities.

ACUTE AND CHRONIC TREATMENT

- Identify and treat secondary infections aggressively to allow a full immune response to the viral infection.
- FeLV associated lymphoma may be treated with chemotherapy agents with more success than the treatment of FeLV-associated leukemias. (See Lymphoma, Cat (Multicentric), p 650; Leukemias, Acute, p 632; Leukemias, Chronic, p 634.)
- Severe nonregenerative anemia may be managed with blood transfusions to provide time for an effective immune response against the virus. (See Transfusion Therapy and Collection Techniques for Blood Banking.)
- Neutropenia may respond to immunosuppressive doses of prednisone (e.g., 1–2 mg/kg PO q 12h, tapering to lowest effective dose and avoiding adverse effects), or may transiently respond to human granulocyte colony stimulating factor (G-CSF 5 μg/kg q 12h SQ). Antibodies that develop against G-CSF limit its use.
- Antiviral agents such as zidovudine and PMEA (9-[2-(phosphonomethoxy)ethyl] adenine) have been used for treating FeLV. These drugs are most effective when given within 96 hours of exposure to the virus. Treatment of viremic cats may result in a decrease in clinical illness but does not clear the infection. Side effects may be severe and treatment has not been shown to clearly prevent progression of disease.
- Use of the immune stimulant interferon-α has been shown to prevent infection when given before viral exposure, but has not been extensively used in patients with clinical illness.

RECOMMENDED MONITORING

The health of FeLV-positive cats should be monitored on a regular basis for early detection of secondary infections and the development of hematologic abnormalities.

PROGNOSIS AND OUTCOME

- The prognosis for an otherwise healthy cat with positive FeLV ELISA and IFA results is guarded for survival beyond 3 years after infection. However, the quality of life is usually excellent, and some cats may live to their full life expectancy.
- The prognosis for cats that develop lymphoma, leukemia, or myelodysplasia secondary to FeLV is guarded to poor. Cats with lymphoma may experience a remission and an improved quality of life with chemotherapy for a median of 6 months. However, cats with leukemia, severe anemia, and myelodysplasia respond poorly to therapy.

PEARLS & CONSIDERATIONS

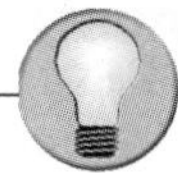

COMMENTS

- A cat is considered to be permanently infected with FeLV if ELISA and IFA tests are both positive.
- FeLV vaccine uses a different FeLV viral protein (glycoprotein 70) than the one screened for by the ELISA and IFA tests. Therefore prior vaccination cannot cause a false-positive result.
- The rate of FeLV infection has dramatically dropped due to aggressive testing, client education, and vaccination.

PREVENTION

- Vaccination is efficacious in cats at risk for exposure to the virus.
- The FeLV vaccine has been associated with the development of injection site sarcomas in cats.
- Vaccinate cats that are at risk of exposure to FeLV low in the left hind limb. Indoor closed cat households do not require FeLV vaccination.
- In cats with FeLV, prevention of common contagious and inflammatory diseases, and vaccination for rabies and FVRCP.
- Cats should remain indoors to prevent exposure to contagious diseases. Stressful situations should be minimized.
- Young kittens should not be introduced into a household with a FeLV-positive cat.

CLIENT EDUCATION

- Advise clients of the benefits of keeping cats indoors to prevent exposure to infectious diseases
- Test new kittens for FeLV and FIV before introduction into a multicat household

SUGGESTED READING

American Association of Feline Practitioners. 2005 Report on Feline Retrovirus Testing and Management: www.aafponline.org/resources/practice_guidelines.htm.

American Association of Feline Practitioners. 2000 Report of the American Association of Feline Practitioners and Academy of Feline Medicine Advisory Panel on Feline Vaccines: www.aafponline.org/resources/practice_guidelines.htm.

Cotter SM: Feline viral neoplasia. In Greene CE (ed): *Infectious Diseases of the Dog and Cat*. St. Louis, WB Saunders, 1998, pp 71-92.

www.aafponline.org/resources/practice_guidelines.htm.

AUTHOR: **KATHRYN TAYLOR**

EDITOR: **DOUGLASS K. MACINTIRE**

Feline Lower Urinary Tract Signs, Idiopathic

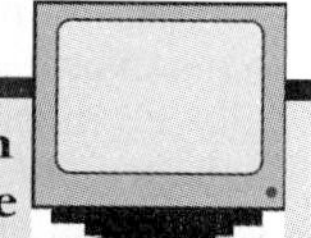

Client Education Sheet on Website

BASIC INFORMATION

DEFINITION

Idiopathic lower urinary tract signs (LUTS) include straining, hematuria, pollakiuria (frequent passage of small amounts of urine), and periuria (urinations in inappropriate locations) in cats. Urethral obstruction is discussed further in Urethral Obstruction, p 1120; Urethral Obstruction (Feline): Medical Management, p 1319.

SYNONYM(S)

Feline lower urinary tract disease (FLUTD)
Feline urologic syndrome (FUS)
Idiopathic cystitis

EPIDEMIOLOGY

SPECIES, AGE, SEX: LUTS can affect cats of either sex at any age from 6 weeks to 16 years.

GENETICS AND BREED PREDISPOSITION: No specific genetic link is known, and epigenetic familial factors (e.g., quality of maternal care) may play a role. Siamese cats have been reported to be at reduced risk of LUTS, whereas Persians and long-haired cats may be at increased risk.

RISK FACTORS: Neutering, indoor housing, increased weight, decreased activity, multicat households.

GEOGRAPHY AND SEASONALITY: None proven.

ASSOCIATED CONDITIONS AND DISORDERS: Cats with LUTS also may be at increased risk for separation anxiety disorder and other behavioral abnormalities (fear, nervousness, aggression), dilated cardiomyopathy, and obesity. The reason(s) for these associations has not been well studied.

CLINICAL PRESENTATION

HISTORY, CHIEF COMPLAINT

- The most common history is abrupt onset of clinical signs.
- The complaint most likely to elicit veterinary care is periuria (urinations in inappropriate locations).

PHYSICAL EXAM FINDINGS

- The most common presentation is of a young adult (2 to 6 years old), neutered, cat housed indoors.
- The cat usually is anxious and may be aggressive. The bladder usually is small and hard to palpate, and it is difficult to obtain urine from.

ETIOLOGY AND PATHOPHYSIOLOGY

- The etiology in all cases is not known, although a subset of patients appears to have a congenital disorder of the stress response system that results in persistent sensitization of the system, and reduced adrenocortical function (which normally serves as a brake on the system).
- This sensitivity may be unmasked by cat-perceived threats in the environment, such as unpredictable owner schedules, conflict with other animals, and impoverished environments.
- In these patients, presenting serum cortisol concentrations usually are low, reflect-

ing decreased adrenal reserve in the presence of enhanced sympathetic drive.

- The enhanced sympathetic drive may reduce epithelial tight junction integrity, resulting in increased exposure of afferent neurons to environmental stimuli. When this occurs in the bladder of a cat with an activated stress response system, LUTS may result.

DIAGNOSIS

DIFFERENTIAL DIAGNOSIS

- There is a 10–20% chance of urolithiasis; calcium oxalate and struvite are the most common stones identified.
- There is a 5–10% chance of behavioral disorder.
- There is a 5–10% chance of anatomic defect.
- There is a 1–5% chance of urinary tract infection.

INITIAL DATABASE

- History, presentation, and physical examination often are sufficient to make the clinical diagnosis in cats presented for an initial episode if the urethra is not obstructed.
- In complicated initial presentations and recurrent cases, radiography of the *entire* (the distal urethra often is not included, which can result in missing important information) lower urinary tract and urinalysis may be performed for ruling out the most common alternative diagnoses, although the sensitivity and specificity of urinalysis results are rather low.

ADVANCED OR CONFIRMATORY TESTING

Cystoscopy to identify lesions and/or computed tomography to evaluate adrenal size are rarely indicated or necessary

TREATMENT

THERAPEUTIC GOAL(S)

- Rule out obstruction
- Relieve pain
- Reduce stress

ACUTE GENERAL TREATMENT

If the cat is obstructed, relieve the obstruction, reestablish urine flow, and correct fluid, electrolyte, and acid-base imbalances.

- Obtain and submit samples for serum biochemistry, complete blood count, and urinalysis; it is not necessary to evaluate the results before treating obstructed cats that present with urethral obstruction and severe systemic signs.
- Resuscitate moribund cats with intravenous fluids and correct serious electrolyte and acid-base disturbances before anesthesia for placement of a urinary catheter.
    - Obtain an electrocardiogram of all systemically ill cats with urethral obstruction, as rescue from the cardiotoxic effects of severe hyperkalemia may be necessary even before laboratory values for serum potassium (K^+) return.
    - Rescue in critical hyperkalemia may include use of K^+ poor solutions (lactated Ringer's solution or sodium chloride), intravenous administration of 1–2 mEq/kg BW sodium bicarbonate, or *slow* intravenous administration of 2–10 ml of 10% calcium gluconate (monitor electrocardiogram for slowing of heart rate of 10% or more, warranting termination of calcium administration).
- Decompress the bladder by cystocentesis *before* attempting to pass a urinary catheter.
    - Insert a 22- or 23-gauge butterfly needle into the bladder wall midway between the apex and urethral outflow and directed caudoventrally.
    - If a longer needle is necessary, it can be attached to an extension set and urine removed using a syringe.
    - Palpate the bladder during drainage to empty it as completely as possible.
    - Rare complications include extravasation of urine into the peritoneal cavity and damage to the bladder wall.
    - This procedure may be sufficient to restore normal urine flow.
- Pass a catheter only if necessary.
    - General anesthesia is needed to allow proper manipulation of the penis to pass the catheter. The combination of intravenous ketamine and diazepam does not provide adequate relaxation for some cats. Isoflurane gas administered by facemask generally provides adequate sedation and urethral relaxation, although propofol infusion also can be used.
    - If a plug or urethrolith is retrieved, it should be submitted for quantitative analysis.
    - An indwelling urinary catheter (e.g., 3.5 French red rubber feeding tube-type) is placed in cats with pronounced azotemia or poor urinary stream after catheter placement. An indwelling urinary catheter also is used for cats with very large bladders at presentation, as they are more likely to develop detrusor atony.
- Manage cats medically unless future recurrent obstructions occur.
    - For most, analgesics (Table I-6) and appropriate fluid therapy are indicated. Some α-blocking drugs (e.g., phenoxybenzamine) have not been shown to be effective. They act on the proximal feline urethra, whereas most obstructions in cats involve the distal urethra.
    - Monitor urine output frequently in severely ill cats; those that recover from severe postrenal uremia generally undergo a substantial postobstructive diuresis (>2.0 ml/kg/hr shortly after relief of obstruction and rehydration). During this period, it is essential to give sufficient intravenous fluids to replace the volume lost as urine. The diuresis declines to normal during 2 to 5 days.
- The role of glucocorticoids (e.g., prednisone), prostaglandin analogs (e.g., misoprostol), and nonsteroidal anti-inflammatory drugs (e.g., aspirin) remains poorly defined and none of these drugs has been shown to be an effective treatment for acute LUTS.
- A perineal urethrostomy may be needed in severe recurrent cases.
    - This surgery increases the risks of bacterial urinary tract infections, however, and postoperative strictures are a potential complication.
    - Clients need to be made aware that this surgery does not correct the underlying problem, and that recurrent episodes of urolithiasis and LUTS still can occur.

CHRONIC TREATMENT

- Step 1: Environmental enrichment (EE).
    - Provide at least one food bowl, one water bowl, and one litter box per cat, plus one. Locate these resources in quiet places where the cat is not startled during use.
    - Provide opportunities for the cat to hide safely, and to explore its environment. Placing "perches" at windows so the cat can look outside, and structures the cat can climb on seem to be important parts of EE.
    - Provide a regularly scheduled time for petting, play, and/or trick-teaching, working toward at least 10 minutes a day.
    - Identify and resolve intercat conflict to the extent possible.
    - If ineffective, proceed to step 2.
- Step 2: Step 1 plus consider use of pheromones (Feliway). If ineffective, proceed to step 3.
- Step 3: Steps 1 and 2 plus consider use of a tricyclic agent such as clomipramine or amitriptyline at the lowest effective dose possible (see Table I-6). These drugs should be used only after steps 1 and 2 have been implemented and the cat is so severely affected that it continues to have recurrences.

POSSIBLE COMPLICATIONS

- When introducing EE, offer changes to the cat (e.g., new food in a separate bowl rather than in place of the

TABLE I-6 **Drugs commonly used for cats with LUTS**

Acute analgesic drugs	Dose	Potential Side Effects
Butorphanol (Torbugesic)	0.2–0.4 mg/kg IV. IM, SQ q 8h (IV: use lower end of dose range)	Sedation
Buprenorphine (Buprenex)	0.01–0.02 mg/kg IM, IV, or SQ q 8–12h; 0.015 mg/kg PO q 8–12h (anecdotal)	
Fentanyl (Duragesic) patch	25 μg/hr	Respiratory depression, bradycardia
Bladder/urethral contractility		
Acepromazine (PromAce)	0.05 mg/kg SQ q 8h	Sedation, hypotension
Prazosin (Minipress)	0.5 mg per cat PO q 12h	
Phenoxybenzamine (Dibenzyline)	2.5 mg PO q 12h	Hypotension
Bethanechol (Urecholine)	2.5–5 mg PO q 12h	Salivation, vomiting, diarrhea
Chronic analgesic/anxiolytic		
Clomipramine (Anafranil)	0.5 mg/kg PO q 24h	Sedation; anticholinergic effects
Amitriptyline (Elavil)	5–12.5 mg PO q 12–24h	Sedation; weight gain; urine retention; urolith formation
Buspirone (BuSpar)	2.5–5 mg PO q 12h	Rare but sedation or other neurologic effects

familiar diet) to avoid precipitating a threat response. Make changes the client wants to make, if possible, to secure support and adherence to the EE effort. Make changes sequentially.

- When tricyclic drugs are used, they should be tapered slowly over at least 2 weeks to avoid adverse reactions.

RECOMMENDED MONITORING

Liver and kidney function should be assessed before use of tricyclic drugs, and at least annually in young animals if therapy is extended

PROGNOSIS AND OUTCOME

Depends on cat, client, and environment:

- Cat:
  - Genetic predisposition
  - Duration of the problem
  - Frequency of occurrences
  - Number of areas and different types of surfaces soiled
- Client:
  - Ability to identify modifiable causes
  - Strength of bond to affected cat
  - Willingness to pay for treatment
  - Amount of time to devote to solution
  - Willingness to accept and use medications
- Environment:
  - Number of cats in the household
  - Number of affected cats
  - Practicality of allowing limited outdoor access
  - Ability to rearrange the environment

PEARLS & CONSIDERATIONS

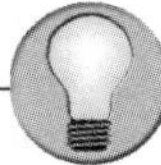

COMMENTS

In our experience, EE often is sufficient to suppress clinical signs and should be offered to all owners of cats exclusively housed indoors.

PREVENTION

EE recommendations should be provided to *all* owners of indoor cats, not just those with a clinical problem.

CLIENT EDUCATION

Client-oriented information is available at www.indoorcat.org.

SUGGESTED READING

Westropp J, Buffington CAT, Chew DJ: Lower urinary tract disorders. In Ettinger SJ, Feldman EC (eds): *Textbook of Veterinary Internal Medicine*, ed 6. St. Louis, Elsevier-Saunders, 2005.

Westropp JL, Buffington CAT: Feline idiopathic cystitis: current understanding of pathophysiology and management. *Vet Clin North Am Small Anim Pract* 34:1043, 2004.

Westropp J, Welk K, Buffington CAT: Adrenal abnormalities in cats with feline interstitial cystitis. *J Urol* 169:258, 2003.

AUTHOR & EDITOR: **C. A. TONY BUFFINGTON**

Feline Symmetric Alopecia

BASIC INFORMATION

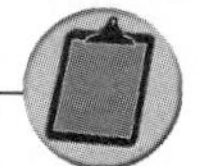

DEFINITION

Symmetric hair loss that may be congenital, or acquired and secondary to pruritus, and/or behavioral influences

EPIDEMIOLOGY

SPECIES, AGE, SEX

- Congenital: young
- Acquired: atopy; young adult
- Endocrine, tumor: middle-aged to older

GENETICS AND BREED PREDISPOSITION

- Alopecia universalis: sphinx cats
- Hereditary hypotrichosis: Siamese, devon rex, Burmese
- Follicular dysplasia: cornish rex
- Psychogenic alopecia: Siamese, Abyssinian, Burmese more common; any breed can be affected

RISK FACTORS: Multicat households; catteries/cats that venture outdoors; exotic breeds.

CONTAGION AND ZOONOSIS: Some parasitic and fungal etiologies are both zoonotic and contagious.

GEOGRAPHY AND SEASONALITY: Parasites have seasonal and geographic variations (e.g., fleas prefer warmer weather, increased humidity).

CLINICAL PRESENTATION

DISEASE FORMS/SUBTYPES

- Congenital
- Acquired (pruritic, behavioral, endocrine)

HISTORY, CHIEF COMPLAINT: Chief complaint: hair loss; overgrooming (not always noted by owners, even in patients that are actually pruritic); hyperthyroid cats may be polyphagic, underweight, and have an anxious disposition.

PHYSICAL EXAM FINDINGS

- Bilaterally symmetric hair loss
- Primary pruritic:
  - Alopecia/barbering of ventrum, dorsum, and legs (both antebrachia and hind legs) is common. Facial excoriations, ceruminous otitis, or crusted papules ("miliary dermatitis") raise index of suspicion. Excoriations secondary to the self-trauma may be noted.
- Secondary to underlying disorder:
  - Endocrine: variable amount of scaling (seborrhea sicca); coat may appear dull and dry. Hyperadrenocorticism (rare in cats): thin skin, pendulous abdomen, and 50% of cases may experience skin fragility syndrome (skin tears easily with gentle traction).
  - Paraneoplastic (e.g., pancreatic carcinoma, bile duct carcinoma): ventral abdominal alopecia and thin skin that appears "shiny." Limbs may be affected as well.
  - Anal sac disorders: ventral abdominal alopecia, hair loss at the base of the tail.
  - Cystitis/gastrointestinal disease: ventral abdominal alopecia.
  - Dermatophytosis: variable. Patient may present with alopecia, seborrhea, miliary dermatitis, erythematous scaling macules, or patches.
  - Behavioral: "barbered" hairs with no primary lesions. Head and neck usually unaffected.

ETIOLOGY AND PATHOPHYSIOLOGY

- Pruritus: overgrooming
- Genetic: malformation/absence of hairs
- Fungal: mycotic destruction of hair shaft
- Endocrine: telogenization of hair follicles
- Medical: self-trauma secondary to discomfort (cystitis, gastrointestinal); tumor
- Behavioral: compulsive; anxiety

DIAGNOSIS

DIFFERENTIAL DIAGNOSIS

- Congenital (all nonpruritic; differentiate based on breed predisposition, clinical presentation, and biopsy/histopathology):
  - Alopecia universalis (affected individuals are born without hair)
  - Hereditary hypotrichosis (affected individuals are born with a thin haircoat progressing to alopecia)
  - Follicular dysplasia (ongoing hair thinning progressing to alopecia)
- Acquired:
  - Pruritic:
    - Parasitic (flea, *Demodex gatoi*, *Cheyletiella*, *Otodectes*, *Notoedres*, scabies, *Trombicula*, *Felicola subrostratus*)
    - Fungal
    - Food allergy
    - Atopy
  - Nonpruritic:
    - Telogen/anagen effluvium
    - Endocrinopathy (hyperthyroidism, hypothyroidism: iatrogenic, spontaneous [very rare]; hyperadrenocorticism: iatrogenic, acquired [rare])
    - Tumor (cutaneous T-cell lymphoma, paraneoplastic syndrome, thymoma, hypereosinophilic syndrome)
    - Cystitis
    - Inflammatory bowel disease
    - Anal sacculitis
    - Behavioral: compulsive, anxiety
    - Neurologic: hyperesthesia

INITIAL DATABASE

- Comprehensive ectoparasite examination (flea combing, skin scrapings, trichograms)
- Trichography: examination of hair tips to determine if hair loss is self-inflicted
- Fungal culture (dermatophyte test medium)
- Anal sac expression

ADVANCED OR CONFIRMATORY TESTING

- Complete blood count: eosinophilia may support a diagnosis of a hypersensitivity/parasite
- Serum biochemical profile: metabolic disease
- Urinalysis: metabolic disease, ventral abdominal alopecia (cystitis)
- Thyroid hormone evaluation
- 8 to 12 week *exclusive* elimination dietary trial
- Intradermal and/or serum allergy testing
- Feline leukemia virus and feline immunodeficiency virus testing
- Abdominal ultrasound/thoracic and abdominal radiographs (paraneoplastic, thymoma)
- Histopathologic study may be helpful in the diagnosis of endocrinopathy, tumor, paraneoplastic syndrome, and follicular dysplasia. Histopathologic findings consistent with normal skin are supportive of a behavioral diagnosis but are not pathognomonic; behavioral cause (psychogenic alopecia) is a diagnosis of exclusion

TREATMENT

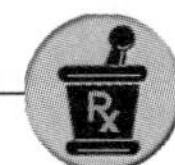

THERAPEUTIC GOAL(S)

Where present:

- Eliminate/control pruritus
- Treat medical conditions/normalize hormone levels
- Address behavioral problem ± psychotropic drugs

ACUTE GENERAL TREATMENT

Specific parasiticide or broad-spectrum antiparasitic therapy:

- Ectoparasiticide response trial (broad-spectrum parasiticide such as selamectin or imidacloprid/moxidectin for 6 to 8 weeks, ± lime sulfur [LymDip] for *D. gatoi*).
- Express anal sacs. External digital pressure is used in cats (versus intrarectal digital expression in dogs).
- Elizabethan collar to separate self-trauma from hair loss.

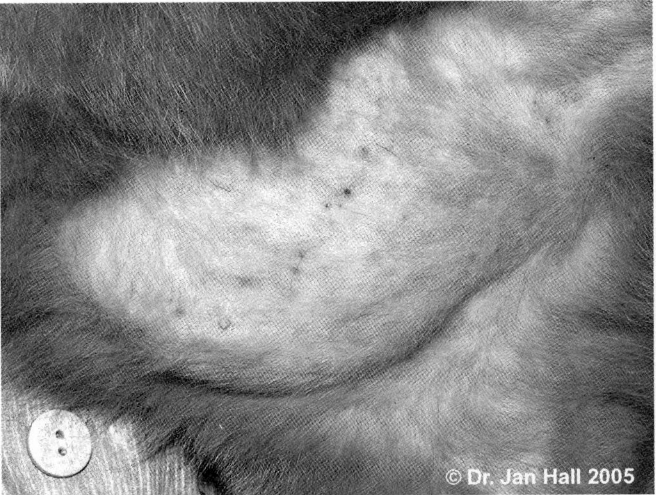

FIGURE I-71 Alopecia on the ventral abdomen of a 4-year-old domestic short-haired cat. The underlying cause of the excessive abdominal licking noted was recurrent anal gland impaction. This problem resolved once the underlying disorder was corrected. Courtesy of Dr. Jan A. Hall.

CHRONIC TREATMENT

- Atopy:
  - Appropriate anti-inflammatory: corticosteroids (prednisone or prednisolone: 1-2 mg/kg/day initially, decreasing to lowest possible dose and frequency; or methylprednisolone acetate (Depo-Medrol) 20 mg/cat IM (maximum q 4 weeks).
  - Allergen-specific immunotherapy, antihistamines, fatty acid supplementation (see Atopy, p 96).
- Food allergy: hypoallergenic diet.
- Dermatophytosis: appropriate antifungal therapy (see Dermatophytosis, p 285).
- Hyperthyroidism: appropriate therapy (see Hyperthyroidism, p 552).
- Behavioral: treat compulsive or anxiety disorder (see Behavioral Problems, Miscellaneous, p 126).

POSSIBLE COMPLICATIONS

Long-term corticosteroid use: diabetes mellitus, iatrogenic hyperadrenocorticism

PROGNOSIS AND OUTCOME

Uncomplicated etiologies carry a better prognosis for control (atopy) and possibly cure (fungal, parasitic, food), but many cases can involve more than one etiology and require a well planned diagnostic protocol and excellent client compliance.

PEARLS & CONSIDERATIONS

COMMENTS

- Absence of parasites on physical examination does not preclude their presence. Consider empiric parasiticide therapeutic trials.
- Important to rule out food allergy in the chronic, continual, nonseasonal patient.

SUGGESTED READING

O'Dair HA, Foster AP: Focal and generalized alopecia. *Vet Clin North Am Small Animal Pract* 24(4):851-870, 1995.

Scott DW, Miller WH, Griffin CE: *Small Animal Dermatology*, ed 6. Toronto, WB Saunders, 2001, pp 900-911.

AUTHOR: **STEPHEN WAISGLASS**
EDITOR: **JAN A. HALL**

Fever of Unknown Origin

BASIC INFORMATION

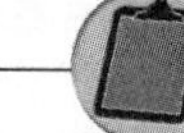

DEFINITION

- Fever is defined as a higher than normal body temperature (>102.5°F [>39.1°C]) due to altered thermoregulatory mechanisms in the hypothalamus.
- Fever of unknown origin (FUO) is a fever that does not resolve spontaneously and for which no obvious cause is identified.
- The normal range of body temperatures in calm, normal individuals in a cool environment is 100.2-102.5°F (37.8-39.1°C) in the dog and 100.5-102.5°F (38.0-39.1°C) in the cat.

SYNONYM(S)

Pyrexia

Fever is a subset of hyperthermia, not a synonym. Nonfebrile hyperthermia (e.g., physical exertion, heat stroke, muscle fasciculations) does not involve alterations in the hypothalamic thermoregulatory mechanisms and is not treated with antipyretic drugs.

EPIDEMIOLOGY

SPECIES, AGE, SEX

- Any age, breed, or sex.
- Young dogs may be more likely to have infectious causes.
- Older dogs may be more likely to have neoplastic causes.

GENETICS AND BREED PREDISPOSITION

- Shar-pei: idiopathic, possible cytokine abnormality
- Weimaraner: neutrophil function deficiency
- Irish setter: leukocyte adhesion deficiency

RISK FACTORS

- Immunosuppression
- Exposure to infectious agents or vectors
- Travel to endemic areas of disease

CONTAGION AND ZOONOSIS: Risk varies, dependent on causative agent.

GEOGRAPHY AND SEASONALITY: Some regions are endemic for particular infectious diseases. See individual specific topics.

CLINICAL PRESENTATION

HISTORY, CHIEF COMPLAINT: Will vary with organ systems involved and causative agent but usually associated with nonspecific clinical signs such as lethargy, depression, and anorexia.

PHYSICAL EXAM FINDINGS

- A complete physical exam in all patients with FUO must include rectal exam (dog), fundic exam (dog, cat), oral exam (dog, cat), meticulous examination of the skin (dog, cat) and, if indicated by initial findings, orthopedic and/or neurologic exams (dog, cat)
- Fever:
  - Individual (haircoat, anxiety) and environmental (ambient temperature) influences may raise the body temperature of normal, healthy dogs and cats, and must be considered when interpreting a patient's temperature.
- Depression
- Lethargy
- Tachycardia
- Hyperpnea
- Dehydration
- Lymphadenopathy with infectious or neoplastic disease
- Neck or back pain or central signs with meningitis, meningoencephalitis, diskospondylitis
- Joint pain or swelling with monoarthritis or polyarthritis
- Heart murmur may indicate bacterial endocarditis
- Chorioretinitis or hemorrhage suggestive of infectious cause
- Localized swelling and/or pain with wounds or abscesses

ETIOLOGY AND PATHOPHYSIOLOGY

- Pathophysiology:
  - The hypothalamus is responsible for thermoregulation. Fever occurs when the hypothalamic setpoint is reset to higher than normal.
  - Inflammation and bacterial endotoxins increase the hypothalamic set point by causing the release of endogenous pyrogens such as interleukin (IL)-1, IL-6, and tumor necrosis factor-α.
- Etiology:
  - Infectious:
    - Localized or systemic bacterial infections (dog, cat): diskospondylitis, osteomyelitis, bacterial endocarditis, septic arthritis, prostatitis, pyelonephritis, septic meningitis, cholangiohepatitis, abscesses, pyothorax, peritonitis, pneumonia, pyometra, catheter site infections.

- Specific bacterial infections: leptospirosis (dog), borreliosis (dog), brucellosis (dog), mycobacterial infections (dog, cat), bartonellosis (dog, cat), hemotrophic *Mycoplasma* (*Haemobartonella*) (dog, cat), tularemia (dog, cat), salmonellosis (dog, cat).
- Viral: canine distemper virus (dog), parvovirus/panleukopenia (dog/cat), feline leukemia (FeLV) (cat), feline immunodeficiency virus (FIV) (cat), feline infectious peritonitis (cat).
- Rickettsial: ehrlichiosis/anaplasmosis (dog, cat), Rocky Mountain spotted fever (*Rickettsia rickettsii*) (dog).
- Fungal (dog, cat): histoplasmosis, blastomycosis, coccidioidomycosis cryptococcosis, aspergillosis
- Protozoal: babesiosis (dog), leishmaniasis (dog), trypanosomiasis (dog), hepatozoonosis (dog), toxoplasmosis (dog, cat), cytauxzoonosis (cat).
- Immune mediated: immune-mediated polyarthritis (dog, cat), systemic lupus erythematosus (SLE) (dog, cat), rheumatoid arthritis (dog), vasculitis (dog, cat), meningitis (dog), pemphigus (dog, cat), immune-mediated hemolytic anemia (IMHA) (dog, cat), immune-mediated thrombocytopenia (ITP; dog, cat), transfusion reaction (dog, cat).
- Neoplastic (dog, cat): lymphoma, leukemia, multiple myeloma, solid necrotic tumors.
- Other (dog, cat):
  - Pancreatitis.
  - Drug induced (tetracyclines, penicillins, sulfas), toxins, metabolic bone disorders, hyperthyroidism, tissue necrosis.

DIAGNOSIS

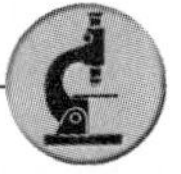

DIFFERENTIAL DIAGNOSIS

Rule out nonpyrogenic causes of an elevated body temperature (heat stroke, overexertion, muscle fasciculations, etc.)

INITIAL DATABASE

- Complete blood count (CBC), chemistry profile, urinalysis: results will vary with organ system involvement
- Urine bacterial culture and sensitivity should be performed in all cases of FUO even if urine sediment is inactive. Helpful with detection of pyelonephritis or prostatitis
- FeLV antigen and FIV antibody tests in all cats

ADVANCED OR CONFIRMATORY TESTING

Further laboratory testing depends on history, physical exam findings, and minimum database results.

- Laboratory tests:
  - Serial blood cultures: to detect bacteremia associated with diskospondylitis, endocarditis, or other foci of infection. A negative culture does not rule out bacteremia (intermittent bacterial showering).
  - Specific serologic tests: antibody titers or antigen tests are obtained for evidence of infectious disease. If infectious disease is suspected and initial titers are negative, repeat in 2 to 4 weeks.
  - Polymerase chain reaction testing for specific infectious agents.
  - Fungal cultures and/or serologic study.
  - Cultures of cerebrospinal fluid (CSF) or synovial fluid.
  - Immune tests: antinuclear antibody test if suspected SLE; Coombs' test if suspicion of IMHA or immune-mediated thrombocytopenia (ITP); serum protein electrophoresis.
- Imaging:
  - Thoracic radiographs: to evaluate for evidence of neoplasia, effusions, or pulmonary infiltrates.
  - Abdominal radiographs: evaluate for abdominal masses, effusions, free gas.
  - Spinal and long bone radiographs: examine for evidence of diskospondylitis, osteomyelitis, periosteal proliferation.
  - Abdominal ultrasound: rule out pyelonephritis, prostatitis, or pyometra; identify ± aspirate any enlarged abdominal organs or masses (unless highly vascular or bleeding disorder).
  - Echocardiogram: identify vegetative valvular lesions associated with bacterial endocarditis.
  - Computed tomography/magnetic resonance imaging often indicated before CSF tap to rule out an intracranial mass and decrease risk of herniation.
- Diagnostic procedures:
  - Arthrocentesis: polyarthritis.
  - Cytologic study of enlarged lymph nodes or affected organs: neoplasia or identification of infectious agents.
  - Bone marrow aspirates and/or biopsy: if CBC changes are reflective of bone marrow involvement or neoplasia is suspected.
  - CSF tap if neurologic signs (± fundic exam) suggest meningoencephalitis or meningitis.
  - Muscle biopsy: hepatozoonosis.
  - Abdominocentesis: peritonitis and pancreatitis.
  - Transtracheal wash or bronchoalveolar lavage if respiratory involvement.

TREATMENT

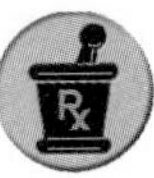

THERAPEUTIC GOAL(S)

- The goal in all cases of FUO is to obtain a specific diagnosis and treat accordingly.
- A therapeutic trial should be initiated only when a specific diagnosis cannot be ascertained.

ACUTE GENERAL TREATMENT

- Intravenous crystalloid fluid therapy at 1.5 to 2 times maintenance for fevers where temperature >103.5°F (>39.7°C).
- Mechanical cooling methods such as cool water baths or fans at temperatures >106°F (>41.1°C).
- Antipyretic agents (e.g., nonsteroidal anti-inflammatories [NSAIDs], to be given only when animal is fully hydrated) may be considered if temperature exceeds 106°F and does not respond to fluids and cooling.
  - Antipyretic drugs should be reserved only for patients with fevers >105°F (40.6°C) and those that have failed to respond to fluids and mechanical cooling, as they can mask the effects of other therapies and can be associated with adverse effects such as gastrointestinal ulceration and hepatic and/or renal toxicity.
- Patients with persistent fevers <105°F (40.6°C) should be treated with supportive care, including IV fluids and mechanical cooling.

CHRONIC TREATMENT

- Antibiotic trials:
  - Broad-spectrum antibiotic therapy may be initiated after all culture specimens have been collected.
  - Therapy should be based on the agents most likely present, their known antibiotic sensitivity, and the organ or system affected.
  - Commonly used empiric antibiotics include amoxicillin-clavulanate 10–20 mg/kg PO q 8–12h, or cephalexin 22 mg/kg PO q 8h or 30 mg/kg PO q 12h, or, if tick-borne diseases are suspected, doxycycline 10 mg/kg PO q 24h or 5 mg/kg PO q 12h. The actual recommendation depends on the previously listed factors.
- Glucocorticoid trials (duration: 24 to 72 hours):
  - Used when immune-mediated disease is suspected.
  - Should be used only when infectious disease has been ruled out.
  - A dramatic response (fever reduction) should be seen within 24 to 48 hours.
  - Examples: prednisone 1 mg/kg PO q 12h, or dexamethasone 0.2 mg/kg IV q 24h; doses for longer term use are adjusted based on the specific underlying cause.

DRUG INTERACTIONS

The use of NSAIDs in combination with glucocorticoids should be avoided.

POSSIBLE COMPLICATIONS

- Drug therapy trials without a definitive diagnosis may interfere with future diagnosis and may exacerbate an undiagnosed condition that may be life threatening.
- Glucocorticoids may lead to immunosuppression or may mask clinical signs due to their anti-inflammatory effects.

RECOMMENDED MONITORING

Monitor temperature at least every 12 hours. Response to trial therapy may be nonspecific or coincidental, so monitoring should continue for a sufficient time to confirm that resolution of the fever can be attributed to selected therapy.

PROGNOSIS AND OUTCOME

Dependent on specific cause

PEARLS & CONSIDERATIONS

COMMENTS

- Infectious disease, immune-mediated conditions, and neoplasia account for more than 75% of FUO cases.
- With aggressive diagnostic testing, usually only 10% of FUO cases are considered idiopathic.
- Immune-mediated polyarthritis will frequently *not* be associated with detectable joint swelling; therefore arthrocentesis is indicated in all FUO cases where no underlying cause has been identified.

PREVENTION

- Ectoparasite prevention may reduce risk of vector-borne disease transmission.
- Indoor pets are less likely to be exposed to vector-borne diseases.
- Vaccination against specific disease agents for high-risk pets.
- Yearly retroviral testing and vaccination in high-risk cats.
- Routine screening of geriatric pets to facilitate early diagnosis and treatment of cancer.

CLIENT EDUCATION

- Animals may serve as sentinels for infections or transmit some infections to humans (zoonoses).
- Exposure to vectors may increase risk of disease transmission.

SUGGESTED READING

Lunn KF: Fever of unknown origin: a systematic approach to diagnosis. *Compend Cont Ed* 23(11):976-992, 2001.

Nelson RW, Couto CG: Fever of undetermined origin. *Small Animal Internal Medicine*. St. Louis, Mosby, 1998, pp 1222-1225.

AUTHORS: **NICOLE PACIFICO, ADAM BIRKENHEUER**

EDITOR: **ETIENNE CÔTÉ**

Fibrocartilaginous Embolism

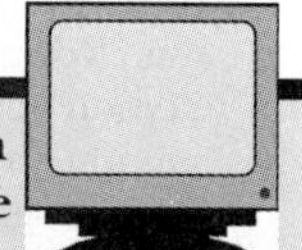

Client Education Sheet on Website

BASIC INFORMATION

DEFINITION

Fibrocartilaginous embolism (FCE) is a syndrome of acute spinal cord, and rarely brainstem, infarction and subsequent necrosis secondary to embolization of arterial and/or venous vasculature within the central nervous system. Although it is unconfirmed at this time, it is suspected that the embolus originates from the nucleus pulposus of the intervertebral disk.

SYNONYM(S)

Fibrocartilaginous embolic encephalomyelopathy

Fibrocartilaginous embolic myelopathy

EPIDEMIOLOGY

SPECIES, AGE, SEX: FCE has been described in dogs, cats, horses, pigs, sheep, turkeys, cattle, and humans. Male dogs may be at higher risk than females, and middle-aged dogs (3 to 6 years) are most commonly affected.

GENETICS AND BREED PREDISPOSITION: FCE most commonly affects nonchondrodystrophoid, large to giant breeds of dogs. Breeds at risk include Labrador retrievers, German shepherds, golden retrievers, Great Danes, and Doberman pinschers. Miniature schnauzers and Shetland sheepdogs can also be affected. FCE has not been reported in chondrodystrophoid breeds with degenerative disk disease.

RISK FACTORS: There may be a history of mild trauma and/or vigorous exercise before the onset of clinical signs of FCE.

ASSOCIATED CONDITIONS AND DISORDERS: Concurrent Hansen type II intervertebral disk disease (fibroid degeneration of the nucleus pulposus) may be present in the affected animal.

CLINICAL PRESENTATION

HISTORY, CHIEF COMPLAINT: Dogs with FCE will present with neurologic deficits that reflect the severity of the infarction and ischemia, as well as the location of the lesion within the central nervous system. The onset of FCE is peracute to acute, and clinical signs generally stabilize within 24 hours, after which the disease is often nonprogressive. This disease is nonpainful, although the affected dog may yelp or cry out at the onset of signs.

PHYSICAL EXAM FINDINGS

- The patient's neurologic deficits depend on the level of spinal cord affected, and clinical findings are consistent with a focal myelopathy.
- If the brachial plexus or lumbosacral intumescence is involved, lower motor neuron signs will predominate; if the C1-C5 or T3-L3 segments are involved, upper motor neuron signs will prevail.
- Nociception and proprioception may also be affected.
- Brainstem involvement can occur, in which case cranial nerve deficits, change in the level of consciousness, and/or cardiorespiratory difficulty may be seen.
- Spinal hyperesthesia is not a consistent finding.
- FCE is often lateralizing, and should be suspected in a patient with the peracute to acute onset of nonpainful, nonprogressive, lateralizing/asymmetric focal myelopathy.

ETIOLOGY AND PATHOPHYSIOLOGY

- FCE is thought to affect large, nonchondrodystrophoid dogs because their nucleus pulposus remains soft and gelatinous longer relative to chondrodystrophoid dogs, and can extrude along tears or fissures in the annulus fibrosus. If ejection pressure of the nucleus pulposus exceeds arterial blood pressure, the material may penetrate the vasculature.

- Histopathologically, the nature of the embolus is similar to that of the nucleus pulposus of the intervertebral disk. Thus the intervertebral disk is thought to be the origin of the embolus. Several theories have been proposed to explain the presence of disk material in the vasculature:
  - Chronic inflammation (such as type II intervertebral disk disease) may induce neovascularization of the intervertebral disk. With increased intradiskal pressure, the nucleus pulposus could extrude into this arterial system and into the radicular artery, causing embolization and subsequent ischemia and necrosis of the spinal cord.
  - Embryonic vasculature of the annulus fibrosus may persist, and the nucleus pulposus could herniate into this arterial system with an increase in intradiskal pressure.
  - The fibrocartilaginous material could extrude directly into an artery (radicular, vertebral, or ventral spinal). However, these arteries have thick, muscular walls, and one would expect to see evidence of hemorrhage if such damage occurred (hemorrhage has not been documented consistently on postmortem examination of dogs with FCE).
  - The disk material could herniate into the vertebral venous sinuses and enter the arterial system in a retrograde manner, induced by a Vasalva maneuver (trauma, exercise, coughing, straining) in which increased intra-abdominal pressure would induce retrograde blood flow, despite the presence of valves in the radicular veins.
- Another theory postulates that the source of the fibrocartilage is endothelial metaplasia.

DIAGNOSIS

DIFFERENTIAL DIAGNOSIS

- Other causes of embolism:
  - Sepsis
  - Leukemia
  - Polycythemia
  - *Dirofilaria immitis* microfilaria
  - Hyperviscosity or hyperlipidemia
  - Fat embolism
- Intervertebral disk disease (IVDD)
- Spinal trauma
- Focal myelitis
- Spinal neoplasia
- Diskospondylitis
- Vertebral osteomyelitis

INITIAL DATABASE

- Antemortem diagnosis is made based on history, clinical presentation, and the exclusion of other differential diagnoses.
- Complete blood count, serum biochemistry profile, and urinalysis: results usually within normal limits.
- Survey radiographs will usually be within normal limits.

ADVANCED OR CONFIRMATORY TESTING

- Cerebrospinal fluid (CSF) analysis may be within normal limits, or it may reveal mild, nonspecific changes, including pleocytosis and increased protein content. CSF analysis is not sufficiently sensitive or specific for the diagnosis of FCE, but it can be useful to rule out other causes of focal myelopathy.
- Myelography may be within normal limits, or it may reveal focal intramedullary swelling. This can be useful to rule out causes of myelopathy that produce spinal cord compression (e.g., IVDD).
- Magnetic resonance imaging is the imaging modality of choice in diagnosing FCE. Initially, evidence of intramedullary spinal cord swelling may be seen (hyperintense signal on T2-weighted images, and hypointense signal on T1-weighted images. Later, the findings may be consistent with ischemia, with increased intensity noted at the infarcted level on T2-weighted images.
- A definitive diagnosis of FCE can be made only with histopathologic examination of the spinal cord, usually performed at postmortem examination. Grossly, the outside of the spinal cord may appear to be normal, or it may be swollen and/or hemorrhagic. Hemorrhage, infarction, and necrosis may be noted on transverse sections of the spinal cord. Microscopically, gitter cells, axonal degeneration, and emboli within the veins or arteries of the parenchyma can be seen. The embolized material has the same histologic characteristics as the fibrocartilage found within the intervertebral disk.

TREATMENT

THERAPEUTIC GOAL(S)

- Nursing and supportive care
- Physical therapy and rehabilitation

ACUTE GENERAL TREATMENT

- Because FCE is not a compressive lesion, surgical decompression is not indicated. In addition, because the fibrocartilaginous material occludes microscopic blood vessels, surgical removal of the embolus should not be attempted.
- The embolus is composed of fibrocartilaginous material and not blood; thus attempts at medical dissolution with fibrinolytic therapy are unsuccessful.
- Good nursing care is crucial. For patients with urinary incontinence, it is important to prevent an atonic urinary bladder; bladder expression or catheterization is necessary. In addition, patients with urinary and/or fecal incontinence must be kept clean and dry. The recumbent patient needs to be placed on appropriate bedding and rotated frequently or placed in a sling to prevent the formation of pressure sores. Nutritional and intravenous fluid support may be indicated in a patient who cannot maintain adequate nutrition per os.
- Free radical scavenger drugs may prevent secondary ischemic complications, including edema and hemorrhage. Although controversial, corticosteroids may be given only if the patient presents within 6 hours of the initial insult (e.g., methylprednisolone sodium succinate 30 mg/kg slowly IV once, then 15 mg/kg slowly IV 2 hours later). If corticosteroids are given, it is imperative to provide gastric protectants to reduce the risk of gastrointestinal ulceration (e.g., famotidine [0.5–1 mg/kg IV q 12h] and/or misoprostol [2–8 μg/kg PO q 8–12h] and/or omeprazole [0.7 mg/kg PO q 24h]). Corticosteroid therapy is contraindicated in the patient who presents longer than 6 hours after the initial insult.

CHRONIC TREATMENT

The patient will benefit from physical therapy and rehabilitation. Physical therapy can be instituted immediately, and modalities include passive range of motion exercises, massage, hydrotherapy, and electrical stimulation.

POSSIBLE COMPLICATIONS

Complications, including the development of decubital ulcers and pneumonia, can arise secondary to the patient's recumbency.

RECOMMENDED MONITORING

Observation of respiratory effort and onset of cough, pulse oximetry, and lung auscultation are recommended to monitor for the development of pneumonia.

PROGNOSIS AND OUTCOME

- The presence of unilateral spinal cord damage yields a better prognosis than a transverse myelopathy.
- Lower motor neuron deficits suggest destruction of the ventral gray matter of the cervicothoracic or lumbosacral intumescence and yield a guarded to poor prognosis.
- Upper motor neuron deficits indicate a better prognosis.

- The absence of deep pain perception lends a poor prognosis, and this may be the most important prognostic indicator with FCE.
- Animals that display a functional recovery within the first 1 to 2 weeks after insult have a better prognosis. After this time period, it is less likely for further improvements to appear.
- The patient should be evaluated frequently with neurologic examinations during the first 12 hours after the insult to detect signs of ascending or descending myelomalacia. If evidence of myelomalacia is present (i.e., rapidly progressive deterioration of the spinal cord), the prognosis is grave.
- The patient with nonprogressive, lateralizing signs, intact deep pain perception, and no evidence of spinal cord swelling on diagnostic imaging has a relatively good prognosis compared with the patient with symmetric lower motor neuron deficits, absent deep pain perception, and CSF changes.

PEARLS & CONSIDERATIONS

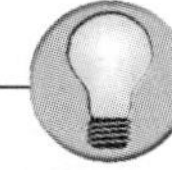

COMMENTS

One should be highly suspicious of FCE in the patient with a peracute to acute onset of nonpainful, nonprogressive, lateralizing focal myelopathy.

CLIENT EDUCATION

Clients must be advised of the intensive nursing and supportive care required of animals with FCE. The client should also have a commitment to rehabilitation and physical therapy, which can be time-consuming and costly.

SUGGESTED READING

Axlund TW, et al: Fibrocartilaginous embolic encephalomyelopathy of the brainstem and midcervical spinal cord in a dog. *J Vet Intern Med* 18:765, 2004.

Cauzinille L: Fibrocartilaginous embolism in dogs. *Vet Clin North Am Small Anim Pract* 30(1):155, 2000.

Dewey CW: Myelopathies: Disorders of the spinal cord. In Dewey CW (ed): *A Practical Guide to Canine and Feline Neurology*. Ames, IA, Iowa State Press, 2003, pp 321–323.

Gandini G, et al: Fibrocartilaginous embolism in 75 dogs: Clinical findings and factors influencing the recovery rate. *J Small Anim Pract* 44:76, 2003.

Han JJ, et al: Fibrocartilaginous embolism: an uncommon cause of spinal cord infarction: A case report and review of the literature. *Arch Phys Med Rehabil* 85:153, 2004.

Naiman JL: Fatal nucleus pulposus embolism of spinal cord after trauma. *Neurology* 11:83, 1961.

Neer TM: Fibrocartilaginous emboli. *Vet Clin North Am Small Anim Pract* 22(4):1017, 1992.

Tefend MB, Dewey CW: Nursing care for patients with neurologic disease. In Dewey CW (ed): *A Practical Guide to Canine and Feline Neurology*. Ames, IA, Iowa State Press, 2003, pp 517–539.

AUTHORS: **TODD W. AXLUND, JILL NARAK**
EDITOR: **CURTIS W. DEWEY**

Fibrosarcoma

BASIC INFORMATION

DEFINITION

A primary, malignant neoplasm of fibrous tissue. Fibrosarcoma is most common in the skin, subcutaneous tissue, and the oral cavity, but can occur anywhere, including the spleen.

EPIDEMIOLOGY

SPECIES, AGE, SEX: Fibrosarcomas are more common in middle-aged to older dogs and cats. Vaccine-site sarcomas have many similarities and are discussed separately (see Vaccine-Site Sarcoma, p 1136).
GENETICS AND BREED PREDISPOSITION: Genetic factors are not well defined in dogs or cats.
RISK FACTORS: Prior irradiation and metal implants have been implicated as a cause for fibrosarcomas.

CLINICAL PRESENTATION

DISEASE FORMS/SUBTYPES
- The most common form of fibrosarcoma in dogs is a solitary mass, typically found on the head, limbs, or oral cavity.
- Sarcomas that are histologically low-grade but biologically high-grade (malignant behavior) are an uncommon variant of fibrosarcoma found in the maxilla and mandible in large breed dogs.

HISTORY, CHIEF COMPLAINT: Most animals present for a progressive mass noticed by the owner or clinical signs related to the location of the tumor (e.g., oral and splenic tumors).
PHYSICAL EXAM FINDINGS
- Fibrosarcoma often appears as a firm, palpable mass in the subcutaneous or deep tissues; occasionally hairless or ulcerated. Oral fibrosarcoma often appears as a flat, ulcerated mass on the hard palate.
- Regional lymphadenomegaly may be present secondary to inflammation or, rarely, lymph node metastasis.
- Dogs with a splenic fibrosarcoma may present with abdominal mass, pain, or enlargement.

ETIOLOGY AND PATHOPHYSIOLOGY

- Fibrosarcomas are spontaneously occurring in most cases in dogs.
- Pathology caused by fibrosarcomas depends on the location of the primary tumor.

DIAGNOSIS

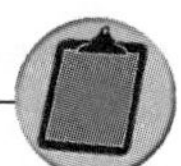

DIFFERENTIAL DIAGNOSIS

- Other soft tissue sarcomas
- Other skin and subcutaneous tumors:
  - Mast cell tumors, etc.
- Other oral tumors (epulis, melanoma, squamous cell carcinoma)
- Benign or non-neoplastic masses:
  - Benign tumor (e.g., lipoma)
  - Abscess

INITIAL DATABASE

- Fine-needle aspiration and cytologic study may help identify the tumor type before other diagnostics.
- Three view thoracic radiographs to rule out pulmonary metastases.
- Radiographs of the affected area may reveal involvement of underlying bone.
- Abdominal ultrasound to identify splenic tumors and rule out metastasis.

ADVANCED OR CONFIRMATORY TESTING

- Biopsy of mass:
  - The definitive diagnosis of fibrosarcoma is based on histopathologic evaluation of tumor tissue.
  - Special stains may be necessary to differentiate fibrosarcoma from other soft tissue sarcomas, especially poorly differentiated tumors.
- Computed tomography or magnetic resonance imaging may be necessary to delineate the local extent of the tumor and to plan for surgery or radiation therapy.
- Histopathologic grade of the tumor is necessary for determining the prognosis and treatment of most soft tissue sarcomas (see Soft Tissue Sarcoma, p 1016).

TREATMENT

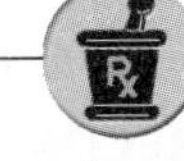

THERAPEUTIC GOAL(S)

Complete eradication of the primary tumor

ACUTE AND CHRONIC TREATMENT

- Chemotherapy may be indicated for tumors of the spleen or high-grade tumors (see Soft Tissue Sarcoma, p 1016).
- Aggressive surgical resection, radiation therapy, and/or chemotherapy may be used for treatment of fibrosarcoma (see Soft Tissue Sarcoma, p 1016 for specific details).

POSSIBLE COMPLICATIONS

Complications of treatment for fibrosarcomas depend on the types of treatments and the location of the primary tumor (see Soft Tissue Sarcoma, p 1016)

RECOMMENDED MONITORING

After appropriate local treatment, follow-up examination should be done on a routine basis to monitor for recurrence and metastasis. High-grade tumors may require more frequent monitoring for metastases during and after chemotherapy administration.

- Dogs that are likely to develop metastasis (splenic tumors, high-grade tumors) should be monitored closely (every 2 to 3 months) with physical exam, lymph node palpation, and thoracic radiographs.
- Dogs with low- or intermediate-grade tumors that have adequate local treatment should have physical examinations every 2 to 3 months or more frequently depending on risk of side effects from treatment. Thoracic radiographs could be done less frequently (6 months and 1 year after therapy).

PROGNOSIS AND OUTCOME

- A combination of radiation therapy and surgery has resulted in long-term tumor control in 86% of dogs with fibrosarcoma in peripheral sites and 54% of fibrosarcomas from all sites including the oral cavity.
- Radiation alone has resulted in 1-year tumor control rates of 33% and therefore is not typically recommended for fibrosarcomas. However, this statistic may underestimate efficacy, as it is derived from studies that used suboptimal radiation dose schedules.
- In certain situations where surgery is not indicated (e.g., nonresectable tumors or metastatic disease), radiation may be used to provide some degree of tumor control.
- Prognosis is excellent for low- to intermediate-grade fibrosarcomas with appropriate local treatment. This includes either surgical resection with clean histopathologic margins or incomplete resection combined with radiation therapy.
- Information is limited regarding prognosis for high-grade fibrosarcomas, but it is considered to be guarded based on the increased likelihood for metastases.
- Dogs with splenic fibrosarcomas are more likely to develop metastases and therefore have a poor prognosis.

PEARLS & CONSIDERATIONS

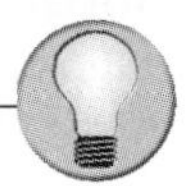

COMMENTS

Many animals with fibrosarcoma are successfully treated with wide surgical excision of the tumor. Animals with tumors that are difficult to treat in this manner (oral sarcomas, grade 3 sarcomas, nonresectable tumors, etc.) should be referred for consultation with a specialist (surgeon, oncologist, or radiation oncologist) to develop a multimodality treatment approach.

CLIENT EDUCATION

Pet owners can be educated to monitor their pets for the occurrence of tissue masses such as fibrosarcomas. Early detection and treatment may allow for less aggressive treatments with fewer side effects.

SUGGESTED READING

MacEwen EG, Powers BE, Macy D, Withrow SJ: Soft tissue sarcomas. In Withrow SJ, MacEwen EG (eds): *Small Animal Clinical Oncology*. Philadelphia, WB Saunders, 2001, pp 283-304.

AUTHOR: **JOHN FARRELLY**
EDITOR: **KENNETH M. RASSNICK**

Flail Chest

BASIC INFORMATION

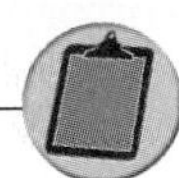

DEFINITION

Two or more adjacent rib fractures at two or more sites on each rib. The fractures result in chest wall segment instability, and therefore in asynchronous chest wall movement during respiration.

SYNONYM(S)

Flail segment
Multiple rib fractures

EPIDEMIOLOGY

SPECIES, AGE, SEX: Young male animals that tend to exhibit roaming behavior are more likely to be involved in traumatic events.

RISK FACTORS: Unmonitored activity (e.g., outdoor cats, dogs walked off leash, free-roaming animals)

ASSOCIATED CONDITIONS AND DISORDERS

- Pulmonary contusions
- Diaphragmatic hernia
- Pneumothorax
- Hemothorax

CLINICAL PRESENTATION

HISTORY, CHIEF COMPLAINT

- Trauma
  - Hit by car
  - Bite wound
- Increased respiratory rate and effort
- External thoracic skin wounds

PHYSICAL EXAM FINDINGS

- Increased respiratory rate and effort
- Paradoxical movement of the flail segment during respiration:
  - Flail segment moves inward during inspiration and outward during expiration
- Concurrent injuries are common:
  - Skin lacerations
  - Other fractures

ETIOLOGY AND PATHOPHYSIOLOGY

- Trauma results in two or more fractures per rib on two or more adjacent ribs.
- Hypoxemia due to abnormal pulmonary airflow (traditional model). Air from the lung in proximity to the flail chest segment flows to the opposite lung during inspiration and then back to the lung in proximity to the flail chest during expiration. This abnormal airflow provides no effective contribution to ventilation and is essentially an increase in dead space.
- Recent evidence indicates that hypoxemia and respiratory distress arise pri-

marily from pulmonary contusions associated with pneumothorax and not from abnormal airflow.

DIAGNOSIS

DIFFERENTIAL DIAGNOSIS

Pathologic rib fractures due to neoplasia or osteomyelitis (very rare)

INITIAL DATABASE

- Thoracic radiographs:
  - Lateral and dorsoventral views required, as fractures may be apparent on only one view
  - If dyspnea is severe, horizontal beam technique may be preferable (less restraint of patient, recumbency not necessary)
- Complete blood count, serum chemistry panel, urinalysis: generally unremarkable unless abdominal or other organs are affected or there is preexisting illness

ADVANCED OR CONFIRMATORY TESTING

Arterial blood gas analysis:

- May help to confirm a clinical suspicion of hypoxemia.
- Serial analysis may be useful to monitor trends.
- Hypoxemia (PaO_2 <80 mmHg) is common.
- In severe cases, hypoventilation may develop (pCO_2 >50 mmHg).

TREATMENT

THERAPEUTIC GOAL(S)

- Normalize oxygenation and control pain
- Surgical stabilization is rarely required

ACUTE GENERAL TREATMENT

- Pain control is key as hypoventilation will contribute to decreased blood oxygenation.
- Local nerve blocks, systemic opioids (e.g., oxymorphone or hydromorphone 0.05-0.1 mg/kg IV q 4-6h, or buprenorphine 0.005-0.02 mg/kg IV, SQ, or IM) and nonsteroidal anti-inflammatory drugs (e.g., carprofen 2-3 mg/kg PO or SQ q 12h) may be used.
- Oxygen supplementation often necessary (nasal oxygen, oxygen mask, oxygen cage). See Oxygen Supplementation, p 1292.
- Pneumothorax management:
  - Intensity of treatment determined mainly by degree of patient dyspnea.
    - Arterial oxygen concentration (PaO_2) and oxygen saturation may be more informative if patient is obtunded.
    - Radiographic extent of pneumothorax may suggest that dyspnea is of some other origin (e.g., pain, pulmonary contusion) if pneumothorax is radiographically mild.
  - Treatment options, in increasing order of intensity, include monitoring only, oxygen supplementation (see p 1292), thoracocentesis (see p 1308), chest tube placement (see p 1210), and thoracotomy (if large segments of rib are perforating the lung).
- Mechanical ventilation may be necessary with patients unresponsive to oxygen supplementation:
  - Response to oxygen supplementation is best assessed clinically by evaluating patient respiratory rate and effort.
  - However, pulse oximetry reading <88-90% or an arterial blood gas oxygen level (PaO_2) <60 mmHg with supplemental oxygen is an indication for mechanical ventilation.
- Surgery is rarely required:
  - Flail chest segments resulting from bite wounds may be stabilized when the bite wounds are repaired.
- Chest wraps are unlikely to be of benefit and may be detrimental.

POSSIBLE COMPLICATIONS

- Hypoventilation associated with pain
- Pneumothorax associated with rib segments piercing lung parenchyma

RECOMMENDED MONITORING

- Electrocardiogram if ventricular arrhythmias noted.
- Monitor respiratory rate and effort closely; use this information to guide decisions regarding oxygen supplementation, thoracentesis, or chest tube placement.
- Signs of pain may include restlessness, tachycardia, anorexia, and excessive vocalization.

PROGNOSIS AND OUTCOME

Good with adequate supportive care and if no other concurrent traumatic injuries

PEARLS & CONSIDERATIONS

COMMENTS

Hypoxemia surrounding flail chest more commonly reflects the underlying pulmonary contusion rather than chest wall instability

PREVENTION

- Keep animals indoors and confined to a leash
- Neutering may prevent roaming behavior

CLIENT EDUCATION

Don't let animals roam

SUGGESTED READING

Olsen D, et al: Clinical management of flail chest in dogs and cats: A retrospective study of 24 cases (1989-1999). *J Am Anim Hosp Assoc* 38:315-320, 2002.

AUTHOR: **THOMAS J. WALKER**
EDITOR: **ELIZABETH ROZANSKI**

Flatulence and Borborygmi

BASIC INFORMATION

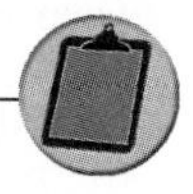

DEFINITION

- Flatulence is the excessive formation of gas in the stomach or intestine.
- Borborygmus is the rumbling noise caused by the propulsion of gas through the intestine.

SYNONYM(S)

Flatus (flatulence)

EPIDEMIOLOGY

SPECIES, AGE, SEX: More prevalent in dogs than cats.

GENETICS AND BREED PREDISPOSITION: Brachycephalic breeds are predisposed.

RISK FACTORS

- Diet
- Gastrointestinal (GI) tract disease

ASSOCIATED CONDITIONS AND DISORDERS: More prevalent in brachycephalic dogs, working and sporting dogs, and greedy eaters due to increased aerophagia (borborygmus).

CLINICAL PRESENTATION

HISTORY, CHIEF COMPLAINT

- May be associated with flatus as detected by owner—also belching, borborygmus, and abdominal distention
- May be associated with other signs of GI disease: vomiting, diarrhea, weight loss

PHYSICAL EXAM FINDINGS

- Generally unremarkable.
- Palpation of gas in the intestines is not in itself an abnormal finding.
- Mild abdominal discomfort may be caused from intestinal distention. If excessive, fermentation may be associated with severe distention of the GI tract and signs of colic and shock.

ETIOLOGY AND PATHOPHYSIOLOGY

- Gas occurs naturally in the GI tract and is caused by:
  - Aerophagia (the major cause: 17 ml of air accompanies 10 ml of swallowed water in humans).
  - Interaction of gastric acid and alkaline food.
  - Diffusion from blood.
  - Bacterial metabolism and fermentation (especially in the colon).
- Gas is removed from the GI tract by passage through the esophagus (belching) or anus (flatus), diffusion into the blood, or utilization by bacteria. Intestinal transit time for gas is 15 to 35 minutes.
- Causes of excessive GI gas:
  - Excessive aerophagia: brachycephalic breeds, vigorous exercise, competitive eating habits.
  - Excessive bacterial fermentation: dietary substances—nonabsorbable oligosaccharides (enzyme to split to monosaccharides is not present) (e.g., soy beans, legumes, rapidly fermentable fibers [pectin]).
  - Gastrointestinal disease: maldigestion and malabsorption—large amounts of malassimilated substances are available for fermentation, especially with lactose-containing foods as lactase is lost with adulthood. Adult dogs are lactose intolerant.
- Most natural intestinal gas is odorless: Aerophagia and dietary carbohydrates are the major contributors to intestinal gas volume, 99% of which is odorless. Sulfur-containing gases cause the foul odor and are produced by cruciferous vegetables, onions, high-protein diets and endogenous mucin, and some bile acids.

DIAGNOSIS

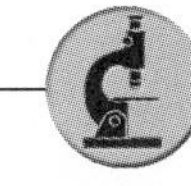

DIFFERENTIAL DIAGNOSIS

- Abdominal distention (organomegaly, ascites)
- Malassimilation and malabsorption
- Aerophagia
- Cats with flatulence will generally have underlying GI tract disease: inflammatory bowel disease, food sensitivity

INITIAL DATABASE

Laboratory testing is required only if additional GI signs are also present.

TREATMENT

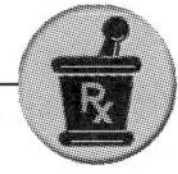

THERAPEUTIC GOAL(S)

- If severe gas accumulation is present, emergency therapy to relieve GI distention and control colic may be indicated.
- Decrease the amount of gas produced in the GI tract.
- Reduce the foul odor of the flatus.

ACUTE GENERAL TREATMENT

Acute treatment would be required only with severe gastric or intestinal distention. Then supportive therapy for colic pain and for shock, as well as decompression, would be required.

CHRONIC TREATMENT

MANAGEMENT

- Control aerophagia
  - Feeding management: specific foods, feeding frequency, competitive eating habits, relationship of feeding to exercise
  - Surgical correction of upper airway obstruction syndrome in brachycephalics
- Decrease bacterial fermentation
  - Decrease substrate/dietary management:
    - Limit undigested food and fiber that support bacterial fermentation
    - Highly digestible diets: small frequent meals (decreased residue in colon)
    - Avoid diets containing legumes: soybean products, pea fiber, etc.
    - Rice as a preferential source of carbohydrate decreases fermentation
  - Diagnose and treat underlying GI disorders
- Increase activity and exercise

MEDICAL TREATMENT: Carminatives are preparations that relieve flatulence. Management is the first step. Medical intervention is indicated only in intractable cases.

- Ingestion of activated charcoal has *not* been proven effective in humans.
- Bismuth subsalicylate: antibacterial and antiendotoxic properties. Dose-dependent efficacy, high frequency dosing, contraindicated at higher doses in cats.
- Zinc acetate (1% total diet): reduces malodor of flatus.
- Simethicone: antifoaming agent, no real effect.
- Combination treatment: activated charcoal, *Yucca schidigera,* and zinc acetate result in a significant decrease in flatulence.
- Pancreatic enzyme replacements may be used in cases with exocrine pancreatic insufficiency and may also be effective with other causes of excessive GI bacterial fermentation.

DRUG INTERACTIONS

Vitamin and mineral supplements can alter intestinal microbial activity.

RECOMMENDED MONITORING

- Progression of clinical signs may warrant an evaluation for GI disease
- Intermittent relapses usually indicate dietary indiscretion

PROGNOSIS AND OUTCOME

Prognosis for control is good in most cases

PEARLS & CONSIDERATIONS

COMMENTS

"After trying empirical therapy for pets with chronic flatulence, sound advice for the client is to always stand upwind of the patient and keep windows open." (Roudebush, Lorenz)

SUGGESTED READING

Giffard C, et al: Administration of charcoal, *Yucca schidigera*, and zinc acetate to reduce malodorous flatulence in dogs. *J Am Vet Med Assoc* 218(6):892, 2001.

Lorenz M: Flatulence in small animals. In Kirk RW (ed): *Current Veterinary Therapy IV.* Philadelphia, WB Saunders, 1974, pp 96-99.

Roudebush P: Flatulence: Causes and management options. *Compend of Contin Educ* 23(12):1075, 2001.

AUTHOR: **LIESEL VAN DER MERWE**

EDITOR: **ETIENNE CÔTÉ**

Flea Bite Allergy

Client Education Sheet on Website

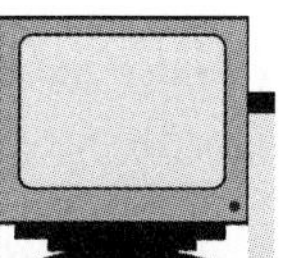

BASIC INFORMATION

DEFINITION

Development of hypersensitivity reaction(s) and subsequent skin lesions accompanied by variable pruritus in response to exposure to flea salivary antigens

SYNONYM(S)

Flea allergy dermatitis (FAD)
Flea bite hypersensitivity

EPIDEMIOLOGY

SPECIES, AGE, SEX

- Dogs: no sex predilection. Develops at any age, but is most common in 3- to 5-year-olds and rare if less than 6 months old
- Cats: no age or sex predilections reported

GENETICS AND BREED PREDISPOSITION

- Dogs: breed predilections not well established. Increased incidence suggested in setters, fox terriers, Pekingese, spaniels, chow chows, and long-coated dogs.
- Cats: no breed predilections reported.

RISK FACTORS

- Genetic predisposition to develop allergic dermatitis.
- Dogs: intermittent flea exposure.
- Cats: persistent flea exposure.
- Atopic patients are at greater risk for flea bite allergy.

GEOGRAPHY AND SEASONALITY

- Diagnosed worldwide, wherever fleas reside
- Seasonal in climates with cold winters
- Continuous in warm, humid climates
- Nonseasonal when indoor infestation is present

ASSOCIATED CONDITIONS AND DISORDERS

- Infestation with *Dipylidium caninum*
- Gastric trichobezoars associated with excessive grooming
- Secondary bacterial pyoderma
- Secondary seborrhea

CLINICAL PRESENTATION

DISEASE FORMS/SUBTYPES

- Canine flea bite allergy:
  - Pruritic, papular dermatitis
  - Acute moist dermatitis ("hot spot")
  - Fibropruritic nodules in chronic cases
- Feline flea bite allergy:
  - Pruritic papulocrustous dermatitis ("miliary dermatitis")
  - Symmetric self-induced alopecia
  - Eosinophilic granuloma complex

HISTORY, CHIEF COMPLAINT

- Dogs: acute onset of moderate-severe pruritus. Hair loss and malodor in longer-standing cases. Clients may report live fleas on their pet or experience flea bites themselves.
- Cats: hair loss, pruritus, excessive grooming, vomiting hairballs, or small crusted papules noted under the haircoat. Lip ulcers, raised plaques or granulomas may be noted. Fleas are less commonly observed than in dogs.

PHYSICAL EXAM FINDINGS

Dogs:

- Papulocrustous lesions, varying degrees of alopecia, erythema, and excoriations. Most commonly affected regions: dorsal lumbosacral region, tailhead, and caudomedial thighs. Ventral abdomen, especially near the umbilical area, flanks, and neck may also be affected
- Well-demarcated moist, erythematous, exudative skin lesions with alopecia
- Lichenification, lattice pattern hyperpigmentation, seborrhea
- Poor body condition, weight loss, worn incisor teeth
- ± Fleas, flea excreta ("flea dirt")

Cats:

- Hair loss on the caudodorsal abdomen or symmetrically on the ventral abdomen and lateral flanks
- Erythematous crusted papules around the neck and on the lumbosacral region
- Small postinflammatory melanotic macules
- Lesions consistent with eosinophilic granuloma complex (indolent ulcer, eosinophilic plaque, eosinophilic granuloma)
- Excoriations, crusts
- Weight loss, poor body condition, peripheral lymphadenopathy
- ± Fleas, flea excreta ("flea dirt")

ETIOLOGY AND PATHOPHYSIOLOGY

- Repeated exposure to flea salivary antigens induces development of various hypersensitivity reactions:
  - Type I (immediate/anaphylactic) hypersensitivity (dogs, cats)
  - Cutaneous basophil hypersensitivity (dogs)
  - Type IV (delayed/cell-mediated) hypersensitivity (dogs, cats)
  - Late-phase IgE-mediated reactions (dogs)
- Hypersensitivity reactions, when recurrent or persistent, may become more intense, and be triggered with progressively less antigen (flea saliva).

DIAGNOSIS

The diagnosis is based almost entirely on history and physical exam findings. Even in the absence of live fleas or flea excreta, physical signs as described warrant empiric antiflea treatment before or while pursuing advanced diagnostic testing for other causes of pruritus.

DIFFERENTIAL DIAGNOSIS

- Dogs, cats:
  - Other hypersensitivities (atopy, foods, intestinal parasites, drugs)
  - Ectoparasitic dermatoses
  - Bacterial folliculitis
- Dogs:
  - *Malassezia* dermatitis
- Cats:
  - Dermatophytosis

INITIAL DATABASE

- History
- Physical examination findings
- ± Observation of fleas, excreta

ADVANCED OR CONFIRMATORY TESTING

- Intradermal testing with 1:1000 w/v aqueous solution of whole flea antigen
- Enzyme-linked immunosorbent assay serologic allergen screening for flea saliva antigens
- Response to flea eradication

TREATMENT

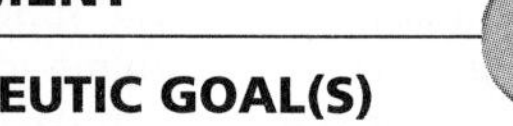

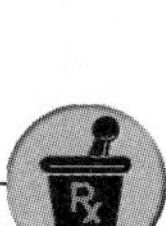

THERAPEUTIC GOAL(S)

- Relief of pruritus
- Elimination of flea exposure

ACUTE GENERAL TREATMENT

- Corticosteroids:
  - Dogs: Prednisone/prednisolone 1 mg/kg PO daily for 5 to 7 days, then taper
  - Cats:
    - Prednisolone 2.2 mg/kg PO daily for 5 to 7 days, then taper
    - Methylprednisolone injectable 5 mg/kg or 20 mg per cat IM or SQ. Multiple risks with use (diabetes mellitus, iatrogenic hyperadrenocorticism, etc.)
- Topical flea adulticide:
  - Permethrin sprays/spot applications (Active-3)
  - Imidacloprid (Advantage)
  - Fipronil (Frontline)
  - Selamectin (Revolution)

- Oral flea adulticide
  - Nitenpyram (Capstar)
- Specific therapy of any secondary infections, seborrhea (see Seborrhea, p 987)

CHRONIC TREATMENT

Integrated flea management: essential for eradication of the problem.

- Ongoing use of topical flea adulticide.
- Insect growth regulators: methoprene, pyriproxyfen, others. Note: some products are formulated for spraying the patient; others are for treating the environment.
- Insect development inhibitors: lufenuron (Program) oral, monthly.
- Environmental control.
  - Identify "point sources" of infestation
  - Cleaning or frequent vacuuming
  - Organic debris removal outdoors
  - Use of an approved insect growth regulator premise spray
- Immunotherapy is experimental at this time.

POSSIBLE COMPLICATIONS

- Neurotoxicity with the use of pyrethrins, permethrins in cats
- Diabetes mellitus, iatrogenic hyperadrenocorticism (glucocorticoids, especially sustained-release injections)

RECOMMENDED MONITORING

Routine flea combing

PROGNOSIS AND OUTCOME

Good with long-term management.

PEARLS & CONSIDERATIONS

COMMENTS

- Clients may not recognize excessive grooming as a manifestation of pruritus.
- Trichograms (microscopic examination of hair plucks) confirm self-induced alopecia: broken ends of hair shafts.
- Excessive grooming decreases live flea population.

PREVENTION

- Avoidance of flea bites prevents disease recurrence
- Continued integrated flea control is mandatory

CLIENT EDUCATION

- Progressive disease unless fleas are eradicated
- Preventable, not curable, disease
- Treatment of all in-contact pets is mandatory

SUGGESTED READING

Bevier DE: Flea allergy dermatitis. In Campbell KL (ed): *Small Animal Dermatology Secrets*. Philadelphia, Hanley & Belfus, 2004, pp 208–213.

Reedy LM, Miller WH, Willemse T: Flea bite hypersensitivity. In *Allergic Skin Diseases of Dogs and Cats*. Philadelphia, WB Saunders, 1997, pp 202–225.

Scott DW, Miller WH, Griffin CE: Skin immune system and allergic diseases. In *Muller and Kirk's Small Animal Dermatology*, ed 6. Philadelphia, WB Saunders, 2001, pp 627–635.

AUTHOR: **STEPHANIE R. BRUNER**

EDITOR: **JAN A. HALL**

Follicular Dysplasia and Pattern Alopecia (Canine)

BASIC INFORMATION

DEFINITION

- Follicular dysplasias are noninflammatory disorders of the haircoat that result in hair loss and altered coat quality. An underlying genetic predisposition for abnormal follicular development has been noted in specific breeds.
- Pattern alopecia is a relatively common, likely heritable, noninflammatory alopecic disorder affecting either the pinnae and/or ventrum of specific breeds.

SYNONYM(S)

Follicular dysplasia: canine recurrent flank alopecia (see Recurrent Flank Alopecia, Canine, p 945), alopecia X (see Alopecia X, p 53), color dilution alopecia (formerly color mutant alopecia), blue Doberman syndrome, black hair follicular dysplasia, follicular dysplasia of specific breeds (Irish water spaniels, Portuguese water dogs, red and black Doberman, Chesapeake bay retriever, etc.)

Pattern alopecia: canine pattern alopecia

EPIDEMIOLOGY

SPECIES, AGE, SEX

- These disorders affect dogs of either sex and of any reproductive status.
- Color dilution alopecia, black hair follicular dysplasia, and pattern baldness are disorders of early onset (usually before 1 year of age).
- Non-color-linked follicular dysplasias usually start during adulthood.

GENETICS AND BREED PREDISPOSITION

- Color dilution alopecia (CDA): seen in several breeds with dilute coat colors such as in blue Doberman pinscher, dachshund, Great Dane, Yorkshire terrier, and Chihuahua.
- Black hair follicular dysplasia (BHFD): recognized in several bi- or tri-colored breeds such as the saluki, basset hound, as well as mixed breeds, but can also be seen in solid-colored (black) breeds.
- Pattern alopecia (ventral type): seen in dogs with fine short coats such as dachshunds, Chihuahuas, miniature pinschers, whippets, greyhounds, Boston terriers, and boxers.

CLINICAL PRESENTATION

DISEASE FORMS/SUBTYPES

- Distinct types of follicular dysplasia have been described in the Irish water spaniel, Portuguese water dog, red and black Doberman pinscher, and Chesapeake Bay retriever.
- The two main forms of pattern alopecia are the ventral type and the pinnal type.

HISTORY, CHIEF COMPLAINT: Dogs born with a normal haircoat are presented for evaluation of a gradual thinning of the haircoat.

PHYSICAL EXAM FINDINGS

- CDA: progressive alopecia involving exclusively hair follicles in the dilute areas, usually starting around 6 months of age (light blue) but as late as 2 to 3 years of age (steel blue Doberman). The rate of hair loss is variable, but most light-colored dogs are almost completely alopecic by 2 to 3 years of age. These dogs are prone to follicular plugging and secondary recurrent bacterial folliculitis that can aggravate the hair loss and may cause pruritus.
- BHFD: progressive alopecia and excessive scaling, exclusively involving the

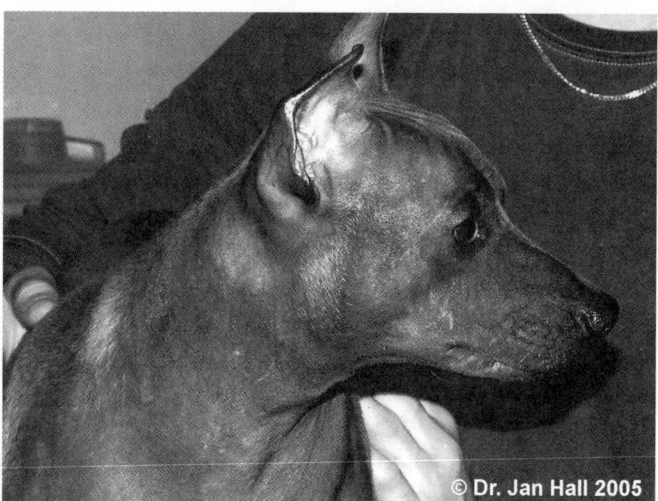

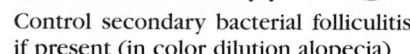

FIGURE I-72 Follicular dysplasia in a 1-year-old male miniature pinscher. Courtesy of Dr. Jan A. Hall.

black-haired areas, seen as early as 4 weeks of age.

- Pattern alopecia (pinnal type): progressive alopecia of the ear pinnae, starting around 6 months of age.
- Pattern alopecia (ventral type): progressive alopecia developing within the caudal auricular region, along the ventral neck, thorax and abdomen, and caudal thighs, starting around 6 months of age.

ETIOLOGY AND PATHOPHYSIOLOGY

- Follicular dysplasia can be divided histologically into categories in which the hair cycle is abnormal (canine recurrent flank alopecia, alopecia X) and those in which there are abnormalities in the process of melanization of the pilosebaceous units (color dilution alopecia, BHFD).
- All forms of follicular dyplasia and pattern baldness are most likely genetically determined.
- In color dilution alopecia, an inherited autosomal recessive disorder of melanosome transportation has been demonstrated.

DIAGNOSIS

DIFFERENTIAL DIAGNOSIS

- Endocrinopathies
- Other follicular dysplasias
- Infectious process (pyoderma, demodicosis, dermatophytosis) in some clinical presentations

INITIAL DATABASE

- Diagnosis is based on history, clinical findings, and ruling out other differentials
- Trichogram: large melanin clumps along the hair shaft, causing distortion and fracture of the hair, in color dilution alopecia and black hair follicular dysplasia

ADVANCED OR CONFIRMATORY TESTING

Dermatohistopathologic evaluation: dilated and cystic hair follicles with melanin clumping in follicular basal cells, hair bulbs, hair shafts, follicular lumen in color dilution alopecia, and BHFD. Follicular miniaturization in pattern baldness.

TREATMENT

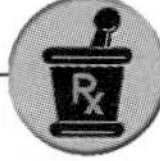

THERAPEUTIC GOAL(S)

- Control secondary bacterial folliculitis if present (in color dilution alopecia)
- Hair regrowth

GENERAL TREATMENT

Anecdotal evidence exists for the efficacy of melatonin at 3-6 mg/kg PO q 8-12h for 1 to 2 months to stimulate hair growth. Reported in both pattern alopecia and in color dilution alopecia.

PROGNOSIS AND OUTCOME

- These entities are incurable, genetically based dermatoses.
- Affected dogs are healthy otherwise with the exception of secondary pyoderma in color dilution alopecia.

PEARLS & CONSIDERATIONS

COMMENTS

- The early onset, pattern-linked alopecia (pattern alopecia), color link (color dilution alopecia, BHFD), and/ or breed predisposition make the diagnosis straightforward in many cases.
- The main impact of these disorders is cosmetic, rather than medical, unless secondary infection or sunburn occurs.

SUGGESTED READING

Cerundolo R, et al:An analysis of factors underlying hypotrichosis and alopecia in Irish water spaniels in the United Kingdom. *Vet Dermatol* 11:107, 2000.

Miller WH: Follicular dysplasia of the Portuguese water dogs. *Vet Dermatol* 6:67-74, 1995.

Scott DW, Miller WH, Griffin CE: *Muller and Kirk's Small Animal Dermatology*, ed 6. Philadelphia, WB Saunders. 2001, pp 959-973.

AUTHOR: **MANON PARADIS**

EDITOR: **JAN A. HALL**

Food Allergy, Dermatologic

Client Education Sheet on Website

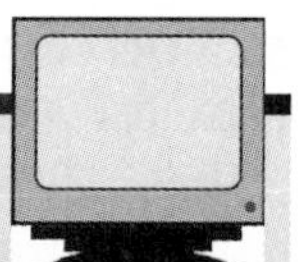

BASIC INFORMATION

DEFINITION

An abnormal response to an ingested food or food additive that produces clinical signs, most commonly pruritus, affecting the skin

SYNONYM(S)

The preferred term is *dermatologic adverse reaction to food*. The terms *food allergy* or *food hypersensitivity* are often incorrectly used synonymously with adverse food reaction. These terms more accurately refer specifically to the subcategory of adverse food reactions that have an immunologic basis. The term *food intolerance*, also encompassed within dermatologic adverse reaction to food, is reserved for the subcategory of adverse food reactions without an immunologic basis and includes metabolic food reactions, food poisoning, food idiosyncrasies, and pharmacologic reactions to food.

EPIDEMIOLOGY

SPECIES, AGE, SEX

- Dogs: from 4 months to 14 years:
  - Up to one-third of cases occur in dogs less than 1 year old
  - No sex predilection
- Cats: from 6 months to 12 years:
  - 50% develop signs by 2 years
  - No sex predilection

GENETICS AND BREED PREDISPOSITION

- Dogs: Some authors propose that the cocker spaniel, springer spaniel, Labrador retriever, collie, miniature schnauzer, Chinese shar-pei, West Highland white terrier, Wheaten terrier, boxer, dachshund, dalmatian, Lhasa apso, German shepherd, and golden retriever are at increased risk.
- Cats: the Siamese cat may be at increased risk.

RISK FACTORS: Risk factors include certain foods or food ingredients, poorly digestible proteins, any disease that increases intestinal mucosal permeability, selective IgA deficiency, certain breeds, age (<1 year), and concurrent allergic disease.

GEOGRAPHY AND SEASONALITY: Nonseasonal.

ASSOCIATED CONDITIONS AND DISORDERS

- 20-30% of cases have concurrent atopy or flea allergy dermatitis.
- 10-15% of cases may have concurrent gastrointestinal (GI) signs such as vomiting and/or diarrhea.
- Secondary infections with bacteria and yeast are common.

CLINICAL PRESENTATION

HISTORY, CHIEF COMPLAINT

- The chief complaint is of nonseasonal pruritus, recurrent pyoderma or otitis externa.
- There may be a history of a poor response to glucocorticoid therapy.
- Adverse food reactions with an immunologic component (food allergy, food hypersensitivity) usually develop after prolonged exposure to a food allergen, whereas food intolerance may occur after a single exposure, as immune mechanisms are not involved.

PHYSICAL EXAM FINDINGS

- No classic pattern exists
- Dogs:
  - Lesion distribution: feet, face, axillae, perineal region, inguinal region, rump, and ears.
  - 25% may show only otitis externa (Fig. I-73).
  - Lesions may consist of papules, pustules, wheals, angioedema, erythema, ulcers, excoriations, lichenification, alopecia, scales, crust, acute moist pyotraumatic dermatitis.
- Cats:
  - Lesion distribution: usually centered around the head and neck but may be generalized.
  - Manifestations may consist of generalized pruritus without lesions; miliary dermatitis; pruritus with self-trauma centered around the head, neck, and ears; self-induced alopecia; scaling dermatoses; lesions of the eosinophilic granuloma complex; angioedema; urticaria; conjunctivitis.

ETIOLOGY AND PATHOPHYSIOLOGY

- A variety of etiologies are proposed to cause dermatologic adverse food reactions.
- The majority are attributed to food allergies; however, immunologic tests are rarely performed to confirm this suspicion.
- Common food allergens in dogs include beef, dairy products, wheat, eggs, chicken, lamb, and soy. Common food allergens in cats include beef, dairy products, and fish.
- Food allergies are thought to be the result of primarily a type I hypersensitivity reaction, although type III and IV reactions have also been proposed.
- Several host defenses exist to prevent the absorption of intact allergens from the GI tract, including effective digestion, intestinal peristalsis, an intact intestinal mucus layer, tight junctions between mucosal cells, and mucosal IgA. The small amounts of food proteins that do cross the intestinal mucosa activate T-suppressor cells and stimulate an immune response in the gut-associated lymphoid tissue that leads to tolerance. A defect in any of these defense mechanisms may lead to sensitization of the immune system and the development of a food allergy.
- Idiosyncratic adverse reactions to food and food additives, such as erythema multiforme, are suspected to occur in animals, although this has not been proven.
- Some foods contain products that may directly produce a pharmacologic effect. Scromboid fish such as tuna, mackerel, skipjack, and bonito contain vasoactive amines such as histamine, and have been reported to cause adverse reactions in cats and dogs. Cadeverine, another vasoactive amine, may exacerbate adverse food reactions by inhibiting histamine metabolism.

DIAGNOSIS

DIFFERENTIAL DIAGNOSIS

- Ectoparasites (*Sarcoptes, Demodex* (uncommonly), *Cheyletiella, Notoedres, Otodectes,* fleas, lice)
- Bacterial folliculitis (*Staphylococcus intermedius*)
- *Malassezia* dermatitis
- Other hypersensitivity disorders (atopy, flea bite hypersensitivity, other ectoparasite hypersensitivities, intestinal parasite hypersensitivity, contact hypersensitivity, drug hypersensitivity)
- Dermatophytosis (ringworm)
- Seborrheic skin diseases
- Behavioral disorders (feline psychogenic alopecia, flank sucking, tail-biting, self-nursing)
- Neoplasia (mast cell tumor, epitheliotropic lymphoma)

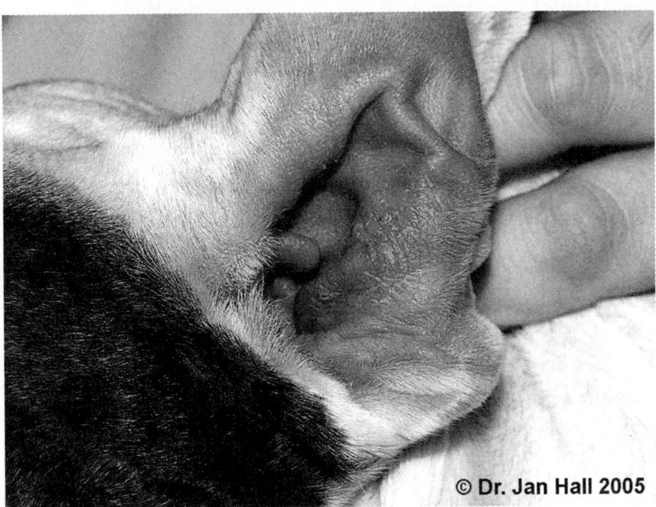

FIGURE I-73 Otitis externa in a boxer dog with food allergy. Note the extensive erythema affecting the inner surface of the pinna. Courtesy of Dr. Jan A. Hall.

INITIAL DATABASE

- Cytologic evaluation: Secondary microbial infections with bacteria and yeast are common. Acetate tape, direct impression smears, and superficial skin scrapings are appropriate methods for obtaining cytologic samples. Ears and interdigital and intertriginous regions are commonly affected. The significance of any secondary microbial infection is determined by assessing the patient's response to appropriate antimicrobial therapy.
- Skin scrapings: Deep, focal skin scrapes should be used to detect *Demodex* mites, while broad superficial scrapes may be more beneficial in detecting *Sarcoptes*. Note: the *Sarcoptes* mite may not be detected on skin scrapings, and *Sarcoptes* infestation requires a trial course of appropriate therapy to be fully ruled out when the index of suspicion for infection is high.
- Examination for fleas/flea comb: While the presence of fleas, flea dirt, or tapeworms raises the index of suspicion, flea allergy dermatitis should be fully ruled out by treatment with an appropriate adulticidal flea control product in patients presenting with pruritic skin disease.
- Elimination diet: this is the only useful test for confirming the diagnosis of adverse food reaction. Current serologic tests correlate poorly with the true offending allergen. The ideal diet should be nutritionally adequate and use a single highly digestible protein source or protein hydrolysate, avoiding additives and vasoactive amines. The exact protein source is not important, but it should be one to which the animal has not been previously exposed. This diet should be fed exclusively for 10 to 12 weeks, ensuring that treats, flavored heartworm preventives, table scraps, and any other source of food are also eliminated from the diet. A significant decrease in pruritus is typically seen within 4 to 6 weeks, but may take up to 12 weeks. Properly prepared home-cooked diets are an alternative to commercial products, although it may be challenging to ensure that they are nutritionally balanced (this requirement may be waived for the duration of the diet trial as long as the patient appears to be maintaining body condition).

ADVANCED OR CONFIRMATORY TESTING

Dietary challenge: This is a necessary step to confirm the diagnosis. The original diet is fed back to the animal for 10 to 14 days. In most cases of true adverse food reaction there is an exacerbation in pruritus within 3 to 7 days, but it may take up to 14 days. Once the pruritus is under control again, individual ingredients may be fed for 14 days each to determine which ingredients caused the adverse reaction. In most cases only one or two substances are the cause of the adverse reaction.

TREATMENT

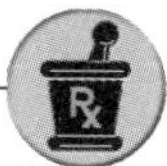

THERAPEUTIC GOAL(S)

Elimination of pruritus

ACUTE GENERAL TREATMENT

- Manage any secondary microbial infection with appropriate antimicrobial therapy.
- Avoid feeding the offending food.
- Topical or systemic antipruritic therapy may be necessary initially to control self-trauma. Corticosteroid use should be avoided where possible, as it may mask other conditions and make it more difficult to assess response to the elimination diet trial.

CHRONIC TREATMENT

The patient may be maintained on a balanced home-cooked or commercial elimination diet, or provocative testing with individual ingredients may be used for determining which dietary components can be tolerated.

PROGNOSIS AND OUTCOME

The prognosis is excellent with avoidance of offending foods

PEARLS & CONSIDERATIONS

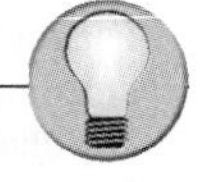

COMMENTS

- The first step when dealing with any suspect dermatologic adverse food reaction is to make sure that other causes of pruritus have been ruled out.
- In some cases a single elimination trial may be insufficient and a second elimination trial using an alternative commercial novel protein or hydrolysed protein source or a novel protein home-cooked diet may be required to see improvement.

SUGGESTED READING

Jackson HA: Diagnostic techniques in dermatology: The investigation and diagnosis of adverse food reactions in dogs and cats. *Clin Techn Small Anim Pract* 16:4, 2001.

Roudebush P, Guilford WG, Shanley KJ: Adverse reactions to food. In Hand MS, Thatcher CD, Remillard RL, Roudebush P (eds): *Small Animal Clinical Nutrition*, ed 4. Marceline, Mark Morris Institute, 2000, pp 431–453.

Scott DW, Miller WH, Griffin CE: Skin immune system and allergic skin diseases. In Scott DW, Miller WH, Griffin CE (eds): *Muller and Kirk's Small Animal Dermatology*, ed 6. Philadelphia, WB Saunders, 2001, pp 615–627.

AUTHOR: **ANDREW LOWE**
EDITOR: **JAN A. HALL**

Food Allergy, Gastrointestinal

Client Education Sheet on Website

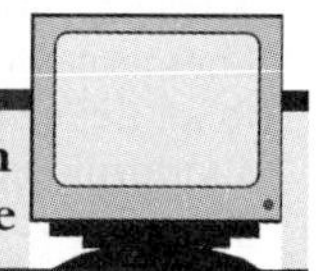

BASIC INFORMATION

DEFINITION

Food allergy and food intolerance are repeatable adverse reactions to specific dietary components that respond to exclusion of the causative agent. Food allergy is immune-mediated, whereas food intolerance is not.

SYNONYM(S)

Dietary/food hypersensitivity

EPIDEMIOLOGY

SPECIES, AGE, SEX

- Dogs and cats
- Age 4 months to 14 years; typically <1 or >5 years old

GENETICS AND BREED PREDISPOSITION

- Dogs: cocker spaniel, springer spaniel, Labrador retriever, collie, miniature schnauzer, shar-pei, West Highland white terrier, Wheaten terrier, boxer, dachshund, dalmatian, Lhasa apso, German shepherd, and golden retriever at increased risk
- Irish setter, soft-coated Wheaten terrier: familial gluten-sensitive enteropathy
- Cats: Siamese and Siamese-cross

RISK FACTORS

- Increased intestinal permeability (e.g., viral enteritis, inflammatory bowel disease [IBD])
- Immunoglobulin (Ig) A deficiency
- Allergic disease

- Repeated exposure to novel proteins in young animals

GEOGRAPHY AND SEASONALITY: Usually nonseasonal, as the provocative agent is typically part of the normal diet.

ASSOCIATED CONDITIONS AND DISORDERS

- Gastrointestinal (GI): antibiotic-responsive enteritis (small intestinal bacterial overgrowth), IBD, exocrine pancreatic insufficiency, pancreatitis, chronic gastritis, gastroesophageal reflux, lymphangiectasia
- Skin disease: food allergy, dermatologic (see Food Allergy, Dermatologic, p 396), atopic dermatitis (see Atopy, p 96)

CLINICAL PRESENTATION

HISTORY, CHIEF COMPLAINT

- Vomiting, weight loss, intermittent signs of abdominal pain, soft feces, diarrhea, flatulence, increased frequency of defecation, irritable demeanor, and/or concurrent cutaneous signs.
- The allergen(s) typically have been ingested for months to years before signs develop. If an allergen is ingested intermittently, the owner may note an association between ingestion and occurrence of signs.

PHYSICAL EXAM FINDINGS

- Systemic: thin body condition, decreased appetite, weight loss, lethargy, urticaria/angioedema/anaphylaxis.
- GI-specific: abdominal distention, diarrhea.
- Skin: pruritic (face, neck, ears, ventral trunk, and feet) otitis externa, uritica, or angioedema. In cats, self-inflicted alopecia or miliary dermatitis may be observed.
- Allergic conjunctivitis possible.

ETIOLOGY AND PATHOPHYSIOLOGY

- Food allergens + altered GI mucosal barrier or poor oral tolerance
- Gliadin in gluten portion of wheat, barley, or rye serves as potent antigen (see Gluten-Sensitive Enteropathy, p 444)
- Abnormal immunologic response (often IgE mediated)
- Immediate and/or delayed hypersensitivity reaction
- Altered GI structure and function (any level of GI tract from stomach to large intestine)

DIAGNOSIS

Dietary hypersensitivity is diagnosed based on negative results of routine diagnostic tests, GI biopsy results indicating inflammation (if biopsy performed), and positive response to an elimination food trial. An accurate diagnosis depends on ensuring that: (1) an elimination diet is truly novel (complete dietary history elicited by veterinarian and provided by owner, and all ingredients ever ingested are eliminated during the trial), (2) client compliance is optimal, and (3) confounding factors (e.g., treatment with antibiotics or corticosteroids) do not occur concurrently.

DIFFERENTIAL DIAGNOSIS

- Any chronic GI disorder (e.g., lymphangiectasia, IBD, lymphoma, enteritis [bacterial, viral, fungal])
- Dietary indiscretion
- Pancreatic disease (pancreatitis, exocrine pancreatic insufficiency [EPI])
- Liver disease
- Hyperthyroidism (cats)
- Metabolic/endocrine (diabetes mellitus, hypoadrenocorticism, acid/base or electrolyte disturbances)

INITIAL DATABASE

- Dietary history:
  - Thoroughly evaluate the current diet, including regular food, treats, snacks, human food, scraps, flavored medications, and anything else ingested; read all ingredient labels
- Complete blood count: often unremarkable; mild anemia of chronic disease, increased eosinophils or basophils possible
- Serum biochemistry profile: nonspecific changes
- Urinalysis: nonspecific; dogs with chronic inflammatory diseases, IBD, etc., may have concurrent proteinuria (protein-losing nephropathy)
- Fecal flotation and smear: rule out parasitism
- Feline immunodeficiency virus/feline leukemia virus testing in cats
- Serum T4/thyroid profile: for hyperthyroidism in cats

ADVANCED OR CONFIRMATORY TESTING

- Elimination food trial: diagnostic test of choice; both diagnostic and therapeutic.
- Intradermal skin or serum allergen testing (patients with concurrent cutaneous signs); both skin and serum tests for specific food allergens are unreliable.
- Abdominal radiography and ultrasonography to rule out other causes of GI disease (e.g., evidence of obstruction, masses, infiltration, non-GI abdominal lesions); findings usually unremarkable.
- Endoscopy with biopsy and histopathologic evaluation of GI mucosa to rule out other structural GI diseases. With food allergy, as with IBD, nonspecific increases in lymphocytes, plasma cells, or eosinophils in the lamina propria are found; confirmation requires favorable response to dietary modification.
- Serum trypsin-like immunoreactivity (rule out EPI).
- Serum bile acids: hepatopathies. Severe GI disease may falsely lower serum bile acid concentrations.

TREATMENT

THERAPEUTIC GOAL(S)

- Control clinical signs. Usually achievable solely by eliminating the provocative dietary component(s).
  - Feed a limited number of protein sources (with high digestibility) such as novel protein sources, or protein hydrolysate-containing diet
  - Avoidance of wheat, barley, or rye ingredients (gluten-induced enteropathy)
- Long-term control. Feed a satisfactory diet not containing the provocative component(s); most owners prefer a commercial diet. Must be sustainable for months to years. Identify treats without the allergen.

ACUTE AND CHRONIC TREATMENT

- Elimination food trial lasting 4 to 8 weeks:
  - Provide a single, specific food, ideally with a novel protein (e.g., venison, duck, or other meat not found in foods previously eaten by the pet) and carbohydrate source. Commercial or home-made limited antigen, or hydrolyzed protein, diets may be used. Many commercial limited antigen diets are available; selection is based on patient's current diet and avoidance of known provocative ingredients. Commercial limited antigen diet may be preferred by some, but home-prepared limited antigen diets are the gold standard (if the owner can feed the diet exclusively for up to 8 weeks).
  - *No* other food (or supplements, treats, chewable medications, or other consumables) may be consumed during the trial. Because the problem is immune-mediated, even a single violation can reactivate hypersensitivity.
  - Client compliance is essential. Both deliberate (e.g., treats, human foods and snacks, etc.) and inadvertent (e.g., chewable heartworm tablets) violations of the trial must be avoided.
- GI signs typically start to abate within days, and substantial improvement usually occurs within 4 weeks:
  - Although partial improvement is expected within 4 weeks, up to 8 weeks may be needed before significant abatement of clinical signs occurs.
  - Absence of clinical improvement after 8 weeks of strict diet adherence makes food allergy extremely unlikely.

- Skin lesions may take 8 weeks or longer to resolve, although significant improvement is seen within 8 weeks in the vast majority of cases.
- Concurrent treatment with corticosteroids (prednisone 1-2 mg/kg orally q 24h, tapering to lowest effective dose and stopping if signs resolve; prednisolone is preferred for cats) is often necessary, but will invalidate conclusions if implemented during the trial.
    - If a positive response to the diet is seen, a food challenge is performed to confirm the diagnosis, and to unambiguously identify the provocative antigen. Additional ingredients are added individually until the signs recur. Clients often are reluctant to do this, but if the patient becomes allergic to the current hypoallergenic diet, there is no way to identify which specific ingredient was allergenic to permit rational choice of an alternative diet.
    - Challenge with the regular food(s) usually results in recrudescence of clinical signs within hours to a few days.
    - Any diet without allergens identified via provocative challenge may be fed, even regular commercial diets.
    - Absence of signs within 14 days of continuous provocative challenge makes any improvement during the trial unlikely to have resulted from diet therapy.

POSSIBLE COMPLICATIONS

- Inappetence, weight loss
- Nutritional-related problems if imbalanced home-made food used
- Intestinal neoplasia (lymphoma) as consequence of chronic GI inflammation

RECOMMENDED MONITORING

If clinical improvement and resolution of clinical signs occur with the trial diet, diagnosis of food sensitivity is confirmed by recurrence of the same clinical signs (provocative challenge) after reintroduction of the original diet (including all treats, snacks, flavored medications, etc.)

PROGNOSIS AND OUTCOME

Good prognosis if offending foods or ingredients are identified and eliminated from the diet

PEARLS & CONSIDERATIONS

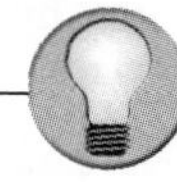

COMMENTS

- Food hypersensitivity should be a differential diagnosis in almost all animals presenting with chronic GI signs.
- Although it can be difficult to convince owners to complete a strict food trial for 4 to 8 weeks, they should be encouraged to do so, as food sensitivity is a "good" disease (i.e., entirely curable by simply changing the diet).
- Using a food diary during the elimination trial helps the owner monitor clinical response and compliance.

CLIENT EDUCATION

- Human food sources, snacks, treats, and food for other animals (e.g., dog having access to cat food) can be an allergen.
- Provide a handout listing all items the animal may not ingest during the food trial to be read by all household members.
- Contact the owner during the first week of the food trial to check that the elimination diet has been started, provide support, and address any problems that may have arisen (e.g., patient will not eat the food).

SUGGESTED READING

Buffington CAT, Holloway C, Abood SK: *Manual of Veterinary Dietetics*. St. Louis, Elsevier, 2004, pp 118–121.

De Weck AL, et al: Dog allergy, a model for allergy genetics. *Int Arch Allergy Immunol* 113:55, 1997.

Hall EJ: Dietary sensitivity. In Bonagura JD (ed): *Kirk's Current Veterinary Therapy (XIII)*. Philadelphia, WB Saunders, 2000, pp 632–637.

Jackson HA, Hammerberg B: Evaluation of a spontaneous canine model of immunoglobulin E-mediated food hypersensitivity: Dynamic changes in serum and fecal immunoglobulin E values relative to dietary change. *Comp Med* 52:316–321, 2002.

Leistra MHG, et al: Evaluation of selected-protein-source diets for management of dogs with adverse reactions to foods. *J Am Vet Med Assoc* 219:1411–1414, 2001.

Olsen ME, et al: Hypersensitivity to dietary antigens in atopic dogs. In Reinhart GA, Carey DP (eds): *Recent Advances in Canine and Feline Nutrition*, vol 3. Wilmington, DE, Orange Frazer Press, 2000, pp 69–77.

Roudebush P, Guilford WG, Shanley KV: Adverse reactions to food. In Hand MS, Thatcher CD, Remillard RL, Roudebush P (eds): *Small Animal Clinical Nutrition*, ed 4. Topeka, KS, Mark Morris Institute, 2000, pp 431–453.

AUTHORS: **ANDREW HILLIER, PHILIP ROUDEBUSH**

EDITORS: **C. A. TONY BUFFINGTON, DEBRA L. ZORAN**

Footpad Disorders

BASIC INFORMATION

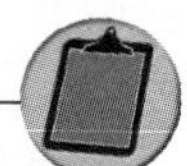

DEFINITION

Pathologic condition involving the footpad skin

EPIDEMIOLOGY

SPECIES, AGE, SEX

- Dogs and cats
- Less than 1 year of age: hereditary footpad hyperkeratosis, collagen disorder of the footpads of German shepherds, familial vasculopathies, acrodermatitis, and junctional and dystrophic epidermolysis bullosa
- Older dogs: superficial necrolytic dermatitis (also called hepatocutaneous syndrome, necrolytic migratory erythema, or metabolic epidermal necrosis) and epitheliotropic lymphoma

GENETICS AND BREED PREDISPOSITION

- Vitiligo: Siamese cats and Belgian Groenendael dogs
- Footpad hyperkeratosis: Irish terriers (probable autosomal recessive) and Dogue de Bordeaux
- Collagen disorders of the footpads: German shepherds
- Familial vasculopathy: German shepherds and Jack Russell terriers
- Acral mutilation syndrome (probable autosomal recessive): German shorthaired and English pointers, English springer spaniels, and French spaniels
- Dermatomyositis: Beauceron dogs (footpad lesions)
- Uveodermatologic syndrome: Akitas, Alaskan malamutes, and Siberian huskies
- Zinc responsive dermatosis: Alaskan malamutes (genetic defect involving enteric zinc absorption) and Siberian huskies
- Systemic and cutaneous (discoid) lupus erythematosus (SLE, DLE): collies, Shetland sheepdogs, and German shepherds

GEOGRAPHY AND SEASONALITY: Leishmaniasis in endemic areas.

ASSOCIATED CONDITIONS AND DISORDERS

- Footpad calcinosis cutis: renal failure or hyperparathyroidism.

- Systemic lupus erythematosus: systemic signs depending on the organs involved.
- Superficial necrolytic dermatitis (hepatocutaneous syndrome): hepatopathy or glucagon-producing pancreatic tumor.
- Feline paraneoplastic alopecia: pancreatic carcinoma or bile duct carcinoma.
- Xanthomatosis in cats can be associated with diabetes mellitus.
- Feline plasma cell pododermatitis: concurrent feline immunodeficiency virus (FIV) infection possible; associated renal glomerulonephritis and amyloidosis also reported.
- Uveodermatologic syndrome: granulomatous uveitis.
- Cutaneous horns have been reported in cats with feline leukemia virus (FeLV) infection.

CLINICAL PRESENTATION

HISTORY, CHIEF COMPLAINT: Skin lesions located on one or multiple footpads. The owner may also notice self-trauma and lameness. In addition, foot involvement may be part of a more generalized condition.

PHYSICAL EXAM FINDINGS

- Number of feet affected. Lesions on multiple feet (see Associated Conditions and Disorders above) versus on one foot only (neoplasia, trauma, infection).
- Depending on the disease, several changes can be present on the footpads:
    - Swelling and inflammation
    - Hyperkeratosis
    - Cracking and fissuring
    - Ulcers
    - Depigmentation or hyperpigmentation
    - Draining tracts
    - Change in footpad texture

ETIOLOGY AND PATHOPHYSIOLOGY

Footpad lesions can arise following various pathomechanisms, including:

- Contact with an irritant or corrosive substance, which can result in skin injury and inflammation.
- Development of antibodies or activated lymphocytes against normal body constituents (autoimmune diseases), or against inciting antigens (drugs, bacteria, viruses), causing tissue damage.
- Altered process of keratinization (proliferation/differentiation/desquamation) resulting in hyperkeratosis.
- Defective melanin production or a destruction of melanocytes, leading to pigment disorders. Moreover, a disorder at the basal epidermal cell level can result in hypopigmentation.
- In addition to primary etiologies, self-trauma and secondary bacterial infection can result in footpad lesions.

DIAGNOSIS

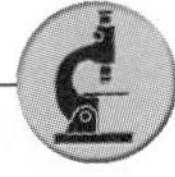

DIFFERENTIAL DIAGNOSIS

- Environmental: trauma, irritant contact dermatitis, calcinosis cutis caused by percutaneous penetration of calcium salts, and thallium toxicosis.
- Hereditary: see Genetics and Breed Predisposition above.
- Allergic/immune-mediated:
    - Dog: pemphigus foliaceus, DLE, SLE, vasculitis, toxic epidermal necrolysis, erythema multiforme, cryoglobulinemia and cryofibrinogenemia (cold agglutinin disease), bullous pemphigoid, epidermolysis bullosa aquisita, uveodermatologic syndrome, and drug reactions.
    - Cat: eosinophilic granuloma complex, pemphigus foliaceus, SLE, erythema multiforme, toxic epidermal necrolysis, vasculitis, cryoglobulinemia and cryofibrinogenemia (cold agglutinin disease), drug reactions, and plasma cell pododermatitis.
- Nutritional: zinc responsive dermatosis.
- Endocrine/metabolic:
    - Dog: superficial necrolytic dermatitis (hepatocutaneous syndrome) and footpad calcinosis cutis (often associated with chronic renal failure or parathyroid hyperplasia).
    - Cat: paraneoplastic alopecia and xanthomatosis (idiopathic or associated with diabetes mellitus).
- Neoplastic: epitheliotropic cutaneous lymphoma, squamous cell carcinoma, fibrosarcomas, mast cell tumors, etc.
- Infectious: canine distemper, cowpoxvirus infection in cats, subcutaneous or systemic mycotic infections, canine papillomatosis, and hookworm and *Pelodera* dermatitis.
- Miscellaneous: noninflammatory hypomelanosis (vitiligo) or hypermelanosis (lentigo in orange cats), cutaneous horns, idiopathic footpad hyperkeratotis seen in older dogs, and idiopathic sterile granulomas and pyogranulomas.

INITIAL DATABASE

- History and general examination are very important in the diagnostic process.
- Cytology of any exudates: bacteria, inflammatory cells, acantholytic keratinocytes (pemphigus), and fungal organisms.
- Complete blood count/biochemistry panel/urinalysis: results variable, depending on suspected cause.
- Thoracic/abdominal imaging, if relevant, to confirm systemic disease (e.g., superficial necrolytic dermatitis [hepatocutaneous syndrome]) or to stage tumors.

ADVANCED OR CONFIRMATORY TESTING

- Skin biopsies for histopathology and possibly immunofluorescence or immunohistochemical stainings
- Endocrine tests and serology depending on suspected disease
- Coombs' test: cold agglutinin disease
- Antinuclear antibody test (ANA): positive in virtually all patients with SLE

TREATMENT

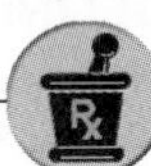

THERAPEUTIC GOAL(S)

- Permanent cure or control of the disease
- Sometimes palliative treatment (e.g., malignancy)

ACUTE GENERAL TREATMENT

- Depends on etiology of the lesion and possible secondary infection

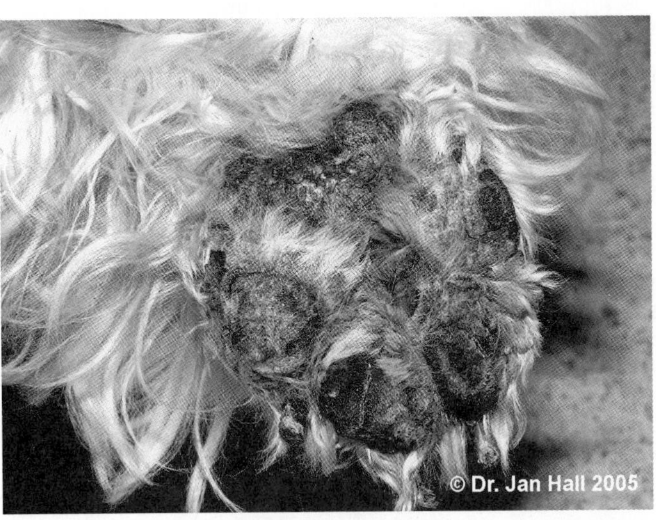

FIGURE I-74 Hyperkeratosis of the footpads in a 10-year-old, male, castrated cocker spaniel with superficial necrolytic dermatitis (hepatocutaneous syndrome). Courtesy of Dr. Jan A. Hall.

DISEASES AND DISORDERS

- Foot soaks or bandages sometimes useful
  - Hyperkeratotic lesions: warm water foot soaks for 5 to 10 minutes, followed by application of a softening agent (e.g., petroleum jelly). The owners should be warned that this can be messy.
  - For more severe hyperkeratosis, daily foot soaks in 50% propylene glycol. Improvement is expected within a few days. Lifelong maintenance therapy (1 to 2 times weekly as needed) is often required.
  - Draining lesions can benefit from foot soaks in warm water with added Epsom salts (magnesium sulfate) (30 ml/L) for 10 minutes q 12-24h, until draining stops.
- Surgery can be considered for some diseases: excision of cutaneous horns and other tumors, surgical debridement of devitalized tissues
- Medication varies depending on underlying cause

CHRONIC TREATMENT

Dependent on the underlying disease

PROGNOSIS AND OUTCOME

Will vary according to the disease

PEARLS & CONSIDERATIONS

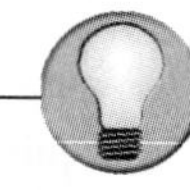

COMMENTS

- Successful therapy is based on identifying the underlying cause.
- Skin biopsies are often needed for the diagnosis of footpad disorders.

PREVENTION

Advise against breeding of animals with hereditary diseases

SUGGESTED READING

Guaguère E, et al: Feline pododermatoses. *Vet Dermatol* 3:1-12, 1992.

Scott DW, Miller WH, Griffin CE: Bacterial skin diseases. In *Muller and Kirk's Small Animal Dermatology*, ed 6. Philadelphia, Saunders, 2001, pp 304-306.

White SD: Pododermatitis. *Vet Dermatol* 1:1-18, 1989.

AUTHOR: **NADIA PAGÉ**

EDITOR: **JAN A. HALL**

Foreign Body, Esophageal

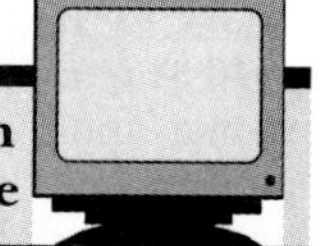

Client Education Sheet on Website

BASIC INFORMATION

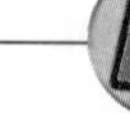

DEFINITION

Any solid object that lodges in the esophagus despite esophageal peristalsis

EPIDEMIOLOGY

SPECIES, AGE, SEX: Dogs and cats of any age or sex.

GENETICS AND BREED PREDISPOSITION: Smaller dogs and cats seem to be affected more commonly.

RISK FACTORS: Feeding bones.

ASSOCIATED CONDITIONS AND DISORDERS

- Esophagitis is common.
- Esophageal perforation can cause septic mediastinitis, pyothorax, and/or pneumothorax.

CLINICAL PRESENTATION

DISEASE FORMS/SUBTYPES

- Nonpenetrating foreign objects (main concerns: esophagitis, aspiration pneumonia)
- Penetrating foreign objects (main concerns: mediastinitis, pyothorax, esophagitis, aspiration pneumonia)

HISTORY, CHIEF COMPLAINT

- Acute onset of regurgitation is very suggestive.
  - Distinguish acute vomiting (active abdominal contractions leading to expulsion of food) from acute regurgitation (passive evacuation of food from the esophagus out of the mouth).
- Anorexia and ptyalism often occur (especially in cats).
- Some patients drink water but will not attempt to eat solid food.
- Dyspnea, nonspecific signs including lethargy and anorexia, and/or signs suggesting general discomfort may be seen if perforation occurs.
- Rarely, pressure of foreign object on trachea causes coughing or choking.

PHYSICAL EXAM FINDINGS

- Ptyalism occasionally noticed during exam
- Dysphagia or gagging may be seen during exam
- Dyspnea/fever sometimes seen secondary to perforation and mediastinitis/pleuritis

ETIOLOGY AND PATHOPHYSIOLOGY

- Bones are the most common cause in dogs.
- Other causes include food boluses, fishhooks, rawhide treats, and dental chew toys.
- Hairballs or medications (pills) are important in cats.

DIAGNOSIS

DIFFERENTIAL DIAGNOSIS

Regurgitation:

- Esophagitis
- Megaesophagus (idiopathic)
- Megaesophagus (secondary to systemic disease)
- Megaesophagus (pediatric: transient, congenital)
- Esophageal mass
- Esophageal stricture
- Vascular ring anomaly

INITIAL DATABASE

- Complete blood count and serum biochemistry panel: to look for evidence of inflammation and to prepare for anesthesia
- Plain thoracic radiographs:
  - Differentiate esophageal foreign body from megaesophagus (often generalized, as opposed to esophageal dilation associated with foreign body, which, when present, is seen cranial to the foreign body) and other thoracic masses (assess location relative to esophagus using at least two radiographic views).
  - Most foreign objects will be seen with good quality films, but poultry bones may be relatively radiolucent, requiring excellent technique for detection.
  - Evidence of pneumothorax and pleural effusion: both are suggestive of esophageal perforation.
  - Esophageal foreign objects can look like lung lesions radiographically.
  - Assess for complications: aspiration pneumonia and/or evidence of perforation (mediastinal widening, pleural effusion suggesting mediastinitis or pleuritis/pyothorax, respectively).
- Contrast esophageal radiographs:
  - Seldom needed and usually only obscure visualization during endoscopy.
  - Risk of aspiration of contrast material.

ADVANCED OR CONFIRMATORY TESTING

Esophagoscopy:
- Definitive differentiation of esophageal foreign body from esophagitis.
- With good technique, the foreign object can virtually always be seen.

TREATMENT

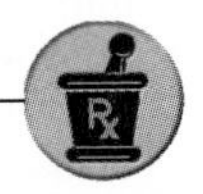

THERAPEUTIC GOAL(S)

Remove the foreign object and resolve any complications (e.g., esophagitis or perforation with resulting pulmonary disease or sepsis)

ACUTE GENERAL TREATMENT

- Esophagoscopy to remove foreign object and determine degree of esophagitis.
    - If foreign object cannot be removed, then it can sometimes be pushed into the stomach where it is removed surgically or allowed to dissolve.
- Surgery if endoscopy is unsuccessful at removing the foreign object.
- Prokinetics (e.g., metoclopramide 0.2-0.4 mg/kg IM or SC PO q 8h) and/or antacid (famotidine 0.5-1 mg/kg IV, IM, SC, or PO q 12-24h or omeprazole (0.7-1 mg/kg PO q 12-24h) to treat esophagitis (see Esophagitis, p 366).
- Place gastrostomy feeding tube if severe esophagitis is present.
- Appropriate treatment of pulmonary disease/pleuritis if a perforation occurs.

CHRONIC TREATMENT

Mechanical dilation of consequent stricture formation, if necessary (see Esophageal Stricture, p 363)

POSSIBLE COMPLICATIONS

- Cicatrix leading to partial or complete esophageal obstruction
- Esophageal perforation leading to septic pleuritis/mediastinitis

PROGNOSIS AND OUTCOME

- Good if there is no perforation and esophagitis is not severe
- Good to guarded if severe esophagitis is likely to cause severe stricture
- Guarded to poor if perforation has caused severe septic mediastinitis or pleuritis

PEARLS & CONSIDERATIONS

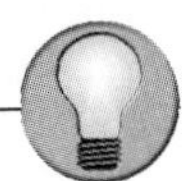

COMMENTS

- Rigid endoscopes are usually more effective than flexible ones in removing foreign objects.
- If a contrast esophagram is required, use a water-soluble iodide contrast agent; do not use barium.

PREVENTION

- Avoid feeding bones.
- Be careful about allowing dogs to have/swallow rawhide chews.
- Use caution when dogs are in the area around baited fish hooks.
- Do not medicate cats with dry tablets or capsules; follow the medication with water or food.

SUGGESTED READING

Houlton JEF, et al: Thoracic oesophageal foreign bodies in the dog: A review of ninety cases. *J Small Anim Pract* 26:521, 1985.

Michels GM, et al: Endoscopic and surgical retrieval of fishhooks from the stomach and esophagus in dogs and cats: 75 cases 1977-1993. *J Am Vet Med Assoc* 207(9):1194, 1995.

Spielman BL, et al: Esophageal foreign body in dogs: A retrospective study of 23 cases. *J Am Anim Hosp Assoc* 28:570, 1992.

AUTHOR: **MICHAEL WILLARD**
EDITOR: **DEBRA L. ZORAN**

Foreign Body, Linear Gastrointestinal

BASIC INFORMATION

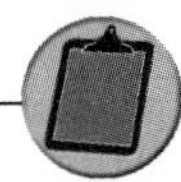

DEFINITION

Ingestion of a linear object that lodges in the proximal alimentary system (commonly under the tongue or at the pylorus) and causes plication of intestines along the length of the object

SYNONYM(S)

String foreign body

EPIDEMIOLOGY

SPECIES, AGE, SEX
- Young animals are at risk for foreign object ingestion.
- Linear foreign body is a more common diagnosis in cats than dogs.
- Dogs with linear foreign bodies are generally older than cats.
- Cats frequently present with string or thread ingestion, while dogs ingest fabric such as clothing or carpet.

RISK FACTORS: Some animals are more prone to ingesting foreign objects than others (individual behavior) irrespective of age.

GEOGRAPHY AND SEASONALITY: December to January: ingestion of Christmas tree "icicles" (long, thin strips of foil-like plastic) or ribbons.

CLINICAL PRESENTATION

HISTORY, CHIEF COMPLAINT
- Owners may witness object ingestion.
- String may be visualized protruding from the anus.
- Clinical signs vary with duration of foreign body ingestion, as well as presence of a partial or complete obstruction.
- Vomiting, anorexia, ptyalism, depression, and weight loss (if chronic) are typical clinical signs.

PHYSICAL EXAM FINDINGS
- Thorough examination at the base of the tongue should be performed to inspect for anchored foreign material.
    - In cats, elevation of the base of the tongue is best accomplished by depressing the mandible using an index finger for pressure on the lower incisors to open the mouth, and externally pressing upward (dorsally) between the bodies of the mandible using the thumb of the same hand.
    - In dogs or cats, a complete examination may require sedation or general anesthesia.
- Painful and bunched intestines may be detected with careful abdominal palpation.
- Dehydration, depression, or shock; severe with complete obstruction or peritonitis.

ETIOLOGY AND PATHOPHYSIOLOGY

- Anchoring of ingested linear material around base of tongue, at the pylorus, or in the proximal intestinal tract.
    - Without an anchor point, ingested linear foreign bodies may pass through the gastrointestinal (GI) tract without complication.
- Peristalsis results in plication of intestines along the length of the fixed material.

- Obstruction of intestinal tract results.
- Due to peristalsis, continued sawing action of the foreign material along mesenteric border may result in intestinal erosion and perforation and the development of peritonitis.
- Presence of an associated intussusception is possible.

DIAGNOSIS

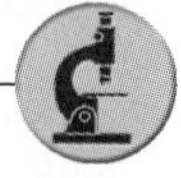

DIFFERENTIAL DIAGNOSIS

- All other causes of intestinal obstruction such as neoplasia, intussusception, granuloma, stricture, adhesions, or volvulus
- Ileus

INITIAL DATABASE

- Complete blood count: normal or shows evidence of inflammation/sepsis due to peritonitis (leukocytosis with increased band neutrophil count, toxic changes in neutrophils).
- Serum chemistry profile:
  - Hypokalemia associated with vomiting, anorexia.
  - Hypoglycemia associated with peritonitis.
  - Azotemia associated with dehydration.
- Urinalysis:
  - Unremarkable. Normal or elevated specific gravity is expected in azotemic, dehydrated patients.
- Abdominal radiographs:
  - Characteristic findings include plication of intestines or eccentric or "comma shaped" intraluminal gas bubbles.
  - Dogs may be more likely than cats to have characteristic radiographic findings allowing the diagnosis of linear foreign body to be made via radiography.
- Abdominocentesis with fluid evaluation should be performed if peritonitis is suspected.

ADVANCED OR CONFIRMATORY TESTING

- Contrast radiography or abdominal ultrasound may be used if survey radiographic findings are inconclusive (Fig. I-75).
- Abdominal ultrasound:
  - May document a tortuous path of the proximal intestine as well as presence of an intraluminal linear object.
  - May document associated disorders such as an intussusception or peritonitis.
  - However, limited efficacy when gas or barium is present in the intestine.
- Noniodinated contrast material is often recommended for upper GI radiographic contrast series, as up to 16% of cats and 41% of dogs may have perforation of the intestinal tract.
  - However, the advantage of iodine (will be resorbed from the peritoneal cavity if perforation exists, unlike barium) must be weighed against its reduced degree of contrast, foul taste (compliance), and the access to any spilled barium at the time of laparotomy because surgical intervention is indicated if perforation is confirmed.

TREATMENT

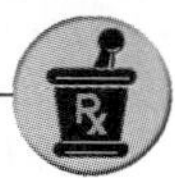

THERAPEUTIC GOAL(S)

- Correct dehydration and electrolyte imbalances
- Remove obstructing foreign body:
  - Although conservative treatment in the cat has been reported, the high likelihood of perforation and the associated morbidity of peritonitis dictate that these cases be treated as surgical emergencies.
  - Conservative treatment is not described in the dog due to the high risk of development of peritonitis.

ACUTE GENERAL TREATMENT

- Intravenous fluid therapy with electrolyte (potassium) supplementation according to need.
- Prophylactic antibiotics:
  - Cefazolin, 22 mg/kg IV q 2h during the perioperative period.
- Surgical intervention includes thorough inspection of the entire intestinal tract for evidence of perforation.
- If the linear foreign body is fixed around the base of the tongue, it should be cut at this point.
- Foreign material is removed through a single or multiple enterotomies.
- Gastrostomy is performed to remove any foreign material trapped in the stomach, particularly at the pylorus.

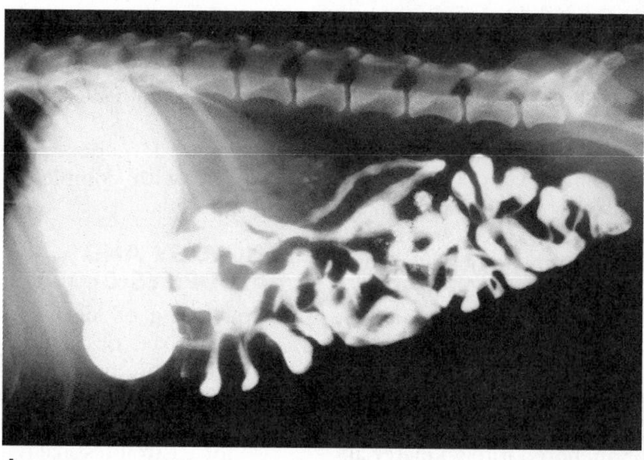

A

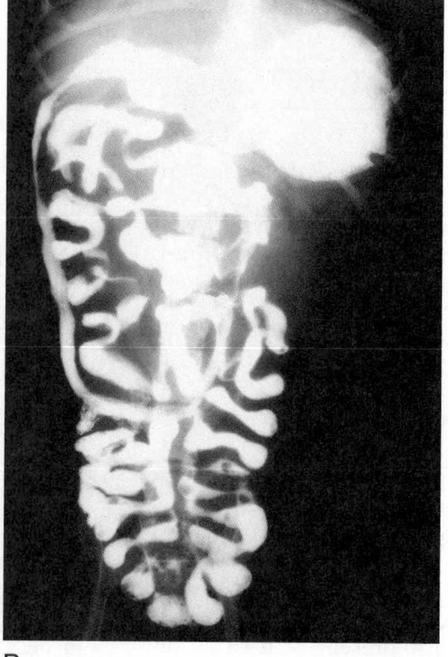

B

FIGURE I-75 Lateral **A**, and ventrodorsal **B**, radiographic projections of an upper gastrointestinal (UGI) barium study. This patient had a gastrointestinal linear foreign body. The characteristic teardrop-shaped appearance of small intestinal segments is seen. Courtesy of Dr. Richard Walshaw.

- Single enterotomy removal using a red rubber catheter has been reported for use when no intestinal perforations are present.
  - This technique involves a single duodenal enterotomy with attachment of a red rubber catheter to the linear object. The enterotomy is closed and the catheter with attached object is advanced distally until removed from rectum.
- If any necrosis, perforation, or intussusception of the intestines is present, a resection and anastomosis should be performed.
- Omentum or serosal patch may be placed to reinforce suture line.
- Change gloves and surgical instruments prior to abdominal lavage and closure.

CHRONIC TREATMENT

Postoperative considerations:

- Continue rehydration and daily electrolyte monitoring
- NPO 12 hours after enterotomy, 12 to 24 hours after resection and anastomosis
- Administer GI protectants or antiemetics as needed

POSSIBLE COMPLICATIONS

- Dehiscence; animals should be monitored in hospital for 48 to 72 hours postoperatively for signs of peritonitis. Risk factors include presence of preoperative peritonitis, serum albumin concentration <2.5 g/dl, and presence of a foreign body (vs. neoplastic disease).
- Ileus.
- Short bowel syndrome; unlikely if less than 70% of small intestine resected.
- Stricture.
- Reoccurrence.

RECOMMENDED MONITORING

The following parameters should be monitored q 6-12h until discharge from hospital:

- Body temperature
- Blood glucose
- Electrolytes
- Hematocrit and total solids
- Presence of abdominal pain

PROGNOSIS AND OUTCOME

- Delay in surgical intervention may increase risk of perforation and peritonitis.
- Presence of peritonitis or free abdominal gas on radiographs is associated with increased rate of mortality in the dog.
- Morbidity and mortality are 50% higher for dogs than cats.

PEARLS & CONSIDERATIONS

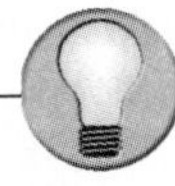

COMMENTS

- Do not put forceful traction on the linear object before or during surgery as this may cause iatrogenic laceration of the mesenteric border of the small intestine.
- Consider placing an intraoperative feeding tube (esophagostomy, gastrostomy, or gastrojejunostomy tube) in these patients based on preoperative nutritional status, degree of patient debilitation, or anticipated postoperative anorexia.

SUGGESTED READING

Anderson S, et al: Single enterotomy removal of gastrointestinal linear foreign bodies. *J Am Anim Hosp Assoc* 28:487, 1992.

Basher A, et al: Conservative versus surgical management of gastrointestinal linear foreign bodies in the cat. *Vet Surg* 16:135, 1987.

Evans K, et al: Gastrointestinal linear foreign bodies in 32 dogs: A retrospective evaluation and feline comparison. *J Am Anim Hosp Assoc* 30:445, 1994.

Macphail C: Gastrointestinal obstruction. *Clin Tech Small Anim Pract* 17(4):178-183, 2002.

AUTHOR: **JANET KOVAK**

EDITOR: **RICHARD WALSHAW**

Foreign Body, Oral

BASIC INFORMATION

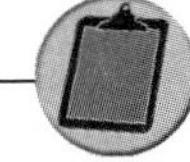

DEFINITION

Foreign object lodged or embedded in the oral cavity

EPIDEMIOLOGY

SPECIES, AGE, SEX: Dog and cat, either sex. Potentially more of a problem in younger animals.

RISK FACTORS

- Habit of chewing on foreign objects:
  - Bones, sticks, string
- Longer-haired dogs playing or running in grassy/wooded areas
- Interacting with a porcupine

ASSOCIATED CONDITIONS AND DISORDERS

- Retrobulbar abscess
- Submandibular/intermandibular abscess
- Necrosis of intraoral structures
- Linear foreign body gastrointestinal obstruction

CLINICAL PRESENTATION

HISTORY, CHIEF COMPLAINT

- Dog playing or running in grassy or wooded area
- Dog seen interacting with porcupine
- Animal seen chewing on foreign object
- Signs of oral discomfort (pawing at mouth, face rubbing, reluctance to eat hard food)
- Facial swelling:
  - Exophthalmos
  - Strabismus
- Nonspecific signs:
  - Depression, anorexia, vomiting

PHYSICAL EXAM FINDINGS

- Nonspecific findings:
  - Depression, pyrexia, dehydration
- Reluctance to open/discomfort on opening mouth
- Facial swelling:
  - Exophthalmos
  - Strabismus
  - Submandibular/intermandibular swelling
- Halitosis
- Oral discharge (hemorrhagic, purulent)
- Findings related to the foreign body:
  - Bone or stick lodged across hard palate, between premolars/molars; or encircling mandible (short segment of large diameter bone)
  - Burrs stuck in lingual, palatine, gingival mucosa
  - String foreign body around base of tongue
  - Porcupine quills in and around muzzle and oral cavity
- Penetrating oral injury:
  - Possibly associated with external facial swelling
- Findings associated with gastrointestinal linear foreign body:
  - Abdominal palpation:
    - Pain
    - Plicated intestines

DISEASES AND DISORDERS

ETIOLOGY AND PATHOPHYSIOLOGY

- Foreign body penetration of the oral cavity may result in abscess formation in the surrounding tissues.
  - Retrobulbar
  - Submandibular/intermandibular
- Foreign body lodged between the maxillary premolars/molars can cause necrosis of the underlying palatine mucosa and palatine bone.
  - Development of oronasal fistula
- Burrs embedded in the oral mucosa—may incite granulomatous reaction.
  - Focal: mass
  - Diffuse: across the whole surface of the tongue
- Linear foreign bodies caught around the base of the tongue can become embedded into the tongue.
  - Can be difficult to identify
  - Can cause a significant inflammatory/granulomatous reaction

DIAGNOSIS

DIFFERENTIAL DIAGNOSIS

- Oral mass:
  - Neoplasia
- Facial swelling:
  - Neoplasia
  - Salivary mucocele

INITIAL DATABASE

- Complete blood count:
  - Neutrophilia associated with inflammation or infection
- Fine-needle aspiration of facial swelling:
  - Cytology to determine etiology
  - Microbiologic culture and sensitivity testing:
    - Aerobic and anaerobic
- Ultrasound examination:
  - Exophthalmos
  - Facial swelling
    - Abscess versus neoplasia

ADVANCED OR CONFIRMATORY TESTING

- Histopathologic examination of oral mass
  - Foreign body granuloma versus neoplasia
- Computed tomography or magnetic resonance imaging: extent of abscess/granulomas

TREATMENT

THERAPEUTIC GOAL(S)

- Remove foreign body
- Resolve associated chronic inflammation/abscess/tissue destruction
- If linear foreign body:
  - Relieve gastrointestinal obstruction

ACUTE GENERAL TREATMENT

Following induction of general anesthesia:

- Oral examination:
  - Routine (foreign material may be found incidentally).
  - Because could not be performed in awake patient (e.g., fractious behavior, physical obstruction).
- Radiographs:
  - Radio-opaque foreign body.
  - Soft tissue swelling (abscess).
  - Destruction of underlying bone.
- Removal of foreign body from oral cavity:
  - Porcupine quills: grasp at base (nearest to skin) with forceps and extract with a gentle twisting motion.
  - Bone or stick: if tightly wedged, may be easier to remove by cutting (e.g., with Stryker saw) first.
  - Release linear foreign body caught around base of tongue.
- Burrs embedded in oral mucosa:
  - Surgical debridement to remove plant material and chronic granulomatous lesions.
    - Open wounds will rapidly be covered by proliferating mucosa.
- Surgical exploration, debridement, and lavage of abscess pocket(s):
  - Retrobulbar area explored through incision in oral mucosa just caudal to last upper molar tooth or through existing penetrating wound.
- Provide postoperative drainage until abscess has resolved:
  - Submandibular/intermandibular.

Antibiotic therapy for bacterial infection:

- Long-term therapy based on results of microbiologic culture and sensitivity tests
- Empiric therapy until results available:
  - Cefazolin 22 mg/kg IV q 6h, if animal receiving IV fluids and unable to take oral medications; or
  - Amoxicillin 10–20 mg/kg PO q 12h.

CHRONIC TREATMENT

- Antibiotic therapy (see Acute General Treatment above) until resolution of infection.
- If lesions or wounds that would prevent oral feeding are present in the oral cavity, it will be necessary to provide alternative route for nutrition and antibiotic administration.
  - Esophagostomy tube (see Feeding Tube Placement: Esophagostomy Tube, p 1243) or PEG tube (see Feeding Tube Placement: Percutaneous Endoscopic Gastrostomy [PEG], p 1247)
  - Reexamine oral cavity in 10 to 14 days:
    - If healed, patient can return to oral feeding and tube can be removed
- Reconstructive surgery of damage caused to oral cavity by foreign body:
  - Oronasal fistula

POSSIBLE COMPLICATIONS

- Failure to remove foreign body:
  - Persistent/recurrent abscess
  - Development of draining tract
- Development of late-onset tissue necrosis:
  - Osteomyelitis
  - Oronasal fistula

RECOMMENDED MONITORING

- Repeat visits to veterinarian as necessary.
  - To ensure oral lesions or wounds heal.
  - To ensure that abscess has resolved.
    - Drain removal
  - To remove feeding tube once oral problems have healed.
- Observe for recurrence of abscess and development of draining tract.

PROGNOSIS AND OUTCOME

- Usually good, provided that:
  - All foreign material removed
  - Abscess pockets adequately drained
- Recurrent problems likely to occur, or chronic draining tract develop, if:
  - Failure to remove all foreign material:
    - Porcupine quills
  - Late-onset tissue necrosis develops:
    - Oronasal fistula
    - Osteomyelitis

PEARLS & CONSIDERATIONS

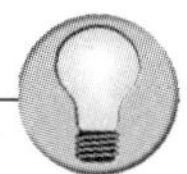

COMMENTS

In situations where multiple foreign bodies are present in the oral cavity (porcupine quills, burrs), it is essential to ensure that a thorough examination is performed, extending throughout the entire pharynx, to ensure that all foreign material is removed.

PREVENTION

Avoid situations that could lead to foreign bodies injuring or becoming lodged in the oral cavity

CLIENT EDUCATION

- Do not let animals play with or chew on objects such as sticks that could cause penetrating oral injuries, or linear objects (fishing line, yarn, etc.) that could act as linear foreign bodies.
- Do not let dogs interact with porcupines.

SUGGESTED READING

Harvey CE: In *Veterinary Dentistry*. Philadelphia, WB Saunders, 1985, p 186.

AUTHOR & EDITOR: **RICHARD WALSHAW**

Foreign Body, Respiratory Tract

BASIC INFORMATION

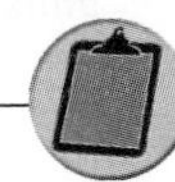

DEFINITION

Inhaled, penetrating, or migrating objects that cause obstruction or inflammation of the respiratory tract

SYNONYM(S)

Migrating foreign body
Nasal foreign body
Tracheal/bronchial foreign body

EPIDEMIOLOGY

SPECIES, AGE, SEX: Dogs and cats can be affected. May be more prevalent in young or active animals.

GENETICS AND BREED PREDISPOSITION

- Pyothorax secondary to aspiration of grass awn is most common in medium to large hunting/sporting dogs.
- Small dogs are more prone to bone foreign body in the nasopharynx.

GEOGRAPHY AND SEASONALITY: May be more common in hunting season or in areas with oat/cereal fields or grass awns ("foxtails").

ASSOCIATED CONDITIONS AND DISORDERS

- Aspergillosis or bacterial rhinitis with chronic intranasal foreign body
- Focal tracheal stenosis with chronic intratracheal foreign body (granuloma)
- Lobar pneumonia with a foreign body in a bronchus
- Bronchoesophageal fistula with penetration of esophageal foreign body through bronchus
- Pyothorax with thoracic migration of foreign body into or through pleural space

CLINICAL PRESENTATION

DISEASE FORMS/SUBTYPES

- Rhinitis
- Tracheitis or tracheobronchial obstruction
- Pyothorax (empyema)

HISTORY, CHIEF COMPLAINT

- Nasal foreign body:
  - Acute onset of sneezing
  - Pawing at face
  - Discomfort
  - Unilateral serosanguineous nasal discharge progressing to mucopurulent nasal discharge
- Nasopharyngeal foreign body:
  - Stridor
  - Sneezing
  - Halitosis possible with chronicity
- Tracheal/bronchial foreign body:
  - Acute onset of coughing, dyspnea
  - Halitosis
  - Hemoptysis
  - Retching/vomiting may occur
  - Exercise intolerance or cyanosis if severe obstruction
  - Temporary response to antibiotics in chronic cases
- Intrathoracic foreign body:
  - Anorexia
  - Lethargy
  - Weight loss
  - Fever
  - Increased respiratory effort
  - Poor performance

PHYSICAL EXAM FINDINGS

- Nasal foreign body:
  - Decreased air movement through one nostril. Assessment:
    - By differentially occluding each nostril one at a time and either listening closely for air flow, or watching for movement of an object held in the expected path of air flow (wisp of cotton ball, or of the pet's hair)
    - By holding a glass microscope slide in front of the nostrils and observing for fogging of the glass
  - Nasal discharge: either unilateral or bilateral
  - Possibly ocular discharge
- Nasopharyngeal foreign body:
  - Stertor
  - Halitosis
  - Reverse sneezing
- Tracheal/bronchial foreign body:
  - Cough
  - Dyspnea, which can be inspiratory and expiratory and worsens with degree of obstruction
  - Stridor
  - High frequency wheezes with partial obstruction
  - Cyanosis
  - Collapse
  - Acute death with complete obstruction is possible
- Intrathoracic foreign body (signs reflect pyothorax most often—see Pyothorax, p 935):
  - Fever
  - Increased inspiratory effort
  - Muffled heart sounds
  - Respiratory sounds muffled ventrally on thoracic auscultation
  - Pleural fluid line on percussion
  - Thorax may be noncompressible in cats with pyothorax

ETIOLOGY AND PATHOPHYSIOLOGY

- Nasopharyngeal foreign body is usually bone in dogs.
- Inhalation most common path of entry for nasal, tracheal, bronchial, thoracic foreign bodies.
  - Grass awns (cereal ears) and other plant material most common foreign objects
  - Plant material aspirated into lungs may migrate into pleural space (see Pyothorax, p 935; Pneumothorax, p 866)
- Sharp esophageal or gastric foreign bodies may migrate into lungs or pleural space.
- Local inflammatory reaction and contamination may result in secondary bacterial or fungal infection.

DIAGNOSIS

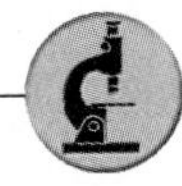

DIFFERENTIAL DIAGNOSIS

- Nasal foreign body:
  - Neoplasia
  - Aspergillosis
  - Lymphocytic-plasmacytic rhinitis
  - Nasal mites
  - Bacterial rhinitis
  - Dental disease
- Nasopharyngeal foreign body:
  - Polyp
  - Granuloma
  - Neoplasia
  - Rhinitis
- Tracheal/bronchial foreign body:
  - Laryngeal paralysis
  - Tracheal collapse
  - Elongated soft palate
  - Trauma
  - Neoplasia
  - Infection
- Lung or intrapleural foreign body:
  - Bronchopneumonia
  - Pyothorax from trauma or systemic disease
  - Neoplasia

INITIAL DATABASE

- Complete blood count.
  - Neutrophilic leukocytosis, possibly with left shift; with pyothorax, secondary bronchopneumonia, or severe secondary rhinitis.
  - Eosinophilia with tracheobronchial grass awns.
- Serum biochemistry profile and urinalysis often unremarkable with nasal, nasopharyngeal, or airway foreign bodies.
  - With pyothorax from pleural foreign bodies, hypoalbuminemia, hypoglycemia, or proteinuria may be seen.

- Radiographs: findings other than radiopaque foreign body may include:
  - Nasal foreign body:
    - Increased intranasal soft tissue opacity.
    - Local bone destruction with chronic disease.
  - Tracheal foreign body:
    - Increased airway soft tissue/fluid opacity on cervical or thoracic films.
  - Bronchial foreign body:
    - Ill-defined peribronchial radiopacity.
  - Lung or bronchial foreign body:
    - Lung consolidation with secondary bronchopneumonia.
  - Intrapleural foreign body:
    - Pleural effusion.
    - Collapsed lung lobes.
    - Spontaneous pneumothorax may occur with penetrating or migrating thoracic foreign bodies (see Pneumothorax, p 866; Pyothorax, p 935).
- Cytologic evaluation/culture of nasal cavity to identify organisms associated with secondary rhinitis.
- Neutrophilia on transtracheal wash cytologic study with tracheobronchial foreign body.
- Pyothorax: inflammatory exudates (degenerate neutrophils ± bacteria) on cytologic study of pleural fluid obtained by thoracocentesis. Macrophages and plasma cells increase with chronicity.
  - Common organisms cultured from pyothorax: obligate anaerobes (*Fusobacterium*), *Nocardia asteroides*, *Actinomyces* in dogs; anaerobes, *Pasteurella multocida* in cats.

ADVANCED OR CONFIRMATORY TESTING

- Nasopharyngeal foreign bodies may be visible with soft palate retraction during oropharyngeal exam with patient under anesthesia.
- Endoscopy is generally diagnostic for tracheal foreign bodies and some bronchial foreign bodies (may be obscured by mucopurulent exudates).
- Intranasal foreign bodies may be visible with anterior rigid scope or posterior flexible scope, although nasal discharge may obscure view.
  - Nasal flushing (see p 1283) removes discharge to improve visualization.
- Computed tomography of nasal cavity: mucosal thickening, focal bone thickening and destruction; may not differentiate foreign body rhinitis from nasal aspergillosis.
- Contrast rhinography or bronchography may outline radiolucent foreign body.

TREATMENT

THERAPEUTIC GOAL(S)

- Resolve dyspnea or airway obstruction
- Treat secondary infection

ACUTE GENERAL TREATMENT

- Oxygen supplementation (see p 1292).
- Sedation if extremely stressed (i.e., such that the anxiety is contributing to dyspnea) (acepromazine 0.1–0.5 mg total dose IM or IV if young and not systemically ill; butorphanol 0.2–0.4 mg/kg IV may be given additionally q 2–4h as needed).
- Rehydrate as needed.
- Thoracocentesis if respiratory compromise from pyothorax.
- Immediate anesthesia and foreign body removal if trachea completely obstructed.
  - Tracheostomy (see p 1310) may be needed for short-term airway management.
- If possible, nonsurgical removal of nasal, laryngeal, tracheal, and some bronchial foreign bodies.
  - Foreign bodies often removed endoscopically with forceps, basket retrievers. Suctioning and flushing (using very small volumes of infused saline to remove mucus) improve visualization and may remove small pieces.
  - Some tracheal foreign bodies removed with vacuum suction or passage of balloon (Fogarty) catheter beyond foreign body and then inflation and retraction of balloon.
- Rhinotomy (dorsal or ventral), tracheotomy, bronchotomy, or lung lobectomy for nonretrievable intraluminal foreign bodies.
  - Lobectomy if lung lobe consolidation. Histopathologic evaluation and culture (aerobic and anaerobic) of excised tissue.
  - Anesthetic/oxygen delivery via contralateral bronchus intubation recommended for unilateral bronchotomy. Total IV anesthesia with endotracheal or endobronchial oxygen delivery if gas leakage expected.
- Lung lobectomy if bronchopneumonia secondary to foreign body or bronchoesophageal fistula.
- Bilateral thoracostomy tubes, or thoracotomy (median sternotomy for generalized disease), and thoracic lavage/drainage for pyothorax.
  - Lavage through large diameter chest tubes with sterile, warm isotonic fluids (20 ml/kg) 2 to 4 times/day for 5 to 7 days.
  - Surgical exploration if intrathoracic mass, consolidated lung lobe, pneumothorax, or no improvement.
- For pyothorax or bronchopneumonia, broad-spectrum antibiotics.

CHRONIC TREATMENT

- Antibiotic therapy for secondary infections, based on culture/sensitivity.
  - Ampicillin or amoxicillin plus clavulanic acid 12.5–20 mg/kg PO q 12h for obligate anaerobes, *Pasteurella* spp., *Actinomyces* spp.
  - Trimethoprim sulfa 10–15 mg/kg PO q 12h (possibly higher, but may increase risk of adverse effects) or amikacin for *Nocardia* spp.
  - For pyothorax, antibiotics are administered for 1 to 2 months.
- Bronchodilators (e.g., aminophylline 10 mg/kg PO q 8h) for 3 to 5 days after endoscopic removal of bronchial foreign bodies.

POSSIBLE COMPLICATIONS

- Inability to oxygenate during endoscopy or surgery
- Increased severity of obstruction with flushing, foreign body manipulation, or endoscopic trauma (mucosal swelling)
- Pulmonary abscess or recurrent pyothorax if migrating foreign body remains or inappropriate antibiotic therapy used
- Chronic rhinitis possible if turbinates are removed during rhinotomy

RECOMMENDED MONITORING

- Tracheal/bronchial/lung/thoracic foreign bodies: Repeat radiographs or endoscopy if clinical signs recur.
- Pyothorax or pneumonia: Repeat radiographs 1 week after discontinuing antibiotics or if clinical signs recur.

PROGNOSIS AND OUTCOME

- Outcome excellent if patient survives foreign body extraction and secondary infections are treated appropriately.
  - Bronchopulmonary abscess develops with foreign body migration if tracheobronchial grass awn present for more than 2 weeks.
- Complication and mortality rates higher with chronicity.
- Tracheobronchial plant material can fragment, requiring multiple endoscopic episodes for complete removal.

PEARLS & CONSIDERATIONS

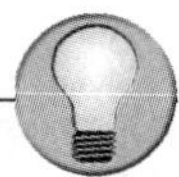

COMMENTS

- Some nasal foreign bodies can be removed with vigorous flushing (see Nasal Flush, p 1283). Make sure endotracheal cuff is properly inflated.
- Right bronchial system more likely to be affected by inhaled bronchial foreign body because of direct tracheobronchial path.
- Grass awns usually migrate to multiple sites, including pericardial sac, in dogs with pyothorax.
- If sulfur granules or branching filamentous gram-positive rods (suspicion of *Actinomyces* infection) are seen during

cytologic examination of the pleural fluid, consider long-term treatment (4 to 6 weeks) with antibiotics.

CLIENT EDUCATION

- Acute onset of coughing in high performance sporting dogs during hunting or harvest season may indicate tracheobronchial foreign body.
- Provide indestructible bones and toys that are appropriately sized for the dog.

SUGGESTED READING

Lotti U, Niebauer GW: Tracheobronchial foreign bodies of plant origin in 153 hunting dogs. *Compend Contin Educ Pract Vet* 14:900–904, 1992.

Saunders JH, et al: Diagnostic value of computed tomography in dogs with chronic nasal disease. *Vet Radiol Ultrasound* 44:409–413, 2003.

Scott JA, Macintire DK: Canine pyothorax: clinical presentation, diagnosis, and treatment. *Compend Contin Educ Pract Vet* 25:180, 2003.

AUTHOR: **KAREN M. TOBIAS**
EDITOR: **RANCE K. SELLON**

Fracture Disease

BASIC INFORMATION

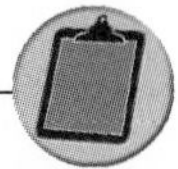

DEFINITION

Fracture disease includes muscle contracture, implant failure, inadequate bone union, and joint disease. These result in abnormal limb function (Fig. I-76).

SYNONYM(S)

Fracture complications

EPIDEMIOLOGY

SPECIES, AGE, SEX: Muscle contracture is most common in young dogs with distal femoral or humeral fractures.

RISK FACTORS
- Limb trauma
- Poor surgical technique

ASSOCIATED CONDITIONS AND DISORDERS: Trauma to other body systems.

CLINICAL PRESENTATION

DISEASE FORMS/SUBTYPES: Quadriceps contracture, joint ankylosis.

HISTORY, CHIEF COMPLAINT: Lack of normal limb function after fracture repair.

PHYSICAL EXAM FINDINGS: Lameness, disuse atrophy of skeletal muscle, decreased range of motion of affected joint(s), draining tracts, nonhealing surgery site.

ETIOLOGY AND PATHOPHYSIOLOGY

- Severe soft tissue damage from injury/surgery and subsequent fibrosis
- Incongruent articular cartilage after joint fracture repair
- Inadequate postoperative rehabilitation to enhance limb function
- Nerve injury preventing use of limb
- Inappropriate use of implants during repair
- Excessive or unrestricted patient activity after surgery

DIAGNOSIS

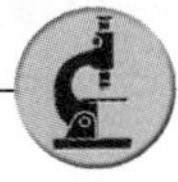

DIFFERENTIAL DIAGNOSIS

- Bone neoplasia
- Joint luxation
- Osteomyelitis
- Joint infection

INITIAL DATABASE

- Orthopedic and neurologic exams to evaluate limb function
- Orthogonal view radiography of affected bone(s)
- Complete blood count, chemistry panel, urinanalysis, electrocardiogram based on patient American Society of Anesthesiologists classification (see p 1334)

ADVANCED OR CONFIRMATORY TESTING

- Muscle biopsy
- Electromyography
- Nerve conduction studies

TREATMENT

THERAPEUTIC GOAL(S)

Restoration of limb function(s)

ACUTE GENERAL TREATMENT

- Accurate joint reconstruction
- Adequate alignment and stable fixation of long bone fracture(s)
- Gentle, aseptic surgical technique; avoidance of excessive soft tissue dissection
- Initiation of physical therapy immediately after fracture repair
- Use of analgesics to alleviate patient discomfort and enhance movement

CHRONIC TREATMENT

- Replacement of failed implants and restabilization of fracture(s)
- Resection of scar tissue to regain joint range of motion
- Intensive postoperative rehabilitation (see Physical Rehabilitation, p 1300)

POSSIBLE COMPLICATIONS

Limb dysfunction: muscle atrophy, tissue fibrosis, degenerative joint disease

RECOMMENDED MONITORING

- Physical therapy immediately after fracture repair to maintain joint(s) range of motion
- Serial radiography to evaluate bone healing
- Serial physical examinations to evaluate limb function

PROGNOSIS AND OUTCOME

- Poor if joint ankylosis or muscle contracture occurs.
- Poor if irreversible nerve damage.
- Joint fusion or limb amputation may be required in failed cases.

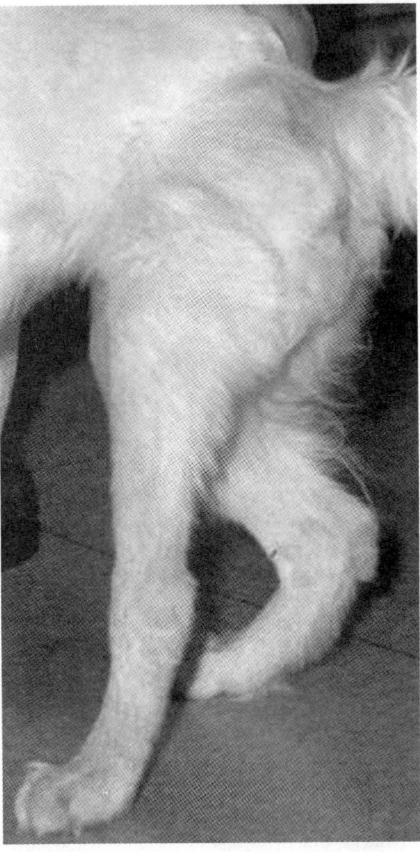

FIGURE I-76 A 1-year-old, mixed-breed dog with quadriceps contracture after distal femoral fracture repair and no physical therapy to retain stifle joint range of motion. Note hyperextension of limb.

PEARLS & CONSIDERATIONS

COMMENTS

- Prevention is essential and easier than therapy.
- Avoid external splintage for humeral and femoral fractures.
- Consider case referral to an orthopedic specialist.

PREVENTION

- Proper implant usage and fracture fixation allowing postoperative ambulation.
- Anatomic joint surface reconstruction is a key goal.
- Avoid reliance on external coaptation to stabilize fractures.
- Use postoperative physical therapy to maintain limb function.

CLIENT EDUCATION

- Patients must be controlled after fracture fixation to prevent loss of implants' stability.
- Physical therapy is necessary after surgery.
- Frequent recheck examinations are required to assess limb function and bone healing.

SUGGESTED READING

Hulse DA, Hohnson AL: Fundamentals of orthopaedic surgery and fracture management. In Fossum TW (ed): *Small Animal Surgery*, ed 2. St. Louis, Mosby, 2002, pp 821–900.

Montgomery R, Fitch R: Muscle and tendon disorders. In Slatter D (ed): *Textbook of Small Animal Surgery*, ed 3. Philadelphia, WB Saunders, 2003, pp 2266–2267.

AUTHOR: **JAMES D. LINCOLN**
EDITOR: **JOSEPH HARARI**

Fractures of the Femur

BASIC INFORMATION

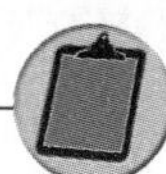

DEFINITION

Fractures of the femur may be classified as proximal (physis, femoral head or neck, trochanter), midshaft (diaphyseal), or distal (supracondylar, condylar)

SYNONYM(S)

Capital (head) physeal fracture: "slipped" capital epiphysis or physis

EPIDEMIOLOGY

RISK FACTORS: Trauma to the caudal trunk or hind limbs.

CLINICAL PRESENTATION

HISTORY, CHIEF COMPLAINT

- Trauma to the caudal trunk/limb:
  - Motor vehicle accident
  - High-velocity impact
  - Falls
- Femoral capital physeal fractures in cats may occur without a history of trauma

PHYSICAL EXAM FINDINGS

- Lameness
- Swelling, bruising, or shortening of limb
- Crepitation/pain at hip/stifle joint
- Loss of sensation to medial (femoral nerve) or lateral (sciatic nerve) digits

ETIOLOGY AND PATHOPHYSIOLOGY

- Most common (45%) long-bone fracture
- Concurrent injuries to abdominal wall or organs, pelvis, and lumbar spine are common
- Capital physeal fracture (immature animals) disrupts ascending vessels and compromises healing
- Extensive hemorrhage with midshaft fractures contributes to shock

DIAGNOSIS

DIFFERENTIAL DIAGNOSIS

- Coxofemoral luxation
- Acetabular/pelvic fracture
- Spinal trauma
- Neoplasia (pathologic fracture)

INITIAL DATABASE

- Craniocaudal and lateral radiographs of affected hind limb and pelvis ± lumbar spine
- Abdominal and thoracic radiographs if whole-body trauma
- Complete blood count/serum biochemistry panel dictated by systemic signs and patient stability
- Evaluation of medial/lateral sensations of digits
- Comprehensive neurologic exam

ADVANCED OR CONFIRMATORY TESTING

Biopsy if pathologic fracture suspected

TREATMENT

THERAPEUTIC GOAL(S)

- Restoration of limb function and alignment
- Reconstruction if articular surface involved

ACUTE GENERAL TREATMENT

- External coaptation (casts, splints, etc.) is usually ineffective and carries a high likelihood of inducing complications.
- Fractures involving the joint space require accurate joint reconstruction.
- Midshaft fractures are stabilized with bone plate/screws, external fixator, interlocking nail, intramedullary pins/cerclage, or plate/rod.
- Condylar fractures are repaired with lag screws, pins.
- Trochanteric fractures are repaired with pin and tension-band wiring or lag screws to counteract pull of gluteal muscles.
- Femoral neck fractures are repaired with multiple small pins, lag screw(s).
- Femoral head/neck ostectomy can be performed for neck and capital physeal fractures in cats and small dogs.

CHRONIC TREATMENT

- Restricted activity until radiographs at 4 to 6 weeks to assess healing
- Radiograph early for suspected complications
- Femoral head/neck resection for failed proximal repairs

POSSIBLE COMPLICATIONS

- Malunion, nonunion (inadequate fixation)
- Degenerative joint disease (articular fractures)
- Sciatic nerve damage (retrograde intramedullary pin placement)
- Decreased hip motion with femoral head ostectomy
- Implant failure
- Infection
- Quadriceps contracture and inability to flex the stifle (young dogs with midshaft and distal femoral fractures)
- Limb shortening

RECOMMENDED MONITORING

- Lameness evaluation every 4 weeks for 2 to 3 months
- Evaluate distal fractures 2 weeks postrepair to assess stifle mobility

- Radiography every 4 to 6 weeks to evaluate fracture healing and implant stability

PROGNOSIS AND OUTCOME

- Based on severity of injury and presence or absence of complications (nerve damage, infection, etc.).
- Associated neuropraxia (temporary nerve damage): may need 2 to 12 weeks to assess for functional recovery.
- Good to excellent for nonarticular lesions treated with appropriate surgical intervention.
- Quadriceps contracture requires physical therapy or surgical intervention.

PEARLS & CONSIDERATIONS

COMMENTS

- Additional orthopedic injuries of the same or other limbs are common.
- Initial proprioceptive deficits of the affected limb can be due to pain, shock, and fracture edema, and not a spinal injury.

SUGGESTED READING

Simpson DJ, Lewis DD: Fractures of the femur. In Slatter D (ed): *Textbook of Small Animal Surgery*, ed 3. Philadelphia, WB Saunders, 2003, pp 2059–2086.

AUTHOR: **MARY E. SOMERVILLE**
EDITOR: **JOSEPH HARARI**

Fractures of the Humerus

BASIC INFORMATION

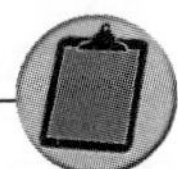

DEFINITION

Humeral fractures involve the proximal physis, greater tubercle, metaphysis, diaphysis, supracondylar region, or condyle.

EPIDEMIOLOGY

GENETICS AND BREED PREDISPOSITION: Spaniel breeds have a higher incidence of condylar fractures.
RISK FACTORS
- Forelimb trauma from gunshot injuries, falls, or motor vehicle accidents
- Focal bone lesions (e.g., osteosarcoma or other bone neoplasm) or diffuse bone disease (e.g., nutritional, metabolic, or inherited) in cases of pathologic fractures

CLINICAL PRESENTATION

HISTORY, CHIEF COMPLAINT: Severe trauma to the forelimb.
PHYSICAL EXAM FINDINGS: Non-weight-bearing lameness with swelling, pain, instability of the humerus.

ETIOLOGY AND PATHOPHYSIOLOGY

- Thoracic wall, cardiopulmonary, and brachial plexus injuries may be present.
- Most fractures involve the middle or distal third segments.
- Condylar fractures involve the lateral portion more frequently than the medial; can be due to incomplete ossification in young dogs.
- Humeral fractures not caused by severe trauma may be pathologic fractures; these fractures are difficult to treat and may heal very slowly or not at all.

DIAGNOSIS

DIFFERENTIAL DIAGNOSIS

- Brachial plexus injury
- Pathologic fractures secondary to neoplasia
- Elbow or shoulder luxation
- Cervical spinal cord disease (disk herniation, tumor, etc.)

INITIAL DATABASE

- Complete blood count and chemistry panel based on American Society of Anesthesiologists patient classification (see p 1334)
- Mediolateral and craniocaudal radiographs of the bone
- Electrocardiogram and thoracic radiography
- Establish presence of deep pain perception and voluntary motor function in the limb

TREATMENT

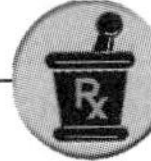

THERAPEUTIC GOAL(S)

- Fracture stabilization
- Elbow joint congruency

ACUTE GENERAL TREATMENT

- Minimally displaced fractures in young animals that do not involve a joint space may be treated with external coaptation such as a spica splint.
- Most humeral fractures require surgical treatment with open reduction and internal/external fixations:
    - Physeal and metaphyseal fractures require stabilization with divergent pins.
    - Fractures of the greater tubercle require tension band wiring.
    - Diaphyseal fractures require stabilization with a plate/screws, plate/rod, interlocking nail or external fixation.
    - Supracondylar fractures require stabilization with cross-pinning, plate/screws, or plate/rod fixation.
    - Condylar fractures require stabilization with a lag screw and an antirotational Kirschner wire or small pin.

CHRONIC TREATMENT

- A carpal flexion bandage may be placed to prevent weight-bearing for the first 2 to 3 weeks.
- A spica bandage can also be used for limiting postoperative forelimb motion.
- Exercise restriction until radiographs confirm good fracture healing.
- Elbow range of motion exercises multiple times daily maintain joint mobility.

POSSIBLE COMPLICATIONS

- Iatrogenic damage to the radial nerve with mid-diaphyseal fracture repair
- Degenerative joint disease with condylar fractures
- Infection
- Implant failure

RECOMMENDED MONITORING

- Suture removal and examination at 2 postoperative weeks
- Physical and radiographic examinations at 4 to 6 and 8 to 10 postoperative weeks to evaluate limb functions and bone healing

PROGNOSIS AND OUTCOME

- Good to excellent with proper bone realignment, joint congruency, healing, and rehabilitation, along with minimal trauma occurring to soft tissue structures (nerves, vessels, muscles)

- Guarded to poor with pathologic humeral fractures; healing is delayed or clinically nonexistent, pain often persists, and surgical repair is difficult or contraindicated (leading to amputation or euthanasia)

PEARLS & CONSIDERATIONS

COMMENTS

- Because cardiopulmonary injury may be present, patients should be stabilized before surgery/anesthesia.
- Intraoperatively, an osteotomy of the olecranon will improve visualization/reduction of a supracondylar or bicondylar fracture.
- Condylar fractures are difficult to identify on a single (lateral) radiographic projection.
- A disproportionately mild degree of trauma as a cause for humeral fracture should prompt the suspicion of a pathologic fracture and underlying bone disease.

SUGGESTED READING

Piermattei DL, Flo GL: Fractures of the humerus. In *Brinker, Piermattei, and Flo's Handbook of Small Animal Orthopedics and Fracture Repair*, ed 3. Philadelphia, WB Saunders, 1997, pp 261–287.

Tomlinson JL: Fractures of the humerus. In Slatter D (ed): *Textbook of Small Animal Surgery*, ed 3. Philadelphia, WB Saunders, 2002, pp 1905–1918.

AUTHOR: **RAVIV J. BALFOUR**
EDITOR: **JOSEPH HARARI**

Fractures of the Mandible and Maxilla

BASIC INFORMATION

DEFINITION

- Mandibular fractures can involve either the horizontal body, or vertical ramus of the mandible; separation of the mandibular symphysis also can occur. The *condyle* is the articular surface at the caudal-most aspect of the mandible.
- Maxillary fractures can involve the incisive, nasal, frontal, maxillary, palatine, zygomatic, or temporal bones.

SYNONYM(S)

Jaw fractures
Maxillofacial fracture(s)

EPIDEMIOLOGY

SPECIES, AGE, SEX

- Traumatic jaw fractures are more likely in younger animals. Pathologic jaw fractures are more likely in older animals.
- Mandibular fractures are more common than maxillary fractures.
- In dogs, areas near the mandibular canine and molar teeth are often involved.
- In cats, the region of the mandibular symphysis and the condylar process are often involved.

GENETICS AND BREED PREDISPOSITION: Mandibular fractures in dogs occur more often in smaller breeds.

RISK FACTORS

- Traumatic fracture: vehicular trauma, bites, kicks, hits, high-rise falls, gunshots, and secondary to tooth extraction
- Pathologic fracture: advanced periodontitis, neoplasia, metabolic disease

ASSOCIATED CONDITIONS AND DISORDERS: Dental trauma (tooth fracture and displacement injury), temporomandibular joint luxation, soft tissue injuries to structures of the head.

CLINICAL PRESENTATION

HISTORY, CHIEF COMPLAINT

- Head trauma
- Malocclusion noted by owner
- Recent dental procedure

PHYSICAL EXAM FINDINGS: Malocclusion, inability to close the mouth, swelling, bruising of face/oral cavity, tongue extrusion, nasal discharge, stertor, dysphagia, blood-tinged saliva, drooling, palpable or visible fracture line.

ETIOLOGY AND PATHOPHYSIOLOGY

- Symphyseal separation/perisymphyseal fracture: most common mandibular injury in cats.
- The most common sites for mandibular fracture in dogs are the areas near the last premolar (fourth premolar) and first and second molars, followed by the area just caudal to the canine tooth.
- Concurrent injuries to the head, thorax, or both are common and may require urgent treatment and delay surgical repair of maxillary/mandibular fractures.
- Surgical repair should avoid damage to mandibular canal, which contains the inferior alveolar nerve, artery, and vein.
- In small dogs, tooth roots often reach into the ventral mandibular cortex and leave little bone farther ventrally.
- Favorable versus unfavorable mandibular fractures:
  - Favorable mandibular fracture: oblique fracture line running in a rostroventral direction. Relatively stable: muscle forces hold fracture segments in apposition.
  - Unfavorable mandibular fracture: oblique fracture line running in a caudoventral direction. Unstable: muscle forces lead to displacement of fracture segments.

DIAGNOSIS

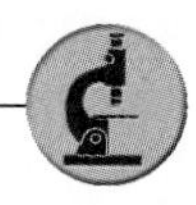

DIFFERENTIAL DIAGNOSIS

- Trigeminal neuritis/neuropathy (cranial nerve V)
- Temporomandibular joint luxation
- Primary dental/periodontal disease
- Neoplasia

INITIAL DATABASE

- Complete blood count/serum chemistry panel: generally unremarkable.
- Skull radiographs of stable, sedated patient can provide limited information.
- Open-mouth, oblique, lateral and ventrodorsal views, and intraoral dental radiographs are preferred, but general anesthesia is usually necessary.
- Thoracic/abdominal radiographs to delineate other traumatic lesions.
- Cranial nerve exam.

ADVANCED OR CONFIRMATORY TESTING

Computed tomography provides high resolution for maxillary and caudal mandibular fractures.

TREATMENT

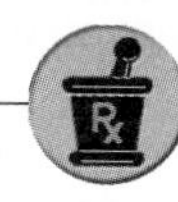

THERAPEUTIC GOAL(S)

- Provide analgesia (See Local Anesthesia and Regional Anesthesia, p 1274)
- Restore dental occlusion
- Restore oral functions

ACUTE GENERAL TREATMENT

- Teeth may need to be removed to allow occlusion or closure of soft-tissue defects.
- Mandible:
  - Body:

- Muzzle in stable or minimally displaced fracture. Muzzle should be flexible (nylon or tape) and be sufficiently snug to immobilize fracture while still allowing the patient to drink water and lick liquid food. Mandibular fractures in animals <6 to 12 months old usually do not require any treatment other than suturing of torn soft tissues and placing a tape muzzle for 2 to 3 weeks.
- Interdental wiring and intraoral acrylic or composite splint.
- Intraosseous/interfragmentary wiring (Figs. I-77–I-79).
- Circumferential wire for symphyseal separation/perisymphyseal fracture.
- Percutaneous external fixation.
- Bone plating.

◦ Ramus:
- Fractures rarely require any particular treatment beyond muzzling (snug tape muzzle, through which the patient can still drink). The muscle forces (temporal, masseter, and medial/lateral pterygoid muscles) hold the fracture segments in apposition.
- If the mandible is displaced, resulting in malocclusion, treatment is required and can include noninvasive techniques first (maxillomandibular fixation, such as fabrication of a composite bridge between maxillary and mandibular canine teeth) before placing intraosseous wiring or bone plates (See Figs. I-77–I-79).

◦ Condylar fractures may require condylectomy if there is progressive difficulty in opening mouth.

- Maxilla:
  - ◦ Interdental wiring and intraoral acrylic or composite splint, intraosseous wiring, bone plating.
  - ◦ Midline palatal separation: primary (surgical) closure if no tension; interarcade wiring with or without acrylic/composite splints if severe distraction.
- Incisive and maxillary bones: interfragmentary wires, acrylic splints/composites, bone plates.
- Adjunctive treatment: broad-spectrum antibiotic therapy (e.g., amoxicillin-clavulanate 13.75 mg/kg PO q 12h) for 1 to 2 weeks when encountering open fractures.

CHRONIC TREATMENT

- Teeth causing mild malocclusion can be filed or removed.
- Tape muzzles are removed in 2 to 6 weeks, bonding composites in 6 to 8 weeks.
- Partial mandibulectomy can be done for chronic nonunions.
- Oronasal fistulas may need secondary or delayed closure.
- Nutritional support during healing (blenderize food into liquid slurry, or place esophagostomy tube while patient is under general anesthesia).
- Adjunctive treatment: oral instillation of dilute chlorhexidine solution or gel for 2 to 4 weeks; brushing of teeth and intraoral splints.

POSSIBLE COMPLICATIONS

- Malocclusion
- Damage to dental structures
- Soft-tissue infection
- Osteomyelitis/sequestrum
- Implant failure
- Delayed union, nonunion
- Oronasal fistula
- Temporomandibular joint dysfunction
- Local pyoderma due to muzzle (transient)
- Malnutrition (very uncommon)

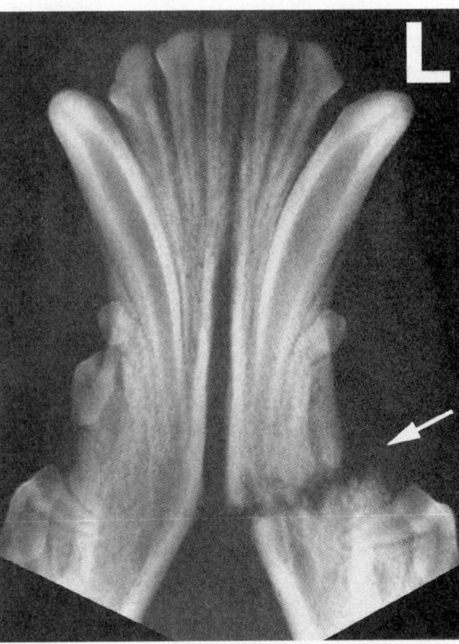

FIGURE I-77 An 8-month-old dog presented for evaluation and treatment of a left mandibular fracture between the first premolar and third premolar (*arrow*). The second premolar is missing. The radiograph is arranged in labial mounting; rostral is toward the top of the image, and the patient's left is on the right of the image. Courtesy of Dr. Alexander M. Reiter, University of Pennsylvania.

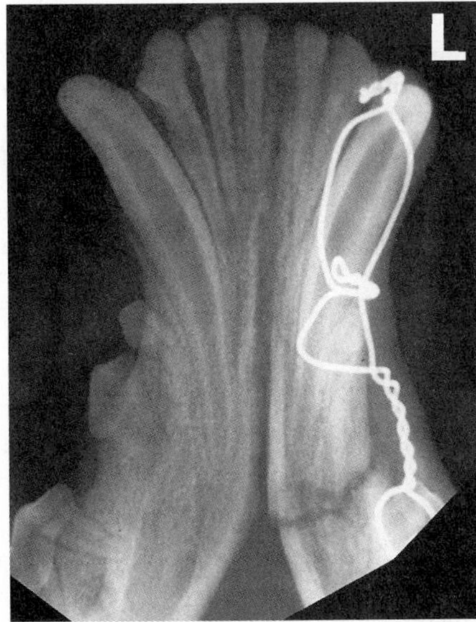

A

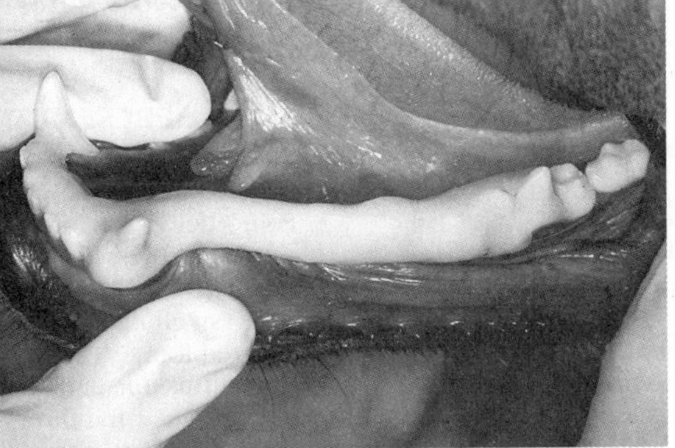

B

FIGURE I-78 **A,** Intraoperative radiograph of the same patient as in Fig. I-77. The fracture was first reduced with interdental wiring. **B,** Open-mouth view of the same patient; rostral is to the left. An intraoral splint was then fabricated covering the wire and tooth crowns. Courtesy of Dr. Alexander M. Reiter, University of Pennsylvania.

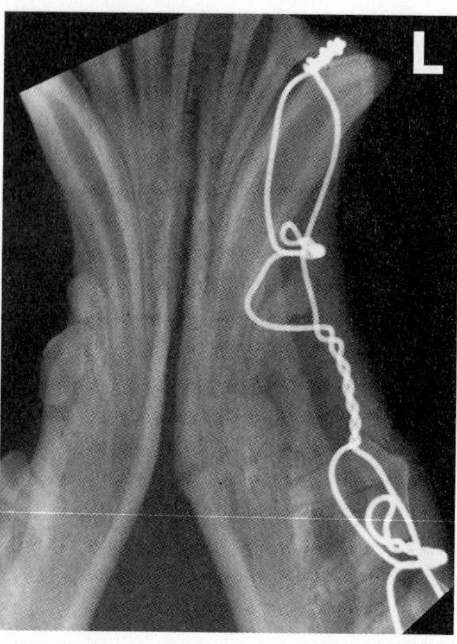

FIGURE I-79 A 5-week reexamination; the fracture site healed nicely; splint and wire were removed, and root canal therapy of the nonvital left mandibular canine tooth was performed (not shown). Courtesy of Dr. Alexander M. Reiter, University of Pennsylvania.

RECOMMENDED MONITORING

- Body weight (monitor adequate nutrition).
- Recheck at postoperative 2 weeks; remove skin sutures.
- Radiographs at 4 to 8 weeks to evaluate bone healing.
- Interdental wires, intraoral splints, and external fixators are removed after fracture healing. Bone implants may be left in place if soft tissue damage and osseous abnormalities are absent.
- Teeth in fracture lines require radiographic monitoring in 6 to 12 months to determine pulp vitality.

PROGNOSIS AND OUTCOME

- Good to excellent if proper occlusion is established.
- Fractures with tooth loss and severe periodontitis may heal slowly by fibrous union.

PEARLS & CONSIDERATIONS

COMMENTS

- Teeth in the fracture line should be preserved whenever possible, as they contribute to stability and alignment; should be removed if severely loose, fractured, or diseased.
- Administration of inhaled anesthetics via a pharyngostomy or temporary tracheostomy will aid with proper bone/teeth alignment during surgery.
- An esophageal feeding tube will reduce stress on repair(s), aid healing, and provide nutrition.
- Plates must have exact bone contour or malocclusion will result.
- Minimally displaced maxillary fractures and fractures of the mandibular ramus may not require surgery.
- The mandible is a curved and small bone, containing neurovascular structures in its mandibular canal. Thus, intramedullary pinning is inappropriate, as it does not provide rotational stability and causes damage to nerves and vessels that supply teeth and lips.

SUGGESTED READING

Davidson JR, Bauer MS: Fractures of the mandible and maxilla. *Vet Clin North Am Small Anim Pract* 22:109, 1992.

Verstraete F: Maxillofacial fractures. In Slatter D (ed): *Textbook of Small Animal Surgery*, ed 3. Philadelphia, WB Saunders, 2003, pp 2190–2207.

AUTHORS: **MARY E. SOMERVILLE, ALEXANDER M. REITER**

EDITORS: **JOSEPH HARARI, ALEXANDER M. REITER**

Fractures of the Metacarpus and Metatarsus

BASIC INFORMATION

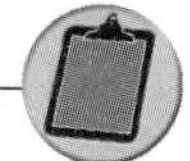

DEFINITION

Metacarpal and metatarsal fractures involve the proximal base, body, or distal head of the metacarpal or metatarsal bone.

SYNONYM(S)

Fracture of the paw

EPIDEMIOLOGY

SPECIES, AGE, SEX

- Young, athletic dogs are at increased risk
- Male racing dogs have a greater incidence of injury (increased muscle mass and late growth plate closure)

RISK FACTORS

- Direct trauma.
- Repetitive stress from racing (greyhounds) in a counterclockwise direction causing fatigue fractures of the right medial and left lateral metacarpal bones. Poor training and nutritional deficiencies increase the risk and severity of these fractures.

ASSOCIATED CONDITIONS AND DISORDERS: Carpal hyperextension (concurrent damage to the carpometacarpal ligaments).

CLINICAL PRESENTATION

HISTORY, CHIEF COMPLAINT

- Acute lameness
- Poor racing performance and subsequent lameness

PHYSICAL EXAM FINDINGS

- Pain, swelling, and crepitus of the affected foot
- Joint effusion, palpable dorsally, with intra-articular fractures
- Valgus (lateral) or varus (medial) displacement if the fracture involves the collateral ligament insertion on metacarpus (MC)/metatarsus (MT) II or V

ETIOLOGY AND PATHOPHYSIOLOGY

- Fractures usually involve the weight-bearing bones (MC/MT III, IV).
- These fractures account for approximately 5% of all long bone fractures. In the front leg, MC II and IV are most frequently affected; in the rear leg, MT III is most often involved.

DIAGNOSIS

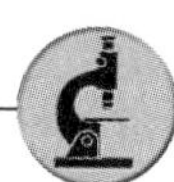

DIFFERENTIAL DIAGNOSIS

- Joint luxation
- Sesamoid bone fracture
- Cellulitis, stress periostitis, or foreign body

INITIAL DATABASE

- Lateral and craniocaudal radiographs
- Stress radiographs of the carpus and digits, if an intra-articular fracture or collateral ligament damage is suspected

- Complete blood count, serum biochemistry panel, and urinalysis based on the American Society of Anesthesiologists (see p 1334) patient classification

ADVANCED OR CONFIRMATORY TESTING

Thermography or bone scintigraphy for stress fractures or suspected lesions not identified with radiography

TREATMENT

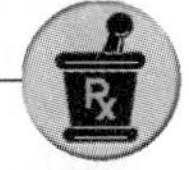

THERAPEUTIC GOAL(S)

Fracture stabilization for bone healing and early return to normal ambulation, and to minimize degenerative joint disease

ACUTE GENERAL TREATMENT

- A cast or molded splint is recommended for:
  - Nondisplaced proximal fractures.
  - Incomplete stress fractures in greyhounds.
  - Simple shaft fractures involving one or two bones, provided one of the central weight-bearing bones (III or IV) is intact.
- Surgical repair (internal fixation) is recommended for:
  - Displaced proximal fractures; lag screw or tension band wire fixation.
  - Simple shaft fractures involving two or more metacarpals/metatarsals. Long oblique fractures are stabilized with lag screw or cerclage wire. If all four bones are fractured, small intramedullary pins or K wires are used for providing axial alignment.
  - Comminuted or severly displaced large shaft fractures are treated with a 1.5- to 2.5-mm bone plate.
  - Distal intra-articular fractures with instability of the metacarpophalangeal or metatarsophalangeal joint are treated with a lag screw or interfragmentary wire.
- Other indications for internal fixation included nonunions, malunions, and simple fractures in large breed, working dogs.

CHRONIC TREATMENT

Most metacarpal and metatarsal fracture repairs are supported postoperatively with a molded splint or cast for 4 weeks. Exercise restriction is maintained for another 4 weeks.

- If a cast or splint is the primary method of fixation, it is removed after clinical union (6 weeks in young animals, longer in older patients). Exercise restriction is maintained for another 3 to 4 weeks.

POSSIBLE COMPLICATIONS

- Healing may be delayed in unstable or highly comminuted fractures.
- Poor fracture alignment, inadequate fixation, and premature implant failure may result in a malunion or nonunion.
- Intra-articular fractures or incorrect pin placement can damage the articular cartilage and interfere with joint motion, resulting in degenerative joint disease and chronic lameness.

RECOMMENDED MONITORING

Periodic physical and radiographic examinations until healing achieved

PROGNOSIS AND OUTCOME

- Good for simple fractures with adequate reduction and fixation
- Guarded for articular, highly displaced, or comminuted fractures

PEARLS & CONSIDERATIONS

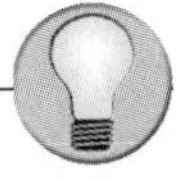

COMMENTS

- Implants are removed if causing a clinical problem after healing.
- External splints require diligent monitoring to prevent iatrogenic skin injury.

SUGGESTED READING

Boemo C: Injuries of the metacarpus and metatarsus. In Bloomberg MS, Dee JF, Taylor RA (eds): *Canine Sports Medicine and Surgery*. Philadelphia, WB Saunders, 1998, pp 150-164.

Brinker WO, Piermattei DL, Flo GL: Fractures of the carpus, metacarpus, and phalanges. In Brinker WO, Piermattei DL, Flo GL (eds): *Handbook of Small Animal Orthopedics and Fracture Treatment*, ed 3. Philadelphia, WB Saunders, 1997, pp 344-394, 607-658.

AUTHOR: **ELIZABETH J. LAING**

EDITOR: **JOSEPH HARARI**

Fractures of the Pelvis

BASIC INFORMATION

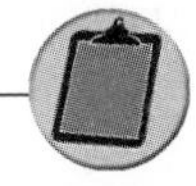

DEFINITION

Pelvic fractures include ilial, ischial, pubic and acetabular fractures; sacroiliac luxation and sacral fractures are also often included.

EPIDEMIOLOGY

Active, outdoor, sexually intact, roaming animals are most likely to be injured by motor vehicles.

RISK FACTORS

- Motor vehicle trauma and falling injuries (e.g., high-rise apartment buildings)
- Also can occur in racing dogs (greyhounds) as a spontaneous acetabular fracture

ASSOCIATED CONDITIONS AND DISORDERS: Multisystemic polytrauma, especially urologic.

CLINICAL PRESENTATION

DISEASE FORMS/SUBTYPES

- Blunt force trauma in pets
- Racing injury (acetabular fracture) in greyhounds

HISTORY, CHIEF COMPLAINT: Severe hind limb trauma from motor vehicle accident or fall.

PHYSICAL EXAM FINDINGS

- Lameness in one or both pelvic limbs, nonambulatory patient
- Palpable crepitus and/or pain on manipulation of leg(s)
- Palpable deformity of the pelvic canal during rectal examination

ETIOLOGY AND PATHOPHYSIOLOGY

- Very common sequela to blunt force trauma.
- Normal boxlike pelvic structure accounts for frequency of injuries affecting two or more sites in the pelvis.
- Direct blows to the greater trochanter of the femur may cause an isolated impaction fracture of the adjacent acetabulum, with protrusion of the femoral head through the medial acetabular wall into the pelvic canal.

DIAGNOSIS

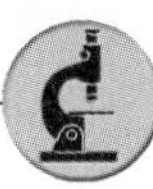

DIFFERENTIAL DIAGNOSIS

- Spinal fracture/luxation and spinal cord injury
- Long bone fracture in pelvic limb
- Coxofemoral luxation(s)

INITIAL DATABASE

- Thoracic and abdominal radiographs
- Neurologic examination
- Complete blood count, serum biochemistry panel, and urinalysis (especially before sedation or anesthesia)
- Electrocardiogram

ADVANCED OR CONFIRMATORY TESTING

- Multiple view radiographs (lateral, obliqued lateral(s), ventrodorsal) for assessment of the two hemipelves, sacroiliac joint, sacrum, tail, and distal lumbar spine. Heavy sedation/general anesthesia usually required
- Computed tomography to assess extent of injuries, identify sacral fractures
- Urinary tract imaging (e.g., contrast radiography) as needed to evaluate disrupted ureter(s), urinary bladder, or urethra

TREATMENT

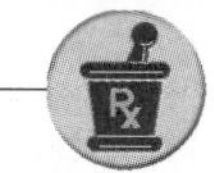

THERAPEUTIC GOAL(S)

- Elimination of pain
- Restoration of normal ambulation
- Restoration of pelvic canal diameter
- Prevention of secondary injuries to nerves from unstable or malunion of bone fragments

ACUTE GENERAL TREATMENT

- Analgesia.
- Ensure patent/functional urinary conduit.
- Surgery delayed until patient is adequately stabilized.
- Injuries affecting the transmission of weight-bearing forces from the limb to the spine usually require surgery. These injuries involve acetabular, iliac, sacroiliac, and sacral disruptions.
  - Acetabular fractures are stabilized with plate/screws or pins/wires/screws, and methylmethacrylate.
  - Iliac fractures are stabilized with plate/screws.
  - Sacroiliac and sacral body injuries are stabilized with screws/pins.
- Patient size, degree of displacement, inherent stability, risk of secondary nerve injuries, and presence of other injuries help determine which injuries can be managed operatively versus conservatively (cage rest).

CHRONIC TREATMENT

- Confinement and sling support for 1 to 2 months, analgesics as needed.
- Monitor for delayed signs of abdominal trauma (e.g., biliary disruption/leakage, delayed manifestations of lower urinary tract rupture) and cardiac complications (myocarditis/ventricular dysrhythmia).

POSSIBLE COMPLICATIONS

- Malunions resulting in pelvic canal compromise, with secondary constipation/megacolon or dystocia
- Malunions or callus formation resulting in sciatic nerve impingement or entrapment, with neuropraxia
- Urethral damage or rupture
- Coxofemoral osteoarthritis (acetabular fractures)
- Persistent neurologic deficits
- Persistent lameness or gait alteration
- Iatrogenic sciatic nerve injury
- Ventral abdominal hernia secondary to prepubic tendon avulsion or displaced pubic fracture

RECOMMENDED MONITORING

- Periodic radiographs to assess fracture healing
- Periodic clinical examinations including rectal palpation to assess improvement/resolution, function, and comfort
- Electromyography as needed in patients with peripheral nerve injuries/dysfunction

PROGNOSIS AND OUTCOME

- Increased risk for prolonged or persistent disability with fractures of the acetabulum or fractures associated with nerve injuries.
- Improved prognosis for return to function when injuries that involve the sacrum, sacroiliac joint, ilium, or acetabulum are treated with anatomic reduction and rigid fixation of bone fragments.

PEARLS & CONSIDERATIONS

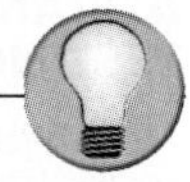

COMMENTS

- Look for secondary injuries to the pelvic girdle (sacroiliac joints, sacral wings, and sacral body) with any diagnosis of pelvic fracture. Use oblique radiographic views to isolate the hemipelves.
- Acetabular fractures require accurate reconstruction of the articular surface to reduce the risk of osteoarthritis.
- If acetabular repair cannot be achieved or if disabling osteoarthritis develops, a salvage surgery (hip replacement or femoral head/neck excision) usually is needed for a functional result.

PREVENTION

Reduce free roaming by use of leashes, fences, neutering, and window screens

CLIENT EDUCATION

- Proper confinement/activity restriction during healing and recovery.
- Pets with acetabular fractures may require an acute or delayed salvage-type surgery (femoral head/neck resection).

SUGGESTED READING

Olmstead ML: Fractures of the bones of the hind limb. In Olmstead ML (ed): *Small Animal Orthopedics*. St. Louis, Mosby, 1995, pp 219–228.

Piermattei DL, Flo GL: *Brinker, Piermattei and Flo's Handbook of Small Animal Orthopedics and Fracture Repair*, ed 3. Philadelphia, WB Saunders, 1997, pp 395–421.

Tomlinson JL: Fractures of the pelvis. In Slatter DH (ed): *Textbook of Small Animal Surgery*, ed 3. Philadelphia, WB Saunders, 2003, pp 1989–2001.

AUTHOR: **JAMES M. FINGEROTH**
EDITOR: **JOSEPH HARARI**

Fractures of the Radius and Ulna

BASIC INFORMATION

DEFINITION

Fractures of the radius involve the head, shaft, or medial styloid process; fractures of the ulna involve the olecranon, shaft, or lateral styloid process.

EPIDEMIOLOGY

SPECIES, AGE, SEX: Dogs and cats of either sex or any age.

RISK FACTORS: Forelimb trauma.

CLINICAL PRESENTATION

HISTORY, CHIEF COMPLAINT: Trauma from motor vehicle/firearm accidents, falls, and fights causing forelimb lameness.

PHYSICAL EXAM FINDINGS: Variable degrees of lameness, soft tissue swelling, bruising, and open wounds associated with an antebrachial injury.

ETIOLOGY AND PATHOPHYSIOLOGY

- Nearly 20% of all fractures in dogs and cats involve the radius and ulna.
- The radius is the primary weight-bearing bone and is the most often stabilized; conversely, ulnar fractures can realign during repair of the radius and will heal in situ.
- The radius and ulna are a paired bone system connected by annular, collateral, and interosseous ligaments. Therefore growth plate trauma and disturbed growth in either bone will cause a forelimb deformation (see Angular Limb Deformities, p 71).
- Diminished vascularity in the distal aspect of the bones in small and toy breeds will cause impaired bone healing.

DIAGNOSIS

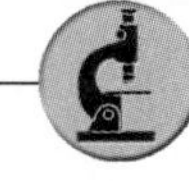

DIFFERENTIAL DIAGNOSIS

- Elbow joint luxations
- Humeral condyle fractures
- Carpal luxations and fractures
- Radial nerve or brachial plexus injury

INITIAL DATABASE

- Complete blood count, chemistry panel, electrocardiogram, thoracic radiography based on patient's American Society of Anesthesiologists patient classification (see p 1334)
- Standard craniocaudal and mediolateral radiographic projections of forelimb

TREATMENT

THERAPEUTIC GOAL(S)

- Anatomic or functional realignment of fractures to maintain proximal and distal joint (elbow and carpus) congruency and parallelism
- Tension band stabilization (pins, wires, or bone plate/screws) of olecranon fractures to neutralize distraction by the triceps muscles
- Tension band pinning/wiring or screw fixation of styloid process fractures to provide collateral ligament support

ACUTE GENERAL TREATMENT

- First aid: external heavy bandage support to limit soft tissue swelling, reduce bone fragment motion, provide limb support, and cover open wounds.
- Lavage, debridement, and deep microbial culture and sensitivity assay of open, contaminated lesions.
- Antibiotic (therapeutic or prophylactic), analgesic, and nonsteroidal anti-inflammatory therapies as indicated.
- Radial shaft fractures are stabilized with bone plate/screws applied cranially, or external skeletal fixation (ESF) with percutaneous pins applied mediolaterally (type 2) or angled craniocaudally (type 1b).
- Fresh autogenous cancellous graft tissue or commercially available allograft should be used for enhancing fracture healing (see Bone Grafting, p 1194).
- Severely displaced ulnar fractures in large dogs can be stabilized with an intramedullary pin or bone plate/screws.
- Proximal ulnar fracture(s) with cranial displacement of the radial head (Monteggia fracture) requires reduction and stabilization of the bones with screws or small pins and suturing of the annular ligament.
- Casting of radius/ulnar fractures can only be recommended for minimally displaced, stable lesions in young, non–small-breed dogs.

CHRONIC TREATMENT

After surgical intervention: bandage support, sometimes with caudal splintage, and controlled exercise until radiographic and clinical evidence of bone union

POSSIBLE COMPLICATIONS

- Implant failure, stress protection (osteopenia), and cold conduction with the use of bone plate and screws for stabilization of radial fractures
- Pin tract sepsis and instability with ESF pins and frames
- Poor healing of distal radial and ulnar fractures in small, toy breeds

RECOMMENDED MONITORING

Clinical and radiographic evaluations 4 to 6 and 10 to 12 weeks after surgery

PROGNOSIS AND OUTCOME

- Bone plates/screws and ESF yield the most consistent clinical recoveries and return of limb functions.
- Casts are effective for minimally displaced fractures in young, healthy patients.
- Intramedullary pinning of the radius causes malunions and carpal joint damage.

PEARLS & CONSIDERATIONS

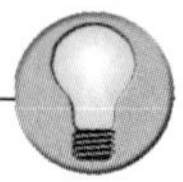

COMMENTS

- Irreparable proximal or distal lesions of the radius and ulna may require arthrodesis of the adjacent joint (elbow or carpus) to salvage the limb.
- ESF can be used in a minimally invasive or closed approach to preserve the soft tissues during a "biologic" surgical approach.
- Patients with ESF require more intensive postoperative care than those treated with a bone plate/screws.
- Plate removal is sometimes required after bone union in dogs that are lame due to cold conduction or have radiographic evidence of osteopenia under the implant.
- Toy breed dogs with distal radial/ulnar fractures often have unsatisfactory healing without surgical intervention (i.e., plating).

SUGGESTED READING

Boudrieau RJ: Fractures of the radius and ulna. In Slatter D (ed): *Textbook of Small Animal Surgery*, ed 3. Philadelphia, WB Saunders, 2002, pp 1953–1973.

Larsen LJ, et al: Bone plate fixation of distal radius and ulna fractures in small and miniature breed dogs. *J Am Anim Hosp Assoc* 35:243, 1999.

Piermattei DL, Flo GL: Fractures of the radius and ulna. In *Brinker, Piermattei, and Flo's Handbook of Small Animal Orthopedics and Fracture Repair*, ed 3. Philadelphia, WB Saunders, 1997, pp 321–343.

AUTHOR & EDITOR: **JOSEPH HARARI**

Fractures of the Scapula

BASIC INFORMATION

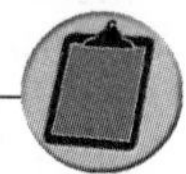

DEFINITION

Scapular fractures involve the spine, body, neck, or glenoid regions of the bone

EPIDEMIOLOGY

SPECIES, AGE, SEX: Dogs and cats of either sex and any age.

RISK FACTORS: Trauma to the proximal aspect of the forelimb.

CLINICAL PRESENTATION

HISTORY, CHIEF COMPLAINT: Forelimb trauma secondary to motor vehicle/firearm accidents, falls, or fighting.

PHYSICAL EXAM FINDINGS: Variable degree of lameness. Swelling, bruising, open wounds around scapula. Pain during palpation of shoulder joint.

ETIOLOGY AND PATHOPHYSIOLOGY

- Uncommon fractures representing 0.5–2.5% of all fractures treated at referral hospitals.
- Can be associated with regional injury to cervicothoracic spine, thoracic structures (pulmonary contusions, pneumothorax), and brachial plexus.
- Extensive medial and lateral musculature provide soft tissue support and extraosseous vascularity to fractured bone segments.
- Fractures are classified based on location: body, spine, neck, and glenoid *or* stable/unstable extra-articular versus intra-articular lesions.

DIAGNOSIS

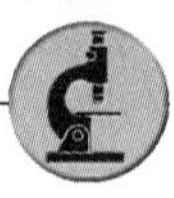

DIFFERENTIAL DIAGNOSIS

- Shoulder luxation
- Dorsal displacement of the scapula

INITIAL DATABASE

- Mediolateral and caudocranial radiographic projections of proximal aspect of limb
- Complete blood count and serum chemistry panel based on American Society of Anesthesiologists patient classification (see p 1334)
- Electrocardiogram and thoracic radiography

ADVANCED OR CONFIRMATORY TESTING

Distoproximal, axial radiographic projection with limb pulled caudally delineates occult lesions

TREATMENT

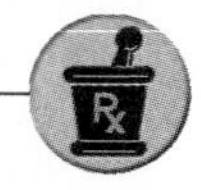

THERAPEUTIC GOAL(S)

- Fracture stabilization for bone healing
- Maintenance of glenoid (joint) congruency

ACUTE GENERAL TREATMENT

- Minimally displaced, nonarticular fractures can be stabilized for 1 month with external bandage support such as a Velpeau sling or spica splint.
- Displaced, malaligned, nonarticular, or glenoid (joint) lesions require internal support with implants.
- Spine or body fractures are stabilized with orthopedic wire or bone plate/screws.
- Neck fractures are stabilized with small pins or bone plate/screws.
- Glenoid fractures require alignment of joint surface and are stabilized with screws or pins.
- Avulsions of the acromion process or supraglenoid tubercle require tension band wiring to counteract distraction by the deltoideus and biceps muscles, respectively.

CHRONIC TREATMENT

- Bandage support for 4 to 6 weeks for comminuted lesions and tenuous fixations
- Controlled ambulation and passive flexion/extension exercises to maintain muscle tone and joint motion for 6 weeks until radiography confirms bone healing

POSSIBLE COMPLICATIONS

- Suprascapular nerve damage with neck fracture or surgical repair
- Malalignment of fractured bone segments
- Degenerative joint disease with glenoid fractures
- Infection
- Implant failure

RECOMMENDED MONITORING

- Lameness evaluation 1 to 3 months after injury and treatment
- Radiography at 6 to 10 weeks to evaluate fracture healing

PROGNOSIS AND OUTCOME

- Based on severity of injury
- Good to excellent for nonarticular lesions

PEARLS & CONSIDERATIONS

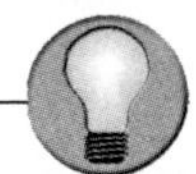

COMMENTS

- Scapular fractures can be missed if lameness is mild or ambulation is not evaluated at hospital admission (e.g., patient is carried in).
- Fractures are often identified during thoracic radiography of trauma patients.
- Suprascapular nerve damage is characterized by atrophy of supraspinatus and infraspinatus muscles.
- Scapular fractures tend to heal well due to abundant periosseous vascularity and cancellous bone supply distally.

SUGGESTED READING

Jerram RM, et al: Scapular fractures in dogs. *Comp Contin Educ Prac Vet* 20:1254, 1998.

Parker RB: Scapula. In Slatter D (ed): *Textbook of Small Animal Surgery*, ed 3. Philadelphia, WB Saunders, 2002, pp 1891-1897.

Piermattei DL, Flo GL: Fractures of the scapula. In *Brinker, Piermattei, and Flo's Handbook of Small Animal Orthopedics and Fracture Repair*, ed 3. Philadelphia, WB Saunders, 1997, pp 221-227.

AUTHOR & EDITOR: **JOSEPH HARARI**

Fractures of the Spine/Luxations of the Spine

BASIC INFORMATION

DEFINITION

Disorders primarily due to trauma and causing spinal instability, spinal cord damage, or spinal nerve damage

SYNONYM(S)

Broken back (thoracolumbar)
Broken neck (cervical)
Spinal dislocations
Spinal fractures

EPIDEMIOLOGY

SPECIES, AGE, SEX: Any dog or cat, but most commonly younger animals.
RISK FACTORS: Trauma. Focal or diffuse bone demineralization (primary or secondary vertebral column neoplasia, infection, chronic phosphorus and calcium imbalances, osteoporosis, nutritional secondary hyperparathyroidism).

CLINICAL PRESENTATION

HISTORY, CHIEF COMPLAINT

- Trauma (e.g., hit by car)
- Spinal pain, swelling, or deformity
- Weakness or inability to stand/walk

PHYSICAL EXAM FINDINGS

- Signs of hypovolemic/hypotensive shock in acute trauma patients.
- Guarding of neck, arched back, spinal hyperpathia and/or deformation.
- Crepitus, excessive spinal movement in unstable fractures.
- Neurologic deficits depend on localization and severity of lesion (proprioceptive deficits); monoparesis, paraparesis, or tetraparesis; upper motor neuron (UMN) or lower motor neuron (LMN) signs; loss of central recognition of pain; areflexia; ipsilateral Horner's syndrome; enlarged UMN or LMN bladder.
- Spinal reflexes for fractures involving spinal cord segments:
  - C1-C5: UMN to the front and UMN to the hind limbs
  - C6-T2: LMN to the front and UMN to the hind limbs
  - T3-L3: Normoreflexia to the front and UMN to the hind limbs
  - L4-S3: Normoreflexia to the front and LMN to the hind limbs

ETIOLOGY AND PATHOPHYSIOLOGY

- Traumatic vertebral fractures result from forces causing spinal hyperextension, hyperflexion, compression, and/or rotation.
- Fractures occur most commonly at the craniocervical, cervicothoracic, thoracolumbar, and lumbosacral junctions.
- A decrease in spinal canal diameter may cause mechanical injury to nervous tissue.
- Secondary pathophysiologic events include ischemia, hemorrhage, alteration in blood flow to the spinal cord, and edema. These secondary effects are often more harmful than the initial mechanical injury.

DIAGNOSIS

DIFFERENTIAL DIAGNOSIS

Intervertebral disk disease, meningomyelitis, diskospondylitis, vertebral osteomyelitis, congenital malformations, spinal neoplasia

INITIAL DATABASE

- Complete blood count, serum chemistry, urinalysis, thoracic and abdominal radiographs: generally unremarkable.
- Spinal survey radiographs to detect discontinuity and fracture lines of vertebral column, malalignment of intervertebral space, and/or articular facets.
- In cooperative patients, initial radiographs should be taken without sedation or anesthesia.

ADVANCED OR CONFIRMATORY TESTING

- Spinal radiographs of anesthetized, stable patients permit more accurate positioning and characterization of lesions (e.g., for surgical planning). Care must be taken to avoid iatrogenic exacerbation of injury when handling the anesthetized patient.
- Myelogram or computed tomogram to exclude compression of spinal cord by herniated disk material or bone fragments (Fig. I-80).

TREATMENT

THERAPEUTIC GOAL(S)

- Stabilization of patients in shock
- Temporary and definitive fracture stabilization
- Pain management and physical rehabilitation

ACUTE GENERAL TREATMENT

- Initial medical management:
  - Shock treatment in trauma patients.
  - Tape thoracolumbar fracture patients to rigid board and apply neck brace to patients with cervical fractures to minimize further spinal cord damage. Sedate fractious or agitated patients.
  - Methylprednisolone sodium succinate: 30 mg/kg bodyweight once IV.
  - Pain management with opiates or nonsteroidal anti-inflammatory drugs.
- Definitive treatment:
  - Decision of nonsurgical (strict confinement, neck or back brace, and pain management) versus surgical management (surgical spinal cord and nerve root decompression, fracture reduction and subsequent stabilization with implants) is based on initial neurologic status, serial reevaluations, spinal stability, and presence of concurrent injuries.
  - Unstable injuries result from lamina, pedicle, dorsal spinous process, and articular facet fractures and supraspinous/interspinous ligament tears.
  - Stable injuries result from disk protrusion, ventral longitudinal ligament rupture, avulsion of ventral vertebral body.
- Nonsurgical management for patients with mild neurologic signs (pain, proprioceptive and motor deficits) and/or stable fractures that respond to medical management.
- Surgery for patients with more severe neurologic signs (uncontrollable pain, minimal motor function, paresis or plegia), with unstable fractures or lesions not improving with medical management.
  - Stabilization with internal implants: pins, wires, plates, or screws.
  - Methylmethacrylate can be used for solidifying implants.
  - External fixators have been used less frequently.

CHRONIC TREATMENT

- Strict cage rest until radiographic evidence of healing
- Supportive care: appropriate bedding with traction, food and water near immobilized patients or hand feeding, bladder expressions in patients without bladder control
- Physical rehabilitation: assisted standing and walking, aquatherapy, gait and proprioceptive training

DRUG INTERACTIONS

Do not give steroidal and nonsteroidal anti-inflammatory medications simultaneously

POSSIBLE COMPLICATIONS

- Respiratory arrest due to cervical fractures
- Hemorrhage
- Neurologic deterioration
- Myelomalacia

- Infection
- Implant failure

RECOMMENDED MONITORING

- Serial neurologic evaluations
- Respiratory monitoring with cervical fractures and trauma patients

PROGNOSIS AND OUTCOME

- Mild neurologic deficits: good prognosis
- More severe neurologic deficits: fair to guarded prognosis
- Severed spinal cord or areflexia: grave prognosis
- Perioperative mortality for surgical stabilization of cervical vertebral fractures is 36%. Nonsurgical treatment often provides reasonable outcome

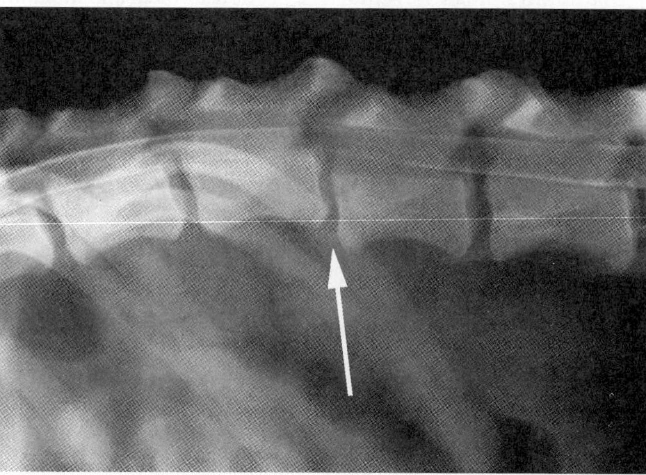

FIGURE I-80 Lateral view of the canine thoracolumbar spine during myelography. Note the subluxation between L1 and L2 vertebrae (*arrow*), widening of the L1–L2 articular facet space, and disruption of the flow of the contrast agent.

PEARLS & CONSIDERATIONS

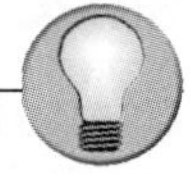

COMMENTS

- Up to 20% of patients with traumatic spinal fractures have a second fracture.
- Radiographs may not reflect maximal spinal displacement. Therefore, neurologic evaluation is often more helpful than radiographic evaluation for prognosis.

CLIENT EDUCATION

Care for paralyzed patients is laborious. It can take months until improvement is observed and return to function cannot be guaranteed.

SUGGESTED READING

Sturges BK, LeCouteur RA: Vertebral fractures and luxations. In Slatter D (ed): *Textbook of Small Animal Surgery*. Philadelphia, Elsevier, 2003, pp 1244-1261.

AUTHOR: **SUSANNE K. LAUER**
EDITOR: **JOSEPH HARARI**

Fractures of the Tibia and Fibula

BASIC INFORMATION

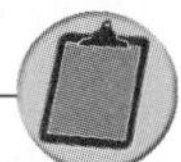

DEFINITION

Fractures of the tibia and fibula include avulsion of the tibial tuberosity, separation of the proximal or distal tibial physis, tibial shaft fractures, and fractures of the medial or lateral malleolus of the tibia.

EPIDEMIOLOGY

SPECIES, AGE, SEX: Tuberosity avulsions and physeal fractures occur in immature animals.

RISK FACTORS

- Direct trauma
- Torsional athletic injuries
- Bone tumors or metabolic bone disease

CLINICAL PRESENTATION

HISTORY, CHIEF COMPLAINT: Acute lameness secondary to trauma.

PHYSICAL EXAM FINDINGS

- Pain, swelling, and crepitus at the fracture site
- Stifle joint effusion with proximal physeal and tuberosity avulsion fractures
- Tarsocrural (hock) instability due to medial or lateral malleolar fractures

ETIOLOGY AND PATHOPHYSIOLOGY

- Tibial fractures account for 20% of all long-bone fractures.
- Due to sparse soft tissue coverage, tibial fractures are often open.
- Most fibular fractures occur with tibial fractures and are not repaired unless stability of the stifle or hock is compromised.

DIAGNOSIS

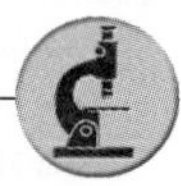

DIFFERENTIAL DIAGNOSIS

- Osteochondrosis of the tibial tuberosity
- Bone neoplasia
- Stifle or hock luxation

INITIAL DATABASE

- Craniocaudal and lateral radiographs, including both the stifle and hock.
- In growing animals (open physes), radiographs of the contralateral leg will help differentiate traumatic physeal injury from the normal appearance of an open physis/growth plate.
- Stress radiography (general anesthesia) to identify a nondisplaced malleolar fracture or collateral ligament injury.
- Complete blood count, serum chemistry panel, and urinalysis based on patient stability and American Society of Anesthesiologists patient classification (see p 1334).

TREATMENT

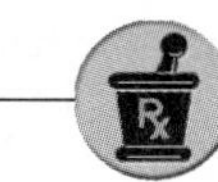

THERAPEUTIC GOAL(S)

Fracture stabilization for rapid bone healing and early return to normal ambulation, without compromising bone growth

ACUTE GENERAL TREATMENT

- Nonsurgical treatment (if patient will tolerate splinting and exercise restriction):
  - Minimally displaced, stable proximal tibial shaft or physeal fractures are

treated with external immobilization for 3 to 6 weeks.
  - Minimally displaced, stable tibial shaft fractures may be treated with external casting or splinting, especially if the fibula is intact and can act as an internal splint.
  - Incomplete or nondisplaced malleolar fractures usually heal with external splinting.
- Surgical treatment:
  - Tibial tuberosity avulsions are treated with a tension band wire technique.
  - Displaced or unstable proximal tibial shaft or physeal fractures are treated with small cross pins, cancellous bone screws, or a small buttress plate.
  - Proximal fibular fractures are stabilized with a bone screw or tension band wire technique to preserve the insertion of the lateral collateral ligament.
  - For multiple or complex tibial shaft fractures, or for large and active dogs requiring more rigid support, treatments include intramedullary pinning, intramedullary nails, bone plates, and external fixators.
  - In highly comminuted shaft fractures, rigid fixation (e.g., bone plating) is used for spanning the fracture site and providing spatial alignment of the fracture ends without disturbing their soft tissue attachments (biologic osteosynthesis). This preserves the vascular supply to the fracture bed and fosters new bone growth.
  - Displaced or unstable malleolar fractures require accurate fixation with a cancellous screw or two small cross pins.

CHRONIC TREATMENT

- Cast or splint used as the primary fixation is removed once radiographic signs of healing are evident.
  - Usually 6 to 12 weeks depending on patient age.
  - Younger patients heal more quickly.
  - Exercise restriction is continued another 3 to 4 weeks.
- Bone plates are removed after bone union (5 to 12 months) in patients with discomfort or cold intolerance.
- Intramedullary pins are removed after healing to prevent later damage to the stifle articular cartilage.
- Implants used for stabilizing physeal fractures are removed after healing to avoid premature physeal closure.

POSSIBLE COMPLICATIONS

- Delayed union or nonunion
- Patellar luxation following poorly reduced tibial tuberosity avulsion fractures
- Degenerative joint disease (intra-articular fractures or implants)
- Osteomyelitis (open or highly comminuted fractures, or poor surgical asepsis)
- Growth disturbances causing limb shortening or angular limb deformity

RECOMMENDED MONITORING

Monthly physical and radiographic examinations until clinical recovery

PROGNOSIS AND OUTCOME

Simple fractures usually heal more quickly and with fewer complications than articular or highly comminuted fractures.

PEARLS & CONSIDERATIONS

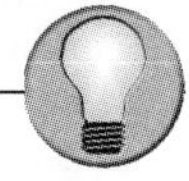

COMMENTS

Normograde intramedullary pinning of the tibia is preferred over retrograde pinning to avoid iatrogenic femoral condyle, cruciate ligament, or meniscal damage.

SUGGESTED READING

Brinker WO, Piermattei DL, Flo GL: Fractures of the tibia and fibula. In Brinker WO, Piermattei DL, Flo GL (eds): *Handbook of Small Animal Orthopedics and Fracture Treatment*, ed 3. Philadelphia, WB Saunders, 1997, pp 581-606.

AUTHOR: **ELIZABETH J. LAING**
EDITOR: **JOSEPH HARARI**

Frostbite

BASIC INFORMATION

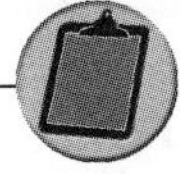

DEFINITION

Tissue damage caused by exposure to cold temperatures or cold agents; effects may be reversible with reheating, or may cause necrosis and be irreversible

SYNONYM(S)

Avascular necrosis

EPIDEMIOLOGY

SPECIES, AGE, SEX

- Any animal exposed to cold environmental temperatures, especially if the body temperature drops below 34°C (93°F). Young animals outdoors, or those in poor body condition, are more at risk.
- Affected tissues often include the tail, testicles, and pinna of ears.

GENETICS AND BREED PREDISPOSITION: Hairless or short-haired breeds of dogs and cats are predisposed.

RISK FACTORS: Low ambient temperatures.

GEOGRAPHY AND SEASONALITY: Winter months in temperate to cold climates.

ASSOCIATED CONDITIONS AND DISORDERS: Hypothermia.

CLINICAL PRESENTATION

HISTORY, CHIEF COMPLAINT

- History of exposure to cold temperatures or agents.
- The owner's observations will depend on the time course since the cold injury occurred.
- Animals may be presented for evaluation of acute injury (e.g., hit by car) and white, waxy skin or injury may not be noticed until later stages when tissue sloughing is occurring.

PHYSICAL EXAM FINDINGS

- Dependent on extent of exposed parts of the body:
  - Mild cold injury to the extremities may go undetected (toe tips, ear tips, tail tip).
  - Very extensive regional cold injury may be evident as a frozen limb or other severe cold injury.
- Acutely affected animals have pale areas of skin that are cool to the touch, with or without freezing of deeper tissues.
- Affected body parts may appear numb or hyperesthetic, and cyanosis may be evident.
- As the affected area thaws, the tissue may become reddened and swollen:
  - Depending on the extent of affected tissue, the thawing process may be associated with signs of intense pain.
- Affected skin may blister.
- Days after the frostbite has occurred, the tissues may appear shrunken and discolored, and may begin to slough if necrotic. Days to weeks after injury, alopecia and sloughing may occur.

ETIOLOGY AND PATHOPHYSIOLOGY

- Cold induces vasoconstriction to affected tissue, as well as endothelial damage and thrombosis.
- Freezing results in crystallization of extracellular fluid that results in a fluid

shift from the cell to the extracellular space. The change in electrolyte concentration within the cell then leads to change in cellular proteins.
- Lack of nutrients as well as direct cellular damage results in local tissue damage.

DIAGNOSIS

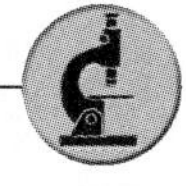

DIFFERENTIAL DIAGNOSIS

Burn injuries may appear similar

INITIAL DATABASE

- None required
- Routine labwork if systemic illness
- Imaging and further evaluation as dictated by other disorders or injuries (e.g., if frostbite is caused by cold exposure after the patient was hit by a car)

TREATMENT

THERAPEUTIC GOAL(S)

- Prevent further damage to tissues from continued cold exposure or self-trauma
- Prevent secondary infection
- Allow damaged tissue to declare itself before extensive debridement or amputation

ACUTE GENERAL TREATMENT

- Ensure further contact with source of cold is prevented
- Apply warm compresses gently to the area
  - Do not rub or massage, which could cause further tissue damage
- Immerse affected areas if possible in warm (102–104°F or 39–40°C) water
  - Avoid warmer temperatures that may potentiate tissue injury
- Dry affected areas: apply light noncompressive bandages if integrity of skin is not intact
- Administer prophylactic antibiotics if appropriate (e.g., cefazolin 22 mg/kg IV q 8h)
  - Infected wound or sloughing tissue

CHRONIC TREATMENT

- Prevent further exposure of the tissue to freezing, particularly during the healing process.
- Assess necrotic tissue conservatively.
  - Do not amputate or debride large areas early on in the healing process unless signs of infection or sepsis are present.
  - Necrotic tissue can act as a protective covering; often, when necrotic tissue is removed, deeper tissue is healing.
- Tissue damaged by frostbite will likely be more susceptible to cold injury in the future.

POSSIBLE COMPLICATIONS

- Tissue necrosis
- Infection

PROGNOSIS AND OUTCOME

- Variable depending on amount of tissue affected:
  - Extremities (ear tips, toes, tail tip) may slough or require amputation without affecting quality of life or longevity.
  - More substantial frostbite (e.g., limbs) carry a greater risk of systemic complications such as infection and therefore a more guarded prognosis.
- Hypothermia may complicate frostbite and alter the prognosis depending on severity.

PEARLS & CONSIDERATIONS

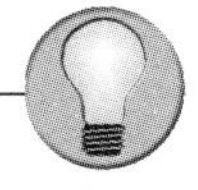

PREVENTION

- Avoid exposure to very low ambient temperature
- Bring animals indoors during periods of low ambient temperature

SUGGESTED READING

Swaim SF: Trauma to the skin and subcutaneous tissues of dogs and cats. *Vet Clin North Am Small Anim Pract* 10(3):599–618, 1980.

AUTHOR: **KIRSTEN AARBO**
EDITOR: **ELIZABETH ROZANSKI**

Gallbladder Rupture

BASIC INFORMATION

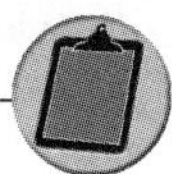

DEFINITION

Loss of gallbladder wall integrity

EPIDEMIOLOGY

SPECIES, AGE, SEX: Dogs:
- Associated with trauma:
  - Younger dogs (mean 2.8 years)
- Associated with intrinsic gallbladder disease:
  - Middle-aged dogs (mean 8.1 years)

GENETICS AND BREED PREDISPOSITION: Associated with gallbladder mucocele.
- Shetland sheepdogs and possibly cocker spaniels are overrepresented.

ASSOCIATED CONDITIONS AND DISORDERS: Dogs:
- Cholelithiasis, cholecystitis, bile peritonitis, sepsis
- Hypothyroidism and hyperadrenocorticism:
  - May predispose a subset of dogs to gallbladder infarction/rupture

CLINICAL PRESENTATION

DISEASE FORMS/SUBTYPES
- Necrotizing cholecystitis/gallbladder infarction:
  - Without rupture
  - With hepatic and omental adhesions and possibly fistulae to other abdominal structures
  - With gallbladder perforation and diffuse peritonitis
- Gallbladder perforation associated with penetrating trauma and subsequent bile peritonitis

HISTORY, CHIEF COMPLAINT
- Nonspecific signs. Vomiting, anorexia, weakness, polydipsia, polyuria, weight loss. Often chronic (duration from onset of signs to presentation: up to 1 month; mean =12 days)
- Some owners may notice icterus, discolored urine (bilirubinuria)

PHYSICAL EXAM FINDINGS
- Icterus: very common (77% of bile peritonitis cases)
- Abdominal distention: common (65% of bile peritonitis cases), may be subtle
- Signs of abdominal pain
- Pyrexia
- Shock

ETIOLOGY AND PATHOPHYSIOLOGY

- Causes of gallbladder rupture:
  - Necrotizing cholecystitis
  - Gallbladder infarction
  - Penetrating trauma
  - Inadequate choleresis due to excessively thick bile, defective gallbladder contractility, and/or altered outflow
- Gallbladder rupture may result in the development of septic peritonitis (see Peritonitis, p 838) or nonseptic peritonitis (see Peritonitis, p 838).
- Lack of bile secretion into the intestine results in:

- Lack of digestion and absorption of fat and fat-soluble vitamins, most importantly vitamin K (coagulopathy)

DIAGNOSIS

DIFFERENTIAL DIAGNOSIS

- Icterus:
  - Hyperbilirubinemia due to hemolysis:
    - Immune-mediated hemolytic anemia and other diseases causing severe intravascular hemolysis
  - Hepatic diseases:
    - Cholangiohepatitis, cirrhosis, neoplasia, copper and other toxins
  - Extrahepatic bilary obstruction:
    - Choleliths
    - Pancreatitis
    - Cholangitis
    - Neoplasia
    - Stricture
  - Biliary leakage from other parts of the biliary system:
    - Traumatic rupture of the common or hepatic ducts
- Abdominal distention (if icterus not apparent):
  - Septic peritonitis:
    - Gastrointestinal perforation
    - Penetrating trauma
  - Uroabdomen
  - Hemoabdomen:
    - Ruptured mass/viscus
    - Bleeding disorder
  - Abdominal organ dilation/enlargement:
    - Gastric dilation/volvulus
    - Mesenteric volvulus
    - Splenic torsion
    - Overeating
    - Hyperadrenocorticism
  - Intra-abdominal abscess:
    - Severe pancreatitis
    - Hepatic abscess
    - Ruptured prostatic abscess
    - Ruptured pyometra
  - Portal hypertension
  - Congestive heart failure (right-sided)

INITIAL DATABASE

- Complete blood count:
  - Inflammatory leukogram
  - Degenerative left shift with toxic changes:
    - Septic bile peritonitis
- Serum biochemistry profile:
  - Elevated bilirubin concentration (virtually all)
  - Elevated liver enzymes concentration (virtually all cases)
  - Hypokalemia
- Survey abdominal radiographs:
  - Increased opacity/loss of detail in anterior abdomen
  - Cholelithiasis (in dogs, 14–48% are radiopaque)
  - Generalized loss of abdominal detail/fluid:
    - Bile peritonitis

ADVANCED OR CONFIRMATORY TESTING

- Abdominal ultrasound examination:
  - Evaluate gallbladder:
    - Wall thickness and integrity:
      - Cholecystitis
    - Contents:
      - Choleliths
      - Mucocele
    - Presence of attached omentum
    - Surrounding fluid, suggesting either bile peritonitis or unrelated (e.g., other differential diagnoses)
- Peritoneal fluid analysis (obtained during abdominal ultrasound examination):
  - Bilirubin concentration: Bilirubin concentration greater than twice that of serum bilirubin is diagnostic of bile peritonitis.
  - Cytologic study and bacterial culture and sensitivity testing (aerobic and anaerobic):
    - Septic peritonitis
- Coagulation profile (prothrombin time is first to be abnormal with vitamin K deficiency/malabsorption)

TREATMENT

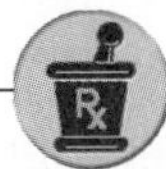

THERAPEUTIC GOAL(S)

- Correction of fluid deficits
- Normalization of serum electrolyte concentrations
- Normalization of coagulation status before surgery
- Surgical removal of ruptured gallbladder once patient is stabilized
- Treatment of bile peritonitis
- Postoperative nutritional support

ACUTE GENERAL TREATMENT

- Rehydation: intravenous administration of balanced electrolyte solution
- Parenteral antibiotics effective against gram negative bacteria and anaerobes
  - Empiric therapy:
    - Cefoxitin, 22 mg/kg IV q 2h perioperatively, then q 6h
    - Metronidazole, 10–15 mg/kg IV q 12h
    - Enrofloxacin, 2.5–5 mg/kg IV q 12h (q 24h in cats)
  - Specific, long-term therapy based on culture and sensitivity test results
- Possible administration of fresh-frozen plasma: see Transfusions, p 1098:
  - Hypoproteinemia
  - Possible coagulopathy
- Vitamin K administration: 2.5 mg/kg SC q 12h × 3 days, then weekly
- Exploratory laparotomy once animal is stabilized:
  - Cholecystectomy
  - Ensure patency of biliary system
  - Aerobic and anaerobic microbiologic culture of peritoneal fluid
  - Treatment of bile peritonitis:
    - Septic → open abdominal drainage
- Nutritional support (see Parenteral Nutrition, p 1296; Feeding Tube Placement: Percutaneous Endoscopic Gastrostomy [PEG], p 1247):
  - Placement of feeding tube if indicated

CHRONIC TREATMENT

Maintenance of bile flow: Ursodeoxycholic acid 10–15 mg/kg/day PO. Only after biliary obstruction is definitively ruled out/corrected, because stimulates gallbladder contraction

POSSIBLE COMPLICATIONS

- Ongoing/recurrent bile leakage
- Failure to resolve septic bile peritonitis:
  - Endotoxemia
  - Sepsis
- Biliary obstruction:
  - Recurrence of cholelithiasis
- Pancreatitis

RECOMMENDED MONITORING

- Clinical and laboratory parameters assessing perfusion including capillary refill time, pulse rate and quality, blood pressure, urine output, arterial pH and lactate concentrations
- Respiratory function
- Serum liver enzymes and bilirubin concentrations
- Coagulation profile

PROGNOSIS AND OUTCOME

- Guarded to fair in animals with aseptic bile peritonitis
- Poor to guarded in animals with septic bile peritonitis

PEARLS & CONSIDERATIONS

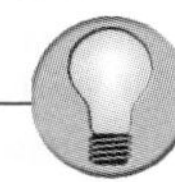

COMMENTS

In dogs and cats with bile peritonitis:

- The peripheral white blood cell count is significantly lower in survivors (mean = 20,608/μl) compared with nonsurvivors (mean = 35,715/μl).
- The immature neutrophil count is significantly lower in survivors (mean = 686/μl) than in nonsurvivors (mean = 4852/μl).

SUGGESTED READING

Church EM, et al: Surgical treatment of 23 dogs with necrotizing cholecystitis. *J Am Anim Hosp Assoc* 24:305, 1988.

Holt DE, et al: Canine gallbladder infarction. *Vet Pathol* 41:416, 2004.

Ludwig LL, et al: Surgical treatment of bile peritonitis in 24 dogs and 2 cats: A retrospective study (1987–1994). *Vet Surg* 26:90, 1997.

AUTHOR: **DAVID HOLT**

EDITOR: **RICHARD WALSHAW**

Gallops and Other Extra Heart Sounds

BASIC INFORMATION

DEFINITION

- Extra heart sounds are classified as noises other than the normal first and second heart sounds that are heard during auscultation of the heart. They must be distinguished from premature cardiac beats.
  - Normally, only the S_1S_2 sounds are heard when auscultating the heart of the dog or cat.
  - Other extra heart sounds heard within the cardiac cycle include sounds that occur within the normal cardiac cycle due to pathologic conditions (gallop sounds), splitting of the normal heart sounds, and extracardiac rubbing sounds.
- *Gallop sounds* are intensified extra heart sounds (third or fourth or both: summation) occurring during the diastolic phase of the cardiac cycle.
  - The sounds are the result of the flow of blood into the ventricles during active ventricular filling (S_3) or atrial contraction (S_4).
  - With advanced heart disease, when ventricular emptying is inadequate, these sounds emerge and may be auscultated (lub-dub-[thud]).
  - The term *gallop* relates to these sounds because when audible to the ear, the combination of the first two normal heart sounds (S_1S_2) and the additional diastolic sound mimics that of a galloping horse.
  - Gallop sounds indicate ventricular systolic and/or diastolic dysfunction and are usually an indication of congestive heart failure.
- Other extra heart sounds that can be confused with the gallop include *split heart sounds* and *systolic clicks*.
  - *Split heart sounds* occur with asynchronous closure of the atrioventricular valves (split S_1) or semilunar valves (split S_2).
    - Split S_1: normal in medium and large-breed individuals.
    - Split S_2: usually from delayed pulmonic valve closure (pulmonary hypertension, heartworm disease, etc.).
  - *Systolic clicks* are usually high frequency sounds (i.e., the third heart sound is similar to the normal heart sounds) heard during systole.
    - They tend to move toward and then away from the first heart sound.
    - They are usually heard best with the diaphragm of the stethoscope in contrast to the *gallop* sound, which is a lower frequency sound heard better with the bell.
    - The *systolic click* may be single or multiple. It also may come and go between consecutive cardiac cycles.
    - Although not necessarily an indication of developing mitral valve disease, it usually is an indication that weakness of the mitral apparatus is present to some degree.

SYNONYM(S)

- "Gallop rhythm" is synonymous with gallop sound and is a poor term, because the actual cardiac rhythm (electrocardiogram) is unaffected by gallops.
- Gallop sound: third heart sound (S_3), fourth heart sound (S_4), diastolic heart sound, protodiastolic heart sound, presystolic heart sound, summation diastolic heart sound.

EPIDEMIOLOGY

SPECIES, AGE, SEX: Any.

RISK FACTORS

- Gallops:
  - Congestive heart failure
  - Systolic and diastolic ventricular dysfunction
- Systolic clicks:
  - Developing or early mitral valvular insufficiency
- Split heart sounds:
  - Increased aortic or pulmonary artery pressures (causing splitting sounds due to delayed aortic or pulmonic valve closure under specific circumstances)

CLINICAL PRESENTATION

HISTORY, CHIEF COMPLAINT

- Clinical signs relating to heart failure are associated with gallop sounds.
- Split sounds may be incidental findings or may be noted in a patient with signs of pulmonary hypertension, such as syncope or dyspnea (split S_2).
- Systolic clicks are not associated with clinical signs.

PHYSICAL EXAM FINDINGS

- A third heart sound with accentuated low frequency and that mimics a horse galloping best describes a gallop sound.
  - This sound is low frequency, heard best with the bell of the stethoscope, and usually over the mitral or tricuspid valve area.
  - The sound is likely to be associated with other signs of heart failure such as dyspnea, tachypnea, and tachycardia. A concurrent heart murmur is common.
- Third heart sounds occurring at a slow rate are not likely to be gallop rhythms and, like all third heart sounds, must be differentiated from systolic clicks and split heart sounds.
  - Systolic clicks are higher frequency sounds heard with the diaphragm of the stethoscope over the point of maximal intensity on the thorax. The sound may be consistent or variable and may be single or multiple. It can easily mimic a gallop sound except in frequency (click is higher-pitched).
  - Split heart sounds are usually heard cranially and left over the aortic and pulmonic valve regions (split S_2). They tend to be higher frequency sounds heard best with the diaphragm of the stethoscope.

ETIOLOGY AND PATHOPHYSIOLOGY

- Systolic failure: increased end diastolic ventricular pressures and volume
- Diastolic failure: increased E and A wave size in diastole on echocardiographic examination of the heart
- Systolic clicks: unidentified. Possibly early mitral valve prolapse
- Split heart sounds: pressure alterations within the heart and great vessels, causing early or delayed valve closure

DIAGNOSIS

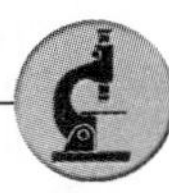

DIFFERENTIAL DIAGNOSIS

See Definition above

INITIAL DATABASE

- Gallop sounds: thoracic radiographs, echocardiography
- Split S_1: none
- Split S_2: heartworm antigen test, echocardiography, thoracic radiographs
- Systolic click: echocardiography and thoracic radiographs, or monitor with physical exam only, depending on clinical presentation and client desires

ADVANCED OR CONFIRMATORY TESTING

Cardiac evaluation (auscultation, radiography, electrocardiography, laboratory analyses, echocardiography) usually is sufficient to identify the specific abnormality causing the extra heart sound

TREATMENT

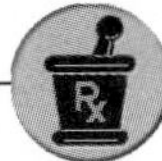

THERAPEUTIC GOAL(S)

Extra heart sounds in and of themselves are *not* treated. Attention is directed to identifying and, if needed, treating, the inciting cause.

PROGNOSIS AND OUTCOME

Variable, depending on cause

PEARLS & CONSIDERATIONS

COMMENTS

Unlike other extra heart sounds, gallops are disproportionately louder when auscultated with the bell of the stethoscope and generally indicate concurrent congestive heart failure.

SUGGESTED READING

Fox P, Sisson D, Moise S: *Canine and Feline Cardiology*, ed 2. Philadelphia, WB Saunders, 1998.

AUTHOR: **STEPHEN J. ETTINGER**
EDITOR: **ETIENNE CÔTÉ**

Garbage Toxicosis

BASIC INFORMATION

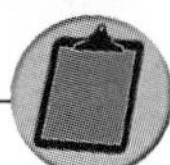

DEFINITION

Gastroenteritis, or hemorrhagic gastroenteritis, caused by the ingestion of food or garbage that is contaminated with bacteria or preformed bacterial toxins; tremors or seizures can occur due to presence of tremorgenic mycotoxins

SYNONYM(S)

Bacterial food poisoning
Carrion toxicosis
Garbage gut
Song bird fever

EPIDEMIOLOGY

SPECIES, AGE, SEX

- Potentially all animals; dogs are more likely to ingest spoiled foods.
- Cats who hunt and consume birds may develop song bird fever.

RISK FACTORS

- Roaming animals
- Dogs fed food considered unfit for human consumption
- Raw food diets

CONTAGION AND ZOONOSIS

- Disease transmissable between animals due to habits of licking and sniffing.
- Dogs also might eat vomitus or feces containing bacteria or bacterial toxins.
- Zoonotic transmission possible, especially in young children or people with compromised immune systems.

GEOGRAPHY AND SEASONALITY: Disease common during warmer months, or year round in tropical and subtropical regions.

ASSOCIATED CONDITIONS AND DISORDERS

- Botulism
- Tremorgenic mycotoxicosis

CLINICAL PRESENTATION

HISTORY, CHIEF COMPLAINT

- History of exposure to carrion or garbage or raw food diets
- Clinical signs within 15 minutes to 6 hours postingestion; diarrhea can be delayed for 48 hours
- Severe vomiting, diarrhea, lethargy, anorexia

PHYSICAL EXAM FINDINGS

- Vomiting
- Signs of abdominal pain
- Abdominal distention from gas
- Foul smelling feces, watery or bloody diarrhea
- Fever
- Ataxia
- Weak pulse, muddy mucous membranes, increased capillary refill time, shock
- Hypothermia as the shock state progresses

ETIOLOGY AND PATHOPHYSIOLOGY

- *Streptococcus* spp., *Salmonella* spp., *Bacillus* spp., *Escherichia coli*, and *Clostridium perfringens* are the most common bacteria involved.
- Endotoxemia and enterotoxemia are possible.
- Via different mechanisms, endotoxins produce circulatory shock, collapse, and death.
- Tremors, seizures, hyperthermia may occur from tremorgenic mycotoxins.
- Gastrointestinal (GI) epithelial cells irritated/eroded:
  - Permeability disturbed, initiating vomiting, GI hemorrhage, fluid and electrolyte loss.
  - Normal absorptive capabilities of the gut may be disrupted.
  - Stasis and GI dilation with gas accumulation follows.
  - GI stasis encourages growth of gram-negative bacteria, which liberate endotoxin.

DIAGNOSIS

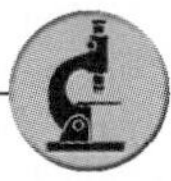

DIFFERENTIAL DIAGNOSIS

- Viral gastroenteritis
- Hemorrhagic gastroenteritis
- Acute pancreatitis
- Acute hepatopathies
- Other toxins causing hemorrhagic gastroenteritis including arsenic, salmon poisoning, sago palm

INITIAL DATABASE

- Complete blood count and serum chemistry profile: nonspecific changes
- Abdominal radiographs
- Monitor blood glucose (hypoglycemia associated with endotoxemia)

ADVANCED OR CONFIRMATORY TESTING

- Bacterial fecal culture is of mixed value (healthy animals often have cultures that are positive for "pathogenic" bacteria)
- Blood culture if sepsis is suspected
- Serologic identification of staphylococcal or clostridial toxins

TREATMENT

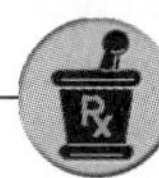

THERAPEUTIC GOAL(S)

- Limit absorption of bacterial toxins
- Correct fluid and electrolyte imbalances
- Prevent shock and secondary pancreatic hypoperfusion

- Control bacterial proliferation
- Supportive care to prevent secondary infection and dehydration

ACUTE GENERAL TREATMENT

- Induction of vomiting (hydrogen peroxide 3%: 1-2 ml/kg [maximum 45 ml total] PO once, or syrup of ipecac: 2-6 ml total dose PO once, or apomorphine 0.04 mg/kg IV or instilled in conjunctival sac and rinsed out when vomiting begins) in animals with a known recent exposure but no clinical signs.
- Activated charcoal 1-3 g/kg PO (dose according to packaging label of product; e.g., 10 ml of activated charcoal suspension PO made from 2 g activated charcoal suspended in 10 ml tap water).
- Appropriate fluid and electrolyte therapy.
- Antibiotics. Injectable aminoglycosides generally contraindicated because of synergistic action with endotoxins in depressing the myocardium. Oral aminoglycosides (streptomycin 5-10 mg/kg PO q 12h, or neomycin 10-20 mg/kg PO q 8-12h) work well. Metronidazole 25 mg/kg PO q 12h (for an absolute maximum of 5 days at this dose) can also be used.
- Gastrointestinal protectants such as sucralfate 1/4 to 1 one-gram tablet PO q 8h.
- Treat shock.
- Appropriate treatment if disseminated intravascular coagulation occurs, e.g., including heparin 75 IU SQ q 8h (see Disseminated Intravascular Coagulation, p 313).
- Control tremors and seizures with methocarbamol (55-220 mg/kg IV; repeat as needed; max dose 330 mg/kg/day) or diazepam (0.5-2 mg/kg IV; repeat as needed) in cases involving tremorgenic mycotoxins.
- Profuse, persistent vomiting after the toxin has been expelled may be controlled with metoclopramide 0.2-0.4 mg/kg IM or SC q 8h.

CHRONIC TREATMENT

Bland diet

POSSIBLE COMPLICATIONS

- Chronic diarrhea with clostridial enteritis
- Pancreatitis, malabsorption syndromes with repeated episodes of garbage toxicosis

RECOMMENDED MONITORING

- Temperature
- Heart rate
- Blood pressure
- Glucose
- Complete blood count

PROGNOSIS AND OUTCOME

- Prognosis good provided shock does not occur
- Poor or guarded if endotoxemic shock

PEARLS & CONSIDERATIONS

COMMENTS

- Clinical signs resolve in 3 to 5 days.
- The term *song bird fever* arises from the source of intoxication, namely the decayed carcasses of song birds that cats hunt.
- If a cat has known song bird fever, routine antibiotics are not recommended, as this tends to alter normal gut flora, allowing colonization by *Salmonella*.
- Consumption of decomposing organic material, moldy refrigerated foods, cottage cheese, cream cheese, moldy walnuts can cause tremors and seizures due to contamination with tremorgenic mycotoxins such as penitrem A and roquefortine.

PREVENTION

- Prevent roaming and scavenging
- Feed fresh, high-quality food

CLIENT EDUCATION

- Discuss nutrition
- Discuss potentially zoonotic aspects of raw diets

SUGGESTED READING

Beasley VR, et al: Garbage toxicosis—carrion toxicoses—bacterial food poisoning. In Beasley VR, et al: *A Systems Affected Approach to Veterinary Toxicology*. Urbana, IL, University of Illinois, 1999, pp 738-741.

Freeman LM, Michel KE: Evaluation of raw food diets for dogs. *J Am Vet Med Assoc* 218:705-709, 2001.

Lejeune JT, Hancock DD: Public health concerns associated with feeding raw meat diets to dogs. *J Am Vet Med Assoc* 219:1222-1225, 2001.

AUTHOR: **CHARLOTTE MEANS**
EDITOR: **SAFDAR A. KHAN**

Gastric Dilatation/Volvulus

BASIC INFORMATION

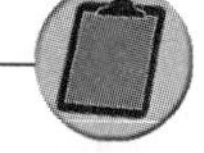

DEFINITION

Rotation of the stomach on its mesenteric axis associated with gastric distention

SYNONYM(S)

Bloat
Gastric torsion
GDV

EPIDEMIOLOGY

SPECIES, AGE, SEX: Older dogs (>7 years) are at greatest risk. Rarely reported in cats.

GENETICS AND BREED PREDISPOSITION

- Large- and giant-breed dogs.
- Purebred dogs at greater risk than mixed breeds.
- Having a first-degree relative with gastric dilatation/volvulus (GDV) is associated with an increased risk.
- The most commonly affected breeds are the Great Dane, weimaraner, Saint Bernard, Gordon setter, Irish setter, Doberman pinscher, Old English sheepdog, and standard poodle. Bassett hound is at greatest risk among smaller breeds.

RISK FACTORS: Increased risk may be associated with:

- Narrow and deep thoracic cavity
- Long hepatogastric ligament
- Once-daily feeding
- Rapid ingestion of food
- Exercise after eating
- Consumption of large volumes of food or water
- Stress
- Fearful temperament
- Being underweight
- Eating from a raised feeding bowl

GEOGRAPHY AND SEASONALITY: One report in the United States has found an increased incidence in the months of November, December, and January.

ASSOCIATED CONDITIONS AND DISORDERS: Inflammatory bowel disease.

CLINICAL PRESENTATION

HISTORY, CHIEF COMPLAINT

- Abdominal distention
- Abdominal pain
- Ptyalism
- Retching or vomiting (may be nonproductive)
- Acute collapse

PHYSICAL EXAM FINDINGS

- Abdominal distention and tympany:
  - Simultaneous auscultation and percussion of the abdomen may reveal a tympanitic sound, indicating the presence of a taut, gas-filled viscus (stomach).
- Splenomegaly
- Clinical signs of hypovolemic shock: weak pulses, tachycardia, pale mucous membranes, prolonged capillary refill time, dyspnea

ETIOLOGY AND PATHOPHYSIOLOGY

- The pylorus moves ventrally and from right to left, becoming displaced between the esophagus and stomach.
- The rotation may be 90 to 360 degrees.
- Gastric dilation occurs due to failure of eructation and pyloric outflow obstruction. This occurs before or after gastric rotation.
- The distended stomach results in caudal vena cava and portal vein compression, causing decreased venous return to the heart.
- Decreased venous return results in decreased cardiac output, decreased arterial blood pressure, and myocardial ischemia.
- Myocardial ischemia causes cardiac arrhythmias.
- Increased intraluminal gastric pressure, portal hypertension, and avulsion of the short gastric vessels, associated with volvulus, compromise blood flow to the gastric wall. Gastric necrosis and perforation can result.
- Portal vein compression/hypertension causes sequestration of splanchnic blood and decreased ability to clear gram-negative endotoxins.
- Endotoxemia further potentiates hypotension and decreased cardiac output.
- Pressure on the diaphragm, decreased lung perfusion, and decreased lung compliance cause respiratory dysfunction and exacerbate tissue hypoxia.

DIAGNOSIS

DIFFERENTIAL DIAGNOSIS

- Gastric bloat associated with overeating
- Mesenteric volvulus
- Splenic torsion
- Diaphragmatic hernia with stomach herniation

INITIAL DATABASE

- Abdominal radiographs (Fig. I-81):
  - Right lateral view is preferred
  - Shows gas-filled pylorus cranial and dorsal to the fundus ("popeye sign," "C sign," or "double bubble")
  - Free abdominal air suggests gastric perforation
- Quick assessment tests:
  - Packed cell volume/total solids (PCV/TS): often increased due to hypovolemia
  - Serum electrolyte and glucose concentrations: hypokalemia and hypoglycemia may be seen
  - Acid-base analysis: metabolic acidosis frequently seen due to lactic acidosis
- Coagulation panel and platelet count: thrombocytopenia, increased prothrombin time/activated partial thromboplastin time/fibrinogen concentration and/or fibrin degradation product concentration associated with disseminated intravascular coagulation
- Electrocardiogram (ECG): ventricular arrhythmias are common

ADVANCED OR CONFIRMATORY TESTING

- Diagnosis confirmed at surgery
- Measurement of lactic acid concentration may assist in determining prognosis
  - Lactic acid (lactate) concentration >6.0 mmol/L associated with gastric necrosis and increased mortality

TREATMENT

THERAPEUTIC GOAL(S)

- Treat hypovolemic shock and endotoxemia
- Provide gastric decompression
- Correct stomach position at surgery
- Remove devitalized stomach and/or spleen
- Perform gastropexy to prevent recurrence

ACUTE GENERAL TREATMENT

- Place large-bore intravenous catheters in both cephalic veins and infuse isotonic crystalloids, hypertonic saline, colloids, or a combination of these fluids at shock dosages, as dictated by clinical state.
- Prophylactic antibiotic therapy.
- Decompress the stomach by orogastric intubation (see Gastric Intubation, Gavage, Lavage, p 1258).
- If orogastric intubation is not possible and patient has visible abdominal distention with a radiographically confirmed GDV, perform percutaneous trocarization of the stomach.
  - Aseptically clip and prepare an area at least 4 × 4 in. (10 × 10 cm) on the left lateral or dorsolateral abdomen, just caudal to the last rib and over the region of most obvious distention.
  - Identify a point that is within the prepared area and that is ventral to the hypaxial muscles and caudal to the last rib.
  - Using a large-bore needle (e.g., 14 or 12 gauge) directed ventrally and slightly cranially, penetrate all layers of the body wall and stomach. When successful, the procedure should produce a hissing sound associated with a release of fetid-smelling gas through the needle.
- Immediate surgery to return stomach to a normal position.
  - Placing traction on the pylorus and elevating it while putting downward pressure on the fundus will aid derotation in a counterclockwise direction.
  - Evaluate stomach and spleen for irreversible vascular compromise and necrosis.
  - Perform partial or complete splenectomy if splenic necrosis, infarction, or torsion. Perform resection or invagination of necrotic areas of stomach.
  - Perform gastropexy of pyloric antrum to the right body wall.
- Medical treatment alone (repeated intubation, trocarization) has been uniformly disappointing.

CHRONIC TREATMENT

- Postoperative potassium supplementation if hypokalemic.
  - Do not exceed 0.5 mEq/kg/hr IV.
- If ventricular arrhythmias are noted on the ECG:
  - Is hypokalemia present? If so, institute potassium replacement immediately.
    - Ventricular arrhythmias are caused by hypokalemia.
    - Ventricular arrhythmias are refractory to treatment with lidocaine, procainamide, and other antiarrhythmics when hypokalemia is present.
  - Is there anemia, hypoxemia, or acidosis? Many ventricular arrhythmias will resolve spontaneously if these systemic disturbances are corrected.
  - Is the rate rapid (>160 bpm), or is the pulse weak, despite addressing the systemic disturbances already mentioned? If so, consider treatment with lidocaine (see Ventricular Arrhythmias [Premature Ventricular Complexes, Ventricular Tachycardia], p 1148).
- Treat peritonitis if gastric perforation has occurred (fluids, antibiotics, abdominal lavage ± drainage). (See Peritonitis, Septic, p 840.)
- Treat gastric ulceration with H_2 receptor antagonists:
  - Famotidine 0.5-1 mg/kg IV, IM, SC, or PO q 12-24h; or
  - Ranitidine 0.5-2 mg/kg IV, IM, SC, or PO q 8-12h.
    - Ranitidine also has promotility properties similar to those of metoclopramide.
- Prevent future gastric dilation:
  - Feed two to four small meals a day; restrict exercise before and after meals; avoid stress during feeding.
- Use drugs that increase gastric motility (i.e., metoclopramide 0.2-0.4 mg/kg

PO, SC, or IM q 6h, or cisapride 0.1-0.5 mg/kg PO q 8h) if recurrent bloating occurs after gastropexy without evidence of gastric outflow obstruction.
- Pain management.

DRUG INTERACTIONS

Lidocaine toxicity may occur at lower doses if given concurrently with cimetidine.

POSSIBLE COMPLICATIONS

- Cardiac arrhythmias
- Reperfusion injury
- Gastric necrosis with peritonitis if devitalized tissue not removed
- Gastric ulceration
- Disseminated intravascular coagulation
- Aspiration pneumonia
- Recurrence of dilation
- Recurrence of volvulus if inadequate gastropexy

RECOMMENDED MONITORING

- ECG: ventricular arrhythmias common within 36 hours of surgery
- Electrolyte concentrations: hypokalemia
- Blood glucose concentration: hypoglycemia
- PCV/TS: hemoconcentration indicates need for increased fluid therapy
- Physical parameters: mucous membrane color, capillary refill, pulse quality, temperature, respiratory effort, lung auscultation, abdominal distention, bruising

PROGNOSIS AND OUTCOME

- Approximately 15% mortality rate for patients with GDV treated surgically
- Gastric necrosis and need for gastric resection are associated with >30% mortality
- Recurrence rates for GDV with gastropexy <10%
- Serum lactate level in dogs with GDV:
  - 99% survival if <6 mmol/L
  - 58% survival if >6 mmol/L

PEARLS & CONSIDERATIONS

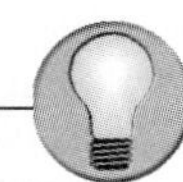

COMMENTS

- Begin fluid resuscitation before abdominal radiography.
- Do not assume the stomach is not rotated just because a stomach tube can be passed.
- Assess suspect areas of stomach for viability 10 to 15 minutes after derotation by palpation, evaluating blood flow and stomach wall color. If stomach wall is green or gray, this area will need to be resected.
- Ventricular arrhythmias have not been shown to worsen prognosis. Rather, they may identify arrhythmogenic disturbances (commonly in GDV: hypokalemia, anemia, or acidosis) that must be corrected for the arrhythmia to resolve.

PREVENTION

- Feed several small meals a day
- Avoid stress during feeding
- Do not elevate feeding bowl during eating
- Restrict exercise before and after meals
- Do not breed dogs if history of GDV
- Prophylactic gastropexy in breeds at high risk

SUGGESTED READING

Brockman DJ, et al: Canine gastric dilatation volvulus syndrome in a veterinary critical care unit: 295 cases (1986-1992). *J Am Vet Med Assoc* 207:460, 1995.

De Papp E, et al: Plasma lactate concentration as a predictor of gastric necrosis and survival among dogs with gastric dilatation-volvulus: 102 cases (1995-1998). *J Am Vet Med Assoc* 215:49, 1999.

Glickman LT, et al: Nondietary risk factors for gastric dilatation-volvulus in large and giant-breed dogs. *J Am Vet Med Assoc* 217:1492, 2000.

Glickman LT, et al: A prospective study of survival and recurrence following the acute gastric dilatation volvulus syndrome in 136 dogs. *J Am Vet Med Assoc* 34:253,1998.

AUTHOR: **LORI LUDWIG**

EDITOR: **RICHARD WALSHAW**

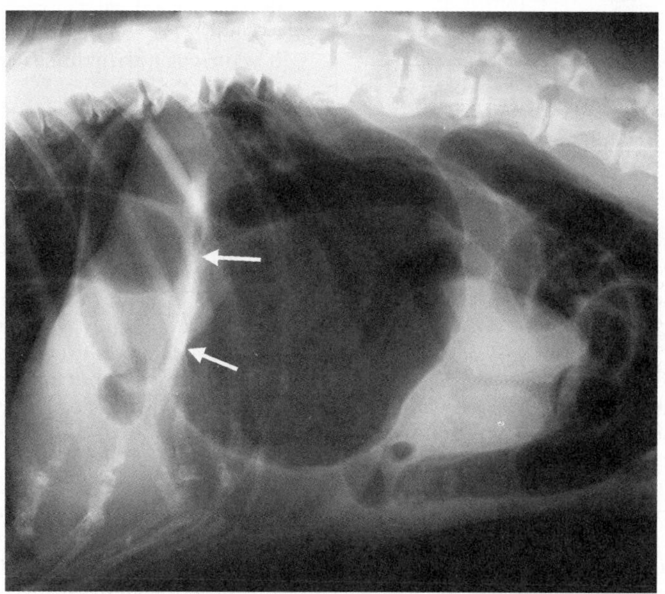

FIGURE I-81 Lateral abdominal radiograph of a dog with gastric dilation/volvulus. The characteristic septation (*arrows*) of the gastric shadow is seen; the displaced, gas-filled antrum is cranial to the arrows (to the left on this image), whereas the gas-filled fundus is caudal (the arrows are within it). A gas-filled esophagus, and evidence of ileus in the form of distended, gas-filled small intestine, are also present. Courtesy of Dr. Richard Walshaw.

Gastric Neoplasia

BASIC INFORMATION

DEFINITION

Benign or malignant tumors of epithelial, lymphoid, or mesenchymal origin. These tumors affect gastric function, are often painful, and may cause secondary systemic effects such as electrolyte disturbances, anemia, and weight loss.

SYNONYM(S)

Gastric adenocarcinoma
Gastric adenoma, gastric polyps (benign)
Gastric carcinoma
Gastric extramedullary plasmacytoma
Gastric lymphoma
Gastrointestinal stromal tumor (GIST)
Leiomyoma
Leiomyosarcoma
Scirrhous carcinoma of the stomach

EPIDEMIOLOGY

SPECIES, AGE, SEX

- In dogs, gastric tumors account for <1% of all malignancies:
  - Median age for adenocarcinoma is 10 years
  - Median age for leiomyomas and GIST is 11 years
- In cats, gastric tumors are most commonly lymphoma, which occurs in cats >7 years old.

GENETICS AND BREED PREDISPOSITION: Breed predisposition:

- Gastric adenocarcinomas: rough collies, Staffordshire terriers, Belgian shepherds, and chows (may be familial).
- Leiomyoma and GISTs: German shepherds.
- GISTs are associated with activating mutation of the c-kit receptor tyrosine kinase oncogene.

RISK FACTORS: Gastric adenocarcinomas:

- Chronic nitrosamine exposure experimentally.
- Association of gastric carcinoma and lymphoma with chronic inflammation from *Helicobacter pylori* infection in people, unproven in companion animals.

CONTAGION AND ZOONOSIS

- *Helicobacter* spp. organisms may be frequently found in normal dogs and cats, but significance is undetermined.
- Zoonotic potential exists for *H. pylori*, but the prevalence of infection in animals is low.

ASSOCIATED CONDITIONS AND DISORDERS: Gastric lymphoma in cats is generally not associated with retroviral infection (feline leukemia virua, feline immunodeficiency virus).

CLINICAL PRESENTATION

HISTORY, CHIEF COMPLAINT

- Chronic vomiting
- Hematemesis/melena
- Anorexia, weight loss
- Depression and lethargy, pain or restlessness

PHYSICAL EXAM FINDINGS: May include some or all of the following:

- Physical exam may be normal
- Poor body condition score (e.g., body condition score 1/9–2/9)
- Pale mucous membranes, signs of anemia
- Abdominal mass
- Abdominal pain

ETIOLOGY AND PATHOPHYSIOLOGY

- Chronic vomiting may result in weight loss, electrolye imbalance
- Anemia secondary to chronic gastrointestinal (GI) bleeding may be hypochromic, microcytic due to iron depletion
- Panhypoproteinemia due to GI blood loss
- Hypoglycemia may occur due to insulin-like growth factor II release from smooth muscle tumors

DIAGNOSIS

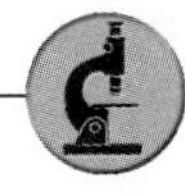

DIFFERENTIAL DIAGNOSIS

Any gastrointestinal or systemic cause of chronic vomiting may mimic gastric neoplasia:

- Gastric foreign body
- Gastric ulceration
- Granulomatous gastritis
- Chronic pancreatitis
- Systemic disease associated with chronic vomiting (renal, hepatic, diabetic ketoacidosis)

INITIAL DATABASE

Complete blood count, serum chemistry panel with electrolytes, urinalysis: frequently normal or changes are nonspecific and secondary to GI electrolyte or blood losses (nonregenerative anemia, increased blood urea nitrogen, normal creatinine, normal urine specific gravity).

- Three-dimensional view thoracic staging radiographs (metastasis).
- Abdominal ultrasound evaluation: to assess gastric wall changes often not seen on routine radiographs, and to rule out other causes of vomiting (pancreatitis, liver disease, etc.).
- Positive contrast gastrogram: assessment for outflow obstruction; does not differentiate neoplasia from other infiltrative diseases such as pythiosis.
- Ultrasound guided fine needle aspiration cytology: if a gastric wall abnormality or lymphadenopathy is present. Lymphoma exfoliates most readily; GIST or gastric muscle tumors do not.
- Endoscopic biopsy: Histopathologic diagnosis is essential for treatment and prognosis. Endoscopy rapidly and effectively provides mucosal tissue specimens, but if the tumor is in the gastric muscular or serosal layers, results may be inadequate, requiring surgical biopsy.
- Surgical biopsy: Exploratory surgery provides opportunity for both diagnosis and treatment (surgical removal of the affected region).

ADVANCED OR CONFIRMATORY TESTING

Diagnosis is confirmed by biopsy with histopathology:

- Immunohistochemical stains for c-kit in GIST
- Cytokeratin, vimentin immunohistochemistry for undifferentiated tumors
- Immunophenotyping for lymphoma

TREATMENT

THERAPEUTIC GOAL(S)

Benign gastric lesions may be cured surgically, as can early diagnosed low-grade malignancy. Other surgical goals might be to relieve gastric obstruction, or to remove tumors that are painful or bleeding for palliation. Chemotherapy is potentially helpful in prolonging survival, although malignant gastric tumors are typically incurable.

ACUTE GENERAL TREATMENT

- Antiemetics (dolasetron 0.3 mg/kg q 12–24h IV, SC, metoclopramide 0.2–0.4 mg/kg q 8h, PO, IV, if no obstruction is present), gastroprotectants (famotidine 0.5 mg/kg IV, PO q 12h).
- Rehydration with intravenous fluids.
- Antibiotics for *Helicobacter* infection, if indicated.
- Blood transfusion and hematinic therapy as indicated for nonregenerative iron-deficiency anemia.
- Analgesic management as indicated by clinical signs.
- Diet modification to easily digested, high-energy content food.
- Parenteral alimentation as indicated (if the patient has not eaten for >3 days or will not be able or willing to eat after surgery).

CHRONIC TREATMENT

- Gastric tumor resection often results in motility disorders.
  - May require motility modifiers (metoclopramide 0.2–0.4 mg/kg IV, PO q 8h, cisapride 0.25 mg/kg q 24h PO)
- Chronic antiemetic therapy may be required.
- Chemotherapy with doxorubicin, platinum agents, or antimetabolites may prove helpful.
- Systemic chemotherapy for gastric lymphoma provides remission and prolonged survival (see Lymphoma, Gastrointestinal, p 661).

POSSIBLE COMPLICATIONS

- Surgical wound dehiscence with secondary peritonitis, pneumoperitoneum
- Chemotherapy-induced leukopenia might predispose to infection
- Chemotherapy-induced thrombocytopenia might increase gastric hemorrhage
- Chemotherapy might result in gastric performation of transmural lesions

RECOMMENDED MONITORING

- Postoperative follow-up with chest radiographs and abdominal ultrasound for signs of recurrence or metastasis on a 1- to 2-month basis for 1 year
- Monitor complete blood count for recovery from nonregenerative anemia
- Monitor for signs of dissemination of alimentary lymphoma

PROGNOSIS AND OUTCOME

- Favorable for benign lesions (adenomas, leiomyomas), although complete resection of mesenchymal tumors is unlikely

- Poor for adenocarcinoma, carcinoma, GIST, especially when metastatic:
  - These dogs generally do not live beyond 6 months with therapy
- Guarded to fair for focal mass presentation of lymphoma
- Guarded for diffuse or multicentric alimentary lymphoma, as these lesions typically regress slowly and may have an indolent course, but are ultimately incurable

PEARLS & CONSIDERATIONS

COMMENTS

- Gastric carcinoma is associated with early lymphatic spread. Lymph nodes detected on ultrasound can be used for diagnosis and prognosis.
- Gastric carcinomas may overexpress cyclooxygenase-2; nonsteroidal anti-inflammatory drugs (piroxicam 0.3 mg/kg PO q 24h) may be palliative.
- Scirrhous carcinoma is rapidly fatal.

SUGGESTED READING

Frost D, Lasota J, Miettinen M: Gastrointestinal stromal tumors and leiomyomas in the dog: A histopathologic, immunohistochemical and molecular genetic study of 50 cases. *Vet Pathol* 40:42, 2003.

Gualtieri M, Monzeglio MG, Scanziani E: Gastric neoplasia. *Vet Clin North Am Small Anim Pract* 29:415, 1999.

AUTHOR: **BARBARA E. KITCHELL**
EDITOR: **DEBRA L. ZORAN**

Gastric Parasites

BASIC INFORMATION

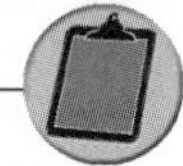

DEFINITION

Nematode parasites of the stomach affecting dogs and cats

EPIDEMIOLOGY

SPECIES, AGE, SEX: *Physaloptera* spp. infect dogs and cats. *Ollulanus tricuspis* is found exclusively in the cat. There is no age or sex predisposition.

RISK FACTORS
- Dogs and cats that habitually ingest the intermediate host (crickets, beetles, cockroaches) or transport hosts (e.g., rodents and snakes) for *Physaloptera* spp. are at greater risk of infection.
- Multicat households are a risk factor for *Ollulanus* spp. infection.

CONTAGION AND ZOONOSIS: These are not zoonotic diseases. *Ollulanus* spp. is spread from cat to cat in the vomitus.

GEOGRAPHY AND SEASONALITY: Worldwide.

CLINICAL PRESENTATION

HISTORY, CHIEF COMPLAINT: Chronic vomiting is the chief complaint for both parasitic infections. A good appetite is usually retained, and weight loss is usually insignificant, particularly for *Physaloptera* spp. infections. Cats with *Ollulanus* spp. infection may have chronic weight loss. The duration of signs may be from a few days to many months.

PHYSICAL EXAM FINDINGS: Typically, there are no significant abnormal findings on physical examination. Chronic weight loss may develop in cats.

ETIOLOGY AND PATHOPHYSIOLOGY

- *Physaloptera* spp., most commonly *P. rara*. They range in length from 1 to 6 cm, although most are 1 to 2 cm.
  - Subclinical infections are believed to occur in many animals, but chronic vomiting due to gastritis or penetration of parasite into the gastric wall is the typical pathophysiologic presentation.
  - Intermediate hosts: beetles and crickets.
- *Ollulanus tricuspis*. Size range is 0.7 to 1.0 mm long.
  - Presence *of Ollulanus* trisuspis may induce gastric irritation and inflammation, or in severe cases a chronic fibrosing gastritis; however, infections with the parasite can also be inapparent.
  - Life cycle is direct: infection from eating vomitus containing larvae.

DIAGNOSIS

DIFFERENTIAL DIAGNOSIS

- Dietary indiscretion
- Food intolerance or hypersensitivity/allergy
- Gastric foreign body
- *Helicobacter* gastritis
- Drugs or toxins (nonsteroidal anti-inflammatory drugs, antibiotics, plants, lead)
- Idiopathic gastritis (lymphoplasmacytic, eosinophilic)
- Pyloric antral hypertrophy
- Pythiosis

INITIAL DATABASE

- Complete blood count, serum biochemistry profile, and urinalysis are usually normal, although a rare dog or cat may have peripheral eosinophilia.
- Fecal flotation is usually negative. On rare occasions the translucent eggs of *Physaloptera* spp. may be identified.
- Abdominal radiographs are normal.
- Abdominal ultrasound is normal.
- Microscopic examination of the vomitus may yield the presence of *Ollulanus* spp.

ADVANCED OR CONFIRMATORY TESTING

- In many cases of unconfirmed *Physaloptera*- or *Ollulanus*-associated gastritis, empiric anthelminthic treatment is highly effective, and advanced testing may be unnecessary.
- Gastroscopy is the only method to reliably identify the presence of *Physaloptera* spp. in the stomach.
- *Ollulanus* spp. can be identified from microscopic examination of vomitus, squash preps, or touch preps of gastric mucosal biopsies (endoscopy or surgery), or on histologic evaluation of the biopsies (less reliable).

TREATMENT

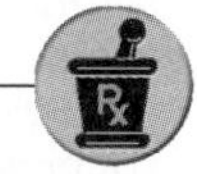

THERAPEUTIC GOAL(S)

Removal of the parasite rapidly resolves vomiting

ACUTE GENERAL TREATMENT

- Mechanical removal of *Physaloptera* spp. resolves clinical signs
- Anthelminthics for *Physaloptera* spp.:
  - Pyrantel: 5 mg/kg PO (dog), 20 mg/kg PO (cat). Using a higher dose in dogs (10–15 mg/kg) and repeating in 2 to 3 weeks may yield a higher response rate.
  - Fenbendazole: 50 mg/kg/day PO for 3 days is reportedly effective (dog, cat). This author uses 75 mg/kg/day PO for 5 days in dogs.
  - Ivermectin: may be effective at 200 µg/kg PO (dog, cat). Not for use in ivermectin-sensitive breeds.
- Anthelminthics for *Ollulanus tricuspis*:
  - Fenbendazole: 50 mg/kg/day PO for 3 days.

- Pyrantel: 20 mg/kg PO, repeat in 2 to 3 weeks.

POSSIBLE COMPLICATIONS

Fenbendazole is not labeled for use in cats, and may be associated with idiosyncratic hepatotoxicity with high doses or prolonged use.

PROGNOSIS AND OUTCOME

The prognosis for complete resolution of chronic vomiting is excellent. Reinfection with *Physaloptera* spp. is likely in most cases as repeated ingestion of intermediate and transport hosts occurs. Treatment of all cats in a household for *O. tricuspis* should eliminate the parasite.

PEARLS & CONSIDERATIONS

COMMENTS

- At gastroscopy, the presence of small erosions or pin-point hemorrhages on the gastric mucosa should prompt a careful inspection for *Physaloptera* spp.
- The elusive nature of the parasites, the minimal severity of clinical signs, and the expense of endoscopy all warrant a therapeutic trial with an anthelminthic before advanced diagnostic testing. Gastric parasites may still be found after a failed therapeutic trial.

PREVENTION

Block access to intermediate hosts or transport hosts

SUGGESTED READING

Guilford WG, Strombeck DR: Chronic gastric diseases: Parasitic gastritis. In Guilford WG, et al (eds): *Strombeck's Small Animal Gastroenterology*, ed 3. Philadelphia, WB Saunders, 1996, pp 285–286.

Theisen SK, et al: *Physaloptera* infection in 18 dogs with intermittent vomiting. *J Am Anim Hosp Assoc* 34:74–78, 1998.

AUTHOR: **KENNETH R. HARKIN**

EDITOR: **DEBRA L. ZORAN**

Gastric Ulcer

BASIC INFORMATION

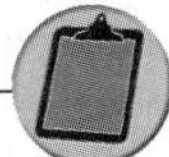

DEFINITION

Disruption of the gastric mucosa as a result of coagulative necrosis that breeches the muscularis layer and exposes the submucosa or deeper layers of the stomach wall

EPIDEMIOLOGY

SPECIES, AGE, SEX: Dogs and cats. No age, sex, or breed predisposition.

RISK FACTORS

- Iatrogenic: administration of cyclooxygenase (COX) inhibitors, other nonsteroidal anti-inflammatory drugs (NSAIDs), or corticosteroids.
- Hypergastrinemia due to any number of causes.
- Severe hypovolemia or ischemia (shock) leads to reduced gastrointestinal (GI) blood flow and increased risk of gastritis/ulcer.

CLINICAL PRESENTATION

HISTORY, CHIEF COMPLAINT

- Vomiting, hematemesis, melena are common complaints.
- Inappetence or anorexia and hypersalivation are variably seen.
- Acute encephalopathic signs (e.g., stupor, seizures, or drooling in cats) may be observed in patients with concurrent severe liver disease.

PHYSICAL EXAM FINDINGS

- Generally nonspecific.
- Abdominal pain, either on palpation or manifested as a "praying" position, is possible.
- Pale mucous membranes and circulatory shock possible with severe bleeding or with gastric perforation.

ETIOLOGY AND PATHOPHYSIOLOGY

- Primary gastroduodenal diseases (e.g., toxins or foreign bodies, chronic gastritis, *Helicobacter* spp. infection, inflammatory bowel disease, neoplasia [mastocytosis, lymphoma, adenocarcinoma, or gastrinoma], pyloric outflow obstruction).
- Gastric hyperacidity disorders (e.g., gastrinomas, hypergastrinemia due to drugs).
- Drug-induced ulcers (e.g., COX inhibitors, other NSAIDs, corticosteroids).
- Other metabolic, endocrine, or systemic causes (e.g., pancreatitis, disseminated intravascular coagulation, hypoadrenocorticism, chronic renal failure, liver failure, hypovolemic/septic shock, neurologic diseases, especially intervertebral disk disease, or stress).
- The causes of ulceration are similar to those of gastritis and erosion, but for unknown reasons the reparative mechanisms of the mucosa are overwhelmed, resulting in deep indolent lesions.
- The process of ulcer healing starts as the necrotic mucosa sloughs and granulation tissue fills the ulcer. Mucus and bicarbonate are actively secreted by the neighboring mucosa to protect the ulcer. Granulation tissue eventually organizes, a connective tissue bed develops, and epithelial tissues finally slide across the surface to reepithelialize it. Glandular structures are the last to repopulate the denuded area.
- Reduced gastric acid secretion facilitates this process, both by decreasing tissue damage from acid, and by decreasing further damage from pepsin, which is less active at higher pH.

DIAGNOSIS

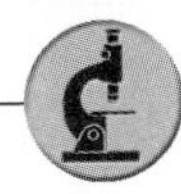

DIFFERENTIAL DIAGNOSIS

- Acute vomiting:
  - Dietary indiscretion
  - Parasites
  - *Helicobacter* gastritis
  - Foreign bodies
  - Pancreatitis
  - Other acute metabolic conditions (renal failure, hypercalcemia, etc.)
- Hematemesis:
  - Coagulopathies or lack of platelets (number or function)
  - Ingested blood (nasopharyngeal, oral, esophageal, or pulmonary bleeding)
  - Hemorrhagic gastroenteritis (all causes of severe gastrointestinal erosion)
- Melena:
  - All causes of hematemesis
  - Intestinal neoplasia
  - Intestinal parasites (hookworm)
  - Intestinal ischemia
  - Inflammatory bowel disease or other infiltrative enteropathies
- Abdominal pain:
  - Hepatitis
  - Splenomegaly/splenic rupture/torsion
  - Intestinal obstruction
  - Acute renal failure
  - Intussusception/mesenteric torsion
  - Peritonitis
  - Pancreatitis

INITIAL DATABASE

- Rectal examination should be performed to assess presence of melena.
- Complete blood count (CBC), serum biochemistry profile, urinalysis: important to identify underlying cause of gastric ulceration, and are especially

needed if hematemesis or melena is present.
  - CBC may show anemia (regenerative if acute, or nonregenerative if chronic, and microcytic, hypochromic nonregenerative if associated with iron deficiency from chronic blood loss), neutrophilia (± left shift if associated with perforation), hypoproteinemia or low platelets.
  - Serum biochemistry profile may show an elevated blood urea nitrogen (BUN)/creatinine ratio or identify conditions that are associated with ulcers (renal failure, etc.).
  - Urinalysis: essential for differentiating BUN elevation due to renal failure (urine specific gravity 1.008–1.020) from BUN elevation due to prerenal causes (urine specific gravity >1.035).
- Fecal occult blood test has limited utility.
  - O-tolidine-based tests are significantly more specific (0/108 false-positive results in healthy dogs) than guaiac-based tests (64/108 false-positive results in same dogs).
- Imaging studies.
  - Plain radiographs cannot confirm gastric ulceration. However, if perforation has occurred, loss of detail (suggesting peritonitis or free abdominal fluid) or free peritoneal gas may be present.
    - Standing lateral films are useful to localize free air in the abdomen if present.
  - Contrast radiographs may identify a mucosal filling defect.
  - Ultrasonography may show local gastric wall thickening, loss of normal layering, the presence of a wall defect or "crater," fluid accumulation in the stomach, and diminished gastric motility. In animals with perforation due to the ulcer, there may be evidence of free fluid in the abdomen.

ADVANCED OR CONFIRMATORY TESTING

- Serum gastrin levels may help diagnose gastrinoma (see Gastrinoma, p 433), but the animal must not have been on histamine-2 receptor blockers or proton pump inhibitors before testing.
- If a gastrointestinal perforation is suspected, abdominocentesis is indicated. If free fluid can be obtained during the ultrasound examination, that is often sufficient. However, a diagnostic peritoneal lavage may be needed to obtain samples if the perforation is relatively recent and the fluid accumulation is minimal.
- Gastroscopy: preferred for confirmation of gastric ulcer and tissue sampling; however, if a perforation is suspected, endoscopic examination is contraindicated as it will increase abdominal contamination
  - A solitary ulcer in an otherwise normal stomach should raise the suspicion of gastric neoplasia, especially if the edges and surrounding mucosa are thickened.
  - NSAID-induced ulcers can be solitary, but the surrounding mucosa is usually not normal due to the generalized mucosal disease (gastritis and other erosions are common).
  - Multiple diffuse small ulcers can be seen with NSAIDs, uremia, liver disease, mastocytosis, gastrinoma, and possibly *Helicobacter* gastritis.
  - Biopsies should be obtained from the ulcer periphery to avoid perforation. Repeated biopsies from the same site may improve the likelihood of identifying neoplasia. However, in some cases, endoscopic biopsies will not be adequate for diagnosis (the neoplastic tissue is deeper than the superficial mucosal tissues that are sampled with endoscopic biopsies) and laparotomy is required for full-thickness biopsies.

TREATMENT

THERAPEUTIC GOAL(S)

- Remove primary cause
- Promote healing
- Stabilization of patient with circulatory collapse from massive bleed or perforation

ACUTE GENERAL TREATMENT

- Supportive care:
  - Intravenous fluids, antibiotics, antiemetics, and opioid analgesics may be required for the patient with severe vomiting that has resulted in dehydration and electrolyte disturbances.
  - Blood transfusion for the patient with severe anemia as a result of massive bleeding.
- Surgery:
  - Surgical resection is indicated when the ulcer appears deeply penetrating (volcano crater appearance), is bleeding continuously, has perforated, or is very large and fails to heal.
  - Surgical exploration may identify the etiology (neoplasia) and allow resection of the mass/ulcer.
- Medical:
  - H_2 blockers:
    - Famotidine: 0.5–1 mg/kg PO, IV, or SC q12–24h.
    - Ranitidine: 1–4 mg/kg PO, IV, or SC q 8–12h.
    - Cimetidine: 5–10 mg/kg PO, IV, or SC q 6–8h.
  - Proton pump inhibitor: reduces gastric acid by >90% (not for use in cats):
    - Omeprazole: 0.7 mg/kg PO q 24h (alternately 20 mg/dog).
    - Esomeprazole (Nexium): 1 mg/kg PO q 24h.
    - Lansoprazole (Pravacid): 1 mg/kg IV q 24h.
  - Prostaglandin E_2-inhibitor: drug of choice for prevention/treatment of NSAID-induced ulcers. Not for use in cats:
    - Misoprostol: 3–5 μg/kg PO q 8h.
  - Sucralfate: mucosal protectant. Dissolve in 6 to 10 ml of water before administration; is most effective if administered in an acidic environment (give 1 to 2 hours before acid-blocking drugs):
    - Dogs: 0.5–1 g PO q 8h.
    - Cats: 0.25 g PO q 8h.
  - Antiemetics: use as needed to control emesis:
    - Metoclopramide: 0.2–0.4 mg/kg PO or SC q 8h.
    - Dolasetron: 0.3 mg/kg IV q 12–24h.

CHRONIC TREATMENT

Misoprostol is indicated for preventing ulcers in dogs that need to be on NSAIDs (e.g., arthritis) but are prone to developing ulcers.

DRUG INTERACTIONS

- Cimetidine and ranitidine inhibit a subset of the cytochrome P-450 enzyme systems and may delay metabolism of some drugs.
- The dose of ranitidine must be altered (reduced) in dogs with renal failure.

POSSIBLE COMPLICATIONS

The most important complications of gastric ulceration are blood loss anemia (can be severe, requiring transfusions) and perforation, resulting in septic peritonitis and shock.

RECOMMENDED MONITORING

In dogs or cats with acute hematemesis, the packed cell volume/total protein must be monitored to determine if a blood transfusion or surgical intervention is needed.

PROGNOSIS AND OUTCOME

The prognosis for most gastric ulcers is good, unless the underlying etiology is not identified or cannot be addressed.

PEARLS & CONSIDERATIONS

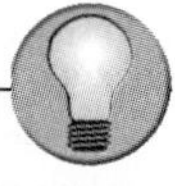

COMMENTS

- Careful endoscopic evaluation of the lesser curvature of the stomach is critical for identification of gastric adenocarcinoma.

- Patients with GI bleeding often have BUN elevations with normal creatinine, concentrated urine, and normal renal function.
- The combination of an H_2 blocker with sucralfate is frequently used in the belief that healing is improved with the combination. A study in people comparing ranitidine to ranitidine-sucralfate showed no benefit from using the combination.
- Proton pump inhibitors (e.g., omeprazole) are the only effective means of completely reducing acid secretion. H_2 blockers are much less potent, and of the group, only famotidine has been shown in dogs to adequately decrease gastric acid levels.

PREVENTION

Careful administration of NSAIDs, or use of NSAIDs with COX-2 selective properties, to minimize the risk of ulceration

CLIENT EDUCATION

- Advise clients of the dangers of consistent NSAID use, and provide them with signs to watch for what may indicate gastritis or ulcer formation.
- Advise clients about the potential dangers of over-the-counter NSAIDs in dogs and cats, as some of the most potent ulcerogenic drugs in dogs are ibuprofen, regular aspirin, and naproxen.
- Advise clients about the risk of potentially life-threatening complications from any over-the-counter NSAID given to cats.

SUGGESTED READING

Boothe DM: Gastrointestinal pharmacology. *Vet Clin North Amer Small Anim Pract* 29(2):343–376, 1999.

Rice JE, et al: Effects of diet on fecal occult blood testing in healthy dogs. *Can J Vet Res* 58:134–137, 1994.

AUTHOR: **KENNETH R. HARKIN**

EDITOR: **DEBRA L. ZORAN**

Gastrinoma

BASIC INFORMATION

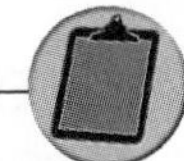

DEFINITION

Malignant neuroendocrine tumor of the pancreatic Langerhans islet D cells that secretes excessive amounts of gastrin

SYNONYM(S)

Zollinger-Ellison syndrome

EPIDEMIOLOGY

SPECIES, AGE, SEX

- Dogs: average age 8.2 years (range 3.5 to 12 years). Cats: average age 10 to 12 years.
- Female dogs and cats may be at a slightly higher risk than males.

GENETICS AND BREED PREDISPOSITION: No breed predisposition is known.

CLINICAL PRESENTATION

HISTORY, CHIEF COMPLAINT

- Associated with gastrointestinal ulceration:
  - Chronic vomiting (most common)
  - Anorexia or ravenous appetite
  - Weight loss
  - Depression
  - Lethargy
  - Diarrhea
  - Polydipsia
  - Obstipation
  - Hematemesis
  - Melena
  - Pale mucous membranes
  - Abdominal pain
- Associated with perforating ulcer and peritonitis:
  - Collapse
  - Acute abdomen (pain)
  - Shock

PHYSICAL EXAM FINDINGS

- Nonspecific findings: lethargy, depression, poor body condition
- Pale mucous membranes
- Melena on rectal exam or apparent on rectal thermometer
- Palpable abdominal mass reported in one cat
- May be unremarkable

ETIOLOGY AND PATHOPHYSIOLOGY

Pancreatic Langerhans islet D cells secrete excessive gastrin, resulting in hypersecretion of gastric acid by the stomach wall parietal cells. Gastric mucosal hypertrophy, gastrointestinal ulceration, esophagitis, and malassimilation secondary to enzyme inactivation and bile salt precipitation follow.

DIAGNOSIS

DIFFERENTIAL DIAGNOSIS

- Refractory gastritis/gastric ulcer disease
- Inflammatory bowel disease
- Gastrointestinal tract neoplasia
- Chronic pancreatitis

INITIAL DATABASE

- Complete blood count: regenerative anemia due to gastrointestinal bleeding; neutrophilia associated with gastrointestinal ulceration.
- Serum chemistry panel and electrolytes: hypoalbuminemia and hypoproteinemia due to protein loss through gastroduodenal ulcerations. Chronic vomiting may result in hypokalemia, hyponatremia, and hypochloremia. Metabolic alkalosis, with or without aciduria, is consistent with a gastric outflow obstruction, which may be present in some cases. Metastasis to the liver may result in bilirubinemia and elevated liver enzymes.
- Abdominal radiographs: loss of abdominal detail if gastrointestinal perforation has occurred; otherwise, they are generally unremarkable. Contrast radiographs may reveal deep ulcers, prominent gastric rugae, or gastric outflow obstruction in some cases.
- Three view thoracic radiographs: usually are within normal limits. Metastatic lesions usually occur late in the course of the disease.
- Abdominal ultrasound: thickened gastric wall or pylorus, evidence of metastatic disease to the liver or lymph nodes.

ADVANCED OR CONFIRMATORY TESTING

- Endoscopy: esophagitis, gastric or duodenal ulceration, hypertrophy of gastric mucosa are evident on visual inspection. Histopathologic evaluation: rugae often appear normal, suggesting submucosal or muscular hypertrophy; duodenal villous blunting and ulceration is supportive of chronic hyperacidity but not diagnostic of gastrinoma.
- Basal gastric acid secretion: increased in more than 80% of human gastrinoma patients. Of the four reported dogs tested, all values were low.
- Basal serum gastrin concentration: best survey test in humans (increased in 98% of human gastrinoma patients). Correlates with dog and cat disease, but can also be elevated in nonfasting sample, renal failure, gastric outflow obstruction, pyloric stenosis, gastric dilatation and volvulus, atrophic gastritis, chronic gastritis, small intestine resection, hepatic disease, drug administration (H_2 blockers, proton pump

inhibitors), immunoproliferative enteropathy of basenji dogs, and possibly *Helicobacter* spp. infection.
- Secretin stimulation test (2-4 U/kg IV, samples at 0.2, 5, 10, and 20 minutes postinjection): preferred provocative test for the diagnosis of gastrinoma in humans (gastrin levels greater than 200 pm/ml diagnostic in humans). Data regarding the procedure and its interpretation are limited in dogs and cats.
- Calcium stimulation test: data regarding the procedure and its interpretation are limited in dogs and cats (may be risky).
- ^{111}Iridium-octreotide or -pentetreoctide: somatostatin analogs bind to receptors expressed on gastrinomas and have facilitated localizing metastatic lesions in one dog.
- Histopathologic evaluation with immunohistochemistries or radioimmunoassay of extracts from the gastrinoma allow for a definitive diagnosis.
- Electron microscopy may also be used for detecting pancreatic Langerhans D cell intracytoplasmic secretory granules that are found in gastrinomas.

TREATMENT

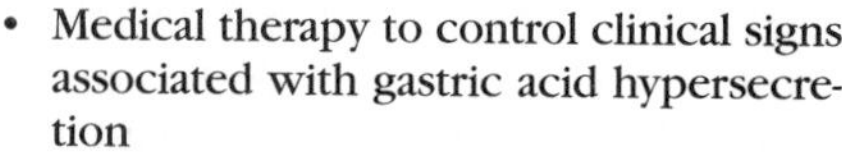

THERAPEUTIC GOAL(S)

- Medical therapy to control clinical signs associated with gastric acid hypersecretion
- Surgical reduction of gastrinoma and metastatic lesions is palliative

ACUTE GENERAL TREATMENT

- Intravenous fluids and electrolyte therapy to correct abnormalities associated with vomiting
- Control gastric hyperacidity:
  - H_2 receptor antagonists (cimetidine 10 mg/kg IV, IM, SC, or PO q 8h; ranitidine 0.5-2 mg/kg IM, SC, PO [IV may cause vomiting] q 8-12h; famotidine 0.2-1 mg/kg IV, IM, SC, or PO q 12-24h; or nizatidine 2.5-5 mg/kg PO q 24h)
  - H^+, K^+-ATPase (proton pump) inhibitors (omeprazole 0.7-1 mg/kg PO q 12-24h)
  - Somatostatin analog (octreotide 10-40 mg [per dog] q 8-12h)
- Promote healing:
  - Sucralfate 0.25-1 g per dog PO q 6-12h
  - Misoprostol 1-5 5 µg/kg PO q 8h
- Surgical and medical management for gastrointestinal ulceration/perforation

CHRONIC TREATMENT

- Acute treatment management, along with antiemetics
- Surgical debulking of the primary and metastatic lesions decreases clinical signs associated with gastrinomas

POSSIBLE COMPLICATIONS

Gastrointestinal ulceration/perforation if hyperacidity is not controlled

RECOMMENDED MONITORING

According to clinical signs

PROGNOSIS AND OUTCOME

- Poor due to high rate of metastasis.
- Animals that are managed medically and surgically live 1 week to 18 months (mean, 4.8 months).

PEARLS & CONSIDERATIONS

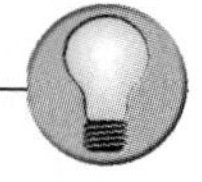

COMMENTS

A palpable abdominal mass or one that is visualized either at ultrasound or at surgery is uncommon with gastrinoma.

CLIENT EDUCATION

- Monitor for recurrence of clinical signs
- Rapid deterioration is possible if gastrointestinal perforation occurs

SUGGESTED READING

Hoenerhoff M, et al: Concurrent gastrinoma and somatostatinoma in a 10-year-old Portuguese water dog. *J Comp Pathol* 130:313, 2004.

Simpson K, et al: Diagnosis and treatment of gastrinoma. *Semin Vet Med Surg Small Anim* 12:274, 1997.

AUTHOR: **M. RAQUEL BROWN**

EDITOR: **DEBRA L. ZORAN**

Gastroenteritis: Acute, Nonspecific

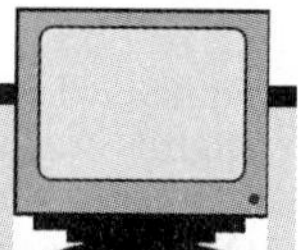

BASIC INFORMATION

DEFINITION

Sudden onset of self-limiting vomiting and/or diarrhea, caused by inflammation and/or mucosal damage from usually unknown insult to the stomach or intestines

SYNONYM(S)

Acute gastritis
Dietary indiscretion
Enteritis
"Garbage enteritis"

EPIDEMIOLOGY

SPECIES, AGE, SEX: Cats and dogs of any age; more common in dogs and young animals due to tendency for indiscriminate eating habits.

RISK FACTORS: Roaming behavior (greater possibility of indiscriminate ingestion).

ASSOCIATED CONDITIONS AND DISORDERS: In severe cases: dehydration, hypokalemia, hypochloremia, metabolic acidosis.

CLINICAL PRESENTATION

HISTORY, CHIEF COMPLAINT
- Acute onset of vomiting and/or diarrhea.
- Anorexia, lethargy are possible, but cases frequently involve no other clinical signs and the patient otherwise feels well.
- Owner may be aware of ingestion of garbage or spoiled food, table food, or nonfood items (rocks, wood, bones, etc.) before onset of signs.

PHYSICAL EXAM FINDINGS
- Usually unremarkable
- Normal vital parameters (temperature, heart rate, respiratory rate, pulse quality, blood pressure)
- Possible dehydration
- Palpation: absent to minimal discomfort, no anatomic abnormalities

ETIOLOGY AND PATHOPHYSIOLOGY

- Etiology is often not determined.
- Clinical signs are caused by ingestion of substances that disrupt gastrointestinal mucosal barrier and cause irritation, inflammation, or motility disturbance.
- Diagnosis usually based on history, no identifiable cause and response to supportive therapy.
- Dietary factors are most commonly associated with this condition (dietary indiscretion, spoiled food, food intolerance, consumption of garbage, fermentation products, plants, foreign material, or hair).
- Toxins and drugs may also cause acute, nonspecific gastroenteritis (antibiotics, nonsteroidal anti-inflammatory drugs [NSAIDs], corticosteroids, chemicals).
- Gastrointestinal infection with bacteria or bacterial toxins and parasites can result in mild, nonspecific signs that are

impossible to overtly distinguish from dietary indiscretion.

DIAGNOSIS

DIFFERENTIAL DIAGNOSIS

- Any cause of acute vomiting or diarrhea
- Infection: parasitic, bacterial, viral
- Drugs and toxins: drugs (NSAIDs, corticosteroids), heavy metal (zinc, lead), household chemicals (ethylene glycol, herbicides, pesticides, cleaning agents), plants (grass, mushrooms)
- Foreign body ingestion
- Systemic diseases: hypoadrenocorticism, liver disease, renal failure, pancreatitis

INITIAL DATABASE

- Extensive diagnostics usually not necessary if patient is bright, alert, and minimally dehydrated
- Complete blood count: stress leukogram common; polycythemia and hyperproteinemia possible if the patient is dehydrated
- Serum biochemistry profile: mild electrolyte abnormalities (e.g., hypokalemia, hypochloremia, metabolic alkalosis)
- Urinalysis: high specific gravity (>1.035) with hydration
- Fecal cytologic evaluation (flotation, direct smear): within normal limits
- Radiographs: generally unremarkable; fluid-filled bowel, ileus possible

TREATMENT

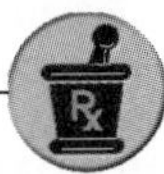

THERAPEUTIC GOAL(S)

- Provide supportive therapy until gastrointestinal (GI) tract returns to normal
- Remove underlying cause if known

ACUTE GENERAL TREATMENT

- Nothing by mouth (NPO) for 12 to 48 hours.
- Frequent small quantities of oral fluids may be offered if vomiting is infrequent.
- Subcutaneous crystalloids may be used for animals with mild dehydration deficits.
- Intravenous fluids are required if patient is moderately or severely dehydrated or has any evidence of hypovolemia.
- After vomiting has ceased for 12 hours, offer small amounts of water or ice cubes.
- Initial diet should be easily digestible starch, low protein, and low fat (such as cooked rice with cottage cheese or boiled chicken).
- Gastric acid–reducing drugs (H_2 blockers: famotidine [0.5 mg/kg PO, IV, or SC q 24h], ranitidine [0.5–2 mg/kg PO or SC q 12h], cimetidine [10 mg/kg PO, IV, or SC q 6–8h]): indicated if hematemesis or melena is present.
- Antiemetics: usually not necessary; metoclopramide (0.2–0.4 mg/kg SC q 8–12h) or phenothiazine derivatives (chlorpromazine, prochlorperazine) are good first choices if needed. Metoclopramide is contraindicated if obstruction is present.
- Protectants/adsorbants: bismuth subsalicylate (1 ml/4 kg PO up to q 4–6h), kaolin-pectin, activated charcoal and aluminum-, magnesium-, or barium-containing products are often used for coating GI mucosa and binding bacteria and their toxins.
- Anticholinergics (e.g., atropine, propantheline) are not recommended.
- Antibiotics are not indicated unless there is evidence of a bacterial cause or breech of GI mucosal integrity (hematemesis or melena).

DRUG INTERACTIONS

- High-dose phenothiazine derivative antiemetics (e.g., chlorpromazine, prochlorperazine) can cause or exacerbate hypotension, especially in dehydrated or hypovolemic patients.
- Bismuth subsalicylate should be used cautiously, especially in cats, due to generation of salicylate (aspirin) in intestine.
- Bismuth subsalicylate will normally cause stool to turn black in color, which can be mistaken for melena.

RECOMMENDED MONITORING

- Vital parameters
- Frequency, volume, and character of diarrhea and vomiting

PROGNOSIS AND OUTCOME

Prognosis is excellent; this disorder usually resolves 24 to 48 hours after onset of signs

PEARLS & CONSIDERATIONS

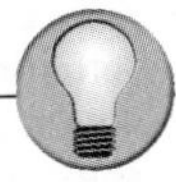

COMMENTS

- If vomiting is not frequent, foregoing antiemetics allows better assessment of response to supportive therapy. If no response occurs within 1 to 2 days, other differentials should be investigated.
- Animals with marked dehydration or hypovolemia at presentation should have more detailed diagnostic evaluation; acute nonspecific gastroenteritis rarely produces severe systemic signs.

SUGGESTED READING

Webb C, Twedt DC: Canine gastritis. *Vet Clin North Am Small Anim Pract* 33(5):969–985, v–vi, 2003.

AUTHOR: **AMIE KOENIG**
EDITOR: **DEBRA L. ZORAN**

Gastrointestinal Endocrine Disease

BASIC INFORMATION

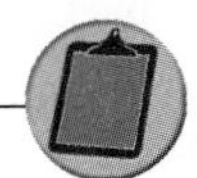

DEFINITION

Gastrointestinal (GI) endocrine disease occurs as a result of a tumor of one or more hormone-secreting cells in the GI tract. Insulinoma is discussed elsewhere (see Insulinoma, p 598); see Gastrinoma, p 433 for additional details concerning gastrinoma.

SYNONYM(S)

General: amine precursor uptake and decarboxylation (APUD) tumors; APUDoma
Specific: gastrinoma (Zollinger-Ellison syndrome), VIPoma (Verner-Morrison syndrome)

EPIDEMIOLOGY

SPECIES, AGE, SEX

- Gastrinoma: rare; middle-aged to old dogs and cats
- Glucagonoma: rare; middle-aged to old dogs; not reported in cats
- Carcinoid syndrome: rare; middle-aged to old dogs and cats

ASSOCIATED CONDITIONS AND DISORDERS: Hepatocutaneous syndrome (necrolytic migratory erythema) and diabetes mellitus: glucagonoma.

CLINICAL PRESENTATION

DISEASE FORMS/SUBTYPES

- Gastrinoma: gastrin

- Glucagonoma: glucagon
- Carcinoid syndrome: serotonin
- Somatostatinomas*: somatostatin
- Pancreatic polypeptide-oma*: pancreatic polypeptide
- VIPoma*: vasoactive intestinal polypeptide

HISTORY, CHIEF COMPLAINT

- Gastrinoma: vomiting, weight loss, anorexia, diarrhea
- Glucagonoma: ulcerative dermatitis, diarrhea, lethargy, weight loss, inappetance, possible polyuria and polydipsia
- Carcinoid syndrome: often no overt clinical signs; possible abdominal pain, vomiting, weight loss, anorexia

PHYSICAL EXAM FINDINGS

- Gastrinoma: weight loss, lethargy, abdominal pain, pale mucous membranes, melena, and/or collapse and shock as a result of GI ulceration
- Glucagonoma: ulcerative dermatitis, lethargy
- Carcinoid syndrome: no specific findings; possible anorexia, weight loss, acute abdomen due to obstruction

ETIOLOGY AND PATHOPHYSIOLOGY

- Specialized endocrine cells that secrete peptides are found throughout the GI tract.
- Neoplasia of these cells results in excess secretion of the hormone(s).
- Clinical signs occur as a result of the specific hormone oversecretion.

DIAGNOSIS

DIFFERENTIAL DIAGNOSIS

See Vomiting, pp 1157–1160; Weight Loss, p 1162; Diarrhea (Acute), p 294; Acute Abdomen, p 29; Ulcerative and Erosive Skin Disorders, p 1108; Hepatocutaneous Syndrome, p 506

INITIAL DATABASE

- The diagnosis is made based on appropriate clinical signs and immunohistochemical staining of the tumor
- A complete blood count, serum biochemical profile, and urinalysis should be evaluated to help rule out other diagnoses.
    - Mild hyperglycemia, increased liver enzymes, hypoalbuminemia, and possible glucosuria may be seen with glucagonoma.
    - A regenerative or iron-deficiency anemia, possible leukocytosis, hypoproteinemia, and increased liver enzymes may be seen with gastrinoma.
    - Results are usually normal with carcinoid syndrome.
- Radiographs and ultrasound results are usually normal but may help identify the primary tumor or metastatic lesions.

ADVANCED OR CONFIRMATORY TESTING

- Glucagonoma: Increased plasma glucagon concentrations (in the absence of other diseases causing hyperglucagonemia), histopathology of skin lesions, and hypoaminoacidemia are supportive. Results of liver function tests are normal (versus abnormal function with hepatocutaneous syndrome).
- Gastrinoma: Increased fasting serum gastrin concentration (in the absence of other diseases causing hypergastrinemia) and gastric hyperacidity; GI ulceration and/or increased gastric rugal folds seen with endoscopy or contrast radiography; and excessive response to a gastrin-secretagogue (secretin or calcium) are supportive.
- Carcinoid syndrome: Increased serotonin metabolites (5-hydroxyindoleacetic acid) in urine are supportive.
- Confirmation requires immunohistochemical staining of the tumor.

TREATMENT

THERAPEUTIC GOAL(S)

- Removal of tumor
- Management of associated clinical signs

ACUTE GENERAL TREATMENT

- Fluid and electrolyte abnormalities should be corrected if present.
- Gastrinoma: treat hyperacidity and GI ulceration (see Gastric Ulcer, p 431).
- Surgical removal of the primary tumor and any visible metastasis, if possible. With gastrinoma, ulcer excision may also be needed.
- If the pancreas is manipulated during surgery, treat postoperatively for pancreatitis (see Pancreatitis, pp 794–798).

CHRONIC TREATMENT

- Because of the high incidence of metastasis at the time of diagnosis, surgery is not often curative and subsequent medical management is needed.
- Gastrinoma: treat hyperacidity and GI ulcerations (see above); somatostatin analog treatment (octreotide: 2 μg/kg SQ q 12h up to 10–20 μg/kg SQ q 8h) can be tried.
- Glucagonoma: amino acid supplementation (eggs, prescription diets, possible IV amino acid infusion) has been suggested but is unproven; manage skin lesions (see Hepatocutaneous Syndrome, p 506, Ulcerative and Erosive Skin Disorders, p 1108); octreotide (6 μg/kg SQ q 8h) can be tried.
- Effective chemotherapy for these tumors has not been reported in the dog and cat.

POSSIBLE COMPLICATIONS

The most common postoperative complication is pancreatitis in dogs.

RECOMMENDED MONITORING

Monitor recurrence of clinical signs

PROGNOSIS AND OUTCOME

- Glucagonoma: poor if concurrent advanced liver disease (mean 5 months) or metastasis
- Gastrinoma: poor long-term prognosis because metastasis is present in 70% of cases at time of diagnosis (mean 8 months)
- Carcinoid syndrome: many are clinically silent and are found postmortem. Prognosis is guarded if metastatic disease is present

PEARLS & CONSIDERATIONS

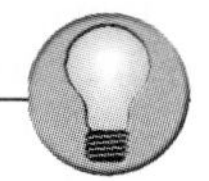

COMMENTS

These are complex tumors and very difficult to diagnose; referral to a specialist center is advised.

SUGGESTED READING

Feldman EC, Nelson RW: Gastrinoma, glucagonoma, and other APUDomas. In Feldman EC, Nelson RW (eds): *Canine and Feline Endocrinology and Reproduction*, ed 3. Philadelphia, WB Saunders, 2004, pp 645–658.

Johnson SE: Pancreatic APUDomas. *Semin Vet Med Surg Small Anim Pract* 4:202–211, 1989.

AUTHOR: **NINETTE KELLER**

EDITOR: **SHERRI IHLE**

Gastrointestinal Obstruction: Foreign Body or Neoplasia

BASIC INFORMATION

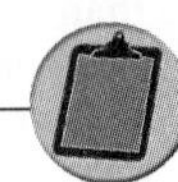

DEFINITION

Disorder caused by a foreign object or mass that partially or completely occludes the intestinal lumen

SYNONYM(S)

Intraluminal obstruction

EPIDEMIOLOGY

RISK FACTORS

- Younger animals are at greater risk for dietary indiscretion and therefore foreign body ingestion.
- Some animals are more prone to ingesting foreign objects than others (individual behavior) irrespective of age.
- Older animals are at greater risk for development of neoplasia.

ASSOCIATED CONDITIONS AND DISORDERS: Animals with diseases that cause pica may be more at risk for foreign object ingestion.

CLINICAL PRESENTATION

HISTORY, CHIEF COMPLAINT

- Vomiting, anorexia, and depression are common primary complaints.
- Severity of clinical signs varies depending on duration and location of obstruction.
- Proximal and complete obstructions are generally associated with more severe clinical signs of illness.
- Distal or partial obstructions may be associated with vague and chronic signs such as intermittent vomiting, anorexia, weight loss, or diarrhea. When associated with gastrointestinal (GI) obstruction, diarrhea is usually scant and not profuse.

PHYSICAL EXAM FINDINGS

- Abdominal splinting or signs of pain on palpation may be noted.
- Mass or foreign object may be identified with careful palpation.
- Dehydration, depression or shock; severe in proximal and complete obstructions.

ETIOLOGY AND PATHOPHYSIOLOGY

- Mechanical obstruction of the intestinal lumen causes fluid and gas accumulation proximal to the foreign object or mass.
- Duodenal and proximal jejunal obstruction is often associated with acute and severe signs.
- Persistent vomiting and loss of gastric secretions associated with proximal obstructions may lead to electrolyte imbalances (hypochloremic metabolic alkalosis).
- Lymphatic and capillary stasis cause intestinal wall edema.
- Impaired intestinal mucosal barrier allows bacterial translocation potentially resulting in endotoxemia and sepsis.
- High intraluminal pressure causes intestinal wall ischemia that may progress to necrosis and peritonitis.

DIAGNOSIS

The diagnosis is suspected based on history and physical examination, is supported by radiographic findings, and is confirmed surgically.

DIFFERENTIAL DIAGNOSIS

- Foreign body
- Mass
- Intussusception
- Linear foreign body
- Trichobezoar
- Intestinal volvulus or torsion
- Stricture or adhesions
- Functional obstruction (i.e., ileus)
- Infectious disease of the GI tract (e.g., parvoviral or coronaviral enteritis)
- Intoxication

INITIAL DATABASE

- Complete blood count, serum biochemistry profile, and urinalysis.
  - Evidence of dehydration (e.g., blood urea nitrogen, creatinine elevations with urine specific gravity >1.030; hemoconcentration/elevated packed cell volume).
  - Electrolyte imbalances (hypochloremia, hypokalemia).
  - Metabolic alkalosis with proximal obstruction; metabolic acidosis with hypoperfusion, sepsis secondary to peritonitis, or other systemic effects.
- Abdominal radiographs:
  - Radiopaque foreign objects may be visualized.
  - Fluid or gas distended intestinal loops.
  - Pathologic dilation of intestinal loops: bowel lumen should not exceed the diameter of twice the width of a rib or be greater than 1.6 times the height of the fifth lumbar vertebra (Figs. I-82 and I-83).
  - Radiographs that demonstrate a foreign body must be recent (minutes or hours before induction of general anesthesia, or better still, retaken just after induction) if surgery is planned. A gastric or duodenal foreign body can be displaced into the esophagus during anesthetic induction, while an intestinal foreign body may have been defecated since the original radiographs were taken.

ADVANCED OR CONFIRMATORY TESTING

- Contrast radiographs (see Upper Gastrointestinal Radiographic Contrast Series, p 1316; Foreign Body, Linear Gastrointestine, p 403).
  - Barium sulfate suspension for upper GI study unless perforation suspected.
    - If perforation suspected, consider using nonionic iodinated contrast medium or other diagnostic techniques (centesis, lavage).
  - Barium enema.
    - For assessing an obstructive pattern in the distal intestine.
    - For differentiating small bowel from large bowel if it is not clear whether a gas-filled viscus is a pathologically distended segment of small intestine or the normal colon.
- Abdominocentesis and fluid analysis if perforation/peritonitis suspected.
- Abdominal ultrasound.
  - Identification of small amounts of free fluid.
  - Localization of free fluid for accurate centesis.
- Diagnostic peritoneal lavage.
  - If peritonitis is suspected but centesis is unrewarding.
  - Limited efficacy.
- Thoracic radiographs in older animals with suspected neoplasia.

TREATMENT

THERAPEUTIC GOAL(S)

- Correct dehydration and electrolyte abnormalities with intravenous fluid administration
- Exploratory laparotomy is indicated to relieve the obstruction

ACUTE GENERAL TREATMENT

- Exploratory laparotomy for foreign body retrieval or mass resection.
- An enterotomy may suffice for acute foreign body removal; if intestinal viability is questionable, perform a resection and anastomosis.
- Wide margin (4 to 8 cm) resection and anastomosis should be performed if neoplastic disease is suspected based on the gross appearance of the lesion. In this case, also perform lymph node and liver biopsies.
- Omentum or serosal patch may be placed to reinforce suture line.
- Change gloves and surgical instruments before abdominal lavage and closure to minimize contamination.

- Administer prophylactic antibiotics.
  - Cefazolin, 22 mg/kg IV q 2h during the perioperative period.
- Obtain gastric, small intestinal, and liver biopsies, even if GI tract appears grossly normal. Biopsy any abnormal-looking organ. Future course of illness may evolve in such a way as to make these specimens essential for diagnosis.

CHRONIC TREATMENT

Postoperative considerations

- Continue rehydration and daily electrolyte monitoring. Treat accordingly (especially hypokalemia arising from dilution [IV fluids] and anorexia).
- Nothing by mouth (NPO) 12 hours postenterotomy, 12 to 24 hours postresection and anastomosis.
- Administer GI protectants as needed.
  - Famotidine 0.5-1 mg/kg IV, IM, SC, or PO q 12-24h; or
  - Ranitidine 0.5-2 mg/kg IV, IM, SC, or PO q 8-12h.
    - Ranitidine also has promotility properties similar to those of metoclopramide.
- Administer antiemetics as needed.
  - Contraindicated before resolution of obstruction.
  - Metoclopramide 0.2-0.4 mg/kg PO, SC, or IM q 6h; or
  - Cisapride 0.1-0.5 mg/kg PO q 8h.

POSSIBLE COMPLICATIONS

- Dehiscence: animals should be monitored in hospital for 48 to 72 hours in the postoperative period for signs of peritonitis. Risk factors include presence of preoperative peritonitis, serum albumin concentration <2.5 g/dl, and presence of a foreign body (vs. neoplastic disease).
- Ileus.
- Short bowel syndrome: unlikely if less than 70% of small intestine resected.
- Stricture.
- Recurrence.

RECOMMENDED MONITORING

- The following parameters should be monitored daily until discharge from hospital:
  - Body temperature
  - Blood glucose
  - Electrolytes
  - Abdominal pain
- The patient should be eating and not vomiting:
  - If anorexia or vomiting persists after surgery, consider performing abdominocentesis and complete blood cell count to evaluate for possible development of peritonitis

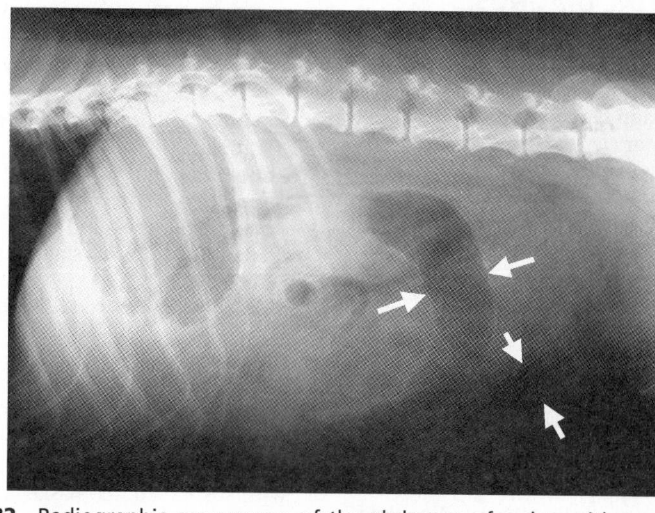

FIGURE I-82 Radiographic appearance of the abdomen of a dog with small intestinal obstruction, lateral view. A small intestinal segment is markedly distended with gas (*arrows*) and another is markedly distended with fluid/soft tissue (*short arrows*). Courtesy of Dr. Richard Walshaw.

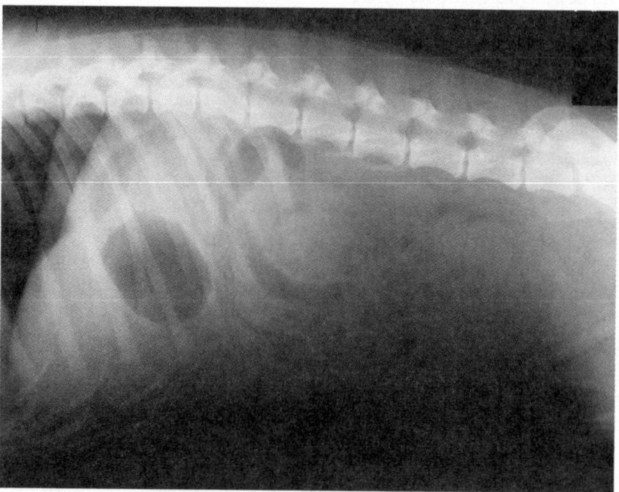

FIGURE I-83 Radiographic appearance of a 5-year-old Labrador dog (different dog from Fig. I-82), also with small intestinal obstruction; lateral view. Several loops of gas-distended intestine are present. Exploratory laparotomy revealed a mid-jejunal obstruction caused by a foreign body (corn cob). Courtesy of Dr. Patricia Rose.

PROGNOSIS AND OUTCOME

- A good prognosis may be expected for acute disease, while those animals with preoperative debilitation or shock should be given a more guarded prognosis.
- Prognosis for neoplastic disease depends on histopathologic grade, evidence of metastasis, and completeness of surgical excision. Lymphosarcoma and adenocarcinoma are the most frequently encountered intestinal tumors.

PEARLS & CONSIDERATIONS

COMMENTS

Consider placing an intraoperative feeding tube (esophagostomy, gastrostomy, or gastrojejunostomy tube) in these patients based on preoperative nutritional status, degree of patient debilitation, or anticipated postoperative anorexia.

SUGGESTED READING

Fossum TW, Hedlund CS: Gastric and intestinal surgery. *Vet Clin North Am Small Anim Pract* 33:1117, 2003.

Graham JP, et al: Quantitative estimation of intestinal dilation as a predictor of obstruction in the dog. *J Small Anim Pract* 39:521, 1998.

Macphail C: Gastrointestinal obstruction. *Clin Tech Small Anim Pract* 17:178, 2002.

Ralphs CS, et al: Risk factors for leakage following intestinal anastomosis in dogs and cats: 115 cases (1991-2000). *J Am Vet Med Assoc* 223:73, 2003.

AUTHOR: **JANET KOVAK**

EDITOR: **RICHARD WALSHAW**

Giardiasis

Client Education Sheet on Website

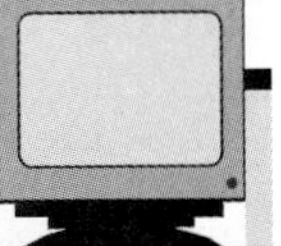

BASIC INFORMATION

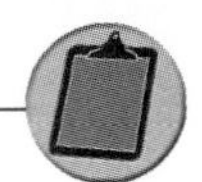

DEFINITION

Giardia lamblia is a flagellate protozoan parasite that can be found in the intestinal tract of humans and most domestic animals. Giardiasis can cause protracted intermittent diarrhea in some individuals but can exist as a latent infection in others.

EPIDEMIOLOGY

SPECIES, AGE, SEX: Can affect humans and most domestic animals. Younger animals may be more susceptible.

RISK FACTORS: Immunodeficient adults, young animals, and animals confined in large groups are at increased risk.

CONTAGION AND ZOONOSIS: *Giardia* isolates do not appear to be highly host specific; zoonosis from dogs and cats to people should be considered possible.

CLINICAL PRESENTATION

HISTORY, CHIEF COMPLAINT

- Most infections produce no clinical signs.
- If diarrhea results, it can be acute and short lived, intermittent, or chronic.
- Steatorrhea or weight loss may be observed.
- Emesis, fever, and anorexia may occur but are not typical.
- Signs consistent with either acute or chronic large bowel diarrhea occur in cats.

PHYSICAL EXAM FINDINGS: No specific abnormalities.

ETIOLOGY AND PATHOPHYSIOLOGY

- The *Giardia* life cycle is direct. Cysts are ingested and excyst in the duodenum, each cyst producing two motile trophozoites that replicate within the lumen of the small intestine. Before being shed in feces, the trophozoite encysts. On excretion, the cysts are infective to another host. Cysts can survive for days to weeks in a cool, moist environment.
- Trophozoites are thought to cause sloughing of intestinal epithelial cells, resulting in blunting of the intestinal villi and subsequent reduction in absorptive surface area causing malabsorption.
- Abnormalities in cellular and humoral immune system likely predispose individuals to clinical infection.
- Immunosuppressive drugs may predispose to clinical infection.

DIAGNOSIS

DIFFERENTIAL DIAGNOSIS

- Intestinal parasitism
- Idiopathic inflammatory bowel disease
- Maldigestion secondary to pancreatic exocrine insufficiency
- Neoplastic intestinal disease (i.e., lymphoma)
- Infectious intestinal disease (viral, bacterial, fungal)
- Food intolerance or dietary indiscretion (acute cases)

INITIAL DATABASE

- Fecal suspension: observation of trophozoites in fresh feces.
  - Feces mixed with a drop of saline and examined microscopically at 40 × under a coverslip with the condenser in the lowest position.
  - Positive result is definitive; negative result does not rule out infection.
- Fecal flotation: zinc sulphate concentration technique. Sensitivity is increased by examining two or more fresh fecal samples obtained over 3 to 5 days. If samples are shipped for testing, they should be maintained at 4°C.

ADVANCED OR CONFIRMATORY TESTING

- Enzyme-linked immunosorbent assay (ELISA) kits to identify fecal *Giardia* antigens. Fresh, frozen, or formalin-preserved feces suitable. Sensitivity of one ELISA is similar to the sensitivity of two or more fecal samples tested using zinc sulfate concentration.
- Direct immunofluorescent testing. This test detects *Giardia* cysts in feces. Feces should be preserved in 10% formalin before being shipped to the laboratory.

TREATMENT

THERAPEUTIC GOAL(S)

- Eliminate clinical signs of *Giardia* infection including diarrhea and weight loss
- Eliminate shedding of infective cysts

ACUTE GENERAL TREATMENT

- Fenbendazole (50 mg/kg PO q 24h for 3 days): 90–100% effective in eliminating cysts in feces of dogs.
- Fenbendazole (25 mg/kg PO q 12h for 7 days) is safe and effective in the cat.
- Metronidazole (15–30 mg/kg PO q 12–24h for 5 to 7 days [dogs]; 10–25 mg/kg PO q 12–24h for 5 to 7 days [cat]) as second choice. Less effective than fenbendazole.
- *Giardia* vaccination has not been shown to be an effective treatment.

CHRONIC TREATMENT

- Autoinfection from fecal material adhered to the haircoat or cysts in a moist, cold environment is possible due to short prepatent period (resulting in cysts being infective, including autoinfective, when excreted in the feces).
- Reinfection is probable in catteries and kennels due to environmental contamination.
- Allowing the environment to dry, cleaning contaminated surfaces with disinfectants containing quarternary ammonium, bathing animals, and retreating before returning to the clean environment are important in preventing reinfection.

POSSIBLE COMPLICATIONS

- Mild diarrhea is a possible side effect with fenbendazole.
- Albendazole (alternative to fenbendazole): myelosuppression, hepatotoxicity (especially in cats) and suspected teratogen. Not recommended.

PROGNOSIS AND OUTCOME

- Prognosis variable; many individuals may be cured with prompt diagnosis and appropriate treatment, but recurrent clinical signs due to persistent infection are well documented.
- Because treatment efficacy has been evaluated based on the elimination of cysts from the feces rather than on removal of organisms from the intestinal tract, cure rates are not known.

PEARLS & CONSIDERATIONS

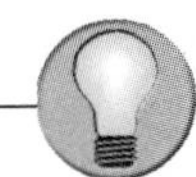

COMMENTS

- Empiric fenbendazole treatment is recommended in dogs with diarrhea, to address both *Giardia* and occult whipworm infection as possible underlying causes.
- The *Giardia* vaccine may be effective in reducing fecal shedding of cysts in dogs but is ineffective in prevention of infection. In a study of cats, the vaccine was ineffective for both.

SUGGESTED READING

Barr SC: Enteric protozoal infections. In Greene CE (ed): *Infectious Disease of the Dog and Cat*, ed 2. Philadelphia, WB Saunders, 1998, pp 482-486.

Guilford WG, et al: Gastrointestinal tract infections, parasites and toxicoses. In Guilford GW, et al (eds): *Strombeck's Small Animal Gastroenterology*. Philadelphia, WB Saunders, 1996, pp 411-432.

AUTHOR: **LAURA J. SMALLWOOD**
EDITOR: **DEBRA L. ZORAN**

Glaucoma

Client Education Sheet on Website

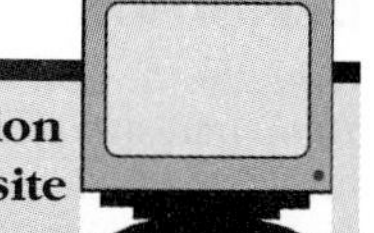

BASIC INFORMATION

DEFINITION

- The glaucomas are a group of diseases characterized by visual impairment and blindness from damage to the retina and optic nerve from increased intraocular pressure (IOP).
- Glaucoma may be the result of primary eye disease (i.e., abnormalities of the drainage/iridocorneal angle; *primary glaucoma*), secondary to other eye diseases (*secondary glaucoma*), or, less commonly, the result of anomalies of the anterior segment of the eye (*congenital glaucoma*).
- The overall prevalence of the primary glaucomas in dogs in North America is 0.9%, while that of the secondary glaucomas in dogs is 0.8%.

SYNONYM(S)

Buphthalmos
Megaloglobus (enlargement of the globe secondary to elevated IOP)

EPIDEMIOLOGY

SPECIES, AGE, SEX

- Dogs and cats:
  - Typically no sex predisposition.
  - Variable age of onset depending on underlying cause.
- *Primary glaucoma:*
  - Mainly affects middle-aged to older dogs (3 to 12 years; average age 8 years); rare in cats.
  - In some breeds of dogs, primary glaucoma occurs more frequently in females.
- *Secondary glaucoma* due to:
  - Lens luxation: usually affects young to middle-aged dogs (3 to 7 years); older cats.
  - Intraocular neoplasia: usually older animals (>7 years).
- *Congenital glaucoma:*
  - Young animals; elevation in IOP develops soon after birth.

GENETICS AND BREED PREDISPOSITION

- *Primary glaucoma*:
  - Dogs: affects about 20 breeds.
  - Top breeds of dogs affected between 1994 and 2002 include American cocker spaniel, basset hound, chow chow, shar-pei, Boston terrier, wire fox terrier, Norwegian elkhound, Siberian husky, cairn terrier, and miniature poodle.
  - Primary open angle glaucoma is inherited in the beagle as an autosomal recessive trait.
  - Primary closed angle glaucoma in the Welsh springer spaniel and Great Dane appears inherited as an autosomal dominant trait with variable expression.
  - Cats: Siamese breed may have inherited primary glaucoma.
- *Secondary glaucoma* from lens luxation: terrier breeds.

RISK FACTORS

- *Primary glaucoma*:
  - Breed predisposition.
  - Abnormalities of the iridocorneal angle (often termed *pectinate ligament dysplasia*) may narrow the opening to the sclerociliary cleft and increase the probability of glaucoma (dogs).
- *Secondary glaucoma*:
  - Anterior uveitis due to:
    - Cataract formation (common in dogs).
    - Systemic bacterial and mycotic diseases (dogs and cats).
    - Feline leukemia and feline immunodeficiency viruses (cats).
  - Lens luxation (see Lens Luxation, p 628).
  - Intraocular neoplasia (see Intraocular Neoplasia, p 603).
  - Hyphema (see Hyphema, p 560).
  - Uveal cysts (see Uveal Cysts, p 1133).

CLINICAL PRESENTATION

DISEASE FORMS/SUBTYPES: Glaucoma may be classified based on:

- Cause: primary, secondary, or congenital
- Duration: acute (vision potential) versus chronic (typically blind, buphthalmic eye)

HISTORY, CHIEF COMPLAINT: Transient or constant red or cloudy eye with any or all of the following:

- Variable ocular pain (usually present when IOP exceeds 40 mmHg), manifesting as unwillingness to be handled around the face or head, or blepharospasm.
- Bumping into objects or other manifestations of visual impairment or blindness.
- Increased green shine from eye (i.e., tapetal reflection from dilated pupil).
- Enlargement of the globe (buphthalmos).

PHYSICAL EXAM FINDINGS: Unilateral or bilateral ocular changes; initially unilateral with primary glaucoma:

- Corneal edema (typically diffuse)
- Episcleral hyperemia (tortuous episcleral vessels)
- Dilated pupil and sluggish to absent pupillary light reflexes
- Possible lens subluxation/luxation
- Variable optic nerve and retinal degeneration (see Retinal Degeneration, p 963)
- Corneal stria (breaks in Descemet's membrane appearing as white lines within cornea; rare)

ETIOLOGY AND PATHOPHYSIOLOGY

- Impediment to aqueous humor outflow causing elevated IOP.
- Elevated IOP can damage the retina (retinal ganglion cells) and optic nerve head by reducing retinal, choroidal, and optic nerve head blood flow and axoplasmic flow in the optic nerve head.
- Onset and severity of these glaucomatous changes appear influenced by the duration and extent of the IOP elevation.
- About 50% of first eyes of dogs presented with the primary glaucomas are blind at initial ophthalmic examination.

DIAGNOSIS

DIFFERENTIAL DIAGNOSIS

Glaucoma must be differentiated from other causes of red eye, including:

- Anterior uveitis
- Severe conjunctivitis
- Episcleritis/scleritis

INITIAL DATABASE

Complete ophthalmic examination including:

- Tonometry (the measurement of IOP): the most important diagnostic test
  - Schiøtz indentation tonometry (requires conversion of value from instrument to mmHg using human calibration chart accompanying instrument or dog/cat calibration chart).
  - Applanation tonometry (e.g., Tonopen).
  - Normal IOP values range from 15-25 mmHg; >30 mmHg = glaucoma (dogs and cats).

ADVANCED OR CONFIRMATORY TESTING

- Referral to veterinary ophthalmologist for:
  - Additional or multiple tonometric measurements
  - Gonioscopy (direct observation of the iridocorneal angle)
  - Ophthalmoscopy of the ocular fundus (posterior segment of the eye including retina and optic nerve)
- Ocular ultrasound if ocular media opaque and prevents evaluation of deeper ocular structures; helps rule out concurrent ocular abnormalities (i.e., lens luxation; retinal detachment)

TREATMENT

THERAPEUTIC GOAL(S)

- Lower IOP of affected eye to:
  - Maintain vision for as long as possible
  - Eliminate ocular pain
- Prophylactic therapy of the fellow eye with IOP-lowering drugs to delay onset of glaucoma from about 6 months (without prophylactic treatment) to 30 months (with prophylactic treatment) (*primary glaucoma*).
- Without tonometry, potential glaucoma patients should be referred to a veterinary ophthalmologist (as an emergency) for IOP measurement.

ACUTE GENERAL TREATMENT

Medical:

- Regardless of the type of glaucoma, the following may be administered initially and then long term if indicated:
  - Topical β-adrenergic antagonists or blockers (0.5% timolol or 0.5% betaxolol, usually q 8h); *and*
  - Topical or systemic carbonic anhydrase inhibitors (topical: 2% dorzolamide or 1% brinzolamide q 8h; oral: methazolamide 5 mg/kg q 12h).
- Mannitol (1-2 g/kg IV over 20 minutes) to rapidly lower IOP (first effects in 1 to 2 hours; maximum effect in 4 to 6 hours; and duration of about 8 to 10 hours) when there is a chance for return of vision (e.g., acute primary glaucoma).
- Topical (1% q 6h) and/or systemic (1-2 mg/kg PO q 24h) prednisolone is indicated when anterior uveitis is also present, unless an infectious cause for the uveitis is documented or strongly suspected (see Uveitis, p 1134).

CHRONIC TREATMENT

- Medical:
  - Topical prostaglandins (PGF analogs 0.005% lantanoprost; 0.03% brimatoprost; or 0.004% travoprost q12-24h) (used for primary glaucoma in dogs; not effective in the feline glaucomas).
  - ± Topical and/or systemic prednisolone (when anterior uveitis also present; taper to lowest effective dose).
  - In all of the breed-related *primary glaucomas*, the disease continues to progress (even though IOP may be controlled) and often combinations of several topical and systemic IOP-lowering drugs or surgery (see below) are eventually necessary.
- Surgical:
  - Anterior chamber shunts and laser cyclophotocoagulation are procedures offered by most veterinary ophthalmologists to prolong vision and prevent ocular pain.
  - Removal of the lens (referrable procedure; glaucoma secondary to lens luxation, see p 628).
  - End-stage blind and buphthalmic glaucomatous globes may be treated by:
    - Enucleation.
    - Evisceration and intrascleral prosthesis.
    - Intravitreal gentamicin injection.
    - Enucleation or evisceration and implant surgeries should be followed with histopathologic examination of the removed tissue, to help determine cause of glaucoma (i.e., primary vs. secondary) and prognosis for fellow eye.

DRUG INTERACTIONS

- Topical β-adrenergic blockers may lower heart rate and blood pressure, and may cause bronchoconstriction in the small breeds of dogs and cats.
- Systemic carbonic anhydrase inhibitors in dogs and cats may cause metabolic acidosis and electrolyte imbalances as evidenced by depression (perhaps related to hypokalemia), and in dogs, vomiting and diarrhea that require drug cessation.
- Topical prostaglandins often cause conjunctival hyperemia within minutes after instillation that gradually declines over an hour or so, and miosis that persists with the IOP reduction.
- Mannitol, an osmotic diuretic, should be avoided in patients with heart disease (risk of fluid overload/iatrogenic pulmonary edema).

POSSIBLE COMPLICATIONS

With poor or inadequate control of IOP, any or all of the following may occur:

- Buphthalmos (see Ocular Size Abnormalities, p 763) causing increased corneal exposure ±:
  - Recurrent corneal ulceration
  - Corneal vascularization
  - Corneal pigmentation
- Lens luxation/subluxation (see Lens Luxation, p 628)
- Optic nerve and retinal degeneration (see Retinal Degeneration, p 963)
- Blindness

RECOMMENDED MONITORING

- Regular re-examinations with tonometry (see Initial Database above) (i.e., monthly once IOP control initially achieved) are necessary to control IOP (should be maintained at levels of ≤ 20-25 mmHg) and maintain vision for as long as possible.
- As the glaucoma progresses, increased frequency and/or additional topical and systemic drugs to lower IOP are usually necessary.

PROGNOSIS AND OUTCOME

- Variable depending on underlying cause.
- Prognosis is usually poor for the first eye presented with the primary glaucomas in dogs because the disease is often advanced and refractory to medical therapy.
- Prognosis for the fellow eye is better, and prophylactic therapy with a β-adrenergic blocker or prostaglandin can significantly delay the onset of glaucoma for up to about 30 months.

PEARLS & CONSIDERATIONS

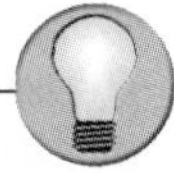

COMMENTS

- Patients with dilated pupils, corneal edema, and conjunctival hyperemia require tonometry to estimate IOP.
- Clinical management of the glaucomas is difficult; therefore referral of these cases to a veterinary ophthalmologist is advised.
- Medical therapy of the glaucomas is expensive and is often required long-term.
- Buphthalmos indicates chronic glaucoma, whereas acute glaucoma, with its potentially better prognosis for vision, presents episcleral injection, and almost never buphthalmos.
- Even in a permanently blind, persistently glaucomatous eye, treatment (e.g., evisceration and implant, or enucleation) is generally indicated to remove the source of chronic intense pain.

- Digital pressure (pressing on the eyes through closed eyelids) cannot be used for accurately assessing intraocular pressure.

PREVENTION

The benefits of periodic tonometry in breeds and/or eyes at risk are unknown but should be considered.

CLIENT EDUCATION

- The primary glaucomas in the dog are concentrated in about 20 breeds.
- Of the secondary glaucomas in the dog, about 80% are related to cataract formation and lens-induced uveitis.
- Dogs with cataracts that are not surgical candidates require periodic eye examinations and tonometry indefinitely.

SUGGESTED READING

Gelatt KN, MacKay EO: Prevalence of the breed-related glaucomas in the pure-bred dogs in North America. *Vet Ophthalmol* 7:97, 2004.

Gelatt KN, MacKay EO: The secondary glaucomas in the dog in North America. *Vet Ophthalmol* 7:245, 2004.

Gelatt KN, Brooks DE: The canine glaucomas. In Gelatt KN (ed): *Veterinary Ophthalmology*, ed 3. Baltimore, Lippincott/Williams & Wilkins, 1999, pp 701-754.

AUTHOR: **KIRK N. GELATT**
EDITOR: **CHERYL L. CULLEN**

Glomerulonephritis

BASIC INFORMATION

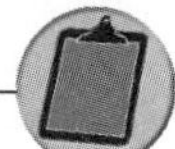

DEFINITION

Glomerulonephritis is a common cause of proteinuria due to immune complex deposition in the glomeruli and resultant inflammation. The condition is often idiopathic, but it can result from inflammatory, infectious, or neoplastic disease processes.

EPIDEMIOLOGY

SPECIES, AGE, SEX: Dogs affected more often than cats, with no gender predilection. While animals of any age may be affected, most are middle-aged or older at diagnosis.

GENETICS AND BREED PREDISPOSITION: Membranoproliferative glomerulonephritis

- Bernese mountain dogs
- Labrador retrievers and golden retrievers with positive *Borrelia* titers

RISK FACTORS

- Chronic bacterial infections (e.g., pyoderma, endocarditis, pyelonephritis, borreliosis, bartonellosis, mycoplasmal polyarthritis)
- Fungal infection (e.g., coccidioidomycosis)
- Parasitic (e.g., heartworm disease)
- Rickettsial disease (e.g., ehrlichiosis)
- Protozoal infection (e.g., babesiosis, hepatozoonosis, leishmaniasis, trypanosomiasis)
- Viral disease (e.g., feline immunodeficiency virus, feline leukemia virus, canine adenovirus)
- Neoplasia (e.g., mastocytosis, leukemia, lymphoma, systemic histiocytosis)
- Immune-mediated disease (e.g., polyarthritis, pemphigus, systemic lupus erythematosus)
- Chronic inflammatory disease (e.g., inflammatory bowel disease, pancreatitis, cholangiohepatitis)
- Corticosteroid excess
- Trimethoprim-sulfa therapy
- Congenital C3 deficiency

CONTAGION AND ZOONOSIS: Some causes of secondary glomerulonephritis are zoonotic (e.g., leptospirosis, leishmaniasis).

GEOGRAPHY AND SEASONALITY: Several causes of secondary glomerulonephritis have specific geographic distributions (e.g., borreliosis in the northeastern and north central United States).

ASSOCIATED CONDITIONS AND DISORDERS

- Protein-losing nephropathy
- Nephrotic syndrome
- Chronic renal failure
- Hypertension
- Hyperlipidemia
- Thromboembolic disease, including pulmonary thromboembolism

CLINICAL PRESENTATION

DISEASE FORMS/SUBTYPES: Morphologic classification: histopathologic (clinical correlates to therapy and prognosis not as well developed as in human nephrology).

- Membranoproliferative glomerulonephritis: most common
  - Type I: mesangiocapillary glomerulonephritis associated with infectious disease, it is the most common type
  - Type II: dense deposit disease
- Proliferative glomerulonephritis: relatively rare

HISTORY, CHIEF COMPLAINT: Clinical signs may be absent. When signs are present, they may be due to renal failure (see Chronic Renal Failure, Overt ["Symptomatic"], p 205), nephrotic syndrome (see Nephrotic Syndrome, p 749), or to the underlying disease responsible for glomerulonephritis:

- Vomiting
- Lethargy
- Anorexia
- Weight loss
- Peripheral edema
- Pendulous abdomen (ascites)
- Polyuria/polydipsia
- Halitosis (uremia)
- Dyspnea/panting
- Blindness (systemic hypertension)
- Signs associated with underlying infectious, inflammatory, or neoplastic disease

PHYSICAL EXAM FINDINGS: Clinical findings may be absent or may include:

- Weight loss
- Dehydration
- Poor haircoat
- Signs associated with hypoalbuminemia:
  - Peripheral edema
  - Ascites (pure transudate)
  - Pleural effusion (rare)
- Signs associated with uremia:
  - Oral ulceration
  - Halitosis (uremia)
- Pallor (either due to anemia [chronic disease, renal failure] or poor perfusion [severe illness])
- Lipid corneal deposits
- Retinal hemorrhage/detachment (systemic hypertension)
- Kidneys may be normal sized or small
- Other findings related to underlying disease

ETIOLOGY AND PATHOPHYSIOLOGY

- Immune complexes are formed or trapped in the glomeruli. While it is often a primary process (idiopathic), there are many infectious, inflammatory, endocrine, or neoplastic conditions that can provide the antigen to which antibody is produced, resulting in secondary immune complex formation.
- Glomerular immune complexes initiate an inflammatory cascade. Inflammation directly damages the glomerulus, neutralizes glomerular endothelial electrical charge, and results in vasoconstriction

and decreased glomerular filtration. The glomerulus responds to these insults with cellular proliferation.
- Albumin and similarly sized proteins are lost in the urine and may result in hypoalbuminemia and the nephrotic syndrome (see Nephrotic Syndrome, p 749). Eventually, tubular function is lost as well, resulting in azotemia and uremia.

DIAGNOSIS

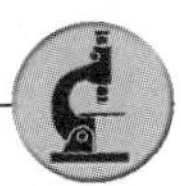

DIFFERENTIAL DIAGNOSIS

Proteinuria:
- Preglomerular (e.g., Bence Jones proteinuria, exercise, hemolysis, fever, seizure)
- Glomerular
  - Glomerulonephritis
  - Amyloidosis
  - Glomerulosclerosis, including chronic renal failure
  - Familial renal disease
- Postglomerular (e.g., urinary tract infection, neoplasia, urolithiasis)

INITIAL DATABASE

- Retinal exam. Tortuous retinal vessels, retinal hemorrhages (acute or chronic), or retinal detachments are possible (both a result of systemic hypertension).
- Blood pressure. Systemic hypertension (repeatable systolic readings >180 mmHg in calm environment) is commonly noted.
- Complete blood count (CBC): often unremarkable. Nonregenerative anemia, leukocytosis (if inflammatory disease is present).
- Serum biochemical profile:
  - Hypoalbuminemia with normal globulin level.
  - Hypercholesterolemia.
  - Hypocalcemia (relative, due to hypoalbuminemia).
  - Azotemia, hyperphosphatemia, hyperamylasemia, metabolic acidosis (in advanced disease).
- Urinalysis: proteinuria, variable urine concentration, sometimes hematuria.
  - Proteinuria must be interpreted in light of urine concentration and urine sediment examination.
  - Dipstick measure of proteinuria should be confirmed by sulfosalicylic acid test (SSA) method or quantitative measures (e.g., urine protein: creatinine ratio).
  - Significant proteinuria may often precede loss of urine concentration or azotemia.
- Urine culture: indicated in all cases.
- Thoracic radiographs: unremarkable. Evidence of underlying disease (neoplasia, chronic infectious or inflammatory disease) or pulmonary thromboembolism occasionally identified.
- Abdominal radiographs: often unremarkable. Kidneys may be small. May identify evidence of underlying disease (neoplasia, chronic infectious or inflammatory disease), or unremarkable.
- Abdominal ultrasound: hyperechoic, small kidneys, decreased corticomedullary distinction, evidence of underlying disease (neoplasia, chronic infectious or inflammatory disease), or unremarkable.

ADVANCED OR CONFIRMATORY TESTING

- Urine protein:creatinine ratio:
  - Cannot be interpreted as indicating glomerular protein loss if urine sediment is active.
  - Normal for dogs <0.5, cats <0.4. Most animals with glomerulonephritis or amyloidosis have ratios >2.0.
- Microalbuminuria testing:
  - Assay for the presence of microalbuminuria does not provide additional benefit in animals with elevated protein:creatinine ratio. These assays detect very small quantities of urine albumin that would be missed on routine dipstick and are thus redundant when significant proteinuria has been identified.
- Renal biopsy is the only definitive means of diagnosis of glomerulonephritis, allowing morphologic classification of disease, and identifying type and location of immunoglobulin. Cortical tissue examined by light microscopy, immunofluorescence, and electron microscopy.
- Determining serum antithrombin III concentrations may help quantify risk of thromboembolic disease (<80% suggests increased risk).
- A variety of other tests may be indicated in a search for an underlying cause of glomerulonephritis. The choice of tests depends on history and physical exam, results of initial evaluation (CBC, serum biochemistry, imaging studies), geographic region, and environmental exposures. Common examples include:
  - Serologic study for heartworm, Borreliosis, feline leukemia virus, feline immunodeficiency virus, *E. canis,* coccidioidomycosis.
  - Antinuclear antibody tests, rheumatoid factor.
  - Arthrocentesis, echocardiography, bone marrow aspirates, thoracic radiographs.
  - Adrenocorticotropic hormone stimulation or low-dose dexamethasone suppression tests.
  - Species specific pancreatic lipase, trypsin-like immunoreactivity.

TREATMENT

THERAPEUTIC GOAL(S)

- Decrease proteinuria
- Decrease embolic risk
- Address hypertension
- Manage renal failure if present

ACUTE GENERAL TREATMENT

- Address underlying disease conditions directly.
- If respirations are compromised by large-volume pleural effusion or severe ascites, thoracocentesis and/or abdominocentesis is indicated. Diuretic drugs are largely ineffective for rapid mobilization of body-cavity fluid.
- Oxygen support may be required for animals with pulmonary thromboembolism.
- Proteinuria may be diminished through the use of angiotensin-converting enzyme inhibitors (ACEI; for dogs, enalapril 0.5 mg/kg PO q 12-24h; benazepril 0.25 mg/kg PO q 24h). These drugs may reduce hypertension but can worsen azotemia.
- If hypertension persists despite ACEI, calcium channel blockers are indicated (amlodipine 0.05-0.5 mg/kg PO q 24h dog; 0.625 mg/cat PO q 12-24h).
- Anticoagulant therapy to reduce the risk of thromboembolic disease. Heparin is not effective due to loss of antithrombin.
  - Aspirin 0.5 mg/kg q 12h PO in the dog.
  - Coumadin initial dose is 0.1-0.2 mg/kg PO q 24h.
    - With coumadin, the prothrombin time should be monitored and dose adjusted until 1.5 to 2.5 times normal.
    - Protein-bound drug; therefore very difficult to titrate the dose effectively in patients with hypoalbuminemia, and not generally recommended unless benefit outweighs risk (e.g., prior embolic event while on aspirin).
- Uremic animals may require fluid diuresis (see Chronic Renal Failure, Overt ["Symptomatic"], p 205). Hypoalbuminemia may result in edema, in which case colloidal support may be necessary.
  - Hetastarch 10-20 ml/kg/day IV.
  - Dextrans. Use with caution due to reported link to renal failure.
  - Large volumes of species-specific plasma or human albumin. Expensive and short-lived effect.

CHRONIC TREATMENT

- Moderate dietary restriction of protein (2-3 g/kg/day for dog; 4 g/kg/day for cat), phosphorus, and sodium are recommended. A variety of commercial or homemade diets can be used (e.g., Hill's k/d, Eukanuba Early Stage, Eukanuba

Advanced stage, Purina NF). Diet changes are best made when animal is not uremic, to avoid food aversions.
- Omega-3 fatty acid supplementation may be renoprotective, decrease inflammation and proteinuria, and decrease cholesterol. Many commercial renal diets are so supplemented.
- Clinical signs of uremia and electrolyte and acid-base disorders are addressed as for chronic renal failure (see Chronic Renal Failure, Occult ["Asymptomatic"], p 204; Chronic Renal Failure, Overt ["Symptomatic"], p 205).
- Glucocorticoids and cyclosporine are ineffective in the treatment of idiopathic glomerulonephritis and may increase thromboembolic potential (glucocorticoids) or worsen renal protein loss (cyclosporine). Therefore they should be used only when documented autoimmune disease is present (e.g., systemic lupus erythematosus).

DRUG INTERACTIONS

- Angiotensin-converting enzyme (ACE) inhibitors may cause hypotension when combined with diuretics or other vasodilators.
- Nonsteroidal anti-inflammatory agents may reduce efficacy of ACE inhibitors.

POSSIBLE COMPLICATIONS

- Third space retention of fluids
- Worsening renal azotemia as a result of ACE inhibitor use (uncommon)
- Hypotension secondary to ACE inhibitor and calcium channel blocker
- Worsening of renal azotemia with dextran use
- Thromboembolic disease as a result of antithrombin and protein C level abnormalities
- Bleeding tendency from aspirin, warfarin use
- Gastrointestinal ulceration as a result of azotemia or aspirin therapy

RECOMMENDED MONITORING

Stable animals are monitored every 3 to 4 months. Rechecks should be more frequent if changes are made in therapy or when indicated by changing clinical signs.

- Physical examination
- Urine protein:creatinine ratio
- Serum blood urea nitrogen/creatinine/phosphorus
- Serum albumin
- Blood pressure
- Urinalysis/culture

PROGNOSIS AND OUTCOME

- Prognosis is best when an underlying disease can be identified and eliminated.
- When elimination of an underlying disease is not possible, survival is variable but disease is usually progressive over months to 1 to 2 years.
- In dogs, prognosis for glomerulonephritis in general is better than for renal amyloidosis.
- Prognosis is worse when azotemia/uremia is/are present at diagnosis.
- Prognosis is worse for cats than dogs.
- Prognosis is poor for dogs where glomerulonephritis is associated with borreliosis.

PEARLS & CONSIDERATIONS

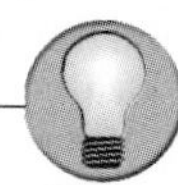

COMMENTS

- Investigation of potential underlying diseases can become expensive. Clinical judgment should guide the choice of ancillary tests for each animal.
- Once protein losing nephropathy is identified, renal biopsy is useful primarily as a prognostic tool. Although biopsy is required to distinguish the type of glomerular disease, therapy is often similar for each type.

PREVENTION

- Ectoparasite prophylaxis
- Heartworm prophylaxis

CLIENT EDUCATION

- Diligent rechecks are very important.
- Finding an underlying disease process may mean a better prognosis for the pet.

SUGGESTED READING

Grant DC, et al: Glomerulonephritis in dogs and cats: glomerular function, pathophysiology, and clinical signs. *Compendium* 23:739–747, 2001.

Grant DC, et al: Glomerulonephritis in dogs and cats: diagnosis and treatment. *Compendium* 23:798–804, 2001.

Vaden SL: Glomerular diseases. In Ettinger SJ, Feldman EC (eds): *Textbook of Veterinary Internal Medicine*, ed 6. Philadelphia, Elsevier Saunders, 2005, pp 1786–1800.

Grauer GF, et al: Effects of enalapril versus placebo as a treatment for canine idiopathic glomerulonephritis. *J Vet Intern Med* 14:526, 2000.

AUTHOR: **ANNE M. DALBY**
EDITOR: **LEAH A. COHN**

Gluten-Sensitive Enteropathy

BASIC INFORMATION

DEFINITION

A chronic, small intestinal disease triggered in susceptible animals by the ingestion of gluten, a protein found in wheat

SYNONYM(S)

Celiac disease (humans)
Gliadin enteropathy
GSE
Wheat-sensitive enteropathy

EPIDEMIOLOGY

SPECIES, AGE, SEX

- Uncommon disorder in dogs
- Can potentially occur in cats, but not well documented
- Disease is first seen in young animals (4 to 7 months old) after weaning
- No gender predisposition described

GENETICS AND BREED PREDISPOSITION: Irish setter, Samoyed, soft-coated Wheaten terrier (SCWT), but potentially any breed. In SCWT, gluten-sensitive enteropathy may be part of a spectrum of small intestinal disease, as resolution of clinical signs does not occur with dietary restriction.

RISK FACTORS

- Exposure to gluten-containing grains after weaning
- Immunologic small bowel disease may lead to secondary gluten sensitivity

ASSOCIATED CONDITIONS AND DISORDERS: None reported conclusively. Humans with gluten-sensitive enteropathy may also suffer from gluten-sensitive skin disease (dermatitis herpetiformis).

CLINICAL PRESENTATION

DISEASE FORMS/SUBTYPES

- Chronic intermittent gastrointestinal signs (diarrhea is most common)
- Ill-thrift but lack of overt gastrointestinal signs may indicate subclinical enteropathy

HISTORY, CHIEF COMPLAINT: Chronic intermittent diarrhea with weight loss or failure to thrive.

PHYSICAL EXAM FINDINGS

- Thin and/or stunted dog

- Poor body and coat condition
- Intermittent or persistent small bowel diarrhea

ETIOLOGY AND PATHOPHYSIOLOGY

- Gliadins are antigenic proteins that make up part of gluten, the main protein of wheat and related proteins in rye and barley.
- Other proteins of flour from various grains have different degrees of antigenicity: secalins (rye), hordeins (barley), and avenins (oats) are also implicated in gluten-sensitive enteropathy, whereas oryzeins (rice) and zeins (corn) do not exacerbate this disorder.
- These peptides cause intestinal damage, probably by an immune-mediated mechanism.
- An underlying defect in the intestinal mucosal barrier of Irish setters is reported and may predispose to this disease. This predisposition may be related to MHC gene expression.
- Serum antibody reactivity to gluten and serum immune complexes has not been demonstrated in dogs.
- The age of exposure to, and dose of, gluten, may modulate the expression of the disease.

DIAGNOSIS

DIFFERENTIAL DIAGNOSIS

- Other dietary sensitivities/hypersensitivities
- Idiopathic inflammatory bowel disease (IBD)
- Antibiotic-responsive diarrhea (small intestinal bacterial overgrowth)
- Exocrine pancreatic insufficiency (EPI)
- Intestinal parasitism (e.g., giardiasis)
- Atypic hypoadrenocorticism
- Chronic intussusception
- Any cause of malabsorption (e.g., lymphangiectasia)

INITIAL DATABASE

- Complete blood count, serum biochemistry profile, urinalysis: usually unremarkable
- Fecal parasite examination
- Normal trypsin-like immunoreactivity: rule out EPI
- Abdominal radiographs and ultrasound are typically unremarkable

ADVANCED OR CONFIRMATORY TESTING

- Serum folate and cobalamin levels are variable; often normal, but decreased serum folate is the most common abnormality.
- Intestinal biopsy shows nonspecific changes of villous atrophy and intraepithelial lymphocyte infiltration, but similar changes are seen in other dietary sensitivities and idiopathic IBD.
- Serologic tests cannot reliably diagnose this condition, although reductions in fecal IgE excretion during a gluten-free diet trial have been reported in SCWT.
- Conclusive diagnosis: proof of gluten sensitivity depends on demonstration of resolution of signs and histologic changes on a gluten-free diet (typically 2 to 4 weeks), and relapse when challenged with gluten.

TREATMENT

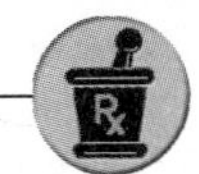

THERAPEUTIC GOAL(S)

Complete resolution of clinical signs through elimination of gluten-containing grains (wheat, rye, barley, oats, buckwheat) from diet, treats, supplements, and chewable/flavored medications

ACUTE GENERAL TREATMENT

Feed a diet lacking wheat and other gluten-containing related cereals

CHRONIC TREATMENT

- Feed a diet lacking wheat gluten and related cereals.
- Evaluate for other causes of small bowel diarrhea if response to dietary modification is suboptimal.
- Other approaches to control of intestinal inflammation include treatment with n-3 fatty acids, and novel immunosuppressive therapy with pentoxyfylline (a phosphodiesterase inhibitor that inhibits tumor necrosis factor-α expression).

POSSIBLE COMPLICATIONS

Potential for nutritional deficiencies with homemade diets

RECOMMENDED MONITORING

Centered on response to treatment (resolution of clinical signs) and physical exam (body weight, quality of coat, etc.)

PROGNOSIS AND OUTCOME

Good to excellent in dogs that respond to strict gluten-free diet

PEARLS & CONSIDERATIONS

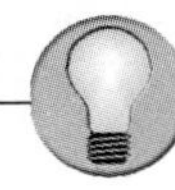

COMMENTS

- This is predominantly a disease of young Irish setter dogs/puppies.
- Consider the development of gluten-sensitive enteropathy as a potential complication to underlying immunologic small bowel disease (IBD, protein-losing enteropathy).
- Gluten sensitivity has not been recorded in cats and is probably quite rare in dogs.
- Be aware that owner noncompliance may be a common cause of treatment failure.

PREVENTION

- Selective breeding, as condition is probably familial
- Feeding a gluten-free diet will prevent disease

CLIENT EDUCATION

- Awareness of gluten content of various foodstuffs
- Monitor for recurrence of clinical signs
- Lifetime careful attention to diet may be required, although some affected dogs may develop tolerance over time

SUGGESTED READING

Elwood CM, et al: Expression of gluten sensitive enteropathy (GSE) of Irish setter dogs may be age dependent. *J Vet Intern Med* 15:274, 2001.

Hall EJ, Batt RM: Development of wheat-sensitive enteropathy in Irish setters: morphological changes. *Am J Vet Res* 51:978, 1990.

Hall EJ, Simpson KW: Diseases of the small intestine. In Ettinger SJ, Feldman EC (eds): *Textbook of Veterinary Internal Medicine*, ed 5. Philadelphia, WB Saunders, 2000, pp 1182-1238.

Vaden SL, et al: Gluten administration provokes mucosal mononuclear cell infiltration, but does not increase intestinal permeability in soft-coated Wheaten terriers (SCWT). *J Vet Intern Med* 12:202, 1998.

AUTHORS: **EDWARD J. HALL, E. KELLY NITSCHE**

EDITOR: **DEBRA L. ZORAN**

Granulomatous Enteritis/Colitis

BASIC INFORMATION

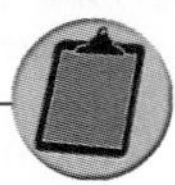

DEFINITION

Denotes persistent (>3 weeks) signs of colonic inflammation caused by mucosal infiltration with macrophages. Affected animals have large bowel diarrhea and will also show systemic signs of fever, anorexia, and weight loss.

SYNONYM(S)

"Boxer colitis" when referring to the inflammatory bowel disease (IBD) variant histiocytic ulcerative colitis (HUC). Histiocytic-ulcerative colitis is characterized by mucosal infiltrates of PAS-positive histiocytes.

EPIDEMIOLOGY

SPECIES, AGE, SEX: HUC appears to be more prevalent in young, male dogs. Granulomatous colitis of any cause is much less common in cats than in dogs.
GENETICS AND BREED PREDISPOSITION: Boxers are predisposed to HUC.
GEOGRAPHY AND SEASONALITY: Midwestern and southern United States for gastrointestinal (GI) histoplasmosis.
ASSOCIATED CONDITIONS AND DISORDERS: HUC is recognized as a severe IBD variant that is much less common than lymphocytic-plasmacytic colitis.

CLINICAL PRESENTATION

DISEASE FORMS/SUBTYPES

- Histiocytic ulcerative colitis: IBD variant characterized by mucosal infiltration with PAS-positive histiocytes
- Infectious causes for granulomatous colitis: includes both systemic fungal infections caused by *Histoplasma capsulatum* and *Pythium insidiosum*, and algal infection caused by *Prototheca* spp.

HISTORY, CHIEF COMPLAINT

- Persistent large bowel diarrhea: tenesmus (straining to defecate), increased frequency of defecation, mucoid feces, and fresh (red) blood.
- Cachexia, anorexia, and weight loss are frequently observed with granulomatous colitis, which is in sharp contrast to other causes of colonic inflammation.

PHYSICAL EXAM FINDINGS: Fever, cachexia, weight loss, and peripheral/mesenteric lymphadenopathy are observed with infectious causes. Dogs with HUC may not have mesenteric lymphadenopathy. Ocular signs (uveitis) and/or neurologic abnormalities (e.g., paresis, head tilt, ataxia) are often reported with *Prototheca* spp. infection.

ETIOLOGY AND PATHOPHYSIOLOGY

- HUC: a severe but uncommon IBD variant.
- Infiltrative mucosal disease caused by fungal or algal agents resulting in granulomatous colonic inflammation. Dissemination to other organ systems is common with systemic mycotic and algal infections.

DIAGNOSIS

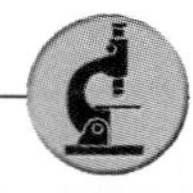

DIFFERENTIAL DIAGNOSIS

- Specific causes: see Etiology and Pathophysiology above
- Other differential diagnoses: severe colonic IBD, neoplasia

INITIAL DATABASE

- Complete blood count, serum biochemistry, urinalysis, and fecal tests are indicated to evaluate involvement of diverse organ systems.
- Exfoliative cytology (e.g., rectal scrape) is a useful tool for confirming the presence of *Histoplasma* organisms contained within colonic macrophages.
- Serologic assays (enzyme-linked immunosorbent assay [ELISA]) for fungal agents are unreliable.
- Abdominal imaging (survey radiographs, contrast radiography, and/or ultrasonography) will identify diffuse colonic wall thickening, loss of wall layering, and/or mesenteric lymphadenopathy.

ADVANCED OR CONFIRMATORY TESTING

- Polymerase chain reaction or ELISA techniques on serum or tissues will confirm *Pythium* spp. infection.
- Mucosal biopsy obtained endoscopically or surgically will demonstrate the presence of PAS-positive histiocytes, or granulomatous inflammation with infectious organisms.
- Oculocentesis may detect *Prototheca* spp. organisms in animals with ocular lesions.

TREATMENT

THERAPEUTIC GOAL(S)

- Treatment requires a specific definitive diagnosis determined by mucosal biopsy.
- Surgical excision of diseased tissues (if possible) is required for pythiosis.
- Dietary management includes the supplementation with sources of soluble fiber, which bind colonic irritants, normalize dysmotility, and promote colonic epithelial repair and renewal.

CHRONIC TREATMENT

- Treat HUC using a combination of diet and oral enrofloxacin (5 mg/kg PO q 24h for 14 days) alone or in combination with metronidazole or amoxicillin. Anti-inflammatory therapy with mesalamine (10–20 mg/kg q 8h) may be beneficial.
- Nutrition: low-fat, fiber-enriched, and highly digestible commercial ration. In some instances, a restricted-antigen (e.g., elimination) diet may be helpful.
- Supplementation with increased n-3:n-6 fatty acids to reduce mucosal inflammation.
- If the animal will not eat a commercial fiber-containing diet, addition of fiber (small to moderate amounts of soluble fiber [Metamucil sprinkled on the food at a dosage of 1–2 teaspoons/10 kg body weight per feeding]) to the regular diet.
- Infection with *Histoplasma* spp. requires antifungal therapy with itraconazole and/or amphotericin B (see Histoplasmosis, p 525).
- Aggressive surgical resection will be required for animals infected with *Pythium* spp.
- There is no effective therapy for protothecosis.

POSSIBLE COMPLICATIONS

- Cure is often not possible in animals with pythiosis or protothecosis. These animals will likely die regardless of therapy.
- Animals having GI histoplasmosis and treated with amphotericin B are at risk for drug-induced renal disease.

RECOMMENDED MONITORING

- Rechecks are required at 2- to 4-week intervals initially in animals with HUC. Gradual drug reduction may occur as clinical signs lessen.
- Monitor renal function in animals treated with amphotericin B.

PROGNOSIS AND OUTCOME

- HUC carries a guarded prognosis, although recent studies suggest that dogs may respond completely.
- GI histoplasmosis carries a guarded prognosis; however, most animals respond favorably to antifungal therapy in spite of disease burden.

- Granulomatous colitis caused by *Pythium* spp. and *Prototheca* spp. carries a poor prognosis.

PEARLS & CONSIDERATIONS

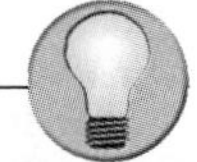

COMMENTS

- Major causes for granulomatous colitis include infectious and infiltrative disorders.
- A thorough diagnostic evaluation is warranted to rule out the varied causes for colonic inflammation.
- Colonoscopy with mucosal biopsy is imperative for diagnosis.

CLIENT EDUCATION

Dietary modification to a diet suitable for colonic disease may be required for the life of the pet.

SUGGESTED READING

Hostutler RA, et al: Antibiotic-responsive histiocytic ulcerative colitis in 9 dogs. *J Vet Intern Med* 18:499, 2004.

Washabau RJ, et al: Diseases of the large intestines. In Ettinger SJ, Feldman EC (eds): *Textbook of Veterinary Internal Medicine*, ed 6. Philadelphia, WB Saunders, 2005, pp 1378–1408.

AUTHOR: **ALBERT E. JERGENS**

EDITOR: **DEBRA L. ZORAN**

Granulomatous Meningoencephalomyelitis

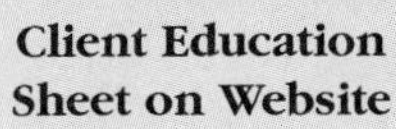

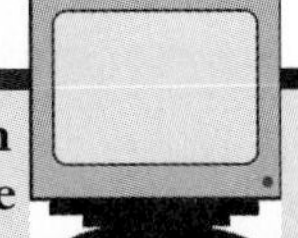

Client Education Sheet on Website

BASIC INFORMATION

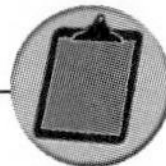

DEFINITION

A common, idiopathic, inflammatory, noninfectious meningoencephalomyelitis of dogs, the definitive diagnosis of which is dependent on characteristic histopathologic features

EPIDEMIOLOGY

SPECIES, AGE, SEX: Any age and either sex can be affected by granulomatous meningoencephalomyelitis (GME). This is a canine disease, being virtually nonexistent in cats. The median age is 5 years and there appears to be a female predominance.

GENETICS AND BREED PREDISPOSITION: The genetics of GME are unknown. Small-breed dogs (e.g., poodles, terriers) are predisposed, although larger breeds are occasionally affected.

CLINICAL PRESENTATION

DISEASE FORMS/SUBTYPES: Three forms of GME have been described:

- Multifocal (disseminated)
- Focal
- Ocular (uncommon)

HISTORY, CHIEF COMPLAINT

- The history and chief complaint are reflective of the form of GME and the particular region or regions of the central nervous system involved.
- Central vestibular dysfunction is a common presentation for dogs with GME.
- Other common complaints include seizures, abnormal mental status, neck pain, and nonambulatory status.
- Dogs with multifocal and ocular forms of GME tend to have acute onset of clinical signs.
- Multifocal GME is usually rapidly progressive.

PHYSICAL EXAM FINDINGS

- Patients with GME are occasionally febrile on presentation.
- There are usually no other abnormalities on general physical examination.
- Neurologic abnormalities depend on the form of GME affecting the patient. Clinical evidence of forebrain, brainstem, cerebellar, and cervical spinal cord dysfunction are prominent, either alone or in combination.

ETIOLOGY AND PATHOPHYSIOLOGY

The etiology of GME is unknown. However, there is strong evidence that this is an autoimmune disorder, most likely a T-cell mediated, delayed-type (type IV) hypersensitivity reaction.

DIAGNOSIS

DIFFERENTIAL DIAGNOSIS

- Necrotizing encephalitis
- Infectious meningoencephalitis
- Neoplasia
- Caudal occipital malformation syndrome
- Intracranial intra-arachnoid cyst (quadrigeminal cyst)

INITIAL DATABASE

A working clinical diagnosis of GME is dependent on imaging and cerebrospinal fluid [CSF] analysis:

- Computed tomography, magnetic resonance imaging: Most cases exhibit contrast-enhancing lesions with white matter predominance.
- Characteristic CSF findings are a sterile, mixed cell (primarily mononuclear) pleocytosis with elevated protein levels.

ADVANCED OR CONFIRMATORY TESTING

Definitive diagnosis of GME is dependent on histopathologic examination of brain and/or spinal cord parenchymal lesions, which are uncommonly obtained in the clinical setting.

TREATMENT

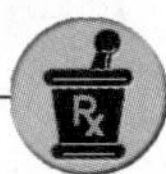

THERAPEUTIC GOAL(S)

- Suppression of the inflammatory process
- Recovery of functional neurologic status.
- Pain management
- Seizure control, if seizures are part of the clinical picture

ACUTE GENERAL TREATMENT

- The standard treatment for GME has traditionally been immunosuppressive doses of glucocorticoids (e.g., prednisone, 1–2 mg/kg PO q 12h).
- Other suggested treatments include procarbazine (PO), cytosine arabinoside (SQ), and leflunomide.
- If the patient is seizuring, intravenous diazepam can be administered while starting a maintenance anticonvulsant drug.

CHRONIC TREATMENT

- One or more of the previously mentioned drugs are continued indefinitely.
- A maintenance anticonvulsant without sedative tendencies and without the side effects of polyuria and polydipsia is recommended for seizure control (e.g., felbamate, zonisamide).
- Radiation therapy has shown to be beneficial in cases of focal GME.

POSSIBLE COMPLICATIONS

- Typical glucocorticoid side effects are to be expected.
- Procarbazine and cytosine arabinoside may cause bone marrow suppression.

RECOMMENDED MONITORING

Complete blood counts should be evaluated for dogs receiving immunosuppressive/chemotherapeutic agents (e.g., cytosine arabinoside, procarbazine) every week for the initial month of therapy, then weekly thereafter.

PROGNOSIS AND OUTCOME

The prognosis for GME treated with glucocorticoids alone has been evaluated for focal and multifocal forms of the disease:

- The overall median survival is 14 days.
- The median survival for focal GME is 114 days, and for multifocal GME is 8 days.
- Dogs with focal GME treated with radiation therapy have a median survival of more than 400 days.
- In a recent report, it was found that dogs with GME treated with a combination of glucocorticoids and procarbazine had a median survival time of 15 months.

PEARLS & CONSIDERATIONS

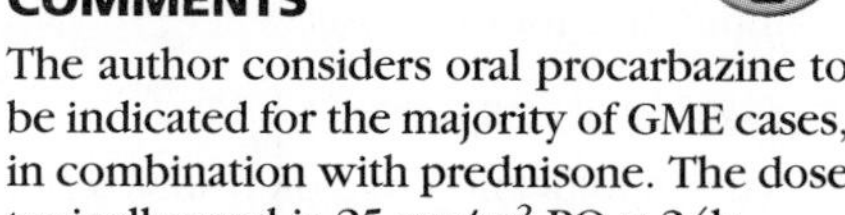

COMMENTS

The author considers oral procarbazine to be indicated for the majority of GME cases, in combination with prednisone. The dose typically used is 25 mg/m^2 PO q 24h.

SUGGESTED READING

Dewey CW: Encephalopathies: disorders of the brain. In Dewey CW (ed): *A Practical Guide to Canine and Feline Neurology*. Ames, IA, Iowa State Press, 2003, pp 99–178.

Kipar A, et al: Immunohistochemical characterization of inflammatory cells in brains of dogs with granulomatous meningoencephalomyelitis. *Vet Pathol* 35:43, 1998.

Munana KR, et al: Prognostic factors for dogs with granulomatous meningoencephalomyelitis: 42 cases (1982–1996). *J Am Vet Med Assoc* 212:1902, 1998.

Cuddon PA, et al: New treatments for granulomatous meningoencephalomyelitis. *Proc 20th ACVIM Forum*, 2002, pp 319–321.

Coates JR, et al: Procarbazine for treatment of suspected granulomatous meningoencephalomyelitis: 20 cases (1998–2004). *J Vet Intern Med* (abstract) in press, 2005.

AUTHOR & EDITOR: **CURTIS W. DEWEY**

Grapes and Raisins Toxicosis

BASIC INFORMATION

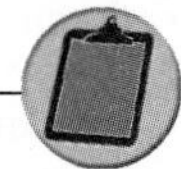

DEFINITION

Acute renal failure (ARF) following ingestion of grapes (*Vitis* spp.) or raisins

SYNONYM(S)

Vitis spp. toxicosis

EPIDEMIOLOGY

SPECIES, AGE, SEX

- Documented in dogs only
- Anecdotally reported in cats, ferrets
- No known age or sex predisposition; all breeds susceptible
- Ingestion of grapes or raisins does not consistently cause acute renal failure in all dogs

RISK FACTORS: Animals with prior renal or heart disease may be at increased risk of developing ARF.

GEOGRAPHY AND SEASONALITY: Toxicity can occur anytime throughout the year.

CLINICAL PRESENTATION

HISTORY, CHIEF COMPLAINT

- History of exposure
- Evidence of grapes/raisins in vomitus or stool
- Most common clinical signs include vomiting, lethargy, anorexia, diarrhea, decreased urine output, signs of abdominal pain, ataxia, and weakness
- Vomiting, lethargy, anorexia within 24 hours; vomiting is usually seen within 12 hours after ingestion

PHYSICAL EXAM FINDINGS

- Dehydration
- Signs of abdominal pain in some dogs
- Lethargy

ETIOLOGY AND PATHOPHYSIOLOGY

- Etiology unknown.
- Renal tubular necrosis is a consistent histopathologic finding (Fig. I-84).
- Tubular basement membrane remains intact, providing possibility for recovery. Evidence of tubular regeneration may be present in some dogs.
- Mineralization of kidneys, gastric mucosa, myocardium, lungs, and blood vessels.

DIAGNOSIS

DIFFERENTIAL DIAGNOSIS

Rule out other causes of ARF:

- Ethylene glycol
- Leptospirosis
- Bacterial pyelonephritis
- Lily toxicosis in cats
- Iatrogenic/medication nephrotoxicity (e.g., aminoglycoside antibiotics)
- Renal thromboembolism (usually accompanied by thromboembolism of other aortic branches)

INITIAL DATABASE

- Serum chemistry profile, complete blood count, calcium × phosphorus product (Ca × P):
  - Azotemia, hyperphosphatemia, elevated Ca × P (>60 if measured in mg/dl) almost always present; hypercalcemia frequent
  - Serum creatinine, phosphorus, and Ca × P can elevate in less than 24 hours
  - Blood urea nitrogen and calcium may be slower to elevate (1 to 3 days)
- Urinalysis before giving fluids:
  - Urine specific gravity <1.030
  - Glucosuria, proteinuria
  - Cylindruria (casts)
- Radiographs: abnormalities fairly uncommon:
  - Increased renal size
  - Metastatic mineralization

ADVANCED OR CONFIRMATORY TESTING

- Ultrasonography to assess kidneys and pancreas
- Renal biopsy may help determine prognosis

TREATMENT

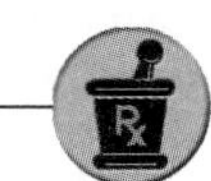

THERAPEUTIC GOAL(S)

- Decontamination (emesis and activated charcoal)
- Supportive care (fluid diuresis, nutritional support, vomiting and seizure control, etc.)
- Treat anuria/oliguria

ACUTE GENERAL TREATMENT

- Decontamination of patient:
  - Emesis: useful 6 to 12 hours after exposure (see Vomiting, Induction of, p 1328).
  - Activated charcoal: useful 12 to 24 hours after exposure.
- Fluid diuresis:
  - Fluid diuresis for 48 hours in animals not showing clinical signs may prevent ARF.
  - Treat signs of ARF as needed (see p 32). Currently no unique treatment identified. If concurrent hypercal-

cemia, consider using 0.9% normal saline.

- Treat anuria/oliguria:
  - Correct dehydration first.
  - Mannitol: 0.25–0.5 g/kg IV over 3 to 5 minutes or constant rate infusion (CRI) of 2–5 ml/min of 5–10% mannitol in lactated Ringer's solution.
  - Furosemide: 2–4 mg/kg IV or 6 mg/kg if needed q 8h; or combine 1 mg/kg/hr furosemide (CRI or IV boluses) with dopamine CRI.
  - Dopamine: 2–5 kg/min IV CRI. Efficacy in ARF questioned, and may cause nausea.
  - Hemodialysis or peritoneal dialysis may be useful in some cases.

CHRONIC TREATMENT

Ongoing supportive care based on initial severity, response to treatments, individual's intrinsic ability to compensate, and extent of permanent renal injury

POSSIBLE COMPLICATIONS

- Uremia-related neurologic signs (seizures, ataxia)
- Metastatic mineralization (renal, cardiac, vascular, pulmonary)
- Pancreatitis

RECOMMENDED MONITORING

- Baseline blood urea nitrogen, creatinine, calcium, phosphorus, Ca × P, potassium, total protein, hematocrit, daily at first then as needed
- Urine output
- Signs of overhydration (respiratory character/effort, body weight)
- Acidosis

PROGNOSIS AND OUTCOME

- Of 43 dogs, 53% recovered with treatment, 12% died, and 35% were euthanized.
- Oliguria/anuria, ataxia and weakness indicate poor prognosis.
- Higher calcium and Ca × P indicates poor prognosis.

PEARLS & CONSIDERATIONS

COMMENTS

- Raisins at 0.1 oz/kg and grapes (10 to 12 grapes in an 8-kg dog) have led to ARF.
- Not all dogs that ingest raisins or grapes develop ARF.
- Raisins are 4.5 times more concentrated than grapes on an oz per oz basis.
- Treatment may be required for days to weeks.

PREVENTION

Keep raisins and grapes out of dogs' reach

CLIENT EDUCATION

- Do not feed grapes or raisins to dogs.
- Treatment may be extensive and expensive, and may be associated with a guarded prognosis.

SUGGESTED READING

Mazzaferro EM, et al: Acute renal failure associated with raisin or grape ingestion in 4 dogs. *J Vet Emerg Crit Care* 14(3):203–212, 2004.

Eubig PA, et al: Acute renal failure in dogs after the ingestion of grapes or raisins: A retrospective evaluation of 43 dogs (1992–2002). *J Vet Intern Med* 19:663–674, 2005.

AUTHOR: **PAUL A. EUBIG**
EDITOR: **SAFDAR A. KHAN**

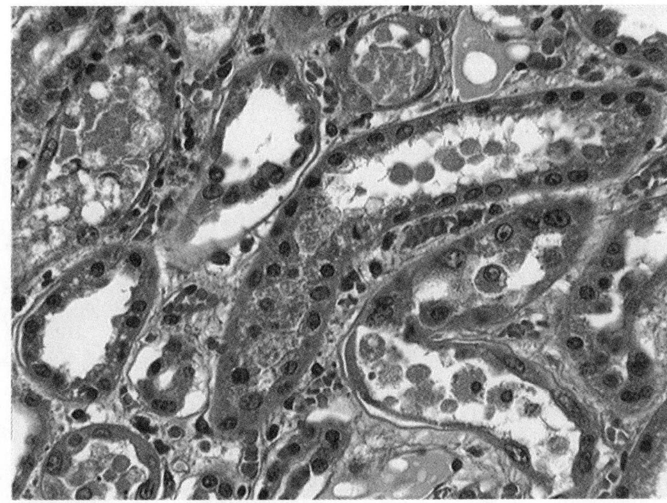

FIGURE I-84 Histologic evaluation of renal specimen from a patient with toxicosis due to grapes/raisins, demonstrating renal tubular necrosis. Courtesy of Dr. Carla Morrow, University of Illinois.

Gunshot Injuries

BASIC INFORMATION

DEFINITION

Penetrating or perforating wound caused by a bullet/pellet(s)

SYNONYM(S)

Bullet wound
Gunshot wound

EPIDEMIOLOGY

SPECIES, AGE, SEX: Dogs: young (<3 years), intact males.

GENETICS AND BREED PREDISPOSITION: German shepherd dogs, pit bull terrier mixes, Rottweilers, Doberman pinschers, and mastiffs are overrepresented.

- Perceived nature of these breeds?
- Their use as security and police dogs?

RISK FACTORS: Young, intact male dogs allowed to roam unsupervised.

GEOGRAPHY AND SEASONALITY

- High-velocity handgun injuries
  - High population density areas
  - Summer heat wave
- High-velocity rifle injuries
  - Deer, elk, and moose hunting seasons
- Low-velocity shotgun injuries with slug projectiles
  - Deer hunting season
- Low-velocity shot injuries
  - Bird hunting season

CLINICAL PRESENTATION

DISEASE FORMS/SUBTYPES: Dependent on area of body injured:

- Extremities/face:
  - Soft tissue injury

- Fractures
- Thorax:
  - Pneumothorax
  - Hemothorax
  - Cardiac perforation
- Abdomen:
  - Penetration/perforation of viscera→ hemoabdomen and/or peritonitis

HISTORY, CHIEF COMPLAINT

- Gunshot injury seen/known to have occurred.
- Entry, ± exit, wound(s) noted by owner.

PHYSICAL EXAM FINDINGS

- Variable, depending on the location of the injury:
  - See Disease Forms/Subtypes above
- Entry, ± exit, wound(s):
  - May be small and easily overlooked:
    - Careful examination required, including extensive clipping of hair in long-haired breeds
  - Massive soft tissue trauma may be present
- Evidence of blood loss:
  - Overt hemorrhage
  - Pale mucous membranes, shock
- Presence of secondary injuries:
  - Perforating forelimb injury with secondary penetrating thoracic injury
  - Perforating hind limb/perineal injury with perforating abdominal trauma

ETIOLOGY AND PATHOPHYSIOLOGY

Gunshot wounds are not "sterilized" by the bullet as it passes through tissues.

- Wound infection due to:
  - Skin bacteria carried into the wound
  - Gastrointestinal (GI) flora leaking into the abdomen

DIAGNOSIS

DIFFERENTIAL DIAGNOSIS

Penetrating wounds due to other causes:

- Sticks, sharp yard/outdoors objects
- Arrows
- Blade weapons
- Bite wounds

INITIAL DATABASE

- Complete blood count, serum chemistry profile, urinalysis: may reflect stress (e.g., stress leukogram), or infection if wound is more than several hours old.
- Survey radiographs (Fig. I-85):
  - Site of primary injury(ies).
  - Thorax, abdomen, if indicated
    - Potential secondary injury from perforating gunshot wound
- Abdominal ultrasound examination:
  - Integrity of viscera
  - Peritoneal fluid accumulation (see Advanced or Confirmatory Testing below)

ADVANCED OR CONFIRMATORY TESTING

Abdominocentesis:

- Ultrasound guided
- Fluid analysis, cytology, and Gram staining:
  - Urine
  - Bile
  - Intestinal contents
- Bacterial culture and sensitivity testing (both aerobic and anaerobic): if septic peritonitis is suspected:
  - Intestinal contents
  - Bile

TREATMENT

THERAPEUTIC GOAL(S)

- Stabilize patient: treat shock, provide pain relief.
- Address life-threatening injuries: hemorrhage, GI perforation, tension pneumothorax.
- Address wounds: debridement, lavage, and bandages.
- Support fractures.

ACUTE GENERAL TREATMENT

- Patient stabilization:
  - Intravenous fluid therapy:
    - Crystalloids
    - Colloids
  - Blood products:
    - Whole blood transfusion (see Transfusion Reactions, p 1098) to replace losses if hemorrhage significant
  - Thoracocentesis indicated if:
    - Pneumothorax: tension
    - Hemothorax
- Initial wound care:
  - Control hemorrhage.
  - Protect tissues from further damage.
    - Preparation and lavage
    - Temporary sterile dressing
    - For wound lavage and sterile dressings: wear gloves to avoid contamination of wound with hospital bacteria
- Temporary fracture stabilization:
  - Robert Jones bandage.
- Pain management:
  - A pure opioid agonist, such as morphine, is preferable due to good analgesic activity, mild to moderate effects on hemodynamic stability and ability to be reversed.
  - Generally, partial agonists (e.g., buprenorphine) and agonist/antagonists (e.g., butorphanol) are inadequate for control of pain caused by gunshot wounds.
- Emergency abdominal surgery once patient stabilized. Indications for surgery:
  - Pneumoperitoneum or bacteria present in abdominal fluid indicating GI perforation.
  - Evidence of active bleeding that is not controllable with pressure dressings.
  - Pneumothorax.
  - Hemothorax.

CHRONIC TREATMENT

- Definitive fracture repair.
- Open wound management. Soft tissue damage and loss of blood supply in the areas surrounding the projectile path can progress to tissue necrosis. Sterile dressings and open wound management will allow tissue viability to be declared. Less extensive debridement is typically required than may be evident initially.
- Definitive wound repair/reconstruction.

POSSIBLE COMPLICATIONS

- Fracture delayed/non-union
  - Bone sequestration due to vascular damage
  - Osteomyelitis
- Problems with wound healing/reconstruction
  - Soft tissue necrosis
  - Open fracture sites
- Death
  - Irreparable organ damage
  - Sepsis/septic peritonitis
  - Disseminated intravascular coagulation

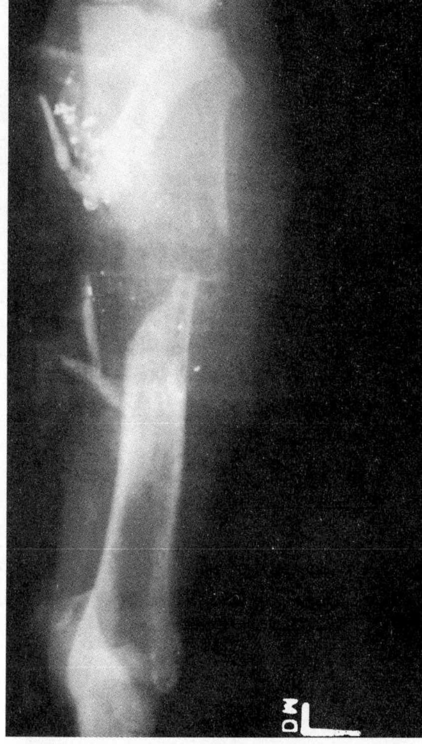

FIGURE I-85 Gunshot injury to the tibia in a dog. A comminuted fracture is present, with extensive bone fragmenting of the proximal third of the tibia, metallic foreign material (bullet remnants), and extensive soft tissue trauma. Courtesy of Dr. Richard Walshaw.

RECOMMENDED MONITORING

Dependent on extent/site of injuries:

- Acute phase:
  - Continuous/frequent intensive care monitoring until patient is stable
- Chronic phase:
  - Wound healing:
    - Open wound management:
      - Daily to every 2- to 3-day bandage changes; interval is based on degree of exudation
    - Reconstructed wound:
      - Dependent on method of reconstruction
  - Fracture healing:
    - Follow-up radiographs 6 to 12 weeks

PROGNOSIS AND OUTCOME

- Depends almost entirely on the extent of injury and presence/absence of complications.
- Aggressive management of hemodynamic abnormalities and penetrating wounds to body cavities can positively affect outcome.
- Generally, injuries to the vertebral column and penetrating abdominal and chest wounds carry a worse prognosis.

PEARLS & CONSIDERATIONS

COMMENTS

- All perforating gunshot wounds to the abdomen require surgical exploration to assess organ damage and to manage peritonitis.
- High velocity, penetrating gunshot wounds are *not* usually amenable to conservative, outpatient treatment. The patient should be stabilized with intravenous fluids and pain management, and referred for definitive treatment if intensive trauma management, surgery, and 24-hour nursing care are not available on site.
- Thoracic injuries do not generally require surgical exploration unless there is evidence of large vessel damage or if tension pneumothorax persists despite chest tube placement.
- Lead poisoning generally does not occur with projectiles that remain embedded in soft tissues indefinitely. If a bullet or other projectile is not interfering with normal function, it is not necessary to remove it.

SUGGESTED READING

Fullingham RJ, et al: Characteristics and management of gunshot wounds in dogs and cats: 84 cases (1986–1995). *J Am Vet Med Assoc* 210:5, 1997.

Pavletic MM: Projectile injuries. In Pavletic MM (ed): *Atlas of Small Animal Reconstructive Surgery*, ed 2. Philadelphia, WB Saunders, 1999.

AUTHORS: **HEIDI HOTTINGER, JENIFER G. SHEEHY**

EDITOR: **RICHARD WALSHAW**

Halitosis, Dental/Nondental

BASIC INFORMATION

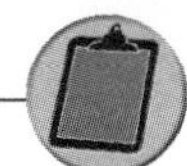

DEFINITION

Halitosis refers to an offensive odor emanating from the oral cavity, which may arise from intraoral or extraoral causes.

SYNONYM(S)

Bad breath

Oral malodor

EPIDEMIOLOGY

RISK FACTORS

- The epithelial surfaces of the oral cavity are exposed to, and ripe for contact with, pathogens, traumatic sources, and constant abrasion with ingestion.
- Risk factors for halitosis include:
  - Retention of plaque and food debris
  - Nonhealing wounds due to trauma, foreign bodies, and surgical procedures or associated with oral cancer
  - Systemic infections
  - Diabetic ketoacidosis
  - End-stage renal failure or hepatic dysfunction
  - Viral or immune-mediated disease

ASSOCIATED CONDITIONS AND DISORDERS

- Intraoral causes of halitosis may be associated with tumors of the oral cavity that outgrow their blood supply and become necrotic (e.g., malignant melanoma).
  - Other causes are canine ulcerative stomatitis and feline gingivostomatitis.
- Extraoral causes of halitosis include "mouth breathing" associated with brachycephalic head conformation, bronchitis, bronchopneumonia, gastroesophageal reflux, dermatologic conditions such as lip fold pyoderma, uremic stomatitis, ketoacidosis from uncontrolled diabetes mellitus, hyperammonemia due to liver failure, anal sac and perineal diseases and associated grooming/licking, infectious diseases such as leptospirosis, and viral diseases in cats. Immune-mediated disorders such as drug eruptions, systemic lupus erythematosus, and other bullous autoimmune diseases may also have malodorous oral manifestations.

CLINICAL PRESENTATION

HISTORY, CHIEF COMPLAINT: Halitosis is a leading concern of pet owners, as it may change the relationship with the beloved pet.

PHYSICAL EXAM FINDINGS: The physical examination including the oral evaluation will be variable depending on the underlying disease process. For example, oral manifestations associated with leptospirosis are variable depending on the serovar, and may include petechiae, oral hemorrhages, ulceration, glossitis with necrosis, and sloughing of the tongue.

ETIOLOGY AND PATHOPHYSIOLOGY

Dependent on the underlying pathologic process

DIAGNOSIS

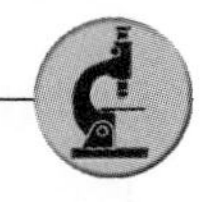

DIFFERENTIAL DIAGNOSIS

The *DAMNIT* scheme can be used as a guide to differential diagnosis:

- *D*evelopmental, degenerative: congenital or acquired palatal defects
- *A*utoimmune, allergic, anatomic: pemphigus vulgaris, systemic lupus erythematosus, erythema multiforme, "mouth breathing" of brachycephalic breeds
- *M*etabolic, mechanical: diabetic ketoacidosis, azotemia, hyperammonemia
- *N*utritional, neoplastic: gastrointestinal reflux; oral, pharyngeal, or esophageal neoplasia; dietary indiscretion/consumption of spoiled food
- *I*nfectious, inflammatory or idiopathic: leptospirosis, fungal diseases, lip fold pyoderma, bronchitis, bronchopneumonia, periodontal disease, gingival hyperplasia, ulcerative stomatitis, feline gingivostomatitis complex, feline leukemia virus, feline immunodeficiency virus, feline calicivirus, feline herpesvirus

- Toxic, traumatic: toxic epidermal necrolysis, malocclusion, fractures, bone sequestra, foreign bodies or neoplasms

INITIAL DATABASE

Sensory evaluation and complete physical examination

ADVANCED OR CONFIRMATORY TESTING

- Complete blood count, chemistry panel, and urinalysis as dictated by history and clinical signs
- Viral testing: feline leukemia, feline immunodeficiency, herpes, calicivirus
- Oral examination with patient under general anesthesia:
    - In the absence of systemic, or readily identifiable, intraoral causes of halitosis
    - Biopsy and histopathologic evaluation as needed
- Case-specific advanced diagnostics
- Identify and quantify volatile sulfur compounds or volatile organic compounds with gas chromatography, mass spectroscopy, and sulfide meters

TREATMENT

THERAPEUTIC GOAL(S)

Establish a breath that is free from offensive odors

ACUTE GENERAL TREATMENT

- Improve oral hygiene via professional periodontal treatment and pay specific attention to treatment of intraoral causes of halitosis.
- Establish the diagnosis for extraoral causes of halitosis and treat specifically.

CHRONIC TREATMENT

- Maintain a healthy periodontium via routine oral home care and professional periodontal treatment as individually indicated.
- Utilization of oral home care products and diets known to diminish plaque and calculus accumulation and reduce gingival inflammation (www.vohc.org).
- Treat the specific systemic disease process causing halitosis.

PROGNOSIS AND OUTCOME

Dependent on the underlying cause

PEARLS & CONSIDERATIONS

COMMENTS

A nonmalodorous oral cavity improves the human-animal bond, as well as the pet's general health and well-being.

PREVENTION

- Routine veterinary assessment including a thorough oral examination
- Complete blood count, chemistry panel, urinalysis, and viral testing
- Professional periodontal treatment

CLIENT EDUCATION

- The oral cavity can be easily assessed by most owners.
- Halitosis is obvious, abnormal, and requires appropriate veterinary intervention.
- Oral home care is important to general health.

SUGGESTED READING

Anderson JG: Approach to diagnosis of canine oral lesions. *Comp Cont Educ Pract Vet* 13(8):1215, 1991.

Clarke DE: Clinical and microbiological effects of oral zinc ascorbate gel in cats. *J Vet Dent* 18(4):177, 2001.

Hennet P, et al: Oral malodor in dogs: measurement using a sulfide monitor. *J Vet Dent* 12(3):101, 1995.

Hennet P, et al: Oral malodor measurements on a [sic] tooth surface of dogs with gingivitis. *Am J Vet Res* 59(3):255, 1998.

Pedersen NC: Inflammatory oral cavity diseases of the cat. *Vet Clin North Am* 22(6):1323, 1992.

Veterinary Oral Health Council (VOHC): www.vohc.org.

Tonzetich J: Production and origin of oral malodor: A review of mechanism and methods of analysis. *J Periodontol* 48:13, 1977.

AUTHOR: **JAMIE G. ANDERSON**

EDITOR: **ALEXANDER M. REITER**

Head Tilt

BASIC INFORMATION

DEFINITION

Tilting of the head in a clockwise or counterclockwise direction along the long axis of the body. The head may be tilted due to a disorder of balance (vestibular disease) or due to discomfort from a dermatologic problem (acute moist dermatitis of the lateral face, or otitis externa). Head tilt due to an orthopedic problem (torticollis) is rare in small animals.

EPIDEMIOLOGY

SPECIES, AGE, SEX: Idiopathic vestibular disease: dogs >8 years; any age in cats.

GENETICS AND BREED PREDISPOSITION

- Otitis externa/dermatitis: usually "floppy"-eared breeds of dogs (e.g., spaniels, retrievers)
- Congenital vestibular disease (uncommon): Doberman pinscher, cocker spaniel, German shepherd, others

GEOGRAPHY AND SEASONALITY: Idiopathic vestibular disease in cats: may predominate in late summer/early fall.

ASSOCIATED CONDITIONS AND DISORDERS

- If head tilt is of vestibular origin, concurrent nystagmus, ataxia, circling, and/or vomiting may occur.
- If head tilt is associated with otitis externa/dermatitis, concurrent vigorous head shaking is common.

CLINICAL PRESENTATION

DISEASE FORMS/SUBTYPES

- Vestibular disease (peripheral or central)
- Associated with discomfort (e.g., otitis externa or dermatitis ventral to the ear)

HISTORY, CHIEF COMPLAINT

- Head tilt associated with idiopathic vestibular disease: usually acute onset:
    - Vomiting, followed by head tilt, ataxia and circling/rolling for the next 1 to 2 hours.
    - Owners may not report nystagmus.
- Head tilt associated with otitis externa/dermatitis:
    - Signs of pain of the affected ear/dermatitis lesion.
    - Scratching of ear/affected skin.
    - Rubbing of face on the floor.

PHYSICAL EXAM FINDINGS

- Head tilt associated with peripheral vestibular disease (one or more may be present):
    - Head tilt is always toward the side of the lesion.
    - Nystagmus (horizontal or rotary) with fast phase away from the side of the head tilt. See Nystagmus, p 759.
    - Circling.
    - Ataxia with falling to the side of the head tilt.
- Head tilt associated with central vestibular disease (one or more may be present):
    - Head tilt is toward the side of the lesion.
    - Nystagmus (horizontal, rotary, or vertical) with fast phase away from the

side of the head tilt. See Nystagmus, p 759.
- Circling.
- Ataxia.
- Propriocepive deficits, motor weakness on the side of the lesion.
- Rarely, central vestibular disease may cause paradoxical signs (the head tilt is away from the side of the lesion).
  - Proprioceptive deficits indicate the true side of the lesion (ipsilateral).
- Other cranial nerve deficits (V, VI, VII).

- Head tilt associated with otitis externa/dermatitis:
  - Otitis externa (frequently suppurative).
  - Moist dermatitis ("hot spot") just ventral to the ear but covered by the pinna.

ETIOLOGY AND PATHOPHYSIOLOGY

- Peripheral vestibular disease:
  - Idiopathic
  - Infection (otitis media/interna)
  - Neoplasia
  - Hypothyroidism (rare)
  - Post middle ear surgery
  - Intoxication (e.g., aminoglycoside antibiotics; rare)
  - Congenital/hereditary
- Central vestibular disease:
  - Infection
  - Inflammation
  - Neoplasia
  - Trauma
- Otitis externa/dermatitis:
  - Dogs: secondary to atopy, food hypersensitivity/allergy, hypothyroidism
  - Bacterial
  - Yeast
  - Mites (cats)

DIAGNOSIS

INITIAL DATABASE

- Complete blood count, serum chemistry profile, and urinalysis: usually normal
- Otoscopic exam:
  - Evidence of otitis externa, polyp, blood (head trauma) are possible.
  - Careful examination may reveal fluid in the middle ear with infectious causes.
- Tympanic bulla radiographs
- In otitis externa, consider evaluation for atopy, food hypersensitivity/allergy, and hypothyroidism

ADVANCED OR CONFIRMATORY TESTING

- Serum thyroid assays if cutaneous, biochemical, or other signs suggesting hypothyroidism are present (dogs).
- Magnetic resonance imaging or computed tomography if inner ear or intracranial lesion is suspected.
- Cerebrospinal fluid analysis if intracranial disease is considered.

TREATMENT

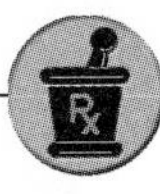

THERAPEUTIC GOAL(S)

- Improve the clinical condition by decreasing nausea, anorexia
- Treat primary cause when possible

ACUTE GENERAL TREATMENT

- Vestibular:
  - No specific therapy is available for treatment of idiopathic vestibular syndrome in dogs or cats.
    - Glucocorticoids do not appear to help.
  - Other specific causes will require treatment based on etiology.
  - It may be difficult for the animal to walk or stand, so good nursing care including ability for the animal to get to food and water as well as appropriate care to prevent urine or fecal scalding are very important.
- Dermatologic:
  - In cases of moist dermatitis, clipping the hair of the affected area and gentle cleaning with an antiseptic are recommended. See Acute Moist Dermatitis, p 31.

PROGNOSIS AND OUTCOME

- Vestibular:
  - The prognosis for idiopathic vestibular disease is excellent (dog and cat), but recurrence is possible.
  - With idiopathic vestibular disease, a head tilt may remain after resolution of all other signs.
  - The prognosis for neoplasia and all causes of central vestibular nystagmus is guarded to poor, depending on the exact cause, ability to treat, and response to therapy.
- Dermatologic:
  - The prognosis for otitis externa is good, but chronic cases may require advanced treatment or occasionally surgery.
  - Moist dermatitis ventral to ear has an excellent prognosis.

PEARLS & CONSIDERATIONS

COMMENTS

- In a majority of cases in dogs and cats, acute onset head tilt is caused by idiopathic peripheral disease and will resolve spontaneously in 1 to 2 weeks.
- Idiopathic vestibular disease is a diagnosis of exclusion.
- Nearly all central vestibular disease cases will have other central nervous system signs (proprioceptive defects, weakness, other cranial nerve involvement).

CLIENT EDUCATION

- When idiopathic vestibular disease is the primary consideration, the owners need to know that the problem will usually resolve with time.
- Otitis externa may become a chronic problem and owners should be advised that rechecks are needed even if the animal appears normal.

SUGGESTED READING

Lorenz M, Kornegay J: Ataxia of the head and the limbs. In Lorenz M, Kornegay J (eds): *Handbood of Veterinary Neurology*. Philadelphia, WB Saunders, 2004, pp 219-243.

Radlinsky M, Mason D: Disease of the ear. In Ettinger S, Feldman E (eds): *Textbook of Veterinary Internal Medicine*. St. Louis, Elsevier Saunders, 2005, pp 1171-1180.

AUTHOR: **JAMES B. MILLER**

EDITOR: **ETIENNE CÔTÉ**

Head Trauma

BASIC INFORMATION

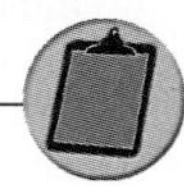

DEFINITION

Traumatic injury resulting in damage to intracranial structures

EPIDEMIOLOGY

SPECIES, AGE, SEX: Animals of any age or breed. Young animals may be overrepresented (lifestyle, increased risk of traumatic injury).

ASSOCIATED CONDITIONS AND DISORDERS

- Animals with traumatic brain injury may have traumatic injuries affecting other body systems (e.g., intra-abdominal hemorrhage, pulmonary contusions, fractures).
- Patients with a history of head trauma may be at risk for future seizure disorders.

CLINICAL PRESENTATION

HISTORY, CHIEF COMPLAINT

- History of traumatic event
- Owners may report loss of consciousness, inappropriate behavior, or seizure activity

PHYSICAL EXAM FINDINGS

- Signs of shock (e.g., tachycardia, hypotension, pale mucous membranes) may be present.
- Neurologic exam: indicators of intracranial injury:
  - Pupil asymmetry, abnormal pupil reactivity (excluding ocular trauma). Dilated unresponsive pupils (in the absence of ocular trauma or atropine) indicate severe neurologic injury and a poor outcome.
  - Diminished or absent oculocephalic (doll's eye) reflex.
  - Postural reaction deficits (may be due to spinal injury; note remainder of neurologic findings).
  - Diminished or altered consciousness (may be due to shock; note remainder of physical exam).
- Skull fractures may be palpable.
- Respiratory, musculoskeletal, and other body systems may show signs of traumatic injury.

ETIOLOGY AND PATHOPHYSIOLOGY

- Cerebral blood flow is mainly determined by blood pressure.
  - Autoregulation maintains blood flow to brain over a variety of pressures.
    - Autoregulation is lost when systolic blood pressure is below 50 or above 150 mmHg.
    - Loss of autoregulation also occurs during neuronal injury.
      - Blood pressure then becomes paramount in determining blood flow to the brain.
    - Cerebral perfusion pressure (CPP) is used for estimating cerebral blood flow (CBF).
    - CPP is determined by mean arterial pressure (MAP) and intracranial pressure (ICP).
      - CPP = MAP − ICP.
        - As intracranial pressure rises, cerebral perfusion decreases.
        - As MAP decreases, CPP also decreases.
- Trauma can result in primary or secondary insults to the brain.
  - Primary injury.
    - Occurs at the time of incident.
    - Result of hemorrhage and direct injury to neuronal tissue.
  - Secondary injury.
    - Consequence of the primary insult.
    - Can occur hours or days after initial insult.
    - Cascade of event that results in energy depletion, free radical injury, and cytokine activation leading to neuronal cell death and cerebral edema.
    - Treatment modalities are aimed at preventing or limiting the secondary effects.
    - If allowed to progress, secondary injury and worsening cerebral edema results in rising intracranial pressure, worsening neurologic injury, and eventually death.

DIAGNOSIS

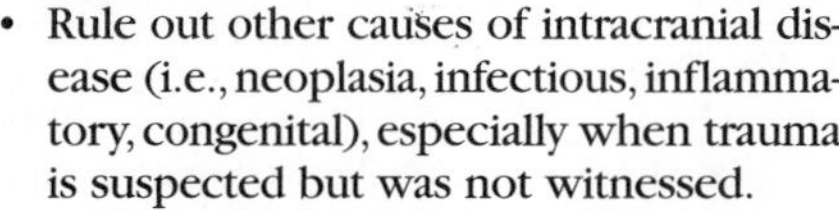

DIFFERENTIAL DIAGNOSIS

- Rule out other causes of intracranial disease (i.e., neoplasia, infectious, inflammatory, congenital), especially when trauma is suspected but was not witnessed.
- Animals in shock may manifest altered consciousness without neurologic damage. Await full neurologic assessment until initial stabilization has been completed.
- Metabolic diseases (e.g., hypoglycemia, liver disease) may also affect neurologic exam and should be considered as differentials if no traumatic event is reported or if the history is uncertain.

INITIAL DATABASE

- Baseline tests (packed cell volume/total solids, blood glucose, blood urea nitrogen): initial assessment of some metabolic causes of altered mentation
  - Consider transfusion if necessary to support adequate oxygen delivery to tissues.
  - Avoid hyperglycemia, which may be associated with poor outcome in head injury.
  - If azotemic or dehydrated, diuretics (mannitol/furosemide) should be used with caution if at all; tissue perfusion (normotension) is most important.
- Blood pressure: hypotension, hypertension
  - Identify and correct hypotension.
  - Systemic hypertension may be seen with elevated intracranial pressures or a consequence of pain or anxiety.
- Blood gas or pulse oximetry
  - Identify hypoxemia (e.g., PaO_2 <80 mmHg when breathing room air) to provide supplemental oxygen.
  - Identify and correct hypercarbia (elevated $PaCO_2$).
- Heart rate/electrocardiogram
  - Sinus tachycardia common with shock or volume depletion; ventricular arrhythmias possible (see Ventricular Arrhythmias [Premature Ventricular Complexes, Ventricular Tachycardia], p 1148).
  - Bradycardia may be seen with elevated ICP and in a comatose patient, suggests brain herniation.
- Neurologic assessment including pupil reactivity and size, cranial nerve function, postural reflexes, and level of consciousness (see Neurologic Examination, p 1286)
  - Localize lesion and rate the severity of injury.

ADVANCED OR CONFIRMATORY TESTING

- Radiographs
  - May be useful in identifying skull fractures.
  - Of limited value in the overall assessment of intracranial injury.
- Computed tomography (CT)
  - Ideal imaging modality if available.
  - Evaluate for skull fractures, hemorrhage, or other injuries.
- ICP monitoring
  - Useful for directing therapies and limiting consequences of elevated intracranial pressures.
  - May also be prognostic.
  - Infrequently used in veterinary medicine.
    - Requires skill and advanced care.

TREATMENT

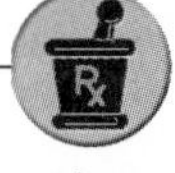

THERAPEUTIC GOAL(S)

- Maintain mean blood pressure above 60 mmHg (generally signifies that systolic blood pressure >90 mmHg):

- Essential in management of head trauma.
- Intravenous fluids: dosage according to need (maintenance vs. correction of hypotension).
  - Crystalloids (e.g., 0.9% NaCl, or lactated Ringer's solution) at shock doses IV (60–90 ml/kg for dog, 45–60 ml/kg for cat), unless renal/cardiovascular/dilutional contraindication.
    - Administer to effect in restoration of adequate blood pressure.
    - Concurrent use of colloids or hypertonic saline may limit cerebral edema that can occur with aggressive fluid administration.
    - Avoid fluids with excessive free water (maintenance fluids, 5% dextrose in water, 0.45% saline).
  - Colloids, e.g., hetastarch, pentastarch, dextran-70 (10–20 ml/kg/day IV).
    - Oncotic effect draws free water from the interstitium into the vasculature.
    - May potentiate effects of lower molecular weight substances (i.e., mannitol).
    - Useful for intravascular support with limited fluid volumes.
  - Hypertonic saline (7.5%) (4 ml/kg IV slowly).
    - Osmotic action to draw fluid from cerebral interstitium.
    - Effect short-lived.
      - Can combine with colloids for longer-lasting effect.
    - May also limit other secondary effects of head injury.
      - Improve microcirculatory blood flow.
      - Decrease neuroexcitotoxicity and intracellular calcium accumulation.
      - Immunomodulatory effects resulting in decreased inflammatory response.
    - Only used if patient is hydrated.
- Decrease intracranial pressure:
  - Mannitol (0.5–1 g/kg IV q 6–8h; limit to three bolus injections/24-hr period).
    - Osmotic diuretic.
    - Increases intravascular osmolarity and draws fluid in from cerebral tissue.
    - Free radical scavenging properties.
    - Decreases blood viscosity, increases cerebral blood flow.
    - Potential adverse effects.
      - Diuresis may decrease blood volume and consequently blood pressure.
        - Ensure adequate blood pressure and volume status before administration.
      - May result in "reverse osmotic shift."
        - In areas of hemorrhage, mannitol may leak into interstitium, pull fluid along, and worsen cerebral edema.
        - The effects of mannitol on lowering ICP may outweigh these potential effects on damaged areas.
  - Furosemide (2–5 mg/kg IV in coordination with mannitol).
    - Decreases production of cerebrospinal fluid and causes diuresis.
    - May potentiate effects of mannitol and decrease ICP.
    - Diuretic action may also worsen volume contraction and lead to hypovolemia.
- Maintain adequate oxygenation:
  - Important to ensure adequate nutrient delivery to neuronal tissue.
  - Provide supplemental oxygen as needed.
    - Also, ensure adequate oxygen carrying capacity (Hgb) and delivery (adequate blood pressure, see Maintain mean blood pressure, above).
- Miscellaneous therapies:
  - Surgery:
    - Craniotomy may be indicated for removal of hematomas, control of hemorrhage, in the case of depressed skull fractures or for removal of penetrating objects.
    - Results in a substantial decrease in ICP (15% with craniotomy and an additional 65% reduction with durotomy) and is superior in relief of elevated ICP compared to any medical therapy.
    - CT is useful for evaluation of injuries and determining need for surgical intervention.
  - Hyperventilation:
    - Has been advocated in head injury, although its use is controversial.
    - Lowers CO_2.
      - Resultant vasoconstriction decreases cerebral perfusion pressure and decreases ICP.
      - Decreased perfusion to brain parenchyma may have deleterious consequences.
    - Current recommendation: ventilate patient so as to maintain $PaCO_2$ between 30 and 35 mmHg.
  - Barbiturates:
    - Can use pentobarbital to effect.
      - 4–16 mg/kg IV titrated for induction.
      - 0.2–1 mg/kg/hr thereafter to maintain sedation.
    - Decrease cerebral metabolic rate.
    - Leads to vasoconstriction and decreases ICP.
    - Studies evaluating efficacy controversial.
      - May cause respiratory or cardiac depression, which is severely problematic in the head-injured patient.
      - If used, intensive nursing care is essential to monitor respiration (intubation and mechanical ventilation may be necessary), as well as blood pressure and temperature.
      - Often discussed as "last resort."
      - May be beneficial for seizure control or in an extremely agitated animal.
  - Hypothermia:
    - Results in decreased cerebral metabolic rate, decreased cerebral perfusion via reflex vasoconstriction, and consequently decreases ICP.
    - May also limit secondary brain injury by limiting neuroexcitatory activities and suppression of local inflammatory response.
    - Can be associated with coagulation abnormalities, cardiac disturbances, and hypotension.
    - Moderate hypothermia (32–33°C) has been reported to be efficacious in human trials and animal models of brain injury.
      - Clinical use in veterinary patients is uncertain.
  - Glucocorticoids:
    - Methylprednisolone sodium succinate (30 mg/kg slow IV over 10 minutes) after initial resuscitation may be best choice.
    - Use of steroids in head injury is highly controversial.
      - Human studies have failed to show benefit with glucocorticoid administration.
    - Potential benefits due to anti-inflammatory and free radical scavenging effects.
    - May be associated with several complications (hyperglycemia, gastric ulceration, decreased wound healing, and infection).

ACUTE GENERAL TREATMENT

- Initial therapy should address the "ABCs":
  - *A*irway:
    - May need intubation if depressed mentation or if mechanical ventilation is needed.
  - *B*reathing:
    - Ensure adequate oxygenation.
    - Supplement as needed.
  - *C*irculation:
    - Ensure adequate volume status and maintain normal blood pressure.
    - Fluid therapy as indicated (see above).
- Assess neurologic status:
  - Repeated examination may aid in the evaluation of efficacy of therapy.
  - Imaging (CT scan) may be helpful in assessing injury.

- Therapy to decrease intracranial pressure if indicated.

POSSIBLE COMPLICATIONS

- Infection
  - Aspiration pneumonia
  - Nosocomial infection
- Seizures
- Renal failure
  - Related to hypotension and hypovolemia
    - May be exacerbated by administration of diuretics.
- Persistent neurologic deficits

RECOMMENDED MONITORING

- Serial neurologic examination
- Monitor oxygenation (arterial blood gas/pulse oximetry)
- Ensure adequate blood pressure
- Monitor electrolytes (especially if mannitol/diuretics are used)
- Maintain euglycemia
- Monitor urine production
  - Specific gravity may be helpful in determining volume status

PROGNOSIS AND OUTCOME

- Prognosis is dependent on severity and type of injury:
  - Fair to good with minor, nonprogressive injury.
  - Severely injured animals have poorer short-term recovery rates and may have longer rehabilitation/recovery periods if they survive.
- Modified Glasgow Coma Score (MGCS) (see Box I-1) has been used for scoring injury severity in head trauma and has been correlated to outcome.

BOX I-1 Modified Glasgow Coma Score

Motor Activity	
Normal gait, normal spinal reflexes	6
Hemiparesis, tetraparesis, or decerebrate activity	5
Recumbent, intermittent extensor rigidity	4
Recumbent, constant extensor rigidity	3
Recumbent, constant extensor rigidity with opisthotonus	2
Recumbent, hypotonia of muscles, depressed or absent spinal reflexes	1
Brainstem Reflexes	
Normal pupillary light reflexes and oculocephalic reflexes	6
Slow pupillary light reflexes and normal to reduced oculocephalic reflexes	5
Bilateral unresponsive miosis with normal to reduced oculocephalic reflexes	4
Pinpoint pupils with reduced to absent oculocephalic reflexes	3
Unilateral unresponsive mydrisasis with reduced to absent oculocephalic reflexes	2
Bilateral unresponsive mydriasis with reduced to absent oculocephalic reflexes	1
Level of Consciousness	
Occasional periods of alertness, responsive to environment	6
Depression or delirium, capable of responding to environment but response may be inappropriate	5
Stupor, responsive to visual stimuli	4
Stupor, responsive to auditory stimuli	3
Stupor, responsive only to repeated noxious stimuli	2
Coma, unresponsive to repeated noxious stimuli	1

Total: _____

Assessment

Good prognosis	15–18
Guarded prognosis	9–14
Grave prognosis	3–8

PEARLS & CONSIDERATIONS

COMMENTS

- Head trauma is a common and serious injury in dogs and cats.
- Clinicians must recognize the signs of progressive neurologic injury.
  - The MGCS may be helpful as a monitoring tool (Box I-1).

CLIENT EDUCATION

- Clients must be informed of the potential for long recovery periods with more severely injured animals.
- Clients should also be made aware of the need for intensive treatment and monitoring of animals with head injury.
- The MGCS may be helpful in quantitating injury severity in order to provide the client with a prognosis.

SUGGESTED READING

Dewey CW: Emergency management of the head trauma patient. Principles and practice. *Vet Clin North Am Small Anim Pract* 30:207, 2000.

Platt SR, Radaelli ST, McDonnell JJ: The prognostic value of the Modified Glasgow Coma Scale in head trauma in dogs. *J Vet Intern Med* 15:581, 2001.

Proulx J, Dhupa N: Severe brain injury. Part I. Pathophysiology. *Compend Contin Educ Pract Vet* 20:897, 1998.

Proulx J, Dhupa N: Severe brain injury. Part II. Therapy. *Compend Contin Educ Pract Vet* 20:993, 1998.

AUTHOR: **ELIZABETH M. STREETER**

EDITOR: **ELIZABETH ROZANSKI**

Heart Base Tumor

BASIC INFORMATION

DEFINITION

A general term used for designating any mass located at the base of the heart in association with the ascending aorta and pulmonary trunk but without right atrial involvement. These masses have a variable rate of growth and metastasis, and almost always cause clinical signs.

SYNONYM(S)

Chemoreceptor cell tumors (chemodectoma, aortic body tumor, non chromaffin paragangliomas)

Ectopic thyroid carcinomas

EPIDEMIOLOGY

SPECIES, AGE

- Dogs: mean age 10.3 years (range 5.2 to 14.5 years), males may be overrepresented
- Cats: reported but rare

GENETICS AND BREED PREDISPOSITION

- Brachycephalic breeds may be predisposed.
- Chemodectomas occur more commonly in medium- to smaller-breed dogs than in large-breed dogs.

RISK FACTORS: Chronic hypoxemia may be a contributing factor.

ASSOCIATED CONDITIONS AND DISORDERS: Metastasis is rare and late in occurrence.

CLINICAL PRESENTATION

DISEASE FORMS/SUBTYPES

- Chemodectomas: arise from specialized neuroepithelial cells within the adventitia of the aortic arch. The majority of heart base masses in dogs are chemodectomas.
- Ectopic thyroid carcinomas: usually nonfunctional; adenomas or carcinomas; represent 5–10% of heart base tumors in dogs.

HISTORY, CHIEF COMPLAINT: Typically due to pericardial effusion elaborated by the mass and causing cardiac tamponade.

- Acute collapse.
- Nonspecific signs for weeks to months including lethargy, cough, dyspnea, abdominal distention, inappetence, episodic weakness, weight loss.
- Occasionally incidental finding such as an enlarged cardiac silhouette on thoracic radiographs.
- Owners may report signs associated with right-sided heart failure (abdominal enlargement perceived as weight gain by owners, exercise intolerance, increased respiratory rate).

PHYSICAL EXAM FINDINGS: Findings associated with pericardial effusion, including weak peripheral pulses, muffled heart sounds, and/or abdominal distention. Signs of lower respiratory tract dysfunction and/or signs of right-sided congestive heart failure (ascites, hepatomegaly, tachypnea, jugular distention/pulsation) may also be present.

ETIOLOGY AND PATHOPHYSIOLOGY

- Benign, nonfunctional tumors that produce clinical signs as a result of their space occupying nature and vascularity. Chemodectomas, may be large and may have produced only modest amounts of pericardial effusion at the time of diagnosis.
- Slowly progressive; occasionally invasive into local vasculature. Metastasis occurs rarely.
- Pericardial effusion causing cardiac tamponade.
- Right-sided congestive heart failure (secondary to pressure on the atrium or venae cavae).

DIAGNOSIS

DIFFERENTIAL DIAGNOSIS

- Other intrapericardial masses or infiltrations (right atrial tumors/hemangiosarcoma, mesothelioma, lymphoma)
- Benign/idiopathic pericardial effusion

INITIAL DATABASE

- Chest radiographs: a globoid cardiac silhouette in most but not all cases of pericardial effusion (80%).
- Electrocardiogram: normal sinus rhythm or sinus tachycardia. Ventricular arrhythmias common. Electrical alternans is suggestive of, but is an insensitive indicator for, pericardial effusion.
- Complete blood count, serum biochemistry profile, urinalysis: often unremarkable.

ADVANCED OR CONFIRMATORY TESTING

- Echocardiography: diagnostic test of choice. Chemodectomas originate around the aortic root, most commonly from the left cranial aspect of the aorta, and lie between the aorta and the main pulmonary artery. Ectopic thyroid carcinomas can be found attached to the ascending aorta.
- Cytologic evaluation of the pericardial effusion is not generally useful, as neoplasms that cause heart base tumors typically do not easily exfoliate cells.

TREATMENT

THERAPEUTIC GOAL(S)

- Relieve pericardial effusion
- Treat signs of right-sided heart failure

ACUTE GENERAL TREATMENT

- Pericardiocentesis (see Pericardiocentesis, p 1298) is essential when cardiac tamponade is present, but may not be necessary if only mild effusion is present and not causing hemodynamic effects.
- Diuretics are contraindicated in acute treatment.

CHRONIC TREATMENT

- Repeated pericardiocentesis.
- Diuretics (furosemide 1 mg/kg PO, IV, IM q 12h; spironolactone 1 mg/kg PO q 12h) have been advocated by some in an attempt to delay effusion recurrence.
- Pericardectomy in patients with recurrent pericardial effusion.

POSSIBLE COMPLICATIONS

- Surgical resection of the mass carries substantial risks because of the location and vascularity of these masses.
- Most heart base tumors are benign, with adenomas far more common than carcinomas. Malignant masses tend to invade local vessels or lymphatics and less frequently establish distant metastatic sites.

RECOMMENDED MONITORING

Recurrent pericardial effusion

PROGNOSIS AND OUTCOME

Dogs with heart base tumors that undergo pericardectomy tend to have longer survival times (mean 661 ± 170 days) than dogs that are treated with medications and repeated pericardiocenteses alone (mean 129 ± 51 days).

PEARLS & CONSIDERATIONS

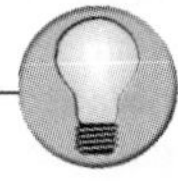

COMMENTS

Unfortunately, cytologic study of pericardial fluid and fine-needle aspiration are unlikely to be diagnostic. Signalment (breed) and characteristic location at the heart base may lead to a greater suspicion of heart base tumor and the possibility of a better prognosis than with other cardiac tumors such as hemangiosarcoma. Decision to proceed with pericardectomy may be difficult for clients without a histopathologic diagnosis.

CLIENT EDUCATION

- Repeated pericardiocentesis and pericardectomy are both palliative and not curative.
- Pericardectomy will likely lead to longer survival time with fewer clinical signs in the interim.

SUGGESTED READING

Kittleson MD, Kienle RD: *Small Animal Cardiovascular Medicine*. St. Louis, Mosby, 1998, pp 418–432.

Tobias A: Pericardial disorders. In Ettinger S, Feldman E (eds): *Textbook of Veterinary Internal Medicine*. St. Louis, Elsevier Saunders, 2005, pp 1115–1116.

Vicari ED, et al: Survival times and prognostic indicators for dogs with heart base masses: 25 cases (1986–1999). *JAVMA* 219:4, 2001.

AUTHOR: **ERIN D. VICARI**

EDITOR: **ETIENNE CÔTÉ**

Heart Failure, Acute/Decompensated

Client Education Sheet on Website

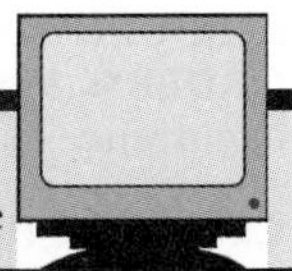

BASIC INFORMATION

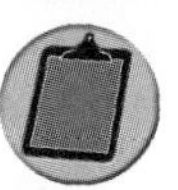

DEFINITION

Acute (or decompensated) congestive heart failure (HF) is characterized by the sudden onset of clinical signs associated with pulmonary edema or cavitary effusions that develop as a consequence of heart disease. Most often, acute/decompensated HF is associated with worsening cardiac performance in patients with chronic heart disease.

SYNONYM(S)

Acute congestive heart failure
Decompensated heart disease
Overt heart failure

EPIDEMIOLOGY

SPECIES, AGE, SEX: Signalment reflects predispositions for the causative heart disorder. Examples:
- Geriatric small-breed dogs: chronic mitral/tricuspid regurgitation (myxomatous valve disease)
- Cats: hypertrophic cardiomyopathy (HCM)

GENETICS AND BREED PREDISPOSITION
- Dilated cardiomyopathy (DCM): Doberman pinschers, Great Danes, Irish wolfhounds, and other large- and giant-breed dogs
- Mitral/tricuspid myxomatous valve disease: Cavalier King Charles spaniels, dachshunds, many others
- HCM: inherited in Maine coon cats; it is possible that feline HCM generally is a genetic disease

RISK FACTORS
- In patients with underlying heart disease:
  - Dietary sodium excess
  - Acute intravascular volume load (e.g., parenteral fluids)
  - Possibly corticosteroids (HCM cats)
  - Possibly ketamine/tiletamine (HCM cats)
- Electrocardiographic, echocardiographic variables: predictive of likelihood of future HF in Doberman pinschers with DCM

CLINICAL PRESENTATION

DISEASE FORMS/SUBTYPES
- Left-sided HF results in pulmonary edema.
- Right-sided HF causes ascites and sometimes concurrent pleural effusion.
- In cats, pleural effusion may result from left- and/or right-sided heart disease.

HISTORY, CHIEF COMPLAINT
- Respiratory signs predominate. Specifically, the characteristic manifestations include tachypnea, dyspnea, and, in the dog, cough. Heart failure seldom causes coughing in cats.
- Clients may report that the patient appears to be uncomfortable, restless, or unwilling to lie down.

PHYSICAL EXAM FINDINGS
- Tachycardia is a relatively consistent, although nonspecific, finding in dogs with HF. Heart rate of cats with acute HF differs little from heart rate of healthy cats.
- The presence of respiratory sinus arrhythmia is generally inconsistent with acute HF; other explanations for the clinical signs should be considered.
- In patients with pulmonary edema, tachypnea and respiratory distress are usually apparent during the physical examination.
- Dogs with acute HF due to mitral or tricuspid regurgitation due to myxomatous valve disease have a cardiac murmur; usually the murmur is loud (≥III/VI).
- An audible, low-frequency third or fourth heart sound—a gallop—reflects high atrial pressures and reduced ventricular compliance. Relatively specific marker of acute HF.

ETIOLOGY AND PATHOPHYSIOLOGY

- Congestive signs result when high venous pressures cause the development of edema) or cavitary effusions.
- In dogs, HF that results primarily from systolic dysfunction—failure of the ventricle to completely empty—is most common.
- HF in cats usually results from diseases that impair ventricular filling (diastolic dysfunction).
- HF is associated with neuroendocrine activation that temporarily maintains perfusion pressure and cardiac output through vasoconstriction and increases in heart rate and contractility.
- In patients with systolic dysfunction, systemic vascular resistance rises disproportionately, causing a detrimental increase in afterload; this explains the beneficial effect of vasodilators.

DIAGNOSIS

DIFFERENTIAL DIAGNOSIS

Other causes of respiratory distress and/or cough:
- Chronic sterile bronchitis
- Collapsing trachea
- Allergic airway disease
- Pleural effusion
- Intrathoracic mass
- Pneumonia
- Pneumothorax

INITIAL DATABASE

- Thoracic radiographs: radiographic findings of left atrial enlargement together with pulmonary opacities is diagnostic of left-sided HF.
- Electrocardiography (ECG) is indicated when arrhythmias complicate the presentation.
- Serum biochemistry profile and urinalysis: in all cases, preferrably before initiating treatment.

ADVANCED OR CONFIRMATORY TESTING

Echocardiography defines the causative disorder

TREATMENT

THERAPEUTIC GOAL(S)

- Restore ventilatory function by eliminating lung edema or pleural effusion
- In some cases, improve cardiac performance

ACUTE GENERAL TREATMENT

- Rest.
- Judicious/minimal restraint, and other measures for reducing anxiety, are essential.
- Furosemide: diuretic of choice in acute HF. Dose and dosage interval are best determined by clinical response.
  - Initially: relatively high dose (2-6 mg/kg IV, IM).
  - If no overt (e.g., respiratory) evidence of effect, this dose can be repeated within 45 to 60 minutes.
  - If respiratory rate and effort decrease: 1-2 mg/kg IV or IM q 1-4h until respirations normalize.
  - The effect of furosemide is rapid but short-lived; low doses at short intervals are recommended to limit adverse effects.
  - In general, cats require lower doses than do dogs.
- Supplementary oxygen.
- Morphine (0.05-0.3 mg/kg SC, IM, or IV) should be considered for dogs that are anxious from respiratory distress.
- Thoracocentesis if physical or radiographic findings indicate that pleural effusion is likely responsible for respiratory distress.
- Transdermal nitroglycerin (0.5-3 cm q 12h) may reduce venous pressures. Efficacy undetermined.

- Patients with systolic dysfunction may benefit from intravenous administration of nitroprusside (0.5–15 μg/kg/min) and/or dobutamine (2–15 μg/kg/min) constant rate infusion. Careful monitoring required.
- IV or SC fluid administration is generally contraindicated unless used as a vehicle for the administration of drugs or electrolytes.
- Angiotensin-converting enzyme inhibitors, other diuretics, etc.: considered once patient is stable. See Heart Failure, Chronic, below.

POSSIBLE COMPLICATIONS

- Hypovolemia/impaired renal perfusion due to excessive diuresis
- Hypotension

RECOMMENDED MONITORING

- Frequent monitoring of vital signs, mucous membranes, body weight.
- ECG if arrhythmias.
- Flow-directed (Swan-Ganz) pulmonary artery catheterization and/or arterial cannula can be considered for hemodynamic monitoring of severely affected dogs admitted to an intensive care unit.

PROGNOSIS AND OUTCOME

- Most patients presented for first treatment of acute HF respond promptly to conservative therapy consisting of rest, supplemental oxygen, furosemide, and in some cases, nitroglycerin.
- Despite favorable initial response, HF is generally associated with a poor long-term prognosis unless the causative disorder is curable.

PEARLS & CONSIDERATIONS

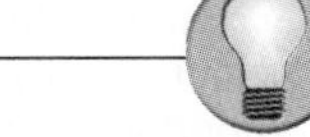

COMMENTS

- Although ancillary therapy including vasodilators and inotropes may speed recovery from acute HF, most patients that are destined to recover respond to conservative management.
- Response to empiric therapy is diagnostically useful; when treatment is based on a presumptive diagnosis, failure to respond to diuresis suggests the possibility that clinical signs are due to primary respiratory tract disease or that the patient has medically refractory HF.

CLIENT EDUCATION

Chronic medical therapy is generally required even after apparent recovery from HF

SUGGESTED READING

Sisson D, Kittleson MD: Management of heart failure: Principles of treatment, therapeutic strategies, and pharmacology. In Fox PR, Sisson D, Moise NS (eds): *Textbook of Canine and Feline Cardiology*, ed 2. Philadelphia, WB Saunders, 1999, pp 216–250.

AUTHOR: **JONATHAN A. ABBOTT**
EDITOR: **ETIENNE CÔTÉ**

Heart Failure, Chronic

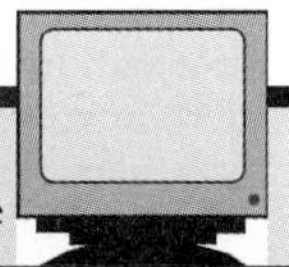

Client Education Sheet on Website

BASIC INFORMATION

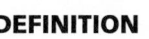

DEFINITION

Heart failure is a syndrome that results from impaired filling or emptying of the heart. Because veterinary patients cannot offer subjective observations—the perception of breathlessness during exertion for example—the presence of cardiogenic edema or cavitary effusions is used as an objective criterion for the diagnosis. Unfortunately, when the causative disorder cannot be definitively treated, cardiac dysfunction is generally progressive even after signs associated with clinical decompensation have resolved. For the purpose of this article, the term *chronic heart failure* (HF) is used for describing the clinical status of patients who have at some time developed congestion due to heart disease.

SYNONYM(S)

Congestive heart failure

EPIDEMIOLOGY

SPECIES, AGE, SEX: Signalment reflects predispositions for the causative heart disorder.

- Geriatric small-breed dogs: chronic mitral and tricuspid regurgitation due to myxomatous valve disease.
- Adult large- and giant-breed dogs: dilated cardiomyopathy (DCM).
- Cats: hypertrophic cardiomyopathy (HCM; males > females), restrictive/unclassified cardiomyopathy.

GENETICS AND BREED PREDISPOSITION

- DCM: Doberman pinschers, Great Danes, Irish wolfhounds, and other large- and giant-breed dogs.
- Mitral and tricuspid regurgitation due to chronic myxomatous valve disease: geriatric small-breed dogs including Cavalier King Charles spaniels, dachshunds, and many others.
- HCM: inherited in Maine coon cats and it is possible that feline HCM generally is a genetic disease.

RISK FACTORS: Electrocardiographic and echocardiographic variables that predict the development of HF in Doberman pinschers have been described. In Irish wolfhounds and other giant-breed dogs, atrial fibrillation sometimes precedes the development of chronic HF. Other than those related to signalment, risk factors for the development of chronic HF in other animals have not been identified.

CLINICAL PRESENTATION

DISEASE FORMS/SUBTYPES

- Left-sided HF results in pulmonary edema.
- Right-sided HF causes ascites and sometimes concurrent pleural effusion.
- In cats, pleural effusion apparently results from left- or right-sided HF; ascites is uncommon.

HISTORY, CHIEF COMPLAINT: By definition, patients with chronic HF previously have had clinically apparent congestion. Clinical signs such as respiratory distress have improved or resolved with initial treatment, but signs such as progressive abdominal distention, syncope, lethargy, and weight loss may persist. Patients with chronic heart failure are subject to episodes of acute/decompensated heart failure.

PHYSICAL EXAM FINDINGS

- Patients with chronic HF due to mitral/tricuspid myxomatous valve disease have a cardiac murmur; usually the murmur is loud, and its intensity is generally not affected by treatment.
- An audible third or fourth heart sound, a gallop, reflects high atrial pressures and reduced ventricular compliance. Regardless of underlying disease, it is a relatively specific marker of HF.

ETIOLOGY AND PATHOPHYSIOLOGY

- Congestive signs result when high venous pressures cause the development of edema or cavitary effusions.
- In dogs, HF that results primarily from systolic dysfunction—failure of the

ventricle to completely empty—is most common.

- HF in cats usually results from diseases that impair ventricular filling; diastolic ventricular pressures are abnormally high when ventricular volume is normal or small.
- High filling pressures are reflected upstream to the venous circulation, resulting in edema or pleural effusion.
- HF is associated with neuroendocrine activation: specifically, impaired cardiac performance leads to increased activity of the renin-angiotensin-aldosterone system (RAAS) and the adrenergic nervous system (ANS).
- Angiotensin II (ATII) is the biologically active product of a biochemical cascade for which the final step is catalyzed by angiotensin-converting enzyme (ACE).
- ATII is a vasoconstrictor, but it also stimulates the release of aldosterone, augments activity of the ANS, and acts as a cardiomyotrophic factor.
- Activation of the RAAS and ANS serves to temporarily maintain perfusion pressure and cardiac output.
- Vasoconstriction increases vascular resistance so that blood pressure is maintained when cardiac output is subnormal. In patients with mitral/tricuspid myxomatous valve disease or DCM, vascular resistance is high, causing a detrimental increase in afterload; this partly explains the beneficial effect of vasodilators.
- Activation of the ANS increases heart rate and inotropy (myocardial contractility).
- Renal retention of salt and water supports the failing heart through increases in preload. However, these increases in intravascular volume result in high venous pressures with potential consequences of edema or cavitary effusions.
- It is now generally accepted that neuroendocrine activation associated with cardiac dysfunction is initially beneficial, but ultimately detrimental and contributes importantly to the pathogenesis of progressive cardiac dysfunction. Current therapies for chronic HF reflect this conceptual framework.

DIAGNOSIS

DIFFERENTIAL DIAGNOSIS

Other causes of respiratory distress, cough, abdominal distention, lethargy, inappetence, and weight loss (cardiac cachexia)

INITIAL DATABASE

- Thoracic radiography:
  - Left atrial enlargement with pulmonary opacities is diagnostic of decompensated left-sided HF. See Heart Failure, Acute/Decompensated, p 458.
  - With diuretic treatment of decompensated HF, clinical improvement is usually rapid (minutes to hours), but radiographic resolution of pulmonary infiltrates may take 12 to 24 hours.
  - Cats commonly develop pleural effusion in association with left-sided cardiac disease.
- Ascites (and rarely, peripheral edema) associated with imaging evidence of substantive right-sided disease is diagnostic of decompensated right-sided HF.
- Electrocardiography (ECG) is indicated when arrhythmias complicate the presentation. Atrial fibrillation is commonly associated with heart failure in large-breed dogs, but tachyarrhythmia of virtually any type may complicate the presentation of heart failure. See Heart Failure, Acute/Decompensated, p 458.
- Serum biochemistry profiles: provide useful ancillary information and are important in monitoring the effects of therapy (especially renal and electrolyte effects).

ADVANCED OR CONFIRMATORY TESTING

Echocardiography generally provides the diagnosis of the underlying cardiac lesion. However, echocardiography does not identify the consequences of heart disease. HF is not an echocardiographic diagnosis, it is a clinical diagnosis that is usually based on radiographic findings. Echocardiography is complementary to physical examination and thoracic radiography but does not replace them.

TREATMENT

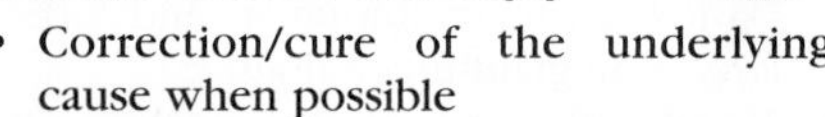

THERAPEUTIC GOAL(S)

- Correction/cure of the underlying cause when possible
- In all cases, increase in quality and duration of life

CHRONIC TREATMENT

- Diuretics. Furosemide is the most effective agent for management of congestive signs.
  - In dogs, a dose of 1 mg/kg PO q 12h is often initially adequate when given concurrently with ancillary agents such as ACE inhibitors. Cats with HF generally require lower initial doses (0.5-1 mg/kg PO q 12-24).
  - Furosemide is used first, but over time, if recurrence of signs warrants more diuretic, other less potent diuretics such as chlorothiazides (2-4 mg/kg PO q 12h) or spironolactone (1-2 mg/kg PO q 12h [dog]) can be added. Doing so allows for synergistic diuretic action: Different diuretics act in different parts of the nephron, which minimizes the negative effects of long-term (weeks or more) administration of high doses of a single diuretic (e.g., >3-4 mg/kg q 8-12h furosemide).
  - Diuretic dose should be determined by clinical response; the optimal dose is the lowest one that eliminates congestive signs.
  - Excessive diuresis may decrease renal perfusion, creates electrolyte imbalances, and contributes to potentially harmful neuroendocrine activation.
  - Most patients require lifelong diuretic administration; progression of the underlying disorder generally necessitates increases in furosemide dose and/or the use of additional diuretics.
  - Furosemide administration sometimes can be tapered or temporarily discontinued in cats with hypertrophic or restrictive/unclassified cardiomyopathy.
- ACE inhibitors partially blunt the effects of RAAS activation and reduce afterload.
  - ACE inhibition has proven benefits for patients with chronic HF caused by systolic dysfunction; preliminary evidence suggests a benefit for patients with chronic HF caused by diastolic dysfunction (e.g., cats with HF caused by hypertrophic or restrictive/unclassified cardiomyopathy).
  - Of the ACE inhibitors, veterinary experience is greatest with enalapril (0.5 mg/kg PO q 12-24h [dog]), benazepril (0.25-0.5 mg/kg PO q 24h [dog], 0.5-1 mg/kg PO q 24h [cat]) and ramipril (0.125 mg/kg PO q 24h [dog]).
- Digoxin:
  - 0.22 mg/m^2 PO q 12h [dog]; 0.03125 mg/cat PO q 48h.
  - Weak positive inotrope that has potentially beneficial neuroendocrine effects; digoxin inhibits adrenergic activity and increases vagal tone.
  - Important in management of patients with both systolic dysfunction (e.g., dilated cardiomyopathy) and atrial fibrillation; benefit to patients with sinus rhythm is controversial. Digoxin is generally contraindicated in HCM.
- Pimobendan (0.1-0.3 mg/kg PO q 12h administered when stomach is empty) is a phosphodiesterase inhibitor that acts as an "inodilator"; it is not currently licensed in the United States but has a role in the management of systolic dysfunction.
- β-Blockers (BB). There is experimental evidence that supports the use of low-dose BB in dogs with systolic dysfunction (e.g., dilated cardiomyopathy, advanced mitral/tricuspid endocardiosis).
  - BB are negative inotropes that can provoke clinical decompensation (induce acute HF) if given at an inappropriately high initial dose or if the

dose is increased too quickly; dose must be gradually titrated over weeks from a low initial dose to a target dose.
  - BB are never started before a patient's pulmonary edema has resolved.
  - BB are a nonstandard therapy for dogs with systolic dysfunction; they should be used only with caution and careful monitoring. An initial dose ≤0.1 mg/kg PO q 12h is probably reasonable for carvedilol. A slightly higher initial dose of metoprolol (0.1–0.2 mg/kg PO q 12h) may be appropriate.
- Spironolactone (1–2 mg/kg PO q 12h [dog]).
  - In chronic HF, excess aldosterone may contribute to the development of myocardial fibrosis.
  - Spironolactone is an aldosterone antagonist, and as such it may limit the detrimental effects of hyperaldosteronemia; careful monitoring of electrolytes is advised.
- Moderate dietary sodium restriction generally is indicated. If palatable to the patient, low-sodium diets may reduce diuretic requirements.

POSSIBLE COMPLICATIONS

- "Cardiorenal syndrome": azotemia associated with diuretic administration and diminished cardiac performance.
- When azotemia is encountered in patients receiving furosemide and ACE inhibitors, *furosemide* is first decreased by 50% provided the patient is free of congestive signs. If creatinine does not decrease, diuretic therapy is discontinued again, provided congestive signs are not evident. Only if this is unsuccessful, is the ACE inhibitor discontinued. ACE inhibitors can increase stroke volume, but in contrast, diuretic therapy serves primarily to limit congestive signs.
- There are, unfortunately, few alternatives for patients that develop clinical signs specifically due to azotemia when congestive signs are present concurrently; this may reflect medically intractable heart failure. However, caution must be exercised, as "overinterpretation" of radiographs can lead to inappropriately high diuretic doses, volume depletion, and azotemia.

RECOMMENDED MONITORING

- Serum urea, creatinine, and electrolytes
- Serum digoxin concentration

PROGNOSIS AND OUTCOME

Despite favorable initial response, heart failure is generally associated with a poor long-term prognosis unless the causative disorder is curable

PEARLS & CONSIDERATIONS

COMMENTS

- Current therapy of heart failure reflects the understanding that activation of the ANS and RAAS is central to the pathogenesis of the syndrome.
- When the causative disorder is not curable, chronic HF is a progressive and terminal syndrome. Therefore attempts to identify a correctable cause are important; some patients with dilated cardiomyopathy respond to supplementation with neutraceuticals such as taurine and L-carnitine.

PREVENTION

- In patients with clinically silent dilated cardiomyopathy, the onset of heart failure may be delayed by the administration of ACE inhibitors and BB.
- Evidence that medical therapy slows the progression of mitral/tricuspid myxomatous valve disease or HCM is currently lacking.

CLIENT EDUCATION

Management of the veterinary patient with chronic HF requires careful monitoring and relatively frequent adjustment of medical therapy.

SUGGESTED READING

Sisson D, Kittleson MD: Management of heart failure: Principles of treatment, therapeutic strategies, and pharmacology. In Fox PR, Sisson D, Moise NS (eds): *Textbook of Canine and Feline Cardiology*, ed 2. Philadelphia, WB Saunders, 1999, pp 216–250.

AUTHOR: **JONATHAN A. ABBOTT**
EDITOR: **ETIENNE CÔTÉ**

Heart Murmurs

BASIC INFORMATION

DEFINITION

Normal blood flow is laminar in nature and is very quiet. When smooth laminar flow is altered, turbulence develops and, as a result, murmurs occur. This can be most easily likened to a slow-flowing wide river. Suddenly a large obstruction such as a large boulder is placed in the river and now the quiet river becomes a turbulent, noisy one as the water flows around and about the rock.

EPIDEMIOLOGY

SPECIES, AGE, SEX

- Dogs and cats of any age and either sex
- "Benign" heart murmurs of puppies and kittens: <4 months old
  - Soft (III/VI or less)*
  - Systolic*
  - Point of maximal intensity: left hemithorax*
  - May be abolished with increase in heart rate or change in body position

GENETICS AND BREED PREDISPOSITION: Many underlying congenital heart malformations and adult-onset cardiac disorders.

RISK FACTORS

- Heart murmurs are associated with congenital or acquired diseases of the heart (myocardium, valves, endocardium) and great vessels.
- Heart murmurs also are associated with noncardiac entities such as fever, anemia, hyperthyroidism, extreme thinness or obesity, and pregnancy. These murmurs are always systolic and soft (≤III/VI).
- Physiologic (functional) murmurs are rare in dogs and cats: a murmur is present in the absence of any cardiac or systemic abnormalities.
- Murmurs may also be identified in the veins and arteries under circumstances that cause nonlaminar flow, such as arteriovenous fistulas.
- Systemic infection may cause bacterial endocarditis (see Endocarditis, Infective, p 344).

*Can also occur with murmurs caused by congenital heart malformations.

CLINICAL PRESENTATION

HISTORY, CHIEF COMPLAINT

- Heart murmurs noted during a routine examination in a patient that is other-

wise well. The goal is to identify the cause of the murmur.
- Heart murmurs noted in a patient that is systemically ill (e.g., anemic). The goal is to ascertain whether the murmur is caused by the illness, or whether an underlying heart problem is coexistent (e.g., endocarditis).
- Heart murmurs noted in patients with signs suggesting heart disease (dyspnea, exercise intolerance, collapse, signs of thromboembolism). The murmur is a clue that these vague signs may be caused by a heart problem; cardiac diagnostic testing is indicated.

PHYSICAL EXAM FINDINGS
- Murmurs should be identified during the physical examination. Using the stethoscope, the examiner thoroughly auscults the dog or cat's thorax, first using the diaphragm and then the bell of the instrument. All four valve areas—mitral, tricuspid, pulmonic, and aortic regions—are ausculted, listening for abnormalities of the heart rate and rhythm as well as alterations in the heart sounds (see Gallops and Other Extra Heart Sounds, p 424). If a murmur exists, it needs to be identified with respect to timing, intensity, and musical tonality, as well as noting where the murmur is heard on the thorax and if the sounds spread to other parts of the thorax or into the jugular region of the neck.
- Murmurs are first identified as to their intensity, using a grading system of VI maximum with a I/VI being the least intense and barely heard, II/VI being just heard with the stethoscope, III/VI being easily distinguished; IV/VI being intense but without a palpable thrill; V/VI being loud, intense, and associated with a precordial (thoracic wall) vibration or thrill on the thorax, where it is auscultated and a VI/VI being so loud that it is heard with the stethoscope off the thorax and also is so intense that a thoracic thrill is present.
- The murmur is identified as to when it occurs—in systole, diastole, or in both of these physiologic periods of the heart cycle (continuous). Murmurs are also noted as being early, mid, or late (systole or diastole) and are then characterized by their musical quality or tone; they may be high frequency, mid range, or low frequency.

ETIOLOGY AND PATHOPHYSIOLOGY
- Systolic murmurs are associated with congenital conditions (subaortic stenosis, pulmonic stenosis, septal defects, atrioventricular dysplasia, tetralogy of Fallot, and other less common congenital lesions).
- Systolic murmurs also are auscultated with acquired conditions including mitral endocardiosis (insufficiency), cardiomyopathies, anemia, fever, hyperthyroid heart disease, heartworm disease, and endocarditis.
- Diastolic murmurs are unusual in small animal medicine but are associated with mitral stenosis, aortic valvular insufficiency, or pulmonic valvular insufficiency.
- Systolic and diastolic murmurs together (continuous murmurs) are most commonly observed with patent ductus arteriosus or arteriovenous fistula.

DIAGNOSIS

DIFFERENTIAL DIAGNOSIS
Heart murmurs must be differentiated from breath sounds. In animals with particularly noisy breathing, respiratory distress, or anxiety, the breath sounds may be confused with heart murmurs due to the noise occurring from the thorax or upper respiratory system during auscultation.

INITIAL DATABASE
- Thoracic radiographs and echocardiography: evaluation of primary heart disorders
- Complete blood count, serum chemistry panel, urinalysis, serum thyroxine level, abdominal imaging: as indicated for systemic disorders

TREATMENT

THERAPEUTIC GOAL(S)
Treatment of heart murmurs is not an option. The veterinarian must identify the murmur first, then the cause of the murmur, and then make associations with the disease condition present. Just because there is a murmur does not mean that the animal requires therapy. Similarly, the intensity of the murmur is not necessarily directly related to the severity of the disease. That is the goal of determining the cause of the problem.

PROGNOSIS AND OUTCOME

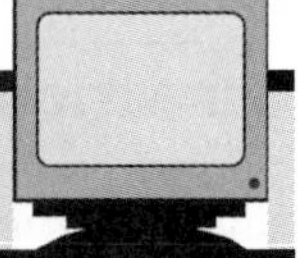

Highly variable. The prognosis of a patient with a heart murmur is influenced by the disorder causing the murmur, not by the murmur itself.

SUGGESTED READING

Fox P, Sisson D, Moise S: *Canine and Feline Cardiology*, ed 2. Philadelphia, WB Saunders, 1998

AUTHOR: **STEPHEN J. ETTINGER**
EDITOR: **ETIENNE CÔTÉ**

Heartworm Disease, Cat

Client Education Sheet on Website

BASIC INFORMATION

DEFINITION
Heartworm disease is the clinicopathologic manifestation of infestation with *Dirofilaria immitis*, an intravascular parasite that resides in the pulmonary arteries, the right side of the heart, and venae cavae. This infestation results in pneumonitis, pulmonary endarteritis, pulmonary thromboembolism (PTE), and uncommonly, pulmonary hypertension (PH) with/without cor pulmonale.

SYNONYM(S)
Heartworm disease (HWD)
Heartworm infection (HWI)

EPIDEMIOLOGY
SPECIES, AGE, SEX
- Felids are atypic hosts for this canine parasite.
- There is no age predilection (range 1 to 17 years).
- Male cats generally have an increased risk of exposure and have a higher incidence than females when infected experimentally.

RISK FACTORS
- Cats not receiving heartworm (HW) preventative in endemic areas are at risk, with varying seasonal individual risk determined by season of the year and geographic location.
- Outdoor cats are predisposed, but indoor cats are also at risk (up to a third of cats with HWD are indoor cats).
- Feline leukemia virus and feline immunodeficiency virus are not predisposing factors.

CONTAGION AND ZOONOSIS: See Heartworm Disease, Dog, p 465.

GEOGRAPHY AND SEASONALITY

- The frequency of feline HW infection correlates with that of dogs in the same geographic region, but at a lower incidence (infection rate is 5–20% that of the dog).
- Reported worldwide and is endemic throughout most parts of the United States.
- HW transmission is unlikely in regions or seasons where the ambient temperature does not average over 65° F during a 30-day period.
- Prevalence: in shelter cats (up to 14%) and 9% in pet cats presented for cardiorespiratory signs (26% of these cats were HW antibody positive, indicating HW exposure). Nationwide in the United States, exposure rate likely exceeds 12%.
- Clinical signs associated with early infection occur in late fall and early winter.

ASSOCIATED CONDITIONS AND DISORDERS

- Aberrant migration of larvae more common in cats (neurologic, dermatologic, and ophthalmic complications).
- Pulmonary thromboembolism (PTE) may be due to dead worms (natural or pharmacologic death) or intravascular thrombi formed in response to the infection resulting in vascular occlusion, infarction, and sometimes acute respiratory death.
- Pulmonary edema, often fulminant, possibly representing acute respiratory distress syndrome (ARDS). This may result acutely after worm death.
- Eosinophilic pneumonitis with cough, wheezing, dyspnea.
- Congestive heart failure (CHF) is uncommon; signs of right-heart failure occur, usually a pleural effusion (either hydrothorax or chylothorax) and/or ascites.

CLINICAL PRESENTATION

DISEASE FORMS/SUBTYPES

- Clinical classification: (1) no clinical signs, (2) acute or peracute, and (3) chronic (most common).
- Most feline HW infections are occult infections, defined as an infection in which microfilaria are not detectable; microfilaremia in cats is uncommon (<20%), inconsistent, and transient.

HISTORY, CHIEF COMPLAINT

- Many cats with HW infection show no clinical signs (28% in one study).
- Chronic signs usually predominate (cough [38%], dyspnea [48%], vomiting, anorexia, weight loss, lethargy, exercise intolerance, and rarely, right-sided CHF).
- Acute signs include tachypnea/dyspnea secondary to PTE or severe pneumonitis or ARDS. Sudden death occurs in approximately 10%.

PHYSICAL EXAM FINDINGS

- Usually nonspecific. There appears to be no correlation between the clinical signs, physical examination, and radiographic changes.
- Adventitial lung sounds may be present.
- An audible heart murmur and/or gallop rhythm is uncommon and CHF is rare. Jugular venous distention, dyspnea, diminished lung sounds, and, rarely, ascites may be detected if CHF is present.

ETIOLOGY AND PATHOPHYSIOLOGY

- Female mosquitoes serve as intermediate hosts after feeding on microfilaria-positive dogs.
- Being an atypic host, cats have an inherent resistance.
  - Lower worm burdens (usually fewer than 6, typically 1 to 3).
  - Shortened worm patency period.
  - High frequency of amicrofilaremia or low microfilaria counts.
  - Shortened lifespan of adult heartworms (2 to 3 years).
- Disease severity is determined in part by the number of adult HW and the host's response to live and dead heartworms.
  - Pulmonary response is more severe in cats when compared to dogs.
- Initiation of pulmonary disease is approximately 3 months after initial infection when L5 larvae arrive in the caudal lobar pulmonary arteries.
- Response of the pulmonary arteries, pulmonary parenchyma, and air spaces.
  - Eosinophilic infiltrates predominate.
  - Pulmonary arterial medial and intimal hypertrophy with or without thrombosis, often resulting in obliteration of the vascular lumen
  - Altered vascular permeability allows plasma leakage, producing noncardiogenic pulmonary edema (ARDS).
  - Chronic changes can result in diminished pulmonary function, hypoxemia, dyspnea, and cough.
- Acute or sudden death is typically associated with worm death and respiratory failure.
  - Lungs are considered to be the "shock organ" in feline HW disease.
    - Immune-mediated reaction to HW antigens produces bronchiolar and bronchial constriction, pulmonary congestion and interstitial edema, acute inflammatory interstitial disease, superficial pulmonary hemorrhage, and periarterial hemorrhage with subsequent fatal respiratory failure.
  - Heartworm embolism.
    - Smaller feline pulmonary arterial tree with less collateral circulation is more susceptible to worm embolization with subsequent pulmonary infarction.
    - May contribute to episodes of dyspnea and/or sudden death.

DIAGNOSIS

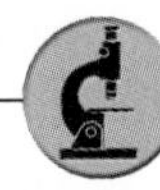

DIFFERENTIAL DIAGNOSIS

- Cat with respiratory signs:
  - Lung worms (*Aelurostrongylus abstrusus*)
  - *Paragonimus kellicotti* infection
  - Bronchitis or asthma
  - Pleural effusions (pyothorax, hydrothorax, chylothorax, or neoplastic)
  - Pneumothorax
- Cat with neurologic signs (brain or spinal cord):
  - Various inflammatory, ischemic, neoplastic or degenerative diseases of central nervous system
- Cat with gastrointestinal (GI) signs:
  - Various systemic diseases such as primary GI disease, neoplasia, hyperthyroidism, and renal failure

INITIAL DATABASE

- Complete blood count, chemistry profile, urinalysis.
  - Mild nonregenerative anemia or eosinophilia in about 33%.
  - Basophilia is highly suggestive, but rare.
- Tracheal wash or bronchoalveolar lavage may contain eosinophils without the presence of peripheral eosinophilia.
- Fecal examination for lung parasites (flotation, sedimentation, Baermann procedure).
- Electrocardiography may demonstrate a right axis shift and/or atrial or ventricular arrhythmias in severe cases (uncommon).
- Imaging:
  - Thoracic radiographs (variable findings depending on duration of infection and HW infection severity).
    - Enlarged and, sometimes torturous, truncated caudal pulmonary arteries. Right heart enlargement, common in dogs, is unusual in cats.
    - Patchy mixed interstitial-alveolar pattern with perivascular infiltrates (primarily in caudal lung lobes).
    - Radiographic vascular findings are transient.
    - Mimics asthma with bronchovascular pattern and pulmonary hyperinflation.

ADVANCED OR CONFIRMATORY TESTING

- The diagnosis of HW infestation/disease in cats can be difficult and often requires an elevated index of suspicion and a battery of diagnostic tests.
- Microfilaria: Most cats are amicrofilaremic. Filter and modified Knott's tests preferred over wet direct blood smear. A positive result is diagnostic.
- HW antibody tests:
  - Used in the detection of exposure to HW.

- Used for ruling out HW infection in cats with compatible signs.
  - Up to 14% of cats with HW infection are antibody-negative.
  - A total of 2% of these antibody-negative cats are HW antigen positive.
- HW antigen tests (enzyme-linked immunosorbent assay and immunochromatographic; assess for antigen elaborate by adult female HW) are specific, and some are semiquantative. A positive result is diagnostic.
  - High number of false-negative results due to low female worm burdens or immature infections.
  - Clinical signs can occur *before* the presence of detectable HW antigen.
- Echocardiography:
  - Dilated pulmonary arteries.
  - Parallel linear hyperechoic densities in pulmonary arteries, the right heart and/or the venae cavae.
  - HW found with echocardiography in 78% of nine naturally infected cats in one study.

TREATMENT

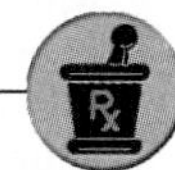

THERAPEUTIC GOAL(S)

- Address complications
- Prevent future infection
- Adulticide therapy is generally not recommended

ACUTE GENERAL TREATMENT

- Cats with HW infection should receive HW preventive medication (see Chronic Treatment, below) and short-term corticosteroids (prednisone 1-2 mg/kg PO q 8-48h) can be used for managing respiratory signs.
- Emergency therapy for acute dyspnea:
  - Oxygen therapy (oxygen cage at 40% O_2 or nasal insufflation at 50-100 ml/kg).
  - Cage rest.
  - Corticosteroids (dexamethasone 1 mg/kg IV or IM or prednisolone sodium succinate 50-100 mg/cat IV).
  - Bronchodilator therapy (aminophylline 6.6 mg/kg IM q 12h).
  - Antithrombotic therapy: aspirin (80 mg PO q 72h) is controversial.
- Worm embolectomy.
  - Can be considered, although mortality rates in one report (2 of 5) thought to be unacceptable.
- Microfilaricide therapy.
  - No agent is currently FDA-approved for the elimination of microfilaria.
  - The authors' recommendation for microfilaricidal therapy is to initiate macrolide prophylactic therapy at the time of diagnosis.
    - Ivermectin (Heartguard): 25 μg/kg PO monthly, or
    - Selamectin (Revolution): 6-12 mg/kg topically monthly, or
    - Milbemycin (Interceptor): 2 mg/kg PO monthly.
      - Preventive doses are microfilaricidal.
      - Patients with microfilaria should be hospitalized, pretreated with diphenhydramine and dexamethasone, and observed for 8 hours for adverse reactions.

CHRONIC TREATMENT

- Preventive therapy:
  - Ivermectin (Heartguard): 25 μg/kg PO monthly.
  - Selamectin (Revolution): 6-12 mg/kg topically monthly.
  - Milbemycin (Interceptor): 2 mg/kg PO monthly.
    - Preventive doses are microfilaricidal; risk of analphylactic reaction in cats with microfilaria (although infrequent due to low microfilarial numbers).
- CHF:
  - Conventional therapy, individualized to patient needs:
    - Furosemide (2-3 mg/kg PO q 8-12h).
    - Spironolactone (1-2 mg/kg PO q 12-24h).
    - Angiotensin-converting enzyme inhibitor (enalapril 0.5 mg/kg PO q 12-24h).
    - Periodic abdominocentesis/thoracocentesis.
    - Oxygen therapy.
    - Extreme exercise restriction.
    - Amlodipine (0.1-0.2 mg/kg PO q 24h).
- Eosinophilic pneumonitis:
  - Corticosteroids (prednisone 2 mg/kg/day, tapering over 4 weeks; reinstitute as needed at lowest q 48h dosage that maintains the cat free of clinical signs).
  - Bronchodilators (optional; aminophylline 6.6 mg/kg IM q 12h).

PROGNOSIS AND OUTCOME

- Good in mild to moderate HW infestations.
  - For more patients that survive the initial insult, the median survival time may be much greater than 1 year.
- Fair to guarded in severe cases.
- Overall, prognosis similar to hypertrophic cardiomyopathy, which shares a median age of diagnosis with HW infection of ~6 years.

PEARLS & CONSIDERATIONS

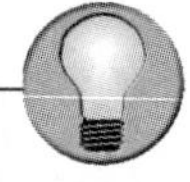

COMMENTS

- Preventive therapy is indicated in cats that are in HW-endemic areas.
- Adulticide therapy is generally not recommended.
- Diagnosis may be difficult, requiring a high index of suspicion and multiple tests including HW antibody tests, HW antigen tests, thoracic radiography, and echocardiography.

CLIENT EDUCATION

- HW infection is a preventable disease.
- Most preventatives are broad spectrum antiparasitic drugs.
- Importance of year-round preventatives. Issues of compliance.

SUGGESTED READING

Atkins CE: Feline heartworm disease. In Ettinger SJ, Feldman EC (eds): *Textbook of Veterinary Internal Medicine*, ed 6. Philadelphia, WB Saunders, 2005, pp 1137-1144.

Berdoulay P, et al: Comparison of serological tests for the detection of natural heartworm infection in cats. *J Am Anim Hosp Assoc* 40:376-384, 2004.

Dillon R: Feline heartworm disease. In Fox P, Sisson D, Moise NS (eds): *Textbook of Canine and Feline Cardiology, Principles and Clinical Practice*. Philadelphia, WB Saunders, 1999, pp 702-726.

Levy JK, et al: Prevalence and risk factors for heartworm infection in cats from northern Florida. *J Am Anim Hosp Assoc* 39:533-537, 2003.

AUTHORS: **KEITH NELSON STRICKLAND, CLARKE E. ATKINS**

EDITOR: **ETIENNE CÔTÉ**

Heartworm Disease, Dog

Client Education Sheet on Website

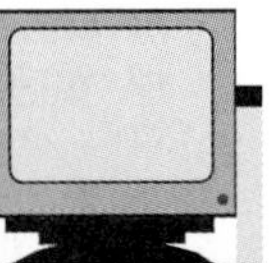

BASIC INFORMATION

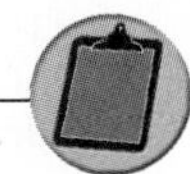

DEFINITION

- Heartworm disease is the clinicopathologic manifestation of infestation with *Dirofilaria immitis*, an intravascular parasite that resides in the pulmonary arteries, the right side of the heart, and venae cavae. It results in pneumonitis, pulmonary endarteritis, pulmonary hypertension (PH), pulmonary thromboembolism (PTE), and/ or cor pulmonale.
- An occult heartworm (HW) infection is defined as an infection in which microfilaria are not detectable in blood.

SYNONYM(S)

Heartworm (HW) infection

EPIDEMIOLOGY

SPECIES, AGE, SEX

- Wild and domestic canids are the natural host, but other species can be infected. All ages are susceptible to HW infestation (not typically seen in patients <12 months old).
- Most dogs are 3 to 6 years old when diagnosed with HW infection.

GENETICS AND BREED PREDISPOSITION

- Sporting breeds are predisposed.
- Caval syndrome occurs most commonly in spring and early summer in middle-aged males housed outdoors.

RISK FACTORS

- Dogs not receiving HW preventative in endemic areas are at risk, with varying seasonal individual risk determined by season of the year and geographic location. Most dogs become infected in July and August.
- The risk of HW infection is correlated with the signalment and the lifestyle of the dog. Outdoor dogs are up to five times more likely to become infected. Most studies suggest that males are up to four times more likely to become infected than females. The type of haircoat apparently does not affect the likelihood of HW infection.

CONTAGION AND ZOONOSIS: Human infections are rare (typically with aberrant migration).

GEOGRAPHY AND SEASONALITY

- Throughout the United States, especially within 150 miles of the Gulf of Mexico and Atlantic coastlines and along the Mississippi River and its tributaries.
- Also endemic in Australia, Japan, and some Mediterranean countries.
- HW transmission is unlikely in regions or seasons where the ambient temperature does not average more than 65° F during a 30-day period.

ASSOCIATED CONDITIONS AND DISORDERS

- Aberrant migration of larvae can result in neurologic, dermatologic, and ophthalmic complications.
- Retrograde migration of part of the worm burden into the right atrium and cavae can result in the caval syndrome (common in highly endemic areas), a serious complication involving entanglement of the worm mass in the tricuspid valve apparatus causing intravascular hemolysis, an acute-onset murmur of tricuspid regurgitation, and signs of forward (hypoperfusion) and backward (congestive) heart failure.
- PTE may be due to dead worms (natural or pharmacologic death) or intravascular thrombi formed in response to the infection.
- PH can occur secondary to pulmonary vascular disease and may result in congestive heart failure (CHF), hemoptysis, and exercise intolerance.
- CHF (uncommon) with signs of right-heart failure (ascites and occasionally pleural effusion).
- Allergic pneumonitis (somewhat common) and eosinophilic granulomatosis (rare).
- Glomerulonephritis (virtually all dogs with HW infection).

CLINICAL PRESENTATION

DISEASE FORMS/SUBTYPES: Classification of HW disease. Class 1: few or no overt clinical signs, Class 2: moderate clinical signs, Class 3: severe clinical signs, and Class 4: caval syndrome.

HISTORY, CHIEF COMPLAINT

- Most dogs with HW infection are in class 1 and show no clinical signs. HW infection is detected as part of routine blood screening.
- When clinical signs exist, coughing is the most common complaint.
- Other complaints include exercise intolerance, weight loss, syncope or collapse, and manifestations of right-sided congestive heart failure (abdominal distention with ascites, hepatosplenomegaly) induced by pulmonary hypertension.
- Acute dyspnea secondary to PTE.

PHYSICAL EXAM FINDINGS

- Dogs not showing overt clinical signs to the owner usually have no abnormal physical examination findings.
- Spontaneous or inducible cough possible upon tracheal palpation.
- A split second (S_2) heart sound may be heard with pulmonary hypertension.
- Jugular venous pulsations and a right apical holosystolic murmur indicate tricuspid regurgitation (a harsh sounding murmur is often present with caval syndrome).
- Palpable fluid wave (ballotment) if abdominal distention (ascites) and jugular venous distention if CHF.
- Discolored urine (from hemoglobinuria), murmur of tricuspid regurgitation, tachypnea/dyspnea, collapse, and right-sided CHF and/or left-sided forward failure indicate caval syndrome.

ETIOLOGY AND PATHOPHYSIOLOGY

- Female mosquitoes serve as intermediate hosts after feeding on microfilaria-positive dogs.
- Microfilaria develop within the mosquito into L3 larvae and can infect another dog within 2 to 2.5 weeks.
- Patent infection (microfilaremia) occurs 6 to 7 months after inoculation of susceptible host by infective (L3) larvae.
- Occult (amicrofilaremic) infections exist due to a prepatent infection, immune-mediated microfilarial destruction, unisex infections, or chronic macrolide administration at prophylactic dosages.
- Disease severity is determined in part by the number of adult HW and the host's response to live and dead heartworms and amount of exercise.
- Response of the pulmonary arteries:
    - Damage from direct contact and other mechanisms (e.g., immune-mediated) to vessel intima.
    - Villous proliferation of the intima and subintimal smooth muscle.
    - Pulmonary hypertension: results from obstruction to blood flow (PTE) and reduced vascular compliance induced by endothelial and medial thickening and probably biological incompetence (failure of damaged vessels to respond to vasodilatory stimuli).
    - Results in dilated pulmonary arteries that can be tortuous and truncated.
- Response of the pulmonary parenchyma:
    - Deposition of HW antigen within the microvasculature causes parenchymal immune/allergic reactions (periarterial edema and inflammation).
    - Corticosteroid-responsive allergic pneumonitis in 14% of HW infections.

- Severe chronic HW infection causes irreversible pulmonary fibrosis with PH.
- Cardiac response:
  - Right ventricular enlargement secondary to moderate-severe PH and subsequent tricuspid regurgitation and myocardial failure.
  - Right-sided congestive heart failure (ascites) in up to 50% of severe HW infections.
- Systemic response:
  - Renal: glomerulonephritis, proteinuria, hypoalbuminemia, and decreased antithrombin III (increases thromboembolic risk).

DIAGNOSIS

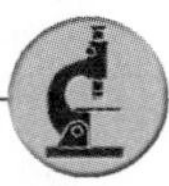

DIFFERENTIAL DIAGNOSIS

- Microfilaria: *Dipetalonema reconditum* microfilaria are shorter, are more narrow, and have a blunted head when compared to *D. immitis* microfilaria.
- Coughing: primary bronchointerstitial disease, collapsing trachea, infectious tracheobronchitis, pneumonia, left-sided congestive heart failure.
- Pulmonary hypertension: PTE (due to other causes); chronic pulmonary disease; cyanotic, right-to-left shunting cardiac disease such as patent ductus arteriosus and ventricular septal defect with primary or secondary PH; and primary PH.
- Congestive heart failure: primary or secondary myocardial failure, chronic congenital or acquired valvular disease.
- Pulmonary granulomas: primary and metastatic neoplasia.

INITIAL DATABASE

- Complete blood count, serum biochemistry profile, urinalysis: evidence of hemolysis and hemoglobinuria if class 4 (caval syndrome). Pathologic proteinuria common due to glomerulonephritis; may be reversible with treatment.
- Electrocardiography may demonstrate a right axis shift (prominent S-waves in leads I, II, III, and V3 indicating PH and right ventricular enlargement) and/or atrial or ventricular arrhythmias in moderate to severe cases.
- Imaging:
  - Thoracic radiographs (variable findings depending on HW infection severity):
    - Dilated and sometimes tortuous, truncated pulmonary arteries
    - Patchy mixed interstitial-alveolar pattern with perivascular infiltrates demonstrated primarily in caudal lung lobes
    - Right heart enlargement
    - Enlarged caudal vena cava if CHF is present or imminent

ADVANCED OR CONFIRMATORY TESTING

- HW antigen tests (enzyme-linked immunosorbent assay and immunochromatographic) are the diagnostic test of choice. They are specific, sensitive, and some are semiquantitative.
  - False-negative results with low female worm burdens or immature infections.
- Microfilaria: filter and modified Knott's tests preferred over wet direct blood smear.
  - Only indicated if no historic macrolide heartworm prophylaxis and patent infection is suspected.
  - Indicated to ascertain presence of microfilaria in dogs with HW infection before institution of therapy.
- Echocardiography for moderate to severe HW infection to assess PH and caval syndrome:
  - Dilated pulmonary arteries.
  - Parallel linear hyperechoic densities in pulmonary arteries (and sometimes the right heart and venae cavae) with large worm burdens.
  - Right ventricular eccentric and concentric hypertrophy with flattened ventricular septum in severe cases.
  - High velocity tricuspid regurgitation or pulmonic insufficiency on echo-Doppler with PH.

TREATMENT

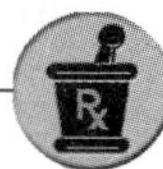

THERAPEUTIC GOAL(S)

- Eliminate worm burden and microfilaria (if present)
- Address complications
- Prevent future infection

ACUTE GENERAL TREATMENT

- Pulmonary thromboembolism:
  - Oxygen therapy (oxygen cage at 40% O_2 or nasal insufflation at 50–100 ml/kg).
  - Cage rest.
  - Corticosteroids (prednisone: 1 mg/kg PO q 24h for 7 to 10 days).
  - Antithrombotic therapy (aspirin 2.5–5 mg/kg PO q 12h or heparin 75 IU/kg SQ q 8h for 5 to 7 days or until the platelet count normalizes) is controversial.
- Allergic pneumonitis: cage rest and corticosteroids (prednisone: 1 mg/kg PO q 24h for 7 to 10 days).
- Adulticide therapy:
  - Melarsomine (Immiticide):
    - Up to 96% efficacy after two doses; 50% of worm burden killed after a single dose.
    - Plan A Melarsomine administered once at 2.5 mg/kg IM followed by two injections at 2.5 mg/kg, 24h apart, given 1 to 3 months later (authors' preference).
    - Plan B Melarsomine administered as two 2.5 mg/kg IM injections, given 24 hours apart.
    - Strict adherence to manufacturer's instructions for intramuscular injection of arsenical agent.
    - Consider corticosteroids (prednisone 1 mg/kg PO q 24h) or administration of a nonsteroidal anti-inflammatory drug (NSAID) at manufacturer's recommended dosage at the time of IM injections to reduce injection site inflammation.
    - Exercise restriction for 6 to 8 weeks.
  - Macrolides as adulticides:
    - Ivermectin and selamectin have a 40–100% efficacy against young HW infections when administered continuously for 18 to 31 months, respectively.
    - Milbemycin: modest adulticide activity.
    - Pulmonary and vascular manifestations of HW infection still result during macrolide adulticide therapy.
    - Reserved for cases in which financial constraints or concurrent medical problems prohibit melarsomine therapy.
- Worm embolectomy:
  - Blind or fluoroscopically guided surgical removal of HW from the venae cavae and right heart with alligator forceps, an endoscopic basket retrieval device, or loop snare device.
- Microfilaricide therapy:
  - No agent is currently FDA-approved for the elimination of microfilaria.
  - Macrolide therapy:
    - Ivermectin: 0.05 mg/kg (about eight times the preventive dose). Ivermectin (Ivomec) diluted 1:9 in propylene glycol or sterile water administered orally at 1 ml/20 kg. Strongly discouraged by the American Heartworm Society.
    - Milbemycin: 0.5–0.99 mg/kg PO (same as preventative dose).
  - Adverse reactions in approximately 10%:
    - Shock, depression, hypothermia, and vomiting.
    - Fluid and corticosteroid (dexamethasone 2–4 mg/kg IV) therapy if severe.
    - Diphenhydramine (2 mg/kg IM) and dexamethasone (0.25 mg/kg IV) administered prophylactically to prevent adverse reactions.
  - The authors' recommendation for microfilaricidal therapy is to initiate routine macrolide prophylactic therapy at the time of diagnosis before adulticide therapy.
    - Ivermectin, selamectin, or milbemycin may be used (see Chronic Treatment below). Patients should be

hospitalized, pretreated as described above using diphenhydramine and dexamethasone, and observed for 8 hours for adverse reactions.

CHRONIC TREATMENT

- Preventive therapy:
  - Wide window of efficacy with up to 2-month "reachback effect" (elimination of larvae that have been in the dog for 2 months).
    - "Reachback effect" can be extended to 3 months with continuous 12-month administration.
  - Ivermectin (Heartguard): 0.006-0.012 mg/kg PO monthly; or
  - Selamectin (Revolution): 6-12 mg/kg topically monthly; or
  - Milbemycin (Interceptor): 500-999 mg/kg PO monthly; or
  - Moxidectin oral and Proheart 6 (currently unavailable).
    - Preventive doses are microfilaricidal; see above for precautions.
- Congestive heart failure:
  - Conventional therapy: individualized based on features of each case:
    - Furosemide (2-3 mg/kg PO q 8-12h).
    - Spironolactone (1-2 mg/kg PO q 12-24h).
    - ACE inhibitor (enalapril 0.5 mg/kg PO q 12-24h).
    - Digoxin (0.005 mg/kg PO q 12h, based on lean weight): optional unless refractory or atrial fibrillation present.
    - Periodic abdominocentesis.
- Pulmonary hypertension:
  - Oxygen therapy.
  - Extreme exercise restriction.
  - Vasodilators (requires careful monitoring for systemic hypotension):
    - Diltiazem (1-2 mg/kg PO q 8h); or
    - Amlodipine (0.1-0.2 mg/kg PO q 24h); or
    - Others (hydralazine and sildenafil).
    - Adulticidal therapy when deemed safe.

POSSIBLE COMPLICATIONS

- Injection site inflammation (adulticide)
- PTE

PROGNOSIS AND OUTCOME

- Good in mild to moderate HW infections
- Fair to guarded in severe cases
- Poor to grave even with treatment in caval syndrome, severe PTE, and CHF

PEARLS & CONSIDERATIONS

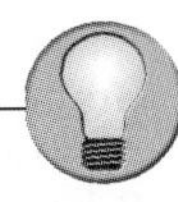

COMMENTS

- Virtually all infected dogs are candidates for adulticide therapy (exception: surgical removal of worms in class 4/caval syndrome patients).
- Macrolide "slow kill" adulticide method is easier but does not prevent pathologic response, and potentially permanent or life-threatening lesions, from HW infection.
- Exercise restriction is an extremely important part of HW infection therapy.

CLIENT EDUCATION

- HW infection is a preventable disease.
- Most preventives are broad spectrum antiparasitic drugs.
- Importance of year-round preventives:
  - "Reach-back effect"
  - Adulticidal effect
  - Other parasiticidal effects
  - Issues of compliance

SUGGESTED READING

Atkins CE: Canine heartworm disease. In Ettinger SJ, Feldman EC (eds): *Textbook of Veterinary Internal Medicine*, ed 6. St. Louis: Elsevier Saunders, 2005, 1118-1136.

Calvert CA, Rawlings CA, McCall JW: Canine heartworm disease. In Fox P, Sisson D, Moise NS (eds): *Textbook of Canine and Feline Cardiology, Principles and Clinical Practice*. Philadelphia, WB Saunders, 1999, pp 702-726.

AUTHORS: **KEITH NELSON STRICKLAND, CLARKE E. ATKINS**

EDITOR: **ETIENNE CÔTÉ**

Heat Stroke/Hyperthermia

BASIC INFORMATION

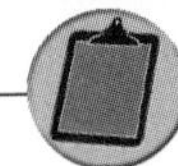

DEFINITION

- Hyperthermia: elevation of the core body temperature.
- Hyperthermia may occur as a result of exposure to endogenous pyrogens (i.e., it is a fever) or it may be the result of excessive external (heat stroke) or internal (muscle fasciculations, seizures) heat.

EPIDEMIOLOGY

SPECIES, AGE, SEX

- Dogs.
- Pediatric or geriatric animals are at higher risk.

GENETICS AND BREED PREDISPOSITION: Increased likelihood in:

- Brachycephalic breeds
- Overweight animals
- Dark-colored dogs

RISK FACTORS

- Excessive muscle fasciculations:
  - Status epilepticus
  - Metaldehyde intoxication
  - Hypocalcemic tetany
- Excessive external heat/inadequate heat dissipation:
  - Exposure to high ambient temperatures.
  - Vigorous exercise
- Endogenous pyrogens:
  - Sepsis
  - Febrile paraneoplastic syndrome
- Other:
  - Drugs
  - Central nervous system lesions

GEOGRAPHY AND SEASONALITY: More common in early summer before acclimatization occurs.

CLINICAL PRESENTATION

HISTORY, CHIEF COMPLAINT

- Excessive panting
- Collapse, inability to rise
- Vomiting, diarrhea
- Patient may be found in enclosed areas (e.g., cars, clothes dryers)
- Seizures/tremors

PHYSICAL EXAM FINDINGS

- Elevated rectal temperature:
  - Generally >40°C (104°F)
  - Note that emergency treatment by owner before arrival may falsely lower the rectal temperature (no longer represents core body temperature)
- Altered mental status
- Hyperemic mucous membranes
- Increased respiratory effort and loud upper airway sounds
- Petechiae

ETIOLOGY AND PATHOPHYSIOLOGY

- Elevation of core body temperature results in activation of the inflammatory system and production of cytokines.
- Endothelial injury results from both direct damage from heat and damage

from the inflammatory system, and further upregulates the production of cytokines.
- Microvascular thrombosis, coagulation, and fibrinolysis occur, and may culminate in disseminated intravascular thrombosis.
- Direct damage to the blood-brain barrier may result in cerebral edema.
- Malignant hyperthermia is an extremely rare genetically based disorder involving rapid-onset hyperthermia, usually triggered by such specific agents as halothane or succinylcholine.

DIAGNOSIS

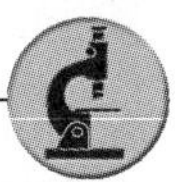

DIFFERENTIAL DIAGNOSIS

Hyperthermia:
- Heat stroke
- Fever

INITIAL DATABASE

- Complete physical exam including neurologic examination
  - In heat stroke, mental status is important prognostically, as dogs that are obtunded are less likely to survive.
- Packed cell volume/total solids, blood glucose, electrolytes
- Prothrombin time, activated partial thromboplastin time, platelet count
- Complete blood count (CBC), serum chemistry panel, urinalysis

TREATMENT

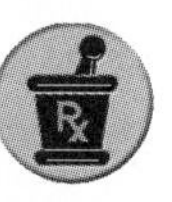

THERAPEUTIC GOAL(S)

- Lower the body temperature to an acceptable range.
- Determine etiology and treat underlying cause.
  - This may be as simple as removing the animal from the source of heat.
  - However, other disorders may be contributing to hyperthermia.
    - Upper airway obstruction
    - Ingested toxins
    - Other
- Manage complications such as disseminated intravascular coagulation (DIC) or cerebral edema.

ACUTE GENERAL TREATMENT

- Remove animal from source of heat.
- Initiate cooling with cool water pads and room temperature intravenous fluids.
  - Iced intravenous fluids cause vasoconstriction and may provide little to no benefit.
- Avoid hypothermia: stop cooling efforts when temperature reaches 39°C (103°F).
- Treat other systemic abnormalities such as hypoglycemia if present.
- Mannitol (20% injectable solution [200 mg/ml]: 0.5-1 g/kg given IV slowly over 15 to 20 minutes) may be used if increased intracranial pressure is suspected.
- Seizure activity should be managed with diazepam 0.2-0.5 mg/kg IV repeated up to three times; if ineffective, either phenobarbital (4 mg/kg IV q 30 minutes up to 16 mg/kg) or propofol continuous rate infusion (CRI) (6 mg/kg IV bolus followed by 0.1-0.2 mg/kg/min).
- Ventricular arrhythmias should be managed if clinical indicated with lidocaine (2 mg/kg IV bolus, then 50 µg/kg/min CRI) (see Ventricular Arrhythmias [Premature Ventricular Complexes, Ventricular Tachycardia], p 1148).

POSSIBLE COMPLICATIONS

- Disseminated intravascular coagulation.
- Cerebral edema.
- Bone marrow dysfunction may result in leukopenia and circulating nucleated red blood cells.

RECOMMENDED MONITORING

- Repeat physical and neurologic examination
- CBC and serum chemistry panel
- Platelet count
- Clotting times

PROGNOSIS AND OUTCOME

Highly variable: good to grave, depending on severity of clinical presentation, occurrence of secondary complications, and response to treatment.

PEARLS & CONSIDERATIONS

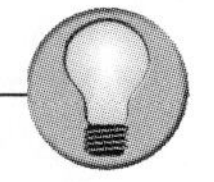

COMMENTS

- Aggressive early cooling warranted
- Avoid hypothermia
- Multiple organ failure including DIC is possible

PREVENTION

Avoid exposing the animal to high ambient temperature

CLIENT EDUCATION

- Educate clients regarding animals left in hot cars and environments.
- Clinical signs such as weakness and panting in hot weather may be an emergency; institute cooling measures and consult a veterinarian.

SUGGESTED READING

Drobatz KJ, Macintire DK: Heat-induced illness in dogs: 42 cases (1976-1993). *J Am Vet Med Assoc* 209(11):1984-1899, 1996.

AUTHOR: **KIRSTEN AARBO**
EDITOR: **ELIZABETH ROZANSKI**

Helicobacter Gastritis

BASIC INFORMATION

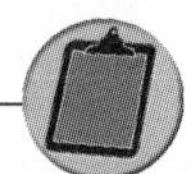

DEFINITION

Inflammation of the stomach as a result of infection with any one of several pathogenic *Helicobacter* spp. bacteria

EPIDEMIOLOGY

SPECIES, AGE, SEX: Dogs and cats can be infected. There is no breed, age, or sex predisposition.

RISK FACTORS: Environmental conditions may play a role, as higher infection rates are found in shelter and colony dog and cats as compared to pets.

CONTAGION AND ZOONOSIS
- The mode of transmission is unknown, although oral-oral and fecal-oral routes may occur. Vector transmission (flies) may occur. Water-borne infections may be important in certain areas' supplies. *Helicobacter* gastritis has zoonotic potential.
- One of the most important reasons for concern about *Helicobacter* infections in dogs and cats is the zoonotic potential for transmission to humans. Careful consideration is warranted due to the association of human *Helicobacter pylori* infection with human peptic ulcer disease and an increased risk of gastric cancer; however, most evidence suggests this potential is very low, and while several species of *Helicobacter* may affect

dogs and cats, *H. pylori* is very uncommonly isolated from cats and has not been isolated from dogs.
- Anthroponosis (human-to-animal) transmission is likely in cats.

CLINICAL PRESENTATION

HISTORY, CHIEF COMPLAINT

- Chronic vomiting, intermittent inappetence, and pica may be seen.
- Hematemesis and melena may be seen if gastric ulceration develops.

PHYSICAL EXAM FINDINGS: There are no specific findings on physical examination suggestive of *Helicobacter* gastritis.

ETIOLOGY AND PATHOPHYSIOLOGY

- Multiple species of *Helicobacter* have been isolated from dogs and cats:
  - Dog: *H. felis, H. bizzozeronii, H. salomonis, H. bilis, H. heilmannii,* and *Flexispira rappini*.
  - Cat: *H. felis, H. pamatensis, H. pylori, H. heilmanii*. Approximately 41–100% of healthy cats, and 57–100% of vomiting cats, have *Helicobacter*-like organisms.
- Pathogenicity is variable.
- Gastritis, erosion, and ulceration occur as a consequence of ammonia production (the bacteria produce urease) and other secretory products of the organism that damage epithelial cells and induce gastric acid secretion.

DIAGNOSIS

DIFFERENTIAL DIAGNOSIS

- Primary gastric diseases causing vomiting:
  - Food hypersensitivity/allergy or intolerance
  - Gastric parasites
  - Chronic idiopathic gastritis (lymphoplasmacytic or eosinophilic, atrophic, hypertrophic)
  - Foreign body
  - Gastric neoplasia
- Nongastric diseases causing vomiting:
  - Systemic diseases (hypoadrenocorticism, hyperthyroidism, heartworm disease, renal disease, liver disease, neoplasia)
  - Inflammatory bowel disease
  - Drug therapy

INITIAL DATABASE

Complete blood count, serum biochemistry profile, urinalysis, and fecal flotation are normal in *Helicobacter* gastritis, but are indicated to identify other (systemic) causes of vomiting.

ADVANCED OR CONFIRMATORY TESTING

- Noninvasive studies:
  - Serologic study: not commercially available; specificity of 95% and sensitivity of 79% when enzyme-linked immunosorbent assay and immunoblotting were used in combination.
  - Urea breath or blood test: requires a radiolabeled-urea test meal; may be useful for monitoring successful therapy. Limited to specialty facilities.
- Invasive studies:
  - Biopsy (endoscopic or surgical) and histology: Warthin-Starry silver stains, Giemsa, or toluidine blue improve identification over routine H&E staining. Squash preps stained with Diff-Quik are useful for rapid identification.
  - Rapid urease testing: performed on endoscopic biopsies in a urea broth with phenol red as a pH indicator. Results in 1 to 3 hours (up to 24 hours).
  - Culture: least sensitive method, difficult to culture. Can identify antimicrobial sensitivity.
  - Polymerase chain reaction on gastric biopsies: high sensitivity and specificity; not widely available.

TREATMENT

The identification of *Helicobacter* organisms or other evidence of helicobacteriosis in dogs and cats warrants treatment if signs of gastritis are present, and there is concurrent evidence of chronic gastritis.

THERAPEUTIC GOAL(S)

Eradication of the organism should be the goal for long-term resolution of clinical signs.

ACUTE AND CHRONIC TREATMENT

- Triple therapy: amoxicillin 20 mg/kg PO q 12h, metronidazole 10 mg/kg PO q 12h, and clarithromycin 7.5 mg/kg PO q 12h for 14 days (first choice).
- Various combinations of antibiotics (amoxicillin, metronidazole, doxycycline, clarithromycin) and antacid drugs (famotidine, omeprazole) are reported.
- It should be noted that although combination antibiotic therapy is the treatment of choice, a recent study revealed there is no proof that this therapy eradicates the organisms. Therefore an animal that has received treatment cannot be assumed to be free of *Helicobacter*.

PROGNOSIS AND OUTCOME

The prognosis is good for initial resolution of clinical signs if the gastritis is due to *Helicobacter* spp. infection. The chance for recurrence is high owing to failure to eradicate the infection or reinfection.

PEARLS & CONSIDERATIONS

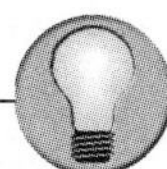

COMMENTS

The identification of *Helicobacter*-like organisms on gastric biopsies is not a definitive diagnosis, as many otherwise healthy dogs and cats carry this organism. In the absence of other causes of gastritis and vomiting, a therapeutic trial is warranted in these patients. When gastric inflammation is mild and colonization by the organism is low, the veterinarian should remain suspicious of other causes of chronic vomiting.

CLIENT EDUCATION

Avoid being licked on the face, sharing utensils, or other forms of oral-oral (or fecal-oral) contact with affected animals.

SUGGESTED READING

Blaser MJ: The bacteria behind ulcers. *Scientific American* February:104–107, 1996.

Neiger R, Simpson KW: *Helicobacter* infection in dogs and cats: Facts and fiction. *J Vet Intern Med* 14:125–133, 2000.

Leib MS, Duncan RB: Diagnosing gastric *Helicobacter* infections in dogs and cats. *Comp Cont Ed* 27:221–228, 2005.

AUTHOR: **KENNETH R. HARKIN**

EDITOR: **DEBRA L. ZORAN**

Hemangiopericytoma

BASIC INFORMATION

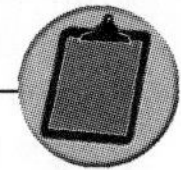

DEFINITION

A locally invasive, slowly progressive tumor that occurs most commonly on the limbs of large-breed dogs and that carries a fair to good prognosis with either complete excision or incomplete excision combined with radiation therapy

SYNONYM(S)

Malignant schwannoma
Neurofibrosarcoma
Peripheral nerve sheath tumor

EPIDEMIOLOGY

SPECIES, AGE, SEX: Common in middle-aged to older dogs. It is rare in cats.
GENETICS AND BREED PREDISPOSITION: Large-breed dogs may be overrepresented.

CLINICAL PRESENTATION

HISTORY, CHIEF COMPLAINT: Most animals are presented for evaluation of a progressive mass noticed by the owner. Pets with hemangiopericytoma in certain locations may be presented because of clinical signs related to the location of the tumor (e.g., limb tumors may result in lameness).
PHYSICAL EXAM FINDINGS

- Visible or palpable mass, more commonly on the limbs (any location on the limbs).
- Mass is usually firm and fixed to underlying tissues. Occasionally, the mass can be hairless or ulcerated.
- Regional lymphadenopathy may be present secondary to inflammation caused by the tumor or, rarely, lymph node metastasis.
- The remainder of the physical examination typically is unremarkable.

ETIOLOGY AND PATHOPHYSIOLOGY

- Hemangiopericytoma has some histologic features similar to the tumor of the same name in humans, but the actual cell of origin of this tumor is disputed.
- Hemangiopericytomas are spontaneously occurring in most cases in dogs.
- Disturbance caused by hemangiopericytomas depends on the location of the primary tumor and the invasion into and destruction of surrounding normal structures.
- Hemangiopericytomas are typically slow growing and slow to metastasize. Over time they can invade into surrounding soft tissue structures.
- It is still unclear whether hemangiopericytomas, schwannomas, and nerve sheath tumors are identical, or related but distinct tumors.

DIAGNOSIS

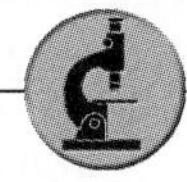

DIFFERENTIAL DIAGNOSIS

- Other soft tissue sarcomas
    - Fibrosarcoma
    - Malignant fibrous histiocytoma
    - Others
- Mast cell tumors
- Other skin and subcutaneous tumors
- Benign or non-neoplastic masses
    - Benign tumor (e.g., lipoma)
    - Abscess
    - Elbow hygroma

INITIAL DATABASE

- Fine-needle aspiration and cytologic evaluation may help identify the tumor type before other diagnostics.
- Three-view thoracic radiographs to rule out pulmonary metastases.
- Radiographs of the affected area may rarely reveal involvement of underlying bone.

ADVANCED OR CONFIRMATORY TESTING

- Biopsy is the diagnostic procedure of choice.
    - Definitive diagnosis of hemangiopericytoma is based on histopathologic evaluation of the tumor tissue.
    - Biopsy is typically excisional, with removal of the entire tumor if possible, or removal of the greatest feasible extent of tumor mass if not entirely resectable.
    - Incisional biopsy may be performed to obtain the diagnosis before treatment, especially in cases where multiple treatment modalities might be necessary (e.g., preoperative radiation).
    - Occasionally, special stains may be necessary to differentiate hemangiopericytoma from other types of soft tissue sarcomas, especially with poorly differentiated tumors.
- Computed tomography or magnetic resonance imaging may be necessary to delineate the local extent of the tumor and to plan for surgery or radiation therapy.
- Histopathologic grade of the tumor is necessary for determining the prognosis and treatment of most soft tissue sarcomas (Soft Tissue Sarcoma, p 1016). Although most hemangiopericytomas are low to intermediate grade, high-grade tumors can occur and may be more likely to metastasize.

TREATMENT

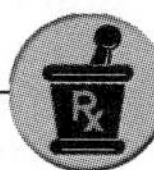

THERAPEUTIC GOAL(S)

Complete eradication of the primary tumor

ACUTE AND CHRONIC TREATMENT

- Aggressive surgical resection (aim: 3 cm margins; often not possible, especially on distal limb). Radiation therapy, and/or chemotherapy may be used (see section on Soft Tissue Sarcoma, p 1016).
- Tumors that are incompletely resected or cannot be surgically resected (e.g., highly invasive or metastatic) may be treated with a combination of radiation therapy and surgery, which is associated with favorable long-term outcomes.
- Radiation therapy alone provides good long-term outcomes, although tumor control rates are higher with combined surgery-radiation therapy.
- Chemotherapy may be indicated for hemangiopericytomas that are high grade based on histologic features.

POSSIBLE COMPLICATIONS

Complications of treatment for hemangiopericytomas depend on the types of treatments and the location of the primary tumor (see Soft Tissue Sarcoma, p 1016).

RECOMMENDED MONITORING

- Following appropriate local treatment of the primary tumor, routine follow-up examination is indicated to monitor for local recurrence and also for metastasis. High-grade tumors may require more frequent monitoring for metastases during and after chemotherapy administration.
    - Dogs that are likely to develop metastasis (splenic tumors, high-grade tumors) should be monitored closely (every 2 to 3 months) with physical exam, including lymph node palpation and thoracic radiographs.
    - Dogs with low or intermediate grade tumors that have adequate treatment should have physical examinations done every 2 to 3 months or more frequently depending on risk of side effects from treatment. Thoracic radiographs could be done less frequently (6 months and 1 year after therapy).

PROGNOSIS AND OUTCOME

- Prognosis is excellent for most hemangiopericytomas with appropriate treatment. This includes either complete surgical resection with clean histopathologic margins or incomplete resection combined with radiation therapy.
    - Combined surgery-radiation therapy treatment results in long-term tumor control in 86% of dogs with hemangiopericytoma. Survival times for dogs with hemangiopericytoma treated this way were >5 years with 85% tumor free at 3 years.
    - Radiation therapy alone has resulted in 1-year tumor control rates of up to 75% at higher doses. However, these studies used suboptimal radiation dose schedules. In certain situations where surgery is not indicated, radiation may be used to provide some degree of tumor control.
- High-grade hemangiopericytoma is rare and information is limited regarding prognosis.

PEARLS & CONSIDERATIONS

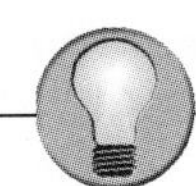

COMMENTS

Despite uncertainty about the cell of origin for these tumors, hemangiopericytoma, peripheral nerve sheath tumor, schwannoma, and neurofibrosarcoma generally have the same biologic behavior and should be treated in the same way.

CLIENT EDUCATION

Pet owners can be educated to monitor their pets for the occurrence of masses under the skin and have such masses evaluated in a timely fashion. Early detection may allow for easier treatment via surgery and may help avoid the need for radiation therapy.

SUGGESTED READING

MacEwen EG, Powers BE, Macy D, Withrow SJ: Soft tissue sarcomas. In Withrow SJ, MacEwen EG (eds): *Small Animal Clinical Oncology*. Philadelphia, WB Saunders, 2001, pp 283-304.

AUTHOR: **JOHN FARRELLY**
EDITOR: **KENNETH M. RASSNICK**

Hemangiosarcoma

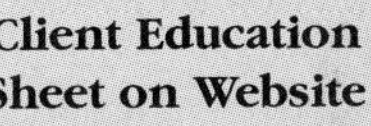

Client Education Sheet on Website

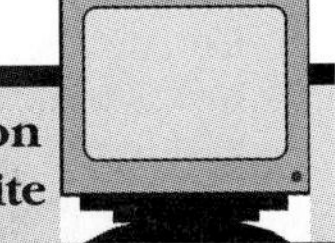

BASIC INFORMATION

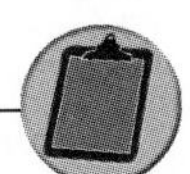

DEFINITION

A malignant, highly metastatic tumor arising from vascular endothelial cells. Cardiac hemangiosarcoma is discussed in detail separately (see Hemangiosarcoma, Cardiac, p 473).

SYNONYM(S)

HSA
Angiosarcoma
Malignant hemangioendothelioma

EPIDEMIOLOGY

SPECIES, AGE, SEX

- Feline: 8 to 10 year median, males > females. Uncommon
- Canine: common
    - Cutaneous: adults (range 4-10+ years), no sex predilection
    - Noncutaneous: 8-10 year median, no sex predilection

GENETICS AND BREED PREDISPOSITION

- Feline: no genetics or specific breed predisposition known
- Canine:
    - Cutaneous: no genetics known, although breeds with short-haired coats are predisposed (e.g., whippets, pit bulls, dalmatians)
    - Noncutaneous: no genetics known; tend to be large-breed dogs such as German shepherds and golden retrievers

RISK FACTORS

- Feline: none known
- Canine:
    - Cutaneous: Dermal hemangiosarcoma arises on nonhaired skin and is associated with ultraviolet (UV) light exposure. Subcutaneous hemangiosarcoma arises in haired skin and is not associated with UV exposure.
    - Noncutaneous: none known, but breed predisposition suggests a genetic etiology.

ASSOCIATED CONDITIONS AND DISORDERS

- Feline: none known
- Canine:
    - Cutaneous: UV exposure may also predispose to cutaneous hemangioma or squamous cell carcinoma.
    - Noncutaneous:
        - With either splenic, hepatic, or right atrial/auricular appendage HSA, potentially life-threatening hemorrhage can occur. Occasionally, large subcutaneous hemangiosarcoma tumors may bleed.
        - Pericardial effusion can result in potentially fatal cardiac tamponade.
        - Splenic, hepatic, and right atrial/auricular appendage HSA are associated with cardiac arrhythmias.
        - In any patient with hemangiosarcoma, disseminated intravascular coagulation (DIC) may arise in conjunction with thrombocytopenia and triggering of the coagulation cascade by the formation of abnormal (tumor-related) vascular channels.

CLINICAL PRESENTATION

DISEASE FORMS/SUBTYPES

- Feline: Subcutaneous and splenic lesions are most common, but hemangiosarcoma can arise anywhere in the body including such diverse tissues as bone, gastrointestinal (GI) tract, and skin.
- Canine:
    - Cutaneous: Tends to arise on lightly haired areas such as the ventral abdomen. Tumors that are <5 cm in diameter and confined to the dermis are classified as stage I. Tumors that are >5 cm in diameter or invade subcutaneous or deeper tissues are classified as stage II.
    - Noncutaneous: Splenic lesions are most common, followed by HSA of the right atrial/auricular appendage (see Hemangiosarcoma, Cardiac, p 473) and skin. Primary HSA of the liver can occasionally occur, but most often, hepatic lesions are metastases from another site. As with cats, hemangiosarcoma can arise anywhere.

HISTORY, CHIEF COMPLAINT

- Feline:
    - Cutaneous: Bleeding from the mass, in a patient that is otherwise well, may be the chief complaint.
    - Noncutaneous: Typically, nonspecific signs such as inappetance/anorexia, weight loss, lethargy, and vomiting are the basis for seeking veterinary attention.
- Canine:
    - Cutaneous: history of extensive sunlight exposure and development of one or more cutaneous masses.
    - Noncutaneous: often nonspecific complaints (e.g., mild exercise intolerance, mild decrease in appetite, weight loss) commonly attributed at

first to "old age," environmental change (weather), etc., but then culminating in subacute (days before presentation) or acute (hours before presentation) deterioration with lethargy, weakness, tachypnea, inappetence/anorexia, and/or abdominal distention. Acute onset of weakness, or collapse, is often mentioned, likely associated with tumor rupture and hemorrhage. Collapse may be self-resolving by the time the patient is presented for veterinary attention, but physical signs of hemorrhage, abdominal mass, or arrhythmia persist.

PHYSICAL EXAM FINDINGS

- Feline: Cutaneous or subcutaneous lesions are typically readily identified on physical examination. Visceral disease is often evident on abdominal palpation. Other possible findings include pale mucous membranes, weak pulses.
- Canine:
  - Cutaneous: single or multiple cutaneous tumors, typically on the ventral abdomen. Usually raised, hairless, smooth, and dark red lesions, although they may also appear as polypoid, hairless lesions that are the same color as surrounding skin.
  - Noncutaneous:
    - Most often, findings are related to tumor rupture and hemorrhage into a body cavity. The most common physical findings therefore include lethargy, pale mucous membranes, abdominal fluid wave, sinus tachycardia (reflex), and weak pulses.
    - A palpable intra-abdominal mass is often present, and such masses should be palpated with great care to avoid further damaging any fragile blood vessels on the surface of the neoplasm and inducing further hemorrhage.
    - Soft heart sounds, cardiac arrhythmia, and signs of circulatory failure may be present either as a result of a ruptured abdominal hemangiosarcoma, as a result of cardiac hemangiosarcoma and subsequent pericardial effusion, or both.

ETIOLOGY AND PATHOPHYSIOLOGY

- Cutaneous hemangiosarcoma is associated with UV light exposure. Cutaneous hemangiosarcoma is unlikely to metastasize and is not usually associated with underlying visceral disease/involvement; subcutaneous hemangiosarcoma may metastasize and may be a marker for underlying visceral disease/involvement.
- Malignant vascular endothelial cells form abnormal vascular channels.
- Microangiopathic disease (abnormal blood vessels in the neoplasm) results in red blood cell morphology changes and DIC.
- Tumor rupture leads to anemia, weakness, and inappetence/anorexia.
- Metastatic disease occurs within the lungs, mesentery, and throughout the body.
- Death is due to uncontrollable bleeding from tumor rupture.

DIAGNOSIS

DIFFERENTIAL DIAGNOSIS

- Feline (subcutaneous): abscess, other neoplasia such as injection-site sarcoma, fibrosarcoma
- Feline (splenic): splenic mast cell tumor, lymphoma, nodular hyperplasia, other sarcoma
- Canine (cutaneous): hemangioma, soft tissue sarcoma
- Canine (splenic): splenic torsion, lymphoma, hemangioma, hematoma, extramedullary hematopoeisis, nodular regeneration, other sarcoma
- Canine (hepatic): hepatocellular adenoma/adenocarcinoma, hematoma

INITIAL DATABASE

- Careful abdominal palpation, assessment for a fluid wave.
- Auscult heart and check for synchronous pulses.
- Complete blood count, chemistry profile, urinalysis, coagulation profile.
  - Anemia (regenerative or nonregenerative, depending on acuity) and hypoproteinemia are common due to blood loss (e.g., abdominal hemorrhage).
  - Schistocytosis may be noted as a result of microangiopathic damage of red blood cells traveling through abnormal vessels in the neoplasm.
- Thoracic and abdominal radiographs.
  - Mass effect is commonly apparent on abdominal radiographs; detail may be obscured by abdominal effusion.
  - Pulmonary metastasis of hemangiosarcoma can involve many (hundreds to thousands of) 1- to 2-mm nodules, which appear radiographically in the lungs as an interstitial pattern.
  - Cardiac silhouette may be enlarged (globoid), indicating pericardial effusion.
  - Lack of globoid cardiac silhouette does not rule out pericardial effusion.
  - Cardiac silhouette rarely affected by presence of a mass lesion.
  - See Hemangiosarcoma, Cardiac, p 473.
- Abdominal ultrasound if suspected splenic or hepatic (abdominal effusion/distention, abdominal mass). Utility of ultrasound for patients with a palpable abdominal mass:
  - Confirm presence of the mass, its organ of origin, and likelihood of resectability.
  - Identify lesions suggesting metastasis.
  - Identify abdominal fluid and, if small in volume, guide needle abdominocentesis.
  - Identify internal structure of mass, indicating feasibility of fine-needle aspiration/core biopsy (mixed echogenicity and high vascularity contraindicate these procedures in hemangiosarcoma).
- Echocardiography if cardiac. Small hemangiosarcoma masses may be too small to visualize with echo while still producing hemodynamically severe pericardial effusion.
- Electrocardiogram if an arrhythmia is present on physical exam, and if splenic involvement, cardiac involvement, or recent hemorrhage is evident.
- Fine-needle aspiration cytology of regional lymph node in patients with cutaneous HSA.

ADVANCED OR CONFIRMATORY TESTING

- Surgical biopsy is the gold standard for diagnosis. The entire spleen should be submitted; some laboratories request it to be shipped chilled on ice (not frozen), whereas others request it be fixed in 10:1 ratio of formalin:tumor for 24 to 48 hours, after which the fixed tissues can be sent to the laboratory in a small amount of formalin.
- Fine-needle aspiration cytology or cytologic evaluation of hemorrhagic fluids is rarely diagnostic. Fine-needle aspiration cytology of visceral masses may result in hemorrhage and is not recommended in cases of suspected splenic, cardiac, and any other noncutaneous form of hemangiosarcoma (see Pearls & Considerations below).

TREATMENT

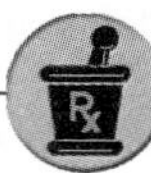

THERAPEUTIC GOAL(S)

- Reduce tumor burden and prevent/minimize future hemorrhagic episodes
- Control metastatic disease
- Prolong survival

ACUTE GENERAL TREATMENT

- Cutaneous (either species):
  - Surgery to remove tumor
- Noncutaneous (either species):
  - If evidence of recent or ongoing hemorrhage: IV fluids ± oxygen ± transfusion (see Hemoabdomen, p 477)
  - Pericardiocentesis (see Pericardiocentesis, p 1298) if pericardial effusion causing cardiac tamponade is present
  - Once stable, surgery to remove the tumor or pericardectomy to prevent recurrence of tamponade

CHRONIC TREATMENT

- Feline and canine (cutaneous): Surgery alone may be curative in most patients with dermal HSA. Margins should be at least 1 to 3 cm wide and 1 or more fascial planes deep.

- Feline and canine (noncutaneous and stage II cutaneous HSA):
  - Chemotherapy with a protocol of five doses of doxorubicin (dog, 30 mg/m^2 IV; cat, 25 mg/m^2 IV) given every 3 weeks. Special handling requirements and potentially severe or life-threatening adverse patient effects exist with this chemotherapeutic drug; these concerns, and rapid evolution of protocols, warrant consultation with/referral to an oncologist.
  - Consider adjuvant radiation therapy for patients with incompletely excised subcutaneous stage II HSA.

POSSIBLE COMPLICATIONS

- General doxorubicin toxicities: myelosuppression, GI upset
- Specific doxorubicin toxicities: allergic reaction during administration, perivascular sloughing with drug extravasation, cumulative myocardial toxicity (dogs) and heart failure, cumulative renal toxicity (cats)

RECOMMENDED MONITORING

- Feline and canine (cutaneous): recheck physical examination every 3 to 4 months
- Feline and canine (noncutaneous): weekly complete blood count initially, thoracic radiographs every 1 to 2 months, abdominal ultrasound every 1 to 2 months

PROGNOSIS AND OUTCOME

- Feline and canine (cutaneous): <30% of patients with dermal (stage I) HSA will develop metastases, so complete surgical excision can be curative
- Feline and canine (noncutaneous and stage II cutaneous):
  - Highly metastatic, so when treated with surgery alone, median survival may be only 2 to 3 months. There are occasional reports of patients surviving several months, but survival up to or beyond 1 year is very uncommon.
  - If all grossly detectable neoplastic tissue can be removed surgically, adjuvant chemotherapy may extend survival to a median time of 6 months.
  - If grossly apparent neoplastic tissue persists in postoperative period, median survival time approximates 2 months.
  - Adjuvant radiation therapy can be considered for patients with incompletely excised stage II cutaneous hemangiosarcoma, but limited data prevent any clear conclusions regarding benefit.

PEARLS & CONSIDERATIONS

COMMENTS

- Hemangiosarcoma is a locally aggressive, highly metastatic tumor that most often arises within the spleen, right atrium, or skin in dogs.
- Most often hemangiosarcoma of the liver is due to metastatic disease since primary hepatic hemangiosarcoma is uncommon.
- Nodules of ectopic splenic tissue on the omentum, and regenerative hepatic nodules, are benign, dark red/brown tissue nodules that must not be misinterpreted as hemangiosarcoma metastases during laparotomy in a patient with a splenic mass. Biopsy is advised to avoid misdiagnosis.
- Although rare in cats, this tumor has a similarly aggressive biologic behavior.
- Fine-needle aspiration/cytologic evaluation and core biopsy are often unrewarding due to poor cellular yield and blood dilution, and both carry the real possibility of causing rupture of the tumor and potentially life-threatening hemorrhage. These procedures are therefore *contraindicated* for evaluation of masses when hemangiosarcoma is on the differential diagnosis list: masses of splenic, hepatic, renal, or cardiac origin that, on ultrasound exam, are of mixed echogenicity and may be highly vascularized based upon color flow Doppler assessment.
- Fine-needle aspiration and cytologic evaluation may be considered for evaluation of skin masses for which hemangiosarcoma is on the differential diagnosis list, but diagnostic yield may be limited for the same reasons.
- Cutaneous hemangiosarcoma in both dogs and cats has a less metastatic behavior and surgical excision may be curative.
- Even with doxorubicin chemotherapy, reported survivals are short in both species. The best chemotherapy protocol for the treatment of hemangiosarcoma remains unknown, as no randomized clinical trials have compared reported protocols. Combining doxorubicin with cyclophosphamide appears to be well tolerated and may provide longer survival times than doxorubicin alone. Adding vincristine to a doxorubicin and cyclophosphamide protocol is associated with more significant toxicity than with doxorubicin and cyclophosphamide or doxorubicin alone. Alkylating agents such as lomustine and ifosfamide may prove to have activity against this disease; however, large studies documenting efficacy are lacking. Immunotherapy appears to be of benefit, but no effective immunotherapies are commercially available.

PREVENTION

The development of cutaneous hemangiosarcoma is related to UV light exposure. Minimize sun exposure in animals with white or thin haircoats.

SUGGESTED READING

Smith A: Hemangiosarcoma in dogs and cats. *Vet Clin Small Anim* 33:533-552, 2003.

Sorenmo KU, et al: Efficacy and toxicity of a dose-intensified doxorubicin protocol in canine hemangiosarcoma. *J Vet Intern Med* 18:209-213, 2004.

Ward H, et al: Cutaneous hemangiosarcoma in 25 dogs: A retrospective study. *J Vet Intern Med* 8:345-348, 1994.

AUTHOR: **RUTHANNE CHUN**
EDITOR: **KENNETH M. RASSNICK**

Hemangiosarcoma, Cardiac

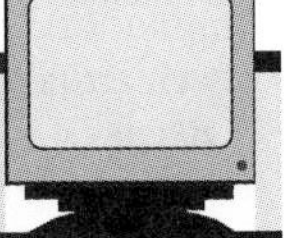

Client Education Sheet on Website

BASIC INFORMATION

DEFINITION

Malignancy of vascular endothelial origin involving cardiac tissue as either a primary or metastatic site. The neoplasm usually is located in the right auricle but may be seen also in the atria and ventricles. Regardless of location, it usually causes a hemorrhagic pericardial effusion.

EPIDEMIOLOGY

SPECIES, AGE, SEX

- Dogs: older adults; both sexes
- Extremely rare in the cat

GENETICS AND BREED PREDISPOSITIONS: Dogs: Genetics unknown, but golden retriever, German shepherd, rottweilers, greyhounds, and other large-breed dogs are overrepresented. Cats: rarely.

RISK FACTORS: Dogs: most common reason for pericardial effusion.

CLINICAL PRESENTATION

DISEASE FORMS/SUBTYPES

- Cardiac tamponade due to intrapericardial hemorrhage from the tumor site
- Occasionally can be an incidental finding on echocardiography without associated clinical signs

HISTORY, CHIEF COMPLAINT: Three forms of presenting complaints (some overlap/combination possible):

- Acute collapse with pallor; may have partially resolved over preceding hours or days
- General malaise, lethargy, anorexia, exercise intolerance
- Visible abdominal distention

PHYSICAL EXAM FINDINGS

- Tachycardia, muffled heart sounds, thready/weak pulse, abdominal distention.
- In some cases: jugular distention, pulsus paradoxus, positive hepatojugular reflux.

ETIOLOGY AND PATHOPHYSIOLOGY

- *Primary*: usually seen as right atrial/auricular infiltration of neoplastic cells that grow on the epicardial surface and ultimately cause rupture of superficial myocardial vessels of varying sizes, triggering bleeding into the pericardial space. The result is cardiac tamponade when intrapericardial pressure exceeds right atrial and ventricular filling pressures.
- *Systemic:* seen as metastatic site from primary involvement of liver or spleen.

DIAGNOSIS

DIFFERENTIAL DIAGNOSIS

Other causes of pericardial effusion:

- Idiopathic benign pericardial effusion
- Other tumors such as chemodectoma, mesothelioma, lymphoma
- Hemopericardium (atrial rupture, anticoagulant rodenticide intoxication)
- Exudative/infectious pericarditis
- Congestive heart failure (right-sided)
- Diaphragmaticopericardial-peritoneal hernia
- Hydropericardium due to hypoalbuminemia
- Pericardial cysts
- Diseases that cause radiographic enlargement of the cardiac silhouette (dilated cardiomyopathy, severe, advanced atrioventricular endocardiosis/valvular heart disease, severe right ventricular enlargement)

INITIAL DATABASE

- Complete blood count: regenerative anemia.
- Serum chemistry: usually unremarkable unless hepatic involvement.
- Electrocardiogram: electrical alternans (25% of the time), diminished R wave amplitudes (50% of the time), arrhythmias (rare).
- Thoracic/abdominal radiographs: enlarged globoid cardiac silhouette possible (80% of time), caudal vena caval distention, pleural effusion, ascites, hepatomegaly. With hemangiosarcoma, multifocal pulmonary metastases may appear as an interstitial pattern.
- Echocardiography: most accurate diagnostic test.
  - Confirm presence of fluid accumulation between the epicardium and the pericardium.
  - Right atrial wall collapse ("sail sign"; the right atrial wall motion seen in pericardial tamponade resembles a sail flapping in the wind).
  - Diastolic collapse of RV wall if severe tamponade.
  - Tumor mass or blood clot from bleeding tumor may be seen bobbing in fluid adjacent to, or involving, a thickened (infiltrated) right atrial/auricular wall.
  - Diminished right atrium, right ventricle, left ventricle volume.
  - Swinging motion of the heart within the anechoic pericardial fluid.
  - Mass seen occasionally within the right atrium; absence of mass does not exclude hemangiosarcoma because of limitations of imaging right auricle with routine (transthoracic) echocardiography.
  - Doppler evaluation of pulmonic flow shows large variation in beat to beat peak velocities.
- Abdominal ultrasonography: evaluate liver, spleen, omentum for presence of primary neoplasia.

ADVANCED OR CONFIRMATORY TESTING

- Pericardial fluid cytology.
  - Typically indicates extensive bleeding and minimal exfoliation.
  - Mainly useful to exclude infectious pericardial effusion and lymphoma.
  - Cytologic evaluation alone is highly unreliable: 74% of malignancies not detected; 13% of benign pericarditis cases erroneously classified as malignant.
- Pericardial fluid pH: controversial. One study indicated pericardial pH ≥7.0 as highly indicative of neoplasia and pericardial pH <7.0 as highly indicative of benign effusion, whereas another study showed no such differentiation.
- Serum troponin-1 (elevation suggests hemangiosarcoma). This blood test may be performed locally at a human hospital (human assay is accurate in dogs) or may be performed at referral veterinary laboratories (e.g., contact Veterinary Medical Teaching Hospital, University of Florida Health Science Center, PO Box 100103, Gainesville, FL 32610-0103, 352-392-4700 ext 4400).
- Contrast computed tomography/cardiac magnetic resonance imaging: investigational.

TREATMENT

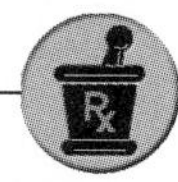

THERAPEUTIC GOAL(S)

Relief of tamponade (palliative treatment)

ACUTE GENERAL TREATMENT

- Pericardiocentesis and drainage of accumulated effusion (see p 1298)
- Diuretics: contraindicated in acute pericardial effusion/cardiac tamponade

CHRONIC TREATMENT

- Subtotal pericardectomy (usually performed following second event of tamponade)
- Right auricular ablation: removal of tumor mass (difficult and may not prolong life)
- Right auricular ablation plus chemotherapy (see Prognosis and Outcome below)
- Repeated pericardiocenteses

POSSIBLE COMPLICATIONS

- Almost all cases have pulmonary metastasis at time of initial diagnosis even though they may not be detected by thoracic radiography
- Additional tumor sites: liver, spleen, skin, ventricle, brain, kidney

RECOMMENDED MONITORING

- Echocardiography 24 hours after pericardiocentesis; 1 week after pericardiocentesis, monthly thereafter
- Thoracic radiographs monthly

PROGNOSIS AND OUTCOME

- Poor to grave: most patients have recurrent bleeding from the tumor site requiring repeat pericardiocentesis; metastatic disease usually present
- Right auricular ablation plus chemotherapy: may prolong life (median survival in 8 dogs with right auricular ablation alone: 42 days, versus in 8 other dogs with right auricular ablation plus chemotherapy: 175 days)

PEARLS & CONSIDERATIONS

COMMENTS

- Life expectancy <6 months.

- Often the mass seen bobbing around within the pericardial fluid is actually an organized blood clot associated with tumor tissue invading the right atrial/auricular wall.

CLIENT EDUCATION

- Watch for recurrent signs associated with return of tamponade
- Watch for signs of respiratory embarrassment associated with pulmonary metastasis

RECOMMENDED READING

Edwards NJ: The diagnostic value of pericardial fluid pH determination. *J Am Anim Hosp Assoc* 32(1):63–67, 1996.

Fine DM, Tobias AH, Jacob KA: Use of pericardial fluid pH to distinguish between idiopathic and neoplastic effusions. *J Vet Intern Med* 17(4):525–529, 2003.

Kienle RD: Pericardial disease and cardiac neoplasia. In Kittleson MD, Kienle RD (eds): *Small Animal Cardiovascular Medicine.* St. Louis, Mosby, 1998, pp 413–432.

Sisson D, Thomas WP: Pericardial disease and cardiac tumors. In Fox PR, Sisson D, Moise NS (eds): *Textbook of Canine and Feline Cardiology*. Philadelphia, WB Saunders, 1999, pp 679–701.

Weisse C, et al: Survival times in dogs with right atrial hemangiosarcoma treated by means of surgical resection with or without adjuvant chemotherapy: 23 cases (1986–2000). *J Am Vet Med Assoc* 226(4):575–579, 2005.

AUTHOR: **N. JOEL EDWARDS**
EDITOR: **ETIENNE CÔTÉ**

Hematochezia

BASIC INFORMATION

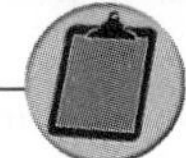

DEFINITION

The presence of bright red streaks of blood on the surface of, or admixed into, the stool

EPIDEMIOLOGY

SPECIES, AGE, SEX

- Dependent on underlying cause
- Older animals: neoplasia
- Younger animals: parasites

RISK FACTORS: The most common risk factor for hematochezia is colitis. Neoplasia is less commonly responsible. Coagulopathies are a rare cause of hematochezia.

ASSOCIATED CONDITIONS AND DISORDERS: Clinically significant anemia very uncommonly occurs as a result of hematochezia.

CLINICAL PRESENTATION

HISTORY, CHIEF COMPLAINT

- Animals presenting with hematochezia will also commonly present with mucus in the stool, straining, and difficulty defecating; all are manifestations of colonic disease.
- Animals with hematochezia rarely present signs of systemic illness.

PHYSICAL EXAM FINDINGS

- These animals generally look clinically healthy. Involuntary weight loss should *not* be present, and if it is, severe colonic disease (e.g., infiltrative disease) or complications of colonic disease (e.g., malignancy) should be investigated.
- The perianal area may be soiled with blood, fecal material, and/or mucus.
- The anus may be inflamed and ulcerated.
- A mass (neoplasm), swelling (anal gland abscess), or fissure (perianal fistula) around the anus may be visible.
- A rectal examination can confirm the presence of hematochezia and is essential in any patient with a presenting complaint of hematochezia.

ETIOLOGY AND PATHOPHYSIOLOGY

Blood most commonly originates from the anus, rectum, and/or descending colon.

DIAGNOSIS

DIFFERENTIAL DIAGNOSIS

- Diseases involving the anus:
  - Anal sacculitis/abscess
  - Perianal fistula
  - Neoplasia (anal sac tumor)
  - Perineal hernia
  - Rectal stricture
  - Trauma
  - Foreign body
- Diseases involving the rectum and colon:
  - Proctitis
  - Colitis:
    - Idiopathic
    - Inflammatory
    - Infectious (*Campylobacter, Clostridium*)
    - Stress
  - Parasites:
    - Hookworms, whipworms, coccidia, roundworms
  - Neoplasia:
    - Benign: rectal polyp
    - Malignant: lymphoma, carcinoma
  - Rectal prolapse
  - Mucosal trauma (foreign body, hair balls, enemas)
  - Dexamethasone administration (especially in the presence of intervertebral disk disease)
  - Coagulation disorders (usually accompanied by bleeding from other sites)

INITIAL DATABASE

- Rectal examination including anal sac palpation
- Fecal examination for parasites
- Fecal smear, culture, *Clostridium* toxin detection
- Response to trial therapy (see Acute General Treatment below)

ADVANCED OR CONFIRMATORY TESTING

Advanced testing should be considered in patients with systemic signs of illness, persistent or recurrent episodes of hematochezia. Tests are selected based on history, physical exam, and initial database results:

- Complete blood count
- Serum biochemistry profile
- Urinalysis
- Coagulation profile
- Abdominal radiographs
- Abdominal ultrasound
- Colonoscopy

TREATMENT

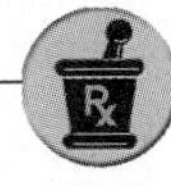

THERAPEUTIC GOAL(S)

Identification and management of the underlying disease

ACUTE GENERAL TREATMENT

- Nonspecific trial therapy can be attempted in an animal without systemic signs:
  - Diet containing fermentable fiber
  - Broad-spectrum dewormer (e.g., fenbendazole 50 mg/kg PO q 24h × 5 days)
  - Trial course of metronidazole (e.g., 10–25 mg/kg PO q 12h × 7 days maximum)
- Dependent on the underlying disease:
  - Perianal fistulas: immunosuppressive therapy
  - Infectious colitis: *Clostridium*: metronidazole, amoxicillin, *Campylobacter*: tylosin
  - Neoplasia: surgical excision, chemotherapy, radiation therapy
  - Stricture: surgery
  - Perianal hernia: surgical correction

CHRONIC TREATMENT

- Dependent on the underlying disease
- Colitis: see Colitis, Acute, p 222; Colitis, Chronic, p 223

POSSIBLE COMPLICATIONS

Perforated colon:
- Neoplasia
- Dexamethasone therapy (especially in the presence of intervertebral disk disease)

PROGNOSIS AND OUTCOME

Dependent on underlying disease

PEARLS & CONSIDERATIONS

COMMENTS

Hematochezia should not be confused with melena, which refers to the presence of dark, tarry stool caused by digested blood from the upper digestive tract or small intestine.

SUGGESTED READING

Kelly KM: Melena and hematochezia. In Ettinger SJ, Feldman EC (eds): *Textbook of Veterinary Internal Medicine*, ed 6. St. Louis, WB Saunders, 2005, pp 141–143.

Tams T: Gastrointestinal symptoms. In *Handbook of Small Animal Gastroenterology*, ed 2. St. Louis, WB Saunders, 2003, pp 31–32.

AUTHOR: **MARILYN DUNN**
EDITOR: **ETIENNE CÔTÉ**

Hematuria

BASIC INFORMATION

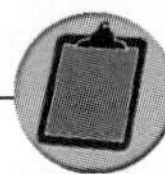

DEFINITION

The presence of blood (gross or microscopic) in the urine

SYNONYM(S)

Bloody urine

EPIDEMIOLOGY

SPECIES, AGE, SEX: Dogs or cats of either gender and any age may develop hematuria for a variety of benign or pathologic reasons.

GENETICS AND BREED PREDISPOSITION: Welsh corgi (renal telangiectasia).

RISK FACTORS
- Conditions predisposing to urolithiasis or urinary tract infection
- Anticoagulants
- Hereditary coagulopathies
- Cyclophosphamide administration
- Trauma

ASSOCIATED CONDITIONS AND DISORDERS
- Hemostatic defects
- Urinary or genital tract trauma, neoplasia, inflammation, or infection
- Urolithiasis
- Acute renal failure
- Glomerulonephritis
- Vascular malformation
- Proestrus
- Renal infarcts
- Feline lower urinary tract signs/disease
- Parasitic cystitis (*Capillaria plica*)

CLINICAL PRESENTATION

DISEASE FORMS/SUBTYPES
- Macroscopic hematuria: grossly discolored, bloody urine
- Microscopic hematuria: >5 red blood cells (RBCs)/hpf without overt urine discoloration

HISTORY, CHIEF COMPLAINT
- Gross hematuria may occur at initiation of urination, throughout urination, or at the end of urination:
  - Initial hematuria: lower urinary tract or reproductive origin
  - Total hematuria: origin anywhere along urinary/reproductive tract
  - Terminal hematuria: upper urinary tract, bladder origin
- Depending on causation, any of the following may be reported:
  - Red, pink, or brown urine (macroscopic) (see also Discolored Urine, p 309)
  - Dysuria/stranguria (suggestive of lower urinary tract disorders)
  - Pollakiuria (suggestive of lower urinary tract disorders)
  - Bloody discharge from penis or vulva unassociated with urination (suggestive of genital origin)
  - Abdominal pain
  - Systemic signs (e.g., lethargy, anorexia, vomiting) suggestive of upper urinary disorders, obstruction, or rupture

PHYSICAL EXAM FINDINGS: Depending on etiology, findings may include:
- Palpable renal/bladder/urethral mass effect
- Prostatomegaly
- Abdominal pain
- Bleeding unrelated to the urinary/genital tract (e.g., petechiae, ecchymosis, epistaxis) suggesting systemic bleeding disorder

ETIOLOGY AND PATHOPHYSIOLOGY

- Primary (coagulation factors) or secondary (platelet) hemostatic defects or vasculitis may result in hematuria in the absence of urinary or reproductive disorders.
- Bleeding anywhere along the length of the urinary tract or from the reproductive tract may cause hematuria.
- A variety of inflammatory, infectious, neoplastic, traumatic, or toxic insults may result in hematuria.
- Vascular malformations (e.g., telangiectasia) are a rare but important cause of marked hematuria.

DIAGNOSIS

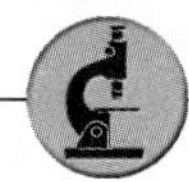

DIFFERENTIAL DIAGNOSIS

Pigmenturia
- Hemoglobinuria
- Myoglobinuria

INITIAL DATABASE

- History reviewed for drugs/toxins (e.g., cyclophosphamide, phenols) or iatrogenic procedures (e.g., urinary catheterization, cystocentesis) that might induce hematuria.
  - If microscopic hematuria is observed after cystocentesis, later evaluation of a voided sample is warranted.
- Rectal examination: prostate, intrapelvic urethra.
- Digital vaginal exam/cytologic evaluation if vulvar bleeding between urinations.
- Urinalysis: Hematuria differentiated from hemoglobinuria, myoglobinuria, or pigmenturia (all of which discolor urine and may produce a positive blood result by urine dipstick) by presence of intact RBC on microscopic exam (hematuria only).
  - Cystocentesis is avoided if coagulopathy, ascites, peritonitis, or neoplastic bladder disease is possible.
  - Urethral catheterization: detection of urethral calculi/mass, urine collection.

- Hematuria in samples obtained by catheterization or cystocentesis suggests origin is kidney(s), ureter(s), or bladder. Conversely, if RBC absent from these samples but present in voided urine, source of bleeding is likely urethra or reproductive tract.
- Complete blood count: thrombocytopenia suggests hemostatic defect; neutrophilia suggests upper urinary infection/inflammation; anemia may correlate to degree of blood loss.
- Serum biochemical profile: azotemia and hyperkalemia suggest renal disease or urinary obstruction/rupture.
- Urine culture.
- Abdominal radiographs: shape and size of kidneys, bladder, prostate evaluated. Radiopaque stones may be observed.
- Abdominal (urinary and genital) ultrasound: Renal parenchyma, bladder wall and luminal content, prostate, uterus, and portions of ureters/urethra evaluated.

ADVANCED OR CONFIRMATORY TESTING

- If coagulopathy is suspected, platelet count, bleeding time, prothrombin time, activated partial thromboplastin time, and/or activated coagulation time are indicated.
- Excretory urographic contrast studies (see Excretory Urogram, p 1241) may delineate masses, stones, or tears in the urinary tract.
- Cystoscopy may identify source of bleeding from vagina, urethra, bladder, or either kidney/ureter.
- Traumatic catheterization for cytology or urethral/bladder mass.
- Consider biopsy of kidney, bladder, prostate, urethra as appropriate.
- Bladder tumor antigen test unreliable in the face of hematuria.

TREATMENT

THERAPEUTIC GOAL(S)

Address underlying cause of hematuria

ACUTE GENERAL TREATMENT

Treatment entirely dependent on causation:

- Coagulopathy is addressed directly.
- Traumatic injury may require supportive care alone or surgical intervention.
- Urinary calculi are treated via medical dissolution and/or mechanical removal, depending on type and location of stone.
- Urinary tract or reproductive infections are treated with appropriate antibiotics.
- Neoplastic disease may require surgical intervention (e.g., unilateral renal carcinoma) or chemotherapy (e.g., transitional cell carcinoma).
- Drugs (e.g., cyclophosphamide, nonsteroidal anti-inflammatory drugs) that might induce hematuria disallowed.
- Rarely, renal hematuria may lead to blood loss sufficient to warrant transfusion.

CHRONIC TREATMENT

Dependent on cause

POSSIBLE COMPLICATIONS

Rarely, blood clots lead to ureteral or urethral obstruction.

RECOMMENDED MONITORING

Dependent on cause

PROGNOSIS AND OUTCOME

Dependent on cause

PEARLS & CONSIDERATIONS

COMMENTS

- Generally, hematuria is a sign of underlying disease rather than a primary disorder.
- Renal telangiectasia is an uncommon hereditary condition in Welsh corgi dogs resulting in potentially profound renal bleeding due to vascular malformations. Diagnosis depends on biopsy, and organs other than the kidney may be involved.
- Benign essential hematuria is an uncommon disorder of young dogs in which no cause for profound, persistent hematuria can be identified. Often it occurs unilaterally; removal of the affected kidney is curative.

SUGGESTED READING

Moore FM, et al: Telangiectasia of Pembroke Welsh corgi dogs. *Vet Pathol* 20:203, 1983.

Forrester SD. Diagnostic approach to hematuria in dogs and cats. *Vet Clinics North Am Small Anim Pract* 34:849, 2004.

Kaufman AC, et al: Benign essential hematuria in dogs. *Comp Contin Educ Pract Vet* 16:1317, 1994.

AUTHOR & EDITOR: **LEAH A. COHN**

Hemoabdomen

BASIC INFORMATION

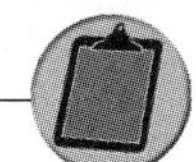

DEFINITION

Hemoabdomen is characterized by the presence of free blood within the peritoneal cavity.

SYNONYM(S)

Hemoperitoneum

EPIDEMIOLOGY

SPECIES, AGE, SEX: Signalment will vary with the underlying cause. Young dogs are more likely to develop hemoabdomen secondary to trauma. Older large-breed dogs without a history of trauma often develop hemoabdomen due to a ruptured splenic or hepatic mass such as hemangiosarcoma.

GENETICS AND BREED PREDISPOSITION: Large-breed older dogs are predisposed to hemangiosarcoma.

RISK FACTORS: Dogs that roam may ingest anticoagulant rodenticides.

ASSOCIATED CONDITIONS AND DISORDERS: Animals with hemangiosarcoma can develop pericardial effusion due to rupture of a metastatic right atrial hemangiosarcoma.

CLINICAL PRESENTATION

HISTORY, CHIEF COMPLAINT

- Historic findings can range from episodes of acute collapse to mild lethargy. Some dogs will present for evaluation of gastrointestinal signs such as vomiting or a distended abdomen. Many dogs have a history of weakness or collapse during the weeks before presentation. Presumptively, this indicates a prior hemorrhagic episode.
- Some, but not all, dogs with anticoagulant rodenticide toxicity will have a history of ingestion of the poison. Anticoagulant rodenticide intoxication much more commonly results in hemothorax, mediastinal, or subcutaneous bleeding rather than hemoabdomen.

PHYSICAL EXAM FINDINGS

- Most physical examination findings are referable to blood loss and hemorrhagic shock. The clinical signs will vary depending on the severity of shock. Dogs may have pale mucous membranes, tachypnea, tachycardia, and bounding pulses. An abdominal fluid wave may be present. In some

cases, a discrete abdominal mass may be palpable.
- A traumatic cause for hemoabdomen may be apparent due to the presence of additional injuries.
- Animals with anticoagulant rodenticide toxicity may have bruising at venipuncture sites.

ETIOLOGY AND PATHOPHYSIOLOGY

- In dogs without a history of trauma and a normal coagulation profile, hemangiosarcoma is the most likely diagnosis.
- Benign splenic hematomas account for a substantial proportion of canine splenic masses in general, but comprise only 5–10% of the splenic masses seen in dogs with hemoabdomen.

DIAGNOSIS

DIFFERENTIAL DIAGNOSIS

- Ruptured hemangiosarcoma
- Ruptured splenic hematoma
- Other ruptured abdominal mass
- Trauma
- Anticoagulant rodenticide toxicity

INITIAL DATABASE

- Packed cell volume and serum total protein
- Prothrombin time and activated partial thromboplastin time
- Complete blood count (CBC) with manual platelet count
- Serum biochemical profile
- Abdominocentesis:
  - Nonclotting bloody effusion: if neoplasia or coagulopathy.
  - Bloody effusion with clots: if trauma; rarely, with voluminous bleed from mass.

ADVANCED OR CONFIRMATORY TESTING

- Abdominal ultrasound to identify the source of hemorrhage in dogs with hemangiosarcoma and splenic hematoma.
- Abdominal radiography may be minimally helpful in the presence of free abdominal fluid.
- Whenever possible, thoracic radiographs and echocardiography should be performed before surgery in dogs with hemoabdomen and an abdominal mass (rule out metastasis/poor prognosis).
- Blood rodenticide levels can be performed in cases of suspected toxicity.

TREATMENT

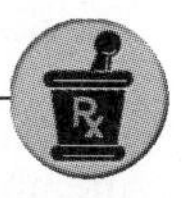

THERAPEUTIC GOAL(S)

- Initial treatment should be directed toward establishing cardiovascular stability.
- Further treatment should focus on preventing ongoing hemorrhage.

ACUTE GENERAL TREATMENT

- Intravenous fluids as indicated by the patient's cardiovascular status.
- Blood transfusion in patients with a packed cell volume less than 20–25% that are hemodynamically unstable (e.g., concurrent hypotension, hemorrhagic shock, or rapid sustained ventricular arrhythmia).
- Patients with a coagulopathy should be treated with 15 ml/kg of fresh frozen plasma or 30 ml/kg of fresh whole blood.
- Emergent laparotomy is indicated in dogs with ongoing hemorrhage.
- Dogs with abdominal neoplasia benefit from surgical removal of the bleeding tumor once they are hemodynamically stable, although postoperative survival times may only be in the weeks to months range depending on the nature of the neoplasm.

CHRONIC TREATMENT

- Patients with neoplasia may benefit from chemotherapy.
- Anticoagulant rodenticide toxicity: vitamin K_1 5 mg/kg SC, then 2.5 mg/kg/day PO for 2 to 6 weeks as indicated by the specific toxin ingested.

POSSIBLE COMPLICATIONS

- Ongoing hemorrhage.
- Some splenic or liver masses have metastasized by the time of laparotomy, and the masses may not be resectable.
- Severe ventricular arrhythmia may develop, and may require therapy.

RECOMMENDED MONITORING

- Cardiac electrocardiogram monitoring is indicated due to the high frequency of arrhythmia in dogs with splenic disease.
- Frequent reassessment of the packed cell volume/total solids is warranted in the initial, urgent setting.
- Coagulation times should be rechecked after the completion of plasma transfusions.
- Specific long-term monitoring depends on cause. Typically, dogs with hemoabdomen are reassessed within 10 postoperative days (history, physical examination, CBC; other tests based on these findings and original etiology), and again 2 to 4 weeks later barring complications.

PROGNOSIS AND OUTCOME

- Often, exact prognosis is only determined in the postoperative period with histopathologic assessment of biopsies.
- Dogs with hemangiosarcoma have a poor prognosis, with an average survival of 3 to 6 months with surgical treatment and 2 to 3 weeks without surgery.
- Dogs with splenic hematomas may be cured with splenectomy.
- Traumatic hemoabdomen usually responds well to supportive nonoperative management.

PEARLS & CONSIDERATIONS

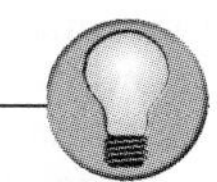

COMMENTS

- In patients with acute hemorrhage, the serum total protein will fall before the packed cell volume.
- It is essential to submit large sections of spleen (or the entire spleen) for histopathologic analysis of splenic masses. Otherwise, some splenic biopsies that are interpreted by the pathologist as a hematoma are actually hemangiosarcoma, as the tumor is small and there is a massive hematoma surrounding it.
- Benign splenic hematomas account for a large proportion of canine splenic masses in general, but hematomas make up only 5–10% of the splenic masses seen in dogs with hemoabdomen.
- Any collapsed large-breed dog should be evaluated for a possible hemoabdomen.

PREVENTION

Keep dogs confined or supervised to prevent trauma and rodenticide intoxication

CLIENT EDUCATION

Advise owner to present older dogs with lethargy for evaluation in a timely fashion

SUGGESTED READING

Pintar J, et al: Acute nontraumatic hemoabdomen in the dog: A retrospective analysis of 39 cases (1987–2001). *J Am Anim Hosp Assoc* 39:518–522, 2003.

Prymak C, et al: Epidemiologic, clinical, pathologic, and prognostic characteristics of splenic hemangiosarcoma and splenic hematoma in dogs: 217 cases (1985). *J Am Vet Med Assoc* 193:706–712, 1988.

AUTHOR: **SCOTT P. SHAW**
EDITOR: **ELIZABETH ROZANSKI**

Hemobartonellosis, Feline

BASIC INFORMATION

DEFINITION

A parasitic infection of feline red blood cells (RBCs) with *Mycoplasma haemofelis* or *Mycoplasma haemominutum*, parasites previously known collectively as *Haemobartonella felis*. The disease is characterized clinically by cyclical episodes of fever and hemolytic anemia.

SYNONYM(S)

Feline hemotropic mycoplasmosis
Feline infectious anemia

EPIDEMIOLOGY

SPECIES, AGE, SEX: Domestic and wild felines of all ages.

RISK FACTORS

- Access to outdoors and other cats: young intact males overrepresented, presumably due to roaming and fighting.
- A history of cat bite abscess often precedes hemobartonellosis by a few weeks.
- Exposure to fleas and ticks.
- Deficient vaccine history has been associated with hemobartonellosis.
- Underlying feline leukemia (FeLV) infection.
- Immunosuppression.

CONTAGION AND ZOONOSIS

- Transmitted vertically from queen to kitten; unknown if route is transplacental, transmammary, or due to exposure to blood during parturition
- Transmitted horizontally from cat to cat via arthropod vectors (fleas, ticks, possibly mosquitoes), bite wounds, or blood transfusion
- No known risk to humans

GEOGRAPHY AND SEASONALITY: Worldwide.

CLINICAL PRESENTATION

DISEASE FORMS/SUBTYPES

- Acute, chronic, or subclinical
- Clinical signs dependent on anemia (severity and rate of development)

HISTORY, CHIEF COMPLAINT

- Acute: sudden death, weakness, depression, collapse, pale mucous membranes, tachypnea, anorexia, ± vomiting
- Chronic: lethargy, anorexia, weight loss
- Subclinical: no abnormalities reported; parasite is an incidental finding

PHYSICAL EXAM FINDINGS

- Acute: pale mucous membranes most commonly; fever, tachypnea, tachycardia, mental depression, weakness, ± splenomegaly possible; rarely icteric mucous membranes
- Chronic: pale mucous membranes, poor body condition, normal mentation and strength, ± splenomegaly, ± fever

ETIOLOGY AND PATHOPHYSIOLOGY

- Causative agents are two species of feline hemotropic *Mycoplasmas*:
  - *Mycoplasma haemofelis*, formerly known as *Haemobartonella felis* large form
  - *Mycoplasma haemominutum*, formerly known as *Haemobartonella felis* small form
- Previously considered rickettsiae, but recent reclassification based on 16S ribosomal RNA sequencing has demonstrated greater sequence homology with mycoplasmas.
- Transmission via blood-sucking arthropods (fleas, ticks).
- Organisms parasitize RBC membranes, causing RBC destruction and thus regenerative hemolytic anemia. Proposed mechanisms: increased RBC fragility and decreased life span; erythrophagocytosis by spleen, liver, lungs, bone marrow; immune-mediated destruction by antibodies and complement. Majority of hemolysis is extravascular.
- Clinical disease is typified by cyclical bouts of parasitemia, resultant anemia, transient recovery, recrudescence, eventual conversion to a carrier state.
- *M. haemofelis* is more pathogenic. *M. haemominutum* often is subclinical. Coinfection with both species typically causes worse clinical disease.
- Underlying immune deficiency or coexistent illness should be suspected in cases with overt clinical signs.

DIAGNOSIS

DIFFERENTIAL DIAGNOSIS

- Primary immune-mediated hemolytic anemia
- Heinz body anemia (acetaminophen toxicity, zinc toxicity, diabetic ketoacidosis, hepatic lipidosis, ingestion of onions or baby food containing onion powder) (Fig. I-86)
- Cytauxzoonosis
- External or internal blood loss
- FeLV infection

INITIAL DATABASE

- Blood smear: visual identification of organism:
  - Nonrefractile basophilic cocci, rods or ring-forms on margins of red cells.
  - Organisms are found on blood smears in fewer than 50% of infections. Lack of identification does not rule out disease.
  - For optimal recognition, a thin blood smear should be made immediately after blood collection and stained with Romanowsky stains. New methylene blue stain highlights feline reticulocytes, which are easily mistaken for organisms.
  - False-positive results are common due to confusion with Howell-Jolly bodies, Heinz bodies, stain, or refractile artifacts.
- Complete blood count: regenerative anemia, macrocytic normochromic red cells, ± mild to moderate neutrophilia and monocytosis are typical.
- Serum biochemistry profile: typically unremarkable; hyperbilirubinemia uncommon despite hemolysis, occasional elevations in alanine aminotransferase, alkaline phosphatase (ALP).
- Urinalysis: unremarkable.
- Abdominal imaging: changes are minimal. Diffuse, mild to marked splenomegaly possible. Imaging is generally indicated to identify predisposing/complicating factors.
- FeLV testing: to rule out coinfection.

ADVANCED OR CONFIRMATORY TESTING

- Culture not possible. Hemotropic mycoplasmas will not grow in vitro.
- On the horizon: polymerase chain reaction identification developed but not yet commercially available.

TREATMENT

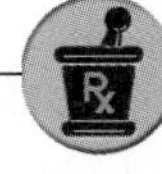

THERAPEUTIC GOAL(S)

Resolution of acute clinical parasitemia and restoration of red cell volume

ACUTE GENERAL TREATMENT

- Supportive care:
  - Blood transfusion or oxygen-carrying compounds for severe anemia (see Transfusion Reactions, p 1098)
  - IV crystalloid fluid replacement as needed
  - Nutritional support in anorectic animals
- Doxycycline/tetracyclines are the drugs of choice for clearing parasitemia. Doxycycline 5-10 mg/kg PO q 12h for 14 to 21 days. Tetracycline 20 mg/kg PO q 12-24h for 14 to 21 days.
- Fluoroquinolones may also be effective. Enrofloxacin 5 mg/kg PO q 24h for 14 to 21 days.

- Penicillins/amoxicillins/macrolides have not demonstrated efficacy.
- Immunosuppressive doses of glucocorticoids for a few days may decrease erythrophagocytosis and red cell removal.

CHRONIC TREATMENT

Treatment is ineffective and unnecessary for carrier individuals (no clinical signs). No drugs have been identified that effectively clear the carrier state.

DRUG INTERACTIONS

- Fluoroquinolones given at high doses may cause blindness in cats.
- Doxycycline: esophagitis/esophageal strictures in cats. Follow doxycycline administration with a small amount of butter, soft margarine, or water to ensure passage into the stomach.

RECOMMENDED MONITORING

Packed cell volume or complete blood counts

PROGNOSIS AND OUTCOME

Severity of infection varies from subclinical to life-threatening. Prognosis is generally good with intensive supportive care and appropriate antibiotic treatment. Infections can recrudesce with stress or other disease.

PEARLS & CONSIDERATIONS

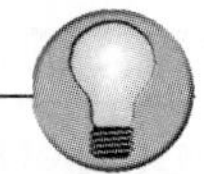

COMMENTS

Affected cats are carriers for life and may have recrudescence of disease during stressful events or other illnesses.

PREVENTION

- To decrease risk of exposure, confine cats indoors or reduce contact with other felines, especially feral populations
- Neuter to decrease roaming and fighting in outside cats
- Practice effective flea and tick control

SUGGESTED READING

Messick J: Hemotrophic mycoplasmas (hemoplasmas): a review and new insights into pathogenic potential. *Vet Clin Pathol* 33:1, 2004.

Sykes JE: Feline hemotropic mycoplasmosis. *Vet Clin North Am Small Anim Pract* 33:4, 2003.

Tasker S: Feline infectious anemia. In Chandler EA, Gaskell CJ, Gaskell RM (eds): *Feline Medicine and Therapeutics*. Oxford UK, Blackwell Publishing, 2004, pp 669-678.

AUTHOR: **SHANNON T. STROUP**
EDITOR: **DOUGLASS K. MACINTIRE**

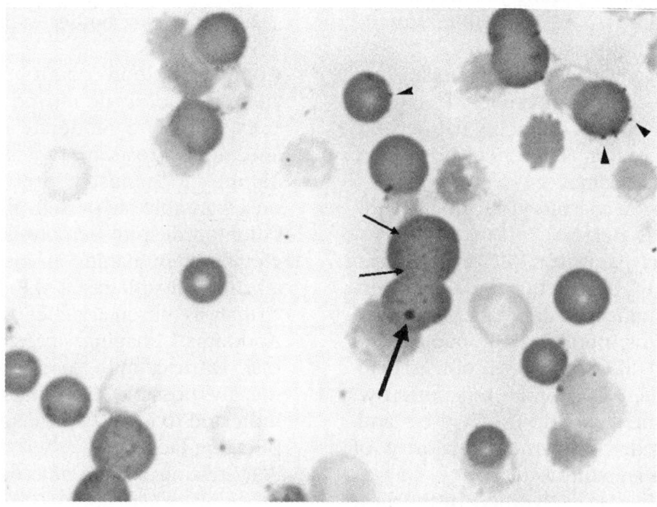

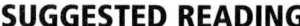

FIGURE I-86 Hematologic differential diagnosis. The larger Howell-Jolly body (*large arrow*) or multiple punctuate appearance of basophilic stippling (seen throughout the two red cells in the center of the image [*small arrows*]) should not be mistaken for *M. felis* (*many arrowheads*). Courtesy of Department of Clinical Pathology, Atlantic Veterinary College; reproduced with permission.

Hemolytic-Uremic Syndrome

BASIC INFORMATION

DEFINITION

An uncommon, severe disease characterized by microangiopathic hemolytic anemia, acute renal failure, and thrombocytopenia. This disease in humans is usually associated with enterohemorrhagic *Escherichia coli* (EHEC) infections and diarrhea, but other infectious organisms have been implicated. A similar syndrome has been reported in dogs and cats.

SYNONYM(S)

Alabama rot
Cutaneous and renal glomerular vasculopathy (CRGV) of greyhounds
Greenetrack disease
HUS

EPIDEMIOLOGY

SPECIES, AGE, SEX

- Mainly dogs; very rare in cats
- No age or sex predilection

GENETICS AND BREED PREDISPOSITION: Reported most frequently and originally in racing greyhounds. Some genetic predispositions possible, because outbreaks in affected kennels are often noted among littermates.

RISK FACTORS: A diet including inappropriately cooked meat may predispose to EHEC infections.

CONTAGION AND ZOONOSIS: Contaminated beef ingestion is most widely responsible for hemolytic-uremic syndrome (HUS) in humans, and common-source exposure could occur in pets. In humans, HUS has been reported from sepsis associated with dog bites and pneumococcal infections transmitted from human to human.

GEOGRAPHY AND SEASONALITY: First noted in Alabama dog racing tracks.

ASSOCIATED CONDITIONS AND DISORDERS: Similar condition noted in some cats after renal transplantation.

CLINICAL PRESENTATION

DISEASE FORMS/SUBTYPES: HUS and cutaneous/renal glomerular vasculopathy are similar, although HUS typically does not have the cutaneous lesions associated with CRGV.

HISTORY, CHIEF COMPLAINT

- History may include feeding raw or undercooked beef. Usually the initial complaint is hemorrhagic diarrhea, although not always reported.

- Lethargy or cutaneous lesions may be the primary complaint as well as vomiting, limb edema, and anorexia.

PHYSICAL EXAM FINDINGS

- In CRGV, cutaneous lesions are multifocal erythematous swellings commonly located on the tarsus, stifle, medial thigh, and rarely forelimb. Lesions may become ulcerated with serosanguinous discharge.
- Physical findings common to both CRGV and HUS include those typical of anemia and acute renal failure, with hemoglobinuria often present.

ETIOLOGY AND PATHOPHYSIOLOGY

- EHEC 0157:H7 producing *Shigella* toxin.
- Other infectious diseases could cause similar syndromes. In humans pneumoccal pneumonia, other gram-negative bacteria, and postrenal transplants have been documented.
- Sepsis/dissemination of toxin causes vasculitis, leading to microangiopathic hemolytic anemia, acute renal failure, and in some cases cutaneous lesions.
- Glomerular disease noted in cutaneous and renal glomerular vasculopathy.

DIAGNOSIS

DIFFERENTIAL DIAGNOSIS

- Leptospirosis, sepsis, systemic inflammatory diseases
- Any disease causing acute renal failure or vasculitis
- Immune-mediated hemolytic anemia

INITIAL DATABASE

- Complete blood count, serum biochemistry profile, urinalysis
  - Anemia, presence of schistocytes, and thrombocytopenia are typical.
    - Ensure adequate platelet count if renal biopsy is being considered
  - Azotemia and isosthenuria may precede, coexist with, or be absent. Generally, increased blood urea nitrogen, creatinine, and phosphorus are seen.
  - Proteinuria possible with glomerular disease (cutaneous and renal glomerular vasculopathy).
  - Hemoglobinuria commonly is present (discolored urine; positive blood result on dipstick but no erythrocytes on sediment exam).
- Coagulation panel with D-dimer or fibrin/fibrinogen degradation product (FDP) analysis: evidence of thrombosis (e.g., increased FDP) common
- Urine culture: rule out urinary infection as cause of proteinuria
- Arterial blood pressure measurement: rule out systemic hypertension associated with renal disease

ADVANCED OR CONFIRMATORY TESTING

- Abdominal ultrasound ± renal biopsy. Assess blood pressure and platelet count first
- Skin biopsy of representative lesions
- Culture of diarrhea for EHEC 0157:H7

TREATMENT

THERAPEUTIC GOAL(S)

- Maintenance or return of urine output
- Appropriate antibiotic therapy
- Supportive care

ACUTE GENERAL TREATMENT

- Treat oliguric or anuric renal failure intensively (see Acute Renal Failure, p 1298)
  - Correct dehydration
  - Transfusion if severe anemia (hematocrit <20%)
  - If urine output deficient and blood pressure adequate, attempt to increase urine output with either mannitol (0.5 g/kg IV over 30 minutes) or if volume overloaded dopamine (2-5 μg/kg/min IV) and furosemide (0.2-0.5 mg/kg/hr IV constant rate infusion)
- Other therapy tailored to cause (i.e., antibiotics for gram-negative sepsis such as enrofloxacin 10-20 mg/kg IV, IM, or PO q 24h in dogs; maximum 5 mg/kg/day in cats)

CHRONIC TREATMENT

Hypertension may be treated with amlodipine (0.5-1 mg/kg PO q 24h).

POSSIBLE COMPLICATIONS

- Hemorrhage from severe thrombocytopenia or disseminated intravascular coagulation
- Bacterial translocation and sepsis from hemorrhagic diarrhea
- Hypertension
- Chronic glomerulonephritis/protein-losing nephropathy
- Poorly healing cutaneous lesions

RECOMMENDED MONITORING

- Renal values on serum chemistry (blood urea nitrogen, creatinine, electrolytes)
- Hematocrit
- Urine output
- Blood pressure

PROGNOSIS AND OUTCOME

- Often fatal disease
- Survivors may have chronic renal failure or glomerular disease

PEARLS & CONSIDERATIONS

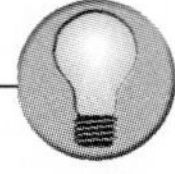

COMMENTS

- More causes of this syndrome are being seen in human medicine and in common diseases that stimulate systemic inflammation and vasculitis.
- Early intensive therapy is the key to survival and perhaps prevention once initial sign of hemorrhagic diarrhea is noted.

PREVENTION

For the cases initiated by ingestion of EHEC 0157:H7, prevention occurs by removal of inadequately cooked beef from diet

SUGGESTED READING

Aronson LR, et al: Possible hemolytic uremic syndrome in three cats after renal transplantation and cyclosporine therapy. *Vet Surg* 28(3):135-140, 1999.

Carpenter JL, et al: Idiopathic cutaneous and renal glomerular vasculopathy of greyhounds. *Vet Pathol* 25(6):401-407, 1988.

Holloway S, et al: Hemolytic uremic syndrome in dogs. *J Vet Intern Med* 7(4):220-227, 1993.

Kruth SA: Gram-negative bacterial infections. In Greene CE (ed): *Infectious Disease of the Dog and Cat*. Philadelphia, WB Saunders, 1998, pp 217-221.

AUTHOR: **JEFFERY SIMMONS**
EDITOR: **DOUGLASS K. MACINTIRE**

Hemophilias and Other Hereditary Coagulation Factor Deficiencies

BASIC INFORMATION

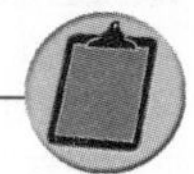

DEFINITION

Congenital hemostatic defects caused by mutations that impair the production of active clotting factors

SYNONYM(S)

Specific defects are classified by the deficient factor, with alternate names in common use for factors I, II, VIII, and IX:

Deficient factor	Alternate name
Fibrinogen (factor I)	Dysfibrinogenemia, hypofibrinogenemia
Factor II	Prothrombin deficiency
Factor VII	Proconvertin or extrinsic factor deficiency
Factor VIII	Hemophilia A or classic hemophilia
Factor IX	Hemophilia B or Christmas disease
Factor X	Stuart Prower deficiency
Factor XI	Hemophilia C
Factor XII	Hageman trait

EPIDEMIOLOGY

SPECIES, AGE, SEX

- Dogs and cats: severe bleeding disorders typically manifest by 6 to 12 months old
- Males almost exclusively affected: hemophilia A and B (factor VIII and factor IX deficiencies)
- Males and females equally affected: all other factor deficiencies

GENETICS AND BREED PREDISPOSITION

- X-linked recessive inheritance pattern: hemophilias A and B
- Autosomal recessive (or incomplete dominant): all other factor deficiencies
- Breed predisposition:
  - Dogs: Hemophilia A is the most common hereditary coagulation defect and may develop in any purebred or mixed-breed dog (presumably due to de novo mutations). A mild to moderate form of hemophilia A has been propagated widely in German shepherds. Less common defects: factor VII deficiency in beagles, factor X deficiency in Jack Russell terriers, factor XI deficiency in Kerry blue terriers.
  - Cats: hemophilia A and B in any breed and domestic cats. Factor XII deficiency is the most common hereditary factor deficiency in domestic and Siamese cats. Combined deficiency of factors II, VII, IX, and X in Devon rex cats.
  - Note: mutations causing factor deficiencies can arise in any breed.

CLINICAL PRESENTATION

DISEASE FORMS/SUBTYPES

- Severe bleeding tendency: deficiencies of factors I, II, VIII, IX, and X
- Mild to moderate bleeding tendency: deficiencies of factors VII, XI, and some forms of factor VIII and IX deficiency
- No clinical signs: factor XII deficiency

HISTORY, CHIEF COMPLAINT

- Severe forms: spontaneous and recurrent hematoma formation, bleeding into body cavities, lameness due to hemarthrosis, prolonged and potentially fatal bleeding from loss of deciduous teeth or minor wounds
- Mild forms: few spontaneous or severe bleeds, abnormal bleeding typically observed after surgical or traumatic injury

PHYSICAL EXAM FINDINGS

- Abnormal hemorrhage:
  - Manifestations of hemorrhage into body cavities or potential spaces (hemarthrosis, hematoma, hemoabdomen, hemothorax, central nervous system hemorrhage)
  - Bleeding from traumatic/surgical wounds
  - Occasionally epistaxis or intraocular bleeds
- Pallor (blood loss anemia)

ETIOLOGY AND PATHOPHYSIOLOGY

- Specific factor deficiencies are caused by mutations in the corresponding coagulation factor genes.
- De novo mutations occur most often in the factor VIII gene.
- Mutations causing mild to moderate clinical signs are more likely to become widely propagated in a breed or line.
- Although factor XII deficiency causes prolongation of the activated clotting time (ACT) and activated partial thromboplastin time (aPTT) coagulation screening tests, it does *not* cause a clinical bleeding tendency.

DIAGNOSIS

DIFFERENTIAL DIAGNOSIS

- Acquired coagulation disorder (e.g., rodenticide intoxication, liver disease, disseminated intravascular coagulation)
- Thrombocytopenia
- Hereditary platelet function defect or von Willebrand disease
- Bleeding caused by tissue injury or infiltrative disorder
- Defect of fibrinolysis

INITIAL DATABASE

- Thorough physical exam to define site(s) of hemorrhage. Hemorrhage from more than a single site suggests a hemostatic defect, ratherr than blood loss from damaged or diseased blood vessels.
- Baseline hematocrit and plasma protein.
- Platelet count: usually normal unless brisk hemorrhage (platelet loss).
- Point-of-care coagulation screening tests (*, markedly abnormal):
  - ACT: prolonged (factors I, II, VIII, IX, X, XI, and XII deficiencies) or normal (factor VII deficiency).
  - aPTT: prolonged (factors I, II, VIII, IX, X, XI*, and XII* deficiencies) or normal (factor VII deficiency).
  - Prothrombin time (PT): prolonged (factors I, II, VII, and X deficiencies) or normal (factors VIII, IX, XI, and XII deficiencies).
- Laboratory coagulation panel:
  - aPTT, PT: as above.
  - Fibrinogen: low (factor I deficiency), normal for others.
  - Thrombin clotting time: prolonged (factor I deficiency), normal for others.

ADVANCED OR CONFIRMATORY TESTING

Definitive diagnosis based on identifying low levels of specific coagulation factors:

- Clottable fibrinogen (factor I)
- Coagulant activity assays (factors II through XII)

TREATMENT

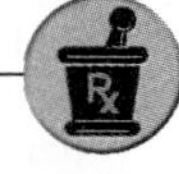

THERAPEUTIC GOAL(S)

- Control active bleeding with transfusion therapy and supportive medical care
- Minimize frequency of induced bleeding by avoiding surgery and trauma

ACUTE GENERAL TREATMENT

- Transfusion to supply hemostatic levels of the deficient factor:
  - Use of plasma components reduces risk of volume overload or red cell sensitization while maximizing factor replacement
  - Fresh frozen plasma (10–12 ml/kg):
    - "Broad spectrum" replacement therapy for fibrinogen and factors II through XI deficiencies
  - Cryoprecipitate (unit dosage varies for different suppliers):

  - Replacement therapy for fibrinogen defects and factor VIII deficiency
- Cryopoor plasma or cryosupernatant (10–12 ml/kg):
  - Replacement therapy for factors II, VII, IX, X, and XI deficiencies
- Replacment of red cells for severe blood loss anemia:
  - Fresh whole blood (≈12 to 20 ml/kg) or packed red cells (≈6–12 ml/kg) (see Transfusion Reactions, p 1098 for specific information)

CHRONIC TREATMENT

- Intermittent transfusion as needed to control hemorrhagic events
- Preoperative transfusion to prevent abnormal bleeding
- Avoidance of unnecessary invasive procedures

DRUG INTERACTIONS

Avoid drugs with anticoagulant or antiplatelet effects:

- Nonsteroidal anti-inflammatory drugs (NSAIDs)
- Sulfonamides
- Heparin, coumadin
- Plasma expanders
- Estrogens
- Cytotoxic drugs

POSSIBLE COMPLICATIONS

- Red cell sensitization causing transfusion reactions:
  - Transfuse plasma components when possible
  - Feline transfusion: donor and recipient must be type-matched for any transfusion
  - Canine transfusion: after the first red cell transfusion, perform crossmatch before subsequent transfusions
- Development of inhibitory antifactor antibodies (rare complication)

RECOMMENDED MONITORING

Adequate factor replacement is demonstrated by:

- Cessation of active bleeding
- Stabilization of hematocrit/plasma protein
- Resolution of lameness and hematoma

PROGNOSIS AND OUTCOME

- Mild to moderate factor deficiencies: good quality of life possible; patient may require occasional transfusion
- Severe factor deficiencies: fair to poor prognosis due to recurrent bleeds and dependence on repeated transfusion; acute fatal bleeds may occur

PEARLS & CONSIDERATIONS

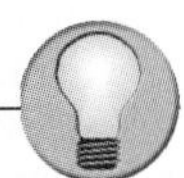

COMMENTS

- Hemophilia A (factor VIII deficiency) is the primary ruleout for abnormal bleeding in young male dogs and cats.
- Feline factor XII deficiency does not cause a clinical bleeding diathesis and is typically identified in the course of preoperative work-up for an acquired disease process.
- Aspirin's anticoagulant properties are due to irreversible acetylation of platelet cyclooxygenase (COX)-1, lasting for the lifespan of the platelet. COX-2–nhibiting NSAIDs (e.g., carprofen, etodolac, ketoprofen) also have some inhibitory effect on COX-1, but the effect does not persist after drug withdrawal.

PREVENTION

- Factor-deficient dogs and cats should never be used for breeding.
- Familial testing is indicated to identify asymptomatic carriers before they are bred.

CLIENT EDUCATION

Definitive diagnosis aids in determining prognosis, selecting appropriate transfusion therapy, and genetic counseling

SUGGESTED READING

Brooks MB: A review of canine inherited bleeding disorders: Biochemical and molecular strategies for disease characterization and carrier detection. *J Hered* 90:112, 1999.

AUTHOR: **MARJORY B. BROOKS**
EDITOR: **SUSAN M. COTLER**

Hemoptysis

BASIC INFORMATION

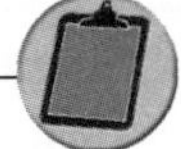

DEFINITION

Expectoration or coughing up of blood or blood-stained sputum from the respiratory tract

EPIDEMIOLO\GY

SPECIES, AGE, SEX

- Dependent on underlying cause
- Young pure-breed animals: coagulopathies
- Young to middle-aged animals: infectious diseases, trauma
- Older animals: neoplasia

GENETICS AND BREED PREDISPOSITIONS: von Willebrand disease (many canine breeds; cats: Himalayan), hemophilia (dogs: many breeds; cats: British shorthair, Siamese).

RISK FACTORS

- Coagulopathies:
  - Immune-mediated disease: young to middle-aged, small to medium female dogs
  - Rickettsial disease: dogs living in or traveling to endemic areas
  - Thrombasthenia: otter hounds
  - Thrombopathia: basset hounds
  - von Willebrand disease: Doberman pinschers, Airedales, German shepherds, Scottish terriers, Chesapeake Bay retrievers, and many other breeds; cats
  - Hemophilia A: German shepherds and many other breeds; cats
  - Hemophilia B: cairn terriers, coonhounds, St. Bernards, and other breeds; cats
- Pulmonary thromboembolism:
  - Neoplasia
  - Hyperadrenocorticism
  - Cardiac disease
  - Immune-mediated hemolytic anemia

CONTAGION AND ZOONOSIS: Systemic fungal infections (risk of common-source infection).

CLINICAL PRESENTATION

HISTORY, CHIEF COMPLAINT (SOME OR ALL MAY BE PRESENT)

- Coughing up of blood: usually foamy consistency
- Hematemesis: from swallowing blood from the respiratory tract
- With coagulopathy: hematochezia, melena, hematuria, or hemorrhage from other areas of the body
- With pulmonary disease: coughing, exercise intolerance, dyspnea, syncope

PHYSICAL EXAM FINDINGS

- Melena: from swallowing blood
- Nasal hemorrhage
- With coagulopathy: possibly petechiae, ecchymoses, hematomas, hematochezia, melena, hematuria, retinal hemorrhages

ETIOLOGY AND PATHOPHYSIOLOGY

- Coagulopathy:
  - Thrombocytopenia:
    - Immune-mediated disease: idiopathic disease, systemic lupus erythematosus, drug reaction
    - Rickettsial disease: ehrlichiosis, Rocky Mountain spotted fever
    - Bone marrow disease: neoplasia, aplastic anemia, infectious (fungal, rickettsial, or viral)
    - Disseminated intravascular coagulation (DIC)
  - Thrombopathia:
    - Congenital: von Willebrand disease, thrombasthenia, thrombopathia
    - Acquired: nonsteroidal anti-inflammatory drugs; hyperglobulinemia (*Ehrlichia,* multiple myeloma); uremia; DIC
  - Coagulation factor defect:
    - Congenital: hemophilia A (factor VIIIc deficiency) and hemophilia B (factor IX deficiency)
    - Acquired: anticoagulant rodenticide (warfarin) intoxication, hepatobiliary disease, DIC
- Pulmonary disease:
  - Pulmonary hypertension
  - Pulmonary thromboembolism
  - Trauma
  - Bronchiectasis
  - Infection: fungal (blastomycosis, histoplasmosis, coccidioidomycosis), bacterial, or parasitic (*Paragonimus kellicotti*, *Capillaria aerophila*, *Aelurostrongylus abstrusus*)
  - Neoplasia: primary or secondary
  - Lung lobe torsion
- Cardiovascular disease:
  - Heartworm
  - Cardiogenic pulmonary edema
  - Arteriovenous fistula

DIAGNOSIS

DIFFERENTIAL DIAGNOSIS

See Etiology and Pathophysiology above

INITIAL DATABASE

- Complete blood count:
  - Anemia: if enough hemorrhage has occurred
  - Thrombocytopenia
  - Neutrophilia: stress; infection; neoplasia
  - Pancytopenia: bone marrow disease
- Urinalysis:
  - Usually normal
  - Hematuria with coagulopathy
  - Avoid sampling by cystocentesis until coagulation status is known
- Serum biochemistry profile:
  - Hypoproteinemia: if enough hemorrhage has occurred
  - High blood urea nitrogen with normal creatinine: possible, owing to gastrointestinal blood
  - Hyperglobulinemia: ehrlichiosis, multiple myeloma
  - High alanine aminotransferase, aspartate aminotransferase, and total bilirubin: severe hepatic disease with coagulopathy possible

ADVANCED OR CONFIRMATORY TESTING

- Other laboratory tests:
  - Coagulation profile: prolonged times with coagulation factor defects; normal with thrombocytopenia and thrombopathia
  - Platelet function testing (e.g., bleeding time, von Willebrand factor analysis): for suspected coagulopathy despite normal platelet count and coagulation profile
  - *Ehrlichia* and Rocky Mountain spotted fever titers/polymerase chain reaction
  - Blood gas analysis (pulmonary disease)
- Diagnostic imaging:
  - Thoracic radiographs-pulmonary/cardiac disease, thoracic trauma, metastatic disease
  - Computed tomography scan: more sensitive than radiographs for some diseases, but requires general anesthesia
  - Echocardiography
- Other diagnostic procedures:
  - Bronchoscopy: examine lower airways, remove foreign bodies, bronchoalveolar lavage
  - Cytologic and histopathologic examination and bacterial and fungal culture and sensitivity testing: lung tissue sample
  - Fine-needle aspirate/lung biopsy: pulmonary masses
  - Scintigraphy: ventilation-perfusion scan

TREATMENT

THERAPEUTIC GOAL(S)

- Stop the hemorrhage
- Treat primary cause

ACUTE GENERAL TREATMENT

- Establish a patent airway
- Oxygen supplementation
- Minimize activity or stimuli that precipitate hemorrhage episodes
- Whole blood or packed red blood cell transfusion: may be needed with severe anemia

SPECIFIC TREATMENT

- Coagulopathy (see Transfusion Reactions, p 1098):
  - von Willebrand disease: plasma or cryoprecipitate for acute bleeding
  - Hemophilia A: plasma or cryoprecipitate for acute bleeding; no long-term treatment
  - Hemophilia B: plasma for acute bleeding; no long-term treatment
  - Anticoagulant rodenticide intoxication: plasma for acute bleeding
  - Liver disease and DIC: treat and support the underlying cause; plasma may be beneficial
  - Discontinue all nonsteroidal anti-inflammatory drugs
- Pulmonary disease:
  - Pulmonary hypertension: treat underlying etiology
  - Pulmonary thromboembolism: treat underlying etiology
  - Infection: treat specific infectious etiology
  - Neoplasia: surgery
  - Lung lobe torsion: surgery
- Cardiovascular disease:
  - Heartworm: specific therapy
  - Cardiogenic pulmonary edema: diuretics, venodilators, oxygen supplementation
  - Arteriovenous fistula: surgery

POSSIBLE COMPLICATIONS

- Anemia
- Collapse state
- Respiratory failure

RECOMMENDED MONITORING

- Hematocrit
- Platelet count with thrombocytopenia
- Coagulation profile with coagulation factor defects
- Blood pressure with hypertension
- Monitor clinical signs

PROGNOSIS AND OUTCOME

Dependent on cause

PEARLS & CONSIDERATIONS

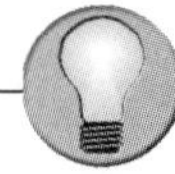

COMMENTS

- Hemoptysis not a diagnosis but a clinical sign
- Consider systemic diseases and cardiovascular diseases, as well as primary pulmonary conditions

CLIENT EDUCATION

Monitor for recurrence of presenting signs (coughing up of blood, presence of blood-stained sputum)

RECOMMENDED READING

Gieger T: Bleeding disorders: Epistaxis and hemoptysis. In Ettinger SJ, Feldman EC (eds): *Textbook of Veterinary Internal Medicine*, ed 6. Philadelphia, WB Saunders, 2006, pp 225–231.

AUTHOR: **REMO LOBETTI**
EDITOR: **ETIENNE CÔTÉ**

Hemorrhage

BASIC INFORMATION

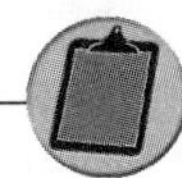

DEFINITION

- The loss of blood from the vascular space into surrounding tissues or from body surfaces
- Clinical signs of hemorrhage result from one of two general mechanisms:
  - Blood loss from damaged or diseased blood vessels
  - Bleeding diatheses: defects causing failure of normal hemostatic processes

SYNONYM(S)

Bleeding

EPIDEMIOLOGY

SPECIES, AGE, SEX: Dogs and cats of all breeds and either sex may be affected, with specific predilections depending on underlying cause. Blood vessel defects are generally acquired disorders, whereas bleeding diatheses may be hereditary traits (e.g., Von Willebrand disease) or acquired disorders (e.g., coagulopathy of rodenticide poisoning).

GENETICS AND BREED PREDISPOSITION: See Hemophilias and Other Hereditary Coagulation Factor Deficiencies, p 482; Platelet Dysfunction, p 856; von Willebrand Disease, p 1160.

RISK FACTORS: See Hemophilias and Other Hereditary Coagulation Factor Deficiencies, p 482; Platelet Dysfunction, p 856; von Willebrand Disease, p 1160.

ASSOCIATED CONDITIONS AND DISORDERS

- Blood vessel defects typically arise from:
  - Traumatic or surgical injuries
  - Inflammatory or neoplastic conditions causing vessel erosion and infiltration
- Bleeding diatheses are classified as:
  - Failure of platelet plug formation (primary hemostatic defects)
  - Failure of fibrin clot formation (secondary hemostatic defects = coagulopathies)
- Disease conditions such as hypertension, anemia, and hyperviscosity alter the normal flow properties of blood (hemorrheology) and are associated with hemorrhage from retinal vessels

CLINICAL PRESENTATION

DISEASE FORMS/SUBTYPES: Subtype classification based on:

- Duration: acute versus chronic hemorrhage
- Location: focal or regional versus multiple anatomic sites
- Tissue or vessel involvement: capillary bleeding versus hemorrhage into joint space, body cavities
  - Primary hemostatic defects (failure of platelet plug formation [e.g., from thrombocytopenia or platelet dysfunction] cause signs of hemorrhage involving capillaries and small vessels [arterioles, venules], clinically evident as petechiae, ecchymoses, bleeding from mucosal surfaces, and nonspecific bleeding from surgical and traumatic wounds)
  - Secondary hemostatic defects (coagulopathies; failure of fibrin clot formation [e.g., from coagulation factor deficiency]) generally cause spontaneous hemorrhage into body cavities or potential spaces (i.e., pleural space, intramuscular tissue planes), resulting in hemothorax, hemoabdomen, hematoma formation, and nonspecific bleeding from surgical and traumatic wounds

HISTORY, CHIEF COMPLAINT: Depends on underlying cause. Frank hemorrhage, hematoma formation, and petechiae are obvious signs that may prompt owners to seek veterinary care. Additional signs include pallor and collapse due to acute hemorrhagic shock, or gradual onset of weakness due to chronic blood loss anemia.

PHYSICAL EXAM FINDINGS

- Physical exam alone may differentiate vessel defects from systemic bleeding diatheses:
  - Frank hemorrhage due to traumatic or surgical blood vessel injury, or vessel infiltration due to solid tissue tumors or inflammatory mass lesions, may be obvious on physical exam or via ancillary diagnostics (endoscopy, radiography).
  - Petechiae evident on cutaneous or mucosal surfaces or funduscopic exam indicate primary hemostatic defect.
  - Retinal hemorrhage and alterations of the normal retinal vasculature may result from abnormal blood flow (hemorrheologic defects, such as systemic hypertension, hyperviscosity, and anemia).
- Other signs are nonspecific:
  - Epistaxis, hematuria, melena, hematemesis.
  - Hemothorax, hemoabdomen.
- Hemorrhage from multiple anatomic sites and/or recurrent episodes are suggestive of a bleeding diathesis rather than blood vessel defects.

ETIOLOGY AND PATHOPHYSIOLOGY

- Blood vessel defects: physical disruption, as described in Physical Exam Findings above
- Bleeding diatheses:
  - Acquired primary hemostatic defects:
    - Thrombocytopenia is the most common bleeding diathesis.
    - Platelet dysfunction.
  - Hereditary primary hemostatic defects:
    - Platelet dysfunction/thrombopathia.
    - von Willebrand disease.
  - Acquired coagulopathies (secondary hemostatic defects):
    - Vitamin K deficiencies (anticoagulant rodenticide intoxication, biliary obstruction, chronic oral antibiotic administration, coumadin overdose, neonatal).
    - Hepatic synthetic failure (hepatic necrosis, atrophy, portosystemic shunts).
    - Consumptive coagulopathy (disseminated intravascular coagulation [DIC]).
    - Drug toxicities, envenomation, complication of heparin, hetastarch, dextran, fibrinolytic drug therapy.
  - Hereditary coagulopathies (secondary hemostatic defects):
    - Hemophilia.
    - Autosomal factor deficiencies.

DIAGNOSIS

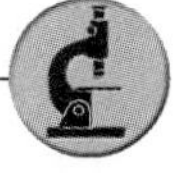

DIFFERENTIAL DIAGNOSIS

Blood vessel defect versus bleeding diathesis:

- Initial physical exam and imaging studies may define the site and cause of vessel defects.
- If a vessel defect cannot be defined on initial exam, blood pressure measurement and screening tests to rule out bleeding diatheses must be performed *before* performing invasive procedures.

INITIAL DATABASE

- Thorough physical exam to define nature and location of hemorrhage
- Baseline hematocrit and plasma protein
- Platelet count
- Blood pressure measurement:
  - Normal in calm setting, awake and resting patient, repeatable measures using Doppler: systolic <180 mmHg (dog, cat).
  - Hypertension and other cause(s) of hemorrhage may coexist.

- Coagulation screening tests: if evidence points to bleeding diathesis:
  - Activated clotting time (ACT):
    - Expected time to fibrin clot end-point ≤120 seconds (dogs and cats).
    - Deficiencies of the intrinsic and common pathway factors cause prolongation of the ACT.
    - Normal values should be established for each test method.
  - Activated partial thromboplastin time (aPTT):
    - The aPTT, like ACT, is sensitive to deficiencies of intrinsic and common pathway factors; however, aPTT is generally a more specific and reproducible test than the ACT.
    - Long aPTT is seen in hereditary coagulopathies, such as hemophilia, and in combined factor deficiencies such as rodenticide intoxication and DIC.
    - Prolongation of aPTT, to a target value of 1.5 to 2 times baseline, is used for adjusting unfractionated heparin dosage.
    - Hemorrhage caused by blood vessel defects or primary hemostatic defects (platelet abnormalities) should not produce abnormal aPTT results.
  - Prothrombin time (PT):
    - Test is sensitive to deficiencies of extrinsic and common pathway factors.
    - Specific prolongation of PT is an indication of factor VII deficiency. Because factor VII is vitamin K-dependent with short plasma half-life (3 to 6 hours), prolongation of PT develops in conditions causing vitamin K deficiency. Prolonged or severe vitamin K deficiency (e.g., anticoagulant rodenticide, severe hepatopathy) impairs activation of all vitamin K–dependent factors and results in prolongation of aPTT (and ACT), in addition to PT.
    - The anticoagulant effect of coumadin and its dosage adjustments are based on prolongation of PT and its standardized derivative, the international normalized ratio (INR).
    - PIVKA (proteins induced by vitamin K absence or antagonism) testing performed using the Thrombotest assay provides equivalent information as the PT.
    - Hemorrhage caused by blood vessel defects or primary hemostatic defects (platelet abnormalities) should not produce abnormal PT results.
  - Thrombin clotting time (TCT) and fibrinogen:
    - Detect a lack of clottable fibrinogen.
    - Long TCT and low fibrinogen develop in patients with severe hepatic insufficiency, causing synthetic failure or hemorrhagic DIC causing depletion of fibrinogen.
    - Vitamin K deficiency does not prolong TCT or decrease fibrinogen values.
    - Hemorrhage caused by blood vessel defects or primary hemostatic defects (platelet abnormalities) should not produce abnormal TCT or fibrinogen results.
- Coagulopathies cause prolongation of one or more coagulation screening tests:
  - The pattern of abnormalities depends on which factor or groups of factors are deficient (Fig. I-87; see Hemophilias and Other Hereditary Coagulation Factor Deficiencies, p 482).
  - Expected coagulation screening test results for common coagulopathies:
    - Vitamin K deficiencies (see Etiology and Pathophysiology above) impair activation of factors II, VII, IX, and X. Coagulation panel reveals prolongation of ACT, aPTT, and PT (but fibrinogen and TCT are normal). Anticoagulant rodenticide toxicity causes severe factor deficiencies, with resultant marked prolongation of clotting times in patients with active hemorrhage.
    - Severe hepatic synthetic failure causes deficiencies of all factors and fibrinogen. ACT, aPTT, PT, TCT are long and fibrinogen is low.
    - Hemorrhagic DIC typically results in depletion of all factors and fibrinogen. Mild to severe prolongation of clotting times and low fibrinogen accompany hemorrhagic DIC. In contrast, high fibrinogen may accompany thrombotic DIC and other hypercoagulable syndromes.
    - Hemorrhage due to anticoagulant drug overdose or envenomation causes factor inhibition or fibrinogen depletion. All coagulation screening tests will detect severe drug overdose; however aPTT and PT are differentially sensitive to unfractionated heparin and coumadin levels, respectively.

ADVANCED OR CONFIRMATORY TESTING

Based on results of initial database:

- Thrombocytopenia work-up may include repeat evaluation, including fresh blood smears, to rule out collection/laboratory artifact; bone marrow, spleen, and lymph node aspiration and cytologic evaluation; serologic evaluation to detect evidence of pathogens; platelet-associated antibody testing.
- Evaluation for platelet dysfunction (see Platelet Dysfunction, p 856).
- Ancillary diagnostics to differentiate coagulopathies include specific coagulation factor analyses, determinations of antithrombin activity and fibrin breakdown products, and drug detection (e.g., heparin or coumadin levels).

THERAPEUTIC GOAL(S)

- Control active bleeding
- Collect pretreatment samples to perform screening and confirmatory tests
- Stabilize patient with one or more of the following: local wound care, supportive medical therapy, transfusion therapy

ACUTE GENERAL TREATMENT

- Hemorrhagic/hypovolemic shock:
  - Volume replacement: intravenous fluid therapy
  - Red cell replacement (see Transfusion Reactions, p 1098)
- Blood vessel injuries:
  - Control bleeding after visualization of the damaged vessels (physical examination, endoscopic examination, ultrasound examination, or surgical exploration)
- Bleeding diatheses:
  - Identify and correct the underlying cause of acquired bleeding diatheses
  - Transfusion if needed to correct hereditary defects or pending response to medical management

CHRONIC TREATMENT

Depends on underlying cause of hemorrhage

DRUG INTERACTIONS

Avoid drugs with anticoagulant or antiplatelet effects:

- Nonsteroidal anti-inflammatory drugs
- Sulfonamides
- Heparin, coumadin
- Plasma expanders
- Estrogens
- Cytotoxic drugs

POSSIBLE COMPLICATIONS

- Uncontrolled hemorrhage and hemorrhagic shock are potentially fatal conditions.
- Chronic hemorrhage may result in iron deficiency anemia, requiring iron supplementation for appropriate bone marrow response.

RECOMMENDED MONITORING

Resolution of hemorrhage is demonstrated by:

- Cessation of active bleeding
- Fading of petechiae, absence of development of new lesions
- Stabilization and normalization of hematocrit/plasma protein
- Correction of low platelet count and/or long clotting times

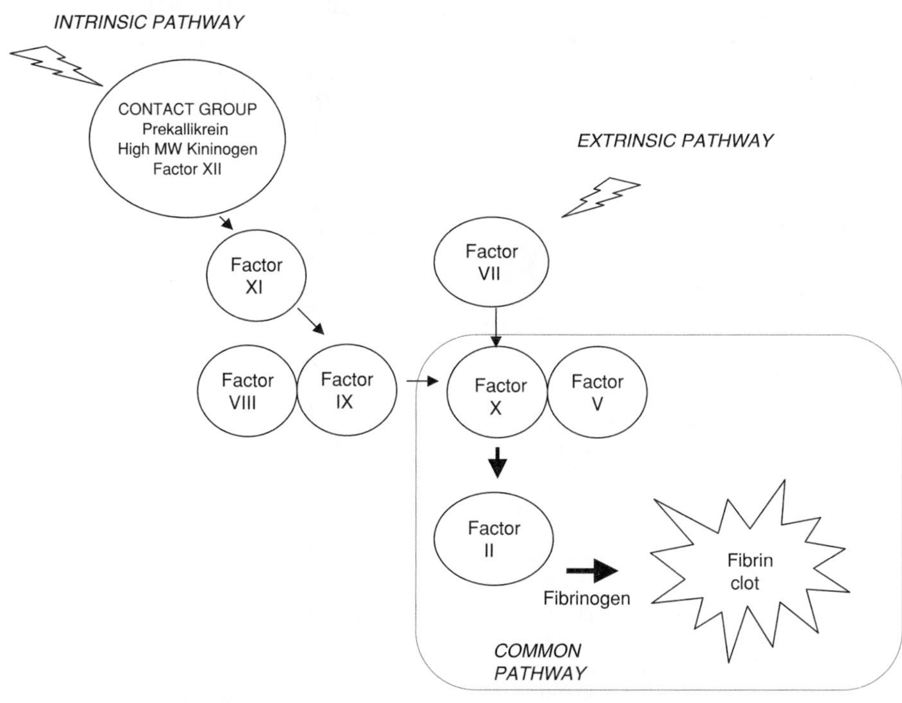

FIGURE I-87 The coagulation cascade.

PROGNOSIS AND OUTCOME

Depends on:
- Initial stabilization and correction of hemorrhagic shock
- Ability to identify and correct vessel defect or cause of acquired bleeding diatheses
- Ability to diagnose and manage hereditary bleeding diatheses

PEARLS & CONSIDERATIONS

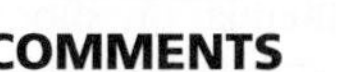

COMMENTS

- Blood vessel injury or infiltration is by far the most common cause of hemorrhage.
- Screening for common bleeding diatheses by performing platelet count and ACT (or point-of-care aPTT and PT) is indicated early in the diagnostic workup of patients with hemorrhage.
- Anticoagulant rodenticide intoxication is a common acquired coagulopathy. Vitamin K therapy (vitamin K_1, 2 mg/kg/day PO or SQ) should be initiated pending results of coagulation screening, regardless of confirmed history of product ingestion. Patients with severe hemorrhage at initial presentation should receive plasma transfusion in addition to vitamin K.
  - Most commercial rodenticides are long-acting. Vitamin K_1 therapy should be continued for 4 to 6 weeks to prevent rebleeding after an initial hemorrhagic event. The dose can be tapered by half at 2-week intervals.
- Results of coagulation tests (PT, aPTT) that are below the normal range do not indicate hypercoagulability.

SUGGESTED READING

Tseng LW, Hughes D, Giger U: Evaluation of a point-of-care coagulation analyzer for measurement of prothrombin time, activated partial thromboplastin time, and activated clotting time in dogs. *Am J Vet Res* 62:1455–1460, 2001.

Brooks M: Coagulation and thrombosis. In Ettinger SJ, Feldman EC (eds): *Textbook of Veterinary Internal Medicine*, ed 5. Philadelphia, WB Saunders, 2000, pp 1829–1841.

AUTHOR: **MARJORY B. BROOKS**
EDITOR: **SUSAN M. COTLER**

Hemorrhagic Gastroenteritis

BASIC INFORMATION

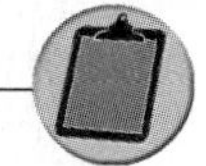

DEFINITION

Acute loss of mucosal integrity leading to hematemesis and hemorrhagic diarrhea with rapid development of hypovolemia and shock

SYNONYM(S)

Acute hemorrhagic enteritis
Acute hemorrhagic enteropathy
Acute intestinal hemorrhagic syndrome
HGE

EPIDEMIOLOGY

SPECIES, AGE, SEX: Canine, usually young (mean of 5 years).

GENETICS AND BREED PREDISPOSITION: Hemorrhagic gastroenteritis (HGE) can occur in any breed; most common in toy and small-breed dogs (miniature schnauzer, poodles).

RISK FACTORS: None known; most dogs are otherwise healthy.

CONTAGION AND ZOONOSIS: Possible association with *Clostridium* spp. or *Escherichia coli* bacteria.

GEOGRAPHY AND SEASONALITY: More prevalent in urban dogs.

CLINICAL PRESENTATION

HISTORY, CHIEF COMPLAINT
- Anorexia
- Lethargy
- Acute onset of vomiting followed by diarrhea (diarrhea may start as hemorrhagic and strawberry jam-like, or it may progress from watery, blood-free stool to hemorrhagic)

PHYSICAL EXAM FINDINGS
- Vital parameters: Pulse rate and quality, hydration, mucous membrane color,

and capillary refill time (CRT) are all normal early in disease. With progression, signs of hypovolemic shock develop, including tachycardia, pallor, prolonged CRT, and poor pulse quality.
- Abdominal palpation: mild discomfort, fluid-filled bowel loops, colon may be distended, doughy, and uncomfortable.
- Rectal examination: fresh dark blood or strawberry jam-like feces.

ETIOLOGY AND PATHOPHYSIOLOGY

- Cause unknown, but an anaphylactic reaction to unidentified antigens has been implicated.
- *Clostridium perfringens* and *E. coli* infections have been associated, likely not causative
- Peracute, massive increase in intestinal permeability results in extravasation of fluid, proteins, and red blood cells into intestinal wall and lumen.
- Hypovolemia and splenic contraction contribute to hemoconcentration, but gastrointestinal loss of proteins exceeds loss of blood cells. Therefore polycythemia is not matched with concurrent increase in serum total protein.
- If untreated, disease can progress to hypovolemic shock and death.

DIAGNOSIS

DIFFERENTIAL DIAGNOSIS

For clinical presentation:
- Infectious: viral (parvovirus) or bacterial (*Salmonella*, *Campylobacter enteritidis*)
- Dietary indiscretion, foreign body, toxicity
- Hypoadrenocorticism
- Ischemic injury: intestinal volvulus, intussusception, other causes of hypovolemic or endotoxic shock
- Pancreatitis
- Neoplasia
- Coagulopathy

INITIAL DATABASE

- Elevated hematocrit (50–80%) with normal to low total protein is hallmark finding
- Complete blood count: most commonly normal or stress leukogram but a neutrophilia with a left shift or degenerative left shift may be present; platelet count may be decreased
- Serum biochemistry profile: may show increased blood urea nitrogen, alanine aminotransferase, hypokalemia, and normal to mildly decreased albumin and total protein levels
- Urinalysis: unremarkable
- Coagulation profile: usually normal early on; may show abnormalities if condition progresses to disseminated intravascular coagulation (DIC)
- Fecal smear and microscopic exam: increased numbers of red cells, organisms consistent with clostridial spores ("safety pins") may be present; negative for parasites
- Parvovirus enzyme-linked immunosorbent assay: negative
- Abdominal radiographs: signs of ileus

TREATMENT

THERAPEUTIC GOAL(S)

- Replace and maintain intravascular volume
- Supportive care

ACUTE GENERAL TREATMENT

- Nothing by mouth (NPO) for 12 to 48 hours.
- Initiate volume resuscitation with IV fluid therapy:
  - Balanced replacement electrolyte solution (crystalloids [e.g., Normosol-R, lactated Ringer's, Plasmalyte, 0.9% NaCl]). If hypovolemic shock is present, calculate a shock dose of crystalloids (90 ml/kg), bolus one fourth to one third of the shock dose over 20 to 30 minutes, then reassess and repeat as necessary.
  - Colloids (e.g., Hetastarch or Dextran 70; 10–20 ml/kg/day IV, titrated based on response) may be used for marked hypoproteinemia or shock unresponsive to crystalloid infusion.
  - Continue fluids at a rate necessary to replace dehydration deficits and ongoing losses, to meet maintenance requirements and maintain vascular volume.
- Antibiotics (e.g., ampicillin, 22 mg/kg IV q 8h): recommended given the potential for bacterial translocation across the intestinal epithelium and the possible relation with *Clostridium* sp. For severely affected patients, an aminoglycoside (e.g., amikacin 15 mg/kg IV q24 h) can be added only once volume resuscitation and rehydration are completed. Enrofloxacin (5–10 mg/kg IM or slow IV q 24h) is an alternative choice for coverage of gram-negative infections.
- Antiemetics and prokinetics are generally not needed but can be used for persistent vomiting.
- Small amounts of a bland, low-fat, low-fiber food are offered once vomiting has ceased and should be continued for several days.

DRUG INTERACTIONS

To reduce risk of nephrotoxicity, aminoglycosides should be used with care and only after hypovolemia and dehydration have been corrected.

POSSIBLE COMPLICATIONS

- Condition may progress to hypovolemic shock, DIC, and death if not treated promptly and aggressively.
- Neurologic signs occur from shock and hemoconcentration with "sludging" of blood in capillaries.
- Cardiac arrhythmias can occur secondary to shock, hypoxemia, and reperfusion injury.

RECOMMENDED MONITORING

- Monitor vital parameters (temperature, heart rate, mucous membranes, CRT, pulse quality, blood pressure) and ongoing fluid losses every 2 to 4 hours.
- Hematocrit and total solids every 4 to 6 hours.
- If clinical signs persist >24 hours, electrolyte disturbances may become important.

PROGNOSIS AND OUTCOME

- Recovery is usually rapid and complete over 1 to 2 days.
- Condition can progress quickly to shock and death without aggressive fluid therapy.
- A total of 10% of affected dogs may die despite therapy.

PEARLS & CONSIDERATIONS

COMMENTS

- The most common term for the disease, hemorrhagic gastroenteritis, incorrectly implies presence of gastrointestinal inflammation.
- Of all the differentials for acute gastroenteritis, HGE is classically identified by the markedly elevated hematocrit and normal to slightly low total protein.
- With aggressive intravenous fluid therapy, outcome for HGE is favorable

CLIENT EDUCATION

A total of 10–15% of dogs will have repeated episodes of HGE.

SUGGESTED READING

Strombeck DR, Guilford WG: Acute hemorrhagic enteropathy (hemorrhagic gastroenteritis: HGE). In Guilford WG, et al (eds): *Strombeck's Small Animal Gastroenterology*. Philadelphia, WB Saunders, 1996, pp 433–435.

AUTHOR: **AMIE KOENIG**
EDITOR: **DEBRA L. ZORAN**

Hepatic Encephalopathy

BASIC INFORMATION

DEFINITION

A reversible metabolic central nervous system (CNS) disturbance secondary to hepatic disease

EPIDEMIOLOGY

SPECIES, AGE, SEX

- Dogs and cats
- Congenital hepatic vascular disease: young
- Acquired hepatic disease: middle-aged to older

GENETICS AND BREED PREDISPOSITIONS

- Hepatic vascular disease: several breed predispositions (see Portosystemic Shunts, p 880)
- Acquired liver disease: copper storage diseases (Bedlington terrier, West Highland white terrier, Labrador, dalmatian; see Hepatitis [Chronic, Idiopathic] of Dogs, p 503; Hepatitis [Chronic] of Doberman Pinscher Dogs, p 500; Hepatitis [Chronic] of Cocker Spaniel Dogs, p 499)

RISK FACTORS

- Acute hepatic disease
- Hepatotoxic drugs and toxins
- Congenital hepatic vascular disease:
  - Single portosystemic vascular anomalies
  - Primary hypoplasia of the portal veins (microvascular dysplasia)
  - Hepatic arteriovenous fistula
- Multiple acquired portosystemic shunts secondary to portal hypertension from chronic hepatic disease

CLINICAL PRESENTATION

HISTORY, CHIEF COMPLAINT

Historic signs of liver disease typically are episodic, involving three systems:

- Neurologic: diffuse cerebral disturbance: lethargy, poor appetite, aimless wandering, head pressing, disorientation, seizures, blindness, depression, stupor, coma, behavioral changes. Poor anesthesia tolerance/ prolonged recovery.
- Gastrointestinal (GI): vomiting, diarrhea, poor weight gain, ptyalism (cats).
- Urinary: polyuria and polydipsia, stranguria, pollakiuria, dysuria, and/or hematuria associated with ammonia biurate uroliths.
- GI and/or urinary signs may be part of the history in patients with hepatic encephalopathy.

PHYSICAL EXAMINATION

- Signs of diffuse cerebral disease but may be subclinical at the time of examination due to the episodic nature of hepatic encephalopathy.
- Variable neurologic signs, but often multifocal or difficult to localize. Deficits are symmetric because systemic effects on CNS are diffuse.
  - Circling, when present, is broad (wide radius, may change directions), and is associated with disorientation and propulsive, aimless pacing, in contrast to vestibular circling (small radius, same direction, mentation often normal).
  - Congenital vascular disease patients may have stunted growth.
  - Cats with congenital portosystemic shunts often have copper-colored irises.
- Acquired hepatic disease: ascites, icterus.
- Acute hepatic failure: initial neuroexcitatory behavior (restlessness, agitation, seizure) progressing to more neuroinhibitory states (depression, coma).
- Hepatic arteriovenous fistula: a continuous murmur may be ausculted on the cranioventral abdomen.

ETIOLOGY AND PATHOPHYSIOLOGY

Complex multifactorial etiology:

- Associated with the accumulation of neurologic toxins most likely of gut origin that escape hepatic detoxification due to shunting of blood away from the portal vasculature into the systemic vasculature.
- GI toxins derived primarily from bacterial metabolism of proteinaceous waste.
  - Ammonia generation in the colon
  - Endogenous benzodiazepine-like substances
- Alterations in inhibitory (γ-aminobutyric acid) and excitatory (glutamate) neurotransmitter balance playing a secondary role.
- Low-grade cerebral edema due to astrocyte detoxification of ammonia to glutamine may also play a role in the development of chronic hepatic encephalopathy associated with portosystemic shunting.
- Pathophysiology of encephalopathy associated with acute hepatic failure is distinct from chronic hepatic encephalopathy, and is complicated by the development of overt intracranial hypertension with cerebral edema secondary to alterations in the blood-brain barrier, disturbances in cerebral blood flow, and the release of neurotoxic substances by the necrotic liver, and frequently is complicated by neuroglycopenia.

DIAGNOSIS

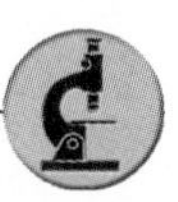

DIFFERENTIAL DIAGNOSIS

- Neurologic signs: Hypoglycemia, lead toxicity, congenital CNS malformation such as hydrocephalus or storage disease, infectious encephalitis/meningitis (e.g., feline infectious peritonitis infection, toxoplasmosis, neosporosis, canine distemper encephalitis), granulomatous meningoencephalitis, CNS neoplasia, thiamine deficiency (cats).
- Chronic GI or urinary signs may mimic primary GI disease or suggest primary genitourinary or endocrine disorders.

INITIAL DATABASE

- Complete blood count: microcytosis, poikilocytosis (cats)
- Serum biochemistry profile:
  - Hepatic vascular disease: may be normal or show mild hypoalbuminemia, low blood urea nitrogen, mild increases in serum alanine aminotransferase and serum alkaline phosphatase (ALP) (some elevation of ALP in young animals may be normal bone isoenzyme), hypocholesterolemia, hypoglycemia (especially in young toy breeds)
  - Acquired hepatic disease: hypoalbuminemia, moderate to severe increases in all serum hepatic enzyme activities, ± hyperbilirubinemia, hypercholesterolemia or hypocholesterolemia, hypoglycemia (with acute hepatic failure)
- Urinalysis: isosthenuria common; ammonia biurate crystalluria, hematuria, pyuria, bacturia possible

ANCILLARY OR CONFIRMATORY TESTING

CLINICAL PATHOLOGY

- Total serum bile acids: sensitive for the detection of congenital or acquired portosystemic shunting (2-hour postprandial sample more sensitive)
- Blood ammonia: specific indicator of hepatic encephalopathy but can be normal even during overt hepatic encephalopathy. Ammonia tolerance test more sensitive to detect hepatic encephalopathy but may induce severe neurologic signs
- Urinary bile acids: less sensitive than serum bile acids in the dog (but may be more convenient)
- Abdominal effusion: pure or modified transudate

IMAGING

- Abdominal ultrasound:

- Portosystemic vascular anomaly: identification of a vascular communication between the intrahepatic or extrahepatic portal circulation and the systemic vasculature, (see Portosystemic Shunts, p 880), microhepatica, renomegaly, urolithiasis
- Primary hypoplasia of the portal veins (see Microvascular Dysplasia, Hepatic, p 705): ± microhepatica, ± abdominal effusion, may be unremarkable
- Hepatoarteriovenous fistula: identification of fistula, ± abdominal effusion
- Chronic hepatitis/hepatopathies, cirrhotic/fibrosing liver disease: microhepatica, possible nodular liver with cirrhosis, abdominal effusion; visualization of multiple portosystemic shunts may be difficult

- Rectal technetium scans (see Enema: Scintigraphic [Radionuclide], p 1237):
  - Abnormal with single or multiple portosystemic shunts and normal with primary hypoplasia of the portal veins without portal hypertension (microvascular dysplasia)

HISTOPATHOLOGY

- Hepatic histopathology:
  - Same pattern of changes (arteriolar proliferation, hepatic atrophy, attenuation of portal vasculature, lobular collapse) seen with all forms of hepatic vascular disease
  - Chronic hepatic disease often shows variable inflammation and fibrosis ± the presence of regenerative nodules
  - Acute hepatic disease: variable but most often accompanied by hepatic necrosis/apoptosis
- Brain histopathology: Alzheimer's type II changes in astrocytes with chronic hepatic encephalopathy, cerebral edema with acute hepatic failure

TREATMENT

THERAPEUTIC GOAL(S)

- Lower levels of circulating neurotoxins by modulating GI protein metabolism
- Maintain optimum nutritional plane
- Control precipitating factors

ACUTE GENERAL TREATMENT

- Nothing per os, if stupor or coma is present.
- Address fluid and electrolyte imbalances, avoid lactated solutions with acute hepatic failure, sodium restrict fluids with ascites, potassium and glucose supplementation as needed, B vitamins (especially thiamine and cobalamin in cats).
- Medications that increase GI protein tolerance.
  - Lactulose: drug of choice. Nonabsorbable disaccharide broken down by colonic bacteria into short-chain fatty acids.Traps soluble NH_3 as NH_4^+, which is nonabsorbable and thus excreted in the feces. Alters bacterial metabolism so that less ammonia is generated.
    - Titrated from an initial dose of 0.5 to 1.0 ml/kg PO q 8-12h to dose that produces 3 to 4 soft stools per day. If stupor or coma is present, may be given rectally in a retention enema (see Enema [Retention, Evacuation], p 1236).
  - Antibiotics:
    - Alter bacterial metabolism, synergistic with lactulose.
    - Metronidazole (7.5 mg/kg PO q 8-12h, low dose to avoid neurotoxicity secondary to decreased hepatic metabolism of the antibiotic); or
    - Neomycin (10-22 mg/kg PO q 12h) (may be difficult to obtain; can be given orally or as a retention enema) or amoxicillin (22 mg/kg PO q 12h).
- Seizures: control seizure activity:
  - Barbiturates (e.g., phenobarbital 6-10 mg/kg slowly IV to effect); the patient should be monitored closely for respiratory depression.
- If patient is seizuring due to hepatic encephalopathy from acute liver injury: Cerebral edema is likely, and the prognosis is grave (seizures often refractory to treatment).
  - Mannitol (0.5 g/kg given IV over 10 to 15 minutes).
  - Infusion of *N*-acetylcysteine (140 mg/kg IV initially followed by 70 mg/kg as needed) may correct disturbances in microcirculation.
  - Corticosteroids of no benefit and may be detrimental.
  - Monitor closely (q 4h) for hypoglycemia, may require infusion of high concentrations of dextrose-containing solutions.
- Control precipitating factors:
  - Oral protein loading: gastrointestinal hemorrhage, high protein meals.
  - Catabolic conditions such as infections, dehydration, azotemia.
  - Alkalosis with hypokalemia: increases renal ammonia production.
  - Synergistic neural inhibition with sedatives, tranquilizers, or anesthetic agents; use these with caution, if at all (e.g., diazepam).
  - Constipation
  - Transfusion with stored blood products containing high ammonia concentrations.

CHRONIC TREATMENT

- Medications to increase GI protein tolerance are first line therapy (see Acute General Treatment above)
- Diet:
  - Adequate calories to avoid catabolism of muscle, which is highly ammongenic and may make control of hepatic encephalopathy difficult.
  - Modulation of protein content: high-quality protein derived preferably from plant and dairy products. Start with diet containing minimum daily protein requirements (cat: 6.5 g/100 kcal; dog: 5.1 g/100 kcal) in combination with medications to increase protein tolerance and decrease protein only if necessary.
  - Increase fiber content.
  - Vitamin supplementation: thiamine in cats (50-100 mg PO daily), vitamin K (if associated coagulopathy) initially parenterally (0.5 mg/kg SQ q 12h) for 5 to 7 days then once weekly.
  - Sodium restriction necessary only with ascites: 0.04-0.05 g/100 kcal.

DRUG INTERACTIONS

- Neuroinhibitory drugs (e.g., sedatives, anesthetics, and tranquilizers) should be used cautiously, as they may potentiate the neuroinhibition of hepatic encephalopathy.
- Avoid drugs that depend heavily on hepatic metabolism and/or excretion, if possible.

RECOMMENDED MONITORING

- Blood ammonia concentration
- Mentation and appetite at home
- Body weight and body condition score
- Serum albumin

PROGNOSIS AND OUTCOME

Depends on nature of underlying liver disease causing encephalopathy:

- Hepatic vascular disease (portosystemic shunt, microvascular dysplasia, arteriovenous fistula): In general, the clinical signs of hepatic encephalopathy due to congenital hepatic vascular disease respond quickly and fully to appropriate drug and dietary intervention. Long-term prognosis depends on whether the congenital intrahepatic or extrahepatic shunt can be fully attenuated or the arteriovenous fistula can be resected (in which case signs of hepatic encephalopathy typically abate) and whether these conditions are complicated by primary hypoplasia of the portal veins (microvascular dysplasia), which ensures the continued shunting of blood from the portal circulation.
- Acquired chronic hepatic disease: Clinical signs of hepatic encephalopathy generally abate with proper intervention, but the long-term prognosis depends on the severity of the underlying hepatic disorder. Generally, patients with signs of severe hepatic encephalopathy due to acquired hepatic diseases have a very poor prognosis, unless the underlying disease can be reversed.

- Acute liver failure: Encephalopathy generally is more refractory to therapy, probably reflecting a more complex underlying cerebral lesion or process. Encephalopathy progressing to coma or stupor (grade 3-4) is considered a grave prognostic sign and is one of the criteria used for determining the need for transplantation in human patients.

PEARLS & CONSIDERATIONS

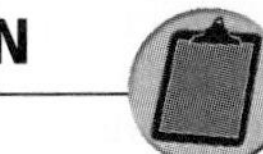

COMMENTS

- Normal blood ammonia concentration does not rule out the presence of hepatic encephalopathy.
- Initial treatment of hepatic encephalopathy involves steps to increase dietary protein tolerance (nonabsorbable disaccharides and antibiotics) in combination with dietary protein modulation but not excessive restriction.
- Be aware of common comorbid conditions that can complicate the control of hepatic encephalopathy such as GI bleeding, dehydration, hypokalemia, azotemia, constipation, and alkalosis.
- Encephalopathy accompanying acute hepatic failure differs from that accompanying congenital vascular disorders or chronic hepatic failure in that it involves the development of overt cerebral edema and an initial neuroexcitatory state that is often refractory to therapeutic intervention. In addition, patients with signs of severe hepatic encephalopathy due to acquired hepatic diseases have a very poor prognosis.
- Propofol is useful for controlling hepatic encephalopathy-induced status epilepticus. Because they are metabolized hepatically, small doses may be used and have a longer duration of action. Maintain an anesthetized state for several hours before tapering and observing for recurrence. Monitor for apnea during use.

CLIENT EDUCATION

Hepatic encephalopathy is an episodic, chronic condition that cannot be cured but can be controlled with strict adherence to dietary modulation and drug therapy.

SUGGESTED READING

Haussinger D, et al: Hepatic encephalopathy in chronic liver disease: A clinical manifestation of astrocyte swelling and low grade cerebral edema. *J Hepatol* 32:1035-1038, 2000.

Maddison JE: Hepatic encephalopathy: Current concepts of pathogenesis. *J Vet Intern Med* 6:341-353, 1992.

AUTHOR: **CYNTHIA R. L. WEBSTER**
EDITOR: **KEITH P. RICHTER**

Hepatic Injury, Acute

BASIC INFORMATION

DEFINITION

Sudden insult to the liver, which if severe enough to compromise at least 70-80% of functional hepatic tissue, results in fulminant hepatic failure

SYNONYM(S)

Acute hepatic failure
Fulminant hepatic failure

EPIDEMIOLOGY

SPECIES, AGE, SEX: Dogs and cats; no age or sex predilection.
RISK FACTORS: Drug administration; free roaming animals with access to potential hepatotoxins (chemicals and pesticides, pond water—"blue-green algae," poisonous mushrooms, cycad palms).
CONTAGION AND ZOONOSIS: Infectious diseases (see Etiology and Pathophysiology below) for dog-to-dog or cat-to-cat transmission; leptospirosis (dog-to-human).
GEOGRAPHY AND SEASONALITY: Cycad palm toxicosis (dogs): southern United States and Hawaii; fungal: Mississippi and Ohio River Valley (dogs: histoplasmosis), southwestern United States (dogs: coccidioidomycosis). Blue-green algae hepatotoxicity (dogs): late summer or early fall.

CLINICAL PRESENTATION

DISEASE FORMS/SUBTYPES
- Unexpected finding of increased liver enzymes/bilirubin detected on routine biochemistries (mild hepatic injury or reactive hepatopathy secondary to systemic disorder)
- Clinical and biochemical evidence of acute hepatic failure (fulminant hepatic failure). Findings reflect general hepatic dysfunction rather than specific underlying cause

HISTORY, CHIEF COMPLAINT
- History of recent drug administration (prescription, over-the-counter, herbals, or dietary supplements *may be implicated*) or exposure to other potential hepatotoxins
- Acute onset of anorexia, lethargy, vomiting, and diarrhea in previously healthy animal
- Other signs: polyuria/polydipsia, hepatic encephalopathy; signs of extrahepatic or multisystemic disease dependent on underlying cause

PHYSICAL EXAM FINDINGS
- Dehydration, icterus/jaundice, excessive bleeding (hematemesis, melena, hemorrhages of skin or mucous membranes), hepatic encephalopathy
- Other findings dependent on specific cause (e.g., fever: consider infectious causes or secondary to acute pancreatitis; signs of abdominal pain: acute pancreatitis, cholangitis, liver abscess, acute swelling, and stretching of liver capsule [nonspecific])

ETIOLOGY AND PATHOPHYSIOLOGY

- Drugs and anesthetics:
  - Hepatic reactions may be dose-related and predictable (e.g., acetaminophen) or idiosyncratic (most drugs). Usually acute but may be chronic (phenobarbital, primidone, lomustine).
  - Acetaminophen (dogs and cats), amiodarone (dogs), azathioprine (dogs), carprofen, and other nonsteroidal anti-inflammatory drugs (NSAIDs) (dogs), clonazepam (cats), danazol (dogs), diazepam (cats), glipizide (cats), griseofulvin (cats), halothane (dogs), itraconazole (dogs and cats), ketoconazole (dogs and cats), lomustine (dogs), nitrofurantoin (dogs), methimazole (cats), methoxyflurane (dogs), mitotane (dogs), oxibendazole (dogs), phenobarbital (dogs), primidone (dogs), potentiated sulfonamides (dogs), stanozolol (cats), tetracycline (dogs and cats), thiacetarsamide (dogs).
  - Idiosyncratic reaction can occur with *any* drug. Diagnosis is presumptive; cannot be proven. Do not rechallenge with suspect drug. Withdrawal of hepatotoxic drug can result in improvement or resolution of hepatic injury (within days to weeks), depending on severity of lesion.
- Biologic substances:
  - Aflatoxin (contaminated dog food).
  - Amanita mushrooms.
  - Blue-green algae.
  - Sago palms.
  - Hornet stings.
  - Pennyroyal oil.
- Chemicals and toxins:
  - Carbon tetrachloride.
  - Dimethylnitrosamine.
  - Metals (e.g., copper, lead, iron, zinc).

- Organochloride pesticides.
- Many others.
- Infectious agents:
  - Viral: infectious canine hepatitis, canine herpesvirus, feline infectious peritonitis, virulent feline calicivirus.
  - Bacterial: leptospirosis, liver abscess, cholangitis/cholangiohepatitis.
  - Fungal: histoplasmosis, coccidioidomycosis, others.
  - Protozoal: *Toxoplasma gondii*, *Babesia* spp., *Cytauxzoon felis*, *Bartonella* spp.
  - Rickettsial: *Ehrlichia* spp., *Rickettsia rickettsiae.*
- Systemic or metabolic disorders:
  - Acute pancreatitis.
  - Extrahepatic infection, septicemia, endotoxemia.
  - Hemolytic anemia.
  - Inflammatory bowel disease.
  - Feline hepatic lipidosis.
- Miscellaneous causes of liver injury:
  - Trauma.
  - Heat stroke.
  - Liver lobe torsion.
  - Shock.
  - Surgical hypotension and hypoxia.

DIAGNOSIS

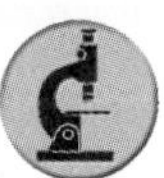

DIFFERENTIAL DIAGNOSIS

- For acute hepatic injury accompanied by jaundice/icterus/hyperbilirubinemia:
  - Prehepatic causes (hemolytic anemia).
  - Posthepatic causes (biliary obstruction).
- Chronic hepatic disease. Recent decompensation of chronic hepatic disease may mimic acute hepatic injury:
  - Determine if subtle signs of chronic illness (weight loss, poor body condition) are present.
  - Findings of ascites, small liver, and hypoalbuminemia suggest chronic rather than acute disease.
  - Chronic liver disease in the final phases of decompensation may not warrant the same aggressive therapeutic approach as acute hepatic failure because the long-term prognosis is poor.

INITIAL DATABASE

- Routine hematologic and biochemical evaluation:
  - Inflammatory complete blood count (infectious diseases, acute pancreatitis, extrahepatic infections with secondary reactive hepatopathy); also for ruling out hemolytic anemia as cause of jaundice.
  - Serum biochemistry profile, urinalysis: increased serum alanine aminotransferase, especially with hepatic necrosis, and alkaline phosphatase.
  - Hyperbilirubinemia/bilirubinuria.
  - Increased serum bile acids.
  - Hypoglycemia (like hyperammonemia and coagulopathy) suggests severe hepatic dysfunction.
  - Hypoalbuminemia suggests chronic rather than acute disease.
  - Azotemia: consider dehydration or concurrent renal damage (leptospirosis, NSAIDs).
  - Other findings depend on underlying systemic disorder.
  - Urinalysis: small degrees of bilirubinuria may be normal in dogs, because dogs can conjugate bilirubin renally. In cats, all bilirubinuria is considered pathologic.
- Imaging:
  - Abdominal radiographs: liver normal or increased in size.
  - Abdominal ultrasound: liver normal or increased in size; variable changes in echogenicity; hypoechoic mass possible (abscess). Evaluate gallbladder and bile ducts to rule out disorders other than acute hepatic injury as a cause of jaundice/icterus, such as posthepatic disorders including extrahepatic biliary tract disease (gallbladder mucocele, cholecystitis, cholelithiasis) or obstruction (distended gallbladder and bile ducts). Evaluate pancreas for acute pancreatitis; other findings dependent on underlying multisystemic or extrahepatic disorder.

ADVANCED OR CONFIRMATORY TESTING

- Liver biopsy:
  - Characterize hepatic lesion histologically; hepatic necrosis most common lesion associated with fulminant hepatic failure; differentiate acute from chronic (fibrosis, nodular regeneration). May provide specific diagnosis (infectious diseases)
- Fine-needle aspiration and cytologic evaluation of the liver: rapid screening for mycoses, neoplasia, feline hepatic lipidosis; abscess (ultrasound-guided), but accuracy is poor for many hepatic diseases
- Bacterial cultures: aerobic and anaerobic of liver and bile (cholangitis, abscess)
- Serum antibody titers for infectious diseases (leptospirosis, mycoses, toxoplasmosis, others)
- Tests to evaluate for systemic or extrahepatic disorders (pancreatic lipase immunoreactivity for acute pancreatitis; thoracic radiographs for systemic fungal infection, toxoplasmosis, metastatic neoplasia)

TREATMENT

THERAPEUTIC GOAL(S)

- Provide supportive therapy to allow adequate time for hepatic regeneration and repair
- Prevent or control complications of liver failure
- Treat underlying cause when possible

ACUTE GENERAL TREATMENT

- IV fluid therapy with balanced electrolyte solution; supplement with KCl using conventional sliding scale (20–40 mEq/L to start); maintain normoglycemia by adding 2.5–5% dextrose to fluids. Avoid alkalosis in hepatic encephalopathy (give 0.9% saline rather than lactated Ringer's solution).
- Treat underlying cause when possible; discontinue any suspect drug; start amoxicillin or penicillin for empiric treatment of suspected leptospirosis (dogs), or broad-spectrum systemic antibiotics for sepsis.
- Give *N*-acetylcysteine as a glutathione source/antioxidant for treatment of acetaminophen toxicity at 140 mg/kg (10% or 20% solution diluted at least 1:2 with saline) IV over 20 to 30 minutes through 0.25 μm nonpyrogenic filter; then 70 mg/kg IV or PO q 6h for 7 treatments. May also be beneficial for treatment of other drug-induced injuries (carprofen, potentiated sulfonamides, diazepam, methimazole, others) or organic solvents and heavy metal toxicity.
- Other hepatoprotective therapy (empiric therapy):
  - S-adenosylmethionine (SAMe) 20 mg/kg/day PO as a glutathione source
  - Silybin (milk thistle) protective against Amanita mushroom toxicity in an experimental study in dogs at 50 mg/kg IV. Oral dose for dogs 20–50 mg/kg of 60–80% silybin but poor absorption
  - Vitamin E (15 IU/kg/day PO) as an antioxidant
- Treatment for hepatic encephalopathy (if present) using a high-quality low-protein diet, lactulose (0.1–0.5 ml/kg PO q 12h, adjusted to achieve loose fecal consistency), and/or intestinal antibiotics such as metronidazole (7.5–10 mg/kg PO q 12h) or amoxicillin-clavulanate (15 mg/kg PO q 12h). (See Hepatic Encephalopathy, p 489.)

CHRONIC TREATMENT

- Provide adequate dietary protein and calories. Do not restrict dietary protein unless hepatic encephalopathy is present (see Hepatic Encephalopathy, p 489); choose non-meat-protein sources such as dairy (e.g., cottage cheese) and eggs.
- Consider empiric oral hepatoprotective therapy (SAMe, silybin, or Vitamin E) until evidence of hepatic injury resolves.
- Glucocorticoids are generally not warranted.

DRUG INTERACTIONS

Avoid drugs that require hepatic metabolism

POSSIBLE COMPLICATIONS

- Hepatic encephalopathy
- Hypoglycemia
- Coagulopathy and anemia
- Gastrointestinal ulceration
- Septicemia

RECOMMENDED MONITORING

- Serum biochemistry profiles
- Blood glucose
- Serum bile acids
- Packed cell volume/total protein (anemia/bleeding)

PROGNOSIS AND OUTCOME

- If patient presents with signs of advanced liver failure (e.g., hepatic encephalopathy, coagulopathy, hypoglycemia), the prognosis is guarded
- For milder hepatic injury, complete recovery is possible, especially when underlying cause is detected and treated

PEARLS & CONSIDERATIONS

COMMENTS

- Clinical and laboratory features reflect general hepatic failure; they are not specific for underlying cause of hepatic injury
- Always consider an adverse drug reaction as the cause of acute hepatic injury or failure, as discontinuing suspect drug can result in improved hepatic function

PREVENTION

- Vaccinate for infectious diseases (e.g., infectious canine hepatitis, leptospirosis)
- Monitor liver enzymes when prescribing a drug with potential to cause hepatotoxicity; promptly discontinue if enzyme elevations arise
- Avoid reexposure of patient to drug suspected to have caused hepatic reaction

SUGGESTED READING

Scherk MA, Center SA: Toxic, metabolic, infectious, and neoplastic liver diseases. In Ettinger SJ, Feldman EC (eds): *Textbook of Veterinary Internal Medicine*. St. Louis, Elsevier Saunders, 2005, pp 1464–1478.

AUTHOR: **SUSAN E. JOHNSON**
EDITOR: **KEITH P. RICHTER**

Hepatic Lipidosis

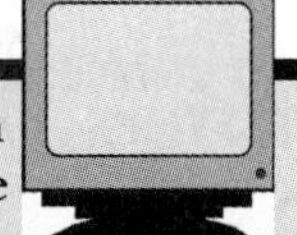

Client Education Sheet on Website

BASIC INFORMATION

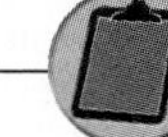

DEFINITION

Excessive accumulation of fat (triglyceride) in the liver, which is associated with severe intrahepatic cholestasis and hepatic dysfunction

SYNONYM(S)

Fatty liver syndrome
Feline hepatic lipidosis (FHL)
Idiopathic hepatic lipidosis

EPIDEMIOLOGY

SPECIES, AGE, SEX: Cats; middle-aged or older; no gender predilection.

GENETICS AND BREED PREDISPOSITION: No breed predilection.

RISK FACTORS: Obesity before onset of anorexia; prior stressful event (boarding, surgery, change in living arrangements, diet change) preceding anorexia; systemic diseases associated with anorexia and a catabolic state.

ASSOCIATED CONDITIONS AND DISORDERS: Cholangitis, pancreatitis, inflammatory bowel disease, systemic neoplasia, diabetes mellitus, toxin- or drug-induced injury (stanozolol, tetracyclines), and many other systemic disorders associated with anorexia and weight loss.

CLINICAL PRESENTATION

DISEASE FORMS/SUBTYPES

- Idiopathic hepatic lipidosis: primary disorder of unknown cause
- Secondary hepatic lipidosis: associated with inciting cause (see Associated Conditions and Disorders above)

HISTORY, CHIEF COMPLAINT: Prolonged anorexia, often several weeks in duration; rapid weight loss (often >25% of body weight). History of stressful event (see Risk Factors above), or nonhepatic diseases associated with anorexia. Other signs: lethargy, depression, sporadic vomiting, constipation, or diarrhea.

PHYSICAL EXAM FINDINGS: Jaundice, hepatomegaly, dehydration, muscle wasting, seborrhea. Pale mucous membranes, weight loss. Overt findings of hepatic encephalopathy (ptyalism, severe depression, stupor) or bleeding are uncommon and indicate severe liver failure. Head or neck ventroflexion may occur with severe electrolyte imbalances (hypokalemia, hypophosphatemia) or thiamine deficiency.

ETIOLOGY AND PATHOPHYSIOLOGY

- Cats have higher nutritional requirements for protein, essential amino acids, and essential fatty acids than do dogs.
- Systemically ill cats have a propensity for accumulating fat in their hepatocytes.
- Profound anorexia and stress may be associated with hormonal (catecholamines, other) alterations that influence fat metabolism and predispose to peripheral fat mobilization and hepatic fat uptake.
- Obese cats appear unable to adapt to metabolism of fat for energy during starvation. The exact metabolic or biochemical aberrations in cats with hepatic lipidosis are unknown.
- However, there appears to be an imbalance between mobilization of peripheral fat, hepatic use of fatty acids for energy, and hepatic dispersal of triglycerides.
- Lipid accumulation is not directly toxic to liver but is a marker for an underlying metabolic disorder.

DIAGNOSIS

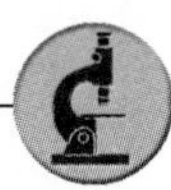

DIFFERENTIAL DIAGNOSIS

- Cholangitis/cholangiohepatitis
- Pancreatitis
- Hepatic manifestations of feline infectious peritonitis
- Hepatic neoplasia
- Drug- or toxin-induced hepatic injury
- Extrahepatic bile duct obstruction

INITIAL DATABASE

- Complete blood count:
  - Normocytic, normochromic anemia.
  - Poikilocytosis (acanthocytes and elliptocytes).
  - Hemolysis (secondary to hypophosphatemia or Heinz bodies).
  - Mature neutrophilia and lymphopenia (stress response).
- Serum biochemistry profile:
  - Alkaline phosphatase (ALP): moderate to marked increases. Earliest biochemical change; precedes hyperbilirubinemia.
  - Alanine aminotransferase (ALT): mild to moderate increases.
  - γ-Glutamyltransferase (GGT): normal to mild increase (as opposed to increased GGT seen with other feline cholestatic disorders). The finding of a greater magnitude of ele-

vation of ALP compared with GGT is highly suggestive of feline hepatic lipidosis.
    - Hyperbilirubinemia.
    - Hyperammonemia, hypoalbuminemia, hypoglycemia (severe hepatic dysfunction).
- Urinalysis: may show bilirubinuria (always abnormal in the cat)
- Coagulation abnormalities (prothrombin time and proteins induced by vitamin K antagonism increased; hypofibrinogenemia)
- Abdominal radiographs: normal to increased liver size
- Abdominal ultrasound: normal to increased liver size; diffusely hyperechoic parenchyma. Ascites rare. Evaluate for concurrent pancreatitis or other disorders causing secondary hepatic lipidosis
- Bile acids: usually elevated (not necessary to measure if hyperbilirubinemia is present)

ADVANCED OR CONFIRMATORY TESTING

- Fine-needle aspiration and cytologic evalvation of the liver are preferred over liver biopsy (less invasive, allows presumptive diagnosis of hepatic lipidosis). However, cytologic evaluation is not accurate in diagnosing other hepatopathies, and therefore these may be missed. In hepatic lipidosis, cytologic evaluation reveals vacuolated hepatocytes without inflammation. Correction of any coagulopathy with vitamin K_1 prior to performing liver aspirate or biopsy is essential. However, clotting studies do not necessarily predict bleeding tendency after liver aspirate or biopsy.
- Liver biopsy provides definitive diagnosis. Not routinely performed when fine-needle aspirate and cytologic study provide the diagnosis, unless there is failure to respond to therapy for hepatic lipidosis or a high level of suspicion of other primary hepatic disorder(s) exists. With hepatic lipidosis, the biopsy sample typically is a pale tan color and floats in formalin. Biopsy results show severe vacuolization of hepatocytes (>50% of acinar unit involved). Inflammation and necrosis absent. Vacuoles stain positive for fat with oil red O.
- Consider serum feline pancreatic lipase immunoreactivity to evaluate for concurrent feline pancreatitis (see Pancreatitis, Cat, p 794). Consider serum cobalamin (vitamin B_{12}) levels if underlying primary intestinal disorder suspected.
- Evaluate for underlying systemic disorder as necessary.

TREATMENT

THERAPEUTIC GOAL(S)

- Correct fluid and electrolyte abnormalities
- Control complications of liver failure
- Give nutritional support to provide adequate calorie and protein intake
- Treat underlying systemic disorder if identified

ACUTE GENERAL TREATMENT

- Initial fluid therapy: intravenous balanced electrolyte solution supplemented with KCl using conventional sliding scale (20–40 mEq/L). Monitor serum potassium twice daily initially and readjust as needed; avoid lactated Ringer's solution (impaired lactate metabolism in severe hepatic lipidosis); avoid dextrose supplementation unless hypoglycemic (promotes hepatic lipid deposition).
- Vitamin K_1 (0.5–1.5 mg/kg SC q 12h for three injections) for coagulopathy.
- Water-soluble vitamin supplementation:
    - B-complex vitamins (added to fluids: 1–2 ml/L).
    - Cobalamin (vitamin B_{12}): 250 µg SC initially while awaiting serum cobalamin levels. If decreased serum cobalamin is documented (primary intestinal disease), continue with 250 µg SC once weekly.
    - Thiamine supplementation (if severe ventroflexion of neck): 50–100 mg PO/cat/day for 1 week.
- Blood transfusion as needed for anemia.
- Nasogastric tube feeding of Clinicare (Abbott Veterinary Diets) for initial 24 to 48 hours, before placing gastrostomy or esophagostomy tube for long-term feeding. This will allow initial stabilization prior to general anesthesia for long-term feeding tube placement.

CHRONIC TREATMENT

- Place gastrostomy or esophagostomy tube (by least invasive method possible) (see Feeding Tube Placement: Esophagostomy Tube, p 1243; Feeding Tube Placement: Percutaneous Endoscopic Gastrostomy [PEG], p 1247).
    - Feed Maximum Calorie (The Iams Co.), Prescription Diet a/d (Hill's Pet Nutrition), or other complete and balanced feline diet. Do not restrict dietary protein unless overt signs of hepatic encephalopathy are present.
    - Provide 40–60 kcal/kg/day. Start with 1/4 to 1/2 of daily requirements given through tube and divided into 4 to 6 feedings. Gradually increase to daily requirements over 3 to 4 days.
    - If vomiting occurs, consider metoclopramide (0.4 mg/kg q 8h SC or through the tube, 30 minutes before feeding), cisapride (1 mg/kg q 8h through the tube), prochlorperazine (0.5 mg/kg SQ q 8h), or tube feedings by slow constant rate infusion. Be sure that any tablet-formulated medications are ground to a fine powder before being administered through the tube; otherwise, there is a risk of tube occlusion.
    - Tube feeding usually required for 3 to 6 weeks (or longer in some cases), pending clinical and biochemical improvement.
    - Do not remove tube until cat eating on its own for at least a week.
- Other dietary supplements used empirically:
    - L-carnitine 250–500 mg PO q 24h (essential cofactor for fatty acid oxidation; relative carnitine deficiency in hepatic lipidosis?).
    - Taurine 250–500 mg PO q 24h for initial 7 to 10 days (plasma levels have been found to be decreased in many cats with hepatic lipidosis; required for bile acid conjugation).
    - Vitamin E (water soluble form) 50–100 units/cat PO q 24h (antioxidant).
    - S-Adenosylmethionine (SAMe; Denosyl SD4; Nutramax Labs) 20 mg/kg PO q 24h (glutathione source). Do not give through the tube (would disrupt enteric coating).

POSSIBLE COMPLICATIONS

- Hepatic encephalopathy (see Hepatic Encephalopathy, p 489 for further details):
    - Manage hepatic encephalopathy with lactulose (0.25–0.5 ml/kg q 8h PO) combined with one of the following antibiotics (neomycin 22 mg/kg q 8h PO, amoxicillin 22 mg/kg q 12h PO, amoxicillin-clavulanate 15 mg/kg q 12h PO, or metronidazole 7.5 mg/kg q 12h PO). Restrict dietary protein.
- Hypophosphatemia (see Refeeding Syndrome, p 948):
    - Monitor serum phosphorus. Supplement with potassium phosphate if phosphorus < 2.0 mg/dl (this severe degree of hypophosphatemia causes hemolysis) at a rate of 0.01–0.03 mmol/kg/ hr, placed in calcium-free fluids and infused over a 6- to 12-hour period. Repeat serum phosphorus q 6h initially; avoid hyperphosphatemia and hypocalcemia. Reduce KCl supplementation based on the amount of potassium delivered as potassium phosphate.
- Heinz body hemolysis:
    - Cats with hepatic lipidosis have decreased hepatic glutathione and are at risk for red blood cell oxidant injury/Heinz body hemolysis. For crisis situation, provide glutathione

source as *N*-acetylcysteine 140 mg/kg (20% solution diluted at least 1:2 with saline) IV over 20 to 30 minutes through 0.25 μm nonpyrogenic filter; then 70 mg/kg IV q 8-12h depending on clinical signs). When enteral feeding is established, switch to SAMe 20 mg/kg PO q 24h (do not give through the tube so the enteric coating is not disrupted) as a glutathione source.

- Hypomagnesemia:
  - Monitor serum magnesium. Supplement if Mg <1.2 mg/dl. Magnesium sulfate (8.13 mEq/g) and magnesium chloride (9.25 mEq/g) salts available in 50% solution; dilute to a concentration of 20% or less in 5% dextrose in water. Give 0.75-1.0 mEq/kg/day constant rate infusion.

RECOMMENDED MONITORING

Biochemical improvement (decreases in bilirubin, ALP, ALT) usually seen within 1 to 2 weeks of initiating tube feeding. Normalization may take several weeks.

PROGNOSIS AND OUTCOME

- Early diagnosis is key to successful management.
- Recovery in approximately 60-85% of cases. If the cat survives the initial few days, the prognosis for complete recovery is excellent.
- Poorer prognosis with concurrent pancreatitis.

PEARLS & CONSIDERATIONS

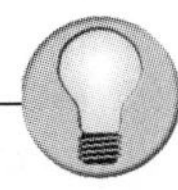

COMMENTS

- Oral appetite stimulants usually are inadequate for aggressive nutritional support required for feline hepatic lipidosis therapy. Oral diazepam is associated with idiosyncratic hepatic necrosis in cats.
- Correct fluid and electrolyte imbalances before anesthesia for tube placement.
- In critically ill cats with hepatic lipidosis, the stress of general anesthesia may be fatal. Therefore initial feeding through a nasogastric tube (placed in awake state) before anesthesia for long-term feeding tube placement is recommended. Once the patient is more stable, anesthesia for long-term feeding tube placement can be more safely accomplished.
- Establishing the diagnosis, identifying any underlying causes (which may require long-term treatment), and initial management (often requires several days of hospitalization, including anesthesia and feeding tube placement) can be costly, time-consuming, but ultimately rewarding.
- Evaluate for underlying systemic disorder (feline hepatic lipidosis may be secondary).

PREVENTION

- Do not switch obese cats to unpalatable diet for weight loss. Consider smaller amounts of favorite food given in parallel (not mixed in) with a weight-loss diet to avoid reducing appetite while allowing the cat to become accustomed to the new food.
- L-carnitine (250 mg/cat PO q 24h) may improve fatty acid oxidation in obese cats undergoing weight loss but won't prevent hepatic lipidosis.

CLIENT EDUCATION

- Tube feeding for 3 to 6 weeks (or longer) at home will be required for recovery.
- Recurrence is unlikely unless an underlying, chronic cause is present; the owner should take care to not allow cat to become anorexic again.

SUGGESTED READING

Center SA: Feline hepatic lipidosis. *Vet Clin Small Anim* 35:225, 2005.

Cornelius LM, et al: CVT Update: therapy for hepatic lipidosis. In Bonagura JD (ed): *Kirk's Current Veterinary Therapy XIII Small Animal Practice*. Philadelphia, WB Saunders, 2000, pp 686-690.

AUTHOR: **SUSAN E. JOHNSON**
EDITOR: **KEITH P. RICHTER**

Hepatic Neoplasia (Malignant)

BASIC INFORMATION

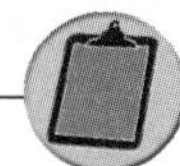

DEFINITION

- Primary malignant neoplasm of the liver or biliary tract.
- Epithelial origin: hepatocellular carcinoma (most common), hepatocellular adenoma/hepatoma, biliary carcinoma, biliary adenoma, hepatic carcinoid.
- Mesenchymal origin: hemangiosarcoma and leiomyosarcoma are the most common.
- Hemolymphatic tumors: lymphoma (dogs, cats) and myeloproliferative disorders (cats). Hepatic lymphoma may be part of multicentric disease or the primary site.
- Metastatic hepatic neoplasia (hemangiosarcoma, histiocytic sarcoma, islet cell carcinoma, pancreatic adenocarcinoma, intestinal adenocarcinoma, leiomyosarcoma, mammary carcinoma, transitional cell carcinoma, renal carcinoma, pheochromocytoma, and others).

SYNONYM(S)

Biliary adenoma: biliary cystadenoma in cats
Biliary carcinoma: cholangiocarcinoma, biliary cystadenocarcinoma

EPIDEMIOLOGY

SPECIES, AGE, SEX

- Primary hepatobiliary tumors are uncommon but occur in both dogs (0.6-1.3% of all canine neoplasms) and cats (1-2.9% of all feline neoplasms).
- Hepatocellular carcinoma is the most common primary liver tumor in dogs, accounting for more than half of all hepatobiliary tumors.
- Biliary carcinomas and adenomas are the most common primary hepatic tumors in cats. Biliary tumors are uncommon in dogs.
- Occur primarily in older animals (average age 10 to 12 years).

GENETICS AND BREED PREDISPOSITION

- No breed predilection for dogs.
- Domestic shorthair cats may have a higher rate of development of hepatic neoplasia than purebred cats.

RISK FACTORS

- Potential causes include aflatoxins, diethylnitrosamine, dichlorobenzidine, aramite, liver flukes (*Clonorchis* spp., *Platynosomum concinnum*), and radioactive compounds such as strontium 90 and cesium 144.
- Biliary carcinoma can occur in juvenile cats with feline leukemia virus infection.
- In humans, hepatitis B and C and cirrhosis are common risk factors for hepatocellular carcinoma. A similar association with viruses is not known to occur in dogs. Cirrhosis was only found in 7% of dogs with hepatocellular carcinoma.

CONTAGION AND ZOONOSIS: As opposed to humans, no association with viral infection has been found.

ASSOCIATED CONDITIONS AND DISORDERS

- Paraneoplastic hypoglycemia is occasionally noted in dogs with hepato-

cellular carcinoma (up to 38% of cases) and less frequently in dogs with hepatocellular adenoma, leiomyosarcoma, and hemangiosarcoma. Serum insulin concentrations are normal to decreased. Potential mechanisms of hypoglycemia include excess use of glucose by the tumor, release of insulin-like factors from the tumor, release of other substances such as somatostatin from the tumor, and secondary hepatic parenchymal destruction with impaired glycogenolysis or gluconeogenesis.
- Bile duct obstruction, coagulopathies, and hepatic encephalopathy are uncommon.
- Myasthenia gravis was associated with biliary carcinoma in one report.

CLINICAL PRESENTATION

DISEASE FORMS/SUBTYPES

- Hepatocellular carcinoma. There are three gross morphologic subtypes: massive, nodular, and diffuse.
  - Massive hepatocellular carcinoma, defined as a large tumor affecting a single liver lobe, represents 53-84% of the cases.The nodular form occurs in 16-25% and the diffuse form in 0-19% of the cases.
- Biliary carcinoma. Also occurs as massive, nodular, or diffuse forms in dogs. The massive form occurs in 37-46%, nodular in 0-21%, and diffuse in 17-54% of the cases. Biliary carcinomas can also be extrahepatic within the bile ducts or within the gallbladder.
- Hepatic carcinoid. A primary neuroendocrine tumor that is uncommon and is typified by aggressive biologic behavior and is most commonly diffuse with early metastasis.

HISTORY, CHIEF COMPLAINT: Clinical signs are usually vague and nonspecific. Anorexia, lethargy, weight loss, polydipsia, polyuria, vomiting, and abdomianl distention are the most common presenting complaints. Less frequent presenting problems are jaundice, diarrhea, excessive bleeding, and signs of central nervous system dysfunction due to hepatic encephalopathy, hypoglyemia, or central nervous system metastases.

PHYSICAL EXAM FINDINGS

- The most common finding in dogs and cats with primary hepatic tumors is a palpable cranial abdominal mass or marked hepatomegaly.
- Ascites or hemoabdomen may also contribute to abdominal distention.
- Pale mucous membranes due to anemia, jaundice, cachexia, and weakness are other potential findings.

ETIOLOGY AND PATHOPHYSIOLOGY

- Etiology unknown.
- Metastasis of canine hepatocellular carcinoma has been reported in 4.8-61% of the cases. Massive hepatocellular carcinoma generally has a low potential for metastasis.
  - Extrahepatic metastases occur more commonly with biliary carcinoma, with metastasis occurring in 56-88% of the cases.
  - Hepatic carcinoids and sarcomas have the highest metastatic rates with metastasis occurring in 86-93% of cases. Metastasis is most commonly to hepatic lymph nodes, the peritoneal cavity, and lungs, although widespread metastases can occur.
- Less is known about the metastatic rate of feline malignant hepatobiliary tumors, with estimates of metastasis in 56-67% of cases; diffuse intraperitoneal involvement is the most common manifestation.

DIAGNOSIS

DIFFERENTIAL DIAGNOSIS

- Metastatic hepatic neoplasia
- Hepatic nodular hyperplasia
- Diffuse hepatomegaly (e.g., vacuolar hepatopathy, hepatic congestion, lipidosis)
- Hepatic regenerative hyperplasia, cirrhosis (presence of nodular regeneration)
- Hepatobiliary cysts
- Hepatic abscess

INITIAL DATABASE

Complete blood count: variable anemia and leukocytosis, pancytopenia may be seen with hematopoietic or lymphoid malignancies that involve the bone marrow and that secondarily involve the liver.
- Coagulation profile: prolonged prothrombin times and activated partial thromboplastin times are not common (when coagulopathies occur, they are most common with hepatic hemangiosarcoma).
- Serum chemistry profile: mild to marked increases in liver enzymes: alanine aminotransferase (ALT), aspartate aminotransferase (AST), and alkaline phosphatase, hyperbilirubinemia (uncommon in dogs with primary hepatic neoplasia, more common in dogs with metastatic liver disease, occurs in one-third of cats with primary liver tumors). Other quite variable biochemical abnormalities include hypoalbuminemia, hyperglobulinemia, and hypoglycemia.
- Serum bile acids: elevated in 50-75% of cases with the magnitude of elevation often being small.
- Abdominal radiographs: symmetric or asymmetric hepatomegaly, ascites, and caudolateral gastric displacement.
- Three-view thoracic radiographs: evaluate for pulmonary metastasis.
- Abdominal ultrasound: very useful for evaluation of the liver when primary or metastatic hepatic neoplasia is suspected:
  - Hepatocellular carcinoma usually appears as a focal hyperechoic or mixed echogenic mass.
  - Primary or metastatic neoplasia often appears as focal or multifocal hypoechoic or mixed echogenic lesions.
  - "Target" lesions, consisting of an echogenic center surrounded by a more sonolucent rim, are often neoplastic.
  - Hyperplastic nodules are usually multifocal hyperechoic lesions, although hypoechoic or mixed echogenic lesions can occur.
  - The ultrasonographic appearance of hepatic lymphoma is quite variable, ranging from normal to mild diffuse hyperechogenicity or hypoechogenicity, multifocal hypoechoic lesions, or mixed echogenic target lesions.

ADVANCED OR CONFIRMATORY TESTING

- Ultrasound guided percutaneous fine-needle aspirate for cytology. Cytologic evaluation can correctly diagnose neoplasia in up to 62% of patients with liver tumors, although it is often unreliable. Cytologic evaluation is most useful for the diagnosis of diffuse hemolymphatic tumors such as lymphoma, myeloproliferative disease, and mast cell tumors.There is low risk with fine-needle aspiration.
- Ultrasound-guided percutaneous core needle biopsy versus laparoscopic biopsy for histopathologic evaluation of liver tissue (confirmatory). Needle biopsies are generally accurate, but due to the small size of the biopsy samples, differentiation of nodular hyperplasia from primary hepatic neoplasia may be difficult and sometimes a larger biopsy specimen obtained via laparoscopy or labarotomy is necessary. Laparoscopy allows for larger biopsy samples and is also useful for staging (observe peritoneal surface and lymph nodes for infiltration or other abnormalities).
- Peritoneal fluid cytology in animals that have ascites may reveal neoplastic cells, especially in advanced cases, although often ascites is a modified transudate without exfoliation of neoplastic cells.
- Abdominal computed tomography (CT) scan or magnetic resonance imaging (MRI) could be considered for lesion characterization and staging. MRI has been shown to be useful for differentiating benign from malignant focal hepatic lesions in dogs.
- α-Fetoprotein is an oncofetal glycoprotein that is a useful serum tumor marker for human hepatocellular carcinoma. It was shown to be elevated significantly in 55% of dogs with biliary carcinoma and 75% of dogs with hepatocellular car-

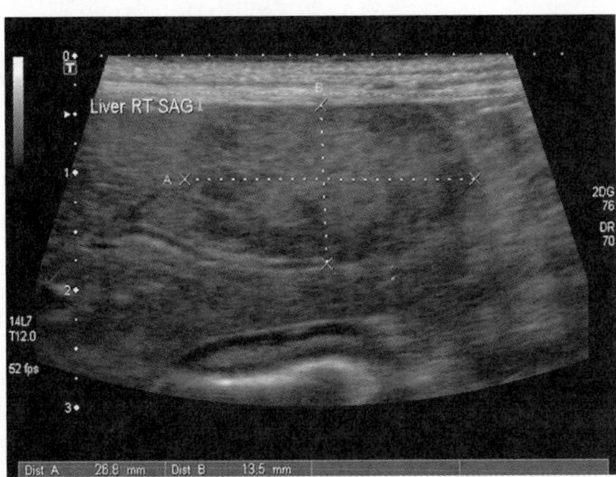

FIGURE I-88 Hepatocellular carcinoma. Solitary well circumscribed complex echogenic liver mass.

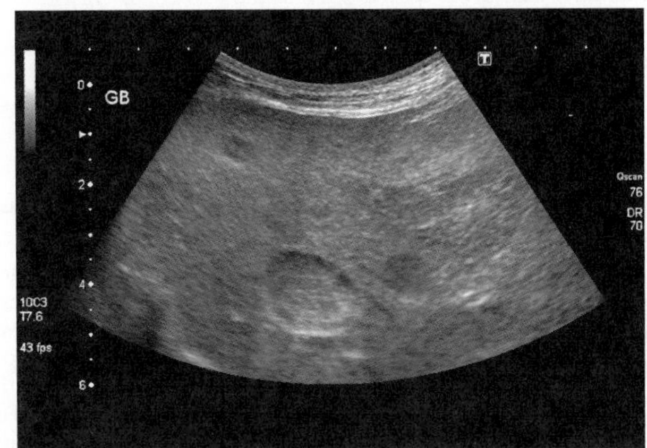

FIGURE I-89 Metastatic carcinoma. Multiple hypoechoic liver lesions. The larger structure at the bottom of the image is the gallbladder containing inspissated bile.

cinoma, but not in dogs with other primary or metastatic hepatic tumors or other types of liver disease. This assay is not readily available in most veterinary laboratories at this time.

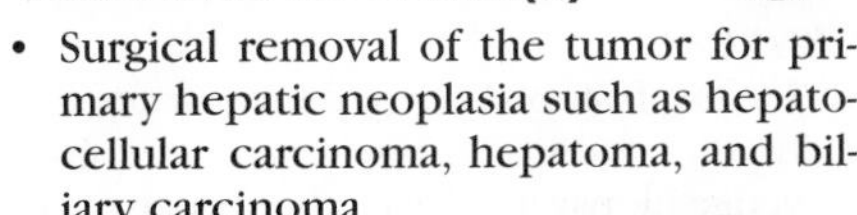

TREATMENT

THERAPEUTIC GOAL(S)

- Surgical removal of the tumor for primary hepatic neoplasia such as hepatocellular carcinoma, hepatoma, and biliary carcinoma
- Chemotherapy for hepatic lymphoma and hepatic mast cell tumor
- Palliative therapy for metastatic hepatic cancer

ACUTE GENERAL TREATMENT

- Supportive therapy for paraneoplastic hypoglycemia, coagulopathies, or hepatic encephalopathy.
- Liver lobectomy for primary hepatic tumors involving a single lobe. Fewer biliary carcinomas can be resected due to the higher percentage that are multifocal or metastatic at presentation.
- Treatment options are very limited for nodular, diffuse, and metastatic liver cancer.

CHRONIC TREATMENT

- Chemotherapy for hepatic lymphoma, mast cell tumor, myeloproliferative disease, and possibly for hemangiosarcoma.
- No effective chemotherapy or radiation therapy protocols have been reported for primary hepatic tumors.
- Several chemotherapy drugs have been used anecdotally (carboplatin, gemcitabine, mitoxantrone, doxorubicin, 5-fluorouracil), although efficacy has not been proven. Given the poor response in humans with hepatobiliary cancer, it is unlikely that systemic chemotherapy with the currently available agents will play a major role in the treatment of hepatobiliary cancer in dogs and or cats.
  - Chemoresistance may be due to expression of P-glycoprotein, which is associated with multidrug resistance, and/or the presence of detoxification enzymes contained in hepatocytes.
- Newer treatment modalities such as intra-arterial chemotherapy, transarterial chemoembolization, percutaneous ethanol injection, microwave coagulation, and immunotherapeutic strategies may be applicable in veterinary patients.

POSSIBLE COMPLICATIONS

- Hemorrhage is the most common surgical complication. Blood products should be available in the event that a transfusion is necessary.
- Although not common, hypoglycemia is a potential transient complication of extensive partial hepatectomy.

RECOMMENDED MONITORING

After removal of primary liver tumors, follow-up abdominal ultrasound and three-view thoracic radiographs are recommended every 3 to 6 months for 1 to 2 years.

PROGNOSIS AND OUTCOME

- For massive hepatocellular carcinoma treated by liver lobectomy, the prognosis is good with a complete excision, with average survival times of more than a year and many patients being cured.
- The median survival time for massive hepatocellular carcinoma treated with liver lobectomy is >1460 days, with high serum ALT and AST activity and right-sided tumors conveying a worse prognosis.
- The prognosis for nodular or diffuse hepatocellular carcinoma is poor.
- Biliary carcinoma, hepatic carcinoids, and hepatic sarcomas have a worse prognosis, as they are commonly nodular or diffuse, resistant to chemotherapy, and have high metastatic rates.
- Hepatic lymphoma has a variable prognosis depending on the grade and response to chemotherapy.
- The liver is a common site of metastasis for a variety of cancers, and metastatic liver disease has a poor prognosis.

PEARLS & CONSIDERATIONS

COMMENTS

- The most common primary hepatobiliary tumor in dogs is a massive hepatocellular carcinoma.
- With liver lobectomy providing a complete excision of massive hepatocellular carcinoma, long-term survival or cure is common.

SUGGESTED READING

Johnson, SE: Chronic hepatic disorders: In Ettinger SJ, Feldman EC (eds): *Textbook of Veterinary Internal Medicine*, ed 5. Philadelphia, WB Saunders, 2000, pp 1320–1325.

Mayhew PD, et al: Massive hepatocellular carcinoma in dogs: 48 cases (1992–2002). *J Am Vet Med Assoc* 225:1225–1230, 2004.

Withrow SJ: Cancer of the gastrointestinal tract: heptobiliary tumors. In Withrow SJ, MacEwen EG (eds): *Small Animal Clinical Oncology*, ed 3. Philadelphia, WB Saunders, 2001, pp 327–334.

AUTHOR: **STEVE HILL**
EDITOR: **KEITH P. RICHTER**

Hepatic Nodules (Benign): Adenoma, Nodular Hyperplasia, and Nodular Regeneration

BASIC INFORMATION

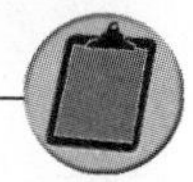

DEFINITION

- Hepatic adenoma: benign neoplasia of hepatocytes
- Nodular hyperplasia: discrete accumulation of hyperplastic hepatocytes surrounded by normal hepatocytes
- Nodular regeneration: discrete accumulation of hyperplastic hepatocytes surrounded by abnormal hepatocellular parenchyma, particularly fibrotic changes

SYNONYM(S)

Nodular hyperplasia: hyperplastic nodules
Nodular regeneration: regenerative nodules

EPIDEMIOLOGY

SPECIES, AGE, SEX

- Hepatic adenomas: rare tumors in dogs and cats; patients usually >10 years old
- Nodular hyperplasia: common lesion in old dogs. Incidence in dogs >14 years old: 70–100%
- Nodular regeneration: seen in dogs with acquired parenchymal hepatic disease. Middle-aged to older dogs

GENETICS AND BREED PREDISPOSITION: Nodular regeneration: Seen in breeds predisposed to chronic hepatitis (Doberman pinscher, cocker spaniel, Labrador retriever) and copper storage hepatopathy (Bedlington terrier, West Highland white terrier, Skye terrier).

RISK FACTORS: Nodular regeneration: chronic hepatic disease, cirrhotic/fibrosing liver disease.

CLINICAL PRESENTATION

HISTORY, CHIEF COMPLAINT

- Nodular hyperplasia: incidental finding, no clinical signs
- Adenoma: incidental finding, no clinical signs; rarely, abdominal discomfort or rupture with hemoperitoneum or abscessation with signs of chronic infection
- Nodular regeneration: see sections on chronic hepatic diseases (Cirrhotic/Fibrosing Liver Disease, p 210; Hepatitis [Chronic] of Cocker Spaniel Dogs, p 499; Hepatitis [Chronic] of Doberman Pinscher Dogs, p 500; Hepatitis [Chronic, Idiopathic] of Dogs, p 503)

PHYSICAL EXAMINATION

- Hepatic adenoma: rarely abdominal pain, inappetence, ascites (if ruptured)
- Nodular hyperplasia: normal exam
- Nodular regeneration: see sections on chronic hepatic disease (Cirrhotic/Fibrosing Liver Disease, p 210; Hepatitis [Chronic] of Cocker Spaniel Dogs, p 499; Hepatitis [Chronic] of Doberman Pinscher Dogs, p 500; Hepatitis [Chronic, Idiopathic] of Dogs, p 503)

ETIOLOGY AND PATHOPHYSIOLOGY

- Nodular hyperplasia: unknown; may be associated with nutritional factors, or a result of focal areas of ischemia. Not preneoplastic
- Adenoma: unknown; may be associated with chronic inflammation or hepatotoxicity
- Nodular regeneration: compensatory response of the liver to chronic injury

DIAGNOSIS

DIFFERENTIAL DIAGNOSIS

- Nodular hyperplasia:
  - Primary or metastatic hepatic neoplasia
  - Cirrhosis with nodular regeneration
  - Vacuolar hepatopathy
- Adenoma:
  - Nodular hyperplasia
  - Primary or metastatic hepatic neoplasia
  - Hepatic abscess
- Nodular regeneration:
  - Nodular hyperplasia
  - Metastatic hepatic neoplasia
  - Vacuolar hepatopathy

INITIAL DATABASE

NODULAR HYPERPLASIA

- Commonly associated with mild to moderate increases in serum alkaline phosphatase (ALP), less commonly with mild increases in serum alanine transaminase (ALT) and aspartate aminotransferase (AST).
- Serum bile acids usually normal.
- Abdominal ultrasonography reveals single to multiple lesions with highly variable appearance. Easily mistaken for primary or metastatic neoplasia or nodular regeneration.

HEPATIC ADENOMA

- Variable increases in ALP, ALT, and AST.
- Serum bile acids usually normal.
  - Leukocytosis ± monocytosis if necrotic regions within adenomas.
  - Anemia if adenoma rupture and hemoperitoneum.
- Radiographs may identify a mass in the cranial abdomen or rarely a gas pocket in a necrotic region.
- Abdominal ultrasonography demonstrates a solitary mass with variable echogenicity that may contain cystic cavities and/or blood- or gas-filled spaces. Ascites seen with with rupture and hemoperitoneum.

NODULAR REGENERATION

- Serum bile acids usually abnormal
- See section on chronic hepatic disease (Cirrhotic/Fibrosing Liver Disease, p 210; Hepatitis [Chronic] of Cocker Spaniel Dogs, p 499; Hepatitis [Chronic] of Doberman Pinscher Dogs, p 500; Hepatitis [Chronic, Idiopathic] of Dogs, p 503)

ADVANCED OR CONFIRMATORY TESTS

GENERAL

- Hepatic histopathology differentiates the three conditions but often requires wedge biopsy, as adjacent hepatic tissue is necessary to make a definitive diagnosis.
- Fine-needle aspiration or single needle biopsies of these focal lesions may result in misdiagnosis of hepatic vacuolar hepatopathy.
- Magnetic resonance imaging of focal hepatic masses may provide better discrimination of these lesions (future direction).

SPECIFIC

- Nodular hyperplasia:
  - Well-circumscribed expansive nodule usually <3 cm containing hyperplastic hepatocytes that often contain cytoplasmic vacuoles and are loosely organized into hepatic cords with discernable portal tracts.
  - Nodules surrounded by normal hepatic parenchyma.
  - Lipogranulomas are a common associated finding.
- Adenoma:
  - Well-circumscribed expansive nodule of variable size containing hyperplastic, but well-differentiated hepatocytes arranged in cords that are 1 to 2 cells thick with a conspicuous absence of portal tracts.
  - Adenomas are surrounded by normal hepatic parenchyma.
- Nodular regeneration:
  - Similar histologic appearance as nodular hyperplasia, but surrounding hepatic parenchyma is abnormal, most often with mixed inflammation and fibrosis.

TREATMENT

THERAPEUTIC GOAL(S)

Determine if the focal lesions present on abdominal ultrasound, which may or may not be accompanied by increases in serum hepatic enzyme activity, require any therapeutic intervention

ACUTE GENERAL TREATMENT

- Nodular hyperplasia:
  - No treatment necessary
- Adenoma:
  - No treatment necessary for small masses not associated with clinical signs
  - Surgical excision for large masses causing abdominal discomfort or for those associated with abscessation or hemorrhage
- Nodular regeneration:
  - See sections on chronic hepatic disease (Cirrhotic/Fibrosing Liver Disease, p 210; Hepatitis [Chronic] of Cocker Spaniel Dogs, see below; Hepatitis [Chronic] of Doberman Pinscher Dogs, p 500; Hepatitis [Chronic, Idiopathic] of Dogs, p 503)

RECOMMENDED MONITORING

Sequential monitoring of serum hepatic enzyme activity and abdominal ultrasonography q 4-6 months

PROGNOSIS AND OUTCOME

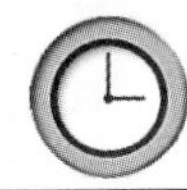

- Nodular hyperplasia or adenoma: excellent long-term prognosis
- Nodular regeneration: see Cirrhotic/ Fibrosing Hepatic Disease, p 210

PEARLS & CONSIDERATIONS

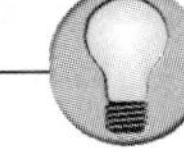

COMMENTS

- Nodular hyperplasia is primarily of clinical concern for two reasons:
  - It is a common cause of increased serum ALP in older dogs.
  - The ultrasonographic appearance may mimic primary or metastatic hepatic neoplasia.
- Differentiation of the three conditions usually requires hepatic wedge biopsy (obtained via laparoscopy or surgery).

SUGGESTED READING

Clifford CA, et al: Magnetic resonance imaging of focal splenic and hepatic lesions in the dog. *J Vet Intern Med* 18:330–338, 2004.

Hammer AS, Sikkema DA: Hepatic neoplasia in the dog and cat. *Vet Clin North Am Small Anim Pract* 25:419–435, 1995.

Prause LC, Twedt D: Hepatic nodular hyperplasia. In Bonagura JD (ed): *Kirk's Current Veterinary Therapy XIII*. Philadelphia, WB Saunders, 2000, 675–676.

AUTHOR: **CYNTHIA R. L. WEBSTER**
EDITOR: **KEITH P. RICHTER**

Hepatitis (Chronic) of Cocker Spaniel Dogs

BASIC INFORMATION

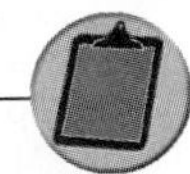

DEFINITION

A progressive chronic inflammatory liver disease distinct to cocker spaniels

SYNONYM(S)

Chronic hepatitis
Chronic idiopathic hepatitis

EPIDEMIOLOGY

SPECIES, AGE, SEX: English and American cocker spaniels are affected. Most are diagnosed between the ages of 2 to 6 years. Male dogs are overrepresented.
GENETICS AND BREED PREDISPOSITION: The high incidence in this breed suggests a genetic predisposition, but the mode of genetic transmission is unknown. Certain lines of dogs seem to be more affected.

CLINICAL PRESENTATION

DISEASE FORMS/SUBTYPES
- Subclinical hepatitis
- Clinical hepatitis

HISTORY, CHIEF COMPLAINT
- Dogs with subclinical hepatitis show no overt signs.
- Historic signs of early clinical hepatitis are often vague and may be associated with intermittent gastrointestinal signs and weight loss.
- When clinical hepatitis progresses to liver failure some or all of the following historic signs may occur:
  - Polydipsia, polyuria
  - Weight loss
  - Abdominal distention
  - Altered mental status associated with hepatic encephalopathy

PHYSICAL EXAM FINDINGS: With clinical hepatitis some or all of the following may be found:
- Weight loss
- Icterus
- Ascites
- Signs of hepatic encephalopathy
- Hemorrhage

ETIOLOGY AND PATHOPHYSIOLOGY

- The etiology is unknown.
- The hepatitis may be associated with abnormal accumulation of α-1 antitrypsin (also called α-1 protease inhibitor) in hepatocytes.
- Hepatic copper accumulation is not a consistent feature.

DIAGNOSIS

DIFFERENTIAL DIAGNOSIS

- Hepatic disease from other causes
- Nonhepatic conditions associated with abnormal liver enzymes

INITIAL DATABASE

- Subclinical disease:
  - Elevation in serum alanine aminotransferase (ALT)
- Clinical disease:
  - Elevation in serum ALT, aspartate aminotransferase (AST), γ-glutamyl transferase, and alkaline phosphatase
  - Elevated serum bile acid concentrations
- Advanced disease:
  - Elevation in serum total bilirubin concentration
  - Low serum albumin, blood urea nitrogen, and glucose concentration
  - Abnormal clotting times

ADVANCED OR CONFIRMATORY TESTING

- Abdominal radiographs: microhepatica ± signs of ascites (loss of serosal detail).
- Ultrasound: microhepatica with altered parenchymal echogenicity, ± ascites, ± vascular changes associated with portal hypertension.
- Surgery or laparoscopy: small liver; micronodular and fibrotic in advanced clinical disease.
- Liver histopathology: subclinical disease is associated with infiltration of mononuclear inflammatory cells into portal and parenchymal areas; clinical disease has evidence of active hepatitis

with areas of piecemeal and bridging necrosis.
- Histochemical staining for α-1 antitrypsin may show globoid accumulations within hepatocytes.
- Hepatic metal quantitative analysis: Hepatic copper is usually normal but secondary increases in copper may occur. Hepatic iron is increased secondary to chronic inflammation; zinc concentrations may be reduced.

TREATMENT

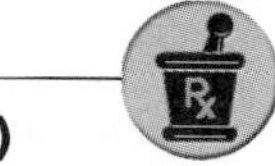

THERAPEUTIC GOAL(S)

- To slow the progression of the liver disease in subclinical cases
- Provide specific therapy for the chronic hepatitis
- Provide liver support treating complications of liver disease such as hepatic encephalopathy, ascites, gastrointestinal ulceration, and nutritional imbalance

ACUTE GENERAL TREATMENT

- Fluid support
- Treatment of hepatic encephalopathy (see Hepatic Encephalopathy, p 489)
- Coagulopathies or sepsis are treated as they occur (see Hepatitis [Chronic, Idiopathic] of Dogs, p 503)

CHRONIC TREATMENT

- Subclinical and early clinical hepatitis (see Hepatitis [Chronic, Idiopathic] of Dogs, p 503):
  - Glucocorticoid therapy (prednisone or prednisolone 2 mg/kg PO q 24-48h) may be beneficial in slowing inflammatory component of the liver disease.
  - Ensure adequate nutrient intake.
  - Provide liver support with antioxidants (vitamin E, 10 IU/kg PO q 24h; s-adenosylmethionine, 20 mg/kg PO q 24h), antifibrotics (colchicine, 0.03 mg/kg PO q 24h), or ursodeoxycholic acid (15 mg/kg PO q 24h).
  - If secondary copper accumulation occurs, chelator or zinc therapy should be used (see Hepatopathy, Copper-Associated, p 509).
- Advanced clinical hepatitis (see Hepatopathy, Copper-Associated, p 509):
  - Treatment for hepatic encephalopathy using a high-quality, low-protein diet, lactulose (0.1-0.5 ml/kg PO q 12h, titrated to achieve loose fecal consistency) and/or intestinal antibiotics (metronidazole, 7.5-10 mg/kg PO q 12h; or amoxicillin-clavulanate, 15 mg/kg PO q 12h). See Hepatic Encephalopathy, p 489.
  - Ascites therapy using spironolactone (1 mg/kg PO q 12h) or furosemide (0.5-2 mg/kg PO q 12h).
  - Gastric ulceration using ranitidine (2 mg/kg PO q 12h).

DRUG INTERACTIONS

Avoid drugs that require hepatic metabolism

POSSIBLE COMPLICATIONS

Glucocorticoids may precipitate ascites, hepatic encephalopathy, and early death in advanced cases.

RECOMMENDED MONITORING

- Young dogs should have periodic liver enzymes measured as screening test to help identify affected dogs.
- Routine complete blood count, serum biochemistry profile, and urinalysis to monitor disease progression, remission, or complications.
- Periodic liver biopsies (yearly) are the best means of evaluating the stage and progression of the disease during therapy.

PROGNOSIS AND OUTCOME

- Diagnosis and appropriate therapy in subclinical cases may slow progression of disease
- Clinical hepatitis denotes advanced disease and the long-term prognosis is guarded

PEARLS & CONSIDERATIONS

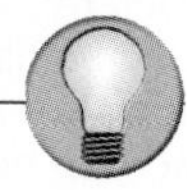

COMMENTS

- The first abnormality observed in young subclinical dogs is an increase in serum ALT activity. Unexplained elevated ALT activities in this breed should be investigated.
- The disease continues to be explored; there is little objective information on chronic hepatitis in cocker spaniels.
- The prognosis is poor when the disease is advanced.

CLIENT EDUCATION

- The incidence and genetic mode of inheritance are unknown. Affected dogs or related dogs should not be used for breeding.
- Screening laboratory enzymes in young dogs will lead to an early diagnosis and may improved prognosis with therapy.

SUGGESTED READING

Anderson M, et al: Breed, sex, and age distribution in dogs with chronic liver disease: A demographic study. *J Small Anim Pract* 32:1-5, 1991.

Center SA: Chronic liver diseases. In Guilford WG, et al (eds): *Strombeck's Small Animal Gastroenterology*. Philadelphia, WB Saunders, 1996, pp 766-801.

Hardy RM: Chronic hepatitis in dogs: A syndrome. *Compend Contin Educ Pract Vet* 8:904-913, 1986.

AUTHOR: **DAVID C. TWEDT**

EDITOR: **KEITH P. RICHTER**

Hepatitis (Chronic) of Doberman Pinscher Dogs

BASIC INFORMATION

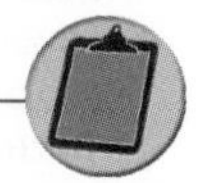

DEFINITION

A progressive chronic inflammatory liver disease associated with hepatic copper accumulation distinct to Doberman pinschers

SYNONYM(S)

Chronic active hepatitis in Doberman pinschers

Copper-associated chronic hepatitis

Doberman hepatitis

EPIDEMIOLOGY

SPECIES, AGE, SEX: Doberman pinschers. Most are diagnosed between the ages of 2 and 6 years. Most are females.

GENETICS AND BREED PREDISPOSITION

- The high incidence in this breed suggests a genetic predisposition.
- Occurrence in this breed may have a prevalence of 2-20% depending on clinical reports.
- Mode of genetic transmission is unknown.

CLINICAL PRESENTATION

DISEASE FORMS/SUBTYPES

- Subclinical hepatitis
- Clinical hepatitis

HISTORY, CHIEF COMPLAINT

- Dogs with subclinical hepatitis show no clinical signs; the disease is discov-

ered incidentally (e.g., diagnostic work-up triggered by liver enzyme elevation on serum biochemistry panel or microhepatica on abdominal imaging).
- Historic signs of early clinical hepatitis are often vague and may be associated with intermittent gastrointestinal signs and weight loss.
- When clinical hepatitis progresses to liver failure, some or all of the following historic signs may occur:
  - Polydipsia, polyuria
  - Weight loss
  - Abdominal distention
  - Altered mental status associated with hepatic encephalopathy
- In advanced disease, the patient may have a rapid deterioration.

PHYSICAL EXAM FINDINGS: With clinical hepatitis some or all of the following may be found:
- Weight loss
- Icterus
- Ascites
- Signs of hepatic encephalopathy (depression/drowsiness, propulsive pacing, seizures) (see Hepatic Encephalopathy, p 489)
- Evidence of hemorrhage (gastrointestinal, overt)

ETIOLOGY AND PATHOPHYSIOLOGY
- The etiology and mode of genetic transmission are unknown.
- Hepatic copper accumulation occurs in affected dogs and is believed to play a role in the disease.
- Studies suggest there may be a defect in biliary copper excretion.
- Inappropriate major histocompatability complex class II antigen expression in affected dogs also suggests there may also be an autoimmune component in this condition.

DIAGNOSIS

DIFFERENTIAL DIAGNOSIS
- Hepatic disease from other causes
- Nonhepatic conditions associated with abnormal liver enzymes

INITIAL DATABASE
- Subclinical disease:
  - Elevation in serum alanine aminotransferase (ALT) first, followed by increases in other liver enzymes
- Clinical disease:
  - Elevation in serum ALT, aspartate aminotransferase, γ-glutamyl transferase, and alkaline phosphatase
  - Abnormal serum bile acid concentrations
- Advanced disease with loss of liver function: some or all of the following abnormalities may result:
  - Elevation in serum total bilirubin concentration
  - Low serum albumin, blood urea nitrogen, and glucose concentrations
  - Abnormal clotting times

ADVANCED OR CONFIRMATORY TESTING
- Abdominal radiographs show a small liver ± evidence of ascites (loss of serosal detail, abdominal distention).
- Abdominal ultrasound may demonstrate:
  - A small liver with altered parenchymal echogenicity. Findings vary from normal appearance (in early disease) to heterogeneous mottling, microhepatica with nodular changes, and an irregular surface.
  - Ascites which, on centesis, may be a pure transudate or a modified transudate; the cellularity is not usually helpful diagnostically.
  - Vascular changes (e.g., multiple extrahepatic portosystemic shunts) associated with portal hypertension.
- Surgery or laparoscopy: The liver may appear normal in subclinical disease or may be small, micronodular, macronodular, and/or fibrotic in clinical disease.
- Liver biopsy and histopathology:
  - Large biopsies (obtained via laparoscopy or laparotomy) are preferred over needle core biopsies or fine-needle aspirates due to superior diagnostic accuracy.
  - Subclinical disease is associated with infiltration of mononuclear inflammatory cells into portal and parenchymal areas, and clinical disease is associated with evidence of active hepatitis including areas of piecemeal and bridging necrosis.
  - Bridging fibrosis and/or cirrhosis with nodular regeneration eventually occur.
  - Histochemical staining for copper and iron are positive.
- Hepatic metal quantitative analysis: Hepatic copper ranges from 400 to 2000 μg/g dry weight liver (normal <400 μg/g). Hepatic iron (thought to be secondary to chronic inflammation and not diagnostic of this disease specifically) ranges from 1500 to 7000 μg/g dry weight liver.

TREATMENT

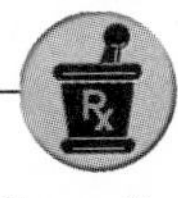

THERAPEUTIC GOAL(S)
- Slow the progression of the liver disease in subclinical cases
- Provide specific therapy for the chronic hepatitis and copper accumulation
- Provide supportive treatment specifically aimed at controlling or avoiding complications of liver disease, including hepatic encephalopathy, ascites, gastrointestinal ulceration, and nutritional imbalance

ACUTE GENERAL TREATMENT
- Subclinical and early clinical hepatitis with high copper concentrations (>600 μg/g liver).
  - d-Penicillamine or trientine (15 mg/kg PO q 12h) for 2 to 4 months or longer after measuring hepatic copper concentrations. Liver lesions improve as a result of lowering copper concentrations. Chelator therapy use should be based on identifying the characteristic histopathologic lesions and hepatic copper concentrations.
  - Glucocorticoid therapy (prednisone or prednisolone 2–4 mg/kg PO q 24–48h) may be beneficial in slowing inflammatory component of the liver disease.
  - Ensure adequate nutrient intake.
- Advanced clinical hepatitis (see Hepatitis [Chronic, Idiopathic] of Dogs, p 503).
  - Treatment for hepatic encephalopathy using a high-quality, low-protein diet, lactulose (0.1–0.5 ml/kg PO q 12h, adjusted to achieve loose fecal consistency) and/or intestinal antibiotics (e.g., neomycin 20 mg/kg PO q 8h, metronidazole 7.5 mg/kg PO q 12h, or amoxicillin-clavulanate 15 mg/kg PO q 12h).
  - Treatment for ascites
    - If very voluminous ("tense," producing marked abdominal distention, discomfort, inappetence, and possibly dyspnea), consider abdominal drainage/centesis (see Abdominal Drainage, p 1176).
    - Smaller amounts of ascites are either not treated, or are treated with diuretics (spironolactone 1 mg/kg PO q 12h and/or furosemide 0.5–2 mg/kg PO q 12h).
  - Treatment for gastric ulceration: ranitidine (2 mg/kg PO q 12h) or omeprazole (0.5–1 mg/kg PO q 24h).

CHRONIC TREATMENT
- Copper chelation to maintain hepatic concentrations near normal.
  - After adequate chelation, zinc acetate may be used for blocking enteric copper uptake. Adequate chelation is most accurately determined by rebiopsy; if rebiopsy is not possible, the change from chelation therapy to zinc therapy is generally warranted after 6 to 12 months of treatment, if the dog is doing well clinically with improving biochemical parameters.
  - Zinc acetate: 100 mg of elemental zinc PO q 12h as loading dose for 2 months, then 50 mg PO q 12h.
  - Zinc dose should be adjusted to keep serum zinc concentrations between 200 and 800 μg/dl. Note: blood samples for zinc levels must be drawn into specific tubes (navy top), because standard rubber tops contain zinc.

- Anti-inflammatory therapy using prednisolone or prednisone (2 mg/kg PO q 24h).
  - The dosage is often tapered to an alternate day therapy once there is clinical improvement.
  - Glucocorticoids cause a secondary steroid hepatopathy and monitoring liver enzymes is generally not helpful. However, there should be a decline in serum bilirubin concentration and an increase in serum albumin concentration as the patient improves.
  - With ascites, dexamethasone (0.2 mg/kg PO q 24h) should be used instead to avoid mineralocorticoid effect.

For glucocorticoid-intolerant animals or when additional immunomodulation is desired, azathioprine (2 mg/kg PO q 24h for 1 week then q 48h) can be given alone or in combination with glucocorticoids.

- Ascites: long-term management:
  - In the hydrated patient, diuretics (see previous) also may be used long-term, either alone or as an adjunct to abdominal drainage, to delay the recurrence of ascites.
  - Repeated abdominocentesis (when ascites becomes large-volume/tense, and causes lethargy/inappetence) is also possible for long-term management of ascites.
- Diet is important to supply adequate calories. Palatability is important in advanced cases. Dietary protein is restricted only with protein intolerance (hepatic encephalopathy). Feed a high-quality, moderate protein content diet given in small multiple feedings. Milk and vegetable protein sources are better for avoiding hepatic encephalopathy than meat protein-based diets. Fermentable fiber may also be beneficial in controlling hepatic encephalopathy.
- General liver support may include ursodeoxycholic acid (15 mg/kg PO q 24h), antioxidants (vitamin E, 10–15 IU/kg PO q 24h; s-adenosylmethionine, 20 mg/kg PO q 24h), and antifibrotics (colchicine, 0.03 mg/kg PO q 24h). (See Hepatitis [Chronic, Idiopathic] of Dogs, p 503.)

DRUG INTERACTIONS

- Penicillamine and zinc should not be given together, as the penicillamine may chelate the zinc.
- Animals with hepatic failure are anesthetic risks. Barbiturates should be avoided and benzodiazepines should be used with care. Isoflurane or sevoflurane are the gas anesthetics of choice. Propofol, although hepatically metabolized, may be administered to effect (usually requiring a small fraction of normal doses) for controlling seizures due to hepatic encephalopathy.
- Lidocaine, theophylline, propranolol, captopril, and tetracyclines should be avoided.
- Diuretics may worsen hepatic encephalopathy, promote dehydration or metabolic alkalosis, and should be used only in otherwise stable patients for the long-term delay of return of ascites, or for concurrent conditions (e.g., congestive heart failure).
- Nonsteroidal anti-inflammatory drugs may exacerbate gastrointestinal ulceration.
- Avoid drugs that require hepatic metabolism or alter hepatic biotransformation (e.g., cimetidine). Glucocorticoids may cause sodium retention, promote gastrointestinal ulceration, or precipitate hepatic failure with advanced disease.

POSSIBLE COMPLICATIONS

- Glucocorticoids may precipitate ascites, hepatic encephalopathy, and early death in advanced cases. Therefore, if ascites develops shortly after starting prednisone, consider switching to dexamethasone. If gastrointestinal ulceration develops, it should be addressed as discussed previously.
- Penicillamine and zinc should be given on an empty stomach but may cause vomiting. *The risk of vomiting may be reduced by beginning penicillamine at the low end of the dosage range and titrating up.* Zinc overdose may cause hemolysis, although the doses required to reach toxic levels are extremely high (many times higher than the therapeutic dose).

RECOMMENDED MONITORING

- Complete blood count, serum biochemistry profile, and urinalysis for disease progression, remission, or complications.
- Periodic liver biopsies are the best means of evaluating the stage and progression of the disease during therapy.

PROGNOSIS AND OUTCOME

- Diagnosis and appropriate therapy in subclinical cases may delay or lessen the disease for years
- Overt clinical manifestations of hepatitis denote advanced disease, and the long-term prognosis is guarded

PEARLS & CONSIDERATIONS

COMMENTS

- The first abnormality observed in young subclinically affected dogs is an increase in serum ALT activities and therefore unexplained ALT activities should be investigated.
- Copper reduction and immunomodulation appear to be helpful; however, clinical studies evaluating therapy are limited.
- While the diagnosis is confirmed with a liver biopsy, the treatment and prognosis depend mainly on whether the disease is subclinical (incidental finding, no clinical signs) or clinically overt (presence of advanced signs of liver disease, including encephalopathy and portal hypertension).

CLIENT EDUCATION

- The incidence and genetic mode of inheritance are unknown. Affected dogs or related dogs should not be used for breeding.
- Screening laboratory enzymes in young dogs will lead to an early diagnosis and improved prognosis with therapy. Since the disease is common in the Doberman breed, all dogs should undergo yearly or biannual blood biochemical screening after 2 years of age.

SUGGESTED READING

Mandigers PJJ, et al: Improvement in liver pathology after 4 months of d-penicillamine in 5 Doberman pinschers with subclinical hepatitis. *J Vet Intern Med* 19:40–43, 2004.

Speeti M, et al: Subclinical versus clinical hepatitis in the Doberman: Evaluation of changes in blood parameters. *J Small Anim Pract* 37:465–470, 1996.

AUTHOR: **DAVID C. TWEDT**
EDITOR: **KEITH P. RICHTER**

Hepatitis (Chronic, Idiopathic) of Dogs

Client Education Sheet on Website

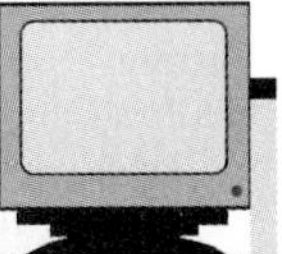

BASIC INFORMATION

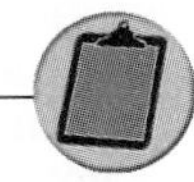

DEFINITION

Chronic progressive hepatic disorder of unknown etiology, characterized by parenchymal inflammation, hepatocyte necrosis, and variable fibrosis

SYNONYM(S)

Chronic active hepatitis
Chronic hepatitis
Chronic hepatopathy

EPIDEMIOLOGY

SPECIES, AGE, SEX: Middle-aged dogs 3 to 10 years of age (mean: 7 years). Females are overrepresented.

GENETICS AND BREED PREDISPOSITION: Breed predispositions occur in the Labrador retriever, standard poodle, cocker spaniel (see Hepatitis [Chronic] of Cocker Spaniel Dogs, p 499) and Scottish terrier. There is also chronic hepatitis-associated genetic-based copper accumulation (see Hepatopathy, Copper-Associated, p 509) observed in the Bedlington terrier, West Highland white terrier, Doberman pinscher (see Hepatitis [Chronic] of Doberman Pinscher Dogs), Skye terrier, and keeshond.

RISK FACTORS: Drug therapy (including phenobarbital, nonsteroidal anti-inflammatory or other drugs), infectious agents such as leptospirosis, and post-toxin induced hepatic damage may result in hepatitis, which eventually may progress to chronic hepatitis.

CONTAGION AND ZOONOSIS: Leptospirosis, infectious canine hepatitis, and canine adenovirus are associated with chronic hepatitis and potentially are contagious (all three) and zoonotic (leptospirosis).

ASSOCIATED CONDITIONS AND DISORDERS: Hepatic inflammation can occur secondary to disorders such as pancreatitis, peritonitis, or inflammatory bowel disease. The type and character of inflammation in the liver is different from typical progressive idiopathic chronic hepatitis: In these disorders, the inflammation is usually mild, confined to the portal triads, and there is an absence of fibrosis.

CLINICAL PRESENTATION

DISEASE FORMS/SUBTYPES: Chronic hepatitis is a progressive disease associated with several clinical stages:

- Subclinical hepatitis associated only with abnormal serum liver enzyme levels
- Clinical hepatitis
- Cirrhosis and hepatic failure

HISTORY, CHIEF COMPLAINT: Historic signs for clinical disease will vary based on the extent of liver damage and include the following:

- Subclinical:
  - None
- Either clinical hepatitis or cirrhosis/hepatic failure:
  - Vomiting
  - Anorexia
  - Weight loss
  - Lethargy
  - Polyuria or polydipsia
  - Signs associated with hepatic encephalopathy
- Cirrhosis/hepatic failure:
  - Abdominal distention from ascites

PHYSICAL EXAM FINDINGS: Physical findings will vary with the severity of the disease:

- Subclinical dogs appear normal.
- Abnormal findings in clinically ill dogs include:
  - Icterus
  - Poor body condition
  - Hepatic encephalopathy
  - Ascites (mainly in cirrhosis/hepatic failure)

ETIOLOGY AND PATHOPHYSIOLOGY

- In most cases etiology is unknown.
- Infectious causes including leptospirosis, canine adenovirus-1 (infectious canine hepatitis) infection, *Bartonella* spp. infection, as well as other possible infectious agents.
- Immune-mediated mechanisms may be responsible, but this has been poorly documented in the dog.
- Drug-associated chronic hepatitis from anticonvulsants, nonsteroidal anti-inflammatory drugs (NSAIDs), trimethoprim-sulfa antibiotics, and oxibendazole. It is possible that any drug has potential to cause liver disease.
- Copper-associated liver disease due to defective copper metabolism.
- Other conditions such as aflatoxins, chemicals, or other environmental factors may be responsible.

DIAGNOSIS

DIFFERENTIAL DIAGNOSIS

- Acute hepatitis
- Hepatic neoplasia
- Pancreatitis
- Reactive hepatopathies secondary to systemic or metabolic disease and gastrointestinal (GI) disease
- Congenital portosystemic shunts

INITIAL DATABASE

- Complete blood count (CBC): nonregenerative anemia, variable white blood cell count.
- Serum biochemistry profile: increased liver enzyme levels, including alanine aminotransferase (ALT), aspartate aminotransferase (AST), alkaline phosphatase (ALP), and γ-glutamyl transferase (GGT). In advanced disease increased total bilirubin concentration, and decreased albumin, glucose, blood urea nitrogen, and/or cholesterol concentrations may occur. Hyperglobulinemia is often observed.
- Urinalysis: bilirubinuria, variable specific gravity, and sometimes ammonium biurate crystalluria associated with hyperammonemia.
- Abdominal radiographs: small liver and possibly signs of ascites in advanced disease (cirrhosis/hepatic failure).

ADVANCED OR CONFIRMATORY TESTING

- Elevated serum bile acid concentrations.
- Elevated plasma ammonia concentrations or ammonia tolerance test (variable results).
- Coagulation tests: prothrombin time (PT), activated partial thromboplastin time (aPTT), and proteins inducted by vitamin K antagonism (PIVKA). Of these, the PIVKA test is the most sensitive. With advanced disease, these become abnormal and reflect severe liver dysfunction.
- Abdominal ultrasonography: variable hepatic parenchymal changes. Microhepatica, nodular liver, and ascites (normal diameter caudal vena cava and hepatic veins help to rule out right-sided heart failure as cause of ascites) in late stage disease (cirrhosis/hepatic failure).
- Serologic testing for antinuclear antibody (ANA) titer and infectious agents such as *Leptospira interrogans*, *Bartonella* spp., or other specific tests where indicated.
- Abdominocentesis in patients with ascites may reveal either a pure transudate or modified transudate.
- Surgery or laparoscopy: The liver may appear normal in subclinical disease or may be small, nodular, and fibrotic/firm in advanced clinical disease.

- Liver biopsy and histopathologic evaluation:
  - Large biopsies (obtained via laparoscopy or laparotomy) are preferred over needle core biopsies or fine-needle aspirates due to superior diagnostic accuracy.
  - Subclinical disease is associated with infiltration of mononuclear inflammatory cells into portal and parenchymal areas.
  - Clinical disease has evidence of active hepatitis with areas of piecemeal and bridging necrosis.
  - With cirrhosis, extensive fibrosis and nodular regeneration are present.
  - Histochemical staining for copper and iron are often positive.
- Hepatic metal quantitative analysis: Hepatic copper can accumulate secondary to the liver disease and concentrations often range from 600–1500 μg/g dry weight liver (normal <400 μg/g). Hepatic iron is often elevated and zinc concentrations are frequently subnormal.

TREATMENT

THERAPEUTIC GOAL(S)

- Remove the inciting etiology if identified
- Provide optimal nutrition
- Stop the progression of ongoing hepatitis
- Provide for optimal hepatic support
- Treat specific complications as they occur

ACUTE GENERAL TREATMENT

Acute complications of chronic hepatitis should be treated as they occur. Commonly used treatments during acute management of idiopathic chronic hepatitis include:

- Fluid therapy to correct deficits and electrolyte losses. Supplemental dextrose (2.5–5%) is recommended; limit sodium with ascites (e.g., switch to low-sodium, isotonic maintenance fluid when patient is hydrated [e.g., Plasmalyte 56 + 5% dextrose, with potassium supplementation]).
- Dextrans, plasma, or albumin infusions may be used for improving oncotic pressure.
  - Plasma advantages include presence of albumin (contributes positively to protein balance), presence of coagulation factors, and persistence in the circulation (versus protein losing enteropathy or nephropathy, where the transfused proteins may be lost quickly); drawbacks include cost and short shelf life (fresh) or need to freeze (fresh frozen).
- Gastric ulceration managed using sucralfate (0.5–1 gm PO q 8h) and ranitidine (2 mg/kg PO q 12h). Avoid cimetidine or proton pump inhibitors due to hepatic metabolism.
- Hepatic encephalopathy treatment using cleansing enemas or retention enemas (betadine diluted 1:10 or lactulose diluted 1:3). Chronic management involves low protein diets, lactulose, and neomycin (see Hepatic Encephalopathy, p 489).
- Coagulopathies are treated with fresh frozen plasma or fresh whole blood if there is clinical evidence of overt bleeding.
- Ascites treated with abdominocentesis if abdomen is tense and the animal is uncomfortable. (See Abdominocentesis, p 1178; Abdominal Drainage, p 1176.) Diuretics are less effective and possibly associated with greater side effects in the acute stages of mobilizing ascitic fluid.
- Sepsis is treated with appropriate antibiotics (see Sepsis and Septic Shock, p 996).

CHRONIC TREATMENT

- Diet is important to supply adequate calories. Palatability is important in advanced cases. Dietary protein is restricted only with protein intolerance (hepatic encephalopathy). Feed a high-quality moderate protein content diet given in small multiple feedings. Milk and vegetable protein sources are more beneficial in hepatic encephalopathy than meat protein-based diets. Fermentable fiber may also be beneficial in controlling hepatic encephalopathy.
- Anti-inflammatory therapy using prednisolone or prednisone (2 mg/kg PO q 24h). The dosage is often tapered to an alternate day therapy once there is clinical improvement. Corticosteroids cause a secondary steroid hepatopathy and monitoring liver enzymes is generally not helpful. However, there should be a decline in serum bilirubin concentration and an increase in serum albumin concentration as the patient improves. With ascites, dexamethasone (0.2 mg/kg PO q 24–48h) should be used instead to avoid mineralocorticoid effect. For corticosteroid intolerant animals or when additional immunomodulation is desired azathioprine (2 mg/kg q 24h for 1 week, then q 48h) can be given alone or in combination with glucocorticoids.
- Copper chelation is indicated if hepatic copper concentrations are greater than 1000 μg/g dry liver weight. D-penicillamine or trientine (10–15 mg/kg PO q 12h) is administered to remove copper. Following chelation, chronic zinc supplementation is used for blocking GI absorption of copper.
- Zinc has antioxidant and antifibrotic effects. Hepatic zinc deficiency occurs in advanced liver disease and supplementation is indicated at 2–3 mg/kg PO q 24h. Higher doses of zinc will block intestinal copper absorption (see Hepatopathy, Copper-Associated, p 509).
- Ursodeoxycholic acid (10–15 mg PO q 24h) has immunomodulatory, antioxidant, hepatoprotective, and choleretic effects.
- Antifibrotic drug colchicine (0.03 mg/kg PO q 24h) inhibits collagen formation. However, few studies report its use in dogs. Side effects are often GI.
- Antioxidant therapy is used as adjunct liver support. Selection of one or several antioxidants is suggested including vitamin E (10 IU/kg PO q 24h), S-adenosylmethionine (20 mg/kg PO q 24h or q 48h), milk thistle (silybin the active isomer at 5 mg/kg PO q 12h), or others could be used.
- Ascites:
  - Medical treatment involves diuretics for long-term chronic management. Spironolactone (0.5–1 mg/kg PO q 12h) or furosemide (0.5–2 mg/kg PO q 12h) or combination of both drugs as needed.
  - Centesis/drainage may be performed intermittently as needed for comfort when patients develop tense ascites (very large volumes of abdominal fluid).

DRUG INTERACTIONS

- Avoid drugs that require hepatic metabolism or alter hepatic biotransformation (e.g., cimetidine). Glucocorticoids may cause sodium retention, promote GI ulceration, or precipitate hepatic failure with advanced disease.
- Penicillamine and zinc should not be given together as the penicillamine may chelate the zinc.
- Animals with hepatic failure are anesthetic risks. Barbiturates should be avoided and benzodiazepines should be used with care. Isoflurane or sevoflurane are the gas anesthetics of choice. Propofol, although hepatically metabolized, may be administered to effect (usually requiring a small fraction of normal doses) for controlling seizures due to hepatic encephalopathy.
- Lidocaine, theophylline, propranolol, captopril and tetracyclines should be avoided if possible.
- Diuretics may worsen hepatic encephalopathy, promote dehydration or metabolic alkalosis, and should be used only in otherwise stable patients for the long-term delay of return of ascites, or for concurrent conditions (e.g., congestive heart failure).
- Nonsteroidal anti-inflammatory drugs may exacerbate GI ulceration.

POSSIBLE COMPLICATIONS

- Hepatic encephalopathy
- Ascites
- GI ulceration
- Sepsis
- Disseminated intravascular coagulation
- Hepatic failure and death

RECOMMENDED MONITORING

- Monitor general condition, body weight, and behavior
- Periodic evaluation of laboratory tests (CBC and serum biochemical profile)

PROGNOSIS AND OUTCOME

- Guarded to fair based on clinical signs at the time of diagnosis and extent of liver damage as determined grossly and histopathologically.
- Most dogs are diagnosed when clinical signs occur, which is usually associated with advanced hepatitis and a guarded prognosis.
- When severe signs of liver failure occur, such as ascites, hepatic encephalopathy, and hypoalbuminemia, the prognosis is grave.
- Early diagnosis and therapy will prolong survival, but limited studies are available on survival times.

PEARLS & CONSIDERATIONS

COMMENTS

- The first clue to chronic hepatitis is unexplained abnormal serum liver enzyme levels.
- Because of the great reserve capacity of the liver, signs of liver failure do not occur until the disease is advanced.
- Therapy in early stages of hepatitis may prolong survival.

CLIENT EDUCATION

- A complete cure is unlikely.
- Medication is generally lifelong but may prolong quality of life and survival times.
- There are few studies evaluating therapy for chronic hepatitis in the dog and repeat liver biopsies are recommended to monitor response to therapy.

SUGGESTED READING

Dill-Mackay E: Chronic hepatitis in dogs. *Vet Clin North Am Small Anim Pract* 25:387-398, 1995.

Fuentealba C, et al: Chronic hepatitis: retrospective study in 34 dogs. *Can Vet J* 38:365-373, 1997.

Sevelius E: Diagnosis and prognosis of chronic hepatitis and cirrhosis in dogs. *J Small Anim Pract* 36:521-528, 1995.

Strombeck DR, et al: Effects of corticosteroid treatment on survival time in dogs with chronic hepatitis: 151 cases. *J Am Vet Med Assoc* 9:1109-1117, 1988.

AUTHOR: **DAVID C. TWEDT**
EDITOR: **KEITH P. RICHTER**

Hepatitis, Infectious Canine

BASIC INFORMATION

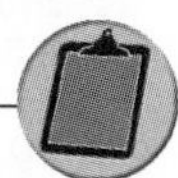

DEFINITION

A specific form of liver disease caused by canine adenovirus-1 (CAV-1, similar to human adenovirus) that can cause acute death or chronic hepatitis. Infectious canine hepatitis (ICH) is uncommon in well-vaccinated dog populations.

SYNONYM(S)

"Blue eye"
ICH

EPIDEMIOLOGY

SPECIES, AGE, SEX: Dogs, coyotes, foxes, and bears can be infected. Usually the disease is seen in dogs less than 1 year old, but dogs of any age that are unvaccinated can be affected.

RISK FACTORS: Nonvaccinated dogs.

CONTAGION AND ZOONOSIS

- Dog-to-dog transmission occurs directly (oronasal infection from secretions of infected animals—urine, feces, etc.)
- Not zoonotic

ASSOCIATED CONDITIONS AND DISORDERS: Chronic hepatitis may occur if the animal survives the initial viremic stage.

CLINICAL PRESENTATION

HISTORY, CHIEF COMPLAINT

- Animals usually have a poor vaccination history on presentation.
- During the acute viremic stage, animals can become moribund and die within a few hours.
- After the acute viremic stage, animals typically present with vomiting, diarrhea, and/or abdominal pain.

PHYSICAL EXAM FINDINGS

- Fever, cervical lymphadenopathy, tachycardia, tachypnea, abdominal tenderness, hepatomegaly.
- Icterus and abdominal distention may be seen in advanced cases.
- Anterior uveitis and corneal edema ("blue eye") are hallmarks.
- Central nervous system signs consistent with hepatic encephalopathy or viral encephalitis, including depression, seizures, disorientation, coma.
- Signs of coagulopathy: petechial and ecchymotic hemorrhages, epistaxis, excessive bleeding from venipuncture sites.

ETIOLOGY AND PATHOPHYSIOLOGY

- Adenovirus-1 is transmitted by oronasal exposure to secretions of infected animals, notably urine. It can also be transmitted by fomites, and ectoparasites can harbor CAV-1.
- The virus initially localizes in the tonsils after exposure. From the tonsils, it disseminates to regional lymph nodes and then through the thoracic duct to the systemic circulation.
- Virus is found in body tissues and secretions, including urine, feces, and saliva, 4 to 8 days postinfection.
- The virus is found in many tissues, including the kidneys 10 to 14 days postinfection; it is secreted in the urine for 6 to 9 months postinfection.
- Predilection for hepatic parenchymal cells (causing acute hepatic injury/necrosis) and vascular endothelial cells (multiple organ injury).
- Cytotoxic effects of the virus cause the initial cellular injury to the eye, liver, and kidney.
- Subclinical infections are widespread, predominantly in dogs with circulating antibody at the time of infection.

DIAGNOSIS

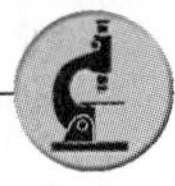

DIFFERENTIAL DIAGNOSIS

- Liver diseases:
  - Portosystemic shunts
  - Leptospirosis
  - Toxins
  - Copper hepatopathy
  - Cholelithiasis/cholangitis
  - Gallbladder rupture
- Pancreatitis
- Canine distemper

INITIAL DATABASE

- Complete blood count/serum biochemistry profile.
  - Neutropenia and lymphopenia initially, then rebound neutrophilia and lymphocytosis.
  - ALT and alkaline phosphatase elevation for 14 days postinfection, then decline unless chronic hepatitis occurs. With chronic hepatitis, signs of hepatic synthetic failure (hypoglycemia hypoalbuminemia, low blood urea nitrogen) may be present.
- Urinalysis: proteinuria.
- Coagulation panel: Changes are most often seen in the viremic stage and include thrombocytopenia, prolongation of prothrombin time, activated par-

tial thromboplastin time, and thrombin time (TT).
- Serum bile acids (postprandial): often elevated with hepatic encephalopathy.

ADVANCED OR CONFIRMATORY TESTING

- Cytologic (aspirates, impression smears) or histologic examination of liver: characteristic inclusion bodies (Cowdry type A).
- Cerebrospinal fluid: usually normal.
- Bone marrow aspirate: decreased megakaryocytes during viremic stage.
- Serologic testing (complement fixation, immunodiffusion, enzyme-linked immunosorbent assay), virus isolation, and immunofluorescent testing are available, but an accurate clinical diagnosis is generally possible without these tests.
- Similarly, the virus can be cultured from any body tissue 5 days postinfection; the kidney is the most persistent site.

TREATMENT

THERAPEUTIC GOAL(S)

Treatment is mostly supportive and nonspecific in nature

ACUTE GENERAL TREATMENT

- Fluid therapy
- Correction of coagulation disturbances with fresh frozen plasma or whole blood (see Transfusion Therapy and Collection Techniques for Blood Banking, p 1312)
- Management of hypoglycemia: intravenous glucose 0.5 g/kg IV bolus (= 1 ml 50% dextrose/kg body weight; before administration, must be diluted with 5 to 10 ml sterile water/ml 50% dextrose to avoid phlebitis/perivascular irritation) followed by 2.5-5% dextrose infused in balanced electrolyte solution
- Lactulose for animals exhibiting neurologic signs (0.5 ml/kg PO q 8h)

CHRONIC TREATMENT

If chronic hepatitis results, the following therapy may be considered (see also Cirrhotic/Fibrosing Liver Disease, p 210; Hepatic Encephalopathy, p 489):

- Diet: protein-restricted diet in animals with hepatic encephalopathy. All other animals should be given a high carbohydrate, moderate fat diet. Dietary fiber has been shown to bind bile acids and aid in their removal; therefore, psyllium 1-3 tsp/day can be added to the diet.
- Prednisone or prednisolone: 1-2 mg/kg PO q 24h. After clinical improvement, taper the dose to 0.5mg/kg/ day, then every other day.
- Colchicine 0.03 mg/kg PO q 24h may help to decrease formation of hepatic fibrosis.
- Vitamin E: 50-400 IU PO q 24h.
- S-Adenososylmethionine (SAMe): 20 mg/kg PO q 24h.
- Milk thistle: 50-250 mg/kg PO q 12h.

POSSIBLE COMPLICATIONS

- Pyelonephritis
- Disseminated intravascular coagulation
- Glaucoma

RECOMMENDED MONITORING

For chronic hepatitis:

- Serum bile acids
- Repeat liver biopsy 6 months after starting treatment

PROGNOSIS AND OUTCOME

- Prognosis for acute, fulminant infection is grave: animals often die within hours.
- Long-term prognosis for chronic hepatitis secondary to adenovirus-1 is guarded.
  - Animals with hypoalbuminemia, hypoglycemia, and coagulopathies usually die within 1 week of diagnosis.

PEARLS & CONSIDERATIONS

PREVENTION

- Routine vaccination (D*H*LPP) provides protection against infectious canine hepatitis.
- Modified live vaccine using CAV-2 isolates is used for preventing infectious canine hepatitis. The CAV-2 MLV vaccine has reduced side effects (corneal edema, fever) compared to the CAV-1 vaccine.
- A routine initial series, followed by a booster at one year and then every 3 years, is recommended.

SUGGESTED READING

Boomkens SY, et al: Hepatitis with special reference to dogs. A review on the pathogenesis and infectious etiologies, including unpublished results of recent own studies. *Vet Q* 26:3, 2004.

Caudell D, et al: Diagnosis of infectious canine hepatitis virus (CAV-1) infection in puppies with encephalopathy. *J Vet Diagn Invest* 17:1, 2005.

Greene CE: Infectious canine hepatitis and canine acidophil cell hepatitis. In Greene CE (ed): *Infectious Diseases of the Dog and Cat*, ed 2. Philadelphia, WB Saunders, 2000, pp 22-28.

AUTHOR: **KHRISTEN J. CARLSON**
EDITOR: **DOUGLASS K. MACINTIRE**

Hepatocutaneous Syndrome

BASIC INFORMATION

DEFINITION

A progressive and debilitating cutaneous disorder commonly associated with advanced hepatic disease and rarely with a glucagon-secreting pancreatic tumor

SYNONYM(S)

Superficial necrolytic dermatitis
Necrolytic migratory erythema
Diabetic dermatopathy
Metabolic epidermal necrosis
Glucagonoma syndrome

EPIDEMIOLOGY

SPECIES, AGE, SEX

- Dogs
- Middle-aged to geriatric animals
- No gender predisposition

RISK FACTORS: Ingestion of mycotoxins; history of administration of phenobarbital, primidone, phenytoin, or combination of these drugs.

ASSOCIATED CONDITIONS AND DISORDERS

- Non-neoplastic: idiopathic vacuolar hepatopathy, cirrhosis, diabetes mellitus
- Paraneoplastic: glucagon-producing pancreatic adenocarcinoma, glucagon-secreting liver metastases, hyperglucagonemia

CLINICAL PRESENTATION

HISTORY, CHIEF COMPLAINT: Owners usually observe footpad lesions first, as dermatologic changes may precede onset of clinical signs of internal disease. Lethargy, inappetence, weight loss, lameness, reluctance to walk, pedal pain, and pruritus are frequently reported. Other chief complaints may include polyuria and polydipsia. Dermatitis may wax and wane.

PHYSICAL EXAM FINDINGS: Physical examination may reveal regional lymphadenopathy and hyperthermia. Lesions in majority of affected dogs are characterized by thickening, fissuring, and crusting of footpads, and interdigital erythema. Crusts, erosions, and ulcers can affect pinnae, mucocutaneous junctions (oral cavity, eyes, anus and genitalia), elbows and pressure points, ventral abdominal and inguinal regions.

ETIOLOGY AND PATHOPHYSIOLOGY

- Unknown.
- Keratinocyte degeneration and epidermal edema may result from cellular starvation or some other epidermal imbalance. Proposed pathogeneses include deficiencies of essential fatty acids, hypoaminoacidemia, and deficiencies in zinc and biotin.
- Hepatic impairment is also a possible mechanism.

DIAGNOSIS

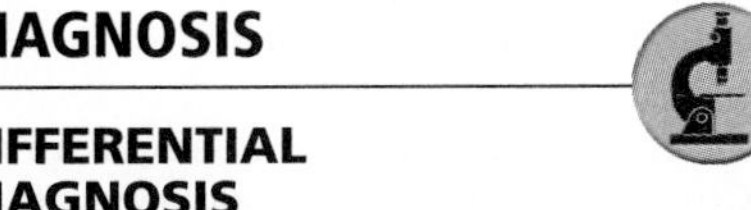

DIFFERENTIAL DIAGNOSIS

- Autoimmune/immune mediated causes: pemphigus foliaceus, drug-induced pemphigus, systemic lupus erythematosus, paraneoplastic pemphigus, cutaneous vasculitis, erythema multiforme, toxic epidermal necrolysis
- Infectious causes: bacterial (pyoderma), fungal (dermatophytosis, *Malassezia* dermatitis), protozoal (leishmaniasis)
- Parasitic causes: demodicosis
- Nutritional causes: zinc-responsive dermatosis
- Neoplastic causes: epitheliotropic lymphoma
- Idiopathic: nasodigital hyperkeratosis

INITIAL DATABASE

- Skin cytologic evaluation often indicates a secondary surface pyoderma and/or *Malassezia* dermatitis.
- Hematology: nonregenerative anemia, leukocytosis.
- Serum biochemistry profile: elevated alkaline phosphatase and alanine aminotransferase, hypoalbuminemia, hyperglycemia.
- Fasting and postprandial bile acid values are frequently elevated.
- Urinalysis: glucosuria in some cases.

ADVANCED OR CONFIRMATORY TESTING

- Skin biopsy: epidermis has a "French flag" (i.e., red-white-blue layers) appearance:
  - Upper layer (stratum corneum): *red* (eosinophilic), parakeratotic hyperkeratosis, crust
  - Middle layer (stratum spinosum): *white* (pale), edema, and necrosis of the keratinocytes
  - Deep layer (stratum basale): *blue* (basophilic), hyperplasia
  - Clefting (ulceration) at level of middle layer may occur and a mixed inflammatory infiltrate may occupy the dermis.
- Abdominal ultrasonographic findings are characterized by hypoechoic nodules with a hyperechoic trabecular network throughout the liver, resulting in a "honeycomb" or "Swiss cheese" pattern of the hepatic parenchyma.
- Ultrasound-guided hepatic biopsy (first perform platelet count, arterial blood pressure, and clotting panel to assess bleeding risk): hepatic neoplasia or idiopathic vacuolar hepatopathy (characterized by nodular hyperplasia and hepatocyte vacuolar degeneration adjacent to areas of parenchymal collapse).
- Complete plasma amino acids (hypoaminoacidemia) testing is available at Amino Acid Analysis Laboratory Service (University of California, Davis). Contact laboratory for sample handling and cost (www.vetmed.ucdavis.edu/vmb/aal/aal.html).
- Due to lack of specificity, utility of plasma glucagon (hyperglucagonemia) and serum insulin (hyperinsulinemia) testing is limited.

TREATMENT

THERAPEUTIC GOAL(S)

- Supportive, nonspecific therapy for the dermatologic manifestations
- Management of internal disease process: may require hospitalization
- Neoplasia: surgical removal of neoplasm if possible or chemotherapy if indicated

ACUTE AND CHRONIC TREATMENT

- Dermatologic treatment:
  - Hydrotherapy and keratolytic shampoo therapy.
  - Treat secondary bacterial and fungal infections with appropriate therapy (avoid systemic azole antifungal therapy because of potential hepatotoxicity).
  - Topical glucocorticoid (e.g., 1% hydrocortisone cream) q 12h. Oral glucocorticoid use may predispose to diabetes.
  - Oral essential fatty acid and zinc supplementation (zinc methionine, 1.5 mg/kg q 24h PO, Zinpro).
- Internal disease:
  - High-quality, high-protein diet. Suitable commercial diets include Hill's Prescription Diet l/d or Eukanuba Nutritional Stress/Maximum Calorie Formula. Adding three hard-boiled entire eggs per day may also be beneficial.
  - Oral amino-acid supplementation: (Promod). 1 scoop/10 kg q24 h PO.
  - Intravenous amino-acid infusions (Aminosyn, Abbott Laboratories) as a hypertonic 10% amino-acid crystalline solution. About 500 ml/dog or 25 ml/ kg body weight (empiric dosages) over 6 to 8 hours. Repeat every 7 to 14 days based on response.
    - Some dermatologists recommend three treatments the first week, followed by once or twice weekly thereafter. Most patients will demonstrate clinical improvement within 5 to 10 days.
    - Monitor for signs of encephalopathy (slow down infusion rate if indicated).
    - Because of the high osmolality of this solution, a central (jugular) venous catheter is recommended to avoid thrombophlebitis.
    - A mixed amino-acid/electrolyte solution (Procalamine, B. Braun) is advocated as an alternative product. Advantages of the latter include lower cost and lesser hypertonicity (can therefore be injected in peripheral veins).
  - Oral nutraceutical S-adenosylmethionine 90–225 mg/dog PO q 24h (SAMe, Denosyl SD-4, Zentonil, S-Adenosyl) can attenuate liver damage.
  - Insulin therapy and dietary management (as appropriate).

PROGNOSIS AND OUTCOME

Guarded to poor, particularly in patients with idiopathic vacuolar hepatopathy (e.g., dogs with hepatocutaneous syndrome and a history of phenobarbital administration are often euthanized within 12 weeks of diagnosis, despite drug discontinuation)

PEARLS & CONSIDERATIONS

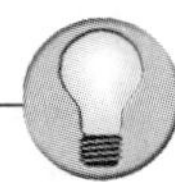

COMMENTS

In dogs, this disorder occurs more commonly in association with a non-neoplastic hepatopathy, giving rise to the familiar name of hepatocutaneous syndrome.

SUGGESTED READING

Byrne KP: Metabolic epidermal necrosis: Hepatocutaneous syndrome. *Vet Clin North Am Small Anim Pract* 29:1337, 1999.

Jacobson LS, et al: Hepatic ultrasonography and pathological findings in dogs with hepatocutaneous syndrome: New concepts. *J Vet Intern Med* 9(6):399, 1995.

March PA, et al: Superficial necrolytic dermatitis in 11 dogs with a history of phenobarbital administration (1995–2002). *J Vet Intern Med* 18:65, 2004.

Outerbridge CA, et al: Plasma amino acid concentrations in 36 dogs with histologically confirmed superficial necrolytic dermatitis. *Vet Dermatol* 13:177, 2002.

Scott DW, et al: Necrolytic migratory erythema. In *Kirk and Muller Small Animal Dermatology*, ed 6. Philadelphia, WB Saunders, 2001, pp 868–873.

AUTHOR: **VINCENT E. DEFALQUE**
EDITOR: **JAN A. HALL**

Hepatomegaly

BASIC INFORMATION

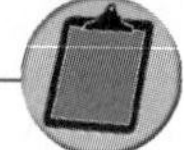

DEFINITION

Liver enlargement

EPIDEMIOLOGY

SPECIES, AGE, SEX: Observed in both dogs and cats. Hepatomegaly is more frequently observed in middle-aged to older animals due to age-related prevalence of associated disease processes. However, younger animals can also present with hepatomegaly (e.g., with feline infectious peritonitis [FIP], congenital veno-occlusive disease, infectious disease, lymphoma).

GENETICS AND BREED PREDISPOSITIONS

- Dogs: Doberman pinschers (inflammatory liver disease), cocker spaniels, Labrador retrievers, Skye terriers; Labrador retrievers (tricuspid dysplasia causing right-sided heart failure)
- Cats: Abyssinians (amyloidosis), Asian breeds (FIP)

CLINICAL PRESENTATION

HISTORY/CHIEF COMPLAINT: Depends on etiology:

- Can be an incidental finding
- Abdominal distention
- Polyuria, polydipsia
- Anorexia, lethargy/weight loss
- Exercise intolerance
- Vomiting/diarrhea
- Pale mucous membranes
- Hepatic encephalopathy
- Coagulopathy
- Cutaneous disease/hair loss/poor haircoat

PHYSICAL EXAM FINDINGS

- Abdominal distention.
- Palpable cranial organomegaly.
- Ascites.
- Icterus.
- Concurrent hepatosplenomegaly suggests a multicentric neoplastic, passive congestive, systemic inflammatory/infectious, or anemia-inducing process, or unrelated disorders.

ETIOLOGY AND PATHOPHYSIOLOGY

Hepatomegaly is caused by inflammation, infiltration, congestion/obstruction, infection, or hyperplasia of the liver.

DIAGNOSIS

DIFFERENTIAL DIAGNOSIS

- Inflammatory diseases of the liver:
  - Cholangitis/cholangiohepatitis complex (cats)
  - Cirrhosis (end stage usually produces microhepatica, not hepatomegaly)
  - Abscess
  - Neoplasia
  - Chronic active hepatitis (idiopathic chronic hepatitis) (dogs)
  - Canine breed-specific hepatopathies
- Neoplastic/cystic diseases:
  - Lymphoma, biliary cystadenoma, bile duct carcinoma, hemangiosarcoma, metastatic neoplasia
  - Hepatocellular carcinoma, hepatoma (enlargement of a single lobe)
  - Malignant histiocytosis
  - Diffuse mast cell tumor
  - Parenchymal/biliary cysts
- Extrahepatic obstruction:
  - Pancreatitis
  - Cholelithiasis (rare in dogs and cats)
  - Bile duct neoplasia
  - Biliary mucocele
  - Inspissated bile syndrome of cats
- Metabolic disease:
  - Diabetes mellitus (lipid accumulation)
  - Hepatic lipidosis (cats)
  - Amyloidosis (Abyssinian/Chinese shar-pei)
  - Storage disease (rare in cats and dogs)
  - Hyperadrenocorticism (dogs/glycogen accumulation)
- Drugs:
  - Glucocorticoids
  - Phenobarbital
- Infectious disease (many cause hepatosplenomegaly due to systemic immune stimulation):
  - Bacterial, rickettsial, protozoal, fungal
  - Liver abscess (enlargement localized to a single lobe)
  - FIP
  - Erythrocyte parasitism (*Mycoplasma haemofelis*/hemobartonellosis, *Babesia* spp.)
- Immune-mediated disease (hepatosplenomegaly common due to systemic immune stimulation):
  - Immune-mediated hemolytic anemia (IMHA)
  - Immune-mediated thrombocytopenia (ITP)
  - Systemic lupus erythematosus
  - Vasculitis
  - Any systemic immune-mediated disease
- Congestion (often associated with ascites):
  - Right-sided heart failure
  - Budd-Chiari syndrome/veno-occlusive disease (rare)
  - Liver lobe torsion (rare)
- Intoxications
- Benign conditions:
  - Nodular hyperplasia (older dogs)
  - Nodular regeneration (associated with severe liver disease)
  - Extramedullary hematopoiesis
  - Individual variation (pseudohepatomegaly)
- Radiographic differential diagnosis for hepatomegaly:
  - Cranial abdominal mass, marked splenomegaly, ascites, dyspnea (caudal displacement of liver), youth (nonmineralized distal ribs gives false impression of liver protruding beyond costal arch)

INITIAL DATABASE

- Complete blood count, chemistry profile, urinalysis, and culture
- Abdominal radiographs (most accurate assessment of liver size)
- Abdominal ultrasound
- Thoracic radiographs (cardiac structures, metastatic disease)

ADVANCED/CONFIRMATORY TESTING

- Coagulation profile (prothrombin time/activated partial thromboplastin time/platelet count), buccal mucosal bleeding time
- Preprandial and postprandial serum bile acids
- Urine bile acids

- Serum ammonia (poor specificity/sensitivity)
- Liver aspirate or biopsy for histopathologic evaluation and culture (aerobic/anaerobic)
- Copper quantification of biopsy specimen
- Amylase/lipase/pancreatic lipase immunoreactivity
- Adrenocorticotropic hormone (ACTH) stimulation, ACTH level, low-dose dexamethasone suppression test
- Antinuclear antibody test
- Infectious disease titers/polymerase chain reaction (PCR)
- FIP serology
- Echocardiography/central venous pressure
- Abdominocentesis (if ascites)
- Abdominal computed tomography
- Venography (Budd-Chiari, veno-occlusive disease)
- D-dimer (thromboembolic disease)
- Bone marrow aspirate (immune-mediated hemolytic anemia/immune-mediated thrombocytopenia, lymphoma staging)

TREATMENT

THERAPEUTIC GOAL(S)

Treat specifically on the basis of an established diagnosis. Hepatomegaly is a sign, not an etiology. Suppress the disease process/manage the metabolic condition/treat any infectious or immune-mediated disease with appropriate medication or surgical intervention.

GENERAL TREATMENT

- Inflammatory diseases:
  - Immunosuppressant therapy (i.e., glucocorticoids, azathioprine, cyclosporine)
  - Antioxidant therapy (S-adenosylmethionine, silymarin, zinc, vitamin E)
  - Immune-modulatory medications; ursodeoxycholate, metronidazole
  - Antifibrotics: colchicine, *d*-penicillamine, methotrexate
  - Antibiotics: metronidazole, amoxicillin, cephalexin, enrofloxacin
  - Gastric protectants
  - Vitamins: carnitine (lipidosis), vitamin C, vitamin E, zinc, vitamin K (if coagulopathy)
  - Dietary therapy
  - Treatment for hepatic encephalopathy: lactulose, neomycin, metronidazole
  - Management for ascites (abdominocentesis/abdominal drainage; diuretics: spironolactone)
  - Fluid therapy
- Neoplastic diseases: surgery/chemotherapy
- Extrahepatic obstruction: supportive care, surgery
- Metabolic diseases:
  - Insulin therapy
  - Colchicine/dimethylsulfoxide for amyloidosis
  - Aggressive feeding (hepatic lipidosis)
  - Lysodren/trilostane/ketoconazole for hyperadrenocorticism
- Infectious diseases:
  - Treatment depends on the organism
- Immune-mediated diseases:
  - Immunosuppressant therapy/depends on the disorder
- Congestion:
  - Treatment depends on the cause

RECOMMENDED MONITORING

Dictated by the disease process. Examples include liver enzyme profile 1 to 2 weeks postdiagnosis, then monthly for 3 months, then every 3 to 4 months; repeat serum or urine bile acids/liver aspirate or biopsy at 6- to 12-month intervals; ACTH-stimulation every 3 to 6 months; convalescent infectious disease titers/PCR at 4-week to 6-month intervals.

PROGNOSIS AND OUTCOME

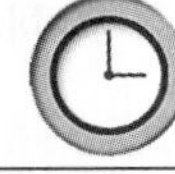

Varies with the cause of each disease

PEARLS & CONSIDERATIONS

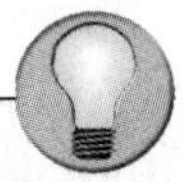

COMMENTS

- Bile acids are an unnecessary test in an icteric patient (rare exception: an icteric patient that is suspected of having both hemolysis and hepatobiliary disease concurrently, where bile acids can help differentiate).
- Fine-needle aspiration and cytologic evaluation of the liver does not reliably assess hepatic structure or function, even with diffuse hepatopathies.
- A normal serum bile acids result in a patient with progressively increasing liver enzymes does not preclude the need for liver biopsy.
- Cats with hepatic lipidosis tend to have greater bleeding after liver biopsy tendency than those with other diseases.
- An abnormal urine bile acids test result should be confirmed with serum bile acids measurement before liver biopsy.
- In cats, most diseases of the liver (including cirrhosis) result in hepatomegaly, whereas in dogs this is not necessarily the case.
- Ursodeoxycholate (e.g., Actigall) therapy can interfere with the interpretation of the urine bile acids test.

RECOMMENDED READING

Bravo AA, Sheth SG, Chopra S: Liver biopsy. *N Engl J Med* 344(7):495–500, 2001.

Center SA: Diagnostic procedures for evaluation of hepatic disease. In Guilford WG, et al (eds): *Strombeck's Small Animal Gastroenterology*, ed 3. Philadelphia, WB Saunders, 1996, pp 130–188.

Trainor D, et al: Urine sulfated and nonsulfated bile acids as a diagnostic test for liver disease in cats. *J Vet Intern Med* 17:145–153, 2003.

AUTHOR: **MAUREEN CARROLL**
EDITOR: **ETIENNE CÔTÉ**

Hepatopathy, Copper-Associated

BASIC INFORMATION

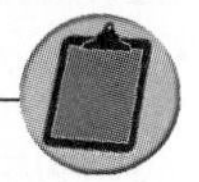

DEFINITION

Accumulation of copper within hepatocytes that leads to hepatotoxicity

EPIDEMIOLOGY

SPECIES, AGE AND SEX: Primarily in dogs; rare in cats. Copper accumulates slowly, so clinical signs are typically not present until middle age.

GENETICS AND BREED PREDISPOSITION

- Autosomal recessive in Bedlington terriers
- Predisposition in dalmatians, West Highland white terriers, and Skye terriers
- Possible association in doberman pinschers
- Reported in other canine breeds, but it is unknown if copper accumulation is the cause or effect of hepatopathy

CLINICAL PRESENTATION

DISEASE FORM/SUBTYPES

- Subclinical

- Chronic inflammatory liver disease/cirrhosis
- Acute hepatic failure with hemolytic anemia (rare)

HISTORY, CHIEF COMPLAINT, AND PHYSICAL EXAMINATION FINDINGS: Patients usually present with features of chronic hepatic disease such as lethargy, vomiting, abdominal distention, or encephalopathy (see Cirrhotic/Fibrosing Liver Disease, p 210), or less commonly with acute hepatic failure (see Hepatic Injury, Acute, p 491) and hemolytic anemia (see Anemia, Hemolytic, p 64).

ETIOLOGY AND PATHOPHYSIOLOGY

- Copper homeostasis maintained by biliary excretion of excess copper.
- Copper is absorbed from ingesta in the small intestine and extracted by hepatocytes.
- Chaperoned around the hepatocyte by a number of proteins before being either released into the serum or excreted in bile. A small amount is stored in lysosomes.
- Abnormal hepatic copper accumulation occurs due to primary inborn error of metabolism or secondary to acquired cholestatic liver disease.
  - In Bedlingtons, copper accumulates in lysosmes due to a genetic defect in the Murr 1 gene, a protein required for the final stages of copper excretion into the bile. When the storage capacity of the lysosomes is exceeded, copper breaks out into the cytoplasm, where it is toxic.
- Excess copper damages hepatocytes by inducing the formation of free radicals.
- Genetic basis for copper accumulation in other breeds is unknown.
- Secondary copper accumulation is due to a generalized impairment in biliary excretion (i.e., cholestasis).

DIAGNOSIS

DIFFERENTIAL DIAGNOSIS

- Chronic:
  - Infectious, immune, or toxic causes of inflammatory hepatic disease
  - Hepatic neoplasia
  - Congenital portosystemic shunts
- Acute:
  - Infectious, immune, drug, or toxin (zinc) induced hemolytic anemia
  - Exposure to hepatotoxic drugs or environmental toxins
  - Infectious canine hepatitis, leptospirosis

INITIAL DATABASE

See Hepatic Injury, Acute, p 491; Hepatitis (Chronic, Idiopathic) of Dogs, p 503; Cirrhotic/Fibrosing Liver Disease, p 210; Anemia, Hemolytic, p 64

ADVANCED OR CONFIRMATORY TESTING

- Determination of hepatic copper concentration:
  - Quantitative analysis on hepatic wedge or needle biopsies.
  - Qualitative analysis by rhodanine or rubeanic acid staining of histopathology slide. Permits determination of copper distribution within the hepatic lobule.
    - Normal hepatic copper levels from 200–400 µg/g dry weight (DW).
    - Secondary copper accumulation levels <1000–2000 µg/g DW.
    - Copper >2000 µg/g dry weight suggests a primary copper abnormality.
    - In Bedlingtons, copper levels gradually increase with age, with levels reported from 850–12,000 µg/g DW.
    - In West Highland white terriers, copper accumulation does not correlate as well with age (levels up to 3500 µg/g DW reported).
- Histopathology:
  - In Bedlingtons, copper initially accumulates centrilobularly.
    - Initial finding is centrilobular hepatocellular vacuolation followed by degeneration/necrosis and finally inflammation and fibrosis. Progresses to become more panlobular eventually with periportal orientation. Findings can mimic idiopathic chronic hepatitis.
  - In secondary copper accumulation, copper staining located primarily in areas of inflammation or degeneration.
- Genetic test, microsatellite marker (C04107) available to screen Bedlingtons, but may miss disease in some pedigrees. No test for Murr 1 mutation available.

TREATMENT

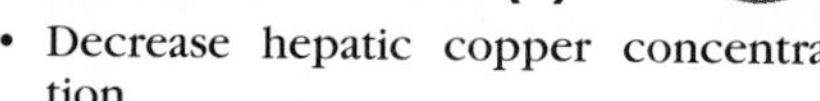

THERAPEUTIC GOAL(S)

- Decrease hepatic copper concentration
- Decrease copper absorption

ACUTE GENERAL TREATMENT

Manage the complications of acute or chronic hepatic disease (see Hepatic Injury, Acute, p 491; Cirrhotic/Fibrosing Liver Disease, p 210; Hepatic Encephalopathy, p 489)

CHRONIC TREATMENT

- See Cirrhotic/Fibrosing Liver Disease, p 210; Hepatic Encephalopathy, p 489.
- Copper chelators, for initial decoppering of liver and maintenance therapy.
  - Penicillamine (10–15 mg/kg PO q 12h). Increases urinary copper excretion. Works slowly (removes ~900 µg/g per year), so that copper levels take several months to years to decrease. Vomiting is a common side effect; therefore, begin at low end of dosage range and titrate upward.
  - Trientine (10–15 mg/kg PO q 12h). Increases urinary copper excretion and may also block intestinal uptake. Fewer side effects than penicillamine.
  - Give all medications on an empty stomach followed by a water bolus.
- Inhibit intestinal copper absorption, maintenance therapy.
  - Zinc (100 mg elemental zinc PO q 12h). Induces intestinal metallothionein, a protein that binds copper, keeping it sequestered within the enterocyte and thus preventing copper absorption. May be combined with chelators (separate administration by 2 hours). Side effects include gastritis, hemolytic anemia, and iron deficiency. Keep serum zinc levels <600 µg/dl to avoid hemolysis. Effective zinc levels are >200 µg/dl.
- Reduce dietary intake of copper.
  - Avoid shellfish, nuts, chocolate, mushrooms, and organ meats. Check water supply if not public. Most veterinary diets do not contain excessive copper levels.
- Antioxidants.
  - Induction of oxidant stress is central to copper-induced hepatic damage.
  - Vitamin E supplementation (200–400 IU PO q 24h).
  - S-Adenosylmethionine (20 mg/kg PO q 24h).

RECOMMENDED MONITORING

Serum enzymes every 4 to 6 months

PROGNOSIS AND OUTCOME

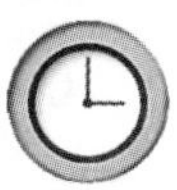

- Subclinical disease: excellent with therapy.
- Chronic: depends on stage. Mild to moderate inflammatory disease: good. Severe inflammatory disease/cirrhosis: guarded.
- Acute: grave.

PEARLS & CONSIDERATIONS

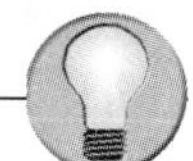

COMMENTS

- All Bedlington terriers should be tested at 1 year of age by determination of hepatic copper concentration and/or genetic testing. Affected dogs should not be bred.
- All dogs with chronic inflammatory hepatitis, particularly West Highland white terriers, Doberman pinschers, Skye terriers, and dalmatians, should have hepatic copper analysis, and if concentrations

are >1000–2000 μg/g DW, they should be treated to decrease hepatic copper.

SUGGESTED READING

Fuentealba IC, Aburto A: Animal models of copper-associated disease. *Comparative Hepatology* 2:1–12, 2003.

Thornberg L: A perspective on copper and liver disease in the dog. *J Vet Diagn Invest* 12:101–110, 2000.

AUTHOR: **CYNTHIA R. L. WEBSTER**
EDITOR: **KEITH P. RICHTER**

Hepatozoonosis

BASIC INFORMATION

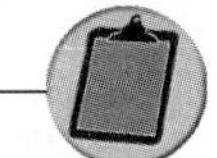

DEFINITION

Protozoal disease of dogs transmitted by ticks that has a gametocyte stage in white blood cells and a cystic stage in host tissues

SYNONYM(S)

Hepatozoon canis and *Hepatozoon americanum* are the two species that infect dogs.

EPIDEMIOLOGY

SPECIES, AGE, SEX: No age or sex predilection; usually outdoor dogs. Also reported in foxes, coyotes, jackals, hyenas, bobcats, ocelots.

RISK FACTORS: Outdoor dogs in endemic areas. History of tick exposure. Ingestion of deer carcass or other mammal with ticks.

CONTAGION AND ZOONOSIS: No reported human cases.

GEOGRAPHY AND SEASONALITY

- *H. canis* is endemic in Southern Europe, the Middle East, Africa, and South America.
- *H. americanum* is endemic in the Gulf Coast area of the United States and now ranges from Oklahoma to Florida.
- Most cases present in the summer and fall.

ASSOCIATED CONDITIONS AND DISORDERS

- *H canis*: usually subclinical unless there is other disease or immunosuppression
- *H americanum*: pyogranulomatous myositis

CLINICAL PRESENTATION

DISEASE FORMS/SUBTYPES

- *H. canis*: usually show no overt clinical signs
- *H. americanum*: chronic wasting disease characterized by waxing and waning muscle pain and fever

HISTORY, CHIEF COMPLAINT

- *H. canis*: finding gametocytes on blood smear. Dogs usually show no overt clinical signs.
- *H. americanum*: depression, reluctance to move, stiff gait, mucopurulent ocular discharge, weight loss. Dogs may have history of ingesting a deer carcass 3 to 4 weeks before developing clinical signs. Some dogs develop transient bloody diarrhea before signs of muscle pain and fever begin.

PHYSICAL EXAM FINDINGS: Fever, mucopurulent ocular discharge, hyperesthesia, neck-guarding, stiffness, ataxia, unwillingness to rise, cachexia, muscle wasting (*H. americanum*).

ETIOLOGY AND PATHOPHYSIOLOGY

- The parasite has a complex life cycle. The definitive host of *H. canis* is the brown dog tick, *Rhipicephalus sanguineus*, and for *H. americanum* it is the Gulf Coast tick, *Amblyomma maculatum*. The dog must ingest the infected tick.
- Sporozoites are released and penetrate the dog's gut. These are phagocytized by macrophages and distributed throughout the body to form schizonts, or "cysts."
- The organisms replicate inside the cyst until it ruptures and merozoites are released. *H. canis* cysts are primarily in the lymph nodes and spleen. *H. americanum* cysts are primarily in skeletal muscle.
- When the merozoites are released, an intense inflammatory reaction occurs, resulting in painful myositis and fever (*H. americanum*).

DIAGNOSIS

DIFFERENTIAL DIAGNOSIS

- Meningitis
- Diskospondylitis
- Polyarthritis
- Pyometra
- Other tick-borne diseases

INITIAL DATABASE

- Complete blood count (CBC) may reveal extreme leukocytosis (20,000–200,000 cells/μl; typically mature neutrophilia with left shift possible) and mild nonregenerative anemia. Platelet count is usually normal. Thrombocytopenia may indicate coinfection with other tick-borne disease.
- Serum chemistry profile: hypoalbuminemia, hyperglobulinemia, elevated serum alkaline phosphatase, low glucose, low blood urea nitrogen are possible.
- Long-bone radiographs: periosteal proliferation secondary to adjacent muscle inflammation is possible.
- Dogs with chronic disease may develop glomerulonephritis with an increased urine protein:creatinine ratio.
- Blood smear or buffy coat smear may reveal gametocytes in circulating white blood cells.

ADVANCED OR CONFIRMATORY TESTING

- Immunofluorescent antibody and polymerase chain reaction tests available for *H. canis* (in Israel).
- PCR test for *H. americanum* available through Auburn University Molecular Diagnostics Lab (http://www.vetmed.auburn.edu/index.pl/molecular_diagnostics).
- Definitive diagnosis usually made by finding organisms in muscle biopsy. Any muscle can be sampled but rear limb muscles are most commonly used.

TREATMENT

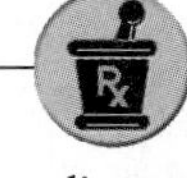

THERAPEUTIC GOAL(S)

Acute antiprotozoal therapy eradicates circulating organisms. Chronic therapy is necessary to prevent relapses from continued release of merozoites from tissue cysts.

ACUTE GENERAL TREATMENT

- For *H. americanum*, "combination therapy" for 2 weeks: trimethoprim-sulfadiazine (15 mg/kg PO q 12h), clindamycin (10 mg/kg PO q 8h), and pyrimethamine (0.25 mg/kg PO q 24h).
- For *H. canis*: imidocarb (5 mg/kg SC repeated every 14 days until parasitemia has resolved).
- Nonsteroidal anti-inflammatory drugs at standard doses for muscle pain.

- Doxycycline (5-10 mg/kg q 12-24h PO). May be required if there is coinfection with other tick-borne diseases.
- IV fluids may be needed for hypoglycemia and dehydration.

CHRONIC TREATMENT

Decoquinate (Deccox 22.7 g/lb Premix, Alphama, Fort Lee, NJ) at a dosage of 10-20 mg/kg or 0.5-1 tsp/10 kg mixed in food q 12h for 2 years will inhibit development of merozoites released from tissue cysts, thereby preventing reinfection of the dog and cyclic bouts of illness.

POSSIBLE COMPLICATIONS

Severely affected dogs may require repeated administration of "combination therapy" if relapses are clinically severe.

RECOMMENDED MONITORING

Repeat CBC and physical examination in 2 weeks. If fever, muscle pain, or marked leukocytosis is present, continue combination therapy for 2 more weeks.

PROGNOSIS AND OUTCOME

- Without treatment, American hepatozoonosis is usually fatal within several months.
- With antiprotozoal combination therapy alone, relapses occur requiring repeated therapy. Relapses become more frequent and refractory to treatment. Death usually occurs within 1 year of the initial diagnosis.
- Long-term cure (>5 years) has been achieved with combination therapy followed by long-term decoquinate therapy.

PEARLS & CONSIDERATIONS

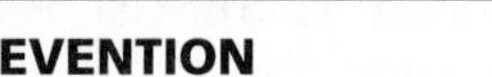

PREVENTION

- Effective tick-control with a topical acaricide and a repellent collar is recommended.
- Clients should not allow dogs to eat dead animals that may harbor ticks (e.g., deer carcasses).

CLIENT EDUCATION

- Clean matted eyes with a warm, moist towel as needed.
- Provide soft bedding.
- Bring food and water to dogs that are nonambulatory.
- Continue all medications for recommended duration. Stopping decoquinate too early can result in reinfestation of the dog and exacerbation of the disease.

SUGGESTED READING

Macintire DK, Vincent-Johnson NA: Canine hepatozoonosis. In Bonagura JD (ed): *Kirk's Current Veterinary Therapy XIII Small Animal Practice*. Philadelphia, WB Saunders, pp 310-313, 2000.

Vincent-Johnson NA: American canine hepatozoonosis. *Vet Clin Small Anim* 33:905-920, 2003.

AUTHOR & EDITOR: **DOUGLASS K. MACINTIRE**

Herbicide (Phenoxy, Others) Toxicosis

BASIC INFORMATION

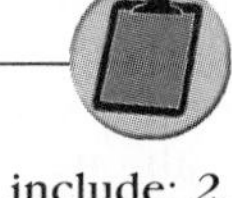

DEFINITION

- Phenoxy-type herbicides include: *2, 4-D* (2,4-dichlorophenoxyacetic acid), *MCPA* (2-methyl-4-chlorophenoxyacetic acid), *MCPP* [2-(4 chloro-2-methoxy) propionic acid], and *dicamba* (3, 6-dichloro-2-methoxybenzoic acid).
- Commonly used in a residential setting (lawns, along fences), and available through lawn care professionals or local retail outlets.
- Available as concentrates or ready-to-use products. Most exposures in animals occur due to walking through a recently treated yard (dermal and oral exposure), or chewing and puncturing the container to produce a spill situation.

SYNONYM(S)

Phenoxy herbicides

EPIDEMIOLOGY

SPECIES, AGE, SEX

- Dogs most commonly involved; outdoor cats on occasion.
- Younger, more inquisitive or active dogs more likely to be exposed. Dogs lick, or sometimes "graze," an herbicide-treated area.
- Cats exposed subsequent to running through a freshly treated area, then ingesting the product through grooming.

GENETICS AND BREED PREDISPOSITION: Dogs eliminate chlorophenoxy compounds (e.g., 2,4-D, MCPA) slowly due to saturation of the renal organic anion system, which can prolong urinary excretion and extend recovery times.

RISK FACTORS

- Pre-existing debilitation or chronic renal failure.
- Pets exposed to concentrated products are typically of greater concern.

GEOGRAPHY AND SEASONALITY: Spring and summer provide greater opportunity for accidental exposure.

CLINICAL PRESENTATION

DISEASE FORMS/SUBTYPES

- Most cases involve ready-to-use products, are acute in nature (onset of signs <1-4 hours after exposure), and are restricted to mild, self-limiting hypersalivation, nausea, excessive licking, hacking, retching, vomiting, and diarrhea. Systemic effects not expected in these cases.
- Much less commonly, exposure to concentrated products in substantial amounts can cause systemic absorption, and subsequent gastritis, myotonia, paresis, generalized muscle weakness, ataxia, and seizures.

HISTORY, CHIEF COMPLAINT

- Most common: patient was on a treated lawn; drooling, vomiting, gagging, hacking, coughing, lethargy, refusal to eat within 4 hours of exposure
- Licking furniture or other inanimate objects, due to the contact irritant nature of the product

PHYSICAL EXAM FINDINGS

- Routine presentation: hypersalivation, increased cough/gag reflex, soft abdomen; vital signs typically within normal limits
- With substantial ingestion of concentrate (rare): protracted vomiting, generalized muscle stiffness or generalized decrease in muscle tone, ataxia, diarrhea, clinical lethargy/depression, and dehydration

ETIOLOGY AND PATHOPHYSIOLOGY

- Local contact physical irritant effect in most cases (due to normally low-end use concentrations of active ingredients and surfactants).
- Consumption of concentrates may lead to systemic absorbtion and in very large doses may uncouple oxidative phosphorylation, induce systemic metabolic acidosis, cause hepatic and renal toxicity, and cause gastrointestinal ulceration and bleeding. Death is rarely encountered.

DIAGNOSIS

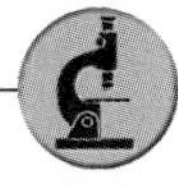

DIFFERENTIAL DIAGNOSIS

- Lawn grass or nontoxic outdoor plant ingestion
- Mild oral mucosal or dental trauma
- Bufo toad ingestion (acute, transient hypersalivation effect)
- Exposure to cleaning agents, petroleum distillates, etc.
- Marijuana, macadamia nuts toxicosis

INITIAL DATABASE

- No significant serum biochemical changes expected with exposure to routine ready-to-use products
- With systemic effects (paresis, ataxia, myotonia), serum biochemical changes may include:
  - ± Azotemia
  - ± Increased liver enzymes
  - ± Increased creatine kinase
  - ± Myoglobinuria
  - ± Metabolic acidosis

ADVANCED OR CONFIRMATORY TESTING

- Rarely needed or done
- Antemortem: chilled vomitus, serum, urine, for toxicology herbicide screen within 48 to 72 hours postexposure. Suspect product container
- Postmortem: liver, kidney, muscle, and brain, chilled or frozen for toxicology herbicide screen. Suspect product container would be helpful

TREATMENT

THERAPEUTIC GOAL(S)

- Decontamination of patient
- Supportive care

ACUTE GENERAL TREATMENT

- Decontamination of patient:
  - Oral rinsing with water or milk, to dilute, flush, and dampen the contact irritant effect to the gastrointestinal mucosa.
  - Bathe with water and mild liquid detergent solution for dermal exposure.
  - Inducing emesis and/or activated charcoal procedures are generally not beneficial or indicated, due to rapid absorption; may be considered if concentrated products are involved.
- Supportive care:
  - Intravenous fluids.
  - Urine trapping (alkaline diuresis) to enhance chlorophenoxy excretion, and decrease the risk of renal failure due to rhabdomyolysis; beneficial if systemic involvement. Consider 1-2 mEq/kg of sodium bicarbonate added to fluids, maintain a urine pH of 7.5. Monitor acid-base status closely.
  - Forced saline diuresis alone is not likely to enhance clearance of the chemical.
  - Gastrointestinal protectants if needed (see Gastric Ulcer, p 431).

POSSIBLE COMPLICATIONS

- Metabolic acidosis (rare).
- Renal and hepatic complications (rare).
- A controversial literature report (Hayes, et al., 1991) suggesting a modest increase in the incidence of lymphoma in dogs exposed to 2,4-D treated lawns is considered suspect in terms of accuracy by many toxicology experts.

RECOMMENDED MONITORING

Animals with systemic effects:

- Serum renal and hepatic values
- Acid-base status

PROGNOSIS AND OUTCOME

- Excellent; self-limiting signs usually resolve in 12 to 24 hours.
- Good with systemic effects; signs resolve within 24 to 96 hours; long-term adverse health effects are rare.

PEARLS & CONSIDERATIONS

COMMENTS

- Other common herbicides dogs and cats are exposed to include *glyphosate* (Roundup) and *pendimethalin*. These herbicides also have low order of toxicity and most exposures result in mild self-limiting gastrointestinal signs.
- Most exposures to phenoxy-type herbicides involve exposure to very low concentrations (<1% active ingredient) on treated lawns, and therefore are of low-risk concern.
- "Weed and feed" lawn care products contain a herbicide (weed) and fertilizer (feed) component. Typically, low risk is expected from accidental exposures to these products, unless an insecticide component has been added.
- No significant exposure or risk of acute toxicity if animal eats treated grass or goes in the treated yard after the spray had already dried (within a few hours).

PREVENTION

Keep product containers locked and away from animals.

CLIENT EDUCATION

- Always read the label and follow label directions before applying any herbicide.
- Allow adequate drying time before allowing pets to re-enter.

SUGGESTED READING

Hayes HM, et al: A case control study of canine malignant lymphoma: Positive association with dog owners' use of 2,4-dichlorophenoxyacetic acid herbicides. *Natl Cancer Inst* 83,1226-1231, 1991.

Yeary R: Miscellaneous herbicides, fungicides, and nematocides. In Peterson ME, Talcott PA (eds): *Small Animal Toxicology*. Philadelphia, WB Saunders, 2001, pp 505-515.

AUTHOR: **MICHAEL W. KNIGHT**
EDITOR: **SAFDAR A. KHAN**

Herpesviral Keratitis in Cats

BASIC INFORMATION

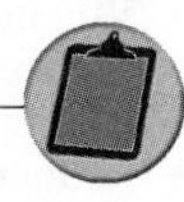

DEFINITION

- Corneal inflammation associated with feline herpesvirus type 1 (FHV-1) infection
- Sometimes divided into ulcerative and nonulcerative (or stromal) keratitis or into an overlapping pair of epidemiologically relevant categories: primary and recrudescent herpesviral keratitis

SYNONYM(S)

Herpetic keratitis
Feline viral rhinotracheitis: FHV-1, FVR

EPIDEMIOLOGY

SPECIES, AGE, SEX

- FHV-1 is highly species-specific.
- Domestic and wild cats of any age may be affected.
- Young kittens undergoing primary exposure usually display ulcerative disease, and older cats undergoing

viral reactivation may experience ulcerative or nonulcerative recrudescent disease.
- Both genders affected equally.

GENETICS AND BREED PREDISPOSITION
- No breed predilection has been proven.
- Individual variation in susceptibility to recrudescent herpetic keratitis suggests immunologic predisposition.

RISK FACTORS
- Stresses such as rehousing, intercurrent disease, or pregnancy/parturition/lactation
- Corticosteroid administration
- Multicat households or shelters
- Inadequate vaccination

CONTAGION AND ZOONOSIS
- Highly contagious among cats
- Not zoonotic

GEOGRAPHY AND SEASONALITY
- Worldwide viral distribution without seasonality
- Due to susceptibility of kittens, trends in disease prevalence may be noted in association with feline breeding seasons

ASSOCIATED CONDITIONS AND DISORDERS
- FHV-1 also causes conjunctivitis, dermatitis, and may cause anterior uveitis.
- FHV-1 is associated with corneal sequestra and eosinophilic keratitis.

CLINICAL PRESENTATION

DISEASE FORMS/SUBTYPES
- Ulcerative keratitis (seen most often upon initial exposure but also in recurrent forms)
- Nonulcerative keratitis (seen most often in chronic primary or recurrent forms)

HISTORY, CHIEF COMPLAINT
- Ocular discharge
- Blepharospasm (squinting)
- Corneal opacification
- Upper respiratory signs may be seen, including nasal congestion, sneezing, and serous or mucopurulent nasal discharge
- Ocular signs are typically bilateral in primary disease but often unilateral during recrudescences

PHYSICAL EXAM FINDINGS
- Ocular discharge (serous, mucoid, purulent, sanguineous, or dry and crusty)
- Blepharospasm
- Deep or superficial corneal vascularization, ulceration (dendritic early; usually geographic by time of presentation)
- Corneal opacification due to white blood cell infiltration and/or corneal edema and/or scarring
- Conjunctival or episcleral injection
- Chemosis (conjunctival edema)
- Blepharoedema
- Reflex uveitis (e.g., miotic pupil; aqueous flare and/or inflamatory cells in the anterior chamber)

ETIOLOGY AND PATHOPHYSIOLOGY
- FHV-1 is a ubiquitous virus.
- Infection causes usually self-limiting primary disease in essentially all cats infected with the virus.
- Approximately 80% of affected cats become latently infected for life.
- Periodic reactivation occurs in about half of these.
- Periodic recrudescent disease occurs in a minority of cats.

DIAGNOSIS

DIFFERENTIAL DIAGNOSIS
- There are no other recognized primary feline corneal pathogens.
- *Chlamydophila felis* (formerly *Chlamydia psittaci*) causes conjunctivitis but is not known to cause keratitis.
- Feline calicivirus is not a primary corneoconjunctival pathogen but rather causes lesions of the oral and pharyngeal mucosa.
- Noninfectious corneal disease (immune-mediated, neoplastic, dry-eye, foreign body, traumatic) is uncommon in cats compared to dogs.

INITIAL DATABASE
- Thorough ophthalmic examination including fluorescein stain
- Corneal or conjunctival cytologic evaluation will eliminate eosinophilic keratoconjunctivitis
  - However, herpesviral inclusions are seen extremely rarely.

ADVANCED OR CONFIRMATORY TESTING
- Corneal or conjunctival cytologic evaluation will assist in the diagnosis or exclusion of eosinophillic keratoconjunctivitis; however herpesviral inclusions are seen extremely rarely in any herpetic disease.
- Serologic evaluation is not useful because of vaccination and widespread (97%) seroprevalence.

TREATMENT

THERAPEUTIC GOAL(S)
- Inhibit viral replication
- Prevent secondary bacterial colonization of corneal ulcers
- Minimize recurrences

ACUTE GENERAL TREATMENT
- Cats with respiratory signs may need supportive care.
- Cats with ulcerative keratitis require a topical broad-spectrum antibiotic.
- Consider a topical antiviral for chronic or severe signs. Topical antiviral agents (e.g., idoxuridine, trifluridine, vidarabine) are virostatic and must be administered at least 4 to 6 times daily.
- Consider oral administration of lysine (500 mg PO q 12h: lifelong treatment) to inhibit viral replication.
- Use systemic antiviral agents (e.g., acyclovir) with extreme care if at all, due to toxicity.
- Avoid topical or systemic corticosteroid administration.

CHRONIC TREATMENT
- Consider lysine to reduce recurrences
- Avoid topical or systemic corticosteroid administration

POSSIBLE COMPLICATIONS
- Topical antiviral agents are epitheliotoxic.
- Valacyclovir is toxic to cats.

RECOMMENDED MONITORING
- Frequent ophthalmic examinations, especially of ulcerative keratitis
- Monitor complete blood count and serum biochemistry panels if systemic antiviral agents are used

PROGNOSIS AND OUTCOME

- Primary disease is self-limiting in most cats.
- A minority experience chronic and/or recrudescent disease.
- Treat recurrences early and aggressively.
- Secondary bacterial invasion of corneal ulcers can cause globe perforation.
- Chronic stromal herpetic keratitis is painful and can be blinding due to corneal scarring.

PEARLS & CONSIDERATIONS

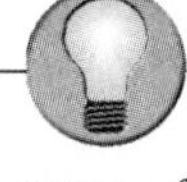

COMMENTS
- FHV-1 is the most common cause of ulcerative and nonulcerative keratitis in cats.
- Diagnostic testing is confounded by latency and low viral shedding.
- Topical antiviral agents must be administered frequently to be effective.
- Treat recurrences early and aggressively.

PREVENTION
- Vaccination lessens signs but may not reduce recurrences or establishment of latency
- Reduction of known stresses is useful

CLIENT EDUCATION
- Minimize known stresses
- Early recognition and therapy of recrudescent disease are important

SUGGESTED READING

Nasisse MP, et al: Experimental ocular herpesvirus infection in the cat. Sites of virus replication, clinical features and effects of corticosteroid administration. *Invest Ophthalmol Vis Sci* 30:1758, 1989.

Stiles J, et al: Effect of oral administration of L-lysine on conjunctivitis caused by feline herpesvirus in cats. *Am J Vet Res* 63:99, 2002.

AUTHOR: **DAVID J. MAGGS**
EDITOR: **CHERYL L. CULLEN**

Herpesvirus, Dog

BASIC INFORMATION

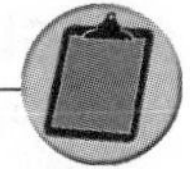

DEFINITION

Canine herpesvirus infections are viral infections that are specific to canids and that can result in four possible clinical outcomes: respiratory distress from nasal/upper airway infection, ranging from mild to severe; abortion; vaginitis; and neonatal puppy deaths up to 3 weeks of age.

SYNONYM(S)

Canine herpesvirus type 1 (CHV-1)
Dog herpes
Neonatal herpes

EPIDEMIOLOGY

SPECIES, AGE, SEX: Canids; domestic dogs; wild canidae. All ages susceptible to infection, with pregnant dams and neonatal puppies the most susceptible to canine herpesvirus-induced disease.

RISK FACTORS: There are eight risk factors: age, mating experience, reproductive cycle, breeding kennel, kennel size, breeding management (use of nonresident males), kennel cough, and kennel hygiene.

CONTAGION AND ZOONOSIS
- Highly contagious among canids only
- Fomites such as dog chew toys may play an important role; common food bowls may contribute to spread
- Direct contact via saliva and urogenital secretions are the most efficient mode of transmission. The virus is readily inactivated outside the body by heat, drying, disinfectants (diluted bleach)
- Not zoonotic

GEOGRAPHY AND SEASONALITY: Occurs worldwide. No seasonal prevalence.

ASSOCIATED CONDITIONS AND DISORDERS: Long-term latency; carrier dogs; stress and pregnancy-associated reexacerbation of clinical signs and viral shedding.

CLINICAL PRESENTATION

DISEASE FORMS/SUBTYPES
- Dogs, usually <2 years old presented for evaluation of acute to chronic respiratory distress (upper airway).
- Dam aborts litter, usually with 100% puppy mortality.
- Dam infects her litter during whelping, usually 80–100% puppy mortality.
- Naïve dam gives birth to naïve litter, and secondary contact with canine herpesvisrus-shedding dog carries virus back to litter. Mortality rate varies from 25–80% depending on virus challenge dose, age of puppies, and body temperature of puppies.
- Dam or sire presented for evaluation of papulovesicular lesions of the genital tract.

HISTORY, CHIEF COMPLAINT: Affected puppies: acute onset of puppies crying; less than 3 weeks old; abdominal tenderness; rapid progression to death.

PHYSICAL EXAM FINDINGS: Puppies appear lethargic, fail to nurse; decreased body weight; soft, yellow-green feces; no fever; rhinitis possible, with serous/mucopurulent/hemorrhagic nasal discharge; mucosal petechiae common. Puppies lose consciousness and may have opisthotonos and seizures before death.

ETIOLOGY AND PATHOPHYSIOLOGY

- Canine herpesvirus is a primary viral infection, either localized (mucosal) in adult, immunocompetent dogs, or systemic in naïve pregnant dams and neonatal puppies.
- Canine herpesvirus has a predilection for lymphoid and neural cells, both of which may become latently infected (no mature viral production), but a dog remains a potential shedder if the virus is reexacerbated due to stress (e.g., pregnancy, corticosteroids, irradiation).
- The optimal temperature for canine herpesvirus replication is 33-35°C (i.e., the temperature of the outer genital and upper respiratory tracts).

DIAGNOSIS

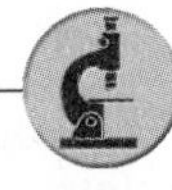

DIFFERENTIAL DIAGNOSIS

- Acute onset respiratory signs/respiratory distress of upper airway origin: canine adenovirus type 2; canine parainfluenza; *Bordetella bronchiseptica*; upper airway foreign body.
- Reproductive disease: brucellosis; *Streptococcus* spp.; canine distemper virus; neosporosis; toxoplasmosis.

INITIAL DATABASE

Complete blood count, serum biochemistry profile, urinalysis: Hematologic and biochemical values are usually nonspecific. However, a marked thrombocytopenia may be observed. A marked increase in the alanine aminotransferase activity may be found in affected neonatal puppies.

ADVANCED OR CONFIRMATORY TESTING

- Antemortem testing:
  - Serology on affected adult dogs (titers equal to or greater than 1:2 indicate exposure/infection). Antibody titers do not correlate with active viral shedding.
  - Virus isolation from nasal/urogenital swabs indicates infection and shedding.
  - Polymerase chain reaction (PCR) on whole blood indicates infection and probable latency.
- Postmortem testing (aborted/neonatally dead puppies):
  - Virus isolation from lung, bronchiolar lymph nodes, liver, kidney, and spleen.
  - Histopathologic evaluation of lung, liver, kidney, spleen, small intestine, and brain. Depending on the stage of cellular infection and method of fixation, basophilic or acidophilic intranuclear inclusions may be noted. These intranuclear inclusion bodies are considered pathognomonic for canine herpesvirus, which is important, as there is no canine herpesvirus immunohistochemistry commercially available. PCR can also be done on the aforementioned selected tissues but is usually reserved for determining latency.

TREATMENT

THERAPEUTIC GOAL(S)

Treatment of neonatal puppies with canine herpesvirus-induced disease is usually not recommended because of rapid progression, poor prognosis, and the potential for cerebellar and retinal dysplasias in surviving puppies

ACUTE GENERAL TREATMENT

- If only a portion of the litter demonstrates overt signs, the remaining littermates can be treated with immune serum (2 ml of serum from a dog with known anti-CHV titer, given intraperitoneally).
- Neonates can also be maintained in an environment with high humidity (up to 55%), and elevated room temps of 36.6-37.7°C (98-100°F). Because canine herpesvirus is naturally temperature sensitive, raising the pup's body temperature by artificial heating early in the course of the infection may have therapeutic value.

PROGNOSIS AND OUTCOME

- Unaffected neonatal puppies from an affected litter have a good prognosis.
- Dams that abort or have a naïve litter that subsequently becomes infected by a secondary source of canine herpesvirus commonly seroconvert, and will subsequently have normal litters. Canine herpesvirus immunity will be passed onto litters via colostrum. Colostral immunity, which persists to 8 weeks, will prevent clinical signs in the puppies, but will not prevent against (latent) infection.

PEARLS & CONSIDERATIONS

COMMENTS

Canine herpesvirus is a manageable infection and a preventable disease (see Prevention and Client Education below).

PREVENTION

- Good hygiene: cleanliness of dam, rigorous handwashing or use of gloves by handlers, and warmth and cleanliness of immediate puppy environment.
- No vaccine (United States). A European product has been licensed with good results reported when used prebreeding.

CLIENT EDUCATION

- Planned exposure of young (>6 months) puppies to older dogs to "naturally immunize" them before breeding and whelping. This induced latent infection rarely becomes overt, and if it does, 6-week quarantine is advised.
- Maintenance of a strict quarantine period to work within the "6-week danger period" (3 weeks before and 3 weeks after whelping).
- Maintaining ambient body temperature to minimize risk of hypothermia. CHV is very heat sensitive.

SUGGESTED READING

Evermann JF: Canine herpesvirus infection: update on risk factors and control measures. *Veterinary Forum* (May):32-37, 2005.

Morresey PR: Reproductive effects of canine herpesvirus. *Compend Cont Educ Prac Vet* 26:804-811, 2004.

Ronsse V, et al: Risk factors and reproductive disorders associated with canine herpesvirus-1 (CHV-1). *Theriogenology* 61:619-636, 2004.

AUTHOR: **JAMES F. EVERMANN**
EDITOR: **MICHELLE A. KUTZLER**

Hiatal Hernia/Gastroesophageal Intussusception

BASIC INFORMATION

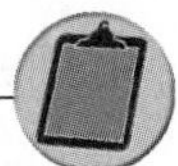

DEFINITION

- Hiatal hernia:
  - Protrusion of the abdominal esophagus, gastroesophageal junction, cardia, or gastric fundus through the esophageal hiatus of the diaphragm into the caudal mediastinum
- Gastroesophageal intussusception:
  - Invagination of the cardia into the terminal esophagus through the hiatus

EPIDEMIOLOGY

SPECIES, AGE, SEX

- Congenital hiatal hernia:
  - Primarily dogs
  - Before 1 year of age
- Acquired hiatal hernia:
  - Dogs or cats of any age

GENETICS AND BREED PREDISPOSITION: Shar-pei and brachycephalic breeds (e.g., bulldog) may be predisposed to hiatal hernia.

RISK FACTOR: Trauma.

ASSOCIATED CONDITIONS AND DISORDERS

- Esophageal hypomotility
- Gastroesophageal reflux/esophagitis

CLINICAL PRESENTATION

DISEASE FORMS/SUBTYPES

- Sliding or axial, hiatal hernia:
  - Longitudinal displacement of the abdominal esophagus, gastroesophageal junction, or stomach into the caudal mediastinum.
- Paraesophageal hernia:
  - Gastroesophageal junction remains caudal to the hiatus and the fundus of the stomach protrudes adjacent to and parallel to the gastroesophageal junction through the hiatus.
- Gastroesophageal intussusception (rare):
  - Cardia invaginates into the terminal esophagus and through the hiatus.
  - Associated with acute obstruction and severe clinical signs in dogs.

HISTORY, CHIEF COMPLAINT

- Absence of clinical signs:
  - Incidental finding on thoracic radiograph (50% of hiatal hernia cases; smaller proportion of gastroesophageal intussusception cases).
- Intermittent signs with sliding hernia. Typically:
  - Regurgitation, dysphagia, ptyalism, and weight loss.
  - Respiratory difficulty, hematemesis, and vomiting may occur.

PHYSICAL EXAM FINDINGS

- May be unremarkable
- If clinical signs are present, they may include:
  - Thin body condition
  - Dehydration
- Ptyalism
- Fever, harsh lung sounds, cough, dyspnea
- Possible aspiration pneumonia

ETIOLOGY AND PATHOPHYSIOLOGY

ETIOLOGY

- Congenital hiatal hernia:
  - Abnormal diaphragmatic esophageal hiatus (too large, or phrenicoesophageal ligament looser than normal)
- Trauma:
  - Esophageal hiatal enlargement and/or stretching of phrenicoesophageal ligament

MECHANISM

- Loss of normal anatomic relationship:
  - Adversely affects the normal high pressure zone at the gastroesophageal junction, causing reflux esophagitis
- Primary or secondary esophageal motility disorders and megaesophagus can exacerbate signs.

- Brachycephalic upper airway obstruction:
  - May result in abnormally low intrapleural pressure during inspiration causing hiatal herniation/gastroesophageal reflux
- Large hernias may allow other abdominal organs to enter the caudal mediastinum.

DIAGNOSIS

DIFFERENTIAL DIAGNOSIS

- Megaesophagus
- Esophageal foreign body, stricture, or mass

INITIAL DATABASE

- Complete blood count:
  - Neutrophilia with toxic changes and/or left shift, associated with inflammation/infection: suspect aspiration pneumonia
- Serum biochemistry profile:
  - Hypoproteinemia possible (malnutrition)
- Diagnostic imaging:
  - Survey thoracic radiographs
    - Increased density/mass lesion in the caudodorsal mediastinum (Fig. I-90). Highly characteristic of these disorders
    - Can be within normal limits if sliding hernia

ADVANCED OR CONFIRMATORY TESTING

- Fluoroscopy with a positive contrast esophagram:
  - Evaluate esophageal size and motility.
  - Identify sliding hernia
    - Application of external abdominal pressure during fluoroscopy may aid in diagnosis of sliding hernia
- Esophagoscopy:
  - Assess presence/severity of esophagitis
  - Gastroesophageal intussusception: confirm diagnosis

TREATMENT

THERAPEUTIC GOAL(S)

- Hiatal hernia:
  - Prevent regurgitation and gastroesophageal reflux
  - Ensure adequate nutritional intake
  - Aggressively treat aspiration pneumonia if present
  - Surgical correction for patients that fail to respond to medical management within 30 days
- Gastroesophageal intussusception:
  - Surgical reduction of intussusception
  - Prevent recurrence

ACUTE GENERAL TREATMENT

- Medical management:
  - Correction of fluid and electrolyte deficits if present
  - Aggressive treatment of aspiration pneumonia (see Pneumonia, Aspiration, p 862)
  - Nutritional support:
    - Upright feeding of small, frequent meals to promote normal function of the esophagus/gastroesophageal junction
    - Feeding (percutaneous endogastric) tube if oral intake inadequate (see Feeding Tube Placement: Percutaneous Endoscopic Gastrostomy [PEG], p 1247)
  - Treatment of gastroesophageal reflux/esophagitis (see p 366)
- Surgical management: patients showing clinical signs referable to hernia/intussusception:
  - Reduction of hiatal hernia/gastroesophageal intussusception
  - Closure of esophageal hiatus to a normal size
  - Gastropexy to prevent recurrence

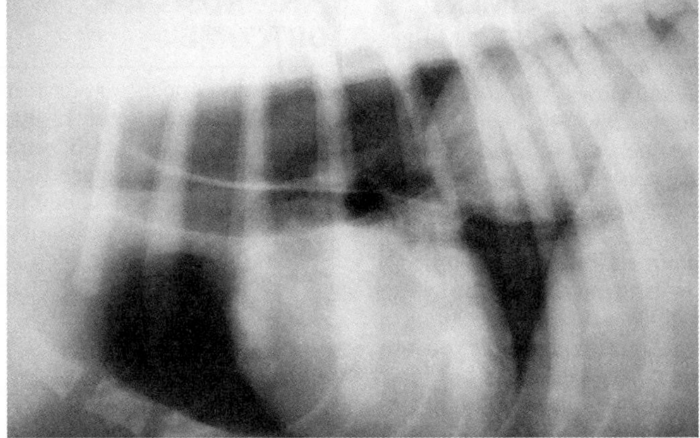

FIGURE I-90 Lateral thoracic radiograph of a dog demonstrating a large soft tissue mass located characteristically in the caudodorsal thorax due to gastroesophageal intussusception. The dog suffered strangulation injury when it became caught in a snare. Also visible is an air-filled esophagus, which demonstrates both sides of the dorsal tracheal membrane ("tracheal stripe sign"). A differential diagnosis for the radiographic appearance of the mass lesion is primary lung tumor. Courtesy of Dr. Richard Walshaw.

CHRONIC TREATMENT

- Continuation of feeding regimen
- Continuation of treatment of gastroesophageal reflux/esophagitis
- Surgical correction of hiatal hernia in patients that do not respond to medical management within 30 days

POSSIBLE COMPLICATIONS

- Failure of medical management to adequately resolve problem
- Recurrence of hiatal hernia after surgical correction
- Development of esophageal stricture secondary to gastroesophageal reflux/esophagitis

RECOMMENDED MONITORING

Follow-up positive contrast esophogram (4 to 6 weeks):

- Demonstrate resolution of:
  - Hiatal hernia/gastroesophageal intussusception
  - Gastroesophageal reflux
- Assess esophageal motility
- Determine whether continuation of feeding regimen and treatment of gastroesophageal reflux/esophagitis still necessary

PROGNOSIS AND OUTCOME

- Good prognosis:
  - If the patient has no or mild clinical signs
  - With surgical intervention in the absence of aspiration pneumonia
- Poor prognosis associated with:
  - Resistant aspiration pneumonia
  - Severe esophagitis/stricture

PEARLS & CONSIDERATIONS

COMMENTS

- Treatment for esophagitis should be continued postoperatively in any patient undergoing surgical correction of hiatal hernia.
- Aspiration pneumonia must be treated aggressively prior to considering surgical intervention.

SUGGESTED READING

Lorinson D, et al: Long-term outcome of medical and surgical treatment of hiatal hernias in dogs and cats: 27 cases (1978–1996). *J Am Vet Med Assoc* 213:381, 1998.

Tams TR: Diseases of the esophagus. In Tams TR (ed): *Handbook of Small Animal Gastroenterology*. St. Louis, WB Saunders, 2003, pp 118–157.

AUTHOR: **MARYANN G. RADLINSKY**
EDITOR: **RICHARD WALSHAW**

High-Rise Syndrome

BASIC INFORMATION

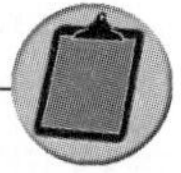

DEFINITION

Description of a triad of facial, thoracic, and limb injuries sustained by an animal that falls from a height of one or more stories; the term was originally coined in reference to cats, associated primarily with falls from a height of two or more stories.

SYNONYM(S)

High-flyer syndrome (in humans)
Jumper's syndrome

EPIDEMIOLOGY

SPECIES, AGE, SEX: The syndrome predominantly affects cats less than 3 years old. Similarly, most dogs subjected to extreme deceleration trauma are less than 5 years old. There is no sex predilection in either species.

RISK FACTORS

- Urban areas
- Tall buildings
- Open windows and balcony doors; roofs

GEOGRAPHY AND SEASONALITY: Falls occur more frequently in summer, followed by autumn, when windows and balcony doors are open and outdoor play is a factor.

CLINICAL PRESENTATION

HISTORY, CHIEF COMPLAINT: Falling from window sills, narrow ledges, balconies, and roofs.

PHYSICAL EXAM FINDINGS

- Mandibular symphysis separation and perisymphyseal fracture; split hard palate; epistaxis; fractured upper canine teeth (with or without pulp exposure) and upper fourth premolar teeth (traumatic hemisection between mesiobuccal and mesiopalatal crown-root segments); temporomandibular joint luxation; zygomatic arch fracture; facial wounds
- Dyspnea due to pulmonary contusion, pneumothorax, and/or pain
- Limb fractures
- Hematuria due to blunt abdominal trauma
- Spinal injuries; cranial neurologic abnormalities
- Soft tissue abrasions

ETIOLOGY AND PATHOPHYSIOLOGY

- Jumping during play or while chasing a squirrel, bird, insect, or other animal
- Slipping while walking on the edge of a balcony railing or window
- Range of heights fallen by cats (2 to 32 stories) and humans (1 to 20 stories) is high, compared to that by dogs (1 to 6 stories)

DIAGNOSIS

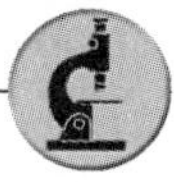

DIFFERENTIAL DIAGNOSIS

- Hit-by-car trauma
- Hit by a blunt object
- Kicked by an ungulate animal
- Fights with other animals
- Foreign body penetration
- Gunshot trauma

INITIAL DATABASE

- Orthopedic and neurologic examination
- Complete blood count, serum biochemistry panel, urinalysis
- Full mouth (intraoral) dental radiographs
- Radiographs of the head, temporomandibular joints, and bullae
- Radiographs of thorax, abdomen, spine, and limbs

ADVANCED OR CONFIRMATORY TESTING

Computed tomography of head and spine

TREATMENT

THERAPEUTIC GOAL(S)

- Stabilize animal.
- Preserve normal anatomy and function. Orthopedic manipulations or surgical procedures may initially need to be delayed, with adjunctive pain control, if the patient is systemically unstable at the time of presentation.

ACUTE GENERAL TREATMENT

- Initial treatment for shock (fluid therapy) and thoracic injury (thoracocentesis if pneumothorax) followed by orthopedic/neurologic examination. Further treatment, if sedation or general anesthesia is required, depends on the successful outcome of this initial stabilization.
- Surgical treatment of skeletal injuries.
- Cerclage wiring for perisymphyseal fracture/symphyseal separation.
- Extraction of teeth with pulp exposure or displacement injury.
- Fresh midline clefts of the hard palate: approximation of the displaced bony structures with digital pressure and suturing of the torn palatal soft tissues in a simple interrupted or mattress pattern; these clefts may also heal spontaneously in 2 to 4 weeks with conservative management, but the benefit of initial surgical management outweighs the risk of developing a persistent oronasal communication; if the separation is extensive, interarcade fixation may be required.
- Temporomandibular joint luxation: conservative reduction with a pencil.
- Nutritional support: soft food; esophagostomy tubes are rarely necessary.

CHRONIC TREATMENT

- If response to emergency treatment is poor, visceral injury (abdominal and thoracic) with possible hemorrhage should be considered and pursued diagnostically.
- Chronic oronasal communication: medially positioned double flaps with releasing incisions along dental arch or overlapping double flaps.
- Temporomandibular joint injury (chronic luxation or ankylosis): unilateral or bilateral condylectomy.
- Extraction or endodontic therapy of teeth with pulp exposure.

POSSIBLE COMPLICATIONS

- Chronic oronasal communication
- Temporomandibular joint ankylosis in very young animals with difficulty or inability to open the mouth
- Chylothorax

RECOMMENDED MONITORING

- In-patient monitoring until discharge
- Reexamination and removal of skin sutures in 2 weeks
- Removal of cerclage wire around mandibles in 4 to 5 weeks

PROGNOSIS AND OUTCOME

- Good prognosis for survival and return to normal function for ~90% of cats.
- Most dogs falling >6 stories may not survive and hence are not brought to the hospital and assessed in case series studies; spinal injuries increase with increasing height of fall due to landing of dogs on their back or in a vertical position.

PEARLS & CONSIDERATIONS

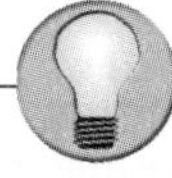

COMMENTS

Number and severity of injuries increase with increasing height of fall; others reported that the association between injuries and height of fall follows a curvilinear pattern.

CLIENT EDUCATION

Close windows and balcony doors in the presence of animals

SUGGESTED READING

Gordon LE, et al: High-rise syndrome in dogs: 81 cases (1985–1991). *J Am Vet Med Assoc* 202:118, 1993.

Papazoglou LG, et al: High-rise syndrome in cats: 207 cases (1988–1998). *Aust Vet Practit* 31:98, 2001.

Vnuk D, et al: Feline high-rise syndrome: 119 cases (1998–2001). *J Feline Med Surg* 6:305, 2004.

Whitney WO, Mehlhaff CJ: High-rise syndrome in cats. *J Am Vet Med Assoc* 191:1399, 1987.

AUTHOR & EDITOR: **ALEXANDER M. REITER**

Hip Dysplasia

BASIC INFORMATION

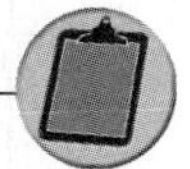

DEFINITION

An abnormal development of the coxofemoral joint characterized by partial or complete luxation of the femoral head in young patients, and mild to severe degenerative joint disease (DJD) in mature patients

EPIDEMIOLOGY

SPECIES, AGE, SEX

- Most common in young (3 to 12 months) and mature dogs
- Less frequent in cats

GENETICS AND BREED PREDISPOSITION

- Most common in large and giant canine breeds
- May be more common in the Maine coon cat

RISK FACTORS

- Rapid weight gain and growth associated with excessive caloric intake
- Factors causing synovial inflammation of the coxofemoral joint
- Trauma to the coxofemoral joint

ASSOCIATED CONDITIONS AND DISORDERS: Affected animals concurrently may have other genetically predisposed or developmental conditions such as:

- Elbow dysplasia
- Osteochondrosis
- Stifle disease
- Panosteitis
- Hypertrophic osteodystrophy

CLINICAL PRESENTATION

DISEASE FORMS/SUBTYPES

- Juvenile:
  - Acetabular dysplasia
  - Abnormal femoral neck angles of inclination and anteversion
- Mature:
  - Joint degeneration

HISTORY, CHIEF COMPLAINT

- Juvenile patients have a history of rear leg lameness characterized by:
  - "Bunny-hopping" gait
  - Unilateral or bilateral pelvic limb lameness
  - Difficulty rising
  - Change in jumping behavior
  - Exercise intolerance
  - Description of an audible "clicking" when rising or walking
- Mature patients have a history of lameness associated with coxofemoral osteoarthritis.

PHYSICAL EXAM FINDINGS

- Juvenile patient:
  - Pain during caudal extension, external rotation and abduction of the coxofemoral joint
  - Hip joint laxity (positive Ortolani sign) characterized by dorsal subluxation of the femoral head with the limb adducted followed by a palpable click with reduction of the femoral head when the limb is abducted
    - Angle of reduction is the measured point at which the femoral head slips back into the acetabulum as the limb is abducted
    - Angle of subluxation is the measured point at which the femoral head slips out of the acetabulum as the limb is then adducted
  - Poor pelvic limb musculature
  - Abnormal pelvic limb conformation (tarsal hyperextension)
  - Patient may have more of an arched spine appearance, as weight is shifted forward onto the forelimbs
  - Narrow pelvic limb stance
- Mature patient:
  - Pain during extension, external rotation and abduction of the hip
  - Decreased joint range of motion
  - Joint crepitation
  - Ortolani sign is lost as pericapsular fibrosis limits femoral head movements
  - Hind limb muscle atrophy

ETIOLOGY AND PATHOPHYSIOLOGY

- A combination of genetic and environmental factors lead to hip joint laxity resulting in joint instability and abnormal progression of endochondral ossification.
- Puppies with a genetic predisposition to canine hip dysplasia are born with hips that are grossly normal. Changes in the hip joint begin within the first few weeks after birth.
- Lameness and gait abnormalities usually appear at time of growth between 3 and 8 months old.

DIAGNOSIS

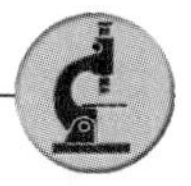

DIFFERENTIAL DIAGNOSIS

- Panosteitis
- Osteochondrosis
- Physeal fractures of the femoral head
- Hypertrophic osteodystrophy
- Partial or complete cranial cruciate ligament injury
- Lumbosacral disease
- Polyarthritis
- Bone neoplasia
- Rickettsial and fungal disease (geographic)

INITIAL DATABASE

- Complete blood count, serum biochemical profile, urinalysis: generally unremarkable.
- Rickettsial and/or fungal titers: to rule out other causes of lameness (polyarthritis, bone lesions).
- Palpation of hip joints for Ortolani sign (displacement and reseating of the femoral head as the limb is taken from adduction to abduction; easiest to perform if dog is in dorsal recumbency), calculation of angles of subluxation and reduction.
  - May require sedation/anesthesia
- Lateral and ventrodorsal pelvic radiographs (Fig. I-91).
  - Orthopedic Foundation for Animals (OFA) and/or PennHip positioning to quantitate hip joint laxity

ADVANCED OR CONFIRMATORY TESTING

- Dorsal acetabular rim (DAR) view radiography
- Calculation of femoral neck inclination and anteversion angles
- Computed tomography

TREATMENT

THERAPEUTIC GOAL(S)

Relieve pain and improve function through biomechanical stabilization of the hip joint

ACUTE GENERAL TREATMENT

- Medical management:
  - Nonsteroidal anti-inflammatory drugs (NSAIDs):
    - Aspirin 10–25 mg/kg PO q 8–24h; or
    - Carprofen 2 mg/kg PO q 12h; or
    - Etodolac 10–15 mg/kg PO q 24h; or
    - Deracoxib 1–2 mg/kg PO q 24h (may use 3 to 4 mg/kg PO q 24h for first 7 days only); or
    - Meloxicam 0.1 mg/kg PO q 24h; or
    - Tepoxalin 10 mg/kg PO q 24h (new product, objective data pending); or
    - Others.
- Surgical management:
  - Juvenile pubic symphysiodesis:
    - In immature patients (14 to 20 weeks of age).
    - To increase acetabular coverage of the femoral head; prevents osteoarthritis.
  - Intertrochanteric osteotomy (ITO):
    - In immature dogs.
    - Limited to dogs with abnormal femoral neck angles.
    - Some surgeons question the efficacy of this procedure.
  - Triple pelvic osteotomy (TPO):
    - In young dogs without DJD.
    - To increase acetabular coverage of the femoral head and prevent osteoarthritis.
  - DAR arthroplasty:
    - In young dogs.
    - To augment/enhance the supportive dorsal acetabular rim.
  - Total hip replacement (THR):
    - In mature dogs.
    - To replace degenerative joint structures with synthetic components.
  - Femoral head and neck ostectomy (FHO):
    - Young to mature dogs.
    - To reduce degenerative bone contact and form a pseudoarthrosis.
    - Once a patient has undergone this procedure, THR can no longer be performed on that joint.

CHRONIC TREATMENT

- Medical management:
  - NSAID drugs as listed under Acute General Treatment above.
  - A chondroprotective agent:
    - Polysulfated glycosaminoglycan 5 mg/kg IM once weekly × 4 to 6 weeks; or
    - Pentosan polysulfate (from beechwood hemicellulose) 3 mg/kg SC once weekly; or
    - Oral formulations (glucosamine, chondroitin sulphate, hyaluronan): according to formulation/labeled instructions.
  - Nutrition (energy restricted diet, as appropriate).
  - Weight control.
  - Exercise moderation.
- Surgical management:
  - FHO or THR are performed in mature animals with chronic disease (joint degeneration) unresponsive to medical therapies.

POSSIBLE COMPLICATIONS

- Medical management:
  - Gastrointestinal, hepatic, renal, or other systemic reactions from NSAID therapy
  - Continued progression of DJD
  - Failure of medical management to control pain
- Surgical management:
  - Nerve and/or urinary tract damage from TPO surgery
  - Implant failure
  - Osteomyelitis
  - Hip luxation or femoral fracture with THR
  - Poor limb usage after FHO due to patient obesity, muscular atony

RECOMMENDED MONITORING

- Basic laboratory monitoring of patients on NSAID therapy
- Weight, exercise levels, and clinical signs as dictated by the patient
- Radiographic monitoring if clinical signs progress

PROGNOSIS AND OUTCOME

- The majority of patients will function at a pain-free high level of activity with appropriate medical and surgical intervention.
- Postoperative rehabilitation is critical for clinical recovery.

PEARLS & CONSIDERATIONS

COMMENTS

- Bilateral lameness may be difficult to recognize.
- A total of 60–75% of juvenile patients who are lame due to hip joint laxity and are treated with medical management may return to acceptable clinical function with maturity.
- Radiographic signs do not always correlate with clinical signs.
- FHO excludes further surgical procedures such as THR.
- Routine radiographic monitoring of the clinically stable patient is generally not necessary.
- *Editor's note:* Practitioners should consider consultation and referral with an orthopedic surgeon; ITO and DAR arthroplasty are controversial.

PREVENTION

- Screening and control of breeding animals for hip dysplasia:
  - Avoid breeding animals not receiving "normal" or excellent/good ratings by OFA or PennHip evaluation schemes.
  - Controversy exists regarding which of the two systems is "best"; OFA evaluation has been the traditional

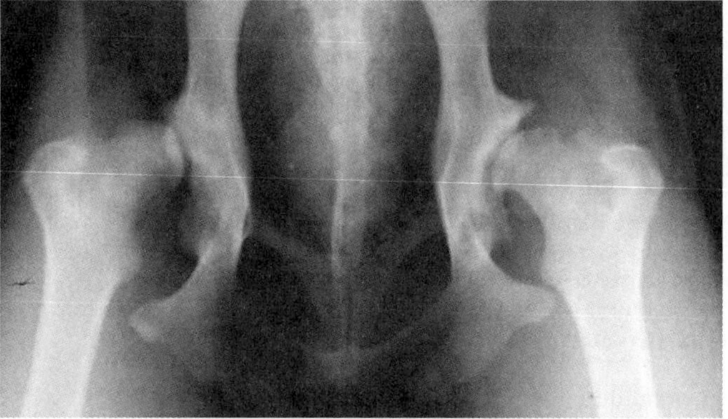

FIGURE I-91 Ventrodorsal projection of severely dysplastic hips in a 16-month-old retriever cross dog. Radiographic abnormalities include subluxation of the femoral heads and remodeling of the shallow acetabula and femoral necks. This dog would be a candidate for total hip replacement or femoral head/neck excisions based on numerous clinical parameters described in the text.

and simpler methodology, whereas the PennHip approach is regarded as more sensitive in detecting loose hips without arthritic changes. This latter evaluation requires course enrollment and certification of the attending veterinarian.

- Avoid high-energy diets in young, rapidly growing large-dog breeds

CLIENT EDUCATION

- Knowledge and careful screening of genetic history on potential pets
- Early sterilization of affected dogs
- Minimize the phenotypic expression of the disease in affected dogs through diet, exercise, and medical management

SUGGESTED READING

Johnson AL, Hulse DA: Hip dysplasia. In Fossum TW (ed): *Small Animal Surgery*, ed 2. St. Louis, Mosby, 2002, pp 1093–1102.

Schultz KS, Dejardin LM: Surgical treatment of canine hip dysplasia. In Slatter D (ed): *Textbook of Small Animal Surgery*, ed 3. Philadelphia, WB Saunders, 2002, pp 2029–2059.

Slocum B, Slocum TD: Hip. In Bojrab MJ (ed): *Current Techniques in Small Animal Surgery*, ed 4. Baltimore, Williams & Wilkins, 1998, pp 1127–1186.

AUTHORS: **JAMES P. BOULAY, BARBARA R. GORES**

EDITOR: **JOSEPH HARARI**

Hip Luxation

BASIC INFORMATION

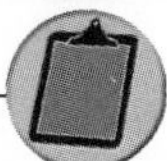

DEFINITION

- Dislocation of the femoral head relative to the acetabulum, most frequently in a craniodorsal direction
- Luxation: complete displacement of the femoral head relative to the acetabulum
- Subluxation: partial or incomplete dislocation of the femoral head relative to the acetabulum (i.e., joint incongruity exists)

SYNONYM(S)

Coxofemoral luxation
Dislocated hip

EPIDEMIOLOGY

RISK FACTORS: Dogs with hip dysplasia are at risk for luxation secondary to minor trauma.

ASSOCIATED CONDITIONS AND DISORDERS: Pelvic and proximal femoral fractures.

CLINICAL PRESENTATION

DISEASE FORMS/SUBTYPES: Craniodorsal luxation most common; caudoventral is uncommon.

HISTORY, CHIEF COMPLAINT

- Trauma (falls, vehicular) causing acute non–weight-bearing lameness
- Intermittent lameness in chronic cases with unrecognized trauma

PHYSICAL EXAM FINDINGS

- Variable lameness
- With craniodorsal luxation, leg appears shortened, stifle rotated externally, and tarsus internally
- Palpation of hip reveals swelling, pain, crepitus, and abnormal position of greater trochanter

ETIOLOGY AND PATHOPHYSIOLOGY

Traumatic coxofemoral luxations comprise 90% of all luxations in small animals.

- With craniodorsal luxation, femoral head is driven dorsally over the acetabular rim:
  - Both femoral head ligament and joint capsule are torn
  - Avulsion fracture associated with ligament can occur
  - Gluteal muscle contractions exacerbate craniodorsal displacement of proximal femur
- With ventral luxation, transverse acetabular ligament is ruptured

DIAGNOSIS

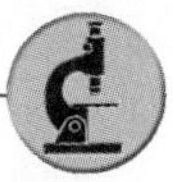

DIFFERENTIAL DIAGNOSIS

Subluxation due to hip dysplasia, femoral capital physeal fracture, femoral neck fracture, acetabular fracture

INITIAL DATABASE

- Physical examination: findings as described previously (see Physical Exam Findings above)
- Complete blood count/serum chemistry panel/urinalysis and thoracic/abdominal radiographs based on patient stability and the American Society of Anesthesiologists' classification (see p 1334)
- Limb and pelvis examinations plus orthogonal view radiography to confirm the diagnosis and determine concomitant or inciting disorders (Figs. I-92 and I-93)

TREATMENT

THERAPEUTIC GOAL(S)

- With acute injury of normal joint, goal is closed or open anatomic joint reduction/stabilization.
- With abnormal or chronic normal joint, goal is to save limb and treat joint by femoral head osteotomy (FHO), total hip replacement (THR), or triple pelvic osteotomy (TPO).

ACUTE GENERAL TREATMENT

- Closed reduction and Ehmer sling application if:
  - Duration of injury is <48 hours, and
  - Hip is otherwise structurally normal, and
  - Patient is sufficiently stable to undergo general anesthesia
- With patient in lateral recumbency (unaffected side down), the upper (affected) limb is externally rotated (toes out), abducted (lifted, as a male dog lifts the leg to urinate), and then internally rotated (toes in) while manual pressure on trochanter guides head into acetabulum.
- After reduction, extensive range of motion maneuvers are performed to force soft tissue out of acetabulum and test joint stability.
- Open reduction is performed in failed or unstable closed reductions in a patient with normal coxofemoral joint.
- Extra-articular techniques include suture between origin of greater trochanter and rectus femoris muscle, iliofemoral suture, synthetic sutures to replace capsule, capsulorrhaphy, or De Vita pinning (controversial).
- Intra-articular techniques (see Fig. I-93): toggle pinning, fascia lata loop, sacrotuberal ligament transposition.
- Triple pelvic osteotomy can be performed for mildly dysplastic, immature dogs with no degenerative joint changes.
- For chronic injuries, open reduction is difficult due to muscular contraction and tissue fibrosis; cartilage degeneration exists. FHO or THR may be required in place of primary repairs.

CHRONIC TREATMENT

- Physical rehabilitation to maintain muscle tone, joint health, and overall limb functions.

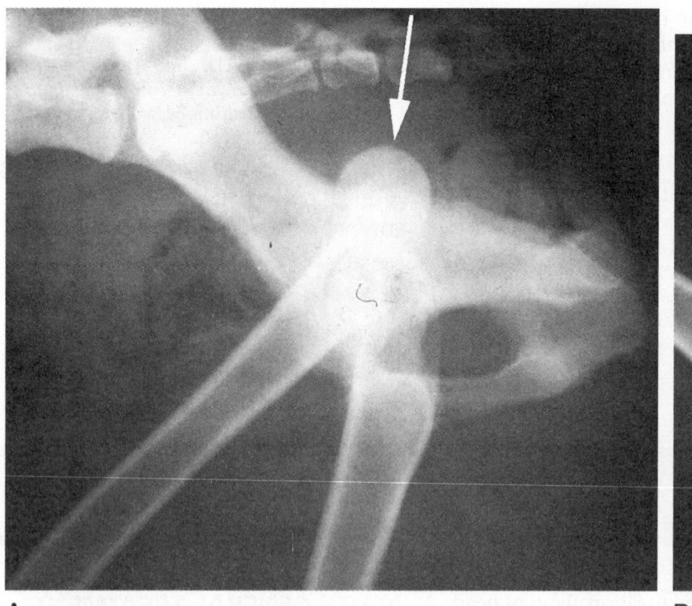

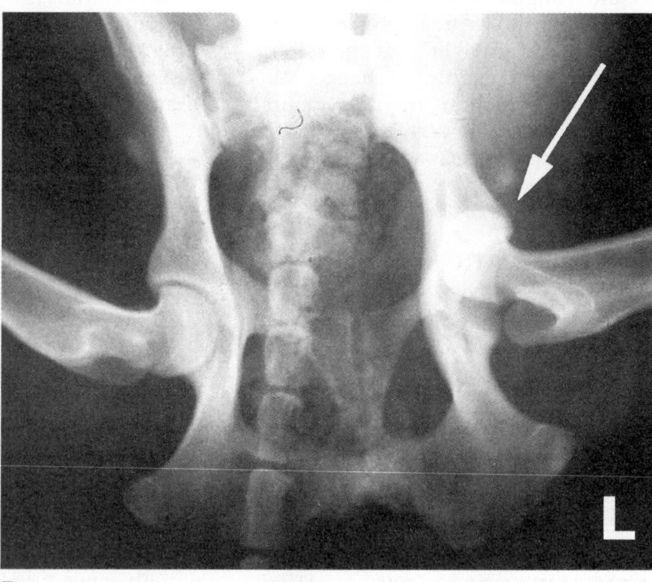

FIGURE I-92 **A**, Lateral and **B**, ventrodorsal projections of a craniodorsal luxation of the left hip joint. Note dorsal and cranial displacement of the femoral head relative to the acetabulum *(arrows)*.

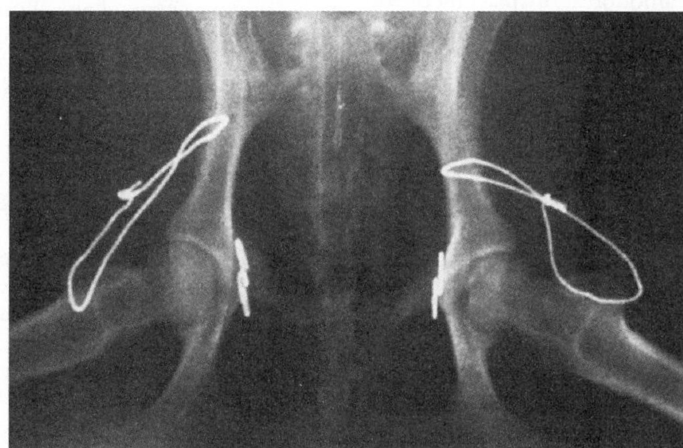

FIGURE I-93 Postoperative ventrodorsal projection of the hip joints of an obese, 45-kg dog treated for traumatic bilateral hip luxation. Bilateral toggle pins and greater-trochanter-to-ilium wires were used for stabilizing the injuries.

- Controlled activity to avoid relaxation, implant failures.
- Nonsteroidal anti-inflammatory drugs (NSAIDs) as needed to reduce pain and inflammation:
    - Aspirin 10–25 mg/kg PO q 8–24h; or
    - Carprofen 2 mg/kg PO q 12h; or
    - Etodolac 10–15 mg/kg PO q 24h; or
    - Deracoxib 1–2 mg/kg PO q 24h (may use 3–4 mg/kg PO q 24h for first 7 days only); or
    - Meloxicam 0.1 mg/kg PO q 24h; or
    - Meclofenamic acid 1.1 mg/kg, PO q 24h after eating, for 5 days maximum; or
    - Tepoxalin 10 mg/kg PO q 24h (new product, objective data pending); or
    - Others.

POSSIBLE COMPLICATIONS

- Reluxation
- Implant failure
- Degenerative joint disease
- Infection

RECOMMENDED MONITORING

- For closed reduction:
    - Frequent sling evaluations and removal 7 to 10 days postapplication
    - Limited activity for 1 month
    - Radiography after sling application and if lameness recurs
- For open repairs:
    - Restricted ambulation 1 to 2 months
    - Radiography if lameness recurs and based on fixation method

PROGNOSIS AND OUTCOME

- Variable with closed reduction: 50% fail due to technical error or unrecognized joint disease
- Good to excellent with most operative procedures of acute injuries (i.e., previously normal joint)
- Guarded for dysplastic hips unless TPO, FHO, THR performed

PEARLS & CONSIDERATIONS

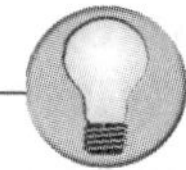

COMMENTS

- With normal hips, reduction/stabilization is preferred over FHO for all patient sizes.
- Extensive joint capsule and ligament damage impede successful closed reduction.
- Femoral head ligament avulsion fractures are often not recognized radiographically.

SUGGESTED READING

Haburjak JJ, et al: Treatment of traumatic coxofemoral luxation with triple pelvic osteotomy in 19 dogs (1987–1999). *Vet Comp Orthop Traumtol* 14:69, 2001.

Holsworth IG, DeCamp CE: Coxofemoral luxation. In Slatter D (ed): *Textbook of Small Animal Surgery*, ed 3. Philadelphia, WB Saunders, 2002, pp 2002–2008.

Kilic E, et al: Transposition of the sacrotuberous ligament for the treatment of coxofemoral luxation in dogs. *J Small Anim Pract* 43:341, 2002.

Piermattei DL, Flo GL: The hip joint. In *Brinker, Piermattei, and Flo's Handbook of Small Animal Orthopedics and Fracture Repair*, ed 3. Philadelphia, WB Saunders, 1997, pp 422–433.

Shani J, et al: Stabilization of traumatic coxofemoral luxation with an extra-capsular suture from the greater trochanter to the origin of the rectus femoris. *Vet Comp Orthop Traumatol* 17:12, 2004.

AUTHORS: **JONATHAN SHANI, JOSEPH HARARI**

EDITOR: **JOSEPH HARARI**

Histiocytic Diseases

BASIC INFORMATION

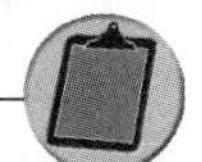

DEFINITION

A complex group of syndromes resulting from an accumulation of histiocytes, which are cells of macrophage or dendritic origin. Recent work suggests a primarily dendritic origin of these histiocytes. Syndromes overlap, diverge, and converge but can be simplified into the following groups:

- Benign tumors:
  - Histiocytoma: spontaneously regressing skin tumor common in young animals.
  - Idiopathic periadnexal multinodular granulomatous dermatitis.
- Reactive histiocytic disorders:
  - Cutaneous histiocytosis: a benign accumulation of histiocytes in the skin, with predilection for the nasal planum, head, and neck.
  - Systemic histiocytosis: similar to cutaneous histiocytosis but characterized by lymph node involvement.
- Malignant histiocytic neoplasia:
  - Malignant histiocytosis: simultaneous multiorgan involvement.
  - Histiocytic sarcoma: begins as a focal lesion and may disseminate, then difficult to differentiate from malignant histiocytosis.
  - Malignant fibrous histiocytoma: focal lesion, behaves as soft tissue sarcoma with three histologic subtypes (see Malignant Fibrous Histiocytoma, p 667).

These disease syndromes share many common features, though clinical and histologic aspects may help differentiate each one. Malignant histiocytosis and disseminated histiocytic sarcoma may be a continuum or even the same disease. Similarly, systemic histiocytosis and malignant histiocytosis may be a continuum, as both have multiorgan involvement and are progressive and poorly responsive to therapy. Malignant fibrous histiocytosis may be a focal form of histiocytic sarcoma, and also has been described as a group of several soft tissue sarcomas (e.g., muscle tumors) that have a unifying characteristic of histiocytic and multinucleated giant cell infiltrate.

SYNONYM(S)

- Histiocytic sarcoma (disseminated): malignant histiocytosis (though some texts describe disseminated histiocytic sarcoma as having features of both malignant histiocytosis and malignant fibrous histiocytoma).
- Histiocytic sarcoma (focal) may be the same as malignant fibrous histiocytoma in some texts, and is sometimes called giant cell tumor of soft parts or of bone.

EPIDEMIOLOGY

SPECIES, AGE, SEX

- Histiocytic diseases have predominantly been reported in dogs, but reports exist in cats (malignant histiocytosis, malignant fibrous histiocytoma), cattle (malignant histiocytosis, malignant fibrous histiocytoma), and people.
- Reports in cats are few, but malignant fibrous histiocytoma is one type of vaccine-associated sarcoma.
- Cutaneous histiocytosis can occur in younger dogs, systemic histiocytosis and malignant histiocytosis in middle-aged dogs (median age 6 years), and malignant fibrous histiocytoma in middle-aged to older dogs.
- Equal prevalence in males and females.

GENETICS AND BREED PREDISPOSITION: Bernese mountain dogs are predisposed to many types of histiocytic disease, though as a breed they are not as commonly reported in malignant fibrous histiocytoma. In Bernese mountain dogs, heritability is polygenic and almost certainly *not* autosomal or sex-linked. Approximately 25% of all tumors in Bernese mountain dogs are histiocytic neoplasms. Other breeds that are overrepresented in histiocytic diseases include golden retrievers, flat-coated retrievers, rottweilers, and Doberman pinschers.

RISK FACTORS: For cats, vaccination may predispose to malignant fibrous histiocytoma.

GEOGRAPHY AND SEASONALITY: In the original description of histiocytosis in Bernese mountain dogs, most of the affected dogs came from Switzerland, where the breed originated. Cases have now been reported in dogs born in the United States and the United Kingdom. There is no reported seasonality.

CLINICAL PRESENTATION

DISEASE FORMS/SUBTYPES

- As detailed above, histiocytic diseases can be divided in different ways but ultimately are either local or diffuse, and reactive, benign, or malignant.
- Malignant fibrous histiocytoma has three subtypes: storiform-pleomorphic (mesenchymal tissue with histiocytic infiltrate, the most common form in dogs), inflammatory (most common in the spleen of dogs), and giant cell (the most common type in cats).

HISTORY, CHIEF COMPLAINT

- Most dogs are presented for signs referable to the primary tumor.
- Dogs with cutaneous histiocytosis and systemic histiocytosis are typically presented for evaluation of skin lesions.
- Systemic histiocytosis can have orbital involvement and patients may be presented for evaluation of ocular signs.
- Dogs with malignant fibrous histiocytoma are usually presented for evaluation of a soft tissue mass, or lameness if the joint tissues or bones are involved.
- Malignant histiocytosis is a much more insidious disease, since masses are primarily visceral (spleen, liver, bone marrow, lymph nodes, lungs). Cutaneous and subcutaneous masses are uncommon with malignant histiocytosis. These dogs and cats are often presented for evaluation of nonspecific systemic signs such as lethargy and anorexia/weight loss.

PHYSICAL EXAM FINDINGS

- Focal lesions typically involve a palpable mass, often on the extremities. If the mass is subarticular, lameness may be prominent, especially with bone involvement.
- A prominent spleen may be palpated with splenic malignant fibrous histiocytoma or with splenic involvement of malignant histiocytosis.
- Dogs with malignant histiocytosis often have significant pulmonary involvement and may be dyspneic with advanced disease.

- With systemic histiocytosis, skin lesions may be seen on the nasal planum, muzzle, flank, and scrotum as well as the periocular tissues. Skin lesions in cutaneous histiocytosis and systemic histiocytosis are typically nodular to plaque-like.
- Generalized lymphadenopathy may be appreciated with systemic histiocytosis and malignant histiocytosis, and enlargement of the draining lymph node may be found with malignant fibrous histiocytoma.

ETIOLOGY AND PATHOPHYSIOLOGY

- Largely unknown in dogs, although polygenic inheritance has been shown in Bernese mountain dogs.
- Malignant fibrous histiocytoma in cats possibly resulting from vaccination is covered elsewhere under vaccine-associated sarcomas (see Vaccine-Site Sarcoma, p 1136).

DIAGNOSIS

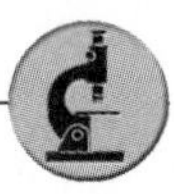

DIFFERENTIAL DIAGNOSIS

- Granulomatous disease
- Lymphoma
- Poorly differentiated mast cell tumor
- Anaplastic sarcoma or carcinoma
- Other soft tissue sarcomas (malignant fibrous histiocytoma)

INITIAL DATABASE

- Complete blood count, serum chemistry profile, and urinalysis. No characteristic or specific findings with histiocytic diseases
- Fine-needle aspiration of accessible masses and lymph nodes with cytology (look for multinucleated giant cells and erythrophagocytosis by macrophages)
- Biopsy of affected tissue
- Radiography of affected area if bony involvement is suspected
- Thoracic radiography to evaluate pulmonary parenchyma for nodules (often large)
- Abdominal ultrasound to screen for visceral involvement
- Bone marrow aspiration and cytology if suspect systemic disease

ADVANCED OR CONFIRMATORY TESTING

- Computed tomography scan of affected area if focal and considering resection
- Immunohistochemistry on biopsy tissue (see Pearls & Considerations below)

TREATMENT

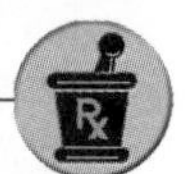

THERAPEUTIC GOAL(S)

Resection (focal disease) or regression (systemic disease) of measurable lesions

ACUTE GENERAL TREATMENT

- Patients with malignant histiocytosis having significant erythrophagocytosis may require red blood cell transfusion, ideally in conjunction with initiation of therapy to abort red cell loss.
- Dyspneic patients with malignant histiocytosis may benefit temporarily from oxygen therapy, but the prognosis is grave when the disease has reached the point of producing respiratory compromise.

CHRONIC TREATMENT

- Reactive histiocytoses are typically treated with immunosuppressive therapy. Initially prednisone is used (2 mg/kg PO q 24h until clinical response is noted, then a slow taper of 1 mg/kg PO q 24h for one month, 0.5 mg/kg PO q 24h for one month, 0.5 mg/kg PO q 48h for 3 months, then stop or maintain at lowest effective dose). If no response is noted within 1 month of prednisone therapy, or if lesions relapse and no longer respond to prednisone, then azathioprine may be added at 2 mg/kg PO q 24h with the same taper schedule.
- Systemic malignant histiocytic diseases are poorly responsive to therapy and remissions, if achieved, are typically short-lived.
  - Therapies attempted include: chemotherapy (doxorubicin-based, CCNU) and TALL104 therapy (cytotoxic T-lymphocytes)
- Focal malignant histiocytic diseases respond well to surgical resection (amputation if joint or bone affected or if complete resection with limb salvage impossible) ± irradiation.

RECOMMENDED MONITORING

- The involved site(s) should be monitored closely via regular observation and diagnostic imaging as appropriate.
- Three-view thoracic radiographs, and physical examination including lymph node palpation and examination of the site, should be performed every 3 months for the first year after diagnosis for malignant fibrous histiocytoma and every 4 to 6 months thereafter.

PROGNOSIS AND OUTCOME

- Cutaneous histiocytosis: good; may regress spontaneously or respond to immunosuppressive doses of prednisone.
- Systemic histiocytosis, malignant histiocytosis, and disseminated histiocytic sarcoma: poor. Systemic histiocytosis may wax and wane but is ultimately progressive, whereas malignant histiocytosis is rapidly progressive. Dogs are typically euthanized for their disease in both cases. Malignant histiocytosis is considered uniformly fatal. Survival of dogs with systemic histiocytosis ranges from months to years. Few dogs with malignant histiocytosis or disseminated histiocytic sarcoma live beyond 4 months. Prognosis to date for cats with malignant histiocytosis is similarly grave and response to therapy has been poor.
- Malignant fibrous histiocytoma or focal histiocytic sarcoma: good if low-grade and local control is achieved with surgery ± radiation.

PEARLS & CONSIDERATIONS

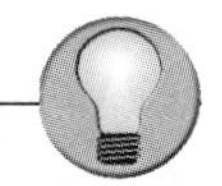

COMMENTS

The following clinical and pathologic differences can help differentiate histiocytic syndromes:

- Clinical findings/behavior:
  - Malignant histiocytosis is a multiorgan disease, typically arising from internal sites, including viscera, whereas systemic histiocytosis involves skin and lymph nodes with occasional internal sites.
  - Systemic histiocytosis may wax and wane but ultimately progresses, whereas malignant histiocytosis is rapidly progressive.
  - Cutaneous histiocytosis is limited to the skin and does not lead to malignant histiocytosis.
  - When malignant fibrous histiocytoma occurs in the viscera, the spleen is the most common location.
  - Malignant fibrous histiocytoma can metastasize to the lymph nodes, especially the giant cell variant, which is unusual for sarcomas.
- Histopathology:
  - Malignant histiocytosis exhibits a greater degree of cellular atypia than systemic histiocytosis.
  - Malignant histiocytosis often exhibits erythrocytophagia and sometimes leukocytophagia.
  - Multinucleated giant cells can be seen in malignant histiocytosis and in malignant fibrous histiocytoma, but malignant fibrous histiocytoma has more spindloid cells.
- Immunohistochemistry:
  - CD 18+, CD 3–, and CD 79a– are the three immunohistochemical stains and the pattern most useful for diagnosing dendritic cell origin and ruling out lymphoma.
  - Dendritic cells should be CD 1+ and macrophages should be CD 1–.
  - Malignant histiocytic diseases should be CD 4– and reactive CD 4+.

PREVENTION

Because histiocytic diseases are often inherited, careful documentation of pedigrees for affected animals is crucial to the eventual control by selective breeding. Inheritance of histiocytosis in Bernese mountain dogs has been calculated at a moderate 0.298, suggesting that careful breeding could be effective at eliminating this disease. This means that 29.8% of the risk of developing histiocytosis in the population of Bernese mountain dogs is attributable to genetic differences among individuals. The remainder of the risk is environmental, though specific factors have not been identified.

CLIENT EDUCATION

- Owners should contact the breeder or source of affected animals.
- An overtly (phenotypically) normal breeding pair of Bernese mountain dogs with one affected offspring will produce, on average, one in seven puppies that will ultimately succumb to histiocytosis.

SUGGESTED READING

Affolter VK, Moore PF: Localized and disseminated histiocytic sarcoma of dendritic cell origin in dogs. *Vet Pathol* 39:74-83, 2002.

Canine histiocytosis overview: www.histiocytosis.ucdavis.edu.

Kraje AC, et al: Malignant histiocytosis in 3 cats. *J Vet Intern Med* 15:252-256, 2001.

Padgett GA, et al: Inheritance of histiocytosis in Bernese Mountain Dogs. *J Sm An Prac* 36:93-98, 1995.

Vail DM: Histiocytic disorders. In Withrow SJ, MacEwen EG (eds): *Small Animal Clinical Oncology*, ed 3. Philadelphia, WB Saunders, 2001, pp 667-671.

AUTHOR: **KIM A. SELTING**

EDITOR: **KENNETH M. RASSNICK**

Histoplasmosis

BASIC INFORMATION

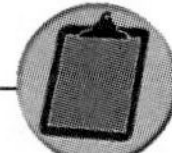

DEFINITION

A systemic fungal disease, affecting both companion animals and humans, caused by the soil-dwelling dimorphic fungus *Histoplasma capsulatum*

EPIDEMIOLOGY

SPECIES, AGE, SEX

- Dogs and cats are both affected and are equally likely to develop histoplasmosis once exposed.
- Most dogs with histoplasmosis are young adult, large-breed dogs. There is no apparent sex predilection; however, some believe males are slightly predisposed.
- Most cats with histoplasmosis are young (<4 years). Females may be more commonly affected.

GENETICS AND BREED PREDISPOSITION

- Although there are no dog breeds identified as being definitively predisposed to developing histoplasmosis, some sporting (hunting) breeds may be overrepresented. This observation may be a result of greater risk of environmental exposure rather than a hereditary characteristic.
- There is no apparent breed predilection in cats.

RISK FACTORS

- Outdoor activities in endemic areas
- Contact with nitrogen-rich organic material such as moist soil containing bird (classically, starling, but many bird species are implicated) or bat excrement

CONTAGION AND ZOONOSIS: As with other systemic mycoses, transmission of histoplasmosis from animal to human has not been reported except via inhalation of fungal spores in infected soil. However, humans are susceptible to the disease if exposed to the mycelial stage (e.g., common-source infections, where humans and dogs are infected simultaneously).

GEOGRAPHY AND SEASONALITY: *H. capsulatum* is endemic to many temperate and subtropical regions of the world (Fig. I-94). In the United States, histoplasmosis occurs most commonly in the Missouri, Mississippi, and Ohio River valleys.

H. capsulatum may thrive in nonendemic regions, however, if soil conditions change so as to favor fungal growth.

CLINICAL PRESENTATION

DISEASE FORMS/SUBTYPES: Disease may remain confined to the lungs or to the gastrointestinal (GI) tract, or may become disseminated (commonly with GI involvement).

HISTORY, CHIEF COMPLAINT

- Clinical signs are determined by the major organ system(s) affected. Clients should be carefully questioned about recent travel with their pets to endemic areas in the preceding 1 to 2 months.
- Nonspecific signs of disease are common (especially in cats) and typically include depression, anorexia, and weight loss. Clients may notice labored breathing in dogs and cats with pulmonary histoplasmosis. Dogs with GI involvement may exhibit signs consistent with small and/or large bowel diarrhea, melena/hematochezia, tenesmus, and recent weight loss. Signs of GI involvement in cats are less readily identifiable versus those in dogs, and may manifest merely as weight loss and anorexia.

PHYSICAL EXAM FINDINGS

- Dyspnea, tachypnea, coughing, abnormal lung sounds
- Poor body condition/emaciation
- Fever
- Hepatomegaly, splenomegaly, or both in some cases of disseminated disease
- Ocular and dermal lesions rarely occur

ETIOLOGY AND PATHOPHYSIOLOGY

- The mycelial stage (the stage that occurs in soil and that results in production of spores [microconidia and macroconidia]) of *H. capsulatum* is responsible for mammalian infections. Exposure probably most commonly occurs by inhaling microconidia, which are small enough to reach the lower airways. It is speculated that less commonly, oral exposure can result in disease, as evidenced by some animals developing only GI signs.
- After microconidia are inhaled, they convert to the yeast form in the small airways of the lower respiratory tract, where they reproduce by budding.
- The organisms are phagocytosed by host mononuclear cells, in which they undergo further replication. Disease at this point may remain limited to the respiratory system or become generalized due to the potential of lymphatic and/or hematogenous dissemination of the organism within mononuclear phagocytic cells.
- Dissemination to the GI tract, lymph nodes, spleen, liver, and bone marrow occurs most commonly. The organism load in infected tissues is generally high, and affected tissues counter with a granulomatous inflammatory response.

DIAGNOSIS

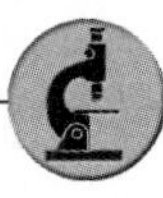

DIFFERENTIAL DIAGNOSIS

- Other systemic mycoses (e.g., blastomycosis, cryptococcosis, coccidioidomycosis)
- Neoplasia

INITIAL DATABASE

- Complete blood count (CBC):
  - Nonregenerative anemia (the most consistent, albeit nonspecific, finding with histoplasmosis). Likely secondary to chronic disease, bone marrow infiltration, and/or GI blood loss.
  - Leukocyte parameters are variably affected, and thrombocytopenia may be present.
  - Intracellular organisms may be (very rarely) observed on blood smears.
- Serum chemistry profile: Variable abnormalities may be present depending on organ system(s) involved. Commonly observed abnormalities include hypoalbuminemia, elevated liver enzyme activity, and hypercalcemia.
- Radiography:
  - Dogs and cats with active pulmonary histoplasmosis often exhibit a nodular interstitial pattern on thoracic radiographs consistent with mycotic pneumonia.
  - Similarly, tracheobronchial lymphadenopathy is commonly observed.
  - Pleural effusion may occasionally be present and obscure the aforementioned radiographic findings.
  - Osseous lesions are rarely observed, but when present, they consist of a mixed pattern of osteolysis and osteoproliferation.

ADVANCED OR CONFIRMATORY TESTING

- Fine-needle aspiration and cytology:
  - Usually provides a definitive antemortem diagnosis.
  - The organisms are usually observed within phagocytic cells and appear as single to multiple round bodies with a basophilic center and clear, thin outer rim.
  - Tissues most rewarding for obtaining a diagnostic sample in the dog include rectal scrapings, colonic biopsy imprints, and aspirates of bone marrow, liver, spleen, lung, and lymph nodes, depending on the extent of disease.
    - Organ enlargement and ease of access determine which organs are sampled.
    - A rectal scraping can be obtained in dogs by using a gloved finger to advance a small curette (e.g., of the type used for uterine curetting or bone marrow harvesting), with which the rectal mucosa is gently scraped. The sample is smeared on a microscope slide and examined microscopically. When properly done, the procedure is painless.
  - In cats, tissues that may successfully be sampled include bone marrow, lung, and lymph nodes.
- Histologic analysis of biopsy specimens may be necessary if cytologic testing results are inconclusive.
- Serologic testing is not recommended due to the unreliability of current immunodiagnostic tests.

TREATMENT

THERAPEUTIC GOAL(S)

- Treatment has focused on clearing *H. capsulatum* infection with oral azole antifungal agents. Duration of treatment depends on the severity of disease and the patient's response to therapy. Typically, animals are treated with oral antifungals for at least 4 to 6 months.
- If central nervous system involvement or ocular lesions are present, fluconazole is recommended due to its better penetration of these tissues.
- Ketoconazole can also be used, but due to its relatively lower efficacy against *H. capsulatum* compared to itraconazole or fluconazole and the potential for adverse side effects, it is typically reserved for cases where cost of treatment is a limiting factor.

ACUTE GENERAL TREATMENT

- Azole drugs (mild cases):
  - For mild cases (local involvement only, no overt respiratory signs, patient is eating and is not debilitated).
  - Itraconazole (10 mg/kg PO q 12-24h); or
  - Fluconazole (2.5-5 mg/kg PO q 12-24h for dogs; 50 mg/animal PO q 8h for cats).
  - Treatment should be initiated as early as possible in the disease process to improve the probability of preventing dissemination.
- Azole drug + amphotericin B (severe cases):
  - For severe disseminated histoplasmosis or fulminant pulmonary or GI disease, combination therapy of an oral azole with parenteral amphotericin B should be considered (various protocols).
  - The drugs are started concomitantly, with the azole continued past cessation of amphotericin B therapy.
  - Sample protocol for amphotericin B. Dog: 0.5 mg/kg IV 3 times weekly up to 60 days or until signs of toxicity, usually renal. Cat: 0.25 mg/kg IV 3 times weekly or until signs of toxicity, usually renal.
  - Sample protocol for lipid-soluble amphotericin B (lower risk of renal toxicity) for dogs and cats: 1 mg/kg

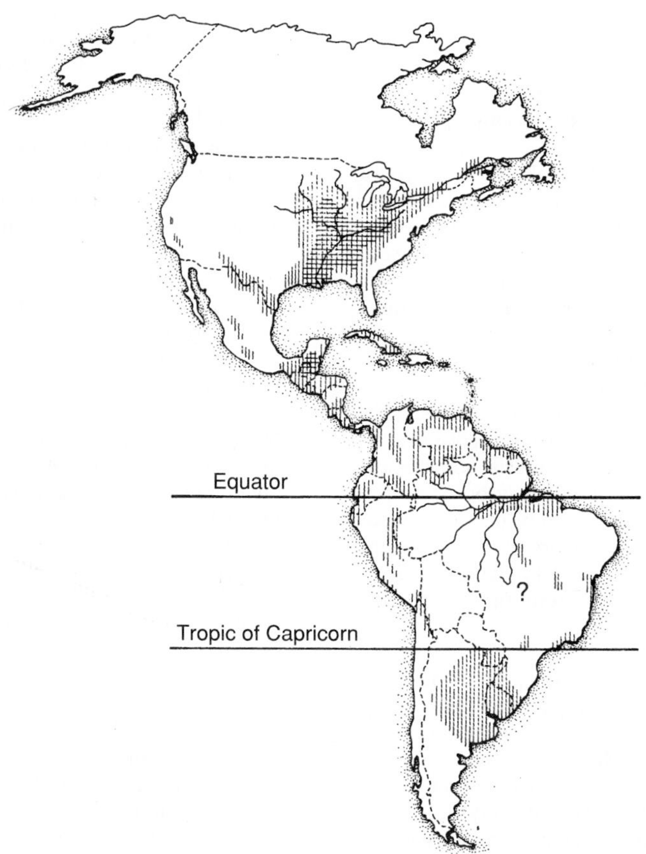

FIGURE I-94 Geographic area in which histoplasmosis is endemic. Areas of highest prevalence are cross-hatched. From Rippon JW: *Medical Mycology*, ed 3. Philadelphia, WB Saunders, 1988. Reprinted with permission.

IV 3 times weekly × 60 days or until signs of toxicity.
- Amphotericin B is fungicidal (vs. azoles, which are fungistatic) but is limited by its high risk of progressive renal toxicity (ensure patient is well hydrated and undergoing diuresis during treatment; monitor daily blood urea nitrogen and creatinine during treatment and stop treatment if >50% increase in either parameter), the potentially severe perivascular reaction or sloughing elicited by extravasation, and the possibility of anaphylaxis.

CHRONIC TREATMENT

Itraconazole or fluconazole should be administered orally for at least 4 to 6 months.

POSSIBLE COMPLICATIONS

Renal failure with amphotericin B

RECOMMENDED MONITORING

Response to treatment is monitored by periodically assessing CBC and serum chemistry values, observing for improvement in body condition, and monitoring for resolution of radiographic lesions.

PROGNOSIS AND OUTCOME

- Prognosis may vary from guarded to good depending on the extent of disease.
- Disease limited to the lungs typically carries a better prognosis compared to GI or disseminated histoplasmosis.

PEARLS & CONSIDERATIONS

COMMENTS

- Depending on the degree of *H. capsulatum* infection, some patients may be successfully treated with oral antifungals alone. Alternatively, some patients may be critically ill and require more intense combination therapy and supportive care. The need for fluid and nutritional support should not be overlooked in these patients.
- Ketoconazole and itraconazole are drugs that should always be administered with food; bioavailability of these drugs is optimized in the presence of ingesta, and given on an empty stomach, these medications may be less than 60% bioavailable.
- Therapeutic drug monitoring (serum level measurement) is available for ketoconazole and itraconazole.

PREVENTION

There is no effective vaccine against *H. capsulatum*. Disease is best prevented by avoiding contact with contaminated soil in endemic areas.

SUGGESTED READING

Kerl ME: Update on canine and feline fungal diseases. In Macintire DK, Breitschwerdt EB (eds): *The Veterinary Clinics of North America, Small Animal Practice: Emerging and Re-emerging Infectious Diseases.* Philadelphia, WB Saunders, 2003, pp 721–747.

Wolf AM: Histoplasmosis. In Greene CE (ed): *Infectious Diseases of the Dog and Cat,* ed 2. Philadephia, WB Saunders, 1998, pp 378–383.

AUTHOR: **JODI D. SMITH**
EDITOR: **DOUGLASS K. MACINTIRE**

Hit by Car

BASIC INFORMATION

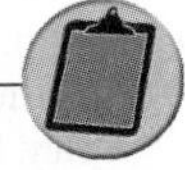

DEFINITION

Trauma sustained as a result of direct impact from a car, truck, or other motorized vehicle

SYNONYM(S)

HBC
Vehicular trauma
Blunt vehicular trauma
Motor vehicle accident
Road traffic accident

EPIDEMIOLOGY

SPECIES, AGE, SEX: Dogs and cats of any age, breed, or sex can be affected.
RISK FACTORS: Some studies suggest that young, male dogs and cats are at increased risk.
ASSOCIATED CONDITIONS AND DISORDERS: Hypovolemic shock, hemorrhage, fractures, neurologic deficits, ocular lesions, skin abrasions/lacerations.

CLINICAL PRESENTATION

HISTORY, CHIEF COMPLAINT
- The accident may be witnessed.
  - The animal may be found near the side of the road.
- Primary complaints include acute collapse, difficulty breathing, lacerations, lameness, and suspected fractures.
- If the accident is witnessed, it is important to determine:
  - Primary location of impact on the animal's body
  - Whether the animal was seen walking after the accident
  - Other signs the owner has noticed since the accident

PHYSICAL EXAM FINDINGS: Dependent on site and extent of injuries:
- Altered mentation (dull, depressed, comatose), ocular injuries, and/or skull fractures with head trauma
- Tachycardia (usually sinus) reflecting pain, hypovolemia, hypotension, or combinations thereof:
  - Sinus tachycardia is essentially never treated with antitachycardic drugs (β-blockers, calcium channel blockers, etc.) because it almost always represents a physiologic response. Rather, the underlying cause needs to be indentified and treated.
- Increased respiratory rate and effort (pulmonary contusions, pneumothorax, pain)
- Skin lacerations:
  - Often associated with incrusted debris or road/tire marking, increasing the suspicion of hit by car in an animal with an uncertain history.
- Fractures
- Other specific injuries reflective of the site of the impact

ETIOLOGY AND PATHOPHYSIOLOGY

- Physiologic response to trauma is complex, involving catecholamine and hormone release.
- Goal of physiologic response is to maintain oxygen delivery to the heart and brain at expense of other tissues (e.g., skeletal muscle, abdominal viscera).
- Initial response results in clinical signs of early/compensatory shock:
  - Tachycardia
  - Tachypnea
  - Increased capillary refill time
  - Bounding femoral pulses
- Compensatory phase of shock has high energy demands and if untreated can rapidly progress to decompensatory (terminal) phase of shock.
- Continued reduction in oxygen delivery to tissues results in clinical signs of decompensatory (terminal) shock:

- Bradycardia
- Pale mucous membranes
- Weak femoral pulses
- Hypotension
- Cardiopulmonary arrest

DIAGNOSIS

DIFFERENTIAL DIAGNOSIS

- Metabolic causes of shock (e.g., sepsis, endocrine, heat stroke)
- Other causes of trauma (e.g., kicks, fall from height, bite wounds)

INITIAL DATABASE

- Triage:
  - A wide spectrum of patient states can result when an animal is hit by a vehicle.
    - Rapid assessment of neurologic (mentation, ability to ambulate), cardiorespiratory (dyspnea, respiratory arrest, palpable heartbeat and pulse), skeletal (fractures), and pain parameters determines the immediate intensity of diagnostic and treatment efforts.
    - An interim prognosis based on a brief but thorough physical examination may often dictate the extent to which an owner wishes to support the patient's diagnostic testing and treatment.
- Packed cell volume/total solids (PCV/TS):
  - Can be normal in a hit-by-car patient even with acute hemorrhage.
  - Decrease may take hours but is more rapid if intravenous fluids are administered (dilution).
  - Serial monitoring of PCV/TS 1 to 2 hours after admission and every 4 to 6 hours is recommended to detect changes associated with hemorrhage.
- Blood glucose, electrolytes, venous or arterial blood gas, lactate measurement if available, complete blood count, serum chemistry profile, urinalysis.
- Electrocardiogram:
  - Monitor arrhythmias (especially ventricular; occasionally premature atrial complexes, atrial fibrillation, or others).
  - Monitor heart rate during fluid resuscitation. Heart rate in dogs will often decrease with successful correction of hypovolemia through fluid resuscitation (e.g., initial heart rate 180-200 beats/min decreasing to 100-130 in a medium- to large-breed dog).
- Blood pressure.
- Blood lactate concentration.
  - Can determine if lactic acidosis is present (e.g., from prolonged hypoperfusion associated with shock).
  - Blood lactate level should return to normal once adequate perfusion is restored with intravascular volume replacement.
- Survey radiographs of chest, abdomen, ± axial or appendicular skeletal system structures as dictated by physical findings.
- Pulse oximetry:
  - Assess oxygenation (possibility of pulmonary contusions or pneumothorax if desaturation [i.e., if <90-93% O_2 saturation]).

ADVANCED OR CONFIRMATORY TESTING

- Radiographic contrast studies to assess integrity of urinary tract if indicated
- Advanced neuroimaging modalities such as computed tomography or magnetic resonance imaging to better define skull and brain injuries

TREATMENT

THERAPEUTIC GOAL(S)

- Rapid restoration of effective circulating volume with bolus intravenous fluid administration
- Stabilization of life-threatening respiratory compromise
- Identification of ongoing blood loss that may require surgical intervention
- Identification of internal injuries (e.g., organ rupture, diaphragmatic hernia)
- Pain management of musculoskeletal injuries, including appropriate bandaging of fractures

ACUTE GENERAL TREATMENT

- Bolus intravenous crystalloid fluid administration up to 90 ml/kg/hr in dogs and up to 45 ml/kg/hr in cats; may start with 25 ml/kg bolus over 5 minutes and repeat as necessary.
- Bolus intravenous colloid administration (dosages vary with different colloids) if crystalloids do not restore cardiovascular function.
- Consider hypertonic fluid therapy (e.g., hypertonic saline [7% NaCl 2-6 ml/kg slow IV; acceptable to inject into peripheral or central IV catheter; follow with isotonic crystalloids such as lactated Ringer's]) in cases of head trauma and/or hemorrhagic shock
- Packed red blood cells or fresh whole blood transfusion in cases of severe hemorrhagic shock (see Transfusion Reactions, p 1098).
- Supplemental oxygen administration in cases of respiratory compromise or head trauma (see Oxygen Supplementation, p 1292).
- Use of sterile bandages to cover wounds, including appropriate bandaging of fractures (definitive wound and fracture repair often not possible until cardiovascular and respiratory systems are stabilized).
- Pain management with systemic narcotics when cardiovascular stability achieved.
  - Options include:
    - Hydromorphone 0.05-0.1 mg/kg IM, IV q 4-6h; or
    - Morphine (dogs) 0.5-1.0 mg/kg SQ, IM q 4-6h; or
    - Fentanyl constant rate IV infusion 0.0012-0.0036 mg/kg/hr; or
    - Morphine-ketamine combination constant rate infusion; can mix together in syringe or bag diluted in 0.9% saline or lactated Ringer's solution:
      - Morphine 0.5 mg/kg IM initial loading dose then 0.12-0.36 mg/kg/hr IV.
      - Ketamine 0.25-0.5 mg/kg IV initial loading dose then 0.12-1.2 mg/kg/hr IV.
- Antibiotics (topical or systemic for superficial or deep wounds, respectively) as needed.

POSSIBLE COMPLICATIONS

- Thoracic injuries including rib fractures, pneumothorax, hemothorax, pulmonary contusions, and diaphragmatic hernias
- Abdominal injuries including body wall hernias and hollow and solid organ rupture
- Musculoskeletal injuries (fractures, luxations, ligament injuries)
- Integument injuries (lacerations, degloving wounds, others)
- Traumatic brain or spinal cord injury
- Peripheral nerve damage (sciatic nerve injury, brachial plexus avulsion, others)

RECOMMENDED MONITORING

- Physical parameters including heart rate, respiratory rate/effort, mucous membrane color, body temperature, and blood pressure
- Oxygenation assessment using pulse oximetry and or arterial blood gas measurement as needed
- PCV/TS to assess for blood loss, recheck of other blood work indicated by baseline values and clinical course
- Urination:
  - Frequency, estimated amount and character
  - May need to place urinary catheter if concerned about urine output or integrity of urinary tract
  - Note that patients with ruptured urinary bladder may still pass urine and may also have a palpable bladder; suspect bladder rupture if ascites, abdominal distention, hematuria, pelvic fractures, or lethargy with hyperkalemia are present

PROGNOSIS AND OUTCOME

- Reported survival rate in dogs is 82-87%; reported survival rate in cats is 84%
- In one study:
  - Death most commonly resulted from intrathoracic and intra-abdominal injuries
  - Most of the dogs that were euthanized had central nervous system injury

PEARLS & CONSIDERATIONS

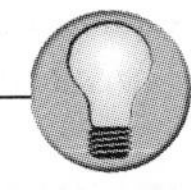

COMMENTS

- Tachycardia, tachypnea, hyperemia/injected mucous membranes, and bounding femoral pulses are signs of early, compensatory shock and require immediate treatment.
- Acute blood loss causes a decrease in the plasma TS before a drop in the PCV because splenic and hepatic contraction replace lost red cells; if blood loss continues the PCV will decrease rapidly.
- Thoracic radiographs are recommended in all cases, especially dogs requiring general anesthesia and surgical repair of fractures, as prevalence of thoracic wall and pulmonary trauma was reported as 39% in one study.
- Uroabdomen may be predicted with an abnormal abdominal fluid creatinine concentration to peripheral blood creatinine ratio of >2:1 or an abnormal potassium concentration to peripheral blood potassium concentration of >1.4:1.
- In rare cases, injuries to gastrointestinal tract or biliary tract are undetectable for several days.

PREVENTION

- Keep cats housed indoors
- Walk dogs on a leash at all times
- Check fences and other enclosure systems frequently for damage
- Do not allow dogs to sleep or lie in driveways

SUGGESTED READING

Day T: Shock syndromes in veterinary medicine. In DiBartola S (ed): *Fluid Therapy in Small Animal Practice*. Philadelphia, WB Saunders, 2000, pp 428-447.

Devey JJ, Crowe DT: The physiologic response to trauma. *Compend Contin Educ Pract Vet* 45 (8):962-977, 1997.

Kolata RJ, Johnston DE: Motor vehicle accidents in urban dogs: A study of 600 cases. *J Am Vet Med Assoc* 167(10):938-941, 1975.

Powell LL, Rozanski EA, Tidwell AS, Rush JE: A retrospective analysis of pulmonary contusion secondary to motor vehicle accidents in 143 dogs. *J Vet Emer Crit Care* 9 (3):127-136, 1999.

Rochlitz I: Study of factors that may predispose domestic cats to road traffic accidents: part 1. *Vet Rec* 153 (18):549-553, 2003.

Rochlitz I: Clinical study of cats injured and killed in road traffic accidents in Cambridgeshire. *J Small Anim Pract* 45 (8):390-394, 2004.

Schmiedt C, Tobias KM, Otto CM: Evaluation of abdominal fluid: peripheral blood creatinine and potassium ratios for diagnosis of uroperitoneum in dogs. *J Vet Emer Crit Care* 11 (4):275-280, 2001.

Spackman CJ, Caywood DD, Feeney DA, Johnston GR: Thoracic wall and pulmonary trauma in dogs sustaining fractures as a result of motor vehicle accidents. *J Am Vet Med Assoc* 185 (9):975-977, 1984.

AUTHOR: **JENNIFER L. HOLM**

EDITOR: **ELIZABETH ROZANSKI**

Hookworm Infection

BASIC INFORMATION

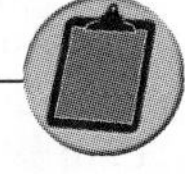

DEFINITION

Infection with nematode parasites of dogs and cats that infest the gastrointestinal tract and cause blood loss anemia

EPIDEMIOLOGY

SPECIES, AGE, SEX

- Cats: *Ancylostoma tubaeforme, Ancylostoma braziliense, Uncinaria stenocephala* (rare).
- Dogs: *Ancylostoma caninum*. Less commonly *Uncinaria stenocephala, Ancylostoma braziliense*.
- Young animals of both species are primarily affected.
- No sex predilection.

RISK FACTORS: Because hookworms cause gastrointestinal blood loss anemia, animals with smaller blood volumes, such as puppies and kittens, are at greater risk for clinically significant compromise with high worm burdens. Puppies born to bitches with poor husbandry are at increased risk, especially from 2 to 8 weeks old.

CONTAGION AND ZOONOSIS

- Contagion:
  - Via soil contamination and vertical transmission from the bitch to offspring.
  - Arrested larvae in the female dog become reactivated during pregnancy and migrate to the placenta and mammary glands, where they are transmitted to pups.
  - There is not a similar transplacental or transmammary transmission of *A. tubaeforme* in the cat.
  - Cats are infected via ingestion or skin penetration.
- Zoonosis:
  - *A. braziliense,* and less commonly *A. caninum,* can cause cutaneous larval migrans in humans.
  - Infective larvae penetrate and migrate through the skin, causing elevated winding tracts that cause intense pruritus.

GEOGRAPHY AND SEASONALITY

- *Ancylostoma tubaeforme*: worldwide.
- *Ancylostoma caninum*: worldwide subtropical and temperate regions.
- *Ancylostoma braziliense*: tropical and subtropical climates in North and South America, Africa; near coastlines.
- *Uncinaria stenocephala*: temperate to cooler climates, North and Central America, Europe, Asia.
- Eggs only develop into infective larvae above 15°C, so infection occurs primarily in warmer months in temperate regions.

ASSOCIATED CONDITIONS AND DISORDERS: Coinfection with other nematodes is common in young animals.

CLINICAL PRESENTATION

HISTORY, CHIEF COMPLAINT

- Weight loss
- Lethargy
- Polydipsia
- Poor growth and unthriftiness (puppies/kittens)
- Melena
- Diarrhea
- Ova may be found incidentally on fecal exam

PHYSICAL EXAM FINDINGS

- Pale mucous membranes are the hallmark, given the bloodsucking characteristics of hookworms
- Poor body condition and haircoat
- Melena on rectal exam
- Heart murmur due to anemia (systolic, left-sided, soft [grade III/VI or less])
- Tachycardia, tachypnea, weakness or obtundation if in hemorrhagic shock
- Clinical signs vary based on degree of blood loss and chronicity of parasitism
- Physical exam may be normal if worm burden is low

ETIOLOGY AND PATHOPHYSIOLOGY

- Hookworms attach to the small intestinal mucosa. Host blood travels through hookworm gut, providing oxygen and nutrients to the worm. Attached worms essentially mimic open blood vessels, causing persistent gastrointestinal hemorrhage.
- *Ancylostoma caninum* is most pathogenic: It consumes more of the host's blood than the other hookworms. *Uncinaria* rarely causes clinical disease or significant anemia.
- Life cycles among species are similar. Prepatent periods (incubation period, from the time of ingestion to the appearance of ova in feces) vary from 12 to 28 days depending on species.
  - Inoculation occurs via oral ingestion or skin penetration from infective larvae in the environment. Puppies are infected via transmammary or transplacental transmission.
    - Oral: swallowed infective larvae penetrate stomach and intestinal wall, where they become arrested in submucosa or other tissues, are reactivated, and return to intestine to attach to mucosa
    - Skin: larvae penetrate skin, migrate through lungs and up trachea, are swallowed, and ultimately attach to intestinal wall

DIAGNOSIS

DIFFERENTIAL DIAGNOSIS

- Foreign body ingestion
- Canine parvovirus (puppies)
- Gastrointestinal ulceration
- Gastrointestinal neoplasia (older animals)
- Anemia due to hemolysis
- Anemia due to ectoparasites
  - Fleas
  - Ticks

INITIAL DATABASE

- Fecal flotation: diagnostic test of choice:
  - Eggs of *Ancylostoma* and *Uncinaria* species are similar in appearance. Characteristic ova are ellipsoidal and morulated.
- Complete blood count:
  - Regenerative anemia (most cases).
  - Nonregenerative anemia with microcytic hypochromic red cells may occur due to chronic gastrointestinal blood loss and subsequent iron deficiency.
  - Eosinophilia.
- Serum biochemistry profile:
  - Hypoproteinemia/hypoalbuminemia.
  - Hyponatremia/hypochloremia in polydipsic animals.
- Urinalysis: generally unremarkable

TREATMENT

THERAPEUTIC GOAL(S)

- Removal of worms is curative
- Focus on volume expansion and oxygen delivery for severe cases (e.g., patients in hemorrhagic shock)

ACUTE GENERAL TREATMENT

- Transfuse severely anemic or compromised patients with blood products or oxygen-carrying fluids. A dosage of 20 ml/kg whole blood or polymerized bovine hemoglobin (Oxyglobin) is usually effective. See Transfusion Therapy and Collection Techniques for Blood Banking, p 1312.
- Iron supplementation may be required in patients with prolonged or profound gastrointestinal blood loss.
  - For severe iron-deficiency anemia: Iron dextran, 10-20 mg/kg IM once (dogs), 50 mg/animal IM once (cats), followed by oral supplementation.
  - Ferrous sulfate, 100-300 mg/animal PO once daily (dogs) 50-100 mg/animal PO once daily (cats). May cause gastric irritation; should be given with food.
- Anthelminthics should be administered once every 2 weeks to puppies and kittens until adolescence (≈ 6 months of age). Infected adults usually require only one to two treatments:
  - Pyrantel pamoate, 5-10 mg/kg PO; or
  - Febantel, 10-15 mg/kg PO (higher dose in younger animals); or
  - Fenbendazole, 50 mg/kg PO q 24h for 3 days; or
  - Ivermectin, 200 µg/kg PO or SQ (beware risks; see Ivermectin Toxicosis, p 610).

CHRONIC TREATMENT

- Repeat dewormings necessary to prevent reinfection. Resistance to infection increases with age and exposure.
- Deworm every 2 to 3 weeks.
- To prevent passage of infective larvae from lactating bitches to puppies, treat with 50 mg/kg of fenbendazole daily from day 40 of gestation to day 14 of lactation.

RECOMMENDED MONITORING

- Acute anemia: monitor hematocrit, reticulocyte counts
- Repeat fecal flotations

PROGNOSIS AND OUTCOME

Prognosis excellent with removal of parasites in compensated infection, but is guarded in cases of acute, severe anemia

PEARLS & CONSIDERATIONS

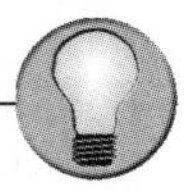

COMMENTS

Peak blood loss from hookworm infestation occurs before eggs are shed in feces. A negative fecal examination should not rule out hookworm disease, especially in very young puppies or kittens that present with evidence of anemia and shock.

PREVENTION

- Sodium borate applied to gravel or concrete will control hookworm larvae in the environment.
- Best prevention is regular administration of anthelminthics. Commercial heartworm preventives containing ivermectin/pyrantel pamoate, milbemycin, and selamectin have simultaneous anthelminthic properties for monthly control of hookworms in adult dogs and cats. Note that selamectin does not control hookworms in dogs, but is efficacious in cats, at heartworm preventive doses.

SUGGESTED READING

Bowman DD, Hendrix CM, Lindsay DS, Barr SC: Ancylostomatoidea. In Bowman DD, Hendrix CM, Lindsay DS, Barr SC (eds): *Feline Clinical Parasitology*. Ames, IA, Iowa State University Press, 2002, pp 242-257.

Bowman DD: Superfamily ancylostomatoidea. In Bowman DD (ed): *Georgi's Parasitology for Veterinarians*. Philadelphia, WB Saunders, 1999, pp 178-184.

AUTHOR: **SHANNON T. STROUP**
EDITOR: **DOUGLASS K. MACINTIRE**

Hormone-Responsive Urinary Incontinence

Client Education Sheet on Website

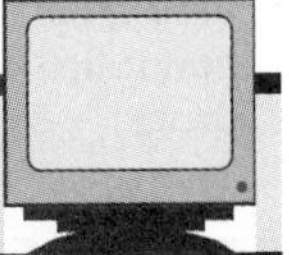

BASIC INFORMATION

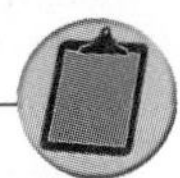

DEFINITION

Hormone-responsive urinary incontinence is a condition causing involuntary voiding of urine due to decreased urethral sphincter tone

SYNONYM(S)

Estrogen-responsive incontinence
Hormone responsive urethral incompetence
Spay incontinence
Urethral sphincter mechanism incompetence

EPIDEMIOLOGY

SPECIES, AGE, SEX: Middle-aged female dogs predominantly affected, although hormone responsive incontinence occurs rarely in neutered males. Onset of incontinence may be months to years after ovariohysterectomy (OHE).

GENETICS AND BREED PREDISPOSITION: Usually medium- to large-breed dogs. A positive association between tail docking and hormone responsive incontinence has been demonstrated. Overrepresented breeds include:

- Boxer
- Doberman pinscher
- German shepherd
- Old English sheepdog
- Rottweiler
- Springer spaniel
- Weimaraner

RISK FACTORS: Intrapelvic bladder, short urethra, and obesity. Any cause of polyuria may initiate or exacerbate clinical signs.

CLINICAL PRESENTATION

HISTORY, CHIEF COMPLAINT

- Urinary incontinence, often most evident during rest (i.e., patients leave "puddles" after sleeping)
- Excessive licking of perineum
- Dogs retain ability to produce normal voluntary urine stream

PHYSICAL EXAM FINDINGS

- Usually unremarkable. Complete neurologic examination should be conducted, including evaluation of tail and anal tone.
- Observed episode of urination is normal; bladder will empty nearly completely after voluntary voiding.
- Perineal urine staining or perivulvar dermatitis sometimes observed.

ETIOLOGY AND PATHOPHYSIOLOGY

- The vast majority of neutered dogs remain continent. It is unclear why only a minority of neutered bitches develop hormone responsive urinary incontinence
- Sex hormones apparently sensitize the internal urethral sphincter to the effects of α-adrenergic stimulation.
- The bladder may be positioned in a relatively caudal position in neutered bitches, lessening the intra-abdominal pressures on the urethra that help maintain urethral closure.

DIAGNOSIS

DIFFERENTIAL DIAGNOSIS

- For inappropriate urination, distinguish between urinary incontinence and pollakiuria, polyuria, or behavioral disorders.
- Differentials for urinary incontinence: lower motor neuron disease/peripheral neuropathy; upper motor neuron disease; dysautonomia; urge incontinence; partial urethral obstruction; and congenital and acquired urinary tract structural defects (ectopic ureter[s], vaginal stricture/stenosis, urethrovaginal fistula).

INITIAL DATABASE

- Complete neurologic examination: normal
- Complete blood count and serum biochemistry profile: unremarkable
- Complete urinalysis: may show evidence of secondary urinary tract infection
- Urine culture: rule out urinary tract infection
- Abdominal radiographs or ultrasound of urinary structures: unremarkable, or bladder may display intrapelvic positioning

ADVANCED OR CONFIRMATORY TESTING

- Contrast studies and/or cystoscopy: rule out structural causes of urinary incontinence
- Urethral pressure profile and/or leak point pressure (requires specialized equipment/expertise): objectively identifies urethral sphincter incompetence
- Response to therapy is often used to aid diagnosis, but response may require dosage adjustment over weeks

TREATMENT

THERAPEUTIC GOAL(S)

Reduce frequency and amount of involuntary voiding of urine

ACUTE GENERAL TREATMENT

- If polyuria is identified, the cause should be sought and treatment instituted (underlying cause is likely not hormone-responsive incontinence alone or at all).
- Medical therapy with phenylpropanolamine or estrogen compounds.
- Treatment of secondary urinary tract infection with appropriate antimicrobials.

CHRONIC TREATMENT

- Phenylpropanolamine is an α-agonist sympathomimetic used for increasing internal urethral sphincter tone. Dose: 1-1.5 mg/kg PO q 8h. Use with caution, or avoid, if systemic hypertension, heart disease, cardiac arrhythmias, or central nervous system disease. Discontinue if anxiety, hyperactivity, or tachycardia.
- Diethylstilbestrol (DES) is a synthetic estrogen that increases sensitivity of internal urethral sphincter to catecholamines. Dosage is empiric, with reduction in frequency and dose to least possible that controls clinical signs. Starting dose: 0.1 mg (small dog), 0.3 mg (medium dog), or 0.7 mg (large dog) total daily dose PO q 24h for 3 to 5 days, then the same dose is given q 5-8 days as needed to control incontinence.
- Conjugated estrogens (e.g., Premarin 20 μg/kg PO q 4 days) has been used in place of DES.
- AVOID estradiol cypionate due to increased risk of marrow suppression.
- Testosterone cypionate (2.2 mg/kg IM q 30 days) can be used in castrated males (phenylpropanolamine preferred).
- Hormones may be administered concurrently with phenylpropanolamine when incontinence persists despite therapy (synergistic actions).
- Surgical therapies (e.g., periurethral injections of Teflon, bladder repositioning) used for refractory patients.

POSSIBLE COMPLICATIONS

- Secondary urinary tract infection
- Hormone therapy may cause adverse reactions; estrogen compounds (e.g., bone marrow suppression), testosterone (e.g., prostatomegaly, behavioral changes)
- Phenylpropanolamine may cause adverse reactions (e.g., hyperactivity, hypertension)

RECOMMENDED MONITORING

- Periodic urinalysis with Gram stain of sediment/bacterial culture and sensitivity if incontinence persists
- Periodic monitoring of blood pressure in dogs treated with phenylpropanolamine

- Periodic monitoring of complete blood count in dogs treated with estrogen drugs

PROGNOSIS AND OUTCOME

Most dogs respond to medical therapy with improvement or resolution of clinical signs. Some dogs require more than a single type of medication, and ancillary surgical procedures may be required in rare cases.

PEARLS & CONSIDERATIONS

COMMENTS

- Hormone responsive urinary incontinence is a common cause of urinary incontinence.
- Diagnosis usually based on clinical presentation, ruling out other common causes of incontinence, and response to therapy.
- Minimal evaluation includes neurologic examination, observation of urination and palpation of bladder afterwards, urinalysis and urine culture, and imaging of the urinary tract with radiographs or ultrasound.

PREVENTION

Hormone responsive incontinence occurs in only a small percentage of ovariohysterectomized bitches. There is little evidence that early neutering increases likelihood of developing incontinence.

SUGGESTED READING

Atalan G, et al: Ultrasonographic assessment of bladder neck mobility in continent bitches and bitches with urinary incontinence attributable to urethral sphincter mechanism incompetence. *Am J Vet Res* 59:673-679, 1998.

Holt PE, et al: Association in bitches between breed, size, neutering and docking, and acquired urinary incontinence due to incompetence of the urethral sphincter mechanism. *Vet Record* 133:177-180, 1993.

Rawlings C, et al: Evaluation of colposuspension for treatment of incontinence in spayed female dogs. *J Am Vet Med Assoc* 219:770-775, 2001.

AUTHOR & EDITOR: **LEAH A. COHN**

Horner's Syndrome

BASIC INFORMATION

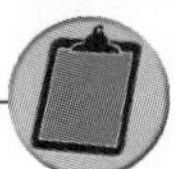

DEFINITION

Manifestations of loss of sympathetic innervation to the eye. Signs are miosis (small pupil), ptosis (dropped upper eyelid, causing a smaller palpebral fissure), enophthalmos, and protrusion of the third eyelid (Fig. I-95).

EPIDEMIOLOGY

SPECIES, AGE, SEX: Dogs and cats of any age and either sex.

GENETICS AND BREED PREDISPOSITION: Male golden retrievers may be overrepresented (of 155 dogs with Horner's syndrome in one study, 110 were golden retrievers; idiopathic Horner's syndrome was present in 100 of them, 95 were male).

RISK FACTORS: Blunt trauma (e.g., hit by car), other cervical/thoracic spinal cord damage (fibrocartilaginous embolization, intervertebral disk disease) or infiltration (lymphosarcoma), surgical trauma or neoplastic infiltration of the neck (affecting the sympathetic trunk), intracranial neoplasia, otitis media or other middle ear lesions, retrobulbar inflammation or mass.

ASSOCIATED CONDITIONS AND DISORDERS: Exposure keratitis. The inability to blink normally is mostly compensated for by the third eyelid, but a band of desiccated cornea may occur across the central cornea.

CLINICAL PRESENTATION

HISTORY, CHIEF COMPLAINT

- Signs referable to the underlying cause (Table I-7)
- Trauma (e.g., hit by car) is the most common historically identifiable cause in dogs and cats
- Ocular signs observed by the owner in an animal that is otherwise well (dogs: idiopathic)

PHYSICAL EXAM FINDINGS

- Enophthalmos (retracted/sunken globe)
- Ptosis
- Miosis
- Third eyelid protrusion
- Other associated signs may be present, depending on the location of the inciting lesion (see Table I-7)

ETIOLOGY AND PATHOPHYSIOLOGY

- Physical interference with/interruption of sympathetic fibers (see Table I-7).
- An immune-mediated mechanism has been speculated as a possible cause for idiopathic Horner's syndrome.

DIAGNOSIS

DIFFERENTIAL DIAGNOSIS

History and physical exam are generally sufficient for differentiation:

- Ocular trauma causing miosis
- Phthisis bulbi causing protrusion of the third eyelid and a small palpebral fissure

INITIAL DATABASE

- Otoscopic examination: all cases
- Thoracic and lateral cervical radiographs: all cases

ADVANCED OR CONFIRMATORY TESTING

- Further evaluation: as dictated by history, physical exam, and initial database results
- Pharmacologic testing. Suggested protocol:
  - Topical 10% phenylephrine solution: 1 drop applied to affected eye
  - Mydriasis occurs in <20 minutes when lesion is postganglionic
  - Mydriasis occurs in 20 to 45 minutes when lesion is preganglionic
  - Mydriasis occurs in >45 minutes when lesion is central/UMN
  - Results have been inconsistent; reliability of test is controversial

TREATMENT

THERAPEUTIC GOAL(S)

Treat underlying cause, if any

ACUTE AND CHRONIC TREATMENT

Horner's syndrome is not treated; it is a sign that may indicate an underlying lesion that may require treatment.

TABLE I-7 **Localizing Lesions in Horner's syndrome**

Location	Common Etiologies	Neuron Affected	Commonly Associated Signs
Hypothalamus	Neoplasia,* infection	UMN	Altered behavior, thermoregulation, endocrine function, appetite, drinking
Brainstem	Neoplasia,* trauma, infection	UMN	Altered consciousness: cranial nerve deficits, motor deficits, dyspnea
Cervical spinal cord	Trauma, neoplasia, FCE	UMN	Tetraparesis/plegia, hemiparesis/plegia, UMN signs in all four limbs if cranial lesion, LMN signs in thoracic limbs with UMN signs in pelvic limbs if caudal cervical lesion
T1-T3 spinal cord	Trauma,* neoplasia,* FCE	UMN	Thoracic limb paresis/paralysis with LMN thoracic limb signs, pelvic limb paresis/paralysis with UMN thoracic limb signs
T1-T3 ventral nerve roots	Brachial plexus avulsion,* neurofibroma	Preganglionic	Brachial plexus paresis/paralysis of the ipsilateral limb
Cranial thoracic sympathetic trunk	Lymphoma, neurofibroma, thoracic disease	Preganglionic	Respiratory distress; no other signs if confined to the trunk
Cervical sympathetic trunk	Trauma, iatrogenic, neoplasia	Preganglionic	May be none if unilateral; may interfere with laryngeal or esophageal function from vagal involvement
Middle ear	Otitis media,* neoplasia	Postganglionic	Head tilt, nystagmus, and/or facial paralysis
Cavernous sinus	Neoplasia, vascular disease	Postganglionic	Internal, external, or complete ophthalmoplegia (may produce mydriasis rather than miosis)
Orbital disease	Abscess, neoplasia, contusion, pseudotumor	Postganglionic	Exophthalmos, discomfort, optic nerve or oculomotor deficits

*Most common.
FCE, fibrocartilaginous emboli; LMN, lower motor neuron; UMN, upper motor neuron.
Modified from Collins BK, O'Brien D: Autonomic dysfunction of the eye. *Semin Vet Med Surg Small Anim* 5:24-36, 1990. Reprinted with permission.

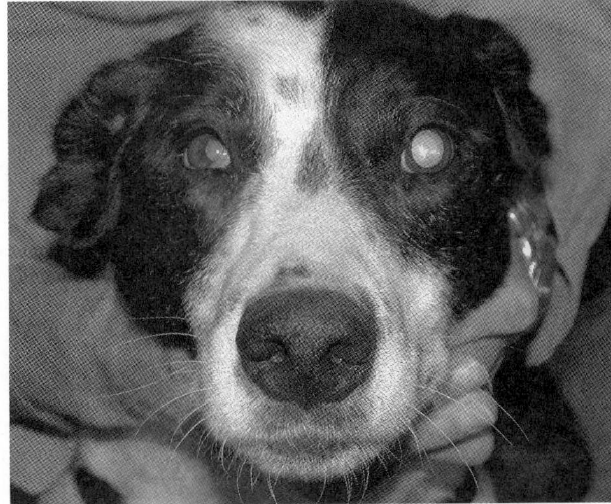

FIGURE I-95 Right-sided Horner's syndrome in a 9-year-old Pointer-cross dog. Note right-sided ptosis, miosis, and protruding third eyelid caused by enophthalmos. The hematocrit was 75% and pathologic proteinuria was present, leading to a suspicion of thromboembolic disease as the cause of the Horner's syndrome.

PROGNOSIS AND OUTCOME

- The prognosis depends on the resolution of the underlying cause. Patients with chest trauma have quicker resolution (days-weeks) than do patients with idiopathic or iatrogenic causes.
- In idiopathic Horner's syndrome, essentially all patients have resolution of the signs of Horner' syndrome within 6 months after diagnosis.

PEARLS & CONSIDERATIONS

COMMENTS

- Approximately 50% of cases of Horner's syndrome in dogs are idiopathic, and the syndrome generally resolves without treatment in <6 months.
- In cats, a cause is virtually always found: Idiopathic Horner's syndrome is very rare.
- Strictly speaking, Horner's syndrome also affects the surface of the face and neck (causing erythema/flushing of the skin) and the nasal mucosa (causing congestion), but these manifestations usually have no clinical significance.
- Pharmacologic testing to determine the site of the lesion has produced inconsistent results.

SUGGESTED READING

Boydell P: Idiopathic Horner's syndrome in the golden retriever. *J Small Anim Pract* 36:382-384, 1995.

Collins BK, O'Brien D: Autonomic dysfunction of the eye. *Semin Vet Med Surg Small Anim* 5:24-36, 1990.

de Lahunta A: *Veterinary Neuroanatomy and Clinical Neurology*, ed 2. Philadelphia, WB Saunders, 1983.

Kern TJ, et al: Horner's syndrome in dogs and cats: 100 cases (1975-1985). *J Am Vet Med Assoc* 195:369-373, 1989.

Morgan RV, et al: Horner's syndrome in dogs and cats: 49 cases (1980-1986). *J Am Vet Med Assoc* 194:1096-1099, 1989.

AUTHOR: **ETIENNE CÔTÉ**

EDITOR: **CURTIS W. DEWEY**

Hydrocephalus

BASIC INFORMATION

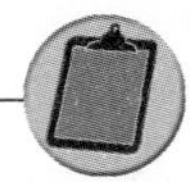

DEFINITION

An increase in volume of cerebrospinal fluid (CSF) within the ventricular system of the brain that causes signs of encephalopathy

EPIDEMIOLOGY

SPECIES, AGE, SEX

- Congenital: dog, cat <6 months old
- Acquired: any

GENETICS AND BREED PREDISPOSITION

- Toy breeds: Chihuahua, toy poodle, Pomeranian, Lhasa apso, pug, Pekingese, and cairn, Yorkshire, Manchester, and Maltese terriers
- Brachycephalic breeds: Boston terrier, bulldog
- Autosomal-recessive inheritance in Siamese cats

RISK FACTORS

- Often represents a secondary manifestation of a developmental (Chiari malformation) or an acquired (neoplasia, inflammatory) disorder
- Vitamin A deficiency, toxicosis (cats: griseofulvin during pregnancy); infectious (cats: panleukopenia, feline infectious peritonitis; dogs: parainfluenza)

ASSOCIATED CONDITIONS AND DISORDERS: Small birth size, short gestation periods, high stress at birth (dystocia).

CLINICAL PRESENTATION

DISEASE FORMS/SUBTYPES

- Congenital: animal is born with clinical signs; usually associated with fusion of mesencephalic aqueduct
- Acquired: caused by obstructive insults at any age, i.e., infection, trauma, neoplasia

HISTORY, CHIEF COMPLAINT

- Changes in mentation: dullness, disorientation, stupor
- Behavioral abnormalities: inability to learn (e.g., litter box use), loss of housebreaking, compulsive activities, aggression
- Seizures

PHYSICAL EXAM FINDINGS

- Domed-shaped head and persistent fontanelle are possible
- Eye position will manifest ventrolateral deviation
- Neurologic examination: mentation changes; gait abnormalities may manifest as dysmetria, ataxia, circling, aimless wandering; central blindness; and seizure activity

ETIOLOGY AND PATHOPHYSIOLOGY

- Pathologic changes include focal destruction of the ependymal lining, compromise of cerebral vasculature, damage to periventricular white matter, and injury to neurons.
- Secondary calvarial abnormalities depend on the stage of ossification at onset of fluid accumulation.
- Ventriculomegaly results from obstruction within the ventricular system, overproduction of CSF, or insufficient absorption of CSF at the arachnoid villi.
- Congenital:
  - Fusion of the rostral colliculi causing mesencephalic aqueductal stenosis. There is no other active disease process.
- Acquired:
  - Exposure to teratogenic drugs, chemicals, and viral diseases during gestation.
  - Obstruction of ventricular system by neoplastic mass, hemorrhage, or inflammation.
  - Hydrocephalus also may be a component of other anomalous disorders (i.e., Chiari malformation, Dandy-Walker syndrome, lissencephaly).

DIAGNOSIS

DIFFERENTIAL DIAGNOSIS

- Hydrocephalus usually will manifest signs of forebrain dysfunction.
- Encephalopathies:
  - Degenerative disorders: storage diseases, leukodystrophies, multisystem atrophy
  - Anomalies (congenital)
  - Metabolic: hepatic encephalopathy
  - Neoplasia
  - Inflammatory: infectious, noninfectious, breed specific
  - Idiopathic: arachnoidal cysts
  - Trauma
  - Toxin exposure

INITIAL DATABASE

- Signalment
- Neurologic examination
- Complete blood count, serum biochemistry profile, urinalysis: generally unremarkable
- Serologic evaluation: to rule out other disorders, if appropriate
- Skull radiography: decreased prominence of normal calvarial convolutions

ADVANCED OR CONFIRMATORY TESTING

- Ultrasonography: through persistent fontanelles
- Advanced imaging:
  - Computed tomography
  - Magnetic resonance imaging
- CSF analysis: to rule out other disorders, if appropriate
- Electroencephalography

TREATMENT

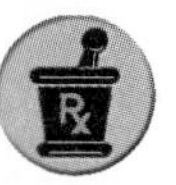

THERAPEUTIC GOAL(S)

- Therapy is aimed at decreasing CSF production and shunting of CSF into another body cavity. Patients that show an acute deterioration of neurologic signs require immediate treatment.
- Choice of treatment is influenced by physical status, size of patient, clinical signs, and underlying cause of hydrocephalus.

ACUTE GENERAL TREATMENT

- Medical:
  - Prednisone (↓ CSF production):
    - 0.25–0.5 mg/kg PO q 12–24h, then tapered to lowest effective dose.
  - Furosemide (↓ CSF production; Na-K cotransport inhibition):
    - 0.5–2.0 mg/kg PO q 12–24h.
  - Acetazolamide (↓ CSF production; carbonic anhydrase inhibition):
    - 10 mg/kg PO q 8h.
  - Omeprazole (↓ CSF production; proton pump inhibition):
    - 0.7 mg/kg PO q 24h.
- Surgical: advocated if clinical signs do not improve within 2 to 3 weeks:
  - Ventriculoperitoneal shunt
  - Ventriculoatrial shunt

CHRONIC TREATMENT

- Continue supportive medical therapy
- Antiepileptic drug therapy for seizure control

DRUG INTERACTIONS

Prolonged use of glucocorticoids and acetazolamide may cause potassium depletion and other systemic disorders.

POSSIBLE COMPLICATIONS

- Generally, medical therapy may result in only transient improvement of clinical signs.
- Complications of shunt place include mechanical and functional obstruction, infections, overshunting.

RECOMMENDED MONITORING

- Signs of acute decompensation: coma, seizures, behavior changes
- Seizure control

DISEASES AND DISORDERS

PROGNOSIS AND OUTCOME

- Congenital: guarded. Prognosis also is influenced by coexistence of other neural abnormalities
- Acquired: prognosis depends on underlying cause

PEARLS & CONSIDERATIONS

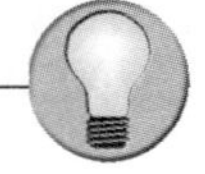

COMMENTS

- Every attempt is made to determine the underlying cause.
- Early shunt placement is advocated to lessen residual neurologic and behavioral deficits.

PREVENTION

Limit prenatal exposure to toxins, viral infections, and vaccines.

CLIENT EDUCATION

- Clinical signs of acute decompensation
- Guarded prognosis and likelihood of residual neurologic deficits with therapy
- Importance of maintaining the pet in a protective environment

SUGGESTED READING

Coates JR, Sullivan SA: Congenital cranial and intracranial malformations. In August JR (ed): *Consultations in Feline Internal Medicine*, ed 4. Philadelphia, WB Saunders, 2001, pp 413–423.

Dewey CW: Encephalopathies: Disorders of the brain. In Dewey CW (ed): *A Practical Guide to Canine and Feline Neurology*, Ames, IA, Iowa State Press, 2003, pp 99–178.

Harrington ML, Bagley RS, Moore MP: Hydrocephalus. *Vet Clin North Am Small Anim Pract* 26:843, 1996.

Simpson ST: Hydrocephalus. In Kirk RW (ed): *Kirk's Current Veterinary Therapy X: Small Animal Practice*, Philadelphia, WB Saunders, 1989, pp. 842–847.

AUTHOR: **JOAN R. COATES**
EDITOR: **CURTIS W. DEWEY**

Hydronephrosis

BASIC INFORMATION

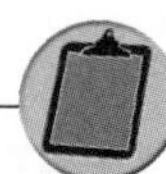

DEFINITION

Dilation of the renal pelvis and calices (pyelectasia) in one or both kidneys, typically as a result of ureteral (or rarely urethral) obstruction, resulting in atrophy of the renal parenchyma

EPIDEMIOLOGY

SPECIES, AGE, SEX: More common in dogs than cats; no age or sex predilection.

RISK FACTORS: Any cause of ureteral (or urethral) obstruction, whether mechanical or functional:
- Bladder atonia/hypotonia
- Blood clots
- Celiotomy (inadvertent ligation or fibrotic entrapment of ureter)
- Congenital ureteral stenosis or stricture
- Ectopic ureter
- Prostatic carcinoma
- Reflex dyssynergia
- Retroperitoneal mass/fibrosis
- Trauma
- Ureteral fibroepithelial polyps
- Urinary tract neoplasia
- Urolithiasis

ASSOCIATED CONDITIONS AND DISORDERS
- Renal Failure
- Uremia
- Hypertension
- Urinary tract infection

CLINICAL PRESENTATION

DISEASE FORMS/SUBTYPES
- Reversible or irreversible
- Unilateral or bilateral

HISTORY, CHIEF COMPLAINT: Often clinically normal. Signs can include:
- Anorexia
- Vomiting
- Vague abdominal pain
- Polydipsia/polyuria
- Hematuria
- Pollakiuria, stranguria, dysuria
- Oliguria or anuria (urethral obstruction or, rarely, bilateral ureteral obstruction)

PHYSICAL EXAM FINDINGS: Often normal. Abnormalities may include:
- Abdominal discomfort (severity related to rate of onset of obstruction rather than degree of obstruction)
- Renomegaly
- Distended bladder (if urethral obstruction)
- Abdominal mass (kidney, bladder, prostate, granuloma)
- Urethral mass (via rectal palpation)
- Prostatomegaly
- Dehydration
- Halitosis (due to uremia)
- Oral ulcerations (due to uremia)

ETIOLOGY AND PATHOPHYSIOLOGY

- Illness varies depending on whether obstruction is unilateral or bilateral, completeness and duration of obstruction, and preexisting renal function.
- Clinical signs can be absent, chronic, or acute; acute signs are more likely when obstruction is complete.
- Obstruction results in increased hydrostatic pressure in renal pelvis, collecting ducts, and distal tubules causing tubular dilatation with flattening of the tubular cells.
- Concurrently, renal vasculature and blood supply are compromised. Renal blood flow progressively decreases, arterioles constrict, capillary pressure decreases, and many arterioles collapse resulting in parenchymal atrophy.
- Changes may become irreversible after 14 to 45 days.

DIAGNOSIS

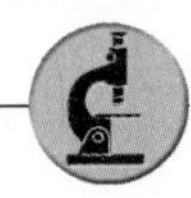

DIFFERENTIAL DIAGNOSIS

- Pyelectasia: pyelonephritis, iatrogenic fluid diuresis (mild)
- Renomegaly: renal cyst(s), perinephric pseudocyst, neoplasia (e.g., renal adenocarcinoma, lymphoma), amyloidosis, granuloma, perinephric abscess, feline infectious peritonitis, hematoma, compensatory hypertrophy (unilateral)

INITIAL DATABASE

- Digital rectal examination: lesions of the urethra and bladder trigone
- Urethral catheterization: if obstruction suspected
- Complete blood count: unremarkable. Neutrophilia possible if concurrent pyelonephritis
- Serum biochemical profile: depending on degree of obstruction and/or nephron loss, azotemia, hyperphosphatemia, hyperkalemia, metabolic acidosis, increased anion gap
- Urinalysis: isosthenuria (e.g., if >66% nephron loss), sometimes hematuria, pyuria
- Urine culture and sensitivity (C&S)
- Blood pressure
- Abdominal radiographs: often, renomegaly. Additional findings may include:
  - Urolithiasis
  - Urinary bladder distension
  - Prostatomegaly
  - Abdominal mass effect
  - Loss of contrast in retroperitoneal space
  - Loss of abdominal detail
- Abdominal ultrasound: pyelectasia Additional findings may include:
  - Loss of medullary parenchyma

- Hydroureter
- Uroliths
- Masses in ureter, bladder, prostate, or urethra

ADVANCED OR CONFIRMATORY TESTING

- Excretory urography (EU)/intravenous pyelography (IVP); to assess perfusion of each kidney/percutaneous nephropyelography (see Excretory Urogram, p 1241)
  - Pyelectasia
  - Ureteral dilatation or lack of filling (EU only)
- Renal scintigraphy
  - Affected kidney contributes little to glomerular filtration rate
- Other testing is aimed at characterizing underlying cause of hydronephrosis (e.g., quantitative analysis of uroliths, imaging studies to localize neurologic lesions contributing to reflex dyssynergia)

TREATMENT

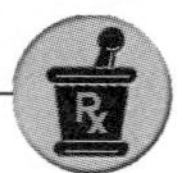

THERAPEUTIC GOAL(S)

- Relieve urinary obstruction if possible
- Address azotemia/uremia, and electrolyte and acid-base disorders
- Address concurrent infection
- Provide analgesia

ACUTE GENERAL TREATMENT

- Relieve urinary obstruction (see Urethral Obstruction, p 1120; Ureteral Obstruction, p 1118)
- Crystalloid fluid therapy for azotemia (see Acute Renal Failure, p 32; Chronic Renal Failure, Overt ["Symptomatic"], p 205):
  - Initial rate of 120 ml/kg IV q 24h if no concurrent heart disease, hypoalbuminemia, or vasculitis; adjust based on dehydration/hypovolemia
  - Postobstructive diuresis may require "ins and outs" method of fluid therapy (rate adjustments based on measured urine output)
- Analgesia for abdominal pain (e.g., buprenorphine 0.01 mg/kg IM, IV, or SQ q 6-8h)
- Address electrolyte disorders, acidosis (see Urethral Obstruction, p 1120; Ureteral Obstruction, p 1118; Acute Renal Failure, p 32)
- Address uremia (see Acute Renal Failure, p 32; Chronic Renal Failure, Overt ["Symptomatic"], p 205)

CHRONIC TREATMENT

- Antibiotics if indicated by results of urine C&S:
  - If infection cannot be cured medically, nephrectomy may be indicated if contralateral renal function is preserved.
- Address underlying cause of structural or functional urinary obstruction (e.g., therapeutic or prophylactic/dietary measures for urolithiasis, pharmacologic therapy of bladder atonia, reflex dyssynergia)

POSSIBLE COMPLICATIONS

- Renal failure
- Urinary tract infection
- Urinary rupture and uroabdomen (septic peritonitis if urinary tract is infected)

RECOMMENDED MONITORING

- Ultrasound is repeated several weeks after urinary obstruction relieved. If hydronephrosis persists after 6 weeks, changes are likely to be permanent.
- Animals with permanent hydronephrosis are monitored as for chronic renal failure (see Chronic Renal Failure, Occult ["Asymptomatic"], [p 204] and Overt ["Symptomatic"], [p 205]) with periodic urinalysis and culture, assessment of azotemia, electrolytes, and packed cell volume. Azotemic animals are monitored more intensively than nonazotemic animals.

PROGNOSIS AND OUTCOME

- Dependent on extent of renal damage, underlying cause and resolution of cause, duration, and concurrent infection
- Structural kidney changes may be irreversible

PEARLS & CONSIDERATIONS

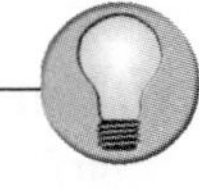

COMMENTS

- Hydronephrosis is a consequence of obstructive urinary tract disease rather than a primary disease.
- Hydronephrosis can lead to renal failure, or may be manifest only as subclinical pyelectasia.

PREVENTION

Strategies that limit the formation of uroliths are important for patients that have already demonstrated a predisposition to urolithiasis or those with known risk factors.

CLIENT EDUCATION

Urinary tract obstruction is life threatening. Stranguria or signs of systemic illness should prompt immediate veterinary attention.

SUGGESTED READING

Osborne CA, Finco DR: *Canine and Feline Nephrology and Urology*. Baltimore, Williams & Wilkins, 1995, pp 474-482.

Steffey MA, et al: Congenital ectopic ureters in a continent male dog and cat. *J Am Vet Med Assoc* 224:1607, 2004.

AUTHORS: **ADAM MORDECAI, RANCE K. SELLON**

EDITOR: **LEAH A. COHN**

Hygroma, Elbow

BASIC INFORMATION

DEFINITION

Fluid-filled (serum) cavity between skin and bony prominence (olecranon)

SYNONYM(S)

Elbow seroma

Olecranon bursitis (incorrect term, as tendon bursa is not involved)

EPIDEMIOLOGY

SPECIES, AGE, SEX: Dogs: any age, either sex.

GENETICS AND BREED PREDISPOSITION: Large-breed, heavy dogs.

RISK FACTORS

- Insufficient callus over elbow
- Thin skin
- Small amount of subcutaneous fat
- Chronic pressure trauma to elbow
- Lying on hard surfaces

ASSOCIATED CONDITIONS AND DISORDERS: Orthopedic problems (hip dysplasia) that increase trauma to skin and other soft tissues overlying the elbows as dog rises or lies down.

CLINICAL PRESENTATION

HISTORY, CHIEF COMPLAINT

- Gradually enlarging, fluid-filled swelling over point of elbow
  - Initially soft, then more turgid as fluid accumulates

- Ulceration of overlying skin may develop if continued trauma

PHYSICAL EXAM FINDINGS: Fluid-filled, fluctuant, to turgid swelling over the point of the elbow:

- Unilateral or bilateral

ETIOLOGY AND PATHOPHYSIOLOGY

- Caused by chronic, repetitive pressure and trauma to the elbow
- Serum accumulates in subcutaneous space superficial to triceps fascia over the olecranon
- Over time, fibrous proliferation occurs, causing nonpitting, nonpainful thickening of skin and subcutis

DIAGNOSIS

DIFFERENTIAL DIAGNOSIS

- Abscess
- Neoplasia

INITIAL DATABASE

- If indicated, presurgical complete blood count, serum chemistry profile, urinalysis
- Fine-needle aspiration cytologic evaluation with or without bacterial culture and sensitivity:
  - Rule out abscess, neoplasia
- Radiographs of elbow:
  - Rule out underlying orthopedic problems:
    - Degenerative joint disease, olecranon fracture

TREATMENT

THERAPEUTIC GOAL(S)

- Drainage of fluid
- Healing of fibrous tissue surfaces together to prevent reformation

ACUTE GENERAL TREATMENT

Three suggested methods of treatment (see references):

- Aseptic aspiration of fluid and pressure coaptation bandage
  - Rarely successful for larger or chronic hygromas
- Penrose drainage and padded bandage
- Suture obliteration and padded bandage

CHRONIC TREATMENT

- Padded bandage must remain in place for at least 4 weeks to allow the fibrous tissue surfaces to heal together and thereby obliterate the subcutaneous space in which fluid could accumulate.
- Dog should be restricted from lying on hard surfaces.
  - Suitable padded bedding should be provided.
- Elbow(s) should be padded until healing and adequate protective callus have developed.

POSSIBLE COMPLICATIONS

- Recurrence
  - Penrose drain removed too soon
  - Inadequate period of bandaging to allow fibrous healing to occur
  - Suitable padded bedding not provided after bandages have been removed
- Infection
  - Repeated needle drainage
  - Inadequate sterile surgical technique
  - Inadequate protective bandage over Penrose drains
- Development of a chronic nonhealing ulcer over olecranon
  - Infected hygroma
  - Dehiscence of suture line after surgery
  - Continued trauma to hygroma

RECOMMENDED MONITORING

- See Chronic Treatment above
- Observe elbow area for evidence of:
  - Recurrence of the hygroma
  - Infection of the overlying skin
  - Development of necrosis/ulceration of the overlying skin
- Be aware that problem may develop on other elbow if preventive measures are not taken

PROGNOSIS AND OUTCOME

- Good with appropriate treatment
- Poor if:
  - Hygroma becomes infected
  - Dehiscence of suture line occurs
  - Nonhealing ulcer develops
- May require extensive reconstructive surgery to correct these problems

PEARLS & CONSIDERATIONS

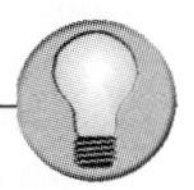

COMMENTS

Do not attempt surgical excision of the hygroma.

- Successful primary closure is difficult to achieve with excision, due to tension and motion at surgical site; high risk of complications

PREVENTION

- Dog should be restricted from lying on hard surfaces:
  - Especially if other orthopedic problems are present that restrict the dog's ability to rise and lie down
  - Suitable padded bedding should be provided
- Elbow(s) should be padded until adequate protective callus has developed

CLIENT EDUCATION

Seek veterinary care and advise as soon as hygroma develops:

- Easier to treat and less risk of complications if treated early (e.g., before infection)

SUGGESTED READING

Johnston DE: Hygroma of the elbow in dogs. *J Am Vet Med Assoc* 167:213, 1975.

Swaim SF, Henderson RA: Wounds on the limbs. In *Small Animal Wound Management*. Philadelphia, Lea & Febiger, 1990, pp 181–188.

AUTHOR & EDITOR: **RICHARD WALSHAW**

Hyperadrenocorticism

Client Education Sheet on Website

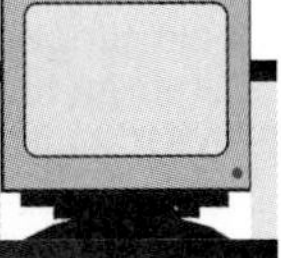

BASIC INFORMATION

DEFINITION

Syndrome caused by an excess of one or more adrenal steroids (i.e., cortisol, mineralocorticoids, adrenal androgens) but most commonly cortisol. Adrenal carcinoma (see Adrenal Neoplasia [Adenoma/Carcinoma], p 43), hyperaldosteronism (see Hyperaldosteronism, Primary, p 541), excessive adrenal sex hormone production (see Aberrant Adrenocortical Disease [Increased Adrenal Sex Hormone Production], p 5), and cases with ambiguous characteristics possibly suggesting hyperadrenocorticism (see Hyperadrenocorticism Suspect/Conflicting Results, p 540) are discussed in greater detail under their respective headings.

SYNONYM(S)

HAC

Canine Cushing's syndrome: hypercortisolemia

Cushing's disease: hypercortisolemia secondary to excessive adrenocorticotropic hormone (ACTH) secretion from the pituitary gland

EPIDEMIOLOGY

SPECIES, AGE, SEX

- Most common in dogs. Rare in cats
- Dogs: middle-aged/old. Rare in dogs <6 years. Slight female predisposition
- Cats: middle-aged/old (median 10.7 years); no sex predilection

GENETICS AND BREED PREDISPOSITION

- Dogs:
  - Pituitary-dependent hyperadrenocorticism (PDH): 75% weigh <20 kg. Beagles, boxers, dachshunds, German shepherds, poodles, and terriers are overrepresented
  - Adrenal tumor hyperadrenocorticism (ATH): 50% weigh >20 kg. Dachshunds, German shepherds, Labrador retrievers, poodles, and terriers are overrepresented
- Cats: none

ASSOCIATED CONDITIONS AND DISORDERS

- Urinary tract infections
- Urinary calculi
- Hypertension
- Diabetes mellitus
- Sudden acquired retinal degeneration
- Glomerular disease
- Pancreatitis
- Neurologic signs with pituitary macroadenoma
- Thrombosis and pulmonary thromboembolism

CLINICAL PRESENTATION

DISEASE FORMS/SUBTYPES

- PDH: 80-85% of cases
- ATH: 15-20% of cases
- Iatrogenic: due to glucocorticoid administration

HISTORY, CHIEF COMPLAINT

- Dogs: polyuria, polydipsia, polyphagia, pendulous abdomen, excessive bruising, panting, alopecia, clitoral hypertrophy, testicular atrophy, anestrus, weakness/lethargy, exercise intolerance, muscle atrophy, obesity
- Cats: polyuria, polydipsia, polyphagia, pendulous abdomen, unkempt haircoat, alopecia, fragile (easily torn) skin, lethargy, muscle wasting, obesity

PHYSICAL EXAM FINDINGS

- Dogs: thin skin, bilaterally symmetric alopecia, hepatomegaly, pyoderma, abdominal enlargement, clitoral hypertrophy, testicular atrophy, bruising, muscle wasting, seborrhea, calcinosis cutis, hyperpigmentation, comedones
- Cats: pendulous abdomen, unkempt haircoat, alopecia, fragile (easily torn) skin, muscle wasting, obesity

ETIOLOGY AND PATHOPHYSIOLOGY

- PDH:
  - Approximately 80-90% caused by a pituitary microadenoma (<10 mm in diameter).
  - Pituitary carcinomas, macroadenomas, and corticotroph hyperplasia are rare.
  - Excessive ACTH secretion from the pituitary gland stimulates the adrenal glands (zonae fasciculata and reticularis of the adrenal cortex) (see Fig. I-101) to produce excessive amounts of cortisol, resulting in adrenal hypertrophy.
  - The abnormal pituitary cells become less sensitive to inhibition by cortisol, continuing to secrete ACTH despite hypercortisolemia.
- ATH: See Adrenal Neoplasia (Adenoma/Carcinoma), p 43.
- Iatrogenic: Exogenous corticosteroids decrease pituitary ACTH secretion (with eventual adrenocortical atrophy), but clinical signs occur as a result of hypercortisolemia.
- Cortisol/glucocorticoids interfere with antidiuretic hormone release (causing polyuria with secondary polydipsia), stimulate protein catabolism (causing muscle loss, weakness, pendulous abdomen, polyphagia), cause hypertension (and secondary proteinuria, associated with low circulating levels of antithrombin III), and compromise normal processes of the skin (causing bilaterally symmetrical alopecia, pyoderma, and/or comedone formation).

DIAGNOSIS

DIFFERENTIAL DIAGNOSIS

- See Polyuria/Polydipsia, p 878
- See Polyphagia, p 877
- See Alopecia, p 52

INITIAL DATABASE

- Complete blood count: mature neutrophilia, monocytosis, lymphopenia, eosinopenia, thrombocytosis
- Serum biochemical profile:
  - Dog: increased alkaline phosphatase (ALP), hypercholesterolemia, hyperglycemia (usually mild)
  - Cat: hyperglycemia (80% have concurrent diabetes mellitus), hypercholesterolemia, increased alanine aminotransferase (ALT), increased ALP (30% of cases)
- Urinalysis and bacterial culture: specific gravity <1.020, proteinuria common, infection in 40-50% of cases regardless of urine sediment
- Abdominal radiographs: hepatomegaly, cystic calculi, mineralized adrenal gland, and/or osteopenia
- Thoracic radiographs (three views): possible metastasis (if adrenal tumor), hypovascular lungs and alveolar infiltrates (secondary thromboembolism), and airway mineralization
- Blood pressure: possible hypertension
- Fundic examination: possible retinal hemorrhage

ADVANCED OR CONFIRMATORY TESTING

- To identify HAC:
  - ACTH stimulation test:
    - Will not differentiate PDH from ATH.
    - A 15% chance of false-positive results with chronic nonadrenal illness, so adrenal testing should be postponed if other disease is present.
    - Sensitivity: dogs: PDH 87%, ATH 60%; cats: 81% for both PDH and ATH.
    - Specificity: 85-90% (dogs).
    - Only test that will identify iatrogenic HAC.
    - Protocol: cortisol measured in blood collected before and 1 to 2 hours after administration of exogenous ACTH. Test times vary depending on the ACTH product used; consult laboratory for protocol details.
      - A poststimulation cortisol concentration greater than 25 μg/dl (690 μmol/L) is suspicious for HAC; >30 μg/dl (830 μmol/L) is usually diagnostic for HAC.
  - Low-dose dexamethasone suppression test (LDDS):
    - Can confirm HAC and in some cases discriminate between PDH and ATH.
    - A 50% chance of false-positive results with nonadrenal illness, so adrenal testing should be postponed if other disease is present.
    - Sensitivity: dogs: 85-95%; cats: 80%.
    - Specificity 70-75% (dogs).
    - Protocol:
      - Dogs: cortisol measured in blood collected before and 4 and 8 hours after administration of dexamethasone (0.01 mg/kg IV).
        - Normal: suppression of serum cortisol concentration (<1.4 μg/dl (40 μmol/L) at both 4 and 8 hours.
        - Dogs with HAC: inadequate cortisol suppression (cortisol >1.4 μg/dl [40 μmol/L]) at 8 hours.

- Dogs with ATH: inadequate cortisol suppression at either time point.
- Dogs with PDH: 35% will not suppress at either time point; 65% will show one of three patterns of suppression:
  - 8-hour cortisol concentration > reference range but <50% of basal value.
  - 4-hour cortisol concentration <50% of basal value or < reference range; 8-hour cortisol > 1.4 mg/dl (40 mmol/L).
  - 4-hour cortisol concentration <1.4 mg/dl, 8-hour cortisol >1.4 mg/dl (40 mmol/L).
- Cats: protocol as for dogs except the dexamethasone dose is 0.1 mg/kg IV.
  - Between 65% and 90% of cats with PDH and 100% of ATH have inadequate cortisol suppression at this dose.
- Random fluctuations in cortisol concentrations can be seen with ATH.
- Urine cortisol:creatinine ratio:
  - Between 90% and 100% sensitive for both dogs and cats; <10-15% chance of dog having HAC if ratio is normal. False-positive results very common (75% dogs with nonadrenal illness have ratio consistent with HAC).
  - Protocol: owner collects morning urine (at home), which is submitted for cortisol and creatinine measurement.
- To differentiate PDH from ATH once a diagnosis of HAC has been established:
  - In some cases, the LDDS results will identify PDH (see preceding discussion).
  - High-dose dexamethasone suppression test (HDDS):
    - Protocol: cortisol measured in blood collected before and 4 and 8 hours after administration of dexamethasone (dogs: 0.1 mg/kg IV; cats: 1.0 mg/kg IV).
      - Dogs with PDH: suppression of cortisol concentrations (<50% of basal concentrations or <1.4 µg/dl [40 µmol/L]) at 4 or 8 hours. However, 24-35% of dogs with PDH fail to suppress HDDS and need a further discriminating test.
      - Dogs with ATH: inadequate suppression, although random fluctuations in cortisol concentrations can be seen. Partial or unclear result warrants other test (e.g., ultrasonography).
  - Endogenous ACTH concentrations:
    - Low in dogs with ATH and high in dogs with PDH.
    - ACTH is very labile in plasma and the hormone degrades rapidly if not handled correctly, so nondiagnostic samples can result.
  - Abdominal ultrasonography: normal adrenal thickness: 3-7.5 mm.
    - PDH: bilaterally symmetric enlargement of the adrenal glands. 5-10% will have nodular hyperplasia.
    - ATH: unilateral adrenal enlargement with a small contralateral adrenal.
  - Computed tomography or magnetic resonance imaging: used for pituitary imaging (pituitary macroadenoma) or abdominal imaging (adrenal size, tumor invasion).

TREATMENT

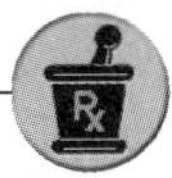

THERAPEUTIC GOAL(S)

- Resolution of clinical signs
- For medical therapy: cortisol concentrations within the basal reference range on both the pre- and post-ACTH stimulation samples

ACUTE GENERAL TREATMENT

By definition, hyperadrenocorticism is a chronic, slowly progressive disease. Therefore acute treatment is not indicated.

CHRONIC TREATMENT

- Medical therapy: mitotane, trilostane, ketoconazole, L-deprenyl:
  - Mitotane (o,p'-DDD, Lysodren):
    - Selectively destroys glucocorticoid-producing zones of the adrenal gland.
    - Protocol:
      - PDH:
        - See treatment algorithm (Hyperadrenocorticism, p 1543)
        - The owner should always have prednisone (0.2 mg/kg/day) available for home administration if needed.
      - ATH: See Adrenal Neoplasia (Adenoma/Carcinoma), p 43.
    - Adverse effects: vomiting, hypocortisolism, complete hypoadrenocorticism (uncommon).
- Ketoconazole:
  - Inhibits adrenal synthesis of cortisol.
  - Protocol: See treatment algorithm, p 1543.
  - Only effective in 50% of PDH and ATH cases.
  - May be used short term to control signs of HAC before surgery for ATH.
  - Adverse effects: anorexia, vomiting, diarrhea, lethargy, hepatopathy.
- Trilostane (Vetoryl):
  - Currently not available in the United States; registered treatment for PDH in Europe.
  - Inhibits cortisol synthesis.
  - Dogs with PDH:
    - Protocol: See treatment algorithm, p 1543.
    - By the end of 6 months, doses can range from 4-16 mg/kg/day.
    - Some dogs require twice-a-day therapy.
  - Adverse effects: hypocortisolism.
- L-Deprenyl (selegiline, Anipryl):
  - Decreases ACTH secretion by increasing dopaminergic tone to the hypothalamic-pituitary axis.
  - Initial reports by Deprenyl Animal Health Inc. showed 75-80% efficacy, but two independent studies showed poor efficacy.
  - Protocol: See treatment algorithm, p 1543.
  - If no response is seen after 2 to 3 months, the diagnosis of hyperadrenocorticism should be reassessed and, if confirmed, another treatment should be used.
- Medical treatment is difficult in cats. Mitotane, ketoconazole, and trilostane (6-10 mg/kg) are reported to have mixed results, but information is limited. Metyrapone (65 mg/kg PO q 12h) and aminoglutethimide (6 mg/kg PO q 12h) have also been tried.
- Surgical therapy:
  - Hypophysectomy has been described in both dogs and cats but is not widely available.
  - Bilateral adrenalectomy is the treatment of choice for PDH in cats.
  - Unilateral adrenalectomy is the treatment of choice for adrenal neoplasia in dogs and cats (see Adrenal Neoplasia [Adenoma/Carcinoma], p 43).
- Radiation therapy (cobalt teletherapy or linear accelerator): for pituitary macroadenomas.

DRUG INTERACTIONS

- Mitotane: increases barbiturate and warfarin metabolism; additive depressive effects with central nervous system depressants; insulin requirements in diabetic dogs may decrease; spironolactone may block mitotane's actions.
- Ketoconazole—antacids and H_2 blockers may decrease absorption; decreases theophylline and increases cyclosporine concentrations; increases anticoagulant effects of warfarin.
- L-Deprenyl: interacts with selective serotonin reuptake inhibitors, tricyclic antidepressants, meperidine.
- Trilostane: avoid concurrent use of other treatments of HAC.

POSSIBLE COMPLICATIONS

- Medical treatment: see adverse effects listed after each drug in Chronic Treatment above
- Adrenalectomy: see Adrenal Neoplasia (Adenoma/Carcinoma), p 43

RECOMMENDED MONITORING

- See Chronic Treatment above and Algorithm for Treatment of Hyperadrenocorticism, p 1543.

- At home: owner monitors clinical signs; treated patients may require short-term prednisone supplementation (0.2 mg/kg/day) during stressful situations.

PROGNOSIS AND OUTCOME

Dogs:
- PDH: mitotane therapy median survival, 20 months; average, 30 months
- ATH: see Adrenal Neoplasia (Adenoma/Carcinoma), p 43

PEARLS & CONSIDERATIONS

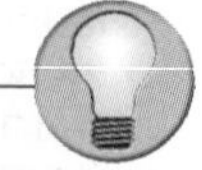

COMMENTS

- For all endocrine tests, consult your laboratory concerning specific test protocols and guidelines for interpretation.
- LDDS test requires very small volumes of dexamethasone; measure carefully and/or dilute for accurate dosing.
- Before medical therapy and during induction therapy, the owner must quantify water and food intake.
- No dog with a decreased appetite should receive mitotane.
- During induction therapy have the owner feed one-third the normal food intake twice a day so that any reduction in appetite is obvious.
- Mitotane should be given after the dog's meal to enhance absorption and to confirm that all food is eaten.
- Never induce a dog in hospital, as food and water intake is usually reduced.
- Daily phone contact with owners is recommended during induction therapy.

CLIENT EDUCATION

Clients must be educated as to the risks of medical therapy and be able to recognize clinical signs of hypoadrenocorticism.

SUGGESTED READING

Feldman EC, Nelson RW: Hyperadrenocorticism. In Feldman EC, Nelson RW: *Canine and Feline Endocrinology and Reproduction*, ed 3. Philadelphia, WB Saunders, 2004; pp 252–357.

AUTHOR: **KATE HILL**
EDITOR: **SHERRI IHLE**

Hyperadrenocorticism Suspect/Conflicting Results

BASIC INFORMATION

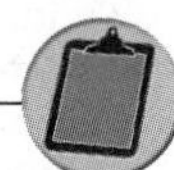

DEFINITION

Some of the clinical signs of hyperadrenocorticism (Cushing's disease) are present and/or biochemical test results are suggestive of hyperadrenocorticism, but there are conflicting results with other clinical features or with cortisol testing

EPIDEMIOLOGY

SPECIES, AGE, SEX: Middle-aged or older dogs.

CLINICAL PRESENTATION

DISEASE FORMS/SUBTYPES: One clinical sign (e.g., polyuria/polydipsia, endocrine alopecia, systemic hypertension), one biochemical abnormality (e.g., increased alkaline phosphatase concentration, proteinuria), or one other finding (e.g., vacuolar hepatopathy on biopsy) suggests hyperadrenocorticism, but other results are normal or contradictory.

HISTORY, CHIEF COMPLAINT
- The absence of any overt clinical signs of hyperadrenocorticism makes the diagnosis of hyperadrenocorticism extremely unlikely. Specifically, a dog showing no polyuria, no polydipsia, and no polyphagia almost certainly does not have hyperadrenocorticism.
  - Example: If hyperadrenocorticism is suspected only because of incidentally discovered elevated liver value[s] on a preanesthetic screen, a disease process other than hyperadrenocorticism is almost always the cause of the liver value elevation.
- If anorexia, vomiting, and/or diarrhea are present, a diagnosis other than hyperadrenocorticism is likely (exception: if undergoing treatment with o'p-DDD).
- Polyphagia, one of the common signs of hyperadrenocorticism, also is very common in healthy, gluttonous dogs. The history therefore should assess whether appetite has increased in the preceding weeks to months despite no change in diet (more consistent with hyperadrenocorticism) or has always been voracious.
- Panting, which is noted in dogs with hyperadrenocorticism, is a common chief complaint in dogs with many disorders that occur more commonly than hyperadrenocorticism, including obesity, hyperthermia, anxiety, pain, and acid-base disorders.
- Seasonal, anxiety-related, or other environmental changes commonly increase water consumption in dogs without producing true polydipsia. Normal daily water consumption: <70 ml/kg/day (dogs; higher in dogs <4 kg), <250 ml/day (average-size cat).
- Dogs first presented for evaluation of critical, severe clinical signs virtually never have hyperadrenocorticism (exception: severe complications of hyperadrenocorticism treatment).

PHYSICAL EXAM FINDINGS
- "Textbook" hyperadrenocorticism appearance (potbellied, thin-skinned, symmetrically alopecic dog with comedones) is not present in all patients with hyperadrenocorticism.
- Similarly, these typical features may be found in patients with diseases other than hyperadrenocorticism (see Aberrant Adrenocortical Disease [Increased Adrenal Sex Hormone Production], p 5).
- Therefore, suggestive physical findings should be correlated to history, and if hyperadrenocorticism remains likely, testing to evaluate both hyperadrenocorticism and aberrant adrenocortical disease (see Hyperadrenocorticism, p 537; Aberrant Adrenocortical Disease [Increased Adrenal Sex Hormone Production], p 5) may be warranted.

ETIOLOGY AND PATHOPHYSIOLOGY

- Hyperadrenocorticism is a slowly-progressive disease that produces clinical signs gradually and chronically.
- The prevalence of complications such as thromboembolic disease and systemic hypertension prior to the onset of overt clinical signs (polyuria/polydipsia, polyphagia) is not known.
- Other endocrine disorders, particularly aberrant adrenocortical disease (see p 5), may mimic hyperadrenocorticism clinically.
- Therefore, the diagnosis of hyperadrenocorticism, and the decision to treat, cannot be based on a single abnormality (be it historic, physical, or biochemical) alone.

DIAGNOSIS

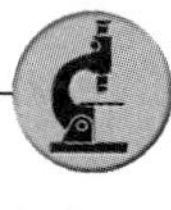

DIFFERENTIAL DIAGNOSIS

Depends on the clinical signs and biochemical abnormalities seen:

- Polyuria/polydipsia (see Polyuria/Polydipsia, p 878)
- Polyphagia (see Polyphagia, p 877)
- Alopecia (see Alopecia, p 52)
- Proteinuria (see Protein-Losing Nephropathy, p 900; Glomerulonephritis, p 442; Amyloidosis, p 57), secondary to other systemic disease
- Hypertension (see Systemic Hypertension, p 1058)
- Alkaline phosphatase elevation

INITIAL DATABASE

- Revisit a detailed history and physical examination to identify any previously missed signs or findings that would support hyperadrenocorticism or another disorder.
- Complete blood count (CBC), serum biochemistry, urinalysis with urine culture, systemic blood pressure, fundic examination (see Hyperadrenocorticism, p 537 for typical findings).

ADVANCED OR CONFIRMATORY TESTING

- Adrenocorticotropic hormone (ACTH) stimulation test with adrenal sex hormone panel (see Aberrant Adrenocortical Disease [Increased Adrenal Sex Hormone Production], p 5).
  - ACTH stimulation test is abnormal in 60-87% of dogs with hyperadrenocorticism.
- Low dose dexamethasone suppression test (see Hyperadrenocorticism, p 537).
  - Abnormal in 85-95% of dogs with hyperadrenocorticism, provided dogs with signs of systemic illness such as anorexia or gastrointestinal signs are not tested (systemic illness falsifies results and precludes treatment for hyperadrenocorticism anyway).
- Urine cortisol:creatinine ratio (see Hyperadrenocorticism, p 537).
  - Highly sensitive (90-100% of dogs with hyperadrenocorticism have elevated result, and normal result means <15% likelihood of hyperadrenoocticism) but poorly specific (many other disorders elevate results).
- Abdominal ultrasound: See Hyperadrenocorticism, p 537 for findings supportive of hyperadrenocorticism; with nonadrenal disease, findings will vary with the primary disease.
- Urine protein:creatinine ratio if proteinuria is present and urine culture is negative. Commonly elevated in hyperadrenocorticism.

TREATMENT

THERAPEUTIC GOAL(S)

- Hyperadrenocorticism is a disease characterized by overt physical manifestations. Therefore:
  - Treatment for hyperadrenocorticism should ONLY be instituted when clinical signs consistent with the disease are present and should not be based solely on laboratory test results. None of the tests of the hypothalamic-pituitary-adrenal axis have 100% sensitivity or specificity and all available information needs to be critically evaluated.
  - If cortisol testing is suggestive of hyperadrenocorticism but there are no clinical signs associated with the disease, either look for other underlying illnesses that could result in increased cortisol concentrations or have the owner monitor for signs of hyperadrenocorticism (e.g., increased water intake, polyphagia).
- If nonadrenal disease is identified, it should be treated and possible hyperadrenocorticism reassessed at a later time if clinical signs persist.

ACUTE GENERAL TREATMENT

- Virtually by definition, hyperadrenocorticism does not warrant acute treatment. Patients in whom the diagnosis is unclear may benefit from watchful waiting, given the potential negative effects of adrenal suppression (see Hyperadrenocorticism, p 537).
- Proteinuria (see Protein-Losing Nephropathy, p 900).
- Hypertension (see Systemic Hypertension, p 1058).

CHRONIC TREATMENT

Treat for hyperadrenocorticism (see Hyperadrenocorticism, p 537) if history, physical exam, and diagnostic testing together support the diagnosis

POSSIBLE COMPLICATIONS

Hypocortisolism, or full hypoadrenocorticism, if hyperadrenocorticism is mistakenly diagnosed and treated

RECOMMENDED MONITORING

- Home: owner to monitor clinical signs (e.g., polyuria/polydipsia, polyphagia).
- In-hospital:
  - Reevaluate a physical examination, history, and serum biochemical profile ± urinalysis and systolic blood pressure q 2-3 months to identify any new signs or abnormalities.
  - If proteinuria: assess UP:UC q 2-3 months.
- If/when clinical signs of hyperadrenocorticism develop, repeat a CBC, serum biochemical profile, urinalysis (± urine culture), and cortisol testing prior to instituting treatment.

PROGNOSIS AND OUTCOME

Dependent on the disease present (see Hyperadrenocorticism, p 537, or the specific chapter)

PEARLS & CONSIDERATIONS

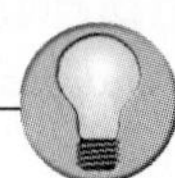

COMMENTS

Because of the number of different combination of signs and test results that can be seen, these can be challenging cases. Controversy exists even among specialists as to exactly which patients should be treated and when.

SUGGESTED READING

Feldman EC, Nelson RW: Hyperadrenocorticism. In Feldman EC, Nelson RW: *Canine and Feline Endocrinology and Reproduction*, ed 3. Philadelphia, WB Saunders, 2004; pp 252-357.

AUTHOR: **KATE HILL**
EDITOR: **SHERRI IHLE**

Hyperaldosteronism, Primary

BASIC INFORMATION

DEFINITION

Autonomous secretion of aldosterone by abnormal zona glomerulosa tissue within the adrenal gland

SYNONYM(S)

Conn's syndrome

EPIDEMIOLOGY

SPECIES, AGE, SEX

- Rare disease of dogs and cats
- Older animals (>8 years)
- No sex predilection

ASSOCIATED CONDITIONS AND DISORDERS: Hypokalemia; occasionally systemic hypertension.

CLINICAL PRESENTATION

DISEASE FORMS/SUBTYPES

- Adrenal tumor
- Bilateral adrenal hyperplasia

HISTORY, CHIEF COMPLAINT: Weakness (may be episodic), lethargy, polyuria/polydipsia, stiff gait, nocturia, loss of vision.

PHYSICAL EXAM FINDINGS: Generalized muscular weakness, cervical ventroflexion (cats), stiff gait, muscle pain, retinal hemorrhages, and/or detachment.

ETIOLOGY AND PATHOPHYSIOLOGY

- Occurs as a result of an aldosterone-secreting adrenal tumor (adenoma or adenocarcinoma) or hyperplasia of the adrenal zona glomerulosa.
- Circulating hyperaldosteronemia leads to increased renal potassium excretion (causing hypokalemia) and increased renal sodium and water resorption (often without overt effects unless renal disease or heart disease is present). The renin system is suppressed.
- Clinical signs result from serum hypokalemia and associated muscle weakness, and hypertension due to extracellular fluid volume expansion.

DIAGNOSIS

DIFFERENTIAL DIAGNOSIS

- Adrenal enlargement or mass:
  - Cortisol or sex-hormone-secreting adrenal tumor
  - Pheochromocytoma
  - Nonsecretory adrenal mass (see Adrenal Mass, Incidental, p 42)
- For hyperaldosteronemia:
  - Secondary to renal failure, heart failure, or severe hepatic dysfunction
- For severe, highly refractory hypokalemia:
  - Hypomagnesemia

INITIAL DATABASE

- Complete blood count, serum biochemical profile, urinalysis: severe hypokalemia (often <3 mEq/L), normal or slightly increased sodium concentration, minimally concentrated urine.
- Abdominal ultrasound: possible unilateral adrenal mass ± intra-abdominal metastasis. Cats with primary hyperaldosteronism secondary to micronodular adrenal hyperplasia may have grossly normal adrenal glands on abdominal imaging.
- Thoracic radiographs: possible metastasis from adrenal adenocarcinoma.
- Systolic arterial blood pressure: usually increased.
- Blood gas analysis: metabolic alkalosis.

ADVANCED OR CONFIRMATORY TESTING

- Plasma aldosterone concentrations (PAC): usually markedly increased.
- Plasma renin concentrations (PRC): may be decreased or within the normal reference range. In theory, an increased plasma renin concentration excludes a diagnosis of primary hyperaldosteronism.
- An increased PAC:PRC ratio may be useful in establishing the diagnosis in those animals without markedly elevated aldosterone concentrations.
- Computed tomographic scan can be used for detecting subtle changes within the adrenal cortex and to better delineate in the preoperative phase the extent of the adrenal mass.

TREATMENT

THERAPEUTIC GOAL(S)

- Normalization of serum potassium concentration and arterial blood pressure
- Surgical excision of abnormal adrenal tissue

ACUTE GENERAL TREATMENT

- Correct hypokalemia: oral supplementation of potassium (mild hypokalemia) or intravenous administration of potassium-supplemented fluids at a rate of potassium delivery not to exceed 0.5 mEq/L/hr.
- Manage hypertension: see Systemic Hypertension, p 1058.
- Spironolactone, an aldosterone antagonist, may be effective alone for control of both hypokalemia and systemic hypertension, at a dose of 1-2 mg/kg PO q 12h.

CHRONIC TREATMENT

Surgical excision of the adrenal tumor is recommended if there is no evidence of abdominal or thoracic metastasis.

DRUG INTERACTIONS

Hyperkalemia can occur if spironolactone is used concurrently with other potassium-sparing diuretics or with angiotensin-converting enzyme inhibitors.

POSSIBLE COMPLICATIONS

- The major potential complication of unilateral adrenalectomy is perioperative hemorrhage
- There are no reports of postoperative hypoaldosteronism occurring after excision of an aldosterone-secreting adrenal tumor

RECOMMENDED MONITORING

- Successful surgical management of primary hyperaldosteronism should result in resolution of hypokalemia and hypertension and normalization of serum aldosterone concentrations.
- If chronic medical management is undertaken, serial electrolyte and blood pressure monitoring is recommended.

PROGNOSIS AND OUTCOME

- There are few reported cases of primary hyperaldosteronism in dogs and cats. Prognosis is fair to guarded in cases of adrenal adenocarcinoma, as metastasis can occur. Medical management of patients with inoperable disease may achieve good short-term control of hypokalemia and systemic hypertension.
- Animals with successfully removed adenomas or adrenal hyperplasia are likely to have a good outcome.
- Data concerning survival times are limited. Reported long-term survival times in cats and dogs with surgical management range from 1 to 4 years. There are reports of cats surviving up to 9 months with medical management.

PEARLS & CONSIDERATIONS

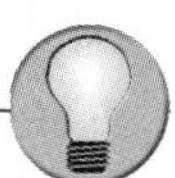

COMMENTS

- In a series of cats with primary hyperaldosteronism secondary to adrenal micronodular hyperplasia, progressive renal insufficiency was observed despite medical management of the hyperaldosteronism and was thought to be a consequence of hyperaldosteronism. Serial monitoring of renal function in these cats is recommended.
- Hyperaldosteronism is an important differential diagnosis for highly refractory hypokalemia.

SUGGESTED READING

Feldman EC, Nelson RW: Primary mineralocorticoid excess: primary hyperaldosteronism. In Feldman EC, Nelson RW: *Canine and Feline Endocrinology and Reproduction,* ed 3. St. Louis, WB Saunders, 2004, pp 351-353.

Feldman EC, Nelson RW: Primary hyperaldosteronism in cats (aldosterone-secreting adrenal tumor). In Feldman EC, Nelson RW: *Canine and Feline Endocrinology and Reproduction,* ed 3. St. Louis, WB Saunders, 2004, pp 389-391.

Javadi S, et al: Primary hyperaldosteronism, a mediator of progressive renal disease in cats. *Domest Anim Endocrinol* 28:85-104, 2005.

AUTHOR: **SARAH L. NAIDOO**

EDITOR: **SHERRI IHLE**

Hypercalcemia

BASIC INFORMATION

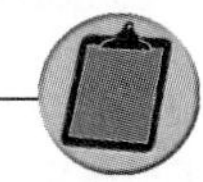

DEFINITION

Elevation in serum calcium concentration

EPIDEMIOLOGY

SPECIES, AGE, SEX

- Hypercalcemia can occur in dogs or cats of either gender and any age; depends on the underlying cause.
- Normal young dogs, cats <6 months old: commonly show mild, incidental hypercalcemia.

GENETICS AND BREED PREDISPOSITION: Depends on etiology.

RISK FACTORS: Depends on etiology.

CONTAGION AND ZOONOSIS: Rarely relevant. Common-source infections possible with systemic mycoses.

GEOGRAPHY AND SEASONALITY: Granulomatous diseases (systemic mycoses, schistosomiasis): specific geographic distributions.

ASSOCIATED CONDITIONS AND DISORDERS: Renal failure (potentially irreversible).

CLINICAL PRESENTATION

HISTORY, CHIEF COMPLAINT

- Polyuria/polydipsia
- Malaise: lethargy, weakness, inappetence
- Other signs depend on underlying problem
- In dogs with hypercalcemia and azotemia: renal failure with secondary hypercalcemia is more likely if the patient is lethargic, inappetent, and overtly ill, whereas dogs with primary hypercalcemia (e.g., hyperparathyroidism) and secondary renal effects more commonly feel well despite moderate/marked hypercalcemia

PHYSICAL EXAM FINDINGS

- Generally reflective of the underlying cause. For example, lymphadenopathy is possible with lymphoma, other malignancies, or granulomatous/fungal disease.
- No physical finding is pathognomonic for a specific cause of hypercalcemia.
- Rectal palpation: Up to 30% of anal sac adenocarcinomas are found incidentally, emphasizing the importance of rectal palpation as a routine part of physical examination of dogs.

ETIOLOGY AND PATHOPHYSIOLOGY

- Normal range of serum total calcium concentration:
  - Dog: 8.5-11.0 mg/dl [2.12-2.98 mmol/L].
  - Cat: 8.0-10.5 mg/dl [2.00-2.90 mmol/L].
- Dystrophic, soft-tissue mineralization is more likely to occur if the product of calcium X phosphorus concentrations (in mg/dl) >70.
- Approximately 50% of circulating calcium is ionized, 40% is protein-bound (mostly to albumin), and 10% is bound to other molecules (lactate, citrate, etc.).
- Mechanisms of causative disorders:
  - Primary hyperparathyroidism: elevated parathyroid hormone concentrations activate osteoclastic resorption of calcium from bone, renal conservation, and intestinal absorption.
  - Hypercalcemia of malignancy: neoplastic cells elaborate parathyroid hormone-related protein (PTHrP; actions similar to parathyroid hormone [PTH]). Less commonly, bone tumors cause hypercalcemia through local erosive effects.
  - Granulomatous disease: elaboration of PTHrP-like substances.
  - Idiopathic hypercalcemia of cats.
  - Chronic renal failure: hemoconcentration, reduced calcium excretion, renal secondary hyperparathyroidism.
  - Vitamin D toxicosis (rodenticide or human prescription medications, e.g., calcipotriene): heightened vitamin D-mediated intestinal calcium absorption, renal calcium conservation.
  - Youth: normal bone growth.

DIAGNOSIS

DIFFERENTIAL DIAGNOSIS

- Dogs: see Etiology and Pathophysiology above.
- In hypercalcemic cats, malignancy (30%), renal failure (25%), and urolithiasis (15%) are recognized associations in addition to idiopathic hypercalcemia and other less common disorders such as primary hyperparathyroidism.

INITIAL DATABASE

- Complete blood count: changes depend on underlying cause
- Serum chemistry panel:
  - Blood urea nitrogen, creatinine: elevation common; prerenal or renal.
  - Potassium: elevation suggests hypoadrenocorticism, acute renal failure, or artifact (common; remeasure with green top tube sample).
  - Concomitant hypophosphatemia: suggests primary hyperparathyroidism, hypercalcemia of malignancy; concomitant hyperphosphatemia suggests chronic renal failure, vitamin D toxicosis, hypoadrenocorticism.
- Urinalysis:
  - Isosthenuria with concurrent azotemia and hypercalcemia suggests renal failure, hypoadrenocorticism, or blood and urine samples drawn at different times (no conclusions possible if blood and urine are not obtained simultaneously).
- Thoracic radiographs:
  - Metastatic disease or sternal lymphadenopathy may suggest neoplasia (rule out fungal disease, if appropriate).
- Abdominal imaging (ultrasound ± radiographs):
  - Lesions suggesting malignancy (lymphadenopathy, hepatosplenomegaly, possible metastases).
  - Uroliths (calcium phosphate, calcium oxalate, or both) and bladder wall thickening due to chronic infection: common in canine hyperparathyroidism.
  - Assess renal structure. Renal dystrophic mineralization due to chronic severe hypercalcemia usually is not apparent radiographically or ultrasonographically.

ADVANCED OR CONFIRMATORY TESTING

- Ionized calcium: biologically active component of serum calcium. Elevated with primary hyperparathyroidism, hypercalcemia of malignancy, and vitamin D toxicosis, but normal or low with chronic renal failure, hypoadrenocorticism, or granulomatous/fungal diseases.
- Serum PTH and PTHrP concentrations: PTH should be undetectable in response to hypercalcemia of any cause. PTH values within reference range or higher (and ionized hypercalcemia) suggest primary hyperparathyroidism.
- Serum vitamin D concentrations: if suspect rodenticide intoxication.
- Cervical ultrasound: ultrasound examination of the neck by a skilled ultrasonographer may identify a mass on one or more parathyroid gland(s).
- Confirmatory testing based on abnormalities identified (e.g., fine-needle aspiration of enlarged lymph node[s]).

TREATMENT

THERAPEUTIC GOAL(S)

- Rapid lowering of serum calcium concentration if very elevated (avoidance of permanent renal or other soft tissue mineralization)
- Treatment of underlying cause

ACUTE GENERAL TREATMENT

- *Primary*: most efficacious:
  - IV fluid therapy (calcium free; e.g., avoid lactated Ringer's solution).
    - Dilution of serum calcium concentration, improvement in renal perfusion and glomerular filtration rate.
    - Rate of 100–150 ml/kg/day (twice maintenance) plus any dehydration deficit (ml replacement = % dehydration [5 to 15] × body weight [kg] × 10) should be administered over the first 24 hours assuming no heart disease, oliguria, or other factor predisposing to intolerance of volume load; adjust according to clinical signs.
  - Furosemide: 2–3 mg/kg IV q 4–8h. Calciuric diuretic (unlike thiazide diuretics or spironolactone, which do not promote calcium excretion). Prolonged use in hypercalcemic patients with renal insufficiency is not recommended, especially if the patient is anorexic and not receiving IV fluids.
  - Glucocorticoids: prednisone 1–2 mg/kg PO q 12h or dexamethasone 0.1–0.2 mg/kg PO q 12h. Decrease intestinal calcium absorption, increase renal calcium excretion. Since lymphoma is common cause of hypercalcemia, and glucocorticoids can interfere with a definitive diagnosis, diagnostic samples should be obtained before (e.g., lymph node aspirates) or within a maximum of 24 hours after the first dose of prednisone (e.g., for procedures requiring general anesthesia or referral, such as bone marrow aspirate, liver or intestinal biopsy, etc.).
- *Secondary*: generally less efficacious:
  - Calcitonin: 4–6 IU/kg SC q 8–12h.
  - Pamidronate: 1.3 mg/kg in 150 ml 0.9% NaCl, infused over 2 hours; may repeat in 1 week.

CHRONIC TREATMENT

Treatment of the inciting cause

POSSIBLE COMPLICATIONS

- Renal failure
- Overcorrection (hypocalcemia)

RECOMMENDED MONITORING

- Serum total and ionized calcium
- Renal parameters
- Serum electrolytes

PROGNOSIS AND OUTCOME

- Variable; excellent with hyperparathyroidism if treated appropriately (secondary renal failure is rare) to poor with other disorders (e.g., end-stage chronic renal failure)
- Specific prognosis depends on ability to achieve normocalcemia rapidly and to correct underlying cause

PEARLS & CONSIDERATIONS

COMMENTS

- Correcting total calcium concentration for hypoalbuminemia or hyperalbuminemia is not reliable (measure serum ionized calcium instead).
- Oral consumption of calcium (e.g., calcium carbonate) alone can virtually never cause hypercalcemia.

SUGGESTED READING

Feldman EC, Nelson RW: Hypercalcemia and primary hyperparathyroidism. In Feldman EC, Nelson RW (eds): *Textbook of Canine and Feline Endocrinology and Reproduction*, ed 3. St. Louis: Elsevier Saunders, 2004, pp 660–715.

AUTHOR: **EDWARD C. FELDMAN**
EDITOR: **ETIENNE CÔTÉ**

Hyperemia

BASIC INFORMATION

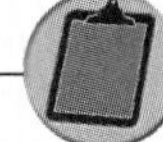

DEFINITION

- Active hyperemia: an increased volume of blood in an affected tissue or area due to arterial and arteriolar dilation
- Passive hyperemia: increased volume of blood in an affected tissue or area due to obstruction of blood outflow

SYNONYM(S)

Active hyperemia: arterial hyperemia, reactive hyperemia, engorgement, flushing, erythema, injected mucous membranes

Passive hyperemia: venous hyperemia, congestion

EPIDEMIOLOGY

SPECIES, AGE, SEX: No species, age, or sex predilection except as dependent on underlying etiology.

RISK FACTORS

- Increased tissue metabolic demand (e.g., fever, physical exertion)
- Vascular occlusion: extravascular or intravascular

GEOGRAPHY AND SEASONALITY: Vasodilatory cooling related to high environmental heat is a normal manifestation of hyperemia.

CLINICAL PRESENTATION

DISEASE FORMS/SUBTYPES

- Primary complaint:
  - Obvious extravascular occlusion such as limb constriction
  - Gross tissue changes
- Secondary finding:
  - Clinical sign noted in addition to other, associated abnormal findings
  - Incidental finding of no clinical significance (e.g., due to anxiety, physical activity, or hot weather)
- Hyperemia may also be classified as active or passive, or as regional or generalized.

HISTORY, CHIEF COMPLAINT

- Highly variable depending on underlying cause
- Examples (generalized hyperemia):
  - Recent exposure to allergen (insect bite, vaccine, food allergen, other)
  - Exposure to infectious agent
  - Exposure to high environmental temperature (enclosed in car during hot weather, other)
  - Anxiety, restlessness (e.g., pheochromocytoma, mast cell disease, polycythemia)
  - None (incidental finding during routine examination)

PHYSICAL EXAM FINDINGS

- Since hyperemia is a clinical sign and not a disease entity, specific physical findings are dependent on the underlying etiology.
- Generalized hyperemia:
  - Tachycardia, tachypnea, hyperthermia
  - Increased respiratory effort, cyanosis
  - Shortened capillary refill time evaluation
  - Weakness, collapse
  - Episodic increased levels of activity
- Localized hyperemia:
  - Regional dermal redness

- Possible swelling and/or pain in the region

ETIOLOGY AND PATHOPHYSIOLOGY

Arteriolar dilation due to sympathetic neurogenic mechanisms or exposure to or release of local or systemic vasoactive substances such as adenosine or nitric oxide in response to altered blood flow

DIAGNOSIS

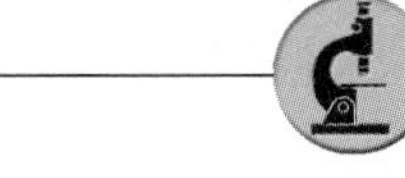

DIFFERENTIAL DIAGNOSIS

- Any condition causing redness, swelling, or inflammation such as infectious, inflammatory, immune-mediated, neurogenic, toxic, allergic
- Any cause of hyperthermia such as environmental, exercise, infectious, inflammatory, immune-mediated, neurogenic, toxicity
- Rebound vasodilation after ischemic crisis such as external constriction, embolic occlusion
- Altered perfusion states such as severe hypotension and hypotensive crises such as cardiac arrest
- Decreased venous return states: cardiac, hepatic, venous occlusion
- Episodic hyperemia: mast cell tumor, pheochromocytoma (Figs. I-96 and I-97)
- Acute contact dermatitis
- Congenital: teleangiectasis
- Vasculitis
- Carbon monoxide intoxication
- Polycythemia
- Acute allergic reaction, drug reaction

INITIAL DATABASE

- Temperature, heart rate, respiration rate
  - Hyperthermia warrants consideration of true fever (infectious, inflammatory, neoplastic causes; see Fever of Unknown Origin, p 386) versus environmental hyperthermia (hot weather, thick haircoat, anxiety, etc.).
- Diascopy: superficial lesions blanch with external pressure, such as with a glass slide
  - This simple maneuver helps confirm whether hyperemia is present (versus normal for the animal).

ADVANCED OR CONFIRMATORY TESTING

Use of these tests depends on determination of need. For example, in animals that are otherwise well (routine exam), behavioral agitation/anxiety, benign environmental hyperthermia, and exercise are common causes of hyperemia that generally do not warrant further evaluation.

- Blood pressure measurements
  - Systemic
  - Localized (if suspect embolic occlusion)
- Complete blood count (infectious, inflammatory, neoplastic, polycythemia)
- Serum biochemistry panel (hepatic, renal elevations)
- Radiographs: organomegaly, neoplasia
- Neurologic evaluation (in cases of suspected intoxication or other systemic disorders with neurologic effects)
- Abdominal ultrasound (neoplasm, infection/abscess, chronic passive congestion)
- Echocardiogram (endocarditis, other)
- Computed tomography or magnetic resonance imaging for embolism evaluation
- Aspirates and/or biopsies: masses/lesions
- Tick-borne disease titers
- Blood gas analysis
- Co-oximetry: carbon monoxide intoxication

TREATMENT

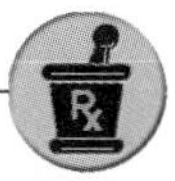

THERAPEUTIC GOAL(S)

- Resolution of underlying etiology
- Restoration of adequate perfusion
- Delivery of oxygen and other nutrients to the tissues

ACUTE GENERAL TREATMENT

- Supportive, as needed: analgesia, oxygen, restoration of perfusion, cooling of affected region
- Identification of etiology

CHRONIC TREATMENT

Treatment as appropriate for underlying etiology

POSSIBLE COMPLICATIONS

- Reperfusion injury
- Tissue necrosis

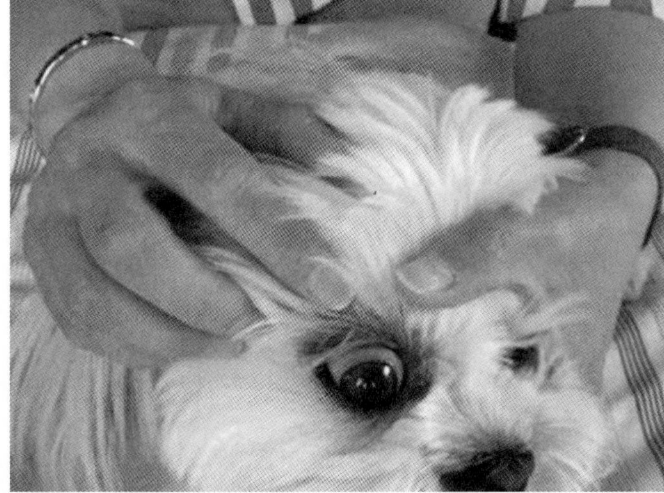

FIGURE I-96 Conjunctival hyperemia in a 5-year-old shih tzu; image taken from digital movie clip obtained by the owner at home. The chief complaint was episodic restlessness and generalized hyperemia, noted intermittently by the owner for a period of weeks. Courtesy of Dr. Etienne Côté.

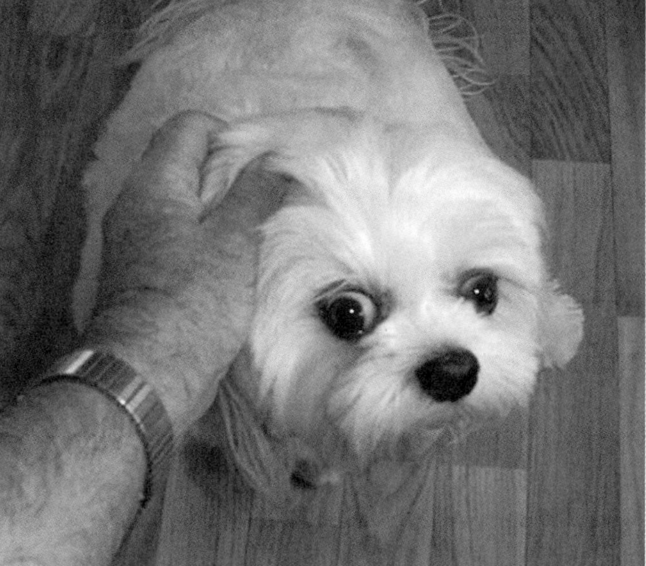

FIGURE I-97 Same patient as in Fig. I-96, normal appearance. There was absence of hyperemia most of the time at home, and hyperemia was not present in the veterinary hospital. Subsequently, fine-needle aspiration of a subcutaneous mass was consistent with mast cell tumor, and surgical excision of the mass led to complete resolution of episodes of hyperemia and restlessness. Courtesy of Dr. Etienne Côté.

PROGNOSIS AND OUTCOME

Highly variable depending on underlying etiology

PEARLS & CONSIDERATIONS

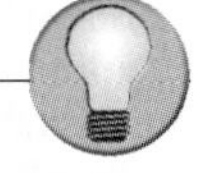

COMMENTS

- Presenting signs (true chief complaint, versus routine visit for preventive/annual exam) are extremely valuable in determining the importance of a patient's hyperemia.
- Intermittent/episodic hyperemia associated with behavioral changes, cardiac arrhythmias, or other systemic signs should arouse the suspicion of mast cell tumor or pheochromocytoma.

SUGGESTED READING

Guyton AC, Hall JE: *Textbook of Medical Physiology. Local Control of Blood Flow by the Tissues; and Humoral Regulation*, ed 10. Philadelphia, WB Saunders, 2000, pp 175-183.

Iida K, et al: Delayed hyperemia causing intracranial hypertension after cardiopulmonary resuscitation. *Crit Care Med* 25:971-976, 1997.

Lima I, et al: The peripheral perfusion index in reactive hyperemia in critically ill patients. *Crit Care* 8(Suppl 1): P53, 2004.

Locke-Bohannon LG, et al: Canine pheochromocytoma: diagnosis and management. *Comp Cont Ed Pract Vet* 23:807-815, 2001.

AUTHORS: **LISA M. ABBOTT, ADAM J. REISS**

EDITOR: **ETIENNE CÔTÉ**

Hyperkalemia

BASIC INFORMATION

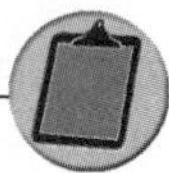

DEFINITION

A serum potassium concentration in excess of 5.5 mEq/L. Amounts exceeding 7.5 mEq/L are potentially harmful.

EPIDEMIOLOGY AND DEMOGRAPHICS

SPECIES, AGE, SEX: Any patient can be affected.

GENETICS AND BREED PREDISPOSITION

- Actual hyperkalemia: standard poodles with Addison's disease
- Pseudohyperkalemia:
  - Akita
  - English springer spaniel with phosphofructokinase deficiency

RISK FACTORS

- Renal impairment
- Urinary obstruction
- Urinary bladder rupture
- Hypoadrenocorticism
- Mineral acid metabolic acidosis
- Excess intake

ASSOCIATED CONDITIONS AND DISORDERS: Bradycardia.

CLINICAL PRESENTATION

DISEASE FORMS/SUBTYPES: Acute and chronic.

HISTORY, CHIEF COMPLAINT

- Acute: dramatic and life-threatening; produces diffuse muscle weakness, mental depression, anorexia. Stranguria accompanies lower urinary outflow obstructions. Vomiting common with acute renal failure and hypoadrenocorticism.
- Chronic: slower in onset and not as dramatic. Decreased appetite, weight loss, intermittent vomiting and diarrhea can occur.

PHYSICAL EXAM FINDINGS

- Generalized muscle weakness
- Weak pulse
- Prolonged capillary refill time
- Bradycardia
- Irregular heart rate

ETIOLOGY AND PATHOPHYSIOLOGY

ETIOLOGY (THREE GENERAL CAUSES)

- Increased potassium intake
- Potassium translocation *from the intracellular to the extracelluar fluid space*:
  - Mineral-acid–caused metabolic acidosis
  - Insulin deficiency
  - Catecholamine increases
  - Hypertonicity
  - Massive tissue destruction (rare in dogs and cats)
- Decreased excretion:
  - Hypoaldosteronism
  - Acute renal failure
  - Urinary bladder rupture or outflow obstruction
  - Type 4 renal tubular acidosis
  - Certain drugs (uncommon)

PATHOPHYSIOLOGY

- Affects primarily skeletal and cardiac muscle tissues
- Life-threatening effects on heart:
  - Depressed excitability and conduction velocity
  - Secondary to persistent depolarization and inactivation of the sodium channels within the cell membranes causing cardiac conduction abnormalities
- Skeletal muscle weakness occurs

DIAGNOSIS

- Abnormal electrocardiogram (ECG) patterns: peaked or depressed T wave, decreased R wave and P-wave amplitudes, prolongation of PR interval, eventual disappearance of P wave, widening of QRS complexes, heart blocks, aberrant atrioventricular conduction, and eventually ventricular fibrillation or asystole (Fig. I-98).
- Confirmed with laboratory serum potassium quantitation

DIFFERENTIAL DIAGNOSIS

Physical:

- Any cause of hypovolemic shock
- Primary underlying myocardial disease

INITIAL DATABASE

- Thorough history and physical examination.
- Complete blood count
- Serum biochemistry profile:
  - Serum electrolytes: elevated potassium (by definition); sodium may be concurrently low with hypoadrenocorticism, enteritis, renal disease, or pregnancy; chloride.
  - Blood urea nitrogen, creatinine: elevated with prerenal (e.g., hypoadrenocorticism), renal, or postrenal (e.g., urethral obstruction or urinary bladder rupture) azotemia.
  - Total CO_2/HCO_3^- decreased with metabolic acidosis.
  - Glucose: may be decreased in hypoadrenocorticism, sepsis.
- Urinalysis: isosthenuria concurrent with azotemia in renal failure or in hypoadrenocorticism.
- Blood gas: pH, HCO_3^-, or TCO_2 helpful.
- Abdominal imaging.

TREATMENT

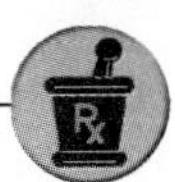

THERAPEUTIC GOAL(S)

- Antagonize myocardiotoxicity
- Treat the underlying cause
- Stop drugs known to increase the serum potassium concentration

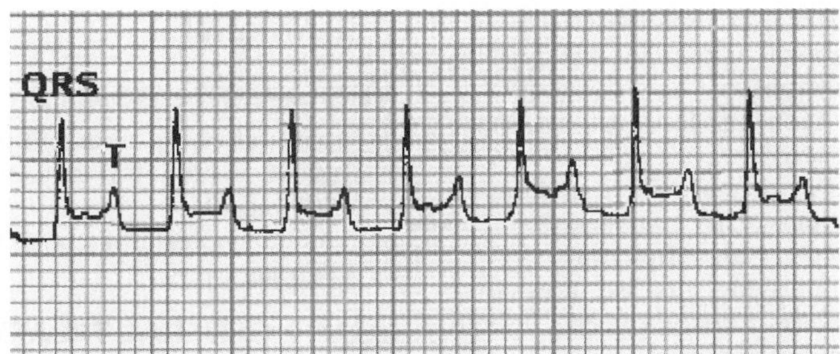

FIGURE I-98 ECG from a cat with urethral obstruction and hyperkalemia (serum $K^+ = 7.1$ mEq/L) showing atrial standstill. No P waves are seen, but the R-R rhythm is regular, typical of atrial standstill. The heart rate is 210/min, demonstrating that in cats, unlike dogs, a rapid heart rate is still consistent with hyperkalemia. There is mild ST segment elevation, suggesting myocardial hypoxia. Lead V2, 25 mm/sec, 1 cm = 1 mV.

ACUTE TREATMENT

- Calcium gluconate 10% solution (0.5–1.5 ml/kg IV) immediately antagonizes myocardiotoxicity without actually lowering serum potassium concentration
- Lowering the serum potassium:
  - Sodium bicarbonate, 1–2 mEq/kg IV bolus
  - Regular insulin and glucose, give 0.25–0.5 units of insulin/kg IV, covering each unit of insulin administered with 2 g dextrose (2 g = 4 ml 50% dextrose)
- ECG monitoring
- Treat the underlying cause
- Repeat serum potassium measurement

CHRONIC TREATMENT

Treat any underlying disease:

- Hypoadrenocorticism (see p 537): desoxycorticosterone pivalate and prednisone
- Renal tubular acidosis type 4: furosemide
- Chronic renal disease: fluid therapy or dialysis

DRUG INTERACTIONS

Can impair potassium excretion

POSSIBLE COMPLICATIONS

Cardiac arrest, death

RECOMMENDED MONITORING

- Periodic serum sodium and potassium monitoring with hypoadrenocorticism
- Follow-up renal evaluations

PROGNOSIS AND OUTCOME

- Guarded for renal failure
- Good for hypoadrenocorticism

PEARLS & CONSIDERATIONS

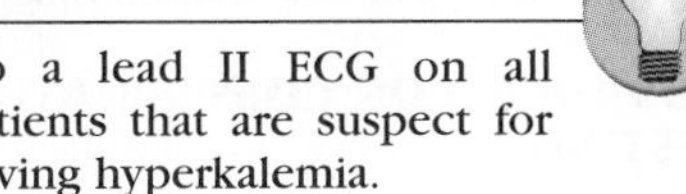

- Do a lead II ECG on all patients that are suspect for having hyperkalemia.
- Calcium gluconate IV works within a few minutes, sodium bicarbonate IV works within 15 minutes, and regular insulin and dextrose works within 30 minutes.
- Other causes of pseudohyperkalemia: thrombocytosis, very high white blood cell counts, blood samples put in ethylenediamine tetraacetic acid (EDTA) tubes.
- In cats, hyperkalemia does not always cause bradycardia; hyperkalemic cats may be tachycardic, even with severe hyperkalemia.
- On an ECG, peaked T waves are often normal; the transition from normal T wave to peaked T wave, however, is very suggestive of evolving hyperkalemia.

PREVENTION

Timely treatment of predisposing cause

CLIENT EDUCATION

Become acquainted with the early signs of the primary disorder

SUGGESTED READING

DiBartola SP, DeMorais HA: Disorders of potassium-hypokalemia and hyperkalemia. In DiBartola SP (ed): *Fluid Therapy in Small Animal Practice*, ed 2. Philadelphia, WB Saunders, 2000, pp 83–107.

Dierks DB, et al: Electrocardiographic manifestations: electrolyte abnormalities. *J Emerg Med* 27:153–160, 2004.

AUTHOR: **MICHAEL SCHAER**
EDITOR: **ETIENNE CÔTÉ**

Hyperlipidemia

BASIC INFORMATION

DEFINITION

- Increased fasting blood cholesterol and/or triglycerides (TG) concentrations
- Occurs under one of three circumstances: postprandially, as a primary defect in lipoprotein metabolism, or as a sequela to systemic disease that alters lipid metabolism

SYNONYM(S)

Hyperlipoproteinemia
Lipemia

EPIDEMIOLOGY

SPECIES, AGE, SEX

- Primary: middle-aged/older (dogs); variable age of onset (cats)
- Secondary: varies with primary cause

GENETICS AND BREED PREDISPOSITION

- Idiopathic hypertriglyceridemia: miniature schnauzers, beagles
- Idiopathic hypercholesterolemia: Doberman pinschers, rottweilers

RISK FACTORS

- Obesity (dogs)
- Drugs: glucocorticoids, megestrol acetate (cats)
- High-fat diets
- Hypothyroidism
- Hyperadrenocorticism
- Pancreatitis
- Diabetes mellitus
- Protein-losing nephropathy
- Cholestasis

ASSOCIATED CONDITIONS AND DISORDERS

- Pancreatitis
- Seizures
- Xanthomas (cutaneous nodules/plaques composed of lipid-containing histiocytes)
- Peripheral neuropathy
- Behavior changes

CLINICAL PRESENTATION

DISEASE FORMS/SUBTYPES

- Primary hyperlipidemia:
  - Dogs:
    - Idiopathic hyperlipidemia/idiopathic hypertriglyceridemia
      - Increased very low density lipoproteins (VLDL)
      - Usually increased chylomicra (CM)
      - ± Mild hypercholesterolemia
    - Idiopathic hyperchylomicronemia
      - Increased TG and CM
    - Idiopathic hypercholesterolemia
  - Cats:
    - Familial hyperchylomicronemia:
      - Increased CM and VLDL
      - Inactive lipoprotein lipase
    - Primary hypercholesterolemia
- Secondary hyperlipidemia: see Risk Factors above

HISTORY, CHIEF COMPLAINT

- Clinical signs, when present, are the result of hypertriglyceridemia; hypercholesterolemia virtually never causes clinical signs
- Dogs: vomiting, diarrhea, abdominal discomfort (pancreatitis), seizures, anorexia, lethargy
- Cats: cutaneous/subcutaneous masses (xanthomas), lameness (neuropathy)

PHYSICAL EXAM FINDINGS

- Hypertriglyceridemia
  - Dogs: signs of abdominal discomfort, hepatosplenomegaly, lipemia retinalis, lipemic aqueous humor
  - Cats: xanthomas, decreased reflexes (peripheral neuropathy), pale mucous membranes, lipemia retinalis, lipid keratopathy, lipemic aqueous humor
- Hypercholesterolemia
  - Dogs: lipemia retinalis, lipid keratopathy, arcus lipoides corneae

ETIOLOGY AND PATHOPHYSIOLOGY

- Lipoproteins
  - Lipids (TG and cholesterol) do not circulate free in circulation; rather, they are complexed in varying proportions as circulating particles called lipoproteins.
  - Four major types (listed in decreasing order of TG concentration and increasing order of cholesterol concentration in the lipoprotein particle):
    - CM
    - VLDL
    - Low-density lipoproteins
    - High-density lipoproteins
- Hyperlipidemia
  - From excessive dietary lipid, excessive endogenous lipid production/mobilization, and/or impaired lipid clearance from blood.
  - Types:
    - Postprandial hyperlipidemia:
      - CM in circulation 2 to 10 hours after fatty meal
    - Primary hyperlipidemia:
      - Inborn error in lipoprotein metabolism
        - Lack of lipoprotein lipase activity
        - Absence of surface apolipoproteins (CII)
    - Secondary hyperlipidemia:
      - Underlying disease (see Risk Factors above) causing altered lipid metabolism.

DIAGNOSIS

DIFFERENTIAL DIAGNOSIS

Hyperlipidemia diagnosis: increased serum cholesterol and/or TG concentrations. Persistent increase after >12-hour fast indicates disease

INITIAL DATABASE

- Complete blood count, serum biochemical profile (including serum cholesterol and TG concentrations), urinalysis:
  - Perform after >12-hour fast
  - Identify causes of secondary hyperlipidemia
- Subsequently, consider:
  - Tests for hypothyroidism (see Hypothyroidism, p 575)
  - Tests for hyperadrenocorticism (see Hyperadrenocorticism, p 537)
  - Urine protein:creatitine ratio
  - Abdominal ultrasound
  - Serum trypsin-like immunoreactivity

ADVANCED OR CONFIRMATORY TESTING

If a cause of secondary hyperlipidemia is not found, additional tests may help define the primary hyperlipidemia.

- CM test: Lipemic serum is left undisturbed for 12 hours at 4°C.
  - If CM are present they will form a surface "cream layer," suggesting a disorder of CM metabolism such as idiopathic hyperchylomicronemia. A nonfasting sample is an important differential.
  - If the sample remains turbid, VLDL retention (and, therefore, a secondary hyperlipidemia such as that due to diabetes mellitus) is likely.
- Lipoprotein electrophoresis, ultracentrifugation, and precipitation tests can be useful but are not routinely available.
- Lipoprotein lipase activity can be assessed by measuring TG (± lipoprotein) concentrations before and 15 minutes after heparin (dog: 90 IU/kg IV; cat: 40 IU/kg IV) administration. If no change, lipoprotein lipase inactivity is suspected.

TREATMENT

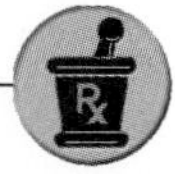

THERAPEUTIC GOAL(S)

- Treat underlying disease if present
- Reduce fasting TG concentrations to <500 mg/dl
- Reduce cholesterol concentrations to <500 mg/dl

ACUTE GENERAL TREATMENT

Treat underlying diseases

CHRONIC TREATMENT

- Hypertriglyceridemia
  - Dietary fat restriction (dog: <20% metabolizable energy [ME]; cat: <25% ME).
  - Marine fish oils: 10-60 mg/kg/day PO (dogs).
  - Gemfibrozil*:100-300 mg PO q 12h (dogs); 7.5 mg/kg PO q 12h (cats).
  - Niacin 100 mg/day (dogs) and clofibrate* have also been used.
- Hypercholesterolemia
  - Cholestyramine: 1 to 2 g PO q 12h (dogs).

DRUG INTERACTIONS

Unknown

POSSIBLE COMPLICATIONS

- Cholestyramine may cause constipation and hypertriglyceridemia.
- Side effects are common with niacin (vomiting, diarrhea, erythema, pruritus, hepatopathy).
- Potential side effects of gemfibrozil: abdominal discomfort, vomiting, diarrhea, hepatopathy.

RECOMMENDED MONITORING

- Monitor plasma triglycerides 1 month after initiation of low-fat diet
- Monitor hematologic/biochemical parameters with gemfibrozil, niacin, or clofibrate
- Monitor plasma TG with cholestyramine

PROGNOSIS AND OUTCOME

- Successful management depends on adequate control of underlying diseases and reduction of plasma lipid concentrations.
- Cats with peripheral neuropathies:
  - Clinical signs generally resolve within 4 to 12 weeks of instituting diet change

PEARLS & CONSIDERATIONS

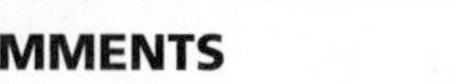

COMMENTS

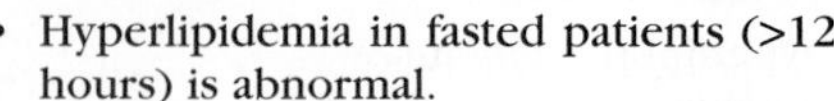

- Hyperlipidemia in fasted patients (>12 hours) is abnormal.

*Use with caution pending further evaluation.

- Hypertriglyceridemia often signals underlying disease.
- Lipemic plasma is an indication of hypertriglyceridemia, not hypercholesterolemia.
- Hypercholesterolemia may indicate the presence of an underlying disorder but rarely causes significant clinical disease.

PREVENTION

- Treat predisposing disorders
- Monitor TG concentrations in susceptible breeds

SUGGESTED READING

Barrie J, Watson TDG: Hyperlipidemia. In Bonagura JD: *Current Veterinary Therapy XII Small Animal Practice*. Philadelphia, WB Saunders, 1995, pp 430–434.

Bauer JE: Hyperlipidemias. In Ettinger SJ, Feldman EC: *Textbook of Veterinary Internal Medicine*. Philadelphia, WB Saunders, 2000, pp 283–292.

Ford RB: Canine hyperlipidemia. In Ettinger SJ, Feldman EC (eds): *Textbook of Veterinary Internal Medicine*. Philadelphia, WB Saunders, 1995, pp 1414–1419.

Jones B: Feline hyperlipidemia. In Ettinger SJ, Feldman EC (eds): *Textbook of Veterinary Internal Medicine*. Philadelphia, WB Saunders, 1995, pp 1410–1414.

AUTHOR: **ANDREA NICASTRO**
EDITOR: **SHERRI IHLE**

Hypernatremia

BASIC INFORMATION

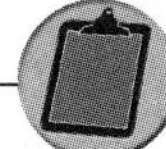

DEFINITION

A serum sodium concentration >158 mEq/L in dogs or >165mEq/L in cats, which represents a deficit of water in relation to the body's sodium stores. Hypernatremia can result from a net water loss or a hypertonic sodium gain.

EPIDEMIOLOGY

SPECIES, AGE, SEX: Dogs and cats of any age and either sex.

GENETICS AND BREED PREDISPOSITION: Primary hypodipsia in miniature schnauzers.

RISK FACTORS: Inadequate access to water, fever, high ambient temperature, altered mental status.

CLINICAL PRESENTATION

DISEASE FORMS/SUBTYPES

- *Pure water deficit*: a net water loss in the absence of sodium deficit; majority of water loss is from the intracellular fluid compartment
- *Hypotonic fluid loss:* water loss along with sodium loss; most common form encountered in veterinary medicine
- *Impermeant solute gain*

HISTORY, CHIEF COMPLAINT

- Often discovered incidentally.
- When present, signs of hypernatremia largely reflect central nervous system dysfunction.
- Severity of signs correlates positively with the degree of hypernatremia and rapidity of onset.

PHYSICAL EXAM FINDINGS

- Primarily neurologic signs: seen when plasma sodium is >170 mEq/L. Signs are due to movement of water out of brain cells.
- Tachypnea, muscular weakness, restlessness, ataxia, seizure, coma. Polydipsia may occur initially, but dissipates as disease progresses.
- With hypotonic fluid loss, signs of volume depletion (hypotension, dehydration) may be present.
- With impermeant solute gain (rare), signs of volume overload (overhydration: serous nasal discharge, dyspnea from pulmonary edema) may be present.
- Other findings depend on underlying condition.

ETIOLOGY AND PATHOPHYSIOLOGY

- *Pure water deficit*: a net water loss from the body in the absence of sodium deficit; majority of water loss is from the intracellular fluid compartment
  - Causes include:
    - Unreplaced insensible losses
    - Hypodipsia: primary hypodipsia in miniature schnauzers
    - Neurogenic diabetes insipidus: post-traumatic, neoplastic, idiopathic, meningitis, encephalitis, hypoxic or ischemic encephalopathy
    - Nephrogenic diabetes insipidus: renal disease, hypercalcemia, hypokalemia
- *Hypotonic fluid loss:* water loss along with some degree of sodium loss
  - Causes include:
    - Renal: loop diuretics, osmotic diuretics, post obstructive diuresis
    - Polyuric phase of acute tubular necrosis, intrinsic renal disease
    - Gastrointestinal: vomiting, diarrhea, osmotic cathartics
    - Cutaneous: burns
- *Impermeant solute gain*
  - Causes include:
    - Administration of hypertonic sodium bicarbonate, sodium chloride, or hypertonic fluid
    - Ingestion of table salt or salt water
    - Hyperaldosteronism or hyperadrenocorticism

DIAGNOSIS

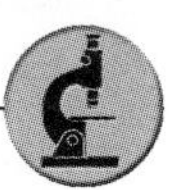

DIFFERENTIAL DIAGNOSIS

See Etiology and Pathophysiology above

INITIAL DATABASE

- Complete blood count, serum biochemistry profile, urinalysis. By definition, identifies hypernatremia. Provides further information regarding possible underlying causes (e.g., renal parameters)
- Serum osmolality (calculated or measured)
  - Elevated with hypernatremia of any cause; sodium is the main determinant of serum osmolality
  - Serial measurement possible for monitoring of response to treatment
  - Advantage over serum sodium measurement alone: measurement of otherwise undetected high-osmolality molecules (e.g., ethylene glycol)

ADVANCED OR CONFIRMATORY TESTING

As dictated by history, physical exam findings, and preliminary tests. May include adrenocorticotropic hormone stimulation test, thyroid profile, imaging studies of the brain, etc.

TREATMENT

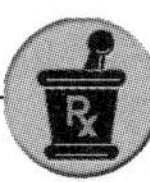

THERAPEUTIC GOAL(S)

- Replace water and electrolytes, restore effective circulating volume and treat underlying cause. Rate of correction depends on whether hypernatremia was acute in onset (began within the previous 24 hours, as with recent administration of hypertonic saline) or chronic or unknown in time of onset (vast majority; hypernatremia is known or suspected to

have begun >24 hours earlier, as with most naturally occurring hypernatremia).
- Acute: replace at a rate such that the decrease in serum sodium does not exceed 1 mEq/L/hr and does not exceed 24 mEq/L/day
- Chronic or unknown: replace at a rate such that the decrease in serum sodium does not exceed 0.5 mEq/L/hr and does not exceed 12 mEq/L/day

- The cornerstone of successful treatment is frequent monitoring of the patient's mentation and serum sodium concentration.

ACUTE GENERAL TREATMENT

- *Pure water loss*: calculate water deficit. Replace the deficit over 24 to 48 hours with 5% dextrose in water, not exceeding limit (see Possible Complications below).
  - Water deficit (L) = body weight (kg) × 0.6 × [(present serum Na/previous serum Na)-1].
  - Administer calculated water deficit over the recommended timeframe for acute or chronic hypernatremia.
  - Total body water is normally 60% of body weight. This percentage can be increased in pediatric/neonates or can be decreased in cachectic animals.
- *Hypotonic fluid loss:* replace with a limited amount of isotonic crystalloids to improve hemodynamic parameters. Once improved/stabilized, switch to a hypotonic solution and administer/titrate based on monitoring, not exceeding limit.
- *Gain of impermeant solute*: 5% dextrose diuresis and administer/titrate based on monitoring, not exceeding limit (see Possible Complications below).
- *Persistent hypernatremia despite fluid therapy adjustments:*
  - Central diabetes insipidus: dDAVP 1 μg/kg SQ q 8-12h or Aqueous vasopressin 1-2 U/cat or 3-5 U/dog q 24-48h
  - Nephrogenic diabetes insipidus: thiazide diuretics

CHRONIC TREATMENT

- Reove offending drugs
- Treat underlying condition

POSSIBLE COMPLICATIONS

Rapid correction of hypernatremia can lead to cerebral edema as excess water moves into brain cells. The signs of cerebral edema may not be seen for 2 to 3 days postcorrection of hypernatremia. Edema is more likely to occur in patients with prolonged hyperosmolality and aggressive hypotonic fluid replacement.

RECOMMENDED MONITORING

Check serum electrolytes q 4-8h

PROGNOSIS AND OUTCOME

Mortality varies according to the severity of hypernatremia, rapidity of onset, and underlying condition

PEARLS & CONSIDERATIONS

COMMENTS

When correcting hypernatremia, the rate of decrease of blood/serum sodium concentration must not exceed 0.5 mEq/L/hr.

- Decreasing sodium concentration at a rate >0.5 mEq/L/hr risks complications such as cerebral edema.
- Exception: up to 1 mEq/L/hr is possible if hypernatremia is known to have begun within 24 hours (e.g., hypertonic saline administration).

PREVENTION

- Ensure adequate drinking water access, prevent excessive drinking of salt water or consumption of pure salt.
- Do not administer table salt as an emetic in cases of toxin ingestion. Use hydrogen peroxide or syrup of ipecac instead.

SUGGESTED READING

DiBartola SP: Disorders of sodium and water: hypernatremia and hyponatremia. In diBartola SP, de Morais HSA (eds): *Fluid Therapy in Small Animal Practice*, ed 2. Philadelphia, WB Saunders, 2000, pp 45-72.

Temo K, et al: Hypernatremia in critically ill cats: pathophysiology. *Compend Cont Ed Pract Vet* 26:422-433, 2004.

Temo K, et al. Hypernatremia in critically ill cats: evaluation and treatment. *Compendium Cont Ed Pract Vet* 26:434-445, 2004.

AUTHORS: **MELISSA MARSHALL, ANN MARIE MANNING**

EDITOR: **ETIENNE CÔTÉ**

Hyperparathyroidism, Primary

BASIC INFORMATION

DEFINITION

An uncommon disease of dogs caused by increased synthesis and secretion of parathyroid hormone (PTH). The source of increased PTH is autonomously functioning parathyroid cells due to parathyroid adenoma, hyperplasia, or carcinoma. (See Renal Secondary Hyperparathyroidism, p 956; Nutritional Secondary Hyperparathyroidism, p 758 for more details.)

EPIDEMIOLOGY

SPECIES, AGE, SEX

- Older dogs predominantly. No gender predilection.
- Rare in cats. Typically older cats are affected.

GENETICS AND BREED PREDISPOSITION

- Any breed.
- Genetic predisposition suspected in keeshonds.
- Hereditary neonatal primary hyperparathyroidism (PHPTH) has been reported in two German shepherd dogs.

CLINICAL PRESENTATION

HISTORY/CHIEF COMPLAINT

- Renal, gastrointestinal, and neurologic presenting signs are most common and may include:
  - Polyuria/polydipsia; lower urinary tract signs (caused by infection or cystic calculi) including pollakiuria, stranguria, and hematuria
  - Inappetence, vomiting
  - Weakness, lethargy
- Some affected animals may have no clinical signs; hypercalcemia is an incidental finding.

PHYSICAL EXAM FINDINGS

- Physical examination is typically unremarkable.
- A parathyroid mass is not usually palpable in dogs. Parathyroid masses may be palpable in the ventral neck of cats.

ETIOLOGY AND PATHOPHYSIOLOGY

ETIOLOGY: PHPTH is most often due to a solitary parathyroid adenoma. Less common causes include hyperplasia of one or more glands, or rarely, parathyroid carcinoma.

PATHOPHYSIOLOGY: In normal animals, serum PTH concentration is controlled by ionized calcium via negative feedback. In PHPTH, the gland(s) function autonomously and feedback inhibition is lost.

- Increased serum PTH concentrations cause hypercalcemia and hypophosphatemia.
- Clinical signs are due to hypercalcemia (see Hypercalcemia, p 543).

DIAGNOSIS

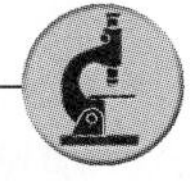

DIFFERENTIAL DIAGNOSIS

Hypercalcemia (see Hypercalcemia, p 543)

INITIAL DATABASE

- Complete blood count, serum biochemical profile, urinalysis, urine culture: Hypercalcemia, low or low-normal phosphorus concentration, and isosthenuria are typical. With prolonged or severe hypercalcemia (causing secondary renal calcification), azotemia and hyperphosphatemia may be present, although this is uncommon with PHPTH.
- Confirm hypercalcemia by repeating the test on a new sample and/or measure the serum ionized calcium concentration if possible.
- Abdominal radiographs: possible cystic calculi.
- Other tests to rule out more common of causes of hypercalcemia, particularly hypercalcemia of malignancy, may include thoracic and abdominal radiographs, abdominal ultrasound, aspiration of lymph nodes and/or bone marrow.
- Ultrasonography of the neck to evaluate the parathyroid glands requires an experienced ultrasonographer and sensitive ultrasound equipment.

ADVANCED OR CONFIRMATORY TESTING

- Concurrent serum ionized calcium and PTH concentrations: Increased serum PTH concentration with high serum ionized calcium concentration supports a diagnosis of PHPTH.
- A serum PTH concentration within the reference range is inappropriate with concurrent increased ionized calcium concentration; thus in a patient with increased ionized calcium, a serum PTH concentration that is normal can also be compatible with a diagnosis of PHPTH.
- Diagnosis is confirmed by exploratory surgery of the neck.

TREATMENT

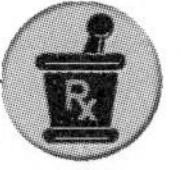

THERAPEUTIC GOAL(S)

- Remove affected parathyroid gland(s)
- Where indicated, nonspecific therapy for hypercalcemia pending definitive diagnosis or surgery
- Remove cystic calculi

ACUTE GENERAL TREATMENT

- Nonspecific treatment of hypercalcemia while awaiting a definitive diagnosis or surgery (see Hypercalcemia, p 543).
- Surgical exploration of the neck with removal of the affected parathyroid gland(s). Most often a solitary parathyroid mass is easily identified and removed. If evaluation/identification of affected glands is difficult, removal of all four parathyroid glands and both thyroid glands is considered (rare).
- Newer therapies (percutaneous ultrasound-guided ethanol ablation or radiofrequency heat ablation) are less invasive but technically challenging and still require general anesthesia. Postprocedural hypocalcemia is still possible. Results are promising but variable.

CHRONIC TREATMENT

- Surgical therapy is curative in most patients, so chronic therapy is not required.
- If all four parathyroid glands are removed, lifelong vitamin D and thyroid hormone replacement are indicated. (See Hypoparathyroidism, Primary, p 568, and Hypothyroidism, p 575, concerning therapy.)

POSSIBLE COMPLICATIONS

The most important complication is postoperative hypocalcemia.

- Unaffected glands often atrophy with prolonged increased serum PTH concentrations. After removal of the affected gland(s), serum PTH and calcium may decline more rapidly than normal glands can recover.
- Hospitalization is recommended for at least 5 days after surgery to minimize physical activity, monitor for signs of hypocalcemia and to monitor serum calcium concentrations at least q 12-24h.
- Treatment must be individualized.
    - In general, if serum calcium concentration <14 mg/dl (3.5 mmol/L) before surgery, postoperative hypocalcemia is unlikely. Treatment (vitamin D ± calcium) is recommended only if total calcium falls below 8.5 mg/dl (2.1 mmol/L), if the rate of decline of calcium after surgery is very rapid (e.g., >25% in 1 day), or if clinical signs of hypocalcemia occur.
    - If presurgical serum calcium concentration >14 mg/dl (3.5 mmol/L), prophylactic treatment with vitamin D and calcium is begun the morning of surgery.
    - If presurgical serum calcium concentration >18 mg/dl (4.5 mmol/L), prophylactic treatment with vitamin D and calcium is begun 36 hours before surgery.
    - See Hypoparathyroidism, Primary, p 568, for details of vitamin D and calcium treatment.
    - Goal of therapy: keep the serum calcium concentration in the slightly low/low-normal range (8-9.5 mg/dL; 2-2.4 mmol/L) to prevent clinical signs of hypocalcemia while stimulating recovery of function in atrophied parathyroid glands.
        - If only one to three parathyroid glands were removed, vitamin D can be tapered over 3 to 6 months by gradually increasing the interval between doses (approximately 1 day every 2 to 3 weeks based on serum calcium levels). Vitamin D can be discontinued when the dosing interval is 7 days and the serum calcium concentration is stable.

RECOMMENDED MONITORING

After discontinuation of vitamin D, evaluation of serum calcium concentration is recommended every 3 to 6 months. Although rare, PHPTH recurrences may be observed even longer than 12 months after successful surgery.

PROGNOSIS AND OUTCOME

Prognosis is excellent following surgery

PEARLS & CONSIDERATIONS

COMMENTS

Referral is indicated if the attending clinician is unfamiliar with thyroid/parathyroid evaluation and surgery, or if 24-hour care and in-house serum calcium monitoring cannot be provided during the immediate postoperative period

SUGGESTED READING

Hypercalcemia and primary hyperparathyroidism. In Feldman EC, Nelson RW (eds): *Canine and Feline Endocrinology and Reproduction,* ed 3. Philadelphia, WB Saunders, 2004, pp 661-715.

Long CD, et al: Percutaneous ultrasound-guided chemical parathyroid ablation for treatment of primary hyperparathyroidism in dogs. *J Am Vet Med Assoc* 215:217-221, 1999.

Pollard RE, et al: Percutaneous ultrasonographically guided radiofrequency heat ablation for treatment of primary hyperparathyroidism in dogs. *J Am Vet Med Assoc* 218:1106-1110, 2001.

AUTHOR: **CARY L. M. BASSETT**

EDITOR: **SHERRI IHLE**

Hyperthyroidism

Client Education Sheet on Website

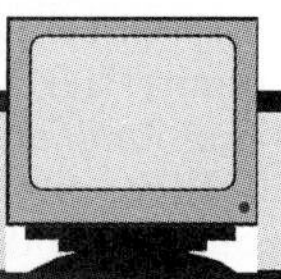

BASIC INFORMATION

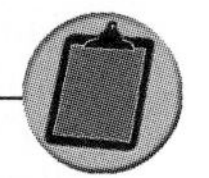

DEFINITION

The clinical condition that results from continued excessive secretion of thyroid hormones (thyroxine and triiodothyronine) by the thyroid gland

SYNONYM(S)

Thyrotoxicosis

EPIDEMIOLOGY

SPECIES, AGE, SEX

- Older cats; range is 4 to 20+ years, but 95% of cats diagnosed with hyperthyroidism are >8 years old
- No sex predilection

GENETICS AND BREED PREDISPOSITION: Purebred cats are significantly less likely to be hyperthyroid than domestic/mixed breeds.

RISK FACTORS: Possibly canned food and ectoparasiticide exposure.

ASSOCIATED CONDITIONS AND DISORDERS

- Concentric cardiac hypertrophy (ventricular thickening)
- Systemic hypertension
- Hyperthyroidism and associated hypertension may mask underlying renal dysfunction

CLINICAL PRESENTATION

DISEASE FORMS/SUBTYPES: Apathetic hyperthyroidism (10%): cat has decreased appetite, lethargy, and occasionally weight gain.

HISTORY, CHIEF COMPLAINT

- Polydipsia and polyuria
- Polyphagia
- Weight loss despite good appetite
- Hyperactivity, nervousness
- Vomiting and/or diarrhea
- Tachypnea/panting
- Weakness, lethargy
- Decreased grooming activity
- Heat avoidance or seeking cool areas

PHYSICAL EXAM FINDINGS

- Poor body condition
- Unkempt haircoat
- Dehydration
- Tachycardia
  - Systolic heart murmur
  - Arrhythmia
- Abnormal retinal examination (tortuous retinal blood vessels, retinal tears, retinal detachment)
- Palpable thyroid gland(s)

ETIOLOGY AND PATHOPHYSIOLOGY

- Benign thyroid neoplasia or adenomatous hyperplasia of one (30%) or both (70%) thyroid lobes is most common.
- Thyroid carcinoma is found in <2% of hyperthyroid cats.
- Although many theories have been proposed, no studies have adequately demonstrated an etiology for feline hyperthyroidism.
- Canine hyperthyroidism is the result of a functional thyroid carcinoma (see Thyroid Carcinoma [Canine], p 1083).

DIAGNOSIS

DIFFERENTIAL DIAGNOSIS

- For polyphagia with weight loss in an adult/geriatric cat: diabetes mellitus, inflammatory bowel disease, gastrointestinal lymphoma; rarely in cats: hyperadrenocorticism, glomerulonephritis/protein-losing nephropathy.
- For Polyuria/Polydipsia, see p 878.
- For Polyphagia, see p 877.
- For Weight Loss, see p 1162.
- For Vomiting, Chronic, see p 1158.
- For Diarrhea, Chronic, see p 297.
- For arrhythmias/tachycardia/murmur:
  - Primary idiopathic hypertrophic cardiomyopathy (see Hypertrophic Cardiomyopathy, p 554)
  - Restrictive cardiomyopathy (see Restrictive/Unclassified Cardiomyopathy, Feline, p 961)

INITIAL DATABASE

- Complete blood count (CBC), serum biochemical profile, urinalysis: possible stress leukogram and mild erythrocytosis; increase in liver enzymes common; increased blood urea nitrogen (BUN) and creatinine, phosphorus, and bilirubin less common; urine specific gravity results vary.
- Serum total thyroxine (TT_4) measurement: usually increased, although values are sometimes in the upper half of the reference range, especially if concurrent disease is present ("euthyroid sick"-like effect).
- Thoracic radiographs: cardiomegaly common; possible pulmonary edema, and/or pleural effusion.
- Systemic blood pressure measurement: hypertension (systolic blood pressure repeatedly >200 mmHg in calm environment) is common.
- Electrocardiogram, if an arrhythmia or other signs of heart disease are present: sinus tachycardia is most common; atrial or ventricular arrhythmias are possible but uncommon.

ADVANCED OR CONFIRMATORY TESTING

- Serum TT_4 (increased) is often diagnostic. If TT_4 is in the normal range but the thyroid gland is palpable and/or signs suggestive of hyperthyroidism are present, one of the following tests can be considered:
  - Reevaluate the TT_4 in a few weeks (if clinical signs are mild).
  - Serum free T_4 by equilibrium dialysis (FT_4ED): increased FT_4ED in conjunction with a high normal TT_4 supports a diagnosis of hyperthyroidism.
  - T3 suppression test: generally replaced by FT_4ED, but may be used if FT_4ED results are equivocal.
    - Procedure: Collect a serum sample for T_3 and TT_4 measurement. Have owner give T_3 (25 µg/cat PO q 8h) for 2 days. On the morning of day 3, administer a final dose of T_3 and 2 to 3 hours later get a second blood sample for T_3 and TT_4.
    - Interpretation: For most laboratories, a TT_4 > 1.5 µg/dl (20 mmol/L) is consistent with hyperthyroidism. Consult your laboratory for specific interpretation.
    - Drawback: failure in owner compliance gives false positive result.
  - Thyroid-stimulating hormone (TSH) and thyrotropin-releasing hormone (TRH) response tests have also been used but are of more limited diagnostic use due to poor differentiation of hyperthyroid and euthyroid cats, especially if concurrent disease is present.
- Radionuclide (technetium-99m) thyroid scan can be used for determining whether one or both thyroid glands are involved, and whether ectopic functional thyroid tissue is present. These points are perhaps of greatest concern if surgical thyroidectomy is contemplated (completeness of excision).
- Echocardiography (cats): can identify left ventricular thickening. If it is symmetric (whole left ventricle is thickened), either hyperthyroidism or unrelated, idiopathic hypertrophic cardiomyopathy (HCM) may be the cause. If it is asymmetric (e.g., interventricular sep-

tum is thicker than left ventricular free wall, or vice-versa), then idiopathic HCM is contributory and hyperthyroidism alone cannot be causative.

TREATMENT

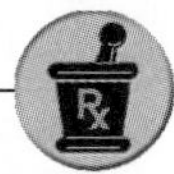

THERAPEUTIC GOAL(S)

- Ideally, to return serum thyroid hormone levels to normal and resolve clinical signs indefinitely.
- The clinical therapeutic goal is to encourage weight gain and improve body condition and haircoat, as well as decrease polyuria, polydipsia, and polyphagia, with the overall goal of maximizing quality of life. Depending on renal function, achieving this goal may or may not include returning the serum thyroid hormone levels to normal.

ACUTE GENERAL TREATMENT

- Hyperthyroidism is a chronic disease, so urgent acute treatment usually is not needed.
- Concurrent congestive heart failure may require immediate intervention (see Heart Failure, Acute/Decompensated, p 458).
- "Thyroid storm": intense sympathetic discharge usually in response to restraint or other stressful trigger.
  - Managed most effectively through prevention (calm environment, cautious/gentle restraint).
  - If thyroid storm occurs, immediately ensure as calm and quiet an environment as possible, while initiating supportive management of complications that occur (may include any or all of the following: see Heart Failure, Acute/Decompensated, p 458; severe tachycardia [best treated through calming environment, possibly mild sedation but not with acepromazine]; severe bradycardia [very conservative doses of atropine, e.g., 0.01-0.02 mg/kg IV once]; severe systemic hypertension [calming environment]).
  - Thyroid storm may be acutely fatal and must be prevented through gentle handling of hyperthyroid cats, who often are hyperesthetic and fractious.

CHRONIC TREATMENT

- There are three general treatment options:
  - Medical (daily antithyroid medication)
  - Surgical thyroidectomy
  - Radioactive iodine treatment
  - See Hyperthyroidism algorithm, p 1544
- Cats often have renal dysfunction that is not identifiable at the time of diagnosis of hyperthyroidism. Once antithyroid therapy is initiated, the renal dysfunction is unmasked. Therefore a trial of antithyroid medication (10 to 14 days or longer), with monitoring of renal parameters, is recommended before treatment with a more permanent and costly modality (i.e., surgery or radioactive iodine).
- Medical treatment:
  - Thioureylene antithyroid drugs suppress thyroid hormone production. Methimazole (5 mg/cat PO q 8-12h) or carbimazole (5 mg/cat PO q 8h; currently not available in North America) are most commonly used. The dosage is adjusted so that serum TT_4 concentrations are in the lower half of the reference range.
  - Discontinuation of the medication will result in return of clinical signs, so client compliance is essential.
  - Potential side effects of methimazole include anorexia/vomiting, lethargy, pruritus of the head and neck (and self-induced trauma), hepatoxicity (uncommon), thrombocytopenia (uncommon), agranulocytosis (uncommon), and immune-mediated hemolytic anemia (rare). If hemorrhage, icterus, or severe neutropenia occurs, drug administration must be stopped and an alternative treatment initiated.
  - Other medical treatments that have been used include potassium iodate and calcium ipodate, but these are considered only for short-term use before a more definitive treatment in patients who cannot tolerate methimazole or carbamizole.
  - A β-blocker (e.g., atenolol 6.25 mg/cat PO q 12h) is used if severe sinus tachycardia (>260 beats/min) persists despite euthyroidism, or if antithyroid drugs need to be stopped (e.g., in preparation for radioiodine).
- Thyroidectomy:
  - Potentially curative.
  - Eliminates grossly abnormal thyroid tissue, but ectopic tissue may remain if radionuclide imaging is bypassed.
  - Unilateral thyroidectomy: contralateral thyroid gland can eventually become hyperplastic or adenomatous (recurrent hyperthyroidism).
  - Medical treatment is recommended for several weeks before surgery (assess euthyroid renal function, improve metabolic and cardiac status before administering anesthetic).
  - Bilateral thyroidectomy: may involve loss of several or all parathyroids. Postoperative monitoring of serum calcium is required; if indicated, treat as for hypoparathyroidism (see Hypoparathyroidism, Primary, p 568).
  - Other possible postoperative complications include Horner's syndrome (see Horner's Syndrome, p 532) and laryngeal paralysis (see Laryngeal Paralysis, p 619).
- Radioactive iodine (^{131}I) therapy:
  - This is considered the best treatment option for long-term control and possible cure of hyperthyroidism, provided that during a trial of medical antithyroid therapy, serum BUN and creatinine are normal or urine specific gravity >1.035.
  - Treatment renders all hyperfunctional thyroid tissue, including ectopic tissue, nonfunctional.
  - Disadvantages: Special handling facilities and post-therapy isolation for several days to weeks are required. The length of isolation is dependent upon the facility. Prior to therapy, the cat must be eating and able to tolerate the required period of time in isolation.
  - The necessity of discontinuing medical antithyroid drugs before treatment is controversial. Consult the facility administering the radiotherapy.

RECOMMENDED MONITORING

- Medical therapy: exam including body weight, CBC, serum biochemical profile, urine specific gravity, TT4 at 2 weeks; if normal, reassess q 6 months or if adverse effect or recurrent signs of hyperthyroidism occur.
- Thyroidectomy: exam including body weight, postoperative monitoring of serum calcium if bilateral thyroidectomy; CBC, serum biochemical profile, urinalysis and TT4 at 2 weeks, then monitor TT4 q 3-6 months.
- Radioactive iodine therapy: exam including body weight, CBC, serum biochemical profile, urinalysis, and TT4 2 weeks after treatment, then monitor TT4 q 3-6 months.

PROGNOSIS AND OUTCOME

- With successful radioactive iodine therapy or thyroidectomy the short-term prognosis is excellent and long-term prognosis is good. Cure may be obtained in many cases.
  - These patients are older at the time of diagnosis, and other conditions may be present or soon develop; thus, length of survival has been documented to be approximately 2 years postdiagnosis regardless of the type of therapy chosen.
- With the presence of renal dysfunction the short-term prognosis is good, but the long-term prognosis is guarded to poor, as both hyperthyroidism and renal dysfunction are progressive illnesses and treatments may be mutually antagonistic.

PEARLS & CONSIDERATIONS

COMMENTS

Concurrent hyperthyroidism and chronic renal failure should be treated according to which disorder is predominantly responsible for clinical signs:

- Hyperthyroid cats with polyphagia, weight loss, and/or hyperactivity who are also incidentally found to be azotemic should be treated for hyperthyroidism. Chronic renal failure is monitored and managed secondarily (see Chronic Renal Failure, Occult ["Asymptomatic"], p 204).
- Cats with chronic renal failure and overt anorexia, dehydration, uremic oral ulcers, and/or vomiting who are also incidentally found to be hyperthyroid should be treated for chronic renal failure (see Chronic Renal Failure, Occult ["Asymptomatic"], p 204). In these cases, hyperthyroidism is monitored and generally not treated unless it is causing characteristic signs.
- Cats with no clinical signs attributable to either chronic renal failure or hyperthyroidism but who are found to have both syndromes incidentally on routine laboratory testing should be monitored periodically (see Reccommended Monitoring above) and not treated specifically for either disorder, other than preventive measures (e.g., nutrition).
- Cats with clinical signs of both chronic renal failure and hyperthyroidism may require medical treatment for chronic renal failure and "partial treatment" of hyperthyroidism (i.e., medical treatment to lower the T4 somewhat, but still above the normal range).

SUGGESTED READING

Feldman EC, Nelson RW: Feline hyperthyroidism (thyrotoxicosis). In Feldman EC, Nelson RW (eds): *Canine and Feline Endocrinology and Reproduction.* Philadelphia, WB Saunders, 2004, pp 152–218.

Mooney CT: Hyperthyroidism. In Ettinger SJ, Feldman EC (eds): *Textbook of Veterinary Internal Medicine.* St. Louis, Elsevier, 2005, pp 1544–1560.

Olczak J, et al: Multivariate analysis of risk factors for feline hyperthyroidism in New Zealand. *N Z Vet J* 53(1):53–58, 2005.

AUTHOR: **KRISTI L. GRAHAM**
EDITOR: **SHERRI IHLE**

Hypertrophic Cardiomyopathy

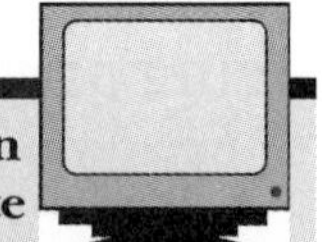

Client Education Sheet on Website

BASIC INFORMATION

DEFINITION

A form of heart disease characterized by concentric hypertrophy (increased wall thickness) of the left ventricle in the absence of other secondary causes such as hypertension, aortic stenosis, or hyperthyroidism

SYNONYM(S)

Idiopathic hypertrophic cardiomyopathy (HCM)

Hypertrophic obstructive cardiomyopathy (HOCM): if systolic anterior motion of the mitral valve is present, obstructing left ventricular outflow tract

EPIDEMIOLOGY

SPECIES, AGE, SEX: The most common heart disease of cats. Age ranges from juvenile to aged; often purebred cats may develop hypertrophic cardiomyopathy (HCM) at an earlier age. Males are more commonly reported, but there is no sex-linked heritability.

GENETICS AND BREED PREDISPOSITION

- Autosomal-dominant heritability with incomplete penetrance in a family of Maine coon cats, caused by a missense mutation of the sarcomeric protein, myosin binding protein C.
- Autosomal-dominant heritability in a family of American shorthair cats.
- Other breeds predisposed: ragdolls, British shorthair, Norwegian forest cat, Turkish van, Scottish fold, and Rex. However, domestic shorthair cats remain the most common type of cat diagnosed with HCM.

ASSOCIATED CONDITIONS AND DISORDERS: Congestive heart failure (CHF), aortic thromboembolism.

CLINICAL PRESENTATION

HISTORY, CHIEF COMPLAINT

- Often, cats show no clinical signs and HCM is discovered incidentally (e.g., murmur on physical exam).
- Respiratory abnormalities: tachypnea, dyspnea, open mouth breathing, uncommonly cough.
- Nonspecific: lethargy, anorexia, vomiting.
- Lameness or unable to move limb (aortic thromboembolism).
- Sudden death.

PHYSICAL EXAM FINDINGS

- Systolic murmur (80% of cases)
- Gallop heart sound (S4 heart sound)
- Arrhythmia: premature beats, irregular rhythm (20–70% of cats)
- Respiratory abnormalities: tachypnea, dyspnea, increased adventitious lung sounds, ventrally dampened lung sounds if pleural effusion
- If arterial thromboembolism: cyanotic nail beds and toe pads, absent pulses of that limb, contracted and painful muscles, paresis or plegia of limb

ETIOLOGY AND PATHOPHYSIOLOGY

- Myocyte dysfunction due to primary sarcomeric defect; remaining sarcomeres develop compensatory, concentric hypertrophy.
- Diastolic dysfunction (impaired relaxation and increased myocardial stiffness) caused by concentric hypertrophy and myocardial fibrosis.
- Elevated left ventricular filling pressure leads to elevated left atrial and pulmonary venous pressure, and development of CHF (pleural effusion and pulmonary edema).
- Left atrial thrombus may form due to sluggish blood flow in the dilated left atrium, and can lead to arterial thromboembolism.

DIAGNOSIS

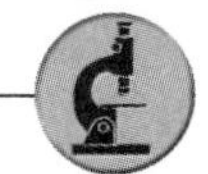

DIFFERENTIAL DIAGNOSIS

Echocardiographically, hypertrophic cardiomyopathy is a diagnosis of exclusion, after other causes of left ventricular thickening have been ruled out:

- Hyperthyroidism
- Systemic hypertension
- Subaortic stenosis
- Acromegaly

INITIAL DATABASE

- Echocardiogram: interventricular septum or left ventricular free wall end diastolic thickness ≥6 mm. Papillary hypertrophy often present and is a subjective determination. End systolic cavity obliteration may be seen. Systolic anterior motion (SAM) of the mitral valve may be seen, confirming HOCM; color flow Doppler shows left ventricular outflow tract/aortic turbulence and mitral regurgitation. Degree of obstruction caused by SAM is determined by continuous wave Doppler measurement of the aortic blood flow velocity using the left apical five-chamber view. Left atrial enlargement is determined by two-dimensional

measurements of left atrial diameter and aortic diameter in diastole using the right parasternal short-axis view at the level of the aortic valve. Left atrial to aortic ratio ≥1.5 denotes left atrial enlargement.
- Electrocardiogram (ECG): supraventricular or ventricular premature complexes possible. Atrial fibrillation is rare but may be seen with severe left atrial dilation. Left axis deviation (mean electrical axis 0 to -90 degrees) or increased QRS amplitude >1 mV may indicate left ventricular hypertrophy.
- Clinicopathologic evaluation: complete blood count, serum biochemistry profile, urinalysis unremarkable unless arterial thromboembolism (see Aortic Thromboembolism, Feline, p 78).
- Serum T4 and systolic blood pressure are important to evaluate for secondary causes of concentric left ventricular hypertrophy.
- Thoracic radiographs: Often normal if no left atrial enlargement. More severe cases may show left atrial enlargement, distended pulmonary veins, and if CHF is present, patchy interstitial to alveolar infiltrates often of caudal lung lobes and accessory lung lobe, although no pattern of distribution is typical; pleural effusion also is possible.

ADVANCED OR CONFIRMATORY TESTING

- Tissue Doppler imaging echocardiography using pulsed wave Doppler or color M-mode derived myocardial velocity gradients may be useful to identify diastolic dysfunction and monitor for potential beneficial therapeutic effects or progression of disease.
- Plasma brain natriuretic peptide (BNP) often is markedly elevated in cats with severe HCM and CHF. Many cats with compensated HCM may also have elevated BNP. Radioimmunoassay is limited to a few research laboratories and not on a commercial basis; no point of care test yet available for cats.

TREATMENT

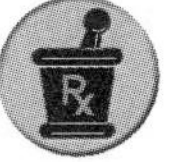

THERAPEUTIC GOAL(S)

- Treatment of CHF: reduce the pleural effusion or pulmonary edema accumulation
- Antihypertrophic treatment in attempts to reduce the concentric hypertrophy of the left ventricle
- Reduce SAM, which will reduce the pressure overload of the left ventricle and reduce mitral regurgitation
- Antiarrhythmic treatment if severe arrhythmias such as ventricular tachycardia, supraventricular tachycardia, or atrial fibrillation
- Anticoagulant therapy in animals with high risk of arterial thromboembolism or in animals having suffered arterial thromboembolism

ACUTE GENERAL TREATMENT

Acute decompensated CHF (see Heart Failure, Acute/Decompensated, p 458):
- Thoracocentesis if large amount of pleural effusion is present.
- Oxygen therapy in oxygen cage, minimize stress.
- Furosemide 2-3 mg/kg IV, SQ, or IM q 2-6h as needed to reduce resting respiratory rate to <50/min. Careful to avoid excessive dehydration or renal failure. Sharply reduce dosing frequency as soon as positive response.
- Nitroglycerin: unproven if beneficial effects of venodilation, but not likely to cause harm. Dose: 1/8-1/4" of 2% topical cream q 4-6h for first 24 hours.

CHRONIC TREATMENT

- Reduce SAM: atenolol or diltiazem
  - Atenolol 6.25-12.5 mg per cat PO q 12h. Start at the low dose, recheck heart rate (HR) and murmur intensity in 1 to 2 weeks, then increase to 12.5 mg PO q 12h if HR remains >170 bpm or if SAM severity by continuous wave Doppler echocardiography or murmur intensity not improved. Do not increase atenolol if HR <130 bpm.
  - Diltiazem: less effective than atenolol in reducing SAM.
    - Diltiazem 7.5 mg per cat PO q 8h.
    - Sustained release diltiazem:
      - Dilacor XR 30 mg PO q 12h (60-mg tablets).
      - Cardizem CD (180-mg capsules) 10 mg/kg PO q 24h.
  - Antihypertrophic treatment for moderate to severe left ventricular hypertrophy (wall thickness ≥7 mm).
    - Atenolol or diltiazem at doses written previously; may reduce hypertrophy in some cases; controversial.
    - Angiotensin-converting enzyme (ACE) inhibitors not likely to be of benefit in early compensated HCM; controversial.
- Chronic CHF:
  - Furosemide 1-4 mg/kg PO q 8-24h.
  - ACE inhibitor:
    - Enalapril 0.5 mg/kg PO q 12h; ramipril, lisinopril, or benazepril 0.5 mg/kg PO q 24h.
- Chronic refractory CHF:
  - Addition of second diuretic: hydrochlorothiazide (1-4 mg/kg PO q 12h) ± spironolactone (1-2 mg/kg PO q 24h q 12h).
  - Low salt diet if palatable.
  - ± Potassium supplement if hypokalemic.
- Anticoagulation for prevention of arterial thromboembolism
  - One baby aspirin (81 mg ASA) or 5 mg PO q 3 days.
  - Low-molecular-weight heparin: 1 mg/kg SQ q 12h; pharmacokinetics and optimal dosing are still under investigation.
  - Consider clopidogrel as a platelet inhibitor.
- Antiarrhythmic therapy if supraventricular tachycardia, ventricular tachycardia, or atrial fibrillation with rapid ventricular response rate

DRUG INTERACTIONS

- Diuretics and ACE inhibitors may exacerbate renal dysfunction.
- Concurrent use of β-blockers and calcium channel blockers is generally contraindicated as they may cause profound negative chronotropic ± negative inotropic effects.

POSSIBLE COMPLICATIONS

- Prerenal azotemia and hypokalemia during treatment with diuretics; diuretics may also exacerbate underlying renal dysfunction and cause renal azotemia.
- Cats receiving high doses of diuretics are often mild to moderately azotemic but often maintain reasonable quality of life.
- ACE inhibitors may cause acute renal azotemia, which may reverse after discontinuation of the ACE inhibitor and supportive care.

RECOMMENDED MONITORING

- Baseline serum renal panel and urinalysis; repeat renal panel twice daily during acute CHF treatment.
- Repeat renal panel 1 to 2 weeks after initiation of treatment with ACE inhibitor. If significant azotemia occurs, decrease or discontinue the ACE inhibitor, and if possible decrease the diuretic, and recheck renal panel.
- Thoracic radiographs to assess therapeutic efficacy of diuretics in resolving the CHF; intermittent recheck radiographs q 2-4 months once stabilized.
- Echocardiogram: depending on severity of HCM q 3-12 months. If recent pulmonary edema or pleural effusion, recheck echocardiogram to assess for left atrial dilation to support the diagnosis of CHF. Monitor left atrial size as risk factor for development of CHF or arterial thromboembolism. Monitor left ventricular (LV) hypertrophy to assess possible progression of disease or assess potential antihypertrophic therapeutic effects. To evaluate for therapeutic reduction in SAM, repeat echocardiogram 1 to 2 weeks after therapy.
- If systemic hypertension or hyperthyroidism is present, a recheck echocardiogram 3 to 4 months after cat is normotensive or euthyroid should show regression of LV hypertrophy. If hypertrophy is still present, the cat has

concurrent HCM or there is incomplete control of the systemic disorder.
- If arrhythmia is present, recheck ECG to assess response to antiarrhythmic therapy.

PROGNOSIS AND OUTCOME

- Fair to good prognosis for cats with mild nonprogressive HCM. Cats with HCM and no clinical signs have a median survival >5 years.
- Young male cats and ragdoll cats with significant left ventricular hypertrophy often progress more rapidly and die from their disease.
- Severe HCM and CHF: poor long-term prognosis, median survival of 3 months, although highly variable with survival times over 2 years in some individuals.
- Severe HCM and arterial thromboembolism: poor prognosis, median survival of 2 months, but highly variable.

PEARLS & CONSIDERATIONS

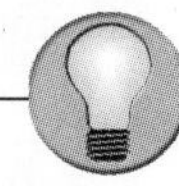

COMMENTS

- Wide range of severity and progression of HCM in individual cats.
- In a recent multicenter, prospective, randomized and blinded study, neither ACE inhibitors, atenolol, nor diltiazem was shown to improve survival in cats with severe HCM and CHF or arterial thromboembolism.
- Avoidance of long-acting corticosteroid injections, as they may result in development of CHF in cats with moderate to severe HCM.
- Anesthetic considerations: avoidance of high fluid rates. Consider induction with midazolam and propofol or with etomidate; maintenance with isoflurane or propofol.

CLIENT EDUCATION

- In cats with CHF, teaching clients to monitor resting respiratory rate is helpful, and when rates are consistently >40 breaths per minute to contact the veterinarian.
- Risk of sudden death and arterial thromboembolism. Difficulty in preventing arterial thrombolism when severe underlying cardiac disease is present.

SUGGESTED READING

Atkins CE, et al: Risk factors, clinical signs, and survival in cats with a clinical diagnosis of idiopathic hypertrophic cardiomyopathy: 74 cases (1985-1989). *J Am Vet Med Assoc* 201:613, 1992.

Kittleson MD: Feline myocardial disease. In Ettinger SJ, Feldman EC (eds): *Textbook of Veterinary Internal Medicine*. Philadelphia, WB Saunders, 2005, pp 1087-1104.

Rush JE, et al: Population and survival characteristics of cats with hypertrophic cardiomyopathy: 260 cases (1990-1999). *J Am Vet Med Assoc* 220:202, 2002.

AUTHOR: **KRISTIN MACDONALD**
EDITOR: **ETIENNE CÔTÉ**

Hypertrophic Osteodystrophy

BASIC INFORMATION

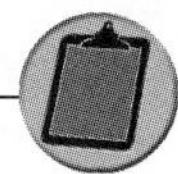

DEFINITION

A disease of the long bones of young, rapidly growing dogs, causing disruption of metaphyseal trabeculae

SYNONYM(S)

Barlow's disease
Canine skeletal scurvy
HOD
Hypovitaminosis C
Idiopathic osteodystrophy
Metaphyseal osteopathy
Moeller-Barlow disease
Osteodystrophy types I and II

EPIDEMIOLOGY

SPECIES, AGE, SEX: Canine, range 2 to 8 months; males more commonly affected.
GENETICS AND BREED PREDISPOSITION: Large breeds.
RISK FACTORS: Rapid rate of growth.

CLINICAL PRESENTATION

DISEASE FORMS/SUBTYPES

- Acute
- Occasionally peracute

HISTORY, CHIEF COMPLAINT

- An acute onset of soft tissue swelling of the distal forelimbs or occasionally of the distal hindlimbs
- Low-grade lameness of short duration
- Peracute refusal to stand, anorexia, signs of pain

PHYSICAL EXAM FINDINGS

- Febrile, 104°F (40°C) or higher
- Swollen, hot limb with moderate pain
- Peracute cases can show lethargy, dehydration, and severe pain on palpation of the swollen extremities

ETIOLOGY AND PATHOPHYSIOLOGY

- Unknown
- Definitely not a deficiency of vitamin C, or an excess of vitamin D, dietary minerals, or caloric intake
- Unproven link to canine distemper virus
- Disturbance of metaphyseal blood supply causing delayed ossification of the physeal hypertrophic zone

DIAGNOSIS

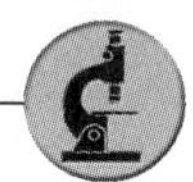

DIFFERENTIAL DIAGNOSIS

Radiographic:

- Panosteitis
- Septic arthritis
- Rickets (failure to calcify the cartilaginous matrix of the growth plate)

INITIAL DATABASE

- Plain radiographs; pathognomonic pseudophyseal line adjacent to the physis on the metaphyseal side ("scorbutic line") (Fig. I-99)
- Complete blood count, biochemistry profile, and urinaylsis are invariably unremarkable
- Rare hypocalcemia of unknown significance

ADVANCED OR CONFIRMATORY TESTING

Arthrocentesis: increased volume of transparent, straw-colored fluid with normal viscosity and increased numbers of neutrophils. Otherwise normal

TREATMENT

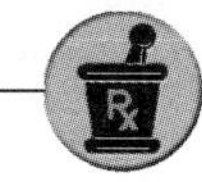

THERAPEUTIC GOAL(S)

Pain relief and supportive care

ACUTE GENERAL TREATMENT

- Nonsteroidal anti-inflammatory medication (e.g., carprofen, meloxicam, or deracoxib)
- Rest, confinement, soft bedding, turning every 4 to 6 hours if nonambulatory
- Severe cases require more intensive management including the use of intravenous glucocorticoids (rule out possibility of bacterial infection first), intravenous fluids, and nutritional support

CHRONIC TREATMENT

- Do not supplement with vitamin C, D, or minerals
- Correct the use of inappropriate diet:
  - Use a lower calorie puppy food

- Feed an amount that will achieve a thin or lean body condition score so as to minimize load on the developing skeleton until the dog reaches skeletal maturity

POSSIBLE COMPLICATIONS

Relapses can occur until the patient reaches skeletal maturity

PROGNOSIS AND OUTCOME

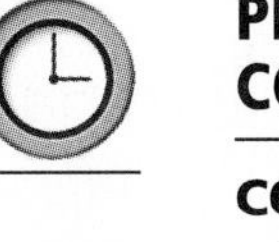

- Good
- Despite expected complete resolution, some owners may elect euthanasia in severe cases or following multiple relapses
- Diaphyseal deformities of the affected long bones may persist

PEARLS & CONSIDERATIONS

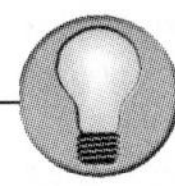

COMMENTS

- Radiographic changes are pathognomonic
- Relapses and permanent bone deformities can occur

SUGGESTED READING

Bellah JR: Hypertrophic osteodsytrophy. In Bojrab MJ (ed): *Disease Mechanisms in Small Animal Surgery*. Philadelphia, Lea and Febiger, 1993, pp 858–864.

Montgomery R: Miscellaneous orthopaedic diseases. In Slatter D (ed): *Textbook of Small Animal Surgery*. Philadelphia, WB Saunders, 2003, pp 2251–2252.

AUTHOR: **NICHOLAS J. TROUT**
EDITOR: **ETIENNE CÔTÉ**

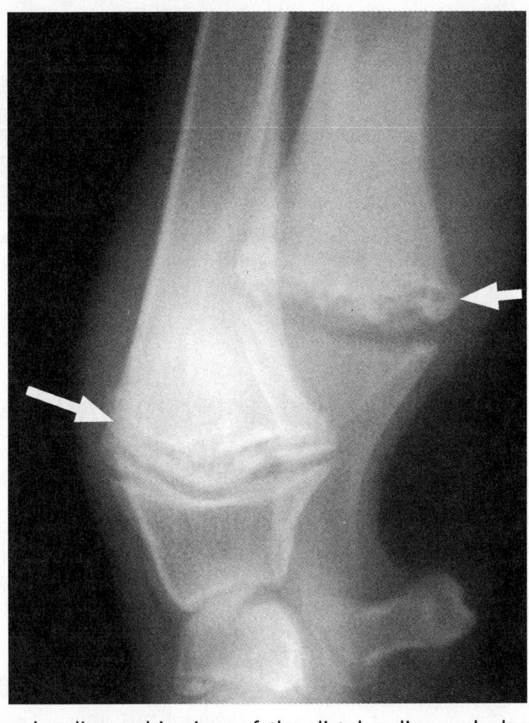

FIGURE I-99 Lateral radiographic view of the distal radius and ulna of a 4-month-old Great Dane puppy with hypertrophic osteodystrophy (HOD). Note the radiolucent lines ("scorbutic lines," *arrows*) parallel to the epiphyseal growth plates and antebrachiocarpal joint, characteristic of HOD.

Hypertrophic Osteopathy

BASIC INFORMATION

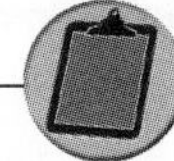

DEFINITION

A periosteal reaction in the distal extremities of the limbs secondary to a mass in the thorax or abdomen

SYNONYM(S)

HO
Hypertrophic pulmonary osteoarthropathy (HPOA)
Hypertrophic pulmonary osteopathy
Marie's disease
Pulmonary osteoarthropathy

EPIDEMIOLOGY

SPECIES, AGE, SEX: Mainly dogs, rare in cats. Older animals, since this disorder is often associated with neoplasia.

GENETICS AND BREED PREDISPOSITION: Large breeds of dogs.

ASSOCIATED CONDITIONS AND DISORDERS

- Thoracic mass (e.g., primary pulmonary neoplasia, metastatic pulmonary neoplasia, pulmonary abscess, esophageal carcinoma, *Spirocerca lupi* granuloma)
- Heartworm disease
- Canine tuberculosis
- Abdominal mass (e.g., rhabdomyosarcoma of the bladder, liver adenocarcinoma, prostatic adenocarcinoma)

CLINICAL PRESENTATION

HISTORY, CHIEF COMPLAINT

- Acute or gradual swelling of limbs, especially forelimbs
- Lethargy, low-grade lameness or reluctance to move
- Incidental finding secondary to a thoracic or abdominal mass

PHYSICAL EXAM FINDINGS

- Swollen, hard extremities (e.g., distal long bones)

- Occasional pitting edema
- Decreased movement in joints secondary to soft tissue swelling

ETIOLOGY AND PATHOPHYSIOLOGY

- Unknown
- Autonomic neurovascular reflex increasing peripheral blood flow causing periosteal congestion and new bone formation is speculated

DIAGNOSIS

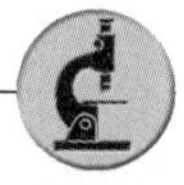

DIFFERENTIAL DIAGNOSIS

Radiographic:

- Primary bone neoplasia
- Secondary bone neoplasia
- Fungal bone disease
- Panosteitis

INITIAL DATABASE

- Complete blood count: thrombocytopenia occasionally seen, unknown cause
- Serum biochemistry profile and urinaylsis, unremarkable or related to thoracic or abdominal mass
- Plain radiographs of extremities (Fig. I-100); palisades of periosteal new bone on phalanges, metacarpi, metatarsi progressing to tibia/fibula, radius/ulna
- Thoracic radiographs
- Abdominal radiographs

ADVANCED OR CONFIRMATORY TESTING

- Thoracic ultrasonography
- Abdominal ultrasonography

TREATMENT

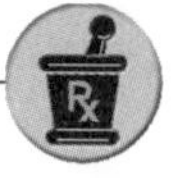

THERAPEUTIC GOAL(S)

Treat the underlying thoracic or abdominal disease

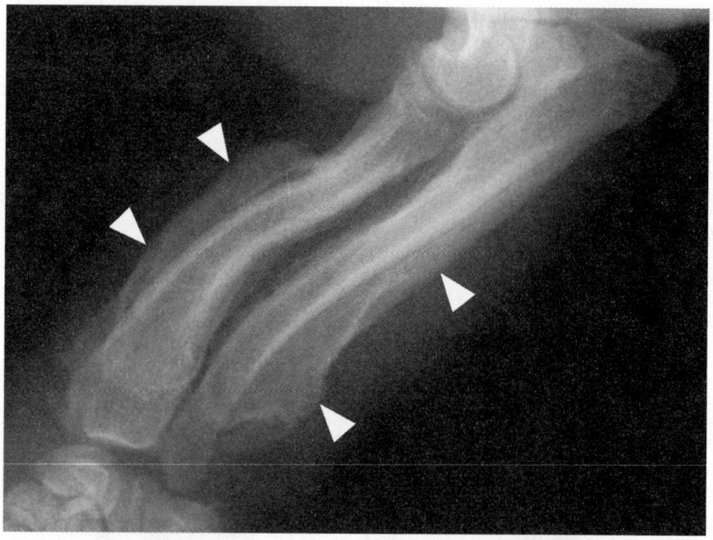

FIGURE I-100 Lateral radiograph of the radius and ulna of a 9-year-old female spayed Dachshund dog with pulmonary carcinoma. Note the exuberant periosteal reaction (*arrowheads*), typical of hypertrophic osteopathy.

ACUTE GENERAL TREATMENT

Biopsy or definitive thoracic or abdominal surgery to treat the primary disease

RECOMMENDED MONITORING

Follow-up radiographs of extremities to evaluate bone remodelling

PROGNOSIS AND OUTCOME

- Determined by the underlying thoracic or abdominal mass.
- After treatment of the primary disease, clinical signs may continue for 1 to 2 weeks. Bone lesions can take months to remodel, even with correction of the underlying disorder, and are not known to be fully reversible.

PEARLS & CONSIDERATIONS

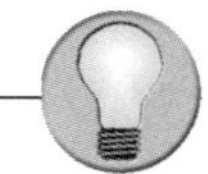

COMMENTS

Swelling of the distal extremities of an older dog with radiographic evidence of characteristic palisading periosteal reaction calls for thoracic and abdominal radiographs in search of an underlying primary lesion.

SUGGESTED READING

Halliwell WH: Tumorlike lesions of bone. In Bojrab MJ (ed): *Disease Mechanisms in Small Animal Surgery*. Philadelphia, Lea & Febiger, 1993, pp 933–934.

Montgomery R: Miscellaneous orthopaedic diseases. In Slatter D (ed): *Textbook of Small Animal Surgery*. Philadelphia, WB Saunders, 2003, p 2251.

AUTHOR: **NICHOLAS J. TROUT**

EDITOR: **ETIENNE CÔTÉ**

Hyperviscosity Syndrome

BASIC INFORMATION

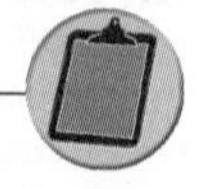

DEFINITION

Constellation of clinical signs that occur secondary to elevated blood viscosity

EPIDEMIOLOGY

SPECIES, AGE, SEX: Dogs more frequently than cats; middle-aged to older.

ASSOCIATED CONDITIONS AND DISORDERS: Several sequlae can occur with hyperviscosity syndrome:

- Volume overload and congestive heart failure
- Azotemia results from decreased renal perfusion, infiltrative renal lesions, or associated hypercalcemia
- Immune suppression and secondary infection
- Pathologic fractures from infiltrative bone lesions
- Neurologic signs from sludging of blood
- Coagulopathy from platelet and coagulation factor inhibition

CLINICAL PRESENTATION

HISTORY, CHIEF COMPLAINT: Variable combinations and severity of nonspecific signs: lethargy, weakness, weight loss, polyuria/polydipsia, neurologic deficits, and blindness. Occasionally a patient will be noted to manifest a bleeding disorder, or blood is noted to be thick and difficult to draw via phlebotomy.

PHYSICAL EXAM FINDINGS: Ocular changes (retinal vessel engorgement/tortuosity, retinal hemorrhage or detachment, papilledema), epistaxis, mucosal hemorrhage or ecchymoses, or lymphadenopathy may be present.

ETIOLOGY AND PATHOPHYSIOLOGY

- Hyperviscosity syndrome may be caused by one of several hematological conditions.
- Blood viscosity is a function of the concentration and composition of its components.
- A marked increase in plasma proteins (for example, monoclonal immunoglobulin in myeloma) or cellular constituents (for example, white blood cells in acute leukemia) will raise the overall blood viscosity. This leads to sludging of the microcirculation and a variety of clinical manifestations as described previously.
- Hyperviscosity may present insidiously with vague, nonspecific signs, or acutely, with neurologic signs.

DIAGNOSIS

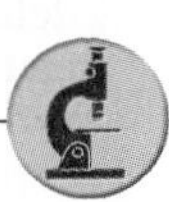

DIFFERENTIAL DIAGNOSIS

- Multiple myeloma (IgG or IgA)
- Waldenström's macroglobulinemia (IgM)
- Plasma cell leukemia
- Lymphoma
- Chronic lymphocytic leukemia
- Feline infectious peritonitis
- Amyloidosis
- Ehrlichiosis
- Primary polycythemia
- Secondary polycythemia:
  - Hypoxemia (right-to-left patent ductus arteriosus, elevated altitude, pulmonary disease)
  - Neoplasia (renal tumors, rarely sarcomas)

INITIAL DATABASE

- Complete blood count (CBC), platelet count: variable findings, including mild to moderate anemia with chronic lymphocytic leukemia, Waldenström's macroglobulinemia, multiple myeloma, feline infectious peritonitis, amyloidosis; or markedly elevated hematocrit (i.e., >60%) with polycythemia.
- Serum biochemistry profile: hyperglobulinemia if hyperviscosity related to Waldenström's macroglobulinemia, multiple myeloma, feline infectious peritonitis, amyloidosis, or ehrlichiosis; possibly present with chronic lymphocytic leukemia.
- Urinalysis: no specific findings. Bence Jones proteins are not detected on routine urinalysis.
- Retinal exam: Retinal arteries may be enlarged or tortuous; signs of uveitis or chorioretinitis may be present in feline infectious peritonitis.
- Arterial blood pressure: Systemic hypertension may be a sequela of hyperglobulinemia.
- Chest radiographs: Lytic bone lesions can be observed with multiple myeloma, or metastatic disease in lymphoma; heavy interstitial or bronchiolar patterns possible in secondary polycythemia.
- Abdominal ultrasound:
  - Diffuse hepatosplenomegaly or lymphadenopathy may be present with lymphoma, ehlichiosis, multiple myeloma (mainly splenomegaly)
  - Renal mass (source of excess erythropoietin) possibly identified in secondary polycythemia

ADVANCED OR CONFIRMATORY TESTING

- Serum protein electrophoresis: monoclonal protein spike commonly present with chronic lymphocytic leukemia, Waldenström's macroglobulinemia, multiple myeloma or plasma cell leukemia; more often polyclonal with feline infectious peritonitis, amyloidosis, or ehrlichiosis but occasionally can be monoclonal.
- Bence Jones proteinuria expected if hyperglobulinemia is cause of hyperviscosity.
  - Excessive immunoglobulin light chains excreted in urine.
  - May be present with multiple myeloma, chronic lymphocytic leukemia, Waldenström's macroglobulinemia, or plasma cell leukemia.
- Urine electrophoresis: may reveal monoclonal spike in cases of chronic lymphocytic leukemia, Waldenström's macroglobulinemia, multiple myeloma, or plasma cell leukemia.
- Coagulation profile: Bleeding disorder, especially platelet dysfunction, may occur with hyperglobulinemia.
- Bone marrow aspirate ± core biopsy: >20% plasma cells in multiple myeloma or plasma cell leukemia.
- Pulse oximetry or arterial blood gas: to document hypoxemia if it is the cause of secondary polycythemia.
- Echocardiogram: could reveal right ventricular hypertrophy and possibly the shunt itself in secondary polycythemia caused by right-to-left cardiac shunts.
- *Ehrlichia canis* titers.
- *Leishmania* direct agglutination test.

TREATMENT

THERAPEUTIC GOAL(S)

- Identify and treat primary disease process
- Ensure patient is adequately hydrated, oxygenated, and producing urine

ACUTE GENERAL TREATMENT

Acute treatment may require plasmapheresis or phlebotomy to decrease Hct to <60% (10-20 ml/kg, with replacement of equivalent volume of isotonic crystalloid fluids) to decrease blood viscosity and alleviate neurologic or ophthalmic signs. When hyperglobulinemia is the cause of hyperviscosity, the withdrawn blood can be centrifuged and the autologous red cells autotransfused.

CHRONIC TREATMENT

- Treatment of the underlying disorder (e.g., chemotherapy for leukemias, lymphoma, multiple myeloma; doxycycline for ehrlichiosis).
- Repeated plasmapheresis for Waldenström's macroglobulinemia.
- Intermittent phlebotomy for secondary polycythemia. A total of 10-20 ml/kg in one day, repeated on an as-needed basis as clinical signs and polycythemia recurrence dictate.
- For polycythemia, first decrease the Hct to <60% using phlebotomy, then use hydroxyurea 30-50 mg/kg PO q 24h initially for 7 to 10 days followed by 30-50 mg/kg 2 or 3 times weekly as needed to maintain Hct <60%. Monitor CBC for signs of myelotoxicity.

RECOMMENDED MONITORING

- For hyperviscosity caused by polycythemia: monitor hematocrit.
- For hyperviscosity caused by hyperglobulinemia, monitor total protein, albumin, and globulin; repeated serum electrophoresis can be used for monitoring multiple myeloma.

PROGNOSIS AND OUTCOME

Guarded, dependent on underlying disease process

PEARLS & CONSIDERATIONS

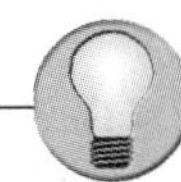

COMMENTS

- Use corticosteroids cautiously, as biopsy or bone marrow results may be affected.
- Patients with hyperglobulinemia are predisposed to infection and corticosteroids suppress the immune system.

SUGGESTED READING

Gaschen FP, Teske E: Paraneoplastic syndrome. In Ettinger SJ, Feldman EC (eds): *Textbook of Veterinary Internal Medicine,* ed 6. St. Louis, Elsevier Saunders, 2005, pp 789-795.

Hohenhaus AE: Syndromes of hyperglobulinemia: diagnosis and therapy. In Bonagura: *Kirk's Current Veterinary Therapy XII*. Philadelphia, WB Saunders, 1995, pp 523-530.

AUTHOR: **JONATHAN BACH**
EDITOR: **SUSAN M. COTTER**

Hyphema

BASIC INFORMATION

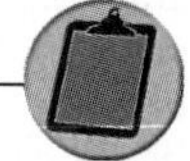

DEFINITION

Blood in the anterior chamber

SYNONYM(S)

"Eight ball" hemorrhage

EPIDEMIOLOGY

SPECIES, AGE, SEX: Dogs and cats; any age or sex.

GENETICS AND BREED PREDISPOSITION: Dependent on the cause:
- Genetic coagulopathies
- Breed predisposition to retinal detachments (see Retinal Detachment, p 965)
- Inherited congenital ocular defects (e.g., collie eye anomaly; persistent hyperplastic primary vitreous syndromes)

RISK FACTORS
- Stimuli for ocular vascularization:
  - Chronic retinal detachments (see Retinal Detachment, p 965)
  - Intraocular neoplasia (see Intraocular Neoplasia, p 603)
  - Glaucoma, p 440
- Animals at increased risk of ocular trauma (e.g., blind animals; hunting dogs)
- Systemic diseases causing vasculopathies and/or coagulopathies (see Systemic Hypertension, p 1058):
  - Systemic hypertension (see Systemic Hypertension, p 1058)
  - Infectious diseases:
    - Feline leukemia virus (FeLV) infection and feline coronavirus/feline infectious peritonitis infection (FIP) in cats (see Feline Leukemia Virus Infection, p 380; Feline Infectious Peritonitis, p 378)
    - Rickettsial diseases (see Ehrlichiosis, Canine Monocytic, p 334; Rocky Mountain Spotted Fever, p 975)
  - Immune-mediated diseases:
    - Thrombocytopenia (see Thrombocytopenia, Immune-Mediated, p 1079)
    - Anemia (see Anemia, Immune-Mediated Hemolytic, p 66)
  - Toxicities:
    - Anticoagulant (see Anticoagulant Rodenticide Toxicosis, p 76)

CONTAGION AND ZOONOSES: Depends on underlying cause (e.g., FeLV and FIP transmitted cat-to-cat).

CLINICAL PRESENTATION

DISEASE FORMS/SUBTYPES
- Acute:
  - Varying degrees of blood are present in the eye.
  - When the blood is unclotted and the animal is quiet, blood settles ventrally producing a meniscus.
  - Appearance may vary.
    - When activity level is increased, settled blood may disperse and appear worse.
- Chronic:
  - Clot formation may become dark or black ("eight ball hemorrhage").
  - If glaucoma occurs, blood staining of the cornea may develop.

HISTORY, CHIEF COMPLAINT
- Reflective of underlying cause (see Risk Factors above)
- Blood or redness in the eye

PHYSICAL EXAM FINDINGS
- Ocular:
  - Varying degrees of blood in the anterior chamber
  - May see fibrin clots with erythocyte entrapment
  - Conjunctival injection is often present, indicating an associated anterior uveitis (see Uveitis, p 1134)
  - Corneal edema
  - Intraocular pressure (IOP):
    - May be reduced (i.e., acute; uveitis)
    - May be elevated (i.e., chronic; secondary glaucoma)
- General physical examination:
  - Search for evidence of systemic disease

ETIOLOGY AND PATHOPHYSIOLOGY

- Neovascularization in the eye is fragile and often results in spontaneous hyphema.
- Blood in the anterior chamber is immediately diluted with aqueous humor and usually undergoes rapid fibrinolysis from tissue plasminogen activator that is produced by the iris. This may lyse the clot adjacent to the iris, but leave a clot in the pupil.

DIAGNOSIS

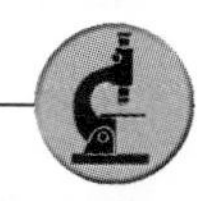

DIFFERENTIAL DIAGNOSIS

- Intense corneal vascularization (see Corneal Vascularization, p 249)
- Rubeosis iridis: new blood vessel growth on the surface of the iris (see Uveitis, p 1134)

INITIAL DATABASE

- Ocular:
  - Examine periocular region for evidence of trauma; examine contralateral eye for lesions in both anterior and posterior segments.
  - Pupillary light and dazzle reflexes, menace response, for vision prognosis.
  - Fluorescein stain and examine cornea/sclera for evidence of perforating injury.
  - If possible, examine iris for evidence of inflammation and assess pupil size (see Uveitis, p 1134).
  - Measure IOP to assess for signs of uveitis (i.e., hypotony or low IOP [IOP <10 mmHg]) versus glaucoma (IOP >30 mmHg).
- Physical examination:
  - Examine mucous membranes and skin for petechiae.
  - Palpate abdominal organs and lymph nodes for organomegaly and/or lymphadenopathy suggestive of neoplastic and/or infectious diseases.
  - Auscult chest.
- Ocular ultrasound: for cause of bleeding such as retinal detachment, intraocular neoplasia, or foreign body.
- Complete blood count, chemistry profile, and urinalysis for evidence of systemic disease.
- Systemic blood pressure to test for hypertension (see Systemic Hypertension, p 1058).

ADVANCED OR CONFIRMATORY TESTING

- Coagulation profile
- Infectious disease titers or tests

- Fine-needle aspirates/biopsy of organomegaly or enlarged lymph nodes

TREATMENT

THERAPEUTIC GOAL(S)

- Correction of underlying cause
- Resorption of erythrocytes and fibrin from the anterior chamber

ACUTE GENERAL TREATMENT

- Restricted activity in cases of clotting disorders
- Treat anterior uveitis with topical corticosteroids
  - *Only* if no lesions of the corneal surface
  - For example, prednisolone acetate 1% or dexamethasone 0.1% q 6-8h
- If pupil is not dilated and IOP is normal or low (<15-20 mmHg), topical atropine 1% solution q 12h
- If IOP >20 mmHg, topical or systemic carbonic anhydrase inhibitors (see Glaucoma, p 440)
- Trauma: surgery to repair corneal and/or scleral defects (see Corneal/Scleral Trauma, p 244)

CHRONIC TREATMENT

- Traumatic hyphema:
  - *Clotted* hyphema may be dissolved with injection of 25 µg of tissue plasminogen activator into the anterior chamber (referable procedure) within 3 to 4 days of the hemorrhage; risk of rebleeding
- Uncontrollable uveitis and/or secondary glaucoma:
  - Enucleation (globe removal) or evisceration and prosthesis (globe salvage)
- Surgical removal of blood from anterior chamber rarely indicated (referable procedure)

DRUG INTERACTIONS

Nonsteroidal anti-inflammatory drugs are usually avoided

POSSIBLE COMPLICATIONS

- Rebleeding
- Glaucoma
- Vision loss

RECOMMENDED MONITORING

Reexamine in 48 to 72 hours for resorption of blood and changes in IOP

PROGNOSIS AND OUTCOME

- Dependent on removal or control of underlying cause.
- Traumatic hyphema of less than half of the anterior chamber typically improves spontaneously.
- Hyphemas greater than three fourths of the chamber have guarded prognosis.
- Prognosis for vision in traumatic hyphema is usually determined by the initial trauma and the associated ocular injury.
- Globes with chronic uveitis and/or glaucoma require enucleation or evisceration and prosthesis.

PEARLS & CONSIDERATIONS

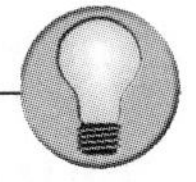

COMMENTS

- Almost every instance of hyphema is thought, by the owner, to be caused by trauma.
- Rule out other causes before confirming traumatic hyphema.

PREVENTION

- Avoid situations that predispose the animal to trauma.
- Ensure toxins such as warfarin are out of reach of animals.
- Avoid breeding dogs and cats with predisposing genetic diseases.

CLIENT EDUCATION

Resorption of hyphema is highly variable and difficult to predict

SUGGESTED READING

Komaromy AM, et al: Hyphema. Part I. Pathophysiologic considerations. *Compend Cont Educ Pract Vet* 21:1064, 1999.

Komaromy AM, et al: Hyphema. Part II. Diagnosis and treatment. *Compend Cont Educ Pract Vet* 22:74, 2000.

AUTHOR: **CHARLES L. MARTIN**

EDITOR: **CHERYL L. CULLEN**

Hypoadrenocorticism

Client Education Sheet on Website

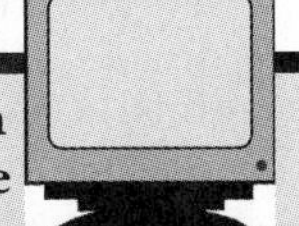

BASIC INFORMATION

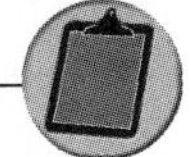

DEFINITION

An endocrine disorder of dogs, and very rarely of cats, caused by adrenocortical insufficiency. Systemic clinical signs are often vague initially and may become life-threatening, mainly due to hyperkalemia, when the diagnosis and treatment are delayed.

SYNONYM(S)

Addison's disease

EPIDEMIOLOGY

SPECIES, AGE, SEX

- Most common in young/middle-aged, female dogs, but any age, gender, or breed may be affected
- Very uncommon in cats

GENETICS AND BREED PREDISPOSITION

- Increased risk: Great Danes, West Highland white terriers, bearded collies, poodles, rottweilers, and basset hounds
- Genetic/familial predisposition suggested in standard poodles, Labrador retrievers, Portugese water dogs, and bearded collies

CLINICAL PRESENTATION

DISEASE FORMS/SUBTYPES: "Typical" versus "atypical" hypoadrenocorticism. "Typical" hypoadrenocorticism: signs of both glucocorticoid and mineralocorticoid deficiency. "Atypical" hypoadrenocorticism: only signs of glucocorticoid deficiency are present.

HISTORY/CHIEF COMPLAINT

- Clinical signs classically are waxing and waning over weeks or months (sometimes only apparent to owners in retrospect), possibly with worsening in "stressful" situations (e.g., travel, kenneling). Severity ranges from a mild, progressive, intermittent course early on, to a culmination in an acute, life-threatening crisis.
- Dogs: weakness, lethargy, anorexia, vomiting, diarrhea (possibly with melena or hematochezia), weight loss, trembling, polyuria/polydipsia (PU/PD), regurgitation, and collapse. Rarely, seizures may occur due to hypoglycemia.
- Cats: anorexia, weight loss, lethargy; vomiting and PU/PD are uncommon.

PHYSICAL EXAM FINDINGS

- Exam may be unremarkable, and the diagnosis suspected only from incidental blood test (electrolyte/albumin/blood urea nitrogen [BUN]) or radiographic (megaesophagus) abnormalities.

- Depression, weakness, dehydration, abdominal pain and melena are possible.
- In crisis, bradycardia (from hyperkalemia), weak pulses, and hypothermia may also be seen.

ETIOLOGY AND PATHOPHYSIOLOGY

ETIOLOGY

- Primary hypoadrenocorticism: most commonly due to idiopathic or immune-mediated destruction of the adrenal cortices. Other uncommon causes of adrenocortical destruction: granulomatous disease (histoplasmosis, blastomycosis, tuberculosis); infarction; neoplasia; adrenocortical amyloidosis; drugs (e.g., mitotane).
- Secondary hypoadrenocorticism (spontaneous): destructive lesions or congenital defects of the hypothalamus or pituitary result in decreased secretion of corticotrophin-releasing factor or adrenocorticotropic hormone (ACTH), respectively. Very rare.
- Secondary hypoadrenocorticism (iatrogenic): administration of exogenous corticosteroids suppresses normal ACTH production, resulting in adrenal gland atrophy; sudden cessation of exogenous corticosteroid administration then produces hypoadrenocorticism.

PATHOPHYSIOLOGY

- Clinical signs and laboratory findings reflect the absence of normal activities of glucocorticoids and mineralocorticoids.
- Hypoadrenocorticism affecting all layers of the adrenal cortex ("typical"; electrolytes are abnormal) is much more common than hypoadrenocorticism affecting only glucocorticoid synthesis ("atypical"; electrolytes are normal) (Fig. I-101).
- Consequences of glucocorticoid (cortisone) deficiency:
  - Malaise, lethargy.
  - Gastrointestinal (GI) signs (anorexia, vomiting, diarrhea, abdominal pain, melena, weight loss, regurgitation).
  - Hypoglycemia.
  - Absence of a stress leukogram in a very ill patient (failure of glucocorticoid-induced neutrophil release and lymphocyte reduction), mild anemia.
- Consequences of mineralocorticoid (aldosterone) deficiency:
  - Decreased renal sodium, chloride (and consequently water) resorption resulting in hyponatremia, hypochloremia, and volume depletion/dehydration. Hyponatremia results in hypovolemia, hypotension, decreased cardiac output and poor tissue perfusion, solute diuresis and medullary solute washout; consequences include prerenal azotemia, metabolic acidosis, weakness, microcardia, depression, decreased urine concentrating ability, and PU/PD.
  - Decreased renal potassium excretion resulting in hyperkalemia (see Hyperkalemia, p 546).
  - Metabolic acidosis due to decreased renal hydrogen ion excretion.
- Additional reported findings for which a mechanism is not clearly defined include hypercalcemia, hypoalbuminemia, and megaesophagus.

DIAGNOSIS

DIFFERENTIAL DIAGNOSIS

- History/chief complaint: primary gastrointestinal disease, intoxication, pancreatitis, renal disease, liver disease
- Hyperkalemia (see p 546)
- Hyponatremia (see p 567)
- Hypercalcemia (see p 543)
- Hypoglycemia

INITIAL DATABASE

- Complete blood count, serum biochemical profile, urinalysis:
  - "Typical" hypoadrenocorticism (common): normocytic, normochromic nonregenerative anemia; absence of stress leukogram; hyponatremia; hypochloremia; hyperkalemia; metabolic acidosis and prerenal azotemia. Hypoglycemia, hypercalcemia, hypoalbuminemia, and isosthenuria are also possible. A decreased Na:K ratio supports a tentative diagnosis but is *not* pathognomonic and cannot be used for making a definitive diagnosis.
  - "Atypic" hypoadrenocorticism: possible normocytic, normochromic anemia; no stress leukogram, possible hypoglycemia. Electrolyte levels are normal.
- Electrocardiogram: changes consistent with hyperkalemia possible, especially loss of P waves (atrial standstill) (see Hyperkalemia, p 546).
- Thoracic radiographs: microcardia common; signs of megaesophagus ± aspiration pneumonia possible.

ADVANCED OR CONFIRMATORY TESTING

- ACTH stimulation test is the definitive diagnostic test for hypoadrenocorticism. Basal serum cortisol concentration may be low normal to low and fails to increase after ACTH administration.
  - Protocol 1: (a) blood sample for preACTH cortisol level; (b) synthetic aqueous ACTH (cosyntropin, Cortrosyn) 250 μg/dog IM or IV; (c) blood sample 60 minutes later (post-ACTH cortisol level).
  - Protocol 2: (a) blood sample for pre-ACTH cortisol level; (b) ACTH gel 2.2 IU/kg IM; (c) blood sample 2 hours later (post-ACTH cortisol level). Anecdotal reports indicate sporadic variability in ACTH gel efficacy.
  - Protocol 3: (a) blood sample for pre-ACTH cortisol level; (b) synthetic aqueous ACTH (cosyntropin, Cortrosyn) 5 μg/kg IV; (c) blood sample 60 minutes later (post-ACTH cortisol level).
  - The low-dose protocol (#3) is as effective as the high-dose protocol and is more widely used with rising costs of cosyntropin.
  - Synthetic ACTH (cosyntropin) may be stored in plastic syringes in a standard domestic freezer (−20°C) for 6 months without loss of efficacy.
- Endogenous ACTH can be measured to differentiate secondary (decreased ACTH) from early primary hypoadrenocorticism (increased ACTH) if atypical hypoadrenocorticism is present.

TREATMENT

THERAPEUTIC GOAL(S)

- Acute: treat life-threatening conditions (hypotension, hypovolemia, hyperkalemia, hypoglycemia, acidosis)
- Chronic: provide physiologic replacement of deficient hormones

ACUTE GENERAL TREATMENT

Treat hypoadrenocorticism suspects (severe, typical clinical and laboratory abnormalities) as if they have hypoadrenocorticism; delaying treatment until ACTH stimulation results are available may result in the death of the patient.

- Normal saline (0.9% NaCl) IV:
  - This is a critical component of therapy; it addresses hypovolemia, hypotension, hyperkalemia, hyponatremia, and azotemia.
  - Dogs: 40–80 ml/kg/hr IV for 1 to 2 hours, then 90–120 ml/kg/day for 1 to 2 days; switch to a balanced electrolyte solution (e.g., lactated Ringer's solution) when electrolytes are within reference ranges.
  - Cats: administer 40 ml/kg IV over 2 to 4 hours to rehydrate, then 65 ml/kg/day.
- Fluid therapy is the primary treatment for hyperkalemia and acidosis.
  - If hyperkalemia is life threatening (serum concentration >8.0 mEq/L and/or electrocardiographic findings), may need sodium bicarbonate, insulin/glucose or calcium gluconate (see Hyperkalemia, p 546).
  - If acidosis is severe (serum bicarbonate <12 mEq/L) consider bicarbonate therapy:
    - Base deficit (mEq/L) = 25 − patient's blood [HCO_3^-]. If blood gas results are not available and

patient is severely ill, assume base deficit = 10 mEq/L: Total dose $NaHCO_3$ (mEq/L) = body weight in kg × 0.3 × base deficit. Give 25% of total dose in IV fluids over first 6 to 8 hours, then reassess and repeat if blood HCO_3^- still <12 mEq/L.

- Glucocorticoid administration:
  - Dexamethasone sodium phosphate: rapid-acting and is not detected by cortisol assay (ACTH stimulation test). Initially administer 0.5-1 mg/kg IV once, *or* 0.05-0.1 mg/kg q 12h in IV solution (dogs) or 0.1-2 mg/kg IV initially then q 6-12h (cats).
  - Alternatively, prednisone sodium succinate (4-20 mg/kg over 2 to 4 minutes initially, then q 2-6h) can be administered but only *after* completion of the ACTH stimulation test.
- Hypoglycemia: add dextrose to IV fluids to make 2.5-5% dextrose concentration.
- Once life-saving treatment has been initiated, perform ACTH stimulation test.
- Administer mineralocorticoids (see Chronic Treatment below) *after* completion of the ACTH stimulation test. Desoxycorticosterone pivalate (DOCP) reported to be safe in dogs subsequently shown not to have hypoadrenocorticism.
- Monitor urine production.
- Monitor electrolytes and glucose q 8-12h until normal.
- Maintain fluid therapy until patient is eating.
- Use injectable dexamethasone until oral prednisone can be instituted.

CHRONIC TREATMENT

- Lifelong supplementation with glucocorticoids and mineralocorticoids (primary hypoadrenocorticism) or with glucocorticoids alone (secondary or atypical hypoadrenocorticism) is required.
- Glucocorticoid supplementation: prednisone—0.22 mg/kg PO q 12h initially then taper to 0.2-0.25 mg/kg PO q 24-48h depending on individual needs.
  - Increased prednisone (0.25-1 mg/kg PO q 12h) may be required during times of stress (e.g., travel, kenneling, visitors, new pet or child). Taper to usual maintenance dose once the event has resolved.
  - Patients receiving fludrocortisone acetate may not require additional daily glucocorticoid therapy, but those receiving DOCP almost always do.
- Mineralocorticoid supplementation:
  - Fludrocortisone acetate
    - Dogs: 0.01 mg/kg PO q 12h initially; dose often needs to be increased over first 6 to 18 months based on serum electrolyte concentrations.
    - Cats: 0.05-0.1 mg PO q 12h initially; adjust based on serum electrolyte concentrations.
  - DOCP: 2.2 mg/kg SQ or IM q ~25 days. Measure serum electrolytes on days 12 and 25 after initial treatment. Adjust dose and dosing interval based on results. If hyperkalemia and hyponatremia exist on day 12, increase the next dose by 5-10%. If electrolytes are normal at 12 days but abnormal at 25 days, shorten the dosing interval. Once dose and dosing interval are determined, clients can be taught to give DOCP at home.
- Salt supplementation: indicated if high fludrocortisone doses are required for normal serum electrolyte concentrations.

POSSIBLE COMPLICATIONS

- With Addisonian crises, death can occur if treatment is not prompt and intensive.
- Side effects of prolonged excessive prednisone and/or fludrocortisone treatment can include PU/PD and other mild signs of iatrogenic hyperadrenocorticism.

RECOMMENDED MONITORING

- Serum electrolytes, BUN, glucose: 7 and 14 days after diagnosis (can coincide with day 12 after DOCP injection).

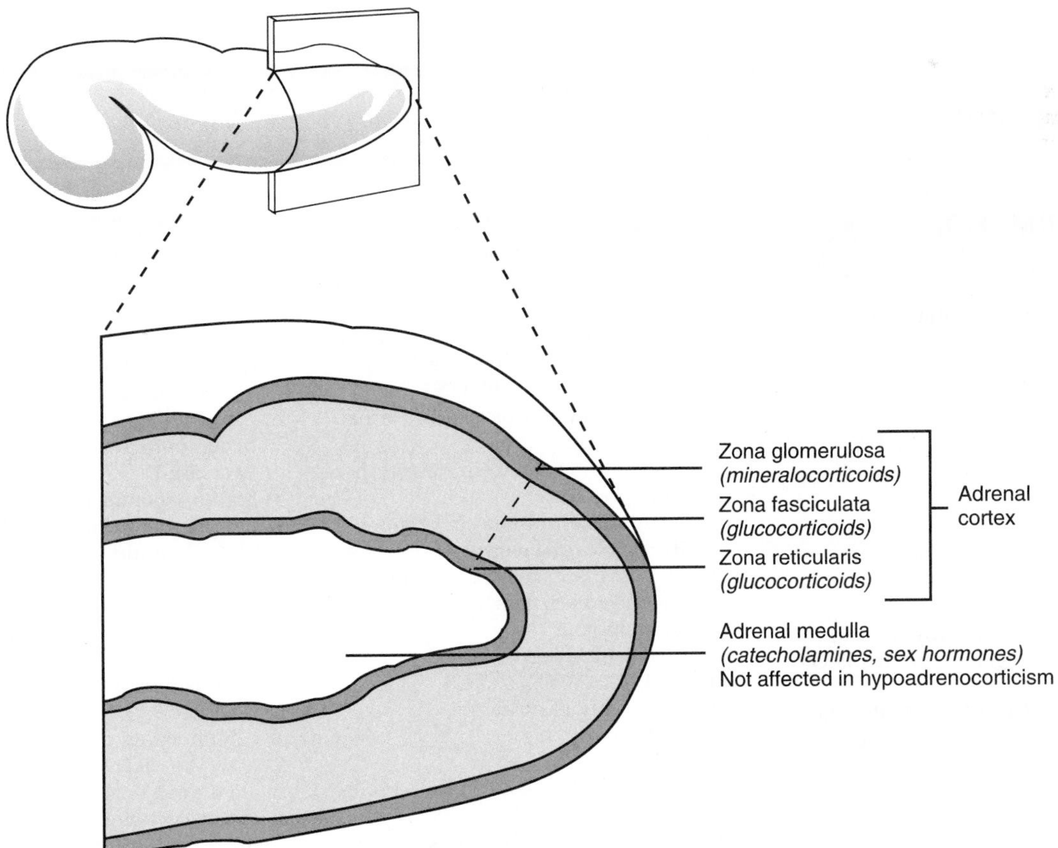

FIGURE I-101 Cross section of the adrenal gland demonstrating the zones of the adrenal gland and the hormones produced by each.

- Once electrolytes stabilize, recheck monthly for 3 to 6 months, then q 3-6 months.
- Once the treatment regimen is established and the dog is well, recheck electrolytes q 6-12 months for dose adjustments based on changing body weight.
- Subsequent ACTH stimulation testing is of no use (glucocorticoid interference).

PROGNOSIS AND OUTCOME

- With treatment and monitoring, prognosis is excellent and a normal lifespan is expected.
- BUN and creatinine elevations with concurrent isosthenuria should not be taken to indicate renal failure and thus do not necessarily influence the prognosis (see Pearls & Considerations below).

PEARLS & CONSIDERATIONS

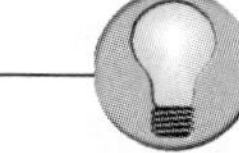

COMMENTS

- This disease can mimic others that are more common (acute renal failure, hepatic disease, GI disease) and the diagnosis of hypoadrenocorticism is commonly missed initially. The complete blood count can provide a valuable clue: absence of a stress leukogram in an ill animal is inappropriate and suggests hypoadrenocorticism.
- Dogs commonly show marked improvement within 24 hours with appropriate treatment. However, lack of sudden improvement while awaiting ACTH stimulation test results, even with aggressive initial treatment, does *not* prove the absence of hypoadrenocorticism. Cats have a slower initial response to treatment and may stay weak and lethargic for 3 to 5 days despite appropriate treatment.
- A common cause of pseudohyperkalemia is normal in vitro blood clotting (platelet activation releases potassium); it is easily ruled out by remeasuring blood potassium on a sample drawn into a green top tube (heparin).
- Hypoadrenocorticism, hypoaldosteronism, and diabetes insipidus are three disorders that may produce azotemia and isosthenuria without permanent renal lesions. Therefore renal function (and renal prognosis) in patients with hypoadrenocorticism can best be determined only after recovery.
- The physiologic dose of glucocorticoids (e.g., prednisolone 0.25 mg/kg PO q 24h) is a small fraction of the more commonly used anti-inflammatory dose.

CLIENT EDUCATION

It is important to educate clients that this disease requires lifelong treatment, and that failure to administer therapy may result in a life-threatening crisis.

SUGGESTED READING

Frank LA, et al: Comparison of serum cortisol concentrations in clinically normal dogs after administration of freshly reconstituted versus reconstituted and stored frozen cosyntropin. *J Am Vet Med Assoc* 212:1569–1571, 1998.

Kerl ME, et al: Evaluation of a low-dose synthetic adrenocorticotropic hormone stimulation test in clinically normal dogs and dogs with naturally developing hyperadrenocorticism. *J Am Vet Med Assoc* 214:1497–1501, 1999.

Kintzer PP, et al: Treatment and long-term follow-up of 205 dogs with hypoadrenocorticism. *J Vet Intern Med* 11:43-49, 1997.

Parnell NK, et al: Hypoadrenocorticism as the primary manifestation of lymphoma in two cats. *J Am Vet Med Assoc* 214(8):1208–1211, 1999.

Sadek D, et al: Atypical Addison's disease in the dog: a retrospective study of 14 cases. *J Am Anim Hosp Assoc* 32:159–163, 1996.

AUTHOR: **CARY L. M. BASSETT**
EDITOR: **SHERRI IHLE**

Hypocalcemia

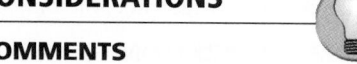

BASIC INFORMATION

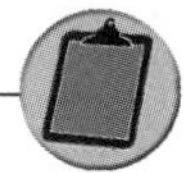

DEFINITION

A reduction of blood calcium concentration below normal

EPIDEMIOLOGY

SPECIES, AGE, SEX

- Dogs and cats of either sex and any age can be affected; exact predispositions depend on underlying causes.
- Hypoparathyroidism occurs mainly in female (65%), middle-aged dogs.
- Puerperal tetany (eclampsia) occurs in small lactating bitches.
- Older cats undergoing thyroidectomy are at risk of iatrogenic parathyroidectomy.

GENETICS AND BREED PREDISPOSITION: Hypoparathyroidism in dogs: toy poodles, miniature schnauzers, Labrador retrievers, German shepherds, dachshunds, terriers.

CLINICAL PRESENTATION

DISEASE FORMS/SUBTYPES

- Animal presented with signs relating to hypocalcemia
- Incidental finding on bloodwork, animal presented for another problem

HISTORY, CHIEF COMPLAINT

- Abrupt onset of neurologic and/or neuromuscular signs
- Signs may be intermittent despite persistent hypocalcemia:
  - Focal/generalized muscle tremors
  - Stiff, stilted, rigid gait
  - Nervousness, excessive panting
  - Generalized seizures, tetany
  - Facial rubbing
  - Ear twitching (cats)

PHYSICAL EXAM FINDINGS

- Muscle rigidity, tremors
- Tense abdomen
- Stiff gait
- Tachyarrhythmias, soft heart sounds, weak pulse
- Raised nictitating membranes (cats)
- Physical exam can be normal

ETIOLOGY AND PATHOPHYSIOLOGY

- Calcium homeostasis: 50% of total circulating calcium is ionized (biologically active form), 40% is bound to albumin (storage form), 10% is complexed to anions (storage form).
- Clinical signs of hypocalcemia will occur *only* when the ionized form is decreased.
- Serum calcium is tightly regulated by parathyroid hormone (PTH), vitamin D, and calcitonin.
- PTH increases serum calcium by:
  - Increasing osteoclastic bone resorption of calcium and phosphorus.
  - Increasing calcium and decreasing phosphorus resorption from renal tubules.
  - Stimulating conversion of vitamin D to its active form by the renal enzyme 1-α-hydroxylase.
- Inactive vitamin D is absorbed in the intestine, transported to the liver where it is hydroxylated to 25-

dihydroxy vitamin D, then transported to the kidney where it is hydroxylated by 1-α-hydroxylase to the active metabolite 1,25-dihydroxy vitamin D (calcitriol).

- Vitamin D increases serum calcium and phosphorus by:
  - Increasing intestinal absorption of calcium, phosphorus and magnesium from the intestine.
  - Facilitating PTH-induced bone resorption.
  - Increasing renal tubular resorption of calcium and phosphorus.
- Calcitonin decreases serum calcium and phosphorus by:
  - Blocking bone resorption.
  - Decreasing renal tubular resorption of calcium and phosphorus.

DIAGNOSIS

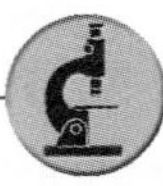

DIFFERENTIAL DIAGNOSIS

- Parathyroid-related:
  - Primary hypoparathyroidism (immune-mediated, idiopathic, surgical complication post-thyroidectomy in cats)
- Acute/chronic renal failure
- Puerperal tetany (eclampsia)
- Acute pancreatitis
- Ethylene glycol toxicity
- Hypomagnesemia
- Vitamin D deficiency
- Hypoalbuminemia (total serum [calcium] is low but ionized serum [calcium] is normal)
- Phosphate-containing enemas
- Laboratory error

INITIAL DATABASE

- Complete serum biochemistry profile: identifies hypocalcemia.
- Serum ionized calcium: differentiates between absolute hypocalcemia and relative (i.e., metabolically insignificant) hypocalcemia.
- Serum magnesium: identifies hypomagnesemia.
- Electrocardiogram.

ADVANCED OR CONFIRMATORY TESTING

- Serum parathyroid hormone concentration
- Serum vitamin D concentration

TREATMENT

THERAPEUTIC GOAL(S)

Increase serum calcium concentration above the threshold responsible for clinical signs:

- Total calcium above 6–7 mg/dl (1.5–1.75 mmol/L)
- Ionized calcium above 2.4–2.8 mg/dl (0.6–0.7 mmol/L)

ACUTE GENERAL TREATMENT

- Intravenous calcium infusion:
  - Administer 10% calcium gluconate IV at a dose of 0.5–1.5 ml/kg or 5–15 mg/kg slowly, to effect, over 15 to 30 minutes.
  - Electrographic monitoring is recommended during IV calcium administration.
  - The infusion should be slowed/discontinued if bradycardia, ventricular premature complexes, or shortening of the Q-T interval is observed.
- Once clinical signs have improved, continue parenteral calcium administration. Calcium can be given either as a continuous intravenous infusion at 60–90 mg/kg/day of elemental calcium (10% calcium gluconate contains 9.3 mg/ml of elemental calcium) or as a subcutaneous bolus every 6 to 8 hours at a dose of 1–2 ml/kg of 10% calcium gluconate. Calcium gluconate must be diluted 1:1 in saline before being administered subcutaneously.

CHRONIC TREATMENT

- Vitamin D: calcitriol is the form of vitamin D recommended for maintenance therapy (rapid onset of action, short half-life, does not require hepatic/renal transformation).
  - Loading dose: 0.02–0.03 μg/kg/day divided q 12h PO for 4 days.
  - Maintenance dose: 0.005–0.015 μg/kg/day divided q 12h.
  - Maximal effect is seen 1 to 4 days after initiation of treatment. Maintenance dose should be adjusted to obtain normocalcemia.
- Calcium supplementation: calcium carbonate (1 g = 20 mEq calcium) is recommended at a dose of 25 mg/kg q 8–12h PO. Dose should be adjusted to obtain normocalcemia.
  - Once normocalcemia is achieved, the dose of oral calcium can be slowly decreased and stopped. Vitamin D must be continued until the underlying disorder is corrected.
- Therapy with synthetic PTH is not currently available.

POSSIBLE COMPLICATIONS

Subcutaneous calcium administration has been associated with the development of calcinosis cutis and therefore the IV route may be preferable.

RECOMMENDED MONITORING

Monitor total serum calcium: target level 8–9.5 mg/dl (just below reference range).

PROGNOSIS AND OUTCOME

Dependent on the underlying disease

PEARLS & CONSIDERATIONS

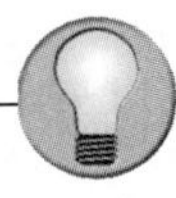

COMMENTS

- Calcium must not be measured on ethylenediamine tetraacetic acid-anticoagulated (EDTA) blood. EDTA will chelate the calcium falsely lowering its value. Therefore, avoid lavender-top tubes for serum calcium measurement.
- Avoid the use of calcium chloride for injections or infusions, as it is very caustic.
- Hypoalbuminemia may cause a mild decrease in the protein-bound fraction of calcium, thus resulting in a mildly decreased total serum calcium. Ionized calcium remains normal.
- Correcting the calcium value to compensate for albumin is not valid in dogs or cats; ionized calcium measurement is accurate.

CLIENT EDUCATION

The owner should be informed of clinical signs associated with hypocalcemia to ensure early and rapid detection.

SUGGESTED READING

Feldman EC, Nelson RW: Hypocalcemia and primary hypoparathyroidism. In *Canine and Feline Endocrinology and Reproduction*, ed 3. St. Louis, WB Saunders, 2004, pp 716–741.

Feldman EC: Disorders of the parathyroid gland. In Ettinger SJ, Feldman EC (eds): *Textbook of Veterinary Internal Medicine*, ed 6. St. Louis, WB Saunders, 2005, pp 1508–1535.

Henderson AK, et al: Hypoparathyroidism: pathophysiology and diagnosis. *Comp Cont Educ Pract* 27(4):270–279, 2005.

Henderson AK, et al: Hypoparathyroidism: treatment. *Comp Cont Educ Pract* 27(4):280–287, 2005.

AUTHOR: **MARILYN DUNN**

EDITOR: **ETIENNE CÔTÉ**

Hypokalemia

BASIC INFORMATION

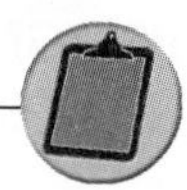

DEFINITION

Serum potassium concentration <3.5 mEq/L

EPIDEMIOLOGY

SPECIES, AGE, SEX: Cats are more likely to show clinical signs than dogs.
- Cats: signs may be seen when serum potassium is between 3.0 and 3.5 mEq/L.
- Dogs: signs may not be evident until serum potassium is <2.5 mEq/L.

GENETICS AND BREED PREDISPOSITION: A familial, inherited (assumed autosomal recessive) hypokalemic myopathy has been reported in 2- to 12-month-old Burmese kittens.

RISK FACTORS: Cats: dietary factors, such as potassium-depleted, acidifying, magnesium-restricted, and/or high-protein diets. Canned feline diets have now been modified to reduce this risk.

CLINICAL PRESENTATION

DISEASE FORMS/SUBTYPES
- Musculoskeletal:
  - Generalized muscle weakness
  - Polymyopathy: increased serum creatine kinase, electromyographic abnormalities (most notable in cats)
- Cardiovascular:
  - Variable clinical expression
- Renal:
  - Chronic tubulointerstitial nephritis, impaired renal function, azotemia (most notable in cats)
- GI (paralytic ileus):
  - Rare in dogs and cat
  - Abdominal distention
  - Constipation

HISTORY, CHIEF COMPLAINT
- Many dogs and cats have no obvious signs.
- Generalized skeletal muscle weakness: most common complaint.
- Hypokalemic polymyopathy in cats: flaccid ventroflexion of neck, forelimb hypermetria, broad-based stance in hind limbs.
- Polyuria, polydipsia, decreased urine concentrating ability.
- Vomiting; diarrhea, or constipation.

PHYSICAL EXAM FINDINGS
- Musculoskeletal
  - Generalized skeletal muscle weakness
  - Cats with polymyopathy: flaccid ventroflexion of neck, forelimb hypermetria, broad-based stance in hind limbs
- Cardiovascular
  - Arrhythmias
  - Abnormalities often only detectable by electrocardiography
- GI (paralytic ileus)
  - Rare in dogs and cats
  - Abdominal distention
  - Constipation

ETIOLOGY AND PATHOPHYSIOLOGY

- Increased potassium loss in urine:
  - Chronic renal failure (cats)
  - Diet-induced hypokalemic nephropathy (cats)
  - Renal tubular acidosis
  - Postobstructive diuresis (cats with urethral obstruction)
  - Diuretic administration
  - Dialysis
  - Hyperaldosteronism
  - Hyperadrenocorticism
- Increased potassium loss via GI tract:
  - Vomiting
  - Diarrhea
- Increased potassium sequestration into cells (translocation from extracellular to intracellular fluid) may occur with alkalemia, insulin release, catecholamine release:
  - Alkalemia: potassium ions enter cells in exchange for hydrogen ions
  - Insulin: promotes uptake of glucose and potassium by hepatocytes and skeletal muscle cells
  - Severe illness: stress leads to epinephrine release, which contributes to hypokalemia
- Decreased potassium dietary intake:
  - Uncommon; may be a contributing factor
- Iatrogenic:
  - Fluid therapy, insulin therapy, bicarbonate therapy, loop and thiazide diuretics, enemas, parenteral nutrition
- Combinations of factors:
  - Diabetic ketoacidosis

DIAGNOSIS

DIFFERENTIAL DIAGNOSIS

See Etiology and Pathophysiology above

INITIAL DATABASE

- Complete blood count: no specific abnormality
- Serum biochemistry profile: establish diagnosis
- Urinalysis

ADVANCED OR CONFIRMATORY TESTING

- Do 24-hour urine potassium excretion (confirmation of excess renal potassium excretion)
- ACTH stimulation; low-dose dexamethasone suppression (hyperadrenocorticism)
- Serum aldosterone levels, abdominal ultrasound exam (hyperaldosteronism)
- Electrocardiography:
  - Hypokalemia delays ventricular repolarization, increases duration of action potential, increases automaticity
  - Supraventricular and ventricular arrhythmias may be seen
  - Decreased T wave amplitude and ST segment depression (often seen in human patients) are not consistent findings in dogs and cats
- Echocardiography:
  - Decreased myocardial contractility
  - Decreased cardiac output

TREATMENT

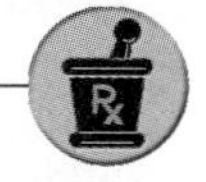

THERAPEUTIC GOAL(S)

- Reestablish normal serum potassium levels, while avoiding hyperkalemia
- Maintain normal serum potassium levels long-term
- Therapy indicated if serum potassium <3.0 mEq/L, or clinical signs of hypokalemia evident, or serum potassium loss expected

ACUTE GENERAL TREATMENT

- Potassium chloride (KCl) administered IV at a rate not to exceed 0.5 mEq/kg/hr.
- In dogs and cats with normal renal function, maintenance potassium concentration should be approximately 20 mEq/L of fluids, given at a rate of 40 ml/kg/day IV.
- Concentration of potassium in IV fluids should not exceed 60 mEq/L (in most cases); higher concentrations can cause pain and sclerosis of peripheral veins.
- Although IV administration is preferred, KCl can be given subcutaneously as long as potassium concentration in fluids is less than 30 mEq/L.
- In mildly affected patients, oral potassium gluconate (Kaon Elixir, Tumil-K) may be the only therapy required; starting dose is 0.33–1 mEq/kg q 8h.

CHRONIC TREATMENT

Once serum potassium is in normal range, oral potassium gluconate is continued at a maintenance dosage of 0.5 mEq/kg PO q 12h until inciting cause is eliminated

DRUG INTERACTIONS

Using potassium supplementation along with angiotensin-converting enzyme inhibitors, potassium-sparing diuretics (e.g., spironolactone), prostaglandin inhibitors, or β-blockers may result in hyperkalemia.

POSSIBLE COMPLICATIONS

Cardiac arrhythmias

RECOMMENDED MONITORING

During acute treatment phase, adjustments in IV potassium therapy should be based on serum potassium concentration measured once or twice a day

PROGNOSIS AND OUTCOME

- Clinical signs usually resolve within 1 to 5 days after correction of hypokalemia
- Depending on cause, long-term oral potassium supplementation may be required

PEARLS & CONSIDERATIONS

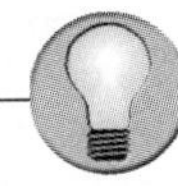

COMMENTS

- Clinical signs associated with hypokalemia are seen more commonly in cats than in dogs.
- Chronic renal failure is the most common condition associated with hypokalemia in cats; approximately 20–30% of cats with chronic renal failure are hypokalemic at presentation.
- Most dogs with chronic renal failure have normal serum potassium concentrations.
- A common iatrogenic cause of hypokalemia is IV administration of potassium-deficient fluids to anorectic patients; solutions used for maintenance fluid therapy should contain 15 to 30 mEq potassium/L to avoid this complication.

SUGGESTED READING

DiBartola SP, de Morais HA: Disorders of potassium: hypokalemia and hyperkalemia. In DiBartola SP (ed): *Fluid Therapy in Small Animal Practice*, ed 2. Philadelphia, WB Saunders, 2000, pp 83–107.

Dow SW, et al: Potassium depletion in cats: hypokalemic polymyopathy. *J Am Vet Med Assoc* 191:1563–1568, 1987.

AUTHOR: **MICHAEL BERNSTEIN**

EDITOR: **ETIENNE CÔTÉ**

Hyponatremia

BASIC INFORMATION

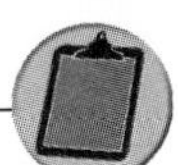

DEFINITION

Low serum sodium (<125 mEq/L) with plasma hypoosmolality; it may be associated with low, normal, or high plasma tonicity

EPIDEMIOLOGY

SPECIES, AGE, SEX: Dogs and cats: no breed or sex predilection.

GENETICS AND BREED PREDISPOSITION: None.

RISK FACTORS

- Renal insufficiency
- Excessive water intake
- Hypoadrenocorticism
- Severe liver disease or end-stage heart failure

ASSOCIATED CONDITIONS AND DISORDERS: Osmotic demyelination syndrome (neurologic signs).

CLINICAL PRESENTATION

DISEASE FORMS/SUBTYPES

- Clinical signs are related to the rapidity of onset rather than to severity of hyponatremia or hypoosmolality
- Signs in humans are often seen with acute levels less than 120 mEq/L or a drop at a rate greater than 0.5 mEq/L/hr
- Can lead to cerebral edema
- Clinical signs may be absent in chronic cases

HISTORY, CHIEF COMPLAINT

- Mild lethargy
- Nausea and vomiting
- Abdominal distention
- Weight gain
- Seizures, incoordination, and coma

PHYSICAL EXAM FINDINGS

- Patient can exhibit signs of dehydration including decreased skin turgor and tacky mucous membranes
- Signs of third spacing such as ascites or edema
- Hypovolemia with weak pulses, tachycardia, prolonged capillary refill time

ETIOLOGY AND PATHOPHYSIOLOGY

- Hypotonic (dilutional) hyponatremia:
  - Excess of water relative to existing sodium stores.
  - Most commonly due to impaired renal excretion of water.
  - Other causes include congestive heart failure, severe liver disease, nephrotic syndrome.
  - Except for renal disease, characterized by high plasma concentrations of arginine vasopressin (antidiuretic hormone) despite hypotonicity.
  - Ascites or edema is common.
  - Excessive water intake may also be a cause.
- Isotonic hyponatremia:
  - Associated with volume depletion (hypovolemia).
  - Causes include loss of fluid via gastrointestinal tract, loss into third spaces (peritoneal effusion, pleural effusion) and renal loss.
  - Hypotonicity with loss of hypotonic fluid results from:
    - A decrease in glomerular filtration rate increases isosmotic resorption of sodium and water in the proximal tubules and decreases delivery of tubular fluid to the distal diluting sites.
    - Volume depletion causes vasopressin release, which impairs water excretion.
    - Stimulation of thirst due to the volume depletion, which causes the animal to drink water.
- Hypertonic (translocational) hyponatremia:
  - Hyperglycemia.
  - Retention of hypertonic mannitol in patients with renal insufficiency.
- Pseudohyponatremia.

DIAGNOSIS

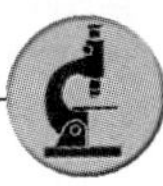

DIFFERENTIAL DIAGNOSIS

Pseudohyponatremia:

- Obtain plasma osmolality; hypernatremic patients with normal osmolality have pseudohyponatremia.
- Pseudohyponatremia is a laboratory artifact that may be seen with hyperlipidemia and severe hyperproteinemia.

INITIAL DATABASE

- Complete blood count
- Serum biochemistry profile and urinalysis
- Abdominal and thoracic radiographs
- Abdominal ultrasound
- Calculated serum osmolality

ADVANCED OR CONFIRMATORY TESTING

- Thyroid panel
- Adrenocorticotropic hormone stimulation
- Abdominocentesis or thoracocentesis with fluid analysis

TREATMENT

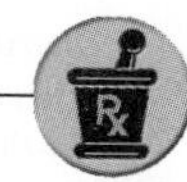

THERAPEUTIC GOAL(S)

- Diagnose and manage underlying disease
- If clinical signs are present, increase sodium concentration and osmolality

ACUTE GENERAL TREATMENT

- Aim to increase serum sodium concentrations by a maximum of 2-3 mEq/hr.
- The use of conventional crystalloids such as lactated Ringer's solution or 0.9% saline is recommended.
- Restore volume if patient is hypovolemic.
- Treatment of underlying cause if systemic disorder.

CHRONIC TREATMENT

- Aim to increase serum sodium concentration by 0.7 mEq/hr.
- Management/resolution of systemic disorder if present.
- Mild water restriction with serum sodium concentration monitoring can be effective.
- Edematous patients should be treated with a combination of sodium-restricted diet, saline, and diuretics.
- Do not correct at a rate of greater than 12-15 mEq/L/day.

POSSIBLE COMPLICATIONS

- Increasing the rate faster than the body can compensate by restoring organic osmolytes can lead to brain dehydration (rapid shifts in osmolality will cause disorders of the central nervous system secondary to dehydration of the brain).
- Brain injury causes osmotic demyelination syndrome, which leads to cerebral edema, seizures, and other neurologic signs.

RECOMMENDED MONITORING

Frequent monitoring of electrolytes including serum sodium and potassium concentrations

PROGNOSIS AND OUTCOME

Good, provided underlying problem can be reversed or eliminated, and overly rapid correction is avoided

PEARLS & CONSIDERATIONS

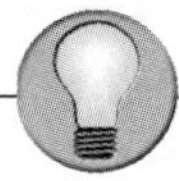

COMMENTS

When treating acute hyponatremia, correction can be made as quickly as the hyponatremia developed (i.e., if the sodium dropped in 24 hours, it can be entirely corrected in 24 hours).

CLIENT EDUCATION

Related to underlying disease

SUGGESTED READING

Bissett SA, Lamb M, Ward CR: Hyponatremia and hyperkalemia associated with peritoneal effusion in four cats. *J Am Vet Med Assoc* 218:1590-1592, 2001.

DiBartola, S: Hyponatremia. *Vet Clin North Am Small Anim Pract* 28:515-532, 1998.

Dibartola S: Disorders of sodium and water: hypernatremia and hyponatremia. *Fluid Therapy in Small Animal Practice,* ed 2. Philadelphia, WB Saunders, 2000, pp 45-71.

AUTHORS: **YONAIRA CORTÉS, ANN MARIE MANNING**

EDITOR: **ETIENNE CÔTÉ**

Hypoparathyroidism, Primary

BASIC INFORMATION

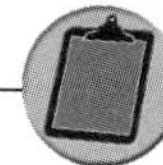

DEFINITION

An absolute or relative deficiency of parathyroid hormone (PTH) from parathyroid gland destruction or atrophy, causing hypocalcemia

EPIDEMIOLOGY

SPECIES, AGE, SEX

- Uncommon disorder in dogs and cats
- Dogs: any age, breed, or sex may be affected
- Cats: any age or breed; male predominance

CLINICAL PRESENTATION

HISTORY/CHIEF COMPLAINT

- Sporadic or episodic signs, all related to hypocalcemia (see Hypocalcemia, p 564):
  - Muscle tremors or twitching that may be focal or diffuse, and may worsen with exercise or excitement
  - Facial rubbing
  - Biting or licking paws
  - Seizures
  - Stiff gait, rear leg muscle pain/cramping
  - Behavior changes (restless, nervous, anxious, aggressive, reluctant to be touched)
  - Decreased activity
- Less common signs: weakness, vomiting, diarrhea, and weight loss

PHYSICAL EXAM FINDINGS

- Neuromuscular signs (see History/Chief Complaint above); raised nictitating membranes possible (cats).
- Additional findings may include nonfebrile hyperthermia (from muscle fasciculations), tense abdomen, thin body condition, or cataracts.
- Physical examination may be normal.

ETIOLOGY AND PATHOPHYSIOLOGY

ETIOLOGY

- Naturally occurring disease is suspected to be due to immune-mediated destruction or idiopathic atrophy of the parathyroid glands.

PATHOPHYSIOLOGY

- In normal animals, PTH secretion is controlled by ionized calcium concentrations via negative feedback, but with hypoparathyroidism the parathyroid glands are unable to respond to hypocalcemia.
- Loss of PTH results in sustained, potentially severe hypocalcemia and hyperphosphatemia.
  - Hypocalcemia results from decreased resorption of calcium from bone, decreased intestinal absorption of calcium, and increased renal excretion of calcium.
  - Hyperphosphatemia occurs due to decreased renal phosphate excretion.

DIAGNOSIS

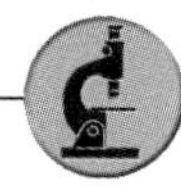

DIFFERENTIAL DIAGNOSIS

Hypocalcemia (see Hypocalcemia, p 564)

INITIAL DATABASE

- Complete blood count, serum biochemical profile, urinalysis: hypocalcemia and hyperphosphatemia
- Confirm hypocalcemia:

TABLE I-8 **Vitamin D Preparations**

Preparation	Daily Dose	Time to Maximal Effect	Time Required for Toxicity Relief
Vitamin D_2 (ergocalciferol)	Initial: 4000–6000 U/kg PO q 24h Maintenance: 1000–2000 U/kg PO q 24h to q week	5–21 days	1–18 weeks
Dihydrotachysterol	Initial: 0.02–0.03 mg/kg PO q 24h Maintenance: 0.01–0.02 mg/kg PO q 24–48h	1–7 days	1–3 weeks
Vitamin D_1 (calcitriol)	Approximately 0.02–0.06 ug/kg PO q 24h	1–4 days	1–14 days

- Repeat calcium measurement on a separate blood sample to confirm hypocalcemia.
- Calculate "corrected" serum calcium to account for changes in total calcium due to serum protein values (see Hypocalcemia, p 564) (not applicable in cats) or preferably, measure serum ionized calcium concentration.

ADVANCED OR CONFIRMATORY TESTING

- Primary hypoparathyroidism is confirmed by evaluating concurrent serum ionized calcium and PTH concentrations; both will usually be decreased.
- A low-normal serum PTH concentration is inappropriate if ionized calcium concentration is low; thus in a patient with low ionized calcium, a serum PTH concentration that is either decreased or low-normal is compatible with a diagnosis of primary hypoparathyroidism.

TREATMENT

THERAPEUTIC GOAL(S)

- Increase serum calcium concentrations above the threshold for clinical signs and maintain them just below or at the low end of the reference range (i.e., 8–9.5 mg/dl [2–2.4 mmol/L]).
- "Overtreatment" resulting in hypercalcemia must be avoided.

ACUTE GENERAL TREATMENT

For hypocalcemic tetany: see Hypocalcemia, p 564

CHRONIC TREATMENT

- Subacute/early chronic treatment:
  - Oral vitamin D:
    - Three forms available: See Table I-8 below.
    - Quicker- and shorter-acting forms (and therefore easier to use for dosage adjustments) are more expensive.
  - Oral calcium:
    - Dose: 0.5–2 g calcium PO q 12h (dogs); 0.25–0.5 g calcium PO q 12h (cats).
    - The amount of elemental calcium per tablet varies with the preparation.
    - Once the serum calcium concentration is stable and the dog is eating well, oral calcium supplementation can be tapered over 2 to 3 weeks and then discontinued, as dietary calcium is adequate for most dogs.
  - Parenteral calcium administration is usually needed during the time it takes for oral vitamin D and oral calcium supplementation to take effect:
    - Calcium gluconate SQ q 6–8h (initial doses as for Acute General Treatment in Hypocalcemia (see p 564); dilute one part calcium to 2–4 parts saline) or continuous IV calcium infusion (60–90 mg/kg q 24h; do not add to bicarbonate-containing fluids). Do NOT give calcium chloride SQ as perivascular administration can cause tissue necrosis and sloughing.
    - Monitor serum calcium concentrations q 12–24h and adjust dose to maintain serum calcium concentration between 8–9.5 mg/dL (2.0–2.4 mmol/L). When serum calcium concentrations have been consistently above 8 mg/dL (2 mmol/L) for 48 hours, parenteral calcium can be tapered and discontinued over 3 to 7 days by increasing the dosing interval.
- Maintenance/long-term chronic treatment:
  - Vitamin D can be tapered over 3 to 6 months by gradually increasing the interval between doses (by approximately 1 day every 2 to 3 weeks based on serum calcium concentrations). Vitamin D should be tapered to the lowest dose (i.e., longest dosing interval) possible to maintain stable serum calcium concentrations. Lifelong therapy with vitamin D is necessary with primary hypoparathyroidism.

POSSIBLE COMPLICATIONS

- Overzealous treatment with vitamin D may result in hypercalcemia. Hypercalcemia in conjunction with hyperphosphatemia puts animals at risk for soft tissue (including renal) mineralization.
- Although SQ calcium gluconate is generally deemed safe, severe, extensive calcinosis cutis with pyogranulomatous dermatitis, dermoepidermal separation, and epidermal necrosis has been reported following SQ administration of calcium gluconate for primary hypoparathyroidism. The author is aware of at least one additional similar anecdotal report.

RECOMMENDED MONITORING

- During the immediate post-tetanic phase, patients should be observed 24 hours/day for seizures and other clinical signs of hypocalcemia.
- Serum calcium and phosphorus concentrations should initially be measured at least q 12–24h, then with decreasing frequency as serum calcium concentration stabilizes. When patients are stable with maintenance oral vitamin D therapy, evaluation of serum calcium and phosphorus concentrations is recommended q 3–6 months.

PROGNOSIS AND OUTCOME

With careful treatment and monitoring, prognosis is excellent

PEARLS & CONSIDERATIONS

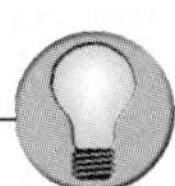

COMMENTS

Referral is indicated if 24-hour care and in-house serum calcium monitoring cannot be provided during the immediate post-tetanic period

CLIENT EDUCATION

Treatment must be lifelong for dogs with naturally-occurring hypoparathyroidism

SUGGESTED READING

Hypocalcemia and primary hypoparathyroidism. In Feldman and Nelson (eds): *Canine and Feline Endocrinology and Reproduction*. Philadelphia, WB Saunders, pp 716–742.

Schaer M, Ginn P, Fox L, Leon J, Ramirez F: Severe calcinosis cutis associated with treatment of hypoparathyroidism in a dog. *J Am Anim Hosp Assoc* 37:364–369, 2001.

AUTHOR: **CARY L. M. BASSETT**
EDITOR: **SHERRI IHLE**

Hypoplastic Trachea

BASIC INFORMATION

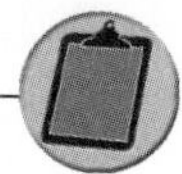

DEFINITION

Congenital abnormal narrowing of the tracheal lumen

SYNONYM(S)

Congenital tracheal stenosis
Tracheal hypoplasia
Wheezer syndrome

EPIDEMIOLOGY

SPECIES, AGE, SEX: Dogs <1 year old; 2:1 males:females. Not reported in cats.
GENETICS AND BREED PREDISPOSITION: Bulldogs, Boston terriers, and boxers are predisposed. Also reported as a recessive trait in Husky mix puppies with blue eyes and partially white faces.
ASSOCIATED CONDITIONS AND DISORDERS: Brachycephalic syndrome (elongated soft palate in 43%, stenotic nares in 22%). Other congenital anomalies (pulmonic or aortic stenosis, megaesophagus) or respiratory abnormalities (bronchopneumonia, laryngeal paralysis, everted laryngeal saccules) may be present.

CLINICAL PRESENTATION

HISTORY, CHIEF COMPLAINT

- Dyspnea, respiratory distress
- Stridor
- Exercise intolerance, lethargy
- Coughing
- Gagging
- Syncope
- Recurrent respiratory infections with poor response to treatment
- Incidental finding in approximately 10% of affected dogs

PHYSICAL EXAM FINDINGS

- Physical examination can be unremarkable
- Abnormalities attributable to dyspnea or bronchopneumonia:
  - Cough
  - Stridor (inspiratory, may be high-pitched or gasping sounds)
  - Increased lung sounds
  - Fever
  - Lethargy
  - Increased respiratory rate and effort

ETIOLOGY AND PATHOPHYSIOLOGY

- Trachea develops with cartilaginous rings apposed or overlapped and dorsal membrane narrow or absent, narrowing the tracheal lumen.
- With narrowed tracheal lumen, linear air velocity and tracheal resistance increase, increasing work of respiration.

DIAGNOSIS

DIFFERENTIAL DIAGNOSIS

- Elongated soft palate
- Everted laryngeal saccules
- Stenotic nares
- Laryngeal paralysis or collapse
- Tracheal collapse
- Any cause of bronchopneumonia or tracheobronchitis

INITIAL DATABASE

- Complete blood count: inflammatory leukogram possible if bronchopneumonia present
- Serum biochemistry panel and urinalysis: usually normal
- Thoracic radiographs:
  - Diffusely narrowed tracheal lumen
  - Bronchopneumonia in approximately 8% of cases

ADVANCED OR CONFIRMATORY TESTING

- Decrease in tracheal diameter on lateral thoracic radiograph:
  - TD:TI ratio is the ratio of tracheal diameter (TD) at the level of the thoracic inlet to the thoracic inlet diameter (TI, distance from the ventral aspect of the vertebral column at the midpoint of the first rib to the closest point on the inner surface of the manubrium).
  - For dogs over 6 months, normal TD:TI = 0.18 for nonbrachycephalic breeds, 0.21 for nonbulldog brachycephalic breeds, and 0.14 for bulldogs.
  - Ratios lower than these indicate tracheal stenosis (assuming a diffuse, not focal, narrowing).
- Tracheoscopy/bronchoscopy or transtracheal wash for cytology, culture and sensitivity in dogs with nonresponsive bronchopneumonia.
- Histopathologic evaluation: generally not beneficial:
  - Overlap or apposition of tracheal rings.
  - Dorsal membrane folded, narrowed, or absent.

TREATMENT

THERAPEUTIC GOAL(S)

- Treat secondary infection
- Reduce respiratory effort

ACUTE GENERAL TREATMENT

- Oxygen
- Sedation (e.g., acepromazine 0.03-0.05 mg/kg IV [e.g., 0.25-0.5 mg (0.025-0.05 ml) total dose for medium-size dog] with butorphanol 0.2-0.4 mg/kg IV q 2-4h as needed) if dyspneic or hyperpneic
- If bronchopneumonia is present, broad-spectrum antibiotic treatment based on results of culture and sensitivity

CHRONIC TREATMENT

- Reduce weight if obese
- Limit exercise, reduce stress
- Correct associated respiratory defects (see Brachycephalic Airway Syndrome, p 149; Laryngeal Paralysis, p 619)

POSSIBLE COMPLICATIONS

Death from severe respiratory distress or bronchopneumonia

RECOMMENDED MONITORING

Repeat thoracic films in 1 to 2 weeks in dogs with bronchopneumonia:

- Radiographic improvement of bronchopneumonia can lag several days behind clinical improvement

PROGNOSIS AND OUTCOME

Mortality rate (death or euthanasia) 50% and often reflects associated respiratory disease or other defects (megaesophagus, cardiac disease)

PEARLS & CONSIDERATIONS

COMMENTS

- Dyspnea is not necessarily related to the degree of tracheal lumen diameter narrowing in dogs with tracheal hypoplasia.
- Some degree of diffuse increase in tracheal diameter may be seen after clinical improvement; this increase in diameter is attributed to reduced tracheal mucosal edema.

PREVENTION

There are no means of preventing this disease. Affected animals should not be bred.

CLIENT EDUCATION

- Consider thoracic radiographs of bulldogs, boxers, Boston terriers before breeding
- Affected dogs have lifelong risk of respiratory infections and dyspnea

SUGGESTED READING

Coyne BE, Fingland RB: Hypoplasia of the trachea in dogs: 103 cases (1974-1990). *J Am Vet Med Assoc* 201:768, 1992.
van Pelt RW: Confirming tracheal hypoplasia in Husky-mix puppies. *Vet Med* 83:266, 1988.

AUTHOR: **KAREN M. TOBIAS**
EDITOR: **RANCE K. SELLON**

Hypopyon

BASIC INFORMATION

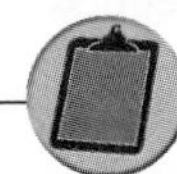

DEFINITION

Accumulation of white blood cells in the anterior chamber of the eye

SYNONYM(S)

Pus in the anterior chamber

EPIDEMIOLOGY

SPECIES, AGE, SEX: Dogs and cats; any age or sex.

RISK FACTORS

- Severe anterior uveitis of any cause (see Uveitis, p 1134)
- Lymphosarcoma (see Intraocular Neoplasia, p 603)

GEOGRAPHY AND SEASONALITY: Generally none except some forms of infectious uveitis.

ASSOCIATED CONDITIONS AND DISORDERS

- Anterior uveitis is usually present concurrently.
- Animals affected with anterior uveitis may have associated systemic signs.
- Intraocular lymphosarcoma (see Intraocular Neoplasia, p 603).
- Infected corneal ulcers.
- Endophthalmitis (i.e., inflammation of the uveal tract and anterior and posterior compartments of the eye).
- Panophthalmitis (i.e., inflammation of the uveal tract and anterior and posterior compartments of the eye and extension of the inflammation into the orbit).

CLINICAL PRESENTATION

DISEASE FORMS/SUBTYPES

- Early forms of incipient hypopyon may be recognized by cells floating in anterior chamber.
- Keratic precipitates are forms of white blood cell aggregates in which multiple, round to ovoid, gray to yellowish opacities are noted on the posterior cornea.
- Gross hypopyon is recognized as ventral accumulation or complete filling of anterior chamber with white to yellow opacity.

HISTORY, CHIEF COMPLAINT

- White to yellow opacity inside the eye
- Conjunctival injection
- Signs of uveitis (see Uveitis, p 1134)

PHYSICAL EXAM FINDINGS

- Dependent on the underlying cause.
- Varying degrees of a creamy white "keel boat" opacity in the anterior chamber.
- Other signs of anterior uveitis (see Uveitis, p 1134).
- Corneal ulceration may be present (see Corneal Ulceration, p 246).

ETIOLOGY AND PATHOPHYSIOLOGY

- Numerous causes of uveitis (see Uveitis, p 1134) result in inflammatory breakdown of blood-aqueous barrier allowing white blood cells into anterior chamber by:
  - Strong leukotaxic stimulus such as intraocular bacterial or fungal infection
  - Corneal infections producing inflammatory mediators that diffuse into anterior chamber
- Leukemias and intraocular lymphosarcoma may be associated with white blood cell accumulation in the anterior chamber.

DIAGNOSIS

DIFFERENTIAL DIAGNOSIS

- Lipids in the anterior chamber are milky/white but invariably diffuse.
- Fibrin in anterior chamber; generally irregular clot rather than ventrally located fluid line.

INITIAL DATABASE

- Thorough ocular and physical examinations to search for a source of sepsis or for a malignancy either locally in or on the eye, or systemically.
- Corneal swab for cytology and culture in cases of infected corneal ulcers.
- Complete blood count, chemistry profile, urinalysis for evidence of systemic disease if no ocular cause of hypopyon is found.
- If disease is so severe as to preclude posterior segment examination, ocular ultrasound is indicated to detect evidence of endophthalmitis, foreign bodies, neoplasia.
- Aspiration of anterior chamber (anterior chamber/aqueous centesis) for culture and cytologic evaluation (referable procedure).
  - In eyes with *mild* hypopyon, or those associated with corneal disease, centesis is often not performed because the signs are often ameliorated by the time the culture results are known, or the cornea is a better source for culturing.

ADVANCED OR CONFIRMATORY TESTING

If cause for hypopyon is anterior uveitis of systemic origin, appropriate systemic work-up is advised (see Uveitis, p 1134)

TREATMENT

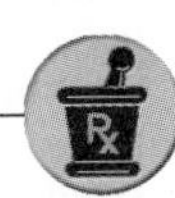

THERAPEUTIC GOAL(S)

Treat the underlying disease; hypopyon itself is *not* treated

ACUTE GENERAL TREATMENT

- Frequent, topical broad-spectrum antibiotic (i.e., fluoroquinolones q 4h, either second generation [e.g., ciprofloxacin, ofloxacin] or third generation [e.g., levofloxacin]).
  - Anterior chamber sepsis may not be present, but the risk is too great to delay initiation of antibiotics
- Systemic broad-spectrum bactericidal antibiotics (e.g., amoxicillin-clavulanic acid, 13.75 mg/kg PO q 12h).
- Topical 1% atropine sufficient to maintain pupil dilation (q 6-24h depending on severity of disease).
- Nonsteroidal anti-inflammatory drugs (NSAIDs) for uveitis:
  - Topical (flurbiprofen or diclofenac q 4-6h depending on severity of disease), and/or
  - Systemic (meloxicam 0.2 mg/kg SQ loading dose and 0.1 mg/kg PO q 24h [dog]; ketoprofen 2 mg/kg SQ loading dose and 1 mg/kg PO q 24h for 4 days [cat])

CHRONIC TREATMENT

Therapy may be modified to include corticosteroids depending on cause and/or culture results:

- Topical prednisolone acetate 1% or dexamethasone 0.1% q 4-12h depending on the severity of disease, and if corneal cause ruled out.
- Systemic prednisone: 0.5-2 mg/kg/day (dog); 1-3 mg/kg/day (cat); tapered over 10 to 14 days; use only if various systemic infectious causes of hypopyon ruled out.
- Do not use systemic NSAIDs and systemic glucocorticoids simultaneously (gastrointestinal ulceration).

POSSIBLE COMPLICATIONS

- Topical or systemic corticosteroids contraindicated if corneal ulceration/infection is the cause of hypopyon.
- Topical or systemic corticosteroids may be contraindicated with bacterial or fungal infections, but indicated with viral or lymphosarcoma-associated hypopyon.
- Secondary glaucoma (see Glaucoma, p 440).
- Blindness and enucleation are potential sequelae in cases due to sepsis.

RECOMMENDED MONITORING

- Monitor intraocular pressure to detect secondary glaucoma.
- If bacterial sepsis is suspected, initial ocular monitoring should be either daily or more frequently if significant inflammation is present.
- Frequency of rechecks dictated by severity of disease and response to treatment.

PROGNOSIS AND OUTCOME

- Prognosis variable, depending on underlying disease and response to treatment.
- Hypopyon improves rapidly with successful therapy of underlying cause.

PEARLS & CONSIDERATIONS

COMMENTS

- Most cases of hypopyon are culture-negative, but the risk for rapid structural damage to the eye is too great to withhold antibiotics until culture results are known.
- Generally, hypopyon produces minimal sequela.
- Hypopyon may be overlooked when mild (often occupies < 20% of anterior chamber), as the third eyelid may hinder visualization.

CLIENT EDUCATION

Blindness and enucleation are potential sequelae depending on the cause.

SUGGESTED READING

Martin CL: Anterior uvea and anterior chamber. In *Ophthalmic Disease in Veterinary Medicine*. London, Manson Publishing, 2005, pp 298–336.

Ramsay A, Lightman S: Hypopyon uveitis. *Surv Ophthalmol* 46:1, 2001.

AUTHOR: **CHARLES L. MARTIN**

EDITOR: **CHERYL L. CULLEN**

Hypotension, Systemic

BASIC INFORMATION

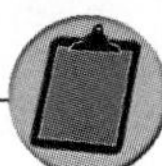

DEFINITION

A mean systemic arterial pressure <60 mmHg and a systolic pressure <80 mmHg

SYNONYM(S)

Low blood pressure

EPIDEMIOLOGY

SPECIES, AGE, SEX: Affects all species, ages, and sexes. The underlying disease may have a breed, sex, and age predilection.

ASSOCIATED CONDITIONS AND DISORDERS: Hypotension is associated with multiple disease processes (see Etiology and Pathophysiology below).

CLINICAL PRESENTATION

HISTORY, CHIEF COMPLAINT: Patients will have a history of lethargy, collapse, weakness, and/or decreased appetite. There may also be clinical signs related to the primary disease process (e.g., dyspnea/cough in a dog with hypotension due to critical congestive heart failure).

PHYSICAL EXAM FINDINGS

- Depression, weak pulses, pale mucous membranes, and delayed capillary refill time.
- Dogs will likely be tachycardic, whereas cats may display tachycardia or bradycardia.

ETIOLOGY AND PATHOPHYSIOLOGY

- There are multiple causes of hypotension:
  - Cardiac dysfunction:
    - Cardiomyopathies (dilated, hypertrophic, unclassified)
    - Pericardial effusion
    - Arrhythmias
    - Drug suppression of cardiac contractility (e.g., anesthetics, β-blockers)
  - Hypovolemia:
    - Hemorrhage
    - Gastrointestinal fluid losses
    - Burns
    - Urinary loss
    - Hypoadrenocorticism
  - Decreased vascular tone:
    - Sepsis
    - Anaphylaxis
    - Drugs (e.g., phenothiazines, angiotensin-converting enzyme (ACE) inhibitors, calcium channel blockers, nitroprusside)
- The body responds to a decrease in blood pressure in much the same way irrespective of cause.
- Decreased blood pressure causes the carotid sinus and aortic body receptors to respond, resulting in stimulation of the sympathetic nervous system, release of antidiuretic hormone (vasopressin) and adrenocorticotropic hormone from the pituitary, and release of catecholamines from the adrenal medulla.
- The renin-angiotensin-aldosterone system is stimulated: decreased arterial blood pressure elicits renin release from the juxtaglomerular cells of the kidney. In turn, renin transforms circulating angiotensinogen (α2-macroglobulin from liver) to angiotensin I, which is activated to the powerful vasoconstrictor angiotensin II by the ACE.
- These mechanisms lead to retention of sodium and water, vasoconstriction, and increased cardiac output, which all help to maintain blood pressure.

DIAGNOSIS

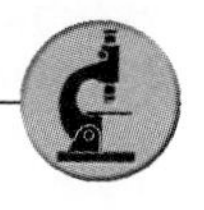

DIFFERENTIAL DIAGNOSIS

See Etiology and Pathophysiology above

INITIAL DATABASE

- Complete blood count (e.g., high or low white cell count if patient has underlying sepsis).
- Serum biochemistry profile: Azotemia is common and may be renal or prerenal; other abnormalities (e.g., liver enzyme elevations) may similarly be related to the causes, or may be the effects, of hypotension.
- Indirect or direct arterial blood pressure: diagnostic test of choice for confirming and monitoring hypotension.
- Thoracic and abdominal radiographs (evidence of pulmonary infiltrates [edema, hemorrhage, metastases], pneumonia, trauma, or effusions).
- Abdominocentesis: to assess the nature of a patient's effusion (e.g., hemorrhage), if present.

ADVANCED OR CONFIRMATORY TESTING

- Echocardiography to assess cardiac structure and function
- Abdominal ultrasound to assess for cause of abdominal effusion
- Computed tomography

TREATMENT

THERAPEUTIC GOAL(S)

The primary goal is to treat the underlying disease. If this goal cannot be achieved promptly or if results of treatment may not be immediate, restoration of blood pressure using other intravenous fluids or vasopressors may be necessary.

ACUTE GENERAL TREATMENT

- Volume replacement: selected according to type of fluid lost:
  - Crystalloids (lactated Ringer's solution, 0.9% NaCl): 40-90 ml/kg IV to effect.
  - Synthetic colloids: 5-20 ml/kg IV to effect.
  - Hypertonic saline: 4-6 ml/kg IV to effect (avoid if patient is dehydrated).
  - Blood, plasma (see Transfusion Therapy and Collection Techniques for Blood Banking, p 1312).
- Positive inotropic support: considered only after hydration is normalized, and used only if low cardiac contractility is documented. Short-term use (minutes-hours):
  - Dobutamine IV:
    - Dogs: 5-20 μg/kg/min.
    - Cats: 2.5-5 μg/kg/min.
- Vasopressors IV: only after hydration is normalized:
  - Dopamine: 7-20 μg/kg/min; or
  - Norepinephrine: 0.05-1 μg/kg/min; or
  - Epinephrine: 0.1-1 μg/kg/min; or
  - Vasopressin: 0.8 U/min.
- Pericardiocentesis if pericardial effusion is present

CHRONIC TREATMENT

Treatment of the underlying cause (e.g., locate and stop source of hemorrhage, IV antibiotics for sepsis)

DRUG INTERACTIONS

Use of multiple vasopressors may lead to intense vasoconstriction that could result in organ ischemia. Catecholamines may precipitate cardiac arrhythmias.

POSSIBLE COMPLICATIONS

Complications related to severe or protracted hypotension include:

- Renal failure
- Loss of gastrointestinal integrity with absorption of bacteria and bacterial toxins
- Myocardial dysfunction
- Brain ischemia
- Loss of vascular tone

RECOMMENDED MONITORING

- Monitor blood pressure either indirectly (cuff) or directly (arterial line) until blood pressure has normalized.
- If hypovolemia is present then can utilize central venous pressure (CVP) as an indicator of volume status; if the CVP is less than 5 cmH_2O then more fluids should be given. Adequate fluid resuscitation is present if the CVP is between 5 and 10 cmH_2O. Exception: heart disease affecting the left ventricle or mitral valve, where volume-overload pulmonary edema can occur despite normal CVP.
- Monitor for signs of end-organ damage (e.g., urine output).
- If hemorrhage is suspected monitor hematocrit and total solids.
- Monitor ECG if arrhythmias are the cause of hypotension.

PROGNOSIS AND OUTCOME

- Prognosis depends on the cause of hypotension.
- In most patients, hypotension will respond to intravenous fluid therapy.
- Nonresponsive hypotension implies a poor prognosis, with multiple organ dysfunction a likely outcome.

PEARLS & CONSIDERATIONS

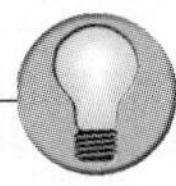

COMMENTS

- Hypotension is a serious consequence of multiple disease processes.
- Persistent hypotension implies ongoing hemorrhage, systemic vasodilation, or capillary leakage.
- Prompt identification and treatment of the underlying cause is essential to a successful outcome.

SUGGESTED READING

Macintire DK: Hypotension. In *Textbook of Veterinary Internal Medicine: Diseases of the Dog and Cat*, ed 5. Vol. 1. Philadelphia, WB Saunders, 2000, pp 183-186.

AUTHOR: **BENJAMIN DAVIDSON**
EDITOR: **ELIZABETH ROZANSKI**

Hypothermia

BASIC INFORMATION

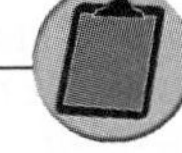

DEFINITION

Body temperature below 99.5°F (37.5°C) in the dog and 100°F (37.8°C) in the cat

EPIDEMIOLOGY

SPECIES, AGE, SEX: Any species, any age, and either sex can be affected.

RISK FACTORS

- Very old, very young animals
- Short-haired animals
- General anesthesia
- Cold environment
- Cardiac disease

CLINICAL PRESENTATION

DISEASE FORMS/SUBTYPES

- Mild hypothermia: 90.0-99.5°F (32.2°C-37.5°C)
- Moderate hypothermia: 82°F-90°F (27.8°C-32.2°C)
- Severe hypothermia: <82°F (27.8°C)

HISTORY, CHIEF COMPLAINT

- Weak or collapsed patient
- Exposure to cold environmental temperatures or general anesthesia

PHYSICAL EXAM FINDINGS

- Shivering
- Weakness
- Ataxia
- Cardiac arrhythmia
- Coma

ETIOLOGY AND PATHOPHYSIOLOGY

- Initial compensation for hypothermia: peripheral vasoconstriction, shivering, piloerection
- Respiratory rate and effort:
  - Increased with mild hypothermia.
  - Decreased with moderate to severe hypothermia (central and reflex-mediated respiratory depression).
- Cardiovascular effects:
  - Mild hypothermia initially increases heart rate and cardiac output.
  - Moderate hypothermia may produce bradycardia and, rarely, Osborn waves (positive electrocardiographic [ECG] deflection after S wave).
  - Severe hypothermia can cause cardiac arrest from ventricular fibrillation.
- Central nervous system:
  - Muscle shivering, stupor, unconsciousness, and coma.
- Gastrointestinal effects:
  - Ulceration.
  - Mild to severe pancreatitis.
- Renal effects:
  - Cold-induced diuresis can result in severe hypovolemia.

- Severely decreased renal perfusion can lead to ischemic tubular necrosis.
- Clinicopathologic changes:
  - Lactic acidosis due to tissue ischemia.
  - Leukopenia and thrombocytopenia (splenic sequestration).
  - Hyperglycemia.
  - Glucosuria.
  - Hyperkalemia.
  - Disseminated intravascular coagulopathy.

DIAGNOSIS

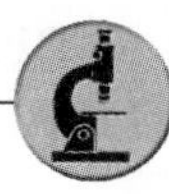

DIFFERENTIAL DIAGNOSIS

- Exposure to cold environment
- Pathologic hypothermia:
  - Hypoglycemia (puppies and kittens, endocrine diseases)
  - Hypothyroidism
  - Anesthesia
  - Severe, advanced cardiac disease (malperfusion)
  - Head trauma, brain disease

INITIAL DATABASE

- Documentation of rectal temperature <99.5°F (37.5°C)
- Packed cell volume, total solids, serum electrolytes

ADVANCED OR CONFIRMATORY TESTING

ECG:

- Sinus bradycardia: common, usually not treated beyond rewarming.
- Ventricular arrhythmias are common (see Ventricular Arrhythmias, p 1149).
- Mild changes (PR, QT, QRS prolongation). Osborn waves possible but less common.

TREATMENT

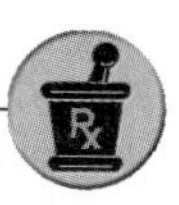

THERAPEUTIC GOAL(S)

- Restoring of core body temperature to normal range
- Treatment of hypothermia varies with:
  - Degree of hypothermia
  - Underlying systemic diseases (cardiovascular, neurologic)

ACUTE GENERAL TREATMENT

- Place intravenous catheter.
- In the unconscious patient, endotracheal intubation and oxygen supplementation (reduce risk of aspiration pneumonia and arrhythmias).
- Monitor urine output.
- Continuous ECG: to monitor for ventricular arrhythmias.
  - If unconscious patient and ventricular arrhythmias, prepare for ventricular fibrillation (requires defibrillation). The cold heart is relatively resistant to defibrillation. Rewarm patient and retry defibrillation.
  - The hypothermic heart hardly responds to antiarrhythmic drugs until a temperature of 86°F (30°C) is reached. Lidocaine is generally ineffective and procainamide is associated with increased ventricular fibrillation in humans.
  - Bradyarrhythmia does not respond to atropine, but resolves with rewarming.
- After addressing acute life-threatening problems, the patient needs to be assessed for the predisposing cause of hypothermia.
- Most hypothermic patients are dehydrated. Administer warm (body temperature) intravenous fluids. Fluid rate needs to be monitored closely due to decreased heart function and severe peripheral vasoconstriction. Start as a bolus of 5 to 11 ml/kg and titrate up as needed.
- Rewarming:
  - Depending on severity of hypothermia, three methods are useful.
    - Passive external rewarming. Use in mild to moderate hypothermia.
      - Animal is wrapped in blankets to prevent further loss of heat
    - Active external rewarming. Use for moderate to severe hypothermia
      - Apply heat (warm water bags, heating pads, warm incubator, bair hugger) to patient's torso.
    - Active internal rewarming. Generally used in severe hypothermia with temperature <86°F (30°C) or for animals that did not respond to other treatments.
    - Gastric, colon, and urinary bladder lavage with 109°F (42.8°C) warm 0.9% NaCl.
    - Peritoneal dialysis with warm 0.9% NaCl at a rate of 10–20 ml/kg and an exchange rate of every 30 minutes.
    - Increase inspired air temperature for animals on a ventilator.

POSSIBLE COMPLICATIONS

During the rewarming process, the extremities reduce vasoconstriction and sequestered cold blood mixes with the central circulation. Relatively warm core blood now perfuses the cold peripheral tissues. These two mechanisms cause "afterdrop," a decrease in body temperature during the rewarming process.

RECOMMENDED MONITORING

- ECG for ventricular arrhythmias during rewarming.
- Serum potassium levels during rewarming.
- Neurologic status during rewarming. Increased intracranial pressure may develop due to ischemic injury, cold-induced edema, or from osmotic gradients.
- Monitor fluid administration with urine output, blood pressure, central venous pressure, and respiratory effort.
- Monitor serum creatinine and blood urea nitrogen to ensure normal kidney function.

PROGNOSIS AND OUTCOME

Depending on severity of hypothermia, good to guarded prognosis

PEARLS & CONSIDERATIONS

COMMENTS

- Rewarming procedures should be tapered when the body temperature is still slightly below normal, to avoid overshooting (causing hyperthermia).
- Unconscious or debilitated patients are unable to move away from a heat source and meticulous monitoring (e.g., body temperature q 15–60 min) is essential during initial rewarming of these individuals. Burns and hyperthermic deaths have been recorded as a result of inadequate monitoring.

PREVENTION

- Avoid exposure to low environmental temperature
- Avoid prolonged general anesthesia

CLIENT EDUCATION

Keep pets indoors or in a protected environment during cold weather

RECOMMENDED READING

Ahn AH: Approach to the hypothermic patient. In Bonagura JD (ed): *Kirk's Current Veterinary Therapy XII*. Philadelphia, WB Saunders, 1995, pp 157–161.

AUTHOR: **CARSTEN BANDT**
EDITOR: **ELIZABETH ROZANSKI**

Hypothyroidism

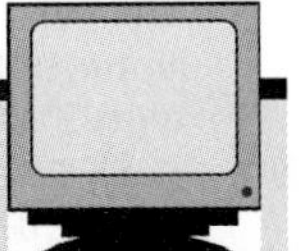

Client Education Sheet on Website

BASIC INFORMATION

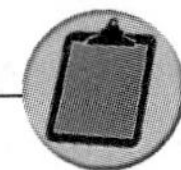

DEFINITION

The clinical syndrome that occurs as a result of decreased circulating levels of serum thyroid hormones (thyroxine [T_4] and triiodothyronine [T_3])

SYNONYM(S)

Congenital hypothyroidism: cretinism

EPIDEMIOLOGY

SPECIES, AGE, SEX

- Dogs:
  - Middle-aged at onset; range is 2 to 9 years of age.
  - No sex predilection.
- Cats:
  - Spontaneous hypothyroidism is very rare.
  - Iatrogenic disease: middle-aged or older.

GENETICS AND BREED PREDISPOSITION

Dogs:

- Can occur in any breed, including mixed breeds
- Reported to be more prevalent in boxers, dachshunds, Doberman pinschers, golden retrievers, Great Danes, Irish setters, miniature schnauzers, poodles, and a number of other breeds

ASSOCIATED CONDITIONS AND DISORDERS: Can occur as part of an autoimmune polyglandular syndrome (rare) along with hypoadrenocorticism or diabetes mellitus.

CLINICAL PRESENTATION

DISEASE FORMS/SUBTYPES

- Congenital hypothyroidism (cretinism); rare
- Primary hypothyroidism (most common): disruption or atrophy of the thyroid glands
- Secondary hypothyroidism (rare): inadequate pituitary secretion of thyroid-stimulating hormone (TSH)

HISTORY, CHIEF COMPLAINT

- Acquired disease:
  - Signs are often nonspecific and gradual in onset.
  - Metabolic: weight gain, lethargy, mental dullness, exercise intolerance/inactivity, and cold intolerance are common.
  - Dermatologic: alopecia (bilaterally symmetric truncal) or thin hair, hyperkeratosis, seborrhea, hyperpigmentation, otitis, "rat tail," and pyoderma are often present, with alopecia or thin hair most common.
  - Reproductive (uncommon): persistent anestrus, infertility, and decreased libido.
  - Neuromuscular: weakness/exercise intolerance are sometimes seen; other signs (ataxia, seizures, facial drooping/paralysis, head tilt/circling [vestibular signs], and stridor/change in bark [laryngeal paralysis]) are uncommon.
- Cretinism: disproportionate dwarfism, short limbs, persistent "puppy coat" or alopecia/thin dull hair, broad head, thick protruding tongue, mental dullness/retardation, delayed dental eruption, constipation

PHYSICAL EXAM FINDINGS

- Exam findings are similar to signs described by the owners.
- Additional findings (uncommon) may include ocular changes (corneal lipid deposits most common), bradycardia or other arrhythmias, constipation, decreased spinal reflexes, and decreased conscious proprioception.

ETIOLOGY AND PATHOPHYSIOLOGY

- Primary hypothyroidism is most common and is usually due to lymphocytic thyroiditis or idiopathic thyroid gland atrophy. Less common causes include follicular cell hyperplasia and infiltrative neoplasia.
- Secondary hypothyroidism is rare. Decreased TSH secretion leads to atrophy of the follicular cells of the thyroid gland. Loss of normal TSH secretion can occur as a result of a congenital pituitary malformation, pituitary neoplasia, or suppression of pituitary thyrotropic cells (most commonly from excess glucocorticoids [exogenous or endogenous hyperadrenocorticism]). Reversibility is possible if glucocorticoid concentrations are returned to normal.
- Tertiary hypothyroidism (decreased secretion of thyrotropin-releasing hormone [TRH]) has not been reported in the dog.
- Iatrogenic hypothyroidism can occur as a result of antithyroid medications (e.g., methimazole), bilateral thyroidectomy, or 131 iodine therapy. (See Hyperthyroidism, p 552.)
- Clinical signs reflect the widespread metabolic effects of thyroid hormones.
- A wide range of concurrent illnesses and nonthyroidal medications (e.g., glucocorticoids, phenobarbital, sulfonamides, carprofen, clomipramine) also affect circulating thyroid hormone concentrations, but not to the extent of producing clinical hypothyroidism.

DIAGNOSIS

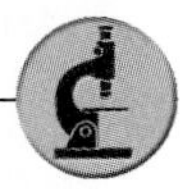

DIFFERENTIAL DIAGNOSIS

- Alopecia (see Alopecia, p 52)
- Seborrhea (see Seborrhea, p 987)
- Obesity/weight gain (see Obesity, p 761)

INITIAL DATABASE

- Complete blood count, serum biochemical profile, urinalysis: Hypercholesterolemia is most common and must be differentiated from normal postprandial hypercholesterolemia. A mild normocytic, normochromic, nonregenerative anemia; fasting hyperlipidemia/ hypertriglyceridemia; mild increases in liver enzymes; and a mild increase in creatine kinase may also be seen.
- Basal serum total thyroxine concentration (TT_4):
  - Includes both free (<1%) and protein-bound (>99%) T_4.
  - Sensitivity: 89–100%; specificity: 75–82%; accuracy: 85%.
  - If TT_4 is in the middle or upper end of the reference range, hypothyroidism is generally ruled out.
    - An exception is the presence of antithyroid antibodies that interfere with the assay.
    - If clinical signs strongly suggest hypothyroidism and TT_4 is normal, then free thyroxine concentration by equilibrium dialysis (FT_4ED), anti-T_4 antibody, and thyroglobulin autoantibody concentrations should be measured.
  - If TT_4 is low or is at the low end of the reference range, it may be due to hypothyroidism, concurrent illness, medications, or may be normal (euthyroid).
- Basal serum free thyroxine concentration by equilibrium dialysis (FT_4ED):
  - Measures just the free (i.e., metabolically available) T_4.
  - An assay based on equilibrium dialysis should be used; it is more time-intensive and expensive, but much more accurate, than radioimmunoassay.
  - Sensitivity: 80–98%; specificity 93–94%; accuracy: 95%.
  - Most accurate single hormone test for the diagnosis of hypothyroidism.
- Basal serum TSH concentration:
  - A validated canine TSH assay should be used.

- The test should not be evaluated alone, but is best used in conjunction with TT_4 and/or FT_4ED results.
  - TSH and TT_4: sensitivity: 63–67%; specificity: 98–100%; accuracy: 82–88%.
  - TSH and FT_4ED: sensitivity: 74%; specificity: 98%; accuracy: 86%.
  - Increased TSH in conjunction with decreased TT_4 or FT_4ED is strongly supportive of hypothyroidism.
  - A normal TSH in conjunction with decreased TT_4 or FT_4ED does not rule out hypothyroidism.
- Also see the Hypothyroidism algorithm, page 1375.

ADVANCED OR CONFIRMATORY TESTING

- If basal thyroid hormone concentrations do not rule in or rule out hypothyroidism, a few options exist:
  - TSH stimulation test.
    - Protocol:
      - Many protocols reported.
      - 0.1 units/kg (maximum 5 units) medical grade bovine TSH IV; evaluate serum TT_4 concentrations in preadministration and 6-hour postadministration samples.
    - Interpretation:
      - If both results are below the reference range, hypothyroidism is present.
      - If post-TSH TT_4 concentration is >3 ug/dl, the dog is euthyroid.
      - Results in between these parameters are equivocal; consider retesting 1 to 2 months later.
    - The availability of medical-grade, bovine TSH is limited, and both medical-grade bovine and recombinant human TSH are expensive.
  - TRH stimulation test.
    - Originally designed to identify secondary hypothyroidism, when the availability of bovine TSH became very limited, this test was used in place of the TSH stimulation test. However, it is less reliable and so is uncommonly used.
    - Protocols: several available.
      - 200 ug TRH/dog IV with evaluation of TT_4 (± TSH) pre-TRH administration and 4-hours post-TRH administration.
      - Interpretation:
        - 4-hour post-TRH TT_4 concentration >2 ug/dl (and/or a relative increase in cTSH of 100% at 30 minutes post-TRH administration) is normal.
        - A post-TRH TT_4 concentration below the reference range is seen with hypothyroidism, but some normal (i.e., euthyroid) dogs also do not respond to TRH.
  - Response to therapy.
  - Serum thyroglobulin antibodies: increased levels suggest lymphocytic thyroiditis. However, lymphocytic thyroiditis does not always lead to, or correlate with, the presence of hypothyroidism.
  - Serum thyroid hormone antibodies: if present, can interfere with testing and lead to spuriously high or low T_4 results, depending on the T_4 assay used.
  - Histopathologic evaluation of skin biopsies: Vacuolated or hypertrophied erector pili muscles, increased dermal mucin, and a thickened dermis are consistent with hypothyroidism. A variety of other nonspecific changes supportive of an endocrinopathy may also be present.

TREATMENT

THERAPEUTIC GOAL(S)

- Return basal serum thyroxine levels to normal
- Eliminate or minimize presenting clinical signs

ACUTE GENERAL TREATMENT

- Hypothyroidism is generally a chronic condition that does not require acute therapy.
- Myxedema coma (rare): levothyroxine for injection 5ug/kg IV q 12h until oral administration possible.

CHRONIC TREATMENT

Oral thyroid supplementation:

- Levothyroxine sodium (synthetic T_4):
  - Initial dose: 0.02 mg/kg PO q 12h. Maximum dose: 0.8 mg/dog q 12h.
  - If concurrent heart failure, renal failure, liver disease, hypoadrenocorticism, or diabetes is present, the initial dose should be decreased by 25–50%, then slowly increased over the following 2 to 4 months. Also, hypothyroidism is rarely life-threatening, so the concurrent disease should be controlled first before treatment of the hypothyroidism is pursued.
  - A brand name preparation for animal use should be used as bioavailability of generic forms can vary.
  - Adjust dose based on clinical response and serum TT_4 concentrations. (See Recommended Monitoring below.)
  - Absorption kinetics vary between brands, so serum concentrations should be reassessed if the levothyroxine brand is changed.
- Liothyronine sodium (synthetic T_3):
  - Rarely indicated.
  - Consider only if a dog with confirmed hypothyroidism has failed to respond clinically, has normalized serum TT_4 concentrations, and at least two brands of levothyroxine have been tried.
  - Initial dosage is 4 to 6 ug/kg PO q 8h.
- Combination products (levothyroxine and liothyronine) are not recommended.

POSSIBLE COMPLICATIONS

Iatrogenic hyperthyroidism

RECOMMENDED MONITORING

- A physical examination and serum thyroxine concentration (4 to 6 hours postpill) should be evaluated at 4 weeks, then q 6–8 weeks for 6 to 8 months, then q 6–12 months.
  - Serum TT_4 concentrations (4 to 6 hours postpill) should be in the upper half of the normal range.
- Monitoring clinical signs: expected evolution of response.
  - An increase in alertness and activity commonly is seen within 1 to 2 weeks.
  - Neurologic improvement may begin within the first month, but several months may be needed for full resolution.
  - Dermatologic improvement often takes 1 to 4 months
  - Resolution of reproductive manifestations may take several months.
- If major clinical improvement is not seen in 3 months despite normal serum TT_4 concentrations, a concurrent as-yet-unidentified disease should be considered.

PROGNOSIS AND OUTCOME

- Primary hypothyroidism: long-term prognosis is good to excellent for return to function
- Secondary hypothyroidism: long-term prognosis is usually guarded since pituitary neoplasia is the most common underlying cause

PEARLS & CONSIDERATIONS

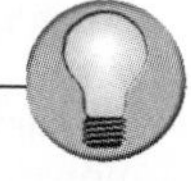

COMMENTS

- The presence of nonthyroidal illness can make it difficult to obtain a definitive diagnosis of hypothyroidism. "Sick euthyroid syndrome" describes the condition that occurs when nonthyroidal illness results in a decrease in the basal TT_4 (and less commonly, FT_4ED) concentrations.
- Subnormal TT_4 concentrations are not an immediate indication for supplementation with levothyroxine may at times be deleterious. The history and physical exam must be critically evaluated both for features supportive of hypothyroidism and for signs of other illness that could be causing the sick euthyroid syndrome. In the latter case,

resolution/treatment of nonthyroidal illness returns TT_4 concentrations to normal.
- Obesity is much more prevalent (21–40% of the North American pet dog population is, or may become, obese) than hypothyroidism (0.2% of dog population, possibly higher). Therefore, obese body condition can only be attributed to hypothyroidism in a small fraction of cases.

SUGGESTED READING

Feldman EC, Nelson RW: Hypothyroidism. In Feldman EC, Nelson RW (eds): *Canine and Feline Endocrinology and Reproduction.* Philadelphia, WB Saunders, 2004, pp 86-151.
Scott-Moncrieff JC, Guptill-Yoran L: Hypothyroidism. In Ettinger SJ, Feldman EC (eds): *Textbook of Veterinary Internal Medicine.* St. Louis, Elsevier Inc., 2005, pp 1535-1544.

AUTHOR: **KRISTI L. GRAHAM**
EDITOR: **SHERRI IHLE**

Icterus

BASIC INFORMATION

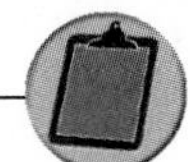

DEFINITION

Yellow discoloration of the skin and mucous membranes

SYNONYM(S)

Jaundice

EPIDEMIOLOGY

SPECIES, AGE, SEX: Dependent on underlying cause (i.e., hepatobiliary disease, hemolytic anemia). Observed in both dogs and cats of any age.

GENETICS AND BREED PREDISPOSITION FOR PRIMARY LIVER DISEASE
- Dogs: Doberman pinschers (inflammatory liver disease), cocker spaniels, Labrador retrievers, Skye terriers.
- Cats: Abyssinian (amyloidosis), Asian breeds (feline infectious peritonitis).

GENETICS AND BREED PREDISPOSITION FOR HEMOLYTIC ANEMIA: American cocker spaniel, English springer spaniel, Old English sheepdog, Irish setter, poodle.

CLINICAL PRESENTATION

HISTORY, CHIEF COMPLAINT
- Hepatobiliary disease:
  - Anorexia, lethargy/weight loss
  - Vomiting/diarrhea
  - Abdominal distention
  - Cranial abdominal pain
  - Polyuria, polydipsia
  - Orange discoloration to the urine
  - Encephalopathy
- Hemolytic anemia:
  - Pallor
  - Anorexia
  - Lethargy, weakness, exercise intolerance
  - Vomiting
  - Orange discoloration to urine
  - Pigmenturia (dark red/brown) if intravascular hemolysis
  - Syncope/collapse

PHYSICAL EXAM FINDINGS
- Yellow discoloration of skin, mucous membranes (gingival, nictitans, sclera, etc.)
- Hepatobiliary disease:
  - Abdominal distention
    - Cranial abdominal organomegaly
    - Ascites
  - Dehydration
  - Halitosis
- Hemolysis:
  - Pale mucous membranes
  - Sinus tachycardia, ventricular arrhythmia
  - Fever
  - Respiratory difficulty if pulmonary thromboembolism (PTE)

ETIOLOGY AND PATHOPHYSIOLOGY

- Prehepatic icterus: increase in production of bilirubin due to presentation of excessive amount of heme (e.g., hemolysis).
- Hepatic icterus: abnormality in hepatic bilirubin uptake, conjugation, or excretion.
- Posthepatic icterus: extrahepatic biliary system obstruction (bile duct system, gallbladder).

DIAGNOSIS

DIFFERENTIAL DIAGNOSIS

- Hepatobiliary disease:
  - Inflammatory/immune-mediated/infectious:
    - Idiopathic chronic hepatitis (dogs).
    - Cholangiohepatitis of cats (suppurative/neutrophilic).
    - Cholangiohepatitis of cats (lymphocytic).
    - Secondary to bacterial translocation from the gastrointestinal system.
    - Leptospirosis (dogs).
  - Hepatic lipidosis (cats).
  - Neoplastic:
    - Lymphoma, hepatocellular carcinoma, hemangiosarcoma, biliary carcinoma, other.
  - Extrahepatic obstruction:
    - Pancreatitis
    - Cholelithiasis (rare in dogs and cats)
    - Bile duct neoplasia
    - Biliary mucocele
    - Inspissated bile syndrome (cats)
  - Cholestatic drug injury:
    - Acetaminophen, azathioprine, diazepam, phenobarbital, sulfonamide, many others.
  - Extrahepatic sepsis: coliform septicemia most common resulting in cholestasis:
    - Endotoxin and acute phase reactants interfere with transport of bile acids into canaliculi.
  - Anoxia: can lead to cholestasis.
- Hemolytic anemia:
  - Idiopathic immune-mediated hemolytic anemia.
  - Associated with other immune disorders:
    - Inflammatory bowel disease.
    - Systemic lupus erythematosus.
  - Infectious:
    - Ehrlichiosis, Rocky Mountain spotted fever, leptospirosis, babesiosis, hemobartonellosis (*Mycoplasma haemofelis*).
    - Viral: feline leukemia virus.
    - Bacterial: any chronic infection.
  - Neoplasia: lymphoma, common association; any form of neoplasia.
  - Microangiopathic hemolysis: commonly associated with hemangiosarcoma, heartworm, disseminated intravascular coagulation (DIC), vasculitis.
  - Drug reaction: postvaccinal, sulfonamides, many others.
  - Erythrocyte membrane fragility/oxidative damage:
    - Abyssinian, Somali cats (osmotic fragility).
    - Hypophosphatemia (phosphorus <1.5 mg/dl).
    - Oxidative damage (intoxications):
      - Onions (dogs)
      - Acetaminophen (cats)
      - Zinc
  - Red blood cell (RBC) enzyme deficiencies: phosphofructokinase deficiency (English springer spaniel),

pyruvate kinase deficiency (Basenji and others), stomatocytosis of malamutes.

INITIAL DATABASE

- Complete blood count:
  - Evaluation of plasma in PCV tube is more sensitive for icterus (seen at bilirubin = 1–1.5 mg/dl) than mucous membranes (icterus when bilirubin ≥2 mg/dl).
- Serum biochemical profile:
  - Alkaline phosphatase is always elevated in cholestatic disease causing icterus.
  - Liver enzymes may be elevated due to hypoxemia of severe anemia.
- Urinalysis and culture
- Abdominal radiographs
- Abdominal ultrasound
- Thoracic radiographs

ADVANCED OR CONFIRMATORY TESTING

- Hepatobiliary:
  - Prothrombin time (PT)/activated partial thromboplastin time (APTT)/ platelet count.
  - Liver aspirate or biopsy for histopathologic evaluation and culture.
  - Amylase/lipase/pancreatic lipase immunoreactivity.
  - Infectious disease titers.
  - Serial blood cultures, body fluid cultures if suspect sepsis.
- Hemolysis:
  - Whole blood smear (spherocytes).
  - Reticulocyte count.
  - PT/APTT platelet count to rule out bleeding disorder, disseminated intravascular coagulation (DIC).
  - Antinuclear antibody test.
  - Direct Coombs' test (false-negative results common).
  - Slide agglutination test.
  - Infectious disease titers/polymerase chain reaction (PCR) (see Etiology and Pathophysiology above).
  - PCR for RBC enzyme deficiencies.
  - Arterial blood gas.
  - D-dimer (to rule out PTE associated with hemolytic anemia; high sensitivity, low specificity).
  - Bone marrow aspirate (evaluate for erythrophagocytosis, differentiate from myelodysplasia, pure red cell aplasia, lymphoma).
  - Fecal occult blood to differentiate hemolysis from gastrointestinal blood loss.

TREATMENT

THERAPEUTIC GOAL(S)

- Hepatobiliary disease:
  - Suppress or eliminate the disease process
  - Manage the metabolic condition
- Hemolysis:
  - Treat inciting cause (e.g., drug withdrawal, toxin removal)
  - Suppress immune system if indicated
  - Treat complications such as PTE, DIC

GENERAL TREATMENT

Because icterus is a clinical sign, not a disease entity, appropriate management depends on identification and treatment of the underlying cause.

POSSIBLE COMPLICATIONS

- PTE: very common with immune-mediated hemolytic anemia.
  - Oxygen/heparinization if PTE suspected
- Persistent/worsening anemia.
  - RBC transfusion reactions (cross-matching important)
- Hepatic Encephalopathy, p 489.
- Gastric Ulcer, p 431.

PROGNOSIS AND OUTCOME

- Varies with the cause of each disease.
- Extrahepatic sepsis: mortality rate usually quite high.
- Hemolytic anemia:
  - Prognosis good if inciting cause can be removed.
  - Idiopathic immune-mediated hemolytic anemia: 40–70% mortality rate; prognosis worse with intravascular hemolysis.

PEARLS & CONSIDERATIONS

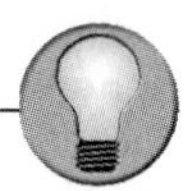

COMMENTS

- Bilirubin concentrations are usually above 2.0 mg/dl to result in clinical icterus.
- The purpose of measuring serum bile acids is to assess liver function. Therefore, bile acids are an unnecessary diagnostic test in an icteric patient with a normal PCV.
- PTE diagnosis is sometimes difficult: low PaO_2 on an arterial blood gas that is drawn during oxygen therapy is suggestive. High-velocity tricuspid regurgitation also suggestive if a murmur is present. D-dimer for thombolysis: high sensitivity but poor specificity (i.e., many false-positive results for unrelated conditions).
- Portosystemic shunts do not cause icterus, unless a complicating factor (e.g., other concurrent hepatopathy) also is present
- Subtle icterus may be difficult to detect (or "icterus" may incorrectly be detected in a normal patient) when the physical examination is performed in a room illuminated with fluorescent tube lighting.
- Ultra low-dose aspirin may become a new therapeutic to replace heparin in the prevention of PTE.
- Hemolytic anemia can be associated with immune-mediated thrombocytopenia (often referred to as Evans syndrome).
- Blood transfusions can suppress the reticulocyte response.

RECOMMENDED READING

Center SA: Diagnostic procedures for evaluation of hepatic disease. In Guilford WG, et al (eds): *Strombeck's Small Animal Gastroenterology*, ed 3. Philadelphia, WB Saunders, 1996, pp 130–188;Table 8-7, p 150.

McCullough S: Immune-mediated hemolytic anemia: Understanding the nemesis. *Vet Clin North Am Small Anim Pract* 33(6):1295–1315, 2003.

AUTHOR: **MAUREEN CARROLL**

EDITOR: **ETIENNE CÔTÉ**

Idiopathic Tremor Syndrome

BASIC INFORMATION

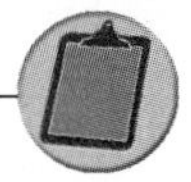

DEFINITION

- A brain disorder of unknown etiology that causes spontaneous generalized tremors and that is responsive to immunosuppressive doses of corticosteroids.
- *Tremor* refers to a rhythmic oscillatory involuntary movement in the body.

SYNONYM(S)

Corticosteroid responsive tremor syndrome

White shaker dog syndrome (a poor term, as approximately half of the dogs with idiopathic tremor syndrome do not have a white coat)

EPIDEMIOLOGY

SPECIES, AGE, SEX: The majority of the dogs affected with this syndrome are young (<5 years) and of small breeds (<15 kg).

GENETICS AND BREED PREDISPOSITION: White dogs, including the West Highland white terrier and Maltese, are overrepresented, although any breed may be affected.

CLINICAL PRESENTATION

HISTORY, CHIEF COMPLAINT

- Owners typically notice an acute onset of a fine, whole-body tremor that often worsens with exercise, stress, and excitement and lessens with rest or sleep.
- The course of the disease is nonprogressive.

PHYSICAL EXAM FINDINGS

- The most notable finding is a fine, whole-body tremor.
- Additional findings may include poor menace responses, head tilt, nystagmus, paresis, tetraparesis, ataxia, seizure activity, and an elevated rectal temperature.

ETIOLOGY AND PATHOPHYSIOLOGY

The exact etiology is unknown but may be the result of an autoimmune-mediated disruption of neurotransmitter metabolism in the central nervous system (CNS), with a decreased conversion of tyrosine to dopamine. Dopamine is an important neurotransmitter for the regulation of movement.

DIAGNOSIS

DIFFERENTIAL DIAGNOSIS

- Congenital abnormal myelin formation (e.g., hypomyelination, dysmyelination)
- Toxicosis (e.g., penitrem A produced by *Penicillium* in moldy foods, hexachlorophene, and organophosphates)
- Metabolic conditions (e.g., hepatic or uremic encephalopathies)
- Cerebellar disease

INITIAL DATABASE

A clinical diagnosis generally is reached on the basis of signalment, history, and physical exam findings.

- Basic blood work (complete blood count, serum chemistry panel) is typically within normal limits.

ADVANCED OR CONFIRMATORY TESTING

- Cerebrospinal fluid analysis is helpful in differentiating idiopathic tremor syndrome from other inflammatory diseases:
  - Results may include minimal to moderate nonsuppurative pleocytosis (lymphocytic, with mean white blood cell count being approximately 16 cell/μL).
  - This is in contrast to the polymorphonuclear pleocytosis associated with mycotic and bacterial encephalitis and the mixed-cell pleocytosis seen in granulomatous meningoencephalitis and protozoal diseases.
  - The protein concentration is often high in cases of idiopathic tremor syndrome.
- Magnetic resonance imaging of the brain is typically normal.
- Histopathology:
  - Histopathologic lesions are not seen in all dogs with idiopathic tremor syndrome.
  - Abnormalities may include diffuse, mild meningoencephalitis, with mild perivascular cuffing and lymphocytic infiltrates throughout the CNS, especially in the cerebellum.

TREATMENT

THERAPEUTIC GOAL(S)

The goal of therapy is to eliminate tremors. Tremors often return in a more mild fashion and are associated with excitement.

ACUTE GENERAL TREATMENT

Treatment consists of immunosuppressive doses of corticosteroids (i.e., prednisone 1-2 mg/kg PO q 12h). Clinical signs often decrease within the first few days of treatment.

CHRONIC TREATMENT

- Once tremors are fully controlled, the dose of prednisone should be gradually decreased over 1 to 3 months.
- Occasionally, dogs need to be kept on low doses or alternate day therapy to control tremors.
- Additional tremor control can be achieved with oral diazepam (0.2 mg/kg PO q 8h).

PROGNOSIS AND OUTCOME

Excellent

PEARLS & CONSIDERATIONS

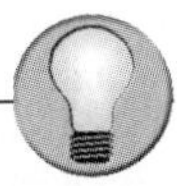

COMMENTS

The synonym "White shaker dog syndrome" is a poor term, as approximately half of the dogs with idiopathic tremor syndrome do not have a white coat.

SUGGESTED READING

Bagley RS, et al: Generalized tremors in Maltese Dogs: Clinical findings in seven cases. *J Am Anim Hosp Assoc* 29:141-145, 1993.

Sanders G, Bagley RS: Cerebellar diseases and tremor syndromes. In Dewey CW (ed): *A Practical Guide to Canine and Feline Neurology*. Ames, IA, Iowa State Press, 2003, pp 270-271.

Wagner SO, et al: Generalized tremors in dogs: 24 cases (1984-1995). *J Am Vet Med Assoc* 221:731-735, 1997.

Yamaya Y, et al: A case of shaker dog disease in a miniature dachshund. *J Vet Med Sci* 66(9):1159-1160, 2004.

AUTHOR: **KERRY SMITH BAILEY**
EDITOR: **CURTIS W. DEWEY**

Immunodeficiency Syndromes, Cat

BASIC INFORMATION

DEFINITION

Conditions resulting from a defective immune response. The condition may be primary from an inherited defect, or secondary to another disease process or infection. It may be specific, with a defect in either B or T lymphocyte function, or nonspecific, due to a defect in phagocytic cell function or skin or mucosal integrity.

SYNONYM(S)

Immune or immunologic deficiency

EPIDEMIOLOGY

SPECIES, AGE, SEX

- One rare nonspecific defect is seen in young Persian cats with Chédiak-Higashi disease syndrome.
- All other known specific immunologic defects in cats are acquired and sec-

ondary to retroviral (feline leukemia virus [FeLV], feline immunodeficiency virus [FIV]) infections. These infections can occur at any age and either gender, although young cats are most susceptible to FeLV infection.

GENETICS AND BREED PREDISPOSITION: Persian cats with a dilute smoke gray coat color and yellow irises may have Chédiak-Higashi syndrome.

RISK FACTORS

- Greater FeLV propagation in crowded multicat households or shelters.
- FIV occurs primarily in adult, outdoor, intact male cats.
- Either virus can be easily spread through blood as in transfusions.

CONTAGION AND ZOONOSIS

- FeLV is spread through contact with saliva, respiratory secretions, and milk. Kittens less than 4 months old are most at risk from queens or other cats.
- FIV is less contagious and is spread primarily through bite wounds.
- No known zoonotic risk.

GEOGRAPHY AND SEASONALITY: Both viruses have worldwide distribution. FIV is more prevalent in countries where cats routinely roam outdoors. FeLV has decreased in prevalence in countries where testing and vaccination have been used.

ASSOCIATED CONDITIONS AND DISORDERS

- Chédiak-Higashi syndrome: slight increased risk for bacterial infections. Bleeding tendencies are also more common with this disease.
- FeLV can cause hematologic neoplasia, myelosuppression, immune-mediated diseases.
- FIV is less pathogenic, and more likely associated with stomatitis or neurologic disorders.
- Both FeLV and FIV cause immunodeficiency, which can result in opportunistic infections.
- Almost any infection can occur in cats infected with FeLV or FIV.
  - Examples include: bacterial (stomatitis, pyoderma), fungal (dermatophytosis, cryptococcosis), protozoal (toxoplasmosis, cryptosporidiosis), viral (FIP, panleukopenia), and *Mycoplasma haemofelis* infection (formerly hemobartonellosis).
  - Some infections may be abnormally persistent or recurrent.
  - Some infections also may be secondary to neutropenia (more common with FeLV than FIV).

CLINICAL PRESENTATION

HISTORY, CHIEF COMPLAINT: Signs may be vague such as weight loss and lethargy, or may be referable to the specific infection that occurs. Common clinical signs are salivation or dysphagia from stomatitis, chronic nasal discharge from bacterial or viral rhinitis, or diarrhea from enteritis.

PHYSICAL EXAM FINDINGS

- Stomatitis (lymphocytic-plasmacytic proliferative type): more commonly associated with FIV than FeLV (FIV > FeLV).
- Signs of neurologic disorders, especially dementia or twitching: FIV > FeLV.
- Gingivitis: FeLV > FIV.
- Anemia: FeLV > FIV.
- Lymphadenopathy (reactive; may be caused by bartonellosis): FeLV > FIV.

ETIOLOGY AND PATHOPHYSIOLOGY

- FeLV/FIV (retroviral)-associated immune deficiency.
  - The subset of lymphocytes most affected by retroviral infection is the CD4 helper T-cell. The ratio of CD4 to CD8 is also decreased.
  - Also described with FeLV: secondary decreased ability of B cells to respond to new antigens.
  - Thymic atrophy in neonatal kittens can cause "fading kitten syndrome."
  - FIV is much less pathogenic than is FeLV. Many cats infected with FIV can live for many years without signs of illness. See Feline Immunodeficiency Virus Infection, p 376; Feline Leukemia Virus Infection, p 380.
- Neither FeLV nor FIV causes cytopathic changes or inflammation in tissues. Thus if a fever is present, a second infectious agent is likely to be the cause.
- Chédiak-Higashi-associated immune deficiency (rare disorder).
  - Abnormal neutrophil granules with abnormal function and survival. Bleeding tendencies are a result of platelet function defects.

DIAGNOSIS

DIFFERENTIAL DIAGNOSIS

- Any unusual, persistent, or recurring infection in any cat might be secondary to a retroviral infection.
- Neutropenia can also be caused by other primary bone marrow disease, drugs, toxins, or may be secondary to an overwhelming infection.

INITIAL DATABASE

- Complete blood count (CBC) to evaluate for anemia, neutropenia, or thrombocytopenia.
  - FeLV/FIV: anemia, neutropenia, or thrombocytopenia. Persistent lymphopenia may occur but is nonspecific.
  - Chédiak-Higashi syndrome produces characteristic large granules in neutrophils.
- Urinalysis to evaluate for proteinuria or infection.
- Serum biochemistry profile: usually unremarkable, and rarely, will reflect visceral organ involvement with opportunistic infections (e.g., pyelonephritis, bacterial translocation via portal circulation). Serum globulin level may be normal or elevated.
- FeLV (antigen) and FIV (antibody) enzyme-linked immunosorbent assay (ELISA) blood tests are excellent for initial screening.
  - Maternal antibody and vaccination interfere with FIV test, but not FeLV.

ADVANCED OR CONFIRMATORY TESTING

- A positive ELISA in a cat with signs compatible with an immunodeficiency syndrome is likely to be accurate. A positive test in a healthy cat without known risk factors is more likely to be a false positive, and should be confirmed by immunofluorescent antibody testing (IFA-FeLV) or Western blot (WB-FIV).
- Polymerase chain reaction testing is somewhat variable between labs, and not needed in most situations.
- Specific testing for other infectious diseases as needed (e.g., serologic titers, bacterial culture and sensitivity for purulent/septic processes).
- Bone marrow aspirate and biopsy if cytopenias are present or abnormal cells are circulating.
- Testing of CD4 counts not readily available, nor prognostic, as not all cats with low counts develop infections.
- When compared to a normal cat, microscopic examination of the shaft of a hair plucked from a cat with Chédiak-Higashi syndrome reveals large, clumped melanin granules.

TREATMENT

THERAPEUTIC GOAL(S)

- FeLV/FIV-associated immunodeficiency:
  - Maintain good nutrition and husbandry including core vaccinations
  - Keep infected cats indoors for their own protection, as well as to protect other cats
  - Treat any secondary infections early and aggressively
- Chediak-Higashi–associated immunodeficiency:
  - Treat secondary infections as they arise; prophylactic treatment if surgery or trauma (bleeding)

ACUTE GENERAL TREATMENT

- Find and treat any infections as quickly and thoroughly as possible
- Use supportive care and nutritional support as needed
- No value in FeLV/FIV vaccines for infected cats

CHRONIC TREATMENT

- No drug has proven efficacy in eliminating feline retroviruses. Anecdotal benefit has been reported for oral human α-interferon (IFN), *Propionibacterium acnes*, acemannan, *Staph* protein A, and PIND-ORF, but so far none of these has been shown to be effective either in decreasing viral replication or prolonging survival in limited controlled clinical trials.
- Recently IFN-omega improved clinical signs and 1-year survival in some cats, but another study in FIV-infection showed no benefit.
- Azidothymidine (AZT) at a dose of 5 mg/kg q 12h SQ caused improvement in clinical signs of stomatitis compared to placebo in a group of FeLV-infected cats. No decrease in virus was shown. Anemia can result from long-term use of AZT.

DRUG INTERACTIONS

Avoid corticosteroids or other immunosuppressive drugs unless absolutely needed. They may increase the risk of infections.

POSSIBLE COMPLICATIONS

- Inability to eradicate some infections
- Bone marrow failure, myelodysplasia, or hematopoietic malignancy, especially from FeLV

RECOMMENDED MONITORING

Monitor weight since weight loss is often an early sign of complications. Also monitor appetite and activity. Once or twice yearly, CBCs might detect a problem, but healthy FeLV-infected cats generally have normal counts except for lymphopenia.

PROGNOSIS AND OUTCOME

- Previous studies showing 50% mortality for FeLV infection in 2 years and 80% in 3 years were done with multicat households where risks of secondary infections were high. For a single indoor cat, the prognosis is guarded, but better than these figures indicate.
- Many FIV-positive cats will survive for many years without developing signs of illness if they are kept indoors.

PEARLS & CONSIDERATIONS

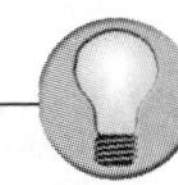

COMMENTS

- Although FeLV and FIV cause immunosuppression, most secondary infections can be treated successfully.
- Keeping these cats indoors and separated from ill or young cats (especially cats with signs of respiratory disease, skin disease, or diarrhea) will protect them from the majority of these infections.

PREVENTION

- FeLV: test kittens at 8 weeks. If negative and from a high-risk environment, repeat in 4 weeks. Isolate FeLV-negative kittens until they are more than 4 months old and have some natural resistance to FeLV.
- FIV test result can be positive from maternal antibody. Kittens testing positive should be retested after 5 months of age. Young kittens are rarely actually infected with FIV.
- FIV, FeLV: vaccinate only cats at risk (outdoor cats with exposure to other cats, or those in multicat households). Neutered male cats are less likely to fight with other cats.

CLIENT EDUCATION

- Explain the benefits of keeping cats indoors. Never introduce new cats without testing. Indoor cats do not need to be vaccinated against retroviruses.
- For multicat households with endemic FeLV infection, isolate or remove positive cats, vaccinate the rest, and do not bring in new cats. Retest negative cats 3 months later. Repeat until all are negative.
- Spread of virus requires carrier cats, as the virus does not survive outside of the cat.

SUGGESTED READING

Hartman K: Feline immunodeficiency virus. In Ettinger SJ, Feldman EC (eds): *Textbook of Veterinary Internal Medicine*, ed 6. St. Louis, Elsevier Saunders, 2005, pp 659–662.

Levy JK, Crawford PC: Feline leukemia virus. In Ettinger SJ, Feldman EC (eds): *Textbook of Veterinary Internal Medicine*, ed 6. St. Louis, Elsevier Saunders, 2005, pp 653–659.

AUTHOR & EDITOR: **SUSAN M. COTTER**

Immunodeficiency Syndromes, Dog

BASIC INFORMATION

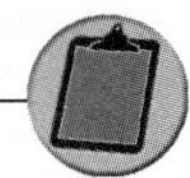

DEFINITION

Primary immunodeficiency syndrome: an inherited defect involving either the humoral (B-cell), cell-mediated (T-cell) immune system, a combination of the two, or the phagocytic system.

SYNONYM(S)

- Cell-mediated (T-cell) immunodeficiency disorder
- Combined (B-cell and T-cell) immunodeficiency disorder
- Functional phagocytic immunodeficiency disorder
- Humoral (B-cell) immunodeficiency disorder

EPIDEMIOLOGY

SPECIES, AGE, SEX

- Signs first manifest around 8 to 12 weeks of age when the protective effects of maternal antibody are lost.
- No sex predilection except for sex-linked severe combined immunodeficiency syndrome (X-SCID)—males.

GENETICS AND BREED PREDISPOSITION

- Humoral (B-cell) immunodeficiency disorder:
  - Selective IgA deficiency: German shepherd, shar-pei, and beagle.
  - Complement deficiency: Brittany spaniel.
- Cell-mediated (T-cell) immunodeficiency disorder:
  - Thymic hypoplasia: dwarf weimaraner.
- Combined (B-cell and T-cell) immunodeficiency disorder:
  - SCID: Jack Russell terrier.
  - X-SCID: bassett hound, Cardigan Welsh Corgi.
- Functional phagocytic immunodeficiency disorder:
  - Canine leukocyte adhesion disorder (CLAD): Irish setter.
  - Weimaraner immunodeficiency syndrome: Weimaraner.

CONTAGION AND ZOONOSIS: Most opportunistic infections that affect immunocompromised individuals are overgrowths or infections with organisms that otherwise are not pathogenic to immunocompetent hosts. However, immunocompromised animals are also more susceptible than normal individuals to infection with organisms that are potentially zoonotic (e.g., dermatophytosis) or contagious to other dogs (e.g., respiratory tract pathogens).

HISTORY, CHIEF COMPLAINT: Recurrent infections that may or may not respond to appropriate therapy. Type of infection may vary with defect in the immune system.

PHYSICAL EXAM FINDINGS

- Humoral (B-cell) immunodeficiency disorder: physical exam findings are largely unremarkable; however, some patients may present with signs associated with chronic/recurring infections; increased incidence of chronic respiratory, skin, and intestinal infections.
- Cell-mediated (T-cell) immunodeficiency disorder: absence of palpable lymph nodes, tonsils are not visible. Affected dogs typically have signs of growth retardation and unthriftiness as compared to the other puppies within the litter.
- Combined (B-cell and T-cell) immunodeficiency disorder: similar findings as for humoral and cell-mediated immunodeficiency disorder.
- Functional phagocytic immunodeficiency disorder: fever, generalized lymphadenopathy, dermatitis, pododermatitis, gingivitis, osteomyelitis; striking absence of pus formation and poor wound healing.

ETIOLOGY AND PATHOPHYSIOLOGY

- Humoral (B-cell) immunodeficiency: decreased concentrations or absence of certain immunoglobulins with increased susceptibility to bacterial infections.
  - IgA deficiency: mode of inheritance is unknown. Epidemiologic studies show that puppies born to dams with IgA deficiency are at increased risk of developing upper respiratory infections as compared to puppies from dams with normal IgA concentrations.
  - Complement deficiency: autosomal recessive mode of inheritance; dogs that are homozygous for the trait have no detectable C3, required for opsonization of bacteria.
- Cell-mediated (T-cell) immunodeficiency: affected animals have either low numbers of, or nonfunctional, T-cells. Findings include a small thymus and lack of lymph nodes, tonsils, and Peyer's patches on postmortem examination. Affected animals are at increased risk for infections with intracellular bacterial, fungal, protozoal, and viral organisms.
- Combined (B-cell and T-cell) immunodeficiency:
  - SCID: autosomal recessive: affected individuals are unable to mount an appropriate antigen-specific immune response due to a lack of DNA–protein kinase (DNA-PK) activity; DNA-PK is required for lymphocyte precursors to mature.
  - X-SCID: sex-linked mutation in the γ chain of the interleukin-2 (IL-2) receptor that is required for normal B-cell and T-cell function; affected male puppies are able to synthesize IgM, but IgG concentrations are significantly reduced and IgA is not detectable.
- Functional phagocytic immunodeficiency: affected animals have an increased risk for systemic or superficial infections with pyogenic microorganisms.
  - Weimaraner immunodeficiency syndrome: inherited, exact mechanism unknown; neutrophil dysfunction at the site of the lesion. However, there also appears to be a failure to produce IgA and IgG.
  - CLAD: deficiency of leukocyte surface glycoprotein (B_2 integrin) associated with leukocyte adherence and egress into affected tissues; failure to express B_2 integrin CD18.

DIAGNOSIS

DIFFERENTIAL DIAGNOSIS

Affected puppies present with varying, often nonspecific clinical signs and common recurrent infections. It is the recurrence of the infections and the poor response to therapy that warrant further investigation of a primary immunodeficiency syndrome.

- Humoral immunodeficiency: varies based on presenting complaint.
  - Upper respiratory infection: *Bordetella bronchiseptica*.
  - Primary ciliary dyskinesia.
  - Otitis.
  - Stomatitis.
  - Staphylococcal dermatitis.
  - Atopic dermatitis.
- Cell-mediated immunodeficiency:
  - Fungal (e.g., cryptococcosis, aspergillosis, blastomycosis, dermatophytosis).
  - Protozoal (e.g., toxoplasmosis, giardiasis).
  - Viral infections can be seen after vaccination with modified live virus vaccine.
  - Intracellular bacteria (e.g., mycobacterial infections).
- Combined immunodeficiency:
  - Affected animals are susceptible to bacterial, viral, fungal, and protozoal agents.
- Functional phagocytic immunodeficiency:
  - Sepsis.
  - Bacteremia.
  - Pelger-Huët: hyposegmentation of nuclei in granulocytes and monocytes; persistent degenerative left shift without toxic change or any signs of illness (it is only an incidental finding).
  - Other infectious disease that would cause a neutrophilic leukocytosis with a left shift.

INITIAL DATABASE

Appropriate diagnostic testing based on clinical presentation.

- Complete blood count, serum chemistry profile, urinalysis with culture and sensitivity, fecal examination, thoracic radiographs.
- Humoral (B-cell) immunodeficiency disorder: minimum database within normal limits.
- Cell-mediated (T-cell) immunodeficiency disorder: normal/decreased lymphocyte count.
- Combined (B-cell and T-cell) immunodeficiency disorder: normal/decreased lymphocyte count (average 1000/µl); possibly low total protein due to low globulin levels; agammaglobulinemia (protein electrophoresis).
- Functional phagocytic immunodeficiency disorder: persistent leukocytosis with regenerative left shift; neutrophil count >200,000/µl.

ADVANCED OR CONFIRMATORY TESTING

- Specific tests performed should be geared toward the clinical presentation and tailored to the suspected immunodeficiency. Commonly considered tests include:
  - Abdominal ultrasound.
  - Transtracheal wash with culture and sensitivity.
  - Bone marrow aspirate or core biopsy.
  - Lymph node biopsy.
  - Lesional biopsy: with CLAD, biopsy of lesion shows bacteria and possibly necrosis, but no infiltration of neutrophils.
- Humoral immunodeficiency:
  - Serum protein electrophoresis: to evaluate immunoglobulin concentrations.
  - Serum immunoglobulin quantitation.
  - Quantitation of serum C3 for C3 deficiency.
- Cell-mediated immunodeficiency:
  - Lymphocyte transformation (blastogenesis): evaluates the ability of the T-cell to proliferate after stimulation.
  - Measurement of growth hormone or insulin-like growth factor-1 if dwarfism is suspected (testing generally available only in research laboratories).
- Functional phagocytic immunodeficiency:
  - Bactericidal assays: measure the ability of neutrophils to kill bacteria.
  - Polymerase chain reaction (PCR): to identify affected, normal, or carrier animals.

TREATMENT

A substantial degree of variation in severity may exist for a given immunodeficiency syndrome. Therefore, treatment intensity, treatment success, and prognosis are individually variable and must be determined case by case. Some individuals require minimal or no treatment, whereas in others, euthanasia is the most humane option.

THERAPEUTIC GOAL(S)

Control opportunistic infections with antimicrobials and supportive care; hospitalize when necessary

ACUTE GENERAL TREATMENT

Supportive care to treat opportunistic infections:

- For example, antibiotics for confirmed bacterial infections. Empiric antibiotics may be used initially, pending culture and sensitivity results. Antibiotic type should be selected based on suspected bacterial population of involved site. Examples:
  - Skin: gram-positive bacteria most common; consider cephalosporins (e.g., cephalexin or cefadroxil 22 mg/kg PO q 8-12h) or penicillins (e.g., amoxicillin 22 mg/kg PO q 8h or ampicillin 22 mg/kg IV q 8h).
  - Oral cavity and respiratory tract: mixed populations. Consider fluoroquinolones (enrofloxacin 5 mg/kg PO or slow IV q 12h), β-lactamase resistant penicillins (e.g., amoxicillin-clavulanate 10-20 mg/kg PO q 12h), or macrolides (e.g., azithromycin 5-10 mg/kg PO q 24h × 1 to 5 days).
- Due to strong possibility of opportunistic fungal, viral, and protozoal infections, empiric antibiotic therapy may be inadequate or may select for resistant strains of bacteria; diagnostic samples for culture should be obtained before initiating antibiotic treatment, and judicious antibiotic use is warranted.
- Nebulization and coupage for bacterial pneumonia (see Pneumonia, Bacterial, p 863).
- Disinfection of cutaneous wounds with diluted (0.05%) chlorhexidine solution.
  - With standard 4% chlorhexidine solution, dilute 1 part chlorhexidine to 80 parts water to obtain 0.05% concentration.
  - The same concentration may be used as an ear wash in opportunistic otitis and as an oral antiseptic rinse in cases of stomatitis.

CHRONIC TREATMENT

- Humoral immunodeficiency:
  - Nonspecific supportive therapy tailored toward treating recurrent microbial infections.
- Cell-mediated immunodeficiency:
  - Supportive care with frequent monitoring for opportunistic infections and then proceed with aggressive treatment when warranted.
  - Dwarf weimaraners respond to thymosin fraction 5 therapy (1 mg/kg SC q 24h for 7 days).
- Combined (B-cell and T-cell) immunodeficiency:
  - Bone marrow transplantation.
- Phagocytic immunodeficiency:
  - Bone marrow transplantation.

POSSIBLE COMPLICATIONS

- Sepsis
- Recurring and resistant infections

RECOMMENDED MONITORING

Monitoring of appetite, activity, temperature, and complete blood counts can aid in the early detection of infection.

PROGNOSIS AND OUTCOME

- Humoral immunodeficiency:
  - Fair to good.
- Cell-mediated immunodeficiency:
  - Poor.
- Combined (B-cell and T-cell) immunodeficiency:
  - Poor: affected animals usually die between 2 and 4 months of age from systemic bacterial or viral infections.
- Phagocytic immunodeficiency:
  - Poor.

PEARLS & CONSIDERATIONS

COMMENTS

The diseases listed here are all severe and have a poor/guarded prognosis, but they are rare.

PREVENTION

The most important aspect of controlling the prevalence of the immunodeficiency syndromes that affect dogs of predisposed breeds is by client education and appropriate genetic screening of potential breeding pairs when molecular testing is possible.

CLIENT EDUCATION

It is important to discuss with the client that the affected dogs will not be cured, the disease is heritable, and other puppies of the same litter may be affected. Affected puppies are at an extremely high risk for secondary infections and should avoid other ill animals.

SUGGESTED READING

Brockus CW: Leukocyte disorders. In Ettinger S, Feldman E (eds): *Textbook of Veterinary Internal Medicine*. St. Louis, Elsevier Saunders, 2005, pp 1941-1943.

Felsburg P: Hereditary and acquired immunodeficiencies. In Bonagura J (ed): *Kirks Current Veterinary Therapy XIII*. Philadelphia, WB Saunders, 2000, pp 516-520.

Felsburg P: Overview of the immune system and immunodeficiency diseases. *Vet Clin North Am* 24(4):629-653, 1994.

AUTHOR: **TRACEY A. ROSSI**
EDITOR: **SUSAN M. COTTER**

Inappropriate Elimination, Cat

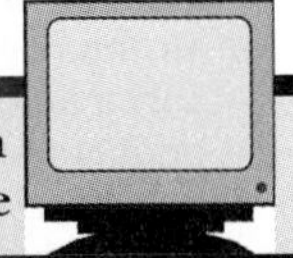

Client Education Sheet on Website

BASIC INFORMATION

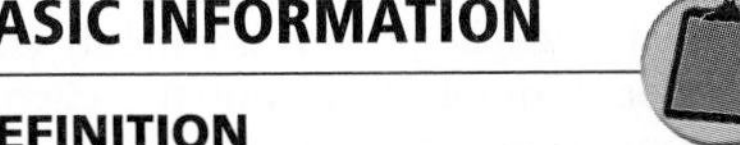

DEFINITION

- Situation characterized by the use of inappropriate or undesirable areas (locations or surfaces) for elimination of urine or feces. "Inappropriate" elimination is often normal for the species but is undesirable to clients.
- Urinary incontinence: passage of urine without awareness, due to a medical problem. Very rare in cats.
- Marking: passage of urine or feces involving social interaction. Very common in cats.

SYNONYM(S)

Toileting problems

EPIDEMIOLOGY

SPECIES, AGE, SEX

- Urine spraying: Sexually intact animals > neutered animals. Possibly males > females.
- Marking behaviors—which need not involve spraying—may develop at sexual maturity (~6 months) if they pertain to sexual advertisement, or at social maturity (~24-48 months) if they pertain to social organization, relative roles in social relationships, or stress or distress.

GENETICS AND BREED PREDISPOSITION: Long-haired cats: possibly overrepresented with substrate (surface onto which a cat eliminates) aversions.

RISK FACTORS

- Risk factors for elimination preferences and aversions include:
  - Dirty litter and/or litter boxes

- Litter boxes that are too small and discourage active digging and exploration
- Litter boxes that are too high for cats to enter readily
- Styles (covered) and placement (in closets) that allow the cat using the litter box to be trapped by a child, another cat, a dog, etc.
- Placement of boxes in locations that the cats cannot reach because of pain (arthritis), access (doors closed), or social factors (being chased by the new puppy)
- Entrapment of odors by lids of covered boxes placed in areas without adequate ventilation
- Illness of any cat in the household that causes changes in bladder and bowel function

• Risk factors for marking are based on social stress and distress. Stressors can include:
  - Addition of another pet
  - Loss of a pet
  - Change in the composition of the human household
  - Change in the "stress" level of the household (e.g., illness, changes in jobs)
  - Visitation by an outside cat
  - Illness or change of relationships between cats in the household (e.g., that concomitant with social maturity)
  - True intercat aggression

GEOGRAPHY AND SEASONALITY: Marking behaviors may intensify in spring, when more animals are let outside, visit indoor animals, and scents aerosolize. Marking increases in frequency when females enter estrus.

ASSOCIATED CONDITIONS AND DISORDERS: Coexistent intercat aggression is common; identifying relative victims and aggressors is essential to resolving the social conflict and fixing the toileting complaints.

CLINICAL PRESENTATION

DISEASE FORMS/SUBTYPES

- Inappropriate elimination: three classes of problems:
  - Substrate (texture/surface) preferences or aversions. The amounts of urine or feces are small and distributed over areas associated with social stimuli.
  - Location preferences or aversions for urination or defecation. As for substrate.
  - In marking involving sprayed urine (spraying), the cat treads on its front feet, raises its tail, quivering the tip, and sprays urine vertically. If the cat is not backed against a vertical surface, sprayed urine makes a linear pattern on horizontal surfaces. Nonspraying marking involves elimination of small amounts of urine or feces in areas that have social, not tactile, significance.
- These can all be normal behaviors in free-ranging cats; spraying is part of a normal signaling repertoire in cats.

HISTORY, CHIEF COMPLAINT: Clients find urine or feces in locations that they find unacceptable.

PHYSICAL EXAM FINDINGS

- Unremarkable.
- Findings suggesting lower urinary tract disease, gastrointestinal problems, or other nonbehavioral disorder warrant a diagnostic medical evaluation.

ETIOLOGY AND PATHOPHYSIOLOGY

- Behavior is normal for the species but unacceptable to clients and/or coexists with intercat aggression or other behavioral disorder.
- Association between spraying and crystalluria, or inappropriate urination and defecation with impacted anal sacs, remains speculative.

DIAGNOSIS

DIFFERENTIAL DIAGNOSIS

- Feline lower urinary tract signs/disease
- Bacterial cystitis
- Urethral obstruction
- Diabetes mellitus
- Cognitive dysfunction
- Hyperthyroidism
- Lower motor neuron disease
- Enteritis/colitis
- Parasitemia

INITIAL DATABASE

- Inappropriate urination: complete blood count (CBC), serum biochemistry profile, urinalysis with culture, thyroid profile (if >6 years old).
- Inappropriate defecation: fecal flotation and direct smear, thyroid profile (if >6 years old).
- Before initiating psychotropic medications: CBC, serum biochemistry profile, urinalysis, thyroid profile (if >6 years old).

ADVANCED OR CONFIRMATORY TESTING

To identify the nature of inappropriate elimination, and any concurrent issues (e.g., intercat aggression), client observations are essential. Videotaping interactions between cats in a multicat household may be extremely informative, especially if the client is unable to determine which cat is eliminating inappropriately, and/or is unable to understand social interactions and dynamics between the cats.

TREATMENT

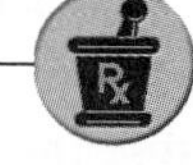

THERAPEUTIC GOAL(S)

- Appropriate and reliable use of intended substrates for elimination
- Aimed at addressing substrate (surface or texture) preferences and location preferences and at identifying and managing concurrent behavioral disorders (e.g., intercat aggression) that can contribute to inappropriate elimination

ACUTE AND CHRONIC TREATMENT

- Identify previously preferred substrates and locations, and replicate these.
- Ensure that there is at least one more litter box than the number of cats.
- Ensure that the litter boxes are at least 1.5 cat body lengths long. This is larger than virtually all commercially available litter boxes for cats, but rigorous research has indicated that this is the size preferred by cats.
- Identify locations where the cat spends the most time and place boxes accordingly.
- Ensure that the clients are complying with an appropriate cleaning regimen:
  - Scoop litter multiple times daily.
  - Totally dump litter including the recyclable multicat litters two to three times a week, depending on the number of cats using them.
  - Wash, rinse, and dry the litter box at least weekly.
  - Avoid liners and scented litters.
  - Ensure that covered litter boxes have good ventilation, if they must be used.
- Use good odor eliminations (e.g., Anti-Icky-Poo [AIP]) on all substrates where urine or feces has been inappropriately deposited.
- Identify potential stressors or conflicts in the household (e.g., intercat aggression) and redress them. The most common of these may be relationships between cats in the household. Intercat aggression is a serious concern if:
  - One cat is avoiding one or more other cats.
  - One cat consistently leaves the room or a preferred resting spot when one or more other cats enter.
  - One cat cannot or does not eat or drink in the presence of the others.
  - One cat is inapparent and always hiding.
  - One cat is hyperreactive to any noise or tactile stimuli.

If any of these conditions can be identified, ensure that the clients separate the afflicted cats when they are not supervised. The more timid cat should have free-range; the more aggressive cat should be confined in a space that is not highly contested or desirable (e.g., not the client's bedroom or the kitchen).

- If anxiety and aggression are involved, benzodiazepines (BZD), tricyclic antidepressants (TCAs), or serotonin specific reuptake inhibitors (SSRIs) may be useful treatments for the anxious/aggressive cat.
  - TCAs: amitriptyline or nortriptyline (0.5-1.0 mg/kg PO q 12-24h × 30 days, minimum); clomipramine (0.5 mg/kg PO q 24h × minimum 60 days).

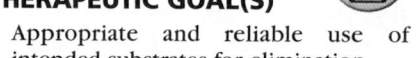

- SSRIs: fluoxetine or paroxetine (0.5 mg/kg PO q 24h × minimum 60 days).
- BZD: diazepam or oxazepam (0.2-0.4 mg/kg PO q12-24h × minimum 30 days); alprazolam (0.01-0.025 mg/kg PO q 12-24h, or as needed q 4-5h for panic).
- BZD are helpful primarily in behavior modification programs involving food reward (e.g., teaching cats that have problems with each other to tolerate each other).
- TCAs and SSRIs can be extremely useful in helping to overcome aversions and to address the anxiety involved in marking behaviors and in intercat aggression.

- If the toileting issue is associated with intercat aggression and the victim needs to become more outgoing, buspirone (0.5-1.0 mg/kg PO q 24h × 60 days, minimum), can be a good drug of choice, but it may act, in part, by rendering the afflicted cat sufficiently confident to engage in social interactions that could result in a true, physical fight, which clients need to monitor and address if it occurs.
- If more animals are added to the household, clients should expect social upheaval.
- Attention should be paid to the victimized cat before the other cats.
- Litter box hygiene must be meticulous and lifelong.
- Outdoor or visitor cats should be kept to a minimum or excluded.
- Consider allowing the cat to be an indoor/outdoor cat, if all else fails.

POSSIBLE COMPLICATIONS

- BZD: hyperexcitability (rare), severe hepatotoxicity (rare), potential abuse by clients.
- Cats treated with monoamine oxidase inhibitors (some flea and tick collars) should not be treated with TCAs or SSRIs.

RECOMMENDED MONITORING

Exam and laboratory tests at least every 6 to 12 months if taking medications.

PROGNOSIS AND OUTCOME

- Without treatment, the prognosis is guarded. Inappropriate elimination is the single most common reason cats in North America are euthanized or relinquished.
- Clients maintain cats in their household for an average of 2 years after a complaint has been identified, but the more obvious inappropriate urination or spraying is to the client, the more likely he or she is to be intolerant of it.
- Prognosis is improved by early diagnosis, comprehensive treatment, attentive client monitoring, and open communication between clinician and client.

PEARLS & CONSIDERATIONS

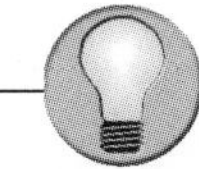

COMMENTS

In the absence of meeting the cat's needs, attempts to constrain the cat to eliminate in places, on substrates, or in modes preferred by the client will likely result in a worsening of the problem.

PREVENTION

- Meeting the cat's needs, whether this involves providing sweater boxes or canine litter boxes, providing multiple boxes, or grouping cats by temperament, is the single best way to prevent elimination problems.
- Veterinarians should screen for elimination problems as a routine part of every appointment, and should encourage clients to call at the first sign of any "accident." Because elimination is a complex behavior in cats, waiting to discuss the issue may result in the death or relinquishment of the cat.

CLIENT EDUCATION

- Treatment of behavioral conditions is an ongoing process, often for the life of the pet. Relapses may occur with treatment discontinuation or with added stressors.
- Physical illness is also a stressor and may promote a behavioral elimination problem where previously none existed.

SUGGESTED READING

Cameron ME, et al: A study of environmental and behavioral factors that may be associated with feline idiopathic cystitis. *J Small Anim Pract* 45:144-147, 2004.

Ciribassi J, et al: Comparative bioavailability of fluoxetine after transdermal and oral administration to healthy cats. *Am J Vet Res* 64:994-998, 2003.

King JN, et al: Determination of the dosage of clomipramine for the treatment of urine spraying in cats. *J Am Vet Med Assoc* 225:881-887, 2004.

Wright JC, Amoss RT: Prevalence of house soiling and aggression in kittens during the first year after adoption from a humane society. *J Am Vet Med Assoc* 224:1790-1795, 2004.

AUTHOR & EDITOR: **KAREN L. OVERALL**

Inappropriate Elimination, Dog

Client Education Sheet on Website

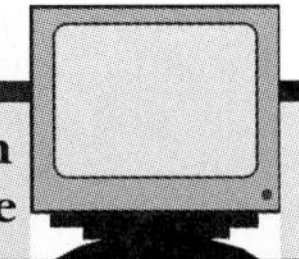

BASIC INFORMATION

DEFINITION

- Urination or defecation, in a location other than areas acceptable to the client.
- Marking: urination (or less commonly defecation) for hierarchial purposes, or as part of an anxiety disorder. Usually involves small amounts of urine deposited in several places, often vertical surfaces.
- Incontinence: inadvertent passage of urine or feces as a clinical manifestation of illness.

SYNONYM(S)

Housesoiling
Incomplete housebreaking
Incomplete housetraining
Soiling
Toileting issues

EPIDEMIOLOGY

SPECIES, AGE, SEX

- Can affect dogs of any age and either sex.
- Sexually intact dogs may have increased rates of urine marking.
- Puppies do not have the physical abilities to inhibit elimination and the cognitive abilities to make associations with preferred substrate (i.e., surface onto which they eliminate) until about 8.5 weeks old. Between 7 and 9 weeks of age is the ideal age to housetrain a dog.
- Older dogs, particularly those who are female and were neutered young, may experience incontinence associated with joint laxity and decreased urethral sphincter tone with age. These problems are medical disorders, not behavioral abnormalities.

GENETICS AND BREED PREDISPOSITION: Owners of toy breed dogs may claim increased difficulty with housetraining. Due to their size and the relatively small amount of damage done by "accidents," small dogs may not be strictly supervised or confined until fully housetrained as would be larger dogs. More important, clients may not appreciate that small dogs have bladders the size of a grape, whereas mid-sized dogs have bladders the size of an orange. Small bladder size, coupled with the proportionally greater metabolic rate that accompanies smaller body size, mean that smaller dogs need more frequent access to appropriate areas for elimination. Specific data with respect to any breed and familial tendencies for marking behaviors do not exist at this time.

RISK FACTORS

- Sexually intact status.
- Presence of intact animals, especially if in estrus (provokes urinary marking by neutered animals).
- Rehomed street and kennel dogs (may never have learned to inhibit their elimination behaviors, and will have to learn inhibition and appropriate substrate and location preferences as adults).
- Urinary and fecal marking and increased urgency can be nonspecific signs associated with anxiety disorders. Many dogs with chronic generalized anxiety disorder, for example, have sporadic or chronic diarrhea. Any dog given a diagnosis of "inflammatory bowel disease" should be fully screened for behavioral problems.

CONTAGION AND ZOONOSIS: If the inappropriate elimination is due to incomplete housetraining, marking by other dogs in the household may occur. The role of olfactory stimulation and social communication in elimination complaints cannot be overstated.

GEOGRAPHY AND SEASONALITY

- Weather may factor into a dog's willingness to eliminate outside, especially if the dog is small and/or becomes cold easily. Snow and ice should be cleared in a way that allows access and traction.
- Dogs should be exposed to a variety of surfaces/substrates (e.g., grass, cement, sand, stones, sawdust) that will meet the seasonal and lifestyle requirements in which the dog is expected to live. Elimination disorders may be caused by some dogs' rigid and singular substrate preferences (e.g., grass for a dog living where snowfall is the rule).

CLINICAL PRESENTATION

DISEASE FORMS/SUBTYPES: The house soiling may involve inappropriate urination, inappropriate defecation, marking with urine, marking with feces, or a combination. Not all urinary marking is vertical. Both males and females can use a variety of positions to mark, and leg-cocking is more associated with unfamiliar social stimuli than with sex-based behaviors.

HISTORY, CHIEF COMPLAINT

- Client finds urine or feces inside the home.
- Client may report that the dog was taken out and returned to eliminate in the house.
- Information on volume, frequency, appearance, and when the housesoiling occurs is critical in determining underlying cause.

PHYSICAL EXAM FINDINGS

- Findings should be unremarkable in cases with a behavioral etiology (including rectal palpation).
- Abnormal physical exam findings should raise the possibility of medical disorders causing urinary or fecal incontinence (see Incontinence, Fecal, p 588; Incontinence, Urinary, p 589).

ETIOLOGY AND PATHOPHYSIOLOGY

- Inappropriate elimination is a nonspecific sign that may be "normal" (e.g., incomplete housetraining) or abnormal and associated either with medical disorders (see Incontinence, Fecal, p 588; Incontinence, Urinary, p 589) or with behavioral disturbances and specifically with anxiety disorders.
- Any condition that triggers a fight or flight response can lead to involuntary voiding that may be misinterpreted by the client as purposeful, malicious, or vengeful.
- While partly associated with reproduction, marking is largely a social behavior and likely to provide information about identity, sex, age, physical condition, and diet of the dog depositing the urine or feces.
- Olfactory stimulation for normal elimination and marking behaviors is extremely important to dogs and poorly understood by humans.
- Meeting the individual dog's age- and size-specific needs is the key to understanding the root of housesoiling and therefore to addressing it.

DIAGNOSIS

DIFFERENTIAL DIAGNOSIS

- Behavioral differential diagnoses:
  - Incomplete housetraining: occurs regardless of client presence or absence, large volume of urine is voided. Normal stool is deposited. Certain areas of the house may be sought preferentially.
  - "Submissive" or excitement urination: occurs upon greeting a person or when the dog is excited. The dog often crouches down and starts to roll over when approached.
  - Marking behaviors: urine marking typically involves small quantities in several locations in the absence of another medical problem. Urine may be deposited in vertical (most common), horizontal, or a combination of surfaces. Fecal marking is less well understood, but small amounts of feces are deposited in response to the presence of unfamiliar animals. Texture and content of feces changes with frequency of marking.
  - Separation anxiety (see Separation Anxiety, p 993).
  - Storm phobia (see Phobias, p 847).
  - Panic disorder.
  - Generalized anxiety disorder.
- Medical differential diagnoses:
  - See Incontinence, Fecal, p 588; Incontinence, Urinary, p 589.

INITIAL DATABASE

Complete blood count, serum chemistry panel, thyroid function evaluation, urinalysis, and fecal flotation to assess possible etiologies for polyuria, pollakiuria, and abnormal stool consistency that may lead to inappropriate voiding.

ADVANCED OR CONFIRMATORY TESTING

- As dictated by physical exam and initial database findings.
- Once any medical disorders are resolved, a behavioral diagnosis and treatment plan can be pursued if the inappropriate elimination persists, because the inciting causes may be medical but the maintenance causes may be behavioral.

TREATMENT

THERAPEUTIC GOAL(S)

Treat underlying medical disorder(s). If inappropriate elimination persists address behavioral sequelae to restore housetraining. Refer to sections on separation anxiety and phobias for treatment of anxiety-related elimination.

ACUTE GENERAL TREATMENT

- Incomplete housetraining: Fully confine or supervise when indoors, using a leash or crate. If the dog is "caught" eliminating, calmly take outside to the chosen elimination area, allow the dog to finish, and praise lavishly. Take to eliminate after eating, after play, after any slowing in play, and after awakening. Any yelling or punishment is likely to hasten the voiding process and is counterproductive.
- Submissive or excitement urination: Owner should maintain an emotionally

"low" approach, especially when greeting the dog. It may be necessary to ignore the dog until it is very calm and then guide it outside to greet after elimination. Cornerstones of successful treatment are to keep the dog's bladder empty through frequent, well-timed walks outside to eliminate, and to use positive methods and rewards for teaching the dog to sit without leaking or cringing.

CHRONIC TREATMENT

- Clients should be advised against punishing after the fact. This makes no sense to the dog and may force it to housesoil out of sight, eliminating the opportunity to praise for correct behavior.
- For "submissive" urination, use rule structures that guide the pet to learn what behaviors are considered correct in the home and in social interactions. This approach lessens the dog's need to signal submission with urination.
- For excitement urination, teaching the dog that calm behaviors like sitting and lying down to get praise and attention will lessen overall reactivity and encourage the dog to react calmly.
- For both excitement and "submissive" urination, it is important to praise body postures associated with a happier, calmer, more confident, less uncertain dog.
- For small dogs with high metabolisms, or less agile or ill dogs, canine litter boxes may be a good solution, especially in urban areas. Accustoming the dog to the substrate to be used in the box at an early age may help.
- For marking behaviors within the house, it is important to address the social interactions between the animals. Screening for overt and covert aggressions and other anxiety-related conditions in all of the household pets should be undertaken (see Aggression, Dog, p 46).
- For marking behaviors outside the house, exposure to other stimuli is the only management possible.
- For intact male dogs who become distracted in the presence of female urine: a problem for many working (e.g., service, assistance, explosives detection) dogs, castration as early in the development of the marking behavior as is possible largely resolves the situation in most cases. There is a learned component to any elimination concern, and the longer the problem has been ongoing without redress, the less likely neutering, alone, is to fix the problem.
- Because of the learning component, veterinarians should screen all dogs at all visits for elimination complaints. Early redress decreases the impact of the learning component.

POSSIBLE COMPLICATIONS

Punishment will either be useless in fixing the problem or will make the problem worse. The latter is particularly true if any anxiety is involved in the elimination.

PROGNOSIS AND OUTCOME

- Prognosis is excellent in cases of incomplete housetraining or "submissive" or excitement elimination, as long as proper identification of underlying cause and thorough behavior modification are carried out.
- Prognosis for problematic marking behaviors is excellent if the associated behavioral concerns of the household are competently addressed.
- Prognosis is guarded for an adult male dog that has urine-marked for his entire life. The learning component is likely far more important at this stage than is the hormonal component.

PEARLS & CONSIDERATIONS

COMMENTS

- Abuse of puppies and abuse of human children often starts with abusive behavior surrounding housetraining/toilet training. Veterinarians should be aware of the signs (see Abuse, p 14).
- Lack of attention to the dog's need is the most common reason for poor housetraining or other nonmarking elimination problems in dogs.
- Fecal marking and increased urgency (e.g., sporadic diarrhea) can be nonspecific signs associated with anxiety disorders rather than primary gastrointestinal disease. Any dog given a diagnosis of inflammatory bowel disease should be fully screened for behavioral problems.

PREVENTION

- Frequent exercise every day. Taking a dog out twice daily often is insufficient. Encourage clients to think of how often they eliminate every day and to understand the dog's metabolism is just like theirs.
- Ensure that dogs are not outside only for the purpose of elimination. If this is so they may delay eliminating outside to have more opportunity to experience outdoor stimuli, and may then eliminate indoors.
- Reward dogs for eliminating outside with play, freedom, exercise, praise, interaction with other dogs, and time to smell their canine world.

CLIENT EDUCATION

- Client education is key to preventing and fixing these problems. All veterinary practices should have handouts (available from numerous texts and sources) that explain how to housetrain dogs and a designated staff member should be responsible for implementing and following up on such training.
- Quick screening at each veterinary visit for elimination complaints and other behavioral concerns saves lives. Veterinarians need to know that clients are unlikely to share behavioral information and questions unless prompted to do so.

SUGGESTED READING

Houpt KA: Housesoiling by dogs. In Horwitz D, Mills D, Heath S (eds): *BSAVA Manual of Canine and Feline Behavioral Medicine*. BSAVA, 2002, pp 90–96.

Overall KL: Canine behavioral disorders. In Morgan RV, Bright RM, Swartout MS (eds): *Handbook of Small Animal Practice*. Philadelphia, WB Saunders, 2003, pp 1149–1162.

Overall KL: *Clinical Behavioral Medicine for Small Animals*. St. Louis, Mosby, 1997.

AUTHOR: **SORAYA V. JUARBE-DIAZ**

EDITOR: **KAREN L. OVERALL**

Incontinence, Fecal

BASIC INFORMATION

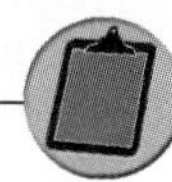

DEFINITION

Inability to retain feces

EPIDEMIOLOGY

SPECIES, AGE, SEX

- Young animals: inappropriate house-training, congenital disorders.
- Old animals: senility/cognitive dysfunction, neoplasia.

GENETICS AND BREED PREDISPOSITION

- German shepherd: degenerative lumbosacral stenosis, perianal fistulas.
- English bulldogs, Manx cats: congenital spinal malformations.

RISK FACTORS

- Perineal surgery
- Pelvic or lumbosacral trauma
- Perianal diseases
- Tail avulsion fractures

ASSOCIATED CONDITIONS AND DISORDERS: Urinary incontinence

CLINICAL PRESENTATION

DISEASE FORMS/SUBTYPES

- Anal sphincter incontinence
  - Non-neurogenic
  - Neurogenic
- Reservoir incontinence
- Behavior
- Sundry

HISTORY, CHIEF COMPLAINT

- Sphincter incontinence:
  - Unaware of fecal elimination; unassociated with defecation behavior.
  - Small amounts of ± normal feces dribble out, especially when intra-abdominal pressure increases suddenly (e.g., coughing).
  - Paraparesis.
  - Urinary incontinence may be present.
  - Perineal soiling.
- Reservoir incontinence:
  - Animal aware of incontinence; defecation behavior present, but is unable to control the time and place of elimination.
  - Abnormal feces, suggestive of recto-colonic disease (diarrhea, mucoid, hematochezia).
  - Defecation associated with signs of rectocolonic disease (tenesmus, dyschezia).
- Behavior:
  - Housesoiling with normal feces and defecation.
  - Destructive behavior.

PHYSICAL EXAM FINDINGS

- Sphincter incontinence:
  - Non-neurogenic:
    - Perineal/anal sphincter tumors, erosions, fistulas, trauma, anal sac disease.
  - Neurogenic:
    - Decreased anal tone.
    - Abnormal bulbocavernosus, rectal inflation, or anal reflexes.
    - Loss of tail tone and voluntary movement.
    - Spinal, lumbosacral pain.
    - Hyperesthesia of hind limbs or perineum.
    - Lower motor neuron signs (paresis/paralysis with decreased muscle tone, decreased spinal reflexes). Or upper motor (increased spinal reflexes, ataxia).
    - Abnormal behavior or mentation.
- Reservoir incontinence:
  - Abnormal feces: mucoid, bloody, and/or parasites.
  - Rectal masses, mucosal changes, pain on digital rectal examination.
  - Signs of gastrointestinal disease (weight loss, anorexia, vomiting).
- Behavior: normal physical exam.

ETIOLOGY AND PATHOPHYSIOLOGY

- Sphincter incontinence: diseases of the anal sphincter or adjacent structures.
  - Non-neurogenic: anatomic disruption of the anal sphincter preventing functional seal. Anal tone and reflexes normal.
  - Neurogenic:
    - Peripheral: sphincter dysfunction due to inadequate sensory or motor nerve supply, normal sphincter anatomy.
    - Central: loss of subconscious or conscious modification of reflex defecation.
- Reservoir incontinence: diseases of the colon/rectum:
  - Diseases impairing colonic-rectal compliance, capacity or causing irritation.
  - Normal sphincter anatomy and neural supply.
  - Altered fecal consistency: feces enter into rectum too rapidly for normal control to take place.
  - Urge incontinence, "overflow incontinence": liquid feces seep around constipated fecal material.

DIAGNOSIS

DIFFERENTIAL DIAGNOSIS

- Sphincter incontinence:
  - Non-neurogenic:
    - Damage to the levator ani, coccygeal, internal and external anal sphincters
    - Perianal trauma, tumors, infections, fistulas; perineal surgery, hernias
  - Neurogenic sphincter incompetence:
    - Cauda equina syndrome
    - Spinal cord disease: trauma, neoplasia, compressive lesions, degenerative conditions
    - Autonomic dysfunction: dysautonomia
    - Peripheral neuropathies
    - Myopathies
    - Cerebral conditions
- Reservoir incontinence:
  - Inflammatory (colitis, proctitis) and noninflammatory (neoplasia) colorectal disease
  - Diets or diseases causing diarrhea or constipation
- Behavior:
  - Inadequate or inappropriate house-training
  - Cognitive dysfunction
  - Conditions affecting locomotion: inability/unwillingness to walk to the elimination area (e.g., severe arthritic pain)
  - Separation anxiety, litter box aversion, location preferences/aversions, inadequate privacy
- Sundry: rectovaginal fistulas

INITIAL DATABASE

- Physical examination including perineal and digital rectal examination
- Fecal analysis
- Complete neurologic examination, especially:
  - Bulbocavernosus, anal and rectal inflation reflexes
  - Perineal and tail sensation
  - Anal sphincter and tail tone
- Complete blood count
- Serum biochemistry panel
- Urinalysis ± culture and sensitivity

ADVANCED OR CONFIRMATORY TESTING

- Sphincter incontinence:
  - Electromyography of the lumbosacral, paraspinal, levator ani, coccygeal, and anal sphincter muscles
  - Nerve conduction velocity assessment
  - Muscle and nerve biopsies
  - Spinal radiographs ± myelography, epidurography
  - Spinal computed tomography, magnetic resonance imaging
  - Cerebrospinal fluid analysis

- Reservoir incontinence:
  - Colonoscopy, proctoscopy
  - Rectal-colonic mucosal biopsy: cytology, histopathology

TREATMENT

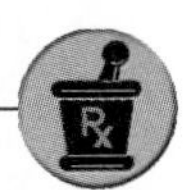

THERAPEUTIC GOAL(S)

- Treat the primary cause
- Supportive care

ACUTE GENERAL TREATMENT

Generally not required. Acute treatment of the underlying cause (e.g., constipation, perianal fistula, neurogenic disorders), rather than fecal incontinence itself, may be necessary.

CHRONIC TREATMENT

- Low-residue diet
- Intestinal motility altering agents: loperamide, diphenoxylate
- Maintain low intrarectal pressures
  - Warm water enemas ± laxatives (lactulose): may help decrease inappropriate fecal dribbling by keeping rectum empty in some cases
  - Frequent opportunities to defecate if some control is present
  - Induction of reflex defecation: warm moist washcloth on anus/perineum
- Prevent fecal scalding (clip and clean perineum, intermittent tail wrap if longhaired, barrier cream)
- Change in environment to make incontinence more acceptable
- Surgical:
  - Anorectal reconstruction
  - Silicon elastomer sling
  - Neosphincter
  - Fecal diversion procedures: colonostomy
  - Semitendinous muscle transfer flap

POSSIBLE COMPLICATIONS

- Fecal soiling predisposes to perineal dermatitis and urinary tract infections (females)
- Constipation possible with motility-modifying medication

RECOMMENDED MONITORING

Medical management must be regarded as a therapeutic trial.

PROGNOSIS AND OUTCOME

- Guarded to poor with:
  - Many neurogenic sphincter causes (degenerative neuropathies, dysautonomia, lumbosacral stenosis)
  - Severe anal sphincter lesions
  - Underlying cause not found
- Fair to good with:
  - Controlled rectocolonic disease
  - Behavioral causes

PEARLS & CONSIDERATIONS

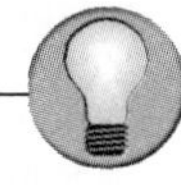

COMMENTS

- Determination of the type of fecal incontinence (neurogenic, non-neurogenic, reservoir, behavioral, sundry) is critical to accurate evaluation, treatment, and prognosis. Determining the type of fecal incontinence is mainly dependent on obtaining a detailed history and performing a complete physical examination.
- Fecal incontinence is a common reason for client requested euthanasia.
- Response and client satisfaction are highly variable and based on client expectation and ability.

PREVENTION

Precise and atraumatic technique when performing perineal surgery

CLIENT EDUCATION

Discuss prognosis and complications early with clients to avoid unrealistic expectations

SUGGESTED READING

Guilford WG: Fecal incontinence in dogs and cats. *Compend Contin Educ Pract Vet* 12:313, 1990.

AUTHOR: **FRANK KETTNER**
EDITOR: **ETIENNE CÔTÉ**

Incontinence, Urinary

BASIC INFORMATION

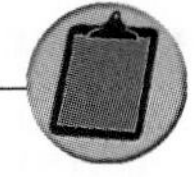

DEFINITION

Lack of voluntary control over the passage of urine

EPIDEMIOLOGY

SPECIES, AGE, SEX

- With young animals, congenital disorders are more likely.
- Female dogs: older, spayed females are prone to incontinence due to urethral incompetence.

GENETICS AND BREED PREDISPOSITION

- Ectopic ureter: Siberian huskies, miniature and standard poodles, Labrador retrievers, Newfoundland, fox terriers, West Highland white terriers, collies, and Welsh Corgis.

CLINICAL PRESENTATION

HISTORY, CHIEF COMPLAINT

- Dribbling urine.
- Incontinence while sleeping: a hallmark of urethral incompetence in spayed female dogs.

PHYSICAL EXAM FINDINGS

- Urine staining or scalding in perineum.
- Neurologic deficits.
- Bladder should be palpated before and after urination.
- Bladder expression:
  - Easy: decreased outflow resistance.
  - Difficult: normal or increased outflow resistance.
- Rectal examination
  - Urethral thickening (inflammation or infiltration).
  - Prostatomegaly (see Prostatomegaly, p 899).
  - Bladder trigone abnormalities.

ETIOLOGY AND PATHOPHYSIOLOGY

- Neurogenic:
  - Lower motor neuron (LMN; lesion at S1-S3 spinal cord segment, or peripheral nerve disorder)
  - Upper motor neuron (UMN; lesion cranial to sacral spinal cord segment S1)
- Non-neurogenic:
  - Anatomic
  - Functional

DIAGNOSIS

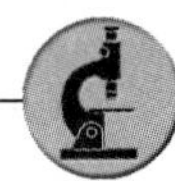

DIFFERENTIAL DIAGNOSIS

- Neurogenic:
  - LMN disorder (S1-S3 segment or peripheral nerve disorder).
    - Sacral fracture/malformation.
    - Trauma to pelvic nerve.
    - Lumbosacral disease.
  - UMN disorder (cranial to S1). Usually characterized by urine retention; overflow incontinence can occur.
    - Intervertebral disk disease.
    - Spinal trauma.
    - Fibrocartilaginous embolization.
    - Spinal neoplasia.

- Non-neurogenic:
  - Hormone responsive incontinence/urethral sphincter mechanism incompetence:
    - Most common cause in adult, female dogs.
  - Urge incontinence/detrusor hyperspasticity:
    - Associated with lower urinary tract signs.
  - Anatomic abnormalities:
    - Ectopic ureters.
    - Patent urachus.
    - Vaginal stricture.

INITIAL DATABASE

- Neurologic examination:
  - UMN.
    - Firm, difficult to express bladder.
  - LMN.
    - Flaccid, easily expressed bladder.
    - Decreased/absent anal tone, bulbospongiosus reflex, perineal sensation.
  - Pain on tail lift: associated with lumbosacral disease.
  - Pain on spinal palpation; ataxia, proprioceptive deficits: associated with intervertebral disk disease.
- Laboratory tests:
  - Urinalysis:
    - Cystocentesis preferred.
    - Pyuria suggests infection of inflammation, leading to increased urge.
    - Hematuria suggests inflammation or neoplasia.
  - Urine culture and sensitivity.
  - Complete blood count (CBC)/serum biochemistry panel.

ADVANCED OR CONFIRMATORY TESTING

- Diagnostic imaging:
  - Abdominal radiographs/ultrasound: structural lesions.
  - Cystourethrography/vaginography: radiolucent defects.
  - Spinal radiography/myelogram/computed tomography/magnetic resonance imaging: spinal cord lesions.
- Endoscopy:
  - Direct visualization of ectopic ureters and other anatomic defects.
  - Evaluate, and if indicated, biopsy vaginal vault and mucosa of urethra and bladder.
- Urodynamic studies: urethral pressure profilometry.
  - Measure pressure, volume, and flow in the urethra and bladder. Improves localization of anatomic site of dysfunction.
  - Generally only available at referral/research facilities.
  - Should be considered in patients refractory to treatment.

TREATMENT

THERAPEUTIC GOAL(S)

- Correct underlying anatomic defect.
- Treat any coexisting or secondary conditions (urinary tract infection, neurologic disease).
- Pharmacologic therapy is the mainstay of treatment of incontinence in dogs.

CHRONIC TREATMENT

- When an underlying disorder is present (e.g, urinary tract infection, prostatic disease, urethral neoplasia), treatment is directed at improvement or resolution of this primary cause.
- If no underlying disorder is found and the patient is an adult female spayed dog with a history consistent with urethral incompetence, the following treatments may be considered.
- α-Agonists:
  - Phenylpropanolamine (PPA) used as first line treatment.
    - When given at 1.1-1.5 mg/kg PO q 8h, effective in 85–90% of female dogs with urethral incompetence.
  - Pseudoephedrine and ephredrine.
    - Generally used when PPA is not available.
    - While efficacy appears to be similar to PPA, not as well researched.
    - Incidence of side effects may be higher than with PPA.
- Reproductive hormones/estrogen:
  - Diethylstilbestrol (DES).
    - 0.1-0.2 mg/kg PO q 24h for 5 days, then the same dose PO 1-2 times per week.
    - Efficacy of 50-65% in female dogs with urethral incompetence.
    - Excessive doses associated with bone marrow suppression—monitor CBCs.
  - Estriol
    - Recently evaluated as a substitute to DES.
    - Dosage is 2 mg PO/day for 7 days, then reduced at weekly intervals to minimum effective dose.
    - Studies are limited, but bone marrow suppression has not been reported.
    - Efficacy and safety need to be further evaluated.
- Surgical and endoscopic therapies:
  - Colposuspension/urethropexy:
    - Resolves incontinence in 50% of dogs.
    - Remaining patients may respond to medication.
  - Bulking agents:
    - Endoscopic injection of Teflon or collagen bulking agents into periurethral tissue.
    - Repeat injections may be needed for satisfactory results.
    - Success rates of approximately 50% have been reported in preliminary studies.

PROGNOSIS AND OUTCOME

- Outcome for dogs and cats with correctable structural abnormalities is good to excellent.
- Treatment is generally successful with urethral incompetence, although dosage adjustment is often required.
- Although not an inherently life-threatening disorder, urinary incontinence may lead to the consideration of euthanasia in refractory cases.

PEARLS & CONSIDERATIONS

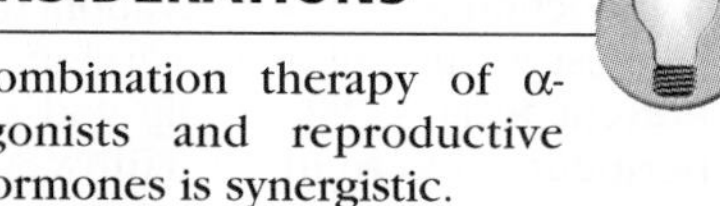

- Combination therapy of α-agonists and reproductive hormones is synergistic.
- Female dogs resistant to single agent therapy should receive combination therapy.
- Treatment failure with PPA may result from inadequate dosing. Studies show 3 times a day therapy is effective, but owners may only administer twice a day.
- Multiple therapies may be needed to control refractory patients.

SUGGESTED READING

Adams LG, Syme HM: Canine lower urinary tract diseases. In Ettinger SJ, Feldman EC (eds): *Textbook of Veterinary Internal Medicine,* ed 6. St. Louis, Elsevier, 2005, pp 1850–1874.

Hoelzler MG, Lidbetter DA: Surgical management of urinary incontinence. *Vet Clin North Am Small Anim Pract* 34(4):1057–1073, 2004.

Lane IF: Treating urinary incontinence. *Vet Med* 98(1):58–64, 2003.

Scott L, Leddy M, Bernay F, Davot JL: Evaluation of phenylpropanolamine in the treatment of urethral sphincter mechanism incompetence in the bitch. *J Small Anim Pract* 43(11):493–496, 2002.

AUTHOR: **CLAIRE WEIGAND**

EDITOR: **ETIENNE CÔTÉ**

Infertility, Female Dog

BASIC INFORMATION

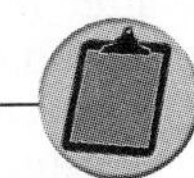

DEFINITION

The failure to ovulate, to accept the male, to become pregnant, to maintain pregnancy, or to deliver live puppies at term

SYNONYM(S)

Infecundity
Sterility

EPIDEMIOLOGY

SPECIES, AGE, SEX: Canine, anytime after puberty (6 months and older), female.

GENETICS AND BREED PREDISPOSITION: Infertility is more prevalent in inbred families of purebred dogs. There is no documented breed predisposition, but there is anecdotal information indicating that some breeds of dogs have poor fertility (e.g., Norwich terriers, some sight hounds).

RISK FACTORS

- Advancing age of bitches at times of attempted breeding can decrease fertility. Many conformation show bitches and many performance and racing bitches are bred past peak fertility, which is 2 to 4 years of age for the canine female.
- Poor or incomplete breeding management is responsible for most apparent infertility in the bitch (see Breeding Management, p 153).
- Previous hormone therapy, abnormal hormone concentrations, and uterine disease also increase the risk of infertility.
- Anestrus, silent heat, persistent estrus, irregular estrus, abnormal sexual behavior, uterine disease, hypoluteoidism, and structural abnormalities of the female reproductive tract are all conditions associated with infertility.
- Systemic disease may result in changes in the general health of the bitch that can interfere with normal fertility.

CONTAGION AND ZOONOSIS: Infertility itself is not contagious. Several bacterial and viral agents contributing to infertility are contagious and can be spread both orally and venereally. These agents include but are not limited to β-hemolytic *Streptococcus*, *Mycoplasma*, and *Ureaplasma* spp., and herpesvirus. The most significant canine venereal disease is *Brucella canis*, which has zoonotic potential, especially through contact with vaginal discharge, aborted fetuses, urine, or semen. Contrary to popular belief, brucellosis is spread dog-to-dog orally as frequently as venereally. The organisms are shed in very high numbers in vaginal discharge and can be found in the urine of infected animals.

GEOGRAPHY AND SEASONALITY: Female domestic dogs are nonseasonal with the exception of the basenji that only enters proestrus in the late summer/early fall.

CLINICAL PRESENTATION

DISEASE FORMS/SUBTYPES: Breeding management issues, abnormalities of the estrous cycle, uterine abnormalities.

HISTORY, CHIEF COMPLAINT: Varies with the client: *history is the most important tool in the approach to infertility.* Important issues to ask about are:

- General health history: What is the vaccination status of the bitch? What medications is she currently receiving? What medications including vitamins and herbal supplements has she received in the past? Include heartworm preventative and any topical medications.
- Housing details: kennel, home, indoor, outdoor, and number of bitches in the household.
- What was the bitch's age at her first cycle?
- Length of each cycle from onset of vulvar swelling to diestrus cytology.
- What is the bitch's cycle interval? Details of cycle: onset of vulvar swelling and vulvar discharge, onset of estrous behavior (flagging), dates of mating.
- Method of mating: natural service or artificial insemination by bitch owner, stud owner, or veterinarian?
- Was the bitch artificially inseminated with fresh, chilled, or frozen semen? Was the semen deposited into the vagina or the uterus?
    - Stud dog status: Is the male proven? If so when was his last litter of puppies born? Has he had a semen evaluation? How old is the male? Has his semen been cultured?
- What are the dates of *B. canis* serology for both the bitch and the stud dog?
- What was the method of pregnancy diagnosis: palpation, endocrinology, ultrasound, or radiographs?
- Were hormone assays performed during the cycle? Was vaginal cytology and/or progesterone testing performed to time the breedings? If progesterone testing was done, was it quantitative or qualitative?
- Was the bitch being campaigned or under any other stressful event such as a new home?
- Is there a history in infertility in the pedigree?

PHYSICAL EXAM FINDINGS: Physical examination is usually within normal limits. Special attention should be paid to the external genitalia and to the mammary glands.

- Digital vaginal examination: to assess the patency and accessibility of the vulva and caudal vagina.
- Vaginal examinations may be difficult in toy breed bitches that are anestrous at the time of the examination.
- Vaginal septae and circumferential strictures may interfere with natural service and may interfere with artificial insemination into the vagina as well.
- The mammary glands are visually inspected and palpated.

ETIOLOGY AND PATHOPHYSIOLOGY

- Mistimed breeding is by far the most common cause of infertility.
- Ovarian dysfunction: abnormalities in ovulation and maintenance of the corpus luteum, persistent estrus, and primary anestrus.
- Uterine dysfunction: lesions of the uterus (cystic endometrial hyperplasia/pyometra), subclinical uterine infection, shortened interestrous interval resulting in implantation failure. The canine uterus requires 130 to 150 days following the onset of proestrus for endometrial repair to occur.

DIAGNOSIS

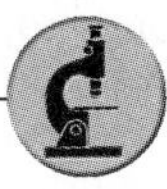

DIFFERENTIAL DIAGNOSIS

Pregnancy loss, ovulation failure, silent heat, or stud dog infertility

INITIAL DATABASE

Complete blood count, serum biochemistry profile, thyroid panel, *B. canis* serology, vaginal cytology, vaginal culture if in estrus or if discharge present

ADVANCED OR CONFIRMATORY TESTING

- Vaginoscopy, progesterone testing, ultrasonography of the uterus and ovaries, ovarian or uterine biopsy in select cases.
- Herpesvirus serology or biopsy with histopathologic evaluation of tissue could be used in select cases.
- In cases of primary anestrus, it is wise to karyotype the bitch to assess her actual chromosomal makeup. Trisomy X, XO females, and other abnormal chromosome combinations have been reported.

TREATMENT

THERAPEUTIC GOAL(S)

Treat the underlying cause of the infertility, which is usually breeding management.

ACUTE GENERAL TREATMENT

- In the case of shortened interestrous interval, the drug mibolerone, a synthetic androgen formerly manufactured by the Upjohn Company, has been used effectively to lengthen the interestrous interval. The drug is currently available through some compounding pharmacies.
- Use appropriate antibiotic therapy for uterine infection and prostaglandin therapy for cystic endometrial hyperplasia/pyometra.
- For persistent estrus either gonadotropin-releasing hormone or human chorionic gonadotropin may be used in an attempt to induce ovulation.
- There is no reliable therapy to induce fertile estrus in the bitch. There are many protocols in use with varying outcomes; however, no controlled studies have been published. For documented premature luteolysis, progestin supplementation may be warranted. Drugs used include Regumate, (altrenogest), megestrol acetate, and progesterone in oil. The client should be warned that this is extra label use and has the potential for masculinization of female fetuses.

DRUG INTERACTIONS

Use care in the selection of any medication used in a breeding bitch. For example, topical corticosteroids can be absorbed systemically and are not recommended. Use reference list for appropriate drug selection in pregnancy.

RECOMMENDED MONITORING

Confirm pregnancy using ultrasonography at 30 days postbreeding. One can measure progesterone levels at that time and weekly if there is any indication of variability in fetal vesicle size or fetal loss.

PROGNOSIS AND OUTCOME

Good to excellent for clients who will comply with breeding management recommendations. Guarded for bitches with uterine disease and for bitches with ovarian dysfunction.

PEARLS & CONSIDERATIONS

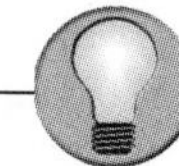

COMMENTS

Infertility of the stud dog is the second most common cause of female infertility after improper breeding management. Be sure that the stud dog is producing adequate numbers of motile and morphologically normal sperm and that the semen is inseminated properly.

PREVENTION

Planning, planning, and planning. Because the bitch has limited opportunities to successfully produce a litter, each desired breeding requires commitment of time, resources, and money by the client.

CLIENT EDUCATION

- Suggest a reproductive work-up before the next anticipated estrous cycle. Once the cycle begins, start vaginal cytologic evaluation as early as the third day of the cycle, obtain a vaginal culture early in the estrous cycle, and begin progesterone testing once vaginal cytologic study indicates greater than 75% cornification. Try to identify the luteinizing hormone peak by using the progesterone concentration of 2 ng/ml. Most bitches ovulate 2 days after reaching a progesterone concentration of 2 ng/ml. Ovulation occurs at progesterone levels of 4-10 ng/ml. Because the bitch ovulates a primary oocyte, litter size is greatest with breeding occurring 2 days after ovulation. Stress the importance of semen quality, sperm numbers, morphology, and motility for good fertility. To confirm infertility or pregnancy loss, ultrasonography is a vital tool.
- Failure to cycle is often a failure to observe the bitch adequately for physical changes consistent with proestrus. The client should blot the vulva daily to detect vaginal discharge and change in vulvar size and shape. Monthly progesterone assays are a valid method to detect ovulatory but unobserved estrus.

SUGGESTED READING

Edens M, et al: Breeding management in the bitch and queen. In *Small Animal Theriogenology*. St. Louis, Butterworth Heinemann, 2003, pp 33-60.

Gobello C, et al: Noninfectious spontaneous pregnancy loss in bitches. *Compendium* 24(10):778-783, 2002.

Johnston S, et al: Clinical approach to infertility in the bitch. In *Canine and Feline Theriogenology*. Philadelphia, WB Saunders, 2001, pp 257-273.

Peña FJ, et al: Mismating and abortion in bitches: The preattachment period. *Compendium* 24(5):400-408, 2002.

Ronsse V, et al: Risk factors and reproductive disorders associated with canine herpesvirus-1 (CHV-1). *Theriogenology* 61:619-636, 2004.

AUTHOR: **FRANCES O. SMITH**

EDITOR: **MICHELLE A. KUTZLER**

Infertility, Male: Abnormalities of the Spermiogram

BASIC INFORMATION

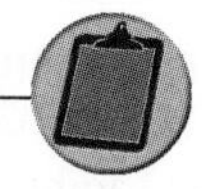

DEFINITION

- Three major categories of derangements may occur, either alone or in combination:
  - Asthenozoospermia: decreased numbers of progressively motile spermatozoa per ejaculate (<30-50%).
  - Teratozoospermia: increased numbers of morphologically abnormal spermatozoa per ejaculate (>40-50%).
  - Oligozoospermia: abnormally low numbers of spermatozoa per ejaculate (<200 million spermatozoa/ml or <22 million spermatozoa/kg body weight in the dog; or <5 million total spermatozoa in the tom).

EPIDEMIOLOGY

SPECIES, AGE, SEX: Canine or feline, intact males, any age.

GENETICS AND BREED PREDISPOSITION: Some etiologies may have a hereditary component.

CONTAGION AND ZOONOSIS: *Brucella canis* possible (see Brucellosis, Dog, p 162).

GEOGRAPHY AND SEASONALITY: Lower total number of spermatozoa and lower percentage of morphologically normal spermatozoa in summer months in North American dogs.

ASSOCIATED CONDITIONS AND DISORDERS: May be associated with poor libido.

CLINICAL PRESENTATION

DISEASE FORMS/SUBTYPES

- Mild to severe
- Transient or chronic depending on etiology

HISTORY, CHIEF COMPLAINT

- Either prior history of normal fertility followed by a decline in fertility, or consistently poor fertility.

- Recent episode of malaise or fever is possible.
- Prior history of physical training where performance-enhancing drugs could have been administered.
- History of bloody penile or preputial discharge or pain with ejaculation.
- History of chronic respiratory disease (asthenozoospermia).

PHYSICAL EXAM FINDINGS

- ± Fever.
- Libido may be normal or decreased.
- Testes may be small and soft or normal in size and consistency.
- Testes, epididymides, or spermatic cords may be enlarged (inflammation or neoplasia), and/or thickened.
- Scrotum may be enlarged or thickened (dermatitis, trauma, or fluid accumulation).
- Prostate may be enlarged (symmetric or asymmetric).
- In dogs with asthenozoospermia caused by primary ciliary dyskinesia/immotile cilia syndrome, additional signs may include nasal discharge, cough, and/or hydrocephalus (open fontanelle, domed calvaria) or situs inversus (spleen is palpated on the right side of the abdomen; heartbeat is loudest on right hemithorax).

ETIOLOGY AND PATHOPHYSIOLOGY

- Causes (all categories):
  - Infectious or inflammatory (orchitis, epididymitis, prostatitis including infection with *B. canis*, mycoplasmas or other aerobic bacteria, or feline infectious peritonitis [FIP]).
  - Scrotal hyperthermia (due to fever, obesity with increased intrascrotal fat, hydrocele, hematocele, or neoplasia).
  - Toxin exposure or exogenous drug administration (corticosteroids, anabolic steroids, other steroid hormones, gonadotropin-releasing hormone (GnRH) agonist/antagonists, chemotherapeutic agents).
  - Testicular degeneration (primary or secondary).
  - Immune mediated (lymphocyctic thyroiditis or spermatozoal autoantibodies).
  - Unilateral or partial epididymal or tubular obstruction (granuloma, spermatocele).
  - Congenital.
- Additional causes (specific to individual categories):
  - Primary ciliary dyskinesia with abnormal spermatozoal midpiece formation (asthenozoospermia).
  - Prostatic disease: benign prostatic hyperplasia or squamous metaplasia (oligozoospermia, asthenozoospermia).
  - Neoplasia (oligozoospermia).
  - Hyperadrenocorticism (oligozoospermia).

DIAGNOSIS

DIFFERENTIAL DIAGNOSIS

- Asthenozoospermia:
  - Contaminated or improperly washed ejaculate collection equipment (e.g., disinfectant residues)
  - Excessive use of lubricants
  - Prolonged exposure of ejaculate to latex
  - Urine contamination of the ejaculate
  - Infrequent ejaculate collection with accumulation of dead sperm in the epididymis and/or vas deferens
- Teratozoospermia:
  - Poor handling of semen after collection (especially if coiled tails or detached heads are present)
  - Improper microscopic interpretation
  - Prolonged sexual abstinence (increases in detached heads) or overuse (increases in cytoplasmic droplets)
- Oligozoospermia:
  - Retrograde ejaculation
  - Fear or apprehension of mating (i.e., presence of dominant female, timid male, first time breeding)
  - Overuse of males resulting in depletion of epididymal sperm reserves

INITIAL DATABASE

- Physical examination including palpation of the scrotal contents, the spermatic cords, and prostate.
- Semen collection and evaluation (including motility, morphology, concentration, volume) and libido evaluation.
- Seminal and prostatic fluid cytology and culture (see Prostatic Massage, p 1303).
- Complete blood count, serum biochemistry panel, urinalysis.
- Serology: *B. canis*, feline coronavirus/FIP.

ADVANCED OR CONFIRMATORY TESTING

- All categories:
  - Scrotal and prostatic ultrasonography for structural lesions.
  - Endocrine testing: baseline testosterone, estradiol, and follicle-stimulating hormone concentrations.
  - Endocrine stimulation testing:
    - Administer 2.2-3.3 μg/kg GnRH IM or 44 IU/kg human chorionic gonadotropin (hCG) IM in dogs with baseline testosterone and luteinizing hormone (LH) and then sample for LH—10 minutes postinjection and testosterone—1 hour postinjection; or
    - 250-500 IU hCG IM or IV or 25 μg GnRH IM in toms with baseline testosterone and poststimulation samples taken 2 and 4 hours later for hCG or 1 hour after GnRH.
    - Normal response: a minimum of a twofold to fourfold increase in testosterone concentrations.
    - Negligible or inappropriate response indicates either a primary testicular lesion or a lesion of the hypothalamic-pituitary axis resulting in failed feedback loop mechanisms.
  - Testicular biopsy or aspirate to be considered if noninvasive testing is unrewarding or if a structural lesion (e.g., mass) is present.
- Asthenozoospermia:
  - Radiography of the thorax, respiratory tract cultures, biopsy and electron microscopy of nasal or respiratory epithelium or spermatozoal midpieces for evaluation for primary ciliary dyskinesia (see Primary Ciliary Dyskinesia, p 889).
  - Examination of the ejaculate for pH and/or presence of urine crystals, indicating urine contamination.
- Teratozoospermia:
  - Detailed morphologic examination using special staining and microscopic techniques such as Spermac, Toluidine blue, or Coomassie blue stains, phase contrast, differential interference contrast or electron microscopy.
- Oligozoospermia:
  - Urinalysis after ejaculation to assess for retrograde ejaculation. Sample may be obtained by cystocentesis or catheterization.
  - Seminal plasma alkaline phosphatase concentrations, to confirm that ejaculation actually occurred.

TREATMENT

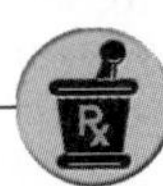

THERAPEUTIC GOAL(S)

- Increase the number of total sperm, the number of total motile cells, and/or the number of normal cells per ejaculate.
- Manage the use of the male to maximize fertility.

ACUTE GENERAL TREATMENT

- All:
  - Bacterial infections should be treated with appropriate antibiotics based on culture and sensitivity. Individuals positively confirmed to be infected with brucellosis should also be neutered.
  - Hemicastration for unilateral inflammatory, obstructive, or neoplastic conditions.
  - Cats that meet the clinical and laboratory criteria for FIP should be removed from catteries/multicat environments (See Feline Infectious Peritonitis, p 378).
- Asthenozoospermia:
  - Careful cleaning and rinsing (at least twice with distilled water) and drying of artificial insemination equipment.

- Sparing use of nonspermicidal lubricants.
- Have males urinate immediately prior to collection to avoid urine contamination of ejaculate.
- Teratozoospermia:
  - With scrotal overheating, waiting a minimum of 65 days from onset of insult should result in return to normal spermatozoal morphology.
  - Weight reduction in obese males.
- Oligozoospermia:
  - With scrotal overheating, waiting a minimum of 65 days from onset of insult should result in return to normal spermatozoal morphology.
  - For retrograde ejaculation: in dogs, phenylpropanolamine (1.1 mg/kg PO q 8-12h) or pseudoephedrine (0.2-0.4 mg/kg PO q 8h or 1 to 3 hours before breeding).
  - Weight reduction in obese males.
  - Positive reinforcement for behavioral issues.

CHRONIC TREATMENT

- Asthenozoospermia:
  - Centrifugation of the ejaculate in cases of urine contamination, followed by reextension with semen extender.
  - Depo-Testosterone enanthate (testosterone) plus pregnant mare serum gonadotropin (PMSG) every 2 weeks for 6 weeks has been advocated but dosages, efficacy, and safety have not been established (50 mg/dog testosterone enanthate + 250 IU/dog PMSG have been used successfully in 15 kg dogs).
- Teratozoopermia, oligospermia ± asthenozoospermia:
  - If testicular degeneration is present, long-term administration of GnRH (3.3 μg/kg) IM once weekly or hCG (500-1000 IU IM) every 2 weeks in dogs; or hCG 250-500 IU IM every 2 weeks in dogs has shown some positive effects.

RECOMMENDED MONITORING

- Routine (monthly) microscopic reevaluation of the spermiogram and reassessment of endocrine function as indicated, beginning 2 to 3 months after initiation of treatment.
- Monitor pregnancy rates and litter size.

PROGNOSIS AND OUTCOME

The prognosis for fertility is guarded if no response to treatment occurs within 3 months, poor if no response to treatment occurs within 6 months, and grave if no response to treatment occurs within a year.

PEARLS & CONSIDERATIONS

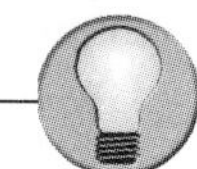

COMMENTS

- Optimize available sperm:
  - Accurate breeding management and ovulation timing.
  - Reduce the number of matings per cycle.
  - Use of transcervical or surgical insemination (surgical insemination preferred).
  - Breeding to young, fertile females.
- Avoid overuse:
  - Do not collect more than every other day.
  - Collection of males 7 to 10 days before anticipated matings, in animals that have had prolonged abstinence, to flush the ejaculatory tract of dead sperm.
  - Avoid strict raw meat diets as they may result in amino acid or vitamin/mineral deficiencies.

PREVENTION

- Brucellosis screening biannually (dogs).
- Coronavirus/FIP screening of all new entries into catteries (seronegative cats can be introduced into coronavirus-free catteries; seropositive cats and/or catteries with endemic coronavirus carry a variable risk of developing FIP).

SUGGESTED READING

Johnston SD, et al: Clinical approach to infertility in the male dog. In *Canine and Feline Theriogenology*. Philadelphia, WB Saunders, 2001, pp 381-382.

Kawakami E, et al: Changes in plasma testosterone and testicular transferrin concentration, testicular histology and semen quality after treatment of testosterone-depot plus PMSG to 3 dogs with asthenozoospermia. *J Vet Med Sci* 62(2):203-206, 2000.

Kawakami E, et al: Changes in plasma LH and testosterone levels and semen quality after a single injection of hCG in two dogs with spermatogenic dysfunction. *J Vet Med Sci* 60(6):765-767, 1998.

Meyers-Wallen VN: Clinical approach to infertile male dogs with sperm in the ejaculate. *Vet Clin North Am Small Anim Pract* 21:609-633, 1991.

Purswell BJ, Wilcke JR: Response to GnRH by the intact male dog: Testosterone, LH, and FSH levels. Proceedings of the 2nd International Symposium on Canine and Feline Reproduction, Liege, Belgium, pp 112-113, 1992.

AUTHOR: **CHERYL LOPATE**

EDITOR: **MICHELLE A. KUTZLER**

Inflammatory Bowel Disease

Client Education Sheet on Website

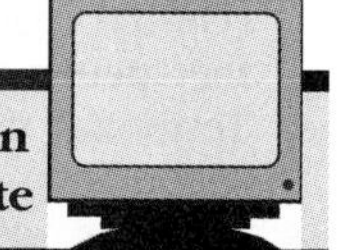

BASIC INFORMATION

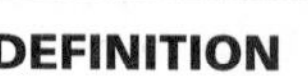

DEFINITION

A chronic disease (typically >3 weeks) associated with gastrointestinal (GI) signs and histologic evidence of idiopathic inflammation of the lamina propria of the small or large intestine

SYNONYM(S)

Eosinophilic enteritis
Granulomatous enterocolitis
Histiocytic ulcerative colitis (see also Granulomatous Enteritis/Colitis, p 446)
Lymphocytic-plasmacytic colitis
Lymphocytic-plasmacytic enteritis

EPIDEMIOLOGY

SPECIES, AGE, SEX: Dogs: any age possible, more common in middle-aged or older, both sexes affected. Cats: small intestinal form more common in older cats, colonic disease more common in young to middle-aged cats.

GENETICS AND BREED PREDISPOSITION: Dogs: common in the German shepherd, boxer, and Chinese shar-pei. Hereditary forms in the soft coated Wheaten terrier, Irish setters, basenji, and lundehund.

ASSOCIATED CONDITIONS AND DISORDERS: Soft coated Wheaten terriers commonly have concurrent protein losing nephropathy.

CLINICAL PRESENTATION

HISTORY, CHIEF COMPLAINT

- Clinical signs vary depending on the segment of the GI tract affected and the duration of disease, to include:
  - Anorexia, polyphagia
  - Vomiting, hematemesis

- Diarrhea (liquid to soft-formed, possibly with mucus)
- Weight loss (this may be the only sign in some animals)
- Patients with mild forms of inflammatory bowel disease (IBD) may present with intermittent, nonprogressive GI signs.
- Severe forms may cause persistent vomiting, protein-losing enteropathy (PLE) (hypoalbuminemia not attributable to hepatic, renal, or dermatologic disease), marked weight loss (>20% body weight), and melena or chronic diarrhea.

PHYSICAL EXAM FINDINGS

- Poor body condition, poor hair coat possible.
- Thickened GI loops and/or enlarged mesenteric lymph nodes.
- Ascites, tachypnea, seizures possible in dogs with severe PLE.
- In milder cases, physical exam may be unremarkable.

ETIOLOGY AND PATHOPHYSIOLOGY

- Hypersensitivity to bacteria and/or food antigens is suspected, but regardless of inciting cause for inflammation, endogenous flora is major player in augmentation of the inflammatory process in IBD.
- Defect in mucosal tolerance mechanisms of gut-associated lymphoid tissue is key.
- Protein loss may occur from inflammatory exudation, ulceration, or abnormal mucosal permeability.

DIAGNOSIS

DIFFERENTIAL DIAGNOSIS

- Differentials for the clinical syndrome (e.g., weight loss with altered appetite):
  - Dogs: GI foreign body/obstruction, intestinal neoplasia, infiltrative diseases (fungal, pythiosis), pancreatic disease (chronic pancreatitis, exocrine pancreatic insufficiency), protein-losing nephropathy, chronic hepatopathy.
  - Cats: as described above, plus feline infectious peritonitis, hyperthyroidism.
- Differentials that may result in GI signs and histologic evidence of GI inflammation; these must be ruled out prior to a diagnosis of idiopathic IBD:
  - Bacterial GI infections (*Escherichia coli*, *Salmonella*, *Yersinia*, *Campylobacter*, *Clostridium*).
  - Occult intestinal parasitism.
  - Mycoses in endemic regions.
  - Dietary hypersensitivity.
- Differentials to consider for PLE:
  - Dogs: intestinal lymphangiectasia (often occurs concurrently with IBD, particularly in the Yorkshire terrier breed), GI lymphoma, histoplasmosis, intussusception.
  - Cats: GI lymphoma.

INITIAL DATABASE

- Complete blood count and serum biochemical findings are inconsistent.
  - Patients with severe IBD or PLE may have elevated liver enzymes, hypoalbuminemia/hypocholesterolemia, and hypocalcemia.
- Serum bile acids testing and urinalysis indicated to rule out concurrent liver disease and protein losing nephropathy, respectively.
- Multiple fecal flotations and empiric deworming are recommended in all cases.
- Abdominal radiographic findings often nonspecific. Intestinal wall thickness cannot be determined from plain radiographs.
- Abdominal ultrasound recommended to screen for focal lesions, pancreatic disease, and occasionally intestinal thickening and lymphadenopathy.
- Serum trypsin-like immunoreactivity, cobalamin, and folate concentrations are recommended to identify concurrent pancreatic disease and cobalamin deficiency (especially in cats).

ADVANCED OR CONFIRMATORY TESTING

Biopsies are necessary for diagnosis and may be collected surgically or endoscopically:

- When collecting endoscopic biopsies, a minimum of eight intestinal biopsies from each anatomic site is recommended.
- The presence of submucosa and subvillous lamina proprial tissue should be noted (apparent to skilled operator on gross visual inspection; confirmed histologically); otherwise, samples may have been too superficial.
- Specimens submitted should contain at least two samples free of crush artifact, oriented so the mucosal portion of several contiguous villi are included.
- Significant variation in pathologic interpretation of intestinal biopsies is possible; diagnosis is ultimately based on integration of clinical and histopathologic findings, exclusion of other causes for observed clinical signs, and response to therapy.

TREATMENT

THERAPEUTIC GOAL(S)

- Stabilization of body weight and amelioration of GI signs
- Minimization of adverse medication side effects

ACUTE GENERAL TREATMENT

- Ensure the following has been done before instituting immunosuppressive therapy for IBD:
  - Empiric deworming, e.g., with fenbendazole 50 mg/kg PO q 24h × 3 days (dogs, cats).
  - Control gut exposure to dietary antigens (feed an elemental/novel protein/low antigen diet). Several food trials may be required.
  - Minimize gut exposure to bacterial antigens, either with probiotics, antimicrobial therapy, or combination therapy. Two to three antibiotic trials may be required. Commonly used antimicrobials for dogs with IBD are metronidazole (10 mg/kg PO q 12h), tylosin (10-20 mg/kg PO q 12h), tetracycline (20 mg/kg PO q 8h on an empty stomach), or enrofloxacin (5-10 mg/kg PO q 24h), the latter particularly for histiocytic ulcerative colitis. In cats, metronidazole (10-15 mg/kg PO q 12h for 2 weeks, then reduce to 10 mg/kg q 12-24h), or tylosin (10-20 mg/kg PO q 12h) are common choices.
  - Feeding a high-fiber diet (commercial, or adding fiber, such as psyllium 1-2 teaspoons/10 kg at each feeding) is recommended with large bowel disease.
- In cases with severe clinical signs or PLE, immunosuppressive medications are appropriate:
  - Prednisone is the most commonly utilized agent (1 mg/kg PO q 12h in dogs, 2 mg/kg PO q 12h in cats; taper to lowest effective dose).
    - Cats may respond more favorably to methylprednisolone (4 mg/cat PO q 12-24h).
  - Budesonide is reputed to have fewer systemic side effects due to extensive first pass metabolism, and may be utilized in cats with corticosteroid intolerance (e.g., diabetes mellitus). Average dog dose highly variable (1-9 mg PO/dog/day), cats: 1 mg PO/cat/day, recompounded).
  - Mesalamine/olsalazine (5-ASA) may be selected for use instead of steroids in dogs with colonic disease (17.5-25 mg/kg PO q 12h). Sulfasalazine is an older drug with similar effects, but the sulfa side effects preclude long-term use.
  - Cytotoxic immunosuppressants can be added if there is a poor response to the preceding regimen. Azathioprine is best tolerated in dogs (2 mg/kg PO every other day), and chlorambucil is the agent of choice in cats (1 mg PO/cat every other day). Monitor for potential neutropenia and opportunistic infections with either medication.

- Patients with PLE can be at increased risk for thromboembolism. Low-dose aspirin (0.5 mg/kg PO q 12h in dogs; 81 mg PO every third day in cats) is recommended if antithrombin levels are low. Gastroprotection with omeprazole (1 mg/kg/day) or famotidine (0.5 mg/kg/day) is recommended.
- Elemental enteral diets, parenteral nutrition, and colloidal osmotic agents, such as plasma or synthetic colloidal solutions, may be required in severely ill patients.

CHRONIC TREATMENT

- Minimize doses of immunosuppressive therapies by attempting to identify well-tolerated foods and antimicrobial/motility modifying medications.
- Cobalamin supplementation (250 μg/cat/week, 25 μg/kg/week in dogs) is required in some cases.

POSSIBLE COMPLICATIONS

- GI ulceration associated with high doses of prednisone.
- Long-term therapy with high doses of prednisone is also associated with significant, and often dose limiting, side effects (e.g., diabetes, hepatopathy).
- Immunosuppressive medications predispose animals to secondary infections.

RECOMMENDED MONITORING

Regular evaluation of the body weight, serum albumin concentration, and overall clinical condition are recommended

PROGNOSIS AND OUTCOME

- Short-term prognosis is antectodally good to excellent in mild to moderate cases of IBD. Limited response data are available, but response rate is likely greater than 75%. Long-term survival data are not available.
- In severe cases of IBD, the prognosis is guarded, depending on the response to therapy. Negative prognostic indicators include severe hypoalbuminemia, malnutrition, or vomiting prohibiting enteral nutrition.
- Treatment failures may be due to incorrect diagnosis (cats with lymphoma, poor disease localization, inadequate biopsy quality), severe disease, or presence of concurrent disease.

PEARLS & CONSIDERATIONS

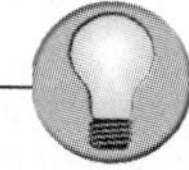

COMMENTS

- IBD is a diagnosis of exclusion, and is only considered once other underlying causes for histologically confirmed GI inflammation have been ruled out.
- Collection of high-quality biopsy samples for histologic evaluation is essential.
- In cases that do not respond as expected, consider rebiopsy, as lymphoma can be missed.

CLIENT EDUCATION

- The long-term treatment goal is to identify and eliminate underlying causes for inflammation to minimize doses of immunosuppressive medications.
- Several diet changes and antimicrobial trials may be needed before achievement of this goal, and variables should be minimized (e.g., dietary indiscretion during food trials).

SUGGESTED READING

Baez JL, et al: Radiographic, ultrasonographic, and endoscopic findings in cats with inflammatory bowel disease of the stomach and small intestine: 33 cases (1990–1997). *J Am Vet Med Assoc* 215:349–354, 1999.

Jergens AE, et al: Idiopathic inflammatory bowel disease in dogs and cats: 84 cases (1987–1990). *J Am Vet Med Assoc* 201:1603–1608, 1992.

Willard MD, et al: Interobserver variation among histopathologic evaluations of intestinal tissues from dogs and cats. *J Am Vet Med Assoc* 220:1177–1182, 2002.

AUTHOR: **POLLY B. PETERSON**

EDITOR: **DEBRA L. ZORAN**

Inguinal Hernia

BASIC INFORMATION

DEFINITION

Protrusion of an organ or tissues through a weakened inguinal ring

EPIDEMIOLOGY

SPECIES, AGE, SEX: Acquired inguinal hernia: middle-aged intact female dogs.

GENETICS AND BREED PREDISPOSITION

- Dogs: predisposed breeds:
  - Basenji, Pekingese, poodle, basset hound, cairn terrier, Cavalier King Charles spaniel, Chihuahua, cocker spaniel, dachshund, Pomeranian, Maltese, West Highland white terrier.
- Congenital:
  - Males: testicular descent may delay narrowing of inguinal ring.
- Heritability:
  - May be polygenic in cocker spaniels and dachshunds.
- No breed predilection for acquired inguinal hernia.

RISK FACTORS

- Obesity
- Trauma
- Pregnancy

ASSOCIATED CONDITIONS AND DISORDERS

- Umbilical hernia
- Perineal hernia

CLINICAL PRESENTATION

DISEASE FORMS/SUBTYPES

- Indirect inguinal hernia:
  - Abdominal viscera enter the cavity of the vaginal process.
  - Males: scrotal hernias.
- Direct inguinal hernia:
  - More common form in small animals.
  - Organs pass through inguinal rings adjacent to the normal evagination of the vaginal process.
  - Usually large.
  - Usually not associated with incarceration/strangulation.
- Congenital inguinal hernia:
  - Rare in dogs and cats.
  - May coexist with umbilical hernia.
- Acquired inguinal hernia:
  - More common in dogs and cats.

HISTORY, CHIEF COMPLAINT

- Chief complaint generally involves one of two categories: either the owner has noticed an inguinal enlargement incidentally, or there are systemic signs of illness due to abdominal organ entrapment/strangulation within the hernia.
- Indirect inguinal hernia in male dogs: often causes organ dysfunction:
  - Vaginal process narrows considerably at the inguinal ring (→ organ incarceration/strangulation).
- Direct inguinal hernia usually larger:
  - Less commonly associated with clinical problems.
- If organ incarceration in hernia: small intestinal, bladder, or uterine entrapment:
  - Abdominal pain, vomiting, dysuria, vaginal discharge/hemorrhage may be noted.
- Vomiting, abdominal pain, or depression:

   - Vomiting for several days' duration is predictive of strangulated, nonviable small intestine.
   - Overall, risk of strangulated intestines is <5% of cases of inguinal hernia.

PHYSICAL EXAM FINDINGS: Vary with size of the hernia and its contents:

- Uncomplicated inguinal hernia:
   - Soft, painless unilateral or bilateral mass.
   - Mass reducible into abdomen.
   - Enlarged inguinal ring palpable.
   - May appear more caudally in the female.
- Complicated inguinal hernia:
   - Firm, nonreducible inguinal mass.
   - Painful on palpation.
   - Bruising/erythema of overlying tissues.

ETIOLOGY AND PATHOPHYSIOLOGY

- Nontraumatic inguinal hernia:
   - Anatomic: Females may be predisposed:
      - Entrance to the vaginal process remains open.
      - Inguinal canal is shorter and larger in diameter.
   - Hormonal:
      - Most inguinal hernias become clinically apparent during estrus or pregnancy.
      - Inguinal hernias occur less frequently in spayed females.
         - Estrogen may play a role in development of inguinal hernias (alters strength and character of connective tissue).
   - Nutritional/metabolic:
      - Weakening of abdominal wall.
      - Obesity:
         - Increased intra-abdominal pressure.
         - Fat forced into the inguinal canals.
            - Dilation of canal and vaginal process.
- Blunt abdominal/pelvic trauma:
   - Disruption/weakening of caudal abdominal muscles.
   - Enlargement of inguinal canal.

DIAGNOSIS

The diagnosis usually is established based on physical examination alone.

DIFFERENTIAL DIAGNOSIS

- Perineal hernia: hernia is adjacent to anus.
- Scrotal hernia (male): most dogs with inguinal hernias present with a fluctuant, painless, unilateral or bilateral mass, whereas scrotal hernias usually appear as a firm cordlike mass that extends into the scrotum.
- Mammary neoplasia or mastitis: firm, enlarged, possibly painful mammary gland(s).
- Hematoma: ecchymosis; nonreducible (gentle pressure only).
- Abscess: may be inflamed; nonreducible (gentle pressure only).

INITIAL DATABASE

- Complete blood count, serum biochemistry profile, urinalysis:
   - If systemic clinical signs exist
   - Preoperative screening
- Avoid fine-needle aspirate, unless performed with ultrasound guidance:
   - Risk of perforation of intestinal loop or gravid uterus

ADVANCED OR CONFIRMATORY TESTING

- Survey abdominal radiographs:
   - Displaced gravid uterus, small or large intestine, urinary bladder, or spleen
   - Loss of intra-abdominal detail in the caudal abdominal and inguinal regions
- Contrast radiography:
   - Cystogram to determine position of bladder
- Ultrasound examination:
   - Determine position of organs in abdomen and contents of hernia

TREATMENT

- All inguinal hernias should be corrected at the time of diagnosis, regardless of size. Delay may make surgery more difficult and increase the risk of complications (visceral strangulation, devitalization, and rupture).
- Inability to reduce strangulated organs, particularly the bladder, intestines, or uterus; clinical signs of peritonitis; and pain are indications for immediate surgical intervention.

THERAPEUTIC GOAL(S)

- Reestablish normal inguinal ring and canal anatomy
- Prevent recurrence of herniation
- Resect nonviable viscera

ACUTE GENERAL TREATMENT

- Treatment for inguinal hernia is herniorrhaphy:
   - Performed at the time of diagnosis:
      - Prevent complications
      - Improve ease of surgical repair
   - Tension-free apposition of tissue and ligation of the hernia sac
- Ovariohysterectomy in intact female

POSSIBLE COMPLICATIONS

- Hernia associated:
   - Incarceration/strangulation of abdominal organ(s):
      - Peritonitis, cellulitis
   - Edema, pain
- Associated with the surgical repair:
   - Hematoma/seroma:
      - Inadequate hemostasis, excessive tissue dissection, excessive activity after repair
   - Infection:
      - Herniorrhaphy site
      - Peritonitis
   - Swelling or edema caused by incorporation of neurovascular bundle into repair
   - Overall postoperative complication rate for herniorrhaphy: 17%

RECOMMENDED MONITORING

- Postoperative exercise restriction for 10 to 14 days
- Surgical site should be monitored for swelling and discharge

PROGNOSIS AND OUTCOME

- Excellent in uncomplicated inguinal hernia with successful repair.
- Prognosis may be less favorable in complicated cases.
   - Intestinal incarceration/strangulation, peritonitis, pyometra.
- There is no information in the literature to suggest that these hernias close spontaneously.

PEARLS & CONSIDERATIONS

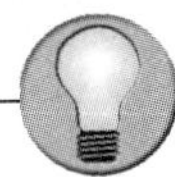

COMMENTS

- Inguinal hernias are most commonly seen in middle-aged, intact female dogs.
- Prompt repair is recommended to minimize complications.
   - Surgical repair is easier with smaller hernias.
- Proper postoperative pain control and exercise restriction are necessary for good outcome.

PREVENTION

- Ovariohysterectomy may decrease risk
- Obesity may increase risk
- Dogs that have nontraumatic inguinal hernia should not be used for breeding purposes

CLIENT EDUCATION

- Proper weight management is recommended.
- Nonbreeding female dogs should be neutered.

SUGGESTED READING

Smeak DD: Abdominal hernias. In Slatter D (ed): *Textbook of Small Animal Surgery*, ed 3. Philadelphia, WB Saunders, 2003, pp 452–455.

Waters DJ, Roy RG, Stone EA: A retrospective study of inguinal hernia in 35 dogs. *Vet Surg* 22: 44–49, 1993.

AUTHOR: **ELLEN B. DAVIDSON DOMNICK**
EDITOR: **RICHARD WALSHAW**

Insulinoma

BASIC INFORMATION

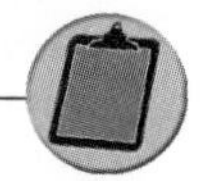

DEFINITION

A functional pancreatic β-cell tumor that secretes excess insulin causing clinical signs associated with hypoglycemia

SYNONYM(S)

β-Cell tumor
Hyperinsulinism
Insulin-secreting tumor
Islet cell adenocarcinoma
Islet cell tumor

EPIDEMIOLOGY

SPECIES, AGE, SEX

- Dogs: uncommon; middle-aged to older (mean 10 years, range 3-14 years); no sex predilection; most reports are of medium to large breed dogs.
- Cats: rare; older (mean 14.7 years, range 12-17 years); no sex predilection.

GENETICS AND BREED PREDISPOSITION

- Dogs: increased incidence suggested for Labrador retrievers, golden retrievers, Irish setters, boxers, German shepherds, standard poodles, fox terriers, and collies.
- Cats: three of four reported cases were Siamese cats.

ASSOCIATED CONDITIONS AND DISORDERS: Obesity.

CLINICAL PRESENTATION

HISTORY, CHIEF COMPLAINT

- Dogs: seizures (48-62%), weakness (40%), and collapse (30-40%) are most common.
  - Ataxia, disorientation, mental dullness, tremors/muscle fasciculations, polyphagia, nervousness may also be seen.
- Cats: seizures, weakness, ataxia, and muscle twitching.

PHYSICAL EXAM FINDINGS

- Usually unremarkable.
- Obesity/overweight is seen in some dogs.
- Signs listed under History, Chief Complaint above may be found if significant hypoglycemia is present at the time of presentation.

ETIOLOGY AND PATHOPHYSIOLOGY

- In normal animals, when blood glucose concentrations decrease below 60 mg/dl (3.2 mmol/L), insulin secretion stops and epinephrine and glucagon are released to help return the blood glucose concentration to normal.
  - Cortisol and growth hormone have more chronic antihypoglycemic effects.
- In animals with insulinoma the neoplastic β-cells do not respond appropriately, but continue to secrete insulin despite hypoglycemia.
- The excess insulin causes increased glucose uptake and use, and decreased hepatic glucose production.
- The clinical signs of insulinoma are the result of neuroglycopenia and/or hypoglycemia-induced release of catecholamines.
- In dogs, insulinoma develops within the right and left pancreatic lobes with equal frequency. Solitary nodules are most common, but multiple nodules and occult nodules can also occur.
- Insulinomas are notorious for masking their malignant tendencies in the dog. Virtually all β-cell tumors in dogs are malignant, and up to 64% have metastatic lesions at the time of surgery. Metastasis to the liver, regional lymph nodes, and omentum is most common.

DIAGNOSIS

DIFFERENTIAL DIAGNOSIS

- Fasting hypoglycemia:
  - Endocrine (i.e., hypopituitarism, hypoadrenocorticism, glucagon deficiency)
  - Hepatic (i.e., vascular shunts, glycogen storage diseases, cirrhosis)
  - Pregnancy
  - Neonatal and juvenile hypoglycemia
  - Sepsis
  - Uremia
  - Severe polycythemia
  - Extrapancreatic tumors (e.g., hepatocellular carcinoma, leiomyosarcoma)
  - Insulin overdose
- Seizures (see Seizures, p 990)
- Collapse/weakness (see Collapse, p 225)
- Tremors/twitching (see Tremors and Myoclonus, p 1102)

INITIAL DATABASE

- Appropriate clinical signs, hypoglycemia and concurrent hyperinsulinemia, and the presence of a pancreatic tumor support the diagnosis. Immunocytochemical staining of the tumor is confirmatory.
- Complete blood count, serum chemistry profile, and urinalysis may show hypoglycemia or may be normal.
  - A normal blood glucose concentration does not rule out an insulinoma.
- Simultaneous measurement of serum glucose and insulin concentrations should be made when the blood glucose concentration is less than 60 mg/dl (3.2 mmol/L).
  - At this blood glucose concentration, insulin secretion is normally suppressed.
- If insulinoma is suspected but the blood glucose concentration is normal, fast the patient and assess a blood glucose concentration every 1 to 2 hours, with collection of a sample for concurrent insulin measurement when hypoglycemia occurs.
- A low serum fructosamine concentration can also provide evidence of chronic/recurrent hypoglycemia.
- Hyperinsulinemia during hypoglycemia is supportive of the diagnosis of insulinoma.
  - An insulin concentration in the middle to upper-normal range (in the face of hypoglycemia) is also suggestive, but not diagnostic, of insulinoma.
- Amended and other insulin:glucose ratios do not improve diagnostic accuracy.
- Thoracic and abdominal radiographs are usually normal with insulinoma but may help identify other disorders causing hypoglycemia.
  - Insulinomas rarely metastasize to the lungs.
- Abdominal ultrasound may be helpful (tumor visible in 30-50% of affected dogs), but should be used in conjunction with other diagnostic tests.

ADVANCED OR CONFIRMATORY TESTING

- Histologic evaluation and immunohistochemical staining of the tumor is confirmatory.
- Abdominal computed tomography scan or magnetic resonance imaging can identify the location of the tumor in up to 70% of cases.

TREATMENT

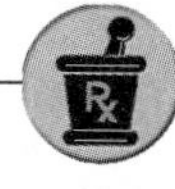

THERAPEUTIC GOAL(S)

- Remove the tumor, if possible
- Control clinical signs

ACUTE GENERAL TREATMENT

- Emergency therapy:
  - If signs are present but the patient is able to eat, feed a small meal (see Chronic Treatment below).
  - If seizure or severe collapse/weakness is present, administer intravenous dextrose bolus (1-2 ml/kg of 50% dextrose solution diluted with saline in the ratio 5 parts saline:1

part 50% dextrose, IV). Follow with an infusion of 2.5-5% dextrose IV, or if the patient is able to eat, feed a small meal.
  - If seizures persist, also administer diazepam 0.5-1 mg/kg IV or another anticonvulsant medication (see Seizures, p 990).
- Surgery:
  - Remove the tumor if possible.
  - Perform a partial pancreatectomy for multiple adenomas or if a nodule cannot be palpated.
    - Insulinomas have no predisposition for one lobe of the pancreas over the other.
- After surgery, treat for potential pancreatitis (see Pancreatitis, Dog, p 796; Pancreatitis, Cat, p 794).

CHRONIC TREATMENT

- Because metastasis is common, signs often continue or recur after surgery and require long-term management.
- Dietary therapy: Feed 4 to 6 small meals/day of a diet high in protein, fat, and complex carbohydrates. Simple sugars, often found in semimoist pet foods, should be avoided.
- Limit exercise.
- When frequent feedings no longer control the signs, prednisone (0.25 mg/kg q 12h) can be added. This dose can be increased up to 2 mg/kg q 12h if needed.
- When frequent feedings and prednisone no longer control the signs, or signs of iatrogenic hyperadrenocorticism are causing problems, diazoxide (5 mg/kg PO q 12h with a gradual increase up to a maximum of 40 mg/kg divided q 8-12h) can be added to the treatment regimen. This drug inhibits insulin release, enhances glycogenolysis and gluconeogenesis, and decreases glucose tissue uptake.
- When these treatments are no longer effective, the following treatments may be considered:
  - Octreotide (somatostatin analog): 10-50 μg/dog SQ q 8-12h; questionable efficacy reported.
  - Streptozotocin: This drug selectively destroys β-cells but is extremely nephrotoxic. If used, a 3-hour diuresis with 0.9% saline is done before drug administration (500 mg streptozocin/m^2 IV in 0.9% saline over 2 hours) and for 2 hours after the streptozocin infusion. This may be repeated every 3 weeks until hypoglycemia resolves or adverse reactions occur.
  - Alloxan: This drug also selectively destroys β-cells but is nephrotoxic and may cause sudden acute respiratory distress syndrome. If used (65 mg/kg IV), concurrent fluid therapy is needed.

POSSIBLE COMPLICATIONS

- The most common postoperative complication is pancreatitis in dogs.
- Recurrent or progressive episodes of hypoglycemia may occur due to residual and/or metastatic disease.
- Iatrogenic hyperadrenocorticism may result from prednisone therapy.
- Anorexia, vomiting, and ptyalism are uncommon potential side effects of diazoxide therapy.
- Renal failure can occur with streptozotocin or alloxan therapy.

RECOMMENDED MONITORING

- At home: return or progression of clinical signs of hypoglycemia.
- In hospital: serum glucose concentrations.

PROGNOSIS AND OUTCOME

- Malignancy is common and many patients have metastases at time of surgery.
- Surgery improves survival time.
- Dogs: median survival time of 12 months after surgery. Younger dogs have shorter survival times. Only 20% of dogs with metastatic disease live longer than 1 year.
- Cats: median survival time of 6 months.

PEARLS & CONSIDERATIONS

COMMENTS

- Insulinoma, although rare, is the most common islet cell tumor in small animals.
- Treatment of insulinoma is generally palliative and improves the quality of life for most patients.
- There is no predisposition for one lobe of the pancreas over the other.
- Recommend referral to a specialty center as surgery and perioperative management can be complicated.

CLIENT EDUCATION

The owner should be aware of the clinical signs of hypoglycemia and seek immediate veterinary attention if they occur.

SUGGESTED READING

Feldman EC, Nelson RW: Beta-cell neoplasia: Insulinoma. In Feldman EC, Nelson RW (eds): *Canine and Feline Endocrinology and Reproduction*, ed 3. Philadelphia, WB Saunders, 2004, pp 616-644.

Lurye JC, Behrend N: Endocrine tumors. *Vet Clin North Am Small Anim Pract* 31:1083, 2001.

Meleo KA, Caplan ER: Treatment of insulinoma in the dog, cat and ferret. In Kirk RW, Bonagura JD (eds): *Current Veterinary Therapy XIII*. Philadelphia, WB Saunders, 2000, pp 357-361.

Steiner JM, Bruyette DS: Canine insulinoma. *Comp Cont Educ Pract Vet* 18:13, 1996.

AUTHOR: **NINETTE KELLER**

EDITOR: **SHERRI IHLE**

Interstitial Lung Diseases

BASIC INFORMATION

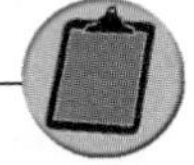

DEFINITION

A heterogeneous group of lung diseases centered around the pulmonary interstitium, and that result from exaggerated inflammatory and/or reparative (fibrotic) responses to inhaled or hematogenous insults

SYNONYM(S)

Examples of interstitial lung diseases (ILDs) include:

Asbestosis

Bronchiolitis obliterans with organizing pneumonia (BOOP)

Eosinophilic pneumonia

Hypersensitivity pneumonitis

Idiopathic pulmonary fibrosis

Lymphocytic interstitial pneumonia

Silicosis

EPIDEMIOLOGY

SPECIES, AGE, SEX

- Dogs or cats; usually middle-aged to older
- No sex predisposition

GENETICS AND BREED PREDISPOSITION: Some specific syndromes have a breed predisposition:

- Pulmonary fibrosis in West Highland white terriers and Staffordshire bull terriers

- Hypereosinophilic syndrome with eosinophilic pneumonia in rottweilers

RISK FACTORS: Generally unknown. Exceptions may include:
- Pulmonary toxicant drugs (e.g., bleomycin)
- Inhaled chemical fumes
- Mineral fibers
- Dusts
- Allergens

ASSOCIATED CONDITIONS AND DISORDERS
- Eosinophilic pneumonia may occur alone, or as part of the hypereosinophilic syndrome.
- Lymphocytic interstitial pneumonia has only been reported in cats with feline immunodeficiency virus infection.

CLINICAL PRESENTATION

DISEASE FORMS/SUBTYPES: Most are chronic diseases, although some may present in an acute fulminating form.

HISTORY, CHIEF COMPLAINT
- Respiratory signs can include:
  - Cough
  - Tachypnea
  - Respiratory distress
  - Exercise intolerance
  - Hemoptysis
- Nonrespiratory signs can include:
  - Fever
  - Lethargy
  - Anorexia
  - Weight loss

PHYSICAL EXAM FINDINGS
- Spontaneous or elicited cough:
  - May be productive or nonproductive
- Crackles are possible
- Increased respiratory rate and/or effort
- Fever
- Poor body condition

ETIOLOGY AND PATHOPHYSIOLOGY

- Disease is believed to result from injury to the alveolar epithelial cells, leading to a cycle of inflammation and host reparative responses that proceed unchecked.
  - In humans, injury can be triggered by:
    - Inhalation of toxins, irritants, or allergens
    - Vascular damage from drugs
    - Collagen-related vascular diseases
    - Systemic immune-mediated diseases
    - Infection
    - Neoplasia
  - Many veterinary cases are idiopathic.
- Alveolar epithelial cell injury leads to:
  - Inflammatory cell influx.
  - Release of proinflammatory and fibrogenic mediators.
  - Deposition of extracellular matrix.
  - Structural changes including fibrosis.
- Idiopathic pulmonary fibrosis appears to be a fibroproliferative disorder that can originate independent of inflammation (i.e., inflammation is secondary).
  - Injured alveolar epithelial cells are still critical for triggering and sustaining fibrogenesis.

DIAGNOSIS

DIFFERENTIAL DIAGNOSIS

- Physical examination (cough/respiratory distress):
  - Other airway diseases (e.g., chronic bronchitis, eosinophilic bronchitis)
  - Pneumonia (infectious, aspiration, foreign body)
  - Neoplasia
  - Pulmonary thromboembolism
  - Cardiogenic or noncardiogenic pulmonary edema
  - Pleural effusion/pneumothorax
- Radiographic:
  - Infectious pneumonia (bacterial, fungal, viral, protozoal, parasitic)
  - Noncardiogenic pulmonary edema
  - Neoplasia

INITIAL DATABASE

- Complete blood count:
  - Inflammatory leukogram and eosinophilia possible
- Thoracic radiographs:
  - Interstitial, alveolar, or bronchointerstitial patterns
  - Interstitial nodules
  - Hypoinflation of the lungs
  - Hilar lymphadenopathy: possible
  - Right-sided cardiomegaly from cor pulmonale: possible
- Arterial blood gas may show:
  - Hypoxemia
  - Hypocarbia
- Fecal float or sedimentation (Baermann): respiratory parasites.
- Serologic study: infectious agents endemic to the patient's area.

ADVANCED OR CONFIRMATORY TESTING

- Computed tomography provides more specific information on the extent, pattern, and location of disease
- Bronchoscopy, bronchoalveolar lavage, and fine-needle aspiration (all for cytologic evaluation and culture) can provide evidence of underlying infection or neoplasia only when microorganisms or neoplastic cells are identified:
  - Nonspecific inflammatory cells or poor cellularity is seen with ILDs
- Lung biopsy is the only definitive means for diagnosis:
  - Can be performed by a key-hole technique, thoracoscopy, or thoracotomy
  - Special stains are indicated to rule out infectious agents

TREATMENT

THERAPEUTIC GOAL(S)

- Remove or treat the inciting cause if it can be identified
- Break the cycle of ongoing inflammation and fibrosis

ACUTE GENERAL TREATMENT

Oxygen may be necessary for hypoxemic patients.

CHRONIC TREATMENT

- Remove any potential inciting cause:
  - Discontinue use of any drug not immediately critical for the patient's health.
  - Minimize exposure to inhalant fumes, chemicals, or dusts.
- For eosinophilic pneumonias, treat underlying etiology (e.g., heartworm, other parasites, or fungi) if identified; if none found, treat with immunosuppressive doses of glucocorticoids.
- For most other ILDs, immunosuppression is indicated (provided infection is definitively ruled out), starting with glucocorticoids (e.g., prednisone 1-2 mg/kg PO q 12h).
  - Empirically, other immunosuppressive drugs have also been tried in refractory cases.
    - Azathioprine (dogs, 1-2 mg/kg PO q 24h for 10 to 14 days, then q 48h).
    - Cyclophosphamide (50 mg/m^2 PO q 24h for 3 to 4 days/week).
    - Cyclosporine (3-5 mg/kg PO q 12h; monitor trough concentrations).

POSSIBLE COMPLICATIONS

- Decompensation during and after bronchoscopy or lung biopsy, especially in patients with a significant degree of respiratory compromise at rest
- Immunosuppression can predispose to secondary infections.
  - After lung biopsy, allow the incision to heal before immunosuppressive medication administration

RECOMMENDED MONITORING

- Clinical signs
- Physical examination
- Arterial blood gas (if significant respiratory compromise)
- Thoracic radiographs

PROGNOSIS AND OUTCOME

- For eosinophilic pneumonia, with appropriate treatment, prognosis is fair to excellent.
- For BOOP, if the insult is removed and the animal responds well clinically and radiographically to glucocorticoids, the prognosis is good.
  - Relapse is common if glucocorticoids are tapered too quickly.
  - For animals with BOOP that do not respond well to therapy, prognosis is guarded to poor.
- For other ILDs, including idiopathic pulmonary fibrosis, prognosis depends

on stage of the disease and rapidity of progression.
- In general, long-term outcome is guarded to poor.

PEARLS & CONSIDERATIONS

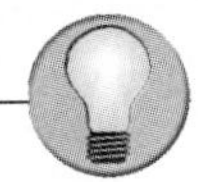

COMMENTS

- Lung biopsy is critical for appropriate diagnosis of interstitial lung diseases.
- Pulmonary crackles on auscultation are common with interstitial fibrosis and therefore are not exclusive to pulmonary edema.

CLIENT EDUCATION

Over time, most of the interstitial lung diseases are associated with permanent architectural changes, and treatment cannot reverse fibrosis. The likelihood that clinical signs will resolve depends on the balance of "active" inflammatory and reparative events, which can be addressed, versus fibrosis, which cannot.

SUGGESTED READING

Cohn LA, et al: Identification and characterization of an idiopathic pulmonary fibrosis-like condition in cats. *J Vet Intern Med* 18:632, 2004.

Norris CR, et al: Comparison of results of thoracic radiography, cytologic evaluation of bronchoalveolar lavage fluid, and histologic evaluation of lung specimens in dogs with respiratory tract disease: 16 cases (1996–2000). *J Am Vet Med Assoc* 218:1456, 2001.

Norris CR, et al: Use of keyhole lung biopsy for diagnosis of interstitial lung diseases in dogs and cats: 13 cases (1988-2001). *J Am Vet Med Assoc* 221:1453, 2002.

Norris CR, et al: Eosinophilic pneumonia. In King LG (ed): *Textbook of Respiratory Disease in Dogs and Cats*. St. Louis, WB Saunders, 2004, pp 541–547.

AUTHOR: **CAROL REINERO**
EDITOR: **RANCE K. SELLON**

Intervertebral Disk Disease

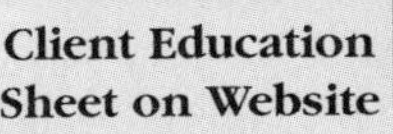

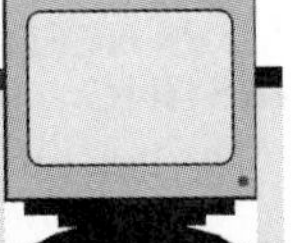

Client Education Sheet on Website

BASIC INFORMATION

DEFINITION

Degeneration and protrusion or extrusion of disk material into the vertebral canal causing a variety of clinical signs ranging from pain to paralysis

SYNONYM(S)

Disk disease
Herniated disk
IVDD

EPIDEMIOLOGY

SPECIES, AGE, SEX: Primarily dogs, 3 to 6 years (chondrodystrophic breeds) or 8 to 10 years (nonchondrodystrophic breeds), no predilection.

GENETICS AND BREED PREDISPOSITION
- Chondrodystrophic breeds: dachshunds, Pekingese, shih tzus, beagles, poodles.
- Nonchondrodystrophic breeds: German shepherds, Labradors.

RISK FACTORS: Premature disk degeneration (chondrodystrophic dogs), trauma.

CLINICAL PRESENTATION

DISEASE FORMS/SUBTYPES: Cervical disk disease, thoracolumbar disk disease.

HISTORY, CHIEF COMPLAINT
- Periodic, recurrent episodes or sudden occurrence of problems associated with neck or lower back.
- Cervical disease: neck pain and stiffness, weak front limb(s) ambulation.
- Thoracolumbar disease: arched, painful back; hind limbs weakness; or collapse.

PHYSICAL EXAM FINDINGS
- Cervical disk disease: neck pain; stiff, contracted neck muscles; front limb lameness or weakness. Reflexes may be abnormal.
- Thoracolumbar disk disease: thoracolumbar kyphosis (hunched posture), pain, abdominal tenseness, abnormal hind limb reflexes, abnormal urination, hind limb weakness, ataxia, or paralysis.

ETIOLOGY AND PATHOPHYSIOLOGY

- Chondrodystrophic dogs: early degeneration of disks characterized by changes in glycosaminoglycan, water, collagen, and proteoglycan contents. Reduced hydroelasticity leads to explosive, dorsal extrusion of calcified nucleus pulposus through annulus fibrosis (Hansen type 1 extrusion). Pressure, inflammation, and subsequent neural tissue destruction from ruptured disk onto spinal cord and nerves produce neurologic signs ranging from pain to paralysis.
- Nonchondrodystrophic dogs: slower fibroid metaplasia of disks produces gradual dehydration changes and subsequent bulging of the annulus fibrosus (Hansen type 2 protrusion). A chronic, compressive myelopathy may be present versus acute, severe pathologic changes seen with a type 1 lesion.
- Loss of neurologic function in dogs with intervertebral disk disease (IVDD) is based on the severity of neuropathologic lesions and type of nerve fibers affected. Large, myelinated fibers mediating conscious proprioception are initially affected, followed by intermediate voluntary motor fibers, and last, smaller fibers mediating pain perception. Spinal pain and discomfort originate from changes to nociceptors in the annulus or meninges, or secondarily due to muscular contractions.

DIAGNOSIS

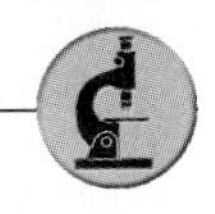

DIFFERENTIAL DIAGNOSIS

Spinal fracture, luxation, neoplasia, embolism, or inflammation

INITIAL DATABASE

- Neurologic examination (see Neurologic Examination, p 1286):
  - Findings are consistent with a single focal spinal cord lesion (e.g., mentation and cranial nerve responses are within normal limits).
  - Deficits help to localize the lesion:
    - Upper motor neuron signs in forelimbs and hind limbs: C1-C5 lesion.
    - Lower motor neuron signs in forelimbs, upper motor neuron signs in hind limbs: C6-T2 (cervical intumescence) lesion.
    - Forelimbs normal, upper motor neuron signs in hind limbs: T3-L3 lesion.
    - Forelimbs normal, lower motor neuron signs in hind limbs: L4-S1 lesion.
  - Location of deficits helps determine the site of the lesion, but does *not* confirm that intervertebral disk disease is the cause.
- Complete blood count, serum biochemistry panel, urinalysis (chronic dysuria).
- Survey radiography of heavily sedated patient will rule out fractures, luxations, and bone neoplasia and provide suggestive evidence of narrowed disk space. Calcified disks in situ are abnormal, but may not be clinically significant (Fig I-102).

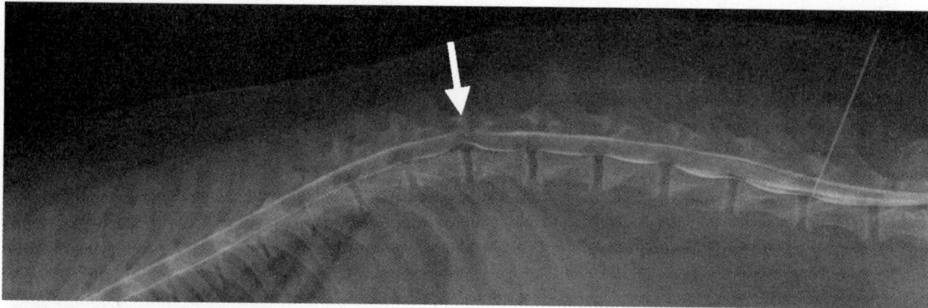

FIGURE I-102 Myelogram in a dog with intervertebral disk disease, lateral view. The myelographic needle is in the L5-L6 interspace. A dorsal deviation in the contrast column is seen at T13-L1, consistent with disk protrusion (*arrow*). As an incidental finding, mineralization of the nucleus pulposus is seen in several intervertebral disks (T10-T11, T12-T13, L5-L6). Courtesy of Dr. LeeAnn Pack.

ADVANCED OR CONFIRMATORY TESTING

- Myelography (see Fig I-102; see Myelography, p 1280) or magnetic resonance imaging (MRI) will reveal location of spinal cord compression due to disk extrusion or protrusion. MRI is more sensitive in delineating a lesion, although confounding, clinically insignificant sites of cord impingement may be present on any imaging study.
- The most common sites of cervical IVDD are C2-C3 and C3-C4; the most common sites of thoracolumbar IVDD are T12-T13 and T13-L1.
- Cerebrospinal fluid analysis to rule out inflammatory, septic, or neoplastic condition if negative imaging findings.

TREATMENT

THERAPEUTIC GOAL(S)

Reverse neurologic dysfunction by reducing pressure on, and inflammation in, the spinal cord.

ACUTE GENERAL TREATMENT

- Based on the severity and history of neurologic dysfunction.
- Initial cases of pain and no motor dysfunction: corticosteroids *or* nonsteroidal anti-inflammatory drugs (NSAIDs), narcotic analgesics, muscle relaxants, and strict cage confinement for 3 to 4 weeks.
- Corticosteroids:
  - Methylprednisolone (Solu-Medrol) 30 mg/kg IV once within 12 hours of onset of clinical signs, or
  - Dexamethasone (Azium) 0.5–1 mg/kg IV or IM once, or
  - Prednisolone 0.5–1 mg/kg PO q 24h for 5 days then tapered dose for 1 to 2 weeks.
- Muscle relaxant:
  - Methocarbamol (Robaxin) 15–22 mg/kg PO q 8h.
- NSAIDs:
  - Carprofen (Rimadyl) 2 mg/kg PO q 12h, or
  - Deracoxib (Deramaxx) 2–4 mg/kg PO q 24h, or
  - Etodolac (Etogesic) 10–15 mg/kg PO q 24h, or
  - Meloxicam (Metacam) 0.1 mg/kg PO q 24h.
- Narcotic analgesics:
  - Butorphanol (Torbugesic) 0.5–1 mg/kg PO q 6–8h.
  - Buprenorphine (Buprenex) 5–15 μg/kg IM, IV q 12h.
  - Morphine 0.5–1 mg/kg IM or SQ q 6–8h.
  - Fentanyl transdermal patch 25 μg (5–15 kg), 50 μg (15–30 kg), 75 μg (30–50 kg).
- Cases with: recurrent episodes of neck or back pain uncontrolled by medication, and/or neurologic signs (gait alterations, proprioception/motor/pain perception deficits) should have decompressive surgery based on myelographic or MRI findings:
  - Ventral slot (cervical) or dorsolateral hemilaminectomy (back) with fenestration of adjacent sites.
- Cervical disk fenestration to alleviate pain is a controversial procedure.
- Chemonucleolysis (direct intradiscal injection of enzymes) has been infrequently described in the veterinary literature.
- Acupuncture has been used for alleviating pain, but will have no direct effect on a compressive spinal cord lesion.
- Chiropractic maneuvers are highly controversial and may worsen neurologic status.

CHRONIC TREATMENT

- Reducing anti-inflammatory medications and analgesics during the first 1 to 3 postoperative weeks.
- Padded rest areas, slings for assisted ambulation, hydrotherapy for cleanliness and to stimulate ambulation, bladder/bowel assistance.
- Control of body weight to avoid obesity.
- Avoidance of jumping activities that stress the spine.
- Physical rehabilitation (see Physical Rehabilitation, p 1300) exercises to strengthen spinal musculature.

DRUG INTERACTIONS

Concurrent usage of corticosteroids and NSAIDs may lead to gastrointestinal ulceration. Therefore these two classes of medications should *not* be combined.

POSSIBLE COMPLICATIONS

- Gastrointestinal ulceration or iatrogenic hyperadrenocorticism due to excessive usage of corticosteroids.
- Intraoperative hemorrhage or cardiopulmonary arrest due to iatrogenic spinal cord trauma during ventral cervical decompression.
- Worsened neurologic status due to iatrogenic spinal cord trauma during bone drilling or secondary embolism after surgery.

RECOMMENDED MONITORING

Pain level, comfort, bladder/bowel evacuations, evidence of pressure sores, and neurologic status should be assessed daily until patient has recovered (ambulatory, pain-free, normal eliminations)

PROGNOSIS AND OUTCOME

- In general, patients have a good prognosis for functional recovery 2 to 6 weeks after surgery assuming intact pain perception preoperatively, no medical or surgical complications, and adequate postoperative rehabilitation. Patients with paralysis (no motor or sensory functions) for several days or longer before surgery have a poorer prognosis.
- Patients treated conservatively may have recurrence rates of clinical signs ranging from 30–50%. Avoidance of obesity and jumping activities, and implementation of physical rehabilitation therapy, may reduce these rates.

PEARLS & CONSIDERATIONS

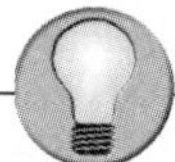

COMMENTS

- Strict cage rest is critical for recovery in nonsurgical patients treated with analgesics and anti-inflammatory medications. Physical therapy, weight control, and avoidance of jumping activities may alleviate future need for surgery.
- In cases of chronic paralysis, decompressive surgery can be performed for diagnostic (durotomy and cord examination for myelomalacia) and possible therapeutic benefits.

PREVENTION

Avoidance of obesity and jumping activities for chondrodystrophic breeds

CLIENT EDUCATION

See Prevention above

SUGGESTED READING

Seim HB: Surgery of the cervical and thoracolumbar spine. In Fossum TW (ed): *Small Animal Surgery*, ed 2. St. Louis, Mosby, 2002, pp 1213–1301.

Sharp NJ, Wheeler SJ: Cervical disc disease and thoracolumbar disc disease. In Sharp NJ, Wheeler SJ (eds): *Small Animal Spinal Disorders*, ed 2. St. Louis, Elsevier, 2005, pp 93–160.

Toombs JP, Waters DJ: Intervertebral disc disease. In Slatter D (ed): *Textbook of Small Animal Surgery*, ed 3. Philadelphia, WB Saunders, 2003, pp 1193–1209.

AUTHOR & EDITOR: **JOSEPH HARARI**

Intraocular Neoplasia

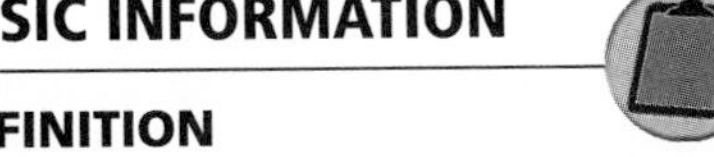

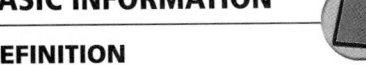

BASIC INFORMATION

DEFINITION

A primary intraocular neoplasm arises from the vascular intraocular tunic (iris, ciliary body, choroid). In cats, primary undifferentiated sarcoma arises from an undetermined cell population, most likely lens epithelium. Secondary intraocular neoplasia occurs through metastasis or (rarely) by extension from adjacent tissues.

SYNONYM(S)

Ocular tumor
Tumor of the globe or eye
Ciliary body adenoma/adenocarcinoma
Intraocular sarcoma
Medulloepithelioma
Uveal (iris/ciliary body) melanoma or melanocytoma (Note: Melanomas of the limbus or uvea/iris in dogs are almost always benign and therefore are appropriately called melanocytomas, which are benign tumors of melanocyte origin)

EPIDEMIOLOGY

SPECIES, AGE, SEX

- Melanoma/melanocytoma affects dogs and cats, usually older adults (>7 years old), although it may also be seen in young dogs <4 years old.
- Medulloepithelioma usually affects animals 1 to 4 years of age.
- Primary sarcoma occurs only in cats of any age.
- There is no sex predilection for any intraocular neoplasm.
- Neoplasia metastatic to the eye follows the signalment expected for the primary neoplasm.

GENETICS AND BREED PREDISPOSITION

- Uveal melanoma: Labrador retrievers (known), golden retrievers, German shepherds (suspected).
- Mode of inheritance is not defined but is suspected to be autosomal dominant.

ASSOCIATED CONDITIONS AND DISORDERS: Secondary to intraocular neoplasia: uveitis, glaucoma, retinal detachment, intraocular hemorrhage.

CLINICAL PRESENTATION

HISTORY, CHIEF COMPLAINT

- Change in appearance of the eye: redness, cloudiness, swelling, darkening of iris, development of a mass.
- Pain, blepharospasm.
- Loss of vision.

PHYSICAL EXAM FINDINGS: Findings associated directly with the tumor:

- Mass that may be pigmented (melanoma/melanocytoma) (Fig. I-103) or pink in color (more likely ciliary body adenoma/adenocarcinoma) (Fig. I-104) or a metastatic neoplasia (Fig. I-105) within the iris or pupil. Not all mela-

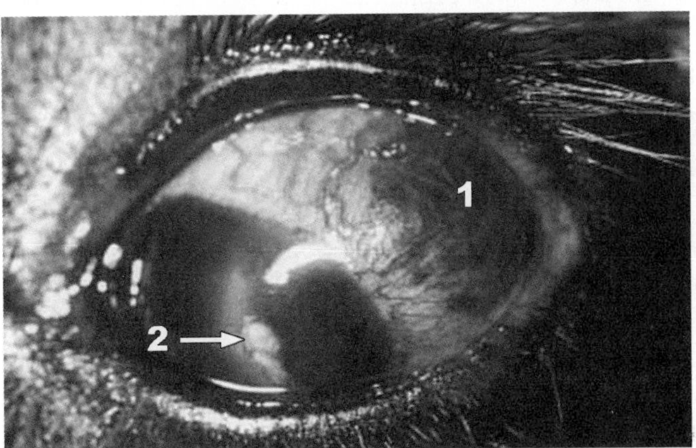

FIGURE I-103 Uveal melanoma in a dog. (1) Corneal and extrascleral extension. (2) White area of calcific corneal degeneration overlying the central to paracentral cornea and at the leading edge of the corneal extension. Enucleation is recommended.

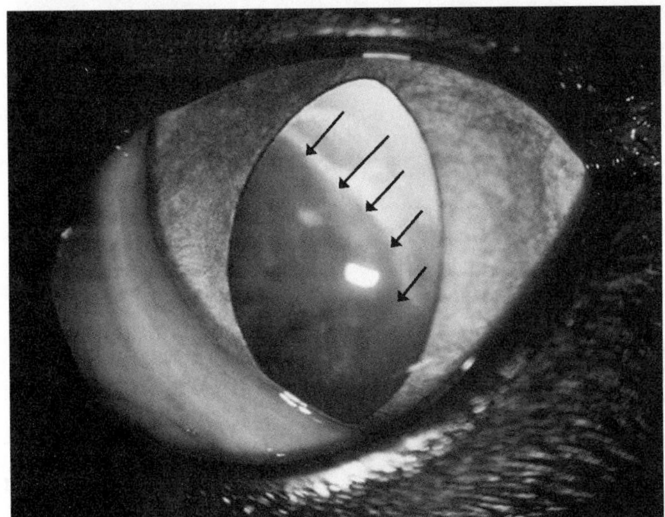

FIGURE I-104 Large mass visible within the pupil in a cat (lateral-most margin of mass outlined by *arrows*). This appearance is typical of a ciliary body adenoma/adenocarcinoma, but ocular metastasis from a distant site is also possible.

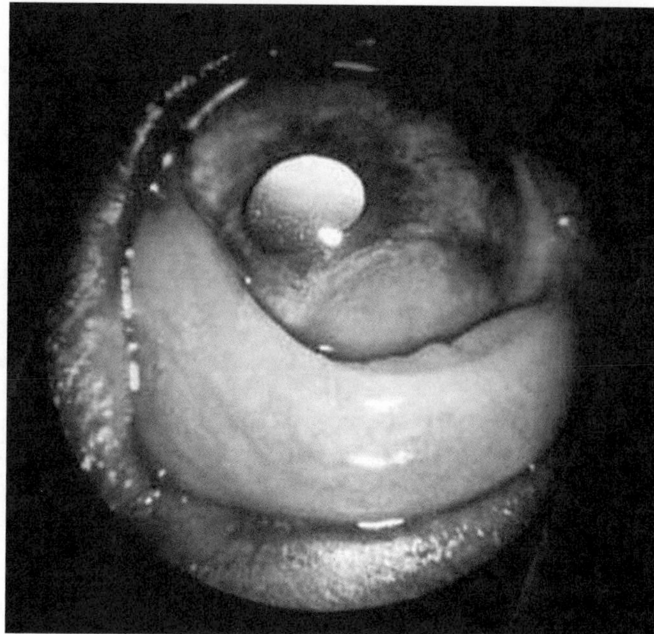

FIGURE I-105 Lymphosarcoma metastatic to the iris and third eyelid in a dog. Diagnosis was made by biopsy of the third eyelid. Courtesy of Dr. Robert L. Peiffer, Jr.

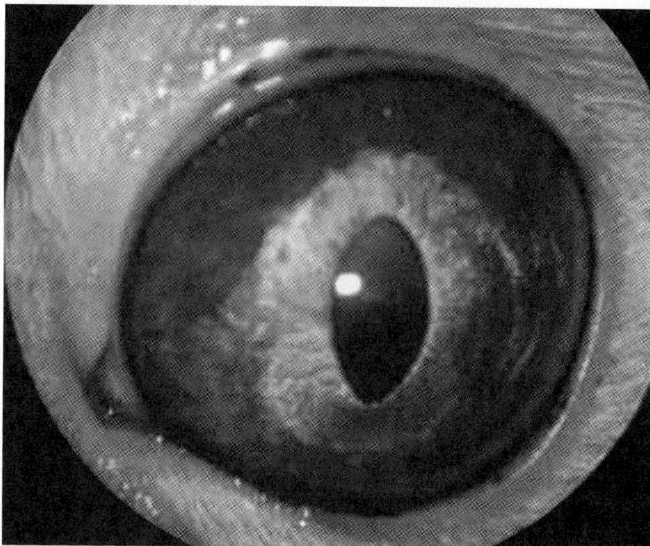

FIGURE I-106 Diffuse iris melanoma in a cat. Note the raised "velvety" dark appearance of the circumferentially affected outer iris distinguishing this from benign iris hyperpigmentation, which appears nonraised and does not appear velvety. Enucleation is recommended.

nomas are pigmented and not all are pigmented masses.

- Extension of mass through sclera (see Fig. I-103).
- Diffuse hyperpigmentation of iris, which is seen more often in cats (Fig. I-106).
- Dyscoria, anisocoria.
- Shallow anterior chamber.
- Intraocular hemorrhage.
- Displacement of lens.

Findings associated with secondary glaucoma/uveitis (see Glaucoma, p 440; Uveitis, p 1134):

- Elevated intraocular pressure.
- Fixed, dilated pupil.
- Corneal edema.
- Scleral injection.
- Aqueous flare.
- Hyphema.
- Lens luxation.
- If chronic, retinal degeneration and peripapillary hyperpigmentation.

ETIOLOGY AND PATHOPHYSIOLOGY

- Primary intraocular neoplasms:
  - The most common primary intraocular neoplasm of dogs and cats is uveal melanoma.
  - Clinicians should not misdiagnose benign uveal cyst (see Uveal Cysts, p 1133) as a melanoma or other neoplasm.
  - Ciliary body adenoma or adenocarcinoma occurs commonly in dogs but is rare in cats.
    - Proliferation of uveal melanocytes or ciliary body epithelium, cause unknown.
    - Melanoma originates most commonly in the anterior uvea (iris and ciliary body), unlike humans, where most are of choroidal origin.
    - Primary tumors in dogs are benign and, although locally invasive, rarely metastasize.
    - Ciliary body tumors rarely metastasize.
    - Uveal melanoma in cats may metastasize.
- Primary undifferentiated intraocular sarcoma in cats:
  - Second most frequent primary intraocular tumor in cats.
  - Occurs months to years after blunt or penetrating trauma to the eye.
  - Damage to lens epithelium is implicated as initiating factor.
  - Frequently metastasize.
- Secondary intraocular neoplasms:
  - Hematogenous metastasis accounts for most secondary intraocular tumors.
  - Lymphosarcoma is the most frequent secondary intraocular tumor in the dog and cat.
    - Anterior uveal disease (e.g., uveitis and/or an intraocular mass) occurs in nearly all affected eyes.
  - Hemangiosarcoma has been reported to be the second most common metastatic intraocular neoplasm in the dog.

DIAGNOSIS

DIFFERENTIAL DIAGNOSIS

- Uveal/iris cyst
- Diffuse iris melanocytosis, hyperpigmentation
- Granulomatous uveitis with accumulation of inflammatory nodules within iris stroma
- Other causes of uveitis, glaucoma, intraocular hemorrhage

INITIAL DATABASE

- Ophthalmic examination including evaluation of vision and pupillary light reflexes and measurement of intraocular pressure.
- Direct visualization of mass may allow conclusive diagnosis.
- Ocular ultrasonography may confirm and delineate mass that cannot be

directly visualized because of location or lack of clarity of media. Tumor appears as a hyperechoic mass within iris or ciliary body and may be difficult to differentiate from organized hemorrhage.
- Systemic evaluation to rule out metastatic disease (complete blood count, serum biochemistry panel, urinalysis, and thoracic and abdominal radiographs).

ADVANCED OR CONFIRMATORY TESTING

- Aqueocentesis may not be diagnostic because tumors often do not exfoliate cells into the aqueous; most valuable for lymphosarcoma.
- Fine-needle aspirate of mass is often nondiagnostic due to inadequate size of sample.
- Biopsy of mass may be accompanied by hemorrhage.

TREATMENT

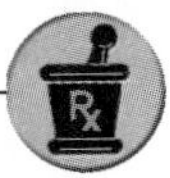

THERAPEUTIC GOAL(S)

- Prevent progressive growth of tumor and thereby preserve vision and comfort
- Alleviate discomfort caused by secondary glaucoma in blind eye

ACUTE GENERAL TREATMENT

- Assessment of vision is a primary factor in determining treatment recommendation.
  - If eye has functional vision, laser treatment should be considered for localized lesions.
  - If eye is blind, enucleation is recommended.
- For malignant melanoma and sarcoma in cats, enucleation is advisable.
- Primary intraocular neoplasms:
  - Enucleation is indicated for eyes that are irreversibly blind and painful due to secondary glaucoma.
  - Due to their metastatic potential, iris melanoma and primary sarcoma in cats should be treated with enucleation.
  - Conservative monitoring only may be justified in older dogs based on likely slow growth of primary tumor.
  - Sector iridectomy may provide incomplete excision and is often accompanied by hemorrhage and secondary glaucoma; this procedure may be the only surgical option for attempting to salvage the globe for nonpigmented tumors because a diode laser is only effective at ablating pigmented tissues.
  - Diode laser treatment, transcorneally or through a limbal incision, is effective for relatively focal pigmented uveal tumors.
- Secondary intraocular neoplasms:
  - Treatment is directed at primary neoplasm, if possible. If systemic prognosis warrants, enucleation may be indicated for comfort.

POSSIBLE COMPLICATIONS

- Laser treatment of large lesions may be accompanied by significant inflammation and may precipitate secondary glaucoma.
- Regrowth of tumor is possible following laser treatment.

RECOMMENDED MONITORING

Long-term monitoring (every 3 to 4 months for the first year, then less frequently thereafter) is indicated after laser treatment to detect recurrent growth of the tumor at the site of the laser treatment or elsewhere within the eye.

PROGNOSIS AND OUTCOME

- Primary neoplasms of the iris and ciliary body in dogs (i.e., uveal melanomas and ciliary body adenomas/adenocarcinomas) are nearly always benign and very rarely metastasize.
- Iris melanomas in cats are malignant tumors and may metastasize.
- Primary intraocular sarcomas in cats are locally aggressive and often metastasize.

PEARLS & CONSIDERATIONS

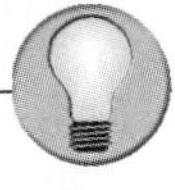

COMMENTS

Not all melanomas are pigmented and not all pigmented masses are melanomas.

PREVENTION

Iris melanoma in dogs: avoid breeding affected or closely related individuals.

SUGGESTED READING

Cook CS, Wilkie DA: Treatment of presumed iris melanoma in dogs by diode laser photocoagulation: 23 cases. *Vet Ophthalmol* 2:217, 1999.

Dubielzig RR: Ocular neoplasia in small animals. *Vet Clin North Am Sm Anim Pract* 20:837, 1990.

Guiliano EA, et al: A matched observational study of canine survival with primary intraocular melanocytic neoplasia. *Vet Ophthalmol* 2:185, 1999.

Kalishman JB, et al: A matched observational study of survival in cats with enucleation due to diffuse iris melanoma. *Vet Ophthalmol* 1:25, 1998.

AUTHOR: **CYNTHIA S. COOK**
EDITOR: **CHERYL L. CULLEN**

Intussusception

BASIC INFORMATION

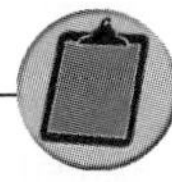

DEFINITION

- Invagination of one segment of the gastrointestinal (GI) tract into the lumen of an adjacent segment
- *Intussusceptum* is the invaginated segment and the *intussuscipiens* is the outer or enveloping segment

SYNONYM(S)

Intestinal telescoping

Enteroenteric intussusception: also called intestinal intussusception

EPIDEMIOLOGY

SPECIES, AGE, SEX

- Intestinal intussusception usually occurs in animals <1 year unless associated with neoplasia.
- Gastroesophageal intussusception is most common in dogs <3 months old.
- No sex predilection.

GENETICS AND BREED PREDISPOSITION: Siamese cats, German shepherds, and shar-peis may be predisposed.

RISK FACTORS: Infectious gastroenteritis (parasitic, bacterial or viral); foreign body ingestion; intestinal mass/neoplasia; previous surgery; peritonitis; organophosphate intoxication.

CLINICAL PRESENTATION

DISEASE FORMS/SUBTYPES

- Any of the following sites can be involved: gastroesophageal, pylorogastric, enteroenteric, enterocolic.
- Intussusception most commonly occurs in direction of normal peristalsis with intussusceptum as proximal segment, but reverse can also occur (e.g., gastroesophageal intussusception).
- More than one site can be involved, or two invaginations may occur at the same site.

HISTORY, CHIEF COMPLAINT

- Diarrhea, vomiting, anorexia, lethargy, and weight loss.
- Respiratory distress if gastroesophageal intussusception.
- Signs can be acute or chronic.

PHYSICAL EXAM FINDINGS

- Palpable, sausage-shaped abdominal mass.
- Signs of pain on abdominal palpation.
- Dehydration, tachycardia (more severe signs associated with more proximal obstruction).
- Intussusception may protrude from anus.

ETIOLOGY AND PATHOPHYSIOLOGY

- Proposed cause is a lack of homogeneity within the bowel wall or lack of mechanical linkage between adjacent segments of the bowel, resulting in an alteration of intestinal pliability or motility.
- Intussusception produces partial or complete intestinal obstruction.
- Increased intraluminal pressure and kinking causes collapse of mesenteric blood vessels. Avulsion of vessels can also occur.
- Bowel wall becomes edematous and may become ischemic.
- Necrosis of the bowel wall with leakage of contents contained by a fibrin seal between the layers of the intussusception may occur. If leakage is not contained, peritonitis develops.

DIAGNOSIS

Enteroenteric (intestinal) intussusception is suspected at the time of abdominal palpation in a patient with consistent history and physical signs. Confirmation is obtained at the time of surgery, although preoperative abdominal ultrasound may be highly suggestive (Fig. I-107).

DIFFERENTIAL DIAGNOSIS

- Gastroenteritis associated with infection or dietary indiscretion
- Intestinal obstruction associated with foreign body, neoplasia, abscess, or granuloma
- Physiologic ileus
- Rectal prolapse if intussusception protruding through anus (see Rectal Prolapse, p 943)

INITIAL DATABASE

- Complete blood cell count may show evidence of a stress leukogram or anemia.
- Serum chemistry profile may show evidence of dehydration, electrolyte abnormalities, or hypoproteinemia.
- Abdominal radiographs: fluid or gas distended intestinal loops. Mass effect (sausage shape) of the intussusception.
- Thoracic radiographs: soft tissue density within esophagus if gastroesophageal intussusception.
- Fecal flotation: indicated in all cases of intussusception, to assess possible parasitic causes.

ADVANCED OR CONFIRMATORY TESTING

- Contrast radiography with upper GI radiographic contrast study or barium enema: filling defect caused by intussusceptum seen within intussuscipiens.
- Ultrasonography: concentric rings seen in transverse plane ("target sign", see Fig. I-107).

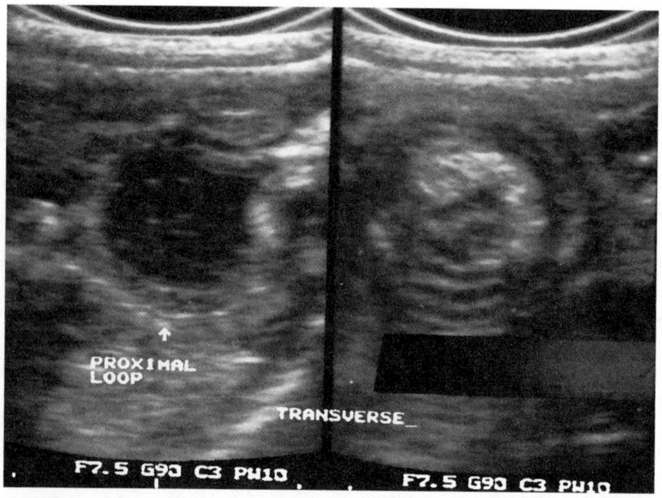

TREATMENT

THERAPEUTIC GOAL(S)

- Stabilize hemodynamic status
- Attempt to reduce intussusception
- Perform resection and anastomosis if unable to reduce intussusception, if a mass is present, or if there is devitalized bowel
- Prevent recurrence by treating underlying cause of intussusception or performing enteroplication or gastropexy

ACUTE GENERAL TREATMENT

- Intravenous fluid and electrolyte therapy
- Perioperative antibiotics:
  - Cefazolin, 22 mg/kg IV q 2h during the perioperative period
- Enteroenteric or enterocolic intussusceptions: at the time of surgical exploration, reduce intussusception by applying pressure to intussuscipiens while *gently* pulling on intussusceptum:
  - Resection and anastomosis if unable to reduce intussusception, a mass is present, or there is nonviable bowel
- With enteroenteric intussusception, perform enteroplication if recurrence appears likely based on inability to correct underlying disease
- With gastroesophageal intussusception, perform gastropexy of fundus and pylorus to prevent recurrence

CHRONIC TREATMENT

- Opioid analgesia after surgery may decrease risk of recurrence.
- Treat infectious enteritis that may have caused intussusception.
- Antibiotics should be continued after surgery if peritonitis is present.
- Enteroplication if not performed at first surgery and postoperative intussusception recurs.

POSSIBLE COMPLICATIONS

- Recurrence of intussusception
- Peritonitis associated with bowel rupture
- Leakage or dehiscence of intestinal suture line
- Entrapment and strangulation of bowel between enteroplication sutures
- Foreign body entrapment in bend of intestine created by enteroplication

RECOMMENDED MONITORING

- Monitor hydration status and serum electrolyte concentrations.
- Monitor for signs of intestinal suture line dehiscence and peritonitis (increased body temperature, abdominal pain, hypoglycemia).
- If clinical signs recur after surgery, repeat imaging to evaluate for possible recurrence of intussusception or complication associated with enteroplication.

FIGURE I-107 Ultrasound appearance of small intestinal intussusception. Left panel: dilated, poorly motile jejunum located proximal to the intussusception. Right panel: the characteristic multilayered, "target" appearance of intussuscepted small intestine. A horizontal bar below the intussuscepted bowel is artifactual. Courtesy of Dr. Richard Walshaw.

PROGNOSIS AND OUTCOME

- Depends on cause, location, and duration of intussusception.
  - Good if fluid and electrolyte abnormalities are corrected and there is immediate surgical intervention.
  - Patients with proximal GI tract intussusception, generalized peritonitis, or underlying malignant intestinal neoplasia have a worse prognosis.
- Up to 25% recurrence is reported if enteroplication is not performed in association with surgical correction of intestinal intussusception.
- Severe complications are associated with enteroplication in 19% of dogs.

PEARLS & CONSIDERATIONS

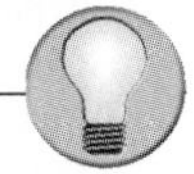

COMMENTS

For each patient, the risk of recurrence must be weighed against the risk of complications associated with enteroplication.

- The decision is based largely on whether an underlying cause that can be corrected has been identified.
- If enteroplication is performed, create gentle loops along entire length of small intestine (from duodenocolic ligament to ileocolic junction.) Sutures 5–10 cm apart.

SUGGESTED READING

Applewhite AA, et al: Complications of enteroplication for the prevention of intussusception recurrence in dogs: 35 cases (1989–1999). *J Am Vet Med Assoc* 219:1415, 2001.

Applewhite AA, et al: Diagnosis and treatment of intussusceptions in dogs. *Compend Contin Educ Pract Vet* 24:110, 2002.

Bellinger CR, et al: Intussusception in 12 cats. *J Small Anim Pract* 35:295, 1994.

AUTHOR: **LORI LUDWIG**

EDITOR: **RICHARD WALSHAW**

Ionophore Toxicosis

BASIC INFORMATION

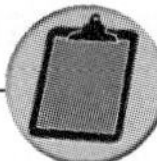

DEFINITION

- Ionophores are antiparasitic fermentation products of *Streptomyces* fungi. They are used primarily as feed additives to increase feed efficiency and weight gain, and as coccidiostats, in ruminants and poultry.
- Toxicity results from accidental ingestion of livestock or poultry feed containing ionophores and is characterized by acute central nervous system (CNS) dysfunction within 12 hours of large ingestions, and signs relating mainly to muscle damage within 24 to 96 hours of smaller ingestions.

SYNONYM(S)

Some of the commonly available ionophores are:

Monensin (Rumensin, Coban)
Lasalocid (Bovatec, Avatec)
Salinomycin (Sacox, Bio-Cox)
Narasin (Monteban)
Semduramicin (Aviax)
Laidlomycin propionate (Cattlyst)

EPIDEMIOLOGY

SPECIES, AGE, SEX

- All animals susceptible; dogs mainly involved compared to cats.
- Dogs are attracted to livestock or poultry feed that may contain the ionophore. Cats rarely attracted to these products.

GENETICS AND BREED PREDISPOSITION: Farm dogs have greater access to ionophore-containing poultry or cattle feed.

RISK FACTORS

- Ionophore premix formulations (concentrated) are much more dangerous than ready-to-feed products.
- Patients with underlying cardiac or myopathic conditions could be at heightened risk.

CLINICAL PRESENTATION

DISEASE FORMS/SUBTYPES

- Acute onset from high doses (<12 hours): acute CNS depression, ataxia, recumbency.
- Subacute onset from lower doses (24 to 96 hours): generalized weakness, lethargy, anorexia.
- Duration of effect: acute exposures, 2 to 10 days. Significant muscle involvement may produce permanent myopathy to variable degree.

HISTORY, CHIEF COMPLAINT

- History of exposure to ionophore (livestock or poultry feed).
- Combination of possible access to ionophore and acute onset of progressive CNS depression, hind limb or full body weakness, or collapse.
- Anorexia, diarrhea.

PHYSICAL EXAM FINDINGS

- As listed above, plus ataxia, quadriplegia, hyporeflexia, tachypnea/dyspnea, tachycardia/arrhythmia, hyperthermia, tongue laxity
- Urine discoloration (myoglobin)

ETIOLOGY AND PATHOPHYSIOLOGY

Ionophore-induced cation transport across cell membranes results in intracellular calcium overload, mitochondrial disruption, catecholamine release, skeletal and myocardial muscle ischemia, necrosis and fibrosis, and acute renal tubular failure from myoglobin deposition.

DIAGNOSIS

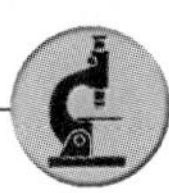

DIFFERENTIAL DIAGNOSIS

- Other intoxications (e.g., ivermectin, amitraz, bromethalin, macadamia nuts, alcohols, muscle relaxants [e.g., baclofen], hypoglycemic agents [e.g., xylitol, artificial sweetener], cardiac glycosides, sedatives, or painkillers [e.g., opioids, barbiturates, benzodiazepines, phenothiazines], and phenoxy herbicides)
- Rhabdomyolysis
- Neuromuscular disease (botulism, myasthenia gravis, polyradiculoneuritis, tick paralysis)
- Hypoadrenocorticism

INITIAL DATABASE

- Baseline serum chemistries and electrolytes, including calcium.
- Electrocardiogram (ECG; early indicator of myocardial involvement). ECG alterations (S-T segment depression, atrial fibrillation, paroxysmal atrial tachycardia), sinus tachycardia.
- Baseline and monitor enzymes of skeletal and cardiac muscle origin: creatine kinase (CK), aspartate aminotransferase (AST), and lactate dehydrogenase (LDH). Cardiac: CK_2 (MB), CK_3 (MM), LDH_1 (H_4). Skeletal: CK_3, LDH_5 (M_4). Also note increase in alanine aminotransferase. CK is the most sensitive indicator, noted within 4 to 6 hours of acute insult, maximum at 6 to 12 hours. AST rises more slowly, may persist for several days. LDH is less dramatic, reaches maximum levels within 48 to 72 hours.
- Myoglobin (serum and urine). Absent in serum/urine of the healthy animal,

released rapidly from damaged muscle tissue; sensitive indicator of myonecrosis.
- Cardiac troponin T: specific and sensitive indicator in humans, potential for use in diagnosing this form of myocardial disease in mammalian species.
- Hematocrit, total solid
- Blood pressure
- Arterial blood gas

ADVANCED OR CONFIRMATORY TESTING

- Feed analysis may help determine ionophore concentration and dose consumed by the animal.
- On gross necropsy, sanguineous pericardial effusion may be present.
- Histopathologic exam of tissues: various stages of focal myocyte degeneration, vacuolation, necrosis, and fibrosis.

TREATMENT

THERAPEUTIC GOAL(S)

- Reduce gut absorption
- Supportive care

ACUTE GENERAL TREATMENT

- Reduce gut absorption:
  - Induce emesis (dogs) if exposure is within 2 hours (see Vomiting, Induction of, p 1328).
  - Activated charcoal with a cathartic (1-4 g/kg PO, repeat in 6 to 8 hours if initial exposure is high).
- Supportive care:
  - Intravenous fluids 0.9% saline, typically at 1.5 to 2 times maintenance rate; caution if exhibiting cardiopulmonary signs. Ensure adequate perfusion to avoid/reduce renal tubular damage (myoglobin-associated), and assist compensation of expected low-moderate degree of acidosis.
  - Urine alkalinization with sodium bicarbonate to reduce myoglobin deposition in renal tubules is controversial, but not necessarily contraindicated; ensure acid-base, electrolyte, and cardiac monitoring.
  - Treat cardiac abnormalities as indicated from abnormal ECG tracings (see Ventricular Arrhythmias, p 1148); caution: lidocaine may potentiate monensin toxicity.
  - Correct electrolyte imbalances; assess and manage expected metabolic acidosis.
  - Oxygen support as indicated from pulse oximetry readings and pulmonary condition.
  - Dialysis benefit unknown, but may be indicated if severe renal failure is of concern.
  - Calcium channel blockers, calcium antagonists or modulators are *not* recommended.

CHRONIC TREATMENT

Patient should not be stressed (minimize activity) and should be rested for several weeks (muscle recovery).

DRUG INTERACTIONS

Concurrent administration of chloramphenicol, tiamulin, erythromycin, sulfonamides, or cardiac glycosides is contraindicated: can potentiate ionophore toxicosis.

POSSIBLE COMPLICATIONS

Cardiac or skeletal muscle fibrosis, vacuolization of peripheral sensory and motor nerves possible.

RECOMMENDED MONITORING

- Selected cardiac, renal, acid-base, and muscle chemistries
- ECG

PROGNOSIS AND OUTCOME

- Poor if extensive damage to skeletal or cardiac muscle occurs.
- The relative degree of myofibrosis will determine the long-term prognosis.
- May require retirement of high performance patients (e.g., breeding, sporting, trial dogs).

PEARLS & CONSIDERATIONS

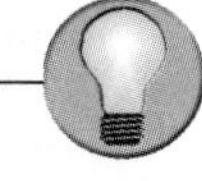

COMMENTS

- Occurrence of ionophore toxicity in dogs and cats is low.
- Monensin: canine acute oral LD50 = 10-20 mg/kg. Lasalocid: field cases reported at 166-210 mg/kg/day of dog food (10-15 mg/kg/day of lasalocid). Salinomycin: reported oral toxicity in cats at 440 mg/kg in cat food.
- Relay (secondary) toxicosis has been reported in dogs consuming dead chickens containing ionophores (lasalocid).
- Intoxication from accidental ionophore adulteration of dog food has also been reported.

PREVENTION

Do not allow dogs and cats to enter cattle or poultry farms where ionophores are stored or being fed.

SUGGESTED READING

Hall J: Ionophores. In Peterson ME, Talcott PA (eds): *Small Animal Toxicology*. Philadelphia, WB Saunders, 2001, pp 516-523.

Bender HS: Muscle. In Latimer KS, Mahaffey EA, Prasse KW (eds): *Duncan & Prasse's Veterinary Laboratory Medicine Clinical Pathology*, ed 4. Ames, IA, Iowa State Press, 2003, pp 260-269.

AUTHOR: **MICHAEL W. KNIGHT**

EDITOR: **SAFDAR A. KHAN**

Iris Abnormalities

BASIC INFORMATION

DEFINITION

Iris abnormalities include any change in the color, character, or appearance of the iris including acquired changes secondary to *anterior uveitis*, *neoplasia*, or *cyst* formation, as well as developmental changes (e.g., persistent pupillary membranes [PPMs]). Definitions of other relevant terms include those for *rubeosis iridis* (blood vessel formation on the surface of the iris) and *synechia* (adhesion of iris-to-cornea [anterior] or iris-to-lens [posterior]).

SYNONYM(S)

Uveal disease

EPIDEMIOLOGY

SPECIES, AGE, SEX

- Dogs and cats.
- Typically, *anterior uveitis* does not demonstrate age or sex predisposition.
- *Anterior uveal neoplasia* usually is seen in middle-aged to older animals.
- *Uveal cysts* most frequently are found in middle-aged to older animals (rare in cats).
- *PPMs* are seen congenitally; usually atrophy by 6 weeks of age in most puppies but, if not, PPMs may be detected in all age groups (rare in cats).

GENETICS AND BREED PREDISPOSITION

- *Uveal melanoma* has a suspected genetic predisposition in the Labrador retriever, golden retriever, and German shepherd.

- *Uveal cysts*: breeds, see Uveal Cysts, p 1133.
- Heritable cause suspected for PPMs in basenjis, Pembroke Welsh Corgis, chow chows, mastiffs, and others.

CLINICAL PRESENTATION

DISEASE FORMS/SUBTYPES

- Uveitis (see Uveitis, p 1134)
- Uveal neoplasia (see Intraocular Neoplasia, p 603)
- Uveal cysts (see Uveal Cysts, p 1133)
- PPMs

HISTORY, CHIEF COMPLAINT

- Variable depending on cause.
- Anterior uveitis (see Uveitis, p 1134): any or all of the following:
  - Change in color and/or appearance of iris:
    - Increased or decreased pigmentation.
    - Blood vessels or hemorrhage on iridal surface.
    - Change in pupil shape.
- Uveal neoplasia (see Intraocular Neoplasia, p 603): any or all of the following:
  - Change in color of iris (usually to dark brown or fleshy).
  - Growth/mass inside eye.
  - Blood inside eye (e.g., hyphema; see Hyphema, p 560).
- Uveal cysts (see Uveal Cysts, p 1133): any or all of the following:
  - Usually incidental findings.
  - Pigmented, oval, or spherical mass(es) inside eye.
- PPMs: any or all of the following:
  - Usually incidental findings.
  - Cloudiness of eye.
  - Cloudiness/opacities in pupil.

PHYSICAL EXAM FINDINGS

- See History, Chief Complaint above.
- PPMs: any or all of the following:
  - Single or multiple fine strands (rarely sheets) of iris tissue originating from the iris collarette and inserting on:
    - Adjacent iris; typically benign, incidental finding.
    - Anterior lens; often associated with anterior capsular cataracts.
    - Corneal endothelium; associated with varying degrees of corneal scarring and/or edema.
    - Iris sheets; most severe form (sheet of tissue bridging pupil); associated with vision impairment.

ETIOLOGY AND PATHOPHYSIOLOGY

- The uveal tract (or vascular layer) of the eye is composed of the iris, ciliary body, and choroid. The iris is the most anterior of these and is a thin diaphragm containing blood vessels, connective tissue, melanocytes, and two muscles—the iris sphincter and the iris dilator. In the center of the iridal diaphragm is a circular aperture, the pupil.
- Anterior uveitis (see Uveitis, p 1134).
- Uveal neoplasia (see Intraocular Neoplasia, p 603).
- Uveal cysts (see Uveal Cysts, p 1133).
- PPMs: nonvascular remnants of the tunica vasculosa lentis, which appear as iris strands or sheets, originating in the iris collarette (midway point between iris base and pupillary margin). PPMs extend across the iris to insert on adjacent iris, lens, or cornea. When they insert on lens or cornea, opacification of these structures may occur. PPMs are a developmental defect that may have a heritable component in some breeds.

DIAGNOSIS

DIFFERENTIAL DIAGNOSIS

- Discoloration of iris:
  - Pigmentation:
    - Uveal melanoma (variable appearance in the dog [focal] versus cat [mainly diffuse]; solid tissue; may cause dyscoria [misshapen/distorted pupil] and/or anisocoria [unequal or asymmetric pupils])
    - Uveal cyst (round to ovoid; single or multiple; often translucent) (see Uveal Cysts, p 1133)
    - Chronic anterior uveitis
  - Depigmentation:
    - Chronic anterior uveitis
    - Uveal neoplasm
  - Reddening:
    - Rubeosis iridis
    - Iridal hemorrhage
    - Uveal neoplasm
- Iris mass:
  - Uveal neoplasm
  - Uveal cyst
- Iris strands:
  - PPMs (arise from iris collarette; typically fine strands)
  - Synechiae (anterior: typically arise from base of iris or pupillary margin; posterior: arise from pupillary margin or posterior aspect of iris; often result in dyscoria [abnormal pupil shape])

INITIAL DATABASE

- Complete ophthalmic examination
- Variable depending on underlying condition

ADVANCED OR CONFIRMATORY TESTING

Variable depending on underlying condition:

- Ocular ultrasound (differentiate uveal neoplasm from cyst)

TREATMENT

THERAPEUTIC GOAL(S)

Dependent on underlying condition

ACUTE GENERAL TREATMENT

- Directed at underlying condition and, when possible, cause (see Uveitis, p 1134; Intraocular Neoplasia, p 603; Uveal Cysts, p 1133).
- PPMs do not generally require treatment unless substantial corneal and/or lens opacification is present:
  - Iris-to-cornea PPMs may cause significant corneal edema, which may benefit from topical 5% hypertonic saline ophthalmic solution or ointment q 6-12h; continued long-term if clinical improvement noted.
  - Iris-to-lens PPMs can lead to cataract formation; if cataract is causing vision impairment, cataract surgery may be warranted (see Cataracts, p 182).

POSSIBLE COMPLICATIONS

- Variable depending on underlying condition.
- Cataracts and corneal edema associated with PPMs are rarely progressive.

PROGNOSIS AND OUTCOME

- Prognosis varies widely depending on underlying condition.
- Prognosis for *anterior uveitis* depends on severity at presentation, individual variation on severity and frequency of recurrences, and client compliance.
- Primary intraocular neoplasia usually carries a poor prognosis for saving eye, but good prognosis for systemic health.
- Uveal cysts and PPMs rarely cause problems with vision or ocular comfort.

PEARLS & CONSIDERATIONS

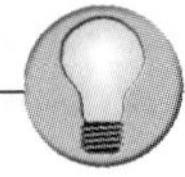

COMMENTS

- Most iridal abnormalities can be readily diagnosed on basis of clinical signs
- Anterior uveitis requires immediate therapeutic intervention

PREVENTION

Avoid breeding affected or closely related dogs predisposed to breed-related iris abnormalities

SUGGESTED READING

Grahn BH, Cullen CL, Peiffer RL: Uvea. In: *Veterinary Ophthalmology Essentials*. Philadelphia, Butterworth Heinemann, 2004, pp 123-135.

AUTHOR: **STEVEN R. HOLLINGSWORTH**
EDITOR: **CHERYL L. CULLEN**

Ivermectin Toxicosis

BASIC INFORMATION

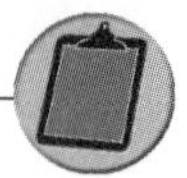

DEFINITION

Clinical syndrome associated with exposure to the macrocyclic lactone antiparasitic drug ivermectin

EPIDEMIOLOGY

SPECIES, AGE, SEX

- Very young animals may be at increased risk: immature blood-brain barrier.
- Dogs more likely to be involved; however, some sensitive cats may show clinical signs at the recommended doses.

GENETICS AND BREED PREDISPOSITION: A defect in p-glycoprotein multidrug transporter in the blood-brain barrier has been identified as an autosomal recessive trait (MDR-1 gene mutation) in some individuals of several dog breeds including collies, Shetland sheepdogs, Australian shepherds, English shepherds, and Old English sheepdogs. This defect allows ivermectin to pass into the central nervous system (CNS) at relatively low dosages, resulting in toxicosis.

RISK FACTORS

- Use of large animal formulations in small animals holds risks of dilution errors and accidental overdosage
- Animals with preexisting CNS disease or disruption of the blood brain barrier (e.g., due to trauma) may be at increased risk of toxicosis

CLINICAL PRESENTATION

DISEASE FORMS/SUBTYPES

- Acute: onset of signs within 4 to 12 hours of exposure
- Subacute: onset of signs within 48 to 96 hours; especially with exposure by injection or after multiple daily doses

HISTORY, CHIEF COMPLAINT

- History of exposure to ivermectin-containing product
- Depression, disorientation, vocalization, stupor, ataxia, tremors, vomiting, anorexia, recumbency, blindness, coma, seizure, death

PHYSICAL EXAM FINDINGS

- Mydriasis (bilateral) ± blindness (clinical: pupillary light reflexes generally intact)
- CNS depression: mild to stupor or coma
- Ataxia (proprioceptive)
- Disorientation
- Hypersalivation
- Tremors
- ± Bradycardia
- ± Vomiting
- ± Seizures
- Hypothermia (recumbency) or hyperthermia (tremor/seizure)

ETIOLOGY AND PATHOPHYSIOLOGY

Macrocyclic lactones enhance the release of γ-aminobutyric acid (GABA), an inhibitory neurotransmitter:

- In insects, GABA-mediated neurons are present throughout the peripheral nervous system, and enhanced GABA release results in paralysis.
- In mammals, GABA-mediated neurons are restricted to the CNS and in normal mammals the blood-brain barrier excludes ivermectin at therapeutic dosages.
- In overdose situations, or in mammals with blood-brain barrier defects, ivermectin enters the CNS and exerts an inhibitory effect, resulting in CNS depression.

DIAGNOSIS

DIFFERENTIAL DIAGNOSIS

- Other intoxications (marijuana, benzodiazepines, barbiturates, ethylene glycol, isoxazole mushrooms)
- Brain neoplasia
- Encephalitis
- Hepatic encephalopathy

INITIAL DATABASE

- Neurologic exam (see Neurologic Examination, p 1286). Asymmetric neurologic deficits are *inconsistent* with intoxication.
- No specific clinical pathologic alterations expected.
- Baseline complete blood count, serum chemistry profile, urinalysis, postprandial bile acids (± thoracic/abdominal diagnostic imaging) to rule out other possible etiologies.

ADVANCED OR CONFIRMATORY TESTING

- In comatose animals, temporary return to consciousness after physostigmine administration (1 mg/40 lb or 0.06 mg/kg IV) supports a diagnosis of ivermectin toxicosis.
    - Not necessarily confirmatory, as physostigmine can reverse depression from many CNS depressants.
    - Physostigmine should be used with care; may trigger seizure activity.
- Ivermectin sensitivity testing (presence of MDR-1 mutant gene) is available from the Washington State University College of Veterinary Medicine Clinical Pharmacology Laboratory (Phone/FAX 509-335-3745). A cheek brush sample is sent for analysis.
- Ivermectin can be detected in liver, adipose tissue, brain, or serum.
    - Serum levels may not correlate well with clinical signs, however.

TREATMENT

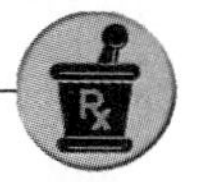

THERAPEUTIC GOAL(S)

- Manage life-threatening conditions
- Provide supportive care
- Decrease absorption/enhance elimination
- Nursing care for comatose animals

ACUTE GENERAL TREATMENT

- Manage seizures (see Seizures, p 990):
    - Diazepam (0.25-2 mg/kg IV) for seizures.
        - Gas anesthetics, propofol if diazepam ineffective.
        - Avoid barbiturates due to residual CNS depression.
    - Minimize sensory stimuli.
- Manage comatose animals:
    - Maintain airway; assist respiration as needed.
    - Thermoregulation essential.
    - Tube feeding may be necessary.
    - Atropine (0.01-0.02 mg/kg IV) for bradycardia.
    - Frequent turning to prevent decubital ulcers.
    - Urinary catheter to avoid urine scald.
    - Physostigmine 1 mg/40 lb or 0.06 mg/kg IV:
        - Only for severely affected animals.
            - Can induce seizures in mildly affected animals.
        - Duration of action 30 to 90 minutes.
        - May allow time for feeding animal.
        - Does not shorten recovery time.
- Decontamination of patients:
    - Emesis (see Vomiting, Induction of, p 1328).
        - Not recommended in animals already showing clinical signs, due to risk of aspiration.
    - Gastric lavage (see Gastric Intubation, Gavage, Lavage, p 1258).
        - For large ingestions.
    - Activated charcoal:
        - Initial dose: 1-4 g/kg PO or labeled dosage of commercial product.
        - Repeat administration q 8-12h in animals showing overt signs.
        - Subsequent doses: ½ initial dosage is used, to avoid osmotic fluid shifts and hypernatremia.

DISEASES AND DISORDERS

CHRONIC TREATMENT

- Multidose-activated charcoal
- Nursing care:
  - Frequent turning
  - Prevent urine scald
  - Thermoregulation
  - Nutritional and fluid support

DRUG INTERACTIONS

Avoid drugs that may contribute to CNS depression (e.g., barbiturates)

POSSIBLE COMPLICATIONS

- Decubital ulcers
- Aspiration of activated charcoal or food

RECOMMENDED MONITORING

- Respiration
- Body temperature
- Heart rate
- Fluid/electrolyte balance

PROGNOSIS AND OUTCOME

- No specific antidote
- Prognosis depends on dose, relative individual sensitivity, and provision of good nursing care:
  - Animals surviving >24 hours have reasonable prognosis even though supportive care may be necessary for days or possibly weeks

PEARLS & CONSIDERATIONS

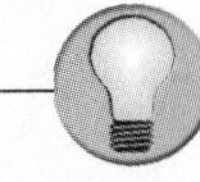

COMMENTS

- Other macrocyclic lactones with similar mechanisms of action and clinical effects include milbemycin, moxidectin, selamectin, doramectin, eprinomectin, and abamectin.
- In general, doses up to 10 times the recommended *heartworm preventive doses* of milbemycin and ivermectin are well tolerated, even by sensitive (e.g., p-glycoprotein defective) dogs.
- Toxic dose of ivermectin in collies and other sensitive breeds ranges between 0.1 and 0.2 mg/kg (15 to 30 times the therapeutic heartworm preventative dose, but equal to the doses sometimes recommended for dermatologic or heartworm microfilaricide treatment) and 2.5-40 mg/kg (>200 times) in beagles.
- Because ivermectin is eliminated primarily through the bile and undergoes enterohepatic recirculation, activated charcoal can be of benefit even if the exposure was parenteral.
- Animals on repeated high doses of ivermectin for dermatologic or other reasons should be closely monitored for mydriasis or ataxia that may develop after several doses.

PREVENTION

- Avoid large animal products (concentration: 10 mg/ml or 10,000 μg/ml) in companion animals to avoid risk of dilution errors.
- Keep dogs out of area while horses are being dewormed to prevent accidental exposure of dogs to spilled product.

SUGGESTED READING

Plumlee KH: Antiparasitic agents. In Peterson ME, Talcott PA (eds): *Small Animal Toxicology*. Philadelphia, WB Saunders, 2001, pp 531-536.

Roder JD: Antiparasiticals. In Plumlee KH (ed): *Clinical Veterinary Toxicology*. St. Louis, Mosby, 2004, pp 302-305.

AUTHOR: **SHARON M. GWALTNEY-BRANT**
EDITOR: **SAFDAR A. KHAN**

Juvenile Cellulitis

BASIC INFORMATION

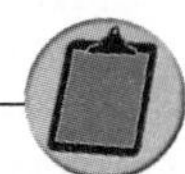

DEFINITION

An uncommon vesiculopustular to granulomatous skin disease primarily affecting dogs less than 4 months old. The pinnae, face, and mandibular lymph nodes are typically involved.

SYNONYM(S)

Juvenile pyoderma
Puppy strangles

EPIDEMIOLOGY

SPECIES, AGE, SEX: Young puppies of either sex between 3 weeks and 4 months old are typically affected, although confirmed cases in young adults have been reported. One or more puppies in the same litter may be affected.

GENETICS AND BREED PREDISPOSITION: Many breeds, including mixed breeds, may develop this disease but golden retrievers, dachshunds, and Gordon setters appear predisposed. A hereditary component is proposed. The exact mode of inheritance has not been established.

CLINICAL PRESENTATION

HISTORY, CHIEF COMPLAINT: Early in the course of the disease, an affected puppy develops an acutely swollen face, in particular the muzzle, lips, and eyelids. Marked mandibular lymphadenopathy, with or without prescapular (superficial cervical) lymphadenopathy, is usually present even in the absence of cutaneous lesions.

PHYSICAL EXAM FINDINGS

- Acute swelling of face noted initially.
- Within 24 to 48 hours, vesicles and pustules appear around mouth, eyes, and muzzle (Figs. I-108 and I-109). Lesions rapidly develop into a serous to purulent exudative dermatitis with or without fistulation.
- Severe purulent bilateral otitis externa with edematous pinnae is common.
- Marked regional (mandibular and prescapular) to diffuse lymphadenopathy is common. Fistulation of lymph nodes is variable.
- Affected skin is frequently painful but rarely pruritic.
- Rarely, fluctuant subcutaneous nodules with or without fistulation develop on the trunk, preputial, or perineal regions.
- Approximately 50% of puppies are lethargic. Anorexia, pyrexia, and joint pain (sterile suppurative arthritis) are inconsistent findings.

ETIOLOGY AND PATHOPHYSIOLOGY

- The etiology and pathogenesis of juvenile cellulitis are unknown, although immune dysfunction is suspected.
- Bacterial invasion is not considered to be the primary cause, and any evidence of infection usually reflects secondary pyoderma.

DIAGNOSIS

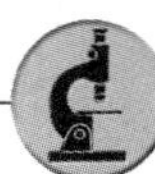

DIFFERENTIAL DIAGNOSIS

- Demodicosis
- Chin acne
- Deep pyoderma

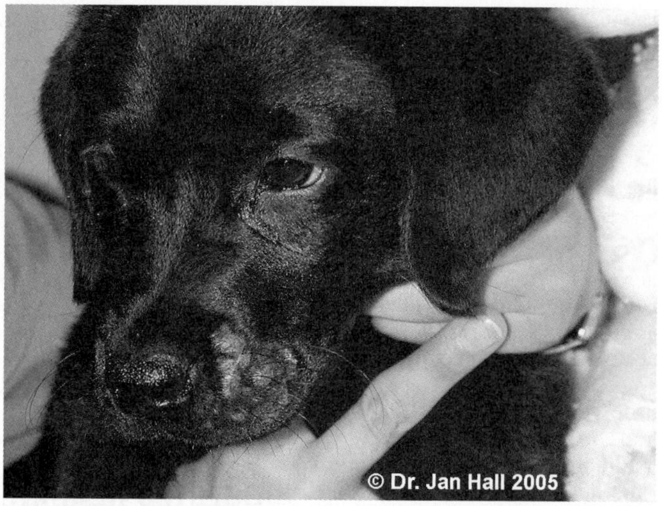

FIGURE I-108 Pustules affecting the muzzle of an 8-week-old female spayed Labrador retriever puppy with juvenile cellulitis. Courtesy of Dr. Jan A. Hall.

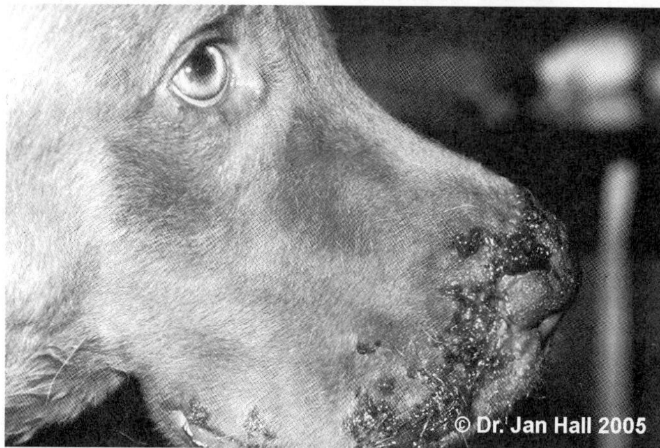

FIGURE I-109 Pustules, crusts, and exudative dermatitis affecting the muzzle of a 2-year-old male castrated Labrador retriever with adult-onset juvenile cellulitis. Courtesy of Dr. Jan A. Hall.

- Drug eruption (cutaneous drug reaction)
- Angioedema

INITIAL DATABASE

- Impression cytology of pustule: numerous neutrophils and macrophages (pyogranulomatous inflammation) without bacteria
- Skin scrapings/hair plucks

ADVANCED OR CONFIRMATORY TESTING

These additional diagnostic tests may be performed, but in most cases the diagnosis is made on the basis of signalment (young dog), history, and physical examination.

- Anaerobic or aerobic bacterial culture and sensitivity: usually sterile.
- Skin biopsy: multiple discrete or confluent granulomas and pyogranulomas composed of nodular clusters of large epithelioid macrophages with variably sized neutrophilic centers.
- Excisional lymph node biopsy: pyogranulomatous lymphadenitis.

TREATMENT

THERAPEUTIC GOAL(S)

Rapid and aggressive treatment to reduce risk of scarring alopecia

ACUTE GENERAL TREATMENT

- Warm water soaks to remove crusts and exudate.
- Topical astringents such as 2% aluminum acetate (Burow's solution) applied q 12h.
- Prednisone (2 mg/kg PO q 24h, total dose can be divided q 12h) until lesions resolve (approximately 1 to 4 weeks), then reduce to 2 mg/kg PO q 48h for 2 weeks, then taper off prednisone over the next 2 to 3 weeks.
- Some dogs respond better to dexamethasone (0.2 mg/kg PO q 24h). Gradually taper dosage (similar to prednisone).
- Bactericidal antibiotics for 3 to 4 weeks required if cytologic or clinical evidence of secondary pyoderma present.

PROGNOSIS AND OUTCOME

Prognosis is good; however, scarring may be extensive in severe cases.

PEARLS & CONSIDERATIONS

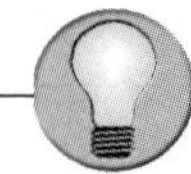

COMMENTS

- Taper corticosteroids gradually (over a few weeks) to reduce the risk of relapse.
- Adult dogs and dogs with panniculitis require a longer treatment interval.

SUGGESTED READING

Hutchings SM: Juvenile cellulitis in a puppy. *Can Vet J* 44:418, 2003.

Scott DW, Miller WH, Griffin CE. In Scott DW, Miller WH, Griffin CE (eds): *Muller and Kirk's Small Animal Dermatology*, ed 6. Philadelphia, WB Saunders, 2001, pp 1163–1167.

AUTHOR: **JOCELYN WELLINGTON**
EDITOR: **JAN A. HALL**

Juvenile Polyarteritis (Beagle Pain Syndrome)

BASIC INFORMATION

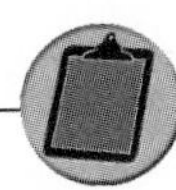

DEFINITION

Systemic necrotizing vasculitis most often reported in young beagles. The neurologic aspects of this disorder are discussed in greater detail under Steroid Responsive Meningitis-Arteritis, p 1037.

SYNONYM(S)

Canine juvenile polyarteritis syndrome
Canine pain syndrome
Juvenile polyarteritis
Necrotizing vasculitis
Steroid-responsive meningitis-arteritis (SRMA)

EPIDEMIOLOGY

SPECIES, AGE, SEX

- Seen most often in young (<12 months) beagles
- Also affects young (8 to 18 months) dogs of other breeds
- No sex predilection

GENETICS AND BREED PREDISPOSITION

- Colonies of research beagles.
- Beagle, Bernese mountain dog, German shorthair pointer overrepresented. May be inherited in the beagle.
- Reported in Toller retriever, boxer, occasionally other breeds.

GEOGRAPHY AND SEASONALITY

- Occurs worldwide
- Incidence may be higher in the spring

ASSOCIATED CONDITIONS AND DISORDERS: Concurrent arthritis sometimes occurs.

CLINICAL PRESENTATION

DISEASE FORMS/SUBTYPES

- Acute form (typical)
- Atypical, protracted form

HISTORY, CHIEF COMPLAINT

- Acute to gradual onset of hunched posture, guarding of the neck, reluctance to move, cervical rigidity.
- Paresis may occur.
- Signs may be episodic: persist for 2 to 7 days and then resolve.
- After several relapses without therapy, patients may develop the protracted form with progressive worsening of neurologic dysfunction.

PHYSICAL EXAM FINDINGS

- Cervical pain and rigidity with an associated hunched posture and unwillingness to move.
- Generalized hyperesthesia.
- Fever.
- Anorexia.
- Weakness.
- With the atypical/protracted form, patients may have proprioceptive deficits, ataxia, paraparesis, or quadraparesis.
- Cranial nerve deficits rarely reported.
- Nonspecific signs such as lethargy, malaise, and depression common.

ETIOLOGY AND PATHOPHYSIOLOGY

- Systemic necrotizing vasculitis with severe subarachnoid hemorrhages throughout spinal cord and brainstem.
- Intimal thickening and fibrinoid necrosis of the tunica media of small to medium-size arteries result in occlusion and thrombosis that may cause neural ischemia and pain.
- Vessels of the cervical spinal cord leptomeninges, cranial mediastinum, and coronary arteries may be involved.
- Mechanism is believed to be immune mediated; may be triggered by an environmental factor that has yet to be identified.
- Genetic or hereditary component suspected in beagles.

DIAGNOSIS

DIFFERENTIAL DIAGNOSIS

- Bacterial meningitis: rule out with cerebrospinal fluid (CSF) analysis and culture.
- Granulomatous and infectious meningoencephalomyelitis.
- Polyarthritis.
- Polymyositis.
- Diskospondylitis: rule out with diagnostic imaging.
- Cervical disk disease, disk herniation: rule out with diagnostic imaging.
- Spinal cord trauma: rule out with diagnostic imaging, history.
- Protozoal infection: rule out with muscle biopsy, serology.

INITIAL DATABASE

- Complete blood count: mild, nonregenerative anemia, leukocytosis, neutrophilia.
- Serum biochemistry profile: hypoalbuminemia possible.
- Urinalysis: proteinuria possible.
- Thoracic, abdominal, cervical radiographs: normal.

ADVANCED OR CONFIRMATORY TESTING

- Synovial fluid analysis: neutrophilic inflammation typical; negative culture.
- Cerebrospinal fluid (CSF) analysis: characteristic findings include erythrophagocytosis, neutrophilic pleocytosis, increased protein; negative culture. In protracted cases, protein content is either slightly elevated or normal with a mild to moderate mixed pleocytosis.
- Brain magnetic resonance imaging and computed tomography: usually normal.
- Systemic and intrathecal IgA levels elevated in acute and atypical/protracted forms.
- Histopathologic evaluation of tissues: severe necrotizing vasculitis, perivasculitis, and thrombosis of small to medium-sized vessels in the leptomeninges of the cervical spinal cord, cranial mediastinum, coronary arteries, and other affected organs.

TREATMENT

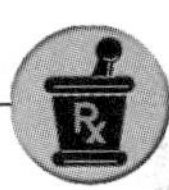

THERAPEUTIC GOAL(S)

- Resolution of clinical signs with remission
- Signs should resolve in 24 to 48 hours with corticosteroid therapy

ACUTE GENERAL TREATMENT

- Fluid therapy may be needed if patient is anorexic
- Restrict activity
- Prednisone therapy; start at 1-2 mg/kg PO, IM, or SC q 12h

CHRONIC TREATMENT

- Taper corticosteroids to the minimum dose that controls clinical signs (usually 0.25-0.5 mg/kg q 48h) over 6 months
- Azathioprine (1.5-2 mg/kg PO q 48h) for patients who do not respond to prednisone

DRUG INTERACTIONS

Do not use corticosteroids and nonsteroidal anti-inflammatory drugs together

POSSIBLE COMPLICATIONS

- Gastrointestinal (GI) upset and GI ulceration/bleeding, polyuria, polydipsia, polyphagia, Cushingoid syndrome as adverse effects of corticosteroid therapy.
- Infections possible, secondary to chronic immunosuppression.
- Bone marrow toxicity and hepatic failure are possible adverse effects of azathioprine therapy.

RECOMMENDED MONITORING

- CBC, serum chemistry profile, urinalysis every 4 to 6 weeks to monitor for inflammation and organ dysfunction.
- Monitor for neck pain (sign of possible recurrence) and GI bleeding.
- Repeat CSF tap every 4 to 6 weeks at the beginning of therapy to help guide corticosteroid therapy. Once CSF is normal and clinical signs remain absent, weaning can commence.

PROGNOSIS AND OUTCOME

- Good prognosis for acute cases if treated promptly and intensively.
- Disease can spontaneously resolve when patient is 12 to 18 months old.
- Prognosis more guarded with protracted cases due to frequent relapses.
- Some patients do not respond to further therapy after relapses.
- Some patients need continuous therapy to control clinical signs.

PEARLS & CONSIDERATIONS

COMMENTS

- Early diagnosis and aggressive treatment result in the best outcome.
- Adverse effects of corticosteroid therapy may be unacceptable to some clients. Azathioprine should be used for its steroid-sparing effects in these cases.

CLIENT EDUCATION

Although patients usually respond to therapy for the acute form, relapses can be common, and some patients require long-term or indefinite treatment to control clinical signs

SUGGESTED READING

Scott-Moncrieff JCR, et al: Systemic necrotizing vasculitis in nine young beagles. *J Am Vet Med Assoc* 201:1553–1558, 1992.

Tipold A: Juvenile polyarteritis (beagle pain syndrome). In Tilley LP (ed): *The 5-Minute Veterinary Consultant Canine and Feline*, ed 2. Philadelphia, Lippincott, Williams & Wilkins, 2000, p 877.

Tipold A: Steroid-responsive meningitis-arteritis in dogs. In Bonagura JD (ed): *Kirk's Current Veterinary Therapy XIII*. Philadelphia, WB Saunders, 2000, pp 978–981.

AUTHOR: **KIMBERLY B. WINTERS**
EDITOR: **SUSAN M. COTTER**

Keratoconjunctivitis Sicca

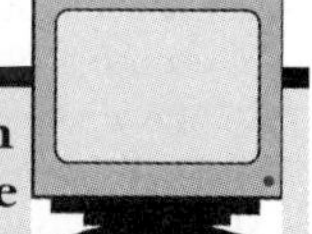

Client Education Sheet on Website

BASIC INFORMATION

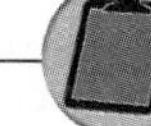

DEFINITION

Inflammation of the cornea and conjunctiva secondary to a deficiency in the aqueous portion of the tear film

SYNONYM(S)

KCS
Dry eye
Quantitative tear film abnormality
Xerophthalmia

EPIDEMIOLOGY

SPECIES, AGE, SEX

- Common in dogs; rare in cats.
- Age of onset variable depending on underlying cause.
- Increased predisposition reported for both neutered male and female dogs, and female West Highland white terrier.

GENETICS AND BREED PREDISPOSITION: Predisposed breeds (dogs): English bulldog, West Highland white terrier, Lhasa apso, pug, American cocker spaniel, Pekingese, Yorkshire terrier, shih tzu, miniature schnauzer, Boston terrier, dachshund, Chihuahua, German shepherd, Doberman pinscher.

RISK FACTORS

- Breed predisposition.
- Medications (see Etiology and Pathophysiology below).
- Removal of gland of the third eyelid.
- Metabolic disorders (see Etiology and Pathophysiology below).
- Infectious diseases (see Etiology and Pathophysiology below).
- Systemic immune-mediated disease (e.g., see Systemic Lupus Erythematosus, p 1061).

CONTAGION AND ZOONOSIS: Infectious causes (e.g., canine distemper; feline herpesvirus-1) are contagious.

CLINICAL PRESENTATION

HISTORY, CHIEF COMPLAINT

- "Red" eye
- Ocular pain
- Mucoid to mucopurulent ocular discharge

PHYSICAL EXAM FINDINGS

- Systemic: generally unremarkable.
- Ophthalmic:
    - Mucoid to mucopurulent ocular discharge
    - Conjunctival hyperemia and chemosis
    - Blepharospasm
    - Protrusion of the third eyelid
    - Dry/lackluster corneal appearance
    - Signs of keratitis with chronicity:
        - Corneal vascularization (see Corneal Vascularization, p 249).
        - Corneal pigmentation (see Corneal Pigmentation, p 242).
        - Corneal ulceration (see Corneal Ulceration, p 246).
    - Blepharitis
    - Periocular dermatitis secondary to exudates and/or self-trauma
    - Vision impairment with chronic disease
- Cats often show fewer clinical signs than dogs.

ETIOLOGY AND PATHOPHYSIOLOGY

- Immune-mediated adenitis: most common (dogs).
- Congenital: lacrimal gland hypoplasia.
- Drug-induced: general or topical anesthesia and atropine (transient KCS).
- Drug-toxicity: some systemic medications (e.g., sulfonamide therapy; phenazopyridine; 5-aminosalicylic acid; etodolac) may cause transient or permanent KCS.
- Iatrogenic: removal of the gland of the third eyelid increases risk of developing KCS, especially in predisposed breeds.
- Infectious disease (e.g., canine distemper [see Distemper, Canine, p 315]; feline herpesvirus-1 [see Herpesviral Keratitis in Cats, p 513]).
- Metabolic disease (e.g., hypothyroidism [see Hypothyroidism, p 575]; hyperadrenocorticism [see Hyperadrenocorticism, p 537]; diabetes mellitus [see Diabetes Mellitus, p 289]).
- Neurogenic: may occur with facial nerve paralysis and denervation of parasympathetic fibers innervating the gland, or following ocular proptosis (see Proptosis of the Globe, p 893).
- Chronic blepharoconjunctivitis due to obstruction of lacrimal ductules secondary to chemosis or ascending infection into lacrimal gland.
- Chronic conjunctivitis (e.g., FHV-1; see Herpesviral Keratitis in Cats, p 513).
- Irradiation: when primary beam near or on periocular region.
- Breed predisposition (dogs).

DIAGNOSIS

DIFFERENTIAL DIAGNOSIS

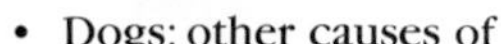

- Dogs: other causes of :
  - Conjunctivitis (see Conjunctivitis: Dogs, p 233).
  - Corneal vascularization (see Corneal Vascularization, p 249) or pigmentation (see Corneal Pigmentation, p 242).
  - Corneal exposure (e.g., lagophthalmos): a common cause of misdiagnosis of "KCS."
  - Corneal ulceration (see Corneal Ulceration, p 246).
  - Blepharitis.
- Cats: other causes of keratoconjunctivitis:
  - FHV-1 conjunctivitis/keratitis.
  - Proliferative (eosinophilic) keratoconjunctivitis.

INITIAL DATABASE

Complete ophthalmic examination including:

- Schirmer tear test (STT).
  - Normal: ≥15 mm/min in dogs; variable in cats.
  - Early or subclinical KCS: 11–14 mm/min.
  - Mild to moderate KCS: 6–10 mm/min.
  - Severe KCS: ≤5 mm/min.
- Fluorescein dye application: secondary corneal ulceration is common.
- Intraocular pressures: normal ≥10–15 mmHg and ≤25 mmHg. Applanation tonometry: 20 ± 5 mmHg.

ADVANCED OR CONFIRMATORY TESTING

Other quantitative test:

- Phenol red-thread tear test.
  - Dogs: normal 34.15 ± 4.45 mm/15 seconds.
  - Cats: normal 23.04 ± 2.23 mm/15 seconds.

TREATMENT

THERAPEUTIC GOAL(S)

- Stimulate tear production
- Stabilize the tear film
- Eliminate ocular pain:
  - Control extraocular inflammation (conjunctivitis and nonulcerative keratitis)
  - Treat secondary bacterial infections
  - Treat corneal ulceration (see Corneal Ulceration, p 246) if present

ACUTE GENERAL TREATMENT

- Lacrimostimulants:
  - Cyclosporine-A (CsA) 0.2 % ointment or 0.5–2% solution q 8–12h.
- Lacrimomimetics (tear substitutes and stabilizers) q 4–6h (e.g., hyaluronic acid 0.4%).
- Antimicrobials if secondary bacterial conjunctivitis and/or corneal ulceration:
  - Topical broad-spectrum antibiotic (e.g., triple-antibiotic solution q 6–8h).
- Anti-inflammatories if severe conjunctivitis and/or corneal vascularization/pigmentation:
  - Dexamethasone 0.1% solution q 6–8h; if corneal ulceration is not present.

CHRONIC TREATMENT

Lacrimostimulants:

- Cyclosporine-A (CsA) 0.2 % ointment or 0.5–2% solution q 8–24h (typically q 12h).
  - For STT values that remain ≤ 10 mm/min after 3 to 4 weeks of treatment, CsA may be increased to q 8h.
  - CsA should not be decreased until STT values are ≥ 20 mm/min.
  - CsA may be decreased to q 24h if favorable response occurs.
- Tacrolimus 0.03–0.02% ointment or solution q 12h.
  - Used if no response to CsA after 3 to 6 weeks of treatment.
  - Studies evaluating long-term safety have not been performed.
- Some ophthalmologists advocate increasing the concentration of the lacrimostimulant if there is no response (i.e., 0.2% CsA ointment to 2% CsA solution).
- Pilocarpine: 1 drop 2% pilocarpine/10 kg body weight on food q 12h, gradually increasing by 1 drop increments until increased tearing or systemic side effects (e.g., vomiting; diarrhea; anorexia; salivation; bradycardia) (primarily effective in neurogenic KCS).
- Consider parotid duct transposition if no response to lacrimostimulants.

POSSIBLE COMPLICATIONS

- Corneal ulceration
- Vision impairment from progressive corneal vascularization/pigmentation (uncontrolled KCS)

RECOMMENDED MONITORING

- Variable depending on underlying cause.
- Complete ophthalmic examination with STT and corneal fluorescein staining performed every 3 to 4 weeks initially.
- Rechecks performed every 4 to 6 weeks until KCS controlled, then every 3 to 4 months.

PROGNOSIS AND OUTCOME

Variable depending on underlying cause

PEARLS & CONSIDERATIONS

COMMENTS

- Immune-mediated KCS usually requires lifelong treatment.
- Some forms of KCS may require transient treatment until tear production returns (e.g., atropine; topical anesthesia).
- May take weeks to months of therapy before determining if favorable response to lacrimostimulants.

PREVENTION

Breeds predisposed to KCS: avoid breeding affected or closely related dogs.

CLIENT EDUCATION

Immune-mediated KCS is a chronic disorder that is manageable but not curable; usually requires lifelong treatment.

SUGGESTED READING

Kaswan R, et al: Topical application of cyclosporine in the management of keratoconjunctivitis sicca in dogs. *J Am Anim Hosp Assoc* 26:269, 1990.

Martin CL: Lacrimal system. In Martin CL (ed): *Ophthalmic Disease in Veterinary Medicine*. London, Manson Publishing, Ltd, 2005, pp 219–240.

AUTHOR: **PHILLIP A. MOORE**

EDITOR: **CHERYL L. CULLEN**

Lameness

BASIC INFORMATION

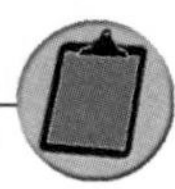

DEFINITION

Alteration of gait caused by structural or functional abnormality in one or more limbs

SYNONYM(S)

Favoring leg
Limp

EPIDEMIOLOGY

RISK FACTORS

- Obesity
- Overnutrition during growth
- Trauma
- Genetics

ASSOCIATED CONDITIONS AND DISORDERS

- Neurologic disorders
- Metabolic disorders
- Neoplasia
- Certain infectious diseases

CLINICAL PRESENTATION

DISEASE FORMS/SUBTYPES: Lameness is most often secondary to pain. However, lameness also commonly occurs secondary to neurologic, mechanical, metabolic, or endocrine dysfunction.

HISTORY, CHIEF COMPLAINT: Thorough history is critical:

- Determine which limb is affected
- Abnormal gait or limping observed by owner
- Difficulty rising
- Improves or worsens with exercise
- Holding leg up
- Shifting leg lameness
- Acute or gradual onset
- Progression over time

PHYSICAL EXAM FINDINGS

- Complete general physical looking for any evidence of systemic abnormalities (e.g., fever)
- Complete orthopedic and neurologic examination (see Orthopedic Examination, p 1290; Neurologic Examination, p 1286)
- Observation at a walk and trot for gait abnormalities to help localize the limb that is affected:
    - Failing to bear full weight on limb
    - Short stride
    - Head bob (down on normal limb and up on affected limb, to decrease weight bearing) with forelimb lameness
    - Toeing in or out
    - Dragging feet or scuffing nails
    - Bunny hopping (hind-limb weakness)
    - Stumbling
    - Ataxia
    - Hypermetria
- When both hind limbs are affected, weight may be shifted onto forelimbs, resulting in arched posture and abduction of the elbows
- Complete orthopedic examination (see Orthopedic Examination, p 1290; Neurologic Examination, p 1286) must include assessment of:
    - Abnormal posture
    - Joint effusion
    - Bone, joint pain, or muscle pain
    - Muscle atrophy
    - Thickening or bony prominences at or near joints
    - Crepitus
    - Abnormal range of motion in joints

ETIOLOGY AND PATHOPHYSIOLOGY

- Lameness secondary to pain from the musculoskeletal system: pain causes decreased weight bearing of the affected limb, and shortness of stride. Severe acute pain may cause non–weight-bearing on affected limb.
- Mechanical lameness: may be caused by abnormal length, or angulation of bones, joints, ligaments, or tendons.
- Endocrine-related lameness: Hyperadrenocorticism may cause myopathy, and diabetes mellitus may cause peripheral neuropathy.
- Neurologic disorders may cause ataxia, paresis, or pain, manifesting as lameness.

DIAGNOSIS

DIFFERENTIAL DIAGNOSIS

- Immature (<12 months) dogs and cats*:
    - Forelimb:
        - Trauma (soft tissue, bone, joint)*
        - Osteochondritis dissecans (OCD) of the shoulder
        - OCD of the elbow
        - Ununited anconeal process (UAP; component of "elbow dysplasia")
        - Fragmented medial coronoid process (FMCP; component of "elbow dysplasia")
        - Elbow incongruity
        - Avulsion of flexor muscles
        - Premature growth plate closure
        - Retained cartilage core
        - Panosteitis
        - Hypertrophic osteodystrophy (HOD)
        - Infection (local or systemic)*
        - Nutritional imbalance*
        - Congenital abnormalities* (i.e., radial agenesis, congenital elbow luxation)
        - Atlantoaxial instability
    - Hind limb:
        - Trauma*
        - Hip dysplasia
        - OCD stifle
        - OCD hock
        - Patellar luxation*
        - Avulsion of long digital extensor
        - Aseptic necrosis of femoral head
        - Panosteitis
        - HOD
        - Infection (local or systemic)*
        - Nutritional imbalance*
        - Congenital abnormalities* (tibial agenesis in cats)
- Mature (>12 months) dogs and cats*:
    - Forelimb:
        - Trauma*
        - Elbow luxation
        - Shoulder luxation
        - Degenerative joint disease*
        - Bicipital tenosynovitis
        - Contracture of infraspinatus or supraspinatus
        - Mineralization of supraspinatus tendon
        - Elbow incongruity
        - Cervical disk disease*
        - Brachial plexus injury*
        - Inflammatory joint disease*
        - Polyneuritis
        - Polymyositis
        - Infection (local or systemic)*
        - Neoplasia of bone or soft tissue*
    - Hind limb:
        - Trauma*
        - Hip luxation*
        - Stifle luxation*
        - Patellar luxation*
        - Superficial digital flexor luxation
        - Hip dysplasia
        - Degenerative joint disease*
        - Cruciate ligament disease*
        - Avulsion of long digital extensor tendon
        - Panosteitis
        - Iliopsoas muscle injury
        - Thoracolumbar disk disease
        - Lumbosacral disease
        - Inflammatory joint disease*
        - Achilles tendon injury*
        - Polyneuritis
        - Polymyositis
        - Hypertrophic osteoarthropathy
        - Aortic thromboembolism*
        - Infection (local or systemic)*
        - Neoplasia of bone or soft tissue*

INITIAL DATABASE

- Complete orthopedic and neurologic examination
- Radiographs of affected limb(s)

*Consider differential diagnosis in cats.

ADVANCED OR CONFIRMATORY TESTING

- Complete blood count
- Serum biochemistry panel
- Urinalysis
- Arthrocentesis (see Arthrocentesis, p 1183)
  - Can aid in distinguishing degenerative joint disease from infectious or inflammatory or immune-mediated joint disease
  - Culture and sensitivity: joint fluid should be cultured in blood culture medium for highest yield
- Immunologic testing: rheumatoid factor, antinuclear antibody test
- Serologic evaluation for infectious disease (Lyme disease, Rocky Mountain spotted fever, ehrlichiosis)
- Ultrasound of tendons or muscles
- Computed tomography (CT) or magnetic resonance imaging (MRI): CT is most useful for bones and joints, whereas MRI is most useful for soft tissue and spinal disease
- Arthroscopy: can be used for both diagnostic and therapeutic purposes
- Arthrotomy
- Soft tissue or bone biopsy
- Force plate and gait analysis
- Nuclear scintigraphy: used for localizing disease such as a difficult to diagnose lameness or metastatic tumors
- Electromyography (EMG) (see Electromyography [EMG] and Nerve Conduction Velocity [NCV], p 1231): useful for evaluating neuromuscular conditions
- Muscle or nerve biopsy (see Muscle and Nerve Biopsy, p 1279)

TREATMENT

THERAPEUTIC GOAL(S)

Alleviate source of pain and treat underlying disorder

ACUTE GENERAL TREATMENT

Lameness is a clinical sign, not a specific disease. Therefore treatment is based on determining the underlying cause.

CHRONIC TREATMENT

- Depends on underlying cause
- Adjunctive/supportive treatment:
  - Weight loss if indicated
  - Exercise moderation
  - Nutraceuticals: chondroitin and glucosamine supplementation
  - Glycosaminoglycans
  - Nonsteroidal anti-inflammatory drugs (NSAIDs) such as meloxicam, deracoxib, firocoxib, or carprofen
  - Prescription diet for joint disease

DRUG INTERACTIONS

Glucocorticoids potentiate the gastrointestinal ulcerogenic effects of nonsteroidal anti-inflammatory drugs (NSAIDs); this combination is contraindicated.

POSSIBLE COMPLICATIONS

NSAIDs may be associated with gastrointestinal irritation in some patients. They should also be used cautiously in animals with preexisting renal disease.

RECOMMENDED MONITORING

Repeat examination if response to therapy is not appropriate or if lameness progresses

PROGNOSIS AND OUTCOME

- Highly variable, depending on underlying cause of lameness.
- For example, most cases of panosteitis in growing dogs resolve spontaneously over time (prognosis excellent), whereas lameness due to osteosarcoma of a long bone has a poor long-term prognosis.

PEARLS & CONSIDERATIONS

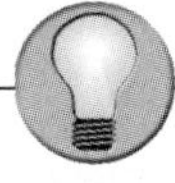

COMMENTS

Attention to signalment, history, and thorough examination are essential for generating "short" list of differential diagnoses

PREVENTION

Weight management has been proven to reduce the incidence and severity of osteoarthritis and clinical signs in patients with orthopedic disease.

SUGGESTED READING

Bardet JF: Lameness in dogs and lameness in cats. In Ettinger SJ (ed): *Textbook of Veterinary Internal Medicine*, ed 3. Philadelphia, WB Saunders, 1989, pp 165–179.

Hulse DA, Johnson AL: Orthopedic examination. In *Small Animal Surgery*. St. Louis, Mosby, 1997, pp 719–729.

AUTHOR: **DAVID A. PUERTO**
EDITOR: **ETIENNE CÔTÉ**

Laryngeal Masses

BASIC INFORMATION

DEFINITION

Proliferation of laryngeal tissues due to benign or malignant processes

EPIDEMIOLOGY

SPECIES, AGE, SEX

- Laryngeal masses are rare in dogs and cats, but occur most often in middle-aged to older animals.
- Benign lesions may be seen in younger animals.
- There is a higher incidence of laryngeal tumors in male dogs and cats.

ASSOCIATED CONDITIONS AND DISORDERS: Laryngeal masses can lead to acute or chronic upper airway obstruction.

CLINICAL PRESENTATION

DISEASE FORMS/SUBTYPES: Benign or malignant masses

HISTORY, CHIEF COMPLAINT

- Acute or progressive history of inspiratory stridor
- Voice change
- Dyspnea
- Cough
- Exercise intolerance
- Gagging and/or dysphagia
- Ptyalism
- Cyanosis
- Collapse
- Mass in the neck

PHYSICAL EXAM FINDINGS

- May be normal, with mass as an incidental finding at time of endotracheal intubation
- Inspiratory dyspnea, with gasping if severe
- Inspiratory stridor
- Palpable mass in the ventral laryngeal area in some
- Coughing and/or gagging due to laryngeal compression
- Weakness

ETIOLOGY AND PATHOPHYSIOLOGY

- Laryngeal tumors cause luminal obstruction by external compression or internal obstruction
- Primary:
  - Benign:
    - Oncocytoma
    - Laryngeal cyst
    - Laryngeal polyp

        - Rhabdomyoma
        - Lipoma
    - Malignant:
        - Squamous cell carcinoma (most common)
        - Mast cell tumor
        - Fibrosarcoma
        - Rhabdomyosarcoma
        - Lymphoma
        - Osteosarcoma
        - Melanoma
        - Mixed cell tumor
- Metastatic:
    - Lymphosarcoma
    - Plasma cell tumor
    - Thyroid neoplasia

DIAGNOSIS

DIFFERENTIAL DIAGNOSIS

- Laryngeal paralysis (dogs > cats)
- Laryngeal collapse
- Elongated soft palate (dogs, especially brachycephalic)
- Nasopharyneal polyp (cats)
- Pharyngeal or laryngeal foreign body
- Granulomatous masses

INITIAL DATABASE

- Results of a complete blood count, biochemistry panel, and urinalysis are usually unremarkable.
- Cervical radiographs may show a soft-tissue density in the area of the larynx leading to laryngeal distortion or decreased laryngeal luminal space. The normal larynx of dogs, especially if mineralized, should not be confused with an abnormality (foreign body or other).
- Thoracic radiographs may have evidence of metastasis or aspiration pneumonia.

ADVANCED OR CONFIRMATORY TESTING

- *Note*: Patients with large laryngeal masses may be at the cusp of respiratory collapse despite showing only moderate dyspnea (inspiratory).
    - These patients may be unable to recover from anesthesia without respiratory distress/suffocation. Therefore, before sedation/anesthesia for evaluation of the upper airway in patients suspected of having airway obstruction:
        - An appropriate-size endotracheal tube must be available.
        - A tracheostomy kit should be available.
        - Hair should be clipped from the ventral neck (preparation for tracheostomy if needed).
        - A contingency plan should be discussed with the owner if the mass is nonresectable (e.g., recover with tracheostomy versus euthanize on the table).
- Laryngoscopy with animal under general anesthesia to directly visualize the mass.
- Tissue biopsy specimen can be obtained by open surgical technique or endoscopically.
    - Masses may also be aspirated for cytology.
- Ultrasound may help visualize the mass and aid fine-needle aspiration.
- Computed tomography or magnetic resonance imaging can better show the extent of the mass and possible involvement of other regional structures.

TREATMENT

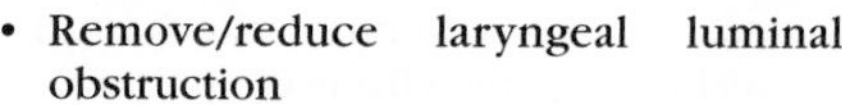

THERAPEUTIC GOAL(S)

- Remove/reduce laryngeal luminal obstruction
- Treatment depends on the extent of the lesion and type of mass

ACUTE GENERAL TREATMENT

Stabilize the patient:

- Oxygen by face mask, oxygen cage, or nasal cannula if needed
- Tracheostomy if in severe distress from near complete obstruction (see Tracheostomy, p 1310)

CHRONIC TREATMENT

- Small, benign lesions may be surgically excised by submucosal resection or partial laryngectomy.
- Large invasive lesions or malignant tumors are best removed surgically by total laryngectomy combined with a permanent tracheostomy.
    - Permanent tracheostomy can palliate signs of respiratory distress in nonresectable cases or cases managed conservatively. Rarely successful in small individuals (cats, small dogs), as tracheal lumen becomes recurrently obstructed with secretions.
- Certain tumors may be better treated with radiation therapy. Consultation with an oncologist can be beneficial.

POSSIBLE COMPLICATIONS

- Postoperative swelling
- Dysphagia and/or gagging
- Pharyngeal dehiscence
- Laryngeal stenosis/webbing
- Hypoparathyroidism/hypothyroidism (if removed during laryngectomy)
- Tumor recurrence or metastasis
- Obstruction or self-trauma of tracheostoma

RECOMMENDED MONITORING

- Monitor closely for upper airway obstruction due to postoperative pharyngeal swelling
- Withhold water and food for at least 24 to 48 hours in the postoperative period
- Exercise should be restricted for 2 to 4 weeks
- Routine laryngoscopic reevaluation is recommended to identify tumor recurrence or laryngeal stenosis
- Periodic physical and radiographic evaluation is recommended to check for recurrence or metastasis

PROGNOSIS AND OUTCOME

- The prognosis is good for benign lesions if complete resection is possible.
- Prognosis for malignant laryngeal tumors is guarded:
    - Advanced disease is often present at the time of diagnosis.
    - May not be surgically resectable.

PEARLS & CONSIDERATIONS

COMMENTS

- A CO_2 laser works well for surgical dissection and results in less inflammation and hemorrhage.
    - When using a laser, make sure the endotracheal tube is protected from the laser beam.
- Some patients may benefit from placement of a feeding tube for postoperative nutritional support.

CLIENT EDUCATION

Vocalization is lost after total laryngectomy

SUGGESTED READING

Saik JE, et al: Canine and feline laryngeal neoplasia: A 10-year survey. *J Am Anim Hosp Assoc* 22:359, 1986.

Withrow SJ: Tumors of the respiratory system. In Withrow SJ, MacEwen EG (eds): *Small Animal Clinical Oncology*. Philadelphia, WB Saunders, 1996, p 268.

AUTHOR: **MICHAEL B. MISON**
EDITOR: **RANCE K. SELLON**

Laryngeal Paralysis

Client Education Sheet on Website

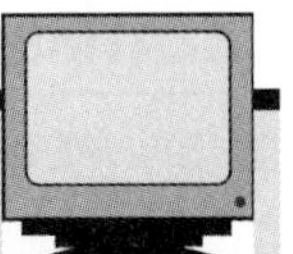

BASIC INFORMATION

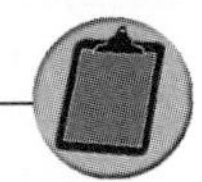

DEFINITION

Lack of abduction of arytenoid cartilages and vocal folds secondary to dysfunction of either the cricoarytenoideus dorsalis muscle or the recurrent laryngeal nerve

EPIDEMIOLOGY

SPECIES, AGE, SEX

- Dogs and cats
- Male dogs: affected 2 to 4 times more often than females; no gender predilection in cats
- Congenital form: animals <1 year old
- Acquired form: middle-aged/older dogs (mean: 9 years)

GENETICS AND BREED PREDISPOSITION

- Commonly reported in Labrador and golden retrievers, other large/giant breeds. No breed predilection in cats
- Inherited (autosomal dominant): Bouvier des Flandres
- Congenital: Bouvier des Flandres, bull terriers, dalmatians, rottweilers, Siberian huskies

RISK FACTORS

- Damage to the recurrent laryngeal nerve (blunt trauma, thoracic or cervical surgery)
- Any polyneuropathy or polymyopathy can potentially cause laryngeal paralysis:
  - Myasthenia gravis
  - Immune-mediated
  - Hypothyroidism
    - Cause-effect relationship not established

GEOGRAPHY AND SEASONALITY: Hot weather (panting) may increase severity of clinical signs.

ASSOCIATED CONDITIONS AND DISORDERS

- An elongated soft palate may develop with chronic increased inspiratory effort.
- Weakness and muscle wasting may be present in chronically affected dogs.
- Dysphagia or megaesophagus possible in dogs with polymyopathy or polyneuropathy.
- Aspiration pneumonia can develop secondary to dysphagia or laryngeal dysfunction.
- Noncardiogenic pulmonary edema/acute respiratory distress syndrome with vigorous inspiration against upper airway obstruction.

CLINICAL PRESENTATION

DISEASE FORMS/SUBTYPES

- Unilateral:
  - Clinical signs mild or absent except in performance animals
- Bilateral:
  - Clinical signs apparent in most animals

HISTORY, CHIEF COMPLAINT

- Early:
  - Voice change
  - Coughing, gagging when eating
- With progression:
  - Inspiratory stridor
  - Exercise intolerance, associated with respiratory noise and/or breathlessness
  - Dyspnea
  - Tachypnea
- Severely affected animals may show:
  - Dyspnea at rest
  - Cyanosis
  - Collapse
  - Hyperthermia
  - Death

PHYSICAL EXAM FINDINGS

- Unremarkable in early stages
- With disease progression, one may see:
  - Increased inspiratory effort, inspiratory stridor
    - These hallmark signs often are characterized by open-mouth, gasping respirations (in contrast to reverse sneezing), and improvement or total resolution at rest compared to during exertion.
  - Increased upper airway sounds (referred on thoracic auscultation)
  - Coughing or gagging
    - Laryngeal compression may induce coughing/gagging or increased respiratory sounds.
  - Weakness
  - Muscle atrophy, neurologic deficits if peripheral neuropathy/myopathy is present

ETIOLOGY AND PATHOPHYSIOLOGY

- Causes:
  - Nucleus ambiguus degeneration (Bouvier, Siberian husky/Alaskan malamute crosses)
  - Peripheral nerve death (dalmatian, rottweiler)
  - Idiopathic: most common cause of acquired
  - Intrathoracic, peritracheal, or laryngeal masses or foreign bodies
  - Other acquired causes include trauma to recurrent laryngeal nerve, polymyopathy, polyneuropathy, myasthenia gravis
- Whatever the cause, recurrent laryngeal nerve dysfunction results in loss of function to all intrinsic muscles of the larynx except the cricothyroid, causing inability to abduct arytenoids during inspiration or adduct arytenoids during swallowing.
  - With increased inspiratory pressure, arytenoids draw inward, collapsing the airway during inhalation ("paradoxical movement")

DIAGNOSIS

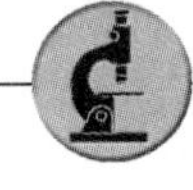

DIFFERENTIAL DIAGNOSIS

- Elongated soft palate
- Collapsing trachea
- Laryngeal collapse
- Reverse sneezing
- Laryngeal mass or other laryngeal obstruction

INITIAL DATABASE

- Results of a complete blood count, biochemistry panel, and urinalysis are usually unremarkable except with systemic disease or dehydration
- Thoracic radiographs:
  - Normal
  - Age-related interstitial changes
  - Aspiration pneumonia
- Esophageal dilation or lack of peristalsis on fluoroscopic contrast esophagram: if concurrent esophageal motility disorder
- Low total T4 or free T4 with normal/increased thyroid-stimulating hormone: hypothyroidism

ADVANCED OR CONFIRMATORY TESTING

- Definitive diagnosis with laryngoscopy (see Laryngeal, Pharyngeal, or Oral Examination, p 1272):
  - May be performed without sedation/anesthesia during dyspneic crisis
  - Otherwise, light anesthetic plane (thiopental or acepromazine/butorphanol/isoflurane)
  - If no motion, administer doxapram HCl (1.1-2.2 mg/kg IV):
    - If laryngeal paralysis is present, no motion or paradoxical motion (inward collapse on inhalation, blown open on exhalation) will be evident
- In patients with polymyopathy or polyneuropathy, electromyography or nerve conduction velocities may be abnormal
- Patients may have antibodies to acetylcholine receptors if myasthenia gravis is present
- May visualize lack of arytenoid movement on cervical ultrasound

TREATMENT

THERAPEUTIC GOAL(S)

- Stabilize patient
- Reduce/resolve respiratory distress

ACUTE GENERAL TREATMENT

- Oxygen
- Reduce laryngeal edema (dexamethasone 0.2–1.0 mg/kg IV q 12h or furosemide 2.2–4.4 mg/kg IV)
- Sedation (acepromazine 0.025–0.05 mg/kg with butorphanol 0.2–0.4 mg/kg IV q 2–4h as needed)
- Cool hyperthermic patients

CHRONIC TREATMENT

- Nonsurgical: rarely sufficient long-term without surgery:
  - Weight loss
  - Exercise restriction
  - Stress reduction
  - Treatment of underlying diseases
- Surgical:
  - Unilateral arytenoid lateralization recommended, as higher complication rates are seen with other surgical options (permanent tracheostomy, vocal fold excision, partial laryngectomy, castellated laryngofissure, muscle-nerve pedicle transposition)
  - Dogs with laryngeal muscle fibrosis and arytenoid cartilage fusion from trauma may require permanent tracheostomy

POSSIBLE COMPLICATIONS

- Postoperative aspiration pneumonia: most common serious complication.
- Coughing/gagging: common, especially with drinking.
- Dyspnea may recur if suture breaks after unilateral arytenoid lateralization.
- Advanced age; temporary tracheostomy placement; postoperative megaesophagus; concurrent respiratory tract, esophageal, neurologic, or neoplastic disease; or bilateral arytenoid lateralization increase risk of postoperative complications and death.

RECOMMENDED MONITORING

- Monitor for respiratory distress 12 to 24 hours after surgery
- Avoid morphine or heavy sedation (may increase risk of aspiration during recovery)
- Exercise restriction and reduce barking for 1 to 2 months after surgery
- Reevaluate laryngeal function and repeat chest films as needed if clinical signs recur

PROGNOSIS AND OUTCOME

- Poor with polyneuropathy (rottweiler, dalmatian, others)
- Poor in dogs <10 kg that have undergone unilateral arytenoid lateralization

PEARLS & CONSIDERATIONS

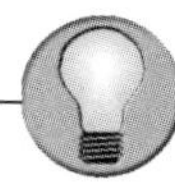

COMMENTS

- Videoendoscopy improves visualization during laryngeal exam
- Laryngeal function is inhibited in normal dogs with some anesthetic combinations (acepromazine/thiopental, acepromazine/propofol, ketamine/diazepam)
- Nonsurgical management is recommended in mildly affected dogs because of high postoperative complication rates associated with surgical treatments

PREVENTION

There is no means of preventing the development of this disease. Affected animals, especially those reflecting predisposed breeds, should not be bred.

CLIENT EDUCATION

- Dogs with polyneuropathy/polymyopathy are poor surgical candidates.
- Upper airway noise, change in/loss of bark, and coughing often persist after surgery.
- There is a lifelong risk of aspiration pneumonia after surgery.

SUGGESTED READING

Jackson AM, et al: Effects of various anesthetic agents on laryngeal motion during laryngoscopy in normal dogs. *Vet Surg* 33:102–106, 2004.

Macphail CM, Monnet E: Outcome and postoperative complications in dogs undergoing surgical treatment of laryngeal paralysis: 140 cases (1985–1998). *J Am Vet Med Assoc* 218:1949–1956, 2001.

Schacter S, Norris CR: Laryngeal paralysis in cats: 16 cases (1990–1999). *J Am Vet Med Assoc* 216:1100–1103, 2000.

Tobias KM, et al: Effects of doxapram HCl on laryngeal function of normal dogs and dogs with naturally occurring laryngeal paralysis. *Vet Anaesth Analg* 31:258–263, 2004.

AUTHOR: **KAREN M. TOBIAS**
EDITOR: **RANCE K. SELLON**

Laryngeal Trauma

BASIC INFORMATION

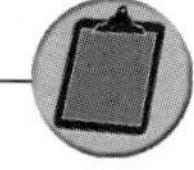

DEFINITION

Trauma resulting in disruption of, or damage to, laryngeal structures (thyroid, cricoid, and arytenoid cartilages) and surrounding soft tissues

EPIDEMIOLOGY

SPECIES, AGE, SEX: Dogs and cats; no age or sex predilection.

RISK FACTORS

- Animals that are outside unsupervised have increased risk for trauma in general
- Anesthesia with intubation
- Long-term intubation for positive pressure ventilation
- Bronchoscopy

ASSOCIATED CONDITIONS AND DISORDERS

- Polytrauma: head trauma, respiratory compromise, cardiovascular shock.
- Laryngeal laceration can result in subcutaneous emphysema, pneumomediastinum, and potentially, pneumothorax and pneumoretroperitoneum.

CLINICAL PRESENTATION

HISTORY, CHIEF COMPLAINT

- Acute onset of dyspnea with upper airway stridor
- Possible: history of witnessed trauma (e.g., bite wounds, penetrating missile, choking), recent prolonged intubation, or difficult intubation or bronchoscopy
- The patient can have had a change of voice and/or dysphagia

PHYSICAL EXAM FINDINGS

- Tachypnea, dyspnea
- Upper airway noise (stridor), usually more prominent on inspiration but can be both inspiratory and expiratory
- Mucous membranes: pallor or cyanosis possible
- Thoracic auscultation: referred upper airway noise; harsh lung sounds, crackles (with either noncardiogenic

pulmonary edema or aspiration pneumonia)
- Subcutaneous emphysema may be present in cervical region with penetrating wounds, such as bite, gunshot, or arrow wounds or with laryngeal fracture and laceration
- Hyperthermia (dogs: inability to pant)

ETIOLOGY AND PATHOPHYSIOLOGY

- Rough or difficult intubation, or prolonged intubation, can cause trauma to the mucosa, arytenoids, and vocal folds, resulting in hyperemia or edema, ulceration, and granulation tissue formation.
- Bite wounds or projectile missiles can cause penetrating or crush injury to the cartilages or recurrent laryngeal nerves.
- Airway lumen can be drastically reduced if cartilages are crushed (e.g., choke chains) or with swelling of, or hemorrhage into, the surrounding soft tissues (e.g., stick foreign bodies).
- Decreased ventilation from airway compromise: hypoxemia ± hypercarbia.
- Worsened hypoxemia (from ventilation-perfusion mismatch) if blood is aspirated into lungs, or with noncardiogenic pulmonary edema from airway obstruction.

DIAGNOSIS

DIFFERENTIAL DIAGNOSIS

- Foreign body in airway
- Insect sting/bite or other allergic reaction
- Trauma to caudal pharynx or trachea
- Laryngeal paralysis
- Laryngeal/pharyngeal mass (neoplasm, granuloma)
- Pharyngeal mucocele

INITIAL DATABASE

- Complete blood count, serum biochemistry profile, urinalysis: usually unremarkable
- Pulse oximetry/arterial blood gas analysis:
  - Hypoxemia
  - Hypercarbia if severe airway obstruction is present
- Cervical radiographs:
  - Look for fractures, dislocations, or asymmetry in hyoid apparatus
  - Subcutaneous emphysema
- Thoracic radiographs:
  - Pneumomediastinum, pneumothorax
  - Concurrent thoracic trauma (e.g., rib fracture)
  - Look for noncardiogenic pulmonary edema secondary to airway obstruction
- Laryngoscopy under general anesthesia (can be performed after tracheostomy, which allows for stabilization of patient):
  - Evaluate symmetry and function of laryngeal structures
  - Look for hematomas, exposed cartilage, foreign body, or flaps of laryngeal mucosa

ADVANCED OR CONFIRMATORY TESTING

- Tracheoscopy/bronchoscopy (can be performed after tracheostomy, if needed):
  - Evaluate larynx beyond the arytenoids
  - Examine lower airways for evidence of trauma or foreign body
- Esophagoscopy: rule out concurrent esophageal injury

TREATMENT

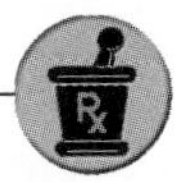

THERAPEUTIC GOAL(S)

- Initial stabilization: ensure patent airway and provide cardiovascular support for adequate tissue perfusion
- Treat concurrent life-threatening injuries
- Definitive repair, or permanent tracheostomy if necessary, to provide long-term airway

ACUTE GENERAL TREATMENT

- Oxygen supplementation.
- Intubation, if needed.
- Emergency tracheostomy (see Tracheostomy, p 1310), if unable to pass endotracheal tube.
- Treat cardiovascular compromise (IV catheter, fluids).
- Surgical exploration and repair, if indicated. Approach: midline ventral thyrotomy or through thyroid cartilage fracture:
  - Mucosal flaps: trim, appose edges.
  - Reduce and immobilize cartilage fractures to prevent stenosis.
  - Intraluminal stents can be used for preventing adhesions, collapse, and other complications.
  - Mitomycin C, applied topically, has been reported to reduce granulation tissue and stenosis after surgical repair of laryngeal trauma.
  - Unilateral arytenoid lateralization (tieback) if traumatic laryngeal paralysis without fractures, or if arytenoid avulsion.
- Postoperative care:
  - Antibiotics after obtaining cultures from contaminated wounds; continue 3 to 4 weeks in the postoperative period. Empiric selections while awaiting culture results could include:
    - Ampicillin 22 mg/kg IV q 8h and enrofloxacin 10 mg/kg slow IV or PO q 24h in dogs (5 mg/kg q 24h in cats)
    - Clindamycin 10 mg/kg IV or PO q 8h and either amoxicillin/clavulanic acid 15 mg/kg PO q 12h or enrofloxacin, as listed above
  - Corticosteroids (dexamethasone sodium phosphate, 0.1-0.2 mg/kg IV) at time of surgery to reduce inflammation; may repeat q 12-24h for first 24 to 48 hours.

CHRONIC TREATMENT

- Intraluminal stents will require second surgery 3 to 4 weeks later to remove stent.
- Permanent tracheostomy may be required if severe damage to larynx has occurred.

POSSIBLE COMPLICATIONS

- Respiratory arrest if complete obstruction
- Stenosis or stricture over the ensuing 1 to 2 weeks resulting in secondary airway compromise
- Obstruction of temporary or permanent tracheostomy site with mucus
- Laryngeal paralysis
- Infection

RECOMMENDED MONITORING

- Vital signs and frequent auscultation during initial admission and in the perioperative period
- Tracheostomy care
- Pulse oximetry and/or arterial blood gas analysis
- Respiratory rate and effort, respiratory noise, and exercise tolerance, during and after the recovery stage

PROGNOSIS AND OUTCOME

- Depends on severity of trauma and time to diagnosis and treatment.
- If severe laryngeal trauma is present and veterinary care can be quickly obtained, permanent tracheostomy can allow for fair to good prognosis (with the exception of cats and very small dogs, where stoma obstruction with mucus may be recurrent and severe).

PEARLS & CONSIDERATIONS

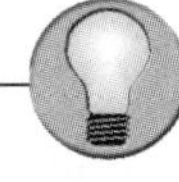

COMMENTS

- Early temporary tracheostomy: stabilizes patient, and allows imaging including laryngoscopy, endoscopic examination, radiographs, and computed tomography.
- Surgical exploration/repair must occur early, optimally within 24 hours after injury.
- Surgical exploration is necessary if:
  - Airway obstruction is severe enough to require temporary tracheostomy
  - There is emphysema in the cervical region and/or pneumomediastinum

- There is exposed cartilage within the lumen of the larynx
- The laryngeal cartilage is fractured

PREVENTION

- Selection of appropriate endotracheal tube size and endoscope size along with use of lubrication will prevent iatrogenic trauma.
- Long-term intubation for positive pressure ventilation can be maintained by temporary tracheostomy to prevent laryngeal damage.

SUGGESTED READING

Correa AJ, et al: Inhibition of subglottic stenosis with mitomycin-C in the canine model. *Ann Otol Rhinol Laryngol* 108:1053, 1999.

Manus AG: Canine epihyoid fractures. *J Am Vet Med* 147:129, 1965.

Nelson AW: Laryngeal trauma and stenosis. In Slatter D (ed): *Textbook of Small Animal Surgery,* ed 3. Philadelphia, WB Saunders, 2003, pp 845-857.

AUTHOR: **LORI S. WADDELL**
EDITOR: **RANCE K. SELLON**

Lead Toxicosis

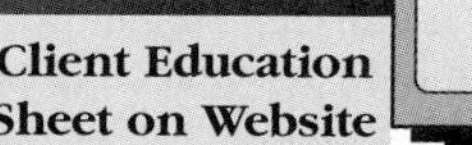
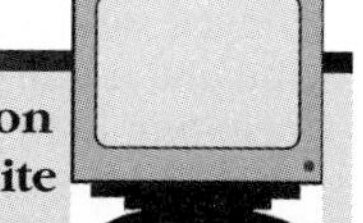

Client Education Sheet on Website

BASIC INFORMATION

DEFINITION

Syndrome produced due to exposure to injurious amounts of lead. Exposure is usually by ingestion, and clinical signs predominantly manifest as neurologic or, less commonly, acute gastrointestinal changes.

SYNONYM(S)

Lead poisoning
Plumbism

EPIDEMIOLOGY

SPECIES, AGE, SEX

- Cats are at increased risk due to grooming habits in areas contaminated with lead-laden particles (e.g., during home remodeling with exposure to flakes of lead-based paint).
- Immature animals can absorb more lead from the gastrointestinal (GI) tract than adults.
- Lead crosses the blood-brain barrier more readily in immature animals than in adults.
- Juvenile dogs are more likely to be involved due to their tendency to lick, mouth, and chew objects that may contain lead or be painted with lead-based paint.

RISK FACTORS

- Lead absorption can be increased in animals deficient in calcium, zinc, iron, or vitamin D.
- Animals living in homes containing paint formulated before 1977 may be at increased risk of exposure, especially during times of home remodeling/renovations.

CONTAGION AND ZOONOSIS: Common-source lead exposure can occur in animals and humans. The owners of animals with lead intoxication should be made aware of the possible risks of human lead toxicosis, especially to infants and young children who may chew on or swallow lead objects (e.g., curtain weights, fishing weights, older painted toys).

CLINICAL PRESENTATION

DISEASE FORMS/SUBTYPES

- Acute toxicosis occurs after a single toxic dose of lead.
- Chronic toxicosis occurs after repeated exposures over time leading to accumulation of lead in the body, and it is the more commonly observed clinical entity.

HISTORY, CHIEF COMPLAINT

- Exposure to lead-containing products.
- Recent remodeling in older residences or agricultural outbuildings increases suspicion.
- Acute toxicosis: acute onset of anorexia and neurologic signs.
- Chronic toxicosis: insidious onset of vomiting, diarrhea, anorexia, abdominal discomfort, regurgitation (uncommon; due to megaesophagus) in cats but not dogs, lethargy, weight loss, anemia, behavior changes and/or intermittent seizures.

PHYSICAL EXAM FINDINGS

- Acute toxicosis:
  - Lethargy
  - Anorexia
  - Aberrant behavior
  - Ataxia
  - Tremors
  - Seizures
- Chronic toxicosis:
  - Weight loss
  - Anorexia
  - Lethargy
  - Vomiting
  - Diarrhea
  - Aberrant behavior
  - Intermittent seizures
  - Pallor (anemia)

ETIOLOGY AND PATHOPHYSIOLOGY

- Inhibition of enzymes associated with heme production results in microcytic, hypochromic, regenerative anemia with presence of nucleated red blood cells (RBCs) and, possibly, basophilic stippling
- Competition with calcium ions results in storage of lead in bones, alteration of nerve and muscle transmission, and displacement of calcium from calcium-binding proteins.
- Inhibition of membrane-associated enzymes (e.g., sodium-potassium pumps) can result in increased RBC fragility and renal tubular epithelial injury.
- Lead may interfere with γ-aminobutyric acid production or activity in the central nervous system (CNS) resulting in loss of inhibitory impulses leading to seizures.

DIAGNOSIS

DIFFERENTIAL DIAGNOSIS

- Sterile encephalitides (e.g., granulomatous encephalitis)
- Viral encephalidities (canine distemper, rabies)
- *Toxoplasma* encephalitis
- Hepatic encephalopathy
- Idiopathic epilepsy
- Brain neoplasm

INITIAL DATABASE

- Clinical pathology:
  - Complete blood count (hematologic abnormalities more common in chronic toxicosis):
    - Nucleated RBC (nRBC) counts of 5-40 nRBC/100 white blood cells (WBCs) consistent with lead toxicity:
      - If >40 nRBC/100 WBCs, rule out myeloproliferative disorders.
      - nRBCs are present in approximately 54% of dogs with lead intoxication.
    - Microcytic, hypochromic, regenerative anemias. Anemia is present in approximately 8% of dogs with lead intoxication.
    - Basophilic stippling in dogs can be suggestive of lead toxicosis:
      - Differentiate from RBC parasites (e.g., *Babesia*).
      - Not a consistent finding; present in approximately 25% of dogs with lead intoxication.

- ± Anisocytosis, poikilocytosis, polychromasia, echinocytosis, target cells.
- ± Mature leukocytosis.
  - Serum bile acids (paired samples: after 12 hour fast [preprandial] and 2 hours postprandial): to help rule out hepatic encephalopathy due to portosystemic shunting.
- Radiography:
  - Radiopaque material/objects in GI tract or joint space:
    - Absence does not rule out lead toxicosis.
    - Presence of metallic material in GI tract is noted in approximately 20% of dogs with lead intoxication.
  - "Lead lines" in epiphyses possible but not common.
- Serum chemistry profile, urinalysis:
  - No specific abnormalities expected.

ADVANCED OR CONFIRMATORY TESTING

- Neurologic examination:
  - Mental dullness, depression are most common changes.
  - Asymmetric (lateralizing) neurologic deficits are inconsistent with lead intoxication and should suggest other diagnoses.
- Blood lead levels (BLL): whole blood (acceptable anticoagulants: heparin [green top tube] or ethylenediamine tetraacetic acid (EDTA) [purple top tube]).
  - Levels >0.35–0.40 ppm (35–40 μg/dl) are suggestive of lead toxicosis.
    - With appropriate clinical signs BLL >35 μg/dl are diagnostic of lead toxicosis.
  - BLL between 0.1 and 0.35 ppm (1–35 μg/dl) suggest significant exposure and with appropriate clinical signs are suggestive of lead toxicosis.
  - Normal background BLL usually <0.1 ppm (10 μg/dl).
  - BLL not reflective of total body burden; may not correlate to severity of clinical signs.
  - In chronic toxicoses, BLL may not be appreciably high due to distribution of lead into body compartments (e.g., bone).

TREATMENT

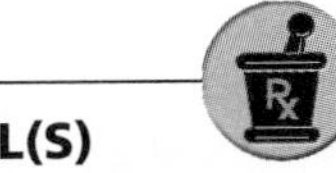

THERAPEUTIC GOAL(S)

- Manage life-threatening clinical signs
- Remove lead from GI tract
- Administer chelation therapy
- Provide supportive care
- Prevent reexposure

ACUTE GENERAL TREATMENT

- Manage seizures:
  - Diazepam 0.5–2 mg/kg IV to effect.
  - If seizures intractable with diazepam alone: phenobarbital 2–10 mg/kg IV to effect.
  - Consider IV diazepam constant rate infusion (0.1–0.5 mg/kg in 5% dextrose [D_5W] at maintenance rate, titrated to effect) for persistently refractory seizures.
  - Pentobarbital (3–15 mg/kg IV to effect), propofol (0.1–0.6 mg/kg/min), or gas anesthesia are additional treatment considerations for persistently refractory seizures not responding to the treatments listed previously.
- Correct fluid and electrolyte abnormalities as needed.
- Remove macroscopic lead from GI tract. It is essential to accomplish this before chelation.
  - Chelators (except succimer) will enhance absorption of lead from the GI tract.
  - Emesis, gastrostomy, cathartics, enemas, whole bowel irrigation may be used for removing lead from GI tract.
    - Activated charcoal does not adsorb lead well and is not helpful.
    - Magnesium sulfate (125–250 mg/kg PO) may precipitate lead in GI tract and reduce its systemic absorption.
- Chelation:
  - Most lead chelators are nephrotoxic.
    - Monitor renal values and maintain adequate hydration.
  - Monitor progress of chelation therapy by monitoring blood lead levels; decline is first expected around 5 days after initiating chelation.
  - If signs persist and levels have not dropped after several days of chelation therapy, patient reassessment is necessary, to be sure reexposure is not occurring (e.g., through environment, or GI lead foreign body).
  - Succimer (meso-2,3 dimercaptosuccinic acid, DMSA): treatment of choice in most cases.
    - Least nephrotoxic chelator.
    - Can be administered orally or rectally.
    - Less likely to bind essential minerals.
    - Does not increase absorption of lead from GI tract.
    - Dogs: 10 mg/kg PO or per rectum q 8h for 10 days.
  - Calcium disodium ethylene diamine tetraacetate (Ca EDTA): mostly replaced by succimer, except in patients with intractable vomiting or other situations in which parenteral treatment is preferred.
    - Dogs: 25 mg/kg SQ q 6h, diluted in 5% dextrose, for 2 to 5 days.
      - A 5-day rest is recommended if additional doses needed.
    - Cats: 27.5 mg/kg in 15 ml of 5% dextrose SQ q 6h for 5 days.
  - Dimercaprol (British anti-Lewisite, BAL): mainly of historic interest. Replaced by others (above).
    - Adsorbs lead from RBCs.
    - Increases urinary and biliary excretion.
    - Painful on injection.
    - Nephrotoxic; contraindicated in hepatic dysfuctions.
    - Administer 3–6 mg/kg IM q 6–8h for 2 days.
  - Penicillamine: mainly of historic interest. Replaced by others already listed.
    - Nephrotoxic; maintain adequate hydration.
    - Binds essential minerals (copper, iron zinc).
    - May cause vomiting (premedicate with dimenhydrinate 2–4 mg/kg PO).
    - Dogs: 8–35 mg/kg PO q 6–8h for 1 to 2 weeks.
- Supportive care:
  - Maintain hydration and nutrition.
  - Manage GI signs.
- Prevent reexposure:
  - Identify and remove lead source from environment.

CHRONIC TREATMENT

- Management of CNS signs, if persistent (e.g., seizures)
- Management of renal injury, if present

POSSIBLE COMPLICATIONS

Severe neurologic injury may be permanent.

RECOMMENDED MONITORING

- Complete blood count
- Packed cell volume
- Hydration
- Renal values
- Blood lead levels. Generally, one round of chelation therapy is given, followed by reassessment:
  - If lead levels are still elevated *and* clinical signs are still present, consider second round of chelation therapy.
  - If lead levels are still elevated but patient is clinically normal, monitor without repeating chelation.

PROGNOSIS AND OUTCOME

- Animals with mild to moderate signs have favorable prognosis with treatment.
- Blood lead levels may rebound within 2 weeks of cessation of chelation due to redistribution of lead from body stores (e.g., bone). If clinical signs recur at that time, then redosing with chelator is recommended, but if no signs occur, then just monitoring lead levels q 14 days is acceptable to verify that the levels are continuing to fall.

PEARLS & CONSIDERATIONS

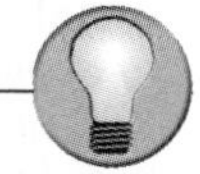

COMMENTS

- Lead embedded in soft tissues is not a significant source of lead toxicosis.
- Lead in joint spaces or areas of active inflammation may undergo systemic absorption.
- Lead stored in bones may be mobilized during times of increased bone resorption (e.g., lactation, fractures) and can result in delayed toxicosis.
- If chelator therapy is not working, either the lead toxicosis is not being addressed or, more likely, the patient is continuing to be exposed to the source of lead.

PREVENTION

Remove lead objects and lead-based paint from pet's environment

CLIENT EDUCATION

Keep pets out of areas where home renovations/remodeling is occurring.

SUGGESTED READING

Casteel WE: Lead. In Peterson ME, Talcott PA (eds): *Small Animal Toxicology*. Philadelphia, WB Saunders, 2001, pp 537–547.

Gwaltney-Brant SM: Lead. In Plumlee KH (ed): *Veterinary Clinical Toxicology*. St. Louis, Mosby, 2004, pp 205–210.

AUTHOR: **SHARON M. GWALTNEY-BRANT**

EDITOR: **SAFDAR A. KHAN**

Left Bundle Branch Block

BASIC INFORMATION

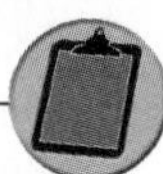

DEFINITION

An intracardiac conduction disturbance sometimes associated with left ventricular enlargement. There is failure of normal (rapid) conduction from the bundle of His through the left bundle branch to the Purkinje fibers in the left ventricle. Conduction to the left ventricle still occurs, but is very slow because it must travel from muscle cell to muscle cell. This results in a marked delay in conduction to the left ventricle and the QRS complex becomes wider on the electrocardiogram (ECG).

EPIDEMIOLOGY

SPECIES, AGE, SEX: Dogs and cats of either sex and any age

RISK FACTORS: Left ventricular enlargement, particularly left ventricular dilation

CLINICAL PRESENTATION

DISEASE FORMS/SUBTYPES

- Intermittence: in some cases, left bundle branch block (LBBB) may occur only when the heart rate surpasses a certain individual threshold (heart rate dependent).
- Left anterior fascicular block:
  - Historically, it was believed the left bundle branched into anterior and posterior fascicles, and that left anterior fascicular block was implicated in causing a marked left axis deviation on the surface ECG, with only slight prolongation of left ventricular depolarization.
  - However, the left bundle does not branch into two distinct fascicles in dogs and cats making this extrapolation inaccurate.
  - Still, a marked left axis deviation in cats, which has been called left anterior fascicular block by some, has often been observed both in cats with hypertrophic cardiac disease and in normal cats.
  - Thus, it is important to recognize this pattern of left axis deviation (tall R wave in leads I and aVL, S wave present in leads II, III, and aVF), although the name of left anterior fascicular block is inappropriate.

HISTORY, CHIEF COMPLAINT: Reflective of the underlying structural heart disease. Chief complaints range in severity from none (uncommon; left bundle branch block is an infrequent incidental finding on ECG) to decompensated states of heart disease, such as congestive heart failure (dyspnea, lethargy, abdominal distention possible) or syncope.

PHYSICAL EXAM FINDINGS

- Typically LBBB is clinically silent. However, in some individuals, split heart sounds may be present due to prolonged left ventricular ejection time and delayed closure of the mitral valve (causing a split first heart sound).
- LBBB does not alter the rhythm of the heartbeat or the pulse.
- Findings relating to underlying structural heart disease (heart murmur, arrhythmia, gallop sound, dyspnea) are common.

ETIOLOGY AND PATHOPHYSIOLOGY

LBBB usually indicates significant underlying cardiac disease such as:

- Cardiomyopathy
- Congenital heart disease, in particular subaortic stenosis
- Cardiac ischemia
- Certain drug toxicities (doxorubicin)

DIAGNOSIS

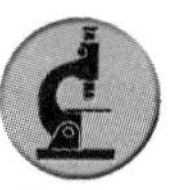

DIFFERENTIAL DIAGNOSIS

Wide QRS complex(es) on ECG:

- Left ventricular hypertrophy
- Ventricular ectopy (premature ventricular complexes, ventricular tachycardia)
- Ventricular escape rhythm
- ± Motion artifact

INITIAL DATABASE

Electrocardiography is the definitive diagnostic test. Electrocardiographic characteristics of LBBB:

- Prolonged QRS complex duration (canine >0.07 sec, feline >0.06 sec) (Fig. I-110)

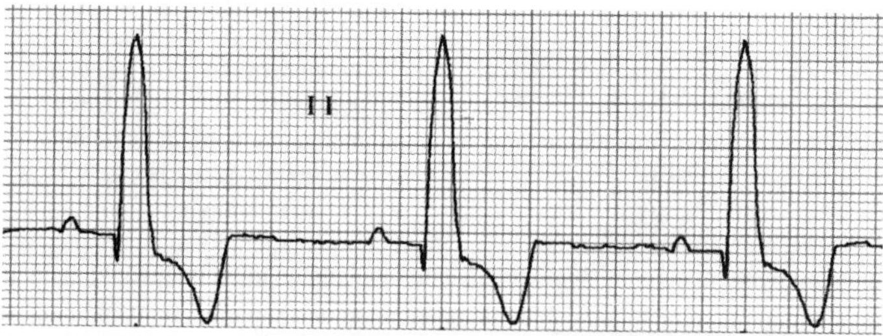

FIGURE I-110 Lead II ECG showing normal sinus rhythm with left bundle branch block. The QRS duration is 0.1 seconds (normal <0.06). The heart rate is 90 beats/min. 50 mm/sec, 1 cm = 1 mV.

- Wide and positive QRS complexes in leads I, II, III, aVF and left precordial leads (CV_6LL [V2] and CV_6LU [V4])
- Negative QRS complexes in leads aVR and CV_5RL (rV2)

ADVANCED OR CONFIRMATORY TESTING

- Thoracic radiographs to evaluate for left ventricular enlargement
- Echocardiogram to assess heart structure and function

TREATMENT

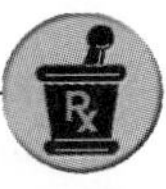

THERAPEUTIC GOAL(S)

- LBBB does not result in any hemodynamic sequelae by itself, and therefore does not require specific treatment.
- However, LBBB is often associated with underlying structural heart disease. Treatment of this underlying condition is indicated if present.

POSSIBLE COMPLICATIONS

Complete block of both the right and left bundle branches produces complete (third-degree) atrioventricular block

PEARLS & CONSIDERATIONS

COMMENTS

- The bizarre QRS morphology seen with bundle branch block can be confused with premature ventricular complexes or ventricular tachycardia (ventricular ectopy).
  - If P waves are present and the PR interval is consistent for every heartbeat, the complex is likely coming from a supraventricular site (and the bizarre QRS morphology is due to bundle branch block rather than ventricular ectopy). However sometimes P waves are buried and not visible, although the rhythm is supraventricular in origin (particularly with tachycardias).
  - Because most dogs with heart rates <140 beats/min have sinus arrhythmia and some degree of irregularity to the heart rhythm, examining the regularity of rhythm can be a helpful clue. A regularly irregular (cyclically varying) rhythm with QRS complexes that are all wide, bizarre, but identical to each other, suggests respiratory sinus arrhythmia with bundle branch block. By contrast, when ventricular ectopy such as ventricular tachycardia produces wide, bizarre QRS complexes that are all of the same shape, the rhythm is often regular (same R-R interval).
- In human patients with heart failure, the presence of a LBBB indicates significant dysynchrony of ventricular contraction. Cardiac resynchronization, by means of biventricular pacing, results in clinical benefits. This therapy may be used in veterinary patients in the future.

SUGGESTED READING

Kittleson MD: Electrocardiography: Basic concepts, diagnosis of chamber enlargement, and intraventricular conduction disturbances. In Kittleson MD, Kienle RD (eds): *Small Animal Cardiovascular Medicine*. Philadelphia, Mosby, 1998, pp 90–94.

Miller MS, Tilley LP, Smith FWK, Fox PR: Electrocardiography. In Fox PR, Sisson D, Moise NS (eds): *Textbook of Canine and Feline Cardiology*. Philadelphia, WB Saunders, 1999, pp 84–86.

Tilley LP: Left bundle branch block. In Tilley LP (ed): *Essentials of Canine and Feline Electrocardiography*. Philadelphia, Lea & Febiger, 1992, pp 75–77.

AUTHOR: **MEG SLEEPER**

EDITOR: **ETIENNE CÔTÉ**

Leiomyoma, Leiomyosarcoma

BASIC INFORMATION

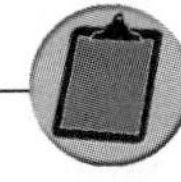

DEFINITION

- Leiomyoma: benign tumor of smooth muscle origin
- Leiomyosarcoma: malignant tumor of smooth muscle origin
- Either can be found wherever smooth muscle is present. Most common sites: gastrointestinal (GI) tract, spleen, genital tract

SYNONYM(S)

Smooth muscle tumors

EPIDEMIOLOGY

SPECIES, AGE, SEX: Uncommon in dogs and rare in cats.

- Leiomyoma: gastric: mean age 16 years (dogs).
- Leiomyoma: colonic: median age 12 years (dogs).
- Leiomyosarcoma: GI: median age 10.5–12 years (dogs).
- Leiomyo(sarco)ma: genital, urinary tract, or intestinal: female > male.

GENETICS AND BREED PREDISPOSITION: Leiomyosarcoma: more common in large breed dogs, notably in German shepherds (intestinal).

ASSOCIATED CONDITIONS AND DISORDERS: Paraneoplastic syndromes:

- Hypoglycemia
- Nephrogenic diabetes insipidus (one dog with intestinal leiomyosarcoma)
- Polycythemia due to elevated plasma erythropoietin levels (one dog with cecal leiomyosarcoma)

CLINICAL PRESENTATION

HISTORY, CHIEF COMPLAINT

- GI leiomyoma:
  - Incidental finding during endoscopy or necropsy. Occasionally, tenesmus or dyschezia if rectal, or regurgitation, if gastroesophageal.
- GI leiomyosarcoma:
  - Signs referable to the GI tract, including chronic vomiting, weight loss, melena, hematemesis, gastric dilation, or regurgitation.
- Peripheral leiomyosarcoma: progressive mass noticed by the owner.
- Rarely, animals with leiomyosarcoma first present with signs related to paraneoplastic hypoglycemia.

PHYSICAL EXAM FINDINGS

- Abdominal mass possible with any visceral leiomyo(sarco)ma.
- Signs of peritonitis possible as a result of intestinal rupture, especially with cecal leiomyosarcoma.
- Abdominal pain, distended loops of bowel, and/or mass palpable per rectum in some cases.
- Subcutaneous mass with peripheral leiomyosarcoma.
- Physical exam may be unremarkable, especially with leiomyoma.

ETIOLOGY AND PATHOPHYSIOLOGY

- Both leiomyomas and leiomyosarcomas have been associated with paraneoplastic hypoglycemia. Potential mechanisms: excessive glucose metabolism by the tumor, diminished hepatic gluconeogenic capacity due to hepatic damage by the tumor, associated peritonitis, or due to production of insulin-like growth

factors by the tumor. Those tumors associated with production of insulin-like growth factors have been associated with long-term disease-free intervals or cure as a result of resection of the tumor.
- Although not confirmed, leiomyosarcomas in the female urogenital organs are thought to develop secondary to hormonal stimulation.

DIAGNOSIS

DIFFERENTIAL DIAGNOSIS

- GI: foreign body, enteritis causing ileus, other GI neoplasm, GI granuloma (fungal, other), GI inflammation/infiltration, renal disease, hepatic disease
- Other sites: other neoplasms (benign or malignant), abscess, granuloma, hematoma

INITIAL DATABASE

- Complete blood count: 63% of dogs are anemic.
- Serum biochemistry panel: 50% are hypoglycemic.
- Three-view thoracic radiographs: usually within normal limits.
- Abdominal radiographs: may reveal GI mass, evidence of lymphadenopathy, changes consistent with peritonitis, or no abnormalities.
- Abdominal ultrasound: 66% have evidence of an abdominal mass. Lymphadenopathy may also be noted.
- Fine-needle aspirate cytologic evaluation, if possible, may help identify the tumor type before invasive diagnostic testing (biopsy).

ADVANCED OR CONFIRMATORY TESTING

- GI contrast radiography (e.g., barium series) may confirm intestinal obstruction or an intestinal mass.
- The gold standard for diagnosis is biopsy with histopathologic evaluation, preferably surgically (rather than endoscopically) to resect the entire neoplasm if possible. Histopathologic grade may be prognostic.

TREATMENT

THERAPEUTIC GOAL(S)

Surgical resection of the entire tumor

ACUTE GENERAL TREATMENT

Stabilization of systemic effects: hypoglycemia, anemia (e.g., due to GI hemorrhage), electrolyte and acid-base disturbances (e.g., due to chronic vomiting).

CHRONIC TREATMENT

- Complete surgical resection:
  - Curative of leiomyoma, and leiomyosarcoma in the absence of metastases.
  - Even with gross metastatic disease, surgical resection of leiomyosarcomas can afford long-term survival.
  - Suspected metastatic lesions should be biopsied for staging purposes.
- Dogs with metastasis or a high likelihood of metastasis (based on tumor location; see Prognosis and Outcome below) can be considered candidates for chemotherapy, although no studies have shown promising efficacy of chemotherapy against these tumors.

POSSIBLE COMPLICATIONS

- Variable, depending on the types of treatments and the location of the primary tumor.
- A 50% rate of localized peritonitis associated with tumor rupture has been reported.

RECOMMENDED MONITORING

- According to clinical signs.
- Exam and three-view thoracic radiographs and abdominal ultrasound q 3 months for postoperative GI leiomyosarcoma patients. Exact frequency based on clinical signs and tumor location (see Prognosis and Outcome below).

PROGNOSIS AND OUTCOME

Prognosis depends on the location of the tumor:

- Dogs with hepatic leiomyosarcoma frequently develop metastases and have a grave prognosis.
- Dogs with gastric or intestinal leiomyosarcomas may have metastatic rates >54%, but many can have a good prognosis, even with confirmed metastasis (e.g., median survival 21.7 months for those surviving the perioperative period, including dogs with metastatic disease); 1-year survival rate 75%, 2-year survival rate 66%, and 3-year survival rate 60%.
- Dogs with cecal leiomyosarcomas may have a lower metastatic rate (10%) and better overall prognosis. Most dogs with successful resection of the cecal tumor eventually die of causes unrelated to the tumor.
- Colorectal leiomyomas: mean survival 31.6 months.

PEARLS & CONSIDERATIONS

COMMENTS

- Leiomyosarcomas most commonly occur in the cecum and jejunum. They are the second most common intestinal tumor in dogs.
- Even with metastatic disease, including gross hepatic and mesenteric involvement apparent at laparotomy, GI leiomyosarcoma is associated with a fair life expectancy (mean: 2 years) postoperatively.

CLIENT EDUCATION

If leiomyosarcoma: monitor for signs indicating recurrence or abdominal metastasis (e.g., vomiting, diarrhea, abdominal distention, and abdominal pain).

SUGGESTED READING

Cohn M, et al: Gastrointestinal leiomyosarcoma in 14 dogs. *J Vet Intern Med* 17:107, 2004.

Grooters A, et al: Canine gastric leiomyoma. *Compend Contin Educ Pract Vet* 17:1485, 1995.

Kapatkin AS, et al: Leiomyosarcoma in dogs: 44 cases (1983-1988). *J Am Vet Med Assoc* 201:1077-1079, 1992.

McPherron M, et al: Colorectal leiomyomas in seven dogs. *J Am Anim Hosp Assoc* 28:43, 1992.

Withrow SJ: Cancer of the gastrointestinal tract. In Withrow SJ, MacEwen EG (eds): *Small Animal Clinical Oncology*. Philadelphia, WB Saunders, 2001, pp 305-334.

AUTHORS: **M. RAQUEL BROWN, JOHN FARRELLY**

EDITORS: **KENNETH M. RASSNICK, DEBRA L. ZORAN**

Leishmaniasis

BASIC INFORMATION

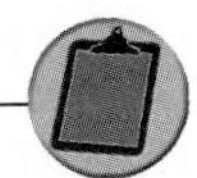

DEFINITION

Leishmaniasis is a vector-borne zoonotic disease that is endemic in the Mediterranean region and South America (70 countries worldwide) and has recently been found in dogs in the United States.

EPIDEMIOLOGY

SPECIES, AGE, SEX: Dogs, foxes, jackals, humans in endemic areas.

GENETICS AND BREED PREDISPOSITION: Most dogs with leishmaniasis in the United States have been foxhounds.

RISK FACTORS: Dogs that have traveled to endemic areas (Middle East, Southern Europe, South and Central America); foxhounds; outdoor dogs living in areas where sandfly is endemic.

CONTAGION AND ZOONOSIS: Dogs may be an important reservoir for human disease. In people, the disease occurs most commonly in infants, children, and immunosuppressed or malnourished individuals.

GEOGRAPHY AND SEASONALITY: Disease is limited to temperate, warm, humid areas where the sandfly lives. The sandfly vector in the Old World is *Phlebotomus* spp. and in the New World *Lutzomyia* spp.

ASSOCIATED CONDITIONS AND DISORDERS
- Skin lesions: alopecia; ulceration of face, pinnae, or limbs
- Glomerulonephritis
- Ocular lesions: keratoconjunctivitis sicca (KCS), uveitis
- Lymphadenopathy

CLINICAL PRESENTATION

DISEASE FORMS/SUBTYPES: Skin, eyes, kidneys, lameness, chronic weight loss.

HISTORY, CHIEF COMPLAINT: Chronic weight loss, exercise intolerance, lymphadenopathy, skin lesions, eye lesions, lameness, epistaxis.

PHYSICAL EXAM FINDINGS
- Lymphadenopathy
- Splenomegaly
- Ulcerative lesions of pinnae, face, and limbs
- Ocular discharge secondary to KCS
- Miosis, photophobia secondary to uveitis

ETIOLOGY AND PATHOPHYSIOLOGY

- *Leishmania donovani infantum* is the cause of human and canine visceral leishmaniasis in Europe, the Middle East, Africa, Asia, China, and the Americas. A similar parasite, *L. chagasi*, is found in Latin America. The worldwide annual death rate in humans is 57,000.
- The parasite's life cycle is diphasic (vector and host phases). Promastigotes develop in the gut of the sandfly and migrate to the proboscis. They are transmitted to the mammal host during a blood meal and are phagocytized by macrophages. Inside the macrophage, they become amastigotes and multiply by binary fission until the macrophage ruptures, and the amastigotes are disseminated throughout the body.

DIAGNOSIS

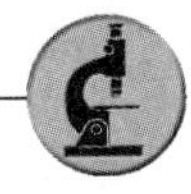

DIFFERENTIAL DIAGNOSIS

- Tick-borne diseases: Rocky Mountain spotted fever, borreliosis, ehrlichiosis
- Leptospirosis
- Dirofilariasis
- Pyoderma
- Immune-mediated vasculitis, glomerulonephritis
- Demodicosis
- Lymphosarcoma
- Malnutrition, poor husbandry

INITIAL DATABASE

- Complete blood count: may show leukocytosis, nonregenerative anemia
- Serum chemistry profile: hyperglobulinemia, ± azotemia
- Cytologic evaluation of lymph node, splenic, and bone marrow aspirates may reveal organisms
- Urinalysis: may reveal isosthenuria and proteinuria secondary to immunoproliferative glomerulonephritis
  - Urine protein:creatinine ratio may be elevated (>1)

ADVANCED OR CONFIRMATORY TESTING

Histopathologic evaluation and immunohistochemical staining of skin biopsies may reveal organisms.
- Serologic tests: titers >1:32 indicate exposure; titers >1:200 are consistent with active infection.
- Polymerase chain reaction (PCR) test: most sensitive test. Will detect subclinically infected dogs.

TREATMENT

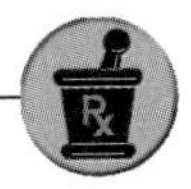

THERAPEUTIC GOAL(S)

Treatment is controversial because the parasite is rarely eliminated, and treated dogs remain asymptomatic carriers with the potential for harboring a zoonotic disease.

ACUTE GENERAL TREATMENT

- Sodium stibogluconate (Pentostam: available from the Centers for Disease Control and Prevention in Atlanta, GA) 30 mg/kg q 24h IV or SC for 3 to 4 weeks; *or*
- Meglumine antimonite (Glucantime): 100 mg/kg IV q 24h for 3 to 4 weeks.
- Allopurinol (20 mg/kg/day PO) for 1 week a month can prevent relapse when added to the antimonials. For the first 3 to 4 weeks, allopurinol is given at a dose of 15-20 mg/kg PO q 12h.

CHRONIC TREATMENT

- Dogs with renal insufficiency and protein-losing nephropathy do not respond well to therapy.
- Euthanasia should be considered in dogs with chronic poorly responsive disease or in households with young children or immunosuppressed people.

RECOMMENDED MONITORING

Negative PCR or declining titers 60 days post-treatment

PROGNOSIS AND OUTCOME

Prognosis is guarded due to inability to completely eradicate the organism

PEARLS & CONSIDERATIONS

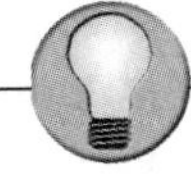

PREVENTION

- There is no vaccine available.
- Insecticidal collars and insect repellent may prevent vector transmission.
- Vector control through environmental spraying may minimize spread of disease.
- If possible, keep pet dogs inside during dawn and dusk, the feeding times of the sandfly.

CLIENT EDUCATION

- Leishmaniasis is a zoonotic disease that can be fatal in humans.
- Leishmaniasis does not respond very well to treatment.
- Leishmaniasis is often a chronic disease in dogs that may not be manifested for years after the initial exposure.

SUGGESTED READING

Rosypal BS, Zajac AM, Lindsay DS: Canine visceral leishmaniasis and its emergence in the United States. *Vet Clin Small Anim* 33:921-937, 2003.

AUTHOR & EDITOR: **DOUGLASS K. MACINTIRE**

Lens Luxation

BASIC INFORMATION

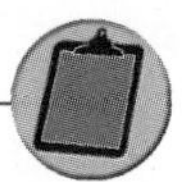

DEFINITION

Complete dislocation of the lens, anteriorly (into the anterior chamber) or posteriorly (into the posterior segment/vitreous), from its normal position. Occurs as a result of abnormal development or degeneration (*primary*: usually bilateral, inherited condition in dogs), or rupture or degeneration (*secondary*: acquired) of the lens zonules (fibers from the ciliary body that hold the lens in place).

SYNONYM(S)

Lens subluxation: partial dislocation of the lens

EPIDEMIOLOGY

SPECIES, AGE, SEX

- *Primary*: occurs most commonly in middle-aged dogs
- *Secondary*: dogs and cats; any age
- No sex predilection

GENETICS AND BREED PREDISPOSITION

- *Primary*: terrier breeds predisposed; typically between 3 and 7 years old
- German shepherd, border collie, and some spaniels may also be predisposed

RISK FACTORS: See Etiology and Pathophysiology below.

ASSOCIATED CONDITIONS AND DISORDERS

- Anterior uveitis
- Cataract
- Corneal endothelial-associated edema (anterior luxation)
- Glaucoma
- Vitreous degeneration
- Intraocular neoplasia
- Retinal detachment

CLINICAL PRESENTATION

HISTORY, CHIEF COMPLAINT

- Signs of ocular pain in cases of anterior lens luxation including tearing, redness, and squinting/blepharospasm
- Visible ocular changes noted by the owner, depending on the visual status of the contralateral eye)

PHYSICAL EXAM FINDINGS

- Systemic: generally unremarkable
- Ophthalmic:
  - Anterior chamber depth abnormal: shallow with anterior luxation; deep with posterior luxation.
  - Iridodonesis (trembling of the iris).
  - Phacodonesis (trembling of the lens).
  - Aphakic crescent (portion of pupil no longer containing the lens).
  - Retina visualized without an ophthalmoscope (i.e., with penlight or transilluminator).
  - Focal or diffuse corneal edema from mechanical damage to corneal endothelium with anterior luxation.
  - Glaucoma (see Glaucoma, p 440) can result in secondary lens luxation by buphthalmus; conversely, primary lens luxation can also result in secondary glaucoma.
  - Cataract: with chronic lens luxation.
  - Blindness from cataract, glaucoma, retinal detachment.

ETIOLOGY AND PATHOPHYSIOLOGY

- *Primary* lens luxation occurs as a result of an inherited, progressive defect in the lens zonules.
- *Secondary* lens luxation occurs as a result of degeneration and/or stretching of the lens zonules; causes include:
  - Chronic anterior uveitis (see Uveitis, p 1134)
  - Glaucoma with associated buphthalmus (see Glaucoma, p 440)
  - Intraocular neoplasia (see Intraocular Neoplasia, p 603)
  - Hypermature cataract (see Cataracts, p 182)
  - Severe ocular trauma (results in other significant ocular damage; see Corneal/Scleral Trauma, p 244)
  - Age-related

DIAGNOSIS

DIFFERENTIAL DIAGNOSIS

- Glaucoma (see Glaucoma, p 440)
- Anterior uveitis (see Uveitis, p 1134)

INITIAL DATABASE

Complete ophthalmic examination including:

- Menace response and pupillary light reflexes.
- Intraocular pressure (IOP): normal = 10–18 mmHg with Tonopen.
- Penlight or slit-beam examination to determine if the lens luxation is primary or secondary, evaluate depth of anterior chamber, and assess cornea, lens, and vitreous for opacities.
- Direct or indirect ophthalmoscopy to evaluate the posterior segment for retinal detachment (see Retinal Detachment, p 965), and optic nerve and retinal degeneration (see Retinal Degeneration, p 963).

ADVANCED OR CONFIRMATORY TESTING

Ocular ultrasound if opacities of the lens or transmitting media prevent complete examination.

TREATMENT

THERAPEUTIC GOAL(S)

- Remove anterior lens luxation or lens subluxation early to avoid secondary complications.
- Remove posterior lens luxation *or* prevent lens from entering anterior chamber by constriction of the pupil.

ACUTE GENERAL TREATMENT

Primary:

- Acute anterior lens luxation is considered an emergency.
- Determine IOP; treat if pressure elevated (see Glaucoma, p 440).
- Prompt referral of acute anterior lens luxation to a veterinary ophthalmologist for surgical lens removal (lensectomy):
  - Intracapsular lens extraction (entire lens removed) ± intraocular lens sutured in place to restore emmetropia (normal vision, neither far-nor near-sighted; without an intraocular lens implant animals are 14 diopters hyperopic [far-sighted] with abnormal vision).
  - If lens only subluxated, phacoemulsification (ultrasonic fragmentation of the lens) may be attempted.
- If referral is not possible and the lens is luxated anteriorly, consider pupil dilation and intravenous mannitol to shrink the vitreous and shift the lens into the vitreous (see Glaucoma, p 440).
- If lens luxation is posterior, consider use of a miotic (e.g., prostaglandin analog; see Glaucoma, p 440) to constrict the pupil and thus restrict lens movement; consider referral for surgery.

Secondary: treat underlying cause.

CHRONIC TREATMENT

See Cataracts, p 182

POSSIBLE COMPLICATIONS

See Cataracts, p 182

RECOMMENDED MONITORING

- See Cataracts, p 182
- Contralateral eye should be monitored for lens position and anterior chamber vitreous presentation in predisposed breeds with unilateral lens luxation

PROGNOSIS AND OUTCOME

- Variable depending on underlying cause, duration, and extent of the lens displacement, and location of the lens (anterior versus posterior).

- Most common complications are glaucoma and retinal detachment; in some reports, complication rate may be as high as 50%.
- Early surgical intervention, while the lens is subluxated, will increase success.

PEARLS & CONSIDERATIONS

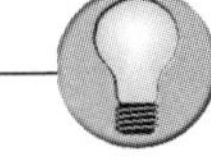

COMMENTS

- Early referral and prompt surgical intervention before onset of complete luxation and secondary glaucoma will improve success.
- Terriers affected with lens luxation, regardless of severity, should not be used for breeding.

PREVENTION

- Dilated ophthalmic examination of all individuals of predisposed breeds, to detect early phacodonesis and anterior vitreous presentation (presence of vitreous rostral to the lens).
- Complete examination of the contralateral eye, especially in breeds with primary lens luxation.
- Avoid head shaking behaviors such as toys or rough playing in animals with phacodonesis or primary lens luxation in one eye.
- Do not breed animals with primary lens luxation.

CLIENT EDUCATION

- Breed predisposition and predilection for bilateral involvement in terriers.
- With or without surgical intervention, affected eyes are at increased risk for retinal detachment and glaucoma.
- Animals undergoing surgical removal of the lens and that do not receive an intraocular lens implant have vision that, in human equivalence, is worse than 20/400, and corresponds to being "legally blind."

SUGGESTED READING

Colitz CMH: Diseases of the lens and vitreous. In Morgan RV, Bright RM, Swartout MS (eds): *Handbook of Small Animal Practice*. Philadelphia, WB Saunders, 2003, pp 995–1003.

Wilkie DA, Gilmour M: Diseases of the lens. In Birchard SJ, Sherding RG (eds): *Saunders Manual of Small Animal Practice*. Philadelphia, WB Saunders, 2000, pp 1342–1346.

AUTHOR: **DAVID A. WILKIE**

EDITOR: **CHERYL L. CULLEN**

Leptospirosis

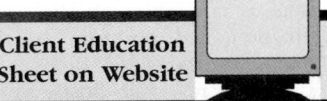

Client Education Sheet on Website

BASIC INFORMATION

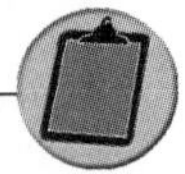

DEFINITION

Leptospirosis is a zoonotic infection caused by different subtypes (serovars) of the spirochetes *Leptospira interrogans* and *L. kirschneri*. There are at least eight serovars (*L. interrogans:* autumnalis, bataviae, bratislava, canicola, hardjo, icterohaemorrhagiae, pomona; *L. kirschneri*: grippotyphosa [previously part of *L. interrogans*]) infectious to dogs and cats causing variable degrees of renal and liver disease.

EPIDEMIOLOGY

SPECIES, AGE, SEX

- Dogs. Cats have been experimentally infected.
- Middle-aged, male dogs are more commonly affected.

GENETICS AND BREED PREDISPOSITION: Leptospirosis is more common in large-breed, male dogs. This may be less genetic and more behavioral (roaming, leading to exposure) in causality.

RISK FACTORS

- Typically considered a rural disease; however, dogs in urban and suburban environments are at risk.
- Increased risk associated with exposure to raw sewage or contaminated water.
- Areas with high concentrations of maintenance hosts (e.g., rats, raccoons, opossum, depending on the serovar) lead to higher risk.

CONTAGION AND ZOONOSIS: Leptospires are transmitted both directly and indirectly to other mammals (including humans). Direct transmission may be through contact with urine, venereal and placental transfer, bite wounds, or ingestion of infected tissues. Indirect transmission may be through exposure to contaminated water, soil, bedding, or food sources. Due to the potential zoonosis, extreme caution should be used when handling suspected leptospirosis cases (dogs with signs of acute hepatopathy or acute renal injury/acute renal failure). In particular, good hygiene practices are essential, gloves should be worn whenever handling these dogs, and bedding and waste should be removed appropriately.

GEOGRAPHY AND SEASONALITY: There is a worldwide distribution. The organisms can survive in the environment in warm, moist areas and prefer alkaline soil. In tropical regions, incidence is year round. In temperate climates, incidence in warmer months predominates. However, though freezing reduces environmental load, shedding from maintenance hosts lasts months to years.

CLINICAL PRESENTATION

DISEASE FORMS/SUBTYPES

- Peracute, acute, subacute, or chronic forms.
- There is also some variability depending on the serovar, age of animal, and immunity of animal.

HISTORY, CHIEF COMPLAINT

- Peracute form: sudden death with few clinical signs associated with massive leptospiremia; very uncommon.
- Acute form: lethargy, anorexia, shivering, muscle tenderness, vomiting.
- Subacute form: lethargy, anorexia, vomiting, polydipsia, reluctance to move, and lumbar pain.
- Chronic form: polyuria and polydipsia, possible icterus or inappetence.

PHYSICAL EXAM FINDINGS

- General:
  - Fever.
  - Dehydration progression to hypovolemic shock with reflex tachycardia.
  - Injected oral and conjunctival mucous membranes.
  - Petechial and ecchymotic hemorrhages.
  - Rhinitis.
  - Increased lung sounds, and abdominal pain among others.
- Additional physical signs depend on the form that is present:
  - Most cases involve shock and manifestations of renal disease.
  - Variable signs of liver involvement are noted, with potential for overt signs of liver failure (e.g., icterus).
  - Gastrointestinal (GI) signs are more common than in other causes of renal failure.
  - Rarely, pulmonary disease is noted with labored breathing and coughing.

ETIOLOGY AND PATHOPHYSIOLOGY

- Leptospires enter abraded skin or mucous membranes.
- They multiply in blood and disseminate widely to tissues such as kidney, liver, spleen, central nervous system, eyes, and genital tract.
- The pathogenetic mechanism may involve toxin formation.
- Infection may cause severe vasculitis in some cases. Renal disease results from leptospiral colonization of, and proliferation in, renal tubular epithelial cells.
- Hepatic disease is variable depending on serovar and animal. Icterohaemorrhagiae and pomona most commonly appear with severe hepatic dysfunction. Younger animals are also more prone to develop hepatic disease. Grippotyphosa has been implicated in causing chronic active hepatitis/idiopathic chronic hepatitis.
- There may be more than one serovar present in an infected animal.
- Central nervous system involvement in dogs is rare, although stiffness, disorientation, and posterior paresis have been reported.
- Common reservoir hosts, by serovar: autumnalis (mouse), bataviae (dog, mouse, rat), bratislava (rat, pig, ± horse), canicola (dog), grippotyphosa (opossum, raccoon, skunk, vole), hardjo (cow), icterohaemorrhagiae (rat), pomona (cow, opossum, pig, skunk).

DIAGNOSIS

DIFFERENTIAL DIAGNOSIS

- Other causes of acute renal failure (e.g., toxin, pyelonephritis, severe shock) (see Acute Renal Failure, p 32).
- Other causes of vasculitis (e.g., sepsis, rickettsial diseases, pancreatitis with systemic inflammatory response syndrome).
- Other causes of hepatic dysfunction (e.g., bacterial cholangiohepatitis, toxin, idiopathic chronic hepatitis, cirrhotic/fibrosing liver disease).
- One of the difficulties in diagnosing leptospirosis is the variability of clinical signs. As such, it is found as a differential diagnosis for many different patients.

INITIAL DATABASE

- Complete blood count: often inflammatory leukogram, with or without a left shift, variable degrees of anemia, and potentially thrombocytopenia, especially if vasculitis and disseminated intravascular coagulation (DIC) are present.
- Serum biochemistry profile:
  - Azotemia, hyperphosphatemia, and hypocalcemia are common.
  - Electrolyte disturbances associated with GI and renal disease (hyponatremia, hypochloremia, and hypokalemia), metabolic acidosis.
  - Hypoalbuminemia may be present in cases with vasculitis or chronic liver dysfunction.
  - Increased alkaline phosphatase, alanine transferase, aspartate transferase, and bilirubin usually peak at 6 to 8 days after the onset of disease. Creatinine kinase, amylase, and lipase may also be increased.
- Urinalysis:
  - Caution when handling specimen: zoonotic risk.
  - Glucosuria, proteinuria, granular casts, pyuria, and hematuria may be present with variable concentrating ability.
  - Oliguria is common and complete anuria may be noted despite adequate hydration (anuric acute renal failure).
- Abdominal radiographs: renomegaly possible.
- Thoracic radiographs: some patients have interstitial, nodular, or even patchy alveolar infiltrates.
- Abdominal ultrasonography: possible renomegaly, "medullary rim sign" (hyperechoic concentric ring), perinephric effusion.
- Arterial blood pressure: in hypovolemic patients (hypotension) or patients with ongoing renal disease (hypertension).

ADVANCED OR CONFIRMATORY TESTING

- Microscopic agglutination test (MAT): diagnostic test of choice.
  - In animals showing compatible clinical signs, any of the following is generally considered diagnostic of leptospirosis.
    - Titer >1:800 in unvaccinated animal.
    - Titer >1:3200 in vaccinated animal.
    - Paired titers 2 to 4 weeks apart, with fourfold rise from first to second titer.
- Enzyme-linked immunosorbent assay tests are not specific and results should be confirmed by MAT.
- Darkfield microscopy may demonstrate leptospires in a fresh wet mount of urine. This test is poorly sensitive (intermittent shedding means frequent false-negative results) and not routinely used.
- Culturing of leptospires is difficult and rarely attempted.
- Fluorescent antibody techniques exist for fluid and tissues as well as polymerase chain reaction techniques. These are not widely available.
- Histopathologic examination of renal tissue is nonspecific: lymphoplasmacytic tubulointerstitial nephritis. Organisms may be identified using special stains, however.

TREATMENT

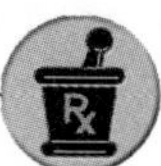

THERAPEUTIC GOAL(S)

- Treat bacteremia/leptospiremia
- Maintain renal perfusion and urine output to diminish or prevent renal injury
- Eliminate bacteria to prevent shedding to environment

ACUTE GENERAL TREATMENT

- Penicillin antibiotics are recommended for bacteremia (crystalline/transparent formulations for IV use).
  - Penicillin sodium: 20,000 IU/kg IV q 4h; or
  - Ampicillin 22 mg/kg IV or PO q 8h; or
  - Amoxicillin 22 mg/kg IV or PO q 8h.
- Initial management of renal injury: fluid therapy. Target is rapid rehydration without volume overload.
  - Correct dehydration over first 12 hours.
  - If clinical dehydration is not noted, initial fluid therapy should involve administration of 3-5% of body weight in isotonic crystalloid fluids (e.g., Plasmalyte 56 with 5% dextrose, but lactated Ringer's solution or 0.9% sodium chloride may be used).
  - Thereafter, matching fluid input with urine output should be the goal.
  - Fluid dose may need to be reduced, and/or more intensive monitoring performed (e.g., central venous pressure measurement; see Central Venous Pressure Monitoring, p 1206) in patients with heart disease or systemic hypertension.
- If urine output still less than 1 ml/kg/h after fluid therapy and adequate blood pressure (>90 mmHg systolic), then further medical management for acute renal failure (see Acute Renal Failure, p 32) is warranted. If ineffective, hemodialysis or peritoneal dialysis may be warranted.
- H_2 blockers are commonly used for uremic gastritis: famotidine 0.5-1 mg/kg IV q 24h, ranitidine 2.2 mg/kg IM, SC, or slow IV (to avoid nausea) q 12h, or cimetidine 10 mg/kg IV q 6-12h.

CHRONIC TREATMENT

To eliminate leptospires from tissues, doxycycline 5 mg PO q 12h for 2 weeks is recommended.

RECOMMENDED MONITORING

- Serum electrolyte levels are often abnormal and therapy may need to be tailored according to nature and severity of imbalance.
- Hypertension may occur, requiring modification of fluid therapy (e.g., switch from isotonic replacement-type fluid to isotonic maintenance-type fluid, if hydration is normal) or treatment (see Systemic Hypertension, p 1058).

- Urine output monitoring is essential in patients with acute renal failure; mainly prognostic.

PROGNOSIS AND OUTCOME

- Survival rates with leptospirosis are reported as 70–85%, including patients requiring and receiving hemodialysis.
- Chronic renal and liver dysfunctions are common sequelae in patients that survive acute leptospirosis.

PEARLS & CONSIDERATIONS

COMMENTS

- Leptospirosis should be considered in any case of acute renal failure, fever of unknown origin, and acute or chronic liver disease.
- Aggressive early therapy is important both for the patient's benefit and to reduce the risk of zoonosis. Empiric therapy with high-dose penicillin is recommended in acute illness while awaiting confirmatory test results.
- Serovars icterohaemorrhagiae and pomona: liver disease > renal disease. Serovars canicola and grippotyphosa: renal disease > liver disease.

PREVENTION

- The conventional vaccination for leptospirosis is a killed bacterin that protects against icterohaemorrhagiae and canicola.
- A newer vaccination is available that protects against icterohaemorrhagiae, canicola, pomona, and grippotyphosa.
- No vaccine protects against other serovars.
- Initially, three vaccinations should be given every 3 to 4 weeks. *Leptospira* titers are present for only 3 to 6 months; therefore vaccinations should be considered at least twice yearly in endemic areas.
- Adverse reactions have been reported with disproportionate frequency with leptospirosis vaccines. Dachshunds may be predisposed. Vaccination should be reserved for patients at reasonable risk. Patients with a history of intolerance should either not receive the vaccine, or be premedicated with antihistamines (e.g., diphenhydramine 2 mg/kg IM once) and glucocorticoids (e.g., dexamethasone 0.2 mg/kg IM once) 15 to 30 minutes before vaccination.

CLIENT EDUCATION

- Leptospirosis is often seen following heavy rains in endemic areas that are frequented by wildlife carriers.
- Dogs should not be allowed to drink from pools of stagnant water.

SUGGESTED READING

Greene CE, et al: Leptospirosis. In *Infectious Diseases of the Dog and Cat*, ed 2. Philadelphia, WB Saunders, 1998, pp 273–281.

Hartmann K, Greene CE: Diseases caused by systemic bacterial infections. In Ettinger SJ, Feldman EC (eds): *Textbook of Veterinary Internal Medicine,* ed 6. St. Louis, Elsevier Saunders, 2005, pp 616–631.

Langston CE, et al: Leptospirosis. A re-emerging zoonotic disease. *Vet Clin North Am Small Anim Pract* 33(4):791–807, 2003.

AUTHOR: **JEFFERY SIMMONS**
EDITOR: **DOUGLASS K. MACINTIRE**

Lethargy

BASIC INFORMATION

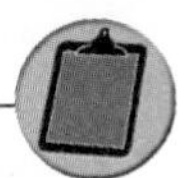

DEFINITION

Inert or apathetic state; lack of interest and/or energy; morbid drowsiness

SYNONYM(S)

"Depressed"
"Not himself/herself"
Others

EPIDEMIOLOGY

SPECIES, AGE, SEX: Any patient.

ASSOCIATED CONDITIONS AND DISORDERS: Any disease process affecting any organ system, if sufficiently severe (systemic and/or direct intracranial involvement) can cause lethargy.

CLINICAL PRESENTATION

HISTORY, CHIEF COMPLAINT

- The owner presents the pet due to a period of decreased activity, depressed mentation, and/or associated loss of appetite.
- A detailed history includes information as to the pet's water intake, presence or absence of vomiting/diarrhea, and whether the pet is eating. Additional useful information includes the pet's exercise level in the preceding days, whether other pets are affected, current medication history, and vaccination and deworming status.

PHYSICAL EXAMINATION

- Temperature, pulse, and respiratory rate: comparison to normal to look for early signs of shock.
- Examination of the mouth for severe dental disease and mucous membrane, color. Capillary refill time to assess peripheral perfusion.
- Palpation of all lymph nodes for enlargement, suggesting hyperplasia (e.g., inflammation) or infiltration (e.g., neoplastic).
- Chest auscultation must include listening to 3 to 5 breath sounds in each of a few quadrants of the chest as well as heart auscultation. Evaluate the pulse while auscultating the heart.
- Abdominal palpation must be methodical. It focuses on quadrants within the abdomen, involving specific palpation of individual organs. The examination includes palpating the small intestine a second time for a foreign body/mass or for fluid accumulation.
- Rectal examination: to check for perianal masses, to assess the prostate, and to collect feces for a fecal flotation.
- Manipulation of the neck for pain and palpation of the whole spine. Simultaneous palpation of the abdomen is important, as pressure on hyperpathic points in the spine always causes abdominal tensing.
- Manipulation of all joints.

ETIOLOGY AND PATHOPHYSIOLOGY

- Direct central nervous system (CNS) insult (inflammatory, vascular, neoplastic, other)
- More commonly, lethargy is the result of systemic disturbances with CNS effects, such as:
  - Inflammation: cytokine effects
  - Vascular: decreased perfusion
  - Metabolic: hypoglycemia, electrolyte disturbance, acid-base imbalance
  - Environmental: hyperthermia/hypothermia
  - Many others

DIAGNOSIS

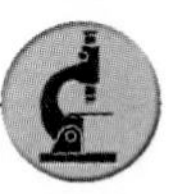

DIFFERENTIAL DIAGNOSIS

Any disease process (metabolic, infectious, neoplastic, traumatic, vascular, degenerative)

INITIAL DATABASE

Minimum database on each case:

- Return to/repeat the physical exam (most important diagnostic test in these cases)
- Urinalysis
- Blood smear: evidence of infection versus inflammation and platelet count
- Fecal flotation

ADVANCED OR CONFIRMATORY TESTING

- Complete blood count, serum biochemistry profile.
- The minimum database and physical exam orient the selection of additional tests. The more tests are performed, however, the greater the likelihood of a false-positive result.
- Thoracic radiographs (two views).
- Abdominal ultrasound and/or radiographs.

TREATMENT

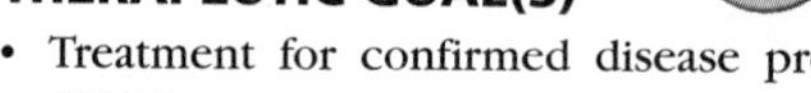

THERAPEUTIC GOAL(S)

- Treatment for confirmed disease processes.
- Antibiotics are reserved for confirmed or highly suspected bacterial disease.
- Withholding of glucocorticoids unless their need has been proven. Glucocorticoids complicate many further diagnostics and can cause clinical deterioration if used inappropriately.

ACUTE AND CHRONIC TREATMENT

- If no trigger is found after the history, physical exam, and initial database, and the pet is not very ill, treat empirically and send the pet home (e.g., in patients with gastrointestinal signs, using intestinal formula diet and asking owner to watch and return if pet is no better).
- Antibiotics are only considered if the blood smear shows signs of infection or if there is fever *with a second sign of infection* (e.g., blood in the feces).
- Specific aspects of treatment are guided by results of the minimum database and advanced testing:
  - Fluids if dehydrated
  - Analgesics if needed

POSSIBLE COMPLICATIONS

Lack of communication. It is essential to explain to the owner that an underlying trigger exists and must be found to provide optimal treatment.

PROGNOSIS AND OUTCOME

Highly variable, depending on the underlying cause of lethargy

PEARLS & CONSIDERATIONS

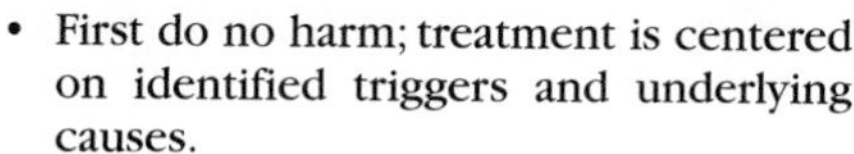

COMMENTS

- First do no harm; treatment is centered on identified triggers and underlying causes.
- More than 35% of sick pets presented to veterinary clinics have acute gastrointestinal upsets.
- Confident presentation of information is essential. Otherwise, owners can mistakenly sense uncertainty rather than a logical stepwise approach to a biologic system.

SUGGESTED READING

Osborne CA: The problem-orientated medical system. Improve knowledge, wisdom and understanding of patient care. *Vet Clin North Am Small Anim Pract* 13(4):745–753, 1983.

AUTHOR: **DAVID MILLER**
EDITOR: **ETIENNE CÔTÉ**

Leukemias, Acute

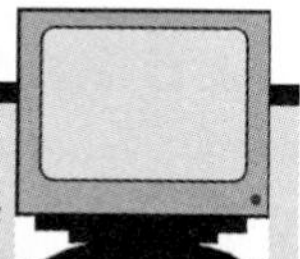

Client Education Sheet on Website

BASIC INFORMATION

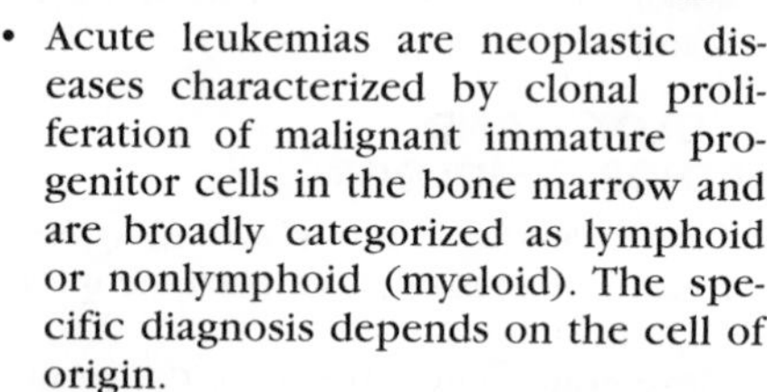

DEFINITION

- Acute leukemias are neoplastic diseases characterized by clonal proliferation of malignant immature progenitor cells in the bone marrow and are broadly categorized as lymphoid or nonlymphoid (myeloid). The specific diagnosis depends on the cell of origin.
- Acute lymphoblastic leukemias (ALL) involve the proliferation of lymphoblasts and prolymphocytes.
- Acute nonlymphoblastic leukemias, also called acute myeloid leukemias (AML), involve the proliferation of myeloid cells and include myeloid, monocytic, megakaryocytic, and erythrocytic leukemias. Nonlymphoid leukemias and myelodysplastic syndromes in veterinary patients are classified according to the Animal Leukemia Study Group modified version of the French-American-British system used in humans.

EPIDEMIOLOGY

SPECIES, AGE, SEX

- Young cats and dogs (median 4 to 5 years) are more commonly affected.
- ALL: In a study of acute leukemias in dogs, 45% had ALL.
- AML: rare. No age, breed, or sex predilections in dogs. In cats, possible male predilection. Frequency of types of AML has varied among studies, but M1 is most common.

RISK FACTORS: FeLV infection: 60–80% of cats with ALL are FeLV positive and ≥90% of cats with AML are FeLV positive.

ASSOCIATED CONDITIONS AND DISORDERS

- ALL in dogs: paraneoplastic hypercalemia
- AML in cats: myelofibrosis, hypercalcemia, glomerulonephritis

CLINICAL PRESENTATION

DISEASE FORMS/SUBTYPES

- Acute lymphoblastic leukemia:
  - B-cell origin: common in dogs.
  - T-cell origin: most common type in cats.
  - Large granular cell origin: common in dogs.
- Acute myeloid leukemias (classified based on bone marrow nucleated cell population):
  - Acute undifferentiated leukemia (AUL): ≥30% of bone marrow nucleated cells are blasts of uncertain lineage.
  - M1: Myeloblastic leukemia without maturation ≥30% of marrow nucleated cells are myeloblasts, ≤10% of nonerythroid cells are maturing granulocytes.
  - M2: Myeloblastic leukemia with maturation ≥30% of marrow nucleated cells are myeloblasts, >10% of nonerythroid cells are maturing granulocytes.
  - M3: promyelocytic leukemia ≥30% of marrow nucleated cells are myeloblasts, >10% of nonerythroid cells are maturing granulocytes, predominantly atypic promyelocytes. Has not been reported in animals.
  - M4: acute myelomonocytic leukemia ≥30% of marrow nucleated cells are

myeloblasts and monoblasts and differentiated granulocytes and monocytes each represent >20% of nonerythroid cells.
  - M5: monoblastic/monocytic leukemia ≥30% of marrow nucleated cells are monoblasts or promonocytes.
  - M6: erythroleukemia ≥50% of marrow nucleated cells are erythroid precursors and ≥30% of nonerythroid cells are myeloblasts and monoblasts or ≥30% of bone marrow nucleated cells are rubriblasts, myeloblasts, and monoblasts.
  - M6-Er: erythremic myelosis ≥50% of marrow nucleated cells are erythroid precursors and ≥30% are erythroblasts.
  - M7: megakaryoblastic leukemia ≥30% of marrow nucleated cells are megakaryoblasts.

HISTORY, CHIEF COMPLAINT

- Acute onset of nonspecific signs such as lethargy, weakness, loss of appetite, and weight loss.
- Hemorrhage (e.g., epistaxis or petechiae) may be noted.
- Lameness due to bone pain is possible.

PHYSICAL EXAM FINDINGS

- Lethargy, weakness, pallor, weight loss, and dehydration are common.
- Fever due to secondary infection.
- Tachypnea/dyspnea and tachycardia may be noted secondary to anemia.
- Hepatomegaly and splenomegaly are common.
- Lymphadenomegaly is uncommon.
- Evidence of hemorrhage secondary to thrombocytopenia (petechiae, ecchymoses, epistaxis, intestinal bleeding).
- Ocular lesions (hyphema, uveitis, chorioretinitis, retinal detachment, chemosis, and conjunctivitis).

ETIOLOGY AND PATHOPHYSIOLOGY

- Leukemic cells infiltrate the marrow, crowding the normal bone marrow cells, changing the marrow microenvironment, and secreting suppressor factors (myelophthisis). This results in decreased normal hematopoiesis, causing anemia, neutropenia, and thrombocytopenia. Cytopenias may result in weakness, secondary infections, and hemorrhage.
- Hepatic and splenic infiltration with leukemic cells is common, resulting in organomegaly, abdominal distention, and contributing to loss of appetite. Other sites may be involved, including lymph nodes, nervous system, kidneys, and gastrointestinal tract. Organ infiltration results in signs referable to failure of that organ or nonspecific signs such as malaise and gastrointestinal disturbances.

DIAGNOSIS

The diagnosis may be made on a peripheral blood smear (high numbers of circulating blast cells), but the definitive diagnosis is made on the bone marrow in a majority of cases of acute leukemia in dogs and cats.

DIFFERENTIAL DIAGNOSIS

- Stage V lymphoma
- Ehrlichiosis

INITIAL DATABASE

- Laboratory tests:
  - Complete blood count (CBC) and peripheral blood smear may reveal a leukocytosis with circulating blasts and cytopenias of other cells. Nonregenerative anemia and thrombocytopenia are common and may be severe. *Aleukemic* or *subleukemic* patients have normal or low white blood cell counts with no or some circulating blasts, respectively.
  - Serum chemistry profile and urinalysis to evaluate overall health and look for evidence of paraneoplastic syndromes.
  - FeLV/feline immunodeficiency virus ELISA test for all cats. Consider polymerase chain reaction test for FeLV using bone marrow (submit marrow sample in EDTA [lavender top tube]).
  - Rickettsial titers are indicated if in endemic area, history of tick exposure, or other compatible features.
- Bone marrow cytology (if unable to obtain a diagnostic sample, a core biopsy is indicated):
  - If the blast cell count is ≥30% of all nucleated cells in the bone marrow, a diagnosis of acute leukemia can be made.
- Fine-needle aspiration and cytology of enlarged peripheral lymph nodes may reveal infiltration with blasts.
- Imaging is performed to stage patients with leukemias and evaluate overall health:
  - Thoracic radiography.
  - Abdominal ultrasonography.

ADVANCED OR CONFIRMATORY TESTING

Special stains/diagnostics:

- Blast cells are frequently difficult to distinguish based on morphologic criteria alone.
- Cytochemical, immunocytochemical, immunohistochemical staining or flow cytometry are often needed to distinguish lymphoid from nonlymphoid leukemias and allow subclassification of AML.

TREATMENT

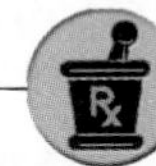

THERAPEUTIC GOAL(S)

- Eradicate leukemic cells
- Restore normal hematopoiesis
- Support patient until blood cell counts normalize

ACUTE GENERAL TREATMENT

- Intensive supportive care is important in patients with acute leukemias:
  - Broad-spectrum antibiotic therapy for treating/preventing secondary infections (see Chemotherapy: Adverse Reactions, p 189).
  - Intravenous fluid therapy for patients with infection, fever, or decreased appetite.
  - Situations that might result in hemorrhage (e.g., jugular vein venipuncture or catheterization) should be avoided if severe thrombocytopenia is present.
  - Transfusions as needed. See Transfusion Therapy and Collection Techniques for Blood Banking, p 1312.
  - Nutritional support for patients with decreased appetite.
- Chemotherapeutic agents are used for eradicating leukemia cells (induce remission). Clinically significant myelosuppression is expected because of myelophthisis. Hospitalization for supportive care during the induction period is indicated. Special handling requirements and potentially severe or life-threatening adverse patient effects exist with these chemotherapeutic drugs; these concerns and rapid evolution of protocols warrant consultation with/referral to an oncologist.
  - ALL: Treatment is generally with standard chemotherapy protocols for lymphoma (see Lymphoma Chemotherapy Treatment Tables, Dog, p 655). Agents include prednisone, vincristine, cyclophosphamide, doxorubicin, and L-asparaginase.
  - AML: Chemotherapy protocols generally include cytosine arabinoside and doxorubicin. Agents such as 6-thioguanine, mitoxantrone, cyclophosphamide, busulfan, melphalan, vincristine, vinblastine, prednisone, and L-asparaginase have also been used. To date, results with chemotherapy have been disappointing.

CHRONIC TREATMENT

Patients responding to treatment will likely receive chemotherapy for the rest of their lives.

POSSIBLE COMPLICATIONS

- Myelosuppression:
  - Neutropenia: sepsis
  - Thrombocytopenia: hemorrhage
  - Anemia requiring transfusion

- Gastrointestinal toxicity: vomiting, diarrhea, lethargy, loss of appetite

RECOMMENDED MONITORING

- Physical examinations and CBC: weekly to every other week, more frequently if needed during the induction period. To monitor remission status and myelosuppression due to therapy.
- Serum chemistry profile: every 2 months to monitor renal and liver status, electrolytes, etc. More frequently if indicated.

PROGNOSIS AND OUTCOME

In general, the prognosis for acute leukemias is poor. Because many patients are euthanized at diagnosis and acute leukemias are relatively uncommon, there is limited information available regarding treatment outcomes. Most patients are clinically ill at presentation and if left untreated or given supportive care only, survival times are generally less than 2 to 4 weeks.

- ALL: For dogs, the response rate to chemotherapy is about 30-50% and the average survival is about 2 to 4 months. For cats, a remission rate of 65% for a median of 7 months has been reported. If chemotherapy is not an option, prednisone may be palliative.
- AML: Treatments attempted to date have done little to alter the course of the disease and prognosis is grave for cats and dogs.

PEARLS & CONSIDERATIONS

COMMENTS

- Patients with acute leukemias present with an acute onset of nonspecific signs. Bone marrow cytologic evaluation and a peripheral blood smear will generally provide a diagnosis, but special diagnostics may be needed to classify the specific type of leukemia.
- Because acute leukemias progress rapidly, if owners are interested in pursuing treatment, consultation with an oncologist and treatment for ALL should be initiated while waiting for the results of special diagnostics.
- Owners should be advised of the poor prognosis and the potential for complications with treatment of acute leukemias.
- Supportive care may help reduce complications with treatment.
- With better characterization of acute leukemias and new treatments based on treatments in human oncology, the treatment and prognosis of dogs and cats with acute leukemias may be improved in the future.

SUGGESTED READING

Jacobs RM, Messick JB, Valli VE: Tumors of the hemolymphatic system. In Meuten DJ (ed): *Tumors in Domestic Animals,* ed 4. Ames, IA, Iowa State Press, 2002, pp 119-198.

Moore AS, Ogilvie GK: Bone marrow disorders. In Ogilvie GK, Moore AS (eds): *Feline Oncology, A Comprehensive Guide to Compassionate Care.* Trenton, NJ, Veterinary Learning Systems, 2001, pp 222-224.

Vail EM, MacEwen EG, Young KM: Canine lymphoma and lymphoid leukemias. In Withrow SJ, MacEwen EG (eds): *Small Animal Clinical Oncology,* ed 3. Philadelphia, 2001, pp 558-590.

Vernau W, Moore PF: An immunophenotypic study of canine leukemias and preliminary assessment of clonality by polymerase chain reaction. *Vet Immunol Immunopathol* 69:145-164, 1999.

AUTHOR: **NICOLE C. NORTHRUP**
EDITOR: **KENNETH M. RASSNICK**

Leukemias, Chronic

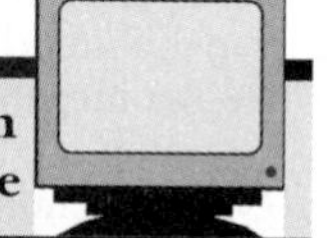

BASIC INFORMATION

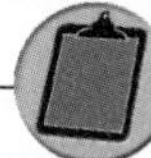

DEFINITION

Chronic leukemias are neoplastic diseases characterized by clonal proliferation of malignant mature hematopoietic cells in the bone marrow. They are categorized as lymphoid or myeloid. Chronic lymphocytic leukemias (CLL) involve the proliferation of mature lymphocytes. Chronic myeloid (myelogenous) leukemias (CML) involve the proliferation of myeloid cells and include myeloid, monocytic, myelomonocytic, basophilic, mastocytic, megakaryocytic, and erythrocytic leukemias.

EPIDEMIOLOGY

SPECIES, AGE, SEX: Typically older dogs and cats but can occur at any age.

GENETICS AND BREED PREDISPOSITION: Mast cell leukemia (MCL): associated with derangement of KIT receptor or its ligand (stem cell factor) in dogs and humans.

RISK FACTORS: In contrast to acute lymphocytic leukemia, most cats with CLL are not infected with feline leukemia virus (FeLV) or feline immunodeficiency virus (FIV).

ASSOCIATED CONDITIONS AND DISORDERS

- CLL: monoclonal gammopathy, hyperviscosity syndrome
- CML: myelofibrosis
- Chronic basophilic leukemia (CBL) and MCL: hyperhistaminemia resulting in urticarial rashes and gastrointestinal (GI) signs/ulceration
- PV: hyperviscosity syndrome

CLINICAL PRESENTATION

DISEASE FORMS/SUBTYPES

- Chronic lymphocytic leukemia:
  - T-cell: 73% canine CLL
  - B-Cell: 25% canine CLL
  - Granular lymphocyte CLL (GL CLL; cytotoxic T-cells or natural killer cells): 54% canine CLL; suspected to originate in the spleen
- Chronic myeloid leukemias:
  - CMoL: chronic monocytic leukemia
  - CMML: chronic myelomonocytic leukemia
  - CML: chronic myeloid (granulocytic) leukemia
  - CEL: chronic eosinophilic leukemia
  - CBL: chronic basophilic leukemia
  - MCL: mast cell leukemia
  - PV: primary erythrocytosis (polycythemia vera)
  - MM: megakaryocytic myelosis (essential thrombocythemia)

HISTORY, CHIEF COMPLAINT

- Insidious onset of increased peripheral blood count of affected cell line.
- Initially no clinical signs.
- Later, nonspecific signs (lethargy, loss of appetite, weight loss) and signs associated with cytopenias (weakness, hemorrhage, infection).
- PV (rarely CLL) can cause neurologic signs (seizures, behavior changes, blindness, ataxia) due to hyperviscosity. Polyuria/polydipsia also possible.
- CEL in cats usually results in gastrointestinal (GI) signs due to infiltration.
- Some forms of CML frequently cause clinical signs due to production of cytokines or other factors (e.g., CBL, MCL: GI signs due to histamine).

PHYSICAL EXAM FINDINGS

- Initially, normal physical examination.
- Hepatomegaly/splenomegaly common as disease progresses.
- Lymphadenomegaly frequently present in dogs with CLL.
- Brick-red mucous membranes and neurologic signs are possible with PV.

- Palpable GI wall thickening possible with CEL and MCL.
- Fundic examination: large, tortuous retinal vessels and retinal hemorrhages possible in dogs with PV.

ETIOLOGY AND PATHOPHYSIOLOGY

- Chronic leukemias arise from neoplastic transformation of a pluripotent stem cell in the marrow or spleen.
- They are insidious, with gradual increases in marrow and peripheral blood cell counts of the leukemic cell type. Bone marrow infiltration may eventually result in myelophthisis (crowding of normal cells, changes in the marrow microenvironment, and secretion of suppressor factors) or myelofibrosis. These conditions result in anemia, neutropenia, and thrombocytopenia.
- Hepatic and splenic infiltration with leukemic cells is gradual, resulting in organomegaly, abdominal distention, and loss of appetite. Organ infiltration and dysfunction are possible in chronic stages or with transformation to acute leukemias.
- Transformation into a blast phase (acute leukemias) may be seen in the terminal stages of chronic leukemias.

DIAGNOSIS

The diagnosis rests on bone marrow cytologic findings, but a high degree of suspicion often is raised when an extremely high count of one cell line is noted on the complete blood count (CBC).

DIFFERENTIAL DIAGNOSIS

- Based on the type of cell(s) with elevated counts on CBC and bone marrow cytology
- Lymphocytes:
  - CLL
  - Small cell or large granular cell lymphoma
  - Ehrlichiosis
  - Chronic antigenic stimulation (e.g., inflammatory bowel disease, cholangiohepatitis)
  - Vaccination
  - Stress/epinephrine in young cats
  - Hypoadrenocorticism
- Neutrophils:
  - CML
  - Infection
  - Leukemoid reaction secondary to immune-mediated disease
  - Rebound following myelosuppressive drugs or chemical or viral insult to the bone marrow
  - Paraneoplastic syndrome (lymphoma, others)
- Monocytes:
  - CMoL
  - CMML
  - Chronic infection/inflammation
  - Granulomatous disease
- Eosinophils:
  - CEL
  - Hypereosinophilic syndrome (HES; difficult to distinguish from CEL; may be a variant of the same disease)
  - Parasites (gastrointestinal, dirofilariasis, other)
  - Eosinophilic granuloma complex
  - Mast cell neoplasia
  - Feline asthma
  - Eosinophilic enteritis
- Basophils:
  - CBL
  - Mast cell neoplasia
  - Dirofilariasis
- Mast cells:
  - MCL
  - Systemic mast cell tumor
  - Allergies
  - Dermatitis
  - Parasites
  - Parvoviral infection (dogs)
  - Regenerative anemias
- Platelets:
  - Megakaryocytic myelosis
  - Hyperadrenocorticism
  - Iron deficiency
  - Postsplenectomy
  - Chronic inflammatory disorders
  - Acute infection
- Erythrocytes:
  - Relative erythrocytosis:
    - Dehydration
    - Diuretics, cardiac medications
    - Breed variation (sight hounds)
  - Absolute erythrocytosis:
    - PV
    - Chronic hypoxemia (right-to-left cardiac shunts, chronic respiratory disease, high altitude)
    - Paraneoplastic production of erythropoietin (renal tumors, others)
    - Splenic contraction

INITIAL DATABASE

- Laboratory tests:
  - CBC and blood smear reveal a high count of the leukemic cell type. Cell counts can be very high (hundreds of thousands and higher); for PV, PCV typically ranges from 60% to ≥80%. Both mature and immature forms of affected cell line may be present. Cytopenias are not generally observed until leukemic cell counts are very high.
  - Serum biochemistry profile and urinalysis to evaluate overall health and look for paraneoplastic syndromes.
  - FeLV/FIV ELISA for cats, ± FeLV polymerase chain reaction (PCR) on bone marrow.
- Bone marrow cytology (if unable to obtain diagnostic sample, core biopsy is indicated):
  - Infiltration of bone marrow with leukemic cell type and its precursors is diagnostic.
- Cytologic evaluation of enlarged peripheral lymph nodes may reveal leukemic cells.
- Imaging for staging and to evaluate overall health and identify concurrent abnormalities:
  - Thoracic radiography.
  - Abdominal ultrasonography.

ADVANCED OR CONFIRMATORY TESTING

- Chronic leukemias are diagnosed by cell morphology. Additional tests may be needed to rule out differential diagnoses (see Differential Diagnosis above). If noted early in the course of the disease, repeat CBC and bone marrow cytology may be needed to confirm or refute the diagnosis.
- For CLL, immunophenotyping can characterize the cell of origin, which may help to better define prognosis in the future. PCR for antigen receptor gene rearrangement can be used for differentiating from lymphoid hyperplasia.

TREATMENT

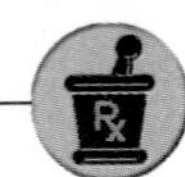

THERAPEUTIC GOAL(S)

- Eradicate leukemic cells
- Restore normal hematopoiesis
- Support patient until blood cell counts normalize

ACUTE GENERAL TREATMENT

- Supportive care may or may not be necessary with chronic leukemias.
  - Broad-spectrum antibiotics for treating/preventing secondary infections:
    - For prophylaxis, a common choice is sufadiazine-trimethoprim 15 mg/kg PO q 12h for dogs. Cats do not usually need prophylactic antibiotics.
    - If fever or overt infection is present, intravenous broad-spectrum antibiotics based on culture and sensitivity (preferred, if available) or empiric use of personal preferred combination are indicated. Example: a combination of either a cephalosporin (e.g., cefazolin 22 mg/kg IV q 8h slow bolus) or a penicillin (e.g., ampicillin 22 mg/kg IV q 8h slow bolus) together with either an aminoglycoside (e.g., amikacin 20 mg/kg IV q 24h [only in hydrated patient without renal dysfunction; can cause renal injury]) or a fluoroquinolone (e.g., enrofloxacin 5 mg/kg diluted 1:1 in sterile water and given as a slow IV bolus q 12h [dogs; in cats, limit to 5 mg/kg/day or less to reduce risk of retinal toxicity/permanent blindness]).

- Intravenous fluids for patients with infection, fever, or decreased appetite.
- Avoid jugular venipuncture or catheterization if severe thrombocytopenia.
- Transfusions as needed (see Transfusion Therapy and Collection Techniques for Blood Banking, p 1312).
- Nutritional support (see Parenteral Nutrition, p 1296).

- Chemotherapeutic agents are used for eradicating leukemia cells. Response is slower and more durable than for acute leukemias. Special handling requirements and potentially severe adverse effects exist for these drugs. Consultation with oncologist is recommended for most current treatment options.
  - CLL: Treatment recommended if patients have clinical signs, cytopenias, or lymphocyte counts >60,000/μl. Treat with prednisone (dogs: 40 mg/m² PO once daily for 7 days and then every other day; cats: similar dosage but ongoing daily dosing) and chlorambucil (6–8 mg/m² PO every other day). Some protocols add vincristine (0.7 mg/m² IV) during the first 1 to 4 weeks. When these drugs fail, other drugs for lymphoma may be used.
  - CML: Treatment depends on diagnosis.
    - PV, CML, and CEL: treated with prednisone (dogs: 40 mg/m² PO once daily for 7 days and then every other day; cats: similar dosage but continued daily dosing) and hydroxyurea (dogs: 30 mg/kg PO once daily for 7 to 10 days, then 15 mg/kg PO once daily; cats: 125 mg PO twice per week. All dosages are adjusted long term based on response). PV may be able to be managed with phlebotomy and fluid replacement initially. Busulfan has also been used in the treatment of CML, but a recommended dosage has not been established.

CHRONIC TREATMENT

Patients responding to treatment will receive chemotherapy for the rest of their lives or until they develop bone marrow toxicity.

POSSIBLE COMPLICATIONS

- Myelosuppression: neutropenia, thrombocytopenia.
- Chronic bone marrow toxicity is possible with chronic alkylating agent therapy (chlorambucil, cyclophosphamide).
- Hydroxyurea can cause methemoglobinemia in cats. It can also cause anemia and skin/hair/nail changes.
- Gastrointestinal toxicity.

RECOMMENDED MONITORING

- Will depend on diagnosis and how severely patient is affected.
- Physical examinations: weekly or more frequently if needed in induction period. Monthly once on chronic maintenance therapy.
- CBC: weekly or more frequently if needed during the induction period. Monthly once on chronic maintenance therapy. To monitor remission status, myelosuppression, and chronic bone marrow injury.
- Serum biochemistry profile, urinalysis (free catch if risk of hemorrhage): 2 to 3 times a year to monitor overall health, paraneoplastic syndromes, and toxicity. More frequently if indicated.

PROGNOSIS AND OUTCOME

In general, the prognosis for chronic leukemias is better than acute leukemias because of the indolent nature of chronic leukemias.

- CLL: Progresses slowly. Responsive to chemotherapy. Survival times of 1 to 3 years expected for dogs and suspected to be similar for cats. If it transforms into lymphoma/acute leukemia (as indicated typically by the recurrence of clinical signs and appearance of blast cells on a blood smear), the prognosis is poor.
- CML: Depends on type. There is little or no information describing the prognosis for some of these conditions.
  - CML/CBL: Some dogs may live 1 year or more with treatment.
  - PV: Survival times of >1 to >6 years reported.
  - CEL: In cats, not very responsive to treatment. Survival times of a few months. Unclear if dogs develop CEL, but if they do, it may respond to prednisone.

PEARLS & CONSIDERATIONS

COMMENTS

- Chronic leukemias have a slow onset and often progress slowly. Patients are initially clinically normal and then show nonspecific signs.
- Diagnosis is based on identifying proliferating mature hematopoietic cells in the blood and bone marrow.
- Patients with chronic leukemias can enjoy long survival times.

SUGGESTED READING

Messick JB: Chronic myeloid leukemias. In Feldman BF, Zinkl JG, Jain NC (eds): *Schalm's Veterinary Hematology,* ed 5. Baltimore, Lippincott, Williams & Wilkins, 2000, pp 733–739.

Moore AS, Ogilvie GK: Bone marrow disorders. In Ogilvie GK, Moore AS (eds): *Feline Oncology, A Comprehensive Guide to Compassionate Care.* Trenton, NJ, Veterinary Learning Systems, 2001, pp 222–224.

Vail EM, MacEwen EG, Young KM: Canine lymphoma and lymphoid leukemias. In Withrow SJ, MacEwen EG (eds): *Small Animal Clinical Oncology,* ed 3. Philadelphia, 2001, pp 558–590.

Workman HC, Vernau W: Chronic lymphocytic leukemia in dogs and cats: The veterinary perspective. *Vet Clin North Am Small Anim Pract* 33:1379–1399, 2003.

Young KM, MacEwen EG: Canine myeloproliferative disorders. In Withrow SJ, MacEwen EG (eds): *Small Animal Clinical Oncology,* ed 3. Philadelphia, 2001, pp 611–626.

AUTHOR: **NICOLE C. NORTHRUP**
EDITOR: **KENNETH M. RASSNICK**

Licking (Excessive) and Similar Behavioral Disorders

BASIC INFORMATION

DEFINITION

Self-directed, repetitive, purposeless behaviors derived from otherwise normal processes such as grooming

SYNONYM(S)

Acral lick dermatitis, lick granuloma (see also Acral Lick Dermatitis, p 24)
Obsessive-compulsive disorders (OCD)
Psychogenic alopecia

EPIDEMIOLOGY

SPECIES, AGE, SEX: Age of onset usually overlaps with social maturity (dogs: 12 to 36 months old; cats: 24 to 48 months old).

RISK FACTORS

- Pain
- Anxiety

- Illness or injury that changes sensory function

ASSOCIATED CONDITIONS AND DISORDERS: Coexisting anxiety-related conditions are common.

CLINICAL PRESENTATION

HISTORY, CHIEF COMPLAINT: Persistent chewing or licking of the skin and hair.

PHYSICAL EXAM FINDINGS

- Hair loss and discoloration occuring only on parts of the body that can be reached by the teeth and tongue.
  - In cats it is especially evident around the sides and rump, hind limbs, and groin. Thus, the head and back of neck may still have normal haircoat.
  - Usually the alopecia is nonsymmetric and the skin may look normal.
- Evidence of self-mutilation may be apparent.

ETIOLOGY AND PATHOPHYSIOLOGY

- Normal adult cats spend about 30-50% of their time awake grooming.
- The anatomic focus of obsessive-compulsive disorders appears to be the limbic system:
  - Dopaminergic, serotonergic, and opioid pathways are thought to be involved in compulsive and self-injurious behaviors.
  - Aberrant serotonin metabolism and possibly endorphin metabolism are also thought to contribute.
  - Lowered serotonin and increased dopamine levels are associated with some obsessive-compulsive disorders.

DIAGNOSIS

DIFFERENTIAL DIAGNOSIS

- Pruritic skin disease
- External parasites
- Endocrine disorders causing alopecia
- Feline lower urinary tract signs/disease: a common cause of cats' chewing or plucking at the abdomen
- Pain associated with any condition including trauma or infection
- Normal response to environmental change (transient)

INITIAL DATABASE

- Behavioral examination (see p 1188).
- Dermatologic examination revealing no evidence of dermatologic causes, such as atopy, external parasites, or food allergy.
- Complete blood count, serum biochemistry profile, thyroid profile (depending on signs), urinalysis: no abnormalities expected. Baseline evaluation before medication.
- Microscopic examination of plucked hair for evidence of shear, as expected with excessive grooming. Hair that is lost due to endocrine conditions has visible telogen bulbs.

ADVANCED OR CONFIRMATORY TESTING

Videotaping. If the cat or dog appears to exhibit odd behavior, videotaping at home by the clients is indicated. Thus, behaviors that are out of context, or that are excessive in frequency, intensity, or duration, and those that are interfering with social functioning, can be identified early, when it is easier to treat them.

TREATMENT

THERAPEUTIC GOAL(S)

- Minimize or resolve the licking, chewing, or barbering of the hair and skin.
- Remove or minimize the cause of the anxiety if possible.

ACUTE GENERAL TREATMENT

- Treatment of underlying medical problems, such as elimination of fleas, or resolution of food allergy
- Remove or minimize the cause of the anxiety if possible
- Provide a regular predictable routine, such as feed and play at a set time each day

CHRONIC TREATMENT

Treatment involves altering the neurochemical as well as the physical environment.

- Anxiolytic medication has also proved useful in some cases:
  - Tricyclic antidepressants (TCAs).
    - Cats:
      - Amitriptyline (0.5-1 mg/kg PO q 12-24h average of 5-10 mg/cat PO q 24h, start at the lowest dose and increase after 10 days if no response).
      - Clomipramine (0.5 mg/kg PO q 24h).
      - Doxepin (0.5-1.0 mg/kg PO q 12-24h).
    - Dogs:
      - Amitriptyline (1-2 mg/kg PO q 12h).
      - Clomipramine (1-2 mg/kg PO q 12h 2 weeks, then 3 mg/kg PO q 12h).
      - Doxepin 3-5 mg/kg PO q 12-24h.
  - Selective serotonin reuptake inhibitors.
    - Cats:
      - Fluoxetine (0.5 mg/kg PO q 24h).
      - Paroxetine (2.5 mg/cat PO q 24h).
    - Dogs:
      - Fluoxetine (1 mg/kg PO q 12-24h).
  - Benzodiazepines such as diazepam (0.2-0.4 mg/kg PO q 12h; average of 1-2 mg/cat PO q 12h) or oxazepam (0.2-0.5 mg/kg PO q 12-24h) are effective in some cats.
  - Termination of these medications, if deemed necessary, should be via slow taper when treatment has been chronic (months).
- Punishment is not effective in changing behavior. It serves to further increase the anxiety, as well as impede learning of nonanxious behavior.

DRUG INTERACTIONS

TCAs and selective serotonin reuptake inhibitors should not be used concurrently with monoamine oxidase inhibitors such as those present in medications or some flea and tick collars.

POSSIBLE COMPLICATIONS

May progress and/or coexist with other anxiety-related disorders such as panic disorder. Referral to a veterinary behaviorist should be considered.

RECOMMENDED MONITORING

- Response to treatment should be monitored every 4 to 6 weeks
- Any patient taking psychotropic medication should undergo full medical and laboratory evaluations q 6-12 months, or as needed based on clinical signs

PROGNOSIS AND OUTCOME

- Prognosis is variable and improves with greater owner commitment, success in determining underlying cause, and management of underlying problem(s).
- Prognosis deteriorates with increased length of time the disorder is left untreated.

PEARLS & CONSIDERATIONS

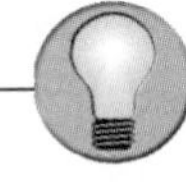

COMMENTS

Avoid punishing the behavior as it may increase the anxiety and arousal and exacerbate the behavior.

PREVENTION

- Early intervention and redirection of concerning behaviors may be useful for cats and dogs without a genetic propensity for the development of such conditions.
- Research has shown that even in cats with familial patterns of obsessive-compulsive disorder, the specific behaviors

involved do not attain the level of diagnosis until some social stressor (e.g., a move, the loss or addition of a pet or human) is involved. Clients should undergo anticipatory guidance when life-change events occur or are planned to occur.

CLIENT EDUCATION

- Monitor and record the occurrence of the behavior, to assess progression over time
- Once identified, these conditions will usually require lifelong treatment for control

SUGGESTED READING

Overall KL: *Clinical Behavioral Medicine for Small Animals*. St. Louis, Mosby, 1997.

Overall KL, Dunham AE: Clinical features and outcome in dogs and cats with obsessive-compulsive disorder: 126 cases (1989–2000). *J Am Vet Med Assoc* 221:1445–1452, 2002.

Seksel K, Lindeman MJ: The use of clomipramine in the treatment of anxiety-related and obsessive-compulsive disorders in dogs. *Aust Vet J* 79:252–256, 2001.

AUTHOR: **KERSTI SEKSEL**
EDITOR: **KAREN L. OVERALL**

Lily Toxicosis

BASIC INFORMATION

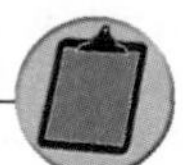

DEFINITION

Lilies are a family of flowering, ornamental plants that are known to cause acute renal failure when ingested by cats.

SYNONYM(S)

Lilies toxic to cats include:
Day lilies (*Hemerocallis* sp.)
Easter lilies (*Lilium longiflorum*)
Rubrum or Japanese showy lilies (*L. speciosum, L. landifolium*)
Stargazer lily (*L. auratum*)
Tiger lilies (*L. tigrinum*)
There are many new *Lilium* varieties developed each year. All *Lilium* or *Hemerocallis* species should be considered toxic.

EPIDEMIOLOGY

SPECIES, AGE, SEX: Lily toxicity has only been reported in cats.
GENETICS AND BREED PREDISPOSITION: All breeds, ages, and sexes of cats are susceptible.
RISK FACTORS: Younger cats may be more likely to eat plant material.
GEOGRAPHY AND SEASONALITY

- Easter lilies are most commonly sold in March and April. Other lilies are found year round.
- Lilies grow naturally along the Pacific Coast of the United States. Lilies are frequently cultivated as garden plants or houseplants.

CLINICAL PRESENTATION

HISTORY, CHIEF COMPLAINT

- History of plant ingestion and/or presence of lilies in owner's home. Cats typically present vomiting (plant material may be present in the vomitus), anorexic, and lethargic.
- Signs usually develop within 12 hours after exposure (range: 2 hours to 5 days).
- Polyuria, polydipsia, and acute renal failure develop within 36 to 72 hours postingestion.

PHYSICAL EXAM FINDINGS

- Unremarkable if ingestion was recent. Initial signs of vomiting, anorexia, and lethargy may appear to resolve without treatment.
- Signs progressing to oliguria and anuria, dehydration, lethargy, and vomiting. Some cats also show vocalization, adipsia, drooling, tremors, ataxia, weakness, and seizures.
- Evidence of pancreatitis may be present.

ETIOLOGY AND PATHOPHYSIOLOGY

- Peak incidence during Christmas and Easter holidays, as lilies are popular holiday ornamentals.
- Lilies have large, showy, funnel-shaped flowers. The plants grow from bulbs, and have erect stems 30–250 cm high. Lilies are frequently included in bouquets and floral arrangements. Day lilies are often grown in gardens.
- Intoxication is via ingestion. Mechanism of action is unknown. Toxin is believed to be a water-soluble fraction. All parts of the plant are considered toxic, including pollen.
- A single bite, or even exposure to pollen only, can cause the clinical syndrome.

DIAGNOSIS

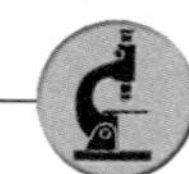

DIFFERENTIAL DIAGNOSIS

- Other intoxications that cause acute renal failure, including ethylene glycol, nonsteroidal anti-inflammatory drugs, cholecalciferol or calcipotriene, oxalic acid, and nephrotoxic antibiotics.
- Acute glomerulonephritis (e.g., feline infectious peritonitis, autoimmune disease-related).
- Renal thromboembolism.
- Acute-on-chronic renal failure (e.g., pyelonephritis, renal lymphoma, polycystic renal disease).

INITIAL DATABASE

- Serum biochemistry panel: azotemia (blood urea nitrogen [BUN] >34 mg/dl and creatinine is often disproportionately elevated), hyperkalemia, and hyperphosphatemia are common. Occasionally, hypercalcemia.
- Urinalysis: isosthenuria, epithelial granular casts, and glucosuria in the absence of hyperglycemia are typical findings.

ADVANCED OR CONFIRMATORY TESTING

- Histologically, the renal lesion generally includes acute necrosis of proximal convoluted tubules. Renal tubular mineralization may be present.
- Pancreatic acinar cells may show degeneration.
- Ultrasound can be used for measuring renal size and cortical thickness, and to rule out other causes of acute renal failure.
- Renal biopsy may help determine extent of renal damage and prognosis (rarely done, since history and exclusion of other causes are usually sufficient).

TREATMENT

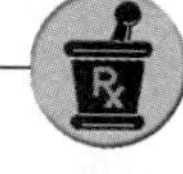

THERAPEUTIC GOAL(S)

- Decontamination of patient
- Prevent development/progression of acute renal failure
- Supportive care

ACUTE GENERAL TREATMENT

- Decontamination of patient (no clinical signs):
  - Emesis: In cats with recent ingestion (within a few hours) and not showing clinical signs, induce vomiting (see Vomiting, Induction of, p 1328) and give activated charcoal 1–4 g/kg PO. Protect airway with cuffed endotracheal tube if patient is unconscious.
- Prevent/slow development of renal failure (if cat is suspected or known to have

ingested lilies in the preceding 2 days). IMPORTANT: Treatment is implemented regardless of whether or not signs are present:
 - Intravenous fluids: diuresis for a minimum of 48 to 72 hours at twice maintenance fluids plus volume deficit (adjust based on hydration, fluid volume tolerance, and response to treatment). IV fluids should be continued until azotemia resolves. In some cases, this may mean days to weeks of treatment.
 - Monitor urine output in azotemic patients. If oliguria is present (urine production <0.25 ml/kg/h), furosemide (2.2-4.4 mg/kg IV q 8-12h) may increase urine output.
 - Treat hyperkalemia if present (see Hyperkalemia, p 546).
- Supportive care:
 - Control seizures with diazepam (0.5-2 mg/kg IV prn).
 - Persistent nausea: consider metoclopramide 0.1-0.5 mg/kg SQ q 6-12h if gastrointestinal obstruction has been ruled out.
 - Abdominal pain may be managed with opiates, such as butorphanol 0.1-0.2 mg/kg IV.
 - Peritoneal dialysis or hemodialysis possibly oriented toward renal transplantation if response is positive, can be considered if renal failure develops.

RECOMMENDED MONITORING

- Serum biochemistry profile baseline, 24, 48, and 72 hours (especially electrolytes and renal values). Recheck BUN and creatinine daily during clinical syndrome or for 72 hours if no abnormalities are seen.
- Urinalysis (baseline, 24, 48, 72 hours): ensure isosthenuria/hyposthenuria as sign of adequate fluid diuresis.
- If azotemia develops, monitor urine output.
- Monitor for fluid overload: respiratory character, onset of gallop sound on cardiac auscultation, central venous pressure if possible.

PROGNOSIS AND OUTCOME

- If treatment is initiated within 18 hours of ingestion, before onset of renal failure, prognosis is good.
- Prognosis after renal failure has developed is guarded to poor.

PEARLS & CONSIDERATIONS

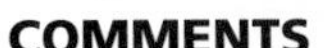

COMMENTS

- Even when vomiting is mild and self-limiting, the presence of plant material in vomitus makes it critical to initiate treatment, including intravenous fluids, to avoid subsequent renal failure.
- Lily toxicosis is high on the differential list for any cat with acute renal failure and an extremely high serum creatinine level.
- Neither lily-of-the-valley (*Convallaria majalis*) nor peace lily (*Spathiphyllum* spp.) belong to the *Lilium* or *Hemerocallis* genera. They are not true lilies and do not cause acute renal damage in cats.

PREVENTION

Do not keep any *Lilium* or *Hemerocallis* species in the cat's environment

CLIENT EDUCATION

Clients should make sure plants are safe before bringing them into a cat's environment.

SUGGESTED READING

Hadley RH, et al: A retrospective study of day lily toxicosis in cats. *Vet Human Toxicol* 45:38-39, 2003.

Richardson JA: Lily toxicosis in cats. *Standards of Care* 4:5-8, 2002.

Rumbeiha WK, et al: A comprehensive study of Easter lily poisoning in cats. *J Vet Diagn Invest* 16:527-541, 2004.

AUTHOR: **CHARLOTTE MEANS**

EDITOR: **SAFDAR A. KHAN**

Liposarcoma

BASIC INFORMATION

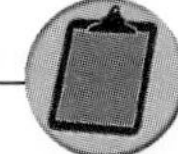

DEFINITION

A primary malignant neoplasm of adipocytes. Can occur anywhere in the body but more commonly found in the skin and subcutaneous tissue

EPIDEMIOLOGY

SPECIES, AGE, SEX: Liposarcomas are uncommon in dogs and rare in cats. They are more common in older dogs (10 years of age average), but can occur at any age. They have been reported at vaccine sites in cats. No sex predilection has been reported.

GENETICS AND BREED PREDISPOSITION: No breed predilection has been reported.

RISK FACTORS: Liposarcomas have been reported in previously irradiated tissues, at the site of a glass foreign body, and at the site of an injected microchip. The limited number of cases suggests that these factors may have a small impact on the risk of developing liposarcoma.

CLINICAL PRESENTATION

DISEASE FORMS/SUBTYPES: Liposarcomas have different pathologic subtypes, but these have not been shown to have prognostic significance. This tumor type has been reported at vaccine-sites in cats (see Vaccine-Site Sarcoma, p 1136).

HISTORY, CHIEF COMPLAINT

- Dogs with liposarcoma in the skin and subcutaneous tissue usually present for evaluation of a progressively growing mass noticed by the owner.
- Dogs with abdominal liposarcoma often present for evaluation of signs related to an abdominal mass.

PHYSICAL EXAM FINDINGS

- Liposarcoma in the skin and subcutaneous tissue often presents as a firm, palpable mass.
- Regional lymphadenopathy may be present secondary to inflammation or, rarely, lymph node metastasis.
- Dogs with an abdominal liposarcoma may present with abdominal mass, pain, or enlargement.

ETIOLOGY AND PATHOPHYSIOLOGY

- Liposarcomas are thought to be spontaneously occurring in most cases in dogs. However there are reports of tumors developing at the site of foreign bodies.
- Pathologic changes caused by liposarcomas depend on the location of the primary tumor and the invasion into and destruction of surrounding normal structures.
- Liposarcomas are not thought to be malignantly transformed lipomas.
- Liposarcomas may grow rapidly.

DIAGNOSIS

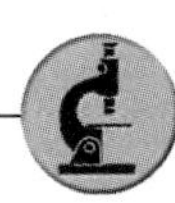

DIFFERENTIAL DIAGNOSIS

- Other skin and subcutaneous tumors:
 - Soft tissue sarcomas

- Mast cell tumor
- Others
- Other splenic tumors:
  - Hemangiosarcoma
  - Lymphoma
  - Others

INITIAL DATABASE

- Fine-needle aspirate cytology may help identify the tumor type before other diagnostics.
- Three-view thoracic radiographs to rule out pulmonary metastases.
- Radiographs of the affected area may reveal involvement of underlying bone.

ADVANCED OR CONFIRMATORY TESTING

- Computed tomography or magnetic resonance imaging may be necessary to delineate the local extent of the tumor and to plan for surgery or radiation therapy.
- Biopsy. Definitive diagnosis is based on histopathologic examination of tissue. Special stains may be necessary to differentiate liposarcoma from other soft tissue sarcomas, especially poorly differentiated tumors.

TREATMENT

THERAPEUTIC GOAL(S)

- Complete eradication of the primary tumor.
- Prevention or delay of the development of metastases in some cases. For example, chemotherapy may be indicated to prevent or delay metastases or in dogs with high-grade tumors or tumors that have already metastasized.

ACUTE GENERAL TREATMENT

- Aggressive surgical resection, radiation therapy, and/or chemotherapy may be used for treatment of liposarcoma (see Soft Tissue Sarcoma, p 1016).
- Although response of liposarcomas to radiation and chemotherapy has not been determined, these treatments may be useful as adjuvant therapy.

POSSIBLE COMPLICATIONS

Complications of treatment for liposarcomas depend on the types of treatments and the location of the primary tumor (see Soft Tissue Sarcoma, p 1016).

RECOMMENDED MONITORING

After appropriate local treatment, follow-up examination should be done on a routine basis to monitor for recurrence (every 2 to 3 months) and metastasis (including thoracic radiographs at 6 months and 1 year). High-grade tumors may require more frequent monitoring for metastases during and after chemotherapy administration.

PROGNOSIS AND OUTCOME

- Early studies reported metastasis to multiple sites (liver, lung, bone). However, in a recent retrospective study of 56 dogs, very few dogs died as a result of metastasis. Dogs in this study had a median survival of almost 2 years, and dogs that had wide excision of their tumor had a median survival >3 years.
- Surgical excision with a clean histopathologic margin may not be adequate for local tumor control in some dogs with liposarcoma, based on a recurrence rate of 31% for dogs with clean margins.

PEARLS & CONSIDERATIONS

COMMENTS

Fine-needle aspirate cytologic evaluation of skin and subcutaneous masses should always be evaluated microscopically. Aspirate of liposarcoma may give "fatty" appearing fluid, which could falsely be interpreted as indicating lipoma or subcutaneous fat. However, liposarcoma can be readily differentiated from benign tumors of adipocytes such as lipoma or infiltrative lipoma with routine microscopic (cytologic) evaluation of smears.

PREVENTION

The individual case of liposarcoma developing at the site of an implanted microchip does not warrant concern about an increased risk of tumors caused by microchips.

CLIENT EDUCATION

Pet owners can be educated to monitor their pets for masses and have them evaluated in a timely fashion. Early detection may allow for easier treatment via surgery and may help avoid the need for radiation therapy.

SUGGESTED READING

Baez JL, et al: Liposarcoma in dogs: 56 cases (1989–2000). *J Am Vet Med Assoc* 224:887–891, 2004.

AUTHOR: **JOHN FARRELLY**

EDITOR: **KENNETH M. RASSNICK**

Lumbosacral Stenosis, Degenerative

BASIC INFORMATION

DEFINITION

- A variety of pathologic conditions (malformation, growth disturbance, degeneration, compressive myelopathy, inflammation, infection, subluxation, ischemia) of the lumbosacral vertebral segments and related soft tissues.
- The most common clinical presentation involves degenerative lumbosacral stenosis.

SYNONYM(S)

Cauda equina syndrome
Lumbosacral spondylopathy
Spondylolisthesis

EPIDEMIOLOGY

SPECIES, AGE, SEX: Middle-aged, medium- to large-breed, male dogs overrepresented.

GENETICS AND BREED PREDISPOSITION: German shepherds are predisposed.

RISK FACTORS: Working dogs: increased risk.

CLINICAL PRESENTATION

HISTORY, CHIEF COMPLAINT

Some or all may be present:

- Signs of caudal lumbar pain
- Pelvic limb weakness/dragging
- Exercise intolerance/reluctance to exercise (especially jumping, rising, climbing stairs)
- Unilateral or bilateral pelvic limb lameness
- Paresthesia of the perineum and/or extremities (manifested by licking or chewing)
- Tail paresis/paralysis
- Urinary/fecal incontinence

PHYSICAL EXAM FINDINGS: Some or all may be present:

- Pain on hind limb or tail hyperextension
- Pain when digital pressure is applied to dorsal sacral/caudal lumbar vertebrae, with or without simultaneous lifting of the pubis
- Pain on rectal palpation of L7-S1 disk space

- Abnormal hind limb conscious proprioceptive response (monoparesis or paraparesis)
- Reduced hind limb flexor reflex (especially hock flexion)
- Exaggerated patellar reflex (pseudo-hyperreflexia)
- Unilateral or bilateral atrophy of sciatic-innervated muscles (hamstring, gastrocnemius, cranial tibial). Reduced perineal reflex
- Poor anal and urethral sphincter tone.
- Atonic bladder
- Decreased tail sensation

ETIOLOGY AND PATHOPHYSIOLOGY

- Large biomechanical forces are placed on the lumbosacral joint, which acts like a "hinge" between the stiff pelvis and the mobile spine. Presumably, the mechanical stress in the lumbosacral joint leads to early disk degeneration, destabilization of the disk space, and dorsal protrusion of the disk.
- Osteophytes may form adjacent to the unstable disk space and contribute to spinal canal stenosis along with the bulging disk, hyperplastic soft tissues, and sacral subluxation.

DIAGNOSIS

DIFFERENTIAL DIAGNOSIS

- Lumbosacral diskospondylitis
- Spinal cord, spinal nerve, or vertebral neoplasia
- Thoracolumbar disk disease
- Spinal trauma
- Degenerative myelopathy
- Coxofemoral arthritis/hip dysplasia
- Cranial cruciate disease
- Pelvic/sacral fracture(s)
- Fibrotic myopathy (semitendinosus, gracilis muscles)
- Prostatic disease

INITIAL DATABASE

- Complete blood count, serum biochemistry panel, urinalysis (older dogs).
- Survey radiographs (heavy sedation/general anesthesia) with evacuated colon, to rule out differential diagnoses (trauma, diskospondylitis). Radiographic changes associated with degenerative lumbosacral stenosis:
  - L7-S1 disk space narrowing.
  - Lumbosacral end-plate sclerosis, spondylosis deformans.
  - Ventral sacral subluxation.
  - Lumbosacral disk mineralization.
  - Note: These changes may also be identified in clinically unaffected dogs.

ADVANCED OR CONFIRMATORY TESTING

- Magnetic resonance imaging (MRI) is extremely useful for evaluating disk degeneration or nerve root compression (soft tissue) (Fig. I-111).
- Computed tomography gives excellent bone detail and can provide cross-sectional imaging. The soft tissue imaging is inferior to MRI, however.
- Myelography. Useful if the dural sac extends beyond the lumbosacral area. Contrast filling of the epidural space may be inconsistent and hard to interpret.
- Diskography. May demonstrate disk protrusion. Note: a normal disk can be injected with less than 0.2 ml contrast agent and a degenerated disk can often easily receive 1 to 3 ml.
- Electromyography (EMG) may delineate denervation. Normal EMG does not rule out lumbosacral stenosis.

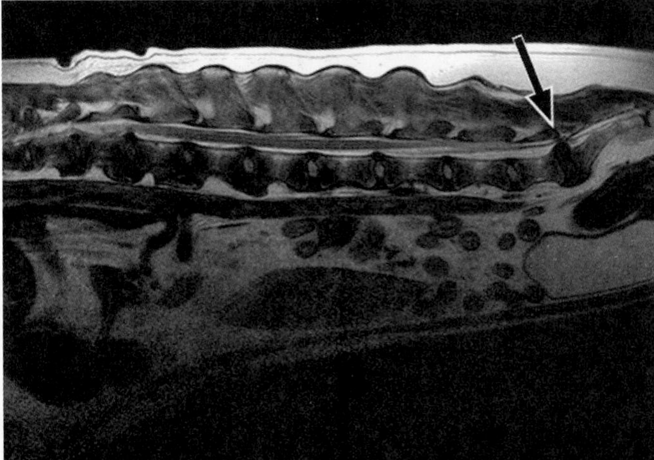

FIGURE I-111 Sagittal T2-weighted MRI of the lumbosacral spine of a mature dog with degenerative lumbosacral stenosis; cranial is to the left. The disk at the LS junction (*arrow*) is protruding into the spinal canal and shows low signal intensity consistent with degeneration.

TREATMENT

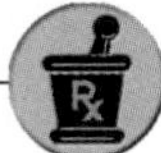

THERAPEUTIC GOAL(S)

- Pain relief
- Return to function

ACUTE GENERAL TREATMENT

- Conservative management: Strict rest (4 to 6 weeks), then gradually increased activity over 4 to 6 weeks. Anti-inflammatory/analgesic medication to control pain as needed. Consider codeine 1 mg/kg every 6 to 12 hours PO in combination with carprofen, or other nonsteroidal anti-inflammatory drug.
- Dogs with continuous pain or neurologic dysfunction are surgical candidates. Surgical treatment most frequently consists of spinal canal/nerve roots decompression through a dorsal laminectomy and, sometimes, foraminotomy.
- Distraction and stabilization of unstable LS space is possible with facet joint transarticular screws, in combination with decompression. May decrease the risk of recurrence.

CHRONIC TREATMENT

- Strict confinement necessary for 8 to 12 weeks after surgery, followed by gradual return to function over 2 months. Early excessive exercise associated with less favorable outcome.
- Sling support may be necessary in the early postoperative period. Urinary bladder management is imperative until there is normal voluntary voiding.

POSSIBLE COMPLICATIONS

- Laminectomy scarring
- Implant failure

PROGNOSIS AND OUTCOME

- Decompressive surgery provides a good to excellent long-term outcome in 78% to 97% of cases.
- Working dogs return to full function in 41-78% of cases.
- Recurrence rates have been reported as 3% in a population of primarily pet dogs, whereas more active or working dogs show recurrence rates of 18-54%. A second surgery can be beneficial in cases with recurrent clinical signs.
- Urinary or fecally incontinent dogs have less favorable outcomes.

PEARLS & CONSIDERATIONS

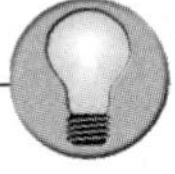

COMMENTS

- Transitional lumbosacral vertebrae and sacral osteochondrosis have been asso-

ciated with lumbosacral stenosis, but can also occur in normal dogs.
- Lumbosacral diskospondylitis can be difficult to distinguish from degenerative lumbosacral stenosis. In cases with osteolytic or severly proliferative changes, urine, blood and, if surgery is performed, the removed disk, should be submitted for bacterial and fungal culture.

SUGGESTED READING

Danielsson F, Sjostrom L: Surgical treatment of degenerative lumbosacral stenosis in dogs. *Vet Surg* 28:91, 1999.

De Risio L, et al: Predictors of outcome after dorsal decompressive laminectomy for degenerative lumbosacral stenosis in dogs: 69 cases (1987-1997). *J Am Vet Med Assoc* 219:624, 2001.

Sjostrom L: Lumbosacral disorders. Degenerative lumbosacral stenosis: Surgical decompression. In Slatter D (ed): *Textbook of Small Animal Surgery*, ed 3. Philadelphia, WB Saunders, 2003, pp 1227-1237.

AUTHOR: **BOEL A. FRANSSON**
EDITOR: **JOSEPH HARARI**

Lung Lobe Torsion

BASIC INFORMATION

DEFINITION

A rotation of a lung lobe along its long axis, with twisting of the bronchus and pulmonary vessels at the hilus

EPIDEMIOLOGY

SPECIES, AGE, SEX: Reported in dogs and cats, although rare in cats. Middle-aged dogs are more commonly affected. There is no gender predilection.

GENETICS AND BREED PREDISPOSITION
- Dogs with deep, narrow chests have a higher incidence.
  - Afghan hounds are overrepresented.
- Has been reported in small-breed dogs.

RISK FACTORS: Preexisting conditions leading to atelectasis of lung lobes such as:
- Pleural effusion
- Pneumothorax
- Trauma
- Surgical manipulation.

ASSOCIATED CONDITIONS AND DISORDERS
- Usually associated with massive pleural effusion.
- Associated with chronic respiratory disease, trauma, chylothorax, thoracic surgery, or neoplasia.

CLINICAL PRESENTATION

HISTORY, CHIEF COMPLAINT
- History of pneumothorax, pneumonia, or trauma
- Dyspnea
- Coughing
- Hemoptysis
- Anorexia with weight loss
- Exercise intolerance

PHYSICAL EXAM FINDINGS
- Muffled heart and lung sounds
- Crackles
- Coughing
- Hemoptysis
- Dyspnea

ETIOLOGY AND PATHOPHYSIOLOGY

- Spontaneous lung lobe torsion can occur.
- Any mechanism that increases the mobility of a lung lobe can lead to the development of torsion.
- Torsion of a lung lobe leads to venous congestion from occlusion of twisted pulmonary veins of the affected lobe and lung consolidation.
  - Persistent venous congestion leads to pleural effusion.

DIAGNOSIS

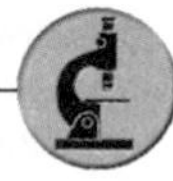

DIFFERENTIAL DIAGNOSIS

- Other causes of pleural effusion:
  - Hydrothorax
  - Hemothorax
  - Chylothorax
  - Pyothorax
- Pneumonia
- Pulmonary thromboembolism
- Pulmonary contusion
- Pulmonary neoplasia
- Pulmonary atelectasis
- Diaphragmatic hernia

INITIAL DATABASE

- Results of complete blood count, biochemistry panel, and urinalysis are variable.
  - Stress or inflammatory leukogram is possible.
- Analysis of pleural fluid may reveal a sterile, inflammatory serosanguineous effusion or chyle.
- Thoracic radiographs show pleural effusion and lung consolidation.
  - Large volume pleural effusions may obscure lung atelectasis. Therefore repeating radiographs after thoracocentesis is important.
- Thoracic ultrasound reveals "hepatization" of the torsed lung lobe, with fluid-filled bronchi having an appearance similar to hepatic vessels and fluid-filled pulmonary parenchyma resembling normal liver.

ADVANCED OR CONFIRMATORY TESTING

Rarely needed or used
- Bronchoscopy may demonstrate an obstructed orifice of the main bronchus supplying the affected lobe.
  - Bronchial mucosa may appear folded and edematous.
- Thoracic computed tomography may demonstrate anatomic alterations of the affected bronchus that suggest lung lobe torsion.
- For some patients, the diagnosis is confirmed at thoracotomy.

TREATMENT

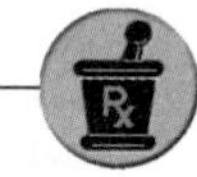

THERAPEUTIC GOAL(S)

- Improve respiratory function and stabilize the patient
- Lobectomy of the affected lobe

ACUTE GENERAL TREATMENT

- Thoracocentesis (see Thoracocentesis, p 1308)
- Oxygen by face mask, nasal cannula, or oxygen cage (see Oxygen Supplementation, p 1292)
- Fluid therapy as needed based on patient status, physical examination, and laboratory parameters

CHRONIC TREATMENT

- This is a surgical condition; spontaneous resolution is rare.
- Lobectomy of the affected lobe is the treatment of choice.

POSSIBLE COMPLICATIONS

- Torsion of another lung lobe is possible.
- Lung lobe torsion may lead to chylothorax.

RECOMMENDED MONITORING

- Vital signs
- Respiratory pattern
- Resolution of pleural effusion:
  - Thoracic radiographs.
  - Volume of fluid aspirated from chest tube in the postoperative period.
    - 1 ml/kg/day of fluid production is expected from the presence of the chest tube alone.
- Postoperative pain

PROGNOSIS AND OUTCOME

The prognosis is good if lung lobectomy is performed.

PEARLS & CONSIDERATIONS

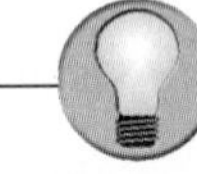

COMMENTS

- Any lobe can torse, but the right cranial and middle lung lobes are more frequently affected.
- Air bronchograms can be seen in affected lobes early in the process, but bronchial air is absorbed and replaced by fluid within 2 to 3 days.
- During lobectomy, clamp the affected pedicle with noncrushing forceps before derotation to help prevent release of toxins into the bloodstream.
- The use of automated stapling devices (TA-30 V3) simplifies the surgery and decreases surgery time.
- Submit excised lung for culture and histologic examination.

CLIENT EDUCATION

Animals with concurrent chylothorax may have a poorer prognosis.

SUGGESTED READING

Gelzer AR, et al: Accessory lung lobe torsion and chylothorax in an Afghan hound. *J Am Anim Hosp Assoc* 33(2):171–176, 1997.

Neath PJ, Brockman DJ, King LG: Lung lobe torsion in dogs: 22 cases (1981–1999). *J Am Vet Med Assoc* 217(7):1041–1044, 2000.

Siems JJ, Jakovljevic S, Van Alstine W: Radiographic diagnosis: Lung lobe torsion. *Vet Radiol Ultrasound* 39(5):418–420, 1998.

AUTHOR: **MICHAEL B. MISON**
EDITOR: **RANCE K. SELLON**

Lung Parasites

BASIC INFORMATION

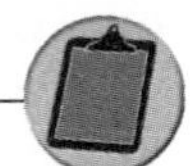

DEFINITION

Infestation of major airways or pulmonary alveoli with parasites such as *Oslerus osleri*, *Paragonimus kellicotti*, *Capillaria aerophila*, *Filaroides hirthi*, *Crenosoma vulpis*, or *Aelurostrongylus abstrusus*

SYNONYM(S)

Lungworms
O. osleri formerly was *F. osleri*

EPIDEMIOLOGY

SPECIES, AGE, SEX

- Dogs and cats:
  - Common parasites in dogs include *O. osleri*, *C. aerophila*, and *F. hirthi*.
  - Common parasites in cats include *P. kellicotti*, *C. aerophila*, and *A. abstrusus*.
- Clinical signs are most common in younger animals, but can be seen in animals of any age.
- No sex predisposition.

RISK FACTORS: Dogs clinically affected by *F. hirthi* often have concurrent immune system compromise.

GEOGRAPHY AND SEASONALITY: The fluke *P. kellicotti* is most often found in the southeast, Midwest, and Great Lakes regions due to the prevalence of the snail and crayfish intermediate hosts. *Crenosoma vulpis* is highly prevalent in Atlantic Canada (red fox reservoir).

ASSOCIATED CONDITIONS AND DISORDERS

- Eosinophilic pneumonia
- Pneumothorax

CLINICAL PRESENTATION

HISTORY, CHIEF COMPLAINT

- Infestation can be an incidental finding.
- Cough.
- Wheezes.
- Exercise intolerance.
  - Respiratory distress may be noted if pneumothorax is present.

PHYSICAL EXAM FINDINGS

- Cough may be elicited on tracheal palpation. However, this sign is nonspecific, and tracheal palpation may also elicit coughing in patients with other tracheal disorders, bronchial disorders, or pulmonary parenchymal diseases.
- Thoracic auscultation is usually unremarkable.
  - Wheezes or crackles can be heard in severely affected animals.

ETIOLOGY AND PATHOPHYSIOLOGY

- *O. osleri*:
  - Obtained via direct transmission (ingestion) of larvae in regurgitated food, feces, or saliva.
  - Adults live in carina and mainstem bronchi and cause local, nodular inflammation and fibrosis.
- *P. kellicotti*:
  - Obtained via ingestion of snail or crayfish intermediate host.
  - Adult flukes live in a subpleural cyst that communicates with a bronchus.
    - Rupture of cyst/bulla in patients with *P. kellicotti* can cause pneumothorax.
- *C. aerophila*:
  - Obtained via direct transmission (ingestion) of eggs in respiratory secretions or feces or by ingestion of earthworm intermediate host.
  - Adults live in bronchial mucosa.
- *F. hirthi*:
  - Obtained via ingestion of larvae in feces.
  - Adult worms live in lung parenchyma (alveoli and terminal airways).
- *A. abstrusus*:
  - Obtained via ingestion of snail or slug intermediate host or paratenic host such as birds and rodents.
  - Adults live in terminal bronchioles.
- Clinical signs reflect immune and inflammatory responses to parasites.

DIAGNOSIS

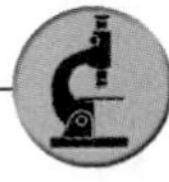

DIFFERENTIAL DIAGNOSIS

- Sterile chronic bronchitis
- Infectious tracheobronchitis
- Asthma
- Pulmonary edema
- Bacterial or fungal pneumonia
- Pulmonary metastatic disease
- Pneumothorax
- Eosinophilic bronchopneumopathy/pulmonary infiltrates with eosinophils

INITIAL DATABASE

- Thoracic radiographic abnormalities based on the causative organism:
  - *O. osleri*: tracheal and bronchial nodules.
  - *P. kellicotti*:
    - Solid or cavitary mass lesion, most commonly in the right caudal lobe.
    - Bulla may also be present.

- Pneumothorax.
- A bronchial or interstitial lung pattern is possible.
  - *C. aerophila*: normal or bronchial to bronchointerstitial pattern.
  - *A. abstrusus*: bronchial to diffuse miliary or nodular interstitial pattern.
  - *F. hirthi*: nodular interstitial pattern or alveolar infiltrates.
- No specific changes may be seen on complete blood count, serum biochemistry panel, or urinalysis.
  - Occasionally, eosinophilia is present, representing nonspecific parasitic infection or mucous membrane inflammation.

ADVANCED OR CONFIRMATORY TESTING

- Transtracheal or bronchial washes may demonstrate larvae or eggs.
- Bronchoscopy to identify nodules of *O. osleri*.
- Fecal examination may show eggs or larvae:
  - Zinc sulfate flotation or Baermann technique is recommended for identification of ova or larvae, respectively, of *O. osleri, A. abstrusus*, and *F. hirthi*.
  - Fecal flotations can identify *C. aerophila* ova.
  - High-density fecal flotation or fecal sedimentation is preferred for identification of *P. kellicotti* ova.

TREATMENT

THERAPEUTIC GOAL(S)

Eliminate infestation and decrease clinical signs secondary to inflammation

ACUTE GENERAL TREATMENT

- With severe respiratory signs (rare), oxygen administration may be necessary.
  - Although secondary inflammation is often seen with infection, corticosteroid therapy (anti-inflammatory doses) should be reserved for severe cases.
- Thoracocentesis for pneumothorax.
- Paraciticidal drugs:
  - Fenbendazole 50 mg/kg PO q 24h for 10 to 14 days can be used for all.
  - Other approaches include:
    - *O. osleri*:
      - Ivermectin 0.4 mg/kg PO, SQ every 3 weeks for 4 treatments.
    - *P. kellicotti*
      - Praziquantel 25 mg/kg PO q 8h for 3 days.
    - *F. hirthi*
      - Albendazole 25-50 mg/kg PO q 12h for 5 days, repeat in 3 weeks.

POSSIBLE COMPLICATIONS

Certain breeds of dogs (such as collies) should not be treated with ivermectin without testing for MDR (multiple drug resistance) gene mutations (see Ivermectin Toxicosis, p 610). Albendazole may cause bone marrow toxicity.

RECOMMENDED MONITORING

- Clinical signs
- Thoracic radiographs
- Fecal examinations

PROGNOSIS AND OUTCOME

The prognosis depends on degree of clinical signs and extent of disease, and is generally good for recovery with appropriate treatment.

PEARLS & CONSIDERATIONS

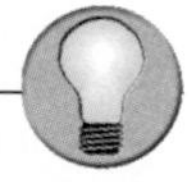

COMMENTS

Lung parasites should be considered in any young animal presenting for coughing and with radiographic evidence of interstitial or bronchial lung disease.

PREVENTION

Limit exposure to intermediate hosts

CLIENT EDUCATION

Reinfection is possible unless pets are limited in opportunities to ingest known paratenic hosts.

SUGGESTED READING

Hawkins EC: Diseases of pulmonary parenchyma. In Nelson RW, Couto CG (eds): *Small Animal Internal Medicine*. St. Louis, Mosby, 2003, pp 302–303.

Hawkins EC: Disorders of the trachea and bronchi. In Nelson RW, Couto CG (eds): *Small Animal Internal Medicine*. St. Louis, Mosby, 2003, pp 297–298.

Nelson OL, Sellon RK: Pulmonary parenchymal disease. In Ettinger SJ, Feldman EC (eds): *Textbook of Veterinary Internal Medicine*. St. Louis, Elsevier Saunders, 2005, pp 1254–1256.

AUTHOR: **LAURA G. RIDGE**
EDITOR: **RANCE K. SELLON**

Lymphadenopathy

BASIC INFORMATION

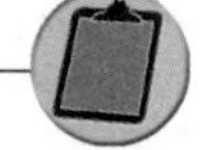

DEFINITION

Enlargement of a solitary, a regional group of, or all lymph nodes

SYNONYM(S)

Lymphadenomegaly

EPIDEMIOLOGY

SPECIES, AGE, SEX: Dogs and cats, any age, either sex.

GENETICS AND BREED PREDISPOSITION: Dogs: bullmastiff, rottweiler, retrievers, other breeds: lymphoma.

RISK FACTORS: Exposure to ticks and other vectors: infectious diseases.

CONTAGION AND ZOONOSIS: Exercise caution when aspirating lymph nodes, especially in animals with fungal disease (zoonosis via needlestick injury).

GEOGRAPHY AND SEASONALITY: Tick vectors are more prevalent in summer in the tropics. Many infectious agents have specific geographic areas of prevalence.

CLINICAL PRESENTATION

DISEASE FORMS/SUBTYPES: Solitary/regional versus generalized.

HISTORY, CHIEF COMPLAINT

- History: visits to geographic areas where certain infectious diseases are endemic.
- Clinical signs generally reflect the underlying disorder and are not directly caused by the lymphadenopathy.
  - Exception: if lymph node enlargement is marked: mechanical obstruction may cause dysphagia, respiratory stridor, regurgitation, cranial vena cava syndrome, swollen limb(s), and dyschezia.

PHYSICAL EXAM FINDINGS

- Evaluate all accessible lymph nodes during physical examination; the following nodes are readily palpable in dogs and cats (Table I-8):
  - Mandibular, prescapular (superficial cervical), axillary, superficial inguinal, and popliteal.
  - Node pain, erythema, heat, adherence of node to underlying tissue suggest lymphadenitis.

TABLE I-8 Selected Superficial Lymph Nodes of the Dog and Associated Anatomic Regions of Lymphatic Drainage

Lymph node (and alternative name)	Location	Distribution of lymphatics contributing to the node
Submandibular (mandibular)*	Ventral to the angle of the mandible; subcutaneous and mobile (versus mandibular salivary glands, which are deeper, fixed structures)	Most structures of the head, except for the external ear and some parts of the skin of the dorsal muzzle.
Prescapular (superficial cervical)*	Medial and dorsal to the point of the shoulder	Skin of the head, neck, and forelimb
Axillary	Dorsal to deep pectoral muscle and at the dorsal-most aspect of medial forelimb	Thoracic wall, deep structures of the forelimb
Inguinal (superficial inguinal)	Caudoventral abdomen, immediately caudal to the fifth mammary gland	Mammary glands, prepuce, scrotum, vulva, ventral abdominal wall up to the umbilicus
Popliteal*	Caudal surface of stifle (femorotibial joint)	All parts of the hind limb distal to the node
Sublumbar (medial or external iliac)	Trifurcation of aorta (dorsal surface of pelvic canal/abdomen); may be palpable per rectum	Genital system, caudal part of the urinary and digestive systems, pelvis, hind limbs, and dorsal half of the abdomen.

*Nodes that are normally palpable in the healthy dog.

- Patients with lymphadenopathy may show signs of systemic illness from underlying disease.
  - Signs generally are vague and include general malaise, pyrexia, anorexia, weight loss, lethargy and polyuria/ polydipsia; lacking diagnostic specificity.
- Patients with chronic leukemias, postvaccinal lymphadenopathies, and early lymphoma generally show subtle signs or no clinical signs at all.
- Evaluate for overtly apparent inciting causes.
  - For example, lesions of the foot (dermatosis, foreign body, neoplasm) if a single node proximal to a limb is enlarged.
- Fat surrounding lymph nodes is a common impostor for lymphadenopathy; the animal's overall body condition needs to be considered when suspecting lymphadenopathy.

ETIOLOGY AND PATHOPHYSIOLOGY

- Lymph nodes enlarge due to the proliferation of normal cells within them or to infiltration with either normal or abnormal cells.
- Reactive hyperplasia:
  - Proliferation of lymphocytes and plasma cells in response to antigens arriving through afferent lymphatics.
  - Occurs mostly in response to inflammation in the tissues drained by the lymph node.
  - After vaccination.
  - Immune-mediated diseases.
- Lymphadenitis:
  - Migration of inflammatory cells into the node, usually caused by infection (bacterial, rickettsial, fungal, parasitic, viral).
- Neoplasia:
  - Primary: lymphoma.
  - Secondary: carcinomas, melanomas, sarcomas, mast cell tumors.
- Extramedullary hematopoiesis (rare).
- Vascular changes: edema, congestion (rare).

DIAGNOSIS

DIFFERENTIAL DIAGNOSIS

- Generalized:
  - Reactive: systemic inflammation (infectious or noninfectious).
  - Lymphoma (most common), systemic mastocytosis, leukemia, multiple myeloma.
  - Nonspecific hyperplasia (mainly cats).
  - Rickettsial diseases.
  - Parasitic diseases.
  - Systemic fungal infections.
- Solitary or regional:
  - Superficial:
    - Abcessation (lymphadenitis)
    - Wounds, tick bites, and other inflammatory causes in the drained region
    - Metastatic neoplasia
  - Deep (visceral):
    - Systemic mycoses
    - Metastatic neoplasia

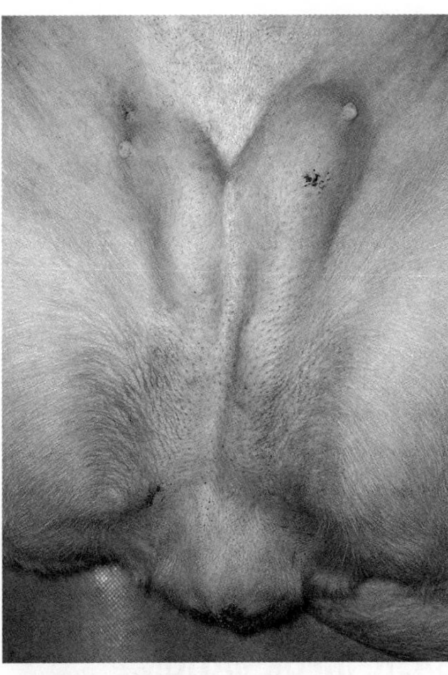

FIGURE I-112 Caudal ventral abdomen of a female dog; cranial is toward the top of the image. Marked, bilateral superficial inguinal lymph node enlargement is evident in this dog with vulvar inflammation. The caudal fifth (inguinal) mammary glands are normal and not palpable in this dog.

INITIAL DATABASE

- Review history for visits to areas where specific infectious diseases are prevalent.
- Complete blood count:
  - Anemia:
    - Anemia of chronic disease: inflammatory, infectious, or neoplastic disorders.
    - Hemolytic: hemoparasitic lymphadenopathies.
    - Nonregenerative: chronic ehrlichiosis, feline leukemia (FeLV), feline immunodeficiency virus (FIV), bone marrow neoplasia.
  - Circulating blasts: lymphoma, acute leukemia.
  - Eosinophilia: allergic, parasitic.
  - Neutrophilia: lymphadenitis, lymph node hyperplasia or neoplasia, depending on the degree of systemic involvement.
  - Thrombocytopenia: ehrlichiosis, lymphoma.
- Serum biochemistry profile:
  - Hypercalcemia: lymphoma, multiple myeloma, anal sac adenocarcinoma if sublumbar nodes are enlarged.

- ◦ Hyperglobulinemia: neoplasia, ehrlichiosis, chronic inflammatory diseases.
- Imaging: radiographs, computed tomography, and ultrasound to search for neoplasia and determine the extent of lymph node involvement.

ADVANCED OR CONFIRMATORY TESTING

- Fine-needle aspiration of lymph nodes allows classification of the disease process and frequently yields etiologic agents in infectious etiologies.
- Excisional lymph node biopsy (usually popliteal node) and histopathologic evaluation sometimes is necessary to confirm the diagnosis, especially in neoplasia and to perform immunophenotyping in lymphoma for prognostication.
- Aspiration and cytologic evaluation of spleen, liver, bone marrow.
- Test cats for FeLV, FIV.
- Antibody tests for agents such as *Blastomyces* or *Ehrlichia*.

TREATMENT

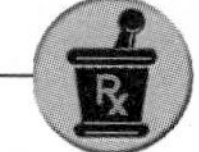

THERAPEUTIC GOAL(S)

- Generalized lymphadenopathy: Treat the underlying condition.
- Single node involvement: Treat the process in the area drained by the lymph node.

ACUTE GENERAL TREATMENT

Prompt therapy in cases where lymph nodes obstruct the airway or vessels.

CHRONIC TREATMENT

Chemotherapy protocols for lymphoma (see Lymphoma, Dog [Multicentric], p 658; Lymphoma, Cat [Multicentric], p 650; Lymphoma Chemotherapy Treatment Tables, Dog, p 655; Lymphoma Chemotherapy Treatment Tables, Cat, p 654)

POSSIBLE COMPLICATIONS

Acute tumor lysis syndrome (see Acute Tumor Lysis Syndrome, p 36)

RECOMMENDED MONITORING

Imaging to monitor response to therapy or detect recurrence of neoplasia

PROGNOSIS AND OUTCOME

Variable; determined by underlying cause

PEARLS & CONSIDERATIONS

COMMENTS

- Most dogs and cats with lymphadenopathy have lymph nodes that are firm, irregular, painless, nonadherent to underlying tissue and not warm to the touch.
- Nodes that are softer, warm, painful, and adherent to underlying tissue denote lymphadenitis.
- Metastatic lesions or lymphoma with extracapsular invasion of nodes are adherent to underlying tissue.
- Marked generalized lymphadenopathy (5 to 10 times enlarged) occurs almost exclusively in dogs with lymphoma or in cats with lymphoma or lymph node hyperplasia.
- Sublumbar lymph nodes can be palpated per rectum in small and medium-breed dogs.
- Lymphoma is a cytologic diagnosis (rarely, if ever, need to confirm with lymph node biopsy).

PREVENTION

Tick and flea control

CLIENT EDUCATION

Parasite control and early presentation for veterinary care

SUGGESTED READING

Couto CG: Lymphadenopathy and splenomegaly. In Nelson RW, Couto CG (eds): *Small Animal Internal Medicine*. St. Louis, Mosby, 2003, pp 1200–1209.

Day MJ, Whitbread TJ: Pathological diagnoses in dogs with lymph node enlargement. *Vet Record* 136:72, 1988.

Moore FM, et al: Distinctive peripheral lymph node hyperplasia of young cats. *Vet Pathol* 23:386, 1986.

AUTHOR: **JOHAN P. SCHOEMAN**
EDITOR: **ETIENNE CÔTÉ**

Lymphangiectasia/Protein-Losing Enteropathy

Client Education Sheet on Website

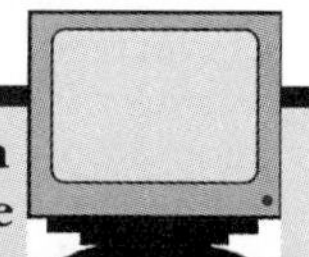

BASIC INFORMATION

DEFINITION

- Lymphangiectasia: dilation of the lacteals of the intestinal villi commonly resulting in protein-losing enteropathy (PLE).
- PLE: primary or secondary gastrointestinal (GI) disease resulting in nonselective loss of protein through the GI tract and hypoalbuminemia. Lymphangiectasia is one type of PLE.

EPIDEMIOLOGY

SPECIES, AGE, SEX

- Dogs are affected more commonly than cats.
- Age predilection dependant on underlying cause.
    - ◦ Yorkshire terriers with PLE caused by inflammatory bowel disease tend to be young to middle-aged.
- No gender predisposition.

GENETICS AND BREED PREDISPOSITION

- Basenji predisposed to immunoproliferative enteropathy.
- Lundehund predisposed to intestinal lymphangiectasia.
- Soft-coated Wheaten terrier predisposed to PLE and protein-losing nephropathy.
- Yorkshire terrier predisposed to inflammatory bowel disease and intestinal lymphangiectasia.
- Shar-peis have recently been reported to have PLE with intestinal inflammation.
- Rottweilers may also be predisposed to PLE from a variety of causes.

RISK FACTORS: Dependent on underlying cause of PLE.

CONTAGION AND ZOONOSIS: Dependent on underlying cause.

ASSOCIATED CONDITIONS AND DISORDERS

- Lymphangiectasia may be associated with primary GI disturbance affecting lacteals and lymphatics of the GI tract only, or may be caused by a disturbance of lymphatics much further "upstream," including the thoracic duct or other lymphatics in the abdomen.
- Any GI disorder may result in PLE and clinical signs identical to those of dogs with lymphangiectasia.
- Liver disease, especially associated with portal hypertension, hypoalbumenia, and coagulopathies.

- Right-sided congestive heart failure, which results in ascites and hypoalbuminemia may result in a PLE:
  - Pericardial disease resulting in cardiac tamponade
  - Cranial vena cava syndrome

CLINICAL PRESENTATION

HISTORY, CHIEF COMPLAINT

- Patients may show no overt clinical signs, with hypoalbuminemia found incidentally on screening tests.
- Variable clinical signs depending on underlying disease process.
- Weight loss commonly occurs and may be the only clinical sign.
- Intermittent vomiting.
- Chronic, small bowel diarrhea may or may not be present.
- Anorexia.
- Abdominal distention may be apparent if ascites is present.
- Respiratory distress possible with pleural effusion or pulmonary thromboembolism.
- Rare neurologic signs (i.e., seizures) or lameness due to thromboembolic disease.

PHYSICAL EXAM FINDINGS

- Weight loss, emaciation
- Thickened intestinal loops possibly apparent on abdominal palpation
- Ascites
- Peripheral edema
- Dyspnea or tachypnea with pleural effusion and/or pulmonary thromboembolism

ETIOLOGY AND PATHOPHYSIOLOGY

- Primary GI disease results in signs including vomiting, diarrhea, weight loss, and anorexia, the degree of which is determined by the extent of bowel affected.
- Hypoalbuminemia occurs when the loss of protein from the GI tract exceeds albumin synthesis by the liver.
  - Abnormal lymphatic drainage from lymphatic obstruction or elevated venous pressures result in protein leakage into the intestine.
  - Loss of the mucosal barrier and increased intestinal permeability with some diseases also result in leakage of protein into the intestinal lumen.
- Hypoalbuminemia results in decreased oncotic pressure and leakage of fluid into interstitial spaces, causing peripheral edema, ascites, and/or pleural effusion.
- Loss of anticoagulant proteins, including antithrombin, results in a prothrombotic state and predisposes to thromboembolic disease.

DIAGNOSIS

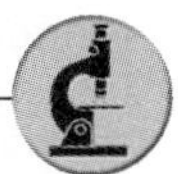

DIFFERENTIAL DIAGNOSIS

Differential diagnosis for lymphangiectasia and its associated PLE syndrome:

- Other protein-losing enteropathies
- Severe cutaneous disease resulting in hypoalbuminemia (e.g., massive burns)
- Protein-losing nephropathy:
  - Glomerulonephritis
  - Glomerular amyloidosis
  - Glomerulosclerosis
- Liver disease resulting in decreased albumin synthesis

INITIAL DATABASE

- Serum biochemistry profile:
  - Hypoalbuminemia is the hallmark of all PLEs including lymphangiectasia.
  - Globulins often are also decreased resulting in panhypoproteinemia but this finding is variable:
    - Inflammatory diseases such as immunoproliferative enteropathy in basenjis or histoplasmosis may produce elevated globulins resulting in normal total protein despite hypoalbuminemia.
  - Hypocholesterolemia, hypocalcemia (ionized and total), and hypomagnesemia also are common findings.
  - Liver enzymes may be slightly elevated with various GI diseases:
    - Serum bile acids are required to help rule out hepatic insufficiency as cause of hypoalbuminemia.
- Complete blood count:
  - Lymphopenia common.
  - Anemia possible, especially if GI ulceration is cause of PLE.
- Urinalysis is required to rule out proteinuria as cause of hypoalbuminemia:
  - Urine protein-to-creatinine ratio will help determine significance of any proteinuria. Normal <0.6.
- Abdominal radiographs often demonstrate loss of serosal detail due to ascites:
  - Underlying cause, such as an abdominal mass or foreign body, may also be apparent.
- Thoracic radiographs often show pleural effusion due to hypoalbuminemia:
  - Changes related to underlying etiology, such as pericardial disease, fungal disease, or metastatic neoplasia, may be seen.
- Abdominal ultrasound:
  - Thickened intestinal walls may be present, with or without normal layering.
  - Evaluation must include scanning for focal intestinal lesions that may not be accessible with endoscopy.
  - Lymphadenopathy is commonly detected.
- Fluid analysis of ascites is consistent with pure transudate.

ADVANCED OR CONFIRMATORY TESTING

- Canine fecal α_1-proteinase inhibitor can be assayed to confirm the presence of PLE:
  - α_1-Proteinase inhibitor is a protein similar in size to albumin so it is lost in the feces with albumin in protein-losing states.
  - Since it is an inhibitor of proteases, it is not degraded and can be measured in the feces to confirm PLE.
  - Three separate voided fecal samples are collected into calibrated fecal tubes supplied by the laboratory (GI laboratory, Texas A&M University) for analysis.
  - Primary use is confirming PLE in the presence of coexisting protein-losing nephropathy or liver disease.
- Microscopic examination of feces, including fecal flotations and direct smears, to identify intestinal parasites.
- Rectal scrapings can be performed and examined cytologically for histoplasmosis or lymphoma.
- Intestinal biopsies are necessary for diagnosis:
  - Intestinal biopsy can be performed with endoscopy, laparoscopy, or exploratory laparotomy.
  - General anesthesia can be a major risk in hypoalbuminemic patients and fluid and electrolyte imbalances should be stabilized before anesthesia.
  - In severely hypoalbuminemic patients, colloid therapy should be instituted before procurement of biopsy samples to reduce the degree of intestinal edema, as this can greatly interfere with the quality of biopsies (this is particulary important in endoscopic biopsy procedures) and with healing of biopsy sites (especially if surgical biopsies are obtained).
  - Endoscopy is minimally invasive and allows evaluation of intestinal mucosa for ulceration or dilated lacteals as well as collection of biopsy samples from stomach, duodenum, ileum, and colon.
  - Exploratory laparotomy allows visualization of abdomen and serosal surface of intestine with collection of full-thickness biopsies but carries a greater risk of infection or dehiscence, especially with hypoalbuminemic state.
  - Feeding corn oil or a fatty meal the night before laparotomy can increase the possibility of visualizing dilated lacteals or lymphatic ducts.

TREATMENT

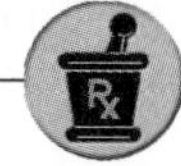

THERAPEUTIC GOAL(S)

- Treat underlying cause of lymphangiectasia and the resultant PLE
- Control peripheral edema and third space fluid accumulation
- Provide positive nutritional balance
- Control complications of hypoalbuminemia

ACUTE GENERAL TREATMENT

- Colloid support to improve fluid balance and minimize extravascular fluid accumulation:
  - Synthetic colloids, such as Hetastarch, improve oncotic pressure to decrease edema and ascites formation.
  - Fresh frozen plasma also improves oncotic pressure, and also supplies coagulation proteins, including antithrombin, to decrease the risk of thromboembolism, and albumin, which may be used for tissue repair.
  - Crystalloid support as necessary for fluid and electrolyte balance but should be given with colloid support to minimize extravascular fluid accumulation.
- Abdominocentesis/thoracocentesis:
  - Abdominocentesis or thoracocentesis is required if the patient is exhibiting respiratory distress due to body cavity effusion. See Abdominocentesis, p 1178; Thoracocentesis, p 1308; Abdominal Drainage, p 1176.
- Total parental nutrition or partial parenteral nutrition will help provide initial nutritional support pending diagnosis and may be essential in patients with severe intestinal lymphangiectasia that are unable to absorb nutrients. See Parenteral Nutrition, p 1296.

CHRONIC TREATMENT

- Effective treatment of lymphangiectasia requires treating the underlying cause, which is rarely possible with primary lymphangiectasia.
- Dietary therapy:
  - Ultra-low fat, easily digestible diets should be fed to patients with intestinal lymphangiectasia to minimize fat malabsorption and lymph accumulation. Hypoallergenic or low-residue diets may be fed to patients with concurrent inflammatory bowel disease to decrease the inflammatory response in the intestine; however, many hypoallergenic diets are not low enough in fat to be tolerated by lymphangiectasia patients. In these dogs, hydrolyzed diets or homemade, novel antigen diets that are ultra low in fat will be needed.
- Immunosuppressive agents should be used for decreasing inflammation associated with inflammatory bowel disease and intestinal lymphangiectasia:
  - Corticosteroid therapy decreases lipogranuloma formation that may obstruct intestinal lymphatics (e.g., prednisone 1-2 mg/kg PO q 12-24h, tapering to lowest effective dosage after 7 to 14 days or once control of clinical signs is achieved).
  - Corticosteroids as well as other immunosuppressive agents such as azathioprine, cyclosporine, or chlorambucil, are often necessary to effectively manage lymphangiectasia.
- Antibiotic therapy using metronidazole (e.g., 15 mg/kg PO q 12h × 1 week) or tylosin (5-10 mg/kg PO × 1 week) may help control secondary bacterial disturbances that occur as a result of lymphangiectasia.
- Thromboembolism prophylaxis is warranted (e.g., aspirin 0.5 mg/kg PO q 12h). Heparin therapy is expected to be suboptimal or ineffective with PLEs, as it acts by potentiating antithrombin III, and antithrombin III deficiency is the main cause of hypercoagulability in PLE.

POSSIBLE COMPLICATIONS

- Thromboembolic disease:
  - Patients may present with lameness, neurologic signs, or respiratory distress secondary to thromboembolic disease.
- Respiratory distress:
  - Patients may exhibit respiratory distress from severe ascites or pleural effusion necessitating abdominocentesis or thoracocentesis.
  - Pulmonary thromboembolism associated with the PLE of lymphangiectasia may also result in respiratory distress.

RECOMMENDED MONITORING

- Monitor third space or tissue fluid accumulation.
- Monitor albumin levels.
  - Unlike many other gastrointestinal diseases, PLE can be monitored objectively if no other disease processes are contributing to hypoalbuminemia.

PROGNOSIS AND OUTCOME

Long-term prognosis for dogs with PLE secondary to lymphangiectasia or inflammatory bowel disease is guarded to fair.

- Basenjis with immunoproliferative enteropathy have a guarded to poor prognosis.
- Yorkshire terriers also have a guarded prognosis as their inflammatory bowel disease or lymphangiectasia is often difficult to control.

PEARLS & CONSIDERATIONS

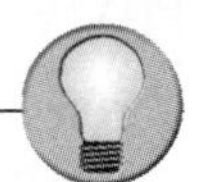

CLIENT EDUCATION

- Clients should be warned that intestinal lymphangiectasia and inflammatory bowel disease are usually lifetime problems requiring occasional adjustments to therapy.
- Dietary recommendations need to be strictly followed to minimize the chances of relapse.

SUGGESTED READING

Kimmel SE, et al: Hypomagnesemia and hypocalcemia associated with protein-losing enteropathy in Yorkshire terriers: Five cases (1992-1998). *J Am Vet Med Assoc* 217: 703-706, 2000.

Peterson PB, Willard MD: Protein-losing enteropathies. *Vet Clin Small Anim* 33:1061, 2003.

AUTHOR: **CHRISTOPHER J. JONES**
EDITOR: **DEBRA L. ZORAN**

Lymphedema

BASIC INFORMATION

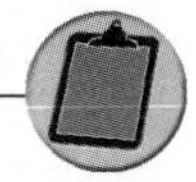

DEFINITION

Lymphedema is a swelling of protein-rich interstitial fluid caused by impaired lymphatic function. The condition can be localized, regional, or widespread. Lymphedema is classified as primary (developmental) or secondary in origin.

SYNONYM(S)

While not specific for lymphedema, other terms include:
Anasarca
Pitting edema
Subcutaneous edema
Ventral edema

EPIDEMIOLOGY

SPECIES, AGE, SEX: Lymphedema can affect dogs or cats. Primary lymphedema is most common in puppies and young dogs. Secondary lymphedema can affect animals of any age.

GENETICS AND BREED PREDISPOSITION: Primary lymphedema has been observed in English bulldogs, Labrador retrievers, and other purebred and mixed-breed dogs. Idiopathic lymphedema may be more common in giant breeds such as Irish wolfhounds.

RISK FACTORS: Primary lymphedema is developmental in origin; diseases that obstruct, invade, or destroy normal lymphatic drainage mechanisms predispose to secondary lymphedema.

ASSOCIATED CONDITIONS AND DISORDERS

- Neoplasm
- Trauma
- Infections
- Surgery
- Radiation therapy

CLINICAL PRESENTATION

DISEASE FORMS/SUBTYPES

- Localized involving a limb, intermandibular space, or ventral thorax
- Bilateral pelvic or forelimb lymphedema
- Generalized lymphedema (that may include pleural or peritoneal effusions)

HISTORY, CHIEF COMPLAINT

- In developmental lymphedema, the typical presentation is nonpainful, bilateral, pitting edema of the pelvic limbs. Generalized fluid retention is rare.
- In secondary lymphedema, there is nonpainful or painful swelling of the limb(s), ventral thorax, or intermandibular space.
- In generalized cases, respiratory distress may be related to pleural effusion.

PHYSICAL EXAM FINDINGS

- Nonpainful or painful swelling(s). In primary lymphedema pain typically indicates secondary infection.
- Regional lymph nodes may be underdeveloped or enlarged.
- Isolated swellings with pain or inflammation suggest cellulitis, trauma, or neoplasia.
- Intermandibular edema with normal jugular venous pressure is suggestive of lymphatic obstruction; with jugular distention, vena caval thrombosis or compression is more likely.
- Chronic lymphedema or that associated with lymphangitis may produce firm, nonpitting swellings, skin ulceration, or oozing of serum across the skin.

ETIOLOGY AND PATHOPHYSIOLOGY

- Lymph is produced by ultrafiltration of capillary blood and normally returns to the bloodstream across the venous end of capillaries and via lymphatic channels and lymph nodes. Lymph traverses the thoracic or lymphatic ducts to reach the systemic venous circulation.
- Malformation of the lymphatic system, lymphangitis, widespread obstruction to lymph drainage, or infiltration of regional lymph nodes can cause accumulation of high-molecular-weight protein and edema. Interstitial protein and fluid accumulation can initiate an inflammatory reaction and fibrosis.
- Progressive accumulation of lymphatic fluid leads to palpable swelling and impairs oxygen delivery, wound healing, and local resistance to infection.
- Gravitational forces influence the accumulation of tissue lymph.
- Lymphedema may be variable, pitting, nonpitting, or fibrotic in nature. These are well-recognized stages in human patients, and also may be observed in dogs or cats with chronic lymphedema.
- Strictly speaking, lymphedema stems from impaired lymphatic drainage. Subcutaneous edema also can be caused by reduced capillary oncotic pressure (hypoalbuminemia), increased vascular permeability, or elevated capillary hydrostatic pressure from venous obstruction, arteriovenous (AV) fistula, or right-sided congestive heart failure.

DIAGNOSIS

DIFFERENTIAL DIAGNOSIS

Lymphedema must be distinguished from other causes of tissue swelling, including:

- Overinfusion of sodium intravenous crystalloid; migration of subcutaneous fluids
- AV fistula
- Venous obstruction or thrombophlebitis
- Hypoproteinemia
- Localized infection
- Vasculitis
- Insect bites
- Postinfarction edema
- Right-sided congestive heart failure
- Cellulitis, abscess, or localized infection
- Infectious or immune-mediated skin disorders with secondary edema
- Chylous effusion
- Localized neoplasm
- Lymphatic tumors: lymphangioma and lymphangiosarcoma

INITIAL DATABASE

- Careful inspection of regional systemic veins
- Auscultation over swellings for bruit (continuous murmur) of AV fistula
- Rectal examination to identify mass lesions
- Complete blood count, serum biochemical panel, and urinalysis
- Chest radiographs: evaluate for heart disease, mediastinal mass, and pleural effusion
- Abdominal radiographs or ultrasonography: identify iliac lymphadenopathy or pelvic mass lesion
- Cytologic examination of regional lymph nodes or tissue fluid

ADVANCED OR CONFIRMATORY TESTING

- Culture and sensitivity (in cases of lymphangitis)
- Duplex Doppler ultrasonography to identify venous obstruction or AV fistula
- Lymphoscintigraphy or lymphangiography: advanced radiologic methods may demonstrate normal or abnormal lymphatic drainage
- Computed tomography to identify regional mass lesions

TREATMENT

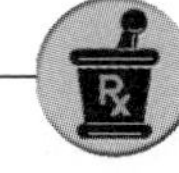

THERAPEUTIC GOAL(S)

- Correct the underlying disorder if possible
- Prevent or treat infections
- Protect swollen tissues from injury; consider lightly compressive bandages
- Improve macrophage function to reduce protein-rich edema
- Treat associated pain

ACUTE GENERAL TREATMENT

- Antibiotic treatment of infections
- Pain management for tense lymphedema or infection

CHRONIC TREATMENT

- Soft compression bandages (may not be well tolerated)
- Controlled exercise to enhance venous return
- Long-term use of benzopyrones, such as rutin, to enhance macrophage function and proteolysis
- Advanced surgical techniques are of uncertain value: consult with a surgical specialist

POSSIBLE COMPLICATIONS

Recurrent infection is likely even in cases of resolved primary lymphedema

RECOMMENDED MONITORING

- Limb size, firmness, and associated pain
- Use of affected limbs

PROGNOSIS AND OUTCOME

- Spontaneous resolution or marked improvement in some dogs with primary lymphedema
- Death or euthanasia related to complications of lymphedema
- Spontaneous death in puppies with generalized anasarca

PEARLS & CONSIDERATIONS

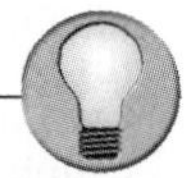

COMMENTS

- In primary lymphedema the swelling is typically caudal and bilateral; regional lymph nodes are difficult to find (whereas in healthy puppies superficial lymph nodes are prominent).
- A subtle pleural effusion in a dog with limb edema is suggestive of a more generalized lymphatic disorder (or hypoalbuminemia).
- When pelvic limb edema is caused by right heart failure, also expect ascites.
- A radiologist may be informative regarding advanced imaging methods.

CLIENT EDUCATION

- Observe the swelling for discharge, odor, or inability to use a limb
- Constitutional signs (anorexia, lethargy, fever) should prompt reevaluation

SUGGESTED READING

Fox PR, Petrie JP, Hohenhaus AE: Peripheral vascular disease. In Ettinger SJ, Feldman E (eds): *Textbook of Veterinary Internal Medicine*, ed 6. Philadelphia, Elsevier Saunders, 2005, pp 1145–1165.

AUTHOR: **JOHN D. BONAGURA**
EDITOR: **ETIENNE CÔTÉ**

Lymphoma, Cat (Multicentric)

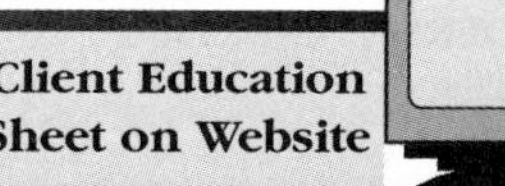

Client Education Sheet on Website

BASIC INFORMATION

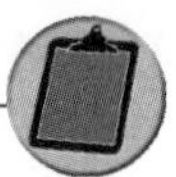

DEFINITION

A systemic malignant neoplasm of lymphoid origin

SYNONYM(S)

Lymphosarcoma
Malignant lymphoma

EPIDEMIOLOGY

SPECIES, AGE, SEX

- Lymphoma is the most common hematopoietic malignancy in the cat.
- May be less common than in the past, coincident with decreases in feline leukemia virus (FeLV) infection rates.
- May develop at any age.
- Siamese cats may be at increased risk for developing certain forms of lymphoma.

RISK FACTORS

- FeLV, and possibly feline immunodeficiency virus, infection are risk factors for the development of lymphoma.
  - FeLV status influences age and anatomic location at which lymphoma develops.
- Household exposure to environmental tobacco smoke (i.e., "second-hand smoke") increases the risk.
  - In one study, cats exposed to tobacco smoke had a 2.4-fold increased risk of lymphoma.
  - Risk increased with duration of exposure, years of exposure, and number of smokers in the house.

CLINICAL PRESENTATION

DISEASE FORMS/SUBTYPES

- Histologic grade:
  - High-grade, or lymphoblastic, lymphoma: most common; rapid onset and progression; affected cells are large and similar in appearance to lymphoblasts.
  - Low-grade, or lymphocytic, lymphoma: most often reported with gastrointestinal (GI) lymphoma; chronic insidious onset; affected cells are well-differentiated and similar in appearance to small lymphocytes.
- Anatomic distribution:
  - Multicentric: typically lymph node, spleen, or liver involvement; presenting signs and physical exam findings vary with organ(s) affected.
  - Alimentary (GI) (see also Lymphoma, Gastrointestinal, p 661): older cats; majority are FeLV negative; presenting signs include anorexia, weight loss, vomiting, diarrhea; physical examination may reveal palpable abdominal mass.
  - Mediastinal: young cats; most are FeLV infected; thymus, mediastinal and sternal lymph nodes may be involved; presenting signs include dyspnea, tachypnea; physical exam may reveal a noncompressible anterior mediastinum and also be suggestive of pleural effusion.
  - Renal: presenting sign is acute renal failure which may completely resolve with chemotherapy; physical exam reveals marked bilateral renomegaly; high rate of central nervous system relapse.
  - Spinal: affected cats are often FeLV infected; presenting sign is hind limb paraparesis; many will have malignant lymphoblasts concurrently in bone marrow. See also Lymphoma, Central Nervous System, p 652; Spinal Cord Neoplasia, p 1022.
  - Nasal: unique form of lymphoma, as it is often localized and may be treated best with radiation therapy.

HISTORY, CHIEF COMPLAINT

- Highly variable presentation (see Disease Forms/Subtypes above).
- Generalized peripheral lymphadenopathy, as is common in dogs with lymphoma, is rare in cats with lymphoma.

PHYSICAL EXAM FINDINGS: Physical exam findings vary and are reflective of organs involved (see Disease Forms/Subtypes above).

ETIOLOGY AND PATHOPHYSIOLOGY

- Rapid onset and disease progression
- Low-grade lymphoma, as reported with alimentary disease, may have chronic history

DIAGNOSIS

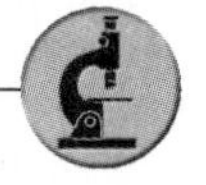

DIFFERENTIAL DIAGNOSIS

- Other neoplasms (e.g., leukemia, mast cell tumor)
- Multicentric: other neoplasms (e.g., mast cell tumor), cholangitis-cholangiohepatitis and other hepatopathies, pancreatitis
- Mediastinal: other neoplasms (e.g., thymoma, mesothelioma), heart disease, pyothorax, feline infectious peritonitis, diaphragmatic hernia
- Renal: acute renal failure, other renal failure, polycystic kidney disease
- Nasal: other neoplasms (e.g., adenocarcinoma), rhinitis, inflammatory polyps, cryptococcosis

INITIAL DATABASE

- Complete blood count. To identify anemia and/or other cytopenias that may develop secondary to lymphoblast infiltration in the marrow (leukemia) or secondary to immune-mediated destruction.
- Serum biochemistry panel. To identify liver or renal abnormalities that may develop secondary to organ involvement and may alter ability to eliminate chemotherapeutic drugs.
- Urinalysis ± urine culture. To further evaluate renal function, and to identify any occult urinary tract infection before chemotherapy.

- FeLV serology. FeLV antigenemia is associated with certain forms of lymphoma and may be prognostic (see Prognosis and Outcome below).
- Aspiration cytologic evaluation of affected organ(s). To identify lymphoblasts.

ADVANCED OR CONFIRMATORY TESTING

- Biopsy of affected organ(s). For definitive diagnosis and histologic grading.
- Thoracic radiographs. To identify lymphadenopathy, mediastinal mass, pulmonary involvement.
- Abdominal ultrasound examination. To identify changes consistent with hepatic, splenic, renal, or gastrointestinal involvement, lymphadenopathy.
- Bone marrow aspiration cytology. To identify marrow involvement and/or develop better understanding of etiology of a patient's cytopenias.
- Phenotyping (flow cytometry, immunocytochemistry, immunohistochemistry, polymerase chain reaction). To determine B- versus T-cell origin.

TREATMENT

THERAPEUTIC GOAL(S)

Chemotherapy is standard therapy for feline lymphoma. The objective goal of treatment is complete remission of the cancer while maintaining the subjective goal of an excellent quality of life for the patient.

ACUTE GENERAL TREATMENT

- Special handling requirements and potentially severe or life-threatening adverse patient effects exist with many of these chemotherapeutic drugs; these concerns, and rapid evolution of protocols, warrant consultation with/referral to an oncologist.
- Reports on single agent chemotherapy, including prednisone, doxorubicin, and mitoxantrone describe response rates ranging from 9-40% with remission durations ranging from 3 to 12 months. Prednisone may be used as a single agent, but its use before the initiation of other chemotherapy should be avoided, as this may decrease rate and duration of response to other agents.
  - Prednisone (20-40 mg/m² PO q 24-48h): mean survival of 1 month with spinal lymphoma.
  - Doxorubicin (25 mg/m² or 1 mg/kg IV q 21 days): 26% complete remission rate for median duration of 3 months.
- Improved remission rates and duration are achieved with combination chemotherapy. Numerous protocols are reported with variations in scheduling, drug dosages, and dose intensity, although most utilize induction followed by maintenance chemotherapy. The most commonly used agents in these protocols include prednisone, L-asparaginase, vincristine, cyclophosphamide, and doxorubicin. (See also Lymphoma Chemotherapy Treatment Tables, Cat, p 654, and Dog, p 655.) Complete response rates range from approximately 50-75% with remission durations of approximately 5 to 9 months. Options can include one of the following:
  - Cyclophosphamide, Vincristine (Oncovin), Prednisone (COP): 47-79% complete remission rate for median duration of 2.8 to 8.4 months; or
  - COP induction + doxorubicin maintenance: 47% complete remission rate for median duration of 9.4 months; or
  - Combination (cyclophosphamide, vincristine, prednisone, L-asparaginase, doxorubicin): 67% complete remission rate for median duration of 4.9 months; or
  - Combination (cyclophosphamide, vincristine, prednisone, L-asparaginase, doxorubicin, methotrexate): 38% complete remission rate for median duration of 9.2 months with alimentary lymphoma. Given the chronic indolent course of low-grade lymphoma, oral chemotherapy consisting of chlorambucil and prednisone may be more appropriate than intensive injectable chemotherapy for this group of cats.
    - Chlorambucil (6-8 mg/m² PO q 48h) and prednisone (20-40 mg/m² PO q 24-48h): 69% complete remission rate for median duration of 20.5 months in cats with low-grade alimentary lymphoma.
- Radiation therapy may be considered for nasal lymphoma.
  - Disease-free intervals of 6 to 69 months are reported after radiation therapy.
  - It has been suggested that radiation therapy, chemotherapy, or a combination of both modalities yield comparable survival times.

POSSIBLE COMPLICATIONS

- Systemic chemotherapy targets rapidly dividing cells. Due to their rapid and often abnormal division and defective repair mechanisms, tumor cells can be destroyed by chemotherapy.
- Some normal tissues have a high rate of cell turnover (GI mucosa, bone marrow, hair) and may be sensitive to chemotherapy, although unlike cancer cells, these normal tissues are able to repair chemotherapy-induced damage. Potential side effects of chemotherapy include GI upset 2 to 4 days after treatment, myelosuppression 7 to 10 days after treatment, and loss of whiskers.

RECOMMENDED MONITORING

- Regular monitoring of remission status.
  - Complete remission: disappearance of all clinical evidence of cancer.
  - Partial remission: decrease in volume of cancer by ≥50% without decrease to completely normal size.
  - Stable disease: decrease in volume of cancer by <50% or increase in volume of cancer by <25%.
  - Progressive disease increase in cancer volume by ≥25% or appearance of new lesions.
- Complete blood count (including differential) monitoring if administration of chemotherapy.

PROGNOSIS AND OUTCOME

Several prognostic factors may help predict an individual's response to treatment:

- Stage
- Substage (*a* is better than *b*)
- Anatomic site of disease (mediastinal lymphoma may have a higher complete remission rate than other anatomic sites; nasal lymphoma has among the longest survival times)
- FeLV status; FeLV status does not appear to influence rates of response to chemotherapy, but FeLV-positive cats have significantly shorter remission and survival times, possibly due in part to concurrent FeLV-related diseases

TABLE I-9 **Body Weight to Body Surface Area (BSA) Correlation for Cats**

Weight—kg (*lb*)	BSA (m²)
2 (*4.5*)	0.159
2.5 (*5.5*)	0.184
3 (*6.5*)	0.208
3.5 (*7.75*)	0.231
4 (*8.75*)	0.252
4.5 (*10*)	0.273
5 (*11*)	0.292
5.5 (*12.25*)	0.311
6 (*13.25*)	0.33
6.5 (*14.25*)	0.348
7 (*15.5*)	0.366
7.5 (*16.5*)	0.383
8 (*17.5*)	0.4
8.5 (*18.75*)	0.416
9 (*19.75*)	0.432
9.5 (*21*)	0.449
10 (*22*)	0.464

PEARLS & CONSIDERATIONS

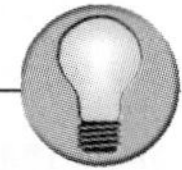

COMMENTS

Lymphoma is a common feline malignancy. The majority of cats achieve complete remission with chemotherapy, and treatment can be rewarding for both the pet owner and veterinarian. A variety of prognostic factors have been identified that may help predict an individual's response to treatment and guide the decision whether or not to pursue treatment. An understanding of the relative efficacy and potential toxicoses of the various protocols aids in determining the best treatment protocol for an individual patient.

SUGGESTED READING

Ogilvie GK, Moore AS: Lymphoma. In *Feline Oncology*. Trenton, NJ, Veterinary Learning Systems Co., Inc., 2001, pp 191-219.

Vail DM, MacEwen EG, Young KM: Feline lymphoma and lymphoid leukemias. In Withrow SJ, MacEwen EG (eds): *Small Animal Clinical Oncology*. Philadelphia, WB Saunders, 2001, pp 590-611.

AUTHOR: **LAUREL E. WILLIAMS**
EDITOR: **KENNETH M. RASSNICK**

Lymphoma, Central Nervous System

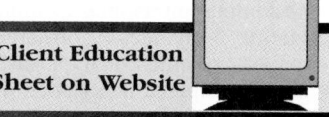

BASIC INFORMATION

DEFINITION

Lymphoma is a hematopoietic tumor originating from lymphoreticular cells. Central nervous system (CNS) lymphoma may be primary, occurring only within the CNS; or secondary, presenting as part of multicentric disease.

SYNONYM(S)

Lymphosarcoma

EPIDEMIOLOGY

SPECIES, AGE, SEX

- In dogs, the reported incidence of lymphoma ranges from 13 to 24 per 100,000 dogs.
  - Involvement of the CNS is uncommon, but the true incidence is not known.
  - There is no breed, age, or sex predilection.
- In cats, the reported incidence of lymphoma is 200 per 100,000 cats.
  - CNS involvement occurs in 5-10% of cases.
  - Although spinal cord involvement has been thought to be more common, a recent study found intracranial involvement to predominate. This may be a reflection of the decrease in the incidence of feline leukemia virus (FeLV) (see Associated Conditions and Disorders).
  - Cats of any age can be affected; those infected with FeLV tend to be younger (<5 years old).
  - A slight male predilection has been reported, likely reflecting the epidemiology of FeLV infection.
  - Domestic short-haired cats are most commonly affected, followed by domestic long-haired and Siamese cats.

ASSOCIATED CONDITIONS AND DISORDERS

- Feline leukemia virus (FeLV)
  - Approximately 20-25% of cats infected with the FeLV will eventually develop lymphoma.
  - The relative risk of lymphoma in FeLV-positive cats is 60 times that of FeLV-negative cats.
  - Approximately 90% of cats with spinal cord lymphoma test positive for FeLV. Most cats with brain lymphoma test negative.
- Feline immunodeficiency virus (FIV)
  - The relative risk of lymphoma in cats infected with FIV is 5 times that of noninfected cats.
  - FIV has been reported in association with CNS lymphoma, but many cats are not tested and the true contribution of FIV is not known.

CLINICAL PRESENTATION

DISEASE FORMS/SUBTYPES

- CNS lymphoma can be primary or secondary (see Definition).
  - In dogs, primary CNS lymphoma is uncommon. In cats, primary CNS lymphoma rarely occurs intracranially but accounts for up to 25% of spinal lymphomas.
  - In dogs, lymph nodes, liver, spleen, and bone marrow are among the sites affected concurrently. Up to 25-50% of dogs with CNS involvement do not have neurologic signs at initial diagnosis; neurologic signs instead develop when the cancer relapses.
  - In cats, bone marrow (often without circulating lymphoblasts), kidney, and liver are among the sites affected concurrently. Most cats present with neurologic signs at the time of initial diagnosis, but up to 50% of cats with renal lymphoma relapse with CNS involvement.
- CNS lymphoma can be categorized based on anatomic site.
  - Intracranial disease usually affects the prosencephalon (cerebrum and thalamus). A focal intraparenchymal mass is most common, followed by infiltration of the meninges. Rarely, intravascular localization is seen.
  - Cranial nerve involvement is more common in cats than dogs. Involvement of cranial nerves III-VIII has been reported. Tumors may extend along the floor of the cranial fossa to involve multiple nerves and compress the adjacent brain.
  - Spinal lymphoma lesions are usually solitary extradural masses compressing the thoracic or lumbar segments of the cord. Multifocal masses have been reported. Meningeal infiltration and extension into the subarachnoid space occur occasionally. Intramedullary lesions are uncommon.
  - Brachial plexus involvement may occur in both dogs and cats. Lesions may extend through the subarachnoid space and invade the spinal cord.

HISTORY, CHIEF COMPLAINT: Most patients present for neurologic abnormalities that are acute in onset and rapidly progressive.

- Patients with intracranial involvement commonly present for seizures, circling, blindness, behavior changes, and/or elevated third eyelid.
- Patients with spinal involvement present for ataxia and paresis/paralysis.

PHYSICAL EXAM FINDINGS

- Focal lesions in the cerebrum or thalamus are associated with seizures, behavior changes, blindness, conscious proprioceptive deficits with a normal gait, and circling.
- The clinical signs associated with cranial nerve deficits depend on the specific nerve(s) affected.
- Depending on the segments involved, spinal cord lesions can result in upper motor neuron signs (stiff ataxic gait, conscious proprioceptive deficits, spastic paresis/paralysis, hyperreflexia) and/or

lower motor neuron signs (short-strided gait, flaccid paresis/paralysis, hyporeflexia).
  - Signs may be bilateral but usually are asymmetric.
  - Focal hyperesthesia is also common.
- Brachial plexus tumors present with unilateral sensory and motor deficits based on the specific nerve roots affected.

ETIOLOGY AND PATHOPHYSIOLOGY

Etiology is unknown

DIAGNOSIS

DIFFERENTIAL DIAGNOSIS

- Intracranial lesions: other primary brain tumors (meningioma, glioma, ependymoma), toxoplasmosis, neosporosis, granulomatous meningoencephalitis (dogs), ischemic encephalopathy (cats)
- Spinal lesions: intervertebral disk disease, diskospondylitis, abscess, fibrocartilaginous emboli, spinal tumors (meningioma, nephroblastoma), vertebral tumors (osteosarcoma, chondrosarcoma, myeloma), feline infectious peritonitis virus (cats)
- Peripheral nerve lesions: neurofibroma, neurofibrosarcoma, trauma/avulsion, trigeminal neuritis (dogs)

INITIAL DATABASE

- Complete neurologic examination.
- Complete blood count (CBC), serum chemistry panel, urinalysis: usually unremarkable.
- FeLV/FIV serology (cats).
- Thoracic radiographs, abdominal ultrasound, and bone marrow aspiration: Screening for evidence of lymphoma in other organ systems may allow a diagnosis to be reached rapidly and less invasively.

ADVANCED OR CONFIRMATORY TESTING

- Advanced imaging of intracranial lesions:
  - Computed tomography (CT) identifies most but not all mass lesions caused by lymphoma. Lesions are characterized by a solitary ring-enhancing mass effect.
  - Magnetic resonance imaging (MRI) provides superior soft tissue detail compared to CT, and may be particularly beneficial for visualizing small focal lesions, diffusely infiltrative lesions, and intravascular CNS lymphoma.
- Advanced imaging of spinal lesions:
  - Plain radiographs are usually normal, but bony lysis occasionally is seen if lymphoma invades the adjacent vertebra(e).
  - Myelography accurately identifies spinal lesions and confirms extradural involvement, although normal results are occasionally obtained.
  - MRI may become the imaging modality of choice, but large-scale results have not yet been reported.
- Cerebrospinal fluid (CSF) analysis:
  - CSF usually is clear and colorless with an elevated cell count (mixed pleocytosis) and elevated protein content.
  - Neoplastic lymphoblasts are identified in up to 50% of cats with brain involvement, and 25% of cats with spinal cord involvement. They reportedly are identified in most dogs with either brain or spinal cord involvement but this is not uniformly accepted.
- To reach a definitive diagnosis, histopathology or cytology is required. For CNS lesions, this usually requires surgery or specialized equipment (fluoroscopy, stereotactic biopsy instruments). If possible, obtaining biopsy samples from other affected organs is preferable.

TREATMENT

THERAPEUTIC GOAL(S)

Complete remission: complete resolution of all clinical signs

ACUTE GENERAL TREATMENT

- Few reports on treatment exist, and optimum regimen(s) is/are not yet known.
- Lymphoma is usually a systemic disease, and therefore systemic chemotherapy is recommended.
  - Several protocols exist. The most commonly used protocols include the drugs L-asparaginase, vincristine, cyclophosphamide, doxorubicin, and prednisone. See Lymphoma, Dog (Multicentric), p 658; Lymphoma Chemotherapy Treatment Tables, Dog, p 655, and Cat, p 654 for dose and usage. Because these drugs are not routinely included in front-line lymphoma chemotherapy protocols, consultation with an oncologist may be warranted.
  - For tumors infiltrating the brain or spinal cord parenchyma, the ability of the drugs to penetrate the blood-brain barrier is of concern.
    - CCNU (lomustine) and cytosine arabinoside both cross this barrier and achieve therapeutic levels within the CNS; inclusion of these drugs into treatment protocols is reasonable. See Lymphoma, Cutaneous, p 657 for dose and usage.
    - Most spinal tumors are extradural; the blood-brain barrier should not interfere with the treatment of these tumors.
  - Single-agent prednisone may be used as a palliative treatment.
- Radiation therapy used in combination with chemotherapy may improve outcome.
  - Lymphocytes are exquisitely sensitive to radiation therapy, and rapid shrinkage of compressive tumors is often possible.
  - Radiation treatment fields may be focal, but more commonly include the entire brain and spinal cord.
- Surgery is indicated only when a biopsy is needed to confirm the diagnosis of lymphoma, or when rapid decompression of the brain or spinal cord is needed and radiation therapy is unavailable.

PROGNOSIS AND OUTCOME

- There is little information regarding the prognosis for dogs and cats with CNS lymphoma. Relatively few animals have been treated, and reported protocols are less aggressive than those currently recommended.
- The prognosis for dogs with CNS lymphoma is very guarded.
  - When treated with systemic chemotherapy, with or without radiation therapy, dogs have had reported survival times ranging from 1 to 3 months.
  - Prognosis may not always be as guarded as initially reported. One of the author's patients, diagnosed with secondary CNS lymphoma and treated with chemotherapy, lived almost 2 years from the time of initial diagnosis. Another dog with primary CNS lymphoma, treated with surgery and adjuvant CCNU, lived almost 1 year from the time of surgery.
- Reported survival times for cats with intracranial CNS lymphoma are up to 7 months.
  - Survival times were longer when a combination of radiation therapy and chemotherapy was used.
- For cats with spinal lymphoma treated with chemotherapy, remission rates are approximately 50%. Remission durations are typically 3 to 5 months, but some individuals may remain in remission for >1 year.
  - Cats that test positive for FeLV have remission rates similar to those for cats that test negative, but remission durations and survival times are significantly shorter.
  - FeLV is also associated with several other secondary problems, including blood dyscrasias and infectious diseases, which can make prognosis even more guarded.

PEARLS & CONSIDERATIONS

COMMENTS

- If a cat tests positive for FeLV or FIV, the owner should be educated about these diseases and all other cats in the household should be tested.
- Most spinal lymphoma is extradural; therefore, the blood-brain barrier should not interfere with the treatment of these tumors

SUGGESTED READING

Couto CG, et al: Central nervous system lymphosarcoma in the dog. *J Am Vet Med Assoc* 184:809, 1984.

Lane SB et al: Feline spinal lymphosarcoma: A retrospective evaluation of 23 cats. *J Vet Intern Med* 8:99, 1994.

Noonan M, Kline KL, Meleo K: Lymphoma of the central nervous system: A retrospective study of 18 cats. *Comp Contin Educ* 19:497, 1997.

Rosin A: Neurologic disease associated with lymphosarcoma in ten dogs. *J Am Vet Med Assoc* 181:50, 1982.

Spodnick GJ, et al: Spinal lymphoma in cats: 21 cases (1976–1989). *J Am Vet Med Assoc* 200:373, 1992.

AUTHOR: **DENNIS B. BAILEY**

EDITOR: **KENNETH M. RASSNICK**

Lymphoma Chemotherapy Treatment Tables, Cat

Client Education Sheet on Website

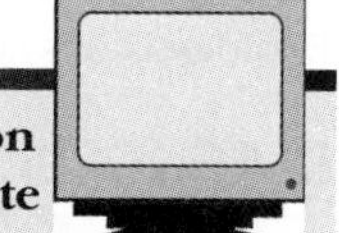

Special handing requirements and potentially severe or life-threatening adverse patient effects exist with many of these chemotherapeutic drugs; these concerns, and rapid evolution of protocols, warrant consultation with/referral to an oncologist.

TABLE I-10 COP Protocol for Cats

Week	1	2	3	4	5	6	7	8	9	10*
CBC	•	•	•	•			•			
CTX	•			•			•			•
VCR	•	•	•	•			•			•
PRED	•	•	•	•	•	•	•	•	•	•

*Continue with 3-week treatment cycle as long as complete remission persists.

CBC: complete blood count, to identify cytopenias that could contraindicate treatment. CTX, cyclophosphamide 200–250 mg/m² IV or PO single weekly dose; VCR, vincristine 0.5 mg/m² IV; PRED, prednisone 5–10 mg PO q 24h continuously.

Body surface area (m²): see Table I-9, Lymphoma, Cat (Multicentric), p 650.

TABLE I-11 Combination Protocol for Cats

Week	1	2	3	4	5	6	8	10	12	14
CBC	•	•	•	•	•	•	•	•		•
PRED	•	•	•	•	•	•	•	•	•	•
L-ASP	•									
VCR	•			•			•		•	
CTX		•			•			•		
DOX			•			•				
MTX										•

CBC: complete blood count, to identify cytopenias that could contraindicate treatment. PRED, prednisone 5–10 mg PO q 24h continuously; L-ASP, L-asparaginase 400 IU/kg SQ or IM; VCR, vincristine 0.025 mg/kg IV; CTX, cyclophosphamide 10 mg/kg single weekly dose IV; DOX, doxorubicin 20–25 mg/m² IV; MTX, methotrexate 0.5–0.8 mg/kg IV.

Weeks 1 through 6 are induction chemotherapy and following weeks are maintenance chemotherapy. The maintenance chemotherapy cycle (weeks 8 to 14) is repeated continuously for 12 months; the same drugs are then administered at 3-week intervals instead of 2-week intervals for 6 months, followed by monthly intervals for another 6 months.

Body surface area (m²): see Table I-9, Lymphoma, Cat (Multicentric), p 650.

BOX I-2 CBC Monitoring Guidelines: Cats

Dosage reduction:

- If neutrophils ≤1000 cells/μl on any complete blood count (CBC) → decrease dosage of causative agent by 25% for future treatments and begin empiric prophylactic antibiotics (e.g., amoxicillin-clavulanate 11–22 mg/kg PO q 12h) and consider additional supportive care and diagnostic testing if cat is overtly ill.
- If platelets ≤50,000 cells/μl on any CBC → decrease dosage of causative agent by 25% for future treatments.

Treatment delay:

- If neutrophils ≤2000 cells/μl on day treatment is due → postpone treatment, recheck CBC in 7 days, and resume treatment when neutrophil count is >2000 cells/μl.
- If platelets ≤50,000 cells/μl on day treatment is due → postpone treatment, recheck CBC in 7 days, and resume treatment when neutrophil count is >50,000 cells/μl.

Lymphoma Chemotherapy Treatment Tables, Dog

AUTHOR: **LAUREL E. WILLIAMS**
EDITOR: **KENNETH M. RASSNICK**

Client Education Sheet on Website

TABLE I-12 COP Protocol for Dogs

Week	1	2	3	4	5	6	7	8	9	10*
CBC	•	•	•	•			•			
CTX	•			•			•			•
VCR	•	•	•	•			•			•
PRED	•	•	•	•	•	•	•	•	•	•

*Continue with 3-week treatment cycle as long as complete remission persists.

CBC: complete blood count, to identify cytopenias that could contraindicate treatment. CTX, cyclophosphamide 200–250 mg/m^2 IV or PO single weekly dose (if cystitis occurs, substitute with chlorambucil at 1.4 mg/kg PO q 3 weeks [same interval as intended for cyclophosphamide]); VCR, vincristine 0.7 mg/m^2 IV; PRED, prednisone 30 mg/m^2 PO q 24h for 7 days, then 30 mg/m^2 PO q 48h continuously.

TABLE I-13 Madison-Wisconsin Protocol for Dogs

Week	1	2 3	4	5	6	7	8	9	11	13	15	17	
CBC	•	•	•	•	•	•	•	•	•	•	•		•
PRED	•	•	•	•									
L-ASP	•												
VCR	•		•			•		•		•		•	
CTX		•					•				•		
DOX				•					•				
MTX													•

CBC: complete blood count, to identify cytopenias that could contraindicate treatment. PRED, prednisone 2 mg/kg PO q 24h for 7 days (week 1), then 1.5 mg/kg PO q 24h for 7 days (week 2), then 1 mg/kg PO q 24h for 7 days (week 3), then 0.5 mg/kg PO q 24h for 7 days (week 4); L-ASP, L-asparaginase 400 IU/kg SQ or IM, to a maximum dose of 10,000 IU per administration; VCR, vincristine 0.5–0.7 mg/m^2 IV; CTX, cyclophosphamide 200 mg/m^2 IV single weekly dose (if cystitis occurs or if in complete remission at week 13, substitute with chlorambucil at 1.4 mg/kg PO instead, at the same interval as intended for cyclophosphamide) DOX, doxorubicin 30 mg/m^2 IV for dogs >15 kg or 1 mg/kg IV for dogs weighing <15 kg; MTX, methotrexate 0.5–0.8 mg/kg IV.

Weeks 1–9 are induction chemotherapy and weeks following are maintenance chemotherapy. The maintenance chemotherapy (weeks 11–17) are repeated. Doxorubicin is given one cycle and methotrexate is given the next cycle. Upon reaching the maximum cumulative dose of doxorubicin (180 mg/m^2), the doxorubicin is discontinued and methotrexate is given during the last week of the cycle. After week 25, the biweekly treatments are given every 3 weeks. After week 49, treatments instead can be given every 4 weeks. Chemotherapy is stopped at 168 weeks (3 years) if the dog is in complete remission.

TABLE I-14 NCACTP Protocol for Dogs

Week	1	2	3	4	5	6	7	8	9	10	11	12	13	14	15	16
CBC	•	•	•	•	•	•	•	•	•	•	•		•	•	•	•
PRED	•	•	•													
L-ASP	•															
VCR	•	•			•	•			•	•						
DOX			•				•				•					
CTX					•				•							
RT (cranial)													•			
RT (caudal)																•

CBC: complete blood count, to identify cytopenias that could contraindicate treatment. PRED, prednisone 30 mg/m² PO q 24h for 7 days, then 20 mg/m² PO q 24h for 7 days, then 10 mg/m² PO q 24h for 7 days; L-ASP, L-asparaginase 400 IU/kg SQ, to a maximum dose of 10,000 IU per administration; VCR, vincristine 0.7 mg/m² IV; DOX, doxorubicin 30 mg/m² IV for dogs weighing >15 kgs and 1 mg/kg IV for dogs weighing <15 kg; CTX, cyclophosphamide 200 mg/m² IV (if cystitis occurs, substitute with chlorambucil at 1.4 mg/kg PO instead, at the same interval as intended for cyclophosphamide]); RT, half-body radiation therapy given in two consecutive daily 4 Gy fractions.

TABLE I-15 VELCAP-S Protocol

Week	1	2	3	4	5	6	7	8	9	10	11	12
CBC	•	•	•	•	•	•	•	•	•	•	•	•
PRED	•	•	•	•	•	•	•	•	•	•	•	•
VCR	•	•	•				•					•
DOX				•					•			
CTX							•					•
L-ASP							•	•	•			

CBC: complete blood count, to identify cytopenias that could contraindicate treatment. PRED, prednisone 40 mg/m² PO q 24h for 7 days, then q 48h; VCR, vincristine 0.75 mg/m² IV; DOX, doxorubicin 25 mg/m² IV; CTX, cyclophosphamide 200 mg/m² PO (if cystitis occurs, substitute chlorambucil instead at 15 mg/m² PO daily for 4 consecutive days on same schedule); L-asparaginase 10,000 IU/m² IM, to a maximum dose of 10,000 IU per administration.

TABLE I-16 VELCAP-S Maintenance Protocol (used if first remission duration was <16 weeks from last induction chemotherapy, begins following repeat of initial 12-week protocol)

Week	15	18	21	24	25	27
CBC	•	•	•	•	•	•
PRED	•	•	•	•	•	•
VCR	•	•	•			•
DOX		•				•
CTX	•		•	•		
L-ASP				•	•	

CBC: complete blood count, to identify cytopenias that could contraindicate treatment. PRED, prednisone 40 mg/m² PO q 48h; VCR, vincristine 0.75 mg/m² IV; DOX, doxorubicin 25 mg/m² IV; CTX, cyclophosphamide 200 mg/m² PO (if cystitis occurs, substitute chlorambucil at 15 mg/m² PO daily for 4 consecutive days on same schedule); L-ASP, L-asparaginase 10,000 IU/m² IM, to a maximum dose of 10,000 IU per administration. From week 30, repeat weeks 12-18 every 9 weeks until week 52, then treatments are given every 4 weeks to week 78.

BOX I-3 CBC Monitoring Guidelines: Dogs

Dosage reduction:
- If neutrophils ≤1000 cells/μl on any CBC → decrease dosage of causative agent by 25% for future treatments and begin empiric prophylactic antibiotics (e.g., amoxicillin-clavulanate 11–22 mg/kg PO q 12h) and consider additional supportive care and diagnostic testing if animal is overtly ill.
- If platelets ≤50,000 cells/μl on any CBC → decrease dosage of causative agent by 25% for future treatments.

Treatment delay:
- If neutrophils ≤2000 cells/μl on day treatment is due → postpone treatment, recheck CBC in 7 days, and resume treatment when neutrophil count is >2000 cells/μl.
- If platelets ≤50,000 cells/μl on day treatment is due → postpone treatment, recheck CBC in 7 days, and resume treatment when neutrophil count is >50,000 cells/μl.

AUTHOR: **LAUREL E. WILLIAMS**
EDITOR: **KENNETH M. RASSNICK**

Lymphoma, Cutaneous

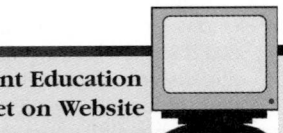

Client Education Sheet on Website

BASIC INFORMATION

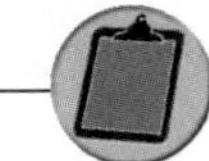

DEFINITION

A malignant neoplasm of lymphoid origin involving the skin or oral cavity. It may be primary, or secondary to other forms of lymphoma

SYNONYM(S)

Epitheliotropic lymphoma
Mycosis fungoides

EPIDEMIOLOGY

SPECIES, AGE, SEX

- Uncommon in dogs and rare in cats
- Usually affects older animals
- No gender predisposition

ASSOCIATED CONDITIONS AND DISORDERS: Sézary syndrome, a concurrent tumor cell population in peripheral blood.

CLINICAL PRESENTATION

DISEASE FORMS/SUBTYPES

- Epitheliotropic lymphoma: the more common form; lesions most commonly involve epidermis, superficial dermis, and periadnexa; oral mucosal form also described; T-cell origin; characteristic histologic feature is Pautrier's microabscesses (small aggregates of epitheliotropic lymphoid tumor cells in epidermis); protracted clinical course.
- Nonepitheliotropic lymphoma: uncommon; subcutaneous nodules; B-cell origin; more rapid onset and progression.

HISTORY, CHIEF COMPLAINT

- Epitheliotropic lymphoma may be divided into three stages:
  - Premycotic stage: erythematous lesions with varying degrees of depigmentation and alopecia over the trunk and neck which may progress to other body locations.
  - Mycotic stage: erythematous, raised, firm plaques which may be ulcerated and exudative.
  - Tumor stage: progressive thickening and proliferation of plaque lesions with ulceration; lymph node and/or other organ involvement possible.
- Nonepitheliotropic lymphoma in dogs presents as rapidly progressing and frequently multiple subcutaneous nodules.
- Cutaneous lymphoma in cats presents as progressive solitary or disseminated ulcerated plaques or nodules.

PHYSICAL EXAM FINDINGS

- Typical presentation of epitheliotropic lymphoma involves chronic, progressive, generalized exfoliative dermatitis with crusting, ulceration, and alopecia.
- Epitheliotropic lymphoma may present as solitary or multiple ulcerated plaques or nodules involving oral mucosa.
- Variably sized subcutaneous nodules are characteristic of nonepitheliotropic lymphoma.
- In cats, plaquelike lesions are most common; nodules and erythroderma are also possible; solitary lesions may be present initially with additional lesions developing as the disease progresses.

ETIOLOGY AND PATHOPHYSIOLOGY

Neoplastic lymphocytes in epitheliotropic lymphoma are T cells; CD3 and CD8 phenotype most common in dogs.

DIAGNOSIS

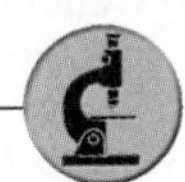

DIFFERENTIAL DIAGNOSIS

- Immune-mediated disease (e.g., pemphigus vulgaris, bullous phemphigoid, discoid lupus erythematosus)
- Allergic skin disease with pyoderma
- Infectious disease (e.g., dermatophytosis)

INITIAL DATABASE

- Complete blood count, serum biochemistry panel, urinalysis: typically unremarkable. Occasionally, circulating lymphoblasts may be present, consistent with Sézary syndrome.
- Skin biopsy: test of choice for establishing the definitive diagnosis of cutaneous lymphoma.

ADVANCED OR CONFIRMATORY TESTING

- Lymph node aspiration cytologic evaluation: to assess enlarged lymph nodes for lymphoma infiltration versus inflammation/reaction if severe dermatopathy
- Thoracic radiographs: to assess for pulmonary infiltration, intrathoracic lymph node enlargement
- Abdominal ultrasound: to identify changes consistent with hepatic or splenic involvement, lymphadenopathy, or other sites of lymphoma
- Bone marrow aspiration cytologic evaluation: to identify bone marrow involvement, particularly in cases with suspected Sézary syndrome (prognostic value)
- Phenotyping (flow cytometry, immunocytochemistry, immunohistochemistry): if uncertainty exists regarding the histologic diagnosis

TREATMENT

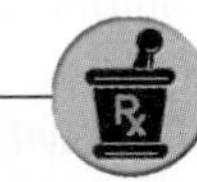

THERAPEUTIC GOAL(S)

Complete remission with resolution of lesions

ACUTE GENERAL TREATMENT

Canine epitheliotropic lymphoma:

- Oral differentiating agents:
  - Vitamin A analogs (isotretinoin 1-3 mg/kg PO q 24h): 45% response rate for 5 to 15 months.
- Topical agents:
  - Nitrogen mustard (25% solution applied once daily): anecdotal response reported; use is *not recommended* due to concern over human contact dermatitis and carcinogen exposure.
- Radiation therapy:
  - Total skin electron beam therapy may prove beneficial; however, current limited availability precludes wide application.
  - Other forms of radiation therapy may benefit patients with localized oral lesions or those with more generalized disease needing palliation of specific discrete skin lesions.
- Chemotherapy: Special handling requirements and potentially severe or life-threatening adverse patient effects exist with many of these chemotherapeutic drugs; these concerns, and rapid evolution of protocols, warrant consultation with/ referral to an oncologist. Chemotherapeutic drug options may include:
  - CCNU (lomustine; 60-70 mg/m^2 PO q 21 days): 15-30% CR rate and 50-60% PR rate for median duration of 3 to 4 months; or
  - Prednisone alone (20-40 mg/m^2 PO q 24-48h): 25-35% response rate.
  - Combination chemotherapy (see Lymphoma, Dog [Multicentric], p 658) has limited activity; response durations range from 2 to 16 weeks.
- Surgery:
  - May be beneficial for patients with solitary resectable oral lesions.
- Canine nonepitheliotropic lymphoma:
- Treat as for other forms of canine multicentric lymphoma.
- Feline cutaneous lymphoma:
- Consider treatment as for canine epitheliotropic lymphoma.

POSSIBLE COMPLICATIONS

See Lymphoma, Dog (Multicentric), p 658

RECOMMENDED MONITORING

Regular monitoring of remission status (see Lymphoma, Dog [Multicentric], p 658)

PROGNOSIS AND OUTCOME

Biologic behavior and response to treatment vary widely. Solitary epitheliotropic lymphoma oral lesions may respond well to local therapy (surgery, radiation therapy). Generalized epitheliotropic lymphoma may benefit from chemotherapy, and early results from the administration of oral CCNU are promising.

PEARLS & CONSIDERATIONS

COMMENTS

- Although rapid complete responses to treatment are uncommon and standard therapy in human medicine (topical chemotherapy or total skin electron-beam therapy) is not currently feasible in veterinary medicine, CCNU alone or in combination with prednisone may be considered a reasonable option for veterinary patients with epitheliotropic lymphoma.
- Most cases of cutaneous lymphoma are epitheliotropic, such that the terms cutaneous lymphoma and epitheliotropic lymphoma are often used interchangeably.
- Mycosis fungoides is cutaneous lymphoma, not a fungal disease.

SUGGESTED READING

Gross TL, Ihrke PJ, Walder EJ: Mycosis fungoides. In Gross TL, Ihrke PJ, Walder EJ (eds): *Veterinary Dermatopathology: A Macroscopic and Microscopic Evaluation of Canine and Feline Skin Disease*. St. Louis, Mosby, 1992, pp 158-161.

Ogilvie GK, Moore AS: Cutaneous lymphoma and mycosis fungoides (cutaneous T-cell-like lymphoma). In *Managing the Veterinary Cancer Patient*. Trenton, NJ, Veterinary Learning Systems Co., Inc., 1995, pp 496-499.

Scott DW, Miller WH, Griffen CE: Neoplastic and non-neoplastic tumors. In Scott DW, Miller WH, Griffin CE (eds): *Small Animal Dermatology*. Philadelphia, WB Saunders, 2001, pp 1330-1340.

Vail DM, MacEwen EG, Young KM: Canine lymphoma and lymphoid leukemias and feline lymphoma and leukemias. In Withrow SJ, MacEwen EG (eds): *Small Animal Clinical Oncology*. Philadelphia, WB Saunders, 2001, pp 558-607.

AUTHOR: **LAUREL E. WILLIAMS**
EDITOR: **KENNETH M. RASSNICK**

Lymphoma, Dog (Multicentric)

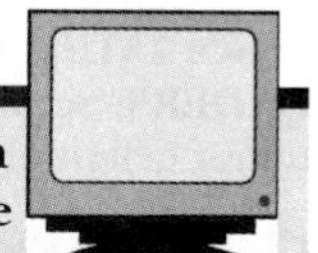

BASIC INFORMATION

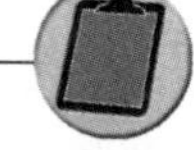

DEFINITION

A systemic malignant neoplasm of lymphoid origin

SYNONYM(S)

Lymphosarcoma
Malignant lymphoma
Non-Hodgkin's lymphoma (human)

EPIDEMIOLOGY

SPECIES, AGE, SEX

- Lymphoma is the most common hematopoietic malignancy in dogs, with an incidence of approximately 25 cases per 100,000 dogs.
- Affected dogs are typically middle-aged, although lymphoma may develop at any age.
- No gender predisposition.

GENETICS AND BREED PREDISPOSITION

- Several breeds are reported to be at increased risk, including golden retrievers, boxers, Scottish terriers, basset hounds, German shepherds, Saint Bernards, Airedales, bulldogs, and poodles.
- Genetic predisposition reported for a pedigree of bull mastiffs and for a family of rottweilers and otter hounds.

RISK FACTORS

- Reported association between herbicide use, particularly 2,4-D, and lymphoma, although a subsequent study failed to confirm this relationship.
- Reported positive association with electromagnetic radiation exposure.
- Residing in industrial areas and use of chemicals by the owners, specifically paints or solvents, are reported to increase risk of lymphoma by 8.5- and 4.6-fold, respectively.

ASSOCIATED CONDITIONS AND DISORDERS: Hypercalcemia secondary to elaboration of parathormone-related protein (PTH-rp) by tumor cells.

CLINICAL PRESENTATION

DISEASE FORMS/SUBTYPES

- Histologic grade:
  - High-grade, or lymphoblastic, lymphoma: most common; rapid onset and progression; affected cells are large and blastic in appearance

- Low-grade, or lymphocytic, lymphoma: rare; chronic insidious onset; affected cells are well-differentiated and similar in appearance to small lymphocytes
- Stage:
  - See Table I-17

HISTORY, CHIEF COMPLAINT

- Most typical presentation is generalized lymphadenopathy
- Owners usually report rapid increases in lymph node size over days to a few short weeks
- Lymph nodes are generally nonpainful and dogs usually appear otherwise healthy in the early stages of disease
- Some patients present for evaluation of nonspecific signs such as anorexia, weight loss, vomiting, diarrhea, dyspnea, and fever

PHYSICAL EXAM FINDINGS

- Marked generalized lymphadenopathy is the most common physical exam finding, although occasionally dogs will present with only single lymph node or regional lymph node enlargement.
- Hepatosplenomegaly may be noted in dogs with visceral involvement.
- Other physical exam findings, including dyspnea, fever, and neurologic signs, may be reflective of other organ involvement.

ETIOLOGY AND PATHOPHYSIOLOGY

- Rapid onset and disease progression
- If untreated, most dogs succumb to disease within 1 to 2 months

DIAGNOSIS

DIFFERENTIAL DIAGNOSIS

- Infectious diseases (e.g., Rocky Mountain spotted fever, ehrlichiosis, leptospirosis, bartonellosis)
- Sepsis
- Pyoderma causing lymphadenopathy
- Other neoplasms (e.g., leukemia, malignant histiocytosis)

INITIAL DATABASE

- Complete blood count. To identify anemia, thrombocytopenia (due to lymphoblast infiltration in the marrow or secondary to immune-mediated destruction), neutropenia, or the presence of circulating lymphoblasts (= leukemia).
- Serum biochemistry panel. To identify paraneoplastic hypercalcemia; to identify liver or renal value abnormalities which suggest organ involvement and may alter ability to metabolize chemotherapeutic agents.
- Urinalysis ± urine culture and sensitivity. To identify urinary tract infections as may be present secondary to immunocompromise; to identify isosthenuria which, if associated with azotemia, suggests renal failure (e.g., hypercalcemia-induced).
- Lymph node (or affected organ) aspiration cytology. May provide a definitive diagnosis of lymphoma.

ADVANCED OR CONFIRMATORY TESTING

- If lymphoma is identified cytologically, the following tests are indicated as part of routine staging in all cases of lymphoma, prior to initiation of chemotherapy:
  - Lymph node biopsy. For definitive diagnosis, histologic grading, and possibly for immunophenotyping.
  - Thoracic radiographs. To identify lymphadenopathy, cranial mediastinal mass, pulmonary involvement.
  - Abdominal ultrasound exam. To identify changes consistent with hepatic or splenic involvement, lymphadenopathy, or other sites of lymphoma.
  - Bone marrow aspiration cytology. To identify marrow involvement and/or develop better understanding of etiology of any cytopenias.
  - Phenotyping (flow cytometry, immunocytochemistry, immunohistochemistry, PCR). To determine B-cell versus T-cell origin (prognosis worse with T-cell).
- If financial restrictions prohibit these tests, one may elect to omit certain tests (e.g., if CBC results are unremarkable, one may elect not to perform a bone marrow aspirate) as long as the client understands that sites of disease may be missed and staging will be less certain.

TREATMENT

THERAPEUTIC GOAL(S)

Chemotherapy is standard therapy for the treatment of canine lymphoma. The objective goal of treatment is complete remission (CR) of the cancer while maintaining the subjective goal of an excellent quality of life for the patient.

ACUTE AND CHRONIC TREATMENT

- Special handling requirements and potentially severe or life-threatening adverse patient effects exist with many of these chemotherapeutic drugs; these concerns, and rapid evolution of protocols, warrant consultation with/referral to an oncologist.
- Reports on single-agent chemotherapy including prednisone, L-asparaginase, cyclophosphamide, and doxorubicin describe response rates ranging from 20–80% with remission durations of approximately 1 to 6 months. While prednisone may be used as a single agent, its use prior to the initiation of other chemotherapy should be avoided since this may decrease response rate and duration to other agents.
  - Prednisone: (20–40 mg/m^2 PO q 24–48h) approximately 50% of dogs achieve a complete or partial remission for duration of 2 to 3 months
  - Doxorubicin: (30 mg/m^2 IV q 21 days) 50–75% complete remission rate for 4 to 6 months
- Improved remission rates and duration are achieved with combination chemotherapy. Numerous protocols are reported with variations in scheduling, drug dosages, and dose intensity, although most utilize induction followed by maintenance chemotherapy. The most commonly used agents in these protocols include prednisone, L-asparaginase, vincristine, cyclophosphamide, and doxorubicin. Complete response rates range from approximately 65–90% with remission durations of approximately 6 to 11 months. (See Lymphoma Chemotherapy Treatment Tables, Dog, p 655.) Options can include one of the following:
  - COP (see Table I-13): 70–75% complete remission rate for median duration of 3.3 to 6 months; or
  - AMC protocol: 77% complete remission rate for median duration of 8.8 months; or
  - UMW protocol (see Table I-14): 84% complete remission rate for median duration of 8.4 months; or
  - ACOPA1: 76% complete remission rate for median duration of 11 months; or
  - ACOPA2: 65% complete remission rate for median duration of 9 months; or
  - VELCAP-L (see Table I-15): 69% complete remission rate for median duration of 13 months.

TABLE I-17 **Lymphoma Staging**

Stage	Characteristics
I	Single lymph node
II	Multiple regional lymph nodes
III	Generalized lymphadenopathy
IV	Hepatic and/or splenic involvement (with or without generalized lymphadenopathy)
V	Involvement of bone marrow, blood, and/or any nonlymphoid organ (± stages I-IV)
Substage a	No overt clinical signs of disease
Substage b	Overt clinical signs of disease are present

- Recent studies suggest that discontinuous chemotherapy protocols provide comparable remission duration to more traditional protocols relying on induction followed by maintenance chemotherapy.
  - VELCAP-S (see Table I-16): 68% complete remission rate for median duration of 10 months.
  - Modified UMW protocol: 92% complete remission rate for duration of 9.4 months.
- Chemotherapy remains standard therapy; however, its use in combination with other treatment modalities, such as radiation therapy, is being investigated with the hope of improving remission rates and duration. Early results suggest that half-body radiation therapy after induction chemotherapy is well tolerated and may increase remission duration compared to conventional protocols utilizing chemotherapy alone.
  - NCACTP protocol (see Table I-14): 78% complete remission rate for median duration of 16 months.
- Low-grade lymphoma: Given the chronic indolent course of low-grade lymphoma, oral chemotherapy consisting of chlorambucil (6–8 mg/m^2 PO q 48h) and prednisone (20–40 mg/m^2 PO q 24–48h) may be more appropriate than intensive injectable chemotherapy for this group of dogs.
- When a patient relapses and no longer responds to front-line chemotherapy, rescue chemotherapy can be considered.
  - MOPP: 30–35% complete remission rate and 35–50% partial remission rate for median duration of 1 to 2 months; or
  - Doxorubicin/DTIC: 35–80% complete remission rate for median duration of 3 months; or
  - CCNU: 25% complete and partial remission rate for median duration of 3 months.

POSSIBLE COMPLICATIONS

- Systemic chemotherapy targets rapidly dividing cells. Due to their rapid and often abnormal division and defective repair mechanisms, tumor cells can be destroyed by chemotherapy.
- Some normal tissues have a high rate of cell turnover (gastrointestinal mucosa, bone marrow, hair) and may be sensitive to chemotherapy, although unlike cancer cells, these normal tissues are able to repair chemotherapy-induced damage. Potential side effects of chemotherapy include gastrointestinal upset 2 to 4 days following treatment, myelosuppression 7 to 10 days after treatment, and hair loss in breeds with continuously growing haircoats (e.g., poodle, Lhasa apso, Old English sheepdog, many terrier breeds). See Chemotherapy: Adverse Reactions, p 189.

TABLE I-18 Body Weight to Body Surface Area (BSA) Correlation for Dogs

Weight—kg *(lb)*	BSA (m^2)
0.5 *(1)*	0.06
1 *(2)*	0.1
2 *(4.5)*	0.15
3 *(6.5)*	0.2
4 *(9)*	0.25
5 *(11)*	0.29
6 *(13)*	0.33
7 *(15.5)*	0.36
8 *(17.5)*	0.40
9 *(20)*	0.43
10 *(22)*	0.46
11 *(24.5)*	0.49
12 *(26.5)*	0.52
13 *(28.5)*	0.55
14 *(31)*	0.58
15 *(33)*	0.6
16 *(35)*	0.63
17 *(37.5)*	0.66
18 *(39.5)*	0.69
19 *(42)*	0.71
20 *(44)*	0.74
21 *(46)*	0.76
22 *(48.5)*	0.78
23 *(50.5)*	0.81
24 *(53)*	0.83
25 *(55)*	0.85
26 *(57)*	0.88
27 *(59.5)*	0.9
28 *(61.5)*	0.92
29 *(64)*	0.94
30 *(66)*	0.96
31 *(68)*	0.99
32 *(70.5)*	1.01
33 *(72.5)*	1.03
34 *(75)*	1.05
35 *(77)*	1.07
36 *(79)*	1.09
37 *(81.5)*	1.11
38 *(83.5)*	1.13
39 *(86)*	1.15
40 *(88)*	1.17
41 *(90)*	1.19
42 *(92.5)*	1.21
43 *(94.5)*	1.23
44 *(97)*	1.25
45 *(99)*	1.26
46 *(101)*	1.28
47 *(103.5)*	1.3
48 *(105.5)*	1.32
49 *(108)*	1.34
50 *(110)*	1.36
51 *(112)*	1.39
52 *(114.5)*	1.41
53 *(116.5)*	1.43
54 *(119)*	1.44
55 *(121)*	1.46
56 *(123)*	1.48
57 *(125.5)*	1.5
58 *(127.5)*	1.51
59 *(130)*	1.53
60 *(132)*	1.55
61 *(134)*	1.57
62 *(136.5)*	1.58
63 *(138.5)*	1.6
64 *(141)*	1.62
65 *(143)*	1.64
66 *(145)*	1.65
67 *(147.5)*	1.67
68 *(149.5)*	1.68
69 *(152)*	1.7
70 *(154)*	1.72
71 *(156)*	1.74
72 *(158.5)*	1.75
73 *(160.5)*	1.77
74 *(163)*	1.78
75 *(165)*	1.8
76 *(167)*	1.81
77 *(169.5)*	1.83
78 *(171.5)*	1.84
79 *(174)*	1.86
80 *(176.5)*	1.88

RECOMMENDED MONITORING

- Regular monitoring of remission status.
  - CR: disappearance of all clinical evidence of cancer.
  - PR: decrease in volume of cancer by ≥50% without decrease to completely normal size.
  - Stable disease (SD): decrease in volume of cancer by <50% or increase in volume of cancer by <25%.
  - Progressive disease (PD): increase in cancer volume by ≥25% or appearance of new lesions.
- Complete blood count (including differential) monitoring after administration of chemotherapy. See Chemotherapy: Adverse Reactions, p 189.

PROGNOSIS AND OUTCOME

Several prognostic factors have been identified that may help predict an individual's response to treatment:

- Gender (females better than males)
- Weight (small dogs better than large dogs, although possibly influenced by dosing regimen)
- Histologic grade (high-grade lymphoma has a better complete remission rate than low-grade, although low-grade is often associated with comparable survival times with less intensive chemotherapy due to its chronic indolent nature)

- Stage and substage (I, II, or III better than IV or V; *a* better than *b*)
- Phenotype (B-cell better than T cell)
- Hypercalcemia (a negative prognostic indicator, likely due to its association with T-cell phenotype)
- Presence of a mediastinal mass (a negative prognostic indicator, likely due to its association with T-cell phenotype)
- Administration of prior prednisone (negative prognostic indicator, possibly due to induction of multidrug resistance or masking of higher-stage disease)
- Other factors conferring a more negative prognosis: AgNOR staining, chromosomal aberrations, age, anorexia, fever, dyspnea, thrombocytopenia, hypoalbuminemia, and chronic inflammatory disease

PEARLS & CONSIDERATIONS

COMMENTS

- Lymphoma is a common canine malignancy.
- The majority of dogs with lymphoma achieve complete remission when treated with chemotherapy, and treatment can be very rewarding for both the pet owner and veterinarian.
- A variety of prognostic factors have been identified that may help predict an individual's response to treatment and guide the decision whether or not to pursue treatment.
- An understanding of the relative efficacy and potential toxicoses of the various protocols aids in determining the best treatment protocol for an individual animal.
- Differentiation of cell type (phenotype) is mainly prognostic. B-cell lymphoma carries a more favorable prognosis than T-cell lymphoma ("B is better"), and B-cell lymphoma makes up the majority of cases of lymphoma in dogs.

SUGGESTED READING

Ogilvie GK, Moore AS: Lymphoma in dogs. In *Managing the Veterinary Cancer Patient*. Trenton, NJ, Veterinary Learning Systems Co., Inc., 1995, pp 229–249.

Vail DM, MacEwen EG, Young KM: Canine lymphoma and lymphoid leukemias. In Withrow SJ, MacEwen EG (eds): *Small Animal Clinical Oncology*. Philadelphia, WB Saunders, 2001, pp 558–590.

AUTHOR: **LAUREL E. WILLIAMS**

EDITOR: **KENNETH M. RASSNICK**

Lymphoma, Gastrointestinal

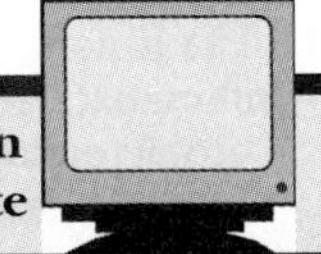

Client Education Sheet on Website

BASIC INFORMATION

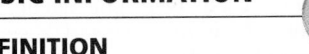

DEFINITION

Gastrointestinal lymphomas (GI LSA) are malignant tumors of lymphoid cell origin that can arise at any location within the gastrointestinal tract, including the stomach, small intestine, colon and rectum. Lesions may be of B-, T-, or large granular lymphocyte subtype, a distinction that is important prognostically.

SYNONYM(S)

Alimentary lymphoma
Alimentary lymphosarcoma
Gut-associated lymphoid tissue (GALT) lymphoma
Large granular lymphocyte lymphoma
Mucosal associated lymphoid tissue (MALT) lymphoma
Neoplasm of globule leukocytes

EPIDEMIOLOGY

SPECIES, AGE, SEX: GI LSA is the second most common form of lymphoid malignancy in dogs (after multicentric lymphoma), accounting for 5–7% of all LSA.

- Dogs with gastrointestinal lymphosarcoma are middle-aged to older (mean 7.7 years in one study).
- No sex predisposition is reported.
- In the cat, the alimentary form of LSA is currently the most prevalent anatomic form, since feline leukemia virus (FeLV) infection as a cause of mediastinal and multicentric LSA in young cats has been largely curtailed by vaccination and management strategies.
    - Cats with GI LSA are typically older (7 to 10 years) although the disorder can occur in much older and also younger cats.
- No sex predisposition is noted in cats.

GENETICS AND BREED PREDISPOSITION

- Dog breeds predisposed include boxers, shar-peis, golden retrievers, springer spaniels, Doberman pinschers, Labrador retrievers, and German shepherds.
- No breed predisposition is noted in cats.

RISK FACTORS: Etiology of most cases of alimentary LSA is unknown.

- Chronic inflammatory bowel disease is a predisposing factor.
- Epidemiologic studies implicate exposure to phenoxy herbicides (2,4-D) and environmental cigarette smoke in lymphomagenesis.
- *Helicobacter pylori* infection is implicated in human GI LSA, but that association has not been established in veterinary medicine.
- Underlying immune disorders may predispose.

CONTAGION AND ZOONOSIS: No infectious or zoonotic cause is known in dogs. In cats, retroviral infection with FeLV and/or FIV is rarely found associated with GI lymphomagenesis.

ASSOCIATED CONDITIONS AND DISORDERS

- Anemia and panhypoproteinemia may occur secondary to chronic GI blood loss.
- Hypercalcemia may be associated with canine GI LSA but is rare in cats.
- LSA metastatic to the liver may be associated with elevated liver enzymes and biliary obstructive disorders.

CLINICAL PRESENTATION

DISEASE FORMS/SUBTYPES

- Lymphoma of the gastrointestinal tract may be of B-, T-, or large granular lymphocyte (LGL) type. LGL lymphomas are typically of T-cell origin, although they can represent a null cell phenotype of natural killer (NK) cells.
- Lesions may be focal masses or diffusely infiltrative throughout the gut.
- Lesions may be submucosal, epitheliotropic, or transmural.
- GI LSA may be a low-grade disease of cellular accumulation due to impaired apoptosis, as in human MALT lymphoma, or may be high-grade with rapid cell replication.

HISTORY, CHIEF COMPLAINT: GI LSA is associated with gastrointestinal signs including:

- Evidence of malassimilation such as weight loss
- Anorexia
- Vomiting and diarrhea
- Melena, hematemesis, hematochezia

PHYSICAL EXAM FINDINGS

- On physical exam, these animals typically are thin and ill-kempt, especially cats.
- Signs of anemia (lethargy or weakness, hyperpnea, tachycardia) or hypercalcemia (muscle tremors) may be evident.
- Palpable abdominal masses and intraabdominal lymphadenomegaly may be noted.

- Hepatosplenomegaly may be present.
- In cases of diffuse intestinal infiltration, turgid, thickened intestinal walls may be palpated.
- Physical examination may be within normal limits.

ETIOLOGY AND PATHOPHYSIOLOGY

Most lymphomas are thought to arise secondary to abnormal somatic cell DNA recombination events, which may be random or may be induced by retroviral infection, environmental carcinogen exposure, or chronic infection/inflammation that increases lymphoid cell population expansion.

DIAGNOSIS

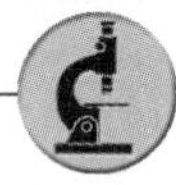

DIFFERENTIAL DIAGNOSIS

Depending on the form and location of the LSA lesion(s):

- Inflammatory bowel disease
- Chronic endoparasitism
- GI foreign body or intussusception
- Chronic pancreatitis (especially cats)
- Other causes of liver disease such as hepatitis, cholangiohepatitis, toxic hepatopathy, or feline hepatic lipidosis
- Benign GI disease such as gastric ulcer, polyp, or adenoma
- Other GI tumors including mast cell disease, adenocarcinoma, and mesenchymal tumors
- Granulomatous bowel disease secondary to bacterial (i.e., mycobacterium) or fungal infection (i.e., histoplasmosis)

INITIAL DATABASE

- Minimum database: complete blood count, serum chemistry panel, urinalysis, fecal examination for parasites, *Giardia* antigen test, thyroid assay in cats, FeLV/feline immunodeficiency virus (FIV) testing in cats
- Evaluation for chronic pancreatic or GI disease (trypsin-like immunoreactivity [TLI], cobalamin/folate, or pancreatic lipase immunoreactivity [PLI])
- Three-view thoracic radiographs
- Abdominal ultrasonography with guided fine-needle aspiration cytology

ADVANCED OR CONFIRMATORY TESTING

- Endoscopy for biopsy of gastric, duodenal, or colorectal lesions.
- Diagnosis is made histologically on endoscopic or full thickness surgical biopsies of affected tissues (gut, lymph nodes, etc.).
- Tumor staging for extent of systemic involvement:
  - Radiographs and ultrasound as described previously.
  - Bone marrow evaluation for staging and/or as indicated by cytopenias.
  - Peripheral node aspiration or biopsy for staging and/or as indicated for lymphadenomegaly.
- Immunohistochemical phenotyping for B-, T-, or LGL subtypes:
  - CD3 for T-cell subset.
  - CD79a or CD20 for B-cell disease.
  - CD3 and CD57 for LGL subtype.
  - Polymerase chain reaction for monoclonality by B-cell (IG gene rearrangement) or T-cell (T-cell receptor gene rearrangement) clonal expansion rather than polyclonal lesions seen in lymphoplasmacytic enteritis.

TREATMENT

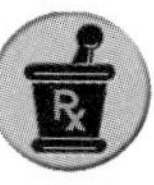

THERAPEUTIC GOAL(S)

- Focal GI LSA lesions can be surgically cured by excision with complete margins, when neoplastic cells have not yet disseminated.
- It is extremely unlikely that dogs and cats with diffuse, nodal, or visceral organ involvement will be cured.
- For most cases the goal is to prolong life with good quality, while avoiding adverse effects to therapy.

ACUTE GENERAL TREATMENT

General supportive care includes:

- Rehydration and restoring electrolyte homeostasis.
- Managing anemia with transfusions and hematinics as indicated by clinical condition.
- Antibiotic and emergency management for peritonitis.
- Analgesic management as indicated for pain in obstructive lesions or peritonitis.
- Promotility agents are contraindicated in obstructive disease.
- Management of hypercalcemia of malignancy by IV fluid and furosemide (1-2 mg/kg IV or PO q 12-24h) diuresis, possibly calcitonin (4-8 IU/kg IV, IM, or SQ q 12h) acutely. Management of hypercalcemia by treating the underlying malignancy should be started (corticosteroids, chemotherapy) only *after* the cytologic or histopathologic diagnosis of GI LSA is established, as treatment with corticosteroids or other lympholytic agents can compromise detection of lymphoma lesions.

CHRONIC TREATMENT

- Curative therapy for focal GI LSA lesions is through complete surgical excision.
  - Because of the high likelihood of systemic or local spread, these animals are followed with a course of lymphoma chemotherapy.
- Low-intensity radiation therapy may be palliative for refractory GI LSA.
- Chemotherapy is generally the treatment of choice for GI LSA.
- A number of chemotherapy protocols have been used to treat GI LSA, which include (see Lymphoma Chemotherapy Treatment Tables, Dog, p 655, and Cat, p 654):
  - For high-grade disease, the University of Madison-Wisconsin protocol involves:
    - Rotating sequential treatment with vincristine, L-asparaginase, prednisone, cyclophosphamide, doxorubicin over 25 weeks.
    - A concurrent combination form of this multidrug protocol called COPLA is less dose-intense, and thus has lower adverse effects for metabolically compromised patients.
    - CHOP therapy (cyclophosphamide, doxorubicin, vincristine, prednisone) may also be effective.
    - Single-agent doxorubicin, mitoxantrone, ifosfamide, or CCNU and combination therapy with doxorubicin/dacarbazine have been used as rescue agents for refractory or relapsed disease, with limited success.
  - For low-grade disease, treatment with milder chemotherapy protocols may be helpful in prolonging life with good quality. Low-grade protocols include:
    - Chlorambucil and prednisolone.
    - COP (cyclophosphamide, vincristine, and prednisone).

POSSIBLE COMPLICATIONS

- Surgical wound dehiscence with secondary peritonitis, pneumoperitoneum.
- Chemotherapy-induced leukopenia might predispose to infection.
- Chemotherapy-induced thrombocytopenia might increase tumor hemorrhage.
- Chemotherapy might result in perforation of transmural lesions.

RECOMMENDED MONITORING

- Ultrasonography is most sensitive for detecting intra-abdominal metastasis or recurrence, and may identify small amounts of peritoneal fluid as the first manifestation of peritonitis in cases of bowel rupture.
- Periodic restaging (physical examination monthly, laboratory evaluation, thoracic radiographs, abdominal ultrasound examination every other month) for patients in complete remission after surgical excision or completion of dose-intense

therapy with CHOP or University of Wisconsin-Madison protocol.

PROGNOSIS AND OUTCOME

GI LSA is a serious, life-threatening illness, but because of the widely differing biologic behaviors of various subtypes, predicting therapeutic response and duration of survival is difficult for individual cases.

- In general, low-grade disease is indolent and associated with longer survival than high-grade disease, depending on extent of disease at the time of diagnosis.
- T-cell phenotype is generally less responsive and associated with shorter survival duration than B-cell disease.
- Historically, median survivals for extranodal T-cell lymphomas were typically 6 months or less.
- Recent advances in aggressive multidrug combination chemotherapy protocols have resulted in longer survivals for dogs with T-cell LSA. In a cohort of dogs treated with high-grade combination chemotherapy, median duration of first remission ranged from 9 to 12 months, with survival medians out to 22 months for different disease subsets. Median duration of first remission for dogs with B-cell LSA was 12 months, whereas survival was 17 months in this study.
- Cats with low-grade GI LSA treated with minimal therapy may survive for years.

PEARLS & CONSIDERATIONS

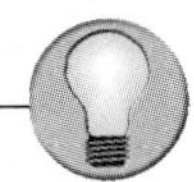

COMMENTS

- Full-thickness surgical biopsies may be necessary to establish a diagnosis of small intestinal LSA as endoscopic access is limited to the duodenum or ileum. Fine-needle aspiration cytology of intestinal wall is possible, but low-grade LSA is difficult to differentiate from reactive lymphocyte expansion.
- In general, the underlying cause of refractory diarrhea should be pursued aggressively, as GI LSA is an important differential diagnosis.
- Treatment with corticosteroids may impede the accurate diagnosis of LSA, as lymphoblasts will be rapidly lysed.

PREVENTION

- Aggressive management of lymphoplasmacytic enteritis is recommended, as some of these inflammatory bowel disease patients will progress to develop GI LSA.
- Managing endoparasitism and food allergies is theoretically important, but proof of benefit has not been established.
- Limiting exposure to lawn and agricultural chemicals and second-hand smoke is likely beneficial, but beyond these theoretical benefits, no specific preventive measures are known.

SUGGESTED READING

Coyle KH, Steinberg H: Characterization of lymphocytes in canine gastrointestinal lymphoma. *Vet Pathol* 41:141, 2004.

Richter KP: Feline gastrointestinal lymphoma. *Vet Clin North Am Small Anim Pract* 33:1083, 2003.

Zwahlen CH, et al: Results of chemotherapy for cats with alimentary malignant lymphoma: 21 cases (1993-1997). *J Am Vet Med Assoc* 213:1144,1998.

AUTHOR: **BARBARA E. KITCHELL**

EDITOR: **DEBRA L. ZORAN**

Macadamia Nut Toxicosis

BASIC INFORMATION

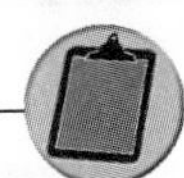

DEFINITION

Acute and often self-limiting toxicosis of dogs resulting from ingestion of macadamia nuts. It is characterized by paresis, depression, vomiting, ataxia, tremors, hyperthermia, abdominal pain, lameness, and/or stiffness. Toxicosis can occur after ingestion of commercially available macadamia nuts or macadamia nut–containing cookies or candies.

EPIDEMIOLOGY

SPECIES, AGE, SEX

- Currently, the syndrome has been described in dogs only.
- Dogs of all breeds, ages, and sexes are susceptible.

RISK FACTORS

- Dogs develop signs of toxicity after ingesting 2.2.-62.4 g/kg macadamia nuts.
- Dogs will readily eat large amounts of chocolate-coated macadamia nuts.

GEOGRAPHY AND SEASONALITY

- Macadamia nuts are obtained from *Macadamia integrifolia* and *Macadamia tetraphylla* trees mostly cultivated in Hawaii in the United States.
- Toxicosis can occur year-round, although it is more likely to occur during holiday seasons.

CLINICAL PRESENTATION

DISEASE FORMS/SUBTYPES

- Severity and onset of signs will depend on amount of macadamia nuts ingested.
- Majority of dogs show clinical signs within 12 hours after ingestion.
- Clinical signs usually resolve within 24 to 48 hours.

HISTORY, CHIEF COMPLAINT

- History of exposure to macadamia nuts
- Evidence of macadamia nuts in the vomitus or in the stool
- Hind limb weakness, depression, vomiting

PHYSICAL EXAM FINDINGS

- Hind limb weakness with no evidence of central nervous system involvement, musculoskeletal pain, or trauma
  - Rarely, generalized weakness is possible.
  - Forelimb weakness without hind limb weakness is inconsistent with macadamia nut toxicosis.
  - Respiratory muscle paralysis likewise has not been a feature of macadamia nut toxicosis in dogs.
- Mild tremor of hind limbs
- Depression
- Vomiting
- Ataxia
- Hyperthermia

ETIOLOGY AND PATHOPHYSIOLOGY

- Exact cause and mechanism of macadamia nut toxicosis are not clear
- Evidence suggests that the syndrome is dog specific
- Toxic principle in macadamia nuts is not known at this time

DIAGNOSIS

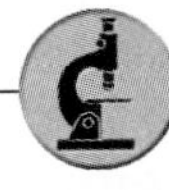

DIFFERENTIAL DIAGNOSIS

- Rule out other toxicoses that can cause hind limb weakness, ataxia, and vomiting:
  - Ethylene glycol
  - Cholinesterase inhibitor pesticides: organophosphates and carbamates
  - Marijuana (dogs)
  - Phenoxy herbicide (2, 4 D)
  - Coral snake bite
  - Bromethalin (dogs)

- Rule out nontoxic causes for hind limb weakness and ataxia (see Paresis, Hind Limb, p 813):
  - Systemic disturbances (e.g., anemia, acid-base or electrolyte abnormalities, cardiac arrhythmias)
  - Neuromuscular disorders (polyradiculoneuritis, myasthenia gravis, tick paralysis, botulism)
  - Orthopedic disorders
  - Trauma

INITIAL DATABASE

- Abdominal radiographs (may show a large amount of ingesta in the gastrointestinal tract).
- Examination of stomach contents for presence of macadamia nuts (if vomiting occurs).
- Rectal palpation may show presence of macadamia nuts in the stool.
- Body temperature.
- A complete medical examination is needed if concurrent ingestion of other harmful compound is suspected and to rule out any preexisting condition.

ADVANCED OR CONFIRMATORY TESTING

Serum biochemistry profile: Mild elevation in serum triglycerides and serum alkaline phosphatase may be noted but is nonspecific.

TREATMENT

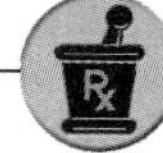

THERAPEUTIC GOAL(S)

- Decontamination of patient
- Supportive therapy

ACUTE GENERAL TREATMENT

- Decontamination of patient:
  - Emesis (in dogs not showing overt clinical signs within 2 to 4 hours after ingestion). See Vomiting, Induction of, p 1328.
    - Apomorphine (0.03-0.04 mg/kg IV or IM, or crush tablet portion with water and instill into conjunctival sac, rinse after emesis).
    - Hydrogen peroxide 3% (2 ml/kg, max 45 ml PO, repeat in 10 to 15 minutes if no vomiting).
  - Activated charcoal:
    - Give after inducing emesis or if a few hours have elapsed after exposure; administer activated charcoal (1-4 g/kg) with a cathartic such as 70% sorbitol (3 ml/kg) orally.
  - Supportive care:
    - Administer IV fluids as needed.
    - Thermoregulation (cold bath, cooling fans if needed).

RECOMMENDED MONITORING

Serum electrolytes, biochemistry profile, and triglycerides in severely affected dogs

PROGNOSIS AND OUTCOME

- Excellent prognosis
- Dogs recover with or without treatment within 24 to 48 hours

PEARLS & CONSIDERATIONS

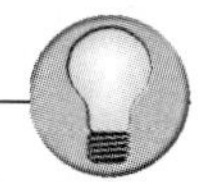

COMMENTS

- Consider concurrent methylxanthine (chocolate) toxicosis if macadamia nuts were covered with chocolate and if large amounts of macadamia have been ingested.
- Mild uncomplicated cases may resolve with home observation for 12 hours.

PREVENTION

Keep macadamia nuts out of reach of dogs

SUGGESTED READING

Hansen SR, Buck WB, Meerdink G, Khan SA: Weakness, tremors, and depression associated with macadamia nuts in dogs. *Vet Human Tox* 42(1):18-21, 2000.

AUTHOR: **MOAZZAM A. KHAN**
EDITOR: **SAFDAR A. KHAN**

Malassezia Dermatitis

BASIC INFORMATION

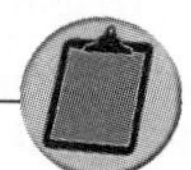

DEFINITION

An extremely common pruritic dermatosis caused by the overgrowth of *Malassezia* spp. yeast. Most infections are caused by the lipophilic organism *Malassezia pachydermatis*.

SYNONYM(S)

Malasseziasis
Yeast infection of the skin

EPIDEMIOLOGY

SPECIES, AGE, SEX: Dogs and cats; any age; either sex.

GENETICS AND BREED PREDISPOSITION: May occur in any breed of dog or cat. Terriers, spaniels, hounds, and shepherd dogs seem predisposed, as many of these breeds are commonly affected with underlying conditions favorable to yeast overgrowth.

RISK FACTORS: Underlying predisposing factors favorable to yeast overgrowth such as excessive sebum production, poor sebum quality, cutaneous moisture accumulation (particularly in skin folds), a disrupted epidermal surface, an altered host immune response, and concurrent dermatoses (e.g. hypersensitivities, endocrinopathies) are risk factors for *Malassezia* dermatitis. Specifically, hypersensitivities (Fig I-113), endocrinopathies, keratinization disorders, folliculitis, ectoparasitism, metabolic diseases, nutritional deficiencies, cutaneous or internal neoplasia, and feline retroviral infections are diseases favorable to yeast overgrowth.

CONTAGION AND ZOONOSIS: *Malassezia* yeasts were transmitted from the contaminated hands of dog-owning healthcare workers to infants in an intensive care nursery, causing mycotic sepsis; therefore *Malassezia* yeast should be considered a potential zoonotic agent especially in immunoincompetent individuals.

GEOGRAPHY AND SEASONALITY: *Malassezia* dermatitis may occur more frequently in humid geographic regions. Animals with underlying seasonal environmental allergies (e.g., atopic dermatitis) may have seasonal exacerbations of *Malassezia* dermatitis.

CLINICAL PRESENTATION

DISEASE FORMS/SUBTYPES

- Localized dermatitis: lesions involving the perioral region, chin, otic canal, ventral neck, axillae, interdigital web, nail fold, perianal area, or ventral tail surface
- Generalized dermatitis: lesions involving several regions as noted

HISTORY, CHIEF COMPLAINT: Intense pruritus is the most consistent reason for owners to seek veterinary care. Other common complaints include a rancid offensive odor; an oily coat; thickened, elephant-like skin; scaling (owners complain of "dandruff"); alopecia; erythroderma; and/or recurrent dermatitis not responsive to antibiotics or glucocorticoids.

PHYSICAL EXAM FINDINGS

- Skin lesions reflect the existing pruritus (excoriations) and seborrhea and are not specific for *Malassezia* dermatitis.
- Intertriginous areas (between skin folds) are typically affected (Fig I-114).

- Lesional skin may be erythematous, hyperpigmented, hyperkeratotic, lichenified, scaly, greasy or dry, alopecic, and saliva-stained.
- Many times, yellow to slate gray seborrheic plaques are evident in skin folds.
- A brown waxy discharge may be present in the nail folds, signifying paronychia.
- Follicular casts (keratosebaceous material adhered to the proximal hair shaft) might be suggestive of an underlying keratinization disorder.

ETIOLOGY AND PATHOPHYSIOLOGY

Malassezia yeasts are part of the normal skin microflora. They become opportunistic invaders when changes occur in the cutaneous microclimate (e.g., lipid composition, relative humidity) or defense mechanisms (e.g., epidermal barrier dysfunction, immunosuppression). Once colonization takes place, yeast may release proteases and lipases that alter the cutaneous surface, allowing for continued yeast overgrowth. In some dogs, specifically atopic ones with cytologic demonstration of the presence of yeast, *Malassezia* might be capable of eliciting a type-1 cutaneous hypersensitivity reaction.

DIAGNOSIS

DIFFERENTIAL DIAGNOSIS

- Hypersensitivities (e.g., environmental/atopic, food, flea, contact)
- Endocrinopathies (e.g., hyperadrenocorticism, hypothyroidism, hyperthyroidism, diabetes mellitus)
- Keratinization disorders (e.g., primary or secondary seborrhea)
- Folliculitis (e.g., demodicosis, dermatophytosis, bacterial)
- Ectoparasitism (e.g., sarcoptic mange, notoedric mange, cheyletiellosis)
- Metabolic diseases (e.g., hepatocutaneous syndrome/superficial necrolytic dermatitis, zinc-responsive dermatosis)
- Nutritional deficiencies
- Cutaneous or internal neoplasia
- Feline retroviral infections (e.g., feline leukemia virus/feline immunodeficiency virus)

INITIAL DATABASE

- Skin cytology:
  - Direct impressions or acetate tape preparations.
  - *Malassezia* are ovoid monopolar budding yeast that resemble the shape of footprints or peanuts. They are 3 to 8 µm in diameter (the same size as, or slightly smaller than, a red blood cell).
  - Best visualized using high power (40×) or oil immersion (100×).
- Multiple skin scrapings to exclude superficial and deep ectoparasites.
- Dermatophyte culture to rule out dermatophytosis.

ADVANCED OR CONFIRMATORY TESTING

- Biopsy and histopathologic analysis:
  - Findings suggestive of *Malassezia* dermatitis, but not specific to *Malassezia* dermatitis, include parakeratotic hyperkeratosis, epidermal hyperplasia, superficial perivascular dermatitis, and possibly eosinophilic microabscesses.
  - Occasionally, yeast may be found in the superficial keratin layer and/or in hair follicles.
  - Other histopathologic findings may represent changes associated with the underlying dermatosis.
  - Loss of surface scale during processing may decrease chance of finding yeast organisms.
- Elimination diet trial to exclude underlying food allergy.
- Intradermal and/or serum allergy testing if history and clinical findings are supportive of atopic dermatitis.
- Complete blood count, serum chemistry panel, and urinalysis to screen for internal diseases.
- Hormonal testing (e.g., screening tests for hyperadrenocorticism, hypothyroidism, and diabetes mellitus).
- Feline retroviral testing.

TREATMENT

THERAPEUTIC GOAL(S)

- Reduce pruritus
- Identify and control concurrent skin diseases or predisposing factors
- Remove surface seborrhea
- Eliminate yeast organisms

ACUTE GENERAL TREATMENT

- Antiseborrheic and antiyeast topical therapies (e.g., sulphur/salicylic acid, benzoyl peroxide, selenium sulfide, boric/acetic acid, miconazole, clotrimazole, ketoconazole, terbinafine, enilconazole, lime sulfur, or chlorhexidine) can be applied daily to weekly depending on the formulation used (e.g., shampoo, solution, lotion, spray, wipe, powder).
- Systemic antifungal therapy may be warranted for severe infections or those not responding to sole topical therapy. Duration of systemic therapy is largely based on clinical and cytologic improvement. Griseofulvin has no effect against *Malassezia* species.
  - Ketoconazole 5-10 mg/kg PO q 12-24h for 15 to 30 days with food.
  - Itraconazole 5-10 mg/kg PO q 24h for 15 to 30 days with (capsules) or without (suspension) food.
  - Fluconazole 2.5-10 mg/kg PO q 24h for 15 to 30 days (generic available in some countries).
  - Terbinafine 30 mg/kg PO q 24h for 15 to 30 days with food.
  - Because dogs with *Malassezia* dermatitis frequently have concurrent staphylococcal pyoderma, treating any secondary bacterial infection with oral antibiotics at an appropriate dose and duration (minimum 21 days) will help improve cutaneous signs.

CHRONIC TREATMENT

- Therapy for underlying predisposing diseases.
- Topical antiseborrheic and/or antiyeast therapy at reduced frequencies of application if possible.
- Azole pulse therapy can be used for remitting and relapsing episodes of *Malassezia* dermatitis as these drugs concentrate in the skin. Typically, the same initial dose is prescribed for 2 consecutive days per week or given daily for 1 week on/1 to 4 weeks off cycles after the initial induction dose described in Acute Treatment above.

DRUG INTERACTIONS

Azole therapy may alter the metabolism or distribution of other prescribed medication by inhibiting cytochrome P-450 metabolizing enzymes and P-glycoprotein transporting pumps. Terbinafine does not inhibit these enzymes.

POSSIBLE COMPLICATIONS

- Idiosyncratic cutaneous adverse reactions to topical therapies (e.g., pruritus, erythroderma, papular rash, pustulation, vesiculation, necrosis, ulceration) may occur on the patient or person applying therapy and must be considered, along with reassessment of possible underlying causes, in "refractory" cases of *Malassezia* dermatitis.
- The patient may have adverse reactions to systemic azoles (e.g., vomiting, diarrhea, hepatotoxicity, vasculitis, lightening of haircoat, pruritus). Ketoconazole may inhibit cortisol synthesis at doses greater than 10 mg/kg/day.

RECOMMENDED MONITORING

- Clinical signs and skin cytology every 2 to 4 weeks during therapy
- Other monitoring recommendations are at the discretion of the clinician based on underlying predisposing diseases

PROGNOSIS AND OUTCOME

- Failure to detect and treat underlying problems will result in partial treatment success, treatment failure, or relapse.

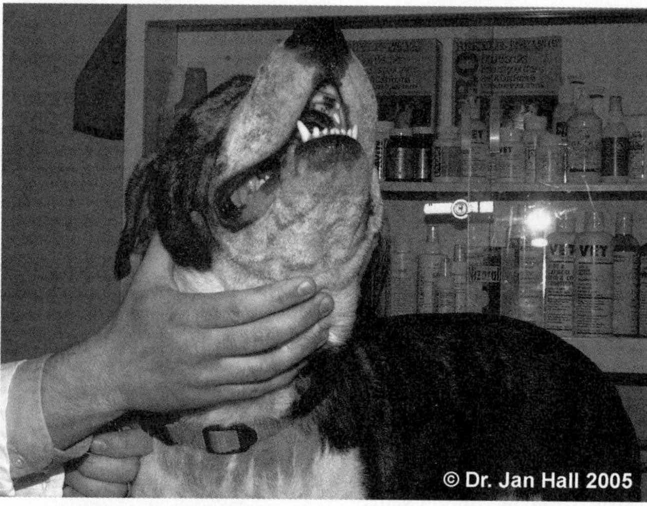

FIGURE I-113 *Malassezia* dermatitis secondary to food allergy in a 2-year-old female spayed American Staffordshire dog. Courtesy of Dr. Jan A. Hall.

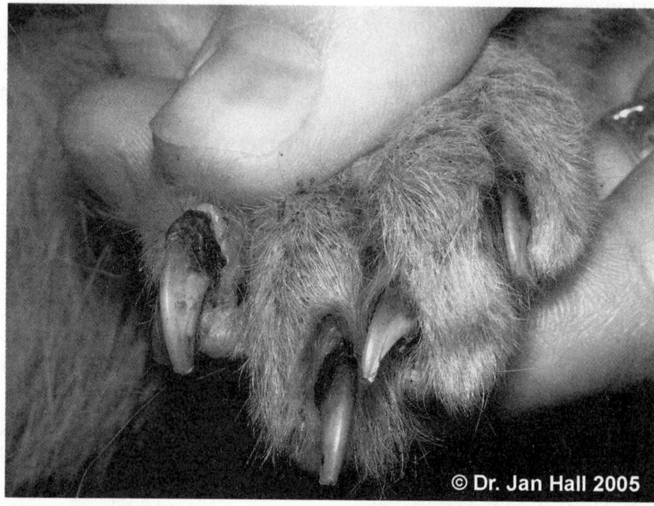

FIGURE I-114 *Malassezia* dermatitis affecting the nail beds secondary to paraneoplastic skin disease in a 15-year-old domestic short-haired cat. Courtesy of Dr. Jan A. Hall.

- For noncurable diseases (e.g., primary keratinization disorders), therapy for *Malassezia* dermatitis may need to be lifelong.

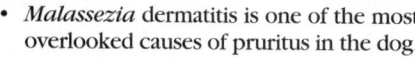

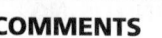

PEARLS & CONSIDERATIONS

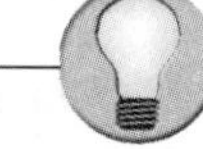

COMMENTS

- *Malassezia* dermatitis is one of the most overlooked causes of pruritus in the dog.
- *Malassezia* dermatitis tends to occur in areas rich in sebaceous glands, high in relative humidity, and commonly associated with allergic dermatitis.
- How many yeast are cytologically significant? Finding any yeast from typical clinical lesions is significant.
- Dogs with atopic dermatitis may be hypersensitive to *Malassezia* resulting in yeast numbers disproportionate to the level of pruritus experienced by the animal.
- Skin culture for *Malassezia* yeast is not recommended in clinical practice, as these organisms are residents on the skin.
- Biopsy with histopathologic evaluation is not considered superior to cytologic evaluation for the diagnosis of *Malassezia* dermatitis (most of the surface scale is lost during biopsy processing), but may be useful in the diagnosis of primary skin disorders in addition to which *Malassezia* dermatitis is a secondary phenomenon.
- Do not use selenium sulfide on cats, as it is too irritating to their skin.
- Enilconazole is not approved for small animal use in some countries.
- Griseofulvin has no effect against *Malassezia* species.
- Cats tend to have gastrointestinal upset with oral ketoconazole, so itraconazole is preferred.
- When given in tablet or capsule form, the azole drugs ketoconazole and itraconazole are best absorbed systemically if administered with food; failure to do so may reduce bioavailability of these important (and expensive) drugs by up to 40%.

PREVENTION

Treating for all underlying predisposing factors favorable to yeast overgrowth.

SUGGESTED READING

Chen T-A, et al: The biology of *Malassezia* organisms and their ability to induce immune responses and skin disease. *Vet Dermatol* 16:4-26, 2005.

Patterson AP, et al: How to diagnose and treat *Malassezia* dermatitis in dogs. *Vet Med* 97:8, 2002.

Rosales MS, et al: Comparison of the clinical efficacy or oral terbinafine and ketoconazole combined with cephalexin in the treatment of *Malassezia* dermatitis in dogs—a pilot study. *Vet Dermatol* 16:171-176, 2005.

AUTHOR: **ADAM P. PATTERSON**
EDITOR: **JAN A. HALL**

Malignant Fibrous Histiocytoma

BASIC INFORMATION

DEFINITION

A primary tumor made up of fibrous and inflammatory cells thought to arise from a primitive mesenchymal cell

SYNONYM(S)

Epithelioid sarcoma
Giant cell fascial sarcoma
Giant cell tumor
Reticulum cell sarcoma

EPIDEMIOLOGY

SPECIES, AGE, SEX: Malignant fibrous histiocytoma is an uncommon tumor of the skin and subcutaneous tissue of dogs and cats, which can also occur in the spleen in dogs. It is not to be mistaken with malignant histiocytosis, a disease of multisystemic histiocytic infiltration (see Histiocytic Diseases, p 523).

GENETICS AND BREED PREDISPOSITION: Golden retrievers and rottweilers may be overrepresented.

CLINICAL PRESENTATION

DISEASE FORMS/SUBTYPES

- Different pathologic types include storiform-pleomorphic, inflammatory, and a giant cell variant. The giant cell variant, which occurs in dogs but is very rare in cats, is associated with metastasis and a poor prognosis.
- Malignant fibrous histiocytoma has been reported at vaccine sites in cats (see Vaccine-Site Sarcoma, p 1136).

HISTORY, CHIEF COMPLAINT

- Pets with malignant fibrous histiocytomas in the skin and subcutaneous tissue usually present for a progressive mass noticed by the owner.
- Dogs with malignant fibrous histiocytomas of the spleen usually present for signs related to an abdominal mass or abdominal hemorrhage.

PHYSICAL EXAM FINDINGS

- Malignant fibrous histiocytomas in the skin and subcutaneous tissue often present as firm, palpable masses. Occasionally they are hairless or ulcerated.
- Regional lymphadenomegaly may be present secondary to inflammation or, rarely, lymph node metastasis.
- Dogs with splenic tumors may present with abdominal mass, pain, or abdominal enlargement.

ETIOLOGY AND PATHOPHYSIOLOGY

- Malignant fibrous histiocytomas are typically firm, slow-growing tumors that commonly infiltrate into surrounding soft tissues and along fascial planes. Overall they have a moderate metastatic potential, but some variants or grades may be more likely to metastasize (see prognosis).
- Lesions caused by malignant fibrous histiocytoma depend on the location of the primary tumor.
- These tumors are considered a separate entity from the other histiocytic diseases. Peripheral tumors can metastasize, but usually to the lungs.

DIAGNOSIS

DIFFERENTIAL DIAGNOSIS

- Other skin and subcutaneous tumors:
  - Soft tissue sarcomas
  - Mast cell tumor
  - Others
- Other splenic tumors:
  - Hemangiosarcoma
  - Lymphoma
  - Others

INITIAL DATABASE

- Fine-needle aspirate cytology may help identify the tumor type before other diagnostics.
- Three view thoracic radiographs to rule out pulmonary metastases.
- Radiographs of the affected area may reveal involvement of underlying bone.
- Abdominal ultrasound to identify splenic tumors and rule out metastasis.

ADVANCED OR CONFIRMATORY TESTING

- Computed tomography or magnetic resonance imaging may be necessary to delineate the local extent of the tumor and to plan for surgery or radiation therapy.
- Biopsy: Diagnosis of malignant fibrous histiocytosis is based on histopathologic evaluation of tissue.
  - Special stains may be necessary to differentiate malignant fibrous histiocytoma from other soft tissue sarcomas, especially poorly differentiated tumors.
  - Care should be taken to differentiate these tumors from other histiocytic tumors, including histiocytic sarcoma and malignant histiocytosis. These other tumors usually have a different prognosis and recommended course of treatment.
  - Histopathologic grade of the tumor is necessary for determining the prognosis and treatment of most soft tissue sarcomas (see Soft Tissue Sarcoma, p 1016).
    - Histopathologic grading typically involves using the general grading system for soft tissue sarcomas based on mitotic rate, percent necrosis, and degree of differentiation.
    - Tumors are graded as low, intermediate, or high grade.
    - In most cases high-grade tumors are larger and more invasive, but gross size and invasiveness cannot be used as a substitute for histopathologic grading.

TREATMENT

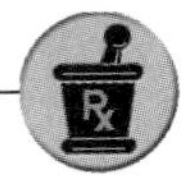

THERAPEUTIC GOAL(S)

Complete eradication of the primary tumor if possible

ACUTE AND CHRONIC TREATMENT

- Aggressive surgical resection, radiation therapy, and/or chemotherapy may be used for treatment (see Soft Tissue Sarcoma, p 1016).
- Chemotherapy may be indicated to delay or prevent metastasis for malignant fibrous histiocytoma affecting the spleen, high-grade tumors, or giant cell variants of malignant fibrous histiocytoma.

POSSIBLE COMPLICATIONS

Complications of treatment depend on the types of treatments and the location of the primary tumor (see Soft Tissue Sarcoma, p 1016).

RECOMMENDED MONITORING

After appropriate local treatment, follow-up examination should be done routinely to monitor for recurrence (every 2 to 3 months) and metastasis (thoracic radiographs at 6 months and 1 year). High-grade tumors may require more frequent monitoring (at least every 2 to 3 months) for metastases during and after chemotherapy administration.

PROGNOSIS AND OUTCOME

- Prognosis is excellent for histologically low to intermediate grade tumors with appropriate treatment. This includes either surgical resection with clean histopathologic margins or incomplete resection combined with radiation therapy.
- Dogs with the giant cell variant of this tumor often have metastases at the time of diagnosis or soon afterward, and prognosis is usually poor despite

treatment. Few cats with this variant develop metastases.
- Dogs with splenic tumors are more likely to develop metastases and therefore have a poor prognosis.
- High-grade malignant fibrous histiocytoma: Like other soft tissue sarcomas, prognosis is considered guarded based on the increased likelihood for metastases.

PEARLS & CONSIDERATIONS

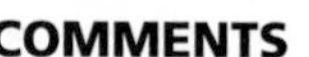

COMMENTS

Aside from the giant cell variant, malignant fibrous histiocytoma should be considered like other soft tissue sarcomas (see Soft Tissue Sarcoma, p 1016) in treatment and prognosis. Tumors at vaccine sites in cats should be treated like vaccine-site sarcomas (see Vaccine-Site Sarcoma, p 1136).

CLIENT EDUCATION

Pet owners can be educated to monitor their pets for palpable or visible masses and have them evaluated in a timely fashion. Early detection may allow for easier treatment via surgery and may help avoid the need for radiation therapy.

SUGGESTED READING

MacEwen EG, Powers BE, Macy D, Withrow SJ: Soft tissue sarcomas. In Withrow SJ, MacEwen EG (eds): *Small Animal Clinical Oncology*. Philadelphia, WB Saunders, 2001, pp 283–304.

Waters CB, et al: Giant cell variant of malignant fibrous histiocytoma in dogs: 10 cases (1986–1993). *J Am Vet Med Assoc* 205:1420–1424, 1994.

AUTHOR: **JOHN FARRELLY**
EDITOR: **KENNETH M. RASSNICK**

Malnutrition

BASIC INFORMATION

DEFINITION

The inappropriate intake of nutrients, resulting in nutritional deficiencies or excesses

EPIDEMIOLOGY

SPECIES, AGE, SEX: Can affect animals of any species, age, lifestage, or lifestyle.

GENETICS AND BREED PREDISPOSITION: An increased prevalence of obesity, resulting from excessive caloric intake, has been associated with basset hounds, beagles, cairn terriers, Cavalier King Charles spaniels, cocker spaniels, long-haired dachshunds, Labrador retrievers, and Shetland sheepdogs.

RISK FACTORS
- Animals fed vegetarian, homemade, or single-food diets may be at risk for multiple nutrient deficiencies.
- Animals with a history of chronic vomiting or diarrhea could have altered digestion or absorption, resulting in decreased nutrient intake.
- Drugs such as corticosteroids, cancer chemotherapeutic agents, antibiotics, or diuretics may adversely affect nutritional homeostasis.
- Neutering, decreased physical activity, age or calorically dense foods may predispose dogs or cats to obesity.

GEOGRAPHY AND SEASONALITY: Inadequate food or water intake during severe weather conditions may result in nutrient deprivation.

ASSOCIATED CONDITIONS AND DISORDERS
- Decreased intake of many nutrients negatively affects immune function.
- Orthopedic problems or diabetes mellitus may be seen in dogs and cats with prolonged excessive food intake.

CLINICAL PRESENTATION

DISEASE FORMS/SUBTYPES
- Weight loss; emaciation; low body condition score (1 on a scale of 1–5; 1 or 2 on a 1–9 scale)
- Weight gain, obesity; high body condition score (4 or 5 on a 1–5 scale; 8 or 9 on a 1–9 scale)

HISTORY, CHIEF COMPLAINT
- Nutrient-deprived animals present with a history of failure to grow, malaise, inappetence, or anorexia.
- Overnourished or obese animals often present with clinical signs associated with lameness or endocrinopathy.

PHYSICAL EXAM FINDINGS
- Nutrient-deprived animals often have a poor physical appearance: thin body condition; dry, coarse haircoat; flaky skin; hyperkeratosis; muscle wasting; broken or missing teeth; skeletal abnormalities; pressure sores; poor wound healing.
- Obese animals also are in poor physical condition with fat deposition over the ribs, hips, tail head, and throughout the abdomen. Some are unable to adequately groom themselves, which can result in an unkempt haircoat, dry skin, skin fold dermatitis, and the inability to walk, run, or jump.

ETIOLOGY AND PATHOPHYSIOLOGY

- Inadequate or excessive nutrient intake results in malnutrition.
- Decreased nutrient intake diminishes immune cell response and production, as well as protein turnover, tissue synthesis, and wound healing.
- Altered drug metabolism results from protein-calorie malnutrition and may increase or decrease both drug efficacy and drug toxicity.
- Although not well documented in hospitalized veterinary patients, malnutrition is thought to increase their morbidity and mortality.

DIAGNOSIS

DIFFERENTIAL DIAGNOSIS

Gastrointestinal disease: protein-losing enteropathy; lymphocytic-plasmacytic enteritis; inflammatory bowel disease; lymphangiectasia; gastrointestinal neoplasia.

INITIAL DATABASE

- A thorough diet history should include sufficient information to purchase all food items necessary to feed the patient exactly as the owner does at home.
- The physical examination should include a body weight, body condition score (1–5 or 1–9 scale), and muscle mass score (1–3 scale).
- Laboratory evaluation plays a limited role in diagnosing nutrition-related problems.

TREATMENT

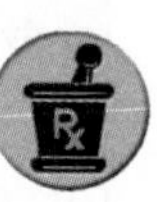

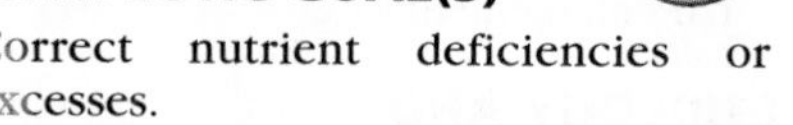

THERAPEUTIC GOAL(S)

- Correct nutrient deficiencies or excesses.
- Attempt to return patient to a normal plane of nutrition and a more appropriate body weight and body condition.

ACUTE GENERAL TREATMENT

- Stabilize patient: Rehydrate and correct electrolyte imbalances as needed before initiating nutritional support.
- Determine if the gastrointestinal tract is functional and how nutrition support is to be delivered (oral, enteral, or parenteral).
- Estimate an initial daily caloric goal for resting energy needs, based upon animal's current weight (rather than an ideal weight), using the equation $97 \times (\text{body weight kg})^{0.655}$ (Table I-19).
- Select a diet or food type that meets the nutritional needs of the patient.
- Determine a feeding regimen that will deliver the estimated caloric goals over a 24-hour period.
- Plan to get the animal eating its own food in its own environment as soon as possible.

CHRONIC TREATMENT

- Identify dietary, animal-related, owner-related, or environmental issue(s) that caused or contributed to the nutritional deficiency or excess.
- Educate owner(s) about nutritional needs of their animal, given the species, age, lifestage, and lifestyle.
- Provide information about, or resources for, complete and balanced homemade diets (e.g., website formulation services, laboratory analyses).
- Provide information and support for owners considering a weight management program for their animal.

DRUG INTERACTIONS

Medical therapies instituted for primary conditions may be altered without adequate nutritional support.

TABLE I-19 Approximate resting energy requirement (±20%) per day

Weight in kg (lbs)	Approximate resting energy requirement (kcal/day)
3 (7)	200
7 (15)	350
10 (22)	430
15 (33)	570
20 (44)	690
30 (66)	900
40 (88)	1100
50 (110)	1260
60 (132)	1420
70 (154)	1570
80 (176)	1710
90 (198)	1850
100 (220)	1980

RECOMMENDED MONITORING

Client education and repeated follow-up are critical for animals enrolled in weight-management programs.

PROGNOSIS AND OUTCOME

- Prognosis is good to excellent with immediate identification and correction of nutrient deficiencies or excesses.
- Prognosis is poor to good with prolonged identification and correction of nutrient deficiencies or excesses.

PEARLS & CONSIDERATIONS

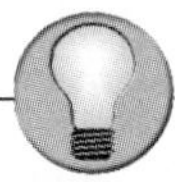

COMMENTS

- Obesity prevention is much easier than obesity management. Client education campaigns should focus on prevention at every well-pet visit.
- Obesity management programs should be directed by veterinarians and delivered by trained, licensed veterinary technicians who are excellent communicators.

PREVENTION

- Complete nutritional assessments should be performed daily on hospitalized patients, to identify malnutrition before it occurs.
- Clients should be educated on the basic nutrient needs of animals, considering species, age, lifestage, and environmental conditions.

CLIENT EDUCATION

- Customized homemade diet formulations can be purchased at www.petdiets.com
- Homemade diet recipes can be analyzed through the Nutrition Laboratory in the Diagnostic Center for Population and Animal Health at Michigan State University: 517-353-9312.

SUGGESTED READING

Buffington T, Holloway C, Abood S: *Manual of Veterinary Dietetics*. St. Louis, Elsevier, 2004.

AUTHOR: **SARAH K. ABOOD**
EDITOR: **C. A. TONY BUFFINGTON**

Malocclusion, Dental/Skeletal

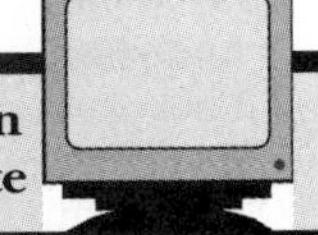

Client Education Sheet on Website

BASIC INFORMATION

DEFINITION

- An abnormal position of the teeth.
- In dental malocclusion, one or several teeth is/are in an abnormal position, whereas in skeletal malocclusion there is a jaw discrepancy.

SYNONYM(S)

Malalignment of teeth

EPIDEMIOLOGY

SPECIES, AGE, SEX: Malocclusion may be seen in all species, of all age groups, and is usually present from the time of eruption of the deciduous or permanent dentition.

GENETICS AND BREED PREDISPOSITION: Occlusal development is determined by genetic and environmental factors. Most brachycephlic animals have malocclusion due to a shortened upper jaw.

RISK FACTORS

- Persistent deciduous teeth
- Facial trauma during tooth and jaw development
- Selective breeding for exaggerated head types

ASSOCIATED CONDITIONS AND DISORDERS

- Discomfort and pain from malocccluding teeth.
- Lingually deviated mandibular canines may lead to oronasal fistula formation.
- Crowded teeth are at risk for early periodontitis from plaque retention.

CLINICAL PRESENTATION

DISEASE FORMS/SUBTYPES: Most commonly seen malocclusions:

- Rostral crossbite (dental or skeletal; one or more upper incisors occlude lingual to the lower incisors)
- Prognathic lower jaw/retrognathic upper jaw (skeletal; lower jaw protrudes rostrally beyond upper jaw)
- Prognathic upper jaw/retrognathic lower jaw (skeletal; upper jaw protrudes rostrally beyond lower jaw)

- Wry bite (skeletal; one upper/lower quadrant is increased/decreased in length compared to the contralateral quadrant)
- Caudal crossbite (dental or skeletal; the lower first molar occludes buccally to the upper fourth premolar)
- Rostroversion/mesioversion of upper canine tooth (dental; the crown of the upper canine is deviated rostrally/mesially)
- Linguoversion of lower canine tooth (dental or skeletal; the crown of the lower canine is instanding and occludes onto the upper canine or into the hard palate)
- Tooth crowding (dental or skeletal)

HISTORY, CHIEF COMPLAINT

- Abnormal incisor occlusion (show and breeding dogs)
- Abnormal tooth position
- Obvious length difference between upper and lower jaws or between left and right

PHYSICAL EXAM FINDINGS

- Normal occlusion:
    - Incisor "scissors bite." The upper incisors are rostral to the lower incisors, and cutting edges of lower incisors occlude onto the cingulum on the palatal surface of upper incisors.
    - Lower canine evenly spaced between upper third incisor and canine.
    - Cusp tips of premolars oppose interdental spaces of opposite arcade with the lower first premolar being most rostral in the dog, and the upper second premolar in the cat.
- Dental malocclusion:
    - One or more teeth are in an abnormal position.
    - No jaw discrepancy.
    - Trauma (to soft tissue or other teeth) may be obvious.
- Skeletal malocclusion:
    - Abnormal incisor relationship.
    - Loss of premolar interdigitation.
    - Incorrect canine occlusion.
    - Jaw length discrepancy may or may not be obvious.

ETIOLOGY AND PATHOPHYSIOLOGY

- Jaw length, tooth bud position, and tooth size are independently inherited. Nonharmonious development of upper and lower jaw and teeth results in malocclusion.
- Persistent deciduous teeth are associated with malpositioned permanent teeth.
- Significant facial trauma at a young age may lead to abnormal development and malocclusion.
- Significant facial trauma at any age may cause changes in jaw relationship.

DIAGNOSIS

DIFFERENTIAL DIAGNOSIS

Skeletal malocclusion versus dental malocclusion

INITIAL DATABASE

- Look for persistent deciduous teeth
- Differentiate between skeletal and dental maloccusion through a thorough occlusal assessment (incisor, canine, and premolar/molar occlusion)

TREATMENT

THERAPEUTIC GOAL(S)

- Pain-free, comfortable animal.
- Functional bite.
- Cosmetic considerations should not play a role.
- Skeletal malocclusion: usually inherited. Therefore breeding of an affected individual is discouraged.

ACUTE GENERAL TREATMENT

- Extract maloccluding deciduous teeth, if they cause discomfort or interfere with jaw growth, as early as possible (6 to 10 weeks of age).
- Treatment options for maloccluding permanent teeth causing trauma to soft tissue or other teeth:
    - Extraction
    - Surgical crown reduction and vital pulp therapy
    - Orthodontic movement
- Linguoversion of lower canines: Verhaert's "rubber ball technique" is useful for young dogs (below age 7 months) with normal jaw relationship and sufficiently wide diasthema between upper third incisor and canine. The dog is stimulated to actively play with a smooth-surfaced hard rubber ball for at least 15 minutes 3 times a day.

POSSIBLE COMPLICATIONS

- Inappropriate extraction technique of deciduous teeth may cause trauma to developing permanent teeth.
- Surgical crown reduction may lead to pulpitis and pulp necrosis.
- Orthodontic treatment usually requires several corrective procedures under general anesthesia and may cause soft tissue trauma from the appliance, tooth ankylosis and root resorption, displacement of anchor tooth, overcorrection of target tooth, avulsion of anchor or target tooth, discomfort, and pain.

RECOMMENDED MONITORING

- Teeth treated by surgical crown reduction should be monitored radiographically after 4 to 6 months and then on a yearly basis.
- During orthodontic treatment, regular monitoring is necessary to assess tooth movement and to recognize possible complications at an early stage.

PROGNOSIS AND OUTCOME

Prognosis is good once a functional bite has been accomplished

PEARLS & CONSIDERATIONS

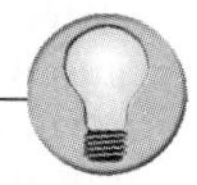

COMMENTS

- Skeletal malocclusion is considered inherited unless a developmental cause (e.g., significant facial trauma) can be identified.
- Dental malocclusions are not considered inherited, unless a familial predisposition exists.
- Ethical considerations: inherited malocclusion should only be corrected orthodontically if the animal is neutered.

PREVENTION

- Do not breed animals with inheritable malocclusion.
- Remove persistent deciduous teeth.

CLIENT EDUCATION

- Neuter animals with skeletal malocclusion (if not "normal" for the breed)
- Institute daily plaque control (toothbrushing)

SUGGESTED READING

Gorrel C: Occlusion and malocclusion. In Gorrel C (ed): *Veterinary Dentistry for the General Practitioner*. Edinburgh, WB Saunders, 2004, pp 35–46.

Hennet P: Orthodontics. In Slatter D (ed): *Textbook of Small Animal Surgery*, ed 3. Philadelphia, WB Saunders, 2003, pp 2686–2695.

AUTHOR: **LEEN VERHAERT**

EDITOR: **ALEXANDER M. REITER**

Mammary Gland Neoplasia, Cat

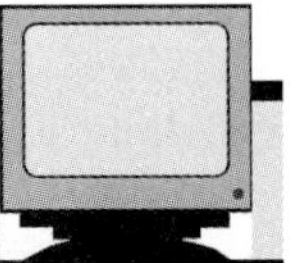

Client Education Sheet on Website

BASIC INFORMATION

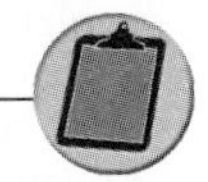

DEFINITION

Mammary gland tumors are benign or malignant neoplasms arising from mammary tissue.

SYNONYM(S)

Mammary cancer
Mammary tumor
Specific mammary neoplasms:
- Adenocarcinoma
- Adenoma/cystadenoma
- Carcinoma
- Duct papilloma
- Fibroadenoma
- Inflammatory carcinoma

EPIDEMIOLOGY

SPECIES, AGE, SEX
- Mammary gland tumors represent less than 20% of all tumors in female cats.
- Incidence ~ 0.25:1000.
- Median age is 10 to 12 years (mean 10.8 years [male], 12.8 years [female]).
- Most common: malignant epithelial carcinoma/adenocarcinoma (female), mammary carcinoma (male).
- Mixed mammary tumors and sarcomas are extremely rare to nonexistent.
- Siamese cats may develop mammary tumors at an earlier age than other cats.
- Mammary tumors are rare in male cats (1-2% of feline mammary carcinomas).

GENETICS AND BREED PREDISPOSITION
- Siamese cats have a twofold risk of developing mammary gland tumors and have a higher incidence of malignant tumors with lymphatic invasion.
- Persian cats may have a higher incidence of benign mammary tumors.

RISK FACTORS: Hormonal factors:
- Ovariohysterectomy reduces the risk of developing mammary tumors by 40-60%.
  - There is little information available regarding the age at which ovariohysterectomy has to be performed to have a protective effect; 6 to 12 months of age advised but unsubstantiated.
- Protective effect of early ovariohysterectomy appears to be much less in cats as compared to dogs.
- Treatment with progesterone and estrogen-progesterone combinations is associated with a threefold increased risk of development of benign and malignant mammary tumors in cats (progesterone treatment: 36% of male cats with mammary carcinoma).

CLINICAL PRESENTATION

DISEASE FORMS/SUBTYPES: Clinical staging:
- Tumor: T1:<1 cm; T2: 1-3 cm; T3:>3 cm.
- Regional lymph node: N0, no metastasis; N1, metastasis detected.
- Distant metastasis: M0, no metastasis; M1, metastasis detected.

Stage Grouping	T	N	M
I	T1	N0	M0
II	T2	N0	M0
III	T1, T2	N1	M0
	T3	N0, N1	M0
IV	T1-3	N0, N1	M1

HISTORY, CHIEF COMPLAINT
- A swelling, "lump," or often ulcerated tissue may be noted in a cat's mammary chain.
- In cases of metastasis or inflammatory carcinoma, cats may be presented due to general signs of illness or specific complaints attributable to a certain site of metastasis (e.g., dyspnea due to pulmonary metastases or effusion).
- Duration of clinical signs is variable, ranging from a few days to several months.

PHYSICAL EXAM FINDINGS
- Clinical signs vary depending on extent and stage of disease.
- More than 50% of cats will have more than one mammary tumor present, and both mammary chains may be affected simultaneously.
- Tumors may be firm on palpation and occasionally fixed to underlying structures.
- Discrete to infiltrative, soft to firm swelling within mammary gland or overlying skin is most common.
- Ulceration is frequently present.
- Can have associated discharge from nipple.
- Regional lymph nodes (inguinal and axillary) may be enlarged or normal on palpation.
- Lymph node enlargement can indicate metastasis or reactive change secondary to inflammation.
- Inflammatory carcinomas occur rarely in cats after mastectomy for mammary carcinoma. These cats present with local erythema, edema, pain, and involvement of the extremities.

ETIOLOGY AND PATHOPHYSIOLOGY

- The vast majority (85-93%) of feline mammary tumors are malignant, with more than 80% of feline mammary tumors classified as adenocarcinoma.
  - Metastasis is common (61%). Preferred sites of metastasis include the lungs (76%), pleura (40%), and lymph nodes (27% or more).
- Inflammatory carcinomas occur rarely in cats after mastectomy for mammary carcinoma.
  - These are aggressive anaplastic carcinomas with considerable inflammatory cell infiltrate and involvement of the skin leading to edema, pain, and rapid metastasis.
- Benign tumors including adenomas, fibroadenomas, and duct papillomas occur uncommonly in cats.

DIAGNOSIS

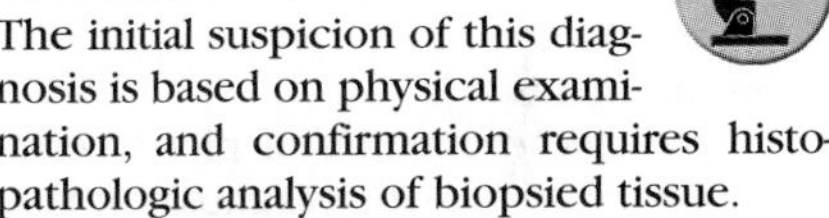

The initial suspicion of this diagnosis is based on physical examination, and confirmation requires histopathologic analysis of biopsied tissue.

DIFFERENTIAL DIAGNOSIS

- Fibroepithelial hyperplasia: involves multiple glands, most often in young intact females and spayed females given progesterone compounds
- Mastitis
- Other cutaneous and subcutaneous tumors
- Inguinal/axillary lymphadenopathy (reactive, neoplastic)
- Inguinal hernia
- Enlarged inguinal fat pad

INITIAL DATABASE

- Physical examination:
  - Measure primary tumor (T)
  - Describe possible signs of invasiveness (ulceration, fixation)
  - Evaluate regional lymph nodes (N): palpation and cytology
- Thoracic radiographs (three views) for pulmonary metastasis.
- Abdominal ultrasound in case of suspected metastasis to abdominal organs or lymph nodes.
- Fine-needle aspiration and cytologic evaluation are of limited utility and generally not recommended. Although seemingly more accurate than in dogs, feline mammary mass aspirates often are not representative of the entire mass, and cytologic criteria of malignancy are not correlated to histologic findings nor clearly defined.
- Complete blood count, serum biochemistry profile, urinalysis, coagulation profile in cases of suspected inflammatory carcinoma.

ADVANCED OR CONFIRMATORY TESTING

- Definitive diagnosis is via biopsy and histopathologic evaluation of mammary masses.
  - Histologic grading scheme is based primarily on mitotic activity, areas of necrosis, and degree of infiltration into soft tissue and vasculature.
  - Because greater than 85% of feline mammary tumors are malignant, histopathologic examination most often is performed on tumor tissue obtained from a radical mastectomy.
  - When fibroepithelial hyperplasia (see Differential Diagnosis above) or other nonmammary tumors are suspected, incisional (wedge) biopsies may be done.
- Lymph node evaluation:
  - In general, the ipsilateral inguinal lymph node should be removed during radical mastectomy and assessed histopathologically.
  - Axillary lymph nodes may be difficult to isolate, but fine-needle aspiration or biopsies can be done if they are enlarged.
- Distant metastasis:
  - Cytologic evaluation of pleural effusion can aid in the diagnosis of thoracic metastatic disease.
  - Advanced imaging (computed tomography, magnetic resonance imaging) may increase diagnostic accuracy of metastatic lesions in the thoracic and abdominal cavities.

TREATMENT

THERAPEUTIC GOAL(S)

- Control local tumor
- Prevent metastasis
- Palliation

ACUTE GENERAL TREATMENT

- Surgery:
  - Radical mastectomy of the affected mammary chain(s) is recommended.
  - In contrast to individual mastectomies or lumpectomies, radical mastectomy significantly reduces the risk for local tumor recurrence.
  - Affected lymph node(s) should be removed along with mammary chain.
  - Fixation of the tumor to underlying muscle or fascia necessitates en bloc removal of these structures.
  - In cats with advanced metastatic disease, local mastectomy to remove ulcerated or infected mammary tumors may be palliative.
  - Inflammatory carcinoma is nonresectable.
- Prolactin inhibitors (e.g., cabergoline) administered before mastectomy are thought by some clinicians to have a positive effect on surgery time and risk of wound dehiscence. These observations await objective confirmation, and such treatment is not currently recommended in feline oncology.

CHRONIC TREATMENT

- Chemotherapy:
  - Single-agent doxorubicin, doxorubicin in combination with cyclophosphamide or single-agent carboplatin may lead to complete and partial responses in cats with metastatic disease or nonresectable mammary gland tumors.
  - Adjuvant chemotherapy using the previously mentioned drugs as single agents or in combination is recommended in cats after radical mastectomy. However, a true survival benefit has yet to be proven.
- Radiation therapy:
  - Radiation to palliate nonresectable disease may be an option in some cats.
- Immunotherapy:
  - Treatment with levamisole, bacterial vaccines, and other immunomodulators has not lead to any improvement in local tumor control or survival.
- Analgesics:
  - Analgesics should be used in cats that present with advanced disease.

POSSIBLE COMPLICATIONS

Inflammatory carcinoma after mastectomy for mammary carcinoma: rare

RECOMMENDED MONITORING

Regular examination of surgical site, local lymph nodes, lung fields

PROGNOSIS AND OUTCOME

- Local recurrence rate: 51–66% (female), 45% (male).
- Prognostic factors for cats with mammary gland carcinomas:
  - Tumor size:
    - >3 cm: median survival of 4 to 6 months (female), 1.6 months (male).
    - 2–3 cm: median survival of 1 to 2 years (female), 5.2 months (male).
    - <2 cm: median survival of >3 years after mastectomy (female), 14 months (male).
  - Type of surgery:
    - Radical mastectomy significantly reduces the risk for local tumor recurrence compared with conservative surgery, but does not appear to improve survival time.
  - Degree of histologic differentiation: high-grade is associated with a shorter survival time.
  - Other unfavorable prognostic factors include old age of the cat and incomplete surgical excision.
- Benign tumors and low-grade malignant tumors may be cured by wide excision.

PEARLS & CONSIDERATIONS

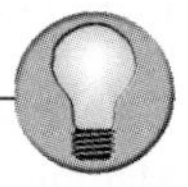

COMMENTS

- Mammary carcinoma in the cat is a highly malignant neoplastic disease that warrants early diagnosis and an aggressive treatment approach.
- Adjuvant chemotherapy should be considered in cats with resectable mammary carcinoma after radical mastectomy.
- In cats with advanced disease, palliative measures including surgery, chemotherapy, radiation, and analgesics may be considered.

PREVENTION

- Castration does not prevent mammary carcinoma in male cats.
- Ovariohysterectomy before age 6 months may reduce the risk but will not prevent mammary carcinoma in female cats.

CLIENT EDUCATION

- Early ovariohysterectomy of queens not intended for breeding
- Regular examination of the mammary chain
- Prompt presentation for veterinary examination when abnormalities are found

SUGGESTED READING

Hayes HM, et al: Epidemiological features of feline mammary carcinoma. *Vet Rec* 108 (22):476–479, 1981.

MacEwen EG, et al: Prognostic factors for feline mammary tumors. *J Am Vet Med Assoc* 185(2):201–204, 1984.

Misdorp W: Tumors of the mammary gland. In Meuten DJ (ed): *Tumors in Domestic Animals,* ed 4. Ames, IA, Iowa State Press, 2002, pp 575–606.

Skorupski KA, et al: Clinical characteristics of mammary carcinoma in male cats. *J Vet Intern Med* 19:52–55, 2005.

AUTHORS: **DANIELA SIMON, BETH A. VALENTINE**

EDITORS: **KENNETH M. RASSNICK, MICHELLE A. KUTZLER**

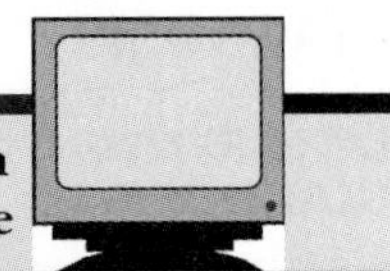

Mammary Gland Neoplasia, Dog

Client Education Sheet on Website

BASIC INFORMATION

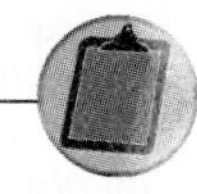

DEFINITION

Mammary gland tumors are benign or malignant neoplasms arising from mammary tissue.

SYNONYM(S)

Mammary cancer, breast cancer
Benign mammary tumors:
- Adenoma/cystadenoma (very common)
- Benign mixed mammary tumor (very common)
- Fibroadenoma (uncommon)

Malignant mammary tumors:
- Adenocarcinoma/cystadenocarcinoma (common)
- Carcinoma (common)
- Inflammatory carcinoma (uncommon)
- Malignant mixed mammary tumor (uncommon)
- Carcinosarcoma (rare)
- Sarcoma (uncommon)

Note: Different pathologic classification schemes exist.

EPIDEMIOLOGY

SPECIES, AGE, SEX
- Mammary gland tumors are the most common tumor in female dogs according to some surveys.
  - Incidence ~2:1000.
  - Due to the common practice of early age ovariohysterectomy (OHE) the incidence has decreased in the United States. In European countries mammary tumors represent 40-50% of all tumors in female dogs.
- Greater prevalence with older age.
- Mammary gland tumors in male dogs are uncommon (approximately 1% of mammary tumors occur in males).

GENETICS AND BREED PREDISPOSITION
- Breeds at increased risk include:
  - Spaniel breeds
  - Pointer breeds
  - Poodles
  - Dachshunds
  - German shepherds
  - Yorkshire terriers
- A genetic factor in the development of mammary tumors seems to be present; however, a specific, common mutation has not been identified. The following genes have been found to be mutated in select canine mammary gland tumors:
  - p53
  - c-erb-2
  - BCRA 1, 2
- Boxer dogs and collies are at lower risk.

RISK FACTORS
- Timing of OHE: the relative risk for developing mammary gland tumors:
  - 0.5% if OHE is performed before the first estrus.
  - 8% if OHE is performed between the first and second estrus.
  - 26% if OHE performed between the second and third estrus.
- Intact females and females neutered after 2 years of age have a sevenfold greater risk of mammary neoplasia compared to those neutered before age 6 months.
- Body condition/diet: reduced risk in dogs with lean body condition at age 9 to 12 months.
- Progesterone treatment: increases the risk for the development of benign and malignant mammary tumors.
- Pregnancy, lactation, pseudo-pregnancy:
  - Unlike people, pregnancy does not afford a protective effect against the development of mammary tumors in dogs.
  - Lactation and pseudo-pregnancy also do not seem to have an influence.

ASSOCIATED CONDITIONS AND DISORDERS: Ovarian cysts, cystic endometrial hyperplasia.

CLINICAL PRESENTATION

DISEASE FORMS/SUBTYPES
- Clinical staging:
  - Tumor: T1, <3 cm; T2, 3-5 cm; T3, >5 cm.
  - Regional lymph node: N0, no metastasis; N1, metastasis detected.
  - Distant metastasis: M0, N0, no metastasis; M1, metastasis detected.

Stage Grouping	T	N	M
I	T1	N0	M0
II	T2	N0	M0
III	T3	N0	M0
IV	T1-3	N1	M0
V	T1-3	N0, N1	M1

- Histologic Staging:

0 Tumor cells limited to ductal tissue.
I Tumor cells limited to ductal/stromal tissue.
II Tumor cells with vascular/lymphatic invasion or regional lymph node metastasis.
III Distant metastasis present.

HISTORY, CHIEF COMPLAINT
- Owners may note a swelling, "lump," or ulceration in their dog's mammary chain, or these may be incidental findings on routine physical examination.
- Duration of clinical signs is highly variable, ranging from days to months.
- In cases of metastasis or inflammatory carcinoma, dogs may be presented due to general signs of illness or specific complaints attributable to a certain site of metastasis (e.g., lameness in cases of bone metastasis).

PHYSICAL EXAM FINDINGS
- Variable depending on extent and stage of the disease.
- Single or multiple nodules may be present. Multiple tumors are common in dogs, and both mammary chains may be affected. Multiple tumor types are common.
- Signs of malignancy include fixation to skin or underlying structures, rapid increase in size, ill-defined borders, ulceration, pain, inflammation or edema.
  - Absence of these signs does not exclude malignancy.
- Inflammatory carcinomas present with diffuse, firm, and painful swelling of the affected gland or chain. The adjacent extremity may be affected. Cutaneous involvement in form of small beadlike nodules may also be found.
- Regional lymph nodes (inguinal and axillary) may be enlarged (due to metastasis or reactive hyperplasia) or normal on palpation. The internal iliac, popliteal, and prescapular nodes may also be affected.

ETIOLOGY AND PATHOPHYSIOLOGY

- Estimates of malignancy rates range from 30-50%.
- Metastasis most common to the lungs.
- Tumors are classified according to their tissue of origin into epithelial, mesenchymal, and mixed tumors.
  - Inflammatory carcinoma is an aggressive anaplastic carcinoma with considerable inflammatory cell infiltrate and involvement of the skin leading to edema, pain, and rapid metastasis.
- Primary mesenchymal mammary tumors (e.g., fibrosarcoma, osteosarcoma) are infrequent. Malignant mesenchymal mammary tumors often behave aggressively with frequent metastasis and a short survival.
- Mixed mammary tumors consist of epithelial, myoepithelial, and mesenchymal tissue Most mixed mammary tumors are benign. Malignant mixed mammary tumors and carcinosarcomas are rare exceptions.

DIAGNOSIS

DIFFERENTIAL DIAGNOSIS

- Mastitis
- Other cutaneous and subcutaneous tumors
- Inguinal/axillary lymphadenopathy (reactive, neoplastic)
- Inguinal hernia

INITIAL DATABASE

- Physical examination:
  - Measure primary tumor (T)
  - Describe possible signs of invasiveness (ulceration, fixation)
  - Evaluation of regional lymph nodes (N): palpation and cytologic study
- Thoracic radiographs (three views)
- Abdominal ultrasound in case of suspected metastasis to abdominal organs or lymph nodes
- Complete blood count, serum biochemistry profile, urinalysis
- Coagulation profile in cases of suspected inflammatory carcinoma (risk of disseminated intravascular coagulation)

ADVANCED OR CONFIRMATORY TESTING

- Excisional biopsy of the tumor and thorough histologic examination are necessary to obtain a definitive diagnosis.
- Fine-needle aspiration cytology is *not* recommended:
  - Poor differentiation between malignant and benign mammary tumors due to their heterogenous composition
- Incisional biopsy also may not represent the whole tumor and is not recommended.
- Lymph node metastasis: Fine-needle aspiration and cytologic evaluation of lymph nodes has been shown to increase diagnostic accuracy of mammary tumor metastasis. Metastases may be present in palpably normal nodes.
- Advanced imaging (computed tomography, magnetic resonance imaging) may be more sensitive to detect metastatic lesions in the thoracic and abdominal cavities and should be considered in cases in which metastasis is strongly suspected but cannot be detected on radiographs or ultrasound.

TREATMENT

THERAPEUTIC GOAL(S)

- Control local tumor
- Prevent metastasis
- Palliation

ACUTE GENERAL TREATMENT

- Mainstay of treatment is surgical excision of the mammary tumor(s) with wide margins (at least 2 cm in all planes if possible).
- Type of surgery (nodulectomy, partial or radical mastectomy) depends on the size, location, and number of tumors present.
  - Type of surgery does not influence survival as long as the entire tumor is removed with histologically clean margins.
- Lumpectomy possible for freely moveable tumors <5 mm, but increases risk of local recurrence of carcinoma.
- Simple or radical (block or unilateral chain resection) mastectomy: Both increase disease-free interval.
- Removal of inguinal lymph node with caudal gland tumors; excise axillary nodes only if metastasis is suspected.
- Inflammatory carcinoma is nonresectable; palliative surgery may be possible in select cases.
- Prolactin inhibitors (e.g., cabergoline) administered before mastectomy are thought by some clinicians to have a positive effect on surgery time and risk of wound dehiscence. These observations await objective confirmation, and such treatment is not currently recommended in canine oncology.

CHRONIC TREATMENT

- Chemotherapy: limited information available.
  - Antitumor activity has been demonstrated in vitro, in select patients with gross metastatic disease, and as adjuvant treatment in a small group of dogs with advanced stage disease. High-risk patients may therefore benefit from adjuvant chemotherapy.
  - Chemotherapeutics studied include doxorubicin (30 mg/m^2 IV), 5-fluoruracil (150 mg/m^2 IV), cyclophosphamide (200 mg/m^2 IV), and platinum compounds (cisplatin 50–70 mg/m^2 IV plus saline diuresis; carboplatin 250–350 mg/m^2 IV). Special handling requirements and potentially severe, life-threatening adverse patient effects exist for these drugs.
  - Consultation with an oncologist for the most current treatment recommendations is indicated.
- OHE at time of mammary tumor surgery: Benefit is controversial, with some studies reporting increased survival and others showing no difference.
- Radiation therapy: limited information available. May be of use in the palliative setting or to improve local control in inoperable cases.
- Antiestrogen therapy (tamoxifen): not recommended. Most anaplastic mammary tumors lack estrogen receptors, so antiestrogen therapy may not be beneficial for most cases in which systemic therapy is indicated. In addition, estrogen-like side effects including vulvar swelling, vaginal discharge, stump pyometra, signs of estrus, and urinary tract infection may occur in dogs treated with antiestrogen drugs.
- Pain medication: Use of analgesics should be considered in the palliative treatment of advanced stage disease or inflammatory carcinoma. Options include nonsteroidal anti-inflammatories (including aspirin 10-25 mg/kg PO q 8-12h, or carprofen 2 mg/kg PO q 12h, or etodolac 10-15 mg/kg PO q 24h, or deracoxib 1-2 mg/kg PO q 24h (may use 3-4 mg/kg PO q 24h for first 7 days only), or meloxicam (0.1 mg/kg PO q 24h).

POSSIBLE COMPLICATIONS

See Chemotherapy: Adverse Reactions, p 189

RECOMMENDED MONITORING

Regular examination of surgical site and local lymph nodes: radiology or other imaging techniques if indicated (e.g., diagnosis of malignancy, respiratory signs, other signs suggestive of internal metastasis)

PROGNOSIS AND OUTCOME

- Dogs with benign mammary tumors are cured by surgical excision as long as histologically clean margins are achieved.
- Prognosis for dogs with malignant mammary gland tumors is extremely variable and ranges from a cure with surgery (especially low-grade malignancy) to rapid recurrence and metastasis within the first year after surgical excision. Prognostic factors include:
  - Tumor size: tumors <3 cm have a better prognosis than tumors >3 cm.
  - Tumor histologic characteristics.
    - Epithelial tumors (adenocarcinomas, cystadenocarcinomas, carcinomas) may have a better prognosis than sarcomas, malignant mixed tumors, and carcinosarcoma. Median survival = 6.5 months (solid carcinoma), 12 months (invasive tumor), 29 months (noninvasive tumor), 10 months (sarcoma), 18 months (carcinosarcoma).
    - Inflammatory carcinomas have a grave prognosis.
    - Anaplastic and high-grade, invasive tumors with stromal or lymphatic or vascular infiltration (histologic stages II–III) carry a worse prognosis than well-differentiated, low-grade or noninvasive lesions.
  - Clinical stage: a worse prognosis is associated with:
    - Large tumors (stages II–V).
    - Lymph node involvement (stages IV–V).
    - Distant metastasis (stage V).
- Disease-free interval of 24 months for malignant tumors = 27–55%.

PEARLS & CONSIDERATIONS

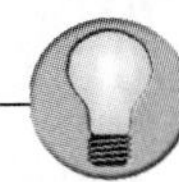

COMMENTS

- Canine mammary tumors represent a heterogenous group of tumors with different prognoses.
- Multicentric mammary tumors occur in >50% of affected dogs; multiple tumor types occurring concurrently or sequentially are common.
- Highest risk patients that will benefit most from postoperative adjuvant chemotherapy still need to be identified; however, these may include patients with advanced clinical stages (II-V), histologic evidence of vascular/lymphatic invasion, or high degree of anaplasia on histopathologic evaluation (histologic stages II-III), or anaplastic histologic tumor features.
- The benefit of OHE at the time of mammary tumor surgery remains controversial; however, a subset of dogs with differentiated, estrogen receptor-positive tumors may indeed benefit from concurrent OHE.

PREVENTION

OHE at age <6 months is not preventive but will significantly reduce risk.

CLIENT EDUCATION

- Early age OHE of bitches not intended for breeding.
- Regular examination of the mammary chain.
- Prompt presentation for veterinary examination if abnormalities are found.

SUGGESTED READING

Karayannopoulo M, et al: Adjuvant post-operative chemotherapy in bitches with mammary cancer. *J Vet Med A Physiol Pathol Clin Med* 48(2):85–89, 2001.

Misdorp W: Tumors of the mammary gland. In Meuten DJ (ed): *Tumors in Domestic Animals,* ed 4. Ames, IA, Iowa State Press, 2002, pp 575–606.

Simon D, et al: Adjuvant treatment of canine invasive malignant mammary gland tumors with doxorubicin and docetaxel (abstract). *J Vet Intern Med* 18: 790–791, 2004.

Sorenmo KU, et al: Effect of spaying and timing of spaying on survival of dogs with mammary carcinoma. *J Vet Intern Med* 14(3):266–270, 2000.

AUTHORS: **DANIELA SIMON, BETH A. VALENTINE**

EDITORS: **KENNETH M. RASSNICK, MICHELLE A. KUTZLER**

Marijuana Toxicosis

BASIC INFORMATION

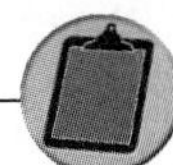

DEFINITION

Acute toxicosis resulting from ingestion of *Cannabis sativa* and characterized by any of the following signs: central nervous system (CNS) depression ataxia, vomiting, hypothermia, bradycardia, hyperreflexia, and possibly coma

SYNONYM(S)

Common street names: *Cannabis sativa,* grass, hashish, hemp (not to be confused with textile hemp, which is THC-deficient), marijuana, Mary Jane, pot, reefer, THC

EPIDEMIOLOGY

SPECIES, AGE, SEX

- Most commonly exposed animals include dogs 96%, cats 3%, other species 1%.
- Dogs exposed are commonly under the age of 5 years.

RISK FACTORS: In humans with a history of seizures, use of marijuana has been associated with lowering the seizure threshold.

CLINICAL PRESENTATION

HISTORY, CHIEF COMPLAINT

- History of exposure to marijuana.
- Ataxia, CNS depression, tremors, vomiting within 15 to 30 minutes of ingestion.
- Specific history of exposure may be withheld by owner due to illicit nature of marijuana.

PHYSICAL EXAM FINDINGS

- Common:
  - Bradycardia
  - Hypothermia (body temperature: 98–99° F [36.7–37.2° C])
  - Mydriasis
  - Vomiting
  - Urinary incontinence
  - Weakness, ataxia
- Possible:
  - Hyperesthesia
  - Hypersalivation
  - Recumbency
  - Tachycardia
  - Tremors
  - Coma

ETIOLOGY AND PATHOPHYSIOLOGY

- Source:
  - Marijuana refers to a mixture of cut, dried flowers, leaves, and stems of the leafy green hemp plant *Cannabis sativa*. It grows in warm, moist climates, or is grown artificially indoors (greenhouses), and can be rolled into cigarettes or in some cases baked into food.
  - Exposure to marijuana in pet animals is mostly accidental, but occasionally is intentional or malicious. Sometimes, drug-detection dogs ingest large amounts of marijuana accidentally.
  - Marijuana is a schedule I control substance commonly used as a recreational drug.
  - It is also used for treating nausea for chemotherapy patients and to decrease intraocular pressure in glaucoma patients.
- Pathophysiology:
  - The predominant psychoactive portion of marijuana is δ-9-tetrahydrocannabinol (THC). THC is believed to act on a unique receptor in the brain that is selective for cannabinoids and is primarily responsible for CNS effects (ataxia and depression).
  - Cannabinoids also enhance CNS formation of norepinephrine, dopamine, and serotonin, and stimulate release of dopamine and enhance γ-aminobutyric acid turnover.
  - When taken orally, THC goes through substantial initial hepatic metabolism (first pass effect). It is highly lipophilic and distributes to brain and other fatty tissues after absorption.
  - Clinical signs in dogs may last 24 to 96 hours.
  - Oral LD50 of THC in rats = 666 mg/kg, mice = 482 mg/kg. Clinical effects of marijuana are seen at much lower doses than this.
  - Concentration of THC in marijuana varies between 1% and 8%.

DIAGNOSIS

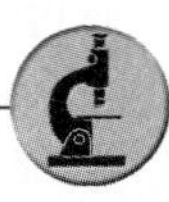

DIFFERENTIAL DIAGNOSIS

Overall, the acuity of onset of clinical signs generally suggests metabolic or toxic CNS disorders, but acute decompensation of primary CNS diseases (e.g., granulomatous meningoencephalitis, neoplasia, others) is possible, especially in an animal that is not closely observed by its owner.

- Hypoglycemia
- Ethylene glycol toxicosis
- Macadamia nuts toxicosis
- Ivermectin toxicosis

INITIAL DATABASE

- Arerial blood pressure (normal or below normal; normal [systolic] >120 mmHg in clinical setting)
- Complete blood count, serum biochemistry panel, urinalysis (to assess for preexisting conditions): no significant changes expected

ADVANCED OR CONFIRMATORY TESTING

- Over-the-counter illicit drug test kits may help confirm exposure in urine during the early course of exposure.
- Rapid analysis at human hospital labs is also an option for confirmation.

TREATMENT

THERAPEUTIC GOAL(S)

- Decontamination of patient
- Supportive care

ACUTE GENERAL TREATMENT

- Decontamination of patient:
  - Emesis: can be induced within 15 to 30 minutes of exposure, as long as no overt clinical signs of toxicosis are present. Use hydrogen peroxide at 2.2 ml/kg PO; max 45 ml. Repeat once if emesis does not occur first time.
  - Apomorphine: not likely to work as an emetic due to strong central antiemetic effect of marijuana.
  - Activated charcoal: very beneficial. Indicated when emesis is absent, in patients with or without clinical signs. In patients with clinical signs or large ingestions, multiple doses can be used every 8 hours to reduce enterohepatic recirculation; 1-3 g/kg or labeled dosage of commercial products.
- Supportive care:
  - IV fluids as needed for dehydration, hypovolemia.
  - Thermoregulation (heating pads for hypothermia).
  - Monitor cardiovascular function. Atropine at a dose of 0.022-0.044 mg/kg IM or SQ can be given for bradycardia in normotensive patients.
  - Control tremors with diazepam at a low dose of 0.25 mg/kg IV.
  - Monitor for signs of aspiration pneumonia in recumbent animals. Pass cuffed endotracheal tube if needed, ensuring a mouth gag/speculum is also used in order to avoid the patient biting and transecting the tube when recovering.
  - Control severe vomiting with metoclopramide at 0.2-0.4 mg/kg q 6h PO, SQ, or IM, once ingested material has been expelled.

DRUG INTERACTIONS

Other CNS depressants (barbiturates, benzodiazepines) may exacerbate signs.

POSSIBLE COMPLICATIONS

Aspiration pneumonia

RECOMMENDED MONITORING

- Heart rate
- Blood pressure
- Body temperature

PROGNOSIS AND OUTCOME

- Excellent with treatment
- Fatalities are extremely rare

PEARLS & CONSIDERATIONS

COMMENTS

A dog presenting with acute onset ataxia, CNS depression, and urinary incontinence that improves with stimulation and then gets worse again with decreased stimulation should be considered highly suspect of marijuana ingestion, until proven otherwise.

SUGGESTED READING

Donaldson CW: Marijuana exposure in animals. *Vet Med* 97:6,2002.

Khan SA: Toxicities from illicit and abused drugs. In Kahn CM (ed): *Merck Veterinary Manual*. Rahway, New Jersey, Merck & Co., Inc., 2005, pp 2537-2541.

Pawel J, Donaldson CW, Gwaltney S: Marijuana toxicosis in dogs 213 cases (1998-2001). *Vet Hum Toxicol* 46:1, 2004.

AUTHOR: **CAROLINE W. DONALDSON**

EDITOR: **SAFDAR A. KHAN**

Mass, Abdominal

BASIC INFORMATION

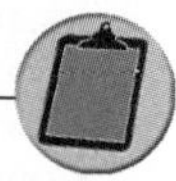

DEFINITION

An abnormal confluence or collection of inflammatory cells, infectious organisms, or neoplastic cells within the abdominal cavity

EPIDEMIOLOGY

SPECIES, AGE, SEX: Any; based on the origin of the mass.

CLINICAL PRESENTATION

HISTORY, CHIEF COMPLAINT

- Variable, from overt illness to incidental discovery on routine exam
- Dependent on organ system affected and systemic involvement

PHYSICAL EXAM FINDINGS

- Specific abdominal findings may include:
  - Distention
  - Pain
  - Palpable mass
  - Fluid
- All dogs with abdominal masses require a digital rectal examination (see Rectal Palpation, p 1304).

ETIOLOGY AND PATHOPHYSIOLOGY

Variable, depending on organ system affected and systemic involvement

DIAGNOSIS

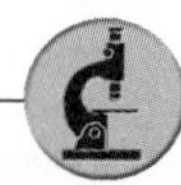

DIFFERENTIAL DIAGNOSIS

Common differential diagnoses for abdominal masses include:

- Spleen: malignant neoplasia (hemangiosarcoma, fibrosarcoma, chondrosarcoma, lymphoma, mastocytosis), benign neoplasia (hemangioma, lipoma), splenic abscess, splenic torsion, hematoma, splenic congestion secondary to drug administration or other toxins, mastocytosis, autoimmune disease, systemic infection/inflammation, normal folded spleen.
- Liver: malignant neoplasia (hepatocellular carcinoma, lymphoma, hemangiosarcoma, mastocytosis, etc.), benign neoplasia (biliary [cyst]adenoma, lipoma, etc.), abscess, hematoma (trauma), chronic passive congestion, regenerative nodular hyperplasia.
- Lymphadenopathy: reactive versus infiltrated.
- Gastrointestinal tract: malignant neoplasia (leiomyosarcoma, adenocarcinoma, etc.), benign neoplasia (adenoma, leiomyoma, etc.), foreign body, intestinal volvulus, trichobezoar, ileus, gastric dilation-volvulus, fecal material.

- Granuloma: secondary to foreign body reaction (retained suture material or gauze), infectious organisms such as protozoa or fungi.
- Pancreas: abscess, hemorrhagic pancreatitis, phlegmon.
- Uterus: uterine torsion, pyometra, mucometra/hydrometra, pregnancy.
- Ovary: cyst, neoplasia (papillary adenoma/adenocarcinoma, granulosa cell tumor, etc.).
- Prostate: benign prostatic hypertrophy, prostatitis, prostatic abscess, prostatic cyst, paraprostatic cyst.
- Testicles: neoplasm of cryptorchid testicle, torsion of cryptorchid testicle.
- Urinary bladder: malignant neoplasia (transitional cell carcinoma, others), cystitis, urolith.
- Kidney: malignant neoplasia (renal cell carcinoma, lymphoma, hemangiosarcoma, etc.), benign neoplasia, polycystic renal disease, toxin ingestion (ethylene glycol), pyelonephritis, hydronephrosis, perirenal pseudocysts.
- Adrenal glands: malignant or benign neoplasia (adenocarcinoma, lymphoma; adenoma).
- Peritoneal cavity and mesentery: cyst, malignant neoplasia (carcinomatosis, mesothelioma), benign neoplasia (lipoma, other).

INITIAL DATABASE

- Complete blood count, serum biochemistry profile, urinalysis: results depend on underlying cause.
  - Avoid cystocentesis if ascites or caudal abdominal mass.
- Urine culture and sensitivity.
- Survey abdominal radiographs.
  - Complementary to ultrasound; may be superior if mass is extremely large or if vertebral involvement is possible.
- Abdominal ultrasound. Helps to determine:
  - Origin of the mass
  - Texture and vascularity of the mass (fine-needle aspirate/core biopsy possible?)
  - Invasiveness of the mass/amenability to surgical removal
  - Presence of free fluid for aspiration and cytologic analysis.
  - Presence of visible lesions consistent with metastasis.

ADVANCED OR CONFIRMATORY TESTING

- Contrast radiographic studies of urogenital tract
- Nuclear scintigraphy (liver, renal)
- Computed tomography
- Magnetic resonance imaging
- Abdominal exploratory celiotomy and tissue sampling for histopathologic examination

TREATMENT

THERAPEUTIC GOAL(S)

Remove mass

- Rationale: pathologic discrete abdominal masses often produce one or more of the following sequelae:
  - Localized or systemic infection
  - Signs of pain or organ dysfunction (mechanical compression)
  - Ongoing growth and subsequent metastasis
  - Death from hemorrhage, metastasis, infection/sepsis, shock, or organ failure

ACUTE GENERAL TREATMENT

- Variable, depending on the origin of the mass.
- The usual treatment of choice for pathologic discrete abdominal masses is surgical removal.

CHRONIC TREATMENT

- Variable, depending on the origin of the mass.
- Adjunct therapy including intravenous fluid therapy, blood products, nutritional supplementation, chemotherapy, or antimicrobial medication administration may be indicated, depending on origin of mass and final histopathologic diagnosis.

POSSIBLE COMPLICATIONS

- Recurrence of infection or neoplasia
- Metastasis
- Hemorrhage
- Shock
- Weight loss, anorexia
- Peritonitis

RECOMMENDED MONITORING

Variable, depending on source of abdominal mass.

PROGNOSIS AND OUTCOME

Variable, depending on source of abdominal mass

PEARLS & CONSIDERATIONS

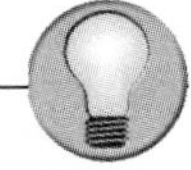

COMMENTS

- Some normal processes (folded spleen, pregnancy) cause an abdominal mass effect and must be ruled out before proceeding to treatment.
- Abdominal masses may be suspected as being pathologic via careful abdominal palpation and abdominal ultrasound and, if so, are definitively diagnosed by surgical exploration and histopathologic examination.
- Nonresectable discrete masses may be treated with alternative therapies depending on the diagnosis; however, prognosis is generally poorer for a patient with a nonresectable mass.

PREVENTION

Variable, depending on the origin of the mass

CLIENT EDUCATION

- Tests, including laboratory evaluation, imaging, and biopsy are necessary in most cases for definitive assessment of an abdominal mass.
- Definitive treatment and outcome for a patient with an abdominal mass are dependent on the origin of the mass, whether the mass is resectable, and if the mass is causing any systemic effects.

SUGGESTED READING

Barthez PY, Marks SL, Woo J, et al: Pheochromocytoma in dogs: 61 cases (1984-1995). *J Vet Intern Med* 11:272-278, 1997.

Barthez PY, Nyland TG, Feldman EC: Ultrasonography of the adrenal glands in the dog, cat, and ferret. *Vet Clin North Am Small Anim Pract* 28:869-885, 1998.

Caruso KJ, Meinkoth JH, Rick L, Cowell RL, et al: A distal colonic mass in a dog. *Vet Clin Pathol* 32:27-30, 2003.

Chastain CB, Panciera D, Waters C: Surgical treatment of adrenocortical tumors: 21 cases (1990-1996). *Small Anim Clin Endocrinol* 11:93-97, 2001.

Crawshaw J, Berg J, Sardinas JC, et al: Prognosis for dogs with nonlymphomatous, small intestinal tumors treated by surgical excision. *J Am Anim Hosp Assoc* 34:451-456, 1998.

Dhaliwal RS, Kitchell BE, Knight BL, et al: Treatment of aggressive testicular tumors in four dogs. *J Am Anim Hosp Assoc* 35:311-318, 1999.

Messick JB, Haddad T, Kitchell B, et al: Abdominal mass in a dog. *Vet Clin Pathol* 30:25-27, 2001.

Muleya JS, Yasuho Y, Munekazu Nakaich M, et al: Appearance of canine abdominal tumors with magnetic resonance imaging using a low field permanent magnet. *Vet Radiol* 38:444-447, 1997.

Prater MR, Bender H, Sponenberg DP: Intra-abdominal mass aspirate from an aged dog. *Vet Clin Pathol* 27:65-66, 1998.

AUTHOR: **ELLEN B. DAVIDSON DOMNICK**
EDITOR: **RICHARD WALSHAW**

Mass: Cutaneous, Subcutaneous

BASIC INFORMATION

DEFINITION

A lump made up of cohering cells in the skin (cutaneous) or soft tissue between the skin and underlying fascia, muscle, or bone

SYNONYM(S)

Bump, growth, lump, nodule, tumor

EPIDEMIOLOGY

SPECIES, AGE, SEX

- Older animals more commonly develop benign and malignant neoplasms.
- Eosinophilic lesions and plasma cell pododermatitis or stomatitis (cats).
- Canine juvenile cellulitis (puppies).
- Histiocytomas and viral papillomas (young dogs).
- Intact male cats are prone to abscesses because of fighting behavior.
- Mammary tumors (intact female dogs).
- Perianal gland tumors (intact male dogs).

GENETICS AND BREED PREDISPOSITION

- Boxers are prone to a variety of benign and malignant neoplasms.
- Keratinous cysts and nodular dermatofibrosis syndrome (German shepherds).
- Idiopathic focal mucinosis (Doberman pinschers).
- Dermatophyte pseudomycetoma (Persian cats).

CONTAGION AND ZOONOSIS: Transmissible venereal tumor is contagious between dogs.

GEOGRAPHY AND SEASONALITY: Transmissible venereal tumor is more prevalent in temperate climates.

ASSOCIATED CONDITIONS AND DISORDERS: Nodular dermatofibrosis syndrome in German shepherds may be associated with renal adenocarcinoma and uterine leiomyoma.

CLINICAL PRESENTATION

HISTORY, CHIEF COMPLAINT

- Most commonly, the pet owner visualizes or feels the mass, but it may be found incidentally by the veterinarian on physical examination.
- Historic information obtained should include:
  - Presence of similar lesions.
  - Rapidity of onset.
  - Evidence of pruritus or pain.
  - Presence of other animals in the household.
  - Possibility of exposure to anticoagulant rodenticides (hematomas).
  - Known trauma.
  - In cats, indoor/outdoor status should be known (increased risk of bite or scratch wounds, foreign bodies, other trauma).

PHYSICAL EXAM FINDINGS

- Characterize the mass in terms of size, shape, location, consistency, depth, ulceration, and whether it is freely movable or pedunculated.
- Examine local lymph nodes and possible sites of metastasis (e.g., lungs, abdomen). Local lymph nodes may be enlarged due to inflammation (i.e., reactive lymph node) or metastasis.
- A complete physical exam is essential to identify any associated abnormalities.

ETIOLOGY AND PATHOPHYSIOLOGY

- A neoplasm is caused by progressive, uncontrolled growth of cells. Unlike benign neoplasms, malignant neoplasia shows a greater degree of anaplasia, and exhibits invasive and metastatic properties. Most have an unknown cause, but some may be induced by irritation, trauma, viruses, vaccinations, or ultraviolet radiation exposure.
- Cysts are accumulation of material (keratin, serum, glandular product) within a membrane, due to idiopathic, traumatic, congenital, follicular, or pilar causes.
- A granuloma is a focal accumulation of mononuclear inflammatory cells due to bacteria, mycoses, mycobacteria, dermatophytes, parasites, endogenous or exogenous foreign objects, allergic, or idiopathic causes. Pyogranulomas also include neutrophilic inflammation.
- Keratoses are solid, circumscribed lesions caused by overproduction of keratin.
- A hamartoma is a benign, disorganized overgrowth of normal cells within a tissue, while a nevus is a hamartoma arising from any skin component.
- A hematoma is local extravasation of blood due to trauma and/or bleeding disorder.
- Abscesses result from a local accumulation of neutrophils and necrotic tissue cells usually secondary to a bacterial or fungal infectious agent.
- Urticaria is a group of wheals in the dermis caused by a hypersensitivity reaction to insect bites, food, irritants, drugs, allergens, or physical stimuli. Angioedema is a hypersensitivity reaction that occurs below the dermis.

DIAGNOSIS

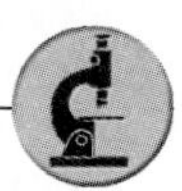

DIFFERENTIAL DIAGNOSIS

- Neoplasm:
  - Benign
  - Malignant:
    - Epithelial
    - Glandular
    - Mesenchymal
    - Round cell
- Pseudoneoplasm:
  - Cyst
  - (Pyo)granuloma
  - Keratoses
  - Hamartoma/nevus
  - Acral lick dermatitis
  - Feline plasma cell pododermatitis or stomatitis
  - Calcinosis cutis
  - Calcinosis circumscripta
  - Canine juvenile cellulitis
  - Nodular sterile panniculitis
  - Idiopathic lichenoid dermatitis (coalescent plaques)
  - Idiopathic focal mucinosis (Doberman pinschers)
  - Eosinophilic lesions:
    - Eosinophilic plaque
    - Indolent ulcer
    - Collagenolytic granuloma
- Hematoma
- Abscess
- Urticaria
- Angioedema
- Normal structures:
  - Lymph node
  - Salivary gland
  - Bulbus glandis (transient preputial "mass" in intact male dogs)

INITIAL DATABASE

- Confirm that the mass is not a normal structure (anatomic location).
- Cytologic examination of samples obtained from a mass via fine-needle aspiration, impression smear, scrape, or swab may provide a diagnosis.
- Fine-needle aspiration cytologic evaluation of a local lymph node may help discern an inflammatory reaction from metastasis.
- Examination for evidence of distant metastasis via three-view thoracic radiographs and/or abdominal ultrasound.
- Preoperative bloodwork (e.g., complete blood count, serum biochemical profile, urinalysis, depending on the age of the patient) if a biopsy is planned.

ADVANCED OR CONFIRMATORY TESTING

Histopathologic evaluation of an incisional or excisional biopsy sample generally is necessary for a definitive diagnosis.

TREATMENT

THERAPEUTIC GOAL(S)

- Eliminate the mass via surgery and/or medical management if possible.
- Known benign neoplasms or pseudoneoplasms may not need to be removed if they are not causing harm to the patient.

ACUTE GENERAL TREATMENT

- Many cutaneous or subcutaneous masses can be successfully removed surgically, and possibly cured if not malignant.
- Drainage and antibacterial therapy, based on culture and sensitivity information, is recommended for most abscesses.
- Medical therapy, without surgical removal, may be appropriate in cases of eosinophilic lesions, urticaria and angioedema, dermatophytic pseudomycetoma, hematomas, and some round cell tumors.

PROGNOSIS AND OUTCOME

- Depends on the diagnosis.
- Many benign growths can be cured with complete surgical removal or appropriate medical therapy.
- Therapy for malignant neoplasms rarely results in a cure, but long remissions can be obtained in many cases.

PEARLS & CONSIDERATIONS

COMMENTS

- Cytologic examination of a sample from a cutaneous or subcutaneous mass obtained by fine-needle aspiration is a simple and inexpensive diagnostic aid that should be recommended in most cases.
- Establishing a diagnosis via physical examination alone, and treating with clinical neglect, can lead to inappropriate patient outcomes.

SUGGESTED READING

Carlotti DN: Cutaneous and subcutaneous lumps, bumps and masses. In Ettinger SJ, Feldman EC (eds): *Textbook of Veterinary Internal Medicine*. St. Louis, Elsevier Saunders, 2005, pp 43–46.

Vail DM, Withrow SJ: Tumors of the skin and subcutaneous tissues. In Withrow SJ, MacEwen EG (eds): *Small Animal Clinical Oncology*. Philadelphia, WB Saunders, 2001, pp 233–260.

AUTHOR: **JEFF D. BAY**
EDITOR: **ETIENNE CÔTÉ**

Mass, Pancreatic

BASIC INFORMATION

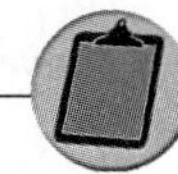

DEFINITION

Mass visualized in the pancreas via ultrasonography or during exploratory celiotomy

EPIDEMIOLOGY

SPECIES, AGE, SEX

- Dogs:
  - Masses associated with pancreatitis: Older intact or spayed females are overrepresented.
  - Endocrine pancreatic neoplasia: Middle-aged to older dogs are overrepresented.
- Cats:
  - Exocrine pancreatic neoplasia: middle-aged to older cats.

RISK FACTORS: Dogs: pancreatitis-associated masses from a high-fat diet.

ASSOCIATED CONDITIONS AND DISORDERS

- Dogs:
  - Pancreatitis-associated masses:
    - Hyperadrenocorticism
    - Diabetes mellitus
    - Hyperlipidemia
    - Biliary obstruction secondary to the mass
  - Exocrine pancreatic neoplasia:
    - Biliary obstruction
    - Paraneoplastic alopecia or panniculitis
  - Endocrine pancreatic mass (insulinoma):
    - Hypoglycemia: weakness, collapse, possibly seizures
- Cats:
  - Exocrine pancreatic neoplasia:
    - Biliary obstruction
    - Paraneoplastic alopecia

CLINICAL PRESENTATION

DISEASE FORMS/SUBTYPES

- Dogs:
  - Associated with pancreatitis:
    - Inflammatory/necrotic mass
    - Abscess
    - Pseudocyst
  - Nodular hyperplasia
  - Neoplasia (primary pancreatic): exocrine (adenocarcinoma) or endocrine (e.g., insulinoma)
  - Metastatic or local extension of another primary neoplasm
  - Icterus secondary to biliary obstruction
- Cats:
  - Associated with pancreatitis
  - Exocrine neoplasia
  - Icterus secondary to biliary obstruction
  - Endocrine neoplasia: extremely rare

HISTORY, CHIEF COMPLAINT

- Pancreatitis: vomiting, anorexia, lethargy, inappetence, diarrhea
- Exocrine neoplasia: similar but may include weight loss
- Secondary biliary obstruction: similar; some owners may also note icterus
- Endocrine neoplasia: weakness, lethargy, altered neurologic state

PHYSICAL EXAM FINDINGS

- Mass may be palpable
- Otherwise, variable depending on etiology of pancreatic mass:
  - Pancreatitis, exocrine pancreatic neoplasia
    - Abdominal pain, dehydration, icterus, palpable abdominal mass, pyrexia
  - Endocrine pancreatic neoplasia
    - Neurologic findings associated with hypoglycemia

ETIOLOGY AND PATHOPHYSIOLOGY

- Pancreatitis (see Pancreatitis, Dog, p 796; Pancreatitis, Cat, p 794).
- Exocrine pancreatic neoplasia: etiology unknown.
- Secondary biliary obstruction: lack of bile secretion into the intestine results in a lack of digestion and absorption of fat and fat-soluble vitamins, most importantly vitamin K; development of significant coagulopathy.
- Endocrine pancreatic neoplasia: inappropriate, excessive insulin secretion leads to persistent, profound hypo-

glycemia (see Insulinoma, p 598; Gastrointestinal Endocrine Disease, p 435).

DIAGNOSIS

DIFFERENTIAL DIAGNOSIS

- Pancreatitis: inflammation, necrosis, abscess, pseudocyst, fibrosis
- Exocrine neoplasm: adenocarcinoma
- Metastasis of another primary neoplasm to the pancreas: gastric or duodenal adenocarcinoma, leiomyosarcoma, lymphoma

INITIAL DATABASE

- CBC: inflammatory leukogram with or without evidence of inflammation (e.g., with pancreatitis): left shift, toxic neutrophil changes.
- Serum biochemistry profile, urinalysis: reflect underlying disorder.
    - Elevated amylase, lipase, ± bilirubin, ± liver enzyme concentrations: pancreatitis.
    - Hypoglycemia: insulinoma.
    - Hyperbilirubinemia, bilirubinuria: secondary biliary obstruction.
- Survey abdominal radiographs:
    - Mass effect in region of pancreas: may displace duodenum laterally, pylorus cranially.
    - Possible increased radiopacity in area of pancreas (pancreatitis).
    - Diffuse granular appearance to abdomen: carcinomatosis.
- Survey thoracic radiographs: help rule out metastatic disease if neoplasia suspected.

ADVANCED OR CONFIRMATORY TESTING

- Abdominal ultrasound examination:
    - Pancreas, morphology/echogenicity of mass:
        - Generalized inflammation of pancreas and surrounding structures: pancreatitis.
        - Fluid-filled mass: pancreatic abscess (mixed echogenicity common), cyst (contents generally anechoic).
        - Solid mass (head of pancreas): exocrine neoplasia.
        - Small, isolated, well-defined mass: insulinoma (hepatic metastases commonly present at time of diagnosis).
    - Evaluation of adjacent organs:
        - Extension of pancreatic disease into duodenum.
            - Inflammation
            - Neoplasia
        - Extension of duodenal disease into pancreas.
            - Neoplasia
        - Evidence of metastatic disease.
            - Regional lymph nodes
            - Liver
            - Carcinomatosis (ascites usually is also present)
    - Evidence of secondary biliary obstruction: any mass, when sufficiently large.
        - Common bile duct dilation.
    - Possible ultrasound-guided fine-needle aspiration (cytologic examination) or needle biopsy of pancreatic mass.
        - Possible metastatic sites:
            - Regional lymph nodes
            - Liver
- Suspected insulinoma:
    - Simultaneous measurement of fasting blood glucose and serum insulin concentrations (see Insulinoma, p 598; Gastrointestinal Endocrine Disease, p 435).

TREATMENT

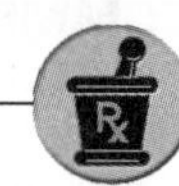

THERAPEUTIC GOAL(S)

Dependent on etiology of pancreatic mass but may include:

- Correction of fluid deficits
- Normalization of serum electrolyte concentrations
- Normalization of coagulation status prior to surgery
- Correction of hypoglycemia (preoperative and postoperative)
- Relief of extrahepatic biliary obstruction
- Nutritional support if indicated (see Parenteral Nutrition, p 1296; Feeding Tube Placement: Percutaneous Endoscopic Jejunostomy [PEJ], p 1249)
    - Animal that has pancreatitis
    - In animals that have undergone extensive pancreatic/duodenal resections, parenteral and enteral nutritional support should be provided postoperatively

ACUTE GENERAL TREATMENT

Dependent on etiology of pancreatic mass but may include:

- Rehydration by IV administration of balanced electrolyte solution and possibly colloid solutions
- Possible administration of fresh frozen plasma (see Transfusion Therapy and Collection Techniques for Blood Banking, p 1312):
    - Hypoproteinemia
    - Possible coagulopathy
- Treat hypoglycemia if present (see Insulinoma, p 598):
    - Addition of dextrose (5%) to IV fluids
    - Change of diet and feeding schedule
    - Corticosteroids
- Vitamin K administration if biliary obstruction (vitamin K1 2.5-5 mg/kg SC or IM, q 12h for 3 days, then once weekly until obstruction relieved)
- Exploratory laparotomy:
    - Identifying pancreatic mass and extent of intra-abdominal disease
    - Removing mass or performing biopsy
    - Draining and omentalizing pancreatic abscess if present
    - Performing biopsy of possible metastatic lesions
    - Correcting biliary obstruction
    - Placing feeding tube for nutritional support (see Parenteral Nutrition, p 1296; Feeding Tube Placement, Percutaneous Endoscopic Jejunostomy [PEJ], p 1249)

POSSIBLE COMPLICATIONS

- Ongoing or recurrent pancreatitis
- Iatrogenically induced pancreatitis
- Persistent hypoglycemia: incomplete removal of primary tumor or functioning metastatic lesions

RECOMMENDED MONITORING

- Dependent on etiology of pancreatic mass but may include:
    - CBC and serum biochemistry profile
    - Blood glucose concentrations
    - Serum amylase and lipase concentrations
- Repeat abdominal ultrasound examination for chronological assessment:
    - Resolution or progression of pancreatic disease
    - Regrowth of pancreatic neoplasm
    - Development of metastatic disease

PROGNOSIS AND OUTCOME

- Fair to guarded in animals with pancreatitis with or without secondary development of abscesses.
- Poor in animals with malignant exocrine pancreatic neoplasia (adenocarcinoma).
- Insulinoma:
    - Persistent hypoglycemia or inability to completely resect all neoplastic disease indicates a poor prognosis.
    - Resolution of hypoglycemia or complete resection of neoplastic disease indicates a good prognosis.

SUGGESTED READING

Jubb KVF: The pancreas. In Jubb KVF, Kennedy PC, Palmer N (eds): *Pathology of Domestic Animals*, vol 2. Orlando, FL, Academic Press, 1985, pp 412–424.

Mayhew PD, et al: Pathogenesis and outcome of extrahepatic biliary obstruction in cats. *J Small Anim Pract*, 43:247, 2002.

Seaman RL: Exocrine pancreatic neoplasia in the cat: A case series. *J Am Anim Hosp Assoc* 40:238, 2004.

AUTHOR: **DAVID HOLT**

EDITOR: **RICHARD WALSHAW**

Mass, Splenic

BASIC INFORMATION

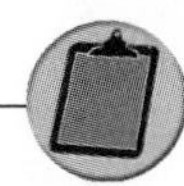

DEFINITION

Diffuse nodular or focal enlargement of the spleen

EPIDEMIOLOGY

SPECIES, AGE, SEX, AND BREED PREDISPOSITION

- Large- to giant-breed, geriatric, male dogs:
  - German shepherds
  - Great Danes
  - Retrievers
- Cats: Splenic lesions are less common and, when present, usually consist of diffuse splenomegaly (see Splenomegaly, p 1027).

ASSOCIATED CONDITIONS AND DISORDERS

- Anemia
- Hemoabdomen
- Disseminated intravascular coagulation (DIC)
- Metastasis

CLINICAL PRESENTATION

DISEASE FORMS/SUBTYPES

- Diffuse, nodular splenic enlargement (multiple masses)
- Focal splenic enlargement (single mass)

HISTORY, CHIEF COMPLAINT

- Incidental finding (no clinical signs)
- Nonspecific signs:
  - Inappetence, lethargy, weight loss, vomiting, diarrhea, discolored urine
- Abdominal enlargement:
  - Obvious mass
- Weakness, collapse

PHYSICAL EXAM FINDINGS: Variable depending on etiology of splenic mass:

- Abdominal distention:
  - Fluid (palpable fluid wave possible)
  - Mass
- Pale mucous membranes, poor or nonpalpable pulses, weakness, tachycardia and tachypnea:
  - Acute blood loss despite normal coagulation (e.g., mass rupture)
  - Bleeding/coagulation disorder
- Nonspecific findings:
  - Fever, dehydration
- Associated findings depending on etiology
  - Peripheral lymphadenopathy
  - Neoplasia elsewhere

ETIOLOGY AND PATHOPHYSIOLOGY

Etiology:

- Diffuse, nodular splenic enlargement (multiple masses):
  - Diffuse neoplasia, for example:
    - Lymphoma
    - Mast cell neoplasia
  - Metastatic neoplasia, for example:
    - Hemangiosarcoma
    - Mast cell neoplasia
- Focal splenic enlargement (single mass):
  - Hematoma
  - Neoplasia
    - Benign, for example:
      - Hemangioma
    - Malignant, for example:
      - Hemangiosarcoma
      - Soft tissue sarcoma

DIAGNOSIS

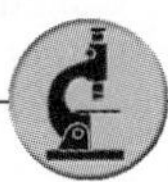

DIFFERENTIAL DIAGNOSIS

Mass arising from/involving another abdominal organ:

- Liver
  - Diffuse hepatomegaly
  - Neoplasia
    - Benign
      - Hepatocellular adenoma
    - Malignant
      - Hepatocellular carcinoma
      - Hemangiosarcoma
- Kidney
  - Neoplasia
    - Renal adenocarcinoma
    - Hemangiosarcoma
  - Hydronephrosis
  - Cyst/polycystic renal disease
  - Perirenal pseudocyst
- Stomach
  - Gastric dilatation/volvulus
- Abdominal cavity
  - Omental mass
- Paraprostatic cyst

INITIAL DATABASE

Some, all, or none of these abnormalities may be present, depending on the case.

- Complete blood count, serum biochemistry profile, urinalysis:
  - Hemorrhage (regenerative anemia, mild panhypoproteinemia)
  - Mass-associated hemolysis (schistocytosis)
  - Paraneoplastic immune-mediated hemolytic anemia (anemia, spherocytosis)
  - Involvement of other organ systems
- Survey abdominal radiographs:
  - Determine if mass appears to be arising from spleen
  - Evidence of other intra-abdominal disease
  - Lymphadenopathy
- Survey thoracic radiographs:
  - Metastatic disease
  - Lymphadenopathy

ADVANCED OR CONFIRMATORY TESTING

- Ultrasound examination:
  - Confirmation of origin of mass
  - Involvement of other organs
  - Metastatic disease
  - Identification of free abdominal fluid for centesis
- Coagulation profile:
  - Hemangiosarcoma potentially can be associated with coagulation disorders
  - Prothrombin time, partial thromboplastin time, platelet count, antithrombin III, fibrin degradation products, D-dimer
- Electrocardiogram (ECG):
  - Ventricular arrhythmias, other arrhythmias
    - Common in dogs with splenic hemangiosarcoma
- Fine-needle aspiration cytology/needle biopsy (ultrasound guided): often contraindicated if splenic mass is highly vascular (poor diagnostic yield, and risk of rupture):
  - Benign versus malignant disease
  - Type of malignancy
    - Primary versus metastatic
  - May be a low yield procedure with certain malignancies (hemangiosarcoma)
    - May only obtain blood
    - Miss focus of neoplastic cells
  - Concern about seeding tumor cells throughout abdominal cavity
- Echocardiography:
  - Rule out presence of cardiac hemangiosarcoma

TREATMENT

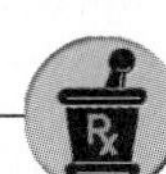

THERAPEUTIC GOAL(S)

- If acute intra-abdominal hemorrhage (e.g., splenic hemangiosarcoma):
  - Support cardiovascular system
  - Prevent exsanguination
  - Aggressively treat any coagulation disorder
  - Specifically treat cardiac arrhythmias, if indicated
- Obtain definitive diagnosis if previous attempts at diagnosis have been unsuccessful

ACUTE GENERAL TREATMENT

Dependent upon etiology of splenic mass:

- Nonsurgically treated splenic masses:
  - Neoplasia—lymphoma, mast cell neoplasia (dog ± cat):
    - Chemotherapy
  - Diffuse metastatic disease—hemangiosarcoma:
    - Palliative, nonsurgical treatment

- Surgically treated splenic masses (splenectomy with histopathologic examination):
  - Benign disease (hematoma, hemangioma)
  - Malignant disease without widespread metastasis (hemangioma, soft tissue sarcoma)
  - Malignant disease with evidence of metastasis, as part of multi-modality treatment plan:
    - Mast cell neoplasia—cat

Prior to splenectomy, if acute intra-abdominal hemorrhage has occurred:

- Support cardiovascular system by replacing intravascular volume and reestablishing peripheral tissue perfusion, replacing blood loss, if significant, and restoring normal cardiac function.
  - Intravenous fluid therapy.
  - Transfusion therapy.
  - Abdominal wrap/gentle abdominal pressure bandage to reduce rate of bleeding if surgery is delayed; ensure ventilation is not compromised.
- Treat any coagulation disorder:
  - Fresh frozen plasma.
  - Fresh whole blood.
- Correct or control cardiac arrhythmias—premature ventricular complexes and ventricular tachycardia (see Ventricular Arrhythmias [Premature Ventricular Complexes, Ventricular Tachycardia], p 1148):
  - In an anemic or hypokalemic patient, correction of these problems often resolves the ventricular arrhythmia without antiarrhythmic drugs.
  - Lidocaine:
    - 2-4 mg/kg, intravenous bolus
    - 50 ug/kg/min continuous rate infusion

CHRONIC TREATMENT

- Continued supportive care in the postoperative period:
  - Intravenous fluid therapy
  - Transfusion therapy
  - Treatment of cardiac arrhythmias
- Long-term treatment dependent upon etiology of splenic mass:
  - Chemotherapy for certain types of neoplasia:
    - Lymphoma
    - Mast cell neoplasia
    - Hemangiosarcoma without gross metastatic disease

DRUG INTERACTIONS

- Avoid thiobarbiturates as part of anesthetic protocol.
  - Cause relaxation of smooth muscle of the splenic capsule.
    - Sequestration of red blood cells (RBCs)
      - Splenic congestion
      - Possible greater difficulty in removing spleen
  - Potentially contraindicated if preexisting ventricular arrhythmias exist.
    - Thiopental causes arrhythmias in approximately 40% of dogs
- Avoid acepromazine or other phenothiazine tranquilizers as part of anesthetic protocol.
  - Cause hypotension via central mechanisms and through α-adrenergic actions.
  - May cause cardiovascular collapse secondary to bradycardia and hypotension.

POSSIBLE COMPLICATIONS

Associated with preoperative rupture of the splenic mass:

- Hypotension
- Hemorrhagic/hypovolemic shock
- Cardiovascular collapse and death

Associated with splenectomy:

- Hemorrhage
- Coagulation disorders
- Sepsis:
  - Loss of white blood cell reservoir
  - Loss of phagocytic function of spleen
- Anemia:
  - Loss of RBC reservoir
  - Decreased hematopoiesis
  - Altered iron metabolism
- Diminished immune function
- Pancreatitis:
  - Inadvertent ligation of pancreatic branch of splenic artery and vein
  - Traumatic handling or retraction of pancreas during splenectomy

RECOMMENDED MONITORING

Postoperative patient monitoring:

- Detection of ongoing hemorrhage:
  - Packed cell volume (PCV), complete blood count
- Maintenance of normovolemia and tissue perfusion:
  - PCV, total solids
  - Urine output
  - Blood pressure
- Continuation/development of cardiac arrhythmias (ventricular premature contractions):
  - ECG monitoring
  - Appropriate treatment, if indicated
    - See Acute General Treatment above.

Long-term monitoring:

- Dependent upon etiology of splenic mass
- May include:
  - Repeat radiographs and ultrasound examination to detect recurrence of malignancy/development of metastasis
  - Monitoring associated with adjuvant chemotherapy:
    - Periodic blood tests
    - Echocardiogram

PROGNOSIS AND OUTCOME

Dependent upon etiology of splenic mass:

- Hemangiosarcoma in dogs:
  - Most common malignant splenic neoplasm.
  - Median survival time postsplenectomy ranges from 10 to 23 weeks.
- Postsplenectomy survival times:
  - 2-month survival times:
    - 83% if non-neoplastic disease
    - 31% if hemangiosarcoma
  - 12-month survival times:
    - 64% if non-neoplastic disease
    - 7% if neoplastic
  - Cats with systemic mastocytosis that undergo splenectomy often have extended survival times and can even be cured.

Preoperatively, dogs with anemia, nucleated RBC, abnormal RBC morphology, or splenic rupture are more likely to have malignant splenic neoplasia. NOTE: These findings should not lead to the definitive conclusion that the splenic mass is due to malignant neoplasia

PEARLS & CONSIDERATIONS

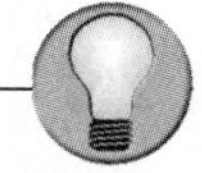

COMMENTS

- In the dog, a splenic mass may be nonneoplastic (hematoma) or a benign (hemangioma) or malignant (hemangiosarcoma) neoplasm. A single biopsy may result in a false-negative diagnosis. Therefore, the *entire* spleen should always be submitted for histopathologic examination.
- It can be difficult to differentiate splenic masses by their gross appearance. Therefore, a diagnosis is always based on histopathologic examination, not on gross appearance.
  - Over 50% of dogs have malignant disease and over 40% have benign disease.
- An echocardiogram is recommended prior to splenectomy to rule out presence of primary cardiac hemangiosarcoma. The splenic hemangiosarcoma may represent metastatic disease.

CLIENT EDUCATION

- Splenic masses may rupture and cause lethal intra-abdominal hemorrhage.
- Over 50% of splenic masses in the dog are malignant neoplasms.
  - Splenectomy does not extend survival time with regard to the malignancy.
  - Splenectomy prevents exsanguinations.
  - Splenectomy improves the quality of life for the patient.

SUGGESTED READING

Johnson KA, Powers BE, Withrow SJ, et al: Splenomegaly in dogs: Predictors of neoplasia and survival after splenectomy. *J Vet Intern Med* 3:160-166, 1989.

Marino DJ, Matthiesen DT, Fox PR, et al: Ventricular arrhythmias in dogs undergoing splenectomy: A prospective study. *Vet Surg* 23: 101-106, 1994.

Pope ER: Spleen. In Bojrab MJ (ed): *Disease Mechanisms in Small Animal Surgery*, ed 2. Philadelphia, Lea & Febiger, 1993, pp 616–620.

Richardson EF, Brown NO: Hematological and biochemical changes and results of aerobic bacteriological culturing in dogs undergoing splenectomy. *J Am Anim Hosp Assoc* 32: 199–210, 1996.

Spangler WL, Kass PH: Pathologic factors affecting post-splenectomy survival in dogs. *J Vet Intern Med* 11:166–171, 1997.

Tillson DM: Surgical techniques—complete and partial splenectomy. In Slatter D (ed): *Textbook of Small Animal Surgery*, ed 3. Philadelphia, Saunders, 2003, pp 1056–1059.

AUTHOR: **ELLEN B. DAVIDSON DOMNICK**
EDITOR: **RICHARD WALSHAW**

Mast Cell Tumors, Cat

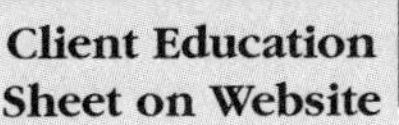

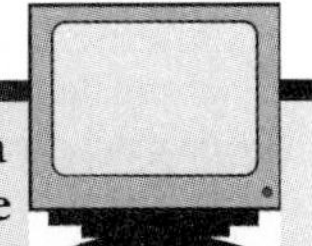

BASIC INFORMATION

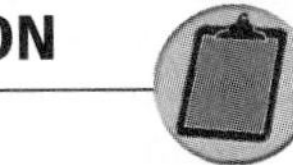

DEFINITION

Feline mast cell tumors are neoplastic accumulations of mast cells in cats. Mast cell tumors (MCTs) produce deleterious effects when the mast cells degranulate, a process resulting in the release of bioactive substances that can produce cutaneous or systemic clinical signs depending on tumor location.

SYNONYM(S)

Mast cell sarcoma
Mastocytoma
Splenic or visceral mastocytosis

EPIDEMIOLOGY

SPECIES, AGE, SEX: MCT is primarily a disease of older cats, although all ages can be affected. Males may be predisposed.
GENETICS AND BREED PREDISPOSITION: Siamese (possibly)
ASSOCIATED CONDITIONS AND DISORDERS: Caused by mast cell degranulation:

- Gastrointestinal ulceration
- Pruritus
- Hypotension

CLINICAL PRESENTATION

DISEASE FORMS/SUBTYPES: In cats, there are two distinct presentations:

- Cutaneous MCTs
- Splenic or visceral MCTs

HISTORY, CHIEF COMPLAINT

- Most cats with cutaneous MCT show no clinical signs, although some lesions are pruritic. MCTs often remain unchanged in size for months or years prior to presentation.
- Most cats with splenic or visceral MCTs display nonspecific signs of illness:
  - Weakness, lethargy.
  - Gastric ulceration–associated anorexia, bruxism, vomiting, diarrhea, weight loss, and melena.

PHYSICAL EXAM FINDINGS

- Although most cutaneous MCTs are found on the head, a thorough examination of the skin is indicated. Tumors are usually alopecic, small (<5 mm), round, and pink or white. Some MCTs are plaque-like.
- Approximately 15% of cats with cutaneous MCTs have concurrent splenic or visceral MCTs.
- Physical exam findings in cats with splenic or visceral MCTs include splenomegaly, ascites, abdominal mass, bowel wall thickening, and mucous membrane pallor secondary to anemia (induced by gastrointestinal ulceration and bleeding, or rarely myelophthisis).

ETIOLOGY AND PATHOPHYSIOLOGY

- Mast cells participate in allergic and inflammatory responses.
- Mast cells contain preformed granules consisting of histamine, heparin, and other cytokines that are released upon activation of the cells (degranulation).
- Mast cell tumors are accumulations of mast cells with malignant potential.
- Cytokine release causes clinical signs.
- Mast cell tumors occur in the skin, spleen, gastrointestinal tract (visceral), or a combination of these sites.
- Mast cell tumors most commonly metastasize to regional lymph nodes followed by spleen, liver, bone marrow, mesenteric lymph nodes, and other cutaneous sites.
- The etiology of feline MCTs is unknown.

DIAGNOSIS

DIFFERENTIAL DIAGNOSIS

- Cutaneous form: histiocytoma, lymphoma, eosinophilic granuloma complex, and lipoma.
- Splenic and visceral forms: splenomegaly: infectious splenitis, lymphoma, myeloproliferative disease, and hemangiosarcoma.
- Visceral lesions: inflammatory bowel disease, lymphoma, intestinal adenocarcinoma or sarcoma, and granulomas.

INITIAL DATABASE

Cutaneous form:

- The diagnosis of MCTs is frequently obtained by fine-needle aspiration of the lesion for cytologic examination.
- Prior to treatment, complete blood count (CBC), serum biochemistry panel, T4, urinalysis, FeLV/FIV test, and a regional lymph node aspirate should be obtained.
- Staging for systemic mast cell disease is indicated prior to surgery in patients with the following:
  - Lymph node metastasis is present.
  - Peritumoral edema or bruising is present.
  - Tumors are recurrent or multiple.
  - There is any suspicion of splenic or visceral MCTs (e.g., splenomegaly).
- Complete staging for metastasis includes CBC, serum biochemistry panel, urinalysis, serum thyroxine (T4) level, FeLV/FIV tests, buffy coat smear, thoracic and abdominal radiographs, abdominal ultrasound, bone marrow aspirate, regional lymph node aspirate or biopsy, and aspirate or biopsy of the primary tumor. Splenic/liver aspirates are indicated if these organs are enlarged or have an abnormal echotexture ultrasonigraphically.

Visceral and splenic forms:

- All cats with the splenic or visceral form of MCTs should have complete staging prior to definitive therapy.

ADVANCED OR CONFIRMATORY TESTING

- Cytologically, mast cells have a round nucleus and intracytoplasmic granules are almost always present.
- The histologic grading system used for canine cutaneous MCTs is not clinically significant in cats.
- CBC abnormalities associated with MCTs can include eosinophilia, basophilia, and regenerative or nonregenerative anemia.
- Normal lymph nodes may contain scattered mast cells; metastasis to regional lymph nodes is documented by the presence of increased numbers or clusters of mast cells in a lymph node draining a MCT.
- The buffy coat smear is more specific in cats than dogs. A positive test supports a diagnosis of mast cell metastasis in cats with MCT.
- The liver, spleen, and bone marrow normally contain a few mast cells; increased

numbers or clusters of mast cells are supportive of MCT metastasis.
- Thoracic radiographs: limited usefulness. Uncommonly, pleural effusion containing mast cells occurs with MCTs, and mediastinal MCTs have been reported.
- Abdominal ultrasound:
  - Affected lymph nodes may be enlarged or irregular.
  - Splenic/hepatic infiltration: hypoechoic lesions throughout the parenchyma, rarely a solitary mass.
  - Gastrointestinal tract lesions may be solitary or diffuse throughout the bowel.

TREATMENT

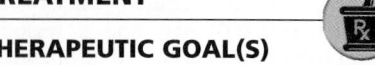

THERAPEUTIC GOAL(S)

In most cases, the goal of therapy is to control the local disease to prevent recurrence and metastasis. In cases presenting with metastasis or nonresectable local disease, the goal is to minimize tumor volume and maintain quality of life.

ACUTE GENERAL TREATMENT

Cutaneous form:
- Treatment options include surgery and radiation therapy.
- Spontaneous resolution is rare.
- Chemotherapy may play a role in some cats with cutaneous MCTs.
- Surgery is the primary treatment for cutaneous MCTs.
  - Wide surgical margins are not as important in cats as in dogs, since recurrence following incomplete excision is uncommon in the cat.
  - All tissue should be submitted for histologic evaluation; margins should be inked prior to placement in formalin.
  - Treatment with antihistamines for at least 48 hours prior to surgery is recommended (reduce effects of mast cell degranulation induced by surgical manipulation of the tumor).
  - Postoperative complications are uncommon; wound healing should be monitored following resection of large, infiltrative MCTs.
- Mast cell tumors in locations that preclude complete excision (i.e., periocular, pinna) are common; radiation therapy with external beam radiation therapy or strontium-90 plesiotherapy may be effective.
- Nonresectable (large/highly invasive/metastatic) tumors may require chemotherapy or radiation therapy prior to or instead of surgery.

Visceral form:
- Surgery is the primary treatment modality for visceral MCTs.
- Exploratory laparotomy is indicated, with incisional liver and mesenteric lymph node biopsies even if the tissue appears normal. Bowel wall masses should be resected if possible.
- Splenectomy is the treatment of choice in cats with splenic MCTs, even if metastasis or cutaneous MCT is present.
- Take care not to excessively manipulate known tumor tissue, since degranulation can result in anaphylaxis and hypotension during surgery.

Chemotherapy for feline MCT:
- The goal of chemotherapy is to delay or prevent metastasis or to attempt cytoreduction in nonresectable tumors or metastases. Chemotherapy for feline MCTs is not well studied. Chemotherapy drugs considered to be effective in the treatment of MCTs include prednisone, vinblastine, and lomustine. Special handling requirements and potentially severe or life-threatening adverse patient effects exist with these chemotherapeutic drugs; these concerns, and rapid evolution of protocols, warrant consultation with/referral to an oncologist.
- Potential indications for chemotherapy in cats with MCTs include: multiple or recurrent cutaneous MCTs, presence of metastasis at the time of diagnosis, or prior to attempting surgical excision in large, infiltrative tumors.

Adjunctive therapies:
- Antihistamines are indicated in cats with MCTs prior to surgical excision or in cases of nonresectable or metastatic disease.
- H_1 blockers = cyproheptadine (2 mg/cat q 12-24h) or diphenhydramine (1-2 mg/kg PO or SC q 12h); cyproheptadine is recommended due to its antiserotonin properties.
- H_2 blockers = ranitidine (1-2 mg/kg PO or SC q 12h) or famotidine (0.5 mg/kg PO or SC q 12-24h).
- Proton pump inhibitors (omeprazole 0.7 mg/kg PO q 24h) are indicated in cats that have developed gastric ulceration.
- Supportive care including nutritional and blood product support and analgesia are indicated perioperatively as needed.

PROGNOSIS AND OUTCOME

- The prognosis for cats with cutaneous MCTs is good; however, some cats will develop multiple cutaneous MCTs, regional lymph node metastasis, or splenic or visceral MCTs.
- Currently there is not a reliable way to predict in which cases this type of progression will occur; client education and frequent rechecks are recommended.
- The prognosis for cats with solitary splenic MCTs is good (median survival time following splenectomy: 12 months [range, 2 to 34 months]).
- For cats with splenic MCTs with other sites involved, the prognosis can be good, and the remaining mast cell disease may resolve following splenectomy. There is no reliable way to predict tumor behavior, so chemotherapy can be considered if metastatic sites do not resolve within 2 months of splenectomy or if clinical signs persist despite splenectomy.
- Primary gastrointestinal MCTs have the poorest prognosis, which may improve if the lesions are surgically resectable. The role of adjuvant chemotherapy is unclear, but should be considered.

PEARLS & CONSIDERATIONS

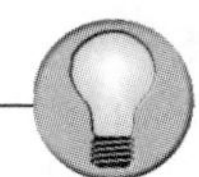

COMMENTS

Many cats with mast cell disease will develop additional MCTs during their lifetime, including cutaneous, splenic, or visceral forms. It is wise to schedule patients for rechecks at least every 4 to 6 months (or more often if indicated) for physical examinations and possibly restaging.

CLIENT EDUCATION

Any new skin masses or signs of illness should be evaluated as soon as possible.

SUGGESTED READING

Molander H, et al: Cutaneous mast cell tumors in cats: 32 cases. *J Am Anim Hosp Assoc* 34: 281, 1998.

Moore AS, Ogilvie GK: Skin tumors. In Ogilvie GK, Moore AS (eds): *Feline Oncology*. Trenton, NJ, Veterinary Learning Systems, 2001, pp 407-412.

Moore AS, Ogilvie GK: Splenic, hepatic, and pancreatic tumors. In Ogilvie GK, Moore AS (eds): *Feline Oncology*. Trenton, NJ, Veterinary Learning Systems, 2001, pp 295-298.

AUTHOR: **TRACY GIEGER**

EDITOR: **KENNETH M. RASSNICK**

Mast Cell Tumors, Dog

Client Education Sheet on Website

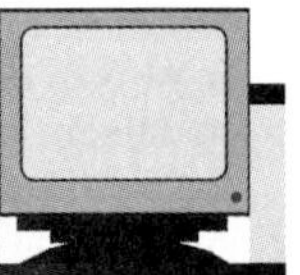

BASIC INFORMATION

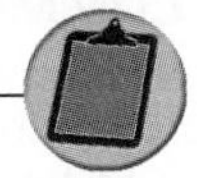

DEFINITION

Canine mast cell tumors (MCTs) are neoplastic accumulations of mast cells in dogs. MCTs produce deleterious effects when the mast cells degranulate, a process resulting in the release of bioactive substances that can produce cutaneous or systemic clinical signs, depending on tumor location.

SYNONYM(S)

Mast cell sarcoma
Mastocytoma
Systemic mastocytosis (metastatic MCT)

EPIDEMIOLOGY

SPECIES, AGE, SEX: No age or sex predilection in dogs.

GENETICS AND BREED PREDISPOSITION: Breeds predisposed to MCT:

- Boxer
- Boston terrier
- Golden retriever
- Labrador retriever
- Pug
- Shar-pei
- Staffordshire bull terrier
- Jack Russell terrier

ASSOCIATED CONDITIONS AND DISORDERS: Caused by mast cell degranulation:

- Gastrointestinal ulceration
- Pruritus
- Hypotension

CLINICAL PRESENTATION

HISTORY, CHIEF COMPLAINT

- Most dogs show no clinical signs and are evaluated due to an incidentally discovered cutaneous or subcutaneous mass. Some lesions are pruritic. MCTs often remain unchanged in size for months to years before presentation.
- Occasionally, dogs are evaluated because of signs related to gastric ulceration (vomiting, diarrhea, weight loss, melena) secondary to histamine-induced gastric acid secretion.

PHYSICAL EXAM FINDINGS

- Mast cell tumors have a highly variable appearance and may be mistaken for lipomas, skin tags, or insect bites. For this reason, skin and subcutaneous masses should always be aspirated and examined cytologically to obtain a diagnosis.
- Some dogs have multiple cutaneous MCTs, so a thorough examination of the entire skin surface is indicated.
- Because of the presence of histamine in mast cell granules, MCTs sometimes shrink and swell intermittently as degranulation (release of granules from the mast cell cytoplasm) occurs. Degranulation can result from manipulation of the tumor or can be spontaneous.
- Because of the presence of heparin in mast cell granules, MCT may bleed excessively when aspirated, but this is rarely clinically significant.
- Peritumoral bruising and edema (Darier's sign) are uncommon but are associated with aggressive-behaving MCT.

ETIOLOGY AND PATHOPHYSIOLOGY

- Mast cells participate in allergic and inflammatory responses. They contain preformed granules consisting of histamine, heparin, and other cytokines that are released on activation of the cells (degranulation).
- Mast cell tumors are accumulations of mast cells with malignant potential.
- Mast cell tumors occur primarily in the skin and subcutaneous tissues, and rarely in extracutaneous sites in dogs.
- Cytokine release causes clinical signs.
- MCTs most commonly metastasize to regional lymph nodes followed by spleen, liver, mesenteric lymph nodes, other cutaneous sites, and bone marrow.
- The etiology of MCT is unknown. Chronic inflammatory skin diseases or mutations in a proto-oncogene, c-KIT, may predispose dogs to mast cell neoplasia.

DIAGNOSIS

DIFFERENTIAL DIAGNOSIS

- Gross appearance and palpation:
  - Hemangiosarcoma, cutaneous
  - Lipoma
  - Phlebectasia
  - Granuloma
  - Abscess
- Cytologically, other round cell tumors (histiocytoma, lymphoma) may have a similar appearance.

INITIAL DATABASE

- MCTs are readily diagnosed cytologically due to their characteristic blue- or purple-staining intracytoplasmic granules.
  - In poorly differentiated MCTs, these granules may not be visible.
- Before surgical excision, a complete blood count (CBC), serum chemistry panel, urinalysis, and a regional lymph node aspirate (regardless of size of the lymph node) should be obtained.
  - CBC abnormalities associated with MCT can include eosinophilia, basophilia, and regenerative or nonregenerative anemia.
- Complete staging for systemic mast cell disease is indicated before surgery in the following patients:
  - Lymph node metastasis is present.
  - Peritumoral edema or bruising is present.
  - Tumors are recurrent.
  - Tumors are located on the prepuce, scrotum, muzzle, digit, pinna or ear canal, or oral mucosa (locations associated with a high rate of metastasis).
- Complete systemic staging to examine for evidence of MCT metastasis includes a CBC, serum chemistry panel, urinalysis, abdominal ultrasound, bone marrow aspiration cytologic study, regional lymph node aspirate or biopsy, and biopsy of the primary tumor.
- Splenic/liver aspirates are indicated if these organs are enlarged or have an abnormal echotexture ultrasonographically.

The buffy coat smear can be part of complete staging for dogs with MCT, but it has a high rate of false positive results and must be interpreted along with other staging tests to confirm metastasis.

ADVANCED OR CONFIRMATORY TESTING

- MCTs are categorized into grades based on their histologic appearance (Patnaik grading system):
  - Grade I = well-differentiated tumors
  - Grade II = intermediately differentiated tumors
  - Grade III = poorly differentiated tumors
- This grading system is the most consistent prognostic indicator for metastasis, disease-free interval, and survival for dogs with MCT. The metastatic rate for grade I and II tumors is less than 10%, and for grade III tumors it is greater than 50%.
- Normal lymph nodes may contain scattered mast cells; increased numbers or clusters of mast cells in a lymph node draining a MCT suggest metastasis.
- The liver, spleen, and bone marrow normally contain a few mast cells, but increased numbers or clusters of mast cells suggest MCT metastasis.

- Thoracic radiographs are of limited usefulness in dogs with MCT. Uncommonly, malignant pleural effusion containing mast cells occurs.
- Abdominal ultrasound:
  - Affected lymph nodes may be enlarged or irregular.
  - Splenic/hepatic infiltration: hypoechoic lesions throughout the parenchyma, rarely a solitary mass.

TREATMENT

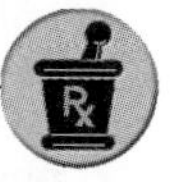

THERAPEUTIC GOAL(S)

- Most cases: to control the local disease, preventing recurrence and metastasis
- With metastasis or nonresectable local disease: to minimize tumor volume and maintain quality of life

ACUTE GENERAL TREATMENT

- Surgery is the primary treatment modality for MCT.
  - For most MCTs, tumors should be surgically excised with 2 cm or greater lateral margins and 1 fascial plane deep to the tumor.
  - All tissue should be submitted for histologic evaluation of grade and margins. Margins should be inked with a marking system before placement in formalin.
  - Histamine blockers are indicated in dogs with MCT before surgical excision or in cases of nonresectable or metastatic disease; H_1 blocker = diphenhydramine (1-2 mg/kg PO or SC q 12h), H_2 blockers = ranitidine (1-2 mg/kg PO or SC q 12h), or famotidine (0.5-1 mg/kg PO or SC q 12h). Proton pump inhibitors (omeprazole 0.5-1 mg/kg PO once daily) are indicated in dogs with MCT and gastric ulceration.
  - Postoperative complications are uncommon, but the patient should be monitored for poor wound healing after resection of large or infiltrative MCT.
- For tumors that are not surgically resectable due to size, invasiveness, or metastasis, chemotherapy or radiation therapy (RT) before or instead of surgery may be indicated.
- Mast cell tumors are responsive to RT.
  - Treating MCT in a microscopic disease setting (i.e., postsurgical resection) yields better results than if treatment is performed in a setting of macroscopic (measurable) disease.
  - Potential indications for RT for mast cell tumors include incompletely excised grade I and II MCT where wider surgical excision is not possible; as an adjunct to surgery and chemotherapy in dogs with grade III MCT; to attempt cytoreduction of nonresectable MCT.
- The goal of chemotherapy is to delay or prevent metastasis or to attempt to cytoreduce or slow progression of nonresectable tumors or metastatic lesions. Potential indications for chemotherapy in dogs with MCT include:
  - Dogs with grade III MCT (because at least 50% will develop metastasis).
  - Dogs with metastasis at diagnosis.
  - Before attempting surgical excision in large, fixed tumors or tumors with peritumoral edema or bruising.
- Chemotherapy drugs considered to be effective in the treatment of MCT include prednisone, vinblastine, and CCNU (lomustine). Special handling requirements and potentially severe or life-threatening adverse patient effects exist with these chemotherapeutic drugs; these concerns, and rapid evolution of protocols, warrant consultation with/referral to an oncologist.

PROGNOSIS AND OUTCOME

- The most significant prognostic indicator for MCT is tumor grade. For dogs with completely excised grade I and II MCT, the prognosis is excellent; approximately 5% of these tumors will recur locally. For dogs with incompletely excised grade I and II tumors, RT provides excellent long-term tumor control, with 80-90% of dogs free of tumor 2 to 5 years after treatment. For dogs with grade III MCT, long-term survival (>1 year) is uncommon due to metastasis and tumor recurrence; however, a recent study suggests that with effective local control, 70% of dogs with grade III tumors were alive 1 year after treatment.
- Tumors located on the prepuce, scrotum, muzzle, digit, pinna and ear canal, and oral mucosa appear to have a higher rate of regional lymph node and possibly distant metastasis versus MCT at other sites.
- Approximately 10-15% of dogs develop additional cutaneous MCTs, which may represent additional primary tumors or metastatic lesions.

PEARLS & CONSIDERATIONS

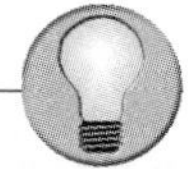

COMMENTS

- At least 10-15% of dogs with MCT will develop additional MCT during their lifetime.
- It is recommended to schedule patients for rechecks including thorough physical examinations every 4 to 6 months (or more often if indicated) to try to detect new masses as soon as possible.
- Grossly, fine-needle aspirates of mast cell tumors look transparent and watery, and are indistinguishable from fat. All fine-needle aspirations must be examined cytologically to differentiate fat from MCT.
- Buffy coat exams frequently are falsely positive and are inferior to bone marrow aspiration and cytologic evaluation for assessing hematologic involvement.
- Due to the occurrence of interpathologist variation when assigning histologic grades to MCT in dogs, the clinician must consider factors including tumor grade, location and size of the tumor, presence of regional and systemic metastasis, and completeness of surgical excision to determine an appropriate treatment plan and prognosis.
- Intralesional therapies such as deionized water or corticosteroids may provide temporary shrinkage of MCT, but are rarely effective for long-term tumor control and are not recommended.

CLIENT EDUCATION

Any new masses on the skin should be evaluated as soon as possible.

SUGGESTED READING

Hahn KA, King GK, Carreras JK: Efficacy of radiation therapy for incompletely resected grade III mast cell tumors in dogs: 31 cases. *J Am Vet Med Assoc* 224:79-82, 2004.

Patnaik AK, Ehler WJ, MacEwen EG: Canine cutaneous mast cell tumor: Morphologic grading and survival time in 83 dogs. *Vet Pathol* 21:469-474, 1984.

Thamm DH, Vail DM: Mast cell tumors. In Withrow SJ, MacEwen EG (eds): *Small Animal Clinical Oncology*. Philadelphia, Saunders, 2001, pp 261-279.

AUTHOR: **TRACY GIEGER**
EDITOR: **KENNETH M. RASSNICK**

Masticatory Muscle Myositis

BASIC INFORMATION

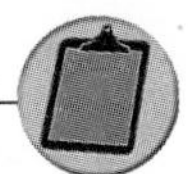

DEFINITION

An immune-mediated, focal, inflammatory myopathy preferentially affecting the muscles of mastication

EPIDEMIOLOGY

SPECIES, AGE, SEX: Dogs of any age, breed, or sex.

GENETICS AND BREED PREDISPOSITION

- German shepherds may be overrepresented.
- In some breeds (e.g., rottweiler, Samoyed, Doberman), inflammation and myofiber destruction can be especially severe.

CLINICAL PRESENTATION

DISEASE FORMS/SUBTYPES: Acute versus chronic.

HISTORY, CHIEF COMPLAINT

- Acutely, ptyalism, dysphagia, exophthalmos, and swelling of the muscles of mastication are common presenting signs. Blindness may occasionally be observed due to compression of the optic nerve by surrounding inflamed musculature.
- In the chronic form, moderate to severe masticatory muscle atrophy, enophthalmos, and inability to fully open the mouth ("pseudo-trismus") are evident.
- The chronic form may develop without the client having observed signs referable to the acute form.

PHYSICAL EXAM FINDINGS

- Acute form: hypertrophy and myalgia of the masseter and temporalis muscles, decreased range of motion in the jaw, fever, lymphadenopathy, depression, and exophthalmia.
- Chronic form: severe masticatory muscle atrophy and inability to fully open the jaw. In rare cases, inability to close the jaw is found.
- In both the acute and chronic forms, the muscles are affected symmetrically bilaterally.

ETIOLOGY AND PATHOPHYSIOLOGY

Masticatory muscle myositis (MMM) is an immune-mediated disorder in which autoantibodies are produced that are directed against specific muscle fibers called 2M.

DIAGNOSIS

DIFFERENTIAL DIAGNOSIS

- Acute stage: orbital/retrobulbar abscess, oral foreign body, extraocular myositis, focal tetanus.
- Chronic stage: ankylosis of the temporomandibular joint, chronic exposure to corticosteroids.

INITIAL DATABASE

- Complete blood count (leukocytosis may be present)
- Serum biochemistry panel (generally unremarkable)
    - Serum creatine phosphokinase level (may be normal or slightly elevated)
- Urinalysis: generally unremarkable
- Oral examination, if possible. Inability to open the jaws even under general anesthesia is a classic finding

ADVANCED OR CONFIRMATORY TESTING

- Demonstration of serum autoantibodies against 2M myofibers. Approximately 81% of dogs with MMM have a positive result.
- Electromyography may show evidence of spontaneous activity (i.e., positive sharp waves, fibrillation potentials).
- Histopathologic evaluation of masseter or temporalis biopsies is necessary for diagnostic and prognostic purposes.

TREATMENT

THERAPEUTIC GOAL(S)

The goal of therapy is to blunt the inflammatory response, prevent muscle fibrosis, and restore normal jaw mobility.

ACUTE GENERAL TREATMENT

Prednisone 1-2 mg/kg PO or SC q 12h usually results in rapid resolution of clinical signs. These treatments should continue for at least 2 weeks, or until jaw function returns to normal. The dose should then be lowered, and alternate day dosing continued for 4 to 6 months.

CHRONIC TREATMENT

- Glucocorticoids (as in Acute General Treatment above) can still be of some benefit in the chronic form of MMM.
- If fibrosis is severe, myotomy of fibrosed muscle may be necessary to allow ingestion of food and water.
    - Traction under anesthesia should *never* be used for forcing the jaws open (e.g., using an orthopedic bone plate bending tool or any leverage tool); mandibular fracture is a recognized and common result.
- In dogs unable to receive corticosteroids, or in dogs receiving elevated doses of corticosteroids such that loss of masticatory muscle mass may be a result of the corticosteroids, azathioprine (1 mg/kg PO q 24-48h) has been used, with or without concurrent lower dose corticosteroids, with variable success.
- In dogs in which none of the treatments described here is successful, placement of a gastrostomy tube (and eventually, a permanent, low-profile gastrostomy tube) can be palliative.

POSSIBLE COMPLICATIONS

- Neutropenia, rare hepatotoxicity: azathioprine.
- Complete inability to open the mouth with end-stage chronic MMM, leading to starvation from inability to prehend.

RECOMMENDED MONITORING

- Physical exam and body weight q 1-2 weeks in acute form; complete blood count (CBC), serum biochemistry profile, serum creatine phosphokinase, urinalysis after 2 to 4 weeks.
- CBC and serum biochemistry profile q 1-6 weeks (shorter interval early in treatment) if receiving azathioprine.

PROGNOSIS AND OUTCOME

- Prognosis for acute MMM that is promptly treated is very good; however, relapses are common.
- The prognosis for chronic MMM is poor. When extensive muscle fibrosis is present, jaw function is rarely restored.

PEARLS & CONSIDERATIONS

COMMENTS

- MMM is a leading differential diagnosis in a dog with symmetrically swollen, painful muscles on the dorsal and lateral head (acute), or in a dog that is physically unable to open its mouth normally (chronic form).
- Using leverage tools to attempt to pry the mouth open with the animal under general anesthesia is contraindicated, as mandibular fracture is a common iatrogenic complication of this procedure.

SUGGESTED READING

Gilmour MA, Morgan RV, Moore FM: Masticatory myopathy in the dog: A retrospective study of 18 cases. *J Am Anim Hosp Assoc* 28:300-306, 1992.

AUTHOR: **GEORGINA BARONE**
EDITOR: **CURTIS W. DEWEY**

Mastitis

BASIC INFORMATION

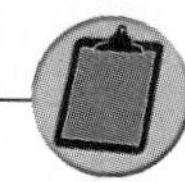

DEFINITION

Inflammation of the mammary gland, commonly with sepsis because the blood-milk barrier often is disrupted

EPIDEMIOLOGY

SPECIES, AGE, SEX: Usually postpartum bitch; uncommon in queens, pseudopregnant bitches, or sterilized bitches.

GENETICS AND BREED PREDISPOSITION: Breeds with short legs and pendulous mammary glands: greater risk of trauma.

RISK FACTORS

- Poor hygiene.
- Trauma (environmental or secondarily to puppies nursing).
- Infections from other sites in the body.
- Older bitches may be at greater risk.
- Sepsis from other infections: bacteria may spread to mammary tissue hematogenously.

CONTAGION AND ZOONOSIS: Most commonly caused by *Escherichia coli*, β-hemolytic streptococci, staphylococci; generally not contagious between bitches if good environmental hygiene. Slight risk of zoonosis if poor hygiene.

ASSOCIATED CONDITIONS AND DISORDERS

- Galactostasis after weaning or overt pseudopregnancy.
- Benign mammary hyperplasia in queens.
- May be associated with mammary neoplasia.

CLINICAL PRESENTATION

DISEASE FORMS/SUBTYPES

- Acute, fulminant
- Chronic, near subclinical

HISTORY, CHIEF COMPLAINT

- Lactating bitch or queen, rarely pseudopregnant bitch.
- Crying puppies or kittens.
- Uncomfortable dam may or may not want to nurse puppies.

PHYSICAL EXAM FINDINGS

- Firm, warm, swollen, often painful mammary gland (one or more).
- Lethargy.
- Dehydration.
- Purulent or discolored milk expressible from gland.
- Gland may abscess, become gangrenous, and rupture (Fig. I-115).
- Possible fever.
- May progress to septic shock.

ETIOLOGY AND PATHOPHYSIOLOGY

- Unknown: possible ascending infection from poor environmental hygiene or traumatic injury from nursing offspring.
- Incidence highest in stimulated mammary gland. This may be due to substrate (milk), open ducts, trauma from nursing and increased trauma because glands are enlarged.

DIAGNOSIS

DIFFERENTIAL DIAGNOSIS

- Mammary adenocarcinoma (inflamed or septic). Usually in older females with no concurrent lactation.
- Galactostasis. Dam not ill, nonseptic.

INITIAL DATABASE

- Complete blood count: leukocytosis with left shift. If acute sepsis, leukopenia is possible.
- Cytologic evaluation of mammary secretions: many toxic neutrophils.

ADVANCED OR CONFIRMATORY TESTING

- Bacterial culture and sensitivity of mammary secretions/milk
  - ± *Mycoplasma* culture (e.g., if poor response to treatment)
- Biopsy of mammary tissue (to rule out cancer and benign mammary hyperplasia)

TREATMENT

THERAPEUTIC GOAL(S)

- Return to normal mammary function.
- Prevention of septicemia.

ACUTE GENERAL TREATMENT

- If mammary necrosis is present or if milk is too contaminated for puppies or kittens, offspring should be removed and the necrotic tissue surgically drained and debrided.
  - Signs include milk that is grossly purulent, malodorous, or markedly discolored, or puppies that are not nursing on their own, or are developing diarrhea, vomiting, or losing weight.
  - Antiprolactin therapy may be administered to stop lactation (cabergoline 5 µg/kg PO q 24h; usually response is seen within 3 to 4 days, and over 80% response by day 7).
- Systemic antibiotic treatment of the dam is required. General guidelines are initially based on Gram stain and on whether pups are still nursing; then use culture and sensitivity results for definitive treatment.
  - Therapeutic goal: significant antibiotic levels in the milk.
  - While awaiting culture results, the choice of antibiotic for initial empiric treatment is limited (e.g., cefadroxil 22 mg/kg PO q 8h or amoxicillin-clavulanic acid 12.75 mg/kg PO q 12h) if the dam's offspring continue to nurse.
  - Nursing puppies and kittens may be negatively impacted by antibiotic concentrations in the dam's milk.
  - Dam nursing neonates:
    - Aerobic bacteria:
      - Gram-negative: cefoxitin 30 mg/kg IV q 6h, or chloramphenicol 40 mg/kg PO q 8h.
      - Gram-positive: first-generation cephalosporins (e.g., cefadroxil 22 mg/kg PO q 8h), or erythromycin (10–20 mg/kg PO q 8h).
    - Anaerobic bacteria: erythromycin, cefoxitin, chloramphenicol.
    - *Mycoplasma*: erythromycin, chloramphenicol.
  - Dam not nursing neonates:
    - Aerobic bacteria:
      - Gram-negative: quinolones (e.g., enrofloxacin 5 mg/kg PO q 12h [5 mg/kg PO q 24h in cats]), or second- or third-generation cephalosporins, (e.g., cefoxitin).
      - Gram-positive: first-generation cephalosporins, amoxicillin/clavulanic acid, or erythromycin.
      - Anaerobic bacteria: penicillin (e.g., procaine penicillin G 20,000 IU/kg IM or SC q 12–24h), metronidazole (15 mg/kg PO q 12h), clindamycin (5–11 mg/kg PO q 12h), erythromycin, or cefoxitin.
      - *Mycoplasma:* tetracyclines (e.g., doxycycline 5 mg/kg PO q 12h), erythromycin, or quinolones.
- Warm packing and ongoing nursing: Unless the gland is necrotic, continued nursing by the offspring and warm packing the affected glands will prevent galactostasis and promote drainage.

CHRONIC TREATMENT

Mastectomy

DRUG INTERACTIONS

Antiprolactinics will stop lactation. Some antibiotics are contraindicated in lactating bitches.

POSSIBLE COMPLICATIONS

Systemic antibiotic therapy in lactating bitches may interfere with normal bacterial colonization of gastrointestinal flora in nursing puppies resulting in diarrhea.

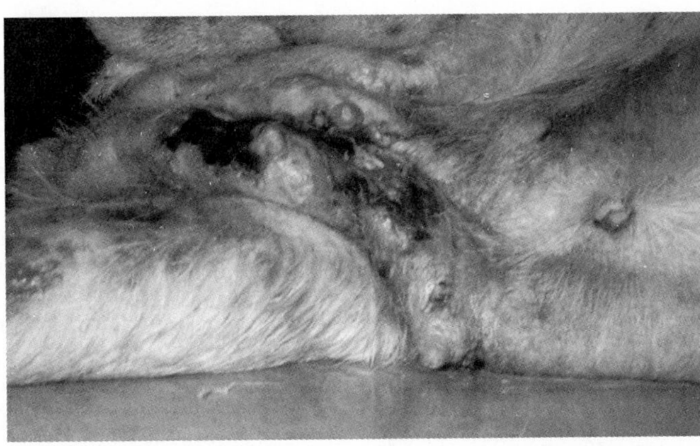

FIGURE I-115 Caudal ventral abdomen of a bitch with severe necrotizing mastitis involving both left and right inguinal and the right caudal abdominal mammary glands. Cranial is to the right. Courtesy of Dr. Michelle A. Kutzler.

RECOMMENDED MONITORING

- Temperature, respiration, and heart rate
- Physical signs of septicemia
- Offspring that are nursing: daily weighing to determine adequate milk intake

PROGNOSIS AND OUTCOME

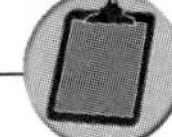

Prognosis is generally good unless sepsis occurs

PEARLS & CONSIDERATIONS

COMMENTS

- Puppies up to 5 weeks old should be allowed access to the dam's food and the bitch should have an area where she can remove herself from puppies (e.g., top of crate, raised platform).
  - Puppies will then start eating solid food for portion of their caloric intake, decreasing the amount of time nursing on mother. Also, the metabolic requirements on the bitch are greatly reduced.
  - Older puppies with teeth nurse more aggressively and can induce both bite and nail trauma to the mammary gland, greatly increasing the risk of inflammation and infection.
- Chronic mastitis has been suspected when puppies fail to thrive. However, subclinical mastitis has not been demonstrated in dogs and cats.

PREVENTION

- Adequate husbandry, particularly clean bedding of mother and offspring
- Keeping mammary glands clean, monitor glands for trauma from pups or kittens claws or teeth

CLIENT EDUCATION

Primarily husbandry issues of proper hygiene and weaning instructions

SUGGESTED READING

Feldman E, Nelson R (eds): *Canine and Feline Endocrinology and Reproduction*. Philadelphia, WB Saunders, 2004.

Johnston SD, et al (eds): *Canine and Feline Theriogenology*. Philadelphia, WB Saunders, 2001.

Nelson RW, Couto CG (eds): *Small Animal Internal Medicine*. St. Louis, Mosby, 2003.

AUTHOR: **MICHAEL E. PETERSON**
EDITOR: **MICHELLE A. KUTZLER**

Mediastinal Disease

BASIC INFORMATION

DEFINITION

Disorders of the mediastinum, the potential space between the right and left lungs

EPIDEMIOLOGY

SPECIES, AGE, SEX: Mediastinal lymphosarcoma: young cats overrepresented.

- Other mediastinal masses more commonly affect middle-aged or older animals.

GENETICS AND BREED PREDISPOSITION: Mediastinal lymphosarcoma: Oriental-breed cats.

RISK FACTORS

- Mediastinal lymphosarcoma: feline leukemia (FeLV; see p 380) infection
- Pneumomediastinum: tracheal laceration/avulsion
- Mediastinitis: esophageal foreign body or rupture

CONTAGION AND ZOONOSIS: FeLV infection.

ASSOCIATED CONDITIONS AND DISORDERS: Mediastinal masses:

- Acquired myasthenia gravis (thymoma)
- Polyuria and polydipsia (lymphosarcoma)

CLINICAL PRESENTATION

DISEASE FORMS/SUBTYPES

- Pneumomediastinum
- Mediastinitis
- Mediastinal masses

HISTORY, CHIEF COMPLAINT

- Pneumomediastinum:
  - History of trauma
  - Recent anesthesia
  - Recent transtracheal wash
  - Recent jugular venipuncture
- Mediastinitis (acute):
  - Obtundation
  - Inappetence
  - Dysphagia
  - Regurgitation
- Mediastinal masses:
  - Inappetence
  - Lethargy
  - Polyuria/polydipsia
  - Dysphagia or regurgitation
  - Cough
  - Dyspnea
  - Facial, neck, and/or forelimb swelling

PHYSICAL EXAM FINDINGS

- Pneumomediastinum:
  - Can be an incidental finding
  - Subcutaneous emphysema (see p 1050)
  - Respiratory signs if severe:
    - Dyspnea
    - Muffled breath sounds
    - Resonant thoracic percussion from pneumothorax
  - Jugular venous distention
  - Shock
- Mediastinitis:
  - Fever
  - Dyspnea, tachypnea, cough
  - Edema of head, neck, forelimbs secondary to cranial vena cava syndrome (see p 256)
  - Dysphagia
  - Regurgitation
  - Thoracic pain
  - Reduced thoracic compressibility
- Mediastinal masses:

- Poor compressibility of cranial thorax (especially cats)
- Cranial vena cava syndrome (see p 256)
- Respiratory or gastrointestinal signs as mentioned previously
- Occasionally paraneoplastic signs:
  - Weakness
  - Stridor if secondary laryngeal paralysis
- Horner's syndrome possible

ETIOLOGY AND PATHOPHYSIOLOGY

- Pneumomediastinum:
  - Air enters from:
    - Penetrating neck wounds.
    - Tracheal laceration.
    - Occasionally from esophageal air leakage.
    - Positive pressure ventilation.
- Mediastinitis:
  - Hematogenous infection.
  - Penetrating wounds and migrating foreign bodies.
  - Extension from surrounding tissues (especially esophagus).
  - Acute mediastinitis (*Staphylococcus* spp., *Streptococcus* spp., *Escherichia coli*, *Corynebacterium* spp.).
  - Chronic bacterial (*Nocardia, Actinomyces, Staphylococcus* spp.) or fungal (histoplasmosis, blastomycosis, cryptococcosis) infection also possible.
    - Clinical signs due to sepsis, pleural effusion, and compression of vascular or respiratory structures.
- Mediastinal masses:
  - Lymphosarcoma, thymoma, thyroid neoplasia, chemodectoma, thymic cysts, granulomas.
  - Clinical signs reflect compression of respiratory, cardiovascular, gastrointestinal structures, possibly pleural effusion, or sometimes neurologic abnormalities (Horner's syndrome, laryngeal paralysis).
  - Occasionally, paraneoplastic syndromes:
    - Hypercalcemia.
    - Myasthenia gravis.

DIAGNOSIS

DIFFERENTIAL DIAGNOSIS

- Pneumomediastinum:
  - Tracheal trauma
  - Pneumothorax
- Mediastinitis:
  - Other causes of sepsis
  - Mediastinal masses/fat/fluid
  - Pleural effusions
- Mediastinal masses:
  - Mediastinitis
  - Pleural space disease
  - Pulmonary masses
  - Thoracic wall masses
  - Mediastinal fat or fluid
  - Normal thymic enlargement (young animals)

INITIAL DATABASE

- Thoracic radiographs:
  - Pneumomediastinum:
    - Visualization of mediastinal vascular structures not normally seen (e.g., branches of aorta): pathognomonic.
    - Subcutaneous emphysema.
  - Mediastinitis and mediastinal masses:
    - Mediastinal widening on dorsoventral or ventrodorsal views.
    - Dorsal displacement of trachea on lateral view possible.
    - Acute mediastinitis may cause no changes.
    - Pleural fluid possible.
    - Gas in fascial planes of neck.
- Abdominal radiographs: pneumoretroperitoneum possible.
- Complete blood count (CBC):
  - Leukocytosis if inflammation.
  - Rarely cytopenias or leukemia.
- Serum biochemistry panel: hypercalcemia possible.
- FeLV test.
- Thoracic ultrasonography: may identify:
  - Presence/structure of masses.
  - Pleural effusion.
  - Lymphadenomegaly.
  - Vascularity/vascular invasiveness of mass (impacts biopsy/excision possibilities).
- Fine-needle aspiration cytology:
  - Risks include hemothorax, pneumothorax, or nondiagnostic sample.
  - If inflammatory: culture (aerobic, anaerobic, *Nocardia, Actinomyces*, ± fungal) indicated.
- Thoracocentesis for cytology and culture if fluid present.

ADVANCED OR CONFIRMATORY TESTING

- Tracheoscopy/bronchoscopy if pneumomediastinum (and patient stable).
- Contrast (water-soluble) esophagram if suspect rupture.
- Esophagoscopy if suspect esophageal disease.
- Cytologic evaluation of respiratory wash samples if underlying pulmonary disease.
- Echocardiography if heart base mass.
- Arterial blood gas to assess respiratory function.
- Computed tomography or magnetic resonance imaging may delineate nature and extent of space-occupying disease.
- Fungal serologic evaluation if possible fungal mediastinitis.
- Biopsy for histopathologic evaluation can be obtained transthoracically (Tru-cut), via thoracoscopy, or via thoracotomy.

TREATMENT

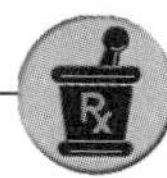

THERAPEUTIC GOAL(S)

Treat underlying disease

ACUTE GENERAL TREATMENT

- Pneumomediastinum:
  - If mild signs, cage rest is sufficient; subcutaneous emphysema typically resolves in approximately 2 weeks.
  - If signs more marked, provide supplemental oxygen.
    - Drain subcutaneous emphysema only if causing discomfort (see Subcutaneous Emphysema, p 1050).
  - If tracheal tear/laceration, consider surgical repair (see Tracheal Avulsion, p 1095).
  - Thoracocentesis if pneumothorax.
- Mediastinitis:
  - Broad-spectrum empiric antimicrobial therapy while culture/sensitivity results are pending.
  - Severe systemic signs may require intravenous fluid therapy.
  - Esophageal laceration/rupture may require surgery.
- Mediastinal masses:
  - Surgery, chemotherapy, radiation therapy, or a combination based on nature of mass.
  - Mediastinal cysts are either drained transthoracically or excised.

CHRONIC TREATMENT

- Pneumomediastinum: cage rest as above.
- Mediastinitis: long-term (minimum 4 to 6 weeks) antimicrobial therapy based on culture and sensitivity results.
  - Fungal mediastinitis may require months of therapy.
  - Large granulomas causing cranial vena cava syndrome may require surgical excision/debulking.
- Mediastinal masses:
  - Chemotherapy or radiation therapy for lymphosarcoma.
  - Radiation therapy for incompletely resected thymoma.

POSSIBLE COMPLICATIONS

- Pneumothorax, pleural effusion, pyothorax from thoracostomy tubes.
- Gastrointestinal and/or myelotoxicity for many chemotherapeutics.
- Individual toxicities for particular drugs:
  - Renal: aminoglycosides, amphotericin B.
  - Hepatic: azole antifungals.
- Surgery entails risks of anesthesia, hemorrhage, infection.

RECOMMENDED MONITORING

- Clinical signs
- Pulse oximetry, arterial blood gases
- Thoracic radiographs
- Pleural fluid volume if thoracostomy tube

- CBC (chemotherapy)
- Serum chemistries for renal and hepatic function depending on antimicrobials administered

PROGNOSIS AND OUTCOME

- Pneumomediastinum: good if underlying disease can be corrected.
- Mediastinitis: variable depending on severity; chronic cases may be hard to resolve.
- Mediastinal masses:
  - Lymphosarcoma: Chemotherapy is usually palliative.
  - Others: surgery for cure or palliation.

PEARLS & CONSIDERATIONS

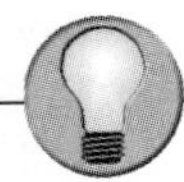

COMMENTS

- Advanced imaging helps define internal structure and extent of mediastinal masses and detect pulmonary metastases.
- In patients at risk of foreign body inhalation (hunting or field trial dogs), consider *Nocardia, Actinomyces* as causes of mediastinitis.

PREVENTION

Avoid iatrogenic tracheal injury associated with:

- Intubating with a stylet
- Overinflation of endotracheal tube cuffs
- Rotating a patient while attached to anesthetic circuit
- Traumatic jugular venipuncture

SUGGESTED READING

Mitchell SL, et al: Tracheal rupture associated with intubation in cats: 20 cases (1996-1998). *J Am Vet Med Assoc* 216:1592, 2000.

Thrall DE: The mediastinum. In Thrall DE (ed): *Textbook of Veterinary Diagnostic Radiology*, ed 3. Philadelphia, WB Saunders, 1998, pp 309-320.

AUTHOR: **GRAHAM SWINNEY**
EDITOR: **RANCE K. SELLON**

Megaesophagus

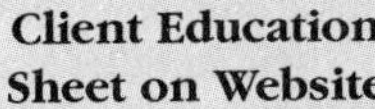

Client Education Sheet on Website

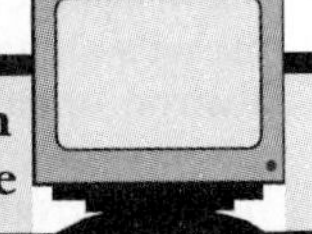

BASIC INFORMATION

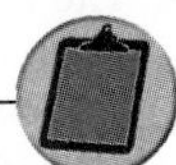

DEFINITION

Obvious dilatation of the esophagus due to weakness of the esophageal musculature from any cause. This is to be distinguished from dilatation of the esophagus orad to an obstruction.

SYNONYM(S)

Esophageal dilatation
Esophageal weakness

EPIDEMIOLOGY

SPECIES, AGE, SEX: Dogs and cats of any age or sex:

- Acquired megaesophagus usually occurs after 3 to 4 years of age.
- Cats are less commonly affected.

GENETICS AND BREED PREDISPOSITION

- For congenital megaesophagus:
  - Cats: Siamese
  - Dogs: German shepherds, Great Danes, Labrador retrievers, miniature schnauzers, Irish setters, shar-peis, fox terriers, Newfoundlands
- For acquired megaesophagus:
  - Dogs: black standard poodles (secondary to hypoadrenocorticism)

RISK FACTORS: Any neuromuscular disease can cause acquired megaesophagus; localized myasthenia gravis is the most commonly identified cause.

ASSOCIATED CONDITIONS AND DISORDERS

- Coughing due to tracheobronchitis or pneumonia secondary to aspiration.
- Aspiration pneumonia is the most common cause of death.

CLINICAL PRESENTATION

DISEASE FORMS/SUBTYPES

- Congenital megaesophagus
- Acquired megaesophagus

HISTORY, CHIEF COMPLAINT

- Regurgitation (must distinguish from vomiting) is the most common complaint.
- Cough (due to aspiration): this is sometimes seen before regurgitation is reported.
- Drooling (due to difficulty swallowing).

PHYSICAL EXAM FINDINGS

- Weight loss or failure to gain weight (if patient is losing excessive calories or has chronic pulmonary infection).
- Pulmonary crackles/easily elicited cough (due to aspiration pneumonia).
- Fever and signs of systemic illness (e.g., anorexia, lethargy) when sepsis from aspiration is present.
- Bellows-like action at thoracic inlet associated with breathing (due to filling and emptying of distended esophagus with air, associated with respirations).
- Nasal discharge (if bronchopneumonia or rhinits secondary to regurgitation is present).

ETIOLOGY AND PATHOPHYSIOLOGY

- Congenital or idiopathic megaesophagus:
  - Considered to involve the loss of peristaltic function.
  - This defect can occur in any part of the neural reflex that controls the pharyngeal and esophageal phases of swallowing, including the sensory receptors, the afferent nerves (glossopharyngeal and vagus), the tractus solitarius (leading to the nucleus solitarius), the swallowing center (near the lateral reticular formation), the lower motor neurons of the nucleus ambiguus, the efferent somatic and parasympathetic nerve fibers in the vagus, the myoneural junction in the esophagus itself, the esophageal striated muscle, and potentially the esophageal smooth muscle.
  - Most evidence suggests that the problem resides in the afferent limb of the reflex arc. This is supported by the fact that dogs with megaesophagus are prone to aspiration pneumonia, which is increased in dogs with loss of the afferent arc (abnormal respiratory reflexes also occur).
- Secondary megaesophagus: etiopathogenesis relates to primary cause:
  - Neurologic (polyradiculoneuritis, dysautonomia, demyelinating neuropathies, lead, etc.).
  - Neuromuscular (botulism, tetanus, myasthenia gravis).
  - Muscular (e.g., toxoplasmosis, polymyositis, systemic lupus erythematosus).
- Other causes of megaesophagus include certain metabolic conditions (hypoadrenocorticism, maybe hypothyroidism).

DIAGNOSIS

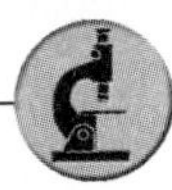

DIFFERENTIAL DIAGNOSIS

- Acquired megaesophagus in the dog:
  - Myasthenia gravis (either generalized or localized)
  - Hypoadrenocorticism

  - Dysautonomia
  - Polymyopathies/polyneuropathies of various causes
  - Lead intoxication
  - Organophosphate intoxication
  - Botulism or tetanus
  - Hypothyroidism (questionable cause)
  - Esophagitis
  - Systemic lupus erythematosus
  - Dermatomyositis
  - Idiopathic
- Acquired megaesophagus in the cat:
  - Dysautonomia
  - Myasthenia gravis
  - Idiopathic (43% of feline cases)

INITIAL DATABASE

- Complete blood count: look for evidence of inflammation consistent with aspiration pneumonia.
- Plain thoracic radiographs: look for megaesophagus (usually seen but is not always obvious) and for pneumonia (especially in right middle lung lobe; *need* ventrodorsal or dorsoventral projection to reliably see this lesion).
- Contrast esophagram using radiographs: if needed.
  - Often not needed, as plain films frequently are confirmatory.
  - Indicated if clinical signs suggest esophageal disease but plain films are equivocal or are interpreted as normal.
  - Can reveal unsuspected esophageal obstruction or segmental weakness.
- Contrast esophagram using fluoroscopy: if needed: will detect megaesophagus missed by radiography, especially if only a segment of the esophagus is affected or if there is only partial loss of muscular tone (see Barium Esophagram, Dynamic, p 1187).

ADVANCED OR CONFIRMATORY TESTING

- Antibodies against acetylcholine receptors (in dogs): when looking for cause of acquired megaesophagus (see Myasthenia Gravis, p 720)
- ACTH-stimulation test (in dogs): when looking for cause of acquired megaesophagus (see Hypoadrenocorticism, p 561)
- Serum creatine kinase determination: various myopathies
- Electromyography/motor nerve conduction velocity (see Electromyography [EMG] and Nerve Conduction Velocity [NCV], p 1231): polymyopathy/polyneuropathy

TREATMENT

THERAPEUTIC GOAL(S)

- Acquired megaesophagus:
  - Find and resolve underlying cause (accomplished in approximately 15-20% of dogs).
  - Treat aspiration pneumonia, if present (see Pneumonia, Aspiration, p 862).
  - If cannot find or treat underlying cause, then treat as idiopathic megaesophagus.
- Idiopathic megaesophagus:
  - Try to minimize regurgitation by modifying feeding practices.
  - Treat aspiration pneumonia when present.

ACUTE GENERAL TREATMENT

- Treat pneumonia, if present (see Pneumonia, Aspiration, p 862).
- Treat underling cause, if found (see Myasthenia Gravis, p 720; Hypoadrenocorticism, p 561).
- Feeding modification:
  - Feed from an elevated platform such that the patient's esophagus approaches a plane perpendicular to the floor, so that gravity aids in food/water emptying from the esophagus into the stomach.
  - Feed different consistencies of food to find which is best tolerated: feeding a gruel is usually the best choice, but some animals fare better if fed canned or solid food or meat balls.
  - Feed several small meals per day (or free choice in the case of dry kibble) to minimize retention of large amounts in esophagus.
- Prokinetic drugs may be tried.
  - Indicated when gastroesophageal reflux is suspected or confirmed, to increase normograde gastric emptying and reduce the volume of acid reflux. Prokinetic drugs are often useful for treating gastric motility disorders, but they do not increase esophageal motility to any clinically appreciable degree.
    - Metoclopramide (0.2-0.4 mg/kg PO, IM, or SC q 8-12h). The increase in lower esophageal sphincter tone described for metoclopramide is not thought to be clinically significant and does not contraindicate usage in megaesophagus.
    - Cisapride (0.1-0.5 mg/kg PO q 8-12h). The cardiac effects noted in humans taking cisapride (QT interval prolongation) have not been noted to be a clinical problem in dogs or cats. Cisapride increases lower esophageal tone.
- Gastric acid-reducing therapy: recommended if gastroesophageal reflux is documented or likely.
  - Omeprazole (1 mg/kg PO q 24h).

CHRONIC TREATMENT

- Ongoing implementation of measures described in acute treatment.
- Treat specific conditions identified as indicated (e.g., hypoadrenocorticism, myasthenia gravis).
- Can place gastrostomy tube to minimize regurgitation of food (especially if waiting for treatment of underlying cause to succeed). (See Feeding Tube Placement: Percutaneous Endoscopic Gastrostomy [PEG], p 1247.)
  - Dog can still swallow and regurgitate saliva, despite gastrostomy tube.

POSSIBLE COMPLICATIONS

- Aspiration pneumonia
- Infected stoma (gastrostomy tube)

PROGNOSIS AND OUTCOME

- If the underlying cause can be found and cured, the outlook is usually good, assuming that the patient does not die first from aspiration pneumonia.
- If the underlying cause cannot be found and treated, the outlook is guarded (at best) and often very poor: Many such patients die of aspiration pnemonia.
- The esophageal function of some dogs with congenital megaesophagus will spontaneously improve over time; however, one cannot predict which patients will improve.

PEARLS & CONSIDERATIONS

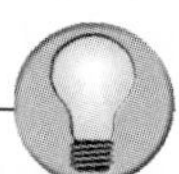

COMMENTS

- Certain drugs used for restraint (e.g., ketamine, xylazine) cause temporary megaesophagus.
- Some dogs with obvious megaesophagus on plain radiographs have normal function during barium-contrast esophagram, and the radiographic megaesophagus will spontaneously disappear.
- Radiography is the preferred way to diagnose megaesophagus; endoscopy is often the preferred way to diagnose esophagitis or the cause of esophageal obstruction, as well as other morphologic changes (e.g., hiatal hernia).
- The severity of radiographic dilation of esophagus is not proportional to severity of regurgitation or aspiration.
- Mild aspiration pneumonia is often missed on lateral radiographs; dorsoventral radiographs are more sensitive for finding this lesion.
- Any unexplained bacterial pneumonia in a dog could be caused by occult esophageal dysfunction; it is often reasonable to perform contrast radiographs looking for esophageal weakness in dogs with pneumonia that do not have esophageal dilation on plain radiographs.
- If a dog with megaesophagus vomits, esophagitis typically occurs due to gas-

tric acid entering and not exiting the esophageal lumen.

- Surgery (cardiomyotomy) is not helpful or indicated in dogs with megaesophagus; true achalasia (which is helped by such surgery) is exceptionally rare in dogs.

PREVENTION

Do not breed animals with known history of producing litters with megaesophagus.

CLIENT EDUCATION

Aspiration pneumonia can occur at any time, even in dogs with mild radiographic signs of megaesophagus.

SUGGESTED READING

Gaynor AR, et al: Risk factors for acquired megaesophagus in dogs. *J Am Vet Med Assoc* 211:1406, 1997.

Mears EA, et al: Canine and feline megaesophagus. *Compend Cont Educ* 19:313-326, 1997.

Moses L, et al: Esophageal motility dysfunction in cats: a study of 44 cases. *J Am Anim Hosp Assoc* 36:309, 2000.

AUTHOR: **MICHAEL WILLARD**
EDITOR: **DEBRA L. ZORAN**

Melanoma (Cutaneous, Digital, Oral)

BASIC INFORMATION

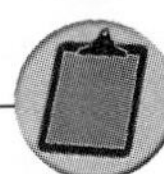

DEFINITION

- Melanoma is a common neoplasm in the dog and is rare in the cat.
- Classification of melanomas by location generally has more clinical utility than by histologic subtype.
- Oral melanomas are uniformly malignant, locally invasive, and highly metastatic (>60%) tumors.
- Subungual (nail bed) melanomas are locally invasive tumors with a lower rate of metastasis (30-60%).
- Cutaneous melanomas are generally (but not always) benign.
- Ocular melanomas are discussed elsewhere in this text (see Intraocular Neoplasia, p 603).

SYNONYM(S)

Malignant melanoma
Melanocytic tumor
Melanocytoma

EPIDEMIOLOGY

SPECIES, AGE, SEX: Melanoma generally occurs in older patients (9 to 12 years).

GENETICS AND BREED PREDISPOSITION

- Predisposed dog breeds include:
  - Doberman pinscher
  - Golden retriever
  - Gordon setter
  - Irish setter
  - Schnauzer, giant
  - Schnauzer, miniature
  - Scottish terrier
- Breed predisposition suggests an underlying genetic mechanism for melanoma in veterinary patients.
- Black dogs may be predisposed, but any color dog may be affected.
- See Prognosis and Outcome below.

CLINICAL PRESENTATION

HISTORY, CHIEF COMPLAINT

- Oral melanoma:
  - Detection of an oral mass by a veterinarian during routine examination or dental prophylaxis (common).
  - After identification of an oral mass by the owner.
  - Recent onset of halitosis and ptyalism.
- Cutaneous or subungual (nail bed) melanomas:
  - Identification of a mass by the owner.

PHYSICAL EXAM FINDINGS

- Examination typically reveals a mass lesion.
- Oral examination should be thorough as some tumors are located at the base of the tongue or in the tonsils.
- Cutaneous and subungual tumors may become ulcerated.
- Melanomas may be pigmented or amelanotic.
- Thorough examination of draining lymph nodes is always indicated, but aspiration cytologic evaluation should be done regardless of physical exam finding.

ETIOLOGY AND PATHOPHYSIOLOGY

- Underlying genetic mutations and ultraviolet light exposure are known etiologic agents in humans.
- Melanomas do not have to arise from pigmented skin.

DIAGNOSIS

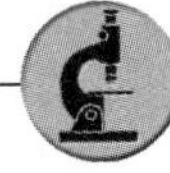

DIFFERENTIAL DIAGNOSIS

- Oral: squamous cell carcinoma, soft tissue sarcoma, epulides
- Cutaneous: any mass lesion of skin (neoplastic or non-neoplastic)
- Subungual: squamous cell carcinoma, nail bed infection

INITIAL DATABASE

Complete blood count, serum biochemistry profile, urinalysis, lymph node aspiration, thoracic radiographs, abdominal ultrasound (in patients with hind limb or caudally located masses)

ADVANCED OR CONFIRMATORY TESTING

- Biopsy and histopathologic examination of tissue.
- Immunohistochemical staining with S-100 or Melan-A may confirm the diagnosis of melanoma in undifferentiated and amelanotic tumors.
- Determination of mitotic index (mitoses/10 high-power fields) may be used for distinguishing benign and malignant canine cutaneous melanomas.
  - Determination of mitotic index requires histopathologic evaluation of tissue and cannot reliably be assessed on fine-needle aspiration/cytology.
  - Tumors with a mitotic index of <3 are typically benign while those ≥3 are generally malignant.

TREATMENT

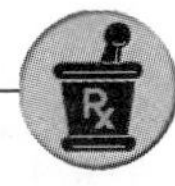

THERAPEUTIC GOAL(S)

- Long-term disease control in patients amenable to definitive therapy.
- Palliation of clinical signs in patients not treated definitively or those with metastatic disease.

ACUTE GENERAL TREATMENT

- Oral melanoma:
  - Radical excision of mass indicated if:
    - Wide surgical margins (>2 cm, including underlying bone) can be obtained, and
    - Patient has no regional lymph node or distant metastasis.
  - Removal of macroscopic (measurable) tumor followed by definitive course of radiation therapy to primary tumor site and regional lymph nodes indicated if:
    - Radical excision is not possible or regional lymph node metastasis is identified; and
    - Patient has no distant metastatic disease.

   - Radiotherapy dosing: see Pearls & Considerations below.
- Definitive course of radiation therapy alone to primary tumor and regional lymph nodes is indicated if:
   - Removal of macroscopic tumor burden is not possible; and
   - Patient has no distant metastatic disease.
- Palliative course of radiation therapy to tumor could be considered if:
   - The patient has distant metastatic disease; and/or
   - Financial or other restrictions preclude definitive therapy with surgery, radiotherapy, or both.
- Chemotherapy indicated for all patients treated definitively with surgery and/or radiotherapy due to high rate of metastatic disease.
   - Systemic therapy with platinum (carboplatin or cisplatin) chemotherapeutic agents given reported activity of carboplatin in dogs with melanoma.
   - Chemotherapy may benefit patients treated with palliative radiotherapy and those with evidence of distant metastasis.

- Subungual (nail bed) melanoma:
   - Radical excision of mass indicated if:
      - Wide surgical margins (>2 cm, to include underlying bone) are possible; and
      - Patient has no distant metastatic disease.
   - Limb amputation should be performed if wide surgical margins cannot be obtained with local resection (i.e., digital amputation).
   - Limb amputation including removal of lymph nodes should be performed in patients with regional lymph node metastasis.
   - Removal of macroscopic (measurable) tumor followed by definitive course of radiotherapy to primary tumor site and regional lymph nodes is indicated if:
      - Digital amputation is not possible or clients decline amputation.
      - If regional lymph node metastasis is identified.
      - Patient has no distant metastatic disease.
   - Palliative course of radiotherapy could be considered if:
      - Patient has distant metastatic disease, and clinical signs associated with local disease result in decreased quality of life for patient.
   - Chemotherapy is indicated for all patients treated definitively with surgery and/or radiotherapy due to the high rate of metastatic disease in patients with subungual melanoma.
      - Refer to oral melanoma section for comments regarding chemotherapy.
- Cutaneous melanoma:
   - Surgical resection is the treatment of choice for benign melanomas (<3 mitoses/10 hpf).
   - Radical excision of malignant cutaneous melanoma (≥3 mitoses/10 hpf) is indicated if:
      - Wide surgical margins (>2 cm) can be obtained; and
      - Patient has no regional lymph node or distant metastatic disease.
   - Removal of macroscopic (measurable) tumor followed by definitive course of radiation therapy to primary tumor site and regional lymph nodes are indicated if:
      - Radical excision is not possible or if regional lymph node metastasis is identified.
      - Patient has no distant metastatic disease.
   - Palliative course of radiation therapy could be considered if:
      - Patient has distant metastatic disease and clinical signs associated with local disease result in decreased quality of life for the patient.
   - Chemotherapy indicated for all patients with malignant cutaneous melanomas treated definitively with surgery and/or radiation therapy.
      - Refer to oral melanoma section for comments regarding chemotherapy.

POSSIBLE COMPLICATIONS

Potential complications of therapy for patients with melanoma are those typically encountered after treatment with surgery, radiation, and chemotherapy.

RECOMMENDED MONITORING

After treatment, patients should be monitored with routine examination (determination of local disease status) and thoracic radiographs (identify metastatic disease).

PROGNOSIS AND OUTCOME

- Oral melanoma:
   - Prognosis:
      - Conservative surgery alone: median survival 3 to 4 months; local recurrence rate >70%.
      - Radical surgery alone: median survival 9 to 10 months; local recurrence rate 20–50%.
      - Radiation therapy for microscopic tumors: median survival 15 months; local recurrence rate 26%.
      - Radiation therapy for macroscopic tumors: response rate 82%; median survival 5 months; local progression/recurrence 45%.
      - Chemotherapy for macroscopic tumors: response rate 28%; efficacy in adjuvant setting unknown.
      - Prognosis for definitively treated feline oral melanoma is not known.
   - Prognostic factors:
      - Most apply to patients treated with radiotherapy.
      - Reported negative prognostic factors include macroscopic tumor burden, caudal tumor location, bone lysis; all oral melanomas should be considered malignant regardless of mitotic index.
      - In one study median survival correlated with the number of negative prognostic factors present: 0 = 21 months; 1 = 11 months; 2 = 5 months; 3 = 3 months.
- Subungual melanoma:
   - Prognosis:
      - Surgical excision (local or limb amputation): median survival 12 months; local recurrence rate 30% (local resection only).
      - Role of radiotherapy and chemotherapy undetermined for this location.
      - Prognostic factors: none identified
      - Prognosis is unknown for feline subungual melanoma.
- Cutaneous melanoma:
   - Prognosis:
      - Surgical excision: median survival 24 months (benign); 7 to 11 months (malignant).
      - Efficacy of radiotherapy and chemotherapy is undetermined for this location.
      - Median survival for feline cutaneous melanoma treated with surgery alone is 12 months.
      - Mitotic index is not uniformly predictive of biologic behavior.
   - Prognostic factors:
      - Mitotic index is the most important prognostic factor: ≥3 indicates malignant tumor.
      - Breed: Doberman pinschers and miniature schnauzers are more likely have benign melanoma (75%); miniature poodles are more likely have malignant melanomas (85%).

PEARLS & CONSIDERATIONS

COMMENTS

- Radiotherapy treatment:
   - Melanoma has a greater capacity for sublethal damage repair and, therefore, is best treated with a hypofractionated (larger doses per fraction) treatment protocol instead of a conventional protocol such as 3Gy doses given in 16 to 19 fractions.
   - Four veterinary protocols for melanoma are: 10Gy × 3; 9Gy × 4;

8Gy × 3; 4Gy × 12. The optimal protocol remains to be determined.
 - As late-responding normal tissues (bone, muscle, central nervous system) are more susceptible to toxicity with larger doses of radiation, large doses (8–10 Gy) should be avoided in patients in which long-term survival (>12 months) is expected.
   - In patients with probable long-term survival (e.g., dog with no negative prognostic factors), a protocol utilizing smaller doses per fraction (4–6 Gy) may be advisable.
   - In patients treated definitively but in which long-term survival is unlikely (e.g., dog with caudally located, macroscopic tumor) or in patients treated palliatively, a protocol utilizing larger doses per fraction is reasonable since long-term survival and, therefore, late-responding tissue toxicity, are unlikely.
- Chemotherapy:
  - In patients failing platinum chemotherapy, there is little information regarding rescue chemotherapy agents for melanoma.
  - Information from the veterinary and human literature may support the use of dacarbazine, melphalan, CCNU, piroxicam, and interferon.

SUGGESTED READING

Bostock DE: Prognosis after surgical excision of canine melanomas. *Vet Pathol* 16:32, 1979.

Marino DJ, et al: Evaluation of dogs with digit masses: 117 cases (1981–1991). *J Am Vet Med Assoc* 207(6):726–728, 1995.

Proulx DR, et al: A retrospective analysis of 140 dogs with oral melanoma treated with external beam radiation. *Vet Radiol Ultrasound* 44(3):352–359, 2003.

Rassnick KM, et al: Use of carboplatin for treatment of dogs with malignant melanoma: 27 cases (1989–2000). *J Am Vet Med Assoc* 218(9):1444–1448, 2001.

AUTHOR: **DAVID R. PROULX**

EDITOR: **KENNETH M. RASSNICK**

Melena

BASIC INFORMATION

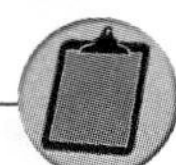

DEFINITION

Dark, tarlike, often foul-smelling stools, as a result of digested blood (specifically oxidized hemoglobin)

EPIDEMIOLOGY

SPECIES, AGE, SEX: Any age, breed, sex.

RISK FACTORS: Anything that will cause hemorrhage into the proximal or mid-gastrointestinal (GI) tract (esophagus, stomach, small intestine) or the mouth, pharynx, nose, or lungs.

CLINICAL PRESENTATION

HISTORY, CHIEF COMPLAINT

- The patient will normally present for signs associated with blood loss (i.e., weakness, pale mucous membranes, bleeding from other sites or due to the melena [foul-smelling flatulence or black tarry feces]).
- Medication history includes those known to have gastrointestinal ulcerogenic potential (e.g., glucocorticoids, nonsteroidal anti-inflammatory drugs [NSAIDs]).
- Intoxication history: known exposure or accessibility of vitamin K antagonists (rodenticides, pharmaceutical) in the environment.
- Specific questions related to potential specific sources of bleeding: coughing, sneezing, vomiting, diarrhea.
- Some patients have a history of recent surgical skin lump removal (possibility of mast cell tumor).
- Rule out false-positive results (cases that do not fulfill the definition):
  - Animals eating meat-based diets.
  - Diets high in iron.
  - Drugs such as salicylates, charcoal, and bismuth.
  - Normal variation.

PHYSICAL EXAM FINDINGS

- Rectal exam to confirm the diagnosis.
- Evaluation for petechial hemorrhages on the mucous membranes and for signs of bleeding on the skin.
- Auscultation of the chest for signs of lung hemorrhage (bronchovesicular sounds that are either louder [interstitial or airway hemorrhage] or softer [pleural effusion]).
- Thorough abdominal palpation: abnormal GI loops or masses.
- Careful examination of the skin for suspect mast cell tumors.
- Additionally, specific aspects of the physical exam will vary depending on the source of bleeding. The blood can originate from the mouth, nose, lungs, pharynx, esophagus, stomach, or small intestine.

ETIOLOGY AND PATHOPHYSIOLOGY

- Blood presented to proximal or mid-GI tract (via any route already mentioned).
- Slow GI transit time of longer than 8 hours (in humans) allows greater degree of oxidation of hemoglobin. Melena occurs based on the duration of the presence of blood in the GI tract, rather than the anatomic site of blood loss.

DIAGNOSIS

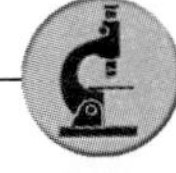

DIFFERENTIAL DIAGNOSIS

- GI bleeding (stomach, small intestine; or large intestine in anorexic animals with slow GI transit time). Examples: hemorrhagic gastroenteritis, foreign body, intussusception, volvulus, inflammatory bowel disease, helminthiasis, or neoplasia.
- Liver or renal failure (coagulopathy or gastric ulceration).
- Pulmonary or upper respiratory tract bleed with swallowing of blood.
- Shock (shock gut).
- Pancreatitis.
- Hypoadrenocorticism.
- Mast cell tumor or rarely gastrinoma.
- High meat-based diet or diet high in iron.
- Drugs such as charcoal and bismuth darken the color of feces but do not signify digested blood.

INITIAL DATABASE

- Recheck history and repeat abdominal palpation
- Complete blood count, serum biochemistry profile (including preprandial and postprandial bile acids if liver disease suspected), urinalysis. Thrombocytopenia may explain, or be a result of, hemorrhage. Microcytosis and hypochromia suggest chronic blood loss.
- Fecal flotation.
- Imaging: survey radiographs of chest and abdomen; abdominal ultrasound.
- Coagulation profile.

ADVANCED OR CONFIRMATORY TESTING

- If still no diagnosis:
  - Repeat abdominal ultrasound exam
  - Thorough nasal and pharyngeal exam [with radiographs]; systemic blood pressure measurement if epistaxis is present
  - Endoscopy
  - Exploratory laparotomy:
    - Biopsy, aspiration, and/or resection of any lesions seen
    - Biopsies of liver, stomach, duodenum, ileum, and jejunum if no macroscopic lesion seen

- If still no diagnosis:
  - Scintigraphy (radiolabeled albumin)
  - Arteriography
  - Small bowel radiographic contrast study

TREATMENT

THERAPEUTIC GOAL(S)

- Control hemorrhage and any secondary complications of hemorrhage
- Cure the trigger

ACUTE GENERAL TREATMENT

- Largely depends on underlying cause
- Identify shock early and treat aggressively with IV fluids
- Blood transfusion—if anemia with resultant clinical signs or for coagulopathy
- Plasma transfusion—for coagulopathy
- Antiemetics and antiulcer therapy as needed
- Stop the inciting medications

DRUG INTERACTIONS

Sucralfate inhibits the absorption of fluoroquinolone antibiotics for up to 8 hours, so patients receiving sucralfate that require quinolone antibiotics should receive the quinolones parenterally, if feasible.

PROGNOSIS AND OUTCOME

Dependent on the trigger

PEARLS & CONSIDERATIONS

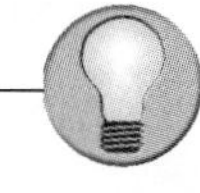

COMMENTS

These cases generally are far more difficult to diagnose than hematochezia cases. A thorough and methodical approach is essential.

CLIENT EDUCATION

Advise all owners on the potential dangers of NSAIDs.

SUGGESTED READING

Kelly K: Melena and hematochezia. In Ettinger S, Feldman E (eds): *Textbook of Veterinary Internal Medicine,* ed 6. St. Louis, Elsevier Saunders, 2005, pp 141-143.

AUTHOR: **DAVID MILLER**
EDITOR: **ETIENNE CÔTÉ**

Meningioma

BASIC INFORMATION

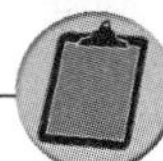

DEFINITION

A neoplasm of the meninges surrounding the brain or spinal cord

EPIDEMIOLOGY

SPECIES, AGE, SEX

- Meningiomas occur in both dogs and cats and usually affect older patients.
- Dogs are usually older than 8 years and females are affected slightly more than males.
- Cats are usually older than 10 years and males are affected slightly more often than females.

GENETICS AND BREED PREDISPOSITION

- In dogs, dolichocephalic breeds are more likely to develop meningiomas than other breeds.
- There is no breed predisposition in cats.

GEOGRAPHY AND SEASONALITY: Reported worldwide.

ASSOCIATED CONDITIONS AND DISORDERS: Meningiomas have been reported to occur in young cats with mucopolysaccharidosis type I.

CLINICAL PRESENTATION

HISTORY, CHIEF COMPLAINT

- Historic findings in general reflect neurologic compromise, but specific signs depend on lesion location.
- Clinical signs are often insidious and progressive; less commonly, acute onset of clinical signs is possible.
- The most common chief complaints for intracranial meningiomas include seizures, circling, behavior change (aggression), altered consciousness, and nonspecific signs such as inappetence and lethargy.
- The most common chief complaints for spinal meningiomas include acute to chronic onset of paresis, ataxia, and neck or back pain.

PHYSICAL EXAM FINDINGS

- Neurologic exam findings vary depending on lesion location.
- Cerebral meningioma: seizures, contralateral menace, and postural reaction deficits, behavior change, contralateral hemiparesis.
- Brainstem meningioma: ipsilateral cranial nerve deficits, hemiparesis or tetraparesis or hemiplegia or tetraplegia, or signs of central vestibular dysfunction.
- Cerebellar meningioma: hypermetria, intention tremors, truncal sway, broad-based stance.
- Spinal meningioma: paresis, ataxia, spinal pain.

ETIOLOGY AND PATHOPHYSIOLOGY

- Etiology is unknown.
- Meningiomas usually occur as solitary masses, but multiple meningiomas are relatively common in cats.
- By definition, they originate on the periphery (neoplastic outgrowths of the meninges), adjacent to cranial or vertebral bone.
- Biologic behavior and histopathologic characteristics are benign; clinical effects are due to space-occupying nature within confines of skull or vertebral canal.
- Most commonly reported in the supratentorial compartment (rostral to the tentorium cerebelli, including the cerebrum and diencephalon) in the brain.
- Tumor tends to invade into the brain parenchyma in dogs, but not in cats.
- Cervical portion of spinal cord is the most commonly affected segment in cases of spinal meningioma, but any location is possible.

DIAGNOSIS

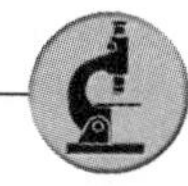

DIFFERENTIAL DIAGNOSIS

- Other brain tumors (e.g., glioma, lymphoma, metastatic tumors)
- Infectious diseases (bacterial, viral, fungal, protozoal)
- Inflammatory diseases (e.g., granulomatous meningoencephalomyelitis)
- Intervertebral disk disease
- Diskospondylitis

INITIAL DATABASE

- Complete blood count/serum biochemical profile/urinalysis: usually normal.
- Survey thoracic and abdominal radiographs should be performed in older patients to rule out extracranial and/or concurrent diseases.

ADVANCED OR CONFIRMATORY TESTING

- Computed tomography or magnetic resonance imaging: mass located outside the brain (Fig. I-116) or spinal cord parenchyma, with marked, often homogeneous, contrast enhancement. Compression of underlying brain or spinal cord is common.
- Cerebrospinal fluid analysis: used as an adjunct to advanced imaging, primarily to rule out encephalitis or myelitis. Results are generally nonspecific with meningioma, and reveal normal to mildly elevated protein. Sterile neutrophilic pleocytosis is relatively common with meningioma but is not pathognomonic.
- Histopathologic evaluation is required for definitive diagnosis. Tissue samples can be obtained via surgical excision or stereotactic brain biopsy.

TREATMENT

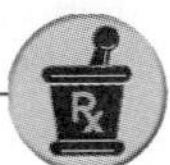

THERAPEUTIC GOAL(S)

Definitive treatment involving surgical excision and/or radiation therapy

ACUTE GENERAL TREATMENT

- Cluster seizures or status epilepticus (see Seizures, p 990): diazepam 0.5 mg/kg IV (can be repeated at 5-minute intervals for a maximum of three doses). If diazepam is initially effective but seizures recur, consider diazepam constant rate infusion (0.25-0.50 mg/kg/hr; shield from light) or loading dose of phenobarbital (16-20 mg/kg IV total dose; monitor for excessive sedation/lethargy, respiratory depression, and cardiovascular depression).
- Cerebral edema/brain herniation: mannitol 0.5 g/kg IV slowly over 15 to 20 minutes; furosemide (2 mg/kg IV) has synergistic effects with mannitol and can be given if needed.

CHRONIC TREATMENT

- Surgical excision for histologic diagnosis and definitive treatment if tumor is accessible.
  - In general, tumors located in superficial (dorsal or lateral) regions of the cerebrum, cerebellum, and spinal cord are the best candidates for surgical excision.
- Radiation therapy: used as an adjunctive treatment to surgery or as a primary treatment.
- Chemotherapy: generally less effective because the blood-brain barrier (BBB) prevents chemotherapeutic agents from entering the brain and spinal cord.
  - There are special handling requirements and potentially life-threatening adverse patient effects associated with these drugs; consultation with an oncologist for appropriate usage and the most current treatment recommendations is indicated.
  - Hydroxyurea (20 mg/kg PO q 24h) crosses the BBB and appears to be effective in dogs as it is in humans with intracranial meningioma. Possible adverse effects include bone marrow suppression (anemia, thrombocytopenia, leukopenia), pulmonary fibrosis, gastrointestinal upset, stomatitis, sloughing of nails, alopecia, and dysuria. Methemoglobinemia has been reported in cats at high dosages (>500 mg).
  - Anecdotally, nitrosourea agents such as lomustine (CCNU; 60-90 mg/m^2 PO q 6 weeks) or carmustine (BCNU 50 mg/m^2 IV q 6 weeks), which can cross the BBB, appear to have some effect; these agents are more specifically used for treating patients with gliomas. The most serious potential adverse effects are bone marrow suppression (anemia, thrombocytopenia, leukopenia) and hepatotoxicity.
- Seizures: Anticonvulsants should be used if more than one seizure occurs every 6 to 8 weeks.
  - Phenobarbital: 2-4 mg/kg PO or IV q 12h.
  - Potassium bromide: 20-50 PO q 24h. Use with caution in cats; frequently causes reversible clinical signs consistent with bronchial asthma, but in rare cases has been fatal.
- Cerebral edema: prednisone 0.5 mg/kg PO q 12h initially then taper to lowest dose that will control clinical signs.

DRUG INTERACTIONS

- Drug interactions or altered metabolism of medications have been reported between corticosteroids and amphotericin B, furosemide, thiazide diuretics, digitalis glycosides, cyclosporine, phenytoin, phenobarbital, and mitotane.
- Corticosteroids should not be given concurrently with nonsteroidal anti-inflammatory drugs or other potentially gastrointestinally ulcerogenic medications.
- Phenobarbital: may cause excessive sedation in patients with intracranial tumors, even at low doses.

POSSIBLE COMPLICATIONS

Progression of clinical signs, including status epilepticus, brain herniation, and sudden death

RECOMMENDED MONITORING

Serial neurologic exam every 4 to 6 weeks. Therapeutic drug monitoring of serum levels of anticonvulsants if relevant.

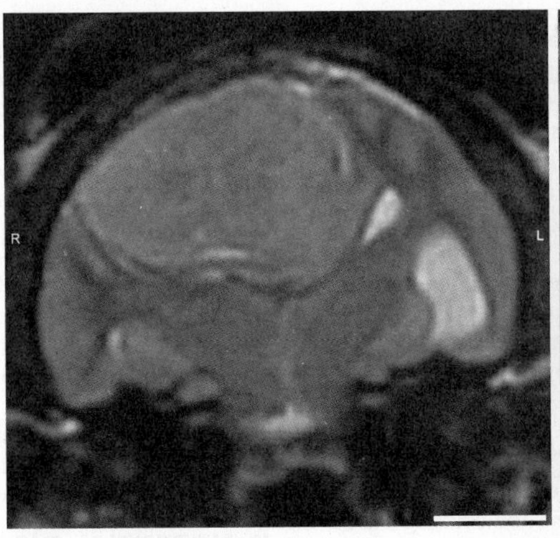

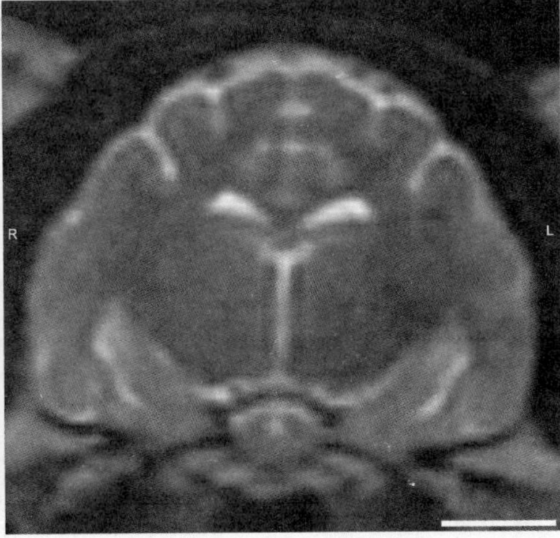

FIGURE I-116 Brain magnetic resonance images of a patient with meningioma (**A,** *left panel*) and a normal patient for comparison (**B,** *right panel*), T2-weighted. The patient's right is on the left of each image. The patient with meningioma has a large, sessile mass originating from the right dorsal calvarium; severe compression and displacement of the right cerebral hemisphere, and midline shift, are seen. Bar = 1 cm.

PROGNOSIS AND OUTCOME

- Dogs: Prognosis is fair in dogs. Median survival time for cerebral meningioma is 5 to 9 months with surgery alone and 16 to 30 months with surgery and radiation therapy. Radiation therapy alone yields a survival time of approximately 6 to 12 months.
- Cats: Prognosis is good after surgical excision, with a median survival time of approximately 2 years with surgical excision alone. Surgical excision can be curative in cats.
- Prognosis for meningiomas in other anatomic locations is fair to guarded.
- Many patients treated with supportive, nonspecific treatments (e.g., anticonvulsants, corticosteroids) are euthanized within 3 months due to progression of clinical signs.
- Dogs with intracranial meningiomas treated with oral hydroxyurea have a mean survival time of approximately 8 months (unpublished data).

PEARLS & CONSIDERATIONS

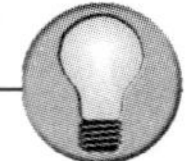

COMMENTS

- Meningiomas are the most common primary brain tumor in dogs and cats.
- Surgical excision followed by radiation therapy provides the longest survival times for dogs.
- Surgical excision alone provides prolonged survival times for cats and may be curative in some cases.
- In canine intracranial meningioma cases with seizure activity, relatively nonsedative anticonvulsant drugs (e.g., felbamate, zonisamide, levetiracetam) should be considered, especially if surgical removal of the tumor is planned. See Seizures, p 990; Epilepsy, Idiopathic, p 351.

CLIENT EDUCATION

- With patients receiving corticosteroids, warn owner of expected side effects (e.g., polyuria, polydipsia, polyphagia, weight gain), and of effects warranting notification (obesity, signs of gastrointestinal ulceration, signs of iatrogenic hyperadrenocorticism).
- Phenobarbital: short-term side effects include sedation/lethargy and pelvic limb weakness and ataxia. Long-term side effects include polyuria, polydipsia, polyphagia, weight gain. Less common adverse effects warranting intervention include hepatotoxicity, blood dyscrasias. See Phenobarbital: Adverse Effects/Toxicosis, p 844.

SUGGESTED READING

Axlund TW, McGlasson ML, Smith AN: Surgery alone or in combination with radiation therapy for treatment of intracranial meningiomas in dogs: 31 cases (1989-2002). *J Am Vet Med Assoc* 221:1597, 2002.

Braund KG, Ribas JL: Central nervous system meningiomas. *Compend Contin Educ Pract Vet* 8:241, 1986.

Brearly MJ, et al: Hypofractionated radiation therapy of brain masses in dogs: A retrospective analysis of survival of 83 cases (1991-1996). *J Vet Intern Med* 13:408, 1999.

Gallagher JG, et al: Prognosis after surgical excision of cerebral meningiomas in cats: 17 cases (1986-1992). *J Am Vet Med Assoc* 203:1437, 1993.

Gordon JE, et al: Results of craniotomy for the treatment of cerebral meningioma in 42 cats. *Vet Surg* 23:94, 1994.

Patnaik AK, Kay WJ, Hurvitz AI: Intracranial meningioma: A comparative pathologic study of 28 dogs. *Vet Pathol* 23:369, 1986.

Theon AP, et al: Influence of tumor cell proliferation and sex hormone receptors on effectiveness of radiation therapy for dogs with incompletely resected meningiomas. *J Am Vet Med Assoc* 216:707, 2000.

Troxel MT, et al: Feline intracranial neoplasia: Retrospective review of 160 cases (1985-2001). *J Vet Intern Med* 17:850, 2003.

AUTHOR: **MARK T. TROXEL**

EDITOR: **CURTIS W. DEWEY**

Mesenteric Volvulus

BASIC INFORMATION

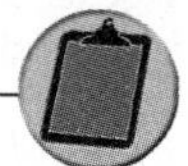

DEFINITION

Mesenteric volvulus is a disorder characterized by a twisting of the intestine around the root of the mesentery, a process that potentially can be rapidly fatal.

SYNONYM(S)

Intestinal volvulus
Mesenteric torsion

EPIDEMIOLOGY

SPECIES, AGE, SEX: Young (<3 years old) adult, male dogs predisposed. Also reported in cats.

GENETICS AND BREED PREDISPOSITION: Large-breed dogs, German shepherds, and English pointers.

ASSOCIATED CONDITIONS AND DISORDERS: Conditions that have been associated with mesenteric volvulus include exocrine pancreatic insufficiency, recent gastrointestinal surgery, gastrointestinal foreign bodies, enteritis, intestinal neoplasia, blunt trauma, and gastric dilatation volvulus (GDV).

CLINICAL PRESENTATION

HISTORY, CHIEF COMPLAINT: Acute onset abdominal distention, pain, vomiting, and hematochezia.

PHYSICAL EXAM FINDINGS

- Physical findings consistent with hypovolemic shock: tachycardia (or bradycardia in cats), weak pulses, pale mucous membranes, prolonged capillary refill time, weakness or collapse.
- Abdominal distention, palpably gas-filled intestinal loops.

ETIOLOGY AND PATHOPHYSIOLOGY

- Twisting of intestine occurs around mesenteric axis or root causing vascular occlusion to the intestines.
- Thin-walled veins and lymphatics become obstructed causing edema in the intestinal wall.
- Blood flow through cranial mesenteric artery and its branches is partially or completely occluded due to twisting.
- Ischemic necrosis of intestine occurs and blood is lost into the intestinal lumen.
- Endotoxins and bacteria translocate into the abdomen through the damaged intestinal mucosa.
- Patients eventually die from circulatory shock and endotoxemia/sepsis.

DIAGNOSIS

The diagnosis is suspected based on physical exam and appearance of abdominal radiographs. Differential diagnoses must be ruled out to the extent possible (e.g., parvoviral testing if appropriate), and confirmation of the diagnosis is made at the time of surgery.

DIFFERENTIAL DIAGNOSIS

Any condition associated with acute abdominal pain or hematochezia and vomiting:

- GDV
- Cecocolic volvulus
- Splenic torsion
- Gastrointestinal obstruction or rupture
- Peritonitis
- Pancreatitis
- Hemorrhagic gastroenteritis
- Parvoviral enteritis

INITIAL DATABASE

- Abdominal radiography: multiple severely distended gas-filled intestinal loops; poor abdominal detail associated with peritoneal fluid (Fig. I-117).
- Complete blood count:
  - Packed cell volume usually normal
- Serum biochemistry profile:
  - Hypoproteinemia, hypokalemia
- Preoperative laboratory evaluation is often limited to on-site tests due to the potentially rapid deterioration of the condition of patients with mesenteric volvulus
- Abdominocentesis with fluid evaluation: modified transudate (early), or septic exudate eventually (with bacterial translocation or peritonitis). With bowel necrosis, the fluid may be dark and fetid.

ADVANCED OR CONFIRMATORY TESTING

Surgical confirmation of diagnosis (Fig. I-118)

TREATMENT

THERAPEUTIC GOAL(S)

- Correct circulatory shock
- Immediate surgery to reduce the twisted mesenteric root
- Resect diseased bowel

ACUTE GENERAL TREATMENT

- Rapid intravenous fluid administration (combination of crystalloids and colloids).
- Treat endotoxemia/sepsis with antibiotics.
  - Third-generation cephalosporin, 22 mg/kg IV q 2h during perioperative period, then q 6h postoperatively.
- Correct electrolyte and acid-base abnormalities with fluid therapy.
- Perform derotation of intestines and monitor for perfusion.
- Resect devitalized bowel.
- Perform thorough exploratory for associated conditions.
- Lavage abdomen and consider postoperative drainage if peritonitis is present.

POSSIBLE COMPLICATIONS

- Septic peritonitis if diseased bowel not removed, contamination of abdomen not cleared or resection and anastomosis site dehiscence
- Reperfusion injury
- Short bowel syndrome if >70% of small intestine resected

RECOMMENDED MONITORING

- Postoperative monitoring of hydration and electrolyte concentrations
- Blood pressure monitoring for hypotension
- Body temperature and blood glucose monitoring for sepsis

PROGNOSIS AND OUTCOME

- Grave prognosis unless volvulus recognized and treated immediately.
- Most reports of mesenteric volvulus cite a 100% mortality rate unless the volvulus is found incidentally during exploratory celiotomy.

PEARLS & CONSIDERATIONS

COMMENTS

- Surgery should not be delayed if an animal presents in shock with multiple gas-filled intestinal loops on radiographs, but parvoviral enteritis should be ruled out.
- Consideration should be given to the use of drugs that block the formation of, or scavenge, oxygen free radicals (i.e., corticosteroids).

SUGGESTED READING

Nemzek JA, et al: Mesenteric volvulus in the dog: A retrospective study. *J Am Anim Hosp Assoc* 29:357, 1993.

Shealy PM, et al: Canine intestinal volvulus: A report of nine new cases. *Vet Surg* 21:15,1992.

Westermarck E, et al: Mesenteric torsion in dogs with exocrine pancreatic insufficiency: 21 cases. *J Am Vet Med Assoc* 55:123, 1989.

AUTHOR: **LORI LUDWIG**
EDITOR: **RICHARD WALSHAW**

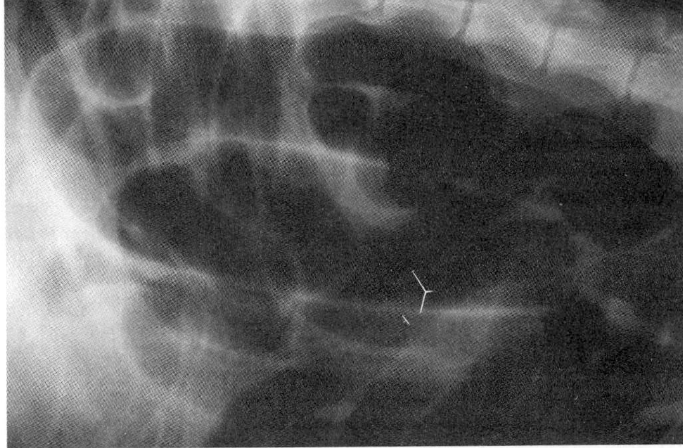

FIGURE I-117 Lateral abdominal radiograph of a dog with mesenteric volvulus. Marked gas distention of bowel is present. A differential diagnosis would be severe enteritis. Courtesy of Dr. Richard Walshaw.

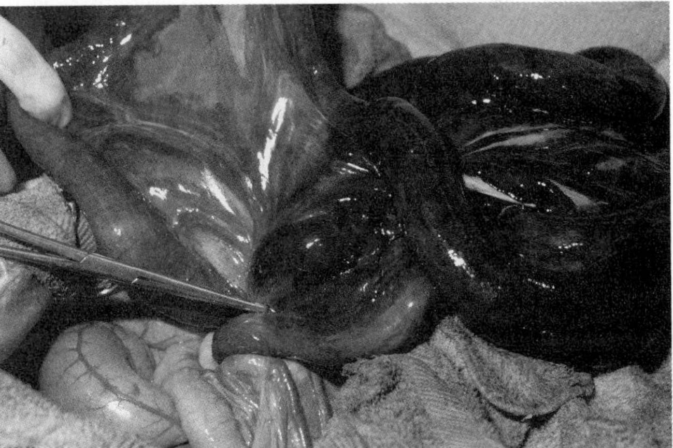

FIGURE I-118 Same dog as in Fig. I-117, gross appearance of the bowel during exploratory laparotomy. The severe discoloration of much of the small intestine, and volvulus of the mesenteric root, are diagnostic. Courtesy of Dr. Richard Walshaw.

Mesocestoides Infection

BASIC INFORMATION

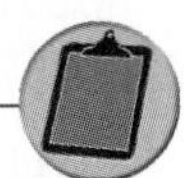

DEFINITION

Infestation with a cestode (tapeworm) of the small intestine of mammals and birds, of which the larval form (tetrathyridium) may infect serous cavities of many animals, particularly canines, causing ascites and pleural effusion

SYNONYM(S)

Mesocestoides lineatus
Mesocestoides corti

EPIDEMIOLOGY

SPECIES, AGE, SEX: Wide host range (reptile, avian, amphibian, and mammals), especially carnivores. Most common in domestic and wild canids. Cats may also be infected.
RISK FACTORS: Hunting and exposure to wildlife.
CONTAGION AND ZOONOSIS: Unknown. Cases have been reported in humans.
GEOGRAPHY AND SEASONALITY: Many parts of the world, including Africa, Asia, and the United States.

CLINICAL PRESENTATION

HISTORY, CHIEF COMPLAINT: Anorexia, respiratory distress, abdominal distention.
PHYSICAL EXAM FINDINGS: Abdominal and pleural effusion.

ETIOLOGY AND PATHOPHYSIOLOGY

- Life cycle involves two intermediate hosts.
- First intermediate host unknown but may be a ground dwelling coprophagous arthropod (oribatid mite, beetle).
- Second intermediate host (reptile, amphibian, bird, rodent, cat) becomes infected by ingestion of the larval form of the first intermediate host.
- The tetrathyridium is the third larval stage and occurs in the peritoneal cavity and musculature.
- Dogs and cats are presumably infected by ingestion of the tetrathyridia within the second intermediate host (i.e., from capturing infected birds, snakes, and small mammals as prey).
- Dogs are the definitive host and may be infected by both adult tapeworms and tetrathyridia.
- Tetrathyridia develop into adult tapeworms within the intestines, which rarely results in clinical disease. Development into adults may take 16 to 20 days in dogs. In cats, development into adults may take longer.
- Some tetrathyridia migrate through the intestinal wall and continue as tetrathyridia within subcutaneous tissues, liver, lungs, retroperitoneal space, or abdominal and thoracic cavities.
- Tetrathyridia may incite a nonpurulent granulomatous inflammatory response on serosal surfaces.

DIAGNOSIS

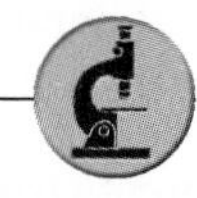

DIFFERENTIAL DIAGNOSIS

Abdominal and pleural effusions: congestive heart failure, portal hypertension, liver disease, hemorrhagic effusions, neoplastic effusions, hypoalbuminemia, septic effusions, chylous effusions. The latter two would be most likely to be confounded grossly with *Mesocestoides*-related effusions (color).

INITIAL DATABASE

- Abdominocentesis or thoracocentesis typically reveals a distinctive thick, opaque white fluid.
- Cytologic evaluation of fluid may show a mixed inflammatory exudate ± hemorrhage and necrosis. Calcareous corpuscles (clear to yellow-gold round to oval structures that are remnant tissues of the cestodes) may be present.
- Tetrathyridia may be found on aspiration of cystic lesions.

ADVANCED OR CONFIRMATORY TESTING

Recovery of organism from peritoneal cavity with identification of cestode DNA via polymerase chain reaction (PCR)

TREATMENT

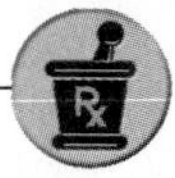

THERAPEUTIC GOAL(S)

- Decrease larva burden
- It may not be possible to completely eliminate organism

ACUTE AND CHRONIC TREATMENT

- Lavage of peritoneal cavity may be helpful to decrease parasite burden.
- Anthelmintics:
  - Praziquantel for adult organisms: 5 mg/kg PO.
  - Fenbendazole for larvae: 100 mg/kg PO q 24h for 28 days. Off-label use. May not clear infection. Side effects (bone marrow, others) possible.

POSSIBLE COMPLICATIONS

Gastrointestinal signs may be seen with antiparasitics.

RECOMMENDED MONITORING

Regular fecal examinations

PROGNOSIS AND OUTCOME

Guarded for infection with tetrathyridia. It may not be possible to completely clear the infection, and signs may recur.

PEARLS & CONSIDERATIONS

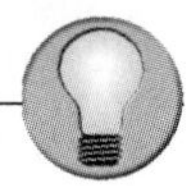

PREVENTION

- Prevent dogs and cats from ingesting second intermediate hosts such as birds, amphibians, reptiles, and rodents
- Regularly deworm

SUGGESTED READING

Bowman DD, Hendrix CM, Lindsay DS, Barr SC (eds): *Feline Clinical Parasitology*. Ames, IA, Iowa State University Press, 2002, pp 199-204.

Caruso KJ, et al: Cytologic diagnosis of peritoneal cestodiasis in dogs caused by *Mesocestoides* sp., *Vet Clin Pathol* 32(2):50-60, 2003.

Crosbie PR, et al: Diagnostic procedures and treatment of 11 dogs with peritoneal infections caused by *Mesocestoides* species. *J Am Vet Med Assoc* 213(11):1578-1583, 1999.

Parker MD: An unusual cause of abdominal distension in a dog. *Vet Med* 189-195, 2002.

Toplu N, Yildiz K, Tunay R: Massive cystic tetrathyridiosis in a dog. *J Small Anim Pract* 45(8): 410-412, 2004.

AUTHOR: **LISA M. TIEBER NIELSON**
EDITOR: **DOUGLASS K. MACINTIRE**

Mesothelioma

Client Education Sheet on Website

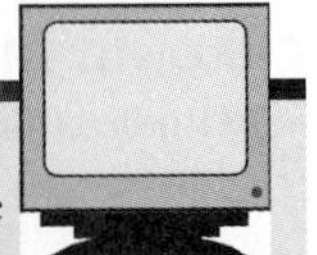

BASIC INFORMATION

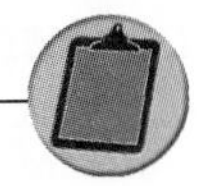

DEFINITION

Mesothelioma is a neoplasm of mesodermal origin that may arise from the pleural, pericardial, or peritoneal surfaces. Also reported from scrotum or tunica vaginalis.

SYNONYM(S)

Malignant mesothelioma

EPIDEMIOLOGY

SPECIES, AGE, SEX

- Dogs > cats
- Generally older age

GENETICS AND BREED PREDISPOSITION: Males (and specifically German shepherd dogs) are overrepresented in the population suffering from sclerosing mesothelioma. Large-breed dogs are affected more commonly.

RISK FACTORS: Possibly asbestos exposure. The type of cancer caused by chronic asbestos exposure in human beings is mesothelioma, and the same histopathologic findings (ferruginous bodies) have been noted in both canine and human mesothelioma.

ASSOCIATED CONDITIONS AND DISORDERS: Pleural, pericardial, and peritoneal effusion with subsequent dyspnea, acute cardiac tamponade and right-sided heart failure, or abdominal distention, respectively.

CLINICAL PRESENTATION

DISEASE FORMS/SUBTYPES

- Mesenchymal form: multiple focal nodules of solid or papillary neoplastic growth; historically, the more common form.
- Sclerosing form: characterized by an intense fibroblastic reaction and thick fibrous adhesions involving all abdominal organs but most markedly centered around the stomach and prostate; uncommonly described in dogs.

HISTORY, CHIEF COMPLAINT

- Patients most commonly are presented for dyspnea or cough.
- This disease should be suspected in any adult patient with:
  - A cough that does not respond to standard treatment for nonspecific respiratory problems, or
  - Evidence of chronic disease and effusion in any body cavity.
- Depending on the anatomic location of the malignancy and the subsequent effusion, the patient may present with dyspnea, cough, weight loss, acute cardiac tamponade and right-sided heart failure, or abdominal distention.

PHYSICAL EXAM FINDINGS

- Dyspnea due to pleural effusion in dogs and cats is usually identified by forceful inspiration and prolonged expiration ("holding its breath").
- In cats, a noncompressible cranial thorax may be detected (differential diagnosis: mediastinal masses such as thymoma or lymphoma).
- Other signs may include tachypnea, open mouth breathing, cyanosis, muffled heart and lung sounds ventrally with increased bronchovesicular sounds dorsally, poor peripheral pulses, jugular distention and abdominal distention.
- In a standing patient, thoracic percussion may reveal a "fluid line" (zone of hyporesonance) ventrally.

ETIOLOGY AND PATHOPHYSIOLOGY

- Mesothelioma involves a malignant transformation of mesothelial cells that line body cavities.
- Pleural, pericardial, and peritoneal effusion from mesothelioma is most likely due to increased capillary permeability (parietal foci) secondary to vasculitis.

DIAGNOSIS

DIFFERENTIAL DIAGNOSIS

- Pleural effusion:
  - Neoplastic effusions secondary to nonmesothelial malignancies (i.e., lymphoma, thymoma, carcinoma, or sarcoma)
  - Pyothorax
  - Chylothorax
  - Congestive heart failure
  - Hemothorax
  - Feline infectious peritonitis (FIP) in cats
  - Vasculitis (any etiology)
- Pericardial effusion:
  - Neoplastic effusions secondary to nonmesothelial malignancies (i.e., hemangiosarcoma, especially in large-breed dogs [as for mesothelioma] including German shepherds, golden retrievers, Labrador retrievers; aortic body tumors such as chemodectomas or nonchromaffin paragangliomas, especially in aged brachycephalic breeds; other heart base tumors such as ectopic thyroid tumors; and metastatic disease, especially carcinoma)
  - Idiopathic/benign sterile pericarditis
  - FIP in cats
  - Vasculitis (any etiology)
- Abdominal effusion:
  - Neoplastic effusions secondary to nonmesothelial malignancies (i.e., disseminated intra-abdominal metastasis, especially carcinoma or hemangiosarcoma)
  - Hypoproteinemia (any cause)
  - Peritonitis
  - Right-sided congestive heart failure
  - FIP in cats
  - Vasculitis (any etiology)

INITIAL DATABASE

- The effusion should be sampled and evaluated with fluid analysis and cytologic assessment.
- Complete blood count (CBC), serum biochemical analysis, and urinalysis.
- These tests should be supplemented with fungal, viral, and parasitic (tick and heartworm) serologic evaluations and microbial (fungal and bacterial) culture as clinical suspicion and history warrant.
- Radiographic studies (especially after removal of as much fluid as possible).
- Ultrasonographic studies (abdomen, heart, and pleural space).

ADVANCED OR CONFIRMATORY TESTING

Definitive diagnosis requires tissue for histopathology. A pH of 7.5 or greater in the effusion immediately at the time of centesis has been associated with malignancy, but accuracy is controversial. A normal fibronectin level in the effusion could help rule out mesothelioma.

TREATMENT

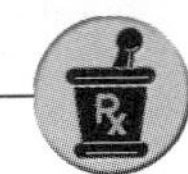

THERAPEUTIC GOAL(S)

Relieve the respiratory or cardiovascular embarrassment

ACUTE GENERAL TREATMENT

Stabilization of the patient by relieving the cardiovascular or respiratory embarrassment is paramount.

- This generally revolves around removal of large-volume effusions, and doing so without delay if clinical signs are severe.
- Oxygen therapy is often indicated before centesis or obtaining blood or urine samples if patients are extremely unstable or volatile in order to prevent acute life-threatening cardiovascular or respiratory decompensation (especially cats).

CHRONIC TREATMENT

- Periodic thoracocentesis or pericardiocentesis can be performed when fluid accumulation or symptoms are slow to return (weeks or more).
- For dogs with pericardial mesothelioma, surgical or thoracoscopic pericardectomy can palliate clinical signs and reduce tumor burden (disease cytoreduction).
- Administration of chemotherapy via intracavitary infusion on an every-3-week schedule can be attempted for long-term control.
- Potential benefits (unproven on a large scale) must be weighed against the real drawbacks of possible adverse reactions to these agents.
- Results suggest intracavitary cisplatin (50–70 mg/m^2 body surface area along with saline fluid diuresis) is effective in some dogs.
- Carboplatin (250–350 mg/m^2 body surface area) has limited intracavitary penetration but can be attempted.
- At this time only small numbers of patients have been evaluated, so efficacy remains unproven.
- Intravenous chemotherapy with cisplatin, carboplatin, or doxorubicin may have a role in some patients.
- Consultation with oncologist for most current treatment recommendations is indicated. However, due to the rarity of this disease, multicenter clinical trials will be required to test and develop effective treatments.

POSSIBLE COMPLICATIONS

Pneumothorax, cardiac puncture, hemopericardium, hemothorax, infection

RECOMMENDED MONITORING

- Hourly for critical (ICU) patients: respiratory rates, degree of dyspnea, blood gases.
- Daily to weekly for outpatients: respiratory rates, quality of life assessments, repeat thoracic radiographs as warranted or required.
- As required per protocol for chemotherapy patients (i.e., CBC), quality of life assessments, repeat thoracic radiographs as warranted or required.

PROGNOSIS AND OUTCOME

- Poor to fair. Survival is dependent on rate of accumulation of the fluid and degree of compensation, which are both variable from patient to patient.
- Many patients are euthanatized at the time of diagnosis.
- For those that are treated, the reported survival time varies considerably from weeks to years.
- Some animals may have a dramatic improvement after pericardiocentesis or thoracocentesis and a prolonged (weeks to months) period without clinical signs while others have a reaccumulation of fluid and return of tamponade or dyspnea within hours or days.
- A good quality of life for months to 1 to 2 years with pericardial or pleural mesothelioma is realistically possible if a good response to the first centesis occurs, and owners are willing to follow up regularly with centesis on an as-needed basis.
- In this author's experience, owners rarely agree to continue with repeat pericardiocentesis after more than 2 or 3 episodes of acute decompensation.

PEARLS & CONSIDERATIONS

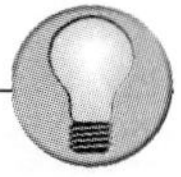

COMMENTS

- Thoracocentesis should be considered before blood or urine sample acquisition or radiographic or ultrasonographic studies in patients that are unstable. The removal of even a small amount of fluid may dramatically relieve the respiratory embarrassment and stabilize the patient.
- Although it shares similarities with mesothelioma in terms of distribution (body cavity surfaces), carcinomatosis refers to seeding of pleural or peritoneal surfaces with malignant carcinoma cells.
- Management of dogs and cats with carcinomatosis may include treatment with intracavitary chemotherapeutics as described for mesothelioma.

CLIENT EDUCATION

Teaching the client to monitor respiratory rate will give both the client and the clinician an objective measure of progression and acuity of decompensation in the patient.

SUGGESTED READING

Garrett LD, MacEwan EG: Mesothelioma. In Withrow SJ, MacEwan EG (eds): *Small Animal Clinical Oncology*, ed 3. Philadelphia, WB Saunders, 2001, pp 656–661.

Glickman LT, et al: Mesothelioma in pet dogs associated with exposure of their owners to asbestos. *Environ Res* 32:305, 1983.

AUTHOR: **CARLOS O. RODRIGUEZ, JR.**
EDITOR: **KENNETH M. RASSNICK**

Metaldehyde Toxicosis

BASIC INFORMATION

DEFINITION

An acute toxicosis manifested by rapid onset of clinical signs such as anxiety, panting, hypersalivation, increasingly vigorous muscle tremors, hyperesthesia, hyperthermia, and seizures. Such uncontrolled signs indicate intoxications that can rapidly become fatal.

SYNONYM(S)

Slug or snail bait poisoning

Metaldehyde-containing baits are formulated as liquid, granules, powder, or pellets.

Ortho Bug-Geta, Corry's Slug and Snail Pellets, Deadline Force II, Dragon Snail and Slug Killer Pellets, Last-Bite Snail and Slug Killer Pellets, Lilly Miller Slug and Snail Bait, Corry's Liquid Slug and Snail Control, Corry's Slug Snail, and Insect Killer are some metaldehyde-containing commercial products.

EPIDEMIOLOGY

SPECIES, AGE, SEX

- Toxic to all species.
- Poisoning seen mostly in dogs.
- All breeds, ages, and sexes susceptible.

RISK FACTORS: Pre-existing hepatopathies may increase sensitivity to the agent.

GEOGRAPHY AND SEASONALITY: Toxicosis can occur anywhere; most common in areas with large populations of snails and slugs (e.g., the North American West Coast [especially California] and East Coast).

CLINICAL PRESENTATION

HISTORY, CHIEF COMPLAINT

- Witnessed or suspected ingestion
- Rapid onset of muscle tremors and seizures

PHYSICAL EXAM FINDINGS

- Rapid, progressively more frequent (or sustained) muscle fasciculations/tremors are characteristic of metaldehyde intoxication, and may progress to extensor rigidity/tetany.
- Secondary hyperthermia, which may be severe (104–108°F), is common. Hyperthermia is not a true fever, but

rather is the result of muscle fasciculations.
- Seizures.
- Concurrent nonspecific signs are common:
  - Tachycardia
  - Tachypnea
  - Hypersalivation
  - Vomiting
  - Diarrhea

ETIOLOGY AND PATHOPHYSIOLOGY

- Metaldehyde is a tetramer of acetaldehyde used as a molluscicide.
- Most poisonings occur in dogs when they consume metaldehyde-containing baits.
- Oral LD50 of metaldehyde in dogs = 100–1000 mg/kg and in cats = 207 mg/kg.
- Clinical signs of toxicosis can be seen within 30 minutes to 5 hours after ingestion.
- Metaldehyde is rapidly absorbed orally.
  - Acetaldehyde is produced upon exposure to gastric (low) pH.
  - Acetaldehyde is presumed to contribute to acidosis and other central nervous system signs such as seizures.
- Minimum toxic dose of metaldehyde in dogs is not known.
  - Consumption of one tablespoon of 2% powder or granular bait will provide approximately 300 mg of metaldehyde; possibly a significant hazard for a 10 kg dog (30 mg/kg of metaldehyde).
- Clinical signs could be due to decreased level of cerebral γ-aminobutyric acid, norepinephrine, and serotonin, which can cause seizures, and increased monoamine oxidase activity, which further decreases serotonin and norepinephrine levels.

DIAGNOSIS

The diagnosis is based almost entirely on geographic location (presence of snails/slugs in region), history, and characteristic physical examination findings. A presumptive diagnosis is generally sufficient to initiate treatment, given the severity of signs in most cases and negative consequences of leaving such signs untreated.

DIFFERENTIAL DIAGNOSIS

- Strychnine Toxicosis (see p 1045).
- Organophosphate and Carbamate Insecticide Toxicosis (see p 775).
- Zinc Phosphide Intoxication (see p 1170).
- Garbage Toxicosis (see p 425).
- Primary central nervous system disease (neoplasia, encephalitis, idiopathic epilepsy, other).

INITIAL DATABASE

- Acid-base status (acidosis may be present)
- Baseline liver enzymes (usually normal)
- Baseline body temperature (commonly 104–108°F)

ADVANCED OR CONFIRMATORY TESTING

- Metaldehyde may be detected in stomach contents, vomitus, serum, liver, and urine
- Acetaldehyde smell (similar to formaldehyde) in the stomach or gastrointestinal tract may help in diagnosis

TREATMENT

THERAPEUTIC GOAL(S)

- Decontamination of patient (remove remaining toxin)
- Control tremors and seizures
- Correct acid/base abnormalities
- Control hyperthermia
- Supportive care

ACUTE GENERAL TREATMENT

- Decontamination of patient:
  - Emesis in patients not showing any clinical signs; useful within 30 minutes of exposure.
    - Hydrogen peroxide 1 ml/kg PO, repeat once in 10 to 20 minutes if needed, maximum dose in largest dogs is 45 ml.
    - Apomorphine 0.04 mg/kg IM or IV, or instill into conjunctival sac part of a crushed tablet dissolved in water.
  - Give activated charcoal after inducing emesis at 1–3 g/kg PO mixed with a cathartic such as magnesium or sodium sulfate 250 mg/kg or sorbitol 1–3 ml/kg; use label dose for commercial preparations; multiple doses may be helpful with large ingestion (caution aspiration risk in vomiting patient).
  - Gastric lavage with large ingestion in symptomatic animals followed by activated charcoal (see Gastric Intubation, Gavage, Lavage, p 1258).
- Control tremors/seizures:
  - Methocarbamol 55–220 mg/kg IV; repeat as needed (maximum dose 330 mg/kg/day).
  - Diazepam 1–2 mg/kg IV; repeat as needed.
  - General anesthesia if no response to above measures.
    - Pentobarbital 10–30 mg/kg IV to effect, repeat as needed, or
    - Propofol up to 5–6 mg/kg slow IV to effect, then constant rate infusion 0.1–0.6 mg/kg/min titrated to effect, and/or
    - Isoflurane inhalant anesthesia.
- Fluid diuresis for hydration, renal perfusion, and diuresis.
- Control hyperthermia (cold bath, fans).
- Control acid-base balance with sodium bicarbonate.

POSSIBLE COMPLICATIONS

- Disseminated intravascular coagulation secondary to prolonged hyperthermia possible.
- Acute hepatic failure in some dogs 2 to 3 days after exposure can occur (uncommonly) when the patient seems to have recovered; monitor closely. (See Hepatic Injury, Acute, p 491.)
- Renal failure due to myoglobinuria (uncommon).

RECOMMENDED MONITORING

- Body temperature
- Liver enzymes for 3 days (baseline, 24, 48, 72 hours)
- Acid-base status

PROGNOSIS AND OUTCOME

- Good with prompt decontamination and control of tremors and seizures
- Guarded with poorly controlled tremors or seizures or prolonged hyperthermia

PEARLS & CONSIDERATIONS

COMMENTS

- Most commercial baits contain 2–5% metaldehyde.
- Some formulations may also contain 5% carbaryl (a carbamate insecticide) along with metaldehyde. See Organophosphate and Carbamate Insecticide Toxicosis, p 775. Toxicity potential of carbaryl is much less compared to metaldehyde.

PREVENTION

- Placement of bait in areas inaccessible to animals
- Use of relatively less toxic baits (e.g., iron-based baits) to control slugs and snails

SUGGESTED READING

Dolder LK: Metaldehyde toxicosis. *Vet Med* 98:213, 2003.

Talcott PA: Metaldehyde. In Plumlee KH (ed): *Clin Vet Toxicol*. St. Louis, Mosby, 2004, pp 182–183.

AUTHOR: **ERIC K. DUNAYER**

EDITOR: **SAFDAR A. KHAN**

Metronidazole Toxicosis

BASIC INFORMATION

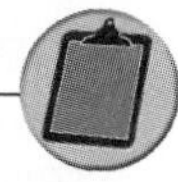

DEFINITION

Neurologic dysfunction due to administration of high doses of the antibiotic metronidazole

SYNONYM(S)

Flagyl toxicosis

EPIDEMIOLOGY

SPECIES, AGE, SEX: Dogs and cats of any age or sex can be affected.
RISK FACTORS: Toxicosis is usually associated with doses of 60 mg/kg/day or higher for 1 week or longer.

CLINICAL PRESENTATION

HISTORY, CHIEF COMPLAINT

- Initial signs in dogs are anorexia and vomiting that progress rapidly to generalized ataxia. Seizures and head tilt are less common.
- Cats suffer a sudden onset of weakness and disorientation, often with seizures.

PHYSICAL EXAM FINDINGS

- Affected dogs typically show severe, generalized ataxia; depression; and vertical nystagmus that changes in frequency with head position. Postural reactions and spinal reflexes are usually normal.
- Affected cats often show ataxia with postural reaction deficits in all limbs, depression or stupor, seizures, and blindness with intact pupillary light reflexes.

ETIOLOGY AND PATHOPHYSIOLOGY

- The cumulative dose may be important in the pathophysiology of neurologic dysfunction, although there seems to be substantial individual susceptibility to signs of toxicity.
- Metronidazole is recommended for two different indications in most drug formularies: at an enteric dose for acute gastrointestinal infections and parasitoses (30-65 mg/kg "divided q 12h" for 5 to 7 days) or at doses for anaerobic bacterial infections (15 mg/kg PO q 12h for days to weeks; lower to 7.5 mg/kg PO q 12h if hepatic dysfunction).
- Common dosage errors (and therefore risk of toxicosis) appear to be:
    - Prescribing the high, enteric dose for >1 week.
    - Overlooking the "divided q 12h" indication and prescribing the high enteric dose q 12h.
    - Failing to reduce the dose in patients with liver disease.
    - Failing to accurately divide the 250-mg tablets in cats or very small dogs, where small differences in tablet fractions correspond to relatively large excesses in dose per kg body weight.

DIAGNOSIS

DIFFERENTIAL DIAGNOSIS

- Encephalitis
- Neoplasia

INITIAL DATABASE

Routine laboratory tests are usually normal, but mild elevations in liver enzymes are possible.

ADVANCED OR CONFIRMATORY TESTING

Diagnosis is based on clinical features, history of metronidazole administration, and recovery on stopping the drug.

TREATMENT

THERAPEUTIC GOAL(S)

The goal of treatment is to stop metronidazole administration and provide supportive care until the signs resolve, usually within 3 to 5 days.

ACUTE GENERAL TREATMENT

- Discontinue the metronidazole.
- Parenteral hydration and nutrition if necessary.
- Antiseizure medication, such as diazepam, as needed.
- Oral diazepam administration (0.5 mg/kg q 8h), may speed recovery from metronidazole toxicosis in dogs, including those that are not showing seizure activity.

RECOMMENDED MONITORING

Clinical response to discontinuation of metronidazole. Deterioration or worsening of clinical signs should prompt evaluation for another diagnosis.

PROGNOSIS AND OUTCOME

The prognosis is excellent with prompt withdrawal of the offending drug. Most patients show improvement within 48 hours, although it may take a week for complete resolution.

PEARLS & CONSIDERATIONS

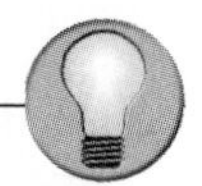

COMMENTS

- Clinicians should consider metronidazole toxicity in any patient developing neurologic signs while taking this antibiotic. With prompt recognition and withdrawal of the offending drug, complete recovery is expected.
- In many instances of intestinal parasitosis, metronidazole may not be the best choice of treatment. Alternative medications (e.g., fenbendazole) have shown greater efficacy and far fewer adverse effects in canine *Giardia* infection, for example.

PREVENTION

Avoid doses of metronidazole higher than 30 mg/kg/day. Some published doses are high enough to cause toxicity.

SUGGESTED READING

Caylor KB, Cassimitis MK: Metronidazole neurotoxicosis in two cats. *J Am Anim Hosp Assoc* 37:258, 2001.

Dow SW, et al: Central nervous system toxicoses associated with metronidazole treatment of dogs: Five cases (1984-1987). *J Am Vet Med Assoc* 195:365, 1989.

Evans J, et al: Diazepam as a treatment for metronidazole toxicosis in dogs: A retrospective study of 21 cases. *J Vet Intern Med* 17:304, 2003.

AUTHOR: **WILLIAM B. THOMAS**
EDITOR: **CURTIS W. DEWEY**

Microvascular Dysplasia, Hepatic

BASIC INFORMATION

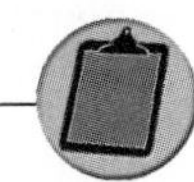

DEFINITION

A congenital disorder of dogs in which there are histologic hepatic vascular abnormalities presumably causing intrahepatic shunting with no demonstrable macroscopic portosystemic shunt (PSS)

SYNONYM(S)

Hepatoportal microvascular dysplasia (HMD)
MD
Microvascular portal dysplasia
Portal vein hypoplasia (with no shunt)

EPIDEMIOLOGY

SPECIES, AGE, SEX

- Primarily dogs; poorly documented in cats.
- Typically affects young adult dogs; clinical signs develop at average age 3 years (can be any age). By contrast, dogs with PSS first develop signs at average age 6 to 18 months.
- Female sex predilection.

GENETICS AND BREED PREDISPOSITION

- Polygenic mode of inheritance suspected in cairn terriers.
- Cairn terriers and Yorkshire terriers predisposed.
- Has been documented in multiple breeds (vast majority are small dogs).

ASSOCIATED CONDITIONS AND DISORDERS: Similar histologic hepatic changes are seen in dogs with PSS.

CLINICAL PRESENTATION

HISTORY, CHIEF COMPLAINT

- Most affected dogs show no clinical signs.
- Severely affected dogs present signs similar to those of dogs with PSS. Signs often wax and wane.
- Clinical signs are typically referrable to the central nervous system (CNS), gastrointestinal (GI) system, or urinary tract.
- CNS (all secondary to hepatic encephalopathy): lethargy, ataxia, weakness, abnormal behavior, abnormal vocalization, ptyalism (more common in cats), head pressing, bumping into objects due to central blindness, incessant pacing or circling, stupor, seizures, or coma.
    - Exacerbation of encephalopathic signs with: high protein meals, GI bleeding, constipation, azotemia, hypokalemia, metabolic alkalosis, tranquilization, and methionine-containing medications.
- GI: intermittent anorexia, vomiting, diarrhea.
- Urinary tract: hematuria, pollakiuria, or dysuria from ammonium urate urolithiasis.

PHYSICAL EXAM FINDINGS

- Usually unremarkable
- Small body stature
- Questionably small liver (inability to palpate liver margins)
- CNS signs (see CNS in History, Chief Complaint above)
- Poor haircoat

ETIOLOGY AND PATHOPHYSIOLOGY

- Shunting is hypothesized to occur through microscopic intrahepatic vessels, but this has not been proven.
- Hepatic encephalopathy (HE) and resultant CNS signs occur from toxins and nutrients absorbed from the intestines, which are thought to bypass metabolism by the liver through the microscopic intrahepatic shunting. (See Hepatic Encephalopathy, p 489).
- High urinary excretion from elevated blood levels of ammonia and uric acid can occasionally result in development of urate urolithiasis (renal, ureteral, bladder).

DIAGNOSIS

DIFFERENTIAL DIAGNOSIS

- CNS signs: infectious disease, toxin, other metabolic encephalopathy (hypoglycemia), idiopathic epilepsy, congenital malformations (e.g., hydrocephalus)
- GI signs: parasitism, foreign body, dietary indiscretion, dietary allergy, intestinal inflammation/infiltration
- Urinary tract signs: urinary tract infection, other calculi

INITIAL DATABASE

- Complete blood count is typically normal. Microcytosis, commonly seen in dogs with PSS, rarely occurs in dogs with hepatic microvascular dysplasia.
- Serum biochemical profile is often normal; however, mild liver enzymes elevations, mildly low blood urea nitrogen have been noted, as have hyperglobulinemia and hypercholesterolemia.
- Coagulation profile: typically normal.
- Urinalysis: usually normal, but ammonium biurate crystalluria, hematuria, or pyuria are possible.
- Abdominal radiographs: usually normal, but occasionally mild microhepatica may be noted.

ADVANCED OR CONFIRMATORY TESTING

- Serum bile acids: Essentially all animals with microvascular dysplasia have elevated postprandial serum bile acid levels; fasting/preprandial may be normal. Mean serum bile acid levels are lower than in dogs with PSS.
- Liver biopsy:
    - Typically reveals hepatic arteriolar hyperplasia, small portal triads, increased smooth muscle thickness of hepatic venules, and an increase in small vascular structures in the periportal area.
    - These findings in association with elevated serum bile acids, in the absence of PSS, are diagnostic for microvascular dysplasia.
    - Certain histologic abnormalities such as portal endothelial cell hyperplasia, Kuppfer cell hyperplasia, and portal vein dilation are considered highly suggestive of hepatic microvascular dysplasia, but this theory is not universally accepted.
    - Many pathologists believe the histological findings in dogs with hepatic microvascular dysplasia are indistinguishable from dogs with PSS.
- Abdominal ultrasound: the liver may be small, and there may be a decreased ease of visualization and number of hepatic vascular structures. No PSS noted.
- Transcolonic portal scintigraphy: This test contrasts hepatic microvascular dysplasia with PSS. There is significant extrahepatic shunting of portal blood past the liver in microvascular dysplasia.
- Mesenteric portography: Negative for shunts in dogs with hepatic microvascular dysplasia where no evidence of extrahepatic shunting is noted. There may also be truncating of the distal hepatic vessels and slow clearance of contrast. This test is typically only available at referral institutions.
- Ideally scintigraphy should be performed first to rule out the need for the more invasive mesenteric portography.

TREATMENT

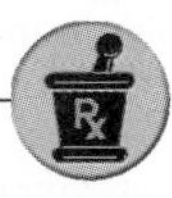

THERAPEUTIC GOAL(S)

Reversal of hepatic encephalopathy through reduction in protein intake, prevention of absorption of toxins from the GI tract and excretion from the kidneys and colon

ACUTE GENERAL TREATMENT

- See Hepatic Encephalopathy, p 489.
    - NPO 24 to 72 hours with moderate to severe hepatic encephalopathy.

- Lactulose (0.25-1.0 ml/kg PO q 8-12h).
- Antibiotic (metronidazole [10-15 mg/kg PO q 12h], amoxicillin [20 mg/kg PO q 12h], amoxicillin-clavulanate [15 mg/kg PO q 12h], or neomycin sulfate [20 mg/kg PO q 8h]).
- IV fluids to correct dehydration and increase renal excretion of toxins such as ammonia.
- With obtundation, stupor, or coma: cleansing lukewarm water enemas followed by retention enema of dilute lactulose (25 ml/kg, 30% lactulose + 70% lukewarm water), left in place for 20 to 30 minutes and repeated q 6h or until signs resolve. Alternative additives are 10% povidone iodine or neomycin sulfate at 20 mg/kg.
- With status epilepticus or seizures: Anticonvulsant medications such as IV propofol, low-dose phenobarbital, or oral potassium bromide (via stomach tube if necessary) may be needed in addition to the other medications and dietary therapy listed previously.

CHRONIC TREATMENT

In animals with overt clinical signs, chronic treatment with a restricted protein diet, lactulose, and/or antibiotic therapy may be required (see Acute General Treatment above).

DRUG INTERACTIONS

Be careful with drugs requiring hepatic metabolism.

POSSIBLE COMPLICATIONS

Sedative and anesthetic agents should be used with caution.

RECOMMENDED MONITORING

- Due to the typical lack of significant clinicopathologic abnormalities, repeat testing is not indicated.
- Serum bile acid levels are typically unchanged with dietary and medical therapy and are not routinely repeated.

PROGNOSIS AND OUTCOME

- Prognosis is good to excellent in patients that have not shown any signs.
- Prognosis is poor to fair in patients with clinical signs.
- Some patients presenting primarily with gastrointestinal signs may lack adequate response to treatment, although the signs do not typically worsen.

PEARLS & CONSIDERATIONS

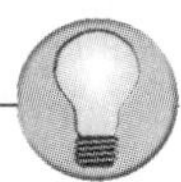

COMMENTS

- Biopsy alone cannot confirm HMD. Macroscopic portosystemic shunts must be ruled out by either transcolonic portal scintigraphy or mesenteric portography.
- Patients not showing any clinical signs and patients diagnosed at a later age with milder increases in serum bile acid levels are more likely to have HMD than PSS.
- Patients with normal complete blood count and serum biochemistry profiles may be more likely to have HMD than PSS.

PREVENTION

Avoid breeding affected dogs of predisposed breeds.

SUGGESTED READING

Christiansen JS, et al: Hepatic microvascular dysplasia in dogs: A retrospective study of 24 cases (1987-1995). *J Am Anim Hosp Assoc* 36:385-389, 2000.

Johnson SE: Chronic hepatic disorders. In Ettinger SJ, Feldman EC (eds): *Textbook of Veterinary Internal Medicine*, ed 2, vol 2. Philadelphia, WB Saunders, 2000, pp 1315-1316.

AUTHOR: **JOHN R. HART, JR.**
EDITOR: **KEITH P. RICHTER**

Mitral/Tricuspid Regurgitation Due to Myxomatous Valve Disease

Client Education Sheet on Website

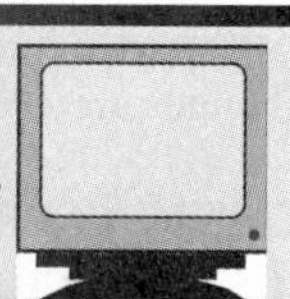

BASIC INFORMATION

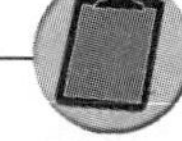

DEFINITION

Pathologic degeneration of the atrioventricular (mitral and tricuspid) heart valves, characterized by accumulation of glycosaminoglycans (myxomatous proliferation), and fibrosis of the valve leaflets and tendinous chords. The valvular degeneration leads to valvular regurgitation and eventually to congestive heart failure (CHF). The condition most commonly involves the mitral valve with or without changes of the tricuspid valve. Isolated tricuspid myxomatous degeneration occurs but is less common.

SYNONYM(S)

Acquired mitral or tricuspid regurgitation or insufficiency
Chronic degenerative valvular disease
Chronic valvular disease
Chronic valvular fibrosis
Endocardiosis
Myxomatous degeneration

EPIDEMIOLOGY

SPECIES, AGE, SEX: The most common cardiac disease in dogs. The prevalence is strongly influenced by age. It is uncommon in young individuals but common in old dogs. Males develop the disease at a younger age than females.

GENETICS AND BREED PREDISPOSITION: Encountered in all breeds, but most common in small to medium-sized breeds: papillons, poodles, Chihuahuas, dachshunds, and Cavalier King Charles spaniels. The age at which the disease develops is inherited as a polygenetic threshold trait (i.e., multiple genes influence the trait and a certain threshold has to be reached before the disease develops). Males have a lower threshold than females, leading to a higher disease prevalence at a given age.

RISK FACTORS: Age, breed, familial disposition, and gender.

ASSOCIATED CONDITIONS AND DISORDERS: Myxomatous degeneration of the semilunar valves (very uncommon in dogs and, when present, seldom of clinical importance).

CLINICAL PRESENTATION

DISEASE FORMS/SUBTYPES

- Incidental finding: no clinical signs of disease caused by the valvular regurgitation.
  - Cardiac auscultation (presence of systolic click [early stage] and/or systolic heart murmur)
  - Cardiomegaly on radiographs

- Electrocardiographic changes: P mitrale and/or P pulmonale, increased R wave amplitude, increased QRS duration
- Valvular regurgitation causing clinical signs of CHF (most commonly left-sided).
- Sudden death may occur but is uncommon, especially in the absence of preceding clinical signs of CHF.

HISTORY, CHIEF COMPLAINT

- Cough (often worse in the morning or evening hours)
- Tachypnea/dyspnea/orthopnea
- Lethargy
- Reduced exercise tolerance
- Syncope
- Anorexia
- Weight loss
- Ascites

PHYSICAL EXAM FINDINGS

- Patients without overt clinical signs:
  - Systolic click (early stage).
  - Systolic heart murmur is present in case of mitral/tricuspid regurgitation. With progression the murmur often increases in duration and intensity.
- Patients showing overt clinical signs:
  - Loud heart murmur, unless there is significant myocardial failure, which may develop because of concurrent myocardial disease or because of chronic volume overload.
  - Tachycardia and loss of respiratory sinus arrhythmia.
  - Arrhythmia and pulse deficit may be present, most commonly supraventricular premature beats or atrial fibrillation.
  - Weak femoral pulse.
  - Prolonged capillary refill time and pale mucous membranes.
  - Tachypnea/dyspnea/orthopnea.
  - Respiratory crackles/rales.
  - Pink froth, i.e., pulmonary edema may be evident in the nostrils and orophraynx in cases with severe CHF.
  - Ascites.

ETIOLOGY AND PATHOPHYSIOLOGY

- Primary inciting factor for the valvular degeneration is unknown.
- Degeneration begins with subendothelial deposition of mucopolysaccaride and areas of fibrosis, which produces ballooning/thickening of the valve leaflet and tendinous chords.
- With progression, the valve lesions cause insufficient coaptation of the leaflets, leading to regurgitation of blood from the ventricle into the atrium.
- Severity and progression of atrioventricular (AV)-valve regurgitation depends on the severity and progression of valve lesions (leaflets and/or tendinous chords).
- Slight to moderate AV-valve regurgitation is often completely compensated for years and is not expected to cause clinical signs of disease.
- Compensatory mechanisms include cardiac dilatation and eccentric hypertrophy, increased force of contraction, increased heart rate, increased pulmonary lymphatic drainage (left-sided AV-valve regurgitation), fluid retention, and neurohormonal modulation of cardiovascular function.
- With progression, the valvular regurgitation can no longer be compensated, leading to reduced cardiac output and increased venous pressures (leading to pulmonary edema if left-sided CHF and to ascites if right-sided).

DIAGNOSIS

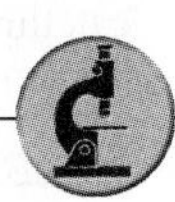

DIFFERENTIAL DIAGNOSIS

- Physical:
  - Other causes of heart murmurs:
    - Secondary mitral regurgitation due to dilated or hypertrophic cardiomyopathy.
    - Congenital heart disease.
    - Vegetative (bacterial) endocarditis.
    - Anemia.
    - Physiologic flow murmur.
  - Other causes of respiratory distress:
    - Primary respiratory disease such as bronchitis, pneumonia, tracheal/bronchial instability, neoplasia, and degenerative disease.
    - Pleural diseases with effusion.
    - Anemia.
    - Metabolic acidosis.
    - Other causes of CHF.
    - Other (noncardiac) causes of pulmonary edema.
  - Other causes of reduced exercise capacity, lethargy, and wasting.
    - Primary diseases of locomotor system, i.e., chronic degenerative joint diseases, intervertebral disk disease.
    - Other systemic or organ-related disease (i.e., renal or hepatic failure, neoplasia, and anemia).
  - Other causes for episodes of weakness and/or syncope:
    - Epilepsy and other causes of seizures.
    - Primary arrhythmia.
    - Other systemic or organ-related disease.
  - Other causes of abdominal distention (unless severe primary tricuspid regurgitation, ascites often does not develop until advanced stages).
- Radiographic:
  - Cardiac enlargement from other heart disease.
  - Increased pulmonary interstitial or alveolar radiopacity due to primary respiratory disease (see under Other Causes for Respiratory Distress), or expiratory radiographs.
  - Normal variation.
- Echocardiographic:
  - Valve abnormality: congenital (e.g., AV-valve dysplasia) or infectious (endocarditis).
  - Increased atrial and ventricular size and secondary regurgitation due to dilated cardiomyopathy or congenital heart disease.

INITIAL DATABASE

- Diagnosis of AV-valve myxomatous degeneration.
  - Echocardiography: detection of thickened/ballooning AV-valve, identification of regurgitant jet (spectral or color Doppler).
- Assessment of disease severity and complications.
  - Auscultation: a low-intensity murmur with or without a systolic click in an otherwise healthy dog usually indicate low disease severity.
  - Echocardiography: atrial and ventricular size, size and velocity of regurgitant jet (reduced velocity indicates high left atrial pressure and severe disease); ventricular motion (fractional shortening) is usually exaggerated in advanced stages, but a normal or reduced motion in the presence of severe regurgitation is indicative of myocardial failure, and evidence of complication.
  - Electrocardiogram: presence of tachyarrhythmia such as atrial fibrillation or ventricular ectopy (usually indicate severe disease, presence of complication, or other cardiac disease).
  - Radiography: cardiac size, presence of pulmonary congestion and edema, exclusion of other (noncardiac) causes for clinical signs of disease.
  - Complete blood count, serum biochemistry panel, urinalysis: usually unremarkable in less severe cases; cases with CHF may have slightly increased liver enzymes and evidence of prerenal azotemia.

ADVANCED OR CONFIRMATORY TESTING

- Serum troponin I level: unremarkable in less severe cases, moderate to severe disease is associated with slightly to moderately increased levels, but significant increases indicate complication or presence of other cardiac disease
- Serum natriuretic peptides (atrial natriuretic peptide [ANP], brain natriuretic peptide [BNP]): levels are often unremarkable in less severe cases. Moderate to severe disease is always associated with increased levels
- Blood culture in case of suspicion of vegetative endocarditis

TREATMENT

THERAPEUTIC GOAL(S)

- Treatment is not indicated in less severe disease without overt clinical signs.
- To alleviate clinical signs and improve quality of life and life expectancy in cases with signs of CHF by evacuating pulmonary edema/ascites and abolishing congestion, improving the hemodynamic situation by controlling heart rate, and reducing the aortic impedance and inotropic support, and protect from detrimental exposure to neurohormones.

ACUTE GENERAL TREATMENT

- Furosemide IV, SC, IM, or PO. Dose is dependent on severity of CHF.
  - Mild to moderate CHF: 2-4 mg/kg q 12-24h.
  - Severe or fulminant CHF: 4-8 mg/kg q 2-6h, preferably IV, IM, or SC.
  - Monitor outcome of treatment by respiratory rate.
- Oxygen supplementation and cage rest to cases with significant dyspnea.
- Additional options in cases with severe fulminant CHF:
  - Nitroglycerin ointment topically in case (applied inside pinna of ear; wear gloves).
  - Arterial vasodilator (hydralazine or sodium nitroprusside). Requires blood pressure monitoring and should be considered only in hospitalized dogs where monitoring by a specialist is available.
- Postive inotrope such as pimobendan at 0.5 mg/kg q 12h PO in cases of myocardial failure.
- Severe ascites may require abdominal paracentesis.

CHRONIC TREATMENT

- Exact composition of medical therapy depends on disease severity and clinical signs. Most dogs with CHF require furosemide, which has traditionally been used together with an angiotensin-converting enzyme inhibitor (ACEI) and digoxin. However, pimobendan has also emerged as adjunct therapy to other heart failure therapy.
- Furosemide PO. Dose depends on severity of heart failure (CHF) but should be kept as low as possible.
  - Mild to moderate CHF: 1 mg/kg q 1-2 days to 3-4 mg/kg q 8h.
  - Moderate to severe CHF: 2-3 mg/kg q 12h or higher.
- Spironolactone at 2 mg/kg q 12-24h PO and/or hydrochlorothiazide at 2-4 mg/kg q 12h PO can be added in cases that require a high dose of furosemide.
- ACEI (i.e., enalapril, benazepril, ramipril). Dose and dose interval dependent on particular ACE-inhibitor used.
- Digoxin at 0.22 mg/m^2 q 12h PO, or lower.
- Pimobendan at 0.5 mg/kg q 12h PO.
- Avoid food with high sodium content.
- Negative inotrope such as β-receptor antagonists or calcium-channel blockers may be required to control ventricular rate in case of atrial fibrillation, but they should be used with caution.
- Avoid strenuous exercise.

DRUG INTERACTIONS

- Furosemide potentiates the effects of an ACE-inhibitor, spironolactone, or a thiazide.
- Nonsteroidal anti-inflammatory drugs should be used with caution in patients receiving furosemide and ACEI.
- The combination of pimobendan and a calcium-channel blocker or a β-receptor antagonist should be avoided.

POSSIBLE COMPLICATIONS

- Dogs initially not showing clinical signs may develop CHF.
- Dogs stabilized by medical therapy may suffer recurrent CHF.
- Dogs with initially left-sided HF may develop biventricular CHF (ascites, pulmonary hypertension).
- Development of arrhythmia, most commonly atrial fibrillation.
- Rupture of first order tendinous chord(s), leading to a flail valve leaflet.
- Atrial tear leading to acquired atrial septal defect or cardiac tamponade.
- Formation of intracardiac thrombus and/or myocardial infarction.

RECOMMENDED MONITORING

- Frequency of reexaminations depends on severity of valvular insufficiency and severity of HF (if present).
- Dogs without signs of CHF:
  - Slight to moderate valvular regurgitation: once every 6 months to once a year.
  - Moderate to severe valvular regurgitation may require more frequent monitoring.
- Dogs with signs of CHF:
  - Once acute CHF has been successfully treated, dogs may often be treated at home.

Reexamination after 1 to 2 weeks of therapy (check for signs of CHF, dehydration, electrolyte balance, renal function and presence of a complication).

Thereafter once every 3 to 6 months.

More severe cases may require more frequent monitoring.

PROGNOSIS AND OUTCOME

- Dogs without signs of CHF:
  - Chronic disease progression. Dogs with low disease severity may sustain for several years before signs of CHF develop.
  - Risk factors for progression from mild to severe: severity of valve lesions, age, and gender.
  - Risk factors for CHF: regurgitant status, left atrial size, natriuretic peptides.
- Dogs with CHF (acute or stabilized):
  - Prognosis depends on age, severity of heart failure, presence of complications or other disease (such as renal failure).
  - Clinical trials indicate a mean survival time from onset of CHF of 8 to 10 months, but may vary from days to years in different dogs.

PEARLS & CONSIDERATIONS

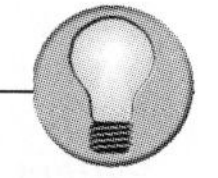

COMMENTS

- If presence of regurgitation is equivocal, the murmur or regurgitant jet may become obvious after stressing the dog slightly.
- Loud musical murmurs are unusual. The intensity of this type of murmur is not related to disease severity.
- Dogs with syncope, related to intermittent atrial arrhythmia, may sometimes be managed by a low dose of digoxin (approximately half recommended dose).
- Mild pleural and/or pericardial effusion may develop because of CHF. More pronounced accumulation of fluid in these locations raises the suspicion of other causes.

PREVENTION

- Because the liability for myxomatous atrioventricular valve degeneration in dogs is inherited, the disease prevalence in affected breeds should be reduced by breeding measures.
- Currently, no medication or management are known to prevent the disease or stop or slow disease progression.

CLIENT EDUCATION

- The disease and expected progression: low disease severity indicates long period without clinical signs; moderate to severe indicates a shorter period.
- If the client is a breeder, inform him/her about the genetics of the disease and impact of the finding on future breeding.
- Appropriate level of exercise (no restrictions for low disease severity, avoid strenuous exercise in moderate to severe cases).
- Signs of CHF.
- How to medicate (if indicated).
- How to monitor resting heart and respiratory rates at home (if indicated).
- Diet (if indicated).

SUGGESTED READING

Häggström J, Kvart C, Pedersen HD: Acquired valvular heart disease. In Ettinger SJ, Feldman E (eds): *Textbook of Veterinary Internal Medicine. Diseases of Dogs and Cats*, ed 6. Philadelphia, WB Saunders, 2005, pp 1020–1037.

Häggström J, et al: New insights into degenerative mitral valve disease in dogs. *Vet Clin North Am Small Anim Pract* 34:1209, 2004.

AUTHOR: **JENS HÄGGSTRÖM**
EDITOR: **ETIENNE CÔTÉ**

Mitral Valve Dysplasia

BASIC INFORMATION

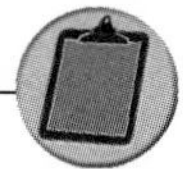

DEFINITION

Congenital malformation of any portion of the mitral valve apparatus (papillary muscles, chordae tendineae, leaflets, annulus) that results in abnormal function

EPIDEMIOLOGY

SPECIES, AGE, SEX: Dogs, cats. Usually identified early in life. Mild defects may be identified later due to a lack of clinical signs and subtle physical findings.

GENETICS AND BREED PREDISPOSITIONS: Dogs: bull terrier, miniature bull terrier, English bulldog, Great Dane, German shepherd, Newfoundland, and Irish setter are predisposed. Cats: unknown.

CLINICAL PRESENTATION

DISEASE FORMS/SUBTYPES: The incidental identification of a heart murmur is common. Alternatively:

- Thoracic radiographs: cardiomegaly.
- Patient presents with clinical signs of congestive heart failure (CHF).
- Echocardiographic identification.
- Electrocardiogram (ECG): may include wide/notched P waves, increased QRS amplitude, atrial arrhythmias.

HISTORY, CHIEF COMPLAINT: With mild defects, there may be no clinical signs. If severe, clinical signs of CHF result.

- Dogs: cough, tachypnea/dyspnea, exercise intolerance, syncope.
- Cats: tachypnea/dyspnea, anorexia, lethargy, thromboembolic disease (ischemic myelopathy, syncope/seizures).

PHYSICAL EXAM FINDINGS: Patient may have no physical findings with mild defects.

- Heart murmur (left apical systolic murmur of variable intensity)
- If CHF is present:
  - Dyspnea/tachypnea, pulmonary crackles, increased bronchovesicular sounds
  - Pale mucous membranes
  - Tachycardia/arrhythmias

ETIOLOGY

Presumed genetic, although specific mutations have not been identified.

PATHOPHYSIOLOGY

- Size of regurgitant orifice determines degree of mitral regurgitation.
- Mitral regurgitation causes increased left atrial size/pressure, which is transmitted to the pulmonary veins.
- Modified transudate emanates from pulmonary veins, overwhelming pulmonary lymphatics and causing pulmonary edema.
- Pulmonary hypertension (PH) may develop (compensatory for CHF or congenital).

DIAGNOSIS

DIFFERENTIAL DIAGNOSIS

- Physical/radiographic: myxomatous valvular degeneration/endocardiosis, vegetative endocarditis, dilated cardiomyopathy, hypertrophic or restrictive/unclassified cardiomyopathy (cats)
- Echocardiographic: myxomatous valvular degeneration, restrictive or unclassified cardiomyopathy (cats)

INITIAL DATABASE

- Echocardiogram: abnormal mitral valve leaflets, abnormal diastolic valve motion, mitral regurgitation. Doppler studies help estimate left atrial pressure, pulmonary artery pressure.
- Thoracic radiographs: cardiomegaly with loss of the caudal cardiac waist (dogs). Pulmonary venous engorgement or pulmonary interstitial infiltrates if CHF. Pulmonary arterial tortuosity/enlargement may be seen with PH.
- ECG: normal, or may show evidence of left atrial enlargement (wide, notched P waves), left ventricular enlargement (increased R-wave amplitude), or atrial arrhythmias.
- Complete blood count, serum biochemistry panel, urinalysis: usually unremarkable.

ADVANCED OR CONFIRMATORY TESTING

Usually not necessary (initial database is sufficient):

- Transesophageal echocardiography to visualize other defects, intra-atrial thrombi.
- Cardiac catheterization may yield quantitative information and help characterize unusual lesions.

TREATMENT

THERAPEUTIC GOAL(S)

Prevent/delay increases in left atrial pressure and CHF

ACUTE GENERAL TREATMENT

- In cases of acute CHF (see Heart Failure, Acute/Decompensated, p 458), therapy should reduce venous congestion (diuretics), inhibit sodium/water retention, and counteract vasoconstriction (ACE-inhibitors, vasodilators).
- Digoxin may be indicated with atrial tachyarrhythmias, myocardial failure, or baroreceptor dysfunction.
- For myocardial failure (advanced/end-stage state characterized by left ventricular hypocontractility), calcium sensitizing agents (pimobendan) are useful but not available worldwide (currently available in Canada, Europe, Australia).

CHRONIC TREATMENT

- As for acute treatment, with doses tailored to the individual patient.
- In cats, antiplatelet and/or anticoagulant therapy for prevention of atrial thrombus formation. Aspirin, coumadin, unfractionated heparin/low-molecular-weight heparins, clopidogrel, and other agents have been advocated for this purpose, but none has demonstrated superior efficacy in controlled clinical trials and all have potential drawbacks. See Aortic Thromboembolism, Feline, p 78 for doses and details.
- Recheck evaluations are essential (monitor renal function, blood pressure, heart rate/rhythm, and left ventricular function).
- Surgical repair/replacement of dysplastic valves is available at selected academic institutions, but benefits do not convincingly outweigh drawbacks (cost, risk of complications).

POSSIBLE COMPLICATIONS

- Recurrent CHF symptoms
- Systemic thromboembolism (cats)

- Syncope (cerebral thromboembolism in cats, tachyarrhythmias, uncontrolled heart failure in dogs)
- Left atrial rupture (dogs)

RECOMMENDED MONITORING

- Serum biochemistry profile, complete blood count, urinalysis and blood pressure before initiation of therapy
- Repeat measurements of serum BUN, creatinine, and electrolytes daily for patients receiving IV therapy, 1 week after initiating oral therapy
- Serial ECG, echocardiography, and thoracic radiographs as dictated by rate of progression

PROGNOSIS AND OUTCOME

- With mild defects and little/no increases in left atrial pressure, prognosis is excellent
- Guarded to poor with moderate/severe dysplasia and CHF

PEARLS & CONSIDERATIONS

CLIENT EDUCATION

- Although a definitive genetic basis is not established, affected individuals should not be used for breeding.
- Recheck evaluations are a necessary part of CHF management.

SUGGESTED READING

Kittleson MD, Kienle RD: Congenital abnormalities of the atrioventricular valves. In Kittleson MD, Kienle RD (eds): *Small Animal Cardiovascular Medicine*. New York, Mosby, 1998, pp 273–281.

AUTHOR: **AARON WEY**
EDITOR: **ETIENNE CÔTÉ**

Mitral Valve Stenosis

BASIC INFORMATION

DEFINITION

A congenital or acquired cardiac disorder characterized by narrowing of the mitral valve orifice. The narrowing is a result of an abnormal mitral valve apparatus; it leads to obstruction of diastolic transmitral inflow, and potentially, left-sided congestive heart failure (CHF).

EPIDEMIOLOGY

SPECIES, AGE, SEX: Dogs and cats. No reported age or sex predilection.

GENETICS AND BREED PREDISPOSITION

- Dogs: bull terrier, Newfoundland (may be predisposed)
- Cats: two Siamese cats reported, but no evidence of breed predisposition

RISK FACTORS

- Predisposed breeds of dogs
- Cardiac valve neoplasia (very rare)

ASSOCIATED CONDITIONS AND DISORDERS

- Dogs (concurrent conditions):
  - Mitral valve dysplasia
  - Subaortic stenosis (SAS)
  - Patent ductus arteriosus (PDA)
  - Pulmonic stenosis
- Dogs and cats (associated conditions):
  - Congestive heart failure
  - Pulmonary hypertension
- Cats (concurrent and associated condition): feline aortic thromboembolism.

CLINICAL PRESENTATION

DISEASE FORMS/SUBTYPES

- Valvular mitral stenosis: involves the mitral valve leaflets (dog and cat)
- Supravalvular mitral stenosis: left atrium is divided by a membrane just above the mitral annulus (cat: see Cor Triatriatum Sinister and Supravalvular Mitral Stenosis, p 238)

HISTORY, CHIEF COMPLAINT

- Exercise intolerance/episodic weakness
- Lethargy
- Cough
- Dyspnea (most common sign in cats)
- Syncope

PHYSICAL EXAM FINDINGS

- Soft (I-III/VI) left apical diastolic murmur (inconsistent)
- Left apical systolic murmur (if mitral regurgitation is present)
- With CHF:
  - Tachycardia
  - Tachypnea
  - Pulmonary crackles and wheezes

ETIOLOGY AND PATHOPHYSIOLOGY

- Congenital (possibly heritable in predisposed breeds)
- Acquired:
  - Bacterial endocarditis (controversial).
  - Intracardiac neoplasia (mitral valve chondrosarcoma reported in a dog).
- Pathophysiology:
  - Obstruction of the transmitral diastolic flow (increase in resistance to blood flow between the left atrium and ventricle).
  - Increase in left atrial, pulmonary vein, and pulmonary capillary pressures.
  - Pulmonary edema formation.
  - Exercise increases left atrial pressure; exercise induced dyspnea/syncope may occur.
  - Pulmonary hypertension may develop due to increased pulmonary capillary pressure.

DIAGNOSIS

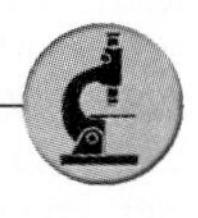

DIFFERENTIAL DIAGNOSIS

- Radiographic/electrocardiographic:
  - Left atrial enlargement: other types of cardiac disease (myxomatous mitral valve disease/endocardiosis, mitral valve dysplasia, dilated cardiomyopathy, subaortic stenosis, patent ductus arteriosus, and, in cats, hypertrophic cardiomyopathy)
- Echocardiographic:
  - Myxomatous mitral valve disease/endocardiosis
  - Mitral valve dysplasia
  - Bacterial endocarditis
  - Intracardiac neoplasia

INITIAL DATABASE

- Thoracic radiographs: left atrial enlargement very common. Signs of pulmonary edema if CHF.
- Electrocardiogram: wide P waves in lead II, supraventricular premature complexes, atrial/supraventricular tachycardia, atrial fibrillation. Increased R wave amplitude in lead II if SAS or PDA is also present.
- Echocardiogram:
  - Two-dimensional mode: left atrial dilation, thickened mitral valve leaflets or supravalvular membrane (cat), decreased mitral valve leaflet excursion, diastolic doming of the leaflets.
  - M mode: thickened mitral valve leaflets, parallel motion of the leaflets, incomplete leaflet separation in diastole, reduced E-F slope; increased LA/Ao ratio.

- Color flow Doppler: diastolic aliased or turbulent flow across the mitral valve. Systolic turbulent flow if mitral regurgitation is present.
- Spectral Doppler: increased early diastolic filling (velocity E wave > 1.1 m/s), prolonged pressure half-time (>50 ms), reduced mitral valve area (MVA).

ADVANCED OR CONFIRMATORY TESTING

- Cardiac catheterization: rarely necessary for confirming diagnosis.
  - Angiogram: thickened and restricted MV leaflets, enlarged left atrium, ± mitral regurgitation.
  - Pressure measurements: increase in left atrial pressure and pulmonary artery pressure, if pulmonary hypertension or CHF is present.
- Transesophageal echocardiography: better visualization of the mitral valve apparatus.

TREATMENT

THERAPEUTIC GOAL(S)

- Control CHF
- Management of supraventricular arrhythmias
- Reduce the severity of the stenosis: surgical therapy

ACUTE GENERAL TREATMENT

- Diuretics: indicated if the patient is in congestive heart failure (see Heart Failure, Acute/Decompensated, p 458)
- Oxygen therapy/supplementation: for dyspneic patients
- Angiotensin-converting enzyme (ACE) inhibitors: reduce preload and afterload (see Heart Failure, Chronic, p 459)
- Digoxin, calcium channel blocker or β-blocker: management of supraventricular arrhythmias (see Atrial Premature Complexes and Atrial/Supraventricular Tachycardia, p 100)

CHRONIC TREATMENT

- Medical therapy:
  - Diuretics, ACE inhibitors, and antiarrhythmics following the acute treatment guidelines.
- Surgical therapy:
  - Open mitral commissurotomy: requires cardiopulmonary bypass (CPB); one encouraging report in the literature.
  - Mitral valve replacement: requires CPB. Postoperative management complications are common.
  - Balloon valvuloplasty: inconsistent results in canine patients; possible damage to the mitral valve apparatus with worsening of mitral regurgitation.

DRUG INTERACTIONS

- Excessive use of diuretics is contraindicated due to the decrease in preload, electrolyte disturbances, prerenal/renal azotemia, and increased risk of digitalis toxicity.
- ACE inhibitor: may reduce glomerular filtration rate and cause azotemia; hypotension may occur when used with diuretics; risk of hyperkalemia when K^+ is supplemented or K^+-sparing diuretics are used concurrently.

POSSIBLE COMPLICATIONS

- Recurrence of signs due to progression of CHF
- Postsurgery: restenosis, coagulation disturbances due to postsurgical management (mitral valve replacement)

RECOMMENDED MONITORING

Recheck examinations should include: thoracic radiographs, serum renal panel including electrolytes, systolic blood pressure measurement, digoxin levels (if applicable), and electrocardiogram.

PROGNOSIS AND OUTCOME

- Long-term prognosis depends on the severity of the stenosis: guarded to poor in severe cases.
- Surgical approach may offer a better outcome in the future.

PEARLS & CONSIDERATIONS

COMMENTS

- Mitral stenosis is a rare cardiac abnormality in dogs and cats.
- A disproportionate number of cases occurs in the bull terrier breed.
- Medical management is relatively unrewarding.
- Surgical approach may offer a better long-term prognosis in the future.

PREVENTION

Do not breed affected animals

CLIENT EDUCATION

- Monitor respiratory rate at rest, exercise tolerance, and appetite
- Advise client not to breed affected animals

SUGGESTED READING

Kittleson MD: Cases in small animal cardiovascular medicine: http://www.vmth.ucdavis.edu/cardio/cases.

Lehmkuhl LB, et al: Mitral stenosis in 15 dogs. *J Vet Intern Med* 8(1):2-17, 1994.

AUTHOR: **JOAO S. ORVALHO**
EDITOR: **ETIENNE CÔTÉ**

Mothball Toxicosis

BASIC INFORMATION

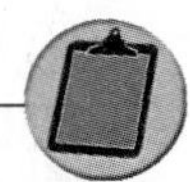

DEFINITION

Adverse reactions, mainly gastrointestinal/hemolytic or gastrointestinal/neurologic, that occur as a result of consuming naphthalene- or paradichlorobenzene-containing mothballs, respectively

SYNONYM(S)

Common brand names of mothballs:

Enoz Old Fashioned Moth Balls (naphthalene 99.9%)

F and B Rabbit and Dog Chaser (naphthalene 15.0%)

Enoz Para Moth Balls (paradichlorobenzene 99.6%)

Garbage Can Deodorizer (paradichlorobenzene 99.75%)

Repel Dog and Cat Repellent (paradichlorobenzene 20.0%)

EPIDEMIOLOGY

SPECIES, AGE, SEX

- Dogs of all breeds, ages, and sexes; dogs more commonly involved than cats.
- Young animals may be more sensitive to naphthalene.
- Cats are considered more sensitive to naphthalene than dogs.

GENETICS AND BREED PREDISPOSITION: Animals deficient in glucose-6-phosphate dehydrogenase (dog breeds such as Akitas, Shiba Inus, and Tosas) may be more susceptible to erythrocyte oxidative damage by naphthalene.

RISK FACTORS: Use of mothballs as repellents.

CLINICAL PRESENTATION

DISEASE FORMS/SUBTYPES

- Naphthalene mothballs
- Paradichlorobenzene mothballs

HISTORY, CHIEF COMPLAINT

- Availability of mothballs in pet's environment
- Acute onset of vomiting, diarrhea, lethargy

PHYSICAL EXAM FINDINGS

- Naphthalene:
  - Listlessness, abdominal pain, inappetence, vomiting, and diarrhea within a few hours after ingestion.
  - Mothball scent on the breath.
  - Evidence of hemolytic anemia (pale mucous membranes, poor capillary refill time, icterus) may not be present until 12 to 48 hours after ingestion with naphthalene mothballs.
- Paradichlorobenzene:
  - Vomiting, diarrhea, lethargy, tremors, and seizures within a few hours after ingestion.

ETIOLOGY AND PATHOPHYSIOLOGY

- The toxin:
  - Naphthalene is found in "old-fashioned" mothballs, and in some moth flakes/crystals. A naphthalene mothball weighs 3.6 g. Acute dose causing hemolysis in dogs = 1525 mg/kg, but a minimum lethal dose as low as 400 mg/kg is reported in dogs.
  - Paradichlorobenzene mothballs are used as cake deodorizers in diaper and garbage pails and in bathrooms.
  - A paradichlorobenzene mothball weighs 5.0 g. Paradichlorobenzene oral LD50 in mouse = 2950 mg/kg, rat = 500 mg/kg.
  - Naphthalene-type mothballs are approximately two times more toxic compared to paradichlorobenzene-type. Ingestion of one mothball for a medium-sized dog (30 lb [14 kg]) can be a potential toxic hazard.
  - According to label claim on some brands, mothballs are occasionally used as animal repellents (rabbits, dogs, cats).
- Pathophysiology:
  - Most cases occur acutely due to accidental ingestion of mothballs.
  - Naphthalene:
    - Naphthalene itself does not cause hemolysis; its metabolites (α- and β-naphtho-quinones) are responsible for hemolysis. Hemolysis and methemoglobinemia occur due to the strong oxidant effect of naphthalene metabolites on red blood cells (RBCs) and the lack of RBC glutathione to prevent these oxidizing effects.
    - Nausea, vomiting, and diarrhea are due to the irritating properties of naphthalene.
  - Paradichlorobenzene:
    - Paradichlorobenzene is an organochlorine insecticide. Other members of this class mainly affect the nervous system and cause tremors, salivation, ataxia, and seizures.

DIAGNOSIS

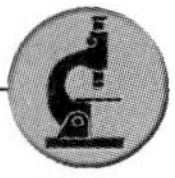

DIFFERENTIAL DIAGNOSIS

- Naphthalene:
  - Other intoxications causing hemolysis (e.g., onions/garlic, zinc, acetaminophen)
  - Immune-mediated hemolytic anemia
  - Erythrocytic parasites
- Paradichlorobenzene:
  - Other intoxications causing tremors/seizures (organophosphate/carbamate, garbage toxicosis, lead, arsenic)
  - Encephalitis (sterile, infectious)
  - Brain neoplasm
  - Idiopathic epilepsy

INITIAL DATABASE

- Naphthalene:
  - Complete blood count (CBC): regenerative anemia due to hemolysis, hemoglobinemia, Heinz bodies (12 to 48 hours after exposure).
  - Serum biochemical changes: elevation in serum bilirubin, increased liver enzymes, increased blood urea nitrogen (BUN) and creatinine.
  - Urinalysis: hemoglobinuria.
- Paradichlorobenzene:
  - No significant CBC or serum biochemistry changes may be noted. Rarely, increases in BUN, serum creatinine, and liver enzymes are possible.

ADVANCED OR CONFIRMATORY TESTING

Naphthalene or its metabolites can be found in urine, stool, or blood, 8 to 24 hours after ingestion. Body fat or liver can also be used for detecting naphthalene.

TREATMENT

THERAPEUTIC GOAL(S)

- Decontamination of patient
- Treat methemoglobinemia (naphthalene)
- Supportive care

ACUTE GENERAL TREATMENT

- Decontamination of patient:
  - Emesis: useful within 1 to 2 hours; do not induce if animal is already vomiting; feed the animal first; 3% hydrogen peroxide (5–10 ml/kg PO, maximum 45 ml in largest dogs; repeat once after 10 to 15 minutes if no vomiting) or apomorphine 0.03 mg/kg IV or 0.04 mg/kg IM, or xylazine (dogs and cats) at 0.05–1 mg/kg IV or IM.
  - Activated charcoal: 2–4 g/kg; mix with 70% sorbitol 1-3 ml/kg and give PO.
- Treat methemoglobinemia:
  - *N*-acetylcysteine (NAC) acts as a precursor to glutathione; may provide some protection to RBCs against oxidative damage; efficacy of NAC in naphthalene toxicosis is not proven; 140 mg/kg slow IV, then 70 mg/kg/dose, q 6h for five doses.
  - Similarly, S-adenosyl methionine (40 mg/kg PO, then 20 mg/kg PO q 24h beginning 24 hours later) has been used as a glutathione donor in a similar setting of Heinz body hemolytic anemia (acetaminophen toxicosis) in a dog.
  - Ascorbic acid (antioxidant effect) at 20–30 mg/kg PO, IM, or IV q 8h.
- Supportive care:
  - Fluid diuresis.
  - Control seizures with diazepam (0.5–2 mg/kg IV prn) for intoxications involving paradichlorobenzene-type mothballs.
  - Blood transfusion if needed (see Transfusion Therapy and Collection Techniques for Blood Banking, p 1312).
  - 1–2 mEq/kg of sodium bicarbonate added to fluids my help reduce renal damage due to hemoglobinuria (assess and monitor acid-base status first).

POSSIBLE COMPLICATIONS

Rare liver or renal damage with paradichlorobenzene

RECOMMENDED MONITORING

- CBC (methemoglobinemia, Heinz body anemia)
- Serum biochemistry profile (serum bilirubin, renal values, and hepatic enzymes)
- Hematocrit
- Urinalysis

PROGNOSIS AND OUTCOME

- Naphthalene: good prognosis with supportive care; poor prognosis if evidence of severe hemolysis, renal or hepatic damage present
- Paradichlorobenezene: good prognosis with supportive care

PEARLS & CONSIDERATIONS

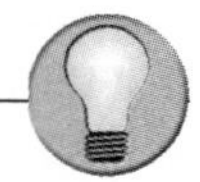

COMMENTS

- Differentiation of the two types of mothballs is difficult because both are white crystalline solids at room temperature and have similar odor.
- Dissolving a mothball in turpentine for 60 minutes can help differentiate between the two types of mothballs. Paradichlorobenezene is more soluble in turpentine than naphthalene. A paradichlorobenezene mothball usually dissolves within 30 to 60 minutes

compared to about ¼ of a naphthalene mothball.

SUGGESTED READING

Kore AM: Common indoor toxicants. In Peterson ME, Talcott PA (eds): *Small Animal Toxicology*. New York, WB Saunders, 2001, p 165.

US Department of Health and Human Services, Agency for Toxic Substances and Disease Registry, Toxicological Profile for Naphthalene, 1-Methylnaphthalene, and 2-Methylnaphthalene, Research Triangle Institute, 1995. Website: http://www.atsdr.cdc.gov/toxprofiles/ tp67.html.

AUTHOR & EDITOR: **SAFDAR A. KHAN**

Mucocele, Salivary

BASIC INFORMATION

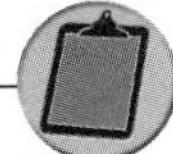

DEFINITION

An accumulation of saliva that has leaked from a salivary gland or its duct into submucosal or subcutaneous tissue. The sublingual gland is most commonly associated with salivary mucoceles.

SYNONYM(S)

Sialocele
Ranula (sublingual salivary mucocele)

EPIDEMIOLOGY

SPECIES, AGE, SEX

- Most often in dogs between 2 and 4 years old
- Incidence: fewer than 20 in 4000 dogs

GENETICS AND BREED PREDISPOSITION: More frequent in German shepherds and miniature poodles.

RISK FACTORS

- Association between oral trauma and activity of young dogs.
- Experimental duct ligation, duct laceration, rupture of the mandibular salivary gland capsule with damage to glandular tissue, and subcutaneous injection of mucocele fluid have not caused salivary mucoceles in healthy dogs, suggesting a developmental predisposition in some dogs.

CLINICAL PRESENTATION

DISEASE FORMS/SUBTYPES

- Sublingual salivary mucocele (ranula): in sublingual tissue. Most common.
- Pharyngeal salivary mucocele: in pharyngeal wall.
- Cervical salivary mucocele: in intermandibular area.
- Zygomatic salivary mucocele: in orbit.

HISTORY, CHIEF COMPLAINT

- The clinical signs associated with salivary mucocele depend on the location of the mucocele.
  - Acute, painful intermandibular swelling: initial stage of cervical mucocele resulting from an inflammatory response. Uncommon presentation.
  - Swelling in the cranial ventral neck region: cervical mucocele at later stages, when inflammation has subsided (more common presentation). Swelling is typically found incidentally by the owner, is slowly enlarging or intermittently large, fluid-filled, and nonpainful.
    - Cranial ventral cervical
    - Sublingual
  - Ptyalism, blood-tinged saliva secondary to masticatory trauma, poor prehension of food and reluctance to eat: can be caused by sublingual mucocele.
  - Dyspnea/dysphagia secondary to pharyngeal obstruction: can be caused by mucocele of the pharyngeal wall.
  - Periorbital mass, and either enophthalmos or exophthalmos depending on the mucocele's exact location and size: can be caused by zygomatic salivary mucoceles (infrequently reported in dogs).

PHYSICAL EXAM FINDINGS

- Fluid-filled, generally painless swelling in the cervical, sublingual, pharyngeal, or periorbital location.
- The patient is otherwise normal with no signs of systemic disease.

ETIOLOGY AND PATHOPHYSIOLOGY

- The lesion is not a cyst but a tissue reaction to extravasation of saliva from the gland/duct complex. The mucocele has a nonepithelial, nonsecretory lining consisting primarily of fibroblasts and capillaries.
- Specific etiology is unknown.
  - Damage to salivary gland or duct, associated with oral/facial trauma appears to contribute via leakage of saliva into adjacent tissues.

DIAGNOSIS

DIFFERENTIAL DIAGNOSIS

- Cyst
- Abscess
- Sialadenitis
- Neoplasia
- Trauma
- Foreign body:
  - Abscess
  - Seroma/hematoma
- Neoplasia

INITIAL DATABASE

- Fine-needle aspiration and cytologic evaluation: Mucocele paracentesis reveals a clear, stringy, sometimes blood-tinged fluid with a very low cellular content.
- Mucin and amylase analyses of the fluid are not reliable diagnostic procedures.
- Placement of patient in exact dorsal recumbency (awake, sedated, or anesthetized) if cervical mucocele appears on the ventral midline:
  - Mucocele usually shifts to the originating side, and is more easily mobile on the originating side, with dog in dorsal recumbency.
  - This important feature is essential for correct identification of the affected side if surgical intervention is contemplated.

ADVANCED OR CONFIRMATORY TESTING

Sialogram: radiographic contrast study of a salivary gland/duct.

- Rarely performed, as careful observation, palpation, and centesis are usually sufficient.
  - The most common indication for sialography is to determine the location of a salivary gland/duct defect in patients with salivary mucocele.
  - Difficult to perform for sublingual gland/duct.

TREATMENT

THERAPEUTIC GOAL(S)

- Complete excision of affected salivary gland(s)
- Drainage of mucocele

ACUTE GENERAL TREATMENT

Needle drainage of mucocele:

- Not recommended:
  - Rapid recurrence and risk of iatrogenic infection

CHRONIC TREATMENT

Surgical removal of involved salivary gland/duct complex:

- Complete surgical excision of affected salivary gland(s) with duct ligation
- Drainage of sialocele/surgical site

POSSIBLE COMPLICATIONS

- It is important to identify and avoid the lingual nerve while completing the dissection and ligating and resecting the mandibular and sublingual gland/duct complex. The lingual nerve is located dorsal and rostral to this gland/duct complex.
- Recurrence of sialocele:
  - Failure to completely excise all affected gland(s):
    - Sublingual
    - Zygomatic
- Seroma/hematoma formation:
  - Failure to appropriately drain sialocele and surgical site

RECOMMENDED MONITORING

Surgical site for evidence of seroma formation

PROGNOSIS AND OUTCOME

Excellent, provided complete excision of gland/duct complex is performed, with appropriate drainage of mucocele.

PEARLS & CONSIDERATIONS

COMMENTS

- Placement of the patient in exact dorsal recumbency can lateralize cervical mucoceles that otherwise hang on the ventral midline, which is essential for knowing which side to approach surgically.
- Sialoliths are concretions of calcium phosphate or calcium carbonate and may occur with chronic mucocele.
- The intimate anatomic association of the sublingual and mandibular salivary glands and their ducts requires resection of both structures when a salivary mucocele affects one of them.
- Surgical removal of both the sublingual and mandibular salivary glands, combined with drainage of the mucocele, has been advocated for treating cervical mucoceles.
- The defect is most often associated with the rostral portion of the sublingual gland/duct complex.

CLIENT EDUCATION

- Complete surgical excision of affected salivary gland(s) with duct ligation is the recommended treatment.
- If left untreated, sialocele may be associated with:
  - Physical problems associated with a large cranial ventral cervical mass.
    - Trauma, ulceration, secondary infection.
  - Dysphagia → sublingual mucocele.
  - Dyspnea/dysphagia → pharyngeal mucocele.
  - Exophthalmos, strabismus, and other ocular complications → zygomatic mucocele.

SUGGESTED READING

Dunning D: Salivary gland. In Slatter D (ed): *Textbook of Small Animal Surgery*, ed 3. Philadelphia, WB Saunders, 2003, pp 558–561.

AUTHORS: **MARK M. SMITH, ELLEN B. DAVIDSON DOMNICK**
EDITORS: **ALEXANDER M. REITER, RICHARD WALSHAW**

Multiple Myeloma and Plasma Cell Tumors

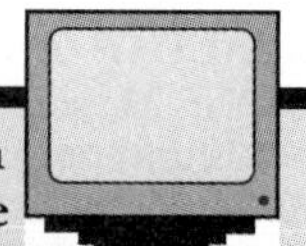

BASIC INFORMATION

DEFINITION

- Multiple myeloma (MM) is a malignant disease of plasma cells derived from one clone in the bone marrow. It is a systemic disease, and multiple bone marrow sites are involved. This disease is characterized by the production of immunoglobulins (Ig) by malignant plasma cells; IgM or IgA in the dog, and IgG in the cat. Waldenström's macroglobulinemia refers to the disease in which IgM is the Ig type produced.
- Plasma cell tumors (PCT) are solitary tumors composed of plasma cells, originating in sites other than the bone marrow (i.e., extramedullary). They can arise from skin, soft tissues, or bone. Serum globulin/Ig levels are often normal in this localized form of disease.

SYNONYM(S)

Plasmacytoma

EPIDEMIOLOGY

SPECIES, AGE, SEX

- Rare in dogs and cats
- Older animals (8 to 10 years)
- Male predominance in noncutaneous PCT, no sex predilection in MM

GENETICS AND BREED PREDISPOSITION

- MM: German shepherd
- PCT:
  - Airedales
  - Cocker spaniels
  - Kerry blue terriers
  - Scottish terriers
  - Standard poodles

ASSOCIATED CONDITIONS AND DISORDERS

Multiple myeloma:

- Hyperviscosity syndrome
- Bence Jones proteinuria
- Pathologic fracture
- Bleeding diathesis
- Increased susceptibility to infection; immunosuppression
- Heart failure
- Renal disease
- Visual/ocular disturbances
- Amyloidosis
- Cryoglobulinemia

CLINICAL PRESENTATION

DISEASE FORMS/SUBTYPES

- Multiple myeloma
- Waldenström's (IgM) macroglobulinemia
- Cutaneous plasma cell tumor
- Extramedullary plasma cell tumor (EMP)
- Solitary osseous plasma cell tumor (SOP)

HISTORY, CHIEF COMPLAINT

- MM:
  - Dogs generally present with lameness or skeletal pain. Bleeding (epistaxis, ecchymoses, mucosal hemorrhage), polyuria and polydipsia, central nervous system signs (seizures, dementia), and visual disturbances may also occur.
  - Cats tend to present with an insidious onset of nonspecific signs (anorexia, weight loss, lethargy). Other signs similar to those seen in dogs may rarely occur.
- Cutaneous PCT:
  - Raised nodule on the trunk, limbs, head, or in the oral cavity.
- EMP:
  - Typically occur in the GI tract and cause signs such as weight loss, anorexia, nausea, vomiting, diarrhea.
- SOP:
  - Occur as a single lesion in bone and can cause bony swellings, lameness, or skeletal pain.

PHYSICAL EXAM FINDINGS

- Skeletal pain, fractures
- Weight loss (MM, EMP)
- Lethargy (MM, EMP)
- Visual disturbances (MM)
- Depression, seizures, abnormal reflexes (MM)
- Epistaxis, gingival bleeding, ecchymoses
- Pallor, weak pulses, heart murmur, increased lung sounds (MM)
- Signs of congestive heart failure such as dyspnea (MM)
- Soft tissue or bony masses

ETIOLOGY AND PATHOPHYSIOLOGY

- Malignant plasma cells produce large amounts of one type of Ig.
- Either the entire immunoglobulin can be produced, or just a portion (e.g., light chain). The Ig or portion is referred to as the M protein, and the concentration is typically proportional to tumor burden in multiple myeloma. Low levels of M proteins are produced in PCT.
- Isolated lesions in bone or diffuse osteopenias are due to areas of proliferating malignant plasma cells. These areas are weakened, and pathologic fractures are common. Bone lesions are uncommon in cats.
- M protein in the blood increases serum viscosity, which causes hyperviscosity syndrome (HVS). HVS is due to sludging of blood in small vessels and it causes ineffective oxygen and nutrient delivery. It is more common with IgM MM (Waldenström's), as the IgM molecule is large. HVS manifests as:
  - Bleeding disorder (due to protein coating of platelets, inhibition of platelet and coagulation factor release, and thrombocytopenia due to bone marrow infiltration).
  - Ocular changes.
  - Congestive heart failure (due to hypertension, myocardial hypoxia, anemia, and increased workload).
  - Mentation changes and peripheral neuropathy (from M protein destruction of myelin).
- The light chain portion of the Ig is also called the Bence Jones protein, and due to its small size, it is filtered by the normal glomerulus. These can be detected in the urine of patients with MM with a specific test (but not on a urine dipstick).
- Renal disease develops due to Bence Jones proteinuria, tumor infiltration into kidney, hypercalcemia, amyloidosis, and decreased renal perfusion.
- Hypercalcemia occurs due to the release of osteoclast activating factor by neoplastic cells.
- Cytopenias develop due to bone marrow infiltration and blood loss due to coagulopathies.
- An increased susceptibility to infection is seen due to the suppression of normal Ig levels, leukopenias, and impaired cell-mediated immunity. Urinary tract infections (UTIs) and pneumonia are the most common manifestations.

DIAGNOSIS

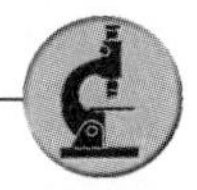

DIFFERENTIAL DIAGNOSIS

Differentials for monoclonal gammopathy: ehrlichiosis, leishmaniasis, feline infectious peritonitis, pyoderma, lymphoma, leukemia, idiopathic (monoclonal gammopathy of unknown significance)

INITIAL DATABASE

- Fundoscopic exam: hemorrhage, retinal detachment, dilated/tortuous vessels
- Complete blood count (CBC): cytopenias, thrombocytopenia
- Serum biochemistry panel may reveal hypercalcemia, elevated total protein, hyperglobulinemia, azotemia
- Urinalysis: infection possible (immunosuppression)

ADVANCED OR CONFIRMATORY TESTING

- MM:
  - For a diagnosis of MM, 2 of the following 4 criteria are needed: monoclonal gammopathy, lytic bone lesions, plasma cell infiltration (>10%) of the bone marrow, and Bence Jones proteinuria.
    - Serum protein electrophoresis: monoclonal gammopathy appears as a spike, typically in the β- or γ-region.
    - Survey radiographs: multiple areas of bony lysis or diffuse osteopenias are frequently found in the vertebrae, scapulae, and long bones in dogs with MM. Pathologic fractures may also be present. These signs are not typically found in cats. A solitary area of lysis is typically seen with SOPs.
    - Bone marrow aspiration: >10% plasma cells are required for the diagnosis of multiple myeloma. Aspiration of multiple sites may be necessary.
    - Heat precipitation, or electrophoresis of urine: identifies Bence Jones proteins. They are not detected on urine dipstick.
  - Serum or urine immunoelectrophoresis: identifies the class of immunoglobulin. (IgG, IgM, IgA). Dogs with multiple myeloma typically produce either IgG or IgM, and cats typically produce IgA.
  - Serum viscosity may be measured in some labs to verify HVS.
- Plasma cell tumor:
  - Tissue biopsy confirmation of cutaneous PCT, EMP, and SOP.

TREATMENT

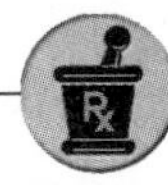

THERAPEUTIC GOAL(S)

- Reduce myeloma cell burden
- Relieve bone pain
- Allow for skeletal healing
- Decrease serum viscosity and Ig levels

ACUTE GENERAL TREATMENT

- Stabilize fractures.
- Surgical excision of plasma cell tumors, if possible. Wide surgical margins generally are not necessary, but the margins should be free of both gross and microscopic evidence of neoplasia (i.e., "clean").
- IV fluids for hydration and diuresis to decrease serum viscosity, azotemia, and hypercalcemia.
- Analgesia for bone pain.
- Plasmapheresis to decrease serum viscosity and remove Bence Jones proteins may be available at some institutions. Therapeutic phlebotomy (with donor red cell transfusion) can possibly achieve a similar effect.
- Antibiotic therapy to treat infections (UTI, pneumonia); prophylactic broad-spectrum antibiotics may be beneficial. Do not use nephrotoxic or bacteriostatic antibiotics.

CHRONIC TREATMENT

- Chemotherapy: melphalan with prednisone is the mainstay of treatment for MM. Cyclophosphamide can also be given initially in cases of widespread disease or severe hypercalcemia, but the benefit is unclear. Chemotherapy can be attempted in cases of cutaneous PCT, EMP, or SOP that are nonresectable or if radiation therapy is not available. However, response information is limited. Other cytotoxic drugs (doxorubicin, vincristine) have been reported to have some activity in the rescue setting for some patients with MM. Consultation with an oncologist for the most current treatment options is recommended.
- Radiation therapy is the treatment of choice for SOP, some incompletely excised PCT and localized MM bony lesions.
- Surgical excision is curative for most cutaneous PCT.

RECOMMENDED MONITORING

- Monitor complete blood counts frequently due to myelosuppressive effects of melphalan. Doses or schedule may need to be adjusted, based on patient response.
- Monitor serum electrophoresis, as size of monoclonal spike is proportional to tumor burden. Plasma globulin level

can also be used for monitoring remission status.
- Monitor for evidence of infection, and treat with antibiotics as needed, due to immunosuppression.

PROGNOSIS AND OUTCOME

- MM:
  - Dogs: when treated with melphalan/ prednisone, response rate is >90%. A good response is defined as 50% reduction of initial M protein level. Long-term prognosis is guarded, as recurrence is inevitable. Median survival time is 540 days with melphalan/prednisone, 220 days for prednisone alone. Negative prognostic factors in dogs include hypercalcemia, Bence Jones proteinuria, and extensive bony lysis.
  - Cats: prognosis is poor; most responses are partial and median survival time is 137 days.
- Cutaneous PCT:
  - Benign biologic behavior: surgical excision is generally curative.
- Extramedullary plasmacytoma (EMP):
  - Frequently metastasize, but long-term survival is possible with surgical excision and chemotherapy and/ or radiation.
- SOP:
  - Eventually progress to MM, but there may be a long disease-free interval. Radiation therapy may provide control for 1 year or more.

PEARLS & CONSIDERATIONS

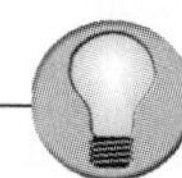

COMMENTS

- Perform serum protein electrophoresis on any animal in which MM is suspected, even if globulin and serum viscosity are normal.
- Use size of monoclonal gammopathy to monitor response to treatment.
- Cats experience more severe myelosuppression from melphalan than dogs.

SUGGESTED READING

Hammer AS, et al: Complications of multiple myeloma. *J Am Anim Hosp Assoc* 30:9–14, 1994.

King AJ, et al: Feline multiple myeloma: Literature review and four case reports. *Aust Vet Pract* 32(4):146–151, 2002.

Matus RE, et al: Prognostic factors for multiple myeloma in the dog. *J Am Vet Med Assoc* 188(11):1288– 1291, 1986.

Rakich PM, et al: Mucocutaneous plasmacytomas in dogs: 75 cases (1980–1987). *J Am Vet Med Assoc* 194(6):803–810, 1989.

Rusbridge C, et al: Vertebral plasma cell tumors in 8 dogs. *J Vet Intern Med* 13:126–133, 1999.

AUTHOR: **ANDREA B. FLORY**

EDITOR: **KENNETH M. RASSNICK**

Multiple Organ Dysfunction Syndrome

BASIC INFORMATION

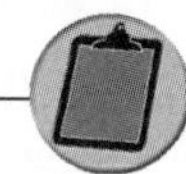

DEFINITION

Failure of two or more organ systems, usually acutely and in association with systemic illness. It commonly represents the end-organ compromise caused by an unchecked systemic inflammatory response syndrome (SIRS).

EPIDEMIOLOGY

SPECIES, AGE, SEX: No predilection for age or sex; dogs appear more commonly affected than cats.

RISK FACTORS: Sepsis, polytrauma (e.g., hit by car), neoplasia.

CLINICAL PRESENTATION

DISEASE FORMS/SUBTYPES: Multiple organ dysfunction syndrome (MODS) is a subset of critical illness; its expression varies according to the organ systems affected.

HISTORY, CHIEF COMPLAINT: Any critical illness and the associated chief complaint may be associated with the development of MODS.

PHYSICAL EXAM FINDINGS

- Physical exam findings are nonspecific and reflect the organ affected.
- Animals are almost invariably collapsed, dull, tachycardic (or possibly bradycardic [cats]), tachypneic, and weak.

ETIOLOGY AND PATHOPHYSIOLOGY

The organ systems that are commonly affected during MODS are the renal, cardiovascular, nervous, respiratory, gastrointestinal, hepatobiliary, and coagulation systems.

- Acute renal failure is a common feature of MODS in people and has been described in hospitalized dogs with critical illness. In this setting, acute renal failure is characterized by serum creatinine >2-3 mg/dl, rising serum creatinine >0.5 mg/dl in 48 hours, or nonphysiologic oliguria.
- The lungs are a common site of organ dysfunction in MODS, manifesting as acute lung injury (ALI) or acute respiratory distress syndrome (ARDS; see Acute Respiratory Distress Syndrome, p 34). ALI is characterized by a PaO_2: FiO_2 ratio between 300 and 200. ARDS is characterized by the presence of acute respiratory distress, bilateral radiographic pulmonary alveolar infiltrates, decreased pulmonary compliance, the absence of left-sided heart failure (pulmonary capillary wedge pressure <18 mmHg), and a PaO_2: FiO_2 ratio of less than 200.
- Gastrointestinal (GI) dysfunction is common in dogs with MODS and can present as ileus, gastric ulceration, vomiting, and diarrhea. Secondary sepsis due to bacterial translocation from the GI tract to the circulation is common and potentially life-threatening.
- Neurologic dysfunction can present as peripheral or central disorders. Animals are usually weak with decreased responsiveness that may progress to stupor or coma.
- Cardiovascular dysfunction may present as decreased cardiac output and hypotension (due to vasodilation, decreased cardiac contractility, etc.), or arrhythmias.
- Hematologic dysfunction produces prolonged coagulation times, decreased fibrinogen concentration, decreased antithrombin III concentration, decreased platelet count, and/or clinical evidence of hemorrhage.
- Hepatic dysfunction manifests with progressive increases in alanine aminotransferase, serum alkaline phosphatase activity, and bilirubin concentration. Hepatic failure can lead to profound coagulopathy.

DIAGNOSIS

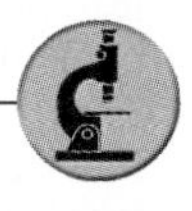

DIFFERENTIAL DIAGNOSIS

Sepsis or SIRS may occur without the failure of multiple organ systems, in which case MODS is not present.

INITIAL DATABASE

- Complete blood count, serum biochemistry profile, urinalysis, coagulation profile: identification of abnormalities listed previously, and abnormalities caused by underlying illness.
- Thoracic radiography, pulse oximetry, and arterial blood gas measurement if respiratory dysfunction.
- Blood pressure: identify hypotension.
- Electrocardiogram: identify cardiac arrhythmias.
- Neurologic exam, to rule out central and peripheral nerve involvement.

TREATMENT

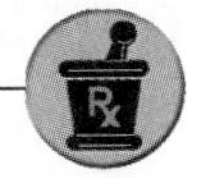

THERAPEUTIC GOAL(S)

Treatment depends on the failing organ system. The overall goals are to stabilize the blood pressure and ensure optimal perfusion of the involved organs (correction of dehydration, treatment of hemodynamically significant arrhythmias).

ACUTE GENERAL TREATMENT

- Respiratory failure:
  Supplemental oxygen and/or positive pressure ventilation.
- Cardiovascular dysfunction:
  - Positive inotropic drugs (dobutamine 5-10 µg/kg/min), and/or vasopressor drugs (dopamine 10-20 µg/kg/min) are used if critically ill, hydrated patients with MODS fail to produce a sufficient arterial blood pressure.
- Coagulopathy:
  - Disseminated intravascular coagulopathy (see Disseminated Intravascular Coagulation, p 313) is the most commonly seen coagulation dysfunction. Goals are to treat the underlying cause while maintaining an adequate hematocrit to ensure oxygen delivery to tissues (treatment with packed red blood cells), and to replace coagulation factors and endogenous anticoagulants (plasma transfusion).
- Renal dysfunction:
  - Goals are to ensure adequate volume status/hydration and blood pressure and to avoid nephrotoxic medications. See Acute Renal Failure, p 32.
- Gastrointestinal dysfunction:
  - Gastroprotectants (e.g., ranitidine 1-2 mg/kg slow IV or famotidine 0.5-1 mg/kg IV q 12 h or omeprazole 0.7 mg/kg PO q 24h) are administered routinely.
  - Prokinetic drugs (ranitidine, or erythromycin 0.5-1 mg/kg PO q 8h, or cisapride 0.1-1 mg/kg PO q 8-12h) are considered if ileus is present without obstruction.
  - Start enteral feedings as soon as possible.

PROGNOSIS AND OUTCOME

Guarded prognosis. Patients with a preexisting organ insufficiency are more likely to develop further organ failures. In people mortality rates depend on the number of organ systems failing. Mortality with one organ system failing is 20%, and will reach almost 100% if four organ systems fail.

PEARLS & CONSIDERATIONS

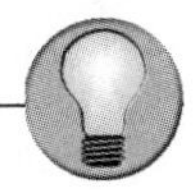

COMMENTS

- MODS should be suspected in any critically ill animal.
- The presence of MODS has prognostic importance (failure of four or more organs is associated with nearly 100% mortality in humans and, by extrapolation, in dogs and cats).
- The onset of MODS is a critical step back in any patient. Critically ill patients should be carefully monitored for the development of signs of failure in a previously unaffected organ, such as new azotemia, icterus, or coagulopathy.
- Rapid appreciation of new-onset abnormalities may permit reversal of organ failure before MODS, and subsequently lead to a better prognosis. For example, development of azotemia may respond to a fluid challenge or therapy with mannitol or dopamine. At the very least, discontinuation of a potentially nephrotoxic agent (e.g., amikacin) in a pet with azotemia is mandatory.

PREVENTION

Rapid identification and correction of sepsis or severe hypovolemia

CLIENT EDUCATION

MODS is a severe complication of disease with guarded to poor outcome.

SUGGESTED READING

Johnson V, et al: Multiple organ dysfunction syndrome. *J Vet Emerg Crit Care* 14(3):158-166, 2004.

AUTHOR: **CARSTEN BANDT**
EDITOR: **ELIZABETH ROZANSKI**

Muscular Dystrophy

BASIC INFORMATION

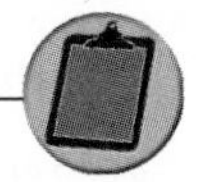

DEFINITION

The muscular dystrophies are a heterogeneous group of rare genetic disorders characterized by deficient or abnormal muscle cytoskeletal proteins. Progressive muscular weakness is the common denominator among the various types of muscular dystrophy (MD).

SYNONYM(S)

There are many forms of muscular dystrophy; the most common terms used in veterinary medicine are:

Duchenne muscular dystrophy (DMD) [a.k.a. Canine X-linked muscular dystrophy (CXMD), Golden retriever muscular dystrophy (GRMD)]

Becker's muscular dystrophy (BMD)

Autosomal recessive muscular dystrophy (ARMD) in Labrador retrievers (previously known as type 2 muscle fiber deficiency)

EPIDEMIOLOGY

SPECIES, AGE, SEX

- The disease is more prevalent in dogs, but has been reported sporadically in cats.
- In dogs with DMD, clinical signs typically begin as early as 6 weeks of age and are progressive.
  - Cats frequently do not demonstrate overt clinical signs until they are ≥ 2 years old.
  - The vast majority of affected animals are male.
- In Labradors with ARMD, clinical signs are generally apparent by 12 to 16 weeks of age. In this form of MD, both males and females may be affected.

GENETICS AND BREED PREDISPOSITION

- DMD, an X-linked disorder, is best described in male golden retrievers, but

has been reported in the male rottweiler, Alaskan malamute, German shorthair pointer, Irish terrier, Samoyed, Groenendaeler shepherd, miniature schnauzer, Brittany spaniel, rat terrier, Pembroke Welsh corgi, Labrador retriever, and in domestic shorthair cats.
- A milder form (BMD) has been described in the Japanese spitz.
- In Labrador retrievers with ARMD, both yellow and black dogs of either sex can be affected.
- Sporadic cases of MD associated with dystrophin defects have been reported in female dogs.

CLINICAL PRESENTATION

DISEASE FORMS/SUBTYPES
- DMD: affects males mainly. Clinical signs often are severe.
- BMD: milder form.
- ARMD: mainly Labrador dogs of either sex.

HISTORY, CHIEF COMPLAINT
- Dogs affected with DMD are stunted.
- Dysphagia and difficulty prehending food can be seen as early as 6 weeks of age. Within weeks, muscle stiffness, "bunny-hopping," exercise intolerance, and muscle atrophy may be observed. Clinical signs typically stabilize by 6 to 8 months of age. Regurgitation due to megaesophagus and diaphragmatic hypertrophy may lead to the development of cough, dyspnea, and respiratory distress due to aspiration pnemonia. Cardiomyopathy may lead to dyspnea, abdominal distention, and other signs of heart failure.
- ARMD: similar weakness, exercise intolerance, and atrophy may be seen but dysphagia is rare, and clinical signs typically occur at a slightly later age.
- Cats with MD may show a predominance of muscle hypertrophy and stiffness. Occasionally dysphagia is evident.

PHYSICAL EXAM FINDINGS
- In DMD, no specific neurologic deficits are found. Affected animals have a characteristic gait, displaying elbow abduction, hock adduction, and lordosis (ventroflexion of the spine). Hypertrophy of specific muscle groups is common, most notably the tongue.
- Dogs affected with ARMD, particularly if clinical signs are severe, will display limb-girdle muscle atrophy, kyphosis (extension/dorsoflexion of the spine), carpal hyperextension, and carpal valgus. In both disorders, myotactic reflexes such as the patellar reflex may be diminished or absent due to severe muscle atrophy.

ETIOLOGY AND PATHOPHYSIOLOGY

- Myofiber cytoskeletal proteins, usually dystrophin, are deficient or absent in DMD.
- Occasionally in DMD, dystrophin-associated or basement membrane proteins are dysfunctional.
- These proteins play a key role in maintaining structural integrity and contractile capability of myofibers. Dystrophin may also play a role in cellular homeostasis.
- The pathophysiology of ARMD is unclear, but likely related to an abnormally positive resting membrane potential in the myocyte.

DIAGNOSIS

DIFFERENTIAL DIAGNOSIS

- Polymyositis (autoimmune or infectious)
- Congenital myotonia
- Nemaline rod myopathy
- Polyneuropathy
- Spinal muscular atrophy
- Exercise-induced collapse of Labrador retrievers
- Progressive ossifying fibrodysplasia (cats)

INITIAL DATABASE

- Creatine kinase levels are markedly elevated in DMD as early as 1 week of age. Elevations peak at 6 to 8 weeks of age and then plateau at approximately 100 × normal. Elevations are less dramatic in ARMD and in female dogs with DMD.
- Thoracic radiographs may reveal evidence of megaesophagus ± aspiration pneumonia.

ADVANCED OR CONFIRMATORY TESTING

- Electromyography (see Electromyography [EMG] and Nerve Conduction Velocity [NCV], p 1231) reveals characteristic pseudomyotonic discharges and occasional fibrillation potentials and positive sharp waves. Abnormalities are evident by 10 weeks of age.
- Muscle biopsy in DMD (see Muscle and Nerve Biopsy, p 1279) typically shows areas of degeneration/mineralization along with areas of regeneration. ARMD is associated with type 2 fiber atrophy.
- Dystrophin deficiency can also be confirmed using immunocytochemistry on biopsy specimens.

TREATMENT

THERAPEUTIC GOAL(S)

- Specific therapies for the muscular dystrophies are lacking.
- Prevention of aspiration pneumonia.

ACUTE GENERAL TREATMENT

- Supportive (e.g., antibiotic therapy and nebulization/coupage for aspiration pneumonia)
- No definitive treatment

PROGNOSIS AND OUTCOME

- The prognosis with DMD is guarded to grave, depending on the severity of clinical signs and whether the animal has megaesophagus or congestive heart failure (both negative prognostic indicators).
- Because clinical signs tend to stabilize within the first year of life, some less severely affected animals may make acceptable house pets and may live for several years until they succumb.
- As with DMD, signs of ARMD tend to plateau between 6 and 12 months of age. Typically signs are mild compared with DMD, so affected Labradors may have a normal lifespan.

PEARLS & CONSIDERATIONS

COMMENTS

Breeders should be advised of the heritable nature of these disorders and remove carriers from the gene pool. Genetic counseling should be sought when an affected animal is identified.

SUGGESTED READING

Dewey C: Myopathies: Disorders of skeletal muscle. In Dewey C (ed): *A Practical Guide to Canine and Feline Neurology*. Ames, IA, Iowa State Press, 2003, pp 414–417.

Klopp LS, Smith BF: Autosomal recessive muscular dystrophy in Labrador retrievers. *Comp Cont Ed Pract Vet* 22:121–129, 2000.

Kornegay JN: Disorders of the skeletal muscles. In Ettinger SJ, Feldman EC (eds): *Textbook of Veterinary Internal Medicine*. Philadelphia, WB Saunders, 1995, pp 727–736.

AUTHOR: **GEORGINA BARONE**
EDITOR: **CURTIS W. DEWEY**

Mushroom Toxicosis

BASIC INFORMATION

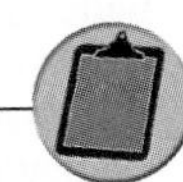

DEFINITION

Clinical condition resulting from ingestion of any of a variety of toxic mushrooms. Toxic syndrome produced depends on mushroom type and amount ingested.

- Gastrointestinal (GI) irritant mushrooms: large variety of species.
- Isoxazole mushrooms: *Amanita gemmata, A. muscaria, A. smithiana, A. strobiliformis,* and *Tricholoma muscarium.*
- Muscarinic mushrooms: *Inocybe* spp., *Clitocybe* spp.
- Hallucinogenic mushrooms: *Psilocybe* spp., *Panaeolus* spp.
- Hepatotoxic mushrooms: *Amanita* spp., *Galerina* spp., *Lepiota* spp.

EPIDEMIOLOGY

SPECIES, AGE, SEX

- All mammalian species are susceptible
- Cats are particularly sensitive to cardiovascular effects of muscarinic mushrooms

GEOGRAPHY AND SEASONALITY

- GI irritant mushroom: wide distribution; large range of fruiting seasons
- Isoxazole mushroom: throughout eastern United States and Pacific Northwest; coniferous and deciduous forests; fruits in spring/early summer then again in fall
- Muscarinic mushroom: wide distribution; forests or fields; fruits in fall, early winter in temperate areas, year round in warm, moist climates
- Hallucinogenic mushroom: wide distribution; Pacific Northwest and Gulf Coast; lawns, gardens, roadsides, open woods; cultivated in homes for recreational use
- Hepatotoxic mushroom: wide distribution throughout United States; wide variation in habitats and fruiting seasons

ASSOCIATED CONDITIONS AND DISORDERS

- GI: acute, self-limiting GI distress
- Isoxazole: acute inebriation followed by coma; generally self-limiting
- Muscarinic: acute muscarinic signs
- Hallucinogenic: acute central nervous system (CNS) signs; generally self-limiting
- Hepatotoxic: acute GI signs, then liver failure in 24 to 72 hours

CLINICAL PRESENTATION

HISTORY, CHIEF COMPLAINT

- History of exposure to a mushroom; presence of mushroom in the vomitus
- GI: vomiting, diarrhea within 4 hours of ingestion
- Isoxazole: vomiting, ataxia, disorientation, sleep/coma within 4 hours of ingestion
- Muscarinic: muscarinic signs (salivation, vomiting, diarrhea, lacrimation, bradycardia) within 4 hours of ingestion
- Hallucinogenic: dysphoria, vocalization within 30 minutes to 2 hours of ingestion
- Hepatotoxic: acute, severe vomiting ± diarrhea within 8 to 24 hours; apparent recovery then return of GI signs; evidence of acute liver failure in 24 to 72 hours; renal failure possible in severe cases

PHYSICAL EXAM FINDINGS

- GI: dehydration possible, but generally unremarkable
- Isoxazole: as described previously
- Muscarinic: as described previously; wet lung sounds
- Hallucinogenic: vocalization, agitation
- Hepatotoxic: GI signs, signs of abdominal pain, icterus, hypotension, hepatomegaly, coma

ETIOLOGY AND PATHOPHYSIOLOGY

- GI: several mechanisms; hypersensitivity, local irritation, induced enzyme deficiencies
- Isoxazole: muscimol mimics γ-aminobutyric acid causing sedation; ibotenic acid acts on glutamate receptors triggering CNS stimulation; combined effects result in hyperesthesia, sedation, intermittent agitation
- Muscarinic: bind muscarinic acetylcholine receptors in parasympathetic nervous system; prolonged duration due to lack of degradation; does not inhibit acetylcholinesterase
- Hallucinogenic: stimulate serotonin and possibly norepinepherine receptors in central and peripheral nervous systems
- Hepatotoxic: interfere with DNA synthesis, protein synthesis resulting in cellular necrosis

DIAGNOSIS

DIFFERENTIAL DIAGNOSIS

- GI, isoxazole, muscarinic, hallucinogenic: parvoviral enteritis, foreign body, garbage toxicosis, encephalitis, organophosphate and carbamate pesticide toxicosis, serotonergic drug toxicosis
- Hepatotoxic: other toxicoses (acetaminophen, iron, blue-green algae, *Cycas* spp.)

INITIAL DATABASE

Complete blood count (CBC), serum biochemistry profile, urinalysis, venous or arterial blood gas measurement:

- Anemia; with hepatotoxic mushrooms: icterus, significant increase in liver enzymes ± bilirubin; hypoglycemia; acidosis.
- Coagulation profile:
  - Coagulopathy possible with severe liver injury
  - Evidence of disseminated intravascular coagulation (hepatotoxic)

ADVANCED OR CONFIRMATORY TESTING

- Radiography: hepatomegaly may be present in cases of hepatotoxic mushroom toxicosis.
- Liver biopsy (hepatotoxic).
- Urine: Muscimol can be detected in urine; turn-around time long, little value in acute cases.

TREATMENT

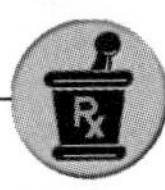

THERAPEUTIC GOAL(S)

- Manage life-threatening conditions
- Decontamination of patient
- Manage clinical signs
- Prevent/manage liver injury
- Supportive care

ACUTE GENERAL TREATMENT

- Manage life-threatening conditions:
  - Control seizures (for isoxazole, hallucinogenic, hepatotoxic).
    - Diazepam (0.5–2 mg/kg IV) for seizures.
      - Barbiturates, gas anesthetics if diazepam is ineffective (see Hepatic Encephalopathy, p 489).
  - Atropine for treating excessive bronchial secretions and bradycardia (muscarinic) 0.04 mg/kg (give 1/4 of dose IV, remainder IM), titrate up as needed.
- Decontamination of patient (only animals showing no clinical signs):
  - Emesis induction (effective in first 8 to 12 hours): see Vomiting, Induction of, p 1328.
  - Gastric lavage (see Gastric Intubation, Gavage, Lavage, p 1258):
    - Consider where emesis is contraindicated (comatose, anesthetized, etc.) or if hepatotoxic mushroom ingestion is suspected.
  - Activated charcoal:
    - 1–4 g/kg or labeled dosage of commercial product given PO, or via stomach tube if patient is uncon-

scious (see Gastric Intubation, Gavage, Lavage, p 1258). Repeat in 8 hours if animal is showing clinical signs of toxicosis, 1/2 original dose.

- Manage clinical signs:
  - Antiemetics (for GI irritant mushroom toxicosis):
    - Metoclopramide 0.2-0.4 mg/kg q 6h PO, SC or IM or 1-2 mg/kg/day as constant rate infusion.
  - Correct fluid/electrolyte/acid-base abnormalities (GI, hepatotoxic).
  - Blood replacement/clotting factors, vitamin K1 for coagulopathy (hepatotoxic).
  - Cyproheptadine (for dysphoria associated with hallucinogenic mushrooms):
    - 1.1 mg/kg PO or rectally q 6-8h prn.
- Prevent/manage liver injury (hepatotoxic mushrooms):
  - *N*-acetylcysteine:
    - 200 mg/kg loading dose then constant rate infusion (CRI) 10 mg/kg/hr.
  - Crystalline (sodium or potassium) penicillin G (interferes with enterohepatic recirculation of hepatotoxins):
    - 0.5-1 million U/kg/day × 3 days as IV CRI.
    - Monitor serum electrolytes as appropriate based on formulation (e.g., sodium, potassium) and adjust therapy if necessary.
    - Do not use procaine penicillin G for intravenous administration (fatal).
  - Silbinin and silymarin (extracts of milk thistle):
    - Not currently available medicinally in the United States; used widely in Europe for *Amanita* toxicosis in humans.
    - 20-30 mg/kg/day IV divided q 6-8h.
    - Over-the-counter products of questionable value.
- Supportive care:
  - Thermoregulation.
  - Dietary support.
  - Confinement for dysphoric, disoriented animals to prevent injury.
  - Pain management.

CHRONIC TREATMENT

- Dietary alterations:
  - High-quality, low-residue protein, fiber diet (hepatotoxic mushrooms)
  - Lactulose, neomycin, or metronidazole (see Hepatic Encephalopathy, p 489)
- S-adenosylmethionine:
  - For chronic liver injury
  - 18 mg/kg/day PO q 24h for 2 to 3 months

POSSIBLE COMPLICATIONS

Hepatic insufficiency ± hepatic encephalopathy

RECOMMENDED MONITORING

- Hydration, electrolytes if severe GI signs
- Hepatotoxic mushrooms:
  - Complete blood count
  - Blood glucose
  - Coagulation parameters
  - Liver enzymes
  - Renal values

PROGNOSIS AND OUTCOME

- GI irritant, isoxazole, muscarinic, and hallucinogenic mushrooms: excellent with supportive care
- Hepatotoxic mushrooms: guarded to poor with hepatotoxicity

PEARLS & CONSIDERATIONS

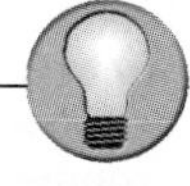

COMMENTS

- Because of difficulty in differentiating between toxic and nontoxic mushrooms, any ingestion of unidentified mushrooms by pets should prompt decontamination procedures (emesis, activated charcoal, etc.).
- Identification of mushrooms is best done by a mycologist; local college biology departments or museums are potentially useful sources of expertise (mycologists).

SUGGESTED READING

Spoerke D: Mushroom exposure. In Peterson ME, Talcott PA (eds): *Small Animal Toxicology*. Philadelphia, WB Saunders, 2001, pp 571-592.

Tegzes JH, Puschner B: Toxic mushrooms. *Vet Clin Small Anim* 32:397-407, 2002.

AUTHOR: **SHARON M. GWALTNEY-BRANT**
EDITOR: **SAFDAR A. KHAN**

Myasthenia Gravis

Client Education Sheet on Website

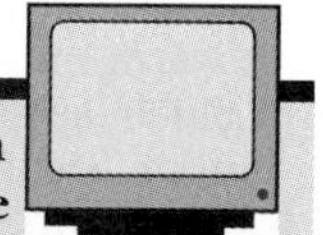

BASIC INFORMATION

DEFINITION

Skeletal muscle weakness due to a decrease of acetylcholine receptors at neuromuscular junctions

EPIDEMIOLOGY

SPECIES, AGE, SEX

- Congenital myasthenia gravis is uncommon and signs occur by 8 weeks of age.
- Acquired myasthenia gravis is fairly common and occurs in adult dogs, with a bimodal age of onset with peaks at 3 and 10 years.
- Acquired myasthenia gravis is uncommon in adult cats.

GENETICS AND BREED PREDISPOSITION

- Congenital myasthenia gravis is inherited as an autosomal recessive trait in Jack Russell terriers and smooth fox terriers, and occurs sporadically in other breeds of dog. It is rare in cats.
- Akitas, terriers, German short-haired pointers, and Chihuahuas have the highest relative risks. German shepherds and golden retrievers are also commonly affected.
- Abyssinians and Somalis are at increased risk of feline-acquired myasthenia gravis.

RISK FACTORS: Methimazole may increase the risk of acquired myasthenia gravis in cats.

ASSOCIATED CONDITIONS AND DISORDERS

- In dogs, associated conditions include hypothyroidism, thymoma and other tumors, hypoadrenocorticism, and thrombocytopenia.
- Thymoma is common in cats with acquired myasthenia gravis.

CLINICAL PRESENTATION

DISEASE FORMS/SUBTYPES

- Acquired: an autoimmune disorder characterized by circulating antibodies against acetylcholine receptors. May occur in generalized, focal, or acute fulminating forms.
- Congenital: an inborn deficiency of muscle acetylcholine receptors.

HISTORY, CHIEF COMPLAINT

- Congenital: generalized limb weakness with or without regurgitation/dysphagia, evident by about 8 weeks of age.
- Generalized acquired: generalized limb weakness that may be precipitated by exercise, with or without regurgitation/dysphagia.

- Focal acquired: dysphagia/regurgitation, or facial weakness with no limb weakness.
- Acute fulminating acquired: acute generalized limb weakness and dyspnea due to respiratory muscle weakness.

PHYSICAL EXAM FINDINGS

- Generalized limb weakness characterized by stiffness, tremor, and short-strided gait that may progress to inability to walk. Weakness may be more severe in the pelvic limbs, is often precipitated by 1 to 2 minutes of exercise, and improves with rest.
- There is no ataxia, and proprioceptive positioning is usually normal when the patient's weight is supported. Muscle atrophy is absent and tendon reflexes are usually preserved.
- Weak palpebral reflex, especially in cats.
- Cats often have neck ventroflexion.
- Abnormal lung sounds and fever possible if concurrent aspiration pneumonia.

ETIOLOGY AND PATHOPHYSIOLOGY

- Congenital myasthenia gravis is caused by mutations in genes coding for the acetylcholine receptor.
- Acquired myasthenia gravis is caused by circulating autoantibodies against the acetylcholine receptor. Factors that initiate the immune response are incompletely understood.

DIAGNOSIS

DIFFERENTIAL DIAGNOSIS

- Myopathies: polymyositis, degenerative myopathies
- Tick paralysis
- Acute idiopathic polyradiculoneuritis
- Botulism
- Polyneuropathy
- Metabolic disorders: hypokalemia, hypoglycemia, hypoadrenocorticism, hyperthyroidism in cats
- Orthopedic diseases: polyarthritis

INITIAL DATABASE

- Complete blood count, serum biochemistry profile, urinalysis to rule out metabolic causes.
- Thoracic radiographs to screen for megaesophagus, aspiration pneumonia.
- Thryoid, adrenal function testing.
- Edrophonium-response test can help diagnose generalized myasthenia gravis. Administer edrophonium chloride (0.1-0.2 mg/kg IV) during weakness. A positive response is obvious improvement in strength within several minutes and suggests the diagnosis. False-negative results are common and false-positive results are possible. Potential side effects include dyspnea due to bronchial constriction and secretions and are treated with atropine.

ADVANCED OR CONFIRMATORY TESTING

- Acetylcholine receptor antibody test. Serologic evaluation to detect antibodies directed against acetylcholine receptors is the gold standard for diagnosis of acquired myasthenia gravis.
- Electrodiagnostic testing (single fiber electromyography and repetitive nerve stimulation) is useful in the diagnosis and in excluding other causes (see Electromyography [EMG] and Nerve Conduction Velocity [NCV], p 1231).
- Definitive diagnosis of congenital myasthenia gravis requires quantification of acetylcholine receptors from muscle biopsy (see Muscle and Nerve Biopsy, p 1279).

TREATMENT

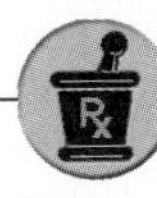

THERAPEUTIC GOAL(S)

- Improve neuromuscular transmission
- Supportive care
- Immunosuppression (acquired form only)

ACUTE GENERAL TREATMENT

- Anticholinesterase drugs. Pyridostigmine (0.5-3.0 mg/kg PO q 8-12h in dogs; 0.25 mg/kg PO q 8-12h in cats). Titrate dose based on weakness and side effects (hypersalivation, vomiting, diarrhea). If dysphagia/regurgitation precludes oral medication, neostigmine (0.04 mg/kg SC q 6h) is an alternative.
- Aspiration pneumonia is treated with antibiotics, nebulization and coupage, and oxygen if necessary (see Pneumonia, Aspiration, p 862).
- Endotracheal intubation and ventilatory support may be necessary for the acute fulminating form or for patients with severe aspiration pneumonia.
- Intravenous fluids as needed.
- Nutritional support as needed: feedings with the head elevated, or placement of a gastrostomy, nasogastric, or pharyngostomy feeding tube (see Feeding Tube Placement: Percutaneous Endoscopic Gastrostomy [PEG], p 1247).

CHRONIC TREATMENT

Immunosupressive therapy (acquired form only) is indicated when there is an inadequate response to anticholinesterase medication. Prednisone is the initial drug of choice (start at 0.5 mg/kg PO q 24h for 1 to 2 weeks then increase to 2-4 mg/kg PO q 24h if needed; gradual taper if possible based on clinical response). Azathioprine or cyclosporine can be added if there is an inadequate response to prednisone or to allow decreased dose of prednisone in patients with severe side effects caused by prednisone.

DRUG INTERACTIONS

- Avoid drugs that impair neuromuscular transmission, including ampicillin, aminoglycosides, and phenothiazines.
- Organophosphates may increase toxicity of anticholinesterase drugs.
- In cats that develop myasthenia gravis while taking methimazole, the methimazole should be discontinued if possible.

POSSIBLE COMPLICATIONS

Aspiration pneumonia is the most common and serious complication in patients with pharyngeal/esophageal weakness.

RECOMMENDED MONITORING

- Client monitors weakness and dysphagia/regurgitation at home daily.
- Monitor anti-acetylcholinesterase antibody titer every 8 weeks in patients with acquired myasthenia gravis because the disease will spontaneously resolve in many patients, usually by 6 to 18 months.

PROGNOSIS AND OUTCOME

- The prognosis for the acquired form is good for patients without pharyngeal/esophageal weakness. Spontaneous remission occurs in almost 90% of affected dogs.
- The prognosis is more guarded in patients with dysphagia/regurgitation because aspiration pneumonia is a common complication and carries an approximately 50% 1-year mortality rate. Spontaneous remission occurs in almost 90% of dogs that survive the acute disease.
- Relapse is rare but can be associated with stress (e.g., surgery) or vaccination.
- The prognosis for the acute fulminating form is grave because most affected dogs die from respiratory failure.

PEARLS & CONSIDERATIONS

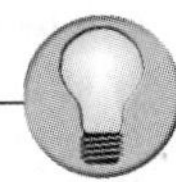

COMMENTS

- Early diagnosis and treatment in an attempt to avoid aspiration pneumonia improves the outcome.
- Serologic testing for antibodies to acetylcholine receptors should be evaluated in any adult dog with unexplained megaesophagus or dysphagia.

SUGGESTED READING

Penderis J: Junctionopathies: Disorders of the neuromuscular junction. In Dewey CW (ed):

A Practical Guide to Canine and Feline Neurology. Ames, IA, Iowa State Press, 2003, pp 463–515.

Shelton GD, et al: Risk factors for acquired myasthenia gravis in cats: 105 cases (1986–1998). *J Am Vet Med Assoc* 215:55, 2000.

Shelton GD, Lindstrom JM: Spontaneous remission in canine myasthenia gravis: Implications for assessing human MG therapies. *Neurology* 57:2139, 2001.

AUTHOR: **WILLIAM B. THOMAS**

EDITOR: **CURTIS W. DEWEY**

Mycobacterial Diseases

BASIC INFORMATION

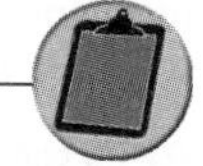

DEFINITION

Infection by any species of *Mycobacterium*

SYNONYM(S)

Atypic mycobacteriosis
Cutaneous tuberculosis
Feline leprosy
Leproid granuloma syndrome
Rapidly growing mycobacterial (RGM) panniculitis

EPIDEMIOLOGY

SPECIES, AGE, SEX

- Tuberculous and leproid forms are rare.
- Opportunistic infections uncommon in cats, rare in dogs.

GENETICS AND BREED PREDISPOSITION: Miniature schnauzers, basset hounds, Siamese cats overrepresented.

RISK FACTORS: Traumatic injuries often precede opportunistic infection.

CONTAGION AND ZOONOSIS

- Zoonotic risk is present with all mycobacterial infections, especially among immunosuppressed people.
- Tuberculous forms are a constant human health threat (especially exudates from cutaneous wounds). Gloves, mask, and eye protection are necessary during wound debridement and care.
- Reverse zoonosis is a common source of infection in animals.
- Common-source exposure is more likely than contagion in leproid and opportunistic forms; however, appropriate caution should be used in handling infected animals and their secretions, exudates, and tissues.
- Urine and feces do not pose a significant zoonotic risk to most immuncompetent people.
- *Mycobacterium tuberculosis* infection (tuberculosis) is a reportable disease from the time of clinical suspicion or diagnosis.

CLINICAL PRESENTATION

DISEASE FORMS/SUBTYPES: Three clinical forms are commonly recognized:

- Tuberculous forms, characterized by skin and internal organ granulomas
- Leproid forms, consisting of regionalized cutaneous nodules
- Opportunistic forms (most prevalent), characterized by spreading, nonhealing subcutaneous lesions

HISTORY, CHIEF COMPLAINT

- Tuberculous forms often are subclinical, or cause skin lesions, weight loss, lethargy, coughing.
- Leproid forms are seen in young cats, with fleshy nodules on the face and forelimbs.
- Opportunistic infections produce nonhealing exudative wound(s). Often there is an associated history of partial response to prior antibiotic therapy, but persistence of the lesions to some degree.

PHYSICAL EXAM FINDINGS

- Tuberculous: systemic signs reflecting the location of visceral granulomata, with/without cutaneous lesions. Involvement of the lungs, spleen, and/or liver is common. In the tuberculous form (very rare) in cats, the gastrointestinal tract may contain granulomata. Mediastinal or mesenteric lymphadenopathy may be noted on imaging.
- Leproid: multiple nonpainful, nonpruritic, fleshy cutaneous nodules, with/without ulceration. Usually, patients are otherwise well.
- Opportunistic: intermittent serous/serosanguineous discharge from spreading skin lesions at sites of prior trauma, especially the inguinal fat pad in cats.

ETIOLOGY AND PATHOPHYSIOLOGY

- Mycobacteria are a large group of acid-fast, aerobic, bacilli, with widely varying pathogenicity.
- Tuberculous species (e.g., *M. tuberculosis, M. bovis*) are facultative intracellular parasites, and none has the dog or cat as the reservoir host.
- Leproid species (*M. leprae, M lepraemurium*) are obligate intracellular parasites, transmitted to cats from rodents.
- Opportunistic species (e.g., *M. avium* complex, *M. smegmatis, M. fortuitum,* etc.) are saprophytes, primarily acquired from water and wet soil across damaged or abraded skin.
- Immune response is insufficient to clear infection, but may confine bacteria within granulomata.

DIAGNOSIS

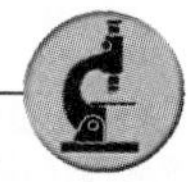

DIFFERENTIAL DIAGNOSIS

- Bacterial folliculitis
- Mycotic infections
- Sterile nodular panniculitis
- Cutaneous neoplasia
- Foreign body reactions
- Drug eruption

INITIAL DATABASE

- Complete blood count/serum biochemistry profile/urinalysis.
  - Hypercalcemia of chronic granulomatous disease is possible and it should not mislead the clinician into a diagnosis of neoplasia.
- Thoracic and abdominal radiographs.
- Cytologic evaluation or biopsy of skin lesions reveals an acid-fast bacillus.

ADVANCED OR CONFIRMATORY TESTING

- Species identification, including antibiotic sensitivity testing, is essential.
- A specialized lab is required (e.g., the National Jewish Center for Immunology and Respiratory Medicine in Denver, Colorado [www.njc.org]).

TREATMENT

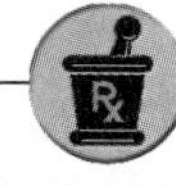

THERAPEUTIC GOAL(S)

- Tuberculous: significant human health threat; treatment may not be recommended.
- Leproid: usually curable with aggressive surgical excision.
- Opportunistic: often curable with long-term treatment.

ACUTE GENERAL TREATMENT

- Surgical excision of leproid granulomata is the treatment of choice.

- Wide surgical debulking of large opportunistic lesions is the first step in long-term management.
- Submit surgical biopsies for species identification.

CHRONIC TREATMENT

- Consultation with an internist specializing in infectious diseases is recommended for drug recommendations; antibiotic resistance is treatment is prevalent, and protocols are evolving rapidly.
- Treatment for tuberculous forms may not be recommended; if treatment is undertaken, combination antibiotic therapy must be administered for a minimum of 6 to 12 months.
- Medical therapy for leproid infections is only indicated with complete surgical excision is not possible.
- Treatment of opportunistic forms, guided by species identification (and sensitivity testing when possible) requires a minimum of 3 months.
- Enrofloxacin, with clarithromycin, gentamicin, or doxycycline, may be acceptable empiric therapy while definitive identification is pending.

POSSIBLE COMPLICATIONS

- Surgical sites prone to dehiscence, and recurrence of infection.
- Risks of drug resistance, toxicosis, or intolerance with long-term antibiotic use.

RECOMMENDED MONITORING

- Reexamination every 2 to 3 weeks for continued effectiveness of therapy.
- Monitor labwork for drug toxicoses.

PROGNOSIS AND OUTCOME

- Recurrence or incomplete clearance is likely.
- Leproid forms have the best prognosis.
- With appropriate, intensive management, outcome of opportunistic infections can be favorable.

PEARLS & CONSIDERATIONS

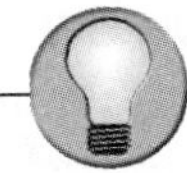

COMMENTS

- Treatment of tuberculous forms may not be recommended (zoonotic risk).
- Significant commitment of owner time and resources is required for positive outcome.
- Accurate species identification and current antimicrobial therapy recommendations are essential.

PREVENTION

- Vaccination with human or large-animal products is not recommended.
- Limiting rodent exposure reduces risk of leproid forms.
- Opportunistic forms are ubiquitous.

SUGGESTED READING

Greene CE, et al: Mycobacterial infections. In Greene CE (ed): *Infectious Diseases of the Dog and Cat*. Philadelphia, WB Saunders, 1998, pp 313–325.

Kaneene JB, et al: Zoonosis update: Tuberculosis. *J Am Vet Med Assoc* 224:685–691, 2004.

Malik R, et al: Infections of the subcutis and skin of cats with rapidly-growing mycobacteria: A review of microbiological and clinical findings. *J Feline Med Surg* 2, 2000.

Malik R, et al: Infections of the subcutis and skin of dogs caused by rapidly-growing mycobacteria. *J Small Anim Pract* 45, 2004.

AUTHOR: **KATE E. CREEVY**
EDITOR: **DOUGLASS K. MACINTIRE**

Mycoplasma/Ureaplasma Infections

BASIC INFORMATION

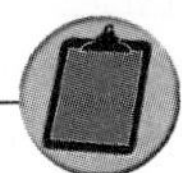

DEFINITION

Infections with small microorganisms of the class Mollicutes, which live on respiratory and urogenital mucosal membranes in many species

EPIDEMIOLOGY

SPECIES, AGE, SEX: Dogs and cats each have a multitude of species, primarily *M. canis* and *M. felis/M. gatae*, respectively.

RISK FACTORS

- Immune suppression
- Underlying disease:
  - General: viral infection, neoplasia, diabetes mellitus
  - Urinary: uroliths, neoplasia, changes in urine concentration or content
  - Pulmonary: aspiration due to laryngeal or esophageal dysfunction, or parenchymal disease (lung parasites, viral infection, neoplasia)

CONTAGION AND ZOONOSIS: Often considered part of the normal flora of upper respiratory, ocular, and urogenital mucosal membranes. There are extremely rare reports of immunocompromised humans with mycoplasmal infections from domestic species.

CLINICAL PRESENTATION

HISTORY, CHIEF COMPLAINT

- Ocular: mucoid ocular discharge, excessive tearing or squinting
- Respiratory: cough, tachypnea, lethargy, anorexia
- Urogenital: dysuria, stranguria, inappropriate elimination, infertility
- Subcutaneous abscesses: lethargy, anorexia, fluctuant subcutaneous swellings or nonhealing open sores
- Joint disease (rare): intermittent lameness, unwillingness to move, lethargy, anorexia, swollen joints

PHYSICAL EXAM FINDINGS

- Mucoid to crusting ocular discharge, epiphora, blepharospasm, hyperemic conjunctiva, chemosis
- Tachypnea or dyspnea, increased airway sounds/wheezes upon auscultation, easily induced cough
- Pain on palpation of bladder
- Subcutaneous abscesses
- Painful or swollen joints

ETIOLOGY AND PATHOPHYSIOLOGY

- *Mycoplasmas/Ureaplasmas* are bacteria that live as normal flora in the upper respiratory tract and distal urethra and cause opportunistic infections in susceptible individuals.
  - Isolation of these bacteria alone is not evidence of infection; concurrent clinical signs and response to treatment must be observed to confirm the diagnosis.
- Pulmonary mycoplasmal infections are presumed to occur due to transfer of organisms from upper respiratory tract to the lungs. Often occurs as part of multiorganism pneumonia, but can be sole causative agent.
- *Mycoplasma* spp. or *Ureaplasma* spp. should not be found in the urinary bladder in health. Urinary tract infections occur due to ascending opportunistic infections. Often found with mixed populations of bacteria.
- Mycoplasmal urinary tract infections in cats and dogs are less common than ureaplasmal infections, due to osmotic fragility of *Mycoplasma* spp.

DISEASES AND DISORDERS

- *Mycoplasma* and *Ureaplasma* spp. have been isolated from vaginal and preputial swabs of infertile dogs; significance is questionable.
- *M. felis* has been associated with conjunctivitis, pneumonia, chronic bronchial disease, and arthritis in cats. Synovitis/arthritis is extremely rare and typically is associated with immunosuppression.

DIAGNOSIS

DIFFERENTIAL DIAGNOSIS

- Urinary tract:
  - Bacterial or fungal urinary tract infection
  - Uroliths
  - Urinary tract neoplasia
- Respiratory:
  - Bacterial pneumonia
  - Viral pneumonia
  - Asthma or allergic lung disease
  - Lung lobe torsion
  - Foreign body
  - Neoplasia
- Ocular infections in cats:
  - Feline herpesvirus-1
  - *Chlamyophila felis* (formerly *Chlamydia psittaci*)
  - Corneal ulcer, trauma, or foreign body

INITIAL DATABASE

- Complete blood count: leukocytosis, neutrophilia, left shift possible.
- Serum biochemistry profile: typically unremarkable.
- Urinalysis:
  - Inflammatory sediment possible.
  - *Mycoplasmas/Ureaplasmas* cannot be seen on sediment exam.
  - Cystocentesis essential, as voided or catheterized urine likely contains normal commensal *Mycoplasma/Ureaplasma* from the distal urethra.
- Urine culture: growth of *Mycoplasma* or *Ureaplasma* spp. Special handling and culture medium are required; contact laboratory prior to sample acquisition.
- Thoracic radiographs: alveolar pattern or areas of consolidation, consistent with pneumonia. Bronchial or interstitial pattern also possible, especially in cats.
- Arthrocentesis: thin, cloudy synovial fluid with many nondegenerate neutrophils.

ADVANCED OR CONFIRMATORY TESTING

- Mycoplasmas cannot be seen with normal stains (they require negative staining with transmission electron microscopy).
- Culture is the best method for identifying these organisms. Requires special media (specify *Mycoplasma/Ureaplasma* culture when requesting).
- Respiratory pathogens should be identified via culture of bronchial wash. Finding *Mycoplasma* in orotracheal/transtracheal washes may be incidental (normal flora). Pure *Mycoplasma* culture more likely indicates true pathogenicity; oropharyngeal contamination typically shows mixed infection with *Mycoplasma* and aerobic bacteria.

TREATMENT

THERAPEUTIC GOAL(S)

Because myco/ureaplasmal infections are typically opportunistic, a thorough search for, and treatment of, underlying disease are imperative.

ACUTE GENERAL TREATMENT

- Urogenital: fluid therapy for dehydrated animals, opioid or nonsteroidal anti-inflammatories for pain, spasm
- Respiratory: oxygen therapy, nebulization and coupage for severe pneumonia
- Ocular
  - Topical ophthalmic tetracycline.
  - Topical ophthalmic pain medications.
  - Systemic antibiotic therapy and pain control are often necessary in addition to topical treatment.

CHRONIC TREATMENT

Systemic antibiotic therapy: options include one of the following:

- Fluoroquinolones: enrofloxacin 10-20 mg/kg (dogs), 5 mg/kg (cats) PO, SQ, slow IV q 24h.
- Doxycycline, 10 mg/kg PO q 12h, or tetracycline 20-30 mg/kg PO q 8h (lower dose for cats).
- Macrolides: azithromycin, 5-10 mg/kg PO q 24h, or erythromycin 10-20 mg/kg PO q 8h.
- Chloramphenicol, 25-50 mg/kg PO q 8h.
- Treatment duration may vary, typically 14-28 days. Treat for 1-2 weeks after resolution of radiographic pneumonia or negative culture.
- Because they lack a cell wall, myco/ureaplasmas are resistant to β-lactam antibiotics (penicillins, cephalosporins). Failure to respond to these antibiotics should suggest possible mycoplasmal infection.

DRUG INTERACTIONS

- Rarely, humans exposed to chloramphenicol can develop a fatal aplastic anemia. Owners *must* be instructed to take appropriate precautions (gloves, hand washing) when administering this medication.
- Erythromycin commonly causes gastrointestinal side effects, such as vomiting, diarrhea, and anorexia.
- Enrofloxacin and other fluoroquinolones may cause blindness in cats at high doses.
- Doxycycline has been reported to cause esophagitis and esophageal strictures in cats, and possibly dogs. To prevent this complication, owners need to follow doxycycline administration with administration of a small amount of butter, soft margarine, or water to ensure passage into the stomach.

RECOMMENDED MONITORING

- Pneumonia: serial radiographs, bronchial lavage cytology and culture
- Urinary: serial cystocentesis urinalysis and culture
- Ocular: recheck ocular exams and fluoroscein staining

PROGNOSIS AND OUTCOME

Mycoplasmas/ureaplasmas are usually quite susceptible to appropriate antibiotic therapy. Prognosis is good with antibiotics and management of underlying disease or concurrent bacterial infection.

PEARLS & CONSIDERATIONS

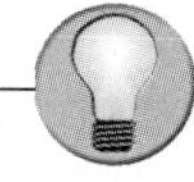

COMMENTS

These organisms are often found in cultures of normal respiratory or urinary tracts, and may be commensals that were inadvertently sampled. A search for other pathogens or underlying disease that have caused enhanced susceptibility to these organisms is essential.

SUGGESTED READING

Gaskell RM, Radford AD, Dawson S: Feline infectious respiratory disease. In Chandler EA, Gaskell CJ, Gaskell RM (eds): *Feline Medicine and Therapeutics*. Denmark, Blackwell Publishing, 2004, pp 577-595.

Greene CE: Mycoplasmal, ureaplasmal, and L-form infections. In Greene CE (ed): *Infectious Diseases of the Dog and Cat*. Philadelphia, WB Saunders, 1998, pp 174-177.

AUTHOR: **SHANNON T. STROUP**
EDITOR: **DOUGLASS K. MACINTIRE**

Myelodysplasia

BASIC INFORMATION

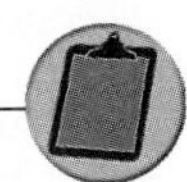

DEFINITION

- Myelodysplasia (MDS) describes a group of bone marrow disorders characterized by peripheral blood cytopenias and a hypercellular to normocellular bone marrow containing less than 30% blast cells. MDS is often considered a precursor of acute myeloid leukemia (AML).
- Morphologic signs of abnormal maturation (dysplasia) are present in the erythroid, myeloid, and/or megakaryocytic cells.

SYNONYM(S)

Ineffective hematopoiesis
MDS
Myelodysplastic syndromes
Refractory cytopenias; preleukemia
Smoldering acute leukemia

EPIDEMIOLOGY

SPECIES, AGE, SEX: MDS has been reported in dogs and cats. MDS is becoming less common in cats as the incidence of feline leukemia virus (FeLV) infection decreases.

RISK FACTORS

- Young cats with FeLV infection.
- Some drugs (chloramphenicol, cephalosporins, melphalan, cyclophosphamide, and vincristine) have been associated with MDS in animals.
- Vitamin B_{12}/folate deficiency.
- Lead toxicity.
- Exposure to radiation.
- Immune-mediated diseases targeting the bone marrow.

CONTAGION AND ZOONOSIS: FeLV: contagious between cats.

CLINICAL PRESENTATION

DISEASE FORMS/SUBTYPES: Myelodysplasia may be primary or secondary. MDS is classified into three subtypes, based on cytologic examination of bone marrow. This classification system does not provide specific prognostic information at this time.

- MDS-ER (erythroid predominant): M:E ratio <1, blasts <30% of nucleated bone marrow cells.
- MDS-RC (refractory cytopenia): M:E ratio >1, nonerythroid blasts <6% of nucleated bone marrow cells.
- MDS-EB (excess blasts): M:E ratio >1, nonerythroid blasts 6–29% of nucleated bone marrow cells.

HISTORY, CHIEF COMPLAINT

- Rapid onset of nonspecific clinical signs including weakness (anemia), lethargy, tachypnea, and decreased or deranged appetite/pica.
- Recurrent/chronic infections if leukopenia
- Bruising/bleeding if thrombocytopenia
- It is important to determine the recent history of drugs administered to the patient.

PHYSICAL EXAM FINDINGS

- Weakness, tachycardia, heart murmurs, and pale mucous membranes may indicate anemia.
- Fever due to secondary infections.
- Epistaxis or petechiae due to thrombocytopenia or abnormal platelet/megakaryocyte maturation.
- Hepatomegaly and splenomegaly are common in cats.
- Pleural effusion has been reported in cats, possibly leading to muffled heart and lung sounds.

ETIOLOGY AND PATHOPHYSIOLOGY

- MDS may be primary (presumably due to mutations in hematopoietic progenitor cells), or secondary (associated with drug therapy or disorders such as lymphoma, myelofibrosis, or immune-mediated anemia/thromobocytopenia).
- A variety of chromosomal abnormalities and mutations in oncogenes and tumor suppressor genes has been identified in humans with MDS, but it is not yet known whether these are present in veterinary patients.
- MDS-associated clonal proliferation, apoptosis, and ineffective hematopoiesis can result in lethal cytopenias, or MDS may progress to acute leukemia.

DIAGNOSIS

DIFFERENTIAL DIAGNOSIS

- Acute leukemias
- Drug-induced bone marrow dyscrasias
- Hyperplasia of recovering bone marrow
- Nonregenerative anemia:
  - Anemia of chronic/inflammatory disease.
  - Anemia of renal disease.
  - Iron-deficiency anemia.
- Neutropenia:
  - Tissue demand.
  - Endotoxemia/sepsis.
  - Immune-mediated destruction.
- Thrombocytopenia:
  - Drug therapy.
  - Immune-mediated destruction.
- Rickettsial (*Ehrlichia* and *Anaplasma* spp., Rocky Mountain spotted fever) organism-induced bone marrow dyscrasias
- Congenital conditions associated with dysplastic features:
  - Miniature and toy poodles: familial nonanemic macrocytosis with dysplastic changes in erythroid precursors.
  - English springer spaniels: congenital dyserythropoiesis, polymyopathy, and cardiac disease.
  - Giant schnauzers: congenital malabsorption of vitamin B_{12} and myelodysplasia.
  - Cavalier King Charles spaniels: idiopathic subclinical thrombocytopenia and dysplastic changes in megakaryocytes and platelets (macroplatelets).

INITIAL DATABASE

- Complete blood count (CBC) and blood smear review: cytopenias and dysplastic blood cell morphology. Blood smear should be reviewed by a clinical pathologist.
  - Nonregenerative anemia (most common) often with many nucleated red blood cells present. Thrombocytopenia and/or leukopenia also are often present.
  - Leukocytes with ringed nuclei, micronuclei, nuclear fragments, or abnormal cytoplasmic granulation.
  - Giant platelets and dwarf megakaryocytes.
- Bone marrow evaluation (biopsy may be necessary as aspirates may be hypocellular or nondiagnostic).
  - Examination of bone marrow is necessary to confirm MDS and identify the subtype.
  - Fewer than 30% of the marrow nucleated cells are blast cells (if >30% blasts are present, the diagnosis is acute myeloid leukemia, and the attendant prognosis is potentially worse).
  - Asynchrony of nuclear and cytoplasmic maturation.
  - Bizarre nuclear morphologies resembling bowling pins, doughnuts, or abnormally small nuclei.
- Serum biochemistry profile and urinalysis to evaluate overall health.
- All cats with MDS should be tested for FeLV and feline immunodeficiency virus (FIV).

ADVANCED OR CONFIRMATORY TESTING

- Cytochemical immunohistochemical stains or flow cytometry may be useful

to rule out myeloid and lymphoid malignancies.
- *Ehrlichia* and *Anaplasma* spp. titers may aid diagnosis of rickettsial disease.
- Serum iron, zinc, lead, and vitamin B_{12}/folate levels.
- Coombs' test may be needed to rule out immune-mediated disease.

TREATMENT

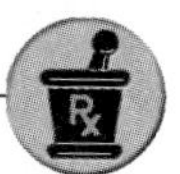

THERAPEUTIC GOAL(S)

- Restore normal hematopoiesis
- Support patient until cytopenias resolve
- Treat underlying cause, if appropriate
- Eradicate neoplastic blast cells and dysplastic cells

ACUTE GENERAL TREATMENT

- Discontinue all drug treatment, especially agents associated with MDS.
- Intensive supportive care may be needed by patients with severe cytopenias.
  - Transfusions (see Transfusion Therapy and Collection Techniques for Blood Banking, p 1312).
  - Antibiotics as indicated for treating/preventing secondary infections.
    - For prophylaxis, a common choice is sufadiazine-trimethoprim 15 mg/kg PO q 12h for dogs. Cats do not usually need prophylactic antibiotics.
    - If fever or overt infection is present, intravenous broad-spectrum antibiotics based on culture and sensitivity (preferred, if available) or empiric use of clinician's preferred combination are indicated. Example: a combination of either a cephalosporin (e.g., cefazolin 22 mg/kg IV q 8h slow bolus) or a penicillin (e.g., ampicillin 22 mg/kg IV q 8h slow bolus) together with either an aminoglycoside (e.g., amikacin 20 mg/kg IV q 24h [only in hydrated patient without renal dysfunction; can cause renal injury]) or a fluoroquinolone (e.g., enrofloxacin 5 mg/kg diluted 1:1 in sterile water and given as a slow IV bolus q 12h [dogs; 5 mg/kg q 24h in cats]).
  - Intravenous fluids for patients with infection, fever, or decreased appetite.
  - Avoid jugular venipuncture or catheterization if severe thrombocytopenia is present.
  - Nutritional support.
- Recombinant granulocyte colony stimulating factor (G-CSF; 5 µg/kg SQ once daily), recombinant human erythropoietin (rh-Epo; Epogen [100 IU/kg SC q 48-72h until hematocrit rises, then q 7 days or as needed to maintain low-normal hematocrit]) and potentially granulocyte-monocyte stimulating factor (GM-CSF) and/or thrombopoietin (currently experimental) may also have a role in treating refractory cytopenias. However, recombinant human cytokines may cause dogs and cats to form cross-reactive neutralizing antibodies to the recombinant products and their own cytokines.
- Immunosuppressive doses of prednisone (2 mg/kg PO q 24h) have been effective for some dogs and cats with refractory cytopenias.
- Low-dose cytosine arabinoside (LD-AraC, 0.7-1.4 mg/kg SC q 24h) has been attempted as a differentiation agent in the management of MDS in nine cats. One complete response was described. LD-AraC administered to a dog with MDS-Er at 10 mg/m^2 SC q 12h for 3 weeks was ineffective.

CHRONIC TREATMENT

- Patients responding to treatment will likely require lifelong therapy.
  - Supportive therapy as indicated (antibiotic therapy, transfusions, hematopoietic cytokines as needed).
  - Hematopoietic cytokines should be discontinued once cell counts are improved to reduce the risk of production of cross-reactive antibodies that could affect the patient's own erythropoietin, G-CSF, GM-CSF, or thrombopoietin.
- Patients with concurrent MDS secondary to drug administration should never receive that drug again.

POSSIBLE COMPLICATIONS

Chronic administration of rh-Epo can result in the production of antibodies that cross-react with feline or canine erythropoietin and cause severe nonregenerative anemia.

RECOMMENDED MONITORING

- Physical examinations and complete blood count: weekly to every other week, more frequently if needed when therapy is initiated. Blood smear review to monitor cytopenias, blasts and other abnormal cell morphology, and possible adverse effects of treatment. If response to therapy is noted, interval may be extended to monthly.
- Serum biochemistry profile: every 2 months to monitor overall health. More frequently if indicated.

PROGNOSIS AND OUTCOME

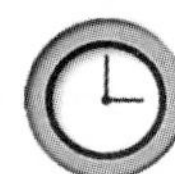

- In general, the prognosis for most animals with MDS is poor, with survival times ranging from a few days to a few months.
  - Primary MDS is considered to be a preneoplastic condition, progressing to acute leukemia in 40-60% of cases. Animals may live a year or more, but eventually succumb to acute myeloid leukemia or bone marrow failure.
  - The prognosis for animals with secondary MDS depends on successful resolution of their underlying disease condition.
- Cats with refractory anemia can enjoy long survival times; however, cats with other types of MDS are typically euthanized due to cytopenias, or may develop AML within 1 week to a few months.
- The prognosis for cats with concurrent MDS and FeLV infection is especially grave; most do not survive 1 week after diagnosis.
- Dogs with MDS-RC may have a better prognosis than those with MDS-EB. In one small study, dogs with refractory anemias lived longer (>6 months) than dogs with other MDS (mean, 2 weeks).
- In general, a high blast count may be associated with a worse prognosis.

PEARLS & CONSIDERATIONS

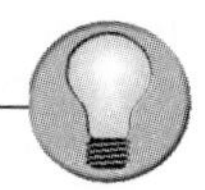

COMMENTS

- Management of MDS is focused on identifying and treating underlying diseases (especially immune-mediated hemolytic anemia and lymphoma in dogs) and supportive care of secondary cytopenias.
- Myelodysplastic syndromes are uncommon diseases, and it can be challenging to accurately diagnose them. When MDS is suspected based on clinical signs and evidence of hematologic abnormalities, bone marrow evaluation is required for definitive diagnosis.
- When considering these conditions, consultations with a veterinary clinical pathologist and a veterinary oncologist are highly recommended.
- Chemotherapy has not been shown to be beneficial for control of MDS or to prevent progression to leukemia.
- Although the overall prognosis for patients with MDS is poor, there is substantial inter-individual variability; some patients can respond well to therapy and enjoy longer survival times.

PREVENTION

All cats should be tested for feline retroviruses (FeLV; also FIV if kitten >6 months old) as kittens.

CLIENT EDUCATION

- Retrovirus-negative cats should be kept inside to prevent them from becoming exposed to cats harboring FeLV or FIV.
- There is a high risk of progression of primary MDS to acute leukemia.

SUGGESTED READING

Blue J: Myelodysplastic syndromes and myelofibrosis. In Feldman BF, Zinkl JG, Jain NC (eds): *Schalm's Veterinary Hematology,* ed 5.

Baltimore, Lippincott, Williams & Wilkins, 2000, pp 682–688.
Brunning RD, et al: Myelodysplastic syndromes. In Jaffe ES, Harris NL, Stein H, Vardiman JW (eds): *Pathology and Genetics of Tumours of Haematopoietic and Lymphoid Tissues.* Lyon, France, IARC Press, 2001, pp 63–73.
Hisasue M, et al: Hematologic abnormalities and outcomes of 16 cats with myelodysplastic syndromes. *J Vet Intern Med* 15:471–477, 2001.
Jacobs RM, et al: Tumors of the hemolymphatic system. In Meuten DJ (ed): *Tumors in Domestic Animals,* ed 4. Ames, IA, Iowa State Press, 2002. pp 193–194.
Weiss DJ, Aird B: Cytologic evaluation of primary and secondary myelodysplastic syndromes in the dog. *Vet Clin Pathol* 30(2):67–75, 2001.
Weiss DJ, Smith SA: Primary myelodysplastic syndromes in dogs. *J Vet Intern Med* 14:491–494, 2000.
Young KM, MacEwen EG: Canine myeloproliferative disorders. In Withrow SJ, MacEwen EG (eds): *Small Animal Clinical Oncology,* ed 3. Philadelphia, WB Saunders, 2001, pp 618–622.

AUTHORS: **BRUCE E. LEROY, JENNIFER E. LOCKE, NICOLE C. NORTHRUP**
EDITORS: **SUSAN M. COTTER, KENNETH M. RASSNICK**

Myiasis

BASIC INFORMATION

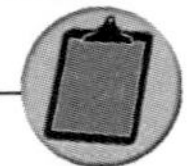

DEFINITION

An infestation of living animals with the larvae (maggots) of dipteran (two-winged) flies. They may cause cutaneous, nasal, or other tissue lesions.

SYNONYM(S)

Maggot infestation

EPIDEMIOLOGY

SPECIES, AGE, SEX: Dogs and cats may be affected. Most of these larvae are relatively species-specific. However, small animals may serve as aberrant hosts when housed near primary hosts. Overall, myiasis occurs without any predilections in age or sex.

RISK FACTORS: Animals living in temperate wet regions known to harbor flies causing myiasis, that are wounded, soiled, debilitated, or weak may be predisposed. Some dipteran larvae can penetrate normal skin.

CONTAGION AND ZOONOSIS: Emerging adult flies are a potential health risk since they serve as fomites for bacteria found in animal waste. People with open wounds could be at risk for myiasis. See Etiology below

GEOGRAPHY AND SEASONALITY: Myiasis has a worldwide distribution; however, larvae-specific infestations do occur in some countries. In the Northern Hemisphere, myiasis occurs during the summer months in temperate moist areas. Screwworm myiasis was eradicated in the United States with the use of sterilized male flies.

CLINICAL PRESENTATION

HISTORY, CHIEF COMPLAINT: A foul, putrid-smelling animal may be the only reason an owner seeks veterinary care. Other owners are well aware that maggots are taking residence in their animal's skin. Occasionally, owners will present an animal because of incontinence, debilitation, or skin fold dermatitis in which invading maggots are an incidental finding.

PHYSICAL EXAM FINDINGS

- Maggot infestation typically occurs in moist locations as those around the eyes, nose, mouth, genitalia, anus, or adjacent to wounded skin. Irregularly ulcerated to crateriform lesions are characteristic.
- Several lesions may coalesce to form large soft tissue defects.
- Tracts dissecting through nearby soft tissue structures may cause fistulation.
- Parasitized skin may present as a focal fistulated subcutaneous nodule.
- Aberrant larval migration can cause signs specific to other tissues.
- Findings associated with incontinence or debilitation (e.g., musculoskeletal, neurologic, or internal disease) might be identified in select cases. Severely infested animals may be in shock.

ETIOLOGY AND PATHOPHYSIOLOGY

- Eggs are laid on the moist skin of debilitated or wounded animals. Emerging larvae (maggots) secrete proteolytic enzymes that liquefy cutaneous tissue creating full-thickness skin defects within hours. Occasionally the initial larval infestation will favor the "strike" of other myiasis-causing flies, resulting in disease propagation.
- Many dipteran flies (e.g., house, stable, horn, and black flies) are capable of infesting the skin of animals with the above risk factors. These flies cause the typical myiases seen in routine small animal practice.
- Blowflies (common in large animals), screwworm flies (reportable in many parts of the world), and flesh flies rarely infest the skin of small animals. However, their presence is alarming due to contagion implications.
- Although more common in rabbits and rodents, *Cuterebra* flies can cause myiasis in companion animals.

DIAGNOSIS

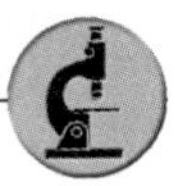

DIFFERENTIAL DIAGNOSIS

Direct visualization of maggots in representative lesions or present on the skin and/or hair excludes other differential diagnoses. Specific species identification is not usually required to treat most cases of myiasis.

INITIAL DATABASE

- Direct visualization of maggots
- Cytologic evaluation of wounded and infested skin to identify secondary bacterial infection

ADVANCED OR CONFIRMATORY TESTING

- Other diagnostic tests are at the discretion of the clinician, but in most patients a complete blood count, biochemistry profile, and urinalysis will be beneficial to exclude concurrent and predisposing conditions.
- Bacterial culture and susceptibility testing for lesions failing to heal rapidly or in septicemic animals.
- Examination of the spiracle and stigmal plates on the maggot can aid in species identification.
- Larvae can be kept until developing adult flies emerge. Flies of severe concern include blowflies, characterized as having a metallic blue or green sheen on the body, and screwworm flies, which have orange-brown eyes and are bluish-green with longitudinal stripes along their thorax. The economic importance of eradication of these flies warrants contacting a regional veterinary office for precautionary identification and confirmation if a suspicion of screwworm myiasis exists.

TREATMENT

THERAPEUTIC GOAL(S)

- Identify and treat underlying conditions
- Remove and kill maggots
- Routine wound care

ACUTE GENERAL TREATMENT

- Stabilize patient if needed (e.g., fluid therapy).
- Clip, clean, and surgically debride lesions (anesthesia required).
- Mechanically remove larvae.
- Apply a non-alcohol-based pyrethrin or pyrethroid (dogs but not cats) spray on lesions to kill maggots.
- Systemically administered avermectins (ivermectin 0.2-0.4 mg/kg PO or SQ, may repeat in 7 to 14 days) for nonherding dog breeds (negative for heartworms) can be used for killing maggots. Caution: susceptible individuals or breeds (see Ivermectin Toxicosis, p 610).
- Anecdotally, oral nitenpyram (Capstar) at routine doses may kill maggots.
- Wound care (e.g., wet to dry bandages to help debride wound).
- House animal in fly-free area (e.g., indoors, screened-in patio).
- Empiric antibiotic therapy for secondary bacterial infection (e.g., cephalexin 22-30 mg/kg PO q 8-12h or clavulanic acid-potentiated amoxicillin 12.5-20 mg/kg PO q 12h for 21 to 30 days).

PROGNOSIS AND OUTCOME

Guarded to good, based on the severity of the problem and predisposing conditions.

PEARLS & CONSIDERATIONS

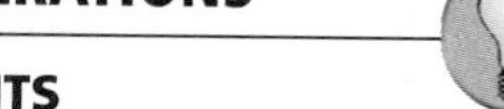

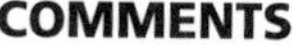

COMMENTS

- Myiasis is a disease of neglect.
- Depending on the country, some types of myiases are reportable.
- Avoid crushing or cutting maggots *in vivo*, as remaining body parts may cause allergic reactions.

CLIENT EDUCATION

Basic hygiene care and early intervention when a pet is debilitated for any reason are essential for preventing myiasis.

SUGGESTED READING

Parasitic skin diseases. In Scott DW, Miller Jr. WH, Griffin CE (eds): *Muller & Kirk's Small Animal Dermatology*, ed 6. Philadelphia, WB Saunders, 2001, pp 423-516.

Urquhart GM, et al: Veterinary entomology. In Urquhart GM, et al (eds): *Veterinary Parasitology*, ed 2. Oxford, Blackwell Science Ltd, 1996, pp 141-206.

AUTHOR: **ADAM P. PATTERSON**
EDITOR: **JAN A. HALL**

Myocarditis

BASIC INFORMATION

DEFINITION

Inflammation of the heart muscle, typically associated with myocytolysis. Myocarditis is a poorly understood group of diseases that can result from a collection of diseases of infectious, chemical, and physical etiologies.

EPIDEMIOLOGY

SPECIES, AGE, SEX: Myocarditis occurs rarely, and is recognized more often in dogs than cats. No age predilection (exception: puppies—parvoviral myocarditis between 3 and 8 weeks of age). No sex predisposition.

RISK FACTORS: Myocarditis can result from an extension of infectious endocarditis; therefore preexisting heart disease, persistent bacteremia, or immune compromise can be considered risk factors. Dogs and cats that roam are at risk for traumatic myocarditis.

GEOGRAPHY AND SEASONALITY: Chagas myocarditis (*Trypanosoma cruzi*): southern United States, Latin America. Lyme myocarditis (*Borrelia burgdorferi*): more common in the northeastern United States.

ASSOCIATED CONDITIONS AND DISORDER: Myocarditis often results in, or coexists with, cardiac arrhythmias (especially ventricular tachyarrhythmias, but occasionally atrial tachyarrhythmias or atrioventricular [AV] block). Myocarditis due to a chronic process, especially persistent infection, may lead to dilated cardiomyopathy.

CLINICAL PRESENTATION

DISEASE FORMS/SUBTYPES: Based on recent discoveries, viral myocarditis has three distinct phases of disease:

- Phase 1: acute myocarditis associated with acute viremia, myocyte necrosis, and macrophage activation.
- Phase 2: subacute myocarditis associated with viral clearing and overzealous immune response by cell-mediated and humoral immunity and cytokine activation.
- Phase 3: chronic myocarditis, or dilated cardiomyopathy, associated with fibrosis, cardiac dilation, and heart failure.

HISTORY, CHIEF COMPLAINT: Presenting complaint can be vague or specific to the cardiovascular system and may include:

- Anorexia.
- Lethargy/exercise intolerance.
- Cough/dyspnea.
- Syncope.
- Sudden death.
- With traumatic myocarditis, a history of the animal's having been hit by a car is common.

PHYSICAL EXAM FINDINGS: Possible findings include:

- Fever.
- Murmur.
- Lymphadenopathy.
- Skeletal muscle weakness.
- Signs of congestive heart failure (usually, phase 3): cough, dyspnea, abnormal breath sounds, weak pulses, pale mucous membranes, ascites, weakness, hepatosplenomegaly, jugular venous distention.
- Arrhythmias: bradyarrhythmia (e.g., AV block) and tachyarrhythmias (ventricular ectopy).
- With traumatic myocarditis, evidence of blunt chest trauma or generalized signs of trauma may be present.

ETIOLOGY AND PATHOPHYSIOLOGY

- Bacterial:
  - *Bacillus piliformis*, *Citrobacter koseri*; streptococcal, staphylococcal, *Bartonella*, *Brucella*, *Leptospira*, and *Salmonella* spp.
- Spirochete:
  - *Borrelia burgdorferi*
- Protozoan:
  - *Trypanosoma cruzi*, *Toxoplasma gondii*, *Neospora caninum*, *Babesia* spp.
- Viral:
  - Parvovirus; panleukopenia (cats)
- Other:
  - Doxorubicin chemotherapy, catecholamines, lead, arsenic, stinging

insect and snake venom, hyperthermia, radiation therapy, blunt or penetrating trauma

DIAGNOSIS

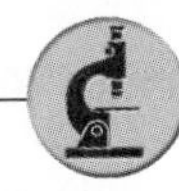

DIFFERENTIAL DIAGNOSIS

- Infectious endocarditis
- Idiopathic dilated cardiomyopathy
- Sepsis

INITIAL DATABASE

- Complete blood count, serum biochemistry profile, urinalysis: inflammatory leukogram possible.
- Blood cultures: for diagnosis of bacterial etiology.
- Cardiac troponin I or other biomarker of cardiac necrosis: serum troponin levels usually are markedly elevated.
- Thoracic radiographs: may show signs of pulmonary edema and cardiomegaly (phase 3).
- Electrocardiogram (ECG): to identify bradyarrhythmias or tachyarrhythmias.
- Echocardiogram: may show cardiac dilation and diminished myocardial function (phase 3).
- Infectious disease serologic tests: *Toxoplasma*, *Neospora*, *Bartonella*; based on geographic location, *Babesia*, Lyme, Chagas, and fungal serologies may be indicated.

ADVANCED OR CONFIRMATORY TESTING

- Endomyocardial biopsy and histopathologic evaluation:
  - Considered the diagnostic gold standard.
  - Rarely performed due to invasive nature.
  - Classic findings include lymphocyte infiltrates with myocyte necrosis (Dallas criteria). Parvovirus inclusion bodies within cardiomyocytes are also possible.
- In acute viremia, parvovirus isolation may be attempted.
- Magnetic resonance imaging is an emerging modality and early studies show high diagnostic accuracy for myocarditis.

TREATMENT

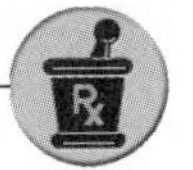

THERAPEUTIC GOAL(S)

- Supportive care is the first line of therapy.
- Treatment of hemodynamically significant arrhythmias.
- Pacemaker implantation for complete AV block.
- Treatment of heart failure by diuretics and vasodilators. Support of cardiac output with positive inotropes may be necessary.
- Treatment with an antimicrobial agent if a bacterial or protozoan etiology is suspected.

ACUTE GENERAL TREATMENT

- If severe ventricular arrhythmias:
  - Lidocaine IV 2 mg/kg bolus, repeat three times if needed for maximum dose of 8 mg/kg.
  - Once acute suppression is achieved with lidocaine bolus, continue with constant rate infusion at 50-75 μg/kg/min.
  - For chronic oral suppression of ventricular arrhythmias, sotalol 2 mg/kg PO q 12h.
- If high-grade second-degree or third-degree AV block:
  - Atropine 0.04 mg/kg SQ.
  - If good heart rate response, can continue atropine q 6h or switch to glycopyrrolate 0.01 mg/kg SQ q 6h.
  - For chronic bradycardia treatment, theophylline 10 mg/kg PO q 8-12h, or terbutaline 2.5-5 mg PO q 8-12h may be beneficial in some cases.
  - If complete or high-grade second-degree AV block is present and there is no response to atropine, consider permanent pacemaker.
- If congestive heart failure (CHF) (pulmonary edema, pleural effusion, ascites): see Heart Failure, Chronic, p 459.
- Antimicrobial therapy:
  - See specific infectious disease topics for recommendations.

CHRONIC TREATMENT

- Conventional CHF therapy is recommended if patient survives acute phase (see Congestive Heart Failure, Chronic, p 459).
- See Ventricular Arrhythmias (Premature Ventricular Complexes, Ventricular Tachycardia), p 1148.

POSSIBLE COMPLICATIONS

- Chronic CHF
- Dilated cardiomyopathy
- Complete AV block

RECOMMENDED MONITORING

- Acute monitoring:
  - Continuous ECG
  - Frequent blood pressure measurement: invasive or noninvasive
  - Dyspnea watch and respiratory rate
- Chronic monitoring:
  - Periodic ECG or Holter monitor
  - Echocardiogram
  - Thoracic radiograph
  - Renal and electrolyte parameters if receiving diuretics
  - Convalescent serologic titers for suspected infectious diseases

PROGNOSIS AND OUTCOME

Because myocarditis is an elusive diagnosis and uncommon disease, good information regarding prognosis and outcome is not known. The possibility of lethal arrhythmia and/or progression to dilated cardiomyopathy and CHF warrant an initial guarded prognosis.

PEARLS & CONSIDERATIONS

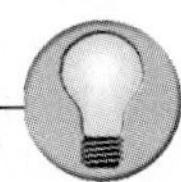

COMMENTS

In the author's clinical experience, myocarditis is strongly suspected when a dog presents with clinical signs attributable to a sudden onset of complex ventricular arrhythmias or complete AV block with no clear underlying etiology.

SUGGESTED READING

Feldman AM, McNamara D: Myocarditis. *N Engl J Med* 343(19):1388-1398, 2000.

Liu PP, Mason JW: Advances in the understanding of myocarditis. *Circulation* 104:1076-1082, 2001.

Meurs KM: Primary myocardial disease in the dog. In Ettingers SJ, Feldman ED (eds): *Textbook of Veterinary Internal Medicine*. St. Louis, Elsevier WB Saunders, 2005, pp 1077-1082.

AUTHOR: **TERESA DEFRANCESCO**
EDITOR: **ETIENNE CÔTÉ**

Nail and Claw Disorders

BASIC INFORMATION

DEFINITION

- Onychodystrophy: toenail deformity caused by abnormal growth
- Onychomadesis: sloughing of the nail
- Onychomycosis: fungal infection of the nail
- Onychorrhexis: brittle nails that tend to split or break
- Paronychia: inflammation of soft tissue around the nail
- Symmetric lupoid onychodystrophy (SLO): a lupus-like condition that causes sloughing (onychomadesis) of multiple nails

EPIDEMIOLOGY

SPECIES, AGE, SEX: Most nail conditions have no specific age or sex predilections other than those listed here:

- SLO: in dogs aged from 3 to 8 years, rare in cats
- Subungual squamous cell carcinoma (SCC): in older dogs
- Subungual melanomas: common in older dogs, rare in older cats
- Onychomycosis: rare in both dogs and cats

GENETICS AND BREED PREDISPOSITION

- Onychorrhexis: often noted in dachshunds
- SLO: often noted in German shepherds
- Subungual SCC: seen in large breeds (75%) and in breeds with a black coat (66%, such as in the black Labrador retriever and black poodle)

RISK FACTORS: Non-neoplastic nail disorders: immunosuppression, feline leukemia virus (FeLV) infection, vascular insult, trauma, improper trimming/care of nails, diabetes mellitus.

CONTAGION AND ZOONOSIS: Dermatophyte infections (*Microsporum canis*, *Microsporum gypseum*, *Trichophyton mentagrophytes*).

ASSOCIATED CONDITIONS AND DISORDERS

- In cats and dogs: hyperadrenocorticism, diabetes mellitus, hypothyroidism, dermatomyositis, arteriovenous fistula, cold-agglutinin disease, drug reaction, vaccine reaction, vasculitis, trauma, leishmaniasis, food allergy, atopy.
- In cats only: hyperthyroidism, primary pulmonary bronchiolar adenocarcinoma, pulmonary SCC, cutaneous SCC with metastasis.

CLINICAL PRESENTATION

HISTORY, CHIEF COMPLAINT

BACTERIAL CLAW INFECTIONS: Signs include chronic licking at affected digit(s), often with associated pain, lameness, and depression.

ONYCHOMYCOSIS

- The paronychia is associated with minimal pain and irritation.
- The history may reflect other areas of cutaneous involvement, zoonosis, and lack of response to antibiotics.

SLO: About 50% of dogs present with pain, and lameness. Others present with observed nail sloughing.

SUBUNGUAL SCC

- Usually only one digit is involved, and the animal may present as a trauma case. A mass is often noted during the nail trim.
- Paronychia, ulceration, and nail loss are commonly associated with a foul odor.

SUBUNGUAL MELANOMA

- Notable proliferation of pigmented to nonpigmented skin originates from the nail bed.
- Pruritus or pain is NOT a common complaint and the mass is typically noted when trimming the nails.

PHYSICAL EXAM FINDINGS

BACTERIAL CLAW INFECTIONS

- Inflammation around the nail bed as well as separation and purulent discharge from the nail
- One or many affected digits
- Fractured claw(s) and associated paronychia, toe swelling, purulent discharge
- Regional lymphadenopathy with fever and possible osteomyelitis
- Other clinical signs of immunocompromising conditions

ONYCHOMYCOSIS

- Paronychia present but less associated pain and irritation
- Typically only one or two affected digits and claws
- Friable and misshapen claws
- Other possible evident areas of cutaneous involvement

SLO

- Separation at the claw bed, frequently with sloughing of one or more claws (onychomadesis).
- Starts with a single abnormal claw on two or more paws; within 2 to 9 weeks, all claws on all four paws are affected.
- Regrowth of short, misshapen, dry, soft, brittle, and crumbling claws.
- Paronychia is UNCOMMON unless a secondary bacterial infection is present.

SUBUNGUAL SCC

- Single, swollen, painful toe with paronychia and associated erosive/ulcerative dermatitis
- Multiple digits affected in black Labradors and black standard poodles
- Pruritic and foul-smelling affected toes
- Misshapen or absent claws

SUBUNGUAL MELANOMA

- Solitary, well-circumscribed, dome-shaped, firm, wartlike growth
- Varies in size from 0.5-10 cm in diameter
- Possibly pigmented or nonpigmented and ulcerated

ETIOLOGY AND PATHOPHYSIOLOGY

BACTERIAL CLAW INFECTION

- Infection is secondary to an underlying etiology (trauma if one or two claws are infected; if many claws are infected, consider hypothyroidism, hyperadrenocorticism, immune-mediated condition [pemphigus], or SLO).
- *Staphyloccoccus intermedius* is the most common bacterium isolated.
- Concurrent demodicosis occurs in both single and multiple digit involvement.
- Leishmaniasis should be considered in endemic areas (the Mediterranean, limited areas in the United States).

ONYCHOMYCOSIS

- *M. canis* in cats
- *T. mentagrophytes* in dogs
- *M. gypseum* and candidiasis (yeast) less common

SYMMETRIC LUPOID ONYCHODYSTROPHY: Currently regarded as an idiopathic condition. SLO may either be a clinical manifestation of many differential diseases or an immune-mediated condition itself. Current emphasis is to look for potential underlying conditions, including hypersensitivity disorders (drug, food, environmental allergens), hormonal and metabolic abnormalities, before committing a pet to lifelong symptomatic therapy.

SUBUNGUAL SCC

- Neoplasm generally originating from the germinal epithelium of the claw
- Reverse also possible (metastasis from a primary pulmonary neoplasm to toe), more common in cats than in dogs

SUBUNGUAL MELANOMA: Malignant proliferation of melanocytes involving the nail beds in older dogs.

DIAGNOSIS

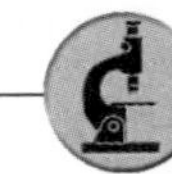

DIFFERENTIAL DIAGNOSIS

SINGLE NAIL AFFECTED
- Trauma-induced condition
- Neoplasia (high-grade mast cell tumors; fibrosarcoma, neurofibrosarcoma, eccrine carcinoma, osteosarcoma, subungual keratoacanthoma)
- Primary pulmonary bronchiolar adenocarcinoma, pulmonary SCC, and cutaneous SCC with metastasis to digits in cats

MULTIPLE NAIL INVOLVEMENT
- Metabolic disease (hypothyroidism, hyperadrenocorticism, zinc-responsive dermatosis, feline hyperthyroidism)
- Immune-mediated diseases (pemphigus complex, bullous pemphigoid, drug eruption, vasculitis, cold-agglutinin disease)

INITIAL DATABASE

- Cytologic examination of claw exudates:
  - Suppurative or pyogranulomatous inflammation with engulfed bacteria: consistent with bacterial claw infection.
  - Evidence of acantholytic cells: indicative of pemphigus.
  - Round cell tumor cells: consistent with melanoma.
- Fungal culture:
  - Indicated if a single nail/nail bed is involved.
  - DermDuets (Sabouraud's dextrose agar and Dermatophyte Test Medium): If color change occurs, a fungal wet mount is indicated to identify causative fungus (*M. canis, M. gypseum, T. mentagrophytes*).
- CBC, serum biochemistry profile, urinalysis:
  - Evidence of systemic conditions (diabetes mellitus, hyperadrenocorticism, systemic lupus erythematosus [SLE]).
- Thyroid profile:
  - Indicated if multiple nails are affected and other consistent clinical signs are present. Hypothyroidism (in dogs) and hyperthyroidism (in cats) as concurrent/causative conditions.
- Elimination diet trial:
  - Indicated if all four feet are affected and other clinical signs (otitis externa, perianal and dorsal lesions, interdigital dermatitis, gastrointestinal disturbances) are noted.
  - Restricted novel or hydrolyzed protein diets (commercial or home-prepared) for a minimum of 8 to 12 weeks before considering a dietary challenge.

ADVANCED OR CONFIRMATORY TESTING

- Bacterial culture and sensitivity (C&S): often *Staphylococcus intermedius*.
- Dermatohistopathologic exam and special stains.
  - SLO: hydropic and lichenoid interface dermatitis.
  - Rule out other immune-mediated conditions (pemphigus, bullous pemphigoid).
  - Identify fungal hyphae and arthrospores or bacterial organisms.
  - About 10% of benign melanomas (identified by histologic examination) behave malignantly.
- Intradermal/serum allergy testing: Some dogs have been reported to respond favorably to allergen specific immunotherapy.
- Antinuclear antibody (ANA) test to rule-in the possibility of a lupus condition.
- FeLV/feline immunodeficiency virus (FIV) serology.
- Radiographs:
  - Rule out osteomyelitis with bacterial claw disease.
  - Bony lysis of P3 and tissue swelling due to neoplasia.
  - Thoracic radiographs: metastasis check (e.g., feline bronchogenic carcinoma).
- Check for metastasis if SCC or melanoma is confirmed by histologic examination.
  - Fine-needle lymph node aspirates, abdominal ultrasound.

TREATMENT

THERAPEUTIC GOAL(S)

- Identify underlying etiology
- Except for cases involving only trauma, continue treatment well beyond clinical resolution (1 to 3 months)

ACUTE AND CHRONIC TREATMENT

NAIL FRACTURE OR AVULSION: The clinician should trim or file (using a Dremel Tool) any fractured nails, using sedation, analgesia, local anesthesia, or general anesthesia as necessary; remove loose claws and bandage foot. In severe conditions or patients with neoplasia, P3 amputation may be necessary.

BACTERIAL CLAW INFECTIONS
- Antibiotic therapy for 2 weeks beyond clinical resolution using cephalosporin (e.g., cephalexin 22 mg/kg PO q 8 or 30 mg/kg PO q 12h), amoxicillin-clavulanate (22 mg/kg PO q 12h), or potentiated sulfonamide (e.g., trimethoprim-sulfa 15 mg/kg PO q 12h).
- Foot scrubs: 2–4% chlorhexidine topical soaks q 12h for 7 days beyond clinical resolution.

ONYCHOMYCOSIS
- Long-term antifungal treatment on a daily or pulse basis (6 months or longer); e.g., 3 days on and 4 days off (ketoconazole) or 1 week on and 1 week off (itraconazole).
- Ketoconazole (10 mg/kg PO q 24h), itraconazole (5–10 mg/kg PO q 24h), fluconazole (5 mg/kg PO q 24h), or terbinafine (10–40 mg/kg PO q 24h) on a continuous or pulse-dosing regimen. The clinician or client must make sure the animal takes the azoles with food for maximal efficacy.
- Treatment is continued 1 to 3 months beyond complete nail regrowth and a negative repeat fungal culture from nail trimmings.
- Topical antifungal products include chlorhexidine, miconazole, clotrimazole, terbinafine, enilconazole, or lime sulfur.

SYMMETRIC LUPOID ONYCHODYSTROPHY: Varying combinations of these treatments are used based on individual response and tolerance.
- Omega-3 fatty acids (36 mg/kg PO q 24h) and omega-6 fatty acids (500–1000 mg PO q 24h) for a minimum of 3 months, then as maintenance therapy.
- Vitamin E (10–20 IU/kg PO q 12h to q 8h) for a minimum of 3 months or longer if improved.
- Novel or hydrolyzed restricted diet for 8 to 12 weeks to eliminate an adverse food reaction as the trigger for the disorder.
- Tetracycline and niacinamide (500 mg of each for dogs >10 kg; 250 mg of each for dogs <10 kg) PO q 8h, until improvement (about 2 to 3 months); then taper the medication monthly. Doxycycline (5–10 mg/kg q 12h) may be substituted for tetracycline.
- Prednisone (2–4 mg/kg PO q 24h induction, weaning based on a favorable response) alone or with azathioprine (2.2 mg/kg PO q 24–48h) as a corticosteroid-sparing agent (monitor for myelosuppression, pancreatitis, opportunistic infection).
- Pentoxifylline (10–30 mg/kg PO q 8–12h) until resolution of lesions; then taper the medication monthly.
- Cyclosporine (2.5–5 mg/kg PO q 12h microemulsion [Atopica, Neoral]) until resolved, then taper to lowest frequency that controls relapse of clinical signs.
- Onychectomy (P3 amputation) as a last resort.

SUBUNGUAL SCC
- Poststaging amputation of the affected digit to the proximal interphalangeal level.
- As SCC is locally invasive and metastasis rate is low, there appears to be no need for adjunctive chemotherapy or radiation therapy.

SUBUNGUAL MELANOMA
- Radical surgical excision of both malignant and benign areas
- Follow-up chemotherapy or radiation therapy

DRUG INTERACTION

Cyclosporine use in conjunction with ketoconazole requires that the daily dose of the former be halved due to ketoconazole's effect on the cP450 enzyme and p-glycoprotein pump.

POSSIBLE COMPLICATIONS

Ketoconazole may cause anorexia, gastric irritation, and hepatic toxicity.

RECOMMENDED MONITORING

Rechecks and monitoring depend on underlying cause

PROGNOSIS AND OUTCOME

Bacterial claw infections

- Generally good for complete resolution
- Protracted course of therapy (about 3 to 6 months) may be necessary to reach this end point
- Response may be influenced by underlying immunosuppressive factors

Onychomycosis

- Prognosis is good to guarded due to incomplete resolution
- May require either P3 amputation or pulse antifungal therapy for life
- Response may be influenced by underlying immunosuppressive factors

SLO

- Chronic and recurrent problem if not treated
- Clinical improvement is usually seen within 3 to 4 months; if not, change therapies
- Nail regrowth is good although nails may be slightly deformed or friable
- Refractory cases may require P3 amputation

Subungual SCC

- Locally invasive with low metastatic potential: regional node or distant metastasis in < 30% of cases
- The 1- and 2-year survival rates are 95% and 75%, respectively, if subungual; rates are 60% and 40%, respectively, if not specifically from the subungual region as determined via a dermatohistopathologic examination.

Subungual melanomas

- Good if benign; poor if malignant. About 50% of dogs die because of distant metastasis.

PEARLS & CONSIDERATIONS

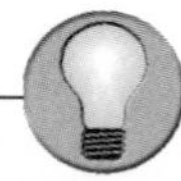

COMMENTS

- When reevaluating the nails, look for normalization of growth patterns at the base of the nail.
- Shortening nails using a nail file or Dremel tool tends to be more readily accepted by pets affected with fragile nails.
- Taper immunomodulatory medications gradually and treat for several months beyond clinical resolution.

PREVENTION

Routine nail care will result in early detection of nail and nail bed disorders

CLIENT EDUCATION

Patience is required as nails grow slowly

SUGGESTED READING

Mueller RS, Rosychuk RAW, Jonas LD: A retrospective study regarding the treatment of lupoid onychodystrophy in 30 dogs and literature review. *J Am Anim Hosp Assoc* 139-150, 2003.

Scott DW, Miller WH, Griffin CE: *Muller and Kirk's Small Animal Dermatology*, ed 6. Philadelphia, WB Saunders, 2001, pp 1190-1200.

Withrow S: *Small Animal Clinical Oncology*. Philadelphia, WB Saunders, 2001, pp 254-255.

AUTHOR: **ANTHONY YU**
EDITOR: **JAN A. HALL**

Narcolepsy

BASIC INFORMATION

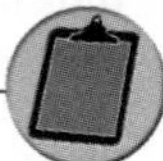

DEFINITION

- A syndrome in which abnormalities in the sleep-wake cycle are manifested as excessive sleepiness and cataplexy.
- Excessive sleepiness is characterized by waxing and waning drowsiness and abrupt onsets of falling asleep.
- Cataplexy is a brief episode of flaccid paralysis, without altered consciousness, that is usually elicited by excitement or emotion.
- Cataplexy is the clinical sign most commonly seen in narcoleptic domestic animals, whereas excessive sleepiness is the more common sign in humans.

EPIDEMIOLOGY

SPECIES, AGE, SEX

- Narcolepsy has been reported in more than 17 canine breeds, cats, cattle, and horses.
- Age of onset of clinical signs is typically between 4 and 24 weeks of age in genetically narcoleptic dogs and between 7 weeks and 7 years in sporadically narcoleptic dogs.
- There is no apparent sex predisposition.

GENETICS AND BREED PREDISPOSITION: Narcolepsy is inherited with autosomal recessive transmission in the Doberman pinscher, Labrador retriever, and dachshund and occurs sporadically in other breeds of dogs. Clinical signs are often most severe in small dog breeds.

CLINICAL PRESENTATION

HISTORY, CHIEF COMPLAINT

- Cataplexy is the most common clinical sign and is manifested by partial to complete paralysis that may involve all muscles or may be restricted to certain limbs or the head and trunk.
  - Consciousness is maintained at the onset of the attack; however, prolonged episodes may lead to rapid eye movement (REM) sleep.
  - The episodes typically occur spontaneously and are usually elicited by excitement, food, or play.
  - There is an abrupt onset as well as termination of the attack, and the attack may be disrupted by a loud noise or stimulation of the animal.
  - Episodes may last a few seconds to more than 30 minutes.
- Excessive sleepiness is characterized by prolonged periods of sleep, difficulty arousing the dog during sleep, and apparent drowsiness throughout the day.
- Sleep attacks, during which the animal is unconscious with closed eyelids and mild twitching of the face and distal limbs, may occur from an awake, active state.

PHYSICAL EXAM FINDINGS: Physical examination and neurologic examination are typically within normal limits, with the exception of any episodes that may occur.

ETIOLOGY AND PATHOPHYSIOLOGY

- The narcolepsy syndrome is associated with a deficit in hypocretin (orexin) neurotransmission.
- Hypocretin is an excitatory peptide neurotransmitter produced in the hypothalamus. It binds to cell membrane receptors in nuclei, such as the locus ceruleus, that are responsible for normal sleep mechanisms. The locus ceruleus is also the source of norepinephrine that regulates REM sleep as an inhibitory mechanism.
- Canine narcoleptics have normal amounts of hypocretin but lack the receptor to which it binds.
- Mutations in hypocretin-receptor-2 gene were found in the familial form (canarc-1), and losses of hypocretin ligand have been associated with sporadic canine narcolepsy.

DIAGNOSIS

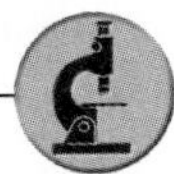

DIFFERENTIAL DIAGNOSIS

Narcolepsy must be distinguished from other paroxysmal disorders, such as epilepsy, syncope, myasthenia gravis, and metabolic disorders (hypoglycemia, hypocalcemia, etc.).

INITIAL DATABASE

Basic clinical pathologic and imaging studies are typically within normal limits.

ADVANCED OR CONFIRMATORY TESTING

- Cerebrospinal fluid may contain a decreased hypocretin-1 concentration (<80 pg/ml; the normal range is 250-350 pg/ml).
- The food-elicited cataplexy test (FECT) is helpful in diagnosing cataplexy and is performed by placing pieces of food at set intervals apart and timing the animal while it consumes the food.
  - A normal animal should be able to consume the food in a short period of time (<45 sec).
  - Narcoleptic animals may need more time (more than 2 min) to consume the food because of partial to complete cataplexy, which is evident on observation of the test.
- Mildly affected animals may need pharmacologic testing to confirm a cataplectic attack.
  - Physostigmine salicylate, a cholinesterase inhibitor that crosses the blood-brain barrier, is given (0.025-0.1 mg/kg IV). Physostigmine increases the chances of spontaneous or elicited cataplectic attacks within 5-15 min in susceptible animals. The side effects of this drug are excessive salivation and diarrhea.

TREATMENT

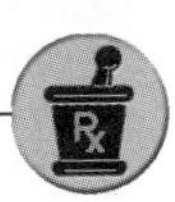

THERAPEUTIC GOAL(S)

A treatment goal is controlling cataplexy because the impact of excessive sleepiness is less in dogs than it is in humans.

CHRONIC TREATMENT

- Cataplexy is treated with tricyclic antidepressants that act by blocking cellular norepinephrine reuptake in the central nervous system.
  - Imipramine (1 mg/kg PO q 8h) has been used successfully in the long-term treatment of cataplexy. Imipramine also blocks serotonin reuptake.
  - Other tricyclic antidepressants used include amitriptyline (2.2-4.4 mg/kg PO q 24h), desipramine and protryptiline.
- Excessive sleepiness is treated with stimulant sympathomimetics such as methylphenidate (0.1 mg/kg PO q 24h) or dextroamphetamine.
- Selegiline (2 mg/kg PO q 24h) is a monoamine oxidase B inhibitor that has been an effective anticataplectic drug through its metabolism to amphetamine and methamphetamine and by increasing dopamine levels in the central nervous system (CNS).

RECOMMENDED MONITORING

Clinicians should order routine blood screening and cardiovascular evaluation prior to and periodically after the initiation of therapy with tricyclic antidepressants.

PROGNOSIS AND OUTCOME

- Cataplectic attacks are generally not life threatening, and although there is no cure, the clinical signs are usually successfully minimized with treatment.
- Some animals may improve with no treatment.

PEARLS & CONSIDERATIONS

COMMENTS

Abrupt withdrawal of medication can lead to increased cataplexy, so clinicians should warn clients not to discontinue medications quickly.

SUGGESTED READING

Coleman ES: Canine narcolepsy and the role of the nervous system. *Comp Cont Ed Pract Vet* 21 (7):641-650, 1999.

Thomas WB: Seizures and narcolepsy. In Dewey CW (ed): *A Practical Guide to Canine and Feline Neurology*. Ames, IA, Iowa State Press, 2003, pp 208-209.

AUTHOR: **KERRY SMITH BAILEY**
EDITOR: **CURTIS W. DEWEY**

Nasal Cutaneous Disorders

BASIC INFORMATION

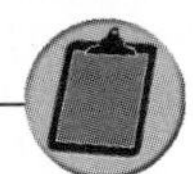

DEFINITION

Dermatoses affecting the bridge of the nose (haired) or the nasal planum (hairless)

EPIDEMIOLOGY

SPECIES, AGE, SEX

- Affects dogs and cats.
- Diseases more likely to appear in dogs younger than 1 year of age: demodicosis, dermatophytosis, dermatomyositis, hereditary nasal parakeratosis, juvenile cellulitis.
- Epitheliotropic (cutaneous) lymphoma is more commonly seen in older dogs.

GENETICS AND BREED PREDISPOSITION

- Nasal parakeratosis: Labrador retrievers (Fig. I-119).
- Zinc-responsive dermatosis: Alaskan malamutes, Siberian huskies.
- Dermatomyositis: collies, Shetland sheepdogs, Beauceron shepherds.
- Uveodermatologic syndrome: Akitas, Samoyeds, Siberian huskies, chow chows.
- Systemic lupus erythematosus (SLE) and cutaneous (discoid) lupus erythematosus (DLE): collies, Shetland sheepdogs, German shepherds.
- Nasal arteritis: Saint Bernards.
- Alopecia and melanoderma: Yorkshire terriers.

- Familial vasculopathy: German shepherds, Scottish terriers.
- Acrodermatitis: bull terriers.
- Lentigo simplex: orange cats.

RISK FACTORS

- Sun exposure can cause or aggravate canine and feline solar dermatitis, DLE, SLE, and pemphigus erythematosus.
- Lack of skin pigmentation can predispose the animal to sun damage.
- Immunosuppression may predispose the animal to infectious diseases.
- Susceptible dogs fed diets high in phytates (high-cereal) or in minerals such as calcium can develop zinc-responsive dermatosis.
- Outdoor animals are more susceptible to contagious diseases.

CONTAGION AND ZOONOSIS

- Dermatophytosis is contagious to other animals and is a zoonotic disease.
- Sporotrichosis (especially feline) has a zoonotic potential.
- Accidental inoculation of *Blastomyces dermatitidis* has been reported in people handling specimens from affected animals.

GEOGRAPHY AND SEASONALITY

- Animals living in sunny climates more commonly develop photoaggravated dermatitis.
- Animals living in areas endemic for leishmaniasis are susceptible to the disease.

ASSOCIATED CONDITIONS AND DISORDERS

- Granulomatous uveitis in uveodermatologic syndrome
- Systemic disease in SLE
- Hepatopathy or glucagon producing pancreatic tumor in hepatocutanous syndrome (superficial necrolytic dermatitis)

CLINICAL PRESENTATION

HISTORY, CHIEF COMPLAINT: Presentation depends on the underlying disease.

- Nonpruritic hair loss confined to the nose (e.g., localized demodicosis, localized dermatophytosis) or with a generalized dermatopathy (e.g., generalized demodicosis, dermatophytosis, endocrine imbalances).
- Pruritus and facial rubbing with secondary nasal alopecia in cases of allergic disease or intranasal foreign bodies (usually accompanied by sneezing and/or nasal discharge).
- Erosions and ulcers in cases of immune-mediated diseases or nodules and plaques (e.g., neoplastic, fungal diseases).
- Signs of systemic illness may be reported concurrently with generalized disorders (e.g., systemic mycoses, systemic lupus erythematosus).

PHYSICAL EXAM FINDINGS

- Depigmentation or hyperpigmentation
- Alopecia
- Erythema
- Papules/pustules/vesicles
- Crusts
- Erosions/ulcers
- Hyperkeratosis (Fig. I-119)
- Nodules/plaques

ETIOLOGY AND PATHOPHYSIOLOGY

Nasal lesions arise following various pathomechanisms, including the following:

- Infectious agents, which induce an immune response from the host, resulting in tissue inflammatory cell infiltrates (folliculitis, furunculosis, granulomatous lesions, etc.).
- Altered keratinization (proliferation, differentiation, or desquamation), resulting in hyperkeratosis.
- The development of antibodies or activated lymphocytes against normal body constituents (autoimmune diseases) or against inciting antigens (drugs, bacteria, viruses), which leads to tissue damage.
- Defective melanin production or a destruction of melanocytes leading to pigment disorders; a disturbance at the basal epidermal cell level can cause hypopigmentation.
- Solar exposure of poorly pigmented nasal skin, resulting in a phototoxic reaction (sunburn); immune-mediated diseases, such as pemphigus erythematosus, SLE, and DLE, can also be photoaggravated.

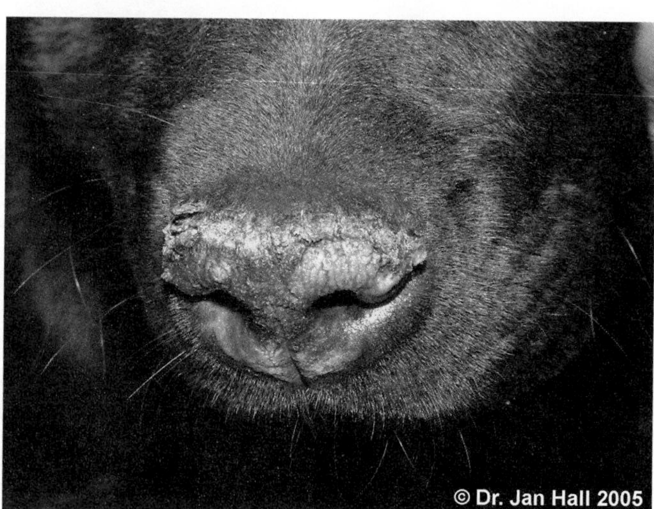

FIGURE I-119 Nasal parakeratosis in a Labrador retriever. Courtesy of Dr. Jan A. Hall.

DIAGNOSIS

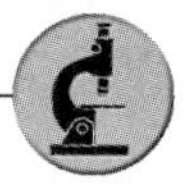

DIFFERENTIAL DIAGNOSIS

- Infectious
  - Bacterial: mucocutaneous pyoderma, nasal pyoderma, feline leprosy.
  - Fungal: dermatophytosis, sporotrichosis, cryptococcosis, blastomycosis, aspergillosis.
  - Parasitic: demodicosis (bridge of the nose).
  - Protozoal: leishmaniasis.
  - Rickettsial: canine Rocky Mountain spotted fever, canine ehrlichiosis.
  - Viral: canine distemper, facial dermatitis associated with herpesvirus infection in cats.
- Immune-mediated: pemphigus foliaceus and erythematosus, SLE, DLE, uveodermatologic syndrome, nasal arteritis, canine eosinophilic furunculosis of the face, feline mosquito bite hypersensitivity.
- Hereditary (see Genetics and Breed Predisposition above).
- Pigmentary: nasal depigmentation ("Dudley nose"), seasonal nasal hypopigmentation ("snow nose"), vitiligo, alopecia and melanoderma, lentigo simplex.
- Metabolic/endocrine: hepatocutaneous syndrome, canine hypothyroidism.
- Nutritional: zinc-responsive dermatosis.
- Environmental/traumatic: canine and feline solar dermatitis, contact dermatitis, local trauma.
- Drug eruption: from topical or systemic administration.
- Neoplastic: squamous cell carcinoma (SCC), basal cell carcinoma, epitheliotropic lymphoma, fibroma, feline "sarcoid," and other such conditions.
- Miscellaneous: idiopathic sterile granulomas and pyogranulomas, cutaneous and systemic histiocytosis, idiopathic nasal hyperkeratosis.

INITIAL DATABASE

Usefulness of different diagnostic tests is based on history and physical examination.

- Skin scrapings: *Demodex* spp.
- Wood's lamp: dermatophytosis (fluorescent strains of *Microsporum canis*).
- Cytologic tests: phagocytized bacteria, inflammatory cells, acantholytic keratinocytes (pemphigus), fungal organisms.
- Complete blood count/serum biochemistry profile/urinalysis: The results depend on underlying cause and are often normal or with nonspecific changes when cause is not systemic.

- Ocular examination: uveitis (uveodermatologic syndrome).
- Thoracic and abdominal imaging, if relevant, to confirm systemic disease or stage tumors.

ADVANCED OR CONFIRMATORY TESTING

- Skin biopsies for histopathologic evaluation and possible immunofluorescence or immunohistochemical staining. Using general anesthesia, nasal planum lesions can be biopsied with a 4-mm biopsy punch. The lesion should be centered in the specimen. If possible, multiple specimens should be taken of primary lesions (e.g., pustules, papules, bullae). Crusted lesions or depigmented lesions can also be useful.
- Culture: bacterial, fungal.
- Antinuclear antibody (ANA) test: positive in virtually all patients with SLE.
- Endocrine testing or serology if relevant.

TREATMENT

THERAPEUTIC GOAL(S)

- Permanent cure or control of the disease
- Sometimes palliative treatment (neoplasia)

ACUTE GENERAL TREATMENT

Treatment depends on the etiology of the lesions. If the animal has undergone prior, recent treatment and a drug reaction is suspected, the animal should avoid contact with the offending medication.

CHRONIC TREATMENT

Infectious diseases may be cured with appropriate treatment. Other diseases may need chronic maintenance treatment.

RECOMMENDED MONITORING

Will depend on the disease and selected medication

PROGNOSIS AND OUTCOME

Variable, depending on the underlying disease

PEARLS & CONSIDERATIONS

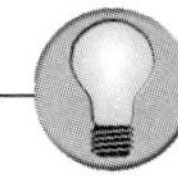

COMMENTS

Skin biopsies are often needed for diagnosis of nasal cutaneous disorders.

PREVENTION

- Prevent sun exposure and use of sunscreens on poorly pigmented animals and/or with photoaggravated diseases.
- Discourage breeding of animals with hereditary diseases.

SUGGESTED READING

Scott DW, Miller WH, Griffin CE: *Muller and Kirk's Small Animal Dermatology*, ed 6. Philadelphia, WB Saunders, 2001.

AUTHOR: **NADIA PAGÉ**
EDITOR: **JAN A. HALL**

Nasal Discharge

BASIC INFORMATION

DEFINITION

- A discharge from the external nares.
- Although usually obvious, the discharge can sometimes be missed due to licking or caudal drainage.
- The underlying etiology of the discharge can be intranasal or extranasal disease.
- The type and duration of the discharge varies with the underlying cause.

EPIDEMIOLOGY

SPECIES, AGE, SEX

- Younger cats may have viral upper respiratory infections (see Upper Respiratory Infection, Feline, p 1115) or nasopharyngeal polyps (see Nasopharyngeal Polyp, p 739).
- Younger unvaccinated dogs are more likely to have canine viral respiratory infections.
- Younger animals may have congenital deformities, such as a cleft palate.
- Older animals are more likely to have neoplastic or dental-related causes of nasal discharge.
- Hunting and working dogs are more likely to have nasal foreign bodies.

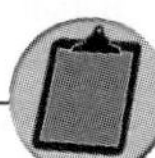

GENETICS AND BREED PREDISPOSITION

- Brachycephalic breeds have upper airway problems that may lead to nasal discharge.
- Dolichocephalic breeds may be more prone to nasal neoplasia.
- Several specific breeds can be affected by primary ciliary dyskinesia (see Primary Ciliary Dyskinesia, p 889) or by cleft palate-cleft lip complex (see Cleft Palate, p 215).

RISK FACTORS

- Lack of adequate immunization against viral respiratory infections
- Exposure to unvaccinated animals and high-density husbandry/housing situations
- Geographic locations where grass awns are ubiquitous
- Dental disease and poor dental care
- Immunosuppression (fungal disease)
- Compromise of nasal mucosa (secondary bacterial infections)
- Outdoor exposure (infection, foreign bodies, trauma)

CONTAGION AND ZOONOSIS: Viral upper and lower respiratory tract infections.
GEOGRAPHY AND SEASONALITY: Geographic locations where grass awns are ubiquitous (dogs) or where there is lush green grass (blade of grass foreign bodies in outdoor cats).
ASSOCIATED CONDITIONS AND DISORDERS: Sneezing.

CLINICAL PRESENTATION

DISEASE FORMS/SUBTYPES: Types of nasal discharge:

- Serous: clear and watery (acellular).
- Mucoid: clear and thick (acellular with high protein content).
- Purulent: yellow-tan and thick (neutrophilic with bacteria).
- Sanguineous: red-tinged (blood mixed with another type of discharge).
- Hemorrhagic (epistaxis): frank red blood.

HISTORY, CHIEF COMPLAINT: Acute onset of paroxysmal sneezing or nasal discharge may suggest nasal foreign bodies or an early viral disease. Husbandry and management predispose animals to certain disorders. Examples: recent boarding or exposure to new animals (viral infections); hunting and geographic location (nasal foreign bodies); pertinent medical history (dental disease, history of neoplasia, immunosuppression); exposure to irritating aerosols (hairspray, paints, etc.); vaccine history (viral respiratory tract infections).
A complete history should include:

- Recent exposure to new or young animals (infectious diseases)
- Environmental risk factors, such as inhaled irritants, foreign bodies, exposure to rodenticides
- Pertinent medical history, such as hypertension, current medications, or a history of neoplasia
- Vaccination status
- Acute versus chronic onset (acute onset more likely to be caused by foreign bodies and early viral infection)

PHYSICAL EXAM FINDINGS

- Serous, mucopurulent, or hemorrhagic discharge that may be unilateral or bilateral
- Concurrently possible, suggesting an intranasal or local problem:
  - Facial deformity
  - Exophthalmos
  - Tooth root abscess, oronasal fistula
  - Ocular discharge (e.g., with local disorders, such as an intranasal mass obstructing the nasolacrimal duct)
  - Pawing at face
- Concurrently possible, suggesting an extranasal or systemic problem:
  - Ocular discharge (e.g., with systemic infections, such as canine distemper)
  - Petechiation, ecchymoses (bleeding disorder)

ETIOLOGY AND PATHOPHYSIOLOGY

- Serous: due to local irritation, early viral infection, allergic rhinitis, or excessive lacrimation.
- Mucoid: due to chronic noninfectious irritation and overproduction of mucus by nasal epithelial cells.
- Purulent: usually due to secondary bacterial infection.
- Sanguineous: due to compromise of the nasal mucosa.
- Hemorrhagic (epistaxis): due to local or systemic causes of bleeding.

DIAGNOSIS

DIFFERENTIAL DIAGNOSIS

- Feline viral upper respiratory tract infections (feline rhinotracheitis, feline calicivirus, *Chlamydia psittaci*)
- Neoplasia (adenocarcinoma, lymphosarcoma, undifferentiated carcinoma, osteosarcoma, chondrosarcoma, fibrosarcoma, transmissible venereal tumor)
- Foreign bodies
- Tooth root abscess, oronasal fistula.
- Nasopharyngeal polyps (cats)
- Canine viral infections (canine distemper virus, canine parainfluenza virus, canine herpesvirus, canine adenovirus, types 1 and 2)
- Mycotic infection (*Aspergillus* spp. in dogs; *Cryptococcus neoformans* in cats)
- Parasitic rhinitis (*Cuterebra* spp., *Pneumonyssoides caninum*, *Linguatala serrata*)
- Bacterial infections (usually secondary)
- Rhinitis (allergic/eosinophilic type I hypersensitivity, lymphoplasmacytic, chronic hyperplastic)
- Congenital defects (cleft palate-cleft lip complex, primary ciliary dyskinesia)
- Trauma
- Inhaled irritants (cat litter dust, aerosols, smoke)
- Epistaxis (local causes: mycotic infections, neoplasia, foreign body, trauma; systemic causes: inherited or acquired coagulopathies, thrombocytopenia, thrombocytopathia, hypertension, vasculitides)

INITIAL DATABASE

- Physical assessment for unilateral versus bilateral nasal disease performed by holding a glass microscope slide close to the external nares while holding the animal's mouth closed. When the animal exhales through the nose, steam will be present asymmetrically or unilaterally (one naris obstructed) or not at all (both nares obstructed). Neoplasia, foreign bodies, and dental disease are often causes of unilateral nasal disease and discharge, while other local and systemic conditions often result in bilateral disease.
- Oral examination to look for hard palate masses.
- Fundic examination to look for evidence of neoplasia, fungal disease, hypertension, and associated retinal hemorrhage.
- Eye globe retropulsion to assess for retrobulbar masses.
- Blood pressure measurement to assess for systemic hypertension.
- Complete blood count (CBC) including platelet count to look for evidence of infection, inflammation, or thrombocytopenia.
- Serum biochemistry profile.
- Feline leukemia and feline immunodeficiency viral testing.
- Thoracic radiographs (pneumonia, metastatic disease); pneumonia commonly causes mucopurulent nasal discharge, and the reverse process (primary nasal discharge causing a secondary pneumonia) virtually never occurs.

ADVANCED OR CONFIRMATORY TESTING

Any of the following may be indicated depending on signalment, history, and preliminary exam findings: Rocky Mountain spotted fever, *Ehrlichia*, and *Bartonella* testing; prothrombin time; partial thromboplastin time; thoracic radiographs; nasal swabs; fungal titer determinations; nasal radiography; computed tomography (CT); rhinoscopy; biopsy; deep tissue cultures; and exploratory rhinotomy.

TREATMENT

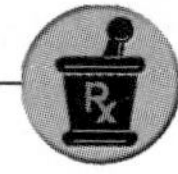

THERAPEUTIC GOAL(S)

- Eliminate underlying etiology of nasal discharge
- Restore normal nasal function
- Reduce pain and discomfort
- Provide supportive care
- Relieve dyspnea, especially in cats that often will not readily breathe with an open mouth

ACUTE GENERAL TREATMENT

- If discharge is causing dyspnea, then oxygen therapy may be needed.
- Treatment for underlying coagulopathy (e.g., vitamin K_1 (0.25–2.5 mg/kg for first-generation rodenticide intoxication or 2.5–5.0 mg/kg for second-generation rodenticide intoxication, SC or PO divided q 12h, 7–21 days, and fresh frozen plasma transfusion).
- Correct dehydration and electrolyte abnormalities as necessary.
- Broad-spectrum antibiotics if secondary nasal/dental infection (bacteria are rarely the primary cause of nasal disease, but secondary infection with normal nasal flora is common) or pneumonia (culture and sensitivity [C&S] test for the lower airways is essential if pneumonia is present). *Bartonella* spp. have been recently implicated as a cause of chronic rhinitis and epistaxis; azithromycin is the drug of choice (5–10 mg/kg PO q 24h; start at 5 mg/kg and, if tolerated, increase by 2.5 mg/kg each day. After 1 week, reduce to q 48h).
- Analgesics if painful (e.g., opiates such as buprenorphine 0.006–0.01 mg/kg IV/IM q 6–8h; nonsteroidal anti-inflammatory drugs [NSAIDs], such as deracoxib 1–2 mg/kg PO q 24h can also be used). Use NSAID analgesics with caution if the animal has a history of concurrent renal, liver, gastrointestinal, or hemostatic disorders.
- Clinicians should remove the animal from environmental agents (e.g., smoke, dust); if not possible, the clinician should introduce measures to reduce exposure (e.g., air filtration systems).
- Clinicians should consider recommending surgery for treating dental disease, neoplasia, nasopharyngeal polyps, cleft palate, foreign bodies, or traumatic causes.
- Rhinoscopy may be useful for removing a foreign body.
- Radiation and/or chemotherapy for neoplasia as appropriate (based on biopsy results).
- Fungal: local or systemic treatment depending on type of mycotic infection.
- Parasitic rhinitis: ivermectin 0.2 mg/kg SC or PO, twice during a 3-week period (treatment reported to be successful).

- Decongestants and cleaning of the nares (e.g., topical pseudoephedrine [pediatric Neo-Synephrine, 1 drop in alternating nares once daily]).

CHRONIC TREATMENT

- Nutrition: cats especially may not eat if unable to smell food. Consider feeding tube (e.g., esophagostomy; see Feeding Tube Placement: Esophagostomy Tube, p 1243) for nutritional support.
- Analgesics.
- Antibiotics for secondary infections.
- In animals with chronic rhinitis, antihistamines, inhaled corticosteroids, and systemic NSAIDs may provide some relief (see Rhinitis, Bacterial, p 970, and Rhinitis, Lymphoplasmacytic, p 971).

POSSIBLE COMPLICATIONS

- Anorexia (especially in cats with severe nasal congestion)
- Keratitis (feline viral upper respiratory infections)
- Upper airway obstruction following extubation after general anesthesia
- Hemorrhage following surgery or rhinoscopy
- Dehiscence of surgical site (e.g., cleft palate)
- Progression of underlying disease

RECOMMENDED MONITORING

- Respiratory rate and effort; ventilation and oxygenation
- Appetite
- Ongoing hemorrhage
- Volume and nature of discharge
- Monitoring as normal for antimicrobials and NSAIDs
- Appropriate laboratory testing or diagnostic imaging (packed cell volume, total solids, prothrombin time/partial thromboplastin time, etc.), depending on underlying disease

PROGNOSIS AND OUTCOME

- Dependent on etiology.
- Good if the underlying problem is canine viral upper respiratory tract infection or foreign body or if the animal has undergone a successful surgery or tooth extraction.
- Guarded for feline chronic viral upper respiratory tract infections; low-grade nasal congestion and discharge, with periodic flare-ups, may become persistent or lifelong.
- Guarded to good for fungal rhinitis, depending on response to therapy.
- Poor if neoplasia is not amenable to surgery and radiation therapy.

PEARLS & CONSIDERATIONS

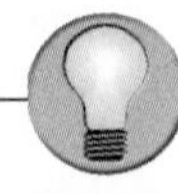

COMMENTS

Determining whether nasal discharge is unilateral or bilateral is a simple but critical first step in diagnosis. Neoplasia, foreign bodies, dental disease, and other conditions are common causes of unilateral nasal disease and discharge, while other local and systemic causes often result in bilateral disease.

PREVENTION

- Isolation of cats with viral infections
- Appropriate vaccination regime and retroviral testing
- Good dental care
- Limited exposure to irritating aerosols or materials

SUGGESTED READING

Doust R, Sullivan M: Nasal discharge, sneezing, and reverse sneezing. In King LG (ed): *Textbook of Respiratory Disease in Dogs and Cats*. St. Louis, WB Saunders, 2004, pp 17–29.

Hawkins EC: Clinical manifestations of nasal disease. In Nelson RW, Couto CG (eds): *Small Animal Internal Medicine*. St. Louis, Mosby, 1998, pp 206–231.

McKiernan BC: Sneezing and nasal discharge. In Ettinger SJ, Feldman EC (eds): *Textbook of Veterinary Internal Medicine*. Philadelphia, WB Saunders, 2000, pp 194–197.

AUTHORS: **ANDREW J. BROWN, ELISE MITTLEMAN, LESLEY G. KING**
EDITOR: **ETIENNE CÔTÉ**

Nasal Neoplasia

BASIC INFORMATION

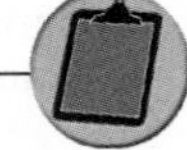

DEFINITION

Neoplastic growth, usually malignant, originating in the nasal passages

SYNONYM(S)

Nasal tumors

EPIDEMIOLOGY

SPECIES, AGE, SEX

- Cats: uncommon (1% of all tumors), with older, neutered male cats most often affected (mean age 8 to 10 years, earliest age 2 years).
- Dogs: nasal tumors represent 1–2.4% of all tumors in dogs. Older dogs (mean 9 to 10 years) most often affected (earliest reported age of 1 year); possible male predilection.

GENETICS AND BREED PREDISPOSITION: Airedale terriers, basset hounds, collies, German shepherds, German shorthaired pointers, keeshonds, and old English sheepdogs are thought to have an increased risk.

RISK FACTORS: Possible, but not consistently proven, risk factors include large size (large breed), dolichocephalicism, urban environment, and exposure to secondhand smoke.

ASSOCIATED CONDITIONS AND DISORDERS: Seizures or behavior changes from direct tumor invasion into the brain are possible. Paraneoplastic hypercalcemia and erythrocytosis are rare.

CLINICAL PRESENTATION

DISEASE FORMS/SUBTYPES

- Malignant tumors:
  - Epithelial:
    - Adenocarcinomas, squamous cell carcinomas, and other carcinomas account for approximately two-thirds of nasal tumors.
  - Mesenchymal:
    - Chondrosarcoma is the most common.
    - Osteosarcoma can occur.
    - Lymphosarcoma is more common in cats.
  - Miscellaneous:
    - Transmissible venereal tumors.
    - Olfactory neuroblastoma.
    - Melanoma.
- Benign tumors:
  - Epithelial or mesenchymal.
  - Inflammatory polyps.

HISTORY, CHIEF COMPLAINT

- Epistaxis (can be intermittent)
- Bilateral or unilateral nasal discharge (can be intermittent)
- Airflow obstruction
- Sneezing or reverse sneezing
- Stertor
- Facial deformity (nasal bones, malpositioned eyes)
- Pain with opening mouth; dysphagia

- Neurologic signs (seizures, mentation, or behavior changes), which are rare but can be the only clinical sign of nasal tumors

PHYSICAL EXAM FINDINGS: Same as chief complaints.

- Airflow obstruction may be detected via a mirror or glass held at the nares or from an occlusion of one nostril at a time while listening to airflow at the opening of the nares.
- Stertor.
- Mandibular lymph node enlargement.
- Diminished ocular retropulsion; pain with ocular retropulsion or opening mouth.
- Altered mentation.
- Physical exam may be unremarkable because dogs and cats frequently lick nasal discharge away.

ETIOLOGY AND PATHOPHYSIOLOGY

Exposure to urban environmental pollution and secondhand smoke, exposure to wood dust, as well as exposure to toxins emitted from boot making and flooring industry work have been weakly linked with the onset of nasal tumors; pollutants filtered in the nasal passages can initiate or promote neoplastic transformation.

DIAGNOSIS

DIFFERENTIAL DIAGNOSIS

- Epistaxis (see Epistaxis, p 354):
  - Inherited or acquired coagulopathies
  - Infectious diseases:
    - Ehrlichiosis
    - Babesiosis
    - Leishmaniasis
    - Rocky Mountain spotted fever
  - Trauma.
- Nasal discharge, obstruction, sneezing or reverse sneezing:
  - Foreign body
  - Granuloma
  - Fungal rhinitis or sinusitis
  - Tooth root abscess
  - Nasal mites
  - Allergic rhinitis

INITIAL DATABASE

- Inflammatory leukogram.
- Mild to moderate anemia that can be nonregenerative or microcytic.
- Hypoproteinemia if severe hemorrhage (uncommon).
- Mandibular lymph node aspiration may show metastasis (10% of cases at diagnosis).
- Thoracic radiographs are usually normal, but metastasis may occasionally be seen.

ADVANCED OR CONFIRMATORY TESTING

- Nasal imaging:
  - Computed tomography (CT) or magnetic resonance imaging (MRI) best identify and define the full extent of a tumor and can aid in distinguishing a tumor mass from fluid and surrounding tissues.
  - Radiographs are less sensitive, but dorsoventral intraoral and rostrocaudal frontal sinus views may identify loss of turbinates and increased density in the normally air-filled sinuses.
  - Imaging should be performed prior to biopsy whenever possible.
- Rhinoscopy may demonstrate a mass in the nasal cavity.
- Biopsy:
  - Blind transnasal core biopsy, with the location determined by previous imaging, provides the best samples.
  - Samples obtained with rhinoscopic guidance may be too small for accurate diagnosis.
  - Rhinotomy may be needed to obtain diagnostic samples, although this procedure is rarely required.

TREATMENT

THERAPEUTIC GOAL(S)

Alleviate signs; cure is possible, but rare

ACUTE GENERAL TREATMENT

- Epistaxis. Treatment measures include:
  - Sedation of the patient.
  - Packing of the nasal passages with gauze or phenylephrine-soaked or epinephrine-soaked gauze.
  - Application of cold compresses to the patient's nose.
  - Ligation of the ipsilateral carotid artery (rarely needed).
- Nasal congestion, discharge:
  - Antimicrobials for secondary bacterial infections, based on a culture and sensitivity (C&S) test.
  - Anti-inflammatory medications (steroidal [e.g., prednisone 1 mg/kg PO q 24-48h] or nonsteroidal [e.g., carprofen 2 mg/kg PO q 12h]) may help, but these should be used cautiously due to the possible risk of adverse effects and should not be used simultaneously in the same patient.

CHRONIC TREATMENT

- External beam radiation therapy is considered definitive therapy.
- Chemotherapy (e.g., cisplatin) may palliate signs for 5 to 6 months without increasing survival.
- Radiation therapy in conjunction with cisplatin does not increase survival over radiation alone.
- Surgery alone does not prolong life and is not recommended.

POSSIBLE COMPLICATIONS

- Radiation damage possible (acute: mucositis, conjunctivitis, and dermatitis; late: effects on eye, brain, and nasal passage)
- Tumor progression can cause neurologic signs

RECOMMENDED MONITORING

Primarily clinical signs; imaging (more than 3 months after radiation) may also be helpful

PROGNOSIS AND OUTCOME

Varies with tumor type (animals with sarcomas generally live longer than those with carcinomas), clinical stage of tumor at time of treatment, and total dose of radiation delivered to the entire tumor. Median survival ranges from 8 to 31 months. Comparison of data from various reports is difficult, limiting its use to offer accurate prognoses.

PEARLS & CONSIDERATIONS

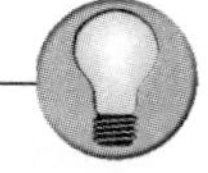

COMMENTS

- Nasal tumors should be considered treatable even though they are not often curable.
- Administration of curative-intent radiation therapy, with possible survival of as little as 8 months, may seem irrational. However, most dogs can survive approximately 1 year. Improvements in radiation therapy have led to decreased side effects; most dogs tolerate therapy and have a good quality life after the treatment.
- Chemotherapy and abbreviated, palliative radiation protocols can bring some relief from signs. Piroxicam (a COX-1 and COX-2 inhibitor) alone (0.3 mg/kg PO q 24h) may improve signs for 4 months or longer (unpublished data) but should not be given concurrently with glucocorticoids or other nonsteroidal anti-inflammatory drugs (NSAIDs) due to gastrointestinal ulceration risk.

SUGGESTED READING

Fox LE, King RR: Cancers of the respiratory system. In Morrison WB (ed): *Cancer in Dogs and Cats*. Baltimore, Williams & Wilkins, 1998, pp 521-527.

Lana SE, et al: Use of radiation and slow release Cisplatin formulation for treatment of canine nasal tumors. *Vet Radiol* 45:577, 2004.

Lana SE, Withrow SJ: Nasal tumors. In Withrow SJ, MacEwen EG (eds): *Small Animal Clinical Oncology*. Philadelphia, WB Saunders, 2001, pp 370-375.

AUTHOR: **JANEAN L. FIDEL**
EDITOR: **RANCE K. SELLON**

Nasopharyngeal Polyp

BASIC INFORMATION

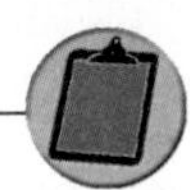

DEFINITION

Non-neoplastic pedunculated mass originating from the middle ear or auditory tube epithelium

SYNONYM(S)

Inflammatory polyp
Middle ear polyp

EPIDEMIOLOGY

SPECIES, AGE, SEX: Primarily in young adult cats.
RISK FACTORS: Proposed: upper respiratory viral infection or any process that obstructs middle ear drainage.
ASSOCIATED CONDITIONS AND DISORDERS
- Otitis media, interna, or externa
- Horner's syndrome

CLINICAL PRESENTATION

DISEASE FORMS/SUBTYPES: Ear (aural) polyp if mass grows into external ear canal instead of nasopharynx.
HISTORY, CHIEF COMPLAINT
- Nasal discharge
- Sneezing
- Stertor
- Dyspnea
- Dysphagia
- Gagging
- Voice change
- Headshaking
- Pawing at ears
- Vestibular signs (otitis media or externa)

PHYSICAL EXAM FINDINGS
- Increased inspiratory noise (often stertor)
- Mucoid to mucopululent nasal discharge (unilateral or bilateral)
- Gagging
- Possible otitis externa
- Head tilt
- Ataxia and nystagmus if inner ear is affected
- Horner's syndrome: miosis, ptosis, enophthalmos, and third eyelid prolapse on affected side

ETIOLOGY AND PATHOPHYSIOLOGY

- Exact etiology is unknown, but proposed causes include inflammatory conditions and congenital persistence of branchial arches.
  - The significance of calicivirus, bacteria, or fungi recovered from polyps is questionable.
- It is suspected that proliferation of the auditory tube or tympanic mucosal epithelium obstructs drainage from the middle ear. The resulting fluid accumulation and inflammation (otitis media), which can extend into the inner ear (otitis interna) or drain through the tympanic membrane (otitis externa), provokes formation of a fibrous polyp.
- Enlarged mass fills the nasopharyngeal region, obstructing caudal nasal drainage and airflow, eventually impeding inspiration and swallowing and causing nasal discharge.

DIAGNOSIS

DIFFERENTIAL DIAGNOSIS

- Neoplasia (e.g., lymphoma, squamous cell carcinoma)
- Infectious rhinitis
- Nasal/nasopharyngeal foreign body
- Nasopharyngeal stenosis
- Laryngeal paralysis
- Granuloma (cryptococcosis)

INITIAL DATABASE

- Results of the complete blood count, biochemistry panel, and urinalysis are usually normal.
- Otoscopic examination:
  - If the animal has otitis media, bulging of tympanic membrane from fluid or mass is noted.
  - The mass may extend through the tympanic membrane and be visible in the external ear canal.
  - If the tympanic membrane has ruptured, the cat will have otitis externa.
- Skull radiographs:
  - Increased soft tissue density in pharynx (lateral view).
  - Evidence of otitis media.
    - Enlarged or thickened bulla containing increased soft tissue density.

ADVANCED OR CONFIRMATORY TESTING

- Oral examination under anesthesia:
  - Palpable mass dorsal to soft palate (exposed by rostral retraction of soft palate with spay hook) or mass protruding into oropharynx.
- Computed tomography:
  - Increased fluid and soft tissue density in bulla.
  - The bulla wall may be thickened or thin and distended.
- Histology:
  - Well-vascularized fibrous tissue is covered by stratified squamous or columnar epithelium.
  - Inflammatory cells, primarily lymphocytes, plasma cells, and macrophages, are present within the stroma.

TREATMENT

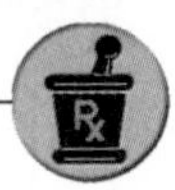

THERAPEUTIC GOAL(S)

- Remove obstructing mass
- Prevent recurrence

ACUTE GENERAL TREATMENT

- Oxygen supplementation (see Oxygen Supplementation, p 1292) if the patient is in respiratory distress.
- Induction of general anesthesia and removal of the polyp using slow steady traction, grasping the polyp at the base of its stalk.
- Ventral bulla osteotomy with removal of the epithelial lining to reduce recurrence rate; culture from the bulla is also indicated at the time of surgery.

CHRONIC TREATMENT

The clinician should administer antibiotics if the diagnosis is otitis media (e.g., amoxicillin with clavulanic acid, 62.5 mg/cat PO q 12h until culture results return).

POSSIBLE COMPLICATIONS

- Horner's syndrome is seen in approximately 80% of cases after a bulla osteotomy and can also occur with polyp traction; it usually resolves within 1 month.
- Otitis interna occurs in approximately 40% of cases following ventral bulla osteotomy; ataxia and head tilt can affect quality of life.

RECOMMENDED MONITORING

- The clinician should reevaluate the animal if clinical signs recur.
- The clinician should repeat otoscopic examination and otic cytologic examination if otitis externa is present.

PROGNOSIS AND OUTCOME

- Polyp regrowth may be seen in 17–50% of cats treated with traction removal alone.
- Ventral bulla osteotomy prevents recurrence in most cats.

PEARLS & CONSIDERATIONS

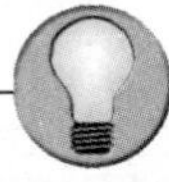

COMMENTS

- Computed tomography (CT) is more sensitive than survey skull radiographs for detecting otitis media.

- For a broad-based mass, the clinician should perform cytologic testing to rule out tonsillar lymphoma.
- The feline tympanic bulla has two chambers; the epithelial lining of both chambers should be removed during the bulla osteotomy.
- Sympathetic fibers are superficial in the feline bulla, making nerve damage and development of Horner's syndrome likely with a bulla osteotomy.

PREVENTION

With traction alone, treatment with prednisone (1–2 mg/kg PO q 24h for 2 weeks after the procedure) may reduce recurrence.

CLIENT EDUCATION

Complications are common, but usually temporary, with a bulla osteotomy.

SUGGESTED READING

Anderson DM, et al: Management of inflammatory polyps in 37 cats. *Vet Rec* 147:684, 2000.

Donnelly KE, Tillson DM: Feline inflammatory polyps and ventral bulla osteotomy. *Compend Contin Educ Pract Vet* 26:446, 2004.

Tobias KM: Management of ear and nasopharyngeal polyps in cats. *Vet Forum* 17:46, 2000.

Veir JK, et al: Feline inflammatory polyps: Historical, clinical, and PCR findings for feline calicivirus and feline herpes virus-1 in 28 cases. *J Fel Med Surg* 4:195, 2002.

AUTHOR: **KAREN M. TOBIAS**
EDITOR: **RANCE K. SELLON**

Nasopharyngeal Stenosis

BASIC INFORMATION

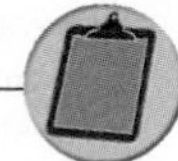

DEFINITION

Formation of a thin fibrous membrane at the internal nasal meatus, resulting in a significant narrowing of the orifice between the caudal nasal cavity and rostral pharynx

EPIDEMIOLOGY

SPECIES, AGE, SEX

- Primarily a disease of cats, although it was reported in a young dog following the surgical correction of choanal atresia.
- Affects cats ranging in age from 8 months to 10 years.

GENETICS AND BREED PREDISPOSITION: No breed predispositions are recognized.

RISK FACTORS: Recurrent upper respiratory tract infections or allergic respiratory disease.

ASSOCIATED CONDITIONS AND DISORDERS: Chronic rhinitis and sinusitis.

CLINICAL PRESENTATION

DISEASE FORMS/SUBTYPES: Congenital stenosis of the internal nasal meatus has been described in the literature. Most cases, however, are acquired.

HISTORY, CHIEF COMPLAINT: Some or all of the following may be present:

- Upper respiratory tract disease:
  - Nasal discharge
  - Nasal stertor
  - Sneezing
- Worsening of the respiratory signs during eating or swallowing
- Poor response to therapy

PHYSICAL EXAM FINDINGS

- Nasal discharge
- Nasal stridor

ETIOLOGY AND PATHOPHYSIOLOGY

In cats, this condition is thought to result from scar formation across the rostral nasopharynx secondary to mucosal ulceration from chronic rhinitis and/or sinusitis. Therefore, the disease is usually associated with recurrent upper respiratory tract infections or allergic disease. Scar formation leads to complete or partial obstruction of the rostral nasopharynx, resulting in the accumulation of nasal secretions within the nasal cavity and consequent nasal stridor and discharge. Affected cats usually show aggravated respiratory signs during eating or swallowing. There is a single report of choanal atresia with secondary rostral nasopharyngeal stenosis in a 20-month-old shih tzu dog. Chronic inflammation from nasopharyngeal foreign bodies in dogs has also been anecdotally associated with the disease.

DIAGNOSIS

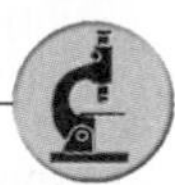

DIFFERENTIAL DIAGNOSIS

- Nasopharyngeal polyps
- Chronic rhinitis or sinusitis
- Foreign body
- Intranasal neoplasia
- Mycotic rhinitis

INITIAL DATABASE

- Complete blood count: normal
- Urinalysis: normal
- Serum biochemistry profile: normal

ADVANCED OR CONFIRMATORY TESTING

- Diagnostic imaging:
  - Nasal radiographs may be normal or may show opacification of turbinate structures due to the accumulation of nasal secretions.
  - Computed tomographic (CT) scan.
- Other diagnostic procedures:
  - Inability to pass a small catheter (3.5 French gauge) gently through the ventral nasal meatus into the pharynx.
  - Visualization of the membrane by use of a retroflexed pediatric bronchoscope or a dental mirror.

TREATMENT

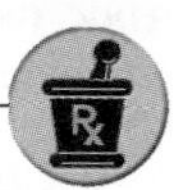

THERAPEUTIC GOAL(S)

Remove the stenotic membrane

ACUTE GENERAL TREATMENT

Removal of the stenotic membrane by:

- Surgical resection
- Dilation/tearing with a valvuloplasty balloon dilation catheter under endoscopic guidance

CHRONIC TREATMENT

Anti-inflammatory doses of corticosteroids after surgery/dilation

POSSIBLE COMPLICATIONS

Recurrence of the stenosis

RECOMMENDED MONITORING

Clinical signs

PROGNOSIS AND OUTCOME

Dependent on the ability to remove and/or tear the membrane causing the stenosis

PEARLS & CONSIDERATIONS

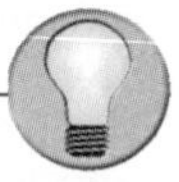

CLIENT EDUCATION

Recurrence is possible

SUGGESTED READING

Henderson SM, et al: Investigation of nasal disease in the cat—A retrospective study of 77 cases. *J Fel Med Surg* 6:245–257, 2004.

Mitten RW: Acquired nasopharyngeal stenosis in cats. In Kirk RW, Bonagura JD (eds): *Current Veterinary Therapy XI*. Philadelphia, WB Saunders, 1992, pp 801–803.

AUTHOR: **REMO LOBETTI**
EDITOR: **RANCE K. SELLON**

Neck Pain

BASIC INFORMATION

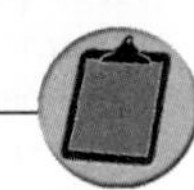

DEFINITION

Sensation of discomfort or distress associated with the cervical spine or surrounding tissues

SYNONYM(S)

Cervical hyperesthesia
Cervical hyperpathia

EPIDEMIOLOGY

GENETICS AND BREED PREDISPOSITION: Atlantoaxial instability: toy breeds:

- Chihuahua, Toy poodle, Pomeranian, Pekingese

Intervertebral disk disease (IVDD): chondrodystrophoid breeds:

- Dachshund, Beagle, Basset, Pekingese, Shih tzu, other breeds

Caudal cervical spondylomyelopathy (CCSM, Wobbler's syndrome):

- Great Dane
- Doberman pinscher
- Many other breeds

Corticosteroid responsive meningitis/arteritis:

- Bernese mountain dog
- Boxer
- Nova Scotia duck tolling retriever

CONTAGION AND ZOONOSIS

- Distemper viral myelitis: dog to dog
- *Brucella canis*-associated diskospondylitis: dog to dog

ASSOCIATED CONDITIONS AND DISORDERS

- Horner's syndrome may be present with caudal cervical spinal lesions.
- Nerve root signature: Holding up of a forelimb may be sign of nerve root pain.

CLINICAL PRESENTATION

DISEASE FORMS/SUBTYPES

- Spinal disease:
  - Congenital: CCSM in young Great Danes, atlantoaxial instability
  - Acquired/degenerative: IVDD, CCSM in Doberman pinschers
  - Traumatic
- Infectious disease: canine distemper myelitis, systemic fungal myelitis, diskospondylitis
- Inflammatory: cranial cervical pain sometimes found with meningitis
- Traumatic: cervical fractures, instability, penetrating pharyngeal or neck wounds
- Neoplastic: spinal tumors, axial skeletal osteosarcoma, nerve sheath tumor, and other such growths

HISTORY, CHIEF COMPLAINT

- Reluctance to rise
- Reluctance to walk on stairs
- Reluctance to jump
- Crying out when changing positions, getting up, or lying down
- Shaking

PHYSICAL EXAM FINDINGS

- Abnormal head posture: holding head down, reluctant to turn head
- Arched neck or back
- Pain on manipulation of the neck
- Pain on palpation of the cervical musculature
- Reluctance to walk
- Abnormal gait if animal is neurologically impaired
- Heat and swelling in cervical tissues
- Hypersalivation, which is possible with pharyngeal injuries
- Fever associated with infections or meningitis
- Root signature (see Root Signature [Nerve], p 976)

ETIOLOGY AND PATHOPHYSIOLOGY

- Various tissues may be the source of neck pain:
  - Epaxial musculature:
    - Traumatic muscle injury.
    - Exertional rhabdomyolosis.
    - Myositis from penetrating injury or foreign body (stick or grass awn migration).
    - Inflammatory myositis: immune mediated, parasitic, bacterial, or protozoal.
  - Spinal column:
    - IVDD: progressive degeneration of intervertebral disk resulting in protrusion or herniation of disk material into the spinal canal. The annulus fibrosus is the portion of the disk that contains pain receptors. Typically affects dogs 3 to 8 years of age but can also occur in cats.
    - Diskospondylitis: bacterial infection of vertebral body end plates; the caudal cervical region is one of the predilection sites.
    - Malformation: CCSM in Great Danes, hemivertebrae, spinal canal stenosis.
    - Instability: Atlantoaxial instability, CCSM, vertebral subluxation, traumatic fracture or luxation.
    - Neoplasia: osteosarcoma, hemangiosarcoma, fibrosarcoma, chondrosarcoma, or metastatic tumors involving the vertebrae.
  - Meninges:
- Inflammatory, parasitic, protozoal, bacterial, and neoplastic lesions:
  - Spinal nerves:
    - Nerve root compression, ischemia.
    - Inflammation: immune mediated, infectious (protozoal, viral, parasitic).
    - Neoplasia.

DIAGNOSIS

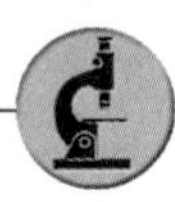

DIFFERENTIAL DIAGNOSIS

Neck pain is a nonspecific clinical sign. Differential diagnosis includes orthopedic, neurologic, and soft tissue problems (see Etiology and Pathophysiology above).

INITIAL DATABASE

- Neurologic examination (see p 1286)
- Complete blood count
- Serum biochemistry panel
- Urinalysis
- Neck radiographs

ADVANCED OR CONFIRMATORY TESTING

- Myelogram, computed tomography (CT), or magnetic resonance imaging (MRI).
  - Very useful for spinal imaging.
  - Myelogram with dynamic views may be useful for diagnosis of CCSM.
  - Myelogram is also useful for IVDD and some spinal tumors.
  - MRI is best for spinal cord and nerve lesions and is becoming more widely used for IVDD.
  - MRI is more sensitive and specific than myelography or CT for identifying the location and potential cause of many spinal lesions.
  - CT is best for evaluating bony lesions: tumors and fractures of the spine.
  - CT can be used as an adjunct to myelography.
- Cerebrospinal fluid (CSF) tap if meningitis or neoplasia is suspected.
- Aspiration or biopsy of abnormal tissues.
- Ultrasound of soft tissues to locate an abscess, a foreign body, a neoplasm, or other such abnormalities.
- Surgical exploration.
  - Histopathologic evaluation of tissue samples.
  - Bacterial culture and sensitivity (C&S).
- Urine culture if there is a concern for diskospondylitis.

TREATMENT

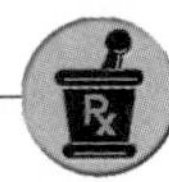

Treatment depends on the underlying cause

THERAPEUTIC GOAL(S)

- Relief of pain

- Immobilization if movement is detrimental or painful
- Treatment of underlying disease process

ACUTE GENERAL TREATMENT

- Animals with acute severe neck pain are often treated with cage rest and medications such as analgesics (hydromorphone 0.1-0.2 mg/kg SQ, IM, or IV, as needed up to q 4h, or butorphanol 0.1-0.2 mg/kg IV, as needed up to q 6h) and/or muscle relaxants (methocarbamol 20-50 mg/kg PO q 8h). Empiric glucocorticoids given prior to ruling out infectious causes can exacerbate infectious diseases.
- If spinal instability is suspected, then the clinician may recommend the use of a neck brace for immobilizing the neck, providing pain relief, and preventing further tissue damage.

CHRONIC TREATMENT

- Nonsteroidal anti-inflammatory drug (NSAID) medications (e.g., carprofen 2 mg/kg PO q 12h, etodolac 10-15 mg/kg PO q 24h, deracoxib 1-2 mg/kg PO q 24h, firocoxib 4-5 mg/kg PO q 24h, or meloxicam 0.1 mg/kg PO q 12h).
- Low-dose corticosteroids: The clinician should taper the medication during periods of improvement.
- Exercise restriction.
- Use of a harness instead of a collar for walks.
- Acupuncture.
- Surgery.

DRUG INTERACTIONS

The clinician should never combine NSAIDs with corticosteroids due to risk of serious or life-threatening gastroenteritis and gastrointestinal ulceration.

POSSIBLE COMPLICATIONS

- Adverse reactions to the medication, especially gastrointestinal ulceration caused by taking corticosteroids and NSAIDs, may occur.
- Pneumonia is a common complication in dogs that have tetraparesis and are recumbent.
- Respiratory obstruction is possible with a neck brace; it is important to adjust the brace so that it fits properly, and the owner and clinician should monitor the animal.
- Paralysis or death is possible with acute spinal injury.

RECOMMENDED MONITORING

Any dog with signs of neck pain should be closely monitored for the development of neurologic conditions, such as ataxia, paresis, paralysis, and respiratory impairment; these conditions suggest a neurologic cause and possibly warrant intensive care and further intervention.

PROGNOSIS AND OUTCOME

Highly variable depending on underlying disease process

PEARLS & CONSIDERATIONS

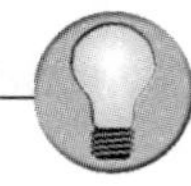

COMMENTS

- Neck pain in certain dog breeds is a very common problem in clinical practice.
- All dogs being considered for nonspecific supportive treatment should have cervical spinal radiographs prior to treatment.
- Cage rest is a critical component of conservative treatment.
- If a dog does not respond appropriately to nonspecific supportive therapy, the clinician should perform further diagnostic testing.

PREVENTION

- Owners should use a harness for walking their dogs.
- The clinician should inform the owner of exercise restrictions.

SUGGESTED READING

Wheeler SJ, Sharp NJ: *Small Animal Spinal Disorders: Diagnosis and Surgery*. Baltimore, Mosby-Wolfe, 1994.

AUTHOR: **DAVID A. PUERTO**
EDITOR: **ETIENNE CÔTÉ**

Neck Ventroflexion

BASIC INFORMATION

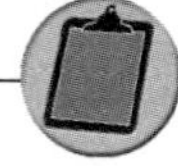

DEFINITION

A syndrome in which the neck is continuously or intermittently maintained in a flexed position due to an inability or unwillingness to extend the neck dorsally or due to involuntary muscular flexion of the neck

EPIDEMIOLOGY

SPECIES, AGE, SEX

- Cats are predominantly affected, but dogs may also show neck ventroflexion.
- Age and sex both vary depending on the underlying cause for the syndrome.
- Cats: hypokalemic polymyopathy, hyperthyroidism.
- Young animals: inherited myopathies.
- Old animals: chronic renal failure.

GENETICS AND BREED PREDISPOSITION

- Burmese cat: hereditary hypokalemic periodic paralysis.
- Devon rex cat: hereditary myopathy.
- Labrador retriever dog: hereditary myopathy.

RISK FACTORS: Hypokalemia, thiamine deficiency, organophosphate toxicity, hyperthyroidism.

ASSOCIATED CONDITIONS AND DISORDERS: Megaesophagus, aspiration pneumonia.

CLINICAL PRESENTATION

DISEASE FORMS/SUBTYPES: The syndrome can be divided into three general categories:

- Neuromuscular weakness
- Neck guarding
- Active flexion

HISTORY, CHIEF COMPLAINT

- Neuromuscular weakness
  - The clinician may or may not notice ventroflexion, and it may be associated with generalized weakness, reluctance or inability to walk, stiff stilted gait, and other signs of systemic illness.
- Neck guarding
  - Clinician may notice mental depression and ataxia. The neck may be held in a fixed position with decreased movement of the head.
- Active flexion
  - The animal may experience seizure-like activity (thiamine deficiency).
  - Dietary history: Raw fish diets are high in thiaminase, causing thiamine deficiency.

PHYSICAL EXAM FINDINGS

- Neuromuscular weakness (Fig. I-120):
  - Generalized or localized neck muscle weakness is possible. Ventroflexion may be episodic or continuous. Exercise or stress may induce weakness or collapse. Muscle pain may be present.
- Neck guarding:
  - Pain on neck manipulation can occur with or without neurologic abnormal-

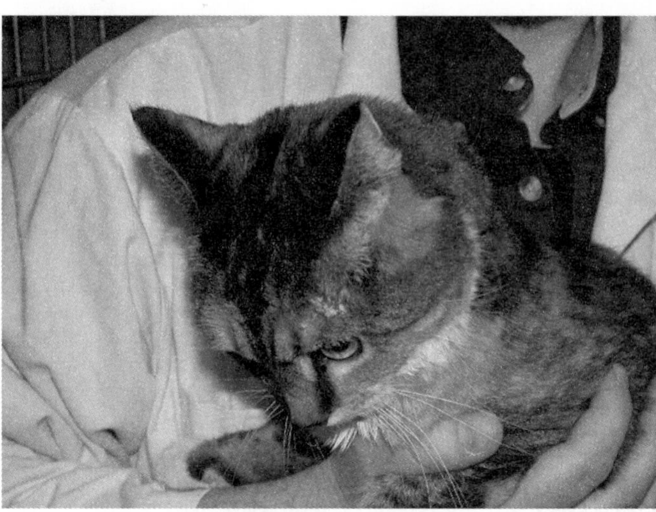

FIGURE. I-120 Seven-year-old female spayed domestic shorthair cat with flaccid ventroflexion of the neck due to severe hypokalemia (serum K^+ = 2.8 mEq/l). Courtesy of Dr. Etienne Côté.

ities, such as ataxia, proprioception abnormalities, and mental depression (cervical orthopedic/neurologic disease). The animal shows resentment or resistance to neck manipulation.

- Active flexion:
  - The animal experiences seizure-like activity, and the neck is actively tucked in under sternum; the clinician may notice increased muscle tone and encephalopathic signs (thiamine deficiency).

ETIOLOGY AND PATHOPHYSIOLOGY

- Weakness: The muscle weakness is such that the neck muscles are unable to lift the head. Ventroflexion of the neck is a hallmark of weakness in cats.
- Neck guarding: Cervical pain may cause an animal to hold the neck in a fixed flexed position (guarding) so that unnecessary head and neck movement is minimized.
- The clinician may notice active contraction of the neck flexor muscles.

DIAGNOSIS

DIFFERENTIAL DIAGNOSIS

- Neck or generalized weakness:
  - Metabolic: hypokalemia (i.e., hypokalemic polymyopathy (see Fig. I-120), hypernatremic myopathy (rare)
  - Toxic (organophosphate toxicosis, botulism, tick paralysis [*Ixodes*, *Dermacentor*], snake bite)
  - Endocrinopathies (hyperthyroidism)
  - Myopathies: Burmese hereditary episodic paralysis/hypokalemic periodic paralysis, Labrador retriever hereditary myopathy, Devon rex myopathy, polymyositis, myasthenia gravis, hyperkalemic periodic paralysis
  - Polyneuropathies: chronic inflammatory demyelinating polyneuropathy
- Neck pain:
  - Polyarthritis
  - Meningitis/meningoencephalitis
  - Cervical-orthopedic diseases: disk herniation, caudal cervical spondylomyelopathy, spondylitis, spinal ankylosis (hypervitaminosis A, mucopolysaccharidosis)
- Active neck flexion:
  - Thiamine deficiency

INITIAL DATABASE

- Complete neurologic examination
- Complete blood count, serum biochemistry panel (biochemistry profile to include blood glucose, creatinine, creatine kinase, sodium, potassium), urinalysis

ADVANCED OR CONFIRMATORY TESTING

- Organophosphate poisoning: serum acetylcholinesterase levels
- Myasthenia gravis: repetitive nerve stimulation, serum acetylcholine receptor antibody titer, edrophonium test
- Hyperthyroidism: serum thyroxine levels
- Polymyopathies/neuropathies: electromyography, nerve conduction velocities, nerve and muscle biopsies, pre-exercise and postexercise electrolyte measurements
- Neck pain with or without neurologic lesions localized to the neck or intracranial region: spinal survey radiographs, cerebrospinal fluid (CSF) analysis, myelogram, cervical computed tomography (CT), and/or magnetic resonance imaging (MRI)
- Urinary fractional excretion of potassium
- Arthrocentesis

TREATMENT

THERAPEUTIC GOAL(S)

Treat the primary disease

ACUTE AND CHRONIC TREATMENT

Depends on the underlying mechanism

POSSIBLE COMPLICATIONS

Complications are usually associated with the underlying primary disease and not with neck ventroflexion per se.

- Megaesophagus with secondary aspiration pneumonia: myasthenia gravis, organophosphate poisoning
- Generalized weakness: decubital ulcers
- Respiratory failure: hypokalemic polymyopathy
- Dysphagia with food accumulation in larynx/pharynx with laryngospasm and asphyxiation: Devon rex

PROGNOSIS AND OUTCOME

Depends on the underlying disease and varies from poor to good

PEARLS & CONSIDERATIONS

COMMENTS

Hypokalemic polymyopathy is probably the most common cause of ventroflexion in cats and must be excluded before an extensive work-up is undertaken.

PREVENTION

- Appropriate amounts of potassium in food and intravenous maintenance fluids
- Appropriate thiamine levels in the diet and correct storage of food to prevent thiamine breakdown
- Correct dosage and application of organophosphate products

SUGGESTED READING

Jones BR: Hypokalemic myopathy in cats. In Bonagura J (ed): *Current Veterinary Therapy XIII*. Philadelphia, WB Saunders, 2000, pp 985–987.

Taboada J, Merchant S: Challenging cases in internal medicine: What's your diagnosis? *Vet Med* 85:932–950, 1990.

AUTHOR: **FRANK KETTNER**
EDITOR: **ETIENNE CÔTÉ**

Necrotizing Encephalitis

BASIC INFORMATION

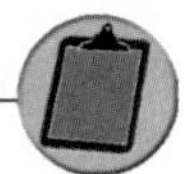

DEFINITION

A unique, nonsuppurative meningoencephalitis resulting in brain parenchymal necrosis; lesions predominate within the cerebral hemispheres

SYNONYM(S)

Pug or Maltese meningoencephalitis
Yorkshire terrier leukoencephalitis

EPIDEMIOLOGY

SPECIES, AGE, SEX: Dogs of either sex ranging in age from 6 months to 7 years have been reported.

GENETICS AND BREED PREDISPOSITION

- Many authors propose a genetic predisposition in pugs, although the exact mode of inheritance is unknown.
- Maltese dogs and Yorkshire terriers are similarly affected, although the distribution of lesions in Yorkies is different than in pug and Maltese dogs.
- The disease has been reported sporadically in other small breeds of dogs, including chihuahuas.
- Because necrotizing encephalitis (NE) is not limited to pugs, clinicians often refer to the condition as NE instead of *pug dog encephalitis*.

RISK FACTORS: Unknown. A number of female dogs with clinical histories of pregnancy or pseudopregnancy prior to the onset of clinical signs have been reported; however, the role, if any, of hormonal factors in the pathogenesis of NE is poorly understood.

CONTAGION AND ZOONOSIS: This disease is not transmissible between animals and poses no known threat of zoonosis. To date, attempts to isolate an infectious agent have been unsuccessful.

CLINICAL PRESENTATION

DISEASE FORMS/SUBTYPES: Forms include acute (<2 weeks) or chronic (4 to 6 months).

HISTORY, CHIEF COMPLAINT: The majority of cases present with generalized seizures, circling, visual deficits, and head pressing. Yorkshire terriers often show signs of a vestibular disturbance (ataxia, head tilt) in addition to the aforementioned signs of proencephalic (forebrain) dysfunction.

PHYSICAL EXAM FINDINGS

- General physical examination is unremarkable
- Neurologic examination reflects the distribution of lesions in the central nervous system (CNS):
    - Signs are frequently asymmetric.
    - When forebrain signs predominate, menace deficits, postural deficits (with a normal gait), nasal hypalgesia, and abnormal mentation may be present.
    - Yorkshire terriers often have signs of central vestibular disease, including abnormal nystagmus, falling, head tilt, and postural deficits.
    - Neck pain is occasionally elicited, secondary to either meningits or forebrain disease.

ETIOLOGY AND PATHOPHYSIOLOGY

- An immune-mediated basis is strongly suspected. Autoantibodies against glial cells have been identified in the cerebrospinal fluid (CSF) and serum of affected pug dogs.
- Selective neuronal necrosis, perivascular mononuclear infiltrates, and foci of malacia and cavitation are seen in both gray and white matter.

DIAGNOSIS

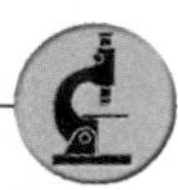

DIFFERENTIAL DIAGNOSIS

- Granulomatous meningoencephalitis (GME)
- Infectious meningoencephalitis (e.g., protozoal, fungal, rickettsial, viral)

INITIAL DATABASE

- Complete blood count and serum chemistry panel results are generally unremarkable.
- Infectious disease titers (*Toxoplasma*, *Neospora*, Rocky Mountain spotted fever, *Ehrlichia*, *Cryptococcus*) can rule out other potential causes of encephalitis.

ADVANCED OR CONFIRMATORY TESTING

- Magnetic resonance imaging (MRI): Findings may include asymmetric ventriculomegaly, cerebral edema, noncontrast enhancing focal or multifocal cavitating lesions, and (rarely) tentorial herniation.
    - In Maltese and pug dogs, the lesions are almost exclusively supratentorial, while in Yorkshire terriers, lesions may also be found in the brainstem.
- CSF analysis: mild-to-moderate lymphocytic pleocytosis and elevated protein.

TREATMENT

THERAPEUTIC GOAL(S)

- Reduction of seizure activity, if present.
- Reduction of inflammation.

ACUTE GENERAL TREATMENT

- Mannitol (1 g/kg IV) in suspected cases of cerebral edema or rapidly deteriorating neurologic status.
- Anticonvulsant therapy, such as with phenobarbital or potassium bromide, is often used.
    - These drugs, however, may cause excessive sedation in cases with structural forebrain disease.
    - Zonisamide (5-10 mg/kg PO q 12h) or felbamate (15 mg/kg PO q 8h) may be preferable choices for controlling seizures without sedative effects.
- Anti-inflammatory therapy, usually prednisone at a dose of 0.5-1.0 mg/kg PO q 12h, may ameliorate clinical signs.

CHRONIC TREATMENT

- Anticonvulsant therapy (as above) is required for life.
- Anti-inflammatory doses of glucocorticosteroids (e.g., prednisone 0.5-1 mg/kg PO q 12h initially, then tapered to q 24h or preferably q 48h for long-term use) are required for life.
- Treatment with mycophenolate mofetil (CellCept) holds promise for treatment of this disorder, but more information and long-term studies are needed before predictions can be made regarding efficacy.

POSSIBLE COMPLICATIONS

With disease progression: seizures

RECOMMENDED MONITORING

Drug monitoring of serum levels (e.g., phenobarbital, KBr) if appropriate

PROGNOSIS AND OUTCOME

Prognosis for long-term survival is grave. Despite therapy, clinical signs progress and seizures become intractable.

PEARLS & CONSIDERATIONS

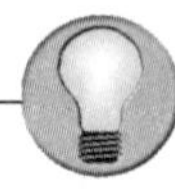

COMMENTS

The majority of dogs with NE die or are euthanized within 6 months of the onset of clinical signs. Clinicians must inform clients of the extremely guarded prognosis of NE.

PREVENTION

Unknown prevention methods

CLIENT EDUCATION

Due to the uncertainty regarding inheritability of this disorder, caution should be exercised when considering breeding relatives of affected dogs.

SUGGESTED READING

Dewey C: Encephalopathies: Disorders of the brain. In Dewey C (ed): *A Practical Guide to Canine and Feline Neurology*. Ames, IA, Iowa State Press, 2003, pp 160–162.

Kuwabara M, et al: Magnetic resonance imaging and histopathology of encephalitis in pug dogs. *J Vet Med Sci* 60:1353, 1998.

Uchida, K, et al: Detection of an autoantibody from pug dogs with necrotizing encephalitis (pug dog encephalitis). *Vet Pathol* 36:301, 1999.

AUTHOR: **GEORGINA BARONE**

EDITOR: **CURTIS W. DEWEY**

Necrotizing Fasciitis

BASIC INFORMATION

DEFINITION

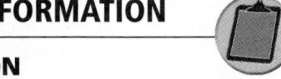

An acute onset of an extremely rapidly progressive streptococcal infection of the subcutis, skin, and fascia, causing coagulation necrosis of affected tissues. Septic shock may also be seen, either at presentation or as a later sequel.

SYNONYM(S)

Flesh-eating bacteria
Flesh-eating disease

EPIDEMIOLOGY

SPECIES, AGE, SEX: The veterinary literature reports only nine canine cases; no data are available on predilections or risk factors.

CONTAGION AND ZOONOSIS: Not known to be directly transmissible to humans. However, the same clinical disease is seen in human beings, involving the same organism. Therefore, strict precautions of hygiene, especially involving exposure to broken skin or mucous membranes, are warranted.

CLINICAL PRESENTATION

DISEASE FORMS/SUBTYPES: Two forms are recognized in humans: Type I infections (about 70% of human cases) are polymicrobial infections, type II infections are single infections with β-hemolytic group A *Streptococcus* (*S. pyogenes*). Type II infections of β-hemolytic group G *Streptococcus* predominate in dogs.

HISTORY, CHIEF COMPLAINT: History of recent minor trauma (e.g., minor laceration, bite) is typical. The injury may be a nonpenetrating wound (e.g., bumping, bruising).

- Some cases present with no trauma history and no external wound.
- Swelling, pain, and lameness may be noted by the owner if the disease is concentrated on a limb.
- Concurrent sepsis results in typical systemic signs, including anorexia, depression, weakness or collapse, and diarrhea.

PHYSICAL EXAM FINDINGS

- Signs include local edematous swelling, erythema, heat, and, often, severe pain.
  - The intensity of pain is characteristically disproportionate to the appearance of the lesion and may be excruciating.
- Overlying skin may appear soft and exudative or present as a hard eschar.
- Systemic signs include pyrexia, tachycardia, and dehydration.
- Septic shock (see Sepsis and Septic Shock, p 996): hypertension or hypotension, hyperthermia or hypothermia, mental depression, profound weakness, vomiting, diarrhea, and petechiae or ecchymoses.

ETIOLOGY AND PATHOPHYSIOLOGY

- Causative organism: Lancefield group G, β-hemolytic *Streptococcus* consistent with *S. canis*.
- Bacterial exotoxins and proteases are believed to be responsible for the local clinical signs and lesions identified by histopathologic examination.
- An extremely rapid course of progression (line of tissue inflammation/edema visibly advances over minutes ± hours) is a hallmark of necrotizing fasciitis, ultimately leading to sepsis and/or the systemic inflammatory response syndrome (SIRS) (see Systemic Inflammatory Response Syndrome, p 1060).

DIAGNOSIS

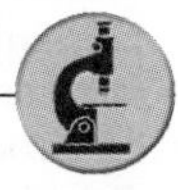

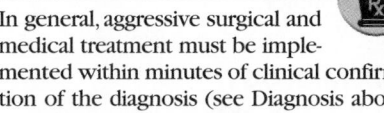

DIFFERENTIAL DIAGNOSIS

Subcutaneous abscess, seroma, or hematoma (secondary to bleeding diathesis); soft tissue or orthopedic trauma, including fractures (suspected based on intense pain), or less compatibly, blunt trauma, bites, and other such inflictions; and envenomation (insect, venomous snake).

INITIAL DATABASE

- Complete blood count, serum biochemistry profile, urinalysis:
  - Nonspecific clinical pathologic abnormalities consistent with severe inflammation.
  - Results often not available before important treatment decisions (e.g., amputation) need to be made.
- Radiographs of affected area to rule out fractures and other lesions as cause of pain.
- Advanced or septic cases have clinical pathologic abnormalities of sepsis and/or disseminated intravascular coagulation (DIC).

ADVANCED OR CONFIRMATORY TESTING

- The fulminant progression of infection requires rapid intervention, which generally precludes extensive diagnostic testing.
- Presumptive diagnosis is based on history, physical exam, absence of other causative lesion (e.g., fractures), and surgical findings. Confirmatory surgical findings:
  - Subcutaneous tissue offers little resistance to blunt (finger) dissection.
  - Copious, foul-smelling, thin, turbid subcutaneous fluid; ± bacteria and degenerate neutrophils present in cytologic test results.
- Definitive diagnosis: histopathologic confirmation of necrotizing fasciitis and bacteriologic isolation of the causative organism.

TREATMENT

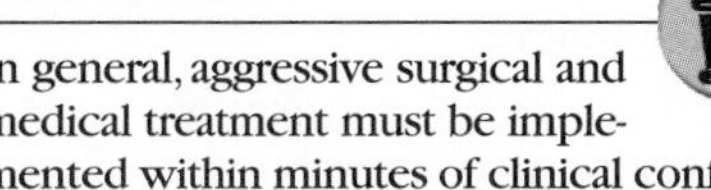

In general, aggressive surgical and medical treatment must be implemented within minutes of clinical confirmation of the diagnosis (see Diagnosis above) before a definitive diagnosis can be reached.

THERAPEUTIC GOAL(S)

- Clinician should recognize and aggressively treat SIRS/septic shock if present.
- Early aggressive surgical debridement is paramount to survival.
- Clinician should recommend appropriate postoperative antibiotic therapy and supportive care.

ACUTE GENERAL TREATMENT

- Immediate aggressive treatment for SIRS and for septic shock if present (see Sepsis and Septic Shock, p 996).
- Early aggressive surgical debridement.
  - The clinician should immediately obtain owner consent for amputation when infection is on a limb and should also inform the owner of the possible need for multiple debridement/reconstructive surgeries and of a guarded prognosis even with treatment.
  - The surgeon performs the amputation when the clinician makes a clinical diagnosis and notices rapid advancement of tissue necrosis.
  - The clinician should debride all affected and questionable tissues and then perform copious lavage with warm isotonic fluids; the addition of chlorhexidine 0.05% may be beneficial, although this outcome is not confirmed.
  - The clinician should bandage the debrided wound (wet-to-dry) until infection is controlled; the bandage should contain a thick absorptive layer and be changed daily (at least).
- Intravenous antibiotics: β-lactamase-resistant antibiotics are generally effective against *S. canis*; a broader spectrum regime may be superior initially because polymicrobial infections may be present.
  - Cefoxitin, 22 mg/kg IV q 6h; *or*
  - Cefazolin or ampicillin, 22 mg/kg IV q 6h, plus enrofloxacin, 20 mg/kg IV q 24h (dogs) or 5 mg/kg q 24h (cats); alternatively, cefazolin or ampicillin as above, plus amikacin, 20 mg/kg IV q 24h (dogs and cats).
- Supportive care:
  - Nutritional support (important).
    - Enteral feeding is preferred over parenteral unless contraindicated.
    - The surgeon can place an esophagostomy (see Feeding Tube Placement: Esophagostomy Tube, p 1243) or a gastrostomy (see Feeding Tube Placement: Percutaneous Endoscopic Gastrostomy [PEG], p 1247) tube during surgery by using separate instrumentation and draping.
    - Feed twice basal requirements.
  - Aggressive analgesia (condition is usually very painful and likely refractory to analgesics).
    - Opioids (examples: morphine sulphate 0.05-0.15 mg/kg/h IV constant rate infusion or buprenorphine 0.02 mg/kg IV q 6h) combined with a nonsteroidal anti-inflammatory drug (NSAID), such as carprofen 2.2 mg/kg IV or PO q 12h.
    - The concern that NSAIDs caused poorer outcomes in humans was unconfirmed in prospective studies.

POSSIBLE COMPLICATIONS

Diagnostic delays allow progression of local necrosis. Further delay or inadequately aggressive early treatment increases risk of sepsis or SIRS.

RECOMMENDED MONITORING

- The clinician should monitor patient for septic shock and DIC and for the progression of the infection, which would indicate the need for further debridement.
- The clinician should monitor the bandage for amount and character of exudate.

PROGNOSIS AND OUTCOME

Negative prognostic factors: delay of surgery, incomplete debridement, and concurrent sepsis. Reported mortality is 17-60% for humans and 12% for dogs based on nine reported cases.

SUGGESTED READING

Miller CW, et al: Streptococcal toxic shock syndrome in dogs. *J Am Vet Med Assoc* 209:1421-1426, 1996.

Naidoo SL, et al: Necrotizing fasciitis: A review. *J Am Anim Hosp Assoc* 41:104-109, 2005.

Prescott JF, et al: Update on canine streptococcal toxic shock syndrome and necrotizing fasciitis. *Can Vet J* 38:241-242, 1997.

Stevens DL: Streptococcal toxic shock syndrome associated with necrotizing fasciitis. *Ann Rev Med* 51:271-288, 2000.

AUTHOR: **MARK W. BOHLING**
EDITOR: **DOUGLASS K. MACINTIRE**

Neonatal Losses

BASIC INFORMATION

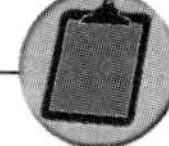

DEFINITION

Life-threatening illness occurring between birth and 4 weeks of age

SYNONYM(S)

Fading kittens
Fading puppies
Stillbirth

EPIDEMIOLOGY

SPECIES, AGE, SEX

- Canine, feline: both sexes.
- Neonatal mortality rates vary from 5-30%. Greatest incidence occurs within the first week of birth.

GENETICS AND BREED PREDISPOSITION: Cats: British shorthair, Scottish fold, Devon Rex, Abyssinian, Birman, Himalayan, Persian, Somali. Purebred puppies and kittens are more prone to congenital and hereditary defects.

RISK FACTORS

- Dam condition
- Premature labor
- Dystocia or fetal distress
- Prolonged labor
- Low birth weight or failure to grow
- Endometritis in the dam
- Congenital anomalies (hereditary, developmental, or teratogenic)
- Malnutrition or nutritional diseases
- Environment
- Parasitism
- Infectious diseases
- Inbreeding
- Tom with blood type A having mated with queen with blood type B

CONTAGION AND ZOONOSIS

- *Brucella canis* infection
- Toxoplasmosis
- Feline leukemia virus (FeLV) or feline immunodeficiency virus (FIV) infections

ASSOCIATED CONDITIONS AND DISORDERS: Failure to thrive (weight loss), diarrhea, persistent crying.

CLINICAL PRESENTATION

HISTORY, CHIEF COMPLAINT

- Low birth weight, low weight gain, and/or failure to gain weight.
- Sudden onset of illness characterized by depression, anorexia, persistent crying, abdominal pain, and failure to suckle. Death can occur in 18-24h depending on the cause.
- Primarily respiratory and gastrointestinal signs in puppies. Clinical signs vary according to the route and time of infection.
- Severity of presenting signs influences survival.

PHYSICAL EXAM FINDINGS

- General: weakness, diarrhea, respiratory distress, dehydration, hypothermia
- Characteristics of neonatal isoerythrolysis in cats: pallor, icterus, tail tip necrosis, tachypnea, discolored urine (hemoglobinuria)

ETIOLOGY AND PATHOPHYSIOLOGY

- Mechanisms:
  - Hypoglycemia, dehydration, and hypothermia are the main mechanisms for neonatal losses in both dogs and cats.
  - Hypothermia also causes ileus at temperatures <96°F.
  - Predisposition to infection depends on: stress, exposure to pathogens, and decrease in systemic immunity due to inadequate colostrum ingestion.
  - The most common route of entry for bacterial organisms is through the umbilicus.
  - Neonatal isoerythrolysis: queens and kittens are of different blood types. Antibodies ingested in the colostrum destroy neonatal red blood cells.
- Causes:
  - Infectious:
    - Neonatal sepsis: *E.coli*, other Gram-negative enteric organisms, β-hemolytic *Streptococcus*, *Staphylococcus*
    - Viral (puppies): canine herpesvirus, canine minute virus (parvovirus type I), canine parvovirus type II (CPV-2), canine distemper virus
    - Viral (kittens): calicivirus, FeLV, FIV, feline panleukopenia virus, feline herpesvirus
    - Enteric: *Campylobacter*, *Salmonella*, *E. coli* spp.
    - Respiratory: disease complex in kittens (rhinotracheitis [feline herpesvirus], calicivirus, *Chlamydophila psittaci*); *Bordetella bronchiseptica* and *Pasturella multocida* in puppies
    - *Mycoplasma*, *Ureaplasma* spp.
    - *Brucella canis* in puppies
    - Parasitic: coccidia, *Giardia*, roundworms, hookworms, *Toxoplasma*, *Neospora*, or *Cryptosporidium*
  - Noninfectious:
    - Environmental: conditions inducing hypothermia, overcrowding, stress, and poor sanitation
    - Nutritional: inadequate nursing inducing hypoglycemia, hypothermia-associated ileus
    - Neonatal isoerythrolysis (feline)
    - Dam-related: dystocia, cannibalism, inadequate nutrition (including taurine deficiency in kittens and lack of milk)
    - Congenital malformations

DIAGNOSIS

DIFFERENTIAL DIAGNOSIS

See Etiology and Pathophysiology above

INITIAL DATABASE

- Complete blood count, serum chemistry profile, urinalysis:
  - Volume of blood withdrawn should be conservative (small body size).
  - Neonates normally have mild serum alkaline phosphatase and phosphorus elevations as well as mild blood urea nitrogen, albumin, globulin, cholesterol, and hematocrit reductions.
- FeLV/FIV test
- Fecal flotation
- Thoracic and abdominal radiographs

ADVANCED OR CONFIRMATORY TESTING

- Urine culture
- Serology: *Brucella canis*, canine herpesvirus, *Toxoplasma*, *Neospora*; polymerase chain reaction (PCR) test is confirmatory for herpesvirus
- Blood typing (purebred cats)
- Virus isolation
- Pleural/abdominal fluid analysis
- Necropsy (e.g., canine herpesvirus: characteristic lesions)

TREATMENT

THERAPEUTIC GOAL(S)

- Supportive care
- Identification and eradication of cause when possible

ACUTE GENERAL TREATMENT

- Management of isoerythrolysis if present (see Anemia, Hemolytic, p 64).
- If immune compromised: Clinician should administer colostrum or avoid this administration if body temperature is <96°F and no suckling reflex is present.
- Neonatal sepsis: broad-spectrum bactericidal antibiotics (e.g., ceftiofur (Naxcel) 2.5 mg/kg SC q 12h for 5 days) with minimal effect on intestinal flora.
- Warmed, balanced crystalloid fluids (lactated Ringer's solution, or Normosol-R and 5% dextrose; 1 ml/30 g body weight IP or IO initially, then as needed based on response).
- Oxygen supplementation: 30–40%.
- Vitamin K1 0.01–0.1 mg SC once (puppies <2 days old have reduced thrombin levels).
- Management of hypoglycemia if present (see Insulinoma, p 598).
- Management of hypokalemia if present (see Hypokalemia, p 566).
- Supported nursing.
- Viral replication might be inhibited by maintaining body temperature above 101–102°F. Clinician should monitor the animal closely to avoid overheating. Incubator should be at a temperature of 85–95°F and relative humidity of 55–65%.

CHRONIC TREATMENT

- Supportive care.
- Commercial milk replacement (Renurse, Esbilac, Just Born, Veta-Lac) if mother's milk is not available. During the first week of life, neonatal caloric requirements are 133 kcal/kg/day; the requirements thereafter are 155 kcal/kg/day for week 2, 175–198 kcal/kg/day for week 3, and 220 kcal/kg/day for week 4.

DRUG INTERACTIONS

- Clinicians should avoid administering pediatric contraindicated drugs (e.g., glucocorticoids, fluoroquinolones, tetracyclines, aminoglycosides, trimethoprim-sulfa, and chloramphenicol).
- Drug absorption, metabolism, and excretion in dog or cat neonates differ from those of adult neonates and vary according to the drug; detailed drug information should be obtained prior to use in neonates.

RECOMMENDED MONITORING

Daily weighing is important. Puppies and kittens should gain weight daily at a rate of 2–7 g per day for each kilogram of anticipated adult weight and should double their birth weight by 10 days of age.

PROGNOSIS AND OUTCOME

Treatment is generally unrewarding for a herpesvirus infection

PEARLS & CONSIDERATIONS

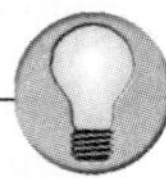

PREVENTION

Clinicians should:

- Avoid administering modified live vaccines during pregnancy.
- Avoid administering teratogenic drugs and chemicals.
- Avoid incompatible matings in cats and should check blood type before breeding.
- Ensure that neonates are ingesting colostrum within the first 24 hours to acquire passive immunity.
- Administer broad-spectrum anthelmintic therapy starting at 3 weeks of age and administer appropriate vaccination protocols.

CLIENT EDUCATION

Prevention and anticipation are the key

SUGGESTED READING

Davidson AP: Approaches to reducing the neonatal mortality in dogs. In Concannon PW, England G, Verstegen J, Linde-Forsberg C (eds): *Recent Advances in Small Animal Reproduction*. Ithaca, NY, International Veterinary Information Service, 2003, A 1226.0303.

Hoskins, Johnny D: *Veterinary Pediatrics. Dogs and Cats from Birth to Six Months*. Philadelphia, WB Saunders, 2001, pp 57-61.

Johnson SD, Root Kustritz MV, Olson PN: *Canine and Feline Theriogenology*. Philadelphia, WB Saunders, 2001, pp 146-167.

Kirk CA: New concepts in pediatric nutrition. *Vet Clin N Am Sm Anim Pract* 31:369, 2001.

Moon PF, Massat BJ, Pascoe PJ: Neonatal critical care. *Vet Clin N Am Sm Anim Pract* 31:343, 2001.

AUTHOR: **VALERIA RICKARD**
EDITOR: **MICHELLE A. KUTZLER**

Nephrolithiasis

BASIC INFORMATION

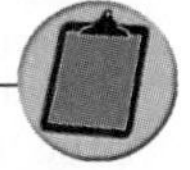

DEFINITION

Deposition of crystallized minerals within the kidney

SYNONYM(S)

Kidney stones
Renal urolithiasis
Renolithiasis

EPIDEMIOLOGY

SPECIES, AGE, SEX

- Feline: male predominance. Bimodal age distribution (1 to 3 years and 11 to 13 years)
- Canine: sex predilection varies (struvite for females; urate for males); middle-aged to older dogs

GENETICS AND BREED PREDISPOSITION

- Feline: Siamese
- Canine breeds overrepresented:
  - Urate: dalmatian, English bulldog, miniature schnauzer, shih tzu, Yorkshire terrier (urate/biurate) (see Urolithiasis, Urate/Biurate, p 1131)
  - Struvite: miniature schnauzer, shih tzu, bichon frise, miniature poodle, cocker spaniel, and Lhasa apso (see Urolithiasis, Struvite, p 1129)
  - Oxalate: miniature schnauzer, Lhasa apso, Yorkshire terrier, bichon frise, Pomeranian, shih tzu, miniature poodle (see Urolithiasis, Oxalate, p 1127)

RISK FACTORS

- Struvite: pyelonephritis
- Calcium oxalate: hyperadrenocorticism, hypercalcemia, diet
- Urate: portosystemic shunt, breed

ASSOCIATED CONDITIONS AND DISORDERS

- Hydronephrosis/hydroureter
- Ureteral obstruction
- Pyelonephritis
- Renal failure

CLINICAL PRESENTATION

DISEASE FORMS/SUBTYPES

- Unilateral or bilateral
- Unobstructed or obstructed (partial or complete)
- Urolith type: calcium oxalate, struvite, urate and other purines, xanthine, silica, cystine, compound/mixed

HISTORY, CHIEF COMPLAINT: Clinical signs may be absent or may include:

- Abdominal pain
- Anorexia
- Depression
- Hematuria
- Pollakiuria
- Polyuria and polydipsia (PU/PD)
- Stranguria
- Vomiting
- Weight loss

PHYSICAL EXAM FINDINGS: Physical examination may be unremarkable or may include identification of:

- Abdominal pain
- Dehydration
- Halitosis/oral ulcers (uremia)
- Ocular changes related to systemic hypertension
- Renomegaly or small kidneys

ETIOLOGY AND PATHOPHYSIOLOGY

- Nephroliths are less common than cystoliths, representing approximately 1-4% of analyzed uroliths. The actual prevalence is likely higher since nephroliths are less frequently removed for analysis.
- The most common nephrolith types in dogs are calcium oxalate (about 40%), struvite (about 33%), and urate (about 12%). The most common nephroliths in cats are calcium oxalate (see Urolithiasis, Oxalate, p 1127).

DIAGNOSIS

DIFFERENTIAL DIAGNOSIS

- Radiodense renal opacities:
  - Nephrocalcinosis
  - Radiodense intestinal content
  - Calcified lymph nodes
  - Calcified adrenal glands
  - Neoplastic mineralization
  - Other ectopic calcification
- Clinical signs:
  - Urolithiasis outside the kidney
  - Feline lower urinary tract signs/disease (FLUTS/D)
  - Pyelonephritis or cystitis
  - Renal failure
  - Urinary tract neoplasia
  - Prostatic disease
  - Causes of hematuria

INITIAL DATABASE

- Complete blood count: often unremarkable
  - Normocytic, normochromic, nonregenerative anemia (chronic renal failure).
  - Leukocytosis ± left shift (pyelonephritis).
- Serum biochemical profile: often unremarkable. Depending on degree of renal dysfunction and/or urinary obstruction, may reveal:
  - Azotemia.
  - Hyperphosphatemia.
  - Hypokalemia/hyperkalemia.
  - Metabolic acidosis.
- Urinalysis:
  - Hematuria.
  - Proteinuria.
  - Pyuria.
  - Bacteruria.
  - Crystalluria.
  - Isosthenuric urine.
- Urine culture and sensitivity (C&S)
- Blood pressure
- Abdominal radiography:
  - Depending on urolith composition, radiopaque density within one or both renal pelvises.
    - Radiopaque: calcium phosphate, calcium oxalate, struvite; small uroliths are difficult to detect radiographically.
    - Radiolucent: urate, cystine.
  - Concurrent ureteral, cystic, or urethral calculi are sometimes present.
  - Enlarged or atrophied kidneys.
- Ultrasound:
  - Acoustic shadowing in renal pelvis.
  - Concurrent pyelectasia or hydronephrosis.

ADVANCED OR CONFIRMATORY TESTING

- If removed, quantitative urolith analysis
- If definitive therapy is anticipated:
  - Nuclear scintigraphic glomerular filtration rate (GFR) to determine

contribution of each kidney to global GFR
  - Intravenous pyelography (IVP) or computerized tomography (CT) to confirm urolith location in kidney

TREATMENT

THERAPEUTIC GOAL(S)

Clinicians should:

- Relieve complete urinary obstruction.
- Address signs of renal failure, including electrolyte and acid-base disorders.
- Address urinary infection, including pyelonephritis.
- Reduce urolith constituent concentrations in urine.
- When possible, institute measures to dissolve uroliths and/or prevent recurrence or growth.

ACUTE GENERAL TREATMENT

- Complete urinary obstruction is rare, but when obstruction is present, it requires surgical intervention.
- Address renal failure, including electrolyte and acid-base disorders (see Chronic Renal Failure, Occult ["Asymptomatic"], p 204; Chronic Renal Failure, Overt ["Symptomatic"], p 205; Acute Renal Failure, p 32).
- Address pyelonephritis (see Pyelonephritis, p 927).

CHRONIC TREATMENT

- Medical dissolution possible for some types of nephrolithiasis (see Urolithiasis, Struvite, p 1129; Urolithiasis, Urate/Biurate, p 1131; Urolithiasis, Other, p 1125).
- Surgical intervention not routinely required.
  - Indications for surgery:
    - Complete obstruction to urine flow.
    - Nephrolith as a nidus for recurrent infection.
    - Nephrolithiasis with concurrent signs of renal failure.
    - Progressive enlargement (despite medical management) accompanied by reduction in renal function or in a solitary functional kidney.
  - Surgical procedures:
    - Nephrotomy.
    - Pyelolithotomy.
    - Nephrectomy.
- Lithotripsy (extracorporeal shock wave, laser, or electrohydraulic):
  - Results in fragmentation or crushing of calculi.
  - Indications similar to those for surgical intervention.
  - Availability limited (e.g., University of Tennessee, Purdue, Tufts).
  - May require multiple treatments depending on shape, size, location, and type of stone.
  - Can cause renal damage.

POSSIBLE COMPLICATIONS

- Nephrolith may lodge in ureter, causing obstructive nephropathy; particularly likely when calculi shrink (e.g., medical dissolution, lithotripsy).
- Surgical trauma of incision and transection of intrarenal vessels may further damage renal parenchyma.
- Some medical conditions may be worsened by calculolytic diets (see Urolithiasis, Struvite, p 1129; Urolithiasis, Urate/Biurate, p 1131).
- Recurrence rates are high, especially for calcium oxalate nephroliths.

RECOMMENDED MONITORING

- Monitoring, including imaging, urinalysis and culture, and serum biochemistry as described for urolithiasis
- Abdominal ultrasound or excretory urography (intravenous pyelography) should be considered in patients with radiolucent stones

PROGNOSIS AND OUTCOME

- Dependent on urolith composition, degree of obstruction, remaining renal function, concurrent infection, and ability to identify and treat underlying cause.
- Surgical intervention does not address causation; recurrence rates are high.

PEARLS & CONSIDERATIONS

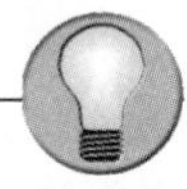

COMMENTS

- Small nephroliths can be incidental findings requiring no therapy.
- Medical management of nephroliths mirrors medical management of cystoliths of identical composition.

PREVENTION

- Clinicians should promote water consumption.
- Clinicians should identify and address risk factors.

CLIENT EDUCATION

Strict adherence to dietary recommendations is crucial

SUGGESTED READING

Ling GV, et al: Renal calculi in dogs and cats: Prevalence, mineral type, breed, age, and gender interrelationships (1981-1993). *J Vet Intern Med* 12:11, 1998.

Ross SJ, et al: Canine and feline nephrolithiasis. Epidemiology, detection, and management, *Vet Clin N Am Small Anim Pract* 29:231, 1999.

AUTHORS: **ADAM MORDECAI, RANCE K. SELLON**

EDITOR: **LEAH A. COHN**

Nephrotic Syndrome

BASIC INFORMATION

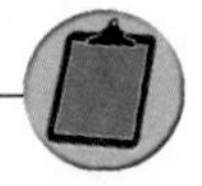

DEFINITION

The presence of pathologic proteinuria, hypoalbuminemia, hypercholesterolemia, and edema

EPIDEMIOLOGY

SPECIES, AGE, SEX

- More common in dogs than in cats
- More common in middle-aged to older dogs (average is about 8.5 years of age)
- For most causes, no sex predilection

GENETICS AND BREED PREDISPOSITION

- Labrador and golden retrievers may be overrepresented.
- Hereditary nephritis: bull terrier, dalmatian, English cocker spaniel, Samoyed, American Eskimo, beagle, mixed breed dog (see Protein-Losing Nephropathy, p 900).
- Amyloidosis: Chinese shar-pei (see Protein-Losing Nephropathy, p 900; Amyloidosis, p 57; Shar-Pei Fever, p 998).

RISK FACTORS: Diseases that can cause glomerular protein loss (e.g., glomerulonephritis, amyloidosis) are invariably the underlying cause of nephrotic syndrome. In turn, neoplasia, infectious, and noninfectious inflammatory diseases predispose an animal to glomerular disease (see Glomerulonephritis, p 442; Protein-Losing Nephropathy, p 900).

CONTAGION AND ZOONOSIS: Some causes are zoonotic (see Glomerulonephritis, p 442).

GEOGRAPHY AND SEASONALITY: Some causes are geographically and/or seasonally restricted (see Glomerulonephritis, p 442).

ASSOCIATED CONDITIONS AND DISORDERS

- Thromboembolic disease
- Chronic renal failure
- Systemic hypertension
- Dyspnea from ascites, pulmonary thromboembolism, or, less commonly, pleural effusion
- Reduced renal perfusion and possibly acute renal failure from decreased plasma oncotic pressure

CLINICAL PRESENTATION

DISEASE FORMS/SUBTYPES: Incomplete nephrotic syndrome: edema absent, which is the most common form.

HISTORY, CHIEF COMPLAINT: Patients may not show overt clinical signs. When present, signs may be nonspecific (e.g., weight loss, lethargy) or caused by:

- Fluid retention (e.g., edema, abdominal distention)
- Renal failure/uremia (e.g., polyuria and polydipsia [PU/PD], vomiting, halitosis)
- Thromboembolism (e.g., dyspnea, collapse)
- Systemic hypertension (e.g., blindness).
- Related to predisposing disease

PHYSICAL EXAM FINDINGS: May be unremarkable. Abnormalities may include:

- Subcutaneous edema, ascites; pleural effusion rare
- Evidence of thromboembolism (e.g., dyspnea, decreased peripheral pulse)
- Evidence of hypertension (e.g., chorioidopathy)
- Evidence of predisposing disease
- Variably sized kidneys

ETIOLOGY AND PATHOPHYSIOLOGY

- Proteinuria is due to altered glomerular capillary wall permselectivity and abnormal (inadequate) filtration of plasma proteins, primarily albumin.
- Hypoalbuminemia develops when the renal loss of plasma proteins exceeds hepatic regenerative capacity.
- The pathogenesis of hypercholesterolemia is complex and incompletely understood. Hypoalbuminemia or decreased oncotic pressure stimulates hepatic protein synthesis, including lipoprotein synthesis, leading to hypercholesterolemia. Altered lipid catabolism may contribute to the condition.
- Sodium retention and decreased plasma oncotic pressure contribute to edema formation.

DIAGNOSIS

DIFFERENTIAL DIAGNOSIS

- The combination of proteinuria, hypoalbuminemia, hypercholesterolemia, and edema is pathognomonic for nephrotic syndrome.
- Most likely with glomerular diseases that cause severe proteinuria: amyloidosis, membranous nephropathy/glomerulonephritis, hereditary nephritis, minimal change disease. (see Protein-Losing Nephropathy, p 900).

INITIAL DATABASE

- Complete blood count, biochemical profile, urinalysis: Clinician should assess renal tubular function (blood urea nitrogen [BUN], creatinine, urine specific gravity), identify evidence of predisposing disease, and rule out other causes of proteinuria (see Glomerulonephritis, p 442; Amyloidosis, p 57; Protein-Losing Nephropathy, p 900).
- Urine culture and sensitivity (C&S).
- Urine protein:creatinine (UPC) ratio: Clinician should confirm nephrotic range proteinuria (UPC > 2) and establish pretreatment baseline.
- Blood pressure measurement: hypertension (systolic >180 mmHg) common.

ADVANCED OR CONFIRMATORY TESTING

- Clinician should identify predisposing diseases with abdominal ultrasound, thoracic radiographs, antinuclear antibody (ANA) serology, and tests for regional infectious diseases.
- Renal biopsy: provides definitive diagnosis of glomerular lesion; should include light, electron, and immunofluorescent microscopic evaluation.

TREATMENT

THERAPEUTIC GOAL(S)

- Reduce magnitude of proteinuria
- Control edema
- Manage uremia, if present
- Control systemic hypertension, if present
- Treat potential underlying disease

ACUTE GENERAL TREATMENT

- Clinician should initiate angiotensin-converting enzyme (ACE) inhibitor therapy: enalapril 0.5 mg/kg PO q 24h to q 12h or benazepril 0.25 mg/kg PO q 24h.
- Address edema and effusion:
  - Abdominocentesis if ascites impinging on ventilation; thoracocentesis rarely required.
  - Appropriate diuretic use:
    - If plasma volume is reduced (e.g., dehydration), diuretics may be ineffective and dangerous, increasing risk of renal failure or thromboembolism.
    - If plasma volume is normal, spironolactone may help delay return of third-spaced fluid and provide benefit of inhibiting aldosterone.
  - Low-level exercise may help mobilize edema.
- Clinician should address components of uremia, if present.
- Plasma and/or synthetic colloids may be needed in uremic crisis, but no long-term benefit has been identified.
- Clinician should initiate aspirin therapy (0.5 mg/kg PO q 12h) if serum albumin is <2.0–2.5 g/dl.
- Clinician should add additional medications as needed to control systemic hypertension (see Systemic Hypertension, p 1058).
- Clinician should treat any concurrent disease.
- Clinician should recommend a diet formulated for renal disease.

CHRONIC TREATMENT

Disease-specific treatment may be indicated on basis of renal biopsy and other test results

DRUG INTERACTIONS

- Hypoalbuminemia will increase the unbound (often active) fraction of highly protein-bound drugs; dosages may need to be adjusted accordingly.
- Warfarin is unsuitable for management of thromboembolism in the face of hypoalbuminemia.

POSSIBLE COMPLICATIONS

- Hypotension from ACE inhibitor and Ca channel blocker
- Bleeding tendency from aspirin (very rare at recommended dose)
- Worsening azotemia as a result of ACE inhibitor administration; possible but rarely clinically relevant
- Exacerbation of ascites/edema following parenteral fluid administration

RECOMMENDED MONITORING

The UPC, urinalysis, blood pressure, serum albumin and creatinine, body weight and condition score should be monitored regularly—weekly to monthly initially. Once stable, the animal should undergo these tests every 3 to 6 months unless changes in therapy are initiated or changes are noted in clinical condition.

PROGNOSIS AND OUTCOME

- Variable but generally guarded.
- Azotemia, systemic hypertension, and marked tubulointerstitial lesions on biopsy may be negative prognostic indicators.

PEARLS & CONSIDERATIONS

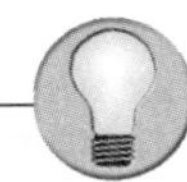

COMMENTS

- Nephrotic syndrome is a complication that can develop in animals with specific types of glomerular diseases. Prompt recognition of nephrotic syndrome is needed because:
  - Nephrotic syndrome is pathognomonic for glomerular disease.
  - The clinical condition can deteriorate rapidly; prompt intervention is warranted.
  - Nephrotic syndrome is a recognized predisposing factor for thromboembolic disease.

PREVENTION

- Urinalyses and urine albumin screening during routine health evaluations may allow early detection.
- Early intervention might prevent the development of nephrotic syndrome.

CLIENT EDUCATION

Rapid deterioration is possible; frequent rechecks are necessary.

SUGGESTED READING

Cook AK, Cowgill LD: Clinical and pathological features of protein-losing glomerular disease in the dog: A review of 137 cases (1985–1992). *J Am Anim Hosp Assoc* 32:313, 1996.

Vaden SL: Glomerular diseases. In Ettinger SJ, Feldman EC (eds): *Textbook of Veterinary Internal Medicine*, ed 6. St. Louis, Elsevier Saunders, 2005, pp 1786–1800.

AUTHOR: **SHELLY VADEN**
EDITOR: **LEAH A. COHN**

Nerve Sheath Tumors

BASIC INFORMATION

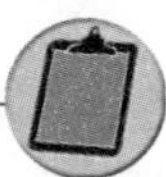

DEFINITION

A benign or malignant tumor of peripheral nerve cell origin. Nerve sheath tumors may affect peripheral nerves, spinal nerve roots, or cranial nerves. Approximately 80% of nerve sheath tumors occur in the brachial plexus region. The remaining 20% involve cranial nerves or other spinal nerve roots. The trigeminal nerve (cranial nerve [CN] V) is the most common cranial nerve affected.

SYNONYM(S)

Nerve root tumor

EPIDEMIOLOGY

SPECIES, AGE, SEX

- Common in dogs, less common in cats
- Reported age range is 3 to 13 years in dogs and 8 to 19 years in cats
- No known sex predilection

CLINICAL PRESENTATION

DISEASE FORMS/SUBTYPES: Nerve sheath tumors include:

- Ganglioneuroma
- Peripheral neuroblastoma
- Paraganglioma
- Peripheral nerve sheath tumors
  - Benign peripheral nerve sheath tumors
    - Schwannoma
    - Neurofibroma
  - Malignant peripheral nerve sheath tumors
    - Malignant schwannoma
    - Neurofibrosarcoma

HISTORY, CHIEF COMPLAINT

- Chronic, progressive lameness or pain
- Muscle atrophy
- Weakness
- Ataxia

PHYSICAL EXAM FINDINGS

- Varies with respect to tumor location and nerve root(s) affected
- Abnormalities *may* include:
  - Localized muscle atrophy
  - Chronic, progressive lameness (commonly in the unilateral forelimb)
  - Asymmetric paresis
  - Proprioceptive deficits
  - Hyporeflexia
  - Sensory deficits
  - Pain on palpation of tumor site (e.g., axilla)
  - Ipsilateral loss of cutaneous trunci reflex (may occur with C8–T1 spinal segments)
  - Ipsilateral Horner's syndrome (may occur with cervical or brachial plexus nerve sheath tumors) (see Brachial Plexus Abnormalities, p 148)

ETIOLOGY AND PATHOPHYSIOLOGY

Undetermined; recent research suggests a point mutation in the *neu* oncogene; however, there is insufficient evidence to determine the consistency of this finding.

DIAGNOSIS

A presumptive diagnosis can be made with history, clinical signs, electrophysiologic studies, and advanced imaging; however, cytologic or histopathologic evaluation is required for definitive diagnosis.

DIFFERENTIAL DIAGNOSIS

- Other soft tissue tumors may invade or compress nerves and result in similar neurologic deficits and imaging appearance (e.g., fibrosarcoma, chondrosarcoma, lymphoma).
- Abscess, granuloma.
- Orthopedic abnormalities (e.g., osteoarthritis, osteochondrosis dessicans [OCD], biceps tenosynovitis).
- Other cranial neuropathies (e.g., tumors of the brainstem or cavernous sinus).
- Other neuropathies (e.g., lateralized disk herniation).
- Traumatic brachial plexus injury.

INITIAL DATABASE

- Neurologic examination.
- Survey radiographs may rule out orthopedic conditions.
  - Clinicians should not overinterpret presence of osteoarthritis; osteoarthritis may be a concurrent condition and not the primary cause for presentation.
- Nerve sheath tumors of spinal nerve roots may show subtle osteolysis at the vertebral foramen.

ADVANCED OR CONFIRMATORY TESTING

- Electrophysiologic studies:
  - Differentiate neurologic from orthopedic conditions
  - Determine specific nerve roots involved; aid in surgical planning
- Cerebrospinal fluid (CSF) evaluation:
  - Occasionally, albuminocytologic dissociation (disproportionate elevation in CSF albumin concentration compared to cellularity)
- Myelography:
  - May indicate local invasion into spinal canal
  - May rule out lateralized disk herniation
- Advanced imaging (computed tomography [CT], magnetic resonance imaging [MRI])
- Fine-needle aspiration for cytologic examination

- Biopsy (percutaneous or surgical excision)
- Tumor staging:
  - Thoracic radiographs
  - Abdominal ultrasound
  - Lymph node aspirates

TREATMENT

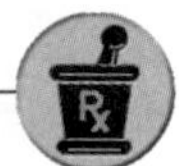

THERAPEUTIC GOAL(S)

- Complete excision, if possible
- Palliative analgesia

ACUTE GENERAL TREATMENT

- Surgical exploratory/excision:
  - Radical excision (i.e., limb amputation, ± hemilaminectomy) provides the optimal chance of complete excision and is recommended in most cases.
- Radiation therapy:
  - Adjunctive to surgical excision.
  - May be used as monotherapy in nonresectable cases.
- Adjunctive chemotherapy:
  - Rarely used as monotherapy.
  - Doxorubicin (dogs, cats), mitoxantrone (dogs, cats), or ifosfamide (dogs).

CHRONIC TREATMENT

- Palliative analgesia.
- Corticosteroids may help alleviate some discomfort and may reduce peritumoral inflammation; however, there is insufficient research to support or refute their use for treating this condition.

DRUG INTERACTIONS

- Concurrent administration of nonsteroidal anti-inflammatory drugs (NSAIDs) and corticosteroids is *not* recommended.
- Other potential drug interactions depend on the specific therapeutic modalities chosen; clinicians should consult appropriate references.

POSSIBLE COMPLICATIONS

- Local invasion into adjacent tissues (e.g., brainstem or spinal cord)
- Metastasis:
  - Metastatic rates for nerve sheath tumors have not been established.
  - The overall metastatic rate for soft tissue sarcomas is 8-17% (dogs) and 0-27% (cats).

RECOMMENDED MONITORING

- Clinicians should monitor for progressive/recurrent neurologic deficits and/or pain.
- Clinicians should monitor for urinary dysfunction and/or respiratory paresis in severe cases (if applicable to localization).

PROGNOSIS AND OUTCOME

- Variable; histopathologic grade, tumor location (e.g., surgical accessibility), and stage are prognostic.
- Although complete excision can be curative, often local invasion into the spinal cord or brainstem has already occurred by the time of diagnosis, making cure unlikely.
  - Recurrence rate is approximately 72%.
  - Time period for clinical signs to reappear following the incomplete excision is typically 5 months (range: 10 days to 14 months).
  - Median survival time is typically 5 to 12 months (range: 0 to 92 months).

PEARLS & CONSIDERATIONS

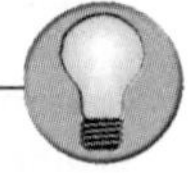

COMMENTS

- Early diagnosis increases the potential for complete excision.
- Orthopedic conditions typically do not produce neurologic deficits; if proprioceptive deficit or localized muscle atrophy is present, a nerve sheath tumor may be the cause.

CLIENT EDUCATION

- Clients should understand the potential for progression/recurrence.
- Clients should be counseled regarding quality of life issues that pertain to their pets.

SUGGESTED READING

Bradley RL, et al: Nerve sheath tumors in the dog. *J Am Anim Hosp Assoc* 18:915-921, 1982.

Brehm DM, et al: A retrospective evaluation of 51 cases of peripheral nerve sheath tumors in the dog. *J Am Anim Hosp Assoc* 31:349-359, 1995.

Targett MP, et al: Tumours involving the nerve sheaths of the forelimb in dogs. *J Small Anim Pract* 34:221-225, 1993.

AUTHOR: **REBECCA A. PACKER**
EDITOR: **CURTIS W. DEWEY**

Neutropenia, Immune-Mediated

BASIC INFORMATION

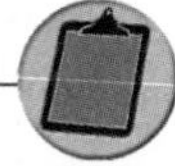

DEFINITION

Antibody-mediated destruction of neutrophils and/or their precursors in the marrow, resulting in an absolute decrease in the number of circulating neutrophils

SYNONYM(S)

Steroid-responsive neutropenia

EPIDEMIOLOGY

SPECIES, AGE, SEX

- Dogs and cats
- Any age or gender

RISK FACTORS: None known. Drugs (phenylbutazone, griseofulvin [cats]) or viruses sometimes implicated.

ASSOCIATED CONDITIONS AND DISORDERS: May be seen with anemia, thrombocytopenia, or pancytopenia (see Anemia, Aplastic, p 62).

CLINICAL PRESENTATION

HISTORY, CHIEF COMPLAINT

- Lethargy or anorexia may be reported by owners.
- Signs may arise from infections, usually bacterial from invasion of normal flora.
- Clinical signs are nonspecific and usually are not helpful in localizing the infection.

PHYSICAL EXAM FINDINGS: Fever and weakness may be the only findings. Sometimes signs of opportunistic infections (e.g., diarrhea or gingivitis) may be present.

ETIOLOGY AND PATHOPHYSIOLOGY

- Idiopathic; not well studied.
- Drugs or infections occasionally cause immune-mediated destruction of neutrophils.

DIAGNOSIS

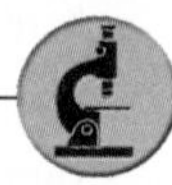

DIFFERENTIAL DIAGNOSIS

- Neutropenia may be the primary problem or it may be secondary to overwhelming infection, and determining which situation exists in a given patient is of paramount importance. Primary, immune-mediated neutropenia is more often associated with thrombocytope-

nia or anemia and clinical signs of variable severity. Secondary neutropenia is usually associated with severe clinical illness, and the count may improve within days of appropriate antibiotic treatment. Primary neutropenia persists after an infection is treated.
- Primary (nonimmune-mediated) neutropenias:
  - Bone marrow abnormality such as aplasia, fibrosis, dysplasia, or neoplasia. Neutropenia occurs first, then thrombocytopenia and anemia.
  - Infections such as parvovirus or ehrlichiosis in dogs and retroviruses (feline leukemia, feline immunodeficiency), or panleukopenia virus in cats.
  - Hyperestrogenism from testicular or ovarian tumors.
- Some normal cats may have neutrophil counts between 1800 and 2500/µl.
- Immune-mediated neutropenia is a diagnosis of exclusion.
- Response to treatment with corticosteroids may allow for retrospective diagnosis of immune-mediated neutropenia.

INITIAL DATABASE

- Complete blood count (CBC): If the neutropenia is associated with other cytopenias, or if it persists for more than 2 to 3 days (if <1000/µl neutrophils) or 1 week (if 1000-2000/µl), a bone marrow aspirate and biopsy are indicated.
- Serum biochemistry profile and possibly thoracic and abdominal radiographs can help clinicians assess for underlying disorders causing secondary (transient) neutropenia, such as neoplasia, or infections.
  - Serum chemistry profile usually unremarkable
  - Possible thoracic radiographic lesions (e.g., mediastinal or pulmonary disease)
- Urinalysis with bacterial culture and sensitivity (C&S) test to evaluate for urinary tract infection.

ADVANCED OR CONFIRMATORY TESTING

- If relevant, abdominal ultrasonography to evaluate for evidence of neoplasia or infection
- Serologic testing for relevant infectious diseases
- No test for antineutrophil antibodies is available currently
- Any concurrent drug therapy should be stopped if possible to rule out immune-mediated neutropenia due to adverse drug reaction

TREATMENT

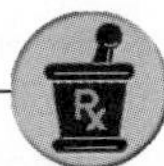

THERAPEUTIC GOAL(S)

- Clinicians should assume that sepsis is present whenever fever and neutropenia are present, regardless of the cause of the neutropenia. Aggressive treatment with IV bactericidal antibiotics is indicated since sepsis may be rapidly fatal.
- Prevention of infection by paying special attention to sterile technique with IV catheters and other invasive procedures.
- Prophylactic antibiotic treatment may be warranted even for afebrile animals with severe neutropenia.
- It is important to weigh risks and benefits and rule out other causes of neutropenia before starting corticosteroid therapy.

ACUTE GENERAL TREATMENT

- Appropriate antibiotics based on a C&S. Empiric antibiotic treatment may be necessary initially (first few days) while bacterial cultures are underway.
  - In severely ill patients, intravenous antibiotics should be used. Options include cefoxitin 30 mg/kg IV q 6-8h or ampicillin 20 mg/kg IV q 8h plus enrofloxacin 5 mg/kg (diluted 1:1 with sterile saline and given slowly IV) q 12h (q 24h in cats).
  - In stable cases, oral trimethoprim-sulfa (15 mg/kg PO q 12h) is often suitable because it preserves normal intestinal anaerobes. Trimethoprim-sulfa has rarely has been implicated as a cause of neutropenia.
- A trial of prednisone at 2 mg/kg PO q 24h may be given ONLY if infectious causes have been ruled out.
- In severe sepsis, consider temporary use of human G-CSF 5 µg/kg SQ q 12h. Antibodies will develop and prevent long-term benefits, however.
- If risk of ehrlichiosis, clinicians can consider doxycycline (5 mg/kg PO q 12h) while awaiting serologic results.

CHRONIC TREATMENT

- Neutrophil count should increase within 1 week of prednisone therapy.
- If there is no response, reassessment of the diagnosis is indicated. If the diagnosis is unchanged, consider human intravenous immunoglobulin (0.5 g/kg slow IV once, and a second dose may be administered after 24 to 48 hours if necessary; risk of anaphylaxis at either time) or cyclosporine (e.g., Neoral, Atopica: 2-5 mg/kg PO q 12h); monitoring of serum levels is recommended (target: 200-500 ng/ml). It is generally best to avoid administering myelosuppressive drugs, such as azathioprine or cyclophosphamide.

POSSIBLE COMPLICATIONS

Sepsis

RECOMMENDED MONITORING

Frequent assessment of body temperature

PROGNOSIS AND OUTCOME

Even with pancytopenia, many dogs under 3 years of age recover. Older dogs are more likely to have other complications, and most do not recover.

PEARLS & CONSIDERATIONS

COMMENTS

- The combination of fever and neutropenia should be considered to be a life-threatening emergency, which warrants obtaining specimens for culture and starting IV antibiotics immediately.
- Cats tolerate neutropenia better than dogs.

CLIENT EDUCATION

Clients can monitor temperature at home. If a fever develops, they must contact their veterinarian immediately for reexamination, reevaluation of CBC, and further diagnostic tests and treatment based on these findings.

SUGGESTED READING

Couto CG: Leukopenia and leukocytosis. In Nelson RW, Couto CG (eds): *Small Animal Internal Medicine*, ed 2. St. Louis, Mosby, 1998, pp 1178-1186.

Schultze AE: Interpretation of canine leukocyte responses. In Feldman BF, Zinkl JG, Jain NC (eds): *Schalm's Veterinary Hematology*, ed 5. Philadelphia, Lippincott Williams & Wilkins, 2000, pp 366-381.

AUTHOR & EDITOR: **SUSAN M. COTTER**

Nicotine Toxicosis

BASIC INFORMATION

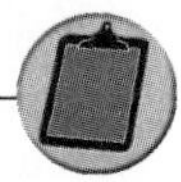

DEFINITION

Intoxication in pets generally due to ingestion of tobacco or related products and manifesting with acute onset of gastrointestinal (GI) signs followed by transient, potentially severe, neurologic dysfunction.

EPIDEMIOLOGY

SPECIES, AGE, SEX: All animals of all ages and sexes are susceptible; dogs are more likely to be involved compared to cats.

RISK FACTORS

- Availability of nicotine-containing products in pet's environment.
- Dogs may be particularly attracted to chewing tobacco containing flavoring agents such as honey, molasses, licorice, syrups, or sugars.

CLINICAL PRESENTATION

HISTORY, CHIEF COMPLAINT

- Evidence of exposure to nicotine-containing products (cigarettes, chewing tobacco, gum).
- Clinical signs occur >1 hour after ingestion; spontaneous vomiting, salivation, and diarrhea.
- Initial central nervous system (CNS) excitation and tachypnea.

PHYSICAL EXAM FINDINGS

- Hypersalivation
- Nausea
- Tenesmus
- Bradycardia (sinus); may be followed by tachycardia
- Shallow, slow respiration, eventually leading to cyanosis, respiratory paralysis
- Neuromuscular weakness, tremors, collapse

ETIOLOGY AND PATHOPHYSIOLOGY

- The toxin:
  - Sources include cigarettes, cigars, chewing tobacco, nicotine gum, skin patches, inhalers, nasal sprays, nicotinic insecticides (nicotine sulfate is available at a concentration of 0.05–4% as insecticide dust or sprays and as a concentrated 40% solution [Black Leaf 40]).
  - Nicotine is a water-soluble alkaloid found primarily in cultivated tobacco (*Nicotiana tabacum*) but also in wild tobacco (*N. attenuata* and *N. trigonophylla*). Tree tobacco (*N. glauca*) contains mostly anabasine (a teratogen) but does contain some nicotine. Indian tobacco (*Lobelia inflata*) contains mostly lobeline (curare-like paralytic) and some nicotine.
- Pathophysiology:
  - Nicotine mimics acetylcholine at sympathetic and parasympathetic ganglia, neuromuscular junctions of skeletal muscle, and at some synapses in the CNS. Low doses cause depolarization and stimulation of receptors similar to acetylcholine. Higher doses cause stimulation, followed by blockade of autonomic ganglia and neuromuscular junctions of skeletal muscle.
  - Cardiovascular stimulation of sympathetic ganglion and adrenal medulla can lead to release of catecholamines.
  - GI effects: Parasympathetic stimulation can lead to increased tone and motility.
  - Death can result from respiratory paralysis.

DIAGNOSIS

DIFFERENTIAL DIAGNOSIS

Other intoxications: strychnine, methylxanthines, tremorigenic mycotoxins/garbage toxicosis, organophosphates/carbamates

INITIAL DATABASE

- Serum chemistry profile: electrolyte abnormalities, azotemia (vomiting, dehydration)
- Blood gas analysis
- Electrocardiogram (ECG): sinus bradycardia or sinus tachycardia most common, ventricular arrhythmias possible

ADVANCED OR CONFIRMATORY TESTING

- Nicotine can be detected in urine, blood, GI contents, vomitus, or lavage washings. Clinicians can contact a veterinary diagnostic laboratory or a human hospital for analysis.
- Necropsy samples: nicotine in liver and kidney.

TREATMENT

THERAPEUTIC GOAL(S)

- Decontamination of patient
- Enhance excretion
- Bradycardia treatment if present
- Supportive care

ACUTE GENERAL TREATMENT

- Decontamination of patient:
  - Decontamination of dermal exposure consists of bathing the patient with liquid dishwashing detergent (wear thick rubber gloves).
  - Induction of emesis is indicated only if the patient is not showing any clinical signs (<1 hour after exposure) (see Vomiting, Induction of, p 1328).
  - Gastric lavage is necessary only if very large doses have been ingested and emesis cannot be induced (comatose animal) (see Gastric Intubation, Gavage, Lavage, p 1258).
  - Activated charcoal 1–4 g/kg PO (repeated doses may be necessary). Clinicians can protect the airway with a cuffed endotracheal tube if the animal is unconscious.
- Enhance excretion:
  - Fluid diuresis.
  - Urine acidification may promote excretion of nicotine, but this should only be done if the acid-base status is monitored. Ammonium chloride (50 mg/kg PO q 6h) or vitamin C (20–30 mg/kg IM or IV q 8h) can be used.
- Treat bradycardia (sinus bradycardia) if present with atropine 0.04 mg/kg SQ, IM, or IV, as needed (prn).
- Supportive care:
  - Oxygen and/or artificial respiration for respiratory difficulty or paralysis.
  - Diazepam for seizures (0.5–2.0 mg/kg IV in dogs and 0.5–1 mg/kg in cats, prn).
  - GI protectants: Clinicans can use sucralfate (0.5–1 g PO q 8h). Antacids are contraindicated because they can increase nicotine absorption.

RECOMMENDED MONITORING

- ECG
- Blood pressure
- Acid-base status
- CNS
- Respiratory system

PROGNOSIS AND OUTCOME

- Poor prognosis with large doses or if artificial ventilation is required
- Prognosis good if animal survives first 4 hours of ingestion

PEARLS & CONSIDERATIONS

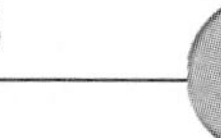

COMMENTS

- In dogs, 10 mg/kg administered orally is considered potentially lethal.
- Clinically significant toxicosis has been reported in dogs at 4 mg (one cigarette in a small- to medium-sized dog).
- Most dogs vomit spontaneously after ingestion, preventing serious toxicosis.

- Nicotine is absorbed more in alkaline pH. In humans, the half-life is 2 hours; excretion occurs via kidneys and is pH dependent.
- Ingestion of approximately 1 mg/kg or more should be considered serious.
- Nicotine from gum has comparatively low bioavailability at about 15%.
- Nicotine content in various products:
  - Cigar: 15–40 mg/cigar
  - Cigarettes: 13–30 mg per one cigarette
  - Low-yield cigarette: 3–8 mg
  - Cigarette butt: 5–7 mg
  - Snuff: 4.6–32 mg/g moist; 12.4–15.6 mg/g dry
  - Nicorette gum: 2 or 4 mg per piece (bioavailability 15%)
  - Nicotrol nasal spray: 10 mg/ml
  - Transdermal patches: 8.3–114 mg/patch
  - Nicotine inhaler: 10 mg/cartridge

PREVENTION

Pet owners should keep nicotine-containing products out of their pets' reach.

SUGGESTED READING

Beasley VR, et al: *Nicotine: A Systems Approach to Veterinary Toxicology*. 1999.

Cheeke PR: *Tobacco (Nicotiana spp)*; *Natural Toxicants in Feeds, Forages, and Poisonous Plants*. Danvile, IL, Interstate Publishers, 1998, pp 383–385.

Hackendahl NC: The dangers of nicotine ingestion in dogs. *Vet Med* 99:218–224, 2004.

National Institute for Occupational Safety and Health: *Registry of Toxic Effects of Chemical Substances*. Cincinnati, OH, National Institute for Occupational Safety and Health,

Rumack BH: *Poisindex® System* (Vol 123). Englewood, CO, Micromedex, 2005.

AUTHOR: **SHARON L. WELCH**
EDITOR: **SAFDAR A. KHAN**

DISEASES AND DISORDERS

Nodular Skin Disorders

BASIC INFORMATION

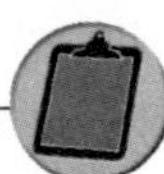

DEFINITION

A large group of diseases that manifest as solid elevated lesions of the skin of >1 cm in diameter, usually as a result of infiltration of inflammatory cells into the dermis or subcutis

EPIDEMIOLOGY

SPECIES, AGE, SEX

- Seen in cats and dogs.
- Neoplastic conditions are more common in mature individuals.
- Juvenile cellulitis: typically seen in dogs 3 to 8 months old (see Juvenile Cellulitis, p 611).
- No sex predilection.

GENETICS AND BREED PREDISPOSITION

- Familial vasculopathy of German shepherd
- Malignant histiocytosis of the Bernese mountain dog
- Sterile nodular panniculitis in dachshunds
- Mucinosis in the shar-pei

RISK FACTORS

- Any disease or medication that causes immune compromise predisposes animals to infections (e.g., feline leukemia virus [FeLV] infection, feline immunodeficiency virus [FIV] infection, hyperadrenocorticism, hypothyroidism, diabetes mellitus).
- Infectious nodular dermatitis: outdoor pets with increased probability of foreign body penetration or bite wound into the subcutis.
- Mineralizing fat necrosis/panniculitis in dogs with pancreatitis or pancreatic carcinomas.

CONTAGION AND ZOONOSIS

- Dermatophytic granuloma: *Microsporum canis* and *Trichophyton mentagrophytes* are potentially contagious to human and other animals.
- Sporotrichosis: Cat to human transmission is extremely high. Dog to human transmission has not yet been described.
- Blastomycosis, coccidioidomycosis, histoplasmosis: risk of zoonosis by aerosol from culture plates; in-house culture is always contraindicated.

GEOGRAPHY AND SEASONALITY: See Blastomycosis, p 133; Histoplasmosis, p 525; Coccidioidomycosis, p 218; Pythiosis and Lagenidiosis, p 937; Protothecosis, p 903.

ASSOCIATED CONDITIONS AND DISORDERS: Cystadenocarcinoma is typically a concurrent finding with nodular dermatofibrosis.

CLINICAL PRESENTATION

HISTORY, CHIEF COMPLAINT: Animals present with acute to chronic onset of single or multiple nodules, with or without draining tracts, and potentially accompanying systemic signs such as anorexia and lethargy.

PHYSICAL EXAM FINDINGS: Lesions are elevations above the epidermal surface of 1 cm or greater in size. They can be solitary to multiple, localized to generalized, hard to fluctuant, draining or intact, and pruritic to nonpruritic, all depending on the underlying etiology. Depending on etiology, systemic signs such as fever may be noted.

ETIOLOGY AND PATHOPHYSIOLOGY

Nodules, larger than papules, that are usually the result of a massive infiltration of inflammatory cells into the dermis or subcutis

DIAGNOSIS

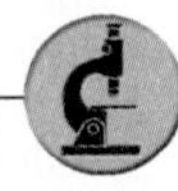

DIFFERENTIAL DIAGNOSIS

- Noninfectious granuloma/pyogranuloma:
  - Idiopathic sterile pyogranuloma/granuloma; sterile nodular panniculitis
  - Juvenile cellulitis
  - Foreign body reaction
  - Acral lick granuloma
  - Sebaceous adenitis
  - Sarcoidosis
  - Histiocytic diseases (cutaneous, systemic)
  - Cutaneous xanthomatosis
- Infectious granuloma/pyogranuloma:
  - Bacterial/botryomycosis, actinomycotic
  - Systemic and subcutaneous fungal, dermatophytic pseudomycetomas
  - Feline leprosy, atypic mycobacteria
  - Leishmaniasis
- Lymphocytic/plasmacytic:
  - Lupus profundus (panniculitis associated with systemic lupus erythematosus [SLE])
  - Vaccine reaction, drug eruption, erythema nodosum
  - Plasma cell pododermatitis
  - Lymphomatoid granulomatosis
  - Pseudolymphoma
  - Epitheliotropic lymphoma
  - Plasmacytoma
- Neutrophilic:
  - Deep pyoderma
  - Familial vasculopathy of German shepherds
  - Abscess
- Eosinophilic:

- Eosinophilic granulomas, insect-bite granulomas
- Dracunculiasis, dirofilariasis
- Pythiosis
- Ruptured hair follicle
- Other fibrosing, dysplastic, or neoplastic cells:
  - Dermoid cyst
  - Acral pruritic nodule/fibropruritic nodule
  - Calcinosis circumscripta
  - Nodular dermatofibrosis
  - Mucinosis
  - Hemangioma, sebaceous gland hyperplasia/adenoma
  - Mast cell tumors

INITIAL DATABASE

- Dermatologic exam to rule out *Cuterebra*, protruding foreign bodies, and any other grossly visible etiologies.
- Skin scrapings to identify possible *Demodex* mites or *Dirofilaria*.
- Impression smears from draining material for cytologic examination.
- Fine-needle aspirate to acquire cells for cytologic examination or discover *Dracunculus* parasite.
- Cytologic examination to help identify any evidence of:
  - Infectious organisms
    - Gram-positive branching filamentous organisms: *Actinomyces* sp. (nonacid-fast); *Nocardia* (partially acid-fast).
    - Diff Quik: yeast or fungal elements of systemic mycoses sometimes detectable.
    - Acid-fast bacilli: atypic mycobacteria, feline lepraemurium.
    - Organisms in foamy macrophages (may be noted).
  - Noninfectious findings
    - Foamy macrophages without evidence of infectious agents often detected with sterile nodular panniculitis.
    - Eosinophils characteristic of eosinophilic granulomas, foreign body reaction, insect bite reactions.
    - Neoplastic cells: round cell tumors (e.g., histiocytes, mast cells, plasmacytoma).
- Surgical excisional biopsies to obtain a deep enough sample to incorporate the panniculus. If using a punch biopsy, clinicians should be certain to double-punch to obtain the subcutaneous fatty tissue.
- Dermatohistopathologic test required to:
  - Differentiate the cellular infiltrate (neutrophils, histiocytes, plasma cells, lymphocytes, eosinophils, multinucleated giant cells, neoplastic cells).
  - Identify the presence of infectious organisms with the aid of special stains (GMS, PAS, Fite's acid-fast).
  - Help direct advanced diagnostics.

ADVANCED OR CONFIRMATORY TESTING

- Clinicians should submit part of a biopsy specimen aseptically for tissue maceration and culture.
- Clinicians should also be certain to notify the laboratory of suspected organisms (adjustments to culture media selection and incubation times; precautions).
  - Bacterial culture and sensitivity (C&S) testing:
    - Aerobic: *Staphylococcus* spp., *Rhodococcus equi*, *Nocardiosis*.
    - Anaerobic: *Actinomycosis*.
  - Atypic mycobacterial culture.
  - Fungal culture (many are biohazards; clinicians should notify the laboratory and not culture these in-house): protothecosis, blastomycosis, histoplasmosis, coccidioidomycosis, cryptococcosis, pythiosis, sporotrichosis, zygomycosis, and phaeohyphomycosis as well as dermatophytic granulomas.
  - Negative cultures support a diagnosis of sterile nodular panniculitis, lupus profundus.
- For the detection of antibody deposition (lupus) and identification of infectious agents that are at times difficult to culture or typically found low in numbers (canine sporotrichosis with direct immunofluorescence [DIF], leishmaniasis with polymerase chain reaction [PCR]):
  - DIF.
  - Immunoperoxidase staining.
  - Immunohistochemistry.
  - Immunostaining with polyclonal BCG antibody (promising method).
  - PCR.
- Serologic testing:
  - *Coccidioides, Blastomyces, Cryptococcus, Histoplasma*
- Additional laboratory tests:
  - FeLV/FIV
  - Antinuclear antibody (lupus profundus, SLE) testing.
  - CBC/serum biochemistry/thyroid profile/urinalysis:
    - Rule-out any metabolic disturbances resulting in immunosuppression.
    - Evidence of concurrent immune-mediated process (e.g., systemic lupus erythematosus [SLE]).
    - Baseline prior to commencing any long-term medications.
- Diagnostic imaging:
  - Radiographs: metastasis or infection dissemination.
  - Abdominal ultrasound: Clinicians should evaluate concurrent factors (pancreatitis, hyperadrenocorticism) and invasion of neoplasms (mast cell tumor, malignant histiocytosis) into abdominal organs.

TREATMENT

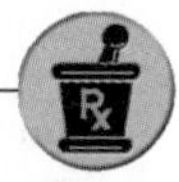

THERAPEUTIC GOAL(S)

Because the group of nodular skin disorders encompasses such a variety of etiologies, treatment is dependent on identification of the specific cause.

ACUTE GENERAL TREATMENT

Etiology dependent

CHRONIC TREATMENT

Etiology dependent

RECOMMENDED MONITORING

Etiology dependent

PROGNOSIS AND OUTCOME

Good to poor depending on the ability to identify and specifically treat the underlying etiology

PEARLS & CONSIDERATIONS

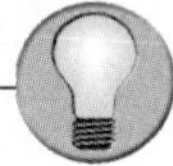

COMMENTS

A thorough and methodical diagnostic protocol is often necessary to confirm a specific cause.

CLIENT EDUCATION

It is better to invest in a diagnostic work-up to identify and treat the specific etiology rather than pursue countless therapeutic trials that often result in minimal response and maximal frustration.

SUGGESTED READING

Scott DW, Miller WH, Griffin CE: *Muller and Kirk's Small Animal Dermatology*, ed 6. Philadelphia, WB Saunders, 2001.

Yager JA, Wilcock BP: *Color Atlas and Text of Surgical Pathology of the Dog and Cat. Volume 1. Dermatopathology and Skin Tumors*. London, Mosby Wolfe, 1994, pp 119-154.

AUTHOR: **ANTHONY YU**

EDITOR: **JAN A. HALL**

Nonsteroidal Anti-Inflammatory Drug Toxicosis

BASIC INFORMATION

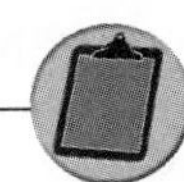

DEFINITION

Toxicosis secondary to acute or chronic administration of a nonsteroidal anti-inflammatory drug (NSAID) and typically characterized by one or more of the following: vomiting; diarrhea; anorexia; lethargy; underlying gastrointestinal (GI) ulceration, bleeding, or perforation; anemia; acute renal failure; or hepatopathy

SYNONYM(S)

Acetic acid derivatives: diclofenac, etodolac (EtoGesic), indomethacin, nabumetone
Cyclooxygenase (COX)-2 inhibitors: celecoxib, deracoxib (Deramaxx)
Fenamic acids: meclofenamic acid
Oxicams: meloxicam (Metacam), piroxicam
Propionic acids: carprofen (Rimadyl), flurbiprofen, ibuprofen, ketoprofen, naproxen
Pyrazalones: phenylbutazone
Salicylic acid derivatives: aspirin, flunixin meglumine

EPIDEMIOLOGY

SPECIES, AGE, SEX

- Cats are generally more sensitive than dogs to adverse effects of NSAIDs.
- All breeds and both sexes are susceptible.
- Elderly and very young animals are at higher risk.

RISK FACTORS

- Pre-existing renal, cardiovascular, or hepatic disease.
- Dehydration, hypotension, and concurrent use of other potentially nephrotoxic drugs.
- Concurrent use of other NSAIDs or corticosteroids: high incidence of severe complications.
- Concurrent use of other highly protein bound drugs that can result in higher active drug levels.
- Hypoalbuminemia.

CLINICAL PRESENTATION

DISEASE FORMS/SUBTYPES

- Acute toxicosis: occurs after ingesting large amounts of an NSAID (usually 5 to 10 times more than the recommended dose).
- Chronic toxicosis: occurs in sensitive animals after NSAID use for days, weeks, or months at recommended doses.

HISTORY, CHIEF COMPLAINT

- History of exposure (acute or chronic) to an NSAID
- Clinical signs typically begin within hours after acute exposure (exception: days or weeks for hepatopathy)
- Vomiting (± hematemesis), anorexia, lethargy, diarrhea (melena)
- Polyuria and polydipsia (PU/PD)

PHYSICAL EXAM FINDINGS

- Variable in severity, from minor digestive upset to life-threatening effects of GI perforation.
- Minor to moderate toxicosis: abdominal pain, vomiting, diarrhea, lethargy, anorexia.
- Severe toxicosis: dehydration, pale mucous membranes, tachycardia, icterus, bruising (aspirin), hyperthermia (aspirin), ataxia, seizures, sudden death.
- Hematemesis is not reliably linked to GI perforation, and absence of hematemesis is not an indicator of absence of perforation.

ETIOLOGY AND PATHOPHYSIOLOGY

- NSAIDs inhibit COX, blocking the production of prostaglandins (analgesic, antipyretic, and anti-inflammatory activity). Adverse effects result from decreased formation of protective prostaglandins and are generally fewer when the branch of the cyclooxygenase pathway that produces mainly inflammatory, nonprotective prostaglandins, COX-2, is inhibited predominantly.
- NSAID hepatopathy: formation of antigenic proteins that trigger an immune-mediated attack against the liver.

DIAGNOSIS

DIFFERENTIAL DIAGNOSIS

Any disease process that can cause GI, renal, or hepatic effects

INITIAL DATABASE

- Complete blood count: anemia from GI hemorrhage (regenerative), leukocytosis (stress or peritonitis)
- Serum chemistry profile: azotemia (prerenal or primary renal insult [usually within 24 to 48 hours after exposure in acute toxicosis]); liver enzyme elevation (hepatopathy)
- Urinalysis: hematuria, glucosuria, pyuria, proteinuria, casts, and isothenuria possible with renal injury

ADVANCED OR CONFIRMATORY TESTING

- Endoscopy: GI ulceration/irritation/perforation
- Histopathologic evaluations:
    - Stomach: irritation/ulceration/hemorrhage; peritonitis if gastric perforation
    - Kidneys: renal tubular or papillary necrosis or interstitial nephritis
    - Liver: multifocal to bridging hepatocellular degeneration and necrosis (apoptosis), with mild to moderate periportal inflammation (neutrophils and lymphocytes)

TREATMENT

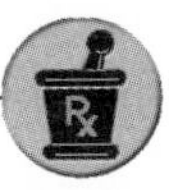

THERAPEUTIC GOAL(S)

- Decontamination of patient
- Preventing/managing GI, renal, and hepatic effects
- Providing supportive care

ACUTE GENERAL TREATMENT

- Decontamination of patient:
    - Emesis induction (see Vomiting, Induction of, p 1328).
    - Activated charcoal: 1-3 g/kg PO with a cathartic, repeated (half dose) q 6-8h to prevent enterohepatic recirculation of NSAID; clinicians should refer to labeled dosage of commercial product.
- Clinicians should prevent/manage GI and renal and hepatic effects:
    - Misoprostol for dogs: 1-3 ug/kg PO q 8h or H_2 receptor antagonists, with two options:
        - Famotidine for dogs and cats: 0.5 mg/kg PO, SC, IM, IV q 12-24h.
        - Cimetidine for dogs and cats: 5-10 mg/kg PO q 6h)
    - Omeprazole for dogs: 0.5-1.0 mg/kg PO q 24h; omeprazole for cats: 0.7 mg/kg PO q 24h.
    - Sucralfate for dogs: 0.5-1 g PO q 8-12h; sucralfate for cats: 0.25-0.5 g PO q 8-12h.
    - Fluid therapy: IV fluids to enhance NSAID excretion at a diuretic rate for at least 48 hr if potential renal toxicity dose has been ingested.
    - For hepatopathy: Clinicians should discontinue the use of NSAID and begin IV fluids; they should also administer vitamin K1 (1-2 mg/kg PO) and control vomiting with metoclopramide (0.2-0.4 mg/kg q 6h PO, SC, or IM or 1-2 mg/kg/day IV as constant rate infusion); SAMe 18 mg/kg PO q 24h for 1-3 months.
- Supportive care:
    - Clinicians should correct fluid losses and electrolyte changes.
    - They should also control seizures with diazepam 1-2 mg/kg IV.
    - Clinicians should administer a blood transfusion if needed.

CHRONIC TREATMENT

Some animals may need long-term therapy for renal or hepatic insufficiency.

DRUG INTERACTIONS

- Corticosteroids or other NSAIDs (increased risk for adverse effects).
- Phenytoin, valproic acid, oral anticoagulants, sulfonamides, sulfonylurea hypoglycemic agents, ketoconazole, methotrexate, fluconazole; increased serum drug levels.
- Aminoglycosides, angiotensin-converting enzyme (ACE) inhibitors, diuretics: increased risk of renal toxicity.

POSSIBLE COMPLICATIONS

- Chronic renal insufficiency
- Hepatopathy
- Peritonitis (perforation)

RECOMMENDED MONITORING

- Blood urea nitrogen, creatinine, urinalysis (baseline, 24, 48, 72 hours in acute cases)
- Liver enzymes (for hepatopathy)

PROGNOSIS AND OUTCOME

- Excellent from mild to moderate gastric irritation/ulceration with appropriate treatment.
- Guarded to poor with GI tract perforation.
- Renal effects of NSAIDs are reversible if discovered early and treated aggressively.
- Recovery from idiosyncratic hepatic toxicity is good when NSAID is discontinued and with supportive care.

PEARLS & CONSIDERATIONS

COMMENTS

- For most NSAIDs, the minimum toxic/lethal dose is unknown. Generally, a single acute ingestion of 5 to 10 times more than the recommended dose could cause potentially severe GI irritation/ulceration in dogs.
- Some NSAIDs (naproxen and meclofenamic acid) have a long half-life due to extensive enterohepatic recirculation in the dog.
- Ibuprofen is not recommended in small animal medicine; it is one of the most commonly reported toxicities.

PREVENTION

Clinicians should inform owners to keep all NSAIDs, especially chewables, out of the reach of pets.

CLIENT EDUCATION

Owners should not give any medications to their pets without consulting a veterinarian first.

SUGGESTED READING

Boothe DM: Nonsteroidal anti-inflammatory drugs. In Boothe DM (ed): *Small Animal Clinical Pharmacology and Therapeutics*. Philadelphia, WB Saunders, 2001, pp 282–295.

Roder JD: Nonsteroidal anti-inflammatory agents. In Plumlee KH (ed): *Clinical Veterinary Toxicology*. St. Louis, Mosby, 2004, pp 282–284.

AUTHOR: **TINA WISMER**
EDITOR: **SAFDAR A. KHAN**

Nutritional Secondary Hyperparathyroidism

BASIC INFORMATION

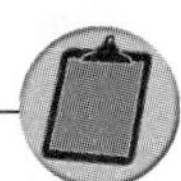

DEFINITION

Chronic elevation of circulating parathyroid hormone (PTH) resulting from low serum ionized calcium concentrations (iCa) due to deficiency of absorbed calcium or vitamin D or due to a calcium:phosphorus (Ca:P) imbalance.

SYNONYM(S)

NSHP
Nutritional osteodystrophy
The term *rickets* describes bony changes consistent with a vitamin D deficiency.

EPIDEMIOLOGY

SPECIES, AGE, SEX: Nutritional secondary hyperparathyroidism (NSHP) is seen in young, growing animals of any sex or species that have been fed an improperly formulated diet; the condition is occasionally seen in older animals.

GENETICS AND BREED PREDISPOSITION: Young, large breed dogs may be at increased risk due to rapid growth rate.

RISK FACTORS

- Animals fed improperly formulated homemade (especially all meat) diets, particularly during growth. Such diets typically contain decreased calcium and/or increased phosphorus, with a Ca:P ratio of ≥1:16 (1:1–2:1 for dogs and 1:1–1.5:1 for cats is recommended), and inadequate vitamin D.
- Exotic pets, since dietary requirements for calcium, phosphorus, and vitamin D are not always known.
- Animals with severe gastrointestinal disease that limits calcium or vitamin D absorption.

GEOGRAPHY AND SEASONALITY: Condition may be more common in winter months in some indoor-housed exotic pets due to decreased exposure to sunlight.

ASSOCIATED CONDITIONS AND DISORDERS: Animals may have decreased bone density or fractures related to increased circulating PTH.

CLINICAL PRESENTATION

DISEASE FORMS/SUBTYPES

- Inadequate dietary calcium or vitamin D concentration or altered dietary Ca:P ratio
- Inadequate absorption of dietary calcium and vitamin D due to intestinal disease

HISTORY, CHIEF COMPLAINT

- History of a homemade diet
- Excessive use of supplements such as meats, vitamins, and minerals
- Reluctance to walk, stiff gait, bone pain, lameness, or limb deformities (pathologic bone fractures); tooth loss; ± neurologic signs if the axial skeleton is involved
- Signs of hypocalcemia: twitching, tremors, stiffness, or seizures (rare)

PHYSICAL EXAM FINDINGS

- Bone palpation may elicit pain; fractures may be noted.
- Swelling of costochondral junctions or metaphyses may be evident.

ETIOLOGY AND PATHOPHYSIOLOGY

- Inadequate calcium absorption decreases iCa, increasing PTH production.
- PTH stimulates renal 1,25-dihydroxyvitamin D (calcitriol, the active metabolite of vitamin D) synthesis and bone resorption and increases renal calcium resorption and phosphorus excretion.
- Calcitriol also stimulates bone resorption to raise iCa into the normal range and decrease PTH production.
- Inadequate absorbed vitamin D decreases calcitriol production, decreasing iCa.
- Excessive PTH production reduces bone density, and pathologic fractures may occur.
- Excess circulating phosphorus also inhibits calcitriol synthesis and can lower iCa by the mass law effect.

DIAGNOSIS

The diagnosis is strongly suspected in young animals with a history of an inadequate diet, radiographic evidence of diffuse bone loss, and pathologic fractures.

DIFFERENTIAL DIAGNOSIS

- Other causes of lameness, bone pain, loss of bone density, or fractures, including congenital problems in young animals.
- Renal secondary hyperparathyroidism (ruled out based on serum biochemistry profile and urinalysis).
- Genetic defects in calcitriol production or utilization (rare). Clinical signs are the same in the absence of compatible diet history or malabsorptive disorder.

INITIAL DATABASE

- Complete blood count and serum biochemical profile: serum total calcium concentration normal to low. Note: Serum phosphorus and alkaline phosphatase may be elevated in normal animals, especially in those who are young and growing.
- Radiography of the skull, axial skeleton, and limbs: diffusely decreased cortical bone density; fractures possible.

ADVANCED OR CONFIRMATORY TESTING

- Measure PTH (increased), iCa (low to normal), and 25-hydroxyvitamin D (25-OH-D is typically low) concentrations to confirm the diagnosis.
- Serum calcitriol determination, although helpful, currently is not readily available.
- Vitamin/mineral analysis of homemade diets may be useful.

TREATMENT

THERAPEUTIC GOAL(S)

To increase intestinal absorption of calcium and vitamin D as well as to decrease PTH production.

ACUTE GENERAL TREATMENT

- Feed a properly formulated diet
- Stop the feeding of all supplements
- Supportive therapy for pain or fractures (cage rest or limited activity as indicated)
- Treatment of malabsorption when present
- Dietary supplementation with oral calcium (25–50 mg/kg/day) if clinical signs of hypocalcemia are present, discontinuing when signs resolve (see Hypocalcemia, p 564)

CHRONIC TREATMENT

- Clinicians should ensure that a properly formulated diet is fed.
- If a homemade diet is fed, a sample of the diet may be sent for vitamin D and mineral analysis.
- Supplemental oral calcium may be indicated in cases of chronic malabsorption.

RECOMMENDED MONITORING

- Clinicians should repeat tests of PTH, iCa, and 25-OH-D concentrations 3 to 4 weeks after initiating treatment. PTH should be decreased and 25-OH-D increased compared to pretreatment values. Clinicians should monitor the animals monthly until levels are normal.
- Clinicians can measure PTH, iCa, and 25-OH-D concentrations every 3 to 4 months, even if secondary hyperparathyroidism has resolved and if intestinal malabsorption is present.
- Clinicians should order repeat radiography tests to assess bone density and fracture healing.

PROGNOSIS AND OUTCOME

- Depends on presence of pathologic fractures, which worsen the prognosis due to pain and a potentially long convalescent period.
- Incidentally discovered NSHP that is due to inappropriate diet typically carries a good prognosis.
- For animals with malabsorption, the prognosis depends on the underlying cause and effectiveness of therapy.

PEARLS & CONSIDERATIONS

PREVENTION

Clinicians should inform owners to:

- Feed their pets nutritionally complete and balanced pet foods rather than improperly formulated homemade diets.
- Avoid supplementing balanced diets with meats, vitamins, or minerals.

CLIENT EDUCATION

- Clinicians should explain skeletal problems associated with deficiencies of calcium or vitamin D or with the excess of phosphorus to clients feeding homemade diets to their pets, especially to young, growing animals.
- Clinicians should have the adequacy of homemade diets verified by a veterinary nutritionist.
- Clinicians should suggest periodic nutrient analysis of homemade diets, especially nutrient analysis, especially for vitamin D and mineral content.

SUGGESTED READING

Cook SD, et al: A quantitative histologic study of osteoporosis produced by nutritional secondary hyperparathyroidism in dogs. *Clin Orthop* 175:105–120, 1983.

DeLay J, Laing J: Nutritional osteodystrophy in puppies fed a BARF diet. *AHL Newsletter* 6(2): 23, 2002.

Gross KL, et al: Nutrients. In Hand MS, Thatcher CD, Remillard RL, Roudebush P (eds): *Small Animal Clinical Nutrition*. Topeka, Mark Morris Institute, 2000, pp 21–110.

Remillard RL: Making pet foods at home. In Hand MS, Thatcher CD, Remillard RL, Roudebush P (eds): *Small Animal Clinical Nutrition*. Topeka, Mark Morris Institute, 2000, pp 163–182.

Schenck, et al: Disorders of calcium. In DiBartola SP (ed): *Fluid Therapy in Small Animal Practice*. St. Louis, Elsevier, 2006, pp 122–194.

Tomsa K, et al: Nutritional secondary hyperparathyroidism in six cats. *J Small Anim Pract* 40(11): 533–539, 1999.

AUTHOR: **PATRICIA A. SCHENCK**

EDITOR: **C. A. TONY BUFFINGTON**

Nystagmus

BASIC INFORMATION

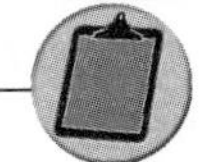

DEFINITION

Repetitive, rapid, and involuntary movement of the globe of the eye in a horizontal, rotary, or vertical manner

SYNONYM(S)

Vestibular nystagmus: jerk nystagmus

EPIDEMIOLOGY

SPECIES, AGE, SEX

- Any age, breed, or sex.
- Idiopathic vestibular disease is more common in older dogs (>8 years) but affects cats of all ages.

GENETICS AND BREED PREDISPOSITION

- Cats: Pendular nystagmus occurs in otherwise normal Siamese cats. Vestibular

nystagmus is a congenital abnormality in Siamese, Tonkinese, and Burmese breeds.
- Dogs: Vestibular nystamus is a congenital abnormality in the Doberman pinscher, cocker spaniel, German shepherd, and other breeds.

GEOGRAPHY AND SEASONALITY: Idiopathic vestibular disease in cats: may predominate in late summer/early fall.

ASSOCIATED CONDITIONS AND DISORDERS: Frequently associated with head tilt, ataxia, circling, vomiting, and anorexia.

CLINICAL PRESENTATION

DISEASE FORMS/SUBTYPES: Types of nystagmus:
- Vestibular nystagmus: The eye movements are faster in one direction than in the other (fast phase and slow phase for each cycle of the nystagmus); also called *jerk nystagmus*.
- Pendular nystagmus: There is no fast or slow phase. Pendular nystagmus is uncommon, is a congenital anomaly, and is not associated with vestibular disease or progression of signs.

HISTORY, CHIEF COMPLAINT
- Vestibular nystagmus usually is acute in onset:
  - The animal may initially exhibit vomiting, followed by vestibular ataxia, circling, or even whole-body rolling.
  - The owners may not notice the nystagmus.
- Much less common are pendular nystagmus or congenital vestibular nystagmus that are present from birth and are not associated with deteriorating vestibular function. The chief complaint is limited to the eye movements.

PHYSICAL EXAM FINDINGS
- Nystagmus due to peripheral vestibular disease (not all signs may be present):
  - Jerk nystagmus (horizontal or rotary) with fast phase away from the side of the vestibular lesion and away from the side of the head tilt.
  - The nystagmus may be difficult to observe, especially in the cat, and may be only observed when the animal's head is changed in position (especially dorsal extension of the neck) or when the animal is placed on its back.
  - Head tilt.
  - Circling.
  - Ataxia with falling to the side of the lesion and to the side of the head tilt.
- Nystagmus due to central vestibular disease (not all signs may be present):
  - Jerk nystagmus (horizontal, rotary, or vertical) with fast phase away from the side of the vestibular lesion and away from the side of the head tilt.
  - Head tilt toward the side of the lesion.
  - Circling.
  - Ataxia.
  - Proprioceptive deficits, motor weakness on the side of the lesion.
  - Central vestibular disease may (rarely) cause paradoxical signs (the nystagmus fast phase is away from the side of the lesion). Proprioceptive deficits indicate the true side of the lesion (ipsilateral).
  - Other cranial nerve deficits (V, VI, VII).

ETIOLOGY AND PATHOPHYSIOLOGY

- The vestibular system allows the body to know its position in space (proprioception) relative to head position, gravity, and linear or rotary acceleration.
- Sensory fibers in the peripheral vestibular system send impulses to the nuclei of cranial nerves III, IV, and VI, coordinating eye movements and allowing the eyes to remain centered on an object until it is beyond the visual field; then, the the eyes are able to jerk back to again center on an object ("watching railroad cars go by").
- Damage to the vestibular system can stimulate these eye movements inappropriately, producing nystagmus.

DIAGNOSIS

DIFFERENTIAL DIAGNOSIS

- Nystagmus from peripheral vestibular disease:
  - Idiopathic
  - Bacterial infection (otitis media/interna)
  - Neoplasia
  - Hypothyroidism (rare)
  - Postsurgery on the middle ear (ear ablation in the dog, removal of polyps in the cat)
  - Congenital or hereditary
- Central vestibular nystagmus:
  - Infection
  - Neoplasia
  - Trauma
- Pendular nystagmus: congenital disease affecting the visual pathway

INITIAL DATABASE

- Complete blood count, serum biochemistry profile, urinalysis: usually unremarkable
- Otoscopic exam
- Otitis externa, polyp, blood (head trauma) possible
- Careful examination may reveal fluid in the middle ear for cases with infectious causes
- Radiographs of the tympanic bullae

ADVANCED OR CONFIRMATORY TESTING

- Magnetic resonance imaging (MRI) or computed tomography (CT) of the middle ear and posterior fossa of the brain.
- Cerebrospinal fluid (CSF) analysis if signs of central vestibular disease are present.
- For cases in which there is no nystagmus but other clinical signs suggest vestibular disease, a postrotary nystagmus evaluation may be performed.
  - The animal is rotated in a circle first in one direction for ten rotations, and the duration of nystagmus is noted.
  - The animal is then rotated in the opposite direction, and the duration the postrotary nystagmus is again noted.
  - Postrotary nystagmus is usually less or absent when the animal is spun away from the side of the lesion.

TREATMENT

THERAPEUTIC GOAL(S)

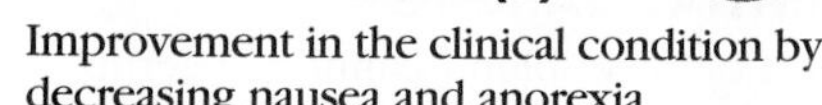

- Improvement in the clinical condition by decreasing nausea and anorexia
- Treatment of the primary cause when possible

ACUTE GENERAL TREATMENT

- Nystagmus is a clinical sign associated with various underlying causes. Therefore, treatment is aimed at the primary disorder.
- Since it may be difficult for the animal to walk or stand, good nursing care is very important: The animal should be able to get to food and water as well as should be cleaned after urinating or defecating so that urine or fecal scalding is avoided.

POSSIBLE COMPLICATIONS

Treatment of otitis with products that contain aminoglycoside antibiotics may be detrimental (ototoxic), particularly if the tympanum is not intact.

PROGNOSIS AND OUTCOME

- The prognosis for idiopathic vestibular disease and nystagmus caused by otitis media/interna are good to excellent for both dogs and cats, but recurrence is possible.
- A head tilt may remain after resolution of all other signs.
- The prognosis for neoplasia and virtually all causes of central vestibular nystagmus is guarded to poor.

PEARLS & CONSIDERATIONS

COMMENTS

- Idiopathic peripheral vestibular disease causes nystagmus in the majority of cases (for cats and dogs); the condition should resolve spontaneously in 1 to 2 weeks.

- Idiopathic vestibular disease is a diagnosis of exclusion.
- Nearly all patients with nystagmus caused by central vestibular disease will have other central nervous system (CNS) signs (proprioceptive defects, weakness, other cranial nerve involvement).

CLIENT EDUCATION

When idiopathic vestibular disease is the primary consideration, the owners need to know that the problem will usually resolve with time.

SUGGESTED READING

Lorenz M, Kornegay J: Ataxia of the head and the limbs. In Lorenz M, Kornegay J (eds): *Handbook of Veterinary Neurology*. Philidelphia, WB Saunders, 2004, pp 219–243.

AUTHOR: **JAMES B. MILLER**
EDITOR: **ETIENNE CÔTÉ**

Obesity

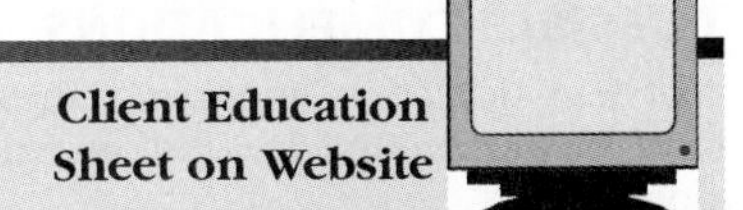

Client Education Sheet on Website

BASIC INFORMATION

DEFINITION

A chronic relapsing disorder associated with excessive accumulation of body fat, resulting in an increase in body weight beyond the limitation of skeletal and physical requirements. Animals with an accumulation of body fat of more than 20% of their moderate body weight for that species and breed are considered obese.

SYNONYM(S)

Fat
Overweight

EPIDEMIOLOGY

SPECIES, AGE, SEX

- Any species
- Both sexes
- Any age (3 months of age until the end of life)

GENETICS AND BREED PREDISPOSITION: Between 30% and 70% of the risk in dogs for obesity is attributable to breed; breeds that are reportedly at increased risk include Labrador retrievers, cairn terriers, cocker spaniels, dachshunds, Shetland sheepdogs, basset hounds, beagles, and cavalier King Charles spaniels.

RISK FACTORS: Genetic predisposition, neutering, multiple pet households, indoor housing, overfeeding, sedentary lifestyle, metabolic disorders.

ASSOCIATED CONDITIONS AND DISORDERS: Some obese animals may be at increased risk for diabetes, joint problems, muscle tears, hip dysplasia, tracheal collapse, skin and heart disorders, complications during anesthesia and surgery, and reduced life expectancy.

CLINICAL PRESENTATION

HISTORY, CHIEF COMPLAINT

- The most common history collected is of a pet that has gradually been gaining weight over a period of years, and the owner has been unaware of the increase.
- Another common history is of acute weight gain over a period of a few months after the animal was switched to a different diet or started on a new medication; the animal could also have gone through a stressful period or could have developed a metabolic disorder.

PHYSICAL EXAM FINDINGS: A body condition score (BCS) of 5/5 is characterized by the following:

- Ribs and other skeletal prominences are difficult to feel under thick fat cover.
- Fat hangs from the abdomen.
- The tail base is thickened.
- The animal does not have an apparent waist when it is viewed from the side or above.
- The animal is markedly broadened when it is viewed from above.

DIAGNOSIS

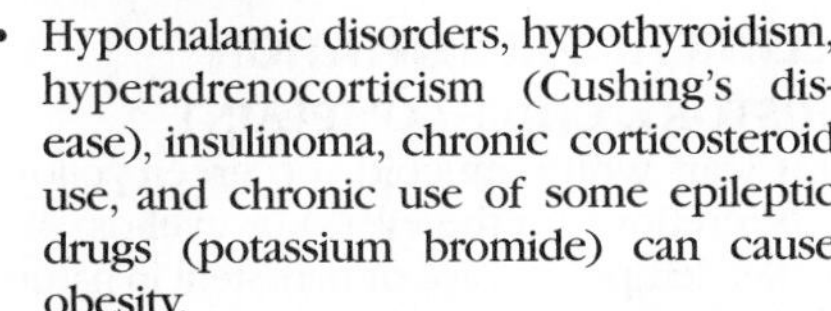

DIFFERENTIAL DIAGNOSIS

- Hypothalamic disorders, hypothyroidism, hyperadrenocorticism (Cushing's disease), insulinoma, chronic corticosteroid use, and chronic use of some epileptic drugs (potassium bromide) can cause obesity.
- Tumors, edema, and ascites may be confused for obesity.

INITIAL DATABASE

- Complete blood count, serum chemistry panel, urinalysis: Clinicians should assess for metabolic diseases that could affect the animal's weight, such as diabetes mellitus, hyperlipidemia, or hypothyroidism.
- Thyroid function studies (TSH, free T4) are used for evaluating the role of hypothyroidism as a cause of obesity (prevalence of hypothyroidism is less than 1% in dogs; rare in cats).

ADVANCED OR CONFIRMATORY TESTING

Radiographic imaging studies are not specific in the diagnosis of obesity but may provide evidence of the extent of fat accumulation in the periphery and in the abdominal and thoracic compartments.

TREATMENT

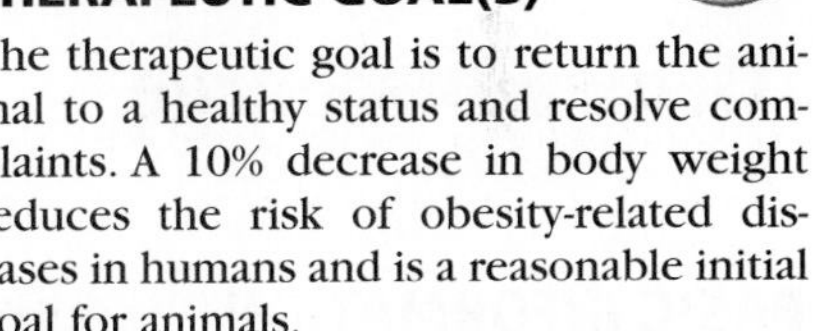

THERAPEUTIC GOAL(S)

The therapeutic goal is to return the animal to a healthy status and resolve complaints. A 10% decrease in body weight reduces the risk of obesity-related diseases in humans and is a reasonable initial goal for animals.

ACUTE GENERAL TREATMENT

Treatment is aimed at weight reduction and risk-factor modification.

- Clinicians should take an accurate diet history; it provides essential information about the food intake of the pet as well as information about the food itself and the related bond between a pet and owner. An accurate diet history can take 30 to 60 minutes to collect.
- The clinician should calculate caloric intake from all sources. Caloric content of human foods is available at the U.S. Department of Agriculture's Web site (http://nal.usda.gov).
- Clinicians should determine weight reduction goal and calories. An initial goal of a 10% weight loss usually is reasonable and can be attained by prescribing an energy deficit of 10 kcal per kilogram of body weight per day through a combination of decreased intake (about 8 kcal/kg/day) and increased activity-induced expenditure (about 2 kcal/kg/day). For example, the owner should encourage the animal to be active 30 minutes every day if the animal can tolerate this comfortably.The clinician and owner can adjust the time and intensity of the activity according to weight loss and the animal's enjoyment.
- The clinician should make sure that the animal completes the dietary plan.
    - The clinician should create the plan with the owner to increase compliance for completion of the plan.

  - Once the owner and clinician agree to a plan, a schedule of follow-ups must be established to provide coaching and monitor progress.
- In all cases, it is crucial to determine the protein, mineral, and vitamin intake of the diet to ensure that changes will not result in nutrient depletion.

DRUG INTERACTIONS

Glucocorticoids, potassium bromide

POSSIBLE COMPLICATIONS

Nutrient depletion, increased anesthetic risk, slower wound healing, hepatic lipidosis (cats)

RECOMMENDED MONITORING

The clinician's first contact with the client occurs 1 week after initial recommendations are made, followed by repeat "check-ins" at 6 weeks, 3 months, 6 months, and 1 year. These appointments permit the clinician to monitor the animal's BCS and weight progress, to make adjustments as needed, and to continue to support and motivate the client.

PROGNOSIS AND OUTCOME

Very good, depending on compliance of owner

PEARLS & CONSIDERATIONS

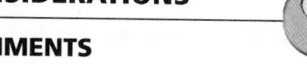

COMMENTS

According to veterinary experience, the critical key to successful obesity therapy is ongoing follow-up and support of the animal and owner's progress.

PREVENTION

Starts with puppies/kittens; clinicians can recommend adjusting feeding after spaying/neutering if needed.

CLIENT EDUCATION

- Clients should be able to assess and feed according to their pet's appropriate BCS.
- Every client should know how many kilocalories a pet food cup or can contains.

SUGGESTED READING

Buffington CAT, Holloway C, Abood S: *Manual of Veterinary Dietetics*. St. Louis, WB Saunders, 2004, pp 109–116.

The Ohio State University Veterinary Hospital Nutrition Support Service: www.nssvet.org.

AUTHOR: **CHERYL A. HOLLOWAY**

EDITOR: **C. A. TONY BUFFINGTON**

Ocular Discharge

BASIC INFORMATION

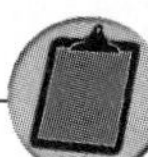

DEFINITION

- Abnormal secretions on or around the eye(s).
- These secretions can be watery (*serous*), contain mucus (*mucoid*), or contain white blood cells, mucus, and bacterial/fungal agents (*mucopurulent*).
- An abnormal overflow of tears down the face is termed *epiphora*.

SYNONYM(S)

Lacrimation: secretion and discharge of tears

Ocular secretion

EPIDEMIOLOGY

SPECIES, AGE, SEX

- Dogs and cats
- Variable age of onset depending on cause.
- No sex predisposition.

GENETICS AND BREED PREDISPOSITION: Depends on cause. Examples:

- Brachycephalic breeds with medial entropion (see Entropion/Ectropion, p 345)
- Breeds predisposed to distichia, ectopic cilia, and trichiasis (see Distichiasis/Ectopic Cilia/Trichiasis, p 317)
- Breeds predisposed to entropion and/or ectropion (see Entropion/Ectropion, p 345)
- Dolichocephalic breeds of dogs with narrow skull conformation and deep medial canthal areas (i.e., medial canthal pocket syndrome)

RISK FACTORS: Outdoor animals prone to infectious causes of conjunctivitis (see Conjunctivitis: Cats, p 231, Dogs, p 233) and ocular trauma (see Corneal/Scleral Trauma, p 244).

CONTAGION AND ZOONOSIS: Certain infectious causes of conjunctivitis are contagious (e.g., feline herpesvirus type-1 [FHV-1]) and/or zoonotic (e.g., chlamydiosis) (see Conjunctivitis: Cats, p 231, Dogs, p 233).

CLINICAL PRESENTATION

HISTORY, CHIEF COMPLAINT

- Clear, white mucoid, or green-yellow secretions on the eye(s) or eyelids
- Sudden, progressive, or persistent in nature

PHYSICAL EXAM FINDINGS: Unilateral or bilateral serous, mucoid, or mucopurulent ocular secretions with one or more of the following:

- Blepharitis: inflammation of the eyelids
- Conjunctivitis (see Conjunctivitis: Cats, p 231, Dogs, p 233)
- Corneal ulceration (see Corneal Ulceration, p 246)
- Keratoconjunctivitis sicca (KCS) (see Keratoconjunctivitis Sicca, p 614)
- Qualitative tear film abnormality (e.g., mucin and/or lipid deficiency)
- Entropion and/or ectropion (see Entropion/Ectropion, p 345)
- Distichiasis/ectopic cilia/trichiasis (see Distichiasis/Ectopic Cilia/Trichiasis, p 317)
- Anterior uveitis (see Uveitis, p 1134)
- Glaucoma (see Glaucoma, p 440)
- Ocular size abnormalities (see Ocular Size Abnormalities, p 763)
- Orbital disease (see Orbital Disease, p 773)
- Blockage of nasolacrimal system (e.g., dacryocystitis) (see Dacryocystitis, p 275)

ETIOLOGY AND PATHOPHYSIOLOGY

- Epiphora (serous discharge):
  - Corneal mechanical irritation:
    - Distichiasis/ectopic cilia/trichiasis
    - Entropion
    - Eyelid agenesis (partial more common than complete): seen in cats
    - Eyelid neoplasia
  - Blockage of nasolacrimal system, congenital:
    - Imperforate lacrimal punctum (dorsal and/or ventral lacrimal puncta/punctum not open; common)
    - Micropunctum (small ventral lacrimal punctum)
    - Nasolacrimal aplasia (lack of opening into nasal cavity; rare)
    - Obstruction of nasolacrimal duct in dogs by dacryops (cysts originating from lacrimal tissue) or nasal cyst
  - Blockage of nasolacrimal system, acquired:
    - Dacryocystitis (inflammation of the nasolacrimal system; see Dacryocystitis p 275)
    - Neoplasia (primary, rare; secondary, more common; e.g., nasal; maxillary sinus)
    - Foreign body

    - Trauma to medial canthus/eyelid involving lacrimal punctum/puncta and/or canaliculus/canaliculi
  - Ocular pain:
    - Conjunctivitis
    - Simple or indolent corneal ulceration (see Corneal Ulceration, p 246)
    - Qualitative tear film abnormality (e.g., mucin and/or lipid deficiency)
    - Anterior uveitis
    - Glaucoma
- Mucoid to mucopurulent discharge:
  - Conjunctivitis
  - KCS
  - Melting/infected corneal ulceration (see Corneal Ulceration, p 246)
  - Orbital abscess/cellulitis (see Orbital Disease, p 773)
  - Dacryocystitis (see Dacryocystitis, p 275)
  - Nasolacrimal foreign body (e.g., grass awn; parasite)

DIAGNOSIS

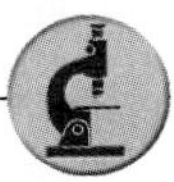

DIFFERENTIAL DIAGNOSIS

- Ocular discharge with "red eye(s)" is often associated with overproduction of tears (i.e., linked with causes of corneal mechanical irritation or ocular pain).
- Ocular discharge with "quiet eye(s)" (no evidence of ocular pain or eyelid swelling/blepharospasm) is often associated with impaired drainage of tears (e.g., congenital or acquired blockage of nasolacrimal system).

INITIAL DATABASE

- Complete ophthalmic examination, including:
  - Schirmer tear test (low with KCS; normal 15-25 mm/min; equivocal if 8-15 mm/min)
  - Fluorescein dye application (corneal dye retention with corneal ulceration; dye exiting nares helps confirm patent nasolacrimal system)
  - Nasolacrimal system flushed if no fluorescein dye exits nares and blockage is therefore suspected
  - Intraocular pressure (IOP) (pressures at >30 mmHg with glaucoma; may be low at <10-15 mmHg with uveitis)
- Conjunctival and/or corneal (if infected corneal ulcer) swabs for:
  - Cytologic examination to determine cell type and possible etiology
  - Culture and sensitivity (C&S): aerobic; if needed, anaerobic and fungal

ADVANCED OR CONFIRMATORY TESTING

- Varies depending on underlying cause
- Blockage of nasolacrimal system can be determined with nasal radiographs and a contrast study of the nasolacrimal system

TREATMENT

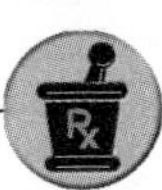

THERAPEUTIC GOAL(S)

Resolution of the ocular discharge

ACUTE GENERAL TREATMENT

- Treat the underlying cause
- Blockage of nasolacrimal system: Treat the primary lesion causing the obstruction (may be difficult to diagnose; if so, consult a veterinary ophthalmologist)

CHRONIC TREATMENT

May be required with certain diseases (e.g., KCS)

POSSIBLE COMPLICATIONS

- Conjunctivitis due to FHV-1 may lead to symblepharon (adhesions of conjunctiva to surrounding tissues), KCS, ulcerative keratitis, and stromal keratitis (see Herpesviral Keratitis in Cats, p 513).
- Chronic epiphora can lead to localized facial dermatitis at the medial canthus.

RECOMMENDED MONITORING

Varies depending on the underlying cause

PROGNOSIS AND OUTCOME

Prognosis is guarded to excellent depending on the underlying cause.

PEARLS & CONSIDERATIONS

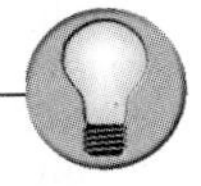

COMMENTS

- Clinicians should perform routine aerobic bacterial C&S tests and submit them in cases of mucopurulent discharge to identify the implicated bacteria or fungus.
- Fungal infections are rare causes of ocular discharge in cats and dogs.
- Serous ocular discharge in cats is common with FHV-1.
- A thorough examination of the ENTIRE conjunctival sac, including dorsally throughout the dorsal surface of the globe and ventrally on both sides of the third eyelid, is necessary to identify any retained foreign material.

CLIENT EDUCATION

At the first sign of abnormal ocular discharge in their pets, owners should consult their veterinarian.

SUGGESTED READING

Gerding PA, Kakoma I: Microbiology of the canine and feline eye. *Vet Clin North Am Small Anim Pract* 20:615, 1990.

Murphy JM: Exfoliative cytologic examination as an aid in diagnosing ocular diseases in the dog and cat. *Sem in Vet Med and Surg (Small Anim)* 3:10, 1988.

AUTHOR: **CHANTALE L. PINARD**

EDITOR: **CHERYL L. CULLEN**

Ocular Size Abnormalities

BASIC INFORMATION

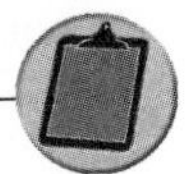

DEFINITION

- May occur in one or both eyes
- Buphthalmos: a larger than normal globe; may be congenital or acquired and is a result of current or past glaucoma
- Microphthalmos: a smaller than normal globe; a congenital condition sometimes associated with other ocular anomalies
- Phthisis bulbi: a shrunken globe; a condition acquired as a result of chronic ocular inflammation (e.g., uveitis or severe ocular trauma)

SYNONYM(S)

Buphthalmia (buphthalmos)
Microphthalmia (microphthalmos)

EPIDEMIOLOGY

SPECIES, AGE, SEX

- No species or sex predispositions.
- Buphthalmos may occur, and microphthalmos does occur, congenitally.
- Phthisis bulbi: no age predisposition.

GENETICS AND BREED PREDISPOSITION: Buphthalmos, secondary to glaucoma, is inherited in several breeds (see Glaucoma, p 440).

Microphthalmos is inherited in miniature schnauzers, Australian shepherds, collies, Shetland sheepdogs, and Doberman pinschers.

ASSOCIATED CONDITIONS AND DISORDERS

- Buphthalmos is associated with:
  - Lagophthalmos (incomplete closure of the eyelids) with or without secondary corneal ulceration (see Corneal Ulceration, p 246)
  - Lens subluxation/luxation (see Lens Luxation, p 628)
- Microphthalmos is associated with:
  - Other congenital ocular anomalies, including cataracts (see Cataracts, p 182) and retinal dysplasia/folds
  - Collie eye anomaly, including choroidal hypoplasia with or without optic nerve coloboma, staphyloma, retinal detachment, and intraocular hemorrhage
- Phthisis bulbi is associated with:
  - Untreated or poorly responsive ocular inflammation (e.g., uveitis or severe ocular trauma)
  - Variable systemic abnormalities depending on cause of uveitis (see Uveitis, p 1134)

CLINICAL PRESENTATION

HISTORY, CHIEF COMPLAINT: Condition is most likely unilateral but can also occur bilaterally.

- Buphthalmos: enlargement of globe during first few months of life (i.e., congenital glaucoma); progressive enlargement of globe and "red eye" (see Glaucoma, p 440)
- Microphthalmos: small eye from birth
- Phthisis bulbi: progressive shrinkage of globe following a "red eye" (see Red Eye, p 946)

PHYSICAL EXAM FINDINGS

- Buphthalmos: larger globe and signs of glaucoma, including:
  - Red eye (congested conjunctival and scleral blood vessels)
  - Diffuse corneal edema with possible striae (white streaks in the cornea from breaks in Descemet's membrane)
  - Corneal vascularization if eyelids cannot close over the enlarged globe (i.e., lagophthalmos)
  - Fixed and dilated pupil
  - Lens subluxation/luxation (see Lens Luxation, p 628)
  - Blindness
- Microphthalmos: smaller globe and the following:
  - Enophthalmos (caudal displacement of the eye) (see Orbital Disease, p 773)
  - Prolapsed third eyelid (see Third Eyelid Abnormalities/Protrusion, p 1077)
  - Other intraocular abnormalities (cataracts, retinal folds/dysplasia)
  - ± Small palpebral fissure (i.e., small opening between the eyelids) or entropion and/or conjunctivitis if eyelids are normal length despite small eye
  - Vision may be normal, reduced, or absent
- Phthisis bulbi: shrunken globe and the following:
  - Enophthalmos (caudal displacement of the eye) (see Orbital Disease, p 773)
  - Prolapsed third eyelid
  - Corneal edema; deep corneal vascularization
  - ± Entropion, conjunctivitis, posterior synechiae, cataract, iris atrophy
  - Vision typically reduced or absent

ETIOLOGY AND PATHOPHYSIOLOGY

- Buphthalmos: result of untreated or poorly managed glaucoma
- Microphthalmos: congenital deficiency of optic vesicle or failure of normal growth and expansion of optic cup; inherited condition
- Phthisis bulbi: acquired condition that possibly follows chronic intraocular inflammation (see Uveitis, p 1134; Glaucoma, p 440; Corneal/Scleral Trauma, p 244)

DIAGNOSIS

DIFFERENTIAL DIAGNOSIS

- Buphthalmos: exophthalmos (see Orbital Disease, p 773)
- Microphthalmos, phthisis bulbi: ruptured globe (see Corneal/Scleral Trauma, p 244)

INITIAL DATABASE

- Complete ophthalmic examination, including:
  - Measurement of intraocular pressure (IOP): may be elevated (>30 mmHg), indicating uncontrolled glaucoma, or normal, with buphthalmos; typically low (<10–15 mmHg) with phthisis bulbi
  - Fluorescein dye application with buphthalmos (there may be positive dye retention, such as with a corneal ulcer)
- Additional tests vary depending on underlying cause

ADVANCED OR CONFIRMATORY TESTING

- Buphthalmos: ocular ultrasound if corneal or ocular media opacification precludes evaluation of intraocular structures (e.g., assess lens for cataracts and globe for intraocular mass)
- Ocular histopathologic examination if enucleation is performed due to blindness and ocular pain (common with buphthalmos)

TREATMENT

THERAPEUTIC GOAL(S)

Controlling ocular pain:

- Buphthalmos:
  - Control increased IOP
  - Prevent corneal ulceration
  - Manage primary or secondary uveitis
- Microphthalmos/phthisis bulbi: prevent chronic ocular irritation from entropion and/or conjunctivitis

No treatment may be required if ocular size abnormalities are not accompanied by evidence of discomfort, inflammation, or elevated IOP.

ACUTE GENERAL TREATMENT

- For buphthalmos (for treatment options, see Glaucoma, p 440), if the animal's globe is blind and if glaucoma remains medically uncontrolled, clinicians should recommend:
  - Enucleation, evisceration with intraocular prosthesis, or chemical ablation of blind eyes with chronic primary glaucoma (see Glaucoma, p 440)
  - Enucleation of eyes with intraocular neoplasia
  - Enucleation of eyes with congenital glaucoma
- For microphthalmos, clinicians should recommend enucleation if eye is blind and entropion or chronic conjunctivitis occurs.
- For phthisis bulbi, clinicians should treat underlying uveitis and advise enucleation if eye is blind and entropion or chronic conjunctivitis occurs.

PROGNOSIS AND OUTCOME

- Prognosis for vision is grave in cases of buphthalmos and advanced phthisis bulbi.
- Depending on the degree of microphthalmos and the presence of other ocular anomalies, the prognosis for vision varies for microphthalmos.

PEARLS & CONSIDERATIONS

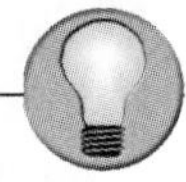

COMMENTS

- Recommendations against breeding animals affected with buphthalmos or microphthalmos if the condition is deemed to be breed-related or inherited in nature.
- Abnormal ocular size requires prompt evaluation and may or may not indicate an immediate need to treat; a proper and complete clinical ophthalmic exam determines the need for intervention (or lack thereof).

CLIENT EDUCATION

Clinicians should advise clients to seek veterinary care for their pets as soon as the eye becomes "red" and/or the eye changes in appearance.

SUGGESTED READING

Moore PA: Examination techniques and interpretation of ophthalmic findings. *Clin Tech Small Anim Pract* 16:1, 2001.

AUTHOR: **CHANTALE L. PINARD**
EDITOR: **CHERYL L. CULLEN**

Oleander Poisoning

BASIC INFORMATION

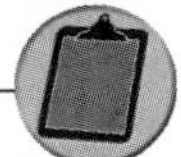

DEFINITION

An acute poisoning that occurs following ingestion of dried or fresh parts of an oleander plant (genus *Nerium* or *Thevitia*). Clinical manifestations are similar to those of digoxin toxicity: gastrointestinal (GI) signs initially, with possible subsequent cardiac arrhythmias.

SYNONYM(S)

Nerium oleander: oleander
Thevitia nerifolia: yellow oleander

EPIDEMIOLOGY

SPECIES, AGE, SEX: Animals of all ages, sexes, and breeds susceptible; dog cases are more common.
RISK FACTORS: Availability of oleander plant in pet's environment.
GEOGRAPHY AND SEASONALITY: Oleander is an ornamental evergreen shrub widely cultivated all over the United States, including California and Florida (Fig. I-121).

CLINICAL PRESENTATION

HISTORY, CHIEF COMPLAINT

- History of exposure to plant.
- Vomiting, with plant material in the vomitus.
- Owners may note lethargy, salivation, signs of abdominal pain, diarrhea, weakness, and tremors.

PHYSICAL EXAM FINDINGS

- See History, Chief Complaint above.
- Cardiac arrhythmias, either tachycardias (premature beats or runs of tachycardia) or bradycardias; a pattern of bradycardia, initially present for 24 hours, followed by tachycardia and ventricular arrhythmia, has been described.
- Central (seizures) and peripheral (tremors, weakness) nervous system effects. Severe intoxications can lead to coma and death.

ETIOLOGY AND PATHOPHYSIOLOGY

Clinical signs usually appear within 6 hours, depending on the amount ingested.

- Oleander contains cardiac glycosides (oleandrin, neriine, etc.) that inhibit the sodium/potassium (Na^+/K^+) ATPase enzyme, which is essential for normal cellular function in multiple body systems, notably the cardiovascular and nervous systems.
- Inhibition of Na^+/K^+ ATPase leads to an abnormal accumulation of potassium outside the cell and sodium inside the cell, producing a cascade of calcium release that results in cardiac arrhythmia and myocardial ischemia or necrosis (in severe cases).
- The toxic effects are indistinguishable from those of digoxin toxicosis in pets receiving digoxin therapeutically.

DIAGNOSIS

DIFFERENTIAL DIAGNOSIS

- Advanced primary heart disease (cardiomyopathy, valvular heart disease, traumatic myocarditis if hit by car, etc.)
- Bradycardias (third-degree atrioventricular block, sick sinus syndrome, atrial standstill/hyperkalemia)
- Systemic causes of ventricular arrhythmias (see Ventricular Arrhythmias, p 1148)
- Exposure to other plants that contain cardiac glycosides (see Cardiac Glycosides-Containing Plant Toxicosis, p 174)

INITIAL DATABASE

- Complete blood count: no significant changes likely.
- Serum chemistry profile: hypokalemia or hyperkalemia possible. Hypokalemia may be particularly detrimental: it fosters ventricular arrhythmia and also makes animals refractory to antiarrhythmics (lidocaine, quinidine, mexiletine, etc.).
- Electrocardiogram (ECG) to determine type of cardiac arrhythmia, if present.

ADVANCED OR CONFIRMATORY TESTING

- Confirmation of oleandrin in body fluids, stomach, and intestinal contents by using TLC and HPLC techniques (available in some veterinary diagnostic laboratories).
- Postmortem examination may reveal fluid in the GI tract and pericardium, possible pulmonary edema, and varying degrees of thrombi and hemorrhages in epicardial surfaces.
- Histologic examination of the heart tissue may reveal evidence of myocardial inflammation, degeneration, and necrosis.

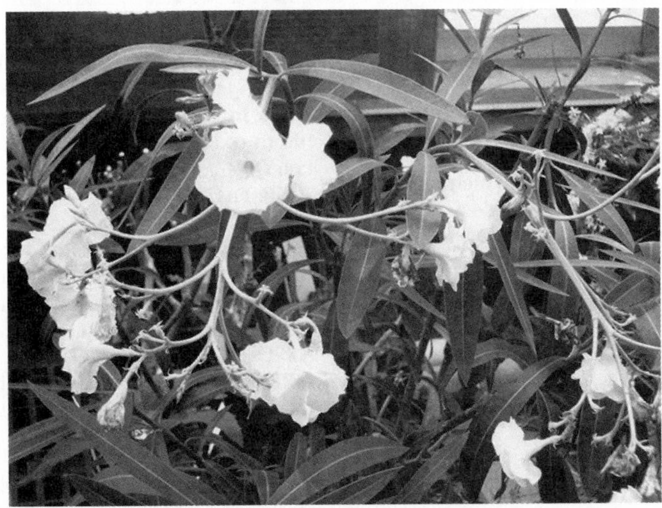

FIGURE I-121 Oleander plant, showing characteristic long, oval, robust leaves and ornamental flowers.

TREATMENT

THERAPEUTIC GOAL(S)

- Decontamination of patient
- Treatment for cardiac arrhythmia if necessary
- Use of specific fluorescent antibodies (FAB, Digibind) in severe cases
- Supportive therapy

ACUTE GENERAL TREATMENT

These guidelines are appropriate for an average adult dog.

- Decontamination of patient:
  - Clinicians should induce emesis if appropriate and within 1 to 2 hours after ingestion (see Vomiting, Induction of, p 1328).
  - Activated charcoal: Clinicians can give the animal charcoal after inducing emesis or if few hours have elapsed after exposure; 1-4 g/kg with a cathartic, such as 70% sorbitol (3 ml/kg) PO.
- Treating cardiac arrhythmias:
  - Sinus bradycardia (see Sinus Bradycardia, p 1005) that occurs within 24 hours of exposure: Clinicians should treat the condition if severe (e.g., heart rate <60-80 beats/min in an awake and standing large- to small-breed dog, respectively) or if the condition is associated with overt signs (e.g., lethargy).
  - Ventricular arrhythmias (see Ventricular Arrhythmias, p 1148).
  - Supraventricular arrhythmias (see Atrial Premature Complexes and Atrial/Supraventricular Tachycardia, p 100): Extremely rapid, persistent supraventricular tachycardias may need to be controlled (e.g., with propranolol 0.1-0.5 mg IV total dose per bolus; no more frequently than 1 bolus q 1-3 min to 5 mg maximum). The goal is to lower heart rate to acceptable level (e.g., by 20%) and not cause an overly rapid suppression.
- Use of specific fluorescent antibodies (FAB, Digibind) in severe cases:
  - IV antidigitalis antibodies; inactivate significant proportion of circulating cardiac glycoside.
  - Extremely expensive (several thousand dollars per dose); reserved for cases in which animals are profoundly ill or manifesting severe arrhythmias and in which cost of treatment is unimportant to the owner (for dosage and details, see Digoxin Toxicity, p 301).
- For supportive care, clinicians should:
  - Administer IV fluids as needed.
  - Treat diarrhea, severe vomiting, and abdominal pain as needed.
  - Correct electrolytes (potassium) if needed.

RECOMMENDED MONITORING

- ECG
- Serum chemistry profile, especially electrolytes

PROGNOSIS AND OUTCOME

- Poor prognosis with severe cardiac arrhythmias; animals are often found dead.
- Clinical signs of toxicity may persist for 24 hours or longer in animals that ultimately survive.

PEARLS & CONSIDERATIONS

COMMENTS

- Animals that survive may have no permanent sequelae or may have sustained myocardial infarcts, causing some degree of permanent cardiac damage (severe intoxications).
- Oleander leaves can be identified by a characteristic venation pattern and stromata; they have a prominent midrib with parallel veins extending to the periphery.
- All parts of oleander are toxic; ingestion of dry leaves/clippings is the most common cause of poisoning in animals.
- As little as 0.005% of an animal's body weight in oleander leaves (e.g., 10 to 12 leaves) may be lethal to an animal.
- Toxicity can occur by drinking water in which oleander was soaked.

PREVENTION

Owners should use extreme caution when growing oleander close to animal housing or on premises.

SUGGESTED READING

Galey FD: Cardiac glycosides. In Plumlee KH (ed): *Clinical Veterinary Toxicology*. Philadelphia, Elsevier (Health Sciences Division), 2004, pp 386-388.

Gwaltney-Brant SM, Rumbeiha WK: Newer antidotal therapies. *Vet Clin Small Anim* 32: 323-339, 2002.

AUTHOR: **MOAZZAM A. KHAN**

EDITOR: **SAFDAR A. KHAN**

Onion or Garlic Toxicosis

BASIC INFORMATION

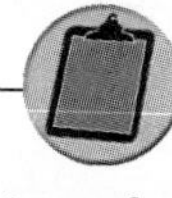

DEFINITION

Intoxication through consumption of a plant in the genus *Allium*, which includes garlic, onions, and chives. Most of these plants are perennial, rhizomatous, or bulbous herbs. Most have a distinctive odor

SYNONYM(S)

Chives
Garlic
Leeks
Onions
Shallots

EPIDEMIOLOGY

SPECIES, AGE, SEX: Cats are more susceptible than dogs.

GENETICS AND BREED PREDISPOSITION: Japanese breeds, such as Akitas, Shiba Inus, and Tosas, are more susceptible to oxidative damage to the red blood cell (RBC).

RISK FACTORS

- Dogs' indiscriminate feeding behavior increases the risk of ingestion.
- Cats likely to be exposed from ingesting foods, like baby food, with onion or garlic powder as a flavoring.

ASSOCIATED CONDITIONS AND DISORDERS: Any cause of oxidative RBC damage, Heinz body anemia, and hemolytic anemia.

CLINICAL PRESENTATION

HISTORY, CHIEF COMPLAINT

- History of exposure to raw, cooked, dried, or powdered onions or garlic.
- Nonspecific lethargy ± vomiting.
- Uncommon chief complaints: halitosis, hypersalivation, or diarrhea.

PHYSICAL EXAM FINDINGS

- Lethargy, weakness, hypersalivation, vomiting, diarrhea, and/or ataxia
- Pale mucous membrane (from hemolysis)
- Coffee-colored urine (from hemoglobinuria)

ETIOLOGY AND PATHOPHYSIOLOGY

- *Allium* spp. contain sulfoxides (which provide the characteristic odor) that are hydrolyzed to thiosulfinates.
- Thiosulfinates decompose to dipropyl sulfide.
- Dipropyl sulfides oxidize RBC membranes, resulting in hemolysis, Heinz

bodies, methemoglobinemia, and anemia.

- Onions can be wild or cultivated.
- Poisoning can result from ingesting raw, dried, powdered, or cooked onions and garlic; cooking or drying does not inactivate the toxic principle.
- Dogs fed onion soup equivalent to 30 g of raw onion/kg q 24h for 3 days developed marked Heinz body anemia. Similarly, a significant increase in Heinz bodies was seen 12 hr after feeding the animals 200 g (1/2 lb) of boiled onions (approximate dose of 17 g onions/kg).
- Dogs given an extract equivalent to 5 g of whole garlic/kg PO q 24h for 7 days developed anemia 9 to 11 days after dosing.
- Generally, most dogs need to eat at least 0.5% body weight to develop onion toxicosis, unless the dog is of a sensitive breed (see Genetics and Breed Predisposition above; Suggested Reading below).

DIAGNOSIS

DIFFERENTIAL DIAGNOSIS

- Other causes of hemolysis or Heinz body anemia (e.g., zinc, benzocaine, acetaminophen, mothballs)
- Blood parasites like *Mycoplasma (Hemobartonella) felis* or *Babesia canis*
- Immune-mediated hemolytic anemia
- Hereditary RBC fragility syndromes

INITIAL DATABASE

- Complete blood count (CBC), serum chemistry profile:
    - Decreased hematocrit, elevated white blood cell count, methemoglobinemia, and Heinz bodies are possible.
    - Smears should be examined for Heinz bodies.
- With methemoglobinemia, serum may be brown and/or blood may fail to turn red when exposed to air.
- Hematologic changes (e.g., hemolysis, Heinz body anemia, methemoglobinemia) may occur as early as 12 hours postingestion, but these generally take 2 to 5 days to develop.
- Urinalysis:
    - Reddish-brown color suggests hemoglobinuria.
        - Urine dipstick will be positive for blood with hemoglobinuria or hematuria.
        - Centrifuged urine will remain reddish-brown with hemoglobinuria, whereas the supernatant of centrifuged urine will clear with hematuria.
- Specific assay for serum methemoglobin is available in central laboratories.

ADVANCED OR CONFIRMATORY TESTING

With necropsy, the tissues may have an onion odor.

TREATMENT

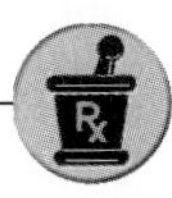

THERAPEUTIC GOAL(S)

Decontamination (induction of vomiting, administration of activated charcoal):

- Removing source of garlic, onion, or chive (*Allium*)
- Supportive care to allow production of new RBCs

ACUTE GENERAL TREATMENT

- Induction of vomiting (see Vomiting, Induction of, p 1328)
- Activated charcoal 1-3 g/kg PO (dose according to packaging label of product, such as 10 ml of activated charcoal suspension PO made from 2 g activated charcoal suspended in 10 ml tap water)
- Oxygen supplementation
- Packed RBC transfusion if necessary
- IV fluids to treat shock and to promote fluid diuresis
- Vomiting and diarrhea controlled as needed

DRUG INTERACTIONS

- Garlic extracts can inhibit serum and liver enzymes and may affect kinetics of drugs dependent on hepatic metabolization.
- There may be a synergistic effect with other drugs inhibiting hepatic metabolism (such as cimetidine, ketoconazole, and fluoxetine).
- Garlic has an antithrombotic effect, and concomitant use of garlic and drugs that alter platelet function is contraindicated (additive effects).

POSSIBLE COMPLICATIONS

- Hemoglobinuria-associated renal tubular damage possible in severe cases.
- Abortions can occur due to severe hypoxemia if a pronounced anemia is present.

RECOMMENDED MONITORING

- CBC
- Methemoglobinemia
- Heinz bodies
- Renal function
- Oxygen saturation

PROGNOSIS AND OUTCOME

- Generally good with prompt veterinary care of animals showing overt clinical signs
- Guarded with severe anemia or secondary renal damage

PEARLS & CONSIDERATIONS

COMMENTS

- Many commercial garlic or onion powder products will list the conversion for a clove of garlic (e.g., 1 tsp of garlic powder equals one clove of garlic).
- One pearl onion weighs about 14 g, a small (2 inches diameter) onion weighs about 56-85 g, a medium onion (3 inches diameter) weighs about 226-255 g, and a large onion (4 inches diameter) weighs about 425-450 g.
- A medium onion yields about 1 cup of coarsely chopped onion.

PREVENTION

- Owners should read labels carefully to see if foods contain onion or garlic powder.
- Owners should keep foods with onion or garlic ingredients out of their pets' reach.

CLIENT EDUCATION

When recommending baby food, clinicians should remind clients to avoid products with garlic or onion powder, especially for cats.

SUGGESTED READING

Lee KW, et al: Hematologic changes associated with the appearance of eccentrocytes after intragastric administration of garlic extract to dogs. *Am J Vet Res* 61:1446-1450, 2000.

Robertson JE, et al: Heinz body formation in cats fed baby food containing onion powder. *J Am Vet Med Assoc* 212:1260-1266, 1998.

Simmons DM: Onion breath. *Vet Tech* 22:424-427, 2001.

Talcott PA: Propyl disulfide. In Plumlee KH (ed): *Clinical Veterinary Toxicology*. St. Louis, Mosby, 2004, pp 408-409.

AUTHOR: **CHARLOTTE MEANS**

EDITOR: **SAFDAR A. KHAN**

Optic Neuritis

BASIC INFORMATION

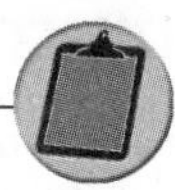

DEFINITION

Optic neuritis is the inflammation of one or both optic nerves, leading to loss of vision. This is an acquired condition that may be primary or secondary to systemic central nervous system (CNS) disease. The optic nerve is surrounded by dura mater and communicates with the subarachnoid space.

SYNONYM(S)

Papillitis (inflammation of the optic disk)

EPIDEMIOLOGY

SPECIES, AGE, SEX

- Dogs and cats
- No sex predisposition
- More commonly seen in middle-aged dogs

ASSOCIATED CONDITIONS AND DISORDERS

- Granulomatous meningoencephalitis (GME) (see Granulomatous Meningoencephalomyelitis, p 447)
- Systemic infectious diseases, including:
  - Systemic mycoses in dogs and cats
  - Feline infectious peritonitis (FIP) (see Feline Infectious Peritonitis, p 378)
  - Canine distemper (see Distemper, Canine, p 315)
  - Toxoplasmosis in dogs and cats (see Toxoplasmosis/Neosporosis, p 1093)
  - Neosporosis in dogs (see Toxoplasmosis/Neosporosis, p 1093)
- Neoplasia: primary or secondary

CLINICAL PRESENTATION

DISEASE FORMS/SUBTYPES: Intraocular, orbital, and/or intracranial:

- Intraocular: inflammation of the optic disk; detected with ophthalmic examination
- Orbital: inflammation of the retrobulbar/orbital portion of the optic nerve; not detectable with ophthalmic examination
- Intracranial: inflammation of the portion of the optic nerve following its exit from the orbit at the optic foramen and to the level of the optic chiasm; not detectable with ophthalmic examination

HISTORY, CHIEF COMPLAINT: Sudden blindness of one or both eyes.

PHYSICAL EXAM FINDINGS

- Blindness if bilateral.
- Absent menace response(s) and absent dazzle reflex(es).
- Fixed and dilated pupil(s).
- Swollen, edematous, and hyperemic optic disk with possible peripheral retinal edema and/or hemorrhages if intraocular portion of optic nerve (i.e., optic disk) is affected.
- Normal appearing optic disk if the inflammation is limited to the orbital and/or intracranial portions of the optic nerve.
- Small, pale optic disk (i.e., optic disk atrophy) in advanced cases.
- Depending on the cause, systemic abnormalities also may be present.

ETIOLOGY AND PATHOPHYSIOLOGY

- Infectious:
  - Canine:
    - Viral: canine distemper (see Distemper, Canine, p 315)
    - Systemic mycoses: see Blastomycosis, p 133; Cryptococcosis, p 259; Histoplasmosis, p 525
    - Protozoal: *Toxoplasma gondii; Neospora caninum* (see Toxoplasmosis/Neosporosis, p 1093)
  - Feline:
    - Viral: FIP
    - Systemic mycoses: cryptococcosis, histoplasmosis
    - Protozoal: *Toxoplasma gondii*
- Neoplastic: feline lymphosarcoma, orbital neoplasia
- Immune-mediated: GME
- Traumatic: leading to orbital cellulitis or abscess
- Nutritional: vitamin A deficiency (rare in dogs and cats)
- Secondary to orbital inflammation, meningitis, scleritis, retinitis, posterior uveitis
- Idiopathic

DIAGNOSIS

DIFFERENTIAL DIAGNOSIS

- Unilateral:
  - Acute primary glaucoma (elevated intraocular pressure [IOP] [>30 mmHg] and signs of glaucoma (see Glaucoma, p 440).
- Bilateral:
  - Sudden acquired retinal degeneration (SARD) in dogs (see Retinal Degeneration, p 963): normal fundic (i.e., posterior segment) examination early on with flatline electroretinogram (ERG), meaning no retinal function, versus ERG waveforms confirming retinal function in acute optic neuritis.
  - Enrofloxacin toxicity in cats: retinal degeneration noted on fundic examination (see Retinal Degeneration, p 963) versus normal-appearing retina with optic neuritis. Exception: If the intraocular portion of optic nerve (i.e., optic disk) is affected with optic neuritis, the clinician may detect peripheral retinal edema and/or hemorrhages.
  - Neoplasm at the optic chiasm (advanced imaging, such as magnetic resonance imaging [MRI], to differentiate from bilateral orbital/intracranial optic neuritis).
  - Cortical (central) blindness (normal pupillary light reflexes; normal fundic examination; possibly additional neurologic abnormalities).
  - Papilledema: edema of the optic nerve head (no blindness).

INITIAL DATABASE

- Complete ophthalmic examination, including:
  - Menace response and dazzle reflex (absent in affected one or both eyes).
  - Pupillary light reflexes (PLRs): if bilateral, pupils typically are fixed and dilated, thus producing negative direct and consensual PLRs; if unilateral, direct PLR absent in affected eye and consensual PLR absent in contralateral eye. Note: Consensual PLR refers to reaction of contralateral eye. For example, an absent consensual PLR in the right eye describes the lack of constriction of the right pupil in response to light shone into the left eye.
  - Assessment of IOP; rule out acute primary glaucoma if IOP >30 mmHg.
  - Examine posterior segment of eye (i.e., fundus) using direct and/or indirect ophthalmoscopy.
- Neurologic examination (see Neurologic Examination, p 1286)

ADVANCED OR CONFIRMATORY TESTING

- ERG to assess retinal function; normal in optic neuritis.
- MRI or computed tomography (CT):
  - May be abnormal, depending on the cause of optic neuritis.
  - Advanced imaging can help detect neoplastic processes along the optic nerve and optic chiasm. If a mass is detected in the retrobulbar optic nerve, exenteration (removal of the globe and all of the orbital contents) could be curative.
- Cerebrospinal fluid (CSF) analysis; may be abnormal, depending on the cause of optic neuritis.
- Visual-evoked potentials to assess optic nerve function; severely diminished with optic neuritis.

TREATMENT

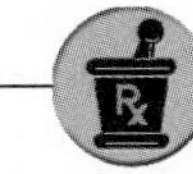

THERAPEUTIC GOAL(S)

- Reduce or eliminate the inflammation of the optic nerve
- Attempt to return vision

ACUTE GENERAL TREATMENT

- Treat the underlying cause if determined
- Idiopathic or traumatic (i.e., noninfectious) etiology: prednisone 1-2 mg/kg PO q 12h for 7-14 days; then 0.5-1 mg/kg PO q 12h for 7-14 days; then gradual decrease to reach a maintenance dosage

CHRONIC TREATMENT

GME: possible lifelong immunosuppressive therapy (see Granulomatous Meningoencephalomyelitis, p 447)

RECOMMENDED MONITORING

Monitor clinical signs (i.e., vision and optic disk with or without secondary retinal lesions if intraocular optic neuritis) within 24 hours of the animal commencing medical treatment(s) and at least weekly for the first month (reassessment intervals will vary depending on the cause and response to treatments)

PROGNOSIS AND OUTCOME

- Prognosis depends on underlying cause.
- Prognosis for return of vision is generally poor, and blindness is usually permanent.
- In cases that do respond to treatment, recurrences may occur if medication is decreased too rapidly or if duration of therapy is inadequate.
- If the animal is untreated or unresponsive to treatment, optic disk atrophy and attenuation of retinal blood vessels (see Retinal Degeneration, p 963) will occur.

PEARLS & CONSIDERATIONS

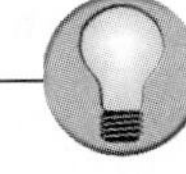

COMMENTS

- Clinicians should immediately refer cases to a veterinary ophthalmologist when optic neuritis is suspected or confirmed.
- Early diagnosis and appropriate, aggressive medical therapy are paramount to limit damage to the optic nerve(s).
- GME is the leading cause of optic neuritis in dogs.

CLIENT EDUCATION

Counsel clients on the high probability of living with a blind dog

SUGGESTED READING

Fischer CA, Jones GT: Optic neuritis in dogs. *J Am Vet Med Assoc* 160:68, 1972.

Nafe LA, Carter JD: Canine optic neuritis. *Compend Contin Pract Vet* 3:978, 1981.

AUTHOR: **CHANTALE L. PINARD**
EDITOR: **CHERYL L. CULLEN**

Oral Neoplasia, Benign

BASIC INFORMATION

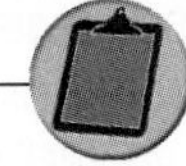

DEFINITION

Neoplastic oral disease that may be locally invasive but does not metastasize to distant sites

SYNONYM(S)

Benign oral tumors

Epulis (plural epulides): general term referring to a gingival mass; has been adapted in veterinary nomenclature to refer to tumors arising from periodontal ligament cells

EPIDEMIOLOGY

SPECIES, AGE, SEX

- Benign oral tumors can occur at any age.
- Oral papillomas usually occur in dogs <2 years old.
- Odontogenic tumors (those arising from tooth-forming tissue) can occur at any age, but tumors in young pets are more likely to be of odontogenic origin.

GENETICS AND BREED PREDISPOSITION

- Epulides: most common in brachycephalic breeds.
- Oral tumors in cats are rarely benign.

CONTAGION AND ZOONOSIS: Oral papillomas in young dogs are caused by species-specific papillomavirus.

ASSOCIATED CONDITIONS AND DISORDERS

- Gingival hyperplasia
- Malignant oral tumors

CLINICAL PRESENTATION

DISEASE FORMS/SUBTYPES

- Dogs: odontogenic tumors, papilloma, osteoma, plasmacytoma, hemangioma.
- Cats: odontogenic tumors, plasmacytoma, hemangioma.
- Odontogenic tumors of periodontal ligament origin are by far the most common benign oral neoplasms in dogs. Historically, epulides have been classified as being fibromatous, ossifying, and acanthomatous. Fibromatous and ossifying epulides are minimally invasive. Ossifying epulides may contain dentin- or cementum-like tissue in a fibrous tissue swelling. Acanthomatous epulis is the most locally invasive. The nomenclature regarding epulides in dogs has changed. Fibromatous and ossifying epulides have been placed under the same heading of peripheral odontogenic fibromas. Based on histologic appearance, acanthomatous epulis is now referred to as canine acanthomatous ameloblastoma.
- Other odontogenic tumors:
  - Ameloblastoma can be characterized as central (intraosseous) or peripheral (extraosseous ameloblastoma). Both can be locally invasive, but central ameloblastoma often exhibits cystic bony changes.
  - Odontoma is not a true tumor. It is considered to be a hamartoma, an accumulation of normal epithelial and mesenchymal odontogenic cells that are arranged in an abnormal manner but allowing for induction of dental hard tissues. A compound odontoma has hard tissues that are produced in a relatively organized manner, producing tooth-like structures (denticles). A complex odontoma produces dental hard tissue that bears no resemblance to a tooth.
  - Feline inductive odontogenic tumor (FIOT), also called inductive fibroameloblastoma, occurs most commonly in the rostral maxilla of cats <2 years of age and may be locally invasive but has not been reported to metastasize.
  - Amyloid-producing odontogenic tumor (APOT), previously referred to as calcifying epithelial odontogenic

tumor (CEOT), may be locally invasive in both dogs and cats but has not been reported to metastasize.

HISTORY, CHIEF COMPLAINT

- Focal swelling of gingiva and/or alveolar mucosa commonly noted as an incidental finding by the client or the veterinarian during routine physical examination.
- Benign oral tumors rarely present with oral bleeding or halitosis unless they are large enough to be traumatized by opposing teeth upon closure of the mouth. Bleeding is a common complaint in dogs with a large acanthomatous ameloblastoma.

PHYSICAL EXAM FINDINGS

- Focal swelling of gingiva and/or alveolar mucosa, often circumscribed and rarely ulcerated.
- Benign tumors that are locally invasive (e.g., canine acanthomatous ameloblastoma) may cause disfigurement from invasion of the maxilla or mandible.
- Displaced but often firmly seated teeth.
- Mandibular lymph nodes are often within normal limits.
- Appetite and activity level are usually unaffected.

ETIOLOGY AND PATHOPHYSIOLOGY

- Etiology is unknown, but genetic predisposition may play a role.
- Some benign masses have been suspected to undergo malignant transformation, though this is thought to be rare.

DIAGNOSIS

DIFFERENTIAL DIAGNOSIS

- Gingival hyperplasia.
- Granulation tissue.
- Scar tissue (chewing lesions from traumatizing buccal or sublingual mucosa).
- Inflammatory swelling due to foreign body.
- Periapical abscess.
- Normal anatomy (e.g., incisive papilla palatal to maxillary incisors; lingual molar gland caudolingual to mandibular first molar teeth in cats): if the mass is located directly on the midline or bilateral, clinicians can consult an anatomy textbook to rule out normal structures before performing a biopsy.
- Malignant oral tumors.
- Craniomandibular osteopathy (CMO): most commonly seen in West Highland white, Scottish, and cairn terriers; mandibular swellings associated with CMO are often bilateral.
- Osteomyelitis/bone sequestrum: usually seen in the incisive bone or bilaterally in the caudal mandible or maxilla; often appears as bony swelling with gingival recession, erosion, and ulceration; exposed bone; and fetid odor. Cocker spaniels and dachshunds may be overrepresented.
- Dentigerous cyst: arising in area of a tooth that has not yet erupted.
- Eosinophilic granuloma: occurring in dogs and cats on tongue, lips, and soft palate.

INITIAL DATABASE

Complete blood count, serum biochemistry profile, urinalysis: generally unremarkable

ADVANCED OR CONFIRMATORY TESTING

- Thoracic radiographs
- Anesthetized oral examination
- Dental radiographs
- Computed tomographic (CT) scan (particularly helpful for maxillary masses)
- Cytologic examination of aspirated oral masses and lymph nodes
- Histopathologic evaluation of incisional or excisional biopsy

TREATMENT

THERAPEUTIC GOAL(S)

- Clinicians can remove the mass and margin of normal surrounding tissue to prevent local recurrence.
- Surgical excision is often possible, but when this is not an option, consider efforts to decrease the rate of growth (radiation, debulking) and pain relief (extraction of teeth impinging upon tumor, pain medications).

ACUTE GENERAL TREATMENT

- Removal of a circumscribed mass to the normal level of the surrounding gingiva will often serve as an adequate biopsy but may not prevent local recurrence. Since peripheral odontogenic fibromas originate from the periodontal ligament, they will likely recur without removal of the tooth and the periodontal ligament lining of its alveolar socket(s).
- Incisional biopsies of large masses are warranted to provide information prior to considering radical surgery.

CHRONIC TREATMENT

- Depending on biopsy results and tumor extent, surgery or radiation therapy may be good long-term options.
- Intralesional chemotherapy has been reported to be successful for treatment of some benign tumors (e.g., canine acanthomatous ameloblastoma). Systemic chemotherapy may be used as an adjunctive therapy but is rarely effective by itself against most oral tumors.
- Radiation therapy offers excellent long-term control for treatment of canine acanthomatous ameloblastoma, but malignant tumors may develop in the irradiated area in up to 20% of dogs.

POSSIBLE COMPLICATIONS

- Recurrence of primary tumor: Benign tumors require complete removal to prevent recurrence.
- Intraoperative or postoperative bleeding.
- Dehiscence of the surgical site: clinicians should avoid using electrocautery because it can obscure histologic examination of margins of excised tissue and increases the likelihood of wound dehiscence, which may carry dire consequences (such as creation of a chronic oronasal fistula); surgeons should use a conventional scalpel blade for surgical resection of oral tumors.
- Sublingual mucocele (ranula) or cervical mucocele may result if rostral mandibulectomy is performed; clinicians can carefully dissect and ligate sublingual and mandibular salivary ducts if they require transection.

RECOMMENDED MONITORING

Clinicians can repeat the oral examination, including head/neck lymph node palpation to monitor for recurrence at 6-month intervals.

PROGNOSIS AND OUTCOME

- Prognosis is good with benign tumors if they are completely resectable.
- When clients are reluctant to pursue surgery, radiation therapy has been documented to provide a good long-term clinical outcome for treatment of canine acanthomatous ameloblastoma.

PEARLS & CONSIDERATIONS

COMMENTS

- Clinicians should perform an incisional biopsy for larger oral masses. Excisional biopsy may be curative but carries the risk of inadequate tumor removal. When submitting excisional biopsies, clinicians should request that the pathologist evaluate margins for presence of neoplastic cells. Clean margins according to histologic examination do not rule out the possibility of recurrence, but animals with clean margins have a better long-term prognosis.
- Dental radiography is invaluable in providing diagnostic and treatment planning information for oral tumors. Benign tumors tend to displace teeth that often remain firmly seated, whereas more aggressive tumors will cause root and alveolar bone resorption, which may manifest as very mobile (floating) teeth. Benign tumors may have a smooth layer of reactive bone surrounding the neoplastic tissue, whereas a malignant tumor often exhibits destruction of cortical bone with formation of a classic "sunburst" appearance.
- Right or left total mandibulectomy (previously referred to as hemimandibulectomy) (Fig. I-122) and maxillectomy surgeries carry with them the

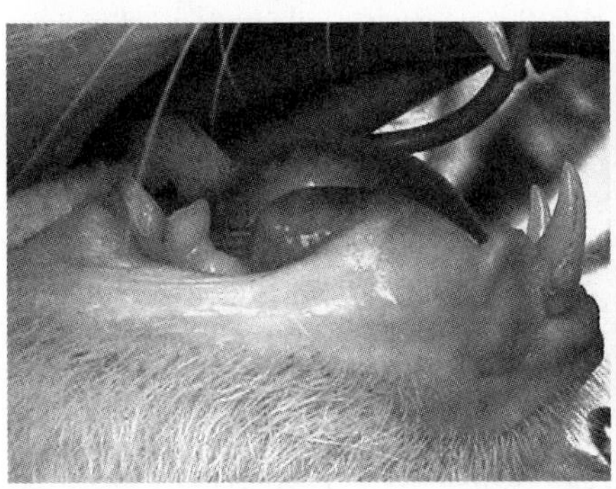

A

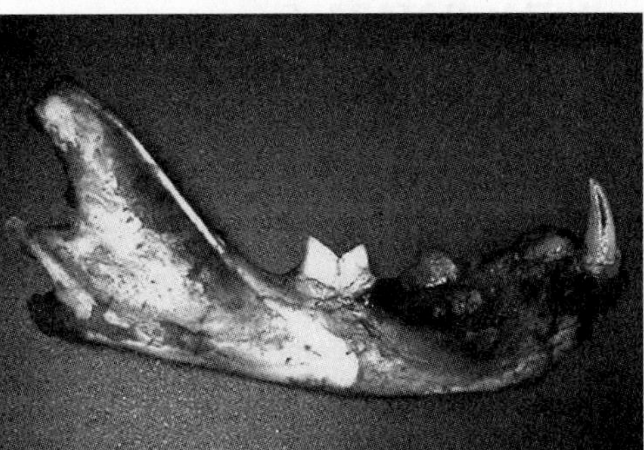

B

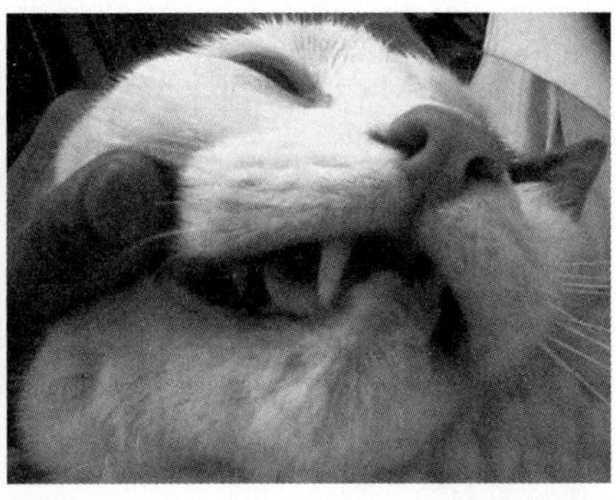

C

FIGURE I-122 **A,** Total mandibulectomy: preoperative image of cat with a right mandibular APOT, which is a benign but locally aggressive neoplasm. **B,** Total mandibulectomy: intraoperative image of resected right mandible from the same cat shown in A. **C,** Total mandibulectomy: postoperative image of same cat presenting several months later for a recheck; excellent healing of the surgical site; no tumor recurrence. Courtesy of Dr. Alexander M. Reiter, University of Pennsylvania.

potential for profuse bleeding. Blood type and cross matching may be warranted preoperatively.

- During excision of oral tumors, sharp dissection is recommended to avoid the risks associated with electrocautery (wound dehiscence, oronasal fistula creation).

CLIENT EDUCATION

- Complete surgical removal of oral tumors provides the best long-term prognosis. Tumors that are detected early are likely to be operable. Clinicians should advise new pet owners to socialize puppies and kittens and allow them to feel comfortable with periodic examination of the oral cavity.
- Animals adapt remarkably well after radical resection of oral tumors, and altered cosmesis is usually well accepted by owners if masticatory function can be restored. Clients should be shown before-and-after pictures of similar surgical cases to ensure their understanding of cosmetic changes.

SUGGESTED READING

Gardner DG: Ameloblastoma in cats: A critical evaluation of the literature and the addition of one example. *J Oral Pathol Med* 27(1): 39–42, 1998.

Gardner DG: Epulides in the dog: A review. *J Oral Pathol Med* 25:32, 1996.

Gardner DG, Dubielzig RR, McGee EV: The so-called calcifying epithelial odontogenic tumour in dogs and cats (amyloid-producing odontogenic tumour). *J Comp Pathol* 111:221–230, 1994.

Harvey C, Emily P: *Small Animal Dentistry*. St. Louis, Mosby, 1993, pp 297–311.

Thrall DE, et al: Malignant tumor formation at the site of previously irradiated acanthomatous epulides in four dogs. *J Am Vet Med Assoc* 178:127, 1981.

Verstraete FJM: *Self-Assessment Colour Review of Veterinary Dentistry*. London, Manson, 1999, pp 25, 67, 193.

AUTHOR: **JOHN R. LEWIS**

EDITOR: **ALEXANDER M. REITER**

Oral Neoplasia, Malignant

BASIC INFORMATION

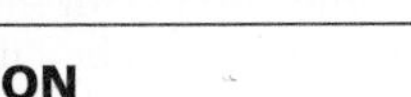

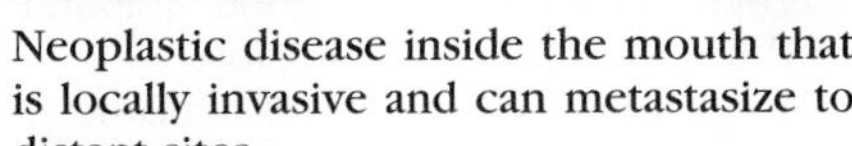

DEFINITION

Neoplastic disease inside the mouth that is locally invasive and can metastasize to distant sites

SYNONYM(S)

Malignant oral tumors

EPIDEMIOLOGY

SPECIES, AGE, SEX

- Malignant oral tumors can occur at any age, but middle-aged and geriatric pets are overrepresented.
- Canine papillary squamous cell carcinoma (SCC) occurs most commonly in adolescent and young adult dogs.
- The most common canine oral tumor is malignant melanoma (melanosarcoma), seen most often in dogs >10 years of age.
- The most common feline oral tumor is SCC, representing 70% of oral tumors in cats. Average age of onset is 10 years, but cats as young as 5 months have been affected. Additional information is presented in Squamous Cell Carcinoma, Oral (Mucosal, Tonsillar), p 1034.

GENETICS AND BREED PREDISPOSITION: Breeds with pigmented oral mucosa may be predisposed to malignant melanoma.

RISK FACTORS: Cats and SCC:

- Exposure to flea collars: associated with a three times increased risk
- High intake of canned cat food: associated with a three times increased risk
- Canned tuna: associated with a three times increased risk

CONTAGION AND ZOONOSIS: Canine transmissible venereal tumor can manifest as a primary or metastatic tumor on the lips, buccal mucosa, and tonsils.

ASSOCIATED CONDITIONS AND DISORDERS

- Gingival hyperplasia
- Benign oral tumors

CLINICAL PRESENTATION

DISEASE FORMS/SUBTYPES

- Dogs: malignant melanoma, SCC, fibrosarcoma, osteosarcoma, osteochondrosarcoma (multilobular tumor of bone), mast cell tumor, hemangiosarcoma, peripheral nerve sheath tumor
- Cats: SCC, fibrosarcoma, osteosarcoma, lymphosarcoma

HISTORY, CHIEF COMPLAINT

- Swelling of mandible or maxilla
- Oral bleeding, halitosis
- Dysphagia if the mass is large enough to affect masticatory function

PHYSICAL EXAM FINDINGS

- Specifics may vary with tumor type:
  - Malignant melanoma is pigmented (melanotic) or nonpigmented (ame-

lanotic) and often lobulated, ulcerative, and friable; necrosis may be present when the tumor outgrows its blood supply.
  - Fibrosarcoma is often smooth and firm and may cause generalized disfigurement but rarely bleeds spontaneously.
  - SCC is firm, pink, and may be proliferative and ulcerative.
  - Osteosarcoma can manifest as a hard diffuse swelling of the maxilla or mandible, but often also exhibits a fleshy, pink or red proliferative component.
  - Osteochondrosarcoma is locally invasive but slow to metastasize usually located at mandibular ramus, caudal maxilla, zygomatic arch, or calvarium.
- Halitosis, oral bleeding, facial/oral swelling.
- Enlarged mandibular lymph nodes possible.
- Appetite and activity level are often unaffected.

ETIOLOGY AND PATHOPHYSIOLOGY

Etiology is unknown, but genetic predisposition may play a role

DIAGNOSIS

DIFFERENTIAL DIAGNOSIS

- Gingival hyperplasia.
- Granulation tissue.
- Scar tissue (chewing lesions from traumatizing buccal or sublingual mucosa).
- Inflammatory swelling due to foreign body.
- Periapical abscess.
- Normal anatomy (e.g., incisive papilla palatal to maxillary incisors; lingual molar gland caudolingual to mandibular first molar teeth in cats): if the mass is located directly on the midline or bilateral, clinicians should consult an anatomy textbook to rule out normal structures before performing a biopsy.
- Benign oral tumors.
- Craniomandibular osteopathy (CMO): most commonly seen in West Highland white, Scottish, and cairn terriers; mandibular swellings associated with CMO are often bilateral.
- Osteomyelitis/bone sequestrum: usually seen in the incisive bone or bilaterally in the caudal mandible or maxilla; often appears as a bony swelling with gingival recession, erosion, and ulceration; exposed bone; and fetid odor. Cocker spaniels and dachshunds may be overrepresented.
- Dentigerous cyst: arising in area of a tooth that has not yet erupted.
- Eosinophilic granuloma: occurring in dogs and cats on tongue, lips, and soft palate.

INITIAL DATABASE

Physical examination, chemistry screen, and complete blood count

ADVANCED OR CONFIRMATORY TESTING

- Thoracic radiographs
- Anesthetized oral examination
- Dental radiographs
- Computed tomographic (CT) scan (particularly helpful for maxillary masses)
- Cytologic examination of oral masses
- Cytologic examination of aspirated material or histopathologic examination of resected lymph nodes
- Histopathologic evaluation of incisional or excisional biopsy

TREATMENT

THERAPEUTIC GOAL(S)

- Clinicians should remove mass and margin of normal surrounding tissue to prevent local recurrence.
- Debulking of aggressive tumors is rarely helpful. If complete removal is not an option, radiation or chemotherapy may decrease rate of growth depending on tumor type.
- Clinicians should stage for metastatic disease and treat accordingly.

ACUTE GENERAL TREATMENT

- Removal of a circumscribed mass to the normal level of the surrounding gingiva will often serve as an adequate biopsy but may not prevent local recurrence. Incisional biopsies of large masses are warranted to provide information prior to performing a radical maxillectomy or mandibulectomy.
- Aspiration and/or resection of head/ neck lymph nodes are warranted for staging of animals with malignant oral tumors.

CHRONIC TREATMENT

- Depending on biopsy results and tumor extent, surgery or radiation therapy may be treatment options. Chemotherapy may be used as an adjunctive therapy but is rarely effective by itself against most oral tumors.
- Radiation therapy offers good long-term control for treatment of microscopic disease, but bulky tumors rarely respond well.
- Piroxicam 0.3 mg/kg PO q 24h in dogs may slow the progression of carcinomas. A dosage has yet to be established in cats. Short-term (10 days) use of piroxicam in cats appears to be safe at 0.3 mg/kg PO q 24h. Further studies are necessary to determine long-term gastrointestinal safety in cats.

DRUG INTERACTIONS

Piroxicam and other nonsteroidal anti-inflammatory drugs (NSAIDs) may cause significant gastric ulceration; clinicians should avoid concurrent use of corticosteroids and consider gastric protectants, such as misoprostol.

POSSIBLE COMPLICATIONS

- Recurrence of primary tumor. To minimize risk, surgeons should remove at least 1 cm of clinically and radiographically healthy tissue surrounding malignant tumors. Fibrosarcoma requires even wider margins.
- Intraoperative or postoperative bleeding.
- Dehiscence of the surgical site: Clinicians should avoid using electrocautery because it can obscure histologic examination of margins of excised tissue and increases the likelihood of wound dehiscence, which may carry dire consequences (such as creation of a chronic oronasal fistula); clinicians should use a conventional scalpel blade for surgical resection of oral tumors.
- Sublingual mucocele (ranula) or cervical mucocele may result if a surgeon performs a rostral mandibulectomy; surgeons should carefully dissect and ligate sublingual and mandibular salivary ducts if they require transection.

RECOMMENDED MONITORING

- Oral examination to monitor for local recurrence 1 month after surgery and at a maximum of 6-month intervals thereafter
- Thoracic radiographs and lymph node palpation should be performed every 6 months

PROGNOSIS AND OUTCOME

- Median survival time for most malignant oral tumors after surgical excision has been 7 to 12 months. However, when surgeons obtain clean surgical margins in the absence of microscopic metastasis, animals can be cured.
- Prognosis with SCC is good if found while still surgically resectable.
- Malignant melanomas >2 cm in diameter have a high incidence of microscopic metastasis at the time of diagnosis.
- Mandibular osteosarcoma has been reported to have a lower metastatic rate and better prognosis than appendicular osteosarcoma.
- Tonsillar SCC carries a grave prognosis, with 98% metastasizing early to regional lymph nodes.

PEARLS & CONSIDERATIONS

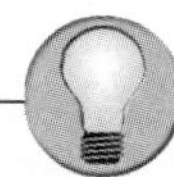

COMMENTS

- Incisional biopsy should be performed for larger oral masses. Excisional biopsy may be curative but carries the risk of inadequate tumor removal. When submitting excisional biopsies, clinicians should request that the pathologist evaluate margins for presence of neoplastic cells. Clean margins according to histologic examination do not rule out the possibility of recurrence, but animals with clean margins have a better long-term prognosis.

- Dental radiography is invaluable in providing diagnostic and treatment planning information for oral tumors. Benign tumors tend to displace teeth that often remain firmly seated, whereas more aggressive tumors will cause root and alveolar bone resorption, which may manifest as very mobile (floating) teeth. Benign tumors may have a smooth layer of reactive bone surrounding the neoplastic tissue, whereas a malignant tumor often exhibits destruction of cortical bone with formation of a classic "sunburst" appearance.
- Right or left total mandibulectomy (previously referred to as hemimandibulectomy) and maxillectomy surgeries carry with them the potential for profuse bleeding. Blood type and cross matching may be warranted preoperatively.
- Pigmentation is not a reliable indicator of tumor type. About 40% of oral malignant melanomas may be amelanotic (unpigmented). Other malignant tumors that are not melanoma may be pigmented if the oral mucosa is normally pigmented.
- Removal of regional lymph nodes is beneficial at the time of oral surgery. A single surgical approach to parotid, mandibular, and retropharyngeal lymph nodes has been described.
- If the biologic nature of a tumor does not match results from histologic examination, clinicians should have the biopsy reread or retaken. A type of fibrosarcoma exists which appears histologically benign but is clinically very aggressive.
- Nonhealing dental extraction sites, particularly in cats, may be a clinical manifestation of SCC; clinicians should biopsy any suspicious tissues at the time of extraction.
- Dehiscence and inappropriate healing often occur when oral surgery is performed on irradiated sites.

PREVENTION

See Risk Factors above

CLIENT EDUCATION

- Complete surgical removal of oral tumors provides the best long-term prognosis. Tumors that are detected early are likely to be operable. Clinicians should advise new pet owners to socialize puppies and kittens and allow them to feel comfortable with periodic examination of the oral cavity.
- Animals adapt remarkably well after radical resection of oral tumors (mandibulectomy or maxillectomy), and altered cosmesis is usually well accepted by owners if masticatory function can be restored. Clients should be shown before-and-after pictures of similar surgical cases to ensure their understanding of cosmetic changes.
- Lymph node aspirates and thoracic radiographs are important for preoperative animal staging, but microscopic metastasis cannot be totally ruled out by these tests.

SUGGESTED READING

Bertone ER, et al: Environmental and lifestyle risk factors for oral squamous cell carcinoma in domestic cats. *J Vet Intern Med* 17(4):557, 2003.

Harvey C, Emily P: *Small Animal Dentistry*. St. Louis, Mosby, 1993, pp 297-311.

Heeb HL, et al: Multiple dose pharmacokinetics and acute safety of piroxicam and cimetidine in the cat. *J Vet Pharmacol Ther* 26(4):259-263, 2003.

Smith MM: Surgical approach for lymph node staging of oral and maxillofacial neoplasms in dogs. *J Am Anim Hosp Assoc* 31(6):514, 1995..

Straw RC, et al: Canine mandibular osteosarcoma: 51 cases (1980-1992). *J Am Anim Hosp Assoc* 32:257-262, 1996.

AUTHOR: **JOHN R. LEWIS**
EDITOR: **ALEXANDER M. REITER**

Orbital Disease

BASIC INFORMATION

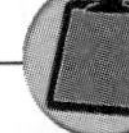

DEFINITION

Orbital diseases encompass several conditions that frequently lead to an abnormal position of the eye within the orbit. These abnormal positions include *exophthalmos* (a forward displacement of the eye), *enophthalmos* (a caudal displacement of the eye), and *strabismus* (a deviation of axis of the resting eye position). Orbital diseases can be congenital or acquired.

SYNONYM(S)

Enophthalmia
Exophthalmia
Retrobulbar disease
Orbital abscess: retrobulbar abscess

EPIDEMIOLOGY

SPECIES, AGE, SEX

- Dogs and cats.
- No sex predisposition.
- Orbital abscess and cellulitis are more common in younger animals.
- Orbital neoplasia are more common in older animals.

GENETICS AND BREED PREDISPOSITION

- Ocular proptosis (see Proptosis of the Globe, p 893) more common in brachycephalic breeds.
- Myositis is more common in German shepherds, weimaraners, golden retrievers, and Labrador retrievers (eosinophilic myositis of the masticatory muscles); golden retrievers (extraocular polymyositis) (see Masticatory Muscle Myositis, p 687).
- Craniomandibular osteopathy in West Highland white terriers.
- Congenital strabismus may be seen in shar-pei dogs as well as in Siamese and some shorthair cats.

RISK FACTORS: Chewing on sticks or other foreign material (orbital abscess).

ASSOCIATED CONDITIONS AND DISORDERS

- Masticatory myositis
- Systemic mycoses (see Blastomycosis, p 133)
- Emaciation
- Dehydration

CLINICAL PRESENTATION

HISTORY, CHIEF COMPLAINT: Sudden, progressive, or congenital change in position of the eye.

PHYSICAL EXAM FINDINGS: Bilateral or unilateral:

- Exophthalmos with any or all of the following:
    - Reduced ability or inability to retropulse the globe within the orbit.
    - Lagophthalmos (incomplete closure of the eyelids) with or without corneal ulceration (see Corneal Ulceration, p 248).
    - Third eyelid protrusion (see Third Eyelid Abnormalities/Protrusion, p 1077).
    - Conjunctival hyperemia, chemosis.
    - Periocular swelling.

- Pain on opening the mouth (orbital abscess/cellulitis; myositis).
- Enophthalmos with any or all of the following:
  - Third eyelid protrusion (see Third Eyelid Abnormalities/Protrusion, p 1077).
  - Ptosis (drooping upper eyelid).
  - Extraocular and/or masticatory muscle atrophy.
  - Entropion.
  - Emaciation may be noted, a component of which (the loss of orbital fat) may be the cause of enophthalmos.
- Strabismus:
  - Deviation of the eye(s): dorsal, ventral, medial, lateral, or a combination of these eye positions.
  - ± Exophthalmos or enophthalmos.
- Variable systemic signs depending on underlying cause
- Inflamed oral mucosa or draining fistula behind the last upper molar with orbital abscess

ETIOLOGY AND PATHOPHYSIOLOGY

- Exophthalmos: caused by space-occupying orbital lesion, caudal to equator of eye:
  - Congenital:
    - Orbital varix, arterial to venous shunts: rare
    - Orbital cysts and dermoids: uncommon
  - Acquired:
    - Ocular proptosis: usually unilateral, peracute, trauma associated (see Proptosis of the Globe, p 893)
    - Orbital abscess/cellulitis: usually unilateral, peracute to acute, painful resistance to ocular retropulsion and mouth manipulation
    - Orbital hemorrhage: secondary to coagulopathy or head trauma.
    - Orbital neoplasia: usually unilateral, progressive, typically not painful, primary or secondary, predominantly malignant
    - Mucocele: unilateral, progressive, arising from zygomatic salivary gland
    - Myositis: bilateral, enophthalmia occuring in late stages
- Enophthalmos: caused by loss of orbital volume or space-occupying lesion rostral to equator of eye:
  - Congenital: microphthalmos (see Ocular Size Abnormalities, p 763)
  - Acquired:
    - Phthisis bulbi (see Ocular Size Abnormalities, p 763)
    - Loss of orbital fat (older animals with weight loss) or muscle
    - Ocular pain
    - Dehydration
    - Horner's syndrome
    - Neoplasia anterior to equator of eye (e.g., rostral orbit)
- Strabismus: typically caused by lesions restricting extraocular muscle mobility or affecting their innervation:
  - Congenital:
    - Unilateral or bilateral, progressive juvenile fibrosis of the medial rectus muscle seen in Chinese shar-pei dogs
    - Bilateral medial strabismus (esotropia) in Siamese cats
  - Acquired:
    - Trauma-induced extraocular muscle avulsion (see Proptosis of the Globe, p 893) or scarring
    - Extraocular muscle scarring from previous inflammation
    - Abnormal innervation of extraocular muscle(s) (e.g., cranial nerve [CN] III, IV, and/or VI lesions)

DIAGNOSIS

DIFFERENTIAL DIAGNOSIS

- Exophthalmos:
  - Buphthalmos, which is marked by enlargement of the eye (see Glaucoma, p 440)
  - Episcleritis/scleritis (see Episcleritis/Scleritis, p 353)
- Enophthalmos: ruptured globe (see Corneal/Scleral Trauma, p 244)

INITIAL DATABASE

- Complete ophthalmic examination (see Ophthalmic Examination, p 1288)
- Complete neurologic examination if strabismus (see Neurologic Examination, p 1286)
- Oral examination (pain and/or purulent drainage if orbital abscess)
- Complete blood count (CBC): may reveal evidence of inflammation (bands, toxic changes in neutrophils) with orbital abscess
- CBC, serum biochemistry profile, urinalysis, skull radiographs, chest radiographs, fine-needle aspirates of submandibular lymph nodes if enlarged, abdominal ultrasound if orbital neoplasia suspected
- Pharmacologic testing (topical 10% phenylephrine) for Horner's syndrome (see Horner's Syndrome, p 532)

ADVANCED OR CONFIRMATORY TESTING

- Ocular/orbital ultrasound if exophthalmos (assess for orbital abscesses or masses)
- Computed tomographic (CT) or magnetic resonance imaging (MRI) scan if orbital masses suspected
- General anesthesia and ultrasound-guided fine-needle aspirates or biopsies for an orbital mass, abscess, or mucocele
- Masticatory (see Muscle and Nerve Biopsy, p 1279) or extraocular muscle biopsies under general anesthesia (e.g., myositis; referrable procedure)

TREATMENT

THERAPEUTIC GOAL(S)

- If possible, return the eye to its normal position.
- Alleviate pain.
- Preserve vision (optic neuropathy and/or retinal detachment may occur with space-occupying orbital lesions).

ACUTE GENERAL TREATMENT

Treat underlying cause:

- Ocular proptosis (see Proptosis of the Globe, p 893).
- Orbital abscess:
  - Suspected if the oral mucosa caudal to last upper molar is abnormal; in such cases, medical stabilization (e.g., rehydration) if necessary, followed by surgical drainage via blunt dissection under general anesthesia, is warranted; obtain samples for culture and sensitivity (C&S), aerobic and anaerobic.
  - Systemic nonsteroidal anti-inflammatory drugs (NSAIDs) for 7 days.
    - Dogs: carprofen 2.2 mg/kg q 12h (may use single loading dose of 4 mg/kg SC once) or meloxicam 0.1 mg/kg PO q 24h (may use single loading dose of 0.2 mg/kg SC or PO once) for 5 days.
    - Cats: tolfenamic acid 4 mg/kg SC, IM, PO q 24h for 3–5 days.
  - Broad-spectrum oral antibiotics for 14 to 21 days (amoxicillin-clavulinic acid 13.5 mg/kg PO q 12h [dogs] or 62.5 mg PO q 12h [cats]).
  - Clinicians should hospitalize animals with supportive treatment for the first postoperative 24 to 48 hours if necessary.
- Orbital neoplasia:
  - Surgical excision (exenteration, orbitotomy, or orbitectomy).
  - Adjunctive radiation therapy or chemotherapy depending on type of neoplasm (consult veterinary oncologist or ophthalmologist).
- Mucocele: Surgical excision typically is curative.
- Myositis: prednisone 1–2 mg/kg PO q 12h, tapered gradually once response to treatment is noted (see Masticatory Muscle Myositis, p 687).

CHRONIC TREATMENT

Myositis: Long-term treatment may be required since relapses can occur.

POSSIBLE COMPLICATIONS

- Permanent strabismus
- Blindness
- Loss of the eye

- Systemic complications possible (potentially severe), depending on extent of disease process

RECOMMENDED MONITORING

Weekly or bimonthly reexamination for inflammatory diseases

PROGNOSIS AND OUTCOME

Varies depending on cause:

- Favorable with orbital abscess if treated adequately
- Guarded with myositis
- Poor with orbital neoplasia

PEARLS & CONSIDERATIONS

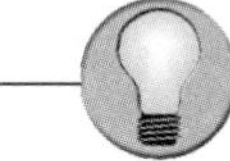

COMMENTS

Orbital disease should be investigated in a timely fashion to alleviate discomfort and to potentially preserve vision.

CLIENT EDUCATION

- Consult a veterinarian as soon as an alteration in position of the eye(s) is noted.
- Relapses can occur with myositis or if an orbital foreign body is not removed.

SUGGESTED READING

Attali-Soussay K, Jegou JP, Clerc B: Retrobulbar tumors in dogs and cats: 25 cases. *Vet Ophthalmol* 4:19–27, 2001.

Speiss BM, Wallin-Hakanson N: Diseases of the canine orbit. In Gelatt KN (ed): *Veterinary Ophthalmology*, ed 3. Philadelphia, Lippincott, Williams & Wilkins, 1999, pp 511–533.

AUTHOR: **CHANTALE L. PINARD**
EDITOR: **CHERYL L. CULLEN**

DISEASES AND DISORDERS

Organophosphate and Carbamate Insecticide Toxicosis

BASIC INFORMATION

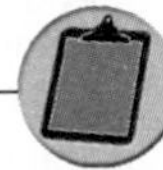

DEFINITION

- Organophosphates (OPs) are aliphatic carbon, cyclic, or heterocyclic phosphate esters.
- Carbamates are cyclic or aliphatic derivatives of carbamic acid.
- Toxicosis results from dermal or oral exposure and is characterized by increased salivation, lacrimation, urinary incontinence, diarrhea, dyspnea, emesis (SLUDDE), bradycardia, tremors, shaking, ataxia, seizures, or death.

SYNONYM(S)

Acetylcholinesterase = cholinesterase

Commonly used carbamates are aldicarb, carbofuran, methomyl, propoxur, and carbaryl (Sevin).

Commonly used OPs are disulfoton, terbufos, phorate, parathion, chlorpyrifos (Dursban), fenthion (Spotton), diazinon, and malathion.

EPIDEMIOLOGY

SPECIES, AGE, SEX

- All breeds and sexes susceptible.
- Very young, elderly, or debilitated animals are more susceptible than healthy adult animals.
- Cats are particularly sensitive to chlorpyrifos; the onset of clinical signs is usually delayed (1 day or more) after exposure, and signs can last 2 to 4 weeks.

RISK FACTORS: Exposure to other acetylcholinesterase inhibitors.

GEOGRAPHY AND SEASONALITY: Toxicosis more common in summer months; can occur year-round in areas where insects flourish throughout the year.

CLINICAL PRESENTATION

HISTORY, CHIEF COMPLAINT

- Dermal or oral exposure to an OP or carbamate
- Recent history (usually within 24 hours prior to onset of clinical signs) of using an OP or carbamate insecticide in the yard or in the house
- Rapid onset of clinical signs (minutes to hours after exposure)
- Salivation, vomiting, diarrhea, lacrimation, dyspnea
- Tremors, muscle weakness, ataxia, seizures

PHYSICAL EXAM FINDINGS

- Muscarinic signs: SLUDDE, miosis, and bradycardia.
- Nicotinic signs: muscle tremors, weakness, and paresis, progressing to paralysis.
- Central nervous system (CNS) signs: hyperactivity, depressed respiration, and seizures.
- Relative predominance of one class of effects over another makes the exact clinical picture variable from one animal to another. For example, CNS hyperactivity may be associated with tachycardia, which overrides the bradycardia classically described as part of muscarinic signs.

ETIOLOGY AND PATHOPHYSIOLOGY

- OPs and carbamates are insecticides commonly used for controlling insects in agriculture, around the home, and on or around animals (e.g., for controlling fleas and ticks). Products containing OPs or carbamates are available as sprays, pour-on solutions, oral anthelmintics, baits, flea collars, dips, and dusts.
- OPs and carbamates are acetylcholinesterase (AChE) inhibitors.
- OPs and carbamates competitively inhibit AChE by binding to its esteric site. Acetylcholine (ACh) then accumulates in the synapse and causes excessive synaptic neurotransmitter activity, leading to mucarinic, nicotinic, or CNS effects. Competitive inhibition of AChE explains the result of confirmatory testing with OP or carbamate toxicosis (low blood AChE level).
- Some OPs undergo "aging," rendering the phosphorylated (inactivated) cholinesterase enzyme very stable so that recovery of AChE activity occurs only through the synthesis of new enzyme. In general, inhibition of AChE by the OPs tends to be irreversible, while inhibition by the carbamates is reversible, which allows a spontaneous regeneration of the enzyme. Therefore, both carbamates and OPs respond initially to atropine, but only carbamates continue to do so. OPs become refractory to atropine treatment when they age.
- Atropine blocks the effects of the excess ACh at the neuromuscular junction. Atropine can only control the muscarinic signs (not the nicotinic signs).
- Death from either OPs or carbamates occurs due to respiratory failure resulting from excessive bronchial secretions, bronchiolar constriction, paralysis of intercostal muscles or diaphragm, or respiratory failure due to CNS effects.
- Cats may not show typical OP toxicosis signs from chlorpyrifos. Clinical signs of anorexia, depression, vomiting, tremors, salivation, ataxia, seizures, and ventroflexion of neck are delayed for 1 to 5 days and can last for 2 to 4 weeks.

DIAGNOSIS

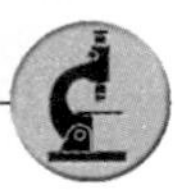

DIFFERENTIAL DIAGNOSIS

- Some Solanaceae family plants; anatoxin-a(s) found in some blue-green algae
- Muscarinic signs: muscarinic mushrooms, tremorgenic mycotoxins

- Nicotinic signs: nicotine, pyrethrins/pyrethroids, strychnine, fluoroacetate (1080), 4-aminopyridine, metaldehyde, zinc phosphide, lead
- CNS signs: any disorder that can cause seizures (see Seizures, p 990)

INITIAL DATABASE

- CBC, urinalysis (usually within normal range)
- Serum biochemistry profile: possible increase in liver and pancreatic enzymes with exposure to some OPs (disulfoton)

ADVANCED OR CONFIRMATORY TESTING

- AChE levels: serum, plasma, or whole blood (preferred), brain, or retina
    - An AChE result that is <50% of normal indicates significant exposure likely, while an AChE activity <25% of normal indicates toxicosis.
    - AChE activity can remain depressed for 6 to 8 weeks (with OPs).
    - Since carbamates are reversible inhibitors of AChE, the results may be normal even in the face of carbamate toxicosis. In such cases, the diagnosis rests on history of exposure and physical exam findings although carbamate levels also may be measured.
- AChE insecticide screen: liver, kidney, gastrointestinal tract contents, and source material to look for specific insecticide

TREATMENT

THERAPEUTIC GOAL(S)

- Treating life-threatening signs
- Decontaminating the animal
- Providing supportive care

ACUTE GENERAL TREATMENT

- Clinicians should treat life-threatening signs if present:
    - Atropine sulfate (dogs/cats: 0.1–0.2 mg/kg one-fourth dose IV and rest of dose IM or SQ) to control the muscarinic signs. The dose can be repeated as needed to control bradycardia and bronchial secretions.
    - Pralidoxime chloride (2-PAM; Protopam) (dogs/cats: 20 mg/kg IM, SC or very slow IV q 12h) is used for controlling the nicotinic signs, although some benefit may be seen with controlling muscarinic and CNS signs as well; 2-PAM should not be used with carbamates since it would not be beneficial: oximes reverse binding of toxin to AChE, but carbamate binding to AChE is inherently reversible. If the animal shows no response after three doses, the clinician should discontinue treatment with 2-PAM. Oximes such as pralidoxime are ineffective once "aging" has occurred. However, the time of aging varies with the compound, so pralidoxime may be effective even days after exposure.
    - Seizure control:
        - Diazepam: 1–2 mg/kg IV, repeat as needed.
        - Phenobarbital: 2–5 mg/kg IV bolus, repeated in 20 minutes up to two times. Clinicians can consider pentobarbital if this is ineffective.
        - Pentobarbital to reach desired effect; repeat as needed.
    - Controlling tremors: methocarbamol 50–100 mg/kg IV. Clinicians can repeat as needed without exceeding more than 330 mg/kg/day.
    - Clinicians can provide oxygen and ventilatory support as needed for animals in respiratory distress.
- Decontamination of the animal:
    - Dermal exposure: Clinicians can bathe the animal with a mild dishwashing liquid and rinse them thoroughly; clinicians should keep the animal warm.
    - Emesis: only in animals *not* showing clinical signs; usually effective within a couple of hours of ingestion.
        - Apomorphine (0.03–0.04 mg/kg IV or IM; clinicians can instead administer a crushed tablet portion with water, instill into conjunctival sac, and rinse following emesis).
        - Hydrogen peroxide 3% (2 ml/kg, max 45 ml PO, repeat in 10–15 minutes if no vomiting).
    - Gastric lavage:
        - Should be considered where a large amount of poison has been ingested or when emesis is contraindicated (comatose) and emesis has not occurred. Clinicians can anesthetize with a short-acting barbiturate and use a cuffed endotracheal tube to protect airway (see Gastric Intubation, Gavage, Lavage, p 1258).
    - Activated charcoal:
        - 1–4 g/kg PO or labeled dosage of commercial product. In animals showing overt clinical signs, repeat in 8 hours (half the original dose).
- Supportive care: IV fluids as needed.

DRUG INTERACTIONS

Clinicians should avoid:

- Enhancing toxicity: phenothiazine tranquilizers, opiates, aminoglycoside antibiotics, theophylline.
- Administering neuromuscular blocking agents: levamisole, succinylcholine, nicotine, and curare can enhance the nicotinic effects of OPs.

POSSIBLE COMPLICATIONS

- Pancreatitis and hepatic disease have occurred in some animals after OP toxicosis.
- Certain OPs can cause a delayed neuropathy within 2 to 3 weeks after acute poisoning. This complication is characterized by hind limb ataxia, hypermetria, and proprioceptive deficits. Chlorpyrifos (experimentally at high doses) is possibly associated with this neuropathy in cats.
- There are usually no long-term effects in animals that recover from acute OP or carbamate toxicosis unless there have been prolonged seizures.

RECOMMENDED MONITORING

- Heart rate
- Respiration
- CNS signs

PROGNOSIS AND OUTCOME

- Prognosis good unless the animal suffers from respiratory distress (excessive bronchial secretions, aspiration pneumonia) or seizures
- Duration of signs depends on treatment, dose, compound, and species of animal

PEARLS & CONSIDERATIONS

COMMENTS

- The main difference of clinical importance between carbamates and OPs is that AChE inhibition is generally irreversible in cases of OP toxicity but reversible in cases of carbamate toxicity. Therefore:
    - Pralidoxime (2-PAM, protopam) is indicated for treatment of OP toxicosis but not carbamate toxicosis (ineffective).
    - Carbamates are generally short-acting.
- SLUDDE signs can occur from several causes. If history of exposure to an anticholinesterase insecticide is not known, a test dose of atropine can be given to determine if the signs are caused by an anticholinesterase (OP or carbamate) insecticide.
    - Clinicians should take a baseline heart rate.
    - They should give a preanesthetic-level dose of atropine (i.e., 0.02 mg/kg IV for dogs and cats) and monitor the animal's response for 15 to 30 minutes.
    - If the heart rate increases and mydriasis occurs, then the muscarinic signs are not due to OP or carbamate toxicosis (it takes approximately 10 times the preanesthetic dose of atropine to resolve signs caused by cholinesterase inhibitor insecticides).
- For dead animals, the clinician can submit half of the brain (sagittal section, frozen) to the lab (put the other half in formalin for histopathologic examina-

tion) but only if rabies is definitively ruled out (otherwise, the material could be hazardous to personnel during opening of skull and handling of tissue).

- Muscarinic signs may be masked by sympathetic stimulation, which can result in the opposite effects (mydriasis, tachycardia, etc.).
- With the availability of safer insecticides for controlling insects, OP and carbamate toxicosis incidences in animals have decreased
- See Table I-20 for toxicity ratings.

PREVENTION

Clinicians should educate clients to keep all insecticides away from pets.

TABLE I-20 **Toxicity Ratings**

Toxicity Rating	LD50	Substances
Highly toxic	<50 mg/kg	Disulfoton, coumaphos, famphur, phorate, terbufos, methomyl, aldicarb
Moderately toxic	50–1000 mg/kg	Acephate, chlorpyrifos, diazinon, carbaryl, phosmet, propoxur
Lower toxicity	>1000 mg/kg	Malathion, tetrachlorvinphos

CLIENT EDUCATION

Pet owners should use insecticides according to label directions.

SUGGESTED READING

The Extension Toxicology Network: http://extoxnet.orst.edu/.

Meerdink GL: Anticholinesterase insecticides. In Plumlee KH (ed): *Clinical Veterinary Toxicology*. St. Louis, Mosby, 2004, pp 178–180.

AUTHOR: **TINA WISMER**
EDITOR: **SAFDAR A. KHAN**

Oronasal Fistula, Acute/Chronic

BASIC INFORMATION

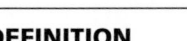

DEFINITION

A connection between the oral and nasal cavities, usually resulting from severe periodontal disease; in dogs, this condition is almost invariably the result of oral disease extending dorsally, and is virtually never caused by nasal disease extending ventrally.

EPIDEMIOLOGY

SPECIES, AGE, SEX: Older small dogs, typically with narrow muzzles. Either sex.
GENETICS AND BREED PREDISPOSITION: Conformation of skull and predisposition to development of periodontal disease. Breeds: miniature poodles, Chihuahuas, Yorkshire terriers, miniature schnauzers, dachshunds.
RISK FACTORS: See Periodontal Disease, p 833.
ASSOCIATED CONDITIONS AND DISORDERS: See Periodontal Disease, p 833.

CLINICAL PRESENTATION

DISEASE FORMS/SUBTYPES: Area of the upper canine tooth is most often affected. Oronasal fistulas are occasionally seen in the premolar area. A fistula may be present even though the tooth is still in place.
HISTORY, CHIEF COMPLAINT

- Chronic: nasal discharge, sneezing, halitosis
- Acute: epistaxis after tooth extraction

PHYSICAL EXAM FINDINGS

- Mucopurulent nasal discharge.
- Typically, the canine tooth has been lost or was previously extracted. A defect is seen at the junction of the palate and mucosa of the lip, with oral epithelium connected to the nasal epithelium; the tissues are healthy (Fig. I-123).
- In the occasional case in which the tooth is still present, the tooth typically is mobile and has severe plaque as well as

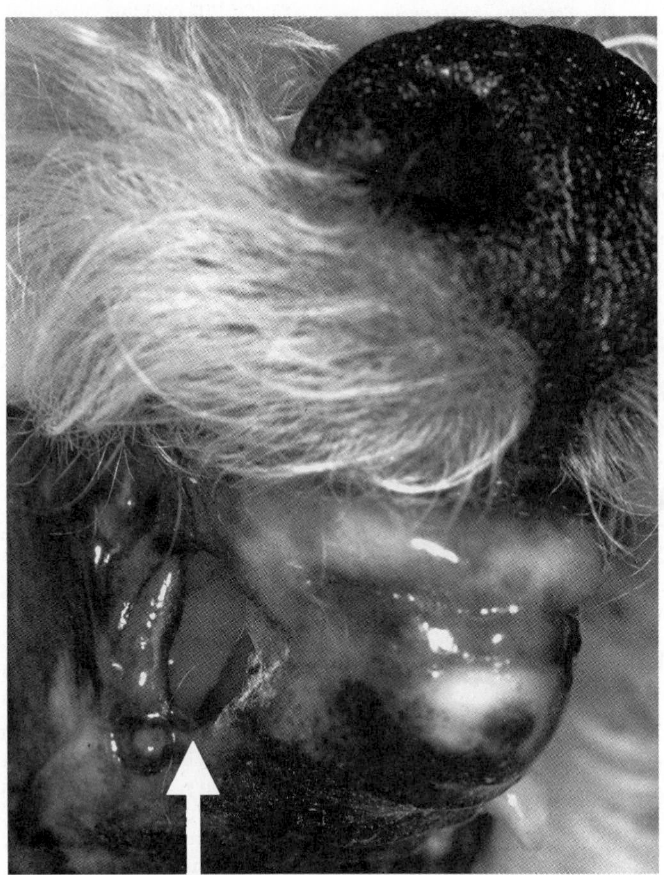

FIGURE I-123 Upper lip retracted to show a chronic oronasal fistula in the area of a missing right upper canine tooth in a dog (*arrow*). The upper incisors and most other upper teeth also are missing in this dog. Courtesy of Dr. Alexander M. Reiter, University of Pennsylvania.

calculus accumulation and deep pockets on periodontal probing (see Fig. I-123).

ETIOLOGY AND PATHOPHYSIOLOGY

Periodontitis results in alveolar bone loss and loss of nasal epithelium separating the oral and nasal cavities.

DIAGNOSIS

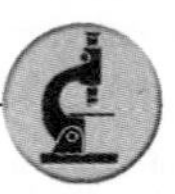

DIFFERENTIAL DIAGNOSIS

Other causes of chronic nasal discharge. Clinicians should ALWAYS remember to thoroughly examine the mouth and teeth of animals with nasal discharge.

INITIAL DATABASE

- Complete blood count, serum chemistry profile, urinalysis (preanesthetic): generally unremarkable
- Thoracic radiographs: if the chief complaint, history, and physical exam findings raise the possibility of metastatic disease or of pneumonia

ADVANCED OR CONFIRMATORY TESTING

- Periodontal probing and dental radiographs will demonstrate the severity of alveolar bone loss.
- If the diagnosis of an oronasal fistula is uncertain, clinicians can inject water (via a syringe nozzle, not by needle) into the questionable area in the mouth while the dog is anesthetized (and while the nose is lower than the cranium) to look for flow of water from the naris.
- Clinicians should check other areas of the mouth because periodontal disease is likely to be generalized and severe.

TREATMENT

THERAPEUTIC GOAL(S)

Clinicians should close the oronasal fistula to prevent continued entry of food or fluid into the nasal cavity.

ACUTE GENERAL TREATMENT

- Under general anesthesia (and after tooth extraction in the area of the oronasal fistula if it is still present), clinicians can gently irrigate the tissue lining of the fistula to remove debris.
- Single buccal-based flap technique: Creation of a flap of buccal mucosa sutured over the defect. The edges of the flap must be gently apposed to freshly incised edges of epithelium and be under no tension following closure. This requires dissection of the buccal mucosa (epithelium and supporting connective tissue) from its maxillary attachments and also requires resection of the epithelium lining the oronasal fistula on the palatal side.
- Double flap technique: Initially, a full-thickness mucoperiosteal palatal flap is raised but remains hinged at the medial margin of the defect. The clinician can overlap the flap to cover the defect (palatine epithelium becomes "nasal" epithelium). Then the clinician can raise a buccal-based flap and advance and suture it over the connective tissue side of the first flap.
- Clinicians should treat periodontal disease in other areas of the mouth. This will often require extraction of other maxillary teeth on the same side; closure of these extraction sites can be combined with closure of the flap covering the oronasal fistula.

POSSIBLE COMPLICATIONS

The major complication is dehiscence: Clinicians should avoid tension as previously described.

PROGNOSIS AND OUTCOME

Excellent

PEARLS & CONSIDERATIONS

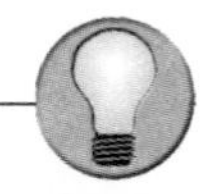

COMMENTS

- Clinicians should always examine the mouth and teeth of animals with nasal discharge.
- If clinicians are kind to the tissue, it will heal readily.

PREVENTION

See Periodontal Disease, p 833

CLIENT EDUCATION

See Periodontal Disease, p 833

SUGGESTED READING

Harvey CE, Emily PP: *Small Animal Dentistry*. St. Louis, Mosby, 1993, pp 345-348.

AUTHOR: **COLIN E. HARVEY**
EDITOR: **ALEXANDER M. REITER**

Osteoarthritis

Client Education Sheet on Website

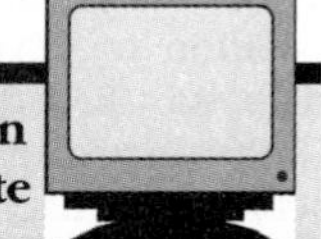

BASIC INFORMATION

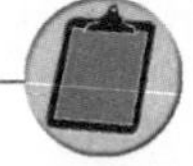

DEFINITION

Progressive, noninflammatory, irreversible deterioration of articular cartilage

SYNONYM(S)

- Degenerative joint disease
- Osteoarthrosis

EPIDEMIOLOGY

SPECIES, AGE, SEX: Increasing prevalence with age.

GENETICS AND BREED PREDISPOSITION: Secondary to:

- Elbow osteochondrosis and dysplasia (rottweilers, Labrador retrievers, Bernese mountain dogs)
- Hip dysplasia (many breeds)
- Patellar luxation (toy breed dogs)
- Arthropathy in Scottish fold cats

RISK FACTORS

- Obesity
- Work duty (dogs)
- Athletics (dogs)

CLINICAL PRESENTATION

DISEASE FORMS/SUBTYPES

- Primary (idiopathic) osteoarthritis: unknown cause; not common in animals
- Secondary osteoarthritis: commonly results from trauma, joint instability, incongruity, immobilization, or osteochondrosis

HISTORY, CHIEF COMPLAINT

- Reluctance to ambulate
- Lameness and stiffness after excessive exercise or prolonged rest
- Irritable behavior when approached or touched

PHYSICAL EXAM FINDINGS

- Stiff or altered gait (e.g., bunny hopping)
- Lameness
- Abnormalities during joint manipulation (flexion and extension): joint pain, crepitus, instability, and/or decreased range of motion
- Joint effusion
- Joint thickening
- Muscle atrophy

ETIOLOGY AND PATHOPHYSIOLOGY

- Joint homeostasis is disrupted by abnormal cartilage and membrane cell functions, nutrition, or joint biomechanics.

- A catabolic imbalance results with chondrocytes unable to replace degraded extracellular matrix (degradation via cytokines and other inflammatory mediators).
- This cycle progresses irreversibly as the weakened biomechanical integrity of articular cartilage potentiates further dysfunction and disease.
- Periarticular fibrosis is a secondary process directed toward stabilizing the joint.

DIAGNOSIS

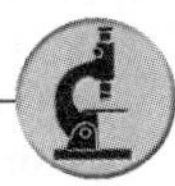

DIFFERENTIAL DIAGNOSIS

- Infectious arthritis (bacterial, spirochetal, bacterial L-forms, mycoplasmal, rickettsial and ehrlichial, viral, fungal, and protozoal)
- Immune-mediated arthritis (erosive arthritis, nonerosive arthritis)
- Neoplasia (synovial cell sarcoma, osteosarcoma)

INITIAL DATABASE

- Clinical examination localizing joint pain
- Radiography: subchondral sclerosis, joint space narrowing, osteophytosis, enthesiophytosis, joint capsule thickening, subchondral bone attrition, intraarticular calcified bodies, soft tissue calcification, or subchondral cysts

ADVANCED OR CONFIRMATORY TESTING

- Arthrocentesis and synovial fluid analysis.
  - Total cell count <5000 nucleated cells/μl; mononuclear cells/macrophages predominate, <10% polymorphonuclear cells; fluid is clear, hazy, or pale yellow with normal to decreased viscosity.
- Computed tomography (CT) may confirm joint incongruity.
- Magnetic resonance imaging (MRI) may identify morphologic cartilage changes.
- Nuclear scintigraphy may help localize osteoarthritis.

TREATMENT

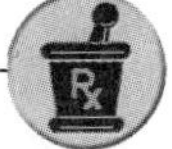

THERAPEUTIC GOAL(S)

- Pain alleviation
- Improved function
- Limiting disease progression
- Facilitating joint reparative process

ACUTE GENERAL TREATMENT

- Surgical treatment for cause of joint degeneration: repair of an articular fracture, removal of osteochondrosis lesion, or stabilization of cruciate deficient stifle
- A nonsteroidal anti-inflammatory drug (NSAID) to reduce inflammatory mediators and pain; the clinician has the choice of one of the following NSAIDs (dogs):
  - Aspirin: 10-25 mg/kg PO, q 8-24h
  - Carprofen: 2 mg/kg PO, q 12h
  - Deracoxib: 1-2 mg/kg PO, q 24h (may use 3-4 mg/kg PO, q 24h for first 7days only)
  - Etodolac: 10-15 mg/kg PO, q 24h
  - Firocoxib: 5 mg/kg PO, q 24h
  - Meloxicam: 0.1 mg/kg PO, q 24h
  - Tepoxalin: 10 mg/kg PO, q 24h
  - Meclofenamic acid: 1.1 mg/kg PO, q 24h after eating, for 5 days maximum
  - Other NSAIDs
- A chondroprotective agent:
  - Polysulfated glycosaminoglycan 5 mg/kg IM once weekly for 4 to 6 weeks (dogs)
  - Pentosan polysulfate (from beechwood hemicellulose) 3 mg/kg SC once weekly (dogs)
  - Oral formulations (glucosamine, chondroitin sulphate, hyaluronan): according to formulation/labeled instructions
- Opioids (e.g., butorphanol 0.5-1 mg/kg PO q 6-8h) or synthetic opiate agonist (e.g., tramadol 1-4 mg/kg PO q 8-12h) if necessary to decrease pain

CHRONIC TREATMENT

- NSAIDs
- Cartilage modifiers
- Weight control if obese
- Physical therapy
- Joint arthroplasty in severely affected hips
- Joint arthrodesis in severely affected joints
- Acupuncture

DRUG INTERACTIONS

- Gastrointestinal irritation, hemorrhage, gastric ulceration, and perforation with NSAIDs
- NSAID-induced nephrotoxicity possible with hypovolemia or preexisting renal disease
- Hepatotoxicity with carprofen
- Decreased platelet aggregation with aspirin therapy

POSSIBLE COMPLICATIONS

Polysulfated glycosaminoglycan is a heparin analog; caution if given with NSAIDs to an animal with a bleeding disorder

RECOMMENDED MONITORING

Clinicians should:

- Quantify muscle mass with palpation and tape measure.
- Measure range of motion during examination with a goniometer.
- Palpate joint effusion and for periarticular fibrosis.
- Monitor joint pain and gait during examination or with force plate analysis.
- Assess serial radiographs.
- Assess animal's attitude, appetite, body condition score, body weight, and activity level.

PROGNOSIS AND OUTCOME

- Osteoarthritis is typically an irreversible, slowly progressive disease.
- Medical and/or surgical treatment may permit a good quality of life.

PEARLS & CONSIDERATIONS

COMMENTS

- Radiographic signs of osteoarthritis may not correlate with clinical signs. Treatment decisions cannot be made on the basis of radiographic findings alone.
- Efficacy of cartilage modifiers not as well documented as NSAIDs.
- Comparative efficacy of NSAIDs is debatable.
- Use of corticosteroids in place of NSAIDs is controversial, but using both together is contraindicated due to severe, potentially life-threatening gastrointestinal ulceration.

PREVENTION

Prompt recognition and early intervention may delay progression of disease

CLIENT EDUCATION

- Treatment is palliative (no "magic bullet"); disease will likely progress.
- Client participation is necessary for long-term management.

SUGGESTED READING

McLaughlin R: Management of chronic osteoarthritis pain. *Vet Clin North Amer: Sm Anim Pract* 30:933-949, 2000.

Pedersen NC, Morgan JP, and Vasseur PB: Joint diseases of dogs and cats. In Ettinger SJ, Feldman EC (eds): *Textbook of Veterinary Internal Medicine*, ed 5. Philadelphia, WB Saunders, 2000, pp 1862-1886.

Todhunter RJ, Johnston SA: Osteoarthritis. In Slatter D (ed): *Textbook of Small Animal Surgery*, ed 3. Philadelphia, WB Saunders, 2003, pp 2208-2246.

AUTHOR: **DEANNA R. WORLEY**

EDITOR: **JOSEPH HARARI**

Osteochondrosis

Client Education Sheet on Website

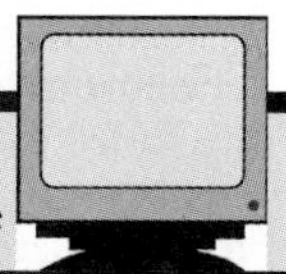

BASIC INFORMATION

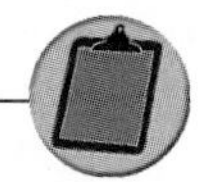

DEFINITION

- Osteochondrosis is an abnormality of endochondral ossification, producing thickened cartilage that is susceptible to injury.
- Osteochondrosis produces a non-painful thickening of cartilage, which may loosen and thus develop into the painful and clinically overt osteochondritis dissecans (OCD).
- In turn, OCD may lead to osteoarthritis (see p 778; also called degenerative joint disease [DJD]), a deterioration of articular cartilage and joint capsule tissues that leads to decreased joint function.

SYNONYM(S)

Osteochondritis

EPIDEMIOLOGY

SPECIES, AGE, SEX

- Fast-growing large- and giant-breed dogs
- More frequent in males
- First signs appear at maximum growth rate (4 to 8 months of age)

GENETICS AND BREED PREDISPOSITION: Predisposition within these breeds is seen in certain blood lines, but the mode of inheritance is unknown:

- Border collie
- German shepherd
- Golden retriever
- Great Danes
- Irish wolfhound
- Labrador retriever
- Newfoundland
- Rottweiler
- Saint Bernard
- Others

RISK FACTORS

- Genetic
- Rapid growth rate
- Excessive intake of calcium (Ca) with or without excess of phosphorus (P) and vitamin D and/or excessive intake of food
- Hormonal effects (i.e., male dogs, calcitonin)
- Increased joint loading and trauma from intense exercise

ASSOCIATED CONDITIONS AND DISORDERS

- Hip dysplasia also occurs in dogs that eat an excessive amount of food.
- Disturbances in endochondral ossification also are seen in the radius curvus syndrome (elbow incongruity) and ununited bone protuberances (anconeal, coronoid, and supraglenoid processes).

CLINICAL PRESENTATION

HISTORY, CHIEF COMPLAINT

- Young dogs with good general health (typically).
- Chief complaint is lameness:
  - Can be unilateral or bilateral
  - Variable degree of lameness
  - Variable duration of lameness
  - May become clinically overt after skeletal maturity
- History may include use of homemade diet or supplemented commercial dog food during the preweaning or post-weaning period.

PHYSICAL EXAM FINDINGS

- Lameness as previously described; may manifest as a short-stepping gait if bilateral
- Joint pain, swelling, crepitus, decreased range of motion during flexion and extension
- Muscle atrophy of the affected limb(s)

ETIOLOGY AND PATHOPHYSIOLOGY

- Excessive intake of food with normal content of Ca, P, and vitamin D, increased Ca intake (with or without increased P intake with normal Ca:P ratio), or increased intake of vitamin D with normal Ca and P intake causes disturbed endochondral ossification in fast-growing (not miniature) dogs.
  - Increased protein intake (as in puppy food) does not disturb endochondral ossification.
- Disturbed endochondral ossification leads to cartilage thickening and retention of cartilage in the physis and articular epiphysis.
- The thickened cartilage impedes the diffusion of nutrients from the synovium.
- Tissue malnutrition, ischemia, and chondrocyte necrosis occur.
- Clefts develop at the junction of viable and nonviable layers.
- During normal joint motion and loading, vertical fissures develop in the articular cartilage and result in the formation of a cartilage flap.
- The flap may remain attached to the remaining cartilage tissue or may completely detach ("joint mouse").
- Inflammatory mediators are released into the synovium, and DJD results.
- Osteochondrosis most commonly affects:
  - Shoulder: caudal humeral head.
  - Elbow: medial humeral condyle.
  - Hock (tibiotarsal joint): medial or lateral trochlear ridges of the talus.
  - Stifle: lateral or medial femoral condyle.

DIAGNOSIS

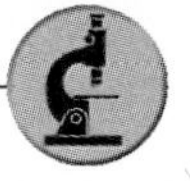

DIFFERENTIAL DIAGNOSIS

- Shoulder joint: humeral or scapular fracture; biceps tenosynovitis
- Elbow joint: fragmented coronoid process, ununited anconeal process, incongruity
- Stifle joint: cranial cruciate ligament rupture or avulsion, extensor tendon avulsion, patella luxation, femoral or tibial fracture
- Hock joint: collateral ligament rupture, fracture
- Radius curvus syndrome: shortening of antebrachium as in chondrodystrophy, curvature due to physeal (Salter type V) fracture

INITIAL DATABASE

- Radiographs of the affected joint:
  - Indentation (flattening or saucer shape of the subchondral bone) at the lesion.
  - Mineralized density within the joint may be present.
  - Varying degrees of osteoarthrosis.
  - Subchondral sclerosis in advanced cases.
  - Multiple orthogonal views may be required for accurate visualization.
- Dietary history including food intake and body condition score.
- Blood Ca, P, and vitamin D concentrations at the time of clinical signs are not diagnostic.

ADVANCED OR CONFIRMATORY TESTING

- Arthrocentesis for synovial fluid analysis when joint swelling or effusion is present. Mild increase in mononuclear cell counts with OCD.
- Contrast radiography, scintigraphy, computed tomography (CT), and magnetic resonance imaging (MRI) are uncommonly indicated.
- Arthroscopy can be used for direct visualization of lesion if radiography inconclusive; can also be used for treatment.

TREATMENT

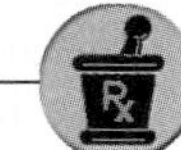

THERAPEUTIC GOAL(S)

- Restoration of joint health
- Elimination discomfort and lameness

- Education of clients to provide satisfactory nutrient intake in growing animals to prevent other joints from developing OCD

ACUTE GENERAL TREATMENT

- Conservative management:
  - Exercise restriction for 6 weeks.
  - Clinicians can choose from the following NSAIDs:
    - Aspirin: 10–25 mg/kg PO q 12h.
    - Carprofen: 2 mg/kg PO q 12h.
    - Etodolac: 10–15 mg/kg PO q 24h.
    - Deracoxib: 1–2 mg/kg PO q 24h.
    - Ketofen 0.25 mg/kg PO q 24h.
    - Meloxicam: 0.1 mg/kg PO q 24h.
    - Tepoxalin: 10 mg/kg PO q 24h (new product, objective data pending).
- Arthrotomy or arthroscopy to remove loose, discolored, thickened, or devitalized cartilage, cartilage flaps, and intra-articular osteochondral fragments.
  - The ridge of the talus is NOT curetted, to avoid creating further joint instability.
  - Curettage and forage (drilling) of the subchondral bone lesion to optimize healing through stimulation of fibrocartilage formation.

CHRONIC TREATMENT

- DJD (also degenerative osteoarthrosis) may occur at a later age; clinicians can treat the condition by preventing overload of the joint (by limiting activity and body weight gain) and administering NSAIDs as listed above.
- Chondroprotective agents:
  - Glucosamine (clinicians should follow label instructions for oral dosing)
  - Chondroitin sulfate (clinicians should follow label instructions for oral dosing)
  - Glycosaminoglycans: 5 mg/kg IM, twice a week
  - Hyaluronan: 3–5 mg intra-articular, once a week
- Limitation/control of activity for 6 weeks after surgery.
- Clinicians can consider supplemental chondroprotective agents and intra-articular hyaluronic acid injections.

DRUG INTERACTIONS

Intra-articular corticosteroid injections increase lesion severity and are contraindicated.

POSSIBLE COMPLICATIONS

- Untreated cartilage flaps irritate the joint and thus cause more DJD. In OCD of the shoulder joint, the flap can loosen and migrate into the biceps tendon sheath.
- Perioperative and postoperative:
  - Seroma formation due to excessive postoperative physical activity
  - Infection
  - Failure to remove all the osteochondral fragments
  - Tibiotarsal joint instability, not only due to aggressive curettage

RECOMMENDED MONITORING

- Multiple joints, including contralateral, may be affected and should be clinically and radiographically evaluated.
- If lameness persists, synovial fluid analysis, radiographs, arthroscopy, CT, or MRI may be indicated.

PROGNOSIS AND OUTCOME

- Shoulder: good after treatment, even in cases with DJD. Most dogs become sound 4 to 8 weeks after surgery.
- Elbow: fair to good when cartilage damage is small in young animals and DJD is minimal. Fair to poor when combined with fragmented coronoid process and/or severe cartilage damage.
- Stifle: variable; a large lesion in a young animal may have a poor prognosis.
- Hock: fair; joint capsule thickening helps stabilize the joint although residual instability will remain, and DJD should be anticipated.

PEARLS & CONSIDERATIONS

COMMENTS

- Although the lameness may be unilateral, osteochondrosis often occurs bilaterally. Radiographs of the contralateral joint are indicated.
- Clinicians should make sure that surgical curettage of the tibiotarsal joint is kept to a minimum to prevent further joint instability.

PREVENTION

- Owners should only breed animals screened for OCD (and other hereditary diseases); affected dogs and their relatives (parents and siblings) should not be bred.
- Animals should avoid excessive intense activity until they are skeletally mature.
- Animals should avoid excessive intake of food, calcium (bones, bone meal, milk, tablets, powder), or vitamin D (drops, tablets, fish diets).
- Owners should avoid *ad libitum* feeding:
  - Volume of food should be based on the animal's body condition score.
  - The lowest risk of diet-induced disease was found in animals whose body condition score was maintained at 2/5 during the period of growth.
  - Owners should only use calculated energy requirements and manufacturer's recommendations as initial starting points for feeding, with amounts adjusted to maintain the desired body condition score.

CLIENT EDUCATION

- Before purchasing a puppy, owners should become familiar with the weaker points of the breed in question.
- When a veterinarian knows that an animal's OCD occurs in high incidence, the veterinarian should inform the owner to buy a puppy of screened parents and preferably from a family with previously screened puppies that do not have any hereditary bone diseases.
- During growth, owners should feed their pets a commercially available dog food with a calcium content of not more than 0.8–1.0% on dry matter base and energy density <4 kcal/g (<17% fat).
  - These percentages may differ with the energy content of the food.
  - Owners should not add supplements.
  - These feeding guidelines are especially important in the preweaning and postweaning periods.
- Owners should give the puppy the time to grow and should not train their dog too heavily or too early.

SUGGESTED READING

Harari J: Osteochondrosis. *Vet Clin North Am Small Anim Pract* 26:1–195, 1998.

Johnson AL Hulse DA: Diseases of the joints. In Fossum T (ed): *Small Animal Surgery*, ed 2. St. Louis, Mosby, 2002, pp 1023–1157.

AUTHORS: **HERMAN A. W. HAZEWINKEL, JOSEPH C. GLENNON**

EDITORS: **JOSEPH HARARI, C. A. TONY BUFFINGTON**

Osteomyelitis

BASIC INFORMATION

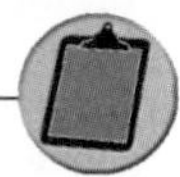

DEFINITION

An acute or chronic inflammatory process of bone secondary to hematogenous or traumatic infection with pyogenic organisms

SYNONYM(S)

Bone infection

EPIDEMIOLOGY

SPECIES, AGE, SEX: Young male dogs for traumatic osteomyelitis.

GENETICS AND BREED PREDISPOSITION: German shepherds for *Aspergillus*.

RISK FACTORS

- Open fractures secondary to trauma, bite wounds, gunshot wounds
- Closed fractures or elective orthopedic procedures with direct or hematogenous contamination
- Extension of soft-tissue infections
- Immune system is compromised, allowing hematogenous dissemination

GEOGRAPHY AND SEASONALITY

- Blastomycosis and histoplasmosis: mid-Atlantic states, south of the Ohio River and east of the Mississippi
- Coccidioidomycosis in the southwestern United States and Central and South Americas
- Actinomycosis associated with migrating grass awns in summer in California and Florida

ASSOCIATED CONDITIONS AND DISORDERS: Periodontitis, bulla osteitis, diskospondylitis, and paronychia, depending on location of infected bone.

CLINICAL PRESENTATION

HISTORY, CHIEF COMPLAINT

- Orthopedic surgery, trauma, or travel (systemic fungal infection) may be in the recent history.
- Owner may have noted lethargy, anorexia, lameness, swelling, signs of pain, and cutaneous draining tracts.

PHYSICAL EXAM FINDINGS

- Acute osteomyelitis: fever, lethargy, anorexia, limb or joint swelling/pain, lameness
- Chronic osteomyelitis: draining tracts or fistulas, normothermia, disuse muscle atrophy, lameness, limb deformity

ETIOLOGY AND PATHOPHYSIOLOGY

- Neonatal osteomyelitis may originate from the umbilicus.
- Acute osteomyelitis presents with clinical signs 2 to 7 days after the surgery.
- Radiographic changes evident 2 weeks after trauma and surgery.
- Glycocalyx (biofilm) is formed on surgical implants after combining with bacteria. This produces a barrier that protects bacteria from antibodies and drugs.
- Between 50% and 60% of cases are monomicrobial, with *Staphylococcus* spp. most common (50%).
- Between 40% and 50% of cases are polymicrobial, with a mixture of aerobes and anaerobes.
- Up to 70% of cases are positive for anaerobes, including *Actinomyces, Clostridium, Bacteroides, Fusobacterium*, and *Peptostreptococcus* spp.
- Other common isolates are *Streptococcus, E. coli, Pasteurella, Pseudomonas, Proteus,* and *Klebsiella* spp.

DIAGNOSIS

DIFFERENTIAL DIAGNOSIS

Bone infarct, neoplasia, cellulitis

INITIAL DATABASE

- Complete blood count, serum biochemistry panel
- Anteriopposterior and mediolateral radiographs of affected bone
- Thorax and abdominal radiographs if fungal etiology suspected
- Arthrocentesis with cytologic examination; culture and sensitivity (C&S) test if joint involvement
- Aerobic and anaerobic C&S tests of deep fine-needle aspirates of tissues

ADVANCED OR CONFIRMATORY TESTING

- Ultrasound may reveal soft-tissue abscess or periosteal elevation
- Contrast fistulogram to localize source or sequestrum
- Computed tomography (CT) and/or magnetic resonance imaging (MRI)
- Radionucleide bone scan with technetium 99m: will detect inflammatory lesions; more specific if performed with leukocytes labeled with gallium 67 or indium 111, and best if animal has a confirmed leukocytosis
- Blood and/or urine cultures if systemic infection suspected

TREATMENT

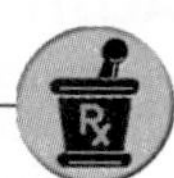

THERAPEUTIC GOAL(S)

- Identify and eliminate the source of the infection
- Stabilize fracture fragments

ACUTE GENERAL TREATMENT

- Acute osteomyelitis requires 4 to 6 weeks of antimicrobials based on C&S results.
- Initial antibiotics may be given IV.
- Since *Staphylococcus* spp. are most common, initial therapy can involve:
    - Clavulanic acid/amoxicillin: 10-20 mg/kg PO q 12h, or
    - Cefazolin: 10-30 mg/kg SQ, IM, or IV q 8h, or
    - Clindamycin: 5-10 mg/kg PO q 12h, or
    - Cloxacillin: 20-40 mg/kg PO q 8h
- Definitive (medium- and long-term) antibiotic selection will depend on results of bacterial C&S.

CHRONIC TREATMENT

- May require surgical exploration and removal of sequestrum with curettage of surrounding bone.
- Removal of loose implants, retention of stable implants, and possibly external fixation if additional stability is needed.
- Infection will not clear unless fracture is stable.
- A cancellous bone graft may be indicated once the infection has subsided.
- Open drainage with lavage or closed drainage with ingress/egress.
- Antibiotic-impregnated polymethylmethacrylate beads.
- Animals should continue antibiotics for minimum of 6 to 8 weeks.

DRUG INTERACTIONS

- Clinicians should avoid administering aminoglycosides to animals with renal disease.
- Clinicians should avoid administering quinolones to skeletally immature dogs (risk of cartilage defects).

POSSIBLE COMPLICATIONS

- Bone abscess
- Bacteremia
- Fracture/limb deformity
- Implant failure(s)
- Cellulitis
- Draining tracts
- Delayed/nonunion

RECOMMENDED MONITORING

- Radiographs at 4 to 6 week intervals to evaluate healing
- Clinicians can aspirate and reculture if animal shows signs of recurrence

PROGNOSIS AND OUTCOME

- Acute osteomyelitis can be eradicated with early aggressive treatment.
- Chronic osteomyelitis can recur within weeks to years after the initial treatment.
- Fungal osteomyelitis may require several months of treatment, and outcome is guarded to poor.
- Involvement of joints may result in osteoarthrosis and limb disuse.

PEARLS & CONSIDERATIONS

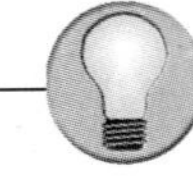

COMMENTS

- Obtaining a culture only from the drainage tract can be confusing because contaminants (skin organisms and gram-negative bacteria) are common.
- Leukocytosis is common with acute disease; typically it is absent with chronic conditions.

PREVENTION

- Aseptic surgical technique
- Appropriate antimicrobial prophylaxis and therapy

CLIENT EDUCATION

Treatment of chronic osteomyelitis can be costly and lengthy.

SUGGESTED READING

Bubenik LJ, Smith MM: Osteomyelitis. In Slatter D (ed): *Textbook of Small Animal Surgery*, ed 3. Philadelphia, WB Saunders, 2003, pp 1862–1875.

Johnson KA. Osteomyelitis. In Birchard SJ, Sherding RG (eds): *Saunders Manual of Small Animal Practice*, ed 2. Philadelphia, WB Saunders, 2000, 1213–1217.

AUTHOR: **MARY E. SOMERVILLE**

EDITOR: **JOSEPH HARARI**

Osteosarcoma

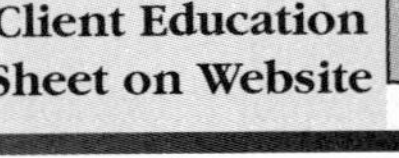

BASIC INFORMATION

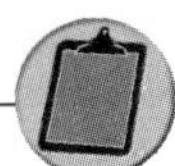

DEFINITION

Osteosarcoma (OSA) is a primary malignant tumor of mesenchymal tissue that always includes the production of bone (osteoid) by malignant osteoblasts. Appendicular OSA refers to the limbs; axial OSA involves any part of the rest of the skeleton.

EPIDEMIOLOGY

SPECIES, AGE, SEX

- In dogs, OSA accounts for up to 85% of all primary bone tumors:
  - Median age is 7 to 9 years, with a smaller peak incidence at 1.5 to 2 years of age.
  - There is no obvious gender predilection.
- In cats, OSA and other primary bone tumors are uncommon. OSA may rarely occur in the soft tissues at sites of previous vaccinations (see Vaccine-Site Sarcoma, p 1136).

GENETICS AND BREED PREDISPOSITION

Large- and giant-breed dogs are predisposed.

- Body size (height and weight) is a more important predictor than breed.
- Compared to small-breed dogs (weighing <10 kg), the risk of OSA is 60 times higher in dogs weighing >30 kg and 8 times higher in dogs weighing 20–30 kg.
- Appendicular OSA accounts for almost 95% of all cases in dogs weighing >40 kg, but only 40–50% of all cases in dogs weighing <15 kg.

CLINICAL PRESENTATION

DISEASE FORMS/SUBTYPES

Approximately 75% of OSA arises from the appendicular skeleton and 25% from the axial skeleton. Rarely, OSA can arise in the soft tissues (called extraskeletal OSA).

- Appendicular: In the forelimb, the distal radius and proximal humerus are most commonly affected. In the hind limb, lesions are evenly distributed between the distal femur, proximal tibia, and distal tibia.
- Axial: In the axial skeleton, the mandible, maxilla, vertebra, and ribs are most commonly affected.

HISTORY, CHIEF COMPLAINT

- Appendicular OSA usually is associated with progressive lameness. Lameness is less commonly acute and severe due to a pathologic fracture. A palpable swelling may or may not be present.
- Axial OSA can present with a variety of signs. Localized swelling with or without pain is common. Tumors arising from the mandible or maxilla can be associated with dysphagia, pain on opening the mouth, or nasal discharge. Vertebral tumors may induce neurologic deficits. Rarely, rib tumors are associated with respiratory signs.
- If pulmonary metastasis is present, the first clinical signs usually are vague, including lethargy and anorexia. The animal may cough, but overt respiratory distress is uncommon. Rarely, lameness develops secondary to hypertrophic osteopathy.

PHYSICAL EXAM FINDINGS

- Dogs with appendicular OSA exhibit lameness of variable severity, ranging from minimal to non-weight-bearing. A palpable swelling may or may not be present.
- Dogs with axial OSA can have variable physical examination findings (see History above). Signs of pain or discomfort are not as consistent as with appendicular tumors. Depending on the size and location of the tumor, a mass may or may not be visible or palpable.

ETIOLOGY AND PATHOPHYSIOLOGY

- Etiology is largely unknown, but it is often hypothesized that minor traumatic events incurred by weight-bearing bones induce mitogenic signals, increasing the probability of mutation and malignant transformation.
- OSA has also been associated with fractures, metallic orthopedic implants, chronic osteomyelitis, bone infarction, osteochondromatosis, and ionizing radiation.

DIAGNOSIS

DIFFERENTIAL DIAGNOSIS

- Other primary bone tumors (chondrosarcoma, fibrosarcoma, hemangiosarcoma).
- Metastatic bone tumors (transitional cell, prostatic, mammary, thyroid, anal sac carcinomas).
- Tumors that locally invade adjacent bone (synovial cell sarcoma; histiocytic sarcoma; oral squamous cell carcinoma [SCC], melanoma, fibrosarcoma, epulides; digital SCC, melanoma).
- Hematopoietic tumors (myeloma, lymphoma). Radiographic lesions typically are purely lytic.
- Bacterial or fungal osteomyelitis.

INITIAL DATABASE

- Radiographic imaging of OSA:
  - Aggressive bony lesions are characterized by one or more of the following radiographic signs:
    - Moth-eaten or permeative destruction.
    - Partial or complete lysis of the bony cortex.
    - Nonhomogenous, interrupted periosteal bone formation.
    - Ill-defined or ragged margin between normal and abnormal bone.
  - Appendicular OSA is usually located in the metaphyseal region of long bones. Extension across joints is uncommon.
- Following a radiographic or histologic diagnosis, animals should be completely staged.
  - Complete blood count, serum biochemistry panel, urinalysis.
  - Three-view thoracic radiographs:
    - About 10-15% of animals will have visible pulmonary metastatic lesions at initial diagnosis.
    - >95% of animals with OSA ultimately develop visible metastatic disease, even if the primary tumor is surgically removed, indicating metastasis has occurred prior to initial presentation.
  - <5% of dogs will have lymph node metastasis. Any enlarged regional lymph nodes should be evaluated with cytologic examination and/or histopathologic examination.

ADVANCED OR CONFIRMATORY TESTING

- Histopathologic examination is required to confirm the diagnosis of OSA.
  - An incisional biopsy can be performed using a Jamshidi bone marrow biopsy needle. Tumors are distinguished from benign lesions with an accuracy of 90%; the specific lesion is diagnosed with an overall accuracy of 80%.
    - Based on radiographic images, biopsy core(s) should be taken from the lesion's center. Samples taken from the periphery are likely to be nondiagnostic, containing only reactive bone.
  - If signalment, history, and initial database all support a diagnosis of OSA, and if the owners are willing to treat aggressively, it is reasonable to surgically remove the local disease (limb spare or amputation), with biopsy submission following surgery.
- CT imaging is recommended for axial tumors to more accurately stage local disease and help with planning surgery and/or radiation therapy.
- Whole-body bone survey radiography is not routinely recommended. Between 5% and 10% of animals will present with bony metastasis, though, and any suspicious lesions or painful areas should be imaged.
- Nuclear scintigraphy using ^{99m}Tc-methylene diphosphonate can be used for assessing the size of the primary tumor prior to a limb-salvage procedure. It also is more sensitive but less specific than survey radiographs for detecting bone metastasis.

TREATMENT

THERAPEUTIC GOAL(S)

- Relief of pain associated with primary tumor
- Prolongation of an animal's disease-free interval and prolongation of survival

ACUTE GENERAL TREATMENT

- Surgical removal of the primary tumor:
  - Amputation is the standard treatment for appendicular OSA. Most animals function well after surgery; osteoarthritis is rarely a contraindication.
  - Several limb-salvage techniques exist, where the neoplastic portion of the affected bone is excised while sparing the remainder of the limb. Candidates should have tumors arising from the distal radius or ulna, and the tumor should involve <50% of the bone with minimal extension into the surrounding soft tissues.
    - Compared to amputation, limb-salvage techniques result in similar survival times but have much higher complication rates (infection, implant failure, local tumor recurrence).
  - For animals with axial OSA, wide surgical excision is recommended whenever possible. Complete excision is often more difficult because of the tumor's proximity to vital structures. When excision is incomplete, adjuvant radiation therapy may help improve local control.
- In the adjuvant setting, IV treatment with cisplatin (50-70 mg/m^2 every 3 weeks along with saline fluid diuresis), carboplatin (250-350 mg/m^2 every 3 weeks), and doxorubicin (30 mg/m^2 every 2 weeks) extend disease-free interval and survival. Special handling requirements and potentially severe or life-threatening adverse effects for animals exist with these chemotherapeutic drugs; these concerns, and rapid evolution of protocols, warrant consultation with/referral to an oncologist.
  - Each drug has been evaluated as a single agent, and there is no definitive evidence that one drug is superior to the others. Platinum drugs may be more efficacious than doxorubicin.
  - Combinations of cisplatin/doxorubicin and carboplatin/doxorubicin have also been evaluated. There is no clear evidence that combination chemotherapy is superior to single-agent therapy.
- Palliative care is indicated for animals with visible metastasis and when owners decline definitive therapy.
  - Oral analgesics, such as a nonsteroidal anti-inflammatory (NSAID). Choices include: aspirin 10-25 mg/kg PO q 8-24h; carprofen 2 mg/kg PO q 12h; etodolac 10-15 mg/kg PO q 24h; deracoxib 1-2 mg/kg PO q 24h (may use 3-4 mg/kg PO q 24h for first 7 days only); meloxicam 0.1 mg/kg PO q 24h. All are occasionally recommended but are rarely sufficient to control pain completely.
  - Other oral analgesic drugs include acetaminophen with codeine (Tylenol #4 [300 mg acetaminophen, 60 mg codeine]) 0.5-2 mg/kg PO q 6-8h with dosing based on codeine, and tramadol (1-2 mg/kg PO q 8-12h).
  - Palliative radiation therapy very effectively controls the pain associated with bony tumors. For animals with appendicular OSA, 75-90% of animals have a noticeable improvement in lameness, with analgesia persisting for a median of 2 to 3 months.
  - Early studies with bisphosphonates, such as pamidronate and zolidronate, are promising.
  - Animals with pulmonary metastasis often benefit from oral glucocorticoids at anti-inflammatory doses, such as prednisone 0.5-1 mg/kg PO q 24h (not to be combined with NSAIDs).

DISEASES AND DISORDERS

RECOMMENDED MONITORING

Clinicians should evaluate animals every 2 to 3 months for evidence of local recurrence and metastatic disease. At a minimum, this includes a thorough physical examination and three-view thoracic radiographs. Imaging of the site of the primary tumor may be indicated as well, depending on location, completeness of excision, and clinical signs.

PROGNOSIS AND OUTCOME

- Most animals with OSA ultimately succumb to the effects of the primary tumor and/or metastatic disease.
- For animals with appendicular OSA:
  - With amputation alone, median survival is 4 to 5 months; the 1-year survival rate is 10%, and the 2-year survival rate is 2%.
  - When amputation or limb-salvage is combined with adjuvant chemotherapy, median survival improves to 10 to 12 months, and the 2-year survival rate improves to 15–25%.
    - Elevated serum alkaline phosphatase is associated with a poor prognosis. In addition, the prognosis may be even more guarded if alkaline phosphatase remains elevated in the postoperative period.
  - With palliative care alone, survival times are up to 4 to 5 months, depending on how well the pain associated with the primary tumor can be controlled.
  - Once metastatic disease is visible, survival times typically are <2 months.
- For most animals with axial OSA, prognosis is similar or more guarded depending on whether the primary tumor can be completely removed surgically.
- Mandibular OSA carries a better prognosis. With mandibulectomy alone, metastatic rate is around 30%, and median survival is around 17 months. There is no evidence that chemotherapy improves outcome.
- Nasal and digital OSA may also have a lower metastatic rate, but information is limited.

PEARLS & CONSIDERATIONS

COMMENTS

- Animals who are non-weight-bearing lame on a limb affected by OSA have already demonstrated the degree to which they will be able to ambulate after amputation.
- Canine OSA has many similarities to human OSA, serving as a useful comparative model.

SUGGESTED READING

Bailey D, Erb H, Williams L, et al: Carboplatin and doxorubicin combination chemotherapy for the treatment of appendicular osteosarcoma in the dog. *J Vet Intern Med* 17:199, 2003.

Heyman SJ, Diefenderfer DL, Goldschmidt MH, et al: Canine axial osteosarcoma: A retrospective study of 116 cases (1986–1989). *Vet Surg* 21:304, 1992.

Spodnick GJ, Berg J, Rand WM, et al: Prognosis for dogs with appendicular osteosarcoma treated by amputation alone: 162 cases (1978–1988). *J Am Vet Med Assoc* 200:995, 1992.

AUTHOR: **DENNIS B. BAILEY**

EDITOR: **KENNETH M. RASSNICK**

Otitis Externa

Client Education Sheet on Website

BASIC INFORMATION

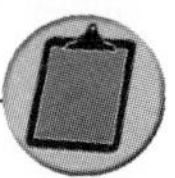

DEFINITION

An acute or chronic inflammatory condition affecting the external ear canal

EPIDEMIOLOGY

SPECIES, AGE, SEX

- Common in dogs, rare in cats
- Dogs: no sex or age predisposition
- Cats: young cats may have ear mites, nasopharyngeal polyps; elderly cats may have neoplasia

GENETICS AND BREED PREDISPOSITION

- Idiopathic glandular hyperplasia: cocker spaniels, springer spaniels
- Hair within ear canal: poodles
- Pendulous pinnae: cocker spaniels, springer spaniels
- Stenotic ear canals: English bulldogs, chow chows, shar-peis

RISK FACTORS

- Frequent swimming
- Excessive ear care

CONTAGION AND ZOONOSIS

- Ear mites (*Otodectes cynotis*): primary cause of 50% feline otitis cases, 5–10% in dogs. Commonly contagious between animals.
- Ear mites are rarely zoonotic, although close contact may cause pruritus on the arms.

GEOGRAPHY AND SEASONALITY

- May be more common in humid environments
- More common in summer months when associated with seasonal environmental allergies (atopy)

ASSOCIATED CONDITIONS AND DISORDERS

- Aural hematoma
- Hypersensitivity disorders
- Seborrheic skin disorders

CLINICAL PRESENTATION

HISTORY, CHIEF COMPLAINT

- Head rubbing, ear scratching, or headshaking common.
- Owners may report discharge from one or both ear canals.
- Head tilt if severe or if otitis media.
- Hearing deficit.
- Potential predisposing or primary factors (e.g., general health, ear care, exposure to water, parasites) should also be explored.
- Evidence of generalized skin disease possible. Foot chewing, face rubbing, or an obvious seasonality may suggest an underlying environmental hypersensitivity.

PHYSICAL EXAM FINDINGS

- Aural pruritus or headshaking.
- Erythema and edema of the ear canal wall.
- Otic discharge: brown coffee grounds (ear mites), brown or gray (complicated by *Malassezia*), white-yellow (ceruminous), yellow-green (complicated by bacteria).
- Erosions and ulcers (if acute).
- Alopecia and excoriations on the pinna.
- Hyperplasia of the ear canal wall, and ceruminous and sebaceous glands leads to stenosis in more chronic cases. Calcification of the auricular cartilages may be noted.
- Hearing deficits.
- Pain when opening the mouth, facial nerve paralysis, head tilt, nystagmus, and Horner's syndrome: suggest otitis media.
- ± Mass within the ear canal.

- ± Signs of generalized skin disease.

ETIOLOGY AND PATHOPHYSIOLOGY

Otitis externa is a multifactorial problem. Its severity depends on the interaction of predisposing, primary, and perpetuating factors:

- Predisposing factors: increase the risk of developing otitis externa, such as conformation (congenital stenosis: shar-pei; excessive hair: poodles), lifestyle (grooming, swimming, excessive ear care), obstructive lesions (neoplasms, polyps), and systemic disease (fever, immune suppression, viruses, debilitation).
- Primary factors: incite the condition, such as foreign bodies, hypersensitivity disorders (atopy, adverse food reactions/food allergy, drug reactions), immune-mediated factors (pemphigus complex), parasites (*Otodectes*), seborrheic disorders (idiopathic seborrhea), and glandular disorders (excessive cerumen/sebum accumulation, sebaceous adenitis).
- Perpetuating factors: prevent the resolution of the problem, such as organism overgrowth (bacteria, yeast), pathologic change (epidermal/glandular hyperplasia, stenosis, calcification, otitis media), and overtreatment with topical ear medications.
- Pathologic changes permanently alter the microclimate within the canal, promoting colonization by opportunistic microorganisms that may produce further inflammation. As the inflammation progresses, dermal fibrosis followed by calcification of the auditory cartilages and osseous metaplasia may be noted, leading to decreased flexibility, progressive stenosis, and finally obstructive ear disease.

DIAGNOSIS

DIFFERENTIAL DIAGNOSIS

The diagnosis of otitis externa and assessment of severity should be based on a thorough history, clinical examination findings, cytologic examination, and, if indicated, the results of bacterial culture.

INITIAL DATABASE

- History and clinical examination of the ear canals and skin. Examination of the vertical and horizontal canal for evidence of ulceration, hyperplasia, or discharge/debris (Fig. I-124). Examination of the tympanic membrane if possible (may require sedation/analgesia or general anesthesia).
- Ear canal cytologic examination (vertical canal: horizontal canal junction) for bacteria, yeast, inflammatory cells, and epithelial cells (acanthocytes in pemphigus foliaceus). Inflammatory cells are an important prognostic indicator and should be assessed at each revisit; considered abnormal, per high-power dry microscopic field (40X): >5 *Malassezia* yeast and/or >25 bacteria (dogs), >12 yeast, and/or >15 bacteria (cats).
- Bacteria or yeast in the cerumen or on epithelial cells with few inflammatory cells present indicates colonization, not infection, and specific antibiotic or antifungal treatment may not be indicated.
- A sample from the inner pinna around the canal orifice with acetate tape can undergo cytologic examination, which may also be useful if secondary *Malassezia* is suspected.
- Bacterial culture, sensitivity, and minimum inhibitory concentrations (MIC): if suspicious bacteria or large numbers of inflammatory cells are noted on a cytologic examination (Fig. I-125).

ADVANCED OR CONFIRMATORY TESTING

- Video otoscopy: facilitates examination of the horizontal canal and tympanic membrane
- Biopsy of the ear canal for histopathologic examination; histologically, epi-

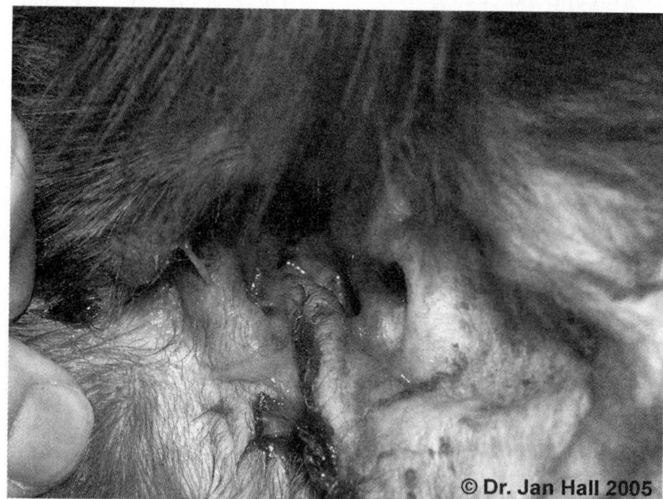

FIGURE I-124 Otitis externa in a 4-year-old Irish setter complicated by bacteria (*Pseudomonas*). Note the purulent material at the canal orifice. A thorough assessment for underlying cause (predisposing, primary, and perpetuating factors) is essential to resolve complicated otitis externa cases. Courtesy of Dr. Jan A. Hall.

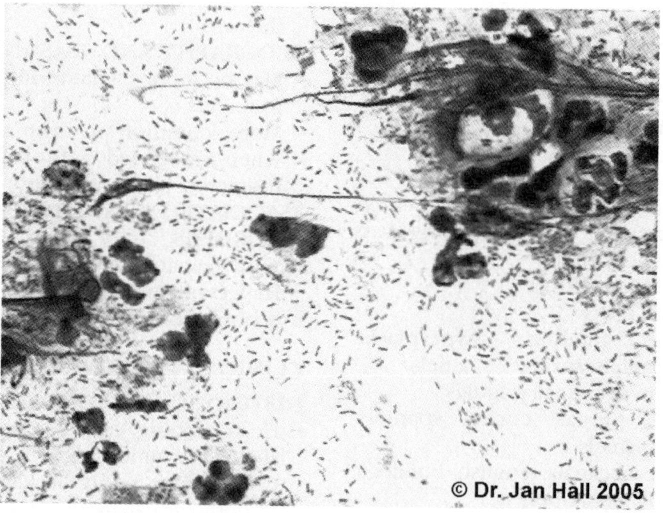

FIGURE I-125 Cytologic examination of the ear canal in a 4-year-old Irish setter with otitis externa. Large numbers of inflammatory cells and bacteria are noted. Bacterial culture confirmed the presence of *Pseudomonas aeruginosa*. Results of ear cytologic examination should be assessed in relation to clinical signs. Courtesy of Dr. Jan A. Hall.

dermal acanthosis with mild to moderate hyperkeratosis, ceruminous gland hyperplasia, ceruminous gland ectasia, and sebaceous gland hyperplasia are noted with a mixed inflammatory infiltrate consisting of lymphocytes, mast cells, and polymorphonuclear cells
- Radiography: failed to diagnose otitis media in 25% of cases in one study
- Computed tomography (CT) and magnetic resonance imaging (MRI) show promise as imaging techniques for the bulla
- Neurologic examination
- Brainstem auditory-evoked response (BAER) testing (hearing examination)
- Allergy testing: elimination diet trial; intradermal or serum allergy testing

TREATMENT

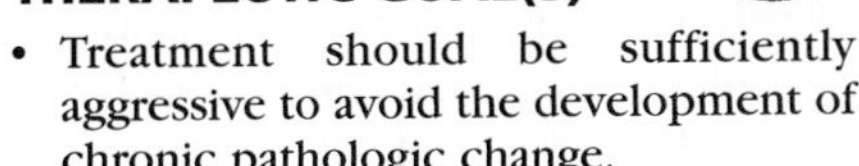

THERAPEUTIC GOAL(S)

- Treatment should be sufficiently aggressive to avoid the development of chronic pathologic change.
- Primary goal: reduction of ear canal inflammation (provides comfort for the animal and may help eliminate secondary organism involvement).
- Clinicians should identify and treat all predisposing and perpetuating factors.

ACUTE GENERAL TREATMENT

- Corticosteroids, topically or systemically, are very beneficial in the treatment of otitis externa and should be first line therapy.
- Corticosteroid therapy has been shown to significantly aid in the elimination of resistant *Pseudomonas* strains through changes in the microclimate that no longer favor the growth of the bacteria.
  - Topical: 1% hydrocortisone in 2% Burow's solution with propylene glycol (generic), flucinolone (Synotic); long-term use may be required to control excessive cerumen production.
  - Systemic: prednisone 1-2 mg/kg PO, q 24h, in a gradually reducing regimen.
  - Triamcinolone acetonide (2 mg/ml solution for injection) injected at 0.1 ml doses into proliferative lesions using a 22-gauge needle.
- Antibiotics:
  - Topical: products containing combinations of neomycin, gentamicin, polymixin B, and enrofloxacin with antifungal agents and/or corticosteroids. Typically administered q 12h for the first week, then q 24h for the second week pending a reevaluation to ensure that the treatment has been effective. Clinicians should use cytologic examinations for assessing response to therapy. Since many products contain corticosteroids, clinical improvement should not necessarily be assumed to be associated with the antibiotic component(s).
  - MIC research suggests that systemic antibiotic therapy may not be helpful and may encourage the overgrowth of resistant strains of bacteria, in particular *Pseudomonas aeruginosa*.
- Antifungal drugs:
  - Topical: proprietary products in combination with antifungal agents and/or corticosteroids.
  - Oral antifungals (given with food): ketoconazole 5-10 mg/kg PO q 12-24h; itraconazole 5 mg/kg PO q 24h; or fluconazole 5-10 mg PO q 24h for 2 to 4 weeks.
- Ear flushing:
  - Flushing debris from the ear canal can be of great benefit. However, flushing should never be attempted in the face of severe inflammation, as it may lead to erosion and ulceration of the ear canal.
  - A warm (body temperature) solution of white vinegar in water (one part of white vinegar to three to five parts water) makes an excellent general flush if well tolerated. This solution appears to be safe in the presence of a ruptured tympanum. Vinegar and water flushing is normally carried out every 2 to 3 days during the treatment protocol. Acidifying ear cleaners may be used in the same way.
  - Tris-EDTA may significantly increase the sensitivity of *Pseudomonas* to topical gentamicin and the other aminoglycosides. The recommended protocol is to flush the canal for 15 minutes prior to topical antibiotic use.

CHRONIC TREATMENT

- Once an ear has reached the obstructive or "end" stage, with complete occlusion of the external ear canal by hyperplastic tissue, surgical intervention and a total ear canal ablation (TECA) and bulla osteotomy may be indicated (Fig. I-126).
- Many obstructive otitis externa cases will respond favorably to medical treatment if it is instituted aggressively. Treatment options include topical 1% hydrocortisone in 2% Burow's solution with propylene glycol or flucinolone (Synotic) for the long-term; if required, the clinician can also administer prednisone—2 mg/kg PO q 24h (then gradually reducing), or cyclosporine (microemulsion, such as Atopica or Neoral) 5 mg/kg PO q 12h.

POSSIBLE COMPLICATIONS

Otitis media and otitis interna may develop if otitis externa is not resolved.

RECOMMENDED MONITORING

Clinicians should reevaluate the animal every 2 weeks; the purpose is to assess response to therapy by noting improvement in clinical findings and performing ear cytologic examination. Monitoring can also include a serum biochemistry profile if using ketoconazole (hepatotoxicity).

PEARLS & CONSIDERATIONS

COMMENTS

Since many ear problems are part of a generalized dermatologic disease, a full

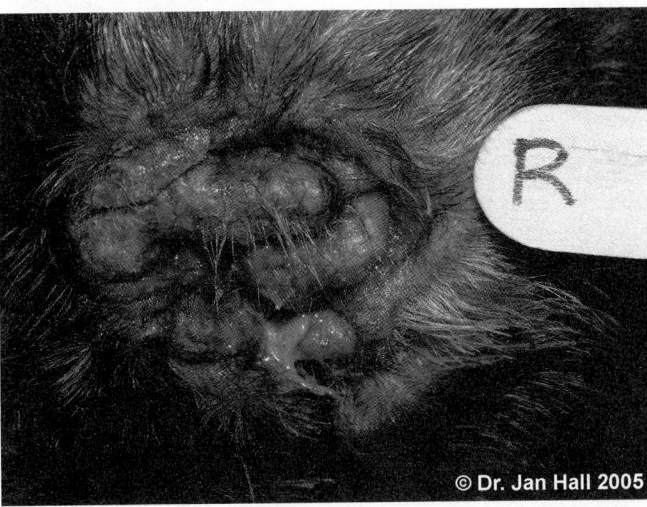

FIGURE I-126 End-stage otitis externa in a cocker spaniel. Note the massive proliferation of epithelial and glandular tissue obliterating the ear canal. Courtesy of Dr. Jan A. Hall.

dermatologic exam is indicated as part of the evaluation.

- Complete resolution of ear problems is very unlikely unless predisposing, primary, and perpetuating factors are identified.
- Dogs with a food allergy may only present with otitis externa.
- Response to therapy should be based on degree of clinical improvement and cytologic examination results.

SUGGESTED READING

Hall JA, et al: Oral cyclosporin in the treatment of end stage ear disease: A pilot study, Proceedings of the 18th Annual Meeting of the American Academy of Veterinary Dermatology/American College of Veterinary Dermatology, Monterey, CA. American Academy of Veterinary Dermatology/American College of Veterinary Dermatology: 217, 2003.

Matousek JL (ed): *Vet Clin North America: Small Animal Practice*. Philadelphia, WB Saunders, 2004.

Scott DW, Miller WH, Griffin CE: *Muller and Kirk's Small Animal Dermatology*. Philadelphia, WB Saunders, 2000, pp 1204-1231.

AUTHOR & EDITOR: **JAN A. HALL**

Ovarian Tumors

BASIC INFORMATION

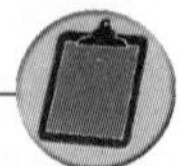

DEFINITION

Ovarian tumors are benign or malignant neoplasms arising from specific ovarian tissue. Tumor classification includes epithelial (adenoma, adenocarcinoma, carcinoma, cyst adenoma, cyst adenocarcinoma), germ cell (dysgerminoma, teratoma, teratocarcinoma), and sex cord (granulosa, Sertoli, Sertoli-Leydig).

SYNONYM(S)

Ovarian adenocarcinoma
Ovarian adenoma
Ovarian carcinoma
Ovarian cyst adenocarcinoma
Ovarian cyst adenoma
Ovarian dysgerminoma
Ovarian granulosa cell tumor
Ovarian Sertoli cell tumor
Ovarian Sertoli-Leydig cell tumor
Ovarian teratocarcinoma
Ovarian teratoma

EPIDEMIOLOGY

SPECIES, AGE, SEX

CANINE, INTACT FEMALES

- Epithelial tumors: 9.6 years (adenomas, 10.5 years; adenocarcinomas, 9.3 years)
- Sex cord tumors: 8 years (granulosa, 7 years; Sertoli, 5 years; Sertoli-Leydig, 12 years)
- Germ cell tumors: 6.4 years (dysgerminoma, 9 years; teratoma, 5 years; teratocarcinoma, 5 years)

INCIDENCE

- Epithelial tumors: 25% of the ovarian neoplasia case reports (adenoma, 21%; adenocarcinoma, 4% of all case reports) and an average of 42% of all the ovarian neoplasia pathologic examination reports (adenoma, 12%; adenocarcinoma, 30%, when neoplasias were subcategorized in the pathologic examination reports, respectively).
- Sex cord tumors: 31% of the ovarian neoplasia case reports (granulosa, 25%; Sertoli, 2%; Leydig, 4% of all case reports) and an average of 42% of all the ovarian neoplasia pathologic examination reports (granulosa, 35%; Sertoli-Leydig, 17%; seminoma, 12%, when neoplasias were subcategorized in the pathologic examination reports, respectively).
- Germ cell tumors: 44% of all the ovarian neoplasia case reports (dysgerminoma, 17%; teratoma, 19%; teratocarinoma, 7% of all case reports, respectively) and an average of 14% of all pathologic examination reports (dysgerminoma, 14%; teratoma, 10%, when neoplasias were subcategorized in the ovarian neoplasia pathologic examination reports, respectively).

FELINE, INTACT FEMALES

- Age
- Epithelial: 10 years (cystadenoma, 10 years)
- Germ cell: 6 years (dysgerminoma, 6 years; teratoma, 8 years)
- Sex cord: 9 years (granulosa, 10 years)

INCIDENCE

- Epithelial: 5% of all pathologic examination reports, no case reports
- Germ cell: 15% of all pathologic examination reports, 50% of case reports
- Sex cord: 31% of all pathologic examination reports, 50% of case reports

ASSOCIATED CONDITIONS AND DISORDERS: Pyometra and/or cystic endometrial hyperplasia are sometimes seen in association with epithelial and sex cord tumors.

CLINICAL PRESENTATION

DISEASE FORMS/SUBTYPES

- Epithelial (adenoma, adenocarcinoma, carcinoma, cyst adenoma, cyst adenocarcinoma)
- Germ cell (dysgerminoma, teratoma, teratocarcinoma)
- Sex cord (granulosa, Sertoli, Sertoli-Leydig)

HISTORY, CHIEF COMPLAINT

- Canine:
    - Abdominal enlargement (adenomas, adenocarcinoma, granulosa cell tumor, dysgerminoma, teratoma, teratocarcinoma)
    - Depression (dysgerminoma, teratocarcinoma)
    - Estrous cycle abnormalities (adenocarcinoma, granulosa cell tumor)
    - Vaginal discharge (adenocarcinoma, granulosa cell tumor)
    - Incidental finding during ovariohysterectomy or necropsy (adenomas, teratoma)
    - No common findings (Sertoli and Sertoli-Leydig cell tumors)
- Feline:
    - Estrous cycle abnormalities (granulosa cell tumor)
    - Depression (granulosa cell tumor)
    - Incidental finding during ovariohysterectomy or necropsy (cystadenoma, dysgerminoma, teratoma)

PHYSICAL EXAM FINDINGS

- Estrus (vaginal smear for cytologic examination)
- Vaginal discharge
- Abdominal enlargement

ETIOLOGY AND PATHOPHYSIOLOGY

Clinical signs can be related to hormone production by sex cord tumors; the signs can also be related to organ impingement by space-occupying masses or metastasis for other types.

DIAGNOSIS

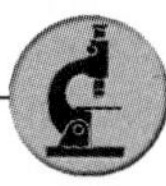

DIFFERENTIAL DIAGNOSIS

- Estrus
- Pyometra
- Gastrointestinal or other intra-abdominal disease

INITIAL DATABASE

- Routine lab tests (complete blood count, urinalysis, serum chemistry panel): generally unremarkable
- Vaginal cytologic examination:
  - Confirmation of estrus
  - Assessment for pyometra or other infection

ADVANCED OR CONFIRMATORY TESTING

- Abdominal radiographs
- Abdominal ultrasound
- Thoracic radiography for metastasis
- Exploratory surgery
- Histopathologic examination of tissue

TREATMENT

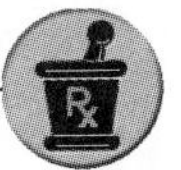

THERAPEUTIC GOAL(S)

Excision of mass

ACUTE GENERAL TREATMENT

Surgeons can perform an ovariohysterectomy. A unilateral ovariectomy has been reported, with a subsequent small litter resulting.

CHRONIC TREATMENT

Uncommon to use chemotherapeutics. However, cisplatin or cyclophosphamide and chlorambucil and nitrosurea have been used for treating metastatic carcinomas, resulting in an average 9-month survival.

POSSIBLE COMPLICATIONS

- Metastasis
- Canine:
  - Epithelial: adenomas and adenocarcinoma in 50% of cases according to pathologic examination reports
  - Sex cord: granulosa in 30% of case reports
  - Germ cell: dysgerminoma is rare; teratoma resulted at a rate of 50% in one study; teratocarcinoma is common
- Feline sex cord: granulosa, lung, liver, and spleen reported

PROGNOSIS AND OUTCOME

Excellent if benign and no metastasis has occurred

PEARLS & CONSIDERATIONS

COMMENTS

May be unilateral or bilateral

SUGGESTED READING

Jergens AE, Shaw DP: Tumors of the canine ovary. *Compend Cont Educ Pract Vet* 9:489, 1987.

Johnston S, Root-Kustritz MV, Olson PNS: Disorders of the canine ovary. In Johnston S, Root-Kustritz MV, Olson PNS (eds): *Canine and Feline Theriogenology*. Philadelphia, WB Saunders, 2001, pp 193–205.

Smith CA: Ovarian disorders of the bitch and queen. In Root-Kustritz MV (ed): *Small Animal Theriogenology*. St. Louis, Butterworth Heinemann, 2003, pp 331–365.

AUTHOR: **BRUCE E. EILTS**
EDITOR: **MICHELLE A. KUTZLER**

Pain

BASIC INFORMATION

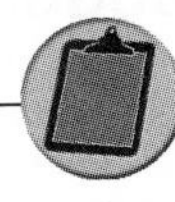

DEFINITION

An unpleasant sensory or emotional experience associated with actual or potential tissue damage

EPIDEMIOLOGY

SPECIES, AGE, SEX: Animals of any species, age, or sex may experience pain although pain thresholds and response characteristics may vary.

ASSOCIATED CONDITIONS AND DISORDERS: The pain intensity does not always correlate with degree of tissue damage. In some cases, there may be no obvious evidence of tissue disruption, and persistence of pain may indicate abnormal processing of input in the central nervous system (CNS). The following are some associated conditions and disorders:

- Trauma
- Surgery
- Degenerative disease processes
- Inflammatory disease processes
- Neoplasia

CLINICAL PRESENTATION

DISEASE FORMS/SUBTYPES

- Physiologic versus pathologic
- Acute versus chronic
- Somatic versus visceral versus neuropathic

HISTORY, CHIEF COMPLAINT

- Humans can report pain as their primary complaint, whereas animals cannot.
- An animal's history will vary depending on the type of pain (i.e., acute versus chronic) and may include an inciting injury.

PHYSICAL EXAM FINDINGS

- Behavioral signs of pain vary considerably among individuals. Common pain-related behaviors in dogs and cats include:
  - Postural changes: arched/hunched back, drooped head
  - Temperament changes: aggression, hiding
  - Vocalization: moaning, howling, purring
  - Locomotor changes: reluctance to move, lameness
  - Others: no interest in food or play, failure to groom
- Physiologic signs associated with stress response (tachycardia, tachypnea, mydriasis, hypertension) may accompany pain but are nonspecific. Clinical signs associated with chronic pain may be very subtle.

ETIOLOGY AND PATHOPHYSIOLOGY

- A noxious stimulus activates specialized nerve endings called nociceptors.
- Nociceptors transduce noxious chemical, mechanical, or thermal stimuli into electrochemical potentials that are transmitted via sensory nerves from affected tissue to spinal cord.
- In the spinal cord dorsal horn, incoming first-order peripheral neurons synapse with ascending spinal neurons that extend to the brainstem.
- Incoming noxious input is modulated at the level of the dorsal horn by other incoming sensory information, descending inhibitory nerve impulses, or pharmacologic interventions.
- In the brainstem, incoming second-order neurons synapse with third-order neurons that form tracts extending to the cerebral cortex, where pain perception ultimately occurs.

DIAGNOSIS

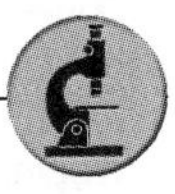

DIFFERENTIAL DIAGNOSIS

- Since animals cannot self-report pain, the veterinarian must *diagnose* it.

- Pain must be differentiated from the following:
  - Distress associated with other factors (restraint, restrictive bandaging, confinement, separation from owners)
  - Dysphoria associated with drugs used to treat pain (particularly opioids, dissociative agents)
- Once a presumptive diagnosis of pain is made, veterinarians should investigate the underlying cause.
- Differential diagnoses of common causes were previously listed under Associated Conditions and Disorders.

INITIAL DATABASE

- Recognition of pain in animals is subjective.
- Veterinarians should follow a routine for evaluation. The veterinarian should:
  - Evaluate the animal's signalment, history, and previous physical exam findings.
  - Observe the animal's behavior from a distance (preferably unobserved by the animal).
  - Observe the animal's behavior during interaction prior to extensive palpation and examination.
  - Gently palpate the body region of interest and evaluate the animal's response.
- Perform serial evaluations and record findings in the animal's medical record.
- Pain should be evaluated as the fourth vital sign (in addition to temperature, pulse, and respiration).
- No predictable changes in routine laboratory tests specifically indicate pain.

TREATMENT

THERAPEUTIC GOAL(S)

- Improve the animal's quality of life while addressing underlying cause of pain if possible.
- If pain is intractable, euthanasia may be most humane option.

ACUTE GENERAL TREATMENT

- Depends on species, pain intensity, underlying cause.
- Acute pain most often is managed pharmacologically.
- Pharmacologic treatment involves one or more of the following:
  - Opioids: morphine, hydromorphone, oxymorphone, fentanyl, buprenorphine, butorphanol
  - Nonsteroidal anti-inflammatory agents (NSAIDs): carprofen, meloxicam, deracoxib
  - Local anesthetics (regional anesthesia techniques, see also Local Anesthesia and Regional Anesthesia, p 1274), lidocaine, bupivacaine
- Utilize the following treatment strategies: *multimodal analgesia*, which is a combination of multiple analgesic drugs or techniques to target different points along the pain pathway; *preemptive analgesia*, which is the administration of analgesic agent(s) prior to noxious insult (i.e., surgery).

CHRONIC TREATMENT

- Dietary changes and nonpharmacologic treatment (e.g., physiotherapy) may be beneficial.
- Treatment typically begins with an oral NSAID and oral opioids added as needed.
- Opioid doses may need to be increased if pain intensifies.
- Adjunctive analgesic agents (tramadol, gabapentin, amantadine) may be added if conventional analgesics fail to manage pain adequately.

DRUG INTERACTIONS

- Opioids reduce anesthetic requirements significantly.
- Certain opioids (e.g., meperidine) may interact with MAO-B inhibitors (e.g., selegiline [L-Deprenyl] or amitraz) and produce "serotonin syndrome."
- There is a significantly increased risk of gastrointestinal toxicity possible when NSAIDs and glucocorticoids are administered concurrently.

PROGNOSIS AND OUTCOME

- Acute pain expected to resolve within period of normal tissue healing.
- When pain persists beyond normal course, veterinarians should suspect persistent disease, injury, or CNS changes and consult a specialist.

PEARLS & CONSIDERATIONS

COMMENTS

For challenging cases, veterinarians should seek advice from a veterinary pain specialist (i.e., an anesthesiologist, surgeon, oncologist, or internist with advanced training in pain management).

PREVENTION

Veterinarians should institute preemptive analgesic protocols when appropriate.

SUGGESTED READING

Gaynor JS, Muir WW III (eds): *Handbook of Veterinary Pain Management*. St. Louis, Mosby, 2002.

Tranquilli WJ, Grimm KA, Lamont LA (eds): *Pain Management for the Small Animal Practitioner*, ed 2. Jackson, WY, Teton NewMedia, 2004.

AUTHOR: **LEIGH A. LAMONT**

EDITOR: **ETIENNE CÔTÉ**

Pallor

BASIC INFORMATION

DEFINITION

Pale mucous membranes

EPIDEMIOLOGY

SPECIES, AGE, SEX

- Depends on underlying cause
- Acetaminophen toxicity: cats > dogs

GENETICS AND BREED PREDISPOSITION: Rare hereditary hemolytic anemias in Abyssinian, Siamese, and Somali cats and in poodle, basenji, and beagle dogs.

CONTAGION AND ZOONOSIS: Feline leukemia virus-associated anemia (cat-to-cat).

CLINICAL PRESENTATION

DISEASE FORMS/SUBTYPES

- Anemia: perfusion is adequate, but circulating red blood cell (RBC) mass is low.
- Shock: perfusion is inadequate, but circulating RBC mass is normal.

HISTORY, CHIEF COMPLAINT

- Weakness
- Tachypnea
- Collapse
- Those due to underlying disease:
  - History of trauma in hypovolemic shock
  - Coughing and dyspnea with cardiogenic shock
  - Lethargy and anorexia with septic shock
- Pale mucous membranes (uncommon as an owner-reported chief complaint)

PHYSICAL EXAM FINDINGS

- Pale mucous membranes of the gingiva, tongue, conjunctiva, anus, penis, and/or vulva.

- Tachypnea, cool mucous membranes, tachycardia, and weakness may be seen with either anemia or shock.
- Capillary refill time (CRT):
  - Unless there is severe anemia, CRT should be normal (<2 sec) in an anemic animal that is not in shock.
  - Animals in shock typically have a prolonged CRT.
- Visualization of stool via rectal examination may find fresh blood or melena in cases with gastrointestinal (GI) hemorrhage.
- Palpation of the extremities (pinnae, paws) reveals a cool temperature with poor perfusion (e.g., shock) but not with anemia alone.

ETIOLOGY AND PATHOPHYSIOLOGY

- Severe blood loss or severe anemia can lead to shock, so both conditions may exist in the same animal.
- Anemia causes pallor due to blood with diminished hemoglobin (i.e., decreased red blood cells) traversing through easily seen capillary beds, creating a pale red color in the mucous membranes.
- Shock leads to poor perfusion of blood through capillary vessels, thus causing pallor. Shock is a peracute condition, but the underlying cause may be chronic in nature.

DIAGNOSIS

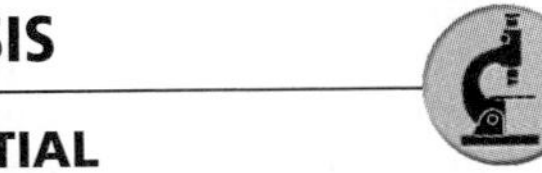

DIFFERENTIAL DIAGNOSIS

There are two major forms of anemia: regenerative and nonregenerative.

- Regenerative anemia:
  - Blood loss/hemorrhage:
    - Trauma
    - Parasitic infestation
    - Coagulopathy
    - GI disease (ulceration, mass, inflammation, infiltration)
    - Abdominal or intrathoracic mass
  - Hemolysis:
    - Primary immune-mediated
    - Fragmentation (disseminated intravascular coagulation [DIC], hemangiosarcoma, heartworm disease, vasculitis)
    - Toxicities (zinc, acetaminophen, onions)
    - RBC parasites
    - Hereditary
- Nonregenerative anemia:
  - Bone marrow disease
  - Chronic renal disease
  - Anemia of chronic disease
  - Feline leukemia virus (FeLV) infection

There are four major types of shock:

- Cardiogenic shock:
  - Severe atrioventricular (AV) valvular endocardiosis
  - Cardiac tamponade secondary to pericardial effusion
  - Dilated cardiomyopathy
  - Hypertrophic cardiomyopathy
  - Heartworm disease
  - Severe dysrhythmia
- Hypovolemic shock:
  - Dehydration
  - Blood loss
  - Hypoadrenocorticism
  - Intoxications
- Traumatic shock
- Septic shock

INITIAL DATABASE

- Packed cell volume (PCV) will help differentiate anemia from shock in most cases. Unless the animal was anemic beforehand, cases of acute shock should have a normal PCV, including those with acute blood loss. Anemic animals, by definition, have a diminished PCV.
- Blood pressure (BP) is usually diminished in cases of shock. Unless the anemia is severe or acute, BP is typically normal in anemic animals.
- Complete blood count, biochemical profile, and urinalysis are warranted in most cases of pallor to assist in determining the underlying cause.

ADVANCED OR CONFIRMATORY TESTING

- Reticulocyte count to characterize type of anemia.
- Evidence of saline-diluted RBC agglutination on a slide suggests an immune-mediated hemolytic anemia, as would a positive Coombs' test result.
- Thoracic radiographs to look for evidence of primary heart disease, trauma (e.g., rib fractures, lung contusions), or an infectious focus causing sepsis (e.g., pneumonia).
- Abdominal radiographs and/or ultrasound to visualize fluid (e.g., blood loss, congestive heart failure), neoplasia, and metallic (zinc) objects in the GI tract.
- Cytologic and/or histopathologic examination of bone marrow to help characterize the amount of regeneration in persistently anemic animals and to look for evidence of primary bone marrow disease (e.g., neoplasia, FeLV).

TREATMENT

THERAPEUTIC GOAL(S)

Stabilization of the animal while the cause of pallor is determined and corrected, if possible

ACUTE GENERAL TREATMENT

- Determined by the underlying cause.
- Patients with severe anemia or acute blood loss may require transfusion of RBC ± plasma (see Transfusion Therapy and Collection Techniques for Blood Banking, p 1312).
- Hypovolemic, traumatic, and septic shock cases are usually treated with vigorous intravenous crystalloids, ± colloids (see Sepsis and Septic Shock, p 996; Shock, Hypovolemic, p 999).
- Cardiogenic shock requires supplemental oxygen and attempts to improve perfusion, such as with pericardiocentesis, positive inotropic, and antidysrhythmic medications as indicated.

CHRONIC TREATMENT

Depends on the underlying cause

RECOMMENDED MONITORING

- PCV in patients with anemia
- CRT and BP in cases of shock

PROGNOSIS AND OUTCOME

- Determined by the underlying cause.
- Many cases of pallor come with a guarded to poor prognosis (e.g., DIC, hemangiosarcoma, FeLV, cardiogenic shock, chronic renal failure), while others may respond much better with proper therapy (e.g., trauma, parasitic infection, hypoadrenocorticism).

PEARLS & CONSIDERATIONS

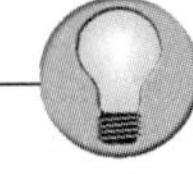

COMMENTS

- Because there are many causes of pallor, the clinician mainly needs to be aware of the differential diagnoses and methods to distinguish anemia from shock.
- Most causes of pallor are serious, thus requiring timely work-up and therapy.

SUGGESTED READING

Cotter SM: A diagnostic approach to anemic patients. *Vet Med* 98:420, 2003.

Morrison WB: Pallor. In Ettinger SJ, Feldman EC (eds): *Textbook of Veterinary Internal Medicine*. St. Louis, Elsevier Saunders, 2005, pp 211–215.

Otto CM: Shock. In Ettinger SJ, Feldman EC (eds): *Textbook of Veterinary Internal Medicine*. St. Louis, Elsevier Saunders, 2005, pp 455–457.

AUTHOR: **JEFF D. BAY**

EDITOR: **ETIENNE CÔTÉ**

Palm (Cycad/Sago) Toxicosis

BASIC INFORMATION

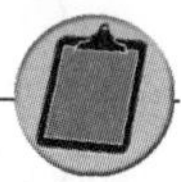

DEFINITION

Acute, potentially fatal toxicity occurring from ingesting cycad palm leaves, seeds, bark, or roots and characterized by vomiting and diarrhea, anorexia, lethargy, acute liver failure (2 to 3 days later), coagulopathies, and neurologic signs.

SYNONYM(S)

Cycad palm/plant: sago palm (true synonyms); includes *Zamia floridana*, *Cycas revoluta*, and *C. circinalis*

EPIDEMIOLOGY

SPECIES, AGE, SEX: All animals are susceptible; most poisoning cases reported in dogs instead of cats.
RISK FACTORS: Presence of palm in the pet's environment.
GEOGRAPHY AND SEASONALITY
- Ornamental plants, indoor; in the southern part of the United States and in Hawaii, sago palms are frequently used for landscaping.
- Toxicity occurs mostly in summer months.

CLINICAL PRESENTATION

HISTORY, CHIEF COMPLAINT
- Exposure to sago palm
- Within 24 hours, onset of vomiting, diarrhea, lethargy, and anorexia; chewed leaves, seeds, plant material may be in vomitus
- Ataxia, weakness, or seizures
- Occurrence or recurrence of lethargy, anorexia, vomiting 2 to 3 days after ingestion due to acute hepatic injury/failure

PHYSICAL EXAM FINDINGS
- As above (see History, Chief Complaint)
- Signs of abdominal pain
- Weak pulse associated with hypovolemia or dehydration
- Petechiae, ecchymoses
- Hypovolemic shock (depressed mentation, weakness/collapse, poor perfusion)
- Central nervous system (CNS) signs: ataxia, seizures

ETIOLOGY AND PATHOPHYSIOLOGY

- Sago palms (cycad plants) are palm-like plants in the family Cycadaceae. These are woody, coarse plants with leaves originating from a thickened stem and are found in dry sandy soils of tropical and subtropical regions throughout the world.
- *C. revoluta* is the most commonly involved species in poisoning cases.
- Toxins: cycasin and methylazoxymethanol, a neurotoxic amino acid, and an unidentified high molecular weight compound.
- The glucose molecule on cycasin is hydrolyzed by the gut bacterial enzyme β-glycosidase, yielding sugars and methylazoxymethanol, which then alkylates DNA and RNA. This process causes hepatotoxic, teratogenic, carcinogenic, and gastrointestinal (GI) effects.
- Azotemia can occur secondary to decreased renal perfusion resulting from systemic hypotension/hypoperfusion.

DIAGNOSIS

DIFFERENTIAL DIAGNOSIS

- Mushroom (Amanita) poisoning
- Blue-green algae toxicosis
- Idiopathic chronic hepatitis
- Viral hepatitis (canine hepatitis virus)
- Iron toxicosis in dogs

INITIAL DATABASE

- Complete blood count (CBC):
  - Leukocytosis (reported: 3500-34,000 cells/μl)
  - Thrombocytopenia: mild and due to blood loss
  - Hyperbilirubinemia (range 1.03-10 mg/dl; reference range 0-0.3 mg/dl)
- Serum biochemistry panel:
  - Increased alanine aminotransferase (ALT; range 128-10,000 IU/L)
  - Increased alkaline phosphatase (ALP; 218-3931 IU/L)
  - Hypoproteinemia
  - Azotemia (prerenal and/or renal)
- Coagulation profile: increased prothrombin time, partial prothromboplastin time due to liver damage
- Urinalysis: glucosuria, bilirubinuria, hematuria possible

ADVANCED OR CONFIRMATORY TESTING

Histopathologic lesions of liver may include marked focal centrolobular and midzonal coagulation necrosis.

TREATMENT

THERAPEUTIC GOAL(S)

- Decontamination of the animal as soon as possible
- Control of CNS and GI signs
- Treatment of liver injury
- Provision of supportive care

ACUTE GENERAL TREATMENT

- Decontaminating the animal:
  - Emesis (see Vomiting, Induction of, p 1328): only in animals not showing clinical signs; may be effective within a couple of hours.
  - Gastric lavage only if a very large dose has been ingested and emesis cannot be induced (e.g., comatose animal).
  - Activated charcoal 1-4 g/kg PO; airway protected with cuffed endotracheal tube if animal is unconscious.
- Controlling CNS and GI signs:
  - Seizures:
    - Diazepam 0.5-2 mg/kg IV as needed.
    - Other anticonvulsants if refractory (see Seizures, p 990).
  - GI signs:
    - Control severe vomiting with metoclopramide (0.1-0.4 mg/kg PO, SC, or IM q 6h).
    - GI protectants, such as famotidine (0.5-1 mg/kg IV q 12-24h) or sucralfate (0.5-1 g for a dog or 125-250 mg for a cat) PO q 8-12h if evidence of gastric ulceration.
- Treating signs of liver damage (see Hepatic Injury, Acute, p 491).
  - Clinicians should monitor and treat secondary effects of acute hepatic failure, such as hepatic encephalopathy (see Hepatic Encephalopathy, p 489), coagulopathy/bleeding tendencies (see Hemorrhage, p 485), and hypoproteinemia (see Transfusion Therapy and Collection Techniques for Blood Banking, p 1312).
  - If liver enzymes are elevated or signs of liver dysfunction are present, oral antibiotics (e.g., neomycin 10-20 mg/kg PO q 6-8h) and lactulose (15-30 ml PO q 6-8h [dogs]; 0.25-1 ml PO q 8-12h [cats]) may help reduce the risk of hepatic encephalopathy.
  - SAM-e (18 mg/kg PO q 48-72h).
  - Vitamin K_1 (3 mg/kg PO, IM, or SC) ± blood transfusions if hemorrhage.
- Providing supportive care
  - IV fluids (may require dextrose supplementation if hypoglycemia).
  - Dietary management if liver injury: optimal/nonmeat protein, without sacrificing appetite.

CHRONIC TREATMENT

SAM-e 18 mg/kg PO every other day to third day for 1 to 3 months if evidence of persistent liver insult (e.g., serum ALT and/or bilirubin elevation)

POSSIBLE COMPLICATIONS

Chronic liver disease (cirrhosis/fibrosis)

RECOMMENDED MONITORING

- CBC
- Serum biochemistry profile, especially liver enzymes (baseline, 24, 48, 72 hours)

- Coagulation panel (prothrombin time [PT], activated partial thromboplastin time [aPTT])
- Hematocrit

PROGNOSIS AND OUTCOME

- Poor prognosis if evidence of severe liver injury
- Good prognosis with early and aggressive treatment

PEARLS & CONSIDERATIONS

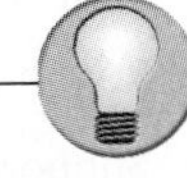

COMMENTS

- All sago palm exposures should be taken seriously because the overall mortality rate in dogs can be 33%.
- All parts are considered toxic, and seeds concentrate more toxins; one to two ingested seeds potentially can be lethal in a medium-sized dog.
- Clinical signs of toxicosis can last from a few days to several weeks depending on the severity of liver injury.

PREVENTION

Owners should keep pets out of areas where sago palm plants are growing.

SUGGESTED READING

Albretsen JC, et al: Cycad palm toxicosis in dogs: 60 cases (1987-1997). *J Am Vet Med Assoc* 213(1):1998, pp 99-101.

AUTHOR & EDITOR: **SAFDAR A. KHAN**

Pancreatic Adenocarcinoma

BASIC INFORMATION

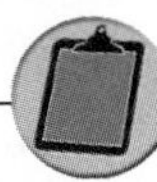

DEFINITION

- Most commonly a malignant, highly metastatic epithelial tumor of the pancreas of ductular or acinar origin.
- Benign pancreatic adenomas occur rarely.
- A few cases of pancreatic sarcoma and lymphoma have been reported. It is questionable whether these tumors are of exocrine pancreatic origin or are metastatic lesions from other primary tumors.

SYNONYM(S)

Exocrine pancreatic neoplasm

EPIDEMIOLOGY

SPECIES, AGE, SEX

- Uncommon tumor of dogs and cats (<0.5% of all cancers)
- Older dogs and cats (dogs median age 9.2 years; cats 8 to 18 years)
- More common in female dogs; no gender predilection in cats

GENETICS AND BREED PREDISPOSITION

- Airedale terriers and spaniel breeds may be at higher risk.
- No breed predilection in cats.

RISK FACTORS

- Unknown.
- Experimentally, N-ethyl-N'-nitro-N-nitrosoguanidine administered intraductally has been shown to induce pancreatic adenocarcinoma.

ASSOCIATED CONDITIONS AND DISORDERS

- Paraneoplastic alopecia in cats
- Bile duct obstruction
- Secondary pancreatitis
- Carcinomatosis with or without ascites and metastasis to distant sites
- Diabetes mellitus (reported in two cats)
- Exocrine pancreatic insufficiency secondary to pancreatic duct obstruction (rare)
- Hepatocutaneous syndrome (in dogs)

CLINICAL PRESENTATION

HISTORY, CHIEF COMPLAINT

- Typically vague and nonspecific: anorexia, weight loss, lethargy, vomiting, constipation, diarrhea, abdominal distention (mass, ascites), and paraneoplastic alopecia (cats).
- Owners may note icterus if the neoplasm is occluding the common bile duct.
- Signs related to metastasis: ascites, dyspnea, lameness/bone pain.
- Signs related to effects of hepatocutaneous syndrome on paws (dogs): reluctance to walk or signs of paw pain when walking.

PHYSICAL EXAM FINDINGS

- Abdominal mass and/or ascites
- Icterus if common bile duct obstruction
- Dyspnea due to pleural effusion or pulmonary metastasis
- Necrolytic pododermatitis/hepatocutaneous syndrome (dogs)

ETIOLOGY AND PATHOPHYSIOLOGY

- Etiology unknown.
- Clinical signs related to local disease (mass), metastatic disease (carcinomatosis and systemic), and metabolic effects.
- The majority of cases have already metastasized to regional or distant sites before the diagnosis can be made.

DIAGNOSIS

DIFFERENTIAL DIAGNOSIS

- Pancreatitis: primary pancreatitis or pancreatitis secondary to the tumor
- Pancreatic pseudocyst
- Pancreatic abscess
- Pancreatic nodular hyperplasia
- Other pancreatic tumors (islet cell tumor, adenoma, sarcoma, and lymphoma)

INITIAL DATABASE

- Complete blood count, serum biochemical profile, and urinalysis:
  - Can be unremarkable.
  - Variable neutrophilia, anemia, hyperbilirubinemia, azotemia, hyperglycemia, and elevations in hepatic enzymes.
  - Serum lipase levels: marked hyperlipasemia may be a noninvasive indicator and biochemical marker for neoplasia of the pancreas; a level of 25 times greater than normal is probably diagnostic for exocrine pancreatic carcinoma.
- Abdominal radiographs: nonspecific; may reveal cranial abdominal mass effect and/or loss of abdominal organ detail due to ascites
- Thoracic radiographs (three views): to evaluate for pulmonary metastasis
- Abdominal ultrasound (high yield):
  - In most cases, a soft tissue mass can be identified in the region of the pancreas. It may not be possible to conclusively identify the mass as pancreatic in origin on the ultrasound exam.
  - Allows identification of metastatic lesions (liver "target lesions," peritoneal masses, lymphadenopathy) and ascites.
  - Metastases are already present in a majority of cases of pancreatic adenocarcinoma and may be visible ultrasonographically.
  - The presence of gross metastatic disease (e.g., on ultrasound) must not be overinterpreted because benign lesions, such as hepatic nodular regeneration/hyperplasia, accessory splenic tissue, and others, can be

present and should not be misidentified as metastases.

ADVANCED OR CONFIRMATORY TESTING

- Cytologic evaluation of ascites may reveal neoplastic cells in some cases (neoplastic cells may not exfoliate).
- Ultrasound-guided percutaneous fine-needle aspirate for cytologic examination (variable yield; neoplastic cells may not exfoliate).
- Ultrasound-guided percutaneous core biopsy, laparoscopic biopsy, or surgical biopsy for histopathologic evaluation of tissue:
    - Cytologic or histologic diagnosis is essential due to the inability to differentiate grossly between pancreatic adenocarcinoma and chronic pancreatitis.
- Pancreatic lipase immunoreactivity (PLI): has not been evaluated with pancreatic neoplasia; increased levels would be expected if there is secondary pancreatitis.
- Abdominal CT scan or MRI (surgical planning and staging).

TREATMENT

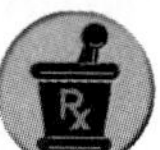

THERAPEUTIC GOAL(S)

- Surgical excision of the tumor may be palliative but is not indicated if metastasis is present (majority of cases).
- Aggressive surgical procedures (complete pancreatectomy or pancreaticoduodenectomy) have been described, but they carry high operative morbidity and mortality without meaningful cure rates.

ACUTE GENERAL TREATMENT

- Supportive therapy if there is secondary pancreatitis.
- Surgery is indicated for solitary masses without evidence of metastasis, although a high metastatic rate makes this situation uncommon.
- Palliative surgery if there is intestinal or biliary obstruction.

CHRONIC TREATMENT

- Chemotherapy or radiation therapy: no effective chemotherapy or radiation therapy protocols have been described.
- Gemcitabine (Gemzar) is approved for the treatment of pancreatic adenocarcinoma in people, and although cures are rare, gemcitabine has improved survival times in human patients. Similar data are not available in dogs.
- Palliation of pain with analgesics.

POSSIBLE COMPLICATIONS

Postoperative pancreatitis; preoperative and perioperative octreotide (Sandostatin, Novartis; 5 ug/kg SQ q 8h) may be protective

PROGNOSIS AND OUTCOME

- Very poor to grave
- Survival time of more than 1 year has not been reported

PEARLS & CONSIDERATIONS

COMMENTS

- Pancreatic adenocarcinoma is an aggressive malignancy with high potential for metastasis and generally no effective treatment.
- Must be differentiated from non-neoplastic pancreatic lesions. It is important to have a cytologic or histologic diagnosis because chronic pancreatitis may closely resemble pancreatic adenocarcinoma.
- Animals with solitary masses without evidence of metastasis are candidates for surgery.

SUGGESTED READING

Seaman RL: Exocrine pancreatic neoplasia in the cat: A case series. *J Am Anim Hosp Assoc* 40:238–245, 2004.

Steiner JM, Williams DA: Poorly recognized diseases of the exocrine pancreas. *ACVIM Forum* 2002, Dallas, Texas.

Withrow SJ: Cancer of the gastrointestinal tract: Exocrine cancer of the pancreas. In Withrow SJ, MacEwen EG (eds): *Small Animal Clinical Oncology*, ed 3. Philadelphia, WB Saunders, 2001, pp 321–323.

Williams DA: Exocrine pancreatic disease. In Ettinger SJ, Feldman EC (eds): *Textbook of Veterinary Internal Medicine*, ed 5. Philadelphia, WB Saunders, 2000, p 1364.

AUTHOR: **STEVE HILL**

EDITOR: **KEITH P. RICHTER**

Pancreatitis, Cat

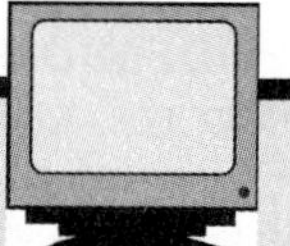

Client Education Sheet on Website

BASIC INFORMATION

DEFINITION

Pancreatitis is an inflammatory condition of the pancreas. Pancreatitis can be acute or chronic, which can only be differentiated histopathologically. In contrast to acute pancreatitis, chronic pancreatitis is associated with permanent changes, such as pancreatic fibrosis and/or atrophy.

EPIDEMIOLOGY

SPECIES, AGE, SEX: No known age or sex predilections for feline pancreatitis.

GENETICS AND BREED PREDISPOSITION: There are no consistently recognized breed predilections for pancreatitis in cats.

RISK FACTORS

- Blunt abdominal trauma
- Hypercalcemia
- Pancreatic hypoperfusion
- Pharmaceuticals: organophosphates and others
    - More than 50 drugs and drug classes have been implicated in causing pancreatitis in humans.
    - Corticosteroids are no longer implicated in humans, and there is no evidence that they cause pancreatitis in cats.
- Hepatic fluke infestation (*Amphimerus pseudofelineus*)
- *Toxoplasma* infection

ASSOCIATED CONDITIONS AND DISORDERS: Cats with chronic pancreatitis often have concurrent inflammatory conditions, such as inflammatory bowel disease (IBD) and/or cholangiohepatitis, a combination referred to as triaditis. There is little scientific evidence to suggest that these concurrent conditions cause pancreatitis.

CLINICAL PRESENTATION

DISEASE FORMS/SUBTYPES

- Acute or chronic
- Mild (not associated with systemic or pancreatic complications) or severe (associated with systemic or pancreatic complications)

HISTORY, CHIEF COMPLAINT

- Vague complaints are typical.
- Lethargy.
- Anorexia.
- Vomiting occurs only in approximately 33% of cases.

PHYSICAL EXAM FINDINGS

- Vague findings.
- Lethargy.
- Dehydration.
- Hypothermia.

- Abdominal pain is only reported in approximately 25% of cases.
- Possible fever.
- Possible icterus.

ETIOLOGY AND PATHOPHYSIOLOGY

- The causes for feline pancreatitis are not well defined. Several risk factors (see previous paragraphs) have been identified.
- There is a common pathogenetic pathway regardless of the initiating cause. Any number of insults can lead to premature activation of trypsinogen to trypsin. Trypsin, in turn, activates more trypsinogen and other pancreatic zymogens. Prematurely activated pancreatic digestive enzymes lead to local and systemic damage and also lead to recruitment of inflammatory cells and cytokine release, leading to further systemic changes.
- In general, premature activation of pancreatic digestive enzymes leads to initiation of pancreatitis, while the inflammatory response leads to progression of the disease and systemic complications.

DIAGNOSIS

DIFFERENTIAL DIAGNOSIS

- Primary acute or chronic gastrointestinal (GI) disorders: infectious, inflammatory, neoplastic, toxic, mechanical, or other conditions
- Acute or chronic metabolic or systemic disorders: hepatic, renal, adrenal, thyroid, systemic, or, less likely, central nervous system (CNS) or heartworm disease

INITIAL DATABASE

- Findings on a complete blood count (CBC) are mostly nonspecific: most commonly observed changes are anemia and leukocytosis.
- Findings on a serum chemistry profile are also mostly nonspecific: elevated serum hepatic enzyme activities, hyperbilirubinemia, hypercholesterolemia, hyperglycemia, azotemia, hypokalemia, hypocalcemia, and hypoalbuminemia.
- Abdominal radiographs are not useful for diagnosing pancreatitis but are useful for ruling out other differential diagnoses.

ADVANCED OR CONFIRMATORY TESTING

- Abdominal ultrasound is useful for the diagnosis of feline pancreatitis.
  - Diagnostic criteria: enlargement of the pancreas, fluid accumulation around the pancreas, pancreatic mass effect, hypoechoic (necrosis) or hyperechoic (fibrosis) pancreas, hyperechoic peripancreatic fat, or dilated pancreatic duct.
  - Resolution of equipment and operator expertise have increased significantly over the last two decades.
  - Clinicians should exercise caution and avoid overdiagnosing pancreatitis.
- Serum amylase and lipase activities are not useful for the diagnosis of feline pancreatitis.
- Serum feline trypsin-like immunoreactivity (fTLI) is specific but not very sensitive (sensitivity 30–60%) for feline pancreatitis. Elevated fTLI strongly suggests pancreatitis, but many cats with pancreatitis may have borderline or normal fTLI results.
- Serum feline pancreatic lipase immunoreactivity (fPLI) concentration.
  - Measures the concentration of pancreatic lipase in serum (there are many other lipases that contribute to the more routinely measured, total serum lipase activity measurement).
  - Reference range: 2.0–6.8 μg/L.
  - Cut-off value for pancreatitis: 12 μg/L.
  - Highly specific for exocrine pancreatic function.
  - Highly sensitive for both acute and chronic pancreatitis.
  - One-time measurement does not allow assessment of disease severity, but serial measurements do allow for monitoring of disease progression in a specific animal.
- Infestation with a hepatic fluke, *A. pseudofelineus*, has been reported as a cause for feline pancreatitis. The prevalence is unknown, but infestation is difficult to diagnose: requires fecal formalin-ethyl acetate sedimentation.

TREATMENT

THERAPEUTIC GOAL(S)

- Treatment of the underlying cause if identified
- Treatment of clinical signs that cause morbidity (e.g., pain)
- Identification and treatment of complications
- Nutritional support

ACUTE GENERAL TREATMENT

- If an underlying cause can be identified, it should be treated appropriately. Examples:
  - The drug history of the animal should be carefully assessed; if the animal has been treated with any medication that has been implicated in causing pancreatitis, the medication should be discontinued.
  - Since infestation with *A. pseudofelineus*, a hepatic fluke, has been reported as a cause for feline pancreatitis and is difficult to diagnose, one option is to routinely treat cats that live in endemic areas of this parasite. Praziquantel (40 mg/kg PO q 24h for 3 days) is reported to be efficacious.
  - In addition, medications that the animal does not necessarily need should be discontinued, or the animal should be switched to a different class of drug with the same or similar effect.
- The mainstay of pancreatitis therapy is supportive care. This includes intensive but judicious fluid therapy and careful monitoring for any signs of ensuing complications. Once a complication has established itself in an animal, treatment of such a complication becomes increasingly difficult.
- Supportive therapy for signs that cause morbidity is also important. Foremost, analgesia is very important.
- Abdominal pain is a key clinical sign in people with pancreatitis and should be assumed to be present in any cat with pancreatitis, whether the sign is clinically apparent. Analgesia can be achieved with intermittent dosing or continuous rate infusion. Acceptable options include one of the following:
  - Meperidine: 2–4 mg/kg IM, as needed (prn); short half-life or adverse effects can be limiting.
  - Butorphanol: 0.1–0.4 mg/kg SQ, IM, or IV.
  - Morphine: 0.05–0.2 mg/kg q 2–6h SQ or IM; may cause dysphoria or nausea.
  - Fentanyl: 0.002–0.003 mg/kg IV once, then if needed, as a constant rate infusion: 0.001–0.004 mg/kg/h IV.
  - Buprenorphine: 0.005–0.01 mg/kg IM or IV.
- Antiemetic therapy can be important. Metoclopramide antagonizes dopamine at the receptor site, which may have a negative impact on pancreatic perfusion and, therefore, is not the first drug of choice. Dolasetron, a 5-HT_3 receptor antagonist, has become available. It has much stronger antiemetic properties than metoclopramide and can be safely used at doses of 0.3 to 0.6 mg/kg IV or SC q 12–24h.
- Recommending nothing per os (NPO), meaning nothing taken orally, used to be standard therapy for cats with pancreatitis. However, nutritional support and, preferably, enteral nutritional support have beneficial effects in animals with pancreatitis. Thus, NPO should only be ordered for animals that are actively vomiting. In animals that are eating and not vomiting, a low-fat diet should be offered in small amounts and given multiple times a day. If the animal vomits and has to be kept NPO, total or partial parenteral nutrition (TPN or PPN) should be considered for nutritional

support. If the animal is not vomiting but has prolonged anorexia, tube feeding (either esophagostomy or percutaneous endoscopic gastrostomy tube) is warranted. Nutritional support is especially important in cats. Many cats with pancreatitis have been partially or fully anorectic for some time before presentation and are thus at increased risk for secondary hepatic lipidosis.

- Antibiotics have failed to show any benefit in human patients with pancreatitis. In addition, infectious complications, which are a common cause for morbidity and mortality in human patients with severe pancreatitis, are rare in cats with pancreatitis. Thus, antibiotic therapy should only be implemented when there is a specific suspicion for a concurrent infectious disease or an infectious complication of pancreatitis.
- Glucocorticoid therapy may be helpful, especially if there is concurrent, histologically confirmed inflammatory bowel disease and/or cholangiohepatitis.
- There is no evidence that any other therapeutic strategy is clinically efficacious in cats with pancreatitis.

CHRONIC TREATMENT

- Cats with chronic pancreatitis often have concurrent inflammatory conditions, such as inflammatory bowel disease (IBD) and/or cholangiohepatitis (known as triaditis). While there is little scientific evidence to suggest that these concurrent conditions cause the pancreatitis, often times the overall health of the animal will improve as these conditions are being appropriately diagnosed and managed.
- Serum calcium and fasting triglyceride concentrations should be measured in cats with pancreatitis, and conditions causing abnormalities in these parameters should be managed if present.
- While there is little evidence that high-fat diets are a cause of pancreatitis in cats, it still seems prudent to place cats with pancreatitis on a low-fat diet.
- Measurement of serum fPLI concentrations can be used for objectively monitoring animals with pancreatitis.
- If animals show signs of chronic abdominal pain (rare in cats), pancreatic enzyme supplementation can be tried (Viokase or Pancreazyme: ½ tsp per cat sprinkled on food q 12h). In human patients with pancreatitis, pancreatic enzyme supplementation does not change the course of the disease itself but does lead to amelioration of abdominal pain and discomfort.

DRUG INTERACTIONS

Any drugs implicated in causing pancreatitis should be avoided. However, corticosteroids, formerly implicated in causing pancreatitis, probably pose little risk of leading to worsening of pancreatitis in cats.

POSSIBLE COMPLICATIONS

- Pancreatic abscessation has not been reported in cats.
- Pancreatitis can lead to extrahepatic biliary obstruction. Most of these obstructions will resolve with supportive care. Approximately 10% of these cases will need surgery to reroute the bile duct.
- Systemic complications may include disseminated intravascular coagulation (DIC), thrombocytopenia, acute renal failure, pleural effusion, and peritonitis. These are rare in cats.

RECOMMENDED MONITORING

- Short-term monitoring: CBC, chemistry profile, coagulation panel, fPLI
- Ultrasound is of little value in monitoring short-term progress
- Long-term monitoring: fPLI

PROGNOSIS AND OUTCOME

The prognosis for cats with pancreatitis is directly related to the severity of disease. Mild disease without pancreatic and systemic complications carries a good prognosis. Severe disease with pancreatic (such as pancreatic necrosis, pancreatic pseudocyst, pancreatic abscess, or other) or systemic (such as renal failure, pulmonary failure, DIC, or other) complications carries a poor to grave prognosis.

PEARLS & CONSIDERATIONS

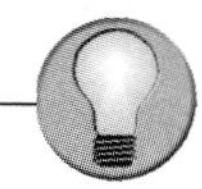

COMMENTS

Pancreatitis is diagnosed with increasing frequency in cats. In addition, immune-mediated pancreatitis has been described with increasing frequency in humans. It is intriguing to speculate that at least some cats with chronic pancreatitis have a similar condition and, like humans with immune-mediated pancreatitis, may benefit from corticosteroid administration.

PREVENTION

There is no known prevention for pancreatitis in cats.

SUGGESTED READING

Steiner JM, Williams DA: Feline exocrine pancreatic disease. In Ettinger SJ, Feldman EC (eds): *Textbook of Veterinary Internal Medicine*, ed 6. St. Louis, Elsevier, WB Saunders, 2005, pp 1489–1492.

AUTHOR: **JÖRG M. STEINER**
EDITOR: **KEITH P. RICHTER**

Pancreatitis, Dog

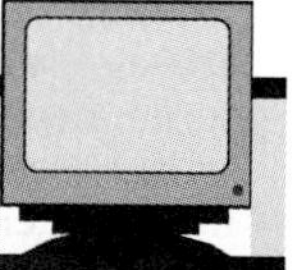

Client Education Sheet on Website

BASIC INFORMATION

DEFINITION

Pancreatitis is an inflammatory condition of the pancreas. Pancreatitis can be acute or chronic, which can only be differentiated histopathologically. In contrast to acute pancreatitis, chronic pancreatitis is associated with permanent changes such as pancreatic fibrosis and/or atrophy.

EPIDEMIOLOGY

SPECIES, AGE, SEX: There are no known age or sex predilections.

GENETICS AND BREED PREDISPOSITION: Miniature schnauzers appear to be more commonly affected; however, the search for a genetic marker has been unsuccessful.

RISK FACTORS

- Dietary indiscretion
- Blunt abdominal trauma
- Hypercalcemia
- Pancreatic hypoperfusion
- Pharmaceuticals: L-asparaginase, azathioprine, potassium bromide, trimethoprim-sulfa, and others:
  - More than 50 drugs and drug classes have been implicated in causing pancreatitis in humans.
  - Corticosteroids are no longer implicated as causing pancreatitis in humans, and there is little evidence that they cause the condition in dogs.

- Hyperlipidemia and disorders of lipid metabolism

ASSOCIATED CONDITIONS AND DISORDERS: Peritonitis (in severe cases).

CLINICAL PRESENTATION

HISTORY, CHIEF COMPLAINT

- History of dietary indiscretion (often high-fat foods)
- Vomiting
- Anorexia
- Weakness
- Abdominal pain
- Diarrhea

PHYSICAL EXAM FINDINGS

- Weakness
- Abdominal pain
- Dehydration
- Fever
- Possible icterus

ETIOLOGY AND PATHOPHYSIOLOGY

- The causes for canine pancreatitis are ill-defined. Several risk factors (see previous paragraphs) have been identified.
- There is a common pathogenetic pathway regardless of the initiating cause. Any number of insults can lead to premature activation of trypsinogen to trypsin. Trypsin, in turn, activates more trypsinogen and other pancreatic zymogens. Prematurely activated pancreatic digestive enzymes lead to local and systemic damage. This process also leads to recruitment of inflammatory cells and cytokine release, causing further systemic changes.
- In general, premature activation of pancreatic digestive enzymes leads to initiation of pancreatitis, while the inflammatory response leads to progression of the disease and systemic complications.

DIAGNOSIS

DIFFERENTIAL DIAGNOSIS

- Primary acute or chronic gastrointestinal disorders: infectious, inflammatory, neoplastic, toxic, mechanical, or other conditions
- Acute or chronic metabolic or systemic disorders: hepatic, renal, adrenal, systemic or thyroid (less likely), reproductive, or central nervous system (CNS) diseases

INITIAL DATABASE

- Findings on a complete blood count (CBC) are mostly nonspecific: most commonly observed changes are thrombocytopenia, neutrophilia with a left shift, and anemia.
- Findings on a serum chemistry profile are also mostly nonspecific: hypochloremia, hypophosphatemia, elevated hepatic enzyme activities, azotemia, hyperbilirubinemia, hypoalbuminemia, hypoglycemia, or hyperglycemia.
- Abdominal radiographs are not useful in diagnosing pancreatitis but are useful in ruling out other differential diagnoses.

ADVANCED OR CONFIRMATORY TESTING

- Abdominal ultrasound is useful for the diagnosis of canine pancreatitis.
  - Diagnostic criteria: enlargement of the pancreas, fluid accumulation around the pancreas, pancreatic mass effect, hypoechoic (necrosis), hyperechoic peripancreatic fat, or dilated pancreatic duct.
  - Resolution of equipment and operator expertise have increased significantly over the last two decades.
  - Clinicians must exercise caution not to overdiagnose pancreatitis.
- Serum amylase and lipase activities have been used for the diagnosis of pancreatitis for several decades.
  - Measurement of serum amylase or serum lipase activities are neither sensitive (approximately 50% sensitivity) nor specific (approximately 50% specificity) for pancreatitis.
  - Only of limited diagnostic usefulness.
  - Result suggestive of pancreatitis when three to five times the upper limit of the reference range.
  - Must be confirmed by other diagnostic tests.
- Serum canine pancreatic lipase immunoreactivity (cPLI) concentration (now measured by the Spec cPL assay).
  - Measures the concentration of pancreatic lipase in serum (there are many other lipases that contribute to serum lipase activity measurement).
  - Reference range: <200 μg/L.
  - Cut-off value for pancreatitis: 400 μg/L.
  - Highly specific for exocrine pancreatic function.
  - Highly sensitive for both acute and chronic pancreatitis.
  - One-time measurement does not allow assessment of disease severity, but serial measurements do allow for monitoring of disease progression in a specific animal.

TREATMENT

THERAPEUTIC GOAL(S)

- Treat the underlying cause if identified
- Treat clinical signs that cause morbidity (e.g., pain, profuse vomiting)
- Identify and treat complications
- Nutritional support

ACUTE GENERAL TREATMENT

- If the clinician can identify an underlying cause, it should be treated appropriately. For example, the drug history of the animal should be carefully assessed, and if the animal has been treated with any medication that has been implicated in causing pancreatitis, the medication should be discontinued. In addition, medications that the animal does not necessarily need should be discontinued or switched to a different class of drug with the same or similar effect.
- The mainstay of pancreatitis therapy is supportive care. This includes aggressive fluid therapy and careful monitoring for any signs of ensuing complications. Once a complication has become established in an animal, treatment of such a complication becomes increasingly difficult.
- Providing supportive therapy for effects of pancreatitis that cause morbidity is also important. Foremost, analgesia is very important.
  - Abdominal pain is a key clinical sign in people with pancreatitis and should be assumed to be present in any dog with pancreatitis, whether or not this is clinically apparent. Analgesia can be achieved with intermittent dosing or continuous rate infusion. Acceptable options include one of the following:
    - Meperidine: 5-10 mg/kg IM or slow IV as needed (prn) (q 1-4h); short half-life can be limiting.
    - Butorphanol: 0.2-0.7 mg/kg SQ, IM, or IV q 3-6h.
    - Morphine: 0.1-1 mg/kg SQ, IM, or IV q 2-6h as needed (prn); may be emetic.
    - Fentanyl: 0.01-0.04 mg/kg SQ, IM, or IV once, then as a constant rate infusion at 0.003-0.006 mg/kg/h; alternatively, may be administered as transdermal patch, which takes >12 hours to be effective.
    - Buprenorphine: 0.01-0.02 mg/kg IM or IV.
  - Antiemetic therapy can be important. Metoclopramide antagonizes dopamine at the receptor site, which may have a negative impact on pancreatic perfusion and, therefore, is not the drug of first choice. Dolasetron, a 5-HT_3 receptor antagonist, has become available. It has much stronger antiemetic properties than metoclopramide and can be safely used at doses of 0.3-0.6 mg/kg IV or SC q 12-24h.
- Recommending nothing per os (NPO), meaning nothing taken orally, for the animal used to be standard therapy for dogs with pancreatitis. However, nutritional support and, preferably, enteral nutritional support have beneficial effects in animals with pancreatitis. Thus, NPO should only be chosen in animals that are actively vomiting. In animals that are eating and not vomiting, a low-fat diet should be chosen in small

amounts and given multiple times a day. If the animal vomits and has to be kept NPO for several days, total or partial parenteral nutrition (TPN or PPN; see Parenteral Nutrition, p 1296) should be considered for nutritional support. Alternatively, jejunostomy tube placement surgically or via endoscopy (see Feeding Tube Placement: Percutaneous Endoscopic Jejunostomy [PEJ], p 1249) can be used for nutritional support.
- Dogs with severe pancreatitis (associated with dehydration, electrolyte and acid-base abnormalities, disseminated intravascular coagulation, and/or other systemic complications) should receive plasma transfusions on a daily basis (10 ml/kg given IV for 1 to 2 hours). While there is little scientific evidence that plasma administration is clinically useful in human patients with pancreatitis, most veterinary gastroenterologists agree that there appears to be a clinical benefit.
- Antibiotics have failed to show any benefit in human patients with pancreatitis. In addition, dogs with pancreatitis do not have the infectious complications of pancreatitis that are commonly seen in humans with the condition. Thus, antibiotic therapy should only be implemented when there is a specific suspicion for a concurrent infectious disease or an infectious complication of pancreatitis.
- There is no evidence that any other therapeutic strategy is clinically efficacious in dogs with pancreatitis.

CHRONIC TREATMENT

- Dogs with chronic pancreatitis should receive a palatable low-fat diet indefinitely (usually for life). In addition, an 18-hour fasting serum triglyceride concentration should be measured, and treatment measures should be employed in hyperlipidemic animals to keep the triglyceride concentration below 500 mg/dl (see Hyperlipidemia, p 547).
- Measurement of serum cPLI concentration can be used for objectively monitoring animals with pancreatitis.
- If animals show signs of chronic abdominal pain, pancreatic enzyme supplementation can be tried (Viokase or Pancreazyme: 1 tsp per 10 kg body weight in food, q 12h). In human patients, pancreatic enzyme supplementation does not change the course of the disease itself but does lead to amelioration of abdominal pain and discomfort.

DRUG INTERACTIONS

Any drugs implicated in causing pancreatitis should be avoided. However, corticosteroids, formerly implicated in causing pancreatitis, probably pose little risk of leading to worsening of pancreatitis in the dog.

POSSIBLE COMPLICATIONS

- A pancreatic pseudocyst (an encapsulated fluid collection in the region of the pancreas) rarely develops in dogs with pancreatitis. Little is known about appropriate management in dogs. In humans, pancreatic pseudocysts are carefully monitored and are only drained if they increase in size.
- Pancreatic abscesses have only been reported in approximately 20 dogs. Most of these were not infected. Surgical removal may be the best option. Aggressive antibiotic therapy should be instituted after draining the abscess, at least until culture results show absence of any infectious organisms.
- Pancreatitis can lead to extrahepatic biliary obstruction. In most cases, the obstruction will resolve with supportive care. Approximately 10% of these cases will need surgery to reroute the bile duct.
- Systemic complications may include disseminated intravascular coagulation (DIC), thrombocytopenia, acute renal failure, pleural effusion, pulmonary emboli, peritonitis, and aspiration pneumonia.

RECOMMENDED MONITORING

- Short-term monitoring: CBC, chemistry profile, coagulation panel, cPLI
- Long-term monitoring: cPLI

PROGNOSIS AND OUTCOME

- The prognosis for dogs with pancreatitis is directly related to the severity of disease. Mild disease without pancreatic and systemic complications carries a good prognosis. Severe disease with pancreatic (e.g., pancreatic necrosis, pancreatic pseudocyst, pancreatic abscess, or other) or systemic (e.g., renal failure, pulmonary failure, DIC, or other) complications carries a poor to grave prognosis.
- There is no commonly accepted scoring system that would allow prediction of the outcome of the disease in a specific animal. Such scoring systems are routinely utilized in human patients with pancreatitis.

PEARLS & CONSIDERATIONS

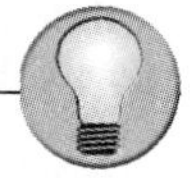

COMMENTS

- Pancreatitis is being diagnosed with increasing frequency in dogs. A recent study has shown histopathologic changes of the exocrine pancreas in most dogs that died for any reason, suggesting that subclinical exocrine pancreatic disease and, more specifically, inflammation are common in dogs. However, at this point, the clinical importance of subclinical pancreatic inflammation in dogs is unknown.
- An appropriate pancreatitis diet should be low in fat. Therefore, an "enteric" diet usually is NOT appropriate since it may not truly be low in fat. Rather, a high-fiber diet, such as a weight-loss or an obesity-prevention diet, is often superior.

PREVENTION

- Avoiding high-fat foods and treats may prevent pancreatitis, especially in animals that have had previous episodes of pancreatitis.
- Eliminating risk factors will aid in the prevention of pancreatitis.

SUGGESTED READING

Williams DA, Steiner JM: Canine pancreatic disease. In Ettinger SJ, Feldman EC (eds): *Textbook of Veterinary Internal Medicine*, ed 6. St. Louis, Elsevier, WB Saunders, 2005, pp 1482–1488.

AUTHOR: **JÖRG M. STEINER**
EDITOR: **KEITH P. RICHTER**

Panleukopenia, Cat

BASIC INFORMATION

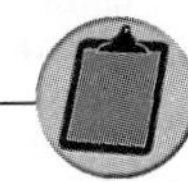

DEFINITION

Highly contagious parvoviral infection of cats; typically causes severe, sometimes fatal, acute gastroenteritis and leukopenia

SYNONYM(S)

Feline infectious enteritis
Feline parvovirus (FPV)

EPIDEMIOLOGY

SPECIES, AGE, SEX

- All Felidae: domestic housecats, tigers, lions, cheetahs
- Also affects raccoons, ferrets, mink, civet cats
- Can affect all susceptible cats, primarily kittens <1 year old; most infections (>75%) are subclinical

RISK FACTORS

- Unvaccinated cats >6–12 weeks old
- Vaccinated kittens 8 to 20 weeks old, when maternal antibodies wane but titers remain high enough to neutralize vaccine-induced antibodies
- Pregnant queens receiving modified live-virus vaccines: risk of kittens with cerebellar hypoplasia

CONTAGION AND ZOONOSIS

- Highly contagious to other cats; quarantine/isolation required.
- Virus is shed in all body secretions, primarily feces. Extremely stable in the environment (up to 1 year). Susceptible cats infected by exposure to infected feces, secretions, or fomites. Can also be transmitted *in utero*; more common in animal shelters, feral populations.
- Does not infect dogs or humans.

GEOGRAPHY AND SEASONALITY: Worldwide; seasonal variations correlate with a greater number of births.

CLINICAL PRESENTATION

DISEASE FORMS/SUBTYPES

- Classical feline enteritis: kittens and susceptible adults
- Silent abortion/fetal death: queens (first trimester)
- Central nervous system (CNS) form: kittens infected *in utero* in second or third trimester or up to 9 days postbirth
  - Virus infects replicating neurons.
  - Neurologic signs are nonprogressive, and affected kittens can still make good pets.

HISTORY, CHIEF COMPLAINT

- Classic enteritis: acute onset:
  - Sudden death, "fading kitten syndrome"
  - Vomiting, anorexia, or diarrhea
  - Extreme lethargy or depression, hiding
- CNS:
  - Queening of mummified fetuses
  - Ataxia and intention tremors noted once kittens start to walk (10 to 14 days old)
  - Altered mentation and dullness (usually not noted until several weeks old)
  - Seizures

PHYSICAL EXAM FINDINGS

- Classic enteritis: kitten is infected with panleukopenia:
  - Fever or hypothermia in severe cases
  - Marked dehydration or hypovolemic shock
  - Vomiting, diarrhea
  - Thickened bowel loops, abdominal discomfort
- CNS form: mother was infected with panleukopenia when pregnant:
  - Cerebellar ataxia, hypermetria, intention tremors
  - Optic nerve hypoplasia, dark foci/folding/streaking of retina
  - Mental dullness, behavior abnormalities

ETIOLOGY AND PATHOPHYSIOLOGY

- Single-stranded nonenveloped DNA virus
- Replicates in rapidly dividing cells; clinical signs reflect destruction of these cells:
  - Lymphoid tissue: lymphopenia, lymph node necrosis
  - Bone marrow: panleukopenia, occasionally other short-lived cell lines (thrombocytes)
  - Intestinal mucosal crypt cells: damage results in malabsorptive diarrhea, increased permeability, increased risk for bacterial translocation
  - Nervous system: cerebellar hypoplasia, hydrocephalus, hydranencephaly, retinal dysplasia from destruction of neural tissue

DIAGNOSIS

DIFFERENTIAL DIAGNOSIS

- Gastroenteritis:
  - Foreign body
  - Other bacterial or viral infections (coronavirus, *Salmonella* spp., *Clostridium* spp.)
  - Inflammatory bowel disease
  - Neoplasia
  - Toxin ingestion
- Leukopenia:
  - Feline leukemia virus (FeLV)
  - *Salmonella* spp.

INITIAL DATABASE

- Complete blood count (CBC): mild anemia, unless severe gastrointestinal (GI) bleeding; leukopenia, especially neutropenia; thrombocytopenia due to bone marrow suppression or disseminated intravascular coagulation (DIC)
- Serum biochemistry profile: often unremarkable; prerenal azotemia, increases in alanine aminotransferase/aspartate aminotransferase/bilirubin possible
- Coagulation panel: may see evidence of DIC
- Radiolography: typically unremarkable

ADVANCED OR CONFIRMATORY TESTING

- Confirmatory laboratory testing is not easily available; therefore, diagnosis is typically made based on history, signalment, clinical signs, and initial laboratory findings.
- Severe gastroenteritis with neutropenia in a 3- to 5-month-old kitten is highly suggestive of FPV infection.
- Confirmatory diagnostic tests for FPV (serologic examination, immunofluorescent antibody testing, polymerase chain reaction [PCR] testing, and virus isolation) are often labor- or time-intensive, expensive, and not readily available.
- Canine parvoviral fecal ELISA test kits can detect FPV antigen. As with vaccination in puppies, false-positive results can occur within 2 weeks of vaccination with modified-live feline panleukopenia vaccine.
- Histologic findings are also similar to those of canine parvovirus.

TREATMENT

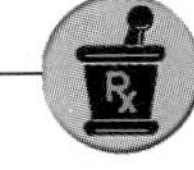

THERAPEUTIC GOAL(S)

- No specific antiviral drug
- Supportive care required during the acute episode

ACUTE GENERAL TREATMENT

Supportive care:

- IV fluids to correct shock, dehydration, and electrolyte abnormalities
- Broad-spectrum antibiotics (e.g., ampicillin 22 mg/kg IV q 8h, and gentamicin 4 mg/kg IV q 24h, only once hydration is normal) to combat secondary bacterial infections
- Withholding of food/water during acute episode to decrease crypt cell division and subsequent viral replication
- Antiemetics (e.g., metoclopramide 0.2–0.4 mg/kg SC q 8h)

- Appetite stimulants or enteral tube feeding during recovery period if anorexia persists
- Vitamin B

CHRONIC TREATMENT

Cats that recover are immune for life.

RECOMMENDED MONITORING

Repeat CBC: rebound leukocytosis (24 to 48 hours). If leukopenia persists, clinicians should rule out other causes (e.g., FeLV).

PROGNOSIS AND OUTCOME

- Guarded for acute gastroenteritis
- Guarded to good for kittens with cerebellar hypoplasia, depending on ability to compensate for deficits; neurologic signs are not treatable but are also nonprogressive
- Grave to poor for kittens with forebrain signs

PEARLS & CONSIDERATIONS

COMMENTS

- Kittens cannot have both neurologic signs and signs of enteritis simultaneously from panleukopenia because neurologic signs occur from *in utero* infection of the dam.
- Routine vaccination has profoundly decreased the incidence of disease. Disease is maintained due to persistence of FPV in the environment and birth of susceptible animals in unvaccinated populations.

PREVENTION

- Modified live vaccines (MLV) are preferred because they are rapid and provide more effective immunity. Clinicians should administer these vaccines after the animal is 8 weeks old to avoid inactivation by maternal antibodies, then every 2 to 4 weeks, and then 1 year later. Initial vaccinations probably provide lifelong immunity, but clinicians should revaccinate triennially per American Association of Feline Practitioners. MLV administered to pregnant queens or kittens less than 4 weeks old may cause cerebellar hypoplasia in the fetuses or kittens.
- Environment: The virus is easily spread via fomites (towels, bowls, shoes) and persists up to 1 year. Disinfection requires 1:32 diluted sodium hypochlorite (bleach), formaldehyde, or glutaraldehyde.

CLIENT EDUCATION

Breeders should vaccinate new, susceptible cats 1 week prior to introduction to cattery.

SUGGESTED READING

Addie D, Thompson H: Feline panleucopenia/feline parvovirus infection. In Chandler EA Gaskell CJ, Gaskell RM (eds): *Feline Medicine and Therapeutics*. Denmark, Blackwell Publishing, 2004, pp 571–575.

Brower AI, Radi C, Toohey-Kurth K: Feline panleukopenia: A diagnostic laboratory's perspective. *Vet Med* 99:8, 2004.

Greene CE: Feline panleukopenia. In Greene CE (ed): *Infectious Diseases of the Dog and Cat*. Philadelphia, WB Saunders, 1998, pp 52–57.

Ikeda Y, et al: Feline host range of canine parvovirus: Recent emergence of new antigenic types in cats. *Emerg Infect Dis* 8:4, 2002.

AUTHOR: **SHANNON T. STROUP**

EDITOR: **DOUGLASS K. MACINTIRE**

Panniculitis

BASIC INFORMATION

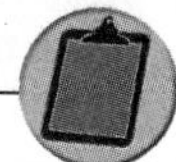

DEFINITION

Inflammation of the subcutaneous adipose tissue

EPIDEMIOLOGY

SPECIES, AGE, SEX: Uncommon in dogs and cats.

GENETICS AND BREED PREDISPOSITION: Sterile nodular panniculitis: dachshunds and also golden retrievers, collies, and miniature poodles.

RISK FACTORS

- Outdoor pets (penetrating foreign body, bite wound): infectious panniculitis
- Immunocompromise (e.g., feline leukemia virus [FeLV], feline immunodeficiency [FIV], or dog that has been receiving glucocorticoids for a long period of time): greater risk of dissemination of infectious organisms
- Recurrent pancreatitis: panniculitis and steatitis
- Pancreatitis or pancreatic carcinomas: mineralizing fat necrosis/panniculitis

CONTAGION AND ZOONOSIS

- Dermatophytic granulomas: *Microsporum canis* and *Trichophyton mentagrophytes* are potentially contagious to other animals and are zoonotic.
- Sporotrichosis: risk of cat to human transmission is extremely high; dog-to-human transmission not yet reported.
- Blastomycosis, coccidioidomycosis, histoplasmosis: risk of zoonosis by aerosol from culture plates; in-house culture is always contraindicated.

GEOGRAPHY AND SEASONALITY: See Blastomycosis, p 133; Histoplasmosis, p 525; Coccidioidomycosis, p 218; Pythiosis and Lagenidiosis, p 937; Protothecosis, p 903.

ASSOCIATED CONDITIONS AND DISORDERS: Interscapular panniculitis may be a precursor of vaccine-associated fibrosarcoma in cats.

CLINICAL PRESENTATION

DISEASE FORMS/SUBTYPES

- Diffuse: Both the lobules and septa (most common in dogs) are involved.
- Septal: The interlobular connective tissue septa are involved (most common in cats).
- Lobular: The fat lobules are affected.

HISTORY, CHIEF COMPLAINT: Acute to chronic onset of single or multiple subcutaneous nodules or draining tracts with potential accompanying systemic signs, such as anorexia and lethargy.

PHYSICAL EXAM FINDINGS

- Lesions typically involve the trunk and may be single or multifocal.
- Subcutaneous nodules to swellings may become cystic and painful, especially prior to rupturing or developing draining tracts.
- Panniculitis and subsequent fat necrosis are characterized by an oily, yellow-brown to blood-tinged discharge.
- Lesions often heal with crusting and scarring.

ETIOLOGY AND PATHOPHYSIOLOGY

- Panniculitis is caused by damage from the aforementioned conditions to lipocytes.
- Result: release of lipids into subcutis, where the lipids undergo hydrolysis to glycerol and fatty acids.
- The fatty acids are potent inflammatory agents, resulting in further inflammation and granulomatous reactions.

DIAGNOSIS

DIFFERENTIAL DIAGNOSIS

- Infectious: bacterial/botryomycosis, actinomycotic, systemic and subcutaneous fungal, dermatophytic pseudomycetomas, feline leprosy, atypical mycobacteria, *Chlamydia* sp.
- Immune-mediated: lupus profundus, erythema nodosum, drug eruption, insect-bite
- Idiopathic: sterile nodular panniculitis
- Trauma with or without foreign body reaction
- Nutritional: vitamin E deficiency (feline nutritional pansteatitis)
- Pancreatitis or pancreatic adenocarcinoma
- Postinjection reaction: corticosteroids, vaccine (rabies)
- Neoplastic: multicentric mast cell tumors, cutaneous lymphosarcoma
- Deep pyoderma/abscess
- Cutaneous cysts
- Drug reaction
- Other cutaneous neoplasia (lipoma, mast cell tumors/cutaneous lymphosarcoma)

INITIAL DATABASE

- Cytologic examination: infectious organisms:
  - Gram-positive branching filamentous organisms: *Actinomyces* sp. (nonacid-fast); *Nocardia* sp. (partially acid-fast).
  - Diff Quik: fungi possible (systemic mycoses).
  - Acid-fast bacilli: atypical mycobacteria, feline lepraemurium.
  - Organisms may be noted within foamy macrophages.
- Full-thickness (skin plus subcutaneous fat) biopsy, and the panniculus must be included; histopathologic analysis:
  - Differentiation of the various patterns (septal, lobular, diffuse).
  - Cellular infiltrate.
  - Infectious organisms (special stains).
  - Severity of lesions (necrosis, fibrosis, vasculitis).

ADVANCED OR CONFIRMATORY TESTING

- Clinicians should submit part of a biopsy specimen aseptically for tissue maceration and culture.
- They should also notify the laboratory of suspected organisms (to make adjustments to culture media selection and incubation times and for precautions taken especially with systemic mycoses):
  - Bacterial culture and sensitivity (C&S) testing.
  - Atypical mycobacterial culture.
  - Fungal culture (not usually for systemic mycoses; other tests are safer).
  - Negative cultures support a diagnosis of sterile nodular panniculitis, lupus profundus.
- Serologic evaluation: systemic mycoses.
- Antinuclear antibody to help detect lupus profundus.
- Direct immunofluorescence testing for *Sporothrix* antigen.
- Abdominal ultrasound: Pancreatic diseases may be a contributing factor (rare).

TREATMENT

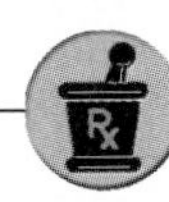

THERAPEUTIC GOAL(S)

- Identification and management of underlying etiology
- Education of clients regarding extended therapeutic protocols, especially when addressing atypical mycobacteria, *Actinomyces*, *Nocardia*, and intermediate/systemic fungal conditions

ACUTE AND CHRONIC TREATMENT

- Surgical excision of solitary lesions.
- Vitamin E (10–20 IU/kg PO q 8–12h); may control mild cases.
- Appropriate antifungal, antibacterial, or antimycobacterial treatment if indicated.
- Sterile panniculitis (rabies vaccine-induced, sterile nodular, lupus profundus).
  - Tetracycline and niacinamide (500 mg of each for dogs >10 kg; 250 mg of each for dogs <10 kg) PO q 8h, until improvement (about 2 to 3 months), then tapering gradually.
  - Pentoxifylline 10–30 mg/kg PO q 8h, until resolved, then tapering gradually.
  - Prednisone 2.2 mg/kg PO q 24h, or methylprednisolone for dogs (1.6 mg/kg PO q 24h) and prednisolone for cats (4.4 mg/kg PO q 24h) until resolution (about 2 to 6 weeks), then gradually tapering.
- Azathioprine 2 mg/kg PO q 24h (dogs) and chlorambucil 0.1–0.2 mg/kg PO q 24h (cats and small dogs): corticosteroid-sparing alternatives for long-term treatment. After a 4- to 8-week lag phase associated with both of these medications, dosage may be q 48h (or less frequent) on alternate days of glucocorticoid use (if still required).
- Dietary elimination trial: adverse food reaction may be a trigger in immune-mediated panniculitis.

DRUG INTERACTIONS

Clinicians should adjust dosage or minimize combination therapy with cytochrome p450/glycoprotein-affecting drugs (e.g., ketoconazole).

POSSIBLE COMPLICATIONS

Glucocorticoid side effects

RECOMMENDED MONITORING

- Schirmer tear test if long-term use of sulfa-based drugs
- Complete blood count, platelet count, serum chemistry profile, and urinalysis if using immunosuppressant agents

PROGNOSIS AND OUTCOME

- Variable, from guarded to good; healed lesions may leave scars.
- Most cases of panniculitis involve lengthy treatment intervals (months).
- Amputation may be a serious consideration to prevent further spread of the disease should traditional therapies provide minimal improvement.

PEARLS & CONSIDERATIONS

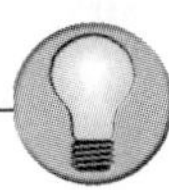

COMMENTS

- An aggressive work-up to identify the underlying etiology leads to the most appropriate and successful treatment plan and outcome.
- Clinicians should review the complexity of the differential diagnoses with clients and ensure that they are willing to pursue prolonged treatment before starting extensive diagnostic testing beyond histologic confirmation.
- Clinicians should obtain and freeze extra serum for future diagnostic tests based on histologic findings.

PREVENTION

- Weight loss for obese animals. Reduces amount of fat to which the body can react; may allow medication discontinuation.
- Owners should minimize pets' access to high-risk areas (swamps, riverbeds) and should rinse/bathe the pet after high-risk area exposure.
- Owner can give their pets routine vitamin E antioxidant.

CLIENT EDUCATION

- Diagnostics can be involved; need to determine infectious versus immune-mediated cause.
- Treatment is generally lengthy, but with appropriate therapy, the prognosis in most cases is positive. Healed lesions may leave scars, however.

SUGGESTED READING

Scott DW, Miller WH, Griffin CE: *Muller and Kirk's Small Animal Dermatology*, ed 6. Philadelphia, WB Saunders, 2001, pp 1156–1162.

Yager JA, Wilcock BP: *Color Atlas and Text of Surgical Pathology of the Dog and Cat. Volume 1. Dermatopathology and Skin Tumors*. London, Mosby-Wolfe, 1994, pp 199–215.

AUTHOR: **ANTHONY YU**
EDITOR: **JAN A. HALL**

Pannus (Chronic Superficial Keratitis)

BASIC INFORMATION

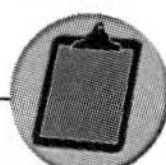

DEFINITION

A typically bilateral, progressive, immune-mediated, inflammatory disease of the cornea that is characterized by the infiltration of vessels and granulation tissue and/or pigmentation

SYNONYM(S)

CSK
Degenerative pannus
German shepherd pannus
Uberreiter's syndrome

EPIDEMIOLOGY

SPECIES, AGE, SEX

- Dogs only
- Age of onset: 2 to 5 years of age; depends on breed and altitude
- No sex predisposition

GENETICS AND BREED PREDISPOSITION

- Primarily affects large-breed dogs; may occur in any breed
- Breed predisposition: German shepherd, greyhound, Belgian Tervuren, Belgian sheepdog, dachshund, border collie, Shetland sheepdog, Siberian husky, Scotch collie, Australian shepherd, miniature pinscher, pointer, dalmatian, English springer spaniel, Airedale terrier

RISK FACTORS

- Breed predisposition
- Ultraviolet radiation exposure
- High altitude

GEOGRAPHY AND SEASONALITY: Increased incidence and severity of disease in geographic regions with high altitude (i.e., elevation of 4500 feet or higher) and intense sunlight. Dogs that live at lower altitudes respond better to therapy (e.g., dogs living in the southeastern part of the United States are less severely affected and respond better to therapy than dogs living in the Rocky Mountains).

CLINICAL PRESENTATION

DISEASE FORMS/SUBTYPES

- Early chronic superficial keratitis (CSK): Lesions occur in the lateral to lateroventral cornea. CSK: The entire cornea may be affected.
- CSK may present as a:
  - Vascular form
  - Pigmentary form
  - Combination of vascular and pigmentary forms in same eye or between eyes

HISTORY, CHIEF COMPLAINT

- Corneal discoloration: rapidly or slowly progressive; reddish and/or brown film covering surface of the eyes
- Progressive loss of vision

PHYSICAL EXAM FINDINGS

- Typically bilateral; often symmetric
- Generally nonulcerative, pinkish-red, vascularized, and/or pigmentary superficial corneal lesions commencing in the lateral to ventrolateral cornea; progressively involving the medial, ventral, and dorsal aspects of the cornea, including the central cornea
- Conjunctivitis present in most cases
- Multifocal, white, crystalline lipid deposits often present at the leading edge of the corneal lesions (see Corneal Lipid Infiltrates, p 241)
- ± Third eyelid involvement as evidenced by pink proliferative lesions and depigmentation along leading edge of third eyelid
- Early CSK:
  - Vascularization and/or pigmentation at the lateral to ventrolateral cornea adjacent to the limbus
  - Progresses centrally
- Chronic CSK:
  - A fleshy lesion (i.e., granulation tissue) with corneal vascularization and/or pigmentation
  - Entire cornea may be affected, predisposing the animal to blindness

ETIOLOGY AND PATHOPHYSIOLOGY

- Immune-mediated disease.
- Ultraviolet radiation exposure at high altitude potentiates the disorder.
- Tissue-specific antigens in the cornea are altered with ultraviolet radiation exposure.
- Dogs with CSK develop a hypersensitivity response to corneal proteins, predisposing them to chronic inflammation.
- CSK is a more rapidly progressive and severe disease in young dogs (<3 years of age).

DIAGNOSIS

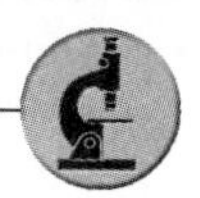

DIFFERENTIAL DIAGNOSIS

Other causes of CSK:

- Corneal vascularization (see Corneal Vascularization, p 249)
- Corneal pigmentation (see Corneal Pigmentation, p 242)

INITIAL DATABASE

Complete ophthalmic examination, including:

- Schirmer tear test (typically normal with CSK)
- Fluorescein dye application (typically no corneal dye retention with CSK but there may be secondary corneal ulceration)
- Intraocular pressures normal (15-25 mmHg) with CSK
- Careful examination of the conjunctiva and cornea

ADVANCED OR CONFIRMATORY TESTING

- Usually not required; CSK is diagnosed by clinical findings, signalment of dog, and ruling out other causes of corneal vascularization and pigmentation.
- Cytologic examination of corneal and conjunctival swabs/scrapings reveals lymphocytes and plasma cells.
- If a keratectomy is performed, histopathologic findings consist of lymphocyte, plasma cell, macrophage, and melanocytic cell infiltrations with corneal vascularization and fibroplasia.

TREATMENT

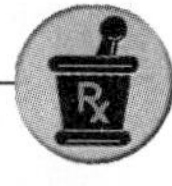

THERAPEUTIC GOAL(S)

- Suppress disease process with aggressive initial treatment
- Improve vision
- Keep disease in remission with maintenance therapy

ACUTE GENERAL TREATMENT

- Topical corticosteroids (dexamethasone 0.1% solution or ointment, or prednisolone acetate 1% suspension) q

6-8h for 3 weeks, followed by slow reduction to a maintenance dose.
- Cyclosporine-A (CsA) 0.2% ointment or 0.5-2% solution topically q 12h.

CHRONIC TREATMENT

- Requires lifelong therapy.
- Maintenance therapy consists of topical corticosteroids and/or CsA once or twice a day.
- Clinicians can maintain remission in some dogs with one daily application of CsA.
- For nonresponsive and severe cases, clinicians can consider:
  - Adjunctive subconjunctival injections of corticosteroids (e.g., methylprednisolone acetate at 4-12 mg or triamcinolone acetonide at 4-12 mg [dose dependent on size of dog]) q 2-3 weeks
  - Referral to veterinary ophthalmologist for:
    - β Irradiation (i.e., strontium-90)
    - Superficial keratectomy

POSSIBLE COMPLICATIONS

- Corneal ulceration (see Corneal Ulceration, p 246); if it occurs, clinicans should discontinue corticosteroid for the animal and commence/continue CsA until corneal ulcer has healed
- Granuloma at site of subconjunctival corticosteroid injection

RECOMMENDED MONITORING

- Response to therapy is monitored every 3 to 4 weeks initially, then every 4 to 6 weeks.
- Once stable, the animal is reevaluated every 3 to 6 months.

PROGNOSIS AND OUTCOME

- CSK is a chronic disorder that typically responds to aggressive medical therapy.
- Maintenance therapy is needed to keep the disease in remission.

PEARLS & CONSIDERATIONS

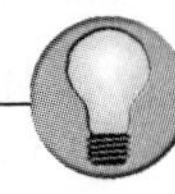

COMMENTS

- A common error in treatment is lack of aggressive therapy in the early stages of disease.
- The disease should be treated aggressively with topical corticosteroids ± CsA, and the frequency should be slowly reduced over weeks to reach a maintenance therapy.
- CSK is a chronic disease that requires lifelong treatment.

PREVENTION

- Owners should limit exposure of pets to ultraviolet light.
- They should also avoid breeding affected or closely related dogs.

CLIENT EDUCATION

- CSK is an immune-mediated disease that is manageable but not curable.
- Lifelong treatment is required.

SUGGESTED READING

Bedford P, Longstaffe J: Corneal pannus (chronic superficial keratitis) in the German shepherd dog. *J Small Anim Pract* 20:41, 1979.

Chavkin MJ, et al: Risk factors for development of chronic superficial keratitis in dogs. *J Am Vet Med Assoc* 204:1630, 1994.

Williams D, et al: Comparison of topical cyclosporine and dexamethasone for the treatment of chronic superficial keratitis in dogs. *Vet Rec* 137:635, 1995.

AUTHOR: **PHILLIP A. MOORE**
EDITOR: **CHERYL L. CULLEN**

Panosteitis

BASIC INFORMATION

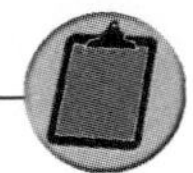

DEFINITION

A spontaneous, self-limiting painful condition of diaphyseal and metaphyseal portions of long bones

SYNONYM(S)

Enostosis
Eosinophilic osteomyelitis
Eosinophilic panosteitis
Juvenile osteomyelitis
Osteomyelitis of young German shepherd dogs

EPIDEMIOLOGY

SPECIES, AGE, SEX

- Young (5 months to 2 years), medium- and large-breed dogs
- Occasionally seen in younger or older dogs and in small breeds
- More common in males than females

GENETICS AND BREED PREDISPOSITION

- German shepherds have been reported to be at highest risk.
- Basset hounds may be overrepresented.

CLINICAL PRESENTATION

HISTORY, CHIEF COMPLAINT

- The hallmark chief complaint is acute, shifting limb lameness of variable severity that typically lasts 1 to 3 weeks (each leg).
- Systemic signs (e.g., anorexia, lethargy) occasionally can be severe and may require nutritional and physical support.

PHYSICAL EXAM FINDINGS

- Orthopedic examination demonstrates pain on deep palpation/firm digital pressure of the diaphyseal and metaphyseal (midshaft and distal) portions of affected bones.
- Frequency: ulna (42%), radius (25%), humerus (14%), femur (11%), and tibia (8%).
- Fever, depression, and anorexia can be seen in more severe (unusual) cases.

ETIOLOGY AND PATHOPHYSIOLOGY

- Panosteitis has an unknown etiology.
- Infectious agents (bacteria, canine distemper virus, modified live viral vaccines) have been suspected but never proven to cause panosteitis.
- Other suggested inciting causes include localized vascular congestion, metabolic diseases, genetic diseases, parasitism, hyperestrinism, and hemophilia.
- Panosteitis is associated with excessive bone remodeling after the death of intramedullary adipocytes and hematopoietic cells. Cell death is attributed to vascular congestion, but the true cause remains unknown.
- The necrotic marrow cells are replaced with fibrous tissue. Woven bone is formed within the fibrous tissue. Endosteal bone formation is a prominent histologic finding with panosteitis.
- Periosteal bone formation is occasionally noted.
- Eventually, endosteal bone resorption occurs, and normal vascularity and marrow adipose tissue are reestablished.

DIAGNOSIS

Based on animal signalment, physical examination findings, and characteristic radiographic changes

DIFFERENTIAL DIAGNOSIS

Infectious diseases (septic arthritis, osteomyelitis), immune-mediated arthropathies, and other developmental bone diseases (hypertrophic osteodystrophy, ununited anconeal process, osteochondrosis, hip dysplasia, etc.)

INITIAL DATABASE

- Anamnesis and physical examination:
  - Pain during deep palpation of the affected bone (diaphysis or metaphysis)
- Radiography:
  - Diagnostic test of choice
  - Characteristic radiographic lesions:
    - Patchy areas of increased intramedullary opacity
    - Increased radiographic lucency near the nutrient foramen of the bone
    - Increased periosteal bone formation
- Characteristic lesions may not be present during acute phase of the disease.
- Radiographs of other nonpainful limbs may also have characteristic lesions.
- Complete blood count (CBC), serum biochemical panel, and urinalysis, as indicated by presence of systemic signs.

TREATMENT

THERAPEUTIC GOAL(S)

Clinicians should provide analgesia during acute phase to permit normal activity with minimal discomfort

ACUTE GENERAL TREATMENT

- Supportive care.
- Nonsteroidal anti-inflammatory drugs (NSAIDs) if ongoing signs of pain:
  - Aspirin: 10–25 mg/kg PO q 24h to q 8h, or
  - Carprofen: 2 mg/kg PO q 12h, or
  - Etodolac: 10–15 mg/kg PO q 24h, or
  - Deracoxib: 1–2 mg/kg PO q 24h (may use 3–4 mg/kg PO q 24h for first 7 days only), or
  - Meloxicam: 0.1 mg/kg PO q 24h, or
  - Meclofenamic acid: 1.1 mg/kg PO q 24h, after eating, or
  - Others
- There is no indication for the use of glucocorticoids in panosteitis.

CHRONIC TREATMENT

- Seldom required since this is a self-limiting condition.
- An occasional, severe case will require use of stronger analgesics (opioids), nutritional support, or short-term hospitalization.

DRUG INTERACTIONS

Gastric ulceration and other side effects may occur with use of NSAIDs; clinicians should check product information.

POSSIBLE COMPLICATIONS

- Arise from treatment rather than disease.
- Gastrointestinal (GI) hemorrhage, ulceration, and perforation (NSAIDs).
- Liver toxicity or failure and renal dysfunction are possible with NSAIDs.
- Coagulation abnormalities are rare with most NSAIDs.

RECOMMENDED MONITORING

- Radiographic examination when other legs become affected.
- Repeated evaluation in dogs with protracted lameness to rule out other developmental bone diseases.
- CBC, biochemical profile, and urinalysis are recommended with long-term NSAID usage.

PROGNOSIS AND OUTCOME

- Disease may last several weeks to months.
- The condition may shift among limbs.
- Long-term prognosis is very good; seldom causes permanent disability.

PEARLS & CONSIDERATIONS

- Panosteitis should be a primary differential diagnosis in any young dog with acute onset of lameness.
- Panosteitis is "self-limiting" in most cases.
- Panosteitis may repeatedly flare up over several months.
- Panosteitis is most common in dogs prone to other developmental orthopedic conditions.
- Nutraceuticals and vitamin supplementation have not been shown to decrease clinical signs, duration, or severity of panosteitis.

CLIENT EDUCATION

- There are potential side effects of NSAID use in dogs.
- Panosteitis can mask other developmental orthopedic conditions.

SUGGESTED READING

Johnson AL, Hulse DA: Diseases of joints. In Fossum TW (ed): *Small Animal Surgery*, ed 2. St. Louis, Mosby, 2002, pp 1169–1170.

Montgomery RD: Miscellaneous orthopaedic diseases. In Slatter D (ed): *Textbook of Small Animal Surgery*, ed 3. Philadelphia, WB Saunders, 2002, pp 2252–2253.

Muir P, Dubielzig RR, Johnson KA: Panosteitis. *Compend Cont Ed Pract Vet* 18:29, 1996.

AUTHOR: **D. MICHAEL TILLSON**

EDITOR: **JOSEPH HARARI**

Panting

BASIC INFORMATION

DEFINITION

- Rapid, shallow breathing with a small tidal volume, usually with the mouth open.
- It is a normal thermoregulatory mechanism in dogs and cats.
- Excessive panting occurs with elevated ambient temperature, exercise, or anxiety (e.g., a visit to the veterinarian's office) in dogs or in the absence of severe ambient temperature elevations in cats.

SYNONYM(S)

Hyperpnea
Hyperventilation
Polypnea
Tachypnea

EPIDEMIOLOGY

SPECIES, AGE, SEX

- Dependent on underlying cause
- Common in normal dogs (thermoregulation, anxiety) but rare in normal cats, except in stressful situations (e.g., car ride)
- Older cats (hyperthyroidism)
- Middle-aged to older dogs, with mild female predominance (hyperadrenocorticism)

RISK FACTORS: Common and physiologic condition with emotional stress in both dogs and cats.

GEOGRAPHY AND SEASONALITY: Summer (normal thermoregulation in dogs).

CLINICAL PRESENTATION

DISEASE FORMS/SUBTYPES: Normal panting due to elevated ambient temperature or anxiety (dogs) versus inappropriate panting due to underlying disease.

HISTORY, CHIEF COMPLAINT
- Increased amount of panting or panting at inappropriate times
- Increased with elevated environmental temperatures and/or humidity
- Perceived evidence of pain
- Glucocorticosteroid or narcotic drug administration
- Polyuria, polydipsia, polyphagia, weight gain (canine hyperadrenocorticism)
- Polyphagia, weight loss, hyperactivity (feline hyperthyroidism)
- Seizures, abnormal mentation (brain disease)
- Exercise intolerance, lethargy, dyspnea (cardiac disease)
- Coughing, dyspnea (cardiac disease, feline bronchial disease)

PHYSICAL EXAM FINDINGS
- Rapid (200–400 breaths/min), shallow breathing without evidence of respiratory distress
- Elevated body temperature if fever or hyperthermia
- Signs of pain
- Truncal hair loss, pot-bellied appearance, hepatomegaly (canine hyperadrenocorticism)
- Enlarged thyroid, tachycardia, heart murmur, or gallop heart sound (feline hyperthyroidism)
- Neurologic deficits (brain disease)
- Heart murmur, tachyarrhythmia (cardiac disease)
- Harsh lung sounds, wheezing (bronchial disease)
- Obesity

ETIOLOGY AND PATHOPHYSIOLOGY
- Primary means of thermoregulation in dogs via evaporative cooling within the mouth and nasal passages; passage of air, blood flow, and secretions are increased in these areas during panting.
- Muscular work of breathing is minimally increased during panting.
- Causes respiratory alkalosis only if prolonged or severe.
- Hyperthyroidism rarely causes panting at rest but commonly with any stress. Possible reasons include respiratory muscle weakness, increased carbon dioxide production, and chemical thermogenesis.
- Hyperadrenocorticism and glucocorticosteroid administration may cause panting because of respiratory muscle weakness, muscle wasting, hepatomegaly, and abdominal fat deposition.
- Pure-agonist narcotics commonly cause dose-dependent panting that is independent of route of administration.
- Cardiac disease and tachyarrythmias may lead to panting due to anxiety or angina.
- Animals with pheochromocytoma may pant because of epinephrine-induced chemical thermogenesis.
- A similar mechanism may be inferred for anxiety-associated panting.
- Hypocalcemia may lead to panting most likely because of anxiety and pain caused by tetany.
- Obese animals fail to lose as much heat through evaporation and radiation, which increases the need for heat loss through panting. Furthermore, the tidal volume may be reduced due to fat deposition in the thorax, further increasing the respiratory rate.

DIAGNOSIS

DIFFERENTIAL DIAGNOSIS
- Elevated ambient temperature, hyperthermia
- Fever
- Anxiety, nervousness
- Pain
- Narcotic administration
- Glucocorticosteroid therapy
- Hyperadrenocorticism
- Hyperthyroidism
- Hypocalcemia
- Pheochromocytoma
- Cardiac disease, tachyarrythmia
- Feline bronchial disease
- Brain disease
- Obesity

INITIAL DATABASE
- Blood pressure (BP): moderate-severe hypertension possible with hyperthyroidism or pheochromocytoma; mild hypertension possible with severe anxiety
- Complete blood count (CBC): possible erythrocytosis, thrombocytosis, leukocytosis, lymphopenia, and eosinopenia in dogs with hyperadrenocorticism
- Serum biochemical profile: elevated alkaline phosphatase (ALP) and cholesterol in dogs with hyperadrenocorticism; elevated liver enzymes in cats with hyperthyroidism; hypocalcemia
- Urinalysis: low specific gravity and/or proteinuria in dogs with hyperadrenocorticism
- Serum T4: elevated in cats with hyperthyroidism
- Thoracic radiographs: heart enlargement ± pulmonary edema, pleural effusion with cardiac disease; bronchiolar lung pattern, lung hyperinflation in feline asthma

ADVANCED OR CONFIRMATORY TESTING
- Arterial blood gas may show respiratory alkalosis (diminished carbon dioxide, elevated pH) in animals with severe panting.
- Hyperadrenocorticism screening via adrenocorticotropic hormone (ACTH) stimulation or low-dose dexamethasone suppression tests if history and initial database are suggestive.
- Abdominal ultrasound to locate adrenal mass(es).
- Electrocardiogram (ECG) and echocardiogram to confirm cardiac disease.
- Bronchial wash cytologic evaluation to confirm feline asthma.
- Brain CT scan or MRI.

TREATMENT

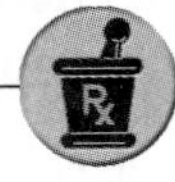

THERAPEUTIC GOAL(S)
Clinicians should treat underlying condition to eliminate excessive panting.

ACUTE GENERAL TREATMENT
Clinicians should:
- Reduce anxiety.
- Control pain if present.
- Decrease ambient temperature if elevated.
- Ensure adequate hydration in animals with elevated body temperature and provide external cooling (e.g., cool water bath, fan, cool water enema, or gastric lavage) in animals with a body temperature above 106°F.
- Discontinue or decrease dose of narcotic or glucocorticosteroid therapy, if possible.
- Manage underlying cause (± antiarrhythmic therapy) for tachyarrhythmias.
- Administer calcium supplementation for hypocalcemic animals.
- Manage underlying cause (± antihypertensive medication) for hypertensive animals with hyperthyroidism or pheochromocytoma.
- Eliminate or control underlying trigger (± glucocorticosteroid and bronchodilator therapy) for feline bronchial disease.

CHRONIC TREATMENT
Clinicians should:
- Start cats with hyperthyroidism on oral or topical methimazole or schedule them for radioactive iodine therapy.
- Treat hyperadrenocorticism with mitotane or adrenalectomy.
- Perform an adrenalectomy for animals with pheochromocytoma.
- Initiate program for weight loss if the animal is obese.

POSSIBLE COMPLICATIONS

Bronchodilator therapy may worsen primary cardiac disease.

PROGNOSIS AND OUTCOME

Highly variable due to range of severity of underlying causes

PEARLS & CONSIDERATIONS

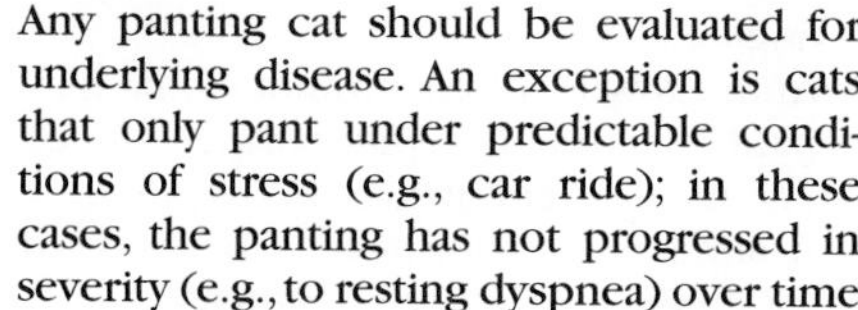

COMMENTS

Any panting cat should be evaluated for underlying disease. An exception is cats that only pant under predictable conditions of stress (e.g., car ride); in these cases, the panting has not progressed in severity (e.g., to resting dyspnea) over time and an initial physical exam has revealed no abnormalities.

SUGGESTED READING

Hackner SG: Panting. In King LG (ed): *Textbook of Respiratory Disease in Dogs and Cats*. St. Louis, WB Saunders, 2004, pp 46–48.

AUTHOR: **JEFF D. BAY**
EDITOR: **ETIENNE CÔTÉ**

Papillomas, Oral and Cutaneous

BASIC INFORMATION

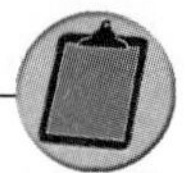

DEFINITION

Benign tumors of the skin and oral cavity caused by site-specific papilloma viruses (see Oral Neoplasia, Benign, p 769)

SYNONYM(S)

Lentiginosis profusa
Papillomas
Pigmented epidermal nevi
Verrucae
Warts

EPIDEMIOLOGY

SPECIES, AGE, SEX

- Young dogs (6 months to 4 years) or immunocompromised adults.
- Cutaneous papillomas are more often seen in males, likely due to their aggressive interactive behavior.

GENETICS AND BREED PREDISPOSITION

- Cutaneous papillomas: cocker spaniels, Kerry blue terriers
- Pigmented sessile papillomas: miniature schnauzers and pugs

RISK FACTORS

- Young and immunologically naive individuals with damaged skin or mucous membranes
- Immunosuppressed individuals (chronic use of glucocorticoids and/or oral cyclosporine)

CONTAGION AND ZOONOSIS: Contagious to other dogs via direct and indirect (fomite) contact but not to humans or cats.

ASSOCIATED CONDITIONS AND DISORDERS

- Hyperadrenocorticism
- Squamous cell carcinoma (SCC)
- Bowen's disease (SCC in situ, cats)

CLINICAL PRESENTATION

HISTORY, CHIEF COMPLAINT

- Oral: owner-observed intraoral nodule(s); oral discomfort, dysphagia, halitosis, and ptyalism possible
- Cutaneous: owner-observed cutaneous growth that often involves a distal extremity and may bleed if scratched or chewed upon; occasional lameness (footpad)

PHYSICAL EXAM FINDINGS

- Multiple growths in the oral cavity (a few millimeters to 1 cm in diameter). Initially develop as smooth white nodules before progressing to gray pedunculated masses with fronds.
- In contrast, cutaneous lesions are normally solitary and can either present as:
  - Pedunculated growth with multiple fronds, found anywhere on the body (head, eyelids, and feet most commonly affected); rarely >1 cm diameter.
  - Inverted papilloma with a small pore opening (ventral trunk and abdomen most common); typically 1–2 cm diameter.
  - Pigmented sessile plaques/nevi/lentigines dispersed in numbers from 3 or 4 up to 80, involving the ventral neck, trunk, and medial surfaces of limbs of pugs and miniature schnauzers (autosomal dominant inheritance).
  - Multiple papillomas affecting the footpads of dogs (digital keratomas). Firm, hyperkeratotic, hornlike growths that occur on multiple footpads, sometimes resulting in lameness as the primary presenting complaint.

ETIOLOGY AND PATHOPHYSIOLOGY

- Papilloma viruses are host-specific and fairly site-specific, nonenveloped, double-stranded DNA viruses that induce proliferative cutaneous and mucosal tumors in dogs.
- Infection requires inoculation via breaks in the epidermal or mucosal barrier by means of direct contact with other infected dogs or iatrogenic transmission through use of contaminated instruments.
- Incubation period is 1 to 8 weeks; regression typically occurs in 1 to 5 months, and lesions may persist for 24 months or more.
- There are at least five types of papilloma virus identified that may infect dogs.

DIAGNOSIS

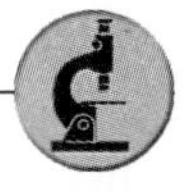

DIFFERENTIAL DIAGNOSIS

- Oral papilloma:
  - Fibromatous epulis
  - Transmissible venereal tumor
  - SCC, especially if ulcerated
- Cutaneous papilloma:
  - Pedunculated with fronds: sebaceous adenoma/hyperplasia
  - Pigmented: melanomas
  - Inverted: intracutaneous cornifying epitheliomas

INITIAL DATABASE

- Oral papillomatosis: clinical appearance is characteristic, followed by dermatohistopathologic examination if a definitive diagnosis is desired.
- Cutaneous papillomatosis is/are not as clinically evident and thus require dermatohistopathologic examination to diagnose the lesion.

ADVANCED OR CONFIRMATORY TESTING

- Immunohistochemistry: avidin-biotin complex method to detect papilloma virus group-specific antigen in tissue.
- Polymerase chain reaction (PCR) to identify cutaneous papillomas.
- Electron microscopy is the gold standard for diagnosis but is primarily used for research or publication purposes.

TREATMENT

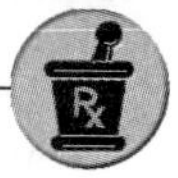

THERAPEUTIC GOAL(S)

Clinicians should:

- Identify and correct any underlying cause of immunosuppression

- Stimulate local immune defenses to self-address the virally induced lesions
- Discontinue use of systemic glucocorticoids or cyclosporine, in particular if oral or cutaneous disease recurs or persists

ACUTE GENERAL TREATMENT

- Lesions may regress spontaneously within 1 to 2 months.
- Some reports explain that crushing of 5 to 15 tumors may induce spontaneous regression.
- Surgical removal: especially if compromising normal body function (airway obstruction, dysphagia) using laser ablation, excision, cryosurgery, or electrosurgery.

CHRONIC TREATMENT

- Interferon (IFN)-α 2a either at immunostimulatory low doses of 1000 IU/ml PO q 24h, or 1.0–1.5 million IU/m^2 SC q 48–72h for 4 to 8 weeks pending response.
- Imiquimod 5% (Aldara) is a topically applied, human-approved immunomodulator that induces interleukin (IL-12), IFN-α, and IFN-γ and activates Langerhans cells at a dosing rate of two to three times weekly to affected areas; irritation is often noted and can sometimes be difficult to differentiate from resolving lesions.

RECOMMENDED MONITORING

- If benign neglect is chosen, clinicians should monitor lesions for ulceration, purulent exudation, and proliferation of growths.
- Clinicians should monitor for potential malignant transformation of affected cells to SCC.

PROGNOSIS AND OUTCOME

- Prognosis usually good.
- Spontaneous regression is likely with subsequent lifelong immunity.

PEARLS & CONSIDERATIONS

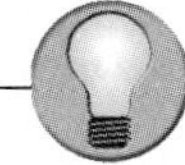

COMMENTS

Once thought to be more of a nuisance often treated by benign neglect with spontaneous regression, persistent lesions should be addressed sooner to minimize the potential metaplasia to SCC.

PREVENTION

- Owners should separate dogs with oral papillomatosis from other susceptible individuals.
- Owners should minimize chronic use of glucocorticoids and cyclosporine.

CLIENT EDUCATION

- Contagious to other dogs but not to humans and cats.
- Clinicians should monitor animals for metaplasia to SCC (rare).

SUGGESTED READING

Scott DW, Miller WH, Griffin CE: *Muller and Kirk's Small Animal Dermatology*, ed 6. Philadelphia, WB Saunders, 2001, pp 1239–1248.

Yager JA, Wilcock BP: *Color Atlas and Text of Surgical Pathology of the Dog and Cat. Volume 1. Dermatopathology and Skin Tumors*. London, Mosby-Wolfe, 1994, pp 249–252.

AUTHOR: **ANTHONY YU**

EDITOR: **JAN A. HALL**

Paraneoplastic Syndromes, Cutaneous

BASIC INFORMATION

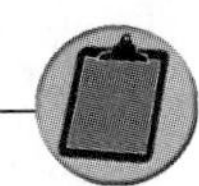

DEFINITION

Non-neoplastic skin lesions that serve as markers for internal neoplasia

SYNONYM(S)

Exfoliative dermatitis
Nodular dermatofibrosis
Paraneoplastic alopecia
Paraneoplastic pemphigus

EPIDEMIOLOGY

SPECIES, AGE, SEX

- Paraneoplastic alopecia: older cats (7 to 16 years)
- Exfoliative dermatitis: middle-aged to old cats
- Nodular dermatofibrosis: middle-aged dogs (3 to 9 years)
- Paraneoplastic pemphigus: dogs

GENETICS AND BREED PREDISPOSITION: Nodular dermatofibrosis: German shepherds; autosomal dominant inheritance.

ASSOCIATED CONDITIONS AND DISORDERS

- Paraneoplastic alopecia: pancreatic carcinoma, bile duct carcinoma
- Exfoliative dermatitis: thymoma
- Nodular dermatofibrosis: renal cystadenocarcinomas/cystadenomas, polycystic kidneys, concurrent uterine leiomyoma
- Paraneoplastic pemphigus: lymphoma, Sertoli cell tumor, mammary carcinoma

CLINICAL PRESENTATION

HISTORY, CHIEF COMPLAINT

- Paraneoplastic alopecia: progressive alopecia, weight loss, lethargy, excessive grooming.
- Exfoliative dermatitis: scaling dermatitis; alopecia; brown, waxy deposits noted on the skin.
- Nodular dermatofibrosis: nodules on the limbs, head.
- Paraneoplastic pemphigus: anorexia, ptyalism, erosive/ulcerative skin, and mucosal lesions.
- These alopecic disorders may be noted as the first manifestations (harbingers) of internal neoplasia. Internal disease is often advanced at the time of presentation, but the chief complaint commonly relates to alopecia.

PHYSICAL EXAM FINDINGS

- Paraneoplastic alopecia (Fig. I-127): nonpruritic symmetrical alopecia on ventrum, legs, face, and neck; glistening skin; fur epilates easily; dry, fissured footpads; erythema; scale; ± dehydration, emaciation
- Exfoliative dermatitis: nonpruritic scaling dermatitis on pinnae, head, generalized; variable alopecia; brown, waxy deposits around mucocutaneous areas, nail beds; variable erythema
- Nodular dermatofibrosis: nonpainful, firm cutaneous nodules on extremities; also present on the head, neck, ventral trunk
- Paraneoplastic pemphigus: depressed attitude; ulcers and erosions of the oral mucosa, mucocutaneous junctions

ETIOLOGY AND PATHOPHYSIOLOGY

- Paraneoplastic alopecia: pathogenesis may involve cytokine production, leading to atrophy of hair follicles.
- Exfoliative dermatosis: a tumor-induced immune-mediated process has been suggested.
- Nodular dermatofibrosis: collagen production within the skin may be stimulated by growth factors produced by the renal tumors; lesions develop separately through a common genetic abnormality, or simultaneous fibrosis of the skin and

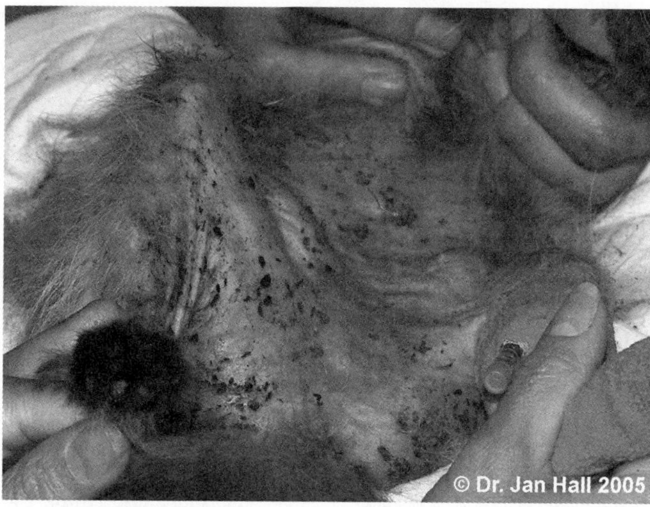

FIGURE I-127 Paraneoplastic alopecia in a 12-year-old Siamese spayed female cat. Note the characteristic glistening appearance to the skin, giving the condition its colloquial name *shiny cat disease*. Courtesy of Dr. Jan A. Hall.

kidneys results in collagenous nevi and renal outflow obstruction.
- Paraneoplastic pemphigus: cross-reactivity between tumor antigen and self-antigen or secretion of excessive immunostimulatory cytokines may be involved.

DIAGNOSIS

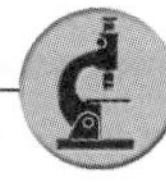

DIFFERENTIAL DIAGNOSIS

- Paraneoplastic alopecia:
  - Demodicosis
  - Dermatophytosis
  - Endocrine (hyperadrenocorticism, hyperthyroidism, hypothyroidism)
  - Immune-mediated (alopecia areata)
  - Neoplasia
  - Telogen effluvium
- Exfoliative dermatosis:
  - Demodicosis
  - Infectious agents (dermatophytosis, bacterial infections, feline leukemia virus [FeLV] infection)
  - Hypersensitivities
  - Cutaneous drug reactions
  - Autoimmune disorders
  - Neoplasia (cutaneous lymphoma)
- Nodular dermatofibrosis:
  - Primary cutaneous neoplasms
- Paraneoplastic pemphigus:
  - Pemphigus vulgaris
  - Bullous pemphigoid
  - Systemic lupus erythematosus
  - Erythema multiforme
  - Toxic epidermal necrolysis
  - Cutaneous lymphoma

INITIAL DATABASE

General database includes complete blood count (CBC), serum biochemical panel, and urinalysis. Nonspecific changes may be noted. FeLV and feline immunodeficiency virus (FIV) serologic examination is indicated in all cats, but these neoplasms are not expected to be associated with seropositive status.

- Paraneoplastic alopecia:
  - Dermatohistopathologic examination: hair follicle atrophy, telogenization, hyperkeratosis, or hypokeratosis
  - Abdominal ultrasonagraphy: liver or pancreatic neoplasia
- Exfoliative dermatosis:
  - Dermatohistopathologic examination: cell poor interface dermatitis with apoptotic keratinocytes in the stratum basal and stratum spinosum layers
  - Thoracic radiographs: mediastinal mass
- Nodular dermatofibrosis:
  - Dermatohistopathologic examination: nodular areas of collagenous hyperplasia
  - Abdominal imaging: renal cysts, renal neoplasms, or uterine neoplasms
- Paraneoplastic pemphigus:
  - Dermatohistopathologic examination: intraepithelial acantholysis, apoptotic keratinocytes, vacuolar interface dermatitis
  - Abdominal and thoracic imaging: primary neoplasm, metastases

ADVANCED OR CONFIRMATORY TESTING

- Paraneoplastic alopecia:
  - Exploratory laparotomy with pancreatic or biliary tract biopsies
- Exfoliative dermatosis:
  - Fine-needle aspiration of the mediastinal mass and cytologic examination
  - Core biopsies of the mediastinal mass
- Nodular dermatofibrosis:
  - Biopsy of renal masses
- Paraneoplastic pemphigus:
  - Biopsy of tumor
  - Indirect immunofluorescence testing:
    - Positive on stratified and nonstratified squamous epithelia
  - Western blot analysis; target antigen proteins include envoplakin (210 kDa), periplakin (190 kDa), desmoglein III (130 kDa), and an unidentified antigen (170 kDa)

TREATMENT

THERAPEUTIC GOAL(S)

- Resolve the primary neoplasm, if possible
- Provide palliative care for dermatologic lesions

ACUTE GENERAL TREATMENT

- Paraneoplastic alopecia: surgical excision of neoplasm, if possible
- Exfoliative dermatosis: surgical excision of thymoma
- Nodular dermatofibrosis: unilateral nephrectomy is rarely curative but is indicated if renal cysts are severe; bilateral renal disease is common
- Paraneoplastic pemphigus: none reported

CHRONIC TREATMENT

Nodular dermatofibrosis: surgical excision of collagenous nevi until end-stage renal failure develops

PROGNOSIS AND OUTCOME

- Paraneoplastic alopecia: grave; euthanasia due to advanced disease
- Exfoliative dermatosis: guarded; outcome depends on complete thymoma removal
- Nodular dermatofibrosis: poor for long-term survival; slowly progressive renal disease; average lifespan: 9 years of age
- Paraneoplastic pemphigus: grave unless neoplasm can be removed; euthanasia for failure to respond to immunosuppression

PEARLS & CONSIDERATIONS

COMMENTS

- Cutaneous clinical signs represent the "tip of the iceberg."
- Internal disease is often advanced at the time of presentation.
- Earlier recognition may improve outcome in some cases.
- Nodular dermatofibrosis may precede clinical signs of renal disease by 3 to 5 years and does not warrant immediate consideration of euthanasia.

SUGGESTED READING

Lemmens P, et al: Paraneoplastic pemphigus in a dog. *Vet Derm* 9:127–134, 1998.

Matousek JL: Paraneoplastic skin diseases. In Campbell KL (ed): *Small Animal Dermatology Secrets*. Philadelphia, Hanley & Belfus, 2004, pp 300–304.
Scott DW, et al: Paraneoplastic acquired alopecias. In *Muller and Kirk's Small Animal Dermatology*, ed 6. Philadelphia, WB Saunders, 2001, pp 902–905.
Turek ME: Cutaneous paraneoplastic syndromes in dogs and cats: A review of the literature. *Vet Derm* 14:279–296, 2003.

AUTHOR: **STEPHANIE R. BRUNER**
EDITOR: **JAN A. HALL**

Paraphimosis

BASIC INFORMATION

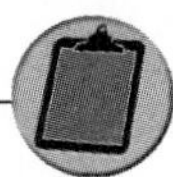

DEFINITION

Inability to retract the penis into the prepuce

EPIDEMIOLOGY

SPECIES, AGE, SEX

- Young, intact male dogs > castrated male dogs; rare in cats
- About 0.3 to 13 years of age (average age 2.9 years)

GENETICS AND BREED PREDISPOSITION

- Boxer, Chihuahua, cocker spaniel, Doberman, German shepherd, German short-haired pointer, Great Pyrenees, labrador retriever, poodle, and mongrels.
- Boxers (n = 4), poodles (n = 2), and mongrels (n = 12) have had more than one case reported.

RISK FACTORS

- Developmental preputial anomalies (e.g., small preputial opening, aplastic or hypoplastic prepuce, hypospadia [urethra opening is on the ventral penis or perineum], male pseudohermaphroditism)
- Infectious (e.g., transmissible venereal tumor, balanoposthitis)
- Neurologic deficits associated with posterior paresis (e.g., intervertebral disk disease [IVDD], spinal tumors)
- Trauma (e.g., os penis fracture)

ASSOCIATED CONDITIONS AND DISORDERS

- Balanoposthitis: inflammation of the glans penis (balanitis) and preputial mucosa (posthitis)
- Phimosis: inability to extrude the penis from the prepuce (paraphimosis occurs 14 times more frequently than phimosis in the dog)
- Priapism: prolonged penile erection with or without sexual arousal

CLINICAL PRESENTATION

DISEASE FORMS/SUBTYPES

- Acute paraphimosis: resolved within 12 hours
- Chronic paraphimosis: may be intermittent or continuous

HISTORY, CHIEF COMPLAINT: History may include recent mating, penile or preputial trauma, masturbation, balanoposthitis, neurologic disease, and/or promazine tranquilizer administration.

PHYSICAL EXAM FINDINGS

- Protrusion of the penis from the prepuce: extent of penile protrusion can vary from only the apex to the entire length of the penis.
- Penile mucosa may be erythematous, dry, inflamed, edematous, ischemic, and painful, which may lead to self-mutilation. Chronic protrusion of the penis may lead to excoriation and subsequent cornification of the mucosa.

ETIOLOGY AND PATHOPHYSIOLOGY

- Most commonly seen with a relatively stenotic preputial orifice or with ineffective preputial musculature that cannot effectively retract the penis into the prepuce.
  - Following sexual excitement or copulation, the engorged penis may become entrapped outside the prepuce (relatively stenotic preputial orifice or preputial constriction) by hair ring or scar tissue, causing penile strangulation, congestion, and paraphimosis.
  - Cranial preputial muscles (paired muscles originating from the cutaneous trunci) draw the prepuce cranially, normally, about 1 cm beyond the tip of the penis.
- About 30% of paraphimosis cases are idiopathic.

DIAGNOSIS

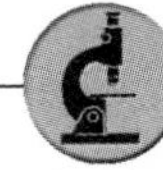

DIFFERENTIAL DIAGNOSIS

- Balanoposthitis
- Phimosis
- Priapism

INITIAL DATABASE

- Physical exam: Clinicans can make a diagnosis by visual inspection and without identifying other urogenital abnormalities.
- Neurologic exam (see Neurologic Examination, p 1286): with specific attention to posterior peripheral motor and sensory function.

ADVANCED OR CONFIRMATORY TESTING

- Electromyography and/or histopathologic evaluation on cranial preputial muscles: to identify abnormal function or cellular architecture; rarely necessary
- Radiography: to identify concomitant os penis fracture

TREATMENT

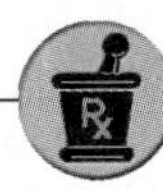

THERAPEUTIC GOAL(S)

- Returning the penis to the preputial cavity before tissue compromise
- Prevention of recurrence

ACUTE GENERAL TREATMENT

- Conservative: Clinicians can reduce the size of the penis via topical cold compresses, topical hyperosmotic solutions (e.g., sugar, honey), and systemic anti-inflammatory therapy (e.g., prednisolone sodium succinate [SoluDeltaCortef] 10 mg/kg slow IV bolus).
- Urinary catheter: to ensure patency of urethra.
- If paraphimosis occurred secondarily to promazine-induced priapism, benzotropine mesylate (0.015 mg/kg IV) should be administered as soon as possible (i.e., within 6 hours of onset of clinical signs).
- Clinicians should carefully remove hair from around the preputial orifice.
- Clinicians can attempt manual replacement of the penis in the preputial sheath using digital pressure after applying copious lubrication to the penile mucosa; if the clinician cannot return the penis to the preputial cavity, emergency surgical intervention is required.

CHRONIC TREATMENT

- To return the penis to the preputial cavity, the preputial orifice may need to be enlarged.

- After retraction within the prepuce, several surgical techniques have been described to maintain the penis within the preputial cavity; these techniques include purse-string suture at the preputial orifice; preputial orifice narrowing; preputial lengthening (preputioplasty); preputial advancement; preputial muscle myorraphy; and phallopexy. None entirely eliminates the possibility of recurrence.
- Chronic recurrence of paraphimosis can be eliminated with amputation of the penis and concurrent scrotal urethrostomy.
- Castration is often performed in conjunction with surgical correction of paraphimosis, but castration alone is not successful in correcting paraphimosis.
- Surgical repair or reconstruction of abnormalities requires a thorough understanding of normal anatomy and basic reconstruction principles.

POSSIBLE COMPLICATIONS

- Erection and ejaculation may be impaired following long-standing paraphimosis.
- Balanoposthitis secondary to phimosis may occur following surgical retention of the penis within the preputial cavity.
- Urethral stricture formation and recurrent urinary tract infections may result following penile amputation.

RECOMMENDED MONITORING

Owners should isolate intact male dogs from female dogs in estrus for at least 4 weeks following occurrence of paraphimosis.

PROGNOSIS AND OUTCOME

The prognosis is good to guarded for resolution of paraphimosis, depending on the severity and duration of clinical signs.

PEARLS & CONSIDERATIONS

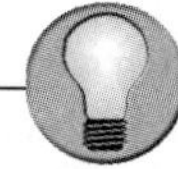

COMMENTS

Dogs with developmental preputial conditions associated with paraphimosis should not be used for breeding.

PREVENTION

- Hairs around the preputial orifice should be kept short in long-haired dogs.
- Following mating or semen collection, application of a topical lubricant to penile mucosa around the preputial opening will prevent inversion of the prepuce during detumescence (natural resolution of erection and penile retraction).

CLIENT EDUCATION

Paraphimosis may occur as a learned behavior secondarily to penile licking (masturbation). Owners should be cautioned not to promote paraphimosis by positive reinforcement.

SUGGESTED READING

Chaffee VW, Knecht CD: Canine paraphimosis: Sequel to inefficient preputial muscles. *Vet Med Small Anim Clin* 70(12):1418–1420, 1975.

Kustritz MV, Olson PN: Theriogenology question of the month. Priapism or paraphimosis. *J Am Vet Med Assoc* 214(10):1483–1484, 1999.

Ndiritu CG: Lesions of the canine penis and prepuce. *Mod Vet Pract* 60(9):1979, 712–715.

Olsen D, Salwei R: Surgical correction of a congenital preputial and penile deformity in a dog. *J Am Anim Hosp Assoc* 37(2):187–192, 2001.

Papazoglou LG: Idiopathic chronic penile protrusion in the dog: A report of six cases. *J Small Anim Pract* 42(10):510–513, 2001.

Root Kustritz MV: Disorders of the canine penis. *Vet Clin North Am Small Anim Pract* 31(2):247–258, vi, 2001.

Somerville ME, Anderson SM: Phallopexy for treatment of paraphimosis in the dog. *J Am Anim Hosp Assoc* 37(4):397–400, 2001.

AUTHOR & EDITOR: **MICHELLE A. KUTZLER**

Paraquat and Diquat Toxicoses

BASIC INFORMATION

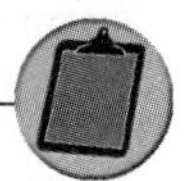

DEFINITION

Paraquat and diquat are herbicides with corrosive properties, causing acute gastrointestinal (GI) signs, abdominal pain, and oral mucosal ulcerations when ingested. Delayed pulmonary toxicity (pulmonary fibrosis) occurs with paraquat toxicosis, and central nervous system (CNS) effects can occur with diquat.

SYNONYM(S)

Paraquat: 1,1′-dimethyl-4,4′-bipyridinium or N,N′-dimethyldipyridyl dichloride

Diquat: 9,10-dihydro-8a,10a-diazoniaphenanthrene dibromide or ethylene dipyridylium dibromide

EPIDEMIOLOGY

SPECIES, AGE, SEX: Dogs are more commonly involved than cats.

GEOGRAPHY AND SEASONALITY: Accidental poisonings are more common during growing seasons; paraquat has been used year-round for malicious poisonings in dogs.

CONTAGION/ZOONOSIS: Paraquat penetrates transcutaneously in animals and humans; users should wear gloves and protective clothing.

CLINICAL PRESENTATION

HISTORY, CHIEF COMPLAINT

- Exposure to paraquat or diquat herbicide
- Clinical signs within hours to days after exposure; with acute ingestions, signs may occur within 2 to 6 hours, whereas the respiratory effects are seen in 3 to 5 days
- Paraquat: vomiting (all cases), lethargy, anorexia, diarrhea; ataxia; eventually, tachypnea and respiratory distress are apparent
- Diquat: vomiting, lethargy, anorexia, diarrhea; ataxia

PHYSICAL EXAM FINDINGS

- Paraquat: Initially, the animal may experience oral, esophageal, and gastric irritation leading to ulceration; abdominal pain; and dermatitis if topical contact; the animal may then experience hypotension, arrhythmias, weakness, and disorientation/depression due to cerebral edema. Onset of cough, dyspnea, and hemoptysis may occur 3 to 14 days after ingestion.
- Diquat: oral/pharyngeal mucosal ulceration, oliguria/anuria, dermal irritation/burns, weakness, coma and rarely, arrhythmias, seizures, and dyspnea due to noncardiogenic pulmonary edema.

ETIOLOGY AND PATHOPHYSIOLOGY

- Paraquat concentrates into lung tissue (type I and II pneumocytes). Free radicals are produced, causing cellular injury (especially pulmonary, GI, renal, and erythrocytic). Cell wall injury leads to mononuclear macrophage activation and, notably, pulmonary fibrosis, which can be fatal 3 to 14 days after ingestion. Paraquat is a restricted-use pesticide (RUP) due to its toxicity; only certified applicators can purchase the product.
- The mechanism of diquat toxicity is similar, but diquat does not accumulate in the lungs (no pulmonary fibrosis);

instead, diquat may cause cerebral hemorrhage, coma, and renal failure.

DIAGNOSIS

DIFFERENTIAL DIAGNOSIS

- Toxicosis involving any caustic or corrosive agent (acids, alkali, cationic detergents, potpourri)
- Uremic ulcers (renal failure)

INITIAL DATABASE

- Paraquat:
  - Complete blood count (CBC): neutrophilia, monocytosis, lymphopenia
  - Serum biochemistry panel: moderate increases in blood urea nitrogen (BUN), aspartate aminotransferase, and alanine aminotransferase in 24 to 96 hours and slight increases in total protein, creatinine, cholesterol, and bilirubin
  - Urinalysis: myoglobinuria (from rhabdomyolysis); proteinuria, hematuria (acute renal injury)
  - Thoracic radiographs: initially normal, progressing to noncardiogenic pulmonary edema (marked interstitial lung pattern); pneumomediastinum is a common, early finding
- Diquat: serum biochemistry panel shows BUN, creatinine elevations (within 24 to 96 hours), and liver enzyme elevations

ADVANCED OR CONFIRMATORY TESTING

- Analysis of vomitus, bait, plasma, blood, tissues, urine: Clinicians should gather samples within 48 hours of exposure because initial excretion is rapid; clinicians should contact the laboratory first.
- Histopathologic lesions:
  - Paraquat: marked pulmonary edema, hemorrhage, congestion, eventually fibrosis; mild hepatic congestion, degeneration; mild renal tubular degeneration, glomerulonephritis
  - Diquat: myocardial necrosis, cerebral hemorrhages, renal tubular damage

TREATMENT

THERAPEUTIC GOAL(S)

- Decontamination of the animal
- Supportive care

ACUTE AND CHRONIC TREATMENT

- No antidote
- Decontamination of the animal
  - Paraquat:
    - Emesis: induction of vomiting as soon as possible after ingestion even though paraquat can be irritating or corrosive to the esophagus; the possible benefits of early removal outweigh the potential risks.
    - Fuller's earth, bentonite (preferred choice over activated charcoal, but most clinics do not carry them), or activated charcoal (1-4 g/kg PO q 4-8h) can be used as an adsorbent and are most useful if given within 4 hours of exposure. Multiple doses are recommended.
    - Clinicians should bathe the entire animal if there is any dermal exposure. Paraquat is absorbed well through abraded or injured skin (wear protective clothing).
    - With ocular exposures, irrigate eyes with copious amounts of tepid water for at least 15 to 30 minutes (see Corneal Ulceration, p 246).
- Supportive care
  - IV fluids.
  - Control pain as needed (e.g., for dogs/cats: 0.005-0.03 mg/kg IV, IM, or SC q 6-12h buprenorphine, or fentanyl patch).
  - Ascorbic acid (antioxidant) 20-30 mg/kg IM, IV, or PO q 8h may be useful.
  - Avoid supplemental oxygen therapy because it increases the formation of superoxide free radicals.
  - Treatment of ventricular arrhythmias (see Ventricular Arrhythmias, p 1148), seizures (see Seizures, p 990), secondary infections, oral ulcers (see Ulcers, Oral Mucosal, p 1110), gastric ulcers (see Gastric Ulcer, p 431), and renal complications (see Acute Renal Failure, p 32) as needed.
  - Positive-pressure ventilation may be used, but lung lesion may become (or may already be) irreversible.
- Diquat
  - Emesis is usually not recommended unless the animal has been exposed to a very large dose of the toxin.
  - Activated charcoal, bentonite clay, or Fuller's earth, same dosage as for paraquat.
  - With dermal exposure, the animal's skin should be immediately washed with soap and water. Diquat can be absorbed through damaged or injured skin, resulting in systemic poisoning. Absorption through intact skin is minimal.
  - Ocular exposures: same treatment as for paraquat.
  - Supportive care: as just described; treatment of chronic renal failure if present.

POSSIBLE COMPLICATIONS

- Paraquat: pneumothorax, pneumopericardium, and subcutaneous emphysema
- Diquat: pneumonia, renal failure

RECOMMENDED MONITORING

- Paraquat: baseline thoracic radiographs and blood gases and serial monitoring for several days (CBC and renal and liver panels)
- Diquat: renal values (monitor for 3 to 4 days with large ingestions) and monitor CBC, liver enzymes, and electrolytes

PROGNOSIS AND OUTCOME

- Paraquat: outcome appears to be related to dose and early intervention (decontamination of animal); poor prognosis for affected animals showing any clinical signs; those that survive the acute toxicosis often succumb to chronic pulmonary fibrosis
- Diquat: good prognosis with early and aggressive treatment

PEARLS & CONSIDERATIONS

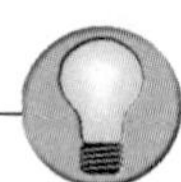

COMMENTS

- Paraquat LD50 (dogs, oral) 25-50 mg/kg.
- Diquat LD50 (dogs, oral) 100 mg/kg.
- Concentration of diquat in most ready-to-use weed and grass killer products is <1%. Systemic effects from these products is highly unlikely with casual exposure (e.g., dog walking through the sprayed area when it was still wet or dog licking the grass after spray) unless large amounts have been ingested from the container.

PREVENTION

Keep animals away from all herbicides until dry; dipyridyl herbicides are rapidly and completely inactivated in the soil.

CLIENT EDUCATION

Follow label directions on all herbicides

SUGGESTED READING

O'Sullivan SP: Paraquat poisoning in the dog. *J Small Anim Pract* 30(6):361-364, 1989.

Shuler CM, et al: Retrospective case series of suspected intentional paraquat poisonings: Diagnostic findings and risk factors for death. *Vet Hum Toxicol Dec* 46(6):313-314, 2004.

http://extoxnet.orst.edu/pips/paraquat.htm.

AUTHOR: **TINA WISMER**

EDITOR: **SAFDAR A. KHAN**

Paresis, Forelimb

BASIC INFORMATION

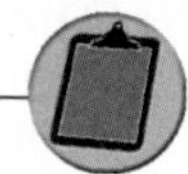

DEFINITION

- Monoparesis: partial loss of motor function to one limb
- Monoplegia/paralysis: complete loss of motor function to one limb

CLINICAL PRESENTATION

HISTORY, CHIEF COMPLAINT: Weakness, lameness, or inability to use a forelimb.

PHYSICAL EXAM FINDINGS

- Lower motor neuron (LMN) signs to the affected limb: weakness and decreased muscle tone
- Variable degree: mild forelimb lameness to complete loss of motor function
- Denervation atrophy of forelimb musculature with chronicity
- Nerve root signature: lameness and pain of affected forelimb caused by entrapment of a nerve root within the brachial plexus (see Brachial Plexus Abnormalities, p 148; Root Signature Nerve, p 976)
- Suspicion of neoplasia if chronic progressive monoparesis, nerve root signature, and denervation atrophy
- Variable exam findings also may include:
  - Horner's syndrome (ipsilateral)
  - Loss of cutaneous trunci reflex (ipsilateral)
  - Palpable mass in axilla
  - Dysesthesia/paresthesia of limb and secondary self-trauma
  - Traumatic injury/fracture

ETIOLOGY AND PATHOPHYSIOLOGY

- Central nervous system (CNS):
  - Lesions affecting spinal cord segments C6–T2 can cause LMN forelimb signs.
  - Flaccid forelimb monoparesis.
  - Basis: injury to LMN cell bodies that innervate forelimb musculature.
  - Usually associated with upper motor neuron signs to ipsilateral pelvic limb.
- Peripheral nervous system:
  - Spinal/peripheral nerve disorders cause sensory and motor dysfunction distal to the lesion (permanent nerve damage or temporary, self-resolving trauma called neuropraxia).
    - Trauma: brachial plexus avulsion and radial nerve injury, as examples.
    - Neoplasia: commonly affected are brachial plexus and dorsal nerve roots.
- Cervicothoracic spinal cord, nerve roots, sympathetic trunk: Horner's syndrome (ipsilateral).
- Lateral thoracic nerve (C8, T1) disruption causes ipsilateral loss of the panniculus reflex.

DIAGNOSIS

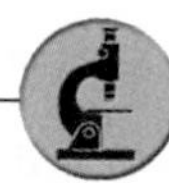

DIFFERENTIAL DIAGNOSIS

- CNS
  - Trauma
  - Vascular
  - Neoplasia
  - Infectious
- Peripheral nervous system
  - Trauma
  - Vascular
  - Neoplasia

INITIAL DATABASE

- Complete blood count (CBC), serum biochemistry panel, urinalysis: generally unremarkable
- Orthopedic and cardiovascular evaluation: rule out concurrent diseases
- Neurologic exam (gait, posture, spinal reflexes; identify sites of sensory loss)
- Forelimb, spinal radiographs (bone fractures, luxations, neoplasia, or infection)

ADVANCED OR CONFIRMATORY TESTING

- Myelogram or MRI to localize unilateral spinal cord compression (intervertebral disk disease [IVDD] or neoplasia)
- CT scan to evaluate for nerve/nerve sheath tumors
- Electrodiagnostics (electromyography, nerve conduction) to localize the dysfunctional spinal cord segment, nerve root, or peripheral nerve
- Surgical exploration (based on imaging results):
  - Biopsy, histopathologic examination for suspected neoplasia
  - Evaluation of type, extent, and severity of nerve injury

TREATMENT

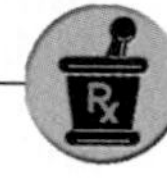

THERAPEUTIC GOAL(S)

- Pain relief
- Return to neurologic function and ambulation

ACUTE GENERAL TREATMENT

- CNS
  - Trauma:
    - Spinal fracture/luxation (see Spinal Cord Trauma, p 1023).
      - Mild/moderate neurologic deficits and stable spine.
        - Medical management.
      - Severe neurologic deficits and/or unstable spine.
        - Referral to neurosurgeon for decompression and stabilization.
    - Intervertebral disk herniation: spinal cord segment C6–T2 (see Intervertebral Disk Disease, p 601).
      - Intravenous methylprednisolone if within 8 hours of injury.
      - Mild neurologic deficits: oral prednisone and methocarbamol for 2 weeks, strict cage confinement for 4 weeks.
      - Moderate/severe neurologic deficits: referral to neurosurgeon for surgical decompression if indicated.
  - Vascular:
    - Fibrocartilaginous embolism (FCE).
      - Methylprednisolone IV if within 8 hours of injury.
  - Neoplasia:
    - Based on tumor location and invasiveness.
  - Infectious:
    - Diskospondylitis.
      - Appropriate antibiotics, analgesics, strict confinement (4 to 6 weeks minimum).
- Peripheral nervous system
  - Trauma:
    - Brachial plexus avulsion (see Brachial Plexus Abnormalities, p 148).
      - Stabilization, assessment for concurrent injuries, prevention of secondary limb trauma; amputation considered if failure to improve in 4 to 6 months or if complications.
    - Peripheral nerve injury.
      - Depends on injury type and severity and the degree of wound contamination.
        - Medical management (wound care, secondary trauma prevention) is recommended for contaminated wounds and compression, crushing, stretching injuries; a minimum 3 months is required for accurate assessment of return to function (see Soft Tissue Trauma of the Extremities, p 1018).
        - Surgical management: referral to neurosurgeon for primary nerve repair (lacerated/entrapped nerve).
  - Neoplasia: Surgical recommendations depend on the location and invasiveness of the tumor.

CHRONIC TREATMENT

- Physical rehabilitation (see Physical Rehabilitation, p 1300); the animal should continue treatment for 3 to 6 months or until it shows signs of reinnervation.
- Adequate protection of an affected limb to prevent secondary trauma and self-mutilation.

POSSIBLE COMPLICATIONS

- Failure to regain adequate function of affected limb
- Local recurrence of nerve root tumors
- Persistent trauma, self-mutilation, or contracture of paretic limb necessitating amputation

RECOMMENDED MONITORING

- Monitoring of limb daily for signs of trauma or self-mutilation
- Serial neurologic examinations for up to 6 months to evaluate limb for reinnervation
- Monitoring for evidence of recurrence of nerve root tumor by physical exam and CT scan if indicated

PROGNOSIS AND OUTCOME

- Largely depends on the neurologic exam at presentation and response to treatment
- Central
  - Intervertebral disk herniation:
    - Fair to excellent if good deep pain perception
    - Guarded to poor with poor deep pain sensation if addressed within 8 hours
    - Poor to grave if poor deep pain sensation and addressed after 8 hours
  - FCE:
    - Approximately 50% chance for return to function of limb
  - Neoplasia:
    - Guarded to poor based on surgical accessibility and follow-up care
- Peripheral
  - Brachial plexus avulsion:
    - Generally poor; often requires amputation
  - Peripheral nerve injuries:
    - Fair to good for mild neurologic deficits, sharp lacerations with prompt surgical repair and short distance from site of injury to end organ
    - Guarded to poor for severe neurologic deficits; stretching, crushing, and avulsion injuries; contaminated wounds with delayed surgical repair; and large distance from site of injury to end organ
  - Nerve sheath tumors:
    - Guarded to poor because local recurrence is common

PEARLS & CONSIDERATIONS

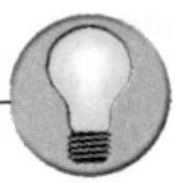

COMMENTS

Brachial plexus avulsions with severe traction on the nerve roots may cause damage to the spinal pathways, resulting in pelvic limb deficits that are generally ipsilateral but can be bilateral.

CLIENT EDUCATION

- Clinicians should inform clients of prognosis, expected duration of forelimb paresis, and potential for failure to regain adequate function of limb, which necessitates amputation.
- Clinicians should perform or recommend physical rehabilitation techniques.

AUTHOR: **DAN POLIDORO**
EDITOR: **ETIENNE CÔTÉ**

Paresis, Hind Limb

BASIC INFORMATION

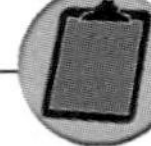

DEFINITION

Paraparesis is defined as partial loss of motor to the pelvic limbs. Paraparalysis or paraplegia is a complete loss of voluntary motor to the pelvic limbs.

EPIDEMIOLOGY

SPECIES, AGE, SEX: Any species, age, or sex can be affected.

GENETICS AND BREED PREDISPOSITION

- Young to middle-aged chondrodystrophoid dogs (e.g., basset hounds, dachshunds, beagles) are predisposed to intervertebral disk disease (IVDD), especially Hansen type I.
- Middle-aged to older nonchondrodystrophoid dogs (e.g., German shepherds) are predisposed to IVDD, especially Hansen type II.
- German shepherds (geriatric) are overrepresented in degenerative myelopathy.

CONTAGION AND ZOONOSIS: In some cases where underlying etiology is infectious (e.g., rabies).

CLINICAL PRESENTATION

DISEASE FORMS/SUBTYPES: Hind limb paresis or paralysis can present as difficulty or inability to use the hind limbs due to weakness, incoordination (ataxia), or spasticity (limb stiffness caused by a neurologic lesion). Weakness suggests a lower motor neuron or neuromuscular lesion, whereas spasticity and ataxia suggest an upper motor neuron lesion.

HISTORY, CHIEF COMPLAINT: Inability to walk on the hind legs.

PHYSICAL EXAM FINDINGS

- Assessment of the femoral pulse; if absent, consider aortic thromboembolism as a diagnosis.
- Palpation of the bones of limbs, pelvis (including rectal exam in dogs), and vertebral column for fractures/luxations.
- Fundic exam: for evidence of multifocal/diffuse central nervous system (CNS) inflammation.
- Neurologic injuries: physical findings depend on severity of lesion.
- Gait varies from mild hind limb ataxia to a nonambulatory status without deep pain perception.
- Spinal reflexes (e.g., patellar):
  - Hyporeflexia: lesion in L4-S2 spinal cord segments
  - Hyperreflexia: lesion in T3-L3 spinal cord segments
- Spinal hyperpathia (back pain on palpation):
  - Presence: may indicate IVDD, neoplasia, or trauma
  - Absence: may indicate embolism or degenerative cord process
- Muscle tone:
  - Increased (spasticity): lesion in T3-L3 spinal cord segments
  - Decreased: lesion in L4-S2 spinal cord segments

ETIOLOGY AND PATHOPHYSIOLOGY

- IVDD (see Intervertebral Disk Disease, p 601):
  - Degenerative disk changes lead to herniation of the nucleus pulposus into the spinal canal.
    - Hansen type I disk rupture: focal, acute myelopathy
    - Hansen type II disk rupture: chronic, progressive disk (annulus) bulging into the spinal canal; chronic, slowly progressive myelopathy
- Fibrocartilaginous embolization:
  - Herniation of disk material into vertebral body and entrance into the venous plexus.
- Degenerative myelopathies:
  - Progressive, diffuse degeneration of spinal cord myelin and axons.

DIAGNOSIS

DIFFERENTIAL DIAGNOSIS

- Acute, nonprogressive: intervertebral disk rupture, fracture/luxation, fibrocartilaginous embolism, aortic thromboembolism
- Acute progressive: intervertebral disk rupture (type I), hemorrhagic myelomalacia, neoplasia, infectious/inflammatory (distemper myelitis; bacterial, protozoal, or fungal myelitis; granulomatous meingoencephalitis; feline infectious peritonitis; diskospondylitis)
- Chronic progressive: IVDD (type II), degenerative myelopathies, neoplasia, infectious/inflammatory (as previously stated)

INITIAL DATABASE

- Complete blood count (CBC), serum biochemistry panel, urinalysis: may reflect stress or underlying infectious cause (less common)
- Complete orthopedic and cardiovascular evaluation to rule out concurrent disease
- Spinal radiographs to evaluate animal for bony lesions, such as fracture, neoplasm, or infection

ADVANCED OR CONFIRMATORY TESTING

- Myelogram or MRI: spinal cord compression secondary to IVDD or neoplasia or changes consistent with infection.
- Cerebrospinal fluid (CSF) analysis: evidence of infection, inflammation, exfoliating neoplasia.
- Serum or CSF titers: to assess for infectious etiologies, especially if initial CSF analysis suggests active inflammation.
- CSF culture if indicated by cytologic examination report.

TREATMENT

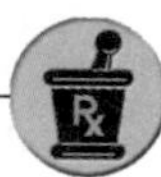

THERAPEUTIC GOAL(S)

- Pain relief.
- Animals should regain neurologic function and ambulation as well as bladder and bowel function.

ACUTE GENERAL TREATMENT

- Acute traumatic spinal cord injuries: clinicians should consider initial methylprednisolone (30 mg/kg IV, then 15 mg/kg IV 2 and 4 hours later; if no improvement, clinicians can consider surgical intervention).
  - Must be given within the first 8 hours to be effective
  - Further evaluation to determine need for surgery
- Mild neurologic deficits secondary to intervertebral disk rupture: consider prednisone (1 mg/kg PO q 12h) and methocarbamol (20 mg/kg PO q 8h) for 2 weeks and strict cage confinement for 4 weeks.
- Evaluation of animals that have moderate to severe neurologic deficits with advanced imaging (myelogram/MRI) and then surgical decompression if indicated; referral to veterinary surgeon or neurosurgeon is recommended.

CHRONIC TREATMENT

Nursing care:

- Preventing pressure sores, urinary tract infections, muscle atrophy
- Hygiene: providing clean, dry, well-padded bedding
- Performing manual urinary bladder expression or catheterization if not voiding normally
- Performing physical rehabilitation exercises as indicated (see Physical Rehabilitation p 1300)

POSSIBLE COMPLICATIONS

Methylprednisolone may cause gastrointestinal (GI) ulceration.

RECOMMENDED MONITORING

- Reevaluation of animal's neurologic function at 4-week intervals; duration of reevaluation is based on the animal's progress.
- If the dog remains nonambulatory after weeks or months, without signs of limbs returning to function, a canine cart is an option.

PROGNOSIS AND OUTCOME

Based on preoperative neurologic exam and underlying disease

- Acute spinal lesion in an animal with good deep pain perception: fair to excellent for return to near normal neurologic function with surgery.
- If deep pain perception is not present: prognosis is guarded to poor if surgical lesion is addressed in the first 8 hours and poor to grave if after 8 hours.
- Chronic spinal cord compression in an animal with good deep pain perception: fair to good prognosis with a prospect of a longer recovery with surgical decompression.
- Nonsurgical spinal cord disease has a variable prognosis depending on underlying etiology.

PEARLS & CONSIDERATIONS

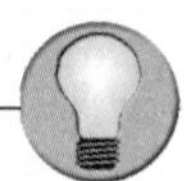

COMMENTS

Immediate referral to a surgeon or neurosurgeon is warranted for an animal that is decompensating neurologically.

CLIENT EDUCATION

- Preoperative prognosis often guarded; potential for prolonged postoperative nursing care.
- It is essential to respect a recommendation of a period of cage rest/confinement.

SUGGESTED READING

Ferriera AJ, Carriera JH, Jaggy A: Thoracolumbar disc disease in 71 paraplegic dogs: Influence of rate of onset and duration of clinical signs on treatment results. *J Small Animal Pract* 43(4):158-163, 2002.

Hart RC, Jerram RM, Schulz KS: Postoperative management of the canine spinal patient. *Compend Contin Educ Pract Vet.* 19(10):1133-1149, 1997.

Simpson ST: Intervertebral disc disease. *Vet Clin North Am Small Anim Pract* 22(4):889-897, 1992.

AUTHOR: **SHARON L. SHIELDS**

EDITOR: **ETIENNE CÔTÉ**

Parturition, Normal

BASIC INFORMATION

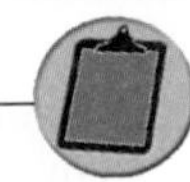

DEFINITION

The act or process of giving birth to puppies or kittens

SYNONYM(S)

Queening: parturition in the queen (female cat)
Whelping: parturition in the bitch

EPIDEMIOLOGY

SPECIES, AGE, SEX

- Canine, adult, female
- Feline, adult, female

ASSOCIATED CONDITIONS AND DISORDERS: Premature parturition.

CLINICAL PRESENTATION

HISTORY, CHIEF COMPLAINT: Bitch or queen uncomfortable about 60 days after breeding; may have vaginal discharge.

PHYSICAL EXAM FINDINGS

- Rectal temperature normal to low normal. Normal temperature ranges: 100.2-102.8°F (37.8-39.3°C) in the bitch, 100.5-102.5°F (38.0-39.2°C) in the queen, with additional variation based on environment, body condition, and other factors
- Slightly increased to normal respiration and heart rates
- Dam may show abdominal contractions
- Examiner may be able to feel puppies or kittens by abdominal palpation

ETIOLOGY AND PATHOPHYSIOLOGY

- Parturition is a normal process of delivering pups or kittens.
- Three stages of whelping:
  - Stage 1: cervical dilation, 3 to 6 hours
  - Stage 2: fetal expulsion, 3 to 6 hours
  - Stage 3: placental expulsion, 5 to 15 minutes
- Dystocia or difficult birth may become an outcome of unproductive abdominal contractions.

DIAGNOSIS

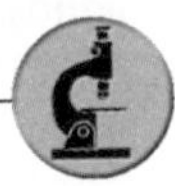

DIFFERENTIAL DIAGNOSIS

- Pseudopregnancy
- Premature birth
- Pyometra

INITIAL DATABASE

- Pups or kittens are present on abdominal palpation
- Confirmation of the presence of fetal skeletons: abdominal radiography after 42 days of gestation
- Evaluation of fetal health: abdominal ultrasonography after about 25 days of pregnancy

ADVANCED OR CONFIRMATORY TESTING

Tocodynamometry can be used for monitoring uterine contractility. An increase in the frequency and amplitude of uterine contractions occurs at the onset of stage 2 parturition.

TREATMENT

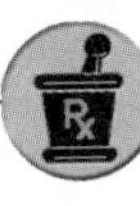

- Bitches and queens with normal parturition do not require any treatment.
- In cases of dystocia, the female should be evaluated for medical or surgical intervention.

THERAPEUTIC GOAL(S)

Delivery of healthy puppies or kittens without compromising mother's health

ACUTE GENERAL TREATMENT

- In normal parturition, treatment is not needed
- If parturition is not normal, see Dystocia, p 327

POSSIBLE COMPLICATIONS

- If the bitch or queen has prolonged abdominal contractions without delivery of a fetus, or appears to be in constant intense pain, she should be evaluated by a clinician. Dystocia (or difficult birth) may be due to inadequate size of birth canal and/or an oversized fetus, birth canal obstruction, or uterine inertia due to hypocalcemia and/or hypoglycemia (see Dystocia, p 327).
- In cases of dystocia, treatment with oxytocin, calcium, and/or glucose products may be indicated if the cervix is open (see Dystocia, p 327).
- Cesarean section if dystocia is not amenable to medical treatment or prophylactically if dystocia is anticipated (e.g., fetal-maternal size mismatch).

RECOMMENDED MONITORING

- Clinicians can monitor the puppy or kitten delivery and be available to assist if needed (e.g., if dystocia occurs, if puppies experience distress).
- Clinicians should make sure a placenta is delivered following each fetus.

PROGNOSIS AND OUTCOME

- Good if parturition is normal
- Fair to guarded in cases of dystocia

PEARLS & CONSIDERATIONS

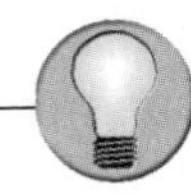

COMMENTS

- As a normal process, animal owners and breeders prefer that the female delivers pups or kittens at home in familiar surroundings.
- Oxytocin treatment to assist delivery process should be used only if the cervix is open.
- Dark-green colored lochia or postpartum vaginal discharge before the delivery of any pups in the bitch is an indication of premature placental separation. The bitch should be evaluated for fetal viability by abdominal ultrasonography and may require a cesarean section to remove fetuses.

PREVENTION

Ovariohysterectomy will prevent pregnancy and parturition from occurring.

CLIENT EDUCATION

For prepartum bitches, the client should monitor the rectal temperature two to three times daily, beginning at 56 days postbreeding. Rectal temperature drops by 1-2°F (hypothermia) about 8 to 12 hours before whelping.

SUGGESTED READING

Johnston S, Root Kustritz M, Olson P: *Canine and Feline Theriogenology*. Philadelphia, WB Saunders, 2001.

AUTHORS: **MUSHTAQ A. MEMON, MICHELLE A. KUTZLER**
EDITOR: **MICHELLE A. KUTZLER**

Parvoviral Enteritis

Client Education Sheet on Website

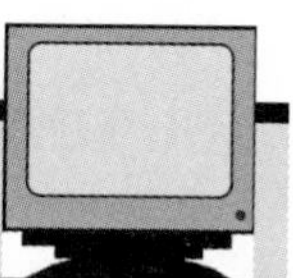

BASIC INFORMATION

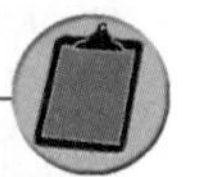

DEFINITION

A viral infection that destroys the crypt cells of the villous epithelium of the small intestine together with lymphocyte depletion and neutropenia, leading to severe enteritis, anorexia, vomiting, hemorrhagic diarrhea, and shock

EPIDEMIOLOGY

SPECIES, AGE, SEX: Dogs only; parvoviral enteritis almost exclusively affects puppies (<8 months old) and unvaccinated adults.

GENETICS AND BREED PREDISPOSITION: Suspected predisposition for Doberman pinscher, rottweiler, pit bull, German shepherd, and dachshund breeds; toy poodles and cocker spaniels have below-normal degree of risk.

RISK FACTORS

- Unvaccinated puppies or pups less than 7 weeks of age with poor maternal immunity; unvaccinated dogs are 12.7 times more likely than vaccinated dogs to develop parvoviral enteritis.
- Exposure to high viral loads.
- Immunosuppression (systemic illness, cancer chemotherapy).

CONTAGION AND ZOONOSIS

- Extremely resistant virus (parvovirus 1 and 2) that can survive more than 7 months in the environment (longer if frozen over winter months) and is resistant to most disinfectants.
    - Diluted bleach (1:32 bleach:water) and quaternary ammonium disinfectants (Parvosol, Roccal-D, quats, and others) effectively kill parvovirus.
- Highly contagious to other dogs via the fecal-oral route.
    - Fecal shedding begins 4 to 5 days after exposure (i.e., before the onset of overt clinical illness, which occurs 6 to 10 days after exposure).
    - Shedding generally occurs for a total of 7 to 10 days, usually ending by day 14 after exposure.
    - An animal that is discharged after successful treatment of parvoviral enteritis has a low risk of contagion to other dogs through feces it passes (for 3 weeks), but there is a high risk of transmitting contagion through fecal staining on the haircoat or in feces or vomit produced at home immediately prior to hospitalization.
- Shedding of vaccine (attenuated live) parvovirus occurs for several days after vaccination; there is no contagion risk, but the shedding may produce a false-positive reaction on fecal ELISA testing for parvovirus.
- Species-specific; no clinically relevant transmission to cats or other species and no zoonotic transmission.

GEOGRAPHY AND SEASONALITY: Occurs worldwide and year-round but is more common in warmer, wetter seasons. Most commonly seen in spring when the majority of puppies are born. However, in a Canadian study, dogs were three times more likely to be admitted with parvoviral enteritis in July, August, or September compared with the rest of the year.

ASSOCIATED CONDITIONS AND DISORDERS

- Helminthiasis, giardiasis, coccidiosis, and coronavirus infections may occur concurrently.
- Clinicians should always suspect sepsis in parvoviral enteritis cases because bacteremia is common: in 90% of dogs that died of parvoviral enteritis, microbial liver or lung cultures revealed growth of *Escherichia coli*.

CLINICAL PRESENTATION

DISEASE FORMS/SUBTYPES: Subclinical, mild, moderate, and severe enteritis.

HISTORY, CHIEF COMPLAINT

- Onset of signs 3 to 14 days after exposure (if known)
- Acute onset of lethargy (often first sign), anorexia, vomiting, and diarrhea (often hemorrhagic)

PHYSICAL EXAM FINDINGS

- Mild cases may be unremarkable.
- Moderate and severely affected puppies are typically lethargic, dehydrated (tacky oral mucous membranes), with palpably fluid filled intestines; abdominal palpation may induce vomiting or retching, and fever and tachycardia are common.
- Severely affected puppies may present in hypovolemic shock, with altered mentation (may be due to septic shock, hypoglycemia), and hypothermia.

ETIOLOGY AND PATHOPHYSIOLOGY

- Parvoviral infection with a 3- to 14-day incubation period
- Parvoviral predilection for rapidly dividing cells
- Destruction of intestinal crypt epithelium, causing sloughing of intestinal mucosa, vomiting, diarrhea, and sepsis from translocation of enteric bacteria into the portal circulation
- Lymphocyte depletion and neutropenia
- Glucose and potassium depletion/loss
- Dehydration and sepsis

DIAGNOSIS

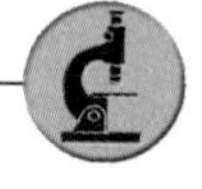

DIFFERENTIAL DIAGNOSIS

- Any severe acute gastroenteritis
- Distemper
- Salmonellosis
- Coronaviral enteritis
- Foreign body/intussusception

INITIAL DATABASE

- ELISA test for parvovirus in feces: diagnostic test of choice.
    - Sensitive and specific
    - False-positive result possible with recent vaccination (beginning 5 days after vaccination and continuing for 1 week)
    - False-negative result possible with fecal sample obtained outside period of shedding or profusely hemorrhagic diarrhea (diluted or complexed antigen fails to react with test antibody)
- Fecal flotation and fecal wet preparation: Concurrent helminthiasis is common.
- Complete blood count (CBC): Leukopenia (neutropenia) is common and supports the need for broad-spectrum antibiotic treatment. If financial restrictions: hematocrit, total solids, and blood smear as a minimum for hematologic examination.
- Serum biochemistry panel: hypokalemia, hypoalbuminemia, and hypoglycemia are common, correctable secondary effects of parvoviral enteritis. Azotemia (often prerenal) and liver enzyme elevations are common. If severe financial restrictions: serum potassium, albumin, and glucose as a minimum for serum biochemistry.
- Urinalysis: generally unremarkable; specific gravity >1.035 confirms prerenal source of azotemia.
- Abdominal radiography: to avoid misdiagnosis (e.g., identify foreign body) and to detect abnormalities secondary to parvoviral enteritis (e.g., obstruction due to intussusception).

ADVANCED OR CONFIRMATORY TESTING

Financial considerations often result in empiric therapy without a confirmed diagnosis beyond fecal ELISA testing. In cases of financial restriction, it is considered more important to direct veterinary costs toward treating the pup rather than toward performing exhaustive diagnostic testing. While doing so carries a risk of missing important information, which the owner must accept, most puppies will recover with supportive care; without treatment, the mortality rate is high.

TREATMENT

THERAPEUTIC GOAL(S)

- Rehydration
- Treatment or prevention of sepsis
- Correction of potassium and glucose levels
- Normalization of blood pressure (BP)
- Cessation of vomiting
- Pain control
- ± Enteral nutrition
- Avoiding iatrogenic complications (e.g., risk of abscess formation with subcutaneous injections in parvovirus cases [especially with neutropenia])

ACUTE GENERAL TREATMENT

See Table I-21 below

CHRONIC TREATMENT

- Continuation of IV fluids, antibiotic therapy, pain control, antiemetic treatment, and nutrition as described in Table I-21 below
- Repeated blood, plasma, colloid, or polymerized hemoglobin (Oxyglobin) transfusions as often as needed
- To control vomiting, after ensuring no obstruction (e.g., intussusception), clinicians can perform the following steps:
  - Step 1: CRI metoclopramide (as previously described).
  - Step 2: add ondansetron (0.5-1 mg/kg IV q 12-24h) or dolasetron (0.6 mg/kg PO q 24h).
  - Step 3: add prochlorperazine (often given as a suppository).
- Diet:
  - High-protein, high-calorie foods (e.g., Eukanuba Max Calorie, Hill's Science Diet A/D) diluted with as little water as possible.
  - It is the author's opinion that a small volume of food is far more important than a low-fat content.
- Deworming:
  - Fenbendazole 50 mg/kg PO q 24h, 3-5 days (if >12 weeks old); or
  - Ivermectin 0.2 mg/kg SC once.

TABLE I-21 Initial Treatment of Parvoviral Enteritis in Puppies

At Admission	• Place IV catheter, administer IV antibiotics (cefazolin 22 mg/kg IV q 8h, or ampicillin 22 mg/kg IV q 6h). If leukopenia: add enrofloxacin 7.5-10 mg/kg slow IV q 24h, or, once patient is rehydrated, gentamicin 6 mg/kg IV q 24h. Fluoroquinolones are potentially contraindicated in young animals and aminoglycosides are contraindicated in hypovolemia/dehydration ◦ Test: hematocrit /total protein/glucose • IV crystalloid fluid bolus (e.g., lactated Ringer's solution 60 ml/kg) if hypovolemic shock
1st 2 Hours	• Calculate fluid needs (i.e., sum of: rehydration + maintenance + ongoing losses for first 12 hours). Note: Rehydration (ml) = % dehydration (expressed as a percent [7% is 7]) × body weight in kg × 10 • Maintenance is 65 ml/kg/day (30 cc/lb/day) • Give 1/4 to 1/2 of amount over first 2 hours to correct intravascular volume and blood pressure (warm fluids to body temperature) • Colloids can be used at 10-20 ml/kg IV over 1 to 4 hours if shock is present or if albumin is low. Recall additional cost of colloids
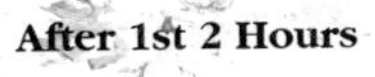 **After 1st 2 Hours**	• Give rest of fluid allotment over next 10 hours ◦ Test hematocrit + total protein + serum potassium + serum/blood glucose • Warm patient on heating pad at this point if needed [not before, as doing so may dilate peripheral vasculature] • Add glucose to fluids if needed (50 ml of 50% dextrose in 1 liter bag = 2.5% or 100 ml of 50% dextrose in 1 liter bag = 5%) • Plasma or polymerized hemoglobin (Oxyglobin) can be administered as an immunotherapy (plasma) and for oncotic pressure. Potentially indicated if plasma albumin <1.5 mg/dl • Blood transfusion or polymerized hemoglobin indicated if status worsening and hematocrit <20%
Approx. 2–3 Hours	• Metoclopramide IV constant rate infusion (CRI) (1-2 mg/kg/day) to treat ileus and/or vomiting • Pain control: Buprenorphine (0.01 mg/kg IV q 6h) or butorphanol (0.1-0.2 mg/kg IV q 4-6h) • Amikacin/gentamicin IV if not already administered and blood pressure has improved, or enrofloxacin if a concern persists regarding nephrotoxicity ◦ Test: blood pressure, palpate for urine in bladder, confirm capillary refill time <2 seconds
Approx. 4–5 Hours	• Start to feed (aim for at least 1/3 of requirements over next 24 hours). Some clinicians will advocate feeding despite vomiting • Calculate energy requirements with formula: kcal = [(body weight (kg) × 30) +70] × illness factor (1.25-1.5) • See main text for added control of vomition and diet
Approx. 12 Hours	• Reassess hydration (weigh patient often): continue rehydration as needed • In pups with large ongoing losses, fluid rates may be very high (5-10 ml/kg/hr). Titrate fluid rate to hydration, perfusion and clinical signs (vomiting and diarrhea)

DRUG INTERACTIONS

- Flunixin meglumine is nephrotoxic and gastric ulcerogenic and should be avoided in animals that are hypovolemic.
- Fluoroquinolones (5 mg/kg q 24h) used for 5 to 8 days should be safe and *not* cause cartilage problems.
- Ivermectin deworming is not advised in debilitated patients.

POSSIBLE COMPLICATIONS

- Intussusception or rectal prolapse
- Septic arthritis or endocarditis
- Acute respiratory distress syndrome
- Pneumonia (embolic, aspiration, or opportunistic [e.g., canine distemper])

RECOMMENDED MONITORING

- Clinicians should monitor the following at admission, after 2 hours of fluid therapy, and then at least on a daily basis in patients that are still ill:
  - Body weight
  - Blood glucose
  - Hematocrit and total solids
  - Serum potassium
- Pediatric sampling tubes and very small quantities of blood should be used. Once the puppy is eating, monitoring should be curtailed or stopped to avoid overinterpretation of results in an animal that is improving.

PROGNOSIS AND OUTCOME

Good with correct therapy. Following the treatment protocol outlined previously, a 93-95% success rate is expected with severely ill, confirmed cases of parvoviral enteritis.

PEARLS & CONSIDERATIONS

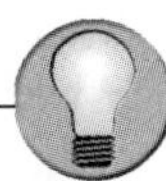

COMMENTS

Essential aspects of management include:

- Normalize hydration, potassium, and glucose
- Control vomiting

- Control pain
- Feed early

PREVENTION

- Ensure adequate vaccination status.
- Owners should limit environmental access for puppies until they are fully vaccinated.
- Dogs that survive parvoviral enteritis generally have immunity to reinfection (lifelong).

CLIENT EDUCATION

- Parvovirus remains in the environment for up to 7 months or more; indoor surfaces should be cleaned and then disinfected with diluted bleach, and only vaccinated adult dogs should be allowed in the dog's immediate environment.
- Serial vaccination of all puppies until at least 12 weeks of age is essential; typical protocols involve vaccination at age 6, 9, 12, and possibly 16 weeks, the latter being for breeds at risk.
- Annual revaccination of adult, and especially geriatric, dogs with a complete history of vaccinations is controversial, since titers remain high for more than 1 year. The debate over the appropriate intervaccination interval in adult dogs remains unresolved, with a recent advisory board recommending vaccination every 3 years.

SUGGESTED READING

Houston DM, et al: Risk factors associated with parvovirus enteritis in dogs: 283 cases (1982-1991). *J Am Vet Med Assoc* 208(4):542-546, 1996.

Mohr AJ, et al: Effect of early enteral nutrition on intestinal permeability, intestinal protein loss, and outcome in dogs with severe parvoviral enteritis. *J Vet Intern Med* 17:791-798, 2003.

Prittie J: Canine parvoviral enteritis: A review of diagnosis, management, and prevention. *J Vet Emerg Crit Care* 14(3):167-176, 2004.

Turk J, et al: Coliform septicemia and pulmonary disease associated with canine parvoviral enteritis: 88 cases (1987-1988). *J Am Vet Med Assoc* 196(5):771-773, 1990.

AUTHOR: **DAVID MILLER**

EDITOR: **ELIZABETH ROZANSKI**

Patellar Luxation

BASIC INFORMATION

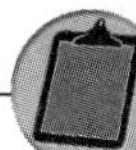

DEFINITION

Medial or lateral displacement of the patella from the femoral trochlear sulcus or groove

SYNONYM(S)

Slipped knee cap

EPIDEMIOLOGY

SPECIES, AGE, SEX

- Primarily seen in dogs; less frequently in cats
- All ages affected; more common in the young dog

GENETICS AND BREED PREDISPOSITION

- All breeds affected; more common in the toy and miniature canine breeds
- Some reports of increased incidence in Devon Rex and Abyssinian cats

RISK FACTORS

- Malalignment of the quadriceps mechanism (hereditary and developmental causes)
- Trauma to the bone or soft tissues of the hind limb
- Systemic diseases resulting in muscle and fascial weaknesses

ASSOCIATED CONDITIONS AND DISORDERS:

- Hip dysplasia in large dogs
- Poor hind limb conformation ("bow-legged" or "cow-hocked")
- Cranial cruciate ligament instability

CLINICAL PRESENTATION

DISEASE FORMS/SUBTYPES

- Medial patellar luxation (MPL):
  - Seen in all breeds; toy and miniature canine breeds and felines most commonly affected
- Lateral patellar luxation (LPL):
  - Seen in all breeds; large and giant canine breeds most commonly affected
- Traumatic luxation:
  - Medial displacement of the patella most common

HISTORY, CHIEF COMPLAINT

- Intermittent, partial to non-weight-bearing lameness of one or both hind limbs
- Transient "skipping" gait when walking or running
- Weakness in jumping or reluctance to jump

PHYSICAL EXAM FINDINGS: Grading system:

- Normal:
  - Patella cannot be manually luxated
  - Normal gait
- Grade I:
  - Patella luxated manually when stifle in extension
  - No clinical signs of lameness
- Grade II:
  - Spontaneous luxation and reduction of the patella occurs
  - Intermittent "skipping" lameness
  - Mild to moderate internal (MPL) or external (LPL) tibial torsion
  - Mild to moderate medial (MPL) or lateral (LPL) deviation of the tibial crest
- Grade III:
  - Patella remains luxated but can be manually reduced with stifle extension
  - Gait varies from skipping to more severe lameness
  - Moderate to severe tibial torsion and tibial crest deviation
  - Shallow distal femoral trochlear groove may be palpable
- Grade IV:
  - Patella is permanently luxated and cannot be manually reduced
  - Non-weight-bearing hind limb lameness or ambulation in a "crouched" position (inability to fully extend the stifles)
  - Severe internal (MPL) or external (LPL) tibial torsion
  - Severe medial (MPL) or lateral (LPL) deviation of the tibial crest
  - Distal femoral trochlear groove is shallow or absent

ETIOLOGY AND PATHOPHYSIOLOGY

- Hereditary and developmental skeletal changes that lead to malalignment of the quadriceps mechanism.
  - Medial patellar luxation.
    - Coxa vara (decreased angle of inclination of the femoral neck).
    - Distal femoral varus and internal torsion.
    - Tibial internal torsion.
    - Shallow femoral trochlear sulcus.
  - Lateral patellar luxation.
    - Coxa valga (increased angle of inclination of the femoral neck).
    - Increased anteversion of the femoral neck.
    - Distal femoral valgus and external torsion.
    - May see external tibial torsion.
- Traumatic disruption of the soft tissue structures supporting the patella.

DISEASES AND DISORDERS

DIAGNOSIS

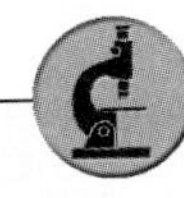

DIFFERENTIAL DIAGNOSIS

- Avascular necrosis of the femoral head (Legg-Calvé-Perthes disease)
- Coxofemoral luxation
- Ligamentous sprain of the stifle
- Muscle strain
- Osteochondrosis of the stifle
- Cranial cruciate ligament rupture (partial or complete)
- Immune-mediated polyarthritis

INITIAL DATABASE

- Complete blood count (CBC), biochemical profile, urinalysis based on signalment: generally unremarkable for patellar luxation alone
- Palpation of the stifle joints for patellar instability
- Radiographs to characterize the femoral and tibial conformation and joint condition:
  - Lateral and craniocaudal radiographs of the femur, stifle, and tibia
  - Need to include the hip and tarsal joints in advanced grades of luxation

ADVANCED OR CONFIRMATORY TESTING

- Calculation of femoral neck inclination and anteversion angles for LPL in large breed dogs
- CT scan with three-dimensional reconstruction

TREATMENT

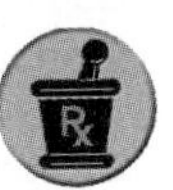

THERAPEUTIC GOAL(S)

- Pain relief and improvement of function through biomechanical realignment of the quadriceps mechanism.
- Stabilization of the patella in the femoral trochlear groove.

ACUTE GENERAL TREATMENT

- Medical management
  - Nonsteroidal anti-inflammatory, drugs (NSAIDs):
    - Aspirin: 10–25 mg/kg PO q 8–24h, or
    - Carprofen: 2 mg/kg PO q 12h, or
    - Etodolac: 10–15 mg/kg PO q 24h, or
    - Deracoxib: 1–2 mg/kg PO q 24h (may use 3–4 mg/kg PO q 24h, for first 7 days only), or
    - Meloxicam: 0.1 mg/kg PO q 24h, or
    - Meclofenamic acid: 1.1 mg/kg, PO q 24h after eating, for 5 days maximum, or
    - Tepoxalin: 10 mg/kg PO q 24h, or
    - Other drugs
- Physical rehabilitation for mild patella luxations (grade I, ± grade II)
  - Exercises to strengthen quadriceps muscle function
- Surgical management
  - Soft tissue reconstruction:
    - Imbrication and release of pericapsular tissues based on direction of luxation
    - Derotational suture from fabella to patella or tibial tuberosity
  - Trochleoplasty to deepen the femoral trochlear groove:
    - Trochlear chondroplasty in immature dogs
    - Trochlear recession sulcoplasty
    - Trochlear abrasion sulcoplasty
  - Tibial tubercle transposition opposite to direction of luxation
  - Femoral or tibial correctional osteotomies

CHRONIC TREATMENT

- Same as in acute cases but may require long-term medical management for the treatment of osteoarthritis.
- One of these chondroprotective agents can be used:
  - Polysulfated glycosaminoglycan 5 mg/kg IM once weekly for 4 to 6 weeks.
  - Pentosan polysulfate (from beechwood hemicellulose) 3 mg/kg SC once weekly.
  - Oral formulations (glucosamine, chondroitin sulfate, hyaluronan): according to formulation/labeled instructions).
- Weight control.
- Exercise moderation.
- It is important to rule out other causes of acute lameness (cruciate ligament injury) in animals with chronic patella luxation.

POSSIBLE COMPLICATIONS

- Medical management:
  - Gastrointestinal (GI), hepatic, renal, or other systemic reactions from NSAIDs
  - Continued progression of degenerative joint disease
  - Failure of medical management to control pain
- Surgical management:
  - Patella reluxation
  - Implant failure

RECOMMENDED MONITORING

- Basic laboratory monitoring of animals on NSAID therapy
- Weight, exercise levels, and clinical signs as dictated by the patient
- Postoperative rehabilitation enhances clinical recovery

PROGNOSIS AND OUTCOME

- Generally good to excellent for return to normal limb function if appropriate techniques are utilized
- Degenerative joint disease progresses despite treatment

PEARLS & CONSIDERATIONS

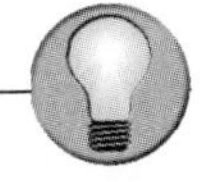

COMMENTS

- Bilateral lameness may be difficult to recognize.
- Severity of lameness may not correlate with grade of patellar luxation.
- In bilateral luxations, the grade of patellar instability may differ between each stifle.
- Soft tissue stabilization techniques alone are not sufficient to stabilize moderate or severe luxations.
- Trochlear recession sulcoplasty (wedge or block) is the preferred method to deepen the femoral trochlear groove because it preserves the articular cartilage.
- In older animals with chronic patellar instability and acutely worsening lameness, always rule out concomitant cranial cruciate ligament rupture.

PREVENTION

Screening and control of breeding animals for prevention of patellar luxation

SUGGESTED READING

Brinker WO, Piermattei DL, Flo GL: Patella luxation. In Brinker WO, Piermattei DL, Flo GL (eds): *Handbook of Small Animal Orthopedics and Fracture Treatment*, ed 3. Philadelphia, WB Saunders, 1997, pp 516-534.

Johnson AL, Hulse DA: Medial and lateral patellar luxation. In Fossum TW (ed): *Small Animal Surgery*, ed 2. St. Louis, Mosby, 2002, pp 1133-1141.

AUTHORS: **JAMES P. BOULAY, BARBARA R. GORES**

EDITOR: **JOSEPH HARARI**

Patent Ductus Arteriosus

Client Education Sheet on Website

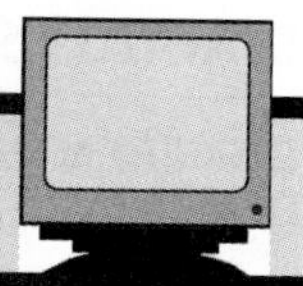

BASIC INFORMATION

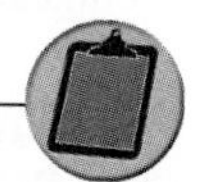

DEFINITION

An arterial shunt between the aorta and pulmonary artery that is normally present in fetuses but should constrict and close within 24 hours after birth. Incomplete closure (patency) results in a variable size channel whose minimum diameter determines the amount and direction of blood flow through the shunt and hence determines the impact on the patient.

SYNONYM(S)

PDA

EPIDEMIOLOGY

SPECIES, AGE, SEX

- All species and any age
- Recognized most frequently in young animals
- Moderate predominance in females
- Occurs much less frequently in cats

GENETICS AND BREED PREDISPOSITION

- Any breed
- Sporadic or heritable defect occurring most frequently in small, relatively nonmuscular dog breeds, such as Maltese, Pomeranians, Yorkshire terriers, Shetland sheepdogs, and toy and miniature poodles

RISK FACTORS: Inbreeding.

GEOGRAPHY AND SEASONALITY: Breed predispositions may vary due to regional differences in the gene pool.

ASSOCIATED CONDITIONS AND DISORDERS

- Arrhythmias
- Congestive heart failure
- Pulmonary hypertension
- Polycythemia

CLINICAL PRESENTATION

DISEASE FORMS/SUBTYPES

- Type 1: small patent ductus arteriosus (PDA)
- Type 2: medium PDA
- Type 3A: large PDA
- Type 3B: large PDA with congestive heart failure
- Type 4: large PDA with pulmonary hypertension and right to left or bidirectional shunt

HISTORY, CHIEF COMPLAINT

- Varies with PDA diameter and age.
- Most often recognized as an incidental heart murmur in a young animal presented for vaccination and not showing overt clinical signs.
- When clinical signs are present, they include exercise intolerance, failure to thrive, and signs of congestive heart failure.

PHYSICAL EXAM FINDINGS: Vary with PDA diameter:

- Type 1, small:
  - Characteristic focal continuous murmur at left heart base
- Type 2, medium:
  - Type 1 signs
  - Continuous murmur audible at apex
  - Precordial thrill at left heart base
- Type 3A, large:
  - Types 1 and 2 signs
  - Bounding pulses
  - Prominent cardiac impulse at left apex
  - Systolic murmur of mitral regurgitation at left apex
- Type 3B, large with congestive heart failure:
  - Types 1, 2, and 3A signs
  - Dyspnea
  - Pulmonary crackles
  - Ascites (occasionally)
  - Arrhythmias, especially atrial fibrillation, possible
- Type 4, large PDA with pulmonary hypertension:
  - No heart murmur
  - Prominent right apical impulse
  - Split second heart sound
  - Caudal cyanosis
  - Hind limb collapse with exercise

ETIOLOGY AND PATHOPHYSIOLOGY

- The principal cause of PDA in dogs is site-specific hypoplasia of ductus smooth muscle coupled with reciprocal excess elastic tissue in the wall of the ductus. In varying degree, the hypoplastic smooth muscle does not encircle the lumen, and muscle contraction does not completely constrict the lumen postpartum.
- Typically, pulmonary vascular resistance decreases after birth and postnatal blood flow through the PDA is from the aorta to the pulmonary artery ("left-to-right type"), causing increased flow through the pulmonary circulation, left atrium, left ventricle, and ascending aorta, resulting in enlargement of these chambers and left ventricular hypertrophy. Established left-to-right types very rarely develop enough pulmonary hypertension to cause reversed PDA flow ("right-to-left type").
- In animals with a large PDA and pulmonary hypertension (type 4, persistent fetal circulation), there is right ventricular hypertrophy; blood flows through the ductus predominantly from the pulmonary artery to the aorta, resulting in caudal cyanosis and systemic polycythemia.

DIAGNOSIS

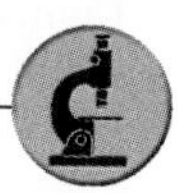

DIFFERENTIAL DIAGNOSIS

Combined abnormalities producing systolic and diastolic heart murmurs, such as a ventricular septal defect and aortic insufficiency due to an unsupported aortic valve cusp.

- Aorticopulmonary window
- Arteriovenous fistula
- Bronchial artery flow in chronic heartworm cor pulmonale
- Tortuous collateral arteries in aortic coarctation or interruption

INITIAL DATABASE

- Thoracic radiographs to assess heart and lung vessel size and lung parenchyma
- Electrocardiogram (ECG) to identify ventricular hypertrophy and arrhythmias
- Packed cell volume to determine presence of anemia or polycythemia

ADVANCED OR CONFIRMATORY TESTING

These tests are optional.

- Two-dimensional echocardiography to determine chamber sizes, wall thickness, and contractility and to identify any concurrent cardiac defects.
- Color Doppler echocardiography to verify turbulent blood flow in the pulmonary artery.
- Spectral Doppler echocardiography to determine flow velocity in the PDA and estimate the aorta-pulmonary artery pressure gradient. If tricuspid and pulmonic insufficiencies are present, respective estimates of right ventricular systolic and pulmonary artery diastolic pressures can be made.

TREATMENT

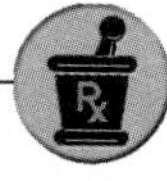

THERAPEUTIC GOAL(S)

- Types 1-3: stop blood flow through the PDA
- Type 4: improve flow characteristics of blood (rheology) by reducing polycythemia

ACUTE GENERAL TREATMENT

- Type 3B: For large PDA, preoperative diuretic and cage rest to alleviate congestive heart failure, then occlusion of PDA are indicated.

- Types 1–3: surgery (Fig. I-128) or transarterial coil (Fig. I-129) to occlude PDA (Table I-22).
- Type 4: phlebotomy to reduce polycythemia.

CHRONIC TREATMENT

Type 4: hydroxyurea to suppress bone marrow, 20–25 mg/kg PO q 12h every other day; titrated based on resulting hematocrit

POSSIBLE COMPLICATIONS

- Refractory congestive heart failure
- Refractory arrhythmias
- Iatrogenic surgical hemorrhage
- Coil embolization into pulmonary artery branch
- Hematoma at transarterial site
- Persistent polycythemia in type 4

RECOMMENDED MONITORING

Nonspecific

PROGNOSIS AND OUTCOME

- Types 1–3A: 98% successful correction and normal lifespan
- Type 3B: 98% initially successful if heart failure and arrhythmia are controlled preoperatively; animal can live for years, but lifespan is usually shortened
- Type 4: May live for years if polycythemia is controlled

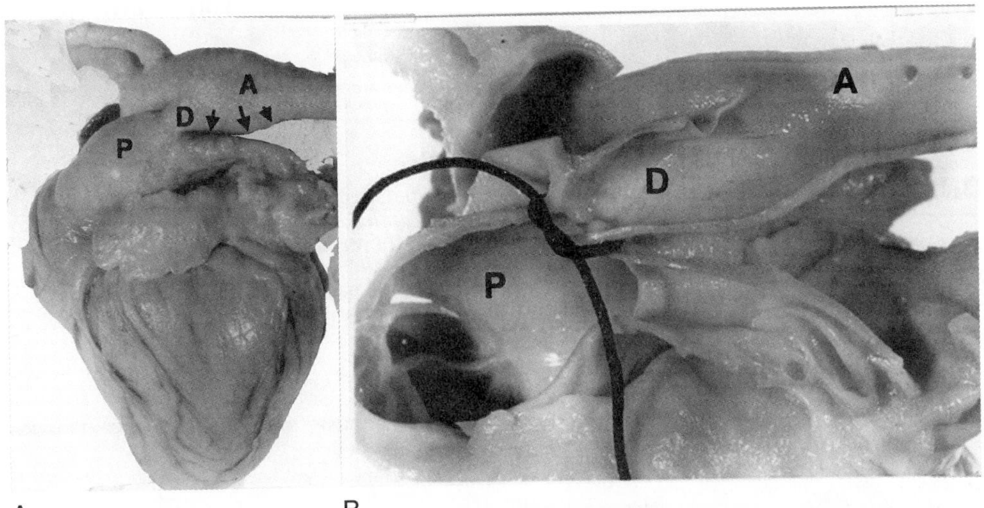

FIGURE I-128 **A**, Photograph of the heart, aorta (*A*), and pulmonary artery (*P*) in a 4-month-old dog with a PDA (*D*) and ductal-aortic aneurysm (*arrows*). **B**, Sagittal section photograph of the great vessels and a ligature demonstrating PDA ligation at surgery. Most of the PDA lies within the wall of the aorta in dogs and constitutes a ductal-aortic aneurysm commonly referred to as a ductus diverticulum. The typical ridge at the pulmonary artery opening limits PDA diameter and determines blood flow through the PDA. Courtesy of Dr. James W. Buchanan, Philadelphia, Pennsylvania.

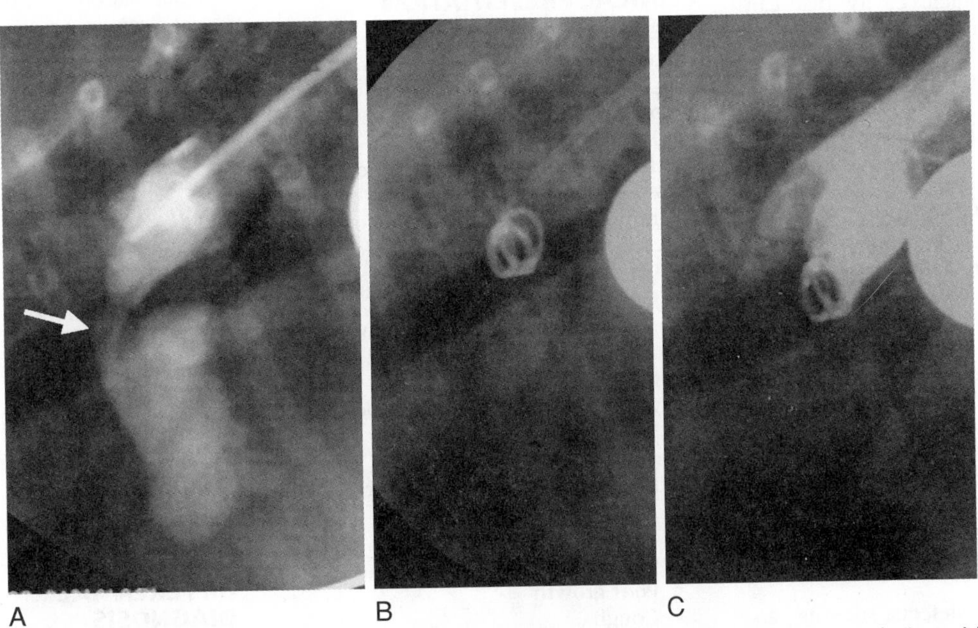

FIGURE I-129 Aortic injection angiograms in a 6-month-old dog with PDA before (**A**) and after (**C**) PDA occlusion with a transarterial coil (**B**). The *arrow* (panel **A**) indicates the narrowest part of the PDA; a properly deployed coil should be placed on the aortic side of this point (as shown in panels **B** and **C**). Courtesy of Dr. James W. Buchanan, Philadelphia, Pennsylvania.

TABLE I-22 Comparison of PDA Occlusion Methods

	Surgery	Coil	Favors
Equipment cost	$1000	$500,000	Surgery
Supply inventory	$1000	$5000	Surgery
Single-use supplies	$100	$500	Surgery
Client charge	$2000	$2000	~
Procedure time	1 hr	1-3 hr	Surgery
Procedure people	2	3	Surgery
Animal size	Any	Limited	Surgery
PDA shape	Any	Limited	Surgery
Success rate	98%	90%	Surgery
Days in hospital	2-3	1-2	Coil
Postoperative monitoring	++	+	Coil
Animal discomfort	+++	+	Coil
Mortality	<2%	<1%	Coil

PEARLS & CONSIDERATIONS

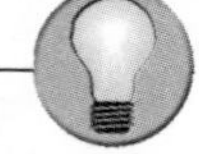

PREVENTION

Owners should avoid breeding affected animals.

SUGGESTED READING

Buchanan JW: Patent ductus arteriosus. In EC Orton (ed): *Advances in Cardiovascular Surgery: Seminars in Veterinary Medicine and Surgery* 9:168–176, 1994.

Buchanan JW: Prevalence of cardiovascular disorders. In Fox P, Sisson D, Moise NS (eds): *Canine and Feline Cardiology*, ed 2. St. Louis, WB Saunders, pp 457–470, 1999.

Buchanan JW: Patent ductus arteriosus: Morphology, pathogenesis, types, and treatment. *J Vet Cardiology* 3:7–16, 2001.

Buchanan JW, Patterson DF: Etiology of patent ductus arteriosus in dogs. *J Vet Intern Med* 17:167–171, 2003.

Buchanan JW: Cardiac surgery for patent ductus arteriosus, persistent right aortic arch, and pulmonic stenosis. University of Pennsylvania, http://cal.vet.upenn. edu/cardiosf.

Buchanan JW: Pulmonary hypertension and patent ductus arteriosus. http://www.vin.com/library/general/JB103pdaRL.htm.

AUTHOR: **JAMES W. BUCHANAN**
EDITOR: **ETIENNE CÔTÉ**

Pectus Excavatum

BASIC INFORMATION

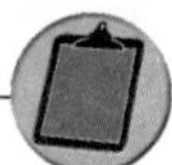

DEFINITION

Congenital dorsoventral narrowing of the thorax or depression of the sternum dorsally into the thoracic cavity that can cause malpositioning or compression of heart and lungs

SYNONYM(S)

Chondrosternal depression
Funnel chest

EPIDEMIOLOGY

SPECIES, AGE, SEX

- More common in cats than dogs.
- No sex predilection.
- While the defect is present at birth, affected animals may not present with clinical complications until secondary disease (e.g., acquired heart disease) develops later in life.

GENETICS AND BREED PREDISPOSITION: The defect is congenital and can be inherited. Brachycephalic dogs are more commonly affected.

ASSOCIATED CONDITIONS AND DISORDERS

- Other congenital defects, such as cardiac defects
- Stunted growth
- Hypoplastic trachea
- "Swimmer's syndrome" (laterally splayed legs as neonate)
- Pneumonia
- Recurrent respiratory infections

CLINICAL PRESENTATION

DISEASE FORMS/SUBTYPES

- Presentation of defect ranges from mild to severe. Severity of thoracic defect does not always correlate to severity of clinical signs, which may be more a reflection of concurrent defects (e.g., cardiac, respiratory).
- Simple cases of pectus excavatum occur in the absence of other congenital anomalies.

HISTORY, CHIEF COMPLAINT

- In many animals, pectus excavatum is found incidentally, and no clinical signs are present.
- Owners may feel that their pet has a defect and seek veterinary advice despite lack of clinical signs.
- When signs occur, they can include:
  - Exercise intolerance
  - Dyspnea
  - Cyanosis
  - Poor growth
  - Cough
  - Inappetence
  - Cachexia
  - Lethargy
  - Weakness
  - Vomiting

PHYSICAL EXAM FINDINGS

- Diagnosis is usually straightforward based on palpation during physical examination of a dorsal defect of caudal sternum, creating sternal concavity.
- Dyspnea, tachypnea, and shallow respirations may be evident at rest or with excitement and minimal exertion.
- Auscultation of a heart murmur or muffled heart and breath sounds are possible.
- Affected animals may be small in stature for age or smaller than their littermates, and exhibit poor condition.

ETIOLOGY AND PATHOPHYSIOLOGY

Congenital malformation of the sternum and costochondral cartilages causes deformation of the thorax and malpositioning of thoracic organs. The exact etiology is unknown.

DIAGNOSIS

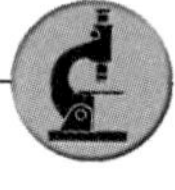

DIFFERENTIAL DIAGNOSIS

- Trauma
- Lordosis of thoracic or thoracolumbar spine

- Differentials must include those for associated abnormalities:
  - Cardiac murmurs indicating cardiac defects must be differentiated from murmurs generated through malpositioning of the heart and great vessels.

INITIAL DATABASE

Thoracic radiographs. Possible findings include:

- Elevated sternum in caudal thorax
- Malformation of sternum and costochondral cartilages
- Decreased thoracic volume
- Displacement of heart and other structures:
  - The heart may falsely appear enlarged because of abnormal positioning and must be differentiated from other causes of true cardiomegaly. Consultation with a radiologist is often warranted.
- Complete diaphragm may be difficult to confirm

ADVANCED OR CONFIRMATORY TESTING

Echocardiography to identify cardiac defects and assess possibility of pleuroperitoneal/pericardioperitoneal hernia; may be very challenging due to chest malformation

TREATMENT

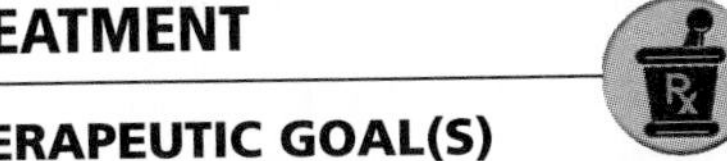

THERAPEUTIC GOAL(S)

- Maximizing of chest capacity to allow normal function and activity
- Treatment of respiratory infections, if present
- Improvement of growth by increasing nutritional plane/assimilation
- Identification and management of concurrent defects

ACUTE GENERAL TREATMENT

- No treatment may be needed for animals without concurrent defects and for whom pectus excavatum is an incidental finding (no clinical signs).
- For severely compromised animals or acute complications:
  - Oxygen supplementation
  - Avoidance of exertion, excitement, and stress
  - Treatment with antibiotics if pneumonia or other infections are suspected or confirmed

CHRONIC TREATMENT

- Incidental/mild cases: daily, gentle, manual, medial-to-lateral chest compressions until the animal is mature (about 9 months of age) to help flatten the chest as the animal grows. External compressing stent may be applied. Chest contour may normalize with growth.
  - The benefits of surgical correction in animals with moderate or severe pectus excavatum and no clinical signs have not been established.
- Moderate/severe clinical signs: surgical application of an external splint. Correction in young animals is generally more successful because the costal cartilages and sternum remain pliable, allowing the thorax to reshape.
  - Optimal age for surgery is variable; a minimum of 8 weeks of age has been recommended.
  - Anesthetic management requires the utmost attention and monitoring.
    - Prevention of hypothermia and hypoglycemia in young animals.
    - Positive-pressure ventilation.
    - Theoretically, reduction of risk for re-expansion pulmonary edema with slow re-expansion of atelectatic lung; often not practical intraoperatively.
    - Avoiding chamber or mask induction if animal is dyspneic.

POSSIBLE COMPLICATIONS

Surgical complications:

- Pneumothorax
- Hemothorax
- Infection
- Re-expansion pulmonary edema

RECOMMENDED MONITORING

- Postoperative monitoring for intrathoracic hemorrhage; immediate postoperative monitoring for pneumothorax
- Monitoring for signs of respiratory infections in untreated or conservatively treated animals

PROGNOSIS AND OUTCOME

- Mild cases without overt clinical signs: excellent prognosis if no other defects are present.
- Prognosis of more severe cases depends on nature of concurrent defects.
- Long-term prognosis is excellent in animals that show clinical signs but have no other defects, provided surgery is performed at a young age. Surgery of older animals may require partial sternectomy.

PEARLS & CONSIDERATIONS

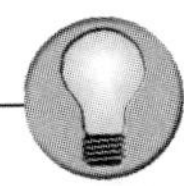

COMMENTS

- Severity of signs at maturity is difficult to predict. If corrective surgery is not possible (cost, unavailability), signs may still lessen spontaneously with growth. Thus, euthanasia should be only considered in the most severe cases when surgery is not possible.
- Puppies and kittens with swimmer's syndrome can benefit from early physical therapy.
- The opposite of pectus excavatum is pectus carinatum (protruding sternum).

PREVENTION

- Spaying or neutering of affected animals once they are stable for elective surgery
- Avoidance of breeding animals with pectus excavatum or the relatives of animals with pectus excavatum

CLIENT EDUCATION

If corrective surgery is not an option, thoracic volume may improve as the animal grows. Outcome is highly variable, and even animals with severe deformities may thrive.

SUGGESTED READING

Fossum TW: Surgery of the lower respiratory system: Lungs and thoracic wall. In Fossum TW (ed): *Small Animal Surgery*. St. Louis, Mosby, 2002, pp 780–784.

AUTHOR: **CHRISTINE L. WILFORD**
EDITOR: **RANCE K. SELLON**

Pemphigus Complex

BASIC INFORMATION

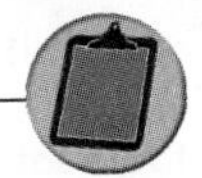

DEFINITION

An uncommon group of autoimmune disorders of the skin or mucous membranes. It is characterized by acantholysis (separation of keratinocytes), producing varying degrees of ulceration, pustules, vesicles, and crusting. Spontaneous and drug-induced forms are known to exist. The most common type is pemphigus foliaceus.

EPIDEMIOLOGY

SPECIES, AGE, SEX: Seen in dogs and cats; more common in middle-aged animals (average age of onset is 5 to 6 years with a range of 0.5 to 16 years).

GENETICS AND BREED PREDISPOSITION

- Pemphigus foliaceus (PF): Akita, chow chow, dachshund, Doberman pinscher, Finnish spitz, schipperke (drug-induced PF in Doberman pinscher and labrador retriever).
- Pemphigus erythematosus (PE): collies and German shepherds.
- Pemphigus vulgaris (PV): no breed or sex predilection.
- Canine benign familial chronic pemphigus has been reported in English setters and their crosses and appears inherited in an autosomal dominant fashion.

RISK FACTORS: PF and PE may be aggravated by sunlight. Some cases of pemphigus are triggered by drug reactions or as a result of chronic diseases, such as allergic dermatitis.

GEOGRAPHY AND SEASONALITY: A lower incidence of canine PF exists in the northeastern part of the United States, and a higher prevalence exists in warmer regions. Seasonal exacerbation of lesions may occur during the warmer months.

ASSOCIATED CONDITIONS AND DISORDERS: Paraneoplastic pemphigus (PNP) in dogs has been associated with underlying neoplasia (lymphoma, thymoma, and, in one case, a Sertoli-cell tumor).

CLINICAL PRESENTATION

DISEASE FORMS/SUBTYPES: Five major types of pemphigus are recognized, listed in decreasing order of frequency of occurrence: pemphigus foliaceus (PF), pemphigus erythematosus (PE), panepidermal pustular pemphigus (PPP), pemphigus vulgaris (PV), and paraneoplastic pemphigus (PNP). A few cases of benign familial pemphigus have been reported in dogs. Pemphigus vegetans has rarely been reported in dogs; it is thought to represent a milder subtype of pemphigus vulgaris.

HISTORY, CHIEF COMPLAINT

- PF: progressive multifocal or generalized truncal skin disease, often with facial and footpad involvement. Degree of pain and pruritus is variable. The initial complaint can be lameness because of footpad disease.
- Cases of PE are presented for facial dermatosis.
- With PV and PNP, disease of the oral cavity is common, and presenting signs include hypersalivation, halitosis, anorexia, and weight loss.
- Fever, anorexia, lethargy, and limb edema are reported in severe cases of pemphigus.

PHYSICAL EXAM FINDINGS

- **PF:** a pustular and crusting dermatitis, with crusts on the trunk being the most common lesion. Inner pinnae and dorsal muzzle are often the first areas affected, and the disease can stay restricted to the face (Fig. I-130). Other commonly involved areas are the feet, footpads, and nail beds (nail beds are affected more often in cats; it is sometimes the only physical exam abnormality). The disease progresses and becomes generalized or multifocal in most cases. Range of lesions noted includes erythematous macules, pustules, dry honey-colored crusts, scales, alopecia, and erosions bordered by collarettes. Secondary bacterial pyoderma (in one-third of PF cases) and peripheral lymphadenopathy are common.
- **PE:** a milder form of PF with crusts, erosions, alopecia, and scales restricted to the nasal and facial regions.
- **PV:** the most severe form of pemphigus, presenting with fragile and transient flaccid vesicles rapidly replaced by large erosions and ulcers. Lesions are first seen on mucosal surfaces and mucocutaneous junctions. Affected areas include oral cavity (70% of cases), inner pinnae, nasal planum, lip margins, genitalia, and anus. Erosions of the nail beds are reported in 14% of the cases. A more localized or milder form of PV has been described in which the disease is restricted to one body area (nail beds, nasal planum, oral cavity).
- **PPP:** not a well-defined entity and could be considered a clinical variant of PF. In PNP, severe erosions and ulcerations of the oral cavity, nose, vulva, as well as haired-skin were seen.

ETIOLOGY AND PATHOPHYSIOLOGY

- Intraepithelial acantholysis (loss of intercellular cohesion between keratinocytes) leading to vesicles/pustules formation related to autoantibodies binding to components of keratinocytes desmosomal desmoglein (Dsg 1 in PF, Dsg 3 in PV).
- The exact mechanism for the development of acantholysis is not completely understood.
- Severity of ulceration and disease is related to the depth of the acantholytic process within the epidermis.
- Serum titers of IgG and IgG4 antikeratinocyte autoantibodies appear to correlate with disease activity and severity of clinical signs.

DIAGNOSIS

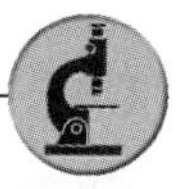

DIFFERENTIAL DIAGNOSIS

- **PF and PNP:** bacterial folliculitis, demodicosis, dermatophytosis, PE, eosinophilic folliculitis and furunculosis, keratinization disorders, cutaneous (discoid) and systemic lupus erythematosus, drug eruptions.
- **PE:** bacterial folliculitis, pemphigus foliaceus, demodicosis, dermatophytosis, cutaneous (discoid) and systemic lupus erythematosus.
- **PV and PPP:** bullous pemphigoid, epidermolysis bullosa acquisita, erythema multiforme, toxic epidermal necrolysis, Stevens-Johnson syndrome, epthelio-tropic lymphoma, ulcerative stomatitis, vesicular cutaneous lupus erythematosus, systemic lupus erythematosus.

INITIAL DATABASE

- Cytologic examination of intact pustules may strongly suggest pemphigus: nondegenerate neutrophils, varying number of eosinophils, and clusters of acantholytic keratinocytes (Fig. I-131).
- Complete blood count (CBC), serum biochemistry profile, urinalysis: often reveal only mild to moderate leukocy-

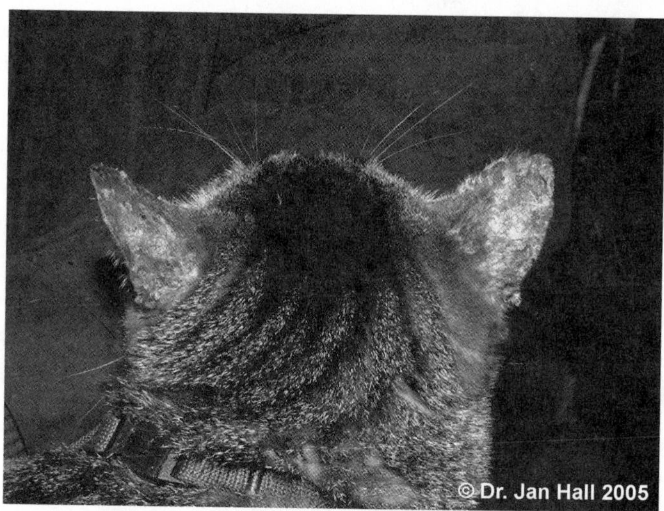

FIGURE I-130 A 3-year-old domestic shorthair castrated male cat with PF affecting the pinnae. Lesions also affected the nail beds, footpads, and lip folds. Courtesy of Dr. Jan A. Hall.

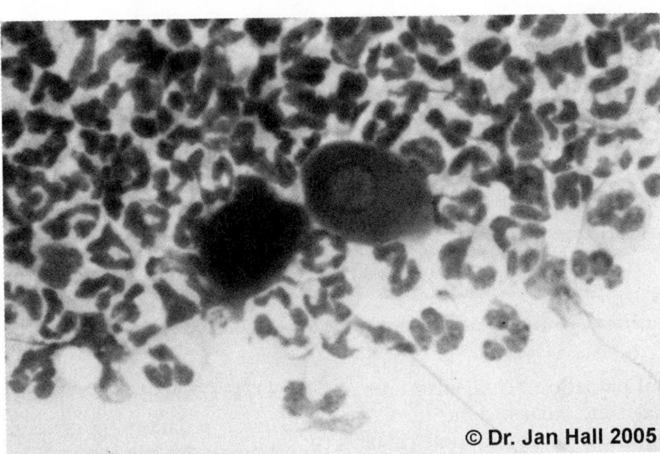

FIGURE I-131 An impression smear of a pustule from a cat with PF showing two acantholytic cells and a background containing numerous degenerative neutrophils. Courtesy of Dr. Jan A. Hall.

tosis with neutrophilia, mild nonregenerative anemia, and hypoalbuminemia

ADVANCED OR CONFIRMATORY TESTING

- Biopsy: histopathologic findings are usually diagnostic and reveal acant holysis and intraepidermal clefting with pustule formation. Lesional epidermal location is related to depth of autoantibody deposition: subcorneal and intragranular in PF and PE; suprabasilar in PV and PPP; panepithelial in PNP.
- Immunohistopathologic examination of skin biopsy (immunohistochemistry and direct immunofluorescence) or serum may be helpful but depends on the sensitivity of the methods being used and previous glucocorticoid administration; not routinely used.

TREATMENT

THERAPEUTIC GOAL(S)

- To implement immunosuppressive therapy that will induce remission without significant side effects.
- There are variable responses to treatment with the different forms of pemphigus.

ACUTE AND CHRONIC TREATMENT

- Systemic glucocorticoids induce remission in most animals.
  - Dogs:
    - Prednisone/prednisolone: 2-4 mg/kg PO q 24h.
  - Cats:
    - Prednisone/prednisolone: 4-8 mg/kg PO q 24h.
    - Dexamethasone: 0.2-0.4 mg/kg PO q 24h.
    - Triamcinolone: 1-2 mg/kg PO q 24h.
- Once remission is attained, the dose of glucocorticoid is very slowly tapered to an alternate-day regimen; the ideal maintenance dose is 1 mg/kg q 48h or less.
- Alternative or concurrent immunosuppressive drugs:
  - Azathioprine: 2.2 mg/kg PO q 24-48h (first choice in dogs, with prednisone/prednisolone, contraindicated in cats).
  - Chlorambucil: 0.1-0.2 mg/kg PO q 24-48h (first choice in cats, with prednisone/prednisolone).
  - Tetracycline and niacinamide: milder or localized cases of PF and PE (250 mg of each PO q 8h for dogs <10 kg; 500 mg PO q 8h for dogs >10 kg).
  - Cyclosporine: 5-10 mg/kg PO q 24h, limited experience (used for treating PF and PV); variable success reported.
  - Mycophenolate mofetil: 7-13 mg/kg PO q 8h, limited experience (used in canine PF); variable success reported.
- Topical therapy is indicated as a sole treatment in some localized form of PF and PE and in conjunction with systemic therapy on more persistent focal areas that remain active despite satisfactory control of the overall disease:
  - Potent topical glucocorticoid initially: fluocinolone acetonide, triamcinolone, betamethasone valerate; when an adequate response occurs, treatment is changed to topical 1-2% hydrocortisone for maintenance.
  - Tacrolimus 0.1%: seems promising for treating both PE and PF.
- Intravenous immunoglobulins (human purified IgG) therapy (IVIg) has been used successfully in a few cases of refractory pemphigus in dogs.
- Supportive therapy for severely affected animals.

POSSIBLE COMPLICATIONS

Euthanasia rate of dogs with PF varies according to one study (25-40%), mostly in the first year of treatment.

RECOMMENDED MONITORING

- Semiannual CBC, serum biochemistry profiles, urinalysis, and urine cultures for all patients receiving long-term oral glucocorticoid with or without concomitant immunosuppressive drugs.
- Azathioprine, chlorambucil, mycophenolate, and other potential myelosuppressives: monitoring to include checking the CBC every 2 to 3 weeks for the first 3 months.

PROGNOSIS AND OUTCOME

- Animals with PE and PF have a better prognosis than those with PV.
- For animals with PF, the average time to improvement with therapy is 6 weeks; average time to remission is 9 months. Mortality is primarily related to complications of therapy during the first year of treatment, and the prognosis improves after 12 months of survival. The 5-year survival rate is 40-70%. Mortality rate in cats with PF: <10% during the 6 months of therapy.
- Of reported cases for animals with PV, 39% died spontaneously or were euthanized because of disease severity, lack of response to treatment, or development of severe adverse effects due to high-dose glucocorticoid therapy. The prognosis for those animals with milder variants of PV appears better.
- Animals with PNP: poor prognosis.

PEARLS & CONSIDERATIONS

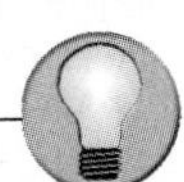

COMMENTS

- There are variable responses to treatment and different prognoses with the different forms of pemphigus. It is therefore essential for clinicians to make a specific diagnosis.
- Although acantholytic cells are characteristic of pemphigus, clinicians may also see these cells in cases of pyoderma and epitheliotrophic lymphoma.
- Clinicians should consider treatment with or prophylactic use of antibiotics during initial immunosuppressive treatment or, in milder cases, prior to starting immunosuppressive therapy.
- Combination therapy (prednisone and azathioprine) as the initial therapy can decrease the maintenance dose of glucocorticoids and reduce associated side effects.

SUGGESTED READING

Preziosi DE, et al: Feline pemphigus foliaceus: A retrospective analysis of 57 cases. *Vet Dermatol* 14:313, 2003.

Rosenkrantz WS: Pemphigus: Current therapy. *Vet Dermatol* 15:90, 2004.
Scott DW, Miller WH, Griffin CE: Pemphigus complex. In Scott DW, Miller WH, Griffin CE (eds): *Muller and Kirk's Small Animal Dermatology*, ed 6. Philadelphia, WB Saunders, 2001, pp 678–693.

AUTHOR: **CAROLINE DE JAHAM**
EDITOR: **JAN A. HALL**

Perianal Fistula

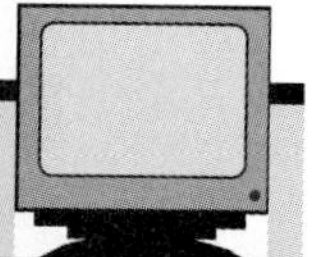

Client Education Sheet on Website

BASIC INFORMATION

DEFINITION

A chronic, inflammatory disease of the tissues surrounding the anus of dogs. The lesions are painful, ulcerative, and sometimes deep and have draining tracts adjacent to the anus. The anus itself is not usually involved.

SYNONYM(S)

Anal furunculosis

EPIDEMIOLOGY

SPECIES, AGE, SEX: Dogs, usually >5 years old; males may be overrepresented.
GENETICS AND BREED PREDISPOSITION: German shepherds and possibly Irish setters are predisposed.
RISK FACTORS: Possibly broad-based tail, low tail carriage, and increased density of apocrine sweat glands in the perianal region.
ASSOCIATED CONDITIONS AND DISORDERS: Possibly caused by a food allergy; manifested as pruritus and/or signs of colitis.

CLINICAL PRESENTATION

HISTORY, CHIEF COMPLAINT: Initially, owners may notice a foul odor or observe that the dog licks its perianal region excessively. As the lesions progress, the dog may have dyschezia, hematochezia, tenesmus, and fecal incontinence; the dog may engage in self-mutilation. In severe cases, inappetence, lethargy, and weight loss are possible.
PHYSICAL EXAM FINDINGS: In mild to moderate cases, physical examination abnormalities are confined to the perianal region. In more severe cases, the dog may also be in poor body condition. Examination of the perianal region may be very difficult in these animals due to pain, and sedation is often necessary. Visual and rectal examinations are indicated:

- Visually, the lesions appear as multiple, ulcerated, draining tracts that may be superficial or extend deeply into the perianal tissues. The lesions may extend 360 degrees around the anus as well as involve the ventrum of the tail base.
- Upon rectal palpation, rectal strictures, loss of anal tone, anal sac rupture or abscessation, and/or roughened rectal mucosa may also be found.

ETIOLOGY AND PATHOPHYSIOLOGY

- An immunologic basis is suspected based on clinical improvement with immunosuppressive drugs as well as a few pathologic studies identifying sterile, chronic inflammatory changes.
- Secondary bacterial infection is common, often due to fecal microflora or skin contaminants.

DIAGNOSIS

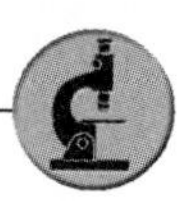

DIFFERENTIAL DIAGNOSIS

- Perianal neoplasia (anal sac adenocarcinoma)
- Anal sac abscessation/rupture
- Trauma (bite wounds)
- Perianal hernia (early phase of fistula, prior to ulcerated lesions)

INITIAL DATABASE

- Complete blood count (CBC), serum chemistry panel, and urinalysis: often within normal limits
- Abdominal radiographs: may show evidence of constipation

ADVANCED OR CONFIRMATORY TESTING

- Contrast radiography may be needed to better delineate the lesion in cases with rectal stricture because a colonoscopy may not be possible if the stricture is profound
- Colonoscopy/proctoscopy: may reveal inflammatory colitis (lymphoplasmacytic), rectal stricture

TREATMENT

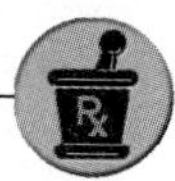

THERAPEUTIC GOAL(S)

- Reduction in number and size of fistulae
- Control of infection
- Treatment of colitis, rectal stricture if present

ACUTE GENERAL TREATMENT

- Under sedation or general anesthesia: clipping of hair, removal of feces and debris, and cleansing of surrounding tissues.
- Enemas and stool softeners may be needed if constipation is present.

CHRONIC TREATMENT

- Immunosuppression is the initial therapy of choice:
  - Cyclosporine: 80–90% success rate; expensive in larger dogs. Starting dose, using emulsion form (Atopica, Neoral): 3–5 mg/kg PO q 12h, adjusted to maintain whole blood trough cyclosporine levels 400–600 ng/ml. Adding ketoconazole (10 mg/kg PO q 24h) allows a reduction in cyclosporine dose to 1 mg/kg PO q 12h, with similar serum levels.
  - Azathioprine (2 mg/kg PO q 24h, for 2 to 4 weeks, then tapered) may be an effective alternative.
  - Prednisone alone (effective in ≤33% of animals): 2 mg/kg PO q 24h, for 2 to 4 weeks as needed for lesion improvement, then gradual taper to 0.5 mg/kg q 48h.
  - Tacrolimus 0.1% topical, applied q 12–24h: resolution of lesions in 50% of dogs.
- Antimicrobials (e.g., cephalexin 22 mg/kg PO q 8–12h) are used as adjunct therapy for perianal dermatitis.
- Dietary therapy has been used in conjunction with immunosuppression. Novel antigen diets have been recommended becuase there is a suspected association with food hypersensitivity. Most important, animals should avoid high-fiber (bulking) diets, and owners should feed highly digestible diets that will result in a softer, smaller stool.
- Stool softeners (e.g., lactulose 0.25–0.5 ml/kg PO q 12h, titrated to stool consistency) as necessary to allow for easier defection.
- Surgery: if medical management does not resolve lesions to an acceptable degree. Use of an Nd:YAG laser and cryotherapy have been reported. Surgical procedures that may be needed include anal sacculectomy,

removal of skin overlying the tracts, debridement of diseased tissue, and rectal pull-through for rectal strictures.
- Balloon dilation of rectal strictures is recommended as first line of therapy because surgical removal of strictures may result in recurrence of strictures or fecal incontence.

DRUG INTERACTIONS

Ketoconazole decreases the catabolism of cyclosporine and is given for this purpose

POSSIBLE COMPLICATIONS

- Recurrence of fistulae with discontinuation of immunosuppressive drugs
- Rectal stricture and constipation secondary to chronic inflammation
- Fecal incontinence secondary to chronicity or surgery

RECOMMENDED MONITORING

- Follow-up examinations of the perianal region every 2 weeks
- Whole blood trough cyclosporine levels
- CBC (risk of cytopenias if azathioprine is being used)

PROGNOSIS AND OUTCOME

- Fair to good prognosis with early treatment
- Long-term prognosis may be guarded with more severe lesions and the need for indefinite medical therapy

PEARLS & CONSIDERATIONS

COMMENTS

Most dogs will respond to medical management but may also require long-term therapy to maintain remission.

CLIENT EDUCATION

Advise clients on the clinical signs and lesions that warrant early intervention if lesions recur

SUGGESTED READING

Ellison GW, Bellah JR, Stubbs WP, van Gilder J: Treatment of perianal fistulas with Nd:YAG laser—Results in twenty cases. *Vet Surg* 24:140-147, 1995.

Harkin KR, Walshaw R, Mullaney TP: Association of perianal fistula and colitis in the German shepherd dog: Response to high-dose prednisone and dietary therapy. *J Am Anim Hosp Assoc* 32:515-520, 1996.

Mathews KA, Sukhiani HR: Randomized controlled trial of cyclosporine for treatment of perianal fistulas in dogs. *J Am Vet Med Assoc* 211:1249-1253, 1997.

Misseghers BS, Binnington AG, Mathews KA: Clinical observations of the treatment of canine perianal fistulas with topical tacrolimus in 10 dogs. *Can Vet J* 41:623-627, 2000.

Patricelli AJ, Hardie RJ, McAnulty JF: Cyclosporine and ketoconazole for the treatment of perianal fistulas in dogs. *J Am Vet Med Assoc* 220:1009-1016, 2002.

Tisdall PLC, Hunt GB, Beck JA, Malik R: Management of perianal fistulae in five dogs using azathioprine and metronidazole prior to surgery. *Aust Vet J* 77:374-378, 1999.

AUTHOR: **LISA E. MOORE**

EDITOR: **DEBRA L. ZORAN**

Pericardial Effusion

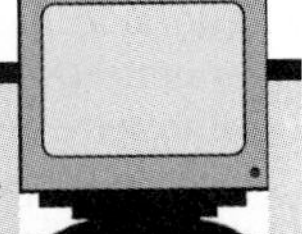

Client Education Sheet on Website

BASIC INFORMATION

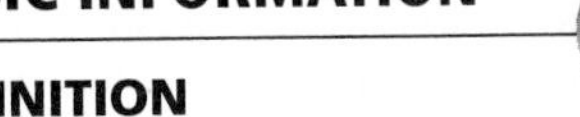

DEFINITION

Pathologic accumulation of fluid (blood, plasma, neoplastic cells, pus, chyle, or combinations) in the pericardial space

SYNONYM(S)

Pericardial fluid accumulation

EPIDEMIOLOGY

SPECIES, AGE, SEX: Dependent on underlying cause; dogs: older adults (neoplastic, idiopathic).

GENETICS AND BREED PREDISPOSITION

- Dogs: golden retrievers, Labrador retrievers, German shepherds, other large breeds (hemangiosarcoma, mesothelioma); boxers, bulldogs (and other brachycephalics), terriers (chemodectoma)
- Cats: rare predispositions. Asian breeds, feline infectious peritonitis (FIP); Maine coon (cardiomyopathy)

RISK FACTORS

- Dogs: mesothelioma associated with asbestosis; speculative link between lymphoma and exposure to volatile chemicals
- Cats: multicat household, FIP

CONTAGION AND ZOONOSIS: Cats: FIP (cat-to-cat only).

CLINICAL PRESENTATION

DISEASE FORMS/SUBTYPES

- Incidental/unexpected finding: no clinical signs caused by pericardial effusion:
  - During echocardiography
  - Cardiomegaly on radiographs
  - Electrocardiogram (ECG) changes: electrical alternans or small QRS complexes
- Cardiac tamponade: pericardial effusion is causing overt signs

HISTORY, CHIEF COMPLAINT

- Acute collapse, usually without loss of consciousness
- Exercise intolerance/episodic weakness
- Abdominal distention
- General discomfort, with or without dyspnea
- Pale mucous membranes

PHYSICAL EXAM FINDINGS

- Tachycardia
- Soft or muffled heart sounds
- Weak pulse
- Abdominal distention possible
- Dyspnea/attenuated lung sounds possible if pleural effusion

ETIOLOGY AND PATHOPHYSIOLOGY

Etiology

- Primary:
  - Neoplasia (hemangiosarcoma [dogs], heart base tumors [chemodectoma, ectopic thyroid carcinoma], mesothelioma, lymphoma)
  - Idiopathic pericardial effusion (dogs)
  - Left atrial rupture
- Systemic:
  - Congestive heart failure (effusion volume usually very small)
  - Infectious (FIP [cats], bacterial [very uncommon])
  - Anticoagulant intoxication
  - Uremia

Mechanism

- Rate and volume of fluid accumulation and pericardial distensibility determine onset of clinical signs.
- When overt signs are present as a result of pericardial effusion, cardiac tamponade exists.
- In general, pericardial effusions caused by systemic processes rarely produce cardiac tamponade (exception: anticoagulant intoxication), whereas pericardial effusions caused by primary lesions within the pericardial space commonly produce cardiac tamponade.

DIAGNOSIS

DIFFERENTIAL DIAGNOSIS

- Physical:
  - Hypovolemia
  - Hypotension
  - Causes of ascites (see Ascites, p 84)
  - Causes of pleural effusion (see Pleural Effusion, p 858)
- Radiographic:
  - Cardiac enlargement from heart disease
  - Expiratory radiograph
  - Normal variation
- Echocardiographic:
  - Pleural effusion
  - Oblique views
- Specific causes can be determined by etiology (previously described)

INITIAL DATABASE

- Echocardiogram: confirmation of the diagnosis and investigation for right atrial/ventricular (hemangiosarcoma) or periaortic (heart base) masses. Right ventricular diastolic collapse is highly indicative of severe cardiac tamponade; right atrial collapse is less specific.
- Thoracic radiographs: large cardiac silhouette (80% of cases), globoid cardiac silhouette (60% of cases), caudal vena cava enlargement; metastatic lesions, pleural effusion.
- Complete blood count (CBC), serum biochemistry panel, and urinalysis are usually unremarkable except with systemic disorders.
- ECG: Electrical alternans is unreliable and only found in 50% of dogs with pericardial effusion.
- Prothrombin time if anticoagulant intoxication is suspected.

ADVANCED OR CONFIRMATORY TESTING

- Pericardial effusion cytologic examination: useful for lymphoma, infectious causes; otherwise, malignant versus benign is totally unreliable with cytologic examination.
- Pericardial effusion pH: generally unreliable, much overlap between benign and malignant.
- Transesophageal echocardiography.
- Serum troponin-I level: elevation is suggestive of hemangiosarcoma.
- Effusion vascular endothelial growth factor (VEGF) concentration: nondiagnostic.

TREATMENT

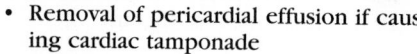

THERAPEUTIC GOAL(S)

- Removal of pericardial effusion if causing cardiac tamponade
- Delaying or eliminating recurrent effusion is a long-term goal

ACUTE GENERAL TREATMENT

- Pericardiocentesis: if cardiac tamponade is present; contraindicated if coagulopathy is a cause of effusion, unless there are critical circulatory effects (severe/periterminal tamponade).
- Abdominal drainage is usually unnecessary if secondary to congestion (resorbs in 24 to 48 hours).
- Treatment of underlying cause if systemic disorder.
- Diuretics contract intravascular volume and, therefore, are contraindicated in treating cardiac tamponade.

CHRONIC TREATMENT

- Management/resolution of systemic disorder if present.
- Recurrent pericardiocentesis if needed.
- Pericardiectomy if recurrent effusion occurs due to idiopathic pericarditis or heart base mass.
- Diuretics are indicated if the animal has congestive heart failure (and secondary pericardial effusion) due to myocardial or valvular heart disease; otherwise, chronic diuretic treatment for delaying recurrence of primary pericardial effusion is controversial.

POSSIBLE COMPLICATIONS

- Recurrent effusion; follow-up echocardiography to assess need for recentesis ± pericardiectomy
- Dyspnea from severe pleural effusion or ascites
- Pericardiocentesis-related (see Pericardiocentesis, p 1298)

RECOMMENDED MONITORING

- Follow-up exam and echocardiography 24 hours after the pericardiocentesis (sooner if poor perfusion): assessment for recurrent effusion
- Follow-up exam and echocardiography 2 to 4 weeks after the pericardiocentesis
- Serial echocardiography and thoracic radiographs as dictated by recurrence

PROGNOSIS AND OUTCOME

- Guarded (average: days to months) with hemangiosarcoma; worse if a mass is seen on the right atrium or if pulmonary metastases exist, but better if nonhemorrhagic ascites is present.
- Guarded to fair with heart base tumors, better if pericardiectomy.
- Guarded to fair with mesothelioma (months to a year or more).
- Guarded to fair with idiopathic (risk of constrictive pericarditis or of mesothelioma).
- Hemorrhagic effusion that recurs in hours to 1 to 2 days after the pericardiocentesis is rarely benign; prognosis is worse.

PEARLS & CONSIDERATIONS

COMMENTS

- Grossly malignant pericardial effusions and benign pericardial effusions can both appear equally hemorrhagic.
- Normal-looking heart on radiographs does not rule out pericardial effusion.
- If a weak pulse, tachycardia, and muffled heart sounds are all present, pericardial effusion is possible, and an echocardiogram is warranted.

CLIENT EDUCATION

- Clients need to monitor for recurrence of presenting signs as described previously.
- Rapid deterioration is possible; rechecks are necessary.

SUGGESTED READING

Dunning D, et al: Analysis of prognostic indicators for dogs with pericardial effusion: 46 cases (1985-1996). *J Am Vet Med Assoc* 212:1276-1280, 1998.

Rush JE, et al: Pericardial disease in the cat: A retrospective evaluation of 66 cases. *J Am Anim Hosp Assoc* 26:39-46, 1990.

AUTHOR & EDITOR: **ETIENNE CÔTÉ**

Pericarditis, Idiopathic Benign

BASIC INFORMATION

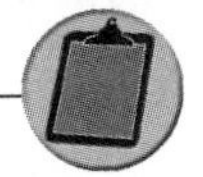

DEFINITION

Non-neoplastic pericardial inflammation and effusion of undetermined etiology frequently accompanied by thickening of the pericardium, epicardial fibrin formation, and adhesions between the serosal layer of the pericardial sac and the epicardium

SYNONYM(S)

Benign pericardial effusion
Hemorrhagic benign pericarditis
Sterile pericarditis

EPIDEMIOLOGY

SPECIES, AGE, SEX

- Species: dog.
- Sex: more common in males.
- Age: middle-aged and older animals; extremely rare in cats.
- Idiopathic benign pericarditis is the second most common cause of pericardial effusion in the dog (after hemangiosarcoma).

GENETICS AND BREED DISPOSITION: Dogs: golden retriever, German shepherd, Saint Bernard, Great Pyrenees, bullmastiff, Lhasa apso, shih tzu.

RISK FACTORS: Associated with immune complex diseases, chronic inflammatory diseases.

CLINICAL PRESENTATION

DISEASE FORMS/SUBTYPES

- Chronic loss of stamina
- Acute cardiac tamponade

HISTORY, CHIEF COMPLAINT

- Exercise intolerance, episodic weakness, lethargy, anorexia, dyspnea, acute collapse, ascites
- Associated with gradual accumulation of pericardial fluid, leading to tamponade

PHYSICAL EXAM FINDINGS

- Tachycardia, muffled heart sounds, thready/weak pulse, abdominal distention
- In some cases: jugular distention, pulsus paradoxus, positive hepatojugular reflux

ETIOLOGY AND PATHOPHYSIOLOGY

- Unknown etiology.
- Generally associated with increasing amounts of sanguineous, inflammatory fluid from damaged blood vessels, lymphatics, mesothelial cells, and microvilli of the serosal layer of the pericardial sac.
- The pericardial sac gradually becomes distended.
- When intrapericardial pressures exceed right atrial filling pressures, tamponade develops, which in turn usually produces overt clinical signs.

DIAGNOSIS

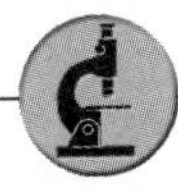

DIFFERENTIAL DIAGNOSIS

- Major differential is cardiac hemangiosarcoma
- Other forms of pericardial disease

INITIAL DATABASE

- Complete blood count (CBC): may show mild anemia, monocytosis, lymphocytosis, mild neutrophilia
- Serum biochemistry profile: usually unremarkable
- Should screen for immune-mediated disease (antinuclear antibody, rheumatoid factor, Coombs' test, thyroid test, serum protein electrophoresis)
- Electrocardiogram (ECG): electrical alternans (25% of the time), diminished R wave amplitudes (50% of the time)
- Thoracic/abdominal radiographs: enlarged globoid cardiac silhouette possible (80% of time), caudal vena caval distention, hepatomegaly, ascites, pleural effusion
- Echocardiography: anechoic fluid surrounding heart, may see fibrin tags in fluid, thickened pericardial sac (occasionally), no tumor mass seen

ADVANCED OR CONFIRMATORY TESTING

- Pericardial fluid cytologic examination:
  - Especially to exclude infectious pericardial effusion and lymphoma.
  - Cytologic examination alone is highly unreliable: 74% of malignancies are not detected, and 13% of benign cases are wrongly identified as malignant.
- Pericardial fluid pH: controversial. One study indicated pericardial pH ≥7.0 as highly indicative of neoplasia and pericardial pH <7.0 as highly indicative of benign effusion; another study showed no statistical ability to differentiate etiology on basis of pH of pericardial fluid.
- Elevated serum troponin-I concentration is inconsistent with benign disease and rather suggests hemangiosarcoma. This blood test may be performed locally at a human hospital (human assay is accurate in dogs) or may be performed in referral veterinary laboratories (e.g., Veterinary Medical Teaching Hospital, University of Florida Health Science Center).
- Lack of evidence for neoplasia of liver or spleen on abdominal ultrasound.
- Contrast CT scan and cardiac MRI: investigational.

TREATMENT

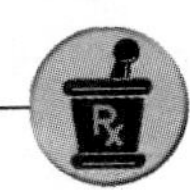

THERAPEUTIC GOAL(S)

Relief of effusion/tamponade

ACUTE GENERAL TREATMENT

- Pericardiocentesis (see Pericardiocentesis, p 1298)
- Diuretics are contraindicated in acute pericardial effusion/cardiac tamponade
- When infectious etiology has been ruled out (effusion cytologic examination ± culture): corticosteroids initially at immunosuppressive doses, taper to anti-inflammatory dosage in 2 weeks

CHRONIC TREATMENT

- Repeat pericardiocentesis
- Subtotal pericardectomy with histopathologic examination

POSSIBLE COMPLICATIONS

May progress to constrictive pericarditis

RECOMMENDED MONITORING

Follow-up echocardiography 24 hours after initial pericardiocentesis and monthly thereafter

PROGNOSIS AND OUTCOME

- Often favorable with initial pericardiocentesis and corticosteroid therapy
- Usually favorable following subtotal pericardectomy

PEARLS & CONSIDERATIONS

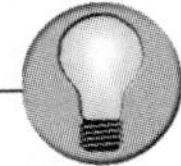

COMMENTS

- Subtotal pericardectomy may lead to development of pleural effusion; initially, postsurgical management may require chest drainage/thoracocentesis.
- Following initial pericardiocentesis, monthly follow-up echocardiograms are advised to evaluate resolution of effusion or subsequent visualization of tumor mass not seen on initial evaluation.
- If effusion/tamponade returns following initial pericardiocentesis, clinicians can consider subtotal pericardectomy

(rather than make repeated attempts at pericardiocentesis) when surgery is an appropriate option, either by thoracotomy or thoracoscopy.
- Differentiation from mesothelioma may be extremely difficult until late in the course or without pericardial tissue histopathologic examination.
- Serum troponin-I concentrations are easily assessed at many local human hospitals (human assay is valid in the dog).

CLIENT EDUCATION

- Clinicians should inform clients that the condition may spontaneously recur after apparent cure.
- Some animals require long-term steroid therapy, risking complications such as iatrogenic hyperadrenocorticism.

SUGGESTED READING

Edwards NJ: The diagnostic value of pericardial fluid pH determination. *J Am Anim Hosp Assoc* 32(1):63–67, 1996.

Fine DM, Tobias AH, Jacob KA: Use of pericardial fluid pH to distinguish between idiopathic and neoplastic effusions. *J Vet Intern Med* 17(4):525–529, 2003.

Kienle RD: Pericardial disease and cardiac neoplasia. In Kittleson MD, Kienle RD (eds): *Small Animal Cardiovascular Medicine*. St. Louis, Mosby, 1998, pp 413–432.

Sisson D, Thomas WP: Pericardial disease and cardiac tumors. In Fox PR, Sisson D, Moise NS (eds): *Textbook of Canine and Feline Cardiology*. Philadelphia, WB Saunders, 1999, pp 679–701.

AUTHOR: **N. JOEL EDWARDS**
EDITOR: **ETIENNE CÔTÉ**

Pericarditis, Infectious

BASIC INFORMATION

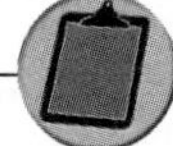

DEFINITION

Inflammation of the parietal and visceral layers of the pericardium due to infectious agent(s)

SYNONYM(S)

Infective pericarditis

EPIDEMIOLOGY

SPECIES, AGE, SEX

- No reported age or sex predilection.
- Dogs: Causative etiology has been identified in 2% of cases diagnosed with pericardial effusion.
- Cats: Causative etiology has been identified in 14% of cases diagnosed with pericardial effusion.

RISK FACTORS

- Local infection (pleural or pulmonary)
- Penetrating trauma
- Migrating foreign body
- Open wounds
- Bacteremia
- Viral infection

CONTAGION AND ZOONOSIS

- Feline infectious peritonitis (FIP), cat-to-cat.
- Tuberculous pericarditis, while uncommon, has been reported (postmortem risk for transmitting the disease from dog to human).
- *Coccidioides immitis* (postmortem risk for transmitting the disease from dog to human).

GEOGRAPHY AND SEASONALITY

- *C. immitis* in the southwestern part of the United States
- Grass awn migration in the western part of the United States

ASSOCIATED CONDITIONS AND DISORDERS

- Pericardial effusion
- Effusive-constrictive pericarditis

CLINICAL PRESENTATION

DISEASE FORMS/SUBTYPES: Virulence of the infectious agent and rate and magnitude of fluid accumulation determine the clinical signs.

HISTORY, CHIEF COMPLAINT

- Weight loss
- Lethargy, weakness
- Dyspnea
- Ascites
- Fever (inconsistent finding)

PHYSICAL EXAM FINDINGS: Reflective of secondary cardiac tamponade or effusive-constrictive pericarditis:

- Jugular vein distention or pulsation
- Weak arterial pulses
- Muffled heart and lung sounds
- Ballotable abdominal fluid wave
- Pale mucous membranes

ETIOLOGY AND PATHOPHYSIOLOGY

- Reported organisms or diseases:
  - *Actinomyces*
  - *Nocardia*
  - *Mycobacterium*
  - *Pasteurella multocida*
  - *C. immitis*
  - *Acremonium*
  - *Leishmania*
  - Tuberculosis
  - Leptospirosis
  - *Streptococcus canis*
  - *Citrobacter* sp.
  - *Pseudomonas* sp.
  - α Hemolytic streptococci
  - Canine distemper virus
- Mixed bacterial infections are common.
- Pathophysiologic examination reflects secondary cardiac tamponade or effusive-constrictive pericarditis:
  - Effusion becomes extensive, and intrapericardial pressure rises.
  - Intrapericardial pressure exceeds intracardiac diastolic pressures, and filling is impaired.
  - Stroke volume is reduced.
  - Central venous pressure increases, and venous return to the right atrium is impaired.
  - Increased venous pressure leads to pleural effusion and ascites. Therefore, pleural effusion or ascites may be due to increased venous pressure or to concurrent infection in those body cavities (cytologic examination to differentiate).

DIAGNOSIS

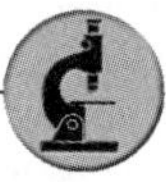

DIFFERENTIAL DIAGNOSIS

- Radiographic:
  - Cardiac enlargement from other types of heart disease
  - Normal variation
- Echocardiographic:
  - Pericardial effusion due to other etiology (i.e., neoplastic, idiopathic)
  - Pleural effusion: many causes (see Pleural Effusion, p 858)

INITIAL DATABASE

- Complete blood count (CBC): ± anemia, ± inflammatory leukogram, ± degenerative left shift
- Serum biochemistry panel: elevated liver enzymes, elevated creatine kinase (CK), decreased albumin

- Thoracic radiographs: mildly to severely enlarged, round cardiac silhouette; caudal vena cava distention; pleural effusion; ± abnormal pulmonary parenchyma if source of infection
- Echocardiogram (ECG): pericardial effusion which may be hyperechoic, ± thickened pericardium, fibrin, ± hyperechoic densities within pericardial space
- ECG changes may be present if effusion is severe: low-voltage complexes, electrical alternans, ST segment changes

ADVANCED OR CONFIRMATORY TESTING

- Cytologic analysis of the effusion:
  - Serosanguineous or bloody.
  - Modified transudate or exudates.
  - Protein content is >2.5 mg/dl; often >3.5 mg/dl.
  - Neutrophils and erythrocytes are predominant cell types.
  - Others: macrophages, reactive mesothelial cells, degenerative neutrophils, etiologic agent.
- Microbial culture of the effusion:
  - Always do both aerobic and anaerobic cultures.
  - Secondary invaders are common with aerobic cultures.
- Histopathologic examination:
  - Lesions dependent on etiology.

TREATMENT

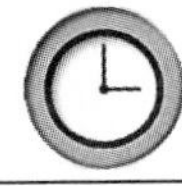

THERAPEUTIC GOAL(S)

- Pericardial effusion is removed if causing cardiac tamponade
- Delaying or eliminating recurrent effusion is a long-term goal:
  - Pericardiectomy
  - Continuous chest drainage after the pericardiectomy
  - Antibiotic therapy

ACUTE GENERAL TREATMENT

- Pericardiocentesis if cardiac tamponade is present
- Thoracocentesis if respiratory compromise
- Abdominocentesis:
  - Usually unnecessary
  - Can be performed if ascites is causing discomfort and/or respiratory compromise

CHRONIC TREATMENT

- Subtotal pericardiectomy:
  - Pericardial window not recommended
  - May require epicardial stripping if pericardium is severely thickened
- Continuous chest drainage after the pericardiectomy
- Aggressive antibiotic therapy based on culture and susceptibility

DRUG INTERACTIONS

Diuretics contraindicated if cardiac tamponade is present:

- Contract intravascular volume
- Reduce venous filling pressure and stroke volume

POSSIBLE COMPLICATIONS

- Infectious effusion can lead to constrictive pericarditis.
- Dyspnea due to pleural effusion or ascites.

RECOMMENDED MONITORING

- Follow-up exam and echocardiography 24 hours after the pericardiocentesis or sooner if poor perfusion.
- Periodic reassessment for recurrent effusion.

PROGNOSIS AND OUTCOME

- If treated aggressively with pericardiectomy, continuous chest drainage, and appropriate antibiotics, prognosis is good in acute phase.
- If the animal is systemically ill and treatment is not aggressive, prognosis is poor.

PEARLS & CONSIDERATIONS

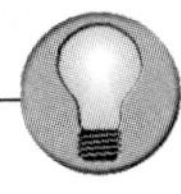

COMMENTS

- Infectious pericarditis is a rare cause of pericardial effusion is dogs and cats.
- A normal cardiac silhouette on radiographs, a negative culture, and the absence of fever may exist in patients with infectious pericarditis.
- Antibiotics concentrate well in pericardial fluid.

PREVENTION

- Minimize foreign body exposure
- Treat local infections, wounds, and bacteremia aggressively
- Minimize viral exposure

CLIENT EDUCATION

- If this disorder is treated aggressively with pericardiectomy, continuous chest drainage, and appropriate antibiotics, prognosis is good in early stages.
- Prognosis worsens with time and degree of fibrosis (scarring).

SUGGESTED READING

Aronson LR, et al: Infectious pericardial effusion in five dogs. *Vet Surg* 24:402-407, 1995.

Berg RJ, et al: Pericardial effusion in the dog: A review of 42 cases. *J Am Anim Hosp Assoc* 20:721-730, 1984.

Calvert CA: Cardiovascular infections. In Greene CE (ed): *Infectious Diseases of the Dog and Cat*. Philadelphia, WB Saunders, 1998, pp 580-581.

AUTHOR: **SARAH J. MILLER**
EDITOR: **ETIENNE CÔTÉ**

Perineal Hernia

BASIC INFORMATION

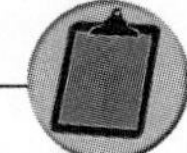

DEFINITION

Weakness and separation of the muscles of the pelvic diaphragm

EPIDEMIOLOGY

SPECIES, AGE, SEX

- Primarily dogs; highest incidence in middle-aged and geriatric intact male dogs
- Rare in cats

GENETICS AND BREED PREDISPOSITION

- Dogs:
  - Reported in many different breeds and mixed breeds
  - Short-tailed breeds may be predisposed
- Cats:
  - Reported in cats with a history of megacolon, feline lower urinary tract signs/disease (FLUTS/D, FUS), or previous perineal surgery
  - Manx cats

RISK FACTORS

- Any condition that causes tenesmus:
  - Prostatomegaly
  - Constipation
- It has been reported that recurrence of perineal hernia was 2.7 times greater in intact dogs than dogs castrated at time of herniorrhaphy.
- Cats:
  - FLUTS/D, FUS
  - Previous perineal urethrostomy

- Megacolon
- Colitis

ASSOCIATED CONDITIONS AND DISORDERS

- Prostatomegaly
- Constipation
- FLUTS/D, FUS

CLINICAL PRESENTATION

HISTORY, CHIEF COMPLAINT

- Tenesmus, constipation
- Unilateral or bilateral perineal swelling lateral to the anus
- Dysuria:
  - Bladder entrapment
  - Common in cats
  - Previous perineal urethrostomy

PHYSICAL EXAM FINDINGS

- Unilateral or bilateral swelling in perineal region lateral, and possibly ventral, to the anus. May contain:
  - Rectal sacculation packed with feces
  - Prostate
  - Bladder
  - Fat
- Rectal palpation:
  - Defect or separation in muscles of the pelvic diaphragm on affected side(s)
  - Rectal sacculation

ETIOLOGY AND PATHOPHYSIOLOGY

- Dog, unknown; possible association with:
  - Tenesmus
    - Constipation, obstipation
    - Prostatomegaly
    - Rectal abnormalities
  - Stranguria
  - Congenital or acquired weakness of the muscles of the pelvic diaphragm
    - Effect of androgens on muscles
  - Neurogenic atrophy of the muscles of the pelvic diaphragm
- Cats: see Risk Factors above

DIAGNOSIS

DIFFERENTIAL DIAGNOSIS

- Colorectal mass
- Pelvic neoplasia
- Prostatic cyst/abscess
- Perianal neoplasia

INITIAL DATABASE

- Complete blood count (CBC), serum biochemistry profile, urinalysis:
  - Presurgical screening
  - Bladder entrapped in hernia
    - Postrenal azotemia
  - Elevated white blood cell count, ± left shift if abscess, cellulitis, strangulation/ischemia of entrapped organs
- External perineal and rectal palpation:
  - Unilateral versus bilateral
  - Contents of hernia:
    - Fecal-filled rectal sacculation
    - Fat
    - Pelvic/abdominal organ (prostate, bladder)
  - Important to rule out neoplasia, prostatic cyst/abscess

ADVANCED OR CONFIRMATORY TESTING

- Survey of abdominal and pelvic radiographs:
  - Position and size of bladder and prostate
  - Contents of hernia
- Ultrasound examination:
  - Position and morphology of bladder and prostate:
    - Underlying prostatic disease

TREATMENT

THERAPEUTIC GOAL(S)

- Repositioning of herniated organs
- Reconstructing pelvic diaphragm:
  - Often a bilateral problem requiring bilateral herniorrhaphy:
    - One side often more obvious than other, but on careful palpation, clinician may note weakening of the pelvic diaphragm
- Preventing recurrence by resolution of underlying causes of tenesmus:
  - Castration to decrease size of prostate

ACUTE GENERAL TREATMENT

- Emergency treatment to relieve urinary obstruction caused by a retroflexed urinary bladder:
  - Perineal cystocentesis
  - Indwelling catheter
- Relief of constipation:
  - Manual evacuation of rectal sacculation
  - Stool softeners/dietary management

CHRONIC TREATMENT

- Prevention of postoperative tenesmus
  - Dietary management
  - Stool softeners
- Identification of cause of constipation, and appropriate treatment
- Identification of cause of prostatomegaly, and appropriate treatment
- Colopexy may be needed to maintain position of bladder in abdomen

POSSIBLE COMPLICATIONS

- Complications associated with perineal hernia:
  - Urinary obstruction
    - Retroflexed bladder (18–25%)
  - Urinary incontinence or bladder atony
    - Damage to pelvic nerves/detrusor muscle
  - Constipation/obstipation
    - Rectal sacculation
- Complications associated with perineal herniorrhaphy:
  - Recurrence (10–46%)
  - Incisional dehiscence and infection (6–26%)
  - Sciatic nerve entrapment
  - Tenesmus or rectal prolapse
    - Compression of rectal sacculation (8–13%)

RECOMMENDED MONITORING

History and physical examination findings consistent with recurrence: perineal swelling, tenesmus, and dysuria

PROGNOSIS AND OUTCOME

- Good to excellent outcome with successful herniorrhaphy and no other concurrent diseases
- Fair to poor if the patient cannot undergo surgical correction, if there is recurrence after appropriate surgical correction, and/or if cannot resolve cause of tenesmus/dysuria

PEARLS & CONSIDERATIONS

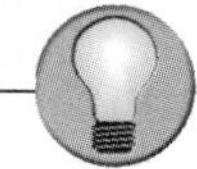

COMMENTS

- Perineal hernia may be a hormonally related disease in the male dog.

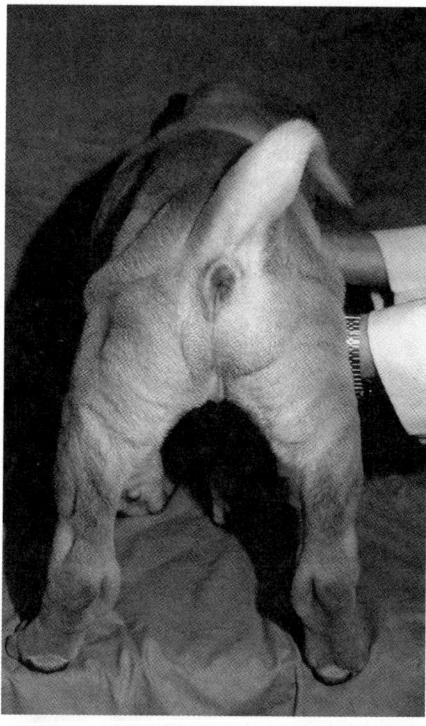

FIGURE I-132 Soft tissue swelling immediately to the right of the anus in a young shar-pei dog. This swelling is characteristic of a perineal hernia. Courtesy of Dr. Richard Walshaw.

- Herniorrhaphy plus castration is the treatment of choice.
- Diagnosis and elimination of underlying causes of tenesmus are important for a successful outcome.

PREVENTION

- Prevention of tenesmus plays a role in retarding the development or progression of perineal hernia.
- Castration reduces or eliminates the risk of prostatomegaly.
- Appropriate diets with increased fiber may help manage constipation.

CLIENT EDUCATION

- Prevention and control of risk factors, such as constipation, prostatomegaly, and colitis
- Surgery is the definitive treatment for perineal hernia

SUGGESTED READING

Hosgood G, Hedlund CS, Dean PW: Perineal herniorrhaphy: Perioperative data from 100 dogs. *J Am Anim Hosp Assoc* 31:331–342, 1995.

Welches CD, Scavelli TD, Aronsohn MG, et al: Perineal hernia in the cat: A retrospective study of 40 cases. *J Am Anim Hosp Assoc* 28:431–438, 1992.

AUTHOR: **ELLEN B. DAVIDSON DOMNICK**
EDITOR: **RICHARD WALSHAW**

Periodontal Disease

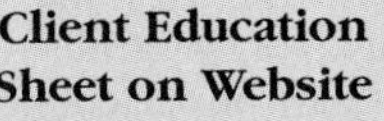

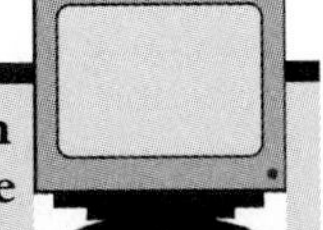

BASIC INFORMATION

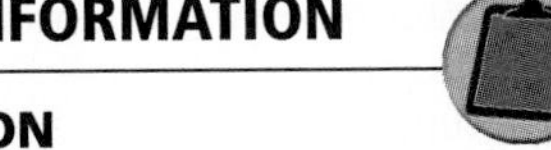

DEFINITION

Plaque-induced inflammation and infection of the gingiva, periodontal ligament and alveolar bone

SYNONYM(S)

Gingivitis (inflammation of gingiva)
Gum disease
Periodontitis (inflammation of the periodontium, which includes gingiva, alveolar bone, periodontal ligament, and cementum)

EPIDEMIOLOGY

SPECIES, AGE, SEX: The most common disease in companion animals. Affects all breeds. Tends to be more common and severe in toy and small breed dogs. Occurs in dogs and cats of any age although the condition is more severe with increasing age.

GENETICS AND BREED PREDISPOSITION: Toy and small breed dogs are particularly prone to severe alveolar bone loss (relatively large teeth compared to small size of jaws, causing crowding of teeth).

RISK FACTORS: Soft food diets.

CONTAGION AND ZOONOSIS: Periodontal disease is an infectious disease; however, all clinically normal animals carry the putative causative organisms in their mouths. There is no evidence of dog/cat to dog/cat or dog/cat to human spread.

GEOGRAPHY AND SEASONALITY: None. Dogs and cats in less developed parts of the world are less prone to develop severe periodontal disease because they have a more varied diet that encourages natural chewing activity.

ASSOCIATED CON833DITIONS AND DISORDERS: Coexists will any other oral conditions and may mask appearance of diseases with a worse prognosis, such as oral neoplasms. Found in almost every animal with stomatitis (see Stomatitis, p 1039). Masks, and is masked by, gingival hyperplasia.

CLINICAL PRESENTATION

DISEASE FORMS/SUBTYPES: Severity of inflammation varies relative to extent of plaque and calculus buildup and to local and general immunologic health (see Stomatitis, p 1039). Maxillary fourth premolar and first molar teeth are typically the most severely affected teeth.

HISTORY, CHIEF COMPLAINT: Halitosis, teeth stained by calculus; gingiva may be swollen, bleeding, or ulcerated.

PHYSICAL EXAM FINDINGS: Consist of signs as described in previous paragraphs. Teeth may be loose or missing. There is often a wide variation in the severity of the disease, which clinicians may note when comparing one part of the mouth with another in the same animal.

ETIOLOGY AND PATHOPHYSIOLOGY

- Caused by bacteria in dental plaque at the gingival margin (primarily gram-negative, anaerobic rods, and spirochetes); exacerbated by accumulation of calculus on the surface of teeth.
- Gingival inflammation leads to destruction of the periodontal ligament and resorption of adjacent alveolar bone, causing gradual loss of attachment of the tooth to the jaw.
- Gingiva may recede in step with worsening bone loss or remain in place with a deepening pocket between the gingiva and root as bone loss worsens.
- Local disease resolves once the teeth are no longer present.

DIAGNOSIS

DIFFERENTIAL DIAGNOSIS

- Any other oral disease; periodontal disease is almost always present when other oral diseases are present.
- Oral tumors may appear as ulcerated gingival lesions; however, unlike tumors, periodontal disease is typically symmetric, and teeth with greater amounts of plaque and calculus deposition are more severely affected.
- Familial gingival hyperplasia of bulldogs, boxers, collies, and some other medium-large dogs; gingiva is firm and symmetric, often irregular in surface contour and may partly or completely cover the tooth crowns. Usually not inflamed or ulcerated (except where extent of overgrowth results in physical injury of gingiva during chewing).
- The abnormalities in periodontal disease are limited to gingiva and alveolar bone in almost all cases; exceptions are considered to be stomatitis cases (see Stomatitis, p 1039). If there is doubt about whether a case is stomatitis or simply a severe case of periodontal disease, clinicians can anesthetize the animal, extract severely affected teeth, scale and polish the remaining teeth, and reexamine the animal in 2 to 3 weeks. If inflammation or ulceration returns, the case is considered to be a stomatitis case.

INITIAL DATABASE

- Awake oral examination. Is the extent of periodontal disease appropriate for the age and diet of the animal? If the extent of inflammation is more severe than would be expected, distant organ or immunopathic disease may be exacerbating the periodontal disease.
- A general physical examination and complete blood count (CBC), serum chemistry profile, and urinalysis are warranted to ensure that the animal is sufficiently healthy to undergo general anesthesia and to rule out distant organ disease (renal, hepatic) that may be exacerbating the oral disease.

ADVANCED OR CONFIRMATORY TESTING

While the animal is under anesthesia, the clinician can perform a detailed oral examination:

1. Visual examination of location, color, and swelling of gingiva.
2. Gentle insertion of a periodontal probe between the gingiva and crown or exposed root to assess the pocket depth (distance between the gingival margin and the bottom of the pocket, normally no more than 2 mm even in a very large dog) and attachment loss (distance between the cementoenamel junction and bottom of the pocket). Note: Because of gingival recession occurring as part of periodontal tissue loss, there may be a considerable difference between pocket depth and attachment loss.
3. Pressure against the side of the tooth determines mobility (assessed on a 0-3 [least to most] mobility index).
4. Dental radiographs are indicated to ensure that remaining bone is healthy, especially when advanced therapy of severely involved teeth is under consideration.

TREATMENT

THERAPEUTIC GOAL(S)

- Removal of the cause: accumulated dental plaque and calculus
- For severely affected teeth: diagnosis and triage of the extent of the disease followed by addressing abnormalities of surrounding bone to stabilize the tooth (if owner is willing to provide long-term home oral hygiene following treatment) *or* extract the tooth
- Prevention of subsequent accumulation of dental plaque and calculus to avoid progression of periodontal disease around remaining teeth

ACUTE GENERAL TREATMENT

- Dental scaling and polishing of all teeth, accompanied by examination of every tooth to assess extent of bone loss and gingiva present.
- For severely affected but retainable teeth (those with periodontal pockets deeper than 5-6 mm and mobility of 1-2), many procedures are available. Which procedure is selected depends on whether the gingival cuff around the tooth is intact, on whether the furcation (space between roots of multirooted teeth) is exposed, on the extent of bone surrounding the root, and on the experience of and equipment and materials available to the veterinarian. Options include gingival flaps or grafts to enhance the gingiva around the tooth and also include using various bone augmentation techniques.
- When more than 50% of the root length (in a single-rooted tooth) or more than 60% of any root in a multirooted tooth is no longer attached to the surrounding alveolar bone or mobility is 2, scaling and polishing are unlikely to provide effective removal of calculus attached to root surfaces; clinicians should consider involved therapy or extraction. When mobility is 3, extraction is the only practical treatment.
- The only guaranteed effective treatment for the animal is extraction; dogs and cats manage very well without teeth.

CHRONIC TREATMENT

Oral hygiene at home to prevent further development of periodontal disease

DRUG INTERACTIONS

Gingival hyperplasia can result from long-term phenytoin or cyclosporine therapy.

POSSIBLE COMPLICATIONS

- Traumatic lesions (typically chronic granulomatous areas) of the caudal buccal mucosa or sublingual tissue resulting from abnormal chewing patterns; the lesions may need to be excised as part of comprehensive periodontal treatment.
- Distant organ disease from periodontitis-related bacteremia or systemic release of inflammatory or bacterial degradation products.
- Pathologic mandibular fracture from extensive bone loss around teeth in toy breed dogs.
- Damage to adjacent organs (jaw, eye, tongue) during extraction procedures.

RECOMMENDED MONITORING

Periodic reexamination: 1 month and 2 to 3 months following involved periodontal surgical procedures to ensure that tissues are responding as expected and that oral hygiene performed at home by owner is effective (if not, clinicians can rescale teeth and make adjustments in home-care regimen). There is a recommended maximum of 6 months between reexaminations following less-involved periodontal surgery, and a maximum of 1 year between reexaminations following scaling and polishing.

PROGNOSIS AND OUTCOME

- Prevention of periodontal disease by plaque and calculus control is very effective.
- Treatment of severe lesions is more problematic as severity of bone loss around the root increases; it is very difficult to create new bone once resorption has occurred, and a tooth that is unstable (mobile) because of insufficient bone surrounding the root(s) will lose more bone as the pressure from the angled, mobile tooth is concentrated on specific areas of bone. Very mobile teeth should always be extracted.
- If teeth have been lost or are extracted because of severe periodontal disease, the tooth that would normally occlude against the missing tooth will be more at risk of plaque and calculus accumulation than teeth with occluding partners present.

PEARLS & CONSIDERATIONS

COMMENTS

- This is a preventable disease if the animal is started on a home oral hygiene program following eruption of permanent teeth.
- The importance of periodontal disease as an insult to the rest of the body is a topic of research; an association has been proven, and the hypothesized cause and effect relationship are under study.
- Meanwhile, an effective prevention program should be built into every animal's wellness program from a young age.
- Oral examination, including assessment of areas of the mouth most severely affected by periodontal disease (maxillary fourth premolars and first molars), does not take much time; clinicians should perform this examination whenever an animal is brought for a veterinary appointment for any reason.
- The Veterinary Oral Health Council (VOHC) provides a standard for efficacy of products marketed as controlling plaque and calculus accumulation and awards its seal of acceptance to products that have been shown to meet its standards.

PREVENTION

Home oral hygiene: Clinicians should educate owners about the combination of brushing or rubbing the tooth surfaces, the use of oral health care products, and offering pets nutritionally complete diets formulated to reduce plaque and calculus accumulation.

CLIENT EDUCATION

Clinicians should teach owners about methods of prevention, as described previously.

SUGGESTED READING

Holmstrom SE, Frost P, Eisner E: *Veterinary Dental Techniques*, ed 3. Philadelphia, WB Saunders, 2004, pp 176-338.

AUTHOR: **COLIN E. HARVEY**
EDITOR: **ALEXANDER M. REITER**

Perirenal Pseudocysts

BASIC INFORMATION

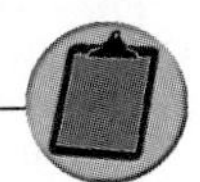

DEFINITION

Collection of fluid (usually transudate, but sometimes urine) between the renal capsule and the kidney. Pseudocysts may be unilateral or bilateral.

SYNONYM(S)

Perinephric pseudocyst
Capsulogenic renal cyst
Capsular cyst
Pararenal pseudocyst
Capsular hydronephrosis
Pseudohydronephrosis

EPIDEMIOLOGY

SPECIES, AGE, SEX

- Rare in cats, extremely rare in dogs.
- Older cats; some reports have shown male cats to be overrepresented.

RISK FACTORS

- Chronic renal failure (transudative pseudocysts)
- Trauma, obstruction, neoplasia (uriniferous pseudocysts)

ASSOCIATED CONDITIONS AND DISORDERS

- Chronic renal failure (transudative perirenal pseudocysts)
- Disruption of renal pelvis or ureter causing urine leakage (uriniferous pseudocysts)

CLINICAL PRESENTATION

HISTORY, CHIEF COMPLAINT

- Usually abdominal enlargement/abdominal mass (noted by owner, or incidental finding during exam)
- Less frequently: weight loss, vomiting, anorexia, polyuria, and polydipsia

PHYSICAL EXAM FINDINGS

- Palpable abdominal mass (renomegaly)
- Thin body condition

ETIOLOGY AND PATHOPHYSIOLOGY

- Incompletely understood pathophysiology.
- Lack of epithelial lining in fibrous sacs means that these are not true cysts.
- Renal interstitial fibrosis may impair venous and lymphatic drainage causing transudate to escape the renal parenchyma and accumulate under the capsule, forming a transudative pseudocyst.
- Uriniferous pseudocysts may form when damage to the renal parenchyma, pelvis, or ureter allows urine to leak between the renal capsule and renal parenchyma.
- The distinction between transudative and uriniferous pseudocysts may be useful with respect to initial management. Transudative pseudocysts suggest chronic renal failure (consider appropriate treatment) whereas uriniferous pseudocysts suggest physical disruption of the integrity of the kidney or proximal ureter (identify and correct source of leakage).

DIAGNOSIS

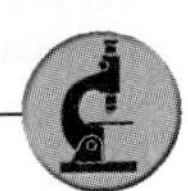

DIFFERENTIAL DIAGNOSIS

For enlarged kidneys: perinephric abscess, renal lymphoma or other neoplasia, ureteral obstruction with hydronephrosis, feline infectious peritonitis, hematoma, polycystic kidney disease, and compensatory hypertrophy (abscess, other neoplasia, ureteral obstruction, hematoma, and compensatory hypertrophy: more commonly unilateral than bilateral)

INITIAL DATABASE

- Complete blood count: possibly nonregenerative anemia of chronic renal failure
- Serum biochemistry profile: usually evidence of mild to moderate renal failure (e.g., azotemia, hyperphosphatemia)
- Urinalysis: isosthenuric or minimally concentrated urine specific gravity
- Urine culture: often positive even in the absence of pyuria
- Abdominal radiographs: unilateral or bilateral renomegaly

ADVANCED OR CONFIRMATORY TESTING

- Abdominal ultrasound: method of choice to confirm diagnosis. Transudative and uriniferous pseudocysts are characterized by an accumulation of completely anechoic fluid between renal parenchyma and capsule. Septations, particulate matter in the perirenal fluid, and other variations suggest a diagnosis other than perirenal pseudocysts.
- Excretory urography if ultrasound unavailable. Decreased renal function may result in poor contrast study. Small risk of contrast-induced renal failure.
- If the diagnosis remains in question after ultrasound, aspiration of anechoic/hypoechoic region for cytologic analysis can differentiate pseudocyst from perinephric abscess, hematoma, or lymphoma.
- Concentration of creatinine will be higher in fluid from uriniferous pseudocysts than concurrent serum creatinine concentration.

TREATMENT

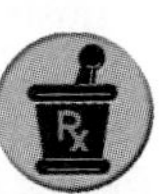

THERAPEUTIC GOAL(S)

- Maintain patient comfort
- Prevent exacerbation of azotemia due to renal and ureteral compression

ACUTE GENERAL TREATMENT

- If transudative pseudocyst, percutaneous drainage
- If uriniferous, identify (i.e., via excretory urography) and correct source of urine leakage

CHRONIC TREATMENT

- Repeated percutaneous drainage of transudative pseudocysts.
- Surgical resection of pseudocyst ± omentopexy.
- Treat existing bacterial cystitis, if present (see Cystitis, Bacterial, p 270).
- With transudative pseudocysts: treat appropriately for chronic renal failure (see Chronic Renal Failure, Occult ["Asymptomatic"], p 204; Chronic Renal Failure, Overt ["Symptomatic"], p 205).
- With uriniferous pseudocysts: consider surgical intervention if necessary.
- In general, nephrectomy should be avoided if possible. May become necessary if persistent ascites develops after surgical resection of pseudocyst.

POSSIBLE COMPLICATIONS

- Urinary tract infection.
- Ascites may be a complication of pseudocyst removal, occasionally necessitating nephrectomy.
- Hydrothorax due to pseudocyst has been reported in a single cat.

RECOMMENDED MONITORING

- Monitor as for chronic renal failure (see Chronic Renal Failure, Occult ["Asymptomatic"], p 204; Chronic Renal Failure, Overt ["Symptomatic"], p 205).
- Repeat ultrasound examination periodically after percutaneous drainage or surgical pseudocyst removal. Frequency of repeat ultrasound depends on rapidity of fluid reaccumulation.

PROGNOSIS AND OUTCOME

- Prognosis variable, generally in the range of months to years.
- Prognosis better if associated chronic renal failure is mild or absent; worse dependent on severity of chronic renal failure.

- Median survival after surgery (capsulectomy): 9 months, with wide range.
- Prognosis apparently worse in cats treated with nephrectomy.
- No clear generalization regarding prognosis in transudative versus uriniferous pseudocysts.

PEARLS & CONSIDERATIONS

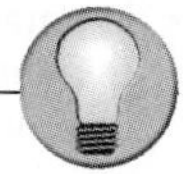

COMMENTS

- The choice between surgical removal of transudative pseudocysts and repeated percutaneous drainage depends on severity of underlying renal failure or disease, concurrent disease, age of the cat, and cost to owner. Cats with severe azotemia, another disease process that makes them a poor anesthetic/surgical candidate, advanced age, or where cost is an issue may be best managed via repeated percutaneous drainage.
- Nephrectomy may result in worsened azotemia in cats and should be reserved for cats that develop persistent ascites after removal of the pseudocyst. Ideally, renal scintigraphy should precede the decision for nephrectomy to determine contribution of kidney to be removed to total glomerular filtration capacity.

SUGGESTED READING

Beck JA, et al: Perirenal pseudocysts in 26 cats. *Aust Vet J* 78(3):166–171, 2000.

Hill TP, Odesnik BJ: Omentalisation of perinephric pseudocysts in a cat. *J Small Anim Pract* 41: 115–118, 2000.

Ochoa VB, et al: Perinephric pseudocysts in the cat: A retrospective study and review of the literature. *J Vet Intern Med* 13:47–55, 1999.

Rishniw M, et al: Hydrothorax secondary to a perinephric pseudocyst in a cat. *Vet Radiol Ultrasound* 39(3):193-196, 1998.

AUTHOR: **JULIENE L. THROOP**

EDITOR: **LEAH A. COHN**

Peritoneopericardial Diaphragmatic Hernia

BASIC INFORMATION

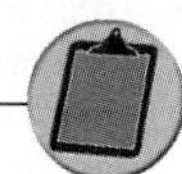

DEFINITION

- Embryologic malformation of the diaphragm resulting in communication between peritoneal and pericardial cavities. It allows herniation of cranial abdominal organs into the pericardial space (from most to least common: liver, gallbladder, small intestine, spleen, stomach).
- Can result in vascular compromise or obstruction of herniated organs and, rarely, cardiac tamponade.

SYNONYM(S)

Pericardioperitoneal diaphragmatic hernia

PPDH

EPIDEMIOLOGY

SPECIES, AGE, SEX

- Peritoneopericardial diaphragmatic hernia (PPDH) is present in dogs and cats.
- Age at diagnosis highly variable (30% diagnosed at >4 years of age).
- No sex predilection.

GENETICS AND BREED PREDISPOSITION

- Not known if hereditary but reported in littermates
- Predisposed breeds: weimaraners, Persians, Himalayans, domestic longhair cats

RISK FACTORS: Possibly systemic illness or toxin exposure affecting pregnant dam.

ASSOCIATED CONDITIONS AND DISORDERS

- Cranioventral abdominal hernias
- Caudal sternal abnormalities (pectus excavatum, malformed or absent sternebrae)
- Ventricular or atrial septal defects, pulmonic stenosis, pericardial cysts

CLINICAL PRESENTATION

HISTORY, CHIEF COMPLAINT

- Often incidental finding with no clinical signs
- Nonspecific signs (lethargy, anorexia, pyrexia, weight loss)
- Respiratory signs (dyspnea, tachypnea, coughing)
- Gastrointestinal (GI) signs (vomiting, diarrhea)
- Rarely, signs of cardiac tamponade and right heart failure (weakness, collapse, ascites, pleural effusion)

PHYSICAL EXAM FINDINGS

- May be normal
- Displaced or absent apical cardiac impulse on thorax
- Muffled or displaced heart sounds
- Cardiac murmur if congenital cardiac defect is also present
- Palpable sternal or cranial abdominal defects
- Inability to palpate cranial abdominal organs if herniated into pericardial space
- Borborygmi (GI sounds) over heart

ETIOLOGY AND PATHOPHYSIOLOGY

- Abnormal development of septum transversum (forms ventral portion of the diaphragm) ± pleuroperitoneal folds (form dorsolateral diaphragm), resulting in an hourglass-like shape of the joined peritoneal and pericardial cavities (that should instead be separate body cavities).
- Peritoneopericardial diaphragmatic hernia is always a congenital abnormality, not an acquired one.

DIAGNOSIS

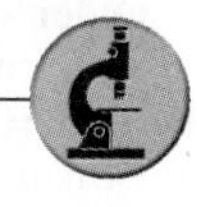

DIFFERENTIAL DIAGNOSIS

- Other causes of generalized cardiomegaly:
  - Pericardial effusion
  - Congenital or acquired cardiac diseases
- True diaphragmatic hernias do not involve the presence of abdominal viscera in the pericardial space.

INITIAL DATABASE

- Complete blood count (CBC) and serum biochemistry panel: no characteristic abnormalities
- Thoracic radiographs (Fig. I-133):
  - Cardiomegaly
  - Dorsal displacement of the trachea
  - Silhouetting of caudal cardiac border with the diaphragm
  - Presence of irregular and heterogeneous radiopacities (soft tissue, fat, gas) within cardiac silhouette
  - Dorsal mesothelial remnant on lateral view in cats: curvilinear soft tissue opacity ventral to caudal vena cava representing dorsal aspect of hernia (Fig. I-134)
  - Sternal deformities
- Abdominal radiographs:
  - Small or absent liver
  - Cranial displacement or absence of stomach or spleen
  - GI gas pattern extending from abdomen into pericardial space

ADVANCED OR CONFIRMATORY TESTING

- Echocardiography: fat or abdominal organs within pericardium, displacing

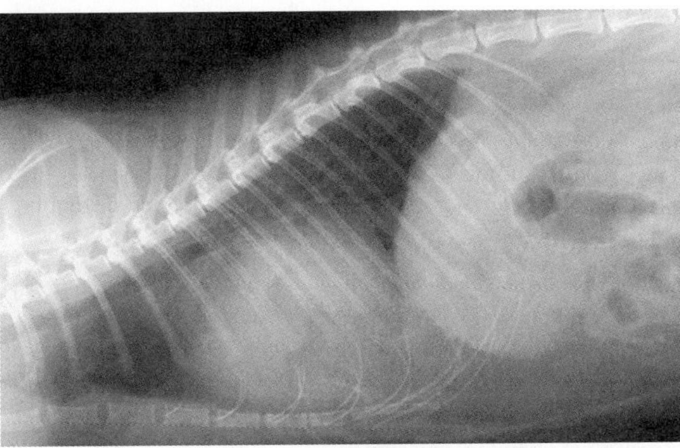

FIGURE I-133 Lateral radiograph of the thorax and cranial abdomen of a cat with PPDH. Note cardiomegaly, irregular soft tissue and fat opacities over the heart, indistinct ventral diaphragm, and small liver. Courtesy of Dr. Stephanie Nykamp.

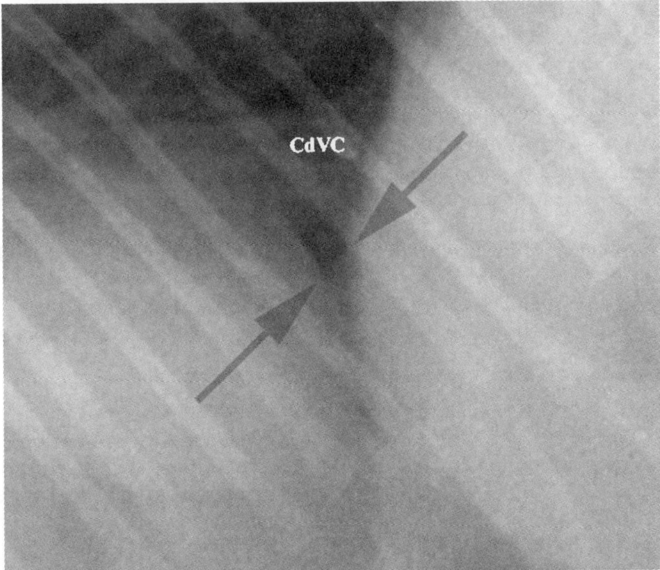

FIGURE I-134 Magnified view of Fig. I-133, showing dorsal mesothelial remnant (between the *arrows*), which is characteristic of PPDH. CdVC: caudal vena cava. Courtesy of Dr. Stephanie Nykamp.

the heart; ± small amount of pericardial effusion.

- Upper GI barium series: may confirm presence of GI segments in pericardial space; often not required for diagnosis.
- Positive contrast peritoneography: 2ml/kg of water-soluble, iodinated radiopaque contrast agent (not barium) injected into peritoneal cavity, followed by elevation of the animal's caudal end and thoracic radiography (contrast may flow into pericardial cavity). Often not required for diagnosis.

TREATMENT

THERAPEUTIC GOAL(S)

- Elimination of clinical signs
- Prevention of vascular compromise or obstruction of organs

ACUTE GENERAL TREATMENT

- Surgical correction via laparotomy: return of all abdominal organs to correct location and closure of the diaphragmatic defect
- Assessment of liver function prior to general anesthesia in order to choose anesthetic protocol accordingly
- It may be appropriate not to pursue surgical repair in some cases (e.g., geriatric animal without clinical signs, small PPDH).

POSSIBLE COMPLICATIONS

- If the PPDH is left uncorrected, the risk of hepatic or splenic incarceration, bowel obstruction, or (rarely) cardiac tamponade and right heart failure persists.
- Surgical complications: difficulty ventilating, hypotension, re-expansion pulmonary edema.

PROGNOSIS AND OUTCOME

- Excellent prognosis with surgical correction.
- Left with an uncorrected PPDH, the patient may remain free of clinical signs, but there is always a risk of complications as listed above.

PEARLS & CONSIDERATIONS

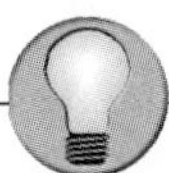

COMMENTS

- PPDH is the most common congenital pericardial disorder in dogs and cats.
- PPDH is a congenital defect (failure of complete separation of the pericardial and abdominal cavities), in contrast to a true diaphragmatic hernia, which is almost always acquired as a result of trauma.
- PPDH is an important rule-out for cardiomegaly and in young animals with cranial abdominal or sternal defects.

SUGGESTED READING

Fossum TW: Surgery of the lower respiratory system: Pleural cavity and diaphragm. In Fossum TW (ed): *Small Animal Surgery*. St. Louis, Mosby, 2002, pp 788–820.

Kienle RD: Pericardial disease and cardiac neoplasia. In Kittleson MD, Kienle RD (eds): *Small Animal Cardiovascular Medicine*. St. Louis, Mosby, 1998, pp 413–432.

Reimer SB, et al: Long-term outcome of cats treated conservatively or surgically for peritoneopericardial diaphragmatic hernia: 66 cases (1987–2002). *J Am Vet Med Assoc* 224:728, 2004.

AUTHOR: **M. LYNNE O'SULLIVAN**

EDITOR: **ETIENNE CÔTÉ**

Peritonitis

BASIC INFORMATION

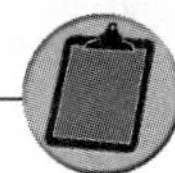

DEFINITION

Inflammation of the peritoneum

EPIDEMIOLOGY

SPECIES, AGE, SEX

- Any species, age, or sex
- Cat: feline infectious peritonitis (FIP)

RISK FACTORS

- Abdominal trauma:
  - Blunt
  - Penetrating
- Intra-abdominal surgery:
  - Gastrointestinal (GI) procedures
- Inflammatory/infectious disease of abdominal organ(s):
  - Cholecystitis/cholangiohepatitis
  - Prostatitis/prostatic abscess
  - Pancreatitis
  - Pyometra
- Cat:
  - Environment that is conducive to transmission of FIP

CONTAGION AND ZOONOSIS: Cat: transmission of coronoavirus FIP is mainly fecal-oral; mutation of coronavirus from less pathogenic form to FIP variant is necessary to cause clinical FIP.

ASSOCIATED CONDITIONS AND DISORDERS

- Sepsis/septic shock
- Coagulopathy/disseminated intravascular coagulation (DIC)
- Systemic inflammatory response syndrome
- Acute respiratory distress syndrome
- Multiple organ dysfunction

CLINICAL PRESENTATION

DISEASE FORMS/SUBTYPES

- Primary versus secondary:
  - Primary
    - Peritoneal inflammation or infection without preexisting intra-abdominal condition:
      - FIP
      - Rare occurrence of bacterial (mycobacteria) and protozoal primary infections
  - Secondary
    - Peritoneal inflammation or infection caused by intra-abdominal pathologic condition:
      - Disruption of hollow viscus
      - Penetrating trauma
      - Organ inflammation/ischemia
      - Iatrogenically induced
- Nonseptic versus septic:
  - Nonseptic
    - Peritoneal inflammation caused by mechanical trauma:
      - Intra-abdominal surgery
    - Sterile foreign material:
      - Urine
      - Bile
      - Iatrogenically introduced: surgical sponge
  - Septic
    - Contamination and subsequent infection of the peritoneal cavity by an infectious agent:
      - Bacteria: most common cause in dog and cat
      - Virus
      - Protozoa

HISTORY, CHIEF COMPLAINT

- History variable depending on underlying cause of peritonitis; may include:
  - Known traumatic event
  - Ingestion of a foreign object
  - Previous abdominal surgery
  - Ongoing or recent treatment for intra-abdominal organ disease
  - Problems urinating or defecating
  - Heat cycle in previous month
- Chief complaint(s) variable depending on underlying cause of peritonitis; may include:
  - Nonspecific complaints:
    - Lethargy, fever, anorexia, vomiting, decreased/no fecal production, diarrhea
  - Complaints related to cause of peritonitis:
    - Wound(s) in abdominal area
    - Urination:
      - Straining to urinate
      - Decreased/no urine production
      - Blood in urine
    - Developing jaundice
    - Vaginal discharge
  - Complaints related to developing peritonitis:
    - Abdominal discomfort:
      - Reluctance to lie down or uncomfortable when lying down
      - "Praying posture"
      - Pain on handling/touching abdomen:
        - May only be subtle (especially in cats)
  - Abdominal distention

PHYSICAL EXAM FINDINGS

- Findings related to peritoneal inflammation
  - Nonspecific findings:
    - Lethargy, fever, dehydration
  - Specific findings:
    - Pain on abdominal palpation
      - Localize to specific region of abdomen if possible
      - May be absent or not dramatic:
        - Even in face of significant peritoneal inflammation
        - Especially in the cat
    - Abdominal distention
    - Fluid
    - Mass
- Findings related to underlying cause of peritonitis
  - Evidence of abdominal trauma:
    - Wound(s)
    - Contusions
    - Disruption of the abdominal wall
  - Linear foreign body caught around tongue base: Clinicians should apply dorsal pressure with thumb externally between mandibles to raise tongue for proper sublingual examination
  - Incision line from previous abdominal surgery
  - Icterus
  - Hematuria, pyuria
  - Purulent or hemorrhagic vaginal discharge
- Findings related to developing sepsis
  - Hyperemia or injected mucous membranes
  - Increased or decreased capillary refill time
  - Tachycardia, tachypnea
  - Hyperdynamic or hypodynamic pulse

ETIOLOGY AND PATHOPHYSIOLOGY

- Peritoneal inflammation: vasculitis, increased capillary permeability
  - Movement of large volumes of fluid into peritoneal cavity
    - Severe hypovolemia or hypovolemic shock
  - Accompanying loss of protein and electrolytes
- Development of coagulation abnormalities due to release of inflammatory mediators and cytokines
  - Hypercoagulable or hypocoagulable state
    - DIC
- If septic, bacterial translocation into the bloodstream
  - Bacteremia
  - Sepsis or septic shock

DIAGNOSIS

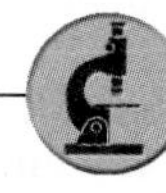

DIFFERENTIAL DIAGNOSIS

- Pain: abdominal, need to rule out non-peritonitis causes:
  - Organ enlargement
  - Organ inflammation
- Pain: nonabdominal, need to rule out:
  - Spinal:
    - Intervertebral disk disease
    - Trauma

- Pelvic:
  - Fracture/dislocation
- Thoracic:
  - Trauma related: rib fractures, diaphragmatic hernia
  - Intrathoracic disease: pleural pain
- Limbs:
  - Joint pain/polyarthritis
- Abdominal distention: fluid:
  - Associated with peritonitis:
    - Refer to fluid analysis for an animal with peritonitis
  - Not associated with peritonitis:
    - Transudate; modified transudate; hemorrhage
- Abdominal distention: mass:
  - Nonperitonitis causes of abdominal mass:
    - Organ enlargement: hepatomegaly, splenomegaly
    - Cyst formation: paraprostatic cyst

INITIAL DATABASE

- Complete blood count (CBC), evidence of:
  - Regenerative left shift: inflammation
  - Degenerative left shift: sepsis
- Serum biochemistry profile:
  - Evidence of cause of peritonitis:
    - Azotemia: uroabdomen versus dehydration (postrenal versus prerenal, respectively)
    - Hyperbilirubinemia: bile peritonitis
  - Assessment of organ function and pathophysiologic effects of the peritonitis:
    - Electrolyte imbalance:
      - Hypokalemia: fluid loss, no intake
      - Hyperkalemia: uroabdomen
    - Hypoproteinemia:
      - Leakage into peritoneal cavity
      - Decreased production
    - Altered blood glucose concentration:
      - Hypoglycemia or hyperglycemia
      - Blood:peritoneal fluid concentration. Blood glucose ≥20 mg/dl higher than peritoneal fluid glucose: highly predictive of septic peritonitis
    - Lactate:
      - Blood:peritoneal fluid lactate concentration difference <−2.0 mmol/L; highly predictive of septic peritonitis in the dog
    - Hyperbilirubinemia:
      - Bile leakage: bile peritonitis
- Urinalysis:
  - Avoid cystocentesis in animals with peritonitis; catheter preferable (indwelling may be desired for monitoring critical cases; contrast cystography for uroperitoneum, etc.)
- Whole abdomen clipping of hair: if possibility of penetrating wound with (e.g., stick, projectile) or without (e.g., tooth, claw) retention of penetrating object
- Survey abdominal radiographs:
  - Findings suggestive of peritonitis:
    - Fluid, causing loss of serosal detail
    - Free gas:
      - Mottling throughout viscera or "gas cap effect" (clearest with horizontal beam radiograph)
    - Ileus
    - Mass(es)
- Ultrasound examination:
  - Integrity of organs
  - Evaluate mass(es)
  - Confirm presence of fluid and obtain sample for analysis (see below)
- Abdominal fluid analysis:
  - Obtain by ultrasound guidance:
    - Preferable to blind abdominocentesis or diagnostic peritoneal lavage
  - Analysis:
    - Glucose, lactate concentrations (see previous text)
    - Urea nitrogen, creatinine concentrations:
      - Fluid:blood creatinine concentration ratio ≥2:1, highly predictive of uroabdomen in the dog
    - Bilirubin concentration:
      - Compare to serum: fluid bilirubin concentration > serum concentration, highly suggestive of bile peritonitis
    - Electrolytes:
      - Fluid:blood potassium concentration ratio ≥1.4:1, highly predictive uroabdomen in the dog
  - Cytologic examination:
    - Neutrophils:
      - Inflammation: increased count, nondegenerative, no intracellular bacteria
      - Septic peritonitis: increased count, toxic changes, intracellular bacteria
    - Plant material: GI leakage
    - Bacteria: Gram stain to aid choice of antibiotic therapy pending culture results
  - Microbiologic culture and sensitivity (C&S) testing:
    - Aerobic and anaerobic

ADVANCED OR CONFIRMATORY TESTING

- Contrast radiographic studies:
  - Uroabdomen: cystography (lower urinary tract) or excretory urography (upper urinary tract; less commonly indicated) to confirm site of disruption prior to surgery
- Coagulation profile: DIC

TREATMENT

THERAPEUTIC GOAL(S)

- Preoperative stabilization of the animal
- Surgical correction if needed
- Postoperative care
- In nonsurgical cases (e.g., feline infectious peritonitis), supportive care and management of the underlying cause

ACUTE AND CHRONIC TREATMENT

- Correction of fluid and electrolyte abnormalities:
  - Hypovolemia
  - Hypokalemia or hyperkalemia:
    - Uroabdomen: hyperkalemia:
      - Potassium-free fluids: 0.9% NaCl (see Hyperkalemia, p 546)
- Blood products if necessary (see Transfusion Reactions, p 1098):
  - Whole blood:
    - Anemia
    - Coagulopathy
  - Packed red cells:
    - Anemia
  - Fresh frozen plasma:
    - Hypoproteinemia
    - Coagulopathy
- Appropriate antimicrobial therapy if septic:
  - Empiric therapy (aerobic and anaerobic coverage):
    - Second-generation cephalosporin:
      - Cefoxitin, 22 mg/kg IV q 2h during the perioperative period, then q 6h
    - Combination therapy:
      - Metronidazole, 10–15 mg/kg IV q 12h; enrofloxacin, 2.5–5 mg/kg (diluted 1:1 in sterile saline and given via slow IV q 12h), and ampicillin, 22 mg/kg IV q 6h
  - Ultimately based on culture results
- Surgical exploration of abdomen to identify and correct underlying cause of peritonitis if appropriate (e.g., evidence of septic peritonitis, or hemorrhage in the absence of systemic bleeding disorder)
  - Thorough lavage of the abdominal cavity
- Consideration of need for postoperative drainage of the abdominal cavity
- Specific sites within the abdomen: drain placement:
  - Pancreatic abscess
  - Prostatic abscess
  - Necrotizing cholecystitis
- Entire abdominal cavity:
  - Open abdominal drainage
- Postoperative intensive care, with continuous monitoring of animal, until peritonitis has resolved

POSSIBLE COMPLICATIONS

See Peritonitis, Septic, p 840; Feline Infectious Peritonitis, p 378; other relevant topics

RECOMMENDED MONITORING

Dependent on cause of peritonitis; see Peritonitis, Septic, p 840; Sepsis and Septic Shock, p 996; Systemic Inflammatory

Response Syndrome, p 1060; Multiple Organ Dysfunction Syndrome, p 716

PROGNOSIS AND OUTCOME

Variable; dependent on underlying cause

PEARLS & CONSIDERATIONS

COMMENTS

In general, septic peritonitis is associated with a poorer prognosis than nonseptic peritonitis. There is a significant difference in survival rates for animals with nonseptic versus septic bile peritonitis.

SUGGESTED READING

Bonczynski JJ, Ludwig LL, Barton LJ, et al: Comparison of peritoneal fluid and peripheral blood pH, bicarbonate, glucose, and lactate concentration as a diagnostic tool for septic peritonitis in dogs and cats. *Vet Surg* 32:161-166, 2003.

King LG: Postoperative complications and prognostic indicators in dogs and cats with septic peritonitis: 23 cases (1989-1992). *J Am Vet Med Assoc* 204:407-414, 1994.

Kirby BM: Peritonitis. In Slatter (ed): *Textbook of Small Animal Surgery*, ed 3. Philadelphia, WB Saunders, 2003, pp 421-429.

Schmiedt C, Tobias KM, Otto CM: Evaluation of abdominal fluid: Peripheral blood creatinine and potassium ratios for diagnosis of uroperitoneum in dogs. *J Vet Emerg Crit Care* 11(4):275-280, 2001.

AUTHOR: **ELLEN B. DAVIDSON DOMNICK**

EDITOR: **RICHARD WALSHAW**

Peritonitis, Septic

BASIC INFORMATION

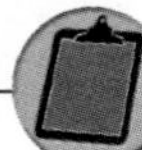

DEFINITION

Peritonitis is the local or generalized inflammation of the peritoneum; a diagnosis of septic peritonitis is based on identification of toxic neutrophils with intracellular bacteria within abdominal fluid.

EPIDEMIOLOGY

SPECIES, AGE, SEX: There is no species or sex predilection; younger animals that are prone to ingesting foreign material and older animals with gastrointestinal (GI) masses that can perforate are predisposed.

RISK FACTORS: Gastrointestinal surgery, gastric dilation, and volvulus with gastric resection.

ASSOCIATED CONDITIONS AND DISORDERS: Neoplasia, linear foreign body, gastric dilation, and volvulus.

CLINICAL PRESENTATION

DISEASE FORMS/SUBTYPE

- GI perforation
- Non-GI perforation of an abdominal organ (e.g., pyometra, prostatic abscesses, hepatic abscess)

HISTORY, CHIEF COMPLAINT

- Lethargy
- Collapse
- Vomiting

PHYSICAL EXAM FINDINGS

- Tachycardia and signs of hypovolemic or septic shock
- Signs of abdominal pain
- Ascites
- Fever
- Altered mentation
- Injected mucous membranes/hyperemia

ETIOLOGY AND PATHOPHYSIOLOGY

- Bacteria gain access to the abdominal cavity. This occurs most frequently via the perforation of the intestinal tract although other internal sources (genitourinary tract, liver) and external sources (penetrating trauma) are possible.
- Infection within the abdominal cavity causes localized inflammation with cellular inflammation and fibrin production.
- The peritoneum responds with increased vascular permeability, cellular infiltration with leukocytes and macrophages, and fibrin deposition.
- With increases in vascular permeability, interstitial fluid may accumulate rapidly.
- Substantial quantities of electrolytes, plasma proteins, and red blood cells (RBCs) may extravasate and be lost through third-spacing in the abdominal cavity.
- This loss may progress to the point of causing hypovolemia, dehydration, severe hemoconcentration, septicemia, and metabolic alterations.

DIAGNOSIS

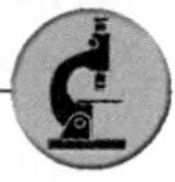

DIFFERENTIAL DIAGNOSIS

Differentiation from other causes of abdominal pain or distention (acute abdomen), such as pain caused by sterile ascites, neoplasia, or sterile pancreatitis (see Acute Abdomen, p 29)

INITIAL DATABASE

- Complete blood count (CBC), serum chemistry panel, urinalysis with culture
  - Urine sample obtained by urethral catheterization if possible; cystocentesis may inadvertently retrieve septic ascitic fluid
- Abdominal radiographs: may document free intra-abdominal air
  - Highly suggestive/specific for septic peritonitis unless air is result of prior abdominal surgery in the preceding week
- Abdominal ultrasound
- Abdominocentesis with fluid analysis, cytologic examination, and culture and sensitivity (C&S) (both aerobic and anaerobic)

ADVANCED OR CONFIRMATORY TESTING

- Clotting profiles (prothrombin time and activated partial thromboplastin time) are useful because many animals with septic peritonitis are septic and thus have coagulopathy.
- Abdominocentesis (see Abdominocentesis, p 1178) and diagnostic peritoneal lavage (see Diagnostic Peritoneal Lavage, p 1225) have been shown to be safe and reliable in evaluating a septic peritonitis.
  - Abdominocentesis: Clinicians can clip the ventral abdomen, aseptically prepare the site, and introduce a 22-gauge needle into the peritoneal cavity just to the right or left of midline (just cranial to the umbilicus). It may help to retrieve fluid by placing two needles simultaneously into the abdominal cavity separated by 2-4 cm.
  - Diagnostic peritoneal lavage: placement of a large bore (12-gauge) 5¼-inch catheter with additional side holes aseptically into the abdomen, followed by instillation of 20 ml/kg body weight of warm (body temperature) sterile saline into the peritoneum using an IV administration set, allowing the fluid to flow with gravity.

The patient is then carefully rolled from side to side to mix the fluid. Finally, a sample is recovered for cytologic examination and for C&S.

- The diagnosis of bacterial peritonitis is based on the presence of toxic degenerate neutrophils with intracellular bacteria in the abdominal fluid.
  - In most cases, the glucose level of the abdominal fluid is at least 20 mg/dl lower than that of the peripheral blood glucose level.

TREATMENT

THERAPEUTIC GOAL(S)

- Animal stabilization
- Identification and correction of underlying cause

ACUTE GENERAL TREATMENT

- Initial treatment must be directed toward stabilization of the metabolic consequences of peritonitis.
- IV fluids (60-90 ml/kg), plasma (10-15 ml/kg), or whole blood may be necessary to maintain cardiac output.
  - Hematocrit to be maintained above 21%
- Exploratory laporatomy is warranted as soon as possible.
  - Stabilization of the patient as much as possible preoperatively
  - Repair of the lesion
  - Biopsy of affected tissues and intraoperative cultures
  - Lavage
  - Closed suction drainage (warranted in almost all cases)
  - Open abdominal drainage if extensive contamination is present
- Broad-spectrum antimicrobial therapy; recommendations include:
  - Ampicillin: 22 mg/kg IV q 6h, + gentamicin 6 mg/kg IV q 24h
    - Gentamicin q 24h is less nephrotoxic than q 12h or q 8h.
    - Gentamicin should not be initiated until the animal is both hydrated and producing urine.
  - Ampicillin: 22 mg/kg IV q 6h, + enrofloxacin 10 mg/kg IV q 24h
    - Enrofloxacin IV should be diluted in saline; use is extralabel.
    - Avoid enrofloxacin at this dose in cats (permanent retinopathy possible).
  - Cefazolin: 22 mg/kg IV q 8h, + gentimicin or enrofloxacin (according to dosage just presented) + metronidazole 10 mg/kg IV q 8h
- Hospital-acquired infections (e.g., dehiscence of enterotomy sites) should be treated based on the sensitivity pattern of the hospital's pathogenic flora.

POSSIBLE COMPLICATIONS

- Sepsis
- Multiple organ dysfunction syndrome
- Dehisence at site of prior repair
- Hypoalbumemia

RECOMMENDED MONITORING

- Hydration status
- Serum total protein and albumin levels
- Serum electrolytes
- Serum/blood glucose level
- Blood pressure (BP)
- Renal function/urine output
- Central venous pressure
- Adequacy of pain control

PROGNOSIS AND OUTCOME

The reported mortality rate for dogs and cats with septic peritonitis ranges from 20-70%. The clinician should inform the owner of the mortality rate prior to surgery.

PEARLS & CONSIDERATIONS

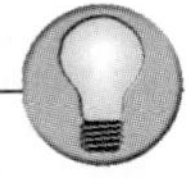

COMMENTS

- Gastric perforations may result in a large amount of free intra-abdominal air without fluid.
- Linear foreign bodies are particularly prone to perforation.

PREVENTION

Good surgical technique is required for abdominal surgery.

SUGGESTED READING

Bonczynski J, et al: Comparison of peritoneal fluid and peripheral blood pH, bicarbonate, glucose, and lactate concentration as a diagnostic tool for septic peritonitis in dogs and cats. *Vet Surg* 32(2):161-166, 2003.

Mueller MG, et al: Use of closed suction drains to treat generalized peritonitis in dogs and cats: 40 cases (1997-1999). *J Am Vet Med Assoc* 219:789-794, 2001.

AUTHOR: **DANNA M. TORRE**

EDITOR: **ELIZABETH ROZANSKI**

Petechiae and Ecchymoses

BASIC INFORMATION

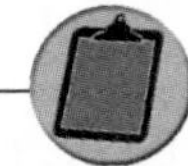

DEFINITION

Manifestations of disorders of the platelet and/or blood vessel wall (primary hemostasis) that can result in bleeding in the skin or mucous membranes to a degree that is out of proportion to the trauma. Petechiae are pinpoint hemorrhages, whereas an ecchymosis is a large area of hemorrhage that can resemble a bruise.

SYNONYM(S)

Bruising

Hemorrhagic diathesis

EPIDEMIOLOGY

SPECIES, AGE, SEX: Dependent on underlying cause:

- Young, purebred animals: von Willebrand disease, thrombasthenia, thrombopathia
- Young to middle-aged animals: infectious diseases, trauma
- Middle-aged animals: acquired immune-mediated diseases
- Older animals: neoplasia

GENETICS AND BREED PREDISPOSITIONS

- von Willebrand disease (doberman pinscher, Airedale, German shepherd, Scottish terrier, Chesapeake Bay retriever, and many other breeds; cats: Himalayan)
- Thrombopathia: basset hounds
- Thrombasthenia: otterhounds
- More common in dogs than in cats

RISK FACTORS

- Thrombocytopenia:
  - Immune-mediated disease: young to middle-aged, small to medium female dogs
  - Rickettsial disease: dogs living in or traveling to endemic areas
  - Bone marrow disease
- Thrombopathia/thrombasthenia:
  - Previous/current administration of nonsteroidal anti-inflammatory drugs (NSAIDs)
  - Metabolic diseases: uremia, liver disease, paraproteinemia/hyperglobulinemia
- Vascular disease:
  - Hyperadrenocorticism
  - Drug reaction
  - Rocky Mountain spotted fever

CLINICAL PRESENTATION

HISTORY, CHIEF COMPLAINT

- Nasal hemorrhage
- Pinpoint to large areas of bleeding on skin and mucous membranes
- Bruising
- Melena
- Hematuria

PHYSICAL EXAM FINDINGS

- Epistaxis

- Melena: from swallowing blood
- Petechiae, ecchymoses, hematochezia, and hematuria

ETIOLOGY AND PATHOPHYSIOLOGY

- Thrombocytopenia:
  - Immune-mediated disease: idiopathic disease, systemic lupus erythematosus (SLE), drug reaction
  - Rickettsial disease: ehrlichiosis, Rocky Mountain spotted fever
  - Bone marrow disease: neoplasia, aplastic anemia, infectious (fungal, rickettsial, or viral)
  - Disseminated intravascular coagulation (DIC)
- Thrombopathia:
  - Congenital: von Willebrand disease, thrombasthenia, thrombopathia
  - Acquired: NSAIDs, hyperglobulinemia (*Ehrlichia,* multiple myeloma), uremia, DIC
- Vascular disease:
  - Vasculitis: immune-mediated and rickettsial diseases
  - Vascular hemostatic defect:
    - Heightened permeability: hyperadrenocorticism
    - Reduced vessel strength: Ehlers-Danlos syndrome
    - Lack of contraction

The conditions just described will all cause capillary hemorrhage, which, unlike clotting factor defects, will result in frank hemorrhage.

DIAGNOSIS

DIFFERENTIAL DIAGNOSIS

- Trauma resulting in areas of bruising
- Hemolytic uremic syndrome
- Cutaneous vasculopathy of greyhounds
- Cutaneous hemangioma or hemagiosarcoma

INITIAL DATABASE

- Complete blood count (CBC):
  - Anemia if enough hemorrhage has occurred
  - RBC fragmentation suggests DIC or other vascular disease
  - Thrombocytopenia
  - Neutrophilia: nonspecific stress, infection, neoplasia
  - Pancytopenia: bone marrow disease
- Urinalysis:
  - Usually normal
  - Isosthenuria with renal disease
  - Hematuria
  - Proteinuria (e.g., with ehrlichosis)
- Serum biochemistry profile:
  - Hypoproteinemia: if enough hemorrhage has occurred
  - Elevated urea with normal creatinine: gastrointestinal (GI) blood
  - Azotemia with renal disease or prerenal causes
  - Hyperglobulinemia with ehrlichiosis, multiple myeloma
  - Elevated ALP activity with hyperadrenocorticism

ADVANCED OR CONFIRMATORY TESTING

- Other laboratory tests:
  - Coagulation profile: prolonged times with DIC; normal with thrombocytopenia and thrombopathia
  - von Willebrand factor analysis
  - Buccal mucosa bleeding time
  - Antinuclear antibody test: SLE
  - Platelet function testing
  - *Ehrlichia* and Rocky Mountain spotted fever titers, polymerase chain reaction (PCR)
- Other diagnostic procedures:
  - Bone marrow aspiration biopsy: with pancytopenia
  - Skin biopsy: vascular disease, cutaneous lesions

TREATMENT

THERAPEUTIC GOAL(S)

Treatment of the primary cause

ACUTE GENERAL TREATMENT

- Restriction of patient's activity or stimuli that precipitate hemorrhage episodes
- Discontinuation of any medications that may alter platelet function
- Blood or platelet transfusions with severe anemia

SPECIFIC TREATMENT

- Immune-suppressive therapy for immune-mediated thrombocytopenia
- von Willebrand disease: plasma or cryoprecipitate for acute bleeding
- Hyperglobulinemia: plasmapheresis
- Vasculitis: doxycycline for rickettsial disease; prednisone for primary immune-mediated diseases

POSSIBLE COMPLICATIONS

- Anemia and collapse state
- Hemorrhage into the brain or other vital organs

RECOMMENDED MONITORING

- Platelet count with thrombocytopenia
- Clinical signs

PROGNOSIS AND OUTCOME

Dependent on cause

PEARLS & CONSIDERATIONS

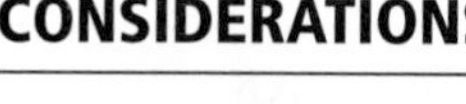

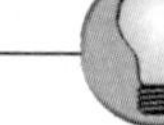

COMMENTS

Petechial hemorrhage is not a diagnosis but a clinical sign

CLIENT EDUCATION

Recurrence of clinical signs

SUGGESTED READING

Callan MB: Epistaxis and hemoptysis. In Ettinger SJ, Feldman EC (eds): *Textbook of Veterinary Internal Medicine*, ed 6. Philadelphia, WB Saunders, 2006, pp 232-235.

De Gopegui RR: Acquired and inherited platelet dysfunction in small animals. *Comp Cont Educ Pract Vet* 20:1039-1052, 1998.

AUTHOR: **REMO LOBETTI**
EDITOR: **ETIENNE CÔTÉ**

Petroleum Distillates/Turpentine Toxicosis

BASIC INFORMATION

DEFINITION

- Toxicosis caused by any of a number of hydrogen- and carbon-containing (HC) chemicals originating from distillation of crude oil/petroleum; a few compounds also originate from steam distillation of plants.
- Toxicosis is usually due to accidental dermal or oral exposure to HC-containing products and is manifested by repeated vomiting, retching, vocalization, lethargy, salivation, anorexia, ataxia, and signs of aspiration pneumonia (wheezing, coughing, dyspnea, panting).

SYNONYM(S)

Petroleum hydrocarbons toxicosis

Examples of hydrocarbon-containing products: naphtha, gasoline, kerosene, paint thinners/strippers, engine cleaners/

degreasers, diesel fuel, heating fuels, lamp and furniture oils, waxes, lubricating oils, grease, paraffin wax, tar, asphalt

Plant distillate examples: turpentine, linseed oil

EPIDEMIOLOGY

SPECIES, AGE, SEX

- Dogs more commonly are exposed than cats.
- Because of grooming behavior, topical exposure in cats can lead to clinically significant oral exposure.

RISK FACTORS

- Free-roaming animals are at higher risk for accidental exposures (open garage, workshop, shed, or construction area).
- Fenced dogs may chew into charcoal lighter fluid containers or lick hydrocarbon spills from a garage floor or work area.

GEOGRAPHY AND SEASONALITY: Warmer months involve an increased use of hydrocarbon distillate-containing products outdoors, with increased opportunities for exposure.

CLINICAL PRESENTATION

HISTORY, CHIEF COMPLAINT

- Evidence or suspicion of exposure to hydrocarbon-containing product
- Onset of clinical signs generally <1-3 hours after exposure
- Owner may note salivation, vomiting, retching, excessive licking motions, and coughing

PHYSICAL EXAM FINDINGS

- Presence of product on the feet, muzzle, or on the trunk
- Hydrocarbon/distillate smell on the coat or breath
- Dermal discomfort (tender and inflamed interdigital or other dermally exposed areas)
- Hyperirritability, agitation, pacing, and crying/whimpering
- Oral exposure: hypersalivation, vomiting, excessive licking motions, hacking, retching, panting, wheezing, coughing, crackling lung sounds
- Ocular: blepharospasm, blepharitis
- Distillate odor on the animal

ETIOLOGY AND PATHOPHYSIOLOGY

- The physical and chemical properties of a particular hydrocarbon determine its toxicity. Hydrocarbons with lower boiling points (more flammable), lower viscosities ("thinner"), and lower surface tensions are more dangerous due to an increased ability to penetrate lipid membranes (increased systemic absorption) and increased ability to "spread" over larger surface areas (providing an increased risk of aspiration).
- Volatile hydrocarbons damage nerve endings and solubilize subdermal/submucosal fat, resulting in acute, generalized pain and discomfort. Systemic absorption can result in dissolution of cellular lipids and cell necrosis with generalized systemic inflammation and congestion. Some specific hydrocarbons can cause more direct organ damage (e.g., benzene causes bone marrow toxicity).

DIAGNOSIS

DIFFERENTIAL DIAGNOSIS

- Acute gastrointestinal (GI) viral and bacterial diseases
- Acute upper and lower respiratory infections
- Organophosphate or carbamate insecticides, zinc phosphide

INITIAL DATABASE

- Complete blood count (CBC): leukocytosis, neutrophilia; possibly septic changes if pneumonia complication; possible hemoconcentration
- Serum biochemistry profile: hypoglycemia possible
- Urinalysis: unremarkable
- Baseline chest radiograph if respiratory involvement (aspiration)
- Pulse oximetry or arterial blood gas measurement if respiratory involvement (aspiration)

ADVANCED OR CONFIRMATORY TESTING

- Simple spot test: vigorously mix warm water and vomitus; distillates will come to the surface; clinicians will note characteristic odor of volatile distillates (e.g., gasoline, charcoal lighter fluid).
- Confirmatory analysis of the distillate is possible but is usually of academic interest and not useful in terms of clinical management; collect samples in airtight containers and refrigerate.

TREATMENT

THERAPEUTIC GOAL(S)

- Minimizing risk of aspiration and pneumonitis
- Prevention of systemic absorption
- General supportive care by bathing with a mild dishwashing detergent solution if exposure is dermal

ACUTE GENERAL TREATMENT

- Emesis, gastric lavage, and administration of activated charcoal are contraindicated due to increased risk of aspiration.
- Oxygen supplementation if the animal is in respiratory distress.
- Mechanical ventilation may be necessary, depending on oxygen concentration and delivery.
- IV fluid support (may begin with 0.9% NaCl; adjustment based on electrolytes, hydration, etc.) to maintain hydration and perfusion; forced diuresis is not effective at eliminating toxins more rapidly.
- Pain control (e.g., butorphanol 0.1-0.2 mg/kg IV or 0.2-0.6 mg/kg IM or SC q 4-8h) because dermal exposure in particular can be painful.
- Corticosteroids: controversial; sometimes considered in aspiration pneumonia, but there is an increased risk of infection; avoid prolonged use.
- Early prophylactic antibiotic use is controversial; hydrocarbon pneumonitis has been reported to be of low risk for bacterial pneumonia complication.
- Broad-spectrum antibiotics (amoxicillin with clavulanate [12-20 mg/kg PO q 12h], second- or third-generation cephalosporins [e.g., cefoxitin 30 mg/kg IV q 8h to q 6h], or fluoroquinolones [e.g., enrofloxacin 5 mg/kg IM or diluted 1:1 in saline and given slowly IV q 12h or q 24h in cats]) for secondary bacterial pneumonia.
- Dermal decontamination, which consists of bathing (including haircoat and feet) with a mild, liquid dishwashing detergent solution and rinsing thoroughly.

CHRONIC TREATMENT

If aspiration pneumonitis: oxygen supplementation, mechanical ventilation as necessary

POSSIBLE COMPLICATIONS

Aspiration and clinical pneumonitis

RECOMMENDED MONITORING

- Chest radiographs as needed
- Arterial blood gas and PaO_2 monitoring in animals that are compromised
- CBC and serum biochemistry profile
- In animals with a pulmonary condition, clinicians can consider tracheal aspirate for a Gram stain or culture to assist with antibiotic selection

PROGNOSIS AND OUTCOME

- Good for cases in which no aspiration pneumonia develops
- Guarded if aspiration occurs; update as needed

PEARLS & CONSIDERATIONS

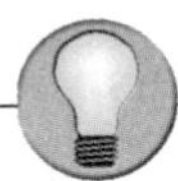

COMMENTS

- "Routine" decontamination measures (emesis, charcoal, gastric lavage) are contraindicated.

- Most commercial or industrial products containing a petroleum distillate carry a rather stern warning "may be harmful or fatal if swallowed." This warning is not specific to the individual product and does not automatically imply a poor prognosis. It is more useful to think in terms of the volatility of the product when reasoning out the relative clinical risk to the animal, with greater volatility carrying a higher risk.
- Aspiration pneumonia caused by exposure to motor oil, transmission oil, waxes, other lubricating oils, grease, paraffin wax, and asphalt is very low. Most of these exposures result in mild self-limiting vomiting, lethargy, and diarrhea.
- Petroleum distillates are listed here in terms of their volatility: tar (least volatile); paraffin wax, lubricating oil, fuel oil, mineral seal oil, kerosene (intermediate); mineral spirits, gasoline, petroleum naphtha, petroleum ether (most volatile).

CLIENT EDUCATION

Owners should keep all products under lock and key and out of reach of pets. Childproof containers are not animal proof.

SUGGESTED READING

Raisbeck MF: Petroleum hydrocarbons. In Peterson ME, Talcott PA (eds): *Small Animal Toxicology*. Philadelphia, WB Saunders, 2001, pp 666–675.

AUTHOR: **MICHAEL W. KNIGHT**
EDITOR: **SAFDAR A. KHAN**

Phenobarbital: Adverse Effects/Toxicoses

BASIC INFORMATION

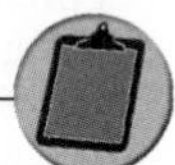

DEFINITION

Adverse, unintended effects resulting from repeated therapeutic doses of phenobarbital (chronic exposure) or from an excessively high dose of phenobarbital (acute exposure caused by accidental ingestion of a prescription drug or a dosage miscalculation). Additional information regarding acute barbiturates toxicosis can be found under Barbiturates Toxicosis, p 115.

EPIDEMIOLOGY

SPECIES, AGE, SEX: All species and ages; both sexes.

CLINICAL PRESENTATION

DISEASE FORMS/SUBTYPES

- Chronic exposure:
  - Central nervous system (CNS) effects: sedation, lethargy, ataxia; hyperactivity, nervousness
  - Polyuria and polydipsia (PU/PD)
  - Polyphagia, weight gain, indiscriminate ingestions
  - Increased serum liver-associated enzymes without clinical signs of liver disease
  - Decreased serum thyroxine (T4) and free T4; ± mildly increased serum thyroid-stimulating hormone (TSH)
  - Hepatotoxicity
  - Blood dyscrasias
  - Hepatocutaneous syndrome
  - Physical dependency
  - Pancreatitis
  - Generalized hypersensitivity reaction
- Acute overdose: adverse CNS effects

HISTORY, CHIEF COMPLAINT: Prescription or possibility of accidental exposure to phenobarbital. Abnormalities of virtually any organ system can be caused by phenobarbital.

PHYSICAL EXAM FINDINGS

- Chronic exposure: one or more of the following may be present:
  - Sedation, ataxia
  - Hyperactivity, nervousness
  - Lethargy, depression
  - Anorexia, vomiting
  - Abdominal pain
  - Icterus, ascites
  - Infection
  - Skin erythema, vesicles, crusted erosions, hyperkeratosis; especially affects footpads, painful
  - Ecchymoses
  - Ulcerations of mouth, mucocutaneous junctions; ear lesions; facial rash; pruritus; swelling of feet and limbs
  - Generalized lymphadenopathy
- Acute overdose:
  - Acute onset of CNS depression, ataxia, weakness, hypothermia, respiratory depression, respiratory arrest, cardiac arrhythmias, hypotension, coma, death
  - Time to onset of signs: 15 minutes to 2 hours
  - Duration of signs: 24 hours to 8 days or longer (dose-dependent)

ETIOLOGY AND PATHOPHYSIOLOGY

- Sedation, PU/PD, polyphagia: direct CNS effects; common after start of drug and often improves within weeks. Sedation is also common with high serum drug concentrations.
- Hyperactivity, nervousness: often associated with low serum drug concentrations.
- Increased serum liver-associated enzymes without clinical liver disease: elevated alkaline phosphatase (ALP) (50% of dogs); alanine aminotransferase (ALT) (25% of dogs); can occur within weeks to months. Other liver enzymes are less commonly elevated. Elevated ALP may be due either to liver abnormalities or to benign induction; elevated ALT most likely due to early liver injury.
- Decreased serum T4: occurs in 40% of dogs and is likely due to increased metabolism and excretion of T4; can occur within weeks. It is generally not associated with clinical signs of hypothyroidism.
- Hepatotoxicity: uncommon but potentially fatal; occurs in dogs (suspected in cats but not documented) and is unpredictable. Usually associated with long-term treatment (months to years) and high serum drug concentrations (>40 μg/ml). Unknown if dose-dependent or idiosyncratic; histopathologic examination reveals hepatic cirrhosis.
- Blood dyscrasias: neutropenia, thrombocytopenia, and/or anemia that often occur within weeks; likely an idiosyncratic or hypersensitivity reaction.
- Hypersensitivity reaction: especially in cats, immunologic mechanism; can affect many organs and often occurs within weeks.
- Physical dependency: can occur within weeks; abrupt discontinuation of drug can precipitate withdrawal seizures.
- Pancreatitis: increased risk with phenobarbital/bromide combination.
- Acute overdose: signs are dose-dependent (ASPCA Animal Poison Control Center information) as shown in Table I-23. Note that any dose leading to coma can also cause death if the animal is left untreated.

DIAGNOSIS

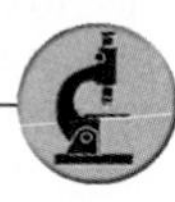

DIFFERENTIAL DIAGNOSIS

Dependent on adverse effects

INITIAL DATABASE

- Serum biochemical profile, CBC
- Serum phenobarbital concentration

TABLE I-23 Signs of Acute Phenobarbital Overdose According to Amount of Drug Intake

Sedation, ataxia:	1-2 mg/kg orally (dogs, cats); any dose IV (dogs, cats)
Recumbent:	12 mg/kg orally (dogs)
Severe CNS signs:	20 mg/kg orally (dogs)
Unconsciousness:	65 mg/kg orally (dogs); 6-10 mg/kg IV (dogs; expect cats similar)
Lethal dose:	110 mg/kg orally (dogs); 125 mg/kg orally (cats)

ADVANCED OR CONFIRMATORY TESTING

- Hepatotoxicity: abdominal radiography/ultrasonography; preprandial and postprandial bile acids; coagulation profile; histopathologic evaluation of biopsy
- Decreased T4: serum TSH concentration
- Pancreatitis: abdominal radiography/ultrasonography; pancreas-specific lipase immunoreactivity
- Blood dyscrasias: bone marrow aspirate
- Dermatopathy: dermatohistopathologic examination
- Acute overdose: analysis of blood, stomach contents, urine, feces for drug

TREATMENT

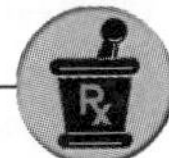

THERAPEUTIC GOAL(S)

- Chronic exposure: If adverse effects are serious, decrease drug dosage or discontinue phenobarbital and initiate alternative anticonvulsant.
- Acute overdose: Stabilize and decontaminate the animal, and then provide supportive care until phenobarbital has been eliminated. Repeated doses of activated charcoal will hasten elimination of the drug from the body.

ACUTE GENERAL TREATMENT

- Chronic exposure:
  - Sedation, PU/PD, polyphagia: If serum drug concentration is excessive, decrease drug dosage.
  - Hyperactivity, nervousness: If drug concentration is low, increase drug dosage.
  - Increased serum liver-associated enzymes without clinical liver disease:
    - If ALP is elevated but other liver-associated enzymes, albumin, and BUN are normal and serum phenobarbital concentration is not excessive, elevation may be due to benign enzyme induction. Monitor the animal and the serum biochemical profile frequently as well as rule out other causes of elevated ALP (e.g., hyperadrenocorticism, corticosteroids).
    - If ALT is greater than two times the upper limit of normal, consider decreasing drug dosage and monitor ALT or can discontinue phenobarbital and initiate alternative anticonvulsant. Discontinue phenobarbital gradually over several weeks to avoid withdrawal-induced seizures. Loading dosages of alternative anticonvulsant may be necessary.
    - If ALT is elevated and BUN and/or albumin are decreased, liver damage is likely. Pursue further diagnostics and discontinue phenobarbital as previously described.
  - Decreased serum T4: Initiate supplemental T4 only if the animal has clinical signs of hypothyroidism.
  - Hepatotoxicity: Discontinue phenobarbital and initiate alternative anticonvulsant. Rapidity of phenobarbital discontinuation depends on severity of liver disease. If the liver is functional and metabolizing phenobarbital, reduce the dose over several weeks. If the liver is severely affected, causing elevated serum drug concentration due to impaired metabolism, phenobarbital may be abruptly discontinued and an alternative anticonvulsant initiated. Monitor the animal's serum phenobarbital concentration daily and treat liver disease.
  - Blood dyscrasias, hypersensitivity reactions, hepatocutaneous syndrome: Discontinue phenobarbital as previously described and initiate alternative anticonvulsant. Treat signs associated with dyscrasia, hypersensitivity, or dermatitis.
  - Pancreatitis: Discontinue the combination of phenobarbital and bromide, then initiate monotherapy with phenobarbital or bromide or an alternative anticonvulsant.
- Acute overdose:
  - Treatment: See Barbiturates Toxicosis, p 115.
  - No specific antidote.

DRUG INTERACTIONS

Drugs that inhibit drug-metabolizing enzymes (e.g., chloramphenicol, cimetidine) can elevate serum phenobarbital concentration and lead to toxicity.

RECOMMENDED MONITORING

- CBC, serum biochemical profile before starting phenobarbital; repeat these tests after 1 to 2 months and every 6 to 12 months or when the animal is ill.
- Monitor the serum phenobarbital concentration 2 weeks after the start of drug and every 6 to 12 months or when the animal is ill or has recurrence of seizures.

PROGNOSIS AND OUTCOME

- With milder adverse effects, prognosis is generally good.
- With serious adverse effects (hepatotoxicity, blood dyscrasias), prognosis can be good if phenobarbital is discontinued early; otherwise, the condition can be fatal.
- Hypersensitivity reactions can resolve within days to weeks of discontinuing the drug.

PEARLS & CONSIDERATIONS

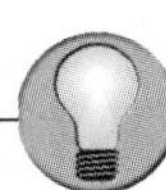

COMMENTS

- Liver failure can cause a rapid rise in serum phenobarbital concentration due to impaired drug metabolism.
- Serum liver-associated enzymes can increase transiently after seizure activity.

PREVENTION

- Maintain serum phenobarbital concentration within the therapeutic range to decrease the risk of adverse effects (dogs 15-40 μg/ml; cats 23-30 μg/ml). Multiply μg/ml by 4.31 to convert to μmol/L.
- Base drug dosage alterations on serum drug concentration. Variation in metabolism of phenobarbital exists between individual animals, resulting in poor correlations between oral dosage of drug and serum drug concentration.

SUGGESTED READING

Berendt M: Epilepsy. In Vite CH (ed): *Braund's Clinical Neurology in Small Animals—Localization, Diagnosis, and Treatment.* New York, International Veterinary Information Service, 2005. www.ivis.org.

AUTHOR: **CYNTHIA GASKILL**
EDITOR: **SAFDAR A. KHAN**

Pheochromocytoma

BASIC INFORMATION

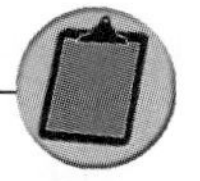

DEFINITION

A chromaffin cell tumor of the adrenal medulla (most common) or extra-adrenal sympathetic ganglia (paragangliomas)

EPIDEMIOLOGY

SPECIES, AGE, SEX

- Dogs: uncommon; middle-aged/old (mean of 11 years; range of 1 to 18 years)
- Cats: rare; old (mean 14.5 years)

ASSOCIATED CONDITIONS AND DISORDERS: May occur as part of multiple endocrine neoplasia syndrome.

CLINICAL PRESENTATION

HISTORY, CHIEF COMPLAINT

- Dogs:
  - Intermittent weakness and collapse are most common. Other clinical signs may include panting/tachypnea, agitation, polyuria and polydipsia (PU/PD), lethargy, vomiting, diarrhea, inappetence/anorexia, sudden blindness, seizures, or sudden death.
  - Signs are often episodic and complicated by the high incidence of concurrent disease.
  - Many animals show no clinical signs, and the diagnosis is made incidentally during abdominal ultrasonography or necropsy.
- Cats: PU/PD, lethargy, and anorexia are most common.

PHYSICAL EXAM FINDINGS

- The physical examination is commonly unremarkable.
- When present, abnormalities may include tachypnea, generalized weakness (often episodic), tachycardia and/or cardiac arrhythmias, and pale mucous membranes; epistaxis, muscle tremors, blindness, retinal hemorrhage/detachment, and signs of abdominal pain are also possible.
- An abdominal mass is not usually palpable.

ETIOLOGY AND PATHOPHYSIOLOGY

- Usually solitary, slow-growing, highly vascular tumors. Rare bilateral pheochromocytomas or adrenal pheochromocytomas with a contralateral adrenocortical tumor have been reported.
- Considered malignant, with local invasion (e.g., caudal vena cava) and metastasis to liver and regional lymph nodes most common.
- Clinical signs result from sporadic oversecretion of catecholamines or local tumor invasion and metastasis.
- Excess catecholamines cause arteriolar vasoconstriction and systemic hypertension, cardiac arrhythmias, mydriasis, increased smooth muscle sphincter tone, and increased hepatic gluconeogenesis and glycogenolysis.

DIAGNOSIS

A presumptive diagnosis rests on identification of concurrent systemic hypertension and an adrenal mass in the affected patient. Definitive diagnosis requires histopathology of the excised adrenal mass or biopsy.

DIFFERENTIAL DIAGNOSIS

- Adrenal mass:
  - Nonfunctional adrenal mass
  - Adrenocortical neoplasia
- Systemic hypertension
- Collapse/weakness
- Sinus tachycardia

INITIAL DATABASE

- Diagnosis requires a high index of suspicion because signs are usually episodic and vague; often not suspected until an adrenal mass is found by ultrasound or during necropsy.
- Complete blood count (CBC), serum biochemical profile, and urinalysis: normal or may show nonspecific changes (mild nonregenerative anemia, mature neutrophilia, increased liver enzymes, hypercholesterolemia, proteinuria).
- Multiple arterial blood pressure (BP) measurements: hypertension (sustained systolic pressure >160 mmHg and/or diastolic pressure >100 mmHg) is common, but normotension does not rule out a pheochromocytoma because tumor catecholamine release is intermittent.
- Abdominal radiographs: often normal but may show a dorsal abdominal mass ± mineralization.
- Thoracic radiographs: may show pulmonary metastasis (10% of dogs), cardiomegaly, or pulmonary edema or congestion (rare).
- Electrocardiogram (ECG): intermittent or sustained tachycardias (sinus tachycardia, ventricular arrhythmias) are common.
- Abdominal ultrasonography: usually unilateral adrenomegaly with normal-size contralateral adrenal gland; may also identify intra-abdominal metastasis or tumor invasion of adjacent structures (see Adrenal Mass, Incidental, p 42).
- Tests for hyperadrenocorticism (see Hyperadrenocorticism, p 537) should be normal, ruling out adrenocortical tumor.

ADVANCED OR CONFIRMATORY TESTING

- Contrast radiography (nonselective venography or excretory urography) for evaluating tumor invasion of the caudal vena cava or kidney, respectively.
- Abdominal CT or MRI: usually shows an adrenal mass and helps identify any local invasion or metastasis.
- Increased serum and urine catecholamines and urinary catecholamine metabolites (e.g., vanillylmandelic acid): confirmatory in humans, but use is limited in veterinary medicine by assay availability, lack of established reference ranges, and the expense and inconvenience of 24-hour urine collection.
- Histopathologic examination and immunohistochemical staining of the excised tumor: required for definitive antemortem diagnosis.

TREATMENT

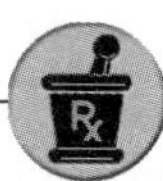

THERAPEUTIC GOAL(S)

- Medical stabilization of the animal
- Surgical excision of the tumor

ACUTE GENERAL TREATMENT

- An α_1-antagonist, phenoxybenzamine (0.25 mg/kg PO q 12h initially, then increased every few days until hypertension controlled) can cause signs of hypotension (lethargy, weakness, syncope) or cause adverse drug reactions (e.g., vomiting); a maximum dosage of 1.5 mg/kg PO q 12h (dogs) (cats: maximum of 0.5 mg/kg PO q 12h) can be reached. Treat the animal for 1 to 3 weeks prior to surgery. Prazosin is an alternative treatment.
- β-Blocker drugs (e.g., atenolol, beginning at 0.5 mg/kg PO q 12h, and titrating up to 1 mg/kg PO q 12h, if needed) may be used for controlling sinus tachycardia but only after α_1-adrenergic blockade has been initiated.

CHRONIC TREATMENT

- Careful anesthetic selection is needed to minimize intraoperative complications. Direct arterial BP and ECG should be monitored during surgery and for at least 24 hours postoperatively.
- If surgical resection is incomplete or not possible, long-term treatment with an α_1-antagonist is required.

DRUG INTERACTIONS

Avoid administering monoamine oxidase inhibitors and metoclopramide, as both may lead to hypertension in these patients.

POSSIBLE COMPLICATIONS

- Sudden blindness, seizures, or even death from a hypertensive crisis.
- Perioperative complications are common and include hypertension, hypotension, arrhythmias, respiratory distress, and hemorrhage. Most animals become normotensive 24 to 48 hours following surgery.

RECOMMENDED MONITORING

- In hospital: monitor BP and central venous pressure perioperatively
- After discharge: assess BP and ECG monthly

PROGNOSIS AND OUTCOME

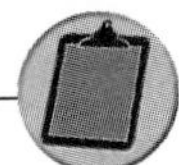

- Prognosis depends on tumor size, metastasis or local tumor invasion, perioperative complications, and the presence of concurrent diseases, which is common (older animals).
- Animals with a surgically excisable tumor have a guarded to good prognosis. If animals survive the immediate postoperative period, a survival time of 18 to 24 months is possible.

PEARLS & CONSIDERATIONS

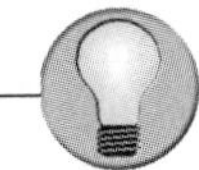

COMMENTS

These tumors are difficult to diagnose antemortem, and perioperative management is complex. Consider referral.

SUGGESTED READING

Barthez PY, et al: Pheochromocytoma in dogs: 61 cases (1984-1995). *J Vet Int Med* 11:272, 1997.

Feldman EC, Nelson RW: Pheochromocytoma and multiple endocrine neoplasia. In Feldman EC, Nelson RW (eds): *Canine and Feline Endocrinology and Reproduction*, ed 3. Philadelphia, WB Saunders, 2004, pp 440-463.

Gilson SD, et al: Pheochromocytoma in 50 dogs. *J Vet Int Med* 8:228, 1994.

Maher ER, McNeil EA: Pheochromocytoma in dogs and cats. *Vet Clin North Am [Small Animal Practice]* 27:359-380, 1997.

AUTHOR: **ELISABETH SNEAD**

EDITOR: **SHERRI IHLE**

Phobias

BASIC INFORMATION

DEFINITION

Behaviors characterized by persistent and extreme anxiety and avoidance, and occurring only in response to specific triggers. The fear response is out of proportion given the objective threat, is beyond voluntary control, and may be preceded by anticipatory anxiety. The sympathetic arousal is excessive and affects the animal's quality of life.

EPIDEMIOLOGY

SPECIES, AGE, SEX: Any age and in both dogs and cats. Phobias can be learned in association with a horrific experience or can be innate and spontaneous. As with most behavioral conditions, phobias most commonly develop during social maturity (about 12 to 36 months [dogs], 24 to 48 months [cats]) when brain neurochemistry is changing.

GENETICS AND BREED PREDISPOSITION: Predispositions suspected, but modes of inheritance and population and breed variability unproven.

RISK FACTORS: Mild signs may exacerbate quickly after exposure to a trigger of large magnitude. The phobia may generalize to multiple triggers that have similar features or appearance (e.g., a mildly noise-phobic dog may start responding severely to loud, rumbling, and rolling noises after a close lightning strike).

CONTAGION AND ZOONOSIS: A young dog that seems well-adjusted and who joins a home with a phobic dog may learn (and/or may react to) some of the behaviors associated with the phobia (e.g., reactive barking), especially if these behaviors engender attention.

In addition, dogs respond to the anxiety level of other dogs and may become anxious because of the information conveyed by the phobic behaviors of the animal. Other pets in a household with an affected individual should be watched carefully for changes in their behavior.

GEOGRAPHY AND SEASONALITY: Noise phobias may first present or exacerbate during holidays that are celebrated with fireworks, gunfire, or cannon blasts. Most cases of thunderstorm/storm phobia follow seasonal weather patterns for the area in which the pet lives. Signs may be most severe where storms are particularly intense or in locations where storms can occur throughout the year.

ASSOCIATED CONDITIONS AND DISORDERS: Comorbidity of thunderstorm phobia and separation anxiety is high. Noise and storm phobias may predispose animals to other anxiety disorders and should be considered serious problems requiring immediate redress and prophylactic treatment. See Separation Anxiety, p 993, for more detailed information on comorbidity.

CLINICAL PRESENTATION

DISEASE FORMS/SUBTYPES: Thunderstorm phobia, noise phobia, neophobia (fear of new objects or circumstances), panic.

HISTORY, CHIEF COMPLAINT

- Exposure to, or anticipation of exposure to, discrete triggering events elicits nonspecific signs of sympathetic arousal (e.g., trembling, shaking, pacing, restlessness, vocalization, mydriasis, piloerection, ptyalism, elimination, anal sac expression, and behaviors associated with avoidance).
- The onset may be acute, with or without an identifiable trigger, or may worsen over time. Repeated events may allow the clients to identify the triggers.
- If escape attempts are interrupted, growling, snarling, lunging, or biting may be elicited.
- The aroused state may stop once the trigger is removed, or it may persist for minutes or hours afterwards.
- When signs occur in the clients' absence, they may miss more subtle signs of the panic (e.g., slightly disarranged furniture, dried saliva on fur or on the ground, destructive chewing or digging).
- Clients' chief complaints may only be destructive behavior, excessive vocalization, or house soiling without awareness of their meaning as markers of anxiety.

PHYSICAL EXAM FINDINGS

- Generally unremarkable exam findings; abnormal wear or damage to teeth, nails, or feet that were injured during escape attempts may be seen (rarely).
- Although uncommon, the pet may be thin due to excessive locomotion associated with pacing and/or decreased

food intake secondary to anxiety. Behavioral data are best collected by obtaining a detailed behavioral history (see Behavioral Assessment, p 1188) and comparing videotapes of the animal when it is and is not distressed to identify potential triggers.

ETIOLOGY AND PATHOPHYSIOLOGY

- Dogs, like humans, may have "susceptibility genes" for the development of problematic anxieties, but these have not yet been identified. Dysfunction or dysregulation of caudate nuclei in the brain has been implicated in some phobic states. Inadequate *in utero* nutrition has also been associated with heightened reactivity. Truly horrific experiences, particularly if they occur during sensitive periods in ontogeny, may render the animal more susceptible to related fears and phobias.
- Cats may remain aroused for 24 to 48 hours after a profound hypothalamic stimulation. With each exposure, the intensity of the response usually worsens until any level of stimulation by the trigger(s) causes the same profound responses.
- The worse the panic, the more insensitive is the animal to physical or social stimuli.

DIAGNOSIS

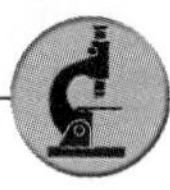

DIFFERENTIAL DIAGNOSIS

- Generalized anxiety disorder (GAD)
- Panic disorder
- Separation anxiety
- Learned fear following a traumatic event
- Attention-seeking behavior

INITIAL DATABASE

- Complete blood count (CBC), serum chemistry profile, urinalysis: generally unremarkable. Assess the possibility of medical conditions that can initiate or contribute to phobic states; also assess hepatic and renal function prior to initiation of psychotropic medication (if indicated).
- Perform additional tests based on history and physical exam findings (e.g., feline leukemia virus [FeLV] and feline immunodeficiency virus [FIV] serologies and serum T4, in most adult cats).

ADVANCED OR CONFIRMATORY TESTING

If signs of neurologic dysfunction are present or develop, a primary behavioral abnormality is virtually never the sole diagnosis; extracranial and intracranial causes should be investigated as appropriate.

TREATMENT

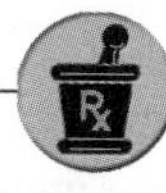

THERAPEUTIC GOAL(S)

A decreased or ablated response to the inciting trigger as evidenced by a reduction in or elimination of overt signs of sympathetic arousal

ACUTE GENERAL TREATMENT

- The owner should help the pet avoid all exposure to the panic-inciting stimulus if it has been identified.
- The owner should reward any spontaneous decrease in reactivity to phobic triggers.
- Anxiolytics, specifically the benzodiazepines (BZD) due to their quick onset of action and specific panicolytic effects, should be prescribed in combination with other psychotropic medications, such as tricyclic antidepressants (TCAs) or selective serotonin reuptake inhibitors (SSRIs).
    - TCA drugs: amitriptyline; dogs, 1-2 mg/kg PO q 12h for a minimum of 30 days; cats, 0.5-1.0 mg/kg PO q12-24h for a minimum of 30 days. First drug of choice in mild cases; inexpensive. Clomipramine (Clomicalm): dogs, 2 mg/kg PO q 12h for a minimum of 8 weeks; cats, 0.5 mg/kg PO q 24h for a minimum of 8 weeks. Most successful when the behaviors have a ritualistic component or elimination component.
    - SSRI drugs: fluoxetine (Prozac); dogs, 1 mg/kg PO q 24h for 8 weeks minimum; cats, 0.5 mg/kg PO q 24h for 8 weeks minimum). Sertraline (Zoloft); dogs, 1 mg/kg PO q 24h for 8 weeks minimum cats, 0.5 mg/kg PO q 24h for 8 weeks minimum can be successful for situations in which other medications have been less helpful.
    - BZD: diazepam or oxazepam at 0.2-0.4 mg/kg PO q12-24h for a minimum 30 days; alprazolam at 0.01-0.025 mg/kg PO q12-24h or q 4-6h for panic, as needed.

CHRONIC TREATMENT

- Owners should teach dogs to relax while making eye contact with them so that this new behavior can be used when the dog encounters a situation about which it is anxious or unsure. Owners can teach their dogs this behavior over time by using positive reinforcement. Owners should learn to monitor facial cues, body postures, pupil size and shape, and respiratory behavior associated with relaxation versus anxiety.
- Avoidance of exposure to the panic-inciting stimulus.
- Desensitization to the triggers can be accomplished if two criteria can be met: if the triggers can be identified and if they can be reproduced faithfully and in a systematic and incremental fashion.
- Owners should continue offering positive reinforcement to their animals for all relaxed and calm behaviors, particularly in the face of phobic triggers.

DRUG INTERACTIONS

- BZDs, TCAs, and SSRIs can all be combined at lower than normal dosages, if needed, but the potential for sedation and interaction must be evaluated.
- TCAs and SSRIs should not be given with monoamine oxidase inhibitors (MAO-Is), which are found in many flea and tick collars and dips and in some medications to treat cognitive dysfunction.
- TCAs can worsen existing cardiac arrhythmias.

POSSIBLE COMPLICATIONS

- Generalization to triggers that are not exact but somewhat similar to the original inciting stimulus (e.g., a thunder-phobic dog that begins to respond to firework displays, progresses to other rolling and booming noises, and then reacts to all loud noises in general).
- BZDs have the potential for drug diversion and abuse by clients.

RECOMMENDED MONITORING

- Animals that take BZDs require a physical exam every 6 months in most U.S. states.The potential for human abuse of the drugs warrants vigilance around refills.
- Performing a yearly CBC, serum chemistry profile, urinalysis, and thyroid screen (bi-yearly in senior and geriatric pets) should be the rule for animals taking other psychotropic medications. Perform ancillary if clinical signs warrant.
- Cardiac monitoring may be recommended if syncope or other suspected cardiac signs are involved in panic.

PROGNOSIS AND OUTCOME

Prognosis is variable and depends on:

- Timeliness of diagnosis (early diagnosis: prognosis more favorable).
- Maintenance of frequent and thorough communication between clinician and client, so treatment can be adjusted according to the animal's response and needs: prognosis more favorable.
- Client factors:
    - Diligence of treatment (comprehensive, persistent treatment plan, and follow-up: prognosis more favorable)
    - Client compliance (good compliance: prognosis more favorable)
- If the best outcome is to be obtained, early intervention is essential.

- If the problem has been ongoing for some time before treatment was sought, treatment may well be lifelong, especially if there are other comorbid anxiety-related conditions.

PEARLS & CONSIDERATIONS

COMMENTS

Because client observations and reports are critical in data collection, it is important to spend time understanding the clients' use of language. Asking clients to describe what they see their pet do, as opposed to their interpretation of the behavior, is key in obtaining behavioral data.

The single best tool for evaluating behavior is observation of the behavior itself. Videocameras make this possible. All practices should have a videocamera that clinicians can use in the practice and can also loan to clients.

PREVENTION

- When selecting breeding stock, clients should assess temperament as well as conformation and medical phenotypes because genetic predisposition is suspected to be a strong contributor to mood disorder development.
- At the first sign of any fearful behavior, clients should watch for any worsening of the behavior and pay attention to possible triggers that might indicate the development of a phobia.
- Veterinarians should screen for fear and phobias as a routine part of every appointment.

CLIENT EDUCATION

- Most behavioral conditions are due to chemical and functional abnormalities of the brain (areas of the limbic system and prefrontal cortex) and, therefore, are not willful acts of disobedience by a vengeful pet.
- Treatment of behavioral conditions is an ongoing process, often for the duration of the pet's life. Relapses may occur with treatment discontinuation or with added stressors.

SUGGESTED READING

Crowell-Davis SL, et al: Use of clomipramine, alprazolam, and behavior modification for the treatment of thunderstorm phobia in dogs. *J Am Vet Med Assoc* 22:744-748, 2003.

Overall KL: Noise phobias in dogs. In Horwitz D, Mills D, Heath S (eds): *BSAVA Manual of Canine and Feline Behavioral Medicine*. United Kingdom, BSAVA, 2002, pp 164-172.

Overall KL, et al: Frequency of nonspecific clinical signs in dogs with separation anxiety, thunderstorm phobia, and noise phobia, alone or in combination. *J Am Vet Med Assoc* 219:467-473, 2001.

AUTHOR: **SORAYA V. JUARBE-DIAZ**
EDITOR: **KAREN L. OVERALL**

Phosphate Enema Toxicosis

BASIC INFORMATION

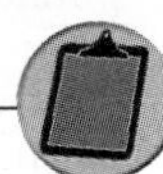

DEFINITION

Administration of sodium phosphate enemas in cats and small-breed dogs can be associated with severe hyperphosphatemia, hypernatremia, and hypocalcemia

SYNONYM(S)

Fleet Enema toxicosis

EPIDEMIOLOGY

SPECIES, AGE, SEX: Younger animals; cats and small breed dogs. Small body size produces a disproportionate ratio of enema fluid to body weight.

RISK FACTORS: Constipation, obstipation, colonic disease, and renal disease may increase the risk for problems from administration of sodium phosphate enemas by decreasing sodium and phosphate excretion (renal disease) or enhancing sodium and phosphate absorption (others).

ASSOCIATED CONDITIONS AND DISORDERS: Hyperphosphatemia, hypernatremia, hypocalcemia (potentially severe/critical).

CLINICAL PRESENTATION

Signs may develop rapidly, within 30 minutes of administration.

HISTORY, CHIEF COMPLAINT: Within 30 minutes to 4 hours of administration of enema, signs that may be apparent include:

- Depression
- Ataxia
- Vomiting
- Diarrhea with or without blood

PHYSICAL EXAM FINDINGS

- Common:
  - Tachycardia
  - Pallor
  - Prolonged capillary refill time
  - Weakness
- Possible:
  - Hyperthermia or hypothermia
  - Tachypnea
  - Tetany
  - Seizure

ETIOLOGY AND PATHOPHYSIOLOGY

- Hypernatremia and hyperphosphatemia can occur after administration of sodium phosphate enemas via massive absorption of sodium and phosphate from the colon. Prolonged retention, overdose, colonic disease (dilation or ulceration), or preexisting electrolyte disturbances as seen with renal failure increase the risk of toxicosis.
- Hypocalcemia occurs if calcium-phosphorus solubility product is exceeded; phosphorus binds and precipitates calcium, leading to hypocalcemia.
- Hyperosmolality.
  - Hypernatremia.
  - Hyperglycemia is only a minor contributor to increased osmolality and is believed to be due to stress release of catecholamines and hypertonicity that alter cellular glucose uptake and metabolism; it can also result from pancreatic insulin release.
- Metabolic acidosis with increased anion gap.

DIAGNOSIS

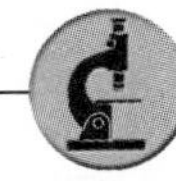

DIFFERENTIAL DIAGNOSIS

See Hypernatremia, p 549; Hypocalcemia, p 564

INITIAL DATABASE

- Complete blood count (CBC): generally unremarkable
- Serum chemistry panel; common abnormalities include:
  - Hyperphosphatemia
  - Hypernatremia
  - Hypocalcemia
  - Hyperkalemia or hypokalemia
  - Metabolic acidosis (decreased HCO_3^-) with increased anion gap
    - Anion gap: $([Na^+] + [K^+]) - ([Cl^-] + [HCO_3^-])$; normal = 12-24 mEq/l.
  - Hyperosmolality
    - Measured directly and also calculated according to formula: 2[Na+] + blood urea nitrogen (BUN) (mg/dl)/2.8 + glucose (mg/dl)/18; result is in milliosmoles per kilogram.

- Normally, and in phosphate enema toxicosis, the difference between calculated and measured values ("osmol gap") should be <10 mOsm/kg.
- Urinalysis: generally unremarkable

TREATMENT

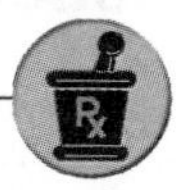

THERAPEUTIC GOAL(S)

- Correct hypernatremia and hypocalcemia
- Address sepsis if present in animals with compromised colonic mucosa

ACUTE GENERAL TREATMENT

- IV fluids to address hypernatremia (see Hypernatremia, p 549).
  - Initial choice: either 5% dextrose in water or 0.45% saline with 2.5% dextrose, with potassium supplementation if hypokalemia is present.
  - Avoid 0.9% saline.
  - Initial rate: one to two times the maintenance rate (30–60 ml/lb/day [65–130 ml/kg/day]), plus a dehydration deficit and ongoing losses compensation if applicable; proceed with caution if the animal has heart disease.
  - Adjustment/change in fluid type and rate based on response and results of ongoing monitoring.
- Calcium gluconate if hypocalcemia-associated tetany is present.
  - Choose the IV route if tetany is severe and/or if hyperthermia is present concurrently.
  - 10% calcium gluconate = 100 mg/ml calcium gluconate. This corresponds to 9.3 mg elemental calcium per milliliter.
  - Give 50–200 mg/kg calcium gluconate (= 0.5–2 ml/kg) slowly IV over a period of 15 to 30 minutes with electrocardiogram (ECG) monitoring, administered to effect. Clinical normality will usually not occur immediately; mild to moderate improvement in signs is sought during the infusion, which warrants stopping administration of the drug.
  - If heart rate decreases significantly, or if an onset of ST segment elevation/depression or QT interval shortening is seen, the infusion must be stopped promptly.
- Calcium gluconate in stable, hypocalcemic animal.
  - 150–250 mg/kg calcium gluconate (1.5–2.5 ml/kg), diluted with two to four times more sterile water and given SC q 6–8h.
- Phosphate-binding agents (e.g., Amphogel 64 mg $Al(OH)_3$/ml or AlternaGEL 120 mg $Al(OH)_3$/ml).
  - 10–30 mg/kg (or higher) PO q 6–12h, based on serum phosphorus levels; may cause inappetence.
- Antibiotics (e.g., ampicillin 22 mg/kg IV q 6–8h, and enrofloxacin 5 mg/kg diluted 1:1 in sterile water and given slowly IV q 12h [q 24h in cats]) in cases with history of colonic disease and suspicion or evidence of sepsis due to translocation of enteric bacteria.

DRUG INTERACTIONS

- Sodium bicarbonate is not recommended unless acidosis is severe because of its hypertonic nature; it may exacerbate hypokalemia and hypocalcemia and may cause metabolic alkalosis.
- Insulin for hyperglycemia is not indicated because spontaneous resolution is expected.

POSSIBLE COMPLICATIONS

Hyperthermia due to ongoing hypocalcemia-induced muscle fasciculations; cerebral edema if hypernatremia is longstanding and then is corrected overly rapidly.

PROGNOSIS AND OUTCOME

- Animals that are treated promptly (when earliest signs are noted or sooner) and thoroughly have a good prognosis: complete recovery is expected.
- Animals that develop central nervous system (CNS) dysfunction and for whom treatment is delayed and/or who develop complications, such as severe hyperthermia due to hypocalcemic tetany, have a guarded and potentially poor prognosis depending on the timing and extent of subsequent treatment.

PEARLS & CONSIDERATIONS

COMMENTS

- Hypernatremia that lasts more than 12 hours may need to be treated as a chronic condition (see Hypernatremia, p 549). In such cases, the serum sodium level may need to be reduced slowly over 48 hours at a rate of not more than 0.5 mEq/l per hour.
- Avoid administration of phosphate-containing enemas to small patients (<10 kg), patients with severe obstipation or suspected/known compromise of the colonic wall, patients with marginal or compromised renal function, or patients with hypernatremia, hyperphosphatemia, or hypocalcemia.
- Several alternative treatments, including purpose-made veterinary dioctyl sulfosuccinate (DSS) enemas, are effective and much safer.
- For injectable calcium, calcium chloride is generally not recommended due to its potentially severe corrosive effects if it leaks perivascularly/subcutaneously.
- Doses for injectable calcium can be listed in milligrams of elemental calcium (Ca^{2+}) or in milligrams of compound (e.g., calcium gluconate, calcium chloride). It is important to be clear which dose is used to avoid overdosing or underdosing. For example, a 10% calcium chloride ($CaCl_2$) solution has 100 mg/ml calcium chloride, which is 27.2 mg Ca^{2+}/ml $CaCl_2$.

CLIENT EDUCATION

Avoid use of phosphate-containing enemas in small animals

SUGGESTED READING

Atkins CE, et al: Clinical, biochemical, acid-base, and electrolyte abnormalities in cats after hypertonic sodium phosphate enema administration. *Am J Vet Res* 46:4, 1985.

Jorgensen LS, et al: Electrolyte abnormalities induced by hypertonic phosphate enemas in two cats. *J Am Vet Med Assoc* 187:12, 1985.

AUTHOR: **CAROLINE W. DONALDSON**

EDITOR: **SAFDAR A. KHAN**

Pilonidal Cyst

BASIC INFORMATION

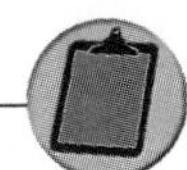

DEFINITION

Tubular skin lesion that extends ventrally from dorsal midline usually as a blind sac, but may connect to dura mater; congenital defect

SYNONYM(S)

Pilonidal sinus
Dermoid cyst
Dermoid sinus

EPIDEMIOLOGY

SPECIES, AGE, SEX: Young dogs, either sex.
GENETICS AND BREED PREDISPOSITION: Primarily Rhodesian Ridgeback; believed to be hereditary (simple recessive gene).

CLINICAL PRESENTATION

DISEASE FORMS/SUBTYPES
- Single or multiple dermal draining tracts
- Subcutaneous cystic mass(es) along dorsal midline

HISTORY, CHIEF COMPLAINT
- Opening in the skin on dorsal midline, with hair protruding from the opening
- Mass in hair on dorsal midline (mass is a concretion of accumulated hair, sebum, and debris overlying the lesion)

PHYSICAL EXAM FINDINGS
- Single or multiple openings in the skin along dorsal midline (Fig. I-135):
  - Occurs precisely on the dorsal midline
  - Hair protruding from opening
  - Cord of tissue palpably extending down through subcutaneous tissue toward the spine:
    - May be confined to subcutaneous tissue
    - Can extend to the spine:
      - Cervical sinus often attached to dorsal spinous process of C2
  - Lumen filled with inspissated sebum, exfoliated keratin, hair (Fig. I-136):
    - May be infected
- Subcutaneous cystic mass and swelling on dorsal midline
- If the cyst is infected and it connects with the spine:
  - Clinical signs associated with myelitis, meningiomyelitis, or encephalitis may be seen:
    - Pain, weakness
    - Neurologic deficits in limbs
    - Seizures

ETIOLOGY AND PATHOPHYSIOLOGY

Congenital neural tube defect:
- Incomplete separation of the skin and neural tube during embryonic development
- Sinus can extend to and connect with dura mater

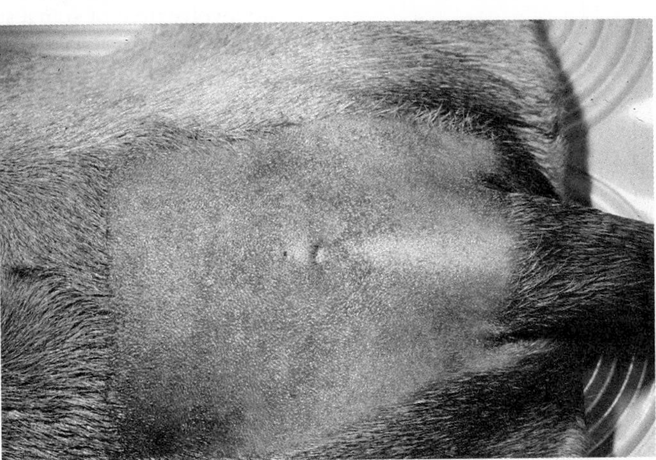

FIGURE I-135 Dorsal lumbosacral region of a Rhodesian Ridgeback dog; cranial is to the left. The appearance of a pore-like opening, and/or a subcutaneous nodule, on the dorsal midline skin is the main physical characteristic of a pilonidal cyst. Courtesy of Dr. Richard Walshaw.

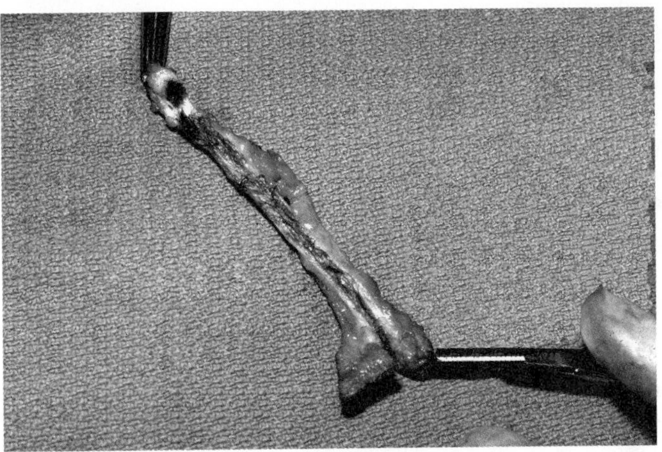

FIGURE I-136 Excised pilonidal cyst from the dog in Fig. I-135. This longitudinal section of the cyst shows its length as well as the haired nature of the cystic tissue. Exterior (skin surface) is at the bottom right; the other extremity of the cyst (upper left of the image) was its deepest point, near the spinal cord. Courtesy of Dr. Richard Walshaw.

DIAGNOSIS

DIFFERENTIAL DIAGNOSIS

- Epidermal inclusion cyst
- Follicular retention cyst
- Sebaceous cyst
- Foreign body
- Abscess
- Hair follicle tumor
- Myiasis

INITIAL DATABASE

Presurgical complete blood count (CBC) and serum chemistry profile

ADVANCED OR CONFIRMATORY TESTING

Rarely necessary because physical findings are usually sufficient:
- Fistulography and myelography:
  - If there is concern about connection to the spine and neurologic signs are present
- Histopathologic examination of excised tissue to confirm diagnosis
- Cytologic examination and microbiologic culture and sensitivity (C&S) testing:
  - If infected
  - If connects to spine

TREATMENT

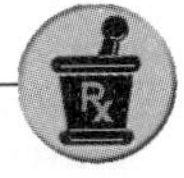

THERAPEUTIC GOAL(S)

Complete excision of sinus tract and cyst

ACUTE AND CHRONIC TREATMENT

Complete surgical resection: strict aseptic technique is essential if sinus extends to dura mater

POSSIBLE COMPLICATIONS

- Recurrence due to incomplete excision:
  - Potential problem if extends to and involves dura mater
  - Development of a chronic draining tract
- Postoperative meningitis:
  - If dura mater involved and surgical wound infection occurs

RECOMMENDED MONITORING

- Monitor the incision site for evidence of recurrent draining tract
- Look for appearance of new lesions:
  - Examine animals for subcutaneous cystic structures

PROGNOSIS AND OUTCOME

- Excellent with complete excision and no involvement of spinal structures
- Guarded if:
  - Neurologic signs are present prior to surgery
  - Dura mater is involved
  - Surgical wound infection develops and dura mater is involved

PEARLS & CONSIDERATIONS

COMMENTS

Avoid clipping, shaving, or cutting a mat of hair located on the dorsal midline without first cleaning and carefully examining the area. Trauma to a pilonidal cyst may lead to subsequent infection and potentially myelitis.

CLIENT EDUCATION

- Common problem in the Rhodesian Ridgeback breed
  - Clients should be aware of this problem if considering purchasing a Rhodesian Ridgeback
  - Believed to be a heritable defect
- Does occur in other purebred dogs

SUGGESTED READING

Angarano DW, Swaim SF: Congenital skin diseases. In Bojrab MJ (ed): *Disease Mechanisms in Small Animal Surgery*, ed 2. Philadelphia, Lea & Febiger, 1993.

Hedlund CS: Surgery of the integumentary system. In Fossum TW (ed): *Small Animal Surgery*, ed 2. St. Louis, Mosby, 2002, pp 194–195.

AUTHOR & EDITOR: **RICHARD WALSHAW**

Pituitary Dwarfism

BASIC INFORMATION

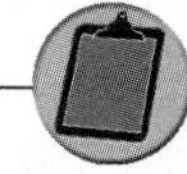

DEFINITION

Congenital growth hormone (GH) deficiency

SYNONYM(S)

Congenital hyposomatotropism

EPIDEMIOLOGY

SPECIES, AGE, SEX

- Dogs and cats
- Signs usually apparent at 2 to 3 months of age
- No gender predilection

GENETICS AND BREED PREDISPOSITION: Inherited as an autosomal recessive trait in the German shepherd and the Karelian bear dog but also occurs in other dog breeds and in cats.

ASSOCIATED CONDITIONS AND DISORDERS: Can occur as part of combined pituitary hormone deficiency with concurrent congenital hypothyroidism (cretinism), hypoadrenocorticism (Addison's disease), and hypogonadism.

CLINICAL PRESENTATION

HISTORY, CHIEF COMPLAINT: Poor growth, stunted stature, alopecia.

PHYSICAL EXAM FINDINGS

- Stunted stature
- Bilaterally symmetric alopecia affecting the trunk, neck, and caudomedial thighs with sparing of the head and extremities
- Soft, wooly haircoat
- Possible hyperpigmention and scaling of exposed skin
- Delayed dental eruption
- Possible open fontanelles

ETIOLOGY AND PATHOPHYSIOLOGY

- Clinical signs result from a deficiency in pituitary production of GH and a resulting deficiency in insulin-like growth factor-1 (IGF-1), which is produced by the liver under the influence of GH.
- Pituitary dwarfism can occur as a result of pressure atrophy of the anterior pituitary gland secondary to congenital cystic enlargement of the craniopharyngeal duct (Rathke's pouch), or due to pituitary hypoplasia secondary to a defect in organogenesis of the pituitary gland.
- Animals with a combined pituitary hormone deficiency may also lack thyroid-stimulating hormone, prolactin, luteinizing hormone, follicular stimulating hormone, and adrenocorticotropic hormone.

DIAGNOSIS

DIFFERENTIAL DIAGNOSIS

See Stunted Growth, p 1047

INITIAL DATABASE

- The diagnosis is based on finding decreased GH or IGF-1 concentrations in conjunction with appropriate clinical signs.
- A complete blood count (CBC), serum biochemical profile, and urinalysis should be performed to help rule out other causes of stunted growth.
  - Results are usually normal.
  - Hypercholesterolemia possible if concurrent hypothyroidism is present.

ADVANCED OR CONFIRMATORY TESTING

- Availability of GH testing is limited.
  - Basal serum GH concentrations may overlap between affected and normal animals and, therefore, should not be used alone as a confirmatory test.
  - GH stimulation (measurement of GH before and 15, 30, 45, 60, and 120 minutes following administration of clonidine [10 ug/kg IV], xylazine [100 ug/kg IV], or GH-releasing hormone [1 ug/kg IV] is more useful than basal GH concentrations. Potential adverse effects of clonidine and xylazine include sedation, bradycardia, hypotension, and collapse. Confirm the protocol with the laboratory prior to performing the test. Pituitary dwarfs will have no increase in GH.
- Basal serum IGF-I concentrations are decreased in dogs with pituitary dwarfism and may be useful when GH measurement is not available. Serum IGF-I levels vary based on breed size; interpretation of results requires consultation with the laboratory performing the assay.

- Screening of animals for combined pituitary hormone deficiency (see Hypothyroidism, p 575; Hypoadrenocorticism, p 561).
- Dermatohistopathologic examination of a skin biopsy shows changes similar to those in other endocrinopathies. A decrease in the quantity and size of dermal elastin fibers suggests pituitary dwarfism.

TREATMENT

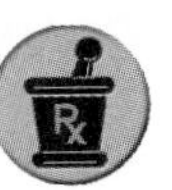

THERAPEUTIC GOAL(S)

- Normalize serum concentrations of IGF-I
- If combined pituitary hormone deficiency is present, also correct thyroxine and cortisol deficiencies

CHRONIC TREATMENT

- Exogenous canine GH is not available.
- Human GH is not effective because dogs form antibodies against it.
- Porcine GH has been used in dogs but can be difficult to obtain.
  - An initial dose of 0.1 IU/kg subcutaneously three times a week for 4 to 6 weeks is recommended, with subsequent adjustment of the dose and interval based on clinical response and plasma IGF-I concentrations.
- With GH therapy, a beneficial response is generally seen within 6 to 8 weeks.
- Progestins may stimulate mammary GH secretion and can be considered as an alternative treatment in dogs.
  - Medroxyprogesterone acetate (2.5-5 mg/kg SQ q 3 weeks, then q 6 weeks) may be used.
  - The efficacy of progestin therapy in affected cats is unknown.

POSSIBLE COMPLICATIONS

- GH supplementation may cause hypersensitivity reactions, carbohydrate intolerance, and overt diabetes mellitus.
- Progestin therapy may cause pyoderma, cystic endometrial hyperplasia in intact females, acromegaly, and diabetes mellitus.

RECOMMENDED MONITORING

- Periodically measure serum glucose and urine glucose levels to monitor for development of serum hyperglycemia and glucosuria associated with diabetes mellitus.
- GH-induced diabetes mellitus can be permanent if GH supplementation is not promptly discontinued.

PROGNOSIS AND OUTCOME

Even with treatment, the long-term prognosis for dogs and cats with pituitary dwarfism is guarded and is dependent on the maintenance of normal IGF-I concentrations and the avoidance of complications of GH or progestin therapy.

PEARLS & CONSIDERATIONS

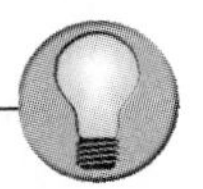

COMMENTS

German shepherd dogs with pituitary dwarfism commonly have concurrent hypothyroidism, but concurrent hypoadrenocorticism is rare.

SUGGESTED READING

Feldman EC, Nelson RW: Disorders of growth hormone. In *Canine and Feline Endocrinology and Reproduction*, ed 3. St. Louis, WB Saunders, 2004, pp 48-59.

AUTHOR: **SARAH L. NAIDOO**
EDITOR: **SHERRI IHLE**

Plague

BASIC INFORMATION

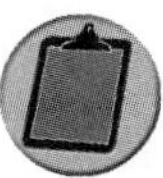

DEFINITION

Bacterial infection with *Yersinia pestis*

SYNONYM(S)

Bubonic plague
Yersiniosis

EPIDEMIOLOGY

SPECIES, AGE, SEX: Cats are most susceptible with no age, sex, or breed predilection. Dogs are resistant to infection.

RISK FACTORS: Cats that hunt and are exposed to wild rodents and fleas are at highest risk for infection.

CONTAGION AND ZOONOSIS: *Y. pestis* is highly contagious and zoonotic; the bacterium is considered a bioterrorism risk. Humans are most commonly infected by flea bites. Cats and other domestic species may temporarily harbor infected fleas. Although rare, humans may be infected through direct contact with infected cats, rabbits, or rodents. Fomites appear to play a minimal role (the organism is sensitive to dessication, temperatures above 105°F (40°C), and routine disinfectants), but hygienic precautions involving gloving, gowning, mask usage, and avoiding contact between discharge/abscess fluid and open cuts or mucosal membranes, and the like, are essential when plague is suspected. Direct transmission of zoonoses to veterinary personnel and cat owners has occurred via the aerosol route (from cats with plague-associated pneumonia). Therefore, in addition to flea elimination, precautions involving protection from respiratory secretions of cats should be implemented when plague is considered possible. A greater degree of human morbidity and mortality also appears to exist with delayed diagnosis, emphasizing the veterinarian's role in public health.

GEOGRAPHY AND SEASONALITY: Foci of plague are most commonly in semi-arid, cooler climates usually adjacent to a desert. Plague is endemic in the western part of the United States, including New Mexico, Arizona, California, and Colorado. Plague is seasonal, with most cases occurring between March and October.

CLINICAL PRESENTATION

DISEASE FORMS/SUBTYPES: Three geographic variants of plague exist (*Y. pestis orientalis, antiqua,* and *mediaevalis*) but are of equal virulence. Of greater clinical relevance, three clinical forms of plague can develop: bubonic, septicemic, and pneumonic.

HISTORY, CHIEF COMPLAINT: Cats may have a history of hunting, ingesting wild rodents, or being exposed to rodent fleas. Clinical signs reported by owners usually are acute and nonspecific, including lethargy, fever, and depression. Some owners may notice swollen lymph nodes or draining cutaneous wounds.

PHYSICAL EXAM FINDINGS: Cats with plague will typically present with a fever (105°F) and depression.

- Bubonic form: Cats have enlarged and often abscessed, draining, or painful lymph nodes, especially around the face and mouth.
- Septicemic form: Cats demonstrate collapse, shock, and other signs attributable to disseminated intravascular coagulation (DIC) with multiorgan involvement.
- Pneumonic form: Cats may cough or sneeze and have nasal discharge and dyspnea. The pneumonic form commonly occurs as a dissemination of the bubonic or septicemic forms.

ETIOLOGY AND PATHOPHYSIOLOGY

- Wild rodents (prairie dogs, squirrels, chipmunks, woodrats, mice) are reservoir hosts.
- Rodent fleas carry the infectious bacteria and transmit the infection to humans and animals through a bite. Domestic species may be infected through ingestion of a reservoir rodent.
- *Y. pestis* replicates within the host mononuclear cells, resulting in the formation of characteristic buboes (abscessed lymph nodes). Alternatively, the infection may develop rapidly into a septicemia with hematogenous spread to multiple organs.

DIAGNOSIS

Presumptive diagnosis is made based on physical examination, relevant history, or suspicion of exposure

DIFFERENTIAL DIAGNOSIS

- Tularemia
- Bite wound abscess
- Other causes of systemic bacterial infection
- Feline panleukopenia virus
- Lymphoma (buboes)

INITIAL DATABASE

- CBC: possible marked leukocytosis
- Gram stain of draining material/fluid: gram-negative coccobacilli
- Chest radiographs: diffuse interstitial pattern or development of abscesses

ADVANCED OR CONFIRMATORY TESTING

- The local public health department can confirm the diagnosis of plague with antigen detection using immunofluorescent antibodies on tissue samples or aspirates.
- Do not attempt an in-house culture of any material from an animal suspected of having *Y. pestis*.

TREATMENT

THERAPEUTIC GOAL(S)

- Treatment must begin prior to definitive diagnosis due to the rapid course of the disease.
- Animals should remain hospitalized and isolated due to the contagious and zoonotic risks.

ACUTE GENERAL TREATMENT

- Stabilization of infected animals that have concurrent dehydration, shock, or other hypovolemic states
- Administration of supplemental oxygen and other critical care measures; these may be necessary depending on the animal's respiratory effort
- Institution of treatment with the antibiotic of choice (gentamicin 6 mg/kg IM or IV q 24h) and brisk rehydration and fluid diuresis as well as monitoring of renal function
- Alternative antibiotics: trimethoprim-sulfonamide, doxycycline, or fluoroquinolones. These may be less effective
- Surgical incision of abscessed lymph nodes for drainage

CHRONIC TREATMENT

Treatment with antibiotics for a minimum of 21 days and continuation beyond resolution of clinical signs

DRUG INTERACTIONS

Gentamicin should not be used in combination with other nephrotoxic, ototoxic, or neurotoxic drugs. Gentamicin must be used carefully when in combination with cephalosporins or nonsteroidal anti-inflammatory drugs (NSAIDs) because of renal effects.

POSSIBLE COMPLICATIONS

Zoonosis

PROGNOSIS AND OUTCOME

Mortality of cats approaches 50%

PEARLS & CONSIDERATIONS

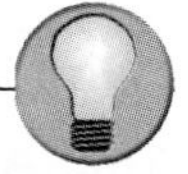

COMMENTS

- Veterinarians who suspect a clinical case of plague should immediately contact the public health department and observe precautions described above.
- People that have been exposed to an infected animal should seek medical advice.

PREVENTION

- Prevent unsupervised outdoor activities
- Apply a flea preventative to cats during high-risk months

CLIENT EDUCATION

- Inform clients of the increased risk of infectious diseases in outdoor cats
- Emphasize proper flea and rodent control

SUGGESTED READING

Macy DW: Plague. In Greene CE (ed): *Infectious Diseases of the Dog and Cat.* St. Louis, WB Saunders, 1998, pp 295–300.

Orloski KA, Lathrop SL: Plague: A veterinary perspective. *J Am Vet Med Assoc* 222(4): 444–448, 2003.

AUTHOR: **KATHRYN TAYLOR**

EDITOR: **DOUGLASS K. MACINTIRE**

Plant Toxicoses

TABLE I-24 **Some Common Garden and Household Toxic Plants**

Botanical Name and Classification	Common Name(s)	Common Clinical Findings and Species Sensitivity
Plants That Cause Central Nervous System (CNS) Stimulation		
Brunfelsia spp.	Yesterday—today and tomorrow	Vomiting/diarrhea (V/D), tremors, and seizures in dogs; some clinical signs may resemble strychnine toxicosis.
Ipomoea spp.	Morning glory	Agitation, tachycardia, hallucination; signs are more likely from the ingestion of the seeds; mostly dogs.
Nicotiana spp.	Tobacco	V/D, lacrimation, agitation, tachycardia, followed by respiratory and cardiovascular (CV) collapse; mostly dogs.

TABLE I-24 **Some Common Garden and Household Toxic Plants—(*Continued*)**

Botanical Name and Classification	Common Name(s)	Common Clinical Findings and Species Sensitivity
Plants That Cause CNS Depression		
Cannabis sativa	Marijuana, pot, mary jane	Sedation, bradycardia, hypothermia, fecal and urinary incontinence; mostly dogs.
Macadamia integrifolia	Macadamia nuts	Depression, hyperthermia, tremors, muscular stiffness, especially in the hind limbs of dogs.
Plants That Cause Mixed CNS Effects		
Ricinus communis	Castor bean	V/D, hemorrhagic enteritis, tremors, seizures/coma, death; renal and liver damage possible; mostly dogs.
Hepatotoxic Plants		
Amanita phalloides	Death cap mushroom	V/D, anorexia, lethargy, acute severe hepatic damage and failure, death; mostly dogs.
Cycas spp., *Zamia* spp.	Sago palm, cycad palm	V/D, hepatic encephalopathy, seizures, hepatic damage and failure, death; mostly dogs.
Cardiotoxic Plants		
Convallaria majalis	Lily of the valley	V/D likely; bradycardia, arrhythmias are possible (cardiac glycosides).
Digitalis purpurea	Foxglove	V/D, lethargy, bradycardia, or tachycardia (any type of arrhythmia); hyperkalemia. Cardiac glycosides.
Kalanchoe spp.	Kalanchoes	V/D, lethargy, diarrhea, arrhythmia, (atrioventricular [AV] block, bradycardia, etc.), paresis; all animals. Cardiac glycosides.
Persea americana	Avocado	Cardiovascular toxicity reported in 1 dog in South Africa; not reported in the United States.
Nerium oleander	Oleander	V/D, bradycardia or tachycardia (any type of arrhythmia); hyperkalemia. Cardiac glycosides.
Phoradendron spp.	Mistletoe	V/D likely; mydriasis, bradycardia; CV collapse is possible (digitalis like).
Rhododendron spp.	Rhododendron, azalea	Most commonly with a small ingestion; V/D; hypotension, bradycardia, conduction disturbances are possible.
Taxus spp.	Yew	V/D likely; tremors, hypotension, bradycardia; onset extremely rapid (minutes to hours).
Plants That Affect the Respiratory System		
Hydrangea macrophylla	Hydrangea	V/D, bloody diarrhea; contains cyanogenic glycosides; cyanide poisoning unlikely, however.
Prunus spp.	Apple, cherry, bitter almond, peach, nectarine	Generally only cause V/D; seeds must be masticated or ingested in large quantities for significant cyanide exposure (seeds contain cyanogenic glycosides).
Nephrotoxic Plants		
Hemerocallis spp.	Day lily	V/D, anorexia, lethargy, acute renal failure (cats).
Lilium spp.	Easter lily, tiger lily, Asiatic lily	V/D, acute renal failure in cats.
Oxalis spp.	Shamrock	Salivation, vomiting, possible renal failure; soluble calcium oxalate crystals.
Rheum spp.	Rhubarb	Salivation, vomiting, possible renal failure; soluble calcium oxalate crystals.
Vitis spp.	Grapes and raisins	V/D, lethargy, acute renal failure, death in dogs.
Plants Causing Hemolysis		
Allium spp.	Onion, garlic, chives	Hemolytic anemia; in cats, dogs.
Plants Affecting the Skin		
Toxicodendron spp.	Poison ivy, poison oak	Small breeds with short-haired coats are more likely to be affected; hyperemia, pruritus possible.
Plants Causing Severe Gastrointestinal (GI) Upset with Potential Systemic Effects		
Amaryllis spp.	Amaryllis, Aztec lily, orchid lily, and others	V/D and lethargy; moderate to severe V/D with ingestion of the bulb; tremors and CV signs (hypotension) also possible.
Colchicum autumnale	Autumn crocus	Severe hemorrhagic enteritis, bone marrow suppression, tremors, seizure, death.
Cycas spp., *Zamia* spp.	Sago palm, cycad palm	Hemorrhagic enteritis, liver necrosis.
Hemerocallis spp.	Day lily	V/D, acute renal failure in cats.
Lilium spp.	Easter lily, tiger lily, Asiatic lilies	V/D, acute renal failure in cats.
Narcissus spp.	Daffodil	V/D and lethargy; moderate to severe V/D with ingestion of the bulb; tremors and CV signs (hypotension) possible.

(*Continued*)

TABLE I-24 **Some Common Garden and Household Toxic Plants—(*Continued*)**

Botanical Name and Classification	Common Name(s)	Common Clinical Findings and Species Sensitivity
Ricinus communis	Castor bean	V/D, hemorrhagic enteritis, tremors, seizures, and coma.
Vitis spp.	Grapes, raisins	V/D, anorexia, lethargy, acute renal failure in 24–72 hr in dogs.
Plants Causing Mild to Moderate GI Upset Without Systemic Effects		
Alocasia antiquorum	Elephant ear	Insoluble calcium oxalate crystals; irritation, drooling, localized inflammation, swelling of mucous membranes of pharynx and tongue; rarely causes dyspnea; may also cause histamine release.
Cyclamen spp.	Cyclamen	Vomiting and diarrhea.
Dieffenbachia	Dumb cane	Insoluble calcium oxalate crystals; salivation, V/D, oral pain.
Dracaena spp.	Corn plant, *Dracaena* plants	V/D sometimes with blood, anorexia, and drooling.
Epipremnum spp.	Golden pothos	Insoluble calcium oxalate crystals; vomiting, salivation, oral pain.
Euphorbia spp.	Poinsettia	Mild V/D.
Hedera helix	English ivy	Mostly V/D, rarely agitation, ataxia, weakness.
Philodendron spp.	Philodendron	Insoluble calcium oxalate crystals.
Phytolacca americana	Pokeweed	V/D common; ingestion of berries may cause red-colored urine.
Schefflera spp.	Schefflera	Insoluble calcium oxalate crystals; V/D, salivation, possible renal damage.
Schlumbergera bridgesii or *truncata*	Christmas cactus	V/D.
Spathiphyllum spp.	Peace lily	Salivation, vomiting, oral pain; insoluble calcium oxalate crystals.
Zantedeschia aethiopica	Calla lily	Salivation, vomiting, oral pain; insoluble calcium oxalate crystals.

AV, atrioventricular; CNS, central nervous system; CV, cardiovascular; GI, gastrointestinal tract; V/D, vomiting and diarrhea.

SUGGESTED READING

Khan CM (ed): *The Merck Veterinary Manual,* ed 9. Whitehouse Station, NJ, Merck & Co, 2005, pp 2432–2505.

Milewski LM, Khan SA: An overview of potentially life-threatening poisonous plants in dogs and cats. *J Vet Emerg Crit Care* 16(1):253, 2006.

AUTHOR: **CAROLINE W. DONALDSON**

EDITOR: **SADFAR A. KHAN**

Platelet Dysfunction

BASIC INFORMATION

DEFINITION

A hemostatic defect caused by impaired platelet activation response. Platelet dysfunction is broadly classified as acquired or hereditary.

SYNONYM(S)

Thrombocytopathia
Thrombopathia

EPIDEMIOLOGY

SPECIES, AGE, SEX

- Acquired: depends on the underlying disease or treatment
- Hereditary: dogs and cats of both sexes; severe defects typically manifest by 1 year of age

GENETICS AND BREED PREDISPOSITION

- All hereditary traits are autosomal, with recessive or unknown expression pattern
- Canine affected breeds: basset hound, boxer, cocker spaniel, collie, German shepherd, Great Pyrenees, otterhound, spitz
- Affected feline breeds: Persian cat, domestic short-haired cat

RISK FACTORS: Acquired platelet dysfunction is associated with systemic disease (anemia, uremia, liver failure, hyperproteinemia), drug therapy (nonsteroidal anti-inflammatory drugs [NSAIDs], heparin, plasma expanders, sulfonamides), and disseminated intravascular coagulation.

CLINICAL PRESENTATION

HISTORY, CHIEF COMPLAINT

- Acquired:
  - Mild to moderate bleeding tendency accompanying a primary disease or drug therapy
  - Hematuria, epistaxis, melena, persistent post-traumatic bleeding
- Hereditary: recurrent mucosal bleeds and ecchymoses, prolonged bleeding from loss of deciduous teeth or minor wounds, blood loss anemia after surgery or trauma

PHYSICAL EXAM FINDINGS

- Petechiae and ecchymoses
- Abnormal bleeding from traumatic/surgical wounds and catheter and venipuncture sites
- Mucosal hemorrhage (epistaxis, gingival hemorrhage, melena, hematuria)

ETIOLOGY AND PATHOPHYSIOLOGY

- Acquired: often multifactorial due to intrinsic changes in platelet metabolism or extrinsic alterations in blood viscosity
  - Platelet effects of NSAIDs, such as aspirin, are irreversible (i.e., effects last as long as the platelet lifespan—several days), whereas others (e.g., colloids/plasma expanders) inhibit platelet function only during the time of administration.

Pathophysiologic classfication of hereditary defects:

- Membrane glycoprotein (GP) disorders. Most common is thrombasthenic thrombasthenia (fibrinogen receptor [GP IIb/IIIa] defects)
- Secretory granule (storage pool) defects
- Signal transduction defects
- Platelet procoagulant deficiency

DIAGNOSIS

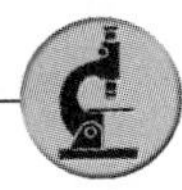

DIFFERENTIAL DIAGNOSIS

- Thrombocytopenia
- Hereditary or acquired coagulation factor deficiencies
- von Willebrand disease
- Vasculopathy or erosive/infiltrative vessel defect
- Defect of fibrinolysis

INITIAL DATABASE

- Physical exam (including funduscopic and rectal exam) to differentiate systemic versus localized or focal site of hemorrhage
- Platelet count: usually normal
- Coagulation screening tests (e.g., activated partial thromboplastin time [aPTT], prothrombin time [PT], activated clotting time [ACT]): usually normal
- Complete blood count (CBC), serum biochemistry profile, urinalysis to define acquired disorders. Avoid cystocentesis
- Thorough history of drug or dietary supplement administration

ADVANCED OR CONFIRMATORY TESTING

- Buccal mucosal bleeding time: usually increased (normal: 2 to 4 minutes)
- Platelet morphology review
- Platelet testing for classification of hereditary defects (may require referral):
  - Clot retraction
  - Platelet aggregation and secretion studies
  - Flow cytometry
  - Electron microscopy
- Mutation detection test (otterhound, Great Pyrenees)

TREATMENT

THERAPEUTIC GOAL(S)

- Control active bleeding with medical or transfusion therapy
- Avoid invasive procedures pending correction of acquired disease (or transfusion)
  - For an acquired dysfunction:
    - Identify and correct underlying disease condition
    - Discontinue or substitute drug therapy
    - Platelet transfusion (although rarely needed)
  - For a hereditary dysfunction:
    - Transfuse sufficient platelets to support hemostasis

ACUTE GENERAL TREATMENT

- Control superficial sites of hemorrhage (gingival or cutaneous wounds).
  - Direct pressure, wound glue, suture, bandage
- Replace red blood cells (RBCs) for severe blood loss anemia (see Transfusion Therapy and Collection Techniques for Blood Banking, p 1312). Adjust initial doses based on hematocrit (HCT) and ongoing loss.
  - Fresh whole blood (e.g., 12–20 ml/kg)
  - Packed cells (e.g., 6–12 ml/kg)
  - Bovine hemoglobin polymer (Oxyglobin) (cats = up to 10 ml/kg; dogs = up to 30 ml/kg)
- Initiate platelet replacement to control systemic bleeding: platelet-rich plasma has a short shelf life (days) and is less widely available and more expensive compared to other blood components. The half-life of transfused platelets is shorter than the half-life of RBCs, but it is still longer than most clotting factors and von Willebrand factor. A single platelet-rich plasma (PRP) transfusion may supply sufficient platelets to form a hemostatic plug, so *in vivo* half-life is not necessarily a limitation of the product.
  - Fresh whole blood (12–20 ml/kg)
  - Platelet-rich plasma (6–12 ml/kg; $>5 \times 10^9$ plat/kg)

CHRONIC TREATMENT

- For hereditary dysfunction:
  - Avoid invasive procedures.
  - Do not administer drugs with antiplatelet effects.
  - Administer a perioperative transfusion to supply platelets.
- For prophylactic treatment:
  - Give platelet-rich plasma to animals with clinically severe hereditary platelet function disorders before any surgical procedure.
  - Consider additional transfusion(s), at 2- to 8-hour intervals; these may be needed for major surgery or if excessive hemorrhage is noted.
  - Administer desmopressin acetate (DDAVP; 1 μg/kg SQ); this may be sufficient to prevent abnormal bleeding due to acquired platelet dysfunction if invasive procedures must be performed. The need for additional transfusions is based on falling HCT and/or abnormal bleeding from the surgical site.

DRUG INTERACTIONS

Judicious use or avoidance of drugs with antiplatelet or anticoagulant effects:

- NSAIDs
- Sulfonamides
- Heparin, warfarin
- Plasma expanders
- Estrogens
- Cytotoxic drugs

RECOMMENDED MONITORING

- Physical exam to monitor external blood loss and petechiae/ecchymoses
- Serial HCT and plasma protein determinations to help identify internal or chronic hemorrhage

PROGNOSIS AND OUTCOME

Acquired dysfunction: good prognosis if underlying disease or drug therapy is reversed.

Hereditary dysfunction:

- Depends on severity of defect.
- Repeated transfusions are required to maintain patients having severe defects.
- Transfusion typically required for any major surgical or traumatic injury.

PEARLS & CONSIDERATIONS

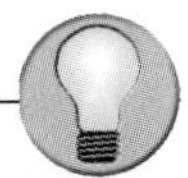

COMMENTS

- Acquired platelet dysfunction is common but rarely causes severe, spontaneous hemorrhage. Animals that are bleeding severely should be evaluated for other potential underlying causes (anticoagulant rodenticide intoxication, severe thrombocytopenia, etc.)
- Hereditary platelet dysfunction is relatively uncommon but is likely underdiagnosed due to the need for referral to document and classify specific traits. Platelet dysfunction belongs on the differential diagnosis of abnormal bleeding in any young dog or cat after common disorders (thrombocytopenia, von Willebrand disease, coagulopathies) have been ruled out.
- Platelets stick to glass, including the inside of anticoagulant-filled blood collection bottles. Therefore, whole blood given to replace platelets should be collected in plastic blood bags.
- The differential diagnoses for animals with persistent bleeding and a normal platelet count, normal PT, and normal aPTT should include platelet function defects, von Willebrand disease, fibrinolytic defects, and diseased or damaged blood vessels.
- The website addresses for some of the veterinary blood banks operating in North America are http://www.hemopet.com/, http://www.midwestabs.com/, http://www.evbb.com/products, html, http://www.ssabb.com/, and http://www.rrc.mb.ca/abb/.

CLIENT EDUCATION

- Owners should avoid giving dietary supplements containing fish oils or

plant alkaloids to any pet with acquired or hereditary platelet dysfunction.
- Platelet function testing may be indicated (before breeding or surgery) for breeds or lines with high prevalence of hereditary thrombopathias.

SUGGESTED READING

Boudreaux MK, Catalfamo JL: Molecular and genetic basis for thrombasthenic thrombopathia in otterhounds. *Am J Vet Res* 62:1979, 2001.

Brooks MB, Catalfamo JL: Platelet disorders and von Willebrand disease. In Ettinger S, Feldman E (eds): *Textbook of Veterinary Internal Medicine*, ed 6. St. Louis, Elsevier, 2004, pp 1918–1929.

AUTHOR: **MARJORY B. BROOKS**
EDITOR: **SUSAN M. COTTER**

Pleural Effusion

BASIC INFORMATION

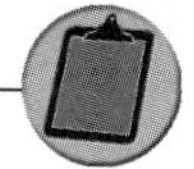

DEFINITION

Accumulation of fluid within the pleural space

SYNONYM(S)

Pleural fluid
Thoracic effusion
Hydrothorax (pure transudate or modified transudate)
Hemothorax (hemorrhage)
Chylothorax (chyle; see Chylothorax, p 208)
Pyothorax (exudate; see Pyothorax, p 935)

EPIDEMIOLOGY

SPECIES, AGE, SEX
- Dogs and cats.
- Pyothorax may be more common in younger cats.
- Pleural effusion secondary to congenital cardiac disease is more common in young animals and pleural effusion secondary to acquired heart disease (including thyrotoxicosis) is more common in middle-aged to older animals.

GENETICS AND BREED PREDISPOSITION
- Pyothorax secondary to aspiration of grass awn is most common in hunting/sporting dogs.
- As a component of congestive heart failure, pleural effusion may occur more commonly in specific breeds predisposed to certain cardiovascular diseases.

RISK FACTORS
- Hydrothorax: heart disease, hypoalbuminemia, neoplasia, lung lobe torsion
- Hemothorax: trauma, intrathoracic neoplasia, anticoagulant toxicity
- Chylothorax: heart disease (cats > dogs), neoplasia, trauma, intestinal lymphangiectasia
- Pyothorax: penetrating injury, inhalation of foreign body (septic); feline infectious peritonitis (FIP) (nonseptic)

CONTAGION AND ZOONOSIS: Based on certain specific causes (e.g., FIP).

CLINICAL PRESENTATION

DISEASE FORMS/SUBTYPES
- Hydrothorax
- Hemothorax
- Chylothorax
- Pyothorax

HISTORY, CHIEF COMPLAINT
- Severity of clinical signs varies with underlying cause, volume of effusion, and rate of fluid accumulation
  - If rate of accumulation is slow, large volumes may be present before clinical signs are apparent (especially cats)
- Restrictive breathing pattern, tachypnea, orthopnea/general discomfort, dyspnea (e.g., abdominal component of respirations) noted by owners
- Lethargy, exercise intolerance
- Cough
- Signs related to underlying disease:
  - Chronic cough
  - Weight loss
  - Inappetence
  - Abdominal effusion
  - Diarrhea
  - Other signs of trauma

PHYSICAL EXAM FINDINGS: In general for pleural effusion:
- Dyspnea, including wide chest excursions, possibly abducted elbows when standing, extension of the neck, reluctance to lie in lateral recumbency, anxious facial expression, and abdominal lift (cats). These animals typically have a prolonged inspiratory phase and very short expiratory phase.
- Muffled heart and lung sounds ventrally.
- Normal to increased bronchovesicular lung sounds (breath sounds) dorsally.
- Ventral hyporesonance with thoracic percussion; a fluid line may be detected.
- Other signs associated with specific underlying cause.

ETIOLOGY AND PATHOPHYSIOLOGY

- Etiology and fluid classification reflect basic pathophysiologic mechanisms of effusion formation:
  - Reduced plasma colloid oncotic pressure (hydrothorax: pure transudate)
    - Hypoalbuminemia: protein loss (renal: glomerulonephritis [GN], amyloidosis; gastrointestinal (GI): inflammatory bowel disease, lymphangiectasia, neoplasia, others) or synthetic failure (chronic hepatopathy)
  - Increased capillary hydrostatic pressure (hydrothorax: usually modified transudate)
    - Congestive heart failure, Budd-Chiari-like syndromes
- Reduced lymphatic drainage/lymphatic obstruction (hydrothorax, chylothorax, or pyothorax: modified transudate to exudate):
  - Thoracic or pulmonary neoplasia
  - Chylothorax
- Increased vascular permeability (pyothorax: exudate):
  - Pyothorax
  - FIP
- Disruption of vascular integrity or hemostatic abnormalities (hemothorax):
  - Rupture of neoplastic mass
  - Coagulopathy
- Respiratory dysfunction can reflect hypoventilation and ventilation:perfusion mismatch

DIAGNOSIS

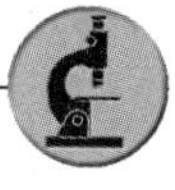

DIFFERENTIAL DIAGNOSIS

- Other pleural space disease:
  - Masses
  - Pneumothorax
  - Constrictive/fibrosing pleuritis (can occur concurrently with pleural effusion—often chylothorax or pyothorax—and typically causes very rounded lung lobe contours that may be difficult to distinguish radiographically from those caused by pleural effusion)
- Pulmonary parenchymal or airway disease
- Thoracic wall disease
- Diaphragmatic hernia
- Neuromuscular disease

INITIAL DATABASE

- In animals with pleural effusion causing severe dyspnea, some clinicians

prefer to perform thoracocentesis first and then take thoracic radiographs.
  - Advantages of centesis first: therapeutic value (removal of effusion), diagnostic value (fluid analysis).
  - Advantage of radiographs first: safety (confirms pleural effusion; can identify displacement of cardiac silhouette, to be avoided during centesis).
- Thoracic radiographs; radiographic signs of pleural effusion vary with fluid volume and can include:
  - Interlobar fissures.
    - Approximately 100 ml of fluid is present in a medium-sized dog if fissure lines are evident.
    - Small volumes may be better appreciated on ventrodorsal views.
  - Impaired heart visualization especially on dorsoventral view.
  - Retraction ("scalloping") of lungs from thoracic wall with interposed fluid opacity.
  - On lateral radiographs, increased opacity dorsal to the sternum and ventral scalloping of lung margins. The lateral view is prone to misinterpretation, and standard two-view thoracic radiography is recommended in all cases.
  - Blunting of lung margins at costophrenic angles (ventrodorsal view).
  - Obscured diaphragm.
  - Widened mediastinum.
  - Fractured ribs, diaphragmatic hernia, and other orthopedic injuries may be present.
  - Pyothorax and chylothorax may cause constrictive pleuritis, preventing full expansion of lungs after thoracocentesis. The lung lobes appear rounded in contour.
  - Evaluation of radiographs post-thoracocentesis for underlying pulmonary disease as visualization of intra-thoracic structures improves.
- Abnormalities depend on etiology; possibilities include:
  - Complete blood count (CBC):
    - Inflammatory leukogram.
    - Thrombocytopenia.
    - Anemia.
  - Biochemical panel:
    - Hypoalbuminemia.
    - Hypoglobulinemia or hyperglobulinemia.
    - Hypoglycemia.
    - Hypocholesterolemia
    - Azotemia.
    - Electrolyte abnormalities.
    - Increased liver enzyme activities.
  - Urinalysis:
    - Proteinuria.
- Thoracocentesis (see p 1308):
  - Fluid in EDTA (lavender top) and plain (red top) tubes for analysis; prepare fresh smears.
  - If pyothorax is suspected, a culture and sensitivity (C&S) is indicated (aerobic and anaerobic in all cases):
    - Most common canine isolates are *Peptostreptococcus*, *Bacteroides* spp., *E.coli*, *Klebsiella pneumoniae*, *Enterobacter*, *Fusobacterium*, *Pasteurella* spp., and *Actinomyces*.
    - Most common in cats are *Bacteroides* spp., *Pasteurella* spp., *Peptostreptococcus, Fusobacterium* spp., and *Actinomyces* spp.
  - Measurement of effusion triglyceride and cholesterol concentration if chylothorax suspected.
  - An effusion albumin:globulin ratio of >0.8 makes FIP unlikely.
- Thoracic ultrasonography:
  - Often performed before thoracocentesis to improve the acoustic window, unless the animal is uncomfortable/dyspneic during restraint for the examination.
  - Can identify mediastinal masses, consolidated lung lobes, pulmonary masses, and abdominal organs in the thoracic cavity with hernias.
  - Can help identify localized fluid for sampling.

ADVANCED OR CONFIRMATORY TESTING

Based on nature of effusion and diagnostic test results to date.

- Hydrothorax: pure transudate (effusion [total protein] <2.5 g/dl).
  - Urine protein:creatinine ratio.
  - Liver function tests.
  - Possibly intestinal biopsies (surgical or endoscopic) if protein-losing enteropathy suspected.
- Hydrothorax: modified transudate (effusion [total protein] 2.5-5.0 g/dl; no cytologic evidence of infection or hemorrhage).
  - Thoracic ultrasound exam.
  - Echocardiography, especially if there are signs of cardiac disease.
  - CT for masses or pulmonary disease.
  - Fine-needle aspirates and cytologic examination of lung or mass if lesion is identified.
  - Thoracoscopy or thoracotomy for pleural or lung biopsy.
- Chylothorax:
  - Lymphangiography is occasionally performed to identify the site of disruption of the thoracic duct if an underlying cause (e.g., congestive heart failure, intestinal lymphangiectasia) has not been identified.
  - Thoracotomy/thoracoscopy.
- Hemothorax:
  - Coagulation profile (PT, PTT, platelet count).
    - If abnormal, toxin screens may sometimes be performed.
    - If normal, imaging (ultrasound and/or CT scan) is indicated, and thoracoscopy/thoracotomy may be warranted if a mass lesion is identified.
- Pyothorax:
  - Careful examination of skin and haircoat (especially in long-haired pets, possibly including extensive shaving of hair over the thorax to improve visualization) for evidence of penetrating injury/foreign body.
  - Postcentesis/postdrainage thoracic radiographs or CT scan to identify masses.
  - Exploratory thoracotomy is indicated if an intrapleural foreign body is suspected. Thoracotomy improves outcome in dogs with pyothorax because pyothorax is often secondary to a migrating foreign body.

TREATMENT

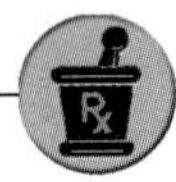

THERAPEUTIC GOAL(S)

- Improve respiratory function
- Identify and correct underlying disease

ACUTE GENERAL TREATMENT

- Oxygen supplementation if dyspnea is present
- Minimize stress
- Thoracocentesis (see Thoracocentesis, p 1308)
- For pyothorax: bilateral (assuming bilateral involvement) thoracostomy tubes (see Chest Tube Placement, p 1210), or thoracotomy and thoracic lavage/drainage:
  - Lavage through large diameter chest tubes with sterile, warm (body temperature) isotonic fluids (10-20 ml/kg) two to four times a day for 5 to 7 days
  - Removal of tubes when fluid production <2 ml/kg/day
- For hemothorax:
  - Blood transfusion if severe anemia
  - Both plasma transfusion (see Transfusion Therapy and Collection Techniques for Blood Banking, p 1312) and vitamin K 2.5-5.0 mg/kg SQ in multiple sites q 12h if anticoagulant rodenticide toxicity (see Anticoagulant Rodenticide Toxicosis, p 76) is identified or suspected as the cause of hemothorax
- Support of circulation and respiratory function if effusion results from trauma

CHRONIC TREATMENT

- For some, correction of the underlying disorder may resolve effusion without thoracocentesis.
- With hypoalbuminemia, cardiac disease, vasculitis, or immune-mediated disease, therapy must be directed at the underlying cause.
- For pyothorax, antimicrobials are necessary but are ineffective without proper drainage.
  - Empiric choices based on Gram stain findings and common organisms (see previous paragraphs); see Pyothorax, p 935.

- If filamentous organisms (*Actinomyces* or *Nocardia*) are identified, ampicillin (22 mg/kg IV q 8h) and trimethoprim-sulfonamide (30 mg/kg PO q 12h) are suitable choices.
- Modify antimicrobial choices based upon results of C&S.
- If using trimethoprim-sulfonamide, a physical exam and monitoring of tear production, hematologic parameters (including CBC), and liver function are indicated.
- Administer antibiotics for 1 to 2 months.
- Consider thoracotomy if there is a poor response to medical therapy over a few days or if pyothorax recurs after antibiotics are discontinued.
    - Some studies suggest better and more rapid resolution with early surgical intervention.
    - Submit any excised tissue for histopathologic examination.

- For hemothorax, consider thoracotomy if there is no evidence of coagulopathy, thrombocytopenia, or trauma and if there is poor/no response to medical treatment.
- Chemotherapy may be indicated when pleural effusion is neoplastic in origin. Confirmation of type of neoplasm (cytologic or histopathologic) is necessary.

POSSIBLE COMPLICATIONS

- Iatrogenic pneumothorax and hemothorax from thoracocentesis or thoracostomy tube.
- Constrictive/fibrosing pleuritis from pyothorax or chylothorax.
- Disseminated intravascular coagulation (DIC) or systemic inflammatory response syndrome from pyothorax.
- Recurrence of pyothorax if migrating foreign body remains or if inappropriate antibiotics are used.
- Complications of thoracocentesis (and corresponding precautions) include:
    - Lung laceration (less likely if needle is introduced and withdrawn without side-to-side or rotatory motions once the needle tip is in the pleural space).
    - Re-expansion pulmonary edema; less likely if large-volume effusions are withdrawn periodically over several hours rather than all at once and more likely with chronic effusions.
    - Pleural shock: a sudden bradycardia of vagal origin caused by needle contact with the pleura (no prevention; responds to immediate administration of atropine 0.04 mg/kg IV).
    - Bronchopleural fistula: when constrictive/fibrosing pleuritis prevents further lung expansion during thoracocentesis and ongoing fluid withdrawal creates excessive negative pressure in the pleural space, a rupture of the bronchial wall into the pleural cavity may occur (possibly less likely to occur if large-volume effusions are withdrawn periodically over several hours rather than all at once, especially if lung lobes are very round, suggesting constrictive/fibrosing pleuritis).

RECOMMENDED MONITORING

- Thoracic radiographs
- Daily cytologic examination and Gram stain of chest tube fluid withdrawn from pyothorax cases to assess antimicrobial response

PROGNOSIS AND OUTCOME

- Varies with cause and severity of underlying disease.
- Pleural effusion may worsen the short-term prognosis of the underlying cause by potentially causing acute respiratory compromise.

PEARLS & CONSIDERATIONS

COMMENTS

- If pleural effusion is suspected, clincians can consider thoracocentesis, which can be both diagnostic and therapeutic, before thoracic radiographs.
    - Drainage of only some fluid can improve respiratory function.
    - First obtain dorsoventral view, which is often sufficient to confirm effusion.
    - Alternatively, a very brief ultrasound evaluation may provide an initial confirmation of pleural effusion, justifying centesis. Radiographs may then be taken more safely after centesis.
    - Thoracic percussion also helps identify pleural effusion and support pre-radiograph thoracocentesis.
- Cats with pleural effusion can be easily stressed by radiographs, so consider thoracocentesis early.
- Hemothorax usually develops from trauma, coagulopathies, or neoplasia.
- Grass awns can be located in multiple sites, including the pericardial sac, in dogs with pyothorax.
- Retrosternal fat and interindividual variation may give the false impression of pleural effusion on lateral radiographic projections of animals without pleural effusion. For this reason, and in order to determine whether the effusion is unilateral or bilateral, standard two-view thoracic radiography is always indicated when pleural effusion is suspected or is known to be present.

PREVENTION

Avoid trauma and exposure to anticoagulant rodenticides

SUGGESTED READING

Forrester SD, et al: Pleural effusions: Pathophysiology and diagnostic considerations. *Compend Contin Educ Pract Vet* 10:121, 1991.

Holtsinger RH, Ellison GW: Spontaneous pneumothorax. *Compend Contin Educ Pract Vet* 17:197, 1995.

Scott JA, Macintire DK: Canine pyothorax: Clinical presentation, diagnosis, and treatment. *Compend Contin Educ Pract Vet* 25:180, 2003.

Waddell LS, et al: Risk factors, prognostic indicators, and outcomes of pyothorax in cats: 80 cases (1986–1999). *J Am Vet Med Assoc* 221:819, 2002.

Walker AL, et al: Bacteria associated with pyothorax of dogs and cats: 98 cases. *J Am Vet Med Assoc* 216:359, 2000.

AUTHOR: **GRAHAM SWINNEY**

EDITOR: **RANCE K. SELLON**

Pneumocystosis

BASIC INFORMATION

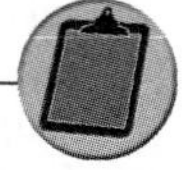

DEFINITION

Infectious opportunistic disease of the lungs associated with immune incompetence

SYNONYM(S)

Pneumocystis carinii pneumonia

EPIDEMIOLOGY

SPECIES, AGE, SEX: Young animals, primarily dogs.

GENETICS AND BREED PREDISPOSITION: Miniature dachshunds, Shetland sheepdogs, and Cavalier King Charles spaniels.

RISK FACTORS

- Congenital or acquired immune suppressive diseases

- Syndrome of common variable immunodeficiency in the miniature dachshund

CONTAGION AND ZOONOSIS: Transmission to an HIV-infected person is possible.

CLINICAL PRESENTATION

HISTORY, CHIEF COMPLAINT: Some or all of the following may prompt an owner to seek veterinary consultation:

- Tachypnea/respiratory distress
- Exercise intolerance
- Weight loss

PHYSICAL EXAM FINDINGS

- Tachypnea
- Respiratory distress
- Poor body condition
- Marked increase in respiratory sounds on thoracic auscultation
- Cyanosis with severe infections

ETIOLOGY AND PATHOPHYSIOLOGY

- Pneumocytosis is caused by *P. carinii*, a saprophyte of the mammalian respiratory tract whose life cycle is completed within the alveolar spaces.
- Based on nucleic acid analysis, the organism is classified as an atypical fungal organism.
- *P. carinii* can be present in low numbers in the pulmonary alveoli of healthy animals and is only associated with pneumonia and respiratory distress when there is immune compromise.
- With immune compromise, *P. carinii* proliferates within the alveoli, resulting in alveolar-capillary blockage and ventilation-perfusion mismatch. Thickening of alveolar septa occurs, but there is rarely extension of the infection into the pulmonary interstitium.

DIAGNOSIS

DIFFERENTIAL DIAGNOSIS

- Other infectious pneumonias:
  - Bacterial
  - Viral
  - Protozoal
  - Mycotic
- Pulmonary fibrosis
- Congestive heart failure

INITIAL DATABASE

- Complete blood count (CBC):
  - Polycythemia
  - Thrombocytosis
  - Mild neutrophilic leukocytosis
  - Eosinophilia and monocytosis in some cases
- Serum biochemistry profile:
  - Normal serum protein levels or a low to low-normal globulin level
- Urinalysis: usually normal.
- Serum protein electrophoresis: hypogammaglobulinemia.
- Thoracic radiographs:
  - Mixed alveolar and interstitial pattern
  - Bronchial pattern
  - Cor pulmonale (right-sided cardiomegaly)

ADVANCED OR CONFIRMATORY TESTING

- Other laboratory tests:
  - Arterial blood gas (ABG) analysis:
    - Hypoxemia
    - Normocapnia to hypocapnia
    - Increased alveolar-arterial (A-a) oxygen gradient
- Serologic tests: available for humans but of uncertain value for dogs.
- Other diagnostic procedures:
  - Definitive antemortem diagnosis of *P. carinii* is established by direct visualization of either the trophozoite or cyst in respiratory washes collected by transtracheal aspiration or bronchoalveolar lavage, needle aspirates, or lung biopsies obtained by thoracotomy or thoracoscopy.
  - Histochemical stains and diagnostic immunohistochemistry tests may facilitate observation of organisms.
  - Polymerase chain reaction (PCR) test on respiratory samples can also document presence of the organisms.

TREATMENT

THERAPEUTIC GOAL(S)

Eradicate infection

ACUTE GENERAL TREATMENT

- Oxygen administration.
- Mucolytics: acetylcysteine (10% or 20% solution) 50 ml/hr for 30-60 minutes q 12h, by nebulization; or bromohexine 1 mg/kg PO q 12h. Administration of bronchodilators beforehand is recommended.
- Bronchodilators: aminophylline 10 mg/kg PO q 8h, or terbutaline 0.625-2.5 mg PO, total dose q 8h.
- Saline nebulization to liquefy hyperviscous mucus and thus promote the removal of secretions from the respiratory tree.

CHRONIC TREATMENT

- Drug of choice: trimethoprim-sulfonamide, 15 mg/kg PO q 8h for 3 weeks
- Pentamidine isethionate: 4 mg/kg IM q 24h for 2 weeks
- Carbutamide: 50 mg/kg IM q 12h for 3 weeks
- Drug combinations: dapsone (1 mg/kg PO q 8h) and pyrimethamine (1 mg/kg PO q 24h)

POSSIBLE COMPLICATIONS

Respiratory failure, respiratory arrest

RECOMMENDED MONITORING

- Thoracic radiographs
- ABG analysis

PROGNOSIS AND OUTCOME

Dependent on severity of infection

PEARLS & CONSIDERATIONS

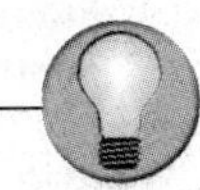

COMMENTS

Infection with *P. carinii* is associated with immunologic defects.

PREVENTION

Because of the probable genetic basis to immune compromise in most animals, owners should not breed affected animals.

CLIENT EDUCATION

- Animals have an underlying immunologic defect.
- May be a zoonosis in HIV-positive animals.

SUGGESTED READING

Lobetti RG: Common variable immunodeficiency in miniature dachshunds affected with *Pneumocystis carinii* pneumonia. *J Vet Diag Invest* 12:39, 2000.

Lobetti RG: Review of *Pneumocystis carinii* infection in miniature dachshunds. *Comp Cont Educ Pract Vet* 23:320, 2001.

AUTHOR: **REMO LOBETTI**
EDITOR: **RANCE K. SELLON**

Pneumonia, Aspiration

Client Education Sheet on Website

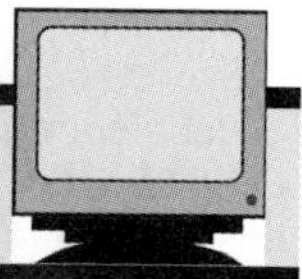

BASIC INFORMATION

DEFINITION

Infection associated with inhalation of oropharyngeal secretions. In veterinary medicine, the term is often used in reference to aspiration pneumonitis, which is chemical injury caused by inhalation of gastric contents (most commonly) or other materials (e.g., barium, mineral oil).

SYNONYM(S)

Aspiration pneumonitis
Mendelson's syndrome

EPIDEMIOLOGY

SPECIES, AGE, SEX: Dogs and cats of either sex and any age.

RISK FACTORS

- Diseases of:
  - Pharynx or larynx (e.g., laryngeal paralysis)
  - Esophagus (e.g., megaesophagus)
  - Stomach or intestine (e.g., pyloric obstruction)
- Forced enteral administration of drugs or foods
- Impaired protective reflexes (e.g., coma, anesthesia, seizure)

ASSOCIATED CONDITIONS AND DISORDERS

- Acquired respiratory distress syndrome
- Bacterial pneumonia
- Hypoxemia
- Lung lobe abscessation
- Pneumothorax
- Shock

CLINICAL PRESENTATION

DISEASE FORMS/SUBTYPES

- Acute or chronic
- Fulminant or insidious

HISTORY, CHIEF COMPLAINT: Clinical signs may be absent or severe; when present, they may include:

- Anorexia
- Collapse
- Cough
- Lethargy
- Respiratory distress
- Others that reflect predisposing cause (e.g., regurgitation, anesthetic episode)

PHYSICAL EXAM FINDINGS: Findings may be absent or severe; when present, they may include:

- Tachypnea
- Inspiratory and expiratory distress
- Auscultatory abnormalities (may be localized):
  - Crackles
  - Wheezes
  - Increased or decreased bronchovesicular sounds
- Cyanosis
- Fever
- Shock
- Others that reflect predisposing cause (e.g., exercise intolerance with myasthenia gravis)

ETIOLOGY AND PATHOPHYSIOLOGY

- Inhalation of particulates or fluid into the larynx and lower respiratory tract triggers injury.
  - Gastric contents are typically sterile, but acid and particulate matter can cause potentially severe damage:
    - Acid causes direct, caustic epithelial damage that is followed by inflammation.
    - Particulate material may obstruct airways.
  - Infection may follow aspiration of colonized oropharyngeal secretions or is a secondary (opportunistic) complication of respiratory damage.
- Severity of injury depends on volume, toxicity, pH, and particulate and pathogen content of aspirated material. Sequelae may include:
  - Airway obstruction.
  - Bronchoconstriction.
  - Pulmonary hemorrhage.
  - Epithelial necrosis.
  - Pulmonary inflammation.

DIAGNOSIS

DIFFERENTIAL DIAGNOSIS

- Infectious pneumonia
- Cardiogenic or noncardiogenic pulmonary edema

INITIAL DATABASE

- Neurologic examination reflects, if present, the underlying neurologic disease
- Complete blood count (CBC): neutrophilic leukocytosis common but not essential (absence does not exclude aspiration pneumonia)
- Serum biochemical profile and urinalysis: no specific changes
- Thoracic radiographs: abnormalities may lag aspiration by up to 24 hours
  - Alveolar or interstitial pattern, or consolidation, in affected lung lobes:
    - Common in the lobes that were dependent at the time of aspiration.
    - If the patient was conscious during aspiration, abnormalities usually occur in the right middle lung lobe or caudal portion of the left cranial lung lobe.

ADVANCED OR CONFIRMATORY TESTING

- Pulse oximetry and/or arterial blood gas (ABG) analyses to assess oxygenation
- Tracheal lavage (submit samples for aerobic culture and sensitivity [C&S]):
  - Neutrophilic inflammation
  - Bacteria possible
  - Hemorrhage
  - Particulates
- Bronchoscopy indicated only if clinician suspects large airway obstruction
- Search for predisposing cause of aspiration (e.g., acetylcholine [Ach] receptor antibody titer for myasthenia gravis-related megaesophagus)

TREATMENT

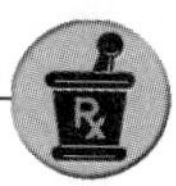

THERAPEUTIC GOAL(S)

- Support oxygenation
- Treat secondary infection
- Prevent recurrence

ACUTE GENERAL TREATMENT

- If aspiration occurs, immediately suction material from pharynx/airways and ensure airway patency.
- If respiratory distress or evidence of hypoxemia exists, administer supplemental oxygen using the lowest effective oxygen concentration (typically, F_IO_2 ~40%).
  - If P_aO_2 <50 mm Hg or if P_aCO_2 >50 mmHg, intubate for positive-pressure ventilation.
- Bronchodilators may relieve bronchospasm (cats especially) (e.g., aminophylline [dose varies with preparation of the medication] or terbutaline [0.01 mg/kg SQ]).
- IV crystalloid fluids may be warranted.
  - Maintenance rate of 60 ml/kg per day after correction of dehydration; more if there are ongoing losses.
  - Rarely, shock occurs, requiring aggressive fluid therapy.
    - Aggressive parenteral fluids may precipitate edema in the damaged lung.
- Antimicrobials are often suggested for these animals since secondary infection is common.
  - Choice ideally based on C&S (tracheal lavage).
  - Initial choice often parenteral, broad-spectrum antibiotics (e.g., combination of ampicillin 22 mg/kg IV q 8h, and enrofloxacin 5 mg/kg 12h [dogs]; 5 mg/kg q 24h [cats]).
- Physiotherapy: coupage, movement.
- Nebulization.
- If aspiration is suspected but respiratory distress is absent, only careful observation may be warranted.

CHRONIC TREATMENT

- Prevent further aspiration or reduce severity of injury from aspiration (see Prevention below)
- Discontinue oxygen when P_aO_2 remains above 65 mm Hg and the animal can breathe comfortably without it
- Continue antibiotics for 3 to 4 weeks or 1 week past radiographic resolution

POSSIBLE COMPLICATIONS

- Administration of high concentrations of oxygen for prolonged periods can contribute to respiratory epithelial injury.
- Parenteral fluids may result in noncardiogenic pulmonary edema.

RECOMMENDED MONITORING

- Oxygenation: depending on severity of disease, q 4-24h until normalized.
- Thoracic radiographs: until abnormalities are resolved with frequency determined by severity of signs and baseline abnormalities; ideally repeated 1 to 2 weeks after discontinuation of antibiotics.
- CBC: rechecked at least weekly until leukocytosis resolved.

PROGNOSIS AND OUTCOME

Depends on volume and character of aspirated material

PEARLS & CONSIDERATIONS

COMMENTS

Because aspiration pneumonia rarely occurs in the absence of an underlying cause, animals should be evaluated for risk factors.

PREVENTION

- Address underlying diseases that predispose the animal to aspiration.
- Fast animals at least 6 hours before general anesthesia, and use properly inflated, cuffed endotracheal tubes during anesthesia.
- For animals at high risk, consider administration of antacids (H2-antagonists, proton pump inhibitors) to increase gastric pH and administration of prokinetic agents (e.g., metoclopramide) to enhance gastric emptying and increase lower esophageal sphincter tone.
- Use caution in forced administration of drugs or foodstuffs.
- Feeding tubes should not cross the lower esophageal sphincter.

CLIENT EDUCATION

When a predisposing cause is not reversible (e.g., idiopathic megaesophagus), repeated aspiration events are common.

SUGGESTED READING

Hawkins EC: Aspiration pneumonia. In Bonagura JD (ed): *Kirk's Current Veterinary Therapy XII*. Philadelphia, WB Saunders, 1995, pp 915-919.

Marik PE: Aspiration pneumonitis and pneumonia: A clinical review. *N Engl J Med* 344:665, 2001.

AUTHOR: **LEAH A. COHN**
EDITOR: **RANCE K. SELLON**

Pneumonia, Bacterial

Client Education Sheet on Website

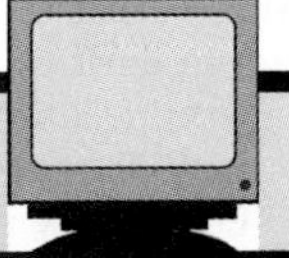

BASIC INFORMATION

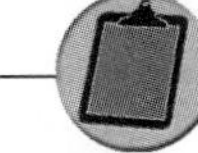

DEFINITION

Inflammation of the lower respiratory tract or interstitium from bacterial infection

EPIDEMIOLOGY

SPECIES, AGE, SEX: No species, age, or gender predilections noted except in cases of bacterial pneumonia secondary to congenital defects (e.g., primary ciliary dyskinesia).

GENETICS AND BREED PREDISPOSITION: No breed or genetic predispositions other than for those associated with underlying primary diseases or associated conditions.

RISK FACTORS: Any disease that comprises respiratory defenses or increases the potential for aspiration.

- Laryngeal disease
  - Laryngeal paralysis post tie-back surgery
  - Laryngeal neoplasia
- Esophageal disease
  - Esophagitis
  - Megaesophagus
  - Esophageal diverticula
- Altered consciousness
- Chronic vomiting
- Bronchial masses or foreign bodies
- Bronchiectasis
- Viral respiratory infection (e.g., distemper)
- Congenital immune deficiencies
- Ciliary dyskinesia

ASSOCIATED CONDITIONS AND DISORDERS

- Sepsis
- Systemic inflammatory response syndrome
- Multiple organ dysfunction syndrome

CLINICAL PRESENTATION

DISEASE FORMS/SUBTYPES: Bronchopneumonia involves inflammation of both airways and alveolar/interstitial compartments.

HISTORY, CHIEF COMPLAINT: Chief complaint may be related to pneumonia or to the predisposing disease:

- Pneumonia:
  - Cough
  - Nasal discharge
  - Sneezing
  - Exercise intolerance
  - Anorexia, lethargy
  - Hemoptysis (uncommon)
- Predisposing disease:
  - Regurgitation
  - Recurrent/persistent infections (usually respiratory, but occasionally other)
- Some animals may exhibit no clinical signs.
- Mild, vague signs (e.g., delayed postoperative recovery, failure to thrive) may be the earliest manifestations of the onset of bacterial pneumonia as a complication of another disorder (e.g., sepsis, systemic inflammatory response syndrome, multiple organ dysfunction syndrome).
- The lack of signs referable to the respiratory system does not exclude the diagnosis.

PHYSICAL EXAM FINDINGS: Variable:

- Cough
- Nasal discharge
- Crackles or wheezes, sometimes focally
- Fever
- Tachypnea
- Increased respiratory effort or overt respiratory distress

The physical examination may be unremarkable or may reflect only signs relating to the underlying predisposing disorder in the presence of mild or moderate bacterial pneumonia. The lack of signs referable to the respiratory system cannot be said to exclude the diagnosis.

ETIOLOGY AND PATHOPHYSIOLOGY

- Bacterial pneumonia is most often a complication of another disease that disrupts mechanical or immunologic

pulmonary clearance and defense mechanisms:
  - Impaired mucociliary clearance.
  - Impaired reflex closure of the glottis.
  - Absent or impaired cough reflex.
  - Abnormal immune function.
    - Innate
    - Acquired
- Bacteria most often enter lungs via airways but can enter hematogenously. With impaired clearance and defense mechanisms, bacteria can proliferate and initiate local inflammatory responses:
  - Common isolates in dogs and cats include gram-negative aerobes, such as *Escherichia coli*, *Klebsiella*, *Bordetella*, *Pasteurella*, and *Staphylococcus* spp.
  - Regionally endemic diseases, such as plague and tularemia, can be causes of primary pneumonia.
- Local inflammatory responses cause pulmonary lesions, impair lung function, and can contribute to respiratory and systemic disease manifestations.

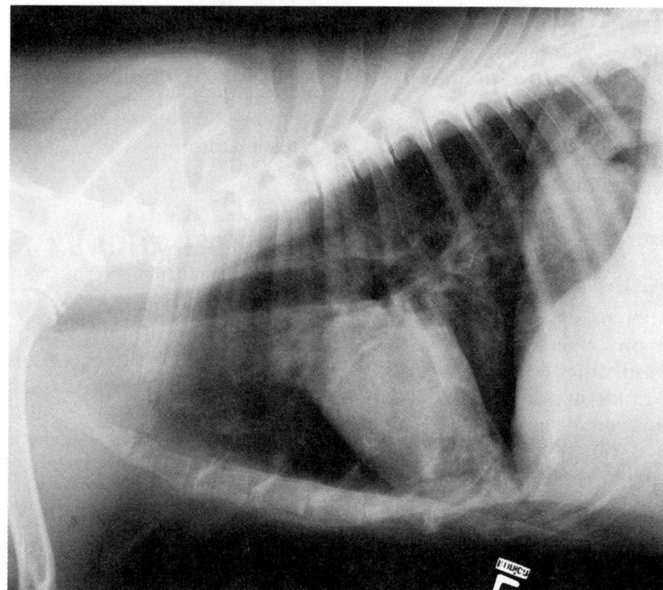

FIGURE I-137 Left lateral thoracic radiograph in a 14-year-old mixed-breed dog with pneumonia. Alveolar infiltrates are visible over the cardiac silhouette (especially the apex) but are not striking. Microcardia is also present, suggesting hypovolemia.

DIAGNOSIS

DIFFERENTIAL DIAGNOSIS

Many diseases share clinical and diagnostic similarities, including:
- Noninfectious inflammatory respiratory diseases
- Pulmonary neoplasia
- Respiratory parasites
- Pulmonary edema

INITIAL DATABASE

- Complete blood count (CBC): inflammatory leukogram (with or without left shift) expected although not seen in all cases.
  - Neutropenia is also possible, especially with severe sepsis. Conversely, bacterial pneumonia can develop secondary to primary neutropenic disorders (e.g., myelosuppression from chemotherapy).
- Serum biochemical profile/urinalysis: often normal.
- Thoracic radiographs:
  - Two or more views (at least one lateral and either a ventrodorsal [VD] or dorsoventral [DV]) are recommended in all cases.
    - Obtaining both right and left lateral-recumbent views can be useful since pneumonia infiltrates may only be apparent in nondependent lung (Figs. I-137, I-138).
  - Alveolar pattern in dependent regions of lung lobes expected in most cases.
    - Right middle lung lobe is commonly affected and may require careful examination on the lateral projection because it overlies the heart.
  - Interstitial patterns, with or without alveolar patterns, are also possible

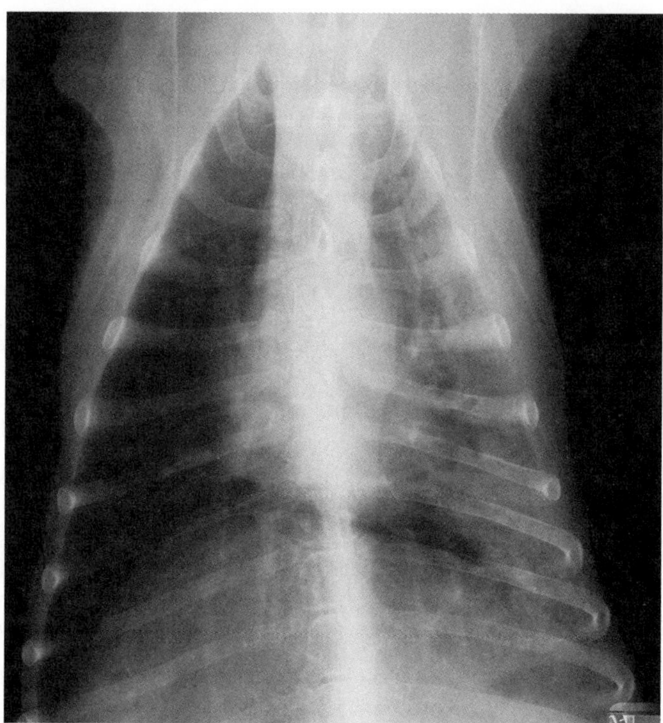

FIGURE I-138 Dorsoventral thoracic radiograph of dog in Fig. I-137. The left-sided alveolar infiltrates are more clearly apparent than in Fig. I-137, where they were obscured by being on the dependent side.

  - In some cases, lobar consolidation will be the prominent radiographic abnormality.
  - Other abnormalities that reflect underlying primary disease (as examples):
    - Megaesophagus.
    - Bronchiectasis.
    - Neoplasia.

ADVANCED OR CONFIRMATORY TESTING

- Confirmatory tests help rule out predisposing diseases/risk factors.
  - Respiratory washes (see Transtracheal Wash, p 1314) and bronchoalveolar lavage (see Bronchoscopy, p 1199).

        - Primarily septic, suppurative inflammation.
            - Bacteria are not always evident in cytologic exams, so clinicians should submit cultures of wash specimens irrespective of cytologic findings.
    - Bronchoscopy (see p 1199).
        - Endobronchial masses or foreign bodies may be evident in some cases.
        - Mucopurulent exudate in airways of affected regions may be seen.
        - Dilated/sacculated airways (bronchiectasis).
    - CT scan: superior delineation of the extent of pneumonia but often not needed when good-quality thoracic radiographs are consistent with the diagnosis.
    - Barium esophagography: if clinician suspects megaesophagus or esophageal motility dysfunction and this condition is not clearly apparent on survey thoracic radiographs.
- Arterial blood gas (ABG) analysis.
    - Hypoxemia and hypocapnea are the most common abnormalities and, when present, generally indicate severe pneumonia or the presence of a complicating factor (e.g., acute respiratory distress syndrome [ARDS]) and therefore a more guarded prognosis.
- Other tests specific for underlying diseases (e.g., serum acetylcholine [Ach]-receptor antibody titers for myasthenia gravis-induced megaesophagus).

TREATMENT

THERAPEUTIC GOAL(S)

- Resolve bacterial infection
- Remove predisposing factors when possible

ACUTE GENERAL TREATMENT

- Broad-spectrum antibiotics.
    - Clinically unstable animals should be treated with broad-spectrum IV antibiotics
        - Ampicillin (22 mg/kg IV q 8h) or cefazolin (22 mg/kg IV q 8h) and either enrofloxacin (3-5 mg/kg IV q 24h [dogs]) or an aminoglycoside, such as amikacin (20 mg/kg SC or IV q 24h); aminoglycosides, however, should not be used in animals that are dehydrated or that have renal compromise.
        - The clinical condition of the animal, if severe, may warrant therapy before obtaining respiratory samples for culture.
    - Clinically stable animals may be treated with oral antibiotics, ideally selected based on culture and sensitivity (C&S) testing. Empiric choices while waiting on results include:
        - Ampicillin or amoxicillin/clavulanate 22 mg/kg q 8h.
        - Trimethoprim-sulfa 15 mg/kg, q 12h.
    - Because of concerns about the pathogenic potential of *Mycoplasma* species in pneumonia, doxycycline 3-5 mg/kg PO q 12h may be considered, particularly for animals that show no response to therapy with other antibiotic choices.
- Saline nebulization several times daily.
- Oxygen (nasal cannula, oxygen cage, face mask) for hypoxemic animals or those in respiratory distress (see Oxygen Supplementation, p 1292).
- IV fluids as needed.
- Bronchodilators as needed.
    - Theophylline: Dosage varies with formulation.
    - Terbutaline: 1.25-5 mg/dog PO q 8h; 0.625 mg/cat PO q 12h, or 0.1-0.2 mg/kg PO q 12h (cat).

CHRONIC TREATMENT

- Thoracic coupage and position changes in recumbent animals
- Identification and management of underlying causes when identified
- Antibiotic therapy continued 1 week beyond clinical and radiographic resolution of infection
    - Lung lobectomy is occasionally needed to resolve infection when extensive single-lobe involvement has failed medical therapy or is associated with recurrent infection
        - Prognosis associated with lobectomy is considered best if done for foreign body pneumonia

POSSIBLE COMPLICATIONS

Lung lobe abscess

RECOMMENDED MONITORING

- Clinical signs (respiratory rate, effort, etc.):
    - Carefully reevaluate animals that are not clinically better within 48 to 72 hours of starting empiric therapy or that deteriorate substantially at any time; consider pursuing more diagnostic tests and/or changing therapy.
- Thoracic radiographs:
    - Radiographic changes can lag as much as 48 hours behind clinical changes.
    - Repeating thoracic radiographs approximately 1 week after cessation of antibiotics may demonstrate focal primary diseases (e.g., neoplasia) not evident on initial radiographs.
- ABG analysis
- CBC

PROGNOSIS AND OUTCOME

Varies with severity of disease and nature of predisposing factors.

- Prognosis for uncomplicated pneumonia is generally good.
- Prognosis for animals with risk factors depends on ability to treat/ resolve the risk factor.
    - Recurrent infections are common in animals with unresolved primary diseases.

PEARLS & CONSIDERATIONS

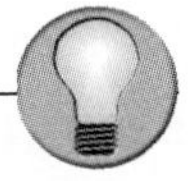

COMMENTS

Bacterial pneumonia should be viewed as a complication of another underlying disease. Therefore, patients should be rigorously evaluated for risk factors if such factors are not immediately apparent.

CLIENT EDUCATION

- Following recommended diagnostic and monitoring suggestions is important for most effective long-term resolution.
- Home treatment may include:
    - Respiratory humidification by inhalation of "cold steam" is best accomplished by having a pet in a closed, nonventilated bathroom (but not in the bath/shower) for 10 to 15 minutes once to three times a day while a warm shower runs.
    - This is often followed by coupage, which is a series of brusque pats to both sides of the chest, performed for 10 to 30 seconds after each humidification session, with the intention of loosening pulmonary secretions and pus to facilitate expectoration.
    - Pet owners should only perform these treatments on the recommendation of a veterinarian because they can make a condition worse if used inappropriately.

SUGGESTED READING

Chandler JC, et al: Mycoplasmal respiratory infections in small animals: 17 cases (1988-1999). *J Am Anim Hosp Assoc* 38:111, 2002.

Ford RB: Bacterial pneumonia. In Bonagura JD (ed): *Current Veterinary Therapy XIII*. Philadelphia, WB Saunders, 2000, pp 812-815.

Fransson BA, et al: Pneumonia after intracranial surgery in dogs. *Vet Surg* 30:432, 2001.

Moses L, et al: Esophageal motility dysfunction in cats: A study of 44 cases. *J Am Anim Hosp Assoc* 36:309, 2000.

Murphy ST, et al: Pulmonary lobectomy in the management of pneumonia in dogs: 59 cases (1972-1994). *J Am Vet Med Assoc* 210:235, 1997.

AUTHOR & EDITOR: **RANCE K. SELLON**

Pneumothorax

BASIC INFORMATION

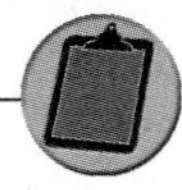

DEFINITION

The accumulation of air within the pleural space

SYNONYM(S)

Collapsed lung

EPIDEMIOLOGY

SPECIES, AGE, SEX: Young, large-breed male dogs are predisposed to trauma and subsequent pneumothorax.

GENETICS AND BREED PREDISPOSITION: Northern breeds (Siberian husky or Alaskan malamute) are predisposed to spontaneous pneumothorax.

RISK FACTORS
- Trauma (hit by car, bite wounds, falls from elevated heights)
- Surgical intervention (cranial abdominal, intervertebral disk, and other surgeries)
- Pleural effusion (centesis leads to pneumothorax)

GEOGRAPHY AND SEASONALITY: Trauma is more common in warmer months.

ASSOCIATED CONDITIONS AND DISORDERS
- Pulmonary contusions
- Diaphragmatic hernia
- Flail chest
- Fracture
- Asthma
- Pleural effusion

CLINICAL PRESENTATION

DISEASE FORMS/SUBTYPES
- Traumatic: due to damage to the pulmonary parenchyma or chest wall
- Spontaneous: due to abnormal pulmonary parenchyma without trauma
- Iatrogenic: due to damage to the lung parenchyma following thoracocentesis for removal of pleural effusion, following aspiration of a pulmonary mass or during surgery

HISTORY, CHIEF COMPLAINT
- Trauma
- Acute onset coughing or tachypnea
- Worsening tachypnea following an intervention

PHYSICAL EXAM FINDINGS
- Dyspnea/increased respiratory effort is the hallmark finding:
  - Expiratory or both expiratory and inspiratory but not inspiratory alone (which would more commonly suggest upper airway disease, not pneumothorax)
  - May be absent in mild cases
- Other evidence of trauma, either blunt (e.g., hit by car) or penetrating (e.g., bite, gunshot, stabbing)
- Dull or muffled lung sounds (auscultation, percussion)

ETIOLOGY AND PATHOPHYSIOLOGY

- Air may enter the pleural space either from damage to the pulmonary parenchyma (e.g., rupture of a pulmonary bleb), which permits the leakage of air from the respiratory system into the pleural space, or via damage to the chest wall, which permits air to rush into the pleural space.
- When the lung parenchyma is normal, small injuries (e.g., needlestick during centesis) heal rapidly.
  - Intrapleural volumes of air of up to 45 ml/kg cause no clinical signs and take about 2 weeks to resorb spontaneously in healthy dogs.
  - Iatrogenic pneumothorax occurring during thoracocentesis is almost invariably associated with chronic effusions (especially chylothorax), diseased lung tissue, or a very inexperienced operator.
- A "tension" pneumothorax is a severe pneumothorax from any cause that results in cardiovascular collapse due to inadequate cardiac filling.
- Rarely, foreign bodies (grass awns, wooden toothpicks, porcupine quills, etc.) may migrate intrathoracically and cause pneumothorax.

DIAGNOSIS

DIFFERENTIAL DIAGNOSIS

Dyspnea in an animal that has undergone trauma:
- Pleural effusion
- Pulmonary contusions
- Primary lung or airway disease
- Pain
- Hypovolemia

INITIAL DATABASE

- Thoracic radiographs are the test of choice; left lateral recumbency is the most sensitive view for detecting small volumes of air in the pleural space.
- Routine laboratory testing (complete blood count [CBC], serum chemistry profile, urinalysis): generally unremarkable.

ADVANCED OR CONFIRMATORY TESTING

- CT scan may be useful in spontaneous pneumothorax.
- Arterial blood gas (ABG) measurement or pulse oximetry: may help elucidate whether dyspnea in a trauma animal with pneumothorax may be in part due to the pneumothorax itself (e.g., PaO_2 <90 mmHg on room air and/or O_2 desaturation <96%) or to pain, hypovolemia, or other conditions associated with trauma. Pulmonary contusions may also cause hypoxemia and desaturation, however.
- Thoracic ultrasound is not usually useful because the air interferes with imaging.
- Analysis of pleural effusion, if present.

TREATMENT

THERAPEUTIC GOAL(S)

- Removal of air from the pleural space
- Encourage the formation of a seal to prevent further leakage

ACUTE GENERAL TREATMENT

- Supplemental oxygen will result in more rapid resolution of a closed (not ongoing) pneumothorax because the trapped air is higher in nitrogen, and if inhaled oxygen is administered, the trapped air will move more quickly down its concentration gradient.
- Traumatic pneumothorax:
  - No clinical signs, identified incidentally on radiographs: no treatment, monitoring is important.
  - Clinical signs: thoracocentesis warranted. If large volumes (>200 ml/kg), no end point, or recurrent pneumothorax, then place thoracostomy tubes (see Chest Tube Placement, p 1210). Apply the "three-strike rule," meaning if three or more thoracocenteses are required within 24 hours following a trauma, a thoracostomy tube should be placed.
- Spontaneous pneumothorax (no trauma):
  - If the clinician suspects a bulla or bleb (no masses on radiographs), a thoracotomy is warranted.
  - If the clinician suspects a necrotic neoplasm, a thoracic CT scan followed by thoracotomy is warranted.
  - If the clinician suspects an underlying feline asthma or chronic bronchitis, conservative therapy may be adequate.
- Iatrogenic:
  - If there are no clinical signs (radiographic diagnosis only), monitoring of the patient is adequate.
  - If the animal is showing clinical signs, repeating the thoracocentesis and monitoring the animal closely are recommended. The animal may require a thoracostomy tube or

exploratory thoracotomy if not responsive. Underlying disease may require specific treatment.

CHRONIC TREATMENT

Correction of the underlying cause, if applicable

POSSIBLE COMPLICATIONS

Ongoing pleural effusion or pneumothorax

RECOMMENDED MONITORING

- Respiratory rate and effort
- Pulse oximetry

PROGNOSIS AND OUTCOME

- Fair to good; often with trauma, the associated injuries are more likely to predict outcome.
- Dyspnea and duration of intensive care are negative prognostic factors in dogs and cats with pneumothorax.

PEARLS & CONSIDERATIONS

COMMENTS

- Traumatic pneumothorax rarely requires surgical correction because most cases rapidly resolve (within 72 hours).
- Spontaneous pneumothorax commonly requires surgical treatment because most cases will not resolve without surgery.

PREVENTION

- Owners should prevent free-roaming of pets.
- Clinicians should use caution when performing a thoracocentesis.

SUGGESTED READING

Kern DA, et al: Radiographic evaluation of induced pneumothorax in the dog. *Vet Radiol Ultrasound* 35:411-417, 1996.

Puerto DA: Surgical and nonsurgical management of and selected risk factors for spontaneous pneumothorax in dogs: 64 cases (1986-1999). *J Am Vet Med Assoc* 220(11):1670-1674, 2002.

White HL, et al: Spontaneous pneumothorax in two cats with small airway disease. *J Am Vet Med Assoc* 222(11):1573-1575, 1547, 2003.

AUTHOR & EDITOR: **ELIZABETH ROZANSKI**

Pododermatitis

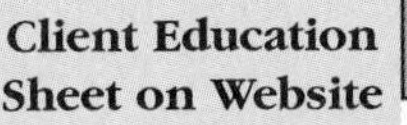

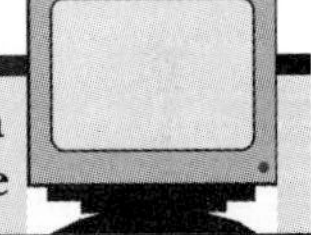

Client Education Sheet on Website

BASIC INFORMATION

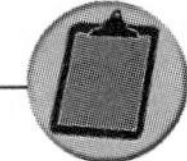

DEFINITION

An inflammatory skin disease affecting the paw

SYNONYM(S)

Interdigital dermatitis
Interdigital pyoderma
Pedal dermatitis

EPIDEMIOLOGY

SPECIES, AGE, SEX

- Pododermatosis is less commonly observed in cats than in dogs. Foot lesions in cats more commonly involve the footpads, claws, and periungual areas, whereas dogs often present with interdigital lesions.
- Dogs and cats of any age or sex can be affected.

GENETICS AND BREED PREDISPOSITION

- Short-haired dog breeds (e.g., English bulldog, Great Dane, basset hound, Mastiff, bull terrier, boxer, dachshund, dalmatian, German short-haired pointer, weimaraner) are more commonly affected (Fig. I-139).
- Long-haired breeds that are more often affected include German shepherds, Labrador retrievers, golden retrievers, Irish setters, and Pekingese dogs.

RISK FACTORS: In cats, immunosuppression, caused by feline leukemia virus (FeLV), feline immunodeficiency virus (FIV), or diabetes mellitus, can predispose to infectious pododermatitis.

CONTAGION AND ZOONOSIS: Dermatophytosis is contagious and zoonotic. Sporotrichosis (especially feline: zoonotic hazard) and blastomycosis (common point-source of infection or accidental inoculation during handling of specimens from affected animals) also may affect humans.

GEOGRAPHY AND SEASONALITY: Atopic dermatitis and allergic or irritant contact dermatitis can be seasonal.

CLINICAL PRESENTATION

HISTORY, CHIEF COMPLAINT: Owners can observe lesions on a single foot or multiple feet. Licking or chewing of the affected areas and lameness may also be noticed. In addition, pododermatitis may be part of a more generalized skin condition.

PHYSICAL EXAM FINDINGS: Lesions can be present on the dorsal and/or the ventral aspects of the feet. One or several interdigital spaces can be affected. Possible lesions include:

- Erythema.
- Nodules.
- Swelling of the feet.
- Interdigital serosanguineous or seropurulent exudates.
- Interdigital bullae or draining tracts.
- Ulcers and erosions.
- Scales and crusts.
- Alopecia.
- Plaques.
- Paronychia.
- Eosinophilic plaques (cat).
- Salivary staining.
- Occasional pitting edema of associated metatarsus or metacarpus.
- Regional lymphadenopathy may be present.

ETIOLOGY AND PATHOPHYSIOLOGY

Pododermatitis can arise following various pathomechanisms, including:

- Contact with irritant substances or physical trauma that can induce skin injury and inflammation.
- Infectious agents that can induce an immune response from the host, resulting in tissue inflammatory cell infiltrates; hormonal imbalances (hypothyroidism, hyperadrenocorticism) can predispose to infectious pododermatitis.
- Allergic disease: self-trauma can result in skin lesions, alopecia, and salivary staining.
- Immune-mediated disorders: the development of antibodies or activated lymphocytes against normal body constituents or inciting antigens (drugs, bacteria, viruses) causes tissue damage.
- Neoplastic cell infiltrates that disturb the normal structure of the skin.

DIAGNOSIS

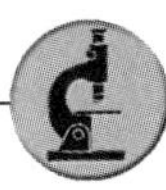

DIFFERENTIAL DIAGNOSIS

- If lesions are restricted to one foot:
  - Foreign bodies, trauma.
  - Neoplasia.
  - Localized bacterial or fungal infection.
  - Osteomyelitis.
- If multiple feet are involved:

- Environmental/traumatic: contact dermatitis to chemicals, clipper burns.
- Infectious: bacterial, fungal (dermatophytosis, *Malassezia* dermatitis, sporotrichosis, mycetoma, blastomycosis, cryptococcosis), parasitic (demodicosis, hookworm and *Pelodera* dermatitis, trombiculosis), rickettsial (canine Rocky Mountain spotted fever), viral (papillomatosis).
- Allergic: food hypersensitivity, atopic dermatitis, contact allergic dermatitis.
- Immune-mediated: pemphigus (foliaceous, erythematosus, vulgaris), bullous pemphigoid, systemic lupus erythematosus (SLE), and cutaneous (discoid) lupus erythematosus (DLE).
- Metabolic/endocrine: superficial necrolytic dermatitis (hepatocutaneous syndrome); hypothyroidism and hyperadrenocorticism can predispose an animal to bacterial or dermatophyte-induced pododermatitis and to adult-onset demodicosis.
- Miscellaneous: behavioral (self-induced lesions), zinc-responsive dermatosis, foreign body reaction (occasionally affects multiple feet), sterile pyogranulomas, nodular dermatofibrosis (German shepherds).

INITIAL DATABASE

Usefulness of different diagnostic tests is based on history and physical examination:

- Skin scrapings: *Demodex* sp.
- Wood's lamp examination: dermatophytosis (fluorescent strains of *Microsporum canis*).
- Cytologic examination: fungal organisms, bacteria, inflammatory cells, acantholytic keratinocytes (pemphigus), neoplastic cells.
- Elimination diet.
- Intradermal skin testing (serologic allergy testing could also be considered): atopy.
- Fecal flotation: hookworm ova.
- Radiographs: osteomyelitis, opaque foreign bodies.
- Complete blood count (CBC), biochemistry panel, urinalysis: results will depend on the underlying cause but are often normal or show nonspecific changes in diseases without systemic involvement.

ADVANCED OR CONFIRMATORY TESTING

- Culture: bacterial, fungal
- Skin biopsy: foreign bodies, demodicosis or other parasites, bacterial or fungal infections, neoplasia, immune-mediated diseases, hepatocutaneous syndrome, zinc responsive dermatosis
- Immunofluorescence or immunohistochemistry testing on biopsy samples: could occasionally be helpful in the diagnosis of autoimmune diseases
- Antinuclear antibody (ANA): positive in virtually all animals with SLE
- Endocrine tests and serology if relevant

TREATMENT

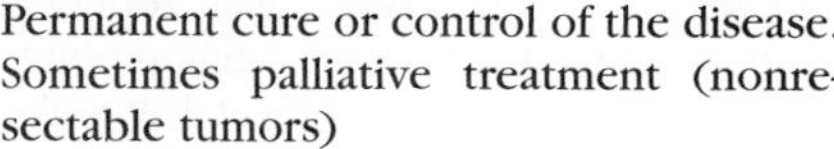

THERAPEUTIC GOAL(S)

Permanent cure or control of the disease. Sometimes palliative treatment (nonresectable tumors)

ACUTE GENERAL TREATMENT

Specifics depend on the underlying cause:

- Minimizing foot trauma.
- Draining lesions can benefit from soaks in a magnesium sulfate (Epsom salt) solution.
- Surgery: neoplastic lesions, surgical exploration (foreign bodies), or debridement.
- Bacterial pododermatitis can necessitate several weeks (8 to 12 weeks) of appropriate systemic antibiotics. The causal organism is often *Staphylococcus intermedius*. An acceptable initial choice is cephalexin 22-30 mg/kg PO q 12h or amoxicillin/clavulanate 12.5-22 mg/kg PO q 12h.
- If other bacteria are involved or the empiric choice of antibiotic does not resolve the infection, the clinician can correct the antibiotic selection based on culture and sensitivity (C&S) results.
- Manage parasitic or fungal infections with appropriate antiparasitic or antifungal medications.
- Atopy often requires management with combination therapy: anti-inflammatory agents, allergen-specific immunotherapy, and antimicrobial drugs to control secondary bacterial or fungal infections.
- Immunosuppressive treatments are usually required for treating immune-mediated diseases.

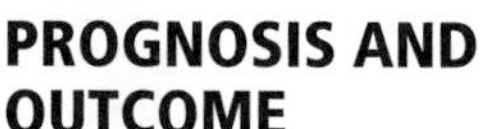

PROGNOSIS AND OUTCOME

Variable, depending on the cause of pododermatitis

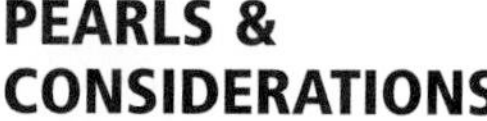

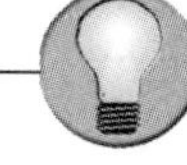

PEARLS & CONSIDERATIONS

COMMENTS

- Interdigital pyoderma can often be a frustrating disease to treat. Even after the resolution of the infection, the remaining fibrosis and scarring may predispose the animal to relapse.
- In severe refractory cases, clinicians may have to consider drastic measures, such as surgery (fusion podoplasty).
- Cases of canine pododermatitis with significant footpad involvement are more commonly seen with autoimmune diseases, drug reactions, zinc-responsive dermatosis, superficial necrolytic dermatitis (hepatocutaneous syndrome), and distemper.

SUGGESTED READING

Scott DW, Miller WH, Griffin CE. *Muller and Kirk's Small Animal Dermatology*, ed 6. Philadelphia, WB Saunders, 2001.

AUTHOR: **NADIA PAGÉ**
EDITOR: **JAN A. HALL**

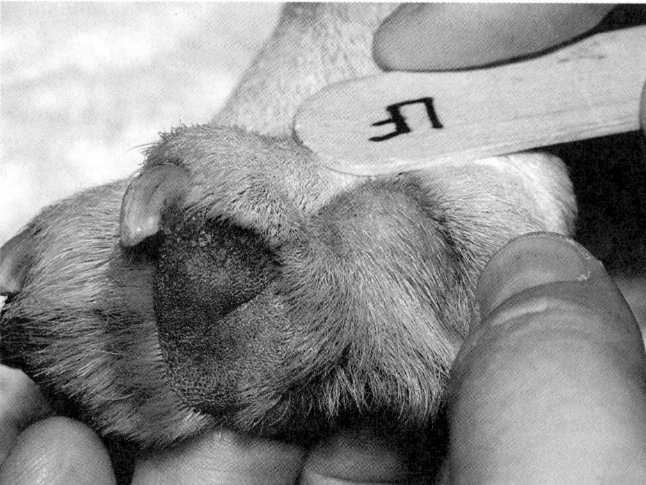

FIGURE I-139 An interdigital cyst associated with interdigital pyoderma in a 3-year-old castrated male English bulldog. The image shows the left forepaw, and the fifth digit is drawn laterally, revealing a fleshy, erythematous interdigital mass. Interdigital cysts can be present on the dorsal and/or the ventral aspects of the feet. One or several interdigital spaces can be affected. Courtesy of Dr. Jan A. Hall.

Poisoning, General Management

BASIC INFORMATION

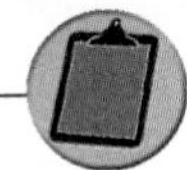

DEFINITION

A poison is a substance that causes death or injury when introduced into or absorbed by a living organism

SYNONYM(S)

Intoxication

EPIDEMIOLOGY

SPECIES, AGE, SEX

- Young animals are more likely to accidentally ingest poisonous materials.
- A cat's unique metabolism may cause it to be predisposed to certain toxicities (e.g., acetaminophen).

RISK FACTORS

- Lack of supervision.
- Access to poisonous materials.
- Individual behavior (some animals routinely ingest materials while others seldom do).
- Poisoning of companion animals is rarely malicious.

CONTAGION AND ZOONOSIS: Several animals may be affected simultaneously from the same source.

CLINICAL PRESENTATION

HISTORY, CHIEF COMPLAINT: The diagnosis of a possible intoxication is most often based upon the animal's history. Key components of the history may include witnessed exposure and characteristic behavior or clinical signs. It is common for owners to believe that their animal has been poisoned when it becomes ill. A thorough history will help to establish the likelihood of poisoning.

Additional important information may include the exact nature of the poison (if known), maximum possible dose ingested, the time elapsed since ingestion, and the time elapsed since clinical signs were first observed.

PHYSICAL EXAM FINDINGS: Highly dependent on the poison involved; common categories of signs include:

- Central nervous system (CNS) alterations and seizures (lead, metaldehyde, organophosphates, carbamates, tremorigenic mycotoxins, alcohol, blue-green algae, marijuana, chocolate, ivermectin)
- Muscle weakness, paresis, and paralysis (coral snakes, black widow spiders, phenoxy herbicides [including 2,4-D], macadamia nuts)
- Acute blindness (horse dewormer medication, salt)
- Oral mucosal lesions (corrosive acids, alkalis, cationic detergents, liquid potpourri, formaldehyde)
- Acute renal failure (ethylene glycol, lily plants)
- Acute hepatic damage or failure (mushrooms, blue-green algae, iron, sago, or cycad palm plants/trees)
- Severe anemia (onions, garlic, naphthalene mothballs, anticoagulant rodenticides, acetaminophen [cats])
- Cardiac arrhythmias (foxglove, lily of the valley, oleander, azalea/rhododendron, and yew plants; bufo toads)
- Gastrointestinal (GI) signs (many, including several already listed; arsenic, castor beans, nitrogen-phosphate-potassium (NPK) fertilizers, zinc oxide, oxalate-containing plants)

ETIOLOGY AND PATHOPHYSIOLOGY

The possibility of poisoning should be considered when a young and otherwise healthy animal exhibits an acute onset of neurologic signs, organ failure, or other systemic signs and after all other common diseases have been ruled out.

DIAGNOSIS

DIFFERENTIAL DIAGNOSIS

Other systemic or metabolic diseases

INITIAL DATABASE

- Packed cell volume/serum total protein.
- Azo stick (blood urea nitrogen).
- Blood glucose.
- Urine specific gravity and dipstick.
- Samples of urine, blood, and gastric contents should be saved for possible toxicologic analysis.

ADVANCED OR CONFIRMATORY TESTING

Serum levels or tissue analysis for specific toxin

TREATMENT

THERAPEUTIC GOAL(S)

- Achieve cardiovascular stability
- Prevent further absorption of the toxin
- Administer antidote, if available

ACUTE GENERAL TREATMENT

- Triage principle: Life-threatening complications need to be addressed first if present. "Start with the animal, not the toxin."
  - Airway support or intubation if respiratory arrest.
  - IV catheter placement if animal is showing systemic signs.
  - Electrocardiographic (ECG), blood pressure (BP), and pulse oximetric monitoring as dictated by physical examination findings.
  - IV fluid and oxygen support as indicated by cardiovascular and respiratory status.
- Decontamination of the patient:
  - Skin: Dermal exposure (i.e., topical pyrethrin exposure) warrants bathing with warm water and a mild dish washing detergent. Care should be taken to prevent hypothermia.
  - Emesis: Consider this treatment if ingestion has occurred within 2 hours of visit. Contraindicated in animals that ingested potentially caustic substances (acids, alkalis, petroleum distillates) or are unable to protect their airway due to depression, seizures, or other neurologic dysfunction. (See Vomiting, Induction of, p 1328.)
  - Gastric lavage: used when emesis is contraindicated due to the animal's inability to protect its airway; requires induction of general anesthesia in conscious animals and intubation of the airway. This procedure involves passage of the distal end of a large bore tube into the stomach; and administration of 5–10 ml/kg of tepid water. The water is then withdrawn through the tube with gravity flow. Lavage is thus repeated until the gastric contents are clear. (See Gastric Intubation, Gavage, Lavage, p 1258.)
  - Activated charcoal: Activated charcoal is the most commonly used general treatment for intoxications; dose: 1–4 g/kg PO (suspension: 5–10 ml/kg PO). It is ineffective in removing heavy metals. Some animals will eat the activated charcoal willingly, but most require orogastric administration. Clinicians must be careful to prevent aspiration pneumonia. Elimination of toxins that undergo enterohepatic circulation may be hastened by additional doses of activated charcoal every 4 to 6 hours for up to 24 hours. Owners must be made aware that the animal will have black stool for several days.
  - Cathartics: accelerate the fecal elimination of toxin. Sorbitol is most commonly used in combination with activated charcoal. Other available cathartics include sodium sulfate, magnesium sulfate or citrate. Contraindications include GI obstruc-

tion, recent bowel surgery, volume depletion, electrolyte imbalance, and the ingestion of a corrosive substance.
  - Fluid diuresis: may be used for accelerating the elimination of toxins that are renally extracted.

METHODS TO INDUCE EMESIS

- Apomorphine (dogs only)
  - Dose: 0.02-0.04 mg/kg. The tablet is placed in the conjunctival fornix and allowed to dissolve. When emesis begins, the tablet is removed and the conjunctiva is lavaged copiously.
  - Onset: 5 minutes.
  - Adverse effects: respiratory depression, protracted vomiting, undesirable CNS excitation; excessive emesis may be reversed with metoclopramide.
- Hydrogen peroxide (3% solution)
  - Dose: 1-2 ml/kg PO, can be repeated once. Emesis is more likely with a full stomach.
  - Onset: 10 minutes.
  - Adverse effects: none known.
- Xylazine (cats only)
  - Dose: 0.5-1.0 mg/kg intramuscularly (IM).
  - Onset: 5 to 10 minutes.
  - Adverse effects: bradycardia, depression; can be reversed with equal volume yohimbine IM.

DRUG INTERACTIONS

Dependent on toxin

POSSIBLE COMPLICATIONS

Dependent on toxin

PROGNOSIS AND OUTCOME

Prognosis will vary depending upon the exact toxin ingested, the total dose ingested, and the severity of clinical signs

PEARLS & CONSIDERATIONS

COMMENTS

- Most of the specific intoxications seen in small animal practice are discussed individually and in detail elsewhere in this book.
- Many poisons cause signs similar to those caused by other common diseases. The diagnosis of toxicity should not be reached without strong historical or physical evidence of exposure.
- National Animal Poison Control Center: 1-900-680-0000 or 1-800-548-2423.

PREVENTION

Owners should prevent their pets from accessing toxins.

CLIENT EDUCATION

Discussions on common poisoning should be made available to clients.

SUGGESTED READING

Plumlee KH: *Clinical Veterinary Toxicology*. St. Louis, Mosby, 2004.

Côté E, Khan SA: Intoxication versus acute, nontoxicologic illness: Differentiaiting the two. In Ettinger SJ, Feldman EC (eds): *Textbook of Veterinary Internal Medicine*, ed 6. St. Louis, Elsevier Saunders, 2005, pp 242-245.

AUTHOR: **SCOTT P. SHAW**

EDITOR: **ELIZABETH ROZANSKI**

Pollakiuria, Stranguria

BASIC INFORMATION

DEFINITION

- Pollakiuria: increased frequency of attempts to urinate
- Stranguria: straining to urinate
- Both are clinical signs of lower urinary tract inflammation, infection, and/or obstruction

CLINICAL PRESENTATION

HISTORY, CHIEF COMPLAINT

- Owners may confuse these clinical signs with inappropriate elimination, polyuria, or tenesmus.
- Other clinical signs can include dysuria and malodorous urine.
- Often pollakiuria/stranguria is the only presenting clinical sign.

PHYSICAL EXAM FINDINGS

- Important to determine if urinary obstruction is the cause.
  - Obstruction: bladder enlarged/firm, nonexpressible, often painful.
  - Nonobstruction: bladder small/soft, expressible; bladder wall may be thickened, often painful as well.
- Bladder should be palpated before and after the patient voids.
  - Uroliths, masses, and bladder wall thickness/irregularities may be assessed more easily in the flaccid bladder.
- Rectal exam may reveal urethral, prostatic, or bladder trigone abnormalities.

ETIOLOGY AND PATHOPHYSIOLOGY

- Any disease that causes lower urinary tract infection (LUTI), inflammation, or obstruction can cause pollakiuria or stranguria.
- Localizes the lesion to the lower urinary tract (bladder, urethra).

DIAGNOSIS

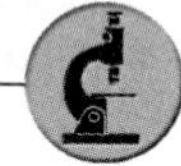

DIFFERENTIAL DIAGNOSIS

- Feline
  - Most common cause is idiopathic feline lower urinary tract signs (FLUTS):
    - Also called feline idiopathic cystitis (FIC), feline lower urinary tract disorder (FLUTD), and feline urologic syndrome (FUS)
  - Primary bacterial infection in cats is rare; infection is present in <2% of cats <10 years of age with lower urinary tract signs
- Canine
  - Most common cause is bacterial cystitis
- Other causes
  - Nonbacterial causes of cystitis:
    - Polypoid: chronic irritation
    - Emphysematous: bacterial fermentation of glucose in devitalized bladder wall
    - Drug induced: usually associated with cyclophosphamide
    - Idiopathic
    - Fungal, algal: uncommon
  - Other bladder diseases:
    - Cystic calculi (uroliths)
    - Neoplasia
  - Prostatic:
    - Neoplasia (transitional cell carcinoma [TCC], adenocarcinoma)
    - Trauma
  - Urethral disease:
    - Urethrorectal fistula
    - Urethral prolapse
    - Urethritis
    - Urethrolithiasis
    - Neoplasia (TCC, squamous cell carcinoma [SCC])
    - Trauma

INITIAL DATABASE

- Complete blood count (CBC) and serum biochemistry panel
  - Metabolic or systemic disease (diabetes mellitus, pyelonephritis, many others)

- Urinalysis
  - Cystocentesis preferred
  - Comparison with free-catch sample may assist in anatomic localization of lesion
- Urine culture and sensitivity (C&S)
  - Cystocentesis preferred
- Abdominal radiographs
  - Mass effect
  - Prostatomegaly
  - Radiopaque calculi
- Abdominal ultrasound
  - Bladder wall thickness.
  - Presence of bladder mass (inflammatory, neoplastic, or blood clot)
  - Architecture of prostate
  - Proximal urethra

ADVANCED OR CONFIRMATORY TESTING

- Advanced imaging
  - Double contrast cystogram
  - Voiding urethrogram
  - Excretory urethrogram
- Cystoscopy
- Voiding urohydropulsion
  - Appropriate if small calculi are present
  - Noninvasive method to collect calculi for chemical anlaysis
- Cystotomy
  - Biopsy of mass
  - Removal of calculi
  - Culture of bladder wall

TREATMENT

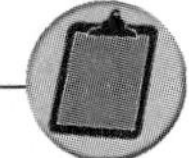

THERAPEUTIC GOAL(S)

- Relieve discomfort associated with LU
- Treat underlying cause

ACUTE GENERAL TREATMENT

- Of greatest immediate concern is urethral obstruction (see Urethral Obstruction, p 1120; Urethral Obstruction [Canine]: Medical Management, p 1318; Urethral Obstruction [Feline]: Medical Management, p 1319).
  - No matter the cause, establish urine flow to prevent life-threatening hyperkalemia if complete obstruction is present (urinary bladder moderately to markedly enlarged).
  - Assess azotemia and potassium level.
  - Gently try to pass a urinary catheter using retrograde hydropulsion if obstruction is met.
  - If catheterization is unsuccessful:
    - Cystocentesis.
      - Relieving pressure may allow urethral catheter to pass.
      - Insert needle relatively caudally (near trigone) and direct it caudodorsally, to minimize risk of contacting devitalized bladder wall.
    - Urethrotomy.
    - Cystostomy tube.
  - Provide fluid and electrolyte support while diagnostic tests are pursued.
    - Consider IV fluid without potassium as first choice until serum potassium level is known (e.g., choose 0.9% NaCl).
- If a bacterial infection is suspected, a C&S is vital for directed antibiotic therapy.

CHRONIC TREATMENT

Dependent on accurate diagnosis of underlying cause

PEARLS & CONSIDERATIONS

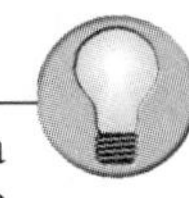

- Pollakiuria and stranguria localize the problem to the lower urinary tract.
- Further diagnostic evaluation is necessary to determine the exact cause of these signs.
- While bacterial infection is the most common cause in dogs, this is rare in cats.
- FLUTS (FLUTD/FUS/FIC) is the most common cause of pollakiuria and stranguria in cats.
- With any episode of pollakiuria or stranguria, urinary obstruction must be ruled out as soon as possible.

SUGGESTED READING

Adams LG, Syme HM: Canine lower urinary tract diseases. In Ettinger SJ, Feldman EC (eds): *Textbook of Veterinary Internal Medicine*, ed 6. St. Louis, Elsevier, 2005, pp 1850–1874.

Lulich JP, Osborne CA: Diseases of the urinary bladder. In Morgan RV, Bright RM, Swartout MS (eds): *Handbook of Small Animal Practice*, ed 4. New York, Saunders/Elsevier, 2003, pp 534–547.

Seguin MA, et al: Persistent urinary tract infections and reinfections in 100 dogs (1989–1999). *J Vet Intern Med* 17(5):622–631, 2003.

Seim HB: Diseases of the urethra. In Morgan RV, Bright RM, Swartout MS (eds): *Handbook of Small Animal Practice*, ed 4. New York, Saunders/Elsevier, 2003, pp 563–569.

Westrop JL, Buffington CAT, Chew D: Feline lower urinary tract diseases. In Ettinger SJ, Feldman EC (eds): *Textbook of Veterinary Internal Medicine*, ed 6. St. Louis, Elsevier, 2005, pp 1828–1850.

AUTHOR: **CLAIRE WEIGAND**
EDITOR: **ETIENNE CÔTÉ**

Polyarthritis

BASIC INFORMATION

DEFINITION

Inflammation of two or more joints

SYNONYM(S)

Rheumatoid arthritis: erosive arthritis

EPIDEMIOLOGY

SPECIES, AGE, SEX: Dependent on underlying cause.

- With idiopathic immune-mediated polyarthritis (IMPA), the age of onset can vary, but many animals are young adults that are 1 to 3 years old.
- With infectious polyarthritis, male dogs are more commonly affected.
- Cats: feline chronic progressive polyarthritis (male > female).

GENETICS AND BREED PREDISPOSITION

- Certain histocompatibility alleles have been associated with rheumatoid arthritis in dogs.
- Idiopathic IMPA is seen more commonly in the Akita and Weimaraner.
- Familial amyloidosis is a cause of polyarthritis in the shar-pei.
- Adverse reaction to sulfonamide drugs, causing polyarthritis: Doberman pinscher.

RISK FACTORS

- Dogs: recent vaccination, treatment with sulphonamide or other antibiotics, exposure to ticks
- Cats: calicivirus vaccination (especially kittens)

ASSOCIATED CONDITIONS AND DISORDERS: IMPA is sometimes associated with systemic lupus erythematosus (SLE) (see Systemic Lupus Erythematosus, p 1061) or drug eruption/hypersensitivity (see Drug Eruption, p 322), secondary infections, and gastrointestinal (GI) disease or neoplasia.

CLINICAL PRESENTATION

DISEASE FORMS/SUBTYPES

- Noninfectious IMPA (nonerosive [idiopathic, SLE, others] or erosive)
  - Canine noninfectious erosive polyarthritis (rheumatoid arthritis)

- Feline progressive polyarthritis: characterized by periosteal new bone formation and bony erosions; either acute (more common, affects young cats) or chronic (less common, slower in onset, affects adult/older cats)
- Infectious arthritis

HISTORY, CHIEF COMPLAINT
- Difficulty walking
- Stiffness, lameness
- Weakness, inability to rise
- Inappetence
- Lethargy, weight loss, vomiting, diarrhea

Animals that have idiopathic IMPA experience a sudden onset of signs with multiple symmetric joint involvement.

PHYSICAL EXAM FINDINGS
- Joint pain, swelling:
  - Characteristic physical finding in polyarthritis.
  - May be difficult to localize source of stiffness; sometimes articular pain may be absent on initial examination.
  - Firm, complete flexion of carpi should be performed whenever polyarthritis is possible; may reveal signs of pain that otherwise would escape notice.
  - Distal, symmetric joint involvement (commonly carpi and tarsi) in IMPA.
  - Usually one but occasionally two or more proximal joints involved with septic bacterial polyarthritis.
- Fever; in some cases of IMPA, pain and joint swelling may be absent and fever may be the only sign.
- Lymphadenopathy.
- Neck pain if meningitis present.

ETIOLOGY AND PATHOPHYSIOLOGY

- Idiopathic nonerosive IMPA is the most common form. The etiology is unknown.
  - Possible mechanisms include immune complex formation in response to a microbial infection with subsequent deposition in joints. Other theories include immune responses to microbial antigens in the joint; genetic predisposition in certain individuals; and molecular mimicry, in which antibodies to certain antigens (from bacteria, viruses, tumors, drugs, or diets) cross-react with joint antigens.
  - Once joint inflammation has occurred, autoantigens, such as altered collagen, are produced that stimulate an immune response, helping to perpetuate the inflammation.
  - The idiopathic nature indicates that the typical case of idiopathic polyarthritis is "uncomplicated" by underlying disease; nevertheless, some cases of IMPA can be seen in association with infections elsewhere in the body (reactive arthritis), such as with GI disease (enteropathic arthritis) or neoplasia (arthritis of malignancy).
- Infectious:
  - Recognized etiologies:
    - Bacterial: borreliosis, ehrlichiosis (especially with *Ehrlichia ewingii*), *Streptococcus*, *Staphylococcus*, *Erysipelothrix*, *Corynebacterium*, *Escherichia coli*, and L-forms.
    - Other: calicivirus, heartworm, *Mycoplasma*, *Leishmania*, *Babesia*, *Hepatozoon*, and systemic fungal infections.
  - May occur following direct penetration of a joint (surgery, trauma, bite wound, arthrocentesis) or from hematogenous spread. Bite wounds are common in cats, whereas hematogenous spread from an unidentified source of infection is common in dogs. Preexisting damage to a joint may aid in the establishment of infection. Single joint involvement is more common, but infection may spread to a second joint; multiple joint involvement is more common with systemic bacterial infections (e.g., bacterial endocarditis [which may also cause IMPA], omphalophlebitis, deep pyoderma, pyelonephritis, diskospondylitis, pyometra, periodontal disease, and prostatitis).
- Vaccines: calicivirus, canine distemper, others; may trigger a nonerosive IMPA.
- Drugs: especially sulfonamide antibiotics but also lincomycin, cephalosporins, penicillins, and others; may act as antigens or combine with haptens to form antigens and trigger a systemic vasculitis, which may manifest as polyarthritis, fever, thrombocytopenia, and other such conditions.
- Autoantibodies to nuclear material (see Systemic Lupus Erythematosus, p 1061).
  - Antibodies to nuclear material, immune complex formation, and subsequent deposition in tissues cause multisystemic disease that commonly manifests with nonerosive polyarthritis, dermatitis, and/or glomerulonephritis (GN).
- Erosive IMPAs include rheumatoid arthritis (rare in the cat) and periosteal proliferative polyarthritis (common in the cat).
  - Rheumatoid arthritis is usually associated with autoantibodies to immunoglobulin G (rheumatoid factor) (see Rheumatoid Arthritis, p 969).
  - Periosteal proliferative polyarthritis is characterized by periosteal new bone formation and bony erosions. It affects young adult cats, often castrated males, and is usually acute in onset. Chronic progressive polyarthritis is a milder form, is insidious in onset, and affects older cats.

DIAGNOSIS

Polyarthritis can be suspected and occasionally diagnosed with history and physical examination alone. Confirmation rests on radiography and arthrocentesis with joint fluid analysis. Successful management of polyarthritis requires that any underlying cause be identified and treated.

DIFFERENTIAL DIAGNOSIS

Man conditions should be ruled out as a cause for inability to walk:
- Neurologic disease (e.g., spinal cord or brain disorders, neuromuscular diseases)
- Muscular disease (e.g., polymyositis)
- Orthopedic disease (e.g., bilateral cranial cruciate ligament rupture, degenerative joint disease)
- Cardiac disease (e.g., pericardial effusion)
- Metabolic disease (e.g., hypoglycemia, hypocalcemia)
- Hematologic disease (e.g., acute blood loss)

INITIAL DATABASE

- Complete blood count (CBC), serum chemistry profile, urinalysis:
  - Anemia and leukocytosis are common in idiopathic polyarthritis but are nonspecific. Further tests are generally needed to rule out underlying diseases.
  - Serum chemistry profile to assess dysfunction in other organs.
  - Proteinuria may be indicative of GN (possible with immune-mediated disease) or amyloidosis.
- Radiographs to distinguish erosive from nonerosive polyarthritis:
  - Erosive polyarthritis is characterized by subchrondral bone destruction, which is seen as an irregular joint surface or "punched-out" erosion of bone at the joint space. In advanced cases of joint deformity, loss of mineralization of the epiphysis and calcification of soft tissues of the joint may be seen.
  - Nonerosive polyarthritis presents no bony radiographic abnormalities; signs of joint effusion and soft tissue swelling may be apparent.

ADVANCED OR CONFIRMATORY TESTING

- Arthrocentesis (see Arthrocentesis, p 1183); two or more joints should be sampled.
  - The tarsi and carpi are especially useful, both because of frequency of involvement and ease of access to the synovial space.
  - Gross appearance: Normal synovial fluid is viscous (tenacious), scant in volume, and clear, whereas synovial fluid of animals with polyarthritis is

generally thin/watery and may be copious (several milliliters) and potentially turbid (more so with infectious/septic polyarthritis).

- Synovial fluid analysis; neutrophils are the predominant cell in inflammatory polyarthritis (distinguishing them from the more common degenerative arthropathies), and total cell counts are always >3000/ul and often 40,000/ul or higher. Cytologic examination is seldom helpful in distinguishing septic from nonseptic arthritis (only occasionally are intracellular, phagocytized organisms seen) although the presence of degenerate or toxic neutrophils is suggestive of septic arthritis.
- Culture: Synovial fluid cultures are usually negative. When clinicians suspect septic arthritis, they should consider a culture of synovial membrane, blood, and/or urine. Special media are needed to culture L-form bacteria and *Mycoplasma*.
- Titers: Lyme disease (*Borrelia burgdorferi*), *Ehrlichia* (especially *canis*, *ewingii*), and *Anaplasma phagocytophila* (formerly *E. equi*).
- Echocardiogram if suspicious of bacterial endocarditis (e.g., heart murmur, especially if new in onset, and/or diastolic) (see Endocarditis, Infective p 344).
- Serum antinuclear antibody if the clinician suspects SLE.
- Serum rheumatoid factor if the clinician suspects rheumatoid arthritis although the test is of limited accuracy.
- Cerebrospinal fluid tap if the clinician suspects meningitis.
- Thoracic radiographs and abdominal ultrasound examination to evaluate for remote infection, GI disease, or neoplasia if suspected.

TREATMENT

THERAPEUTIC GOAL(S)

- Resolution of clinical signs and return of synovial cell counts to <3000/ul
- Gradual withdrawal of immunosuppressive therapy without relapse in cases of IMPA

ACUTE GENERAL TREATMENT

- Doxycycyline 10 mg/kg PO q 24h for 28 days for tick-borne infections, *Mycoplasma*, and L-form bacteria.
- Prednisone 1.1 mg/kg PO q 12h initially for nonerosive and erosive noninfectious IMPA.
- Broad-spectrum antibiotics (e.g., amoxicillin-clavulanate 12.5 mg/kg PO q 12h) or cephalosporins (e.g., cephalexin 22 mg/kg PO q 8h) pending cultures, in suspected or confirmed cases of septic arthritis.
- Surgical joint lavage and drainage sometimes are required for septic arthritis.

CHRONIC TREATMENT

- For IMPA: prednisone 1.1 mg/kg twice daily until resolution of signs (usually 2 weeks), then slowly reduce the dose and administer every other day. Average of 3 to 6 months and sometimes lifelong treatment is required.
- If a high dose of prednisone is required to suppress signs, consider other immunosuppressive drugs, such as azathioprine, cyclophosphamide, gold salts, methotrexate, or leflunomide, to keep clinical signs suppressed while using lower doses of glucocorticoids.
- Septic arthritis: antibiotics required until 2 weeks after infection has resolved; often a minimum of 6 weeks.

DRUG INTERACTIONS

Many drugs can potentially interact negatively with the drug in question; clinicians should consult a formulary for possible interactions.

POSSIBLE COMPLICATIONS

- Secondary infections from immunosuppressive drugs.
- Prednisone has many potential adverse effects including polyuria and polydipsia (PU/PD), polyphagia, panting, weight gain, muscle wasting, and elevated liver enzymes.
- Azathioprine: myelosuppression, hepatotoxicity, acute pancreatitis; avoid in cats.
- Cyclophosphamide: myelosuppression, hemorrhagic cystitis.

RECOMMENDED MONITORING

- Primarily resolution of clinical signs; if uncertainty exists, repeat arthrocentesis to see if cell counts have returned to normal.
- Monthly CBCs are required for animals receiving cyclophosphamide or azathioprine.
- Monitor liver enzymes in animals receiving prednisone.

PROGNOSIS AND OUTCOME

- Nonerosive IMPA: good to guarded. About 30% of cases relapse and may be difficult to control or may require lifelong treatment.
- Juvenile hereditary arthritis of Akitas: very poor. Does not respond to immunosuppressive therapy.
- Calicivirus infection of cats: excellent. Generally resolves in 3 days with supportive care.
- Noninfectious erosive arthritis: guarded. Arthrodesis may improve quality of life.
- Infectious arthritis: provided the condition is nonerosive and the infection can be treated, the prognosis is good.

PEARLS & CONSIDERATIONS

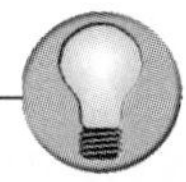

COMMENTS

- Polyarthritis should be suspected in any animal that is reluctant to walk or in any case of fever of unknown origin. Even in the absence of joint pain or swelling, arthrocentesis of multiple joints is indicated in such animals to confirm or refute a diagnosis of IMPA.
- Cats with polyarthritis may be described only as lethargic by owners; polyarthritis might be missed unless cats are observed walking in the exam room.
- Empiric treatment with doxycycline may be considered while completing a work-up.
- The majority of cases of polyarthritis are idiopathic, immune mediated, and nonerosive.

PREVENTION

Tick prevention if relevant (dogs in endemic regions)

CLIENT EDUCATION

- Close monitoring is required while patients are receiving immunosuppressive therapy.
- Relapses are possible.
- Genetic counseling for genetic forms.

SUGGESTED READING

Carro T: Polyarthritis in cats. *Comp Cont Ed Pract Vet* 16:57–67, 1994.

Clements DN, et al: Type 1 immune-mediated polyarthritis in dogs: 39 cases (1997–2002). *J Am Vet Med Assoc* 224:1323–1327, 2004.

Cowell RL, et al: Ehrlichiosis and polyarthritis in three dogs. *J Am Vet Med Assoc* 192: 1093–1099, 1988.

Ellison RS: The cytologic evaluation of synovial fluid. *Semin Vet Med Surg (Small Animal)* 3:133–139, 1988.

Jacques D, et al: A retrospective study of 40 dogs with polyarthritis. *Vet Surg* 31: 428–434, 2002.

AUTHOR: **ORLA MAHONY**

EDITOR: **SUSAN M. COTTER**

Polycystic Kidney Disease

BASIC INFORMATION

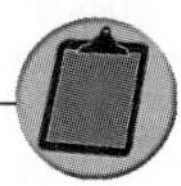

DEFINITION

Inherited cystic renal disease characterized by the presence of at least one cyst in one kidney. Although single cysts are rare, strict definitions of three or more cysts distributed between both kidneys create a risk of underdiagnosis of affected cats.

SYNONYM(S)

PKD

Autosomal dominant polycystic kidney disease (ADPKD)

EPIDEMIOLOGY

SPECIES, AGE, SEX

- Cats of either gender affected. Can be diagnosed at <6 months of age; clinical signs become apparent from 3 to 10 years of age (average 7 years).
- Has been reported uncommonly in dogs.

GENETICS AND BREED PREDISPOSITION

- Persians, Himalayans, long-haired cats, and exotic short-haired cats are commonly affected; increasing numbers of affected short-haired cats documented.
- Inherited as an autosomal dominant trait that is not strictly associated with long haircoat or brachycephalic facial conformation.
- About 40% of all Persians and Persian-related cats are affected.
- Australian bull terriers also affected.

ASSOCIATED CONDITIONS AND DISORDERS

- Polycystic liver disease in dogs and cats
- In Australian bull terriers, may be inherited with hereditary nephritis

CLINICAL PRESENTATION

HISTORY, CHIEF COMPLAINT

- Animals with overt manifestations of illness present for signs of chronic renal failure (CRF): polyuria, polydipsia, anorexia, lethargy, nausea, vomiting, weight loss, poor body condition, etc.
- Young animals presented for screening usually have no clinical signs.

PHYSICAL EXAM FINDINGS

- Early disease: normal renal palpation
- Moderate disease: enlarged kidneys, but contour may be smooth
- Advanced disease: enlarged, irregular kidneys usually bilaterally, although may not be symmetric

ETIOLOGY AND PATHOPHYSIOLOGY

- Cysts present at birth slowly enlarge compressing adjacent renal tissue. When sufficient renal parenchymal damage is present, CRF results. Rate of progression variable.
- Abnormal proteins, polycystin 1, and polycystin 2, are the result of mutations in the polycystic kidney gene. Cysts are abnormal dilations of renal tubules. Any section of the renal tubule may be affected by cyst formation.

DIAGNOSIS

DIFFERENTIAL DIAGNOSIS

For enlarged kidneys: perinephric pseudocysts, renal lymphoma or other neoplasia, ureteral obstruction with hydronephrosis, feline infectious peritonitis, hematoma, perinephric abscess, and compensatory hypertrophy (unilateral)

INITIAL DATABASE

- Overtly healthy-appearing young cats presenting for initial screening: renal ultrasound
- Clinically ill cats: complete blood count, serum biochemistry profile, and urinalysis to assess renal function and identify uremia-associated complications (e.g., hyperphosphatemia, hypokalemia, anemia)
- Blood pressure: especially important in azotemic animals

ADVANCED OR CONFIRMATORY TESTING

- Abdominal ultrasound can establish diagnosis. Cysts are anechoic, spherical structures with smooth, sharply marginated walls and through-transmission. Cysts are easier to identify in cortex than medulla due to normal relative hypoechogenicity of medulla. Ultrasound has 75% sensitivity for diagnosis in cats <16 weeks, and 90% sensitivity in cats at 36 weeks.
- Genetic testing is available for cats >8 weeks old (Veterinary Genetics Laboratory, University of California—Davis: www.vgl.ucdavis.edu). Buccal swab samples can be collected by owner.

TREATMENT

THERAPEUTIC GOAL(S)

- Cats with no clinical signs: remove from breeding program
- Cats with clinical manifestations: treat for CRF

ACUTE GENERAL TREATMENT

No treatment specific for polycystic kidney disease (PKD)—treat for CRF and associated complications

CHRONIC TREATMENT

Same as for CRF (see Chronic Renal Failure, Occult ["Asymptomatic"], p 204; Chronic Renal Failure, Overt ["Symptomatic"], p 205)

POSSIBLE COMPLICATIONS

Cysts can become infected. Alkaline and lipid-soluble antibiotics including fluoroquinolones, clindamycin, chloramphenicol, and trimethoprim-sulfonamide penetrate cysts well.

RECOMMENDED MONITORING

- Cats with no clinical signs: BUN, creatinine, urine specific gravity every 6 to 12 months, to help predict progression to renal failure
- Cats with CRF: monitor as for CRF of any cause

PROGNOSIS AND OUTCOME

- Not all cats with PKD will develop CRF.
- Onset of clinical signs usually occurs after 7 years of age.
- PKD tends to progress more slowly than many other types of CRF. Once CRF develops, long-term prognosis is poor.

PEARLS & CONSIDERATIONS

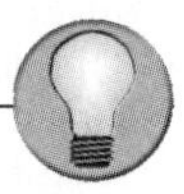

COMMENTS

Although hypertension is very common in people with ADPKD, hypertension is uncommon in overtly healthy cats with PKD.

PREVENTION

Eliminate affected animals from breeding population

CLIENT EDUCATION

- Because PKD is an autosomal dominant trait, 50% of offspring from an affected animal will have PKD. Screening and subsequent removal of positive animals will prevent PKD in offspring.
- Kittens can be screened by ultrasound at >16 weeks, but if negative, screening should be repeated at >10 months of age.
- Genetic screening can be completed at >8 weeks.
- If an individual cat with PKD is important to a breeding program, breed only to PKD-negative cats and screen offspring. Half of the offspring will be affected and should be neutered; the unaffected individuals can be bred.

SUGGESTED READING

Lulich JP, Osborne CA, Polzin DJ: Cystic diseases of the kidney. In Osborne CA, Finco DR (eds): *Canine and Feline Nephrology and Urology*. Baltimore, Williams & Wilkins, 1995, pp 460–470.

Biller DS: Polycystic kidney disease. In August JR (ed): *Consultations in Feline Internal Medicine 2*. Philadelphia, WB Saunders, 1994, pp 325–330.

AUTHOR: **CATHY LANGSTON**
EDITOR: **LEAH A. COHN**

Polycythemia Vera

BASIC INFORMATION

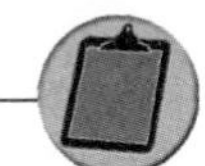

DEFINITION

An inappropriate, absolute increase in red blood cell (RBC) mass as measured by RBC count, hematocrit (HCT), and hemoglobin (Hb) concentration

SYNONYM(S)

Polycythemia rubra vera
Primary erythrocytosis

EPIDEMIOLOGY

SPECIES, AGE, SEX: Usually middle-aged to older dogs or cats.
ASSOCIATED CONDITIONS AND DISORDERS: Hyperviscosity syndrome.

CLINICAL PRESENTATION

HISTORY, CHIEF COMPLAINT

- Neurologic changes (e.g., behavior, motor, or sensory), mental dullness
- Seizures
- Lethargy, exercise, intolerance
- Hemorrhage (e.g., epistaxis, hyphema)

PHYSICAL EXAM FINDINGS: None, one, or many may be present:

- Hyperemic or cyanotic mucous membranes
- Erythema of the skin
- Polyuria and polydipsia (PU/PD)
- Splenomegaly
- Palpable abdominal mass (e.g., spleen or kidney)

ETIOLOGY AND PATHOPHYSIOLOGY

Polycythemia vera:

- Absolute primary erythrocytosis.
- Autonomous production of RBCs (erythropoietin independent).
- Myeloproliferative clonal disease.
- Arises from a multipotent hematopoietic progenitor cell in the bone marrow, resulting in the accumulation of morphologically and functionally normal RBCs.
- Polycythemia may lead to the hyperviscosity syndrome and resultant clinical signs.

DIAGNOSIS

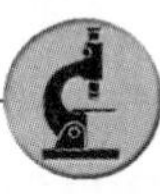

DIFFERENTIAL DIAGNOSIS

- Relative polycythemia (pseudoerythrocytosis):
  - Elevated HCT with normal or decreased RBC mass
  - Decrease in plasma volume associated with severe dehydration and with increased serum total protein (TP) concentration
  - Rarely causes clinical signs of hyperviscosity
- Absolute secondary polycythemia. Erythropoietin dependent. Appropriate or inappropriate response:
  - Appropriate (secondary to decreased tissue oxygenation):
    - High altitude
    - Chronic pulmonary disease
    - Right-to-left cardiovascular shunts (ventricular septal defect, reversed patent ductus arteriosus [PDA], tetralogy of Fallot, atrial septal defect)
    - Hemoglobinopathies (abnormal hemoglobins, methemoglobin reductase deficiency)
  - Inappropriate (normal tissue oxygenation):
    - Renal disease (e.g., polycystic kidney disease, rarely amyloidosis or glomerulonephritis).
    - Renal neoplasia (e.g., lymphoma, nephroblastoma, carcinomas, fibrosarcomas)
    - Other neoplasms (e.g., cecal leiomyosarcoma, hepatic tumors)

INITIAL DATABASE

- Complete blood count (CBC): increased HCT, RBC count, and Hb concentrations with normal total protein concentration. The RBC morphology is normal.
- Serum biochemistry profile, urinalysis: generally unremarkable.
- Arterial blood gas (ABG) analysis: to rule out hypoxia as a cause of secondary polycythemia.
- Abdominal ultrasound:
  - To identify renal masses or other neoplasia as other causes of secondary polycythemia (erythropoietin-producing tumors).
  - Nonspecific signs (hyperechoic kidneys, splenomegaly noted in 25% of cats and 10% of dogs with primary polycythemia).
- Thoracic radiographs:
  - Bronchial or interstitial changes are nonspecific. If thought to cause hypoxemia and secondary polycythemia, ABG measurement is indicated for confirmation.
- Echocardiography:
  - To identify myocardial hypertrophy, right-to-left shunts, or other abnormalities that could cause secondary polycythemia.

ADVANCED OR CONFIRMATORY TESTING

- Measurement of plasma erythropoietin concentration:
  - Generally normal to low in polycythemia vera.
  - Test has low diagnostic specificity; there is substantial overlap with the normal range, and other types of polycythemia (e.g., relative polycythemia) are associated with similar results.
  - Measurement is indicated to help rule out secondary polycythemia (high plasma erythropoietin concentration).
- Bone marrow aspiration and cytologic examination or bone marrow core biopsy:
  - Not useful: cannot distinguish primary from secondary polycythemia.

TREATMENT

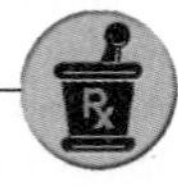

THERAPEUTIC GOAL(S)

Decrease blood viscosity and RBC mass to reduce or resolve clinical signs

ACUTE GENERAL TREATMENT

Initial treatment is phlebotomy:

- 20 ml/kg of blood collected from central vein.
- Avoid hypotension due to volume depletion: due to volume depletion by replacement with equivalent volume of IV 0.9% NaCl.

- Target HCT is <55% in dogs, <50% in cats.
- Replacement of coagulation factors and albumin, if multiple phlebotomies in short period of time (rare). Clinicians can use autologous plasma (centrifuge phlebotomized blood, discard RBCs, and administer plasma) or use allogeneic fresh frozen plasma.

CHRONIC TREATMENT

- Periodic phlebotomies if needed.
- Alternatively, hydroxyurea (Hydrea) 30 mg/kg PO, q 24h, 7 to 10 days, then decrease the dose and increase dosing interval gradually to maintain normal HCT; reduces RBC production. Monitor CBC for myelosuppression.
- Other chemotherapy agents, such as chlorambucil, have been used less often.
- Radioactive phosphorus rarely used in animals.

POSSIBLE COMPLICATIONS

Hydroxyurea can cause myelosuppression. With chronic use, adverse effects including nail sloughing, macrocytosis (increased mean corpuscular volume [MCV]), methemoglobinemia (cats), and induction of secondary tumors, including leukemia, have been reported.

RECOMMENDED MONITORING

- CBC counts weekly at first until HCT stabilizes, then every 4 to 6 weeks
- Physical examination and diagnostic testing as needed; opportunistic infections, myelosuppression, and other complications of varying degrees of concern can occur during treatment with chemotherapeutic agents

PROGNOSIS AND OUTCOME

Polycythemia vera can be successfully managed for years.

PEARLS & CONSIDERATIONS

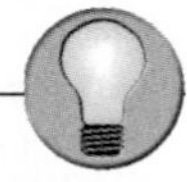

COMMENTS

- The diagnosis is usually made by excluding other causes of polycythemia.
- Most pets tolerate treatment well.

CLIENT EDUCATION

Infections can occur secondary to myelosuppression. Routine follow-up evaluations are necessary during treatment, even when clinical signs are well controlled.

SUGGESTED READING

Couto G: Erythrocytosis. In Nelson RW, Couto CG (eds): *Small Animal Internal Medicine*, ed 3. St. Louis, Mosby, 2003, pp 1170–1172

Ettinger S, Feldman E: Polycythemia vera. In Ettinger SJ, Feldman E (eds): *Textbook of Veterinary Internal Medicine*, ed 6. St. Louis, Elsevier, 2005.

AUTHOR: **PASCALE GRIESSMAYR**

EDITOR: **SUSAN M. COTTER**

Polymyositis, Autoimmune

BASIC INFORMATION

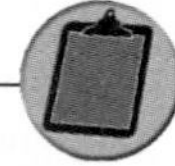

DEFINITION

An autoimmune inflammatory disease of unknown pathogenesis that primarily affects appendicular musculature

EPIDEMIOLOGY

SPECIES, AGE, SEX: Although any breed or age of dog can be affected, the majority of reported cases are middle-aged, large breeds. There is no apparent sex predilection.

GENETICS AND BREED PREDISPOSITION: New foundlands and boxers appear to be overrepresented. New foundlands tend to develop the disease at a younger age than other breeds. A substantial number of boxers with polymyositis may develop the disorder as a preneoplastic condition.

ASSOCIATED CONDITIONS AND DISORDERS: Uncommonly, dogs with autoimmune polymyositis may have concurrent masticatory myositis. This combination is referred to as overlap syndrome. Another uncommon associated condition in dogs with autoimmune polymyositis is thymoma.

CLINICAL PRESENTATION

HISTORY, CHIEF COMPLAINT: Clinical signs may be acute or chronic. The animal's medical history or clinical complaints include generalized weakness (often worsened by exercise), stiff gait, generalized muscle atrophy, dysphonia, myalgia, dysphagia, regurgitation (megaesophagus may be present), fever, and muscle swelling.

PHYSICAL EXAM FINDINGS: Physical examination findings typically concur with the animal's medical history and clinical complaints just described.

ETIOLOGY AND PATHOPHYSIOLOGY

This is an idiopathic autoimmune disorder.

DIAGNOSIS

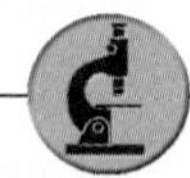

DIFFERENTIAL DIAGNOSIS

- Infectious polymyositis (e.g., toxoplasmosis, neosporosis)
- Overlap syndrome
- Preneoplastic myositis
- Myasthenia gravis

INITIAL DATABASE

- Complete blood count (CBC), serum chemistry profile, urinalysis: elevated aspartate aminotransferase (AST) possible
- Serum creatine kinase: usually elevated, often markedly so
- Electrodiagnostics: electromyogram (EMG) is usually abnormal
- Serology for infectious diseases (e.g., toxoplasmosis, neosporosis)

ADVANCED OR CONFIRMATORY TESTING

Definitive diagnosis of autoimmune polymyositis depends upon muscle biopsy results, in combination with normal (negative) serology test results for potential infectious causes. A nonsuppurative inflammatory infiltrate is typically evident on muscle biopsy (see Muscle and Nerve Biopsy, p 1279). Immunohistochemical staining of muscle tissue can verify immunoglobulin localization to the sarcolemma.

TREATMENT

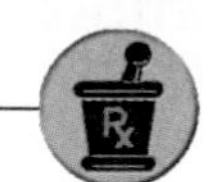

THERAPEUTIC GOAL(S)

The goal of therapy is to achieve clinical remission of myopathic signs.

ACUTE GENERAL TREATMENT

Immunosuppressive doses of prednisone (e.g., 1–2 mg/kg PO q 24h) are generally used as initial therapy.

CHRONIC TREATMENT

- Once clinical remission of signs is achieved, the dosage of prednisone is

slowly tapered over several months and is discontinued if possible.
- If prednisone cannot be effectively tapered or discontinued, alternative immunosuppressive drugs can be instituted (e.g., azathioprine 2 mg/kg PO q 24h for 5 days, then every other day (EOD), or mycophenolate mofetil 5-10 mg/kg PO q 12h).

POSSIBLE COMPLICATIONS
- Either inadequate or excessive immunosuppression
- Drug side effects or complications, including polyuria and polydipsia (PU/PD), polyphagia, weight gain, iatrogenic hyperadrenocorticism (glucocorticoids), bone marrow effects (azathioprine), and others

PROGNOSIS AND OUTCOME

The prognosis is favorable in approximately 80% of cases. Relapses may occur with tapering or discontinuation of immunosuppressive drugs.

PEARLS & CONSIDERATIONS

COMMENTS
When tapering prednisone in cases of autoimmune polymyositis, dose reductions should not be made more frequently than every 4 weeks.

SUGGESTED READING
Cuddon PA, et al: Breed-associated polymyositis of young Newfoundlands. *J Vet Intern Med* 13:239, 1999 (abstract).
Dewey CW: Myopathies: Disorders of skeletal muscle. In Dewey CW (ed): *A Practical Guide to Canine and Feline Neurology*. Ames, IA, Iowa State Press, 2003, pp 413-462.
Evans J, et al: Canine inflammatory myopathies: A clinicopathologic review of 200 cases. *J Vet Intern Med* 18:679, 2004.

AUTHOR & EDITOR: **CURTIS W. DEWEY**

Polyphagia

BASIC INFORMATION

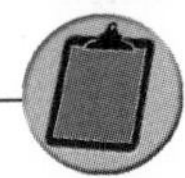

DEFINITION
Increased appetite or frequency of eating. Caloric consumption exceeding expected metabolic requirement

EPIDEMIOLOGY
SPECIES, AGE, SEX
- Dependent on underlying cause. In any age, behavioral polyphagia (gluttony) is possible.
- Cats:
  - Young: parasites, pregnancy, lactation.
  - Adult and geriatric: diabetes mellitus (DM), acromegaly, hyperthyroidism, intestinal infiltration (e.g., inflammatory bowel disease [IBD], gastrointestinal [GI] lymphoma).
- Dogs:
  - Young: parasites, pregnancy, lactation, exocrine pancreatic insufficiency (EPI).
  - Adult: diabetes mellitus, sudden acquired retinal degeneration syndrome (SARDS), hyperadrenocorticism (HAC), IBD, GI lymphoma.
  - Geriatric: diabetes mellitus, SARDS, hyperadrenocorticism (Cushing's disease), IBD, GI lymphoma, hyperthyroidism (rarely).

GENETICS AND BREED PREDISPOSITION: Dogs: EPI—German shepherd; hyperadrenocorticism—poodle, dachshund, terrier.

RISK FACTORS: Risk factors exist for certain diseases that commonly cause polyphagia. Examples include:
- Diabetes mellitus: obesity (cats), concurrent hyperadrenocorticism, concurrent acromegaly
- EPI: severe pancreatitis (rarely)
- hyperadrenocorticism, SARDS, insulinoma

ASSOCIATED CONDITIONS AND DISORDERS: Certain polyphagia-inducing diseases are in turn associated with other disorders.
- Acromegaly: diabetes mellitus, myocardial hypertrophy
- Hyperthyroidism: myocardial hypertrophy, arrhythmias, systemic hypertension, retinal detachment, renal failure, cerebral vascular accident, vomiting, diarrhea, weight loss, thyroid carcinoma (rare)
- DM: hyperlipidemia, pancreatitis, cataracts (dog), urinary tract infection (UTI)
- HAC: hyperlipidemia, diabetes mellitus, pyoderma, calcinosis cutis, UTI, pulmonary thromboembolism, cranial cruciate ligament rupture

CLINICAL PRESENTATION
DISEASE FORMS/SUBTYPES
- Iatrogenic/drug induced (anticonvulsants, benzodiazepines, glucocorticoids, insulin excess, cyproheptadine)
- Primary polyphagia: behavioral, psychogenic, ventromedial hypothalamic lesion
- Secondary polyphagia: increased metabolic rate/physiologic (growth, pregnancy, lactation), hyperthyroidism, acromegaly. Decreased nutrient availability: diabetes mellitus, EPI, parasitism, infiltrative bowel diseases. Hypoglycemia: insulinoma. Miscellaneous: SARDS, hyperadrenocorticism

HISTORY, CHIEF COMPLAINT
- Increased food consumption with:
  - Weight loss: hyperthyroidism, EPI, diabetes mellitus, infiltrative bowel disease, parasitism
  - Weight gain: psychogenic, drug induced, physiologic, acromegaly, hyperadrenocorticism, SARDS, insulinoma
- Polyuria and polydipsia: diabetes mellitus, HAC, acromegaly, hyperthyroidism, SARDS
- Panting: hyperadrenocorticism, SARDS
- Hair loss: hyperadrenocorticism
- Vomiting, diarrhea: hyperthyroidism, EPI, infiltrative bowel disease
- Weakness, seizures: insulinoma, hyperadrenocorticism (rare)

PHYSICAL EXAM FINDINGS
- Disorientation: insulinoma, hyperadrenocorticism (rarely), SARDS, hypothalamic lesions
- Alopecia, comedones: hyperadrenocorticism
- Cataracts: diabetes mellitus
- Dilated pupils: SARDS (initially normal fundic examination)
- Thin to emaciated: EPI, hyperthyroidism, diabetes mellitus, infiltrative bowel disease
- Tachycardia, murmur, arrhythmias: hyperthyroidism
- Panting: hyperadrenocorticism, SARDS, obesity
- Obesity: behavioral, diabetes mellitus (especially cats), SARDS, hyperadrenocorticism, insulinoma
- Hepatomegaly: hyperadrenocorticism, diabetes mellitus

ETIOLOGY AND PATHOPHYSIOLOGY
- Varies with disease
- Primary: damage to satiety center (trauma, infectious, inflammatory, neoplastic)
- Behavioral: may be related to boredom or interindividual variation
- Secondary:
  - Accelerated metabolism
  - Diminished nutrient availability

DIAGNOSIS

DIFFERENTIAL DIAGNOSIS

- Weight loss: poor nutrient quality, owner underfeeding
- Weight gain: physiologic (cold environment, growth, pregnancy)

INITIAL DATABASE

- Complete blood count: anemia (parasites), leukocytosis (hyperadrenocorticism, SARDS), eosinophilia (parasites)
- Serum biochemistry panel: liver enzymes (hyperadrenocorticism, diabetes mellitus, SARDS), glucose (diabetes mellitus, insulinoma)
- Urinalysis: low specific gravity (hyperadrenocorticism, SARDS, hyperthyroidism), glucose (diabetes mellitus), ketones (diabetes mellitus), bacteriuria (hyperadrenocorticism, diabetes mellitus)
- T4: hyperthyroidism

ADVANCED OR CONFIRMATORY TESTING

- Low dose dexamethasone suppression or ACTH stimulation: hyperadrenocorticism
- Ultrasound: pancreatic nodules, adrenal size, thickened bowel, pregnancy
- Computed tomography/magnetic resonance imaging of brain: hypothalamic lesions, pituitary macrotumors
- High dose dexamethasone suppression: discriminates between adrenal-dependent hyperadrenocorticism and pituitary-dependent hyperadrenocorticism; generally replaced by abdominal ultrasound
- Endogenous ACTH level: discriminates between adrenal-dependent hyperadrenocorticism and pituitary-dependent hyperadrenocorticism
- Free T4: may clarify thyroid status that is unclear with total T4
- Technetium-99 thyroid scan: confirm hyperthyroidism, determine bilateral versus unilateral disease

TREATMENT

THERAPEUTIC GOAL(S)

Varies with disease

DRUG INTERACTIONS

With HAC: concurrent phenobarbital and o,p'-DDD (mitotane [Lysodren]) lessens effectiveness of o,p'-DDD

POSSIBLE COMPLICATIONS

- Iatrogenic hypoadrenocorticism (o,p'-DDD treatment)
- Renal insufficiency, hypothyroidism (hyperthyroidism treatment)
- Ketoacidosis (uncontrolled diabetes)

RECOMMENDED MONITORING

- EPI: weight gain
- Diabetes mellitus: clinical signs improving
- Hyperadrenocorticism: clinical signs improving; ACTH stimulation
- Hyperthyroidism: weight gain; lower or normal serum T4 levels

PROGNOSIS AND OUTCOME

Varies with disease

PEARLS & CONSIDERATIONS

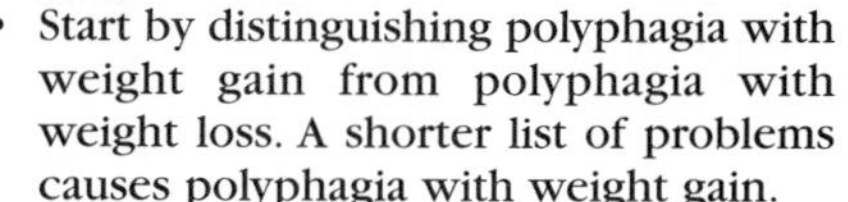

COMMENTS

- Start by distinguishing polyphagia with weight gain from polyphagia with weight loss. A shorter list of problems causes polyphagia with weight gain.
- Thorough history and physical examination will help eliminate many differential diagnoses.

SUGGESTED READING

Behrend E: Polyphagia. In Ettinger SJ, Feldman EC (eds): *Textbook of Veterinary Internal Medicine*, ed 6. St. Louis, Elsevier Saunders, 2005, pp 120–123.

AUTHOR: **DENNIS SPANN**
EDITOR: **ETIENNE CÔTÉ**

Polyuria/Polydipsia

BASIC INFORMATION

DEFINITION

- Polydipsia (PD): excessive consumption of water (>100 ml/kg/day)
- Polyuria (PU): production of excessive volumes of urine (>50 ml/kg/day)

EPIDEMIOLOGY

SPECIES, AGE, SEX: Cats and dogs, any age, either sex.
GENETICS AND BREED PREDISPOSITION: Depends on underlying cause.
CONTAGION AND ZOONOSIS: Depends on underlying cause.
GEOGRAPHY AND SEASONALITY: Depends on underlying cause.
ASSOCIATED CONDITIONS AND DISORDERS: Diet (e.g., formulation [dry kibble versus moist/canned], salt content) will affect water consumption in both normal and ill dogs and cats.

CLINICAL PRESENTATION

DISEASE FORMS/SUBTYPES

- PU with secondary PD
- PD with secondary PU

HISTORY, CHIEF COMPLAINT

- Common chief complaints:
  - Increased frequency and amount of drinking.
    - "Water-starved" behavior (pets actively seeking to drink water from abnormal or typically inaccessible locations) is possible in extreme cases or if owner is restricting water intake.
  - Urination in inappropriate indoor locations.
  - Prolonged duration of individual urinations.
  - Need to change litter with increased frequency (cats).
- Clinicians should initially ask owners whether there has been any change in water consumption, not whether water consumption has increased (to avoid leading the owner's answer).
- It is usually not possible to determine whether PU is primary, with secondary PD, or vice-versa from the history alone.
- History should aim to differentiate PU from pollakiuria, stranguria, inappropriate elimination/urinary incontinence, and urinary marking/spraying.
- Basic environmental questions include duration of time indoors between walks (most normal dogs need to urinate at least every 8 to 12 hours), introduction of new pets or family members (suggesting behavioral changes/marking), new environment (behavior/marking or exposure to toxins), and change in litter type, location, or hygiene (cats).
- Some owners may not be aware of water consumption or urination because the pet mainly lives outdoors; clinicians should view PD in dogs that

are in a hospital setting with initial skepticism because many dogs drink voluminous amounts of water as a result of anxiety or excitement.
- Medication history: glucocorticoids, phenobarbital, diuretics.
- Intoxication history should cover recent and distant potential exposures (ethylene glycol, grapes, raisins, lilies [cats]) and nephrotoxic medications (see Nephrotoxic Drugs and Substances, p 1387).

PHYSICAL EXAM FINDINGS

- Dehydration: consistent with any cause of PU/PD other than psychogenic PD.
- Thin body condition, poor haircoat: consistent with chronic renal failure, chronic liver disease, diabetes mellitus, hyperthyroidism, chronic gastrointestinal (GI) disease.
- Dyspnea, tachypnea: may occur concurrently with metabolic acidosis, severe hypovolemia/shock (many possible causes).
- Panting (excessive): may be noted in dogs whose PU/PD is due to hyperadrenocorticism; also commonly present in animals that have anxiety or that are obese (i.e., nonspecific finding).
- Bilaterally symmetric truncal alopecia: endocrine disease (e.g., hyperadrenocorticism).
- Rectal examination: assess for primary disorders (e.g., adenocarcinoma of the anal sac causing PU/PD via hypercalcemia) and for causes of urinary incontinence other than PU (urethral or trigone thickening, suggesting inflammation or infiltration; prostatitis).
- Vaginal exam: purulent exudative discharge suggests pyometra.
- Abdominal palpation:
  - Kidneys: small (e.g., chronic renal failure) or large (e.g., polycystic kidney disease, renal lymphoma, other renal neoplasia, pyelonephritis).
  - Hepatomegaly (e.g., primary hepatopathies, hyperadrenocorticism, diabetes mellitus, iatrogenic [glucocorticoids, barbiturates], lymphoma causing malignancy-associated hypercalcemia).
  - Splenomegaly (e.g., lymphoma causing malignancy-associated hypercalcemia).
  - Duodenal/jejunal thickening may be palpable with diffuse intestinal infiltrative diseases.
  - Uterine enlargement may be palpable (abdominal palpation must be performed gently because the uterus is potentially friable) with pyometra.
- Cardiac auscultation: heart murmur, third heart sound/gallop, and/or arrhythmia possible with hyperthyroidism.

ETIOLOGY AND PATHOPHYSIOLOGY

- Normal daily water consumption:
  - Dogs: up to 100 ml/kg per day (higher in dogs <4 kg; up to 132 ml/day in dogs that weigh 1 kg).
  - Cats: up to 250 ml per day.
- Mechanisms of PU/PD:
  - Chronic renal failure: overload of glomerular filtrate to remaining functional nephrons presents excessive amounts of urea and sodium to distal tubules, eliciting an osmotic diuresis (primary PU, secondary PD).
  - Pyelonephritis: inflammation of the renal pelvis can destroy the countercurrent concentrating mechanism in the renal medulla (primary PU, secondary PD).
  - Hyperadrenocorticism: suspected secondary antidiuretic hormone (ADH) deficiency (i.e., reversible central diabetes insipidus; primary PD, secondary PU).
  - Liver disease: hypokalemia and compromised renal medullary concentration gradient due to impaired urea synthesis (primary PU, secondary PD); possibly impaired cortisol metabolism (primary PD, secondary PU).
  - Hypokalemia: interferes with renal tubular action of ADH (i.e., reversible nephrogenic diabetes insipidus; primary PU, secondary PD).
  - Hypoadrenocorticism: chronic hyponatremia depletes the renal medullary concentration gradient (primary PU, secondary PD).
  - Diabetes mellitus: glucosuria creates an osmotic diuresis (primary PU, secondary PD).
  - Diabetes insipidus (DI): lack of adequate ADH formation or release at the hypothalamic level (central DI) or ineffective ADH action on the renal collecting tubules (nephrogenic DI). Both central and nephrogenic DI cause a primary PU with secondary PD.
  - Intoxication: osmotic diuresis initially, followed by renal failure (ethylene glycol; both mechanisms cause primary PU, secondary PD). Mechanisms for lily, raisin, grape intoxication: unknown.
  - Psychogenic PD: neurobehavioral changes with secondary renal medullary washout (primary PD, secondary PU).
  - Hyperthyroidism: increased medullary blood flow causing secondary decreased renal medullary concentration gradient; also hypokalemia (both primary PU, secondary PD).
  - Renal medullary washout: usually a secondary effect of other disorders listed here. Decreased renal medullary concentration gradient causes osmotic diuresis (primary PU, secondary PD).
  - Pyometra: *Escherichia coli* endotoxin interferes with ADH action on renal tubules (reversible nephrogenic diabetes insipidus; primary PU, secondary PD).
  - Hypercalcemia: interference of hypercalcemia with renal ADH actions (reversible nephrogenic diabetes insipidus; primary PU, secondary PD).

DIAGNOSIS

DIFFERENTIAL DIAGNOSIS

- PD:
  - Normal water intake (e.g., overinterpretation of seasonal variation)
- PU:
  - Inappropriate elimination/urinary incontinence: poor control of voiding, but overall daily volume of urine is normal
  - Pollakiuria: frequent voiding of small volumes of urine, but overall daily volume is normal
  - Spraying/marking: small amounts of urine are eliminated, usually onto vertical surfaces

INITIAL DATABASE

- Complete blood count (CBC):
  - Anemia of chronic disease.
  - Stress leukogram possible with many disorders that cause PU/PD (though not commonly with hyperadrenocorticism or central or nephrogenic diabetes insipidus).
  - Neutrophilia with evidence of inflammation (band forms, toxic change in neutrophils): rule out pyometra; may not be present with pyelonephritis (counterintuitive).
  - Normal lymphocyte and eosinophil counts in a clinically severely ill dog (i.e., absence of stress leukogram): rule out hypoadrenocorticism.
- Serum chemistry profile:
  - Hyperglycemia: Rule out diabetes mellitus (clinical signs, glucosuria, fructosamine).
  - Increased blood urea nitrogen (BUN), creatinine, with isosthenuria (urine specific gravity [USG] 1.008–1.012): most consistent with renal failure; less commonly, may also occur in animals with normal kidneys that have hypoadrenocorticism or diabetes insipidus.
  - Hypoalbuminemia, low BUN, hypocholesterolemia, hypoglycemia, hyperbilirubinemia (all, or combinations): evaluate for liver failure.
  - Hypercalcemia: Rule out malignancy, primary hyperparathyroidism (both usually have concurrent hypophosphatemia), vitamin D toxicosis, chronic renal disease (cats; phosphorus usually normal or elevated), and other conditions (see Hypercalcemia, p 543). Idiopathic hypercalcemia (cats) is not usually associated with PU/PD.

 - Hyperkalemia with hyponatremia suggests hypoadrenocorticism.
- Urinalysis:
 - Owners should collect a fresh sample prior to the appointment.
 - True PU is almost always associated with dilute urine (USG <1.012), "relatively" dilute urine (USG >1.012 but <1.022), or glucosuria.
 - Concentrated urine (USG >1.025) without glucosuria is inconsistent with PU/PD; other causes to explain clinical signs, such as lower urinary tract disorders, should be sought.
 - Diabetes mellitus causes PU but relatively concentrated urine (USG ≈1.025–1.045), at least in part due to glucosuria.
 - Isosthenuria (USG = 1.008–1.012) can be caused by renal failure (tubules fail to concentrate urine) or by normal free water excretion (e.g., after a normal animal has drunk a large volume of water).
 - Calcium oxalate dihydrate crystals suggest postacute ethylene glycol ingestion.
- Urine culture and sensitivity (C&S): routinely performed in all animals with PU/PD. Urinary tract infection may complicate virtually any cause of PU/PD, may not produce additional overt clinical signs, often escapes diagnosis on urinalysis alone due to dilute urine, and is treatable and curable.
- Serum thyroid hormone levels: Rule out hyperthyroidism (cats >6 years old).

ADVANCED OR CONFIRMATORY TESTING

- Abdominal ultrasound: Evaluate kidneys (renal failure, pyelonephritis, neoplasia); urinary bladder (signs of cystitis, urolithiasis, or mass [e.g., neoplasm] producing pollakiuria or stranguria rather than PU); GI tract (evidence of infiltration); liver (chronic hepatopathies, portosystemic shunt, nonspecific enlargement, and hyperechogenicity [diabetes mellitus, hyperadrenocorticism, others]); adrenal glands (mass; subtle changes related to pituitary-dependent hyperadrenocorticism although 50% of dogs with pituitary-dependent hyperadrenocorticism have structurally normal adrenal glands on ultrasound exam); and uterus (pyometra)
- Radiographs (thoracic, abdominal)
- Others as dictated by specific etiologies suspected

TREATMENT

THERAPEUTIC GOAL(S)

Identification of cause. PU and PD are not diseases but rather are clinical manifestations of primary underlying disorders. Therefore, nonspecific treatment, such as withholding water, is unlikely to succeed and may be dangerous in many/most cases of PU/PD for which an underlying cause has not been sought.

ACUTE GENERAL TREATMENT

Withholding water can be dangerous or life threatening in all cases of PU/PD for which the underlying disease produces primary PU with secondary PD (see Etiology and Pathophysiology above).

POSSIBLE COMPLICATIONS

- Dehydration
- Progression of the primary problem if not identified and addressed

RECOMMENDED MONITORING

Physical examination, including body weight; diagnostic testing as indicated by underlying disease process, results obtained to date, and evolution of case.

PROGNOSIS AND OUTCOME

Highly variable, from excellent to poor, depending on underlying cause and response to treatment.

PEARLS & CONSIDERATIONS

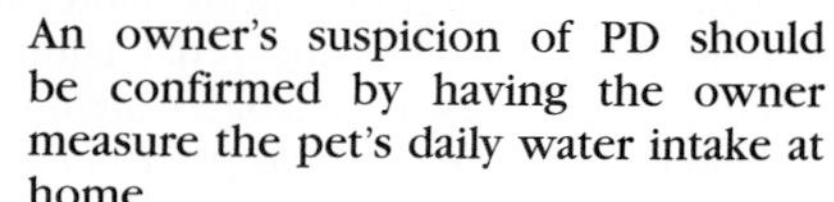

COMMENTS

- An owner's suspicion of PD should be confirmed by having the owner measure the pet's daily water intake at home.
- Isosthenuria (USG = 1.008–1.012) implies that the USG is the same as the specific gravity of plasma. Since dehydrated animals may have hyperosmolar plasma, USG up to 1.020 may still be consistent with isosthenuria in some cases.

SUGGESTED READING

DiBartola SP: Disorders of sodium and water. In DiBartola SP (ed): *Fluid Therapy in Small Animal Practice*, ed 2. Philadelphia, WB Saunders, 2000, pp 45–72.

Feldman EC: Polyuria and polydipsia. In Ettinger SJ, Feldman EC (eds): *Textbook of Veterinary Internal Medicine*, ed 6. St. Louis, Elsevier, WB Saunders, 2005, pp 102–105.

Feldman EC, Nelson RW: Water metabolism and diabetes insipidus. In Feldman EC, Nelson RW (eds): *Canine and Feline Endocrinology and Reproduction*, ed 3. St. Louis, WB Saunders, 2004, pp 2–44.

AUTHOR: **EDWARD C. FELDMAN**
EDITOR: **ETIENNE CÔTÉ**

Portosystemic Shunt

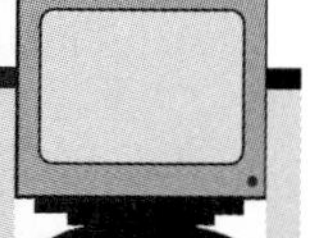

Client Education Sheet on Website

BASIC INFORMATION

DEFINITION

- Macroscopic vascular communication allowing blood flow between the portal and systemic circulation without first passing through the liver
- The shunt can be congenital or acquired

SYNONYM(S)

Portocaval shunt
Portosystemic vascular anomaly
PSS

EPIDEMIOLOGY

SPECIES, AGE, SEX

- Dogs and cats.
- Congenital shunts typically produce clinical signs by 6 months of age; with rare exceptions, most animals are diagnosed by 2 years of age.
- Acquired shunts can occur at any age but typically are noted in middle-aged to older adults.
- Congenital PSS: 2:1 male to female ratio in the cat; in the bichon frisé, the relative risk is 12 times greater in females than males.

GENETICS AND BREED PREDISPOSITION

- Congenital PSS:
 - Inherited in the Maltese terrier and Irish wolfhound and thought to be inherited in the Yorkshire terrier (relative risk: 20 times greater than general dog population).
 - Dogs: golden and Labrador retrievers, Old English sheepdog, Irish wolfhound, Samoyed, bichon frisé, Australian shepherd, and Australian cattle dog (intrahepatic); Yorkshire

terrier, poodle, Maltese, shih tzu, dachshund (extrahepatic).
  - Cat: Persian and Himalayan.
  - Incidence: in cats, 2.5 per 10,000; in dogs, variable reports, ranging from 2.5 to 60 per 10,000.
- Acquired PSS: greater prevalence in breeds with breed-associated chronic hepatopathies (cocker spaniels, Doberman pinschers).

RISK FACTORS: Acquired: chronic hepatic diseases causing portal hypertension.

ASSOCIATED CONDITIONS AND DISORDERS: Hepatic microvascular dysplasia and cryptorchidism.

CLINICAL PRESENTATION

DISEASE FORMS/SUBTYPES

- Congenital versus acquired.
  - Congenital shunts are single, are present from birth, and are usually treated surgically. They are intrahepatic or extrahepatic.
  - Acquired shunts are multiple, occur in the context of chronic liver disease (they are portosystemic anastomoses resulting from chronic portal hypertension), and are not treated surgically because new shunts would arise to replace them. They are always extrahepatic.
- Congenital intrahepatic versus congenital extrahepatic.
  - Intrahepatic: more common in larger breed dogs and more difficult to correct surgically.
  - Extrahepatic: more common in smaller breed dogs and more easily accessed surgically.
  - Cats: either (extrahepatic > intrahepatic).

HISTORY, CHIEF COMPLAINT

- Congenital or acquired.
  - Waxing-waning course of clinical signs is typical.
  - Animals often have only one or a few signs.
- Congenital:
  - Central nervous system (CNS) signs are all secondary to hepatic encephalopathy: lethargy, ataxia, weakness, abnormal behavior, abnormal vocalization, hypersalivation/ptyalism (especially cats), head pressing, bumping into objects due to central blindness, incessant pacing or circling, stupor, seizures, or coma.
  - Gastrointestinal (GI): intermittent anorexia, vomiting, diarrhea or constipation, polyphagia, pica.
  - Urinary tract: hematuria, pollakiuria, or dysuria from ammonium urate urolithiasis.
  - Miscellaneous: stunted growth, polyuria and polydipsia (PU/PD), intense pruritus.
  - High-protein meal, GI bleeding, constipation, azotemia, hypokalemia, metabolic alkalosis, tranquilization, and methionine-containing medications can exacerbate clinical signs.
  - Intolerance to or slow recovery from anesthetic agents or tranquilizers.
  - Incidental findings of microhepatica, ammonium biurate crystalluria, shunt visualization on abdominal ultrasound.
- Acquired: Signs of chronic hepatopathy/liver failure usually predominate.

PHYSICAL EXAM FINDINGS

- Signs: See History, Chief Complaint above.
- Plump kidneys.
- Small body stature.
- Small liver (inability to palpate liver margins).
- Poor haircoat, excoriations if intensely pruritic.
- Copper-colored irises without green or yellow pigment (some cats with congenital shunts).
- Ascites:
  - Since congenital PSSs represent a path of lesser resistance than the normal hepatic vasculature, ascites does not occur. Congenital shunts suspected to be linked with ascites usually cause severe hypoalbuminemia, or a disorder other than congenital PSS is present.
  - Acquired PSSs, since they occur due to portal hypertension, often exist concurrently with ascites.
- Icterus:
  - Does not occur with congenital PSS; if icterus is present, consider another diagnosis (primary hepatobiliary disorder, hemolysis).
  - Commonly observed with chronic liver diseases causing acquired PSS.
- Physical exam can be unremarkable.

ETIOLOGY AND PATHOPHYSIOLOGY

- Congenital shunts are embryonic vessels that failed to regress postnatally. In dogs, persistent ductus venosus is the most common form, whereas in cats, left gastric vein shunting to the caudal vena cava is most common.
- Acquired shunts arise from rudimentary nonfunctional collateral vessels when portal hypertension occurs due to end-stage parenchymal disorders, such as cirrhosis, or severe vascular disorders.
- Hepatic encephalopathy and resultant CNS signs occur with either type of PSS from toxins and nutrients absorbed from the intestines that are allowed to bypass metabolism by the liver and circulate in much higher concentrations than normal. Many of these substances (ammonia, methyl mercaptans, short-chain fatty acids, benzodiazepine-like substances) are directly toxic to the CNS or alter its normal metabolism (see Hepatic Encephalopathy, p 489).
- Reduced hepatic blood flow and lower concentrations of hepatotrophic factors, such as glucagon, insulin, and nutrients, result in microhepatica.
- High levels of urinary excretion from elevated blood levels of ammonia and uric acid can result in development of urate urolithiasis (renal, ureteral, bladder) in up to 50% of cases.

DIAGNOSIS

Congenital PSSs are identified for the purpose of treatment: surgical ligation or occlusion, or transvenous coil occlusion. Acquired PSSs may be identified incidentally in animals with chronic hepatopathies, but their presence does not affect the diagnostic and treatment approach used for managing animals with chronic liver disease.

DIFFERENTIAL DIAGNOSIS

- CNS signs: infectious diseases, toxins, other metabolic encephalopathy (hypoglycemia), idiopathic epilepsy, and congenital malformations (e.g., hydrocephalus).
- GI signs: parasitism, foreign body, dietary indiscretion, dietary allergy, inflammatory/infiltrative intestinal diseases.
- Urinary tract signs: urinary tract infections, other calculi.

INITIAL DATABASE

Tests for acquired shunts are those for underlying chronic hepatopathy.

For congenital PSS:

- Complete blood count (CBC): microcytic normochromic red blood cells (RBCs), mild nonregenerative anemia, target cells are possible.
- Serum biochemistry panel: minor elevation of liver enzymes, low blood urea nitrogen (BUN), hypoglycemia, hypoalb minemia, hypocholesterolemia may be seen.
- Coagulation profile: mild activated partial thromboplastin time elevation, low fibrinogen can be present.
- Urinalysis: isosthenuria or hyposthenuria, ammonium biurate crystalluria, hematuria, or pyuria possible.
- Abdominal radiographs: microhepatica, mild to moderate renomegaly; urate calculi often undetectable unless complexed with magnesium and phosphate.
- Initial testing can be normal in affected animals.

ADVANCED OR CONFIRMATORY TESTING

Tests for acquired shunts are those for underlying chronic hepatopathy.

For congenital PSS:

- Serum bile acids (preprandial and postprandial): Preprandial sample (drawn

after a 12-hour fast) may be normal in 20% of cases. Postprandial sample (drawn 2 hours after a meal) is typically markedly elevated, often over 100 μM/l. False-positive and false-negative results are uncommon; if clinical suspicion persists despite normal postprandial bile acid values, additional testing is warranted.
- Abdominal ultrasound: Skilled clinicians may be able to image a shunting vessel. Intrahepatic shunts are easier to identify than extrahepatic shunts. Other common findings are a small liver and a subjective decrease of hepatic vascular structures.
- Transcolonic portal scintigraphy: identifies excessive shunting of portal blood bypassing the liver; confirms the presence of a shunt but cannot identify its location or differentiate between congenital or acquired shunts. False-negative results can rarely occur, and the test is only available at referral institutions.
- Radiographic mesenteric portography:
  - Performed either intraoperatively or with percutaneous splenic catheterization guided with ultrasound.
  - Test of choice to confirm the presence of a shunt and identify its location.
  - Intrahepatic most likely if the most caudal loop of the shunt, or the point where the shunt diverges from the portal vein, is cranial to vertebra T13.
- Liver biopsy: indicated in all suspected and confirmed PSS cases; typically reveals hepatic arteriolar hyperplasia, small portal triads, increased smooth muscle thickness of hepatic venules, and an increase in small vascular structures in the periportal area in dogs with congenital PSS. If a PSS is absent, these histologic findings are diagnostic for microvascular dysplasia. Many pathologists believe the histologic findings in dogs with hepatic microvascular dysplasia are indistinguishable from dogs with PSS.

TREATMENT

THERAPEUTIC GOAL(S)

- Reversal of hepatic encephalopathy
- Congenital: complete or partial attenuation of congenital shunts, which halts or limits the bypass of blood around the liver and reverses some or all of the signs of hepatic encephalopathy and other clinical signs
- Acquired: management of the underlying liver disease. Acquired PSSs are not treated surgically (other shunts would form to replace them)

ACUTE GENERAL TREATMENT

- See Hepatic Encephalopathy, p 489
- Congenital: supportive care prior to general anesthesia for portography or shunt attenuation/ligation

CHRONIC TREATMENT

Treatment for congenital PSS:
- Primary therapy for congenital PSS is complete or partial shunt attenuation.
  - Preoperative patient preparation is essential and typically involves:
    - Prophylactic medical treatment and nutritional modification for prevention of hepatic encephalopathy for several days or more prior to general anesthesia if the animal's neurologic status is stable.
    - More aggressive or intensive management in cases of severe hepatic encephalopathy (seizures, coma).
    - Identification and treatment of associated abnormalities that could create complications if not addressed (e.g., hypoglycemia, hypoalbuminemia, gastric ulceration).
- With complete shunt ligation or obliteration (e.g., with ameroid constrictor), most animals are able to live normal lives without dietary therapy and medications. Complete ligation may not be possible due to the development of intraoperative portal hypertension, requiring partial ligation only.
- Without surgery or with only partial attenuation, animals may need to be managed chronically with restricted protein diets, lactulose, and/or antibiotic therapy.

DRUG INTERACTIONS

- Be careful with drugs requiring hepatic metabolism
- Congenital portosystemic shunts increase glomerular filtration rate, which may raise the rate of excretion of some medications

POSSIBLE COMPLICATIONS

- Intraoperative and postoperative complications include portal hypertension, hypoglycemia, hemorrhage, and intractable seizures.
- Sedative and anaesthetic agents should be used with caution.

RECOMMENDED MONITORING

Monitoring for congenital PSS:
- Postligation: Monitor for reversal of clinical signs while discontinuing medications and changing to a normal protein diet after 6 to 8 weeks. If clinical signs recur, then repeat colonic scintigraphy to ensure complete shunt attenuation. If scintigraphy indicates continued shunting, repeat portography and consider surgery.
- Partial ligation: Complete closure facilitated by scar tissue formation may occur after 2 to 3 months. If clinical signs recur after termination of medications and low-protein diet, consider repeat colonic scintigraphy after 3 months. If shunting is still present, a second surgery can be considered to attempt complete ligation.
- Perform bile acids testing 6 to 8 weeks postoperatively; bile acid concentrations may decrease dramatically but often continue to be abnormally elevated even with complete attenuation due to the presence of concomitant hepatic microvascular dysplasia.
- Obtain a serum biochemical profile 6 to 8 weeks postoperatively. With complete ligation, serum liver enzyme activities, albumin, and glucose levels will typically normalize.

PROGNOSIS AND OUTCOME

- Excellent long-term prognosis with complete ligation.
- Fair to poor prognosis for cure with partial ligation. Many partially ligated shunts will completely close over time; however, up to 50% of animals with partial ligation will have recurrence of clinical signs.
- Poor prognosis with medical therapy alone. In some animals, clinical signs can be controlled for a few years, but most develop refractory neurologic signs.
- Animals that present later in life with clinical signs (often due to urinary tract calculi) have a good prognosis with surgery.

PEARLS & CONSIDERATIONS

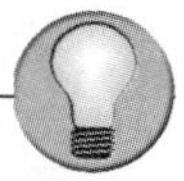

COMMENTS

- Always obtain postprandial bile acid concentrations to increase the sensitivity of the test.
- Consider the congenital portosystemic shunt as a differential diagnosis in any young cat or dog with clinical signs of neurologic disease or with unexplained poor or stunted growth, delayed or difficult anesthetic recovery, waxing and waning appetite or GI signs, or in any animal presenting with urate urolithiasis.
- In unexplained polyuria and polydipsia (PU/PD) in young animals, consider bile acid stimulation testing to assess for a portosystemic shunt.
- Intrahepatic shunts are much more difficult to ligate, either partially or completely, and have a much higher perioperative mortality rate, than extrahepatic shunts. Percutaneous transvenous coil embolization has been performed successfully in dogs with this type of shunt and has a much lower mortality rate.

SUGGESTED READING

Hunt GB: Effect of breed on anatomy of portosystemic shunts resulting from congenital diseases in dogs and cats: A review of 242 cases. *Aust Vet J* 82:746-749, 2004.

Johnson SE: Chronic hepatic disorders. In Ettinger SJ, Feldman EC (eds): *Textbook of Veterinary Internal Medicine*, vol 2, ed 2. Philadelphia, WB Saunders, 2000, pp 1311-1315.

Levy JK, et al: Feline portosystemic vascular shunts. In Bonagura JD (ed): *Kirk's Current Veterinary Therapy, Small Animal Practice XII*. Philadelphia, WB Saunders, 1995, pp 743-748.

AUTHOR: **JOHN R. HART, JR.**
EDITOR: **KEITH P. RICHTER**

Postpartum Management of the Bitch

BASIC INFORMATION

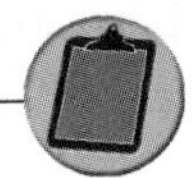

DEFINITION

Care of the female dog and offspring following parturition

SYNONYM(S)

Postparturient care
Postwhelping management

EPIDEMIOLOGY

SPECIES, AGE, SEX: Canine, postpubertal, female.

GENETICS AND BREED PREDISPOSITION: Toy breeds are at a greater risk of developing postparturient hypocalcemia.

RISK FACTORS

- Maiden bitches may not have a good mothering ability and are susceptible to subinvolution of placental sites (SIPS).
- Older bitches are more predisposed to postpartum disorders (e.g., metritis, mastitis).
- Excessively large litters (more than 6 pups for small breeds [<9 kg], more than 9 pups for medium breeds [9-20 kg], more than 10 pups for large breeds [20-40 kg], and more than 12 pups for giant breeds [>40 kg]).

CONTAGION AND ZOONOSIS: Canine herpesvirus, *Brucella canis*, and *Leptospira* spp. organisms may be shed in high concentrations in lochia following late-term abortions.

ASSOCIATED CONDITIONS AND DISORDERS: SIPS, metritis, mastitis, cesarean section.

CLINICAL PRESENTATION

HISTORY, CHIEF COMPLAINT

- Recent whelping
- No complaints unless a postpartum disorder exists

PHYSICAL EXAM FINDINGS: Healthy dam and pups:

- If postpartum problems exist: Exam findings in the dam may reveal depression, inappetence, poor mothering, inadequate lactation (evident by anxious or distressed puppies), prolonged or abnormal vaginal discharge, and engorged or inflamed mammary glands.
    - Rectal temperatures may normally be elevated for 24 to 48 hours postpartum but should not be >103°F.
    - Lochia (vaginal discharge; normal endometrial drainage) can be evident for 4 to 6 weeks postpartum and may last as long as 12 weeks.
        - Typically green-black to brick red and has no significant odor.
        - Abnormal if creamy color or if associated with a foul odor.
    - Mammary glands should be evaluated daily for heat, pain, or changes in consistency.
        - Milk should be white or slightly yellow.
        - Discoloration or purulent discharge is abnormal and suggests mastitis.

ETIOLOGY AND PATHOPHYSIOLOGY

Variable, depending on associated conditions

DIAGNOSIS

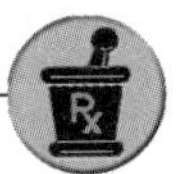

DIFFERENTIAL DIAGNOSIS

- Normal postpartum female
- Prolonged or abnormal appearing vaginal discharge: SIPS, metritis, retained placenta
- Swollen mammary glands: mastitis, galactostasis

INITIAL DATABASE

Not necessary unless bitch shows historic or physical abnormalities.

ADVANCED OR CONFIRMATORY TESTING

- Complete blood count (CBC), serum chemistry panel, fibrinogen: healthy postpartum dams may be slightly anemic with an elevated fibrinogen.
- Vaginal cytologic examination: healthy dams typically have erythrocytes and hemosiderophages present in vaginal discharge for 4 to 6 weeks postpartum.
- Vaginal culture: healthy postpartum dams have positive vaginal bacterial cultures, similar to all healthy bitches.
- Milk cytologic examination, pH, and culture.
- Abdominal ultrasonography.

TREATMENT

THERAPEUTIC GOAL(S)

To wean as many pups as possible

ACUTE GENERAL TREATMENT

- Treatment of associated disorder depends on specific condition; dam may need to be separated from pups (weaning).
- Oxytocin injections are often requested postpartum by breeders.
    - These are no longer considered necessary because suckling puppies have the same effect.
    - Two to 10 units, and up to a maximum of 20 units, may be given to aid in uterine involution if retained placentas are suspected or if the pups are born dead.
- Dog-Appeasing Pheromone diffuser may help to calm nervous or agitated bitches.
- Cooked pumpkin is a useful food additive to help correct diarrhea following placental ingestion.

POSSIBLE COMPLICATIONS

Many therapeutics are excreted into the milk, which can then be ingested at high (even toxic) levels by the nursing offspring; verification is essential prior to prescribing a drug to a lactating bitch.

RECOMMENDED MONITORING

- Physical exam, then diagnostic testing based on findings.
- Exam allows for early detection of periparturient disorders should they arise.

PROGNOSIS AND OUTCOME

- Good prognosis for bitches without associated disorders
- Specific prognosis depends on accompanying disorder

PEARLS & CONSIDERATIONS

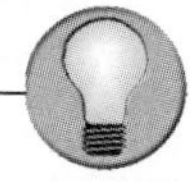

PREVENTION

- A clean, warm environment affording the bitch privacy should be provided postpartum.
- Ambient temperature in the puppy area should be maintained at 75-85°F, with space away from the puppies available for the bitch.
- Attention to hygiene reduces the risk of infection both to the dam and pups.

CLIENT EDUCATION

- Nutrition:
  - It is important during lactation to provide enough energy to the bitch so that she will produce enough milk for the puppies and maintain her own body weight.
  - Small breeds have a higher energy requirement per pound/body weight than larger breeds.
  - First week, one-and-a-half times maintenance; second week, two times maintenance; and third week to weaning, three times maintenance.
  - Good quality, high-energy, easily digested food is recommended.
- Behavior:
  - Owners should not leave first-time mothers and nervous bitches alone with puppies until they are sure the mother will not cannibalize the pups.
  - Typically it takes 2 to 3 days, especially after a cesarean section, before a bitch can be left alone.
  - It may be necessary, initially, to hold the bitch down to allow the puppies to suckle.
  - If the bitch continues to refuse to accept the puppies, she needs to be evaluated for causes such as mastitis (causing mammary pain).
- The bitch may express reluctance to leave the whelping box and her puppies, so food and water may need to be provided in the whelping/nursing box.
  - The bitch should be encouraged to get fresh air and exercise while the whelping box is being cleaned.

SUGGESTED READING

Johnston SD, Root Kustritz MV, Olson PN: Periparturient disorders in the bitch. *Canine and Feline Theriogenology*. Philadelphia, WB Saunders, 2001, pp 129-145.

Lewis LD, Morris ML Jr., Hand MS: Dogs, feeding and care. *Small Animal Clinical Nutrition III*. Topeka, KS, Mark Morris, 1990, pp 6-10.

AUTHOR: **VIVIEN SURMAN**

EDITOR: **MICHELLE A. KUTZLER**

Potpourri Toxicosis

BASIC INFORMATION

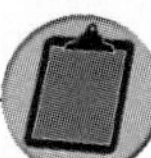

DEFINITION

- Liquid potpourri: combination of essential oils and cationic detergents.
- Acute toxicosis occurs mostly in cats from accidental dermal and oral exposure and is characterized by hypersalivation, vomiting, protrusion of the tongue, dysphagia, corrosive burns on the skin and oral cavity, hyperthermia, muscle weakness, and ataxia.

EPIDEMIOLOGY

SPECIES, AGE, SEX

- All pets of all ages and sexes are susceptible.
- Cats are more sensitive, and grooming behavior can increase toxicity from dermal exposures.

RISK FACTORS: Preexisting liver disease can increase risk of toxicity.

CLINICAL PRESENTATION

HISTORY, CHIEF COMPLAINT

- Dermal and/or oral contact with liquid potpourri
- Clinical signs within minutes to up to 8 hours postexposure
- Lethargy, drooling, vomiting, vocalizing, anorexia, and tongue protrusion

PHYSICAL EXAM FINDINGS

- Liquid potpourri may be felt (oily texture) or smelled on the coat and/or breath.
- Hypersalivation, dysphagia, vomiting (± hematemesis), diarrhea, corrosive burns of the oral, pharyngeal, and/or esophageal mucosa (ulceration could take several hours to appear).
- Hyperthermia.
- Dyspnea, wheezing, abnormal respiratory sounds, aspiration pneumonia, pulmonary edema, hypotension.
- Muscular weakness, ataxia.
- Hair loss (focal), skin erythema, dermatitis, edema, pain, and ulceration (dermal exposure).
- Ocular exposure: mild irritation to severe corneal injury (ulcer).

ETIOLOGY AND PATHOPHYSIOLOGY

- Liquid potpourri is a mixture of essential oils and cationic detergents.
- Essential oils are volatile oils or a mixture of terpenes (complex hydrocarbons) obtained through a distillation process.
- Cationic detergents include quaternary ammonium compounds (benzalkonium and benzethonium chlorides), pyridinium compounds (cetylpyridinium, cetrimonium), quinolinium compounds (dequalinium chloride).
- Cationic detergents (depending on concentration) can be irritating or corrosive to mucous membranes. They can cause local as well as systemic effects. Usually <1% concentration causes irritation to the mucous membrane and >7.5% can cause corrosive injury.
- The exact mechanism responsible for the systemic effects of cationic detergents is not known. Current belief is that these compounds have a ganglionic blocking effect and a curare-like action with the paralysis of the neuromuscular junction of striated muscle.
- The exact mechanism of action for essential oils is unknown. Essential oils can cause mucous membrane irritation and have CNS depressant effects.
- Toxicosis is acute, with signs occurring minutes to a few hours after exposure.

DIAGNOSIS

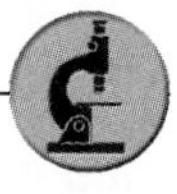

DIFFERENTIAL DIAGNOSIS

- Corrosives (acids, alkali) toxicoses
- Household products (detergents, bleaches, pine oils) toxicoses
- Acetylcholinesterase (AChE) inhibitor pesticides (organophosphates, carbamates) toxicoses
- Upper respiratory tract infection
- Uremic ulcers (renal failure)
- Garbage toxicosis
- Foreign body

INITIAL DATABASE

- Complete blood count (CBC): inflammatory leukogram.
- Serum chemistry profile ± blood gas analysis: Oils causing hepatic damage may produce increased liver enzymes (uncommon) and acid-base or electrolyte abnormalities.

ADVANCED OR CONFIRMATORY TESTING

- Gas chromatography and mass spectrometry (GC/MS) on urine can identify both essential oils and metabolites.
- Necropsy: no characteristic lesions.
- If indicated by clinical findings, endoscopic examination of esophagus and stomach may be considered within 12 to 24 hours to rule out perforation of gastrointestinal (GI) tract.

TREATMENT

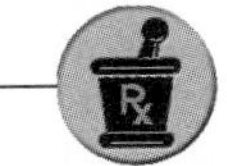

THERAPEUTIC GOAL(S)

- Inform owners to eliminate their pets' contact with liquid potpourri.
- Decrease pain and allow healing of irritated/ulcerated tissue.

ACUTE GENERAL TREATMENT

- Dermal exposure: Immediate bathing of the pet using a mild liquid dishwashing detergent; monitoring for erythema, swelling, pain, or pruritus. Treatment may include administering analgesics, anti-inflammatories, and antibiotics.
- Ocular: Ocular flushing for 20 to 30 minutes with tepid tap water or physiologic saline and fluorescein stain of the cornea to assess for corneal ulceration (see Corneal Ulceration, p 246).
- Oral: Dilution with oral administration of milk or water (dogs: ½ cup [125 ml] per 15 kg; cats: 1-2 tbsp [15-30 ml] per cat; most effective if performed early).
- Emesis, gastric lavage, and activated charcoal are contraindicated (liquid potpourri is a caustic agent).
- Protecting GI mucosa:
  - Sucralfate slurries (dog: 0.5-1 g PO q 8-12h; cat: 0.25-0.5 g PO q 8-12h).
  - H_2 receptor antagonists:
    - Famotidine, dogs/cats: 0.5 mg/kg PO, SC, IM, IV q 12-24h.
    - Cimetidine, dogs/cats: 5-10 mg/kg PO q 6h.
- Pain control: buprenorphine (dogs/cats) 0.005-0.03 mg/kg IV, IM, SC q 6-12h.
- Broad-spectrum antibiotics (for caustic burns).
- Anti-inflammatory medications:
  - Corticosteroids (dexamethasone 0.1-0.2 mg/kg IV or IM q 24h for 3-5 days or prednisolone 0.25-1 mg/kg PO q 24h). Use is controversial; may use for several days if esophageal damage has occurred; appear to help reduce esophageal stricture but concurrently increase risk of opportunistic infection (e.g., pneumonia); concurrent use of broad-spectrum antibiotics unproven to reduce risk.
- IV fluids: most commonly indicated in cases involving anorexia, dehydration, electrolyte imbalances, or hyperthermia.

CHRONIC TREATMENT

- If aspiration pneumonia develops, oxygen and a broad-spectrum antibiotic may be necessary (see Pneumonia, Aspiration, p 862).
- Nutritional support: with severe oral lesions, food prepared as a liquid slurry or soft mashed foods are appropriate; rarely, additional measures (see Feeding Tube Placement: Esophagostomy Tube, p 1243; Feeding Tube Placement: Percutaneous Endoscopic Gastrostomy [PEG], p 1247) are required in severe cases or when concurrent anorexigenic disorders (e.g., hepatic lipidosis) occur.

DRUG INTERACTIONS

Nonsteroidal anti-inflammatory drugs (NSAIDs) or corticosteroids can worsen GI ulcers by reducing protective prostaglandins.

POSSIBLE COMPLICATIONS

- Esophageal stricture/perforation
- Aspiration pneumonia

RECOMMENDED MONITORING

- Body temperature (elevation may indicate pneumonia or other secondary infection)
- White blood cell (WBC) count
- Endoscopic examination of esophagus and stomach if clinical concern of severe mucosal erosion, perforation, or subsequent stricture

PROGNOSIS AND OUTCOME

With supportive care, signs resolve in a few hours to several days, depending on the degree of exposure.

PEARLS & CONSIDERATIONS

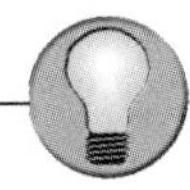

COMMENTS

- Liquid potpourri is rapidly absorbed both orally and dermally.
- Hepatic damage from essential oils in potpourri is possible but very uncommon.
- Dry potpourri contains small amounts of essential oils and is essentially a foreign body risk if ingested.
- Liquid potpourri can cause burns even if the liquid is not hot (chemical burns).

PREVENTION

Owners should keep simmer pots out of the reach of pets.

SUGGESTED READING

Richardson JA: Potpourri hazards in cats. *Vet Med* 94:12, 1999.

AUTHOR: **TINA WISMER**
EDITOR: **SAFDAR A. KHAN**

Pregnancy

BASIC INFORMATION

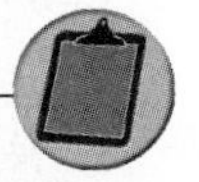

DEFINITION

Gestation length in the bitch is 65 days from the luteinizing hormone (LH) surge (54 to 60 days from the first day of diestrus and 57 to 72 days from breeding). Gestational length in the queen is 64 days from LH surge. Cats are induced ovulators, and the LH surge corresponds to 24 hours following the first breeding date.

SYNONYM(S)

Gestation

EPIDEMIOLOGY

SPECIES, AGE, SEX

- Canine: postpubertal intact female (usually >6 months old)
- Feline: postpubertal intact female (>4-6 months old)

GENETICS AND BREED PREDISPOSITION: Fertility and fecundity are heritable traits. Mixed breeds and outcross matings generally result in higher pregnancy rates and large litter sizes. Litter size is also dependent on maternal size; smaller breeds have fewer pups/kittens.

RISK FACTORS: Intact females exposed to intact males.

GEOGRAPHY AND SEASONALITY: Canine: Most domestic breeds cycle twice yearly irrespective of season with the potential to become pregnant during each estrous cycle. Wolf hybrids cycle annually during the spring (long-day breeders), and basenjis also cycle annually during autumn (short-day breeders).
Feline: Domesticated cats are polyestrous, long-day breeders with seasonal anestrus during the winter months. It is possible

for a queen to have multiple litters each year.

ASSOCIATED CONDITIONS AND DISORDERS

- Insulin resistance (pregnancy-associated diabetes)
- Pregnancy anemia
- Pyometra
- Hydrops (amnion or allantoic)
- Overt false pregnancy/pseudocyesis

CLINICAL PRESENTATION

HISTORY, CHIEF COMPLAINT

- Intentional breeding
- Unintentional breeding
- Unexplained weight gain
- Unexplained mammary development and lactation
- Nesting behavior

PHYSICAL EXAM FINDINGS

- Embryonic vesicles or fetuses palpable abdominally:
  - Embryonic vesicles are palpable approximately 25 to 35 days post-LH surge.
  - Fetuses are palpable approximately 45 days post-LH surge.
- Mammary development and lactation

ETIOLOGY AND PATHOPHYSIOLOGY

- Ovulation occurs 48 hours post-LH surge in dogs and 48 hours postbreeding in cats.
- Fertilization occurs in the uterine tube (ampulla-isthmus junction), and the embryos enter the uterus approximately 10 to 11 days post-LH surge in the bitch (5 to 6 days post-LH surge in the queen).
- Embryos migrate within the uterus and may implant in the horn ipsilateral to ovulation.
- Implantation occurs 15 to 17 days post-LH surge in the bitch (14 to 15 days post-LH surge in the queen).
- Pregnancy is progesterone dependent throughout gestation. Corpora luteal production of progesterone is required for pregnancy maintenance. Prolactin is luteotropic and maintains the corpus luteum during the second half of pregnancy in both dogs and cats.

DIAGNOSIS

DIFFERENTIAL DIAGNOSIS

- Pyometra
- Mucometra
- Overt false pregnancy/pseudocyesis

INITIAL DATABASE

- Abdominal ultrasound (Fig. I-140):
  - Embryonic vesicles can be detected as early as 20 days post-LH surge (16 days post-LH surge in cats).
  - The embryo can be detected after 25 days post-LH surge (see Fig. I-140).
  - False-positives may result from misinterpretation of early pyometra or mucometra.
  - False-negatives may occur in early pregnancy, particularly if the day of the LH surge is unknown.
  - Fetal viability can be readily assessed by evaluating fetal heart rates after 25 days post-LH surge.
  - Gestational age can be determined by fetal measurements and fetal structures.
  - Litter size can only be approximated. Accurate counts are difficult because only segments of the uterus can be seen at a time, resulting in double counting or not visualizing fetuses.
- Serum relaxin: relaxin is a hormone produced by the placenta and is a confirmatory test of pregnancy after 30 days post-LH surge. A commercially available test is labeled for dogs and has been validated for use in cats.
  - False positives may result when relaxin levels remain elevated after fetal death (up to 2 days) or in cases of large ovarian cysts (queens).
  - False-negatives can occur in early pregnancy or in singleton litters that do not generate sufficiently elevated relaxin for detection.
  - Litter size and fetal viability do not correlate well with relaxin concentrations.
- Abdominal radiographs: pregnancy can be diagnosed by visualization of ossified fetal skeletons greater than 45 days post-LH surge.
  - False negatives may occur with small litters if a full colon obscures fetuses.
  - False-negatives may occur prior to 45 days post-LH surge.
  - Fetal loss of viability can be evaluated by fetal posture (appearance of disarticulation), bone juxtaposition (especially skull), and intrafetal presence of gas.
  - Litter size is most reliably estimated by radiographs.

TREATMENT

THERAPEUTIC GOAL(S)

- No treatment is necessary for desired pregnancies.
- In the event of an unwanted pregnancy, pregnancy termination will prevent parturition of term fetuses (see Pregnancy Termination, p 887).

POSSIBLE COMPLICATIONS

- See Dystocia, p 327
- See Abortion (Canine), p 6
- Fetal resorption

RECOMMENDED MONITORING

- Termination of pregnancy should be confirmed by ultrasound examination.
- Serum progesterone levels below 2 ng/ml are incompatible with pregnancy but do not confirm pregnancy loss.

PROGNOSIS AND OUTCOME

Parturition usually occurs without complications.

PEARLS & CONSIDERATIONS

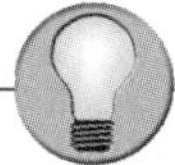

COMMENTS

- Superfecundation: A bitch bred to multiple males can have pups within the same litter that are from different sires.

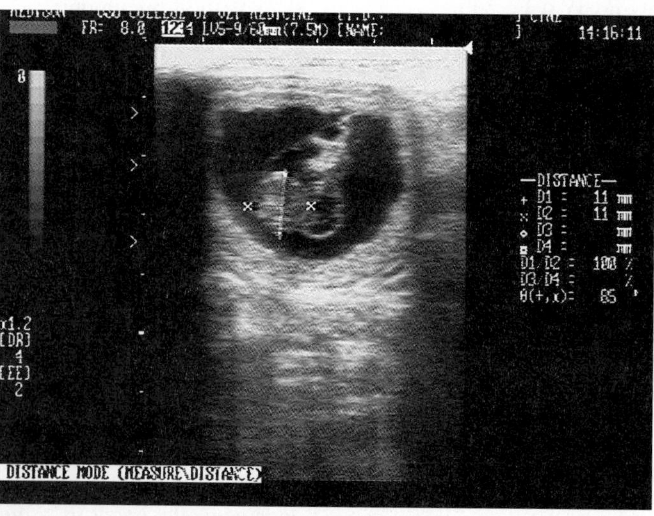

FIGURE I-140 Transabdominal ultrasonogram from a pregnant bitch that illustrates a gestational sac containing a fetus. The body diameter measurement made between the cursors indicates that this fetus is 34 days past the LH surge (31 days before whelping). Courtesy of Dr. Michelle A. Kutzler.

- Elevated serum progesterone does not indicate pregnancy. Progesterone concentrations remain elevated throughout diestrus whether or not pregnancy is established. Progesterone concentrations remain elevated for ≥65 days post-LH surge in the bitch and for 40 days post-LH surge in the queen.

PREVENTION

Preventing unwanted pregnancies: Castration of nonbreeding animals and proper supervision of intact animals.

SUGGESTED READING

Concannon PW, et al: Recent Advances in Small Animal Reproduction. International Veterinary Information Service (IVIS): http://www.ivis.org/advances/Concannon/wanke/chapter_frm.asp, 2001.

Johnson S, Root Kustritz M, Olson P: *Canine and Feline Theriogenology*. Philadelphia, WB Saunders, 2001.

Yeager AE, et al: Ultrasonographic appearance of the uterus: Placenta, fetus, and fetal membranes throughout accurately timed pregnancy in beagles. *Am J Vet Res* 53:342-351, 1992.

AUTHOR: **RICHARD WHEELER**
EDITOR: **MICHELLE A. KUTZLER**

Pregnancy Termination

BASIC INFORMATION

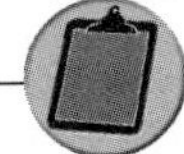

DEFINITION

Elective nonsurgical abortion of a litter prior to 55 days of gestation

SYNONYM(S)

Elective abortion
Mismating/misalliance options

EPIDEMIOLOGY

SPECIES, AGE, SEX: Intact bitches and queens of any age.
RISK FACTORS: Intact cycling females.

CLINICAL PRESENTATION

HISTORY, CHIEF COMPLAINT: Female bred to an unintended male.
PHYSICAL EXAM FINDINGS

- Normal healthy female.
- Abdominal palpation of focal, discrete uterine enlargements during the fourth week of gestation. Accuracy will depend on the expertise of the palpator and the stage of pregnancy.

ETIOLOGY AND PATHOPHYSIOLOGY

- Luteal support (via progesterone production) is required for the entire length of a successful canine or feline pregnancy.
- Pregnancy in the bitch and queen can be terminated by administration of drugs that prematurely lyse the corpora lutea (CL) on the ovary.

DIAGNOSIS

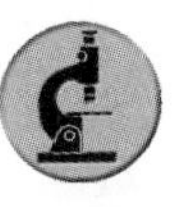

DIFFERENTIAL DIAGNOSIS

- Pseudopregnancy is normal in the bitch after every estrus. Pseudopregnancy in the queen will occur only after an infertile mating or other ovulation induction.
- Pyometra is an enlarged uterus containing purulent intraluminal material during the luteal phase.
- Mucometra/hydrometra is an enlarged uterus containing nonpurulent intraluminal material with varying degrees of mucin content during the luteal phase.

INITIAL DATABASE

- Ultrasonography: earliest detection of pregnancy is 3-4 week postbreeding.
- Radiographs: detection of an enlarged uterus. Radiography will not differentiate between pregnancy and other causes of uterine enlargement until after 42 days of gestation.
- In the pregnant bitch, a serum relaxin assay will be positive after placental implantation has occurred (21 days of gestation until term). See Pregnancy, p 885.

TREATMENT

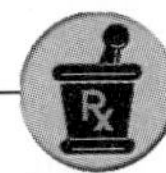

THERAPEUTIC GOAL(S)

- Reduce serum progesterone concentrations to <2 ng/ml by lysis of the CL
- Perform a complete evacuation of the uterus

ACUTE GENERAL TREATMENT

- Depending on the protocol, premature lysis of the CL (luteolysis) can be induced before or after a pregnancy diagnosis has been made.
    - Prostaglandin q 8-12h SQ to effect; usually 3 to 9 days of therapy is needed (canine: dinoprost 0.1-0.25 mg/kg, cloprostenol 1-2.5 ug/kg; feline: dinoprost 0.25-0.5 mg/kg). Prostaglandin therapy can be initiated as soon as day 5 of diestrus, as determined by vaginal cytologic examination, and as late as day 45.
    - Combination of prostaglandin with prolactin inhibitor: prostaglandin SQ q 8h (see dose previously listed), and prolactin inhibitor (bromocriptine 10 ug/kg [0.01 mg/kg] or cabergoline 5 ug/kg [0.005 mg/kg]) PO q 8h, usually 3 to 4 days of therapy needed. Prostaglandin may be needed for an additional 1 to 2 days for complete uterine evacuation. Protocols using prolactin inhibitors are initiated during the second three weeks of pregnancy, during which the clinician is able to verify the diagnosis of pregnancy by palpation or ultrasonography.
    - Prolactin inhibitor in queens: cabergoline 25-50 μg/cat PO q 24h for 3-5 days.

POSSIBLE COMPLICATIONS

- Side effects of prostaglandins include salivation, panting, vomition, defecation/diarrhea, and vocalization in queens. Side effects are limited to the first 30 to 40 minutes after injection. Side effects decrease over time with subsequent injections. Bromocriptine can cause vomiting. The vomiting caused by bromocriptine is seen outside the 30 to 40 minutes after prostaglandin administration. If needed, this vomiting can be controlled by an antiemetic.
- Typical protocols using prostaglandin or prostaglandin plus a prolactin inhibitor are administered from 21 to 42 days of gestation. Some protocols (dinoprost alone at 0.25 mg/kg) can be implemented prior to 21 days of gestation. Incomplete luteolysis may occur when treatment is initiated prior to 21 days of gestation, which results in failure to terminate pregnancy. Serum progesterone must be <2 ng/ml for 48 hours before the pregnancy termination will commence and must stay <2 ng/ml for pregnancy termination to be complete. Rebound of luteal tissue and the subsequent rise of serum progesterone concentrations can occur even after a partial abortion has been obtained. Incomplete luteolysis occurs when treatment is given for an insufficient duration of time. Therefore, baseline serum progesterone concentrations must be documented before cessation of treatment. It is also highly advisable to document the complete evacuation of the uterus ultrasonographically.
- Shortening the luteal phase will shorten the interestrous period. Clients should

be advised to expect the next cycle to occur sooner than normally expected.

RECOMMENDED MONITORING

Ultrasonography and serum progesterone concentrations to verify completion of abortion and uterine evacuation.

PROGNOSIS AND OUTCOME

Good prognosis for future fertility.

PEARLS & CONSIDERATIONS

COMMENTS

- Since >50% of bitches will not be pregnant after a misalliance situation, waiting until the pregnancy is positively diagnosed to begin a protocol to terminate a pregnancy is recommended.
- Using estrogen during estrus has been reported to be a safe and effective method for pregnancy termination
  - Estradiol cypionate: canine, 0.044 mg/kg IM once; feline, 0.25 mg/cat IM once).
  - Estrogen treatment should not be repeated even if the bitch or queen gets bred again during the same estrus.
  - Possible side effects of estrogen treatment include pyometra and severe, irreversible bone marrow suppression (canine).
  - Due to the potential severe side effects of estrogen therapy, client education and specific written permission should be obtained prior to its use.
- The combination protocols using prostaglandin and prolactin inhibitors achieve success more quickly with fewer side effects than using either individually.
- In-house radiography is not an effective tool for monitoring the success of pregnancy termination. In addition, relaxin concentrations do not drop rapidly enough to warrant their use as a monitoring test for pregnancy termination.
- If pregnancy termination protocols are initiated after 50 days of gestation, birth of viable puppies or kittens may occur.

PREVENTION

- Effective physical control of cycling bitch or queen during estrus.
- Ovariectomy or ovariohysterectomy will eliminate the problem permanently.

CLIENT EDUCATION

- Clients should be actively counseled concerning the options available, and the protocol chosen should be the best for the situation.
- In the bitch or queen not intended for breeding, ovariectomy or ovariohysterectomy should be performed as early in gestation as possible.

SUGGESTED READING

Bowen RA, et al: Efficacy and toxicity of estrogens commonly used to terminate canine pregnancy. *J Am Vet Med Assoc* 186:783–788, 1985.

Eilts BE: Pregnancy termination in the bitch and queen. *Clin Tech Small Anim Pract* 17:116–123, 2002.

Feldman EC, et al: Prostaglandin induction of abortion in pregnant bitches after misalliance. *J Am Vet Med Assoc* 202:1855–1858, 1993.

AUTHORS: **BEVERLY J. PURSWELL, KARA A. KOLSTER**

EDITOR: **MICHELLE A. KUTZLER**

Preputial Discharge

BASIC INFORMATION

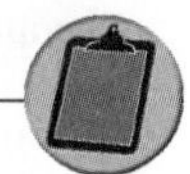

DEFINITION

Discharge through the penile sheath (prepuce) consisting of normal or abnormal secretions of various amounts and types. Discharge can be physiologic or pathologic and either primary or secondary to other reproductive or systemic diseases.

SYNONYM(S)

Purulent or catarrhal posthitis

EPIDEMIOLOGY

SPECIES, AGE, SEX: Canine; prepubertal or adult; normal males or pseudohermaphrodite females.

GENETICS AND BREED PREDISPOSITION: None known; however, the incidence is higher in consanguinous family or certain breeds (i.e., brachycephalic).

RISK FACTORS

- Acquired or congenital penile anatomic abnormalities
- Acquired or iatrogenic hormonal imbalance
- Poor hygiene/kennel management
- Canine herpesvirus type 1 or *Brucella canis* infection
- Prostatic disease
- Anticoagulant rodenticide exposure
- Foreign body exposure (e.g., grass awn)

CONTAGION AND ZOONOSIS: Preputial discharge may be contagious if caused by canine herpesvirus type 1 or *B. canis* (see Brucellosis, Dog, p 162).

CLINICAL PRESENTATION

DISEASE FORMS/SUBTYPES

- Normal: small amount of yellow-white smegma
- Abnormal:
  - Mucoid (hormonal imbalance in prepubertal dogs)
  - Purulent (infection, foreign body)
  - Hemorrhagic (coagulopathy, trauma, neoplasia, prostatic disease, testicular disease)

HISTORY, CHIEF COMPLAINT

- Preputial discharge (observed by owner)
- Preputial licking
- Preputial discomfort/pain if touched
- Additional signs (lethargy, pollakiuria, dysuria) depend upon underlying primary disease

PHYSICAL EXAM FINDINGS: Dependent on cause:

- Preputial anatomic abnormalities
- Preputial or penile lesions
- Pain resulting from inflammation exacerbated during manipulation
- Preputial opening atrophy
- Vesicles (canine herpesvirus type 1)
- Lymphoid follicles (nonspecific)
- Masses (e.g., transmissible venereal tumor [TVT])
- Systemic signs (e.g., lethargy, sluggishness, possibly other sites of bleeding) with anticoagulant rodenticide toxicosis
- Rectal palpation: essential in all adult dogs

ETIOLOGY AND PATHOPHYSIOLOGY

- Young animals: Congenital abnormality, coagulopathy, and hormonal imbalance preceding puberty (diagnosis of exclusion for mucoid discharge in juvenile animal) are the most common causes.
- In mature dogs, potential causes include:
  - Chronic congenital abnormality
  - Infectious disease of the external genitalia (canine herpesvirus type 1 or *B. canis*) or urinary tract or iatrogenic origin (improper antibiotic treatment)
  - Systemic or reproductive tract diseases including prostatic disease and trauma

DISEASES AND DISORDERS

DIAGNOSIS

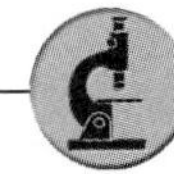

DIFFERENTIAL DIAGNOSIS

- Primary: preputial or penile problem
  - Anatomic abnormality (stenotic opening, phimosis, pseudoparaphimosis or paraphimosis, penile frenulum, adhesion, hypospadias)
  - Trauma (fighting, biting, mating, os penis fracture)
  - Foreign body (e.g., grass awn)
  - Infection (canine herpesvirus type 1 or *B. canis*)
  - Neoplasia (e.g., TVT)
- Secondary: other general or reproductive diseases
  - Prostatic disease
  - Hormonal imbalance (particularly at puberty or associated with Sertoli-cell tumor)
  - Urinary tract infection
  - Urethral neoplasm
  - Bladder disease
  - Coagulopathy

INITIAL DATABASE

- Complete preputial examination, including retraction of the prepuce to caudal to the bulbus glandis; may require sedation or anesthesia if painful
- Coagulation profile and platelet count if hemorrhagic preputial discharge
- Preputial swab for culture and cytologic examination.
  - Normal flora: mixed, including *Escherichia coli*, *Pseudomonas* spp., *Streptococcus* spp., *Pasteurella* spp., *Staphylococcus* spp., *Klebsiella* spp., *Mycoplasma* spp., *Ureaplasma* spp.
  - Antibiotics are not indicated and should not be administered to treat a normal mixed population of preputial bacteria.
  - A heavy growth of a single type of bacteria, associated with clinical signs, suggests infection.

ADVANCED OR CONFIRMATORY TESTING

- Physical examination of the penis at rest and during erection
- Complete systemic and urogenital exam, including urinalysis, prostatic ultrasonography, semen analysis, and possibly urethrography if stranguria/pollakiuria
- *Ureaplasma* spp. and *Mycoplasma* spp. culture
  - Both isolated from the prepuce of 60–85% of normal dogs
  - *Mycoplasma* spp. more prevalent (92–95%) when balanoposthitis is present
  - *Ureaplasma* spp. infection associated with infertility
- Complete blood count (CBC) and serum biochemistry profile if systemic signs of illness are manifested
- Endoscopy of prepuce: if foreign body or mass is suspected but not seen otherwise

TREATMENT

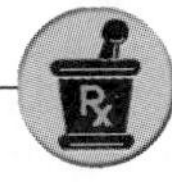

THERAPEUTIC GOAL(S)

Identification and management of cause

ACUTE AND CHRONIC TREATMENT

- Varies depending on the origin and the causal agents.
- In all cases, excessive discharge should be cleansed by flushing with lukewarm (body temperature) saline.
- Selected specific examples:
  - Anatomic defects: surgical correction of the abnormality
  - Hormonal imbalance: benign neglect; antibiotic treatment is contraindicated
  - Preputial foreign body: removal

POSSIBLE COMPLICATIONS

- Primary recurrent and/or chronic infections: urinary tract infections, prostatic disease, orchitis possible
- Canine herpesvirus type 1 and brucellosis: associated with infertility

RECOMMENDED MONITORING

In adult animals, long-term systemic antibiotic treatment is indicated to reduce the risk of complications (e.g., prostatitis, urinary tract infection).

PROGNOSIS AND OUTCOME

- Variable depending on cause
- Generally good in young animals. Fair to guarded in older animals, depending on the origin

PEARLS & CONSIDERATIONS

COMMENTS

- A small amount of yellow-white smegma is normal at the preputial opening of male dogs of any age or neuter status.
- More of an annoyance than a real disease in young animals except if it is of anatomic origin (defect) or systemic (e.g., coagulopathy).
- Preputial discharges generally resolve spontaneously without treatment in young (prepubertal) dogs.
  - Secondary infection is rare except when systemic antibiotics are administered, leading to selection of resistant bacteria.
- Preputial discharges are often of secondary origin in older animals, and identifying the primary cause of the discharge should always be the initial objective after a systematic physical exam of the external genitalia.

SUGGESTED READING

Doig PA, et al: The genital mycoplasma and ureaplasma flora of healthy and diseased dogs. *Can J Comp Med* 45(3):233–823, 1981.

Johnston S, et al: Disorders of the canine penis and prepuce. In Johnston S, Root Kustritz MV, Olson P (eds): *Canine and Feline Theriogenology*. Philadelphia, WB Saunders, 2001, pp 356–367.

Verstegen J: Conditions in the male. In England G, Harvey M (eds): *Manual of Small Animal Reproduction and Neonatalogy*. Cheltenham, United Kingdom, British Small Animal Veterinary Association, 1998, pp 71–82.

AUTHORS: **JOHN VERSTEGEN, KARINE M. ONCLIN**

EDITOR: **MICHELLE A. KUTZLER**

Primary Ciliary Dyskinesia

BASIC INFORMATION

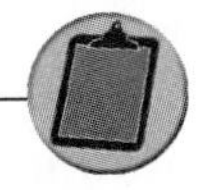

DEFINITION

A rare congenital disorder in which defective ciliary motility leads to impaired mucociliary transport and recurrent respiratory infection

SYNONYM(S)

Immotile cilia syndrome
Kartagener's syndrome
PCD

EPIDEMIOLOGY

SPECIES, AGE, SEX: Young dogs of either sex.

GENETICS AND BREED PREDISPOSITION: Numerous breeds of dogs are affected with primary ciliary dyskinesia (PCD); a monogenic autosomal recessive pattern of inheritance has been demonstrated in Newfoundland dogs and is likely to be present in other breeds as well.

ASSOCIATED CONDITIONS AND DISORDERS

- Rhinitis, sinusitis, and pneumonia occur as a result of PCD.
- Bronchiectasis results from repeated airway infections.
- Defective ciliary function in other organs may lead to male infertility, hydrocephalus, or otitis media.
- Situs inversus (mirror-image reversal of the position of organs in the body) accompanies PCD (Kartagener's syndrome) in a subset of animals.

CLINICAL PRESENTATION

HISTORY, CHIEF COMPLAINT: Young dogs present with signs of recurrent upper and/or lower respiratory tract infection. Nasal discharge, sneeze, and cough are common features, while dyspnea occurs less frequently. Infections often improve dramatically with antibiotic treatment but recur after cessation of antibiotics.

PHYSICAL EXAM FINDINGS

- Bilateral mucopurulent nasal discharge
- Sneezing
- Cough
- Dyspnea with crackles (when pneumonia is present)
- Fever (when pneumonia is present)

ETIOLOGY AND PATHOPHYSIOLOGY

- The mucociliary escalator is the major physical defense of the airways.
- Pathogens and particulates are normally trapped in a layer of mucus overlying the ciliated epithelium.
- Synchronized movement of the cilia propels entrapped particles craniad so that they can be removed from the airways.
- In animals with PCD, there are structural and/or functional defects in the cilia themselves that lead to uncoordinated, asynchronous ciliary motion and ineffective clearance of particles trapped in the mucous layer.
- Failure of the mucociliary escalator results in recurrent bacterial infection of the airways.

DIAGNOSIS

DIFFERENTIAL DIAGNOSIS

- Secondary (acquired) ciliary dyskinesia
  - Primary respiratory infections
  - Inhalation of toxic substances (e.g., smoke)
- Congenital immunodeficiency syndromes
- Chronic bacterial or fungal respiratory infections, either treated inappropriately or from infection with atypical pathogens

INITIAL DATABASE

- Complete blood count (CBC):
  - Neutrophilic leukocytosis possible if pneumonia is present.
- Serum biochemistry: nonspecific
- Thoracic radiographs:
  - Alveolar, bronchiolar, and/or interstitial lung patterns may be observed.
  - Bronchiectasis.
  - Situs inversus is detected in some dogs (apex of the heart points to the right; lung anatomy is reversed on the median plane) and is strongly suggestive of PCD.

ADVANCED OR CONFIRMATORY TESTING

- Semen evaluation: abnormal motility of spermatozoa.
- Tracheal wash or bronchoalveolar lavage: neutrophilic inflammation, often with intracellular bacteria; samples should be cultured.
- Nuclear scintigraphy: 99Tc-macroaggregated albumin is deposited at the carina, and movement is followed with gamma camera for 30 minutes. Isotope fails to move craniad in dogs with congenital or acquired ciliary dysfunction.
- Electron microscopy: ultrastructural defects can be detected on glutaraldehyde-fixed biopsies of nasal or tracheal mucosa, but detection is technically demanding. Thus, samples should be sent to a pathologist with experience in interpretating these biopsies. Alternatively, ciliated epithelium may be cultured *in vitro* and resultant tissues examined by electron microscopy.
- Ciliary beat frequency and synchronization: technically demanding process requiring special equipment allows functional observation of cilia from freshly obtained biopsies; impractical in most instances.

TREATMENT

THERAPEUTIC GOAL(S)

- Minimize damage to airways (bronchiectasis) and lungs from recurrent infection
- Treat bacterial (or rarely, fungal) infections

ACUTE GENERAL TREATMENT

- Appropriate antimicrobial therapy instituted, based ideally on culture and sensitivity (C&S) results from tracheal or bronchial lavage samples
- For dogs with pneumonia:
  - Consider oxygen supplementation if respiratory distress is present in the face of hypoxemia (P_aO_2 <80 mmHg or SpO_2 <94%)
  - Maintain hydration with parenteral fluids as needed
  - Encourage expectoration of mucus from airways via saline nebulization and coupage

CHRONIC TREATMENT

- Repeated courses of antimicrobial drugs are required for recurrent infections.
- Avoidance of treatment with cough suppressants.
- Avoidance of exposure to respiratory irritants, such as cigarette smoke.

POSSIBLE COMPLICATIONS

- Bronchiectasis
- Pneumonia
- Sepsis
- Cor pulmonale
- Reactive systemic amyloidosis

RECOMMENDED MONITORING

- Evaluate thoracic radiographs at least every 6 to 9 months in animals with prior episodes of pneumonia.
- Exacerbations of clinical signs due to lower respiratory disease should prompt tracheal or bronchial lavage for cytologic examination and culture.

PROGNOSIS AND OUTCOME

Dependent on severity of ciliary dysfunction. Illness can range from occasional episodes of upper respiratory infection to severe and frequent bronchopneumonia. Lifespan is usually negatively impacted by the condition.

PEARLS & CONSIDERATIONS

COMMENTS

Even when episodes of pneumonia are rapidly addressed, affected dogs are often euthanized due to the inconvenience and expense of treating recurrent respiratory disease and chronic nasal discharge despite appropriate antimicrobial therapy; these treatments may be a nuisance for owners of affected dogs.

PREVENTION

Affected dogs should not be bred.

CLIENT EDUCATION

Clients should understand that this is an inherited condition that cannot be cured.

SUGGESTED READING

Edwards DF, et al: Primary ciliary dyskinesia in the dog. *Prob Vet Med* 4:291, 1992.

Watson PJ, et al: Primary ciliary dyskinesia in Newfoundland dogs. *Vet Rec* 144:718, 1999.

AUTHOR: **LEAH A. COHN**

EDITOR: **RANCE K. SELLON**

Prolonged Anestrus

BASIC INFORMATION

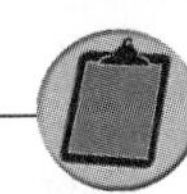

DEFINITION

Duration of interestrous interval >40 weeks

SYNONYM(S)

Primary or secondary anestrus
Prolonged interestrous interval

EPIDEMIOLOGY

SPECIES, AGE, SEX: Female dogs and cats.

- Bitches >12 months old (more common in older bitches)
- Queens >6 months old

GENETICS AND BREED PREDISPOSITION: No breed predilection, but long-haired queens have a tendency to experience delayed puberty.

RISK FACTORS: Previous oophorectomy, exogenous hormonal treatment (including glucocorticoids), hypothyroidism, ovarian disease (cysts or neoplasia), or abnormal karyotype.

GEOGRAPHY AND SEASONALITY

- Bitches are nonseasonally monoestrous, with the exception of the basenji dog that only comes into estrus in the fall. Although the interestrous interval varies among breeds, the normal interval is between 26 and 36 weeks.
- The queen is a seasonally polyestrous long-day breeder with an anestrous period that varies with geographic latitude. Cats are considered long-day breeders, and anestrus usually occurs during the fall and winter months in the northern hemisphere. The normal interestrous interval in queens is 12 to 22 days.

ASSOCIATED CONDITIONS AND DISORDERS: Ambiguous or infantile external genitalia may be associated with an intersex condition or abnormal karyotype.

CLINICAL PRESENTATION

DISEASE FORMS/SUBTYPES

- Primary anestrus: delayed puberty
- Secondary anestrus: increased interestrous interval

HISTORY, CHIEF COMPLAINT: Failure to show external signs of proestrus or estrus (failure to cycle).

PHYSICAL EXAM FINDINGS: Abnormal physical findings may include poor or excessive general body condition, overall immature appearance, ambiguous or infantile external genitalia. The physical examination may be unremarkable.

ETIOLOGY AND PATHOPHYSIOLOGY

- Variable, depending on the cause
- Disruption in the normal cyclical hormonal milieu

DIAGNOSIS

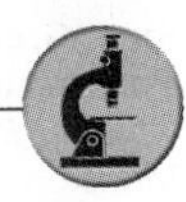

DIFFERENTIAL DIAGNOSIS

- Dogs:
  - Silent heats
  - Abnormalities in sexual differentiation
  - Hyperadrenocorticism
  - Hypothyroidism
  - Pituitary insufficiency
  - Lymphocytic oophoritis
  - Luteal ovarian cyst
  - Ovarian aplasia
  - Ovariohysterectomy
- Cats:
  - Seasonal or lighting changes
  - Pseudopregnancy
  - Disease of reproduction (pyometra, cysts)
  - Diabetes mellitus
  - Silent heat (social stress in cattery)
  - Ovariohysterectomy

INITIAL DATABASE

- Complete blood count (CBC) and serum biochemistry profile for systemic health status
- Assessment of endocrine-related illnesses via thyroid hormone analysis and dexamethasone suppression tests
- Exclusion of silent heats using exfoliative vaginal cytologic examination and serum progesterone determination
- Exclusion of abnormal reproductive tract using abdominal ultrasonography
- Exclusion of abnormal karyotype

ADVANCED OR CONFIRMATORY TESTING

- Confirmation of oophoritis with ovarian histologic examination
- CT scan of pituitary to identify cystic dilation or absence of the gland

TREATMENT

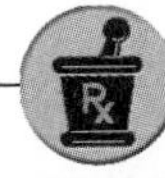

THERAPEUTIC GOAL(S)

Correct insufficiencies or excesses in endocrine hormones (e.g., hyperadrenocorticism)

ACUTE GENERAL TREATMENT

- Observe bitch or queen closely while housing her near an intact male dog or tom
- Monitor serum progesterone concentrations monthly to assess cyclicity (serum progesterone >2 ng/ml for 2 months after each estrus in the normal bitch)
- Cohouse anestrous bitch with cycling bitches to stimulate a "dormitory" effect
- Increase lighting in cattery to 14 hours of light per day

CHRONIC TREATMENT

Estrus induction: There are no approved methods of estrus induction in the dog or cat, but many protocols have been described. The following is a list of possible methods:

- Dogs: After confirming a progesterone concentration <1 ng/ml, administer 1 Ovuplant (deslorelin implant) under the subvestibular mucosa. Proestrus will be initiated in <10 days.
- Cats: Administration of a single injection of human chorionic gonadotropin (hCG), 1000 IU SQ; daily administration of 0.1 ml/kg IM of a solution compounded from adding naloxone powder for injection to 20% calcium gluconate solution to achieve a solution with a concentration of 0.4 mg/ml naloxone.

POSSIBLE COMPLICATIONS

Continued release of deslorelin from the Ovuplant implant may result in pituitary downregulation and premature luteal failure. To prevent premature luteal failure, remove the implant once serum progesterone concentration is >2 ng/ml.

RECOMMENDED MONITORING

- Initially, progesterone concentrations should be measured to determine time for implant removal
- Monitor the bitch and queen for signs of behavioral estrus

PROGNOSIS AND OUTCOME

- With correction of endocrine abnormalities, future reproductive success is not compromised
- If chromosomal abnormality, ovarian aplasia, or autoimmune disease exists, the prognosis for successful return to cyclicity is poor

PEARLS & CONSIDERATIONS

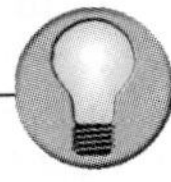

COMMENTS

Evaluation of the entire clinical picture is important:

- Review estrus identification techniques with owner
- Identify medications that the animal is receiving

- Assess the animal's overall metabolic health status
- Evaluate thyroid and adrenal gland function in bitches

PREVENTION

In cats, ensure 14 hours of light exposure daily to induce seasonal cycles.

CLIENT EDUCATION

- Provide training for the client so that he or she can recognize estrus in the animal or discuss outward signs of behavioral estrus for the bitch and queen
- Discuss age as a factor for the absence of cyclicity (prepubertal, photoperiod, and older animals)

SUGGESTED READING

Aiudi G, et al: Induction of fertile estrus in cats by administration of hCG and calcium-naloxone. *J Reprod Fertil Suppl* 57:335-337, 2001.

Johnston S: Infertility in the bitch. In Kirk RW, Bonagura JD (eds): *Current Veterinary Therapy VIII: Small Animal Practice*. Philadelphia, WB Saunders, 1992, pp 954-960.

Johnston SD, Root Kustritz MV, Olson PNS: *Canine and Feline Theriogenology*. Philadelphia, WB Saunders, 2001.

Merck Veterinary Manual website: Reproductive diseases of the female small animal. Available from: http://merckvetmanual.com/mvm/index.jsp?cfile-htm/bc/toc_112000.htm. Accessed July 31, 2006.

Romagnoli S: Clinical approach to infertility in the queen. *J Fel Med Surg* 5:143-146, 2003.

Wright PJ, et al: Suppression of the estrous responses of bitches to the GnRH analogue deslorelin by progestin. *J Reprod Fertil Suppl* 57:263-268, 2001.

AUTHOR: **TIMOTHY M. HAZZARD**

EDITOR: **MICHELLE A. KUTZLER**

Prolonged Estrus

BASIC INFORMATION

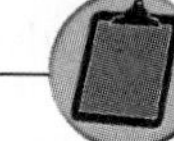

DEFINITION

- Prolonged estrus in the bitch is defined as a combined proestrus and estrus of >6 weeks or a cytologic estrus that lasts for >21 days. The normal interval between the onset of proestrus and ovulation ranges from 5 to 30 days, with most bitches ovulating between 10 and 14 days following the onset of proestrus.
- In the queen, estrus lasting longer than 10 days is considered prolonged.

SYNONYM(S)

Persistent estrus (heat)
Nymphomania

EPIDEMIOLOGY

SPECIES, AGE, SEX: Female dogs and cats >4 months of age.

RISK FACTORS: Young and very old bitches; previous history of follicular cysts; abnormal karyotype.

ASSOCIATED CONDITIONS AND DISORDERS: Secondary to chronic estrogen exposure, bone marrow suppression, uterine disease, and mammary disease may occur.

CLINICAL PRESENTATION

HISTORY, CHIEF COMPLAINT

- More than 21 days (dog) or 10 days (cat) of behavioral estrus.
- Estrous behaviors include receptivity to males, vulvar edema and serosanguineous vaginal discharge (bitch), and lordosis and vocalization (queen).
- Recent use of estradiol cypionate as an abortifacient for unintended breedings is sometimes reported although not recommended.

PHYSICAL EXAM FINDINGS

- Bitch or queen may be in good health.
- Chronic exposure to estrogen can result in disease states manifesting as cystic endometrial hyperplasia-pyometra complex, bone marrow suppression (anemia, agranulocytosis, thrombocytopenia), mammary and uterine neoplasia, as well as endocrinologic alopecia.
- Palpable unilateral abdominal mass (ovarian tumor).

ETIOLOGY AND PATHOPHYSIOLOGY

- Etiology depends on source of persistently circulating estradiol (exogenous or endogenous).
- Estrogen-secreting follicular cysts or granulosa cell tumors can result in persistent estrus.
    - Follicular cysts have been reported to occur in 3-62% of dogs with ovarian cystic disorders.
    - These cysts occur as either single or multiple thin-walled structures that contain a clear, serous fluid.
- In the queen, persistent estrus may result from the overlapping waves of maturing ovarian follicles, resulting in prolonged high concentrations of estradiol.

DIAGNOSIS

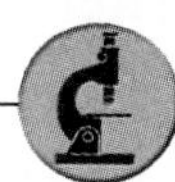

DIFFERENTIAL DIAGNOSIS

- Persistent proestrus
- Split estrus (proestrus without subsequent estrus followed by a normal cycle in about 4 weeks)
- Recurrent estrus (low progesterone or premature luteal failure)
- Pyometra
- Vaginitis
- Coagulopathy

INITIAL DATABASE

- Complete blood count (CBC) (anemia, thrombocytopenia), serum biochemistry profile, urinalysis
- Exfoliative vaginal cytologic examination indicative of estrus: >90% cornification of epithelial cells
- Identification of abnormal ovarian structures using abdominal ultrasonography: anechoic spherical regions in the ovary (follicles) or mixed echogenicity of a tumor

ADVANCED OR CONFIRMATORY TESTING

- Vaginoscopy to rule out foreign body and vaginitis
- Exclusion of abnormal karyotype
- Coagulation panel to rule out coagulopathy

TREATMENT

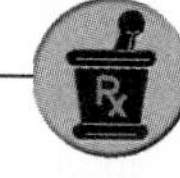

THERAPEUTIC GOAL(S)

Remove source of estradiol

ACUTE GENERAL TREATMENT

- Medical:
    - Follicular cysts in dogs and cats may be treated with gonadotropin-releasing hormone (GnRH; 25 μg IM; use 2.2 μg/kg if >11 kg) or human chorionic gonadotropin (hCG; 500-1000 IU, IM), which results in luteinization of the follicles.
    - Monitor serum progesterone and perform a vaginal cytologic examination weekly following GnRH or hCG administration; monitor for signs of diestrus or anestrus.
- Surgical:
    - When genetic qualities of the dam are not superior, ovariohysterectomy is the treatment of choice following reduction of current hyperestrogenic state.

CHRONIC TREATMENT

If acute medical treatment is not effective, surgical treatment is required.

POSSIBLE COMPLICATIONS

Pyometra sequelae:

- Progesterone promotes endometrial growth and glandular secretion while decreasing myometrial activity. Cystic endometrial hyperplasia and accumulation of uterine secretions ultimately develop and provide an excellent environment for bacterial growth.
- Chronic estradiol production by the cystic follicles up-regulates progesterone receptors in the uterus. This enhances the effect of the progestins produced following treatment to luteinize the cystic follicles.

RECOMMENDED MONITORING

Monitor signs of estrus that should subside within 5 to 7 days of treatment

PROGNOSIS AND OUTCOME

- Recurrence is possible, but prognosis is good if signs of diestrus follow treatment.
- If estrus persists, increased suspicion of neoplasia or abnormal karyotype yields a poorer prognosis for subsequent fertility, and an ovariohysterectomy is indicated.

PEARLS & CONSIDERATIONS

COMMENT

Although ovarian cancer is rare in the bitch or queen, failure of medical treatment to end signs of behavioral estrus or decrease circulating estradiol concentrations greatly increases the possibility of this diagnosis.

PREVENTION

In animals of nonbreeding stock, ovariohysterectomy will prevent reproductive abnormalities and their sequelae.

CLIENT EDUCATION

- Train owners to recognize signs of estrus or discuss outward signs of behavioral estrus for the bitch and queen.
- Clinicians and owners should discuss multiple benefits of spaying nonbreeding stock while young.
- Recurrence is more likely in animals with previous follicular cysts.

SUGGESTED READING

England GCW: Infertility in the bitch and queen. In Noakes DE, Parkinson TJ, England GCW (eds): *Arthur's Veterinary Reproduction and Obstetrics*. Philadelphia, WB Saunders, 2001, pp 639–670.

Fayrer-Hosken RA, et al: Follicular cystic ovaries and cystic endometrial hyperplasia in a bitch. *J Am Vet Med Assoc* 201:107–108, 1992.

Little S: Feline reproduction and breeding management. Cat Fanciers' Association website. Available from: http://cfa.org/articles.reproduction.pdf. Accessed July 31, 2006.

Merck Veterinary Manual website: Follicular cysts. Available from: http://merckvetmanual.com/mvm/index.jsp?cfile=htm/bc/112004.htm. Accessed July 31, 2006.

Meyers-Wallen VN: Persistent estrus in the bitch. In Kirk RW, Bonagura JD (eds): *Current Veterinary Therapy VIII: Small Animal Practice*. Philadelphia, WB Saunders, 1992, pp 963–966.

Noakes DE, et al: Cystic endometrial hyperplasia/pyometra in dogs: A review of the causes and pathogenesis. *J Repro Fert Suppl* 57:395–406, 2001.

AUTHOR: **TIMOTHY M. HAZZARD**
EDITOR: **MICHELLE A. KUTZLER**

Proptosis of the Globe

BASIC INFORMATION

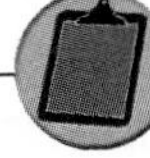

DEFINITION

Forward displacement of the globe (exophthalmos) with posterior entrapment of eyelids

SYNONYM(S)

Globe/ocular proptosis

EPIDEMIOLOGY

GENETICS AND BREED PREDISPOSITION: Brachycephalic breeds of dogs and cats are at higher risk; however, if traumatic forces are sufficient, proptosis can occur in any breed and species.

RISK FACTORS: Traumatic forces to the head (mild for brachycephalic; moderate to severe for mesaticephalic and dolichocephalic breeds).

ASSOCIATED CONDITIONS AND DISORDERS: Retrobulbar mass or severe orbital abscess or cellulitis may predispose the eye to proptosis (see Orbital Disease, p 773).

CLINICAL PRESENTATION

HISTORY, CHIEF COMPLAINT: Caused by peracute event, primarily blunt head trauma (e.g., hit by car, fighting).

PHYSICAL EXAM FINDINGS: Exophthalmos with eyelids entrapped behind eye. Any or all of the following may also be present:

- Conjunctival hyperemia or hemorrhage
- Corneal ulceration (see Corneal Ulceration, p 246)
- Abnormal pupil size: constricted or dilated
- Intraocular inflammation and/or hemorrhage (see Uveitis, p 1134; Hyphema, p 560)
- Ruptured globe
- Avulsion of extraocular muscle(s) (mainly medial and/or ventral oblique recti muscles)
- Optic nerve rupture/transection
- Orbital fractures
- Other fractures
- Neurologic deficits from brain trauma
- Shock
- Diaphragmatic hernia

ETIOLOGY AND PATHOPHYSIOLOGY

- Force(s) applied to the head (i.e., trauma), leading to the forward displacement of the globe and posterior entrapment of eyelids.
- The orbit encircles a lesser proportion of the globe (i.e., is shallower) in brachycephalic individuals, allowing proptosis to occur despite a relatively milder force of trauma.
- The medial rectus is the first extraocular muscle to avulse during trauma (lateral strabismus). Multiple extraocular muscle avulsions produce greater proptosis, which indicates a worse prognosis.

DIAGNOSIS

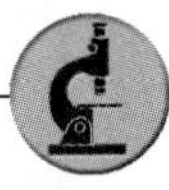

DIFFERENTIAL DIAGNOSIS

- Exophthalmos secondary to orbital abscess (opening mouth may cause pain), benign or malignant orbital mass (opening mouth is rarely painful), congenital vascular anomalies (opening mouth is rarely painful; forward displacement of globe but eyelids are in a normal position; rarely peracute) (see Orbital Disease, p 773).
- Buphthalmos secondary to congenital primary or secondary glaucoma (enlarged globe; eyelids in normal position; rarely acute). Unlike proptosis, is not associated with a blunt traumatic event. (See Ocular Size Abnormalities, p 763.)

INITIAL DATABASE

- Ophthalmic examination, including:
  - Pupillary light reflexes (PLRs). A dilated, unresponsive pupil (both direct and consensual) carries a poor prognosis for the eye because optic nerve avulsion or transection is likely.
  - Fluorescein dye application.
  - Intraocular pressures (>30 mmHg with glaucoma; may be low [<10–15 mmHg] with uveitis). Measurement should only be performed after the globe has been replaced in the orbit, thus releasing the pressure of the eyelids on the globe.
- Chest radiographs if signs of trauma beyond the face and/or if dyspnea.
- Skull radiographs if physical exam raises the possibility of orbital and/or skull fractures (e.g., extensive facial/cranial trauma, bony crepitus, and neurologic compromise, such as obtundation).

TREATMENT

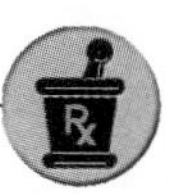

THERAPEUTIC GOAL(S)

- Return eye to proper anatomic location
- Preserve eye and possibly vision if the ocular structures are still viable

ACUTE GENERAL TREATMENT

- Keep cornea lubricated. If surgical correction is not immediately possible (e.g., grave anesthetic risk), hourly topical ointment application (alternate between triple antibiotic q 2h and sterile lubricant q 2h) is recommended.
- Placement of an Elizabethan collar around the animal's neck to prevent self-inflicted trauma.
- Patient stabilization prior to general anesthesia to reposition globe: respiratory and cardiovascular systems most important (see Hit by Car, p 527).
- Repositioning of the globe, with patient under general anesthesia:
  - Lateral canthotomy: 1–2 cm incision at the lateral canthus to relieve pressure on the eyelids
  - Eyelids replaced over globe
  - Two to three horizontal mattress sutures exiting meibomian gland openings (4-0 to 6-0 suture material)
  - Segments of Penrose drain or IV tubing to distribute tension evenly on upper and lower eyelids
  - Simple interrupted sutures to close lateral canthotomy
  - Removal of medial-most sutures in 1 to 2 weeks and lateral-most sutures in 2 to 3 weeks, depending on resolution of exophthalmos
  - Vision, tear production, cornea, and intraocular structures (i.e., lens, retina) assessment within 1 to 2 weeks following surgery

CHRONIC TREATMENT

- Topical atropine in medial canthus q 12h for 3 to 5 days
- Topical triple antibiotic ointment q 6h for 2 weeks
- Nonsteroidal anti-inflammatory drugs (NSAIDs) systemically for 5 to 7 days (e.g., dogs: carprofen 2.2 mg/kg PO q 12h, or meloxicam 0.1 mg/kg PO q 24h; cats: tolfenamic acid 4 mg/kg, SC, IM, or PO q 24h, 3–5 days)
- Broad-spectrum systemic antibiotics for 5 to 7 days (e.g., cephalexin 10–20 mg/kg PO q 8h)
- Placement of an Elizabethan collar until suture removal is performed
- Enucleation if globe is ruptured, optic nerve is transected, and/or three or more extraocular muscles are avulsed
- After repositioning and healing (days/weeks later): enucleation is sometimes still necessary if:
  - Eye is blind and painful (e.g., chronic uveitis)
  - If glaucoma occurs, especially in cats due to risk of post-traumatic intraocular sarcoma (see Intraocular Neoplasia, p 603)

POSSIBLE COMPLICATIONS

- Glaucoma
- Uveitis
- Strabismus (frequently lateral or dorsolateral due to avulsion of medial rectus or medial and ventral oblique recti muscles, respectively; see Orbital Disease, p 773)
- Mydriasis and blindness
- Keratoconjunctivitis sicca (KCS)
- Neurotrophic keratitis (damage to ophthalmic branch of trigeminal nerve supplying cornea, such as in corneal denervation) with chronic corneal ulceration

RECOMMENDED MONITORING

Recheck suture placement 24 to 48 hours postoperatively since the eyelid swelling could have dramatically resolved, thereby causing loosening of sutures.

PROGNOSIS AND OUTCOME

- Varies depending on the extent of trauma
- Most proptosed eyes can be salvaged
- Prognosis for vision varies:
  - Poor to grave (dolichocephalic breeds and cats; dilated unresponsive pupil; marked proptosis [globe displaced several centimeters rostral to the orbit])
  - Guarded to good (brachycephalic breeds)

PEARLS & CONSIDERATIONS

COMMENTS

- True ocular emergency.
- Avoid using topical corticosteroids (corneal ulceration is common).
- A blind comfortable eye can remain and have an excellent cosmetic appearance for the pet.
- In the postoperative stage, avoid excessive pressure around the neck to avoid reproptosis (e.g., use harness instead of collar).

PREVENTION

Permanent partial tarsorrhaphy (surgery to shorten palpebral fissure [length of eyelid opening]) in brachycephalic breeds of dogs

CLIENT EDUCATION

- If globe is replaced but remains blind and painful in the postoperative stage, enucleation or evisceration and intraocular prosthesis are warranted.
- Early enucleation of blind and painful eyes in cats to prevent post-traumatic ocular sarcoma.

SUGGESTED READING

Gilger BC, et al: Traumatic ocular proptosis in dogs and cats: 84 cases (1980–1994). *J Am Vet Med Assoc* 206:1186, 1995.

AUTHOR: **CHANTALE L. PINARD**
EDITOR: **CHERYL L. CULLEN**

Prostatic Cysts

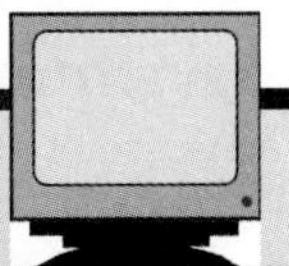

Client Education Sheet on Website

BASIC INFORMATION

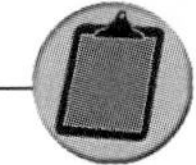

DEFINITION

- Paraprostatic cysts: thin-walled, epithelium-lined, fluid-filled structures outside the prostatic parenchyma
- Prostatic cysts: thin-walled, epithelium-lined structures within the prostatic parenchyma, containing nonpurulent fluid comprised of prostatic glandular secretions

SYNONYM(S)

Prostatic cysts: true or retention cysts

EPIDEMIOLOGY

SPECIES, AGE, SEX: Dogs, predominantly older intact males (rarely seen in neutered males).

GENETICS AND BREED PREDISPOSITION

- Paraprostatic cysts: large-breed dogs predisposed.
- Doberman pinschers have been reported to have a high incidence of all prostatic diseases.

ASSOCIATED DISEASES AND CONDITIONS: Prostatic cysts: result from obstructed prostatic ducts, possibly secondary to benign prostatic hypertrophy (BPH), squamous metaplasia, or neoplasia.

CLINICAL PRESENTATION

HISTORY, CHIEF COMPLAINT (SOME OR ALL MAY BE PRESENT): Signs arise primarily from compression of adjacent structures (tenesmus, dyschezia, ribbon-like feces, dysuria, stranguria) but may also relate to pain or systemic illness and can include:

- Anorexia
- Weakness
- Abdominal distention
- Hematuria
- Dysuria
- Urethral discharge
- Infertility

PHYSICAL EXAM FINDINGS: Some or all may be found:

- Abdominal distention
- Prostatomegaly on rectal exam (asymmetric)
- Urethral/preputial discharge (may be bloody)
- Prostate may be felt as a caudal abdominal mass if severely enlarged

ETIOLOGY AND PATHOPHYSIOLOGY

- Paraprostatic cysts: etiology unknown, thought to be vestiges of müllerian ducts
  - Thin-walled structures, usually craniolateral or caudal to the bladder and prostate
  - Filled with fibrinonecrotic debris
  - Can become secondarily infected
- Prostatic cysts: prostatic ducts become obstructed and then dilate when filled with nonpurulent secretions from the glandular epithelium
  - Can become obstructed due to squamous metaplasia, BPH, or inflammation within the ducts

DIAGNOSIS

DIFFERENTIAL DIAGNOSIS

- Other prostatic disease: prostatic abscess, prostatic neoplasia, prostatitis, BPH
- Lower urinary tract disease: neoplasia (e.g., transitional cell carcinoma), urethral calculi, cystitis
- Colonic disease: colitis, neoplasia (e.g., adenocarcinoma, leiomyosarcoma)
- Caudal abdominal mass of other tissue origin (e.g., fibrosarcoma)

INITIAL DATABASE

- Abdominal radiographs: mild to severe prostatomegaly, possible abdominal mass
  - Paraprostatic cysts may have mineralization within the wall
- Complete blood count, serum biochemistry panel, and urinalysis generally unremarkable

ADVANCED OR CONFIRMATORY TESTING

- Abdominal ultrasound:
  - Paraprostatic cysts: large hypoechoic or anechoic mass, commonly seen craniolateral or caudal to the bladder and prostate
  - Prostatic cysts: large hypoechoic/anechoic mass within the prostate
- Cytology: fine-needle aspiration may be performed to differentiate from an abscess; material within a cyst consists of cellular debris only, without evidence of suppurative inflammation
- Definitive diagnosis may still need to be confirmed at surgery

TREATMENT

THERAPEUTIC GOAL(S)

- Remove or drain the cyst to provide relief from compression of adjacent structures
- Eliminate secondary bacterial infection
- Neuter intact males to minimize risk of recurrence

ACUTE GENERAL TREATMENT

- Prostatic and paraprostatic cysts: traditionally, surgical removal is recommended with/without subtotal prostatectomy and omentalization of the prostate.
- Recent reports of percutaneous ultrasound guided drainage offer promise for less invasive option.
- Castration is recommended for prostatic cysts. If castration is refused, drug therapy (e.g., finasteride 5 mg/dog PO q 24h assuming 10-40 kg body weight) may be an alternative treatment.
- The effect of castration on resolution of paraprostatic cysts is unknown, but castration reduces the risk of future recurrence.

CHRONIC TREATMENT

Antibiotic treatment may be necessary if cyst is secondarily infected; choice should be based on culture results and ability of drug to penetrate into prostate (see Prostatitis, p 897)

POSSIBLE COMPLICATIONS

Possible complications of the cyst and surgery include urinary incontinence, chronic draining tracts, and peritonitis.

RECOMMENDED MONITORING

If percutaneous drainage is used, follow-up ultrasound examinations should be performed approximately monthly until the lesion appears to be resolved.

PROGNOSIS AND OUTCOME

- Guarded.
- Current recommendations regarding omentalizaion of the prostate have decreased complications and improved the prognosis with surgery, but long-term sequelae may still be significant.

PEARLS & CONSIDERATIONS

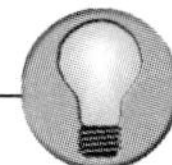

COMMENTS

An anechoic prostatic or paraprostatic mass is strongly suggestive of a cyst, but confirmation of the diagnosis depends on analysis of aspirated contents or of tissue and fluid specimens obtained during prostatic surgery.

PREVENTION

Incidence of prostatic cysts can be greatly decreased by castration of male dogs

CLIENT EDUCATION

When discussing treatment with owners, it is important to warn of the guarded prognosis, long-term problems of possible urinary incontinence, and the possible need for subsequent surgery.

SUGGESTED READING

Boland LE, et al: Ultrasound-guided percutaneous drainage as the primary treatment for prostatic abscesses and cysts in dogs. *J Am Anim Hosp Assoc* 39:151, 2003.

White RA, et al: Intracapsular prostatic omentalization: A new technique for management of prostatic abscesses in dogs. *Vet Surg* 24:390, 1995.

AUTHOR: **LISA BROWNLEE**
EDITOR: **LEAH A. COHN**

Prostatic Neoplasia

Client Education Sheet on Website

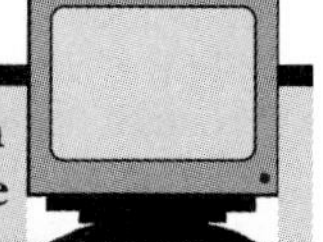

BASIC INFORMATION

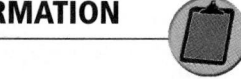

DEFINITION

- Prostatic neoplasia is uncommon in dogs and rare in cats.
- The most common tumor types include adenocarcinoma, urothelial carcinoma, and undifferentiated carcinoma.
- Prostate tumors are locally invasive and highly metastatic.

EPIDEMIOLOGY

SPECIES, AGE, SEX: Prostate tumors occur almost exclusively in dogs; sporadic cases have been reported in cats. Median age at diagnosis in dogs is 10 years.
GENETICS AND BREED PREDISPOSITION: No breed predilection has been reported; middle- to large-breed dogs are more commonly affected.

CLINICAL PRESENTATION

HISTORY, CHIEF COMPLAINT: Clinical signs are often chronic in nature and linked to the urinary tract. These signs most commonly include hematuria, incontinence, and stranguria. Animals with large masses may present with tenesmus caused by compression of the colon by the tumor. Lameness may occur in animals with bone metastasis.
PHYSICAL EXAM FINDINGS: External physical examination is often unremarkable. A large, irregular mass is typically found on rectal palpation. Animals with bone metastasis may display evidence of pain during orthopedic examination of the spine, pelvis, and/or hind limbs.

ETIOLOGY AND PATHOPHYSIOLOGY

- Intact or recently castrated dogs more likely develop adenocarcinoma, while castrated dogs likely develop other tumor types.
- Tumor location often precludes early diagnosis. Most tumors are consequently locally advanced and have metastasized (70–80%) at the time of diagnosis.
- The ultimate metastatic rate for prostate tumors is 85–100%.
- The most common sites for metastasis include lungs (50%), lymph node (30%), and bone (15–45%). The pelvis and lumbosacral spine are the most common sites of bony metastasis.

DIAGNOSIS

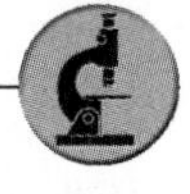

DIFFERENTIAL DIAGNOSIS

- Benign prostatic hyperplasia (BPH)
- Prostatic abscess
- Paraprostatic cyst

INITIAL DATABASE

Complete blood count (CBC), chemistry profile, urinalysis, urine culture, thoracic and abdominal radiographs (including evaluation of bony structures for metastasis), abdominal ultrasound, ± aspirate of regional lymph nodes

ADVANCED OR CONFIRMATORY TESTING

- Biopsy for histopathologic evaluation of tumor tissue.
- Cytologic evaluation of prostatic aspirate or wash may aid in establishing a diagnosis. Histopathologic evaluation of biopsied tissue for confirmation is essential prior to having patients undergo definitive therapy. Percutaneous aspiration or biopsy of the prostate may be associated with a risk of tumor seeding; however, the need to establish a definitive diagnosis usually supersedes the risk of tumor seeding.
- CT scan for surgical or radiation treatment planning.

TREATMENT

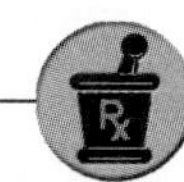

THERAPEUTIC GOAL(S)

- Long-term disease control is the ultimate goal in any animal but is often not possible due to extensive local or metastatic disease.
- In patients with lesions not amenable to definitive therapy, palliation of clinical signs is the primary goal.

ACUTE GENERAL TREATMENT

- Definitive therapy:
  - Curative-intent therapy should only be considered in dogs with no evidence of metastases.
  - Reports describing definitive therapy for dogs with localized prostate tumors are limited. The following treatments could be considered:
    - External beam radiotherapy to prostate ± regional lymph nodes.
    - Partial prostatectomy with preservation of the urethra (animals with focal prostatic lesions).
    - Complete prostatectomy with urethral resection/permanent cystostomy tube placement.
    - Given the high metastatic rate, chemotherapy (e.g., doxorubicin, cisplatin, carboplatin) is indicated in definitively treated animals. The efficacy of chemotherapy has not been established conclusively.
    - Treatment with piroxicam 0.3 mg/kg PO q 24–48h (caution: gastric ulcerogenic potential) may be beneficial in animals with prostatic carcinoma of urothelial origin.
- Palliative therapy:
  - Palliative care should be considered in animals with metastatic disease and those with advanced localized disease not amenable to definitive therapy. The efficacy of palliative treatments has not been established conclusively.
    - Palliative radiotherapy may provide short-term relief from urinary obstruction or other clinical signs resulting from local disease.
    - Permanent cystostomy tube placement/urinary bladder marsupialization may provide relief from urinary obstruction.
    - Castration may provide alleviation of signs in intact dogs with concurrent prostatic hyperplasia.
    - Systemic treatment with chemotherapy and/or piroxicam.

RECOMMENDED MONITORING

Following treatment, recommended monitoring includes routine examination, abdominal ultrasound, and thoracic radiographs; routine monitoring should be undertaken for chemotherapy based on protocol.

PROGNOSIS AND OUTCOME

- Due to the severity of clinical disease (advanced local and distant metastasis), most dogs with clinical signs caused by prostate tumors are euthanized within 1 month of diagnosis.
- The prognosis for definitive therapy is largely unknown with the exception of radiotherapy. Animals treated with a single 30 Gray dose of intraoperative radiation have shown a median survival of 4 months; animals treated with conventional external beam radiotherapy (57 Gray) have shown a median survival of 7 months.

PEARLS & CONSIDERATIONS

COMMENTS

- With rare exception, the prognosis for animals with prostatic tumors is poor; advanced disease at the time of diagnosis is the major causative factor for this poor prognosis.
- Advances in the treatment of dogs with prostate tumors will more likely come from earlier detection rather than improved treatment.

SUGGESTED READING

Bell FW, et al: Clinical and pathologic features of prostatic adenocarcinoma in sexually intact and castrated dogs: 31 cases (1970-1987). *J Am Vet Med Assoc* 199(11):1623-1630, 1991.

Cornell KK, et al: Clinical and pathologic aspects of spontaneous canine prostate carcinoma: A retrospective analysis of 76 cases. *Prostate* 45:173-183, 2000.

Obradovich J, et al: The influence of castration on the development of prostatic carcinoma in the dog. *J Vet Int Med* 1:183-187, 1987.

Proulx DR, et al: Canine prostatic neoplasia: A retrospective analysis of 10 dogs treated with external beam radiation (1989-2001). *Vet Cancer Soc Abstracts* 22:40, 2002.

Turrel JM: Intraoperative radiotherapy of carcinoma of the prostate gland in ten dogs. *J Am Vet Med Assoc* 190(1):48-52, 1987.

AUTHOR: **DAVID R. PROULX**

EDITOR: **KENNETH M. RASSNICK**

Prostatitis

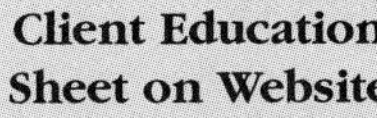

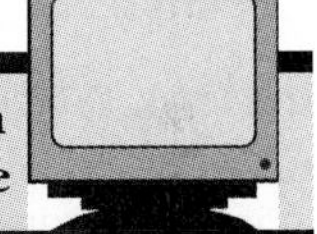

BASIC INFORMATION

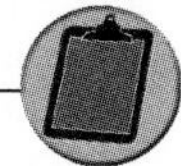

DEFINITION

Inflammation of the prostate, almost always as a consequence of infection

EPIDEMIOLOGY

SPECIES, AGE, SEX

- Can affect any age, but more likely in dogs over 5 years.
- Male cats have prostate glands, but prostatitis is extremely rare in this species.

GENETICS AND BREED PREDISPOSITION

- Doberman pinschers have been reported to have a higher incidence of all prostatic diseases.
- Increased risk reported in the bouvier des Flandres, Scottish terrier, Bernese mountain dog, German pointer, and doberman pinscher.

RISK FACTORS: Intact males are at greatest risk.

CONTAGION AND ZOONOSIS

- Prostatitis can occasionally be caused by *Brucella canis*, a potential zoonotic pathogen, via a hematogenous route.
- The most common organism reported in canine prostatitis is *Escherichia coli*, which gains access to the prostate via an ascending urinary tract infection.

ASSOCIATED DISEASES AND CONDITIONS

- Chronic form of the disease is almost always associated with benign prostatic hypertrophy/hyperplasia (BPH).
- Squamous metaplasia of the parenchymal ducts and prostatic neoplasia are also associated with prostatitis.

CLINICAL PRESENTATION

DISEASE FORMS/SUBTYPES

- Acute prostatitis: often associated with systemic illness:
  - Manifested as severe acute abdominal pain
  - Primarily in young male (usually intact) dogs
  - Prostate is not typically enlarged radiographically or ultrasonographically
- Chronic prostatitis: not associated with systemic illness:
  - Disease is usually occult in the early stages
  - Primarily in older intact male dogs with concurrent BPH
  - Prostate is not painful on palpation
  - Prostate is enlarged radiographically and ultrasonographically

HISTORY, CHIEF COMPLAINT (SOME OR ALL MAY BE PRESENT)

- Signs arise from compression or displacement of adjacent structures, prostatic pain, or systemic illness (sepsis).
- Acute: tenesmus, dysuria, lethargy, anorexia, weakness, stiff gait, hematuria.
  - Over 70% of dogs with acute prostatitis have signs of systemic illness.
- Chronic: clinical signs reported by owner may be minimal.
  - Initially, clinical signs include a recurrent urinary tract infection, preputial discharge, and hemospermia/pyospermia.
  - Depending on duration of illness: tenesmus and/or dysuria.
  - Infertility is weakly correlated with chronic prostatitis.
  - Signs of systemic illness are unlikely in dogs with chronic prostatitis.

PHYSICAL EXAM FINDINGS (SOME OR ALL MAY BE PRESENT)

- Acute prostatitis:
  - Fever
  - Tense, painful abdomen
  - Prostatic pain on rectal exam
  - Abdominal pain
  - Systemic signs of illness such as anorexia and lethargy
- Chronic prostatitis:
  - Urethral/preputial discharge possible (may be hemorrhagic or purulent)
  - Variable rectal examination findings Possibilities include:
    - Prostatomegaly
    - Normal prostatic palpation
    - Minimal prostatic pain

ETIOLOGY AND PATHOPHYSIOLOGY

- Disturbances in normal defense mechanisms (urine flow during micturition, urethral high pressure zone, bactericidal effects of prostatic fluid, and local IgA production) may predispose to prostatitis.
- Bacterial infection may spread to the prostate from elsewhere in the urinary tract, or can be hematogenous.
  - Common bacterial causes of prostatitis: *E. coli*, *Staphylococcus* spp., *Streptococcus* spp., *Proteus* spp., *Pseudomonas* spp., and *B. canis*.

◦ Hypersecretory and cystic degenerative changes that occur with BPH create ideal conditions for bacterial overgrowth. In rare cases, prostatitis can result from nonbacterial organisms (e.g., *Blastomyces*, *Pythium*) that cause systemic disease.

DIAGNOSIS

DIFFERENTIAL DIAGNOSIS

- Other prostatic disease: prostatic abscess, prostatic/paraprostatic cyst, benign prostatic hyperplasia, prostatic neoplasia
- Other lower urinary tract disease: neoplasia, urethral calculi, cystitis
- Colonic disease: colitis, neoplasia
- Mass of other tissue origin (e.g., transitional cell carcinoma, fibrosarcoma)
- Other causes of hemospermia/urospermia

INITIAL DATABASE

- Complete blood count: may have an inflammatory leukogram (more common in acute forms)
- Serum biochemistry profile: generally unremarkable
- Urinalysis: inflammatory sediment present (regardless of method of collection)
- Urine culture: may be positive for bacterial growth
- Abdominal radiographs:
  - Acute: prostate commonly of normal size, but mild to moderate prostatomegaly may be present
  - Chronic: prostate may be normal size or mildly to moderately enlarged; prostatic mineralization is almost always associated with neoplasia
- Abdominal ultrasound: focal or diffuse heterogenous echogenicity, prostatomegaly, cystic changes

ADVANCED OR CONFIRMATORY TESTING

- Prostatic fluid cytology (from ejaculate or prostatic massage): increased erythrocytes and leukocytes; bacteria may be seen within neutrophils (see Prostatic Massage, p 1303).
- Prostatic fluid culture: usually large numbers of one bacterial species cultured.
- Prostatic fine-needle aspiration is also an effective method of obtaining cells for cytology and culture (should not be performed in dogs with systemic illness).
- *B. canis* testing (see Brucellosis, Dog, p 162).

TREATMENT

THERAPEUTIC GOAL(S)

- Eliminate underlying condition (BPH).
- Eliminate infection and clinical signs.
- In some instances maintenance of breeding potential is also important, although not always possible.

ACUTE GENERAL TREATMENT

- Initiate antibiotic therapy.
  - Lipid solubility, pKa, and degree of protein binding affect penetration into the prostate
  - Antibiotics known to readily penetrate the prostatic capsule include:
    - Chloramphenicol 30–50 mg/kg PO q 8h (bacteriostatic)
    - Trimethoprim-sulfadiazine 15 mg/kg PO q 12h (bactericidal)
    - Enrofloxacin 5 mg/kg PO q 12–24h (bactericidal)
- Acute prostatitis:
  - Blood prostate barrier is disrupted
  - Most antibiotics will penetrate
  - Initial choice based on likely organism, then adjusted based on culture and sensitivity (C&S) results
- Chronic prostatitis: antibiotics that can penetrate the intact prostatic capsule (above) must be used and choice is ideally based on C&S.
- Reduction of prostatic size allows infection to be cleared more readily (castration or treatment with drugs that reduce prostate size [e.g., finasteride 5 mg/dog PO q 24h assuming 10–40 kg body weight]).
- Castration is mandatory if *Brucella* is identified. Check local regulatory guidelines for this zoonotic infection.

CHRONIC TREATMENT

- Adjust antibiotic therapy based on culture results.
- Antibiotic therapy should be continued at least 4 to 6 weeks.
- Finasteride therapy should be continued until the dog is castrated.

POSSIBLE COMPLICATIONS

- Antimicrobial side effects (e.g., trimethoprim-sulfamethoxazole may cause anemia, polyarthritis, and keratoconjunctivitis sicca if given long-term; chloramphenicol is associated with bone marrow toxicity; enrofloxacin can cause permanent retinopathy in cats).
- Prostatic abscess formation is a possible sequela of acute prostatitis.
- Decrease in ejaculatory volume from prostatic size reduction.

RECOMMENDED MONITORING

- Prostatic fluid and urine should be cultured 2 weeks after completion of antibiotics, and again 4 weeks later.
- Infection generally will not recur if finasteride is continued.

PROGNOSIS AND OUTCOME

- Prognosis is fair.
- Acute prostatitis is generally more amenable to cure than chronic prostatitis, but systemic illness makes it a more urgent and potentially life threatening disease than chronic prostatitis.

PEARLS & CONSIDERATIONS

- It can never be assumed that *B. canis* is cured, despite aggressive treatment; the owners should be aware of the potential for zoonosis.
- Radiographic evidence of prostatic mineralization can occur with bacterial prostatitis or prostatic neoplasia, but is more common with the latter.
- Castrated dogs are much less likely to develop prostatitis (versus the incidence of prostatic neoplasia, which appears to be unaffected by castration).
- Semen cryopreservation may be considered following resolution of the bacterial infection in a valuable breeding animal so that castration can be performed.

PREVENTION

Castration greatly reduces the risk of prostatitis in dogs.

CLIENT EDUCATION

Warn clients of necessity of treating chronic cases with both an antibiotic and finasteride when castration is not an option.

SUGGESTED READING

Krawiec DR, et al: Study of prostatic disease in dogs: 177 cases (1981–1986). *J Am Vet Med Assoc* 200:1119, 1992.

Kutzler MA, Yeager AE: Prostatic diseases. In Ettinger SJ, Feldman EC (eds): *Textbook of Veterinary Internal Medicine*. St. Louis, Elsevier, 2005, 1809–1818.

AUTHOR: **LISA BROWNLEE**

EDITORS: **MICHELLE A. KUTZLER, LEAH A. COHN**

Prostatomegaly

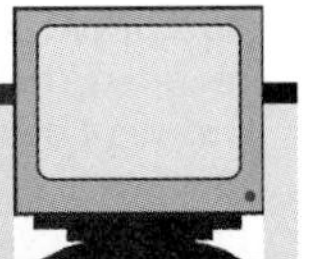

Client Education Sheet on Website

BASIC INFORMATION

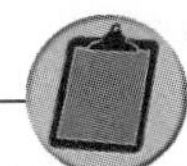

DEFINITION

Increase in volume and mass of prostate gland. Includes benign prostatic hyperplasia/hypertrophy (BPH), prostatitis, prostatic neoplasia, prostatic cyst, prostatic abscess

SYNONYM(S)

BPH is sometimes referred to as prostatomegaly although BPH only represents one cause of prostatic enlargement.

EPIDEMIOLOGY

SPECIES, AGE, SEX

- Canine
- BPH: 60% in intact male dogs >5 years and 95% in intact male dogs >9 years
- Prostatitis: second most common prostatic disorder after BPH in intact male dogs; can occur in castrated dogs secondary to neoplasia
- Prostatic neoplasia: 0.2–0.6% of all canine neoplasias; affects intact and castrated males; mean age: 10 years
- Prostatic cysts: rare; represent 5% of prostatic pathologies
- Prostatic abscesses: rare; severe form of chronic prostatitis or cysts

GENETICS AND BREED PREDISPOSITION: Increased risk of prostatomegaly reported in bouvier des Flandres, Scottish terrier, Bernese mountain dog, German pointer, doberman pinscher.

RISK FACTORS

- Advanced age
- Source of endogenous (intact male) or exogenous (anabolic steroids) androgens, especially for BPH

ASSOCIATED CONDITIONS AND DISORDERS: BPH is often a primary condition that predisposes the prostate gland to further disease (e.g. prostatitis, cyst formation, abscessation).

CLINICAL PRESENTATION

HISTORY, CHIEF COMPLAINT

- Typical clinical signs of prostatic disease include:
  - Bloody discharge from urethra
    - Can be related or unrelated to urination
    - May be purulent in cases of acute prostatitis
  - Dysuria, tenesmus, flat feces
  - In severe cases: hind limb stiffness, signs of back pain
- Additional signs may include:
  - BPH: blood in the semen
  - Prostatitis: recurrent urinary tract infections
  - Prostatic neoplasia: can be associated with signs resulting from metastasis in lumbar vertebrae (signs of back pain), pelvis (gait abnormalities), and lungs (dyspnea, cough)

PHYSICAL EXAM FINDINGS: Fever is usually present in acute prostatitis and abscesses; rectal palpation of the prostate gland may reveal the following prostatic abnormalities:

- BPH: symmetric; not painful and enlarged; middle sulcus is palpable
- Acute prostatitis: might be asymmetric; painful, enlarged
- Chronic prostatitis: asymmetric; usually not painful, might be enlarged
- Cyst: asymmetric; not painful, enlarged; might be fluctuant
- Abscess: asymmetric; might be painful and/or fluctuant, enlarged
- Neoplasia: asymmetric; enlarged, might be painful; adhered to surrounding tissue

ETIOLOGY AND PATHOPHYSIOLOGY

- BPH: multifactorial hormone dependent; BPH predisposes the animal to all other prostatitic diseases with the exception of neoplasia.
- Prostatitis: impaired prostate (due to hyperplasia, metaplasia) is susceptible to infection due to ascension of bacteria of normal urethral flora (hematogenous spread possible). See Prostatitis, p 897.
- Prostatic neoplasia:
  - Adenocarcinoma is the most common form.
  - Infiltrating transitional cell carcinoma possible.
  - Hypothesis: multistep carcinogenesis from normal prostate epithelium to metastatic, androgen-independent prostatic adenocarcinoma.
  - Castration does not initiate tumorigenesis but might favor tumor progression.
- Prostatic cysts: gland obstruction predisposed by BPH; can develop into abscesses.
- Paraprostatic cysts: remnants of paramesonephric ducts; located outside the gland but connected with prostatic tissue.
- Prostatic abscesses: develop as complication of chronic prostatitis or prostatic cysts.

DIAGNOSIS

INITIAL DATABASE

- Ultrasonography:
  - Measurements, volume determination
  - Echogenicity of tissue, distribution of lesions (focal, diffuse, multifocal)
  - Typical appearance of cysts and abscesses confirm diagnosis
  - Changes in regional lymph nodes indicator for neoplasia or infection
  - Allows fine-needle biopsy
- Cytologic/histopathologic evaluation:
  - Fine-needle core biopsy: contraindicated in abscesses and prostatitis (risk of abdominal contamination) and BPH (risk of hemorrhage); indicated in cases of suspected neoplasia (risk of seeding of biopsy tract is possible but generally does not contraindicate procedure)
- Prostatic fluid cytologic evaluation (third fraction of ejaculate): recommended if chronic prostatitis is suspected
- Radiography (abdominal):
  - Prostate location (caudal or cranial of brim of pelvis)
  - Mineralization possible in cases of chronic infections, cyst walls, abscesses, neoplasia
  - Lumbar vertebral and pelvic lesions suggest metastasis
- Complete blood count (CBC), serum chemistry panel, urinalysis:
  - Leukocytosis, neutrophilia, and left shift in acute infections and abscesses
  - Azotemia possible with dehydration or urinary tract obstruction

ADVANCED OR CONFIRMATORY TESTING

- Urinalysis with bacterial culture and sensitivity (C&S) if prostatitis, abscess, or neoplasia is suspected
- See Cystogram, p 1214
- See Prostatic Massage, p 1303

TREATMENT

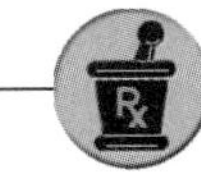

THERAPEUTIC GOAL(S)

BPH: involution of prostate and, therefore, decrease likelihood of secondary problems

ACUTE GENERAL TREATMENT

- BPH: castration if applicable; medical management possible (see Benign Prostatic Hyperplasia, p 128).
- Acute prostatitis and abscesses can be life threatening; immediate antibiotic treatment is indicated (see Prostatitis, p 897).
- Prostatic neoplasia: Treatment is not curative; castration and prostatectomy (associated with major postoperative

complications) have been recommended; no successful chemotherapy protocol exists (see Prostatic Neoplasia, p 896).
- Prostatic cysts: treatment of BPH; surgical removal (omentalization) in severe cases (see Prostatic Cysts, p 895).

CHRONIC TREATMENT

- Castration is method of choice if possible; reduces BPH and therefore decreases likelihood of recurrence of other diseases with the exception of neoplasia
- Long-term medical treatment of BPH also possible but 5α-reductase inhibitors and antiandrogens are costly; discontinuation of treatment will result in recurrence of problem

POSSIBLE COMPLICATIONS

- Surgery: often incomplete removal and recurrence of problem; postoperative complications
- Abscess: rupture, peritonitis

RECOMMENDED MONITORING

- BPH: prostate size should decrease to half the size within 3 weeks of castration; if no response, consider other differentials (e.g., cysts, abscess, neoplasia)
- Cysts: monthly follow-ups
- Prostatitis: recheck prostatic fluid (cytologic examination and quantitative culture) 1 and 4 weeks after termination of antibiotic treatment

PROGNOSIS AND OUTCOME

- BPH: good prognosis as long as treated
- Prostatitis and abscess: favorable if treated aggressively and for a long time (4 to 6 weeks)
- Prostatic neoplasia: grave

PEARLS & CONSIDERATIONS

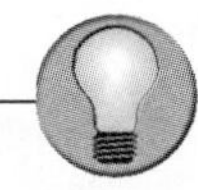

COMMENTS

In cases involving a valuable stud dog, consider medical treatment for BPH for a period of time that is sufficient to cryopreserve dog's sperm; then castrate

PREVENTION

Castration prevents all prostatic diseases except neoplasia.

SUGGESTED READING

Johnston SD, Kamolpatana K, Root-Kustritz MV, Johnston GR: Prostatic disorders in the dog. *Anim Reprod Sci* 60-61:405-415, 2000.

Krawiec DR, Heflin D: Study of prostatic disease in dogs: 177 cases (1981-1986). *J Am Vet Med Assoc* 200(8):1119-1122, 1992.

Teske E, et al: Canine prostate carcinoma: Epidemiological evidence of increased risk in castrated dogs. *Mol Cell Endocrinol* 29;197(1-2):251-255, 2002.

AUTHOR: **NATALI KREKELER**

EDITOR: **MICHELLE A. KUTZLER**

Protein-Losing Nephropathy

Client Education Sheet on Website

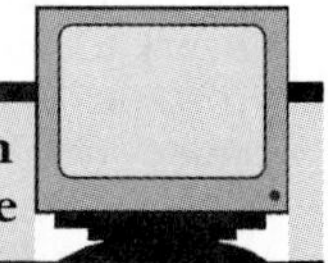

BASIC INFORMATION

DEFINITION

Any condition in which glomerular damage leads to biologically significant loss of plasma proteins. Subsequent nephron loss may lead to chronic or acute renal failure

SYNONYM(S)

PLN

Proteinuric renal failure

EPIDEMIOLOGY

SPECIES, AGE, SEX

- Familial nephropathy:
  - Dog > cats
  - Age at onset of illness varies with breed
  - Sex predilection present for some (see Genetics and Breed Predisposition below)
- Glomerulosclerosis:
  - Either sex
  - Incidence increases with age; average 8 years
- Membranous nephropathy:
  - Either sex
  - Most common protein-losing nephropathy (PLN) in the cat
  - Mean age: cats 3 to 4 years; dogs 7 years
- Minimal change nephropathy:
  - Uncommonly described in dogs and cats
- See Glomerulonephritis, p 442
- See Amyloidosis, p 57

GENETICS AND BREED PREDISPOSITION: Familial nephropathy: inheritance not always defined; typical age of onset of signs is in parentheses.

- Glomerular disease:
  - Bernese mountain dog (2 to 5 years), suspected autosomal recessive inheritance
  - Brittany spaniel (4 to 9 years), autosomal recessive inheritance
  - Rottweiler (<1 year)
  - Soft-coated wheaten terrier (2 to 11 years)
  - Beagle (2 to 8 years)
- Amyloidosis:
  - Beagle (5 to 11 years)
  - English foxhound (5 to 8 years)
  - Shar-pei (1 to 6 years)
  - Abyssinian cat (1 to 5 years), autosomal dominant with incomplete penetrance
  - Oriental shorthair (<5 years)
  - Siamese (<5 years)
- Basement membrane abnormality:
  - Bull terrier (1 to 10 years), autosomal dominant inheritance
  - Doberman pinscher (<1 to 6 years)
  - English cocker spaniel (<2 years), autosomal recessive inheritance
  - Samoyed (<1 year), X-linked dominant (males affected)
- Tubular dysfunction:
  - Basenji (1 to 5 years)
- Membranous nephropathy:
  - Doberman pinscher, possibly (3 to 4 years)

RISK FACTORS

- Corticosteroid excess (iatrogenic, hyperadrenocorticism)
- Systemic hypertension
- Diabetes mellitus
- Chronic infections (bacterial, rickettsial, protozoal, fungal, viral, parasitic)
- Chronic inflammatory disease, including immune-mediated disease
- Neoplasia

CONTAGION AND ZOONOSIS: Some infectious causes of glomerulonephritis (GN) are zoonotic (see Glomerulonephritis, p 442).

GEOGRAPHY AND SEASONALITY: Some infectious causes of GN are geographically and/or seasonally limited (see Glomerulonephritis, p 442).

ASSOCIATED CONDITIONS AND DISORDERS

- Nephrotic syndrome
- Chronic renal failure
- Hypertension
- Hyperlipidemia
- Thromboembolic disease, including pulmonary thromboembolism

CLINICAL PRESENTATION

DISEASE FORMS/SUBTYPES
- GN
- Amyloidosis
- Familial nephropathy
- Glomerulosclerosis
- Membranous nephropathy
- Minimal change disease

HISTORY, CHIEF COMPLAINT: Clinical signs may be absent. Shar-pei dogs may present for lameness and/or fever (see Shar-Pei Fever, p 998). When signs are present, they may be due to renal failure, nephrotic syndrome, or to an underlying disease process:
- Vomiting
- Lethargy
- Anorexia
- Weight loss
- Pendulous abdomen (ascites)
- Edema
- Dyspnea
- Polyuria and polydipsia (PU/PD)
- Blindness (systemic hypertension)
- Halitosis (uremia)

PHYSICAL EXAM FINDINGS: May be unremarkable. Shar-pei dogs may have fever, tibiotarsal joint pain, and joint effusion. Other findings may suggest an underlying disease process. Abnormalities may include those listed in the previous bulleted list or those listed here:
- Dehydration
- Poor haircoat
- Peripheral edema
- Abdominal effusion
- Pleural effusion (rare)
- Pallor
- Oral ulceration
- Lipid corneal deposits
- Retinal hemorrhage/detachment
- Kidneys may be normally sized or small

ETIOLOGY AND PATHOPHYSIOLOGY
- Familial nephropathy:
  - Diverse group of hereditary renal diseases.
  - Defects vary with individual diseases but include familial amyloidosis, failure of tubular protein resorption, and defects in type IV collagen in the glomerular basement membrane.
  - In some cases, nephropathy is associated with other conditions (e.g., food sensitivity [soft-coated wheaten terrier], complement deficiency [Brittany spaniel]).
- Glomerulosclerosis:
  - Results from hyperfiltration in dogs with "typical" chronic renal failure, often as an end-stage lesion.
  - Reported in dogs with familial nephropathy, systemic hypertension, diabetes mellitus, hyperadrenocorticism, and postradiation therapy. Multiple other causes described in people.
  - Sclerosis ultimately leads to altered intraglomerular hemodynamics and progressive renal failure.
- Membranous nephropathy:
  - Immune complex deposition in the glomerular basement membrane without evidence of inflammation.
  - Primary (most common) and secondary forms can be distinguished by the location of the immune complex deposition.
- Minimal change nephropathy
  - Loss of anionic charge in glomerulus leads to selective albumin loss.
  - Because electron microscopy is required for diagnosis, may be underreported in veterinary medicine.
- See Glomerulonephritis, p 442.
- See Amyloidosis, p 57.

DIAGNOSIS

DIFFERENTIAL DIAGNOSIS

Proteinuria
- Preglomerular:
  - Bence Jones proteinuria
  - Exercise
  - Hemolysis
  - Fever
  - Seizure
- Glomerular (i.e., the disorders that can cause protein-losing nephropathy):
  - GN
  - Amyloidosis
  - Glomerulosclerosis
  - Familial nephropathy
  - Minimal change disease
- Postglomerular:
  - Urinary tract infection
  - Acute renal failure
  - Neoplasia (e.g., transitional cell carcinoma, prostatic carcinoma)
  - Urolithiasis
  - Urinary hemorrhage
  - Fanconi syndrome
  - Trauma
  - Endocrine disease (e.g., hyperadrenocorticism)

INITIAL DATABASE
- Retinal exam: hemorrhages (acute or chronic) or retinal detachments are possible (both a result of systemic hypertension).
- Blood pressure (BP): systemic hypertension is possible (systolic BP >180 mmHg, repeatably, in a calm environment).
- Complete blood count (CBC): often unremarkable; nonregenerative anemia, leukocytosis (if inflammatory disease is present).
- Serum biochemical profile:
  - Hypoalbuminemia with normal globulin level.
  - Hypercholesterolemia.
  - Hypocalcemia (due to hypoalbuminemia).
  - Azotemia (in advanced disease).
  - Hyperphosphatemia (in advanced disease).
  - Metabolic acidosis.
- Urinalysis: Proteinuria, variable urine concentration, sometimes hematuria.
  - Proteinuria must be interpreted in light of urine concentration and urine sediment examination.
  - Dipstick measure of proteinuria should be confirmed by sulfosalicylic acid (SSA) method or quantitative measures (e.g., urine protein:creatinine ratio).
  - Proteinuria may be mild in subset of shar-pei dogs and Abyssinians with renal medullary amyloidosis.
  - Significant proteinuria may precede loss of urine concentration or azotemia.
- Urine culture: indicated in all cases.
- Thoracic radiographs: unremarkable. Evidence of underlying disease (neoplasia, chronic infectious or inflammatory disease) or pulmonary thromboembolism occasionally identified.
- Abdominal radiographs: often unremarkable. Kidneys may be large (amyloidosis) or small (chronic GN, sclerosis); may identify evidence of underlying disease (neoplasia, chronic infectious or inflammatory disease).
- Abdominal ultrasound: hyperechoic kidneys (though this is a normal finding in some cats), decreased corticomedullary junction, medullary rim sign, cortical cysts.

ADVANCED OR CONFIRMATORY TESTING
- Microalbuminuria test (early renal disease [ERD] screen) can detect small amounts of urine albumin before dipstick protein is positive:
  - Significance of this test in apparently healthy dogs is not known.
  - May identify animals with familial nephropathy before overt renal damage apparent.
  - Used in humans with diabetes mellitus and hypertension as early indicator of glomerulosclerosis.
- Urine protein:creatinine ratio:
  - Normal ratio <0.5 in dogs and <0.4 in cats.
  - Only useful when urine sediment is inactive.
  - Protein loss tends to be higher in amyloidosis than in GN.
- Urine protein excretion, 24 hours: largely replaced by single-sample protein:creatinine ratio.
- Biopsy of the renal cortex for light microscopy, electron microscopy (EM), or immunofluorescence:
  - Amyloidosis: Congo red stain for amyloid.
  - GN: morphologic description and immunologic classification.

 - Glomerulosclerosis: immunofluorescent microscopy is negative; immunoglobulin and C3 trapping may be present. A segmental increase in mesangial matrix and basement membrane is typically seen.
 - Membranous nephropathy: thickened glomerular basement membrane due to immune complex deposition. Location of immune complexes determined by EM.
 - Minimal change disease: lack of light microscopic glomerular changes; foot process effacement seen on EM.
- Antithrombin levels to determine risk of thromboembolic disease.
- Blood gas analysis: increased alveolar-arterial (A-a) gradient may support ventilation-perfusion mismatch due to pulmonary thromboembolism.
- Search for underlying disease; in addition to causes of GN (see Glomerulonephritis, p 442), causes of glomerulosclerosis should be considered as well (e.g., systemic hypertension, hyperadrenocorticism, diabetes mellitus).

TREATMENT

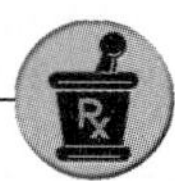

THERAPEUTIC GOAL(S)

- Treat underlying disease if possible
- Reduce proteinuria
- Reduce thromboembolic risk
- Address uremic signs and electrolyte and acid-base disorders

ACUTE GENERAL TREATMENT

- If identified, underlying causes should be addressed directly whenever possible.
- Supportive care for protein-losing nephropathy includes measures to address proteinuria, hypertension, thromboembolic risks, edema formation, and uremia. See Glomerulonephritis, p 442.

CHRONIC TREATMENT

- Identification and treatment of a causative disease provide the best prognosis for affected animals. PLN is often idiopathic or causation cannot be treated (e.g., familial disease). In these cases, supportive, nonspecific measures are employed (see Nephrotic Syndrome, p 749; Glomerulonephritis, p 442; Amyloidosis, p 57).
- Specific treatment for amyloidosis may be attempted (see Amyloidosis, p 57).
- Immunosuppression (glucocorticoids 2 mg/kg PO q 24h) may be useful for membranous nephropathy but only if infectious causes have been ruled out.

DRUG INTERACTIONS

ACE inhibitors may cause hypotension when combined with diuretics or other vasodilators. Nonsteroidal anti-inflammatory drugs (NSAIDs) may reduce efficacy of angiotensin-converting enzyme (ACE) inhibitors.

POSSIBLE COMPLICATIONS

- Third-space retention of fluids/nephrotic syndrome
- Worsening renal azotemia as a result of ACE inhibitor use
- Hypotension secondary to ACE inhibitor and Ca channel blocker
- Worsening of renal azotemia with dextran use
- Thromboembolic disease as a result of abnormal antithrombin and protein C abnormalities
- Bleeding tendency from aspirin, warfarin use
- Gastrointestinal (GI) ulceration as a result of azotemia or aspirin therapy

RECOMMENDED MONITORING

Stable animals may be monitored every 3 to 4 months. Rechecks should be more frequent when changes are made in therapy or when indicated by changes in clinical signs.

- Physical examination
- Urine protein:creatinine ratio
- Serum/blood urea nitrogen (BUN), serum creatinine, and serum phosphorus levels
- Serum albumin
- BP
- Urinalysis and culture

PROGNOSIS AND OUTCOME

- The prognosis of PLN is extremely variable, depending on cause and severity of renal compromise.
- If an underlying disease can be identified and treated, the prognosis may be good.
- If it is not possible to identify or correct an underlying disease process, PLN is usually progressive.
- Animals with PLN may be medically managed for variable periods of time, even when uremic signs develop.
- In general, the prognosis for animals with renal amyloidosis is worse than that of GN.
- Familial renal diseases often begin at a young age and are rapidly progressive with a poor prognosis.
- When glomerulosclerosis is associated with end-stage renal disease, the prognosis is poor.
- Animals with membranous nephropathy may have a better prognosis with appropriate treatment. It is often slowly progressive, and the animal can occasionally go into remission.

PEARLS & CONSIDERATIONS

COMMENTS

- Renal cortical biopsy is the only method to distinguish amyloidosis and GN. While treatment is impacted occasionally, it provides useful prognostic information.
- Shar-pei dogs and Abyssinian cats occasionally have a normal cortical biopsy since the amyloid may be deposited in the renal medulla.

PREVENTION

- Heartworm prophylaxis
- Tick prophylaxis
- Breeder education for dogs and cats with familial disease

CLIENT EDUCATION

Renal biopsy can help to definitively identify the disease process. This may be important for animals with familial renal disease.

SUGGESTED READING

Cook AK, Cowgill LD: Clinical and pathological features of protein-losing glomerular disease in the dog: A review of 137 cases (1985-1992). *J Am Anim Hosp Assoc* 32:313, 1996.

Grant DC, et al: Glomerulonephritis in dogs and cats: Diagnosis and treatment. *Comp Cont Ed Pract Vet* 23:9, 2001.

Grant DC, et al: Glomerulonephritis in dogs and cats: Glomerular function, pathophysiology, and clinical signs. *Comp Cont Ed Pract Vet* 23:8, 2001.

Littman MP, et al: Familial protein-losing enteropathy and protein-losing nephropathy in soft-coated wheaten terriers: 222 cases (1983-1997). *J Vet Intern Med* 14:68, 2000.

AUTHOR: **ANNE M. DALBY**

EDITOR: **LEAH A. COHN**

Protothecosis

BASIC INFORMATION

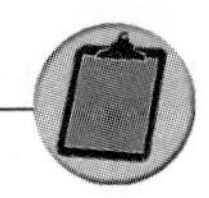

DEFINITION

A multisystemic disease caused by infection with *Prototheca* algal species

EPIDEMIOLOGY

SPECIES, AGE, SEX

- Cats: cutaneous infection.
- Dogs: disseminated infections are more common. Female dogs are overrepresented.

GENETICS AND BREED PREDISPOSITION: Collies and German shepherds appear to be predisposed to infection.

RISK FACTORS: Successful infection requires some degree of immunodeficiency in the host.

CONTAGION AND ZOONOSIS: *Prototheca* is an opportunistic pathogen found in soil, sewage, and tree slime flux. Clinical disease has been reported in multiple animal species including humans. Zoonotic transmission is not recorded, but immunocompromised persons should observe hygienic precautions around affected animals (and the environmental source).

GEOGRAPHY AND SEASONALITY: In North America, most cases are reported in the southeastern United States.

CLINICAL PRESENTATION

HISTORY, CHIEF COMPLAINT

- Colitis-type diarrhea: mucoid, bloody, and foul-smelling; intermittent or protracted. Weight loss possible in chronic cases.
- Many dogs with diarrhea have ocular lesions (owners may note red or cloudy eyes).
- Central nervous system (CNS) signs include depression, stumbling, falling, or head tilt.

PHYSICAL EXAM FINDINGS

- Palpable fluid filled bowel loops and blood on thermometer can be noted.
- Cachexia with muscle atrophy possible.
- Ocular manifestations include conjunctivitis, uveitis, vitreous clouding, and acute blindness due to retinal detachment.
- Neurologic examination findings are consistent with disseminated CNS disease; asymmetric signs of ataxia, head tilt, circling, and paresis are reported in fewer cases.
- Mucocutaneous ulceration, ulcerative, and/or nodular cutaneous lesions: less common.

ETIOLOGY AND PATHOPHYSIOLOGY

- *P. zopfii* and *P. wickerhamii* are the two algae species responsible for clinical disease. Immunosuppression due to concurrent disease, administration of immunosuppressive agents, or genetic predisposition at time of exposure are considered key to development and persistence of infection.
- *Prototheca* organisms can be found in the kidney (where they may cause renal failure), liver, heart, intestine, brain, and eyes of infected animals.

DIAGNOSIS

DIFFERENTIAL DIAGNOSIS

- Bloody diarrhea: parvovirus infection, clostridial infection, salmon poisoning, giardiasis, *Salmonella* enteritis, inflammatory bowel disease/ulcerative colitis, rectal adenocarcinoma, pythiosis, whipworm infection, coagulopathies caused by tick-borne diseases or rodenticide poisoning, and gastrointestinal (GI) lymphoma.
- In dogs with protothecal colitis, ocular lesions, and/or neurologic signs, systemic infectious diseases (e.g., mycoses), and lymphoma are important differential diagnoses.

INITIAL DATABASE

- Complete blood count (CBC) is usually unremarkable. Serum chemistry analysis usually shows mild increases in liver enzymes (alkaline phosphatase [ALP] and alanine aminotransferase [ALT]).
- Urinalysis usually is unremarkable but inflammatory urine sediment may be seen indicating possible renal involvement. Protothecal organisms have been isolated from the urine of dogs with renal failure secondary to renal invasion.
- Fecal analysis consisting of Sheather's flotation and ZnSO4 flotation is indicated in all suspected cases; *Prototheca* is occasionally found this way (many false-negative results).

ADVANCED OR CONFIRMATORY TESTING

- Organisms can be demonstrated in the cytology of a rectal scrape (e.g., obtained with a uterine or bone marrow grafting-type curette) stained with Diff Quik or Wright's stain. Many false-negative results.
- Intestinal biopsy (surgical or endoscopic) may yield a diagnosis when lesser invasive means are unsuccessful.
- A complete ophthalmic examination is indicated in suspected or confirmed cases, since ocular lesions may be missed initially. Organisms can be recovered from vitreous centesis.
- Neurologic examination should be performed on dogs showing CNS signs. Spinal radiographs or CT may be needed in dogs showing paresis. Organisms can be recovered from cerebrospinal fluid, which indicates severe clinical disease and dissemination.
- Culture can be performed on rectal scrape or any biopsy samples.
- Fluorescent antibody testing can differentiate *P. zopfii* from *P. wickerhamii*.

TREATMENT

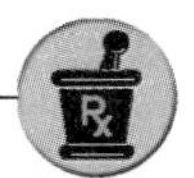

THERAPEUTIC GOAL(S)

- Abort infection
- Reduce or prevent further dissemination of infection particularly to CNS
- Decrease frequency and volume of diarrhea

ACUTE GENERAL TREATMENT

- Initial treatment consists of parenteral fluid therapy.
- Antifungal treatment (amphotericin B with/without one of the following: itraconazole, ketoconazole, tetracycline, doxycycline) is beneficial to prevent immediate dissemination.
- Amphotericin B: Patient must be hydrated. Dose: 0.25-0.5 mg/kg diluted in 5% dextrose and given IV q 48h to total cumulative dose 8-10 mg/kg or first signs of nephrotoxicity (monitor blood urea nitrogen, creatinine daily).
- Liposomal amphotericin B: as above, but SQ and for a shorter time period. Less nephrotoxic but still requires monitoring.

CHRONIC TREATMENT

Tetracycline 25 mg/kg PO q 8h for 30 days, or doxycycline 5-10 mg/kg PO q 24h for 30 days, or ketoconazole or itraconazole 5-10 mg/kg PO q 24h with food for 30 days. Limited or no success in most cases.

DRUG INTERACTIONS

Ketoconazole, itraconazole: vomiting, inappetence, and elevated liver enzymes possible. If such signs occur, the drug therapy should be stopped and liver enzymes evaluated.

POSSIBLE COMPLICATIONS

- Treatment of concurrent infections and secondary *Escherichia coli* and *Clostridium* infections can reduce frequency and volume of diarrhea.
- Metronidazole 7.5-15 mg/kg PO q 12h can be used for *Clostridium* overgrowth.

RECOMMENDED MONITORING

- Monthly monitoring of the success of therapy is recommended.
- Rectal scrapes with cytology and culture, ophthalmologic examinations, CBC, serum chemistry, and urinalysis are recommended.

PROGNOSIS AND OUTCOME

- Prognosis is poor especially with CNS signs, multiple organ involvement, and/or renal failure
- Survival for >1 year has been reported in some animals with only GI and ocular lesions

PEARLS & CONSIDERATIONS

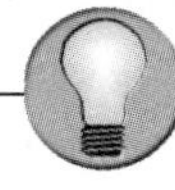

COMMENTS

Prototheca is a ubiquitous organism and only an opportunistic pathogen in the immunocompromised dog. Further immunosuppressive therapy with glucocorticoids or other agents is contraindicated and counterproductive.

PREVENTION

If a potential area of patient exposure can be identified, the patient and possibly humans should be prevented from further contact with this environment.

CLIENT EDUCATION

The disease is not transmissible. However, owners who are immunocompromised should be cautious in handling the feces of infected animals.

SUGGESTED READING

Greene CE: Protothecosis. In CE Greene (ed): *Infectious Diseases of the Dog and Cat.* Philadelphia, WB Saunders, 1998, pp 430–435.

Hollingsworth SR: Canine protothecosis. *Vet Clin North Am (Small An Pract)* 30(5):1091–1101, 2000.

AUTHOR: **SARALYN SMITH-CARR**

EDITOR: **DEBRA L. ZORAN**

Protozoal Enteritides

BASIC INFORMATION

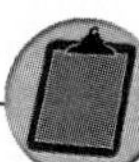

DEFINITION

Infection of the small or large intestine with protozoal organisms; includes giardiasis, trichomoniasis, amebiasis, balantidiasis, coccidiosis

SYNONYM(S)

Balantidium coli (balantidiasis)
Cystoisospora or related organisms (coccidiosis)
Entamoeba histolytica (amebiasis)
Giardia lamblia (giardiasis)
Pentatrichomonas hominis or *Tritrichomonas foetus* (trichomoniasis)

EPIDEMIOLOGY

SPECIES, AGE, SEX

- Giardiasis, trichomoniasis, and amebiasis occur in dogs, cats, humans, and many other domestic species.
- Balantidiasis is common in pigs and can occur in dogs and humans.
- *T. foetus* infection prinicipally causes reproductive problems in cattle but may also cause enteric signs in cats.
- *Cystoisospora* enteritis may affect dogs, cats, pigs, fowl, and other domestic animals.
- Young animals are at higher risk of developing overt, and potentially more severe, clinical signs.

RISK FACTORS: Overcrowding, kennel boarding, unsanitary conditions, and immunosuppression increase the risk of protozoal enteritis.

CONTAGION AND ZOONOSIS

- All of the protozoal organisms are infectious via a fecal-oral route.
- *Cystoisospora* spp.: Each species of the organism is host-specific and cannot be transmitted to other domestic animal species.
- *G. lamblia, B. coli,* and *P. hominis* enteritides pose a known or suspected zoonotic risk.
- *E. histolytica* can be transmitted from humans to dogs or cats but generally not from dogs or cats to humans. Dogs and cats do not shed the infective cyst form of *E. histolytica*.

GEOGRAPHY AND SEASONALITY: Protozoal enteritides are distributed worldwide with increased infection rates in areas of poverty and overcrowding.

ASSOCIATED CONDITIONS AND DISORDERS: Many protozoal enteritides are detected as a secondary infection due to an underlying primary gastrointestinal (GI) disease.

CLINICAL PRESENTATION

DISEASE FORMS/SUBTYPES: Most infections with protozoa are subclinical. However, severe infections or infections in young or immunosuppressed animals may be serious with overt, potentially debilitating clinical signs.

HISTORY, CHIEF COMPLAINT: The most common clinical sign is acute to chronic diarrhea. Some animals may be depressed or occasionally vomit. *G. lamblia* and *Cystoisospora* spp. may cause small or large bowel diarrhea, while other protozoa generally cause only large bowel diarrhea.

PHYSICAL EXAM FINDINGS: Physical examination findings may be nonspecific and include depression, mild to severe dehydration, and discomfort on abdominal palpation with gas or fluid-filled intestinal loops. In milder cases, no physical anormalities may be present.

ETIOLOGY AND PATHOPHYSIOLOGY

- Transmission of protozoal enteritides is fecal-oral.
- Infective cysts are ingested from the environment and commonly from fecally-contaminated water.
- Upon exposure to intestinal enzymes, cysts open releasing trophozoites that mature and attach to the intestinal epithelium.
- *G. lamblia* and *Cystoisospora* spp. remain on the surface of the epithelium, causing damage to the microvilli.
- *Entamoeba* and *Balantidium* spp. may invade the colonic wall causing ulceration.
- *P. hominis* is considered rarely pathogenic.

DIAGNOSIS

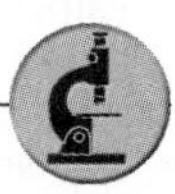

DIFFERENTIAL DIAGNOSIS

- Young dogs: parvoviral, distemper viral, and bacterial enteritides; enteritis caused by parasites (*Toxocara, Ancylostoma, Trichuris* spp.).
- Young cats: feline panleukopenia, feline leukemia virus (FeLV).
- *Sarcocystis* oocysts may be observed on fecal examination; however, this coccidian is not pathogenic in dogs or cats. Herbivores are the intermediate host and develop parasitic cysts in muscle and nervous tissues after consuming the infected feces of dogs.

- *Hammondia* and *Besnoitia* oocysts may be seen on fecal examination. These coccidians are also nonpathogenic.
- Older animals with acute to chronic diarrhea may have a primary intestinal disorder, such as inflammatory bowel disease or neoplasia (dogs and cats), ulcerative colitis (dogs), or feline immunodeficiency virus-associated enteritis (cats).

INITIAL DATABASE

- Direct fecal smear may reveal trophozoites.
- A zinc-sulfate concentration fecal may reveal protozoal cysts.
- A complete blood count (CBC) and chemistry panel are nonspecific but may help rule out other diseases.

ADVANCED OR CONFIRMATORY TESTING

- Multiple fecal examinations may be necessary to find trophozoites or cysts, which may be shed intermittently. Three fecal examinations performed over a period of 3 to 5 days are recommended in challenging cases.
- A therapeutic trial with fenbendazole and metronidazole may be helpful in animals with chronic diarrhea that have multiple negative fecal samples.

TREATMENT

THERAPEUTIC GOAL(S)

- Control clinical signs
- Eradicate the protozoa from the intestinal tract

ACUTE GENERAL TREATMENT

- Fenbendazole 50 mg/kg PO q 24h for 3 to 5 days is the current treatment of choice for giardiasis.
- Metronidazole 10-20 mg/kg PO q 12-24h for 5 to 7 days is an effective treatment for enteritis caused by *Pentatrichomonas, Entamoeba*, and *Balantidium* spp.
- *Cystoisospora* enteritis may be treated with amprolium 110-200 mg/kg PO q 24h (dogs), or 50-60 mg/kg PO q 24h (cats), or sulfadimethoxine for 14 days. Combination therapy may be more effective and allow use of lower doses with fewer side effects.
- There are no effective treatments known at this time for eradication of *T. foetus* in cats. Paromomycin 125-160 mg/kg PO q 12h for 5 days may be effective, but some cases of renal toxicity have been reported with the use of this drug in cats.

PROGNOSIS AND OUTCOME

- Prognosis for most protozoal enteritides is good. Recurrent infection is possible and complete elimination of the organism may be challenging because some protozoa are commensal organisms and opportunistic pathogens.
- The prognosis for elimination of *T. foetus* from cats is guarded although treatment may reduce clinical signs.

PEARLS & CONSIDERATIONS

COMMENTS

- Protozoal enteritides are often secondary infections in adult animals. If appropriate antiprotozoal therapy is not effective, clinicians should seek an underlying disease.
- Protozoal enteritis should not be eliminated as a possible cause of diarrhea in a young animal based on a single negative fecal result.

PREVENTION

Prevention of overcrowding and maintaining a clean environment for young animals will help prevent protozoal infections.

CLIENT EDUCATION

Clients should be advised to seek medical attention if their pet has been diagnosed with protozoal enteritis. *G. lamblia, B. coli*, and *P. hominis* enteritides carry a zoonotic risk.

SUGGESTED READING

Barr SC: Enteric protozoal infections. In Greene CE (ed): *Infectious Diseases of the Dog and Cat*. St. Louis, WB Saunders, 1998, pp 482-491.

Dubey JP, Greene CE: Enteric coccidiosis. In Greene CE (ed): *Infectious Diseases of the Dog and Cat*. St. Louis, WB Saunders, 1998, pp 510-518.

Washabau RJ: Gastrointestinal infectious diseases of dogs and cats. *Western Veterinary Conference*, Las Vegas, NV, Feb. 15-19, 2004. Available from: www.vin.com/Members/Proceedings/Proceedings.plx?CID=WVC2004&O=VIN. Accessed July 31, 2006.

AUTHOR: **KATHRYN TAYLOR**

EDITOR: **DOUGLASS K. MACINTIRE**

Pruritus

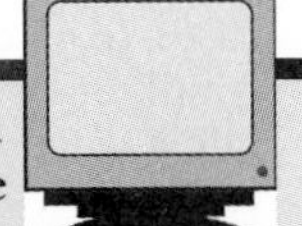

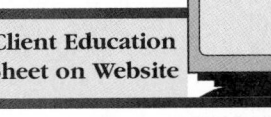

Client Education Sheet on Website

BASIC INFORMATION

DEFINITION

The unpleasant sensation that triggers the desire to scratch, chew, rub, lick, or bite at the skin

SYNONYM(S)

Itch

EPIDEMIOLOGY

SPECIES, AGE, SEX

- Any species
- Sex and age of onset depend on the underlying etiology
- Contagious acarioses: more common in young animals.
- Canine atopy is first seen in young adults (1 to 3 years of age).
- Food allergy may develop at any age.

CLINICAL PRESENTATION

HISTORY, CHIEF COMPLAINT: Animals scratch, chew, rub, lick, or bite at the skin. In addition, cats can be secretive lickers and present only for extensive self-induced alopecia.

PHYSICAL EXAM FINDINGS

- Skin lesions vary according to etiology.
- Self-induced alopecia, excoriation, and erythema are common findings.
- Typically, no primary lesion is noted in canine atopy.
- Papules and/or pustules are noted in infectious or parasitic conditions.
- In cats: miliary dermatitis, eosinophilic granuloma complex, self-induced symmetric alopecia, or self-induced ulcerative facial dermatitis

ETIOLOGY AND PATHOPHYSIOLOGY

- Etiologies of pruritus are numerous.
- For most parasitic infestations, a hypersensitivity reaction develops which is responsible for most, if not all, of the

pruritus (often disproportionate to the number of parasites found).
- Pyoderma and yeast dermatitis are frequent causes of pruritus in dogs but are uncommon in cats.

DIAGNOSIS

DIFFERENTIAL DIAGNOSIS

- Parasitic: fleas, contagious acarioses (*Sarcoptes, Notoedres, Cheyletiella, Otodectes* spp.), lice, and *Trombicula* and *Pelodera* spp.
- Bacterial: staphylococcal pyoderma
- Fungal: *Malassezia* sp. dermatitis and otitis
- Allergic: flea bite hypersensitivity, atopic dermatitis, food hypersensitivity, contact hypersensitivity, drug reaction
- Miscellaneous: calcinosis cutis, cutaneous lymphoma

INITIAL DATABASE

- Complete history and dermatologic exam
- Skin scrapings
- Skin cytologic examination
- Wood's lamp and dermatophyte culture (in cats)

ADVANCED OR CONFIRMATORY TESTING

- Therapeutic trial with broad-spectrum antiparasitic agents (this is an integral part of the case work-up).
- Clinicians occasionally use therapeutic trials with antibiotics or antifungal agents in dogs to document the contribution of bacteria and yeast in the degree of pruritus seen.
- Hypoallergenic dietary trial (ideally using home-cooked novel protein and carbohydrate sources).
- Intradermal skin test. This is the preferred test for atopic dermatitis.
- Skin biopsies are useful in unusual cases (e.g., calcinosis cutis, cutaneous lymphoma). The biopsy may corroborate a diagnosis of allergic skin disease but rarely confirms the specific cause.

TREATMENT

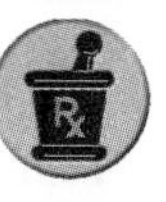

THERAPEUTIC GOAL(S)

- Monotherapy when possible to facilitate interpretation of treatment response.
- When doing therapeutic trials, the best treatment regimen available should be used in order to eradicate parasites or infections, so interpretation of response is clear.

ACUTE GENERAL TREATMENT

An acute intense pruritic episode can be treated with IM or IV short-acting glucocorticoids (dexamethasone sodium phosphate 0.1-0.2 mg/kg) followed by a few days of prednisone or prednisolone at 1 mg/kg PO q 24h. Short-term use of glucocorticoids seldom causes serious problems.

CHRONIC TREATMENT

- Immunotherapy (hyposensitization) should be attempted when possible.
- For long-term management of canine atopy, clinicians must find alternatives to long-term administration of glucocorticoids. In selected cases, however, some dogs can be maintained safely on long-term oral glucocorticoid if the maintenance dose is relatively low and/or if the treatment is intermittent. For example, a maintenance dose of 0.2-0.3 mg/kg q 48h and/or a total annual dose of 30-50 mg/kg or less are rarely responsible for significant side effects.
- A glucocorticoid-antihistamine combination containing prednisolone 2 mg and trimeprazine 5 mg generally controls pruritus better than an equivalent dose of prednisone alone, reducing the risk of glucocorticoid side effects. Recommended induction and maintenance doses of prednisolone are typically 30-40% less than when using prednisone alone, when using a similar treatment regimen (e.g., q 24h administration for a week, then same dose q 48h for a week, then weaning to the lowest possible dose at q 48h).
- Antihistamines, in combination with omega-3 essential fatty acids (EFA), may alleviate pruritus in up to 30% of cases. Oral antihistamines shown to be of benefit for dogs include hydroxyzine 2.2 mg/kg q 8-12h; diphenhydramine 2.2 mg/kg q 8-12h; chlorpheniramine 0.4 mg/kg q 8-12h; clemastine 0.05-0.1 mg/kg q 12h; and amitriptyline 1 mg/kg q 12h. Chlorpheniramine and amitriptyline have also been useful in cats. Drowsiness, lethargy, or nervousness are sometimes noted and can be minimized by reducing frequency of administration and dose. Nonsedating antihistamines have not generally been effective.
- Omega-3 EFA in capsule form as a supplement (eicosapentaenoic acid 30 mg/kg PO, q 24h) or in food may help manage pruritus by decreasing the production of proinflammatory mediators. The optimum ratio of supplementation within the diet appears to lie between 10:1 and 5:1, omega-6/omega-3.
- Cyclosporine microemulsion (e.g., Neoral, Atopica) 5 mg/kg PO q 24h is an effective alternative when glucocorticoids are contraindicated (e.g., diabetes mellitus, pancreatitis).
- In food hypersensitivity, clinicians must find a commercial hypoallergenic diet that maintains the animal free of clinical signs.
- In flea bite hypersensitivity, maintain an effective flea elimination treatment.

RECOMMENDED MONITORING

Animals receiving chronic glucocorticoid therapy should be monitored every 6 months for signs of iatrogenic hyperglucocorticism or other complications (e.g., urinary tract infection, pyoderma).

PROGNOSIS AND OUTCOME

- Varies according to the etiology.
- Excellent for most parasitic and infectious skin problems and food hypersensitivity.
- Atopic dermatitis is an incurable disease that requires long-term management of pruritus.

PEARLS & CONSIDERATIONS

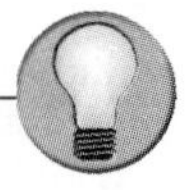

COMMENTS

- Treatment of pruritic dermatoses does not always imply use of antipruritic drugs *sensu stricto*. In fact, antiparasitic drugs, antibiotics, and antifungal drugs (for yeast dermatitis), which are not inherently antipruritic, are among the most useful antipruritic drugs. They have a key role in pruritus management. Superficial pyoderma is a frequent cause of pruritus in dogs.
- Always rule out parasitic and infectious causes of pruritus before administering long-term steroidal or nonsteroidal antipruritic drugs or before initiating a food trial.
- If pruritus is refractory to a usual maintenance dose of glucocorticoid (i.e., >0.5 mg/kg q 48h of prednisone in dogs), consider the following diagnoses: sarcoptic acariosis, yeast dermatitis, pyoderma, food hypersensitivity, calcinosis cutis, contact allergic dermatitis, epitheliotropic lymphoma.
- More than one disease may be contributing to pruritus; for example, dogs with atopic dermatitis often have secondary bacterial and/or yeast skin infections.
- In cats, prednisone is generally not as effective as other glucocorticoids at equivalent doses. Use oral prenisolone, methylprednisolone, dexamethasone, or triamcinolone.

CLIENT EDUCATION

Owners of dogs with canine atopy must be well informed of the chronic and multifaceted aspect of the disease.

SUGGESTED READING

Scott DW, Miller WH, Griffin CE: In *Muller and Kirk's Small Animal Dermatology*, ed 6. Philadelphia, WB Saunders, 2001.

AUTHOR: **MANON PARADIS**
EDITOR: **JAN A. HALL**

Pseudopregnancy

BASIC INFORMATION

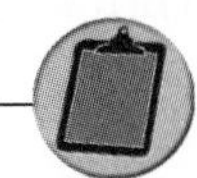

DEFINITION

Pseudopregnancy is a syndrome observed in nonpregnant diestrous or anestrous bitches. It is characterized by different degrees of maternal behavior, mammary gland enlargement, and lactation.

SYNONYM(S)

False pregnancy
Nervous anorexia
Pseudocyesis

EPIDEMIOLOGY

SPECIES, AGE, SEX: Postpubertal female dogs of any age; cats are not commonly affected.

GENETICS AND BREED PREDISPOSITION: Any breed can be affected, although dalmatian, basset hound, and pointer breed dogs are more frequently affected.

RISK FACTORS: Exogenous administration of progestins, diestrous ovariectomy, and hypothyroidism may trigger its occurrence.

ASSOCIATED CONDITIONS AND DISORDERS: Pseudopregnancy can coexist with other diestrous diseases, such as pyometra.

CLINICAL PRESENTATION

DISEASE FORMS/SUBTYPES: Depending on the intensity of clinical signs, pseudopregnancy can be classified as:

- Covert (physiologic although recognizable from the rest of the estrous cycle)
- Overt, which can even become a clinical problem (clinical pseudopregnancy)

HISTORY, CHIEF COMPLAINT: History reveals the occurrence of estrus at 6 to 12 weeks previously without an ensuing pregnancy. The chief complaints mainly focus on mammary problems (engorgement, lactation, licking of the glands) and abnormalities associated with aberrant maternal behavior (nesting, digging, adoption of animals or objects). In addition, the bitch may have depression or anxiety, anorexia, and excessive vocalization (whining).

PHYSICAL EXAM FINDINGS: Physical exam reveals some degree of mammary enlargement, which can vary from turgid nipples to an important engorgement and galactostasis. Mammary enlargement is most evident in the caudal pair of glands. Mammary dermatitis is occasionally present if excessive licking occurs. Mastitis may also be present.

ETIOLOGY AND PATHOPHYSIOLOGY

The high plasma concentration of prolactin at the end of the luteal phase when progesterone concentrations are decreasing is associated with the development and maintenance of pseudopregnancy. Individual and breed sensitivity to these hormonal changes and environmental factors have been hypothesized to influence its occurrence.

DIAGNOSIS

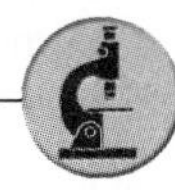

DIFFERENTIAL DIAGNOSIS

- Pregnancy.
- Pyometra.
- Mastitis.
- Mammary tumors.
- Any other cause of anorexia, depression, or anxiety should be ruled out.
- Pseudopregnancy can even coexist with pyometra, mastitis, and mammary tumors.

INITIAL DATABASE

- History and physical findings (as already described)
- Complete blood count (CBC) is normal

ADVANCED OR CONFIRMATORY TESTING

Use ultrasonography or radiography for confirming the absence of pregnancy

TREATMENT

THERAPEUTIC GOAL(S)

- Eliminate or treat predisposing factors, such as exogenous administration of progestins and hypothyroidism
- Avoid stimulation on the mammary glands (e.g., padding [either hot or cold], touching, or licking)
- Discourage maternal behavior, using aversion methods
- Decrease plasma prolactin with dopaminergic agonist or antiserotonergic drugs
- Avoid steroid hormones (progestins/androgens) because they usually postpone the problem and cause many side effects

ACUTE GENERAL TREATMENT

- If necessary, Elizabethan collars can be used for preventing licking and self-milking.
- Administer dopaminergic agonists with food to reduce digestive side effects: cabergoline 5 μg/kg PO q 24h for 5 to 7 days.
- See Mastitis, p 688; Acute Moist Dermatitis, p 31.

CHRONIC TREATMENT

Clinical, chronic, unresponsive, or recurring pseudopregnancy cases should be treated surgically (ovariectomy) after the acute phase of the syndrome has been controlled and during anestrus.

DRUG INTERACTIONS

- Avoid administering phenothiazine drugs during pseudopregnancy because they increase plasma prolactin.
- Do not administer metergoline for anxious and restless bitches because this drug could potentiate pseudopregnancy behavior.

POSSIBLE COMPLICATIONS

- Mammary dermatitis and mastitis are the most frequent complications and may have an influence in perpetuating the problem.
- Repeated episodes of pseudopregnancy have been hypothetically associated with the future development of mammary tumors.

PROGNOSIS AND OUTCOME

Pseudopregnancy typically resolves spontaneously within a few weeks (2 or 3 weeks) from its onset; however, pseudopregnancy can occasionally persist until the next estrous cycle.

PEARLS & CONSIDERATIONS

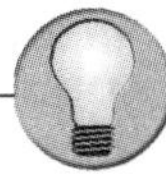

COMMENTS

- Pseudopregnancy is a good indicator of ovulatory estrous cycles.
- Predisposed bitches usually suffer the syndrome after each estrous cycle, with the disorder becoming more severe throughout life.

PREVENTION

- Ovariectomy in predisposed bitches.
- Pregnancy does not prevent future episodes.

CLIENT EDUCATION

Teach clients to recognize pseudopregnancy and to ask for treatment if it becomes clinically relevant.

SUGGESTED READING

Gobello C, et al: Dioestrous ovariectomy: A model to study the role of progesterone in the onset of canine pseudopregnancy. *J Reprod Fertil Suppl* 57:55, 2001.

Gobello, et al: Canine pseudopregnancy: A review. In Concannon PW, et al (eds): *Recent Advances in Small Animal Reproduction*. Ithaca, NY, International Veterinary Information Service, 2001;A1215.0801.

Harvey MJ, et al: A study of the aetiology of pseudopregnancy in the bitch and the effect of cabergoline therapy. *Vet Rec* 17;144(16):433, 1999.

Lawler DF, et al: Influence of restricted food intake on estrous cycles and pseudopregnancies in dogs. *Am J Vet Res* 60(7):820, 1999.

Okkens AC, et al: Plasma prolactin concentration and the effect of metergoline in pseudopregnant Afghan hounds. *Tijdschr Diergeneeskd* 1,125(3):81, 2000.

AUTHOR: **CRISTINA GOBELLO**
EDITOR: **MICHELLE A. KUTZLER**

Pseudorabies

BASIC INFORMATION

DEFINITION

Pseudorabies results from infection with pseudorabies virus (PRV), an alphaherpesvirus in the family Herpesviridae. An economically important disease of swine, pseudorabies is capable of causing subclinical, neurologic, or respiratory disease in pigs and causing severe and almost inevitably fatal central nervous system (CNS) disease in dogs and cats.

SYNONYM(S)

Aujeszky's disease
Mad itch

EPIDEMIOLOGY

SPECIES, AGE, SEX: Dogs and cats are sporadically affected with pseudorabies (uncommon). Pigs are the primary reservoir of the virus because they have become well adapted to the virus and are often only subclinically affected.

RISK FACTORS

- Pets living in areas where pseudorabies virus is enzootic in the swine population
- Feeding raw pork from endemic areas to dogs and cats

CONTAGION AND ZOONOSIS

- Pseudorabies virus may be found in porcine respiratory secretions, saliva, blood, and in the CNS and tonsillar tissues. Dogs and cats are commonly infected via the oral route after ingesting contaminated porcine tissue. Pseudorabies has also reportedly been transmitted to a dog by either biting or being bitten by an infected pig.
- Pseudorabies is not considered a zoonotic disease, but seroconversion does occur.

GEOGRAPHY AND SEASONALITY: Pseudorabies can be found in Europe, Mexico, Brazil, Venezuela, Cuba, New Zealand, Samoa, Southeast Asia, and portions of the United States.

CLINICAL PRESENTATION

HISTORY, CHIEF COMPLAINT: Acute onset and rapid progression of neurologic signs until death occurs (usually within 2 to 3 days of disease onset). Initial signs may include lethargy, depression, restlessness, or aggression and occasionally vomiting and diarrhea. Hypersalivation is commonly noted. Intense pruritus, usually of the head region, is probably the most clinically striking and consistent sign of pseudorabies. Animals will frequently excoriate the skin of the face and ears secondary to violent scratching.

PHYSICAL EXAM FINDINGS

- Pruritus with swelling, erythema, excoriation, or ulceration of the skin secondary to self-mutilation, especially of the face and head
- Altered mentation
- Ptyalism
- Cranial nerve deficits indicative of a brainstem lesion(s)
- Dyspnea
- Seizures

ETIOLOGY AND PATHOPHYSIOLOGY

- Once infection with pseudorabies virus has occurred, the virus travels retrograde along peripheral nerves from the site of inoculation to the CNS.
- Damage to brain parenchyma results from inflammation and interference of normal neuronal function by the virus.
- Microscopic lesions are located almost exclusively in the brainstem. The incubation period for pseudorabies in dogs and cats is 3 to 6 days.

DIAGNOSIS

DIFFERENTIAL DIAGNOSIS

- Rabies
- Canine distemper
- Neurotoxicoses

INITIAL DATABASE

- A provisional diagnosis of pseudorabies is usually made on clinical suspicion of the disease. Confirmatory testing is required for definitive diagnosis.
- There are no characteristic hematologic or biochemical abnormalities associated with pseudorabies.

ADVANCED OR CONFIRMATORY TESTING

- Definitive diagnosis of pseudorabies has classically been made postmortem. Histopathologic abnormalities are generally limited to the brainstem and include perivascular cuffing, multifocal gliosis, neuronal degeneration, and weak eosinophilic inclusions within the nuclei of glial cells and neurons.
- Immunohistochemical techniques can be used to identify viral antigen in fixed tissue sections (brain, tonsils).
- Alternatively, inoculation of cell cultures with brain homogenate for virus isolation can be performed. Cultures are observed for cytologic changes characteristic of herpesvirus infection, and immunofluorescent techniques can be applied to the cultures to identify pseudorabies virus.

TREATMENT

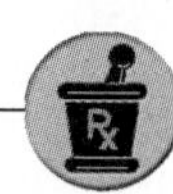

THERAPEUTIC GOAL(S)

With very few exceptions, the treatment of pseudorabies in dogs and cats is futile due to the generally unavoidable fatal outcome. If treatment is initiated, it is aimed at controlling the major clinical signs and providing supportive care until the animal recovers (rare) or dies.

ACUTE GENERAL TREATMENT

- Sedation or anesthesia as required for control of self-mutilation and/or seizures
- IV fluids if needed

PROGNOSIS AND OUTCOME

Grave prognosis; despite treatment, death usually occurs within 2 to 3 days of the onset of clinical signs.

PEARLS & CONSIDERATIONS

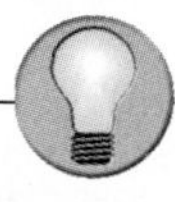

COMMENTS

Vaccination of dogs and cats against pseudorabies virus (usually in endemic areas) is possible but of questionable efficacy in the prevention of disease.

PREVENTION

Preventing contact with infected pigs or contaminated pork products is paramount to the prevention of pseudorabies in dogs and cats.

SUGGESTED READING

Buergelt CD, et al: Pseudorabies in two dogs. *Vet Med* 95:439–442, 2000.

Vandevelde M: Pseudorabies. In Greene CE (ed): *Infectious Diseases of the Dog and Cat*, ed 2. Philadephia, WB Saunders, 1998, pp 126–128.

AUTHOR: **JODI D. SMITH**
EDITOR: **DOUGLASS K. MACINTIRE**

Ptyalism

BASIC INFORMATION

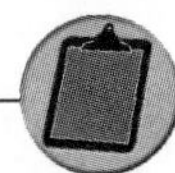

DEFINITION

Production of excessive amounts of saliva, manifesting as drooling

SYNONYM(S)

Hypersalivation
Polysialia
Sialorrhea

EPIDEMIOLOGY

SPECIES, AGE, SEX

- No species, age, or sex predilection except as dependent on underlying etiology
- Young animals: portosystemic shunts, seizure disorders
- Older animals: oral neoplasia, such as malignant melanomas (dogs), and squamous cell carcinoma (SCC) (cats)

GENETICS AND BREED PREDISPOSITION: Predisposition dependent on underlying cause.

RISK FACTORS

- Trauma of oral/pharyngeal region or nerves
- Exposure to toxins
- Esophageal disorders (esophagitis, esophageal obstruction)
- Oral foreign bodies
- Severe dental disease and/or dental abscesses
- Metabolic or physical disorders causing nausea or abdominal pain
- Primary or secondary neurologic disorders affecting saliva production
- Nausea
- Unvaccinated pets exposed to contagious diseases that may cause oral lesions or metabolic disorders

Note: Certain conformations of the lips may allow the excessive leakage of saliva from the sides of the mouth without reflecting an increase in saliva production.

CONTAGION AND ZOONOSIS

- Zoonotic: rabies
- Contagion: viral infections causing oral lesions, such as calicivirus in cats

CLINICAL PRESENTATION

HISTORY, CHIEF COMPLAINT: All or some may be present:

- Dysphagia
- Pawing at mouth
- Halitosis
- Oral discomfort with oral or pharyngeal causes
- Anorexia or weight loss
- Coughing and/or dyspnea (from aspiration pneumonia)
- Gagging or retching with esophageal or gastric causes
- Seizures, facial twitching, behavioral changes possible with intoxications

PHYSICAL EXAM FINDINGS

- Saliva around mouth, salivary staining of fur
- Oral lesions, including masses, foreign bodies, abscesses, stomatitis, gingivitis, or other dental diseases
- Swelling of salivary glands, facial paralysis, atrophy of temporal or facial muscles
- Loss of gag reflex, inability to use tongue, dysphagia
- Mentation changes, seizures, tremors, or anxiety
- Painful abdomen
- Nausea

ETIOLOGY AND PATHOPHYSIOLOGY

- Etiology:
  - Oral lesions: stomatitis, gingivitis, dental disease, neoplasia, foreign bodies.
  - Neurologic: peripheral nerve injury affecting swallowing, movement of tongue, pharynx; central nervous system (CNS) lesions, including neoplasia and infectious disorders such as rabies and feline infectious peritonitis (cats).
  - Neuromuscular disorders (myasthenia gravis causing megaesophagus; masticatory myositis).
  - Metabolic: hepatic disease (portosystemic shunts), renal disease, nausea.
  - Toxins: caustic or noxious substances, pesticides (organophosphates), drugs (marijuana).
  - Immune disease: polymyositis, pemphigus.
  - Pain, anxiety, excitement, fear.
- Pathophysiology:
  - Oral secretions are produced by submandibular, parotid, and sublingual salivary glands. Innervation to salivary glands is controlled by the autonomic nervous system with primary control by the parasympathetic nervous system. Many environmental, physical, or metabolic events may stimulate increased saliva production.

DIAGNOSIS

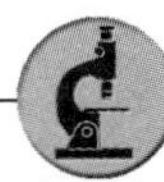

DIFFERENTIAL DIAGNOSIS

Ptyalism must be differentiated from drooling caused by certain conformations of the lips (but in which the amount of saliva produced by the salivary glands is normal). History (ptyalism is usually recent in onset, whereas confirmation-associated drooling is chronic) and physical examination of the lips are generally sufficient for correct identification.

INITIAL DATABASE

- Complete blood count (CBC) to evaluate for anemia and evidence of infectious/inflammatory disease
- Serum biochemistry profile and urinalysis to evaluate for metabolic disorders
- Neurologic exam
- Thoracic, abdominal, and neck/head radiographs

ADVANCED OR CONFIRMATORY TESTING

- Oral examination with sedation or anesthesia
- Serum bile acids if history, exam, and minimum database consistent with liver disorder
- Abdominal ultrasound
- Electroencephalogram (EEG)/CT scan and MRI to evaluate CNS lesions
- Endoscopy to evaluate esophageal or gastric lesions

- Toxin screens
- Specific tests, such as acetylcholine (ACh) receptor antibody testing for myasthenia gravis

TREATMENT

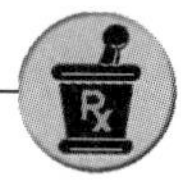

THERAPEUTIC GOAL(S)

Resolution of underlying cause

ACUTE GENERAL TREATMENT

Supportive and nonspecific; possible use of anticholinergics and antinausea or antianxiety medications; identification of underlying etiology and prevention of aspiration

CHRONIC TREATMENT

Treatment as appropriate for underlying etiology. Although surgical ligation or transposition of salivary ducts is sometimes performed in people with ptyalism, this surgery is usually not indicated in animals.

POSSIBLE COMPLICATIONS

- Anticholinergics often cause tachycardia, dry mouth, constipation, and behavioral changes; these require frequent dosing. Antiemetics, such as chlorpromazine, may cause sedation.
- Antisialagogues may reduce salivary output but do not stop salivation.

RECOMMENDED MONITORING

Monitor signs, including coughing, breathing difficulty, and fever, which may suggest aspiration of excessive saliva

PROGNOSIS AND OUTCOME

Fair to guarded prognosis depending on response to treatment of underlying etiology of disorder. Removal of foreign bodies, resolution of dental disease, repair of traumatic injury, and response to detoxification may have very favorable outcomes. Prognosis may be guarded with more serious disease processes, such as immune diseases and neoplasia.

PEARLS & CONSIDERATIONS

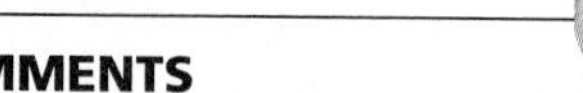

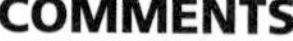

COMMENTS

Ptyalism is usually a sign of a more serious disorder and deserves attention aimed at identifying the underlying cause. In addition, many owners find that their pets' hypersalivation is unacceptable even if caused by minor problems and may cause them to choose euthanasia for the animals.

SUGGESTED READING

Hockstein NG, et al: Sialorrhea: A management challenge. *Am Fam Physician* 69(11): 2628–2634, 2004.

Langdon P, et al: Acquired portosystemic shunting in two cats. *J Am Anim Hosp Assoc* 38(1):21–27, 2002.

Mayhew PD, et al: Trigeminal neuropathy in dogs: A retrospective study of 29 cases (1991–2000). *J Am Anim Hosp Assoc* 38(3):262–270, 2002.

Sherding B: Diagnosis and management of feline esophageal disease. *World Small Animal Veterinary Association World Congress Proceedings,* Vancouver, 2001.

Simpson BS: Canine separation anxiety. *Compend Contin Educ Pract Vet* 22(4):328–338, 2000.

AUTHORS: **DIANA M. SCHROPP, ADAM J. REISS**

EDITOR: **ETIENNE CÔTÉ**

Pulmonary Contusion

BASIC INFORMATION

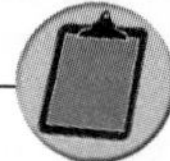

DEFINITION

A pulmonary contusion is a lesion consisting of intrapulmonary hemorrhage and inflammation secondary to blunt trauma

SYNONYM(S)

Traumatic lung injury

EPIDEMIOLOGY

SPECIES, AGE, SEX: Young male dogs are at increased risk of trauma.

GENETICS AND BREED PREDISPOSITION: None; larger dogs are more likely to roam unsupervised.

RISK FACTORS: Free-roaming behavior

GEOGRAPHY AND SEASONALITY: More common in warmer months.

ASSOCIATED CONDITIONS AND DISORDERS

- Pneumothorax
- Diaphragmatic hernia
- Flail chest
- Hit by car (HBC) injury
- Fracture

CLINICAL PRESENTATION

HISTORY, CHIEF COMPLAINT: Traumatic event; increased respiratory rate and effort.

PHYSICAL EXAM FINDINGS

- External evidence of trauma: cutaneous abrasions or lacerations, fractures
- Increased respiratory rate and effort
- Increased bronchovesicular sounds
- Pale mucous membranes
- Tachycardia

ETIOLOGY AND PATHOPHYSIOLOGY

- Trauma results in intraparenchymal pulmonary hemorrhage. Extracapillary hemorrhage results in the recruitment of inflammatory cells and protein into the alveolar and interstitial spaces.
- Pulmonary hemorrhage results in ventilation-perfusion mismatch and subsequent hypoxemia.
- Sequelae of pulmonary contusion may vary from very mild to rapidly fatal.

DIAGNOSIS

Suspected clinically due to association with blunt trauma; clinical confirmation is generally radiographic

DIFFERENTIAL DIAGNOSIS

- Pulmonary hemorrhage (anticoagulant rodenticide, neoplasia)
- Congestive heart failure (pulmonary edema)
- Pneumonia
- Pain (tachypnea)

INITIAL DATABASE

- Thoracic radiographs: document a patchy to diffuse interstitial to alveolar pattern
  - Radiographic changes may lag behind clinical signs.
  - May be indistinguishable from other patchy interstitial infiltrates, especially pulmonary edema in cats.
- Complete blood count (CBC), serum biochemistry profile: generally unremarkable

ADVANCED OR CONFIRMATORY TESTING

- Arterial blood gas (ABG) analysis or pulse oximetry may be useful to characterize the degree of hypoxemia. These are especially useful for determining whether tachypnea is due to pain (results are normal) or pulmonary lesions (hypoxemia commonly observed).
- Central Venous Pressure Monitoring (see p 1206), pulmonary wedge pressure measurement: Assess right- and left-sided vascular pressures, respectively

(helps rule out cardiogenic causes). Pulmonary wedge pressure specifically assesses the propensity for pulmonary edema but is a somewhat cumbersome procedure and is especially challenging in cats and small dogs.

TREATMENT

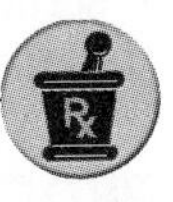

THERAPEUTIC GOAL(S)

- Maintain adequate intravascular volume but avoid overhydration, which may worsen pulmonary contusions
- Provide supplemental oxygen and rest

ACUTE GENERAL TREATMENT

- Judicious administration of IV fluids as needed to maintain perfusion.
  - Administration of boluses of 5-10 ml/kg of crystalloid fluids (e.g., lactated Ringer's solution) until adequate blood pressure (BP) and pulse quality are obtained.
- Administration of supplemental oxygen.
- Evaluation for other associated injuries.
- Note that glucocorticoids, antibiotics, and diuretics are not indicated for treatment of pulmonary contusions.

POSSIBLE COMPLICATIONS

- Infection (rare).
- Respiratory failure.
- Severe pulmonary contusion may require intermittent positive-pressure ventilation with positive end-expiratory pressure (PEEP) and/or may progress to acute respiratory distress syndrome (ARDS) (see Ventilation, Positive Pressure, p 1325).

RECOMMENDED MONITORING

- Hourly respiratory rate and effort
- Pulse oximetry

PROGNOSIS AND OUTCOME

Guarded to good prognosis. Most animals surviving a trip to the hospital will also survive pulmonary contusions with appropriate supportive care. Concurrent injuries (e.g., vertebral body fractures) are more likely to compromise the prognosis; other than very severe cases, pulmonary contusions are generally incidental findings that resolve with supportive care.

PEARLS & CONSIDERATIONS

COMMENTS

Avoid excessive volume resuscitation; administer IV fluids judiciously and adjust the rate frequently based on the animal's response and evolution of the case

PREVENTION

Prevent roaming

CLIENT EDUCATION

Pulmonary contusions are "lung bruises"; the injured animal will often get worse over the first 24 hours and then the lesions regress in the following 48 hours.

SUGGESTED READING

Powell LL, et al: A retrospective analysis of pulmonary contusion secondary to motor vehicle accidents in 143 dogs: 1994-1997. *J Vet Emerg Crit Care* 9:127-136, 1999.

AUTHOR & EDITOR: **ELIZABETH ROZANSKI**

Pulmonary Edema, Cardiogenic

BASIC INFORMATION

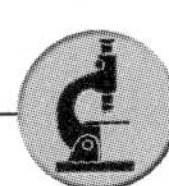

DEFINITION

The extravasation of fluid from the pulmonary vasculature into the interstitial and alveolar spaces as a result of left-sided heart disease

SYNONYM(S)

Congestive heart failure (CHF), left-sided decompensated heart failure
Pulmonary congestion

EPIDEMIOLOGY

SPECIES, AGE, SEX: Dependent on underlying cause.

GENETICS AND BREED PREDISPOSITION

- Certain breeds are predisposed to dilated cardiomyopathy (boxers, Doberman pinchers, Irish wolfhounds, Newfoundlands) or mitral valve endocardiosis (Cavalier King Charles spaniels, small breed dogs).
- Cats are predisposed to cardiomyopathy (Maine coons, Persians, Ragdolls).

CLINICAL PRESENTATION

HISTORY, CHIEF COMPLAINT

- Varies with severity of the fluid accumulation
- Tachypnea or exertional dyspnea
- Dry cough (uncommon in cats)
- Open mouth breathing (cats)
- Difficulty in breathing in lateral recumbency, trouble sleeping

PHYSICAL EXAM FINDINGS

- Auscultation can vary (absence of auscultable abnormalities, or presence of cardiac murmurs, gallop sounds, and arrhythmias).
- Lung sounds: crackles and wheezes possible, during both inspiration and expiration.
- Femoral pulse strength might vary based on cardiac output and arrhythmias.
- Severe cardiogenic pulmonary edema may produce pink tinged secretions from mouth and nares.
- Cyanosis.

ETIOLOGY AND PATHOPHYSIOLOGY

- In cardiogenic pulmonary edema, fluid moves from the pulmonary vasculature to the interstitial space due to elevated hydrostatic pressure in the pulmonary capillaries.
- This is in contrast to noncardiogenic pulmonary edema, in which fluid extravasates as a result of increased pulmonary vascular permeability.
- Elevated pulmonary capillary pressures secondary to left-sided heart failure:
  - Left ventricular volume overload caused by:
    - Primary valve disease (mitral or aortic insufficiency). Causes include myxomatous valve disease/endocardiosis, endocarditis, valve dysplasia, and mitral valve stenosis.
    - Primary heart muscle disease (dilated cardiomyopathy in dogs, various cardiomyopathies in cats).
    - Congenital left-to-right cardiac shunts (patent ductus arteriosus, aorticopulmonary window, atrial septal defect, ventricular septal defect, arteriovenous fistula).
    - Iatrogenic (overzealous fluid therapy).
    - Severe anemia.
  - Left ventricular dysfunction:
    - Arrhythmias.
    - Ischemic disease (rare).
    - Myocarditis.
    - Thyrotoxic cardiac disease.
    - Sepsis.
    - Myocardial toxins (i.e., chemotherapeutic agents such as doxorubicin).
    - Constrictive pericarditis.
    - Obstructive disease of the left atrium (rare): neoplasia, thrombus, cor triatriatum sinister.

DIAGNOSIS

DIFFERENTIAL DIAGNOSIS

Other causes of pulmonary edema (e.g., head trauma, seizures, electrocution) versus other cause for coughing and dyspnea:

- Primary lower respiratory disease (pneumonia, bronchitis, heartworm disease, neoplasia)
- Upper airway disease (collapsing trachea, tracheitis)

INITIAL DATABASE

- Thoracic radiographs: interstitial and/or alveolar infiltrates are present, primarily in the caudal dorsal region (perihilar region in dogs). With severe disease the pulmonary opacities can occur throughout the lung fields. A large cardiac silhouette, particularly left atrial, is common.
- Complete blood count: usually normal. Abnormalities may suggest a noncardiogenic cause (severe anemia, increased white blood cell count may suggest sepsis).
- Serum biochemistry panel: electrolyte abnormalities/azotemia from concurrent renal failure or previous diuretic usage, increased liver enzymes from passive congestion.
- Urinalysis: usually unremarkable except with systemic disorders.
- Electrocardiogram (ECG): sinus tachycardia may be present with ectopic premature contractions (depends on severity of cardiac disease and underlying etiology). The presence of atrial enlargement (wide and/or tall P waves) and left ventricular enlargement (tall R waves) are sensitive (although nonspecific) for chronic chamber enlargements.

ADVANCED OR CONFIRMATORY TESTING

- Echocardiography: cannot identify pulmonary edema but may confirm cardiac cause.
- Right heart catheterization: pulmonary capillary wedge pressure can be measured using a Swan-Ganz cathether: this is a surrogate for left atrial pressure (pressures >20 mmHg are indicative of cardiogenic pulmonary edema).
- Measurement of serum BNP and ANP levels: may help to distinguish between cardiac and noncardiogenic causes of congestive heart failure.

TREATMENT

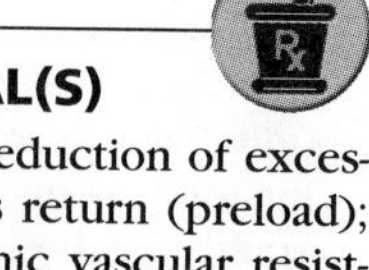

THERAPEUTIC GOAL(S)

Three main goals: (1) reduction of excessive pulmonary venous return (preload); (2) reduction of systemic vascular resistance (afterload); and (3) inotropic support in a subset of patients. See additional information under Heart Failure, Acute/Decompensated, p 458; Heart Failure, Chronic, p 459.

ACUTE GENERAL TREATMENT

- Avoid/reduce stress.
- Oxygenation.
- Intravenous furosemide (2-5 mg/kg in dogs, 2-4 mg/kg in cats) IV q 1-2h until labored respirations and respiratory rate decrease to normal, then decrease the dose of furosemide and frequency of administration based on clinical response. Alternatively for refractory pulmonary edema furosemide can be given as an infusion. Start with a loading bolus at 1 mg/kg, followed by a continuous rate infusion: 0.6-1 mg/kg/h IV until improvement in respiratory rate and effort is noted.
- ± Nitroprusside.
- ± Dobutamine.

CHRONIC TREATMENT

- First line therapy with furosemide (1-4 mg/kg PO q 8-24h) and ACE inhibitor (enalapril 0.5 mg/kg q 12-24h, benazepril 0.25-0.5 mg/kg q 12-24h preferred if renal dysfunction present).
- If refractory pulmonary edema, add spironolactone (1-2 mg/kg q 12-24h), hydrochlorothiazide (2-4 mg/kg q 12h).
- If systolic dysfunction, add inotrope (digoxin 0.005 mg/kg q 12h dog, ¼ of a 0.125 mg tablet q 48-72h, pimobendan 0.25 mg/kg PO q 12h).
- Dietary sodium restriction (sodium <80 mg/100 kcal), potassium salt supplementation as needed.
- See Heart Failure, Chronic, p 459 for further details.

POSSIBLE COMPLICATIONS

Pulmonary edema usually returns despite aggressive medical therapy.

RECOMMENDED MONITORING

- Thoracic radiographs to assess response to therapy. A 12- to 24-hour lag period between clinical improvement and radiographic improvement is common, however.
- Serum electrolytes and renal status.
- Respiratory status.

PROGNOSIS AND OUTCOME

Long-term prognosis is guarded because underlying disease is rarely cured. Exceptions can include correctable congenital defects (patent ductus arteriosus, pulmonic stenosis, others) and taurine-responsive dilated cardiomyopathy.

PEARLS & CONSIDERATIONS

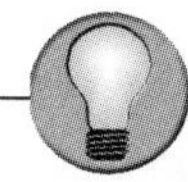

COMMENTS

Owners should monitor respiratory rate at home. If it increases by more than 25% for 2 days in a row, a call to the veterinarian is warranted.

CLIENT EDUCATION

- Monitor for recurrence of presenting signs (see History, Chief Complaint above)
- Rapid deterioration is possible; rechecks necessary

SUGGESTED READING

Fuentes VL: In Abbott JA (ed): *Veterinary Clinics of North America Small Animal Practice*. Philadelphia, WB Saunders, 2004, pp 1145-1155.

Sisson D: Neuroendocrine evaluation of cardiac disease. In Abbott JA (ed): *Veterinary Clinics of North America Small Animal Practice*. Philadelphia, WB Saunders, 2004, pp 1105-1126.

Ware W, Bonagura JD: Pulmonary edema. In Fox PR, Sisson D, Moise NS (eds): *Textbook of Canine and Feline Cardiology*. Philadelphia, WB Saunders, 1999, pp 251-264.

AUTHORS: **MARC S. KRAUS, ANNA R. M. GELZER**

EDITOR: **ETIENNE CÔTÉ**

Pulmonary Edema, Noncardiogenic

BASIC INFORMATION

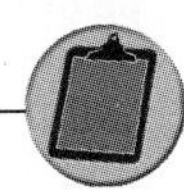

DEFINITION

Fluid accumulation in the pulmonary interstitium and alveoli caused by a disorder other than congestion resulting from heart disease

SYNONYM(S)

Acute respiratory distress syndrome (ARDS)
Neurogenic pulmonary edema

EPIDEMIOLOGY

SPECIES, AGE, SEX: Dogs and cats of any age or sex may be affected.

RISK FACTORS

- Acute upper airway obstruction (laryngeal paralysis, brachycephalic upper airway syndrome, foreign body, mass or infiltration, strangulation, others)
- Electrocution
- Protracted seizures or head trauma
- Other major trauma
- Sepsis or nonseptic systemic inflammatory disease (e.g., pancreatitis)
- Any cause of vasculitis
- Hepatic disease
- Smoke inhalation or other inhaled irritants
- Near-drowning experience

CLINICAL PRESENTATION

HISTORY, CHIEF COMPLAINT

- Cough, tachypnea, and respiratory distress are the most common.
  - Severe edema may cause coughing with expectoration of blood-tinged fluid.
- Other complaints could reflect primary diseases as already mentioned.

PHYSICAL EXAM FINDINGS

- Increased effort noted during inspiration and expiration, from increased lung stiffness.
- Cyanosis with severe alveolar involvement may be present.
- Fine crackles, often at end inspiration and early expiration, in the dorsocaudal lung fields. Coarse crackles throughout inspiration more often indicate airway disease or progression of an interstitial disease into airways.
- Crackles may be absent in early or mild edema.
- Lung sounds may be exceptionally quiet in very severe edema, particularly in cats.
- Cardiac murmurs and arrhythmias do not always indicate that edema is of cardiogenic origin.
- Other clinical signs associated with the underlying disease process may be present.

ETIOLOGY AND PATHOPHYSIOLOGY

- Pulmonary edema causes respiratory distress from arterial hypoxemia secondary to ventilation-perfusion mismatches and, to a lesser extent, diffusion barriers to oxygenation of pulmonary capillary blood.
- Noncardiogenic pulmonary edema arises from three mechanisms:
  - Increased vascular permeability is the most common and is seen with a wide variety of pulmonary and systemic disorders, as already described.
  - Decreased plasma oncotic pressure, most often from hypoalbuminemia. Pleural effusions (transudative) are more common than pulmonary edema in animals with reduced oncotic pressure as a single driving mechanism.
  - Impaired lymphatic drainage is an uncommon etiology that is usually secondary to neoplasia or lymphangitis.
- Regardless of the mechanism, the edema fluid that infiltrates the interstitial and alveolar spaces is rich in protein (same concentration as plasma), in contrast to cardiogenic pulmonary edema that is characterized by protein-poor fluid.
- Cardiogenic pulmonary edema arises most commonly from increased pulmonary venous hydrostatic pressure secondary to left-sided congestive heart failure (see Heart Failure, Acute/Decompensated, p 458; Heart Failure, Chronic, p 459).

DIAGNOSIS

DIFFERENTIAL DIAGNOSIS

Any cause of tachypnea, cough, or pulmonary parenchymal infiltration, such as:

- Pneumonia
- Neoplasia
- Fungal disease
- Protozoal infection (e.g., toxoplasmosis in cats)
- Thromboembolic disease
- Complicated bronchial disease
- Inflammatory respiratory disease (i.e., pulmonary infiltrates with eosinophils/eosinophilic bronchopneumopathy)
- Pulmonary contusions
- Cardiogenic pulmonary edema

INITIAL DATABASE

- Thoracic radiographs: "fluffy" interstitial opacities that may progress to an alveolar pattern.
  - Opacities are most often in the caudodorsal lung fields in animals with edema caused by increased vascular permeability (as well as in cardiogenic edema).
  - The absence of cardiac and pulmonary venous abnormalities can help distinguish cardiogenic from noncardiogenic edema.
- A complete blood count (CBC), biochemical profile, and urinalysis may be helpful in determining underlying causes.
- Historic information may help confirm underlying causes, such as electrocution or near-drowning experience.

ADVANCED OR CONFIRMATORY TESTING

- Respiratory washes do not often yield abnormalities; occasionally, a primary pulmonary disorder is detected.
- Arterial blood gas (ABG) analysis:
  - Hypoxemia
  - Hypocapnia
  - Widened alveolar-arterial (Aa) gradient
- The ratio of protein content of edema fluid (E) to plasma protein content (P) in noncardiogenic edema is 79–90%, while the E:P ratio in cardiogenic edema is typically <50%. Protein may be measured by refractometer or with biochemical methods.

TREATMENT

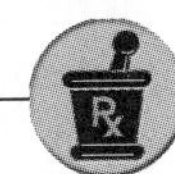

THERAPEUTIC GOAL(S)

- Improve oxygenation
- Minimize stress in severely distressed animals that could experience cardiopulmonary arrest from simple manipulations
- Support respiratory function and provide other supportive care while primary causes are identified and treated

ACUTE GENERAL TREATMENT

- Administer oxygen.
  - Face mask, nasal catheter, or oxygen cage (see Oxygen Supplementation, p 1292)
- Relieve anxiety and minimize unnecessary oxygen consumption.
  - Light sedation if needed:
    - Dogs: morphine, 0.1–1 mg/kg IV
    - Cats and dogs: acepromazine, 0.03–0.05 mg/kg IV, IM, or SQ
- Diuretics may be less beneficial for animals with noncardiogenic pulmonary edema.
  - Furosemide: 2–4 mg/kg IV q 4–12h
- Bronchodilators may combat bronchospasm, enhance mucociliary function, and diminish diaphragmatic fatigue.

- Aminophylline, theophylline: dogs: 5–10 mg/kg PO, IV, IM q 8–12h; cats: 5 mg/kg PO, IV, IM q 8–12h)

CHRONIC TREATMENT

- Specific therapies that address underlying cause.
- Intubation and positive-pressure ventilation may be necessary in severe cases and this constitutes the treatment of choice for critically dyspneic animals with noncardiogenic pulmonary edema caused by a reversible event (e.g., airway obstruction).

POSSIBLE COMPLICATIONS

- Secondary pneumonia.
- Fluid therapy may exacerbate fluid exudation into the pulmonary interstitium and should be administered cautiously, if at all, in animals with pulmonary edema from any cause.
  - Intravenous infusions of vasoactive agents, such as dopamine (2.5–10 ug/kg/min) and dobutamine (2.5–20 ug/kg/min), may help support animals with severe systemic hypotension.

RECOMMENDED MONITORING

- Clinical signs
- Thoracic radiographs
- Blood gas analysis or pulse oximetry
- Underlying disease state

PROGNOSIS AND OUTCOME

- Variable
- Depends upon the severity of the respiratory dysfunction and underlying disorder
- Aggressive treatment and intensive monitoring can improve outcomes

PEARLS & CONSIDERATIONS

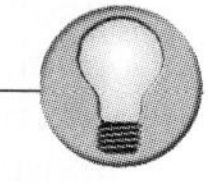

PREVENTION

Avoid leaving unsupervised puppies and kittens in environments where electrical cords could be easily reached

SUGGESTED READING

Drobatz KJ, Saunders HM: Noncardiogenic pulmonary edema. In Bonagura JB (ed): *Current Veterinary Therapy XIII: Small Animal Practice*. Philadelphia, WB Saunders, 2000, pp 810–812.

Myers NC, Wall RE: Pathophysiologic mechanisms of noncardiogenic pulmonary edema. *J Am Vet Med Assoc* 5;207(8):1018–1019, 1995.

Nelson OL, Sellon RK: Pulmonary parenchymal diseases. In Ettinger S, Feldman E (eds): *Textbook of Veterinary Internal Medicine*, ed 6. St. Louis, Elsevier Saunders, 2005, pp 1239–1265.

AUTHOR: **O. LYNNE NELSON**
EDITOR: **RANCE K. SELLON**

Pulmonary Hypertension (Arterial)

BASIC INFORMATION

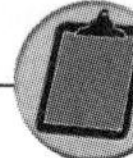

DEFINITION

- Pulmonary arterial hypertension (PH) is defined as increased pulmonary artery pressure, and may be primary (PPH) or secondary. PPH is diagnosed when no underlying cause for PH and histological findings typical for PPH can be identified; a special form of primary PH is persistent fetal circulation or persistent pulmonary hypertension.
- *Cor pulmonale* refers to right ventricular hypertrophy secondary to PH.
- Plexiform pulmonary arteriopathy is the term that describes the typical histologic abnormality found in PPH.

SYNONYM(S)

Pulmonary arterial hypertension: pulmonary hypertension

EPIDEMIOLOGY

SPECIES, AGE, SEX

- Dogs: dependent on underlying cause.
- Cats: data on any cause of PH are scant.

GENETICS AND BREED PREDISPOSITION: In secondary PH depending on underlying cause:

- Mitral endocardiosis in poodles, dachshunds, terriers, and other small breeds
- Chronic obstructive upper airway disease in brachycephalic breeds
- Pulmonary fibrosis in West Highland white terriers

RISK FACTORS

- Nephrotic syndrome, hyperadrenocorticism, immune mediated hemolytic anemia, pancreatitis, neoplasia, heartworm disease are risk factors for pulmonary thromboembolism (PTE)
- Ingestion of snails for infection with *Angiostrongylus vasorum* (French heartworm) in Europe and Newfoundland, Canada
- Septic shock, pancreatitis, other systemic inflammatory states for adult respiratory distress syndrome (ARDS)

GEOGRAPHY AND SEASONALITY

- *Dirofilaria immitis* in endemic areas.
- High altitude (hypobaric hypoxia) causes or contributes to pulmonary hypertension. Dogs living at 2300 m altitude (7500 ft) have a higher mean systolic pulmonary artery pressure (29.5 ± 10.4 mmHg as determined by Doppler evaluation of tricuspid regurgitation) than do dogs living at 700–900 m (2300–3000 ft) altitude (mean pulmonary artery pressure = 17.4 ± 3.9 mmHg determined in the same manner).

CLINICAL PRESENTATION

DISEASE FORMS/SUBTYPES: PH can be acute or chronic; acute PH is usually the result of PTE or ARDS.

HISTORY, CHIEF COMPLAINT

- Depending on underlying cause.
- Signs of PH itself or of the underlying cause may predominate.
- Signs associated with PH include:
  - Exercise intolerance
  - Collapse, syncope (reflex bradycardia caused by high resistance to forward flow from the right ventricle)
  - Dyspnea, coughing
  - Abdominal distention
  - Rear limb weakness in reverse patent dutcus arteriosus (PDA)
  - Right ventricular hypertrophy as incidental finding during echocardiography or electrocardiography

PHYSICAL EXAM FINDINGS

- PPH: exam may be unremarkable. Possible findings include:
  - Pale mucous membranes
  - Tachycardia
  - Weak pulse
  - Signs of right-sided congestive heart failure (distended jugular veins or jugular venous pulse, abdominal distention)
  - Split second heart sound (pulmonic valve closing after aortic valve)
  - Murmur of tricuspid regurgitation (systolic, right-sided)
  - Murmur of pulmonic regurgitation (rare; diastolic and loudest over left heart base)

- Secondary PH: depending on underlying disease, possible findings include:
    - Same as PPH
    - Stertorous breathing in brachycephalic syndrome
    - Cyanosis
    - Dyspnea
    - Loud murmur of mitral regurgitation
    - Increased lung sounds, wheezes, crackles
    - Red oral and conjunctival mucous membranes due to polycythemia in reverse PDA
    - Differential cyanosis in reverse PDA

ETIOLOGY AND PATHOPHYSIOLOGY

- PPH is very rare. Inciting factors may be drugs (experimentally inducible with appetite suppressants), toxins, infections, and genetically determined susceptibility to such injuries.
    - Thrombosis elicited by diseased vessel walls may complicate PPH.
- Secondary PH is a common complication of different cardiac and extracardiac diseases and results from two main mechanisms: increased left atrial pressure and increased pulmonary vascular resistance. Important causes are:
    - Cardiac:
        - Pulmonary venous hypertension due to increased left atrial pressure in left myocardial failure, most common in advanced chronic mitral regurgitation, also in dilated cardiomyopathy
        - Vascular remodeling due to increased pulmonary flow in congenital heart disease (large left-to-right shunts in ventricular septal defect [VSD] and PDA; see Eisenmenger's Syndrome, p 335), possibly more common in cats than in dogs
    - Hypoxic vasoconstriction:
        - Chronic obstructive lower airway disease (bronchitis, emphysema)
        - Chronic obstructive upper airway disease
        - High altitude hypoxia
    - Occlusion of the pulmonary vascular bed:
        - PTE
        - Parasites (*D. immitis, A. vasorum*)
    - Pulmonary parenchymal disease:
        - Pulmonary fibrosis (see Interstitial Lung Diseases, p 599)
        - ARDS
    - Combination of mechanisms, e.g., heartworm infection (*D. immitis, A. vasorum*): obstruction by intravascular parasites, vasculitis, thrombosis, and hypoxic vasoconstriction.

DIAGNOSIS

DIFFERENTIAL DIAGNOSIS

- For right-sided cardiac failure:
    - Congenital cardiac disease: pulmonic stenosis, tricuspid dysplasia, tetralogy of Fallot, tricuspid stenosis, cor triatriatum dexter
    - Acquired cardiovascular disease: severe tricuspid myxomatous valve disease/endocardiosis, right ventricular dilated cardiomyopathy, pericardial effusion
- For right ventricular hypertrophy:
    - Pulmonic stenosis, tetralogy of Fallot

INITIAL DATABASE

- Thoracic radiographs; dorsoventral view is particularly important.
    - Document right ventricular and main pulmonary artery enlargement; somewhat nonspecific, as findings of "reversed D" and "increased sternal contact" on the lateral view are often overinterpreted in normal dogs and cats (expiratory films, rotation of patient, thoracic conformation).
    - Peripheral pulmonary vasculature may be tortuous and enlarged, or may be unremarkable with PPH and PTE.
    - Peripheral pulmonary arterial markings may abruptly stop with PTE.
    - Left atrium is enlarged and pulmonary veins are congested with underlying left ventricular or mitral valve disease.
    - Signs of underlying bronchial, interstitial or alveolar pulmonary disease may be evident.
- Echocardiogram, dual role:
    - Rule in or out causes of PH, including acquired left ventricular heart disease (mitral endocardiosis, dilated cardiomyopathy) and congenital cardiovascular shunt.
    - Confirmation of PH qualitatively and quantitatively:
        - Qualitatively: characteristic two-dimensional and M-mode findings are dilation of right ventricle and atrium, thickening of right ventricular wall and papillary muscles, paradoxical septal motion, and decreased left ventricular chamber size.
        - Quantitatively: Doppler examination is the most useful noninvasive clinical tool to confirm and quantitate severity of PH.
            - Systolic: velocity of tricuspid regurgitation correlates to right ventricular systolic pressure, and therefore, barring pulmonic stenosis, to pulmonary arterial systolic pressure. Normal: <30 mmHg, and higher suggests/indicates PH. The modified Bernoulli equation allows Doppler-derived blood flow velocities to be used for estimating intracardiac pressures: $PG = 4 \times (V_{max})^2$, where PG is the peak pressure gradient between right ventricle and right atrium, in mmHg, and V_{max} is the peak velocity of tricuspid regurgitation (TR), in m/sec. It is assumed that right atrial pressure approximates 0 mmHg during ventricular systole, such that the right atrial:right ventricular systolic PG equals systolic right ventricular pressure.
            - Diastolic pulmonary artery pressure is calculated with Doppler quantification of pulmonary valve insufficiency instead of tricuspid regurgitation; by this method PH is considered to be present when PG calculated based on Doppler-derived is >20 mmHg.
- ECG: document right ventricular hypertrophy (RVH; deep S-waves in leads I, II, III, aVF), right axis deviation, and possible arrhythmias; in acute PH, ECG abnormalities may not be present; in chronic PH, marked PH must be present to cause ECG abnormalities. Less sensitive and specific than echocardiography.
- Serology for *D. immitis* and fecal Baermann for *A. vasorum*.
- Platelet count, coagulation profile, and parameters associated with hypercoagulability (e.g., antithrombin III levels, D-dimer levels) may be abnormal with vasculitis and thrombosis.
- Arterial blood gas analysis: may show hypoxemia in primary respiratory disease or right-to-left cardiovascular shunt.
- Complete blood count, biochemistry panel, urinalysis: may show abnormalities suggestive of parasitic disease (eosinophilia, basophilia), chronic inflammation (hyperglobulinemia), and systemic disease predisposing to PTE (proteinuria, hypoalbuminemia).

ADVANCED OR CONFIRMATORY TESTING

- Contrast ultrasound (microbubbles) of the heart and descending aorta to rule out cardiovascular right-to-left shunt
- Right-sided cardiac catheterization for invasive measurement of pulmonary wedge pressure as an estimate of left atrial pressure, systolic and diastolic pulmonary artery pressure; evaluation of therapeutic intervention
- Pulmonary angiography; tortuous pulmonary arteries indicate PH, perfusion deficits are present in PTE

- Pulmonary ventilation-perfusion scintigraphy to rule out pulmonary thromboembolism
- Pulmonary histopathologic evaluation to confirm PPH

TREATMENT

THERAPEUTIC GOAL(S)

- PPH or secondary PH with signs referable to PH or right ventricular failure: lower pulmonary artery pressure
- Secondary PH: focus should be to correct/improve underlying disease

ACUTE GENERAL TREATMENT

Oxygen therapy (cage or nasal)

CHRONIC TREATMENT

There is no controlled trial documenting efficacy of medical treatment in naturally occurring PH in dogs; thus the following are merely treatment considerations:

- Therapeutic trial with amlodipine (Norvasc) in moderate PH, starting at 0.05 mg/kg PO q 24h and titrating dose based on response and BP (avoid hypotension)
- Anticoagulant therapy with low dose aspirin, 2-5 mg/kg PO q 12h (dog)
- Sildenafil (Viagra) in severe PH, 2-3 mg/kg PO q 8-12h
- Dedicated owner may consider intermittent oxygen therapy at home
- Furosemide, ACE inhibitor, spironolactone in case of overt right-sided congestive heart failure (see Heart Failure, Chronic, p 459)
- Specific treatment of underlying mechanism or disease in secondary PH (see Heart Failure, Chronic, p 459; Eisenmenger's Syndrome, p 335; Pulmonary Thromboembolism, p 920; Heartworm Disease, Dog, p 465; Heartworm Disease, Cat, p 462; Acute Respiratory Distress Syndrome, p 34)

POSSIBLE COMPLICATIONS

- PH: right ventricular failure
- Treatment: systemic arterial hypotension with syncope, prerenal azotemia

RECOMMENDED MONITORING

- Most important are simple clinical parameters: general attitude, exercise tolerance, respiration, severity of ascites
- Systemic blood pressure

PROGNOSIS AND OUTCOME

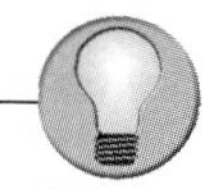

Depends on underlying disease and stage of disease:

- Good in parasitic pulmonary vasculature disease with acute PH
- Moderate in right-to-left cardiovascular shunts, mitral endocardiosis, chronic PH secondary to parasitic pulmonary vasculature disease
- Poor in advanced PPH, advanced pulmonary fibrosis, ARDS, nonparasitic PTE, presence of right-sided heart failure

PEARLS & CONSIDERATIONS

COMMENTS

- Most causes of secondary PH are readily detectable.
- Pulmonary thromboembolism and right-to-left PDA in particular may be missed if not considered.
- PPH is a clinical diagnosis of exclusion and definitive confirmation is available only histologically.
- Newer human drugs to decrease pulmonary artery pressure are very expensive: iloprost = prostaglandin analog for inhalation, and bosentan = endothelin antagonist for oral administration.

CLIENT EDUCATION

In dogs with cardiac disease, travel to higher altitude (above 7000 feet) may aggravate PH to a clinically relevant degree due to hypobaric hypoxia.

SUGGESTED READING

Atkins CE, et al: Pathophysiologic mechanism of cardiac dysfunction in experimentally induced heartworm caval syndrome in dogs: An echocardiographic study. *Am J Vet Res* 49:403-410, 1988.

Glaus TM, et al: Clinical and pathological characterisation of primary pulmonary hypertension in a dog. *Vet Rec* 154:786-789, 2004.

Glaus TM, et al: Non-invasive measurement of the cardiovascular effects of chronic hypoxaemia on dogs living at moderately high altitude. *Vet Rec* 152: 800-803, 2003.

Johnson L, et al: Clinical characteristics of 53 dogs with Doppler-derived evidence of pulmonary hypertension: 1992-1996. *J Vet Intern Med* 13:440-447, 1999.

AUTHOR: **TONY M. GLAUS**
EDITOR: **ETIENNE CÔTÉ**

Pulmonary Infiltrates with Eosinophils

BASIC INFORMATION

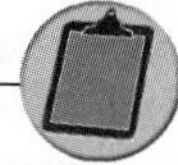

DEFINITION

Idiopathic infiltration of airways, interstitium, and sometimes alveoli and/or nasal cavities with inflammatory infiltrates characterized by a high proportion of eosinophils

SYNONYM(S)

PIE

Canine idiopathic eosinophilic bronchopneumopathy (the most current term)

Eosinophilic bronchopneumopathy

EPIDEMIOLOGY

SPECIES, AGE, SEX: Primarily a disease of dogs of any age with no sex predilection. Cats are not affected.

GENETICS AND BREED PREDISPOSITION: Any breed can be affected although Siberian huskies have been suggested as a breed predisposed to the disease.

CLINICAL PRESENTATION

HISTORY, CHIEF COMPLAINT

- Animals that have pulmonary infiltrates with eosinophils (PIE) most often present with a chronic cough that is unresponsive, or poorly responsive, to antimicrobial therapy. Cough may be intermittent, frequent, or persistent and is usually accompanied by a terminal gag/retch. Affected animals may have very productive coughing to the point of expectoration of respiratory secretions onto the floor or may experience gagging and retching.
- Nasal discharge, which can be serous or mucopurulent, may also be a presenting complaint.
- Exercise intolerance.
- Depression (uncommon).
- Weight loss in affected dogs is more rare.

PHYSICAL EXAM FINDINGS

- Cough
- Crackles, wheezes, and increased bronchovesicular sounds heard during thoracic auscultation
- Tachypnea
- Hyperpnea/Dyspnea
- Fever

ETIOLOGY AND PATHOPHYSIOLOGY

- A hypersensitivity reaction is suspected as the main pathophysiologic process underlying the disease.
- The precipitating cause is rarely identified.

DIAGNOSIS

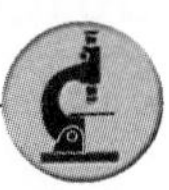

DIFFERENTIAL DIAGNOSIS

Other diseases associated with eosinophilic respiratory inflammation:

- Respiratory parasites (*Oslerus* and *Capillaria* spp., others)
- Respiratory infection (bacterial, fungal)
- Pulmonary neoplasia (primary or metastatic)
- Heartworm infection
- Eosinophilic granulomatosis, which on radiographs appears more as a nodular pulmonary disease

INITIAL DATABASE

- Complete blood count (CBC).
  - Inflammatory leukogram.
  - Peripheral eosinophilia is not always present.
- Serum biochemical profile and urinalysis results are usually normal.
- Thoracic radiographs commonly show bronchial and peribronchiolar patterns; increases in interstitial markings, alveolar patterns, and lobar consolidation or bronchiectasis may also be observed.
- Heartworm test results are negative.
- Fecal examinations (flotation, sedimentation techniques) will be negative for parasites and ova.

ADVANCED OR CONFIRMATORY TESTING

- Bronchoscopic abnormalities:
  - A common finding is green to yellow-green mucus, often abundant, in airways.
  - Airway mucosa may appear reddened, thickened, nodular, or polypoid; airway collapse may be evident during expiration.
- Examination of respiratory washes or brush cytologic examination shows a mix primarily of neutrophils and eosinophils. Infectious agents, neoplastic cells, or evidence of respiratory parasites are not expected with this disease.
- Culture of respiratory washes will be negative for pathogens in some cases; in those that have positive culture results, clinical signs persist in the face of antimicrobial therapy.

TREATMENT

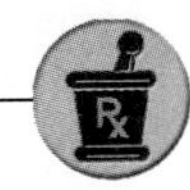

THERAPEUTIC GOAL(S)

- Resolve eosinophilic inflammation
- Address potential inciting causes

ACUTE GENERAL TREATMENT

Immunosuppressive dosage of glucocorticoids (e.g., prednisone 1–2 mg/kg PO q 24h) initially

CHRONIC TREATMENT

Glucocorticoids on a slowly tapering (weeks to months) dosage schedule are often needed for control of clinical signs:

- Clinical signs are likely to recur if glucocorticoids are administered inconsistently or if tapering occurs too quickly.
- Low-dose glucocorticoid therapy may be needed in some animals. Administer the lowest dose q 24–48h to control clinical signs.

POSSIBLE COMPLICATIONS

Side effects of glucocorticoid therapy such as polyuria, polydipsia, and polyphagia are expected in treated animals.

RECOMMENDED MONITORING

- Clinical signs
- Thoracic radiographs

PROGNOSIS AND OUTCOME

- Prognosis is generally good with appropriate doses of glucocorticoids for appropriate periods of time. Some animals may be able to be completely weaned from glucocorticoids.
- Excessively rapid cessation of glucocorticoids may provoke a relapse of clinical signs.

PEARLS & CONSIDERATIONS

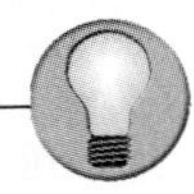

COMMENTS

Hyposensitization against antigens identified by allergy testing has been associated with alleviation of clinical signs or control of clinical signs with smaller doses of glucocorticoids in a small number of reported animals. The amount of clinical benefit derived from hyposensitization and the role of hyposensitization in long-term management need additional investigation; hyposensitization may be a consideration for animals in which side effects of glucocorticoids are unacceptable or intolerable to owners.

PREVENTION

There is no reliable means of preventing this disease.

CLIENT EDUCATION

Clients should understand the importance of consistent treatment with glucocorticoids, particularly during the initial stages of treatment.

SUGGESTED READING

Clercx C, et al: Eosinophilic bronchopneumopathy in dogs. *J Vet Intern Med* 14:282, 2000.

AUTHORS: **RANCE K. SELLON, CÉCILE CLERCX**
EDITOR: **RANCE K. SELLON**

Pulmonary Lymphoid Granulomatosis

BASIC INFORMATION

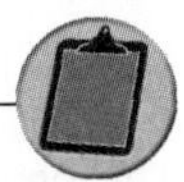

DEFINITION

Rare lymphoproliferative neoplasm in which infiltrates of atypical lymphoid cells develop around and destroy pulmonary blood vessels

SYNONYM(S)

PLG
Lymphomatoid granulomatosis

EPIDEMIOLOGY

SPECIES, AGE, SEX: Rare in dogs and reported in a single cat. Young to middle-aged adults of either gender are typically affected.

ASSOCIATED CONDITIONS AND DISORDERS: Lymphomatoid granulomatosis may be observed in sites other than the lungs, including lymph nodes, liver, heart, spleen, kidneys, pancreas, adrenal gland, or skin.

CLINICAL PRESENTATION

HISTORY, CHIEF COMPLAINT

- Nonproductive cough that is unresponsive to treatment with antimicrobials
- Increased respiratory effort
- Lethargy
- Anorexia and weight loss
- Rarely: fever, lameness, peripheral lymphadenopathy, ascites, or vomiting

PHYSICAL EXAM FINDINGS

- Nonproductive cough
- Tachypnea
- Areas of decreased bronchovesicular lung sounds
- Areas of increased bronchovesicular lung sounds
- Peripheral lymphadenomegaly (occasionally)
- Other sites of infiltration may be identified, including the skin

ETIOLOGY AND PATHOPHYSIOLOGY

- In humans, pulmonary lymphoid granulomatosis (PLG) is considered a precursor to low-grade T-cell lymphoma.
- The disease also seems to be T-cell mediated in the few animals studied to date.
- Infiltrates of atypical lymphocytes are centered on the vasculature. While pulmonary vasculature is most commonly targeted, other lymphatic tissues or solid organs may be affected as well.

DIAGNOSIS

DIFFERENTIAL DIAGNOSIS

- Metastatic pulmonary neoplasia
- Pulmonary lymphoma
- Other primary lung tumors
- Granulomatous fungal pneumonia
- Eosinophilic bronchopneumopathy/pulmonary infiltrates with eosinophils, eosinophilic granulomatosis
- Severe bacterial pneumonia

INITIAL DATABASE

- Complete blood count (CBC): leukocytosis, eosinophilia, and basophilia are common
- Serum biochemistry profile and urinalysis: usually unremarkable
- Heartworm serology: negative
- Thoracic radiographs:
  - Large pulmonary masses or lobar consolidation are typical.
  - An interstitial lung pattern is commonly observed.
  - Tracheobronchial and/or sternal lymph nodes are often enlarged.
  - Pleural effusion is sometimes present.

ADVANCED OR CONFIRMATORY TESTING

- Pulmonary biopsy is the only means of definitive diagnosis. Samples may be obtained via sternal or intercostal thoracotomy, keyhole biopsy, or thoracoscopy.
- Tracheal wash, bronchoalveolar lavage, and fine-needle aspirates may reveal cells suggestive of either inflammation or lymphoma, but cytologic examination cannot confirm a diagnosis of PLG. These tests are, however, useful in ruling out other potential causes of lung disease.

TREATMENT

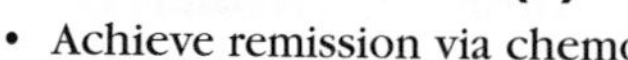

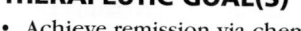

THERAPEUTIC GOAL(S)

- Achieve remission via chemotherapy
- Provide short-term support for hypoxemia if required

ACUTE GENERAL TREATMENT

- If required, oxygen supplementation for hypoxemic animals.
- Chemotherapy protocols (see Lymphoma, Dog [Multicentric], p 658; Lymphoma Chemotherapy Treatment Tables, Dog, p 655) similar to those used for treatment of lymphoma, including the use of cytotoxic agents.
- Glucocorticosteroids alone will seldom produce remission.

CHRONIC TREATMENT

Chemotherapy should proceed as for lymphoma.

POSSIBLE COMPLICATIONS

Extensive and serious adverse reactions, including leukopenia and immune suppression, are possible in response to many chemotherapeutic agents; drug-specific reactions are also possible (e.g., cyclophosphamide-induced sterile hemorrhagic cystitis).

RECOMMENDED MONITORING

- Repeat thoracic radiographs 2 to 3 weeks after initial chemotherapy and periodically thereafter. The interval between radiographs can be prolonged as the duration of remission endures.
- Periodically assess CBC for dogs receiving chemotherapy for lymphoma; other specific tests may be needed depending on the chemotherapeutic agent employed (e.g., cardiac ultrasound for dogs receiving doxorubicin).

PROGNOSIS AND OUTCOME

- Guarded
- Many dogs attain durable remission
- Lymphoma may follow PLG by months to years

PEARLS & CONSIDERATIONS

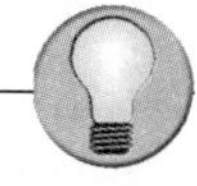

COMMENTS

In humans, PLG is regarded as a slowly progressive precursor to lymphoma.

CLIENT EDUCATION

Owners should understand that even if durable remission is achieved, the disease may progress to lymphoma years later.

SUGGESTED READING

Berry CR, et al: Pulmonary lymphomatoid granulomatosis in seven dogs (1976–1987). *J Vet Intern Med* 4:157, 1990.

Fitzgerald SD, et al: Eight cases of canine lymphomatoid granulomatosis. *Vet Path* 28:241, 1991.

Smith KC, et al: Canine lymphomatoid granulomatosis: An immunophenotypic analysis of three cases. *J Comp Pathol* 115:129, 1996.

Valentine BA, et al: Pulmonary lymphomatoid granulomatosis in a cat. *J Vet Diagn Invest* 12:465, 2000.

AUTHOR: **LEAH A. COHN**

EDITOR: **RANCE K. SELLON**

Pulmonary Nodules

BASIC INFORMATION

DEFINITION

Single or multiple masses of varying sizes occurring in the lung parenchyma. Usually detected radiographically

SYNONYM(S)

Lung nodules

EPIDEMIOLOGY

SPECIES, AGE, SEX

- Dogs: 9–11 years
- Cats: 11–12 years
- Females may be at increased risk

The prevalence of pulmonary nodules in dogs and cats is not known. Pulmonary neoplasms have an average reported incidence rate of 5.6/100,000 in dogs and 2.2/100,000 in cats;

RISK FACTORS: Exposure to secondhand smoke may be a risk factor.

ASSOCIATED CONDITIONS AND DISORDERS: Paraneoplastic syndromes reported to occur secondary to primary or metastatic lung neoplasms:

- Hypertrophic osteopathy
- Hypercalcemia
- Fever
- Elevated ACTH with associated signs of hyperadrenocorticism

CLINICAL PRESENTATION

DISEASE FORMS/SUBTYPES: Most primary lung neoplasms are adenocarcinomas (75%) or carcinomas (20%).

HISTORY, CHIEF COMPLAINT

- Pulmonary nodules or masses may be found incidentally in patients undergoing radiography for other reasons.
- When lung neoplasms cause clinical signs, the most frequent complaints from the owner are cough and dyspnea.
  - Sputum with or without blood or hemoptysis is possible.
  - Other possible signs: fever, weight loss, dysphagia, vomiting, regurgitation, wheezing.
  - Cats often manifest signs related to metastatic disease to their digits as opposed to respiratory signs.

PHYSICAL EXAM FINDINGS

- Physical exam: usually normal.
- Pulmonary nodules due to metastatic disease: physical abnormalities from the primary tumor may be found in other parts of the body.
  - In patients with pulmonary nodules, careful evaluation of the more common sites of origin of tumors that metastasize to the lungs is indicated, including the oral cavity, the area of the thyroid, mammary glands, and toe nails (especially in cats).
  - A rectal exam is indispensable in every dog with pulmonary nodules (assess prostate, anal sacs, bladder/urethra, sublumbar lymph nodes).
- A fundic exam and careful dermatologic evaluation may be helpful in identifying disseminated fungal disease.

ETIOLOGY AND PATHOPHYSIOLOGY

- The main concern with pulmonary nodules is malignancy; neoplasms from virtually any part of the body, including primary lung tumors, may metastasize to the lungs.
- Metastatic neoplasia may reach the lungs via lymphatics or via the bloodstream; both can produce a nodular pulmonary pattern.
- The development of metastasis is a complex, multistep process and failure to complete any of the steps will prevent the development of a metastatic focus. It is estimated that less than 1 in 10^4 neoplastic cells that leaves the primary tumor survives the metastatic cascade. This multistep process includes the induction of neovascularization detachment of the tumor cell from the primary tumor, dissolution of the basement membrane and invasion into the bloodstream, evasion of the host immunity and survival in the bloodstream, margination in a new capillary and attachment to the endothelium, dissolution of the basement membrane and extravasation into the extracellular matrix, survival in the new tissue by evading the host immunity, and finally the induction of neovascularization to support continued growth of the new metastatic focus. This neovascularization begins the process again.

DIAGNOSIS

DIFFERENTIAL DIAGNOSIS

- Solitary lung mass: primary neoplasia, metastatic neoplasia, granuloma, cyst, infarct, localized hemorrhage, focal pneumonia, abscess.
- Multiple pulmonary masses: primary or metastatic neoplasia, fungal disease (blastomycosis, histoplasmosis), pulmonary osteomas (rarely more than 3-4 mm in diameter, and more radiopaque than soft tissue nodules because of mineral composition). Bacterial abscesses and granulomas uncommonly cause multiple pulmonary masses.
- One or more cutaneous or subcutaneous nodules, one or more nipples, and intrahepatic mineralizations can be mistaken for focal pulmonary lesions, especially if only one radiographic projection is made.

INITIAL DATABASE

- Thoracic radiographs: the source of initial identification of pulmonary nodules in most cases (less commonly at surgery or necropsy).
- Complete blood count (CBC), serum biochemistry profile, urinalysis. Typically unremarkable in patients with incidentally discovered pulmonary nodules. Hypercalcemia may occur with neoplasia, fungal, and other granulomatous diseases.
- Pleural effusion, if present, should be sampled and evaluated with fluid analysis, cytology, and, if evidence of infection exists, bacterial culture (aerobic and anaerobic).
- Repeated meticulous physical exam (see above).

ADVANCED OR CONFIRMATORY TESTING

- Thoracic radiographs: 3 views if the lesion was found incidentally.
- Ultrasonographic studies (of the abdomen to screen for primary sites of disease; of the lesion with aspiration for diagnosis if possible).
- Computed tomography (CT) to assess for lesions too small to be identified with plain-film radiography and/or to be used for CT-guided aspirates or biopsies.
- The minimum database should be supplemented with fungal serology and microbial (fungal and bacterial) culture based on clinical suspicion and history.
- Thoracotomy with histopathologic evaluation of biopsy specimens. The hilar lymph nodes and lung lobes should be carefully evaluated and sampled as necessary at the time of thoracotomy.

TREATMENT

THERAPEUTIC GOAL(S)

- Resolution of clinical signs if present.
- Control or elimination of primary disease process (exception: clinically unimportant pulmonary nodules, i.e., pulmonary osteomas).
- Single pulmonary masses are more commonly addressed surgically (focal process).
- Multiple pulmonary masses are usually not addressed surgically, because they typically are part of a generalized process (e.g., neoplastic, fungal). Rather, identifying the underlying cause and systemic (medical) treatment are usually most important.

ACUTE GENERAL TREATMENT

Once a lesion has been identified, surgical excision should be considered.

- Treatment of choice for primary pulmonary neoplasia (single pulmonary nodule in which the diagnosis was established with ultrasound- or CT-guided aspiration or biopsy).
- Surgical excision may be considered for solitary pulmonary nodules/masses of unknown tissue type. The slow-growing nature of some single pulmonary nodules means that other concerns (concurrent illnesses, patient age, etc.) may supersede the need for thoracotomy.
- In specific cases, metastatectomy (excision of metastases) can be performed. Consultation with an oncologist is recommended beforehand.

CHRONIC TREATMENT

Chemotherapy may be attempted for primary pulmonary neoplasia that is deemed unresectable or has evidence of lymphatic metastasis at the time of diagnosis. Options may include doxorubicin, platinum compounds (cisplatin, carboplatin), or vinorelbine. However, chemotherapy is largely unproven in the management of pulmonary tumors.

POSSIBLE COMPLICATIONS

- Hypertrophic osteopathy; typically resolves with removal of pulmonary disease
- Digital metastasis (cats)

RECOMMENDED MONITORING

- Monthly to quarterly radiographs to assess for recurrence, progression
- As required per protocol for chemotherapy patients (i.e., CBC), quality of life assessments

PROGNOSIS AND OUTCOME

- Guarded and extremely variable (median survivals in parentheses)
- Dogs with primary lung tumors:
  - 50% of dogs without clinical signs and having peripheral, solitary, small (<5 cm), well-differentiated, low-grade pulmonary adenocarcinomas without lymph node metastasis or pleural effusion have survivals >1 year (12–20 months).
  - In contrast, median survival is shorter (8 months) for patients with clinical signs referable to the pulmonary nodule/mass, or with a large solitary (>5 cm or 100 cm^3) neoplasm, one that involves an entire lobe, squamous cell carcinoma histologically, or nodal metastasis (1–2 months)
- Cats with primary lung tumors: median survival 4 months after lobectomy. Cats with poorly differentiated tumors or enlarged tracheobronchial lymph nodes: median 2 months

PEARLS & CONSIDERATIONS

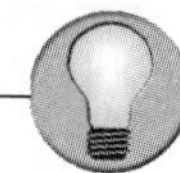

COMMENTS

- Metastatic neoplasia is much more common than primary pulmonary neoplasia.
- One half of patients with newly diagnosed pulmonary neoplasia are deemed inoperable because regional or systemic extension is identified at presentation.
- Pulmonary osteomas are benign mineralizations often identified incidentally on the radiographs of older dogs. The diagnosis of osteoma versus metastasis can be made empirically based on size and relative opacity. The limit of detection for soft tissue lesions in the pulmonary parenchyma is considered to range from 5–10 mm. Because osteomas are of mineral or bone density, they can be identified in the 2–5 mm range.
- In this author's experience, cats with pulmonary metastases tend to show overt signs and have more advanced disease at the time of presentation, and have markedly shorter survival times than dogs.

SUGGESTED READING

Withrow SJ: Tumors of the respiratory system c. lung cancer. In Withrow SJ, MacEwen EG (eds): *Small Animal Clinical Oncology*, ed 3. Philadelphia, WB Saunders, 2001, pp 361–367.

AUTHOR: **CARLOS O. RODRIGUEZ, JR.**
EDITOR: **KENNETH M. RASSNICK**

Pulmonary Thromboembolism

BASIC INFORMATION

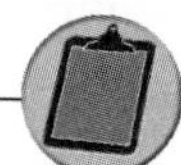

DEFINITION

The occlusion of pulmonary artery or arteriole by a thrombus that forms in a nonpulmonary organ system (i.e., embolism). Localized, or *in situ*, thrombus formation has also come to be included in discussions of pulmonary thromboembolism (PTE). The onset of clinical signs of PTE is often sudden and antemortem diagnosis can be difficult. PTE constitutes a medical emergency.

SYNONYM(S)

Pulmonary embolism
Pulmonary thrombosis

EPIDEMIOLOGY

SPECIES, SEX, AGE

- Dogs: 10 months to 18 years, median age 11 years
- Cats: 2 to 14 years, median age 7 years
- Prevalence in postmortem diagnoses: 0.9% (dogs), 0.06% (cats)

RISK FACTORS: Identifying risk factors is a cornerstone for suspecting and making the diagnosis of PTE.

- Immune-mediated hemolytic anemia (IHA) (autoagglutination *in vivo*)
- Neoplasia (platelets hyperaggregable; collagen exposure; disruption of blood flow; elaboration of paraneoplastic substances)
- Protein-losing nephropathy/enteropathy (loss of antithrombin III [AT III])
- Heartworm disease with or without right atrial or ventricular enlargement (endothelial disruption; sluggish blood flow)
- Jugular catheters (surface for thrombus formation)
- Hyperadrenocorticism (mechanism unknown; possibly loss of AT III)
- Disseminated intravascular coagulation (DIC) (consumption of anticoagulants; activation of coagulation cascade; underlying disorder)
- Vasculitis (endothelial inflammation/damage)
- Pancreatitis (loss of antithrombin III; DIC)
- Sepsis (activation of coagulation cascade)
- Orthopedic procedures such as total hip replacement

ASSOCIATED CONDITIONS AND DISORDERS: Hypoxemia, right-sided congestive heart failure.

CLINICAL PRESENTATION

CHIEF COMPLAINT, HISTORY

- Classically, acute onset dyspnea as a manifestation of massive PTE.
- More often, and less grossly apparent: mild dyspnea and/or normal respirations, when PTE is more gradual, milder, or both.
- Often, the signs of the underlying, triggering disorders may predominate, and dyspnea is insidious in onset.
- Signs of right-sided heart failure (abdominal distention, exercise intolerance) may occasionally be the sign of PTE that prompts owners to seek veterinary attention.

PHYSICAL EXAM FINDINGS

- Dyspnea
- Tachypnea
- Coughing
- Pulmonary crackles/increased bronchial sounds (pulmonary auscultation may be normal)
- Signs of right heart failure (jugular venous distention/pulsation, ascites, pleural effusion)
- Hemoptysis (occasional)
- Weight loss in chronic PTE

ETIOLOGY AND PATHOPHYSIOLOGY

- *In situ* thrombus formation may result from venous stasis/endothelial injury leading to pathologic alteration of metabolism of compounds involved in vascular tone (i.e., endothelin) and coagulation (i.e., thromboxane), as is seen in heartworm disease. (i.e., recruitment of one or more of the components of Virchow's triad: venous stasis, vascular injury, coagulopathy). Alternatively, embolism of thrombi/cells/parasites of nonpulmonary origin may occur. See Risk Factors above.

- Increased pulmonary vascular resistance combines with mechanical occlusion of pulmonary vasculature to decrease pulmonary vascular blood flow (PVBF).
- Decreased PVBF diminishes gas exchange in affected regions and causes ventilation/perfusion mismatch, increased alveolar dead space, and ultimate hypoxemia.
- Note: The lung has a dual blood supply. Bronchial arteries are branches of the aorta which perfuse the lung parenchyma. They are not affected by pulmonary thromboembolism. The pulmonary arteries, which become occluded with thromboemboli in PTE, carry blood from the right ventricle through the lungs for oxygenation. Therefore, even massive pulmonary thromboembolism generally does not cause lung infarction; rather, PTE is life-threatening due to hypoxemia (ventilation:perfusion mismatch).

DIAGNOSIS

DIFFERENTIAL DIAGNOSIS

- Pathologic processes in pulmonary parenchyma (bronchopneumonia, pulmonary edema, neoplasia, parasitism, contusion, hemorrhage)
- Pathologic processes in bronchial system (bronchitis/asthma, acquired or congenital structural abnormalities, neoplasia, obstruction)
- Pathologic processes in pleural space (pleural effusion, restrictive pleuritis, neoplasia)
- Other causes of pulmonary hypertension

INITIAL DATABASE

- Thoracic radiographs (initial test of choice):
  - Proximal pulmonary vascular dilation/distal pulmonary vascular attenuation.
  - Bronchointerstitial pulmonary parenchymal pattern (especially caudodorsal lung fields).
  - Right ventricular/atrial enlargement.
  - ± Pleural effusion.
  - Thoracic radiographs may be normal.
- Echocardiography:
  - Evidence of pulmonary hypertension ± visible thrombus (rare).
- Blood gas analysis:
  - Not specific.
  - Hypoxemia/hypocapnia (hypercapnia if severe).
  - Metabolic acidosis.
  - Elevated alveolar-arterial (A–a) gradient:
    - A–a gradient = $FIO_2(P_b - P_{H_2O}) - (P_aCO_2/R) - P_aO_2$, where:
      - FIO_2 is the fraction of inhaled oxygen (e.g., 0.21 for room air; 0.4 for 40% oxygen; etc.)
      - P_b = barometric pressure (627–643 mmHg)
      - P_{H_2O} = 47 mmHg
      - R = 0.8
      - PaO_2 and pCO_2 are obtained from the arterial blood gas result
    - Normal: <15 mmHg.
    - 15/15 dogs with necropsy-confirmed PTE had elevated A–a gradient.
- Plasma D-dimer concentration:
  - Problems with specificity, but high concentrations (i.e., >2000 ng/ml) consistent with thrombembolic disease in the dog.
- Nuclear ventilation/perfusion scan:
  - There may be problems with staged sensitivity/specificity, although a grossly abnormal scan is supportive of a diagnosis of PTE, while an absolutely normal scan rules PTE down.
- Pulmonary angiography:
  - Most sensitive/specific test.
  - Can document pulmonary vascular occlusion directly.
  - Unstable condition of patient may preclude the required sedation/anesthesia.

TREATMENT

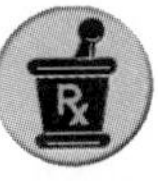

- Oxygen therapy (nasal administration is best).
- Positive end-expiratory pressure ventilation if severe.
- Antithrombotic therapy:
  - Unfractionated heparin acute treatment: 200 U/kg IV, followed by 75-200 U/kg SQ q 6-8h.
  - Warfarin/coumarin compounds for chronic treatment: 0.1 mg/kg PO q 24h.
  - Careful coagulation profile monitoring required. May result in iatrogenic hemorrhage.
- Thrombinolytic therapy (streptokinase, tissue plasminogen activator) may be useful in acute stage.
- Embolectomy is technically feasible in some cases depending upon location of thrombus, but significant morbidity/mortality is associated with this procedure.
- Judicious use of parenteral fluid therapy to maintain systemic blood pressure (careful not to exacerbate cardiac right sided pressure overload).

RECOMMENDED MONITORING

- Respiratory rate, blood gas analysis, and thoracic radiography provide relative indications of response to therapy/deterioration of patient condition.
- Careful monitoring of coagulation times is recommended.
  - For warfarin therapy: 1.5- to 2-fold increase in prothrombin time.

PROGNOSIS AND OUTCOME

Variable depending upon size of thrombus and degree of pulmonary vascular occlusion. Large thrombi resulting in significant occlusion of large portions of the pulmonary vascular bed are associated with a poor prognosis.

SUGGESTED READING

Johnson LR, et al: Pulmonary thromboembolism in 29 dogs: 1985–1995. *J Vet Intern Med* 13:338–345, 1999.

AUTHOR: **BRUCE G. KORNREICH**

EDITOR: **ETIENNE CÔTÉ**

Pulmonic Stenosis

BASIC INFORMATION

DEFINITION

A fixed or dynamic impediment to the ejection of blood from the right ventricle due to abnormal narrowing of the right ventricular outflow tract, pulmonic valve orifice, or main pulmonary artery

SYNONYM(S)

Pulmonic valve dysplasia

EPIDEMIOLOGY

SPECIES, AGE, SEX: Pulmonic stenosis (PS) is the third most common congenital heart defect in dogs. It is an uncommon congenital defect in cats, which are more likely to develop acquired, benign dynamic infundibular RV outflow tract obstructions as adults, most often in association with other systemic or cardiac diseases.

GENETICS AND BREED PREDISPOSITION: Inherited as a polygenic trait or single gene defect with variable penetrance. English bulldog, miniature schnauzer, Chihuahua, Samoyed, miniature pinscher, Labrador retriever, mastiff, beagle, fox terrier, Scottish terrier, West Highland white terrier, other terrier breeds are overrepresented.

ASSOCIATED CONDITIONS AND DISORDERS: Pulmonic stenosis occurs most often as an isolated defect but may be combined with other defects of the conotruncal septum (e.g., tetralogy of Fallot). The tricuspid valve apparatus is concurrently malformed in about one-third of dogs with pulmonic stenosis.

CLINICAL PRESENTATION

DISEASE FORMS/SUBTYPES: Four anatomic types of obstruction can occur: supravalvular, valvular, subvalvular, and infundibular. While the functional consequences of these different types of obstruction are similar, their distinction is important if repair is contemplated.

HISTORY, CHIEF COMPLAINT: Affected animals may show no overt clinical manifestations, or may exhibit exercise intolerance, or syncope. Signs of right heart failure (venous engorgement, hepatomegaly, ascites) commonly develop in severely affected animals.

PHYSICAL EXAM FINDINGS: A systolic ejection murmur is typically best heard at the left heart base, specifically over the pulmonic area. It may also radiate loudly cranially along the sternal border. Arterial pulses are unremarkable unless severe heart failure is present. Jugular distention, jugular pulses, hepatosplenomegaly, and ascites develop with the onset of right heart failure. Cyanosis may be observed when PS is complicated by right-to-left shunting across a patent foramen ovale, or coexisting atrial or ventricular septal defect.

ETIOLOGY AND PATHOPHYSIOLOGY

- Increased resistance to ejection results in concentric RV hypertrophy which develops in proportion to the severity of obstruction.
- The resulting decline in right ventricular diastolic compliance impairs ventricular filling, resulting in elevated right atrial pressure.
- Tricuspid regurgitation from progressive ventricular dilation or concurrent valvular dysplasia further increases right atrial pressure.
- Hypertrophy of the infundibular region of the right ventricular outflow tract may also contribute to outflow tract obstruction, particularly during exercise. This additional mechanism of obstruction can be particularly problematic following surgical valvotomy or balloon valvuloplasty.

DIAGNOSIS

DIFFERENTIAL DIAGNOSIS

Other congenital heart defects causing a systolic murmur, such as subvalvular aortic stenosis, ventricular septal defect, and tetralogy of Fallot

INITIAL DATABASE

- Electrocardiography: RVH is usually evident; right axis deviation, S_1, S_2, S_3 deep S waves in CV_6LU (or V4), CV_6LL (or V2).
- Thoracic radiography: characteristic findings include right ventricular enlargement and dilation of the main pulmonary artery segment. These changes are usually most evident on the dorsoventral view. Pulmonary vasculature is usually normal; however, in severe cases, the lungs may appear hypoperfused.
- Echocardiography: The site of obstruction, severity of RV hypertrophy, and poststenotic dilation of the main pulmonary artery are best demonstrated by the two-dimensional echocardiogram. The pulmonic valve area is best visualized from right parasternal short axis views or from the left cranial parasternal position or by transesophageal echocardiography. Color flow and spectral Doppler studies are useful to confirm the diagnosis and to determine the severity of obstruction. Estimation of peak blood flow velocity through the stenotic area, by Doppler interrogation, permits calculation of the pressure gradient using the modified Bernoulli equation, pressure gradient = $4 \times V^2$.

ADVANCED OR CONFIRMATORY TESTING

Angiocardiography is performed as a prelude to balloon valvuloplasty or surgical repair. Such studies are useful for clarifying the anatomic location of the obstruction, identifying leaflet fusion and thickening, identifying the severity of RV hypertrophy, and verifying the presence of other abnormalities such as hypoplasia of the pulmonic annulus, tricuspid regurgitation, or a patent foramen ovale. Left ventricular angiography or coronary arteriography should be performed when abnormalities of the left heart are suspected or when concurrent developmental abnormalities of the coronary arteries are suspected in boxer dogs and English bulldogs. The hemodynamic severity of outflow tract obstructions is accomplished by measuring the systolic pressure gradient across the lesion and estimating the effective valve orifice area.

TREATMENT

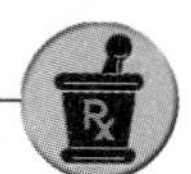

THERAPEUTIC GOAL(S)

Elimination of severe obstructing lesions prior to the development of heart failure

ACUTE GENERAL TREATMENT

- Dogs with mild pulmonic stenosis that is not causing overt manifestations do not require treatment.
- Dogs with such overt manifestations as exercise intolerance, synope, or signs of right heart failure and dogs with severe fixed anatomic obstructions should be referred for surgical repair or balloon valvuloplasty depending on the precise anatomy of the defect and/or presence of concurrent defects.
- Balloon valvuloplasty is the preferred method of treatment when the main abnormality is fusion of the pulmonic leaflets. Surgery is often required to effectively remedy complex lesions with annular hypoplasia and fixed or persistent subvalvular obstruction.
- Dynamic obstructions during stress or exercise can often be effectively palliated by β-receptor blockade. Such therapy is sometimes required following balloon valvuloplasty or surgical repair.

POSSIBLE COMPLICATIONS

Dogs with severe, untreated disease frequently develop progressive right heart enlargement, tricuspid regurgitation, right heart failure, and atrial fibrillation. Sudden death is less common than heart failure but is not uncommon.

RECOMMENDED MONITORING

Color-flow Doppler echocardiography is the most useful tool for assessing dogs with pulmonic stenosis over time. Some lesions that are modest in severity in juvenile animals can become progressively more severe over time. The short- and long-term success of surgery or balloon valvuloplasty is best determined by periodic echocardiographic evaluation. Chest radiographs and electrocardiography are useful for evaluating overall heart size and cardiac arrhythmias, respectively.

PROGNOSIS AND OUTCOME

- Dogs with mild obstructions have a very good prognosis and often reach old age.
- Dogs with severe obstructions (systolic pressure gradient >100 mmHg) have a guarded prognosis as they often develop heart failure or die suddenly.

- Balloon valvuloplasty improves outcome, particularly when the pressure gradients are substantially reduced.
- Restenosis occurs in about 10% of dogs treated by balloon valvuloplasty.

PEARLS & CONSIDERATIONS

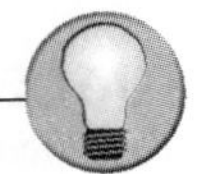

PREVENTION

- Conscientiously performed physical examinations with careful cardiac auscultation are key to early recognition.
- Dogs with confirmed pulmonic stenosis should not be bred.

CLIENT EDUCATION

Owners should be advised of the high likelihood of heart failure or sudden death in animals with severe disease that are not treated. Balloon valvuloplasty and surgical repair are recommended for patients with severe obstructions.

SUGGESTED READING

Johnson MS, et al: Pulmonic stenosis in dogs: balloon dilation improves clinical outcome. *J Vet Intern Med* 18:656, 2004.

Oyama M, Sisson DD, Thomas WP, Bonagura JD: Congenital heart disease. In Ettinger SJ, Feldman E (eds): *Textbook of Veterinary Internal Medicine*, ed 6. Philadelphia, WB Saunders, 2005, pp 972–1021.

Staudte KL, et al: Evaluation of closed pericardial patch grafting for management of severe pulmonic stenosis. *Aust Vet J* 82:33, 2004.

AUTHOR: **D. DAVID SISSON**

EDITOR: **ETIENNE CÔTÉ**

Pulse Abnormalities

BASIC INFORMATION

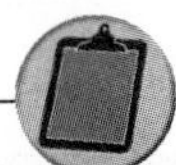

DEFINITION

The arterial pulse is produced by the fluctuation between diastolic and systolic arterial pressure and can be palpated as an impulse in superficial arteries, such as the femoral artery. Pulse deficit refers to a heartbeat that is heard on auscultation or felt on the chest wall but that does not generate a palpable arterial pulse.

SYNONYM(S)

Hyperkinetic pulse: strong, bounding, or "water-hammer" pulse

Hypokinetic pulse: weak or "thready" pulse

EPIDEMIOLOGY

SPECIES, AGE, SEX: Dogs and cats of either sex and any age.

ASSOCIATED CONDITIONS AND DISORDERS

- Reduced pulse amplitude (hypokinetic pulse):
  - Decreased cardiac output (hypovolemia, systolic dysfunction).
  - Left ventricular outflow tract obstruction (aortic stenosis, systolic anterior motion of the mitral valve). The pulse is not transmitted normally to the peripheral arteries; with aortic stenosis, it may be decreased and delayed (*pulsus parvus et tardus*).
- Increased pulse amplitude (hyperkinetic pulse):
  - Increased stroke volume (anemia, pregnancy, increased sympathetic tone, hyperthyroidism, bradyarrhythmias).
  - Decreased diastolic arterial pressure (patent ductus arteriosus, aortic insufficiency). Diastolic runoff through the ductus arteriosus or aortic valve, respectively, causes a greater difference between systolic and diastolic pressures (greater pulse pressure) and a correspondingly stronger pulse.
- Variation in pulse amplitude:
  - Exaggerated effect of respiration: *pulsus paradoxus* (pericardial effusion with cardiac tamponade). The pulse is stronger during expiration and weaker during inspiration.
  - Tachyarrhythmias (atrial fibrillation, ventricular and atrial premature complexes, ventricular tachycardia). Generally, in a given animal with one of these arrhythmias, the pulse becomes weaker with higher heart rates or beats that are more premature.
  - Severe myocardial failure (*pulsus alternans*).
- Regional variation in pulse amplitude:
  - Arterial thromboembolism (feline myocardial disease, infective endocarditis, hypercoagulable states).
- Variation in pulse rhythm:
  - Tachyarrhythmias (atrial fibrillation, premature atrial and ventricular complexes).
  - Bradyarrhythmias (second-degree atrioventricular block).

CLINICAL PRESENTATION

HISTORY, CHIEF COMPLAINT: Highly variable and dependent on underlying cause.

PHYSICAL EXAM FINDINGS

- Systemic or primary cardiac problems may alter the pulse; therefore, a complete physical exam is necessary.
- Femoral pulses are easiest to palpate in cats and dogs.
- Auscultate heart sounds simultaneously (by definition, a pulse deficit exists when heart sounds do not correspond with a palpable peripheral pulse).
- Pulse quality relates mainly to pulse amplitude (also affected by rate of rise of arterial pressure in systole and affected by pulse duration).

ETIOLOGY AND PATHOPHYSIOLOGY

- Pulse pressure: difference between systolic and diastolic blood pressure (BP).
- Variations in left ventricular stroke volume are detected as variation in arterial pulse pressure.
- With premature beats, the weak ventricular contraction may not generate sufficient systolic pressure to open the aortic valve, and no S_2 or pulse is produced (S_1 is still normally heard).
- Variations in stroke volume will also occur with the phase of respiration with cardiac tamponade, where increased filling of the right heart during inspiration leads to decreased filling of the left heart and a reduced pulse pressure.
- *Pulsus alternans* is an uncommon finding characterized by alternate pulses that are very weak or even absent, despite consistent electrical activation (due to abnormal intracellular calcium cycling in myocardial failure).

DIAGNOSIS

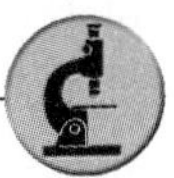

DIFFERENTIAL DIAGNOSIS

- Hypokinetic pulse: obesity, arterial disease/disorder. The combination of hypokinetic pulse and a palpably strong or hyperdynamic heartbeat (apex beat) is strongly suggestive of outflow obstruction (e.g., moderate to marked aortic stenosis or, less commonly, pulmonic stenosis).
- Hyperkinetic pulse: thin body condition.

- Variation in pulse amplitude: normal variation as occurs with respiratory sinus arrhythmia (pulse is stronger after pause).

INITIAL DATABASE

- The presence of pulse deficit should prompt recording of an electrocardiogram.
- The presence of alternate pulse deficits with normal sinus rhythm (*pulsus alternans*) should prompt a thoracic radiographic exam and an echocardiographic exam.

TREATMENT

THERAPEUTIC GOAL(S)

Management of underlying cause

PROGNOSIS AND OUTCOME

Highly variable and dependent on underlying cause

PEARLS & CONSIDERATIONS

COMMENTS

- Palpation of the peripheral arterial pulse can give useful information about stroke volume and cardiac output.
- Palpation of the arterial pulse is not a useful way of detecting systemic hypertension.
- Presence of a hyperkinetic pulse may be more obvious than a diastolic murmur with severe aortic insufficiency (as with infective endocarditis of the aortic valve).
- Pulsus paradoxus is a very helpful finding when cardiac tamponade is suspected but may be difficult to detect if the dog is panting.

SUGGESTED READING

Braunwald E, Perloff JK: Physical examination of the heart and circulation. In Braunwald E, Zipes DP, Peter L, Bonow R (eds): *Braunwald's Heart Disease: A Textbook of Cardiovascular Medicine*. Philadelpia, WB Saunders, 2004, pp 82–85.

AUTHOR: **VIRGINIA LUIS FUENTES**
EDITOR: **ETIENNE CÔTÉ**

Pupil Abnormalities

BASIC INFORMATION

DEFINITION

Abnormalities include pupils that are inappropriately dilated or constricted as well as pupils with distorted shape or form

SYNONYM(S)

Anisocoria: unequal or asymmetric pupils
Dyscoria: misshapen/distorted pupil
Miosis: constricted pupil
Mydriasis: dilated pupil

EPIDEMIOLOGY

SPECIES, AGE, SEX

- Dogs and cats.
- Iris atrophy is a normal change that occurs with aging and is therefore seen in older animals.
- Iris coloboma (absence or defect in iris) is a developmental/heritable condition that is usually noticed initially in young animals, usually dogs.

GENETICS AND BREED PREDISPOSITION: A distorted pupil, such as iris coloboma, is breed-related in dogs. Australian shepherds and dalmatians are overrepresented.

Dilated pupil:

- Cocker spaniels, basset hounds, beagles, Alaskan malamute, chow chows, and Samoyeds are among breeds predisposed to developing primary glaucoma (see Glaucoma, p 440).
- Toy and miniature poodles are predisposed to optic nerve hypoplasia.
- A relatively large number of purebred dogs may demonstrate heritable retinal degeneration; while also reported in cats, the condition is far less common (see Retinal Degeneration, p 963).

CLINICAL PRESENTATION

DISEASE FORMS/SUBTYPES: Conditions that lead to pupil abnormalities can be divided into those that cause:

- Pupillary dilation (mydriasis)
- Pupillary constriction (miosis)
- Abnormal pupil shape (dyscoria)

HISTORY, CHIEF COMPLAINT: The pet's owner may notice abnormalities in pupil size and shape. More likely, animals present for painful, red, or blind eyes; veterinarians then notice the pupil abnormalities.

PHYSICAL EXAM FINDINGS

- Dilated pupil and the following:
  - Scalloping at pupillary margin:
    - Iris coloboma: focal; young animal
    - Iris atrophy: typically multifocal and/or "moth-eaten" effect in iris stroma; typically age-related change (i.e., older animals)
  - Blindness (negative menace response):
    - See Retinal Degeneration, p 963; Retinal Detachment, p 965
    - Optic nerve lesion (e.g., optic nerve hypoplasia, congenital; see Glaucoma, p 440; Optic Neuritis, p 768)
    - Optic chiasmal lesion (see Blindness, p 136)
    - Cerebral lesion (occipital/visual cortex)
  - "Quiet" (i.e., nonred), sighted (visual) eye:
    - Internal ophthalmoplegia, paralysis of the iris and ciliary muscles caused by:
      - Pharmacologic pupillary dilation (e.g., parasympatholytics, such as atropine and topical tropicamide)
      - Iris atrophy
      - Lesions involving the parasympathetic fibers of the oculomotor nerve (cranial nerve [CN] III); relatively rare
    - Fearful animal (i.e., sympathetic stimulation): transient mydriasis; resolves once animal becomes calm
- Constricted pupil and the following:
  - Red eye with or without vision impairment:
    - See Uveitis, p 1134
    - Corneal ulceration (see Corneal Ulceration, p 246) and "axon reflex" miosis through trigeminal and oculomotor nerves (CN V and III)
    - Pharmacologic pupillary constriction (e.g., parasympathomimetic, such as topical pilocarpine, demecarium, or prostaglandin analogs; analogs include latanoprost and travoprost; may cause conjunctival hyperemia)
  - Quiet eye with or without vision impairment:
    - Horner's syndrome: other signs include ptosis (drooping of upper eyelid), enophthalmos (caudal displacement of the eye), and third eyelid protrusion (see Horner's Syndrome, p 532)
- Distorted pupil and the following:
  - Scalloping at pupillary margin:
    - Iris coloboma: focal; young animal
    - Iris atrophy: typically multifocal and/or "moth-eaten" effect in iris

stroma; typically age-related change (i.e., older animals)
  - Red eye with or without vision impairment:
    - Adhesions of iris-to-lens and/or iris-to-cornea (posterior and anterior synechiae, respectively) from current or past anterior uveitis (see Uveitis, p 1134)
    - Iris prolapse through full-thickness corneal lesion (see Corneal/Scleral Trauma, p 244)
    - Iridodonesis (tremulousness of the iris on movement of the eye) noted with loss of iris support subsequent to lens subluxation/luxation (see Lens Luxation, p 628)
- Anisocoria:
  - Primary iridal disease (age-related atrophy); heritable or developmental coloboma, active inflammatory process causing miosis; chronic inflammation leading to degeneration and/or posterior synechia
  - Primary neurologic cause (CN III abnormality, Horner's syndrome, fright response)
  - Pharmacologic agents (miotics, such as pilocarpine; mydriatics, such as atropine and tropicamide)
- Unresponsive pupil(s):
  - Retinal disease (see Blindness, p 136)
  - Optic nerve disease
  - Iridal disease (see Iris Abnormalities, p 608)
  - Pharmacologic agents
  - Posterior synechia secondary to anterior uveitis

DIAGNOSIS

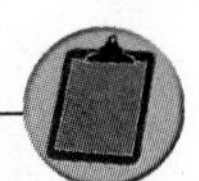

INITIAL DATABASE

Complete ophthalmic examination, including:

- Neuro-ophthalmic examination (i.e., menace response; dazzle, palpebral, pupillary light, and vestibulo-ocular reflexes)
- Fluorescein dye application (miosis commonly occurs in animals with corneal ulceration)
- Intraocular pressures (>30 mmHg with glaucoma; often low [<10–15 mmHg] with uveitis)

ADVANCED OR CONFIRMATORY TESTING

Variable depending on underlying condition:

- Pharmacologic testing (e.g., 10% phenylephrine) for Horner's syndrome
- CT scans, MRIs, and other imaging procedures; cerebrospinal fluid tap for diseases of the neurologic system (e.g., optic neuritis; optic chiasmal lesions) or orbital disorders
- Electroretinogram to assess retinal function (see Retinal Degeneration, p 963)

TREATMENT

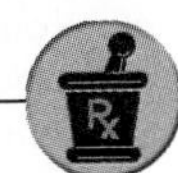

THERAPEUTIC GOAL(S)

- Depend(s) on underlying condition and cause.
- Treatment is either not indicated or not available for iris atrophy, iris coloboma, optic nerve hypoplasia, retinal degeneration, and optic nerve atrophy/degeneration.
- If a specific systemic cause of oculomotor neuropathy, optic neuropathy, anterior uveitis, or Horner's syndrome can be identified, treatment can address the specific cause.

ACUTE AND CHRONIC TREATMENT

Directed at underlying cause

PROGNOSIS AND OUTCOME

- Prognosis varies widely depending on underlying condition and cause.
- Many causes of pupil abnormalities are completely innocuous, while others may be life threatening.

PEARLS & CONSIDERATIONS

COMMENTS

Many pupil abnormalities can be diagnosed with careful consideration of the signalment and the presence or absence of other ophthalmic signs.

CLIENT EDUCATION

- Pupil abnormalities can be an early sign of serious disease.
- Early detection may improve prognosis.

SUGGESTED READING

Grahn BH, Cullen CL, Peiffer RL: Neuro-ophthalmology. In *Veterinary Ophthalmology Essentials*. Philadelphia, Butterworth Heinemann, 2004, pp 200–224.

Scagliotti RH: Comparative neuro-ophthalmology. In Gelatt KN (ed): *Veterinary Ophthalmology*, ed 3. Philadelphia, Lippincott Williams & Wilkins, 1999, pp 1307–1400.

Ocular Disorders Presumed to Be Inherited in Purebred Dogs, ed 3. Genetics Committee of the American College of Veterinary Ophthalmologists, 1999.

AUTHOR: **STEVEN R. HOLLINGSWORTH**
EDITOR: **CHERYL L. CULLEN**

Pustular and Crusting Skin Disorders

BASIC INFORMATION

DEFINITION

Skin diseases associated with pustules and crusting. Pustules are small, circumscribed elevations of the skin filled with pus. Healing or ruptured pustules may form scabs or crusts, the dried accumulation of exudate (blood, pus, serum) over a lost or damaged epidermis.

EPIDEMIOLOGY

SPECIES, AGE, SEX

- Dogs and cats.
- In dogs, dermatophytosis, demodicosis, and impetigo are causes that are more likely in animals <1 year old. Pemphigus is more common in middle-aged adults.
- Drug eruptions may occur at any age.

GENETICS AND BREED PREDISPOSITION

- Subcorneal pustular dermatosis and superficial suppurative necrolytic dermatitis: miniature schnauzer
- Pemphigus foliaceus: Akita, chow chow, dachshund
- Drug eruption (especially to sulfonamides): Doberman pinscher
- Canine linear IgA pustular dermatosis: dachshund

RISK FACTORS

- Pyoderma, the most common cause of pustular and crusting dermatitis in dogs, is almost always secondary to a predisposing skin disease.
- Cats affected with feline immunodeficiency virus (FIV) infection are more susceptible to dermatophytosis.

CONTAGION AND ZOONOSIS: Dermatophytosis is contagious to other animals and is zoonotic.

GEOGRAPHY AND SEASONALITY

- Pemphigus foliaceus and pemphigus erythematosus can be aggravated by exposure to sunlight (see Pemphigus Complex, p 823).

- Pyodermas associated with underlying atopy may have a seasonal occurrence.
- Leishmaniasis is more common in endemic areas.

ASSOCIATED CONDITIONS AND DISORDERS: Bullous impetigo in adult dogs is often associated with immunosuppression (e.g., hyperadrenocorticism, diabetes mellitus, hypothyroidism).

CLINICAL PRESENTATION

HISTORY, CHIEF COMPLAINT

- Pustules are usually short-lived and may go unnoticed. Scaling and crusting are often the dominant presentation.
- Pruritus varies with the etiology. It can be a major presenting complaint in disorders such as pyodermas with underlying allergies or ectoparasitism.
- A variable degree of hair loss may accompany follicular damage.
- Systemic signs of lethargy and anorexia can be part of the presenting picture with pemphigus foliaceus, cutaneous drug eruptions, or superficial suppurative necrolytic dermatitis of the miniature schnauzer.

PHYSICAL EXAM FINDINGS

- Pustules are most commonly yellow. Green pustules may indicate the presence of gram-negative bacteria or marked toxic change. Larger flaccid pustules are more common in the pemphigus complex and bullous impetigo.
- Scales, collarettes, crusts of various color (brown, honey-colored) and texture (adherent, flaky), alopecia, erythema, and focal areas of hyperpigmentation or hyperkeratosis may be noted. Depending on the condition and severity, the extent and location of lesions may be variable.

ETIOLOGY AND PATHOPHYSIOLOGY

Pustules result from a loss of epidermal intercellular cohesion (edema, degeneration, inflammation, autoantibody formation, etc.), causing epidermal or subepidermal cavities that eventually fill with inflammatory cells.

DIAGNOSIS

DIFFERENTIAL DIAGNOSIS

- Infectious: pustules most often have a follicular orientation.
  - Bacterial: pyoderma (bacterial folliculitis*, impetigo*, furunculosis), dermatophilosis
  - Fungal: dermatophytosis
  - Parasitic: demodicosis*, *Pelodera* dermatitis
  - Protozoal: leishmaniasis
- Immune-mediated: pemphigus complex (especially pemphigus foliaceus*), canine eosinophilic folliculitis and furunculosis, canine sterile eosinophilic pustulosis*, subcorneal pustular dermatosis*, and canine linear IgA pustular dermatosis.*
- Drug eruption: superficial suppurative necrolytic dermatitis of schnauzer (associated with shampoo therapy), drug-induced pemphigus foliaceus, and eosinophilic pustulosis (subcorneal to follicular neutrophilic pustulosis).

INITIAL DATABASE

- The medical history of animal is important: presence or absence of pruritus, progression, chronicity, and seasonality to determine etiology.
- Cytologic examination of pustular contents:
  - Bacteria: phagocytized bacteria (often cocci, because staphylococcal organisms are the primary isolates from dogs and cats).
  - Neutrophils: pemphigus complex, subcorneal pustular dermatosis, and canine linear IgA pustular dermatosis are usually sterile and contain numerous intact neutrophils with a variable number of acantholytic keratinocytes (numerous in pemphigus and subcorneal pustular dermatosis; occasional to none in linear IgA dermatosis).
  - Eosinophils: eosinophilic folliculitis/furunculosis and sterile eosinophilic pustulosis contain numerous eosinophils; eosinophils are also associated with superficial pyodermas with parasitic or allergic disorders, deep pyodermas (furunculosis), drug eruptions, and pemphigus foliaceus.
- Skin scrapings: *Demodex* sp.
- Fungal culture: dermatophytosis.
- Complete blood count (CBC), serum biochemistry profile, and urinalysis if disease with systemic involvement is suspected; results are most often unremarkable besides mild to moderate neutrophilic or eosinophilic leukocytosis.

ADVANCED OR CONFIRMATORY TESTING

- Skin biopsies for histopathologic evaluation.
- Bacterial culture and sensitivity (C&S) if indicated: if bacilliform bacteria are noted on cytologic examination results or if there is a poor response to appropriate antibiotic therapy.
- Endocrine tests if clinician suspects underlying endocrinopathy.
- Serology for FIV, feline leukemia virus (FeLV), leishmaniasis.

TREATMENT

THERAPEUTIC GOAL(S)

Permanent cure whenever possible, or control of the disease, with appropriate therapy.

ACUTE AND CHRONIC TREATMENT

Depends on etiology of the disorder:

- Antibiotic therapy: a common empiric choice is cephalexin 22 mg/kg PO q 8–12h; a more specific selection can be made based on results of C&S.
- Antifungal therapy: choice of antifungal (oral versus systemic; specific type) depends on type of mycosis.
- Antiparasitics: choice of medication depends on the parasite identified.

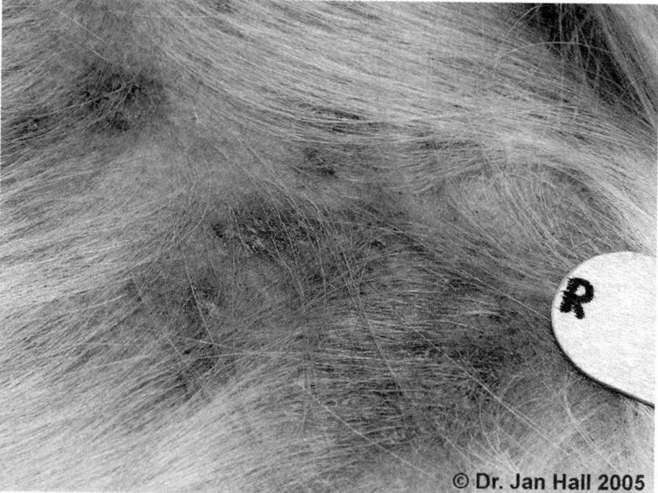

FIGURE I-141 Crusts on the ventral abdomen of a golden retriever with pyoderma. Courtesy of Dr. Jan A. Hall.

*Presence of intact pustules is most commonly noted clinically in these disorders.

- Immunosuppressive dosage of glucocorticoids and/or other immunosuppressive drugs for immune-mediated disorders.

PROGNOSIS AND OUTCOME

Varies according to the disease

PEARLS & CONSIDERATIONS

COMMENTS

- Crusts alone are noted in certain diseases, such as in cornification disorders or zinc-responsive dermatosis.
- Crusts secondary to excoriations are frequent in common disease processes, such as atopic dermatitis, food intolerance, and flea-bite dermatitis.
- The combined presence of crusts and pustules restricts the differential diagnosis, but pustules can be short-lived, and the clinician should perform a careful examination before confirming their absence.
- Treat and rule out the presence of bacterial disease before taking biopsies for histopathologic evaluation.

SUGGESTED READING

Bensignor E: Diagnostic approach to crusting dermatoses. In Gaguère E, Prélaud P (eds): *A Practical Guide to Feline Dermatology*. Lyon, France, Merial, 1999, pp 20.1–20.4.

Scott DW, Miller WH, Griffin CE: Diagnostic methods. In Scott DW, Miller WH, Griffin CE (eds): *Muller and Kirk's Small Animal Dermatology*, ed 6. Philadelphia, WB Saunders, 2001, pp 71–206.

AUTHOR: **CAROLINE DE JAHAM**
EDITOR: **JAN A. HALL**

Pyelonephritis

BASIC INFORMATION

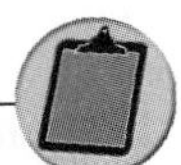

DEFINITION

Inflammation of the renal pelvis and interstitium typically associated with, or originating from, ascending bacterial infection

SYNONYM(S)

Kidney infection
Pyelitis

EPIDEMIOLOGY

SPECIES, AGE, SEX: Dogs and cats are susceptible, with females predisposed; most common in older animals or in younger animals with predisposing cause (e.g., congenital urinary malformations, uroliths).

RISK FACTORS: Dogs and cats:

- Anatomic abnormalities:
  - Ectopic ureter(s)
  - Urethral/ureteral obstruction
  - Hydroureter/hydronephrosis
  - Perineal urethrostomy
  - Urolithiasis
  - Vulvar conformational abnormalities
- Functional abnormalities:
  - Urine retention (>0.25 ml/kg following complete voiding)
  - Urine reflux due to increased intravesicular pressure
  - Isosthenuria or hyposthenuria from any cause
  - Immunocompromise
  - Indwelling urinary catheter
- Lower genitourinary tract infection:
  - Dogs and cats: various bacteria
    - *Escherichia coli* most common isolate in urinary infections
  - Fungal and yeast pyelonephritis possible, especially in immunocompromised animals
  - Bacterial prostatitis: intact male dogs

CONTAGION AND ZOONOSIS: None

ASSOCIATED CONDITIONS AND DISORDERS

- Acute renal failure
- Chronic renal failure
- Hypokalemia (cats)
- Bacterial cystitis
- Urolithiasis (renal or cystic)

CLINICAL PRESENTATION

DISEASE FORMS/SUBTYPES

- Ascending pyelonephritis
- Hematogenous pyelonephritis: rare; may be associated with septicemia

HISTORY, CHIEF COMPLAINT: Clinical signs may be absent; chronic pyelonephritis is a common complicating factor in chronic renal diseases. When present, clinical signs may include:

- Polyuria and polydipsia (PU/PD)
- Fever, malaise (rare)
- Hematuria (with or without stranguria and pollakiuria from concurrent lower urinary tract disorder)
- Pollakiuria, stranguria (if concurrent lower urinary tract disorder)
- Abdominal, lumbar, or general discomfort
- Renomegaly (acute pyelonephritis)
- Renal asymmetry (chronic)
- Recurrent lower urinary infections
- History of predisposing cause may be present (e.g., urinary catheterization, uroliths)

PHYSICAL EXAM FINDINGS: Exam may be normal. Abnormalities, when present, may include:

- Dehydration
- Renomegaly
- Renal asymmetry
- Abdominal/renal/lumbar pain
- Unkempt haircoat
- Oral ulcerations/halitosis (uremia)
- Debris or secretions in the oral cavity (vomitus, saliva)
- Bladder discomfort (if concurrent lower urinary infection)

ETIOLOGY AND PATHOPHYSIOLOGY

- Infectious agent (bacteria, fungus, yeast) usually ascends to renal pelvis from lower urinary tract. The agent rarely infects the kidneys hematogenously.
- Onset may be acute (less common) or insidious (more common).
- Renal response to injury causes clinical signs:
  - Acute infection results in nephritis (renal inflammation), causing renomegaly and renal pain.
  - Acute or chronic infection causes nephrogenic diabetes insipidus via bacterial toxin actions on antidiuretic hormone receptors.
  - Chronic infection results in renal scarring, resulting in smaller than normal kidneys.
- Infection may result in acute renal failure, chronic renal failure, or exacerbation of preexisting chronic renal failure.

DIAGNOSIS

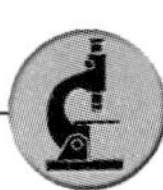

DIFFERENTIAL DIAGNOSIS

- Differential diagnosis of PU/PD (see Polyuria/Polydipsia, p 878)
- PD from psychogenic causes, hyperosmolarity, or alteration of the thirst center (e.g., central nervous system [CNS] neoplasia)

- Osmotic diuresis (e.g., diabetes mellitus, renal glucosuria, drug or toxin)
- Nephrogenic diabetes insipidus (e.g., congenital, electrolyte abnormalities, hormonal abnormalities, renal failure)
- Deficient interstitial concentrating gradient (e.g., medullary washout, hyponatremia, protosystemic shunt)
- Lack of antidiuretic hormone (i.e., central diabetes insipidus)

Note: Pyelonephritis can be a primary cause of renal disease or may occur as a complication of renal failure.

INITIAL DATABASE

- Complete blood count (CBC): may be normal (chronic pyelonephritis) or may show leukocytosis with left shift (acute pyelonephritis); normocytic, normochromic nonregenerative anemia is possible with concurrent chronic renal failure.
- Serum biochemical profile: may be normal (chronic pyelonephritis). Azotemia (elevated blood urea nitrogen [BUN], creatinine, phosphorus), hypokalemia or hyperkalemia, metabolic acidosis (acute or chronic renal failure).
- Urinalysis: isosthenuria; occasionally the animal may experience leukocyte casts (acute pyelonephritis), pyuria, hematuria, bacturia, crystalluria.
- Abdominal radiographs: variable renal shadow (normal, large, or small and irregular). Radiopaque urinary (upper or lower) calculi (suspect struvite) are sometimes present.
- Abdominal ultrasound: Renal pelvic dilation is common; renomegaly or small and irregular kidneys, alterations in renal parenchymal echogenicity also can be present.
- Urine culture prior to treatment whenever suspicion of pyelonephritis exists (even if urine sediment inactive):
  - In occult pyelonephritis, urine culture can be negative.

ADVANCED OR CONFIRMATORY TESTING

- Pyelocentesis (ultrasound guided) to obtain urine for culture; this procedure is uncommonly used. Begin with routine cystocentesis instead and choose pyelocentesis if trying to pinpoint source of infection to one kidney (rarely clinically necessary).
- Excretory urogram and/or cystourethrogram to rule out anatomic abnormalities. Abdominal ultrasound is the preferred first choice instead.
- If clinical signs are compatible, rule out hyperadrenocorticism as a predisposing cause.
- Renal cortex biopsy: typically not helpful to diagnose pyelonephritis due to localization of disease (renal pelvis and interstitium).

TREATMENT

THERAPEUTIC GOAL(S)

- Treatment of renal failure if appropriate (see Acute Renal Failure, p 32; Chronic Renal Failure, Occult ["Asymptomatic"], p 204; Chronic Renal Failure, Overt ["Symptomatic"], p 205)
- Resolution of anatomic or functional abnormalities predisposing to pyelonephritis
- Treatment of infectious causation with appropriate long-term antimicrobial therapy

ACUTE GENERAL TREATMENT

- Antimicrobial therapy:
  - Antibiotic selection is based on culture and antimicrobial susceptibility results.
  - Pending results, or if culture is negative despite clinical suspicion of pyelonephritis, therapy is indicated using an antibiotic that is renally excreted with gram-negative spectrum (fluoroquinolone, augmented penicillin, trimethoprim-sulfa) to reach adequate tissue concentrations. Examples:
    - Fluoroquinolone, such as enrofloxacin 5–20 mg/kg q 12–24h (dogs), or 5 mg/kg q 24h (cats) PO, IM, or diluted 1:1 with sterile saline and given slowly IV.
    - Amoxicillin with clavulanic acid at 22 mg/kg PO q 8–12h.
  - For intact male dogs, it is preferable to select an antimicrobial that will penetrate the blood-prostate barrier (e.g., fluoroquinolone, trimethoprim-sulfa).
  - Antibiotic choice is adjusted based on sensitivity results as they become available.
  - Due to the sluggish rate of medullary blood flow, duration of antibiotic therapy should be greater than that for a simple lower urinary tract infection. Therapy typically lasts 3 to 6 weeks depending on clinical improvement, underlying disease, and follow-up test results.
  - If initial urine sediment was active, a repeat urinalysis about 1 week after starting antibiotic therapy is recommended to ensure resolution of bacturia and pyuria.
  - If predisposing cause cannot be resolved, urine cultures should be repeated regularly to address future infections.
  - Fungal pyelonephritis may be more difficult to eradicate than bacterial pyelonephritis (see Cystitis, Fungal/Algal, p 272).
- Treatment of uremic renal failure starts with isotonic crystalloid fluid therapy (see Acute Renal Failure, p 32; Chronic Renal Failure, Overt ["Symptomatic"], p 205; Chronic Renal Failure, Occult ["Asymptomatic"], p 204).
- Medical therapy for hypokalemia:
  - Occurs commonly in cats with chronic PU/PD.
  - Potassium chloride (KCl) supplementation of IV fluids used for diuresis, based on sliding scale (see Table I-25):
  - Do not exceed a rate of 0.5 mEq KCl/kg per hour for potassium replacement.
  - Recheck potassium levels are indicated at least daily during fluid therapy.
  - When the patient is eating, oral potassium gluconate replacement can be initiated at a starting dose of 2 mEq per cat, q 12h, adjusted as needed based on serial serum potassium measurements.
- Uremic signs are managed as for acute and chronic renal failure (see Acute Renal Failure, p 32; Chronic Renal Failure, Overt ["Symptomatic"], p 205).

CHRONIC TREATMENT

- Maintain fluid balance.
  - Hospitalization is not indicated if the patient is drinking and eating enough to maintain hydration.
  - If the patient is hospitalized for IV fluid therapy, fluids should be tapered slowly over 2 to 3 days and discontinued once hydration is maintained by oral intake.
  - In cats and small dogs, the ability to maintain hydration might require a period of adaptation. Following hospital discharge, SC crystalloid fluid therapy might be indicated q 12–48h (see Acute Renal Failure, p 32; Chronic Renal Failure, Occult ["Asymptomatic"], p 204.
- Identification, treatment, or cure of predisposing cause if possible (e.g.,

TABLE I-25 Potassium Supplementation in Intravenous Fluid Therapy

Serum potassium concentration	Potassium supplementation to IV fluids
Potassium 3.5–5.5 mEq/L	Add 20 mEq KCl/L crystalloid
Potassium 3.0–3.4 mEq/L	Add 30 mEq KCl/L crystalloid
Potassium 2.5–2.9 mEq/L	Add 40 mEq KCl/L crystalloid
Potassium 2.0–2.4 mEq/L	Add 60 mEq KCl/L crystalloid
Potassium <2.0 mEq/L	Add 80 mEq KCl/L crystalloid

hyperadrenocorticism, ectopic ureter, urolithiasis).
- Appropriate nutritional support; a diet restricted/optimized in protein and phosphorus is ideal.
- Other treatments for chronic renal failure as necessary (see Chronic Renal Failure, Overt ["Symptomatic"], p 205; Chronic Renal Failure, Occult ["Asymptomatic"], p 204).

POSSIBLE COMPLICATIONS

- Failure to resolve infection.
- Bacterial resistance is common if there is infection secondary to an underlying process or a structural lesion.

RECOMMENDED MONITORING

- A repeat urine culture 1 to 2 weeks after completion of antibiotics and approximately 1 and 2 months later are indicated to ensure negative culture.
- If predisposing cause cannot be resolved (e.g., chronic renal failure), monitoring should include urinalysis and urine culture every 3 to 6 months to identify recurrence.
- When initial urine culture is negative despite clinical suspicion of pyelonephritis, monitoring should include water consumption daily before and after initiation of antibiotics to assess efficacy of therapy. If water consumption decreases within 2 weeks of antimicrobial therapy, treatment should be continued for a total of 3 to 6 weeks.

PROGNOSIS AND OUTCOME

- Guarded to good depending on ability to correct predisposing cause and antimicrobial susceptibility of pathogen.
- Prognosis for recurrent pyelonephritis is guarded since infections can cause chronic or acute renal failure, and recurrent infections tend to develop multiple antimicrobial resistance over time.

PEARLS & CONSIDERATIONS

COMMENTS

- Pyelonephritis is often difficult to confirm, especially after antimicrobial therapy has been initiated.
- Evidence of renal pelvic dilation (pyelectasia) on ultrasound without other supportive clinical findings might indicate a past infection with permanent renal injury instead of active infection; a differential diagnosis is vigorous IV fluid therapy, which can also cause pyelectasia.
- Chronic pyelonephritis can occur without producing any overt clinical signs and without changes on CBC, serum biochemical profile, or urine sediment exam.
- A urine C&S is warranted in the management of any chronic renal disorder because pyelonephritis may be clinically silent and may be difficult to detect (e.g., diluted urine may give the mistaken appearance of an inactive sediment); however, the condition is treatable, potentially resulting in a reversal of renal tubular damage.

PREVENTION

- Address anatomic or functional abnormalities directly
- Treatment of infections with the appropriate antimicrobial therapy at the correct dose for at least 3 to 6 weeks
- Regular follow-up visits to identify recurrent infections as early as possible

CLIENT EDUCATION

- Owner education regarding signs of lower and upper urinary tract infection before pyelonephritis develops.
- Treatment of resistant strains of bacteria causing pyelonephritis may be costly.
- Chronic renal failure may predispose animals (especially cats) to recurrent renal infections.

SUGGESTED READING

Bartges JW, Barsanti JA: Bacterial urinary tract infections in cats. In Bonagura JD (ed): *Kirk's Current Veterinary Therapy XIII.* Philadelphia, WB Saunders, 2000, pp 880–882.

Cowgill LD, Francey T: Acute uremia. In Ettinger SJ, Feldman EC (eds): *Textbook of Veterinary Internal Medicine*, vol 2, ed 6. St. Louis, Elsevier, 2005, pp 1731–1751.

Newman SJ, et al: Cryptococcal pyelonephritis in a dog. *J Am Vet Med Assoc* 222:180, 2003.

AUTHOR: **MARIE E. KERL**

EDITOR: **LEAH A. COHN**

Pyloric Hypertrophy Syndrome

BASIC INFORMATION

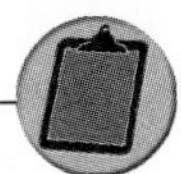

DEFINITION

Stenosis of the gastric outflow tract secondary to one of the following: hypertrophy of the circular muscle of the pylorus, hyperplasia of the mucosa of the pyloric antrum, or combination of muscular and mucosal thickening

SYNONYM(S)

Acquired antral pyloric hypertrophy
Chronic hypertrophic pyloric gastropathy
Hypertrophic gastritis
Pyloric stenosis

EPIDEMIOLOGY

SPECIES, AGE, SEX

- Congenital: dogs and cats, identified sometime after animal starts eating solid food, usually at 4 to 12 months of age
- Acquired: canine, middle-aged (4 to 7 years) and older, usually male

GENETICS AND BREED PREDISPOSITION

- Congenital: brachycephalic breeds including Boston terriers, English bulldogs, boxers, and Siamese cats
- Acquired: small, often Asian-breed dogs including Lhasa apso, shih tzu, Pekingese, and Maltese

ASSOCIATED CONDITIONS AND DISORDERS: Vicious temperament may be associated with acquired form.

CLINICAL PRESENTATION

DISEASE FORMS/SUBTYPES

- Congenital: selective hypertrophy of the circular pyloric muscle
- Acquired: mucosal hypertrophy or combination of mucosal and muscular hypertrophy; mucosal hypertrophy may be focal (polyp) or more generalized involving entire pyloric antrum

HISTORY, CHIEF COMPLAINT

- Chronic vomiting, usually of food several hours after eating; may be projectile
- In congenital form, vomiting begins after animal starts eating solid foods
- Anorexia
- Mild weight loss
- Regurgitation

PHYSICAL EXAM FINDINGS

- Generally unremarkable
- Thin body condition is possible

ETIOLOGY AND PATHOPHYSIOLOGY

- Cause is unknown and genetics of congenital form are not described.
- Excessive secretion of gastrin may stimulate growth of gastric smooth muscle and mucosa of gastric body.

- Some cases of "acquired" form may be slow progression of congenital form.
- Regurgitation can develop secondary to reflux esophagitis or persistent vomiting.
- Paradoxic aciduria possible. Vomiting causes hypovolemia, triggering renal Na^+ resorption. Proximal tubular renal Na^+ resorption requires coresorption of Cl^-, which is scarce in the tubular fluid of hypochloremic, vomiting animals. Therefore, Na^+ resorption occurs in the distal tubule in exchange for excretion of H^+ or K^+ (less so K^+, since these patients are often markedly hypokalemic). The result is aciduria despite metabolic alkalosis ("paradox").

DIAGNOSIS

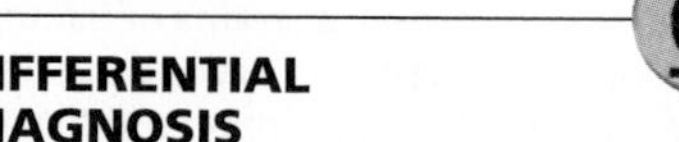

DIFFERENTIAL DIAGNOSIS

- For clinical presentation: other causes of chronic vomiting such as parasitism, viral, bacterial, fungal, or protozoal infection, inflammatory bowel disease, food allergy or intolerance, neoplasia, obstruction, systemic disease (liver disease, renal failure), central nervous system disease, drugs, must be ruled out by a systematic evaluation.
- For imaging findings: infiltrative diseases, such as neoplasia, pythiosis, or other fungal diseases.

INITIAL DATABASE

- Complete blood count, serum biochemistry profile, and urinalysis: often unremarkable but hyponatremic, hypochloremic metabolic alkalosis, and paradoxic aciduria may be present due to vomiting of gastric contents only.
- Radiographs: usually unremarkable. Stomach may be distended with fluid or air. Severe pyloric hypertrophy may occasionally be noted on plain films.
- Ultrasound: mucosal or muscular thickening of pylorus.

ADVANCED OR CONFIRMATORY TESTING

- Contrast radiographs: delayed gastric emptying with thickening of the pylorus, abrupt narrowing of the pyloric canal, or a long wisp of contrast joining the thickened pylorus to the duodenum. Note: purpose-made radiopaque spheres, pellets, or other devices for measurement of gastric motility are often not more useful than routine contrast studies.
- Endoscopy: mucosal hypertrophy with abundant antral folds or polyps with or without erosive lesions. Muscular hypertrophy can be more difficult to appreciate. Either lesion may yield a pylorus that is difficult to intubate with endoscope.
- Celiotomy: thickened pylorus and abundant mucosal folds in the antrum and pylorus.
- Histopathologic evaluation of tissue: mucosa normal or thickened with erosions, edema, and hyperplasia or cystic changes in gastric glands; increased numbers and prominent branching pattern of surface gastric pits; erosions may have lymphocyte and plasma cell infiltration; *Campylobacter*-like organisms have been reported.

TREATMENT

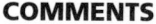

THERAPEUTIC GOAL(S)

Elimination of pyloric canal obstruction caused by the exuberant tissue

ACUTE GENERAL TREATMENT

- Surgery is indicated for both forms of antral pyloric hypertophy syndrome.
- Y-U pyloroplasty is the most common procedure, especially if mucosal hypertrophy is present.
- Gastroduodenal anastomosis (Bilroth I) for cases with extensive mucosal involvement.
- Pyloromyotomy is often ineffective and is not recommended for any type of pyloric hypertrophy other than those cases limited to pyloric muscular hypertrophy.
- Short-term postoperative compromise of gastrointestinal motility may be treated with metoclopramide (0.2-0.4 PO or SC mg/kg q 8-12h).

POSSIBLE COMPLICATIONS

- Potential complications of surgery include infection, leakage, and dehiscence.
- Gastrointestinal motility may be temporarily compromised after surgery.

PROGNOSIS AND OUTCOME

Prognosis is excellent if no postoperative complications occur

PEARLS & CONSIDERATIONS

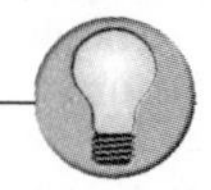

COMMENTS

- Should be suspected in brachycephalic breeds with chronic vomiting.
- Some cases of "pyloric stenosis" may be functional defects rather than anatomic defects.
- Surgery may not improve measured gastric transit time.

SUGGESTED READING

Bellenger CR, et al: Chronic hypertophic pyloric gastropathy in 14 dogs. *Aust Vet J* 67:317-320, 1990.

Fossum TW: Surgery of the digestive system. In Fossum TW, Hedlund CS, et al (eds): *Small Animal Surgery*. St. Louis, Mosby, 2002, pp 360-362.

AUTHOR: **AMIE KOENIG**

EDITOR: **DEBRA L. ZORAN**

Pyoderma

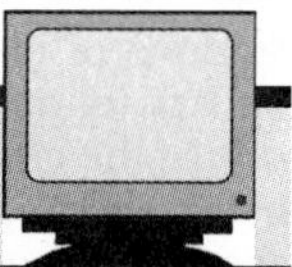

Client Education Sheet on Website

BASIC INFORMATION

DEFINITION

Pyoderma, or bacterial infection of the skin, is one of the most common diseases of dogs. Pyoderma is characterized by the depth of the infection within the skin:

- Surface pyoderma: infection restricted to the surface layer of the epidermis
- Superficial pyoderma: infection involving the epidermis and the infundibular portion of the hair follicle
- Deep pyoderma: bacterial infection extending beyond the hair follicle to involve the dermis and subcutis, which may lead to cellulitis

SYNONYM(S)

Bacterial dermatitis
Staphylococcal pyoderma

EPIDEMIOLOGY

SPECIES, AGE, SEX

- Common in dogs, rare in cats.
- Impetigo: noted in puppies and associated with immunosuppression, poor nutrition, endoparasitism, or poor hygiene.
- Acne is more common in young dogs.
- Feline: deep bacterial infections (cellulitis) are more common in outdoor animals.

GENETICS AND BREED PREDISPOSITION

- Intertrigo (pyoderma between skin folds): English bulldogs
- Mucocutaneous pyoderma: German shepherds

- Idiopathic deep pyoderma: German shepherds
- Acne: short-coated breeds, such as boxers, Doberman pinschers, bulldogs, great Danes, mastiffs, rottweilers, and German short-haired pointers

RISK FACTORS

- Bacterial infections are often secondary to underlying etiologies, such as hypersensitivity skin disease (atopy, food allergy, flea-bite hypersensitivity), endocrinopathies (hypothyroidism, hyperadrenocorticism), parasitic skin disease (*Sarcoptes*, *Demodex* spp.), immune-mediated diseases, or keratinization disorders.
- Deep pyoderma may be associated with underlying immunoincompetence.

CONTAGION AND ZOONOSIS: Approximately 90% of cases are caused by coagulase-positive *Staphylococcus intermedius*, a normal component of canine skin flora. A small number of cases are caused by *S. aureus*, the most common human pathogen. *S. intermedius* is considered nonpathogenic to humans. The gram-negative organisms *Proteus*, *Escherichia coli*, and *Pseudomonas* may act as secondary invaders. Deep pyoderma is occasionally associated with *Actinomyces*, *Nocardia*, mycobacteria, and *Actinobacillus* spp. In cats, *Pasteurella multocida* and β-hemolytic *Streptococcus* are involved.

GEOGRAPHY AND SEASONALITY: High environmental temperatures and humidity predispose animals to superficial pyoderma, which, in turn, may lead to deep pyoderma.

CLINICAL PRESENTATION

DISEASE FORMS/SUBTYPES

- Surface pyoderma:
  - Dog: intertrigo (fold pyoderma), acute moist dermatitis (pyotraumatic dermatitis, hot spots)
- Superficial pyoderma:
  - Dog: impetigo, bacterial folliculitis, mucocutaneous pyoderma, superficial spreading pyoderma
- Deep pyoderma:
  - Dog: canine acne, pyotraumatic furunculosis, nasal folliculitis and furunculosis, interdigital furunculosis/pododermatitis, infected acral lick dermatitis, callus pyoderma, and postgrooming furunculosis; German shepherd pyoderma: a familial idiopathic deep pyoderma
  - Cat: bite wounds, cellulitis, abscess, feline acne

HISTORY, CHIEF COMPLAINT: Animals typically are presented for evaluation of skin changes: pustules, crusts, epidermal collarettes, or hair loss. Pruritus is variable. Animals with deep pyoderma may be experiencing pain.

PHYSICAL EXAM FINDINGS

- Impetigo: small and nonfollicular pustules and crusts on the ventral abdomen.
- Bacterial folliculitis: papules, pustules, and epidermal collarettes (Fig. I-142) with patchy alopecia, producing a "moth-eaten" appearance of the haircoat over the trunk. Resolving lesions may show central hyperpigmentation (footprints).
- Superficial spreading pyoderma: large epidermal collarettes with an erythematous leading edge noted over the trunk; associated exudate may form crusts.
- Canine acne: a chronic disorder affecting the lips and chin of young dogs; characterized by a deep furunculosis and folliculitis, with crusting and scarring.
- Mucocutaneous pyoderma: crusts and erosions affecting the lip margin, eyelid margin, vulva, prepuce, and perianal area.
- Pyotraumatic folliculitis and furunculosis: may occur anywhere on the body depending on underlying cause; atypical acute moist dermatitis with superficial ulceration but also a component of deep folliculitis and occasional furunculosis. Clinically, this lesion may be thickened and plaque-like and have satellite papules and pustules.
- Nasal folliculitis and furunculosis: initially a papular/pustular eruption on the bridge of the nose that progresses to ulceration, crusting, and hemorrhage.
- Interdigital folliculitis/pododermatitis: lesions of the feet; interdigital papules, pustules, and ulceration with draining tracts and fibrosis; alopecia secondary to licking.
- Callus pyoderma: develops over pressure points. Skin is thickened, fibrotic, and hyperpigmented with foci of papules, pustules, and ulceration.
- Postgrooming folliculitis/furunculosis: papular/pustular rash, crust formation, self-induced alopecia.
- German shepherd pyoderma: lesions include ulcerations and draining tracts on the lateral thighs, trunk, lips, and groin.
- Feline acne: comedones, papules, pustules, and alopecia confined to the mandibular and perilabial areas.
- Feline bite wounds/abscess/cellulitis: swelling, pain, and alopecia in the affected area; possible dermal and cutaneous necrosis with ulceration, purulent exudate, and hemorrhage.

ETIOLOGY AND PATHOPHYSIOLOGY

- Canine skin is characterized by a relatively thin stratum corneum, a paucity of intercellular lipids, lack of a follicular plug, and a higher pH than for humans and other domestic species. This predisposes the dog to overgrowth of commensal flora and colonization by potentially pathogenic bacteria. Superficial infection may occur if the integrity of the skin is weakened by trauma or there are changes in surface immunity.
- Deep bacterial infections are generally an extension of a superficial pyoderma. As infection progresses deeper into the hair follicle, rupture of the follicle occurs. This leads to a pyogranulomatous foreign body reaction on the part of the host. This reaction occurs initially in the dermis and is an inflammatory response to keratin, bacterial organisms, and cellular debris.

DIAGNOSIS

DIFFERENTIAL DIAGNOSIS

- Demodicosis
- Dermatophytosis
- Pemphigus foliaceus
- Cutaneous neoplasia: epitheliotropic lymphoma
- Subcutaneous mycoses (deep pyoderma)
- Atypical mycobacterial infections (deep pyoderma)

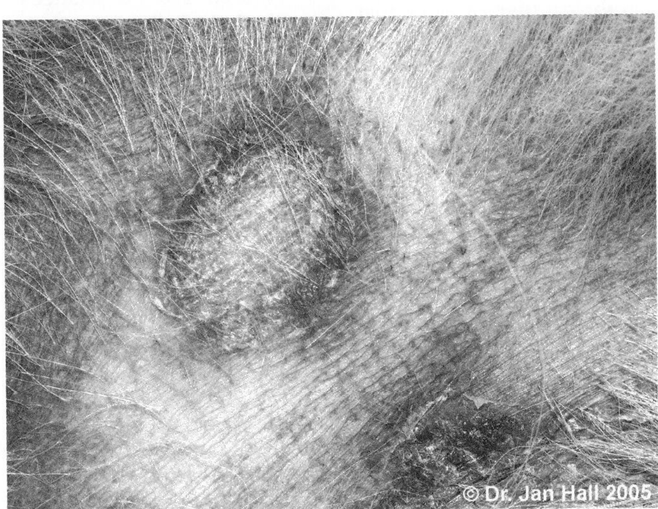

FIGURE I-142 Epidermal collarette on the ventral abdomen of a corgi with pyoderma. Courtesy of Dr. Jan A. Hall.

- Hookworm (deep pyoderma: pododermatitis)
- Foreign body granulomas (deep pyoderma)

INITIAL DATABASE

- Skin scrapings
- Skin cytologic examination: direct smear from pustule reveals bacteria, neutrophils in varying stages of degeneration, and active bacterial phagocytosis
- Fungal culture (dermatophytes)

ADVANCED OR CONFIRMATORY TESTING

- Culture and sensitivity (C&S): not normally employed in superficial pyoderma cases unless there has been a failure to respond to rational antibiotic therapy or bacilli are noted on skin cytologic examination.
- Skin biopsy and histopathologic exam: normally not performed unless cases are not responding to appropriate antibiotic therapy. Findings include intraepidermal neutrophilic pustules or folliculitis.
- Endocrine status; thyroid function and adrenal function tests.
- Allergy testing: intradermal testing, serum allergy testing, and elimination diet trial.

TREATMENT

THERAPEUTIC GOAL(S)

- Elimination of infection.
- Determination of underlying disease factors.

ACUTE GENERAL TREATMENT

TOPICAL THERAPY

- The most commonly used antibacterial agents for topical use are mupirocin (Bactroderm) and fusidic acid (Fucidin). Benzoyl peroxide 5% gels are also available. Shampoo therapy very effectively decreases bacterial skin colonization. Even though topical therapy alone may not be sufficient, it can be very useful as an adjunctive therapy. Shampoo therapy (10 to 15 minutes contact time) with products containing benzoyl peroxide, chlorhexidine, ethyl lactate, and povidone-iodine may improve the condition.
- Clip the fur off affected areas.
- Deep pyoderma: Bathe the animal with Epsom salts (magnesium sulfate) solution or Burow's solution (aluminum acetate) daily.

SYSTEMIC ANTIBIOTIC THERAPY

- Bactericidal antibiotics are recommended for skin infections; however, bacteriostatic drugs may be effective if the animal is not immunocompromised. The chosen drug should have a narrow spectrum to limit the effects on the normal flora of both the skin and gastrointestinal (GI) tract.
- Cases should be treated until the condition plateaus. Minimum duration of 3 to 4 weeks or 7 to 14 days beyond clinical cure. Deep pyoderma may take as long as 12 weeks to resolve.
- The most commonly used antibiotics include (generally monotherapy; all PO):
  - Cephalexin 22-30 mg/kg q 8-12h (most common choice in dogs)
  - Clavulanic acid potentiated amoxicillin 12.5 mg/kg q 12h (most common choice in cats)
  - Clindamycin 5.5-11 mg/kg q 12h
- Other suggested drugs/dosages include (generally monotherapy; all PO):
  - Cefpodoxime 5-10 mg/kg q 24h
  - Cefadroxil 22 mg/kg q 12h
  - Oxacillin 22 mg/kg q 8h
  - Erythromycin 15 mg/kg q 8h (vomiting and diarrhea common)
  - Lincomycin 15-22 mg/kg q 12h
  - Azithromycin 5 mg/kg q 24h
  - Tylosin 10-20 mg/kg q 12h
  - Trimethoprim-sulfa 15-30 mg/kg q 12h (keratoconjunctivitis sicca, drug reactions, hypothyroidism at high doses)
  - Difloxacin 5-10 mg/kg q 12h (not in immature animals)
  - Enrofloxacin 5 mg/kg q 24h (not in immature animals)
  - Marbofloxacin 2 mg/kg q 24h (not in immature animals)
  - Orbifloxacin 2.5 mg/kg q 24h (not in immature animals)
  - Doxycycline 5 mg/kg (day 1), then 2.5 mg/kg q 12h
- Appropriate pain management: meloxicam (Metacam) 0.1 mg/kg PO q 24h.

CHRONIC TREATMENT

- Shampoo therapy.
- Long-term antibiotic therapy. The use of low-dose or pulse administration is controversial because of an increased risk of resistance development. Cephalexin is the only antibiotic recommended for this type of therapy because of a documented lack of resistance development over time. In low-dose continuous therapy, the dose is reduced by half once monthly, until the lowest dose that keeps pyoderma at bay is determined. In intermittent dosing, a full therapeutic dose is administered for 7 to 14 days once monthly.
- Immunomodulatory therapy (Staphage Lysate [SPL; Delmont Laboratories]): 0.5 ml twice weekly SC while receiving a 6-week antibiotic course. Cases should be reevaluated for progress at the end of the first 10 weeks of therapy (end of the first 10-ml treatment vial). The frequency of injections is gradually reduced to once weekly and then every other week after 20 weeks if the pyoderma remains under control.

POSSIBLE COMPLICATIONS

- Many antibiotics occasionally cause vomiting and diarrhea.
- Fluoroquinolones: cartilage damage in growing dogs.
- Potentiated sulfonamides: keratoconjunctivitis sicca, arthritis, uveitis, immune-mediated dermatitis, hepatobiliary disease, decreased thyroid function.
- Benzoyl peroxide gel has to be used with care because it may be irritating with repeated use.
- Drug-induced pemphigus foliaceus.

RECOMMENDED MONITORING

History and physical exam: Assess response to therapy before the antibiotic course is completed.

PROGNOSIS AND OUTCOME

- Superficial pyoderma: good prognosis as long as underlying factors are addressed adequately.
- Deep pyoderma: many cases of deep pyoderma will result in scarring.
- Animals are often immunosuppressed or have other intercurrent diseases.

PEARLS & CONSIDERATIONS

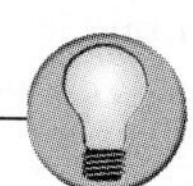

COMMENTS

- Any therapeutic plan for controlling pyoderma without considering underlying predisposing factors is destined to fail.
- Most dermatologists use cephalexin as their first drug choice because it has been shown to be a very effective drug against *S. intermedius* with minimal change in resistance pattern over the years.
- Both pemphigus foliaceus and epitheliotrophic lymphoma may present as a pyoderma that fails to respond to appropriate antibiotic therapy. Skin biopsy is indicated.

CLIENT EDUCATION

Counsel clients concerning the potential chronicity of the disease.

SUGGESTED READING

Scott DW, Miller WH, Griffin CE: *Muller and Kirk's Small Animal Dermatology*, ed 6. Philadelphia, WB Saunders, 2001, pp 274-335.

White SD: Systemic treatment of bacterial skin infection of dogs and cats. *Vet Dermatol* 7(3):133-139, 1996.

AUTHOR: **MICHAEL HANNIGAN**

EDITOR: **JAN A. HALL**

Pyometra

BASIC INFORMATION

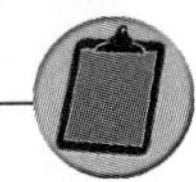

DEFINITION

An accumulation of purulent material within the uterine lumen; derived from the Latin words *pyo*, which means *pus*, and *metrum*, which means *uterus*

SYNONYM(S)

Purulent endometritis
Purulent metritis
Pyo
Pyometritis

EPIDEMIOLOGY

SPECIES, AGE, SEX

- Canine, feline females (more common in bitches than queens)
- Any age after puberty (more common after 9 years of age)

GENETICS AND BREED PREDISPOSITION: A genetic or breed predisposition has not been clearly demonstrated. Anecdotal reports indicate that some lines within a breed may be predisposed.

RISK FACTORS: Age, estrogen or progestin treatment, estrous cycle irregularities, ovarian diseases.

ASSOCIATED CONDITIONS AND DISORDERS

- Sepsis
- Septic shock
- Systemic inflammatory response syndrome (SIRS)
- Multiple organs dysfunction syndrome (MODS)
- Disseminated intravascular coagulation (DIC)
- Acute renal failure
- Acute hepatic injury

CLINICAL PRESENTATION

DISEASE FORMS/SUBTYPES: Open pyometra (mucoid or purulent vulvar discharge, sometimes containing blood); closed pyometra (no vulvar discharge).

HISTORY, CHIEF COMPLAINT

- Diestrus (a few weeks following the end of estrus).
- Anorexia, vomiting.
- Lethargy, depression.
- Polyuria and polydipsia (PU/PD).
- Vaginal discharge may be noted by owner.
- A history of incomplete ovariohysterectomy, previous treatment to induce abortion, or parturition may be present.

PHYSICAL EXAM FINDINGS

- Purulent vaginal discharge is common and should always prompt the consideration of pyometra.
  - Absence of vaginal discharge does not rule out pyometra.
- Abdominal palpation: evidence of abdominal pain and enlarged uterus (may be difficult to palpate if moderate enlargement and/or soft swollen uterus in a tense abdomen).
- Dehydration.
- Fever (or hypothermia if severe, such as in septic shock).
- Red mucous membranes (hyperdynamic stage of sepsis) or pale mucous membranes (septic shock).
- Normal pulse and cardiac auscultation or tachycardia, weak pulse, and cool extremities possible with septic shock.
- Normal respiration or hyperpnea.

ETIOLOGY AND PATHOPHYSIOLOGY

- Pyometra associated with cystic endometrial hyperplasia (CEH):
  - During diestrus, progesterone from the corpora lutea prepares the endometrium for pregnancy by promoting glandular development and secretion as well as hyperplasia of the endometrium.
  - Endometrial hyperplasia may become excessive, and cyst formation may result.
  - Progesterone also reduces myometrial activity and suppresses the immune responses of the uterus.
  - Pyometra results when bacteria colonize the uterus via an ascending infection through the cervix or a hematogenous route.
  - The most commonly isolated bacterium from pyometra is *Escherichia coli*, but *Staphylococcus* spp., *Streptococcus* spp., *Pseudomonas* spp., and *Proteus* spp. have also been reported.
- Pyometra not associated with CEH:
  - A new mechanism for the development of pyometra has been suggested and is termed trophoblastic reaction theory.
  - A subtle (subclinical) bacterial infection within the uterine lumen provides a nidus for reversible endometrial hypertrophy and hyperplasia to occur.
  - The associated increase in glandular secretions exacerbates the infection, leading to a further increase in endometrial gland secretion, which progresses into pyometra.
  - This mechanism may explain the occurrence of pyometra in young bitches.

DIAGNOSIS

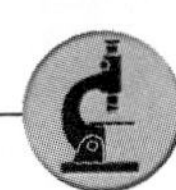

DIFFERENTIAL DIAGNOSIS

- Mucometra (uterine lumen filled with mucoid endometrial gland secretions without infection)
- Pregnancy
- Vaginitis
- Reproductive tract tumors
- Uterine torsion
- Postpartum metritis
- Other systemic diseases resulting in an acute abdomen

INITIAL DATABASE

- Complete blood count (CBC):
  - Mild to moderate normocytic, normochromic anemia (packed cell volume 30-35%).
  - Leukocytosis with left shift and/or toxic changes.
    - Note: About 25% of leukograms are within normal range in pyometra cases.
- Serum biochemistry profile: elevated hepatic and renal values.
- Urinalysis:
  - Cystocentesis is contraindicated in suspected or confirmed pyometra cases.
  - Catheterized or free-catch samples may show evidence of infection, either as a real finding (bacterial cystitis is often concurrent with pyometra) or as an artifact of collection.
- Abdominal radiographs:
  - Distended viscus consistent with enlarged, fluid-filled uterus.
    - Note: Abdominal radiographs will not differentiate between pyometra and pregnancy (less than 45 days of gestation) or mucometra.
- Ultrasonographic examination:
  - Enlarged fluid-filled uterus.
    - Note: easily differentiates from pregnancy; abdominal ultrasound is the method of choice for establishing a diagnosis of pyometra.

ADVANCED OR CONFIRMATORY TESTING

- Open pyometra: cranial vaginal (near external cervical os) culture and sensitivity (C&S)
- Closed pyometra: transcervical endoscopy with uterine sample for C&S
- Gross and histopathologic examination of the surgically removed uterus

TREATMENT

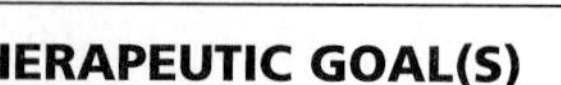

THERAPEUTIC GOAL(S)

Provide supportive care for the animal as needed and treat the uterine infection so that it is eliminated.

ACUTE GENERAL TREATMENT

- General systemic treatment:
  - Stabilization of the animal as needed; treatment for shock and acute renal failure if identified.
  - IV fluid therapy: typically to correct dehydration, using replacement fluids such as lactated Ringer's solution or 0.9% NaCl, with or without colloids. Rate is calculated based on dehydration and ongoing fluid losses.
  - Broad-spectrum antibiotic therapy: oral route is indicated for stable patients; individuals showing systemic signs of illness should receive antibiotics parenterally:
    - Amoxicillin with clavulanic acid 20 mg/kg PO q 8-12h.
    - Enrofloxacin 5 mg/kg PO or diluted 1:1 with saline and given slowly (over 5 minutes) IV q 6-12h as needed based on pain parameters.
    - Cephalexin 22-30 mg/kg PO q 8h.
  - Pain management (e.g., buprenophine 0.01-0.02 mg/kg SQ, IM, IV, q 6-12h as needed based on pain parameters).
- Surgical pyometra treatment:
  - Complete ovariohysterectomy: removal of both ovaries and the entire uterus and cervix.
  - Advantages: rapid resolution of the infection, no possibility of recurrence, treatment of choice for non-breeding animals.
  - Drawbacks: challenging surgery, possible life-threatening situation for the animal, no possibility for future breeding.
- Pharmacologic pyometra treatment:
  - Prostaglandin F-2α (PGF-2α, dinoprost, Lutalyse; Upjohn) administration: low, increasing doses (0.010-0.100 mg/kg SQ q 5-8h for 7-10 days or until uterine evacuation is complete as assessed by frequent ultrasonographic exams.
    - Dopamine agonists: used in conjunction with PGF-2α.
      - Cabergoline (Dostinex) administration: 0.005 mg/kg PO, q 24h for 10 days.
      - Bromocriptine (Parlodel) 0.03 mg/kg PO, q 8-12h for 10 days given orally; adverse effects uncommon at this dose.
      - Used for hastening luteolysis via prolactin inhibition.
    - Progesterone receptor antagonists:
      - Mifepristone (Mifeprex) administration: 2.5 mg/kg PO q 24h for 5 days.
      - Aglepristone (Alizine) administration: 10 mg/kg SQ twice at 24 hours apart.
  - Advantages: possibility of future pregnancy (should only be considered for valuable breeding animals), no risk of surgery.
  - Drawbacks: uterine rupture (increased risk with higher doses of PGF-2α), DIC, recurrence of pyometra (note: to address the risk of DIC, preventive heparin treatment is advised at a dose of 100 U/kg SQ once).

CHRONIC TREATMENT

Chronic renal failure may develop from the acute renal failure due to the formation of an antigen-antibodies complexes within the glomeruli and tubular damage resulting from endotoxemia, which may require lifelong treatment.

DRUG INTERACTIONS

Antiemetic drugs may stimulate prolactin release, which would delay luteolysis and prolong pharmacologic pyometra treatment.

POSSIBLE COMPLICATIONS

- Peritonitis (resulting from uterine rupture)
- Stump pyometra (resulting from incomplete ovariohysterectomy)
- Bacterial cystitis (often concurrent with pyometra)
- Abdominal abscesses (resulting from bacteremia)
- DIC, SIRS, MODS
- Septic shock

RECOMMENDED MONITORING

- Intensive/critical care
- Cardiovascular support with IV fluid therapy
- Pain management
- Monitor for DIC (platelet count, coagulation profile, possibly a D-dimer test) and liver and kidney failure with CBC and chemistry profile
- Ultrasonographic examination of uterus every other day to monitor response to medical treatment

PROGNOSIS AND OUTCOME

- Always guarded, depending on the presence of liver or renal failure.
- Risk of recurrence if medical treatment. It is generally advised to breed the dog during the first subsequent cycle. However, preliminary results show no difference in the incidence of pyometra in medically treated dogs compared to dogs of the same age that did not previously have pyometra.

PEARLS & CONSIDERATIONS

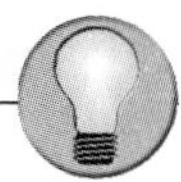

COMMENTS

- Clinical signs are not related to the size of the distended uterus.
  - Septic shock can occur with a uterine lumen distended to 2 cm compared to minimal systemic signs (e.g., inappetence) with a uterine lumen distended to 8 cm.
- Pyometra should always be included as a differential diagnosis in a female dog with an acute abdomen or with non-specific clinical signs.
- A closed pyometra can be a life-threatening condition. Treatment should not be delayed even if the animal appears to be healthy.

PREVENTION

Ovariohysterectomy in females that are not going to breed and in females that have retired from breeding

SUGGESTED READING

Blendiger K, Bostedt H: The age and stage of estrus in bitches with pyometra. Statistical inquiry and interpretive study of the understanding of variability. *Tierarztl Prx* 19:307, 1991.

Blendiger K, et al: Hormonal state and effects of the use of an antiprogestin in bitches with pyometra. *J Reprod Fertil Suppl* 51:317, 1997.

Faldyna M, et al: Immunosuppression in bitches with pyometra. *J Small Anim Pract* 42:5, 2001.

Feldman EC, Nelson RW: Cystic endometrial hyperplasia/pyometra complex. In Feldman EC, Nelson RW (eds): *Canine and Feline Endocrinology and Reproduction*. St. Louis, WB Saunders, 2004, pp 852-867.

Gobello C, et al: A study of two protocols combining aglepristone and cloprostenol to treat open cervix pyometra in the bitch. *Theriogenology* 60:901, 2003

Johnston S, et al: Disorders of the canine uterus and uterine tubes. In Johnston SD, Root-Kustritz MV, Olson PNS (eds): *Canine and Feline Theriogenology*. Philadelphia, WB Saunders, 2000, pp 206-224.

Noakes DE, et al: Cystic endometrial hyperplasia/pyometra in dogs: A review of the causes and pathogenesis. *J Reprod Fertil Suppl* 57: 395, 2001

Nomura K: Induction of canine deciduoma in some reproductive stages with the different conditions of corpora lutea. *J Vet Med Sci* 59:185, 1997.

Nomura K, Nishida A: Histological variations of canine deciduoma induced in non pregnant horn at different stages of unilateral pregnancy. *J Vet Med Sci* 60:623, 1998.

AUTHORS: **KARINE M. ONCLIN, JOHN VERSTEGEN**

EDITOR: **MICHELLE A. KUTZLER**

Pyothorax

BASIC INFORMATION

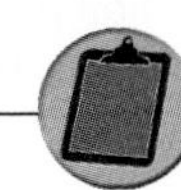

DEFINITION

Accumulation of purulent exudate within the pleural space

SYNONYM(S)

Plural empyema

EPIDEMIOLOGY

SPECIES, AGE, SEX: Dogs and cats:
- Medium and large breeds of dogs overrepresented
- Males of both species overrepresented
- Median age of occurrence is approximately 4 years

GENETICS AND BREED PREDISPOSITION
- Dog: hunting breeds: increased risk of inhaled foreign (plant) material
- Cat: higher risk if from multicat household and if young; no difference if indoor versus outdoor

CLINICAL PRESENTATION

HISTORY, CHIEF COMPLAINT
- Slowly progressive onset of dyspnea, inappetence, weight loss
- Acute decompensation with dyspnea/tachypnea/collapse from pleural effusion

PHYSICAL EXAM FINDINGS
- Respiratory: dyspnea, tachypnea; muffled heart and lung sounds on auscultation (unilateral/bilateral)
- Systemic: depression, weight loss, ± pyrexia, ± pale mucous membranes
- Cats: possible decreased compressibility of cranial thorax on palpation

ETIOLOGY AND PATHOPHYSIOLOGY

- Septic pyothorax (most common): potential routes of infection of the pleural space include:
  - Penetrating/migrating plant material
  - Inhaled plant material
  - Penetrating injury
    - Bite, stab, gunshot wounds
  - Esophageal perforation
    - Foreign body
    - *Spirocerca lupi* infection
  - Hematogenous spread
  - Extension from diskospondylitis
  - Pneumonia or lung abscess
  - Pulmonary or intrathoracic neoplasia
- Pleuritis (and nonseptic pyothorax) can be associated with canine hepatitis, leptospirosis, canine distemper, feline infectious peritonitis, or feline upper respiratory tract infection
- Cats: role of feline immunodeficiency virus (FIV) or feline leukemia virus (FeLV) in development of pyothorax not proven

DIAGNOSIS

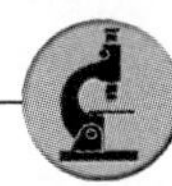

DIFFERENTIAL DIAGNOSIS

- Pulmonary disease:
  - Pneumonia
  - Abscess
- Pleural effusion:
  - Chylothorax
  - Heart failure
  - Hemothorax
  - Idiopathic
- Diaphragmatic hernia
- Intrathoracic neoplasia

INITIAL DATABASE

- Complete blood count (CBC):
  - Usually: neutrophilic leukocytosis with or without a left shift.
  - Possible: leukopenia, thrombocytopenia if sepsis.
- Serum biochemistry profile:
  - Multiple abnormalities (hepatic and renal parameters, electrolytes, hypoalbuminemia, etc.) can occur secondary to sepsis.
- Pleural fluid evaluation (see Thoracocentesis, p 1308):
  - Diagnostic: Obtain fluid for analysis; typically blood-tinged fluid, which may be opaque and often has a foul odor (anaerobes). Macroscopic yellow clumps ("sulfur granules") strongly suggest presence of *Actinomyces*.
- Analysis of pleural fluid:
  - Fluid analysis/cytologic examination: exudate (by definition)
    - Protein >3 g/dl.
    - Nucleated cell count $>7 \times 10^9$/L, often $>30 \times 10^9$/L.
    - Degenerate neutrophils predominate, with macrophages and activated mesothelial cells also present. Intraleukocytic bacteria are diagnostic (septic pyothorax).
  - Gram stain:
    - Guides initial empiric antimicrobial therapy.
      - *Pasteurella* spp. most common in cats; *Escherichia coli* in dogs (both Gram-negative rods).
      - *Actinomyces* (anaerobe) and *Nocardia* (aerobe): both gram-positive short rods and filaments. Important potential pathogens in dogs from regions where grass awn are endemic.
  - Anaerobic and aerobic bacterial culture and sensitivity (C&S).
    - Test of choice for planning long-term antimicrobial therapy.
- Survey thoracic radiographs:
  - Initially to identify pleural effusion.
  - After therapeutic thoracocentesis, to evaluate pleural space, mediastinum, and pulmonary parenchyma for potential cause of pyothorax.
- Thoracic ultrasound examination:
  - Identify masses and evaluate their structure.
  - Identify foreign material in the pleural space if possible (may be very challenging).

ADVANCED OR CONFIRMATORY TESTING

CT scan:
- Potentially identify cause of pyothorax
- Evaluate mass(es) in thoracic cavity and determine if resectable

TREATMENT

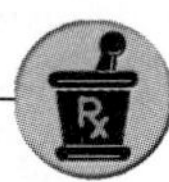

THERAPEUTIC GOAL(S)

- Identify and remove cause of pyothorax
- Treat pyothorax:
  - Debridement, lavage, and establish drainage
  - Long-term antimicrobial therapy based on C&S test results

ACUTE GENERAL TREATMENT

- Stabilization of respiratory compromise:
  - Therapeutic (and diagnostic) thoracocentesis (see Thoracocentesis, p 1308)
  - Oxygen administration
  - Intensive care monitoring
- Correction of fluid and electrolyte deficits
- Antimicrobial therapy:
  - Empiric therapy active against both aerobic and anaerobic bacteria
    - Gram stain results (as previously described)
    - Amoxicillin/ampicillin 22 mg/kg IV or PO q 8h if *Actinomyces* suspected
    - Trimethoprim-sulfa 15 mg/kg PO q 12h, if *Nocardia, E. coli*, or *Pasteurella* suspected
- Medical management:
  - Bilateral thoracostomy tube placement
  - Thoracic lavage every 8 to 12 hours with body-temperature warmed sterile saline
  - Serial cytologic evaluation of pleural fluid to assess success of lavage therapy
    - Improvement includes change from degenerate neutrophils with intracellular or extracellular bacteria to nondegenerate neutrophils without bacteria
- Surgical management:
  - Indicated if:

- Definitive cause identified (foreign body, lung lobe abscess)
- Fluid loculated within the pleural space (lavage cannot access portions of fluid accumulation)
- Animal fails to respond to aggressive medical therapy (4 to 5 days of pleural lavage and antibiotics)
- *Actinomyces* present (notoriously poor response to medical management alone)
- Consists of:
  - Aggressive debridement of the pleural space
  - Removal of underlying cause if identified
  - Thorough intraoperative lavage
  - Postoperative intermittent pleural aspiration, lavage

CHRONIC TREATMENT

- Thoracostomy tube removal based on overt clinical and cytologic resolution of infection
- Long-term antibiotic therapy in all cases:
  - Based on accurate identification of organism(s) involved.
  - Up to 3 months of therapy may be required.

POSSIBLE COMPLICATIONS

Failure to resolve/recurrence of pyothorax:

- Cause not removed
- Failure of medical management:
  - Ineffective pleural lavage
  - Ineffective/inappropriate antibiotic therapy

RECOMMENDED MONITORING

Survey thoracic radiographs:

- At completion of antibiotic therapy
- Periodically (every 3 months)

PROGNOSIS AND OUTCOME

- Surgical management is associated with a better prognosis than medical management in dogs with pyothorax: disease-free at 1 year: 78% (surgical) versus 25% (medical).
- Development of fibrosing pleuritis associated with poor outcome.
- Lower heart rate and hypersalivation: both associated with poorer outcomes in cats.
- Overall, 66% of cats and 80% of dogs can survive if treated appropriately.

PEARLS & CONSIDERATIONS

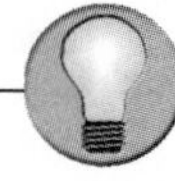

COMMENTS

- Aggressive therapy should start immediately upon diagnosis. Undertreatment is thought to be a major contributor to morbidity/mortality.
- Surgical treatment has been associated with a better outcome than medical treatment alone.
- Bilateral thoracostomy tubes are helpful in aspiration and lavage of the pleural space.
- Antimicrobial therapy should be guided by culture and susceptibility with attention paid to *Actinomyces* and *Nocardia*.
- Obligate anaerobes are common in pyothorax and are present in combination with aerobes; antimicrobial treatment should be aimed at both types of bacteria until culture results are available.

CLIENT EDUCATION

Sporting or hunting dogs may be more at risk for developing pyothorax due their activity and potential interaction with wild animals.

SUGGESTED READING

Rooney MB, et al: Medical and surgical treatment of pyothorax in dogs: 26 cases (1991–2001). *J Am Vet Med Assoc* 221:86, 2002.

Waddell LS, et al: Risk factors, prognostic indicators, and outcome of pyothorax in cats: 80 cases (1986–1999). *J Am Vet Med Assoc* 221:819, 2002.

Walker AL, et al: Bacteria associated with pyothorax of dogs and cats: 98 cases (1989–1998). *J Am Vet Med Assoc* 216:359, 2000.

AUTHOR: **MARYANN G. RADLINSKY**
EDITOR: **RICHARD WALSHAW**

Pyrethrins/Pyrethroids Toxicosis

BASIC INFORMATION

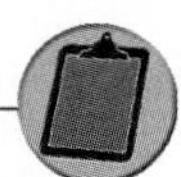

DEFINITION

Pyrethrins (natural) and pyrethroids (synthetic) insecticides are used in numerous household and garden insecticides as well as flea control formulations, such as in aerosols, sprays, dusts, dips granules, shampoos, and spot-on once-a-month products. Toxicity varies in severity depending on the compound involved and route of administration, and is characterized by hypersalivation, tremors, ataxia, vomiting, hyperactivity, and seizures.

SYNONYM(S)

- Agents sold under numerous trade names.
- Different formulations may contain methoprene (an insect growth regulator) or piperonyl butoxide (a synergist).
- Pyrethrins are obtained from *Chrysanthemum* flowers.
  - Examples: cinerin I and II, jasmolin I and II, pyrethrin I and II, pyrethrum.
- Pyrethroids are of two types: type I lacks an α-cyano group; type II possesses an α-cyano group. Type II is more toxic than type I.
  - Examples, type I: allethrin, barthrin, bifenthrin, bioresmethrin, cismethrin, dimethrin, permethrin, phenothrin, resmethrin, tefluthrin, tetramethrin.
  - Examples, type II: acrinathrin, cyfluthrin, cyhalothrin, cypermethrin, cyphenothrin, deltamethrin, esfenvalerate, fenpropathrin, fenvalerate, flumethrin, fluvalinate, lamda-cyhalothrin, tralomethrin.

EPIDEMIOLOGY

SPECIES, AGE, SEX

- Cats are more sensitive than dogs, especially to concentrated permethrin (45–65%) or phenothrin (85%).
- No breed or sex predisposition.

RISK FACTORS: Very young, aged, anemic, or debilitated animals may be at higher risk.

CLINICAL PRESENTATION

DISEASE FORMS/SUBTYPES

- Oral exposure (grooming) may result in mild hypersalivation and vomiting due to carrier.
- Excessive dermal spray may result in paresthesia or tingling due to effect on sensory nerve endings.
- Pyrethrins and type I pyrethroids can cause tremors, ataxia, hyperexicitablilty, and hyperthermia.
- Type II pyrethroids can cause hypersalivation, tremors, rigidity, seizures, ataxia, and coma.

HISTORY, CHIEF COMPLAINT

- History of product use on the animal, in the yard, or in the house
- Hypersalivation, vomiting
- Muscle tremors, ataxia, or seizures

PHYSICAL EXAM FINDINGS
- Hypersalivation
- Muscle tremors
- Hyperthermia followed by hypothermia

ETIOLOGY AND PATHOPHYSIOLOGY
- Agents delay opening and closing of sodium channels, resulting in repetitive nerve discharges.
- Type II pyrethroids cause longer duration of the sodium current in the axon than type I pyrethroids and pyrethrins.
- Type I pyrethroids and pyrethrins cause repetitive discharges and tend to cause tremors and seizures.
- Type II pyrethroids can cause conduction blockage, so weakness and paralysis are possible.

DIAGNOSIS

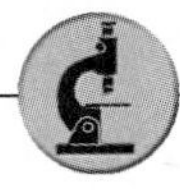

DIFFERENTIAL DIAGNOSIS
- Rule out other agents associated with tremors and seizures:
  - Tremorgenic mycotoxins (see Garbage Toxicosis, p 425)
  - Organphosphate/carbamate toxicosis (see Organophosphate and Carbamate Insecticide Toxicosis, p 775)
  - See Metaldehyde Toxicosis, p 702
  - See Strychnine Toxicosis, p 1045
  - Caffeine toxicosis
  - Organochlorine pesticides
- Also rule out nontoxicologic causes of tremors and/or seizures:
  - Intracranial disorders (neoplasia, encephalitis, trauma, idiopathic epilepsy)
  - Metabolic disorders (hypocalcemia, portosystemic shunt, etc.)

INITIAL DATABASE
- Body temperature
- Renal profile and urinalysis (for myoglobinuria if severe tremors are present)
- Complete blood count (CBC), serum biochemistry profile: no significant changes expected
- Neurologic examination

ADVANCED OR CONFIRMATORY TESTING
Pyrethrins/pyrethroids can be detected in hair, stomach contents, fat, liver, brain, serum, and urine. Presence of insecticide only confirms exposure.

TREATMENT

THERAPEUTIC GOAL(S)
- Decontamination of patient
- Control of central nervous system (CNS) signs
- Supportive care

ACUTE GENERAL TREATMENT
- Decontamination of patient:
  - Bathe the animal in a dilute solution of liquid dishwashing detergent in tap water for dermal exposures and repeat if needed.
  - Induction of vomiting (hydrogen peroxide 3%: 0.25-0.5 ml/kg PO once or syrup of ipecac: 2-6 ml total dose PO once) in animals without overt clinical signs if oral ingestion was significant.
  - Activated charcoal (dose according to packaging label of product; e.g., 10 ml of activated charcoal suspension PO made from 2 g activated charcoal suspended in 10 ml tap water) if oral ingestion significant.
- Control CNS signs:
  - Diazepam 0.5-1.0 mg/kg IV for mild tremors or paresthesia (after bathing).
  - Severe tremors best controlled with methocarbamol 55-220 mg/kg IV to effect.
    - Repeat as needed but do not exceed 330 mg/kg per day.
  - Diazepam is generally not effective for controlling severe tremors.
  - If methocarbamol is ineffective, use phenobarbital, propofol, or isoflurane.
  - Seizure control with diazepam, phenobarbital, propofol, or isoflurane.
- Supportive care:
  - IV fluids (e.g., lactated Ringer's solution to correct dehydration or volume loss, plus maintenance).
  - Atropine 0.01-0.02 mg/kg IV/IM for controlling hypersalivation. Atropine provides no beneficial effect for such signs as tremors or seizures.
  - Regulation of body temperature.

DRUG INTERACTIONS
Concurrent exposure to other pesticides may increase risk of toxicity

POSSIBLE COMPLICATIONS
- Myoglobinuria and acute renal failure due to severe tremors (uncommon)
- Disseminated intravascular coagulation secondary to hyperthermia (uncommon)

PROGNOSIS AND OUTCOME

- Generally good; recovery in 1 to 3 days
- Guarded if tremors not controlled or if seizures develop

PEARLS & CONSIDERATIONS

COMMENTS
- In general, flea products will not cause systemic CNS signs if used according to label.
- Systemic CNS effects unlikely if animals access a sprayed area after it has dried.
- Tremors may last for 3 days. After stabilizing the animal, oral methocarbamol (50-100 mg/kg PO q 6-8h) can be started and the animal can be sent home on discharge.

PREVENTION
- Use products labeled for appropriate species only; do not use dog products on cats.
- Keep pets out of areas being treated with insecticides until the product has dried.

SUGGESTED READING
Volmer PA: Pyrethrins and pyrethroids. In Plumlee KH (ed): *Clinical Veterinary Toxicology*. St. Louis, Mosby, 2004, pp 188-190.

AUTHOR: **ERIC K. DUNAYER**
EDITOR: **SAFDAR A. KHAN**

Pythiosis and Lagenidiosis

BASIC INFORMATION

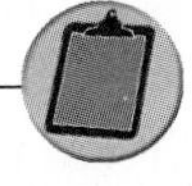

DEFINITION
Pythiosis and lagenidiosis are oomycotic infections of the gastrointestinal (GI) tract (*Pythium*) or skin (*Pythium* and *Lagenidium*) of dogs and cats caused by *Pythium insidiosum* and *Lagenidium* spp.

SYNONYM(S)
Phycomycosis
Swamp cancer

EPIDEMIOLOGY
SPECIES, AGE, SEX: Dogs are affected more often than cats. Dogs (young to middle-aged adults); cats (any age but often less than 1 year old).

GENETICS AND BREED PREDISPOSITION
- Dogs: large breeds, especially outdoor working breeds such as Labrador retriever
- Cats: none known

RISK FACTORS: Recurrent exposure to warm freshwater lakes, swamps, and ponds that may contain *Pythium* or *Lagenidium* zoospores.

CONTAGION AND ZOONOSIS: Motile zoospores found in warm freshwater habitats cause infections in mammalian species including man; no direct contagion or zoonotic potential.

GEOGRAPHY AND SEASONALITY: Endemic in warm, humid regions such as the southern United States and the Gulf coast of Texas. Infections are most often diagnosed in fall, winter, and early spring.

CLINICAL PRESENTATION

DISEASE FORMS/SUBTYPES

- Pythiosis: GI disease, cutaneous disease
- Lagenidiosis: cutaneous disease initially, usually progressing to systemic involvement by the time the diagnosis is established; often affecting large vessels

HISTORY, CHIEF COMPLAINT

- GI infection: weight loss with chronic vomiting and/or diarrhea; dogs usually continue to feel well and have a good appetite
- Cutaneous infection: nonhealing wounds and skin masses

PHYSICAL EXAM FINDINGS

- Dog:
  - GI infection: chronic severe weight loss in an otherwise active alert dog; abdominal mass often palpable
  - Cutaneous infection: chronic nonhealing wounds and invasive masses that contain ulcerated nodules and draining tracts, most often involving the extremities, tailhead, ventral neck, or perineum
- Cat:
  - Nasopharyngeal infection: chronic nasal discharge and upper respiratory signs
  - Cutaneous infection: invasive subcutaneous masses (especially in inguinal, tailhead, and periorbital regions) or ulcerated plaque-like lesions on the extremities
  - GI infection: rare

ETIOLOGY AND PATHOPHYSIOLOGY

- Infection follows exposure of the immunocompetent host to motile zoospores in warm freshwater environments.
- Hyphal growth within affected tissues causes massive inflammation resulting in masses, draining lesions, and regional lymphadenopathy. In the GI tract transmural thickening may result in GI obstruction.
- Any portion of the GI tract may be affected; pylorus, proximal duodenum, and ileocolic junction are affected most often. Mesenteric lymphadenopathy is common.
- Dogs with *Lagenidium* spp. infection have progressive cutaneous or subcutaneous lesions (often multifocal) involving the extremities, mammary region, perineum, or trunk.
- In contrast to *Pythium* infection, dogs with lagenidiosis have lesions in distant sites, including great vessels, sublumbar and inguinal lymph nodes, lung, pulmonary hilus, and cranial mediastinum.

DIAGNOSIS

DIFFERENTIAL DIAGNOSIS

- GI neoplasia
- Pyloric outflow obstruction due to hypertrophy, intussusception
- Zygomycosis and other hyphal fungal infections
- Mycobacterial, nocardial, and actinomycotic infections of skin

INITIAL DATABASE

- Complete blood count: eosinophilia and nonregenerative anemia may be seen.
- Serum biochemistry panel: hyperglobulinemia is common. Hypercalcemia has been reported.
- Abdominal radiographs: abdominal mass effect; evidence of intestinal obstruction.
- Abdominal ultrasound: severe segmental thickening of the GI tract, mesenteric lymphadenopathy.

ADVANCED OR CONFIRMATORY TESTING

- Histopathologic examination of tissue: eosinophilic pyogranulomatous inflammation; *Pythium* hyphae are difficult to visualize on H&E-stained sections while *Lagenidium* hyphae are easier to see.
  - Broad, rarely septate, occasionally branching hyphae seen on silver stains. *Lagenidium* hyphae are much wider than *Pythium* hyphae.
  - Immunohistochemical stains can be used to confirm diagnosis.
- Culture: using fungal media.
- Serology: ELISA and immunoblot assays available from the *Pythium* laboratory at Louisiana State University—sensitive and specific for diagnosis of pythiosis and lagenidiosis and for monitoring response to therapy (titers may decrease to normal in months following successful treatment).

TREATMENT

THERAPEUTIC GOAL(S)

Complete surgical resection if possible, otherwise disease will progress

ACUTE GENERAL TREATMENT

Complete surgical resection is treatment of choice: segmental GI lesions are occasionally completely resectable; if cutaneous lesions are limited to a single extremity, amputation is recommended. Local postoperative recurrence is common.

CHRONIC TREATMENT

- Medical therapy with itraconazole (10 mg/kg PO q 24h) and terbinafine (5-10 mg/kg PO q 24h) is recommended for at least 2 to 3 months after surgery. Fewer than 20% of animals will respond to long-term medical therapy alone. Medical therapy for lagenidiosis is typically ineffective.
- Treatment with a *Pythium* vaccine has been recommended but it has not been well evaluated.

POSSIBLE COMPLICATIONS

Sudden death associated with *Pythium* infarction or invasion of mesenteric vessels or rupture of a *Lagenidium*-induced aneurysm of the aorta or vena cava.

RECOMMENDED MONITORING

ELISA serology should be used for monitoring for response to medical therapy or recurrence after surgical resection.

PROGNOSIS AND OUTCOME

- Pythiosis: fair to guarded if lesions appear surgically resectable; guarded to poor if medical therapy alone is used
- Lagenidiosis: grave

PEARLS & CONSIDERATIONS

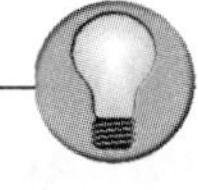

COMMENTS

- GI pythiosis is often mistaken for diffuse neoplasia at surgery.
- Aggressive surgery with wide surgical margins is critical to surgical cure.

CLIENT EDUCATION

Chronic vomiting and weight loss in a dog that spends time in the water in endemic areas should prompt early evaluation for *Pythium* infection.

SUGGESTED READING

Grooters AM: Pythiosis, lagenidiosis, and zygomycosis in small animals. *Vet Clin North Am Small Anim Pract* 33:695, 2003.

Grooters AM, et al: Clinicopathologic findings associated with *Lagenidium* sp. infection in 6 dogs: Initial description of an emerging oomycosis. *J Vet Intern Med* 17:637, 2003.

Thomas RC, Lewis DT: Pythiosis in dogs and cats. *Compend Contin Ed Pract Vet* 20:63, 1998.

AUTHOR: **JOSEPH TABOADA**

EDITOR: **DEBRA L. ZORAN**

Rabies

BASIC INFORMATION

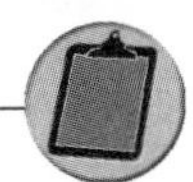

DEFINITION

Fatal polioencephalitis of warm-blooded animals and humans caused by a *Lyssavirus* sp. and generally transmitted by the bite of an infected mammal

SYNONYM(S)

Hydrophobia
Rage

EPIDEMIOLOGY

SPECIES, AGE, SEX: Warm-blooded animals of all ages are susceptible.

- Foxes, coyotes, wolves, and some rodents are highly susceptible.
- Moderately susceptible species include dogs, cats, horses, sheep, goats, and humans.
- Birds and opossums have a low susceptibility.
- Often endemic in wild animals with periodic outbreaks (epizootics).
- In the United States, the most important species-adapted strains are in the fox, raccoon, skunk, and bat.
- Salivary gland infections occur in vampire bats without producing clinical signs in the bats, resulting in prolonged viremia. Insectivorous bats may also be infected.

RISK FACTORS

- Contact with wildlife, especially raccoons, skunks, bats, and foxes
- Lack of vaccination against rabies
- Exposure to aerosols in bat caves
- Modified live-virus rabies vaccines used in immunocompromised animals

CONTAGION AND ZOONOSIS

- Highly zoonotic disease.
- Transmission is most commonly by bite.
    - The risk of human infection is far greater through a rabid animal's bite (5–80%) than a scratch (0.1–1%).

GEOGRAPHY AND SEASONALITY

- Worldwide.
- Rabies-free regions include New Zealand, some Caribbean islands, the British Isles, parts of Scandinavia, Japan, and Hawaii.
- Rabies is a disease of wildlife in the United States.
    - Raccoons: mainly eastern part of the United States.
    - Skunks: mainly in the eastern part of the United States as well as in California and the upper and lower Midwest.
    - Bats: entire United States except Hawaii.
    - Foxes: mainly Alaska, Texas, southwestern part of the United States.
- The dog is the primary species involved in transmission of rabies in the Southern Hemisphere.

CLINICAL PRESENTATION

DISEASE FORMS/SUBTYPES: Clinical signs can be variable but predominantly arise from central nervous system (CNS) dysfunction.

- Prodromal form:
    - Characterized by a change in behavior, which may include anxiety, solitude, and apprehension.
    - Fever may be present.
    - Pruritus may be present at the site of exposure.
    - Lasts 2 to 3 days.
- Paralytic (dumb) form (majority of canine cases, minority of feline cases):
    - Characterized by lethargy, difficulty swallowing, pytalism, voice or bark change, dropped jaw, and lower motor neuron paralysis.
    - Lasts 1 to 7 days, from onset of overt signs to death.
- Furious form (majority of feline cases, minority of canine cases):
    - Characterized by aggression, biting, altered voice, paralysis, seizures, and ataxia.
    - Hyperesthesia and hyper-responsiveness to auditory and visual stimuli are possible.
    - Lasts 2 to 4 days, from onset of overt signs to death.

HISTORY, CHIEF COMPLAINT

- History of wound may or may not be present:
    - Given the pathophysiology of rabies, neurologic clinical signs beginning within 1 week of the occurrence of a wound are extremely unlikely to be related to rabies infection via the wound.
- Behavioral changes are very common and can be varied:
    - Aggression, viciousness, irritability, excitability, nervousness, apprehension, and anxiety.
    - Abnormal or erratic behaviors, such as licking, biting, wandering, disorientation, ataxia, seizures, or paralysis.
- Pytalism and change in bark.
- No clinical signs; exposure is suspected but not confirmed.

PHYSICAL EXAM FINDINGS: Onset of clinical signs is variable in timing: signs occur 2 weeks to several months after exposure. Signs include fever, dropped jaw, pytalism, inability to swallow, mandibular, and laryngeal paralysis. Lower motor neuron limb signs, ataxia, and cranial nerve deficits may be present.

ETIOLOGY AND PATHOPHYSIOLOGY

- Single-stranded RNA virus of the genus *Lyssavirus*, family Rhabdoviridae.
- Transmission:
    - Virus within saliva is transmitted via a wound or mucous membranes.
    - Inhalation of aerosolized virus may occur in exposure to large colonies of bats.
    - Ingestion of infected tissues is also possible but rare.
    - Transmission has also occurred in humans through organ transplantation.
- Virus replicates in local tissues, where it enters neuromuscular junctions and neurotendinal spindles.
    - Virus is vulnerable to immune-mediated destruction (e.g., vaccine-induced) in local tissues but becomes protected once it reaches peripheral nerves or the CNS.
- Spreads by intra-axonal flow through peripheral nerves to the spinal cord and brain. Replicates within the CNS and then moves outward through peripheral, sensory, motor, and cranial nerves.
- Large amount of virus present in salivary glands, where it is shed. Salivary virus excretion begins up to 2 weeks before the onset of neurologic signs.
- The incubation period varies and depends on the innervation at the bite site, the distance of the bite site to the CNS, and the virus variant and amount of virus in the exposure; can range from 2 weeks to as long as 6 months or more.
- Once clinical signs are apparent, death ensues within 10 days.

DIAGNOSIS

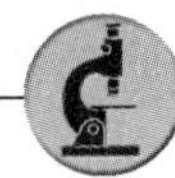

DIFFERENTIAL DIAGNOSIS

- Encephalitis: viral (canine distemper, feline leukemia virus, feline immunodeficiency virus, feline infectious peritonitis), immune-mediated (e.g., granulomatous meningoencephalitis); rarely, protozoal, rickettsial, bacterial, fungal
- Pseudorabies
- Toxicity (e.g., lead)
- Portosystemic shunt
- Hypoglycemia
- Neoplasia
- Trauma
- Causes of ptyalism (see Pytalism, p 909)

INITIAL DATABASE

- The clinical suspicion of rabies is based on history and physical examination.
- Complete blood cell (CBC) count, serum chemistry panel, and urinalysis are not diagnostic.

ADVANCED OR CONFIRMATORY TESTING

- Cerebrospinal fluid (CSF) analysis may show nonspecific increases in protein and leukocytes.
- Direct immunofluorescent antibody (IFA) test of nervous tissue is the confirmatory test of choice.
  - Chill—do not freeze—the body or brain of any dead/euthanized rabies suspect.
  - Immediately submit the brain to a state-approved laboratory for rabies IFA testing.
  - Use extreme caution in obtaining samples and shipping specimens; zoonosis can occur if rabies virus is aerosolized (e.g., when an electric saw is used for opening the skull and proper protection is not used) or is inadvertently inoculated.
- Direct immunofluorescent antibody testing of dermis: skin biopsy of sensory vibrissae of the maxillary area should not be used (false-negative results).

TREATMENT

THERAPEUTIC GOAL(S)

- Invariably fatal; recovery is extraordinarily rare
- No treatment, but suspects must be confined and quarantined

RECOMMENDED MONITORING

- Management of rabies suspects varies with immunization status and local laws. Clinicians should contact the local state veterinarian.
- Most public health laws require a 10-day confined observation period after human exposure from a suspected dog or cat.
  - Virus shedding in saliva before the onset of neurologic signs in infected animals is usually 1 to 5 days but may be up to 13 days.
- All rabies suspects must be securely confined and monitored for behavioral changes and/or neurologic signs suggestive of rabies.
- A healthy dog or cat that bites or scratches an individual should be confined and monitored for 10 days.
  - If clinical signs do not develop within 10 days of bite/scratch, there has been no exposure to rabies virus.
  - If clinical signs consistent with rabies develop during the 10-day quarantine period, euthanize the animal and submit the brain immediately for examination; if infection is thus confirmed within 24 to 48 hours, there is adequate time to begin human postexposure prophylaxis.
- Unvaccinated dogs or cats that are exposed to a known rabid animal or to any bat or wild, carnivorous mammal.
  - Typically, the animals are placed in quarantine for up to 6 months.
  - The animals must be monitored for the onset of clinical signs (with vaccination 1 month prior to release) or euthanized immediately at presentation or at the time of onset of clinical signs consistent with rabies.
- Vaccinated dogs or cats that are exposed to a known rabid animal or to any bat or wild, carnivorous mammal.
  - Immediate revaccination for rabies is indicated.
  - A period of monitoring must follow, typically for 45 days.
- When a dog or cat with an expired rabies vaccination status is exposed to a rabid animal, individual factors will determine the recommended course. Clinicians should contact the state veterinarian.

PROGNOSIS AND OUTCOME

- Fatal
- Cats and dogs will typically succumb within 7 to 10 days after onset of clinical signs
- Rare cases of recovery in dogs, cats, and humans

PEARLS & CONSIDERATIONS

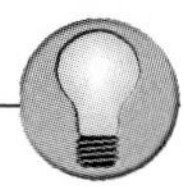

COMMENTS

- If clients are concerned regarding possible or known human exposure to rabies, they must see their physician immediately.
- Clinicians should notify the local public health official.
- Signs take weeks to months to develop after exposure, but once signs are present, death ensues quickly (<2 weeks).

PREVENTION

- All dogs and cats should be vaccinated for rabies after 12 weeks of age, again at 12 months of age, and then every 3 years or yearly depending on state regulations.
- An immediate booster vaccination in immunized dogs and cats exposed to rabies is advised.
- Cats should only receive inactivated vaccines; do not use modified live virus (MLV) vaccines in cats.
- Disinfect contaminated cages, food dishes, and instruments with a diluted solution of 1 part bleach : 32 parts tap water.

CLIENT EDUCATION

- Keep pets from roaming ("leash laws").
- Inform clients of state and local policies.
- Advise the client to bring animal to a veterinarian immediately if exposure is suspected. With human exposure, individuals should immediately contact a physician.

SUGGESTED READING

Centers for Disease Control and Prevention: http://www.cdc.gov/ncidod/dvrd/rabies/.

Greene CE, Dreesen DW: Rabies. In Greene CE (ed): *Infectious Diseases of the Dog and Cat.* Philadelphia, WB Saunders, 1990, pp 114–126.

National Association of State Public Health Veterinarians: Compendium of Animal Rabies Prevention and Control. *J Am Vet Med Assoc* 224(2):216–222, 2004.

Rupprecht CE, Gibbons RV: Prophylaxis against rabies. *N Engl J Med* 351:2626–2635, 2004.

AUTHOR: **LISA M. TIEBER NIELSON**
EDITOR: **DOUGLASS K. MACINTIRE**

Radiation Therapy: Adverse Reactions

BASIC INFORMATION

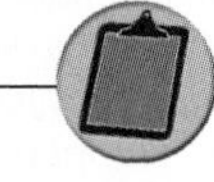

DEFINITION

Radiation reactions are considered acute (or early) if they occur during or shortly after radiation and subside after radiation completion. Reactions with clinical signs that persist over a longer period of time or occur months to years after treatment are considered chronic (or late).

SYNONYM(S)

Acute or chronic radiation reactions
Early or late radiation reactions
Radiation complications

EPIDEMIOLOGY

SPECIES, AGE, SEX: Any patient treated with radiation will be at risk for development of radiation reactions.

RISK FACTORS

- Radiation dose, fraction size, radiation energy, overall treatment time, field size, previous surgery, concurrent administration of chemotherapy, and necrotic or unhealthy tissues may influence a patient's risk for the development of adverse radiation reactions. Cats are less likely to have radiation side effects versus dogs.
- Site-specific risk factors include:
  - Skin: presence of skin folds, tangential radiation fields, poor nutrition, individual differences, use of bolus, use of electron therapy, coincident infection.
  - Head/neck: periodontal disease, coincident infection, concurrent xerostomia.
  - Heart: doxorubicin treatment.

CLINICAL PRESENTATION

DISEASE FORMS/SUBTYPES

- Acute effects: depend on total dose, dose per fraction, and overall treatment time.
- Chronic effects: depend highly on dose per fraction.

HISTORY, CHIEF COMPLAINT: Owners are most likely to report history or complaints in form of physical exam findings listed below.

PHYSICAL EXAM FINDINGS: All physical exam findings are directly related to tissues present within radiation therapy field and usually confined to limits of the radiation treatment field.

- Skin effects:
  - Acute: hyperemia, dry desquamation, moist desquamation, ulceration, necrosis, hair loss, lymphedema, pain.
  - Chronic: telangiectasia, fibrosis, necrosis, lymphedema, hyperpigmentation or hypopigmentation, leukotrichia, loss of pliability/flexibility/range of motion, pain, dry desquamation, chronic wound.
- Head/neck effects:
  - Acute: stomatitis, mucositis, pharyngitis, esophagitis (erythema, edema, confluent or patchy white/yellow membrane formation), xerostomia, dry/cracked lips, ulceration, pain, difficulty swallowing, secondary infection with bacteria or fungi (soft, curd-like white patches), swelling of parotid/submandibular salivary glands, keratitis, keratoconjunctivitis sicca, blepharospasm, periocular crusting, corneal edema.
  - Chronic: osteonecrosis (bone pain, swelling, evidence of infection, exposed bone, nonhealing gingival ulcers), xerostomia, regurgitation, dental caries, keratoconjunctivitis sicca, cataract formation, retinitis, blindness.
- Bone effects (chronic): clinical/radiographic evidence of fracture, necrosis, infection, or secondary tumor.
- Heart effects (acute/chronic): signs relative to pericarditis, chronic constrictive pericarditis, or restrictive cardiomyopathy due to myocardial fibrosis, such as fever, tachycardia, presence of pericardial effusion, cardiac tamponade, pleural effusion, dyspnea, conduction abnormalities, exercise intolerance, subclinical valvular defects.
- Bladder effects (acute/chronic): pain on palpation, clinicopathologic evidence of cystitis (pollakiuria, nocturia, dysuria, hematuria).
- Lung effects (acute/chronic): clinical and radiograph signs compatible with acute pneumonitis and chronic fibrosis (fever, dyspnea, cough, production of sputum, signs of right heart failure if pulmonary hypertension exists). Fibrosis usually, not always, preceded by pneumonitis.
- Colon/rectal effects (acute/chronic): diarrhea secondary to acute enteritis, hematochezia, sense of urgency, chronic diarrhea, proctitis, stricture, fistula formation secondary to chronic colorectal/anorectal injury.
- Central nervous system effects (acute/chronic): signs compatible with location of irradiation field (neurologic deficits, seizures, ataxia, blindness, dementia, somnolence, endocrinopathies).

ETIOLOGY AND PATHOPHYSIOLOGY

- Radiation lesions induced in normal tissues are attributed primarily to loss of specific target cells, or clonogenic cells. Hence, acute effects develop in rapidly renewing tissues, such as skin, gastrointestinal (GI) tract, or bone marrow.
- This target cell theory also applies to vascular damage as the predominant lesion in chronic effects, as endothelial cells are slowly lost to mitotic death.
- In addition, cytokines induced immediately after irradiation have been shown to contribute to the progression of chronic effects.

DIAGNOSIS

DIFFERENTIAL DIAGNOSIS

Few differentials exist for radiation therapy site specific side effects short of progression or recurrence of tumor

INITIAL DATABASE

- Minimum database to rule out metabolic contribution to complications.
- Diagnostic imaging (radiographs, computed tomography, or magnetic resonance imaging) where applicable to determine extent/nature of disease.
- Biopsies where necessary to differentiate tumor recurrence from radiation reaction.
- Clinician-based assessment: Veterinary Radiation Therapy Oncology Group (VRTOG) Acute/Chronic Radiation Scoring Scheme (see reference).

ADVANCED OR CONFIRMATORY TESTING

Generally, not necessary. In people:

- Chronic skin fibrosis measured by tissue compliance meter, ultrasound measurement, or BTC-2000 suction device in humans.
- Xerostomia measured by functional radioisotope imaging, salivary flow output, and patient assessment in humans.
- Pulmonary function tests for confirmation of decreased lung capacity.

TREATMENT

THERAPEUTIC GOAL(S)

- Improving patient quality of life by minimizing pain, establishing return to function, and ruling out tumor recurrence.
- Amelioration of acute side effects may decrease risk of chronic side effects for some tissue types.

ACUTE TREATMENT

- Skin effects:
  - Protect irradiated skin from heat, cold, sunlight, friction, and other sources of irritation.
  - Avoid use of tape.
  - Avoid swimming.
  - Clean moist desquamation with aluminum subacetate (Domeboro) soaks, 1/3 strength hydrogen peroxide (1%), or diluted chlorhexidine solution.
  - Use of skin care products anecdotal, but include: Aquaphor, Collasate, vitamin A/E ointment, aloe vera gel, Theracare, 1% hydrocortisone ointment, silver sulfadiazene.
  - Keep site free of crusts to encourage reepithelialization.
  - Use of ointments preferable to creams or lotions.
  - Bandages promote moist environment and are NOT advised when possible. If necessary, use moisture vapor permeable dressings (Tegaderm).
  - Antibiotic therapy to control infection and anti-inflammatory therapy to decrease inflammation.
  - Pain management and breaks in radiation therapy where necessary.
- Head/neck effects:
  - Stomatitis/mucositis/esophagitis:
    - Maintain good oral hygiene.
    - Use of soft, bland diet with decreased amount, increased frequency, and room temperature. Avoidance of salty, acidic foods.
    - Mouthwashes to cleanse and lubricate the oral cavity (saline, sodium bicarbonate solutions, dilute tea,

dilute hydrogen peroxide; avoid alcohol preparations).
   - Topical anesthetics and coating agents such as viscous lidocaine (xylocaine), sucralfate suspensions, Acemannan-containing gel all proven to ameliorate mucositis. Note: viscous lidocaine may burn initially prior to taking effect.
   - Omega-3 fatty acid, arginine, glutamine, and oral zinc supplementation all proven in humans to ameliorate pathologic or clinical evidence of mucositis.
   - Antibiotics (aerobic gram-negative bacteria most likely) and/or antifungals topically (chlorhexidine rinse with topical suspension of nystatin) or systemically for secondary infections.
   - Narcotic analgesics and nutritional support for severe effects.
  - Xerostomia (dry mouth):
    - Increase fluid intake.
    - Maintain good oral hygiene.
    - Use of salivary substitutes (short-lived) or pilocarpine (Salagen) (may have unacceptable side effects), acupuncture, olive oil rinse, and autotransplantation of salivary gland tissue to site outside radiation field all reported to ameliorate signs in humans.
  - Acute ocular effects: topical antibiotics and steroids if no corneal ulceration present; topical antibiotics and anesthetics if corneal ulceration present; supplementary eye lubrication.
- Acute heart effects: pericarditis managed primarily by prevention. Rest, nonsteroidal anti-inflammatory drugs, and mild diuretics often all that is needed during self-limiting, subclinical resolution. Subtotal parietal pericardiectomy if clinical signs do not resolve.
- Acute bladder effects: maintain patient hydration; increase fluid intake to dilute urine (less irritating). Treat underlying urinary infections, treat bladder spasms (phenazopyridine hydrochloride, Urimax, flavoxate hydrochloride agents, oxybutynin used in human oncology), rule out recurrent tumor.
- Acute lung effects: glucocorticosteroids provide much clinical utility despite lack of published evidence. Rest, oxygen therapy, antibiotics as needed. Supportive care with expectorants and bronchodilators.
- Acute bowel effects: see chronic bowel effects below.
- Acute central nervous system side effects: edema and temporary demyelination usually responsive to anti-inflammatory doses of steroids. Anticonvulsants as necessary.

CHRONIC TREATMENT

- Skin effects:
  - Fibrosis: physical therapy, impedance-controlled microcurrent treatment, hyperbaric oxygen, pain management, glucocorticosteroids in the initial setting (limited usefulness for established fibrosis), pentoxifylline ± vitamin E, and superoxide dismutase all are methods to delay or reduce fibrosis in human oncology. Investigational treatments include decorin (inhibitor of TGF-β), ACE-inhibitors, and interferons.
  - Lymphedema: Manual Lymphatic Drainage (specialized massage with specific stroke duration, orientation, pressure, sequence) combined with compression bandages, exercise, skin care, pressure gradient sleeves, and/or pneumatic pumps method to ameliorate lymphedema in human oncology. Diuretics to cause acute reduction in the initial setting (limited usefulness for long-term due to removal of lymph fluid but NOT proteinaceous debris from interstitial space). Benzopyrones (coumarin), autologous lymphocyte injection, and selenium proven methods to improve resolution in humans. Of interest but less usefulness, glucocorticosteroids, weight management, hyperbaric oxygen, antibiotic therapy, flavonoids, surgical intervention.
- Chronic head/neck effects:
  - Osteonecrosis (a.k.a. osteoradionecrosis): antibiotics, surgical debridement.
  - Esophageal stricture (see Esophageal Stricture, p 363): dilatations and semi-solid diet, feeding tubes, hydrocortisone injection at the stricture site.
  - Xerostomia: see Acute Treatment above.
  - Cataract formation can be treated with surgical removal.
- Chronic bone effects: surgical intervention, antibiotics. Secondary tumor management as needed.
- Chronic heart effects: antipyretics for fever, centesis for tamponade, pericardiectomy if severe. Medical management by veterinary cardiologist.
- Chronic bladder cystitis/fibrosis: see Acute Treatment above. Surgical intervention for fistula formation.
- Pulmonary fibrosis ameliorated by captopril in human oncology. Oxygen and glucocorticosteroids as needed.
- Chronic bowel effects: initial management with increased dietary fiber and diphenoxylate (Lomotil) or loperamide. Addition of opioid analgesics titrated to effect. Topical viscous lidocaine for anorectal irritation. Glucocorticosteroid-containing suppositories (Protofoam, Canasa) for acute inflammation. Sucralfate or short chain fatty acid (butyrate) enemas for bleeding. Topical formalin, topical amifostine, coagulation with electocautery, laser therapy, argon plasma beam coagulation, and hyperbaric oxygen for refractory bleeding in human oncology.
- Late central nervous system side effects: glucocorticosteroids (dexamethasone) ideal in early onset radiation necrosis. May consider surgical resection if area of necrosis is localized.

DRUG INTERACTIONS

Concurrent use of some chemotherapeutics may exacerbate radiation side effects.

POSSIBLE COMPLICATIONS

- Skin effects: progression of moist desquamation to full thickness necrosis and secondary infection necessitating surgical debridement. Unrelenting fibrosis or lymphedema necessitating surgical intervention.
- Oral cavity effects: *Candidia albicans* yeast infection can increase severity of stomatitis/mucositis. Rare reports of trismus (contractions of muscles of mastication) with reduced capacity to open mouth.

RECOMMENDED MONITORING

Advise recheck of patient at 1, 2, 3, 5, 7, 9, and 12 months and every 3 to 6 months post radiation therapy completion.

PROGNOSIS AND OUTCOME

Prognosis for most acute radiation reactions is excellent if managed efficiently and in a timely manner. Prognosis for most late radiation reactions is guarded to poor for complete recovery. Prevention of late radiation reactions is of great concern during radiation therapy planning.

PEARLS & CONSIDERATIONS

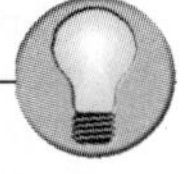

COMMENTS

- Use VRTOG Toxicity Criteria Scale to document reactions.
- This review is not all-inclusive. Consult with veterinary radiation oncologist as need arises.

PREVENTION

- Use of intensity modulated radiation therapy/conformal radiation therapy techniques, to allow increased dose to tumor while also increasing normal tissue sparing.
- Acute skin effects: reduce skin folds, remove bolus where necessary, avoid topical agents immediately prior to radi-

ation therapy, use higher energy radiation, and ensure surgical wounds have healed prior to initiation of radiation therapy.
- Chronic skin effects: early detection and treatment.
- Head/neck effects: preradiation therapy dental prophylaxis and removal of unhealthy teeth to decrease severity of mucositis and risk of osteonecrosis. Amifostine as a radiation protector routinely used to prevent development of xerostomia (dry mouth) in humans. Ocular: tape eyelids open for anterior megavoltage beam fields to the eye to decrease dose to cornea and conjunctiva (otherwise, the eyelids will serve as a site of radiation dose buildup, increasing the radiation dose delivered to the cornea).

CLIENT EDUCATION

- Teach family members when to expect and how to manage acute effects. Promote role of radiation therapist in client education and side effect management.
- Prepare notebook with photographs of radiation side effects as a tool for client education. Use serial photographs to display effects as they heal with time.
- Use handouts describing potential effects and management to encourage client information recall.

SUGGESTED READING

Cox JD, Ang KK: *Radiation Oncology: Rationale, Technique, Results*. St. Louis, Mosby, 2003.

Dow KD, Bucholtz JD, Iwamoto R, Fieler V, Hilderley L: *Nursing Care in Radiation Oncology*. Philadelphia, WB Saunders, 1997.

LaDue T, Klein MK: Toxicity criteria of the veterinary radiation therapy oncology group. *Vet Rad & Ultrasound* 42:475-476, 2001.

AUTHOR: **TRACY A. LADUE**

EDITOR: **KENNETH M. RASSNICK**

Rectal Prolapse

BASIC INFORMATION

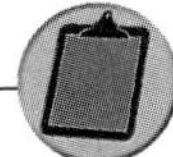

DEFINITION

Rectal prolapse is eversion of the anal mucosa or full-thickness rectal wall through the anal opening.

EPIDEMIOLOGY

SPECIES, AGE, SEX: Can occur at any age, but young dogs and cats are most frequently affected.

GENETICS AND BREED PREDISPOSITION: Manx cats may be predisposed.

RISK FACTORS: Recent perineal surgery

ASSOCIATED CONDITIONS AND DISORDERS: Any condition that causes tenesmus may be associated with rectal prolapse: gastrointestinal (GI) parasitism; neoplasia of the colon, rectum, or anus; rectal foreign bodies; colitis; perineal hernia; prostatic disease; urinary disease; dystocia.

CLINICAL PRESENTATION

DISEASE FORMS/SUBTYPES

- Partial prolapse (mucosa only)
- Complete prolapse (all layers of the rectal wall)

HISTORY, CHIEF COMPLAINT

- Visualization of red tissue protruding from anus
- Straining to defecate or urinate
- Diarrhea

PHYSICAL EXAM FINDINGS

- Partial prolapse: a few millimeters of red, swollen mucosa protruding through anus.
- Complete prolapse: cylindrical mass protruding from anus (Fig. I-143); tissue may be red, ulcerated, or necrotic.
- Other findings consistent with underlying cause for straining (i.e., enlarged prostate, palpable neoplastic mass, etc.).

ETIOLOGY AND PATHOPHYSIOLOGY

- Animal affected by underlying disease that causes straining.
- Repetitively increased intra-abdominal pressure from straining causes weakness of perirectal and perianal connective tissue or muscles, resulting in prolapse.
- Inflammation or edema of mucosa may result in more straining and can exacerbate prolapse.
- Prolapsed tissue may become traumatized or desiccate, resulting in ulceration and necrosis.

DIAGNOSIS

DIFFERENTIAL DIAGNOSIS

- Prolapsed intussusception (Fig. I-144)
- Neoplastic mass protruding from anus

INITIAL DATABASE

- Rectal examination (see Fig. I-144): insert a blunt probe between prolapsed tissue and rectal wall. The probe cannot be passed with rectal prolapse but will pass at least a few centimeters with a prolapsed intussusception.
- Complete blood cell (CBC) count, serum chemistry profile, urinalysis, and urine culture may identify underlying cause of straining and indicate an animal's metabolic status.
- Abdominal radiographs may demonstrate conditions associated with rectal prolapse (i.e., neoplastic masses, prostatomegaly, urinary calculi).
- Fecal analysis for intestinal parasitism.

ADVANCED OR CONFIRMATORY TESTING

- Abdominal ultrasonography to identify associated conditions
- Proctoscopy and biopsy to rule out potential underlying causes (colitis, neoplasia)

TREATMENT

THERAPEUTIC GOAL(S)

- Reduce prolapsed tissue
- Prevent recurrence of prolapse
- Treat underlying cause of straining
- Resect necrotic tissue

ACUTE GENERAL TREATMENT

- Peform acute treatment with patient under general anesthesia to prevent the patient from straining during prolapse reduction.
- Lavage prolapsed tissue with saline and inspect viability.
- Apply lubricant and manually reduce (gentle digital pressure) if tissue is viable.
- Apply dextrose (50%) to tissue to decrease edema and aid in reduction.
- Place purse-string suture around rectum at mucocutaneous junction to maintain reduction. The purse-string suture should be tight enough to prevent prolapse but should still allow for passage of soft stools.
- Perform resection and anastomosis of diseased tissue if tissue is not viable.

CHRONIC TREATMENT

- Maintain purse-string suture for 3 to 5 days and begin treatment of underlying cause of straining.

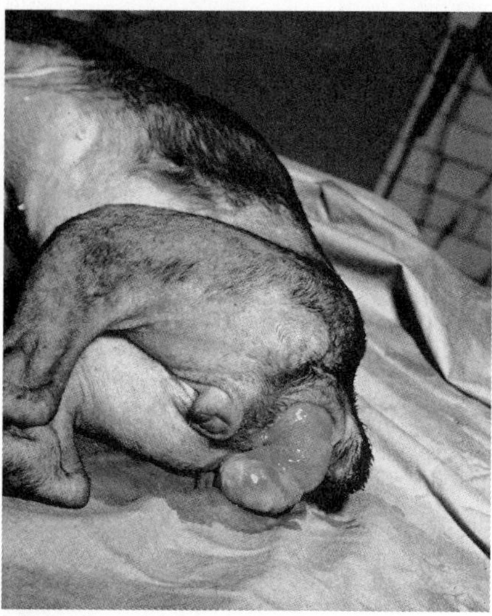

FIGURE I-143 Clinical image of rectal prolapse in a dog. Courtesy of Dr. Richard Walshaw.

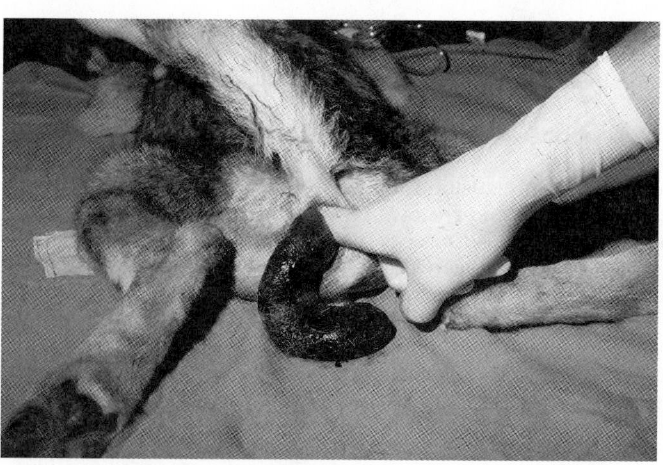

FIGURE I-144 Image of colonic intussusception. This clinical image shows a colonic intussusception, an important differential diagnosis for rectal prolapse. In an animal with a colonic intussusception, a digit may be passed into the rectum, as shown in this anesthetized animal. With rectal prolapse, the bowel is everted at the anus, not within the colon; therefore, such rectal palpation is not possible. Courtesy of Dr. Richard Walshaw.

- If the patient undergoes resection and anastomosis, the animal should receive a low-residue diet and stool softeners are indicated to reduce postoperative straining.
- Perform a colopexy if prolapse repeatedly recurs after appropriate acute treatment.

POSSIBLE COMPLICATIONS

- Continued tenesmus
- Dyschezia, hematochezia
- Recurrent prolapse
- Leakage, dehiscence, and stricture if resection performed

PROGNOSIS AND OUTCOME

Good prognosis if surgically treated and underlying cause treatable

PEARLS & CONSIDERATIONS

COMMENTS

- Place a lubricated finger or small syringe case in rectum while tightening purse-string suture to prevent overtightening.
- Apply a local anesthetic to the rectal tissue after removal of the purse-string suture, which may help prevent recurrence.
- Treat all young animals with rectal prolapse empirically for intestinal parasitism even if fecal flotation result is negative.

SUGGESTED READING

Aronson L: Rectum and anus. In Slatter D (ed): *Textbook of Small Animal Surgery*. Philadelphia, WB Saunders, 2002, pp 682–708.

Popovitch CA, et al: Colopexy as a treatment for rectal prolapse in dogs and cats: A retrospective study of 14 cases. *Vet Surg* 23:115, 1994.

AUTHOR: **LORI LUDWIG**
EDITOR: **RICHARD WALSHAW**

Rectoanal Stricture

BASIC INFORMATION

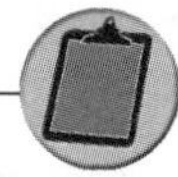

DEFINITION

Narrowing of anal or rectal lumen diameter

SYNONYM(S)

Anorectal stricture

EPIDEMIOLOGY

SPECIES, AGE, SEX: While atresia ani is a congenital stricture that is seen in young puppies and kittens, stricture formation is generally a sequela to disease processes that occur in middle-aged to older animals.

RISK FACTORS: Anal trauma or surgery.

CLINICAL PRESENTATION

HISTORY, CHIEF COMPLAINT

- Tenesmus, diarrhea, hematochezia, and ribbon-like stools.
- Animals with advanced or metastatic malignancy may present with weight loss, anorexia, and lethargy.

PHYSICAL EXAM FINDINGS: Stricture is usually palpable on digital rectal examination.

ETIOLOGY AND PATHOPHYSIOLOGY

- Stricture may be related to a primary infiltrative process such as inflammatory, infectious, or neoplastic disease.
- Stricture formation may also be seen secondary to surgery, penetrating trauma, radiation, or enema administration.

DIAGNOSIS

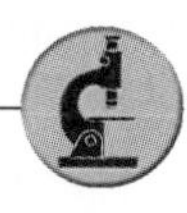

DIFFERENTIAL DIAGNOSIS

Possible causes of anorectal stricture:

- Neoplasia:
  - The most common malignant tumor of the rectum is adenocarcinoma (see Adenocarcinoma, Intestinal/Colonic, p 38).
  - Other tumor types include lymphosarcoma, leiomyosarcoma, and hemangiosarcoma.

- Benign neoplasia may include adenoma, fibroma, or leiomyoma.
- Inflammatory disease, such as colitis.
- Infectious disease: Histoplasmosis has been reported to cause rectal stricture in one dog.
- Trauma.
- Scar formation secondary to surgery (e.g., anal sacculectomy, perianal fistula repair, mass excision), enema, or radiation therapy.

INITIAL DATABASE

- Gentle rectal examination.
- Assessment of location (identifying possible organ of origin), symmetry. (circumferential versus focal), pain, and evidence of metastatis (palpation of sublumbar lymph nodes).
- Complete blood count (CBC), serum chemistry analysis, and urinalysis usually within normal limits.
- Abdominal radiographs:
  - Potential for visualizing area of stenosis as well as megacolon that may be present cranial to stricture
  - Evidence of underlying cause of stricture, metastatic disease (± thoracic radiographs)

ADVANCED OR CONFIRMATORY TESTING

- Contrast radiography may help localize stricture (see Barium Enema, p 1185).
- Abdominal ultrasound can help assess for diffuse metastatic disease.
- Colonoscopy should be used for visualizing extent of stricture formation and to acquire biopsy samples.

TREATMENT

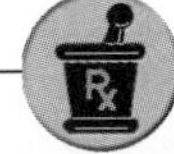

THERAPEUTIC GOAL(S)

Improve narrowed lumen and attain definitive histopathologic diagnosis

ACUTE GENERAL TREATMENT

- With the animal under general anesthesia, mild strictures can be dilated using gentle digital or balloon bougienage.
- Surgical intervention, if possible, is indicated to resect stricture, or cause of stricture, and obtain a definitive biopsy sample:
  - Use a rectal pull-through or dorsal rectal approach.
  - Colostomy has been reported in dogs as an option for rectal obstruction or perforation.

POSSIBLE COMPLICATIONS

Surgical complications include incontinence, dehiscence, infection, and recurrence of stricture or neoplasia.

PROGNOSIS AND OUTCOME

- Prognosis is related to histopathologic findings. Approximately 50% of rectal neoplasms are malignant. Reported outcome for adenocarcinoma is poor.
- Regardless of the underlying etiology, there is a high likelihood for stricture reformation. Multiple surgical procedures may be required to correct the problem.

PEARLS & CONSIDERATIONS

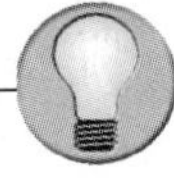

COMMENTS

- It is common to cause iatrogenic tears of the rectum or anus, so care is warranted when performing digital or balloon bougienage.
- If resection of stricture is performed, avoid enema administration for 24 hours prior to surgery to reduce intraoperative fecal contamination (fecal spillage from the anus during surgery).

SUGGESTED READING

Anson LW, et al: A retrospective evaluation of the rectal pull-through technique. Procedure and postoperative complications. *Vet Surg* 17(3):141-146, 1988.

Aronson L: Rectum and anus. In Slatter D (ed): *Textbook of Small Animal Surgery*. Philadelphia, WB Saunders, 2003, p 682.

Hardie E, et al: Use of colostomy to manage rectal disease in dogs. *Vet Surg* 26:270-274, 1997.

Hill LN, et al: Open versus closed bilateral anal sacculectomy for treatment of non-neoplastic anal sac disease in dogs: 95 cases (1969-1994). *J Am Vet Med Assoc* 221(5):662-665, 2002.

Holt D, et al: Clinical use of a dorsal surgical approach to the rectum. *Compend Contin Educ Pract Vet* 13(10):1519-1529, 1991.

AUTHOR: **JANET KOVAK**
EDITOR: **RICHARD WALSHAW**

Recurrent Flank Alopecia, Canine

BASIC INFORMATION

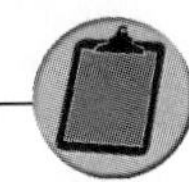

DEFINITION

Skin disorder of unknown etiology characterized by episodes of truncal hair loss with spontaneous regrowth that often occurs on a recurrent basis

SYNONYM(S)

Canine idiopathic cyclic flank alopecia
CRFA
Cyclic follicular dysplasia
Seasonal flank alopecia

EPIDEMIOLOGY

SPECIES, AGE, SEX

- Dogs of either sex and of any reproductive status can be affected.
- Mean age at onset of the first episode is 4 years (range 8 months to 11 years).
- Most dogs have an onset of alopecia between November and March (in the Northern Hemisphere).

GENETICS AND BREED PREDISPOSITION: Boxers may account for approximately half of all cases, but other breeds at high risk include English bulldog, Airedale terrier, and schnauzer (miniature, standard, and giant). Although canine recurrent flank alopecia (CRFA) seems to affect virtually any breed, this condition appears to be rare to absent in the plush-coat Nordic breeds, German shepherd dog, and cocker spaniel.

CLINICAL PRESENTATION

HISTORY, CHIEF COMPLAINT: Fairly abrupt onset of bilateral alopecia affecting the thoracolumbar region.

PHYSICAL EXAM FINDINGS

- Nonscarring alopecia, usually bilaterally symmetric, with well-demarcated borders (Fig. I-145).
- Marked hyperpigmention of the alopecic skin is common.
- The alopecia is usually confined to the thoracolumbar region, but on rare occasions, this condition is seen in association with alopecia on the dorsum of the nose, base of the ears, base of tail, and perineum.
- Spontaneous regrowth of a normal coat occurs in 3 to 8 months (range: 1 to 14 months) in most dogs.
- Most dogs will develop recurrent alopecic episodes every year; however, some dogs have an occasional year when the alopecia does not recur.
- The degree of alopecia is variable, with some dogs developing a virtually iden-

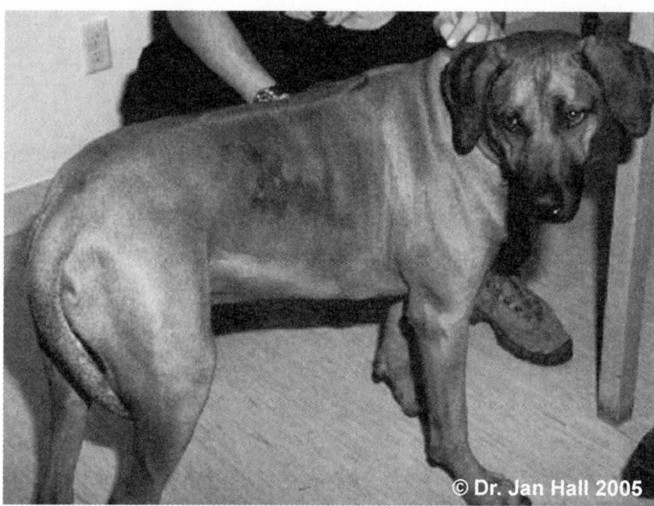

FIGURE I-145 Recurrent seasonal flank alopecia in a Rhodesian Ridgeback. Note the characteristic geographical pattern of alopecia and hyperpigmentation. Courtesy of Dr. Jan A. Hall.

tical hair loss (size and duration) year after year, and other dogs developing larger areas and/or longer episodes of hair loss as years go by.

- In a few cases, hair regrowth may become less complete after several episodes; it may even progress to an end-stage permanent flank alopecia and marked hyperpigmentation.
- Up to 20% of the dogs have only one isolated episode of alopecia during their lifetime.

ETIOLOGY AND PATHOPHYSIOLOGY

- The high incidence in some breeds and the familial character of CRFA suggest a genetic influence.
- The seasonal nature and annual recurrence suggests that photoperiod may be involved. The higher incidence of CRFA at higher latitude (around or north of the 45-degree parallel in the Northern Hemisphere) supports the implication of light exposure in this disorder.

DIAGNOSIS

DIFFERENTIAL DIAGNOSIS

- Hypothyroidism
- Hyperadrenocorticism
- Functional gonadal neoplasm
- Other follicular dysplasias
- Telogen defluxion

INITIAL DATABASE

Diagnosis is based on history, clinical findings, and ruling out other differentials (e.g., exclusion of hypothyroidism in dogs >2 years of age).

ADVANCED OR CONFIRMATORY TESTING

Dermatohistopathologic examination: nonspecific changes of endocrinopathies. In addition, truncated, keratin-filled atrophic primary and secondary hair follicles ("witch's feet") are suggestive but not pathognomonic of CRFA.

TREATMENT

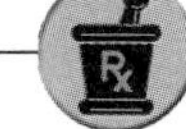

THERAPEUTIC GOAL(S)

Reduce or prevent hair loss

ACUTE AND CHRONIC TREATMENT

- Oral melatonin, administered at the rate of 3-6 mg PO, q 8-12h, for 1 to 2 months, may change the clinical course in up to 50-75% of cases (whether initiated before or shortly after the onset of alopecia).
- To prevent hair loss, administer melatonin 1 to 2 months prior to the expected episode of alopecia.
- To shorten the duration of an existing alopecic episode, start melatonin administration as soon as possible after the onset of alopecia.

PROGNOSIS AND OUTCOME

Dogs affected with CRFA are healthy otherwise, and benign neglect is a valuable therapeutic approach.

PEARLS & CONSIDERATIONS

COMMENTS

The unpredictable course of CRFA and the spontaneous regrowth of hair render the evaluation of any therapeutic agent difficult, whether used for preventing the condition or to shorten an existing episode of alopecia.

SUGGESTED READING

Paradis M: Melatonin therapy in canine alopecia. In Bonagura JD (ed): *Kirk's Current Veterinary Therapy XIII*. Philadelphia, WB Saunders, 2000, pp 546-549.

Paradis M, Cerundolo R: An approach to symmetrical alopecia in the dog. In Foster A, Foil C (eds): *Manual of Small Animal Dermatology*, ed 2. British Small Animal Veterinary Assocation, Ames, IA: Iowa State University Press, 2002, pp 83-93.

AUTHOR: **MANON PARADIS**
EDITOR: **JAN A. HALL**

Red Eye

BASIC INFORMATION

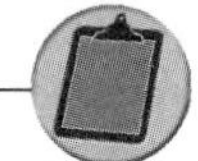

DEFINITION

- Conjunctival, episcleral/scleral, or palpebral hyperemia.
- The term *red eye* does not traditionally apply to redness within the anterior chamber (i.e., hyphema).

SYNONYM(S)

Conjunctival hyperemia
Conjunctival injection
Episcleral/scleral hyperemia
Episcleral/scleral injection

EPIDEMIOLOGY

SPECIES, AGE, SEX: Dogs and cats; no age or gender predisposition.

GENETICS AND BREED PREDISPOSITION: Variable depending on underlying cause.

RISK FACTORS

- Trauma
- Systemic infectious or inflammatory diseases
- Coagulopathy
- Current therapy with potentially irritating topical ophthalmic medications (e.g., pilocarpine; neomycin; prostaglandin analogs; aminoglycosides)

CLINICAL PRESENTATION

HISTORY, CHIEF COMPLAINT: Variable, but may include any or all of the following:

- "Red" eye, by definition
- Blepharospasm
- Ocular discharge
- Cloudiness of eye
- Loss of vision

PHYSICAL EXAM FINDINGS

- Conjunctival vessel hyperemia: diffuse conjunctival redness:
  - Usually indicates ocular surface (i.e., superficial) disease, including:
    - Conjunctivitis.
    - Superficial keratitis (see Corneal Ulceration, p 246; Pannus [Chronic Superficial Keratitis], p 802).
  - Vessels appear to originate in conjunctival fornix and branch as they approach limbus.
- Episcleral/scleral hyperemia: discrete engorgement and tortuosity of episcleral vessels:
  - Usually indicates intraocular disease (see Uveitis, p 1134; Glaucoma, p 440), deep corneal disease (see Corneal Ulceration, p 246), or episcleritis/scleritis (see Episcleritis/Scleritis, p 353).
  - Vessels originate near limbus and follow a deep, straight course toward the conjunctival fornix.
- Both conjunctival and episcleral/scleral vessel injection can occur in the same eye. Ocular discharge and blepharospasm are nonspecific signs; other signs depend on the underlying cause of red eye:
  - Blepharitis; hyperemic, swollen eyelids:
    - ± Mucopurulent ocular discharge.
    - Normal intraocular examination.
  - Conjunctivitis (see Conjunctivitis: Cats, p 231, Dogs, p 233); hyperemic conjunctiva:
    - Chemosis (conjunctival swelling).
    - Ocular discharge.
    - Normal intraocular examination.
  - Keratitis (see Corneal Ulceration, p 246; Pannus [Chronic Superficial Keratitis], p 802):
    - Corneal opacities (see Corneal Discoloration, p 239).
    - Corneal vascularization.
    - Corneal vessels that cross the limbus and branch suggest superficial corneal disease.
    - Vessels that start at the limbus and form a dense straight pattern on cornea suggest deep corneal disease and/or intraocular disease.
    - ± Fluorescein dye retention.
  - Uveitis (see Uveitis, p 1134); any or all of the following:
    - Aqueous cells or flare.
    - Constricted pupil.
    - Abnormal appearance to iris (see Iris Abnormalities, p 608).
    - Hyphema (see Hyphema, p 560).
    - Fibrin clot in anterior chamber.
    - Hypopyon (see Hypopyon, p 571).
    - Low intraocular pressure.
  - Glaucoma (see Glaucoma, p 440):
    - Dilated pupil.
    - Diffuse corneal edema.
    - ± Buphthalmos (see Ocular Size Abnormalities, p 763).
    - Fundic exam: optic disk cupping.
    - Lens luxation (see Lens Luxation, p 628): suggests primary or secondary glaucoma.

ETIOLOGY AND PATHOPHYSIOLOGY

Dilation of conjunctival and/or episcleral/scleral vessels:

- Typically inflammatory response to superficial and/or deep ocular disease.
- May be caused by passive congestion (e.g., large, space-occupying orbital lesion) (see Orbital Disease, p 773).

DIAGNOSIS

DIFFERENTIAL DIAGNOSIS

- Conjunctivitis (see Conjunctivitis: Cats, p 231, Dogs, p 233).
- Corneal ulceration (see Corneal Ulceration, p 246).
- Nonulcerative keratitis (see Keratoconjunctivitis Sicca, p 614; Pannus [Chronic Superficial Keratitis], p 802).
- Uveitis (see Uveitis, p 1134).
- Glaucoma (see Glaucoma, p 440).
- Episcleritis/scleritis (see Episcleritis/Scleritis, p 353).
- Orbital disease (see Orbital Disease, p 773).
- Blepharitis (inflammation of the eyelids).
- A "red" eye may also involve more than one ocular disease (e.g., corneal ulceration with secondary uveitis).

INITIAL DATABASE

Complete ophthalmic examination, including:

- Schirmer tear test; a low result (<5–10 mm/min) indicates KCS.
- Fluorescein dye application; a positive fluorescein dye retention indicates corneal ulceration (see Corneal Ulceration, p 246).
- Intraocular pressure measurement; elevated level (>30 mmHg) is diagnostic of glaucoma, but level is typically low (<10–15 mmHg) with uveitis.

ADVANCED OR CONFIRMATORY TESTING

- Variable depending on results of initial examination and testing (i.e., suspected cause).
- Corneal or conjunctival swabs for cytologic examination with or without culture and sensitivity (C&S) for conjunctivitis, corneal ulcers, keratitis, or blepharitis.
- Complete blood count (CBC), serum chemistry panel, titers for infectious disease; radiography, ultrasonography for certain causes of uveitis (see Uveitis, p 1134).
- Biopsy of lesion and histopathologic exam for refractory or complex blepharitis or episcleritis/scleritis.

TREATMENT

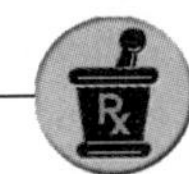

THERAPEUTIC GOAL(S)

- Decrease inflammation.
- Eliminate infection, if present.
- Achieve appropriate intraocular pressure, if abnormal.
- Eliminate ocular pain.
- Maintain vision.

ACUTE GENERAL TREATMENT

- Loss of vision is an emergency that requires immediate determination and treatment of underlying cause; glaucoma, severe uveitis, and severe keratitis should be considered in acute or progressive vision loss (see Blindness, p 136).
- Blepharitis:
  - Determine underlying cause.
  - Animal often needs systemic antibiotic and/or anti-inflammatory therapy(ies).
  - See Demodicosis, p 282; Juvenile Cellulitis, p 611; Pemphigus Complex, p 823.
- See Keratoconjunctivitis Sicca, p 614.
- See Conjunctivitis: Cats, p 231; Dogs, p 233.
- See Corneal Ulceration, p 246.
- See Uveitis, p 1134.
- See Glaucoma, p 440.
- See Episcleritis/Scleritis, p 353.
- See Orbital Disease, p 773.

CHRONIC TREATMENT

Variable depending on underlying condition and cause

POSSIBLE COMPLICATIONS

Variable depending on underlying condition and cause; may include:

- Loss of eye

- Loss of vision
- Worsening of systemic disease

PROGNOSIS AND OUTCOME

- Variable depending on underlying cause
- Lack of vision at presentation is often a poor prognostic indicator (return of vision uncommon)

PEARLS & CONSIDERATIONS

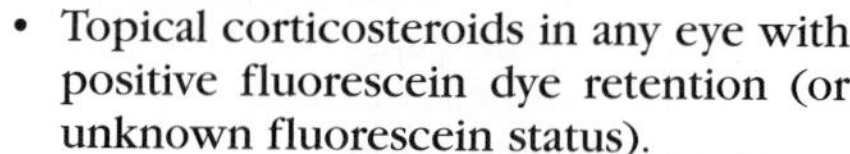

COMMENTS

Clinicians should not use:

- Topical corticosteroids in any eye with positive fluorescein dye retention (or unknown fluorescein status).
- Systemic corticosteroids until preliminary diagnostics are performed or a diagnosis is reached, because these drugs are generally contraindicated for treating infectious systemic disease.

CLIENT EDUCATION

Seek veterinary attention promptly at first sign of red eye because many causes of red eye are globe and/or vision threatening.

SUGGESTED READING

Slatter D: Ocular emergencies. In Slatter D (ed): *Fundamentals of Veterinary Ophthalmology*. Philadelphia, WB Saunders, 2001, pp 562–570.

AUTHOR: **ELLISON BENTLEY**
EDITOR: **CHERYL L. CULLEN**

Refeeding Syndrome

BASIC INFORMATION

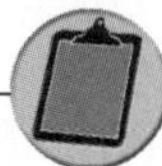

DEFINITION

Fluid and electrolyte abnormalities associated with either enteral or parenteral feeding of previously malnourished animals

EPIDEMIOLOGY

SPECIES, AGE, SEX: Can occur in any malnourished animal; aged and critically ill animals may be at increased risk.
RISK FACTORS: Malnutrition, prolonged starvation, animals receiving supplemental nutritional support, overly aggressive nutritional support of malnourished animals, animals that have neurologic problems and dysphagias, reportedly diabetic ketoacidosis (dogs), and hepatic lipidosis (cats).

CLINICAL PRESENTATION

DISEASE FORMS/SUBTYPES: This is a secondary syndrome. Variable combinations of fluid retention, hypokalemia, hypophosphatemia, and hypomagnesemia may occur within the first 4 days of refeeding by any route. Overt clinical signs tend to become apparent when serum phosphorus <1.5 mg/dl (0.5 mmol/l). Thiamin (vitamin B_1) deficiency has been reported in humans but not in animals with refeeding syndrome.
HISTORY, CHIEF COMPLAINT

- History of aggressive nutrition support in animals that have undergone prolonged anorexia, particularly in the presence of disease.
- Chief complaint depends on the exact pattern of abnormalities in each animal.
- Animals generally are malnourished and undergoing treatment for an illness that requires nutritional support. Therefore, the chief complaint of refeeding syndrome may initially be overshadowed by signs of the primary illness.
- Additional signs of fluid retention (e.g., rapid weight gain), hypokalemia or hypomagnesemia (e.g., weakness), and hypophosphatemia (weakness, lethargy due to hemolytic anemia) may be noted concurrently.

PHYSICAL EXAM FINDINGS: Weakness, weight loss, reduced muscle mass, and signs resulting from primary disease process are all possible physical exam findings. Signs of individual abnormalities vary with the severity and the presence of concurrent illness. Many animals do not show clinical signs until the abnormality is severe; these tend to be primarily related to fluid and electrolyte abnormalities.

- Fluid overload: rapid weight gain ± serous nasal discharge, chemosis, restlessness, shivering, tachycardia, tachypnea, dyspnea, pulmonary crackles, vomiting, and diarrhea.
- Hypokalemia: (serum K^+ <3.5 mEq/L), arrhythmia, ileus, decreased urinary concentrating ability.
- Hypophosphatemia: (serum PO_4^{2-} <1.5 mg/dl), hemolytic anemia, muscle weakness, rhabdomyolysis, renal tubular defects.
- Hypomagnesemia: (serum Mg^{2+} <1 mEq/L), cardiac arrhythmia and electrocardiographic abnormalities, tremors, weakness, tetany, and secondary hypokalemia and hypocalcemia.

ETIOLOGY AND PATHOPHYSIOLOGY

- Disease and malnutrition result in decreased serum levels of glucose. Catecholamines, glucagon, and glucocorticoid hormones increase to maintain serum glucose levels via gluconeogenesis by utilizing fatty acids and protein as precursors.
- Depletion of lean body mass and intracellular electrolytes may result.
- Refeeding allows use of carbohydrates (glucose) as the primary fuel source.
- Carbohydrate intake results in increased insulin secretion. This stimulates cellular uptake of phosphorus for protein synthesis, which can lead to profound hypophosphatemia.
- Feeding can also drive other molecules and electrolytes into the cells, resulting in acute extracellular deficiencies (hypoglycemia, hypomagnesemia, and hypokalemia) and fluid balance abnormalities.

DIAGNOSIS

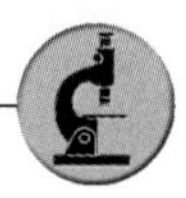

DIFFERENTIAL DIAGNOSIS

- Any disease with prolonged anorexia or resulting malnutrition
- Exacerbation of the primary disease

INITIAL DATABASE

- Body weight
- Serum glucose, albumin
- Blood gas and serum biochemical profile, including electrolyte determinations: hypokalemia, hypophosphatemia, hypomagnesemia are common
- Complete blood count (CBC): generally unremarkable
- Urinalysis

TREATMENT

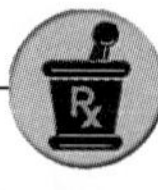

THERAPEUTIC GOAL(S)

- Administer phosphorus supplementation via IV route
- Correct other electrolyte abnormalities via IV route
- Correct acid-base abnormalities

ACUTE GENERAL TREATMENT

- Reduce the rate of feeding by 50%.
- Red blood cell transfusions may be required.

DISEASES AND DISORDERS

- Address electrolyte deficits according to the information in Table I-25.

CHRONIC TREATMENT

Slow increase in the caloric amounts until normal intake returns

POSSIBLE COMPLICATIONS

- Repair of hypokalemia and hypocalcemia in hypomagnesemic animals may depend on magnesium replacement.
- Phosphorus supplementation must be gradual to reduce the risk of renal failure and hypocalcemia.

RECOMMENDED MONITORING

- Body weight taken daily.
- Glucose and electrolyte concentrations q 4-6h until normalized, then daily during enteral or parenteral feeding.
- Hematocrit if hypophosphatemia is present.
- Renal parameters and urine output.

PROGNOSIS AND OUTCOME

Guarded to good depending on underlying problem and severity of the refeeding syndrome.

PEARLS & CONSIDERATIONS

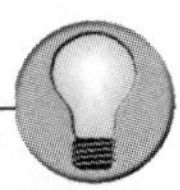

COMMENTS

- Although not common in veterinary animals, a high index of suspicion for the syndrome should be maintained in any depleted animal during the initial period (about 4 days) of refeeding.
- Refeeding syndrome can occur anytime during the first few days of nutritional support or return to food intake and may develop within hours.

PREVENTION

- Correct identified fluid and electrolyte abnormalities before instituting nutritional support.
- Use caution in return to feeding (e.g., start with 25-50% of basal energy requirements).
- Monitor electrolytes, blood gas, and renal parameters daily.
- Recognize that some replacement fluid recommendations assume normal food intake; ill and hospitalized animals often are anorexic.

SUGGESTED READING

Crook MA, et al: The importance of the refeeding syndrome. *Nutrition* 17:285, 2002.

Dibartola SP: *Fluid Therapy in Small Animal Practice*. Philadelphia, WB Saunders, 1992, p 720.

Michel KE: Preventing and managing complications of enteral nutritional support. *Clin Tech Small Anim Pract* 19:49, 2004.

AUTHOR: **ELIZABETH O'TOOLE**

EDITORS: **C. A. TONY BUFFINGTON, DEBRA L. ZORAN**

TABLE I-25 **Recommended Replacement Regimens**

	Hypokalemia	Hypophosphatemia	Hypomagnesemia
Oral (per 100 kcal/day)	2-4 mEq potassium gluconate	100 mg potassium phosphate	5-10 mg magnesium gluconate (not compatible with enteral diets)
IV (amount per kg BW per 24h), as constant rate infusion—never bolus	≤ 12 mEq potassium chloride	0.7-3 mmol potassium phosphate	125 mg magnesium sulfate

Reflex Dyssynergia

BASIC INFORMATION

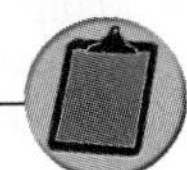

DEFINITION

Upper motor neuron (UMN) dysfunction preventing the bladder and urethra from acting in a coordinated manner during micturition. Sacral spinal cord lesions, diseases associated with the urethra, and an idiopathic condition can each mimic reflex dyssynergia.

SYNONYM(S)

Detrusor-sphincter dyssynergia
Detrusor-sphincter incoordination
Functional urethral obstruction
UMN bladder

EPIDEMIOLOGY

SPECIES, AGE, SEX: Affects dogs and cats of any age depending on causation; an idiopathic dyssynergia-like condition affects predominantly large-breed male dogs.

RISK FACTORS

- Thoracolumbar spinal cord injury/disease
- Dyssynergia-like condition:
  - Following relief of urethral obstruction
  - Sacral spinal cord injury/disease

ASSOCIATED CONDITIONS AND DISORDERS

- Bladder atony/hypotonia
- Urinary tract infection

CLINICAL PRESENTATION

DISEASE FORMS/SUBTYPES

- True reflex dyssynergia: neurogenic suprasacral lesions.
- Dyssynergia-like conditions: neurogenic and non-neurogenic disorders.

HISTORY, CHIEF COMPLAINT

- Frequent attempts at voiding with inability to empty bladder completely.
- Normal initiation of voiding with interruption of urine stream; short spurts of urine followed by cessation of urine flow.
- Animal may strain with no urine produced.

PHYSICAL EXAM FINDINGS

- Bladder expression difficult.
- Clinicians should palpate the bladder before and after voiding: turgid, incomplete emptying of bladder, increased residual urine volume.
- Manual bladder expression in these patients may be difficult.
- Perineal reflex is present or exaggerated.
- Neurologic dysfunction unrelated to urination may be present.
- Rectal and vaginal examinations are indicated to assess structural causes (e.g., sacral vertebral lesion) versus other causes of dysuria (e.g., urethral lith or mass). Anal tone is normal/good.
- Observation of urination: thin, interrupted urine stream.

ETIOLOGY AND PATHOPHYSIOLOGY

- Disordered urinary retention resulting from central nervous system (CNS) lesion located between the pontine micturition center and the sacral spinal cord (suprasacral spinal cord: L7 to brainstem).
- UMN lesion causes a loss of inhibitory pathways (Fig. I-146):

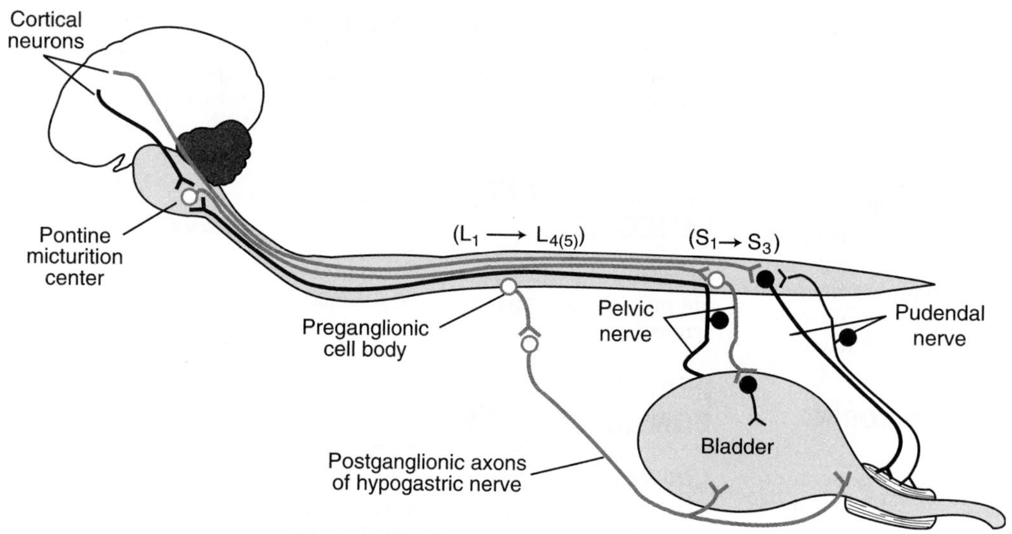

FIGURE I-146 Neurologic pathways to and from the urinary bladder.

- To sympathetic innervation of the internal urethral sphincter (smooth muscle).
- To somatic innervation (pudendal nerve) of the external urethral sphincter (striated muscle).

- Additional factors include increased sensory input (sacral nerves), increased sympathetic output, and bladder neck hypertrophy.
- Neurogenic dyssynergia-like conditions occur when pelvic nerve damage results in weakened detrusor contraction that cannot override urethral sphincter tone.
- In animals with non-neurogenic dyssynergia-like conditions, there is a similar failure of simultaneous relaxation of the internal or external urethral sphincter with detrusor contraction. This may be idiopathic or may follow irritation/disease of the urethra.

DIAGNOSIS

DIFFERENTIAL DIAGNOSIS

- Anatomic urethral obstruction:
  - Intraluminal (e.g., urethral plug/lith, transitional cell carcinoma, urethritis)
  - Extraluminal (e.g., prostatomegaly, pelvic granuloma)
- Functional urethral obstruction (dyssynergia-like conditions):
  - Neurogenic:
    - Sacral spinal cord disease
    - Pelvic plexus injury
    - Cauda equina disease
  - Non-neurogenic:
    - Idiopathic
    - Following relief of urethral obstruction
    - Secondary urinary tract infection
    - Bladder neck obstruction
    - α-Adrenergic agonist administration (e.g., phenylpropanolamine, pseudoephedrine)
    - Myopathic disease
- Bladder wall atony (see Atonic or Hypotonic Urinary Bladder, p 94)

INITIAL DATABASE

- Urethral catheterization: unobstructed. Residual urine volume increased (normal, 0.2–0.4 ml/kg in dogs).
- Rectal examination: good anal tone, no pelvic/urethral mass.
- Neurologic examination, including perineal and bulbocavernosus reflexes:
  - Neuroanatomic lesion localization: spinal cord, usually T3–L3.
- Clinical pathologic examination:
  - Complete bood count (CBC) and serum biochemistry: unremarkable.
  - Urinalysis and urine culture: secondary urinary tract infection common.
- Caudal abdominal and pelvic radiographs, abdominal ultrasound: no urethral obstruction or mass, possible vertebral injury/disease.

ADVANCED OR CONFIRMATORY TESTING

- Contrast urethrography: rule out urethral obstruction.
- Neurodiagnostic procedures: confirm lesion localization, extent of lesion, and suspected cause:
  - Myelography.
  - Epidurography.
  - Electromyography.
  - Somatosensory-evoked response testing.
  - Advanced imaging:
    - MRI
    - CT scan
- Urodynamic procedures:
  - Cystometry: assess bladder function.
  - Urethral pressure profile: assess urethral tone, which is the only means to confirm idiopathic dyssynergia-like condition.
  - Leak point pressure measurement: assess urethral resistance.

TREATMENT

THERAPEUTIC GOAL(S)

- Treat underlying cause.
- Provide supportive therapy: urethral relaxation and detrusor muscle contraction.
- Maintain empty bladder to avoid bladder atony/hypotonia (see Atonic or Hypotonic Urinary Bladder, p 94).

ACUTE GENERAL TREATMENT

- Indwelling urinary catheter (closed-collection system).
- Urethral sphincter relaxation (see Atonic or Hypotonic Urinary Bladder, p 94).
  - Smooth muscle relaxation (α-antagonists):
    - Phenoxybenzamine (dogs: 0.25 mg/kg PO q 8–12h; cats: 1.25–5 mg/cat PO q 12h). Onset of action is delayed up to 4 days. Possible side effects: hypotension, tachycardia, and increased intraocular pressure. Contraindications: cardiovascular disease, glaucoma, and renal failure.
    - Prazosin (dogs: 1 mg/15 kg PO q 8–12h; cats 0.25–0.5 mg/cat PO q 12–24h). Possible side effects: hypotension and mild sedation; contraindications (see phenoxybenzamine above).

- Striated muscle relaxation (skeletal muscle relaxants):
  - Diazepam (dogs: 2-10 mg PO q 8h; cats: 2-5 mg PO q 8h, or 0.2-0.5 mg/kg IV, as needed). Possible side effects: sedation, excitation, and idiosyncratic hepatic necrosis in cats.
  - Methocarbamol (dogs: 15-20 mg/kg PO q 8h; cats: 61-132 mg/kg per day PO, divided q 8-12h). Possible side effects: weakness, sedation, and vomiting.
- May add drugs to stimulate detrusor muscle contraction (see Atonic or Hypotonic Urinary Bladder, p 94).
  - Bethanechol (parasympathomimetic): (dogs: 5-25 mg PO q 8h; cats: 1.25-5 mg PO q 8h). Possible side effects: ptyalism, vomiting, diarrhea, and bronchoconstriction; contraindications: urinary or gastrointestinal (GI) obstruction.
  - Cisapride (prokinetic; enhances acetylcholine release): (dogs: 0.5 mg/kg PO q 8h; cats: 1.25-5 mg/cat PO q 8-12h). Possible side effects: diarrhea and abdominal pain.

CHRONIC TREATMENT

- Resolution of underlying disorder.
- Intermittent bladder catheterization or manual bladder expression.
  - Complete emptying with manual expression may take several attempts; allow the animal to relax between attempts.
- Long-term drug therapy.
- Address secondary urinary infection.

DRUG INTERACTIONS

Start treatment with an α-antagonist (e.g., phenoxybenzamine) at least 3 days prior to bethanechol; bethanechol may enhance urethral sphincter tone (has nonspecific cholinergic effects on the caudal mesenteric ganglia, causing further stimulation to the hypogastric nerve).

RECOMMENDED MONITORING

- Observe voiding activity daily.
- Monitor residual urine volume.
- Perform a periodic urine culture/urinalysis after removal of indwelling catheter and at least every 3 months until condition has resolved.

PROGNOSIS AND OUTCOME

- Good prognosis with resolution of underlying disease but may require weeks to resolve.
- Good prognosis for resolution of dyssynergia-like conditions when underlying cause eliminated (e.g., urethral inflammation).
- Fair prognosis for medical control of idiopathic dyssynergia-like condition.

PEARLS & CONSIDERATIONS

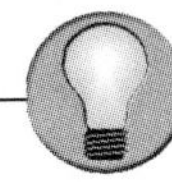

COMMENTS

- Reflex dyssynergia is a common sequela of severe spinal cord injury.
- If prolonged recovery from the spinal cord injury is expected, initiate phenoxybenzamine early (3 to 5 days from initial onset of action).

PREVENTION

Successful management depends on identification and treatment of underlying disorder.

CLIENT EDUCATION

- Manual bladder expression or intermittent catheterization may be required.
- Watch for signs of urinary tract infection (e.g., change in color or odor).

SUGGESTED READING

Barsanti JA, et al: Detrusor-sphincter dyssynergia. *Vet Clin N Am: Sm Anim Pract*, 26:327, 1996.

Fischer JR, Lane IF: Medical treatment of voiding dysfunction in dogs and cats. *Vet Med* 98:67, 2003.

Lane IF: A diagnostic approach to micturition disorders. *Vet Med* 98:49, 2003.

AUTHOR: **JOAN R. COATES**
EDITOR: **LEAH A. COHN**

Regurgitation

BASIC INFORMATION

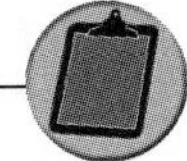

DEFINITION

The passive, retrograde expulsion of food and/or fluid from the esophagus or pharynx into the oral and/or nasal cavities

EPIDEMIOLOGY

SPECIES, AGE, SEX: Congenital causes may cause clinical signs as early as weaning; acquired forms usually in young to middle-aged animals.

GENETICS AND BREED PREDISPOSITION

- Dogs:
  - Wire-haired fox terriers and miniature schnauzers: hereditary megaesophagus.
  - German shepherd, Newfoundland, Great Dane, Irish setter, and shar-pei: familial megaesophagus.
  - German shepherd and Irish setter: vascular ring anomalies.
  - German shepherd: gastroesophageal intussusception.
  - German shepherd, Jack Russell terrier, springer spaniel, Labrador retriever, and Scottish terrier: myasthenia gravis.
  - Shar-pei: hiatal hernia.
  - Medium- to large-breed dogs: hypothyroidism; link to megaesophagus remains anecdotal.
  - Great Dane, rottweiler, standard poodle, and West Highland white terrier (hypoadrenocorticism).
- Cats: Siamese (familial megaesophagus); long-haired breeds (hairballs).

ASSOCIATED CONDITIONS AND DISORDERS: Aspiration pneumonia (most common and serious complication of megaesophagus), rhinitis, esophageal strictures.

CLINICAL PRESENTATION

DISEASE FORMS/SUBTYPES

- Esophageal
- Pharyngeal

HISTORY, CHIEF COMPLAINT

- "Vomiting" is commonly reported by owners of animals that are regurgitating; accordingly, clinicians should question owners about what the animal does when food is ejected from the mouth (more details in Differential Diagnosis below).
- Coughing.
- Dyspnea.
- Weakness.
- Weight loss.

PHYSICAL EXAM FINDINGS: Findings are variable:

- Emaciation
- Weakness
- Esophageal bulge (pressure on abdomen, close nostrils)
- Fever
- Respiratory signs
- Abnormal neurologic examination

ETIOLOGY AND PATHOPHYSIOLOGY

- Regurgitation indicates esophageal or pharyngeal dysfunction due to mechanical obstructive disease or functional (motility) abnormalities such as megaesophagus.

- Esophageal disease:
  - Megaesophagus: primary (idiopathic) or secondary
  - Esophagitis
  - Esophageal obstruction/foreign body
  - Esophageal mass (e.g., *Spirocerca lupi*)
  - Esophageal diverticulum
  - Esophageal stricture/stenosis
  - Vascular ring anomaly
  - Other motility disorder
  - Thoracic neoplasia (e.g., thymoma)
- Pharyngeal disease:
  - Pharyngeal obstruction
- Other alimentary tract disease:
  - Gastroesophageal intussusception
  - Pyloric outflow obstruction
  - Hiatal hernia
- Neuromuscular disease:
  - Myasthenia gravis
  - Botulism
  - Tetanus
  - Anticholinesterase activity (e.g., organophosphate toxicity)
  - Dysautonomia
  - Polyradiculoneuritis
- Immune-mediated:
  - Systemic lupus erythematosus
  - Polymyositis
- Endocrine:
  - Hypothyroidism (speculative)
  - Hypoadrenocorticism

DIAGNOSIS

DIFFERENTIAL DIAGNOSIS

- It is essential to distinguish regurgitation from vomition, since the underlying causes, treatment approaches, and outcomes are generally very different.
- Regurgitation: passive (usually); undigested food (covered by mucus or saliva); sausage shaped; neutral pH; immediately postprandial or delayed (hours). Forceful abdominal compressions leading to ejection of food from the mouth suggest vomiting (see Vomiting, Acute, p 1157; Vomiting, Chronic, p 1158) rather than regurgitation.

INITIAL DATABASE

- Usually normal.
- Complete blood count (CBC): Aspiration pneumonia may occasionally cause leukocytosis.
- Serum chemistry: Some metabolic diseases can result in esophageal dysfunction (i.e., electrolyte imbalance with hypoadrenocorticism).
- Thoracic, pharyngeal, and cervical radiographs: megaesophagus, vascular ring anomaly, foreign bodies, and other such findings.
- Contrast radiography/esophagram.

ADVANCED OR CONFIRMATORY TESTING

- Fluoroscopy.
- Esophagoscopy.
- Esophageal manometry.
- Radiographic scintigraphy to measure transit time.
- Thyroid-stimulating hormone (TSH) test and free t4 test: hypothyroidism.
- Adrenocorticotropic hormone (ACTH) stimulation test: hypoadrenocorticism.
- Antinuclear antibody test: immune-mediated causes.
- Acetylcholine (ACh) receptor antibody test: myasthenia gravis.
- Bioassay techniques: botulism and tetanus.

TREATMENT

THERAPEUTIC GOAL(S)

Successful treatment requires elimination of the underlying cause.

ACUTE GENERAL TREATMENT

- Aspiration pneumonia: appropriate antibiotic therapy and supportive care.
- For esophageal disease other than idiopathic megaesophagus: treat and correct disease (i.e., surgery for removal of foreign bodies).
- For systemic causes of regurgitation: treat underlying disease.

CHRONIC TREATMENT

- Megaesophagus: feed the animal from an upright position and maintain position for another 10 minutes postprandially.
- Individualize the consistency of the diet for each animal.
- Limit activity after feeding.
- Bypass the esophagus with a gastrostomy tube if necessary.
- Motility-modifying drugs are controversial in treating megaesophagus because their efficacy is unproven; increasing lower esophageal tone could hinder the transit of food from esophagus to stomach:
  - Metoclopramide (0.2–0.5 mg/kg PO q 8h or q 12h) increases the lower esophageal sphincter pressure and gastric emptying and reduces gastroesophageal reflux.
  - Cisapride (0.5 mg/kg q 8h or q 12h) increases lower esophageal peristalsis and sphincter pressure (cats > dogs) and accelerates gastric emptying. This drug can be difficult to obtain.

POSSIBLE COMPLICATIONS

- Aspiration pneumonia
- Esophageal rupture due to foreign bodies
- Esophageal stricture formation
- Esophageal reflux

RECOMMENDED MONITORING

- Check for resolution of clinical signs for animals whose causes were systemic.
- Regularly check thoracic radiographs for signs of aspiration pneumonia.

PROGNOSIS AND OUTCOME

Depend greatly on the cause of the regurgitation and presence or absence of complications

PEARLS & CONSIDERATIONS

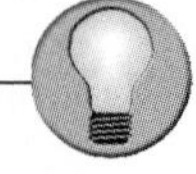

COMMENTS

- Clinicians should make sure the animal is regurgitating and not vomiting.
- Aspiration pneumonia often does not increase the white blood cell (WBC) count, even if extensive.

CLIENT EDUCATION

The owner should be aware of the clinical signs of aspiration pneumonia and seek immediate veterinary attention if they occur.

SUGGESTED READING

Guilford WG, Strombeck DR: Diseases of swallowing. In Strombeck DR (ed): *Strombeck's Small Animal Gastroenterology*. Philadelphia, WB Saunders, 1996, pp 211–238.

Jenkins CC: Dysphagia and regurgitation. In Ettinger SJ (ed): *Textbook of Veterinary Internal Medicine*. Philadelphia, WB Saunders, 2000, pp 114–117.

AUTHOR: **NINETTE KELLER**
EDITOR: **ETIENNE CÔTÉ**

Renal Dysplasia

BASIC INFORMATION

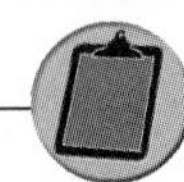

DEFINITION

Disorganized renal development resulting from arrested or anomalous cellular processes

SYNONYM(S)

Familial renal disease
Progressive juvenile nephropathy

EPIDEMIOLOGY

SPECIES, AGE, SEX: Dogs (rarely, cats) of either gender; onset of signs ranges from weeks to years of age, with most animals developing signs prior to 2 years.

GENETICS AND BREED PREDISPOSITION: Familial; reported in a number of common breeds (e.g., golden retriever, cocker spaniel, Lhasa apso, shih tzu) and less common breeds (e.g., Dutch kooiker, Finnish harrier, soft-coated wheaten terrier).

RISK FACTORS: *In-utero* viral infection (e.g., canine herpesvirus, feline panleukopenia).

ASSOCIATED CONDITIONS AND DISORDERS

- Chronic renal failure (CRF)
- Stunted growth
- Renal (fibrous) osteodystrophy
- Systemic hypertension

CLINICAL PRESENTATION

DISEASE FORMS/SUBTYPES

- Familial
- Nonfamilial

HISTORY, CHIEF COMPLAINT: Clinical signs may be absent. When present, abnormalities may include:

- Anestrus
- Anorexia/wasting
- Bone pain
- Depression/lethargy
- Hematuria
- Polyuria and polydipsia (PU/PD)
- Poor wound healing
- Stunted growth
- Vomiting/diarrhea

PHYSICAL EXAM FINDINGS: Physical examination may be unremarkable, but abnormalities can include:

- Calcinosis circumscripta
- Dehydration
- Enlarged mandible/maxillae
- Muscular twitching
- Oral ulceration/halitosis
- Pallor
- Pathologic fracture
- Pliable mandible ("rubber jaw")
- Poor haircoat
- Small kidneys on abdominal palpation
- Small stature/poor body condition

ETIOLOGY AND PATHOPHYSIOLOGY

- The microscopic appearance of kidneys should be mature by 70 days of age (some development and histologic change normally continues during the first 2 months of life). Disorganized parenchymal development with immature or anomalous structures characterizes renal dysplasia with histologic features inappropriate for the animal's age.
- Poorly developed kidneys result in renal failure and eventual death.
- Diminished renal conversion of vitamin D to the active form calcitriol contributes to secondary hyperparathyroidism and subsequent renal osteodystrophy. This complication is more pronounced in juvenile renal disease.

DIAGNOSIS

DIFFERENTIAL DIAGNOSIS

Azotemia:

- Prerenal (e.g., dehydration, hypoadrenocorticism)
- Renal (e.g., acute renal failure or CRF of any cause)
- Postrenal (e.g., urinary obstruction, urinary tract rupture)

INITIAL DATABASE

- Blood pressure (BP) (see Systemic Hypertension, p 1058; Blood Pressure Measurement, p 1191).
- Complete blood count (CBC):
  - Nonregenerative anemia
- Serum biochemical profile:
  - Azotemia
  - Hyperphosphatemia
  - Hypokalemia
  - Hypercalcemia/hypocalcemia
  - Metabolic acidosis
  - Hypercholesterolemia
  - Hypoalbuminemia
- Urinalysis: isosthenuric or minimally concentrated urine, variable hematuria, proteinuria, glucosuria.
- Urine culture and sensitivity (C&S).
- Abdominal radiography:
  - Small kidneys
  - Poor abdominal detail (young age, poor body condition)
  - Soft-tissue mineralization
- Ultrasonography:
  - Small, irregularly shaped kidneys
  - Thin renal cortex
  - Hyperechoic renal parenchyma
  - Poor corticomedullary distinction
  - Soft-tissue mineralization

ADVANCED OR CONFIRMATORY TESTING

- Serum parathyroid hormone (PTH) concentration: initially normal, then rises. Intention is to delay/prevent this rise using calcitriol therapy.
- Serum ionized calcium: to confirm biologically significant hypercalcemia; may be normal initially and then may increase as PTH concentration rises.
- Assessment of glomerular filtration rate: may have a role in evaluating nonazotemic animals suspected of having renal dysplasia.
- Renal histopathologic examination: required to confirm diagnosis.
  - Asynchronous nephron development
  - Immature glomeruli and/or tubules
  - Persistent fetal mesenchyme
  - Persistent metanephric ducts
  - Atypical tubular epithelium
  - Dysontogenetic metaplasia

TREATMENT

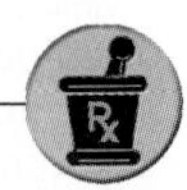

THERAPEUTIC GOAL(S)

- Maintain normal hydration, electrolyte, and acid-base status
- Delay progression of renal failure and its complications
- Address uremic signs
- Minimize proteinuria

ACUTE GENERAL TREATMENT

Acute treatment will address uremia, dehydration, electrolyte, and acid-base disorders (see Chronic Renal Failure, Occult ("Asymptomatic"), p 204; Chronic Renal Failure, Overt ["Symptomatic"], p 205).

CHRONIC TREATMENT

- See Chronic Renal Failure, Occult ("Asymptomatic"), p 204; Chronic Renal Failure, Overt ["Symptomatic"], p 205; Protein-Losing Nephropathy, p 900; Renal Secondary Hyperparathyroidism, p 956.
- Vomiting: Address vomiting promptly (or dehydration may lead to rapid deterioration of renal function). For example, barring evidence of gastrointestinal (GI) obstruction, clinicians can administer metoclopramide 0.2-0.5 mg/kg SC or IM q 8h or ondansetron 0.1-0.2 mg/kg IV q 12h. Provide crystalloid fluid therapy as needed to prevent dehydration.
- Bone pain (renal osteodystrophy): opioids (e.g., full mu agonists [e.g., oxymorphone 0.03-0.2 mg/kg SC, IM, or IV; fentanyl (patch)] or buprenorphine 0.01-0.02 mg/kg SC, IM, or IV, q 6-8h).

Avoid administering nonsteroidal anti-inflammatory drugs (NSAIDs), which have potentially negative renal effects.
- Early calcitriol therapy may delay or prevent bone changes and should be considered before hyperphosphatemia occurs:
  - Initial dose 1.65–3.63 ng/kg (= 0.00165–0.00363 µg/kg) PO q 24h (dogs and cats); dose is adjusted based primarily on serum calcium and phosphorus concentrations (± PTH concentrations).
  - Maintain Ca (mg/dl) × P (mg/dl) product of <70; avoid hypercalcemia; if total calcium elevated, confirm with ionized calcium.
  - Ideally, PTH should be within reference range during treatment. If low, dose is decreased; if high, dose is increased.
  - Calcitriol loses efficacy when phosphorus >8 mg/dl. Typically, calcitriol is used in conjunction with a phosphorus-reducing diet and noncalcium-containing phosphate binders.

DRUG INTERACTIONS

- Vascular calcium channel blockers (amlodipine) and angiotensin-converting enzyme (ACE) inhibitors used concurrently may produce hypotension.
- Phosphate binders can interfere with absorption of orally administered medications.
- To optimize effects of sucralfate, administer it at least 30 minutes prior to acid-reduction therapy.
- Concurrent use of calcitriol and calcium-containing phosphate binders, thiazide diuretic, corticosteroids, and barbiturates should be avoided.

POSSIBLE COMPLICATIONS

- Hypotension may result from use of a calcium channel blocker and/or ACE inhibitors.
- Calcitriol may lead to hypercalcemia and/or ectopic mineralization of tissues.

RECOMMENDED MONITORING

- Monitor calcium and phosphorus levels 2 weeks after beginning calcitriol therapy and at least monthly thereafter for adjusting dosages. Ideally, measure PTH levels prior to and 1 to 2 months after therapy has started.
- The clinician is advised to monitor the animal as he/she would other animals with CRF (see Chronic Renal Failure, Overt ["Symptomatic"], p 205); monitoring includes complete physical examination; measurement of BP; serum biochemistry profiles and blood gas determinations to assess azotemia, electrolyte, and acid-base status; and monitoring for clinical signs suggesting urinary tract infection.

PROGNOSIS AND OUTCOME

- Depends on degree of dysplasia, age at onset of signs, severity of dysfunction at diagnosis, and subsequent treatment.
- It is an irreversible condition; long-term prognosis is poor.

PEARLS & CONSIDERATIONS

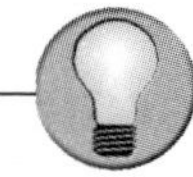

COMMENTS

- Renal dysplasia can occur in any breed of dog or cat.
- There is no specific therapy, but animals are managed as for CRF and its complications.

PREVENTION

- Do not breed affected dogs.
- Inform owners of appropriate vaccination of cats against panleukopenia.

CLIENT EDUCATION

Owners should research breed-associated diseases prior to considering adoption or purchase.

SUGGESTED READING

Greco DS: Congenital and inherited renal disease of small animals. *Vet Clin North Am: Small Anim Pract* 31:393, 2001.

Osborne CA, Finco DR: *Canine and Feline Nephrology and Urology*. Baltimore, Williams & Wilkins, 1995, pp 474–482.

AUTHORS: **ADAM MORDECAI, RANCE K. SELLON**

EDITOR: **LEAH A. COHN**

Renal Neoplasia

BASIC INFORMATION

DEFINITION

Neoplasms arising in the kidney parenchyma of epithelial (carcinoma), mesothelial (sarcoma), or mixed embryonic (nephroblastoma) origin

SYNONYM(S)

Wilms' tumor (nephroblastoma)

EPIDEMIOLOGY

SPECIES, AGE, SEX

- Dogs: older adults; nephroblastomas reported in young dogs.
- Cats: older adults, but young cats may develop feline leukemia (FeLV)-related lymphoma.

GENETICS AND BREED PREDISPOSITION: Nodular dermatofibrosis associated with multiple renal cystadenocarcinomas in German shepherds.

RISK FACTORS

- Dogs: male predominance.
- Cats: FeLV infection associated with renal lymphoma.

CONTAGION AND ZOONOSIS: Cats: FeLV (cat-to-cat).

ASSOCIATED DISEASES AND CONDITIONS: Paraneoplastic polycythemia; nodular dermatofibrosis with renal cystadenocarcinoma.

CLINICAL PRESENTATION

DISEASE FORMS/SUBTYPES

- Primary renal tumors are associated with minimal clinical signs until advanced stage.
- Renal lymphoma in cats may disseminate to the central nervous system (CNS).

HISTORY, CHIEF COMPLAINT (SOME OR ALL MAY BE PRESENT)

- Lethargy
- Hematuria
- Polyuria and polydipsia (PU/PD)
- Inappetence
- Weight loss
- Behavior changes
- Acute collapse
- Abdominal distention
- Flank pain

PHYSICAL EXAM FINDINGS (SOME OR ALL MAY BE PRESENT)

- Nephromegaly
- Abdominal mass
- Pale mucous membranes
- Abdominal distention with fluid wave
- Shock (if actively bleeding)

ETIOLOGY AND PATHOPHYSIOLOGY

- Lymphoma:
  - May occur spontaneously (dogs and cats) or be associated with FeLV (cats)
- Carcinoma:
  - Transitional cell carcinoma, renal cell carcinoma, or adenocarcinoma with tubular or papillary differentiation

- Mass in renal parenchyma leads to hematuria and proteinuria
- Pyuria common; may be secondary to inflammation from tumor or bacterial infection
- Anemia secondary to blood loss (with hypoalbuminemia) or diminished erythropoietin production
- Polycythemia (rare) due to erythropoietin or erythropoietin-like secretion
- Metastasis common (48% at diagnosis)
- Unilateral or bilateral

- Sarcoma:
  - Hemangiosarcoma, fibrosarcoma, renal sarcoma, and spindle-cell sarcomas reported
  - May be metastatic from other site
  - Hematuria common
  - Hypoalbuminemia less common
  - Polycythemia (rare)
  - Flank pain more common
  - Metastasis common
- Nephroblastoma:
  - Anemia
  - Associated with young, but reported in older, dogs
  - Metastasis common
- Benign tumors:
  - Hemangioma most common (dogs)
  - Renal adenomas and leiomyomas most common (cats)

DIAGNOSIS

DIFFERENTIAL DIAGNOSIS

- Physical exam:
  - Abdominal mass ± pain ± ascites:
    - Urinary tract infection, urolithiasis, bladder tumor
    - Mass in spleen, mesenteric lymph node, or retroperitoneal space
    - Ruptured splenic or hepatic mass with hemoperitoneum
    - Abdominal trauma or coagulopathy with peritoneal or retroperitoneal bleeding
    - Renal cysts, perirenal pseudocysts
    - Hydronephrosis
  - Abdominal pain without mass:
    - Pyelonephritis
    - Ethylene glycol ingestion
- Radiographic:
  - Mass in spleen, mesenteric lymph node, or retroperitoneal space
  - Ruptured splenic or hepatic mass with hemoperitoneum
  - Retroperitoneal fluid—blood or urine
  - Renal cyst, perirenal pseudocyst, hydronephrosis
- Ultrasonographic:
  - Renal abscess or granulomas
  - Metastatic neoplasia
- Urinalysis:
  - Urinary tract infection
  - Urolithiasis
  - Ureteral or bladder tumor
  - Idiopathic renal hematuria

INITIAL DATABASE

- Complete blood count (CBC), serum biochemistry profile, urinalysis: anemia or polycythemia, thrombocytopenia, azotemia (prerenal and renal), hypoalbuminemia, proteinuria, hematuria.
- Abdominal radiographs: mass, possibly peritoneal or retroperitoneal fluid.
- Thoracic radiographs: metastasis (up to 48% at diagnosis).
- Abdominal ultrasound: renal mass and possibly metastasis to any abdominal organ including adrenal gland and vena cava.
- Prothrombin time and partial thromboplastin time if suspect disseminated intravascular coagulation.

ADVANCED OR CONFIRMATORY TESTING

- Cytology or biopsy necessary for diagnosis.
- Renal scintigraphy or excretory urogram to assess functional renal mass.
- Veterinary bladder tumor antigen test (V-BTA, Alidex Inc., Redmond, WA) may detect renal pelvic transitional cell carcinoma.
- Echocardiogram if hemangiosarcoma to rule out cardiac mass.
- Cerebrospinal fluid tap and bone marrow aspirate if lymphoma to stage disease.

TREATMENT

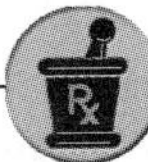

THERAPEUTIC GOAL(S)

- Remove bleeding mass
- Resect primary tumor entirely
- Alleviate clinical signs

ACUTE, GENERAL TREATMENT

- Stabilize with crystalloids, colloids, and oxygen-carrying capacity (oxyglobin or blood products).
- Address renal insufficiency with fluid diuresis.
- Surgically remove bleeding mass.
- Begin chemotherapy with caution in lymphoma. Special handling requirements and potentially severe or life-threatening adverse patient effects exist with many of these chemotherapeutic drugs; these concerns, and rapid evolution of protocols, warrant consultation with/referral to an oncologist.
- COAP chemotherapy protocol for renal lymphoma:
  - L-asparaginase 10,000 U/m^2 IM once on day 1.
  - Cytosine arabinoside 50 mg/m^2 SQ q 12h × 3 days for first week starting day 1.
  - Vincristine 0.5 mg/m^2 IV q 7d starting day 1.
  - Cyclophosphamide 50 mg/m^2 PO q 24h for 4 days each week starting on day 1 if no evidence of cystitis.
  - Prednisone 2 mg/kg PO q 24h for 7 days, then 1 mg/kg PO q 24h thereafter.
- Alleviate pain with opioids.

CHRONIC TREATMENT

- Lymphoma:
  - If remission achieved with COAP protocol, after 6 weeks discontinue multidrug protocol and administer doxorubicin IV at 30 mg/m^2 for dogs >30 kg, or 1mg/kg for dog <30 kg and cats, q 3 weeks.
- Others:
  - No prospective clinical trials exist.
  - Most literature reports are based on doxorubicin or actinomycin-D.
  - Anecdotal reports of response to carboplatin for carcinomas.
  - Carcinomas may express COX-2, which may imply a response to piroxicam 0.3 mg/kg PO q 24h (avoid if azotemia).

DRUG INTERACTIONS

Avoid combining drugs with similar toxicity profiles such as cisplatin and piroxicam.

POSSIBLE COMPLICATIONS

Neutropenia, thrombocytopenia, sepsis, and renal injury secondary to chemotherapy

RECOMMENDED MONITORING

- Monitor CBC prior to every chemotherapy treatment and 7 to 10 days later.
- Monitor blood urea nitrogen, creatinine, and urine specific gravity for renal function.

PROGNOSIS AND OUTCOME

- Benign: good.
- Lymphoma: guarded to poor.
  - Sixty percent remission rate; median duration 4 months (cats).
- Carcinomas: guarded to poor.
  - Reported survivals generally short unless tumor completely resected.
  - Rare survivals >1 year.
- Sarcomas: guarded to poor.
  - Reportedly more aggressive than carcinomas.
- Nephroblastomas: guarded to poor.
  - Rare reports of long survivals.
- Metastatic potential of all tumors is high.
  - Lymphoma metastasis to CNS is lower with cytosine arabinoside in chemotherapy protocol.

- ◦ Chemotherapy effect on metastasis of carcinomas, sarcomas, nephroblastomas unevaluated.

PEARLS & CONSIDERATIONS

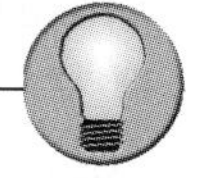

COMMENTS

- Hematuria in the absence of clinical signs warrants an evaluation for renal neoplasia.
- Early detection is critical for successful treatment.
- Definitive diagnosis is necessary for prognosis and therapeutic decisions.
- Complete resection offers best chances for long survival.
- When present, polycythemia usually resolves with nephrectomy.

CLIENT EDUCATION

- Nephrectomy may be palliative and maximize quality of remaining life.
- Signs are subtle and nonspecific, so advanced diagnostics and imaging are most useful early.

SUGGESTED READING

Henry CJ, et al: Primary renal tumours in cats: 19 cases (1992–1998). *J Feline Med Surg* 1:165, 1999.

Klein MK, et al: Canine primary renal neoplasms: A retrospective review of 54 cases. *J Am Anim Hosp* Assoc 24:443, 1987.

Lucke VM, et al: Renal carcinoma in the dog. *Vet Pathol* 13:264, 1976.

AUTHOR: **JEFFREY N. BRYAN**
EDITOR: **LEAH A. COHN**

Renal Secondary Hyperparathyroidism

BASIC INFORMATION

DEFINITION

Renal secondary hyperparathyroidism (RSHP) results from the effects of excessive production of parathyroid hormone (PTH) in animals with chronic kidney/renal failure (CRF).

EPIDEMIOLOGY

SPECIES, AGE, SEX: Any animal with CRF.
RISK FACTORS: CRF.
ASSOCIATED CONDITIONS AND DISORDERS: Hyperphosphatemia, hypocalcemia, and CRF.

CLINICAL PRESENTATION

HISTORY, CHIEF COMPLAINT: History of CRF; chief complaint is usually associated with exacerbation of signs of CRF (see Chronic Renal Failure, Occult ["Asymptomatic"], p 204; Chronic Renal Failure, Overt ["Symptomatic"], p 205).
PHYSICAL EXAM FINDINGS: Variable combinations of signs of CRF (see History, Chief Complaint and relevant cross-references [above]). In cats, parathyroid gland enlargement must be differentiated from thyroid gland enlargement associated with hyperthyroidism. Skull and jaw lesions ("rubber jaw") occasionally occur in growing dogs with RSHP.

ETIOLOGY AND PATHOPHYSIOLOGY

- Declining kidney function increases phosphorus retention, which leads to increased PTH.
  - ◦ Increased circulating phosphorus inhibits renal synthesis of calcitriol, the active form of vitamin D, removing calcitriol-mediated inhibition of PTH synthesis.
- PTH stimulates calcitriol synthesis, which proceeds at the cost of increased PTH.
- Progressive decline in calcitriol synthetic capacity and circulating concentrations reduces calcium (Ca) entry into the circulation from bone and intestine, decreasing serum ionized calcium (Ca_i) concentrations. Excessive PTH rarely results in hypercalcemia (tertiary hyperparathyroidism).

DIAGNOSIS

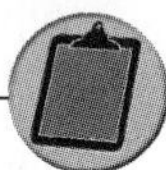

DIFFERENTIAL DIAGNOSIS

- Tertiary hyperparathyroidism
- Hypovitaminosis D

INITIAL DATABASE

- Laboratory assessment of CRF.
- Total serum Ca: usually normal to low, occasionally slightly high; serum Ca_i is more reliable and often does not parallel serum total Ca.

ADVANCED OR CONFIRMATORY TESTING

- Measure serum PTH concentration using the two-site method for intact PTH; contact a veterinary laboratory for sample collection, preparation, and submission instructions (can degrade during transport if not chilled). Increased PTH can occur within normal range (usually upper half) in early phases of CRF.
- Measure Ca_i with PTH to determine the appropriateness of the response.
- Radiography may reveal diffuse bone demineralization. Pathologic fractures are rare. The earliest lesion in facial bones of young growing animals is lamina dura dentes demineralization, seen using high-definition dental technique.
- High-frequency ultrasonography of the neck will reveal parathyroid gland enlargement.

TREATMENT

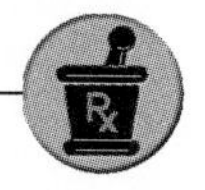

THERAPEUTIC GOAL(S)

- Reduce dietary phosphorus intake.
- Encourage binding of phosphorus in intestine.
- Increase endogenous synthesis of calcitriol.
- Decrease PTH levels.
- Provide exogenous calcitriol.
- Try to reduce the rate of CRF progression.

ACUTE GENERAL TREATMENT

Reduce the animal's phosphorus intake by providing a phosphorus-restricted diet, which ranges in content from 0.4–1.6 mg P/kcal.

CHRONIC TREATMENT

- If restriction of phosphorus intake is inadequate or if phosphorus-restricted diets are refused, provide intestinal phosphorus binders with food, starting at the lowest dose and increasing the dose as necessary to control serum phosphorus at 4 mg/dl; intestinal phosphorus binding effects are greatest when the binder is given with food (increases fecal phosphorus excretion). Options include:
  - ◦ Aluminum hydroxide (30–90 mg/kg per day PO)
  - ◦ Calcium carbonate (90–150 mg/kg per day PO)
  - ◦ Calcium acetate (60–90 mg/kg per day PO)
- Aluminum- and calcium-containing binders can be used in combination to reduce the dose of each, which minimizes the risk of hypercalcemia and aluminium accumulation.
- Prescribe calcitriol (2.5–3.5 ng/kg PO q 24h) after serum P < 6 mg/dl.

- Recommend therapy for animals with CRF as appropriate (see Chronic Renal Failure, Overt ["Symptomatic"], p 205).

DRUG INTERACTIONS

Calcitriol can accentuate soft-tissue mineralization in animals with increased serum Ca_i or phosphorus.

POSSIBLE COMPLICATIONS

- Ionized hypercalcemia (>6 mg/dl in dogs; 5.5 mg/dl in cats); increased total serum Ca occurs in 10–20% of dogs and cats with CRF before treatment; Ca_i may be increased, normal, or low. Hypercalcemia is dangerous only when Ca_i is increased. When:
  - Excessive calcitriol supplementation: give twice the dose every other day or decrease the dose by 50% to decrease Ca absorbtion from the intestine.
  - Inadequate phosphorus intake (rare); increase the animal's phosphorus intake.

RECOMMENDED MONITORING

- Measure PTH and Ca_i (from the same sample) after 1, 3, and 6 months of therapy to determine initial and subsequent adequacy of RSHP control and twice yearly thereafter for stable animals.
- Modify extent of dietary phosphorus restriction, dosage, and types of intestinal phosphorus binders and changes in calcitriol dose on PTH and Ca_i results.
- Measure serum phosphorus to ensure control of hyperphosphatemia.
- Refer animals with persistently increased Ca_i for evaluation of tertiary hyperparathyroidism.
- Monitor the animal's CRF as needed.

PROGNOSIS AND OUTCOME

- Days to weeks of survival if CRF is severe.
- Months to years of survival, but guarded to poor for animals with CRF and uncontrolled RSHP.
- Worse for animals with uncontrollable hyperphosphatemia.
- Survival increases with appropriate PTH-lowering therapy.

PEARLS & CONSIDERATIONS

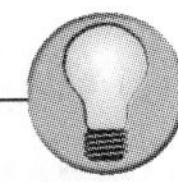

COMMENTS

- Nearly impossible to lower PTH if serum P >6 mg/dl.
- Normal ranges for serum phosphorus levels often include results from growing animals, which are much higher than for adult animals.
- The goal for serum phosphorus during CRF is ≤4 mg/dl versus the upper limit of many normal ranges for adults (<6 mg/dl).

PREVENTION

- Appropriate phosphorus restriction can control or prevent development of RSHP in early CRF.
- Calcitriol can prevent development of parathyroid gland hyperplasia in RSHP.
- Calcitriol treatment is necessary to control RSHP in more advanced CRF.

CLIENT EDUCATION

Medical progress visits will be necessary to monitor the CRF and to determine the adequacy of RSHP control.

SUGGESTED READING

Barber PJ, et al: Effect of dietary phosphate restriction on renal secondary hyperparathyroidism in the cat. *J Small Anim Pract* 40:62, 1999.

Elliott J, et al: Survival of cats with naturally occurring chronic renal failure: Effect of dietary management. *J Small Anim Pract* 41:235, 2000.

Nagode LA, et al: Benefits of calcitriol therapy and serum phosphorus control in dogs and cats with chronic renal failure. *Vet Clin North Amer* 26:1293, 1996.

AUTHOR: **DENNIS J. CHEW**

EDITOR: **C. A. TONY BUFFINGTON**

Renal Tubular Acidosis

BASIC INFORMATION

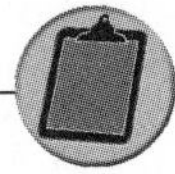

DEFINITION

Renal tubular acidosis (RTA) is a group of renal tubular disorders that result in hyperchloremic metabolic acidosis with a normal glomerular filtration rate.

- The tubular defect may result in decreased tubular resorption of HCO_3^- (proximal RTA) or defective acid secretion (distal RTA).
- Proximal RTA may be recognized along with proximal tubular resorption defects of glucose, phosphate, sodium, potassium, uric acid and amino acids as part of Fanconi syndrome (see Fanconi Syndrome, p 375).

SYNONYM(S)

Classic or type I = proximal RTA.

Type II = distal RTA.

Type IV = hypoaldosteronism or aldosterone resistance causing distal RTA (see Hypoadrenocorticism, p 561).

EPIDEMIOLOGY

SPECIES, AGE, SEX: RTA is rare in both dogs and cats. Age of onset is dependent upon etiology (inherited = 3 to 4 years of age, acquired = any age).

GENETICS AND BREED PREDISPOSITIONS: Dogs: basenjis, border terriers, Norwegian elkhounds (Fanconi syndrome).

CLINICAL PRESENTATION

HISTORY, CHIEF COMPLAINT (SOME OR ALL MAY BE PRESENT)

- Polyuria/polydipsia
- Anorexia
- Lethargy
- Weakness
- Signs consistent with urolithiasis (distal RTA)

PHYSICAL EXAM FINDINGS

- Renomegaly
- Nephrolithiasis/urolithiasis (distal RTA)
- Dehydration
- Poor haircoat
- Muscular weakness
- Bone demineralization

ETIOLOGY AND PATHOPHYSIOLOGY

Etiology

- Inherited: dogs: Fanconi syndrome (see Fanconi Syndrome, p 375).
- Acquired:
  - Any substance that can cause renal tubular toxicity; toxins (e.g., heavy metals, ethylene glycol, 4-pentenoate, maleic acid), drugs (gentamicin, cephalosporins, tetracycline, cisplatin, salicylate).
  - Neoplasia (multiple myeloma).
  - Hypoparathyroidism with concurrent hypovitaminosis D.
  - *E. coli* pyelonephritis (cats).
  - Ischemia-induced renal failure.
  - Hypoaldosteronism or aldosterone resistance (spironolactone).

Pathophysiology

- Proximal RTA:
  - Dysfunction of the proximal tubule leading to decreased bicarbonate resorption.

- ◦ Distal tubular bicarbonate resorption mechanisms are intact.
- ◦ Acidosis is less severe than in distal RTA, since the distal tubule is able to partially compensate.
- Distal RTA:
  - ◦ Impaired hydrogen ion secretion in the collecting ducts.
  - ◦ Urinary acid secretion is decreased, little change in bicarbonate resorption.
  - ◦ Nephrocalcinosis, urolithiasis, bone demineralization, and potassium wasting are possible features.

DIAGNOSIS

DIFFERENTIAL DIAGNOSIS

- *Hyperchloremic metabolic acidosis:* diarrhea, Fanconi syndrome, posthypocapnic metabolic acidosis, dilutional acidosis, hypoadrenocorticism, medications (carbonic anhydrase inhibitors, spironolactone, ammonium chloride).
- *Alkaline urine:* urinary tract infection, postprandial, dietary.

INITIAL DATABASE

- ◦ Complete blood count: typically unremarkable.
- ◦ Serum biochemistry profile: hypokalemia, hyperchloremia, normal anion gap, decreased TCO_2.
  - ◦ Hyperkalemia and hyponatremia may be seen with aldosterone deficiency or resistance.
- Urinalysis: distal RTA = pH >6, proximal RTA = pH <6.
- Urine culture: urinary tract infection with urease producing bacteria must be ruled out.
- Abdominal radiographs: rule out nephrolithiasis or urolithiasis (distal RTA).

ADVANCED OR CONFIRMATORY TESTING

- Blood gas analysis: hyperchloremic metabolic acidosis.
- Glomerular filtration rate: normal.
- Differentiation of proximal and distal RTA (important for therapeutic management):
  - ◦ Urinary fractional excretion of HCO_3^-.
    - ▪ Urine fractional excretion of HCO_3^- is measured after normalization of plasma HCO_3^- with alkali administration.
      - ▫ Normal (<5%) with distal RTA.
      - ▫ Markedly elevated (>15%) with proximal RTA.
  - ◦ Ammonium chloride tolerance test:
    - ▪ Administer 110 mg/kg ammonia chloride PO. Monitor urine pH before and q 1h for 6 hours after administration.
      - ▫ Urine pH should decrease to a minimum of 5.0 and 5.5 after ammonia chloride administration in normal dogs and cats, respectively.
      - ▫ Failure to acidify urine is consistent with distal RTA.

TREATMENT

THERAPEUTIC GOAL(S)

Resolution of acidemia (TCO_2 or HCO_3^- >12 mEq/L) and correction of hypokalemia (if present).

ACUTE AND CHRONIC TREATMENT

- Administration of a mixture of potassium and sodium citrate (1 mEq/kg to >10 mEq/kg q 24h).
- The dose and ratio of potassium to sodium citrate should be titrated to maintain plasma potassium and bicarbonate within the reference ranges, respectively.
- Generally, proximal RTA requires higher alkali dosages than distal RTA.
- Type IV: therapy for hypoaldosteronism or discontinuation of aldosterone inhibitors.

RECOMMENDED MONITORING

Blood gas analysis, urine pH, and serum potassium concentrations should be monitored regularly, with frequency of monitoring tailored according to severity of metabolic disturbance.

PROGNOSIS AND OUTCOME

- Prognosis is variable and dependent upon inciting cause and response to therapy.
- Animals with acquired RTA (especially toxin induced) may have spontaneous resolution. Others may develop progressive chronic renal failure within a few months of diagnosis.
- Animals with complex tubular disorders (i.e., Fanconi syndrome) that have progressed to the point of showing overt clinical signs generally have a poorer prognosis.

PEARLS & CONSIDERATIONS

COMMENTS

- Renal tubular acidosis is a rare condition in small animals (with the exception of basenji dogs).
- Prior to diagnosis of RTA, other more common causes of metabolic acidosis should be definitively ruled out.

SUGGESTED READING

Bartges JW: Disorders of renal tubules. In Ettinger SJ, Feldman EC (eds): *Textbook of Veterinary Internal Medicine*, ed 5. Philadelphia, WB Saunders, 2000, pp 1704–1709.

DiBartola SP: Metabolic acid base disorders. In DiBartola SP (ed): *Fluid Therapy in Small Animal Practice*, ed 2. Philadelphia, WB Saunders, 2000, pp 211–240.

Rose BD, Post TW: *Clinical Physiology of Acid-Base and Electrolyte Disorders*, ed 5. New York, McGraw-Hill, 2001, pp 612–635.

AUTHOR: **AMY E. DECLUE**
EDITOR: **LEAH A. COHN**

Renomegaly

BASIC INFORMATION

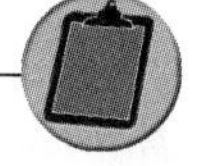

DEFINITION

Unilateral or bilateral enlargement of the kidneys. See Table I-26 for normal anatomic parameters.

SYNONYM(S)

Kidney enlargement
Nephromegaly

EPIDEMIOLOGY

SPECIES, AGE, SEX: Dependent on underlying cause.

GENETICS AND BREED PREDISPOSITION: Persians and other long-haired cats are more commonly affected by polycystic kidney disease, which is inherited in an autosomal-dominant fashion in Persian cats.

RISK FACTORS: Presence of certain infectious diseases (i.e., feline leukemia virus [FeLV], feline infectious peritonitis [FIP], leptospirosis) or disorders that may lead to urinary obstruction (i.e., urolithiasis, neoplasia).

CONTAGION AND ZOONOSIS: Cat-to-cat transmission of FeLV and FIP can occur. Leptospirosis can be transmitted to other animals as well as to humans.

ASSOCIATED CONDITIONS AND DISORDERS: Acute renal failure or chronic renal failure (CRF).

CLINICAL PRESENTATION

DISEASE FORMS/SUBTYPES

- Unilateral or bilateral renal enlargement.
- May be an incidental finding.

HISTORY, CHIEF COMPLAINT

- Lethargy, depression
- Anorexia
- Polyuria and polydipsia (PU/PD)
- Vomiting

PHYSICAL EXAM FINDINGS

- Depression
- Fever
- Palpably enlarged kidneys (unilateral or bilateral)
- Renal or abdominal pain
- Abdominal enlargement
- Pale mucous membranes
- Oral ulcers or erosions
- Halitosis

ETIOLOGY AND PATHOPHYSIOLOGY

- Neoplasia
  - Several primary renal and metastatic tumors can cause unilateral or bilateral renomegaly.
  - Examples include lymphoma (most common in cats and may be related to FeLV; renomegaly is usually bilateral), renal carcinoma (most common in dogs), nephroblastoma, and cystadenocarcinoma (can occur in German shepherds and is associated with dermatofibrosis).
- Inflammation/swelling
  - Infectious causes include FIP (granulomatous inflammation), leptospirosis, and renal abscesses (abscesses usually unilateral).
  - Ethylene glycol intoxication can cause acute bilateral renal swelling and pain.
- Hydronephrosis
  - Unilateral or bilateral ureteral obstruction due to strictures, uroliths, or neoplasia (ureteral or in the bladder trigone).
  - Ectopic ureters.
- Other
  - Polycystic kidney disease: most common in Persian and domestic long-haired cats.
  - Compensatory hypertrophy: unilateral enlargement of remaining kidney following removal of or severe damage to the other.
  - Hematoma: usually unilateral enlargement and following trauma (rare).
  - Portosystemic shunt (increased glomerular filtration rate is often concurrent; both can be reversible with shunt ligation).

DIAGNOSIS

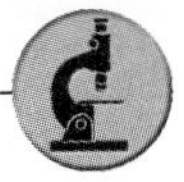

DIFFERENTIAL DIAGNOSIS

- Other causes of abdominal masses or enlargement
- Specific causes (e.g, neoplasia, hydronephrosis, polycystic kidney disease, etc.)

INITIAL DATABASE

- Complete blood count (CBC): Inflammatory leukogram and/or nonregenerative anemia may accompany infectious or neoplastic diseases. Thrombocytopenia may be present with leptospirosis. Polycythemia and/or extreme leukocytosis can occur, although rarely, with some renal neoplasms.
- Serum biochemical profile: Abnormalities are consistent with acute renal failure or CRF (azotemia, hyperphosphatemia, hyperkalemia, or hypokalemia; urine specific gravity less than 1.030 [dogs] or 1.035 [cats]). Hyperglobulinemia is present in some chronic inflammatory disorders (e.g., FIP).
- Urinalysis: proteinuria and hematuria with some neoplastic and inflammatory disorders. Calcium oxalate monohydrate and dihydrate crystals may be observed with ethylene glycol toxicity.
- Abdominal ultrasound (see Table I-26): very effective at differentiating major causes and detecting presence of uroliths.
- Abdominal radiographs (see Table I-26): effective at ruling out other causes of abdominal enlargement/masses and identifying radiopaque uroliths.

ADVANCED OR CONFIRMATORY TESTING

- Urine culture and sensitivity (C&S).
- Serologic evaluation or other diagnostic tests for infectious disease (leptospirosis, FeLV, FIP).
- Thoracic radiographs to rule out metastatic disease.
- Serum or urine ethylene glycol assay.
- Aspirate cytologic examination of renal masses.
- Excretory urography/intravenous pyelography.
- Exploratory laparotomy.

TREATMENT

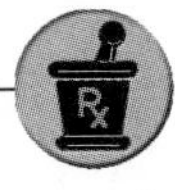

THERAPEUTIC GOAL(S)

- Resolve underlying cause of renomegaly if possible.
- Treat associated disorders (e.g., acute renal failure or CRF).

ACUTE GENERAL TREATMENT

Treat acute renal failure if present and address any related toxicity (i.e., ethylene glycol) or infection (i.e., leptospirosis).

CHRONIC TREATMENT

- Neoplasia: may involve nephrectomy if disease is unilateral with no sign of metastatic disease or chemotherapy if tumor is potentially responsive to drug therapy (e.g., lymphoma).
- Hydronephrosis: correct cause of obstruction or ectopic ureter.

PROGNOSIS AND OUTCOME

Depends on the underlying cause and concurrent disorders (e.g., renal failure).

SUGGESTED READING

Cuypers MD, Grooters AM, Willams J, et al: Renomegaly in dogs and cats. Part I. Differential diagnosis. *Compend Contin Educ Pract Vet* 19:1019–1032, 1997.

AUTHOR: **DARCY H. SHAW**
EDITOR: **ETIENNE CÔTÉ**

TABLE I-26 Characteristic Features of the Kidneys

Feature	Dog	Cat
Type	Unipyramidal (fused pyramids)	Unipyramidal (single pyramids)
Kidney mass as a percentage of body weight	0.6	0.6–1.0
Total nephrons per kidney	415,000	190,000
Kidney length in proportion to length of lumbar vertebra (L2)	2.9	2.7
Kidney width in proportion to length of lumbar vertebra (L2)	1.6	1.7
Ventral displacement in proportion to length of lumbar vertebra (L2)	L: 0.7 R: 0.3	L: 0.7 R: 0.7
Diffusely hyperechoic renal cortex on ultrasound exam	Pathologic	Normal or pathologic

Modified from Christie BA: Anatomy of the urinary system. In Slatter D (ed): Textbook of Small Animal Surgery, ed 3. Philadelphia, WB Saunders, 2003, p 1562.

Resorption Lesions, Feline Odontoclastic (FORL)

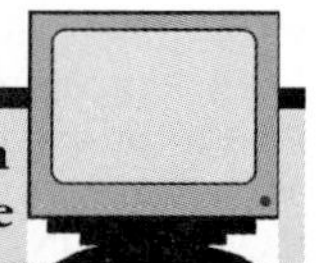

Client Education Sheet on Website

BASIC INFORMATION

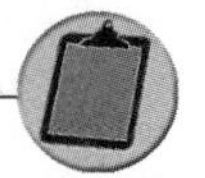

DEFINITION

Loss of tooth substance due to resorption by osteoclast-like cells (odontoclasts)

SYNONYM(S)

Cervical line erosion
External root resorption
Feline caries
Neck lesion
Note: The term *neck lesion* is a topographical distinction only. The terms *erosion* and *caries* are inappropriate because the dental defect is resorptive in nature and is not caused by acidic or bacterial insult.

EPIDEMIOLOGY

SPECIES, AGE, SEX: Resorption can occur in any mammalian permanent tooth, but the condition is seen predominantly in domestic cats 4 years of age and older (feline odontoclastic resorptive lesions [FORL]), with reported prevalence rates ranging between 25% and 75%.
GENETICS AND BREED PREDISPOSITION: There is no obvious breed predisposition, although purebred cats have been reported to develop FORL at a younger age compared to other breeds.
RISK FACTORS

- Periodontal disease
- Trauma from occlusion
- Dietary composition
- Increased vitamin D levels in commercial diets

GEOGRAPHY AND SEASONALITY: Worldwide.
ASSOCIATED CONDITIONS AND DISORDERS: Thickening of bone at the alveolar margin and abnormal extrusion of teeth (particularly canine teeth).

CLINICAL PRESENTATION

DISEASE FORMS/SUBTYPES

- Dentoalveolar ankylosis (fusion between root and bone)
- Root replacement resorption (tooth resorption followed by bone replacement)
- Inflammatory resorption (vascular and inflamed granulation tissue filling a resorptive defect)

HISTORY, CHIEF COMPLAINT: Animals may present with "red spots" on their teeth (crown defect filled with granulation tissue), repetitive lower jaw motions (jaw opening reflex), fractured crowns, and missing teeth; these animals may also have difficulty eating hard food and may refuse to drink cold water. The majority of FORL cases, however, are diagnosed with radiographic examination of teeth.
PHYSICAL EXAM FINDINGS: Oral examination reveals crown defects filled with vascular and inflamed granulation tissue, fractured crowns, root remnants, bulging gingiva in areas of missing teeth, thickening of bone at the alveolar margin, and abnormal extrusion of the canine teeth.

ETIOLOGY AND PATHOPHYSIOLOGY

- Suggested causes include periodontal disease, anatomic peculiarities, mechanical trauma, increased vitamin A intake, abnormal calcium homeostasis, and viruses causing immunosuppression.
- Two investigations have shed new light on the possible etiology and pathophysiology of FORL:
  - Histologic examination of healthy teeth from cats with FORL on other teeth showed periodontal ligament degeneration, hypercementosis, decreased width of the periodontal space, and dentoalveolar ankylosis, indicating that inflammatory cells may not play a primary role in the development of FORL.
  - A prospective study showed that cats with FORL have significantly increased serum levels of 25-hydroxyvitamin D, compared to cats without FORL; these findings indicate that cats with FORL must have had a higher intake of dietary vitamin D, compared to cats without FORL.

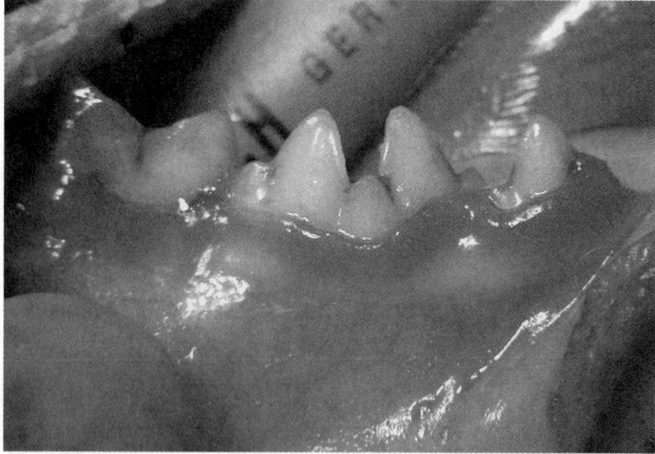

A

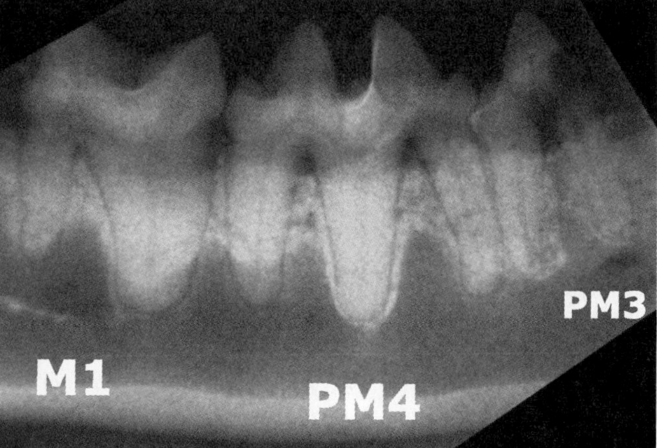

B

FIGURE I-147 **A,** Clinical picture of right mandibular third and fourth premolars and first molar; rostral is to the right. Generalized moderate gingivitis with focalized gingival hyperplasia; possible FORL on third premolar and first molar; fourth premolar shows gemination (division of a tooth bud resulting in the formation of partially or completely separated crowns). **B,** Radiograph of same area. Generalized mild to moderate horizontal alveolar bone loss; FORL on third premolar (PM3; inflammatory resorption near cervical region and furcation; dentoalveolar ankylosis and replacement resorption at distal root) and first molar (M1; inflammatory resorption near cervical region on mesial tooth surface); geminated fourth premolar (PM4) does not show signs of tooth resorption. Courtesy of Dr. Alexander M. Reiter, University of Pennsylvania.

DIAGNOSIS

DIFFERENTIAL DIAGNOSIS

- Periodontal disease
- Fractured teeth
- Root remnants
- Tooth resorption due to local causes (periapical abscess, orthodontic tooth movement, trauma, neoplasia)

INITIAL DATABASE

- Preanesthetic complete blood count (CBC), serum biochemistry profile, urinalysis
- Full-mouth (intraoral) dental radiographs

TREATMENT

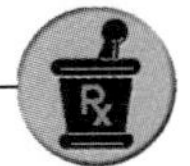

THERAPEUTIC GOAL(S)

- Make the mouth free of pain.
- Preserve masticatory function.
- Prevent abscess formation and local osteomyelitis.

ACUTE GENERAL TREATMENT

- Nonsurgical or surgical extraction of root remnants and FORL-affected teeth.
- Flaps should be closed with synthetic absorbable suture material.
- Administration of antibiotics is not usually necessary after tooth extraction unless another medical condition or extensive tissue trauma at the extraction site is present.
- Pain management: local nerve block(s) intraoperatively (0.3-0.5 ml of 0.5% bupivacaine hydrochloride per block) followed by opioid medications upon extubation (hydromorphone 0.1 mg/kg IM) and opioid medications postoperatively for 2 to 3 days (butorphanol 0.2-0.4 mg/kg PO q 8h; buprenorphine 0.01-0.02 mg/kg buccal transmucosal q 8h); transdermal fentanyl patch (25 μg) if multiple extractions were performed.

POSSIBLE COMPLICATIONS

- Fractured teeth and roots
- Root remnants
- Regional trauma due to improper extraction technique
- Infection
- Future development of FORL on other teeth

RECOMMENDED MONITORING

- Examination in 1 to 2 weeks to evaluate extraction sites
- Clinical examination and full-mouth dental radiography once per year

PROGNOSIS AND OUTCOME

- Excellent for extraction site healing
- Fair with regard to preventing the development of FORL on other teeth

PEARLS & CONSIDERATIONS

COMMENTS

- Usually more than one tooth is affected.
- Dental radiography is an invaluable tool in diagnosing FORL that are missed on clinical examination.

PREVENTION

There is no reliable prevention strategy available at this time.

CLIENT EDUCATION

Inform clients about the likelihood of development of FORL on other teeth and the need for continued clinical and radiographic monitoring.

SUGGESTED READING

Gorrel C, Larsson A: Feline odontoclastic resorptive lesions: Unveiling the early lesion. *J Small Anim Pract* 43:482, 2002.

Reiter AM, et al: Evaluation of calciotropic hormones in cats with odontoclastic resorptive lesions. *Am J Vet Res* 66:1446, 2005.

Reiter AM, et al: Update on the etiology of tooth resorption in domestic cats. *Vet Clin North Am Small Anim Pract* 35:913, 2005.

Reiter AM, Mendoza K: Feline odontoclastic resorptive lesions: An unsolved enigma in veterinary dentistry. *Vet Clin North Am Small Anim Pract* 32:791, 2002.

AUTHOR & EDITOR: **ALEXANDER M. REITER**

Restrictive/Unclassified Cardiomyopathy, Feline

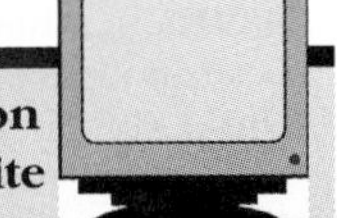

Client Education Sheet on Website

BASIC INFORMATION

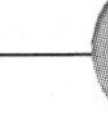

DEFINITION

- Restrictive Cardiomyopathy (RCM): disorder of the myocardium characterized by severe left or biatrial enlargement with normal to slightly thickened ventricular myocardium, normal to slightly reduced ventricular volume, and normal to slightly reduced systolic function. On a two-dimensional echocardiogram, the presence of right and left ventricles of normal dimensions together with moderate to marked biatrial enlargement in the absence of any valvular, shunting, or stenotic lesions are hallmarks of RCM.
- Unclassified cardiomyopathy (UCM): disorder of the myocardium characterized by severe left or biatrial enlargement with mixed ventricular myocardial changes, including areas of thickening mixed with areas of thinning, mild to severe ventricular dilation, and mild to severe systolic dysfunction (decreased ventricular contractility), which could be global or regional.

SYNONYM(S)

- Intermediate-form cardiomyopathy: ICM (UCM)
- Restrictive filling or physiology: ventricular filling is similar to restrictive cardiomyopathy (RCM) but echocardiographic findings reveal abnormal ventricular myocardium

EPIDEMIOLOGY

SPECIES, AGE, SEX

- Feline, middle-aged to older; no apparent sex predilection although a female predominance has been reported.
- Accurate prevalence is difficult to determine due to overlapping diagnostic criteria in the past; however RCM appears to be the second most common myocardial disease in the cat after hypertrophic cardiomyopathy.

GENETICS AND BREED PREDISPOSITION: No definitive breed predilection but may be seen more commonly in certain breeds (Persian, Birman, Balinese, Siamese, Burmese).

ASSOCIATED CONDITIONS AND DISORDERS

- Congestive heart failure (CHF) is commonly seen: left-sided (pulmonary edema) or biventricular (pulmonary edema, pleural effusion, ascites).
- Cardiogenic embolism (systemic arterial thromboembolism) may be more commonly associated with this form of myocardial disease compared to hypertrophic cardiomyopathy.

CLINICAL PRESENTATION

- Primary RCM: idiopathic disorder involving ventricular stiffness and in which ventricular dimensions are normal.
- Secondary RCM: myocardial disorders involving ventricular stiffness and in which ventricular dimensions are abnormal; see Hypertrophic Cardiomyopathy (p 554) and Dilated Cardiomyopathy (p 302). The information presented below will focus on primary RCM.
- Clinical presentation is variable but similar with both types of cardiomyopathy (RCM/UCM).

HISTORY, CHIEF COMPLAINT

- Dyspnea and tachypnea, from pulmonary edema, are most common. Some cats will have ascites and dyspnea from pleural effusion.
- Some cats will present for cardiogenic embolism, with or without concomitant CHF. Some cats will have a history of episodic lameness not associated with trauma.

PHYSICAL EXAM FINDINGS: Can be quite variable but could include:

- Soft systolic murmur (seemingly less common than in hypertrophic cardiomyopathy, presumably because left ventricular outflow tract obstruction and systolic anterior motion of the mitral valve occur less frequently with RCM/UCM).
- Gallop heart sound.
- Muffled heart/lung sounds when pleural effusion is present.
- Pulmonary crackles possible with pulmonary edema.
- Ascites as a manifestation of right-sided CHF.
- Absent femoral arterial pulses, cyanosis of nailbeds, cool paws, and firm, painful gastrocnemius muscles if aortic thromboembolism is present.
- Pulse deficits from arrhythmias.

ETIOLOGY AND PATHOPHYSIOLOGY

- Primary RCM: idiopathic.
- Secondary, noninfiltrative restrictive physiology:
  - Dilated cardiomyopathy.
  - Hypertrophic cardiomyopathy.
  - Diffuse myocardial fibrosis.
- Secondary, infiltrative restrictive physiology:
  - Myocarditis.
- Secondary RCM-endomyocardial form:
  - Endomyocardial fibrosis (idiopathic).
- UCM:
  - Regional or diffuse areas of fibrosis.
  - Regional or diffuse intramural myocardial ischemia (unproven).
- RCM/UCM: similar pathophysiologic effects resulting from excessive ventricular stiffness and, therefore, limitation in ventricular diastolic filling.
  - Severely impaired (restricted) filling of ventricles induces diastolic dysfunction/failure, which results in elevated atrial pressures, pulmonary or systemic venous pressures, and congestion (pulmonary edema and/or ascites, respectively)
  - Systolic function is variable depending upon the underlying cause of the myocardial disease.
  - Dilated atria can allow blood stasis as well as having areas of endocardial fibrosis; both factors can result in mural thrombus formation.
    - Emboli originating from the cardiac thrombi can infarct the terminal aorta, thoracic limbs, kidneys, bowel, or brain.

DIAGNOSIS

DIFFERENTIAL DIAGNOSIS

- Physical
  - Tachypnea/dyspnea
    - Pulmonary disease
    - Pleural disease
    - CHF from other causes
  - Muffled heart/lung sounds
    - Pleural disease
    - Obesity
    - Pneumothorax
  - Pulmonary crackles
    - Pulmonary disease
  - Ascites
    - Abdominal disease (generally more common than CHF as a cause of ascites in cats)
    - Effusive disease (e.g., feline infectious peritonitis, neoplasia, others)
    - CHF from other causes
  - Heart murmur
    - Other cardiac disease
    - Physiologic murmur (i.e., anemia, hyperthyroidism)
  - Caudal paresis/paralysis
    - Neurologic disease
    - Trauma
- Electrocardiogram (ECG)
  - Arrhythmias
    - Other cardiac disease
    - Systemic disease
    - Trauma
- Thoracic radiographs
  - Cardiomegaly
    - Other cardiac disease
    - Pericardial disease
  - Pulmonary infiltrates
    - Pulmonary disease
    - Noncardiogenic pulmonary edema
  - Pleural effusion
    - Pleural disease
    - Neoplastic disease
    - Effusive disease

INITIAL DATABASE

- ECG
  - Arrhythmias are commonly seen.
    - Atrial premature complexes (APCs), ventricular premature complexes (VPCs), atrial fibrillation.
  - Evidence of left ventricular and/or atrial enlargement may be seen.
- Thoracic radiographs
  - Cardiomegaly.
    - Variable: usually left ± right atrial enlargement.
    - Possible left ventricular enlargement.
  - Pulmonary venous congestion/edema.
    - Often present.
  - Pleural effusion.
    - Can be seen.
- Echocardiogram
  - Severe left or biatrial dilation.
  - Relatively normal-appearing ventricles (primary idiopathic RCM or secondary infiltrative restrictive physiology).
  - Hypertrophic segments interspersed with thin segments of the ventricular myocardium with variable systolic function and ventricular dilation (secondary, noninfiltrative restrictive physiology, and UCM).
  - Left atrial thrombi may be seen.
  - Pericardial effusion may be present.
  - By definition, regurgitant valvular lesions, cardiac shunts, and stenotic lesions are absent or insignificant.

ADVANCED OR CONFIRMATORY TESTING

- Spectral Doppler echocardiogram
  - Increased E wave amplitude
  - Shortened E wave deceleration time
  - Reduced A wave amplitude
  - Increased E/A wave ratio
  - Preserved respiratory variability on transtricuspid inflow profile
- Tissue Doppler imaging
  - Reduced Ea and Aa velocities

TREATMENT

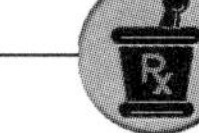

THERAPEUTIC GOAL(S)

- Alleviate CHF
- Delay development of recurrent CHF

ACUTE GENERAL TREATMENT

- See also Heart Failure, Acute/Decompensated, p 458.
- Remove pulmonary edema.
  - Furosemide: 1 mg/kg IV, IM, SQ PRN.
  - Oxygen: 30–40% (via cage, nasal line, hood, etc.).
  - Nitroglycerin: 1/8–1/4" topically on pinna or on unhaired region of ventral abdomen/inguinal area q 6–8h.
- Remove pleural effusion/ascites.
  - Thoracocentesis/abdominocentesis to remove as much as possible.
- Cardiogenic embolism.
  - Reduce thrombus formation.
    - Heparin: 250–350 IU/kg IV, then 250 IU/kg SQ q 8h.
    - Clopidogrel: 75 mg PO once.
  - Thrombolysis (only attempt if able to provide advanced critical care, including monitoring for hemor-

rhage and reperfusion injury/hyperkalemia).
  - Tissue plasminogen activator (t-PA): 0.25–1.0 mg/kg/hr IV, up to 10 mg/kg total.
  - Streptokinase: 90,000 IU IV over first hour, then 45,000 IU q 1h for up to 8 hours.
- There is no known treatment for slowing the progression of, or reversing, idiopathic RCM or UCM.

CHRONIC TREATMENT

- Prevent fluid retention.
  - Furosemide: 1–2 mg/kg PO q 12–24h.
  - ACE inhibitors:
    - Enalapril: 0.25–0.5 mg/kg PO q 12–24h.
    - Benazepril: 0.25–0.5 mg/kg PO q 12–24h.
- Improve cardiac function.
  - Digoxin (if systolic dysfunction [decreased left ventricular contractility] is present): 0.03125 mg PO q 24–48h.
  - β-Blockers (especially if ventricular arrhythmias are present):
    - Atenolol: 6.25–12.5 mg PO q 12–24h.
- Prevent cardiogenic embolism.
  - Antiplatelet agents:
    - Clopidogrel: 18.75 mg PO q 24h.
    - Aspirin: 25 mg/kg PO q 48–72h.
    - Combination clopidogrel and aspirin.
  - Anticoagulants:
    - Low-molecular-weight heparins:
      - Dalteparin: 100 IU/kg SQ q 12–24h; or
      - Enoxaparin: 1.0–1.5 mg/kg SQ q 12–24h.
  - Combination therapy:
    - Clopidogrel + dalteparin OR enoxaparin.

DRUG INTERACTIONS

- Aggressive diuretic administration together with ACE inhibitor therapy can result in acute, reversible renal failure.
- Combined antithrombotics theoretically can confer an increased risk of bleeding, although this has not been seen clinically.

POSSIBLE COMPLICATIONS

- Recurrent, intractable congestive heart failure is most common cause of death.
- Cardiogenic embolism can result in acute decompensation, reduced quality of life, and sudden death.

RECOMMENDED MONITORING

- Owners should watch for onset of dyspnea and possible embolic events.
- Repeated evaluation of thoracic radiographs and echocardiogram to evaluate for progression and alterations to medical therapy.

PROGNOSIS AND OUTCOME

- Guarded to good for treatment of acute CHF
- Guarded for treatment of acute cardiogenic embolism
- Poor to guarded for long-term survival (months to 1 year)

PEARLS & CONSIDERATIONS

COMMENTS

- RCM and UCM are irreversible diseases and the cat is likely to have recurrent CHF episodes even with effective therapy.
- While cardiogenic embolism is a negative prognostic indicator and likely to occur again, many of these cats can do quite well with appropriate therapy and time; owners should at least consider treating such cats.

CLIENT EDUCATION

Owners should watch for onset of dyspnea and possible signs of embolic events.

SUGGESTED READING

Ferasin L, et al: Feline idiopathic cardiomyopathy: A retrospective study of 106 cats (1994-2001). *J Fel Med Surg* 5:151, 2003.

Fox PR: Feline cardiomyopathies. In Fox PR, Sisson DD, Moise NS (eds): *Textbook of Canine and Feline Cardiology*, ed 2. Philadelphia, WB Saunders, 1999, pp 621–678.

AUTHOR: **DANIEL F. HOGAN**
EDITOR: **ETIENNE CÔTÉ**

Retinal Degeneration

BASIC INFORMATION

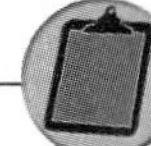

DEFINITION

Deterioration of the retina due to primary inherited retinal disorders or secondary to other intraocular disease (acquired); may be focal, multifocal, or generalized; extent of retinal involvement determines degree of vision impairment

SYNONYM(S)

Retinal atrophy

EPIDEMIOLOGY

SPECIES, AGE, SEX: Affects dogs and cats; age of onset and sex predisposition vary with underlying cause.

- Inherited:
  - Progressive retinal atrophy (PRA): early onset (i.e., dysplasia; ≤12 weeks of age) and late onset (i.e., degeneration; typically detected by 2 to 5 years of age) in dogs and cats.
  - Retinal pigment epithelial dystrophy (RPED); young dogs; uncommon.
- Acquired:
  - Sudden acquired retinal degeneration (SARD) typically affects middle-aged to older dogs; females are predisposed.

GENETICS AND BREED PREDISPOSITION

- Dogs:
  - PRA: autosomal recessive in most predisposed breeds, including poodles, cocker spaniels, Irish setters, and collies.
  - RPED: high frequency in briards.
- Cats: PRA is seen in Abyssinians as autosomal dominant (dysplasia) and autosomal recessive (degeneration).

RISK FACTORS

- Inherited: breed predisposition.
- Acquired:
  - See Uveitis, p 1134.
  - See Retinal Detachment, p 965.
  - See Glaucoma, p 440.
  - See Intraocular Neoplasia, p 603.
  - Nutritional deficiency (e.g., taurine in cats; vitamin A or E in dogs and cats).
  - Toxicity (e.g., idiosyncratic reaction to enrofloxacin, typically at high doses [>5 mg/kg per day], or griseofulvin in cats).
  - Metabolic (e.g., Mucopolysaccharidosis, dogs and cats; see Storage Diseases, p 1041).

ASSOCIATED CONDITIONS AND DISORDERS

- Cataracts
- Retinal detachment
- Systemic diseases causing uveitis (see Uveitis, p 1134)
- See Hyperadrenocorticism, p 537, regarding SARD
- See Dilated Cardiomyopathy, p 302, regarding taurine deficiency in cats

CLINICAL PRESENTATION

DISEASE FORMS/SUBTYPES

- Bilateral or unilateral

- Inherited versus acquired
- Acute onset versus progressive
- Focal, multifocal, generalized

HISTORY, CHIEF COMPLAINT: Variable depending on underlying cause; may be any or all of the following:

- Acute or progressive vision impairment or blindness.
- Red eye and/or other signs of glaucoma (see Glaucoma, p 440) or uveitis (see Uveitis, p 1134).
- Greenish shine to eye (tapetal reflection in dilated pupil).
- "Enlarged eye" (illusional due to dilated pupil or caused by buphthalmos); see Ocular Size Abnormalities, p 763.

PHYSICAL EXAM FINDINGS

- May show no clinical signs if focal.
- Generalized:
  - Often bilateral.
  - Dilated pupils and sluggish to absent pupillary light reflexes (PLRs).
  - Vision disturbances: ranging from impaired night vision (nyctalopia) and/or day vision (hemeralopia) (e.g., PRA) to complete blindness (e.g., SARD; end-stage PRA).
  - With/without signs of:
    - Uveitis (see p 1134).
    - Glaucoma (see p 440).
    - Cataracts (see p 182).
    - Systemic disease (acquired).

ETIOLOGY AND PATHOPHYSIOLOGY

- Inherited:
  - Breed-specific genetic abnormality in photoreceptor metabolism termed PRA:
    - PRA: always bilateral; variable rate of progression; leads to blindness when both rods and cones affected:
      - Early onset: Photoreceptors fail to develop normally (i.e., dysplasia).
      - Late onset: Photoreceptors develop normally but degenerate:
        - Typically rods affected first, causing nyctalopia.
        - Eventually cones also affected, resulting in hemeralopia and blindness.
  - RPED is a genetic abnormality affecting the RPE layer with secondary effects on the neural retina (nine inner retinal layers); uncommon.
- Acquired:
  - SARD is idiopathic; always bilateral; dogs only:
    - Sudden blindness within days or 1 to 2 weeks.
    - Normal fundic examination acutely; when disease is end-stage, generalized retinal degeneration indistinguishable from PRA is present.

DIAGNOSIS

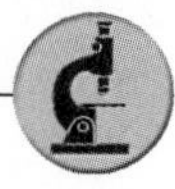

DIFFERENTIAL DIAGNOSIS

- Acute, nonred, quiet-eye blindness (e.g., SARD):
  - Optic neuritis
  - Optic chiasmal lesion
  - Postchiasmal/cortical blindness (pupil size and PLRs usually normal)
- Progressive blindness (e.g., PRA):
  - Slowly progressive cataracts
  - Progressive corneal discoloration
- "Red eye" blindness (e.g., glaucoma):
  - Uveitis
  - Cataracts
  - Lens luxation
  - Complex corneal ulceration
- See Blindness

INITIAL DATABASE

Complete ophthalmic examination, including:

- Menace response, dazzle reflex, direct and consensual PLRs.
- Intraocular pressure (normal: 15-25 mmHg; >30 mmHg indicates glaucoma).
- Direct or indirect ophthalmoscopy to assess the posterior segment of the eye, including:
  - Optic nerve (pale and small with end-stage retinal degeneration).
  - Tapetum (dorsal reflective mirror; hyper-reflective/brighter with retinal degeneration).
  - Nontapetal fundus (typically pigmented and located ventrally; whitish/grey depigmentation and/or mottled hyperpigmentation with retinal degeneration).
    - Retinal vasculature (small arteries and larger veins normally come from the optic disk and course peripherally; with retinal degeneration, the retinal vessels become narrowed and eventually diminish in number; no retinal vessels are discernable with end-stage retinal degeneration).

ADVANCED OR CONFIRMATORY TESTING

- Histopathologic evaluation of eye (when eye blind and painful, enucleation is advised).
- Genetic screening of blood sample for various inherited ocular diseases, including PRA (available for certain breeds).
- Referral is advisable for all cases of blindness of undetermined cause for additional evaluation.
  - Electroretinography (ERG) to assess retinal function:
    - Flatline response (i.e., no retinal function) in SARD.
    - Variable to flatline response in PRA depending on stage of disease.
    - See Blindness, p 136.
    - See Electroretinogram, p 1234.

TREATMENT

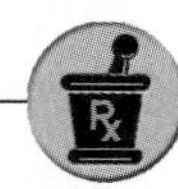

THERAPEUTIC GOAL(S)

Treat underlying cause and preserve vision when possible.

ACUTE GENERAL TREATMENT

- There is no available treatment to reverse retinal degeneration.
- Treat underlying cause, when possible, to prevent progression of acquired retinal degeneration.

POSSIBLE COMPLICATIONS

- Cataracts
- Retinal detachment ± hyphema
- Uveitis ± secondary glaucoma
- Corneal/scleral trauma (see Corneal/Scleral Trauma, p 244) due to vision impairment

RECOMMENDED MONITORING

- Variable depending on underlying cause.
- Clinicians should monitor the animal for secondary cataracts and lens-induced uveitis (see Cataracts, p 182).
- If SARD is suspected but cannot be confirmed with ERG, repeat fundic examinations at 3, 6, and 12 months are indicated for clinical signs of progressive retinal degeneration.

PROGNOSIS AND OUTCOME

- Variable depending on underlying cause.
- Permanent blindness with SARD and PRA.
- Prognosis typically good with focal retinal degeneration due to scarring from previous posterior uveitis and/or retinal detachment, assuming disease process does not recur.

PEARLS & CONSIDERATIONS

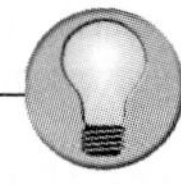

COMMENTS

- There is no available treatment to reverse retinal degeneration.
- Avoid enrofloxacin doses greater than 5 mg/kg per day in cats.

PREVENTION

- Ophthalmic screening of animals used for breeding by a board-certified veterinary ophthalmologist and registration through the Canine Eye Registration Foundation will help to remove PRA-

and RPED-affected animals from the breeding population.

- Genetic testing of blood samples for breed-specific inherited ocular diseases will help detect carrier and affected animals.

CLIENT EDUCATION

- Retinal degeneration alone does not cause ocular pain.
- Animals often adjust well to blindness.

SUGGESTED READING

Genetic testing for various inherited ocular diseases: www.optigen.com/opt9_test.html.

AUTHOR & EDITOR: **CHERYL L. CULLEN**

Retinal Detachment

BASIC INFORMATION

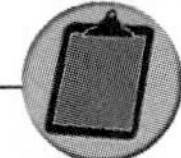

DEFINITION

Separation of the neural retina (inner nine layers) from the underlying retinal pigment epithelium (RPE) as a result of primary inherited retinal disease or secondary to other intraocular disease (acquired); may be focal, multifocal, or complete; extent of retinal involvement determines degree of vision impairment.

SYNONYM(S)

Retinal nonattachment

EPIDEMIOLOGY

SPECIES, AGE, SEX: Affects dogs and cats; age of onset and sex predisposition vary with underlying cause.

- Inherited (dogs):
  - Severe retinal dysplasia: congenital.
  - Collie eye anomaly (CEA): retinal detachments occur in up to 10% of CEA-affected dogs; commonly young pups; may also develop later in life.
- Acquired:
  - Secondary to vitreous degeneration (liquefaction of the vitreous); usually older dogs.
  - Systemic hypertension; typically older animals.

GENETICS AND BREED PREDISPOSITION: Dogs:

- Retinal dysplasia: presumed autosomal recessive in many predisposed breeds, including English springer spaniels, Bedlington terriers, American cocker spaniels, and miniature schnauzers; presumed an incomplete dominant inheritance in breeds with associated skeletal deformities, including Labrador retrievers and Samoyeds.
- CEA: predisposed breeds include collies, Shetland sheepdogs, Border collies, and Australian shepherds.
- Shih tzus are predisposed to vitreous degeneration and rhegmatogenous retinal detachments.

RISK FACTORS

- Inherited: breed predisposition
- Acquired:
  - Ocular trauma (see Corneal/Scleral Trauma, p 244)
  - Uveitis (see p 1134)
  - Glaucoma (see p 440)
  - Cataracts (see p 182)
  - Intraocular Neoplasia (see p 603)
  - Lens Luxation (see p 628)
  - Bleeding disorder (e.g., coagulopathy due to anticoagulant rodenticide intoxication) (see Hemorrhage, p 485)
  - Surgical lens removal (lensectomy)
  - Systemic Hypertension (see p 1058)
  - Old age

ASSOCIATED CONDITIONS AND DISORDERS

- Cataracts
- Hyphema (see p 560)
- Retinal degeneration (see p 963)
- Systemic diseases causing uveitis (see Uveitis, p 1134)
- Diseases causing systemic hypertension (see Systemic Hypertension, p 1058)

CLINICAL PRESENTATION

DISEASE FORMS/SUBTYPES

- Bilateral or unilateral
- Inherited versus acquired
- Rhegmatogenous (retinal tear) versus nonrhegmatogenous
- Focal, multifocal, complete
- Bullous versus flat
- Exudative versus nonexudative
- Tractional

HISTORY, CHIEF COMPLAINT: Similar to retinal degeneration (see Retinal Degeneration, p 963) ± bleeding inside eye.

PHYSICAL EXAM FINDINGS: May produce no clinical signs if detachment is focal or multifocal.

Complete:

- Pupil(s) dilated or fixed and dilated.
- Pupillary light reflex (PLR) decreased (i.e., sluggish and incomplete) or absent.
- ± Anisocoria (asymmetric pupil size, especially if unilateral lesion; only pupil of affected eye is dilated).
- Blindness (variable vision impairment if incomplete).
- Grey-to-white membrane (retina) with blood vessels and/or hemorrhage often visible through pupil behind lens.
- With or without signs of:
  - Uveitis (see Uveitis, p 1134)
  - Hyphema (see Hyphema, p 560)
  - Glaucoma (see Glaucoma, p 440)
  - Cataracts (see Cataracts, p 182)
  - Systemic disease (acquired)

ETIOLOGY AND PATHOPHYSIOLOGY

- A potential space exists between the neural retina and the retinal pigment epithelium (RPE) (subretinal space).
- Exudative/nonexudative:
  - The breakdown of the blood-retinal barrier, allowing the following into the subretinal space:
    - Serous fluid ± hemorrhage (e.g., hypertension; hyperviscosity; vasculitis).
    - Exudative fluid (e.g., posterior uveitis due to systemic bacterial or mycotic infection).
- Rhegmatogenous:
  - Tear in retina allows vitreous to enter the subretinal space (e.g., hypermature cataracts; after lensectomy; CEA; old age or breed predisposition to vitreous degeneration/liquefaction; retinal degeneration).
- Tractional:
  - Fibrous or fibrocellular tissue causing pulling on the retina, with separation of the neural retina from the retinal pigment epithelium (RPE) (e.g., ocular trauma resulting in vitreous hemorrhage; posterior uveitis and hyalitis [inflammation of the vitreous]).
- Causes: see Risk factors above.

DIAGNOSIS

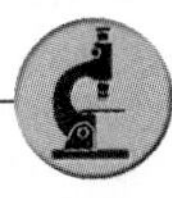

DIFFERENTIAL DIAGNOSIS

Other causes of blindness (see Blindness, p 136)

INITIAL DATABASE

Complete ophthalmic examination, including:

- Menace response, dazzle reflex, direct and consensual PLRs.
- Intraocular pressure (normal: 15-25 mmHg; >30 mmHg indicates glaucoma).

- Direct or indirect ophthalmoscopy to assess the posterior segment of the eye, including:
  - Optic nerve (optic disk hidden under membrane of detached retina with complete rhegmatogenous/ "morning glory" form).
  - Tapetum (dorsal reflective mirror; hyporeflective/greyish, dull discoloration ± hemorrhage with most forms of retinal detachment; hyperreflective/brighter with complete rhegmatogenous form because retina remains attached at/hangs off optic disk and no longer covers underlying tapetum).
  - Nontapetal fundus (typically pigmented and located ventrally; whitish/ grey discoloration ± hemorrhage with retinal detachment).
  - Retinal vasculature (well focused, small arteries and larger veins normally come from the optic disk and course peripherally; with retinal detachment, the blood vessels change their course and become out of focus; blood vessels may be visualized in the pupil behind the lens with certain forms of retinal detachment).

ADVANCED OR CONFIRMATORY TESTING

- Ocular ultrasound if ocular media opaque, preventing evaluation of deeper ocular structures.
- Histopathologic evaluation of eye when eye is blind and painful and enucleation advised.
- Referral is advisable for all cases of blindness of undetermined cause for additional work-up (see Blindness, p 136).

TREATMENT

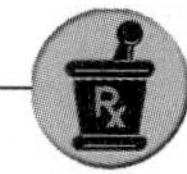

THERAPEUTIC GOAL(S)

Treat underlying cause and restore vision or preserve remaining vision when possible

ACUTE GENERAL TREATMENT

- Variable depending on underlying cause, duration, extent, and type of retinal detachment.
- Treat underlying cause, when possible, to prevent progressive retinal detachment.
- Promptly refer animals with acute blindness of undetermined cause to a veterinary ophthalmologist for early diagnosis and treatment (medical and/or surgical).

POSSIBLE COMPLICATIONS

- Permanent blindness
- Cataracts
- Retinal degeneration (see Retinal Degeneration, p 963)
- Hyphema (see Hyphema, p 560)
- Uveitis ± secondary glaucoma
- Corneal/scleral trauma due to vision impairment (see Corneal/Sceral Trauma, p 245)

RECOMMENDED MONITORING

- Variable depending on underlying cause
- Monitor for secondary cataracts and uveitis ± glaucoma

PROGNOSIS AND OUTCOME

- Variable depending on underlying cause, duration, extent, and type of retinal detachment.
- Prognosis for vision with focal or multifocal forms typically good, especially if underlying cause addressed and does not recur.
- Prognosis for vision with complete retinal detachment typically guarded.

PEARLS & CONSIDERATIONS

COMMENTS

Irreversible retinal degeneration occurs quickly following retinal detachment; therefore, prompt diagnosis and treatment of underlying cause (when possible) are crucial.

PREVENTION

Ophthalmic screening of animals used for breeding by a board-certified veterinary ophthalmologist and registration through the Canine Eye Registration Foundation will help to remove animals with inherited forms of retinal detachment from the breeding population.

CLIENT EDUCATION

- Retinal detachment may indicate systemic disease and may or may not be reversible, depending on cause; therefore, diagnostic testing is advised.
- Animals often adjust well to blindness.

SUGGESTED READING

Vainisi SJ, Wolfer JC: Canine retinal surgery. *Vet Ophthalmol* 7:291–306, 2004.

AUTHOR & EDITOR: **CHERYL L. CULLEN**

Reverse Sneezing

BASIC INFORMATION

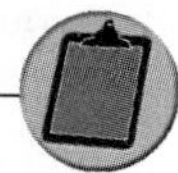

DEFINITION

A paroxysmal and noisy inspiratory effort, localized to the nasopharynx, during which the owner commonly thinks that the animal is suffocating

SYNONYM(S)

Mechanosensitive aspiration reflex

EPIDEMIOLOGY

SPECIES, AGE, SEX: Clinically, reverse sneezing is more commonly seen in dogs of any sex or age, depending on the underlying cause. Reverse sneezing can be experimentally induced in cats.

GENETICS AND BREED PREDISPOSITION

- Idiopathic form: any breed can be affected.
- Secondary to nasal mites: primarily large-breed dogs.
- Secondary to nasal neoplasia: primarily dolichocephalic dogs.

CONTAGION AND ZOONOSIS: Nasal mite (*Pneumonyssoides caninum*): The mode of transmission is not well established.

GEOGRAPHY AND SEASONALITY: Nasal mite: exists worldwide but is especially prevalent in the United States and northern European countries (Norway, Sweden, Finland).

ASSOCIATED CONDITIONS AND DISORDERS: Reverse sneezing can be a normal occurrence in many dogs, but can also be associated with nasal or nasopharyngeal disease (material coming from the nasal cavities, inflammation, abscess, foreign body, tumor, atresia) and nasal mites.

CLINICAL PRESENTATION

DISEASE FORMS/SUBTYPES

- Incidental episodes that do not require any treatment.
- Repeated frequent episodes that are associated with other causes of nasal or nasopharyngeal disease.

HISTORY, CHIEF COMPLAINT

- Incidental episodes of reverse sneezing are typically short in duration (a few seconds to 1 minute) and are generally

self-limiting. Between episodes, the animal is generally normal.
- Frequent episodes of reverse sneezing may be a reflection of underlying disease and thus associated with signs of nasal/nasopharyngeal disease, such as sneezing, nasal discharge, epistaxis, stertor, or others according to the etiology.

PHYSICAL EXAM FINDINGS: Incidental episodes of reverse sneezing: normal physical examination.

Reverse sneezing associated with:
- Nasal/nasopharyngeal inflammation and bacterial infection of various origins:
  - Unilateral or bilateral serous to bloody discharge.
  - Sneezing.
  - Stertor.
  - Decreased or sometimes increased nasal air passage.
  - Systemic signs are rare.
- Nasal tumor:
  - Decreased nasal air passage (unilateral or bilateral).
  - Unilateral or bilateral serous, mucopurulent, or bloody discharge.
  - Sneezing.
  - Stertor.
  - Facial or hard palate deformity (occasionally).
- Nasal aspergillosis:
  - Sneezing.
  - Unilateral serous, mucopurulent, or bloody discharge.
  - Depigmentation of nasal planum.
  - Pain with palpation of facial bones.
  - Increased nasal air passage.
  - Decreased appetite and poor body condition are possible.
- Nasal mite:
  - Sneezing.
  - Reverse sneezing, which may be the only abnormality in some dogs.
  - Nasal discharge.
  - Facial pruritis and hyposmia.

ETIOLOGY AND PATHOPHYSIOLOGY

- Incidental reverse sneezing can be a normal finding.
- Receptors and myelinated trigeminal nerve endings situated in the lateral aspects of the nasopharynx respond to local stimulation, implying a reflex pathway. Any local stimulation can activate the reflex, which causes a strong inspiration of material from the nasopharynx to the oropharynx through a decreased nasopharyngeal opening.

DIAGNOSIS

The diagnosis is based almost exclusively on history: recognition of the characteristically loud, stertorous inspiratory episode that is sudden in onset and in termination and that occurs in an animal that is usually otherwise well.

DIFFERENTIAL DIAGNOSIS

When reverse sneezing occurs frequently (daily or several times a day) and/or is accompanied by other clinical signs, nasal or nasopharyngeal disease is possible:
- Nasal or nasopharyngeal tumor
- Cyst
- Foreign body
- Abscess
- Mycotic infection
- Chronic lymphoplasmocytic rhinitis, sinusitis
- Nasopharyngitis
- Nasal mites

INITIAL DATABASE

- Results of complete blood count (CBC), biochemistry panel, and urinalysis are usually unremarkable.
  - Eosinophilia may be present in some cases of nasal mites.
  - Anemia and hypoproteinemia may be present in animals with nasal or nasopharyngeal disorders that cause heavy and/or repeated bloody discharge.
- Nasal radiographs can be useful for the diagnosis of underlying diseases

ADVANCED OR CONFIRMATORY TESTING

- If the episodes only occur at home (not in the veterinary hospital) and it is unclear whether they are consistent with reverse sneezing, clinicians can make the diagnosis by instructing the owner to videotape the episodes when they occur.
- Direct rhinoscopy results with culture, cytologic, and histopathologic samplings are useful for the diagnosis of primary nasal diseases, while posterior rhinoscopy is needed for the diagnosis of nasopharyngeal diseases.
- CT scans and/or MRIs are useful in the diagnosis of some underlying conditions, such as neoplasia and aspergillosis.

TREATMENT

THERAPEUTIC GOAL(S)

Reduce nasopharyngeal irritation by treating the underlying disorder when possible.

ACUTE GENERAL TREATMENT

Acute episodes of reverse sneezing associated with severe discomfort of the animal can be shortened by opening the dog's mouth and gently pulling on the tongue or giving the animal something to lick or drink.

CHRONIC TREATMENT

- Incidental episodes need no treatment.
- Increased frequency of episodes without any other sign of nasal or nasopharyngeal disease:
  - A short period of nonsteroidal anti-inflammatory drug (NSAID) administration (e.g., ketoprofen 1 mg/kg PO q 24h) may limit repeated reflex induced by local inflammation.
  - Treatment against the nasal mite if present (ivermectin 0.1-0.4 mg/kg [= 100-400 μg/kg] PO or SC three times at 3-week intervals; milbemycin oxime 0.5-1 mg/kg PO once weekly for 3 consecutive weeks).
- Related to nasal or nasopharyngeal disorders: treatment dictated by the underlying condition.

PROGNOSIS AND OUTCOME

- Excellent for incidental episodes and when the underlying cause is nasal mite infestation
- Otherwise variable depending on the underlying etiology

PEARLS & CONSIDERATIONS

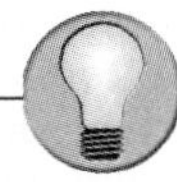

COMMENTS

The presence of clinical signs that suggest nasal or nasopharyngeal disease in conjunction with reverse sneezing should prompt diagnostic testing to detect underlying diseases.

CLIENT EDUCATION

Clients should learn not to worry during acute episodes of reverse sneezing since there is, in fact, no real danger of suffocation.

SUGGESTED READING

Doust R, Sullivan M: Nasal discharge, sneezing, and reverse sneezing. In King L (ed): *Textbook of Respiratory Diseases*. Philadelphia, WB Saunders, 2004, pp19-20.

AUTHOR: **CÉCILE CLERCX**
EDITOR: **RANCE K. SELLON**

Rhabdomyosarcoma

BASIC INFORMATION

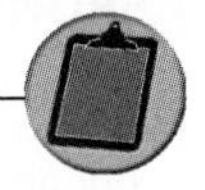

DEFINITION

A primary neoplasm of striated muscle; occurs very uncommonly

EPIDEMIOLOGY

SPECIES, AGE, SEX

- Rare in dogs. When affected, dogs often are <18 months old, but some cases have been reported in older dogs.
- Rare in cats.

GENETICS AND BREED PREDISPOSITION: The young age at diagnosis and occasional presence of more than one tumor suggest a hereditary basis for the disease. However, the low incidence of these tumors makes it difficult to determine genetic or breed predispositions.

CLINICAL PRESENTATION

DISEASE FORMS/SUBTYPES

- Botryoid rhabdomyosarcoma is a rare tumor usually found in the bladder of young, large-breed dogs.
- Other locations reported for rhabdomyosarcoma include the mouth or oropharynx, the tongue, larynx, heart (very rare), and peripheral skeletal muscle.

HISTORY, CHIEF COMPLAINT

- Presenting clinical signs depend on the location of the tumor.
- Dogs with oral and tongue tumors present for evaluation of signs related to an oral mass (halitosis, oral bleeding, discharge, visible mass).
- Dogs with laryngeal tumors may present for evaluation of dysphonia, dysphagia, inspiratory dyspnea, or respiratory distress.
- Tumors in the bladder cause signs attributable to a bladder mass (hematuria, pollakiuria, dysuria).

PHYSICAL EXAM FINDINGS: Physical exam findings vary depending on the location of the primary tumor and are reflected in the presenting complaints.

ETIOLOGY AND PATHOPHYSIOLOGY

- The cell of origin of these tumors is a myocyte in striated muscle.
- Lesions caused by rhabdomyosarcomas depend on the location of the primary tumor and the invasion into and destruction of surrounding normal structures.

DIAGNOSIS

DIFFERENTIAL DIAGNOSIS

Differential diagnosis depends on the location of the primary tumor:

- Bladder: transitional cell carcinoma, other bladder tumors.
- Heart: hemangiosarcoma, aortic body tumors, other cardiac tumors.
- Oral cavity: melanoma, squamous cell carcinoma, fibrosarcoma.

INITIAL DATABASE

- Fine-needle aspirate cytology may help identify the tumor type prior to other diagnostics.
- Three view thoracic radiographs to rule out pulmonary metastases.
- Abdominal ultrasound:
  - To rule out abdominal metastases.
  - Abdominal ultrasonography and echocardiography generally are the diagnostic tests of choice for identifying masses in the bladder or the heart, respectively.

ADVANCED OR CONFIRMATORY TESTING

- Computed tomography (CT) or magnetic resonance imaging (MRI) may be necessary to delineate the local extent of the tumor in some locations (e.g., oropharynx, larynx) and to plan for surgery or radiation therapy.
- Diagnosis is based on histopathologic evaluation of biopsy samples. Special stains may be necessary to differentiate rhabdomyosarcoma from other soft tissue sarcomas, especially poorly differentiated tumors.
  - Bladder tumors often require cystotomy to obtain a suitable biopsy and to attempt surgical excision. Botryoid ("grape-like") rhabdomyosarcoma often has a gross appearance that resembles a cluster of grapes.

TREATMENT

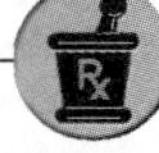

THERAPEUTIC GOAL(S)

- Complete eradication of the primary tumor
- Prevention or delay of the development of metastases if complete eradication is not possible

ACUTE AND CHRONIC TREATMENT

- Treatment of the primary tumor usually involves aggressive surgical resection.
- Radiation therapy has not been investigated for treatment of rhabdomyosaroma. It may be indicated for tumors that cannot be removed with surgery alone. However, the response to radiation is not known.
- Chemotherapy may be indicated for rhabdomyosarcomas. Many cases develop metastases, but chemotherapy traditionally is underutilized and could be beneficial.
- Peripheral rhabdomyosarcomas arising from skeletal muscle should be approached like other peripheral soft tissue sarcomas (see Soft Tissue Sarcoma, p 1016).

POSSIBLE COMPLICATIONS

Complications of treatment for rhabdomyosarcomas depend on the types of treatments and the location of the primary tumor (see Soft Tissue Sarcoma, p 1016).

RECOMMENDED MONITORING

Rhabdomyosarcomas may require more frequent monitoring for metastases (thoracic radiographs, abdominal ultrasound typically q 2-3 months) because of possible high metastatic rates.

PROGNOSIS AND OUTCOME

- Prognosis is guarded to grave for dogs with rhabdomyosarcoma of the bladder, heart, or oral cavity. Many dogs have masses that are not resectable and metastases are common after treatment of the primary tumor.
- Surgical resection has been reported to have a fair prognosis in a few cases. These include a dog with a perianal tumor treated with surgery, radiation, and chemotherapy that developed metastasis at 252 days and two dogs treated with laryngectomy and tracheostomy that lived 18 and 22 months after surgery, but all three of these dogs developed metastasis.
- Prognosis for rhabdomyosarcoma arising from skeletal muscle is not known.

PEARLS & CONSIDERATIONS

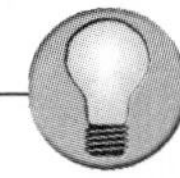

COMMENTS

Young animals that are treated for tumors may be more likely to develop late complications of chemotherapy and radiation (second malignancies, bone necrosis, central nervous system necrosis, radiation-induced tumors). This should be taken into consideration when deciding about treatment for rhabdomyosarcoma in young dogs. However, the poor prognosis for many of these tumors makes late side effects less of a concern.

CLIENT EDUCATION

Clients should be educated to monitor their pets for masses or signs of tumor development, even in young dogs. Early detection may allow for more successful treatment of these tumors.

SUGGESTED READING

MacEwen EG, Powers BE, Macy D, Withrow SJ: Soft tissue sarcomas. In Withrow SJ, MacEwen EG (eds): *Small Animal Clinical Oncology*. Philadelphia, WB Saunders, 2001, pp 283–304.

AUTHOR: **JOHN FARRELLY**
EDITOR: **KENNETH M. RASSNICK**

Rheumatoid Arthritis

BASIC INFORMATION

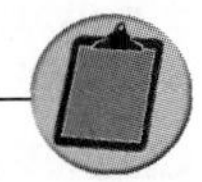

DEFINITION

A progressive, immune-mediated, inflammatory polyarthropathy with erosion of the articular cartilage

SYNONYM(S)

Canine: immune-mediated erosive polyarthritis
Greyhounds: erosive polyarthritis of greyhounds (PG)
Feline: feline chronic progressive polyarthritis (FCPP)

EPIDEMIOLOGY

SPECIES, AGE, SEX

- Rheumatoid arthritis (RA): variable; usually young to middle-aged animals.
- PG: young greyhounds (3 to 30 months of age).
- FCPP: Animals of any age can be affected; most of these are young adult males.

GENETICS AND BREED PREDISPOSITION

- RA: small breeds commonly affected.
- PG: breed specific.
- FCPP: domestic short-haired cats, Persians, Siamese cats.

ASSOCIATED CONDITIONS AND DISORDERS: Dogs:

- Felty's syndrome (FS): RA, splenomegaly, and neutropenia.
- Sjögren's syndrome (SS): nonerosive or erosive polyarthritis, keratoconjunctivitis sicca (KCS), xerostomia.
- Occasional association of RA with amyloidosis.

CLINICAL PRESENTATION

HISTORY, CHIEF COMPLAINT

- Early:
  - Initially indistinguishable from idiopathic polyarthritis.
  - Acute single or multiple leg lameness with anorexia is possible.
  - PG and FCPP: onset often more insidious.
- Later: chronic intermittent lameness; angular deformities secondary to ligamentous damage, mostly in the carpus, metacarpus, tarsus, and metatarsus.

PHYSICAL EXAM FINDINGS

- Joint pain, soft tissue swelling, reduced range of motion, joint crepitus; distal joints most severely affected.
- Low grade fever
- Mild generalized lymphadenopathy

ETIOLOGY AND PATHOPHYSIOLOGY

- Etiology unknown.
- Synovitis arises from a type III (immune complex) hypersensitivity reaction. Synovial lymphocytes and plasma cells produce rheumatoid factors (RFs) (IgM and IgA autoantibodies) directed against altered endogenous IgG.
- Immune complexes activate complement and attract neutrophils (accumulate in the joint fluid).
- Vascular granulation tissue (pannus) erodes the articular cartilage and destroys subchondral bone.
- Inflammation and damage to the joint capsule and collateral ligaments lead to joint instability and angular deformities.
- Electron microscopy: distemper viral particles in synovial macrophages.
- FCPP: unknown etiology; association with feline syncytium-forming virus.

DIAGNOSIS

DIFFERENTIAL DIAGNOSIS

- Idiopathic nonerosive polyarthritis (see Polyarthritis, p 871)
- Bacterial polyarthritis
- Systemic lupus erythematosus
- Reactive polyarthritis
- Neoplasia

INITIAL DATABASE

Complete blood count (CBC), serum biochemistry profile, urinalysis: all typically normal; leukocytosis, neutrophilia, hyperglobulinemia, hyperfibrinogenemia, and proteinuria possible.

ADVANCED OR CONFIRMATORY TESTING

- Radiographs of affected joints: indicated in all cases. Findings vary with duration of illness.
  - Early stage: periarticular swelling; minimal bony changes.
  - Later periarticular osteoporosis, subchondral lucencies ("erosive" changes); joint swelling.
  - Late stage: extensive bone destruction, joint space collapse, subluxations and luxations.
  - FCPP: marked periosteal new bone; focal erosions, especially hocks and carpi.
- Arthrocentesis, synovial fluid analysis: indicated in all cases; thin, cloudy, hypercellular (neutrophils predominate); culture negative; mucin clot test negative.
- Rheumatoid factor (RF): lacks sensitivity/specificity; positive in 20–70% of RA dogs; false positives with other inflammatory diseases; IgA RF more specific and more prevalent with severe erosive disease.
- Synovial biopsy: proliferative synovitis with lymphocytes, plasma cells, and macrophages.

TREATMENT

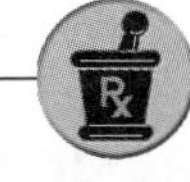

THERAPEUTIC GOAL(S)

A cure is not possible; clinical remission is the goal.

ACUTE GENERAL TREATMENT

- Nonsteroidal anti-inflammatory drugs (NSAIDs) have not proven to be successful. The high doses required for human RA have intolerable gastrointestinal (GI) side effects in dogs.
- Glucocorticoids, in combination with azathioprine, cyclophoshamide, or gold salts, are preferable and often required for remission.
  - Prednisone: 1–2 mg/kg PO q 12h for 2 to 3 weeks. If lameness and synovial fluid inflammation subside, the dose is reduced gradually over 3 to 4 months to lowest dose that maintains remission.
  - Azathioprine: 2 mg/kg PO q 48h (dogs).
  - Cyclophosphamide: 2 mg/kg PO q 24h, four consecutive days weekly.
  - Chrysotherapy (gold salts): requires concurrent use of glucocorticoids.
    - Sodium aurothiomalate:
      - 1 mg/kg IM once weekly for 10 weeks or until clinical remission.

- Give a small test dose first.
- To maintain remission: 1 mg/kg IM q 30 days.
- Auranofin:
  - 0.05–2.0 mg/kg PO q 12h (max. 9 mg per day).
  - Diarrhea common.
- FCPP: combination of glucocorticoids and cyclophosphamide may be of benefit in early stages. Gold salts are highly toxic in cats.
- PG: treatment with NSAIDs, glucocorticoids, or cytotoxic drugs has been unrewarding.

CHRONIC TREATMENT

- Taper prednisone to lowest dose that maintains clinical remission (e.g., 1.0 mg/kg, q 48h or lower). Continue cytotoxic drug-barring adverse effects (e.g., myelosuppression).
  - Evaluate the animal's synovial fluid monthly to guide dose reduction.
  - Monitor CBC and platelet counts frequently to detect myelosuppression from cytotoxic drugs.
- Adjunctive: exercise restriction, weight control.

POSSIBLE COMPLICATIONS

- Long-term glucocorticoids: Cushing's disease.
- Cytotoxic drugs: bone marrow suppression, cystitis from cyclophosphamide.
- Gold salts: fever, thrombocytopenia, leukopenia, dermatitis, glomerulonephritis, stomatitis.
- Avoid administering cytotoxic drugs if the animal has concurrent infections.

RECOMMENDED MONITORING

- Physical exam and joint fluid analysis to assess remission
- CBCs to assess myelosuppression

PROGNOSIS AND OUTCOME

- Poor long-term prognosis.
- Even with appropriate therapy, most animals deteriorate over time.
- Joint pain and instability may necessitate arthrodesis (questionable benefits in joints other than carpus).

PEARLS & CONSIDERATIONS

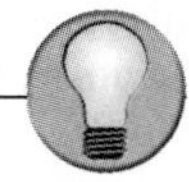

COMMENTS

- RF blood testing is not reliably accurate (positive in only 20–70% of affected dogs; other factors can cause false-positive results); an accurate diagnosis of RA is multifactorial, involving physical exam, radiographs of affected joints, and arthrocentesis.
- RA may initially resemble idiopathic polyarthritis, but eventually joint destruction becomes apparent.

CLIENT EDUCATION

Poor prognosis for cure; progressive disease that requires frequent rechecks

SUGGESTED READING

Bell SC, et al: IgA and IgM rheumatoid factors in canine rheumatoid arthritis. *J Sm Anim Pract* 34:259–264, 1993.

Bennett D, May C: Joint diseases of dogs and cats. In Ettinger SJ, Feldman EC (eds): *Textbook of Veterinary Internal Medicine*, ed 4. Philadelphia, WB Saunders, 1995, pp 2032–2074.

AUTHOR: **LILIAN CORNEJO**
EDITOR: **SUSAN M. COTTER**

Rhinitis, Bacterial

BASIC INFORMATION

DEFINITION

Inflammation of one or both nasal cavities associated with a bacterial infection that is often secondary to a primary nasal disease

EPIDEMIOLOGY

SPECIES, AGE, SEX

- Rhinitis is possible in dogs and cats of all ages and breeds depending on underlying cause.
- Puppies may develop bacterial rhinitis due to congenital abnormalities or immune deficiencies.
- Viral upper respiratory tract infections can lead to rhinitis in cats.

GENETICS AND BREED PREDISPOSITION: Predisposition reflects susceptibility to primary disease processes.

- Toy breeds are more susceptible to rhinitis associated with dental root infections.
- Dolichocephalic breeds of dogs are at risk for acquiring nasal aspergillosis and neoplasia.

RISK FACTORS: Bacterial rhinitis is most often secondary to a primary nasal disease.

- In dogs, primary disorders include:
  - Foreign body (especially active hunting dogs; plant material as foreign body)
  - Dental root infection
  - Congenital abnormalities, such as primary ciliary dyskinesia and soft palate defects
  - Lymphoplasmacytic rhinitis
  - Fungal rhinitis (aspergillosis)
  - Neoplasia
  - Fracture or osteomyelitis of conchae or facial bones from trauma
- In cats, primary diseases include:
  - Viral infection (most common)
  - Nasopharyngeal polyps
  - Neoplasia (carcinomas, lymphosarcoma)
  - Fungal rhinitis (cryptococcosis, less commonly aspergillosis)

CONTAGION AND ZOONOSIS: Kittens in multiple-cat environments have increased risk of viral infections.

ASSOCIATED CONDITIONS AND DISORDERS: Epistaxis and stridor.

CLINICAL PRESENTATION

DISEASE FORMS/SUBTYPES: Acute or recurrent, depending on primary cause.

HISTORY, CHIEF COMPLAINT

- Sneezing
- Nasal discharge
- Sometimes unilateral or bilateral epistaxis
- Head shaking, pawing the nose, snorting (nasal foreign body)
- Halitosis, inappetence (dental disease)

PHYSICAL EXAM FINDINGS

- Unilateral or bilateral mucopurulent nasal discharge
- Decreased (most commonly) or increased air passage through nares
- Enlarged submandibular lymph node(s)
- Evidence of systemic disease is uncommon
- Other signs are possible depending on primary disease

ETIOLOGY AND PATHOPHYSIOLOGY

Nasal turbinates, acting as powerful filters, and mucociliary clearance in the distal third of the nasal cavities are excellent defense mechanisms against infection. Secondary or recurrent bacterial infections develop when a primary nasal disease has impaired these defense mechanisms.

DIAGNOSIS

DIFFERENTIAL DIAGNOSIS

There are many causes of mucopurulent nasal discharge (see Risk Factors above).

INITIAL DATABASE

- Oral and dental examinations, under anesthesia or sedation if needed, to exclude dental disease and palatal defects.
- Plain radiographs of the nasal cavities, sinuses, and dental roots under general anesthesia to identify an inciting cause.
- Bacteriologic cultures are rarely useful because the organisms identified are commonly present in normal individuals and it is the predisposing nasal disease that must be identified and managed.
- Results of complete blood count (CBC), serum biochemistry profile, and urinalysis are often normal.

ADVANCED OR CONFIRMATORY TESTING

Advanced testing is recommended to rule out primary nasal cavity diseases:

- Rhinoscopy (direct and retrograde).
- Cytologic or histologic evaluation of nasal mucosal samples.
- CT or MRI is superior to standard radiography for imaging the nasal cavity.
- Viral culture or polymerase chain reaction (PCR) tests for viral infections of cats.
- Electron microscopy (primary ciliary dyskinesia).

TREATMENT

THERAPEUTIC GOAL(S)

- Identify and treat underlying cause
- Control bacterial infection
- Promote clearance of nasal secretions

ACUTE GENERAL TREATMENT

- Broad-spectrum antibiotics: per os, intranasal, or aerosol delivery as appropriate for the animal for short periods of time (1 week is sufficient in most cases). For example, administer amoxicillin 20 mg/kg PO q 8h; cefadroxil 20 mg/kg PO q 8h; or amoxicillin-clavulanate 15 mg/kg PO q 12h.
- Antibiotics do not need to be selected on the basis of Gram stain or culture and sensitivity (C&S) testing, except in recurrent cases.

CHRONIC TREATMENT

- Intranasal administration of sterile physiologic solution several times a day.
- Mucolytics:
  - N-acetylcysteine has a wide therapeutic range with dosage usually of 5-10 mg/kg and up to 100 mg/kg PO, q 12h.
    - Intranasal or aerosol delivery of 5-20% solution has also been described.
  - Bromhexine hydrochloride (0.5-1 mg/kg PO) or through aerosol delivery.
- Contraindicated treatments: Reduction of inflammation with short-acting corticosteroids and attempts to provide relief with decongestants are not indicated.

POSSIBLE COMPLICATIONS

Inflammation and injury to the ciliated nasal epithelium can decrease mucociliary clearance in the distal third of the nasal cavity and cause turbinate lysis or remodeling (especially in young kittens with severe viral infections or dogs with nasal aspergillosis). This will in turn cause mucus to accumulate and further promote bacterial infection.

RECOMMENDED MONITORING

Clinical signs of the condition

PROGNOSIS AND OUTCOME

Prognosis varies depending on the primary cause.

PEARLS & CONSIDERATIONS

COMMENTS

- Most animals with bacterial rhinitis have another primary nasal cavity disease; therefore, failure to achieve a prompt and sustained response to empiric therapy (or spontaneous resolution) should provoke recommendations for advanced testing.
- Obtaining a diagnosis and implementing specific treatment lessen the likelihood of chronic and irreversible epithelial and turbinate lesions that could otherwise predispose the animal to bacterial rhinitis.

CLIENT EDUCATION

Bacterial rhinitis secondary to a viral upper respiratory infection in cats can be difficult to control in the long term without daily medication administration for extended periods of time.

SUGGESTED READING

Forbes-Lent SE, Hawkins EC: Evaluation of rhinoscopy-assisted mucosal biopsy in diagnosis of nasal disease in dogs: 119 cases (1985-1989). *J Am Vet Med Assoc* 201, 1425, 1992.

Hunt GB, et al: Nasopharyngeal disorders of dogs and cats: A review and retrospective study. *Compendium on Continuing Education for the Practicing Veterinarian* 24, 184, 2002.

AUTHOR: **CÉCILE CLERCX**
EDITOR: **RANCE K. SELLON**

Rhinitis, Lymphoplasmacytic

BASIC INFORMATION

DEFINITION

Chronic, gradually progressive inflammatory nasal disease of unknown etiology characterized by infiltration of the nasal mucosa with lymphocytes and plasma cells

SYNONYM(S)

Chronic idiopathic rhinitis/rhinosinusitis
Chronic inflammatory rhinitis
Immune-mediated rhinitis

EPIDEMIOLOGY

SPECIES, AGE, SEX

- Dogs: any age, although young adult to middle-aged dogs of either sex are considered at risk.
- Cats: young adult to middle-aged cats of either sex.

GENETICS AND BREED PREDISPOSITION: The disease is seen primarily in large-breed dogs, although dachshunds may be predisposed.

RISK FACTORS

- Diseases causing chronic inflammation with epithelial erosion, turbinate lysis, and remodeling, such as long-standing or recurrent infections (e.g., foreign body, aspergillosis), can provoke lymphoplasmacytic nasal infiltrates.
- The idiopathic disease is not associated with an identifiable underlying cause of inflammation.

CLINICAL PRESENTATION

DISEASE FORMS/SUBTYPES: The disease is chronic, sometimes with very mild signs initially, followed by moderate to severe signs.

HISTORY, CHIEF COMPLAINT

- Nasal discharge
- Sneezing

- Stridor
- Reverse sneezing
- Ocular discharge and rubbing at the nose (occasionally)

PHYSICAL EXAM FINDINGS

- Unilateral or bilateral serous, mucoid, or bloody nasal discharge
- Decreased air passage through one or both nares
- Submandibular lymph node enlargement
- General condition is normal

ETIOLOGY AND PATHOPHYSIOLOGY

- Poorly defined but hypothesized to be either a chronic inflammatory response to an inhaled irritant or allergen or an immune-mediated process.
- Chronic inflammation causes loss of epithelium and squamous metaplasia, reduced population of ciliated cells, hyperplasia of subepithelial glands, increased amount of viscid mucus, and impaired ciliary clearance.
- Retention of mucus plugs, inhaled bacteria, and irritable particles maintain and aggravate inflammation.

DIAGNOSIS

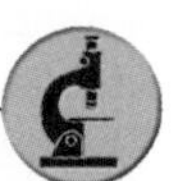

DIFFERENTIAL DIAGNOSIS

Other causes of nasal discharge (see Nasal Discharge, p 735):

- Dogs:
  - Fungal rhinitis
  - Nasal neoplasia
  - Dental disease
  - Foreign bodies
  - Nasal mites
  - Ciliary dyskinesia
- Cats:
  - Chronic viral upper respiratory tract infection
  - Nasopharyngeal polyps
  - Nasopharyngeal stenosis
  - Others as for dogs

INITIAL DATABASE

- Plain radiographs of the nasal cavities, sinuses, and dental roots can help eliminate other structural disorders, such as neoplasia, fungal rhinitis, and dental disease, but cannot confirm the diagnosis.
- Bacterial cultures can be positive or negative; positive cultures rarely reflect a primary role of bacteria in pathogenesis.
- Results of complete blood count (CBC), biochemistry panel, and urinalysis are usually normal.

ADVANCED OR CONFIRMATORY TESTING

- CT scan and/or MRI of the nasal cavities and sinuses can help identify differentials, such as neoplasia, fungal rhinitis, and dental disease, with more accuracy than plain radiographs but cannot confirm the diagnosis.
- Rhinoscopy findings are variable and can include:
  - Copious thick mucus or mucopurulent discharge
  - Mucosal hyperemia
  - Proliferative or thickened nasal mucosa
  - Turbinate lysis or remodeling
  - Pseudopolypoid appearance of mucosa
  - Absence of other causes of nasal discharge (*Aspergillus*, foreign bodies, etc.)
- Histopathologic examination of nasal mucosal biopsies predominantly shows mild to severe lymphoplasmacytic infiltration

TREATMENT

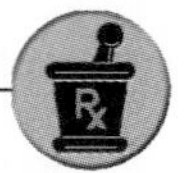

THERAPEUTIC GOAL(S)

- Prevent or reduce inflammation
- Control secondary bacterial infection
- Promote clearance of nasal secretions

ACUTE GENERAL TREATMENT

- Antibiotics are of little benefit unless there is a secondary bacterial infection.
- Glucocorticoids at immunosuppressive dosages:
  - Prednisone 1-2 mg/kg PO q 12h, then gradually tapered to lowest dose that controls clinical signs.
  - Topical (nasal spray, drops, or aerosols) administration of poorly absorbed glucocorticoids (such as fluticasone propionate) may be beneficial without involving secondary effects of systemic glucocorticoid therapy.
  - Many dogs do not respond to glucocorticoid therapy.
- Other anti-inflammatory agents, such as piroxicam, could potentially have some benefit, but efficacy has not been documented.
- In severe nonresponsive cases, consider additional oral immunosuppressive agents:
  - Azathioprine (dogs: 1-2 mg/kg PO q 24h for 10-14 days, then q 48h).
  - Cyclosporine (3-5 mg/kg PO q 12h; monitor therapeutic concentrations).
- Mucolytic drugs:
  - N-acetylcysteine has a wide therapeutic range with dosage usually of 5-10 mg and up to 100 mg/kg PO q 12h.
    - Intranasal or aerosol delivery of 5-20% solution has also been described.
  - Bromhexine hydrochloride (0.5-1 mg/kg PO) or through aerosol delivery.

CHRONIC TREATMENT

- Intranasal saline (drops or aerosol delivery).
- Mucolytics (as noted in previous paragraphs).
- Long-term oral glucocorticoids: Give the lowest dose at the greatest interval needed to control clinical signs.

POSSIBLE COMPLICATIONS

- Secondary bacterial rhinitis
- Chronic sinusitis

RECOMMENDED MONITORING

Identify and treat episodes of secondary bacterial rhinitis accordingly.

PROGNOSIS AND OUTCOME

- Although clinical signs may appear distressing to owners, and although some cases remain refractory to any treatment, the disease is rarely life threatening.
- In the worst cases, maintenance therapy is generally successful in keeping clinical signs mild.
- Treatment must be sustained since relapses frequently occur.
  - A cure is uncommonly obtained; persistence of mild to moderate clinical signs, despite treatment, is common.
- Owners should prevent their pets' exposure to potential exacerbating factors (e.g., cigarette smoke, perfumes).

PEARLS & CONSIDERATIONS

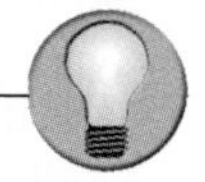

COMMENTS

- Definitive diagnosis is established by elimination of other potential causes of chronic lymphoplasmacytic infiltration of the nasal mucosa, such as chronic aspergillosis, chronic or recurrent infection due to dental disease, primary ciliary dyskinesia, or intranasal neoplasia.
- The disease is chronic and progressive, and cure is rarely achieved.
- There is no therapeutic gold standard.

CLIENT EDUCATION

- Treatment must be sustained since relapses are common.
- Complete cure is rare, but a normal quality of life is expected in most cases.
- Persistence of some degree of clinical signs is expected despite treatment.
- Potential exacerbating factors should be avoided.

SUGGESTED READING

Mackin AJ: Lymphoplasmacytic rhinitis. In King L (ed): *Textbook of Respiratory Diseases*. Philadelphia, WB Saunders, 2004, pp 305-310.

Michiels L, et al: A retrospective study of non-specific rhinitis in 22 cats and the value of nasal cytology and histopathology. *J Feline Med Surg* 5:279, 2003.

Windsor RC, et al: Idiopathic lymphoplasmacytic rhinitis in dogs: 37 cases (1997-2002). *J Am Vet Med Assoc* 224:1952, 2004.

AUTHOR: **CÉCILE CLERCX**

EDITOR: **RANCE K. SELLON**

Rhinosporidiosis

BASIC INFORMATION

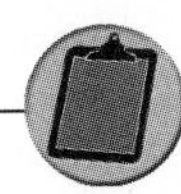

DEFINITION

A fungal infection caused by *Rhinosporidium seeberi*.This organism induces tumor-like growth of epithelial cells. In dogs, this has only been isolated in the nasal cavity. There are no documented cases in cats.

EPIDEMIOLOGY

SPECIES, AGE, SEX

- Species: canine.
- Sex: males > females; whether the condition is behavioral or biologic is unknown.

GENETICS AND BREED PREDISPOSITION: None proven, though large breed dogs tend to be affected.

RISK FACTORS

- Contact with stagnant water
- Nasal mucosal trauma

CONTAGION AND ZOONOSIS

- Humans may be infected from the same environmental point source as dogs.
- No dog-to-dog or dog-to-human infection has been reported.

GEOGRAPHY AND SEASONALITY: Found in the southeastern part of the United States and in other countries; also reported in Ontario and Italy as well as some arid countries.

CLINICAL PRESENTATION

HISTORY, CHIEF COMPLAINT

Presenting complaints include wheezing, sneezing, nasal discharge, or epistaxis.

PHYSICAL EXAM FINDINGS

- Unilateral nasal discharge: mucopurulent.
- Epistaxis.
- Nasal polyps are sometimes visible:
  - Fleshy mass on the nasal mucosa (e.g., in the nostril).
  - Polyp or mass characteristically demonstrates miliary white pinpoint nodules (<0.5 mm in diameter) on its surface. These are sporangia (maturing bodies of the fungus).

ETIOLOGY AND PATHOPHYSIOLOGY

- Infections occur when small spores reach traumatized nasal mucosa. This often occurs in association with contact with stagnant water. However, in humans living in arid countries, the ocular form predominates, potentially with dust as the fomite for inoculation.
- Once the fungal spore reaches the nasal mucosa, it proliferates in epithelial tissue to form sporangia, which can be seen grossly on polyps.
- Polyps are composed of fibrovascular tissue lined by epithelium. Grossly, they can be ulcerated. Exudate associated with polyps contains extruded spores, neutrophils, epithelial cells, and erythrocytes. A mixed inflammatory response throughout the tissues consisting of lymphocytes, plasma cells, and macrophages is also present.

DIAGNOSIS

DIFFERENTIAL DIAGNOSIS

- Other nasal mycoses (i.e., aspergillosis).
- Lymphocytic-plasmacytic rhinitis.
- Parasitic rhinitis (*Pneumonyssoides caninum* or *Capillaria aerophila*).
- Nasal tumors (most commonly squamous cell carcinoma).

INITIAL DATABASE

- Fecal examination (for *C. aerophila*)
- Cytologic examination of exudates
  - Obtained from smears or impression preparations of exudates, ulcerated polyps, and other such sources.
  - Stain using hematoxylin and eosin, Gridley's toluidine blue, Periodic Acid-Schiff, or Grocott's stains, preferably rather than Wright's-type (Diff-Quik) stains.
  - Findings include inflammatory cells (lymphocytes, plasma cells, and macrophages) and identifying spores.
  - Spores are round, walled, and approximately the same diameter as erythrocytes.

ADVANCED OR CONFIRMATORY TESTING

- Rhinoscopy
- Nasal biopsy: for definitive diagnosis if cytologic evaluation was not conclusive
- Skull radiographs or CT scan

TREATMENT

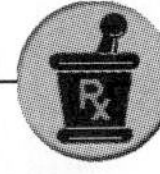

THERAPEUTIC GOAL(S)

Removal of polyps and organisms usually requires surgical excision

ACUTE GENERAL TREATMENT

- Dapsone (1 mg/kg PO q 8h for 2 weeks, then q 12h for 4 months) has been effective with polyp recurrence after initial surgical excision. Possible toxicity (see below) may limit use of the drug.
- Ketoconazole (8.7 mg/kg PO q 8h for 21 days) may be effective if surgery is not an option (elimination of polyps, though possibility of recurrence).

CHRONIC TREATMENT

- Medical therapy may need to be protracted or reinitiated if recurrence of polyps is noted.
- Surgical therapy may also need to be performed again.

DRUG INTERACTIONS

Dapsone and ketoconazole may alter the metabolism of drugs that undergo hepatic biotransformation.

POSSIBLE COMPLICATIONS

- Recurrence is the most common complication.
- Dapsone may cause aplastic anemia, agranulocytosis, cutaneous drug eruption, acute gastrointestinal (GI) signs, and hepatic necrosis.
- Ketoconazole may cause hepatic necrosis and GI signs.

RECOMMENDED MONITORING

- With administration of dapsone, clinicians should monitor complete blood count (CBC) and serum biochemistry profile every 2 to 4 weeks.
- With administration of ketoconazole, clinicians should monitor liver enzymes and bilirubin every 2 to 4 weeks.

PROGNOSIS AND OUTCOME

Surgery may be curative when only one polyp is present. However, recurrence is common, especially with more than one polyp.

PEARLS & CONSIDERATIONS

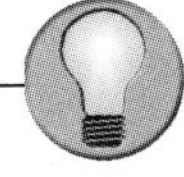

COMMENTS

- Radical surgical excision may be necessary.
- Medical management, while reported, still has questionable utility.

PREVENTION

No specific prevention is available.

SUGGESTED READING

Breitschwerdt EB, et al: Rhinosporidiosis. In Greene CE (ed): *Infectious Disease of the Dog and Cat*. Philadelphia, WB Saunders, 1998, pp 402–404.

Caniatti M, et al: Nasal rhinosporidiosis in dogs: Four cases from Europe and a review of the literature. *Vet Rec* 13:33–338, 1998.

AUTHOR: **JEFFERY SIMMONS**

EDITOR: **DOUGLASS K. MACINTIRE**

Right Bundle Branch Block

BASIC INFORMATION

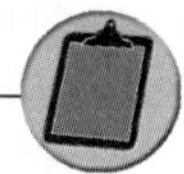

DEFINITION

An intracardiac conduction disturbance involving failure of normal (rapid) conduction from the bundle of His through the right bundle branch to the Purkinje fibers in the right ventricle. The result is a wide, bizarre-appearing QRS complex on the electrocardiogram (ECG) (see Fig. I-148). Right bundle branch block (RBBB) has no clinically meaningful hemodynamic effect on patients and is often a variant of normal. Its main clinical importance lies in the fact that it must not be misinterpreted as a ventricular arrhythmia.

SYNONYM(S)

RBBB

EPIDEMIOLOGY

SPECIES, AGE, SEX: Dogs of any age and either sex; less common in cats.

GENETICS AND BREED PREDISPOSITION: Incomplete RBBB has been recognized in a family of beagles in association with congenital right ventricular structural disease.

ASSOCIATED CONDITIONS AND DISORDERS: RBBB often occurs in normal animals; however, it may be associated with underlying, structural heart diseases such as:

- Cardiomyopathy
- Congenital heart disease
- Heartworm disease

CLINICAL PRESENTATION

DISEASE FORMS/SUBTYPES

- Incomplete or complete RBBB depending on where the block occurs in the right bundle branch.
- Intermittent bundle branch block (left bundle branch block [LBBB] or RBBB) may occur that is heart rate dependent.

HISTORY, CHIEF COMPLAINT: RBBB is an ECG phenomenon only; no overt physical manifestations are expected from RBBB itself.

PHYSICAL EXAM FINDINGS: Typically RBBB is clinically silent and no clinical signs are observed. However, in some individuals split heart sounds may be present due to prolonged right ventricular ejection time and delayed closure of the tricuspid (splitting of the first heart sound) and pulmonic (splitting of the second heart sound) valves. A split second heart sound is most common.

ETIOLOGY AND PATHOPHYSIOLOGY

- With RBBB, impulse formation in the sinoatrial node, atrial depolarization, and passage of the impulse through the AV node all can occur normally; however, distribution of the impulse through the Purkinje fibers in the right ventricle is blocked.
- Conduction to the right ventricle still occurs but is very slow because it must travel from muscle cell to muscle cell.
- This results in a marked delay in conduction to the right ventricle and the QRS complex becomes wide and bizarre on the ECG.
- Additionally, this slow conduction toward the right results in a right axis deviation on the surface ECG.

DIAGNOSIS

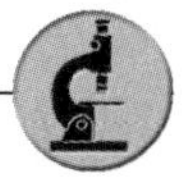

DIFFERENTIAL DIAGNOSIS

- Right ventricular hypertrophy
- Ventricular ectopy
- Ventricular escape rhythm
- Motion artifact

INITIAL DATABASE

By definition, RBBB is an electrocardiographic diagnosis.

- Electrocardiogram characteristics of complete RBBB (see Fig. I-148):
  - Prolonged QRS complex duration (canine: >0.07 second; feline: >0.06 second).
  - Wide and negative QRS complexes with an S wave in leads I, II, III, aVF, and left precordial leads (CV_6LL [V2] and CV_6LU [V4]).
  - Positive QRS complexes in leads aVR, aVL, and CV_5RL (V1 or rV2).
- Electrocardiogram characteristics of incomplete RBBB:
  - When the morphology of the QRS complex as described above is noted, but the QRS duration is normal or only slightly prolonged, incomplete RBBB is suspected. It can be very challenging to differentiate this finding from right

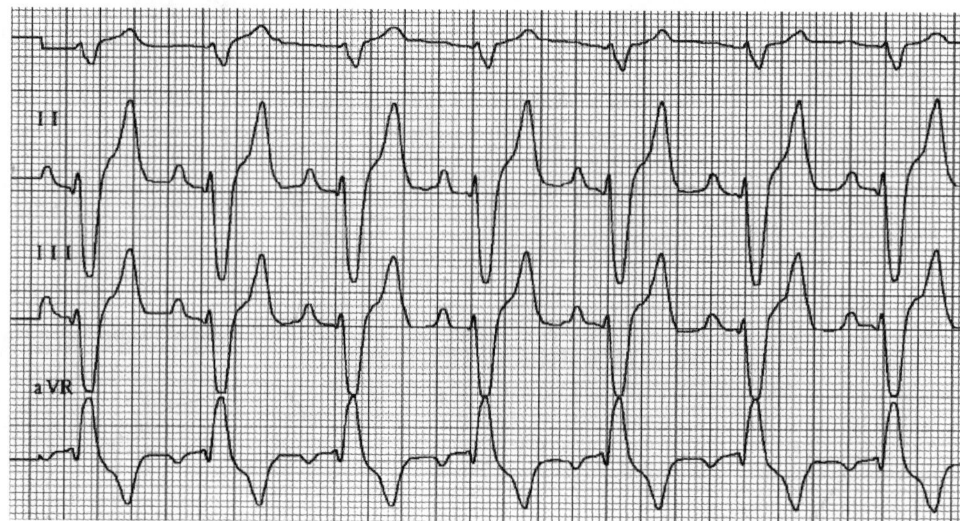

FIGURE I-148 Four-lead ECG (I, II, III, aVR) showing RBBB. Every QRS complex is preceded by a P wave at a repeatable interval, indicating normal conduction from the atria through the AV node to the ventricles. The rhythm is regular (R-R interval is constant) and the heart rate is 150 beats/min. The QRS complexes are wide and bizarre. The ECG diagnosis is normal sinus rhythm with RBBB. 50 mm/sec, 1 cm = 1 mV.

ventricular hypertrophy, and assessment of the ventricle (e.g., echocardiographically) is usually required; if the ventricle is structurally normal, incomplete RBBB is diagnosed by exclusion.

ADVANCED OR CONFIRMATORY TESTING

- Thoracic radiographs to evaluate for right ventricular enlargement.
- Echocardiogram to assess heart structure and function.

TREATMENT

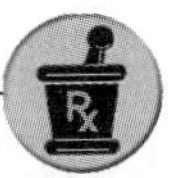

THERAPEUTIC GOAL(S)

- RBBB does not result in clinical or hemodynamic sequelae by itself, and therefore does not require treatment.
- The right bundle branch is anatomically vulnerable to injury and therefore RBBB may be observed in otherwise normal dogs.

POSSIBLE COMPLICATIONS

- Misdiagnosis of RBBB as premature ventricular complexes (PVCs) or ventricular tachcardia can lead to treatment—and toxicosis—with antiarrhythmic drugs.
- Complete block of both the right and left bundle branches produces complete (third degree) atrioventricular block (rare).

PROGNOSIS AND OUTCOME

RBBB is not a progressive or deleterious entity; therefore, the prognosis is good, except when it is associated with structural heart disease in which case the prognosis is the same as that of the underlying disorder.

PEARLS & CONSIDERATIONS

COMMENTS

The bizarre QRS morphology seen with bundle branch block can be confused with ventricular ectopy.

- If P waves are present and the PR is consistent, the complex is likely coming from a supraventricular site (and the bizarre QRS morphology is due to BBB rather than ventricular ectopy). However sometimes P waves are buried and not visible, although the rhythm is supraventricular in origin (particularly with tachycardias). Since most dogs have sinus arrhythmia and some degree of irregularity to the heart rhythm, the regularity of rhythm can be a helpful clue (see Fig. I-152 [p 1005] and Fig. I-185 [p 1148]).
- Supraventricular rhythms (such as sinus rhythm, sinus tachycardia, atrial fibrillation, etc.) respond to vagal maneuvers with slowing of the heart rate, even when RBBB is present. Ventricular arrhythmias do not.

SUGGESTED READING

Kittleson MD: Electrocardiography: basic concepts, diagnosis of chamber enlargement, and intraventricular conduction disturbances. In Kittleson MD, Kienle RD (eds): *Small Animal Cardiovascular Medicine*. Philadelphia, Mosby, 1998, pp 90–94.

Miller MS, Tilley LP, Smith FWK, Fox PR: Electrocardiolgraphy. In Fox PR, Sisson D, Moise NS (eds): *Textbook of Canine and Feline Cardiology*. Philadelphia, WB Saunders, 1999, pp 84–86.

Tilley LP: Left bundle branch block. In Tilley LP (ed): *Essentials of Canine and Feline Electrocardiography*. Philadelphia, Lea & Febiger, 1992, pp 75–77.

AUTHOR: **MEG SLEEPER**
EDITOR: **ETIENNE CÔTÉ**

Rocky Mountain Spotted Fever

BASIC INFORMATION

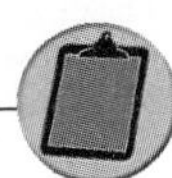

DEFINITION

An acute, potentially life-threatening tick-borne rickettsial disease that affects dogs and people. Clinical signs are vague (lethargy, depression, anorexia, fever; tick exposure), and clinical suspicion justifies treatment, while confirmation is still pending due to the fulminant course of disease in some individuals.

EPIDEMIOLOGY

SPECIES, AGE, SEX

- Species: Dogs and people are primarily affected. Cats have been seropositive but not clinically ill.
- Age: The condition is generally found in young dogs (<2 years), though all ages are represented.

GENETICS AND BREED PREDISPOSITION: Dogs: Purebred dogs (e.g., purebred German shepherds) may be more prone to clinical signs.

RISK FACTORS: Increased risk in animals that are free roaming or that live near wooded areas with higher tick exposure.

CONTAGION AND ZOONOSIS: Direct transmission does not occur from dogs to people. However, dogs are reservoir hosts for the organism and for ticks; increased zoonotic susceptibility may occur in households with infected dogs.

GEOGRAPHY AND SEASONALITY: Rocky Mountain spotted fever (RMSF) is found in North, Central, and South America, with the majority of cases in the United States occurring in the Southeast; disease occurrence is highest in the months of March to October.

ASSOCIATED CONDITIONS AND DISORDERS: Coinfection with other tick-borne diseases, such as ehrlichiosis, can occur.

CLINICAL PRESENTATION

DISEASE FORMS/SUBTYPES

- Clinical and subclinical illness have been reported.
- Clinical disease can be systemic or more localized to various systems (dermatologic, neurologic, ocular).

HISTORY, CHIEF COMPLAINT

- Incubation period can be 2 to 14 days.
- A common feature of RMSF is the vagueness of its initial signs.
- Depression, anorexia, pain, and vomiting are often noted.
- A history of tick exposure or infestation is often noted by the owner.

PHYSICAL EXAM FINDINGS

- Fever: commonly seen within 2 to 3 days of exposure/infection.
- Joint and muscle pain.
- Dyspnea and cough.
- Cutaneous lesions: petechial and ecchymotic hemorrhages (especially on mucous membranes), edema, hyperemia, vesicles, and macules are all possible.

ETIOLOGY AND PATHOPHYSIOLOGY

- *Rickettsia rickettsii* is an obligate intracellular parasite. Ticks become infected by horizontal transmission, transstadially, or transovarial passage. Infection of dogs by affected ticks requires at least 5 to 20 hours from the attachment of the tick. *Dermacentor variabilis* (American dog tick) is the primary vector in the eastern part of the United States and *D. andersoni* (wood tick) is the main vector in the western part of the United States.
- The organism enters the body through the bite of the tick and disseminates via the circulatory system.

- Invasions and replications occur in endothelial cells of small arteries and venules, causing vasculitis, activation of the coagulation cascade, and vasoconstriction.
- These events may cause local necrosis, thrombocytopenia, and increased extracellular fluid accumulation. Plasma loss may cause hypotension subcutaneous, pulmonary, or cerebral edema.
- Organ damage depends on the degree of local damage, most commonly seen in organs with end-arterial circulation, such as the kidneys, brain, heart, and skin. Global effects also may be seen due to severe thrombocytopenia and decreased perfusion as well as systemic inflammation in fulminant cases.

DIAGNOSIS

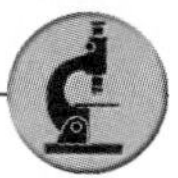

DIFFERENTIAL DIAGNOSIS

Many possibilities exist due to the variety of clinical signs:

- Acute ehrlichiosis
- Babesiosis
- Borreliosis
- Leptospirosis
- Immune-mediated diseases
- Canine distemper
- Bacterial diskospondylitis
- Pneumonia
- Acute renal failure
- Pancreatitis
- Colitis
- Meningitis

INITIAL DATABASE

- Complete blood count (CBC): thrombocytopenia, leukopenia, or leukocytosis; mild to severe anemia
- Serum biochemistry profile: hypoproteinemia, hypoalbuminemia, azotemia, hyponatremia, hypocalcemia, and increased liver enzymes
- Fluid analysis (joint or cerebrospinal fluid [CSF] if affected): mild increase in protein and cells, initially neutrophils and later monocytes

ADVANCED OR CONFIRMATORY TESTING

- Serologic testing: indirect immunofluorescent antibody (IFA) documentation of fourfold or greater increase between acute and convalescent titers or an acute titer of 1:1064 or greater is confirmatory. There can be some cross-reactivity with nonpathogenic rickettsial organisms.
- Direct IFA testing for antigen in tissue biopsy or necropsy samples.
- Polymerase chain reaction (PCR) testing.
- Rickettsial organisms culture (requires a biosafety level-3 lab, not commonly performed).

TREATMENT

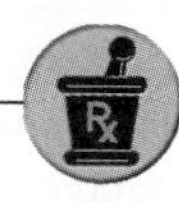

THERAPEUTIC GOAL(S)

- Supportive care of affected organs and wounds
- Removal of organisms

ACUTE GENERAL TREATMENT

- Tetracycline (22 mg/kg PO, IV, q 8h for 14 to 21 days) or doxycycline (5-10 mg/kg PO, IV, q 12h for 14 to 21 days); or
- Chloramphenicol (15-30 mg/kg PO, SC, IV, IM, q 8h for 14 days); or
- Enrofloxacin (5-10 mg/kg PO, slow IV, IM, q 12h for 14 days).
- Prednisolone (1-4 mg/kg PO q 24h) does not potentiate severity in experimental infections and may minimize immune-mediated complications.
- Fluid therapy and other supportive therapies to improve perfusion without increasing extracellular fluid loss.

RECOMMENDED MONITORING

- Repeat serologic testing or monitoring antigen levels in repeat biopsies may help confirm resolution.
- A fourfold increase in acute and convalescent titers is considered diagnostic.
- Following treatment, the titers should decrease after 4 or 5 months.
- Monitoring of platelet levels and coagulation parameters for signs of severe coagulopathy, including disseminated intravascular coagulation.

PROGNOSIS AND OUTCOME

- With early diagnosis, prognosis is usually excellent.
- Delayed diagnosis, fulminant disease, and the use of ineffective antibiotics (penicillins, cephalosporins, etc.) have been shown to increase mortality.

PEARLS & CONSIDERATIONS

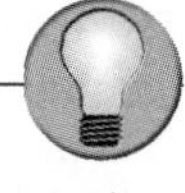

PREVENTION

- Owners should limit outdoor roaming, especially in wooded areas.
- Adequate tick control is ideal.
- Lifelong immunity may follow treated disease.

CLIENT EDUCATION

- RMSF in dogs should be a warning to owners that they may also have been exposed to the agent, though not via zoonosis.
- Care should be taken when removing ticks from pets to minimize human exposure.

SUGGESTED READING

Breitschwerdt EB: The Rickettsioses. In Ettinger SJ, Feldman EC (eds): *Textbook of Veterinary Internal Medicine*. Philadelphia, WB Saunders, 2000, pp 400-401.

Gasser AM, et al: Canine Rocky Mountain spotted fever: A retrospective of 30 cases. *J Amer Animal Hosp Assoc* 37:41-48, 2001.

Greene CE, Breitschwerdt EB: Rocky Mountain spotted fever, Q fever, and typhus. In Greene CE (ed): *Infectious Diseases of Dogs and Cats*. Philadelphia, WB Saunders, 1998, pp 155-162.

Warner RD, Marsh WW: Rocky Mountain spotted fever. *J Amer Vet Med Assoc* 221:1413-1417, 2002.

AUTHOR: **JEFFERY SIMMONS**
EDITOR: **DOUGLASS K. MACINTIRE**

Root Signature (Nerve)

BASIC INFORMATION

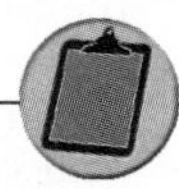

DEFINITION

Non-weight-bearing lameness and pain resulting from disturbances in sensation within a nerve root or sensory nerve of the cervical or lumbosacral intumescence; usually the result of nerve compression

EPIDEMIOLOGY

SPECIES, AGE, SEX: Dependent on underlying cause; dogs: older adults (neoplasia); cats: young adults (lymphoma).

GENETICS AND BREED PREDISPOSITION: Dogs: dachshund, cocker spaniel, beagle, other chondrodystrophoid breeds (intervertebral disk disease [IVDD]); German shepherds (degenerative lumbosacral stenosis).

RISK FACTORS: Cats: multicat household (risk of feline leukemia virus [FeLV]).
CONTAGION AND ZOONOSIS: Cats: FeLV (cat-to-cat).

CLINICAL PRESENTATION

DISEASE FORMS/SUBTYPES

- Acute (IVDD)
- Chronic, progressive (neoplasia)
- Intermittent (degenerative lumbosacral stenosis)

HISTORY, CHIEF COMPLAINT

- Thoracic limbs > pelvic limbs.
- Non–weight-bearing lameness and pain.
- Paravertebral pain.
- Trauma.
- Difficulty rising, reluctance to jump.
- Lack of response to anti-inflammatory medications.

PHYSICAL EXAM FINDINGS

- Non–weight-bearing lameness (limb typically held in flexion).
- Focal hyperesthesia (pain), typically following the dermatomal distribution of the affected nerve. A hallmark of nerve root signature is pain.
- Paresis and hypotonia of the affected limb.
- Neurogenic muscle atrophy if chronic (>1 week).
- Ipsilateral Horner's syndrome (T1-T3).
- Ipsilateral cutaneous trunci deficit (C8, T1).
- Paraspinal pain, resistance to cervical manipulation.
- Axillary or inguinal pain.
- Palpable axillary mass (uncommon).
- Paraparesis, hemiparesis, or tetraparesis if involvement of the spinal cord.
- Evidence of external trauma.

ETIOLOGY AND PATHOPHYSIOLOGY

- Lateralized or foraminal intervertebral disk extrusion.
- Neoplasia (peripheral nerve sheath tumors, lymphoma, primary neural tumors, metastatic).
- Trauma.
- Degenerative lumbosacral stenosis.
- Diskospondylitis.
- Summary: Clinical signs result from a sensory disturbance within the dorsal root or spinal nerve, typically by compression.
- The spinal cord may be affected in all cases, causing long tract signs (e.g., gait deficit distal to the lesion).
- The dorsal longitudinal ligament of the vertebral column is thicker in the cervical region, predisposing animals to lateral disk extrusions at this site.

DIAGNOSIS

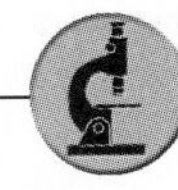

DIFFERENTIAL DIAGNOSIS

- Orthopedic disorders
- Soft-tissue injury

INITIAL DATABASE

- Complete neurologic and orthopedic examinations.
- Vertebral radiographs: rule out orthopedic causes, bony neoplasia, chronic diskospondylitis; may support a diagnosis of IVDD, degenerative lumbosacral stenosis, or nerve sheath neoplasm (enlarged intervertebral foramen).
- Note: Many animals have orthopedic disease unrelated to the clinical signs.

ADVANCED OR CONFIRMATORY TESTING

- Myelography and epidurography: useful for IVDD, degenerative lumbosacral stenosis, nerve sheath neoplasm.
- CT and MRI: permit evaluation of the nerve roots, location of extruded disk material.
- Electromyography (EMG): Changes are present 1 week following denervation of muscle.
- Cerebrospinal fluid (CSF) analysis.
- Biopsy: allows definitive diagnosis of confirmed mass lesions; benefit must be weighed against risk of procedure.
- Surgical exploration.

TREATMENT

THERAPEUTIC GOAL(S)

- Removal of the source of nerve root or spinal nerve impingement
- Provision of the optimal environment for nerve recovery

ACUTE GENERAL TREATMENT

Dependent on underlying cause:

- Surgical decompression for IVDD, degerative lumbosacral stenosis.
- Tumor resection with or without limb amputation and laminectomy for peripheral nerve sheath neoplasm; surgical intervention should be considered early in these cases (reduce extension of tumor/spinal cord involvement).
- Conservative therapy: generally ineffective in relieving pain of cervical IVDD.

CHRONIC TREATMENT

- Attempt conservative therapy (corticosteroids, protection of the distal limb with a boot, physiotherapy) for traumatic injuries. Amputation should be delayed for 6 months if possible to allow for reinnervation.
- Radiation therapy: nerve sheath tumors.
- Lifelong exercise modification: IVDD.
- Physiotherapy: if trauma has compromised limb use.

POSSIBLE COMPLICATIONS

- Persistent or progressive clinical signs
- Recurrence or acute progression of clinical signs (IVDD)
- Self-mutilation associated with dysesthesia
- Distal limb trauma associated with decreased sensation and normal activity
- Surgical complications

RECOMMENDED MONITORING

Follow-up exam and serial diagnostic studies as directed by the animal's clinical progression

PROGNOSIS AND OUTCOME

Dependent on underlying cause:

- Good to excellent (according to clinical signs) with IVDD treated with decompression
- Fair to good (according to clinical signs) with degenerative lumbosacral stenosis
- Guarded to fair with traumatic injury
- Poor with nerve sheath neoplasia

PEARLS & CONSIDERATIONS

COMMENTS

- It can be difficult to distinguish orthopedic from neurologic causes for clinical signs, and both may be present with traumatic injury. Careful examination with particular attention to muscle tone and sensory deficits is important.
- A ruptured cranial cruciate ligament is often mistaken for a lumbar nerve root signature and vice versa.
- Nerve sheath neoplasms are most common in the cervical intumescence (80%).

CLIENT EDUCATION

Monitor for recurrence of clinical signs

SUGGESTED READING

McDonnell J, et al: Neurologic conditions causing lameness in companion animals. *Vet Clin N Am: Sm Anim Pract* 31(1):17-38, 2001.

AUTHORS: **GREG KILBURN, JOLI M. JARBOE**
EDITOR: **ETIENNE CÔTÉ**

Round Cell Tumors

BASIC INFORMATION

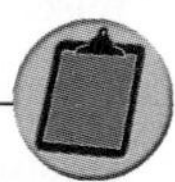

DEFINITION

- Round cell tumors are composed of a homogenous population of cells that have well-defined cytoplasmic margins, are round in shape, and have a round nucleus. Distinct cytologic characteristics of each type of round cell aid in definitive diagnosis.
- Tumor types include lymphoma, mast cell tumor (MCT), transmissible venereal tumor (TVT), histiocytoma, and plasma cell tumor. Malignant melanoma is highly variable in appearance and is often classified as a round cell tumor.
- Round cell tumors can be either malignant (e.g., lymphoma, grade II or III mast cell tumors) or benign (histiocytoma, grade I mast cell tumor).

SYNONYM(S)

Discrete cell tumors

EPIDEMIOLOGY

SPECIES, AGE, SEX

Dependent on tumor type

CLINICAL PRESENTATION

DISEASE FORMS/SUBTYPES

- Lymphoma (malignant lymphoma, lymphosarcoma) is seen in dogs and cats of all ages, and can affect any organ system. In dogs, the most common form involves generalized lymph node infiltration; in cats, the gastrointestinal form prevails.
- Mast cell tumors (mastocytomas, mast cell sarcomas) are seen in dogs and cats. The most common form is skin and subcutaneous masses. In cats, a splenic or visceral form can occur.
- Transmissible venereal tumors (TVT) are transplanted from dog to dog by direct contact. TVT is most commonly seen in intact dogs in the genital regions and oral and nasal cavities.
- Histiocytomas are most commonly seen in young dogs (<3 years age). They are usually small (<2 cm), raised, and alopecic.
- Plasma cell tumors (plasmacytomas) most commonly occur in dogs as skin and subcutaneous masses. The systemic form of plasma cell cancer is multiple myeloma. Plasma cell neoplasia is rare in cats.
- Melanomas are most commonly seen in the skin, oral cavity, and digits of dogs. They are rare in cats.

HISTORY, CHIEF COMPLAINT: Dependent on tumor type.

PHYSICAL EXAM FINDINGS: Dependent on tumor type.

ETIOLOGY AND PATHOPHYSIOLOGY

Dependent on tumor type

DIAGNOSIS

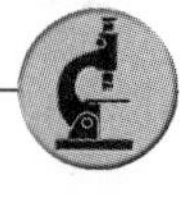

DIFFERENTIAL DIAGNOSIS

Dependent on tumor type (see chapters on specific tumor types)

INITIAL DATABASE

- Cytologic evaluation will confirm the cell type (diagnosis) for many round cell tumors.
- The following cytologic characteristics are commonly seen in these specific cell types:
    - Lymphoma: high nuclear to cytoplasmic ratio; multiple nucleoli; thin rim of dark blue cytoplasm; chromatin is clumped; mitotic figures numerous; in large granular lymphocyte lymphoma (uncommon form of lymphoma seen most commonly in the gastrointestinal tract of cats): red to purple granules are present that are larger and less numerous than granules in MCT.
    - Mast cell tumor: low nuclear to cytoplasmic ratio; nuclear details obscured by pink to purple intracytoplasmic granules that are present in most MCT (in some poorly differentiated MCT, granules are absent); eosinophils are often present.
    - Transmissible venereal tumor: cytoplasmic vacuolation is common and distinctive; chromatin is coarse; nucleoli are prominent; mitotic figures may be seen; inflammatory cells such as lymphocytes and plasma cells may be seen.
    - Histiocytoma: low to intermediate nuclear to cytoplasmic ratio; anisocytosis and anisokaryosis common; the cytoplasm is pale and may contain fine granules; cytoplasmic vacuolation is sometimes seen; mitotic figures are occasionally seen; inflammatory cells are present when tumors are regressing (histiocytomas often spontaneously regress).
    - Plasma cell tumor: perinuclear clear zone adjacent to nucleus; eccentrically positioned nucleus; chromatin is clumped; large amount of dark blue cytoplasm; bi- and tri-nucleation can be seen but does not correlate with the degree of malignancy
    - Melanoma: can have the appearance of an epithelial, mesenchymal, or round cell tumor; green, brown, or black intracytoplasmic granules often seen, but are not always present (absence = amelanotic melanoma).

ADVANCED OR CONFIRMATORY TESTING

- In some cases, the tumor type is not readily distinguished cytologically; a biopsy of the lesion should be submitted for histopathologic analysis. If the cell lineage is still not determined, immunohistochemistry or special stains may be performed.
- Special stains such as toluidine blue or Giemsa can identify granules in MCT.
- Immunohistochemistry involves the use of antibodies directed against specific cell antigens that are markers of individual cell types. These antibodies are linked to dyes that are visualized using a microscope. Examples include: CD3, CD4, CD8 (T lymphocytes); CD21, CD79a (B lymphocytes), Melan A or S-100 (melanocytes).

TREATMENT

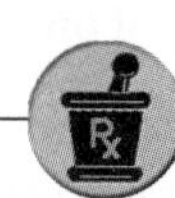

THERAPEUTIC GOAL(S)

Dependent on tumor type

ACUTE AND CHRONIC TREATMENT

Dependent on tumor type

PROGNOSIS AND OUTCOME

Dependent on tumor type

PEARLS & CONSIDERATIONS

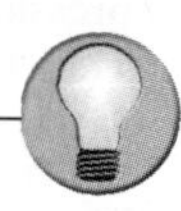

COMMENTS

Round cell tumors are one of three cytologic categories of major tumor types: carcinomas (epithelial tumors), sarcomas (mesenchymal tumors), and round cell tumors. The diagnosis of round cell tumors is generally straightforward with cytology, and treatment, staging, and prognosis are dependent on tumor type.

SUGGESTED READING

DeNicola D, Reagan WJ: Using cytology in the diagnosis of cancer. In Morrison WB (ed): *Cancer in Dogs and Cats*, ed 2. Jackson, WY, Teton New Media, 2002, pp 71–87.

Powers B: Tumour pathology. In Dobson JM, Lascelles BDX (eds): *BSAVA Manual of Canine and Feline Oncology*. Haryana, India, Replika Press, 2003, pp 10–17.

AUTHOR: **TRACY GIEGER**
EDITOR: **KENNETH M. RASSNICK**

Roundworm Infection

BASIC INFORMATION

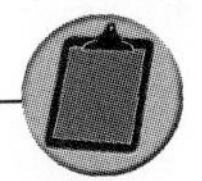

DEFINITION

Infection with a small intestinal roundworm (*Toxocara or Toxascaris* spp.)

SYNONYM(S)

Toxocariasis
Ascarid infection
Infection with *Toxocara canis* (dog) or *T. cati* (cat)
Infection with *T. leonina*

EPIDEMIOLOGY

SPECIES, AGE, SEX: Young puppies and kittens less than 6 months old are most commonly infected; no sex predilection. Clinically significant disease is uncommon in adult dogs and cats. *T. canis* affects dogs, *T. cati* affects cats, and *T. leonina* affects both dogs and cats.

RISK FACTORS: Young animals and pregnant dogs and cats are more susceptible to infection.

CONTAGION AND ZOONOSIS: *Toxocara* spp. eggs within the environment are infective, via ingestion, to people and other dogs and cats. Infection with *Toxocara* spp. is the most common cause of human visceral and ocular larva migrans. Young children are most susceptible. *T. leonina* is not zoonotic.

GEOGRAPHY AND SEASONALITY: *Toxocara* spp. are found worldwide with a higher incidence in lower socioeconomic communities.

ASSOCIATED CONDITIONS AND DISORDERS: Commonly found in association with other intestinal parasites. Intussusception and, with very large worm burdens, intestinal obstruction are possible.

CLINICAL PRESENTATION

DISEASE FORMS/SUBTYPES

- Intestinal infestation is most common.
- Aberrant migration of larvae may rarely cause neurologic or ocular disease.

HISTORY, CHIEF COMPLAINT

- Commonly normal; the parasite is discovered incidentally during a routine fecal examination, or infection is never detected.
- Intestinal: in overt cases, presence of worms in feces or diarrhea, a pot-bellied appearance in young puppies or kittens, or occasional vomiting with or without worms may prompt the owner to seek veterinary attention.

PHYSICAL EXAM FINDINGS: Typically, no physical abnormalities are noted. It has been speculated that essentially all puppies have *Toxocara*. It is possible for young puppies and kittens with severe infections to have a pot-bellied appearance and/or evidence of diarrhea or intestinal obstruction due to worm burden.

ETIOLOGY AND PATHOPHYSIOLOGY

- The primary mode of transmission of *T. canis* is transplacental from the infected bitch to puppies.
- Puppies and kittens may also be infected with *T. canis* or *T. cati*, respectively, by nursing an infected lactating dam or queen (transmammary transmission). The transmammary route is the principal form of transmission in cats.
- Fecal-oral transmission is also a possible route of infection, as is ingestion of other hosts such as rodents.
- After infection, the parasite may migrate through the liver into the lungs (*T. canis* and *T. cati*), within the wall of the gastrointestinal (GI) tract (*T. canis, T. cati*, and *T. leonina*), or somatically within the tissues (*T. canis, T. cati*). Puppies and kittens may begin to shed eggs within 2.5 to 3.5 weeks and generally continue to do so until age 4 to 6 months.
- Eggs are highly resistant and long-lived within the environment. They adhere easily to fomites. Eggs are most susceptible to heat. A 20% bleach solution will decrease the adherence of the eggs but will not kill them.

DIAGNOSIS

DIFFERENTIAL DIAGNOSIS

- Infections with *Ancylostoma caninum* (hookworms), *Trichuris vulpis* (whipworms), *Giardia lamblia*, and coccidia
- Campylobacter enteritis
- Canine parvovirus
- Feline panleukopenia
- Intussusception or foreign body ingestion (if obstruction)

INITIAL DATABASE

Fecal examination should be performed in all puppies and kittens up to 6 months of age. Eggs are easily detected in a simple fecal flotation.

TREATMENT

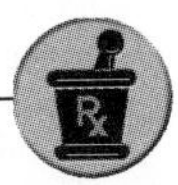

THERAPEUTIC GOAL(S)

Remove infection and prevent environmental contamination and reinfection.

ACUTE GENERAL TREATMENT

- The Center for Disease Control and Prevention (CDC) and Association of Veterinary Parasitologists recommend deworming all puppies beginning at 2 weeks with additional treatments at 4, 6, and 8 weeks of age. Semi-monthly deworming may be continued up to 12 weeks of age. These recommendations aim to reduce zoonotic risk by decreasing environmental parasite burden.
- Deworm kittens at 6 weeks of age and again at 8 and 10 weeks.
- Deworm puppies and kittens monthly after they reach 3 months of age.
- Deworm puppies and kittens even if fecal results are negative to ensure removal of prepatent worms prior to shedding.
- Treat lactating bitches and queens to prevent further transmammary transmission.
- Most deworming medications are effective against ascarids. Pyrantel pamoate (5–10 mg/kg PO; considered safe during pregnancy) is used most widely. Other anthelmintics (e.g., milbemycin oxime, moxidectin, selamectin) have antiascarid activity but are not used in a 2-week protocol as previously described. Ivermectin at parasiticidal doses may be effective (*T. canis* > *T. leonina*), but alternatives with a wider safety margin are preferred.
- Many products used for heartworm prevention are also effective against roundworms.

CHRONIC TREATMENT

Environmental decontamination should be considered in all animals, especially those with repeated infections or adult animals with infection.

DRUG INTERACTIONS

The parasiticidal dose of ivermectin (200 μg/kg) should not be used in collies or other susceptible breeds.

PROGNOSIS AND OUTCOME

Prognosis is excellent for appropriately treated animals

PEARLS & CONSIDERATIONS

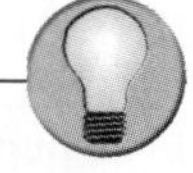

COMMENTS

- All puppies and kittens should be strategically dewormed to prevent environmental contamination and human exposure.
- The zoonotic risk associated with *Toxocara* spp. parasites outweighs their impact on dogs and cats.

PREVENTION

- Treatment of pregnant dogs and cats can decrease the level of transplacental and transmammary infection of puppies and kittens. Common treatment regimes described for dogs include fenbendazole (50 mg/kg) PO once daily from day 40 of gestation to day 14 of lactation or ivermectin (200 μg/kg), once a week from 3 weeks prior to whelping to 3 weeks after whelping.
- Pregnant cats may be treated with topical selamectin (6 mg/kg) 6 weeks and 2 weeks before parturition and 2 weeks and 6 weeks after parturition.

CLIENT EDUCATION

Warn all clients of the risks of exposure to *Toxocara*, especially those clients with young children or those who are immunosuppressed.

SUGGESTED READING

Kazacos KR: Larval migrans from pets and wildlife. In *2002 Tufts Animal Expo Proceedings Online.* North Grafton, MA: www.vin.com/Members/Proceedings.plx?CID=TUFTS2002&O=VIN.

Reinemeyer CR: Canine gastrointestinal parasites. In Bonagura JD (ed): *Kirk's Current Veterinary Therapy XII.* Philadelphia, WB Saunders, 1995, pp 711-716.

AUTHOR: **KATHRYN TAYLOR**

EDITOR: **DOUGLASS K. MACINTIRE**

Salivary Gland Neoplasia

BASIC INFORMATION

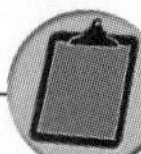

DEFINITION

Neoplasm arising from the salivary gland; typically locally invasive and may metastasize

EPIDEMIOLOGY

SPECIES, AGE, SEX

- Older dogs and cats
- Male cats more commonly affected than females (2:1 ratio)

GENETICS AND BREED PREDISPOSITION

- Dogs: spaniel breeds at increased risk
- Cats: Siamese cats may be predisposed

RISK FACTORS: Unknown. In people, occupational exposure to carcinogens in hair salons and the rubber industry increases risk, as does prior radiation to head and neck; influence of alcohol and tobacco smoke are controversial.

CLINICAL PRESENTATION

DISEASE FORMS/SUBTYPES

- Salivary gland adenocarcinomas
- Squamous cell carcinoma
- Mucoepidermoid carcinoma
- Anaplastic carcinoma
- Complex carcinoma
- Adenomas, myoepitheliomas, and sarcomas are rare

HISTORY, CHIEF COMPLAINT

- Presence of a mass noted by the owner in the pet's upper neck, base of ear, lip, maxilla, or tongue
- Halitosis
- Weight loss
- Inappetence
- Dysphagia
- Exophthalmos
- Sneezing
- Dysphonia

PHYSICAL EXAM FINDINGS

- Palpable mass in the region of the salivary gland
    - The mass is typically not warm or painful (in contrast to sialadenitis).
    - In cats, the mandibular salivary gland is most commonly affected (ventral and medial to the angle of the mandible).
    - In dogs, the parotid salivary gland is most commonly affected (caudal, ventral, and cranial to the external ear canal).
- Halitosis
- Lymphadenomegaly
- Exophthalmos
- Horner's syndrome

ETIOLOGY AND PATHOPHYSIOLOGY

- Unknown etiology.
- Salivary gland tumors are locally invasive and have a low to moderate rate of metastasis. Metastatic rate to regional lymph nodes is 39% for cats and 17% for dogs. The rate of pulmonary metastasis is 16% for cats and 8% for dogs.

DIAGNOSIS

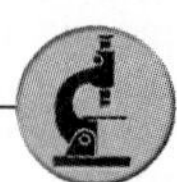

DIFFERENTIAL DIAGNOSIS

- Abscess
- Mucocele
- Sialadenitis
- Lymphoma
- Lymphadenopathy

INITIAL DATABASE

- Fine-needle aspiration and cytologic examination of primary mass, to confirm mass as salivary gland in origin and to differentiate an inflammatory lesion from a neoplasm.
- Fine-needle aspiration and cytologic examination of any enlarged regional lymph nodes, to differentiate reactive from metastatic disease.
- Thoracic radiographs (three views), to screen for pulmonary metastasis.
- Complete blood count, serum biochemical panel, and urinalysis are usually normal and are used as a general health screen prior to therapy.

ADVANCED OR CONFIRMATORY TESTING

- Biopsy with histopathologic evaluation of tissue
- Computed tomography (CT) or magnetic resonance imaging (MRI) to determine feasibility of surgically resecting tumor

TREATMENT

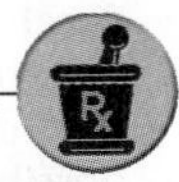

THERAPEUTIC GOAL(S)

- Short-term: relief of discomfort or dysfunction associated with presence of mass
- Long-term: delay of disease progression (slow or prevent local recurrence or metastasis)

ACUTE GENERAL TREATMENT

- Surgical resection of mass when possible
- Adjuvant radiation therapy when mass is narrowly or incompletely excised to prevent local recurrence, or for palliation in cases where mass is nonresectable
- Chemotherapy to delay or prevent metastasis, but no data on efficacy are currently available

CHRONIC TREATMENT

- Antibiotics as needed to control secondary infection if they occur (e.g., cephalexin 22 mg/kg PO q 8h)
- Anti-inflammatory drugs for comfort (e.g., carprofen 2 mg/kg PO q 12h or meloxicam 0.1 mg/kg PO q 24h)

POSSIBLE COMPLICATIONS

Damage to the facial nerve during parotid gland surgery may produce facial paralysis, inability to blink, and exposure keratitis.

RECOMMENDED MONITORING

- Primary tumor site
- Regional lymph nodes
- Thoracic radiographs

PROGNOSIS AND OUTCOME

- Currently, there are only limited data available for dogs and cats with salivary carcinomas. In one study, the median survival time was 550 days in dogs and 516 days in cats. A lower mitotic index was a negative prognostic indicator in cats.
- Adjuvant radiation therapy likely has a role in the treatment of incompletely excised salivary gland tumors, but data to confirm this suspicion are lacking.

PEARLS & CONSIDERATIONS

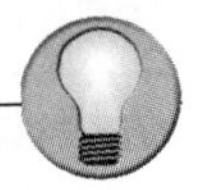

CLIENT EDUCATION

Salivary gland neoplasms are aggressive forms of cancer with a poor long-term prognosis.

SUGGESTED READING

Hammer A, et al: Salivary gland neoplasia in the dog and cat: survival times and prognostic factors. *J Am Anim Hosp Assoc* 37(5):478–482, 2001.

AUTHOR: **LINDA S. FINEMAN**
EDITOR: **KENNETH M. RASSNICK**

Salmon Poisoning

BASIC INFORMATION

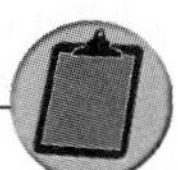

DEFINITION

A febrile rickettsial infection of dogs in the Pacific northwestern United States and Pacific coastal Canada, associated with ingestion of raw fish

SYNONYM(S)

Neorickettsia helminthoeca
Salmon poisoning disease

EPIDEMIOLOGY

SPECIES, AGE, SEX: Dogs: any age, both sexes affected.

RISK FACTORS: Exposure to a fresh brackish stream or beach is commonly elicited in the history.

GEOGRAPHY AND SEASONALITY: Infections are limited to the habitat range of the intermediate snail host (*Oxytrema silicula*) in western British Columbia, Washington, Oregon, northern California, and more sporadically in areas where fish carrying the causative organism, *Neorickettsia helminthoeca*, migrate or are transported. Dogs have the greatest access to dead fish during spawning seasons (late summer to early winter).

CLINICAL PRESENTATION

DISEASE FORMS/SUBTYPES

- Acute, severe febrile illness 5 to 7 days after fish ingestion, often fatal.
- A more moderate illness may be seen as late as 14 to 33 days after exposure, particularly with the Elokomin Fluke Fever disease variant.

HISTORY, CHIEF COMPLAINT

- Acute onset of anorexia, and lethargy associated with fever
- Vomiting and bloody diarrhea common
- Oculonasal discharge occasionally reported

PHYSICAL EXAM FINDINGS

- Fever
- Lymphadenopathy
- Signs of hypovolemic shock (tachycardia, collapse, poor pulse quality)

ETIOLOGY AND PATHOPHYSIOLOGY

- Dogs acquire the causative organism (*N. helminthoeca*), and therefore the disease, from a fluke parasite (*Nanophyteus salmincola*) carried in the kidneys of salmon, and rarely other fish or salamanders.
- Rickettsial infection transmitted when flukes mature in the canine gastrointestinal (GI) tract.
  - Fluke maturation in the GI tract involves release of the rickettsiae, which are taken up into macrophages and disseminate to lymph nodes (especially mesenteric).
  - Replication of the organism actually occurs in the lymph nodes and this is where the lesions are most pronounced (other than the inflammatory response that occurs in the GI mucosa due to the flukes and rickettsiae eliciting an immune response).
- Systemic rickettsial replication results in clinical disease in dogs.

DIAGNOSIS

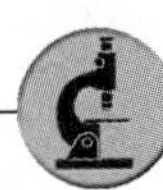

DIFFERENTIAL DIAGNOSIS

- Parvoviral enteritis
- Ehrlichial infections
- Acute gastroenteritis
- Sepsis (e.g., due to foreign body perforation, cholangiohepatitis)
- Pancreatitis
- Neoplasia, especially GI lymphoma

INITIAL DATABASE

- Complete blood count and serum biochemical findings are inconsistent but may include thrombocytopenia, lymphopenia, eosinophilia, hypoalbuminemia, and elevated alkaline phosphatase.
- Operculated fluke eggs are most easily seen on fecal sediment exam, but may be seen on direct smear or fecal flotation.

ADVANCED OR CONFIRMATORY TESTING

- Giemsa-stained lymph node aspirates may reveal intracytoplasmic rickettsial bodies.

- Response to treatment in clinically suspect dogs is the most common method of clinical confirmation.

TREATMENT

THERAPEUTIC GOAL(S)

- Resolution of fever, anorexia, and GI signs, and stabilization of associated cardiovascular shock and systemic illness
- Eradication of the underlying parasite

ACUTE GENERAL TREATMENT

- Hospitalization is recommended for intravenous fluid support and alleviation of vomiting and diarrhea.
- Mild cases: Rickettsial infection can be treated with oral doxycycline (10 mg/kg q 12h) or tetracycline (22 mg/kg q 8h) for 5 to 7 days.
- Severe cases, particularly with vomiting/diarrhea: Parenteral doxycycline (10 mg/kg IV q 12h until oral form is tolerated), oxytetracycline (7 mg/kg IV q 8h × 3 days), or ampicillin (20-30 mg/kg IV q 6h).
- Praziquantel (10-30 mg/kg PO or SQ once) is effective for elimination of the fluke.

PROGNOSIS AND OUTCOME

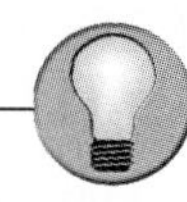

- Prognosis is fair to good in aggressively managed cases; recovery is usually noted within 2 to 3 days after treatment initiation.
- Death is likely within 5 to 10 days if the disease remains untreated.

PEARLS & CONSIDERATIONS

COMMENTS

- Salmon poisoning is an important cause of fever, lymphadenopathy, and severe GI signs in dogs in the Pacific northwestern United States and Pacific coastal Canada.
- Clinical signs are indistinguishable from parvoviral enteritis.
- Fecal direct and sedimentation exams and treatment with doxycycline are recommended in febrile dogs when possible ingestion of raw fish is noted in disease-endemic regions.

PREVENTION

Restrict canine access to raw fish in the Pacific Northwest

CLIENT EDUCATION

Early aggressive treatment is required for salmon poisoning or death is likely.

SUGGESTED READING

Gorham JR, Foreyt WJ: Salmon poisoning disease. In Greene CE (ed): *Infectious Disease of the Dog and Cat*. Philadelphia, WB Saunders, 1998, pp 135-139.

AUTHOR: **POLLY B. PETERSON**
EDITOR: **DEBRA L. ZORAN**

Salmonellosis

BASIC INFORMATION

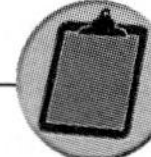

DEFINITION

Infection of susceptible patients with pathogenic *Salmonella* spp.

EPIDEMIOLOGY

SPECIES, AGE, SEX

- Many species can be infected including cats, dogs, and people.
- Cats appear to be more resistant to *Salmonella* infection.
- Younger animals are more commonly affected.

RISK FACTORS

- Young, immunocompromised patients.
- Feeding raw or undercooked meat products or diets.
- Overcrowded, unsanitary, or stressful conditions.
- Concurrent gastrointestinal (GI) infections.
- Antibiotic therapy.

CONTAGION AND ZOONOSIS

- Infected dogs and cats are a major risk to people, especially immunocompromised persons.
- Risk to people increases if pets are eating raw meat diets.
- Undercooked meat is also a risk for people if ingested.

ASSOCIATED CONDITIONS AND DISORDERS: Bacterial endocarditis (cats).

CLINICAL PRESENTATION

DISEASE FORMS/SUBTYPES

- Up to 30% of dogs are subclinical carriers.
- Acute enterocolitis.
- Chronic diarrhea rare.
- Septicemia/endotoxemia.
- Cats may develop chronic, febrile illness.

HISTORY, CHIEF COMPLAINT

- Watery to mucoid diarrhea with or without blood
- Straining or increased urgency to defecate
- Vomiting
- Anorexia and lethargy
- Weight loss

PHYSICAL EXAM FINDINGS

- Fever.
- Abdominal pain.
- Dehydration.
- Pale mucous membranes, tachycardia, tachypnea, weakness, weak pulses if septicemic.

ETIOLOGY AND PATHOPHYSIOLOGY

- *Salmonella* spp: gram-negative, aerobic, motile, non-spore-forming rods from the family Enterobacteriaceae.
- Most common route of transmission is through contact with infected food, water, or fomites.
- Bacterium survives for long periods, up to 6 weeks, in environment.
- Clinical signs occur secondary to mucosal invasion and epithelial injury.
  - *Salmonella* spp. also produce an enterotoxin resulting in secretory diarrhea.
- Organism persists in phagocytic cells of intestinal mucosa and mesenteric lymph nodes, liver, and spleen.
  - Results in persistent shedding for 3 to 6 weeks after infection.
- Bacteremia and endotoxemia may occur in association with mucosal invasion resulting in systemic infection and possibly the systemic inflammatory response syndrome (SIRS).
- Persistence and severity of infection depend on the patient's immune status.

DIAGNOSIS

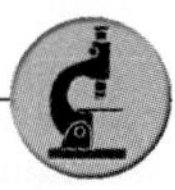

DIFFERENTIAL DIAGNOSIS

- Viral diarrhea: parvovirus, coronavirus, rotavirus.
- Bacterial diarrhea: *Clostridium*, *Campylobacter* enteritides.
- GI parasites.
- Dietary indiscretion.
- Bacterial endocarditis or septicemia due to other causes.

INITIAL DATABASE

Complete blood count and biochemistry profile changes are generally nonspecific.

- Neutropenia with left shift and toxic neutrophils in acute phase.
- Neutrophilia if chronic illness.
- Nonregenerative, possibly hypochromic anemia may be noted.
- Thrombocytopenia in severe cases with septicemia leading to disseminated intravascular coagulation (DIC).
- Hypoproteinemia due to GI loss.

Fecal flotation, direct smear, and parvoviral ELISA test as needed to address differential diagnosis.

ADVANCED OR CONFIRMATORY TESTING

- Fecal bacterial culture:
  - Best results using enrichment broth or selective culture media.
  - Positive fecal culture establishes infection but not necessarily that signs are due to salmonellosis, since subclinical carriers are common.
  - Positive culture from blood, bile, or other normally sterile samples is more strongly indicative of salmonellosis.
  - False negative results are possible since organism grows fastidiously.
- Serologic testing is used in establishing diagnoses in human salmonellosis but is not routinely used in animals.

TREATMENT

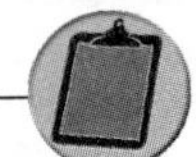

THERAPEUTIC GOAL(S)

- Treat for sepsis and accompanying SIRS if present (see Systemic Inflammatory Response Syndrome, p 1060)
- Prevent exposure to humans

ACUTE GENERAL TREATMENT

- Depends on severity of illness.
- Mild cases are often self-limiting and require only supportive therapy.
- Intravenous fluid support, including plasma or colloids if necessary, recommended if dehydrated or septicemia is present.
- Antibiotic therapy is controversial.
  - May induce carrier state and prolong fecal shedding of organisms.
  - Antibiotics are indicated if hemorrhagic diarrhea is present, if the patient is depressed or febrile, if evidence of sepsis exists, if the patient is immunosuppressed and shows GI signs, or if positive blood cultures are obtained. Duration of treatment corresponds to time to resolution of fever, shock, or other signs of complications.
  - The most effective antibiotics are enrofloxacin (5 mg/kg PO or slow IV q 24h in dogs [4 mg/kg PO or slow IV q 24h in cats]), trimethoprim-sulfa (15 mg/kg PO q 12h), or amoxicillin (22 mg/kg PO q 8h).

RECOMMENDED MONITORING

See Sepsis and Septic Shock, p 996; Systemic Inflammatory Response Syndrome, p 1060

PROGNOSIS AND OUTCOME

- Prognosis for mild cases is good; infections may resolve spontaneously or with supportive care only.
- Prognosis for septicemic patients is guarded; potential disease complications include dehydration, electrolyte imbalances, sepsis, septic shock, SIRS, and DIC.

PEARLS & CONSIDERATIONS

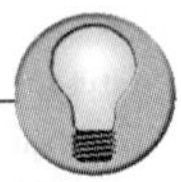

COMMENTS

Patients fed raw food diets are at increased risk of salmonellosis.

- *Salmonella* isolated from 80% of samples of raw food (BARF diet).
- *Salmonella* isolated from 30% of stool samples from dogs fed these diets (thus, there is an increased risk for human exposure and infection).

PREVENTION

- Avoid feeding raw or undercooked meat diets.
- Isolate infected animals and practice good hygiene.

CLIENT EDUCATION

- Owners should be informed that this is a zoonotic disease and humans are very susceptible.
- Avoid eating undercooked meats.

SUGGESTED READING

Greene CE: Salmonellosis. In Greene CE (ed): *Infectious Diseases of the Dog and Cat*. Philadelphia, WB Saunders, 1998, pp 235–240.

Marks SL, Kather EJ: Bacterial-associated diarrhea in the dog: A critical appraisal. *Vet Clin North Am Small Anim Pract* 33:5, 2003.

AUTHOR: **CHRISTOPHER J. JONES**
EDITOR: **DEBRA L. ZORAN**

Salt Toxicosis

BASIC INFORMATION

DEFINITION

Salt (sodium chloride, table salt, or NaCl) toxicosis results when an excessive amount of salt has been ingested and intake of potable water is limited.

SYNONYM(S)

Water deprivation
Sodium ion toxicosis

EPIDEMIOLOGY

SPECIES, AGE, SEX: Dogs (all breeds, both sexes, all ages) are more commonly seen for salt toxicosis than cats.

RISK FACTORS

- Use of table salt as an emetic, a technique which is now contraindicated for this reason
- Availability of homemade play dough in pet's environment
- Swimming and drinking seawater when availability of potable drinking water is limited
- Dehydration (places animals at higher risk)

CLINICAL PRESENTATION

HISTORY, CHIEF COMPLAINT

- Owner description of typical risk factor (see Risk Factors above)
- Lack of drinking water after ingesting excessive amounts of salt
- Polydipsia, vomiting, tremors, and seizures within 1 to 4 hours after ingestion

PHYSICAL EXAM FINDINGS

- Polyuria and polydipsia (PU/PD), vomiting, diarrhea, tremors, seizures
- Dehydration
- Hyperthermia possible if muscle fasciculations are present
- Tachycardia (usually sinus) possible

ETIOLOGY AND PATHOPHYSIOLOGY

- Excessive salt intake can lead to hypernatremia.
- Signs of toxicosis appear when serum sodium is >170 mEq/L (vomiting, polydipsia), and central nervous system

(CNS) signs such as tremors and seizures begin when serum sodium is >180 mEq/L (typical normal range in healthy dogs: 145–157 mEq/L).
- Sources of excess sodium chloride for animals include homemade play dough (modeling clay), table salt used as an emetic, improperly mixed feed or formula, seawater, hypertonic saline solutions, sodium bicarbonate, and sodium phosphate enemas.
- Hypernatremia creates a hypertonic state in the extracellular fluid (ECF). Initially, water shifts from the interstitium to the vasculature and then from intracellular fluid (ICF) to the ECF to maintain equilibrium.
- Excess sodium is irritating to gastrointestinal (GI) mucosa and can cause gastroenteritis and dehydration.
- The CNS is particularly vulnerable due to initial tissue shrinkage as water leaves the ICF or because of subsequent edema formation as water reenters the cerebral spinal fluid (CSF) or neurons.
- An influx of water into the brain results in cerebral edema, seizures, permanent neurologic dysfunction, and possibly death.
- Process: Sodium passively crosses the blood-brain barrier into the CSF. Once in the CSF, excess sodium affects neuronal function by inhibiting anaerobic glycolysis, leading to decreased energy production. Sodium requires active transport to move from the CSF back to the serum; decreased energy production limits this process. The result is water influx into the CSF and neurons, causing cerebral edema and CNS signs.

DIAGNOSIS

DIFFERENTIAL DIAGNOSIS

Rule out other causes of hypernatremia (see Hypernatremia, p 549):
- Excessive water loss:
  - Nephrogenic diabetes insipidus, inadequate water intake, diabetes mellitus, heat stroke; excessive water loss very rarely occurs with acute or chronic renal failure (CRF) or with administration of furosemide or mannitol

INITIAL DATABASE

- Complete blood count (CBC): mature leukocytosis
- Serum biochemistry profile:
  - Hypernatremia; serum sodium >170–180 mEq/L
  - Hyperchloremia
  - Hyperalbuminemia
  - Decreased serum HCO_3^- possible (metabolic acidosis)
  - Azotemia possible (prerenal)
- Thoracic radiographs: pulmonary edema possible

ADVANCED OR CONFIRMATORY TESTING

NaCl can be analyzed in vomitus, food, water; may help determine the source and concentration of NaCl

TREATMENT

THERAPEUTIC GOAL(S)

- Decontaminate the patient
- Replace water and electrolytes
- Facilitate renal excretion of sodium
- Provide supportive care

ACUTE GENERAL TREATMENT

- Decontamination of patient:
  - Emesis: if the animal is not showing clinical signs and it is performed within 30 minutes of ingestion (see Vomiting, Induction of, p 1328).
  - Activated charcoal: does not adsorb NaCl; not indicated.
- Replacement of water and electrolytes:
  - Calculate the amount of free water needed. Free water deficit (liters) = body weight (kg) × 0.6 × ([present serum Na concentration/previous or normal range serum Na concetration] - 1).
  - Replace 50% of the water deficit in the first 24 hours using sterile 5% dextrose solution IV; replace the remaining deficit in the next 24 to 48 hours using the same fluid type (5% dextrose).
  - Do not decrease serum sodium concentration faster than 0.5–1.0 mEq/L/ hr. A rapid drop in serum sodium concentrations can cause water influx into the brain and cerebral edema.
- Facilitation of renal excretion of sodium:
  - 5% dextrose at 3.7 ml/kg/hr IV in dogs can decrease serum sodium at about 1 mEq/L/hr or use 0.45% or 0.9% saline IV or lactated Ringer's solution with 5% dextrose.
  - Furosemide 1–2 mg/kg IM or IV q 6h (correct dehydration first).
- Supportive care:
  - Control seizures with diazepam 0.5–2.0 mg/kg IV, as needed (prn).

POSSIBLE COMPLICATIONS

Permanent CNS damage

RECOMMENDED MONITORING

- Hydration status
- Body weight
- Packed cell volume (PCV)
- Total serum proteins
- CBC
- Serum biochemistry profiles

PROGNOSIS AND OUTCOME

- Poor if serum sodium >180 mEq/L and seizures are present
- Good if treated early and comprehensively

PEARLS & CONSIDERATIONS

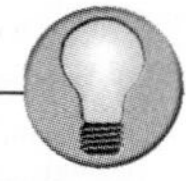

COMMENTS

- Do not decrease serum sodium concentration faster than 0.5–1.0 mEq/L/hr.
- A homemade play dough recipe contains 2 cups of flour, 1 cup of table salt, and 0.5–1 cup of water.
- Minimum lethal dose of NaCl in dog = 4 g/kg; minimum toxic dose = 1.9 g/kg. Equivalences: 1 tsp NaCl = 6 g; 1 lb table salt = 454 g.
- A 10-lb (4.5-kg) dog needs to eat 3.4 tsp of homemade play dough to reach a minimum toxic dose of NaCl.
- In less severely affected animals, frequent access to small amounts of drinking water may be sufficient to lower serum sodium levels.

CLIENT EDUCATION

Do not use NaCl to induce vomiting

SUGGESTED READING

Barr JM, Khan SA, McCullough SM, Volmer PA: Hypernatremia secondary to homemade play dough ingestion in dogs: A review of 14 cases from 1998 to 2001. *J Vet Emerg Crit Care* 14(3):196–202, 2004.

Hardy RM: Hypernatremia. *Vet Clin North Am Small Anim Pract* 19:231–240, 1989.

AUTHOR & EDITOR: **SAFDAR A. KHAN**

Sarcoptic Mange

Client Education Sheet on Website

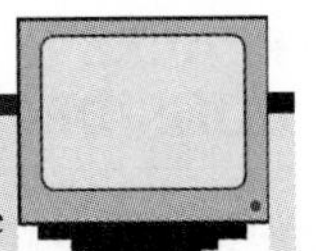

BASIC INFORMATION

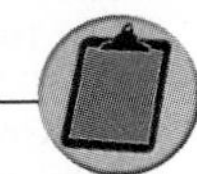

DEFINITION

A nonseasonal, intensely pruritic skin disease caused by *Sarcoptes scabiei* var. *canis*

SYNONYM(S)

Canine scabies
Scabies

EPIDEMIOLOGY

SPECIES, AGE, SEX: Dogs are commonly affected, but humans and cats (although rarely) can be transiently infected.

RISK FACTORS

- Affected animals often have a history of being in an animal shelter, being in contact with stray dogs, or visiting a boarding or grooming facility.
- In multipet households, usually more than one dog is affected.

CONTAGION AND ZOONOSIS: Because sarcoptic mange is a zoonotic disease, humans are at risk if exposed to an infected pet (whether or not overt clinical signs are present in the pet); likewise, a pet may acquire the parasite from an infected human.

CLINICAL PRESENTATION

HISTORY, CHIEF COMPLAINT

- Consider *S. scabiei* when presented with any dog with an apparent sudden onset of intense itching.
- The condition can present as nonseasonal intense pruritus that has responded poorly to corticosteroid therapy; chronic failure to respond to various dermatologic therapies (especially corticosteroids) is a common component of the history, especially if serial skin scrapings have not been done.

PHYSICAL EXAM FINDINGS

- Crusting of the elbows, hocks, and pinnal ear margins may indicate *S. scabiei*.
- Other lesions can include papules, alopecia, erythema, and excoriations.
- With time, lesions may spread over the body, including the ventral abdomen and legs.

ETIOLOGY AND PATHOPHYSIOLOGY

S. scabiei var. *canis* is a superficial burrowing skin mite that secretes allergenic substances, which leads to an intensely pruritic hypersensitivity reaction in sensitized dogs.

DIAGNOSIS

DIFFERENTIAL DIAGNOSIS

- Ectoparasites (*Demodex* [uncommon], *Cheyletiella*, *Notoedres*, and *Otodectes* spp.; fleas, lice).
- Allergies/hypersensitivities (atopy, flea-bite hypersensitivity, other ectoparasite hypersensitivities, adverse food reaction, contact hypersensitivity, drug hypersensitivity).
- Bacterial infections (*Staphylococcus intermedius*).
- Fungal infections (*Malassezia*, ringworm [dermatophytes]).
- Seborrhea.
- Behavioral disorders (psychogenic alopecia, flank sucking, tail-biting, self-nursing).
- Neoplasia (mast cell tumor, epitheliotropic lymphoma).

INITIAL DATABASE

- Look for a reflex scratching action with the hind limb when the edge of the pinna is rubbed (pinnal-pedal reflex), because this is very common in dogs with *S. scabiei*. Treat for *S. scabiei* if this reflex is noted.
- Collect a minimum of three to five broad, deep skin scrapings for microscopic examination from the lesions, especially those at predilection sites. Crusts and papules represent the best areas to scrape. Mites may be hard to find.
- *S. scabiei* mites and/or eggs can also sometimes be identified by fecal flotation.

ADVANCED OR CONFIRMATORY TESTING

An enzyme-linked immunosorbent assay (ELISA) test for sarcoptic mite antigen is available in Europe but not yet available in North America.

TREATMENT

THERAPEUTIC GOAL(S)

- Treatment is geared to thoroughly eradicating the mites.
- All clinically suspected *S. scabiei* cases should be treated regardless of whether mites are found.
- Because the mite is highly contagious, all in-contact animals should be treated (e.g., all animals in the household, regardless of presence or absence of clinical signs).

ACUTE GENERAL TREATMENT

- Selamectin (Revolution; Pfizer) is approved as a topical treatment once every 30 days for one or two treatments, is the current treatment of choice, and can be used in puppies as young as 6 weeks of age.
- Many dermatologists recommend a course of three selamectin treatments at 0, 2, and 6 weeks postdiagnosis.
- Other treatments can include 2% lime sulfur (LymDip; DVM) and 0.025% amitraz (Mitaban; Pfizer) dips every 7 to 24 days for 1 month, but these are discouraged due to the highly contagious and zoonotic nature of this disease.
- Ivermectin (Ivomec Bovine Injection, 10 mg/ml, Merial) at a dose of 0.2–0.4 mg/kg SC two to three times a week at 2-week intervals or PO once weekly for 3 to 4 weeks can be used, but this is not the treatment of choice due to the risk of neurologic side effects.
- Concomitant antibiotic therapy may also be required if secondary pyoderma is present. Cephalexin at a dose of 30 mg/kg PO q 12h for 30 days is a good choice.
- If the dog is severely pruritic, it is permissable to give the animal corticosteroids for a short time if necessary, but only in cases that were confirmed by skin scrapings. Prednisone can be used at 0.25–0.5 mg/kg PO q 12h for the first 2 to 3 days and then weaning down. Longer courses of treatment may be immunosuppressive.

POSSIBLE COMPLICATIONS

In collie breeds and other sensitive breeds, clinical signs of an adverse reaction to ivermectin include hypersalivation, disorientation, ataxia, mydriasis (dilated pupils), coma, and, possibly, death if supportive care is not instituted.

RECOMMENDED MONITORING

- It will take 14 days to see any decrease in the level of pruritus and as long as 3 months for a complete resolution.
- Follow-up skin scrapings are recommended.

PROGNOSIS AND OUTCOME

- Prognosis is good.
- Some increase in pruritus often occurs in the first few days after treatment. This is believed to be associated with an immnunogenic response to the dying mites.

PEARLS & CONSIDERATIONS

COMMENTS

- Look for a reflex when the edge of the pinna is rubbed (pinnal-pedal reflex), because this is very common in dogs with *S. scabiei*. Treat for *S. scabiei* if this reflex is noted.
- It is important to remember that elimination of the mite may not necessarily be the only recommended treatment; based on the presence or absence of secondary pyoderma and extreme pruritus, concurrent antibiotic and, if necessary, short-term corticosteroid therapy may need to be instituted, respectively.
- "Feline scabies" is caused by a different parasite, *Notoedres cati*; however, cats in close contact with dogs affected with sarcoptic mites may also develop transient signs of canine scabies.
- Approximately 30% of dogs with *S. scabiei* will react to the house dust mite antigen.

CLIENT EDUCATION

Humans transiently affected with *S. scabiei* mites may develop a pruritic rash on the arms or trunk. Any suspicion should prompt the client to consult with a physician.

SUGGESTED READING

Curtis CF: Current trends in the treatment of *Sarcoptes*, *Cheyletiella* and *Otodectes* mite infestations in dogs and cats. *Vet Dermatol* 15(2):108–114, 2004.

Scott DW, Miller WH Jr., Griffin CE: In: *Muller and Kirk's Small Animal Dermatology*, ed 6. Philadelphia, WB Saunders, 2001, pp 423–516.

AUTHORS: **JAN A. HALL, AMANDA P. AMARATUNGA**

EDITOR: **JAN A. HALL**

Sebaceous Adenitis

BASIC INFORMATION

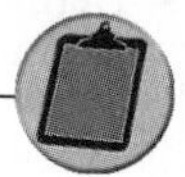

DEFINITION

A poorly understood, suspected heritable, inflammatory skin disorder leading to the destruction of sebaceous glands

SYNONYM(S)

Granulomatous sebaceous adenitis

EPIDEMIOLOGY

SPECIES, AGE, SEX: Uncommon in dogs, rare in cats; more common in young adult to middle-aged dogs (1.5 to 7 years).

GENETICS AND BREED PREDISPOSITION: The condition appears to be inherited at least in the Samoyed, Akita, and standard poodle, where it is considered to have a simple autosomal recessive mode of inheritance. Other breeds more frequently reported are Hungarian Vizsla, German shepherd, Lhasa apso, Hovawart, and Bernese mountain dog.

ASSOCIATED CONDITIONS AND DISORDERS: Seborrhea, bacterial folliculitis, and pruritus.

CLINICAL PRESENTATION

DISEASE FORMS/SUBTYPES

- The condition may appear differently in individual breeds with marked variability depending on severity. Two clinical presentations exist:
  - Generalized sebaceous adenitis (SA): in long-coated breeds, such as the Akita, Samoyed, and the standard poodle
  - Multifocal SA: in short-coated breeds, such as the Hungarian Vizsla (Fig. I-149), and in cats
- SA can also be subclinical and only identifiable by histologic examination in some very mildly affected dogs.

HISTORY, CHIEF COMPLAINT: Progressive areas of hair loss, poor haircoat, excessive scaling, and musty odor are signs. Pruritus is variable but may be marked, especially if a secondary bacterial folliculitis is present.

PHYSICAL EXAM FINDINGS

- Generalized SA: presents with dramatic amounts of scale on the skin, scales adherent to hairs (follicular castings), and coat and skin often dry to the touch. Partial alopecia along the top of the head, back of the neck, and dorsum is observed as the disease progresses. In more chronic cases, hyperkeratotic skin is observed. The dorsal midline and the ears are usually the first and the most affected areas. In the Akita, where the disease can be more severe, fever, anorexia, and lethargy have been reported.
- Multifocal SA: localized areas of alopecia, erythema, and excessive scaling (the scale is characteristically adherent to hairs). The head and extremities appear to be more consistently involved.

ETIOLOGY AND PATHOPHYSIOLOGY

- May be a genetically inherited cell-mediated autoimmune reaction against the sebaceous glands
- Initial defect could be a keratinization disorder or may be a result of abnormalities in cutaneous lipid metabolism that affect sebum production

DIAGNOSIS

DIFFERENTIAL DIAGNOSIS

- Generalized form: keratinization disorders (primary seborrhea, ichthyosis), endocrinopathies, leishmaniasis
- Multifocal form: bacterial folliculitis, demodicosis, dermatophytosis, zinc-responsive dermatosis, pemphigus foliaceus

INITIAL DATABASE

- Skin cytologic examination to assess for presence of secondary bacterial folliculitis
- Skin scrapings: negative
- Dermatophyte culture: negative
- Complete blood count (CBC), serum biochemistry profile, urinalysis, and endocrine function tests: no abnormalities expected

ADVANCED OR CONFIRMATORY TESTING

Histopathologic findings are usually diagnostic. Affected areas show a pyogranulomatous inflammation around the sebaceous glands. Sebaceous glands are in various stages of being destroyed. Marked orthokeratotic hyperkeratosis is present. In late-stage disease, the inflammation resolves, leaving an absence of sebaceous glands.

TREATMENT

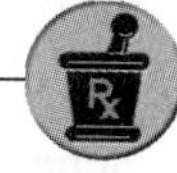

THERAPEUTIC GOAL(S)

- Control recurrent secondary bacterial infections
- Control inflammation and seborrhea
- Promote hair regrowth

ACUTE GENERAL TREATMENT

- Treat bacterial infections with appropriate systemic antibiotic therapy. An acceptable empiric choice initially is cephalexin 22–30 mg/kg PO q 8–12h.
- There is no gold standard for treatment of SA in dogs; a variety of protocols has been published, all with variable efficacy.
- Mild cases: intensive topical therapy leads to effective (although partial in

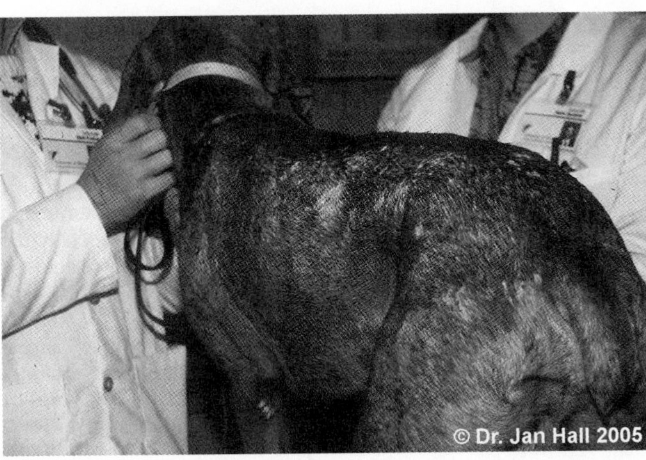

FIGURE I-149 Multifocal areas of alopecia over the dorsal trunk of a 4-year-old spayed Hungarian Vizsla female with sebaceous adenitis. Courtesy of Dr. Jan A. Hall.

most cases) control of scaling: keratolytic shampoos and emollient rinses; weekly baby oil soaks beneficial in some standard poodles. For more stubborn cases, topical application of 50-75% propylene glycol as a rinse daily then decrease frequency as needed.

- For severe or refractory cases:
  - Synthetic retinoid: isotretinoin (Accutane) or acitretin (Soriatane) 1-3 mg/kg PO q 12h until remission; then the lowest, most infrequent dose (reported particularly effective in the Hungarian Vizsla, variable results in other breeds).
  - Cyclosporine microemulsion (Atopica, Neoral): 5 mg/kg PO q 12-24h until remission, then decrease to the lowest most infrequent dose (effectively reduces inflammation and permits hair regrowth).
- Some dogs partially improve with high dosages of fatty acids (omega-3 and omega-6) PO or vitamin A supplementation, 10,000 IU PO q 24h.

DRUG INTERACTION

Drugs that inhibit cytochrome P-450 (ketoconazole, methylprednisolone, etc.) potentiate cyclosporine activity

PROGNOSIS AND OUTCOME

- SA is a cosmetic disorder in most cases; it does not affect general health.
- Lifelong treatments are usually required to control the disease.

PEARLS & CONSIDERATIONS

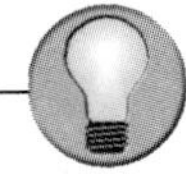

COMMENTS

- Early diagnosis improves prognosis for long-term management.
- No information on the treatment in cats has been published.

PREVENTION

Discourage the breeding of affected animals

CLIENT EDUCATION

The Orthopedic Foundation for Animals (OFA) provides a database and guidelines for assessment and registration on its website: www.offa.org.

SUGGESTED READING

Linek M, et al: Effects of cyclosporine A on clinical and histologic abnormalities in dogs with sebaceous adenitis. *J Am Vet Med Assoc* 226:59, 2005.

Rosser EJ: Therapy for sebaceous adenitis. In Bonagura JD (ed): *Kirk's Current Veterinary Therapy XIII*. Philadelphia, WB Saunders, 2000, pp 572-573.

Scott DW, Miller WH, Griffin CE: Granulomatous sebaceous adenitis. In Scott DW, Miller WH, Griffin CE (eds): *Muller and Kirk's Small Animal Dermatology*, ed 6. Philadelphia, WB Saunders, 2001, pp 1140-1146.

AUTHOR: **CAROLINE DE JAHAM**
EDITOR: **JAN A. HALL**

Seborrhea

BASIC INFORMATION

DEFINITION

A class of scaling skin disorders resulting from primary (congenital) or secondary (acquired) defects in epidermal maturation, desquamation, or sebum production; classified as sicca (dry form) or oleosa (waxy form), although animals typically present with a combination of both forms

SYNONYM(S)

Cornification disorders
Keratinization defects/disorders
Scaling disorders
Seborrheic disorders

EPIDEMIOLOGY

SPECIES, AGE, SEX

- Congenital causes: early in life
- Acquired: middle-aged to older pets

GENETICS AND BREED PREDISPOSITION

- Primary idiopathic seborrhea: basset hound, shar-pei, cocker spaniel, dachshund, Doberman pinscher, English springer spaniel, German shepherd dog, Irish setter, Labrador retriever, West Highland white terrier; Persian cat
- Vitamin A responsive dermatosis: cocker spaniel, Labrador retriever, miniature schnauzer
- Zinc-responsive dermatosis: Alaskan malamute, Siberian husky, Samoyed
- Chin acne: English bulldog, boxer, Doberman pinscher, Great Dane
- Lethal acrodermatitis: bull terrier
- Epidermal dysplasia: West Highland white terrier
- Sebaceous adenitis: Akita, Belgian sheepdog, Samoyed, standard poodle, Hungarian Vizsla
- Lichenoid-psoriasiform dermatosis: springer spaniel
- Acanthosis nigricans: dachshund
- Ichthyosis: golden retriever (Fig. I-150)

RISK FACTORS: Secondary seborrhea: nutritional disorders, microbial dermatitis, endocrinopathies, hypersensitivity disorders, parasitoses, autoimmune disorders, metabolic diseases, malignancies, and low environmental humidity.

CONTAGION AND ZOONOSIS: Most are not contagious, but parasitic and fungal etiologies have contagious and zoonotic potential.

GEOGRAPHY AND SEASONALITY: Seborrhea sicca is more common in the winter (low environmental humidity).

ASSOCIATED CONDITIONS AND DISORDERS: Primary seborrheic disorders may be associated with ceruminous otitis externa.

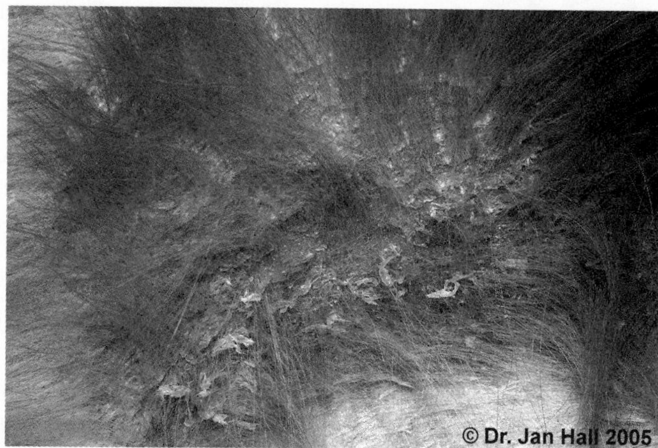

FIGURE I-150 Extensive scaling affecting the inguinal region of a 3-year-old male castrated golden retriever with a mild form of canine ichthyosis. Courtesy of Dr. Jan A. Hall.

CLINICAL PRESENTATION

DISEASE FORMS/SUBTYPES

- Primary (congenital) or secondary (acquired)
- Generalized or localized

HISTORY, CHIEF COMPLAINT: Owners generally present seborrheic pets for evaluation of an unpleasant-appearing haircoat or coat with a foul odor. Specific complaints may include a generalized, dry, waxy, or scaly coat condition, oftentimes associated with a rancid odor. Pruritus is of variable intensity, depending on presence of parasites, dry skin, or secondary bacterial or yeast infection; however, seborrhea may be an incidental finding in some animals.

PHYSICAL EXAM FINDINGS

- Primary: varying degrees of alopecia and dry scale that may be focal, multifocal, or generalized over the trunk. Animals may present with large hyperkeratotic patches of adherent scale. Follicular casts (waxy debris surrounding hair shafts), fronds (clumps of hairs stuck together like a paint brush), or severe "dandruff" with large flakes may be noted.
- Localized seborrheic disorders:
  - Nasal hyperkeratosis of the Labrador retriever: restricted to the nasal planum (unhaired dorsal part of the nose)
  - Nasodigital hyperkeratosis: restricted to nasal planum and digital pads
  - Ear margin dermatosis: alopecia and scaling of distal pinnal margins, possibly associated with fissures
  - Acanthosis nigricans: hyperpigmented, lichenified patches in the axillary region
  - Lichenoid-psoriasiform dermatosis: erythematous papules and plaques involving the ear and the preauricular and periorbital regions; may affect lips, inguinal region, and prepuce
  - Chin acne: papules, pustules, scaling, and crusts affecting the chin only
- Secondary: General physical findings depend on the underlying etiology or vary with the underlying etiology. Cutaneous findings include a dull (or waxy) coat with various combinations of alopecia, scaling, crusting, and excoriations secondary to self-trauma and pyoderma.

ETIOLOGY AND PATHOPHYSIOLOGY

Alteration in epidermal turnover times, maturation processes, and/or desquamation or transepidermal water loss lead to scaling. Other considerations include abnormal apocrine or sebaceous glandular secretions (either in volume or quality).

DIAGNOSIS

DIFFERENTIAL DIAGNOSIS

- Primary causes may be multifocal and generalized or localized:
  - Multifocal and generalized:
    - Primary idiopathic seborrhea
    - Vitamin A–responsive dermatosis
    - Zinc-responsive dermatosis
    - Epidermal dysplasia
    - Schnauzer comedo syndrome
    - Canine ichthyosis
    - Sebaceous adenitis
  - Localized:
    - Chin acne
    - Ear margin dermatosis
    - Nasodigital hyperkeratosis
    - Nasal hyperkeratosis of the Labrador retriever
    - Lichenoid-psoriasiform dermatosis of the English springer spaniel
- Secondary causes include the following:
  - Microbial: pyoderma, *Malassezia*, dermatophytosis
  - Parasitic: flea infestation, cheyletiellosis, sarcoptic mange, demodectic mange, pediculosis
  - Endocrinopathy: hypothyroidism, hyperadrenocorticism, sex hormone imbalance (e.g., sertoli cell tumor)
  - Allergic: food hypersensitivity, atopic dermatitis
  - Management: low environmental humidity, inappropriate topical therapy or frequency, nutritionally inadequate diet (especially if high in phytates, low in fatty acids, high fiber)
  - Metabolic disease (especially liver disease)
  - Immune-mediated disease: pemphigus foliaceus, adverse drug reaction
  - Cutaneous T-cell lymphoma
  - Paraneoplastic disorders

INITIAL DATABASE

- Comprehensive evaluation for ectoparasites (skin scrapings, flea combing, acetate tape preparations, fecal evaluation, ectoparasiticide response trial)
- Skin cytologic examination (to rule out secondary bacterial and yeast involvement)
- Fungal culture (dermatophytosis)
- Complete blood count (CBC), serum biochemical profile, urinalysis (as appropriate, to look for evidence of underlying disease)

ADVANCED OR CONFIRMATORY TESTING

- Skin biopsy: orthokeratotic and parakeratotic hyperkeratosis, with follicular keratosis
- Elimination diet trial to rule out food allergy (if pruritic)
- Intradermal and serum allergy testing for atopy (if pruritic)
- Response to dietary management (if poor quality diet)
- Thyroid function testing
- Adrenal function testing

TREATMENT

THERAPEUTIC GOAL(S)

- Address underlying etiology specifically, if possible
- Control secondary microbial dermatitis
- Control amount of scale produced

ACUTE GENERAL TREATMENT

- Systemic antibiotics, such as cephalexin at 30 mg/kg PO q 12h for at least 2 weeks past resolution of clinical signs or until improvement plateaus (minimum of 4 weeks). Some animals require chronic treatment.
- Essential fatty acid (EFA) oral supplementation (omega-3 and omega-6); rarely provides complete control of seborrhea but may be beneficial as adjunctive therapy.
- Systemic antifungal treatment as needed (see *Malassezia* Dermatitis, p 664; Dermatophytosis, p 285).

- Topical therapy: clipping of haircoat may benefit topical therapy:
  - Antiseborrheic shampoos containing keratolytic or keratoplastic compounds that are used initially two times a week. Good choices of ingredients for dry, scaly coats include sulfur and salicylic acid; decrease frequency as needed.
  - Greasy, scaly skin can be degreased using products containing benzoyl peroxide, selenium sulfide, or tars. These products should always be followed with a conditioner. Note: Shampoos containing benzoyl peroxide are drying and will bleach fabric.
  - Mild dry scaling may respond to moisturizing or hypoallergenic shampoos. Conditioners containing lipids or humectants (agents that help the skin to retain moisture) are beneficial.

CHRONIC TREATMENT

- Generalized disease
  - Primary idiopathic seborrhea: topical therapy as already described; EFA supplementation; antibiotics administered as already described. Consider retinoids; acitretin (Soriatane), 0.5-1.0 mg/kg PO q 24h, or cyclosporine, 5-10 mg/kg PO q 12-24h.
  - Vitamin A-responsive dermatosis: topical therapy and antibiotics as already described; vitamin A 625-800 IU/kg PO q 24h; usually 10,000 IU PO daily, lifelong, for the average cocker spaniel. Improvement is noted by 3 weeks, with remission in 8 to 10 weeks.
  - Zinc-responsive dermatosis: zinc supplementation is recommended at 1-3 mg/kg elemental zinc PO q 24h.
  - Epidermal dysplasia: address any bacterial, yeast, parasitic, atopic, and hypersensitivity reactions. Bathe the animal frequently with keratolytic and keratoplastic shampoos.
  - Schnauzer comedo syndrome: Benzoyl peroxide shampoos help the condition via follicular flushing. Systemic antibiotics (as already described) to control bacterial folliculitis. In some cases, retinoids such as isotretinoin (Accutane), 1-2 mg/kg PO q 24h, may be helpful but can be costly. Wean to alternate day therapy after 4 weeks if a favorable response is noted.
  - Canine ichthyosis: Antiseborrheic shampoos and a topical spray conditioner containing propylene glycol and humectants can be useful. Try isotretinoin (Accutane), 1-2 mg/kg PO q 24h for 8 to 12 weeks, decreasing to alternate day therapy if effective) in more severe cases.
  - Sebaceous adenitis (see also Sebaceous Adenitis, p 986):
    1. EFA supplementation.
    2. Vitamin A: 8000 to 20,000 IU PO q 12h.
    3. Bath oil treatment: ratio of 50:50 bath oil and warm water in a spray bottle. Spray entire coat, working into coat and leaving on for 1 to 2 hours. Shampoo the animal thoroughly with a degreasing unscented dish detergent (while not allowing the detergent to get into the eyes) or a benzoyl peroxide shampoo, scrubbing the skin with a soft brush. Be sure to rinse well and follow with an oil-base conditioner (available in containers that can be used as either a spray or leave-in conditioner). Towel dry. Repeat this treatment weekly for the first month and, if a good response is noted, slowly decrease the frequency.
    4. Antibiotics as indicated.
    5. Consider cyclosporine at 5 mg/kg PO, q 12h (while monitoring blood levels to reduce risk of toxicity).
- Localized disease
  - Chin acne:
    - Dogs: Follicular flushing products containing benzoyl peroxide may be beneficial. Add systemic antibiotics as already described.
    - Cats: Keep region clean. Chlorhexidine skin cleanser or commercially obtained wipes containing boric and acetic acid can be quite useful. Apply mupirocin ointment twice daily *sparingly* and do not allow the cat to clean the area for 5 to 10 minutes (to reduce the potential for nephrotoxicity from the polyethylene base).
  - Ear margin dermatosis: local use of an antiseborrheic shampoo. If inflammation is severe, topical glucocorticoid such as 0.5-1% hydrocortisone may reduce inflammation.
  - Nasal and nasodigital hyperkeratosis: moisturize affected area with water or wet dressings and then apply petrolatum jelly. More severely affected animals may benefit from topical application of an ointment containing salicylic acid and urea, topical application of 50% propylene glycol or topical application of 0.025 or 0.01% tretinoin gel (Retin-A).
  - Lichenoid-psoriasiform dermatosis: The condition may wax and wane despite therapy. Antibiotic therapy may help; cephalexin 30 mg/kg PO q 12h, until condition plateaus (4 to 12 weeks). Glucocorticoids may be used: initially prednisone 2.2 mg/kg PO q 12h, followed by a tapering of the dosage.

DRUG INTERACTIONS

Cyclosporine: Concurrent use of cyclosporine with other P-glycoprotein inhibitors or substrates can increase blood cyclosporine levels. This may be beneficial (e.g., lowers the dose of cyclosporine required by half [q 12-24h] when administered with standard doses of ketoconazole) but can also increase the potential toxicity of some agents.

POSSIBLE COMPLICATIONS

- High fatty acid treatment may increase the potential for gastrointestinal (GI) disturbance or pancreatitis
- Retinoids: keratoconjunctivitis sicca (KCS), conjunctivitis, pruritus, hyperactivity, stiffness, mucocutaneous junction, erythema, vomiting, diarrhea, teratogenicity, elevated liver enzymes
- Cyclosporine: diarrhea, vomiting, anorexia, gingival hyperplasia, and gingivitis; monitor animals for tumors

RECOMMENDED MONITORING

- Vitamin A, retinoids: monitor liver enzymes and tear production.
- Cyclosporine: physical examination (tumor, infection, gingival hyperplasia), urea, creatinine, urinalysis, and liver enzymes; blood pressure (BP) if any history of heart disease. Check trough serum cyclosporine levels if adverse reactions are noted or if there is a poor clinical response. A trough serum level of 500-700 ng/ml has been associated with efficacy.

PROGNOSIS AND OUTCOME

Primary causes often require lifelong therapy; secondary syndromes improve with correction or control of underlying etiology

PEARLS & CONSIDERATIONS

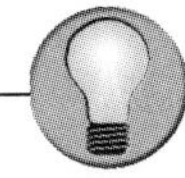

COMMENTS

Control secondary microbial dermatitis and evaluate thoroughly for underlying secondary etiologies before diagnosing a primary seborrheic syndrome

PREVENTION

Animals affected with primary seborrheic syndromes should not be used for breeding.

CLIENT EDUCATION

Concept of control versus cure

SUGGESTED READING

Kwochka KW: Scales, Crusts and Seborrhea. *Proceedings of the Fifth World Congress of*

Veterinary Dermatology, Vienna, Austria 148–156, 2004.

Kwochka KW: Section V: Keratinization disorders. Griffin CE, Kwochka KW, MacDonald JM (eds): *Current Veterinary Dermatology*. St. Louis, Mosby-Yearbook, 1993, pp 167–214.

Scott DW, Miller WH, Griffin CE: *Small Animal Dermatology*, ed 6. Toronto, WB Saunders, 2001, pp 1025–1054.

AUTHOR: **STEPHEN WAISGLASS**
EDITOR: **JAN A. HALL**

Seizures

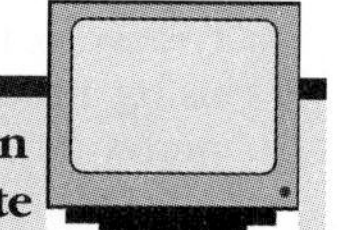

Client Education Sheet on Website

BASIC INFORMATION

DEFINITION

A seizure is the clinical manifestation of abnormal, excessive, and/or hypersynchronous neuronal activity in the cerebral cortex. The location and extent of this abnormal neuronal activity determines the clinical appearance of the seizure. In clinical practice, seizures must be differentiated according to whether they are of extracranial or intracranial origin.

SYNONYM(S)

Convulsion
Epileptic seizure
Ictus

EPIDEMIOLOGY

SPECIES, AGE, SEX

- Both sexes, dogs and cats, all ages
- Dependent on underlying cause
- Dogs: 6 months to 5 years (primary epilepsy); older dogs (brain tumor); young dogs (intoxication, metabolic, malformation)

CLINICAL PRESENTATION

DISEASE FORMS/SUBTYPES

- Focal or partial seizures (previously called *petit mal*): focal or asymmetrical sensory or motor activity affecting any part of the body (e.g., facial twitching, chomping of the mouth); can be associated with autonomic signs (e.g., salivation, vomiting)
    - Simple (no alteration of consciousness) or complex (alteration in mentation)
- Generalized seizures (previously called *grand mal*): diffuse, bilateral motor activity with loss of consciousness
- Status epilepticus: continuous seizure activity lasting for 5 minutes or more or repeated seizures with failure to return to normality in between

HISTORY, CHIEF COMPLAINT

- Any combination of uncontrollable, involuntary, excessive, or reduced motor activity; alteration in consciousness; behavioral disturbance and autonomic signs (e.g., salivation, urination, defecation, piloerection).
- A seizure is transient and starts and ends abruptly.
- Postictal disturbances frequently follow the seizure (e.g., confusion, pacing, blindness, ataxia).
- The motor activity can be bilateral and diffuse (e.g., generalized tonic/clonic seizure) or minor and subtle (e.g., facial twitching).

PHYSICAL EXAM FINDINGS

- The animal is often normal between episodes.
- Complete neurologic examination is mandatory:
    - Presence of any neurologic deficits after complete resolution of the seizure (interictal period) is important. Interictal neurologic deficits are an indication of a structural intracranial lesion, such as inflammation or neoplasm.
    - A patient that shows no interictal neurologic deficits, however, may have either a primary brain disturbance as the cause of seizures or, less likely, an extracranial cause for the seizures.
- Evidence of systemic illness is often present in cases where seizures are the result of intoxication (e.g., bradycardia, gastrointestinal [GI] signs) or metabolic diseases (e.g., anorexia, lethargy, vomiting).

ETIOLOGY AND PATHOPHYSIOLOGY

Etiology:

- Intracranial:
    - Primary (or idiopathic): genetic, common in dogs, rare and poorly documented in cats, possible ion channel mutation.
    - Symptomatic: structural forebrain lesion causing the seizures that include infectious encephalitis (e.g., viral, fungal, other), noninfectious encephalitis (e.g., granulomatous meningoencephalitis, necrotizing meningoencephalitis), brain tumor, vascular insult (e.g., stroke, feline ischemic encephalopathy), head trauma, degenerative diseases (e.g., storage disease), and malformation (e.g., cyst, hydrocephalus).
- Extracranial (or reactive): seizure secondary to a transient systemic or toxic insult to a normal brain. Systemic causes include hypoglycemia (e.g., insulinoma), encephalopathy (e.g., portosystemic shunt), and hypocalcemia (e.g., hypoparathyroidism, eclampsia). Many toxins can cause seizure at the advanced stage (e.g., ethylene glycol, metaldehyde, lead). For most toxins, there is progression from shaking to trembling to, finally, seizuring.

Pathophysiology:

- An alteration in neuronal excitability causes a paroxysmal depolarizing shift (PDS). This PDS may be secondary to inadequate neuronal inhibition (neurotransmitters GABA and glycine) or to excessive neuronal stimulation (neurotransmitters glutamate and aspartate) or can be a combination of both.

DIAGNOSIS

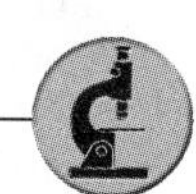

DIFFERENTIAL DIAGNOSIS

- Syncope: sudden loss of consciousness and muscle tone, usually without motor activity and without postictal signs (fast and complete recovery). Onset of syncope is likely to be associated with activity or effort, and clues of a cardiac problem may be present on examination (e.g., heart murmur, arrhythmias).
- Metabolic diseases: Seizures are usually preceded by other signs (e.g., confusion, change in behavior, weakness).
    - Hypoglycemia (e.g., insulinoma): diagnosed rapidly with a simple blood glucose evaluation
    - Hypocalcemia: causes muscle cramping, spasms and fasciculation, and weakness and irritability rather than "true" seizures; diagnosed rapidly with simple blood total calcium or ionized calcium evaluation
    - Hepatic encephalopathy: episodes usually last hours, often associated with food intake
    - Polycythemia: may cause weakness, confusion, collapse, and even a vascular event in the brain; diagnosed rap-

idly with hematocrit > 60–65% (sight hounds >70%)
  - Kidney failure: at advanced stages, evident on physical exam (anuria) and/or blood work and urinalysis (concurrent azotemia and isosthenuria)
- Narcolepsy/cataplexy: animal "falls" asleep but can be awakened; usually associated with excitement or food.
- Sleep disorder: excessive "jerky" movements occurring exclusively during sleep. The animal can be awakened and exhibits normal wakening behavior (i.e., no postictal signs).
- Obsessive/compulsive behavior (e.g., "fly biting"): complex behavior that is usually goal directed and/or can be interrupted; more common in dogs. Affected dogs often have other behavioral problems (e.g., separation anxiety).
- Movement disorders: Focal motor signs are not associated with loss of consciousness or postictal signs. One of these signs is the "head bob," which is occasionally seen in Doberman pinschers, boxers, and bulldogs (movement of the head from side to side or up and down); another sign is dyskinesia in the bichon frise.

INITIAL DATABASE

- Fundic examination: evidence of papilledema (as can be seen with optic neuritis/encephalitis); hypertension, polycythemia, or coagulopathy (retinal hemorrhage, detachment, etc.); systemic infection (ehrlichiosis, toxoplasmosis, neosporosis, fungal disease).
- Complete blood count (CBC), serum biochemistry panel, and urinalysis: evaluate for hypoglycemia, hypocalcemia, signs of liver or kidney disease, anemia, polycythemia, and calcium oxalate monohydrate crystals in antifreeze toxicity.
  - Usually normal in cases of primary brain disease
  - After severe seizures or status epilepticus, hyperglycemia (or, rarely, hypoglycemia if prolonged seizures last for more than 20 minutes), increased liver enzymes (reduced perfusion or congestion), increased creatine kinase (CK; muscular damage or necrosis), and metabolic acidosis can be seen
- Electrocardiogram (ECG): evaluate for arrhythmias.
- Thoracic and abdominal radiographs: usually unremarkable.
- Serum bile acids assay: indicated if hepatic encephalopathy is suspected and/or if a young animal presents with seizures. More than 90% of dogs and cats with portosystemic shunts have abnormal 2-hour postprandial serum bile acid levels.

ADVANCED OR CONFIRMATORY TESTING

- Portable ECG (cardiac event monitor or Holter monitor): if distinction between syncope and seizure is unclear on history and physical exam. Helps rule in (severe tachycardia or severe bradycardia occurs during episode) or rule out (cardiac rhythm is normal during episode) a cardiac arrhythmia as the cause of episodic clinical signs. Important prior to proceeding to general anesthesia, as for advanced imaging or cerebrospinal fluid (CSF) tap.
- Advanced imaging of the brain (MRI or CT scan): brain tumor, multifocal lesions suggestive of inflammation, vascular lesion. MRI is slightly more sensitive. Radiographs of the skull are unrewarding except in cases of head trauma or palpable skull abnormalities.
- CSF analysis: often nonspecific but can be helpful in confirming brain disease or inflammation.
- Serologic testing (e.g., fungal diseases, *Toxoplasma*, *Neospora*, and others; selection based on physical findings and initial database).
- Tests for toxins if exposure (e.g., plasma lead concentration, serum cholinesterase level).
- Electroencephalogram (EEG): limited availability; usefulness has yet to be proven.

TREATMENT

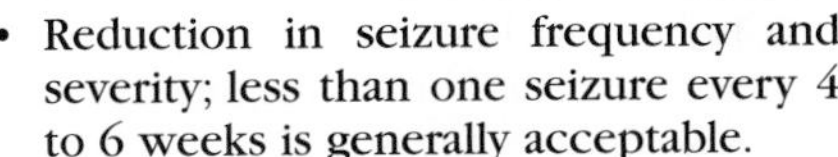

THERAPEUTIC GOAL(S)

- Reduction in seizure frequency and severity; less than one seizure every 4 to 6 weeks is generally acceptable.
- For cluster seizures (more then two seizures per 24 hours) and status epilepticus: stopping the seizures and preventing others.

ACUTE GENERAL TREATMENT

For emergency situations (cluster or status):
- Identify and address any immediately reversible causes:
  - Hypoglycemia (blood or serum glucose <40 mg/dl): administration of dextrose 2 g/kg IV. If using 50% dextrose, this equals 4 ml/kg, which must be diluted with 5 to 10 times as much 0.9% saline or other sterile fluid by volume prior to administration to reduce the risk of phlebitis.
  - Hypocalcemia (blood or serum calcium <6 mg/dl): administration of 10% calcium gluconate IV at a dose of 0.5–1.5 ml/kg or 5–15 mg/kg slowly, to effect, over a 15 to 30 minute period. Monitor ECG for onset of bradycardia, ventricular arrhythmia, or shortening of the QT interval, any of which justifies temporarily stopping the infusion. Total dose is the amount required to stop clinical signs.
  - Dextrose and calcium should not be administered unless a deficiency is documented.
- To stop the seizure and if reversible causes are absent: diazepam 0.5–1.0 mg/kg IV bolus; can be repeated safely if seizure activity persists. Animals receiving phenobarbital may require 2 mg/kg of diazepam. Diazepam lasts only 20 to 30 minutes; further seizure activity must be prevented by one of the following steps.
- To prevent another seizure:
  - Re-evaluate animal's history to ensure that episodes truly are seizures.
  - Identify and control any known causes (e.g., antidote if known intoxication: pralidoxime or atropine for organophosphate; others).
  - Administer loading dose of phenobarbital: IV bolus of 10–20 mg/kg slowly; will reach an optimal serum level immediately; monitor the patient carefully if combined with diazepam.
  - Administer diazepam at a constant rate infusion (CRI): 0.5–1.0 mg/kg/hr; can be added to 0.9% sodium chloride (NaCl) in an in-line burette; reduced by 25% every 4 to 6 hours if the seizures are controlled; do not prepare more than 2 hours at a time because diazepam is adsorbed by plastic and is sensitive to light.
  - Give diazepam boluses: alternative to a CRI; give two IV boluses of 1.0 mg/kg 30 minutes apart followed by an IV bolus of 0.5 mg/kg 30 minutes and 60 minutes later.
- If seizures persist, administer propofol via IV bolus of 1–6 mg/kg to effect followed by a CRI of 2–8 mg/kg/hr; then reduce the dose by 25% every 4 to 6 hours if the seizures are controlled; adequate monitoring is recommended.

CHRONIC TREATMENT

Depends on underlying cause. Initiation of long-term, oral antiepileptic drug therapy (e.g., phenobarbital, potassium bromide) is often required. See also: Epilepsy, Idiopathic, p 351.

DRUG INTERACTIONS

Cimetidine, ranitidine, and chloramphenicol may interfere with the metabolism of phenobarbital.

POSSIBLE COMPLICATIONS

- Seizures may continue despite adequate antiepileptic drug therapy.
- Status epilepticus and death.
- Hyperthermia, noncardiogenic pulmonary edema.
- Neuronal damage if long, severe, or frequent seizures.
- Hypersensitivity to phenobarbital; hepatotoxicity, rare bone marrow aplasia or blood dyscrasia, skin lesions.

RECOMMENDED MONITORING

- Phenobarbital serum level 3 weeks after initiation, change in dosage, signs of toxicity or poor seizure control.
- Bromide level after loading dose (if applicable), 3 to 4 months after initiation and change in dosage; toxicity or poor control.
- CBC and serum biochemistry panel every 6 to 12 months.

PROGNOSIS AND OUTCOME

- Good to guarded, depending on the cause.
- Many patients need lifetime medication and follow-up appointments.

PEARLS & CONSIDERATIONS

COMMENTS

- A structural forebrain lesion, rather than primary epilepsy, should be suspected in seizuring dogs younger than 6 months or older than 5 years, and in seizuring cats.
- Status epilepticus is a medical emergency and needs to be treated aggressively.
- Most animals will need long-term or lifelong treatment, and some animals may be refractory to treatment.

SUGGESTED READING

Lorenz MD, Kornegay JN: Seizures, narcolepsy, and cataplexy. In Oliver JE, Lorenz MD (eds): *Handbook of Veterinary Neurology*. St. Louis, WB Saunders, 2004, pp 323-338.

Platt SR, McDonnell JJ: Status epilepticus: Patient management and pharmacologic therapy. *Compend Contin Educ Pract Vet* 22: 722-728, 2000.

Podell M: Seizures. In Platt SR, Olby NJ (eds): *BSAVA Manual of Canine and Feline Neurology*, ed 3. Gloucester, United Kingdom, British Small Animal Veterinary Association, 2004, pp 97-112.

Understanding your pet's epilepsy: www.canine-epilepsy.net. College of Veterinary Medicine, University of Missouri, 1999.

AUTHOR: **VÉRONIQUE SAMMUT**
EDITOR: **CURTIS W. DEWEY**

Semilunar Valve Insufficiency

BASIC INFORMATION

DEFINITION

Diastolic incompetence of the aortic valve and/or pulmonic valve

SYNONYM(S)

Aortic insufficiency (AI)
Aortic regurgitation (AR)
Pulmonic insufficiency (PI)
Pulmonic regurgitation (PR)

EPIDEMIOLOGY

SPECIES, AGE, SEX: May affect dogs and cats of any age and either sex.

GENETICS AND BREED PREDISPOSITION: Only when associated with an inciting cause (e.g., subaortic stenosis in Newfoundland dogs).

RISK FACTORS

- Aortic insufficiency: subvalvular aortic stenosis, aortic stenosis, ventricular septal defect, tetralogy of Fallot, infectious endocarditis, cardiac catheterization, aortic valve balloon valvuloplasty, aortic dilation
- Pulmonic insufficiency: pulmonic stenosis, patent ductus arteriosus, pulmonary hypertension, infectious endocarditis, heartworm disease, cardiac catheterization, pulmonic valve balloon valvuloplasty

GEOGRAPHY AND SEASONALITY: See Endocarditis, Infective, p 344; Heartworm Disease, Cat, p 462; Heartworm Disease, Dog, p 465.

ASSOCIATED CONDITIONS AND DISORDERS

- Severe AI may cause volume overload of the left ventricle and ultimately may lead to left-sided congestive heart failure. Such severe AI is very rare in dogs and cats.
- Pulmonic insufficiency, even if severe, essentially never produces volume overload of the right ventricle.

CLINICAL PRESENTATION

DISEASE FORMS/SUBTYPES

- Aortic insufficiency:
  - Isolated AI: uncommon
  - Secondary AI: underlying causes: see Risk Factors above
- Pulmonic insufficiency:
  - Isolated trivial PI: relatively common in dogs of all ages and either sex; uncommon in cats
  - Secondary PI: underlying causes: see Risk Factors above

HISTORY, CHIEF COMPLAINT

- Aortic insufficiency:
  - Often an incidental finding; no overt clinical signs
  - If severe: respiratory distress, cough, exercise intolerance, weakness, collapse
  - Signs of the causative cardiac disorder may predominate
- Pulmonic insufficiency:
  - Virtually never associated with clinical signs
  - If severe: respiratory distress, cough, cyanosis, exercise intolerance, weakness, collapse, abdominal distention
  - Signs of the causative disorder may predominate

PHYSICAL EXAM FINDINGS

- Aortic insufficiency:
  - No abnormal findings if AI is trivial to mild
  - If moderate to severe:
    - Cardiac auscultation reveals a soft, low-frequency holodiastolic murmur over the left heart base (4th-5th ICS) with radiation to right hemithorax
    - Bounding peripheral pulses in some instances (dependent upon quantity of AI and underlying etiology)
  - If sufficiently severe to cause congestive heart failure (CHF): dyspnea, cough, pale mucus membranes, lethargy, pulmonary crackles
- Pulmonic insufficiency:
  - No abnormal findings if PI is trivial to moderate
  - If severe, and/or if concurrent pulmonary hypertension:
    - Cardiac auscultation reveals a low-frequency, diastolic/decrescendo murmur over the left heart base (3rd–4th ICS)
  - If sufficiently severe to cause CHF (rarely, under any circumstance, and virtually never without a complicating factor such as pulmonary hypertension):
    - Pulse quality may be decreased
    - Dyspnea, cough, dull lung sounds, abdominal fluid wave, pale mucous membranes, lethargy

ETIOLOGY AND PATHOPHYSIOLOGY

- Isolated semilunar valvular insufficiency:
  - Usually mild, rarely associated with clinical disease (especially PI)
  - Presumed mild congenital valvular malformation
- Aortic valve incompetence secondary to other causes:
  - Subaortic stenosis:
    - Poststenotic turbulence distorts valve endothelium, such that valve closure is ineffective
  - Valvular aortic stenosis (rare), infectious endocarditis:

- Malformed valve leaflets do not coapt/close normally
  - Ventricular septal defect (membranous):
    - Base of aortic valve is poorly supported due to absent basal septal tissue, causing sagging and partial prolapse of the aortic valve in diastole
- Pulmonic valve incompetence secondary to other causes:
  - Pulmonic stenosis: malformed pulmonic valve leaflets do not coapt/close normally
  - Heartworm disease: physical blockage of pulmonic valve closure by worms
- Volume overload and increased end-diastolic ventricular and atrial pressures if AI or PI severe:
  - Predisposes to CHF and, ultimately, myocardial failure

DIAGNOSIS

DIFFERENTIAL DIAGNOSIS

- Normal
- Differentiate isolated semilunar insufficiency from specific causes (see Etiology and Pathophysiology above)

INITIAL DATABASE

- Echocardiogram: confirm diagnosis, identify underlying conditions, and qualitatively assess degree of insufficiency
- Thoracic radiographs: normal if insufficiency mild
  - AI—if moderate to marked: left ventricular enlargement, left atrial enlargement, distended pulmonary veins, pulmonary edema
  - PI—if marked: right ventricular enlargement, pleural effusion, distended caudal vena cava
  - Findings consistent with primary disorder
- Blood pressure: assess hemodynamic consequence of valvular insufficiency
- Complete blood count, serum biochemistry panel, urinalysis usually unremarkable with mild insufficiency but varies with underlying etiology

ADVANCED OR CONFIRMATORY TESTING

- Tests to rule out specific acquired diseases (see Endocarditis, Infective, p 344; Heartworm Disease, Cat, p 462; Heartworm Disease, Dog, p 465)
- Angiogram: confirmation of echocardiographic findings (rarely necessary)

TREATMENT

THERAPEUTIC GOAL(S)

- None, if insufficiency is mild
- Treat primary cause of insufficiency—if applicable
- Manage CHF, if present (see Heart Failure, Acute/Decompensated, p 458; Heart Failure, Chronic, p 459)
- Prevent progressive cardiac remodelling and myocardial failure

ACUTE AND CHRONIC TREATMENT

Dependent on underlying cause and presence or absence of CHF

POSSIBLE COMPLICATIONS

- Refractory CHF
- Systemic hypotension
- Azotemia (especially in patients with preexisting renal compromise and/or those receiving aggressive diuretic therapy)

RECOMMENDED MONITORING

- Systemic blood pressure
- Renal function (with diuretics)
- Serum digoxin levels (measure 6 to 8 hours postadministration)
- Repeat echocardiograms regularly (frequency dependent on the severity of insufficiency)

PROGNOSIS AND OUTCOME

- Excellent for mild to moderate PI and mild AI without evidence of ventricular or atrial dilation
- Guarded to poor for patients with marked AI/PI and CHF

PEARLS & CONSIDERATIONS

COMMENTS

- Auscultation of soft, low-frequency diastolic murmurs may be enhanced by positioning patient in left lateral recumbency and placing stethoscope bell on the dependent side of the chest wall over the heart base.
- The detection of small jets of semilunar valve insufficiency requires a high-quality echocardiograph.
- With increasingly sensitive color-flow Doppler echocardiography, semilunar valve insufficiency can be detected in a progressively larger proportion of the normal dog and cat population; the volume of insufficiency and its impact on the ventricle are most important.

PREVENTION

See Endocarditis, Infective, p 344; Heartworm Disease, Cat, p 462; Heartworm Disease, Dog, p 465

SUGGESTED READING

Darke P, Bonagura JD, Kelly DF: *Color Atlas of Veterinary Cardiology*. Boston, Mosby-Wolfe, 1996, pp 77–79.

Kvart C, Häggström J: Acquired valvular heart disease. In Ettinger JE, Feldman EC (eds): *Veterinary Internal Medicine*, ed 5. Philadelphia, WB Saunders, 2000, pp 787–800.

Nakayama, et al: Prevalence of valvular regurgitation in normal beagle dogs detected by color Doppler echocardiography. *J Vet Med Sci* 56:5, 1994.

AUTHOR: **NATHANIEL FENOLLOSA**
EDITOR: **ETIENNE CÔTÉ**

Separation Anxiety

Client Education Sheet on Website

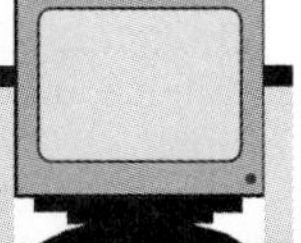

BASIC INFORMATION

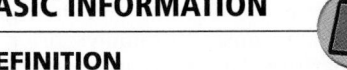

DEFINITION

Physical or behavioral signs of distress exhibited by the animal only in the absence of or lack of access to the client. Distress can manifest with destruction, elimination, vocalization, and salivation

EPIDEMIOLOGY

Prevalence has been estimated at 14% of dogs seen in the average United States private practice.

SPECIES, AGE, SEX: Dogs > cats; age of onset usually overlaps with social maturity (dogs: 12 to 36 months old; cats: 24 to 48 months old).

RISK FACTORS

- Trauma during a client's absence (e.g., fire, burglary) can precipitate a

sudden onset of full-blown separation anxiety.
- Severe illness may lower the threshold for manifestations of an otherwise subclinical state of separation anxiety.
- The popular beliefs that dogs with separation anxiety are "spoiled," are "only dogs," or have never "learned" to be left alone are incorrect.

ASSOCIATED CONDITIONS AND DISORDERS
- Phobias: commonly coexistent
- Probability of separation anxiety, given a diagnosis of storm or noise phobia in a dog: 0.87 and 0.88, respectively (note: a guarantee that the dog has the condition is a probability of 1.00); probability of also having a storm or noise phobia, given a diagnosis of separation anxiety: 0.61 and 0.73, respectively

CLINICAL PRESENTATION

HISTORY, CHIEF COMPLAINT
- Destructive behavior, excessive vocalization, or house soiling are the most common hallmark signs of separation anxiety.
- Specific chief complaints range from minor (a chewed slipper) to major (walls chewed through) destruction, urination, defecation, puddles of saliva, salivary staining, primary self-mutilation (e.g., a chewed leg) or secondary self-mutilation (e.g., injury incurred when breaking out of a crate or through a window).
- Vocalization, while common, is often unrecognized (e.g., no near neighbors).
- Observant clients may see earliest manifestations of separation anxiety begin when signs of impending absence occur (e.g., client putting on a coat, rushing, drinking while moving, alarm clock ringing).
- Dogs with separation anxiety have routinely experienced unexplained diarrhea or have been previously considered as candidates for inflammatory bowel disease.
- Some dogs with separation anxiety freeze and withdraw from all action and interaction when left. These animals are under diagnosed but suffering.

PHYSICAL EXAM FINDINGS: Self-induced during anxiety:
- Broken teeth
- Lingual, nasal, buccal, cutaneous lacerations
- Torn or broken claws
- Abdominal palpation: evidence of ingestion of drywall, plastic, and other such items
- Weight loss possible if chronic condition

ETIOLOGY AND PATHOPHYSIOLOGY
- Multiple mechanisms likely, given the wide variety of anxiety manifestations.
- Greater duration of the disorder may lead to more signs, more intense signs, and worse response to treatment.
- Dogs, like humans, may have "susceptibility genes" for the development of problematic anxieties.

DIAGNOSIS

DIFFERENTIAL DIAGNOSIS
- Generalized anxiety disorder (GAD), panic disorder: Many signs are similar to separation anxiety, but in animals with separation anxiety, signs occur only around or during a pet owner's absence.
- Attention-seeking behavior: Signs occur only in the owner's presence and generally improve with proper management (ignoring the signs while they occur and rewarding good behavior by interacting with the pet).
- Incomplete housetraining: Signs are confined to inappropriate elimination and occur continually (daily for months or more).
- Age-associated destruction and elimination problems (youth or old age).
- Pseudocyesis-like reaction: Destructive behavior is typically confined to bedding, occurs after an ovariohysterectomy, and responds to hormonal supplementation.
- Systemic medical conditions can produce changes in behavior, including hyperthyroidism (cats), hypothyroidism (dogs), neurologic disease (some seizure disorders, rare brain tumors, rabies, etc.), and urinary tract disorders.

INITIAL DATABASE
- A complete and detailed history is the cornerstone of diagnosis.
- The most powerful diagnostic tool for separation anxiety is a videocamera. Animals should be videotaped when left alone.
  - Identification of distressed but nondestructive animals
  - Identification/ruling out provocative stimuli for the destructive animals
  - Assessment of improvement by comparison with a later videotape
- Neurologic exam: no abnormalities expected.
- Complete blood count (CBC), serum biochemistry panel, urinalysis ± thyroid profile: results should be within normal limits.

ADVANCED OR CONFIRMATORY TESTING
If neurologic signs are present or develop, a full neurologic evaluation including spinal fluid analysis and imaging (CT scan or MRI) may be indicated.

TREATMENT

THERAPEUTIC GOAL(S)
The ultimate goal is to change the pet's behavior so that it no longer responds to being left alone with any of the signs of anxiety. Instead, the pet should be calm in these circumstances.

ACUTE GENERAL TREATMENT
- Separation anxiety is a veterinary emergency. Until medications can take effect, or if clients are unwilling to use medication, pets must not be left alone. Options include dog and cat sitters, daycare, boarding, or bringing the pet to work if possible.
- Reward any spontaneous decrease in reactivity.
- Implement behavior modification designed to teach the pet to relax and to substitute a new and calming rule structure for the pet that panics. First, ensure that clients understand what pet anxiety looks like and teach them to avoid rewarding it. Accidental reinforcement of anxiety-related behaviors occurs frequently (e.g., clients arrive home and think their frantic pet is just glad to see them).
- Clients should not respond to any nonspecific sign of anxiety and only engage with the pet if it is sitting calmly and quietly. Talking to the pet calmly can often help to induce future, calmer behaviors. Then, clients can add to the behavior modification by gradually teaching the dog or cat that it can be gradually left for incrementally increasing amounts of time.
- Pets should be rewarded with praise and food treats when calm, and the pace of the behavior modification must proceed at an appropriate rate that will allow improvement. If the pet is distressed, the owner is trying to progress too quickly.
- If panic, noise phobia, or storm phobia coexist, consider: alprazolam (dogs: 0.01–0.1 mg/kg PO q 4–6h, as needed [prn]; cats: 0.0125–0.025 mg/kg PO q 12–24h prn; some published sources recommend a ten-fold higher dose, which is an error) with 0.5–1 dose given 2 hours before the expected provacative event and repeated 30 minutes beforehand. If the pet panics when the owner leaves for work in the morning, he/she can give the pet 0.5–1 dose when awakening in the morning and then give the same dose 30 minutes prior to departure. An alternative (though more sedative and more side effects) is: diazepam (dogs: 0.5–2.0 mg/kg PO q 4–6 h prn; cats: 0.2–0.4 mg/kg PO q 12–24h prn).

CHRONIC TREATMENT

- Dogs should be taught to relax while making eye contact with their owners as a new default behavior when the dogs encounter a situation about which they are anxious or unsure. Clients should learn to monitor facial cues, body postures, pupil size and shape, and respiratory behavior associated with relaxation.
- Avoid exposing dogs to circumstances likely to distress them (e.g., boarding dogs in a kennel if they have never enjoyed or experienced this).
- Desensitization to the triggers can be accomplished if two criteria can be met: the triggers can be identified and they can be reproduced faithfully in a systematic and incremental fashion.
- Dogs and cats should be crated as part of treatment only if they voluntarily and routinely use and enjoy their crates.
- Once the pet has improved, it is important that the owners continue the behavior modification as a consistent and kind rule. A decreased or ablated response to an inciting trigger as evidenced by a reduction in or elimination of somatic signs of sympathetic arousal is the desired goal.
- Once developed, humane treatment of separation anxiety will likely require long-term treatment with antianxiety medications:
    - Amitriptyline: dogs, 1–2 mg/kg PO, q 12h for a minimum of 30 days; cats, 0.5–1.0 mg/kg PO, q12–24h for a minimum of 30 days; tricyclic antidepressant (TCA) drug and first drug of choice in mild cases; inexpensive.
    - Clomipramine (Clomicalm): dogs, up to 3 mg/kg PO q 12h for a minimum of 8 weeks; cats, 0.5 mg/kg PO q 24h for a minimum of 8 weeks; TCA drug and the only medication licensed for use for separation anxiety. Most successful when the behaviors have a ritualistic component or elimination component.
    - Selective serotonin reuptake inhibitor (SSRI) drugs: fluoxetine (Prozac; dogs: 1 mg/kg PO q 24h for 8 weeks, minimum; cats: 0.5 mg/kg PO q 24h for 8 weeks, minimum) or sertraline (Zoloft; dogs: 1+ mg/kg PO, q 24h for 8 weeks, minimum; cats: 0.5 mg/kg PO q 24h for 8 weeks, minimum) can be successful in situations where other medications have been less helpful.
    - The minimal total treatment time for using medication with behavior modification is 4 to 6 months. Drugs should not be stopped too early.

DRUG INTERACTIONS

- Benzodiazepines, TCAs, and SSRIs can all be combined at lower than normal dosages, if needed, but the potential for sedation and interaction must be evaluated.
- TCAs and SSRIs should not be given with monoamine oxidase inhibitors (MAOIs) that are found in many flea and tick collars and dips as well as in some cognitive dysfunction medications.

POSSIBLE COMPLICATIONS

- Abrupt cessation of medications with short half-lives is not recommended for the TCAs and SSRIs; wean over 10 to 14 days.
- TCAs should be used cautiously or not at all in animals with heart disease.
- Cats and dogs receiving serotonergic medications can manifest "serotonin-like syndromes" with hyperactivity, unpredictability, and, ultimately, seizures. This is an extraordinarily rare side effect.

RECOMMENDED MONITORING

- Owners can abuse benzodiazepines. Abuse can be limited by frequent follow-up appointments and not allowing automatic refills.
- Examination, CBC, serum chemistry profile, urinalysis, ± thyroid profile are indicated q 6–12 months for animals receiving long-term medication.
- Clients should learn to monitor heart rate digitally since the first sign of cardiac side effects of medications can be an unremitting tachycardia.

PROGNOSIS AND OUTCOME

- Prognosis is improved by early diagnosis and aggressive treatment and by client compliance. Frequent and thorough communication between clinician and client so the treatment plan can be adjusted according to the animal's response and needs is essential.
- With chronic separation anxiety, treatment may be lifelong, especially if there are other comorbid anxiety-related conditions.

PEARLS & CONSIDERATIONS

COMMENTS

- If a veterinarian is not comfortable treating a case of separation anxiety, the animal should be referred to a specialist (see www.dacvb.org for a listing in the United States).
- Most veterinary staffs have no one with extensive experience in behavior modification. Resources to help inform and train support personnel include the Association of Pet Dog Trainers (www.APDT.com) and the Society of Veterinary Behavioral Technicians (www.SVBT.org).

PREVENTION

- Early intervention for diagnosis and treatment.
- Veterinarians should screen for behavioral problems as a routine part of every appointment. Otherwise, left untreated, separation anxiety worsens.
- When selecting breeding stock, clients should assess both medical and behavioral patterns of the pet's family members.

CLIENT EDUCATION

- Most behavioral conditions are due to chemical and functional abnormalities. These pets are distressed; they are not vindictive, jealous, spoiled, or disobedient.
- Under no circumstances should pets with behavioral problems be "punished," physically "disciplined," or "corrected." These techniques only render the animal more anxious.
- Clients should expect treatment to be long-term (at least 6 months) and possibly lifelong if the condition has been ongoing and/or severe.
- Relapses may occur with treatment discontinuation or with added stressors. When such stressors are anticipated, premedication may be helpful.

SUGGESTED READING

King JN, et al: Results of a follow-up investigation to a clinical trial testing the efficacy of clomipramine in the treatment of separation anxiety in dogs. *Appl Anim Behav Sci* 89:233–242, 2004.

Overall KL, et al: Frequency of nonspecific clinical signs in dogs with separation anxiety, thunderstorm phobia, and noise phobia, alone or in combination. *J Am Vet Med Assoc* 219:467–473, 2001.

Overall KL: Early intervention and prevention of behavior problems: Step 3, dealing with dogs affected with separation anxiety. *Veterinary Forum* 2001:40–53.

Schwartz S: Separation anxiety syndrome in dogs and cats. *J Am Vet Med Assoc* 222:1526–1532, 2003.

AUTHOR & EDITOR: **KAREN L. OVERALL**

Sepsis and Septic Shock

BASIC INFORMATION

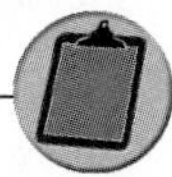

DEFINITION

Sepsis is the occurrence of systemic inflammation in response to infection (see Systemic Inflammatory Response Syndrome, p 1060). It generally implies systemic circulation of infectious agents (e.g., bacteremia). Septic shock is defined as sepsis with concurrent hypotension that is refractory to fluid therapy and requires vasopressor therapy.

EPIDEMIOLOGY

SPECIES, AGE, SEX: Dogs and cats of any age and either sex may develop sepsis or septic shock.

RISK FACTORS

- Animals with established infections
- Animals with diseases resulting in immunosuppression (such as hyper-Adrenocorticism or diabetes mellitus)
- Noninfectious diseases that may predispose an animal to bacteremia include neoplasia, glucocorticoid therapy, trauma, surgery, cytotoxic therapy, IV and urinary tract catheters, burns, and hematologic abnormalities (e.g., leukocyte function defects)

CLINICAL PRESENTATION

DISEASE FORMS/SUBTYPES: Sepsis and early septic shock initially present a hyperdynamic phase characterized by increased metabolic processes: tachycardia, fever, warm extremities, injected mucous membranes, and a bounding pulse. If unchecked, the hyperdynamic phase progresses to a more critical and potentially terminal hypodynamic phase of septic shock, characterized by normothermia or hypothermia, pallor, cool extremities, a weak or absent pulse, and decreased mentation.

HISTORY, CHIEF COMPLAINT: Complaints vary depending on the source of sepsis. Animals with abdominal sources of sepsis may present with vomiting, anorexia, or abdominal pain, while those with thoracic sepsis often present with a history of coughing, labored breathing/ dyspnea, or respiratory distress. Sepsis from an occult source (anywhere in the body) may not produce localizing signs, and some animals with sepsis present with only vague signs of general malaise, such as anorexia and lethargy.

PHYSICAL EXAM FINDINGS

- General:
  - Hyperthermia (>104°F [>40°C]): fever in response to infection (hyperdynamic phase)
  - Hypothermia (<100.4°F [<38°C] in dogs, <100°F [<37.8°C] in cats): advanced stages, usually with visible lethargy, mental depression, or collapse (hypodynamic phase)
  - Tachycardia (although bradycardia may be present in cats with septic shock): by definition, as part of the systemic inflammatory response syndrome
  - Tachypnea, dyspnea: as compensation for metabolic acidosis, as a manifestation of pain, or with primary respiratory disease (e.g., pneumonia) as the source of sepsis/septic shock
  - Pulse and mucous membrane alterations:
    - Injected/red mucous membranes and bounding pulse (hyperdynamic phase)
    - Pale mucous membranes, slow capillary refill time (>3 seconds), weak pulse (hypodynamic phase)
  - Collapse (hyperdynamic or hypodynamic phase)
- Specific signs may indicate the source of infection, such as:
  - Abdominal pain or a distended abdomen (if present, abdominal source of sepsis is suspected)
  - Swollen limb or an infected cutaneous wound

ETIOLOGY AND PATHOPHYSIOLOGY

- Generalized infection leads to the release of inflammatory mediators, including tumor necrosis factor-α (TNF-α), interleukin-1 (IL-1), and IL-6. These and other inflammatory mediators increase microvascular permeability, cause leakage of fluid from the vascular space, and lead to reduced effective circulating volume.
- Excessive nitric oxide production via the inducible nitric oxide synthase pathway results in arterial and venous vasodilation, reduced systemic vascular resistance, and eventually, hypotension. Tachycardia and increased cardiac output occur as compensatory mechanisms for these changes, though these compensatory effects may be negated by reduced myocardial contractility as a result of inflammatory mediators with myocardial depressant properties (e.g., TNF-α).
- Other physiologic changes in sepsis include stimulation of the coagulation cascade, reduction in endogenous anticoagulants such as protein C and antithrombin, hypoalbuminemia from changes in microvascular permeability and reduced production by the liver, and lung injury secondary to atelectasis or acute respiratory distress syndrome (ARDS).
- Ultimately, if left to progress, these serious changes lead to further reduced tissue perfusion and decreased oxygen delivery to tissues. Deprived of oxygen, tissues sustain terminal cellular injury, leading to the development of multiple organ failure (see Multiple Organ Dysfunction Syndrome, p 716) and death.

DIAGNOSIS

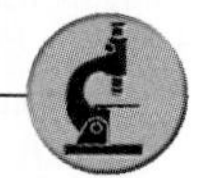

DIFFERENTIAL DIAGNOSIS

Causes of:

- Fever (see Fever of Unknown Origin, p 386)
- Abdominal pain without an infectious basis (pancreatitis, reno/ureterolithiasis, neoplasia)
- Abdominal distention (organomegaly, neoplasia, obesity, gastrointestinal [GI] obstruction, ascites secondary to cirrhosis or right-sided heart failure, hyperadrenocorticism)

INITIAL DATABASE

- Complete blood count (CBC): neutrophilia (medium term) or neutropenia (acute sepsis) and the presence of band forms and toxic changes in neutrophils; thrombocytopenia suggests a hypercoagulable state or early disseminated intravascular coagulation (DIC).
- Serum biochemistry panel:
  - Azotemia (prerenal or renal—correlate to urine specific gravity ≥1.035 or <1.035, respectively).
  - Elevated liver enzymes (alanine aminotransferase [ALT] and aspartate aminotransferase [AST]) often occur secondary to hepatic hypoperfusion, hepatic thromboembolism, or bacterial showering from a compromised GI tract.
  - Hyperbilirubinemia due to sepsis-induced cholestasis or hemolysis (assess hematocrit).
  - Hypoalbuminemia: common due to reduced hepatic synthesis (in favor of acute phase protein production) and to increased microvascular permeability.
  - Hypoglycemia: common (changes in hepatic gluconeogenesis versus insulin-like factor production).
- Elevated lactate is an important marker of hypoperfusion and is often elevated in dogs with sepsis.

- Hyperlactatemia (>3.5 mmol/L) often resolves quickly following initiation of fluid therapy.
- Increasing lactate despite fluid resuscitation is a negative prognostic indicator and should lead the clinician to seek superior treatment modalities or alternate reasons for deteriorating status.

- Urinalysis with culture and sensitivity (C&S) to help rule out genitourinary source of sepsis. Urine is obtained by cystocentesis to prevent contamination, unless pyometra, ascites, or a bleeding disorder is suspected.
- A coagulation profile helps identify animals with coagulopathy including DIC.
- Diagnostic imaging, including chest and abdominal radiographs and/or abdominal ultrasound, are often necessary to further elucidate the source of sepsis.

ADVANCED OR CONFIRMATORY TESTING

- Abdominocentesis (see Abdominocentesis, p 1178) should be performed in animals with abdominal effusion and fever. A neutrophilic effusion with intracellular bacteria is diagnostic of septic effusion, which essentially always warrants surgical intervention. The glucose level of septic abdominal fluid is often <50 mg/dl.
- Thoracocentesis is indicated in animals with pleural effusion and fever to identify septic pleural effusion.
- Echocardiography is indicated in animals whose source of fever is difficult to identify, especially when a new-onset murmur is noted in the absence of anemia. Echocardiographic lesions of the aortic valve are often consistent with bacterial endocarditis; less so mitral valve changes, which may be due either to infection or to sterile myxomatous valve disease/endocardiosis.
- Blood cultures (four samples: aerobic and anaerobic, both drawn at time 0 and 2 hours later) are indicated in any critically ill animal that develops a fever, neutropenia, neutrophilia with a left shift, a new cardiac murmur, or other signs suggestive of sepsis that cannot be explained by a known preexisting condition.
- Arterial blood gas (ABG) measurement often may identify hypoxemia and metabolic acidosis, conditions commonly associated with sepsis and that may be corrected with treatment.

TREATMENT

THERAPEUTIC GOAL(S)

- Hemodynamic resuscitation to correct intravascular volume deficits and to maintain organ perfusion. IV fluids (crystalloids and colloids) are the mainstay of therapy.
- Eradication of the inciting infection using source control measures (e.g., surgery) and systemic antibiotic therapy.
- A future direction and goal is modulation of the inflammatory response with interventions that target its specific mediators. Specific agents to target the inflammatory response are not readily available in veterinary medicine but continue to be a subject of intense research in the field of human medicine.

ACUTE GENERAL TREATMENT

- Antibiotic therapy: It is essential that broad-spectrum IV antibiotics be initiated early for successful treatment of sepsis. Antibiotic therapy should be effective against gram-negative, gram-positive, and anaerobic organisms. Two commonly used empiric combinations are a cephalosporin (cefazolin 22 mg/kg IV q 8h), a fluroquinolone (enrofloxacin 10 mg/kg [5 mg/kg in cats] diluted 1:1 in saline and given slowly IV q 24h), and metronidazole (10 mg/kg given slowly IV q 8h); or ampicillin (22 mg/kg IV q 6h) along with an aminoglycoside (gentamicin 6 mg/kg IV q 24h). Definitive antimicrobial treatment based on C&S, when results become available, replaces empiric therapy of sepsis. Aminoglycosides should not be used in animals that are, or have recently experienced, periods of hypoperfusion or animals with preexisting renal failure.
- Cardiovascular support: Peripheral vasodilation and increased capillary permeability cause profound intravascular fluid deficits (dehydration, hypotension); correction of this deficit by the administration of IV fluids is the mainstay of treatment of the animal that is septic. IV crystalloids (e.g., lactated Ringer's solution, 0.9% NaCl) with or without the addition of a colloid should be administered initially at doses required to correct deficits (up to 90 ml/kg per hour initially in dogs and up to 70 ml/kg per hour in cats) and titrated until end points of fluid resuscitation/fluid therapy are reached, namely normalization of heart rate and blood pressure (BP) and improved mentation, pulse quality, and capillary refill time. When central venous pressure (CVP) measurement is available, fluid therapy should be administered aggressively until CVP = 8-10 cm H_2O. If signs of hypoperfusion persist despite aggressive fluid therapy and correction of dehydration, vasopressor drugs such as dopamine (5-20 μg/kg per minute) may be added and titrated to achieve a mean arterial BP of 60 mmHg. Packed red blood cells (RBCs) or whole blood is indicated if packed cell volume (PCV) < 25% to maximize oxygen content and oxygen delivery to tissues.
- Surgery: After stabilization of the animal, a search for surgically correctable sources of infection is indicated. Surgery is generally performed once hemodynamic stability has been achieved (normalization of heart rate and BP, improved mentation, pulse quality, and capillary refill time) or if hemodynamic stability cannot be achieved despite aggressive supportive treatment and deterioration is expected without intervention. The source of infection is removed if possible. Accumulations of exudates should be removed or drained.
- Coagulation abnormalities: In the absence of prolonged clotting times or thrombocytopenia, heparin (unfractionated: 75 U/kg SQ q 6-8h) may be administered to reduce coagulation cascade activation and help maintain blood flow in the microcirculation (see Disseminated Intravascular Coagulation, p 313).
- Support of organ function: Increased oxygen delivery to the tissues is critical to prevent organ dysfunction. Provide supplemental oxygen if hypoxemia is present, and mechanical ventilation if PaO_2 <60 mmHg despite oxygen supplementation. GI dysfunction may lead to gastric ulcer formation or bacterial translocation; gastric protectants (e.g., famotidine 0.5-1 mg/kg IV q 12h) are routinely administered to reduce the risk of developing a gastric ulcer, while antibiotic therapy (as described previously) addresses bacterial translocation. Renal dysfunction associated with sepsis and septic shock may lead to oliguria and renal failure. Maintenance of mean arterial BP at >60 mmHg using IV fluids and vasopressors may reduce the risk of acute renal failure.
- Nutritional support: After stabilization, nutritional support can be considered. In general, enteral nutrition is considered superior to parenteral nutrition in preservation of gut function and integrity, but parenteral nutrition should be considered in animals that are not expected to begin eating within several days.

POSSIBLE COMPLICATIONS

Recognized complications of sepsis and septic shock include DIC, MODS, acute renal failure, pulmonary thromboembolism, ARDS, and intractable hypotension leading to cardiac arrest.

RECOMMENDED MONITORING

- Heart rate and pulse quality: hourly or as indicated by case evolution
- Respiratory rate, mentation, BP, and central venous pressure: hourly or as dictated by case evolution

- Continuous electrocardiogram (ECG): all animals with ventricular arrhythmias or those that are persistently tachycardic despite therapy
- Hematocrit, total protein, and electrolyte concentrations; body weight; urine output; and fluid cytologic examination from indwelling closed suction drains are evaluated daily
- CBC and biochemistry profile are repeated every 48 hours

PROGNOSIS AND OUTCOME

- Reported mortality from sepsis in animals ranges from 30–70%
- Severity of underlying disease and choice of antibiotic therapy are important factors influencing mortality in animals with sepsis

SUGGESTED READING

Hardie EM: Life-threatening bacterial infection. *Comp Cont Ed Pract Vet* 17:763–777, 1995.

Hotchkiss RS: The pathophysiology and treatment of sepsis. *N Engl J Med* 348:138–150, 2003.

Marshall JC: Sepsis: Current status, future prospects. *Curr Opin Crit Care* 10:250–264, 2004.

AUTHOR: **DANNA M. TORRE**
EDITOR: **ELIZABETH ROZANSKI**

Shar-Pei Fever

BASIC INFORMATION

DEFINITION

A familial, sterile, systemic inflammatory disorder characterized by recurrent fever, swelling of the tibiotarsal joints, and renal amyloidosis

SYNONYM(S)

Familial amyloidosis of Chinese shar-pei dogs

Resembles familial Mediterranean fever of humans

EPIDEMIOLOGY

SPECIES, AGE, SEX: Young adults, 1 to 5 years old.

GENETICS AND BREED PREDISPOSITION: Shar-pei dogs; unknown pattern of inheritance.

ASSOCIATED CONDITIONS AND DISORDERS: Two reports of vasculitis have been associated the condition with shar-pei fever.

CLINICAL PRESENTATION

DISEASE FORMS/SUBTYPES

- Early stage: fever, tibiotarsal (hock) swelling
- Late stage: signs of renal amyloidosis, hepatic amyloidosis, or amyloid deposition in other organs

HISTORY, CHIEF COMPLAINT

- Early stage: signs due to intermittent fever lasting 24 to 36 hours (e.g., lethargy, inappetence)
- Late stage: signs of renal and liver failure; signs include vomiting, anorexia, lethargy, polyuria and polydipsia (PU/PD), and weight loss

PHYSICAL EXAM FINDINGS

- Early stage: fever (103–107°F); palpable swelling of tibiotarsal joints; swollen muzzle may be present
- Late stage:
    - Dehydration, halitosis, weight loss, and other signs of chronic renal failure
    - If nephrotic syndrome is present: ascites, peripheral edema possible; dyspnea may also develop due to pulmonary thromboembolism or rarely from pleural effusion, which is generally small in volume
    - Liver disease; icterus, hepatomegaly, dehydration, weight loss

ETIOLOGY AND PATHOPHYSIOLOGY

- Elevated levels of the cytokine interleukin-6α (IL-6α) are thought to lead to chronic overproduction of acute phase reactant proteins (APP), the precursors of amyloid A.
- Amyloid is then deposited in many organs, and its presence in the kidneys usually leads to renal failure and death. Contrary to other many other disorders causing amyloidosis, which affect the glomerulus predominantly, renal amyloid deposition in shar-pei fever is preferentially in the renal medulla.

DIAGNOSIS

Shar-pei fever is a diagnosis of exclusion. A work-up is directed toward detecting organ damage and to rule out other causes of fever, polyarthritis, azotemia, or liver disease.

DIFFERENTIAL DIAGNOSIS

- See Polyarthritis, p 871
- Lyme disease (see Borreliosis, p 143), ehrlichiosis (see Ehrlichiosis, Canine Granulocytic, p 332)
- Other causes of fever (see Fever of Unknown Origin, p 386)
- Other causes of renal and liver disease

INITIAL DATABASE

- Complete blood count (CBC): may show an inflammatory leukogram and (in the presence of renal failure) nonregenerative anemia.
- Serum biochemistry profile: azotemia (blood urea nitrogen [BUN], creatinine elevation) if renal insufficiency; hypoalbuminemia and hypercholesterolemia with nephrotic syndrome.
- Urinalysis: proteinuria possible. If proteinuria is present, evaluate the condition further with a culture and sensitivity (C&S) to rule out urinary tract infection and with a urine/protein: creatinine ratio to detect pathologic proteinuria, a hallmark of glomerular disease.
- Blood pressure (BP) measurement: rule out systemic hypertension in cases with renal involvement.
- Other tests to consider depending on signs and geographic location: *Borrelia, Ehrlichia*, *Leptospira,* and fungal titers; heartworm test; and survey radiographs to screen for evidence of metastatic or fungal disease.

ADVANCED OR CONFIRMATORY TESTING

- Abdominal ultrasound exam to evaluate kidney, liver, and other abdominal organs and screen for arterial macrothrombi from urinary loss of antithrombin.
- Renal biopsy: While the majority of these animals have moderate to severe amyloid deposition in the renal medulla, a renal biopsy must be limited to the renal cortex (i.e., the biopsy instrument must be oriented parallel to the long axis of the kidney) to avoid lacerating a renal arcuate artery. Approximately two-thirds of animals with shar-pei fever have glomerular deposition of amyloid.
- Consider a liver biopsy (generally safer than renal biopsies), especially if there are clinical and biochemical signs of hepatic dysfunction. Assessment of albumin level, coagulation parameters, and a platelet count must be performed

first and abnormalities corrected prior to biopsy.
- Tissue biopsy is the only way to document the presence of amyloid (using Congo red stains).

TREATMENT

THERAPEUTIC GOAL(S)

- Supportive care during fever episodes
- Attempt to prevent further amyloid deposition and subsequent organ failure

ACUTE GENERAL TREATMENT

- If fever >105°F, the animal may need hospitalization and aggressive management.
- Presentation in early stage: nonsteroidal anti-inflammatory drugs (NSAIDs) for fever (e.g., carprofen 2.2 mg/kg PO q 12h).
- Presentation in late stage: supportive care:
  - IV fluids for rehydration and diuresis if renal failure.
  - Antacids if vomiting, anorexia, or other evidence consistent with uremic gastropathy (e.g., famotidine 0.5 mg/kg PO q 12-24h).
  - Antihypertensives if systemic hypertension (e.g., amlodipine 0.125-0.25 mg/kg PO q 24h).

CHRONIC TREATMENT

- Colchicine 0.03 mg/kg PO q 24h for 2 weeks; if no gastrointestinal (GI) signs, may increase to 0.03 mg/kg PO q 12h.
  - Used in people with familial Mediterranean fever; no controlled trials in shar-pei dogs.
  - Recommend early in the course of the disease to prevent or delay the development of amyloidosis.
- Renal disease: see Glomerulonephritis, p 442; Chronic Renal Failure, Occult ("Asymptomatic"), p 204; Chronic Renal Failure, Overt ("Symptomatic"), p 205.
- Liver disease: dogs respond to supportive care and to colchicine therapy.

DRUG INTERACTIONS

Colchicine given with NSAIDs produces more myelosuppressive effects

POSSIBLE COMPLICATIONS

- Colchicine in humans can cause anorexia, vomiting, diarrhea, renal failure, hepatotoxicity, pancytopenia, and paralysis.
- Vomiting and diarrhea have been reported in dogs taking colchicine and may resolve with dose reduction.

RECOMMENDED MONITORING

Periodic CBC, serum biochemistry profile, and urinalysis with urine protein:creatinine ratio

PROGNOSIS AND OUTCOME

- Early stage: guarded to fair long-term prognosis; colchicine may improve survival
- Late stage: very poor; most dogs die of renal failure, and thromboembolism and hepatic rupture have also been reported

PEARLS & CONSIDERATIONS

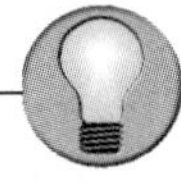

COMMENTS

- Shar-pei dogs with fever episodes are at high risk of developing amyloidosis.
- The most common cause of renal failure in shar-pei dogs is renal amyloidosis.

PREVENTION

- Removal of affected dogs from the breeding pool
- Colchicine treatment may help prevent or delay amyloidosis once early stage of disease is confirmed with biopsy

CLIENT EDUCATION

- Closely monitor temperature of an animal during a fever episode
- Monitor the animal's lab work if treating with colchicine
- Inform the owner of the guarded long-term prognosis

SUGGESTED READING

DiBartola SP, et al: Familial renal amyloidosis in Chinese Shar Pei dogs. *J Am Vet Med Assoc* 197:483-487, 1990.

Loeven KO: Hepatic amyloidosis in two Chinese Shar Pei dogs. *J Am Vet Med Assoc* 204:1212-1216, 1994.

Rivas AL, Tintle L, et al: A canine febrile disorder associated with elevated interleukin-6. *Clinical Immunol Immunopathol* 64:36-45, 1992.

Tintle LJ: Familial Shar Pei fever and familial amyloidosis of Chinese Shar Pei dogs: http://www. royalsharpei. com/amyloidosis. htm.

AUTHOR: **ORLA MAHONY**
EDITOR: **SUSAN M. COTTER**

Shock, Hypovolemic

BASIC INFORMATION

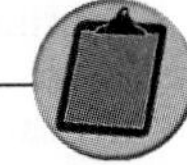

DEFINITION

Inadequate circulating blood volume, resulting in impaired oxygen delivery to tissues

EPIDEMIOLOGY

SPECIES, AGE, SEX

- Dogs are more commonly affected than cats.
- Underlying causes of shock will be more common in different age groups.

RISK FACTORS: Free-roaming dogs and cats are more likely to be traumatized and experience hypovolemic shock.

GEOGRAPHY AND SEASONALITY: Warm weather may increase the risk of free-roaming animals being injured or developing heat stroke.

ASSOCIATED CONDITIONS AND DISORDERS: Intra-abdominal hemangiosarcoma: blood loss; gastric dilatation-volvulus (GDV); maldistributive shock.

CLINICAL PRESENTATION

DISEASE FORMS/SUBTYPES: Subtypes include:

- Hemorrhagic shock
- Traumatic hemorrhagic shock
- Traumatic hypovolemic shock
- Spontaneous neoplastic
- Spontaneous non-neoplastic (e.g., GDV, gastrointestinal [GI] obstruction)

Note: There is minimal or no information in veterinary medicine to correlate subtype with prognosis/outcome.

HISTORY, CHIEF COMPLAINT

- Witnessed or unwitnessed suspected trauma (traumatic hemorrhagic or hypovolemic shock)
- Acute collapse (any nontraumatic type of shock)
- Distended abdomen (hemoabdomen, GDV)
- Vomiting/diarrhea (GDV, primary GI, or as a manifestation of GI hypoperfusion)

PHYSICAL EXAM FINDINGS

- All cases:

- Quiet or dull mentation
- Tachycardia (>150 bpm) or some cats may develop bradycardia
- Weak pulses
- Pale mucous membranes
- Tachypnea

- Possible:
  - Distended abdomen (in cases of hemoabdomen or GDV)
  - Signs of external bleeding
  - Signs of dehydration: enophthalmos, skin tenting, dry mucous membranes

ETIOLOGY AND PATHOPHYSIOLOGY

- Causes of excess vascular volume loss include:
  - Trauma.
  - Ruptured neoplasms.
  - Coagulopathies with hemorrhage into body cavities (e.g., anticoagulant rodenticide toxicity).
  - Vomiting ± diarrhea.
  - Burns.
- Pathophysiology of hypovolemic shock:
  - A decrease in blood volume leads to decreased tissue perfusion.
  - Decreased tissue perfusion leads to a decrease in oxygen supply to cells.
  - Inadequate energy consumption at the cellular level results in a conversion from aerobic to anaerobic metabolism and decreased adenosine triphosphate (ATP) production.
  - Decreased ATP production alters cellular function, leading to alterations in intracellular calcium homeostasis; this process in turn leads to direct cellular injury, enzyme activation, release of reactive oxygen species, and inhibition of oxidative phosphorylation.
  - Cell death can precipitate a cascade of events, such as activation of the coagulation cascade or bacterial translocation in the gut, which then may result in multiorgan damage and death.

DIAGNOSIS

The diagnosis is largely dependent on history and physical examination (suspected possible source[s] of fluid loss) and is confirmed with routine laboratory testing and imaging.

DIFFERENTIAL DIAGNOSIS

Differentials include:

- Septic shock
- Cardiogenic shock
- Neurogenic shock
- Anaphylactic shock

INITIAL DATABASE

- Packed cell volume/total solids (PCV/TS) and blood glucose: Low or decreasing PCV/TS may indicate blood loss.
- Complete blood count (CBC), serum chemistry profile, coagulation profile prothrombin time/activated (thromboplastin time): Prolonged clotting times may indicate internal blood loss as a cause for hypovolemia.
- Blood pressure (BP): Low BP is consistent with hypovolemic shock.
- Abdomino/thoracocentesis with fluid analysis: A positive tap will help elucidate the cause of the hypovolemia (e.g., if blood is obtained, then intracavitary hemorrhage as a cause of the hypovolemia should be considered).
- Abdominal and thoracic radiographs.
- Lactate analysis: An elevated blood lactate (>2.5 mmol/L) supports hypovolemia, but extraneous factors (e.g., struggling during phlebotomy) may raise lactate levels.

ADVANCED OR CONFIRMATORY TESTING

- Abdominal ultrasound
- Histopathologic examination will determine tumor type if neoplasia is the underlying cause

TREATMENT

THERAPEUTIC GOAL(S)

- The primary goal is to restore blood volume, thus increasing tissue perfusion
- Treatment of the underlying disease

ACUTE GENERAL TREATMENT

- The best fluid for restoration depends on:
  - The cause of hypovolemia.
  - The serum electrolyte status of the animal.
  - PCV/TS.
- If the animal is bleeding, fresh whole blood or packed red cells ± plasma is the best replacement fluid.
- Give fluids to reach an adequate BP (systolic arterial pressure > 90 mmHg) and central venous pressure (CVP > 5 cm H_2O).
- Restoration of volume can include the following fluid types:
  - Crystalloids: requires a replacement fluid (e.g., lactated Ringers, 0.9% NaCl):
    - 40-90 ml/kg IV to reach desired effect.
  - Synthetic colloids (e.g.. Hetastarch, Dextran 70):
    - 5-20 ml/kg IV to reach desired effect.
  - Blood (see Transfusion Therapy and Collection Techniques for Blood Banking, p 1312).
  - Plasma: may be required if massive quantities of crystalloids, synthetic colloids, or blood have been given to an animal and the animal has developed a dilutional coagulopathy.
- Locate and control the source of hemorrhage.

POSSIBLE COMPLICATIONS

Complication of prolonged shock include:

- Renal failure
- Loss of GI integrity with absorption of bacteria and bacterial toxins
- Myocardial dysfunction
- Brain ischemia
- Loss of vascular tone
- Disseminated intravascular coagulation
- Acute lung injury
- Sepsis

RECOMMENDED MONITORING

- Monitor BP either indirectly or directly until it has normalized.
- Recognize that persistent hypotension or tachycardia often implies ongoing hemorrhage, systemic vasodilation, or capillary leakage.
- Utilize central venous pressure as an indicator of volume status: If the CVP is less than 5 cm H_2O, then more fluids should be given. Adequate fluid resuscitation is generally present if the CVP is between 5 and 10 cm H_2O.
- Monitor for signs of end-organ damage (e.g., monitor urine output).
- Monitor PCV/TS for evidence of adequate fluid therapy.
- Monitor heart rate: Persistent tachycardia may indicate inadequate fluid loading.

PROGNOSIS AND OUTCOME

- Determined by the cause of the hypovolemia and the rapidity with which the volume deficit has been corrected.
- Prolonged hypotension may cause multiple organ dysfunction, which carries a poor prognosis.

PEARLS & CONSIDERATIONS

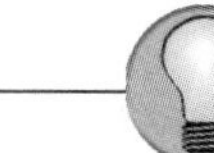

COMMENTS

- Hypovolemic shock is a potentially life-threatening process that requires early identification and treatment.
- Tachycardia (or bradycardia in the cat) together with low BP and a known cause of fluid loss are hallmarks for diagnosis of hypovolemic shock.
- Essential elements for the successful management of hypovolemic shock are identification of the source of fluid loss and reversal/replacement of the fluid loss.
- Treatment of the underlying cause is the key to long-term success.

PREVENTION

Avoid allowing dogs and cats to roam freely.

SUGGESTED READING

Macintire DK: Hypotension. In Ettinger SJ, Feldman EC (eds): *Textbook of Veterinary Internal Medicine.* Philadelphia, WB Saunders, 2000, pp 183–186.

AUTHOR: **BENJAMIN DAVIDSON**
EDITOR: **ELIZABETH ROZANSKI**

Shoulder Luxation

BASIC INFORMATION

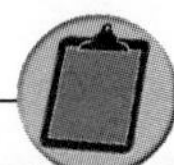

DEFINITION

Traumatic or congenital scapulohumeral luxation

EPIDEMIOLOGY

SPECIES, AGE, SEX: Traumatic luxation can occur in dogs of all sizes and ages; rare in cats.
GENETICS AND BREED PREDISPOSITION: Congenital luxation occurs most often in small dogs. Toy poodles and Shetland sheepdogs appear predisposed.

CLINICAL PRESENTATION

DISEASE FORMS/SUBTYPES: Any direction for traumatic luxation; congenital is usually medial.
HISTORY, CHIEF COMPLAINT: Traumatic luxations cause acute non-weight-bearing lameness. Congenital luxation will cause intermittent or continous lameness of variable degree and associated pain.
PHYSICAL EXAM FINDINGS

- Animals that have gone through trauma experience pain and crepitus during shoulder manipulations. Dogs carry the limb in flexion with the foot externally rotated (medial luxation) or internally rotated (lateral luxation). The greater tubercle is displaced relative to the acromion.
- Dogs with congenital luxation may be comfortable during shoulder manipulation; the joint is luxated and reduced easily.

ETIOLOGY AND PATHOPHYSIOLOGY

- Humerus is medially displaced in 75% of cases.
- Medial luxation in small dogs is congenital and associated with developmental laxity or dysplasia of the glenoid cavity; often occurs bilaterally.
- Medial luxation in large-breed dogs is caused by trauma.
- Lateral luxation is caused by trauma and is associated with disruption of the lateral joint capsule, lateral glenohumeral ligament, and infraspinatus tendon.
- Cranial and caudal luxations are rare and are caused by trauma.

DIAGNOSIS

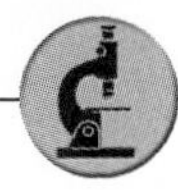

DIFFERENTIAL DIAGNOSIS

- Scapular neck or glenoid fractures
- Fracture of proximal humerus
- Bicipital tenosynovitis
- Supraspinatus degeneration or mineralization
- Osteosarcoma of proximal humerus
- Brachial plexus avulsion
- Nerve root signature in the forelimb

INITIAL DATABASE

- Orthopedic and neurologic evaluations
- Radiography of the scapulohumeral joint, orthogonal views
- Complete blood count (CBC), serum biochemistry panel, urinalysis: in older dogs or trauma cases
- Electrocardiogram (ECG) and thoracic radiographs if trauma is suspected

ADVANCED OR CONFIRMATORY TESTING

- Evaluate shoulder "drawer movement" by cranial, caudal, medial, and lateral displacement of the humerus relative to the scapula
- Test medial instability by abduction of the humerus relative to the scapula
- Stress radiography

TREATMENT

THERAPEUTIC GOAL(S)

Preserve integrity of the scapulohumeral joint or pain-free use of the affected limb

ACUTE GENERAL TREATMENT

- Traumatic luxation without glenoid dysplasia can be reduced closed. If the joint reluxates easily during manipulation or in the postoperative period, surgery is indicated.
- Surgical options in traumatic luxations or congenital luxations with good joint integrity include primary repair of joint capsule/ligaments and stabilization by transposition of the biceps tendon or prosthetic suture repair of the glenohumeral ligament.
- Congenital luxations with glenoid dysplasia are not suitable for closed reduction and require surgery if pain or decreased function of the limb is present. Surgical options include excision arthroplasty and shoulder arthrodesis.

CHRONIC TREATMENT

- Conservatively or surgically (biceps tenodesis, ligament prosthesis) managed dogs are immobilized with a spica splint (lateral luxations) or Velpeau sling (medial luxations) for 10 to 14 days (see Slings, Casts, and Other Forms of Immobilization, p 1306). Exercise is restricted for 4 to 8 weeks after splint or sling removal. Physical therapy with passive range-of-motion exercises and swimming are recommended after immobilization.
- Excision arthroplasty cases should be walked using a leash after surgery. Swimming or other vigorous exercise is encouraged starting 10 days after surgery.
- After shoulder arthrodesis, the limb is immobilized in a spica splint until radiographic signs of fusion are present.

POSSIBLE COMPLICATIONS

- Seroma
- Midsubstance tearing of the biceps tendon after tenodesis
- Articular incongruity after biceps tenodesis causing osteoarthritis
- Suprascapular nerve damage with prosthetic repair
- Fixation failure
- Infection

RECOMMENDED MONITORING

- With conservative management, routine reexamination of the joint is indicated to ensure stable reduction

- Shoulder arthrodesis cases need monthly radiographic examination starting at week 6 until fusion has occurred

PROGNOSIS AND OUTCOME

- Animals with biceps tenodesis have good to excellent outcomes in 60% (three out of five dogs) to 93% (11 out of 12 dogs) of cases. A small number of dogs with prosthetic glenohumeral ligament (GHL) repair have had good and excellent results.
- Salvage procedures are rarely performed and may provide adequate function in small dogs; limb amputation is an option in unilateral cases.

PEARLS & CONSIDERATIONS

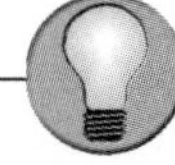

COMMENTS

- A Velpau sling is contraindicated for lateral luxations due to lateral translation of the humeral head
- Radiography helps to identify articular fractures or glenoid dysplasia before joint stabilization is attempted

SUGGESTED READING

Fitch RB, et al: Clinical evaluation of prosthetic medial glenohumeral ligament repair in the dog (ten cases). *Vet Comp Orthop Traumatol* 14:221, 2001.

Piermattei DL, Flo GL: The shoulder joint. In *Brinker, Piermattei, and Flo's Handbook of Small Animal Orthopedics and Fracture Repair*, ed 3. Philadelphia, WB Saunders, 1997, pp 228–260.

Talcott KW, Vasseur PB: Luxation of the scapulohumeral joint. In Slatter D (ed): *Textbook of Small Animal Surgery*, ed 3. Philadelphia, WB Saunders, 2003, pp 1897–1904.

AUTHOR: **BOEL A. FRANSSON**
EDITOR: **JOSEPH HARARI**

Sick Sinus Syndrome

BASIC INFORMATION

DEFINITION

One of the two most common indications for cardiac pacemaker implantation in dogs. It represents diffuse cardiac conduction system disease that displays variable degrees of sinoatrial (SA) nodal dysfunction (sinus bradycardia, sinoatrial block, or sinus arrest) and/or atrioventricular (AV) nodal dysfunction. The subsidiary pacemakers often display depressed automaticity so prolonged episodes of sinus arrest are accompanied by asystole and syncope. Some dogs may display episodes of supraventricular tachycardia alternating with their bradyarrhythmias, producing a so-called brady-tachy syndrome (see Fig. I-152).

SYNONYM(S)

SSS
Bradycardia-tachycardia (brady-tachy) syndrome
Chronotropic incompetence
Lazy sinus syndrome
SA syncope
Sinus node dysfunction
Sluggish sinus syndrome

EPIDEMIOLOGY

SPECIES, AGE, SEX: Small-breed, older dogs.

GENETICS AND BREED PREDISPOSITION: Middle-aged to older female miniature schnauzers are most commonly afflicted. West Highland white terriers and cocker spaniels also appear to be overrepresented.

ASSOCIATED CONDITIONS AND DISORDERS: Sick sinus syndrome (SSS) and chronic degenerative valvular disease often occur in the same animal because of their similar breed and age predispositions, but there is no known link between the two disease processes.

CLINICAL PRESENTATION

HISTORY, CHIEF COMPLAINT

- Most dogs with clinical signs from SSS are presented for episodic weakness or syncopal/seizure-like episodes.
- Some animals with severe, long-standing sinus bradycardia may develop congestive heart failure (CHF) and are presented for the evaluation of coughing, respiratory distress, or exercise intolerance.
- Some dogs are diagnosed with bradyarrhythmias and SSS during routine preventative health examination or prior to dental prophylaxis.

PHYSICAL EXAM FINDINGS

- The classic physical examination findings include a detectable bradyarrhythmia with prolonged episodes of asystole due to sinus arrest without activation of subsidiary (AV or intraventricular) pacemakers.
- Because of the predisposition for SSS to occur in older, small-breed dogs, many will display variable intensity, left apical, systolic murmurs of mitral insufficiency.
- Dogs with brady-tachy syndrome may have paroxysms of tachycardia followed by audible pauses.
- Unfortunately, some animals will have normal physical examinations without evidence of bradyarrhythmias because dogs with SSS may still have some response to the elevated circulating levels of catecholamines associated with visits to the veterinary hospital.

ETIOLOGY AND PATHOPHYSIOLOGY

- To date, the etiologic basis for SSS in dogs has not been determined.
- Fibrosis and fatty infiltration with sclerodegenerative processes have been identified within the sinus node, AV node, and bundle of His in humans with SSS.
- Occlusion or degeneration of the sinus node artery could play an important role in the development of this disease.
- The absence of morphologic abnormalities in some humans with sinus node dysfunction suggests that alterations of neural innervation or neural regulation may contribute to the bradyarrhythmias.
- Autoantibodies to proteins isolated from sinus node cells have been identified in humans, suggesting an immune-mediated process in some cases of sinus node dysfunction.

DIAGNOSIS

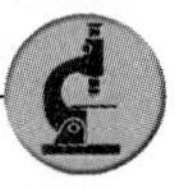

DIFFERENTIAL DIAGNOSIS

- Other bradyarrhythmias:
  - Third-degree AV block
  - Persistent atrial standstill
  - Vagally mediated bradyarrhythmias
  - Metabolic disorders that may slow SA nodal activity:
    - Hyperkalemia, see p 546
    - Hypothermia, see p 573
    - Hypothyroidism, see p 575
    - Hypoadrenocorticism, see p 561
    - Dysautonomia, see p 323
- Seizures of any etiology (see Seizures, p 990)

INITIAL DATABASE

- Electrocardiogram (ECG): characterize the bradyarrhythmia.
  - ECG is the diagnostic test of choice for SSS (Fig. I-151).
  - Although exact criteria have not been established for the diagnosis of

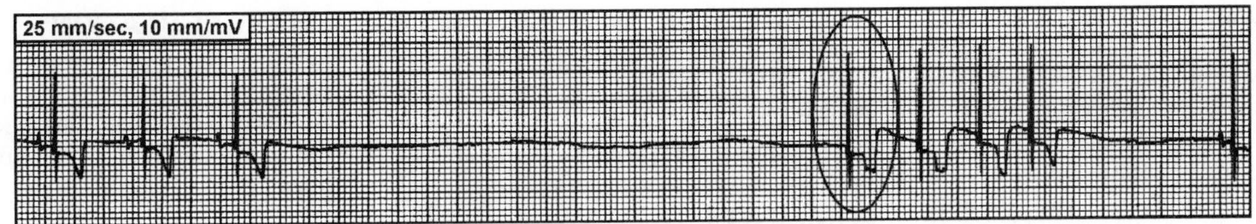

FIGURE I-151 A dog with brady-tachy SSS displays a prolonged period of sinus arrest, followed by a supraventricular escape beat (the circled complex) and a short run of accelerated supraventricular complexes thereafter.

SSS, sinus arrest with or without variable degress of atrioventricular block or supraventricular tachycardia should raise the suspicion of SSS.

- Atropine response test: determine if the bradyarrhythmia is wholly or partially vagally mediated. If the bradyarrhythmia is vagally mediated (i.e., physiologic), the test reveals a positive response in the form of sustained sinus tachycardia; if it is pathologic, the test reveals no change in the ECG.
  - Obtain initial ECG.
  - Adminster atropine 0.04 mg/kg IV.
  - Obtain follow-up ECG 15 minutes later.
  - An increase of at least 50% in the heart rate is expected when the bradycardia is vagally mediated and therefore physiologic but also occurs in a certain number of dogs with SSS. The absence of any response to atropine in a dog with appropriate signalment and clinical signs is strongly suggestive of SSS.
- Complete blood count (CBC), serum chemistry profile, and urinalysis to detect underlying electrolyte imbalances or metabolic disorders that may contribute to bradyarrhythmias or seizures.
- Thoracic radiographs: Cardiomegaly or CHF may develop in the face of longstanding bradyarrhythmias, especially when complicated by valvular disease in older, small-breed dogs.
- Echocardiography to assess the severity of valvular, myocardial, or structural (including neoplastic) cardiac disease if present.

ADVANCED OR CONFIRMATORY TESTING

- Videotaping of episodes by the owner may help to differentiate syncope from seizures if the episodes occur infrequently and are not clearly one or the other based on historic description alone.
- A 24-hour Holter monitor or cardiac event monitor may be indicated in cases where the history, clinical signs, ECG, and atropine response test are inconclusive.

TREATMENT

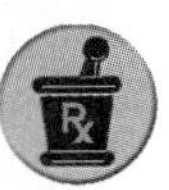

THERAPEUTIC GOAL(S)

- Dogs showing no overt clinical signs (arrhythmia was discovered incidentally): periodic monitoring and client education to detect progression of disease
- Dogs showing overt clinical signs, such as syncope:
  - Bradycardia: increase the heart rate to alleviate the syncopal episodes
  - Brady-tachy syndrome: therapy aimed at reducing the supraventricular tachycardia (see Atrial Premature Complexes and Atrial/Supraventricular Tachycardia, p 100) may be required after resolution of the bradyarrhythmia

ACUTE GENERAL TREATMENT

- Dogs showing no overt clinical signs: in the absence of syncope, significant cardiomegaly or CHF, periodic ECGs, and client education are indicated. General anesthesia should be avoided.
- Dogs showing overt clinical signs:
  - Vagolytic drugs display variable and often temporary efficacy in animals with SSS. One option is to begin with a sympathomimetic followed by a parasympatholytic (anticholinergic) if clinical signs persist.
    - Theophylline: 10 mg/kg PO q 8h.
    - Terbutaline (instead of theophylline): 0.2 mg/kg PO q 8-12h.
    - Propantheline bromide: 0.25 to 0.5 mg/kg PO q 8h.
  - Pacemaker implantaton (see Pacemaker: Transthoracic Cardiac Pacing, p 1294): Dogs with overt clinical signs caused by SSS require artificial pacing if they fail to respond or become refractory to vagolytic drugs.

CHRONIC TREATMENT

- Vagolytic drugs: If animals are responsive, therapy will be maintained lifelong; refractoriness may develop over time, however.
- Pacemaker: In some instances, animals may outlive the battery life and require replacement of the pulse generator.

DRUG INTERACTIONS

- Theophylline:
  - Arrhythmias may develop when used with additional sympathomimetics
  - Cimetidine, erythromycin, allopurinol, thiabendazole, clindamycin, and lincomycin may increase its effects
  - Phenobarbital or phenytoin may decrease its effects
  - Enrofloxacin or ciprofloxacin inhibit the metabolism of theophylline and may promote toxicity
- Terbutaline:
  - Arrhythmias may develop when used with additional sympathomimetics or digitalis glycosides.
  - Tricyclic antidepressants or monoamine oxidase inhibitors (MAOIs) may potentiate the vascular effects
- Propantheline bromide:
  - Antihistamines, procainamide, quinidine, meperidine, benzodiazepines, and phenothiazines may enhance its activity
  - Primidone, disopyramide, nitrates, and long-term corticosteroid use may potentiate its adverse effects
  - May enhance the actions of nitrofurantoin, thiazide diuretics, and sympathomimetics

POSSIBLE COMPLICATIONS

- Tachyarrhythmias, nervousness/anxiety, vomiting, diarrhea, polyuria and polydipsia (PU/PD), and anorexia with administration of sympathomimetics
- Tachyarrhythmias, dry mouth, dry eyes, urinary hesitancy, constipation, and vomiting with administration of anticholinergics such as propantheline bromide
- Pacemakers: lead dislodgement, infection, failure to sense, ventriculoatrial conduction, or skeletal muscle stimulation (if a unipolar pacemaker is implanted)

RECOMMENDED MONITORING

- ECG: periodic monitoring or as dictated by recurrence of syncopal episodes.
  - Animals showing no overt clinical signs: every 3 to 4 months to evaluate for progression of bradyarrhythmia-tachyarrythmia; atropine response test may need to be repeated
  - Animals showing overt clinical signs: whether medical therapy or pacemaker implantation has been performed, ECGs should be repeated every 6 months to assess the long-term response to vagolytic agents or appropriate functionality of the pacemaker.
  - If clinical signs recur, re-examination including ECG is indicated immediately.

- Thoracic radiographs: every 6 months, especially in the face of valvular disease; assessment for progressive cardiomegaly and CHF, assessment of the integrity of the pacemaker.
- Pacemaker interrogation: every 6 months; evaluation of the pacing threshold, lead impedance, and battery life.

PROGNOSIS AND OUTCOME

- The risk of sudden death with SSS appears low, and some animals never develop clinical signs.
- If syncope is present, the episodes tend to increase in frequency over time.
- Medical therapy is usually well tolerated, although the respose is variable and, in some cases, short-lived.
- The prognosis and response to therapy following successful pacemaker implantation are good for animals with SSS. Episodes of syncope tend to resolve, animals become much more suitable anesthetic candidates, and episodes of supraventricular tachycardia can be managed with medications if necessary.

PEARLS & CONSIDERATIONS

COMMENTS

- Seizures and syncope can be very difficult to differentiate.
- SSS should always be on the differential list for older miniature schnauzers, Westies, and cocker spaniels that display seizure-like activity.
- A normal heart rate at the time of examination does not exclude SSS.
- Even in the absence of syncope during Holter monitoring, many animals with SSS display significant and prolonged episodes of sinus arrest. Analysis of the tape is still warranted when no episodes have occurred during the monitoring period.
- While ventricular-based pacemakers readily alleviate the clinical signs, atrial-based pacing may be the most appropriate if AV nodal function is normal.

CLIENT EDUCATION

Artificial pacemaker implantation is most commonly performed via a transvenous approach, therefore markedly reducing the pain and recovery time for older dogs.

SUGGESTED READING

Cote E, Ettinger SJ: Electrocardiography and cardiac arrhythmias. In Ettinger SJ, Feldman EC (eds): *Textbook of Veterinary Internal Medicine*. St. Louis, Elsevier Saunders, 2005, pp 1040–1076.

Moise NS: Pacemaker therapy. In Fox PR, Sisson DD, Moise NS (eds): *Textbook of Canine and Feline Cardiology: Principles and Clinical Practice*. Philadelphia, WB Saunders, 1999, pp 400–425.

Rishniw M, Thomas WP: Bradyarrhythmias. In Bonagura JD (ed): *Kirk's Current Veterinary Therapy XIII Small Animal Practice*. Philadelphia, WB Saunders, 2000, pp 719–725.

AUTHOR: **BARRET J. BULMER**
EDITOR: **ETIENNE CÔTÉ**

Sinus Arrhythmia

BASIC INFORMATION

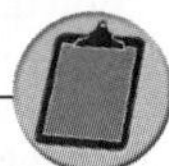

DEFINITION

Sinus arrhythmia is a physiologic, autonomically mediated cyclical change in sinus rate. The P-P intervals are "regularly irregular" due to fluctuations of the autonomic tone that result in phasic changes of the sinus node discharge rate.

SYNONYM(S)

Respiratory sinus arrhythmia

EPIDEMIOLOGY

SPECIES, AGE, SEX

- Common in dogs (physiologic)
- Rare in cats (can be pathologic)

GENETICS AND BREED PREDISPOSITION

- All dog breeds can display sinus arrhythmia.
- Brachycephalic breeds often have the largest variations in R-R interval (bulldog, pug, boxer, Pekinese, Lhasa apso) due to increased inspiratory effort.

CLINICAL PRESENTATION

DISEASE FORMS/SUBTYPES

- Respiratory sinus arrhythmia
  - Physiologic fluctuation associated with respiration
- Nonrespiratory sinus arrhythmia
  - Cyclic change in P-P interval independent of respiration but due to increased vagal tone:
    - Respiratory disease
    - Central nervous system (CNS) disease (increased intracranial pressure)
    - Gastrointestinal (GI) disease

HISTORY, CHIEF COMPLAINT: Respiratory sinus arrhythmia does not cause clinical signs. In animals with nonrespiratory sinus arrhythmia, particularly cats, the chief complaint is related to the underlying disease.

PHYSICAL EXAM FINDINGS

- Normal to "slow-normal" heart rate
- Regularly irregular heart rate by auscultation and pulse palpation
- Also possible:
  - Upper airway noises: stridor, dyspnea, wheezes
  - Neurologic signs: depression
  - GI disturbances

ETIOLOGY AND PATHOPHYSIOLOGY

- Respiratory sinus arrhythmia: Sinus node discharge rate is regulated by the autonomic nervous system. Inspiration causes a decrease in vagal tone and an increase in sympathetic tone, resulting in an increased heart rate. Conversely, on expiration there is an increase in vagal tone and a decrease in sympathetic tone, resulting in a decrease in heart rate.
- Nonrespiratory sinus arrhythmia: Autonomic influences can also cause sinus arrhythmia independent of respiration, slowing the heart rate during periods when parasympathetic tone predominate over sympathetic tone.

DIAGNOSIS

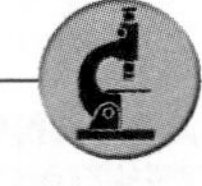

DIFFERENTIAL DIAGNOSIS

- By electrocardiogram (ECG): sinus arrhythmia should be differentiated from (also see Initial Database below):
  - Sick sinus syndrome (SSS): pauses between sinus beats are longer (can be up to several seconds with SSS)
  - Slow atrial fibrillation (no P waves, "irregularly irregular").
  - Transient sinus arrest (intermittent nature of pauses instead of cyclic pattern).
  - Atrial premature contractions (APCs): Underlying rhythm may be a regular sinus rhythm frequently interrupted by APCs. Differentiation: the P wave of an APC may occur inside the preced-

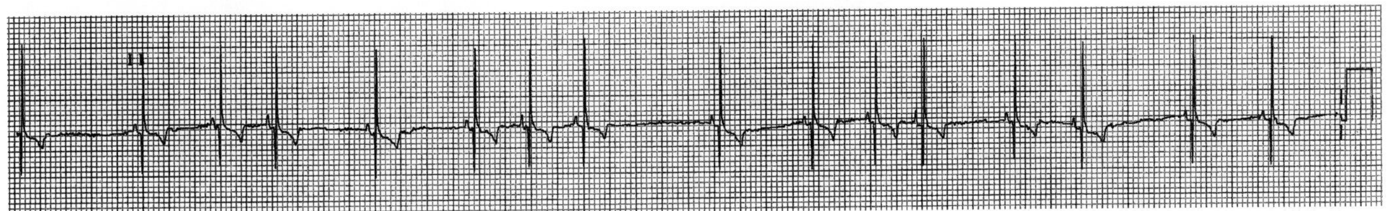

FIGURE I-152 ECG rhythm strip, lead II, 25 mm/sec, 10 mm/mV; healthy dog displaying sinus arrhythmia. The average heart rate is about 95 bpm. The individual RR intervals vary by over 50% (range 0.4–1 sec). There is a wandering pacemaker, demonstrated by the variable amplitude of the P wave (tallest P wave after the shortest RR interval, flattest P wave after the longest RR interval). Since the wandering pacemaker and sinus arrhythmia are both vagally mediated, they often occur together.

ing T wave, but such a degree of prematurity does not occur with sinus arrhythmia; APCs do not occur cyclically in conjuction with the patient's respirations.

- By auscultation alone, sinus arrhythmia may be confused with these pathologic arrhythmias. ECG is important to confirm the diagnosis

INITIAL DATABASE

ECG (Fig. I-152):

- Morphology is similar to normal sinus rhythm.
    - Heart rate is normal to slow (<140 bpm in dogs)
    - P-P interval is variable in a "regularly irregular" fashion
    - Variability in P-P interval is greater than 10%
    - Normal P wave morphology: P wave is followed by a QRS complex in a 1:1 ratio
    - P wave amplitude may vary if wandering pacemaker is present (tall P wave after a short P-P interval, low voltage [short] P wave after a long P-P interval)
- If sinus arrhythmia is concurrent with significant respiratory, CNS, or GI disease, specific diagnostic testing should be recommended based on the relevant abnormalities of the case.

TREATMENT

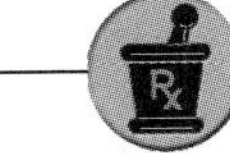

THERAPEUTIC GOAL(S)

Sinus arrhythmia is a physiologic phenomenon and does not warrant therapy.

PROGNOSIS AND OUTCOME

Both are good

PEARLS & CONSIDERATIONS

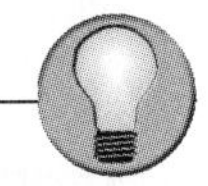

COMMENTS

Sinus arrhythmia is a physiologic phenomenon, most commonly indicative of a healthy cardiovascular system.

SUGGESTED READING

Miller MS, Tilley LP, Smith FWK Jr., Fox PR: Electrocardiography. In Fox PR, Sisson D, Moise NS (eds): *Textbook of Canine and Feline Cardiology*. Philadelphia, WB Saunders, 1999, pp 67-106.

Saul JP, Cohen RJ: Respiratory sinus arrhythmia. In Levy MN, Schwartz PJ (eds): *Vagal Control of the Heart: Experimental Basis and Clinical Implications*. Armonk, NY, Futura Publishing 1994, pp 511-536.

AUTHORS: **ANNA R. M. GELZER, MARC S. KRAUS**

EDITOR: **ETIENNE CÔTÉ**

Sinus Bradycardia

BASIC INFORMATION

DEFINITION

Normal sinus rhythm with heart rate less than 70 bpm in dogs (60 bpm for giant breeds) and less than 120 bpm in cats

EPIDEMIOLOGY

SPECIES, AGE, SEX

- More common in dogs
- No age or sex predilection

GENETICS AND BREED PREDISPOSITION: Physiologic sinus bradycardia is more common in brachycephalic breeds.

RISK FACTORS

- Variations of normal: athletic dogs, brachycephalic conformation
- Disorders: upper airway disease, respiratory disease, gastrointestinal (GI) disease, systemic disease, central nervous system (CNS) disease, hypothermia, hypothyroidism, sinus node dysfunction, feline dilated cardiomyopathy, end-stage heart failure, drug toxicities, inhalation anesthetics

ASSOCIATED CONDITIONS AND DISORDERS: Sinus arrhythmia (normal); sick sinus syndrome (SSS); sinoatrial (SA) block (very rare).

CLINICAL PRESENTATION

DISEASE FORMS/SUBTYPES

- Physiologic: athletes, brachycephalic breeds
- Pathologic: sinus node dysfunction, toxicity, secondary to systemic disease states

HISTORY, CHIEF COMPLAINT

- Often incidental finding: owner auscults/palpates low heart rate.
- Rarely, exercise intolerance; malaise, lethargy, depression; collapse (usually with exertion). When such overt signs occur, they are commonly related to SSS (see Sick Sinus Syndrome, p 1002).

PHYSICAL EXAM FINDINGS

- Cardiac auscultation: reduced heart rate in an alert ± nervous animal:
    - <60-70 bpm in dogs
    - <120 bpm in cats
- Femoral pulse character: may be normal, reduced, or pronounced (depending on underlying etiology and chronicity of bradycardia)
- Malaise, lethargy, depression: if bradycardia is severe

ETIOLOGY AND PATHOPHYSIOLOGY

- Increased vagal tone:
    - Physiologic
        - Brachycephalic conformation
        - Athlete
    - Respiratory disease (upper and/or lower respiratory tract)
    - GI disease: severe vomiting
- CNS disorders:
    - Head trauma
    - Increased intracranial pressure
    - Brainstem lesions
    - Spinal trauma
- Metabolic/systemic disorders:

- Hypothyroidism
- Hypothermia
- Hypoxemia
- Toxicity:
  - Phenothiazines (although phenothiazines may instead induce hypotension and reflex tachycardia)
  - β-Adrenergic receptor antagonists
  - Digitalis
  - Quinidine
  - Narcotics
  - Inhalation anesthetics
- Primary cardiac disease:
  - Sinus node dysfunction (from SSS)
  - End-stage heart failure
  - Feline dilated cardiomyopathy

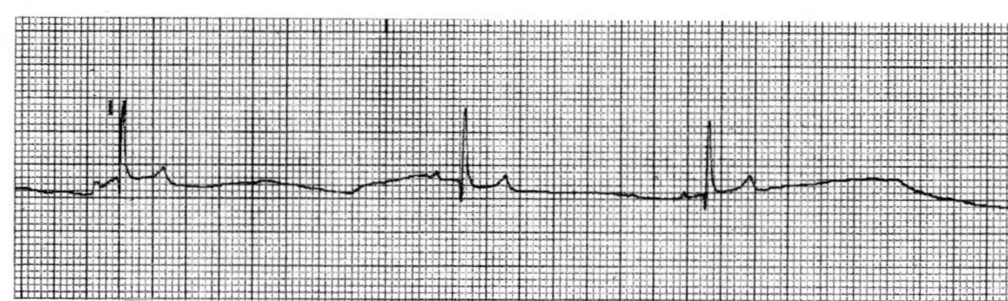

FIGURE I-153 Sinus bradycardia/respiratory sinus arrhythmia. Incidental finding in healthy 5-year-old German shepherd dog. Heart rate = 37 bpm; lead II, 25 mm/sec, 1 cm/mV.

DIAGNOSIS

Once sinus bradycardia is confirmed with an electrocardiogram (ECG), further diagnostic testing is warranted if the patient is showing abnormal systemic signs. If no signs are present, the strong possibility of sinus bradycardia as a normal finding should be considered.

DIFFERENTIAL DIAGNOSIS

- Normal
- Other bradycardias (e.g., atrioventricular [AV] block, atrial standstill)
- Specific causes: see Etiology and Pathophysiology above

INITIAL DATABASE

- ECG: confirm clinical diagnosis (Fig. I-153)
- Complete blood count (CBC), biochemistry panel, urinalysis: may reveal evidence of systemic disease
- Thoracic and abdominal radiographs to identify underlying respiratory, cardiovascular, or GI disorders
- Abdominal ultrasound: to confirm equivocal or subtle abdominal radiographic findings (operator skill dependent)

ADVANCED OR CONFIRMATORY TESTING

- Atropine response test to differentiate between vagally mediated bradyarrhythmias and those arising from a conduction disturbance
- Echocardiography to rule out underlying cardiac disease
- Serum digoxin level (if applicable)
- Complete thyroid hormone panel

TREATMENT

THERAPEUTIC GOAL(S)

- Treatment is rarely necessary
- Increase the animal's heart rate
- Improve the animal's exercise capacity and quality of life

ACUTE GENERAL TREATMENT

- Rarely indicated
- Treat underlying problem (if applicable)
- Discontinue or taper all medications with potential to promote bradycardia
- For animals with sinus bradycardia that are also showing critical clinical signs (recumbency, unconsciousness, etc.):
  - Administer anticholinergic agent IV (atropine sulfate 0.04 mg/kg IV or glycopyrrolate 0.11 mg/kg IV).
  - If anticholinergic therapy is unsuccessful, consider IV constant rate infusion of isoproterenol (0.4 mg in 250 ml saline; slow drip to effect [prime IV line, start slowly, and increase titration based on response]) or dopamine (2 μg/kg per minute).
  - Rarely, emergency cardiac pacing may be required for severe refractory bradycardia.

CHRONIC TREATMENT

- Treat underlying problem (if applicable)
- Discontinue or reduce dosages of all medications with potential to induce bradycardia
- For animals showing overt signs due to the bradycardia:
  - Propantheline bromide (0.2-1 mg/kg PO q 8h) (variable response)
  - Theophylline (10 mg/kg PO q 8h) (variable response)
  - Permanent pacemaker implantation

DRUG INTERACTIONS

- Propantheline bromide: use this drug cautiously in animals with suspected GI disease or autonomic neuropathy, multiple drug interactions
- Theophylline: narrow therapeutic window, to be used cautiously, multiple drug interactions

POSSIBLE COMPLICATIONS

- Medical management failure common when sinus node dysfunction/SSS is present
- Side effects of propantheline bromide or theophylline administration may be problematic

RECOMMENDED MONITORING

- None for physiologic sinus bradycardia not causing clinical signs
- The owner monitors for signs of bradycardia: lethargy, exercise intolerance, malaise, collapse
- Follow-up ECG 1 week after initiation of medical management, then every 1 to 3 months (as directed by clinical course)
- If pacemaker implantation performed, schedule a follow-up visit as directed (see Sick Sinus Syndrome, p 1002)

PROGNOSIS AND OUTCOME

- Physiologic: excellent; by definition, physiologic sinus bradycardia is not associated with clinical disease
- Secondary: dependent on response to treatment of primary disorder
- Sinus node dysfunction/SSS:
  - Chronic response to medical therapy is generally unrewarding
  - Good with pacemaker implantation

PEARLS & CONSIDERATIONS

COMMENTS

- Large- and giant-breed dogs may exhibit normal heart rates as low as 30 to 40 bpm when asleep.
- A life-threatening situation can be the sudden (instantaneous) transition from sinus tachycardia to sinus bradycardia in an unconscious animal, which is associated with impending cardiac arrest.

SUGGESTED READING

Russell LC, Rush JE: Cardiac arrhythmias in systemic disease. In Bonagura JD, Kirk RW (eds): *Kirk's Current Veterinary Therapy XII: Small Animal Practice*. Philadelphia, WB Saunders, 1995, pp 161-166.

Tilley LP: *Essentials of Canine and Feline Electrocardiography: Interpretation and Treatment*, ed 3. Media, Lippincott Williams & Wilkins, 1992.

AUTHOR: **NATHANIEL FENOLLOSA**
EDITOR: **ETIENNE CÔTÉ**

Sinus Tachycardia

BASIC INFORMATION

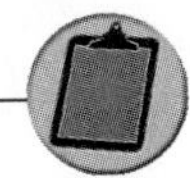

DEFINITION

An accelerated heart rate caused by rapid firing of the sinus node. Sinus tachycardia is a physiologic response to the body's needs rather than a pathologic condition. Sinus tachycardia usually appears and subsides gradually over a few seconds; this characteristic helps set it apart from pathologic tachycardias, which may appear and subside instantaneously.

EPIDEMIOLOGY

SPECIES, AGE, SEX: Definition of sinus tachycardia depends on the species, breed, and age:

- Dogs > 160 bpm:
  - Toy breeds > 180 bpm; giant-breed dogs > 140 bpm; puppies > 200 bpm
- Cats > 240 bpm

CLINICAL PRESENTATION

DISEASE FORMS/SUBTYPES

- Primary physiologic sinus tachycardia:
  - Response to exercise, stress (restraint, anxiety), pain
- Secondary physiologic sinus tachycardia:
  - Response to underlying disease, causing:
    - Fever and infection
    - Shock and hypotension
    - Hypovolemia
    - Anemia
    - Hypoxemia
    - Heart failure and cardiac tamponade
    - Hyperthyroidism
    - Catecholamine excess (e.g., pheochromocytoma)
- Pharmacologic sinus tachycardia:
  - Response to drug administration:
    - Vagolytic drugs (atropine, glycopyrrolate)
    - Sympathomimetic drugs (β-agonists, dopaminergic drugs)
    - Phosphodiesterase inhibitors (aminophylline, theophylline)

HISTORY, CHIEF COMPLAINT: Sinus tachycardia per se does not cause a chief complaint. The chief complaint is typically associated with the respective underlying disease (as already listed).

PHYSICAL EXAM FINDINGS

- Tachycardia
- Also possible:
  - Weak pulse or increased capillary refill time (heart failure/decreased cardiac output)
  - Pale or cyanotic mucous membranes (anemia/hypovolemia or hypoxemia)
  - Fever (infection)
  - Palpable thyroid nodule (feline hyperthyroidism)

ETIOLOGY AND PATHOPHYSIOLOGY

- Sinus tachycardia is a manifestation of the so-called fight or flight response governed by the sympathetic nervous system.
- Activation of the sympathetic nervous system increases the automatic discharge rate of sinoatrial (SA) nodal cells, either directly by activating the β-1 receptors in the SA node or indirectly by stimulating the release of norepinephrine from the adrenal gland into the circulation.
- Transient sinus tachycardia usually occurs during vigorous exercise, anxiety from restraint, fear, or pain.
- Sustained sinus tachycardia is more likely a compensatory phenomenon associated with a decreased cardiac output, hypoxia, or increased metabolic demand (fever, hyperthyroidism).
- Drug-induced sinus tachycardia.

DIAGNOSIS

DIFFERENTIAL DIAGNOSIS

By ECG:

- Any narrow complex supraventricular tachycardia (SVT):
  - Sinus node reentry tachycardia.
  - Ectopic atrial tachycardia (if normal P wave morphology).
  - In fast sinus tachycardia, the P waves cannot be distinguished from the T waves of the previous beat. In those cases, it can be difficult to differentiate sinus tachycardia from AV reentry (bypass tract-mediated supraventricular tachycardia) or AV nodal reentry tachycardia (see the text on vagal maneuver in the Initial Database section below).
  - Atrial flutter with 2:1 or 3:1 conduction.
- Sinus tachycardia with bundle branch block can mimic ventricular tachycardia.

INITIAL DATABASE

- ECG (Fig. I-154):
  - QRS complexes are similar to normal sinus rhythm
  - RR interval is shorter
  - Regular P waves with normal morphology
  - Each P wave is followed by a QRS complex in a 1:1 ratio
  - At very rapid rates, the P waves might become superimposed on the preceding T waves, such that the P waves are obscured by T waves
- Physical tests:
  - Vagal maneuver: A positive response (transient, gradual slowing of sinus tachycardia over a few seconds) may increase the RR interval enough to allow visualization of P waves. Abrupt termination of a tachycardia during a vagal maneuver suggests presence of another type of SVT, such as sinus node reentry or AV node–dependent SVT (see Vagal Maneuver, p 1323)
  - Capillary refill time (peripheral perfusion prolonged in shock or with reduced cardiac output)
- Blood pressure (BP) (hypotension)
- Oxygen saturation (hypoxemia)
- Hematocrit and hemoglobin (anemia)
- Thoracic radiography (cardiomegaly, pulmonary edema, or pleural effusion secondary to congestive heart failure [CHF])
- Echocardiography to check for cause of reduced cardiac output or CHF if present

TREATMENT

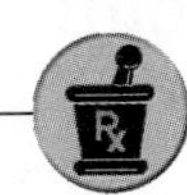

THERAPEUTIC GOAL(S)

- Treat underlying cause of sinus tachycardia (if necessary)
- Medical (β-blockers) reduction of heart rate during sinus tachycardia without knowledge of the underlying disorder can be detrimental since the elevated heart rate might be necessary for maintaining cardiac output

ACUTE GENERAL TREATMENT

Depends on cause of sinus tachycardia:

- Provide calming environment to reduce anxiety
- Administer pain medication if indicated
- Provide oxygen or hemoglobin for hypoxemic or anemic animals
- Administer fluids or vasopressor agents to stabilize blood pressure for animals in shock
- Start antimicrobials (if indicated); reduce fever with cool fluid administration
- Discontinue drugs that are causing sinus tachycardia

CHRONIC TREATMENT

Address the underlying disease and:

- Manage CHF
- Control T4 levels (correct hyperthyroidism)
- Treat other signs

POSSIBLE COMPLICATIONS

- Acute, transient sinus tachycardia can be associated with weakness or syn-

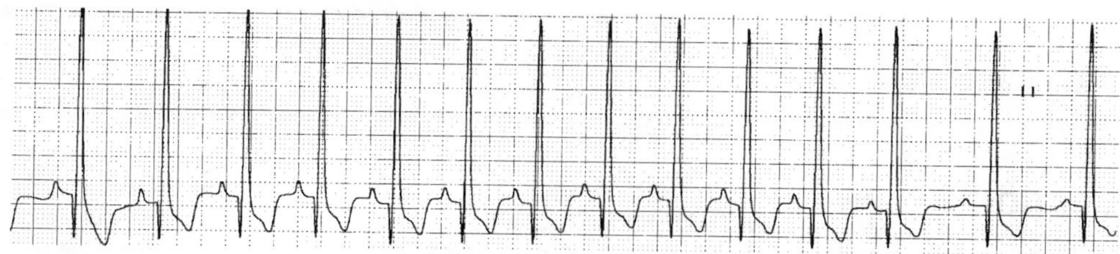

FIGURE I-154 ECG rhythm strip; lead II, 50 mm/sec, 10 mm/mV. Sinus tachycardia in a mixed-breed dog with chronic myxomatous atrioventricular (AV) valve disease. Normal sinus rhythm initially; acceleration to a heart rate of up to 200 bpm (sinus tachycardia) is seen in the middle of the strip, with a gradual slowing down again to 150 bpm (sinus rhythm) toward the end of the strip. The R wave amplitude is tall, indicative of left ventricular enlargement (in this case, secondary to mitral endocardiosis), and there is mild ST segment depression, suggesting myocardial hypoxia. Rapid-onset sinus tachycardia, such as in this example, is usually due to catecholamine release in response to environmental stimuli (stress, excitement, etc.).

cope, particularly in animals with reduced cardiac function (e.g., dilated cardiomyopathy, advanced mitral/tricuspid endocardiosis).
- Chronic sinus tachycardia can cause tachycardia-induced cardiomyopathy.

RECOMMENDED MONITORING

If the underlying cause has been identified and corrected, the sinus tachycardia should resolve.

PROGNOSIS AND OUTCOME

- Prognosis is good if underlying cause can be corrected
- Outcome depends on underlying condition

PEARLS & CONSIDERATIONS

COMMENTS

Sinus tachycardia is a benign "arrhythmia," and usually should be considered a red flag that indicates an underlying cause needs to be investigated. If the heart rate does not slow down, it can be assumed that the underlying cause is not yet addressed adequately.

CLIENT EDUCATION

Avoid excessive stress or vigorous exercise in animals with reduced cardiac output and CHF.

SUGGESTED READING

Moise NS: Diagnosis and management of canine arrhythmias. In Fox PR, Sisson D, Moise NS (eds): *Textbook of Canine and Feline Cardiology*. Philadelphia, WB Saunders, 1999, pp 331–385.

Reiffel JA: Normal sinus rhythm and its variants, sinus node reentry and sinus node dysfunction: mechanisms, recognition, and management. In Podrid PJ, Kowey PR (eds): *Cardiac Arrhythmia*. Philadelphia, Lippincott Williams & Wilkins, 1995, pp 752–767.

AUTHORS: **ANNA R. M. GELZER, MARC S. KRAUS**

EDITOR: **ETIENNE CÔTÉ**

Sinusitis and Other Sinus Disorders

BASIC INFORMATION

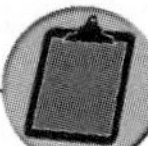

DEFINITION

Mucosal inflammation in, or other diseases of, one or more of the sinuses: either the frontal or the maxillary sinuses in dogs and either the frontal or (less commonly) the sphenoidal sinuses in cats

EPIDEMIOLOGY

SPECIES, AGE, SEX

- Cats:
  - No sex predilection
  - Young to middle-aged animals for chronic idiopathic (rhino) sinusitis
  - Older animals for sinus tumors
  - Any age for trauma
- Dogs:
  - No sex predilection
  - Older dogs for frontal sinusitis associated with tumors
  - Young adults more commonly with aspergillosis
  - Young to middle-aged dogs more often seen with chronic idiopathic sinusitis
  - Any age for trauma

GENETICS AND BREED PREDISPOSITION

- Cats: any breed
- Dogs: primarily dolichocephalic breeds for frontal sinusitis associated with tumors, aspergillosis, or chronic idiopathic sinusitis

ASSOCIATED CONDITIONS AND DISORDERS

- Nasal tumors
- Nasal aspergillosis
- Chronic idiopathic or lymphoplasmacytic rhinosinusitis
- Nasal or frontal sinus trauma
- Abscessation of the roots of the upper fourth premolar tooth (apical dental abscess), causing maxillary sinus empyema
- Feline herpesvirus (rhinotracheitis)

CLINICAL PRESENTATION

DISEASE FORMS/SUBTYPES: See Associated Conditions and Disorders above.

HISTORY, CHIEF COMPLAINT

- Nasal discharge
- Intermittent sneezing
- Focal facial swelling or deformity
- Signs related to local pain
  - Dullness or lethargy
  - Decreased movements of the head
  - Anorexia

PHYSICAL EXAM FINDINGS

- Unilateral nasal discharge of variable nature: mucoid, mucopurulent or blood-tinged; often bloody with nasal neoplasia
- If nasal cavity affected, diminished air flow through nasal passages/nares
- Focal swelling, firm enlargement, facial deformity, and/or pain with atrophy or lysis of the frontal or nasal bones:
  - Depressions, or defects in frontal/nasal bone integrity from osteolysis, may be noted during palpation

- Dogs with maxillary sinusitis from fourth premolar tooth root abscessation may have a swelling or fistulous tract and drainage from ventral to the eye on the affected side
- Enlargement of submandibular lymph nodes is possible
- Percussion of the sinus may induce pain or be associated with reduced resonance

ETIOLOGY AND PATHOPHYSIOLOGY

- Sinusitis is most often secondary to another primary nasal or frontal sinus disease (as already described in Associated Conditions and Disorders above) in which disruption of the normal nasal/sinus anatomy impairs mucociliary clearance or obstructs mucus drainage.
- Due to physical continuity between the chambers, tumors of the frontal sinus can extend into the nasal cavity, and nasal tumors can extend in the frontal sinus.
- Mycotic sinusitis and rhinitis, mostly due to *Aspergillus fumigatus,* can affect both the nasal cavity and sinus or either independently.
- Chronic lymphoplasmacytic inflammation in dogs can be a sequel to bacterial or mycotic infections (even after successful fungal therapy), can be idiopathic, or possibly could be related to an allergic etiology.
- Chronic lymphoplasmacytic inflammation in cats can be a sequel to bacterial, viral (feline upper respiratory tract infection complex), and, although rarely, mycotic infections.
  - Like in dogs, the condition can be idiopathic in cats, possibly related to an allergic etiology.

DIAGNOSIS

DIFFERENTIAL DIAGNOSIS

Nasal diseases of various origins:

- Fungal rhinitis
- Nasal neoplasia
- Dental disease/dental root infection (maxillary sinus)
- Foreign bodies
- Lymphoplasmacytic rhinitis
- Nasal mites
- Chronic viral upper respiratory tract infection in cats

INITIAL DATABASE

- For some cases, plain radiographs of the nasal cavities, sinuses, and dental roots can be helpful in the diagnosis of structural lesions, such as neoplasia, fungal rhinitis/sinusitis, disease, but will not help discriminate among the various causes of nasal/sinus disease in other cases not involving structural changes.
- Results of a complete blood count (CBC), serum biochemical profile, and urinalysis are often normal.
- For cases in which there is swelling or lysis (which can be palpable) of nasal/facial bones or the frontal sinus area, fine-needle aspirate (FNA) cytologic examination can show neoplasia or inflammation.

ADVANCED OR CONFIRMATORY TESTING

- CT scan and/or MRI of the nasal cavities and sinuses can differentiate neoplasia, fungal rhinitis, and dental disease with more accuracy than plain radiographs but will not confirm the diagnosis in all cases (Figs. I-155 and I-156).
- The frontal sinus can be examined by direct rhinoscopy in some dogs, but access to and visualization of the frontal sinus is often possible only in animals with severe turbinate destruction (Figs. I-157 and I-158).
- Trephination of the frontal sinus for examination and biopsy may be necessary to confirm the presence of neoplasia, fungal rhinitis, or inflammation, especially if disease is confined to the frontal sinus. Trephination may also have therapeutic value for cases of fungal rhinitis (see Aspergillosis, p 87).

TREATMENT

THERAPEUTIC GOAL(S)

- Identify and treat the primary disease
- Manage complications of primary nasal/sinus disease

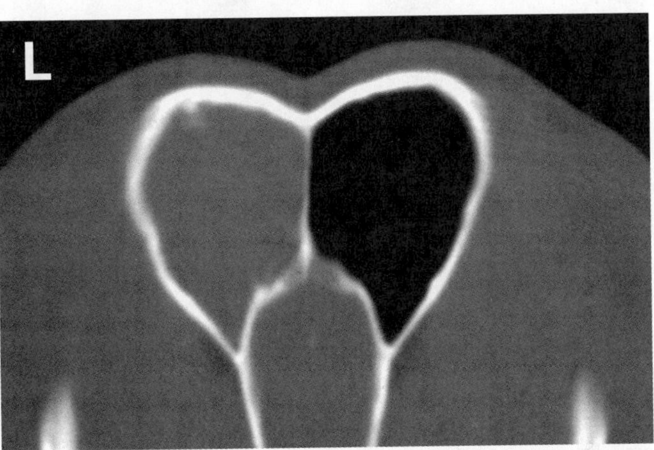

FIGURE I-155 CT scan of a dog with a nasal tumor extending into the left frontal sinus; transverse plane. There is extensive soft tissue/fluid opacification of the left frontal sinus. Sinonasal aspergillosis and a primary tumor of the frontal sinus could have a similar tomographic appearance. Courtesy of Drs. Jimmy H. Saunders and Cécile Clercx, University of Liège.

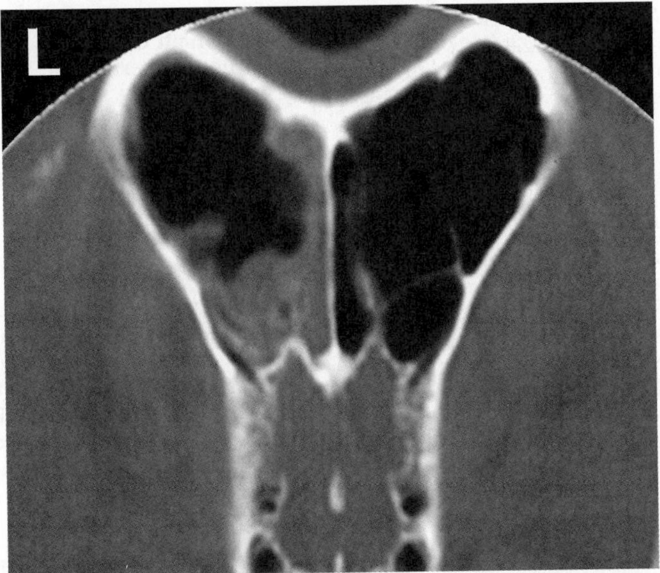

FIGURE I-156 CT scan of a dog with sinonasal aspergillosis; transverse plane. There is regional soft tissue/fluid opacification of the left frontal sinus. Courtesy of Drs. Jimmy H. Saunders and Cécile Clercx, University of Liège.

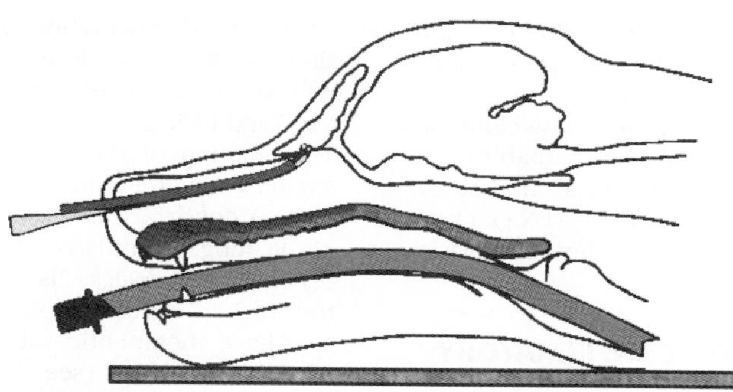

FIGURE I-157 Diagram demonstrating the standard position for endoscopic imaging of the frontal sinuses in the dog. Courtesy of Dr. Cécile Clercx, University of Liège.

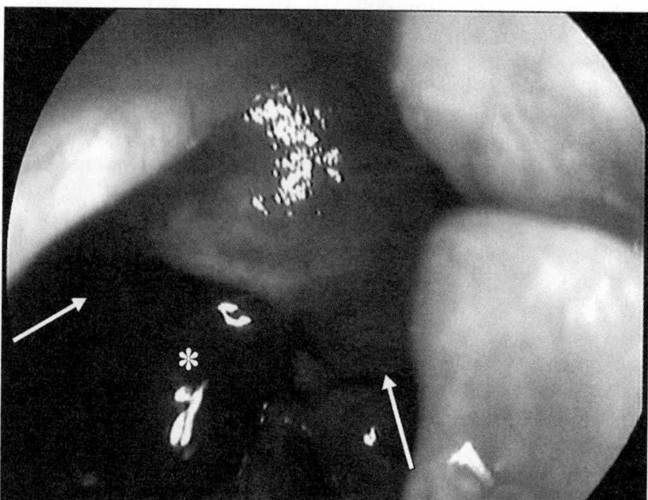

FIGURE I-158 Endoscopic view of the frontal sinus of a dog, as shown in Fig. I-157. A large, smooth convex mass occupies the center of the image (*arrows*), and its appearance strongly suggests neoplasia. An adjacent blood vessel is seen (*asterisk*). Courtesy of Dr. Cécile Clercx, University of Liège.

ACUTE GENERAL TREATMENT

- Direct treatment toward the causal agent:
  - Fungal sinusitis/rhinitis: antimycotic therapy (see Aspergillosis, p 87)
  - Frontal tumors: radiation therapy and, occasionally, surgical resection
  - Traumatic injuries causing fractures of the frontal bone: removal of bone fragments present in the frontal sinus and possibly reconstruction; check patency of the nasofrontal ostium (nasofrontal opening); broad-spectrum antibiotics
  - Apical dental (tooth root) abscess: surgical extraction of the tooth, including roots, or endodontic treatment
- In acute infection, as well as in chronic idiopathic inflammation with episodes of secondary bacterial infections, oral or injectable antibiotics (e.g., amoxicillin 20 mg/kg PO q 8h; cefadroxil 20 mg/kg PO q 8h; or amoxicillin-clavulanate 15 mg/kg PO q 12h) and possibly mucolytics may be needed.
  - The frontal sinus is a combination of several large cavities surrounded by bone; systemically administered drugs often do not achieve high concentrations in the sinus. Even very high dosages of highly soluble drugs, preferred for systemic therapy, may not reach adequate concentrations throughout the entire sinus cavity.
  - Drug nebulization is unproven; the amount of drug delivered into the frontal sinus is unknown.

CHRONIC TREATMENT

In case of concomitant nasal disease, with loss of the protective filter provided by normal turbinates and decreased mucociliary clearance along the distal third of the nasal cavity, recurrent bacterial secondary infections are common and are treated each time with antibiotics and mucolytics, orally or locally (intranasal administration or aerosol delivery).

POSSIBLE COMPLICATIONS

In animals with chronic sinusitis, episodes of bacterial infection can be expected.

RECOMMENDED MONITORING

Monitoring depends on etiology of the condition and persistence of clinical signs. For example, in lymphoplasmacytic inflammation of the frontal sinus after treatment of aspergillosis, diagnostic work-up is warranted in cases of severe recurrence of clinical signs to differentiate between secondary bacterial infection and recurrence of aspergillosis because the latter must be treated with antifungal agents.

PROGNOSIS AND OUTCOME

- Prognosis and outcome depend on the cause, whether the cause can be eliminated or treated accordingly, and depend on whether there are chronic irreversible sequelae of the turbinates and sinus mucosa
- Poor in most frontal sinus tumors, which are mostly malignant
- In chronic sinusitis, total cure is rarely achieved, but response to ongoing therapy is generally good

PEARLS & CONSIDERATIONS

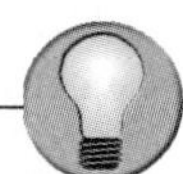

COMMENTS

- In acute cases, quickly find the cause using appropriate diagnostic tests and immediately treat the animal to avoid chronic irreversible sequelae.
- When sinusitis is related to the extension of nasal disease, it is often a chronic condition with consequent remodeling, and total cure is rare; secondary bacterial infections can always occur.

CLIENT EDUCATION

Treatment must be repeated when relapses, which are common in chronic idiopathic sinusitis, occur. The disease will rarely totally resolve, and most of the time, mild clinical signs persist despite treatment. If more severe signs persist, repeating a complete diagnostic evaluation is indicated with the intent of identifying an etiologic cause.

SUGGESTED READING

Norris AM, Laing EJ: Diseases of the nose and sinuses. *Vet Clin N Amer: Small Anim Pract* 15:865–890, 1985.

Saunders JH, et al: Radiographic, magnetic resonance, computed tomographic, and rhinoscopic features of canine nasal aspergillosis. *J Am Vet Med Assoc* 225:1703, 2004.

AUTHOR: **CÉCILE CLERCX**

EDITOR: **RANCE K. SELLON**

Smoke Inhalation

BASIC INFORMATION

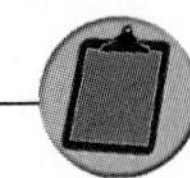

DEFINITION

Inhalation injury due to breathing of harmful gases, vapors, and particulate matter contained in smoke

SYNONYM(S)

Smoke exposure
Smoke toxicity

EPIDEMIOLOGY

RISK FACTORS

- Closed-space fires increase the risk for smoke inhalation
- History of respiratory disease

GEOGRAPHY AND SEASONALITY: More residential fires in winter.

ASSOCIATED CONDITIONS AND DISORDERS: Acute respiratory distress syndrome (ARDS), bacterial pneumonia, systemic inflammatory response syndrome (SIRS).

CLINICAL PRESENTATION

DISEASE FORMS/SUBTYPES

- Inhalation injury generally manifests in three clinical stages:
  - Acute pulmonary insufficiency
  - Pulmonary edema
  - Bronchopneumonia
- Occasionally, smoke inhalation injury may be confined to the nasal passages and pharynx.

HISTORY, CHIEF COMPLAINT

- Complaint of respiratory difficulties following smoke inhalation (respiratory distress, foaming, coughing or gagging)
- Weakness, stupor, or coma following rescue

PHYSICAL EXAM FINDINGS

- Harsh or moist airway sounds, crackles, wheezes, loud laryngeal or tracheal sounds, dyspnea, coughing, tachypnea, short or shallow respirations; in milder cases, signs may be limited to the nasal cavity (inflammation-induced nasal congestion, obstruction to nasal airflow).
- Postural adaptations to respiratory distress may be noted.
- Mentation and motor dysfunction may include ataxia, weakness, depression, stupor, or coma.
- Mucous membranes may be hyperemic (due to carboxyhemoglobin [COHb], cyanide [CN], or vasodilation), pale, or cyanotic.
- Dermatologic findings include smoky smell, singed or burnt hair, soot, or skin lacerations.

ETIOLOGY AND PATHOPHYSIOLOGY

Causes of respiratory injury:

- Thermal damage is usually limited to the upper airway mucosa due to rapid heat dissipation. Steam, soot (particles <2.5 μm), and volatile and explosive gases, however, may also cause thermal injury to lower airways.
- Asphyxiation:
  - Atmospheric oxygen deficit due to combustion.
  - Carbon monoxide (CO) toxicity: tissue hypoxia from COHb formation and subsequent decrease in the oxygen carrying-capacity of blood. A left shift of the oxyhemoglobin-dissociation curve also reduces peripheral oxygen delivery.
  - Combustion of plastics, polyurethane, fiber, rubber, and paper produces cyanide gas, which arrests cellular respiration by binding to cytochrome a3.
  - Methemoglobinemia occurs due to heat denaturation of hemoglobin and release of oxides and nitrites.
- Pulmonary irritants cause direct tissue injury (dependent on particle size, water solubility, and acidity), bronchospasm, and inflammation. Leukocyte activation with cytokine release and nitric oxide upregulation lead to pulmonary vascular hyperpermeability and edema. Pulmonary hypertension and atelectasis due to acute surfactant inactivation contribute to hypoxemia.
  - Impaired macrophage function and decreased mucociliary clearance predispose the animal to bacterial pneumonia.
  - Neurologic dysfunction: central nervous system (CNS) oxygen deprivation.

DIAGNOSIS

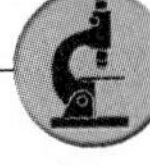

DIFFERENTIAL DIAGNOSIS

- Anaphylaxis
- ARDS
- Asthma (cats)
- Congestive heart failure (CHF) and pulmonary edema
- Pneumonia
- Pneumothorax
- Pulmonary thromboembolism
- Primary CNS disorders

INITIAL DATABASE

- Arterial blood gas (ABG) and pulse oximetry:
  - ABG may confirm hypoxemia, hypercarbia.
  - Less useful for determining tissue oxygenation in the face of carbon monoxide (CO) exposure and methemoglobinemia.
  - With smoke inhalation, pulse oximetry cannot evaluate the severity of hypoxia because of its inability to differentiate between oxygenated hemoglobin and carboxyhemoglobin.
- Complete blood count (CBC):
  - Increased packed cell volume (PCV) (dehydration, splenic contraction). Dogs with a more severe inhalation injury tend to have a higher PCV (mean: 58%) than milder cases (mean: 50%).
  - Neutropenia: pulmonary neutrophil sequestration.
- Serum chemistry profile:
  - May demonstrate hypoxic organ damage (e.g., liver, kidneys).
  - Electrolyte (and lactate) levels can identify a high anion gap acidosis.
- Thoracic radiography:
  - May be normal after initial smoke inhalation but useful to establish a baseline.
  - Findings may include atelectasis, aspiration, and pulmonary edema.

ADVANCED OR CONFIRMATORY TESTING

- Bronchoscopy: may demonstrate the severity of airway damage and indicate impending airway obstruction. A bronchoalveolar lavage (cytologic examination, culture) is helpful in stable animals.
- Transtracheal wash: if infection is suspected.
- Pulmonary function testing: uncommonly used; inhalation injury may decrease functional residual capacity.

TREATMENT

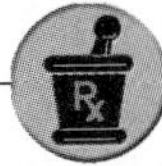

THERAPEUTIC GOAL(S)

- Maintain airway patency and restore normal gas exchange
- Reverse or prevent tissue hypoxia
- Control SIRS
- Prevent neurologic sequelae and postinhalation bacterial pneumonia

ACUTE GENERAL TREATMENT

- High-flow humidified oxygen therapy is crucial to reverse hypoxia and accelerates CO elimination.
  - COHb half-life: 4 hours (room air) versus 1.5 hours (100% oxygen).
- Severe cases: mechanical ventilation with positive end-expiratory pressure (PEEP).

- Administration of IV fluid therapy in hypoxic states and shock to maintain cardiac output. Synthetic colloids (e.g., Hetastarch 10-20 ml/kg IV) may be beneficial to minimize pulmonary edema.
- Blood or plasma transfusions may be necessary (see Transfusion Therapy and Collection Techniques for Blood Banking, p 1312).
- Nebulization of saline and coupage may facilitate clearance of respiratory secretions.
- Nutritional support to preserve body condition and immune status.
- Drug therapy:
    - Smoke inhalation predisposes the animal to secondary bacterial infections; consider broad-spectrum antimicrobials based on appropriate bacterial cultures, or use them if clinical deterioration occurs early in therapy.
    - Corticosteroids: controversial, not recommended. Analgesics (e.g., buprenorphine 0.01 mg/kg IM, IV, or SQ q 6-12h, fentanyl 3-5 μg/kg/hr IV) and nonsteroidal anti-inflammatory drugs (NSAIDs) (meloxicam 0.1-0.2 mg/kg IV, SQ, or PO q 24h; carprofen 2.2 mg/kg PO q 12h [dog]) can relieve inflammation and discomfort.
    - Bronchodilators (albuterol 90 μg inhaler, one to two puffs per large breed dog q 8h, as needed; aminophylline 6-10 mg/kg IM, PO, or diluted IV, q 8h) may alleviate reflex bronchospasm.
    - Specific antidotes include:
    - 20% sodium thiosulfate 30-50 mg/kg IV, q 8-12h, or 1% sodium nitrite 16 mg/kg IV (dog) for CNS toxicity.
    - Reducing agents (1% methylene blue 1-1.5 mg/kg slow IV infusion once (dogs only) to treat methemoglobinemia.

DRUG INTERACTIONS

- Systemic corticosteroids may predispose the animal to bacterial infections.
- Diuretics may decrease intravascular volume without major benefits on pulmonary function and edema.

POSSIBLE COMPLICATIONS

- ARDS and respiratory failure
- Superimposed bacterial infections: common cause of deterioration

RECOMMENDED MONITORING

- Careful monitoring of airway patency, gas exchange, hydration, and cardiovascular function
- Repeat thoracic radiographs

PROGNOSIS AND OUTCOME

- The duration of smoke exposure, type of burn material, and availability of immediate oxygen supplementation impact recovery.
- Severe burns, organ injury, and deteriorating respiratory function within 24 hours carry a poor prognosis.

PEARLS & CONSIDERATIONS

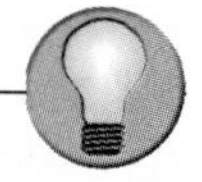

COMMENTS

Substantial pulmonary damage may not manifest until several hours following admission.

SUGGESTED READING

Drobatz KJ, et al: Smoke exposure in dogs: 27 cases (1988-1997). *J Am Vet Med Assoc* 215(9): 1306- 1311, 1999.

Drobatz KJ, et al: Smoke exposure in cats: 22 cases (1986-1997). *J Am Vet Med Assoc* 215(9): 1312-1316, 1999.

Lafferty KA: Smoke inhalation. November 2004: www.emedicine.com.

AUTHOR: **DANIELA BEDENICE**

EDITOR: **ELIZABETH ROZANSKI**

Snakebite

BASIC INFORMATION

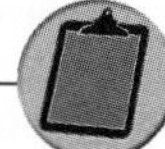

DEFINITION

Injury resulting from a snake biting an animal

SYNONYM(S)

Snake envenomization

EPIDEMIOLOGY

SPECIES, AGE, SEX: Any age or species or either sex.

GENETICS AND BREED PREDISPOSITION: Large-breed, outdoor dogs appear to have an increased risk.

RISK FACTORS

- Environment: exposure to outdoors in warm climates
- Behavior: curiosity

CONTAGION AND ZOONOSIS

- The same snakes that are venomous to dogs and cats are venomous to humans.
- No zoonosis associated with snakebites.

GEOGRAPHY AND SEASONALITY

- There are two main families of venomous snakes: Elapidae and Viperidae.
    - Elapids: coral snakes, cobras, mambas, kraits, and the tiger snake. Found predominantly in the southeastern areas of the United States.
    - Vipers: rattlesnakes (*Crotalus* and *Sistrus* spp.) and cottonmouths and copperheads (*Agkistrodon* spp.); found throughout the United States.
- Increased incidence of bites in summer months (in North America, 90% of bites occur between April and October). Toxicity increased in young or very large snakes during springtime.

ASSOCIATED CONDITIONS AND DISORDERS

- Neurologic dysfunction: elapids
- Local tissue damage and possibly systemic bleeding/coagulation: vipers

CLINICAL PRESENTATION

DISEASE FORMS/SUBTYPES

- Vipers (e.g., rattlesnakes) inflict 99% of the estimated 150,000 annual snake bites of dogs and cats in North America.
- "Dry" bites possible: contain little or no toxic venom (22% of rattlesnake bites are dry; higher proportion in elapids).

HISTORY, CHIEF COMPLAINT

Observed bite

- Dogs: head and neck; cats: abdomen, thorax
- Common scenario: the dog cries out after sniffing in the bushes or behind a rock where snake is hidden

Unobserved bite: facial or neck swelling and pain after being outdoors without supervision

PHYSICAL EXAM FINDINGS

- Fang marks with swelling and bruising around the area may exist. The animal may show signs of mild discomfort to profound hemorrhagic and neurologic alterations. Fang marks are often difficult to find, especially in long-haired or thick-coated dogs and cats.
- Coral snakes:
    - Leave tiny fang or tooth marks with little or no local swelling
    - Signs may be delayed 1 to 7.5 hours
    - Salivation
    - Vomiting
    - Convulsions
    - Quadriplegia
    - Death

- Rattlesnakes (Figs. I-159, I-160)
  - Usually leave two fang marks
  - Swelling
  - Pain
  - Erythema
  - Petechiae or ecchymoses
  - Cyanosis and tissue sloughing

ETIOLOGY AND PATHOPHYSIOLOGY

- Elapid venom is neurotoxic and hemolytic:
  - Signs appear 1 to 7.5 hours after the bite was inflicted and progress rapidly.
  - Signs start with salivation, vomiting, and apprehensive behavior.
  - Signs progress to convulsions, quadriplegia, and eventually may lead to death from respiratory paralysis.
- Crotalid venom is vasculotoxic and necrogenic (Fig. I-160).
  - Bites lead to immediate, regional swelling.
  - Area around the bite may have swelling, pain, erythema, ecchymosis, cyanosis, and tissue sloughing.
  - Bites are most often inflicted on the face and head and occasionally on the paws.
  - In severe cases, the tissue around the fang marks turns black within 30 minutes, and the blood oozing from the site is dark and watery.
  - Swelling typically worsens over the first 24 hours after the bite was inflicted, and the swollen tissue may be similar to a hematoma (occasionally requiring transfusion).

DIAGNOSIS

DIFFERENTIAL DIAGNOSIS

- Other animal attacks
- Scorpion bite
- Insect bite
- Wound of unknown origin
- Intoxication with neurotoxic substance (versus elapid envenomation)

INITIAL DATABASE

- Complete blood count (CBC) with platelet count: may reveal hemoconcentration, leukocytosis, echinocytosis, or thrombocytopenia
- Serum biochemistry profile: may reveal hypokalemia, high creatine kinase
- Urinalysis: may reveal hematuria or myoglobinuria
- Coagulation profile: prolonged activated clotting time (ACT), prothrombin time (PT), partial thromboplastin time (PTT), and increased fibrin(ogen) degradation products (FDPs) possible
- Aerobic and anaerobic bacterial culture and sensitivity (C&S) of the wound

ADVANCED OR CONFIRMATORY TESTING

No test exists that is diagnostic for a snake bite, but echinocytes found on a blood smear are a common finding in animals with envenomation. Echinocytes are "burred" red blood cells (RBCs) that appear soon after envenomation and last 24 to 48 hours. These cells often precede the massive tissue swelling and necrosis that occur with serious bites.

TREATMENT

THERAPEUTIC GOAL(S)

- Management/prevention of hypotension
- Neutralization of venom (minimizing local and systemic effects)
- Prevention of secondary bacterial infection
- Pain management
- Avoidance of iatrogenic complications, particularly during first-aid efforts in the field

ACUTE GENERAL TREATMENT

- All animals that have a snakebite, regardless of apparent stability, should be hospitalized for a minimum of 8 hours to assess for clinical signs that may first manifest during this period.
- IV fluid therapy:
  - First line of therapy to treat hypotension or hypovolemic shock and decreased cardiac output
  - Crystalloids (e.g., lactated Ringer's solution or 0.9% NaCl) at maintenance rates (e.g., 30 ml/lb per day [65 ml/kg per day] plus deficit for extravasated fluid; estimate amount of tissue swelling) if animal is stable or at shock rates (90 ml/lb/hr [200 ml/kg/hr]) if animal is in hypovolemic shock
  - Colloids indicated for animals with hypoalbuminemia; plasma preferred because both albumin and acute phase proteins are administered (see Transfusion Therapy and Collection Techniques for Blood Banking, p 1312)
- Antivenin (polyvalent Crotalidae):
  - Administered immediately for viper bites; increased survival when given closer to time of bite, but beneficial effects noted for at least 60 hours after envenomization
  - A dose of up to 10 to 25 vials is routinely recommended in human cases, but very high cost (up to $300 per vial), reduced availability, smaller animal size, and mild extent of some bites generally limit the number of vials used to one to three
  - Protocol:
    - Reconstitute antivenin (10 ml diluent into lyophilized antivenin). Warm to body temperature (e.g., armpit method) and not warmer.

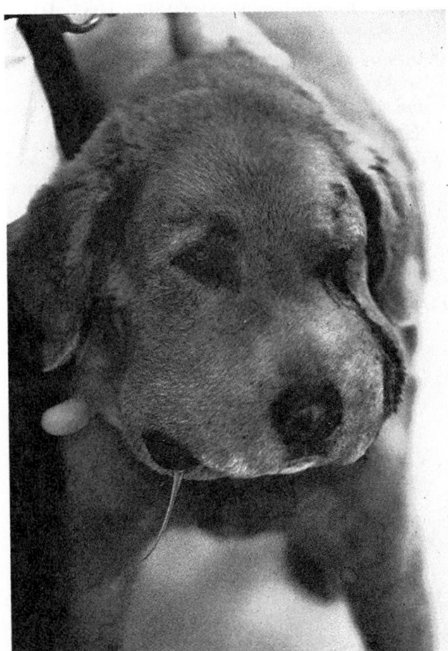

FIGURE I-159 Viper (rattlesnake) bite to a dog's muzzle. Note the marked, diffuse swelling of the face and lips.

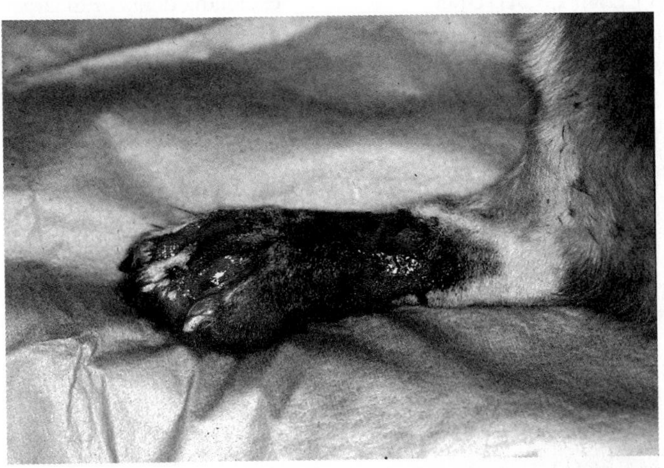

FIGURE I-160 Viper (rattlesnake) bite to a cat's distal forelimb. Note marked swelling, moist exudation, and dark discoloration of the skin, which suggests necrosis.

Gently swirl to dissolve over 10 to 15 minutes and avoid shaking the solution
  - Pretreat the patient (diphenhydramine 2 mg/kg IM)
  - Dilute antivenin into 50–200 ml IV fluids and administer test dose IV (10–20 ml over several minutes) while monitoring for anaphylaxis (see Transfusion Reactions, p 1098; Anaphylaxis, p 60)
  - If no anaphylaxis, administer remainder over 1 hour while continuing to monitor
- Antibiotics: chosen empirically at first while culture results are pending; first- or second-generation cephalosporins (e.g., cefazolin 22 mg/kg IV q 8h)
- Analgesics: opiates for sedation and analgesia while ensuring that the animal does not develop respiratory depression; buprenorphine (0.01 mg/kg IV q 6h) or fentanyl at a constant rate infusion (3 µg/kg IV, then 3–6 µg/kg/hr)
- Corticosteroids: anti-inflammatory doses (e.g., prednisone 0.5 mg/kg per day PO, maximum 5 days) may be of benefit
- Antihistamines: not recommended (have been shown to potentiate the toxicity of venom) except in pretreatment doses prior to antivenin administration
- Urgent airway management (critical from time of presentation to 72 hours later): prepare endotracheal tubes and tracheostomy kits when facial, neck, or tongue bites have occurred, even if swelling is initially unimpressive

CHRONIC TREATMENT

Surgical debridement of necrotic tissue is necessary in some cases

DRUG INTERACTIONS

Antivenin may cause an anaphylactic reaction (see Anaphylaxis, p 60). Monitor vital signs during infusion; if signs of anaphylaxis develop, temporarily stop the infusion and then restart the infusion at a slower rate when signs have subsided.

POSSIBLE COMPLICATIONS

Renal failure may result from myoglobinuria, hemoglobinuria, toxic nephropathy, and hypovolemic shock.

RECOMMENDED MONITORING

Monitor respiratory rate and effort as well as blood pressure (BP), electrocardiogram (ECG), coagulation status and urine output

PROGNOSIS AND OUTCOME

- The prognosis is worse in animals with high-venom burdens, shock, severe cardiac arrhythmias, hematologic complications, and infection.
- Nevertheless, the spectrum of severity is wide, and the majority of dog or cat snakebite victims survive without permanent sequelae if treated early and thoroughly.
- Although death may occur in spite of the timely use of crotalid-specific antivenin, a higher survival rate has been found in dogs that received antivenin than in dogs that did not.

PEARLS & CONSIDERATIONS

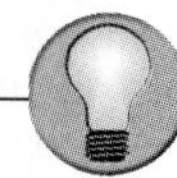

COMMENTS

- With viper bites, marked worsening of tissue swelling in the 24 to 48 hours following the bite is common, even with excellent treatment.
  - Warn owners in advance, to pre-empt their perception that treatment is unsuccessful.
  - Prepare airway mobilization material (endotracheal tube or tracheostomy kit) if the snake bit the animal on the head or neck.
- Ineffective first-aid techniques include tourniquet application, incision and suction of the bite, electroshock of the bite, and hot or cold pack application. These maneuvers can harm the animal by fostering infection.
- Effective first aid involves minimizing exertion immediately after the bite (reducing cutaneous blood flow/venom absorption) and immediate transport to a veterinary hospital for diagnosis and treatment as outlined previously.
- Snakebites on digits or in very small animals may require 50% more antivenin on a body weight basis than bites excluding digits or in larger animals.
  - A relatively small volume of body fluid in smaller animals (higher absolute venom concentrations).
  - Difficulty attaining high antivenin concentrations in digits.
- Rattlesnakes may bite for up to 30 minutes after they are killed, including death by decapitation. Therefore, the body or head of a snake that has bitten and is then killed and transported for identification should be kept in a rigid, closed container, and the head should not be handled directly.

PREVENTION

The best way to prevent snakebites is to avoid snakes.

- Vipers bite in self-defense or when they are surprised (as occurs in veterinary and human medicine), or to immobilize and consume prey, such as small rodents.
- Vipers may strike with unavoidable speed (8 ft/sec) but typically for a distance corresponding only to half the snake's length (e.g., half of 3–5 ft [1–1.6 m]).
- Keeping dogs in enclosed areas with cement walls or keeping dogs on leashes while outside may help prevent contact with snakes.
- Keeping cats indoors will help to prevent their contact with snakes.
- In regions where rattlesnakes are common, courses are offered to try to teach dogs to avoid snakes.
- Bitten dogs and cats cannot be counted on to avoid snakes in the future; repeat victims occur.

CLIENT EDUCATION

Most North American snakes bite when surprised or threatened; vigilance and avoidance of snakes during warm months are the best approach to preventing bite incidents.

SUGGESTED READING

Hackett TB, et al: Clinical findings associated with prairie rattlesnake bites in dogs: 100 cases (1989–1998). *J Am Vet Med Assoc* 220:1675–1680, 2002.

Hudelson S, Hudelson P: Pathophysiology of snake envenomization and evaluation of treatments: Parts I, II, & III, *Compend Contin Educ Pract Vet* 17:889–897, 1035–1040, 1385–1396, 1995.

Peterson ME: Snake bite: Pit vipers and coral snakes. In Peterson ME, Talcott PA (eds): *Small Animal Toxicology*. Philadelphia, WB Saunders, 2001, pp 695–720.

Willey JR, Schaer M: Eastern diamond rattlesnake (*Crotalus adamanteus*) envenomation of dogs: 31 cases (1982–2002). *J Am Anim Hosp Assoc* 41:22–33, 2005.

AUTHOR: **APRIL PAUL**

EDITOR: **ELIZABETH ROZANSKI**

Sneezing

BASIC INFORMATION

DEFINITION

- Sneezing is characterized as explosive expiration of air from the nose for the purpose of clearing the nasopharynx. Sneezing is mediated by a central reflex as a result of stimulation of the nasal mucosa. Occasional sneezing is normal.
- Reverse sneezing is characterized by paroxysmal, forceful, and loud *inspiratory* efforts that are triggered by nasopharyngeal irritation. The syndrome, most commonly seen in small- and toy-breed dogs, is self-limiting and rarely progressive. Reverse sneezing serves to move irritating debris from the nasopharynx into the oropharynx where it can be swallowed.
- All causes of nasal discharge and/or irritation are potential causes of sneezing. The type and duration of the discharge varies with the underlying cause (see Etiology and Pathophysiology below).

EPIDEMIOLOGY

SPECIES, AGE, SEX:

- Young cats may have viral upper respiratory infections or nasopharyngeal polyps.
- Young unvaccinated dogs are more likely to have canine viral respiratory infections.
- Younger animals may have congenital deformities.
- Older animals are more likely to have neoplastic or dental-related causes of nasal discharge and sneezing.
- Hunting and working dogs are more likely to have nasal foreign bodies.

GENETICS AND BREED PREDISPOSITION: Brachycephalic breeds have upper airway problems that may lead to sneezing and/or nasal discharge. Certain breeds can be affected by primary ciliary dyskinesia or by cleft palate-cleft lip complex.

RISK FACTORS

- Lack of adequate immunization against viral respiratory infections
- Exposure to unvaccinated animals and high-density husbandry situations
- Geographic locations where grass awns are ubiquitous
- Dental disease and poor dental care
- Immunosuppression (fungal disease)
- Compromise of nasal mucosa (secondary bacterial infections)

CONTAGION AND ZOONOSIS: Viral upper and lower respiratory tract infections.

GEOGRAPHY AND SEASONALITY: Geographic locations where grass awns are ubiquitous.

ASSOCIATED CONDITIONS AND DISORDERS: Sneezing itself can be a cause of acute nasal trauma.

CLINICAL PRESENTATION

DISEASE FORMS/SUBTYPES: Sneezing versus reverse sneezing.

HISTORY, CHIEF COMPLAINT: Acute onset of paroxysmal sneezing may suggest nasal foreign bodies or early viral disease. Husbandry and management predispose to certain disorders, for example: recent boarding, exposure to new animals, and/or history of inadequate vaccination (viral infections); hunting and geographic location (nasal foreign bodies); pertinent medical history (dental disease, history of neoplasia, immunosuppression); exposure to irritating aerosols (hairspray, paints, etc.) or anticoagulants (rodenticides, pharmaceuticals).

PHYSICAL EXAM FINDINGS

- Serous, mucopurulent, or hemorrhagic discharge that may be unilateral or bilateral
- Facial deformity
- Exophthalmos
- Maxillary swelling dorsal to carnassial tooth (apical dental ["tooth root"] abscess)
- Oronasal fistula
- Ocular discharge
- Petechiation, ecchymoses
- Pawing at face

ETIOLOGY AND PATHOPHYSIOLOGY

All causes of nasal discharge and/or irritation are potential causes of sneezing. Types of nasal discharge:

- Serous: clear and watery (acellular) due to local irritation, early viral infection, allergic rhinitis, or excessive lacrimation
- Mucoid: clear and thicker (acellular with higher protein content) due to chronic noninfectious irritation and overproduction of mucus by nasal epithelial cells
- Purulent: yellow-tan, thick discharge (neutrophilic with bacteria) usually due to secondary bacterial infection
- Sanguineous: red-tinged (blood mixed with another type of discharge) due to compromise of the nasal mucosa
- Hemorrhagic (epistaxis): frank red blood due to local or systemic causes of bleeding

DIAGNOSIS

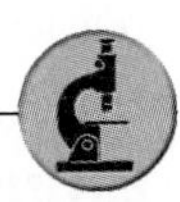

DIFFERENTIAL DIAGNOSIS

- Feline viral upper respiratory tract infections (feline rhinotracheitis, feline calicivirus, *Chlamydophila felis*)
- Neoplasia (adenocarcinoma, lymphosarcoma, undifferentiated carcinoma, osteosarcoma, chondrosarcoma, fibrosarcoma, transmissible venereal tumor)
- Foreign bodies
- Apical dental ("tooth root") abscess
- Oronasal fistula
- Nasopharyngeal polyps
- Canine viral infections (canine distemper virus, canine parainfluenza virus, canine herpesvirus, canine adenovirus types 1 and 2)
- Mycotic infection (*Aspergillus* spp. in dogs; *Cryptococcus neoformans* in cats)
- Parasitic rhinitis (*Cuterebra* spp., *Pneumonyssoides caninum*, *Linguatala serrata*)
- Bacterial infections (usually secondary)
- Rhinitis (allergic/eosinophilic type I hypersensitivity, lymphoplasmacytic, chronic hyperplastic)
- Congenital defects (cleft palate-cleft lip complex, primary ciliary dyskinesis)
- Trauma
- Inhaled irritants (cat litter dust, aerosols, smoke)
- Epistaxis (local causes: mycotic infections, neoplasia, foreign body, trauma. Systemic causes: inherited or acquired coagulopathies, thrombocytopenia, thrombocytopathia, hypertension, vasculitides)

INITIAL DATABASE

- Assessment for unilateral versus bilateral nasal disease by holding a glass microscope slide close to the external nares while the patient breathes on it through its nose (mouth held closed). Presence or absence of steam on the slide suggests unilateral obstruction, bilateral obstruction, or normal air flow. Neoplasia, foreign bodies, and dental disease are often causes of unilateral nasal disease while other local and systemic causes often result in bilateral disease.
- Examination of the oral cavity to look for hard palate masses, fundic examination to look for evidence of neoplasia, fungal disease, or hypertension and associated retinal hemorrhage.
- Eye globe retropulsion ± ocular ultrasound to assess for retrobulbar masses.
- Blood pressure measurement to assess for hypertension.

- Complete blood count including platelet count to look for evidence of infection, inflammation, or thrombocytopenia.
- Serum biochemistry profile, urinalysis.
- Feline leukemia and feline immunodeficiency viral testing.

ADVANCED OR CONFIRMATORY TESTING

Rocky Mountain spotted fever, *Ehrlichia*, and *Bartonella* testing, prothrombin time, partial thromboplastin time, thoracic radiographs, nasal swabs, fungal titer determinations, nasal radiography, computed tomography, rhinoscopy, biopsy, deep tissue cultures, exploratory rhinotomy—as dictated by history, physical exam, and preliminary findings

TREATMENT

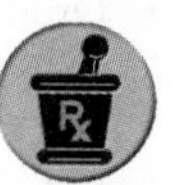

THERAPEUTIC GOAL(S)

- Eliminate underlying etiology of sneezing
- Restore normal nasal function
- Reduce pain and discomfort
- Provide supportive care
- Relieve dyspnea, especially in cats who oftentimes will not readily open mouth breathe

ACUTE GENERAL TREATMENT

- If nasal discharge or nasal mucosal edema is causing dyspnea, then oxygen therapy may be needed.
- Treatment for underlying coagulopathy (e.g., vitamin K_1 [0.25-2.5 mg/kg for first generation rodenticide intoxication or 2.5-5.0 mg/kg for second generation, SC or PO divided q 12h for 7 to 21 days] and fresh frozen plasma).
- Correct dehydration and electrolyte abnormalities as necessary.
- Broad-spectrum antibiotics if secondary nasal or dental infection (bacteria are rarely the primary cause of nasal disease but secondary infection with normal nasal flora is common) or pneumonia (culture and sensitivity from the lower airways is essential if pneumonia is present). *Bartonella* recently has been implicated as a cause of chronic rhinitis and epistaxis, azithromycin is the drug of choice (5-10 mg/kg PO q 24h. Start at 5 mg/kg and if tolerated increase by 2.5 mg/kg each day, to 10 mg/kg limit. After one week reduce to q 48h).
- Analgesics if painful (opiates and/or nonsteroidal anti-inflammatory drugs [NSAIDs]).
- Removal of animal from environmental agents (e.g., smoke, dust, allergens).
- Surgery should be considered for dental disease, neoplasia, nasopharyngeal polyps, cleft palate, foreign bodies, or traumatic causes.
- Rhinoscopy may be useful for removing a foreign body.
- Radiation and/or chemotherapy for neoplasia.
- Fungal: local or systemic treatment.
- Parasitic rhinitis: ivermectin 0.2 mg/kg SC or PO, twice over a 3 week period, is reported to be successful; avoid in breeds susceptible to toxicosis (collies, Shetland sheepdogs, Old English sheepdogs, and others).
- Decongestants and cleaning of the nares (pediatric Neo-synephrine, 1 drop in alternating nares q 24h).

CHRONIC TREATMENT

- Nutrition: cats especially won't eat if unable to smell food; consider feeding tube (e.g., esophagostomy; see Feeding Tube Placement: Esophagostomy Tube, p 1243) for nutritional support
- Analgesics
- Antibiotics for secondary infections
- In animals with chronic rhinitis, antihistamines, inhaled corticosteroids, and systemic NSAIDs may provide some relief

POSSIBLE COMPLICATIONS

- Anorexia (especially in cats with severe nasal congestion)
- Keratitis (feline viral upper respiratory infections)
- Upper airway obstruction following extubation after general anesthesia
- Hemorrhage following surgery or rhinoscopy
- Dehiscence of surgical site (e.g., cleft palate)
- Progression of underlying disease
- Acute nasal trauma due to paroxysmal sneezing in small, short-legged dogs whose noses may hit the floor while sneezing (e.g., dachshunds)

RECOMMENDED MONITORING

- Respiratory rate and effort; ventilation and oxygenation
- Appetite
- Ongoing hemorrhage
- Volume and nature of discharge
- Monitoring as normal for antimicrobials and NSAIDs
- Appropriate laboratory testing or diagnostic imaging, dependent on underlying disease

PROGNOSIS AND OUTCOME

- Dependent on etiology
- Good if the underlying problem is canine viral upper respiratory tract infection, foreign body, successful surgery, teeth extractions
- Guarded for feline chronic viral upper respiratory tract infections
- Guarded to good for fungal rhinitis depending on response to therapy
- Poor if neoplasia is not amenable to surgery and radiation therapy

PEARLS & CONSIDERATIONS

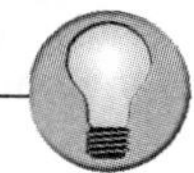

PREVENTION

- Isolation of cats with viral infections
- Appropriate vaccination regime and retroviral testing
- Good dental care
- Limit exposure to irritating aerosols or materials

SUGGESTED READING

Doust R, Sullivan M: Nasal discharge, sneezing and reverse sneezing. In King LG (ed): *Textbook of Respiratory Disease in Dogs and Cats*. St. Louis, Saunders, 2004, pp 17-29.

Hawkins EC: Clinical manifestations of nasal disease. In Nelson RW, Couto CG (eds): *Small Animal Internal Medicine*. St. Louis, Mosby, 1998, pp 206-231.

McKiernan BC: Sneezing and nasal discharge. In Ettinger SJ, Feldman EC (eds): *Textbook of Veterinary Internal Medicine*. Philadelphia, WB Saunders, 2000, pp 194-197.

AUTHORS: **ELISE MITTLEMAN, ANDREW J. BROWN, LESLEY G. KING**

EDITOR: **ETIENNE CÔTÉ**

Soft Tissue Sarcoma

BASIC INFORMATION

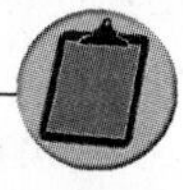

DEFINITION

A group of tumors arising from various mesenchymal tissues, classified together because of a similar biologic behavior and treatment. They include fibrosarcoma, hemangiopericytoma, malignant fibrous histiocytoma, nerve sheath tumor, neurofibrosarcoma, malignant schwannoma, leiomyosarcoma, rhabdomyosarcoma, liposarcoma, myxosarcoma, lymphangiosarcoma, and synovial cell sarcoma. Although it is also a mesenchymal tumor arising from soft tissue, hemangiosarcoma is often excluded from this group because of its aggressive biologic behavior.

SYNONYM(S)

Soft part sarcomas

EPIDEMIOLOGY

SPECIES, AGE, SEX: Common in middle-aged to older dogs. Soft tissue sarcomas at sites other than injection sites are less common in cats.

GENETICS AND BREED PREDISPOSITION: In general, soft tissue sarcomas tend to occur more commonly in larger breeds, but direct inheritance of these tumors has not been reported.

RISK FACTORS

- Certain sarcomas have been associated with metal implants, previous exposure to ionizing radiation, and parasites (*Spirocerca lupi*).
- Sarcomas at injection sites have been described in dogs but are rare.

CONTAGION AND ZOONOSIS: Multiple sarcomas of the head and neck have been reported secondary to combined feline sarcoma virus and feline leukemia virus infection.

ASSOCIATED CONDITIONS AND DISORDERS: Hypoglycemia has been reported as an uncommon paraneoplastic syndrome in dogs with intestinal leiomyosarcoma.

CLINICAL PRESENTATION

HISTORY, CHIEF COMPLAINT

- Most animals present for a progressive mass noticed by the owner.
- Animals with sarcoma in certain locations will be presented because of clinical signs related to the location of the tumor. Dogs with oral tumors often present with a foul odor from the mouth, difficulty eating or prehending food, oral bleeding, or a visible oral mass. Dogs with intestinal sarcomas will often be presented because of signs related to intestinal obstruction including vomiting and diarrhea.

PHYSICAL EXAM FINDINGS

- Visible or palpable mass. Regional lymphadenomegaly may be present secondary to inflammation caused by the tumor or, rarely, lymph node metastasis.
- Sarcomas in specific sites may present with physical exam findings related to the location of the tumor (e.g., abdominal pain, weight loss, dehydration).

ETIOLOGY AND PATHOPHYSIOLOGY

- Soft tissue sarcomas arise spontaneously in dogs and cats. Genetic and environmental factors may be involved in tumor development. However, these factors are poorly understood in companion animals.
- Specific lesions and overt clinical manifestations caused by soft tissue sarcomas depend on the location of the primary tumor and the invasion into and destruction of surrounding normal structures.

DIAGNOSIS

DIFFERENTIAL DIAGNOSIS

- Mast cell tumors
- Other skin and subcutaneous tumors
  - Lipoma, histiocytoma, etc.
- Other masses
  - Abscess

INITIAL DATABASE

- Fine-needle aspiration and cytologic examination may help identify the type of soft tissue sarcoma or differentiate from other tumor types
- Thoracic radiographs to rule out pulmonary metastases
- Radiographs of the affected area may reveal involvement of underlying bone

ADVANCED OR CONFIRMATORY TESTING

- Computed tomography (CT) or magnetic resonance imaging (MRI) may be necessary to delineate the local extent of the tumor and to plan for surgery or radiation therapy
- Diagnosis is based on histopathologic evaluation of tissue. Occasionally, special stains may be necessary to differentiate various types of soft tissue sarcomas, especially with poorly differentiated tumors
- Histopathologic grade of the tumor is necessary for determining the prognosis and treatment of most soft tissue sarcomas

TREATMENT

THERAPEUTIC GOAL(S)

- The goal of treatment for soft tissue sarcomas in dogs or cats is complete eradication of the primary tumor.
- In cases where the tumor cannot be eliminated entirely, the goal of treatment is prevention or delay of the development of metastases.

ACUTE GENERAL TREATMENT

- Surgery
  - Commonly these tumors appear encapsulated at surgery. This can be misleading because the capsule is usually a pseudocapsule made up of compressed tumor cells, and viable tumor cells are often present beyond the extent of the pseudocapsule.
  - Surgery should be aimed at an aggressive resection of the mass with as wide a margin of normal tissue as possible from around the tumor. In situations where this is not possible because of the size and location of the tumor, radiation therapy may be indicated in addition to surgery.
- Radiation therapy
  - May be used prior to surgery in situations where the tumor is not easily resectable due to its location or size. In cases where surgery is attempted first but resection is incomplete based on histologic evaluation, these patients should be treated with radiation therapy after surgery.
- Chemotherapy
  - May be indicated for patients with high-grade tumors, tumors in certain locations, certain tumor types, and in patients that develop metastatic disease.
  - Chemotherapy drugs that have been used for soft tissue sarcoma include doxorubicin, mitoxantrone, platinum drugs, ifosfamide, and combinations of these drugs.
- Hyperthermia
  - Oncologic hyperthermia treatment has been shown to increase response rates for macroscopic tumors that are treated with radiation therapy. However, such treatment has limited availability and recurrence of tumors often occurs rapidly after treatment.

POSSIBLE COMPLICATIONS

Complications of treatments for fibrosarcomas depend on the types of treatments and the location of the primary tumor:

- Surgery may result in wound complications, including infection, dehiscence, or loss of function of a limb.
- Radiation therapy can cause short-term complications in skin and mucosa involved in the radiation field (dermatitis, mucositis). Long-term complications, including bone necrosis and haircoat changes, are uncommon, but are permanent when they do occur. See Radiation Therapy: Adverse Reactions, p 940.
- Chemotherapy complications may include bone marrow suppression, gastrointestinal effects and haircoat changes along with other side effects caused by specific chemotherapy drugs. See Chemotherapy: Adverse Reactions, p 189.

RECOMMENDED MONITORING

Following appropriate local treatment of the primary tumor follow-up examination should be done on a routine basis to monitor for local recurrence and also for metastasis. High-grade tumors may require more frequent monitoring for metastasis during and after chemotherapy administration.

PROGNOSIS AND OUTCOME

Prognosis is variable depending on the type of tumor, location of the primary tumor, clinical stage of the tumor, and the histologic grade of tumor.

- Certain tumor types may have higher metastatic rates (e.g. leiomyosarcoma) or more aggressive local behavior (e.g., histologically low grade, biologically high grade sarcomas of the oral cavity).
- Soft tissue sarcomas located in the abdomen (spleen, intestines) are typically more likely to lead to metastasis.
- Soft tissue sarcomas in certain locations (e.g., oral tumors) may be more difficult to treat with local therapy (surgery or radiation) resulting in lower rates of local disease control.
- Soft tissue sarcomas that are large or have metastasized at the time of diagnosis usually lead to a poor prognosis.
- Histologic grading of canine soft tissue sarcomas is based on: 1) degree of differentiation; 2) mitotic index (0–9 per high power field (HPF), 10–19 per HPF, >20 per HPF); and 3) percent necrosis (0%, <50%, >50%). High-grade (grade 3) tumors are more likely to lead to metastasis. Typical metastatic rates are considered to be 40% for grade 3 tumors, up to 20% for grade 2 tumors, and 10% or less for grade 1 tumors. It is unclear whether this grading scheme is applicable in feline soft tissue sarcomas.

PEARLS & CONSIDERATIONS

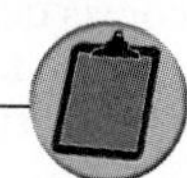

COMMENTS

Many patients with soft tissue sarcomas can be successfully treated with wide surgical excision alone. Patients with soft tissue sarcomas that may be more difficult to treat (oral sarcomas, grade 3 sarcomas, nonresectable tumors, etc.) should be referred for consultation with specialists, including a surgeon, oncologist, or radiation oncologist, to develop a multimodality treatment approach.

PREVENTION

In most cases prevention of soft tissue sarcomas is not possible. Early detection and treatment may result in easier treatment and better prognosis.

CLIENT EDUCATION

Owners should be educated to monitor their pets for the emergence of cutaneous or other masses and have them evaluated in a timely fashion. Early detection may allow for easier treatment via surgery and may help avoid the need for radiation therapy.

SUGGESTED READING

MacEwen EG, Powers BE, Macy D, Withrow SJ: Soft tissue sarcomas. In Withrow SJ, MacEwen EG (eds): *Small Animal Clinical Oncology*. Philadelphia, WB Saunders, 2001, pp 283–304.

AUTHOR: **JOHN FARRELLY**
EDITOR: **KENNETH M. RASSNICK**

Soft Tissue Trauma of the Extremities

BASIC INFORMATION

DEFINITION

Soft-tissue injury to the limbs and tail as the result of external trauma

EPIDEMIOLOGY

SPECIES, AGE, SEX

- Dogs and cats
- No specific age or sex

RISK FACTORS: Dogs and cats that are allowed to roam in unconfined areas without supervision or leash restriction.

GEOGRAPHY AND SEASONALITY: Vehicular trauma is the primary cause of external trauma; dogs and cats are most susceptible to injury in areas with high traffic.

CLINICAL PRESENTATION

DISEASE FORMS/SUBTYPES

- Laceration
- Contusion
- Crushing
- Shearing
- Penetration or perforation
- Avulsion

HISTORY, CHIEF COMPLAINT

- An open wound, bleeding, or swelling to the injured area
- Lameness may be noted in association with a limb injury
- The animal may display pain by vocalization, guarding the injured area, or defensive posturing

PHYSICAL EXAM FINDINGS

- Open wounds (Fig. I-161):
  - Skin laceration
  - Partial or complete loss of skin and underlying tissues
  - Avulsion or partial detachment of skin segments
  - Entry or exit wounds secondary to a bite, projectile, or impalement injury
- Evidence of previous or ongoing hemorrhage
- Intact skin but the presence of contusion (bruising)
- Local swelling as a result of edema, hematoma formation
- Evidence of underlying orthopedic injury:
  - Fracture
  - Joint instability associated with soft tissue trauma
- Pain:
  - Possibly in association with manual examination of the injury
- The overall health status of the animal depends on a variety of factors, including:
  - Body region(s) involved
  - Extent of the trauma
  - Blood loss

ETIOLOGY AND PATHOPHYSIOLOGY

- Wounds are the result of the transfer and absorption of energy by the body. The severity or trauma depends on the exact type of trauma and the area of absorption.
- Lacerations may be the result of contact with a sharp, blade-like object (glass, metal, etc.) or impact against a hard-edged surface. Bite wounds may create an irregular laceration as a result of the cutting and tearing of tissues.
- Crushing wounds are the result of compression; these can result from impact with a heavy object or contact with a mechanical device; the wounds can also be caused by a powerful bite.
- Shearing wounds may be the result of tangential impact with a hard surface, the dragging of a body region on a hard road surface, or entrapment of an extremity beneath the tire of a moving vehicle.
- Avulsion is the result of the tearing or pulling of the skin and adjacent tissues, usually as the result of vehicular trauma or a bite.
- Tissue necrosis is usually associated with a loss of sufficient circulation to sustain the tissues. Crushing wounds can result in significant circulatory compromise; avulsion wounds often result in the stretching and tearing of vessels supplying the tissues.
- Assessment of circulation at the time of injury can be difficult. Progressive loss of circulation can result in vascular stasis, and necrosis that may not be evident for 4 to 5 days after the initial injury.

DIAGNOSIS

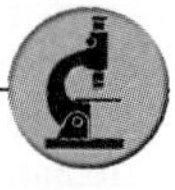

DIFFERENTIAL DIAGNOSIS

Common causes of soft tissue trauma include:

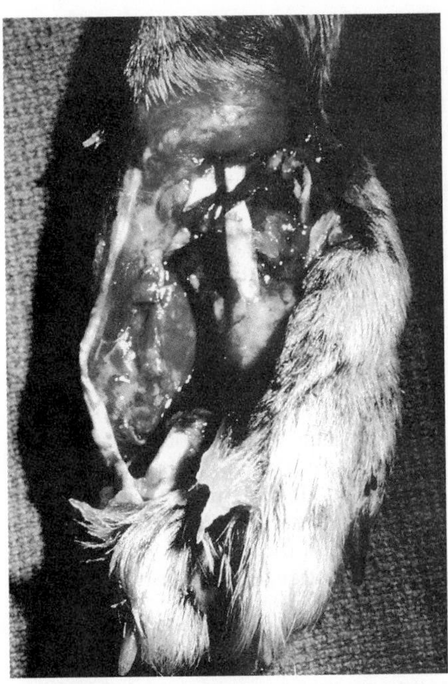

FIGURE I-161 Clinical image of a dog's paw with extensive trauma of the extremity; dorsal view. The dog's paw had been crushed under the wheel of a moving school bus. Multiple open fractures of the metacarpal bones are seen. Courtesy of Dr. Richard Walshaw.

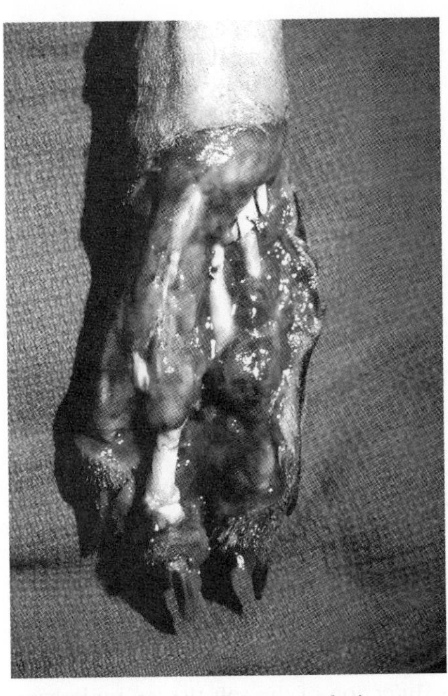

FIGURE I-162 Appearance of the same case as in Fig. I-161 after surgical repair of the fractures (note wires) and intensive wound care; dorsal view. A good granulation bed is present throughout the wound, indicating the viability of underlying tissue and active healing.

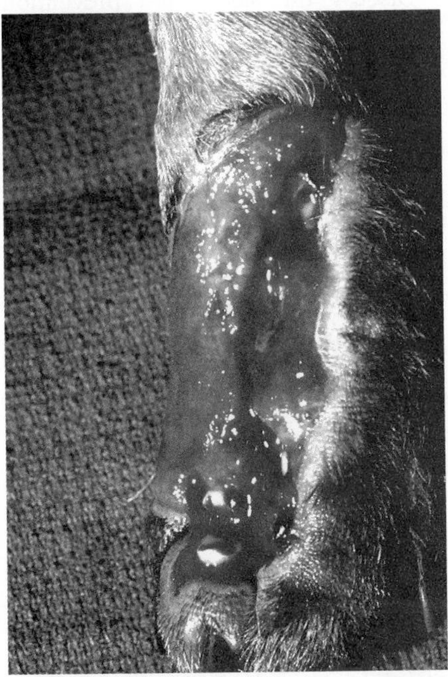

FIGURE I-163 Appearance of the wound in Fig. I-161 after further healing; dorsal view. The granulation bed remains healthy in appearance and is smaller due to wound contraction.

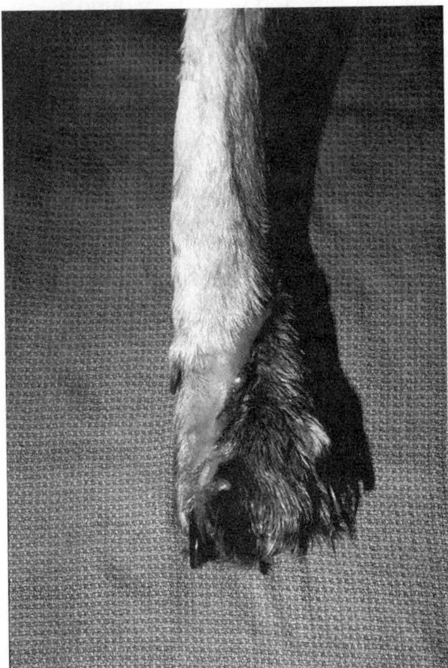

FIGURE I-164 Final appearance of the wound in Fig. I-161 after complete healing; dorsal view. A large cicatrix (scar) is present, but the overall functional result is excellent.

- Vehicular trauma
- Bite wounds
- Penetrating/perforating objects (gunshot, impalement)
- Sharp objects

INITIAL DATABASE

- Complete blood count (CBC) and serum biochemistry profile:
  - Minimum database is indicated
- Radiographs (two views) of the injured area:
  - Rule out underlying orthopedic trauma
- Survey thoracic radiographs:
  - Rule out diaphragmatic hernia, lung contusions, pneumothorax, and other lesions in the face of vehicular trauma

ADVANCED OR CONFIRMATORY TESTING

The severity of trauma will dictate whether additional diagnostic imaging techniques are required

TREATMENT

THERAPEUTIC GOAL(S)

- Ensure that the animal is hemodynamically stable before inducing general anesthesia
- Assess severity of soft tissue and orthopedic trauma
- Assess wound for tissue viability
- Provide definitive wound care and closure
- Prevent or manage infection
- Stabilize local fractures or joint instability

ACUTE GENERAL TREATMENT

- General anesthesia is preferable for definitive wound care
- Initiate systemic antibiotic therapy:
  - Empiric therapy to provide broad aerobic coverage
    - Cefazolin 22 mg/kg IV q 2h during the perioperative period
  - Definitive therapy for infected wounds should be based on the results of microbiologic culture and sensitivity (C&S) testing
- Cover open wounds with a sterile dressing
- Liberally remove fur from around the circumference of a shearing wound
- Povidone iodine or chlorhexidine surgical scrub is used for preparing the skin, alternated with swabbing the area with sterile saline impregnated sponges
- Aseptically drape the wound and remove the sterile cover
- Explore the wound and:
  - Resect nonviable tissue
  - Remove foreign debris
  - Perform copious lavage of the wound with sterile saline to remove contaminants:
    - Chlorhexidine solution (1:40 dilution) or povidone iodine solution (1:9 dilution) may be added to the sterile saline
    - Pressure lavage is useful for removal of contaminants, using a 35-cc syringe and 18-gauge needle
- In the absence of infection and necrotic tissue (absent or resected):
  - Skin borders can be approximated with sutures
  - If significant incisional tension is present, perform partial closure or delayed primary closure

- Joint injury in association with shearing wounds:
  - Repair collateral ligament support using conventional bone screws and braided suture material; stainless steel also may be used
  - Perform copious lavage for open joints; in the absence of infection, the joint capsule can be closed, if feasible
- With extensive bruising and swelling, open wound management should be considered until circulation improves, noted by resolution of these two conditions
- Open wound management varies with the severity of trauma and extent of the wound. Common options include:
  - Wet to dry dressings in the presence of extensive contamination:
    - Wet to dry dressings are primarily used as a form of mechanical debridement
    - With "wet" (exudative, contaminated) wounds, exudation from the wound is intended to adhere to the dressing and thus is removed when the bandage is removed
  - Nonadherent dressing and antimicrobial ointment if a surgically clean wound is achieved:
    - Several topical agents and dressings are currently available for basic wound care
  - Apply a thick, protective bandage over the contact dressing
  - Change bandages one to three times per day depending on the condition of the wound:
    - Wet to dry dressings are normally changed two to three times per day for 3 to 5 days
    - Once infection is neutralized and debridement is complete, apply a nonadherent dressing and topical antimicrobial to the wound
  - In viable wounds, granulation tissue should begin to form as early as 4 to 5 days after injury:
    - As a healthy granulation bed forms, bandage changes can be extended to every second or third day
  - Occlusive dressings can be considered once a healthy granulation bed forms to facilitate epithelization
  - Large open wounds may require closure with skin grafts or skin flaps if contraction and epithelization are not suitable options:
    - In general, wounds less than 90 degrees of the extremity circumference may heal by second intention, often within 6 weeks after injury
- Extensive extremity trauma, especially with concurrent severe circulatory compromise and tissue necrosis, usually necessitates amputation

CHRONIC TREATMENT

- Bandage changes
- Skin grafts or flaps may be needed for shearing wounds with extensive skin loss

POSSIBLE COMPLICATIONS

- Infection of the soft tissues, underlying bone, or exposed joint
- Failure to heal
- Persistent instability of a shearing wound involving a joint
- Associated fracture nonunion

RECOMMENDED MONITORING

Bandage care and periodic wound assessment

PROGNOSIS AND OUTCOME

- Massive trauma to the extremities may necessitate limb amputation
- Progressive loss of circulation may necessitate serial debridement of the wound or eventual amputation
- Many shearing wounds will heal by second intention (Figs. I-162 to I-164)
- Failure to heal usually necessitates wound closure with a skin graft or flap
- Severe joint injury/instability may require eventual arthrodesis
- Loss of the weight-bearing metacarpal or metatarsal pad usually warrants reconstruction, either by digital pad transfer or pad grafts when applicable

PEARLS & CONSIDERATIONS

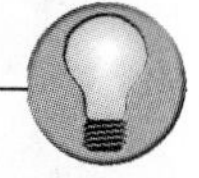

COMMENTS

- Most cases of soft tissue trauma that are presented to veterinarians are relatively simple to manage.
- Confusion occasionally arises with larger wounds, for which the full extent of the injury is difficult to assess at presentation.
- In the face of infection, open wound management usually is the safest option.
  - Daily debridement, lavage, and wound assessment make it possible to assess the progress of the wound and better determine the optimal time to close the skin defect.

PREVENTION

Most wounds occur in pets that are permitted to roam unsupervised. Confining the pet to the house or yard, or accompanying the pet on a leash, dramatically reduces the risks associated with vehicular trauma, bites, and malicious injury.

CLIENT EDUCATION

- Discuss the safety and prevention issues noted above.
- In open wound management, many willing owners can be trained to perform simple bandage changes and manage wound drains. Costs can therefore be reduced.
- The veterinarian's role is one of assessing the progress of healing and deciding upon wound closure options.

SUGGESTED READING

Pavletic MM: *Atlas of Small Animal Reconstructive Surgery*, ed 2. Philadelphia, WB Saunders, 1999, pp 11–130.

Swaim SF, Henderson R: *Small Animal Wound Management*, ed 2. Philadelphia, Williams & Wilkins, 1997, pp 13–87.

AUTHOR: **MICHAEL PAVLETIC**

EDITOR: **RICHARD WALSHAW**

Spider Envenomation

BASIC INFORMATION

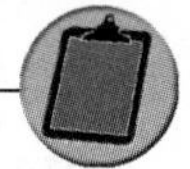

DEFINITION

- Lactrodectism: envenomating bites from widow spiders of the genus *Latrodectus*, resulting in systemic signs including myalgia, weakness, paralysis, and death
- Loxoscelism or necrotic arachnidism: envenomating bites from recluse spiders of the genus *Loxosceles* that result in a severe necrotizing wound and occasional systemic signs

SYNONYM(S)

- Widow spiders:
  - Latrodectism: syndrome associated with widow envenomation.
- Brown recluse spiders:

- Loxoscelism or necrotic arachnidism: syndrome associated with recluse spider bites.

EPIDEMIOLOGY

SPECIES, AGE, SEX

- Very young and aged animals may be more sensitive to the effects of venom.
- Cats are very sensitive to widow bites; mortality can exceed 90%.
- Dogs are more likely than other species to develop systemic effects from brown recluse bites.

RISK FACTORS: Animals with preexisting respiratory conditions may be at increased risk of developing signs from black widow venom due to paralysis of respiratory muscles.

CLINICAL PRESENTATION

HISTORY, CHIEF COMPLAINT

- Witnessed or suspected spider bite
- Specific signs based on species of spider:
  - Little to no local swelling and redness (widow spiders)
  - Reluctance to move due to muscle pain within 2 hours following bite incident (widow spiders)
  - Expanding necrotizing wound (recluse spiders)

PHYSICAL EXAM FINDINGS

- Widow spiders: vomiting, myalgia, rigidity, tachypnea, tremors, ataxia, and atonic paralysis
- Recluse spiders:
  - Red, swollen lesion (bull's-eye lesion) 3 to 8 hours after envenomation
  - Eschar, sloughing of the skin:
    - Lesion can be 1 to 25 cm in size
  - Systemic signs in 24 to 72 hours may include anemia, hematuria, pyrexia, and myalgia

ETIOLOGY AND PATHOPHYSIOLOGY

- Widow spiders:
  - Widow spiders have an hourglass-shaped red or orange marking on the female's abdomen. Male fangs are too short for envenomation.
  - Important *Latrodectus* spp. in the United States:
    - *L. mactans* (black widow spider, southern black widow) found throughout the United States, especially in the South
    - *L. hesperus* (western black widow spider) found in the western part of the United States
    - *L. variolus* (northern widow spider) found in the northern part of the United States
    - *L. bishopi* (red widow spider; red-legged widow spider) found in central and southern Florida
    - *L. geometricus* (brown widow spider) found in Florida
  - α-latrotoxin is the main toxic component of the venom. It causes release and depletion of acetylcholine at motor nerve endings and the release of catecholamines (norepinephrine) at postganglionic sympathetic synapses, resulting in blockade of neurotransmitter release.
- Recluse spiders:
  - Brown recluse spider (*Loxosceles reclusa*) or fiddleback spider (distinctive fiddle-shaped mark on its back) are found in the south-central region of the United States (Texas through Georgia) but can be found as far north as Iowa, central Illinois, and Indiana. These spiders are nocturnal, not aggressive, and can be active in a wide range of temperatures.
  - Mediterranean recluse (*L. rufscens*), the desert recluse (*L. deserta*), and the Arizona recluse (*L. arizonica*) may produce mild necrotic lesions that are not as serious as the brown recluse bite.
  - The spider's venom contains several proteins, polypeptides, and necrotizing enzymes, including hyaluronidase, esterase, alkaline phosphatase, and 5'-ribonucleotide phosphorylase and sphingomyelinase D.
  - These proteins and enzymes work in different ways, causing inflammation, local lesions, coagulation, occlusion of small capillaries, tissue necrosis, depletion of clotting factors (VII, IX, XI, and XII), hemolysis, platelet activation, and thromboembolic disease.

DIAGNOSIS

DIFFERENTIAL DIAGNOSIS

- Widow spiders: bromethalin, macadamia nuts, or marijuana toxicosis
- Recluse spiders: cellulitis, hemolytic anemia, idiopathic thrombocytopenia

INITIAL DATABASE

- The diagnosis is established mainly through history and physical findings
- Complete blood count (CBC): leukocytosis common with widow spiders
- CBC, platelet count, coagulation profile (recluse spiders).

TREATMENT

THERAPEUTIC GOAL(S)

- Control local signs
- Monitor and treat systemic signs
- Provide supportive care

ACUTE GENERAL TREATMENT

- Widow spider:
  - Systemic analgesia:
    - Opioids for severe pain (e.g., hydromorphone 0.1–0.2 mg/kg SQ, IM, or IV once or as needed up to q 2–4h)
    - Nonsteroidal anti-inflammatory drugs (NSAIDs) for moderate pain (e.g., carprofen 1 mg/kg PO, q 12h, or etodolac 10–15 mg/kg PO, q 24h)
  - Muscle relaxants:
    - Diazepam 0.25–1 mg/kg PO q 8h
    - Methocarbamol 20–45 mg/kg PO q 8h; 55–220 mg/kg IV slow, not to exceed 330 mg/kg/day.
  - Respiratory support for hypoventilating animals
  - Black Widow Spider Antivenin (by Merck) can be used in severe or unresponsive cases
  - IV fluids
- Recluse spiders:
  - Diphenhydramine (2.2 mg/kg PO or IM, q 8h) may control pruritus; corticosteroids at anti-inflammatory levels (e.g., prednisone 1–2 mg/kg PO q 24h) can also be used
  - Broad-spectrum antibiotics for secondary infection (e.g., amoxicillin-clavulanate 20 mg/kg PO q 12h)
  - Monitor and measure size of lesion every day
  - Dapsone, a neutrophil migration inhibitor, may limit severity of lesions:
    - In dogs, 1 mg/kg PO q 24h has been suggested
  - Surgical debridement not recommended
  - IV fluids to promote fluid diuresis if hemolysis occurs
  - Packed red blood cells (RBCs) or whole blood for anemia
  - Monitor and treat disseminated intravascular coagulation (DIC) if present

CHRONIC TREATMENT

Manage necrotic lesions as open wounds (recluse spiders).

POSSIBLE COMPLICATIONS

Recluse spider bites can lead to scarring as they heal.

RECOMMENDED MONITORING

CBC, platelet count, and coagulation parameters

PROGNOSIS AND OUTCOME

Fatalities rare in dogs; prognosis is guarded in cats bitten by widow spiders.

PEARLS & CONSIDERATIONS

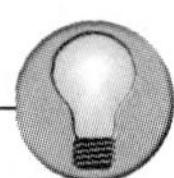

COMMENTS

- Many spiders are capable of inflicting an envenomating bite. In the United States, however, with the exception of

widow and recluse spider bites, most bites will not cause more than a mild, local reaction. Anaphylaxis possible.
- Widow spiders prefer dark places, especially under debris, such as leaf litter or cardboard.

SUGGESTED READING

Arachnology: www.arachnology.be. Useful website for information on and identifying spiders.
Roder JD: Spiders. In Plumlee KH (ed): *Clinical Veterinary Toxicology*. St. Louis, Mosby, 2004, pp 111–113.
Twedt DC, et al: Black widow spider envenomation in a cat. *J Vet Intern Med* 13:613, 1999.

AUTHOR: **ERIC K. DUNAYER**
EDITOR: **SAFDAR A. KHAN**

Spinal Cord Neoplasia

BASIC INFORMATION

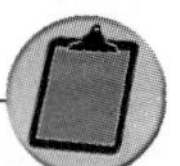

DEFINITION

- Spinal tumors encompass a wide range of cancers.
- Spinal tumors can arise from vertebrae, meninges, or neuroparenchyma.
    - Vertebral neoplasia: osteosarcoma, fibrosarcoma, and hemangiosarcoma, plasma cell tumor/multiple myeloma, lymphoma, cartilaginous exostosis/osteochondroma
    - Meningeal: meningioma
    - Neuroparenchyma: peripheral nerve sheath tumors (PNST), oligodendroglioma, astrocytoma, ganglioma, nephroblastoma, ependymoma
    - Mesenchymal tumors: myxoma/myxosarcoma, histiocytic sarcoma, liposarcoma
- Metastatic neoplasia: prostatic, mammary adenocarcinoma, osteosarcoma, transitional cell carcinoma, melanoma, thyroid carcinoma, pheochromocytoma.

EPIDEMIOLOGY

SPECIES, AGE, SEX

- Canine: middle-aged to older, large-breed dogs
    - Possible male predilection for meningioma (see Meningioma, p 696).
- Feline: lymphoma: young (median age 2 to 3 years). Concurrent feline leukemia (FeLV) infection is common (see Lymphoma, Central Nervous System, p 652).

CLINICAL PRESENTATION

HISTORY, CHIEF COMPLAINT

- Canine: duration of clinical signs prior to diagnosis is longest for intradural/extramedullary, followed by extradural. Shortest duration for intramedullary tumors. Chronic progressive paresis and proprioceptive ataxia (scuffing toes, knuckling, crossing limbs). Mean duration 6 weeks, range 1 day to 1 year.
- Occasionally, acute paresis/plegia—absent voluntary motor function.
- Feline lymphoma: acute onset (often 7 days or less).
    - Hyperesthesia
- Clinical signs relate to neuroanatomic lesion: Lesions affecting the cervical spinal cord present with tetraparesis, while lesions affecting the thoracolumbar spinal cord present with paraparesis.

PHYSICAL EXAM FINDINGS

- Location dependent.
- Often asymmetric.
- C1-C6 spinal cord: tetraparesis/plegia, postural reaction deficits, proprioceptive ataxia, normal to exaggerated myotatic reflexes, normal withdrawal reflexes, normal to increased muscular tone, lack of muscle atrophy in all four limbs.
- C6-T2 spinal cord: tetraparesis/plegia, postural reaction deficits all four limbs, short, choppy gait (forelimbs), decreased withdrawal reflexes, decreased tone, muscle atrophy in thoracic limbs; proprioceptive ataxia, normal to exaggerated myotatic reflexes, normal withdrawal reflexes, normal to increased muscular tone, lack of muscle atrophy in pelvic limbs.
- T3-L3 spinal cord: paraparesis/plegia, proprioceptive ataxia, normal to exaggerated myotatic reflexes, normal withdrawal reflexes, normal to increased muscular tone, lack of muscle atrophy in pelvic limbs; thoracic limbs normal.
- L4-S3: hind limb paraparesis/plegia, short-strided, crouched pelvic limb gait, postural reaction deficits, decreased myotatic and withdrawal reflexes, decreased muscular tone, muscle atrophy in pelvic limbs; decreased perineal reflex, urinary incontinence and/or fecal incontinence, decreased tail function.

ETIOLOGY AND PATHOPHYSIOLOGY

- Unknown
- Canine:
    - Osteosarcoma: secondary to radiation therapy
    - Nephroblastoma: (rare) <2 years old, intradural/extramedullary, between T10 and L2 vertebrae
    - Multiple cartilaginous exostosis/osteochodroma can undergo malignant transformation to osteosarcoma or chondrosarcoma
- Feline lymphoma: FeLV infection

DIAGNOSIS

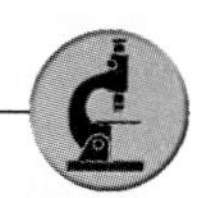

DIFFERENTIAL DIAGNOSIS

- Canine: intervertebral disk herniation, diskospondylitis, infectious meningomyelitis (canine distemper virus [CDV], rabies, fungal, *Neospora caninum*/*Toxoplasma gondii*, bacterial), granulomatous meningoencephalitis, trauma, orthopedic disease, caudal cervical spondylomyelopathy, fibrocartilaginous embolic myelopathy
- Feline: infectious meningomyelitis (feline infectious peritonitis virus, feline immunodeficiency virus [FIV], *Toxoplasma gondii*, rabies, fungal, bacterial), trauma, aortic thromboembolism, intervertebral disk herniation (rare)

INITIAL DATABASE

- Complete blood count, serum biochemical profile, urinalysis, thoracic and abdominal radiographs, survey (plain) radiographs of the vertebral column
- Feline: serologic testing for FeLV, FIV, *Cryptococcus neoformans*, *Toxoplasma gondii*
- Canine: serologic testing for *Cryptococcus neoformans*, *Neospora caninum*, *Toxoplasma gondii*, paired titers (CSF/serum) for CDV

ADVANCED OR CONFIRMATORY TESTING

- Advanced imaging: magnetic resonance imaging (MRI): gold standard for spinal cord; computed tomography (CT); combined CT/myelography, myelography.
    - CT more sensitive for bone abnormalities (lysis or proliferation) than radiographs or MRI
- Cerebrospinal fluid (CSF) analysis
- Fluoroscopic guided needle aspiration of vertebral lesion
- Spinal lymphoma: further staging required. Bone marrow evaluation (60–80% have bone marrow infiltration). Renal, lymph node, and hepatosplenic involvement common
- Presumptive differentials based on anatomic location:

- Vertebral: osteosarcoma, fibrosarcoma, hemangiosarcoma, plasma cell neoplasia, metastatic neoplasia
- Extradural: lymphoma, metastatic neoplasia
- Intradural/extramedullary: PNST, meningioma, nephroblastoma
- Intramedullary: glial cell tumors (astrocytoma, oligodendroglioma), metastatic neoplasia

TREATMENT

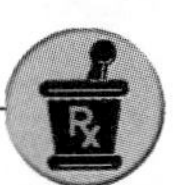

THERAPEUTIC GOAL(S)

Primary goal is to alleviate neurologic deficits by decompression of neural structures

ACUTE GENERAL TREATMENT

- Based on tumor location. However, to date, primary treatment involves surgical debulking.
- Surgical decompression of affected site(s) via hemilaminectomy/dorsal laminectomy.
- Palliation with corticosteroids.

CHRONIC TREATMENT

- Variable depending on tumor type
- Incompletely excised meningioma, neuroparenchymal, and vertebral tumors should receive postoperative radiation therapy
- Spinal lymphoma: systemic chemotherapy, radiation therapy
- Plasma cell tumor/multiple myeloma: systemic chemotherapy, radiation therapy

POSSIBLE COMPLICATIONS

Radiation myelopathy

RECOMMENDED MONITORING

- Periodic neurologic examination
- Repeat imaging studies
- Chemotherapy necessitates hematologic and biochemical monitoring dictated by protocol

PROGNOSIS AND OUTCOME

- Variable based on tumor type, completeness of resection, and severity of neurologic deficits:
  - Patients lacking both motor function and nociception (deep pain perception) have grave prognosis for return of function.
- Canine:
  - Surgical resection alone: In one study of dogs with spinal tumors of various histologic types, overall median survival was 240 days.
  - Surgical resection and postoperative radiation: In one report of 9 dogs (6 with spinal meningiomas), overall median survival was 510 days.
  - Specific tumors:
    - Meningioma: based on degree of resection:
      - Surgical resection: survival ranges from <30 days to 1440 days.
      - Surgery with postoperative radiation survival ranges from 240 to 750 days.
    - Vertebral tumors: osteosarcoma and fibrosarcoma: median survival 135 days (15 days to 600 days).
    - PNST: median survival 203 days (120 to 300 days).
- Feline:
  - Lymphoma (– COP protocol): if complete remission achieved: median 14 weeks; if partial remission achieved: median 6 weeks. Longer remissions may be possible with doxorubicin-containing protocols.

PEARLS & CONSIDERATIONS

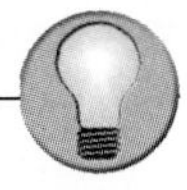

COMMENTS

- Based on imaging studies, the differential diagnosis may be narrowed substantially according to the anatomic location of the lesion.
- Definitive diagnosis requires histopathologic evaluation.
- Long-term remission can be possible regardless of completeness of excision.

SUGGESTED READING

Dernell WS, et al: Outcome following treatment of vertebral tumors in 20 dogs (1986–1995). *J Am Anim Hosp Assoc* 36:245-251, 2000.

Levy MS, et al: Spinal tumors in 37 dogs: clinical outcome and long-term survival (1987–1994). *J Am Anim Hosp Assoc* 33:307–312, 1997.

Luttgen PJ, et al: A retrospective study of twenty-nine spinal tumours in the dog and cat. *J Sm Anim Pract* 21:213-226, 1980.

Siegel S, et al: Postoperative irradiation of spinal cord tumors in 9 dogs. *Vet Radiol & Ultrasound* 37:150–153, 1996.

Spodnick GJ, et al: Spinal lymphoma in cats: 21 cases (1976–1989). *J Am Vet Med Assoc* 200:373–376, 1992.

AUTHOR: **MARC KENT**

EDITOR: **KENNETH M. RASSNICK**

Spinal Cord Trauma

BASIC INFORMATION

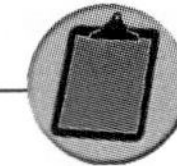

DEFINITION

Acute injury to the spinal cord caused by external trauma

EPIDEMIOLOGY

SPECIES, AGE, SEX

- Common in dogs and cats
- Animals of any age, both sexes, and all breeds can be affected

RISK FACTORS

- Unconfined
- Access to high places such as balconies

CLINICAL PRESENTATION

HISTORY, CHIEF COMPLAINT

- Often documented trauma
- Abrupt onset deficits, usually nonprogressive

PHYSICAL EXAM FINDINGS

- Focal spinal pain
- Neurologic deficits ranging from mild ataxia to paralysis
- Schiff-Sherrington posture (paraplegia with increased extensor tone in the pelvic limbs) possible with thoracic or lumbar injuries
- Presence or absence of deep pain caudal to the injury is the most important prognostic finding
- Signs of other injuries may be present, including chest injury, abdominal injury, head injury, or orthopedic injury

ETIOLOGY AND PATHOPHYSIOLOGY

- Causes include motor vehicle accidents, falls, bite wounds, and gunshot wounds.
- Primary injury is due to initial concussive injury to the cord and any persistent compressive injury due to displaced fracture/luxation, hematoma, or disk extrusion or unstable vertebral segments.
- Secondary injury is caused by metabolic changes, including release of free radicals that lead to progressive damage to cell membranes.

DIAGNOSIS

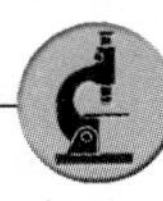

DIFFERENTIAL DIAGNOSIS

- Acute intervertebral disk extrusion
- Pathologic fracture from neoplasia or infection
- Orthopedic injury, such as pelvic fracture
- Fibrocartilaginous embolism

- Ischemic neuromyopathy due to aortic embolus

INITIAL DATABASE

Spinal radiographs: initially perform lateral view only until vertebral instability is ruled out

ADVANCED OR CONFIRMATORY TESTING

Myelography and/or CT scan is indicated if plain radiographs are normal or do not correlate with clinical assessment, and to determine if there is persistent spinal cord compression if surgery is considered.

TREATMENT

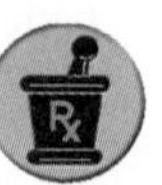

THERAPEUTIC GOAL(S)

- Treat any life-threatening injuries, such as shock
- Prevent further spinal cord injury caused by unstable vertebral injuries
- Minimize secondary injury
- Decompress the spinal cord

ACUTE GENERAL TREATMENT

- General trauma management (e.g., airway, oxygenation, IV fluids as indicated)
- Strap or tape the animal to a rigid board or gurney until an unstable vertebral injury is ruled out
- Analgesics as needed for pain control
- Corticosteroids:
  - Methylprednisolone sodium succinate 30 mg/kg IV within 8 hours of injury
  - 15 mg/kg IV at 2 and 6 hours later, then q 6h for 24 to 48 hours
  - May slightly improve outcome with severe spinal cord injury
  - Starting treatment >8 hours after injury is not effective and may be detrimental
  - Other doses and other corticosteroid preparations are not indicated
- Surgery:
  - Indicated for severe or progressive neurologic deficits and unstable vertebral injury or persistent compression of the spinal cord
  - Hemilaminectomy or dorsal laminectomy
  - Stabilization with pins or screws and bone cement, plates, or modified spinal instrumentation

CHRONIC TREATMENT

- Cage rest for 4 to 6 weeks with a clean, well-padded surface.
- External splints are helpful for cervical and thoracolumbar injuries that do not require surgery.
- Manual bladder expression if urinary incontinence is present.

DRUG INTERACTIONS

Avoid coadministration of corticosteroids and nonsteroidal anti-inflammatory drugs (NSAIDs) (potentially severe gastrointestinal [GI] ulceration)

POSSIBLE COMPLICATIONS

- Decubital ulcers in nonambulatory animals
- Urinary retention in incontinent animals
- Infection in penetrating injuries, especially bite wounds
- Self-mutilation caudal to the site of injury due to paresthesia

RECOMMENDED MONITORING

- Initially evaluate neurologic status daily, including ability to urinate
- Any deterioration indicates possible vertebral instability

PROGNOSIS AND OUTCOME

- Voluntary movement: good prognosis
- Paralysis with intact deep pain perception: guarded prognosis
- Paralysis with loss of deep pain perception: very poor prognosis

PEARLS & CONSIDERATIONS

COMMENTS

- A common mistake is inaccurate assessment of deep pain. When there is no response to pinching with the fingers, use a hemostat to compress the digits or tail. Withdrawal of the limb indicates only an intact reflex arc (peripheral nerve and spinal segments) and does not mean the animal can feel pain. A behavioral response, such as turning the head or vocalization, indicates conscious perception of deep pain.
- Hemodynamic shock can affect testing of deep pain, so if initial test is negative, reassess the animal after resuscitation.

PREVENTION

Do not allow pets to roam freely or have unsupervised access to balconies and other dangerous areas

SUGGESTED READING

Wheeler SJ, Sharp NJH: Trauma. In Wheeler SJ, Sharp NJH: *Small Animal Spinal Disorders: Diagnosis and Surgery*, ed 2. London, Mosby-Wolfe, 2005, pp 171–191.

AUTHOR: **WILLIAM B. THOMAS**
EDITOR: **CURTIS W. DEWEY**

Spirocercosis

BASIC INFORMATION

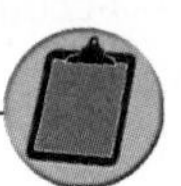

DEFINITION

A disease of dogs that is caused by the nematode *Spirocerca lupi* and is characterized by lesions that can affect the esophagus (with potential for esophageal malignancy), aorta, and vertebrae

SYNONYM(S)

Esophageal worm

EPIDEMIOLOGY

SPECIES, AGE, SEX: Primarily affects dogs. Middle-aged dogs overrepresented; dogs <1 year old unlikely to develop infection.

GENETICS AND BREED PREDISPOSITION: Medium- and large-breed dogs predisposed.

GEOGRAPHY AND SEASONALITY: This parasite is found in the southern United States and many tropical and subtropical regions. In some endemic areas, there is a disproportionately high prevalence in urban dogs compared to rural dogs.

CONTAGION AND ZOONOSIS: This is not a zoonotic disease.

ASSOCIATED DISEASES AND CONDITIONS: Esophageal neoplasia (osteosarcoma, fibrosarcoma) may occur secondary to esophageal granuloma formation from the encysted worms. These dogs may also develop hypertrophic osteopathy. Thoracic aortic aneurysm may occur due to migration of *S. lupi* from the gastrointestinal (GI) tract into the aortic wall. Thoracic vertebral spondylitis has been reported to occur due to migration and granuloma formation.

CLINICAL PRESENTATION

HISTORY, CHIEF COMPLAINT: Vomiting or regurgitation, weakness, respiratory abnormalities, anorexia, melena, paraparesis.

PHYSICAL EXAM FINDINGS: There are no pathognomonic physical examination findings. Physical examination findings are related to the area of the body affected by the parasite. In addition to the chief complaints listed above, the most common abnormalities include weight loss and fever.

ETIOLOGY AND PATHOPHYSIOLOGY

- Spirocercosis is caused by the migration of the nematode *S. lupi*. Carnivores are infected by ingestion of an intermediate host (coprophagous beetles) or other paratenic hosts in which the parasite does not undergo further development during its passage including birds, hedgehogs, lizards, mice, and rabbits.
- Adult *S. lupi* generally live within nodules in the esophagus and stomach. *Spirocerca* eggs pass with feces, where they are ingested by coprophagous beetles.The definitive host may acquire the infection by ingesting the beetle intermediate host or other paratenic host.
- The L3 larvae penetrate the stomach wall of the definitive host and migration occurs within the walls of the gastric arteries to the thoracic aorta. From the aorta they migrate to the esophagus. The prepatent period time from infection of the host to the first ability to detect the infection with diagnostic evaluation is approximately 5 to 6 months.
- Clinically significant lesions are related to the migration route and final destination site of the parasite. The most common scenario is esophageal granuloma formation.

DIAGNOSIS

DIFFERENTIAL DIAGNOSIS

- Regurgitation: other esophageal disorders such as megaesophagus, esophagitis, foreign bodies, esophageal stricture, gastroesophageal reflux disease
- Esophageal mass: esophageal neoplasia, granuloma of other origin
- Vomiting: both GI (inflammatory, infectious, parasitic, neoplastic, dietary) and extra-GI (metabolic, endocrine, pancreatitis) etiologies

INITIAL DATABASE

- Complete blood count, serum biochemical profile, urinalysis: no characteristic abnormalities
  - Anemia (53% of cases) and leukocytosis possible
  - Elevation in serum creatine kinase: most common biochemical abnormality (54% of cases)
- Fecal flotation, performed using high specific gravity (1.36) sodium nitrate solution
  - May reveal characteristic small, elongated eggs
  - Variable yield. Positive result in 29–80% of cases
- Thoracic and abdominal radiographs indicated. May reveal:
  - Esophageal and stomach lesions (soft tissue masses with/without calcification). A mass is typically noted in the caudal esophagus (53% of cases of spirocercosis). Most affected dogs have more than one granuloma, but not all are seen radiographically.
  - Bony changes in the thoracic vertebrae.
  - Evidence of metastasis when esophageal neoplasia is present.
- Limb radiographs in patients with lameness or hard swelling of distal limbs, to assess for hypertrophic osteopathy

ADVANCED OR CONFIRMATORY TESTING

- Esophagoscopy and gastroscopy may allow for visualization of granulomas and for biopsy procedures. In most cases of spirocercosis, endoscopy is the confirmatory diagnostic procedure of choice.
- Thoracic computed tomography (CT) may be useful for identifying esophageal masses and aortic aneurysm.
- Postmortem examination in patients with sudden death or who have been euthanized will also provide a definitive diagnosis.

TREATMENT

THERAPEUTIC GOAL(S)

- Resolution of regurgitation or vomiting
- Prevent development of esophageal neoplasia or hypertrophic osteopathy
- Prevention of sudden death due to rupture of aneurysm

ACUTE AND CHRONIC TREATMENT

- Doramectin (Dectomax, Pfizer) 200 microg/kg SC q 14 days for 3 treatments
  - Treatment of choice
  - Permanent resolution/cure is expected in many or most dogs in 6 weeks' time or less
  - Dogs with persistent lesions after 6 weeks have been treated safely and successfully using doramectin 500 microg/kg PO q 24h × 6 weeks
- Fenbendazole (50 mg/kg PO q 24h 5–7 days) or ivermectin (200–400 μg/kg SC q 14–28 days) have been used for treatment of spirocercosis

DRUG INTERACTIONS/POSSIBLE COMPLICATIONS

Do not use ivermectins in collies, Shetland sheepdogs, Australian shepherds, or other susceptible breeds or individuals

PROGNOSIS AND OUTCOME

Prognosis is variable:

- With appropriate treatment, cure is expected in many or most dogs in 6 weeks' time or less
- However, presence of esophageal neoplasia, aortic aneurysm, or large masses obstructing flow of ingesta worsen the prognosis
- Sixty-three percent of dogs with spirocercosis may die or be euthanized within one month of admission

PEARLS & CONSIDERATIONS

COMMENTS

- In North America and Europe, spirocercosis is a rare disease and is only considered when there is a high index of clinical suspicion.
- The characteristic lesion is a soft tissue mass in the caudal esophagus; radiographically, foreign body ingestion is an important differential diagnosis.
- A minority of dogs develop neoplastic transformation of esophageal granulomas (e.g., 13 out of 14 dogs with spirocercosis had esophageal masses, but only 1 out of 13 had esophageal neoplasia).

PREVENTION

Prevent dogs from eating beetles or paratenic hosts

SUGGESTED READING

Berry WL: *Spirocerca lupi* esophageal granulomas in 7 dogs: resolution after treatment with doramectin. *J Vet Intern Med* 14:609-12, 2000.

Gal A, et al: Aortic thromboembolism associated with *Spirocerca lupi* infection. *Vet Parasitol* 130:331-335, 2005.

Mazaki-Tovi M, et al: Canine spirocercosis: clinical, diagnostic, pathologic, and epidemiologic characterisitcs. *Vet Parasitol* 107: 235-250, 2002.

Ranen E, et al: Spirocercosis-associated esophageal sarcomas in dogs. A retrospective study of 17 cases (1997-2003). *Vet Parasitol* 119:209-221, 2004.

AUTHOR: **STEVEN L. MARKS**
EDITOR: **DEBRA L. ZORAN**

Splenic Torsion

BASIC INFORMATION

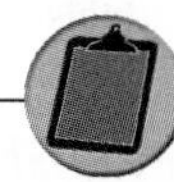

DEFINITION

Twisting of the splenic pedicle, resulting in occlusion and thrombosis of the splenic vasculature and splenic ischemia

EPIDEMIOLOGY

SPECIES, AGE, SEX

Dogs:

- No age predilection
- Males more frequently affected

GENETICS AND BREED PREDISPOSITION: Large-breed, deep-chested dogs (great danes, German shepherds).

RISK FACTORS: Gastric dilatation-volvulus (GDV).

ASSOCIATED CONDITIONS AND DISORDERS

- GDV
- Splenic infarction

CLINICAL PRESENTATION

HISTORY, CHIEF COMPLAINT

- Often vague, nonspecific signs for up to 3 weeks prior to diagnosis:
  - Intermittent vomiting, diarrhea
  - Weakness, depression
  - Anorexia
  - Abdominal distention
  - Weight loss
  - Discolored urine
- Acute collapse
- Previous episode of GDV

PHYSICAL EXAM FINDINGS

- Abdominal distention
- Abdominal mass/splenomegaly
- The following may also be noted:
  - Abdominal pain
  - Fever
  - Dehydration
  - Pale mucous membranes
  - Icterus
- If acute cardiovascular collapse:
  - Tachycardia
  - Pale mucous membranes
  - Prolonged capillary refill time
  - Weak peripheral pulses

ETIOLOGY AND PATHOPHYSIOLOGY

- Etiology unknown:
  - Occurs in large-breed, deep-chested dogs
  - Associated with GDV:
    - Occurs in conjunction with GDV
    - GDV occurs after treatment of splenic torsion
- Proposed theory: repeated stretching of gastrosplenic and splenocolic ligaments resulting in splenic hypermotility

DIAGNOSIS

DIFFERENTIAL DIAGNOSIS

- Splenic neoplasia
- Other causes of splenomegaly (see Splenomegaly, p 1027)
- Neoplasia of other abdominal organs (e.g., liver)
- GDV

INITIAL DATABASE

- Complete blood count (CBC):
  - Anemia
  - Leukocytosis (neutrophilia, monocytosis: stress leukogram common)
- Serum biochemistry profile:
  - Elevated alkaline phosphatase (ALP), alanine aminotransferase (ALT), bilirubin concentrations
- Urinalysis:
  - Hemoglobinuria common
- Diagnostic imaging:
  - Survey abdominal radiographs
    - Splenomegaly (diffuse)
      - May be the only abnormal radiographic finding
      - Often the enlarged spleen may have a "reversed C" shape (Fig. I-165)
      - Abnormal position of spleen in abdomen is common
      - Gas bubbles may be seen in spleen
    - Peritoneal effusion is common and can obscure visceral detail to the point that the findings listed previously are not apparent, requiring abdominal ultrasonography
    - Displacement of the small intestines
  - Abdominal ultrasound examination: indicated in all cases in which splenic torsion is suspected
    - Diffuse splenomegaly, appearing to curve around the hilus
    - Free abdominal fluid is generally present
    - Diffusely hypoechoic spleen: "lacy" appearance of splenic parenchyma
      - Linear echoes separating large, hypoechoic areas. This appearance is a result of vascular congestion (hypoechoic) within the dilated sinusoids and vessels (the walls of which are the framework of the "lace")
      - Thrombi may be visible within the lumen of splenic vessels
    - Doppler color flow
      - Decreased blood flow through splenic veins
      - Lack of flow in regions associated with intravascular thrombi
- Electrocardiogram (ECG) if arrhythmia is noted on exam, if there is suspicion of syncope/collapse, or for postoperative monitoring
  - Possible ventricular arrhythmias

ADVANCED OR CONFIRMATORY TESTING

Coagulation profile: while laboratory evidence of coagulopathy may exist, a clinical bleeding problem is rarely detected

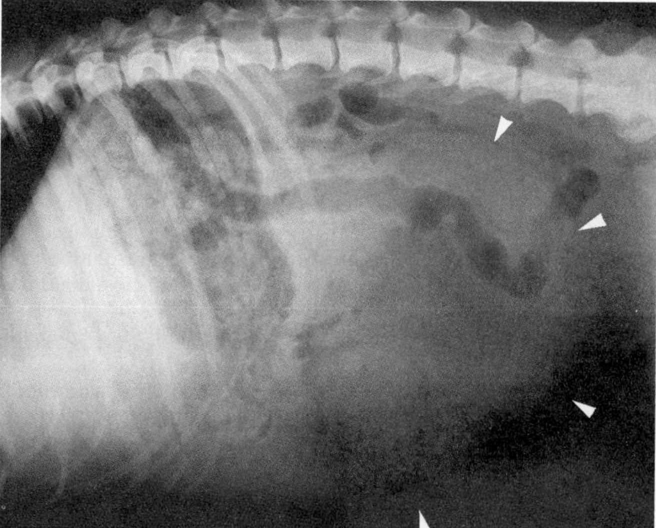

FIGURE I-165 Lateral abdominal radiograph of a dog with splenic torsion. The characteristic "reversed C" shape of the torsed spleen is apparent (*arrowheads*). Courtesy of Dr. Richard Walshaw.

TREATMENT

THERAPEUTIC GOAL(S)

- Patient stabilization
- Splenectomy
- Postoperative supportive care

ACUTE GENERAL TREATMENT

- Preoperative patient stabilization:
  - Correction of fluid deficits and electrolyte imbalance
  - Blood products (see Transfusion Therapy and Collection Techniques for Blood Banking, p 1312)
    - Whole blood if hematocrit <20% or if acute large-volume blood loss
    - Fresh frozen plasma if coagulopathy is present
  - Treatment of cardiac arrhythmias if indicated (see Ventricular Arrhythmias, p 1148)
  - Perioperative antibiotic therapy
    - Cefazolin 22 mg/kg IV q 2h
- Surgical intervention as soon as animal is stable:
  - Splenectomy without untwisting the pedicle
  - Gastropexy
- Postoperative supportive care:
  - Continuation of IV fluid and electrolyte therapy
  - Additional blood products if indicated
  - ECG monitoring
    - Treatment of arrhythmias if indicated

POSSIBLE COMPLICATIONS

- Delay in diagnosis and treatment:
  - Splenic necrosis
  - Peritonitis/sepsis
  - Disseminated intravascular coagulation (DIC)
- Pancreatitis:
  - If distal portion of left limb is involved in torsion of the splenic pedicle

PROGNOSIS AND OUTCOME

Good with early diagnosis and treatment; reported 100% postsurgical survival

PEARLS & CONSIDERATIONS

COMMENTS

- Splenic torsion can occur in association with GDV or as an isolated problem.
- The same type of dog that has the greatest risk of developing GDV also has an increased risk of developing isolated splenic torsion.
- Gastropexy after splenectomy for splenic torsion is indicated to prevent future GDV.

CLIENT EDUCATION

Large-breed, deep-chested dogs that develop vague, nonspecific signs of abdominal problems (as already described in this entry) may have splenic torsion.

SUGGESTED READING

Millis DL, Nemzek J, Riggs C, Walshaw R: Gastric dilatation-volvulus after splenic torsion in two dogs. *J Am Vet Med Assoc* 207(3):314–315, 1995.

Neath PJ, Brockman DJ, Saunders HM: Retrospective analysis of 19 cases of isolated torsion of the splenic pedicle in dogs. *J Small Anim Pract* 38:387–392, 1997.

Saunders HM, Neath PJ, Brockman DJ: B-mode and Doppler ultrasound imaging of the spleen with canine splenic torsion: A retrospective evaluation. *Vet Radiol Ultrasound* 39:349, 1998.

AUTHOR & EDITOR: **RICHARD WALSHAW**

Splenomegaly

BASIC INFORMATION

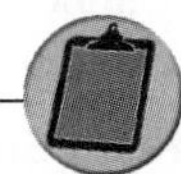

DEFINITION

Enlargement of the spleen—focal or generalized

EPIDEMIOLOGY

GENETICS AND BREED PREDISPOSITION: Dogs:

- German shepherd, Great Dane (gastric dilatation volvulus [GDV] with splenic torsion)
- Boxer (mastocytosis)
- German shepherd, golden retriever, Labrador retriever (hemangiosarcoma)
- German shepherd (systemic mycoses, especially aspergillosis)
- Cocker spaniel (immune-mediated hemolytic anemia)
- Bull mastiff and many others (lymphoma)
- Oriental-breed cats (feline infectious peritonitis [FIP])

RISK FACTORS: Living in endemic tick-borne disease areas.

GEOGRAPHY AND SEASONALITY: Tick-borne diseases: more prevalent in tropical climates and during the summer.

ASSOCIATED CONDITIONS AND DISORDERS

- Diffuse splenomegaly:
  - Infiltration (e.g., lymphoma, mast cell neoplasia, leukemia)
  - Reaction (ehrlichiosis, immune-mediated hemolytic anemia [IMHA], immune-mediated thrombocytopenia [ITP], systemic mycoses)
- Focal splenomegaly (see Mass, Splenic, p 681):
  - Neoplasia (hemangiosarcoma, hematoma, others)
  - Hyperplastic nodule
  - Granuloma (mycoses, other infections)
  - Abscess (bacterial infection)

CLINICAL PRESENTATION

HISTORY, CHIEF COMPLAINT

- Vague and nonspecific: anorexia, lethargy, weight loss
- Related to underlying disease rather than splenomegaly
- Chronic vomition if marked splenic enlargement
- Polyuria/polydipsia: paraneoplastic hypercalcemia

PHYSICAL EXAM FINDINGS

- Palpation of abdominal mass
- Abdominal distention if severe enlargement or hemoabdomen
- Lymph node enlargement: lymphoma, ehrlichiosis, mycoses, autoimmune disorders
- Collapse, pallor, tachycardia: splenic rupture (IMHA, acute babesiosis)
- Petechiae: ITP

ETIOLOGY AND PATHOPHYSIOLOGY

- Generalized splenomegaly
  - Infiltrative disorders
    - Neoplastic: acute and chronic leukemia, systemic mastocytosis (more common in cats), lymphoma, multiple myeloma
    - Non-neoplastic: amyloidosis
  - Congestion
    - Smooth muscle relaxants: barbiturates, halothane anesthesia
    - Splenic torsion (alone or in association with GDV)
    - Right-sided heart failure with portal hypertension
  - Inflammatory/infectious disorders (splenitis)
    - Suppurative: hematogenous dissemination of bacterial infection

- Necrotizing: gas-forming anaerobes associated with splenic torsion
- Eosinophilic: hypereosinophilic syndrome (cats)
- Lymphoplasmacytic: ehrlichiosis, infectious canine hepatitis, babesiosis
- Granulomatous: systemic mycoses
- Pyogranulomatous: FIP
  - Lymphoreticular hyperplasia
    - Chronic bacteremic conditions: diskospondylitis, brucellosis
    - Hemolytic disorders
  - Extramedullary hematopoiesis
- Focal splenomegaly (splenic mass)
  - Neoplastic
    - Hemangiosarcoma, hemangioma, leiomyosarcoma, fibrosarcoma
  - Non-neoplastic
    - Hematoma, abscess, nodular hyperplasia

DIAGNOSIS

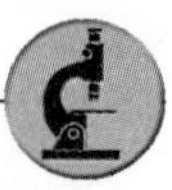

DIFFERENTIAL DIAGNOSIS

- Other cranial abdominal organomegaly
- Other nonspecific abdominal masses

INITIAL DATABASE

- Complete blood count
  - Regenerative anemia: IMHA, splenic rupture, blood parasites
  - Nonregenerative anemia: ehrlichiosis, retroviral infections, neoplastic bone marrow infiltration
  - Pancytopenia: ehrlichiosis, bone marrow infiltration
  - Spherocytosis: IMHA
  - Hemoglobinemia, bilirubinemia: splenic torsion, hemolysis
  - Lymphoblastosis: lymphoma, infections (rarely)
  - Blood parasites: babesiosis, acute ehrlichiosis, feline hemoplasmas (hemobartonellosis/*M. felis*)
  - Thrombocytopenia: ITP, babesiosis, ehrlichiosis and other rickettsial diseases
- Urinalysis
  - Hemoglobinuria, bilirubinuria: hemolytic disease, splenic torsion
- Serum biochemistry profile
  - Hyperglobulinemia: FIP, multiple myeloma, ehrlichiosis
  - Hypercalcemia: lymphoma, multiple myeloma, granulomatous disease
- Imaging
  - Abdominal radiographs: confirm abdominal mass (if sufficiently large)
  - Thoracic radiographs: assess for metastases (take ventrodorsal, left-, and right-lateral views)
  - Abdominal ultrasonography: detect abdominal effusion, define splenic architecture, confirm splenic origin (mass), delineate metastatic abdominal masses
- Retroviral testing (cats)

ADVANCED OR CONFIRMATORY TESTING

- Fine-needle aspiration and cytologic examination to detect infectious agents or predominant inflammatory cell type
  - Not recommended with mixed echogenicity masses (suspicion of hemangiosarcoma) because of risk (may hemorrhage) and poor diagnostic yield (heterogenous tumor)
- Histopathologic examination of tissue after splenectomy or of tissue samples taken at the periphery of large masses
- Bone marrow aspiration
- Exploratory laparotomy
- Computed tomography (abdominal)
- Polymerase chain reaction: *Ehrlichia*, feline hemoplasmas
- Coagulation panel: disseminated intravascular coagulation

TREATMENT

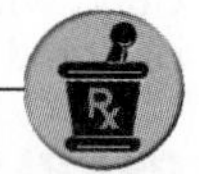

THERAPEUTIC GOAL(S)

Treat the underlying disease process

ACUTE GENERAL TREATMENT

- Doxycycline in ehrlichiosis
- Chemotherapy for certain malignancies
- Splenectomy: splenic torsion, splenic rupture, possibly refractory IMHA (controversial). Rule out bone marrow aplasia first—spleen may be essential for hemopoietic activity
- Diminazene or imidocarb in canine babesiosis

CHRONIC TREATMENT

Doxorubicin-based protocols in hemangiosarcoma

DRUG INTERACTIONS

Do not repeat diminazene within 2 weeks

POSSIBLE COMPLICATIONS

Susceptibility to infectious diseases after splenectomy

RECOMMENDED MONITORING

Monitor for ventricular arrhythmias for up to 3 days after surgery of splenic masses

PROGNOSIS AND OUTCOME

- Good to excellent with uncomplicated infections (babesiosis, ehrlichiosis)
- Guarded to grave in the case of advanced stage (metastatic) hemangiosarcoma
- With splenic masses, prognosis cannot be determined without complete histopathologic evaluation of tissue
  - Hematoma/nodular hyperplasia (55% of splenic masses): 83% alive 2 months postsplenectomy, 64% alive at 1 year. Most deaths/euthanasia due to unrelated causes
  - Hemangiosarcoma (40% of splenic masses): 31% alive 2 months postsplenectomy, 7% at 1 year. Most deaths/euthanasia due to hemangiosarcoma progression

PEARLS & CONSIDERATIONS

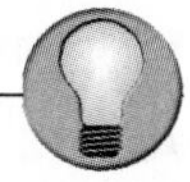

COMMENTS

- Age does not discriminate between neoplastic and non-neoplastic splenic disease.
- Clinical signs are vague.
- A common clinical error is the excessive suspicion of hemangiosarcoma on the basis of a splenic mass as the only abnormality.
- Differentiate splenomegaly from hepatomegaly by ability to move the spleen caudally during abdominal palpation. Raise patient's forelimbs to facilitate examination.
- Dogs with anemia, nucleated red blood cells, abnormal red cell morphology or splenic rupture: greater chance of having splenic neoplasia.
- The spleen is an accessible organ to obtain diagnostic sample in the evaluation of systemic diseases (diffuse splenomegaly).
- For histopathologic examination of splenic masses after splenectomy, a submitted tissue sample should cross from normal tissue to abnormal/mass. Ideally, the whole spleen is submitted fresh on cold packs (not frozen).
- Gross appearance at laparotomy cannot discriminate between hematoma, nodular hyperplasia, hemangioma and hemangiosarcoma, and normal ectopic splenic tissue in abdomen may falsely appear to be metastases—be careful when recommending euthanasia.

PREVENTION

Regular tick control in endemic areas

SUGGESTED READING

Couto CG: Lymphadenopathy and splenomegaly. In Nelson RW, Couto CG (eds): *Small Animal Internal Medicine*. Mosby, 2003, pp 1200–1209.

Neer TM: Clinical approach to splenomegaly in dogs and cats. *Compend Cont Ed Pract Vet* 18:35–48, 1996.

Prymak C, et al: Epidemiologic, clinical, pathologic and prognostic characteristics of splenic hemangiosarcoma and splenic hematoma in dogs: 217 cases. *J Am Vet Med Assoc* 193:706, 1988.

Spangler WL, et al: Prevalence and type of splenic diseases in cats: 455 cases (1985–1991). *J Am Med Assoc* 201:773, 1992.

Spangler WL, et al: Prevalence, type and importance of splenic diseases in dogs: 1480 cases (1985–1989). *J Am Vet Med Assoc* 200:829, 1992.

Spangler WL, Kass PH: Pathologic factors affecting postsplenectomy survival in dogs. *J Vet Intern Med* 11:166–171, 1997.

AUTHOR: **JOHAN P. SCHOEMAN**
EDITOR: **ETIENNE CÔTÉ**

Spongiform Encephalopathies

BASIC INFORMATION

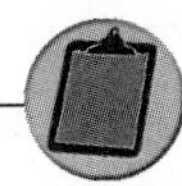

DEFINITION

A heterogeneous group of neurologic diseases having in common histologic spongiform change within the brain. Subdivided as grey matter (vacuolation occurs within neurons or their processes; diseases are heritable or are transmissible) or white matter (vacuolation occurs within the myelin sheaths; caused by heredity or by intoxications)

SYNONYM(S)

Grey matter:
- Transmissible spongiform encephalopathies
- Bovine spongiform encephalopathy (BSE)
- Prion diseases

White matter:
- Spongiform leukoencephalopathies
- Spongy degeneration of white matter (avoids confusion with prion diseases)

EPIDEMIOLOGY

SPECIES, AGE, SEX
- Grey matter:
  - Transmissible: cats >2 years old
  - Hereditary: rottweiler dogs; signs begin at age 6 weeks, progress over 6 to 7 months
- White matter:
  - Acquired: dog/cat, any age and both sexes
  - Hereditary: dogs, cats:
    - Signs begin at 3 to 5 weeks and progress rapidly in silky terriers, Shetland sheepdogs, Samoyeds, and kittens.
    - Signs begin at 4 to 6 months and progress over 6 to 8 months in Labrador retrievers and dalmatians.

GENETICS AND BREED PREDISPOSITION
- Grey matter
  - Hereditary: suspected autosomal recessive in rottweiler dogs
- White matter
  - Hereditary: appears to be autosomal recessive

CONTAGION AND ZOONOSIS
- Grey matter:
  - Transmissible: ingestion of BSE-contaminated meat/byproducts can cause variant Creutzfeldt-Jacob disease in humans and feline spongiform encephalopathy in cats.
  - Transmissible: necropsy requires basic precautions, including gloves and other protective items. Pathologists working with known prion-infected carcasses wear full-body protection, including respirators, but given the newness of these diseases and lengthy incubation time, the necessity of such precautions remains speculative for the clinical veterinary population.

GEOGRAPHY AND SEASONALITY: Grey matter:
- Transmissible: only reported in Europe but could appear anywhere BSE appears
- Hereditary: affected rottweilers have been reported in the United States and Europe

CLINICAL PRESENTATION

HISTORY, CHIEF COMPLAINT
- Grey matter:
  - Transmissible: behavioral changes (timidity or aggression), progressing to ataxia, hypermetria, and hyperesthesia to touch and sound
  - Hereditary: ataxia, paresis, signs of laryngeal paralysis, progression to severe quadriparesis
- White matter:
  - Acquired (see Bromethalin Toxicosis, p 154)
  - Hereditary:
    - Labrador retrievers: hypermetria, spastic paresis, episodes of decerebrate rigidity; progression to quadriplegia
    - Shetland sheepdogs, kittens: motor deficits, altered mentation, seizures

PHYSICAL EXAM FINDINGS
- Grey matter:
  - Transmissible: behavioral changes (timidity or aggression), progressing to ataxia, hypermetria, hyperesthesia to touch and sound
  - Hereditary: ataxia and paresis with normal reflexes (hind limbs > forelimbs), laryngeal paralysis; quadriparesis possible if advanced
- White matter:
  - Acquired (see Bromethalin Toxicosis, p 154)
  - Hereditary: as already described

ETIOLOGY AND PATHOPHYSIOLOGY

- Grey matter:
  - Transmissible: caused by prions, enigmatic infectious proteins. Abnormally folded prion proteins accumulate within neurons as scrapie-associated fibrils and ultimately cause cell death. Cats were infected at the height of the BSE outbreak in Europe in the early 1990s.
  - Hereditary: gene not yet identified.
- White matter:
  - Acquired: toxins that uncouple oxidative phosphorylation, including bromethelin and hexachlorophene.
  - Hereditary: enzyme deficiencies and/or genes not yet identified in dogs or cats.

DIAGNOSIS

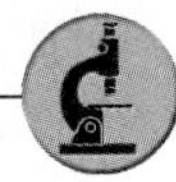

DIFFERENTIAL DIAGNOSIS

CLINICAL
- Grey matter:
  - Transmissible
    - Any cause of diffuse forebrain signs in adult cat
      - Infectious: rabies, feline immunodeficiency virus (FIV), feline infectious peritonitis (FIP), fungal, protozoal
      - Metabolic: hepatic, electrolytes, endocrine
      - Neoplasia: meningioma, astrocytoma, metastatic
      - Toxic: organophosphates, heavy metals
  - Hereditary
    - Any cause of multifocal central nervous system (CNS) or peripheral nerve diseases in young dogs
    - Other hereditary diseases of rottweilers: leukodystrophy, motor neuron disease, neuroaxonal dystrophy
    - Idiopathic laryngeal paralysis
    - Infectious: neosporosis, distemper, tick-borne, fungal
    - Toxic
- White matter:
  - Juvenile onset
    - Any cause of diffuse white matter disease
      - Canine distemper
      - Lysosomal storage diseases or other inborn errors of metabolism
  - Neonatal onset
    - Any cause of diffuse forebrain disease
      - Lysosomal storage diseases or other inborn error of metabolism
      - Hepatic encephalopathy
      - Hypoglycemia

HISTOLOGIC: Like spongiform encephalopathies, lysosomal storage diseases may also show extensive vacuolation of neurons, but unlike spongiform encephalopathies, the vacuoles are lysosomes distended with storage products. In the spongiform encephalopathies, vacuoles appear empty; if intraneuronal, they are not membrane bound.

INITIAL DATABASE

- Neurologic exam:
  - Localize lesion(s)
- Complete blood count (CBC), serum chemistry profile (including bile acids), urinalysis:
  - To rule out metabolic disease and look for evidence of infections
- Brain imaging (CT scan or MRI):
  - To rule out structural disease
  - May see evidence of diffuse increase in water density of grey or white matter
- Cerebrospinal fluid (CSF) analysis:
  - To rule out encephalitis or meningitis

ADVANCED OR CONFIRMATORY TESTING

Ultimate diagnosis is based on histopathologic examination that shows vacuolation in white matter or grey matter

TREATMENT

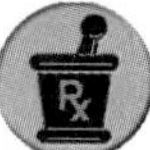

THERAPEUTIC GOAL(S)

- No definitive treatment
- Supportive only (e.g., anticonvulsant drugs for seizures)

ACUTE GENERAL TREATMENT

Mannitol (0.5–1 g/kg slow IV over 15 to 20 minutes) may improve the intramyelinic edema in bromethalin toxicity.

PROGNOSIS AND OUTCOME

- Prognosis for animals with spongiform encephalopathies is guarded to grave.
- Personality changes make animals with transmissible forms potentially dangerous.
- Hereditary forms have been inexorably progressive.
- Toxic spongiform leukoencephalopathies respond poorly to treatment but may recover if dose is low.

PEARLS & CONSIDERATIONS

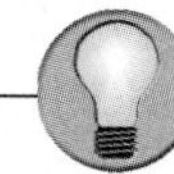

COMMENTS

- The cystic, spongiform appearance is apparent microscopically; it is not apparent to the naked eye and not revealed by such diagnostic tests as MRIs.
- Transmissible spongiform encephalopathies will hopefully remain rare in dogs and cats; however, it is important to recognize them if they should occur because of the public health implications. A necropsy is necessary to confirm a diagnosis of spongiform encephalopathy of grey matter, which should be reported to the appropriate agency.

PREVENTION

Do not feed bovine nervous system or byproducts to cats in BSE endemic areas. Risk from deer with chronic wasting disease is unknown, but it is best to not feed deer nervous system or byproducts to cats.

CLIENT EDUCATION

Educate clients about transmissible spongiform encephalopathies so they can make intelligent choices regarding meat safety rather than being swayed by emotional appeals

SUGGESTED READING

Kortz GD, et al: Neuronal vacuolation and spinocerebellar degeneration in young rottweiler dogs. *Vet Pathology*, 34(4):296–302, 1997.

O'Brien DP, Zachary JF: Clinical features of spongy degeneration of the central nervous system in two Labrador retriever littermates. *J Am Vet Met Assoc* 186(11):1207–1210, 1985.

Wyatt JM, et al: Naturally occurring scrapie-like spongiform encephalopathy in five domestic cats. *Vet Record* 129(11):233–236, 1991.

AUTHOR: **DENNIS P. O'BRIEN**

EDITOR: **CURTIS W. DEWEY**

Sporotrichosis

BASIC INFORMATION

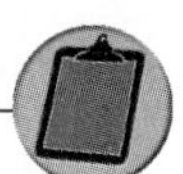

DEFINITION

A mycotic disease caused by *Sporothrix schenckii*. The disease is caused by a dimorphic fungus and clinically manifests with chronic granulomatous skin lesions.

EPIDEMIOLOGY

SPECIES, AGE, SEX

- Dogs and cats
- Young to middle-aged cats and dogs predominate
- Males infected twice as often as females

GENETICS AND BREED PREDISPOSITION: Dogs: most frequently seen in hunting dogs.

RISK FACTORS

- The disease is often associated with puncture wounds, so outdoor roaming dogs are predominantly the ones that develop the disease. In cats, fighting intact males predominate in contracting the disease.
- A higher concentration of organisms exists in soils rich in decaying organic matter, barberry and rose bush thorns, sphagnum moss, tree bark, and mine timbers.
- Immune suppression allows for dissemination
- Punctures and other wounds allow for inoculation

CONTAGION AND ZOONOSIS

- Dog-to-dog or dog-to-human transmission is rare to unlikely due to low numbers of organisms found in lesions.
- Cat-to-cat or cat-to-human transmission is considered possible and is a significant means of zoonotic transmission, especially in immunosuppressed people. This transmission may come from wounds or through contaminated claws. Canine and human cases of sporotrichosis usually are preceded by cases of sporotrichosis in associated cats; feline sporotrichosis may be a harbinger of sporotrichosis in dogs and humans in contact with these cases.

GEOGRAPHY AND SEASONALITY: Worldwide distribution.

CLINICAL PRESENTATION

DISEASE FORMS/SUBTYPES

- Dogs: predominately have cutaneous and cutaneolymphatic forms
- Cats: cutaneous, cutaneolymphatic, and disseminated forms

HISTORY, CHIEF COMPLAINT

- Cutaneous lesions (nodular to ulcerated)
- Possible draining tracts
- Lethargy
- Anorexia

PHYSICAL EXAM FINDINGS

- Fever: suggests possible disseminated disease
- Depression
- Dogs: multinodular lesions on the trunk or head in the dermis or subcutaneous layers:
  - Ulcerations with purulent exudate and crust formation are possible
  - Cutaneolymphatic form usually presents nodules on the distal aspect of one limb with ascending development following lymphatics and lymphadenomegaly

- Cats: About 97% of affected cats have one or multiple skin lesions, commonly on the distal limbs, head, or tail base:
  - Draining puncture wounds, abscesses, or cellulitis
  - Ulcerations, purulent exudate, and large crusted lesions
  - Possible lymphadenomegaly
  - About 44% of affected cats have respiratory tract signs

ETIOLOGY AND PATHOPHYSIOLOGY

- Inoculation of mycelial form of *S. schenckii* into tissues leads to production of the yeast form
- Pyogranulomatous inflammation occurs, with organisms seen in macrophages and neutrophils
- Dissemination occurs through lymphatics and into other organs (spleen, liver, lung, eyes, bones, muscles, central nervous system [CNS])
- Dissemination is rare in dogs but may occur in up to 50% of cats, especially with immune-suppressive dosages of corticosteroids

DIAGNOSIS

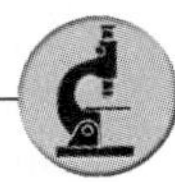

DIFFERENTIAL DIAGNOSIS

- Deep cutaneous bacterial infection, L-form bacterial infection
- Systemic mycosis

INITIAL DATABASE

- Complete blood count (CBC), serum biochemistry profile, urinalysis: anemia, leukocytosis with neutrophilia, hypoalbuminemia, and hyperglobulinemia commonly observed
- Feline leukemia virus (FeLV) and feline immunodeficiency virus (FIV) serologic testing: positive in < 1% and 8% of affected cats, respectively
- Cytologic examination from aspirates, exudates, or skin preps: diagnostic
  - Organism is small (slightly smaller than erythrocytes), is round or oval, and may be difficult (dogs) or easy (cats) to find in exudates

ADVANCED OR CONFIRMATORY TESTING

- Histopathologic examination of nodules: diagnostic.
- Fungal culture: notify laboratory of the possibility of *Sporothrix* organisms due to the infectious nature of sample to humans. Never culture suspected sporotrichosis lesions in-house (zoonosis risk).
- The Centers for Disease Control and Prevention, Atlanta, can perform fluorescent antibody testing on exudates or tissue.

TREATMENT

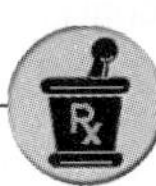

THERAPEUTIC GOAL(S)

Removal of organisms

ACUTE AND CHRONIC TREATMENT

- Dogs; options include one of the following:
  - Supersaturated solution of potassium iodide (SSKI) 40 mg/kg PO q 8h for 30 days beyond apparent cure; or
  - Ketoconazole 5-15 mg/kg PO q 8h for 30 days beyond apparent cure; or
  - Itraconazole 5-10 mg/kg PO q 12-24h for 30 days beyond apparent cure
- Cats:
  - Itraconazole 5-10 mg/kg PO q 12-24h for 30 days beyond apparent cure

POSSIBLE COMPLICATIONS

- SSKI can cause systemic iodination (ocular and nasal discharge, dry haircoat with scaling, vomiting, depression, collapse). If signs are mild, discontinue the medication for 1 week and reinitiate; if signs are severe, change treatment to alternative therapy.
- Ketoconazole can be hepatotoxic, especially in cats.
- Itraconazole has been found to be hepatotoxic in 10% of dogs treated with a dosage of 5 mg/kg q 12h.

RECOMMENDED MONITORING

With itraconazole or ketaconazole administration, monitor liver enzymes every 2 to 4 weeks for duration of therapy

PROGNOSIS AND OUTCOME

- Response of cutaneous or cutaneolymphatic is fair to good. Of 266 cats treated in one study, 68 (26%) were cured.
  - Irrespective of extracutaneous signs or FIV status
- Disseminated disease carries a guarded prognosis.

PEARLS & CONSIDERATIONS

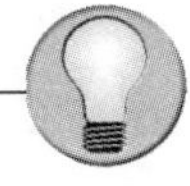

COMMENTS

- Even after treatment is completed, use of immunosuppressive dosages of corticosteroids is contraindicated due to reported recurrence of infection
- Duration of therapy is often 3 months or more
- Cats have been given iodide and ketoconazole, but due to high sensitivity, these are not recommended

PREVENTION

- Limit outdoor roaming, especially in wooded areas
- Castrate male cats to diminish fighting

CLIENT EDUCATION

- Sporotrichosis is a zoonotic disease, especially in cats
- Wear gloves when handling infected animals
- Separation of infected animals from immunosuppressed people is necessary

SUGGESTED READING

Rosser EJ, et al: Sporotrichosis. In Greene CE (ed): *Infectious Diseases of Dogs and Cats*. Philadelphia, WB Saunders, 1998, pp 399-400.

Schubach AO, et al: Epidemic cat-transmitted sporotrichosis (letter). *N Engl J Med* 353:1185-1186, 2005.

Schubach TM, et al: Evaluation of an epidemic of sporotrichosis in cats: 347 cases (1998-2001). *J Am Vet Med Assoc* 224:1623-1629, 2004.

Taboada J: Systemic mycoses. In Ettinger SJ, Feldman EC (eds.): *Textbook of Veterinary Internal Medicine*. Philadelphia, WB Saunders, 2000, pp 471-472.

AUTHOR: **JEFFERY SIMMONS**

EDITOR: **DOUGLASS K. MACINTIRE**

Squamous Cell Carcinoma, Cutaneous (Planum, Aural, Digital)

Client Education Sheet on Website

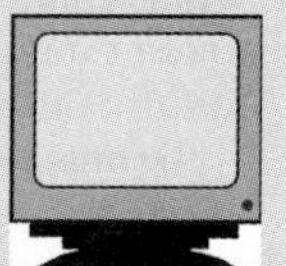

BASIC INFORMATION

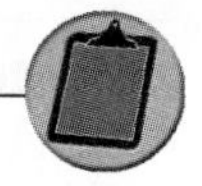

DEFINITION

A malignant tumor arising from squamous epithelium

EPIDEMIOLOGY

SPECIES, AGE, SEX

- Nasal planum (nonhaired, rostral, external part of nose):
  - Dog: rare site
  - Cat: Squamous cell carcinoma (SCC) is the most common tumor in this site; older cats
- Aural: generally occurs in older animals:
  - Dog: SCC is the second most common ear canal tumor (after ceruminous gland adenocarcinoma)
  - Cat: SCC may affect the pinna, often in cats with planum and periocular SCC; may also affect the ear canal, where it is the most common tumor type, equal in frequency to ceruminous gland adenocarcinoma
- Digital:
  - Dog: SCC is one of the most common digital tumors (along with melanoma and mast cell tumor); age between 7 and 11 years
  - Cat: Primary SCC of the digit is very rare (about 10%). Digital carcinomas usually occur as metastasis from a bronchogenic carcinoma in older (mean of 13 years) cats

GENETICS AND BREED PREDISPOSITION

- Planum:
  - Dog: none
  - Cat: lightly pigmented animals; Siamese breed underrepresented
- Aural:
  - Dog: none
  - Cat: in pinna; found in lightly pigmented animals; Siamese breed underrepresented
- Digital:
  - Dog: Approximately 75% are large-breed dogs, with around 70% having black coats. Breeds at increased risk include giant, standard, and miniature schnauzers; Gordon setter; standard and miniature poodles; Scottish terrier; Labrador retriever; rottweiler, and dachshund. Digital SCC involving multiple digits has been reported in three related giant schnauzers and has been observed in other large black dogs, including standard poodles and Labrador retrievers.
  - Cat: none.

RISK FACTORS: Solar exposure in white-coated cats is associated with increased risk of development of nasal planum, pinnal, and periocular SCC.

GEOGRAPHY AND SEASONALITY: High altitude may increase the risk for solar exposure-induced SCC.

CLINICAL PRESENTATION

HISTORY, CHIEF COMPLAINT

- Planum and pinna: Clients may seek veterinary care due to the occurrence of crusted or ulcerated lesions or an actual mass. There may be bleeding or sneezing.
- Aural, external ear canal: There may be a visible mass, ear discharge, odor, pruritus, pain, facial nerve paralysis, head tilt, or circling. Compared to dogs, cats are more likely to present with neurologic signs.
- Digital:
  - Dog: lameness, swelling of digit, abnormal nail growth, fractured nail, licking/chewing at digit; oftentimes animals have a history of chronic nail bed infection treated with multiple different antibiotics with no improvement.
  - Cat: lameness; despite the fact that digital SCC in cats is usually metastatic from an underlying lung tumor, cats rarely have pulmonary signs.

PHYSICAL EXAM FINDINGS

- Planum and pinna: lesion may be proliferative or erosive; thus, mass or crusting and ulcerative lesion may be present. Adjacent lymph node may be enlarged.
- Aural, external ear canal: Otic exam shows raised irregular mass, often ulcerated. Palpation of vertical ear canal may reveal large mass invading the area in late-stage cases.
- Digital:
  - Dog: painful swollen digit with an abnormal or absent toe nail. Ulceration may be present. The draining lymph node may be enlarged.
  - Cat: swollen digit, ulcerated skin with purulent discharge; constant exsheathment, deviation, or loss of nail. About one-third of animals present with multiple digits involved.

ETIOLOGY AND PATHOPHYSIOLOGY

- Planum and pinna: may begin as actinic keratosis and become locally invasive; low metastatic rate
- Aural, external ear canal: locally invasive, more aggressive in cats than dogs; low metastatic rate (about 5-15% in local lymph nodes)
- Digital:
  - Dog: locally invasive with digital (P3) bony destruction, low metastatic rate (5-10% pulmonary; local lymph node metastatic rate not well documented but also rare)
  - Cat: locally invasive with digital (P3) destruction. These are usually metastatic lesions from a pulmonary tumor. Lymph node involvement not documented

DIAGNOSIS

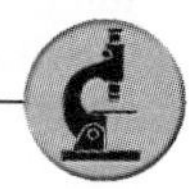

DIFFERENTIAL DIAGNOSIS

- Planum: fungal lesion (particularly *Cryptococcus* in cats), cutaneous lymphoma, mast cell tumor, fibrosarcoma, melanoma, eosinophilic granuloma, immune-mediated dermatopathy
- Aural:
  - Canal: severe hyperplasia in dogs with chronic otitis, ceruminous gland adenocarcinoma, adenoma, papilloma, polyp, plasmacytoma, basal cell tumor, melanoma, granuloma
  - Pinna: consider trauma, frostbite, insect bites; also see Planum above
- Digital:
  - Dog: melanoma, mast cell tumor, soft tissue sarcoma, osteomyelitis, paronychia
  - Cat: usually metastatic lung tumor; bacterial paronychia; other primary tumors much less likely

INITIAL DATABASE

- Dog: all sites (planum, aural, digital): complete blood count (CBC), serum biochemistry profile, urinalysis: unremarkable:
  - Aspirate and cytologic examination from surrounding lymph nodes to assess for metastasis in all cases; unlikely to be positive but an easy test with prognostic value
  - Three-view thoracic radiographs to assess for metastasis; usually negative
  - Fine-needle aspirate (FNA) and cytologic examination of the primary mass; it may be possible to obtain the samples on animal that is awake, but if sedation is needed, plan to biopsy as well
  - Cytologic examination can provide a definitive diagnosis, but at times extreme inflammation of the tumor

can make interpretation of the squamous cells difficult, necessitating a biopsy

- Cat:
  - Planum and aural: see Dog above. Hypercalcemia is rarely seen as paraneoplastic syndrome in ear canal SCC
  - Digital: three-view thoracic radiographs almost always reveal lung neoplasia; usually solitary mass but may be multiple. FNA and cytologic examination of the digital mass can provide a definitive diagnosis, but at times extreme inflammation of the tumor can make interpretation of the epithelial cells difficult. These cells, while usually pulmonary adenocarcinoma in origin, may have some squamous differentiation. FNA of the lung mass can confirm a lung tumor if the digit lesion is nondiagnostic

ADVANCED OR CONFIRMATORY TESTING

- Incisional or excisional biopsy of the primary mass for histopathologic diagnosis
- Radiographs, CT scan, or MRI of lesion to assess for tumor extent, bone involvement, and to plan surgery or radiation therapy

TREATMENT

THERAPEUTIC GOAL(S)

Excision of primary tumor with wide margins is often curative, as indicated by low metastatic rates. Due to location and extent of lesion in many cases, however, wide excision may be difficult or impossible. In cats with digital carcinoma, treatment options are poor due to lesion being metastatic; even palliative digital amputation provides little benefit as rapid progression to other digits and systemic illness occurs.

ACUTE GENERAL TREATMENT

Aggressive surgical resection; if margins are not complete on histologic evaluation, radiation is effective for microscopic disease.

- Planum:
  - Dog: Excising the premaxilla along with the planum in cases with very large masses may provide better cosmesis.
  - Cat: Excision is an excellent option if the tumor is not too extensive along the bridge of the nose or does not involve the lip or surrounding skin. Radiation, photodynamic therapy, cryotherapy, and intralesional chemotherapy (platinum drugs, 5-FU) can be effective for small superficial lesions, with decreasing effectiveness for larger lesions. In one study, six out of six cats with large lesions had complete remission with intralesional carboplatin combined with radiation therapy (median follow-up time 9 months, with median time to recurrence or survival time not yet reached).
- Aural: Total ear canal ablation with bulla osteotomy provides best survival times. In cats, the tumors can invade aggressively into the skull bones.
- Digital:
  - Dog: digital amputation; adjuvant therapy usually unnecessary (for discussion of chemotherapy options, see Squamous Cell Carcinoma, Oral [Mucosal, Tonsillar], p 1034).
  - Cats: therapy unrewarding if metastatic lesion; if thoracic films are normal and only one digit is involved, amputation of the digit is recommended.

CHRONIC TREATMENT

- Cyclooxygenase (COX)-2 expression was shown in 40 out of 40 canine SCC cases, so therapy with piroxicam or other nonsteroidal anti-inflammatory drugs (NSAIDs) may be of benefit.
- Only 9% of feline oral SCC cases and zero out of six cutaneous SCC cases showed COX-2 expression, bringing into question the benefit of using NSAIDs for treatment of the feline disease.

PROGNOSIS AND OUTCOME

- Planum: excellent prognosis for cure if complete surgical resection. Median survival in cats with planum and/or pinna SCC: 673 days with surgery alone.
- Aural, canal: excellent prognosis for cure if treated early; unfortunately, tumors in cats have often progressed massively prior to identification leading to a median survival time of only 3.8 months.
- Digital:
  - Dog: good prognosis with 95% 1-year and 75% 2-year survival rates.
  - Cat: when a metastatic lesion, digital amputation median survival is only 1 to 2 months; if it is a primary digital SCC, reported survival time with surgery is variable (3 weeks to 2 years).

PEARLS & CONSIDERATIONS

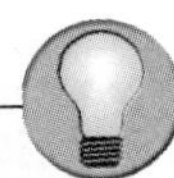

COMMENTS

- Planum: Cosmesis and quality of life after a nosectomy are generally good to excellent with high owner satisfaction. Early treatment, when the lesion is small enough for a surgical cure, is strongly recommended when possible.
- Aural:
  - Canal: Complete ear ablation is needed; simple debulking is inadequate because the tumor will continue to invade inward, making a surgical cure impossible later.
  - Pinna: Preneoplastic changes can extend along the entire edge of the pinna; complete pinnaectomy may be required for cure. If lesion is very small, simple removal of the affected tip of the ear can be considered, with a later decision made according the need for further excision based on histopathologic examination results.
- Digital:
  - Dog: Tumors often go undiagnosed for extensive amounts of time due to treatment for a nail bed infection. Any questionable, nonantibiotic-responsive digital swelling must be biopsied.
  - Cat: Primary digit tumors are very rare; three-view thoracic radiographs are essential prior to surgery, because digital tumors are usually secondary.

PREVENTION

Planum and pinna: limit sun exposure in light-coated cats

SUGGESTED READING

de Vos J, et al: Results from the treatment of advanced-stage squamous cell carcinoma of the nasal planum in cats, using a combination of intralesional carboplatin and superficial radiotherapy: A pilot study. *Vet Compar Onc* 2:75, 2004.

Fidel J, et al: Proton irradiation of feline nasal planum squamous cell carcinomas using an accelerated protocol. *Vet Radiol Ultrasound* 42:569, 2001.

Lascelles BD, et al: Squamous cell carcinoma of the nasal planum in 17 dogs. *Vet Rec* 147:473, 2000.

van der Linde-Sipman JS, et al: Primary and metastatic carcinomas in the digits of cats. *Vet Q* 22:141, 2000.

AUTHOR: **LAURA D. GARRETT**

EDITOR: **KENNETH M. RASSNICK**

Squamous Cell Carcinoma, Oral (Mucosal, Tonsillar)

Client Education Sheet on Website

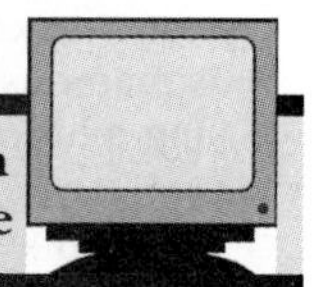

BASIC INFORMATION

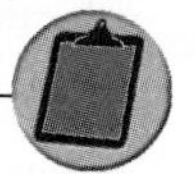

DEFINITION

A malignant tumor arising from squamous epithelium. The information in this entry describes squamous cell carcinoma (SCC) that affects mucosal and intraoral structures; cutaneous SCC is described elsewhere (see Squamous Cell Carcinoma, Cutaneous [Planum, Aural, Digital], p 1032). Other oral tumors are discussed under Oral Neoplasia, Benign, p 769, and Oral Neoplasia, Malignant, p 771.

EPIDEMIOLOGY

SPECIES, AGE, SEX

- Dogs:
  - SCC is one of the three most common malignant oral tumors, with nontonsillar SCC having a prevalence rate of approximately 7 per 100,000 dogs.
  - Gingival area is most frequently affected, followed by lips, tongue, palate, and pharynx.
  - Tonsillar SCC ranges in prevalence depending on the environment (urban dogs are more commonly affected).
  - Middle-aged to older dogs are affected for most oral SCC, and there is no sex predilection.
  - Gingival papillary SCC has been reported in very young (<1 year old) dogs.
- Cats:
  - SCC is the most common oral tumor in cats.
  - SCC makes up about 75% of all feline oral tumors and occurs in the gingival and sublingual area in equal frequency.
  - Older cats are affected; no sex predilection.
  - Tonsillar SCC is very rare in cats.

GENETICS AND BREED PREDISPOSITION

- Dogs: Large dogs may be more likely to develop nontonsillar SCC than small dogs; white dogs may be predisposed to SCC of the tongue.
- Cats: no predisposition.

RISK FACTORS

- Exposure to air pollution may be associated with development of tonsillar SCC in dogs. Gingival SCC has been reported to develop after oral radiation therapy in dogs.
- Oral SCC in cats may be associated with flea collar use, canned cat food or canned tuna consumption, and (possibly) environmental tobacco smoke. In one study, cats with SCC that were exposed to environmental smoke were much more likely to overexpress mutant p53 (a gene that, when mutated, can no longer function in its role as tumor suppressor) than cats with SCC living in nonsmoking environments.

GEOGRAPHY AND SEASONALITY: Tonsillar SCC is about 10 times more likely to occur in dogs living in urban areas versus those living in rural areas.

CLINICAL PRESENTATION

HISTORY, CHIEF COMPLAINT

- Dogs and cats may be presented for evaluation of difficulty eating, reluctance to eat, drooling, halitosis, bloody oral discharge, pawing at mouth, facial mass, oral mass, loose teeth, or weight loss.
- Dogs with tonsillar SCC may also be presented for evaluation of "lumps under jaw" due to large mandibular lymph node metastasis, with no other clinical signs.

PHYSICAL EXAM FINDINGS

- Gingival SCC: swelling or raised mass along gingival margin that may be irregular, ulcerated. Cats can have normal gingiva with the tumor affecting the mandible/maxilla and causing a large swelling in the bone.
- Tonsillar SCC: enlarged mandibular lymph nodes and enlarged irregular tonsils may be seen. Tonsillar enlargement is usually unilateral (see Tonsillar Enlargement, p 1088).
- Sublingual SCC: irregular mass under tongue.

ETIOLOGY AND PATHOPHYSIOLOGY

- Gingival and sublingual SCC: locally invasive with a low metastatic rate (5–10% regional lymph nodes, 3% lung)
- Tonsillar SCC: invasive and highly metastatic (98% regional lymph nodes, 63% lung)

DIAGNOSIS

DIFFERENTIAL DIAGNOSIS

- Gingival mass in a dog: SCC, melanoma, fibrosarcoma, acanthomatous epulis; less likely osteosarcoma, plasma cell tumor, tooth root abscess, fungal disease, other primary tumors
- Gingival mass in a cat: SCC, fibrosarcoma, dental disease; less likely melanoma, other primary tumors
- Tonsillar mass in a dog: SCC, lymphoma; less likely bacterial or fungal infection
- Sublingual mass in a cat: SCC, foreign body, fungal infection, other neoplasia

INITIAL DATABASE

- Complete blood count (CBC), serum biochemistry panel, urinalysis:
  - Dogs: results are generally normal, but tests are still indicated as a general health screen
  - Cats: hypercalcemia may be seen as a paraneoplastic syndrome
- Mandibular lymph node fine-needle aspirates (FNA) and cytologic examination to assess for metastasis in all cases.
- Three-view thoracic radiographs to assess for metastasis.
- Incisional biopsy with histopathologic evaluation of tissue is necessary for a definitive diagnosis. FNA and cytologic examination of the primary mass can provide a definitive diagnosis in some cases; frequently, extreme inflammation of the tumor can make interpretation of the squamous cells difficult.

ADVANCED OR CONFIRMATORY TESTING

Radiographs, CT scan, or MRI of lesion to assess for tumor extent, bone involvement, and to plan surgery or radiation therapy

TREATMENT

THERAPEUTIC GOAL(S)

- Surgery is a critical component for curative intent treatment of SCC; SCC is generally poorly responsive to radiation or chemotherapy. One exception is dogs with small tumors in a rostral oral location that may have a good response to radiation; however, these dogs also are excellent candidates for complete surgical resection.
- Dog: Maxillary and mandibular SCC can be cured with aggressive surgical resection. Radiation for microscopic disease postincomplete resection can extend disease-free interval and survival times. Histologically low-grade SCC of the tongue that is in a rostral location may be cured surgically. Tonsillar SCC can rarely be controlled due to extreme local invasiveness and high metastatic rate. Surgery, radiation, and chemotherapy in a multimodality approach may extend survival times but will not be curative.
- Cat: Maxillary and mandibular SCC are rarely found at a size when surgical

excision is possible; thus, treatment is rarely curative. Multimodality therapy may extend survival times. Sublingual SCC is not amenable to surgical resection, and thus treatment is limited.

ACUTE AND CHRONIC TREATMENT

- Gingival: aggressive resection, including partial mandibulectomy or maxillectomy. Definitive radiation for residual microscopic disease if surgery does not provide tumor-free margins.
- Tongue, dog: if rostral, surgical resection (40–60% of the tongue can be removed with good function, possibly more). Histologic grade predicts metastatic behavior; if high grade, consider chemotherapy.
- Tonsillar: poor treatment options due to invasiveness and metastatic behavior; multimodality therapy: surgical debulking, if possible, of primary mass and involved lymph nodes followed by chemotherapy and radiation may extend survival times.
- Sublingual and gingival, cat: very poor treatment options. Surgical excision usually not feasible. Radiation therapy and photodynamic therapy have been tried with limited success. Gemcitabine as a radiation sensitizer with palliative radiation has shown some short duration responses (50% complete and partial remission, with median duration 42.5 days) but may be associated with significant hematologic and normal tissue toxicity and, thus, cannot be recommended.
- Chemotherapy: Piroxicam (0.3 mg/kg PO once daily; caution regarding gastric ulcerative effects) has some effect against gross SCC in dogs (18% complete and partial remission, 29% stable disease). Cisplatin combined with piroxicam also showed antitumor effect in dogs (55% complete and partial remission, 33% stable disease), but renal toxicity is a significant concern when combining these drugs (about 40% renal toxicoses). Combining these drugs is not recommended.

POSSIBLE COMPLICATIONS

Cats may not tolerate aggressive orofacial surgery very well postoperatively, and placement of feeding tubes may be necessary.

PROGNOSIS AND OUTCOME

- Dogs with rostral SCC: wide surgical resection can be curative.
- Dogs with mandibular or maxillary nonresectable SCC: radiation. Median survival time is 450 days. Control time for dogs with tumors greater than 4 cm diameter is generally shorter.
- Dogs with tonsillar SCC: surgery and radiation. Median survival is 100 days. With surgery, radiation, and chemotherapy (doxorubicin and cisplatin), median survival is 270 days.
- Dogs with lingual SCC: Rostral masses can be cured with wide resection if low grade. Dogs with nonresectable lingual SCC can be treated with radiation therapy, but survival is generally short (i.e., median 4 months), with dogs being euthanized due to local proliferation or metastasis.
- Cats with mandibular SCC:
  - Radiation and mitoxantrone, without surgery: generally poor response; median survival is 180 days
  - Mandibulectomy and radiation; median survival is 14 months; euthanasia usually due to local recurrence
- Cats sublingual: poor response to therapy; survival time <3 months.

PEARLS & CONSIDERATIONS

COMMENTS

- Mandibular, maxillary, and lingual SCC in rostral locations in dogs can be cured with aggressive resection.
- SCC in cats and in other locations in the mouth in dogs is difficult to address due to invasiveness and/or metastasis.
- Multimodality therapy may extend survival times, but quality of life can be an issue with the treatments:
  - Dogs with tonsillar SCC can have pronounced dysphagia and discomfort; surgical debulking may not alleviate clinical signs, and radiation therapy can contribute to local discomfort for several weeks.
  - Cats with mandibular or maxillary SCC can have temporary responses to chemotherapy and radiation, but side effects may necessitate placement of a feeding tube. The occasional cat with a small lesion may have a greatly extended survival time with surgery, radiation, and chemotherapy.
  - Case selection for multimodality treatment is important in both dogs and cats, and owners need to have realistic expectations for the success of the therapy.

SUGGESTED READING

Bertone ER, et al: Environmental and lifestyle risk factors for oral squamous cell carcinoma in domestic cats. *J Vet Intern Med* 17:557, 2003.

Boria PA, et al: Evaluation of cisplatin combined with piroxicam for the treatment of oral malignant melanoma and oral squamous cell carcinoma in dogs. *J Am Vet Med Assoc* 224:388, 2004.

Klein MK: Multimodality therapy for head and neck cancer. *Vet Clin Small Anim* 33:615, 2003.

McEntee M: Summary of results of cancer treatment with radiation therapy. In Morrison WB (ed): *Cancer in Dogs and Cats*, ed 2. Jackson, WY. Teton NewMedia, 2002, pp 412–416.

Snyder LA, et al: p53 expression and environmental tobacco smoke exposure in feline oral squamous cell carcinoma. *Vet Pathol* 41:209, 2004.

AUTHOR: **LAURA D. GARRETT**

EDITOR: **KENNETH M. RASSNICK**

Stab Wounds

BASIC INFORMATION

DEFINITION

- Low-energy impact, penetrating injuries inflicted by sharp instruments such as knives and screwdrivers and resulting in localized tissue trauma.
- This topic covers nonaccidental/malicious injuries causing incised wounds (cuts) and/or stab wounds.

SYNONYM(S)

Knife wounds

EPIDEMIOLOGY

SPECIES, AGE, SEX

- Animals of any signalment.
- Animals sustaining nonaccidental/malicious physical injuries are significantly more likely to be male than female; this gender difference may apply to stab wounds specifically.

GENETICS AND BREED PREDISPOSITION

- Certain breeds (e.g., Staffordshire bull terrier) have been shown to be at markedly greater risk for nonaccidental/malicious physical injuries.
- Conversely, other breeds (e.g., Labrador retriever) are at markedly lower risk.

- Whether these breed predilections apply specifically to stab wounds remains to be proven.

RISK FACTORS

- Stabbing wounds are almost invariably the result of malicious intention, although stab injuries from falls (e.g., onto pointed fenceposts) have also been described.
- Working dogs with exposure to potentially dangerous encounters may be at greater risk
- Outdoor cats

CLINICAL PRESENTATION

HISTORY, CHIEF COMPLAINT

- Usually acute onset of signs.
- Victim may be a working dog recently involved in a violent encounter.
- Unless an act of violence is evident or clear malicious intent is suspected, history may be vague.
- Repeated presentations for treatment of unexplained or poorly explained injuries should raise the suspicion of nonaccidental/malicious injury.
- Chief complaint (e.g., dyspnea, skin laceration, abdominal discomfort) may suggest localization of the wound.
- Animals with a minor, previously unattended wound may present for signs associated with infection.

PHYSICAL EXAM FINDINGS

- Obvious skin laceration
- Fever or hypothermia with infection
- Dyspnea or respiratory distress with lacerations to the chest or neck
- Abdominal distention or discomfort with abdominal wounds
- Tachycardia, tachypnea, and collapse with major hemorrhage

ETIOLOGY AND PATHOPHYSIOLOGY

- Injury reflects the shape and length of the weapon, the location of the injury, and the direction of impact.
- In addition to the initial injury, further injury can result from injudicious removal of the weapon, which may involve twisting and dragging of the blade on its tract out of the wound.
- Penetrating wounds to the thorax or neck may cause cardiovascular collapse if major vascular structures or the heart are involved.
- Tension pneumothorax can result from injury to lung or major airway strictures.
- Penetrating wounds to the abdomen may cause injury to visceral organs, resulting in vascular injury, leakage of intestinal contents, leakage of bile, or leakage of urine.
- Laceration to the diaphragm can result in herniation of visceral organs and potentially bowel strangulation months to years later.
- Penetrating wounds to the head may cause hemorrhage or infection in the brain or eyes.

DIAGNOSIS

DIFFERENTIAL DIAGNOSIS

- Impaling from sticks
- Arrows
- Gunshot wounds
- Hemoabdomen
- Uroabdomen
- Spontaneous pneumothorax
- Sepsis

INITIAL DATABASE

- Complete blood count (CBC), platelet count
- Serum chemistry profile
- Survey radiography
- Abdominal ultrasonography

ADVANCED OR CONFIRMATORY TESTING

As needed, based on extent and location of wound(s):

- CT scan
- MRI
- Selective angiography
- Fistulography
- Wound culture
- Esophagoscopy

TREATMENT

THERAPEUTIC GOAL(S)

- Control blood loss
- Maintain adequate oxygenation and ventilation
- Control infection
- Manage the wound(s)

ACUTE GENERAL TREATMENT

- Control of airway and ventilation
- Cardiovascular resuscitation with IV fluid therapy or blood products
- Surgical exploration via celiotomy if applicable
- Surgical exploration via thoracotomy if applicable
- Surgical exploration of neck if applicable, with consideration of esophascopy to identify esophageal injury
- Debride and close (with a drain) minor stab wounds to the soft tissue
- Broad-spectrum antibiotics

CHRONIC TREATMENT

Short-term antibiotic therapy

POSSIBLE COMPLICATIONS

- Unidentified laceration to the diaphragm will often result in a diaphragmatic hernia days to years later
- Wound sepsis

PROGNOSIS AND OUTCOME

- Depends on localization and severity of injury
- Depends on response to therapy

PEARLS & CONSIDERATIONS

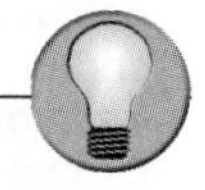

COMMENTS

- Because a stabbing wound is externally small, it may go undetected in an animal with only vague signs. Therefore, close inspection of the skin (including clipping of hair when necessary) is recommended when a small cutaneous wound exists in an ill animal.
- History of a recent interaction involving a sharp instrument should prompt the clinician to perform a thorough search for suspicious injuries.
- Survey radiography or advanced imaging, including CT scan or MRI, may identify internal injuries, such as hematoma, abscess, or subcutaneous emphysema.
- Because removal of an embedded blade may inflict additional tissue trauma, the injured animal should be kept quiet and as immobile as possible in the field; this is immediately followed by presentation of the patient to an emergency service for stabilization and cautious withdrawal of the instrument where radiographic, surgical, and supportive care (e.g., blood transfusion) facilities are available.

SUGGESTED READING

Munro HMC, Thrusfield MV: Battered pets: Nonaccidental physical injuries found in dogs and cats. *J Sm Anim Prac* 42:279-290, 2001.

AUTHORS: **THERESE E. O'TOOLE, ETIENNE CÔTÉ**

EDITOR: **ELIZABETH ROZANSKI**

Steroid Responsive Meningitis-Arteritis

BASIC INFORMATION

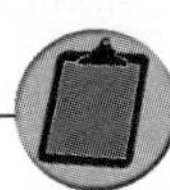

DEFINITION

Steroid responsive meningitis-arteritis (SRMA) is an immune-mediated disorder characterized by inflammation of the meninges and meningeal arteries. The non-neurologic aspects of this disorder are discussed under juvenile polyarteritis (see Juvenile Polyarteritis [Beagle Pain Syndrome], p 613).

SYNONYM(S)

SRMA
Corticosteroid-responsive meningomyelitis
Aseptic meningitis
Beagle pain syndrome
Canine juvenile polyarteritis syndrome
Sterile suppurative meningitis

EPIDEMIOLOGY

SPECIES, AGE, SEX: Young adult dogs (6 to 18 months old), but any age is possible. There is no sex predilection.

GENETICS AND BREED PREDISPOSITION

- Genetic factors are possible, but have not been proven
- Most often diagnosed in boxers, Bernese mountain dogs, and beagles; however, any breed can be affected

RISK FACTORS: No proven risk factors. Immune response may occur secondary to environmental or infectious causes.

CONTAGION AND ZOONOSIS: Not known. Infectious cause has not been demonstrated.

GEOGRAPHY AND SEASONALITY: Reported worldwide. No seasonality.

ASSOCIATED CONDITIONS AND DISORDERS: May occur concurrently in dogs with immune-mediated polyarthritis.

CLINICAL PRESENTATION

DISEASE FORMS/SUBTYPES

- Classical (acute)
- Chronic

HISTORY, CHIEF COMPLAINT

- Classical (acute): cervical hyperesthesia and rigidity, fever, stiff gait, lethargy
- Chronic: as with acute disease, but with additional complaints suggestive of spinal cord dysfunction (proprioceptive deficits, paresis, ataxia)

PHYSICAL EXAM FINDINGS

- Typical of meningitis.
  - Cervical pain and rigidity; stiff, stilted gait; fever; lethargy.
- In more protracted cases: gait abnormalities, proprioceptive deficits, back pain. Other neurologic signs are less commonly reported.

ETIOLOGY AND PATHOPHYSIOLOGY

- Idiopathic: possibly an autoimmune condition.
- Classical (acute): histologic analysis demonstrates moderate to marked meningitis characterized by infiltration of neutrophils, macrophages, lymphocytes, and plasma cells; and degenerative changes and perivascular inflammation of the meningeal arteries. Lesions are most commonly found in the cervical spinal cord.
- Chronic: histologic analysis demonstrates moderate to marked fibrosis and patchy mineralization of the meninges.

DIAGNOSIS

DIFFERENTIAL DIAGNOSIS

- Infectious meningitis (bacterial, viral, protozoal, fungal)
- Diskospondylitis
- Inflammatory, noninfectious meningitis (e.g., granulomatous meningoencephalomyelitis [GME])
- Intervertebral disk disease
- Neoplasia (e.g., spinal meningioma, lymphoma, malignant histiocytosis)

INITIAL DATABASE

- Complete blood count: leukocytosis, neutrophilia with left shift; may be normal in chronic cases
- Serum biochemistry profile: usually normal
- Urinalysis: usually normal
- Survey spinal radiographs: should be normal

ADVANCED OR CONFIRMATORY TESTING

- IgA (serum or cerebrospinal fluid [CSF]) is often elevated and supports the diagnosis.
- CSF analysis often reveals an elevated protein level and white blood cell count with sterile neutrophilic pleocytosis in the acute stage of disease. Chronic cases may have normal CSF or mononuclear pleocytosis.
- CSF culture and sensitivity should be negative.
- Infectious disease titers and/or advanced imaging (magnetic resonance imaging [MRI], computed tomography [CT], myelography) may be required to rule out other diseases.

TREATMENT

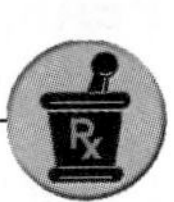

THERAPEUTIC GOAL(S)

Judicious immunosuppression

ACUTE GENERAL TREATMENT

- Prednisone: initially 2 mg/kg PO q 24h for 1 to 2 days, then reduce to 1 mg/kg PO q 24h for 2 to 4 weeks, then slowly taper by 25% every 3 to 4 weeks to lowest effective dose
- Consider gastrointestinal (GI) protective agents (e.g., famotidine 0.5 mg/kg PO or IV q 12-24h, sucralfate 1/4 to 1 g PO q 8h)
- Analgesics (e.g., Tramadol 2 mg/kg PO q 8-12h, or amantadine 2 mg/kg PO q 24h for 4-6 weeks).

CHRONIC TREATMENT

Additional immunosuppressive medications may be required. Consider mycophenolate (CellCept, 5-10 mg/kg PO q 12h), azathioprine (Imuran 2 mg/kg PO q 24h × 5 days then q 48h), or cyclosporine.

DRUG INTERACTIONS

- Drug interactions or altered metabolism of medications have been reported between corticosteroids and amphotericin B, furosemide, thiazide diuretics, digitalis glycosides, cyclosporine, phenytoin, phenobarbital, and mitotane.
- All immunosuppressive drugs carry the risk of excessive immune suppression, and some may have other (e.g., bone marrow suppressant) effects.
- Corticosteroids should not be given concurrently with NSAIDs or other potentially ulcerogenic medications.

POSSIBLE COMPLICATIONS

Corticosteroid side effects—polyuria, polydipsia, polyphagia, weight gain, GI ulceration, iatrogenic hyperadrenocorticism, etc.

RECOMMENDED MONITORING

- Neurologic exam every 4 to 6 weeks
- Ideally, CSF analysis should be repeated every 4 to 6 weeks prior to reduction in medication dosage

PROGNOSIS AND OUTCOME

- Classical (acute): generally good to excellent prognosis if treated early and aggressively
- Chronic: prognosis is fair to guarded due to frequent relapses

- Reports indicate 60% of dogs can be cured. Remaining patients require some level of corticosteroids long-term

PEARLS & CONSIDERATIONS

COMMENTS

- SRMA has a good to excellent prognosis when patients are treated early in disease
- CSF analysis should be performed early in the course of disease

CLIENT EDUCATION

Warn owners of corticosteroid side effects (e.g., polyuria, polydipsia, polyphagia, weight gain, GI ulceration, iatrogenic hyperadrenocorticism)

SUGGESTED READING

Cizinauskas S, Jaggy A, Tipold A: Long-term treatment of dogs with steroid-responsive meningitis-arteritis: clinical, laboratory and therapeutic results. *J Sm Anim Pract* 41:295–301, 2000.

Meric SM, Perman V, Hardy R: Corticosteroid-responsive meningitis in ten dogs. *J Am Anim Hosp Assoc* 21:677–684, 1985.

Tipold A, Jaggy A: Steroid responsive meningitis-arteritis in dogs: Long-term study of 32 cases. *J Sm Anim Pract* 35:311–316, 1994.

AUTHOR: **MARK T. TROXEL**
EDITOR: **CURTIS W. DEWEY**

Stifle Joint Derangement

BASIC INFORMATION

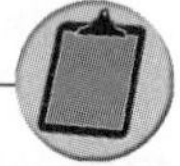

DEFINITION

Complete luxation of the stifle joint in which ligaments, joint capsule, and menisci have been damaged

SYNONYM(S)

Multiple ligament injury of the stifle
Stifle joint luxation

EPIDEMIOLOGY

RISK FACTORS: Trauma from falls, fights, or motor vehicle accidents.

CLINICAL PRESENTATION

HISTORY, CHIEF COMPLAINT: Fall, fighting, or injury caused by a motor vehicle or firearm.

PHYSICAL EXAM FINDINGS

- Non–weight-bearing extremity
- Extreme stifle joint pain
- Thickened or distorted stifle
- Severe joint instability

ETIOLOGY AND PATHOPHYSIOLOGY

- Uncommon condition of the stifle joint; 12% of all cases involving ligament injuries in dogs
- Extreme, unnatural stress applied to joint causing multiple ligamentous failures
- Both cruciate ligaments, at least one collateral ligament, a joint capsule, and one or both menisci are torn or avulsed

DIAGNOSIS

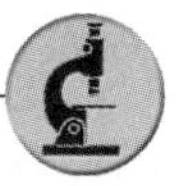

DIFFERENTIAL DIAGNOSIS

Femoral or tibial fractures involving the stifle joint

INITIAL DATABASE

- Orthopedic examination to confirm stifle joint instability; palpation performed with adequate pain management
- Complete blood count (CBC) and serum biochemistry panel based on American Society of Anesthesiologists (ASA) patient classification (see p 1334).
- Thoracic and spinal radiographs when body trauma is suspected
- Craniocaudal and mediolateral radiographs of stifle

TREATMENT

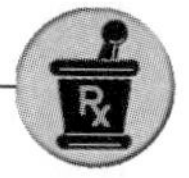

THERAPEUTIC GOAL(S)

Restoration of stifle joint function (congruency, motion) by ligament repair or substitution

ACUTE GENERAL TREATMENT

Surgical intervention:

- Inspect and remove damaged parts of menisci
- Suture meniscal tibial ligaments if torn and menisci are intact
- Debride remnants of cruciate ligaments and use intracapsular or extracapsular repairs
- Primary repair of collateral ligaments or replacement with synthetic sutures
- Restoration of caudal cruciate ligament function is not necessary
- Possible transarticular pinning of the stifle joint for immobilization during initial healing of soft tissues
- Temporary transarticular external skeletal fixation with the joint fixed at normal standing angle

CHRONIC TREATMENT

- External coaptation (soft padded bandage, half splint, or Schroeder-Thomas splint) for 3 to 4 weeks
- Transarticular pin or transarticular external skeletal fixation left in position for at least 3 weeks
- Initially, exercise restriction
- Following removal of external coaptation, physical therapy is initiated to restore joint function(s)
- Increased physical activity (rehabilitation) is allowed as stifle joint function is improving (see Physical Rehabilitation, p 1300)

POSSIBLE COMPLICATIONS

- Persistent stifle joint instability
- Osteoarthritis secondary to trauma and instability
- Reduced range of motion due to fibrosis

RECOMMENDED MONITORING

Monthly monitoring for stifle joint stability and range of motion

PROGNOSIS AND OUTCOME

- Good for restoration of adequate joint function.
- Working or athletic dogs generally do not return to preinjury status.
- If treatment fails, arthrodesis or limb amputation can be considered.

PEARLS & CONSIDERATIONS

COMMENTS

Although prognosis appears grim during initial presentation, appropriate surgical techniques will often result in a satisfactory restoration of function

SUGGESTED READING

Piermattei DL, Flo GL: Luxation of the stifle joint. In Piermattei DL, Flo GL (eds): *Handbook of Small Animal Orthopedics and Fracture Repair*, ed 3. Philadelphia, WB Saunders, 1997, pp 565–568.

Vasseur PB: Stifle joint. In Slatter D (ed): *Textbook of Small Animal* Surgery, ed 3. Philadelphia, WB Saunders, 2003, pp 2119–2122.

AUTHOR: **JAMES D. LINCOLN**
EDITOR: **JOSEPH HARARI**

Stomatitis

BASIC INFORMATION

DEFINITION

Any inflammation of the mouth (stoma); as used in clinical veterinary medicine, the term refers to severe inflammation or ulceration of nongingival tissues

SYNONYM(S)

Lymphocytic-plasmacytic gingivitis
Stomatitis (cats)
Ulcerative stomatitis (dogs)

EPIDEMIOLOGY

SPECIES, AGE, SEX: Cats and dogs; mature animals of many breeds, both sexes.

GENETICS AND BREED PREDISPOSITION

- Cats: no known genetic predisposition, although the condition sometimes is seen in families or group-housed cats (may be viral-associated rather than genetic)
- Dogs: ulcerative stomatitis: familial disorder in Maltese dogs, although no genetic analysis has been reported

RISK FACTORS

- Cats: feline leukemia virus (FeLV) or feline immunodeficiency virus (FIV) infection. Unclear association with calicivirus (which can be isolated from most clinically affected cats, and these calicivirus strains cause acute oral ulcerative infection; however, cats with experimentally induced infection do not go on to develop chronic stomatitis). FIV- and calicivirus-positive cats tend to have more severe disease
- Dogs: none known

CONTAGION AND ZOONOSIS

- Cats and dogs: bacteria (many species, all found in mouths of normal animals)
- Cats: viruses (calicivirus, herpesvirus less commonly), possible source of viral infection to other cats
- No known zoonotic risk

ASSOCIATED CONDITIONS AND DISORDERS: In both cats and dogs, there is very often severe gingivitis. In cats, there are often teeth that have odontoclastic resorptive lesions (ORLs); see Resorption Lesions, Feline Odontoclastic (FORL), p 960.

CLINICAL PRESENTATION

DISEASE FORMS/SUBTYPES

- Cats: symmetric, clinically obvious bright red ulcerated lesions of the buccal mucosa (upper or lower lip) or the area lateral to the palatoglossal fold (Fig. I-166) and sometimes the lateral margins of the tongue or the pharyngeal walls. The association of this condition with "juvenile gingivitis" in cats is unclear (Fig. I-167).
- Dogs: Ulcers are found most often on the upper lip in areas that normally lie against the plaque-laden surfaces of crowns of teeth. In severely affected dogs, lesions are sometimes found on lateral margins of the tongue and on edges of the hard palate adjacent to teeth.

HISTORY, CHIEF COMPLAINT: Cats and dogs: signs of pain on eating or when owner touches the mouth; unkempt coat; drooling from mouth; sometimes weight loss.

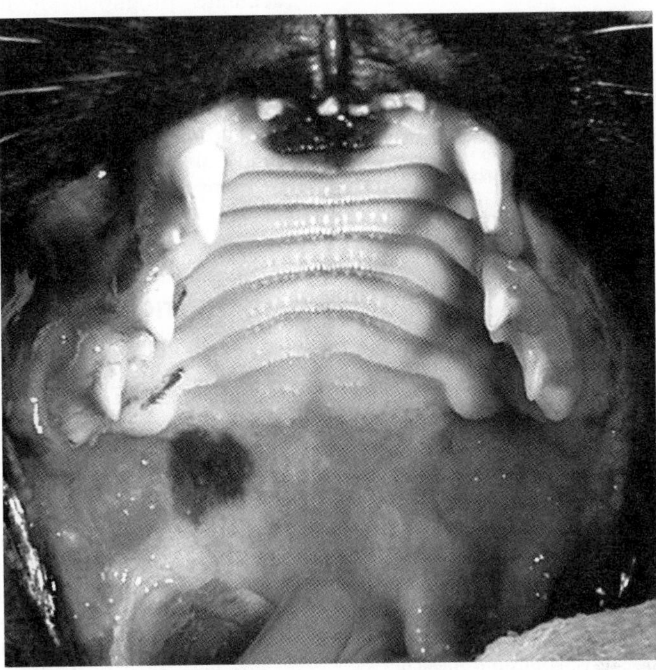

FIGURE I-166 Cat with inflammation of the gingiva, alveolar mucosa, buccal mucosa, and mucosa lateral to the palatoglossal folds. Note that the mucosa of the hard palate is usually not inflamed in cats with stomatitis. Courtesy of Dr. Alexander M. Reiter, University of Pennsylvania.

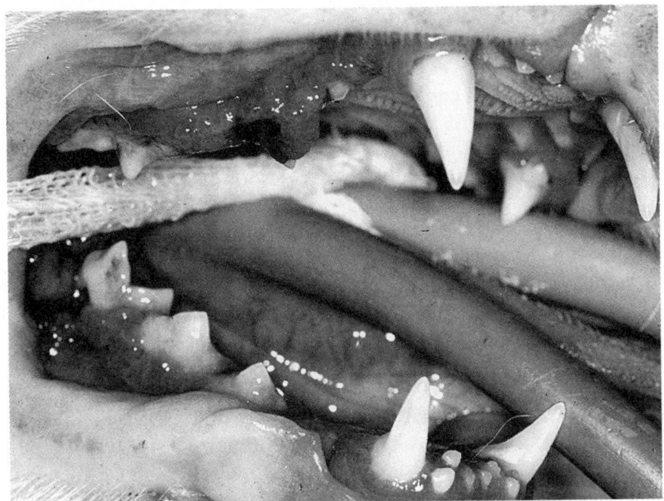

FIGURE I-167 Young cat with inflammation of the gingiva, alveolar mucosa, and buccal mucosa; note the proliferative changes of gingival tissue, entirely covering the crown of the right upper third premolar tooth. Courtesy of Dr. Alexander M. Reiter, University of Pennsylvania.

PHYSICAL EXAM FINDINGS

- Oral lesions as already described
- Cats: rarely any other physical abnormalities, unless the cat is FIV or FeLV positive
- Dogs: rarely any other physical abnormalities

ETIOLOGY AND PATHOPHYSIOLOGY

- Cats: undefined immunopathy (associated with viral infections, as already described).
- Dogs: undefined immunopathy.
- The role of dental plaque bacteria in the etiology of these conditions is unclear. Bacteria clearly play a role in the progression of the disease, and control of oral bacteria can be a critical contributor to successful management. The most reliable treatment in both species is extraction of all teeth in affected areas of the mouth, thus eliminating bacteria-laden dental plaque deposits.
- There has been interest in *Bartonella* spp. as a cause or contributory factor in feline stomatitis cases. As of the time of this writing, there is no evidence that cats with stomatitis are more likely to be *Bartonella*-positive than nonstomatitis cats (nor that they respond to treatment recommended for *Bartonella* infection [e.g., azithromycin]).

DIAGNOSIS

DIFFERENTIAL DIAGNOSIS

- In both species, periodontal disease
- In cats, squamous cell carcinoma (SCC) of the gingival area, lip, or tongue; other neoplasms are much less common
- In cats and dogs, eosinophilic granuloma (though these are typically isolated raised lesions on the tongue, lip, or palate in cats or irregularly protuberant lesions on lateral margins of the tongue and soft palate in dogs)
- In cats, any other disease that can cause emaciation
- In dogs, autoimmune disease (though the location of the lesions is a reliable differentiating factor; typically, autoimmune disease with oral lesions is either confined primarily to the mucocutaneous junctions of the lips or is widespread across the buccal mucosa and hard palate) and neoplasia

INITIAL DATABASE

- Cats: FIV and FeLV tests; complete blood count (CBC), serum chemistry profile, and urinalysis are indicated for ruling out distant organ disease. Total white blood cell (WBC) count may be low, normal, or high, and there is very often hypergammaglobulinemia (largely consisting of antibodies to oral bacteria)
- Dogs: preanesthetic screen

ADVANCED OR CONFIRMATORY TESTING

- Biopsy of representative lesions is often performed in cats. The lesions are usually reported as caused by chronic inflammation, with a mixture of acute and chronic inflammatory cells (particularly lymphocytes and plasma cells). Since this pattern is expected when immune-responsive tissue is exposed to bacteria chronically, this biopsy information is rarely of clinical value (it does not assist the clinician in making a more accurate prognosis or determining treatment).
- In dogs, the characteristic location and appearance of the lesions rarely requires confirmatory biopsy; as for cats, no useful information (other than ruling out other diseases) is provided by biopsy.

TREATMENT

THERAPEUTIC GOAL(S)

Ideally, eliminate the condition. More importantly, reduce the severity and extent of the inflammation so that the animal can eat, drink, and groom.

ACUTE GENERAL TREATMENT

- Cats with large, severe lesions:
  - Antibacterial (e.g., amoxicillin-clavulanate 10–20 mg/kg PO q 12h) and anti-inflammatory (typically a corticosteroid, such as prednisone 0.5–1 mg/kg PO q 24h) treatment and nursing care (nutritional support, grooming), followed 1 to 2 weeks later by anesthesia, oral examination including dental radiographs, extraction of mobile teeth and teeth with odontoclastic resorptive lesions, and thorough scaling/polishing of remaining teeth. Follow with antibacterial treatment for 2 weeks, plus daily oral hygiene home care (chlorhexidine gel, brushing or rubbing the surface of the teeth daily, dental diet as the primary food) as soon as the cat will tolerate it.
  - Reexamine the animal 2 weeks following dental treatment.
  - If the cat is significantly improved, continue the oral hygiene regimen and reexamine the animal in 2 to 3 months.
  - If there is some improvement but there are still areas of severe inflammation, start prednisone treatment (initially 2 mg/kg PO q 24h) and reexamine the animal in another 2 weeks; if there is further improvement, titrate the prednisone dosage to the minimal effective level (alternative: 5.5 mg/kg methylprednisolone or 0.1–0.2 mg/kg triamcinolone SQ once every 4 to 8 weeks).
  - If there is no improvement at all following dental treatment and prednisolone treatment, and there still are teeth in the diseased sections of the mouth, extract all remaining teeth.
  - Lesions will continue in about 20% of cats following extraction of all teeth. Many treatments have been used in severely affected cats, with no agreement on the most successful therapy. Continuous or intermittent corticosteroid, cyclosporine, or gold-salt therapy as well as multiple laser treatment of local lesions are examples.
- Dogs with ulcerative stomatitis:
  - Systemic antibacterial treatment (e.g., amoxicillin-clavulanate 10–20 mg/kg PO q 12h), chlorhexidine gel, and nursing care (soft food) followed 1 to 2 weeks later by anesthesia; oral examination including dental radiographs, extraction of mobile teeth, and thorough scaling/polishing of remaining teeth. Follow with metronidazole treatment (30 mg/kg PO q 24h) for 2 weeks, plus daily oral hygiene home care (brushing or rubbing the surface of the teeth daily, dental diet as the primary food) if the dog will tolerate it.
  - If there is significant improvement, continue the chlorhexidine home care program and reexamine the dog in 1 to 2 months. Excellent plaque control is the key to continued comfort of the dog. Some dogs may start to develop lesions (and oral pain) soon after completion of metronidazole treatment; in such cases, restart metronidazole at 30 mg/kg PO q 24h for 1 to 2 weeks, then gradually reduce dose (continuous treatment at 10 mg/kg PO every other day provides good control in some animals that relapse if metronidazole is completely discontinued).
  - If there is no improvement following the initial treatment regime, extract all remaining teeth, and if necessary, start prednisone treatment at 2 mg/kg PO q 24h, titrating down to the lowest dose/frequency compatible with stability of the animal.

CHRONIC TREATMENT

Chronic or lifelong treatment is often needed for these feline and canine cases.

DRUG INTERACTIONS

Some of the immunosuppressive drugs have severe potential side effects, and the dose/frequency should always be titrated to the minimum dose/frequency that is compatible with the comfort of the animal.

POSSIBLE COMPLICATIONS

The major complication is failure to obtain clinical improvement. Explaining the (poorly understood) nature of the disease and the need for frequent reexaminations and treatment adjustments to the owner is an important contributor to success.

RECOMMENDED MONITORING

Frequent reexaminations, with daily examination of the mouth by the owner.

PROGNOSIS AND OUTCOME

Variable, which is not surprising, given the lack of full understanding of the disease process and the potential side effects of the anti-inflammatory/immunosuppressive medications often required

PEARLS & CONSIDERATIONS

COMMENTS

- There is no magic bullet. Find what works best for a particular animal and stick with it.
- Extraction of teeth should be an early option, not a last resort.
- Bring the owner along while working with the animal.

PREVENTION

Good oral hygiene from an early age may prevent development of disease in at-risk animals. However, these lesions (in both dogs and cats) are often very painful, which makes animal compliance with oral hygiene procedures questionable. Work with the owners and the animals.

CLIENT EDUCATION

The most important considerations are taking time to explain the disease to the owner and listening to the owner to ensure he or she understands what is being said.

SUGGESTED READING

Harvey CE: The oral cavity. In Chandler EA, Gaskell RM, Gaskell CJ (eds): *Feline Medicine and Therapeutics*, ed 3. Oxford, UK, Blackwell Publishing, 2004, pp 379–395.

AUTHOR: **COLIN E. HARVEY**
EDITOR: **ALEXANDER M. REITER**

Storage Diseases

BASIC INFORMATION

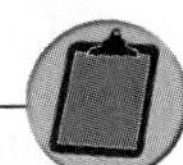

DEFINITION

Disorders that result in the accumulation of a specific substance within tissues, generally due to a congenital deficiency of an enzyme or cofactor necessary for further metabolism of the substance. This discussion will be limited to the lysosomal storage disorders, in which the substance that fails to be processed accumulates in the lysosomes.

SYNONYM(S)

Lysosomal storage disorders
Storage disorders

EPIDEMIOLOGY

SPECIES, AGE, SEX

- Dogs and cats
- Age of onset varies:
  - Signs typically become apparent within the first 6 months of life and continue to progress over 1 to 2 years.
  - For some diseases, signs may not become apparent until much later in life.
- No known sex predilection

GENETICS AND BREED PREDISPOSITION

- Storage disorders generally have an inherited basis but could occur as spontaneous mutations.
- Most have an autosomal recessive patterns of inheritance.
- See Disease Forms/Subtypes below.

RISK FACTORS: Affected relatives or breeds that are at risk.

CLINICAL PRESENTATION

DISEASE FORMS/SUBTYPES

- Sphingolipidoses:
  - Globoid cell leukodystrophy (Krabbe's disease)
    - Most common in West Highland white terriers and cairn terriers
    - Also reported in Pomeranian, miniature poodle, basset hound, beagle, blue tick hound, and domestic short-haired cats
    - Clinical signs: multifocal; predominantly ataxia, pelvic limb paresis/paralysis
  - Gangliosidosis I (GMI) (Norman-Landing disease)
    - Siamese and domestic short-haired cats
    - English springer spaniel, Portuguese water dog, beagle crosses, husky
    - Clinical signs: multifocal; predominantly cerebellar dysfunction; may progress to tetraplegia
  - Gangliosidosis II (GMII) (Derry's disease)
    - Korat, Siamese, domestic short-haired cats
    - German short-haired pointer, Japanese spaniel
    - Clinical signs: multifocal; predominantly cerebellar dysfunction; may progress to tetraplegia
  - Glucocerebrosidase deficiency (Gaucher's disease)
    - Australian silky terriers
    - Clinical signs: multifocal; predominantly cerebellar ataxia, tremors, hyperactivity
  - Sphingomyelinase deficiency, cholesterol transport defect (Neimann-Pick disease)
    - Siamese, Balinese, domestic short-haired cats
    - Miniature poodle
    - Clinical signs: ataxia, head tremors, paraparesis, weight loss, depression
- Glycoproteinoses:
  - Fucosidosis
    - English springer spaniels
    - Clinical signs: predominantly behavioral changes, ataxia, deterioration of vision and hearing, weight loss; possibly loss of bark, dysphagia
  - Mannosidosis
    - Persian, domestic short-haired, domestic long-haired cats
    - Clinical signs include skeletal abnormalities, ataxia, head tremor; possibly gingival hyperplasia
  - Galactosialidosis
    - Schipperke
    - Clinical signs: predominantly ataxia
- Mucopolysaccharidoses:
  - Mucopolysaccharidosis type I (Hurler's syndrome)
    - Domestic short-haired cats
    - Mixed-breed dogs, Plott hounds
    - Clinical signs: predominantly pelvic limb gait disorder without overt neurologic deficits; patients may have hyperextensible joints and plantigrade stance; skeletal and craniofacial abnormalities may be present
  - Mucopolysaccharidosis type II (Hunter's disease)
    - Siamese, domestic short-haired cats
    - Miniature pinscher
  - Mucopolysaccharidosis type III (Sanfilippo's syndrome)

- Type IIIA: Heparan sulfate sulfamidase deficiency
  - Wirehaired dachshunds, New Zealand huntaway dogs
- Type IIIB: *N*-acetyl-α-*D*-glucosaminidase deficiency
  - Schipperkes
- Clinical signs: not well described; predominantly tremors and ataxia
- Mucopolysaccharidosis type VI (Maroteaux-Lamy syndrome)
  - Primarily affects cats
  - Clinical signs: predominantly skeletal malformations (kyphosis, facial deformities); upper motor neuron paraparesis
- Mucopolysaccharidosis type VII
  - β-Glucuronidase deficiency
  - German shepherd dogs, mixed-breed dogs, domestic short-haired cats
  - Clinical signs: not well described; skeletal deformities, ataxia, corneal cloudiness
- Glygogen storage disorders:
  - Glycogenosis type II
    - Lapland dogs
    - Clinical signs: muscular weakness, exercise intolerance, collapse
  - Glycogenosis type III
    - German shepherds, Akitas
    - Clinical signs: predominantly neuromuscular (weakness, exercise intolerance)
  - Glycogenosis type IV
    - Norwegian forest cats
    - Clinical signs: predominantly muscle tremors, weakness, muscle atrophy, contractures; may exhibit neuromuscular weakness or dysphagia
  - Glycogenosis type VII
    - English springer spaniel
    - Clinical signs: not well described; predominantly muscle weakness
  - Mucolipidosis type II
    - Domestic short-haired cats
    - Clinical signs: not well described; may include skeletal malformations
- Other storage disorders:
  - Ceroid lipofuscinosis (CL) type VIII
    - English setter
  - Unclassified CL
    - Reported in numerous dog breeds, including American bulldog, Australian shepherd, Border collie, Chihuahua, cocker spaniel, Australian cattle dog, dalmatian, dachshund, golden retriever, Labrador retriever, miniature schnauzer, Polish Lowland sheepdog, saluki, Tibetan terrier, Yugoslavian sheepdog, Welsh corgi
    - Siamese cats
    - Clinical signs: predominantly diffuse forebrain disease, including behavioral changes, aggression, central blindness; may also exhibit ataxia, head tremor, hypermetria
  - LaFora's disease
    - Miniature wirehaired dachshund, basset hound, beagle, poodle, and mixed-breed dogs

HISTORY, CHIEF COMPLAINT

- Normal at birth.
- Clinical signs typically become apparent within the first 6 months of life and slowly progress over 1 to 2 years.
- Intention tremors are common chief complaints.
- Specific presenting complaints depend on the specific storage disease as already described:
  - Forebrain: may present for behavioral changes, loss of learned behavior, seizures
  - Cerebellum: may present for intention tremors, ataxia, dysmetria
  - Spinal cord or peripheral neuropathy/myopathy: may present for ataxia, weakness, exercise intolerance
- May have history of affected relatives.

PHYSICAL EXAM FINDINGS

- General physical examination is typically unremarkable.
- Neurologic exam findings depend on the specific storage disease; findings may include:
  - Mentation changes (behavioral changes, aggression, loss of learned behavior)
  - Menace deficits, central blindness
  - Gait abnormalities (ataxia, paresis)
  - Proprioceptive deficits
  - Intention tremors
  - Exercise intolerance
- In some cases of the following storage diseases, hepatomegaly (gangliosidosis, glycogenosis types I and III, mannosidosis, mucopolysaccharidoses types I and VII, and sphingomyelinosis) or splenomegaly (mucopolysaccharidosis type I, sphingomyelinosis) have been noted due to accumulation of storage products in the cells of these organs.
- Some subtypes may exhibit skeletal or connective tissue abnormalities (mannosidosis, mucopolysaccharidoses types I and VI, mucolipidosis type II).
- Lens opacification may be present.

ETIOLOGY AND PATHOPHYSIOLOGY

- Mutation causes loss of enzyme function, but the mechanisms by which accumulation of storage product leads to neurologic deficits are not well understood.
  - The substance accumulating may be toxic to cells.
  - The deficient enzyme may result in the lack of important substances downstream.

DIAGNOSIS

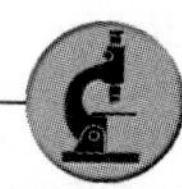

DIFFERENTIAL DIAGNOSIS

Any slowly progressive multifocal or diffuse encephalopathy, cerebellar dysfunction, or neuromuscular dysfunction should be considered as a differential diagnosis.

- Degenerative:
  - Leukodystrophy
  - Neuronal or cerebellar abiotrophy
  - Neuraxonal dystrophy
  - Other breed-related axonopathies and polyneuropathies
- Infectious:
  - Protozoal (e.g., *Neospora caninum, Toxoplasma gondii, Hepatozoon americanum*)
  - Fungal (e.g., *Cryptococcus neoformans, Coccidiodes immitis, Histoplasma capsulatum, Blastomyces dermatitidis*)
  - Viral (e.g., canine distemper virus, feline immunodeficiency virus [FIV] infection, feline leukemia virus [FeLV] infection)
- Noninfectious inflammatory:
  - Necrotizing meningoencephalitis of small-breed dogs
  - Granulomatous meningoencephalomyelitis (GME)
  - Eosinophilic meningoencephalitis
- Metabolic:
  - Organic acidurias (e.g., *L*-2-hydroxyglutaric aciduria in the Staffordshire bull terrier, malonic aciduria in the Maltese)
  - Mitochondrial encephalopathies (e.g., pyruvate dehydrogenase deficiency in Sussex spaniels)
  - Hepatic encephalopathy
- Neoplasia, primary or metastatic
- Toxic (e.g., lead)

INITIAL DATABASE

- Complete blood count (CBC), serum biochemical profile, urinalysis
  - Findings:
    - May reveal leukocytes containing vacuoles or storage product
    - Some storage disorders produce elevated creatine kinase (CK) activity
    - Some disorders show evidence of multiple organs that are affected
  - Performed to rule out other metabolic disorders
- Serologic titers
  - Performed to rule out infectious diseases

ADVANCED OR CONFIRMATORY TESTING

- Supportive diagnostic tests:
  - Cerebrospinal fluid (CSF) analysis
    - Findings:
      - Typically normal.

- Protein level may be elevated; however, nucleated cell count should remain normal (albuminocytologic dissociation).
- Storage products may occasionally be visible in macrophages or lymphocytes.
- Performed to rule out inflammatory disorders.
- MRI tests
  - Findings:
    - Brain atrophy with secondary ventriculomegaly.
    - Diffuse changes in tissue intensity (due to accumulation of storage products).
  - Performed to rule out other structural abnormalities.
- Confirmatory diagnostic tests (only available for certain storage disorders):
  - Urinalysis (specialized testing)
    - Abnormal metabolites may be detected in urine.
    - Oligosaccharides and glycopeptides can be profiled in urine samples using thin-layer chromatography to determine the particular compound that is accumulating and being excreted.
    - Available for most lysosomal storage diseases.
  - Enzymatic assay
    - Measures lysosomal enzyme activity for a panel of known lysosomal enzymes.
    - Performed using whole blood (leukocytes), kidney or liver biopsy samples, or cultured skin fibroblast cells.
    - Assays are available for some enzymes (i.e., some storage diseases), and the level of activity of an affected animal can be compared to an age-matched control.
    - Since these diseases are most commonly autosomal recessive, an affected animal would have significantly decreased enzyme activity (nearly none), and a heterozygous carrier would have 50% of the enzyme activity of a normal (wild-type) homozygous animal.
  - Molecular genetic testing for affected gene (DNA testing)
    - When the specific mutation has been identified, perform genetic testing to confirm the presence of the mutation.
    - The specific genetic mutation responsible for a disease may vary among different species and breeds, so molecular testing is very specific concerning breed and species for any given disease.
    - Genetic tests could exist for any disease in which the specific genetic mutation has been identified, even though these tests may not be available for public use.
    - Consultation with a neurologist and/or laboratory specialist is recommended.
  - Histopathologic evaluation
    - Tissues used:
      - Peripheral nerve, muscle, liver, or lymph node biopsy may be diagnostic in some cases.
      - Brain biopsy guided by CT scan.
      - Postmortem/necropsy.
    - Provides diagnosis of storage disease in most cases but not of a specific deficit.
    - Requires use of special staining techniques to characterize the specific storage product.

TREATMENT

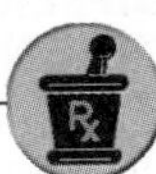

THERAPEUTIC GOAL(S)

- No specific treatment available.
- Limited to supportive care and maintenance of quality of life for as long as possible.
- Future therapeutic options may involve gene therapy or stem cell transplantation.

RECOMMENDED MONITORING

- Progressive neurologic impairment is expected
- Monitoring for quality of life

PROGNOSIS AND OUTCOME

- Grave.
- Short-term survival may be possible because these disorders are generally slowly progressive; however, progression is inevitable.
- Euthanasia is often necessary in the later stages.

PEARLS & CONSIDERATIONS

COMMENTS

- The field of medical genetics is rapidly advancing, and genetic tests and therapies may be available for these disorders in the future.
- Future directions for treatment may eventually include enzyme replacement therapy, as is used for humans who have many of these disorders.
- Consultation with a veterinary neurologist is recommended to obtain the most up-to-date diagnostic and treatment information available.

PREVENTION

- Maintain responsible breeding practices and avoid breeding affected animals.
- Genetic testing is available for a limited number of these storage diseases and may be used for identifying carriers.

CLIENT EDUCATION

- Caution owners about the possibility of personality changes or aggressive behavior associated with these disorders, especially where children may be involved
- Counsel owners concerning the progressive nature of storage disorders and likelihood of eventual euthanasia
- Counsel breeders about the inheritance of the condition and availability of DNA testing

SUGGESTED READING

Coates JR, O'Brien DP: Inherited peripheral neuropathies in dogs and cats. *Vet Clin North Am Small Anim Pract* 34:1361–1401, 2004.

Skelly BJ, et al: Recognition and diagnosis of lysosomal storage diseases in the cat and dog. *J Vet Intern Med* 16:133–141, 2002.

AUTHOR: **REBECCA A. PACKER**

EDITOR: **CURTIS W. DEWEY**

Stridor, Respiratory

BASIC INFORMATION

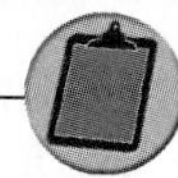

DEFINITION

Stridor: a harsh, high-pitched sound occurring during inspiration due to partial upper airway obstruction

SYNONYM(S)

Stertor (inspiratory noise occurring specifically during sleeping, e.g., snoring)

EPIDEMIOLOGY

SPECIES, AGE, SEX: No predilection given the broad spectrum of possible underlying diseases.

GENETICS AND BREED PREDISPOSITION: Brachycephalic breeds are predisposed to partial upper airway obstruction and stridor.

RISK FACTORS

- Nasal/nasopharyngeal disorders, either through primary obstruction (mass, foreign body, mucosal edema) or secondarily due to obstruction by discharge
- Pharyngeal, laryngeal, and tracheal disorders

ASSOCIATED CONDITIONS AND DISORDERS: Powerful, sustained inspirations against an obstructed upper airway are associated with the development of noncardiogenic pulmonary edema.

CLINICAL PRESENTATION

HISTORY, CHIEF COMPLAINT: Owners may report stridor individually as a chief complaint, or concurrently with other signs suggesting respiratory disease (coughing, nasal discharge, sneezing, dyspnea, epistaxis), pharyngeal disease (gagging, dysphagia), or intermittent complete respiratory obstruction (decreased exercise tolerance, syncope). Clinical signs often may be exacerbated by excitement. Many animals show no clinical signs at rest. Owner may report voice change with laryngeal involvement.

PHYSICAL EXAM FINDINGS

- Stridor of nasal cavity origin: nasal discharge, occlusion of air flow from one or both nostrils, stenotic nares in brachycephalic breeds, stridor disappears with open-mouth breathing, periodontal disease with evidence of tooth root abscessation or tooth loss
- Stridor of pharyngeal, laryngeal, or tracheal origin: coughing, gagging, dyspnea, hyperthermia, open-mouth gasping, unilateral discharge from the ear (sometimes seen in cats with nasopharyngeal polyps)

ETIOLOGY AND PATHOPHYSIOLOGY

- During inspiration, air pressure in the upper airway is low, allowing air to flow in through the nares or mouth and fill the lungs.
- Obstruction narrows airway diameter, causing turbulence proximal to the obstruction during inspiration. The turbulence is audible as stridor.
- Any obstructions of the upper airway can be drawn into the lumen during inspiration (dynamic obstruction), exacerbating the obstruction and causing further airflow turbulence and stridor.
- Stridor may be absent on expiration if the pressure of exhaled air opens the airway (e.g., laryngeal paralysis, other dynamic obstructions).

DIAGNOSIS

DIFFERENTIAL DIAGNOSIS

- Stridor of nasal cavity origin:
  - Brachycephalic syndrome (stenotic nares)
  - Foreign body (nasal)
  - Neoplasia (nasal)
  - Nasopharyngeal polyp
  - Rhinitis (fungal, bacterial, viral, parasitic, tooth root abscess, chronic vomiting or regurgitation)
  - Trauma
  - Coagulopathy
- Stridor of pharyngeal, laryngeal, or tracheal origin:
  - Brachycephalic syndrome (elongated soft palate; everted laryngeal saccules; hypoplastic trachea)
  - Laryngeal paralysis
  - Foreign body (pharyngeal, laryngeal, or tracheal)
  - Neoplasia (pharyngeal, laryngeal, or tracheal)
  - Nasopharyngeal polyp
  - Trauma
  - Coagulopathy
  - Laryngeal or tracheal collapse
  - Tracheal stenosis
  - Extraluminal compression of the trachea (neoplasia, granuloma, cervical lymphadenopathy)

INITIAL DATABASE

- Complete blood count, serum biochemistry profile, and urinalysis to rule out underlying systemic diseases
- Nasal cavity stridor:
  - Assessing airflow through both nostrils using a wisp of cotton ball, or a cold glass slide (warm, moist, expired air fogging the glass if the nasal passage is patent)
- Pharyngeal, laryngeal, and tracheal stridor:
  - Cervical radiographs to rule out laryngeal and tracheal masses and foreign bodies:
    - The normal larynx (especially if mineralized and/or radiographed obliquely) should not be misinterpreted as a foreign body.
  - Thoracic radiographs:
    - Intrathoracic trachea.
    - Lungs (noncardiogenic pulmonary edema; underlying abnormalities, e.g., infection, pulmonary hemorrhage [coagulopathy]).

ADVANCED OR CONFIRMATORY TESTING

- Coagulation profile to rule out coagulopathies
- Nasal cavity stridor:
  - Rhinoscopy with biopsies, cytology, and bacterial culture and sensitivity (aerobic) if discharge is present
  - Computed tomographic scan of nasal cavity and pharynx
  - Dental radiographs (tooth root abscesses)
- Pharyngeal, laryngeal, and tracheal stridor:
  - Laryngoscopy under light general anesthesia to evaluate laryngeal and oral anatomy, and rule out laryngeal paralysis
  - If severe, open-mouth inspiratory dyspnea: it may be possible to visualize the caudal pharynx and larynx with the patient awake (laryngeal paralysis, pharyngeal foreign body, laryngeal/pharyngeal mass) using only a bright light source
  - Pharyngoscopy and tracheoscopy with biopsies, cytology, and bronchoalveolar lavage

TREATMENT

THERAPEUTIC GOAL(S)

Remove or decrease obstruction of the upper airway

ACUTE GENERAL TREATMENT

- Nasal stridor: rarely associated with dyspneic crisis, as dogs and cats will open-mouth breathe to circumvent nasal obstruction.
- Pharyngeal, laryngeal, and tracheal stridor: if associated with severe obstruction, may cause (in increasing order of

severity) severe upper airway dyspnea, cyanosis, collapse, and respiratory arrest.
- Patients with marked respiratory stridor associated with exaggerated, severe inspiratory efforts require immediate attention.
  - Calm environment.
  - Oxygen supplementation if tolerated.
  - Sedation should be considered, especially if the degree of inspiratory dyspnea is severe and the patient is known to otherwise be healthy (e.g., butorphanol 0.05–0.3 mg/kg IV).
- In cases of pharyngeal, laryngeal, or tracheal stridor with deterioration or failure to improve despite the measures described above:
  - If the obstruction is cranial to the mid-cervical trachea and stridor and dyspnea are severe, either anesthesia and endotracheal intubation (see Intubation, Endotracheal p 1269), or a tracheotomy if intubation is not possible (see Tracheostomy, p 1310), should be considered.
  - If the obstruction is caudal to the mid-cervical trachea and stridor and dyspnea are severe despite the treatments mentioned above, immediate preparations should be made for tracheoscopy and/or surgical intervention.
  - If the site of obstruction is unknown, the patient must undergo radiography or direct visualization of the pharynx and larynx to determine the best intervention.

CHRONIC TREATMENT

Correction of underlying causes (as applicable):
- Brachycephalic airway surgery (nasal wedge resection, soft palate resection [staphylectomy], everted laryngeal saccule resection [laryngeal sacculectomy])
- Arytenoid lateralization (laryngeal tie-back surgery) for laryngeal paralysis
- Surgical excision of masses or polyps
- Endoscopic or surgical retrieval of foreign bodies
- Antimicrobial therapy for infectious disease

RECOMMENDED MONITORING

- Respiratory effort improvement/deterioration
- Mucous membrane color (pallor/cyanosis)
- Pulse oximetry and arterial blood gas analysis if debilitated or severely affected patient

PROGNOSIS AND OUTCOME

Dependent on the underlying disease

PEARLS & CONSIDERATIONS

COMMENTS

- Cats are much more reluctant than dogs to breathe with their mouths open. As a result, significant nasal cavity obstruction can cause marked respiratory distress in a cat, whereas a dog would simply pant more to bypass the obstruction.
- Stridor is often exacerbated by excitement and exercise.

SUGGESTED READING

Fingland RB: Obstructive upper airway disorders. In Birchard SJ, Sherding RG (eds): *Saunders Manual of Small Animal Practice*, ed 2. Philadelphia, WB Saunders, 2000, pp 629–641.

Mattson A: Pharyngeal disorders. *Vet Clin N Am: Sm Anim Pract* 24:825–854, 1994.

AUTHOR: **PETER FOLEY**

EDITOR: **ETIENNE CÔTÉ**

Strychnine Toxicosis

BASIC INFORMATION

DEFINITION

A rapid-onset (30 minutes to 2 hours after ingestion), potentially fatal toxicosis characterized by neurologic dysfunction

SYNONYM(S)

Nux vomica

EPIDEMIOLOGY

SPECIES, AGE, SEX
- All animals are susceptible; dogs are more commonly involved than cats.
- Male dogs are more commonly involved.

GENETICS AND BREED PREDISPOSITION: Younger dogs and large-breed dogs, such as German shepherds, are overrepresented.

GEOGRAPHY AND SEASONALITY
- Year-round
- Rural and urban dogs equally affected
- Most cases are reported in the western part of the United States and in the Midwest

CLINICAL PRESENTATION

HISTORY, CHIEF COMPLAINT
- Availability or presence of strychnine-containing bait in pet's environment; evidence of exposure
- Rapid onset of apprehension (30 minutes to 2 hours), nervousness, chewing movements, muscular rigidity, tonic clonic convulsions

PHYSICAL EXAM FINDINGS
- Hyperesthesia, apprehension, nervousness initially
- Severe muscle stiffness, rigidity
- Hyperthermia (>104°F), caused by muscle activity and not febrile in origin
- Sawhorse stance
- Eventually, tetanic seizures (marked by violent, stiff limb movements):
  - Occur spontaneously or may be initiated by external stimuli (touch, sound, sudden bright light)
- Opisthotonos, mydriasis, exophthalmos, and cyanosis may be present before death

ETIOLOGY AND PATHOPHYSIOLOGY

The toxin:
- Strychnine is a bitter indole alkaloid from the seeds of the vine-like, Southeast Asian or Australian trees *Strychnos nux-vomica* and *Strychnos ignatii*.
- Since 1978 in the United States, strychnine has been a restricted-use pesticide and rodenticide (licensed exterminators only) or has been forbidden in certain U.S. states. Over-the-counter preparations contain <0.5% strychnine; preparations used by licensed exterminators may contain up to 5% strychnine.
- Malicious or accidental strychnine toxicosis occurs when nontarget animals ingest strychnine-containing baits.

Pathophysiology:
- Strychnine competitively and reversibly inhibits the inhibitory neurotransmitter glycine at postsynaptic neuronal sites in the spinal cord and medulla. This results in unchecked reflex stimulation of motor neurons affecting all the striated muscles,

resulting in generalized rigidity and tonic-clonic seizures caused by these direct central nervous system (CNS) effects.
- Death usually results from respiratory arrest and exhaustion from prolonged seizuring.

DIAGNOSIS

DIFFERENTIAL DIAGNOSIS

- Other intoxications causing seizures: metaldehyde, tremorgenic mycotoxins/garbage toxicosis, organochlorine, organophosphorus or carbamate pesticides, zinc phosphide, nicotine
- Tetanus
- Hypocalcemic tetany
- Hepatic encephalopathy

INITIAL DATABASE

Due to rapid onset of clinical signs, no specific biochemical changes are expected on presentation other than elevated creatine kinase (CK); metabolic acidosis and myoglobinuria possible

ADVANCED OR CONFIRMATORY TESTING

- On postmortem examination, no characteristic lesions are seen. In cases that have prolonged convulsions before death, agonal hemorrhages of the heart and lungs and cyanotic congestion due to anoxia may be seen.
- Occasionally, poisoned animals may have undigested red or green strychnine-laced grain seeds (wheat, milo, barley) in their stomach.
- Presence of strychnine alkaloid in the vomitus, stomach contents, liver, kidney, or urine is considered diagnostic. In living animals, submit stomach contents (vomitus or stomach washings) or urine early (within the first several hours of exposure). Urine may not contain detectable amounts of strychnine if samples are collected late (1 to 2 days after the exposure). Seal samples (stomach contents, liver, or kidney) in a plastic bag, freeze them, and then submit them to a veterinary diagnostic laboratory for strychnine analysis.

TREATMENT

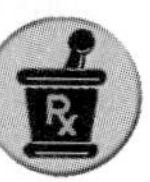

THERAPEUTIC GOAL(S)

- Decontaminate the patient
- Control seizures and prevent asphyxia
- Provide supportive care

ACUTE GENERAL TREATMENT

- Control seizures and prevent asphyxia. Do not attempt to decontaminate patients that are already showing neurologic effects. Control seizures and stabilize the patient first.
  - Anticonvulsants:
    - Diazepam 0.5-1 mg/kg IV has been used with variable success.
    - Pentobarbital sodium 3-15 mg/kg IV to effect; repeated as needed.
    - Isoflurane gas anesthesia: used if seizures are not controlled with the preceding treatment measures.
  - Muscle relaxants:
    - Glycerol guaiacolate (5% solution at 110 mg/kg) can be tried.
    - Methocarbamol 100-200 mg/kg IV; maximum dose of 330 mg/kg per day.
  - Intubate and provide artifical respiration for severely affected animals.
- Decontamination of patient:
  - Emesis (see Vomiting, Induction of, p 1328): useful within 30 minutes and only in patients showing no clinical signs.
  - Gastric lavage: used if emesis cannot be induced or when suspected lethal doses have been ingested; intubate the patient with a cuffed endotracheal tube to reduce aspiration risk if the patient is unconscious.
  - Enterogastric lavage: also called "through and through" lavage; induce general anesthesia (unless patient is already unconscious). Begin with gastric lavage followed by an enema/colonic irrigation under low pressure and continue until fluids exit via the gastric tube; used if known ingestion of potentially lethal dose. Premedication: atropine 0.04 mg/kg IV (to decrease enteric muscle tone, helping fluid flow).
  - Activated charcoal: 2-4 g/kg with a cathartic such as sorbitol (5-10 ml/kg, 3% solution) PO or via stomach tube.
- Supportive care:
  - IV fluid diuresis (24 to 48 hours or longer).
  - Treat hyperthermia if present (see Heat Stroke/Hyperthermia, p 467).
  - Confine the patient in a dark, quiet room.
  - Acidification of urine: Ammonium chloride (100 mg/kg PO q 12h) may help increase urinary excretion of strychnine.

POSSIBLE COMPLICATIONS

- Myoglobinuria and associated renal failure
- Disseminated intravascular coagulation from hyperthermia

RECOMMENDED MONITORING

- Body temperature
- Respiratory rate and character
- Acid-base status

PROGNOSIS AND OUTCOME

- Poor prognosis if status epilepticus
- Good prognosis if seizures are controlled early

PEARLS & CONSIDERATIONS

COMMENTS

- Sporadic strychnine poisoning of animals still occurs.
- Strychnine is ionized in an acidic pH; therefore, it is mainly absorbed from the small intestine, emphasizing the importance of rapid intervention before the onset of signs. Strychnine and its metabolites are mainly excreted in the urine. A toxic dose is eliminated within 24 to 48 hours following exposure.
- Oral lethal dose in dogs is 0.75 mg/kg; for cats, the dose is 2 mg/kg.
- Ingestion of 1.7 g (1/4 tsp) of 0.5% strychnine bait in a 25-lb (11.3-kg) dog could be lethal.

PREVENTION

Do not use strychnine-containing baits in any pet's environment

SUGGESTED READING

Morgan S, et al: Investigating a case of strychnine poisoning. *Vet Med* 82:1044-1047, 1987.

Talcott PA: Strychnine. In Peterson ME, Talcott PA (eds): *Small Animal Toxicology*. Philadelphia, WB Saunders, 2001 pp 741-747.

AUTHOR & EDITOR: **SAFDAR A. KHAN**

Stunted Growth

BASIC INFORMATION

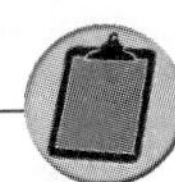

DEFINITION

Slowed or retarded growth rate. Failure to attain expected body size/stature

SYNONYM(S)

Cretinism: congenital hypothyroidism
Delayed growth
Dwarf, runt, poor-doer, unthrifty
Pituitary dwarfism: growth hormone deficiency, hyposomatotropism

EPIDEMIOLOGY

SPECIES, AGE, SEX

- Varies with cause
- Failure to grow is usually recognized by 1 year of age (most noted prior to 2 years)
- Dogs and cats
- First 3 months: growth hormone deficiency, congenital hypothyroidism, cleft palate, congenital megaesophagus, persistent right aortic arch (PRAA), other vascular ring anomaly, parasitism, juvenile hyperparathyroidism
- Under 1 year: juvenile diabetes, portosystemic shunt/microvascular dysplasia, exocrine pancreatic insufficiency, cardiac abnormalities, renal disease, osteochondrodystrophies, ciliary dyskinesia
- Under 2 years: most noted prior to 2 years. Nutritional deficiencies in giant breed dogs might manifest later. Renal diseases, hepatopathies

GENETICS AND BREED PREDISPOSITION

- Pituitary dwarfism: German shepherd, Karelian bear dog, spitz, toy pinscher
- Congenital hypothyroidism: fox terrier, boxer, giant schnauzer, Abyssinian cat
- Osteochondrodysplasia: various, including Labrador retriever, Irish setter
- Cleft palate: shih tzu, bulldog, pointers, Swiss sheepdog, Brittany spaniel
- Congenital megaesophagus: Irish setter, German shepherd, Labrador retriever, miniature schnauzer
- Vascular ring anomaly: German shepherd, Irish setter
- Pancreatic acinar atrophy: German shepherd
- Portosystemic shunt: Havanese, Yorkshire terrier, Maltese, Dandy Dinmont terrier, pug, miniature schnauzer
- Microvascular dysplasia: cairn terrier, and breeds predisposed to portosystemic shunts
- Polycystic kidney disease: cairn terrier, West Highland white terrier, Persian, Himalayan
- Hereditary nephritis: English cocker spaniel, Samoyed
- Renal dysplasia: malamute, chow chow

RISK FACTORS

- Varies with disease
- Most risk factors are not identified except genetic diseases
- Malnutrition: poor quality feed
- Hypothyroidism: maternal exposure to ^{131}I

CONTAGION AND ZOONOSIS: Some intestinal parasites present risks of visceral larval migrans to humans.

ASSOCIATED CONDITIONS AND DISORDERS

- Juvenile diabetes mellitus: pancreatic acinar atrophy and exocrine pancreatic insufficiency
- Pituitary dwarfism: hypoadrenocorticism
- Portosystemic shunt: urate urolithiasis, microvascular dysplasia
- Megaesophagus: myasthenia gravis, vascular ring anomaly
- Cleft palate: middle ear abnormalities

CLINICAL PRESENTATION

DISEASE FORMS/SUBTYPES

- Nutritional
  - Poor feed or insufficient supply
  - Mechanical problems: cleft palate, megaesophagus, PRAA
  - Maldigestion/malabsorption: parasites, intestinal infections (salmonella, histoplasmosis), pancreatic acinar atrophy
- Endocrine
  - Congenital hyposomatotropism, congenital hypothyroidism, juvenile hyperparathyroidism, diabetes mellitus
- Cardiac diseases
  - Patent ductus arteriosus, others
- Metabolic
  - Portosystemic shunt, microvascular dysplasia
  - Renal dysplasia, other nephritis
- Chondrodysplastic

HISTORY, CHIEF COMPLAINT

- May be unnoticed by owner
- Pet lags behind littermates in growth
- Diet history, deworming history, onset and progression of signs are important
- Medication exposure
- Signs of mental dullness
- Polyuria/polydipsia

PHYSICAL EXAM FINDINGS

- Varies with disease. Important distinctions are good versus poor body condition, and proportionate versus disproportionate dwarfism:
  - Hyposomatotropism and chondrodysplastic animals are in good body condition, whereas other disorders lead to poor body condition.
  - Congenitally hypothyroid patients and chondrodysplastic patients are disproportionate dwarfs (limbs are exceptionally short). This is in contrast to proportional dwarfism (e.g., toy poodle), in which the limbs, trunk, and head are of appropriate relative sizes.
- Examine patient for:
  - Mental dullness or disorientation
  - Dwarfism
  - Cleft palate
  - Cough, respiratory distress
  - Heart murmur
  - Bloated abdomen
  - Signs of diarrhea staining coat

ETIOLOGY AND PATHOPHYSIOLOGY

Specific pathophysiologic mechanism varies with disease:

- Inability to ingest, absorb, or utilize nutrients
- Inability to properly execute growth

DIAGNOSIS

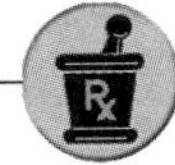

INITIAL DATABASE

- Fecal flotation
- Complete blood count
  - Microcytic anemia: portosystemic shunt, polycythemia
  - Eosinophilia: hypoadrenocorticism, parasitism
  - Lymphocytosis/neutropenia: hypoadrenocorticism
- Serum biochemistry panel
  - Low albumin: exocrine pancreatic insufficiency, portosystemic shunt, infiltrative bowel disease
  - Hyperglycemia: diabetes mellitus
  - Hypoglycemia: hypoadrenocorticism
  - High calcium with normal or low phosphorus: hypoparathyroidism
  - High blood urea nitrogen: renal disease versus prerenal azotemia
- Urinalysis
  - Urine specific gravity <1.035: renal failure, hypothyroidism. May be normal in nonazotemic patient (elimination of free water)
  - Glucose: diabetes mellitus
  - Protein: nephritis, glomerulopathies
  - Casts, infection: nephritis
  - Urate uroliths: portosystemic shunt, microvascular dysplasia
- T4
  - Congenital hypothyroidism

ADVANCED OR CONFIRMATORY TESTING

- Trypsin-like immunoreactivity: pancreatic acinar atrophy/exocrine pancreatic insufficiency

- Urine bacterial culture and sensitivity
- ACTH stimulation test: hypoadrenocorticism
- Abdominal ultrasound: kidney disease, portosystemic shunt
- Scintigraphy: portosystemic shunt, ciliary dyskinesia
- Xylazine stimulation, serum level of insulin-like growth factor: hyposomatotropism

TREATMENT

THERAPEUTIC GOAL(S)

Correct diseases that are reversible

ACUTE GENERAL TREATMENT

Generally not acute presentations

CHRONIC TREATMENT

- Varies with disease
- Examples, depending on disorder: close portosystemic shunt; treat parasitism; improve diet; provide thyroxine, insulin, pancreatic enzyme replacement

POSSIBLE COMPLICATIONS

- Death: patent ductus arteriosus, portosystemic shunt, extreme malnutrition
- Ketoacidosis
- Aspiration pneumonia

RECOMMENDED MONITORING

Frequent physical exams

PROGNOSIS AND OUTCOME

- Guarded. Most of the diseases are serious and irreversible.
- With surgical reversal, normal longevity of portosystemic shunt patients and patent ductus arteriosus patients is possible, as long as underlying microvascular dysplasia and irreversible cardiac changes are not present, respectively.
- Osteochondrodysplastic dogs can fare well but the disorder is irreversible.

PEARLS & CONSIDERATIONS

COMMENTS

- Key to diagnosis is distinction between good and poor thrift, and proportionate and disproportionate dwarfs
- Adequate nutrition and effective deworming should be assured prior to more expensive diagnostics

PREVENTION

Careful attention to genetic lines in purebred dogs

CLIENT EDUCATION

The prognosis varies with the disease

SUGGESTED READING

Greco DS: Congenital and inherited renal disease of small animals. In Davidson AP (ed): *Veterinary Clinics of North America Small Animal Practice*. Philadelphia, WB Saunders, 2001, pp 393–399.

Greco DS: Diagnosis and treatment of juvenile endocrine disorders in puppies and kittens. In Davidson AP (ed): *Veterinary Clinics of North America Small Animal Practice*. Philadelphia, WB Saunders, 2001, pp 400–409.

Ihle SL: Failure to grow. In Ettinger SJ, Feldman EC (eds): *Textbook of Veterinary Internal Medicine*, ed 6. Philadelphia, WB Saunders, 2005, pp 80–83.

AUTHOR: **DENNIS SPANN**
EDITOR: **ETIENNE CÔTÉ**

Subaortic Stenosis

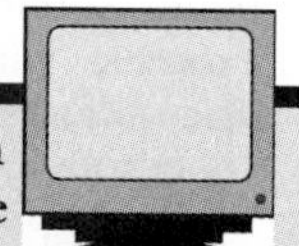

Client Education Sheet on Website

BASIC INFORMATION

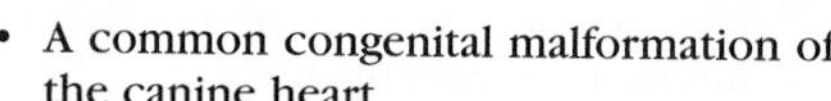

DEFINITION

- A common congenital malformation of the canine heart
- Hallmark: a narrowing of the outflow tract of the left ventricle (the subaortic valvular region)
- May be fixed (fibrous nodule, band, or annulus) or dynamic (systolic anterior motion of the mitral valve, asymmetric septal hypertrophy)

SYNONYM(S)

SAS
Subvalvular aortic stenosis

EPIDEMIOLOGY

SPECIES, AGE, SEX

- First noted in puppies <12 months old.
- The severity of narrowing often is progressive during a puppy's growth, and the true severity of narrowing cannot be determined until the dog is fully grown (at least 1 year old).
- Depending on the study, subaortic stenosis (SAS) is either the most common congenital heart defect of dogs or is second only to patent ductus arteriosus.
- In cats, hypertrophic cardiomyopathy affecting the interventricular septum may produce the same effect of left ventricular outflow obstruction as SAS (see Hypertrophic Cardiomyopathy, p 554).

GENETICS AND BREED PREDISPOSITION

- Large-breed dogs (Newfoundland, golden retriever, rottweiler, boxer, German shepherd, Bouvier des Flandres, and Bernese mountain dogs)
- Hereditary transmission (autosomal dominant with a polygenic pattern) has been demonstrated in the Newfoundland dog
- Cannot be attributed specifically to sire or dam in any breed (no apparent sex linkage)
- Familial predisposition: The risk of having affected offspring increases when one or both parents are affected

ASSOCIATED CONDITIONS AND DISORDERS

- Mild aortic valvular regurgitation/insufficiency: very commonly observed in dogs with SAS.
- Mitral dysplasia, patent ductus arteriosus, and a variety of aortic arch abnormalities have also been associated with some SAS cases.
- Dogs with SAS are predisposed to bacterial endocarditis of the aortic valve.

CLINICAL PRESENTATION

DISEASE FORMS/SUBTYPES: Many distinct malformations are grouped under the heading of SAS.

- Fixed obstruction:
  - Grade 1: small raised nodules of thickened endocardium.
  - Grade 2: narrow ridge of thickened endocardium that partially encircles the left ventricular outflow tract.
  - Grade 3: fibrous band, ridge, or collar completely encircles the left ventricular outflow tract.
  - This grading system is only for gross pathologic findings. It is unrelated to murmur intensity or clinical signs.
- Dynamic obstruction:
  - Systolic anterior motion of the mitral valve:
    - Narrowing of the left ventricular outflow tract and papillary muscle distortion caused by left ventricular hypertrophy slightly distort the mitral valve such that a small amount of mitral regurgitation occurs.
  - Septal hypertrophy or malalignment:

- The left ventricular hypertrophy induced by SAS may itself further contribute to left ventricular outflow obstruction because of hypertrophy of the interventricular septum.
- The aortic arch may be congenitally malaligned in its attachment to the left ventricular outflow tract, resulting in SAS due to protrusion of the interventricular septum into the subvalvular area.

HISTORY, CHIEF COMPLAINT: In most cases, the condition causes a heart murmur in a dog not showing any overt clinical signs. However, severe cases may show:

- Exertional fatigue or syncope
- Congestive heart failure (CHF) (rare)
- Sudden death

PHYSICAL EXAM FINDINGS: Often unremarkable except for a systolic, ejection-type heart murmur, heard loudest in the left cranial thorax (between the third and fifth intercostal spaces) or at the thoracic inlet (immediately lateral to the trachea). Intensity of the heart murmur grossly correlates with severity of disease:
Grades 1 to 3/6 = mildly affected dogs
Grades 4 to 6/6 = severely affected dogs

- Murmur may radiate cranially through the carotid arteries to the neck and head or to the right hemithorax.
- Weak and slow rising femoral pulse (*pulsus parvus et tardus*) in severe cases.
- A diastolic heart murmur is sometimes heard with aortic valve insufficiency.
- Premature beats and pulse deficits (due to ventricular arrhythmias) may be detected, generally with more severe cases.

ETIOLOGY AND PATHOPHYSIOLOGY

The consequence of SAS, regardless of it origin (forms/subtypes as already described), is an increased resistance to the normal left ventricular outflow ("left ventricular pressure overload") that results in:

- An increase in left ventricular systolic pressure and a pressure gradient across the subaortic lesion.
- An increased blood flow velocity through the left ventricular outflow tract.
- Compensatory left ventricular concentric hypertrophy (diffuse, symmetrical thickening of the left ventricle).
- This process may lead to left-sided CHF.

With worsening SAS over time, left ventricular thickening may exceed intramyocardial (coronary) blood supply, which does not grow along with the hypertrophied myocardial cells:

- The result is relative underperfusion of left ventricular tissue and ventricular arrhythmias or, less commonly, myocardial infarction.
- Either process may be responsible for sudden death (common in advanced SAS).

DIAGNOSIS

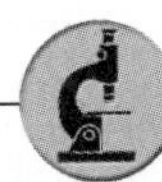

DIFFERENTIAL DIAGNOSIS

- Other systolic heart murmur heard between the second and fifth intercostal spaces:
  - Pulmonic stenosis
  - Tetralogy of Fallot
  - Atrial septal defect
  - Incompletely ausculted patent ductus arteriosus
- High output states:
  - Hyperthyroidism
  - Anemia
  - Fever
  - Exercise (rare); note that physical activity increases the heart rate, which may make apparent a murmur of SAS that was not audible at rest. The distinction between this phenomenon and a benign, exercise-induced heart murmur requires echocardiography
- Juvenile "innocent" heart murmur:
  - Puppies and kittens <6 months old
  - Soft heart murmur, grades 1 to 3/6, short (early to midsystolic, never diastolic or continuous)
  - Often disappears with a change in body position or increase in heart rate
  - Electrocardiogram (ECG), thoracic radiographs, and echocardiogram are normal

INITIAL DATABASE

- ECG:
  - May be normal in mild to moderate cases
  - Left ventricular hypertrophy pattern often present but not striking (increased R wave amplitude in lead II) in moderate to severe cases; unreliable as a screening tool
  - ST segment may be slurred, depressed, or elevated in severe cases (myocardial hypoxia)
  - Ventricular arrhythmias in severe or long-standing cases
- Thoracic radiographs:
  - Often normal; unreliable as a screening tool
  - Variable left-sided cardiomegaly (left ventricular and atrial enlargement), usually only with moderate to severe cases
  - Poststenotic dilatation of the aortic root may be visible in severe cases
- Echocardiogram: (definitive diagnosis):
  - Two-dimensional (2-D):
    - Often normal in mildly affected dogs
    - Subvalvular obstruction lesion or narrowed left ventricular outflow tract
    - Left ventricular concentric hypertrophy (diffuse, symmetrical left ventricular thickening)
    - Variable dilatation of the left atrium
    - Dilated ascending aorta
  - M-Mode:
    - Normal to increased left ventricular fractional shortening (poorly sensitive)
    - Systolic anterior motion of the mitral valve sometimes observed
  - Doppler study:
    - Turbulent, high-velocity systolic signal in the left ventricular outflow tract and aortic root. Normal range = up to 1.7 m/s; "grey zone" = 1.7-2.2 m/s; > 2.2 m/s = highly suggestive of SAS when corresponding murmur and breed are also present
    - Determination of the peak pressure gradient in combination with the indexed effective orifice area (IEOA) roughly estimates the severity of disease; peak pressure gradient = 4 × (Doppler-derived LVOT velocity in m/s)^2
      - 16–40 mmHg = mild SAS
      - 40–100 mmHg = moderate SAS
      - >100 mmHg = severe SAS
      - IEOA <0.6 cm^2/m^2 = severe SAS
    - Diastolic signal of aortic regurgitation is present in most cases of SAS

ADVANCED OR CONFIRMATORY TESTING

Cardiac catheterization and angiography: virtually never used for diagnosis. The procedure is invasive, requires general anesthesia, and provides little additional beneficial information over echocardiography.

TREATMENT

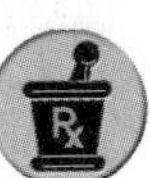

THERAPEUTIC GOAL(S)

- For severe cases:
  - Reduce exercise intolerance
  - Reduce syncopal events/risk of sudden death
- No definitive treatment exists for curing SAS. Excision of the stenotic tissue via open-heart surgery has not yet been shown to provide an outcome that is superior to conservative, medical management.

ACUTE GENERAL TREATMENT

See Ventricular Arrhythmias (Premature Ventricular Complexes, Ventricular Tachycardia), p 1148; Heart Failure, Acute/Decompensated, p 458

CHRONIC TREATMENT

- Mild SAS: no treatment
- Moderate SAS: mild exercise restriction (avoid vigorous activity and swimming [syncope risk]) and β-adrenergic blocking agent to prevent or control ventricular arrhythmias when present:
  - Atenolol 0.25–1.0 mg/kg PO q 12–24h; begin at low dose and increase titration over 2 to 4 weeks until upper end of dose range or signs of intolerance (lethargy, inappetence)

- Severe SAS and SAS of any degree of severity in which syncope has occurred:
  - Open resection of the obstructing lesion is possible
  - Balloon dilation of the stenosis (long-term recurrence will still occur in most cases of severe SAS)
  - β-Adrenergic blocking agent to prevent or control ventricular arrhythmias:
    - Atenolol (as already presented)
    - Exercise restriction (as already described)
- SAS with CHF; see Heart Failure, Acute/Decompensated, p 458

DRUG INTERACTIONS

- Concurrent use of antacids can alter the bioavailability of atenolol.
- Calcium (Ca) channel blockers may cause hypotension and bradycardia when administered together with atenolol.
- Effects of theophylline can be blocked by β-adrenergic blocking agents like propranolol.

POSSIBLE COMPLICATIONS

- Ventricular arrhythmias
- Exertional syncope or sudden death
- Left-sided heart failure
- Aortic valve endocarditis

RECOMMENDED MONITORING

- Control ventricular arrhythmias when present (ambulatory ECG recordings recommended if syncope is noted and for monitoring efficacy of antiarrhythmic treatment if possible); see Holter/Cardiac Event Monitoring, p 1264.
- SAS is a progressive disease; therefore, the final cardiac evaluation should be done at 12 months of age or older to stage the severity of disease.

PROGNOSIS AND OUTCOME

- Favorable: mild to moderate SAS
  - Normal quality of life and longevity in most cases, especially when follow-up visit shows no progression of SAS
- Poor: severe SAS
  - Most dogs die suddenly, usually within the first 3 years of life

PEARLS & CONSIDERATIONS

COMMENTS

- The combination of a ≥ grade 4/6 ejection heart murmur that radiates cranially to the thoracic inlet and over the carotid arteries along with a weak femoral pulse in a puppy is highly suggestive of severe SAS.
- The severity of ventricular arrhythmias detected by extended (24-hour) ambulatory ECG recordings correlates with the severity of disease.
- Dogs with peak pressure gradients > 125 mmHg are very likely to develop serious complications or sudden death.
- Because of the progressive nature of SAS during growth, the lesion/heart murmur may be clinically silent in very young puppies but becomes increasingly prominent at > 2–3 months of age
- Overtly healthy boxer dogs may have systolic murmurs and accelerated left ventricular outflow velocities on Doppler exam without obvious SAS.
  - Grades I–III/VI murmur.
  - No SAS lesion on echocardiography.
  - Differentiation between SAS and the normal state in these dogs is challenging and requires echocardiography (left ventricular thickening, left atrial enlargement, and aortic insufficiency suggest SAS), ECG (ventricular arrhythmia of left ventricular origin suggests SAS), and follow-up exams (progression of these abnormalities and of Doppler-derived pressure gradient suggest SAS).
- Identification of the most mildly affected animals (clinically silent, "carrier"), such as dogs with a soft systolic murmur only apparent at higher heart rates and a structurally normal heart on a 2-D echocardiography, remains extremely challenging. Diagnosis in these cases involves a combination of physical examination, Doppler echocardiography, and tightly controlled follow-up exams (both the animal in question and its siblings or offspring).

PREVENTION

- Vigilance regarding the possible need for antibiotics is important in all SAS cases during periods of anticipated bacteremia (dental procedures, surgery, severe skin disease, other concurrent bacterial disease); avoiding overuse of antibacterials is also important.
- Use breeding dogs that have been screened for SAS.

CLIENT EDUCATION

- In cases of severe SAS, avoid prolonged, vigorous exercise
- Contact breeders to notify them of SAS cases

SUGGESTED READING

Belanger MC, et al: Usefulness of the indexed effective orifice area in the assessment of subaortic stenosis in the dog. *J Vet Intern Med* 15:430, 2001.

Kienle RD, et al: The natural clinical history of canine subaortic stenosis. *J Vet Intern Med* 8:423, 1994.

Kittleson MD, Kienle RD: Aortic stenosis. In *Small Animal Cardiovascular Medicine*. St. Louis, Mosby, 1998, pp 260–272.

Lehmkuhl LB, Bonagura JD: CVT update: Canine subvalvular aortic stenosis. In Bonagura JD (ed): *Kirk's Current Veterinary Therapy XII: Small Animal Practice*. Philadelphia, WB Saunders, 1995, pp 822–830.

Oyama MA, Sisson DD, Thomas WP, Bonagura JD: Congenital heart disease. In Ettinger SJ, Feldman EC (eds): *Textbook of Veterinary Internal Medicine*, ed 6. St. Louis, Elsevier Saunders, 2005, pp 1006–1012.

AUTHOR: **MARIE-CLAUDE BÉLANGER**
EDITOR: **ETIENNE CÔTÉ**

Subcutaneous Emphysema

BASIC INFORMATION

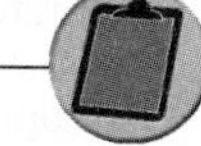

DEFINITION

Accumulation of air in subcutaneous tissues

EPIDEMIOLOGY

SPECIES, AGE, SEX

- More often seen in cats than in dogs
- Cats have a thin dorsal tracheal membrane compared to dogs
- No age or sex predilection

RISK FACTORS

- Endotracheal intubation, especially in cats
- Trauma to airways
- Bite wounds (anaerobic infection of subcutis)
- Surgery of the airways, especially upper airway surgery

ASSOCIATED CONDITIONS AND DISORDERS

- Pneumomediastinum
- Pneumoretroperitoneum
- Pneumopericardium
- Pneumothorax

CLINICAL PRESENTATION

HISTORY, CHIEF COMPLAINT

- History of recent anesthesia with intubation, trauma, or surgery

- History of recent jugular venipuncture, transtracheal aspiration, or other penetrating medical procedure of the neck
- Dyspnea, discomfort
- Rapid onset of swelling of the body, initially around the neck but may progress to total body (Fig. I-168)

PHYSICAL EXAM FINDINGS: Animal may manifest respiratory discomfort. Characteristic crackling sensation on palpation of the skin overlying the trapped air:

- Initially focal (especially around the neck) and progressing rapidly to affect the whole body: suggests airway perforation/rupture as source; dyspnea, discomfort may or may not be present
- Focal in an animal showing signs of severe illness: may suggest infection-related subcutaneous emphysema. A meticulous search for penetrating wounds is indicated

ETIOLOGY AND PATHOPHYSIOLOGY

- A break in the integrity of the airway at any point between the pharynx and terminal bronchioles
- An independent source of gas formation (bacteria) in the subcutis
- Mechanisms: With any of the following three mechanisms, air may remain trapped in the subcutaneous tissues by unidirectional valve action of the airway trauma:
  - Rupture of dorsal tracheal membrane (cats > dogs)
  - Rupture of dorsolateral or ventrolateral tracheal annular ligament
  - Penetrating wound in cervical area

Specific etiologies:

- Related to anesthetic administration of intubation:
  - Overinflation of endotracheal cuff
  - Use of a stiff stylet to guide the endotracheal tube through the larynx causes stylet tip punctures in trachea
  - Manipulation of the head without disconnecting the endotracheal tube
- Surgical
- Traumatic:
  - Bite wounds
  - Lacerations or penetrating foreign objects, including jugular venipuncture and transtracheal aspirates
- Infectious:
  - Inoculation of gas-forming bacteria (e.g., anaerobes) during penetrating injuries such as bite wounds anywhere on the body can produce infection of the subcutis
- Idiopathic

DIAGNOSIS

DIFFERENTIAL DIAGNOSIS

Tracheal avulsion/rupture (radiographs reveal physical separation of the trachea; surgery is required)

INITIAL DATABASE

- Complete blood count (CBC) and serum biochemical profile: generally unremarkable for cases of airway trauma; may show evidence of infection (neutrophilia, left shift, toxic changes) if subcutaneous emphysema is due to anaerobic infection of the subcutis
- Radiographs of neck and thorax show presence of air trapped under the skin (Fig. I-169)

ADVANCED OR CONFIRMATORY TESTING

Tracheoscopy:

- Lesions may be difficult to visualize
- Negative finding does not rule out tracheal trauma as cause for subcutaneous emphysema

TREATMENT

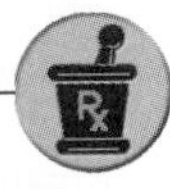

THERAPEUTIC GOAL(S)

Stop further accumulation of subcutaneous air:

- Medical management in mild cases
- Surgical repair in animals with progressive respiratory distress

ACUTE GENERAL TREATMENT

- In animals without respiratory discomfort:
  - Supportive care while awaiting spontaneous absorption of the air
  - Cage rest
- In animals with mild discomfort:
  - Consider light sedation
  - Removal of air via an 18- or 16-gauge needle. Air may be gently massaged toward the needle for evacuation. Needle suction alone may not able to remove the trapped air. Air removal via skin stab incisions is not advised

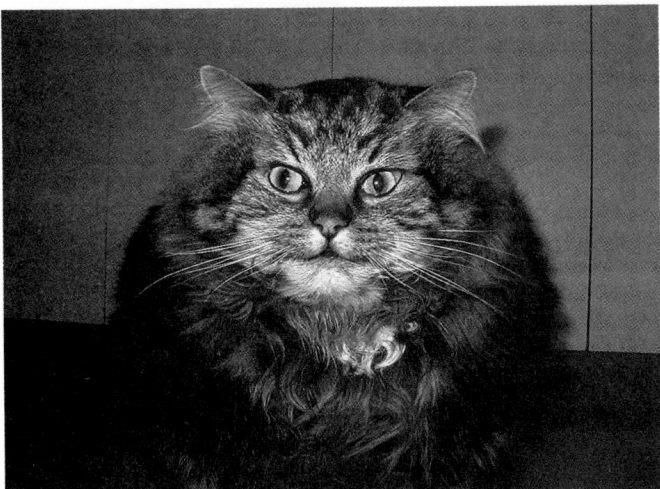

FIGURE I-168 External appearance of a domestic long-haired cat with marked subcutaneous emphysema. Note severe distention of the subcutaneous space, manifesting as a diffusely bloated appearance over the torso but not the head.

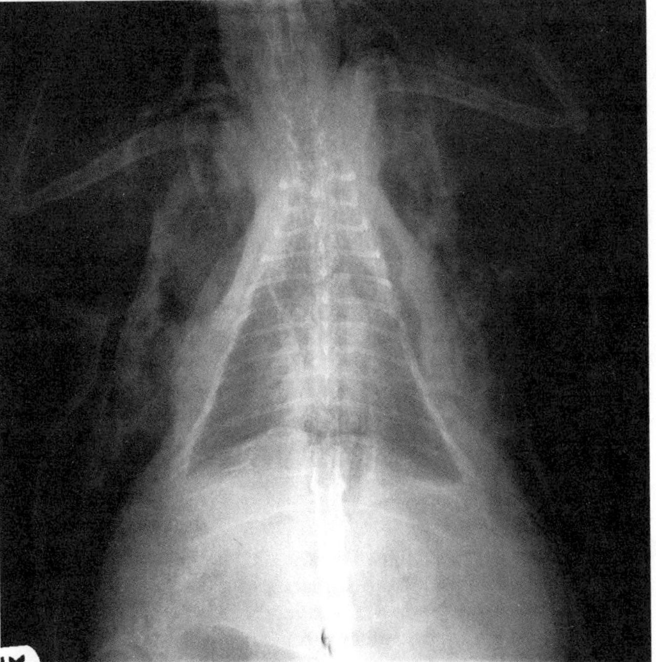

FIGURE I-169 Radiograph taken at the same time as the photo in Fig. I-168. Severe subcutaneous emphysema is apparent as gas lucencies throughout the subcutis.

  - Repeat this procedure to keep the animal comfortable as needed
  - Penrose drains can be placed into the subcutis (similar to treating a subcutaneous abscess) to allow for continuous drainage of air. Generally less labor intensive and more effective than repeated centesis
  - Analgesia (e.g., with butorphanol 0.1-0.3 mg/kg IV q 6-8h)
- In animals with recurrent/refractory subcutaneous emphysema and progressive respiratory distress:
  - If dyspnea is due to compression of the airways by trapped air in the subcutis or mediastinum, trapped air should be allowed to drain, leading to improved respiratory effort
  - Surgical repair of the trachea if conservative measures are inadequate or if radiography suggests tracheal avulsion/rupture
  - Analgesia (e.g., with butorphanol 0.1-0.3 mg/kg IV q 6-8h)

DRUG INTERACTIONS

Avoid subcutaneous drug administration until normalized

POSSIBLE COMPLICATIONS

Depending on the etiology of the subcutaneous emphysema: tracheal rupture, pneumothorax, and pneumoretroperitoneum are possible as is sepsis (if bacterial infection of the subcutis)

RECOMMENDED MONITORING

Evaluate rate and depth of respiration as an indicator for the level of comfort in the animal and consider the need for surgical treatment

PROGNOSIS AND OUTCOME

In animals that do not develop respiratory distress, the prognosis is good, and spontaneous recovery will occur between 3 and 15 days.

PEARLS & CONSIDERATIONS

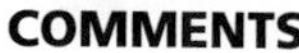

COMMENTS

- Most animals will recover with supportive care and will not require surgery.
- Sloughing of the skin is not a recognized complication of subcutaneous emphysema.
- Some animals show discomfort and pain during the presence of subcutaneous emphysema. Analgesic treatment should be initiated.

PREVENTION

- Prevent overinflation of endotracheal cuffs
- Provide cautious, appropriate jugular venipuncture, especially in cats
- Disconnect endotracheal tubes prior to repositioning of the animal's head

SUGGESTED READING

Hardie EM, et al: Tracheal rupture in cats: 16 cases (1983-1998). *J Am Vet Med Assoc* 214(4):508-512, 1999.

AUTHOR: **HANS GELENS**

EDITOR: **ELIZABETH ROZANSKI**

Subinvolution of Placental Sites

BASIC INFORMATION

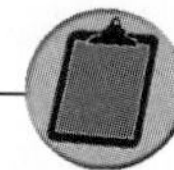

DEFINITION

Delay of the normal uterine involution process in the bitch beyond 12 weeks after whelping, manifesting as persistent bloody vaginal discharge in a dog that is otherwise well

SYNONYM(S)

SIPS

Metrorrhagia (uterine bleeding) postpartum

Placentitis postpartum

EPIDEMIOLOGY

SPECIES, AGE, SEX

- Not often observed clinically; however, in two surveys for which histopathologic examinations of postpartum uteruses were performed, the incidence was 8-21%
- Young bitches, less than 3 years old. Although subinvolution of placental sites (SIPS) can be seen at any age, the condition is more prevalent after the first parturition; no effect of litter size

GENETICS AND BREED PREDISPOSITION: No breed predilection.

RISK FACTORS: Low parity (especially in first pregnancy/litter).

CLINICAL PRESENTATION

HISTORY, CHIEF COMPLAINT

- History of recent whelping
- Likely primiparous bitch (first litter)
- Hemorrhagic vaginal discharge persistent even after pups are weaned
- Persistent postparturient serosanguineous vaginal discharge
- Bitch is in otherwise good health

PHYSICAL EXAM FINDINGS

- Discharge red rather than normal brown lochia
- Slight pallor of mucous membranes if discharge is copious
- Abdominal palpation: pain and uterine enlargement possible
- Physical exam generally reveals an otherwise healthy animal

ETIOLOGY AND PATHOPHYSIOLOGY

- Normally, expulsion of the fetal membranes and lochia takes place in the immediate postpartum period, and a mild serosanguineous discharge may last 3 to 5 weeks after parturition.
- With SIPS, the endometrium and myometrium are invaded by fetal trophoblasts.
- Failure of these cells to regress prevents normal involution, which then results in persistent hemorrhagic vaginal discharge in a bitch that usually has no other clinical signs.

DIAGNOSIS

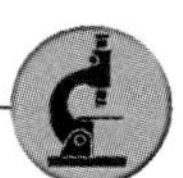

DIFFERENTIAL DIAGNOSIS

- Proestrus
- Metritis
- Cystic endometrial hyperplasia/pyometra
- Vaginitis
- Vulvar, vaginal, or uterine tumor
- Urinary tract hemorrhage (e.g., bacterial cystitis, calculi)
- Coagulopathy
- Brucellosis
- Trauma

INITIAL DATABASE

- Complete blood count (CBC) (note that mild normocytic, normochromic anemia is normal in postpartum bitches)
- Serum biochemistry profile
- Vaginal cytologic examination showing fetal trophoblasts

ADVANCED OR CONFIRMATORY TESTING

- Definitive diagnosis: histologic examination based on biopsy specimen of placental sites (rarely done)

- Vaginoscopy: to distinguish vaginal bleeding from blood derived from the uterus
- Abdominal ultrasound: focal thickenings of the uterine wall and a fluid-distended lumen
- Abdominal radiographs: focal areas of uterine irregularity

TREATMENT

ACUTE GENERAL TREATMENT

- Observation:
  - Erosion through the uterine wall resulting in peritonitis is possible but rare.
- In most cases, SIPS resolves spontaneously.
- Ovariohysterectomy indicated if:
  - Bitch is not intended for future breeding.
  - Hemorrhage is severe.
- Acute, life-threatening uterine bleeding may require blood transfusion.
- Systemic and intrauterine antibiotics may be indicated when metritis or peritonitis is present.

RECOMMENDED MONITORING

Recheck animals showing any signs of systemic illness and look for complications

PROGNOSIS AND OUTCOME

- With spontaneous remission, future reproductive success is not compromised.
- Affected bitches are not predisposed to SIPS in subsequent pregnancies.

SUGGESTED READING

Al-Bassam MA, et al: Involution abnormalities in the postpartum uterus of the bitch. *Vet Path* 18:208, 1981.

Beck AM: Subinvolution of placental sites in a postpartum bitch. A case report. *Cornell Vet* 56:269, 1966.

Dickie MB, et al: Diagnosis and therapy of the subinvolution of placental sites in the bitch. *J Reprod Fertil Suppl* 47:471, 1993.

AUTHOR: **CARLOS GRADIL**

EDITOR: **MICHELLE A. KUTZLER**

Syncope

BASIC INFORMATION

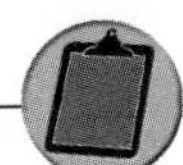

DEFINITION

Sudden and transient loss of consciousness resulting in collapse, followed by spontaneous recovery. The cause is a transient cerebral deficiency of oxygen.

SYNONYM(S)

Faint, collapse

Neurocardiogenic syncope: vasovagal syncope

Tussive syncope: "cough-drop" phenomenon

EPIDEMIOLOGY

SPECIES, AGE, SEX: Dependent on underlying cause: cardiac versus noncardiac causes. Acquired heart disease: middle-aged to older animals; congenital heart disease: young animals.

GENETICS AND BREED PREDISPOSITION

- Dilated cardiomyopathy (Doberman pinscher, boxer, American cocker spaniel, giant-breed dogs)
- Myxomatous AV valvular endocardiosis/degeneration (older small-breed dogs)
- Pulmonic stenosis (English bulldog, fox terrier, miniature schnauzer, boxer, bullmastiff, West Highland white terrier, Samoyed, beagle, Chihuahua, American cocker spaniel, Boykin spaniel)
- Subaortic stenosis (Newfoundland, boxer, golden retriever, German shepherd, rottweiler)
- Right-to-left shunting congenital heart defects (English bulldog, keeshond)
- Hypertrophic cardiomyopathy (Maine coon, Persian, American shorthair, Norwegian forest cat)
- Pericardial effusion (German shepherd, golden retriever)
- Sick sinus syndrome (SSS; miniature schnauzer, dachshund, cocker spaniel, West Highland white terrier)
- Third-degree atrioventricular block (pug, German shepherd, dachshund, Doberman pinscher)
- Supraventricular tachycardia (Labrador retriever)
- Ventricular tachycardia (Doberman pinscher, boxer)
- Tussive syncope (older small-breed dogs with pulmonary disease)
- Neurocardiogenic syncope (boxer, brachycephalic breeds?)

RISK FACTORS

- Autonomic dysfunction (neurocardiogenic syncope)
- Drugs: β-blockers, diuretics, vasodilators (hypotensive syncope)

CLINICAL PRESENTATION

HISTORY, CHIEF COMPLAINT

- Acute collapse, with altered or loss of consciousness
- Either no clinical signs, or staggering or ataxia prior to the event
- Exercise, excitement, or coughing may precipitate the event
- ± Clonic movements
- ± Involuntary urination or defecation
- No postictal phase
- Duration: seconds
- Recovery: complete and rapid

PHYSICAL EXAM FINDINGS: Dependent on underlying disorder(s).

- Cardiac:
  - ± Murmur
  - ± Arrhythmia
  - ± Altered arterial pulse quality
  - ± Pulse deficits
  - ± Cyanotic mucous membranes
  - ± Pulmonary rales or crackles
- Neuro:
  - ± Cranial nerve abnormalities
  - ± Altered reflexes
  - ± Proprioceptive deficits
  - ± Altered mentation
- Upper airway exam:
  - ± Brachycephalic syndrome (i.e., stenotic nares, hypoplastic trachea, everted laryngeal saccules, elongated soft palate)

ETIOLOGY AND PATHOPHYSIOLOGY

- Cardiac:
  - *Bradyarrhythmias*: syncope can result when there is a >6–8 second pause in electrical activity (i.e., failure of subsidiary pacemaker in third-degree AV block, sinus arrest associated with SSS).
  - *Tachyarrhythmias*: rates >300 bpm for >6 seconds (i.e., supraventricular tachycardia (SVT) or ventricular tachycardia) in dogs; cats uncommonly experience syncope with tachyarrhythmias but more so with bradycardias. Heart rate and time necessary for syncope may vary depending on underlying systolic function (i.e., a slower heart rate for a shorter duration may cause syncope in an animal with underlying myocardial or valvular heart disease). Various outcomes include: nonsustained tachyarrhythmia results in a return to sinus rhythm; overdrive suppression leads to sinus arrest; or possibly ventricular fibrillation.

  - *Outflow obstruction* (i.e., pulmonic stenosis, subaortic stenosis, cor pulmonale due to heartworm disease with secondary pulmonary hypertension):
    - Classic theory: exercise results in vasodilation of systemic arterioles. Fixed obstruction to flow results in inadequate increase in cardiac output leading to hypotension and syncope.
    - Alternate theory: contractility, cardiac output, and flow increase through stenosis during exercise. Increased left ventricular systolic pressure causes overstimulation of left ventricular mechanoreceptors. Reflex activation of cardiac afferent vagal fibers results in increased parasympathetic tone to heart and systemic blood vessels, resulting in bradycardia, vasodilation, and subsequent syncope.
  - *Cyanotic heart disease*: (i.e., right-to-left patent ductus arteriosus, tetralogy of Fallot): syncope is due to hypoxia and/or hyperviscosity of blood from polycythemia, or else is from arrhythmias.
  - *Masses obstructing inflow or outflow of blood (rare)*: intracardiac mass lesions reduce cardiac output by restricting blood flow through atrioventricular valves or obstructing a ventricular outflow tract. Pericardial disease compromises cardiac output by interfering with systemic venous return (i.e., pericardial effusion).
  - *Congestive heart failure*: syncope mechanism presumed to be similar to autonomic dysfunction (see below).
- Noncardiac:
  - *Neurologic syncope*: increased intracranial pressure with resultant decrease in cerebral perfusion (i.e., cerebral edema, brain tumors, meningitis, encephalitis, cerebral vascular obstructions, acute bleed). Syncope occurs very rarely, in contrast to seizures, which occur commonly with the same diseases.
  - *Metabolic syncope*: abrupt decrease in oxygen or nutrient delivery (i.e., glucose) to the brain (i.e., oxygen concentration is affected by blood flow, hemoglobin concentration, and oxygen tension). Seizures > syncope.
  - *Tussive syncope*:
    - Proposed mechansisms:
      1. Increased intrathoracic pressure transiently increases intracranial pressure and diminishes cardiac venous return and resultant cardiac output; cerebral blood flow is decreased during paroxysms of coughing.
      2. Coughing stimulates vagal afferent transmission to the vasomotor center in the medulla with subsequent stimulation of vagal efferents to the heart and blood vessels (bradycardia, hypotension).
  - *Autonomic dysfunction*: excessive baroreflex resulting in cardiac inhibition and/or peripheral vasodilation (i.e., neurocardiogenic syncope, carotid sinus sensitivity, carotid body tumor).
  - *Peripheral vasomotor dysfunction*: abnormality of peripheral vasoconstriction, muscle tone, heart rate, and/or respiration, resulting in syncope (postural hypotension).
  - *Undetermined*: ~40% of human syncope cases despite extensive testing; likely similar percentage in veterinary medicine,

DIAGNOSIS

DIFFERENTIAL DIAGNOSIS

- Primary cardiac disease (see above)
- Hypotension (inadequate cardiac output, poor vascular tone)
- Hypoxemia (pulmonary thromboembolism, pulmonary disease, right-to-left shunt)
- Abnormal blood or metabolic constituents (hypoglycemia, hypokalemia, anemia)
- Neoplasia (splenic hemangiosarcoma)
- Neurologic and neuromuscular disorders (epilepsy, structural central nervous system disorders, narcolepsy, myasthenia gravis)

INITIAL DATABASE

- Complete blood count: ± anemia, thrombocytopenia
- Serum biochemistry panel: ± electrolyte abnormalities, ± metabolic derangements
- Urinalysis: ± proteinuria with AT III loss and subsequent hypercoagulable state (thromboembolism)
- Blood pressure: normal result does not rule out transient hypotension
- ± Heartworm antigen test
- ± Microfilaria test
- Thoracic radiographs: ± evidence of structural heart disease, ± pulmonary parenchymal abnormalities (i.e., pulmonary artery abnormalities with heartworm disease, cardiogenic pulmonary edema)
- Echocardiogram: ± congenital or acquired heart disease
- Resting electrocardiogram (ECG): ± rhythm abnormalities
- Neurologic exam: ± neurologic deficits

ADVANCED OR CONFIRMATORY TESTING

- Videotaping: Episodes that are not convincingly syncopal based on history alone (a common problem) and do not occur in the veterinary facility may be evaluated objectively by having the owner videotape them at home.
- Holter monitor: 24-hour ECG; helpful in establishing a diagnosis 42% of the time (see Holter/Cardiac Event Monitoring, p 1264).
- Cardiac event recorder: digital loop recorder that is patient or owner activated, programmed to capture the heart rate and rhythm prior to and after the syncopal episode(s); diagnostic yield 85%.
- Abdominal ultrasound: may be helpful in identification of mass(es).
- Computed tomography/magnetic resonance imaging/cerebrospinal fluid tap: neurologic disease.

TREATMENT

THERAPEUTIC GOAL(S)

- Alleviate syncopal episodes
- Prevent sudden death

ACUTE GENERAL TREATMENT

- Acute treatment is aimed at the underlying cause or at stabilization procedures Blood loss: fluids, blood products, etc.
- Pericardial effusion with cardiac tamponade: pericardiocentesis
- Continuous ECG
- *Bradyarrhythmias*:
  - SSS, third-degree AV block: medical management may be effective if arrhythmia is due to excessive vagal tone and atropine responsive (i.e., anticholinergics (propantheline) and β agonists (terbutaline); see individual diseases for specific treatment recommendations).Temporary pacemaker if bradyarrhythmia is refractory to medical management and animal is showing persistent clinical signs
- *Tachyarrhythmias*:
  - Ventricular tachycardia: oral or intravenous medical management depending on malignancy of the arrhythmia (i.e., oral options: mexiletine, sotalol, atenolol; intravenous options: lidocaine, procainamide, esmolol). See Ventricular Arrhythmias, p 1148. Cautious use of, or avoid, β-blockers in cases with systolic dysfunction/dilated cardiomyopathy

CHRONIC TREATMENT

- Treatment of underlying cause if systemic disorder
- Bradyarrhythmias:
  - Medically refractory SSS, high-grade second-degree AV block, third-degree AV block: permanent pacemaker
- Tachyarrhythmias:
  - Supraventricular tachycardia: calcium channel blocker, β-blocker, digitalis glycosides. See Atrial Premature Complexes and Atrial/Supraventricular Tachycardia, p 100

- Ventricular Tachycardia: see Ventricular Arrhythmias, p 1148
- Severe outflow obstructions:
  - Limit exertion in all cases
  - Subaortic stenosis (SAS): β-blockers if severe (see Subaortic Stenosis, p 1048)
  - Pulmonic stenosis: β-blockers if severe (see Pulmonic Stenosis p, 921)
  - Hypertrophic obstructive cardiomyopathy: β-blocker, calcium channel blocker (see Hypertrophic Cardiomyopathy, p 554)
  - Heartworm disease with secondary pulmonary hypertension: see Heartworm Disease, Cat, p 462; Heartworm Disease, Dog, p 465
- Cyanotic heart disease-induced polycythemia: phlebotomy or hydroxyurea 50 mg/kg PO 2 to 3 times weekly, adjusted based on response
- Congestive heart failure: see Heart Failure, Chronic, p 459
- Neurologic syncope: treatment of underlying cause
- Metabolic syncope: treatment of underlying cause
- Tussive syncope: cough suppressant (e.g., butorphanol 0.1-0.5 mg/kg PO q 8-12h), bronchodilator (aminophylline 10 mg/kg PO q 8h), treatment with diuretics (e.g., furosemide 2 mg/kg IV, SC) if pulmonary edema is present
- Autonomic dysfunction: anticholinergics (e.g., propantheline bromide 0.5-1 mg/kg PO q 8h if bradycardia-related), β-blocker (e.g., atenolol 0.25-1 mg/kg PO q 12h if tachycardia-related). Treatment modalities are aimed at maintaining heart rate and/or preventing sympathetic surge. Medical management fails to address hypotensive component of reflex arc, and animals continue to faint, potentially requiring a pacemaker

DRUG INTERACTIONS

β-Blockers, diuretics, and vasodilators can exacerbate hypotension.

POSSIBLE COMPLICATIONS

Sudden death

RECOMMENDED MONITORING

Serial evaluations as needed to acquire initial database and confirmatory testing

PROGNOSIS AND OUTCOME

- Highly dependent on underlying etiology
- Excellent for bradyarrhythmias treated with pacemaker implantation
- Fair to good with supraventricular tachycardia responsive to medical therapy
- Guarded with ventricular tachycardia treated medically; poor if systolic dysfunction/dilated cardiomyopathy present
- Variable prognosis with outflow obstructions (i.e., severe SAS has a poor long-term prognosis)
- Good with tussive syncope treated medically if cough responds well to therapy
- Good prognosis with autonomic dysfunction. Treatment is usually unrewarding. Fortunately, sudden death is not common
- Poor prognosis: neoplasia

PEARLS & CONSIDERATIONS

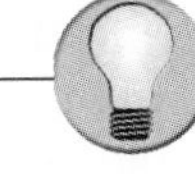

COMMENTS

- Syncopal episodes may be difficult to differentiate from seizures. Videotaping and ECG event monitoring (see Holter/Cardiac Event Monitoring, p 1264) are simple, noninvasive tests that greatly help differentiate between the two.
- Syncope, while uncommon in cats, occasionally occurs with hypertrophic obstructive cardiomyopathy and with bradyarrhythmias (e.g., third-degree AV block).
- In SSS, bradyarrhythmias (e.g., sinus arrest) typically cause syncopal episodes warranting pacemaker therapy prior to addressing tachyarrhythmias (e.g., SVT, see Atrial Premature Complexes and Atrial/Supraventricular Tachycardia, p 100).
- In 40% of human cases, an etiology is never identified; similar percentages are suspected in veterinary medicine.

PREVENTION

- Tussive syncope: cough suppressant, bronchodilator, treatment with diuretics if pulmonary edema is present
- Autonomic dysfunction: anticholinergics, β-blocker

CLIENT EDUCATION

- Treatment and prognosis are dependent on the underlying etiology.
- Sudden death is possible but is dependent on the underlying etiology.

SUGGESTED READING

Beckett SD, et al: Syncopal attacks and sudden death in dogs: mechanisms and etiologies. *J Am Anim Hosp Assoc* 14:378-386, 1978.

Davidow EB, et al: Syncope: pathophysiology and differential diagnosis. *Comp Con Ed Pract Vet* 23(7):609-618, 2001.

Kittleson MD: Syncope. In Kittleson (ed): *Small Animal Cardiovascular Medicine*. St. Louis, Mosby, 1998, pp 495-501.

Rush JE: Syncope and episodic weakness. In Fox PR, Sisson D, Moise NS (eds): *Textbook of Canine and Feline Cardiology*. Philadelphia, Saunders, 1999, pp 446-454.

AUTHOR: **SARAH J. MILLER**

EDITOR: **ETIENNE CÔTÉ**

Syndrome of Inappropriate Antidiuretic Hormone Secretion

BASIC INFORMATION

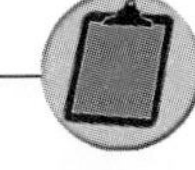

DEFINITION

Release of antidiuretic hormone (ADH) in the absence of normal osmotic or nonosmotic stimuli

SYNONYM(S)

Antidiuretic hormone: vasopressin

Secretion of inappropriate antidiuretic hormone (SIADH)

EPIDEMIOLOGY

SPECIES, AGE, SEX

- Rare disease of the dog
- No gender or age predilection

CLINICAL PRESENTATION

DISEASE FORMS/SUBTYPES

- Idiopathic
- Secondary to an underlying disorder

HISTORY, CHIEF COMPLAINT

- Lethargy
- Inappetence
- Neurologic signs

PHYSICAL EXAM FINDINGS

- Weakness
- Tremors
- Seizures
- No evidence of peripheral edema or ascites
- No evidence of hypovolemia

ETIOLOGY AND PATHOPHYSIOLOGY

- In this syndrome, ADH release occurs independent of normal stimuli due to production of ADH or an analog by a tumor or occurs as an idiopathic phenomenon.
- In dogs, the syndrome of inappropriate antidiuretic hormone secretion (SIADH) has been reported as an idiopathic phenomenon in two cases, secondary to a central nervous system (CNS) disease in two cases (hypothalamic tumor, amebic meningoencephali-

tis), in a dog with heartworm disease, and in a dog with an undifferentiated carcinoma.
- In people, SIADH has been associated with pulmonary disease, cranial disease, malignant neoplasms, and drugs.
- Inappropriate ADH release results in increased water resorption at the renal collecting ducts, which leads to volume expansion and hyponatremia.
- Volume expansion leads to reduced proximal tubular sodium resorption and enhanced natriuresis.
- Neurologic signs secondary to cerebral edema occur as a consequence of volume expansion and hyponatremia.

DIAGNOSIS

DIFFERENTIAL DIAGNOSIS

- Hyponatremia (see Hyponatremia, p 567):
  - Hypoadrenocorticism
  - Diabetes mellitus
  - Gastrointestinal (GI) sodium loss (vomiting, diarrhea)
  - Chronic congestive heart failure
  - Psychogenic polydipsia
  - Artifact (hyperlipidemia)
  - Acute renal failure
  - Severe liver disease
  - Nephrotic syndrome
  - Severe hypothyroidism with myxedema

INITIAL DATABASE

- Complete blood count (CBC), serum biochemical profile, urinalysis: hyponatremia, normal renal parameters
- Thoracic radiographs: possible underlying pulmonary disease, such as primary or metastatic neoplasia
- Adrenocorticotropic hormone (ACTH) stimulation test: normal response

ADVANCED OR CONFIRMATORY TESTING

- Plasma osmolality: decreased (<280-310 mOsm/kg)
- Urine osmolality: inappropriately increased (>100 mOsm/kg) in the face of plasma hypoosmolality and hyponatremia
- Urine sodium concentration: increased despite hyponatremia

TREATMENT

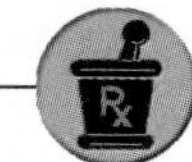

THERAPEUTIC GOAL(S)

- Correction of hyponatremia
- Treatment of underlying disease

ACUTE GENERAL TREATMENT

Severe hyponatremia (<120 mEq/L) should be corrected with IV fluid therapy using conventional crystalloid solutions (0.9% saline, lactated Ringer's solution) to raise serum sodium levels at a rate of less than 0.5 mEq/L/hr.

- Hypertonic saline (3-5%) should be used with caution as it may raise the serum sodium concentrations too rapidly in cases of chronic hyponatremia.
- Administration of furosemide in conjunction with fluid therapy reduces the risk of extracellular fluid (ECF) volume expansion in already overhydrated patients.
- Once serum sodium concentrations have been corrected to >125 mEq/L, water intake may be restricted to a volume less than urine output to promote free water loss and restore normal body fluid volume.

CHRONIC TREATMENT

- Chronic management of SIADH is directed at treating the underlying cause.
- A selective ADH receptor antagonist, OPC-31260 (Otsuka Pharmaceutical, Tokyo), has been reported to palliate signs in a dog with SIADH over a 3-year treatment period (3mg/kg PO q 12h).

POSSIBLE COMPLICATIONS

- Rapid correction of chronic hyponatremia can result in osmotic demyelination syndrome due to brain dehydration as free water moves out of the brain and into the relatively hypertonic serum.
- Clinical signs of osmotic demyelination syndrome occur 3 to 4 days after rapid correction of hyponatremia, are neurologic in nature (lethargy, ataxia, hypermetria, paresis), and may be fatal.

RECOMMENDED MONITORING

Serial monitoring of serum sodium concentration during acute correction phase and periodic monitoring during chronic management

PROGNOSIS AND OUTCOME

Prognosis is dependent on the underlying cause of SIADH

PEARLS & CONSIDERATIONS

COMMENTS

- ADH release may be stimulated by various drugs used during anesthesia (barbiturates, narcotics) and can result in impaired free water excretion and hyponatremia in the postoperative period, similar to what is seen in animals with SIADH. Restriction of water intake is generally sufficient to restore normal water balance in these animals.
- During treatment, never increase serum sodium concentration by more than 0.5 mEq/L/hr (risk of osmotic demyelination syndrome and life-threatening cerebral complications).

SUGGESTED READING

DiBartola SP: Disorders of sodium and water. In Dibartola SP: *Fluid Therapy in Small Animal Practice*, ed 2. Philadelphia, WB Saunders, 2000, pp 64-65.

Feldman EC, Nelson RW: Water metabolism and diabetes insipidus. In Feldman EC, Nelson RW (eds): *Canine and Feline Endocrinology and Reproduction*, ed 3. St. Louis, WB Saunders, 2004, pp 41-42.

AUTHOR: **SARAH L. NAIDOO**
EDITOR: **SHERRI IHLE**

Synovial Cell Sarcoma

BASIC INFORMATION

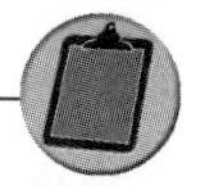

DEFINITION

A malignant tumor in the tissue lining the capsule of a joint

SYNONYM(S)

SCS

Synovial sarcoma

EPIDEMIOLOGY

SPECIES, AGE, SEX: The median reported age is 8.5 years.

GENETICS AND BREED PREDISPOSITION: Golden retrievers seem to be overrepresented.

CLINICAL PRESENTATION

DISEASE FORMS/SUBTYPES: Histopathologically, there are two cell types: epitheloid (synovioblastic) and spindle (fibrosarcomatous) cell types.

HISTORY, CHIEF COMPLAINT: Most animals present with a slow growing mass over a joint and concurrent lameness.

PHYSICAL EXAM FINDINGS: The clinical signs are directly related to the site of involvement and local invasiveness. Physical examination abnormalities include lameness and the presence of a mass near the affected joint. Other lameness-related findings could include stiffness of gait, reduced range of motion, crepitus, joint swelling, and pain. Depending on the duration of disease, joint instability may be present (ligament tear, subluxation). Other nonspecific clinical signs include lethargy, anorexia, and hemiparesis.

ETIOLOGY AND PATHOPHYSIOLOGY

- Synovial cell sarcoma (SCS) is a locally invasive tumor, and underlying bone destruction is common.
- Metastasis to regional lymph nodes, lungs, and other sites occurs in up to 25% of cases.
- In dogs, SCS most frequently involves the stifle and elbow, although other sites have been reported.
- No known etiologic factors.

DIAGNOSIS

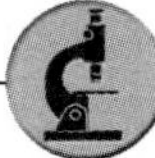

DIFFERENTIAL DIAGNOSIS

- Degenerative joint disease, immune-mediated, or infectious arthritis.
- Other joint tumors reported in dogs include fibrosarcoma, rhabdomyosarcoma, osteosarcoma, malignant fibrous histiocytoma, liposarcoma, hemangiosarcoma, myxoma, malignant giant cell tumor of soft tissue, and undifferentiated sarcoma.
- Histiocytic sarcomas have also been reported in the periarticular tissue of large appendicular joints.
- Histologically, it may be challenging to differentiate SCS from other mesenchymal or epitheloid malignancies. Special immunohistochemical stains are almost always necessary to confirm a diagnosis of SCS.

INITIAL DATABASE

- Fine-needle aspirate (FNA) and cytologic examination of the mass or the affected joint are useful in identifying and differentiating other causes of lameness.
- Regional radiographs of the affected joint are recommended to help rule out other causes of musculoskeletal lameness.
  - Regional radiographic abnormalities include soft tissue swelling; in advanced cases, cortical destruction and periosteal reaction are evident.
  - Radiographic evidence of lysis involving the proximal and distal bones of a joint is suggestive of SCS; however, other soft tissue sarcomas can cross the joint space and will need to be ruled out.
- After a diagnosis of malignancy has been confirmed, the minimum database should include laboratory evaluation of complete blood count (CBC), serum biochemical analysis, urinalysis, three views of thoracic radiographs, and abdominal ultrasound to rule out any abdominal visceral metastasis.

ADVANCED OR CONFIRMATORY TESTING

- If necessary, a CT scan or an MRI can be performed to evaluate the local extension of the causative lesions.
- An immunohistochemistry test is necessary to confirm a histologic diagnosis and differentiate SCS from histiocytic sarcoma and other malignancies; however, reliability of current immunohistochemistry stains may be equivocal. This is due to marked variation in proportions and differentiation of the cellular elements involved with the mesenchymal tissue adjacent to the synovial membrane.
- In cases of SCS, positive histochemical staining for cytokeratin (epithelial marker) and histologic grade may predict outcome and prognosis.

TREATMENT

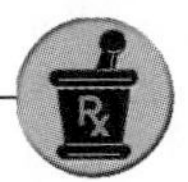

THERAPEUTIC GOAL(S)

Long-term tumor control

ACUTE GENERAL TREATMENT

- Analgesic and nonsteroidal anti-inflammatory drugs (NSAIDs) are often indicated for pain palliation.
- Limb amputation.
- Local resection followed by radiotherapy to the tumor bed can be attempted if the animal is not a candidate for limb amputation. Efficacy of radiotherapy is not known.

CHRONIC TREATMENT

Efficacy of chemotherapy has not been determined for canine SCS. For dogs with high-grade tumors or dogs that present with overt metastasis, adjuvant chemotherapy with drugs, such as doxorubicin, platinum agents, and ifosfamide, may prove beneficial. Consultation with a medical oncologist is recommended.

RECOMMENDED MONITORING

Periodic evaluation for distant metastasis and local recurrence

PROGNOSIS AND OUTCOME

- Clinical outcome is excellent after limb amputation in cases with no gross detectable metastatic disease. A median survival of 28 to 36 months has been reported in dogs treated by means of limb amputation alone, with or without adjuvant chemotherapy.
- It may be possible to better determine the prognosis of dogs with SCS based on certain prognostic factors. Prognostic factors for survival of dogs with SCS treated with amputation include clinical stage (no metastases >48 months; metastases: 3 months), histologic grade (grade I or II: 36 months; grade III: 7 months), and cytokeratin staining (negative: >48 months; positive: 4 months).

PEARLS & CONSIDERATIONS

COMMENTS

- Histopathologically, the majority of cases exhibit a biphasic pattern, resembling both mesenchymal and epitheloid origins. Because of these features, pathologists may have to differentiate between a poorly differentiated carcinoma, histiocytic sarcoma, and SCS.
- SCS is rarely diagnosed in cats. Among the nine reported cases of feline SCS, there have been six reports of malignant SCS and three reports of benign synovioma.

SUGGESTED READING

Craig LE, et al: The diagnosis and prognosis of synovial tumors in dogs: 35 cases. *Vet Pathol* 39:66, 2002.

Fox DB, et al: Canine synovial sarcoma: A retrospective assessment of described prognostic criteria in 16 cases (1994-1999). *J Am Anim Hosp Assoc* 38:347, 2002.

Liptak JM, et al: Metastatic synovial cell sarcoma in two cats. *Veterinary and Comparative Oncology* 2:164, 2004.

Loukopoulos P, et al: Canine biphasic synovial sarcoma: Case report and immunohistochemical characterization. *J Vet Sci* 5:173, 2004.

Vail DM, et al: Evaluation of prognostic factors for dogs with synovial sarcoma: 36 cases (1986-1991). *J Am Vet Med Assoc* 205:1300, 1994.

AUTHOR: **RAVINDER S. DHALIWAL**
EDITOR: **KENNETH M. RASSNICK**

Systemic Hypertension

Client Education Sheet on Website

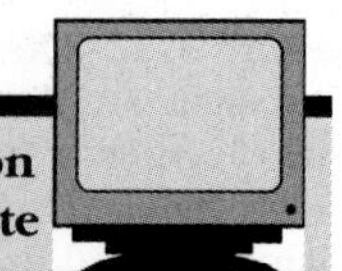

BASIC INFORMATION

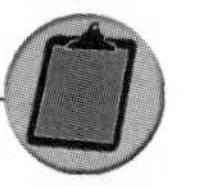

DEFINITION

A sustained elevation in the arterial blood pressure (BP). In dogs and cats, systemic hypertension is suspected if sustained systolic BP >160 mmHg, diastolic BP >95 mmHg, or both.

SYNONYM(S)

Arterial hypertension

EPIDEMIOLOGY

SPECIES, AGE, SEX: Systemic hypertension occurs in both dogs and cats, and there is no significant age or sex predisposition in either species. However, some systemic diseases commonly associated with systemic hypertension (e.g., chronic renal failure, hyperthyroidism) are more common in older animals.

GENETICS AND BREED PREDISPOSITION: There is no breed predisposition in cats. Sighthounds (e.g., deerhounds, Irish wolfhounds) have higher normal BP ranges than other breeds. Although essential hypertension has been diagnosed in one family of dogs, systemic hypertension usually occurs secondary to other diseases and, as such, is not inherited.

ASSOCIATED CONDITIONS AND DISORDERS: Although essential (cause unknown) hypertension is diagnosed in veterinary patients, most cases of systemic hypertension occur as a complication of another systemic disease. In cats, the most common diseases associated with systemic hypertension are chronic renal failure and hyperthyroidism. Many cats with hyperthyroidism have subclinical renal disease; in these animals, it is unclear whether renal disease, hyperthyroidism, or both are responsible for the hypertension. The prevalence of hypertension in cats with diabetes mellitus is still unclear.

In dogs, the diseases most commonly associated with systemic hypertension are chronic renal disease (especially proteinuric renal disease), hyperadrenocorticism, diabetes mellitus, and pheochromocytoma. Less typical causes of systemic hypertension in either species include hyperaldosteronism, acromegaly, and use of hypertensive medications (e.g., phenylpropanolamine, excessive thyroxine supplementation).

CLINICAL PRESENTATION

DISEASE FORMS/SUBTYPES: Systemic hypertension can be diagnosed based on clinical signs (clinical systemic hypertension) or be diagnosed as part of a diagnostic evaluation of a systemic disease, with the animal showing no overt clinical signs (subclinical systemic hypertension).

HISTORY, CHIEF COMPLAINT

- Signs associated with the underlying disease
- Lethargy, changes in activity or appetite, or mentation changes:
  - Owner may interpret the signs as "signs of aging"
- Acute blindness, intraocular hemorrhage
- Intracranial neurologic signs:
  - Generalized seizures
  - Focal facial seizures

PHYSICAL EXAM FINDINGS

- Signs of underlying systemic disease (e.g., signs of renal failure or hyperthyroidism)
- Ocular: vitreal or retinal hemorrhage, retinal detachment, hyphema, vascular tortuosity
- Nervous system: signs of intracranial disease, changes in mentation (usually decreased but may include heightened anxiety), seizures (generalized or focal facial)
- Cardiovascular system: new murmur, typically mitral insufficiency, arrhythmia, gallop sound, left ventricular hypertrophy on echocardiographic examination
- Other: epistaxis

ETIOLOGY AND PATHOPHYSIOLOGY

- The pathophysiology of systemic hypertension is still poorly understood.
- Likely to be multifactorial; individual mechanisms may predominate in some diseases.
  - Abnormalities in renal sodium handling
  - Inappropriate activation of the renin-angiotensin-aldosterone system
  - Inappropriate activation of the sympathetic nervous system
  - Hypersensitivity to the effects of cortisol
  - Blood volume expansion secondary to underlying disease states
- Better understanding of mechanisms in individual diseases is likely to lead to more effective tailoring of therapy.

DIAGNOSIS

DIFFERENTIAL DIAGNOSIS

- Ocular signs: coagulopathies; uveitis; inflammatory, infectious, or neoplastic diseases; trauma
- Neurologic signs: intracranial lesions
- Cardiovascular signs: primary cardiac disease, other secondary cardiac diseases
- Epistaxis: coagulopathies, trauma, neoplasia, fungal rhinitis

INITIAL DATABASE

- Initial diagnostic testing as guided by underlying disease, if known
- BP measurement (see Blood Pressure Measurement, p 1191)
- If systemic hypertension is diagnosed in a patient without known predisposing disease:
  - Dogs: complete blood count (CBC), serum chemistry profile, urinalysis with urine protein analysis if proteinuria is present
  - Cats: CBC, serum chemistry profile, urinalysis, serum thyroxine if patient is ≥10 years old
  - Both species: consider thoracic radiographs or abdominal ultrasound

ADVANCED OR CONFIRMATORY TESTING

Repeated BP measurements over the course of several hours may be needed if animal is excited or very anxious during the first measurement period

TREATMENT

THERAPEUTIC GOAL(S)

- Systemic hypertension with clinical signs present:
  - First priority: prompt reduction of systolic BP to <160 mmHg
  - Second priority: initiating clinical evaluation for causative disease
- Systemic hypertension found in conjunction with causative underlying disease but no clinical signs of hypertension are present:
  - Institute optimal therapy of causative condition
  - Confirm elevated BP values on >1 occasion to lessen the chance of anxiety- or excitement-related elevations of BP
  - If systolic BP >180 mmHg on more than one measurement occasion, begin antihypertensive therapy
  - Systolic BP is 160–180 mmHg on more than one measurement occasion:
    - If underlying disease can be controlled (e.g., hyperthyroidism or hyperadrenocorticism) or cured (e.g., hyperthyroidism if surgery/radioiodine therapy is available), monitor BP during therapy of underlying disease and treat if systolic BP exceeds 180 mmHg on >1

occasion. If hypertension persists when causative disease is controlled or cured, antihypertensive medication is indicated
- If underlying disease is unknown or unlikely to be cured (e.g., chronic renal failure), begin antihypertensive therapy

ACUTE GENERAL TREATMENT

- Discontinue any hypertensive medications
- Emergency antihypertensive therapy for animals with acute ocular or neurologic signs:
  - Dogs: either oral or IV therapy (start at low end of dose and titrate to effect):
    - Nitroprusside: 0.5–5 μg/kg/min as continuous rate infusion IV, or
    - Hydralazine (oral): 0.5–2 mg/kg PO q 12h
  - Cats:
    - Amlodipine: 0.625 mg PO q 24h if cat ≤ 5 kg; 1.25 mg PO q 24h if cat >5 kg, or
    - Hydralazine: 0.5–2 mg/kg PO q 12h

CHRONIC TREATMENT

Dogs: medications from different groups may be added if original medication is not adequate to control hypertension
- Angiotensin-coverting enzyme inhibitors:
  - Enalapril: 0.5 mg/kg PO q 12–24h, or
  - Benazepril: 0.25–0.5 mg/kg PO q 24h
- Calcium (Ca) channel blockers:
  - Amlodipine: 0.01–0.2 mg/kg PO q 12–24h

Cats:
- Ca channel blockers (preferred first line therapy):
  - Amlodipine: 0.625 mg PO q 24h if cat <5 kg; 1.25 mg PO q 24h if cat >5 kg
- β-Receptor antagonists (β-blockers):
  - May be useful addition to amlodipine if hyperthyroidism is present
  - Atenolol: 6.25 mg PO q 24h if cat ≤5 kg; 12.5 mg PO q 24h if cat >5 kg
- Angiotensin-coverting enzyme inhibitors:
  - Usually inadequate as monotherapy but may have additive effects when given with other medications
  - Enalapril: 0.5 mg/kg PO q 12–24h
  - Benazepril: 0.25–0.5 mg/kg PO q 12–24h

DRUG INTERACTIONS

- BP-lowering sedatives (e.g., acepromazine) should be used with caution in animals receiving any antihypertensive medication.
- Two medications from the same drug group should not be used together (e.g., benazepril and enalapril).

POSSIBLE COMPLICATIONS

- Hypotension:
  - Resuscitate as needed
  - Reduce dose of BP medication
  - Reevaluate need for antihypertensive medication
- Uncontrolled hypertension despite drug therapy:
  - Review medications and administration information with caregiver
  - Add medications from other classes if needed
  - Consult a specialist for further additions/modifications if hypertension is not controlled with two antihypertensive medications at upper end of dosing ranges
- Previously controlled hypertension now out of desired target range:
  - Dogs: hypertension may worsen over time, or underlying disease may be inadequately controlled:
    - Ensure optimal therapy of underlying disease
    - Screen for hypertensive medications and check postpill serum thyroxine concentration in animals receiving thyroid supplementation
    - Add additional antihypertensive medications or increase doses of present medications to high end of dosage range, if tolerated
  - Cats: hypertension control is usually stable once achieved. If BP continues to increase over time, treat as recommended in dogs, above

RECOMMENDED MONITORING

- Once the condition is controlled, check BP in hypertensive patients every 3 months
- If doses/medications change, recheck BP in 3 to 5 days after change to ensure efficacy

PROGNOSIS AND OUTCOME

- If retinal detachment has occurred, the retina may reattach, but prognosis for return of vision is poor
- Prognosis for resolution of other clinical signs of hypertension (e.g., focal facial seizures, changes in mentation, hyphema) is favorable if BP can be controlled with medication and underlying diseases can be controlled as well
- Prognosis of systemic hypertension may be affected by prognosis of causative disease

PEARLS & CONSIDERATIONS

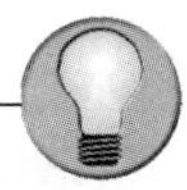

COMMENTS

- Owners may interpret clinical signs of hypertension as "signs of aging," and vigilance regarding monitoring of BP in animals at risk will detect subclinical cases.
- Any dog or cat with a systemic disease known to cause hypertension should have its BP monitored periodically regardless of clinical signs.
- High BP detected in young animals with no risk factors is often spurious.

CLIENT EDUCATION

For optimal patient management, inform clients that:
- Hypertension is usually a complication of another disease rather than primary disease in itself.
- Control of hypertension is necessary to avoid catastrophic ocular or neurologic damage and to minimize ongoing damage to susceptible organs (e.g., kidneys).
- If the underlying disease is not curable, therapy for systemic hypertension is likely to be lifelong.
- Many patients will require >1 medication to adequately control hypertension, and the need for medication may increase over time.

SUGGESTED READING

Brown SA, Henik RA: Therapy for systemic hypertension in dogs and cats. In Bonagura JD (ed): *Kirk's Current Veterinary Therapy XIII: Small Animal Practice*. Philadelphia, WB Saunders, 2000, pp 838–841.

Cowgill LG, Kallet AJ: Recognition and management of hypertension in the dog. In Kirk RW, Bonagura JD (eds): *Current Veterinary Therapy VIII: Small Animal Practice*. Philadelphia, WB Saunders, 1983, pp 1025–1028.

Elliott J, et al: Feline hypertension: Clinical findings and response to antihypertensive treatment in 30 cases. *J Sm Anim Prac* 42:122, 2001.

Maggio FT, et al: Ocular lesions associated with systemic hypertension in cats: 69 cases (1985–1998). *J Am Vet Med Assoc* 217: 695, 2000.

AUTHOR: **REBECCA L. STEPIEN**
EDITOR: **ETIENNE CÔTÉ**

Systemic Inflammatory Response Syndrome

BASIC INFORMATION

DEFINITION

- A systemic dysregulated inflammatory process. It leads to disorders of microcirculation, organ perfusion, and finally to organ dysfunction. Untreated, SIRS leads to multiple organ dysfunction syndrome (MODS) and death.
- Systemic inflammatory response syndrome (SIRS) is defined clinically as the presence of two or more of the following conditions in dogs and cats:
  - Dogs: body temperature >40°C or <38°C; heart rate >120 bpm in a calm, resting dog; hyperventilation or $PaCO_2$ <30 mmHg; and white blood cell (WBC) count >18,000/mm³ or <5000/mm³ or >5% immature (band) forms.
  - Cats: body temperature >40°C or <38°C; heart rate >140 bpm in calm, resting cat; respiratory rate >20 breaths per minute or $PaCO_2$ <28 mmHg; and WBC count >18,000/mm³ or <5000/mm³ or >5% immature (band) forms.
- SIRS is differentiated from sepsis by the fact that no infection can be documented in animals with SIRS.

EPIDEMIOLOGY

SPECIES, AGE, SEX: There are no species, age, or sex predilections.

HISTORY, CHIEF COMPLAINT: May include vague complaints, such as lethargy, anorexia, vomiting, or diarrhea, or may include a specific event (i.e., trauma, burn injury, heat stroke).

PHYSICAL EXAM FINDINGS

- Often varied and may include generalized depression, fever, tachycardia, or tachypnea.
- By definition, findings associated with an underlying inflammatory condition (i.e., pancreatitis, trauma) and two or more of the four criteria already listed are expected in animals with SIRS.
- Specific physical exam findings depend on the underlying cause of the SIRS (e.g., if hit by a car: associated injuries, such as lacerations and fractures, are commonly found).

ETIOLOGY AND PATHOPHYSIOLOGY

- SIRS can arise from a number of etiologic triggers, including pancreatitis, burns, massive trauma (e.g., hit by car, fall from high elevation, attack by other animal), hypovolemic shock, immune reactions (autoimmune disease), heat stroke, and tissue ischemia of various causes.
- Inflammation is a response to infection, antigen challenge, or tissue injury that is designed to eradicate microbes or irritants and to potentiate tissue repair; however, excessive inflammation may lead, via SIRS, to physiologic decompensation, organ dysfunction, and death.
- A balance normally exists among proinflammatory cytokines and anti-inflammatory cytokines; however, for cases in which the proinflammatory response predominates, severe systemic inflammation may ensue as typified by SIRS.
- In addition to high circulating cytokine levels, systemic inflammation is also associated with activation of the clotting cascade and release of vasoactive mediators such as nitric oxide (NO).
  - High systemic cytokine levels may result in myocardial dysfunction, altered intracellular oxygen utilization, and direct inflammatory injury.
  - Activation of the clotting cascade can cause microvascular thrombosis and tissue hypoperfusion.
  - Increased production of NO and metabolites can lead to peripheral vasodilation, decreased peripheral vascular resistance, and hypotension.

DIAGNOSIS

DIFFERENTIAL DIAGNOSIS

- Sepsis: similar historic and physical findings, but systemic inflammation is pinpointed to an infectious cause (usually bacterial) through cytologic examination of tissue or fluid, bacterial culture and sensitivity (C&S), or histopathologic examination of tissue.
- Neoplasia: Paraneoplastic syndromes may mimic SIRS; identification of the primary neoplasm and resolution of signs with treatment rule out SIRS, retrospectively.
- Hypovolemic shock: like SIRS, it may cause tachycardia, tachypnea, and depression or obtundation; unlike SIRS, hypovolemic shock is not associated with fever or inflammatory changes on a complete blood count (CBC). Generally with hypovolemic shock, the extremities are cold to the touch, whereas they may be warm in animals with SIRS.
- Congestive heart failure (CHF): like SIRS, it may cause tachycardia, tachypnea, and respiratory distress. CHF is differentiated by its underlying cardiac problem (physical examination, thoracic radiographs, echocardiography) and typically by fluid retention (e.g., signs of pulmonary edema seen on radiographs).

INITIAL DATABASE

Main goal is to determine the source of the systemic inflammatory response:

- CBC: by definition, will show either a WBC count greater than 18,000 or less than 5000 or will show the presence of greater than 5% band forms (immature neutrophils). Thrombocytopenia and evidence of hemoconcentration may be present.
- Serum biochemistry panel: commonly shows electrolyte abnormalities, hypoalbuminemia, hyperglycemia or hypoglycemia, hyperbilirubinemia, elevated blood urea nitrogen (BUN)/creatinine (azotemia), and/or elevated liver enzymes, depending on the source of the inciting problem and extent of inflammatory response's effects on visceral organs (progression towards MODS).
- Urinalysis: isosthenuria (normal free water excretion versus renal compromise if azotemia is present simultaneously), concentrated urine (if dehydration/hypovolemia and normal renal function), glucosuria (stress, diabetes mellitus), proteinuria (systemic inflammation, urinary tract inflammation, glomerulopathy), and cellular casts (tubular damage) may be seen.
- Urine C&S is indicated in animals with SIRS, even in the absence of an active urine sediment.
- Blood cultures are recommended because the initial clinical picture of SIRS may not immediately be discernable from that of sepsis and septic shock (see Sepsis and Septic Shock, p 996).

ADVANCED OR CONFIRMATORY TESTING

Specific diagnostic tests will depend on etiology of SIRS. For example, if acute pancreatitis is suspected, abdominal radiographs and an abdominal ultrasound examination are warranted.

TREATMENT

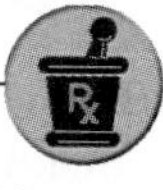

THERAPEUTIC GOAL(S)

- In managing an animal with SIRS, try to achieve three essential treatment principles:
  1. Hemodynamic stability and support of acute life-threatening organ dysfunction
  2. Prolonged support of vital organ function using interventions that minimize iatrogenic injury

3. Modulation of the host-based inflammatory response with interventions that target its specific mediators

- The specific therapeutic goals for treating the systemic inflammatory response syndrome depend on the underlying cause.

ACUTE GENERAL TREATMENT

- IV fluids (crystalloids and colloids) are used for treating hypovolemia and electrolyte abnormalities. During treatment, monitor and maintain electrolytes, BP, and central venous pressure (i.e., mean arterial pressure should be maintained above 60 mmHg, and central venous pressure should be maintained above 5 mmHg). Dextrose-containing solutions may need to be added to the treatment regimen if the patient is hypoglycemic; however, hyperglycemia should probably be avoided because an increase in mortality has been associated with hyperglycemia in humans with critical illness. Blood products (plasma, whole blood, and/or packed red blood cells [RBCs]) may need to be used if continued blood loss is documented (see Transfusion Therapy and Collection Techniques for Blood Banking, p 1312).
- Crystalloid fluids: initial shock dose of 90 ml/kg (dog), 70 ml/kg (cat). Administer this dose IV as a bolus of one-third of the total amount. Then reassess the patient (i.e., measure BP, heart rate) and administer the remainder of the shock dose if the measured parameters have not normalized or substantially improved.
- Colloid fluids: Colloids are useful to use when hypoperfusion and/or hypotension persist and when the shock dose of fluids has already been given as crystalloids. Administer Hetastarch and/or dextran IV either as a bolus or as a constant rate infusion. A dose for initial bolus is 10–20 ml/kg in dogs and 10–15 ml/kg in cats (should be given over 10 to 15 minutes in a cat because it has been associated with nausea). Administer a constant rate infusion of 20 ml/kg per day after the initial bolus if the patient's disease process and cardiovascular status require continued colloid therapy. In humans, coagulopathies have been associated with the use of hetastarch. Therefore, colloids should be used with caution in patients with known coagulopathies.
- Fresh frozen plasma transfusion: dose of 10 ml/kg, at a rate of 4–10 ml/min (infusion should be within 4 hours of thawing plasma/opening bag).
- Whole blood transfusion: dose of 20 ml/kg should be given over 4 hours and can be given faster if the patient requires it due to active bleeding; monitor for transfusion reactions (fever, tachypnea, vomiting) (see Transfusion Therapy and Collection Techniques for Blood Banking, p 1312).
- Packed RBC transfusion: dose of 10 ml/kg, at a rate of over 3 to 4 hours; can be given faster if patient requires the transfusion due to active bleeding or hemolysis; monitor for transfusion reactions (fever, tachypnea, vomiting) (see Transfusion Therapy and Collection Techniques for Blood Banking, p 1312; Transfusion Reactions, p 1098).
- Antimicrobial therapy may be necessary if bacterial translocation or subsequent infections are suspected as possible complications (e.g., transition towards sepsis). Type and dosage of antibiotic depends on suspected source of infection, ideally pending cultures. For example, bacterial translocation from the gastrointestinal (GI) tract, as can occur after prolonged hypotension or a primary GI insult (e.g., parvoviral enteritis), should be treated with a combination of ampicillin 22 mg/kg IV q 8h, and either enrofloxacin 5 mg diluted 1:1 in sterile water and given slowly IV q 12–24h (q 24h maximum in cats due to retinal toxicity risk; never in patients <6 months old), or gentamicin 4 mg/kg IV q 24h (only if renal function is adequate and patient is fully hydrated).
- Corticosteriods are generally contraindicated for patients with SIRS.

PROGNOSIS AND OUTCOME

The prognosis and outcome for SIRS depend on the underlying cause and its severity. If SIRS progresses to sepsis and septic shock, the mortality rate may approach 70%.

PEARLS & CONSIDERATIONS

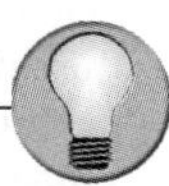

COMMENTS

SIRS caused by a noninfectious etiology may nevertheless progress to sepsis due to development of a nosocomial infection

SUGGESTED READING

Hardie EM: Life-threatening bacterial infection. *Compend Cont Educ Pract Vet* 17(6):763–778, 1995.

AUTHOR: **DANNA M. TORRE**
EDITOR: **ELIZABETH ROZANSKI**

Systemic Lupus Erythematosus

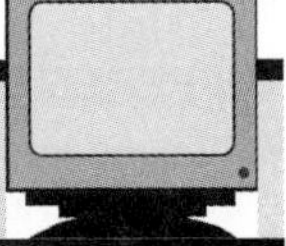

Client Education Sheet on Website

BASIC INFORMATION

DEFINITION

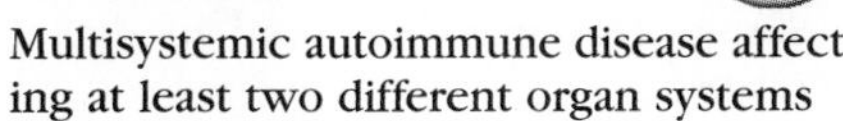

Multisystemic autoimmune disease affecting at least two different organ systems

SYNONYM(S)

SLE
Systemic lupus

EPIDEMIOLOGY

SPECIES, AGE, SEX: More commonly reported in dogs than cats; young to middle-aged animals are predisposed.

GENETICS AND BREED PREDISPOSITION

- Systemic lupus erythematosus (SLE) is clearly inherited in dogs.
- German shepherds may be overrepresented.

GEOGRAPHY AND SEASONALITY: Exposure to UV light may trigger disease flares of the skin.

ASSOCIATED CONDITIONS AND DISORDERS: It is difficult to determine if a concurrent disease is present or instead represents an additional manifestation of SLE.

CLINICAL PRESENTATION

DISEASE FORMS/SUBTYPES: The diagnosis of SLE is made when any three of the following occur concurrently or over any period of time:

- Cutaneous lesions, especially skin exposed to sunlight and/or at mucocutaneous junctions
- Oral ulcers
- Nonseptic, nonerosive polyarthritis
- Glomerulonephritis
- Hemolytic anemia and/or thrombocytopenia
- Leukopenia
- Polymyositis or myocarditis

- Serositis (nonseptic inflammatory effusion in the abdominal, pleural, or pericardial cavity)
- Neurologic disorder (seizures, psychosis, or polyneuritis)
- Significant serum antinuclear antibody (ANA) titer

HISTORY, CHIEF COMPLAINT

- Lameness is the most common primary complaint in dogs.
- Nonspecific lethargy and poor appetite.
- Skin lesions.
- Signs may wax and wane, confusing response to treatment.

PHYSICAL EXAM FINDINGS

- Lameness with swollen, painful joints. The carpi, tarsi, elbows, and stifles are most frequently involved.
- Fever.
- Lymphadenopathy and/or splenomegaly.
- Cutaneous lesions: erythema, scaling, crusting, depigmentation, and alopecia. Lesions may develop on the skin, mucocutaneous junctions, and oral cavity.

ETIOLOGY AND PATHOPHYSIOLOGY

- SLE occurs when a stimulus triggers the appropriate susceptibility genes in a patient.
- Triggering factors may include vaccination, drug administration, stress, infection, or exposure to UV radiation.
- SLE patients produce antibodies directed against a broad range of nuclear, cytoplasmic, and cell membrane molecules; antibodies against the patient's own DNA are measured with the ANA test.

DIAGNOSIS

The diagnosis of SLE is not based on a single test but on the constellation of clinical signs and exclusion of other possible etiologies (see Disease Forms/Subtypes, above).

DIFFERENTIAL DIAGNOSIS

- Tick-borne disease
- Neoplasia and paraneoplastic syndromes
- Bacterial, fungal, or viral infection
- Other immune-mediated diseases

INITIAL DATABASE

- Complete blood count (CBC), including manual differential: may show anemia, leukocytosis, or leukopenia
- Platelet count: may be normal or low
- Serum biochemical profile: abnormalities reflect the site of inflammation (e.g., azotemia and hypoalbuminemia with glomerular involvement)
- Urinalysis: proteinuria is possible
- Urine protein:creatinine ratio
- Urine culture and sensitivity (C&S)
- Skin biopsies: may reveal inflammatory infiltrates at the dermoepidermal junction and vacuolar change in the basal columnar cells
- Radiographs of affected joints: may reveal nonerosive joint swelling
- Arthrocentesis of multiple joints: may reveal sterile neutrophilic inflammation
- Serum ANA titer:
  - Serum ANA are commonly stated as a requirement for the diagnosis of SLE, but the sensitivity and specificity of this test is not known.
  - Normal ranges are determined by individual laboratories.
  - False-positive results can occur with various medications (nonsteroidal anti-inflammatory drugs [NSAIDs], antibiotics, others).
  - False-positive or false-negative results can occur due to variable laboratory standardization, variable quality control, and other factors.
- Lupus erythematosus (LE) cell test: rarely useful
- Thoracic radiographs: may reveal pleural or pericardial effusion (usually subtle)
- Abdominal ultrasonography: usually normal
- Tick-borne disease titers to rule out diseases that can mimic SLE (glomerulonephritis, polyarthritis, hematologic changes, etc.)
- Cats: feline leukemia virus (FeLV) and feline immunodeficiency virus (FIV) serologic tests

ADVANCED OR CONFIRMATORY TESTING

- See Disease Forms/Subtypes above
- Coombs' test: usually negative
- Platelet autoantibodies: rarely useful
- Rheumatoid factor: usually negative
- Immunohistologic evaluation of skin biopsies (immunoperoxidase and immunofluorescent staining): may demonstrate immunoglobulin and complement deposits at the epidermal basement membrane

TREATMENT

THERAPEUTIC GOAL(S)

- Resolve clinical signs
- Prevent progressive renal failure
- Realize that because of the natural waxing and waning of the disease, aggressive therapy may not be indicated for all cases

ACUTE GENERAL TREATMENT

- Prednisone 1 mg/kg PO q 12–24h initially.
- With severe disease, the addition of azathioprine 2.2 mg/kg PO q 24h should be considered.
- Cases with only joint involvement may respond to carprofen 4 mg/kg PO q 24h, or 2 mg/kg PO q 12h; NSAIDs and corticosteroids should not be used together.
- Proteinuria may be lessened with enalapril 0.5 mg/kg PO q 12h, along with dietary protein optimization/restriction.

CHRONIC TREATMENT

- Treat the patient until all clinical and laboratory abnormalities have resolved, then attempt to taper drugs.
- In general, decrease doses by one-half every month, while monitoring clinical and laboratory abnormalities.
- The minimum duration of immunosuppressive therapy is 6 months.
- If signs recur during drug taper, increase level to the previous dose and attempt to taper more slowly.

DRUG INTERACTIONS

- NSAIDs and corticosteroids should not be concurrently administered due to gastrointestinal (GI) ulceration.
- Prolonged administration of azathioprine may cause bone marrow suppression. To reduce the risk, decrease administration to every other day once clinical signs and laboratory abnormalities have resolved.

POSSIBLE COMPLICATIONS

- Progressive renal insufficiency
- Infections (such as urinary tract infection) from long-term immunosuppression

RECOMMENDED MONITORING

- If prednisone is administered, monitor body weight closely and avoid obesity.
- If azathioprine is administered, monitor CBC every 2 weeks while azathioprine is being administered daily. Bone marrow suppression is unusual when azathioprine is tapered to 2.2 mg/kg q 48h; in this case, monitor CBC every 2 to 3 months.
- If immunosuppressive medications are needed chronically, perform a urine culture every 3 months even in the absence of clinical signs of infection.
- Monitor the CBC, serum biochemistry profile, and urinalysis every 3 months once in remission.
- Serum ANA may be useful to detect relapse.

PROGNOSIS AND OUTCOME

- Not well-known; many cases wax and wane
- Good for most cases
- Progressive renal disease indicates guarded prognosis

PEARLS & CONSIDERATIONS

COMMENTS

- The diagnosis of SLE is not based on a single test but on the constellation of clinical signs and exclusion of other possible etiologies.
- Treatment with doxycycline is useful to exclude infectious causes of polyarthropathy.
- Arthrocentesis: perform arthrocentesis on at least three joints, even if not swollen or painful.
- Biopsy of skin lesions must include intact epithelium. Ulcerated lesions are inherently nondiagnostic. Erythematous areas adjacent to ulcers yield the most conclusive results.
- Many animals are euthanized not from progressive disease but due to adverse effects of prednisone. Avoid obesity and routinely monitor for infection of the skin and urinary tract.
- Combination immunosuppressive therapy with azathioprine is often more effective and has fewer adverse effects than prednisone alone.

PREVENTION

- Although a link has not been proven, future vaccinations should be limited to those considered absolutely essential.
- Stressful circumstances should be avoided, if possible, to minimize risk of recurrence.

CLIENT EDUCATION

- Routine monitoring should be scheduled to detect relapse of disease and adverse effects of immunosuppressive medications
- Many dogs live normal lives after the diagnosis

SUGGESTED READING

Day MJ: Systemic lupus erythematosus. In Feldman BF, Zinkl JG, Jain NC (eds): *Schalm's Veterinary Hematology*. Baltimore, Lippincott Williams & Wilkins, 2000, pp 819–826.

Scott DW, et al: Canine lupus erythematosus I. Systemic lupus erythematosus. *J Am Anim Hosp Assoc* 19:461, 1983.

Stone MS: Systemic lupus erythematosus. In Ettinger SJ, Feldman EC (eds): *Textbook of Veterinary Internal Medicine*, ed 6. Philadelphia, Elsevier Saunders, 2005, pp 1952–1957.

AUTHOR: **MICHAEL STONE**

EDITOR: **SUSAN M. COTTER**

Tail Paralysis

BASIC INFORMATION

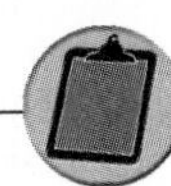

DEFINITION

Severe impairment or loss of tail motor function

EPIDEMIOLOGY

SPECIES, AGE, SEX: Dependent on underlying cause.

GENETICS AND BREED PREDISPOSITION

- Pugs, bulldogs (spina bifida, sacrocaudal dysgenesis)
- Chondrodystrophic breeds (disk herniation)

RISK FACTORS

- Outdoor cats (trauma)
- Cardiomyopathies in cats (aortic thromboembolism)
- Type I disk herniation with severe paraparesis
- Degenerative lumbosacral stenosis (cauda equina syndrome)

ASSOCIATED CONDITIONS AND DISORDERS

- Cutaneous wounds of the tail if sensation is affected
- Tail fracture

CLINICAL PRESENTATION

HISTORY, CHIEF COMPLAINT

- Trauma involving the hind quarters (hit by car, falls, stepped on, etc.)
- Trauma involving traction injury on the tail (exercise-related, malicious, caught in door, etc.)
- Unwillingess to jump up (e.g., lumbosacral diseases)
- Acute onset vocalization and hind limb paresis/paralysis (aortic thromboembolism)

PHYSICAL EXAM FINDINGS

- Impaired tail motility with or without hind limb paresis
- Concurrent fractures of the axial skeleton, pelvis, pelvic limbs, and/or thoracic limbs
- Urinary and/or fecal incontinence, urine- or feces-soiled tail
- Pain originating from the pelvic area
- Weakness, pale mucous membranes, dyspnea (if cat with thromboembolic disease)
- Shock if massive trauma
- Tachycardia, heart murmur, gallop, weak or absent pulses, cyanosis of the pelvic limbs (if feline cardiomyopathy)
- Transverse myelopathy (T3-L3 or L4-S3 or Cd1-Cd5 only)
- Large distended bladder:
    - Easy to empty if spinal lesion involves lumbar intumescence ("lower motor neuron bladder")
    - Difficult to empty if spinal lesion is cranial to lumbar intumescence ("upper motor neuron bladder")
- Rectal exam: painful and might induce sacrocaudal instability if associated with trauma

ETIOLOGY AND PATHOPHYSIOLOGY

- Orthopedic:
    - Spinal/coccygeal fracture
    - Degenerative lumbosacral stenosis
- Neurologic:
    - Spinal malformations
    - Spinal fracture
    - Nerve root avulsion (lumbar intumescence/coccygeal)
    - Disk herniation (with or without paraparesis)
    - Tumor of the spine/spinal canal/cord
- Cardiac/vascular:
    - Feline thromboembolic disease
    - Vascular compromise secondary to trauma (arterial avulsion or thrombosis)
    - Fibrocartilaginous embolism

DIAGNOSIS

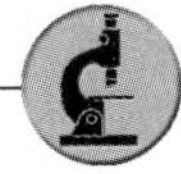

DIFFERENTIAL DIAGNOSIS

- Anomalous (spina bifida, hemivertebra, sacrocaudal dysgenesis, dermoid sinus)
- Degenerative lumbosacral stenosis (stenosis of vertebral canal, type II disk at L7/S1 space, sacral osteochondrosis, instability and misalignment of L7/S1, articular facet arthritis)
- Intervertebral disk disease (type I or type II)
- Spinal trauma/fracture/avulsion
- Vascular (feline thromboembolism, fibrocartilaginous embolism)
- Neoplasia
- Diskospondylitis

INITIAL DATABASE

- Rectal exam to document pain, swelling, instability, mass effect
- Complete neurologic examination to localize the lesion
- Radiographs of the spine including the sacrocaudal region (malformations, fracture/trauma/avulsion, diskospondylitis, osteolytic/osteoproliferative tumor, intervertebral disk disease)
- Complete blood count, serum biochemistry panel, urinalysis depending on patient stability and systemic involvement
- Thoracic radiographs:
    - To evaluate the presence of thoracic lesions secondary to trauma
    - To assess for metastases if neoplasia is suspected
- Ultrasound:
    - Thoracic (for feline cardiomyopathy)
    - Abdominal if suspected pelvic canal tumor

ADVANCED OR CONFIRMATORY TESTING

- Advanced imaging modalities: myelography; computed tomography, magnetic resonance imaging
    - May be indicated for assessing underlying spinal abnormalities
- Electromyography (rare instances of neuromuscular disease)
- Fine-needle aspiration if possible for cytologic evaluation (masses, diskospondylitis)
- Ultrasound guided biopsy (masses)

TREATMENT

THERAPEUTIC GOAL(S)

- Orthopedic or neurologic:
    - Treatment limited to addressing underlying cause if no vascular compromise
    - Amputate tail if vascular compromise
        - Leave 3 to 4 coccygeal vertebrae if well vascularized
        - Amputate to the level of the skin if tail is devascularized
- Cardiac/vascular:
    - Tail amputation if tail is soiled by urine and/or feces or if tail has not revascularized well
    - Address underlying cardiac disease
- Neoplasia:
    - Wide surgical excision if possible
    - Radiation therapy or chemotherapy if indicated and if possible

ACUTE GENERAL TREATMENT

- Treat shock if present
- Treat underlying cardiac cause
- Administer corticosteroids if tail paralysis is secondary to spinal cord/nerve compression (controversial)
    - Methylprednisolone sodium succinate:
        - 30 mg/kg IV, then 15 mg/kg IV 2 and 6 hours later, or
        - 30 mg/kg IV followed by 5.4 mg/kg per hour infusion for 23 hours
    - Dexamethasone: 2 mg/kg IV, then 0.2 mg/kg SC q 8-12h
    - Prednisolone: 0.5-1 mg/kg q 24h
- Once patient is stable, treatment depends on underlying cause

CHRONIC TREATMENT

- Hygiene and topical care to prevent urine/fecal contact dermatitis:
    - Bathing, keeping area dry and clean, clipping of the perianal region, and protective ointment if necessary
- Bladder catheterization if necessary
- Physical therapy for paraparetic patients
- As indicated by underlying cardiac disease

POSSIBLE COMPLICATIONS

- Dependent on therapeutic options
- Beware of corticosteroid administration:
    - Associated with gastrointestinal ulceration, colonic perforation

RECOMMENDED MONITORING

Dependent of primary cause and therapeutic options

PROGNOSIS AND OUTCOME

- Trauma:
    - Intact deep pain perception and normal vascularization: guarded. Generally these patients will regain enough motor activity to avoid lack of hygiene
    - Absence of deep pain for more than 48 hours: poor prognosis for return of motor activity, but good if tail amputated and normal voluntary hind limb activity and bladder control
- Guarded to poor if feline thromboembolic disease

PEARLS & CONSIDERATIONS

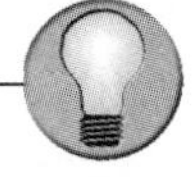

COMMENTS

- The most common causes of tail paralysis are trauma and degenerative lumbosacral stenosis.
    - Prognosis depends on deep pain perception and vascular supply.
    - In dogs and cats, the tail is not essential to life.
        - Tail amputation in patients with normal limb function and bladder control provides an excellent quality of life.
- Beware: pain originating from the pelvic canal (e.g., prostatic abscess, degenerative lumbosacral stenosis) can mimic tail paralysis.

CLIENT EDUCATION

Variable: depends on primary cause of tail paralysis

SUGGESTED READING

De Lahunta A: *Veterinary Neuroanatomy and Clinical Neurology*, ed 2. Philadelphia, WB Saunders, 1983, p 471.

AUTHOR: **BERTRAND LUSSIER**
EDITOR: **ETIENNE CÔTÉ**

Tarsal Trauma

BASIC INFORMATION

DEFINITION

Includes ligament damage, fractures, or shearing injuries

SYNONYM(S)

Tarsal breakdown

EPIDEMIOLOGY

GENETICS AND BREED PREDISPOSITION: Racing greyhounds: central tarsal bone fractures.

RISK FACTORS: Racing or agility activities; distal hind limb trauma.

CLINICAL PRESENTATION

DISEASE FORMS/SUBTYPES: Sprains, fractures, and shearing or degloving wounds; coaptation-related injuries, including pressure sores from casts or splints, dermatitis from soiled bandages, and wound infection or dehiscence from contaminated dressings.

HISTORY, CHIEF COMPLAINT: Hind limb trauma; lameness after competition.

PHYSICAL EXAM FINDINGS

- Lameness
- Swelling

- Open wounds around the tarsus
- Pain or crepitation on palpation of the tarsus
- Gross instability characterized by a plantigrade stance

ETIOLOGY AND PATHOPHYSIOLOGY

- Racing animals on counterclockwise tracks are predisposed to right-sided injuries.
- In racing greyhounds, there is a classic triad of fractures involving the central tarsal bone, calcaneus, and base of metatarsal V.
- In pets, fractures often occur in the calcaneus.

DIAGNOSIS

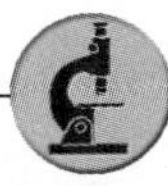

DIFFERENTIAL DIAGNOSIS

- Autoimmune polyarthropathy (systemic lupus erythematosus [SLE], rheumatoid arthritis)
- Infectious (Lyme borreliosis, rickettsial disease)

INITIAL DATABASE

- Mediolateral and dorsopalmar radiographic projections of the tarsus
- Complete blood count (CBC), chemistry panel, and urinalysis based on the animal's stability and the American Society of Anesthesiologists (ASA) classification (p 1334)
- Thoracic/abdominal radiographs, abdominal ultrasound, electrocardiogram (ECG) for animals that have undergone severe trauma

ADVANCED OR CONFIRMATORY TESTING

- Oblique radiography (nondisplaced fractures); skyline views (trochlea of the talus)
- Stress-film radiography (mediolateral radiograph with tarsus manually forced into dorsal and plantar extension and a dorsoplantar radiograph with a medial to lateral stress applied) to identify location of joint instability

TREATMENT

THERAPEUTIC GOAL(S)

- Fractures: stabilization and anatomic reduction
  - Buttress repair of comminuted tarsal bone fractures to prevent joint collapse
- Ligamentous injuries: reestablishment of joint support by repairing collateral ligaments or arthrodesis
- Shearing injuries: wound management

ACUTE GENERAL TREATMENT

Minimally displaced, nonarticular fractures, grade I and most grade II sprains can be stabilized for 6 to 8 weeks with an external splint.

- Luxated joints, intra-articular fractures, and grade III sprains are supported in a modified Robert-Jones bandage until surgery.
- Shearing injuries require initial wound management treatment.
  - Gentle lavage of open wounds using warm saline, lactated Ringer's solution, and dilute chlorhexidine solutions to reduce gross contamination. (Animals are sedated and given analgesics.)
  - Coverage of tissues with moistened (above solutions) gauze sponges useful in debridement (wet-to-dry-bandages) as they are changed daily.
  - Alternatively, direct application of sugar or honey has been used for reducing infection and promoting healing for highly contaminated, traumatic open wounds, but the role of such treatment in the joint is unclear.
  - Final surgical debridement and joint lavage can be performed during orthopedic stabilization surgery.
  - Wounds with healthy granulation tissue, reduced contamination, and early epithelialization can be closed with sutures or covered with a nonadherent dressing and allowed to heal via second intention.

CHRONIC TREATMENT

- Surgical repairs to the tarsus require 6 to 12 weeks of external coaptation (splints or external fixatures) and exercise restriction.
- Collateral ligament disruption requires stabilization with tension band principle (malleolar fractures) or replacement with prosthetic suture.
- Instability of the tarsocrural joint or complete (grade III) plantar tarsal disruption necessitates pantarsal arthrodesis.
- Individual tarsal bone fractures require lag screw fixation, except for lesions of the calcaneus (tension band principle).
- Plantar intertarsal and plantar tarsometatarsal subluxations are unstable in weight-bearing animals and require partial tarsal arthrodesis with pins or small plates (tension band principle).
- Dorsal intertarsal and dorsal tarsometatarsal suluxations are rare and stable (compressed) in weight-bearing animals:
  - Establishing the diagnosis requires stress film radiography.
  - Primary ligament repair or partial tarsal arthrodesis is performed.

POSSIBLE COMPLICATIONS

- Reduction/implant failure
- Delayed or failed arthrodesis
- Wound infection
- Coaptation-related morbidity
- Degenerative joint disease

RECOMMENDED MONITORING

- Lameness evaluation 1 to 3 months following injury and treatment
- Serial radiographic studies to evaluate fracture healing or progression of arthrodesis

PROGNOSIS AND OUTCOME

- Good to excellent for noncompeting dogs
- Variable for return to preinjury status for competing dogs
- Severe shearing injuries with neurovascular compromise may necessitate limb amputation

PEARLS & CONSIDERATIONS

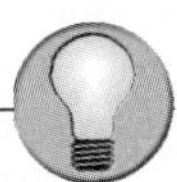

COMMENTS

- When conservatively managed, intra-articular fractures rarely heal with osseous bridging, thus leading to degenerative joint disease.
- Severe shearing injuries are commonly due to motor vehicle trauma. Despite significant damage, acceptable function is possible with various reconstructive efforts (see Soft Tissue Trauma of the Extremities, p 1018).
- In noncompeting animals, solitary intertarsal joint fusion (i.e., calcaneotarsal, calcaneoquartal, quartalmetatarsal) can lead to near normal function.

SUGGESTED READING

Dee JF: Tarsal injuries. In Bloomberg MS, Dee JF, Taylor RA (eds): *Canine Sports Medicine and Surgery*. Philadelphia, WB Saunders, 1998, pp 120–137.

Piermattei DL, Flo GL: Orthopedic injuries of the tarsus. In *Brinker, Piermattei, and Flo's Handbook of Small Animal Orthopedics and Fracture Repair*, ed 3. Philadelphia, WB Saunders, 1997, pp 607–658.

AUTHOR: **JOHN J. HABURJAK**
EDITOR: **JOSEPH HARARI**

Taurine Deficiency

BASIC INFORMATION

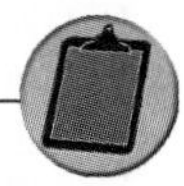

DEFINITION

Inadequate intake or availability of dietary taurine

EPIDEMIOLOGY

SPECIES, AGE, SEX: Taurine is an essential nutrient for cats but not for dogs under most circumstances. Deficiency can occur in cats that cannot meet metabolic needs from dietary sources.

GENETICS AND BREED PREDISPOSITION
- None reported in cats.
- In dogs, isolated occurrences of taurine-deficient dilated cardiomyopathy have been identified in a variety of breeds, including American cocker spaniels, golden retrievers, and possibly Newfoundlands.

RISK FACTORS
- Cats: inadequately supplemented commercial or home-prepared diets
- Dogs: breed predisposition, cystinuria (?), inadequate protein and sulfur-containing amino acid intake, decreased intestinal availability due to taurine binding to fiber

CLINICAL PRESENTATION

DISEASE FORMS/SUBTYPES
- Cats: central retinal degeneration (CRD), reproductive failure, growth retardation, and dilated cardiomyopathy (DCM)
- Dogs: DCM in susceptible breeds or individuals

HISTORY, CHIEF COMPLAINT
- Cats: compatible diet history (poorly formulated commercial or home-prepared diet) is suggestive but not pathognomonic; dyspnea, respiratory distress
- Dogs: exercise intolerance and weight loss progressing to cough, respiratory distress, and eventually ascites; possible diet history of restricted diet (not commonly identified)

PHYSICAL EXAM FINDINGS
- Cats: variable combinations of tachypnea, dyspnea, tachycardia, lethargy, dehydration, and hypothermia; systolic murmur at the apex on the left side, with gallop rhythm in severe cases. Peripheral vasoconstriction may result in cold extremities
- Dogs: similar to cats, tachyarrhythmia

ETIOLOGY AND PATHOPHYSIOLOGY

Taurine is synthesized from methionine and cysteine. It does not occur in proteins but is required for a variety of cellular homeostatic functions. Synthesis occurs in cats (but apparently not dogs) too slowly to maintain taurine balance in the absence of adequate intake. Obligatory loss also occurs in cats and dogs because only taurine can combine with cholesterol during bile salt synthesis, whereas most other species can substitute glycine for taurine.

In cats, excessive taurine-conjugated bile salt loss in feces occurs due to variable combinations of type of diet processing, protein source, changes in location and/or numbers of intestinal microflora, and/or increased secretion of bile salts due to changes in the release of cholecystokinin.

DIAGNOSIS

DIFFERENTIAL DIAGNOSIS

- Idiopathic DCM
- Other causes of myocardial failure

INITIAL DATABASE

- Cats: radiography to determine presence of heart failure (cardiomegaly plus pleural effusion, pulmonary edema, or both). Do not attempt to obtain radiographs of severely dyspneic, struggling patients, because the stress of the procedure may result in the death of the cat
- Dogs: radiography, as for cats; electrocardiographic (ECG) signs include variable combinations of left-sided enlargement, sinus tachycardia, atrial fibrillation, and ventricular tachyarrhythmias

ADVANCED OR CONFIRMATORY TESTING

Echocardiography is the test of choice for diagnosis of DCM; absence of motion of the left ventricular walls, increased end-diastolic diameter, and reduced shortening fraction.

- Blood and/or plasma taurine concentration: for plasma taurine determination
  - Ensure that plasma is separated before the blood is chilled to avoid release of taurine from platelets.
  - Whole blood taurine may be measured by freezing the sample to ensure release of taurine from all the formed elements of the blood. Animals with whole blood taurine concentrations <200 nmol/ml (plasma: <50 nmol/ml) should be switched to diets known to result in higher plasma concentrations. Plasma taurine concentrations fluctuate with food intake, whereas whole blood taurine reflects long-term (weeks to months) intake.

TREATMENT

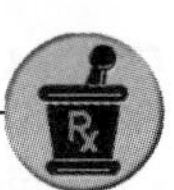

THERAPEUTIC GOAL(S)

- Restore taurine homeostasis
- Improve cardiac function

ACUTE GENERAL TREATMENT

- Supportive care for congestive heart failure (CHF) (see Heart Failure, Chronic, p 459) and arrhythmias
- Taurine supplementation pending confirmation of diagnosis

CHRONIC TREATMENT

- Cats: recommend switching the cat to a satisfactory diet and supplementing with taurine at 250-500 mg PO or in food q 12h for 12-16 weeks or until echocardiographic parameters return to normal
- Dogs: recommend 500 mg taurine PO q 8h (+ L-carnitine 1000 mg PO q 8h if possible) for American cocker spaniels. Change to a diet containing more protein and sulfur-containing amino acids and less fiber

RECOMMENDED MONITORING

- Clinical condition
- Radiography, echocardiography

PROGNOSIS AND OUTCOME

- The prognosis is better when deficiency is identified and treated appropriately before extensive permanent change exists in the myocardium. Clinical signs of advanced heart failure, such as hypothermia or thromboembolism, suggest a poorer prognosis.
- Dogs that improve in conjunction with taurine supplementation become more energetic after a few weeks; they then also show reduction in cardiomegaly and improvement in echocardiographic parameters after 1 to 4 months.

PEARLS & CONSIDERATIONS

COMMENTS

Recovery of function and appetite occur within days to weeks after provision of taurine if deficiency of this amino acid is the cause of the signs. When they occur, reduction in cardiomegaly and improvement in echocardiographic parameters may require 1 to 4 months of supplementation; improvement may permit reduction or discontinuation of cardiac medications.

PREVENTION

Feeding of a properly formulated diet.

CLIENT EDUCATION

Explain the importance of feeding pets a properly formulated diet

SUGGESTED READING

Buffington CAT: Nutritional diseases and nutritional therapy. In Sherding RG (ed): *The Cat: Diseases and Clinical Management*. New York, Churchill Livingstone, 1994, pp 161-190.

Meurs KM: Primary myocardial disease in the dog. In Ettinger SJ, Feldman EC (eds): *Textbook of Veterinary Internal Medicine*. St. Louis, Elsevier Saunders, 2005, pp 1077-1082.

Pion PD: Traditional and nontraditional effective and noneffective therapies for cardiac disease in dogs and cats. *Vet Clin North Am Small An Pract* 34:187, 2004.

AUTHORS: **C. A. TONY BUFFINGTON, KATHRYN M. MEURS**

EDITOR: **C. A. TONY BUFFINGTON**

Temporomandibular Joint Luxation

BASIC INFORMATION

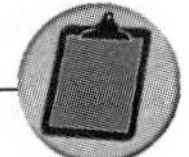

DEFINITION

Complete displacement of the condyle of the mandible out of its corresponding mandibular fossa of the temporal bone

EPIDEMIOLOGY

SPECIES, AGE, SEX: Temporomandibular joint (TMJ) luxation can occur in dogs and cats of any age. Traumatic TMJ luxation with regional fracture is more common in younger cats; no sex predilection.

GENETICS AND BREED PREDISPOSITION: Any breed when associated with trauma; breeds predisposed to TMJ dysplasia: basset hound, dachshund, Irish setter, and possibly also Persian cats.

RISK FACTORS: Trauma, TMJ dysplasia.

CLINICAL PRESENTATION

DISEASE FORMS/SUBTYPES

- Subluxation (partial dislocation of a joint): minimal displacement of the mandibular condyle, which is still situated in its corresponding mandibular fossa of the temporal bone
- Luxation (complete dislocation of a joint):
  - Rostrodorsal: most commonly; usually unilateral
  - Caudal: rarely noted; possibly with fracture of the retroarticular process of the temporal bone
- Luxation, caudal: rarely noted; possible with fracture of the retroarticular process
- Open-mouth jaw locking (see Etiology and Pathophysiology below)

HISTORY, CHIEF COMPLAINT: Owners present animals for inability to close the mouth fully, pain on chewing/yawning, reluctance to play or chew on toys, inappetence, and/or an audible click when opening the mouth. Depending on etiology, progression may be peracute, acute, or chronic.

PHYSICAL EXAM FINDINGS: In rostrodorsal luxation, the lower jaw is shifted to the unaffected side. This malocclusion results in abnormal upper and lower tooth contact, leading to inability to close the mouth fully. Other findings may include decreased range of jaw motion, decreased eye globe retropulsion on the affected side, swelling, crepitation and pain on TMJ palpation, dehydration, and hypersalivation.

ETIOLOGY AND PATHOPHYSIOLOGY

Relevant anatomy:

- Mandibular ramus: vertical part of mandible that lies medial to the zygomatic arch, caudolateral to the orbit
- Mandibular condyle: articular process of the mandible. Articulates with mandibular fossa of the temporal bone to form the temporomandibular joint
- Retroarticular process: process of the temporal bone preventing caudal dislocation of the mandibular condyle
- Coronoid process: dorsal protuberance of the mandibular ramus providing insertion for the temporal muscle

Luxation with/without regional fracture:

- Trauma is the most common inciting cause; TMJ dysplasia may predispose the animal to subluxation/luxation without obvious outside force.
- Luxation in a rostrodorsal direction is most common because the prominent retroarticular process prevents caudoventral movement of the mandibular condyle.
- Due to a more tightly seated mandibular condyle in the mandibular fossa of the temporal bone, cats are more prone to luxation with associated regional fracture. Dogs have a more loosely seated mandibular condyle, and luxations usually occur without regional fracture.
- Cats have a higher incidence of TMJ luxation than dogs due to decreased mandibular symphyseal movement and shorter jaw length.
- In rostrodorsal luxation, the lower jaw will be shifted rostrally and laterally to the unaffected side.

TMJ dysplasia with/without coronoid process displacement:

- Rare congenital or acquired malformation: shallow mandibular fossa, underdeveloped/misshapen retroarticular process, flattened mandibular condyle, and periarticular osteophytosis; abnormal laxity in mandibular symphysis also reported as inciting cause of open-mouth jaw locking
- Open-mouth jaw locking: TMJ subluxation, rotational movement of the mandibular body and locking of coronoid process lateral to zygomatic arch; mouth is locked wide open, and compared to TMJ luxation, there is no tooth-to-tooth contact

DIAGNOSIS

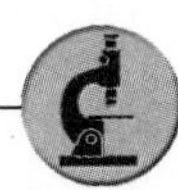

DIFFERENTIAL DIAGNOSIS

- TMJ luxation with/without regional fracture
- TMJ dysplasia with/without coronoid process displacement
- Mandibular neuropraxia (mandibular branch of cranial nerve V)
- Mandibular ramus/zygomatic arch fracture
- Masticatory muscle myositis
- Dental/skeletal malocclusion
- Periorbital/caudal mandibular/caudal maxillary neoplasia
- Foreign body

INITIAL DATABASE

- Complete blood count (CBC) and serum biochemistry panel: generally unremarkable
- Head radiographs: dorsoventral (ventrodorsal), right and left lateral oblique, and open-mouth views that show displacement of the mandibular condyle with/without fracture of associated bone structures

ADVANCED OR CONFIRMATORY TESTING

CT scan:

- The best and most productive imaging modality for assessing TMJ disease

- Subtle abnormalities not identified on radiographs are easily demonstrated on CT scan
- Three-dimensional (3-D) reconstruction beneficial for diagnosis and treatment planning

TREATMENT

THERAPEUTIC GOAL(S)

- Alleviate animal discomfort
- Obtain functional jaw movement

ACUTE GENERAL TREATMENT

Acute TMJ luxation:

- Manual reduction of rostrodorsal luxation:
  - Chemical restraint (sedation or anesthesia).
  - Place a wooden dowel (pencil in small pets) between carnassial teeth of affected side only and gently force the mouth closed until the joint is reduced. Remove the dowel/pencil but keep the mouth closed to maintain joint reduction.
  - Apply a slightly snug tape muzzle for 1 to 3 weeks. The muzzle should be fairly snug but loose enough to allow the animal to lap up water and liquefied food.
  - Recovery from sedation/anesthesia, with particular attention to aspiration (e.g., remove muzzle immediately if vomiting).
- Regional fractures (condylar process of mandible; mandibular fossa/retroarticular process of temporal bone) are usually treated conservatively without surgical intervention. Owners must be warned of possible complications, such as TMJ ankylosis.

CHRONIC TREATMENT

Chronic TMJ luxation:

- Maxillomandibular fixation (applying a muzzle using white medical tape or inserting a composite bridge between upper and lower canines) for 4 to 6 weeks
- Condylectomy and bone fragment resection are indicated for severe regional fractures resulting in TMJ ankylosis and arthrosis

PROGNOSIS AND OUTCOME

Excellent (no regional fracture); fair to poor (regional fracture ± ankylosis, particularly in immature/adolescent animals)

PEARLS & CONSIDERATIONS

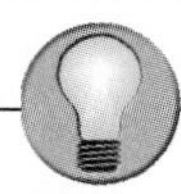

COMMENTS

Do not force the mouth closed in patients presenting with the mouth wide open. Manual correction of open-mouth jaw locking is achieved by opening the mouth a little further, pressing the coronoid process medially, and closing the mouth.

SUGGESTED READING

Capron TM: Traumatic temporomandibular joint luxation: Comparative anatomy of the temporomandibular joint. *Vet Comp Orthop Traumatol* 8:58-60, 1995.

Lantz GC: Surgical correction of unusual temporomandibular joint conditions. *Comp Cont Educ Pract Vet* 13:1570-1576, 1991.

Reiter AM: Symphysiotomy, symphysiectomy, and intermandibular arthrodesis in a cat with open-mouth jaw locking: Case report and literature review. *J Vet Dent* 21: 147-158, 2004.

Schwarz T, et al: Imaging of the canine and feline temporomandibular joint: A review. *Vet Radiol Ultrasound* 43:85-97, 2002.

Ticer JW, Spencer CP: Injury of the temporomandibular joint: Radiographic signs. *J Am Vet Rad Soc* 19:146-156, 1978.

AUTHOR: **JENNIFER E. RAWLINSON**
EDITOR: **ALEXANDER M. REITER**

Tenesmus

BASIC INFORMATION

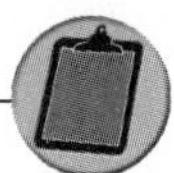

DEFINITION

Ineffectual or painful straining to defecate due to obstruction or inflammatory lesions of distal colon, rectum, or anus

SYNONYM(S)

Straining to defecate

CLINICAL PRESENTATION

HISTORY, CHIEF COMPLAINT

- Frequent posturing to defecate/urinate without producing feces/urine
- Turning around/looking at hind end while attempting to defecate
- Excessive licking/chewing of perineal region
- Flattened, ribbon-like stools
- History of trauma
- Vocalizing (cats most often)
- Inappropriate defecation in the house/outside litter box
- Refusal to defecate (severe pain) and 2^{0} constipation
- Common error in cats: overdiagnosis of "tenesmus" by owner or veterinarian; careful history/observation reveals lower urinary tract signs

PHYSICAL EXAM FINDINGS

- Observe the animal defecate/urinate
- Tail between legs/low carriage, resentment of tail elevation (discomfort)
- Arched back (abdominal or back pain)
- Examine anus/perianal area
  - Erythema of anal/perineal region
  - Perineal fistulas
  - Perineal masses
  - Pseudocoprostasis (anal obstruction due to severe matting of fur with feces)
- Abdominal palpation
  - Mass
  - Signs of discomfort despite gentle palpation
- Rectal palpation. May require sedation/general anesthesia if patients have very painful perineal conditions
  - Perineal hernia
  - Mass
  - Prostatomegaly
  - Pelvic fractures
  - Fecal consistency (constipation, foreign material)
  - Stricture
  - Foreign bodies (e.g., bones, rocks, grass, fur, food wrappers)
  - Cytology (infection, inflammation)
  - Origin of clinical signs unclear? Catheterize urethra/urinary bladder
  - Palpation of anal sacs
    - Impaction
    - Infection, abscess, or rupture
    - Mass

ETIOLOGY AND PATHOPHYSIOLOGY

- Perianal (specifically adjacent to anus) and perineal (whole region between tail and pubis) disorders:
  - Anal sacculitis
  - Anal sac abscess
  - Perianal gland tumours
  - Perineal hernia
  - Perianal fistula
  - Neoplasia: anal sac adenocarcinoma
  - Pseudocoprostasis
- Large bowel:
  - Neoplasia
  - Polyps
  - Rectal granulomas
  - Rectal stricture (non-neoplastic)
  - Constipation

- Colitis/proctitis (1^0 or 2^0 to diarrhea/prolapse)
- Irritable bowel syndrome
- Rectal foreign body (dietary indiscretion)
- Histoplasmosis
- Pythiosis
- Miscellaneous
  - Acute pancreatitis (segmental colitis)
  - 2^0 to chronic small bowel diarrhea
  - Neurologic disorders (intervertebral disk disease, dysautonomia)
- Genitourinary tract: In general, these abnormalities produce disorders of urination rather than tenesmus (careful history and examination for accurate diagnosis):
  - Prostatomegaly
    - Benign prostatic hyperplasia/hypertrophy (BPH)
    - Prostatitis
    - Abscess
    - Neoplasia
  - Paraprostatic cyst
  - Genitourinary neoplasia
- Caudal abdominal cavity disorders:
  - Mass: organ compression
  - Pelvic fractures (misaligned healing of old pelvic fractures)
  - Pelvic osteosarcoma

DIAGNOSIS

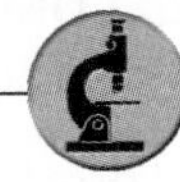

DIFFERENTIAL DIAGNOSIS

See Etiology and Pathophysiology above

INITIAL DATABASE

- Complete blood count, serum biochemical profile, urinalysis: elucidate possible urinary tract or systemic abnormalities
- Radiographs (abdominal/pelvic): constipation, megacolon, prostatomegaly, pelvic fractures, malunion of pelvic fractures, foreign bodies, masses or sublumbar lymphadenopathy
- Abdominal ultrasonography: gastrointestinal (GI)/pelvic mass, ± lymphadenopathy, urogenital tract, GI motility, distention/wall thickening
- Colonoscopy: biopsy mass(es), strictures or infiltrative lesions
- Urogenital system (to exclude impostors for tenesmus):
  - Vaginal examination
  - Ultrasonography and/or urinary tract contrast radiography
  - Urethroscopy/cystoscopy
  - Culture and sensitivity of urine/prostatic fluid
  - Cytology and/or biopsies of urinary tract/prostate
- Neurologic exam (perineal reflex, and tone, presence of lumbosacral/back pain)

TREATMENT

THERAPEUTIC GOAL(S)

- Treat the underlying cause
- Relieve discomfort

ACUTE GENERAL TREATMENT

- Clip fur and gently wash perineal area if needed.
- Hydrotherapy to affected area multiple times per day if indicated.
- Enemas: soften impacted feces if constipation.
- Topical cutaneous glucocorticoids/anesthetics (creams, ointments, suppositories): reduce inflammation/pain.
- Corticosteroid enemas, if severe, noninfectious colitis: budesonide (Entocort) 2-mg dissolvable tablet. Give 1 mg (½ tablet dissolved in enema diluent) per rectum (dose is for most small animals). Budesonide does not reach high concentrations outside the GI-hepatoportal system (high first-pass metabolism), which minimizes systemic glucocorticoid effects.
- Drain/flush anal gland abscesses.
- Cyclosporine (3-5 mg/kg PO q 12h, adjusted based on serum levels) or tacrolimus ointment (0.03-0.1%): perianal fistula.
- Surgery: perineal hernias (repair); colonic or rectal polyps (excision); colonic/rectal/anal sac tumours (resection); rectal strictures (rectal "pull-through").
- Adjunctive chemotherapy and/or palliative therapy with piroxicam (0.3 mg/kg PO q 24-48h) for anal sac adenocarcinomas.

CHRONIC TREATMENT

- Inflammatory lesions of the colon and rectum (histologically confirmed, noninfectious):
  - Systemic glucocorticoids, ± other immunosuppressive drugs (azathioprine, chlorambucil)
  - Topical GI glucocorticoid (budesonide). Available as oral and enema formulations (see Acute Treatment above)
  - Metronidazole (immunomodulating effects)
  - Sulfasalazine (caution in cats: salicylates)
- Other specific treatments based on etiology

POSSIBLE COMPLICATIONS

- Recurrent tenesmus
- Colonic/rectal obstruction causing obstipation
- Rectal prolapse (uncommon; usually young patients <6 months old)
- Surgery: risk of postoperative fecal incontinence

PROGNOSIS AND OUTCOME

- Colonic/rectal inflammatory lesions: often successful (medical therapy)
- Anal sac disease, perineal hernias, wounds within and surrounding the anorectal area: better prognosis than strictures or neoplasia
- Perineal fistulas: improved prognosis with cyclosporine, but costly. Tacrolimus is less expensive, but not as effective

PEARLS & CONSIDERATIONS

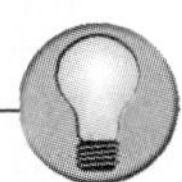

COMMENTS

- Stranguria is a common impostor for tenesmus, especially in cats. Thorough questioning during history-taking, and observation of the animal's elimination process, are essential for avoiding misdiagnosis.
- Tenesmus is a clinical sign, not a disease. Therefore, an underlying cause must be sought.
- Work-up is highly dependent upon:
  - Clear history
  - Observing the animal urinate/defecate

SUGGESTED READING

Guilford WG: Approach to clinical problems in gastroenterology. In Guilford WG, Center SA, Strombeck DR, et al (eds): *Strombeck's Small Animal Gastroenterology*, ed 2. Philadelphia, WB Saunders, 1996, pp 50-76.

Jones B: Constipation, tenesmus, dyschezia, and fecal incontinence. In Ettinger SJ, Feldman EC (eds): *Textbook of Veterinary Internal Medicine Volume I*, ed 5. Philadelphia, WB Saunders, 2000, pp 129-135.

Tams TR: Gastrointestinal symptoms. In Tams TR (ed): *Small Animal Gastroenterology*, ed 2. St. Louis, Saunders (Elsevier).

Willard M: Clinical manifestations of gastrointestinal disorders. In Nelson RW, Couto CG (eds): *Essentials of Small Animal Internal Medicine*, ed 2. St. Louis, Mosby, 1998, pp 346-367.

AUTHOR: **LISA CARIOTO**
EDITOR: **ETIENNE CÔTÉ**

Testicular Tumors

BASIC INFORMATION

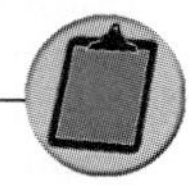

DEFINITION

Neoplasia arising from testicular germ cells or sex-cord stromal cells

SYNONYM(S)

Germ cell: seminoma
Mixed tumors: germ cell-stromal tumors
Sex-cord stromal: interstitial (Leydig) cell tumor; Sertoli (sustentacular) cell tumor

EPIDEMIOLOGY

SPECIES, AGE, SEX:
- Dogs:
  - Incidence: common (75% of all tumors affecting the male urogenital tract)
  - Age: aged patients, most >7 years
  - Equal incidence of seminoma, interstitial cell tumor, are Sertoli cell tumor
- Cats: all tumor types are very rare

GENETICS AND BREED PREDISPOSITION
- Seminoma: all breeds; boxer is predisposed
- Sertoli cell: miniature schnauzers with persistent Müllerian duct syndrome are predisposed

RISK FACTORS:
- Dogs: cryptorchidism
  - Overall risk of testicular tumor development increased 13 to 14 times
  - Risk of Sertoli cell tumor increased 20 times
  - Approximately one-half of Sertoli cell tumors occur in cryptorchid testes
  - Approximately one-third of seminomas occur in cryptorchid testes
- Cats: none identified

ASSOCIATED CONDITIONS AND DISORDERS: Sertoli cell tumor: hyperestrogenism occurs in approximately 20–30% of affected dogs.

CLINICAL PRESENTATION

DISEASE FORMS/SUBTYPES
- Primary: unilateral or bilateral, focal or multifocal
- Metastatic (rare)

HISTORY, CHIEF COMPLAINT
- Testicular enlargement ± atrophy of unaffected testis (most severe associated with Sertoli cell tumor but can occur with other neoplasms, especially larger tumors)
- Sertoli cell tumor: symmetric hair loss, feminization (gynecomastia, attractiveness to other male dogs, pendulous penile sheath, lethargy, loss of libido, redistribution of body fat)

PHYSICAL EXAM FINDINGS: Testicular enlargement ± atrophy of contralateral testis:
- Seminoma: soft to slightly firm texture
- Sertoli cell tumor: very firm texture, discrete mass
- Interstitial cell tumor: soft texture, discrete mass
- Mixed germ cell/stromal tumors: variable texture, generally discrete and focal

Sertoli cell with hyperestrogenism: endocrine dermatopathy, gynecomastia, pendulous penile sheath, redistribution of body fat, marked contralateral testicular atrophy

ETIOLOGY AND PATHOPHYSIOLOGY

Cryptorchidism: altered testicular environment due to increased testicular temperature favors neoplastic transformation of Sertoli cells and, less commonly, germ cells

DIAGNOSIS

DIFFERENTIAL DIAGNOSIS

- Testicular torsion
- Abscess
- Cyst

INITIAL DATABASE

- Complete blood count (CBC): rule out bone marrow suppression due to Sertoli cell tumor-associated hyperestrogenism
- Semen evaluation and/or testicular biopsy with histologic examination of unaffected testis will aid in decision for unilateral or bilateral castration in breeding dogs

ADVANCED OR CONFIRMATORY TESTING

- Ultrasound, all tumor types: hypoechoic or mixed echotexture (Figs. I-170 and I-171).
- Gross pathologic examination of excised testis: seminoma signs include soft to slightly firm testis, homogeneous gray/white glistening appearance, areas of discoloration due to hemorrhage or necrosis possible, focal to multifocal; Sertoli cell tumor signs include very firm testis, discrete, white or gray in color, tan or yellow hemorrhagic areas possible, usually focal; interstitial cell tumor signs include soft testis, discrete, yellow/brown in color, bulges on section, areas of hemorrhage or cystic change common, focal to multifocal; mixed germ cell/stromal tumors signs include variable texture, pale white or gray, generally discrete and focal.
- Bilateral tumors are common, and multiple tumor types are often present within the same testis.
- Histopathologic examination: include spermatic cord to evaluate for local invasion; multiple tumor types can occur in the same testis.

TREATMENT

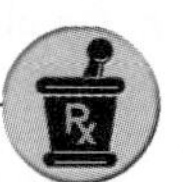

THERAPEUTIC GOAL(S)

Surgical excision

ACUTE GENERAL TREATMENT

- Testicular removal: unilateral castration if contralateral testis is normal to small in size and future breeding with the dog is desired
- Supportive care for dogs with Sertoli cell tumor–associated bone marrow suppression

CHRONIC TREATMENT

Metastastic disease: chemotherapy or radiation therapy for metastatic seminoma

RECOMMENDED MONITORING

- Seminoma, interstitial cell tumor, nonactive Sertoli cell tumor, mixed sex cord/stromal tumor: yearly physical examination
- Sertoli cell tumor with bone marrow suppression: close follow-up for evidence of bacterial septicemia; yearly physical examination

PROGNOSIS AND OUTCOME

- Seminoma: excellent following testicular removal; metastasis is rare
- Sertoli cell tumor: excellent following testicular removal; metastasis is rare, but risk of metastasis is increased for tumors >2 cm diameter
- Interstitial cell tumor: excellent following testicular removal; metastasis is not expected
- Mixed sex cord/stromal tumor: excellent following testicular removal; metastasis is not expected

PEARLS & CONSIDERATIONS

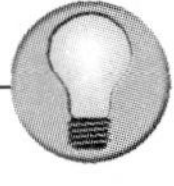

COMMENTS

- Histopathologic examination is needed for determination of tumor type
- Unilateral castration may result in up to 50% hypertrophy of the remaining testis. Return to fertility following uni-

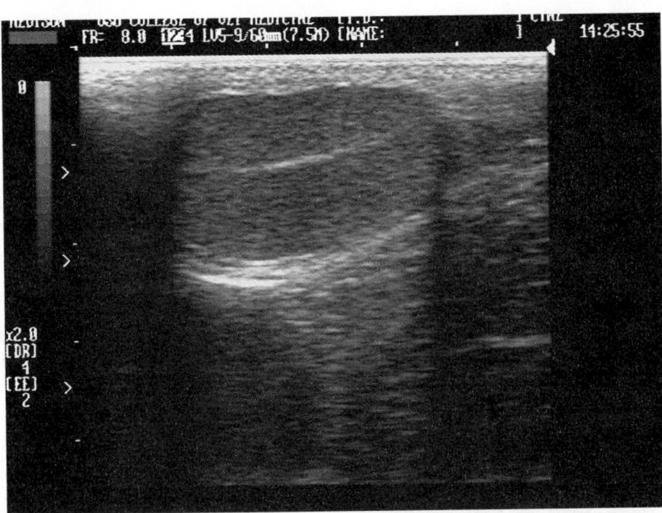

FIGURE I-170 Transscrotal ultrasonogram of the left testis from a normal fertile male dog. The echotexture of the parenchyma is homogeneous with the exception of the hyperechoic mediastinum (rete testis). Courtesy of Dr. Michelle A. Kutzler.

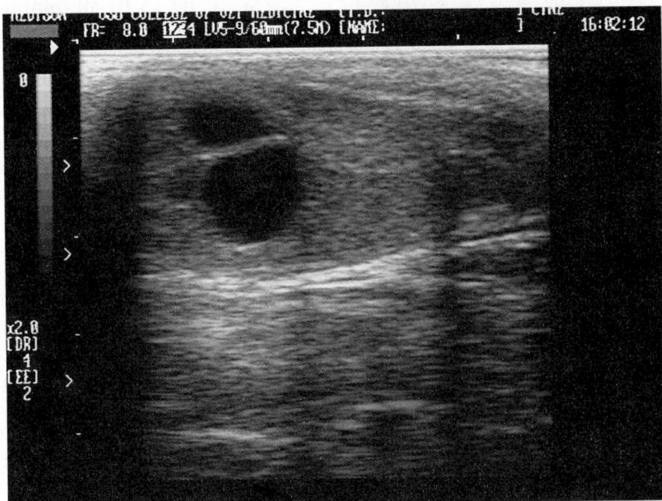

FIGURE I-171 Transscrotal ultrasonogram of the left testis from an infertile male dog. Two anechoic cystic structures are present within the parenchyma on either side of the mediastinum. Differential diagnoses include cystic neoplasia or testicular cyst. Courtesy of Dr. Michelle A. Kutzler.

lateral castration depends on the severity of testicular atrophy secondary to hormonal downregulation as well as the presence of underlying disease (testicular degeneration with loss of spermatogonia)

PREVENTION

Testicular removal, especially of cryptorchid testes

CLIENT EDUCATION

- Regular examination of testes and evaluation of the semen in breeding animals
- Prompt presentation for veterinary examination if an abnormality is detected

SUGGESTED READING

MacLachlan NJ, Kennedy PC: Tumors of the genital systems. In Meuten DJ (ed): *Tumors in Domestic Animals*, ed 4. Ames, IA, Iowa State Press, 2002, pp 561-567.

Morrison WB: Cancers of the reproductive tract. In Morrison WB (ed): *Cancer in Dogs and Cats: Medical and Surgical Management*. Baltimore, MD, Lippincott, Williams & Wilkins, 1998, pp 584-586.

AUTHOR: **BETH A. VALENTINE**
EDITOR: **MICHELLE A. KUTZLER**

Tetanus

BASIC INFORMATION

DEFINITION

An infectious disease caused by a potent neurotoxin. The neurotoxin is produced by the bacterium *Clostridium tetani*, resulting in a sustained tonic contraction of the muscles.

SYNONYM(S)

Lockjaw

EPIDEMIOLOGY

SPECIES, AGE, SEX: All domestic animals are susceptible; cats are more resistant than dogs.
RISK FACTORS: Open wounds; exposure to organism in feces or in the environment.
GEOGRAPHY AND SEASONALITY: Ubiquitous in the environment; no seasonality.

CLINICAL PRESENTATION

DISEASE FORMS/SUBTYPES: Focal versus generalized dependent on inoculation site; the focal form is more common.

HISTORY, CHIEF COMPLAINT

- Cutaneous/soft tissue wound (cut, puncture, surgical [e.g., ovariohysterectomy])
- Progressively worsening gait stiffness

PHYSICAL EXAM FINDINGS

- Extreme sensitivity to tactile and auditory stimulation: mildly to extremely exaggerated reaction to sound or touch
- Characteristic facial expression due to facial muscle spasm: ears held erect (Figs. I-172 and I-173), forehead wrinkled, lips drawn back (risus sardonicus)
- Trismus (teeth clenching)

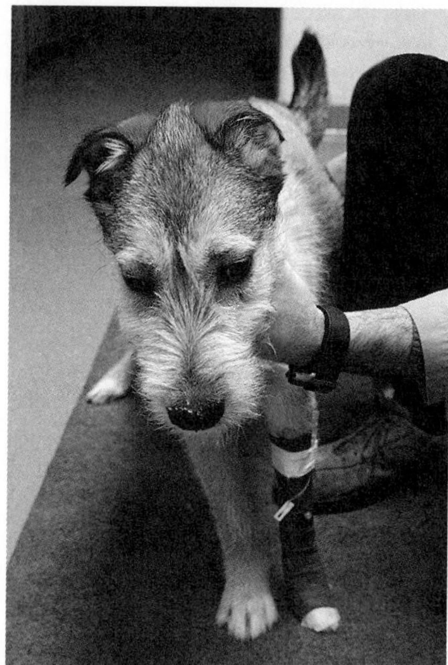

FIGURE I-172 Dog with fulminant tetanus. The contraction of the facial muscles has drawn the ears dorsally; a divergent strabismus is present, and the canthi of the lips are also drawn into a sardonic grin (not seen here). The mouth could not be opened. The extreme rigidity of the limbs explains the stiff, stilted posture.

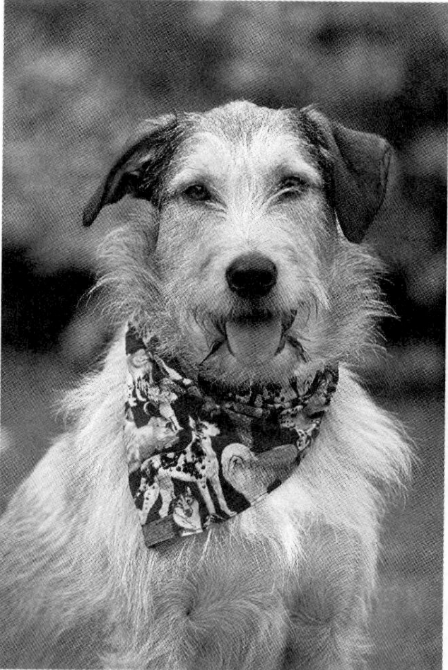

FIGURE I-173 The same dog as in Fig. I-172 after having made a complete recovery. Courtesy of John Sylvester.

- Protrusion of third eyelids, enophthalmos, strabismus, hypersalivation, laryngeal spasm, dysphagia
- Mild hyperthermia due to excessive muscular activity
- Dyspnea, coughing possible from aspiration pneumonia
- Progression to periodic generalized tonic muscle contraction possible
- Death can result from respiratory compromise

ETIOLOGY AND PATHOPHYSIOLOGY

- *C tetani* typically enters the body through wounds.
- A potent neurotoxin (tetanospasmin) is formed in the patient's body during vegetative growth of *C tetani*.
- Tetanospasmin enters the neuromuscular end plate of motor nerves and migrates to the neuronal cell body in the spinal cord or brainstem.
- Tetanospasmin blocks inhibitory neurotransmitter release (glycine, γ-aminobutyric acid [GABA]), facilitating muscle contraction.
- Tetanospasmin's binding to presynaptic sites of inhibitory neurons is irreversible; recovery depends on sprouting of new axon terminals.
- Signs occur within 5 to 10 days of injury but can be delayed up to 3 weeks.
- Wounds close to the head are associated with a more rapid onset of signs than those in the extremeties.

DIAGNOSIS

Tetanus is diagnosed based on clinical signs and history of a recent wound. The source of infection or wounds is not always immediately apparent.

DIFFERENTIAL DIAGNOSIS

Hypocalcemic tetany

INITIAL DATABASE

All the following test results may be seen, but none of these tests is required for a diagnosis of tetanus:

- Complete blood count (CBC): leukocytosis (neutrophilia with left shift)
- Serum biochemistry profile: elevated serum CPK
- Cerebrospinal fluid (CSF) analysis: unremarkable
- Electrocardiogram (ECG): tachyarrhythmias or bradyarrhythmias (atrioventricular [AV] block, sinus arrest) possible
- Thoracic and abdominal imaging: megaesophagus with or without aspiration pneumonia possible; abdominal effusion possible if source of *C tetani* is septic peritonitis (metritis, enteritis, ruptured abscess)
- Muscle biopsy: usually unremarkable.
- Serum antibody titers to tetanus toxin may support the diagnosis (compared to control animals)
- Isolation of *C tetani* from wounds is unrewarding

TREATMENT

THERAPEUTIC GOAL(S)

Resolution of clinical signs; may take days to weeks, depending on form (generalized or localized) and individual response

ACUTE GENERAL TREATMENT

- As much as possible, keep the animal in a quiet, sound-proof area with minimal stimulation.
- Wound debridement and resection of necrotic tissue; wounds are left open (avoid anaerobic conditions).
- Equine antitetanus serum (ATS) (given IM or IV) or human tetanus immunoglobulin (TIG) given IM.
- Tetanus antitoxin (equine):
  - Give the initial test dose 0.1-0.2 ml SC or ID 15 to 30 minutes before IV administration; monitor for anaphylaxis.
  - If no anaphylaxis, therapeutic dose is 2.5-25 IU/kg IV, and continue to monitor for anaphylaxis during and immediately after administration.
  - Intralesional injection appears promising (experimental studies).
  - Antitoxin prevents further toxin binding to axons but does not eliminate currently bound toxin.
- Sedation (e.g., one of the following: diazepam [helps enhance GABA inhibition], phenobarbital, acepromazine, chlorpromazine) is recommended.
- Antibacterial treatment (*C tetani*): sodium or potassium penicillin 20,000-50,000 IU/kg IV q 6h for 10 days and metronidazole 10 mg/kg PO q 8h for 10 days.

CHRONIC TREATMENT

- Physical rehabilitation (see Physical Rehabilitation, p 1300)
- Intensive nursing care to include IV fluids and nasogastric or percutaneous endoscopic gastrostomy (PEG) tube feedings (see Feeding Tube Placement: Nasoesophageal and Nasogastric, p 1245; Feeding Tube Placement: Percutaneous Endoscopic Gastrostomy [PEG], p 1247)
- Prevention of decubital ulcers
- Indwelling urinary catheter

DRUG INTERACTIONS

- Narcotics can depress the respiratory center and may stimulate other areas of the central nervous system (CNS).
- Parasympatholytic drugs, such as atropine, should be avoided in routine cases.

POSSIBLE COMPLICATIONS

- Aspiration pneumonia
- Decubital ulcers
- Respiratory paralysis

RECOMMENDED MONITORING

- Heart and respiratory rates
- Temperature monitoring
- Seizure watch
- Urine output

PROGNOSIS AND OUTCOME

- Guarded; better with mild clinical signs and localized clinical signs.
- In mildly affected animals, normal function usually returns within 3 weeks of the initial treatment.

PEARLS & CONSIDERATIONS

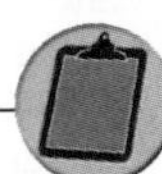

PREVENTION

- Avoid exposure to potential sources of infection
- Routine immunoprophylaxis (tetanus toxoid): not recommended in dogs and cats
- Appropriate (open) care of infected wounds and rational antibiotic therapy

CLIENT EDUCATION

- Treatment of the disease can take weeks, but a cure is possible.
- Seek veterinary attention in cases of open wounds.

SUGGESTED READING

Greene CE: Tetanus. In Greene CE (ed): *Infectious Diseases of the Dog and Cat*. Philadelphia, Elsevier, 2002, pp 267–273.

Oliver JE, Lorenz MD, Kornegay JN: Disorders of involuntary movement. In *Handbook of Veterinary Neurology*, ed 4. Philadelphia, Elsevier, 2004, pp 268–269.

AUTHOR: **KAREN L. KLINE**

EDITOR: **CURTIS W. DEWEY**

Tetralogy of Fallot

BASIC INFORMATION

DEFINITION

Consists of a large (unrestrictive) ventricular septal defect (VSD), pulmonic stenosis (PS), dextropositioned or overriding aorta, and secondary right ventricular hypertrophy. Ventricular outflow obstruction may be subvalvular or valvular.

EPIDEMIOLOGY

SPECIES, AGE, SEX: Tetralogy of Fallot (TF) is a cardiac malformation present at birth. Some dogs and cats survive to maturity (occasionally >5 years).

GENETICS AND BREED PREDISPOSITION: Keeshond, West Highland white terrier, and English bulldog are affected. In the keeshond, three distinct gene loci contribute to conotruncal malformations, the embryologic basis for TF.

ASSOCIATED CONDITIONS AND DISORDERS: Patent ductus arteriosus (PDA) or atrial septal defect (ASD) may be cofindings.

CLINICAL PRESENTATION

DISEASE FORMS/SUBTYPES: Most cases of TF manifest overt clinical signs due to hypoxemia or polycythemia. Right-sided congestive heart failure (CHF) is rare.

HISTORY, CHIEF COMPLAINT

- Cardiac murmur in an apparently healthy puppy or kitten
- Exercise intolerance, often with tachypnea
- Exertional syncope
- Stunted growth

PHYSICAL EXAM FINDINGS

- Systolic murmur over the pulmonic valve area with radiation to the right. A softer murmur may be evident with severe PS, marked polycythemia, or pulmonary atresia.
- Cyanosis may be observed, particularly after exertion.
- Palpable right ventricular precordial heave.

ETIOLOGY AND PATHOPHYSIOLOGY

- TF is a cardiac malformation that causes bidirectional shunting across a large VSD, leading to hypoxemia, cyanosis, secondary polycythemia, and impaired exercise capacity.
- Hyperviscosity syndrome may develop from polycythemia.
- Sudden cardiac death is the typical outcome.

DIAGNOSIS

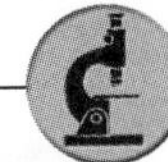

DIFFERENTIAL DIAGNOSIS

- PS with ASD or VSD
- Pulmonary or tricuspid valve atresia
- Severe pulmonary hypertension (Eisenmenger's physiology)
- Other causes of polycythemia (polycythemia vera, renal mass lesions)
- Respiratory diseases

INITIAL DATABASE

- Chest radiographs show right ventricular prominence, straight left auricular border on the dorsoventral projection, and pulmonary hypoperfusion. Radiographs also exclude primary pulmonary causes of cyanosis and respiratory distress.
- The electrocardiogram (ECG) usually shows a right ventricular hypertrophy pattern (or a cranially directed axis).
- Complete blood count (CBC) may demonstrate polycythemia.
- Pulse oximetry (or arterial blood gas [ABG]) testing quantifies oxygen saturation and functional status.

ADVANCED OR CONFIRMATORY TESTING

- Echocardiography with Doppler studies (± contrast echocardiography) is confirmatory
- Cardiac catheterization and angiography are rarely needed

TREATMENT

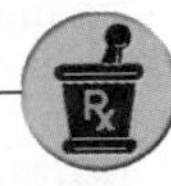

THERAPEUTIC GOAL(S)

- Definitive therapy requires open-heart surgery with cardiopulmonary bypass and is rarely done.
- Palliation involves preventing arterial desaturation and controlling the hematocrit. A slightly higher packed cell volume (PCV) is beneficial for increasing oxygen-carrying capacity and raising systemic vascular resistance.
- Avoid drugs that are vasodilators and reduce systemic vascular resistance (increasing right-to-left shunting).

ACUTE GENERAL TREATMENT

For bouts of dyspnea:

- Enforce rest, providing a cool, well-ventilated or fanned space (prevent overheating).
- Although supplemental oxygen has minimal benefits for patients with right-to-left shunting, it should be provided and the effect on oxygen saturation should be measured by pulse oximetry.
- Sedation with butorphanol may be helpful, but avoid acepromazine.
- Once the patient is stable for handling, measure the PCV; if >68%, perform a

phlebotomy, replacing the removed volume with a balanced crystalloid (100–150% of volume removed).
- If necessary, increase systemic vascular resistance with an α-adrenergic agonist (phenylephrine).

CHRONIC TREATMENT

- Assuming definitive repair is not possible, long-term benefits can be achieved by extracardiac, thoracic surgery. A palliative left-to-right shunt between a systemic artery and the pulmonary artery (e.g., Blalock-Taussig shunt) increases pulmonary blood flow and usually raises arterial oxygen saturation to >90%. Alternatively, "partial" balloon valvuloplasty of the stenotic right ventricular outlet can be considered, provided a residual pulmonary obstruction is maintained to prevent severe left-to-right shunting across the unrestrictive VSD.
- Perform a phlebotomy periodically and maintain PCV <68% (target 62–65% although lower values may be well tolerated).
- Prescribe nonspecific β-blocker propranolol to mitigate dynamic right ventricular outflow tract obstruction (from hypertrophy) while preventing drug-induced vasodilation.
- Consider a trial course of hydroxyurea to suppress the bone marrow when frequent phlebotomies are needed.
- Prescribe low-dose aspirin to animals with surgically created palliative shunts (to impede thrombosis).
- Limit the animal's exercise and avoid high heat-humidity conditions; prevent dehydration.
- Consider pentoxifylline to improve red blood cell (RBC) flexibility in the microcirculation (however, use in animals with TF is completely empiric).

POSSIBLE COMPLICATIONS

- Adverse effects of the aforementioned drugs
- Gradual spontaneous closure or thrombosis of a surgically created palliative shunt
- Acute pulmonary edema from creation of a large palliative shunt or overzealous balloon valvuloplasty for relief of PS
- Paradoxical (right-to-left) thromboembolic episode following venipuncture, causing stroke or coronary embolus

RECOMMENDED MONITORING

- Clinical signs: exercise capacity and respiratory effort at home
- Mucous membrane color and arterial oxygen saturation (oximetry)
- Hematocrit or full CBC with platelet count if the patient is taking hydroxyurea
- Resting heart rate as bradycardia (<60 in dogs or <120 in cats) may indicate overdosage of propranolol
- Pulmonary blood flow in surgically created shunts (by auscultation and echo-Doppler studies of the pulmonary artery)

PROGNOSIS AND OUTCOME

Guarded; most affected dogs and cats will succumb to complications of hypoxia or polycythemia (or will have to be euthanized). Common findings include:
- Bouts of exertional dyspnea or respiratory distress
- Stroke or other signs of hyperviscosity syndrome
- Sudden cardiac death

PEARLS & CONSIDERATIONS

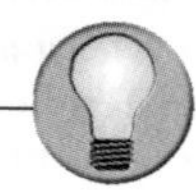

COMMENTS

- Systemic vascular resistance and pulmonary blood flow impact clinical outcome.
- Vigorous exercise, anemia, thyrotoxicosis, and vasodilator drugs increase right-to-left shunting.
- Mild PS or concurrent PDA may reduce clinical signs.
- The magnitude of polycythemia may not correlate with clinical signs.
- Palliative surgery for TF is very challenging and best performed by an experienced thoracic surgeon.

PREVENTION

Do not breed dogs with TF

CLIENT EDUCATION

- Observe exercise capacity, effort and rate of breathing, and general well-being
- Avoid environmental and exercise extremes
- Report progressive signs or syncope
- Provide ventilation (a fan) and water during periods of respiratory distress

SUGGESTED READING

Oyama MA, Sisson DD, Thomas WP, Bonagura JD: Congenital heart disease. In Ettinger SJ, Feldman EC (eds): *Textbook of Veterinary Internal Medicine*, ed 6. Philadelphia, Elsevier Saunders, 2005, pp 972–1021.

AUTHOR: **JOHN D. BONAGURA**
EDITOR: **ETIENNE CÔTÉ**

Tetraplegia/Tetraparesis

BASIC INFORMATION

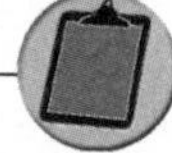

DEFINITION

- *-plegia* signifies complete paralysis
- *-paresis* signifies incomplete paralysis
- Either may manifest with upper motor neuron (UMN) or lower motor neuron (LMN) signs
- Tetraplegia: paralysis of all limbs
- Tetraparesis: incomplete paralysis of all limbs

SYNONYM(S)

Tetraplegia: quadriplegia
Tetraparesis: quadriparesis

EPIDEMIOLOGY

GENETICS AND BREED PREDISPOSITION
- Toy breed dogs: atlantoaxial instability
- Older Doberman pinschers, young Great Danes, and other large-breed dogs: cervical spondylopathy
- Chondrodystrophic dog breeds: cervical intervertebral disk protrusion
- Burmese cats: hypokalemia
- Labrador retrievers: exercise-induced collapse
- Various dog breeds: breed-associated motor neuron diseases
- Various cat/dog breeds: breed-associated muscular dystrophies and myopathies

RISK FACTORS
- Exposure to carrion: botulism (dogs)
- Exposure to toxins (e.g., 2, 4-D herbicide; organophosphates/carbamates)
- Penetrating wounds (tetanus)
- Areas endemic for coral snakes; black widow spiders (*Latrodectus* spp.); *Dermacentor* spp., *Amblyomma* spp., and *Ixodes* spp. of ticks (tick-bite paralysis)

CLINICAL PRESENTATION

HISTORY, CHIEF COMPLAINT: Tetraplegia:
- Inability to bear weight, voluntarily move limbs, or ambulate

Tetraparesis:
- Impaired locomotion, ranging from mild weakness or spasticity (usually with ataxia) to recumbency
- Ability to voluntarily move limbs even if recumbent

Tetraparetic/tetraplegic animals with diseases involving the cerebral cortex and/or brainstem will typically show other abnormal neurologic signs:
- Abnormal mentation and/or seizures (cerebral cortex or diencephalon)
- Dullness, stupor, or coma (brainstem)
- Cranial nerve disturbances (brainstem)
- Abnormal respiratory character (brain, cervical spinal cord)

PHYSICAL EXAM FINDINGS
- Variable (see specific diseases)
- It is important to neuroanatomically localize the lesion (see Neurologic Examination, p 1286)
- Tetraplegia or tetraparesis can be seen with UMN and/or LMN signs
- Symmetry or asymmetry of paresis should be noted because this finding may help narrow the differential diagnosis
- Animals may have UMN or LMN bladder
- Animals with tetraplegia or tetraparesis must have a disease involving one of the following regions:
  - Tetraplegia or tetraparesis with UMN signs to all four limbs (e.g., increased muscle tone and hyperreflexia)
    - Bilateral cerebral cortex
    - Bilateral brainstem (midbrain)
    - Bilateral cervical spinal cord
  - Tetraplegia or tetraparesis with hind limb UMN (as above) and forelimb LMN signs
    - Bilateral C6–T2 spinal cord involvement
  - Tetraplegia or tetraparesis with LMN signs to all four limbs
    - Disease affecting motor neurons of C6–T2 and L4–S2
    - Disease affecting peripheral nerves (motor component) of all four limbs
    - Disease affecting the neuromuscular junction
    - Disease affecting the skeletal muscle
  - If one particular region cannot be logically identified, then the disease process is likely multifocal

ETIOLOGY AND PATHOPHYSIOLOGY
- UMNs are found in the brain and control LMNs.
- LMNs transmit information from the central nervous system (CNS) to an effector organ like skeletal muscle.
- Conditions affecting UMNs and/or their axons result in UMN signs:
  - Paralysis or paresis
  - Normal to increased spinal reflexes
  - Later onset muscle atrophy (disuse atrophy)
  - Normal to increased muscle tone
- Conditions that affect LMNs, their axons, and the neuromuscular junction result in LMN signs:
  - Paralysis or paresis
  - Decreased or absent spinal reflexes
  - Rapid, severe muscle atrophy (neurogenic atrophy)
  - Decreased muscle tone
- Primary or systemic diseases affecting skeletal muscle cause impaired muscular function and can manifest as tetraplegia or tetraparesis.

DIAGNOSIS

DIFFERENTIAL DIAGNOSIS
- Intracranial:
  - Neoplasia
  - Trauma
  - Encephalitis (various causes, including infectious and immune-mediated granulomatous meningoencephalitis [GME] diseases)
  - Hydrocephalus
  - Postictal state
- Cervical spinal cord:
  - Intervertebral disk prolapse
  - Trauma
  - Cervical spondylopathy
  - Atlantoaxial instability
  - Myelitis (various causes, including infectious and immune-mediated [GME] diseases)
  - Osteochondromatosis
  - Synovial or arachnoid cysts
- Peripheral nerves or neuromuscular junction:
  - Tick-bite paralysis
  - Idiopathic polyradiculoneuritis
  - Snake or spider envenomation
  - Myasthenia gravis
  - Botulism
  - Hypothyroidism
  - Various toxins
- Muscle:
  - Immune-mediated polymyositis (primary or secondary to another disease, such as neoplasia)
  - Hypokalemia
  - Endocrine disease (hyperthyroidism [cats], hypothyroidism, hyperadrenocorticism)
  - Various breed-related muscular dystrophies and myopathies

INITIAL DATABASE
- Assess animal stability (some animals may present with impaired respiratory function and/or cardiac arrhythmias)
- Complete physical and neurologic examinations
- Complete blood count (CBC), serum chemistry profile, and urinalysis for assessment of systemic causes and preanesthetic evaluation

ADVANCED OR CONFIRMATORY TESTING
- Plain skull or spinal radiographs
- Cerebral spinal fluid (CSF) analysis
- Myelography
- MRI or CT scan
- Electrodiagnostic and histopathologic evaluation of affected muscle and nerves
- Detection of antibodies to acetylcholine receptors in cases of fulminant myasthenia gravis

TREATMENT

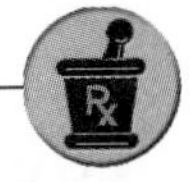

THERAPEUTIC GOAL(S)
- Eliminate inciting cause
- Provide adequate supportive nursing care

ACUTE GENERAL TREATMENT
- Treat underlying condition if possible
- Intensity of nursing care depends on the individual needs of the animal
- Some supportive therapies to be considered:
  - Assisted pulmonary ventilation: if inadequate spontaneous ventilation
  - Caloric intake: hand-feeding, feeding via esophagostomy/gastrostomy tube, or parenteral nutrition
  - Hydration: appropriate fluid therapy
  - Muscle contracture: passive range-of-motion exercises
  - Pressure sores: turn animals frequently and treat the lesions early and aggressively if they occur
  - Urinary bladder (e.g., catheterization) and bowel management (e.g., stool softener)
  - Hygiene: regular cleaning of perineum; ensure animals are kept on clean, dry bedding

CHRONIC TREATMENT
Long-term supportive therapy may be necessary

POSSIBLE COMPLICATIONS
Complications associated with tetraplegia or severe tetraparesis include:
- Pressure sores
- Urinary tract infections with chronic bladder catheterization
- Fecal impaction
- Pneumonia

RECOMMENDED MONITORING
- Complete physical examinations two times per day to identify complications from recumbency
- Regularly scheduled neurologic assessments to monitor disease progression
- Severe or progressive CNS or neuromuscular disease: regular assessment of respiratory function

PROGNOSIS AND OUTCOME

Variable, depending on underlying cause

PEARLS & CONSIDERATIONS

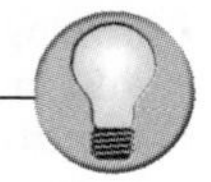

COMMENTS

- Referral to an appropriate treatment center is often necessary.
- Nursing care is often times intensive, extensive, and expensive.

CLIENT EDUCATION

Diseases resulting in tetraplegia or tetraparesis can be costly to diagnose and treat.

SUGGESTED READING

Comparative Neuromuscular Laboratory Website. University of California, San Diego, Department of Pathology, School of Medicine. http://medicine.ucsd.edu/vet_neuromuscular/index.html. Accessed August 9, 2006.

Vite CH, Braund KG (eds): *Braund's Clinical Neurology in Small Animals: Localization, Diagnosis and Treatment*. New York, International Veterinary Information Service: http://www.ivis.org/advances/Vite/toc.asp.

AUTHOR: **AUBREY A. WEBB**
EDITOR: **ETIENNE CÔTÉ**

Thiamin (Vitamin B_1) Deficiency

BASIC INFORMATION

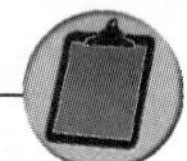

DEFINITION

Inadequate intake of thiamin

SYNONYM(S)

Chastek paralysis (foxes)
Thiamine (British spelling) deficiency

EPIDEMIOLOGY

SPECIES, AGE, SEX: Thiamin is an essential nutrient; deficiency can occur in any mammal that must meet its needs from a dietary source (dogs, cats, and other mammals with similar gastrointestinal [GI] tracts).

RISK FACTORS

- Inadequately supplemented commercial diets
- Overcooked foods
- Consumption of fish containing thiaminase (species of both freshwater fish [e.g., carp, catfish, bass] and saltwater fish [e.g., skipjack, yellow-fin tuna] may contain thiaminase enzymes)

GEOGRAPHY AND SEASONALITY: Areas of high fish consumption and poor-quality diets for pets.

ASSOCIATED CONDITIONS AND DISORDERS: Generalized malnutrition from prolonged consumption of an unsatisfactory diet.

CLINICAL PRESENTATION

HISTORY, CHIEF COMPLAINT: Compatible diet history:

- In dogs, clinical signs can include variable combinations of inappetence progressing to anorexia, depression, weight loss, and vomiting. Musculoskeletal signs include muscular weakness, ataxia, hyperesthesia, ventroflexion of the head, and circling, which may progress to generalized "tonic-clonic" seizures, recumbency, opisthotonus, coma, and death.
- In cats, signs of thiamin deficiency begin with a period of decreased food intake and hypersalivation after 2 to 4 weeks of ingestion of a thiamin-deficient diet. The decreased food intake is distinctive in that cats appear to retain their interest in food but do not consume it. They may be observed sitting with the head positioned over the food dish without eating. This stage is followed in another 2 to 4 weeks by a period of brief tonic convulsive seizures. During this period, ventroflexion of the head and loss of normal righting reflexes may occur. Cats with severe lesions eventually progress to semicoma, may cry persistently, and develop opisthotonus and limb spasticity prior to death.

PHYSICAL EXAM FINDINGS

- In dogs, patellar reflexes usually are increased. Tremors, menace and proprioceptive deficits, and occasionally nystagmus may be observed. Some dogs show signs of hysteria.
- In cats, the pupils may be poorly responsive to light, and the menace response may be absent; retinal veins may be dilated, and retinal hemorrhages may be seen. Ventroflexion of the head, especially when the cat is suspended by the hind limbs, may be present, and the cat may lie in a tight semicircular posture. Handling may precipitate seizure activity.

ETIOLOGY AND PATHOPHYSIOLOGY

- Thiamin is an essential cofactor in intermediary metabolism. It is required for complete metabolism of glucose to carbon dioxide and water by the tricarboxylic acid cycle.
- The precise mechanism by which thiamin deficiency results in the observed clinical signs is not known, but tissues (e.g., nervous and cardiovascular) particularly dependent on glucose and its metabolites for energy are particularly at risk.

DIAGNOSIS

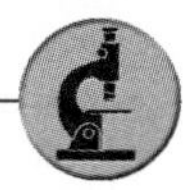

DIFFERENTIAL DIAGNOSIS

- Toxin
- Inflammatory or infectious central nervous system (CNS) disorder
- Multifocal neoplasia
- Metabolic disease

INITIAL DATABASE

- Review diet history
- Question owners about possibility of toxin ingestion
- CBC, serum biochemical profile, and urinalysis to rule out other abnormalities
- Electrocardiogram (ECG): abnormal rate, exaggerated sinus arrhythmia, "notched" P waves, QRS prolongation, elevated ST segment, and flattened or inverted T waves

ADVANCED OR CONFIRMATORY TESTING

- Treat with thiamin; expect rapid response
- Erythrocyte transketolase assay (a local laboratory should be contacted for sample collection procedures and interpretation of results)
- Cerebrospinal fluid (CSF) tap and brain MRI to rule out inflammatory/structural brain disease

TREATMENT

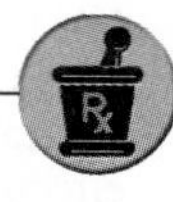

THERAPEUTIC GOAL(S)

Reestablish thiamin homeostasis

ACUTE GENERAL TREATMENT

- Supportive care

- Intramuscular injection of thiamin hydrogen chloride (HCl); doses ranging from 1-20 mg/day have been recommended

CHRONIC TREATMENT

If thiamin deficiency was present, other (subclinical) nutrient deficiencies also are likely to have been present. Providing a diet known to be nutritionally complete is preferred to attempting to repair the defective diet. If this is not possible, consult a veterinary nutritionist to provide an appropriate diet based on available resources.

PROGNOSIS AND OUTCOME

Excellent if identified before the animal becomes agonal

PEARLS & CONSIDERATIONS

COMMENTS

Recovery of function and appetite is rapid (hours) after provision of thiamin if deficiency of this vitamin is the cause of the signs

PREVENTION

Feed a properly formulated diet

CLIENT EDUCATION

Explain the importance of feeding a properly formulated diet

SUGGESTED READING

Buffington CAT: Nutritional diseases and nutritional therapy. In Sherding RG (ed): *The Cat Diseases and Clinical Management.* New York, Churchill Livingstone, 1994, pp 161-190.

Garosi LS, et al: Thiamine deficiency in a dog: Clinical, clinicopathologic, and magnetic resonance imaging findings. *J Vet Intern Med* 17:719, 2003.

AUTHOR & EDITOR: **C. A. TONY BUFFINGTON**

Third Eyelid Abnormalities/Protrusion

BASIC INFORMATION

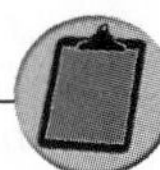

DEFINITION

- *Scrolled cartilage* is an everted scroll-like malformation of the third eyelid.
- *Third eyelid gland prolapse* is a dorsal displacement of the gland from the base of the third eyelid.
- *Protrusion of the third eyelid* is a dorsolateral displacement of a normal third eyelid structure, typically as a result of alteration of ocular or orbital contents, orbital muscular tone, or globe position.
- *Neoplasia of the third eyelid* involves a smooth or irregular mass or diffuse thickening of the third eyelid; adenocarcinoma is reported to be most common; papilloma is second most common.

SYNONYM(S)

Third eyelid: nictitating membrane, membrana nictitans

Scrolled cartilage: everted cartilage, bent cartilage

Third eyelid gland prolapse: cherry eye, Haws syndrome

Third eyelid inflammatory disorders:

- Plasma cell infiltration of the third eyelid: plasmoma, pannus, or chronic superficial keratitis of the third eyelid
- Nodular granulomatous episclerokeratitis of the third eyelid: nodular episcleritis, nodular fasciitis (dogs)
- Proliferative (eosinophilic) keratoconjunctivitis (cats)
- Follicular conjunctivitis: lymphofollicular conjunctivitis

Third eyelid protrusion: elevation of third eyelid

EPIDEMIOLOGY

SPECIES, AGE, SEX

- *Scrolled cartilage*: congenital/early developmental disorder (dogs and cats)
- *Third eyelid gland prolapse*: generally occurs before 2 years of age (dogs and cats)

GENETICS AND BREED PREDISPOSITION

- *Scrolled cartilage*: familial problem in large breeds including basset hound, bloodhound, English setter, German shepherd, Great Dane, Newfoundland, Rhodesian Ridgeback, weimaraner; reported to be a simple recessive trait in Saint Bernard and German shorthaired pointer dogs; uncommon in cats but reported in Burmese
- *Third eyelid gland prolapse*: predisposed breeds include American and English cocker spaniels, English bulldog, beagle, shih tzu (dogs); Burmese (cats)
- Third eyelid inflammatory disorders:
  - Breeds predisposed to plasma cell infiltration include German shepherds, Belgian sheepdog, Borzoi, doberman pinscher, English springer spaniel.
  - Nodular granulomatous episclerokeratitis can involve the third eyelid of all dog breeds, with the collie apparently predisposed.
  - Follicular conjunctivitis affects primarily large breeds of dogs and dogs typically younger than 18 months of age.

ASSOCIATED CONDITIONS AND DISORDERS

Third eyelid inflammation:

- Dogs:
  - Chronic superficial keratitis (see Pannus [Chronic Superficial Keratitis], p 802)
  - Nodular granulomatous episclerokeratitis (limbal lesions) (see Episcleritis/Scleritis, p 353)
  - Follicular conjunctivitis (bulbar conjunctival lesions) (see Conjunctivitis: Dogs, p 233)
- Cats:
  - Proliferative (eosinophilic) keratoconjunctivitis (see Corneal Vascularization, p 249)
  - Feline herpesvirus type 1 infection (see Conjunctivitis: Cats, p 231; Herpesviral Keratitis in Cats, p 513)

Protrusion of the third eyelid:

- Conditions causing alteration of orbital contents:
  - Dehydration
  - Loss of orbital fat from emaciation
  - Temporal muscle atrophy
  - Orbital neoplasia; cystic disease in the orbit; and orbital cellulitis, abscess, or hemorrhage (see Orbital Disease, p 773)
- Conditions associated with alteration in globe size:
  - Microphthalmia (congenital smallness of the eye) (see Ocular Size Abnormalities, p 763)
  - Chronic uveitis or glaucoma or ocular trauma causing phthisis bulbi (shrinkage of the eye) (see Uveitis, p 1134; Glaucoma, p 440)

- Conditions associated with alteration in orbital muscle tone:
  - Tetanus (see p 1071)
  - Strychnine poisoning (see p 1045)
  - Horner's syndrome (see p 532)
- Conditions associated with alteration in globe position:
  - Painful ocular disorders, including:
    - Corneal ulceration (see p 246)
    - Uveitis (see p 1134)
    - Conjunctivitis (see Conjunctivitis: Cats, p 231; Conjunctivitis: Dogs, p 233)
- In cats, also consider dysautonomia or a bilateral chronic idiopathic condition associated with gastrointestinal (GI) parasites, GI malfunction, or feline leukemia virus (FeLV) infection

CLINICAL PRESENTATION

HISTORY, CHIEF COMPLAINT

- Membrane covering part of the eye
- Abnormal appearance of or position of third eyelid or gland of the third eyelid

PHYSICAL EXAM FINDINGS

Scrolled cartilage appears as an anterior folding of the dorsal portion of the third eyelid.

Third eyelid gland prolapse appears as a smooth, moist (mucosa-covered) pink to red mass at the medial canthus protruding over the free margin of the third eyelid; may be unilateral or bilateral.

Third eyelid inflammatory disorders:

- Plasma cell infiltration causes a thickened, pebbly, often depigmented, hyperemic change in appearance of the third eyelid, especially noticable along the free margin of the third eyelid.
- Nodular granulomatous episclerokeratitis lesions of the third eyelid are typically smooth, hyperemic subconjunctival tubular-like swellings along the palpebral surface of the third eyelid.
- Animals with follicular conjunctivitis have an increased number of larger than usual follicles on the bulbar side of the third eyelid in addition to multiple small pink follicles along the bulbar conjunctival surface.

Neoplasia of the third eyelid: typically appears as a smooth to irregular, occasionally ulcerated, pink to red mass at the medial canthus arising from the third eyelid; typically unilateral.

ETIOLOGY AND PATHOPHYSIOLOGY

- *Scrolled cartilage*: differential growth rate of the posterior (caudal) portion of the cartilage compared to that of the anterior (rostral) portion
- *Third eyelid gland prolapse*: may result from weakness of connective tissue attaching the base of the gland to the periorbital structures
- Third eyelid protrusion: Movement of the third eyelid is passive and occurs with:
  - Changes in volume of globe or orbit
  - Secondary globe retraction via retractor bulbi muscle (e.g., ocular pain)
  - Changes in extraocular muscle tone (e.g., Horner's syndrome resulting in a decrease in sympathetic tone; tetanus producing increased extraocular muscle tone)
- Third eyelid inflammatory disorders:
  - Plasma cell infiltration is often associated with chronic superficial keratitis (see Pannus [Chronic Superficial Keratitis], p 802); the inflammatory infiltrate consists of plasma cells and lymphocytes.
  - Nodular granulomatous episclerokeratitis appears to be an immune-mediated disease; lesions are characterized by a chronic granulomatous inflammatory cell response.
  - Follicular conjunctivitis is thought to represent chronic antigenic stimulation.

DIAGNOSIS

The diagnosis of many disorders of the third eyelid rests on careful physical examination of the third eyelid lesions; confirmatory testing is needed in a minority of cases.

DIFFERENTIAL DIAGNOSIS

- *Scrolled cartilage* is diagnosed based on ophthalmic examination revealing a curled or bent third eyelid
- The differential diagnosis for a smooth fleshy mass at the medial canthus in a middle-aged or older dog is neoplasia versus glandular prolapse in a young (<2 year) dog
- Third eyelid protrusion (as previously described)

INITIAL DATABASE

- Characteristic clinical examination findings exist for most lesions involving the third eyelid, as described above
- Definitive diagnosis of mass lesions may require excisional biopsy and histologic examination
- Complete physical and ophthalmic examinations to determine cause of third eyelid protrusion, including:
  - Pupillary light reflexes (PLRs) (e.g., miotic pupil in Horner's syndrome and uveitis)
  - Fluorescein dye application (positive fluorescein stain retention in corneal ulceration)
  - Evaluate globe size (e.g., if small: microphthalmia versus phthisis bulbi)
  - Retropulsion of globe (may be reduced with orbital disease) (see Orbital Disease, p 773)
  - Hydration status
  - Body condition
  - Signs of systemic illness (fever, lethargy, etc.)

ADVANCED OR CONFIRMATORY TESTING

- Variable depending on underlying abnormality
- Imaging studies (ocular or orbital ultrasound, CT scan, MRI) for retrobulbar space-occupying lesions, possibly in conjunction with fine-needle aspirates (FNAs) and cytologic examination and/or biopsy and histologic examination of the orbital mass (see Orbital Disease, p 773)

TREATMENT

THERAPEUTIC GOAL(S)

- Improve the appearance and function of third eyelid structures to as normal as possible to minimize chronic low-grade corneal and conjunctival irritation and associated ocular discharge (*scrolled cartilage* and *third eyelid gland prolapse*)
- Preserve vital tear production from the gland of the third eyelid (*third eyelid gland prolapse*)
- Specific goals depend on the nature of the abnormality

ACUTE GENERAL TREATMENT

- *Scrolled cartilage*: Treatment is surgical, requiring removal of the folded/scrolled portion of the cartilage through the bulbar conjunctival surface of the third eyelid.
- *Third eyelid gland prolapse* requires surgical replacement of the third eyelid gland, which involves:
  - Anchoring the prolapsed gland to the orbital periosteum
  - Burying the prolapsed gland in a pocket created under the conjunctiva of the third eyelid
  - Contraindicated: excision of the gland of the third eyelid. It is associated with significantly decreased tear production and a high incidence of keratoconjunctivitis sicca (KCS) months to years postoperatively
- Third eyelid inflammatory disorders:
  - Treatment of plasma cell infiltrate typically consists of topical (q 6-12h), subconjunctival (q 2-4 weeks initially), or (rarely) systemic corticosteroids; topical cyclosporine A (q 12h) used for a long period of time (see Pannus [Chronic Superficial Keratitis], p 802)
  - Nodular granulomatous episclerokeratitis is generally controllable with the long-term use of topical and/or systemic corticosteroids and/or azathioprine (see Episcleritis/Scleritis, p 353)

- Follicular conjunctivitis is often self-limiting. In severe cases, or those cases that feature unacceptable hyperemia or ocular discharge, irrigation of the conjunctival cul-de-sac with saline and the judicious use of topical corticosteroids are helpful. Mechanical debridement with a gauze square/sponge following instillation of topical anesthesia (e.g., 0.5% proparacaine ophthalmic solution) is described but seldom necessary
- *Neoplasia of the third eyelid* may necessitate surgical removal of the entire third eyelid.

CHRONIC TREATMENT

If the third eyelid and gland are removed for *neoplasia of the third eyelid*, long-term use of topical artificial tear supplements (q 6–12h) with or without topical cyclosporine A (q 12h) may be required, especially if KCS develops.

POSSIBLE COMPLICATIONS

- *Third eyelid gland prolapse*: if uncorrected, chronic exposure of the gland results in glandular hypertrophy, decreased tear production chronic KCS, and ocular discharge
- Use caution with deep passage of suture needle in orbital "tie-down" procedures because perforation of the globe may cause devastating consequences

PROGNOSIS AND OUTCOME

- *Scrolled cartilage*: Following surgery, most third eyelids return to a normal function and appearance; in some cases, surgical removal of the scrolled section still does not produce complete flattening against the globe.
- *Third eyelid gland prolapse*: Although surgical failure (up to 20%) can occur, subsequent repositioning is typically successful.
- Most inflammatory conditions of the third eyelid can be controlled medically; however, recurrence may arise, and maintenance therapy is often necessary.
- Prognosis of third eyelid protrusion depends on the underlying disease process and ranges from excellent (e.g., orbital cellulitis) to grave (malignant orbital neoplasia).
- *Neoplasia of the third eyelid*: Adenocarcinoma is the most common condition and is associated with recurrence following excision; the second most common is papilloma for which local excision is typically curative.

PEARLS & CONSIDERATIONS

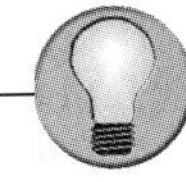

COMMENTS

- The only indication for surgical removal of the third eyelid is neoplasia.
- Be suspicious of *neoplasia of the third eyelid* gland in a middle-aged or older dog rather than *third eyelid gland prolapse*; do not surgically replace the gland in a suspicious animal until confirmed (by FNA and cytologic examination or wedge biopsy and histologic examination) that it is not neoplasia.
- Check the bulbar surface (i.e., underside) of the third eyelid in cases with third eyelid protrusion and cases in which concurrent corneal ulcers are not responding to treatment.

SUGGESTED READING

Barnett KC: Diseases of the nictitating membrane of the dog. *J Small Anim Pract* 19:101, 1978.

Dugan SJ, et al: Clinical and histological evaluation of the prolapsed third eyelid gland in dogs. *J Am Vet Med Assoc* 201:1861, 1992.

Morgan RV, et al: Prolapse of the gland of the third eyelid in dogs: A retrospective study of 89 cases (1980–1990). *J Am Anim Hosp Assoc* 29:56, 1993.

Wilcock B, et al: Adenocarcinoma of the gland of the third eyelid in seven dogs. *J Am Vet Med Assoc* 193:1549, 1988.

AUTHOR: **RICHARD F. QUINN**

EDITOR: **CHERYL L. CULLEN**

Thrombocytopenia, Immune-Mediated

Client Education Sheet on Website

BASIC INFORMATION

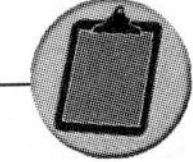

DEFINITION

Thrombocytopenia resulting from idiopathic destruction of platelets. A causative etiologic agent cannot be identified

SYNONYM(S)

Idiopathic thrombocytopenic purpura (ITP)
Immune ITP
IMT
Primary IMT

EPIDEMIOLOGY

SPECIES, AGE, SEX: Dogs are far more frequently affected than cats; reported in male and female dogs from 8 months to 15 years of age with middle-aged females predisposed.

GENETICS AND BREED PREDISPOSITION: Cocker spaniels, old English sheep dogs, German shepherds, and poodles are overrepresented.

ASSOCIATED CONDITIONS AND DISORDERS: Immune-mediated diseases may affect multiple body systems; for example, immune-mediated thrombocytopenia (IMT) may be associated with polyarthritis or proteinuria. Anemia may be due to blood loss (especially gastrointestinal [GI]) or concurrent immune-mediated hemolytic anemia (Evans syndrome).

CLINICAL PRESENTATION

DISEASE FORMS/SUBTYPES: Primary IMT remains idiopathic despite investigation.

Secondary IMT occurs in association with infection, drug therapy, or neoplasia.

HISTORY, CHIEF COMPLAINT: Owners commonly notice bleeding in the skin, from the nose or mouth, or associated with minor trauma. Frank blood in the stool or melena may be detected. The animal may continue to eat and act normally although some cases present with lethargy and weakness. Signs caused by bleeding into vital organs (brain, spinal cord) are an uncommon presentation.

PHYSICAL EXAM FINDINGS

- Petechiae, ecchymoses
- Ocular hemorrhage/hyphema
- GI bleeding, manifesting as melena or hematochezia noted on rectal examination or on a thermometer
- Pale mucous membranes
- Fever: present in less than 20% of cases

ETIOLOGY AND PATHOPHYSIOLOGY

- Immune-mediated thrombocytopenia occurs when a stimulus triggers an animal with the appropriate susceptibility genes.
- The identification and inheritance of predisposing genes are unknown.

- Triggering factors may include vaccination, drug administration, stress, or infection.
- Bleeding does not occur until the platelet count is less than 25,000/μl although bleeding may occur in the face of higher platelet counts if the platelets are dysfunctional (thrombocytopathia).

DIAGNOSIS

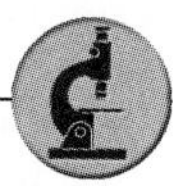

DIFFERENTIAL DIAGNOSIS

- Breed-associated physiologic thrombocytopenia (greyhounds and Cavalier King Charles spaniels)
- Thrombocytopathia (drug-related, inherited, von Willebrand disease) (see Platelet Dysfunction, p 856)
- Tick-borne disease (ehrlichiosis, anaplasmosis, Rocky Mountain spotted fever)
- Splenic disease (neoplasia, torsion, infarction)
- Drug administration (chemotherapy, antibiotics, estrogen, nonsteroidal anti-inflammatory drugs [NSAIDs], albendazole, griseofulvin, propythiouracil, ketoconazole)
- Recent vaccination
- Bacterial sepsis, vasculitis, disseminated intravascular coagulation
- Bone marrow disease (myelofibrosis, myelodysplasia, necrosis, myelophthisis)
- Severe hemorrhage (anticoagulant rodenticide, trauma)
- Cats: feline leukemia virus (FeLV), feline immunodeficiency virus (FIV)

INITIAL DATABASE

- Complete blood count (CBC) with manual differential: usually normal unless excess bleeding causes anemia
- Platelet count: usually <25,000 μl (severe thrombocytopenia)
- Biochemical profile: usually normal
- Urinalysis (voided):
  - Usually normal or may show hematuria
  - Avoid cystocentesis in any severely thrombocytopenic animal
- Coagulation profile: usually normal
- Thoracic radiographs: usually normal
- Abdominal ultrasonography: usually normal or may show mild splenomegaly
- Titers for tick-borne diseases in endemic areas

ADVANCED OR CONFIRMATORY TESTING

- Bone marrow cytologic examination is unnecessary in most cases (only necessary if the animal has concurrent leukopenia or nonregenerative anemia): may show increased or decreased megakaryocytes
- Testing for platelet-bound antibody is unnecessary in most cases

TREATMENT

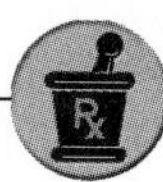

THERAPEUTIC GOAL(S)

- Raise the animal's platelet count to the normal range.
- In some cases, it may be preferable to allow a low grade of thrombocytopenia to persist to decrease medications to tolerable levels.

ACUTE GENERAL TREATMENT

- Prednisone 2.2 mg/kg PO q 24h or divided q 12h (alternative: dexamethasone 0.2 mg/kg IV q 24h or divided at q 12h)
- Vincristine 0.02 mg/kg IV once weekly
- Azathioprine 2.2 mg/kg PO q 24h
- Red blood cell (RBC) transfusions (fresh whole blood, packed cells) given as needed (see Transfusion Therapy and Collection Techniques for Blood Banking, p 1312)
- Platelet transfusions usually are impractical since platelets are immediately destroyed
- Human IV immunoglobulin (0.5 g/kg slow IV q 24h; risk of anaphylaxis) has been effective in refractory cases

CHRONIC TREATMENT

- Discontinue vincristine once platelet count is >50,000 μl or if no response
- Taper prednisone and azathioprine together once platelet count has normalized
- Decrease doses by one-half every month (in general) while monitoring platelet count
- The minimum duration of therapy is 6 months
- Increase to the previous dose and attempt to taper more slowly if the platelet count falls during the drug tapering

DRUG INTERACTIONS

- Extravasation of vincristine must be avoided because it causes severe skin necrosis; use an indwelling IV catheter
- Avoid drugs such as aspirin or other NSAIDs

POSSIBLE COMPLICATIONS

- Avoid the use of cyclophosphamide: hemorrhagic cystitis may be fatal
- Prolonged administration of azathioprine may cause bone marrow suppression: monitor CBC and decrease dosage once platelet count returns to normal

RECOMMENDED MONITORING

- Platelet counts every other day until >50,000 μl, then weekly until normal
- CBC 1 week after starting azathioprine, then every 2 weeks while on daily dosing. Bone marrow suppression is unusual once azathioprine is tapered to 2.2 mg/kg every other day; CBC needs to be monitored only every 2 to 3 months

PROGNOSIS AND OUTCOME

- The prognosis is initially guarded, with fatal bleeding into the brain or spinal cord possible.
- Response often takes 3 to 10 days.
- Once the platelet count normalizes, the prognosis is fair to good.
- Many pets may be completely tapered from immunosuppressive medications although relapse remains possible.

PEARLS & CONSIDERATIONS

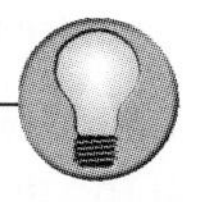

COMMENTS

- The presence of severe thrombocytopenia (<25,000 μl) in an otherwise healthy appearing animal is most likely due to IMT.
- If bleeding is present when the platelet count >25,000 μl, an additional problem, such as clotting factor deficiency, thrombocytopathia, or vasculitis must be present.
- Many animals are euthanized due to adverse effects of prednisone. Strategies to decrease prednisone-induced adverse effects include the avoidance of obesity, substituting prednisone with methylprednisolone or prednisolone, use of an additional immunosuppressive agent and lower glucocorticoid doses, and routine monitoring for infection of the skin and urinary tract.
- Combination immunosuppressive therapy with azathioprine is often more effective and has fewer adverse effects than prednisone alone.

PREVENTION

- Although a link has not been proven, future vaccinations should be limited to those considered absolutely essential.
- Stressful circumstances should be avoided if possible.

CLIENT EDUCATION

- Routine monitoring should be scheduled to detect relapse of disease and side effects of immunosuppressive medications
- Weight must be carefully monitored and obesity avoided

SUGGESTED READING

Lewis DC, Meyers KM: Canine idiopathic thrombocytopenic purpura. *J Vet Internal Med* 10: 207, 1996.

AUTHOR: **MICHAEL STONE**
EDITOR: **SUSAN M. COTTER**

Thymic Hemorrhage

BASIC INFORMATION

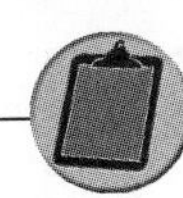

DEFINITION

Accumulation of blood in the parenchyma of the thymus

SYNONYM(S)

Thymic hematoma

EPIDEMIOLOGY

SPECIES, AGE, SEX

- Generally, an uncommon disease that occurs primarily in dogs; rare cases in cats have been reported.
- Thymic hemorrhage has been described predominantly in dogs less than 2 years of age although it has been seen in older dogs.

GENETICS AND BREED PREDISPOSITION: No sex or breed predilections have been identified; however, in some reports, German shepherds have been overrepresented.

RISK FACTORS: Potential risk factors that have been identified include:

- Thoracic trauma
- Exposure to anticoagulant rodenticides
- Thymic neoplasia (uncommon)

ASSOCIATED CONDITIONS AND DISORDERS

- Hemothorax
- Hemopericardium (with heart base thymic remnants)

CLINICAL PRESENTATION

HISTORY, CHIEF COMPLAINT

- Acute onset of lethargy, depression
- Tachypnea
- Increased respiratory effort
- Sudden death

PHYSICAL EXAM FINDINGS

- Mucous membrane pallor
- Tachycardia
- Tachypnea
- Muffled heart sounds and decreased lung sounds ventrally are possible
- Pain with compression of the cranial thorax

ETIOLOGY AND PATHOPHYSIOLOGY

- Intrathymic bleeding secondary to thymic trauma or a coagulation disorder, such as vitamin K rodenticide toxicity, will be the proximate cause identified in some cases.
- The initiating cause may not be identified in some animals.
- Another proposed cause includes bleeding from increased vessel fragility associated with normal thymic involution.

DIAGNOSIS

DIFFERENTIAL DIAGNOSIS

- Other causes of hemothorax, such as:
  - Trauma
  - Anticoagulant rodenticide toxicity
  - Intrathoracic neoplasia
- Other causes of hemopericardium:
  - Heart base tumors
  - Right atrial hemangiosarcoma
  - Pericarditis
- Occult blood loss into other sites, such as the gastrointestinal (GI) tract and urinary tract.

INITIAL DATABASE

- Complete blood count (CBC): anemia; thrombocytopenia has been described in some animals
- Serum biochemical profile: hypoproteinemia (hypoalbuminemia and hypoglobulinemia)
- Thoracic radiographs/ultrasound: pleural effusion or evidence of a soft-tissue density in the mediastinum

ADVANCED OR CONFIRMATORY TESTING

- Thoracocentesis and fluid analysis will confirm hemothorax.
- Prolongations of one-step prothrombin time (PT) and activated partial thromboplastin time (APTT, PTT) will be expected in animals with anticoagulant rodenticide toxicity. These animals may also have increases in serum levels of proteins induced by vitamin K absence or antagonism (PIVKA) and could have high concentrations of specific rodenticides identified in blood samples with toxicologic analysis.
- Cardiac ultrasound and pericardiocentesis can rule out or document the presence of heart base masses/tumors and pericardial effusion (hemopericardium), respectively.

TREATMENT

THERAPEUTIC GOAL(S)

- Identify underlying cause whenever possible
- Provide hemodynamic support

ACUTE GENERAL TREATMENT

- IV fluids (crystalloids, colloids)
- Blood products (whole blood, packed red blood cells [RBCs], and plasma)
- Vitamin K_1 for animals with historic or laboratory features suggestive of anticoagulant rodenticide toxicity

POSSIBLE COMPLICATIONS

Complications of treatment or with the primary disease have not been described for those animals that survive.

RECOMMENDED MONITORING

- Clinical signs
- Packed cell volume (PCV), total protein
- PT, APTT, particularly as vitamin K_1 therapy is discontinued

PROGNOSIS AND OUTCOME

- Most reported cases have been associated with fatal outcomes, probably because of the low clinical suspicion of the disease and delay in diagnosis and treatment.
- Provision of timely, aggressive supportive care in the form of fluids and blood products and administration of vitamin K_1 for animals with known or suspected rodenticide toxicity have been associated with survival of some affected animals.

PEARLS & CONSIDERATIONS

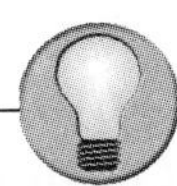

COMMENTS

- Perform thoracic radiographs on young animals with an acute onset of anemia of undetermined origin and consider the diagnosis if there is evidence of a mass or density in the mediastinum or if the animal has pleural effusion (hemothorax).
- When hemorrhage is documented in the absence of a history of trauma, assess coagulation parameters to rule out coagulation disorders.

PREVENTION AND CLIENT EDUCATION

Avoid trauma and exposure to rodenticides

SUGGESTED READING

Coolman BR, et al: Severe idiopathic thymic hemorrhage in two littermate dogs. *J Am Vet Assoc* 205:1152, 1994.

Liggett AD, et al: Thymic hematoma in juvenile dogs associated with anticoagulant rodenticide toxicosis. *J Vet Diagn Invest* 14:416, 2002.

AUTHOR & EDITOR: **RANCE K. SELLON**

Thymoma

BASIC INFORMATION

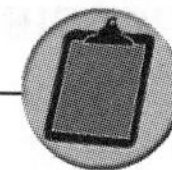

DEFINITION

Primary tumor originating from the thymic epithelium. Clinically, the presenting complaints for animals with thymoma are signs caused by the space-occupying nature of the mediastinal mass or by paraneoplastic syndromes, such as myasthenia gravis.

EPIDEMIOLOGY

SPECIES, AGE, SEX

- Dog: average age is 8 years
- Cat: average age is 9 years

GENETICS AND BREED PREDISPOSITION: Dog: large-breed dogs (Labrador retriever, German shepherd) may be more commonly affected.

ASSOCIATED CONDITIONS AND DISORDERS

- Paraneoplastic syndromes associated with thymoma:
  - Myasthenia gravis
  - Hypercalcemia
  - Immune-mediated syndromes (less common)
    - Polymyositis, dermatitis, and myocarditis
- Cardiac arrhythmias: rare
- Cranial vena cava syndrome: rare

CLINICAL PRESENTATION

HISTORY, CHIEF COMPLAINT

- Respiratory signs: very common chief complaints (dyspnea, coughing); signs may be surprisingly mild given size of thymoma
- Anorexia and weight loss also common
- Weakness:
  - Associated with myasthenia or hypercalcemia
- Regurgitation:
  - If megaesophagus is present

PHYSICAL EXAM FINDINGS

- Respiratory system:
  - Muffled or absent lung and heart sounds:
    - Pleural effusion
    - Space-occupying nature of mass
  - Increased, harsh lung sounds:
    - Aspiration pneumonia
- Weakness: episodic or sustained; associated with loss of muscle tone, decreased spinal reflexes
- Decreased chest wall compliance with cranial thoracic compression:
  - Important physical finding in cats with medium to large thymomas

ETIOLOGY AND PATHOPHYSIOLOGY

- Neoplastic transformation of thymic epithelial cells
- Cranial mediastinal mass ± pleural effusion:
  - Clinical signs of respiratory compromise
- Paraneoplastic syndrome of myasthenia gravis:
  - Result of aberrant immune stimulation

DIAGNOSIS

DIFFERENTIAL DIAGNOSIS

- Thymic lymphoma
- Thymic hyperplasia
- Thymic hemorrhage
- Branchial cyst
- Ectopic thyroid neoplasia
- Mediastinal abscess or granuloma

INITIAL DATABASE

- Complete blood count (CBC), serum biochemical profile, and urinalysis
  - Preoperative evaluation
- Feline leukemia virus (FeLV) and feline immunodeficiency (FIV) serologic testing in cats
- Survey thoracic radiographs (three views) (Figs. I-174 and I-175)
  - Extent of primary neoplasm
  - Evidence of metastasis
  - Evidence of megaesophagus and/or aspiration pneumonia (secondary to myasthenia gravis)
  - Pleural effusion
- Thoracic ultrasound
  - Morphologic examination of mass, including association with/invasion of vascular structures
  - Fine-needle aspirate (FNA) cytologic examination/needle biopsy of mass
    - Rule out lymphoma
  - Collection of pleural fluid (analysis, cytologic examination)
- Survey abdominal radiographs, ultrasound
  - Rule out abdominal organ involvement
    - Lymphoma

ADVANCED OR CONFIRMATORY TESTING

- MRI or CT scan: determine whether surgical excision is a viable treatment option
- Acetylcholine (ACh) receptor antibody titers rule out myasthenia gravis

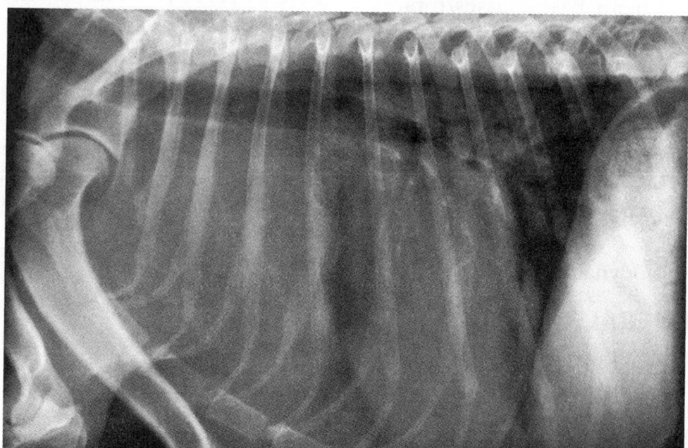

FIGURE I-174 Lateral thoracic radiograph. A large soft-tissue/fluid opacity mass occupies the entire cranial thorax of this dog, elevating the trachea. Courtesy of Dr. Richard Walshaw.

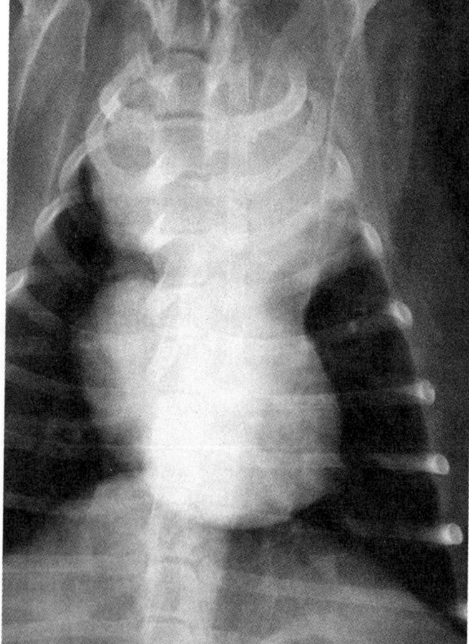

FIGURE I-175 Dorsoventral radiograph of the same dog as in Fig. I-174. The midline location suggests a mediastinal mass. Surgical excision and histopathologic analysis confirmed thymoma. Courtesy of Dr. Richard Walshaw.

TREATMENT

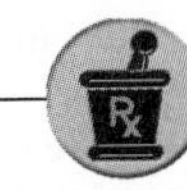

THERAPEUTIC GOAL(S)

Long-term survival and elimination of paraneoplastic syndromes

ACUTE GENERAL TREATMENT

Complete surgical excision: often feasible with thymoma.

- Incomplete surgical excision: more likely when thoracic ultrasonography reveals invasion into or attachment to local vessels. The size of thymoma is not necessarily predictive of complete versus incomplete resection:
  - Chemotherapy
    - Lymphoma protocol
  - Radiation therapy
- Nonresectable masses:
  - Radiation therapy ± chemotherapy
- Myasthenia gravis (see Myasthenia Gravis, p 720):
  - Resolution following complete resection of neoplasm
  - Prednisone
    - 2 mg/kg PO q 24h for 4 weeks, then tapered
  - Hypercalcemia (see Hypercalcemia, p 543)
  - Aspiration pneumonia
    - Antibiotic therapy: based on culture and sensitivity (C&S) testing
- Therapeutic thoracocentesis:
  - If respiratory compromise
  - Preanesthetic animal stabilization

CHRONIC TREATMENT

- Chemotherapy for nonresectable disease
  - Lymphoma protocol (see Lymphoma, Dog [Multicentric], p 658; Lymphoma, Cat [Multicentric], p 650)

POSSIBLE COMPLICATIONS

- Inability to resolve the associated myasthenia gravis:
  - Persistent regurgitation
  - Recurring aspiration pneumonia
- Regrowth of thymoma: occurs in some cases after complete surgical resection as well as cases with incomplete surgical resection. Monitoring is essential regardless of completeness of resection

RECOMMENDED MONITORING

- Following surgical resection (complete or incomplete):
  - Every 3 months (exam, thoracic radiographs) for 1 year, then every 6 months
- If animal is receiving chemotherapy:
  - As determined by protocol

PROGNOSIS AND OUTCOME

- Dog:
  - Resectable thymoma without megaesophagus: over 80% 1-year survival
  - Nonresectable thymoma: poor
  - Presence of myasthenia gravis or megaesophagus: guarded to poor; may resolve over a period of months
- Cat:
  - Resectable thymoma: 2-year median survival

PEARLS & CONSIDERATIONS

COMMENTS

- Adjuvant radiation therapy ± chemotherapy may benefit animals with nonresectable thymoma
- Closely monitor animals for development of aspiration pneumonia and myasthenia gravis after surgery

SUGGESTED READING

Atwater SW, et al: Thymoma in dogs: 23 cases (1980–1991). *J Am Vet Med Assoc* 205:1007, 1994.

Day MJ: Review of thymic pathology in 30 cats and 36 dogs. *J Small Anim Pract* 38:393, 1997.

Gores BR, et al: Surgical treatment of thymoma in cats: 12 cases (1987–1992). *J Am Vet Med Assoc* 204:1782, 1994.

Smith AN, et al: Radiation therapy in the treatment of canine and feline thymomas: A retrospective study (1985–1999). *J Am Anim Hosp Assoc* 37:489, 2001

AUTHOR: **MARYANN G. RADLINSKY**
EDITOR: **RICHARD WALSHAW**

Thyroid Carcinoma (Canine)

BASIC INFORMATION

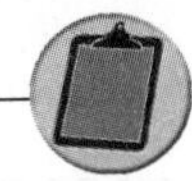

DEFINITION

Malignant neoplasia of the thyroid gland

SYNONYM(S)

Thyroid adenocarcinoma

EPIDEMIOLOGY

SPECIES, AGE, SEX: Median age at diagnosis is 9 to 10 years; no sex predilection.
GENETICS AND BREED PREDISPOSITION: Any breed; beagles, boxers, and golden retrievers may be at increased risk.
RISK FACTORS: Radiation exposure; possibly iodine deficiency or excess.
ASSOCIATED CONDITIONS AND DISORDERS

- Hypothyroidism
- Hyperthyroidism
- May occur as part of multiple endocrine neoplasia syndromes

CLINICAL PRESENTATION

DISEASE FORMS/SUBTYPES

- Histologic classification:
  - Follicular, compact, mixed, or papillary; majority are follicular or mixed
  - Medullary tumors (parafollicular or C cell) are rare
- Functional classification:
  - Hypofunctional (35%), normal function (45–55%), or hyperfunctional (10–20%)

HISTORY, CHIEF COMPLAINT

- Ventral cervical mass, cough, dysphagia, dysphonia, weight loss, dyspnea, regurgitation, polyuria and polydipsia (PU/PD), and vomiting are chief complaints.
- With concurrent hypothyroidism, the patient may manifest lethargy and poor haircoat.
- With concurrent hyperthyroidism, the patient may have polyphagia, restlessness, and tachypnea.
- With medullary carcinoma, the patient may manifest diarrhea and tetany.

PHYSICAL EXAM FINDINGS

- Most findings are the same as signs noted by the owner.
- The normal paired thyroid glands lie lateral to the trachea and just caudal to the larynx. A thyroid carcinoma is generally palpable as a cervical mass that is subcutaneous and usually lateralized, firm, sessile/broad-based, asymmetric, irregular, and nonpainful; may be fixed or movable.
- With concurrent hyperthyroidism, tachycardia is possible.

ETIOLOGY AND PATHOPHYSIOLOGY

- Etiology is unknown.
- Metastasis to the lungs or regional lymph nodes is fairly common. About 30–50% of affected animals have clini-

cally detectable metastasis at the time of diagnosis.
- Even without metastasis, local invasion of vital vascular and neurologic structures, including external carotid artery, external jugular vein, and vagosympathetic trunk, are common. In these cases, full excision is impossible, contributing substantially to morbidity and mortality.
- Unilateral tumors are twice as common as bilateral tumors.
- Ectopic thyroid tissue can occur anywhere from the base of the tongue to the base of the heart.

DIAGNOSIS

DIFFERENTIAL DIAGNOSIS

Cervical mass:
- Other primary tumors: soft-tissue sarcoma, salivary gland adenocarcinoma, parathyroid carcinoma, lymphosarcoma
- Metastatic tumors: oral squamous cell carcinoma (SCC), oral melanoma
- Abscess or granuloma
- Salivary mucocele

INITIAL DATABASE

- Complete blood count (CBC), serum biochemical profile, and urinalysis:
    - Usually normal
    - Mild anemia possible
    - If hypothyroidism: fasting hypercholesterolemia is common
    - If medullary carcinoma: hypocalcemia likely
- Testing of T4, free T4, and endogenous TSH: results depend on functional status of tumor (see Hypothyroidism, p 575; Hyperthyroidism, p 552)
- Thoracic radiographs (three views): possible metastasis
- Fine-needle aspirate (FNA) of regional lymph nodes: possible metastasis
- Cervical ultrasound: extent of tissue invasion and vascularity

ADVANCED OR CONFIRMATORY TESTING

- FNA of the mass:
    - Often difficult to assess cytologically because of heavy contamination with peripheral blood, and neoplastic cells may not exfoliate well.
    - Often bypassed in favor of surgical exploration because bleeding may be extensive.
    - If thyroid cells are seen: it is not possible to differentiate benign versus malignant tumors based on cell characteristics.
- Needle biopsy: greater diagnostic yield than an aspirate but high risk of hemorrhage. This biopsy should not be performed without ultrasound guidance, and even with such guidance, both the owner and animal should be prepared for immediate surgery if intractable bleeding occurs.
- Cervical exploratory surgery for incisional biopsy and histopathologic evaluation.
- Thyroid scintigraphy (99mTc-pertechnetate scan): may identify ectopic thyroid tissue and can help predict radioactive iodine (^{131}I) uptake.
- CT scan with contrast enhancement: assess tissue invasion and feasibility of surgical excision; also useful in planning radiation therapy.

TREATMENT

THERAPEUTIC GOAL(S)

- Surgical removal of tumor
- If complete surgical excision is not possible, halt or slow tumor regrowth and metastasis
- Treatment of any related thyroid dysfunction

GENERAL TREATMENT

- The best treatment option depends on tumor size, mobility, and functionality and whether metastasis is present.
- Nonfixed tumor without metastasis: thyroidectomy.
- Fixed/locally invasive tumor without metastasis: surgical debulking; if debulking is not possible due to the vascularity or extent of invasion, initial radiation therapy may shrink the tumor so that surgical debulking becomes possible.
- Fixed or nonfixed tumor with metastasis: surgical debulking, palliative or definitive radiation therapy.
- Local residual disease: radiation therapy and/or chemotherapy (doxorubicin and/or cisplatin; consult a veterinary oncologist for treatment regimen details).
- Metastatic disease: chemotherapy as already described.
- Use of ^{131}I: can be considered for residual and/or metastatic disease if the thyroid tissue is functional, but higher doses are required than those used for treating benign disease.

CHRONIC TREATMENT

- If the animal does not have hyperthyroidism, T4 supplementation may be helpful; inhibits endogenous TSH secretion, and TSH may stimulate remaining tumor cells
- Methimazole (2.5-5 mg PO q 8h): If hyperthyroidism is present, use for decreasing systemic signs and treatment of thyrotoxicosis prior to definitive treatment

POSSIBLE COMPLICATIONS

- Tumor alone: anemia, hypercalcemia (paraneoplastic), hypocalcemia (medullary carcinoma), respiratory distress, disseminated intravascular coagulation
- Surgery: extensive hemorrhage, laryngeal paralysis, and postoperative hypoparathyroidism and hypothyroidism (if bilateral excision)
- External radiation treatment: pharyngeal mucosal irritation, esophagitis, local alopecia
- Chemotherapy: myelosuppression, cardiotoxicity (doxorubicin), nephrotoxicity (cisplatin)

RECOMMENDED MONITORING

- Bilateral thyroidectomy: monitor serum calcium concentrations for 7 to 10 days
- Chemotherapy: monitoring dependent on protocol used
- General: physical examination, thoracic radiographs, and ± serum T4 concentrations every 3 to 4 months

PROGNOSIS AND OUTCOME

- Usually guarded to poor because of tumor size, local invasion, and relatively high incidence of metastasis; however, tumors with a volume <20 cm^3 are less likely to have metastasized, and surgery may be curative if the tumor is movable.
- Neither chemotherapy nor external beam radiation therapy is curative, but long-term progression-free intervals (>1 year) have been reported in some dogs treated with the latter.

SUGGESTED READING

Adams WH, et al: Treatment of differentiated thyroid carcinoma in 7 dogs utilizing ^{131}I. *Vet Radiol Ultrasound* 36:417-424, 1995.

Klein MK, et al: Treatment of thyroid carcinomas in dogs by surgical resection alone: 20 cases (1981-1989). *J Am Vet Med Assoc* 206:1007-1009, 1995.

Theon AP, et al: Prognostic factors and patterns of treatment failure in dogs with unresectable differentiated thyroid carcinomas treated with megavoltage irradiation. *J Am Vet Med Assoc* 216:1175-1179, 2000.

AUTHOR: **TARA CHAPMAN**
EDITOR: **SHERRI IHLE**

Tick Paralysis

BASIC INFORMATION

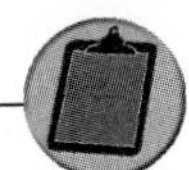

DEFINITION

An acute, rapidly progressive generalized lower motor neuron (LMN) paralysis that results from neuromuscular blockade due to a salivary neurotoxin produced by certain gravid, female tick species

EPIDEMIOLOGY

SPECIES, AGE, SEX

- Any age or breed; both sexes.
- North American tick paralysis (*Dermacentor* ticks) affects dogs but not cats; Australian tick paralysis (*Ixodes* ticks) affects dogs and cats.

GENETICS AND BREED PREDISPOSITION: Any species; incidence is rare in the cat.

RISK FACTORS: Tick exposure.

CONTAGION AND ZOONOSIS: Some ticks may cause tick paralysis in humans; animal-to-animal or zoonotic transmission does not occur.

GEOGRAPHY AND SEASONALITY

- Recognized worldwide; most in-depth reports from the United States and Australia
- Incidence is most frequent in the summer months

CLINICAL PRESENTATION

HISTORY, CHIEF COMPLAINT

- History of hind limb and then forelimb stiff gait that progresses to flaccid paralysis
- Mentation, behavior, and ability to urinate and defecate remain normal

PHYSICAL EXAM FINDINGS: North America (*Dermacentor* spp. ticks):

- Hind limb weakness rapidly progressing to generalized weakness, then complete flaccid paralysis. Tail wag often is preserved.
- Cranial nerve involvement is rare, but nystagmus or mild facial palsy may be observed.
- Pain sensation is preserved, but hyperpathia is rare.
- Voice change and intercostal muscle paresis can be observed, potentially leading to ventilatory failure (respiratory paralysis).

Australia (*Ixodes* spp. ticks):

- Hind limb weakness rapidly progressing to generalized weakness, then complete flaccid paralysis. Tail wag often is preserved.
- Pain sensation is preserved, but hyperpathia is rare.
- Signs of facial paralysis, dysphagia, and megaesophagus are common and may be profound.
- Autonomic signs (mydriasis, peripheral vasoconstriction, arterial and pulmonary hypertension) can be observed. If left undiagnosed, respiratory paralysis and death may ensue.

ETIOLOGY AND PATHOPHYSIOLOGY

- Gravid female tick of the species *D. variabilis* (Eastern wood or dog tick), *D. andersoni* (Rocky Mountain wood tick) in the United States, and *Ixodes holocyclus* in Australia.
- Adult *D. variabilis* and *D. andersoni* female ticks elaborate the neurotoxin; adult female, nymphs, and larvae of *Ixodes* ticks are incriminated.
- The neurotoxin is secreted by the engorged feeding female tick; the toxin either inhibits depolarization in the terminal portions of motor nerves or blocks the release of acetylcholine (ACh) from the motor nerve terminals at the neuromuscular junction.
- The toxin may affect both the motor and sensory nerve fibers by altering ionic fluxes that mediate action potential production.
- In most cases, hind limb weakness begins 5 to 9 days after tick attachment, rapidly followed by generalized weakness and complete flaccid paralysis as well as areflexia within 24 to 72 hours.

DIAGNOSIS

Rests entirely on finding tick(s) in an animal with compatible clinical signs. Delay to finding and removing tick(s) can affect prognosis markedly

DIFFERENTIAL DIAGNOSIS

- Polyradiculoneuritis
- Early stages of botulism
- Fulminant myasthenia gravis

INITIAL DATABASE

- Diagnosed by patient's rapid clinical improvement after tick removal (within 24 hours for *Dermacentor* spp. and return to normalcy in 48 to 72 hours; clinical signs may initially progress for 24 to 48 hours after tick removal for *Ixodes* spp.)
- Exclusion of other causes of rapidly progressive LMN diseases (see Differential Diagnosis above)
- Hematologic and biochemical profiles are usually normal

ADVANCED OR CONFIRMATORY TESTING

- Chest and abdominal radiographs are usually normal (exception: megaesophagus [*Ixodes* spp.])
- Electromyography:
    - Shows no evidence of denervation
    - Amplitude of evoked motor potentials is markedly reduced
    - Repetitive stimulation does not cause further decrement in amplitude
- Nerve conduction velocity (motor and sensory) may be slightly slower; terminal conduction times may be prolonged

TREATMENT

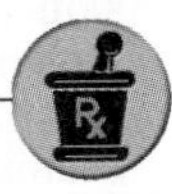

THERAPEUTIC GOAL(S)

Supportive care until the clinical signs resolve

ACUTE GENERAL TREATMENT

- Tick removal can be curative; remember to remove the head since the toxin resides in the salivary glands.
- Insecticide if ticks are not found.
- Whole body shaving if long-haired patient (tick search).
- Hyperimmune serum (0.5-1 ml/kg IV): recommended for binding circulating neurotoxin and preventing further progression in the dog; caution regarding anaphylaxis risk.
- Autonomic dysfunction can be treated with a combination of phenoxybenzamine hydrochloride 1 mg/kg as a 0.1% solution given IV over 15 minutes, q 12-24h, and acepromazine at 0.05-0.10 mg/kg IV q 6-12h.
- Oxygen and ventilatory support necessary for animals with respiratory compromise.

CHRONIC TREATMENT

- Supportive care
- Physical therapy
- Sanitation
- Provision of food and water
- Recurrence is possible with reexposure

DRUG INTERACTIONS

Avoid aminoglycosides (associated with neuromuscular blockade)

POSSIBLE COMPLICATIONS

- Respiratory paralysis (especially with recurrent exposure)
- Decubital ulcers
- Aspiration pneumonia

RECOMMENDED MONITORING

- Respirations
- Urination/defecation
- Progression of signs

PROGNOSIS AND OUTCOME

- Highly dependent on timely identification and removal of tick(s)

- Excellent if rapid removal of *Dermacentor* tick (in United States); fatal if undiagnosed/untreated
- Guarded with *Ixodes* ticks (Australia); fatal if undiagnosed/untreated

PEARLS & CONSIDERATIONS

COMMENTS

- Consider time of the year in the differential diagnosis.
- Note rapid (24 to 72 hours) progression to areflexic flaccid paralysis, which should raise the suspicion of tick paralysis and prompt a meticulous examination of the skin and coat.
- Make sure that whole tick is removed because the toxin lies in the tick's head (salivary glands).
- Make sure that the animal is shaved if heavily furred so that identifying the tick(s) (if present) is easier.

PREVENTION

- Avoid tick exposure
- Use insecticides at appropriate doses
- Avoid reexposure

SUGGESTED READING

Chrisman CL: Hemiplegia, hemiparesis, quadriplegia, quadraparesis, ataxia, and episodic weakness. In Chrisman CL (ed): *Problems in Small Animal Neurology*. Philadelphia, Lea & Febiger, pp 384–385.

Felz MW, Smith CD, Swift TR: A six-year-old girl with tick paralysis. *New Engl J Med* 342:90–94, 2000.

Inzana KD: Peripheral nerve disorders. In Ettinger SJ, Feldman EC (eds): *Textbook of Veterinary Internal Medicine*, ed 6. Philadelphia, Elsevier, 2005, p 893.

Oliver JE, Lorenz MD, Kornegay JN: Teterapresis, hemiparesis, and ataxia. In Oliver JE, Lorenz MD, Kornegay JN (eds): *Handbook of Veterinary Neurology*, ed 4. Philadelphia, Elsevier, 2004, pp 191–192.

Shelton GD: Myasthenia gravis and disorders of neuromuscular transmission. *Vet Clin North Am Small An Pract* 32:189–206, 2002.

AUTHOR: **KAREN L. KLINE**

EDITOR: **CURTIS W. DEWEY**

Ticks

BASIC INFORMATION

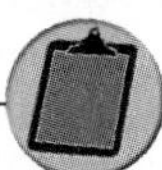

DEFINITION

Ectoparasites that feed on the blood of their hosts and can be divided into hard (ixodid) and soft (argasid) ticks. Ixodid ticks are highly parasitic, produce more progeny, and infest larger areas compared to argasid ticks.

EPIDEMIOLOGY

SPECIES, AGE, SEX: Ixodid ticks (*Ixodes, Dermacentor* spp.) are more commonly found on dogs than on cats.

RISK FACTORS: Canine hunting breeds (greater environmental exposure).

CONTAGION AND ZOONOSIS: Infected animals may act as a source of transmission to other animals and people.

GEOGRAPHY AND SEASONALITY: Ixodid ticks:

- *Ixodes scapularis* (black-legged tick): the Midwest and the northeastern and southeastern parts of the United States (borreliosis [Lyme disease])
- *Dermacentor variabilis* (American dog tick): throughout North America but most commonly found along the Atlantic Coast in areas of shrub and beach grass (Rocky Mountain spotted fever and tick paralysis)
- *Rhipicephalus sanguineus* (brown dog tick): widely distributed throughout North America (babesiosis, *Ehrlichia canis*, and tick paralysis)

Argasid ticks: *Otobius megnini* (spinous ear tick) in North America, South America, India, and South Africa

ASSOCIATED CONDITIONS AND DISORDERS

- Ehrlichiosis
- Babesiosis
- Borreliosis (Lyme disease)
- Rocky Mountain spotted fever
- Tick paralysis

CLINICAL PRESENTATION

DISEASE FORMS/SUBTYPES: Ticks can injure animals by producing tick paralysis through their secretions; causing localized irritation via bites; producing hypersensitivity reactions; and serving as vectors for bacterial, viral, protozoal, and rickettsial diseases.

HISTORY, CHIEF COMPLAINT: Owners note a tick infestation. Generally the patient is either in or has traveled to a tick-infested area.

PHYSICAL EXAM FINDINGS: Presence of ticks noted on the skin. Clinical signs vary from none to the presence of a nodule at the site of tick attachment or systemic signs of tick-borne diseases (ehrlichiosis, Lyme disease, Rocky Mountain spotted fever, babesiosis, tick paralysis). Ticks are most commonly found in the ears or within the interdigital spaces.

ETIOLOGY AND PATHOPHYSIOLOGY

- Heavy infestations can lead to significant blood loss.
- Several types of neurotoxins produced by a variety of ticks affect the lower motor neurons (LMNs) of the spinal cord and cranial nerves and produce a progressive ascending flaccid paralysis (tick paralysis).

DIAGNOSIS

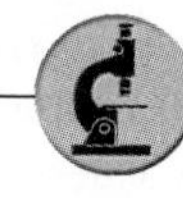

DIFFERENTIAL DIAGNOSIS

Tick-borne systemic disorders:

- Tick paralysis
- Rocky Mountain spotted fever: vector is *D. variabilis*; caused by *R. ricketsii*; causes a necrotizing vasculitis
- Ehrlichiosis: vector is *Rhipicephalus sanguineus*; caused by *Ehrlichia canis* (other species exist also); vasculitis and facial dermatitis
- Lyme disease: vectors are *I. scapularis* and *I. pacificus*; caused by *Borrelia burgdorferi*; in dogs: fever, neurologic signs, polyarthritis

INITIAL DATABASE

- Examine the entire skin for ticks, paying special attention in the ears and between the toes
- Perform a complete physical examination; if clinical signs and history warrant, more specific testing should be done for the various tick-borne diseases

TREATMENT

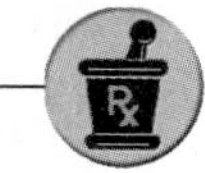

THERAPEUTIC GOAL(S)

- Efficiently remove attached ticks
- Provide environmental control
- Treat localized reactions or transmitted diseases

ACUTE GENERAL TREATMENT

- Tick removal as soon as possible.
    - Soak the tick in alcohol while it is still attached to the animal's skin, then, using a pair of hemostats, grasp the head parts at the surface of the skin and apply firm traction with a gentle twist.
- Effective approved treatments for dogs include fipronil (Frontline) and acaricidal collars containing amitraz

(Preventic). Fipronil (Frontline) may be effective for tick control in cats.

- Repeated spraying of the internal (kennel) and external environments with approved pesticides may be effective for controlling or eliminating infestations with *R. sanguineus*.

PROGNOSIS AND OUTCOME

Prognosis is good, but reinfestation can occur if preventive measures to prevent exposure are not undertaken

PEARLS & CONSIDERATIONS

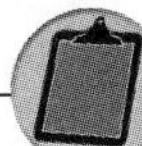

PREVENTION

- Avoid environments with large tick populations.
- May require strict indoor sequestration.
- Selamectin (Revolution) and imidacloprid-permethrin (Advantix) are effective in controlling *D. variabilis* when administered monthly.
- Immunotherapy with a tick vaccine has been proposed.
- Tick habitats can be destroyed by cutting and burning brush and grass, cultivating land, and rotating pastures.
- Grass and shrubbed areas can be treated with appropriately registered pesticides in urban areas; application is done in the spring and repeated once during midsummer.

CLIENT EDUCATION

- Inform clients that tick control/prevention can be challenging because ticks have long lifespans, are widely spread throughout the environment, have incredible reproductive capabilities, and spend short time periods on their hosts.
- Infected animals may act as a source of transmission to people.

SUGGESTED READING

Hoskins JD: Ixodid and argasid ticks. Keys to their identification. In Hoskins JD (ed): *Vet Clin North Am Small An Pract* 21:185–197, 1991.

Scott D, et al: *Muller and Kirk's Small Animal Dermatology*, ed 6. Philadelphia, WB Saunders, 2001, pp 442–445.

AUTHOR: **EDWARD JAZIC**
EDITOR: **JAN A. HALL**

Toad or Lizard Intoxication

BASIC INFORMATION

DEFINITION

Toxicoses associated with exposure to toads of the genus *Bufo*; generally characterized by severe neurologic and cardiovascular effects (hypersalivation, tremors, ataxia, collapse, seizures, cardiac arrhythmias, and death)

EPIDEMIOLOGY

SPECIES, AGE, SEX: Dogs are more likely than cats to be exposed.

GEOGRAPHY AND SEASONALITY: Most cases are seen in Florida.

CLINICAL PRESENTATION

HISTORY, CHIEF COMPLAINT

- Witnessed or suspected exposure (mouthing by the dog or cat)
- Hypersalivation, head shaking
- Sudden onset of collapse, seizures

PHYSICAL EXAM FINDINGS

- Hypersalivation
- Vomiting
- Tachypnea
- Ataxia
- Seizures
- Stupor
- Pale mucous membranes
- Cardiac arrhythmias:
  - Sinus tachycardia
  - Bradycardia; atrioventricular (AV) block

ETIOLOGY AND PATHOPHYSIOLOGY

- Two species of toads have been associated with poisonings:
  - *Bufo marinus* (cane toad, marine toad, giant toad): sizes of 4–9.5 inches (10.1–24.3 cm); found in southern tips of Florida and Texas, much of the Caribbean, and Hawaii
  - *B. alvarius* (Colorado River toad): sizes 3–7 inches (7.6–17.8 cm); found in extreme southeastern California across the southern half of Arizona into extreme southwestern New Mexico
- Modified parotid glands (skin glands) of toads excrete several toxins known as bufogenins, including marinobufagin and bufotoxins
- Action of bufogenins is similar to that of cardiac glycosides (such as digitalis), which inhibit Na^+-K^+-ATPase activity in myocardial cells; this process leads to increased intracellular calcium and blockage of sodium channels, resulting in cardiac arrhythmias
- Secondary toxins in the parotid secretions include bufotenins, serotonin, 5-hydroxytryptophan, or catecholamines and could be responsible for such other signs as gastrointestinal (GI) upset, tremors, hyperthermia, and seizures

DIAGNOSIS

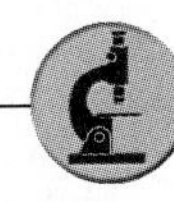

DIFFERENTIAL DIAGNOSIS

- Cardiac glycoside toxicity (e.g., digoxin/digitalis, foxglove, lily of the valley)
- Illicit or prescription drug intoxication

INITIAL DATABASE

- Blood pressure (BP):
  - Hypotension is common and may require treatment
- Electrocardiogram (ECG):
  - Various cardiac arrhythmias
  - Serum potassium:
  - Hypokalemia or hyperkalemia may be present

TREATMENT

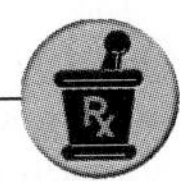

THERAPEUTIC GOAL(S)

- Topical oral ± GI decontamination (depending on whether a toad was mouthed or actually ingested)
- Monitoring and controlling clinical signs

ACUTE GENERAL TREATMENT

- Immediately rinse the patient's mouth with running water for 5 minutes.
- If a toad has been ingested and the animal is not showing overt clinical signs of toxicosis:

- Induction of vomiting:
  - Hydrogen peroxide 3%: 0.25–0.5 ml/kg PO once, or
  - Apomorphine 0.04 mg/kg IV, IM, SQ, or conjunctivally.
- Administration of activated charcoal:
  - Dose according to packaging label of product (e.g., 10 ml of activated charcoal suspension PO made from 2 g activated charcoal suspended in 10 ml tap water).

- IV fluids ± colloids to correct shock and hypotension.
- Correct hyperkalemia or hypokalemia if present (see Hyperkalemia, p 546; Hypokalemia, p 566).
- Control seizures with diazepam (0.5–1 mg/kg IV) or barbiturates as needed.
- Monitor and control arrhythmias:
  - Atropine (0.02–0.04 mg/kg IV/IM for significant bradycardia; do not use atropine to treat the hypersalivation because it can predispose the patient to arrhythmias.
  - Propranolol (0.02–0.06 mg/kg via slow IV) or other beta blocker only for extremely rapid, sustained tachyarrhythmias. Reflex tachycardia may occur secondary to hypotension and must not be suppressed; correct hypotension before treating tachycardia.
  - Lidocaine (2 mg/kg IV bolus followed by 50–80 µg/kg/min constant infusion rate) for ventricular tachyarrhythmias.
- Digibind (Glaxo Wellcome), a digoxin-specific Fab fragment for poorly responsive or deteriorating animals:
  - Determine serum digoxin levels for dosing Digibind.
    - See Digoxin Toxicity, p 301.
  - Due to the high cost and large amounts needed for treatment, treatment with Digibind may be impractical in most cases.

RECOMMENDED MONITORING

- ECG
- Serum potassium

PROGNOSIS AND OUTCOME

Good if signs are mild; guarded if both neurologic and cardiac signs develop

PEARLS & CONSIDERATIONS

COMMENTS

- Exposure to other North American toads such as *B. americanus* (American toad), *B. boreas* (western toad), *B. cognatus* (great plains toad), *B. terrestris* (southern toad), *B. valliceps* (Gulf Coast toad), and *B. woodhousei* (Woodhouse's toad) may result in only mild hypersalivation; severe systemic signs are unlikely.
- Several species of salamanders and newts (e.g., California newt) may contain tetrodotoxin in their skin and muscles. Ingestion can cause vomiting, muscle weakness, ataxia, hypotension, bradycardia, and an ascending paralysis with respiratory arrest. The treatment is centered on supportive care.
- Gila monsters (*Heloderma suspectum*) and the Mexican beaded lizard (*Heloderma horridum*) are two venomous lizards found in North America. Gila monsters are found in the southwestern part of the United States, while the Mexican bead lizard is found in the southwestern part of Mexico and Guatemala. The lizards' bites tend to be defensive; they will hang on after biting, so they can inflict considerable physical damage in addition to envenomation. The venom can cause local pain, weakness, vomiting, muscle fasciculation, hypotension, and tachycardia or anaphylaxis. Treatment consists of wound irrigation, antibiotics, analgesia, and monitoring for systemic signs. Fluids and dopamine may be given for hypotension. Antivenin is not commercially available.

SUGGESTED READING

Eubig PA: *Bufo* species toxicosis: Big toad, big problem. *Vet Med* 96(10):594, 2001.

Peterson ME: Reptiles: Lizards. In Plumlee KH (ed): *Clinical Veterinary Toxicology*. St. Louis, Mosby, 2004, pp 105–106.

Roder JD: Toads. In Plumlee KH (ed): *Clinical Veterinary Toxicology*. St. Louis, Mosby, 2004, p 113.

AUTHOR: **ERIC K. DUNAYER**

EDITOR: **SAFDAR A. KHAN**

Tonsillar Enlargement

BASIC INFORMATION

DEFINITION

Increased size of the palatine tonsils, often with protrusion from the tonsillar fossa

SYNONYM(S)

Palatine tonsillar enlargement

EPIDEMIOLOGY

SPECIES, AGE, SEX: Occasionally seen in dogs; less frequent in cats. No known sex predilection. Acute tonsillitis appears to be more frequent in animals less than 1 year of age.

CONTAGION AND ZOONOSIS

- Group A *Streptococcus pyogenes* ("strep throat" in humans) does not cause signs of tonsillitis in dogs or cats.
- Rates of infection in dogs or cats from contact with infected humans appear low; in rare circumstances, infected dogs or cats not showing clinical signs may serve as a source of reinfection to humans in the household.

CLINICAL PRESENTATION

HISTORY, CHIEF COMPLAINT: Tonsillar enlargement often is an incidental finding; when present, signs may include dysphagia/retching, coughing, ptyalism, and inappetence. The clinical signs of the underlying disease may often be more clinically significant than the signs attributable to tonsillar enlargement.

PHYSICAL EXAM FINDINGS: Bilaterally or unilaterally enlarged palatine tonsils (Figs. I-176 and I-177); with tonsillitis, the tonsils are often bright red and protruding from the tonsillar crypts. There may be petechiae or a purulent exudate on the tonsils or in the tonsillar crypts. Fever is common with infectious disease.

ETIOLOGY AND PATHOPHYSIOLOGY

- Primary tonsillitis: bacterial or viral colonization of the lymphatic tissue of the tonsils. The tonsils are a common portal of entry for enteric bacteria and viruses.
- Secondary tonsillitis: results from chronic pharyngeal irritation, such as recurrent vomiting, regurgitation, or coughing; may also result from chronic pharyngitis secondary to elongated soft palate, immunosuppression from feline immunodeficiency virus (FIV), chronic contamination of the oropharynx with pathogenic bacteria in cases of chronic periodontal disease, or licking of distant infected sites such as skin or anal sacs.

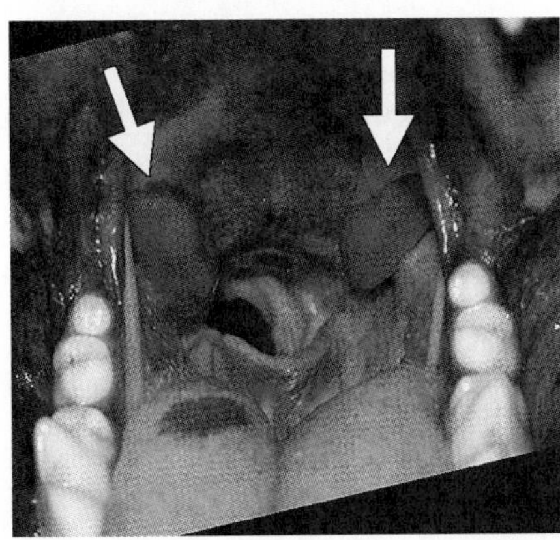

FIGURE I-176 Intraoral view of a dog with marked bilateral enlargement of the tonsils (*arrows*).

- Swallowed foreign bodies such as grass awns or wood splinters may become lodged in the tonsillar crypt.
- Tonsillar cyst: embryonic remnant.
- Neoplasia: squamous cell carcinoma (SCC) or lymphoma may develop from the epithelial or lymphoid components of the tonsils, respectively.

DIAGNOSIS

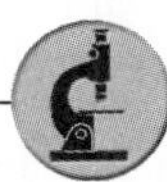

DIFFERENTIAL DIAGNOSIS

Symmetric/bilateral tonsillar enlargement:

- Primary tonsillitis:
  - Bacteria: streptococci, staphylococci, coliforms, canine infectious tracheobronchitis
  - Viruses: feline panleukopenia, canine distemper, infectious canine hepatitis, rabies
  - Parasites: *Pneumonyssium caninum* nasal mites
- Secondary tonsillitis:
  - Pharyngeal irritation: chronic vomiting, regurgitation, or coughing
  - Anatomic abnormalities: elongated soft palate, cleft palate
  - Oropharyngeal contamination: anal sac disease (licking at distant site), pyoderma (licking at distant site), possibly periodontal disease
  - In racing greyhounds, lymphoid hyperplasia of the tonsils and tonsillar enlargement are associated with respiratory disease and poor performance.

Unilateral tonsillar enlargement:

- Foreign body (e.g., grass awn or splinter in tonsillar crypt)

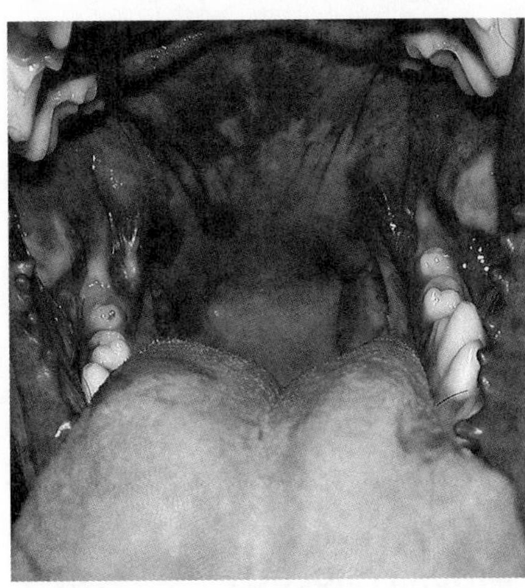

FIGURE I-177 Intraoral view of the tonsils in a normal dog, for comparison to Fig. I-176.

- Tonsillar cyst

Unilateral or symmetric/bilateral tonsillar enlargement:

- Neoplasia: tonsillar lymphoma or SCC

INITIAL DATABASE

- Complete blood count (CBC), serum biochemistry profile, and urinalysis to identify underlying systemic disease
- Feline leukemia virus (FeLV) and FIV testing of cats

ADVANCED OR CONFIRMATORY TESTING

- Bacterial culture and sensitivity (C&S) or virus isolation in cases of primary tonsillitis that fail to respond to routine antibiotics
- General anesthesia and tonsillar fine-needle aspirate (FNA) cytologic examination or biopsy:
  - Specific indications: unilateral tonsillar enlargement or tonsillar enlargement that does not resolve (or worsens) despite identification and treatment of underlying disease

TREATMENT

THERAPEUTIC GOAL(S)

- Treat the underlying disease
- Tonsillectomy is only indicated with the following:
  - Chronic recurrent tonsillitis unresponsive to antibiotic therapy
  - Marked tonsillar enlargement interfering with swallowing or breathing
  - Neoplasia

ACUTE AND CHRONIC TREATMENT

- Primary tonsillitis with no identifiable etiology: broad-spectrum antibiotics if necessary (e.g., ampicillin or amoxicillin at 20 mg/kg PO q 8-12h, 10-14 days).
- Chronic tonsillitis: antibiotic therapy based on C&S results.
- Foreign body retrieval.
- Tonsillar lymphoma: chemotherapy for lymphoma.
- SCC: surgical excision followed by chemotherapy (e.g., doxorubicin or epirubicin and cisplatin or carboplatin) and radiation therapy.
- Incidentally discovered bilateral/symmetric tonsillar enlargement is often most appropriately treated with only monitoring (watchful waiting), while the underlying cause is sought and treated.

PROGNOSIS AND OUTCOME

- Tonsillitis: good prognosis, usually resolves with underlying disease
- Neoplasia: poor long-term prognosis

PEARLS & CONSIDERATIONS

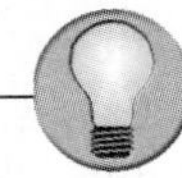

COMMENTS

- Therapeutic intervention for enlarged tonsils is rarely required.
- The most common cause of symmetric/bilateral tonsillar enlargement is a reactive change as part of a systemic process; therefore, diagnostic investigation and treatment should focus on these processes, not on the tonsils.

SUGGESTED READING

DeBowes LJ, et al: Association of periodontal disease and histologic lesions in multiple organs from 45 dogs. *J Vet Dent* 13:57-60, 1996.

Degner DA, et al: Palatine tonsil cyst in a dog. *J Am Vet Med Assoc* 204:1041-1042, 1994.

Dulisch ML: The tonsils. In Slatter D (ed): *Textbook of Small Animal Surgery*, ed 3. Philadelphia, WB Saunders, 2003, pp 1079-1083.

Gunnarsson L, et al: Experimental infection of dogs with the nasal mite *Pneumonyssoides caninum*. *Vet Parasitol* 77:179-186, 1998.

Montague AL, et al: A study of greyhounds with tonsillar enlargement and a history of poor racing performance. *Vet J* 164:106-115, 2002.

AUTHOR: **PETER FOLEY**

EDITOR: **ETIENNE CÔTÉ**

Tooth Displacement Injuries

Client Education Sheet on Website

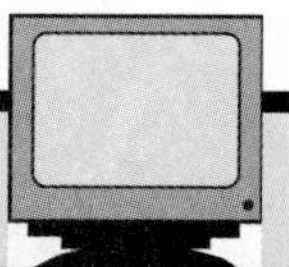

BASIC INFORMATION

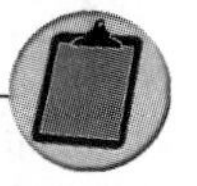

DEFINITION

- Concussion and subluxation: injuries to the periodontal tissues with little or no tooth loosening or displacement and with mild hemorrhage and edema in the periodontal space. Usually do not require treatment
- Luxation: partial displacement of the tooth in an axial (intrusion, extrusion) or lateral direction, usually accompanied by extensive injury to the pulp and periodontal ligament, and (except in case of extrusion) fracture of the alveolar bone as well as soft-tissue laceration
- Avulsion: complete displacement of the tooth out of the alveolus, with total tearing of periodontal fibers and shearing of the pulp neurovascular supply
- Replantation/reimplantation: replacement of the tooth in its alveolar socket

EPIDEMIOLOGY

SPECIES, AGE, SEX

- Uncommon in dogs and cats
- More common in dogs than cats, with lateral luxation following fights with other animals most commonly reported
- Maxillary incisor and canine teeth are most commonly affected

RISK FACTORS

- Loss of attachment due to periodontitis or other diseases causing alveolar bone lysis
- Young age: the alveolar bone and periodontal ligament of teeth of young animals are more resilient than the same tissues of older individuals

ASSOCIATED CONDITIONS AND DISORDERS

- Facial trauma
- Evaluate traumatized animals for any other oral, cranial, thoracic, or abdominal injuries before addressing affected teeth
  - Evaluate teeth adjacent to a displaced tooth for structural defects or abnormal mobility, which may indicate periodontal trauma, root fracture, or bone fracture

CLINICAL PRESENTATION

HISTORY, CHIEF COMPLAINT

- Owners usually report a recent traumatic event and oral hemorrhage
- Anorexia, oral pain, continuous licking, and abnormal facial profile may be present

PHYSICAL EXAM FINDINGS

- Lateral luxation: hemorrhage from the periodontal space, displacement of the tooth crown in a labial direction, alveolar bone fracture, laceration of gingiva and alveolar mucosa
- Extrusive and intrusive luxation: tooth elongation or shortening, with increased or decreased mobility; hemorrhage from the periodontal space
- Avulsion: empty alveolar socket, eventually filled with blood clots and debris

ETIOLOGY AND PATHOPHYSIOLOGY

Impact energy and direction determine type of displacement. A frontal impact may cause concussion or subluxation if mild to moderate or cause luxation or avulsion if severe. A horizontal force usually causes lateral displacement, and an oblique force causes extrusion. Intrusion follows an impact in an axial direction.

DIAGNOSIS

DIFFERENTIAL DIAGNOSIS

- Increased tooth mobility and displacement (lateral luxation): root fracture, bone fracture, neoplasia
- Decreased tooth mobility (intrusive luxation): incomplete tooth eruption, root replacement resorption, dentoalveolar ankylosis
- Tooth elongation (extrusive luxation): buccal bone expansion and idiopathic tooth extrusion
- Missing tooth (avulsion): congenital or acquired (postextraction) missing tooth, unerupted tooth, crown-root fracture with retained root tip

INITIAL DATABASE

- Routine preoperative blood work; no specific associated abnormalities expected
- Dental radiographs of the affected tooth and surrounding tissues; intraoral techniques are preferable over extraoral techniques to avoid superimposition with other structures of the head

TREATMENT

THERAPEUTIC GOAL(S)

- Tooth replantation
- Bone fracture reduction
- Treatment of periodontal and pulpal injuries

ACUTE GENERAL TREATMENT

- Keep avulsed tooth moist in commercial tissue culture media or cold low-fat milk until replantation
- Start systemic tetracycline hydrochloride (20 mg/kg PO q 8h for 4 weeks) or amoxicillin (22 mg/kg PO q 12h for 4 weeks) immediately
- Induce general anesthesia, provided the patient is a suitable anesthetic candidate
- Obtain dental radiographs to evaluate the extent of injury
- Rinse the alveolus and tooth root with sterile saline. Do not scrape the root surface and not use chlorhexidine solution to avoid damage to viable periodontal fibers
- Soak the avulsed tooth in 5% doxycycline solution for 5 minutes before replantation
- Replant the tooth manually, and confirm its position radiographically
- Suture lacerated soft tissues
- After scaling and polishing, splint the replanted tooth to adjacent teeth with or without wire reinforcement using an acid-etch resin technique and cold-cured composite or acrylic resin applied to one to three teeth mesially and distally to the replanted tooth
- Smooth the splint, and check the occlusion before recovery from anesthesia
- Orthodontically move an intruded tooth into position over a few weeks

CHRONIC TREATMENT

- Remove the splint from 1 to 2 weeks (avulsion and extrusion) to 4 to 6 weeks (lateral luxation and intrusion with extensive bone fracture) postreplantation
- Perform standard root canal therapy at the time of splint removal

POSSIBLE COMPLICATIONS

- Pulp necrosis, pulp infection, tooth discoloration, root canal obliteration
- Inflammatory root resorption, replacement resorption, dentoalveolar ankylosis
- Loss of marginal alveolar bone

RECOMMENDED MONITORING

Radiographic follow-ups for several years after replantation

PROGNOSIS AND OUTCOME

- Good prognosis after immediate replantation followed by proper endodontic treatment.
- Poor prognosis after delayed replantation, long-term and rigid splinting, and delayed endodontic treatment.
- In humans, concussion injuries have the best prognosis, followed by the prognoses for subluxation and extrusion. Lateral luxation, intrusion, and

avulsion show the highest incidence of complications.

PEARLS & CONSIDERATIONS

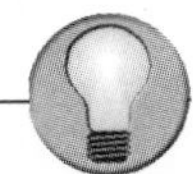

COMMENTS

- Tooth luxation and avulsion are dental emergencies. Immediate replantation and splinting are mandatory for successful treatment.
- Severed pulp tissue may survive for 2 hours in an extraoral environment. Periodontal fibers survive 30 minutes if dry and 1 to 3 hours if kept moistened.
- In most instances, endodontic treatment is necessary after replantation.
- Displaced deciduous teeth should be extracted rather than replanted.
- Extraction of displaced permanent teeth is an alternative to replantation.

CLIENT EDUCATION

- Feed a soft diet and perform daily oral hygiene in patients when an oral splint is in place.
- Discuss the need for endodontic treatment and radiographic follow-ups before tooth replantation is performed.

SUGGESTED READING

Andreasen JO, Andreasen FM: *Textbook and Color Atlas of Traumatic Injuries to the Teeth*, ed 3. Copenhagen, Munksgaard, 1994.
Gracis M, Orsini P: Treatment of traumatic dental luxation in six dogs. *J Vet Dent* 15:65-72, 1998.

AUTHOR: **MARGHERITA GRACIS**
EDITOR: **ALEXANDER M. REITER**

Tooth Fractures

BASIC INFORMATION

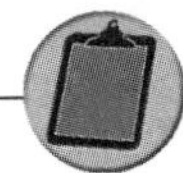

DEFINITION

Fracture of enamel, dentin, and/or cementum associated with trauma

SYNONYM(S)

"Slab" fracture: fracture of the buccal surface of a tooth, most often seen in upper fourth premolars

EPIDEMIOLOGY

SPECIES, AGE, SEX

- Dogs: canines and upper fourth premolar fractures are common
- Cats: fractures may commonly occur in canines or teeth with odontoclastic resorptive lesions are common

RISK FACTORS

- Dogs: chewing on bones, ice cubes, nylon toys, cow hooves, rocks
- Cats: "high-rise syndrome," vehicle trauma, weakening of teeth due to odontoclastic resorptive lesions

ASSOCIATED CONDITIONS AND DISORDERS: Attrition (wear from tooth-to-tooth contact), abrasion (wear due to contact of teeth with nondental materials such as bones), pulpitis (pulpal inflammation), tooth displacement injuries (luxation, avulsion), odontoclastic resorptive lesions (commonly seen in cats), and caries (bacterial infection causing tooth demineralization).

CLINICAL PRESENTATION

DISEASE FORMS/SUBTYPES

- Uncomplicated fracture: without pulp exposure
- Complicated fracture: with pulp exposure
- Crown-root fracture: involving crown and root(s)

HISTORY, CHIEF COMPLAINT

- Tooth fractures are commonly noted as incidental findings on routine physical examination
- History of falls, motor vehicle trauma, fights with other animals, aggressive chewing tendencies, or other trauma

PHYSICAL EXAM FINDINGS

- Animals commonly exhibit no overt clinical signs, especially if the fracture is uncomplicated.
- Complicated fractures may present with oral bleeding.
- Drooling can occur with acute complicated fractures.
- Appetite is rarely affected; chewing on opposite side results in greater calculus accumulation on the affected side.
- Calculus may obscure a fracture of the upper fourth premolar; compare with crown height and shape of the contralateral tooth (Fig. I-178).
- Acute pulp exposure: red spot in tooth defect ± bleeding from exposed pulp, painful on probing (see Fig. I-178).
- Chronic pulp exposure: dark/black spot in tooth defect, asymmetric calculus, regional facial swelling ± draining tracts along mucogingival junction.

ETIOLOGY AND PATHOPHYSIOLOGY

- Uncomplicated fracture: Exposure of dentinal tubules causes sensitivity and allows bacterial access to the pulp. Odontoblasts may respond by forming tertiary dentin, sealing off exposed tubules.
- Complicated fracture: Pulp exposure results in pulpitis and bacterial infection; most will develop periapical disease (e.g., periapical "tooth root" abscess).

DIAGNOSIS

DIFFERENTIAL DIAGNOSIS

- Abrasion/attrition
- Odontoclastic resorptive lesions
- Caries
- Luxation/avulsion

INITIAL DATABASE

- Physical examination
- Complete blood count (CBC), serum chemistry panel, urinalysis: generally unremarkable (preoperative evaluation)

ADVANCED OR CONFIRMATORY TESTING

- Anesthetized oral examination using a dental explorer to determine pulp exposure
- Dental radiographs. Structural crown and/or root defect, arrested root development (open root apex, wider root canal when compared with contralateral tooth), diffuse root canal calcification, apical root resorption, and/or periapical lucency may be seen

TREATMENT

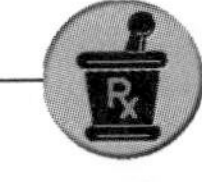

THERAPEUTIC GOAL(S)

Prevent chronic discomfort and infection of endodontic system and periapical tissues

ACUTE GENERAL TREATMENT

- Uncomplicated crown fractures may not require treatment. The patient may benefit from sealing dentinal tubules of exposed dentin with a bonding agent. Fractures extending below the gum line may require periodontal surgery to prevent focal periodontal pocketing.
- Acute complicated crown fracture: vital pulp therapy (partial pulpectomy, direct pulp capping, and restoration) within 48 hours of pulp exposure; administer antibiotics (e.g., ampicillin 22 mg/kg IV q 6h; amoxicillin/clavulanic acid 13.75

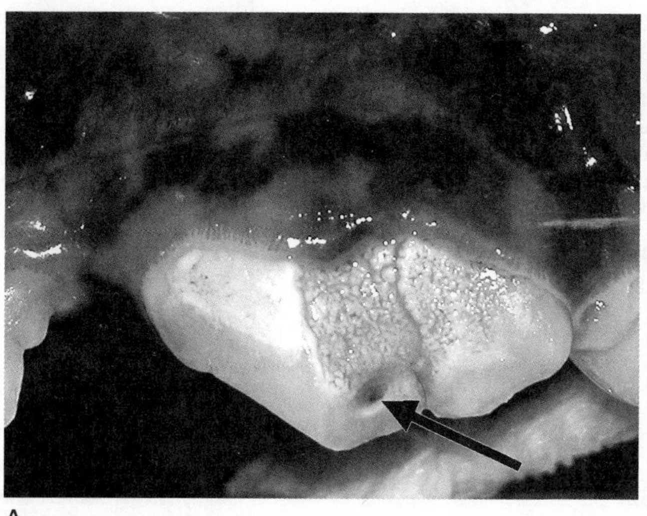

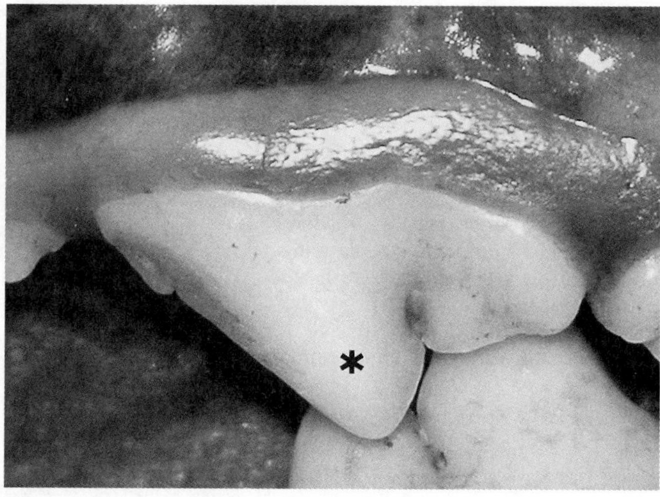

FIGURE I-178 **A,** Slab fracture of left upper fourth premolar tooth in a dog. The main cusp is fractured off; there is pulp exposure (*arrow*) and moderate calculus accumulation. The amount of calculus accumulated indicates that the fracture occurred more than 1 or 2 months prior to the visit; however, the bleeding pulp tissue indicates that the fracture may not be older than 6 to 12 months. **B,** Normal left upper fourth premolar tooth for comparison. The tooth (notably the main cusp [shown by *asterisk*]) is structurally intact; mild calculus accumulation in developmental groove. Courtesy of Dr. Alexander M. Reiter, University of Pennsylvania.

mg/kg PO q 12h × 7 days or clindamycin 5.5 mg/kg PO q 12h × 7 days).

CHRONIC TREATMENT

- Chronic, complicated crown fractures (adults): root canal therapy or extraction (extraction of large, firmly rooted teeth causes more postoperative morbidity than root canal therapy).
- Recently (<2 weeks old) fractured teeth in immature animals (<18 months old) may be treated by vital pulp therapy in an attempt to achieve root lengthening and apical closure (apexogenesis).

POSSIBLE COMPLICATIONS

Uncontrolled force during elevation of crown-root segments can result in:

- Fracture and incomplete removal of the tooth/root, resulting in formation of a tooth root abscess
- Trauma to soft tissues (eye, brain, tongue, salivary gland ducts, and vessels)
- Transposition of tooth/root fragments into the mandibular/infraorbital canal and nasal passages
- Iatrogenic jaw fracture

RECOMMENDED MONITORING

Vital pulp therapy and root canal therapy require follow-up radiography under sedation/anesthesia at 6 months postoperatively and yearly thereafter

PROGNOSIS AND OUTCOME

- In periodontally sound teeth, root canal therapy fails in only 6% of treated roots (depending on the skill of the operator).
- Animals that are likely to continue abusive dental tendencies may benefit from the placement of prosthodontic metal crowns.

PEARLS & CONSIDERATIONS

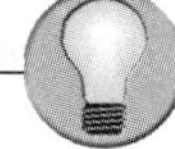

COMMENTS

- A "wait and see" approach to a tooth with pulp exposure is below the standard of care.
- Functionally important teeth should be preserved with endodontic therapy rather than extracted.
- Although root canal therapy can be performed for almost any dog tooth, endodontic therapy in cats is often not feasible due to size, except for the canine teeth.
- Dental radiography is an important diagnostic tool in determining appropriate treatment.

PREVENTION

Discuss appropriate chewing habits during wellness visits. Owners should avoid very hard treats and toys such as real bones, nylon bones, ice cubes, cow hooves, and rocks. Appropriate chew toys will allow for decreased plaque and calculus accumulation without fracturing teeth.

CLIENT EDUCATION

Root canal therapy causes less postoperative discomfort than surgical extraction.

SUGGESTED READING

Clarke DE: Vital pulp therapy for complicated crown fracture of permanent canine teeth in dogs: A three-year retrospective study. *J Vet Dent* 18:117–121, 2001.

Kuntsi-Vaattovaara H, et al: Results of root canal treatment in dogs: 127 cases (1995–2000). *J Am Vet Med Assoc* 220:775–780, 2002.

Niemiec BA: Assessment of vital pulp therapy for nine complicated crown fractures and fifty-four crown reductions in dogs and cats. *J Vet Dent* 18:122–125, 2002.

AUTHOR: **JOHN R. LEWIS**

EDITOR: **ALEXANDER M. REITER**

Toxoplasmosis/Neosporosis

BASIC INFORMATION

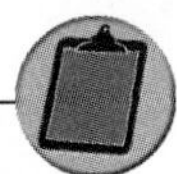

DEFINITION

Infections with obligate intracellular coccidian parasites that infect mammals, including humans

SYNONYM(S)

Toxoplasma gondii
Neospora caninum

EPIDEMIOLOGY

SPECIES, AGE, SEX: Cats and other members of the Felidae family are definitive hosts for *T. gondii*.

- Warm-blooded mammals serve as intermediate hosts.
- More severe disease can affect transplacentally infected kittens.
- Cats of any age can be affected.

N. caninum infections have been seen in dogs, cattle, sheep, goats, horses, and deer but not in cats.

- Cats, rats, and mice have been infected experimentally.
- Dogs are both intermediate and definitive hosts.
- Puppies are more severely affected by disease, but dogs of any age can be affected.
- Cats have demonstrated antibodies to *N. caninum* in field conditions but are not known to develop clinical neosporosis.

GENETICS AND BREED PREDISPOSITION: German short-haired pointers, Labrador retrievers, boxers, golden retrievers, basset hounds, and greyhounds may be more susceptible to neosporosis.

RISK FACTORS: Immunosuppression (e.g., from glucocorticoids or antineoplastic drugs) or concomitant illnesses, such as ehrlichiosis, canine distemper, feline leukemia virus (FeLV), feline immunodeficiency virus (FIV), feline infectious peritonitis (FIP), or *Mycoplasma haemofelis* infection. Immunosuppression is not consistently found in cases of neosporosis. Cutaneous neosporosis was documented in two dogs receiving chronic immunosuppressive therapy.

CONTAGION AND ZOONOSIS: Toxoplasmosis is zoonotic. The zoonotic potential of *N. caninum* is not known.

- A cat without a *T. gondii* antibody titer is at greatest risk for developing oocyst shedding and is a danger to a susceptible owner, especially if it goes outside where it can ingest the intermediate host.
- A healthy cat with a *T. gondii* antibody titer is of little risk to its owner.

GEOGRAPHY AND SEASONALITY

- Worldwide.
- About 30% of cats and dogs in the United States have antibodies against *T. gondii*.
- There is a higher prevalence of antibodies against *N. caninum* in rural or farm dogs than urban dogs.

CLINICAL PRESENTATION

In dogs, the clinical presentation of toxoplasmosis and neosporosis may be identical.

DISEASE FORMS/SUBTYPES

- Unaffected cat (intermittently shedding *T. gondii*)
- Clinically ill dog (toxoplasmosis or neosporosis) or cat (toxoplasmosis)

HISTORY, CHIEF COMPLAINT

Toxoplasmosis:

- Cats with clinical illness commonly present with anorexia, lethargy, respiratory distress, and ocular signs.
- Dogs and cats can present with anorexia, vomiting, diarrhea, weight loss, lethargy, dyspnea, ocular signs, lameness, and signs of central nervous system (CNS) dysfunction (seizures, paresis, cranial nerve deficits).
- Stillborn kittens.

Neosporosis:

- Older dogs may present with dermatitis, respiratory signs (cough, dyspnea), gastrointestinal (GI) signs, or neurologic signs (lameness, seizures).
- In young dogs (<6 months), acute ascending paralysis is typical. Dysphagia, incontinence, and muscle atrophy are also seen.

PHYSICAL EXAM FINDINGS

Toxoplasmosis:

- Prenatally infected kittens: hepatomegaly, ascites, dyspnea, fever, and GI signs.
- Postnatal infection in cats is characterized by uveitis, chorioretinitis, dyspnea, icterus, ascites, vomiting, diarrhea, fever, stiff gait, hyperesthesia, and neurologic deficits (spinal cord or brain).
- As definitive hosts, most cats with *T. gondii* harbor the organism intestinally with no adverse effect and no clinical signs.
- Young dogs (1 year or less) have generalized infections resulting in fever, icterus, dyspnea, and tonsillitis.
- Older dogs more commonly have neuromuscular signs, including muscle atrophy, stiffness, abnormal gait, and multifocal neurologic deficits involving the spinal cord or the brain (seizures, ataxia, lower motor neuron [LMN] signs, cranial nerve deficits).
- Arrhythmias or, rarely, heart failure may be present in some older dogs.

Neosporosis:

- Puppies are more severely affected and show ascending rigid paralysis, with hind limbs worse than forelimbs.
    - Muscle atrophy and stiffness; muscle contractures leading to arthrogryposis and hyperesthesia. Cervical weakness, dysphagia, and variable CNS signs may also be seen.
- Older dogs may have a LMN flaccid paralysis or show multifocal CNS signs (cranial nerve deficits, seizures, blindness).
- Systemic signs include fever, dyspnea, cough, skin lesions, vomiting, icterus, cardiac arrhythmias, megaesophagus, and regurgitation.

ETIOLOGY AND PATHOPHYSIOLOGY

- *T. gondii* exists in three infectious stages: sporozoites, tachyzoites, and bradyzoites.
    - Sporozoites occur in oocysts, which are excreted in a cat's feces, whereas tachyzoites and bradyzoites occur as tissue cysts.
- Transmission can occur through ingestion of infected tissues or ingestion of oocysts in contaminated food or water; transmission can also occur congenitally.
- The enteroepithelial life cycle (and thus, fecal shedding) occurs only in cats.
- Cats are infected by ingestion of intermediate hosts infected with tissue cysts.
    - Bradyzoites are released in the GI tract from tissue cysts during digestion.
    - The bradyzoites penetrate the small intestinal epithelium and initiate asexual stages, eventually forming oocysts. These oocysts are passed in feces.
- The extraintestinal life cycle occurs in all hosts including cats.
    - After ingestion of oocysts or tissue cysts, the organism invades the small intestine and spreads to many extraintestinal tissues through blood and lymph where it causes a focal necrosis. The CNS, muscles, liver, lungs, and eyes are commonly affected.
    - The organism can localize in tissues as cysts, resulting in chronic infection. These cysts may rupture, resulting in clinical relapses during immunosuppression.
- The life cycle of *N. caninum* involves three infectious stages: tachyzoites, tissue cysts found primarily in the CNS, and oocysts.
    - Tissue cysts and tachyzoites are found in intermediate hosts.

- Transmission is suspected to occur through ingestion of shed oocysts, ingestion of infected tissues, and transplacentally.
- Transplacental transmission may be the predominant route in dogs.
- The organism and the associated necrosis may be found in macrophages, polymorphonuclear cells, spinal fluid, and neural cells (brain, spinal cord, peripheral nerves, retina) as well as other cells, causing focal necrosis.

DIAGNOSIS

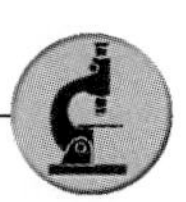

DIFFERENTIAL DIAGNOSIS

- Uveitis: infectious (FeLV, FIV, FIP [coronavirus]), immune-mediated, trauma
- Respiratory signs: feline asthma, pneumonia (bacterial, mycoplasma, parasitic, fungal), pulmonary edema, neoplasia, heartworm disease, trauma
- Hepatic: hepatic lipidosis (cats), cholangiohepatitis (cats), infectious hepatitis, neoplasia, toxic hepatopathy
- GI: infectious (bacterial, viral, parasitic), dietary, endocrine (hypoadrenocorticism), obstructive
- Neurologic signs: meningoencephalitis (FeLV, FIV, FIP; canine distemper; ehrlichiosis; Rocky Mountain spotted fever; rabies; fungal disease; parasitic disease; thiamin deficiency [cats]; immune-mediated disease)
- Neuromuscular: hepatozoonosis, Lyme borreliosis, immune-mediated disease (polyradiculoneuritis, polymyositis)

INITIAL DATABASE

Complete blood count, serum biochemistry profile, urinalysis:

- Nonregenerative anemia, neutrophilic leukocytosis, lymphocytosis, monocytosis, and eosinophilia may be seen with toxoplasmosis.
- Leukopenia characterized by lymphopenia, neutropenia, and degenerative left shift may be seen in cats severely affected with toxoplasmosis.
- Serum biochemistry profile may show elevated alanine aminotransferase (ALT), aspartate aminotransferase (AST), alkaline phosphatase, bilirubin, amylase, lipase, and creatine kinase (CK). Hyperglobulinemia, hypoalbuminemia, and hypoproteinemia may also be present with toxoplasmosis.
- Proteinuria and bilirubinuria may be present in cats with toxoplasmosis.
- Dogs with neosporosis may have elevated CK and AST due to muscle disease.
- Liver enzymes may be elevated with hepatic involvement in neosporosis.

Radiographs:

- Thoracic radiographs may show a diffuse interstitial to alveolar pattern and mild pleural effusion.
- Abdominal radiographs may show hepatomegaly, ascites, masses in the intestines, or mesenteric lymph nodes.

Other tests:

- Fecal examination with Sheather's sugar solution may not reveal oocysts in clinically ill cats.
- Cytologic examination of ascitic fluid, tracheal washes, and pleural fluid may reveal tachyzoites.

ADVANCED OR CONFIRMATORY TESTING

Toxoplasmosis:

- Clinical confirmation comes from serologic testing combined with clinical response to antitoxoplasmosis drugs and exclusion of other causes for clinical signs.
  - Serologic testing (Sabin-Feldman dye test, indirect fluorescent antibody [FA], indirect hemagglutination, latex agglutination, modified agglutination, or enzyme-linked immunosorbent assay [ELISA] tests) showing a fourfold rise in IgG over a 2 to 3 week period, or a high IgM titer, suggest active infection.
  - The presence of a positive IgM may not be reliable; some cats remain IgM positive for years, and other cats may not develop detectable IgM.
  - IgG reflects only past exposure and is unreliable (positive in 30% of the cat population).
- Organism detection: *T. gondii* can be detected using polymerase chain reaction (PCR) on tissue or blood and aqueous humor samples.
- Neosporosis:
  - Serologic testing with indirect FA, ELISA, and direct agglutination tests can confirm neosporosis.
  - Serologic testing can be done on cerebrospinal fluid (CSF).
  - Organism detection with histologic or cytologic examination.
  - *N. caninum* may be found in CSF or tissue samples.
- Both organisms can be grown in cell culture and in mice.
- CSF analysis and aqueous humor may have elevated protein levels and leukocytes in both toxoplasmosis and neosporosis.

TREATMENT

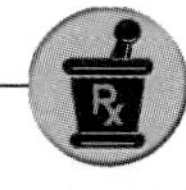

THERAPEUTIC GOAL(S)

Drugs suppress replication of *T. gondii* and are not completely effective at killing the organism. There is limited information for effective treatment of neosporosis.

ACUTE AND CHRONIC TREATMENT

- Toxoplasmosis: Clindamycin is the treatment of choice in dogs and cats.
- Neosporosis should be treated early in the disease with the same drugs used for treating toxoplasmosis. Treatment should continue at least 2 weeks after resolution of clinical signs.
- Clindamycin (dogs): 10–20 mg/kg PO or IM q 12h for at least 2 weeks.
- Clindamycin (cats): 8–17 mg/kg PO or IM q 8–12h for 2 to 4 weeks.
- Alternatively, trimethoprim-sulfonamide: 15 mg/kg PO q 12h for 2 to 4 weeks; can be given concurrently with clindamycin to improve efficacy.
- Uveitis may be treated with topical corticosteroids, barring corneal ulceration.

POSSIBLE COMPLICATIONS

- Clindamycin may cause anorexia, vomiting, and diarrhea with higher doses. *Clostridium difficile* overgrowth has been shown in people.
- Trimethoprim-sulfonamides are associated with bone marrow suppression (anemia, leukopenia, thrombocytopenia), keratoconjunctivitis sicca (KCS), depression, immune-mediated disease, cutaneous drug eruptions, renal failure, GI signs, and hepatotoxicity (especially in Doberman pinschers). Reduce dose of trimethoprim sulfa in renal insufficiency and avoid use in hepatic disease, anemia, leukopenia, and congenital bleeding disorders.

RECOMMENDED MONITORING

Serial recheck examinations at 2 days and 1 week after initiation of therapy and again at 2 weeks after resolution of signs and prior to discontinuation of therapy

PROGNOSIS AND OUTCOME

- In most cases, clinical signs of systemic illness usually begin to resolve within 1 to 2 days after institution of therapy.
- Uveitis should resolve in 1 week with therapy.
- Neuromuscular deficits should partially resolve within 2 weeks of initiation of therapy; however, some signs may be permanent. Animals may survive acute disease if treated aggressively and rapidly; ocular signs respond well to therapy.
- Guarded for complete resolution of neuromuscular signs.

- Clinical improvement is not likely in severe cases of neosporosis with muscle contracture.
- Older puppies (>16 weeks) and adult dogs generally respond better to treatment for *N. caninum*.

PEARLS & CONSIDERATIONS

COMMENTS

- Examine and treat all dogs in a litter for neosporosis if one littermate is diagnosed.
- No drug will clear the organism, and relapses may occur.
- Toxoplasmosis-associated chorioretinitis in cats can be treated with topical glucocorticoids.
- Precautions are often adequate for preventing zoonosis, and immunocompromised individuals need not necessarily be separated from their cats.
- Toxoplasmosis in animals with FIV is most often a reactivation of latent infection rather than a newly acquired one.

PREVENTION

- Clean litter boxes daily (oocysts need 1 to 5 days to sporulate and become infective)
- Disinfect litter boxes with boiling water
- Cover outdoor sandboxes

CLIENT EDUCATION

- Wash hands and surfaces after handling raw meat or cleaning litter boxes.
- Wear gloves when gardening and wash vegetables and hands thoroughly to prevent contamination from soil.
- Do not eat undercooked meat or unpasteurized dairy products.
- Boil drinking water from unreliable sources.
- Pregnant women must avoid contact with soil, cat litter, raw meat, and cats excreting oocysts.

SUGGESTED READING

Dubey JP: Review of *Neospora caninum* and neosporosis in animals. *Korean J Parasit* 41(1):1-16, 2003.

Dubey JP, Lappin MR: Toxoplasmosis and neosporosis. In Greene CE (ed): *Infectious Diseases of the Dog and Cat*. Philadelphia, WB Saunders, 1990, pp 493-509.

La Perle KM, Del Piero F, Carr RF, Harris C, Stromberg PC: Cutaneous neosporosis in two adult dogs on chronic immunosuppressive therapy. *J Vet Diagn Invest* 13(3):252-255, 2001.

AUTHOR: **LISA M. TIEBER NIELSON**

EDITOR: **DOUGLASS K. MACINTIRE**

Tracheal Avulsion

BASIC INFORMATION

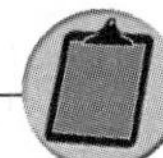

DEFINITION

Disruption of the continuity of or a tear in the trachea

SYNONYM(S)

Tracheal laceration
Tracheal rupture
Tracheal transection

EPIDEMIOLOGY

SPECIES, AGE, SEX: Reported primarily in small dogs and cats; there is no age or gender predilection.

RISK FACTORS

- Choke chains
- Overinflation of an endotracheal tube cuff
- Cervical trauma

ASSOCIATED CONDITIONS AND DISORDERS: Can lead to pneumomediastinum, pneumothorax, and/or subcutaneous emphysema.

CLINICAL PRESENTATION

HISTORY, CHIEF COMPLAINT

- History of trauma or recent general anesthesia and subsequent dyspnea
- Intermittent, continuous, or progressive respiratory distress

PHYSICAL EXAM FINDINGS

- Increased respiratory effort:
  - Decreased heart and breath sounds on thoracic auscultation if pneumothorax is present
- Subcutaneous emphysema: inflated, crepitant subcutaneous space
- Precipitation of severe dyspnea with neck flexion

ETIOLOGY AND PATHOPHYSIOLOGY

- Direct injury to the trachea due to either blunt or penetrating trauma to the cervical or thoracic area.
- Violent hyperextension of the head and neck can lead to stretching of the trachea and may cause tracheal transection.
  - The carina and lungs are a fixed point that is stronger than the tracheal wall.
  - As the trachea is stretched, the intrathoracic trachea ruptures cranial to the carina.
- The dorsal tracheal membrane is the most common location for a tear from overinflation of an endotracheal tube cuff.
- Peritracheal tissues can maintain tracheal continuity.
- Initial dyspnea may persist, worsen, or resolve until subsequent stenosis or displacement causes return of clinical signs.

DIAGNOSIS

DIFFERENTIAL DIAGNOSIS

- Tracheal foreign body
- Collapsing trachea
- Tracheal stenosis
- Tracheal neoplasia or mass
- Laryngeal paralysis
- Laryngeal collapse
- Tracheobronchitis
- Pneumothorax/pneumomediastinum from other causes
- Pulmonary disease

INITIAL DATABASE

- Results of complete blood count (CBC), serum biochemistry panel, and urinalysis are usually unremarkable.
- Radiographs of the neck (lateral view) show discontinuity of the tracheal wall. Site of rupture may be obscured by the humeri or scapulae, requiring retaking of radiographs with the forelimbs repositioned.
- Cervical and/or thoracic radiographs may show peritracheal air accumulation, subcutaneous emphysema, and/or pneumomediastinum.
  - Pneumothorax is rare.
  - Tracheal stenosis can be seen in chronic cases.

ADVANCED OR CONFIRMATORY TESTING

Tracheoscopy is useful in documenting tracheal rupture if a radiographic diagnosis is not definitive.

TREATMENT

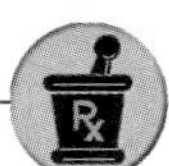

THERAPEUTIC GOAL(S)

- Stabilize animal
- Repair or resect damaged trachea or stenosis to resolve respiratory distress

- Note that surgery is not always needed and follow guidelines for conservative versus surgical management

ACUTE GENERAL TREATMENT

- Oxygen supplementation if dyspnea.
- For animals with respiratory distress, induction of anesthesia or heavy sedation and intubation per os or through a cervical tracheal laceration (if present) are indicated to quickly gain control of the airway.
  - Intubation through a cervical laceration/avulsion is accomplished in similar fashion to tracheostomy.
  - Distal cervical tracheal lacerations may require retrieval of the distal trachea from the thoracic inlet via traction sutures.
- Thoracocentesis may be indicated if pneumothorax is present.
- Prepare the animal for exploration of all structures in the injured area to determine extent of injury and provide the opportunity for primary repair.
- Treat any other additional wounds.
- Antibiotics are indicated especially if traumatic injuries are present.
  - Coverage against skin organisms (*Staphylococcus* or *Streptococcus* spp.) is considered most important.
    - Ampicillin 22 mg/kg PO or IV q 8-12h; cefazolin 22 mg/kg PO or IV q 12h; or clavulanic acid/amoxicillin 12.5-25 mg/kg PO q 8-12h (dogs), 62.5 mg PO q 8-12h (cats).
    - Enrofloxacin 5-20 mg/kg PO or IV q 24h if concerns about gram-negative organisms (maximum 5 mg/kg PO q 24h in cats).

CHRONIC TREATMENT

- Closure and debridement of tracheal laceration
  - Surgery is indicated for repair of tracheal defects if:
    - The cause is from injury associated with contamination (e.g., bite wounds or other penetrating injury)
    - The animal is not improving or getting worse with conservative (nonsurgical) treatment
    - There is stenosis or stricture causing respiratory difficulty
- Resection of damaged or stenotic trachea and anastomosis of normal ends
  - Minimize tension
  - May need to use tracheal tubes/stents
  - Use a tape neck splint to hold the neck in a flexed position to reduce tension on the trachea postoperatively:
    - Try to keep the splint in place for 2 weeks if it is needed

POSSIBLE COMPLICATIONS

- Dehiscence may occur if excessive tracheal suture tension is present.
- Narrowing of the tracheal lumen due to scar tissue may occur secondary to tracheal anastomosis.

RECOMMENDED MONITORING

- Monitor for respiratory distress.
- Drainage of the peritracheal area may be indicated if area is contaminated.
- Small areas of tracheal granulation tissue may be removed through a bronchoscope at periodic examinations during the healing period.
- Removal of tubes/stents is indicated when a healed mucosal surface is present.

PROGNOSIS AND OUTCOME

- Prognosis is good for long-term resolution of clinical signs.
- Stenosis of the tracheal lumen may be a complication postoperatively.

PEARLS & CONSIDERATIONS

COMMENTS

- Trauma is the most common cause of tracheal avulsion in small dogs.
- Overinflation of the endotracheal tube is the most common cause of tracheal rupture in cats.
  - Tracheal tears can occur from overinflation of either low-volume/high-pressure cuffs or high-volume/low-pressure cuffs.

CLIENT EDUCATION

Recurrence of clinical signs is possible due to tracheal stenosis.

SUGGESTED READING

Hardie EM, et al: Tracheal rupture in cats: 16 cases (1983-1998). *J Am Vet Med Assoc* 214:508, 1999.

Nelson AW: Diseases of the trachea and bronchi. In Slatter D (ed): *Textbook of Small Animal Surgery*. Philadelphia, WB Saunders, 2002, pp 864-870.

White RN, Burton CA: Surgical management of intrathoracic tracheal avulsion in cats: Long-term results in nine consecutive cases. *Vet Surg* 29:430, 2000.

AUTHOR: **MICHAEL B. MISON**

EDITOR: **RANCE K. SELLON**

Tracheobronchitis (Infectious): Dogs

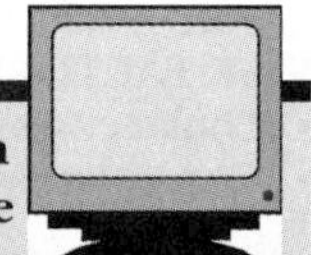

Client Education Sheet on Website

BASIC INFORMATION

DEFINITION

An acute, highly contagious, generally benign respiratory disease complex of dogs. Common manifestations include cough, oculonasal discharge, and occasionally bronchopneumonia. For more information regarding cats, see Upper Respiratory Infection, Feline, p 1115.

SYNONYM(S)

Kennel cough
Canine croup

EPIDEMIOLOGY

SPECIES, AGE, SEX: Common in dogs; puppies more prone to pneumonia. *Bordetella* (see Bordetellosis, p 140) can infect multiple species, including felines, wildlife, and rodents.

RISK FACTORS: Exposure to other dogs; affected animals usually have a history of boarding, grooming, or being in environments with many other dogs (e.g., dog parks, veterinary hospitals).

CONTAGION AND ZOONOSIS

- Highly contagious among canines
- *B. bronchiseptica* zoonosis can occur, mainly in immunocompromised humans

ASSOCIATED CONDITIONS AND DISORDERS: Pneumonia (rare).

CLINICAL PRESENTATION

DISEASE FORMS/SUBTYPES

- Most dogs develop a typical mild "classic" clinical disease characterized by coughing even though the dog is otherwise normal.
- Unvaccinated puppies or adult dogs may develop a more severe disease with bronchopneumonia and rhinitis.

HISTORY, CHIEF COMPLAINT: Classic:

- Sudden onset deep hacking cough often followed by retching.

- Owners often believe the dog has "something stuck in its throat."
- Appetite and demeanor are not affected although excessive coughing may cause mild lethargy.

Bronchopneumonia:
- Nasal and ocular discharge
- Deep cough with retching; can be productive
- Anorexia
- Lethargy
- Dyspnea

PHYSICAL EXAM FINDINGS: Physical exam is often unremarkable in dogs with classic disease, other than an easily inducible cough on tracheal palpation and mild nasal or ocular discharge.

Bronchopneumonia:
- Fever
- Depression
- Tachypnea, dyspnea, cyanosis.
- Wheezes, crackles, rales on lung auscultation

ETIOLOGY AND PATHOPHYSIOLOGY

- Infectious causative agents include *B. bronchiseptica*, canine parainfluenza virus, and canine adenovirus-2 (CAV-2). Clinical disease is often the result of multiagent infections.
- Canine parainfluenza virus (CPIV) damages the respiratory epithelium of the upper respiratory tract and trachea. Alone, it primarily causes a dry cough and serous nasal discharge. Incubation period is 3 to 10 days.
- CAV-2 replicates and damages epithelial cells in the nasopharynx, tonsils, trachea, and unciliated bronchial epithelium. Incubation period is 3 to 6 days.
- *B. bronchiseptica* is a gram-negative coccobacillus that replicates on respiratory ciliary epithelial cells and produces toxins that can paralyze cilia and impair local phagocytosis, allowing colonization by opportunistic pathogens. Incubation period is approximately 6 days.
- *Mycoplasma* spp. infections (see *Mycoplasma/Ureaplasma* Infections, p 723) can develop secondarily and cause bronchopneumonia.
- Transmission of all three primary pathogens is via airborne transmission or oronasal contact.

DIAGNOSIS

DIFFERENTIAL DIAGNOSIS

- Pulmonary signs:
  - Fungal pneumonia
  - Aspiration pneumonia
  - Pulmonary neoplasia
  - Pulmonary thromboembolism
  - Lung lobe torsion
- Cough:
  - Collapsing trachea
  - Chronic bronchitis
  - Heartworm disease
  - Nasopharyngeal foreign body
  - *Oslerus osleri* infection
  - Pulmonary or mediastinal neoplasia
  - Pulmonary edema
  - Left atrial enlargement due to chronic left heart disease

INITIAL DATABASE

- For dogs with a simple cough, diagnosis is typically made according to history, physical examination, and possibly response to therapy.
- For dogs with suspected pulmonary involvement, routine blood and urine tests, thoracic radiographs, and transtracheal wash (see Transtracheal Wash, p 1314) are indicated.
- Complete blood count (CBC), serum biochemistry panel, and urinalysis are often unremarkable, especially in dogs with simple infection. CBC may show an inflammatory leukogram with left shift in complicated bronchopneumonia.
- Thoracic radiographs are usually normal in dogs with cough only. Puppies and adults with pulmonary signs may show diffuse or focal bronchial or alveolar pattern, ± evidence of hyperinflation or atelectastis, or complete lobar consolidation.
- Transtracheal wash cytologic examination is characterized by excessive neutrophils and may demonstrate bacterial colonization.

ADVANCED OR CONFIRMATORY TESTING

Viral isolation from nasopharyngeal or tracheal swabs may demonstrate CPIV or CAV-2 infection although such testing is virtually never necessary or helpful in formulating a treatment plan.

TREATMENT

THERAPEUTIC GOAL(S)

In simple clinical disease, the goal of treatment is cough suppression and prevention of secondary infection; the cough resolves spontaneously, generally in 7 to 10 days.

In bronchopneumonia, the goals are to identify and eradicate bacterial agents involved, decrease cough, improve air movement, and maintain respiratory epithelial health.

ACUTE GENERAL TREATMENT

- In animals with simple clinical disease, antibiotic treatment is often not necessary because most dogs with a healthy immune system can clear the disease on their own.
- Antibiotic selection in bronchopneumonia should be based on culture and sensitivity (C&S) results.
- Empirical antibiotics (while C&S is pending). In bronchopneumonia, appropriate antibiotics are given 7 to 28 days beyond resolution of clinical and radiographic signs, depending on severity of disease. Empirical choices can include one of the following:
  - Amoxicillin/clavulanic acid: 12-25 mg/kg PO q 8-12h.
  - Ampicillin: 30 mg/kg IV or SQ q 6-8h.
  - Azithromycin: 5-10 mg/kg PO q 24h.
  - Trimethoprim-sulfa drugs: 15 mg/kg PO or IV q 12h.
  - Enrofloxacin: 10-20 mg/kg PO, SQ, or IV q 24h.
  - Antibiotics effective against *B. bronchiseptica* include azithromycin, enrofloxacin, and doxycycline 5-10 mg/kg PO q 12h.
- Antitussives:
  - Hydrocodone: 0.22 mg/kg PO q 6-12h as needed (prn).
  - Butorphanol: 0.5 mg/kg PO, SQ, or IM q 6-12h prn.
  - Dextromethorphan: (available in over-the-counter human cough suppressants) 1-2 mg/kg PO q 6-8h. Warn owners to avoid products that contain other ingredients, such as antihistamines and decongestants.
- Dogs with bronchopneumonia may require further therapy, including bronchodilators, aerosol therapy, and supportive care (see Pneumonia, Bacterial, p 861).

PROGNOSIS AND OUTCOME

Prognosis in dogs with simple disease is excellent. Prognosis for those with bronchopneumonia is guarded to good, depending on age of animal and severity of disease

PEARLS & CONSIDERATIONS

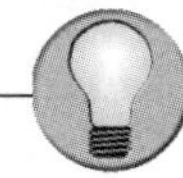

PREVENTION

- Vaccination (CPIV, CAV-2: modified live); part of many commercial combination canine vaccines (DHLPP). CPIV vaccine is also available as intranasal formulation with *Bordetella*.
- Parenteral and intranasal vaccines against *B. bronchiseptica*: duration of immunity is variable and can be short (3 to 6 months).

CLIENT EDUCATION

- To prevent disease, limit exposure to other dogs, especially in high-density populations, such as boarding kennels, shelters, and dog parks.

- If exposure is unavoidable, recommend vaccination 5 to 14 days prior to potential risk.

SUGGESTED READING

Keil DJ, et al: Role of *Bordetella bronchiseptica* in infectious tracheobronchitis in dogs. *J Am Vet Med Assoc* 212: 200–207, 1998.

AUTHOR: **SHANNON T. STROUP**
EDITOR: **DOUGLASS K. MACINTIRE**

Transfusion Reactions

BASIC INFORMATION

DEFINITION

Adverse effect from infusion of blood products; classified as immunologic or nonimmunologic and further categorized as acute (minutes to 48 hours later) or delayed (days to weeks later)

EPIDEMIOLOGY

SPECIES, AGE, SEX: Dogs and cats of any age and either sex.

CLINICAL PRESENTATION

DISEASE FORMS/SUBTYPES

- Acute immunologic:
  - Acute hemolytic transfusion reaction (AHTR): Antibodies to donor red blood cells (RBCs) are present in recipient plasma (incompatible blood type).
  - Nonhemolytic febrile reaction: recipient antibodies against donor leukocyte or protein antigens.
  - Anaphylaxis: recipient hypersensitivity/immune reaction to donor leukocyte, major histocompatibility complex, or protein antigens.
- Acute nonimmunologic:
  - *In-vitro* hemolysis: improper handling of blood (freezing, overheating, mixing with nonisotonic solutions, inappropriate infusion devices).
  - Volume overload: excessively rapid or large volume infusion, particularly in cats, puppies, and small dogs or in those with compromised cardiac or renal function.
  - Contaminated blood: lack of aseptic collection or storage, long transfusion times (>4 hours), and subclinical infection of donor.
  - Citrate toxicity: rapid large volume infusions of whole blood or plasma in small animals or those with liver failure.
  - Hyperammonemia: high ammonia levels in stored blood in animals with hepatic failure.
- Delayed immunologic:
  - Development of antibody that shortens lifespan of transfused RBCs.
  - Occurs within 3 days to several weeks.
- Delayed nonimmunologic:
  - Transmission of infectious diseases from donors.

HISTORY, CHIEF COMPLAINT: Current (acute reaction) or recent (delayed reaction) transfusion of whole blood, packed RBCs, or platelet-rich plasma.

PHYSICAL EXAM FINDINGS: In most instances, the first manifestations of a transfusion reaction include only one or two of the physical signs listed for each. If unnoticed, however, these signs may quickly worsen, with additional signs occurring as the reaction worsens.

- Acute immunologic:
  - RBC: vomiting, fever, anaphylaxis (lethargy, urticaria, pruritus, tachypnea/dyspnea), hemolysis (pallor, tachycardia, weakness), tremors, salivation hypotension (weak pulse), pigmenturia, ventricular arrhythmias, apnea
  - Platelet/leukocyte: fever, vomiting
  - Plasma proteins: urticaria, edema, pruritus, erythema
- Acute nonimmunologic:
  - Contamination: sepsis (fever, weak pulse, tachycardia), hemoglobinuria, vomiting
  - Disseminated intravascular coagulation possible (hemorrhage, thrombosis)
  - Improper collection: *in vitro* hemolysis, vomiting
  - Volume overload: dyspnea, tachypnea, tachycardia, new-onset cough (dry, soft at first), vomiting (rarely)
  - Citrate toxicity: uncommon; vomiting, tremors, tetany
- Delayed immunologic:
  - RBC: recurrence of clinical signs of anemia sooner than expected (shortened RBC survival)
  - Platelet: melena, epistaxis, ecchymoses (thrombocytopenia: post-transfusion purpura)
- Delayed nonimmunologic:
  - Disease transmission; signs reflect pathogen transmitted

ETIOLOGY AND PATHOPHYSIOLOGY

- Immunologic: specific cellular or protein fraction in blood transfused to sensitized recipient:
  - Acute: animals receiving incompatible blood (A/B incompatibility in cats) or dogs sensitized by prior transfusion, usually dog erythrocyte antigen (DEA) 1.1 incompatibility
  - Delayed: previously transfused animals with antibodies to minor RBC antigens
- Nonimmunologic: results from contamination, improper handling, or cytokine activation in the blood product

DIAGNOSIS

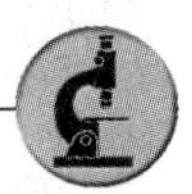

DIFFERENTIAL DIAGNOSIS

- Hemolysis: rule out underlying hemolytic diseases (see Anemia, Hemolytic, p 64)
- Fever: rule out acute hemolytic transfusion reaction, sepsis, underlying inflammatory diseases

INITIAL DATABASE

- Complete blood count (CBC), serum biochemistry panel, urinalysis:
  - Hemoglobinemia (after centrifuging, serum is pink; repeat blood sampling to rule out hemolysis from blood collection)
  - Bilirubinemia (serum often icteric if bilirubin >1 mg/dl [>17 mmol/l])
  - Leukocytosis
- Urinalysis: hemoglobinuria, bilirubinuria
- Hypocalcemia (citrate toxicity). Only ionized calcium is reduced

- Blood pressure (BP) measurement: rule out hypotension
- Thoracic radiographs: if volume overload is suspected (rule out pulmonary edema)

ADVANCED OR CONFIRMATORY TESTING

- Acute hemolytic transfusion reaction: centrifuge recipient blood to check for evidence of hemolysis; repeat major cross match (see Cross-Match and Blood Typing, p 1212); Coombs' test on recipient
- Inspect transfused unit for dark discoloration, clots, air bubbles, or hemolysis to detect contaminated blood; Gram stain and culture (aerobic/anaerobic)
- Examine blood from bag or administration set for *in-vitro* hemolysis

TREATMENT

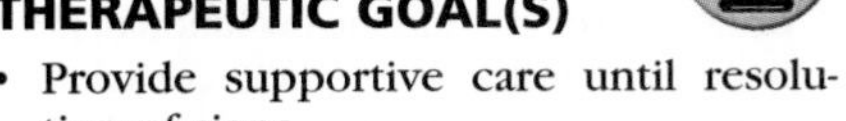

THERAPEUTIC GOAL(S)

- Provide supportive care until resolution of signs
- Identify and correct cause of reaction (when possible)

ACUTE GENERAL TREATMENT

- Acute hemolytic transfusion reaction: stop the transfusion and treat for shock (IV fluids, vasopressor agents if persistent hypotension, ± glucocorticoids)
- Urticaria: antihistamines (e.g., diphenhydramine 2 mg/kg IM) and/or short-acting corticosteroids (e.g., dexamethasone sodium phosphate 0.2 mg/kg slow IV); temporarily halt transfusion until signs resolve
- Nonhemolytic febrile reaction without cardiovascular or respiratory compromise (temperature rise of 2°F [1°C]): slow rate of transfusion. Discontinue if fever persists or worsens
- Volume overload (pulmonary edema): halt transfusion and give IV diuretics (furosemide 2 mg/kg IV) and oxygen
- Sepsis: halt transfusion and obtain samples for culture; IV antibiotics; IV fluids

POSSIBLE COMPLICATIONS

Acute immunologic hemolytic reactions and reactions to infected blood may be severe and require a rapid and intensive response. Most other transfusion reactions, when detected early, respond well to conservative management.

- Acute hemolytic transfusion reaction/contaminated blood: arterial hypotension and shock, renal failure, disseminated intravascular coagulation
- Volume overload: hypoxemia

RECOMMENDED MONITORING

- Monitor attitude, temperature, and vital signs throughout and following the transfusion
- Monitor hematocrit/total protein before and after the transfusion

PROGNOSIS AND OUTCOME

- Stable animals: good with early recognition and intervention
- Severely ill: guarded

PEARLS & CONSIDERATIONS

COMMENTS

- Pretreating with antihistamines or corticosteroids will not prevent immunologic hemolytic reactions.
- Severe reactions usually occur during or shortly after transfusion.
- Most acute hemolytic transfusion reactions can be prevented by using DEA 1.1 negative canine blood donors (in nontyped recipients) and, in cats, using matched blood donors.
- All animals that have been previously transfused need to be crossmatched unless the animal's only other transfusion(s) was/were within the preceding 3 to 5 days.
- Crossmatching detects antibodies against donor RBCs. Nonimmune reactions or reactions due to antibodies attacking white blood cells (WBCs), platelets, or proteins will not be detected by crossmatching.

PREVENTION

- Type all donors, screen for infectious diseases, and use a sterile collection technique.
- Type all recipients if possible.
- Crossmatch all cats and dogs that have had previous transfusions.
- Never use outdated or hemolyzed products.
- Consider the animal's underlying diseases when choosing component and administration rate.
- Follow strict guidelines for storage, handling, and administration of blood products.
- Monitor transfusions carefully.

SUGGESTED READING

Griot-Wenk ME, Giger U: Feline transfusion medicine; Blood types and their clinical importance. *Vet Clin N Am Small An Pract* 25:1305–1323, 1995.

Harrell KA, Kristensen AT: Canine transfusion reactions and their management. *Vet Clin N Am Small An Pract* 25:1333–1361, 1995.

AUTHOR: **LILIAN CORNEJO**
EDITOR: **SUSAN M. COTTER**

Transitional Cell Carcinoma

BASIC INFORMATION

DEFINITION

Epithelial neoplasm arising in the bladder parenchyma

SYNONYM(S)

TCC

EPIDEMIOLOGY

SPECIES, AGE, SEX

- Dogs: typically older adults (median: 11 years), females at higher risk
- Cats: rarely affected. Older adults, males are at increased risk

GENETICS AND BREED PREDISPOSITION: Scottish terriers, Shetland sheepdogs, West Highland white terriers, Wirehaired fox terriers, Airedales, beagles, collies: higher incidence.

RISK FACTORS

- Dogs: exposure to insecticides associated with an increased risk; worsened in the presence of obesity, possibly due to accumulation of "inert ingredients." Cyclophosphamide administration may increase risk
- Cats: possibly associated with chronic urinary tract infection (UTI)

ASSOCIATED DISEASES AND CONDITIONS

- Bacterial UTI
- Hypertrophic osteopathy
- Urethral obstruction
- Bladder atonia/hypotonia

CLINICAL PRESENTATION

DISEASE FORMS/SUBTYPES

- Most common form is invasive cancer into muscularis of bladder trigone

- Early form of superficial cancer may be identified that may be more responsive to therapy

HISTORY, CHIEF COMPLAINT

- Pollakiuria
- Hematuria
- Stranguria
- Tenesmus
- Abdominal pain
- Abdominal distention
- Lameness and joint thickening (associated with hypertrophic osteopathy)

PHYSICAL EXAM FINDINGS

- Abdominal tenderness
- Caudal abdominal mass
- Distended urinary bladder
- Abdominal distention with fluid wave
- Rectal exam:
  - May reveal urethral and/or trigonal mass
  - Essential for ruling out other causes of similar signs (urethrolith, pelvic mass, other)
- Vaginal exam:
  - May reveal extension of tumor to urethral papilla
  - Essential for ruling out other causes of similar signs (distal urethal lith, vaginal mass, foreign body)

ETIOLOGY AND PATHOPHYSIOLOGY

- Most commonly occurs as bladder mass in trigone region, causing signs of lower urinary tract obstruction and often limiting surgical resectability
- Urethral, prostatic involvement: common
- Lymph node metastasis: 15% of cases
- Distant metastasis common (49% at death)
- Metastatic sites include lymph node, lung, liver, kidney, spleen, uterus, gastrointestinal (GI) tract, bone, muscle
- Secondary bacterial UTI common

DIAGNOSIS

DIFFERENTIAL DIAGNOSIS

- Pollakiuria, stranguria, hematuria:
  - UTI
  - Urolithiasis
  - Feline lower urinary tract signs/disease, interstitial cystitis
  - Other bladder tumor (botryoid rhabdomyosarcoma in young, large-breed dogs; leiomyosarcoma)
- Abdominal distention/tenderness or abdominal mass:
  - Mass in spleen, mesenteric lymph node, or retroperitoneal space
  - Ruptured splenic or hepatic mass with hemoperitoneum
  - Abdominal trauma or coagulopathy with uroperitoneum, peritoneal or retroperitoneal bleeding
  - Rectal mass
  - Prostatic abscess, cyst, or neoplasia
  - Pyelonephritis
  - Hydronephrosis or hydroureter
  - Pyometra
- Radiographic:
  - Other bladder neoplasm or radiolucent urolithiasis
  - Ruptured splenic, renal, or hepatic mass with hemoperitoneum
  - Traumatic bladder rupture
- Ultrasonographic:
  - Papillary cystitis
  - Leiomyosarcoma
  - Botryoid rhabdomyosarcoma
- Urinalysis:
  - UTI
  - Urolithiasis
  - Other bladder tumor
  - Idiopathic renal hematuria

INITIAL DATABASE

- Complete blood count (CBC), serum biochemistry profile: no specific findings supporting transitional cell carcinoma (TCC); azotemia or hyperkalemia possible with urethral or ureteral obstruction.
- Urinalysis:
  - Proteinuria and hematuria common.
  - May be complicated by secondary bacterial UTI with pyuria, bacteriuria.
  - Unreliable for TCC diagnosis (poorly exfoliative; TCC cells' cytologic appearance overlaps with reactive change).
- Veterinary bladder tumor antigen (VBTA) test: This test is approximately 85% sensitive for TCC but only 45% specific in the presence of other urinary tract disease. As such, it is a good screening test (negative is likely true negative) but does not confirm the presence of TCC (positive is only somewhat likely to be true positive).
- Abdominal radiographs: bladder mass is possible but unusual. Bladder distention may be seen, and with rupture, peritoneal or retroperitoneal fluid is possible.
- Thoracic radiographs: metastasis may be present. Lesions may be nodular interstitial, unstructured interstitial, cavitated, or alveolar in appearance.
- Abdominal ultrasound: bladder mass or wall thickening with possible metastasis to abdominal organs; prostate or urethra is commonly involved.

ADVANCED OR CONFIRMATORY TESTING

- Cytologic examination or biopsy from ultrasound guided diagnostic catheterization or biopsy from cystoscopy necessary for diagnosis (see Cystoscopy, p 1216)
- Contrast cystography/ureterography may be used for delineating ureteral involvement and impending urethral obstruction (see Cystogram, p 1214)
- Veterinary bladder tumor antigen test does not confirm and only suggests TCC

TREATMENT

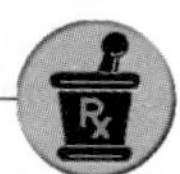

THERAPEUTIC GOAL(S)

- Alleviate clinical signs
- Control primary mass
- Prevent/delay metastasis

ACUTE GENERAL TREATMENT

- Surgically manage urinary bladder rupture if present
- Surgically remove lesions at bladder apex if operable. Surgery may be of greater benefit in cats
- Address complicating bacterial UTI with antibiotics (see Cystitis, Bacterial, p 270)
- Begin chemotherapy to palliate clinical signs and address metastatic disease. Special handling requirements and potential adverse animal effects exist for these drugs. These risks and the evolution of new treatment protocols warrant consultaion with or referral to a veterinary oncologist.
  - Piroxicam 0.3 mg/kg PO once daily if renal function is normal; can be used alone or in combination with the following drugs.
  - Mitoxantrone 5 mg/m^2 IV q 21 days for four cycles.
  - Doxorubicin 30 mg/m^2 IV q 21 days for four cycles (dogs), or 1 mg/kg IV q 21 days (cats and small dogs).
  - Check CBC and blood urea nitrogen (BUN), creatinine, and urine specific gravity prior to each dose; check CBC 1 week later.
  - Cisplatin has been associated with renal compromise in combination with piroxicam.
  - Intravesicular infusions of bacillus Calmette-Guérin (BCG) or thiotepa used in humans have not been very effective in veterinary patients.
- If bladder is distended initially, ensure urinary drainage to avoid overdistention and detrusor hypotonia (see Atonic or Hypotonic Urinary Bladder, p 94)
- Address electrolyte imbalances if present secondary to obstruction (see Urethral Obstruction, p 1120)

CHRONIC TREATMENT

- Continue piroxicam indefinitely
- May repeat mitoxantrone after first four doses if clinical signs recur
- Cumulative doxorubicin doses greater than 180-240 mg/m^2 are associated with increased risk of cardiotoxicity and should be avoided
- Urinary diversion surgery may prolong life if urethral obstruction is imminent

DRUG INTERACTIONS

- Avoid combining drugs with similar toxicity profiles, such as cisplatin and piroxicam

- Piroxicam contraindications: corticosteroids, other nonsteroidal anti-inflammatory drugs (NSAIDs); GI ulceration, renal failure, poor appetite

POSSIBLE COMPLICATIONS

- Neutropenia, thrombocytopenia, sepsis, and renal injury secondary to chemotherapy
- Urethral or ureteral obstruction secondary to tumor growth

RECOMMENDED MONITORING

- Monitor CBC prior to every chemotherapy treatment and 7 to 10 days later
- Monitor BUN, creatinine, and urine specific gravity for renal function every 3 to 12 weeks
- Urine culture and sensitivity every 3 months

PROGNOSIS AND OUTCOME

This disease is locally aggressive with a significant metastatic potential.

- Dogs:
  - Median reported survival for animal treated with piroxicam alone is approximately 6 to 7 months
  - Median reported survival for animal treated with piroxicam and mitoxantrone is approximately 12 months
  - Median reported survival for animal treated with surgery alone is approximately 3½ months
- Cats:
  - Median reported survival for an animal described in one study is approximately 7 months
  - Surgical resection may improve prognosis significantly in cats

PEARLS & CONSIDERATIONS

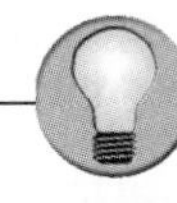

COMMENTS

- Repeated urinary tract signs or infection, especially in older animals, should prompt screening for TCC.
- Early detection is critical for best response to treatment.
- VBTA test may allow early detection in geriatric at-risk breeds of dogs with lower urinary tract signs.
- Definitive diagnosis, necessary for prognosis and therapeutic decisions, requires cytologic examination or biopsy.
- Bacterial UTI is a frequent complication.

CLIENT EDUCATION

- Signs are subtle and nonspecific, so advanced diagnostics and imaging are most useful early.
- Urethral obstruction is often the life-limiting complication, and urinary diversion may be beneficial.

SUGGESTED READING

Henry CJ: Management of transitional cell carcinoma. *Vet Clin North Am* 33:597-613, 2003.

Mutsaers JA, et al: Canine transitional cell carcinoma. *J Vet Intern Med* 17:136-144, 2003.

AUTHOR: **JEFFREY N. BRYAN**

EDITOR: **LEAH A. COHN**

Transmissible Venereal Tumor

BASIC INFORMATION

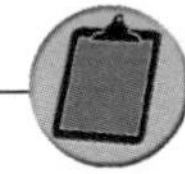

DEFINITION

A contagious, neoplastic disease transmitted by transplantation of viable tumor cells during coitus

SYNONYM(S)

Canine condyloma
Contagious lymphoma
Contagious venereal tumor
Infectious sarcoma
Sticker's sarcoma
Transmissible venereal sarcoma
Venereal granuloma

EPIDEMIOLOGY

SPECIES, AGE, SEX

- Species: canids; dogs, foxes, coyotes, jackals
- Age: mostly young, sexually active animals; average age 4 to 5 years
- Sex: both sexes

GENETICS AND BREED PREDISPOSITION: Higher prevalence in mixed-breed dogs.

RISK FACTORS

- More commonly occurs in free-roaming sexually active dogs
- Grows more rapidly in neonatal or immunosuppressed dogs

CONTAGION AND ZOONOSIS: By definition, transmissible venereal tumor (TVT) is contagious among members of the family Canidae.

GEOGRAPHY AND SEASONALITY

- Worldwide distribution
- Greatest prevalence in tropical and subtropical urban environments

ASSOCIATED CONDITIONS AND DISORDERS

- Urinary tract infections (UTIs) due to presence of TVT in the vestibulovaginal junction (females) and phimosis (males). Both conditions interfere with voiding of urine.
- Tumors are easily traumatized and ulcerated; secondary bacterial infection is a common sequela.

CLINICAL PRESENTATION

HISTORY, CHIEF COMPLAINT

- Initial persistent or intermittent bloody genital discharge (often foul smelling), constant licking, genital malformation, or swelling.
- Eventually, masses can be seen protruding either from vulva or penis.
- Clinical signs of TVT typically last 40 to 100 days but may last longer depending on the tumor size and location, immune status of the animal, and occurrence of secondary bacterial infections.

PHYSICAL EXAM FINDINGS

- Nodular lesions in the external genitalia.
- Solitary or multiple masses progressing to cauliflower-like, papillary, multilobulated, or pedunculated masses.
- Appearance is typically gray or pinkish gray.
- Texture is firm but friable; masses bleed easily when manipulated, resulting in genital bleeding in both sexes.
- In the oronasal presentation, epistaxis and frequent sneezing with bloody catarrhal discharge, halitosis, hypersalivation, dyspnea, loss of teeth, and ulcerative lesions in gingivae and palate.
- In the skin, nodular masses may be ulcerated and regional lymph nodes may be enlarged.

ETIOLOGY AND PATHOPHYSIOLOGY

- Transmitted by coitus; affecting mainly external genital organs and spreading to internal genitalia.
- Transmitted more easily if there are abrasions or breaks in the integrity of the mucosal surface.
- Social behavior, such as licking and sniffing affected areas, can produce extragenital TVT in the skin and eyes and in oral and nasal cavities.
- Metastasis is rare; however, when it occurs, it affects regional lymph nodes, subcutaneous tissues, abdominal and thoracic viscera, brain, pituitary, spleen, and kidneys. Metastatic disease can also

occur without the presence of a primary genital tumor.
- Exact cell origin of TVT is unknown but is presumed to be an undifferentiated round-cell neoplasm of histiocytic origin.
- Chromosome number of tumor cells is 59 ± 5, whereas the normal canine complement is 78.

DIAGNOSIS

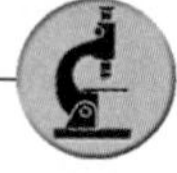

DIFFERENTIAL DIAGNOSIS

- Tumor type is suspected by the history, location, and appearance of the mass.
- Especially when there is no evidence of a primary genital tumor, TVT can be confused with other round cell tumors, such as mast cell tumor, histiocytoma, lymphosarcoma. Also to be considered are malignant melanoma, squamous cell carcinoma (SCC), fibrosarcoma.
- Clinical signs may be similar to those found with prostatitis, estrus, urethritis, and cystitis.

INITIAL DATABASE

Cytologic examination of impression smears stained with Wright's or new methylene blue reveal homogeneous sheets of round to oval cells with prominent nucleoli and small amount of cytoplasm with multiple mitotic figures.

ADVANCED OR CONFIRMATORY TESTING

Definitive diagnosis is by histologic classification of a biopsy specimen (after formalin fixation and staining with hematoxylin and eosin) and immunochemistry testing to determine degree of malignancy.

TREATMENT

THERAPEUTIC GOAL(S)

Elimination of the tumor

ACUTE GENERAL TREATMENT

- The rationale for surgical removal of the tumor is to induce an immune response as well as to mechanically remove the mass. A small TVT may be surgically excised without relapse, but tumor regrowth frequently occurs over a very short period of time following excision of large tumors (>2 cm).
- Chemotherapy with vincristine at 0.5 to 0.7 mg/m^2 of body surface area IV (highly corrosive if extravascular) once weekly for 6 weeks until complete tumor regression is the treatment of choice for metastatic or multifocal TVT.
- Radiation therapy is effective (100% cure with a single radiation dose) when appropriate facilities are available. Spontaneous regression occurs in experimental and clinical cases.

DRUG INTERACTIONS

Severe bronchospasm has been reported in humans when vinca alkaloids are used in combination with mitomycin-C.

POSSIBLE COMPLICATIONS

- Extravasation injuries associated with perivascular injection of vincristine can range from irritation to necrosis and tissue sloughing.
- Combined chemotherapy with vincristine presents more side effects (vomiting, diarrhea, and neutropenia) than vincristine alone.

RECOMMENDED MONITORING

- Monitor for efficacy (tumor reduction)
- Monitor for toxicity using peripheral neuropathic clinical signs; complete blood counts (CBCs) with platelets; and liver tests before, during, and after treatment

PROGNOSIS AND OUTCOME

Despite the location or pattern of metastasis, the prognosis for TVT is excellent with recommended therapy.

PEARLS & CONSIDERATIONS

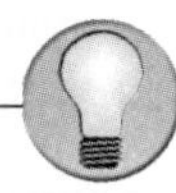

PREVENTION

Pet dogs should avoid contact with stray dogs.

CLIENT EDUCATION

In areas were TVT is endemic, pet dogs should be confined and spayed or neutered to reduce the risk of disease transmission.

SUGGESTED READING

Feldman EC, Nelson RW: Brucellosis and transmissible venereal tumor. In *Canine and Feline Endocrinology and Reproduction*, ed 3. New York, WB Saunders, 2004, pp 924-927.

Gobello C, Corrada Y: Effects of vincristine treatment on semen quality in a dog with a transmissible venereal tumour. *J Small Anim Pract* 43(9):416-417, 2002.

Johnston SD, Root Kustritz MV, Olson PNS: Disorders of the canine penis and prepuce. In *Canine and Feline Theriogenology*. New York, WB Saunders, 2001, pp 356-365

Rogers KS: Transmissible venereal tumor. *Comp Cont Educ Pract Vet* 19:1036-1045, 1997.

Rogers KS, Walker MA, Dillon HB: Transmissible venereal tumor: A retrospective study of 29 cases. *J Am Anim Hosp Assoc* 34:463-470, 1998.

Weir EC, Pond MJ, Duncan JR, Polzin DJ: Extragenital occurrence of transmissible venereal tumor in the dog: Literature review and case reports. *J Am Anim Hosp Assoc* 14:532-536, 1978.

AUTHOR: **ROSA MARÍA PÁRAMO RAMIREZ**

EDITOR: **MICHELLE A. KUTZLER**

Tremors and Myoclonus

BASIC INFORMATION

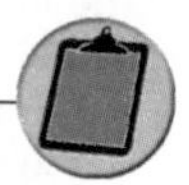

DEFINITION

- Tremor: involuntary oscillating contraction of opposing muscle groups. It may occur during rest or movement and typically disappears during sleep.
- Myoclonus: single or multiple shock-like contractions of a muscle group; may occur singly or repetitively, regularly or irregularly, and does not stop during sleep.

EPIDEMIOLOGY

SPECIES, AGE, SEX

Dependent on underlying cause.
- Dogs: puppies (hypomyelination/dysmyelination, familial myoclonus); young adults (see Idiopathic Tremor Syndrome, p 578); older adults (senile tremors)
- Cats: kittens (hypomyelination)

GENETICS AND BREED PREDISPOSITION

- Dogs:
  - Maltese, West Highland white terriers, other small-breed white or non-white dogs: see Idiopathic Tremor Syndrome, p 578

- Doberman pinscher, English bulldog, Shetland sheepdog: idiopathic head tremors
- Labrador retriever: idiopathic head tremor, familial myoclonus
- Springer spaniel, Samoyed, chow chow, weimaraner, Lurcher, Bernese mountain dog, dalmatian: hypomyelination/dysmyelination
- Scottish terriers: central axonopathy

- Cats:
  - Siamese: hypomyelination

RISK FACTORS: Exposure to tremorgenic drugs or toxins.

CONTAGION AND ZOONOSIS: Dogs: distemper virus (dog-to-dog transmission).

CLINICAL PRESENTATION

DISEASE FORMS/SUBTYPES

- Generalized more common than localized
- Resting tremor
- Action tremor
- Intention tremor

HISTORY, CHIEF COMPLAINT

- Tremor may worsen with exercise and abate with rest or sleep.
- Littermates may be affected.
  - Tremor associated with hypomyelination/dysmyelination typically begins between 12 days and 3 weeks of age. Signs worsen with exercise but often resolve with rest; littermates may be affected.
- Exposure to tremorgenic toxins.
- Insulin therapy for diabetes mellitus, suggesting hypoglycemia.
- Recent (preceding weeks/months) history of respiratory disease, ill thrift, or adoption from a shelter, suggesting canine distemper-associated myoclonus.
- Recent whelping, suggesting hypocalcemia.
- Seizures (must be differentiated from tremor/myoclonus).
- Idiopathic head tremors are episodic and may be confused for partial seizures. They are often precipitated by excitement or particular head positions, and owners may describe a characteristic "yes" or "no" movement of the head and normal consciousness with tremors, in contrast to the tonic-clonic or gum-chewing motions of seizures.
- Scottish terriers with central axonopathy develop tremors and ataxia at 10 to 12 weeks of age.

PHYSICAL AND NEUROLOGIC EXAM FINDINGS

- The presence of tremors or myoclonus may be the only abnormality on the physical or neurologic examination.
- Ataxia, paresis, and proprioceptive deficits may be present, suggesting a central (brain, spinal cord) lesion.
- Seizures, stupor, and coma may be seen concurrently with intoxication or metabolic derangement.
- Ocular tremors and menace deficits often accompany idiopathic tremor syndrome.
- Intention tremor (i.e., tremor precipitated by the onset of voluntary movement, such as responding to a command) if associated with a fine head tremor, dysmetria, and nystagmus, is characteristic of cerebellar disease.
- Pelvic limb tremors in older dogs (senile tremors).

ETIOLOGY AND PATHOPHYSIOLOGY

Primary:

- Idiopathic tremor syndrome: immune-mediated (see Idiopathic Tremor Syndrome, p 578)
- Hypomyelination, dysmyelination: congenital
- Lysosomal storage diseases: congenital
- Cerebellar disease
- Idiopathic head tremors
- Senile tremors

Systemic:

- Intoxication (mycotoxins [see Blue-Green Algae Toxicosis, p 138], hexachlorophene, heavy metals, organophosphates [see Organophosphate and Carbamate Insecticide Toxicosis, p 775], metaldehyde [see Metaldehyde Toxicosis, p 702], pyrethrins [see Pyrethrins/Pyrethroids Toxicosis, p 936], others)
- Drug administration (fentanyl/droperidol, epinephrine, metoclopramide, diphenhydramine, isoproterenol, numerous illicit drugs)
- Metabolic (hypocalcemia, hypoglycemia, hepatic or uremic encephalopathy, hyperthyroidism)
- Infectious (canine distemper)

DIAGNOSIS

A presumptive diagnosis is often made based on the signalment, history, and clinical findings.

DIFFERENTIAL DIAGNOSIS

- Shivering
- Tetany
- Weakness
- Seizure
- Specific causes according to etiology

INITIAL DATABASE

- Complete physical and neurologic examination
- Complete blood cell count (CBC), serum biochemistry, and urinalysis to assess for metabolic etiologies
- Serum T4 (hyperthyroidism in cats)

ADVANCED OR CONFIRMATORY TESTING

Cerebrospinal fluid (CSF) analysis: may be normal or reveal increased numbers of leukocytes (usually lymphocytes) with increased levels of protein, reflecting a nonsuppurative meningoencephalitis

TREATMENT

THERAPEUTIC GOAL(S)

Identify and treat the underlying cause of the tremors

ACUTE GENERAL TREATMENT

- General and/or specific treatment for intoxication.
- Discontinue drug therapy if suspected to be causing tremors.
- Correct metabolic and electrolyte abnormalities.
- Sterile inflammatory tremor syndromes often respond to corticosteroid therapy.

CHRONIC TREATMENT

- Long-term corticosteroid therapy is often necessary for inflammatory tremor syndromes.
- Supportive care aimed at keeping animals safe and ensuring adequate caloric and water intake.

POSSIBLE COMPLICATIONS

Prolonged tremors may result in hyperthermia, hypoglycemia, dehydration, and anorexia.

RECOMMENDED MONITORING

Follow-up exam and serial diagnostic studies as directed by the animal's clinical progression

PROGNOSIS AND OUTCOME

- Tremors associated with idiopathic tremor syndrome usually resolve within days of the initiation of corticosteroid therapy.
  - Treatment should be continued for 2 to 3 months
  - Relapses may occur
- Male springer spaniels with hypomyelination are nonambulatory and generally do not recover.
- Female springer spaniels and other breeds with hypomyelination/dysmyelination usually recover completely between 2 and 12 months of age.
- Idiopathic head tremors may improve and become less frequent over time and rarely cause any clinical dysfunction.
- Senile tremors also generally do not interfere with normal function.
- Central axonopathy in Scottish terriers is progressive and associated with a poor prognosis.
- Lysosomal storage diseases are usually fatal.
- Toxin and drug-induced tremors resolve if the animal survives the initial event.

PEARLS & CONSIDERATIONS

CLIENT EDUCATION

- Owners should be warned that excitement and exercise often precipitate or worsen tremors.
- Many tremor syndromes have a known or suspected inherited basis, and these animals should not be bred.

SUGGESTED READING

Bagley RS: Tremor syndromes in dogs: Diagnosis and treatment. *J Small Anim Pract* 33:485–490, 1991.

Cuddon PA: Tremor syndromes. *Prog Vet Neurol* 3:285–299, 1990.

AUTHORS: **GREG KILBURN, JOLI M. JARBOE**
EDITOR: **ETIENNE CÔTÉ**

Tricuspid Valve Dysplasia

BASIC INFORMATION

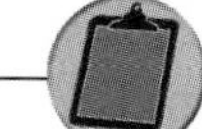

DEFINITION

Congenital cardiac abnormality involving the right atrioventricular (AV) valve (tricuspid valve) and characterized by any or all of the following: thickening of leaflets, foreshortening of chordae tendinae, fusing or underdevelopment of right ventricle (RV) papillary muscles, tethering of particularly the septal leaflet to the underlying ventricular muscle, and redundancy of the parietal leaflet

SYNONYM(S)

Congenital tricuspid valve malformation
Ebstein anomaly
TVD

EPIDEMIOLOGY

SPECIES, AGE, SEX

- Dogs and cats
- Present at birth; however, affected individuals are identified at any age based on when the heart murmur is detected
- Either sex

GENETICS AND BREED PREDISPOSITION

- Identified in several breeds.
- Labrador retrievers are predisposed; autosomal dominant mode of inheritance with reduced penetrance. Affected Labrador retrievers that have been studied thus far (from different families) all had the same susceptibility locus identified, suggesting a founder effect.

ASSOCIATED CONDITIONS AND DISORDERS

- Typically an isolated congenital heart defect.
- Atrial septal defect (ASD), patent foramen ovale, mitral valve dysplasia, ventricular septal defect (VSD), pulmonic stenosis (PS), and patent ductus arteriosus have coexisted.

CLINICAL PRESENTATION

HISTORY, CHIEF COMPLAINT

- Often no clinical signs (heart murmur only)
- Severe forms of the disease cause exercise intolerance, abdominal distention, dyspnea (secondary to pleural effusion), poor appetite, and weight loss

PHYSICAL EXAM FINDINGS

- Right-sided systolic heart murmur of tricuspid regurgitation
- Rarely a soft diastolic murmur of tricuspid stenosis
- Tachycardia possible
- Jugular venous distention and pulsation if severe disease
- Abdominal palpation: hepatomegaly and a peritoneal fluid wave if right-sided congestive heart failure (R-CHF) is present
- Femoral pulses: usually normal; weak with severe disease associated with poor cardiac output
- Lung auscultation: usually normal; muffled lung sounds if pleural effusion
- Mucous membrane color: usually normal; pale with poor cardiac output; cyanotic if concurrent patent foramen ovale or septal defect

ETIOLOGY AND PATHOPHYSIOLOGY

- During embryonic development, tricuspid valve leaflets are almost exclusively derived from ventricular myocardium by a process of undermining the RV inner wall.
- The inner layer of RV myocardium is undermined from the remainder to form a skirt in which perforations appear in the apical portion.
- These perforations enlarge until only the papillary muscles remain and the initially muscular chordae tendinae become fibrous.
- Abnormalities during this process lead to tricuspid valve dysplasia (TVD).

DIFFERENTIAL DIAGNOSIS

- Tricuspid valve endocardiosis/myxomatous valve disease: older dogs; concurrent more severe myxomatous mitral valve disease/endocardiosis generally is present
- Tricuspid valve endocarditis: very rare in dogs and cats, associated with systemic illness and fever (can be waxing and waning); focal valve thickening or vegetation

INITIAL DATABASE

- Echocardiogram:
  - The diagnostic test of choice.
  - Two-dimensional (2-D) mode defines degrees of tricuspid valve leaflet thickening, adherence of the septal leaflet to the interventricular septum, redundancy of the parietal leaflet, presence of hyperechoic fibrous tissue at the annulus resulting in stenosis, and right atrial and right ventricular dilation.
  - Doppler echocardiography documents the presence and degree of tricuspid regurgitation and presence/severity of tricuspid stenosis.
  - Concurrent defects can be identified.
- Thoracic radiographs:
  - Normal in mild disease.
  - Evidence of right atrial and right ventricular enlargement in moderate to severe disease.
  - Enlargement of the caudal vena cava and possible pulmonary hypoperfusion in severe disease.
  - Hepatomegaly and peritoneal effusion can occur in severe cases (such as in R-CHF).
- Electrocardiogram (ECG):
  - Normal in mild disease.
  - May exhibit fragmentation or splintering of the QRS complex with a normal mean electrical axis.
  - Less commonly, classic right axis deviation of the QRS complex as seen with right ventricular dilation.
  - P waves may be tall and wide.
  - May exhibit ventricular pre-excitation or supraventricular tachycardias associated with accessory pathway conduction (see Wolff-Parkinson-White Syndrome, p 1166).

ADVANCED OR CONFIRMATORY TESTING

- Generally not required
- Holter monitoring to document intermittent tachyarrhythmias

TREATMENT

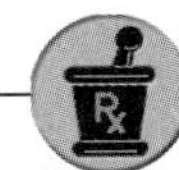

THERAPEUTIC GOAL(S)

- Control R-CHF if present
- Control associated tachyarrhythmias
- Consider surgical valve reconstruction in severe cases

ACUTE GENERAL TREATMENT

- Abdominocentesis (see Abdominocentesis, p 1178) or abdominal drainage (see Abdominal Drainage, p 1176) for severe peritoneal effusion to relieve abdominal pressure that can inhibit diaphragmatic movement
- Cage rest for severe R-CHF
- Antiarrhythmic treatment to control supraventricular tachyarrhythmias acutely

CHRONIC TREATMENT

- Careful diuretic administration for CHF (furosemide 1 mg/kg PO q 8-12h spironolactone 1-2 mg/kg PO q 12h)
- Low-dose angiotensin-converting enzyme (ACE) inhibition may be helpful (e.g., enalapril or benazepril 0.1-0.25 mg/kg PO q 12-24h)
- Digoxin (0.0055 mg/kg PO q 12h, adjusting based on serum digoxin concentrations) for supraventricular tachyarrhythmias
- Exercise restriction
- Nutritional management of cardiac cachexia (adequate calorie intake for disease state, highly digestible foods [see Cachexia, Cardiac, p 168])

DRUG INTERACTIONS

- Be careful about compromising renal perfusion due to excessive diuretic administration and poor forward cardiac output from the disease.
- Spironolactone and ACE inhibitors can theoretically lead to hyperkalemia although concurrent furosemide administration generally causes potassium wasting.

POSSIBLE COMPLICATIONS

- Excessive diuresis causing decreased forward output and weakness
- Electrolyte abnormalities secondary to diuresis
- Hypoalbuminemia secondary to cardiac cachexia and continued peritoneal effusion

RECOMMENDED MONITORING

- Monitor for signs of R-CHF (peritoneal effusion, decreased exercise tolerance, decreasing muscle mass).
- Monitor for tachyarrhythmias (ECG, Holter monitoring if necessary).
- If the animal is receiving a diuretic and other CHF therapy, monitor the serum chemistry profile every 5 to 7 days after medication adjustments are made, and every 2 to 3 months thereafter.

PROGNOSIS AND OUTCOME

- Better than is typically found in the literature
- Dogs with mild disease and even many with moderate disease can live a normal lifespan
- Dogs with severe disease will have shortened lifespans, but some can live several years (5 or more years is possible)

PEARLS & CONSIDERATIONS

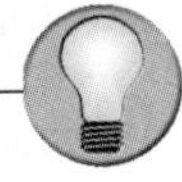

COMMENTS

- Prominent in Labrador retrievers, tricuspid valve dysplasia appears to be inherited as an autosomal dominant trait with reduced penetrance in this breed.
- Carefully auscult dogs over the right precordium to detect this disease.
- Prognosis in animals with isolated TVD is better than initially thought although the lifespan of dogs with severe disease is still shortened.
- Major complications in severe disease include CHF and tachyarrhythmias.
- Concurrent congenital heart defects are not common but, if present, generally worsen the prognosis.

SUGGESTED READING

Andelfinger G, et al: Canine tricuspid valve malformation, a model of human Ebstein anomaly, maps to dog chromosome 9. *J Med Genetics* 40:320-324.

Moise NS: Tricuspid valve dysplasia in the dog. In Bonagura JD (ed): *Kirk's Current Veterinary Therapy XII*. Philadelphia, WB Saunders, 1995, pp 813-816.

AUTHOR: **KATHY WRIGHT**

EDITOR: **ETIENNE CÔTÉ**

Trigeminal Neuritis

BASIC INFORMATION

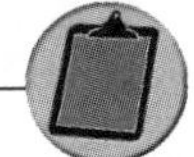

DEFINITION

An idiopathic, self-limiting inflammatory condition that involves the motor and sensory branches of the trigeminal nerve and, on occasion, the sympathetic tract

EPIDEMIOLOGY

SPECIES, AGE, SEX: Dogs most commonly affected; rare in cats.

GENETICS AND BREED PREDISPOSITION: No sex or breed predilection although golden retrievers have been reported to be overrepresented.

CLINICAL PRESENTATION

DISEASE FORMS/SUBTYPES: Bilateral paralysis of the masticatory muscles that primarily affects the mandibular branch of the trigeminal nerve.

HISTORY, CHIEF COMPLAINT: Acute or subacute onset of an inability to close the mouth. The dog cannot prehend food, may hypersalivate, and has difficulty drinking water.

PHYSICAL EXAM FINDINGS

- Bilateral paralysis of the masticatory muscles.
- Affected dogs are bright and alert and do not appear as though they are in pain. They have no other detectable neurologic abnormalities.
- In some cases, there is decreased facial sensation bilaterally, and Horner's syndrome may be observed.
- Trismus/inability to open the mouth does not occur with trigeminal neuritis.

ETIOLOGY AND PATHOPHYSIOLOGY

- The most common neurologic cause of an inability to close the mouth in the dog.
- The etiology is unknown; however, extensive, bilateral nonsuppurative inflammation, demyelination, and, in some cases, axonal degeneration of all portions of the trigeminal nerve and its ganglion, with no brainstem lesions, have been reported at necropsy.
- Complete recovery is observed in 2 to 3 weeks (rarely, may take several months) with no drug therapy being reported as useful.
- Facial sensation is usually preserved. Occasionally, Horner's syndrome may be observed presumably because the postganglionic sympathetic axons

course with the ophthalmic branch of the trigeminal nerve.

DIAGNOSIS

The diagnosis is based on characteristic clinical signs, absence of other neurologic deficits, and elimination of the possibility of orthopedic (mandibular, temporomandibular joint) disorders

DIFFERENTIAL DIAGNOSIS

- Rabies
- Traumatic mandibular injury
- Inflammatory or infectious central nervous system (CNS) disease

INITIAL DATABASE

Complete blood count (CBC), serum chemistry profile, urinalysis: usually within normal limits

ADVANCED OR CONFIRMATORY TESTING

- Cerebrospinal fluid (CSF) analysis may be normal or show mild increases in protein concentration. Lymphocytic pleocytosis is rarely observed.
- Electromyography may reveal increased insertional activity and other mild changes.
- CT scan or MRI of the brain: within normal limits.
- Trigeminal nerve biopsy: not recommended.

TREATMENT

THERAPEUTIC GOAL(S)

Spontaneous activity usually occurs in 2 to 3 weeks with no treatment.

ACUTE GENERAL TREATMENT

- Maintenance of hydration and alimentation is critical.
- Percutaneous gastrostomy may be helpful in severe cases (see Feeding Tube Placement: Percutaneous Endoscopic Gastrostomy [PEG], p 1247).
- Feeding canned food gruel is most helpful since tongue function is maintained.

CHRONIC TREATMENT

Signs will typically resolve spontaneously in 2 to 3 weeks but, in some cases, will take months to totally normalize.

POSSIBLE COMPLICATIONS

- Dehydration
- Weight loss

RECOMMENDED MONITORING

- Hydration status
- Food intake

PROGNOSIS AND OUTCOME

Excellent for recovery

PEARLS & CONSIDERATIONS

COMMENTS

- If signs do not resolve in the 2- to 3-week period, then other differentials need to be considered.
- If sensory deficits are observed, the recovery period may take longer.

CLIENT EDUCATION

- Signs are typically self-limiting and should resolve in 2 to 3 weeks.
- Suggested feeding protocols.

SUGGESTED READING

deLahunta A: General somatic efferent system, special visceral efferent system. In deLahunta A (ed): *Veterinary Neuroanatomy and Clinical Neurology*, ed 2. Philadelphia, WB Saunders, 1983, pp 110–111.

Inzana KD: Peripheral nerve disorders. In Ettinger SJ, Felman EC. (eds): *Textbook of Veterinary Internal Medicine*, ed 6. Philadelphia, Elsevier, 2005, p 900.

Mayhew PD, et al: Trigeminal neuropathy in dogs: A retrospective study of 29 cases (1991–2000). *J Am Anim Hosp Assoc* 38:262, 2002.

Oliver JE, Lorenz MD, Kornegay JN: Disorders of the face, tongue, esophagus, larynx, and hearing. In Oliver JE, Lorenz MD, Kornegay JN (eds): *Handbook of Veterinary Neurology*, ed 4. Philadelphia, Elsevier, 2004, p 249.

AUTHOR: **KAREN L. KLINE**
EDITOR: **CURTIS W. DEWEY**

Tritrichomonas Infection

BASIC INFORMATION

DEFINITION

Infection with an enteric protozoan that has been identified as a cause of large bowel diarrhea in cats

EPIDEMIOLOGY

RISK FACTORS: The predominant risk factor appears to be population density. The infection is most prevalent in cats housed in shelters and catteries and those participating in purebred cat shows.
CONTAGION AND ZOONOSIS: Zoonotic transmission has not been described.

CLINICAL PRESENTATION

HISTORY, CHIEF COMPLAINT: Chronic large bowel diarrhea that is refractory to standard antibiotic or antidiarrheal therapy. The diarrhea is often fetid.
PHYSICAL EXAM FINDINGS: There are no specific physical exam findings. Affected kittens may have a reddened, protruding anal mucosa and may have a thin or unthrifty body condition.

ETIOLOGY AND PATHOPHYSIOLOGY

- *Tritrichomonas foetus* is a single-cell flagellated protozoan found in the colon of domestic cats.
- It does not form cysts but is passed in the feces as a trophozoite.
- Infection occurs by direct transmission.
- The pathophysiologic mechanism has not been described, but, in one case, colonic biopsies revealed severe lymphocytic plasmacytic colitis with multifocal disruption of the surface epithelium.

DIAGNOSIS

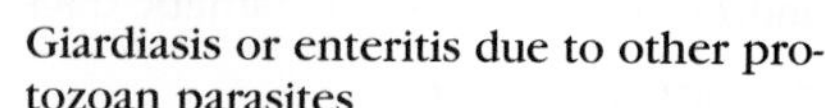

DIFFERENTIAL DIAGNOSIS

- Giardiasis or enteritis due to other protozoan parasites
- Intestinal parasitism
- Idiopathic colitis or inflammatory bowel disease
- Bacterial colitis
- Neoplasia

INITIAL DATABASE

- Microscopic evaluation of fresh fecal preparations for trophozoites; diagnostic test of choice

- ◦ Fecal saline suspension (by mixing a speck of feces with a drop of saline on a microscope slide and covering with coverslip) or fecal smear
- ◦ Motile, ovoid organisms, 10-25-μm long, flagellated
- ◦ Differentiation: unlike *Giardia* spp., trophozoites of *T. foetus* have an undulating membrane and demonstrate directed movement across the slide. *Giardia* spp. form cysts (which may also be seen on fecal suspensions, smears, and flotations) but *T. foetus* does not
- Minimum database (complete blood count [CBC], panel) is typically within normal limits
- Fecal flotation to rule out other parasites
- Imaging (radiographs and ultrasound): generally unremarkable

ADVANCED OR CONFIRMATORY TESTING

- Polymerase chain reaction (PCR) to amplify *T. foetus* rDNA in the feces
- Protozoal culture of feces using the *T. foetus* pouch; rarely indicated or used in the clinical setting

TREATMENT

THERAPEUTIC GOAL(S)

Resolution of diarrhea and eradication of infection

ACUTE AND CHRONIC TREATMENT

- Standard antiprotozoal and antidiarrheal therapies are ineffective for the eradication of *T. foetus* infection and the management of chronic diarrhea associated with this infection.
- Oral ronidazole (a nitroimidazole antimicrobial) 30-50 mg/kg PO q 12h for 2 weeks. Preliminary reports indicate resolution of *T. foetus*-associated diarrhea and eradication of the infection (based on PCR studies); no reported relapses. However, adverse effects (e.g., neurotoxicity) are relatively common with use of ronidazole.

PROGNOSIS AND OUTCOME

- Historically, most cats diagnosed with chronic diarrhea resulting from *T. foetus* infection have had apparent resolution of the diarrhea within 2 years of onset. Chronic *T. foetus* infection following resolution of clinical signs appears to have been common.
- If ronidazole therapy proves to be as effective in large case series as it was initially, the prognosis for treatment is very good.
- There appears to be an inverse correlation between housing density and the interval to the resolution of *T. foetus*-associated diarrhea.

PEARLS & CONSIDERATIONS

COMMENTS

Consider *T. foetus* as a differential diagnosis in cats with chronic large bowel diarrhea, particularly if they are housed with other cats or have come from a shelter or cattery.

SUGGESTED READING

Foster DM, et al: Outcome of cats with diarrhea and *Tritrichomonas foetus* infection. *J Am Vet Med Assoc* 225:888, 2004.

Gookin JL, et al: Prevalence and risk of *T. foetus* infection in cattery cats. *ACVIM Forum Proceedings* 21:16, 2003.

Gookin JL, et al: Efficacy of ronidazole *in vitro* and *in vivo* for treatment of feline *Tritrichomonas foetus* infection [abstract]. *Twenty-Third Annual ACVIM Forum Proceedings* 23:877, 2005, Baltimore, MD.

AUTHOR: **LAURA J. SMALLWOOD**

EDITOR: **DEBRA L. ZORAN**

Tularemia

BASIC INFORMATION

DEFINITION

Acute zoonotic infection caused by gram-negative facultative intracellular bacterium, *Francisella tularensis*

SYNONYM(S)

Rabbit fever
Deerfly fever
Brucella tularensis
Pasteurella tularensis

EPIDEMIOLOGY

SPECIES, AGE, SEX

- Wild and domestic mammals, humans, and birds.
- Cats can be severely affected. Dogs have a mild clinical illness and are uncommonly affected. Puppies and kittens are more susceptible than adults.

RISK FACTORS: Exposure to ticks or wild rabbits or rodents; outdoor cats or hunter cats in endemic areas.

CONTAGION AND ZOONOSIS: Highly zoonotic disease; the infectious dose for humans is less than 100 organisms either inhaled, inoculated, or via conjunctival exposure. Transmission to humans can be through ticks, exposure to tissues of rabbits or rodents, or cat bites or scratches; may be transmitted through dog saliva.

GEOGRAPHY AND SEASONALITY: Throughout the Northern Hemisphere between 20° and 70° latitude.

CLINICAL PRESENTATION

HISTORY, CHIEF COMPLAINT

- Cats may present with severe acute disease approximately 2 to 7 days after exposure
- Dogs may present with anorexia, lethargy, and mucopurulent oculonasal discharge
- Recent contact with rabbits or rabbit carcasses is common

PHYSICAL EXAM FINDINGS

- Cats: frequently severe illness characterized by oral or lingual ulcerations, lymphadenopathy, splenomegaly, hepatomegaly, icterus, fever, depression, and cutaneous abscesses.
- Dogs may have lymphadenopathy, oculonasal discharge, and skin lesions.

ETIOLOGY AND PATHOPHYSIOLOGY

- *F. tularensis* is a small pleomorphic gram-negative intracellular facultative bacillus with two subspecies present in North America.
- Type A (subspecies tularensis) has a rabbit-tick (*Dermacentor variabilis, D. andersoni, D. occidentalis, Amblyomma americanum*) life cycle and is highly virulent for rabbits, humans, and cats.
- Type B (subspecies *holarctica*) is less virulent and is associated with water and the life cycles of aquatic mammals or insects (ticks, mosquitoes).
- Transmission occurs through a tick bite, ingestion of infected rabbits or rodents, or inhalation.
- At the site of inoculation, the organism multiplies and spreads to local lymph nodes. A localized infection and local lymphadenomegaly are often present.

- Bacteremia and multiple organ involvement may follow, particularly in cats and humans.

DIAGNOSIS

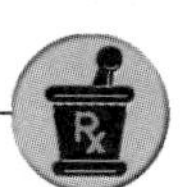

DIFFERENTIAL DIAGNOSIS

- *Yersinia pestis* infection (bubonic plague)
- *Y. pseudotuberculosis* infection

INITIAL DATABASE

- Complete blood cell (CBC) count may show leukopenia with toxic neutrophils
- Serum chemistry panel may show elevated liver enzymes and bilirubin

ADVANCED OR CONFIRMATORY TESTING

- Serologic test results showing an increasing titer with tube agglutination
- Definitive diagnosis: polymerase chain reaction (PCR) or culture of organism from tissue biopsy or aspirate samples (use caution during diagnostic sampling and specimen handling: organism highly zoonotic)

TREATMENT

THERAPEUTIC GOAL(S)

- Cats must be treated early and aggressively.
- Canine cases are often self-limiting, requiring only supportive care.

ACUTE AND CHRONIC TREATMENT

- Supportive therapy to include IV fluids is necessary in acute cases
- Treatments of choice for humans are aminoglycosides (streptomycin or gentamicin). Animals must be adequately hydrated prior to treatment with an aminoglycoside. IV fluid therapy prior to administration is advised
- Bacteriostatic antimicrobials (e.g., tetracycline, chloramphenicol) may be useful but may result in relapses
- Gentamicin 4-8 mg/kg IV, SC, IM q 12-24h in dogs. Ensure hydration and normal renal function prior to treatment to reduce risk of nephrotoxicity
- Streptomycin 10-20 mg/kg IM q 12h in cats and dogs
- Chloramphenicol 25-50 mg/kg IV, IM, SC, PO q 8h in dogs
- Chloramphenicol 50 mg PO or IV q 12h in cats
- Doxycycline 5-10 mg/kg PO or IV q 12-24h

DRUG INTERACTIONS

- Aminoglycosides should not be used with other drugs excreted by the kidneys.
- Chloramphenicol can inhibit hepatic metabolism of several drugs (phenobarbital, cyclophosphamide).

POSSIBLE COMPLICATIONS

- Aminoglycosides are potentially nephrotoxic and ototoxic.
  - Decrease dose of aminoglycoside in animals with renal insufficiency or choose another treatment
- Chloramphenicol may cause fatal aplastic anemia in humans. Wear gloves and wash hands when handling.
- Chloramphenicol may cause a dose-dependent bone marrow suppression in animals and can cause gastrointestinal (GI) signs. Cats are more sensitive to developing adverse reactions. Reduce dose in animals with liver disease.
- Doxycycline may cause GI signs. Esophageal stricture may develop in cats, particularly when pills are halved, and prevention consists of giving a few cc of tap water PO by syringe after each dose.

RECOMMENDED MONITORING

Frequent monitoring of blood urea nitrogen (BUN), creatinine, urine γ-glutamyl transferase (GGT), and urine sediment while on aminoglycosides

PROGNOSIS AND OUTCOME

- Rapidly fatal in cats
- Self-limiting infection in dogs

PEARLS & CONSIDERATIONS

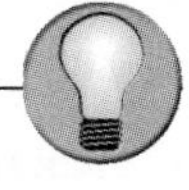

COMMENTS

- May be underreported in dogs due to self-limiting nature
- Highly zoonotic

PREVENTION

- Tick control
- Limit exposure to rabbits
- Neuter cats to prevent hunting and roaming

CLIENT EDUCATION

No recorded transmission from infected dog to humans but the possibility is not excluded

SUGGESTED READING

Kaufmann AF: Tularemia. In Greene CE (ed): *Infectious Diseases of the Dog and Cat.* Philadelphia, WB Saunders, 1998, pp 300-302.

Meinkoth KR, Morton RJ, Meinkoth JH: Naturally occurring tularemia in a dog. *J Am Vet Med Assoc* 225(4):545-547, 2004.

Woods JP, Panciera RJ, Morton RJ: Feline tularemia. *Comp Cont Educ Pract Vet* 20:442-256, 1998.

AUTHOR: **LISA M. TIEBER NIELSON**

EDITOR: **DOUGLASS K. MACINTIRE**

Ulcerative and Erosive Skin Disorders

BASIC INFORMATION

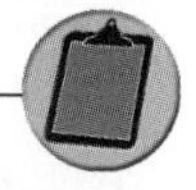

DEFINITION

A cutaneous erosion is a shallow epidermal defect that does not penetrate the basal membrane. Erosions are usually associated with self trauma. A cutaneous ulcer is produced by a break in the continuity of the epidermis with exposure of the underlying dermis. Ulcers are usually a consequence of a deep and serious pathologic process. Healing ulcers typically result in scarring.

EPIDEMIOLOGY

SPECIES, AGE, SEX: Vary according to the underlying pathologic process:

- Some dermatoses are seen more frequently or strictly in one species rather than another (e.g., eosinophilic plaque in cats).
- Young animals are predisposed to genetic defects or infectious diseases, whereas older animals are predisposed to immune-mediated diseases or neoplasia.

GENETICS AND BREED PREDISPOSITION: Some diseases tend to have a genetic basis or are related to anatomic defects (e.g., intertrigo in such breeds as the Chinese shar-pei).

CONTAGION AND ZOONOSIS

- Some skin diseases are more likely to occur in animals kept outdoors (e.g., burns, frostbite, infectious diseases).
- Repeated contact with other animals can increase the risk of animals developing contagious diseases (e.g., herpesvirus

infection). It is important to be aware of affected animals.

CLINICAL PRESENTATION

HISTORY, CHIEF COMPLAINT: A thorough history of the animal is important considering the extensive list of differential diagnoses. Some essential clues help to define the condition:

- It is important to know if the animal travels, is regularly groomed, has a boarding history, or has been in any situation that would increase its risk of developing a certain condition. This information will help to determine which dermatoses are more likely; geographic information (e.g., leishmaniasis in dogs traveling to Europe) and information concerning exposure to contagious disorders (e.g., herpesvirus infection in cats) can be key in making the diagnosis.
- Dietary history (e.g., food allergy).
- Signs of systemic illness (e.g., lethargy, anorexia, lameness, etc.). Presence of such signs narrows the differential diagnosis, and diagnostic methods will be oriented differently (e.g., toward systemic lupus erythematosus [SLE], leishmaniasis, systemic mycoses).
- Prior treatments: response to prior therapy or therapy administered prior to onset of clinical signs allows the inclusion or exclusion of some dermatoses (e.g., drug eruption).

PHYSICAL EXAM FINDINGS

- Dermatologic examination is important for identifying erosive and ulcerative lesions, but a general physical examination is essential to detect signs of systemic diseases.
- The clinician should take note of primary lesions such as vesicles, bullae, and pustules and the distribution of the lesions (e.g., involvement of the mucosa).This information can suggest a specific group of diseases.
- Secondary lesions, such as crusts, are common.
- Exact description of the lesions varies according to the underlying disease.

ETIOLOGY AND PATHOPHYSIOLOGY

Variable, depending on underlying cause.

- Congenital, hereditary, and conformational defects. For example, ulcerations can result from skin friction (e.g., intertrigo) or can be secondary to an abnormal fragility of the dermoepidermal junction (e.g., epidermolysis bullosa).
- Infectious diseases (bacterial, viral, parasitic, fungal, rickettsial): Some organisms infect and lyse keratinocytes (e.g., herpesvirus) or can cause epidermal necrosis secondary to either vasculitis (e.g., canine Rocky Mountain spotted fever) or a substantial inflammatory reaction, leading to ulcerative dermatitis.
- Immune-mediated disorders: Ulcers may follow the rupture of vesicles and bullae caused by the action of antibodies.
- Drug-induced conditions.
- Self-induced lesions.
- Environmental injuries (e.g., coagulation necrosis of the epidermis/dermis associated with thermal or chemical burns results in ulcerations).
- Secondary to systemic diseases (e.g., uremia resulting from renal failure may cause oral ulceration).
- Ischemic disorders: any dermatopathy that interferes with vascular supply of the skin can potentially cause ulcers secondary to skin necrosis.
- Neoplasia: ulcerations noticed in skin tumors, such as cutaneous epitheliotropic lymphoma or squamous cell carcinoma (SCC), are usually secondary to the infiltration of the skin by neoplastic cells and correlate with the aggressiveness of the tumor.
- Idiopathic condition.

DIAGNOSIS

DIFFERENTIAL DIAGNOSIS

- Congenital and hereditary: idiopathic facial dermatitis of Persian and Himalayan cats, aplasia cutis, epidermolysis bullosa (EB), familial canine dermatomyositis
- Infectious diseases: demodicosis, flea bite hypersensitivity, feline mosquito bite hypersensitivity, fly dermatitis; systemic mycoses, sporotrichosis, phaeohyphomycosis, zygomycosis, candidiasis, dermatophyte granuloma, pseudomycetoma, protothecosis, pythiosis, aspergillosis; deep pyoderma, mucocutaneous pyoderma, pyotraumatic dermatitis; feline leukemia virus (FeLV), feline cowpox, feline calicivirus (FCV), feline herpesvirus (FHV); canine Rocky Mountain spotted fever, leishmaniasis
- Immune-mediated disorders: pemphigus, bullous pemphigoid, erythema multiforme, toxic epidermal necrolysis, vasculitis, lupus erythematosus, EB acquisita, cold-agglutinin disease, cutaneous drug eruption
- Self-induced lesions: pruritic dermatoses, psychogenic dermatoses, neuropathies
- Environmental injuries: burns, frostbites
- Systemic diseases: necrolytic migratory erythema, calcinosis cutis, uremia
- Neoplasia: SCC, cutaneous epitheliotropic lymphoma, mast cell tumor, paraneoplastic alopecia
- Conformational dermatoses: intertrigo, pressure sores
- Miscellaneous: feline indolent ulcer, feline eosinophilic plaque, feline plasma cell pododermatitis, feline ulcerative dermatitis with linear subepidermal fibrosis, snakebite

INITIAL DATABASE

- Patient history and physical examination are very important in the diagnostic process
- Cytologic examination of any exudate contents: bacteria, inflammatory cells, acantholytic keratinocytes (pemphigus), fungal organisms
- Complete blood count (CBC), serum biochemistry panel, and urinalysis if systemic signs are observed; type of tests depends on suspected cause

ADVANCED OR CONFIRMATORY TESTING

- Skin biopsies for histopathologic examination are indicated in most cases of ulcerative dermatoses
- Endocrine tests and serologic examination depend on suspected disease
- Coombs' test: cold-agglutinin disease
- Antinuclear antibody (ANA) test: positive in virtually all animals with SLE
- Radiographs and ultrasound, if relevant, to confirm systemic disease or stage tumors

TREATMENT

THERAPEUTIC GOAL(S)

To address the primary cause of the erosions or ulcers

ACUTE GENERAL TREATMENT

- Varies considerably according to the disease.
- Immunosuppressive treatments are required in immune-mediated diseases, while infectious diseases require proper antimicrobial treatment.
- Antiparasitic treatments may be required.
- Neoplastic diseases should be addressed according to the type of tumor.
- Some conformational dermatoses may need surgery to correct the skin defect.
- Supportive care may be required, especially in animals with severe lesions or systemic illness.

PROGNOSIS AND OUTCOME

Good to poor depending of the primary cause of the disease

PEARLS & CONSIDERATIONS

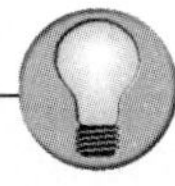

COMMENTS

- Considering the wide range of treatments, make a definitive diagnosis to address correctly the disease and to prevent adverse effects of an improper treatment trial.

- Be aware of the zoonotic potential of some of these diseases.
- Some of these diseases are life threatening.

SUGGESTED READING

Mason IS: Erosions and ulcerations. In Ettinger SJ, Feldman EC (eds): *Textbook of Veterinary Internal Medicine*, ed 6. St. Louis, Elsevier Saunders, 2005, pp 46–50.

Scott DW, Miller WH, Griffin CE: In *Muller and Kirk's Small Animal Dermatology*, ed 6. Philadelphia, WB Saunders, 2001.

AUTHOR: **FRÉDÉRIC SAUVÉ**
EDITOR: **JAN A. HALL**

Ulcers, Oral Mucosal

BASIC INFORMATION

DEFINITION

Focal or multifocal loss of superficial epithelial integrity affecting the oral mucosa

EPIDEMIOLOGY

SPECIES, AGE, SEX: Dogs and cats of either gender and all ages can be affected.

GENETICS AND BREED PREDISPOSITION: Maltese, Cavalier King Charles spaniel, cocker spaniel, and Bouvier des Flandres dogs are predisposed to chronic ulcerative periodontal stomatitis (CUPS). Abyssinian and Somali cats are predisposed to lymphocytic/plasmacytic stomatitis (LPS).

CONTAGION AND ZOONOSIS: Feline leukemia virus (FeLV), feline immunodeficiency virus (FIV), feline herpesvirus (FHV), and feline calicivirus (FCV) in cats are transmissible to other cats. Leptospirosis is transmissible to other animals and human beings.

CLINICAL PRESENTATION

HISTORY, CHIEF COMPLAINT

- Lethargy
- Anorexia
- Behavior change due to oral pain
- Halitosis
- Hypersalivation

PHYSICAL EXAM FINDINGS

- Gingivitis
- Faucitis
- Pharyngitis
- Dental plaque accumulation
- Oral mass
- Buccitis/buccal mucosal ulceration
- Lingual ulceration
- Kissing ulcers: mucosal ulceration (common in CUPS)
- Scar tissue formation on lateral margins of tongue (CUPS)

ETIOLOGY AND PATHOPHYSIOLOGY

- Metabolic causes: renal failure (uremia; common), diabetes mellitus, hypothyroidism, hypoparathyroidism
- Immune-mediated disease: Oral ulcers occur with pemphigus vulgaris (90% of cases), bullous pemphigoid (80% of cases), systemic lupus erythematosus (SLE) (50% of cases), and discoid lupus erythematosus and can also be drug-induced (toxic epidermal necrolysis)
- Infectious: FeLV, FIV, FCV, FHV, leptospirosis (dogs), periodontal disease (dogs and cats)
- Neoplastic: melanoma, squamous cell carcinoma (SCC), fibrosarcoma
- Traumatic: foreign body, electric cord shock, malocclusion, "gum chewer's disease" (chronic chewing of cheek)
- Idiopathic: eosinophilic granuloma (cats, Siberian huskies, Samoyeds), LPS, CUPS
- Miscellaneous: caustic burns (acids), thallium toxicity, protein-calorie malnutrition, riboflavin deficiency

DIAGNOSIS

DIFFERENTIAL DIAGNOSIS

- History, physical and oral exam: can differentiate foreign bodies, malocclusions, toxin/chemical exposure, and electrical burns
- Breed predispositions and response to therapy can help identify idiopathic disorders

INITIAL DATABASE

- Thorough oral examination (may require sedation or general anesthesia)
- Complete blood count (CBC): inflammatory leukogram may be present with infectious or immune-mediated diseases
- Serum biochemical profile: evidence for metabolic disease (e.g., renal failure)
- Urinalysis: urine specific gravity may support a diagnosis of renal failure. Proteinuria may be present if immune-mediated, neoplastic, or infectious disorders cause secondary glomerular damage

ADVANCED OR CONFIRMATORY TESTING

- Serologic titers or other tests (e.g., polymerase chain reaction [PCR]) for infectious agents (e.g., FeLV, herpesvirus) or systemic immune-mediated disease (e.g., antinuclear antibody titer for SLE)
- Thyroid hormone assays
- Thoracic radiographs: evaluation for metastatic disease
- Oral radiographs: evaluation for concurrent osteomyelitis secondary to severe periodontal disease or bony involvement from malignant neoplasia
- Mucosal or gingival biopsy: support for diagnosis of idiopathic, immune-mediated, chronic inflammatory and neoplastic diseases

TREATMENT

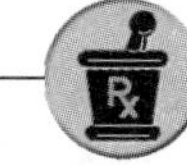

THERAPEUTIC GOAL(S)

Correct underlying cause if possible

ACUTE GENERAL TREATMENT

Supportive therapy:

- Soft diets
- Fluid support (SC or IV) if the patient is dehydrated
- Nutrition: esophagostomy or gastrostomy feeding tubes may be required if oral disease or pain is resulting in steadfast and prolonged anorexia. See Feeding Tube Placement: Nasoesophageal and Nasogastric, p 1245; Feeding Tube Placement: Percutaneous Endoscopic Gastrostomy (PEG), p 1247.

CHRONIC TREATMENT

- For idiopathic conditions (i.e., CUPS, LPS), meticulous dental care to prevent plaque accumulation is necessary. In addition, dental extractions (partial, caudal, or full mouth) may be necessary to remove the source of inflammation.
- Treat metabolic conditions if present.
- Immunosuppressive drug therapy (e.g., corticosteroids, azathioprine) may be required for immune-mediated diseases.
- Antimicrobial therapy may be required to treat secondary periodontal or oral infections.
- Topical solutions (e.g., chlorhexidine solution) to inhibit bacterial growth or to promote improved dental health may be beneficial.

POSSIBLE COMPLICATIONS

Side effects from corticosteroid (e.g., polyuria and polydipsia [PU/PD]) or immunosuppressive medications (e.g., myelosuppression)

RECOMMENDED MONITORING

Dependent on cause and therapies employed

PROGNOSIS AND OUTCOME

- Dependent on underlying cause.
- The idiopathic conditions (CUPS, LPS) can be difficult to treat and require considerable client commitment and compliance.

PEARLS & CONSIDERATIONS

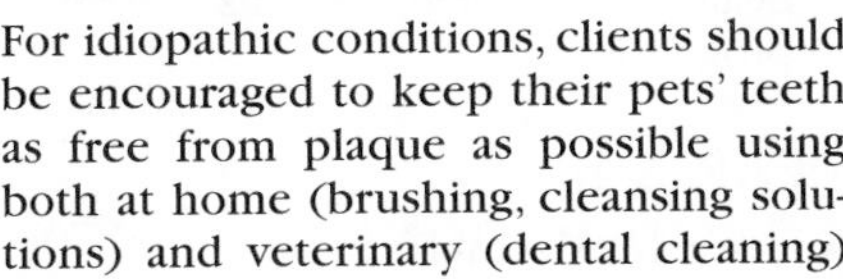

CLIENT EDUCATION

For idiopathic conditions, clients should be encouraged to keep their pets' teeth as free from plaque as possible using both at home (brushing, cleansing solutions) and veterinary (dental cleaning) therapies. See Dental Preventative (Home) Care, p 1221.

SUGGESTED READING

Mason IS: Erosions and ulcerations. In Ettinger SJ, Feldman EC (eds): *Textbook of Veterinary Internal Medicine*, ed 6. St. Louis, Elsevier Saunders, 2005, pp 46–50.

Smith MM: Oral and salivary gland disorders. In Ettinger SJ, Feldman EC (eds): *Textbook of Veterinary Internal Medicine*, ed 6. St. Louis, Elsevier Saunders, 2005, pp 1290–1297.

AUTHOR: **DARCY H. SHAW**

EDITOR: **ETIENNE CÔTÉ**

Umbilical Hernia

BASIC INFORMATION

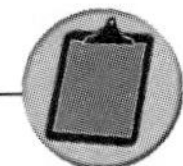

DEFINITION

Full-thickness congenital abdominal wall defect at the umbilicus

EPIDEMIOLOGY

SPECIES, AGE, SEX

- Dogs and cats
- Greater incidence in females of predisposed breeds

GENETICS AND BREED PREDISPOSITION

- Breed predisposition in dogs:
  - Airedale terrier, basenji, Pekingese, pointer, and weimaraner
- Could be an inherited defect:
  - Polygenic inheritance possible

ASSOCIATED CONDITIONS AND DISORDERS

- Fucosidosis, an inherited lysosomal storage disease reported in English springer spaniels
- Cryptorchidism
- Incomplete caudal sternal fusion
- Pericardial peritoneal diaphragmatic hernia
- Exstrophy of the bladder
- Hypospadia
- Imperforate anus

CLINICAL PRESENTATION

DISEASE FORMS/SUBTYPES

- Uncomplicated:
  - Single umbilical hernia without incarceration or strangulation of abdominal contents, concurrent anatomic abnormalities, or multiple hernias.
- Complicated:
  - Presence of multiple hernias; other associated anatomic abnormalities, defects, or diseases; or strangulation or contamination of abdominal contents.
- Omphalocele:
  - Large midline umbilical hernia and skin defect that allow abdominal organs to protrude externally. The umbilical sac is merely a thin transparent membrane (amniotic sac). The membrane is attached to the hernia edges and may rupture easily. Most affected puppies die or are euthanized before treatment is sought.
- Gastroschisis:
  - Grossly similar to omphalocele, but the defect is paramedian.

HISTORY, CHIEF COMPLAINT

- None: incidental finding (most common)
- Soft swelling at umbilicus: may be noticed by some owners
- Systemic signs of illness (anorexia, vomiting, lethargy) are possible if abdominal contents are strangulated

PHYSICAL EXAM FINDINGS

- Protruding mass at the umbilicus:
  - Soft, fluctuant, and reducible, especially if animal is placed in dorsal recumbency
  - Large, firm, and irreducible if contents are incarcerated
- Acute intestinal incarceration or strangulation:
  - Firm, painful mass; vomiting, abdominal pain, signs of sepsis are possible

ETIOLOGY AND PATHOPHYSIOLOGY

- Abdominal wall of the embryo normally is formed by migration of cephalic, caudal, and lateral folds.
- Umbilical aperture remains after normal migration and fusion of the folds.
- Umbilical hernia results when the lateral folds, principally the rectus abdominis muscle and fascia, fail to fuse or have delayed fusion after the midgut relocates in the sixth week of gestation.

DIAGNOSIS

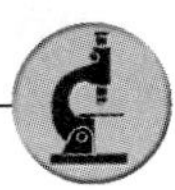

DIFFERENTIAL DIAGNOSIS

Traumatic umbilical hernia: peripartum insult caused by traction on umbilical cord or cutting cord too close to abdominal wall

INITIAL DATABASE

Survey abdominal and thoracic radiographs; only needed if hernia is very large and if other anomalies (diaphragmatic hernia, incomplete sternal fusion, strangulation/incarceration) are present

ADVANCED OR CONFIRMATORY TESTING

Ultrasound examination (uncommonly used; only considered with large and/or incarcerated hernia contents) to determine contents of hernia

TREATMENT

THERAPEUTIC GOAL(S)

- Resolve any existing visceral entrapment
- Reduce or eliminate risk of herniation of abdominal viscera

ACUTE GENERAL TREATMENT

- Conservative treatment:
  - Small hernia (less than the size of the intestine; i.e., the size of a fingertip)
  - Spontaneous closure may occur as late as 6 months of age
- Surgical correction:
  - Large hernia but no associated clinical problems (incarceration of abdominal contents):
    - Elective surgical correction; also repaired when another elective surgical procedure (ovariohysterectomy, orchiectomy) is performed

- Large hernia with evidence of incarcerated or strangulated viscera:
    - Immediate surgical correction
- Omphalocele:
    - Immediate surgical correction to prevent further organ damage or contamination

POSSIBLE COMPLICATIONS

- Dehiscence of repair:
    - Large defect
    - Excess tension on repair
    - Friability of abdominal wall
- Gastroschisis and omphalocele may be associated with early neonatal death:
    - Contamination of abdominal contents
    - Inability to correct defect

RECOMMENDED MONITORING

Counsel owners to watch for enlargement of hernia or acute gastrointestinal (GI) signs in animals that are managed conservatively; onset warrants immediate evaluation and consideration of surgical correction

PROGNOSIS AND OUTCOME

- Excellent with uncomplicated umbilical hernia and successful closure
- Guarded to poor with complicated or open hernia
- Status of animal at presentation and health of herniated contents determine prognosis

PEARLS & CONSIDERATIONS

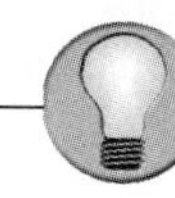

COMMENTS

- There are usually no clinical signs associated with umbilical hernias. Correction is usually an elective procedure.
- Entrapment of abdominal contents can occur with larger hernias.
- Always examine animals with umbilical hernias for additional congenital abnormalities.

PREVENTION

- Consideration should be given to avoiding breeding affected dogs or cats because this condition is usually an inherited defect.
- At the time of the animal's birth, carefully ligate and transect the umbilical cord, without excessive traction, at least 1-2 cm from the neonate's body wall.

CLIENT EDUCATION

- Treatment may be conservative, or a herniorrhaphy may be required to prevent complications.
- Veterinarians should train breeders in proper neonatal care.

SUGGESTED READING

Robinson R: Genetic aspects of umbilical hernia incidence in cats and dogs. *Vet Red* 100:9-10, 1977.

Smeak DD: In Slatter D (ed): *Textbook of Small Animal Surgery*, ed 3. Philadelphia, WB Saunders, 2003, pp 449-50.

AUTHOR: **ELLEN B. DAVIDSON DOMNICK**

EDITOR: **RICHARD WALSHAW**

Unerupted Teeth

BASIC INFORMATION

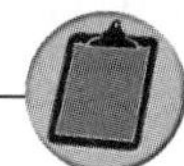

DEFINITION

Teeth that have not emerged into the mouth are unerupted. Clinically, the tooth appears to be missing. Radiographic diagnosis is required.

SYNONYM(S)

Embedded teeth (unerupted for no obvious reason)

Impacted teeth (unerupted because of some interposing tissue, such as an adjacent tooth)

EPIDEMIOLOGY

SPECIES, AGE, SEX: Unerupted teeth occur more commonly in the younger dog and less commonly in cats. They may not be recognized until animals have reached adulthood. There is no sex predilection.

GENETICS AND BREED PREDISPOSITION: Familial delayed eruption does occur in Tibetan and Wheaten terriers, and toy breeds can have overall slower eruption times. Because erupting teeth can be influenced by internal and external causes, a genetic link is suspected but difficult to prove.

RISK FACTORS

- Persistent deciduous teeth (see Deciduous Teeth, Persistent ["Retained"], p 277)
- Regional trauma
- Certain endocrine disorders
- Malnutrition

ASSOCIATED CONDITIONS AND DISORDERS: Dentigerous (tooth-containing) cyst (also called follicular cyst).

CLINICAL PRESENTATION

HISTORY, CHIEF COMPLAINT: Animals present for evaluation of missing teeth, but the majority of unerupted teeth are found incidentally on routine physical examination.

PHYSICAL EXAM FINDINGS: Most animals are in good health. Oral examination reveals an edentulous (toothless) region. Permanent premolars are the most common unerupted teeth, but any tooth can be affected. If a dentigerous cyst is present, a fluctuant soft-tissue swelling may be located in the edentulous region.

ETIOLOGY AND PATHOPHYSIOLOGY

- Complications leading to abnormal tooth eruption are many and varied: primary defects in the eruptive process, genetic/traumatic displacement of the tooth bud, mechanical obstruction from surrounding structures.
- Endocrine abnormalities (hypothyroidism, cretinism, hypogonadism, mongolism, hypopituitarism) can prevent or slow the eruption of teeth.
- Unerupted teeth can incite dentigerous cyst formation: an epithelial-lined soft tissue is attached to the cementoenamel junction of an unerupted tooth with the crown protruding into the fluid-filled cyst, causing pressure resorption of alveolar bone, displacement of adjacent teeth, abscess, and fistulation.

DIAGNOSIS

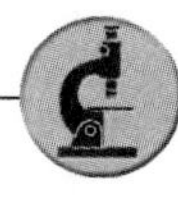

DIFFERENTIAL DIAGNOSIS

Edentulous region:

- Partially erupted, ankylosed, embedded, and impacted teeth
- Presence of an operculum (tough gingival covering preventing tooth eruption)
- Anodontia and hypodontia resulting from a large variety of causes
- Fractured tooth ± retained tooth roots
- Previously extracted tooth

Edentulous region associated with soft tissue swelling:

- Odontoma
- Cyst (e.g., radicular, dentigerous)
- Abscess
- Neoplasia

INITIAL DATABASE

- Complete blood count (CBC), serum biochemistry panel, urinalysis: generally unremarkable

- Full mouth (intraoral) dental radiographs

ADVANCED OR CONFIRMATORY TESTING

CT scan: if associated cystic structure is large and to define surgical margins and/or regions for debridement

TREATMENT

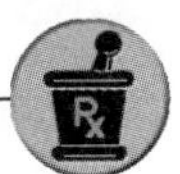

THERAPEUTIC GOAL(S)

- Preserve normal anatomy
- Encourage complete tooth eruption
- Prevent cyst/abscess formation

ACUTE GENERAL TREATMENT

- No treatment if entire tooth is missing on radiographs.
- Unerupted teeth with eruption potential (open tooth root apex on radiographs) can be orthodontically coaxed into position.
- If an operculum is present, dissect gingiva to allow for tooth eruption (operculectomy).
- Surgically extract unerupted teeth without eruption potential to prevent dentigerous cyst development. Curettage of the extraction site is recommended to remove remnant odontogenic tissue. Postoperative radiographs ensure complete removal of all tooth structures.
- If a dentigerous cyst is present, the tooth and cyst are removed *en bloc*. If this is not possible, extensive curettage to remove all epithelial cyst lining is mandatory because small islands of remaining epithelium can lead to cyst reoccurrence or malignant transformation.
- Flaps should be closed with synthetic absorbable suture material.
- Administration of antibiotics is not usually necessary after the extraction procedure unless another medical condition or extensive tissue trauma at the extraction site is present.
- Pain management: local nerve block (0.3-0.5 ml of 0.5% bupivacaine hydrochloride) intraoperatively followed by nonsteroidal anti-inflammatory drugs [NSAIDs] (e.g., deracoxib 2 mg/kg PO q 24h) ± opioid medications (butorphanol 0.2-0.4 mg/kg PO q 4-6h) given postoperatively for 2 to 3 days.

POSSIBLE COMPLICATIONS

- Inability to locate the unerupted tooth
- Extraction of a healthy erupting permanent tooth
- Cyst reoccurrence
- Regional trauma due to improper extraction technique
- Infection

RECOMMENDED MONITORING

- Examination 1 to 2 weeks postoperatively to evaluate extraction sites
- Cyst: examination with radiographs in 6 months

PROGNOSIS AND OUTCOME

- Unerupted teeth with operculectomy: fair for tooth eruption (depends on tooth eruption potential)
- Extracted unerupted teeth: excellent for extraction site healing
- Dentigerous cyst: excellent if all cystic lining is removed

PEARLS & CONSIDERATIONS

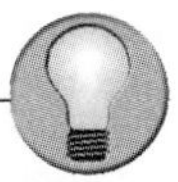

COMMENTS

- No tooth should be considered "missing" without radiographic diagnosis.
- Extraction of unerupted teeth may be unnecessary in older pets (>8-9 years) if there is no radiographic evidence of associated lesions. The odds a dentigerous cyst will form at this age are low.

PREVENTION

- Removal of persistent deciduous teeth
- Early recognition of "missing" teeth in young animals

SUGGESTED READING

Gioso MA, Carvalho VG: Maxillary dentigerous cyst in a cat. *J Vet Dent* 20:28, 2003.

Harvey CE, Emily PP: *Small Animal Dentistry*. St. Louis, Mosby, 1993, pp 276-281.

Mulligan TW, Aller MS, Williams CA: *Atlas of Canine and Feline Dental Radiography*. Trenton, NJ, Veterinary Learning Systems, 1998, pp 91-103, 188-189.

AUTHOR: **JENNIFER E. RAWLINSON**
EDITOR: **ALEXANDER M. REITER**

Upper Airway Obstruction

BASIC INFORMATION

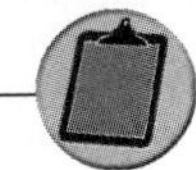

DEFINITION

The inability to move air effectively through trachea, larynx, pharynx, or nose and mouth

SYNONYM(S)

Choking
Occlusion of the upper airway

EPIDEMIOLOGY

SPECIES, AGE, SEX

- No sex predilection.
- Young dogs may be more likely to have foreign objects lodged in their airways.
- Older dogs may be more likely to have tumors or to acquire laryngeal paralysis.
- Young cats may have nasopharyngeal polyps.

GENETICS AND BREED PREDISPOSITION: Short-nosed (brachycephalic) animals are predisposed to airway obstruction.

RISK FACTORS: Environmental factors: excitement, heat, and exercise, especially in animals with physical predisposition (e.g., elongated soft palate, laryngeal paresis).

GEOGRAPHY AND SEASONALITY: More common in warmer climates (heat stress).

ASSOCIATED CONDITIONS AND DISORDERS: Brachycephalic upper airway syndrome, laryngeal paralysis, neoplasia.

CLINICAL PRESENTATION

DISEASE FORMS/SUBTYPES

- Supraglottic structures: "brachycephalic upper airway syndrome," which includes stenoic nares, elongated soft palate, and/or eversion of laryngeal saccules. Laryngeal paralysis (bilateral) may be acquired in older dogs; foreign bodies (pharyngeal) are more common in dogs than cats; laryngeal collapse, laryngeal edema, and nasopharyngeal polyps are common in cats.
- Subglottic structures: tracheal neoplasia, tracheal hypoplasia (the fourth component of brachycephalic upper airway syndrome), tracheal collapse, foreign-body aspiration, trauma.

HISTORY, CHIEF COMPLAINT: Owners often report that their pet appears anxious or agitated, that he or she is having difficulty breathing, and that they can hear loud respiratory noises or a honking cough. Clinical signs can occur more commonly after exercise, excitement, or on a warm day. Animals may have been witnessed aspirating a foreign object.

However, overinterpretation of inhaled foreign bodies as the cause of upper airway obstruction is a mistake that is frequently made by owners. Dogs and cats that have a sudden onset of respiratory signs (e.g., due to pulmonary edema, pleural effusion, or other causes not involving foreign bodies) often may be thought mistakenly by owners to have inhaled a foreign body.

PHYSICAL EXAM FINDINGS: Common findings include noisy and/or stridorous breathing. Hyperthermia may be present due to excessive muscle activity from inspiratory effort. Conformation changes (e.g., short nose) may be present. Often, loud sounds may be ausculted over the trachea and may be referred to the lower airways.

ETIOLOGY AND PATHOPHYSIOLOGY

Most of the resistance to airflow occurs in the upper airways. Any fixed or dynamic obstruction in the upper airways will increase the resistance to breathing and, subsequently, the work of breathing.

Inspiration against a partially or completely closed upper airway may cause flooding of pulmonary alveoli with plasma (i.e., noncardiogenic pulmonary edema due to negative pressure generated in the air space).

DIAGNOSIS

DIFFERENTIAL DIAGNOSIS

- Occasionally, pleural effusion in cats will mimic upper respiratory obstruction.
- Commonly, upper airway obstruction is suspected on physical exam alone, and the differential diagnosis involves determination of the cause of the obstruction rather than the site of the respiratory problem.

INITIAL DATABASE

- Oral examination under sedation is the most important diagnostic test. The clinician should be prepared for an emergent tracheostomy (and possibly positive-pressure ventilation, if noncardiogenic pulmonary edema is present) if needed.
- Other ancillary testing includes radiographs (thoracic and neck), ultrasound, complete blood count (CBC)/serum biochemistry profile, and evaluation of oxygenation (pulse oximetry or arterial blood gas [ABG] analysis).

ADVANCED OR CONFIRMATORY TESTING

Bronchoscopy, fluoroscopy, or CT scan may be useful for evaluating focal lesions or obtaining biopsies or cytologic specimens.

TREATMENT

THERAPEUTIC GOAL(S)

Minimize stress and address the clinical signs until a definitive diagnosis and plan can be made to alleviate the airway problem

ACUTE GENERAL TREATMENT

- Tranquilizers or analgesics, corticosteroids at anti-inflammatory doses, and oxygen supplementation. Secure airway if necessary. See Intubation, Endotracheal, p 1269; Tracheostomy, p 1310.
- If hyperthermia is due to exertion or anxiety (i.e., muscle activity, not true fever), it can respond to physical cooling measures but not to anti-inflammatory drugs (see Heat Stroke/Hyperthermia, p 467).

CHRONIC TREATMENT

Either medical or surgical management of the underlying problem

- Medical: anxiolytics, antitussives, and environmental control
- Surgical: stenoic nares repair; soft palate resection; everted laryngeal saccule resection; abscess drainage; tracheal ring implants; removal of foreign body, tumor, or polyp; permanent tracheostomy; or temporary tracheotomy

POSSIBLE COMPLICATIONS

Postsurgical complications include the recurrence of clinical signs, aspiration pneumonia, noncardiogenic pulmonary edema, and/or respiratory arrest.

RECOMMENDED MONITORING

Monitor respiratory rate/effort and mucous membrane color

PROGNOSIS AND OUTCOME

Depend on the actual underlying problem and the degree of clinical signs

PEARLS & CONSIDERATIONS

COMMENTS

- Up to one-half of the diameter of the airway can be compromised without obvious clinical signs.
- Major errors in the initial treatment include underestimation of the patient's distress, overzealous examination, and performance of diagnostics that are detrimental to the condition of the patient at that time.
- A common radiographic misdiagnosis is the interpretation of a prominent or mineralized (but normal) larynx as a foreign body, especially if the neck is radiographed obliquely.
- Thoracic radiography and positive-pressure ventilation should be planned in case dyspnea and/or hypoxemia persist after relief of upper airway obstruction, as can occur when noncardiogenic pulmonary edema is also present.

PREVENTION

Avoid overexertion; prevent heat stress and know the medical options that are available to help break the cycle of distress and resultant respiratory difficulty

CLIENT EDUCATION

Explain to owners that a brachycephalic animal is predisposed to developing upper airway problems

SUGGESTED READING

Aron DN, et al: Upper airway obstruction. *Vet Clin North Am Small An Pract* 15:891, 1985.

Griffon DJ: Upper airway obstruction in cats: Pathogenesis and clinical signs. *Compend Contin Educ Pract Vet* 22:822, 2000.

Griffon DJ: Upper airway obstruction in cats: Diagnosis and treatment. *Compend Contin Educ Pract Vet* 22:897, 2000.

AUTHOR: **MEGAN WHELAN**

EDITOR: **ELIZABETH ROZANSKI**

Upper Respiratory Infection, Feline

BASIC INFORMATION

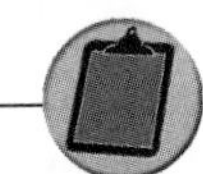

DEFINITION

A complex of viral and bacterial agents can cause upper respiratory tract signs, such as sneezing, nasal congestion, and nasal discharge, in cats. Etiologies include feline herpesvirus (FHV), feline calicivirus (FCV), *Bordetella bronchiseptica*, *Chlamydophila felis*, and, less commonly, feline reovirus, cowpox virus, and mycoplasmas

SYNONYM(S)

Feline infectious respiratory disease
Feline respiratory disease complex
C. felis: previously known as *Chlamydia psittaci*
Feline herpesvirus: feline rhinotracheitis virus

EPIDEMIOLOGY

SPECIES, AGE, SEX: The main causative infectious agents (herpes- and caliciviruses) are confined to the family of Felidae and are typically found in young animals. Mycoplasmas are often found as normal flora in the upper respiratory tract of many species.

RISK FACTORS

- Poor husbandry and overcrowding in catteries or rescue shelters
- Exposure to free-roaming cats in high-density feral populations

CONTAGION AND ZOONOSIS: FHV and FCV are shed in ocular, nasal, and oral secretions and are passed via direct cat-to-cat contact. Both viruses spread easily through susceptible populations and are perpetuated by carrier animals not showing overt signs. Disease can be spread via fomites, such as contaminated cages, bowls, and clothing. FCV can persist in the environment for up to 1 month.

Direct aerosol transmission is actually an unlikely cause of respiratory disease spread due to the small feline tidal lung volume and relatively low numbers of pathogenic organisms in the respiratory volume. Sneezing of nasal-oral secretions, however, may disseminate a virus more readily over a radius of several feet.

GEOGRAPHY AND SEASONALITY: Worldwide and no true seasonality; more cases may be noted in late spring and summer when many susceptible kittens are added to the population.

CLINICAL PRESENTATION

DISEASE FORMS/SUBTYPES: Herpesvirus: in young animals, usually acute, severe upper respiratory signs; in chronic adult cases, often manifests as a chronic conjunctivitis/keratitis without respiratory signs.

Calicivirus: typical upper respiratory signs; isolated highly virulent strains that cause severe systemic disease and death have been noted.

HISTORY, CHIEF COMPLAINT

- General signs of respiratory disease complex include anorexia, lethargy, ocular and nasal discharges, sneezing, epiphora, blepharospasm
- Specific to calicivirus (see Calicivirus, Cat, p 171), Herpesvirus, and *C. felis* (see Herpesviral Keratitis of Cats, p 513; Chlamydiosis, Cat, p 193)

PHYSICAL EXAM FINDINGS: Respiratory disease complex:

- Serous to mucopurulent nasal and ocular discharge
- Epiphora, blepharospasm, chemosis, conjunctival hyperemia
- Fever
- Dyspnea, increased airway sounds, wheezes, cough

In addition:

- Herpesvirus: conjunctivitis, ± dendritic corneal ulcers
- Calicivirus: oral, nasal, lip ulcers, or generalized stomatitis and gingivitis
- Rare severe cases of very virulent calicivirus strains: facial/limb edema, dermal necrosis, vomiting, diarrhea, icterus, petechiae and ecchymoses from disseminated intravascular coagulation, or sudden death
- *B. bronchiseptica*: fever, submandibular lymphadenopathy, and cyanosis/dyspnea in cases of severe bronchopneumonia

ETIOLOGY AND PATHOPHYSIOLOGY

Feline herpesvirus:

- A double-stranded DNA α-herpesvirus specific to those in the family Felidae that attacks mucosal epithelial cells of the soft palate, tonsils, turbinates, cornea, and conjunctiva, leading to multifocal epithelial necrosis and secondary clinical signs. Pulmonary involvement is rare.
- Incubation period is 2 to 6 days; disease usually runs its course in 10 to 20 days.
- Turbinate destruction due to herpesvirus infection may be permanent, and predispose the cat to chronic rhinitis, even in the absence of active infection.
- Chronic conjunctivitis/keratitis can lead to symblepharon, corneal scarring, or keratoconjunctivitis sicca (KCS).
- Essentially all cats infected with FHV become chronic carriers: the virus remains latent in the trigeminal ganglia; however, a smaller proportion of cats are truly susceptible to recrudescence, and these animals act as the FHV reservoir for the feline population. Recrudescence and viral shedding often occur 1 to 3 weeks after a stressful event. Not all recrudescence is accompanied by obvious clinical signs.

Feline calicivirus:

- Small nonenveloped single-stranded RNA viruses; several strains exist that generally cause respiratory signs of varying severity.
- Replicates in oral and respiratory tissues and occasionally in synovial cells and vascular endothelial cells in hemorrhagic strains.
- Oral ulcers are the most prominent lesions associated with calicivirus. Lesions start as vesicles that arise and then rupture due to epithelial cell necrosis and neutrophilic infiltration.
- Lesions in the lungs typically start as isolated alveolar inflammation and progress to focal areas of interstitial pneumonia.
- Synovial cell invasion leads to synovial membrane thickening and joint effusion.
- After acute infection, approximately 50% of cats clear the virus, and 50% become short-term carriers (a period of a few months). Some short-term carriers eventually eliminate the virus completely. A smaller percentage of cats become lifetime carriers, providing a constant source of virus for susceptible cats.
- Cats that recover from illness and clear the virus can become infected again.
- Isolated outbreaks of highly virulent systemic "hemorrhagic" calicivirus have occurred in the past few years. Vaccination has not been protective.

B. bronchiseptica:

- A small aerobic gram-negative coccobacillus that infects multiple species, including cats, dogs, and rabbits.
- Formerly considered opportunistic in cats but recently discovered to cause primary respiratory disease.
- *B. bronchiseptica* adheres to respiratory cilia via fimbriae and causes decreased ciliary function or complete ciliary destruction, effectively paralyzing the mucociliary elevator and allowing further dissemination of *B. bronchiseptica* and other bacterial species. Toxin release causes local and systemic inflammation.

C. felis:

- An obligate intracellular organism that has a cell wall, DNA, and RNA but requires host cell machinery for replication.

- Found as commensal flora on ocular and respiratory mucosa.
- Typically causes mild rhinitis and unilateral conjunctivitis initially, with spread to the other eye within 7 days. Does not affect the cornea.

DIAGNOSIS

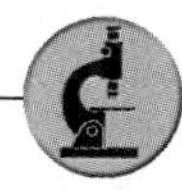

DIFFERENTIAL DIAGNOSIS

- Nasal signs:
  - Nasal neoplasia
  - Nasopharyngeal polyps
  - Periodontal disease
  - Foreign body
  - Fungal infection
  - Structural malformation of nasal passages/sinuses
  - Esophageal motility dysfunction
- Ocular signs:
  - Corneal and/or conjunctival trauma
  - Corneal foreign body
  - Eosinophilic keratoconjunctivitis
  - Neoplasia
  - KCS
  - Uveitis
  - Glaucoma
- Cough or dyspnea:
  - Feline asthma
  - Intrathoracic neoplasia (pulmonary, lymphoid, mediastinal, or pleural)
  - Congestive heart failure (CHF)
  - Pleural effusion of other causes

INITIAL DATABASE

- Complete blood count (CBC): neutrophilia with left shift if secondary bacterial infection is severe. Stress leukogram is possible, and results are often normal.
- Serum biochemistry profile and urinalysis: may reflect dehydration but typically unremarkable. With virulent calicivirus infections, increases in alanine aminotransferase (ALT), creatine kinase (CK), and bilirubin levels and decreased albumin level are possible.
- Thoracic radiographs: assessing for signs of pneumonia in cats with lower respiratory tract signs.
- CT scan of the skull with rhinoscopy and nasal biopsy/culture can help rule out neoplasia, fungal infection, dental disease, nasopharyngeal polyps, and structural deformities as causes of chronic respiratory signs.

ADVANCED OR CONFIRMATORY TESTING

- Diagnosis is typically made based on clinical signs. Specific identification of causative agent is not always necessary but is worthwhile in breeding animals.
- Serologic testing for herpesvirus and calicivirus is unrewarding because of widespread vaccination.
- Virus isolation from nasal, conjunctival, or oropharyngeal swabs is the best diagnostic assay for FHV and FCV. Requires special swabs or media for transport; however, FCV is commonly isolated from the oral/respiratory mucosa of healthy cats, so positive viral culture should be supported by appropriate clinical presentation. Polymerase chain reaction (PCR) for FCV has been developed but is strain dependent and typically only available in research laboratories.
- Conjunctival scrapes may demonstrate basophilic intracytoplasmic inclusions indicative of *C. felis* infection.
- Culture or PCR on conjunctival swabs can also be used to rule out *C. felis*. Special transport medium is required for culture. Serologic testing may also be helpful in the unvaccinated cat because affected animals typically have high titers.
- Transtracheal or bronchoalveolar washes with cytologic examination and culture and sensitivity (C&S) are helpful in isolating *B. bronchiseptica*, *C. felis*, or secondary bacteria as causative agents of pneumonia.
- Cryptococcal antigen titer to rule out cryptococcosis.
- Dynamic contrast esophagram to rule out esophageal motility disorder.

TREATMENT

THERAPEUTIC GOAL(S)

Treatment is typically supportive, with the goal of controlling secondary bacterial infections and maintaining comfort and appetite.

ACUTE GENERAL TREATMENT

- Most cats with upper respiratory infections can and should be managed at home by the owner to decrease pathogen dissemination in the hospital setting.
- Animals that are febrile, dehydrated, severely depressed, or compromised should be treated in the hospital until they are stable and can be sent home. These animals should be isolated from other cats.
  - IV crystalloids and colloids if patients are febrile and/or dehydrated or have evidence of hypovolemia.
  - Broad-spectrum antibiotics (one of the following):
    - Amoxicillin-clavulanate 13.75 mg/kg PO q 12h.
    - Cefadroxil 10-30 mg/kg PO q 8-12h.
    - Cephalexin 22-30 mg/kg PO q 8-12h.
    - Enrofloxacin 5 mg/kg PO q 24h.
  - Antibiotics most effective against specific bacteria (see Bordetellosis, p 140; Chlamydiosis, Cat, p 193):
    - Doxycycline 5 mg/kg PO q 12h, or tetracycline 20 mg/kg PO q 8h
  - Topical ophthalmic preparations:
    - Artificial tears q 2-6h
    - Tetracycline ophthalmics are the treatment of choice for *C. felis* and *Mycoplasma* spp. conjunctivitis and in FHV cats to prevent secondary bacterial infections. Topical tetracyclines can be irritating. Chloramphenicol, erythromycin, or fluoroquinolone topicals are alternative options.
    - Topical or systemic corticosteroids should not be used in suspected FHV keratitis.
    - Typical "triple antibiotic" ophthalmic preparations (neomycin, polymyxin, and bacitracin/gramicidin) are typically ineffective against *C. felis*, *Mycoplasma* spp., and FHV-1.
  - Topical and systemic antiviral drugs for FHV keratitis/conjunctivitis (see Herpesviral Keratitis of Cats, p 513)
  - Appetite stimulants may be necessary:
    - Cyproheptadine 2 mg/cat PO q 12-24h; or
    - Diazepam 0.05-0.15 mg/kg IV q 24h; may cause extreme sedation soon after administration; paradoxically, in some cats, may lead to hyperexcitability and fractiousness.
  - Treatment duration with antibiotics and antivirals should be determined on an individual case basis, but typically 1 to 2 weeks is required while the viral disease runs its course.

CHRONIC TREATMENT

- Feed animals very pungent, highly palatable foods to overcome a decreased sense of smell from nasal infection.
- Home nebulization (putting the cat on a dry surface in a steamy bathroom) may help ease nasal or airway congestion.
- Tube feeding may be necessary in chronic cases with prolonged anorexia.
- Owners should be instructed to cleanse the face, mouth, and nares regularly to minimize accumulation of discharges or saliva.
- Herpesvirus carriers that have bouts of recrudescence can be treated on as-needed basis with L-lysine to decrease severity of outbreaks.

POSSIBLE COMPLICATIONS

FHV keratoconjunctivitis can predispose the animal to KCS.

PROGNOSIS AND OUTCOME

Except in very young or compromised animals or in cases of virulent calicivirus, prognosis is usually good for recovery from acute bouts of respiratory disease.

Some animals develop chronic rhinitis and/or keratoconjunctivitis and will have recurrent bouts of disease that may require lifelong management.

PEARLS & CONSIDERATIONS

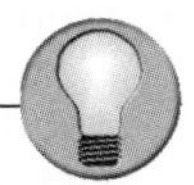

PREVENTION

- Several modified live or killed vaccines are available for protection against herpesvirus and calicivirus. They offer good-to-moderate protection against clinical disease but are not guaranteed to prevent infection or development of a carrier state.
- Modified live vaccines (MLV) may induce a mild form of respiratory disease.
- Vaccines are available for *B. bronchiseptica* and *C. felis*, but because these diseases are relatively benign and easy to treat, the benefit of immunization in most pet cats is questionable. Vaccination may be warranted in cattery or shelter situations.
- Dilute bleach (1 part bleach:32 parts water) is the best disinfectant for preventing FHV and FCV spread in the hospital environment. FCV has shown resistance to common disinfectants, such as quaternary ammonium compounds and chlorhexidine.

SUGGESTED READING

Gaskell R, Dawson S: Feline respiratory disease. In Greene CE (ed): *Infectious Diseases of the Dog and Cat*. Philadelphia, WB Saunders, 1998, pp 97-106.

Gaskell RM, Radford AD, Dawson S: Feline infectious respiratory disease. In Chandler EA, Gaskell CJ, Gaskell RM (eds): *Feline Medicine and Therapeutics*. Denmark, Blackwell Publishing, 2004, pp 577-595.

Hurley KF, Sykes JE: Update on feline calicivirus: New trends. *Vet Clin North Am Small Anim Pract* 33:4, 2003.

AUTHOR: **SHANNON T. STROUP**

EDITOR: **DOUGLASS K. MACINTIRE**

Urachal Diverticulum

BASIC INFORMATION

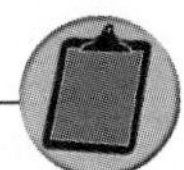

DEFINITION

Embryonic remnant at the apex of the urinary bladder

SYNONYMS

Vesicourachal diverticulum

EPIDEMIOLOGY

SPECIES, AGE, SEX: Dogs and cats.

RISK FACTORS: Microscopic diverticula in cats may be at risk for developing macroscopic diverticula following urinary tract obstruction from any cause.

ASSOCIATED CONDITIONS AND DISORDERS

- Urinary tract infection (UTI)/bacterial cystitis
- Urolithiasis
- Feline lower urinary tract signs/disease (FLUTS/D)

CLINICAL PRESENTATION

DISEASE FORMS/SUBTYPES

- Macroscopic: intramural and extramural
- Microscopic
- Acquired macroscopic

HISTORY, CHIEF COMPLAINT

Clinical signs may be absent. When clinical signs are apparent, they may include:

- Hematuria
- Pollakiuria
- Dysuria
- Stranguria
- Inappropriate elimination
- Systemic illness due to urinary obstruction (rare)

PHYSICAL EXAM FINDINGS: Physical exam may be unremarkable. When present, abnormalities are nonspecific and may include:

- Hematuria (stains on prepuce, vulva, or hocks)
- Painful urinary bladder
- Enlarged turgid bladder with urethral obstruction

ETIOLOGY AND PATHOPHYSIOLOGY

- The urachus is a canal connecting the fetal bladder with the allantois. The urachal lumen normally becomes obliterated during development, but on occasion the lumen remains patent (patent urachus) or the obliteration is incomplete, leaving a remnant diverticulum. Cause of incomplete urachal atrophy is unknown.
- Macroscopic:
  - Most common form in dogs
  - May not be associated with clinical signs
  - May be associated with or predispose the animal to chronic/recurrent UTI and urolithiasis
- Microscopic:
  - Most common form in cats
  - Remnants of urachus at bladder apex that can extend from the level of the submucosa to the subserosa
  - Not associated with clinical signs
- Acquired macroscopic:
  - Microscopic diverticula may become macroscopic secondary to sustained increase in bladder intraluminal pressure
  - May spontaneously regress if the cause of increased bladder pressure is removed

DIAGNOSIS

DIFFERENTIAL DIAGNOSIS

- Neoplasia
- Polyps
- Urolithiasis
- Blood clots

INITIAL DATABASE

- Complete blood count (CBC): unremarkable
- Serum chemistry profile: unremarkable unless urinary obstruction exists (azotemia, hyperkalemia, acidemia)
- Urinalysis: may be unremarkable; sometimes shows pyuria, hematuria, bacturia, or struvite crystalluria
- Urine culture and sensitivity (C&S)
- Abdominal radiographs to rule out radiopaque uroliths

ADVANCED OR CONFIRMATORY TESTING

- Contrast cystography:
  - Positive-contrast cystography
  - Double-contrast cystography (Fig. I-179)
- Ultrasonography
- Cystoscopy
- Exploratory celiotomy and cystotomy

TREATMENT

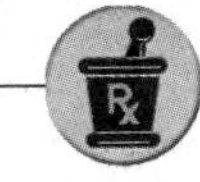

THERAPEUTIC GOAL(S)

- Relieve urinary tract obstruction if present
- Address electrolyte disorders or azotemia due to urinary obstruction if present
- Eliminate bacterial infection if present
- Address urolithiasis if present

ACUTE GENERAL TREATMENT

- Relieve urethral obstruction if present (see Urethral Obstruction [Canine], Medical Management, p 1318; Urethral Obstruction [Feline], Medical Management, p 1319)
- Fluid therapy and correction of electrolyte disturbances (see Urethral Obstruction, p 1118; Feline Lower Urinary Tract Signs, Idiopathic, p 382)

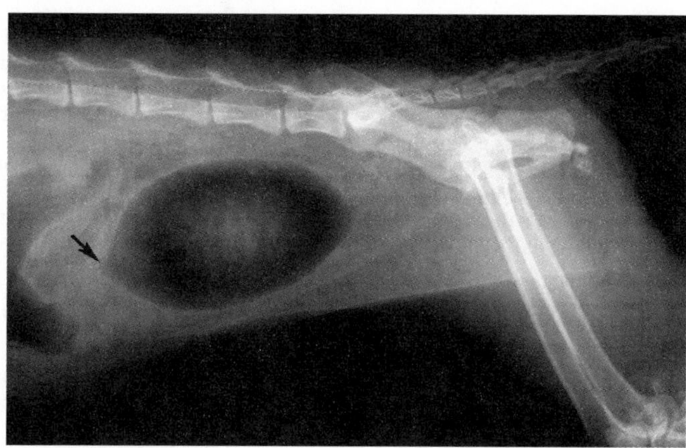

FIGURE I-179 Lateral radiographic projection of a double contrast cystogram performed on a 4-year-old male DSH cat with a history of chronic UTIs. A small "out-pouching" of the bladder wall is present at the apex (*black arrow*). Diagnosis: bladder diverticulum predisposing the animal to chronic cystitis. Courtesy of Dr. Stephanie Essman, University of Missouri.

- Antimicrobial therapy for bacterial cystitis (see Cystitis, Bacterial, p 270)

CHRONIC TREATMENT

- Animals with clinical signs or a urinary infection related to either congenital macroscopic diverticula or nonresolving acquired macroscopic diverticula should undergo surgical resection of the diverticulum.
  - Exploratory celiotomy
  - Ventral midline cystotomy
  - Identification of diverticulum at apex of bladder
  - Excision of diverticulum with elliptical incision
  - Routine closure
- Address chronic feline lower urinary tract signs/disease (see Feline Lower Urinary Tract Signs, Idiopathic, p 382).
- Address urolithiasis.

POSSIBLE COMPLICATIONS

Suture line leakage with peritonitis following surgical excision

RECOMMENDED MONITORING

- Monitor cats with acquired macroscopic diverticula for regression of diverticulum by contrast cystography 2 to 3 weeks after treatment of obstruction and resolution of clinical signs.
- Monitor for recurrence of signs of FLUTS/D (see Feline Lower Urinary Tract Signs, Idiopathic, p 382).

PROGNOSIS AND OUTCOME

- Surgical excision for congenital macroscopic diverticula is curative.
- Acquired macroscopic lesions that spontaneously resolve may recur with repeated episodes of lower urinary tract obstruction.

PEARLS & CONSIDERATIONS

COMMENTS

Patent urachus causes umbilical urine dribbling in neonates and should be corrected surgically.

PREVENTION

Prevention of lower urinary tract obstruction will prevent acquired diverticula formation.

CLIENT EDUCATION

- Recurrent UTI may be a sequela to uncorrected congenital macroscopic diverticula.
- Recurrent or persistent UTI may lead to struvite urolithiasis.

SUGGESTED READING

Waldron DR: Urinary bladder. In Slatter D (ed): *Textbook of Small Animal Surgery*. Philadelphia, WB Saunders, 2003, pp 1629-1637.

AUTHOR: **ERIC R. POPE**
EDITOR: **LEAH A. COHN**

Ureteral Obstruction

BASIC INFORMATION

DEFINITION

Obstruction of urine flow through one or both ureters

EPIDEMIOLOGY

SPECIES, AGE, SEX: Uncommon; affects dogs or cats of any age or sex.

RISK FACTORS

- Intraluminal obstruction (e.g., urolith, trauma, inflammation, fibrosis/stricture, congenital stenosis, blood clots)
- Intramural obstruction (e.g., fibrosis/stenosis, ureterocele, fibroepithelial polyps, proliferative ureteritis, neoplasia)
- Extramural obstruction (e.g., retroperitoneal or pelvic masses, prostatic/bladder neoplasia, inadvertent ligation or fibrotic entrapment of ureter)

ASSOCIATED CONDITIONS AND DISORDERS

- Renal failure
- Uremia
- Hydronephrosis
- Hydroureter
- Pyelonephritis

CLINICAL PRESENTATION

DISEASE FORMS/SUBTYPES

- Partial or complete
- Unilateral or bilateral

HISTORY, CHIEF COMPLAINT: Clinical signs may be absent, especially with unilateral obstruction. When signs are present, some or all of the following may be noted:

- Lethargy/depression
- Anorexia
- Vomiting
- Polyuria and polydipsia (PU/PD)
- Dysuria, stranguria, or pollakiuria
- Hematuria

PHYSICAL EXAM FINDINGS: Physical examination may be normal; abnormalities can include:

- Dehydration
- Poor body condition
- Enlarged kidney(s)
- Abdominal mass
- Prostatomegaly
- Abdominal discomfort (severity related to rate of onset of obstruction rather than degree of obstruction)
- Halitosis (due to uremia)
- Oral ulcerations (due to uremia)
- Fever

- Abdominal fluid wave (if rupture and uroabdomen)

ETIOLOGY AND PATHOPHYSIOLOGY

See Hydronephrosis, p 535

DIAGNOSIS

DIFFERENTIAL DIAGNOSIS

Other causes of renomegaly (see Renomegaly, p 958):

- Renal cyst(s)
- Renal neoplasia
- Granuloma
- Perirenal pseudocyst/abscess
- Feline infectious peritonitis
- Hematoma

INITIAL DATABASE

- Complete blood count (CBC): generally unremarkable:
  - Normocytic, normochromic, nonregenerative anemia (if chronic renal failure or chronic inflammation)
  - Leukocytosis with left shift possible if concurrent pyelonephritis
- Serum biochemical profile: abnormalities depend on degree of obstruction and/or nephron loss:
  - Azotemia
  - Hyperphosphatemia
  - Hyperkalemia
  - Metabolic acidosis
- Urinalysis: commonly abnormal:
  - Isosthenuria
  - Hematuria
  - Pyuria
- Urine culture and sensitivity (C&S): indicated even if sediment is inactive (occult infection)
- Blood pressure (BP)
- Abdominal radiographs: renomegaly common; may identify:
  - Urolithiasis
  - Prostatomegaly
  - Abdominal mass
  - Loss of retroperitoneal/abdominal contrast
  - Distended ureter
  - Mass associated with ureter or bladder

ADVANCED OR CONFIRMATORY TESTING

- Abdominal ultrasound (sensitive and specific):
  - Pyelectasia (dilation of renal pelvis): common
  - Hydronephrosis: common
  - Hydroureter: common
  - Urolithiasis: possible
- Excretory urography (intravenous pyelography [IVP]); percutaneous nephropyelography:
  - Pyelectasia
  - Ureteral dilatation or lack of filling (IVP only)
- Renal scintigraphy:
  - Affected kidney contributes little to overall glomerular filtration rate (GFR)
- Quantitative analysis and culture of uroliths

TREATMENT

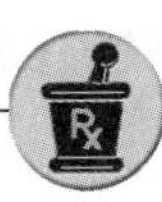

THERAPEUTIC GOAL(S)

- Identify underlying cause and relieve urinary obstruction (ideally)
- Address azotemia/uremia, electrolyte, and acid-base disorders (see Acute Renal Failure, p 32; Chronic Renal Failure, Occult ["Asymptomatic"], p 204; Chronic Renal Failure, Overt ["Symptomatic"], p 205)
- Treat concurrent infection (see Cystitis, Bacterial, p 270)
- Provide analgesia

ACUTE GENERAL TREATMENT

- Correct hydration, acid-base, and electrolyte disorders:
  - Crystalloid fluid therapy for azotemia, dehydration (see Acute Renal Failure, p 32)
    - Initial rate of 120 ml/kg per day unless diuresis contraindicated.
    - Postobstructive diuresis may require the "ins and outs" method of adjustment (rate based on measured urine output).
    - Diuresis may flush out ureterolith.
  - Address electrolyte disorders and acidosis (see Urethral Obstruction, p 1120; Acute Renal Failure, p 32)
  - Consider hemodialysis for stabilization
- Nephrostomy tubes may be used for preventing further renal damage while assessing renal function prior to surgical intervention.
  - Only possible if renal pelvis dilated
  - Placed with ultrasound guidance or via laparotomy
- Analgesia for abdominal pain (e.g., buprenorphine 0.01 mg/kg IM, IV, or SQ q 6–8h).
- Address uremic signs (see Acute Renal Failure, p 32; Chronic Renal Failure, Overt ["Symptomatic"], p 205)

CHRONIC TREATMENT

- Surgical intervention is not always required, especially if adequate renal function is retained and infection is absent.
- Ureteral surgery is indicated for bilateral obstruction or when function of contralateral kidney is impaired; major complication: postoperative ureteral stricture formation. Nuclear scintigraphy provides quantitative assessment of each kidney's contribution to glomerular filtration rate:
  - Ureterotomy: for intraluminal or intramural obstruction in the proximal third of the ureter
  - Ureteroneocystostomy: for resection of distal ureter
  - Ureteroureterostomy: to repair ureter after resection or transection (anastomosis of proximal ureter to distal portion of ureter on ipsilateral side), usually when proximal third cannot be implanted directly into bladder neck
    - Highest incidence of postoperative obstruction
- Nephrectomy: reserved for animals with unilateral obstruction and adequate function in contralateral kidney.
- Antibiotics, if appropriate (e.g., pyelonephritis, bacterial cystitis) based on C&S.
- Therapeutic or prophylactic measures for urolithiasis if present (see Urolithiasis, Oxalate, p 1127; Urolithiasis, Struvite, p 1129; Urolithiasis, Other, p 1125).

POSSIBLE COMPLICATIONS

- Renal failure
- Postoperative ureteral stenosis
- Urinary rupture and uroabdomen

RECOMMENDED MONITORING

- Repeat ultrasound 10 to 12 weeks after treatment. Remaining renal parenchymal changes are likely permanent.
- Animals with permanent hydroureter/hydronephrosis are monitored as for CRF (see Chronic Renal Failure, Occult ["Asymptomatic"], p 204; Chronic Renal Failure, Overt ["Symptomatic"], p 205) with periodic urinalysis and C&S as well as assessment of azotemia, electrolytes, and packed cell volume (PCV). Azotemic animals are monitored more intensively than nonazotemic animals.

PROGNOSIS AND OUTCOME

- Dependent on underlying cause, duration of obstruction, extent of renal parenchymal damage, presence of concurrent infection, and ability to resolve underlying cause.
- Surviving animals, especially cats, may have abnormal renal function.
- Structural renal changes persisting 14 to 45 days or more after relief of ureteral obstruction are generally permanent.
- Complete bilateral obstruction of more than 3 days is fatal without appropriate treatment.

PEARLS & CONSIDERATIONS

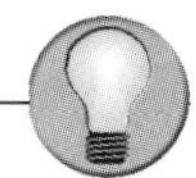

COMMENTS

- Ureteral obstruction is rare but should be considered in the differential diagnosis for renal failure, especially in patients with evidence of nephrolithiasis or pyelonephritis.
- Bilateral ureteral obstruction is rare compared to unilateral obstruction but is life threatening.

PREVENTION

Strategies that limit the formation of urolithiasis (see Urolithiasis, Struvite, p 1129; Urolithiasis, Oxalate, p 1127; Urolithiasis, Other, p 1125)

CLIENT EDUCATION

Strict adherence to dietary recommendations can minimize the risk of ureteral or urethral obstruction due to urolithiasis.

SUGGESTED READING

Hardie EM, et al: Management of ureteral obstruction. *Vet Clin North Am Small Anim Pract* 34:989, 2004.

Kyles AE, et al: Clinical, clinicopathologic, radiographic, and ultrasonographic abnormalities in cats with ureteral calculi: 163 cases. *J Am Vet Med Assoc* 226:6, 2005.

Kyles AE, et al: Management and outcome of cats with ureteral calculi: 153 cases (1984-2002). *J Am Vet Med Assoc* 226:6, 2005.

AUTHORS: **ADAM MORDECAI, RANCE K. SELLON**

EDITOR: **LEAH A. COHN**

Urethral Obstruction

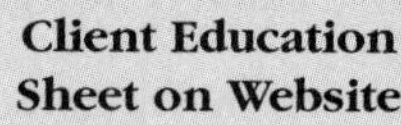

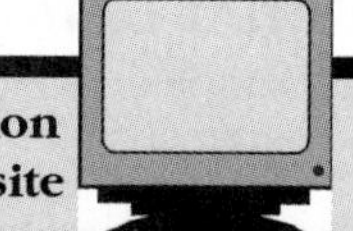

BASIC INFORMATION

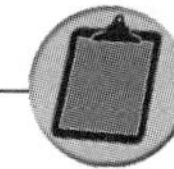

DEFINITION

Lower urinary tract obstruction caused by uroliths or matrix

EPIDEMIOLOGY

SPECIES, AGE, SEX

- Any age
- Males predisposed
- Cats predisposed

GENETICS AND BREED PREDISPOSITION: Certain breeds predisposed to specific urolith formation (e.g., dalmatians: urate uroliths).

RISK FACTORS

- Feline lower urinary tract signs/disease (FLUTS/D)
- Urinary tract infection
- Neoplasia
- Risk factors associated with urolithiasis (see Urolithiasis, Struvite, p 1129; Urolithiasis, Oxalate, p 1127; Urolithiasis, Urate/Biurate, p 1131; Urolithiasis, Other, p 1125)

ASSOCIATED CONDITIONS AND DISORDERS

- Hydronephrosis
- Azotemia/uremia
- Hyperkalemic cardiac dysrhythmia
- Urinary bladder rupture
- Bladder atonia/hypotonia
- Urinary tract infection
- Post obstructive diuresis

CLINICAL PRESENTATION

HISTORY, CHIEF COMPLAINT

- Stranguria
- Anuria/oliguria
- Hematuria
- Lethargy
- Anorexia
- Vocalization
- Restlessness
- Dribbling urine
- Licking prepuce/vulva (urethral discharge)
- Dyschezia
- History of urinary infection or urolithiasis

PHYSICAL EXAM FINDINGS

- Enlarged, turgid urinary bladder
- Abdominal discomfort
- Dribbling urine
- Bloody preputial/vulvar discharge
- Palpable urethral urolith (digital rectal exam in dogs)
- Bradycardia if severe hyperkalemia

ETIOLOGY AND PATHOPHYSIOLOGY

- Urine supersaturation, urinary tract infection, certain disease states, and breed predisposition contribute to urolithiasis.
- In cats especially, urethral plugs may be composed of matrix (cellular debris, virus-like particles, with or without bacteria, urinary crystals).
- Uroliths or plugs can obstruct the urethra; urethral anatomy favors obstruction in males.

DIAGNOSIS

DIFFERENTIAL DIAGNOSIS

- Detrusor atony
- FLUTS/D
- Fungal granulomas
- Reflex dyssynergia
- Trauma (pelvic fracture) with urethral damage, bladder entrapment hernia, penile fracture
- Urethral neoplasia
- Urethral stricture
- Urethral tissue valve/flap
- Urethritis
- Urolithiasis

INITIAL DATABASE

- Complete blood count: unremarkable
- Serum biochemical profile: possible azotemia, hyperkalemia, findings consistent with predisposing conditions
- Urethral catheterization: distinguish functional from structural urethral obstruction, localize structural obstruction, may relieve obstruction and provide urine for analysis
- Urinalysis: possible hematuria, crystalluria, pyuria, epithelial cells, dilute urine, bacturia. Rarely, fungal hyphae or neoplastic cells
- Urine culture: if sample is obtained by catheterization, quantitative culture to distinguish contamination ($<10^3$ CFU/ml) from infection
- Abdominal/pelvic radiographs: distended urinary bladder, possible radiopaque uroliths, renomegaly, ascites
- Abdominal ultrasound: possible uroliths, urinary bladder debris, pyelectasia, ascites
- Electrocardiogram: hyperkalemia signs (absent P waves, wide QRS complexes, bradycardia)

ADVANCED OR CONFIRMATORY TESTING

- Voiding cystourethrogram: determine location of urethral obstruction
- Retrieved uroliths: quantitative analysis, culture
- Other testing for conditions predisposing to urolith formation (e.g., bile acids as screen for portosystemic shunt)

TREATMENT

THERAPEUTIC GOAL(S)

- Relieve urethral obstruction
- Correct uremia, electrolyte abnormalities
- Address predisposing conditions
- Prevent recurrence

ACUTE GENERAL TREATMENT

- Intravenous catheter for crystalloid fluid therapy, correcting electrolyte disorders, and administering sedation/anesthesia.
  - Crystalloid fluids: 5–10 ml/kg/hr during sedation/anesthesia.
  - Thereafter, rate should provide maintenance (60 ml/kg q 24h), correct dehydration, and match postobstructive diuresis losses.
    - Closed urine collection system to identify profound postobstructive diuresis and allows "ins and outs" fluid treatment plan
  - If serum potassium >7 mEq/l, consider calcium gluconate, sodium bicarbonate, or insulin/dextrose therapy (see Acute Renal Failure, p 32; Hyperkalemia, p 546).
- Small plug/urolith at the tip of the penis: remove via gentle massage (cats).
- Urethral catheterization can be attempted without sedation in male dogs; in cats, bitches, or dogs resistant to catheterization, sedation/anesthesia is usually required (see Catheterization, Urethral, p 1205).
- Insert a sterile red rubber catheter or open-ended polypropylene catheter into the urethra to the point of obstruction. Once encountered, retropulse the urolith/debris into the urinary bladder using sterile saline or a 75% sterile saline and 25% sterile water-based-lubricant mixture.
  - In male cats, a sterile 22-gauge, 1-inch intravenous catheter (without stylet) may be used to dislodge urethral plug.
  - The urinary bladder is emptied; if debris is identified, lavage with sterile saline.
- An indwelling urinary catheter attached to a sterile, closed urine collection system is often indicated (e.g., pending correction of anatomic or functional obstruction, in cats with FLUTS/D, or to prevent urolith movement back into urethra following retropulsion and pending cystotomy).
  - For indwelling purposes, polypropylene catheters should be replaced with red rubber or Foley catheters.
  - Ideally, radiographs are obtained to identify remaining radiopaque urethral/bladder uroliths and to evaluate appropriate catheter placement. The catheter should just enter the trigone.
- If a urinary catheter cannot be passed, periodic cystocentesis can be performed in order to temporarily empty the urinary bladder pending definitive treatment.
- See Urethral Obstruction (Canine): Medical Management, p 1318; Urethral Obstruction (Feline): Medical Management, p 1319.

CHRONIC TREATMENT

- Maintain indwelling urinary catheter appropriately (sterile, closed collection system)
  - Typically for 24 to 72 hours in cats with crystalluria or FLUTS/D
- Phenoxybenzamine (dog: 0.25 mg/kg PO q 12h; cat: 2.5 mg/kg PO q 12–24h) may decrease urethral spasm
- Antibiotic therapy based on urine culture/sensitivity; obtain culture when removing catheter
- Address urolithiasis:
  - Diet/medical dissolution possible for some types, but risk of repeated obstruction
  - Consider cystotomy, urohydropulsion (voiding, retrograde), cystoscopic assisted retrieval
- Perineal urethrostomy considered for male cats (or dogs) with recurrent obstruction

POSSIBLE COMPLICATIONS

- Urethral tear
- Urinary bladder rupture
- Urethritis
- Iatrogenic urinary tract infection
- Urethral stricture

RECOMMENDED MONITORING

- Daily bladder palpation during hospitalization after removing urinary catheter
- Repeat urinalysis and urine culture when urinary catheter is removed and again 1 week later
- Monitor as appropriate for urolith type or FLUTD (see Feline Lower Urinary Tract Signs, Idiopathic, p 382)

PROGNOSIS AND OUTCOME

- Urethral obstruction is life-threatening.
- If obstruction is alleviated and electrolyte disorders are addressed, prognosis is good (exception: neoplasia).
- Risk for recurrence is present regardless of cause.

PEARLS & CONSIDERATIONS

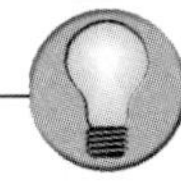

PREVENTION

- Promote water consumption.
- Dietary/medical therapy may be indicated depending on type of urolith identified.
- Predisposing factors for urolith formation should be addressed directly whenever possible.

CLIENT EDUCATION

- Urinary tract obstruction is life threatening. Stranguria or dysuria should prompt immediate veterinary attention.
- Adherence to dietary therapy for urolith dissolution must be strict.

SUGGESTED READING

Bartges JW, et al: Pathophysiology of urethral obstruction. *Vet Clin North Am Small Anim Pract* 26:255, 1996.

Lekcharoensuk C, et al: Evaluation of trends in frequency of urethrostomy for treatment of urethral obstruction in cats. *J Am Vet Med Assoc* 221:502, 2002.

Osborne CA, et al: Medical management of feline urethral obstruction. *Vet Clin North Am Small Anim Pract* 26:483, 1996.

AUTHOR: **ANNE M. DALBY**

EDITOR: **LEAH A. COHN**

Urethral Prolapse

BASIC INFORMATION

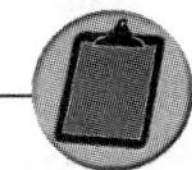

DEFINITION

Prolapse of urethral mucosa from urethral orifice

EPIDEMIOLOGY

SPECIES, AGE, SEX: Young, intact male dogs.

GENETICS AND BREED PREDISPOSITION: English bulldog.

RISK FACTORS

- Intact male dog
- Brachycephalic breed

ASSOCIATED CONDITIONS AND DISORDERS: Brachycephalic airway syndrome.

CLINICAL PRESENTATION

HISTORY, CHIEF COMPLAINT

- Excessive licking of prepuce or penis
- Blood from preputial opening
- Stranguria

PHYSICAL EXAM FINDINGS

- Hemorrhagic discharge from prepuce.
- Red or purple mass protruding from urethral orifice.
- A prolapsed urethra typically appears as a small red bulb of smooth, congested (red) mucosa at the tip of the penis surrounding the urethral opening.

ETIOLOGY AND PATHOPHYSIOLOGY

Possible causes include:

- Excessive sexual excitement
- Masturbation
- Genitourinary infection
- Urolithiasis

Secondary swelling of the prolapsed segment prevents spontaneous reduction.

DIAGNOSIS

DIFFERENTIAL DIAGNOSIS

- Penile trauma
- Urethritis
- Neoplasia (transmissible venereal tumor [TVT])

INITIAL DATABASE

- Presurgical complete blood count (CBC), serum chemistry profile: generally unremarkable
- Urinalysis (cystocentesis) ± microbiologic culture:
  - Rule out associated urinary tract infection (UTI), prostatic disease

ADVANCED OR CONFIRMATORY TESTING

- Impression smear of prolapsed tissue for cytologic examination:
  - Rule out TVT
- Abdominal ultrasound examination:
  - Rule out prostatic disease

TREATMENT

THERAPEUTIC GOAL(S)

- Prevent continued trauma to prolapsed urethral mucosa
- Surgically correct mucosal prolapse

ACUTE GENERAL TREATMENT

Surgical correction of prolapsed urethra:

- Urethropexy technique: inversion of urethral mucosa using several mattress sutures

CHRONIC TREATMENT

- Prevent masturbation in the immediate postoperative period
- Treat UTI, prostatic disease, and urolithiasis if present
- Consider castration to reduce sexual arousal:
  - Dog should not be used for breeding purposes because of genetic predisposition

POSSIBLE COMPLICATIONS

Recurrence of prolapse after surgical correction

RECOMMENDED MONITORING

Observe animals for recurrence of bleeding from prepuce; the signs may indicate recurrence of prolapse

PROGNOSIS AND OUTCOME

Excellent prognosis with appropriate surgical technique

PEARLS & CONSIDERATIONS

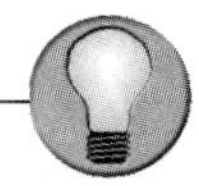

COMMENTS

The hallmark of diagnosis is the physical finding of a red bulb-like mass at the tip of the penis in a patient with stranguria or penile self-trauma.

PREVENTION

- Recognize genetic predisposition for the problem: English bulldog
- Early castration to reduce sexual activity or excitement
- Prevention of masturbation
- Prevention of obesity

CLIENT EDUCATION

- Early castration in predisposed breeds to reduce sexual activity or excitement
- Prevention of masturbation and self-trauma to penis
- Avoid circumstances that would exacerbate respiratory problems in brachycephalic dogs:
  - Obesity
  - Stress
  - Heat, humidity

SUGGESTED READING

Kirsch JA, Hauptman JG, Walshaw R: A urethropexy technique for surgical treatment of urethral prolapse in the male dog. *J Am Anim Hosp Assoc* 38:381-384, 2002

AUTHOR & EDITOR: **RICHARD WALSHAW**

Urinary Bladder and Urethral Rupture

BASIC INFORMATION

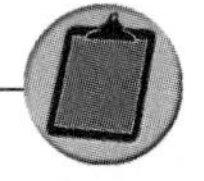

DEFINITION

Traumatic rupture of the urinary bladder and/or urethra

EPIDEMIOLOGY

SPECIES, AGE, SEX: Urethral trauma more common in males.

RISK FACTORS

- Ability to roam freely
- Blunt trauma (e.g., vehicular accident, kicks, falls)
- Penetrating injury (e.g., gunshot wound, cystocentesis)
- Pelvic fracture
- Fracture of the os penis

- Urolithiasis
- Lower urinary tract obstruction
- Urethral catheterization
- Urogenital surgery

ASSOCIATED CONDITIONS AND DISORDERS

- Azotemia
- Hyperkalemia

CLINICAL PRESENTATION

HISTORY, CHIEF COMPLAINT

- Precipitating event (e.g., trauma, penetrating injury)
- Hematuria (common)
- Dysuria (common); ability to produce urine stream does not rule out urinary bladder rupture
- Vomiting
- Depression
- Anorexia
- Abdominal pain
- Urethrocutaneous fistula (chronic)

PHYSICAL EXAM FINDINGS

- Abdominal effusion (especially with bladder rupture)
- Caudal abdominal pain (especially with bladder rupture)
- Dehydration
- Depression
- Dysuria (especially with urethral rupture)
- Halitosis
- Hematuria (especially with urethral rupture)
- Hypovolemia secondary to urine peritonitis/uroabdomen
- Inability to palpate bladder (especially with bladder rupture)
- Pelvic fracture
- Stranguria (especially with urethral rupture)
- Uremic oral ulcers
- Ventral abdominal wall or perineal bruising
- Vomiting

ETIOLOGY AND PATHOPHYSIOLOGY

- Blunt external trauma, penetrating projectiles, perforation by fracture fragments.
- Iatrogenic: secondary to catheterization, cystocentesis, or other diagnostic procedure errors; forceful bladder expression.
- Intraperitoneal accumulation of urine results in chemical peritonitis, azotemia, hyperkalemia, and acidemia; death may occur in 3 to 5 days if animal is left untreated.
- Extraperitoneal accumulation of urine results in cellulitis and tissue death acutely and may result in formation of urethrocutaneous fistulas if the rupture is not treated.
- See Uroabdomen, p 1124.

DIAGNOSIS

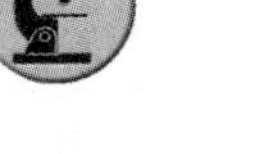

DIFFERENTIAL DIAGNOSIS

- Bladder rupture:
  - Urinary tract infection
  - Urine leakage from upper urinary tract
  - Other causes of peritonitis
- Urethral rupture:
  - Urinary tract obstruction due to urolithiasis, neoplasia, granulomatous urethritis, or prostatic disease
  - Periurethral hematoma or abscess

INITIAL DATABASE

- Complete blood count (CBC):
  - Initially unremarkable, progressing to neutrophilic leukocytosis often with left shift
- Serum biochemical profile:
  - Azotemia
  - Hyperkalemia (may be life threatening; i.e., >8.0 mEq/L)
  - Metabolic acidemia
- Abdominal/pelvic radiographs:
  - Loss of serosal detail
  - Pelvic or os penis fracture
- Abdominocentesis (see Abdominocentesis, p 1178) or peritoneal lavage (see Diagnostic Peritoneal Lavage, p 1225) with fluid analysis:
  - Compare fluid and serum creatinine
- Urethral catheterization: should normally encounter no friction/resistance

ADVANCED OR CONFIRMATORY TESTING

- Positive-contrast urethrocystogram (see Urethrogram, p 1321; Cystogram, p 1214)
- Ultrasonography

TREATMENT

THERAPEUTIC GOAL(S)

- Address fluid, electrolyte, and acid-base disturbances (may be urgent)
- Restore integrity of the urinary tract

ACUTE GENERAL TREATMENT

- Temporary urinary diversion by transurethral catheter or cystostomy tube
- Correct electrolyte and acid-base disturbances:
  - If potassium >7 mEq/L, consider one or more of the following:
    - Regular crystalline insulin (¼ unit/kg IV bolus) with IV dextrose (2 g dextrose/unit insulin over 6 hours IV; 50% dextrose is 0.5 g/ml, 5% dextrose is 0.05 g/ml. Generally administered as 5% dextrose infusion; dextrose concentrations >10% can cause phlebitis).
    - Sodium bicarbonate: 1 mEq/kg IV bolus.
    - Calcium gluconate (10% solution): 1 ml/kg slow IV bolus (cardioprotective). Monitor electrocardiogram (ECG) and stop infusion if bradycardia occurs.
  - If pH <7.1, institute sodium bicarbonate therapy:
    - Calculate bicarbonate deficit: [(0.3) × (BW in kilograms) × (base deficit)]. Base deficit is (24 – patient's HCO_3^-) in milliequivalents per liter.
    - Administer half of deficit in IV fluids over 6 hours.
- Provide crystalloid fluids at an adequate rate:
  - Rehydration: % dehydration* × body weight (kilograms) = deficit (liters); the asterisk sign* for this equation refers to dehydration entered as a decimal, so 10% is 0.1, 7% is 0.07, etc.).
  - Maintenance: 60 ml/kg per day.
  - Ongoing loss: estimate loss from vomiting, third space loss, and other such losses.
- Abdominocentesis or peritoneal lavage to decrease the effects of uroabdomen
- Primary repair of rupture or conservative management by urine diversion until adequate healing occurs:
  - Primary repair:
    - Bladder ruptures due to blunt trauma; complete abdominal exploration
    - Complete urethral transections
  - Conservative management by urine diversion:
    - Small bladder perforations (e.g., from catheter trauma)
    - Incomplete urethral lacerations
    - Bladder rupture: urethral catheter ± peritoneal lavage catheter
    - Urethral rupture: urethral catheter or cystostomy tube

CHRONIC TREATMENT

- Antimicrobial therapy for bacterial cystitis may be necessary after urinary diversion catheter is removed.
- Stricture formation or urethral dehiscence postoperatively may necessitate antepubic urethrostomy.

POSSIBLE COMPLICATIONS

- Urinary tract infection
- Continued leakage after surgical correction
- Urethral stricture

RECOMMENDED MONITORING

- Positive-contrast urethrocystography after conservative management to assess adequacy of healing and identify formation of any strictures
- Observation of animal for dysuria or stranguria
- Urinalysis and/or urine culture after removing urinary diversion catheter

PROGNOSIS AND OUTCOME

- Good to excellent for bladder rupture and incomplete urethral transection
- Guarded to good with complete urethral transection, especially if com-

plicated by urethrocutaneous fistula formation

PEARLS & CONSIDERATIONS

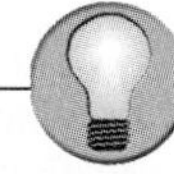

COMMENTS

- Emergency surgery to repair bladder or urethral rupture is rarely necessary if urinary diversion can be established
- Address life-threatening shock and metabolic disorders prior to surgery

PREVENTION

Avoid excessive force during bladder expression or catheterization

CLIENT EDUCATION

- Do not allow pets to roam.
- Dysuria/stranguria can indicate a life-threatening problem and warrant rapid veterinary evaluation.
- Dysuria and/or stranguria after treatment of urinary tract rupture could indicate stricture formation.

SUGGESTED READING

Bjorling DE: The urethra. In Slatter D (ed): *Textbook of Small Animal Surgery*. Philadelphia, WB Saunders, 2003, pp 1638–1651.

Waldron DR: Urinary bladder. In Slatter D (ed): *Textbook of Small Animal Surgery*. Philadelphia, WB Saunders, 2003, pp 1629–1637.

AUTHOR: **ERIC R. POPE**

EDITOR: **LEAH A. COHN**

Uroabdomen

BASIC INFORMATION

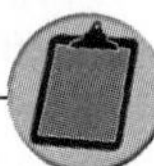

DEFINITION

The accumulation of urine within the peritoneal and/or retroperitoneal spaces caused by leakage from the kidneys, ureters, bladder, or proximal urethra

SYNONYM(S)

Urinary tract rupture
Uroperitoneum

EPIDEMIOLOGY

SPECIES, AGE, SEX: May affect all species and ages and both sexes.

RISK FACTORS: Preexisting compromise of the urinary tract due to urinary obstruction (urolith[s], neoplasia, other), iatrogenic causes (urethral catheterization, aggressive bladder palpation, surgical complication [laceration or ligation of urinary tract]), or abdominal or pelvic trauma (hit by car, pelvic fractures of any cause, penetrating abdominal wounds).

ASSOCIATED CONDITIONS AND DISORDERS

- Hyperkalemia
- Postrenal azotemia

CLINICAL PRESENTATION

HISTORY, CHIEF COMPLAINT

- Lethargy
- Anorexia
- Vomiting
- Discomfort
- Signs identifying or suggesting the underlying cause (e.g., animal was observed being hit by a car, pollakiuria with progressive urethral obstruction due to neoplasia or accumulation of uroliths)
- Urination: ability to pass urine does not rule out urinary tract rupture or uroabdomen; patient may or may not be hematuric

PHYSICAL EXAM FINDINGS

- Dehydration
- Abdominal pain:
  - Lack of signs of abdominal pain does not rule out uroabdomen.
- Lack of a palpable bladder:
  - Palpable bladder does not rule out urinary tract rupture/uroabdomen (small rupture, but still potentially life threatening).
- Bruising (perineum, ventral abdomen, and inguinal region)
- Depression
- Inappropriate bradycardia (from hyperkalemia):
  - Unlike dogs, cats may have severe hyperkalemia and maintain a normal or elevated heart rate.

ETIOLOGY AND PATHOPHYSIOLOGY

Accumulation of urine in the abdominal cavity results in the following consequences:

- Translocation of solutes that are normally higher in urine concentration (urea, creatinine, potassium, hydrogen) across the peritoneal lining into the extracellular fluid spaces and systemic circulation
- Postrenal azotemia
- Metabolic acidosis
- Hyperkalemia
- Chemical peritonitis

DIAGNOSIS

DIFFERENTIAL DIAGNOSIS

- Acute abdomen with gastrointestinal (GI) compromise
- Ascites of other causes (e.g., hypoalbuminemic, cardiogenic, hemorrhagic)
- Acute (oliguric/anuric) renal failure

INITIAL DATABASE

- Complete blood count (CBC): generally unremarkable
- Serum biochemistry profile: moderate or marked blood urea nitrogen (BUN), creatinine, and potassium elevations as well as low HCO_3^- are common
- Urinalysis: cystocentesis not feasible if bladder has collapsed; catheter acceptable if no urethral resistance. Hematuria is most common finding
- Abdominal radiographs: loss of serosal detail
- Abominal ultrasound: free abdominal fluid (anechoic); ultrasound contrast cystography may confirm bladder rupture

ADVANCED OR CONFIRMATORY TESTING

- Abdominal paracentesis, with increased creatinine and potassium of fluid compared with serum
- Positive contrast radiography (cystourethrography [bladder, urethra] or IV excretory urography [kidneys, ureters]). The most sensitive method to confirm urine leakage and localize the site of leakage

TREATMENT

THERAPEUTIC GOAL(S)

- Restore plasma volume
- Treat severe hyperkalemia if present
- Remove the urine from the abdominal cavity and minimize continued leakage into the abdomen
- Provide pain management
- Provide nutritional support
- Surgical correction of the urinary tract defect

ACUTE GENERAL TREATMENT

- Aggressive fluid therapy to treat shock if present and correct severe dehydration:

- Fluid without potassium or lactate is recommended as an initial choice (e.g., 0.9% NaCl, minimum 70-90 ml/kg/day if no renal or cardiac compromise).
- Higher rates are necessary for dehydration correction or diuresis.
- Fluid type and rate are changed later on as necessary based on physical monitoring and serial electrolyte levels.

- If the patient's potassium is greater than 7-8 mEq/L and/or there are clinical (e.g., bradycardia) or electrocardiographic (ECG) (e.g., no P waves in all ECG leads) changes due to hyperkalemia, immediate therapy is recommended (see Hyperkalemia, p 546).
- For animals with lower urinary tract injury and urine accumulation in the peritoneal space:
  - Placement of peritoneal drainage catheter.
  - Placement of urethral catheter (bladder decompression).
  - Placement of prepubic tube cystostomy in animals with severe urethral trauma.
  - Opiods (e.g., butorphanol 0.1-0.3 mg/kg IV) for pain management and sedation for procedures.

CHRONIC TREATMENT

- Fluid therapy to replace ongoing losses, including the presence of postobstructive diuresis
- Surgical correction of the site of leakage

DRUG INTERACTIONS

Do not add potassium chloride (KCl) to IV fluids until serum potassium level is known

POSSIBLE COMPLICATIONS

- Obstruction of the peritoneal drainage catheter with omentum
- Injury to other intra-abdominal structures during placement of peritoneal drainage catheter
- Urethral stricture formation and urinary incontinence

RECOMMENDED MONITORING

- Frequent monitoring of vital signs, including blood pressure (BP)
- ECG monitoring if hyperkalemia
- Fluid input and urine output from both peritoneal drainage and urethral catheters q 4h
- Serum chemistry, venous blood gas (VBG), packed cell volume (PCV) q 8-12h during initial stabilization
- Patient's weight q 12h

PROGNOSIS AND OUTCOME

- Prognosis is good with early diagnosis, aggressive emergency management, and definitive repair.
- The mortality rate is increased in animals with concurrent injuries.

PEARLS & CONSIDERATIONS

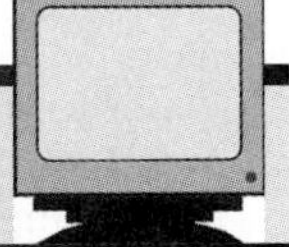

COMMENTS

- Consider uroabdomen in animals with a history of abdominal or pelvic trauma, urinary obstruction, or urethral catheterization.
- A palpable bladder and the ability to void urine do not rule out uroabdomen because animals with urinary tract disruption may continue to urinate.
- The abdominal fluid obtained is serosanguineous and may not look like urine; creatinine and potassium concentrations of the fluid are diagnostic when compared to serum levels.
- Asepsis (urethral and peritoneal drainage catheters, sterile collection system) is essential for preventing complications secondary to infection.
- In dogs and cats, lower urinary tract injuries are more common than renal/ureteral injuries. Therefore, contrast cystography and retrograde urethrography take precedence over intravenous excretory urography.
- Surgical repair is not attempted until the animal has been stabilized with fluid therapy and abdominal drainage.

SUGGESTED READING

Aumann M, et al: Uroperitoneum in cats: 26 cases (1986-1995). *J Am Anim Hosp Assoc* 34:315-324, 1998.

Côté E, et al: Diagnosis of urinary bladder rupture using ultrasound contrast cystography: *In vitro* model and two case-history reports. *Vet Radiol Ultrasound* 43:281-286, 2002.

Feeney DA: Role of imaging in urinary tract emergencies. *Proc Int Vet Emerg Crit Care Soc VII* 414-417, 2000.

Gannon KM, Moses LM: Uroabdomen in dogs and cats. *Comp Cont Educ Pract Vet* 24(8):604-612, 2002.

Mann FA: Acute abdomen: Evaluation and emergency treatment. In Bonagura JD, Dhupa N, Murtaugh RJ (eds): *Kirk's Current Veterinary Therapy XIII: Small Animal Practice*. Philadelphia, WB Saunders, 2000, pp 162-163.

McLoughlin MA: Surgical emergencies of the urinary tract. *Vet Clin North Am Small Anim Pract* 30(3):585-593, 2000.

Schmiedt C, et al: Evaluation of abdominal fluid: Peripheral blood creatinine and potassium ratios for diagnosis of uroperitoneum in dogs. *J Vet Emerg Crit Care Soc* 11(4): 275-280, 2001.

AUTHOR: **KRISTI M. GANNON**

EDITOR: **ELIZABETH ROZANSKI**

Urolithiasis, Other

Client Education Sheet on Website

BASIC INFORMATION

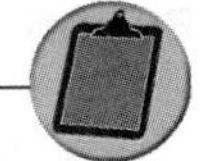

DEFINITION

Organized concretions located in the urinary tract that are composed of cystine, calcium phosphate ($CaPO_4$), or silica

SYNONYM(S)

$CaPO_4$: apatite uroliths
Cystine: cysteine

EPIDEMIOLOGY

SPECIES, AGE, SEX

- Cystine: uncommon in dogs, rare in cats. Onset in middle age. Males are overrepresented.
- $CaPO_4$: uncommon in dogs, rare in cats. Middle aged to older. Gender prevalence varies: brushite—mostly males; hydroxyapatite—either sex; carbonate apatite—female.
- Silica: rare in dogs. Middle aged. Males predominate.

GENETICS AND BREED PREDISPOSITION: Many breeds are affected, and several breeds are overrepresented for each urolith type:

- Cystine: English bulldog, dachshund, mastiff, Newfoundland (cystinuria: autosomal recessive trait), Siamese cats, others
- $CaPO_4$: miniature schnauzer, Yorkshire terrier, shih tzu, others
- Silica: German shepherd, miniature schnauzer, cocker spaniel, others

RISK FACTORS

- Cystine: renal tubular transport defects for cystinuria
- $CaPO_4$: primary hyperparathyroidism, distal renal tubular acidosis, hypercalcemia

GEOGRAPHY AND SEASONALITY: Cystine: prevalence greater in Europe than in the United States.

ASSOCIATED CONDITIONS AND DISORDERS

- Urethral obstruction
- Renal dystrophic mineralization
- A link between cystinuria and taurine-deficient dilated cardiomyopathy has

been proposed in the Newfoundland dog but remains unproven. Cystine is a precursor for taurine synthesis.

CLINICAL PRESENTATION

HISTORY, CHIEF COMPLAINT: Clinical signs may be absent. If present, they may include:

- Hematuria
- Pollakiuria
- Dysuria
- Stranguria
- Inappropriate elimination
- Rarely, systemic illness due to urinary obstruction

PHYSICAL EXAM FINDINGS: Examination may be unremarkable. Abnormalities, if present, may include:

- Hematuria (stains on prepuce, vulva, if present, or hocks)
- Painful urinary bladder
- Palpable cystic calculi
- Palpable urethral calculi (via digital rectal exam)
- Enlarged turgid bladder, if urethral obstruction
- Renomegaly, if secondary hydronephrosis

ETIOLOGY AND PATHOPHYSIOLOGY

- Cystine:
  - Inborn error of metabolism leading to defective renal tubular transport of cystine (± other amino acids) resulting in cystinuria.
- $CaPO_4$:
  - Hypercalcemia is contributory but not necessary.
  - Hypercalciuria may occur without hypercalcemia.
  - Factors decreasing the solubility of calcium salts (e.g., urine pH) or promoting crystallization (e.g., deficient inhibitor substances, epitaxy [concentric layered formation of a stone of mixed composition]) also contribute.
- Silica:
  - Poorly understood. May be associated with ingestion of silica-rich feedstuffs such as rice or soybean hulls.

DIAGNOSIS

DIFFERENTIAL DIAGNOSIS

- Other types of uroliths
- Urinary neoplasia
- Urinary tract infection

INITIAL DATABASE

- Complete blood count: unremarkable
- Serum biochemical profile: hypercalcemia in some animals with $CaPO_4$ uroliths
- Complete urinalysis: hematuria, crystalluria, bacturia, pyuria:
  - Cystine: aciduria to neutral
  - $CaPO_4$: alkiuria (apatite/hydroxyapatite) to neutral to aciduria (brushite)
  - Silica: pH variable (solubility not linked to pH)
- Urine culture and sensitivity
- Abdominal radiographs:
  - Cystine uroliths: radiolucent to slightly radiopaque
  - $CaPO_4$ uroliths: radiopaque
  - Silica uroliths: radiopaque
  - Relative radiopacity: struvite ≈ oxalate ≈ $CaPO_4$ ≈ silica > cystine > urate
- Abdominal ultrasound: confirm/identify radiopaque/radiolucent uroliths, assess kidneys for pyelonephritis, hydronephrosis
- Urethral catheterization: rule out obstruction

ADVANCED OR CONFIRMATORY TESTING

- Contrast cystography/urethrography for radiolucent uroliths
- Urolith quantitative analysis
- Cystoscopy: may facilitate stone removal for analysis and therapy
- Screening tests for cystinuria (Metabolic Screening Laboratory, Veterinary Hospital University of Pennsylvania)
- 24-hour urine assay of calcium excretion
- Specific tests for diagnosis of hypercalcemia (see Hypercalcemia, p 543)

TREATMENT

THERAPEUTIC GOAL(S)

- Remove stones by medical dissolution (cystine) or mechanical removal (any)
- Eliminate urinary tract infection
- Address underlying metabolic disorders (e.g., hypercalcemia, renal tubular defects)
- Prevent recurrence

ACUTE GENERAL TREATMENT

- Relieve urinary tract obstruction
- Antibiotics for documented urinary tract infection; selection based on culture and sensitivity
- Choose between medical dissolution and mechanical calculi removal:
  - Urinary obstruction should be relieved mechanically
  - Mechanical removal allows for urolith analysis, culture
  - Cystine uroliths are amenable to medial dissolution; $CaPO_4$ and silica uroliths are not
  - Medical dissolution: see Chronic Treatment below
- Mechanical removal of calculi:
  - Urohydropropulsion (voiding, retrograde) (see Urethral Obstruction [Canine]: Medical Management, p 1318; Urethral Obstruction [Feline]: Medical Management, p 1319)
    - Avoid performing voiding urohydropropulsion in male cats without perineal urethrostomy
  - Catheter assisted retrieval
  - Cystoscopic assisted retrieval
  - Surgery
  - Lithotripsy

CHRONIC TREATMENT

- Promote water consumption
  - Goal is the production of dilute urine: slows precipitation/concretion of minerals and stone formation
- Cystine uroliths: dissolution may require 1 to 3 months
  - Limit dietary cystine with a restricted protein diet low in methionine (e.g., Hill's u/d)
  - If urine remains acidic, alkalinize with potassium citrate (50-150 mg/kg PO q 12h; dose adjusted to maintain urine pH of 7.0 to 7.5). Avoid sodium bicarbonate
  - Solubility of cystine increased by administration of N-(2-mercaptopropionyl)-glycine (2-MPG). A higher dose (15-20 mg/kg PO q 12h) is used for promoting dissolution of uroliths, while a lower dose (10-15 mg/kg PO q 12h) is used for preventing recurrence. Not evaluated in cats. Although uncommon, adverse reactions can be serious (e.g., aggression, myopathy, proteinuria, spherocytic anemia, thrombocytopenia, increased liver enzymes, dermatopathy)
- $CaPO_4$: address hypercalcemic conditions

POSSIBLE COMPLICATIONS

- Urinary tract obstruction:
  - Hydronephrosis
  - Hydroureter
- Urinary tract infection
- Cystinuric dogs fed protein restricted diets may be at risk of carnitine and taurine deficiency, potentially with risk of dilated cardiomyopathy

RECOMMENDED MONITORING

- Repeat urinalysis 2 weeks after initiation of medical therapy or diet changes, and again every 2 to 4 weeks thereafter to assess for pH, crystals, specific gravity, or evidence of infection. When pH and specific gravity have met goals (specific gravity <1.020, pH as appropriate for urolith type), monitoring frequency can be extended to q 3-6 months for a year, then q 6-12 months.
- Imaging (radiographs for $CaPO_4$ and silica; contrast or ultrasound for cystine) should be repeated after mechanical

removal or q 2–4 weeks during dissolution. Thereafter, imaging should be repeated q 6–12 months.
- Urine should be cultured if signs/uroliths recur or an active urine sediment is identified on urinalysis.

PROGNOSIS AND OUTCOME

Because cystinuria is due to a persistent renal tubular defect, recurrence of cysteine urolithiasis is likely without dietary modification ± 2-MPG

PEARLS & CONSIDERATIONS

COMMENTS

All of these uroliths are rare, and only the cystine urolith can be medically dissolved.

PREVENTION

- Promote water consumption (e.g., canned food, wetted food, water fountains).
- Cystine: restricted protein diet, urine alkalinization as necessary, ± long-term use of 2-MPG.
- $CaPO_4$: address hypercalcemic disorders directly (e.g., surgical correction of hyperparathyroidism). Avoid low calcium diets (paradoxic hypercalciuria). Other therapies (e.g., thiazide diuretics, dietary modifications, acidification of urine) may be warranted in cases with multiple recurrences.
- Silica: avoid feedstuffs high in silica (e.g., rice, soybean hulls).

CLIENT EDUCATION

- Adherence to dietary therapy must be strict for urolith dissolution.
- Animals with metabolic defects should not be bred.
- Urinary tract obstruction is life threatening. Stranguria should prompt immediate veterinary attention.

SUGGESTED READING

Kruger JM, et al: Canine calcium phosphate uroliths. Etiopathogenesis, diagnosis, and management. *Vet Clin North Am Small Anim Pract* 29:141, 1999.

McClain HM, et al: Hypercalcemia and calcium oxalate urolithiasis in cats: A report of five cases. *J Am Anim Hosp Assoc* 35:297, 1999.

Osborne CA, et al: Canine cystine urolithiasis. Cause, detection, treatment, and prevention. *Vet Clin North Am Small Anim Pract* 29:193, 1999.

Osborne CA, et al: Canine silica urolithiasis. Risk factors, detection, treatment, and prevention. *Vet Clin North Am Small Anim Pract* 29:213, 1999.

Sanderson SL, et al: Evaluation of urinary carnitine and taurine excretion in 5 cystinuric dogs with carnitine and taurine deficiency. *J Vet Intern Med* 15:94, 2001.

AUTHORS: **KAREN K. FAUNT, LEAH A. COHN**

EDITOR: **LEAH A. COHN**

Urolithiasis, Oxalate

Client Education Sheet on Website

BASIC INFORMATION

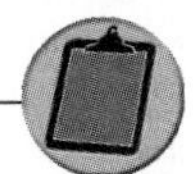

DEFINITION

Organized concretions located in the urinary tract that are composed of calcium oxalate

SYNONYM(S)

Calcium oxalate dihydrate crystals: weddellite

Jack stones

EPIDEMIOLOGY

SPECIES, AGE, SEX

- Dogs:
  - The relative frequency of calcium oxalate urolithiasis has increased over the last 20 years, and they are now the second most common urolith in dogs.
  - They are overwhelmingly the most common cause of nephrolithiasis.
  - Middle-aged to older castrated male dogs are at increased risk for developing calcium oxalate uroliths.
- Cats:
  - Calcium oxalate stones are the most common urolith type in the cat.
  - Incidence is greatest between 7 and 10 years of age, with males accounting for ~60% of affected cats.

GENETICS AND BREED PREDISPOSITION

- Dog breeds at increased risk for developing calcium oxalate stones include the miniature schnauzer, Lhasa apso, Yorkshire terrier, bichon frise, pomeranian, shih tzu, and miniature poodle.
- Cat breeds at increased risk for forming calcium oxalate stones include the ragdoll, British shorthair, foreign shorthair, Himalayan, Havana brown, Scottish fold, Persian, and exotic shorthair.

RISK FACTORS

- Hypercalcemia
- Acidic urine
- Highly concentrated urine
- Infrequent urination
- Primary hyperparathyroidism
- Hyperadrenocorticism
- Chronic metabolic acidosis
- Obesity
- Diets designed to minimize struvite formation in cats

ASSOCIATED CONDITIONS AND DISORDERS: Hypercalcemia (any cause, especially primary hyperparathyroidism), feline lower urinary tract signs/disease/urologic syndrome, hyperadrenocorticism, chronic renal failure.

CLINICAL PRESENTATION

HISTORY, CHIEF COMPLAINT: Clinical signs may be absent. When clinical signs are apparent, they may include:

- Hematuria
- Pollakiuria
- Dysuria
- Stranguria
- Inappropriate elimination
- Rarely, systemic illness due to urinary obstruction
- Polyuria/polydipsia if hypercalcemic

PHYSICAL EXAM FINDINGS: Physical exam may be unremarkable. Abnormalities may include:

- Hematuria (stains on prepuce, vulva, or hocks)
- Painful urinary bladder
- Palpable cystic calculi
- Palpable urethral calculi (via digital rectal exam in dogs)
- Enlarged turgid bladder, if urethral obstruction
- Renomegaly, if secondary hydronephrosis
- Findings associated with predisposing factors (e.g., hyperadrenocorticism: pot bellied appearance, alopecia, hepatomegaly)

ETIOLOGY AND PATHOPHYSIOLOGY

- Hypercalciuria and/or hyperoxaluria promote formation of calcium oxalate urolithiasis.
- Hypercalciuria may result from increased intestinal absorption of calcium, increased renal excretion of calcium, or increased resorption of calcium from bone with or without hypercalcemia.
- Hypercalcemia is identified in ~35% of cats and ~4% of dogs with calcium oxalate urolithiasis.

- Hyperoxaluria in cats may be related to dietary sources, inadequate vitamin B_6, and hepatic enzyme deficiencies.
- Urolith formation is potentiated by diminished concentrations of urinary crystallization inhibitors (e.g., citrate, pyrophosphate, glycosaminoglycans, Tamm-Horsfall mucoprotein).
- Diets with moderate fat and carbohydrate levels are associated with an increased risk of calcium oxalate stone formation, while diets high in moisture with a moderate magnesium, phosphorus, and calcium content result in a diminished risk.

DIAGNOSIS

DIFFERENTIAL DIAGNOSIS

- Other types of uroliths
- Urinary neoplasia
- Urinary tract infection

INITIAL DATABASE

- Complete blood count: unremarkable
- Serum biochemistry profile (including electrolytes):
  - Typically unremarkable.
  - Hypercalcemia or evidence of endocrinopathy may be detected.
  - Urinary tract obstruction results in azotemia, hyperkalemia, and metabolic acidosis.
- Urinalysis: acidic pH unless secondary bacterial infection present; crystalluria; hematuria; pyuria:
  - Storage of urine may lead to precipitation of oxalate crystals (artifact).
  - Urine sediment therefore should be examined within 2 hours of collection.
- Urine culture and sensitivity
- Abdominal/pelvic radiographs: radiopaque calculi most commonly located in bladder, sometimes urethra, ureter, or renal pelvis:
  - Relative radiopacity of uroliths: struvite ≈ oxalate ≈ $CaPO_4$ ≈ silica > cystine > urate.
  - When abdominal radiographs are taken of animals with a chief complaint of stranguria, the perineum must be included in the radiographic field in order to see uroliths located in the urethra.

ADVANCED OR CONFIRMATORY TESTING

- Abdominal ultrasound: confirm location of stones (seldom adds additional benefit to abdominal radiography, since oxalate uroliths are radiopaque), assess kidneys for evidence of pyelonephritis, hydronephrosis
- Urolith (stone) analysis: retrieved stones should be submitted for quantitative analysis (crystallography, x-ray diffraction, infared spectroscopy)
- Urolith (stone) culture
- Cystoscopy: may facilitate stone removal for analysis and therapy (see Cystoscopy, p 1216)
- Specific diagnostic tests may be indicated to confirm predisposing conditions (e.g., parathyroid hormone assay)

TREATMENT

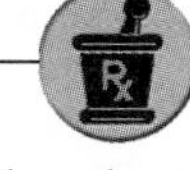

THERAPEUTIC GOAL(S)

- Identify and treat underlying disorder, if present
- Mechanical removal of bladder or urethral calculi
- Treat secondary infection
- Prevent recurrence or growth of uroliths

ACUTE GENERAL TREATMENT

- Relieve urinary tract obstruction. See Urethral Obstruction (Canine): Medical Management, p 1318; Urethral Obstruction (Feline): Medical Management, p 1319.
- Antibiotics if urinary tract infection is present, based on culture and sensitivity.
- If uroliths are found incidentally in the absence of clinical signs, it is reasonable to institute preventive measures to minimize growth of uroliths and to adopt a program of regular follow-up, including periodic urinalysis, urine culture, and radiography.
- Mechanical removal of bladder/urethral calculi producing clinical signs. Radiographs should be repeated afterwards to ensure complete removal.
  - Urohydropropulsion (voiding, retrograde):
    - Avoid voiding urohydropropulsion in male cats without perineal urethrostomy
  - Catheter assisted retrieval
  - Cystoscopic assisted retrieval
  - Surgery
  - Lithotrispy
- Calcium oxalate is the most common type of nephrolith/ureterolith. Because surgical removal of nephroliths may be associated with loss of renal function, it is not uniformly indicated. See Nephrolithiasis, p 748.

CHRONIC TREATMENT

- Determine if underlying disorder (e.g., hyperadrenocorticism, hyperparathyroidism) is present, and treat appropriately
  - For cats with idiopathic hypercalcemia, a diet high in fiber may be beneficial. To simultaneously alkalinize the urine, add potassium citrate (75 mg/kg PO q 12h, adjusted to increase urine pH to 6.5-7.0).
- Initiate measures to prevent recurrence, as described

POSSIBLE COMPLICATIONS

- Urinary tract obstruction
- Hydronephrosis
- Hydroureter
- Chronic renal failure (nephrolithiasis)
- Urinary tract infection
- Diets appropriate for prevention of calcium oxalate urolithiasis may predispose to struvite urolithiasis

RECOMMENDED MONITORING

- Repeat urinalysis q 2 weeks, starting 2 weeks after removal of stones and initiation of dietary changes until pH is between 6.5 and 7.0, specific gravity is between 1.010 and 1.020, and no calcium oxalate crystals are found. If goals are not met, consider adding supplementary therapies (see Prevention below).
- Repeat abdominal radiographs and a urinalysis every 3 to 6 months for the first year, then every 6 to 12 months thereafter to evaluate for recurrence of uroliths.
- Monitor and treat any concurrent conditions such as hypercalcemia.

PROGNOSIS AND OUTCOME

- Recurrence is common; therefore, long-term monitoring and care are required.
- Nephrolithiasis may be associated with diminished renal function.

PEARLS & CONSIDERATIONS

COMMENTS

- Calcium oxalate urolithiasis frequently recurs. Therefore, long-term management and observation are necessary.
- Calcium oxalate crystalluria does not necessarily correlate with the presence of calcium oxalate uroliths.
- Calcium oxalate dihydrate crystals (square envelope, or Maltese cross, shape: ⊠) are more commonly associated with nutritional or artifactual causes, whereas calcium oxalate monohydrate crystals ("picket fence board," or flattened hexagon, shape: ⬭) are more commonly associated with ethylene glycol intoxication.
- Calcium oxalate dihydrate crystalluria can be found in normal urine and does not reliably predict oxalate urolithiasis.
- Large quantities of calcium oxalate dihydrate crystals or large crystal aggregates should prompt evaluation of hyperoxaluric or hypercalciuric conditions.
- The appearance of calcium oxalate monohydrate crystals in a dog presenting with acute renal failure is strongly

suggestive of ethylene glycol intoxication (see Ethylene Glycol Intoxication, p 367).

PREVENTION

- Treat any identified cause of hypercalcemia.
- Initiate measures to prevent recurrence in a stepwise manner, adding the next measure when the first one is found to be insufficient to produce urine with a pH between 6.5 and 7.0, a urine specific gravity between 1.010 and 1.020, or prevent calcium oxalate crystal formation.
  - Promote water consumption (e.g., canned diet, wetted food, water fountains for cats).
  - Provide diet with restricted oxalate, sodium, and protein and which does not acidify the urine. Examples include Royal Canin (Waltham) SO, Hills Pet Nutrition u/d (for dogs) or x/d (for cats), or Eukanuba Moderate pH/O/Feline.
  - Potassium citrate can be added if the urinary pH remains acidic. Initial dose of 50-75 mg/kg PO q 12h is adjusted to maintain urine pH 6.5-7.0.
  - If calcium oxalate crystalluria persists despite prior measures, hydrochlorothiazide (2-4 mg/kg PO q 12h) or vitamin B_6 (2 mg/kg PO q 12h) can be added.
  - Avoid supplementation of vitamins C and D.
- For males with recurrent history of urethral obstruction, consider perineal urethrostomy.

CLIENT EDUCATION

- Adherence to dietary therapy must be strict.
- Urinary tract obstruction is life threatening. Stranguria should prompt immediate veterinary attention.

SUGGESTED READING

Bartges JW, et al: Update: Management of calcium oxalate uroliths in dogs and cats. *Vet Clin North Am Small Anim Pract* 34:969, 2004.

Lekcharoensuk C, et al: Association between dietary factors and calcium oxalate and magnesium ammonium phosphate urolithiasis in cats. *J Am Vet Med Assoc* 219:1228, 2001.

Lekcharoensuk C, et al: Patient and environmental factors associated with calcium oxalate urolithiasis in dogs. *J Am Vet Med Assoc* 217:55, 2000.

AUTHORS: **KAREN K. FAUNT, LEAH A. COHN**
EDITOR: **LEAH A. COHN**

Urolithiasis, Struvite

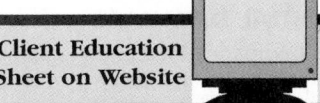
Client Education Sheet on Website

BASIC INFORMATION

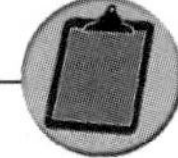

DEFINITION

Organized concretions located in the urinary tract composed of magnesium ammonium phosphate

SYNONYM(S)

Infection stones
Magnesium ammonium phosphate stones
Struvite calculi
Triple phosphate stones
Urease stones

EPIDEMIOLOGY

SPECIES, AGE, SEX

- Dogs:
  - The most common urolith of dogs, struvite uroliths in this species are usually associated with urinary tract infections (UTI) involving urease-producing bacteria.
  - Sterile struvite urolithiasis is rare in dogs.
  - Found at any age, they occur nearly twice as often in females as in males.
- Cats:
  - The second most common urolith of cats, struvite uroliths are typically found in sterile, alkaline urine.
  - Female cats may be at increased risk.
  - Compared to calcium oxalate uroliths (most common in cats), cats with struvite uroliths are generally younger and are more likely to be neutered.

GENETICS AND BREED PREDISPOSITION

- Dogs: Many breeds and breed mixes are affected. Miniature schnauzers, shih tzus, bichon frises, miniature poodles, cocker spaniels, and Lhasa apsos are overrepresented. Cocker spaniels may form sterile struvite uroliths.
- Cats: Commonly affected breeds include the domestic shorthair, foreign shorthair, ragdoll, Chartreux, Oriental shorthair, and Himalayan.

RISK FACTORS

- Dogs:
  - UTI
  - Highly concentrated urine
  - Infrequent urination
- Cats:
  - Highly concentrated urine
  - Alkaline urine
  - Diets high in magnesium

ASSOCIATED CONDITIONS AND DISORDERS

- Dogs: UTI
- Cats: feline lower urinary tract signs/FLUTD/FUS; urethral plugs

CLINICAL PRESENTATION

HISTORY, CHIEF COMPLAINT: Clinical signs may be absent. When clinical signs are apparent, they may include:

- Hematuria
- Pollakiuria
- Dysuria
- Stranguria
- Inappropriate elimination
- Rarely, systemic illness due to urinary obstruction or to ascending infection causing pyelonephritis

PHYSICAL EXAM FINDINGS: Physical exam may be unremarkable. Abnormalities may include:

- Hematuria (stains on prepuce, vulva, or hocks)
- Painful urinary bladder
- Palpable cystic calculi
- Palpable urethral calculi (via digital rectal exam in dogs)
- Enlarged turgid bladder, if urethral obstruction
- Renomegaly, if secondary hydronephrosis

ETIOLOGY AND PATHOPHYSIOLOGY

- Infection associated struvite urolithiasis (mainly dogs):
  - Bacterial urease converts urea to ammonia and bicarbonate.
    - The most common urease-producing pathogens are *Staphylococcus* and *Proteus* spp.
    - Other urease-producing pathogens include *Pseudomonas*, *Klebsiella*, and *Ureaplasma* (urease-producing *Mycoplasma*) spp.
  - Ammonium binds to phosphorus and magnesium, forming struvite crystals.
  - Bicarbonate increases urine pH.
  - Alkalinity decreases solubility of magnesium ammonium phosphate crystals.

- Crystals aggregate with organic material (including viable bacteria) and combine to form stones.
- Decreased presence of glycosaminoglycans.
- Sterile struvite urolithiasis (mainly cats): There appears to be a complex relationship between diet, water intake, individual predisposition and subsequent urine pH and relative supersaturation.
  - Diets high in magnesium, phosphorus, calcium, chloride, and fiber with moderate protein content may predispose to struvite crystal formation.

DIAGNOSIS

DIFFERENTIAL DIAGNOSIS

- Other types of uroliths
- Urinary neoplasia
- Urinary tract infection

INITIAL DATABASE

- Complete blood count: unremarkable
- Serum biochemistry profile (including electrolytes): typically unremarkable unless urinary obstruction.
- Complete urinalysis: alkaline urine pH, bacturia, crystalluria, hematuria, and pyuria are possible findings.
  - Storage of urine may lead to precipitation of struvite crystals. Urine sediment therefore should be examined within 2 hours of collection.
- Urine culture and sensitivity.
- Abdominal radiographs:
  - Radiopaque calculi most commonly located in bladder, sometimes urethra, ureter, or kidney.
  - Struvite calculi are generally radiopaque (radiopacity: struvite ≈ oxalate ≈ $CaPO_4$ ≈ silica > cystine > urate).

ADVANCED OR CONFIRMATORY TESTING

- Abdominal ultrasound: confirm location of stones (seldom adds additional benefit to abdominal radiography), assess kidneys for evidence of pyelonephritis, hydronephrosis
- Urolith (stone) analysis: retrieved stones should be submitted for quantitative analysis (crystallography, x-ray diffraction, infrared spectroscopy) to determine urolith type and the best course of long-term treatment/management
- Urolith (stone) culture: ideally, retrieved stones are cultured, since viable bacteria can be found within the matrix of the stone
- Cystoscopy: may facilitate stone removal for analysis and therapy (see Cystoscopy, p 1216)

TREATMENT

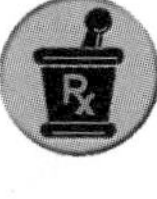

THERAPEUTIC GOAL(S)

- Eliminate UTI
- Remove stones by medical dissolution or mechanical removal
- Prevent recurrence

ACUTE GENERAL TREATMENT

- Relieve urinary tract obstruction (see Urethral Obstruction [Canine]: Medical Management, p 1318; Urethral Obstruction [Feline]: Medical Management, p 1319)
- Antibiotics for urinary tract infection, based on culture and sensitivity results (dogs > cats; see Cystitis, Bacterial, p 270)
- Choose between medial dissolution and mechanical calculi removal:
  - Urinary tract obstruction should be relieved mechanically.
  - Mechanical removal allows for urolith analysis, culture.
  - Even large stones can be amenable to medical dissolution.
  - Provided urethral obstruction is absent, trial of medical dissolution prior to mechanical removal is reasonable; potential drawbacks include risk of obstruction prior to complete dissolution and risk of ineffectiveness with uroliths of mixed composition.
- For medical dissolution, calculytic diets and appropriate antimicrobials are required:
  - Mean time to dissolution is 3 months (less for sterile uroliths).
  - Variety of commercial diets available for struvite dissolution:
    - Hills Pet Nutrition s/d
    - Royal Canin (Waltham) SO
  - Urinalysis and urine culture should be repeated 5 to 7 days after initiating medical therapy. Goals are urine pH <7.0, urine specific gravity 1.010 to 1.020, and negative culture.
  - Medical therapy is continued 1 month beyond radiologic disappearance of uroliths.
  - Small stones may become lodged in the urethra (especially males) during stone dissolution.
- Mechanical removal of calculi:
  - Urohydropropulsion (voiding, retrograde).
    - Avoid performing voiding urohydropropulsion in male cats without perineal urethrostomy
  - Catheter assisted retrieval.
  - Cystoscopic assisted retrieval (see Cystoscopy, p 1216).
  - Surgery.
  - Lithotripsy.
- Promote water consumption (e.g., canned food, wetting dry food, use of water fountains for cats)

CHRONIC TREATMENT

- Predisposing causes of UTI should be addressed (e.g., control glucosuria in diabetic animals, treat hyperadrenocorticism).
- For animals in which UTI is a recurrent problem, chronic prophylactic antimicrobial therapy may be considered after appropriate therapy of recognized infection (see Cystitis, Bacterial, p 270).
- Diets appropriate for prevention of recurrent struvite uroliths can be fed to animals with sterile struvite urolithiasis (e.g., Royal Canin (Waltham) SO; Hills Pet Nutrition c/d or w/d, Eukanuba Low pH/S/Feline).
- Urinary acidifiers are seldom required if the pet is eating an appropriate diet and urinary tract infection is eliminated.
- Ensuring adequate freah water intake is essential to prevent excessively concentrated urine (e.g., use of cat water fountains) (see Feline Lower Urinary Tract Signs, Idiopathic, p 382).

POSSIBLE COMPLICATIONS

- Risk of urethral obstruction during medical dissolution of stones as the stones become small enough to pass into the urethra (males):
  - Urinary tract obstruction
  - Hydronephrosis
  - Hydroureter
- Urinary tract infection due to catheterization
- Diets appropriate for treatment/prevention of struvite urolithiasis may predispose to calcium oxalate urolithiasis
- Long-term feeding of Hills s/d can lead to malnutrition

RECOMMENDED MONITORING

- Repeat radiographs every 2 to 4 weeks during medical dissolution to evaluate the size and number of uroliths.
- If no improvement is seen on radiographs after 4 to 8 weeks, mechanical removal is indicated.
- Repeat urinalysis 5 to 7 days after initiating medical dissolution therapy to ensure pH between 6.5 and 7, specific gravity between 1.010 and 1.020, absent struvite crystals and absent bacturia.
- Ideally, urine culture is repeated 5 to 7 days after initiating medical dissolution therapy to ensure sterile urine.
- Repeat urine culture 5 to 7 days after stopping antibiotics to evaluate for recurrence of infection, then again 3 to 4 weeks later.
- If predisposing causes of bacterial cystitis cannot be corrected, or in animals with sterile struvite urolithiasis, repeat urinalysis every 4 to 6 months.
- If predisposing causes of bacterial cystitis cannot be corrected, or in animals with sterile struvite urolithiasis, repeat abdominal radiographs initially every 3

to 6 months for 1 year then every 6 months thereafter.

PROGNOSIS AND OUTCOME

- Prognosis for dissolution of uroliths is good
- Recurrence of struvite urolithiasis is common

PEARLS & CONSIDERATIONS

COMMENTS

- Struvite urolithiasis in dogs is routinely associated with a urinary tract infection. Elimination of infection is crucial for dissolution of stones with a calculolytic diet.
- Struvite urolithiasis in cats is rarely associated with urinary tract infections; long-term diet modification is often necessary to prevent recurrence.
- If uroliths fail to resolve with medical therapy, consider:
    - Inadequate infection control
    - Failure to comply with diet restrictions
    - Mixed or alternative urolith composition
- Some struvite dissolution diets (e.g., Hills s/d) are inappropriate for long-term use.
- Struvite crystalluria can be found in normal urine and does not reliably predict struvite urolithiasis.

PREVENTION

- Dogs: if urinary infection can be eliminated, long-term diet change is usually not necessary.
- Cats: long-term use of canned struvite management diets (e.g., Waltham SO or Hills Pet Nutrition c/d or w/d) is best if recurrence noted.
- The merit of supplementing with glycosaminoglycans is unknown.

CLIENT EDUCATION

- Adherence to dietary therapy must be strict.
- Urinary tract obstruction is life threatening. Stranguria should prompt immediate veterinary attention.

SUGGESTED READING

Houston DM, et al: Canine urolithiasis: A look at over 16,000 urolith submissions to the Canadian Veterinary Urolith Centre from February 1998 to April 2003. *Can Vet J* 45:225, 2004.

Lekcharoensuk C, et al: Association between dietary factors and calcium oxalate and magnesium ammonium phosphate urolithiasis in cats. *J Am Vet Med Assoc* 219:1228, 2001.

Lekcharoensuk C, et al: Association between patient-related factors and risk of calcium oxalate and magnesium ammonium phosphate urolithiasis in cats. *J Am Vet Med Assoc* 217:520, 2000.

Seaman R, et al: Canine struvite urolithiasis. *Compend Contin Educ Pract Vet* 23:407, 2001.

AUTHORS: **KAREN K. FAUNT, LEAH A. COHN**

EDITOR: **LEAH A. COHN**

Urolithiasis, Urate/Biurate

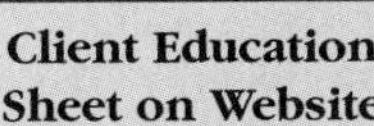

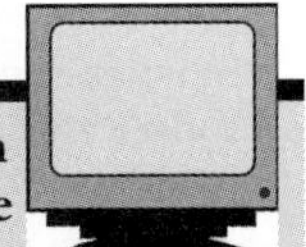

Client Education Sheet on Website

BASIC INFORMATION

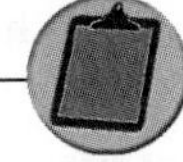

DEFINITION

Organized concretions located in the urinary tract that are composed of uric acid and its salts

SYNONYM(S)

Purine, ammonium urate, or uric acid urolithiasis
Urate and biurate are synonyms
Urate calculi
Urate stones

EPIDEMIOLOGY

SPECIES, AGE, SEX

- Accounting for ~10% of all canine uroliths, they are the most common type in dalmatians. Uncommon in cats.
- Age at diagnosis averages 4.5 years.
- Affected dalmatians are usually male.

GENETICS AND BREED PREDISPOSITION

- All dalmatians are unique in their excretion of uric acid instead of allantoin as an end product of purine metabolism, but only a subset develop urate urolithiasis. The tendency to form uroliths is heritable, although genetics are incompletely understood.
- Predisposed nondalmatian breeds include English bulldog, miniature schnauzer, shih tzu, and Yorkshire terrier.

RISK FACTORS

- Dalmatian breed
- Portosystemic shunt (PSS)
- Hepatic microvascular dysplasia
- Hepatic cirrhosis

ASSOCIATED CONDITIONS AND DISORDERS

- Severe hepatic dysfunction
- Urinary tract infection
- Ureteral or urethral obstruction

CLINICAL PRESENTATION

HISTORY, CHIEF COMPLAINT: Clinical signs may be absent. When apparent, signs may include:

- Stranguria
- Dysuria
- Hematuria
- Pollakiuria
- Inappropriate elimination
- If congenital hepatic disease is present, growth retardation
- If hepatic dysfunction is present, encephalopathy and/or hypoglycemia (e.g., altered mentation, seizures)
- Occasionally, systemic illness due to urinary obstruction

PHYSICAL EXAM FINDINGS: May be unremarkable. When present, abnormalities may include:

- Hematuria (stains on prepuce, vulva, hocks)
- Palpable cystic calculi
- Palpable urethral calculi (via digital rectal exam in dogs)
- Enlarged turgid bladder, if urethral obstruction
- Renomegaly, related to PSS or hydronephrosis
- Small body size if PSS present
- Neurologic deficits related to encephalopathy and/or hypoglycemia if due to congenital hepatic disease

ETIOLOGY AND PATHOPHYSIOLOGY

- Dalmatians:
    - During protein catabolism in normal dogs, purine metabolism normally leads to uric acid oxidation by hepatic uricase with resultant allantoin production.
    - Despite normal uricase activity, dalmatians inadequately convert uric acid to allantoin, resulting in increased urinary excretion of poorly soluble uric acid.

  - Contributing mechanisms may include decreased tubular resorption of uric acid and less activity of urinary crystal inhibiting proteins.
- Non-dalmatian dogs and cats without hepatic dysfunction: unknown
- Animals with hepatic dysfunction: increased renal excretion of uric acid and ammonia resulting from reduced hepatic conversion/urea synthesis

DIAGNOSIS

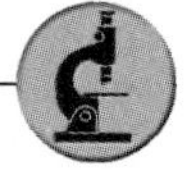

DIFFERENTIAL DIAGNOSIS

- Other types of uroliths
- Urinary neoplasia

INITIAL DATABASE

- Complete blood count: unremarkable. PSS associated with microcytosis
- Serum biochemical profile: may suggest hepatic dysfunction (low blood urea nitrogen, hypoglycemia, hypocholesterolemia, hypoalbuminemia, hyperbilirubinemia if cirrhotic)
- Urinalysis: hematuria, urate crystals, pyuria or bacturia
- Urine culture and sensitivity
- Abdominal radiographs: urate uroliths are poorly seen (radiolucent). Microhepatica suggestive of PSS, cirrhosis
- Abdominal ultrasound: confirm uroliths. May identify PSS, hepatic changes

ADVANCED OR CONFIRMATORY TESTING

- Serum bile acids: rule out hepatic disease
- Contrast cystography/urethrography: localize radiolucent stones (see Cystogram, p 1214; Urethrogram, p 1321)
- Quantitative urolith analysis and culture
- Cystoscopy: may facilitate urolith removal for analysis and therapy (see Cystoscopy, p 1216)

TREATMENT

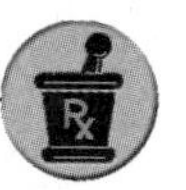

THERAPEUTIC GOAL(S)

- Remove stones medically or mechanically
- Eliminate urinary infection
- Treat hepatic disease
- Prevent recurrence

ACUTE GENERAL TREATMENT

- Relieve urinary obstruction (see Urethral Obstruction [Canine]: Medical Management, p 1318; Urethral Obstruction [Feline]: Medical Management, p 1319)
- Treat hepatic encephalopathy (see Hepatic Encephalopathy, p 489)
- Treat urinary infection (see Cystitis, Bacterial, p 270)
- Choose between medical dissolution (see Chronic Treatment below) and mechanical removal:
  - Urinary obstruction: relieve mechanically
  - Mechanical removal allows for urolith analysis
  - Cats are poorly amenable to medical dissolution of urates
- Mechanical removal:
  - Urohydropropulsion (voiding, retrograde)
    - Avoid performing voiding urohydropropulsion in male cats without perineal urethrostomy
  - Catheter assisted retrieval
  - Cystoscopic retrieval
  - Surgery
  - Lithotripsy

CHRONIC TREATMENT

- Medical dissolution for dogs:
  - Diet low in purine (e.g., Hills u/d, balanced homemade diet)
  - If urine remains acidic, sodium bicarbonate (25-50 mg/kg PO q 12h) or potassium citrate (50-150 mg/kg PO q 12h). Dose adjusted to maintain urine pH of 7.0 to 7.5
  - Allopurinol (10-15 mg/kg PO q 12h) minimizes uric acid production. Use cautiously with renal insufficiency
- Cats: low purine diet (Hills l/d or k/d)
- Animals with hepatic disease:
  - Surgical correction of PSS allows dissolution of uroliths and prevents recurrence
  - If hepatic disease cannot be corrected, institute medical management (including restricted protein diet) and monitor for recurrence
- Promote water consumption (e.g., canned food)

POSSIBLE COMPLICATIONS

- Chronic use of low purine diets may result in cardiomyopathy, perhaps related to carnitine or taurine deficiency.
- Severely protein restricted diets are inappropriate for growing, pregnant, or lactating animals.

RECOMMENDED MONITORING

- Serum biochemical profile and urinalysis 2 weeks after diet change. Goal is urine pH 7 to 7.5, specific gravity <1.020, and absent crystals. Assuming adequate renal function and diet adherence, BUN should be <10 mg/dl. Monitor urinalysis q 2-4 weeks until uroliths resolved and q 3-6 months thereafter.
- Monitor dissolution of uroliths q 2-4 weeks via lower urinary tract contrast studies or ultrasound. Monitor for recurrence in like manner q 3-6 months for a year, then q 6-12 months.

PROGNOSIS AND OUTCOME

- Prognosis for dissolution is good in dogs
- Recurrence is common unless cause resolved (e.g., PSS corrected)

PEARLS & CONSIDERATIONS

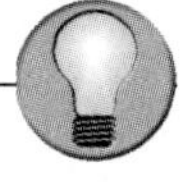

COMMENTS

Nondalmatian dogs and cats with urate uroliths should be evaluated for hepatic disease, even when showing no overt clinical signs of hepatopathy.

PREVENTION

- Avoid high protein diets in at-risk dogs.
- Severely protein restricted diets or allopurinol prior to a first episode of urate urolithiasis is not recommended.
- Heritability of tendency to form urate uroliths suggests breeding affected dalmatians should be avoided.

CLIENT EDUCATION

- Urethral obstruction is life threatening. Stranguria should prompt immediate veterinary attention.
- Adherence to dietary therapy must be strict.
- Implications for heritability in dalmatians should be addressed.

SUGGESTED READING

Bannasch DL, et al: Inheritance of urinary calculi in the dalmatian. *J Vet Intern Med* 18:483, 2004.

Bartges JW, et al: Canine urate urolithiasis. Etiopathogenesis, diagnosis, and management. *Vet Clin North Am Small Anim Pract* 29:161, 1999.

AUTHORS: **KAREN K. FAUNT, LEAH A. COHN**

EDITOR: **LEAH A. COHN**

Uveal Cysts

BASIC INFORMATION

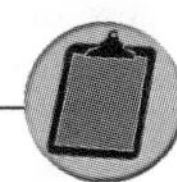

DEFINITION

Generally benign/incidental, round to ovoid, pigmented intraocular structures arising from the iris or ciliary body. They may be seen attached at the pupillary margin and/or the posterior iris, seen free-floating in the anterior chamber, and rarely seen in the vitreous.

SYNONYM(S)

Anterior chamber cysts
Ciliary cysts
Iridociliary cysts
Iris cysts
Pupillary cysts

EPIDEMIOLOGY

SPECIES, AGE, SEX: Dogs, cats, and other domestic species; in dogs, mean age is 6.8 to 9.1 years. No sex predilection.

GENETICS AND BREED PREDISPOSITION

- Dogs: golden retrievers, Labrador retrievers, Boston terriers, Great Danes, rottweilers
- Cats: Siamese (one report)

RISK FACTORS

- Trauma
- Uveitis, especially lens-induced uveitis; uveal cysts may arise as a consequence of uveitis, or uveitis may result as a consequence of the cysts (see Uveitis, p 1134)
- Spontaneous in nature in most cases

ASSOCIATED CONDITIONS AND DISORDERS

- Dogs: uveitis and secondary glaucoma (i.e., glaucoma results as a complication of the cysts) associated with iridociliary cysts in golden retrievers and Great Danes (Fig. I-180)
- Cats: Cysts may be associated with trauma or uveitis

CLINICAL PRESENTATION

DISEASE FORMS/SUBTYPES

- Free-floating cysts within the anterior chamber (see Fig. I-180)
- Cysts attached to the pupillary margin
- Iridociliary cysts
- Rarely cysts in the vitreous

HISTORY, CHIEF COMPLAINT

- Usually incidental findings
- Pigmented intraocular mass
- Signs of uveitis (see Uveitis, p 1134) and glaucoma (see Glaucoma, p 440) in golden retrievers and Great Danes
- Intraocular bleeding (rare)
- Vision impairment

PHYSICAL EXAM FINDINGS

- Single or multiple pigmented masses in anterior chamber, along pupillary margin, posterior to the iris, or rarely in the vitreous.
- Canine uveal cysts are often translucent such that they can be transilluminated (i.e., it is possible to see through them using a strong light source, such as a Finnoff transilluminator), whereas feline uveal cysts may be very dark and difficult to transilluminate.

ETIOLOGY AND PATHOPHYSIOLOGY

- Most are spontaneous in nature but may be associated with previous trauma or anterior uveitis
- Generally arise from the pigmented epithelial layer of the iris or the ciliary body

DIAGNOSIS

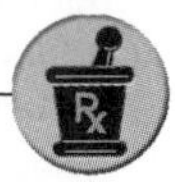

DIFFERENTIAL DIAGNOSIS

- Iridal or anterior uveal melanomas.
- To differentiate uveal cysts (often translucent and thus can be transilluminated) from neoplastic tissue (more dense/opaque and cannot be transilluminated), a strong light source, such as a Finnoff transilluminator, is advised.

INITIAL DATABASE

- Neuro-ophthalmic examination
- Schirmer tear test, intraocular pressure measurement, and fluorescein staining
- Full ocular examination performed with and without mydriasis (topical tropicamide 1%)

ADVANCED OR CONFIRMATORY TESTING

- Ocular ultrasonography may confirm the diagnosis by revealing a cyst's anechoic (fluid-filled) center
- Biopsy of cyst and its contents can be performed, but this is usually not necessary

TREATMENT

THERAPEUTIC GOAL(S)

- Most cases are benign and incidental.
- Cyst removal can be contemplated if the cysts are very large, obstruct the pupillary axis, cause corneal endothelial decompensation (edema), or are associated with iris plateauing and glaucoma.

ACUTE GENERAL TREATMENT

- Laser ablation of cysts with a Nd:YAG or diode laser
- Aspiration of the cyst with a 25- to 27-gauge needle through a limbal paracentesis

CHRONIC TREATMENT

- Usually not necessary unless chronic uveitis or glaucoma is present. Therapy may entail topical steroidal ophthalmic preparations (prednisolone acetate 1% or dexamethasone 0.1%), topical nonsteroidal agents (diclofenac 0.1% or flurbiprofen 0.03%), as well as topical and oral antiglaucoma medications.
- Laser ablation of the cysts or selective laser ablation of the ciliary body to control increased intraocular pressure.

POSSIBLE COMPLICATIONS

- Cyst rupture with adherence to the corneal endothelium or anterior lens capsule
- Mechanical interference with iris function
- Aqueous outflow obstruction:
  - Secondary glaucoma

RECOMMENDED MONITORING

- For most asymptomatic cases, monitor every 6 to 12 months

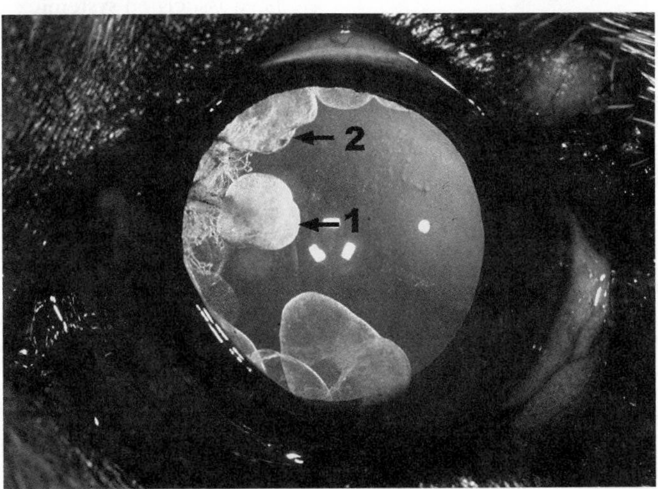

FIGURE I-180 Multiple uveal cysts in a dog located in the anterior chamber (*1*) and posterior to the iris (*2*).

- If the condition is associated with uveitis or glaucoma, recheck every 2 to 4 months or sooner

PROGNOSIS AND OUTCOME

Generally benign condition; of concern in the golden retriever and Great Dane breeds

- According to one report, 46% of the eyes studied in golden retrievers became blind due to glaucoma.

PEARLS & CONSIDERATIONS

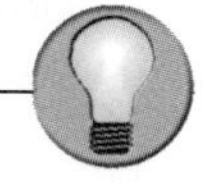

COMMENTS

A strong light source is advised for ocular examination and transillumination (Finnoff transilluminator) to differentiate uveal cysts (often translucent) from neoplastic tissue (more dense/opaque and cannot be transilluminated).

PREVENTION

- Breeds of dogs predisposed to uveal cysts: avoid breeding affected or closely related individuals
- If associated with uveitis, topical anti-inflammatory medications are advised

CLIENT EDUCATION

- Uveal cysts are typically a benign condition, requiring no therapy. Periodic recheck evaluations are advised every 6 to 8 months.
- If the cysts become large, impair vision, or are associated with glaucoma, laser ablation can be considered.

SUGGESTED READING

Corcoran KA, Koch SA: Uveal cysts in dogs: 28 cases (1989-1991). *J Am Vet Med Assoc* 203:545-546, 1993.

Gemensky-Metzler AJ, Wilkie DA, Cook CS: The use of semiconductor diode laser for deflation and coagulation of anterior uveal cysts in dogs, cats, and horses: A report of 20 cases. *Vet Ophthalmol* 7:360-368, 2004.

Sapienza JS, et al: Golden retriever uveitis: 75 cases (1994-1999). *Vet Ophthalmol* 3:241- 246, 2000.

AUTHOR: **JOHN S. SAPIENZA**

EDITOR: **CHERYL L. CULLEN**

Uveitis

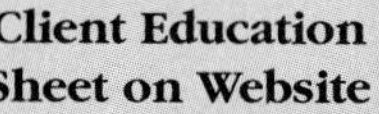

Client Education Sheet on Website

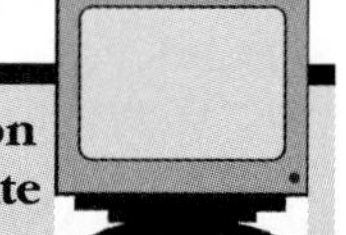

BASIC INFORMATION

DEFINITION

Inflammation of part or all of the uveal tract, including the iris, ciliary body, and choroid (Fig. I-181). May be associated with inflammation of adjacent structures such as the retina, vitreous, sclera, lens, and cornea

SYNONYM(S)

Anterior uveitis: iridocyclitis; cyclitis

Panuveitis (inflammation of the entire uveal tract)

Posterior uveitis: choroiditis; chorioretinitis; retinochoroiditis

EPIDEMIOLOGY

SPECIES, AGE, SEX: Dogs and cats; any age or sex.

GENETICS AND BREED PREDISPOSITION: Many forms of uveitis have a significant immune-mediated component and thus may have a genetic/breed predisposition:

- Uveodermatologic syndrome/Vogt-Koyanagi-Harada (VKH) syndrome: causes granulomatous uveitis and depigmenting dermatitis in dogs, especially Akitas, Samoyeds, and Siberian huskies
- Pigmentary uveitis: associated with pigment dispersion in the anterior chamber in the golden retriever:
  - Uveal cysts (see Uveal Cysts, p 1133) are often seen in conjunction with pigmentary uveitis.

CONTAGION AND ZOONOSIS: A few selected forms of uveitis associated with certain infectious diseases may have contagion and zoonotic potential:

- *Brucella* uveitis (dogs): both contagious and zoonotic implications
- Feline leukemia virus (FeLV), feline infectious peritonitis (FIP), and feline immunodeficiency virus (FIV) infections: contagious between cats
- Toxoplasmosis in cats may have zoonotic potential (see Toxoplasmosis/Neosporosis, p 1093)

GEOGRAPHY AND SEASONALITY: Certain infectious disease etiologies may exhibit seasonality and/or geographic incidence.

ASSOCIATED CONDITIONS AND DISORDERS

- Variable, depending on the underlying cause.
- Uveitis associated with infectious diseases frequently, but not invariably, may have associated systemic signs.
- Immune-mediated causes of uveitis may also have nonocular signs (e.g., dermatologic signs as noted in uveodermatologic syndrome/VKH).

CLINICAL PRESENTATION

DISEASE FORMS/SUBTYPES

- Portion of the uvea involved (anterior: iris and/or ciliary body; posterior: choroid; panuveitis: entire uveal tract)
- Acute versus chronic
- Type of inflammation (i.e., nongranulomatous versus granulomatous; nonsuppurative versus suppurative)
- Cause of the uveitis

HISTORY, CHIEF COMPLAINT

- Variable systemic complaints if caused by systemic disease
- "Red eye"
- Vision problem

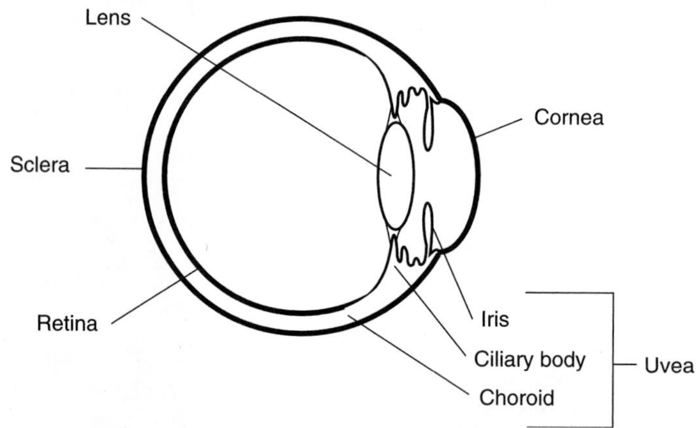

FIGURE I-181 Sagittal section of the globe, showing the anatomic relationships of the uvea to the other parts of the eye.

- Photophobia
- Blepharospasm
- Color changes in interior of eye

PHYSICAL EXAM FINDINGS

- Conjunctiva and episclera:
  - Injection
- Cornea:
  - Corneal edema of varying degrees
  - Corneal vascularization if more chronic
  - Keratic precipitates (forms of white blood cell [WBC] aggregates in which multiple, round to ovoid, gray to yellowish opacities are noted on the posterior cornea)
- Anterior chamber:
  - Aqueous flare (cloudiness of the aqueous humor caused by increased protein levels)
  - Fibrin clots
  - Hyphema
  - Hypopyon
- Iris:
  - Color changes (e.g., blue iris becomes brown, brown iris becomes darker or depigmented)
  - Texture changes (e.g., thickened iris with possible visible neovascularization, such as in rubeosis iridis)
- Pupil:
  - Acute, often miotic; chronic midrange in size
  - Slow to dilate in response to or lack of response to mydriatics, such as to topical 1% tropicamide
  - Focal or diffuse posterior synechia (adhesions of iris-to-lens; e.g., iris bombé, 360 degrees pupillary synechiae impairing aqueous drainage and causing iris to balloon forward)
  - Lack of consensual pupillary light reflex in opposite eye if involved eye is blind
- Lens:
  - Varying degrees of cataract
  - Intraocular pressure (IOP): low unless complicated by secondary glaucoma
- Posterior segment:
  - Posterior uveitis may be accompanied by effusive retinal detachments of varying degrees
  - Vitreal haze due to inflammation in vitreous humor
  - Diffuse or more likely multifocal color changes in the fundus associated with inflammatory infiltrates
  - Optic nerve swelling and hyperemia in some cases

ETIOLOGY AND PATHOPHYSIOLOGY

- All types of uveitis involve tissue damage.
- Clinical signs are attributed to disruption of the blood-ocular barrier (physiologic mechanism that prevents exchange of materials between the blood and the chambers of the eye) and release of numerous chemical mediators following tissue damage.

Etiologies:

- Primary ocular:
  - Blunt and perforating trauma (see Corneal/Scleral Trauma, p 244), including surgical trauma.
  - Corneal ulceration (see Corneal Ulceration, p 246).
  - Lens-induced:
    - Rapidly developing or hypermature cataracts leaking soluble lens proteins into eye causing phacolytic uveitis.
    - Lens capsule rupture causing phacoclastic uveitis.
    - Lens luxation (see Lens Luxation, p 628).
  - Scleritis (see Episcleritis/Scleritis, p 353).
  - Uveal cysts (see Uveal Cysts, p 1133).
  - Primary intraocular neoplasia, such as uveal melanoma (see Intraocular Neoplasia, p 603).
- Systemic:
  - Infectious diseases that are often species-specific:
    - Cats: toxoplasmosis, FIP, FeLV, FIV, systemic mycoses, bartonellosis, tuberculosis, herpesvirus.
    - Dogs: infectious canine hepatitis, ehrlichiosis, Rocky Mountain spotted fever, toxoplasmosis, protothecosis, brucellosis, borreliosis, leptospirosis, leishmaniasis, systemic mycoses.
  - Aberrent metazoan parasites: *Dirofilaria immitis*, ascarids, fly larvae.
  - Secondary intraocular neoplasia (e.g., lymphosarcoma most common).
  - Immune-mediated: uveodermatologic syndrome/VKH.
  - Pigmentary uveitis in golden retrievers.
  - Idiopathic: In the dog, roughly 50–60% of uveitis work-ups fail to identify a definite cause and are probably immune-mediated; in the cat, lymphocytic-plasmacytic uveitis of undetermined cause is common.

DIAGNOSIS

DIFFERENTIAL DIAGNOSIS

Other causes for "red eye":

- Glaucoma
- Conjunctivitis
- Episcleritis/scleritis
- Keratitis
- Orbital disease

INITIAL DATABASE

- Complete ocular examination of both eyes.
  - A patient may have anterior lesions in one eye and posterior lesions in the contralateral eye.
- IOP: glaucoma is a frequent complication of uveitis (see Glaucoma, p 440).
  - Normal range is 10–25 mmHg.
  - A measurement of <10 mmHg is consistent with uveitis; >30 mmHg is consistent with glaucoma.
- Thorough general physical examination and history: systemic causes for uveitis are common.
- Ocular ultrasound is indicated when opaque ocular media preclude thorough examination.
- Unless the cause is obvious, a systemic work-up with CBC, serum biochemistry profile, and urinalysis is indicated.

ADVANCED OR CONFIRMATORY TESTING

- Selected infectious disease titers based on species, geography, and systemic signs
- Chest radiographs for neoplasia and systemic mycoses
- Fine-needle aspirate (FNA)/biopsy of enlarged lymph nodes, abnormal organs
- Anterior chamber/aqueous centesis in selective cases for culture, cytologic examination, and titers (referable procedure)

TREATMENT

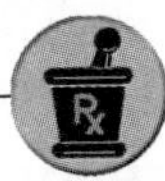

THERAPEUTIC GOAL(S)

- Ameliorate the inflammation before inflammatory sequelae produce blindness
- Alleviate ocular pain
- Eliminate the initiating cause if possible

ACUTE GENERAL TREATMENT

- In general, topical therapies are used for anterior uveitis, whereas systemic therapies are required for effective treatment of posterior uveitis.
- Reduce ocular inflammation with anti-inflammatory drugs:
  - Corticosteroids:
    - Topical and/or systemic depending on severity and location of uveitis.
    - Contraindicated with many infectious etiologies (i.e., systemic mycoses; acute bacterial) and corneal ulceration.
    - Start with frequent dose, q 4–6h, for topical (e.g., prednisolone acetate 1%; dexamethasone 0.1%) and anti-inflammatory doses of systemic drug (e.g., prednisone 1 mg/kg per day).
  - Nonsteroidal anti-inflammatory drugs (NSAIDs):
    - Topical and/or systemic depending on severity and location of uveitis.
    - Topical (flurbiprofen or diclofenac, q 4–6h, depending on severity of disease) and/or systemic (meloxicam: 0.2 mg/kg SQ loading dose and 0.1 mg/kg PO q 24h [dog]; ketoprofen: 2 mg/kg SQ loading dose and 1 mg/kg PO q 24h for 4 days [cat]).
  - Do not use systemic glucocorticoids and systemic NSAIDs concurrently (gastrointestinal [GI] ulceration).
  - Miscellaneous immunosuppresive drugs: severe, recalcitrant forms of

inflammation may necessitate systemic drugs such as azathioprine and cyclosporine.
- Control ocular pain and prevent synechiae:
  - Topical atropine 1% q 6–8h to dilate the pupil (i.e., mydriatic) in acute cases to minimize posterior synechia and to prevent spasms of the ciliary body muscle (i.e., cycloplegic) that contribute to pain.
- Other therapies:
  - Specific therapies.
    - If an infectious agent is the initiating cause, specific anti-infective therapy, such as antibiotics, is indicated.
    - Usually administered by both topical and systemic routes.
    - Broad-spectrum, bactericidal drugs are preferred until sensitivity is known.
  - Tissue plasminogen activator (tPA) injected into the anterior chamber (referable procedure): 25 μg of tPA may release posterior synechia and dramatically dissolve fibrin clots of anterior chamber in animals with acute uveitis.

CHRONIC TREATMENT

- After 7 to 10 days, anti-inflammatory therapy is usually reduced in frequency if the uveitis is significantly reduced but is continued for several weeks at a lower frequency and/or systemic dose.
- Some immune-mediated diseases, such as uveodermatologic syndrome/VKH, are treated indefinitely.
- Most infectious causes are treated for 3 to 4 weeks with antibiotics, although some, such as those caused by *Brucella* spp. and *Leishmania*, may require prolonged therapy.

DRUG INTERACTIONS

Topical NSAIDs may elevate IOP and, if secondary glaucoma develops, may need reevaluation

POSSIBLE COMPLICATIONS

- Blindness (see Blindness, p 136)
- Glaucoma (see Glaucoma, p 440)
- Cataracts (see Cataracts, p 182)
- Synechia resulting in pupil immobility
- Retinal detachment (see Retinal Detachment, p 965)
- Corneal opacity (see Corneal Discoloration, p 239)
- Prolonged ocular hypotony (low IOP)
- Phthisis bulbi (shrinkage of the eye)

RECOMMENDED MONITORING

- Animals with acute, severe forms should be monitored daily until inflammation begins to subside, and then weekly and biweekly.
- IOPs should be monitored:
  - The frequency will depend on the values.
  - As the uveitis subsides and aqueous production normalizes, any outflow restrictions from adhesions/synechia may become manifest and need therapy (see Acute General Treatment above).
- Certain infectious diseases may be monitored by repeat titers.

PROGNOSIS AND OUTCOME

- The prognosis is highly variable depending on severity of inflammation, stage at presentation, and the underlying cause.
- Any significant inflammation of the interior of the eye should have a guarded prognosis for maintenance of ocular function.

PEARLS & CONSIDERATIONS

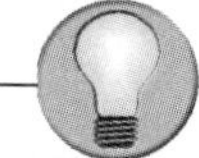

COMMENTS

- Despite extensive medical work-ups, more than 50% of cases of uveitis in the dog are idiopathic and, by default, thought to be immune-mediated conditions.
- In the younger cat, systemic infectious diseases are often implicated; in the older cat, they are often idiopathic (i.e., lymphocytic-plasmacytic).
- Infectious etiologies (*Brucella*, systemic mycoses) may be difficult to clear from the eye despite specific therapy.

PREVENTION

- Minimize infectious diseases through vaccination and restriction of environment
- Surgical removal of cataracts (referable procedure) before becoming mature to hypermature in nature
- Removal of lenses in eyes with vision potential:
  - Perforating injuries that have created lens rupture (specifically, capsular tears of greater than 2 mm)
  - Lens luxation

CLIENT EDUCATION

- Any inflammation of the interior of the eye is potentially serious and can threaten vision.
- Causes of uveitis are multiple and often difficult to pinpoint; nevertheless, it is important to perform laboratory diagnostics in hopes of formulating a specific therapy and to determine the systemic prognosis.

SUGGESTED READING

Lappin MR, et al: Serologic prevalence of selected infectious diseases in cats with uveitis. *J Am Vet Med Assoc* 201:1005, 1992.

Martin CL: Anterior uvea and anterior chamber. In *Ophthalmic Disease in Veterinary Medicine*. London, Manson Publishing, 2005, pp 298–336.

Massa KL, et al: Causes of uveitis in dogs: 102 cases (1989–2000). *Vet Ophthalmol* 5:93, 2002.

AUTHOR: **CHARLES L. MARTIN**

EDITOR: **CHERYL L. CULLEN**

Vaccine-Site Sarcoma

BASIC INFORMATION

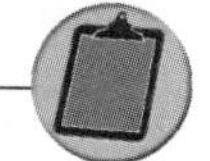

DEFINITION

Tumors arising from mesenchymal tissue secondary to vaccine administration or other injection

SYNONYM(S)

Injection-site sarcoma
Vaccine-associated fibrosarcoma
Vaccine-associated sarcoma

EPIDEMIOLOGY

SPECIES, AGE, SEX

- Almost exclusively found in cats; one report describes similar tumors at injection sites in a small number of dogs.
- Age at the time of tumor development may be less for vaccine-site sarcomas (7 to 9 years) compared with cats that develop sarcomas at nonvaccine sites.

GENETICS AND BREED PREDISPOSITION: No direct inheritance or breed predisposition has been reported.

RISK FACTORS: Previous vaccination or subcutaneous injection weeks to years prior to tumor development

CLINICAL PRESENTATION

DISEASE FORMS/SUBTYPES: Many different tumor types have been identified at vaccination sites in cats, including fibrosarcoma, malignant fibrous histiocytoma, neurofibrosarcoma, nerve sheath tumor, hemangiopericytoma, schwannoma, leiomyosarcoma, rhabdomyosarcoma, undifferentiated sarcoma, osteosarcoma, chondrosarcoma, liposarcoma, and myofibroblastic sarcoma.

HISTORY, CHIEF COMPLAINT

- Cats are usually presented for veterinary attention because their owners have noticed a progressively enlarging mass.
- A vaccination history should be obtained. Often cats with vaccine-site sarcomas will have a prior history of having been vaccinated in a site near the tumor.

PHYSICAL EXAM FINDINGS: Cats usually present with a palpable firm cutaneous mass. Typical locations include the interscapular area, the dorsal lumbar area, the flank, or the lateral thorax. Less commonly they can be found on extremities. Often the mass is hairless and/or ulcerated.

ETIOLOGY AND PATHOPHYSIOLOGY

- Vaccine-site sarcomas have been clearly linked to vaccination with certain inactive vaccines, particularly vaccines that contain aluminum hydroxide adjuvants. It is believed that inflammation at injection sites causes local cell proliferation, which may lead to tumor development.
- Small numbers of case reports and anecdotal reports suggest that these tumors may result from subcutaneous injection of medications or fluids.

DIAGNOSIS

DIFFERENTIAL DIAGNOSIS

- Local inflammatory vaccine reaction
- Other subcutaneous tumor
- Abscess

INITIAL DATABASE

- Fine-needle aspirate (FNA) and cytologic examination may help identify the tumor type prior to other diagnostics
- Thoracic radiographs to rule out pulmonary metastases
- Radiographs of the affected area may reveal involvement of underlying bone

ADVANCED OR CONFIRMATORY TESTING

- Histopathologic examination of an incisional biopsy specimen. Markers that may link the tumor with vaccine administration include peripheral lymphocytic infiltrate or macrophages within the tumor that contain aluminum adjuvant. In the absence of these markers, the location of the tumor, vaccination history, and diagnosis of a sarcoma also can suggest that the tumor was caused by vaccination.
- Simple excisional biopsy is not recommended as a first step in obtaining a diagnosis for this tumor. Reports suggest that aggressive surgical resection or multimodality therapy at the time of the first intervention is more likely to result in local disease control.
- Advanced imaging (i.e., CT scan or MRI) to delineate the local extent of the tumor. Many of these tumors have a peripheral region that is contrast-enhancing with a central, nonenhancing area. They also often have fingerlike projections that extend far into surrounding normal tissues.

TREATMENT

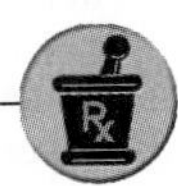

THERAPEUTIC GOAL(S)

- The primary objective of treatment is eradication of the local tumor.
- Prevention or delay of metastasis may play a role in some cats.

ACUTE AND CHRONIC TREATMENT

- Radical surgical excision is the treatment of choice if possible.
  - Tumors on the distal limbs and tail may be successfully treated with amputation alone.
  - Tumors on the trunk are usually not amenable to radical excision. For these cases, a combination of radiation and surgery (excision with as wide a margin as possible based on physical examination and advanced imaging [e.g., CT, MRI]) is usually indicated for the successful treatment of the local tumor.
  - Rarely, surgery with complete excision may be possible and result in adequate local control of the tumor; however, in one report, 31% of cats with complete excision of their tumor based on histopathologically clean margins developed a recurrence.
- Radiation therapy prior to surgery allows for adequate treatment of the microscopic tumor extensions with smaller radiation fields; however, therapy interferes with the histopathologic evaluation of the primary tumor mass and the margins, and it may lead to a slightly greater risk of wound complications after surgery.
- The role of chemotherapy in the treatment of vaccine-site sarcoma is not well-defined. Studies have not shown a definite advantage to using chemotherapy if local therapy (surgery, radiation) is adequate. Nevertheless, many oncologists recommend chemotherapy.
  - Chemotherapy drugs that have been shown to be effective against vaccine-associated sarcomas in cats include doxorubicin/cyclophosphamide, carboplatin, and ifosfamide.

POSSIBLE COMPLICATIONS

- Complications of surgery may include wound dehiscence or infection. The risk of these may be increased in cats that receive radiation therapy prior to surgery although this elevated risk has not been proven in cats.
- Complications of radiation depend on the location of the tumor in relation to critical normal structures (e.g., spinal cord, kidneys) and the amount of radiation delivered to those structures.
- Chemotherapy complications include bone marrow suppression, gastrointestinal (GI) side effects, haircoat changes, as well as side effects specific for individual chemotherapy drugs (see Chemotherapy: Adverse Reactions, p 189).

RECOMMENDED MONITORING

Due to the aggressive local nature of these tumors and the low risk of metastases, long-term monitoring should include:

- Routine examination by a veterinarian to monitor for local recurrence or side effects of treatment
- Routine thoracic radiographs to monitor for pulmonary metastases

PROGNOSIS AND OUTCOME

- Prognosis for a feline vaccine-site sarcoma varies greatly depending on the stage and location of the tumor.
  - Cats with tumors that can be resected with a wide margin of normal tissue (tumors on the tail or distal limbs, small localized tumors) may have an excellent prognosis.
  - Cats with larger tumors that can still be removed with an aggressive surgery and are treated with multimodality therapy (radiation, surgery, and chemotherapy) may still have an excellent prognosis for long-term tumor control; however, some of these cats will still develop metastases or recurrence of the primary tumor.
  - Cats with large nonresectable tumors or metastases at the time of diagnosis have a poor prognosis regardless of the treatments used.
- Another factor shown to affect recurrence of vaccine-site sarcoma is the extent of surgery performed at the first intervention after identification of the tumor. Cats that had the first excision of their tumor at a referral institution had a longer period of time to experience recurrence than cats that had surgery performed by the local veterinarian. This is likely due to the relatively aggressive nature of surgery performed at the referral institution.

PEARLS & CONSIDERATIONS

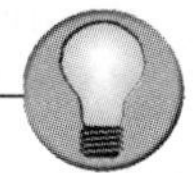

COMMENTS

- Treatment of cats with vaccine-site sarcoma is usually best performed using a team approach. Specialists, including a surgeon, oncologist, and radiation oncologist, should be consulted early in the course of the diagnostics to determine the best multimodality approach for the patient.
- Many different types of sarcoma have been identified at vaccine sites.

PREVENTION

- Early detection of these tumors may lead to more successful treatment.
  - Guidelines have been established by the American Veterinary Medical Association (AVMA) Vaccine Associated Sarcoma Task Force for approaching a cat that has a mass in an injection site after vaccination. According to these guidelines, the following masses should be investigated with an incisional biopsy to determine if further diagnostics or treatment are necessary:
    - A mass that is increasing in size after 1 month postinjection
    - A mass that is >2 cm in diameter
    - A mass that persists >3 months postinjection
- Vaccination of cats in areas of the body that may allow for an aggressive surgical removal if a tumor develops may prevent these tumors from requiring radiation or chemotherapy or from becoming life threatening.
- Critical evaluation of vaccination protocols for animals that have a low risk of contracting infectious disease may help decrease the risk of vaccine-associated sarcomas.

CLIENT EDUCATION

- Educate clients about the risks of tumor development following vaccination as well as other risks of vaccination compared with the benefits of vaccination.
- Clients may also be educated on the importance of examining their cats regularly for new masses to allow for early detection and treatment of these tumors.

SUGGESTED READING

McEntee MC, Page RL: Feline vaccine-associated sarcomas. *J Vet Intern Med* 15:176–182, 2001.

Vaccine-Associated Feline Sarcoma Task Force: *Vaccines and Sarcomas: A Concern for Cat Owners.* Accessed May 2006: http://www.avma.org/VAFSTF/ownbroch.asp.

AUTHOR: **JOHN FARRELLY**

EDITOR: **KENNETH M. RASSNICK**

Vacuolar Hepatopathy

BASIC INFORMATION

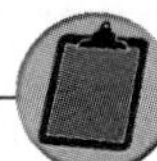

DEFINITION

Benign reversible hepatic lesion of glycogen accumulation that occurs in dogs in response to excess glucocorticoids or as a reactive change secondary to systemic disorders

SYNONYM(S)

Glucocorticoid hepatopathy
Hepatic glycogen accumulation
Steroid hepatopathy

EPIDEMIOLOGY

SPECIES, AGE, SEX: Dogs only; age and sex dependent on underlying cause. Older dogs may have spontaneous hyperadrenocorticism or idiopathic vacuolar hepatopathy.

GENETICS AND BREED PREDISPOSITION

- Poodles, dachshunds, beagles, boxers, terrier breeds: pituitary-dependent hyperadrenocorticism
- German shepherd, Labrador retriever, poodle, dachshund, terrier breeds: functional adrenal tumor
- Scottish terriers: increased adrenal steroids other than cortisol (see Aberrant Adrenocortical Disease [Increased Adrenal Sex Hormone Production], p 5)

RISK FACTORS: Glucocorticoid administration.

ASSOCIATED CONDITIONS AND DISORDERS: Hyperadrenocorticism including atypical forms (increased adrenal steroids other than cortisol, or "aberrant adrenocortical disease"); secondary reactive change associated with chronic stress (>4 weeks) from other systemic inflammatory, infectious, or neoplastic disorders.

CLINICAL PRESENTATION

DISEASE FORMS/SUBTYPES

- Incidental finding of increased serum alkaline phosphatase (ALP) activity; subsequent fine-needle aspirate (FNA) and cytologic examination or liver biopsy show vacuolar change
- Clinical signs of glucocorticoid excess
- Clinical signs of primary systemic disorder

HISTORY, CHIEF COMPLAINT

- For glucocorticoid excess, clinical signs reflect systemic effects of hypercortisolism rather than hepatic disease: polyuria and polydipsia (PU/PD), polyphagia, panting.
- If iatrogenic, a history of glucocorticoid administration (oral, injectable, topical: eyes, ears, skin) within last 3 to 6 months (depends on route, preparation, duration of therapy, and individual sensitivity) is expected.
- Other signs depend on primary systemic disorder.
- The patient may show no clinical signs (incidental finding) or mild polydipsia: idiopathic vacuolar hepatopathy; Scottish terriers.

PHYSICAL EXAM FINDINGS

- For iatrogenic or spontaneous hyperadrenocorticism: hepatomegaly (may be massive); abdominal enlargement, thin haircoat or truncal alopecia, thin skin
- Other findings dependent on primary systemic disorder
- May be unremarkable

ETIOLOGY AND PATHOPHYSIOLOGY

- Excess glucocorticoids (exogenous, or spontaneous hyperadrenocorticism):
  - Dogs are uniquely susceptible to hepatic effects of glucocorticoids
  - Gradual hepatic glycogen accumulation and hepatomegaly occur within the first 2 weeks of daily prednisolone administration
  - Preceded by increased ALP activity
  - Individual variation
  - Lesions identical with exogenous or endogenous corticosteroids
  - Hepatic function is typically normal
  - Reversible
- Aberrant adrenocortical disease ("atypical hyperadrenocorticism"):
  - Increased adrenal steroid hormones other than cortisol (especially progesterone and 17-α hydroxyprogesterone)
  - Progesterone has glucocorticoid-like effects on the liver
- Scottish terriers:
  - Increased adrenal steroid hormones other than cortisol (especially progesterone and 17-α hydroxyprogesterone)
  - Increased ALP (predominantly steroid-induced isoenzyme)

- No overt clinical signs; cause unknown
- Reactive hepatopathy:
  - Common lesion in dogs with other systemic illnesses (including dental disease)
  - Chronic stress (>4 weeks) associated with increased levels of endogenous glucocorticoids
- Hepatic nodular hyperplasia or regeneration:
  - Etiology unknown; may be associated with nutritional factors or the result of focal areas of ischemia
- Idiopathic vacuolar hepatopathy:
  - Excess corticosteroids or other adrenal steroid hormones cannot be documented; absence of systemic disease; usually associated with no clinical signs; clinical significance unknown

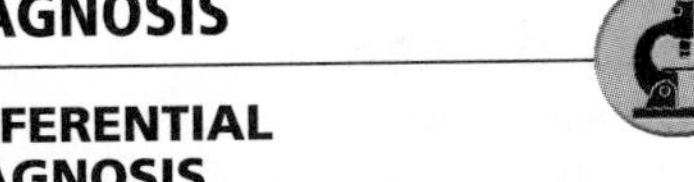

DIAGNOSIS

DIFFERENTIAL DIAGNOSIS

- Other hepatopathies (inflammatory, neoplastic)
- Nodular hyperplasia or regeneration
- Hyperlipidemia:
  - Diabetes mellitus
  - Hypothyroidism
  - Miniature schnauzers, Sheltland sheepdogs, others
- Hepatocutaneous syndrome
- Exocrine pancreatic insufficiency
- Chronic pancreatitis
- Tetracycline administration
- Glycogen or lysosomal storage disease

INITIAL DATABASE

- Complete blood count (CBC): lymphopenia, eosinopenia (excess glucocorticoids); other abnormalities depending on primary systemic disorder
- Serum biochemistry panel: ALP increased, may be marked; predominantly due to steroid-induced isoenzyme of ALP; alanine aminotransferase (ALT) mild to moderate increases (or levels may be normal); increased cholesterol (excess glucocorticoids). Other biochemistry values typically normal (bilirubin, albumin)
- Serum bile acids normal to mildly increased
- Abdominal radiographs: hepatomegaly (may be marked)
- Abdominal ultrasound: diffusely hyperechoic liver; may also be mottled and/or nodular. Adrenomegaly (hyperadrenocorticism)

ADVANCED OR CONFIRMATORY TESTING

- Fine-needle aspirate (FNA) and cytologic evaluation of liver:
  - Ballooned hepatocytes with decreased cytoplasmic density, commonly described as vacuolar hepatopathy
- Liver biopsy and histopathologic evaluation:
  - Patchy distribution of ballooned hepatocytes with decreased cytoplasmic density. Glycogen accumulation is characteristic. Glycogen accumulation can be differentiated from hydropic degeneration with PAS stains for glycogen; oil red O (ORO) stain to differentiate lipid vacuoles
  - No evidence of inflammation, necrosis, or cholestasis
- Rule out spontaneous hyperadrenocorticism:
  - Review clinical history and physical exam
  - Low-dose dexamethasone suppression test or adrenocorticotropic hormone (ACTH) stimulation test to screen for hyperadrenocorticism
  - Endogenous ACTH level, high-dose dexamethasone suppression test, and adrenal gland ultrasonography to differentiate pituitary from adrenal causes
  - Adrenal steroid profile before and after ACTH to diagnose aberrant adrenocortical disease/atypical hyperadrenocorticism or other abnormalities in adrenal steroid hormone production (send profile to Clinical Endocrinology Service, College of Vet Med, University of Tennessee, 2407 River Drive, Room A105, Knoxville, TN 37996; [865] 974-5638)
- Evaluate for other systemic disorders that could cause secondary reactive vacuolar hepatopathy

TREATMENT

THERAPEUTIC GOAL(S)

Focus therapeutic efforts on treating underlying disorder

CHRONIC TREATMENT

- If the patient is receiving high doses of glucocorticoids and is showing clinical signs of hepatic disease (e.g., lethargy or depression, difficult to distinguish from underlying condition), other immunosuppressive drugs such as azathioprine and cyclosporine may be warranted to allow dose reduction of glucocorticoids.
- Idiopathic vacuolar hepatopathy:
  - If no clinical signs are present, treatment may not be warranted.
  - Necessity or clinical effectiveness of hepatoprotective drug therapy (S-adenosylmethionine, vitamin E) unknown.

POSSIBLE COMPLICATIONS

See Hyperadrenocorticism, p 537, for complications involving glucocorticoid excess.

RECOMMENDED MONITORING

Idiopathic vacuolar hepatopathy: because some dogs may eventually develop spontaneous hyperadrenocorticism, monitor for clinical signs and follow up with screening tests (low-dose dexamethasone suppression test or ACTH stimulation) as needed.

PROGNOSIS AND OUTCOME

- Idiopathic vacuolar hepatopathy; vacuolar hepatopathy of Scottish terriers:
  - Benign clinical course
  - Good long-term prognosis
  - Some dogs may eventually develop clinical hyperadrenocorticism
- Exogenous glucocorticoid therapy:
  - Vacuolar hepatopathy is reversible once glucocorticoids are discontinued; may require weeks to months

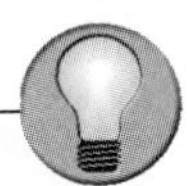

PEARLS & CONSIDERATIONS

COMMENTS

- Diagnostic and therapeutic efforts should be directed at identifying and correcting causes of glucocorticoid excess or primary systemic disorders.
- Hepatic function is typically preserved. If ALT > ALP or if hypoalbuminemia, hyperbilirubinemia, or markedly increased serum bile acids are present, a more serious primary hepatobiliary disorder may be present and should be identified and treated.
- Presence of increased ALP and vacuolar hepatopathy does not preclude continued use of corticosteroids if their administration is necessary. Liver function is generally preserved; benign lesion. Whenever possible, make an attempt to minimize systemic effects of glucocorticoids with alternate day therapy using lowest effective dose possible (prednisolone or prednisone) and/or use other immunosuppressive drugs (azathioprine, cyclosporine).
- Cats that are receiving glucocorticoids (or with hyperadrenocorticism) rarely develop vacuolar hepatopathy.

PREVENTION

If long-term glucocorticoid therapy is necessary, give oral prednisolone or prednisone (rather than oral dexamethasone or injectable long-acting forms) at the lowest dose possible on alternate days to minimize the systemic (including hepatic) effects of glucocorticoids. Also consider administering other immunosuppressive drugs (e.g., azathioprine, cyclosporine) to allow dose reduction of glucocorticoids.

CLIENT EDUCATION

Idiopathic vacuolar hepatopathy appears to be clinically benign.

SUGGESTED READING

Badylak SF, et al: Sequential morphologic and clinicopathologic alterations in dogs with experimentally induced glucocorticoid hepatopathy. *Am J Vet Res* 42:1310, 1981.

Ristic JME, et al: The use of 17-hydroxyprogesterone in the diagnosis of canine hyperadrenocorticism. *J Vet Intern Med* 16:433, 2002.

Twedt D: Breed-associated canine hepatopathies. *Proceedings of the 28th Annual Royal Canine/OSU Symposium for the Treatment of Small Animal Diseases, Gastroenterology* October 16–17, 2004, p 51.

AUTHOR: **SUSAN E. JOHNSON**

EDITOR: **KEITH P. RICHTER**

Vaginal Congenital Abnormalities in the Bitch

BASIC INFORMATION

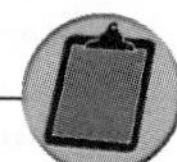

DEFINITION

Malformations that reduce the diameter of the vestibulovaginal junction and may cause secondary infertility, vaginitis, or cystitis include incomplete fusion of the mesonephric ducts, hymenal remnants, hypoplasia of the vestibulovaginal junction, and paramesonephric bands

SYNONYM(S)

Double vagina
Hypoplasia of the vaginal vault
Imperforate hymen
Incomplete perforation of the hymen
Vaginal stenosis
Vaginal stricture

EPIDEMIOLOGY

SPECIES, AGE, SEX

- Congenital vaginal abnormalities are present at birth but are usually undetected until the appearance of clinical signs:
  - Breeding difficulties in sexually intact bitches
  - Cystitis or vaginitis in intact or spayed bitches
- Young adult female dogs are most commonly affected.

ASSOCIATED CONDITIONS AND DISORDERS: Female dogs with ectopic ureters often have coincident congenital vaginal abnormalities.

CLINICAL PRESENTATION

DISEASE FORMS/SUBTYPES

- Difficult breeding
- Vaginitis
- Urinary tract infection (UTI)
- Ectopic ureter(s)

HISTORY, CHIEF COMPLAINT

- Unsuccessful breeding attempts, obvious pain during breeding, avoidance of male during breeding attempts
- Purulent, often recurrent vaginal discharge
- Persistent urinary tract infection that recurs after antibiotic therapy is stopped
- Urine dribbling or leakage after recumbency

PHYSICAL EXAM FINDINGS

- Vaginal discharge may be present.
- Narrowing of vestibulovaginal junction may be apparent during manual vaginal exam (see Vaginal Examination in the Bitch, p 1324).
- Pathologic vestibulovaginal stricture must be differentiated from normal anatomic narrowing that is present at the vestibulovaginal junction.

ETIOLOGY AND PATHOPHYSIOLOGY

- The vagina is derived from fusion of paired mesonephric ducts in the fetus:
  - Incomplete fusion of the mesonephric ducts can result in persistent dorsoventral bands that completely or partially bisect the vagina.
- The vestibule develops from the urogenital sinus:
  - Vestibulovaginal hypoplasia causes concentric narrowing of the vestibulovaginal junction.
- The hymen is an epithelium-covered membrane that separates the vagina from the vestibule:
  - The hymen normally degenerates prior to 6 months of age in dogs.
  - Incomplete dissolution of the hymen can compromise the vestibulovaginal junction.
- Any type of vestibulovaginal stricture can interfere with breeding due to pain produced during penetration by a male dog.
- Anatomic abnormalities of the vestibulovaginal junction can inhibit drainage of vaginal secretions, which predisposes the animal to bacterial proliferation and can lead to vaginitis or ascending UTI.

DIAGNOSIS

DIFFERENTIAL DIAGNOSIS

- Behavioral abnormalities in breeding bitches in estrus who are reluctant to stand for a male.
- Urolithiasis is a much more common cause of chronic UTI.
- Vaginal discharge may be associated with puppy vaginitis, pyometra, traumatic lesions in the vagina, or vaginal foreign bodies.

INITIAL DATABASE

Vaginoscopy using a flexible or rigid endoscope (see Vaginal Examination in the Bitch, p 1324):

- Heavy sedation or general anesthesia is necessary.
- Findings as described previously concerning the etiology of the condition.

ADVANCED OR CONFIRMATORY TESTING

Contrast radiography: retrograde vaginography

- A radiograph of the vestibulovaginal region is taken after instillation of contrast media through a Foley catheter introduced into the vaginal vault while the vulva is manually occluded

TREATMENT

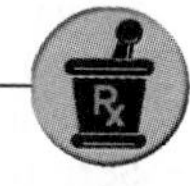

THERAPEUTIC GOAL(S)

Remove obstruction/narrowing at vestibulovaginal junction

ACUTE GENERAL TREATMENT

- Digital dilation of vestibulovaginal junction (effective for treatment of hymenal remnants or mild (membranous) vestibulovaginal stenosis).
- Resection of dorsoventral paramesonephric duct remnants or bands if present.
- For severe (fibrous) vestibulovaginal stenosis: resection and anastomosis of vestibulovaginal junction via an extended episiotomy.
- Dogs with mating difficulties caused by congenital vaginal abnomalities can be treated by artificial insemination and cesarean section if resection/dilation of vaginal stenosis is not possible.

CHRONIC TREATMENT

Antibiotic therapy (based on culture and sensitivity [C&S]) may need to be extended up to 6 weeks after manual or surgical dilation for treatment of ascending UTI if present.

POSSIBLE COMPLICATIONS

- Stricture secondary to resection and anastomosis.
- Inadequate resection does not resolve clinical signs.

RECOMMENDED MONITORING

Observe the animal for recurrence of signs; initial treatment may need to be repeated if stricture occurs secondary to resection or traumatic dilation

PROGNOSIS AND OUTCOME

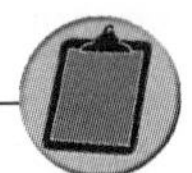

- Prognosis is good if clinical signs are caused by hymenal remnants or mild vaginal stricture
- Prognosis for resolution of clinical signs is fair to good for severe vaginal stricture treated by vestibulovaginal resection and anastomosis

PEARLS & CONSIDERATIONS

COMMENTS

- Do not confuse the normal narrowing at the vestibulovaginal junction with a pathologic condition.
- The diameter of the vestibulovaginal junction must be less than 30% of the diameter of the maximal diameter of the vagina to be considered pathologic.
- If no obvious vestibulovaginal abnormalities are observed during a vaginoscopy for a dog that is suspected of having a congenital abnormality, perform a contrast retrograde vaginography to determine if stricture is present.
- Most congenital vaginal abnormalities do not cause clinical signs.
- Congenital vaginal abnormalities are rarely the primary cause of urinary incontinence.
- Congenital vaginal abnormalities may occur with urethral sphincter mechanism incontinence (estrogen responsive urinary incontinence).

CLIENT EDUCATION

- Breeding bitches that are reluctant to stand for a male may have vestibulovaginal abnormalities that cause painful breeding.
- Older dogs that have purulent vaginal discharge must be examined to rule out pyometra.
- Congenital vaginal anomalies may be present without causing clinical signs.

SUGGESTED READING

Crawford JT, Adams WM: Influence of vestibulovaginal stenosis, pelvic bladder, and recessed vulva on response to treatment for clinical signs of lower urinary tract disease in dogs: 38 cases (1990-1999). *J Am Vet Med Assoc* 221:995, 2002.

Kyles AE, et al: Vestibulovaginal stenosis in dogs: 18 cases (1987-1995). *J Am Vet Med Assoc* 209:1889, 1996.

AUTHOR: **JAMES A. FLANDERS**

EDITOR: **MICHELLE A. KUTZLER**

Vaginal Discharge

BASIC INFORMATION

DEFINITION

- Discharge of substance from the vagina
- May be abnormal or physiologically appropriate

EPIDEMIOLOGY

SPECIES, AGE, SEX

- More common in dogs
- Spayed or intact females
- Frequently associated with pyometra
- Puppy vaginitis: bitches 2 to 10 months old
- Pyometra: more common in cats and dogs > 6 years old

RISK FACTORS: Vaginal stricture or septum, ovarian remnant syndrome, vaginal foreign body, vaginal neoplasia, redundant dorsal vulvar fold, ectopic ureters, mibolerone treatment.

CONTAGION AND ZOONOSIS: Brucellosis, transmissible venereal tumor (TVT).

GEOGRAPHY AND SEASONALITY: Increased risk of vaginal foreign body (e.g., grass awn) in summer or in dry/arid zones.

ASSOCIATED CONDITIONS AND DISORDERS

- Pyometra
- Vulvar fold pyoderma
- Urinary tract infection (UTI)
- Urethritis
- Pseudohermaphroditism
- Hermaphroditism

CLINICAL PRESENTATION

DISEASE FORMS/SUBTYPES

- Primary vaginal infection: uncommon.
- Secondary bacterial infection due to pyometra, foreign body: most common
- Primary inflammatory (lymphoplasmacytic vaginitis) is a rule-out diagnosis

HISTORY, CHIEF COMPLAINT

- Visible vulvar discharge
- Increased genital grooming
- Staining of carpet/bedding
- "Scooting" (rubbing perineum on floor)
- Pollakiuria
- Attracting males
- Hair staining in perineal area
- Lethargy, inappetence in cases of sepsis or hypovolemic shock (e.g., pyometra)
- Polyuria and polydipsia (PU/PD) with pyometra

PHYSICAL EXAM FINDINGS

- Generally, physical abnormalities are restricted to genital tract; exceptions: pyometra with sepsis, or coagulopathy
- Inflamed, moist, red perivulvar skin ± moist or ulcerative pyoderma
- Red ± ulcerated vulvar mucosa; clitoral enlargement
- Classification of discharge type assists diagnostic approach:
    - Color (colorless, brown, green, red)
    - Smell (malodorous or not)
    - Volume (mild, moderate, copious)
- Discharge due to bacterial infection is typically mucoid/mucosanguineous and malodorous;moderate to copious volume
- Discharge due to inflammation is typically white mucoid: clear, mild to moderate volume, and not malodorous
- Rectal palpation (see Rectal Palpation, p 1304) may reveal foreign body or mass
- Digital vaginal examination (see Vaginal Examination in the Bitch, p 1324) reveals discharge; small mucosal nodules (reactive lymphoid tissue) may be palpable with any inflammation
    - Most vaginal strictures should be palpable at the level of the urethral papilla
- Fever, signs of septic shock, distended uterine horns, and/or abdominal discomfort: possible if pyometra
- Petechiae and bleeding of other mucous membranes (nose, gums) may be present with coagulopathy is the cause of vaginal discharge

ETIOLOGY AND PATHOPHYSIOLOGY

- Vaginal discharge in adult animals: commonly from secondary bacterial vagini-

tis due to anatomic abnormalities (stricture, septum) or foreign body.
- Lymphoplasmacytic vaginitis and juvenile "puppy vaginitis": unknown etiology.
- Strictures are associated with chronic vaginitis due to a change in vaginal mucus drainage.

DIAGNOSIS

DIFFERENTIAL DIAGNOSIS

- Pyometra: mucoid/mucosanguineous, malodorous, moderate to copious volume
- Normal vaginal discharge; none should be malodorous:
  - Estrus: hemorrhagic, low volume
  - Parturition: moderate to large volume; hemorrhagic; green, brown
  - Postpartum: low to moderate volume for up to 4 to 6 weeks, green initially then brown
- Puppy vaginitis: white, mucoid, moderate in volume
- Secondary bacterial vaginitis due to stricture: mucoid, blood-tinged discharge; may be malodorous; scant to moderate in volume
- *Brucella canis* infection (abortion): abortion-associated discharge is typically brown, moderate in volume
- Herpesvirus infection (abortion): as for *B. canis*
- Foreign body-associated secondary bacterial vaginitis: see secondary bacterial vaginitis
- Urogenital neoplasia: variable; may be hemorrhagic, serous, or mucoid; scant to moderate in volume
- Coagulopathy: hemorrhagic; volume depends on degree of coagulation impairment
- Lymphoplasmacytic vaginitis: typically low volume, scant, and serous initially; may become mucoid with secondary bacterial infection; occasionally serosanguineous
- Primary bacterial vaginitis (uncommon)
- Urinary tract infection/urethritis
- Dorsal vulvar fold pyoderma: malodor is typically noted from the vulvar area; discharge may be mild to moderate in volume; mucoid and occasionally blood tinged
- Transmissible venereal tumor (TVT): vulvar mass typically noted; associated discharge is typically serosanguineous (see Transmissible Venereal Tumor, p 1101)

INITIAL DATABASE

- Physical examination of vulvar lip conformation, mucosa
- Vaginal cytologic examination
- Complete blood count (CBC): leukocytosis with left shift, toxic changes: common with pyometra
- Serum biochemical analysis: generally unremarkable
- Urinalysis and sediment examination: assess for concurrent UTI. Avoid cystocentesis if there is a possibility of pyometra or coagulopathy
- Ultrasonographic evaluation of genitourinary tract: diagnostic test of choice for pyometra

ADVANCED OR CONFIRMATORY TESTING

- Guarded cranial vaginal aerobic/anaerobic/mycoplasma bacterial culture
- Retrograde double-contrast vaginocystourethrogram
- Cystoscopy and vaginoscopy, including examination of cervix if present: foreign body, congenital malformation, mass
- Vaginal biopsy ± mass biopsy
- Coagulation profile
- Urethral pressure profile

TREATMENT

THERAPEUTIC GOAL(S)

- Restore patient's comfort
- Remove foreign body if present
- Resolve inflammation and infection if present
- Surgically treat anatomic abnormalities
- Prevent recurrence

ACUTE GENERAL TREATMENT

- Evaluate for inciting cause and treat
- Specific surgical therapy as indicated for pyometra
- Administer antimicrobials for pyoderma (e.g., cephalexin 22 mg/kg PO q 8h)
- Oral anti-inflammatories for discomfort, inflammation (e.g., carprofen 2 mg/kg PO q 12h, or meloxicam 0.1 mg/kg PO q 24h)

CHRONIC TREATMENT

- Low-dose oral (e.g., prednisone 0.5 mg/kg PO q 24h) or topical glucocorticoid use for refractory lymphoplasmacytic vaginitis
- Vulvar hygiene (chlorhexidine wipes)
- Vulvar conformational abnormalities: specific surgical therapy once infection is controlled (episioplasty)

POSSIBLE COMPLICATIONS

Chronic estrogen supplementation may cause myelotoxicity.

RECOMMENDED MONITORING

- Clinical response for uncomplicated bacterial vaginitis
- Reexamination and reevaluation if complete resolution is not achieved after 14 days of therapy

PROGNOSIS AND OUTCOME

- Good prognosis for secondary bacterial vaginitis if underlying cause is identified
- Idiopathic lymphoplasmacytic vaginitis is often recurrent but responsive to steroid therapy

PEARLS & CONSIDERATIONS

COMMENTS

- *Always* rule out pyometra in an intact animal with vaginal discharge.
- Normal vaginal flora is mixed (*Escherichia coli*, *Pasteurella multocida*, β-hemolytic strep group G most common); abnormal flora, typically a single isolate and/or heavy growth.
- Vaginal cytologic examination is always helpful to detect discharge due to estrus in the bitch.
- Surgical correction of strictures is not advised; clitorectomy is advised in cases of clitoral hypertrophy.
- *Always* perform rectal palpation.

PREVENTION

Pyometra may be avoided by ovariohysterectomy

CLIENT EDUCATION

- Positive bacterial culture does not indicate disease is present.
- Prebreeding antibiotics do not prevent vaginitis or pyometra.
- Puppy vaginitis is usually self-limiting and does not require antimicrobial treatment; antimicrobial treatment of puppy vaginitis may prolong resolution of the problem.

SUGGESTED READING

Bjurstrom L, et al: Long-term study of aerobic bacteria of the genital tract in breeding bitches. *Am J Vet Res* 53:665, 1992.

Johnson CA: Diagnosis and treatment of chronic vaginitis in the bitch. *Vet Clin North Am Small Anim Pract* 21:523, 1991.

Johnston SD, et al: Disorders of the canine vagina, vestibule, and vulva. In *Canine and Feline Theriogenology*. Philadelphia, WB Saunders, 2001, pp 225–242.

AUTHOR: **SOPHIE A. GRUNDY**
EDITOR: **MICHELLE A. KUTZLER**

Vaginal Hyperplasia

BASIC INFORMATION

DEFINITION

Edematous swelling of the vaginal mucosa cranial to the urethral orifice during the time of estrogen stimulation in the intact bitch. It may progress to vaginal protrusion through the vulvar lips.

SYNONYM(S)

Vaginal edema
Vaginal (fold) prolapse
Vaginal or estrual hypertrophy
Vestibular hyperplasia

EPIDEMIOLOGY

SPECIES, AGE, SEX

- Intact female dogs
- Age range of 7 months to 16 years old

GENETICS AND BREED PREDISPOSITION

- Common in large-breed dogs and less so in small breeds
- Hereditary predisposition is likely
- Breeds predisposed: bulldog, mastiff, boxer, dalmatian, German shepherd, Saint Bernard, Labrador and Chesapeake Bay retrievers, weimaraner, Walker hound, springer spaniel, Airedale terrier, and American pit bull terrier

RISK FACTORS: Young bitch under the influence of estrogen during proestrus or estrus; may occur or recur during diestrus, pregnancy, or parturition.

ASSOCIATED CONDITIONS AND DISORDERS: Markedly prolapsed vaginal tissue is subject to self-mutilation and may be dry, ulcerated, necrotic, and devascularized; possible dysuria or pollakiuria.

CLINICAL PRESENTATION

DISEASE FORMS/SUBTYPES

- Type I: slight to moderate eversion of the vaginal floor cranial to the urethral orifice that is confined to the vestibulum, appearing as a bulge at the perineum.
- Type II: well-developed swelling of the vaginal floor, which may include the lateral vaginal walls, protruding through the vulvar lips. This incomplete prolapse appears dome-shaped.
- Type III: well-developed protrusion of the entire circumference of the vaginal wall through the vulvar lips. This complete prolapse appears doughnut-shaped.

HISTORY, CHIEF COMPLAINT

- Previous occurrence of vaginal hyperplasia
- Onset of proestrus or estrus
- Licking or irritation of the vulva
- Mass protruding from vulva or bulge at the perineum
- Dysuria or pollakiuria
- Failure to allow intromission during breeding
- Tenesmus

PHYSICAL EXAM FINDINGS: Bulge at the perineum or protrusion of a pink dome-shaped or doughnut-shaped mass from vulva; surface of protrusion may be dry, necrotic, or ulcerated. Vaginal examination reveals:

- A urethral orifice located ventrally in all three types.
- A vaginal lumen located dorsally in types I and II but centrally located in type III.
- By contrast, uterine prolapse is distinguished by the presence of tubular masses within the vagina or protruding from the vulva.

ETIOLOGY AND PATHOPHYSIOLOGY

- An exaggerated response of the vaginal mucosa to estrogen (hyperemia, edema, keratinization). The swelling begins as an eversion in the vaginal floor cranial to the urethral orifice.
- Histopathologic examination of affected vaginal tissue is consistent with submucosal edema rather than with hyperplasia or hypertrophy.

DIAGNOSIS

DIFFERENTIAL DIAGNOSIS

- Benign or malignant vaginal neoplasia
- Vaginal polyp
- Vaginal prolapse with concurrent entrapment of visceral organs
- Uterine prolapse
- Urethral neoplasia

INITIAL DATABASE

- Stage of hormonal cycle based on vaginal cytologic examination
- Vaginal examination to locate the urethral orifice, vaginal lumen, origin of the protruding mass, and the size of its base (see Vaginal Examination in the Bitch, p 1324)
- Ensure that the animal is able to urinate

ADVANCED OR CONFIRMATORY TESTING

- Biopsy of vaginal mass confirms diagnosis in nontypical bitches.
- In severe cases, survey radiographs can be used to evaluate for visceral organ involvement; contrast radiography can confirm the location of the urethral orifice and vaginal lumen.

TREATMENT

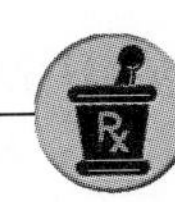

THERAPEUTIC GOAL(S)

- Prevent drying, necrosis, and devitalization of exposed vaginal tissue
- Prevent future recurrence
- Prevent urethral obstruction

ACUTE GENERAL TREATMENT

- Insertion of a urethral catheter to relieve obstruction when present
- Ensuring that vaginal tissue is kept clean
- Topical application of sterile water-soluble lubrication or antibiotic ointment
- Application of an Elizabethan collar or protective pants
- Provision of a clean environment to minimize tissue trauma
- Scheduling an ovariohysterectomy
- Recognition that spontaneous regression at end of estrus is common

CHRONIC TREATMENT

- Ovariohysterectomy prevents recurrence in nonbreeding bitches.
- Surgical excision of prolapsed vaginal tissue in bitches intended for breeding:
  - May prevent recurrence during subsequent estrous cycles or at parturition.
  - Various surgical techniques are described involving circumferential incision at the base of the prolapse.
  - Episiotomy may be needed.
- Manual reduction of prolapsed tissue and placement of stay sutures in the vagina do not prevent recurrence and may cause the bitch discomfort.
- Hysteropexy is an uncommon surgical procedure performed to correct chronic cases involving vaginal prolapse.
- Artificial insemination can be performed in breeding bitches.
- Induction of ovulation during a nonbreeding cycle may hasten regression of vaginal tissue by decreasing estrogenic stimulation: gonadotropin-releasing hormone (2.2 μg/kg IM) or human chorionic gonadotropin (1000 IU, IM, irrespective of body weight as a single injection, or 500 IU, IM, irrespective of body weight and repeated in 48 hours); a 1-week regression follows ovulation. Treatment is ineffective if given after ovulation.

DRUG INTERACTIONS

Avoidance of progestational drugs that contribute to pyometra

POSSIBLE COMPLICATIONS

- Necrosis, infection, and devascularization of vaginal tissue
- Evisceration of abdominal organs
- Urination and defecation difficulties

RECOMMENDED MONITORING

- Monitor viability of prolapsed vaginal tissue
- Evaluate ability to urinate

PROGNOSIS AND OUTCOME

- Good prognosis with ovariohysterectomy
- Recurrence rate is 66% in untreated bitches

PEARLS & CONSIDERATIONS

COMMENTS

Surgical timing and comments:

- If excision of vaginal tissue is performed late estrus or early diestrus, bleeding is minimized.
- If ovariohysterectomy is performed in anestrus (serum progesterone concentrations <2 ng/ml), development of pseudopregnancy is minimized.
- Catheterize urethra during excision of vaginal tissue to help prevent inadvertent urethral trauma.

PREVENTION

- Ovariohysterectomy.
- Surgical excision of redundant vaginal tissue may prevent recurrence during the following cycle.

CLIENT EDUCATION

Discuss heritability and intended plans for the bitch; ovariohysterectomy is the recommendation for nonbreeding bitches.

SUGGESTED READING

Johnston SD: Vaginal prolapse. In Kirk RW (eds): *Current Veterinary Therapy X*. Philadelphia, WB Saunders, 1989, pp 1302–1305.

Manothaiudom K, Johnston SD: Clinical approach to vaginal/vestibular masses in the bitch. *Vet Clin North Am Small Anim Pract* 21(3):509–521, 1991.

Post K, van Haaften B, Okkens AC: An unusual case of canine vaginal hyperplasia. *Can Vet J* 32:38–39, 1991.

Schaefers-Okkens AC: Vaginal edema and vaginal fold prolapse in the bitch, including surgical management. *International Veterinary Information Service* April 10, 2001: www.ivis.org.

AUTHOR: **KRISTINE L. GONZALES**
EDITOR: **MICHELLE A. KUTZLER**

Vascular Ring Anomaly

BASIC INFORMATION

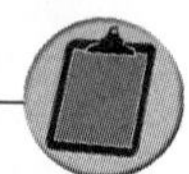

DEFINITION

Congenital malformation of one or more parts of the aortic arch during embryogenesis such that vessels encircle the esophagus and trachea causing chronic compression

SYNONYM(S)

Vascular ring malformation
Persistent right aortic arch (PRAA) (the most common vascular ring anomaly)

EPIDEMIOLOGY

SPECIES, AGE, SEX

- More common in dogs than in cats
- Clinical signs usually develop shortly after weaning
- No sex predilection

GENETICS AND BREED PREDISPOSITION

- The majority of dogs with PRAA are of large breeds (>15 kg expected adult weight).
- German shepherds are overrepresented and, therefore, heritability is suspected.
- Suspected heritability has been reported for greyhounds from one particular kennel.

ASSOCIATED CONDITIONS AND DISORDERS

- Persistent left cranial vena cava and patent ductus arteriosus (PDA) can be associated vascular anomalies.
- Megaesophagus and aspiration pneumonia are secondary problems associated with chronic partial esophageal obstruction.

CLINICAL PRESENTATION

HISTORY, CHIEF COMPLAINT: Most dogs and cats develop clinical signs once they start to ingest solid food because the vascular ring obstructs passage of food down the esophagus. Postprandial regurgitation is the usual presenting complaint, and the majority of cases are diagnosed before 6 months of age. Occasionally, animals may have coughing or respiratory distress because of aspiration pneumonia or tracheal compression.

PHYSICAL EXAM FINDINGS: Animals have a good appetite but may be thin as a result of chronic regurgitation. An enlarged esophagus may occasionally be palpated in the thoracic inlet, especially after eating. In dogs with a concurrent PDA (minority of cases), a continuous left basilar murmur is ausculted; however, in the absence of PDA, cardiac auscultation is normal. Animals with aspiration pneumonia may be febrile with harsh ventral lung sounds.

ETIOLOGY AND PATHOPHYSIOLOGY

- Normal embryogenesis:
  - In the embryo, the great vessels are formed from six aortic arches that connect paired ventral and dorsal aortas. During development, these vessels undergo regression and reconnection that normally result in a left-sided aorta, left-sided ligamentum arteriosum, and normal branching of the brachiocephalic trunk and left subclavian arteries off the ascending aorta.
- Pathophysiology:
  - Developmental anomalies of the great vessels appear to be relatively common; however, these anomalies are only clinically important when the vessels entrap the esophagus and trachea within a vascular ring.
  - Passage of food down the esophagus is impeded by the vascular ring, causing esophageal dilation, food stasis, and regurgitation. Regurgitation with aspiration can cause pneumonia.
- PRAA (most common in dogs):
  - The normal left aortic arch regresses, while the right aortic arch is retained. The left ligamentum arteriosum passes over the esophagus, connecting the right aortic arch to the left-sided pulmonary artery and compressing the esophagus at the base of the heart.
  - PRAA can also occur with an aberrant left subclavian artery. This causes an incomplete ring that dorsally compresses the esophagus (the left subclavian arises from the right aorta and courses dorsally over the esophagus).
- Double aortic arch:
  - Both left and right aortic arches persist, encircling the esophagus and trachea as the two vessels merge to form the descending aorta.

- Persistent right ligamentum arteriosum with normal left aorta is an uncommon cause of a vascular ring anomaly. It is important to note that correction by a left lateral thoracotomy is more difficult for this malformation than for the other vascular ring anomalies.
- An aberrant right subclavian artery with a normal left aorta can cause an incomplete ring because the aberrant vessel courses over and dorsally compresses the esophagus.

DIAGNOSIS

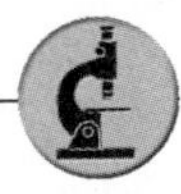

DIFFERENTIAL DIAGNOSIS

- Differential diagnoses for regurgitation include congenital megaesophagus, stricture, foreign body, neoplasia, granuloma, hiatal disorder, and esophageal diverticulum.
- Esophageal stricture is the major differential diagnosis to consider for radiographic esophageal dilation that terminates at the base of the heart.

INITIAL DATABASE

- Thoracic radiographs:
  - The esophagus may appear dilated up to the base of the heart on plain films. Its visualization may be enhanced by residual food (Fig. I-182). Lateral radiographs often show ventral deviation of the trachea cranial to the heart, and the tracheal lumen may be narrowed in this deviated segment (see Fig. I-182).
  - Leftward curvature of the trachea near the cranial border of the heart on the dorsoventral (DV) or ventrodorsal (VD) view reliably differentiates dogs with vascular ring anomalies from dogs with generalized megaesophagus (Fig. I-183). These radiographic findings may obviate the need for a barium esophagram.
- Complete blood count (CBC) is indicated if there is evidence of aspiration pneumonia

ADVANCED OR CONFIRMATORY TESTING

- Barium esophagram: Barium given in food can be used to radiographically outline the focal dilation of the esophagus that narrows at the base of the heart. Although this finding is diagnostic for a vascular ring anomaly, it does not reveal the type of anomaly present.
- Angiography, though logical, is often nondiagnostic or misleading and is generally not beneficial for delineating the anatomy of a vascular ring anomaly.

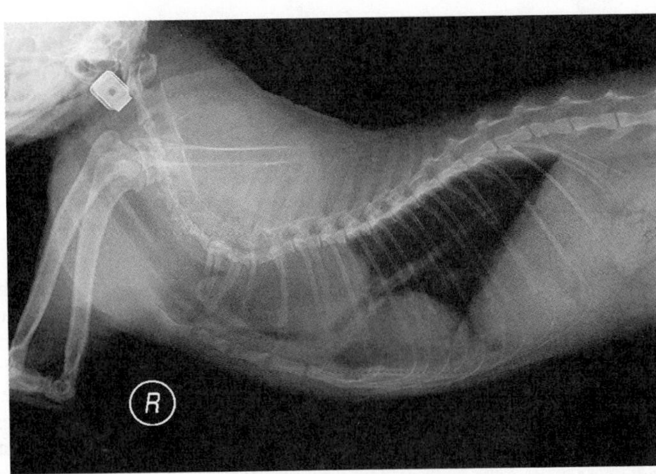

FIGURE I-182 Lateral thoracic radiograph demonstrating marked ventral deviation of the trachea and severe esophageal filling with fluid/soft-tissue opacity material cranial to the carina. The cause was a vascular ring anomaly.

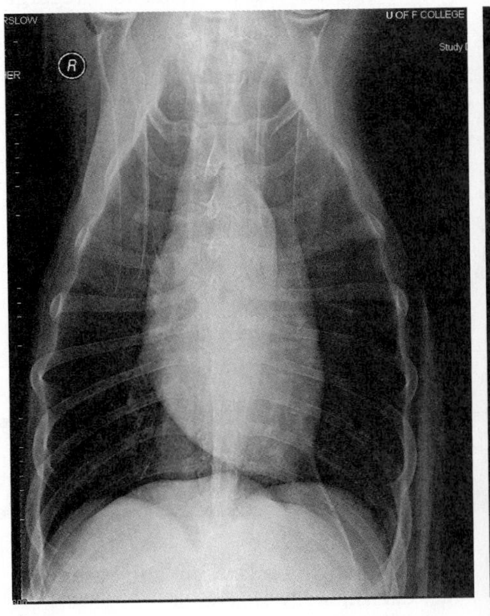

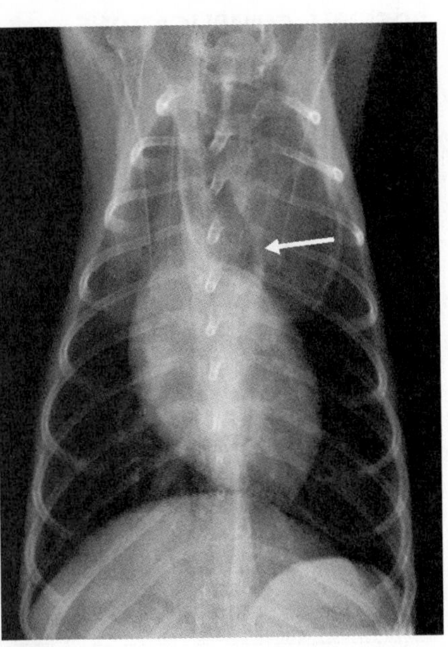

A B

FIGURE I-183 **A**, Ventrodorsal thoracic radiograph of a normal dog. **B**, Ventrodorsal thoracic radiograph of a dog with vascular ring anomaly. Leftward deviation of the trachea (*arrow*) is characteristic of vascular ring anomaly rather than of megaesophagus due to other causes.

TREATMENT

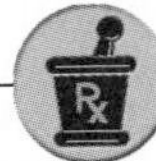

THERAPEUTIC GOAL(S)

- Remove the esophageal constriction by surgical resection and division of the vascular ring
- Decrease or eliminate regurgitation

ACUTE GENERAL TREATMENT

- Severely malnourished animals may require nutritional support prior to surgery. This may involve elevated feedings of slurried food or, in some cases, placement of a gastrostomy tube.
- Young malnourished animals may benefit from fluid therapy with dextrose.
- Animals with aspiration pneumonia require antibiotic therapy prior to surgical intervention.
- Surgical division of the vascular ring:
  - For the vast majority of vascular ring anomalies, the preferred surgical approach is a left fourth intercostal thoracotomy.
  - Ventilation is required after entering the thorax; place a thoracostomy tube after surgery for 24 hours to evacuate air.
  - When the vascular ring is caused by PRAA, the left ligamentum arteriosum is ligated and divided, releasing the constriction on the esophagus.

- When the vascular ring is caused by an aberrant subclavian artery coursing over the esophagus, this artery is ligated and divided. No adverse effects are noted from this ligation as the vertebral artery supplies adequate collateral flow.
- When a double aortic arch is present, the smaller arch is ligated and divided.

CHRONIC TREATMENT

Give slurried food to the animal from an elevated position for several weeks after surgery. After feeding, maintain the animal in a vertical position for 10 minutes. Then introduce solid food from an elevated position. If no regurgitation occurs, most dogs can be returned to a normal feeding regimen 1 to 2 months after surgery.

POSSIBLE COMPLICATIONS

- The most common complication associated with vascular ring anomalies is aspiration pneumonia secondary to regurgitation and aspiration of food material.
- Regurgitation may continue after surgical disruption of the vascular ring because of loss of neuromuscular esophageal function. Some animals may never be able to ingest solid food and may need to be fed a slurry diet indefinitely.

RECOMMENDED MONITORING

Monitor dogs that continue to regurgitate after surgery for signs of aspiration pneumonia.

PROGNOSIS AND OUTCOME

- The prognosis is dependent on the age at the time of surgical therapy, the severity of malnourishment, the presence of aspiration pneumonia, and the degree of esophageal constriction.
- For animals with PRAA, much of the prognosis appears to depend on the length of the ligamentum arteriosum, with a longer ligamentum causing less esophageal compression and therefore milder signs.
- A study found that 6 months after surgery, the majority (92%) of dogs did not regurgitate and the remainder regurgitated only occasionally.

PEARLS & CONSIDERATIONS

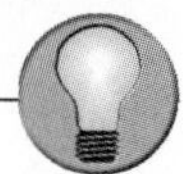

COMMENTS

- Oral passage of a stomach tube into the esophagus by an assistant during surgery can help to locate the stricture and facilitates dissection around the esophagus.
- Intraoperative balloon dilation of the esophagus is particularly helpful to remove constricting fibrous bands after the ring has been resected.

CLIENT EDUCATION

Although the prognosis is good for most dogs following surgical therapy, counsel owners about the potential for continued esophageal dysfunction.

SUGGESTED READING

Buchanan JW: Tracheal signs and associated vascular anomalies in dogs with persistent right aortic arch. *J Vet Intern Med* 18:510–514, 2004.

Buchanan JW: Embryogenesis of the aortic arches and associated abnormalities. http://cal.vet.upenn.edu/cardiosf.

Helphrey ML: Vascular ring anomalies in the dog. *Vet Clin North Am Small Anim Pract* 9(2):207–218, 1979.

Kyles AE: Esophagus. In Slatter DH (ed): *Textbook of Small Animal Surgery*. Philadelphia, WB Saunders, 2003, pp 577–582.

Muldoon MM, et al: Long-term results of surgical correction of persistent right aortic arch in dogs: 25 cases (1980–1995). *J Am Vet Med Assoc* 210(12):1761–1763, 1997.

AUTHORS: **DARCY B. ADIN, CHRISTOPHER A. ADIN**
EDITOR: **ETIENNE CÔTÉ**

Vasculitis, Cutaneous

BASIC INFORMATION

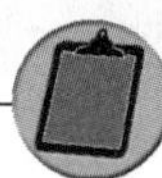

DEFINITION

- A condition characterized by blood vessel damage that results in ischemia of the skin and resultant tissue necrosis
- May be localized, regional, or multifocal to generalized
- Categorized histologically as neutrophilic (leukocytoclastic, nonleukocytoclastic), eosinophilic, lymphocytic, granulomatous, or cell-poor

SYNONYM(S)

Cutaneous vasculopathy
Small vessel necrotizing vasculitis

EPIDEMIOLOGY

GENETICS AND BREED PREDISPOSITION: Any breed, but certain syndromes show breed predisposition:

- Familial cutaneous vasculopathy (autosomal recessive): Jack Russell terrier, Scottish terrier, German shepherd
- Alabama rot: greyhounds
- Thrombovascular pinnal vasculitis: dachshund, weimaraner
- Rabies vaccine injection-site vasculitis: rottweiler, miniature poodle, bichon frise, silky terrier, Yorkshire terrier, Pekingese, Maltese, and miniature pinscher
- Familial canine dermatomyositis: collie, Shetland sheepdog, and Beauceron shepherd

RISK FACTORS

- Drug therapy (oral or injectable)
- Malignancy
- Infection (viral, bacterial, fungal, rickettsial)
- Immune-mediated diseases
- Insect bites
- Food allergy/hypersensitivity

ASSOCIATED CONDITIONS AND DISORDERS:

- Systemic lupus erythematosus (SLE)
- Familial canine dermatomyositis

CLINICAL PRESENTATION

DISEASE FORMS/SUBTYPES: Small vessel necrotizing vasculitis; hypersensitivity vasculitis; large vessel vasculitis. Lesions can be localized, regional, or multifocal to generalized.

HISTORY, CHIEF COMPLAINT: Patients may present with crusted or ulcerative macules or patches that may be a source of self-trauma. Patients with urticarial vasculitis may present with erythematous and often pruritic wheals. These patients are often anorexic and lethargic.

PHYSICAL EXAM FINDINGS

Description of the lesions varies according to the disease. Fever is often present.

- Injection site vasculitis: focal, well demarcated, alopecic, variably hyperkeratotic, and hyperpigmented patch.
- Thrombovascular pinnal vasculitis: notching of pinnal margins at tip and/or well-demarcated ulcers on the concave aspect of the pinna.
- Idiopathic vasculitis: well-demarcated necrosis and ulceration, particularly at the extremities and pressure points; may include edema, alopecia, or crateriform ulcers on the central aspect of the footpads.

- Urticarial vasculitis: generalized pruritus associated with papules, purpura, and wheals.
- Familial canine dermatomyositis: erythema, ulceration, and mild crusting in the young dog. Affected areas include face, pressure points, digits, and tail tip.

ETIOLOGY AND PATHOPHYSIOLOGY

- Suspected type III hypersensitivity although multiple pathomechanisms likely play a role. Antigen-antibody complexes become trapped along the basement membrane of vessel walls and activate the complement cascade.
- Other mechanisms proposed include direct antibody binding to the vessel wall and the release of toxic mediators leading to a bystander reaction.
- In many cases, the exact mechanism is not known.

DIAGNOSIS

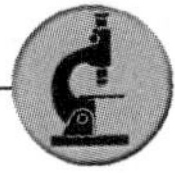

DIFFERENTIAL DIAGNOSIS

- Cold-agglutinin disease
- Disseminated intravascular coagulation
- Frostbite
- Demodicosis (focal lesions)
- Dermatophytosis (focal lesions)

INITIAL DATABASE

- Thorough history to assess risk of drug-induced vasculitis
- Routine complete blood count (CBC), serum biochemical profile, urinalysis: results are typically within normal limits
- Skin scrapings for focal (not ulcerated) lesions
- Diascopy (hemorrhagic lesions do not blanch when a slide is pressed over the top)
- Biopsy: histopathologic evaluation reveals varying degrees of neutrophilic, eosinophilic, lymphocytic, granulomatous, or cell-poor vasculitis

ADVANCED OR CONFIRMATORY TESTING

- Bacterial serologic titers (dogs: *Rickettsia rickettsii*, *Ehrlichia canis*, *Borrelia burgdorferi*)
- Viral serologic titers (cats: feline leukemia virus [FeLV], feline immunodeficiency virus [FIV])
- Coagulation profiles, Coombs' test, antinuclear antibody (ANA) test, and rheumatoid factors test may be indicated based on history, physical exam, and initial database supporting immune-mediated disease
- Blood culture if sepsis is suspected
- Tissue culture of nodular or granulomatous lesions
- Hypoallergenic dietary trial (urticarial form)

TREATMENT

THERAPEUTIC GOAL(S)

- Improve circulation to affected area
- Reduce self-trauma
- Remove inciting cause
- Suppress immune reaction

ACUTE GENERAL TREATMENT

- Discontinue current drug therapies
- Bandage pressure points and keep wounds clean
- Prevent self-trauma (Elizabethan collar)

CHRONIC TREATMENT

One or more may be indicated:

- Pentoxifylline: 20 mg/kg PO q 12h, following a meal
- Tetracycline and niacinamide: >10 kg, 500 mg of each drug q 8h (<10 kg, 250 mg of each drug) for a minimum of 3 months; tapering is based on a favorable response
- Prednisone or prednisolone: 2-4 mg/kg PO q 24h starting dose, tapering based on a favorable response
- Azathioprine (dogs): 2.2 mg/kg PO q 24-48h (with prednisone or prednisolone)
- Chlorambucil (cats): 0.1-0.2 mg/kg PO q 24-48h (with prednisone or prednisolone)
- Dapsone: 1 mg/kg PO q 8h in dogs
- Sulfasalazine: 22-44 mg/kg PO q 8h in dogs
- Cyclosporine: 5 mg/kg PO q 12-24h

POSSIBLE COMPLICATIONS

Tissue necrosis and secondary infection; septicemia

RECOMMENDED MONITORING

- Response to therapy
- Monitor as appropriate for adverse reactions to therapy

PROGNOSIS AND OUTCOME

- Some cases resolve, whereas others are chronic or recurrent. Damage to other organs (renal, neurologic) will also affect prognosis
- Injection site vasculitis: good prognosis though focal alopecia may persist indefinitely
- Thrombovascular pinnal vasculitis: variable response (may wax and wane)
- Idiopathic: may require long-term to indefinite treatment
- Urticarial: dependent on identification of underlying etiology; rule out food allergy
- See Dermatomyositis, p 284

PEARLS & CONSIDERATIONS

COMMENTS

- Multiple skin biopsies for histopathologic evaluation are the key to diagnosis.
- Do not use similar classes of drugs to those preceding development of the disease.
- Monitor closely for adverse reactions to therapy.

PREVENTION

Vaccinate dogs IM if there is a history of rabies vaccine-induced vasculitis; increased risk of an anaphylactic reaction has been suggested

CLIENT EDUCATION

Long-term treatment (4 to 6 months, sometimes indefinitely) is often needed.

SUGGESTED READING

Morris DO, Beale KM: Cutaneous vasculitis and vasculopathy. *Vet Clin North Am Small Anim Pract* 29(6):1325-1335, 1999.

Nichols PR, Morris DO, Beale KM: A retrospective study of canine and feline cutaneous vasculitis. *Vet Dermatol* 12:255-264, 2001.

Scott DW, Miller WH, Griffin CE: *Small Animal Dermatology*, ed 6. Philadelphia, WB Saunders, 2001, pp 742-756.

AUTHOR: **STEPHEN WAISGLASS**

EDITOR: **JAN A. HALL**

Ventricular Arrhythmias (Premature Ventricular Complexes, Ventricular Tachycardia)

BASIC INFORMATION

DEFINITION

- Ventricular arrhythmias are excessive electrical discharges occurring spontaneously and prematurely in the ventricles.
- By definition, the term premature ventricular complex(es) (PVCs) applies to one, two, or three consecutive premature ventricular impulses (Fig. I-184), whereas four or more in a row are defined as ventricular tachycardia (VT) (Fig. I-185).
- By definition, ventricular tachycardia involves a ventricular rate of 180 bpm or more in dogs and 240 bpm or more in cats.
- Strictly speaking, these are ventricular tachyarrhythmias (to distinguish them from ventricular escape rhythms); for simplicity, the term "ventricular arrhythmia" will be used here for designating PVCs and VT.

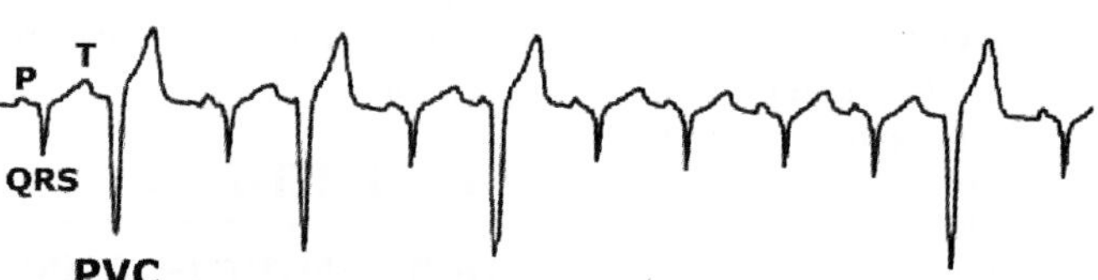

FIGURE I-184 Single premature ventricular complexes (PVCs) and normal heartbeats (P wave, QRS complex, and T wave are indicated) in a cat; lead II. Initially, normal sinus beats alternate with PVCs, a condition called bigeminy. The predominantly negative normal QRS complexes are typical for sinus rhythm in cats.

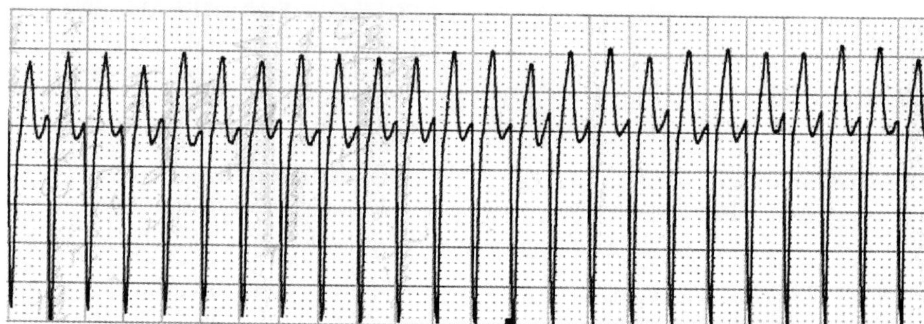

FIGURE I-185 Ventricular tachycardia; lead II, 25 mm/sec, 1 mm/mV. The ventricular tachycardia is monomorphic (PVCs all of the same shape) and rapid (290 bpm) in this critically ill dog with pheochromocytoma.

SYNONYM(S)

Ventricular ectopy
Ventricular extrasystoles
Ventricular tachyarrhythmias
Premature ventricular complexes (PVCs) are synonymous with ventricular premature complexes or contractions (VPCs), premature ventricular depolarizations (VPDs), and similar variations.

EPIDEMIOLOGY

SPECIES, AGE, SEX: Any can be affected.
GENETICS AND BREED PREDISPOSITION

- Boxers: arrhythmogenic cardiomyopathy (see Arrhythmogenic Right Ventricular Cardiomyopathy, p 79; Boxer Cardiomyopathy, p 145)
- Doberman pinschers and other breeds: dilated cardiomyopathy
- German shepherds: inherited ventricular tachycardia of young adults
- Large-breed dogs: splenic masses
- Large-breed dogs (Great Danes, setters, retrievers, and many others): gastric dilatation/volvulus
- Cats (male > female): hypertrophic cardiomyopathy

RISK FACTORS: Outdoor, roaming dogs: traumatic myocarditis (hit by car).
GEOGRAPHY AND SEASONALITY: Chagas' disease: myocarditis (southern parts of the United States and Latin America).
ASSOCIATED CONDITIONS AND DISORDERS: Primary heart disease or any systemic disturbance, if sufficiently severe, can cause ventricular arrhythmias.

CLINICAL PRESENTATION

DISEASE FORMS/SUBTYPES

- Incidental finding
- Clinically overt (e.g., causing syncope)

HISTORY, CHIEF COMPLAINT
Incidental finding (more common):

- Animal is presented for evaluation of a disorder other than syncope (Table I-27)
- Arrhythmia is noted during physical examination or subsequent monitoring

Clinically overt:

- Syncope/episodic collapse
- Episodic stumbling, disorientation, confusion
- Animal may be well (and even playful and active) before and after episodes or may be lethargic, weak, or anorexic

PHYSICAL EXAM FINDINGS:
Incidental finding:

- Physical exam findings reflect the underlying disorder; however, an arrhythmia is noted on physical exam.
- With ventricular tachycardia, the arrhythmia is rapid and may be irregular (usually polymorphic on ECG) or regular (usually monomorphic on ECG).
- Pulse deficit:
  - Premature heartbeat ausculted, without a corresponding palpable pulse for that beat
  - Common with ventricular arrhythmias
  - Depends on the degree of prematurity of PVCs ("How underfilled are the ventricles when the PVC causes them to contract again?")

Clinically overt:

- Wide range of presentations, from clinically normal and alert, if arrhythmia is intermittent to profoundly weak and hemodynamically collapsed with very rapid, sustained ventricular tachycardia (see Fig. I-184)
- Regularity or irregularity and pulse deficit, as for incidental finding (above)

ETIOLOGY AND PATHOPHYSIOLOGY

- Enhanced or abnormal automaticity, microreentry, and triggered activity (early or delayed after depolarizations) are mechanisms that underlie ventricular arrhythmias.
- These mechanisms can be activated or potentiated by systemic disturbances such as those previously listed (see Associated Conditions above).
- The result is one or more spontaneous electrical depolarizations originating prematurely in the ventricles. The prematurity is manifested on the electrocardiogram (ECG) as a shorter R-R interval. The ventricular origin results in a QRS complex that is of

a different shape than a sinus QRS complex.
- A greater degree of prematurity of PVCs (or a higher rate of ventricular tachycardia) reduces the time the ventricles have for filling prior to contracting. Therefore, faster ventricular arrhythmias compromise diastolic filling time more severely and are more likely to produce clinical signs or hemodynamic deterioration (e.g., poor pulse, cerebral hypoperfusion) than slower or infrequent ventricular arrhythmias.

TABLE I-27 **Common Causes of Ventricular Arrhythmias**

Hypokalemia*,**
Hypoxemia (e.g., due to cardiogenic pulmonary edema, pleural effusion, primary lung disease)*
Cardiomyopathy
Gastric dilatation/volvulus*
Traumatic myocarditis/hit by car
Abdominal mass, especially splenic or hepatic*
Advanced valvular heart disease
Hypomagnesemia*,**
Acidosis*
Intoxication (digitalis; oleander, foxglove, lily of the valley, azalea, and yew plants; many over-the-counter, prescription, or illicit drugs)

*Potentially correctable/curable.
**Presence makes ventricular antiarrhythmic drugs such as lidocaine, procainamide, and mexiletine ineffective.

DIAGNOSIS

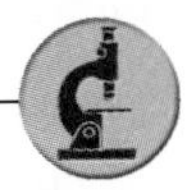

DIFFERENTIAL DIAGNOSIS

- Physical examination:
  - Supraventricular premature beats, marked respiratory sinus arrhythmia
  - Physical auscultation or palpation of premature heartbeats alone cannot differentiate between these and PVCs
- ECG (wide, bizarre, and/or predominantly negative QRS complexes in lead II):
  - Right bundle-branch block
  - Ventricular escape rhythm
  - Right ventricular enlargement
  - Motion artifact

INITIAL DATABASE

ECG remains the gold standard for diagnosis of cardiac arrhythmias. Criteria for ventricular arrhythmias:
- PVC is substantially different from normal sinus QRS complexes.
  - Often, but not always, wide, bizarre, and predominantly negative in lead II (see Figs. I-184 and I-185)
- PVC occurs prematurely. The R-R interval from the preceding normal sinus beat to the PVC is shorter than the interval between two normal sinus beats.
- The T wave following a PVC is different (often larger) than the T wave of a normal sinus beat (see Fig. I-184).
- P waves continue to occur regularly during ventricular arrhythmias, but they are not related to PVCs and often are lost within the PVCs.

ADVANCED OR CONFIRMATORY TESTING

- Ten-lead ECG: improved visualization of certain features of ventricular arrhythmias (e.g., better ability to see P waves not associated with the wide, bizarre QRS complexes of PVCs)
- Complete blood count (CBC), serum biochemistry profile, urinalysis: especially to assess systemic, proarrhythmic abnormalities like hypokalemia (Table I-127)
- Thoracic radiographs: particularly if suspicion of primary cardiac disease, hypoxemia, or thoracic trauma
- Echocardiogram: if a primary cardiac problem is suspected or if no other cause is identified
- Abdominal imaging: if there is suspicion of an abdominal problem or if a primary cause for the arrhythmia is not found
- Arterial blood gas (ABG) analysis: if acid-base or oxygenation abnormalities are suspected

TREATMENT

THERAPEUTIC GOAL(S)

- To control the arrhythmia to such a degree that adequate organ perfusion is present and there is a resolution or control of any arrhythmia-related clinical signs (e.g., syncope).
- The goal is not to abolish every PVC or otherwise try to "normalize" the ECG, because overzealous treatment of arrhythmias may be detrimental.

ACUTE GENERAL TREATMENT

- First, determine if the arrhythmia is a ventricular arrhythmia (PVC, VT) by ruling out common impostors:
  - Right bundle-branch block (a P wave precedes each wide, bizarre QRS complex at a fixed interval)
  - Right axis deviation (a P wave precedes each wide, bizarre QRS complex at a fixed interval)
  - Ventricular escape rhythm (ventricular rate is 30-70 bpm)
  - Motion artifact (sinus rhythm persists inside wide, bizarre deflections)
- Second, identify and address any relevant underlying causes (see Table I-27, above)
- Third, determine if there are overt clinical signs associated with the ventricular arrhythmia (e.g., syncope). If so, antiarrhythmic treatment is warranted.
- Fourth, if the ventricular arrhythmia is sustained at a rapid rate (>180/min in large-breed dogs, >220/ min in small-breed dogs, >260/min in cats) despite the three steps described so far, then treatment should be considered. The following are recognized treatments for ventricular arrhythmias:
  - Lidocaine 1-2 mg/kg (dog) or 0.25-1 mg/kg (cat) IV bolus (can repeat up to three times in 10-15 minutes); can be followed with IV constant rate infusion (CRI) at 40-80 μg/kg/min (dog) or 10-20 μg/kg/min (cat)
    - To make lidocaine CRI: withdraw 25 ml from a 500 ml bag of crystalloid fluid (e.g., lactated Ringer's solution) and replace with 25 ml of 2% lidocaine. Concentration in bag is 1000 μg/ml. Administer IV at usual fluid maintenance rate (66 ml/kg per day) assuming congestive heart failure (CHF) is not present. Infusion at this rate will be 50 μg/kg/min
  - Procainamide 6-15 mg/kg (dog) or 1-2 mg/kg (cat) slow IV bolus; may follow with IV CRI at 25-50 (dog) or 10-20 (cat) μg/kg/min; usually administered instead of lidocaine if lidocaine was ineffective, but both may be given together

CHRONIC TREATMENT

- Ongoing management of the underlying cause
- Oral antiarrhythmic drugs may be used for treating rapid and/or clinically overt (syncopal) ventricular arrhythmia. Options include one of the following:
  - Sotalol: 0.5-2 mg/kg PO q 12h (dogs); 10-20 mg per cat PO q 12h
  - Mexiletine 4-8 mg/kg PO q 12h to q 8h, and atenolol 0.2-0.75 mg/kg PO q 12h (dogs)
  - Amiodarone 10 mg/kg PO q 12h for 1 week (loading), then 5-8 mg/kg PO q 24h (dogs)

- Atenolol (cats) 6.25–12.5 mg per cat PO q 24h to q 12h
- Procainamide sustained release (dogs) has been given at 10–20 mg/kg PO q 8h to q 6h, but variable dissolution of tablets makes pharmacokinetics unpredictable

DRUG INTERACTIONS

Digoxin can cause ventricular arrhythmias. Serum digoxin levels (and risk of toxicity) are increased with concurrent administration of diazepam, erythromycin, quinidine, tetracycline, or verapamil.

POSSIBLE COMPLICATIONS

Uncontrolled ventricular arrhythmias may progress to ventricular flutter and ventricular fibrillation (cardiac arrest); however, normalization of the ECG to sinus rhythm using antiarrhythmic drugs alone has never been shown to improve the prognosis for survival. Therefore, complications can be minimized by treating/correcting inciting factors (see Table I-27) reserving ventricular antiarrhythmic drugs for cases in which overt signs such as syncope are present or in which a very high rate (e.g., >220 bpm in dogs, >260 bpm in cats) is present despite management or correction of the underlying cause.

RECOMMENDED MONITORING

- ECG as dictated by clinical evolution; ranges from continuous ECG with ventricular tachycardia in an unstable animal to periodic ECG or Holter monitoring during visits in stable animals
- Follow-up tests as listed for initial diagnosis to monitor underlying condition

PROGNOSIS AND OUTCOME

- Ventricular arrhythmias that occur at a faster rate are more likely to produce clinical signs and carry a more guarded prognosis than slower ventricular arrhythmias.
- Ventricular arrhythmias that fail to respond to correction of the underlying problem (or for which the underlying problem cannot be corrected) usually indicate cardiac manifestations of a serious problem that carries a guarded short-term prognosis. Long-term prognosis depends on the exact nature of the underlying problem.

PEARLS & CONSIDERATIONS

COMMENTS

- Virtually any disease or disorder, if sufficiently severe to have systemic effects, can cause ventricular arrhythmias.
- Ventricular escape beats and VPCs often look identical. Ventricular escape beats occur at a rate of 40–100 bpm against a background of second- or third-degree AV block or asystole—they are saving the heart from arrest and should never be treated with ventricular antiarrhythmics. By contrast, VPCs are excessive, unwanted ventricular complexes that occur in addition to the heart's usual rhythm.
- The most common correctable underlying causes of ventricular arrhythmias are hypokalemia, hypoxia, gastric dilatation and volvulus, abdominal masses, anemia, metabolic acidosis, and pain.
- The most common treatable but noncorrectable causes of ventricular arrhythmias are cardiomyopathy, degenerative valvular heart disease, and traumatic myocarditis (hit by car).
- Ventricular arrhythmias most commonly are manifestations of an underlying disorder. Attempting to eliminate ventricular arrhythmias with antiarrhythmic drugs in a stable animal is analogous to "shooting the messenger." Rather, the underlying cause needs to be found and addressed. Perhaps no antiarrhythmic drug is as beneficial to a patient with ventricular arrhythmias as is correction of the underlying cause.

PREVENTION

Ventricular arrhythmias are clues to a primary cardiac or systemic disturbance; therefore, preventing them relies on identifying and managing the underlying disease whenever possible.

CLIENT EDUCATION

- Ventricular arrhythmias are serious disturbances of the cardiac rhythm. Their impact can range from minimal to life threatening, and sudden cardiac death is always possible when an animal has a disorder that causes ventricular arrhythmias.
- Antiarrhythmic treatment may help reduce clinical manifestations (e.g., syncope), but no treatment has yet been shown to successfully prevent deterioration or cardiac arrest in patients with ventricular arrhythmias.

SUGGESTED READING

Côté E, Ettinger SJ: Electrocardiography and cardiac arrhythmias. In Ettinger SJ, Feldman EC (eds): *Textbook of Veterinary Internal Medicine*, ed 6. St. Louis, Elsevier, 2005, pp 1040–1076.

Kittleson MD: Diagnosis and treatment of arrhythmias (dysrhythmias). In Kittleson MD, Kienle RD: *Small Animal Cardiovascular Disease*. St. Louis, Mosby, 1998, pp 449–494.

AUTHOR & EDITOR: **ETIENNE CÔTÉ**

Ventricular Septal Defect

BASIC INFORMATION

DEFINITION

Anomalous communication between the right and left ventricles of the heart resulting in interventricular shunting of blood

SYNONYM(S)

Interventricular septal defect
VSD

EPIDEMIOLOGY

SPECIES, AGE, SEX

- Dogs and cats
- Second most common congenital heart defect in cats
- Typically diagnosed at a young age
- No sex predilection

GENETICS AND BREED PREDISPOSITION

- Hereditary in a family of English springer spaniels and keeshonden
- Predisposed breeds: Akita, basset hound, English bulldog, English springer spaniel, keeshonden, Lakeland terrier, West Highland white terrier

ASSOCIATED CONDITIONS AND DISORDERS

- Aortic valvular regurgitation/insufficiency (AI) due to decreased support of aortic valve
- Pulmonic stenosis, overriding aorta, atrial septal defects

CLINICAL PRESENTATION

DISEASE FORMS/SUBTYPES

- In small animals, ventricular septal defects (VSDs) most commonly involve the high membranous septum (below aortic valve on left side, below septal leaflet of tricuspid valve on right side; "perimembranous" VSD)
- Typically, blood shunts through the defect from left to right (L→R)
- A very large VSD or VSD accompanied by other specific defects (e.g., severe pulmonic stenosis or pulmonary hypertension) may produce shunting of blood from right to left (R→L, "reverse shunting"), potentially causing generalized cyanosis

HISTORY, CHIEF COMPLAINT

- Usually there are no overt clinical signs reported by the owner (incidental finding of heart murmur during routine exam)
- If progression to the point of decompensation has occurred, the following may be observed:
  - Exercise intolerance
  - Dyspnea, tachypnea
  - Cough
  - Syncope

PHYSICAL EXAM FINDINGS

- Systolic murmur loudest around the fourth intercostal space (ICS) on the ventral thorax to the right of the sternum (most common) or left base
- If substantial AI is present, a diastolic murmur may be heard on the left cranial thorax (heart base, third ICS)
- Tachycardia, dyspnea, tachypnea, crackles may be apparent if left-sided congestive heart failure (CHF) is present
- R→L shunt: cyanosis, generally no murmur unless another malformation is present (e.g., pulmonic stenosis)

ETIOLOGY AND PATHOPHYSIOLOGY

- Etiology unknown
- Magnitude and direction of shunting and thus clinical consequences depend on size of defect, relative pulmonary and systemic vascular resistances, and presence of other cardiopulmonary defects
- L→R shunting VSD causes volume overload of pulmonary circulation and left side of the heart; ultimately the result may be left-sided CHF and/or pulmonary hypertension
- R→L shunting VSD (much less common) causes systemic arterial hypoxemia

DIAGNOSIS

DIFFERENTIAL DIAGNOSIS

- Other congenital causes of systolic murmurs: aortic/subaortic or pulmonic stenosis, atrioventricular (AV) valve dysplasia, tetralogy of Fallot (of which VSD is one component)
- Acquired heart diseases: acquired AV valve regurgitation (dogs), dilated cardiomyopathy (dogs or cats), hypertrophic cardiomyopathy (cats)

INITIAL DATABASE

- Complete blood count (CBC)/serum biochemistry panel:
  - Typically normal
  - Polycythemia if R→L shunting
- Thoracic radiographs:
  - Normal with small VSD
  - Larger L→R VSD: left-sided cardiomegaly, pulmonary overcirculation, ± pulmonary edema, ± right ventricular enlargement
  - R→L VSD: right-sided cardiomegaly, variable pulmonary artery pattern (e.g., normal to enlarged if pulmonary arterial hypertension; normal or small if pulmonic stenosis)
- Electrocardiogram (ECG):
  - Various arrhythmias (ventricular, supraventricular) possible
  - Left atrial and/or ventricular enlargement if large L→R shunt or right ventricular hypertrophy if R→L shunt
  - ± Wide and/or notched Q wave representing abnormal septal activation
- Echocardiography:
  - May demonstrate a visible defect in intraventricular septum (beware of artifact "septal drop-out")
  - L→R VSD: turbulent jet from left to right ventricle with color Doppler, ± left atrial enlargement, ± left ventricular enlargement
  - Peak velocity (V in m/s) of VSD jet using spectral Doppler reflects the pressure gradient (ΔP [mmHg]) between left and right ventricles according to modified Bernoulli equation ($\Delta P = 4V^2$), which generally speaks to size of defect (i.e., small VSD: V >4.5 m/s; moderate-size VSD: 3 < V <4.5 m/s; large VSD: V <3 m/s). Beware of underestimation of velocity due to erroneous/oblique alignment of Doppler sample
  - R→L VSD: right ventricular hypertrophy, main pulmonary artery dilation
  - ±AI using color and spectral Doppler

ADVANCED OR CONFIRMATORY TESTING

- Contrast echocardiography (bubble study) to confirm R→L shunt
- Cardiac catheterization for angiography, shunt quantification, and measurement of cardiac pressures (virtually never used; mainly preoperative if open-heart surgery)

TREATMENT

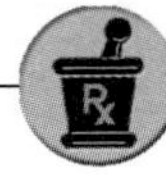

THERAPEUTIC GOAL(S)

- Prevent or eliminate CHF signs
- Decrease shunt volume

ACUTE GENERAL TREATMENT

- No treatment required for small, uncomplicated VSD (i.e., the majority of VSD cases)
- Larger L→R VSD:
  - Surgical repair uncommon (ideally requires cardiac bypass)
  - Pulmonary artery banding is a palliative surgical technique to decrease L→R shunt
  - Arterial vasodilators used with caution to decrease L→R shunt; contraindicated if complex malformations or R→L shunt
  - If CHF present, may use ACE-inhibitors, diuretics, ± pimobendan, ± digoxin (see Heart Failure, Acute/ Decompensated, p 458)
- R→L VSD:
  - Surgical repair contraindicated
  - Phlebotomy to palliate signs and maintain PCV at 55-65%

CHRONIC TREATMENT

- Treatment of CHF as already described (see also Heart Failure, Chronic, p 459)
- Phlebotomy ± hydroxyurea as needed if R→L shunt

POSSIBLE COMPLICATIONS

- Left-sided CHF
- Pulmonary hypertension
- Shunt reversal (R→L) over time (Eisenmenger's complex); rare in dogs and cats

RECOMMENDED MONITORING

- Following diagnosis in puppies/kittens with no clinical signs, examination at 6 months, 1 year, then yearly thereafter
- Frequent monitoring for animals with overt decompensation and treatment

PROGNOSIS AND OUTCOME

- Excellent prognosis for small, uncomplicated VSD
- Guarded prognosis for larger VSD (risk CHF and/or pulmonary hypertension)
- Concurrent substantial AI carries poor prognosis
- Guarded to poor prognosis for R→L shunts; severe exercise limitations

PEARLS & CONSIDERATIONS

COMMENTS

- In L→R shunting VSDs, the right ventricle and pulmonary arterial circulation essentially act as conduits for VSD flow. The left atrium and left ventricle, however, receive increased venous return, resulting in increased diastolic pressures. In addition, effective forward flow into the systemic circulation is reduced as a result of the shunt flow. The latter two points account for the increased left ventricular workload and predominant occurrence of left heart failure, not right heart failure, in L→R VSDs.
- VSD and tricuspid dysplasia are the two main differential diagnoses for a systolic murmur heard best on the right side of the chest in dogs or cats (murmurs due to subaortic stenosis may radiate prominently to the right side in some cases; hypertroptohic cardiomyopathy is another common differential in cats).
- Most VSDs are relatively small, well tolerated, and do not require therapy.

PREVENTION

Genetic basis possible but unproven in the breeds listed previously. Consider discouraging breeding of affected animals

SUGGESTED READING

Bonagura JD, Lehmkuhl LB: Congenital heart disease. In Fox PR, Sisson D, Moise NS (eds): *Textbook of Canine and Feline Cardiology*. Philadelphia, WB Saunders, 1999, pp 471-535.

Kittleson MD: Septal defects. In Kittleson MD, Kienle RD (eds): *Small Animal Cardiovascular Medicine*. St. Louis, Mosby, 1998, pp 231-239.

AUTHOR: **M. LYNNE O'SULLIVAN**

EDITOR: **ETIENNE CÔTÉ**

Vestibular Disease

BASIC INFORMATION

DEFINITION

Diseases affecting the vestibular system of dogs and cats that usually cause clinical signs of head tilt, nystagmus, and/or loss of balance

EPIDEMIOLOGY

SPECIES, AGE, SEX

- Occurs in both dogs and cats
- No sex predisposition reported
- Idiopathic vestibular disease occurs in older dogs (usually >8 years) but in cats of any age
- Encephalitis occurs more often in young adult dogs and cats

GEOGRAPHY AND SEASONALITY: Reported worldwide; no seasonality.

ASSOCIATED CONDITIONS AND DISORDERS: Nausea, vomiting.

CLINICAL PRESENTATION

DISEASE FORMS/SUBTYPES

- Peripheral vestibular disease (PVD): vestibular nerve lesion in inner ear
- Central vestibular disease (CVD): brainstem lesion (medulla)

HISTORY, CHIEF COMPLAINT

- Regardless of the underlying cause, most animals present with a peracute to subacute onset of clinical signs.
- The most common chief complaints are head tilt, nystagmus, and ataxia.
- Acute-onset vestibular disorders may produce such profound dysequilibrium and ataxia that owners are concerned about the animal's having "had a stroke."

PHYSICAL EXAM FINDINGS

- Head tilt, nystagmus, and vestibular ataxia (possibly to the extent of causing recumbency and whole-body rolling) are the hallmarks of vestibular disorders, be they peripheral (inner ear; PVD) or central (brainstem; CVD) in origin.
- Specific physical exam findings are critical for establishing whether the vestibular disease is central or peripheral in origin.
- The most important aspect in localization of a lesion to the central vestibular system is identification of neurologic signs that cannot be attributed to peripheral vestibular disease.
- Mental status:
  - Central: often altered (depression, stupor, or coma)
  - Peripheral: animal should be alert and responsive and can often appear disoriented
- Gait: Vestibular ataxia (falling, veering, leaning, rolling, circling) usually toward the side of the lesion; seen with both CVD and PVD. Hypermetria, intention tremors, and truncal sway may be observed if the cerebellum is affected (central).
- Head tilt: usually toward the side of the lesion; seen with both CVD and PVD.
- Spontaneous nystagmus: usually present with both CVD and PVD. Vertical nystagmus occurs only in animals with CVD, while horizontal or rotary nystagmus can be seen with either PVD or CVD. The fast phase of the nystagmus is usually away from the side of the lesion. Change in direction of the fast phase with altered head positions suggests CVD.
- Cranial nerve deficits: cranial nerve VII (facial nerve) paresis is sometimes seen in animals with PVD due to its proximity to peripheral vestibular structures; cranial nerves V, VI, IX and XII ipsilateral to lesion may be affected in animals with CVD but not PVD.
- Horner's syndrome: possible with PVD but rare with CVD ipsilateral to lesion.
- Postural reaction deficits are commonly seen with CVD but should not be observed with PVD.
- Paradoxical CVD: Lesion location as suggested by clinical signs related to the head (head tilt, nystagmus, etc.) does not match the lesion location suggested by the postural reaction deficits. In this paradoxical situation, the lesion is always ipsilateral to the postural reaction deficits, usually in the ipsilateral side of the cerebellum or caudal cerebellar peduncle. For example, in an animal with a right head tilt and nystagmus with the fast phase to the left, a right-sided lesion is suspected (peripheral or central); however, if postural reaction deficits are observed (must be a central vestibular lesion) and the postural reaction deficits are on the left side, a left-sided central lesion is most likely, especially affecting the cerebellum or caudal cerebellar peduncle on that side because of the paradoxical lateralizing signs.
- Bilateral peripheral vestibular disease: head tilt and nystagmus may not be present; animals may walk with a crouched gait.
- Clinical signs related to disease in other central nervous system (CNS) locations, such as seizures, behavioral changes, hypermetria, intention tremors, and truncal sway, suggest multifocal central neurologic disease.

ETIOLOGY AND PATHOPHYSIOLOGY

- Basic neuroanatomy of the vestibular system:
  - Peripheral: vestibular receptors (semicircular canals, saccule, utricle)

located within the petrous temporal bone and cranial nerve VIII (vestibulocochlear nerve)
 - Central: vestibular nuclei in the dorsal portion of the medulla oblongata, vestibular pathways of the brainstem and spinal cord (medial longitudinal fasciculus, vestibulospinal tracts), vestibular components in the cerebellum, and vestibular pathways through the caudal cerebellar peduncle
- Etiology for idiopathic vestibular disease in dogs and cats is unknown; an immune-mediated mechanism is suspected, but immunosuppressive drugs such as glucocorticoids have not been shown to help

DIAGNOSIS

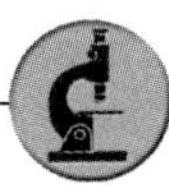

DIFFERENTIAL DIAGNOSIS

- Peripheral vestibular diseases:
  - Otitis media-interna
  - Idiopathic vestibular disease
  - Nasopharyngeal polyps: most commonly found in cats
  - Hypothyroidism: dogs
  - Neoplasia: squamous cell carcinoma (SCC), ceruminous gland adenocarcinoma, and other related conditions
  - Ototoxicity: topical chlorhexidine or iodine; systemic aminoglycosides and other drugs
- Central vestibular diseases:
  - Canine distemper virus (CDV) encephalomyelitis
  - Feline infectious peritonitis (FIP)
  - Rickettsial encephalitis: Rocky Mountain spotted fever (RMSF), ehrlichiosis
  - Fungal encephalitis: *Cryptococcus neoformans* most common; blastomycosis or coccidioidomycosis in certain regions of North America
  - Granulomatous meningoencephalomyelitis (GME)
  - Protozoal encephalitis: *Toxoplasma gondii*, *Neospora caninum*
  - Neoplasia: meningioma, choroid plexus tumor, lymphoma, metastatic neoplasia
  - Metronidazole toxicity
  - Cerebrovascular accident (infarct)

INITIAL DATABASE

- Complete blood count (CBC), serum biochemical analysis, urinalysis: results often normal
- Thyroid hormone analysis: low TT4 and fT4 and elevated thyroid-stimulating hormone (TSH) in dogs with hypothyroidism
- Otoscopic examination: evaluate tympanic membranes for integrity

ADVANCED OR CONFIRMATORY TESTING

- Bulla radiographs: dorsoventral, oblique lateral, and rostroventral-caudodorsal open-mouthed views. Abnormalities include soft-tissue or fluid opacity within the bulla and sclerosis of the tympanic bulla.
- Oropharyngeal and otoscopic examination under general anesthesia to identify nasopharyngeal polyps and otitis media. Abnormalities include soft-tissue or fluid opacity within and sclerosis of the affected tympanic bulla. See Otoscopy (Video), p 1291.
- Brainstem auditory-evoked response (BAER) test may be useful for distinguishing PVD from CVD (see Brainstem Auditory Evoked Response, p 1197).
- CT scan: useful for examination of the middle ear in patients with peripheral vestibular disease. CT scans can also be used for central vestibular disease; however, beam-hardening artifacts in the caudal brain may preclude evaluation of the brainstem, and small lesions may not be visualized (MRI preferable for this location).
- MRI: useful for examination of both the peripheral and central vestibular structures. It provides superior resolution of brain parenchyma.
- Cerebrospinal fluid (CSF) analysis: used as an adjunct to advanced imaging, primarily to rule out encephalitis. In the absence of encephalitis (pleocytosis), results are generally nonspecific and reveal normal to mildly elevated protein. Albuminocytologic dissociation (elevated CSF protein with normal white blood cell [WBC] count) can be seen with infarcts and neoplasia but is not pathognomonic. Neoplastic cells are rarely identified within the CSF; however, the presence of lymphoblasts within the CSF supports a diagnosis of CNS lymphoma. Fungal organisms will occasionally be identified in fungal encephalitis cases.
- Infectious disease titers may be required in certain cases to rule out infectious encephalitis. CSF is the preferred sample for canine distemper virus, FIP, and cryptococcosis. Serum titers are performed for *Toxoplasma* and *Neospora* spp.
- CSF culture and sensitivity (C&S) may be required for ruling out bacterial encephalitis.
- Histopathologic examination is required for definitive diagnosis in many diseases causing structural lesions (e.g., masses). Tissue samples can be obtained via surgical excision or stereotactic brain biopsy.

TREATMENT

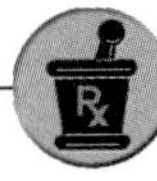

THERAPEUTIC GOAL(S)

Definitive treatment for vestibular disease is based on definitive diagnosis

ACUTE GENERAL TREATMENT

- Meclizine (25 mg PO q 24h in dogs; 12.5 mg PO q 24h in cats) or diazepam (0.1–0.5 mg/kg PO q 8h in dogs) may help alleviate clinical signs of nausea and vomiting. Meclizine causes less sedation than diazepam and can be purchased as an over-the-counter drug. Oral diazepam should be used with extreme caution in cats due to the reported incidence of idiosyncratic hepatic necrosis.
- Idiopathic vestibular disease: Clinical signs improve spontaneously over 1 to 2 weeks; no treatment has been shown to accelerate the natural resolution of the disorder.
- Otitis media-interna: systemic antibiotics ± antifungals for 4 to 6 weeks, ideally based on bacterial C&S. Surgical treatment (bulla osteotomy and total ear canal ablation) may be required to remove infected tissues.
- Nasopharyngeal polyps: bulla osteotomy.
- Hypothyroidism: thyroid supplementation (see Hypothyroidism, p 575).
- Neoplasia: surgical excision may be possible for meningioma and choroid plexus tumors depending on lesion location. Surgical excision of tumors in the middle and inner ear may be possible but is difficult. Radiation therapy may provide some relief of clinical signs, and consultation with an oncologist is recommended in these cases.
- CDV and FIP encephalomyelitis: No specific therapy is available. Nonspecific supportive therapy with antibiotics and corticosteroids may alleviate signs temporarily (see Feline Infectious Peritonitis, p 378).
- Rickettsial encephalitis: doxycycline (5 mg/kg PO q 12h) or chloramphenicol (50 mg/kg PO q 8h) for 3 to 4 weeks.
- Fungal encephalitis: fluconazole (5 mg/kg PO q 12h) penetrates the CNS to a greater degree than other antifungal medications. Itraconazole and amphotericin B can be used with blastomycosis. Oral treatment should be continued for at least 6 months barring adverse reactions and may be required long term to control clinical signs.
- GME: immunosuppressive dose of prednisone, initially at 2 mg/kg PO q 12h for 1 to 2 days, then 1 mg/kg PO q 12h for at least 2 weeks; then slowly taper the drug over 4 to 8 months to reach the minimal effective dose (see Granulomatous Meningoencephalomyelitis, p 447).

- Protozoal encephalitis: clindamycin (10 mg/kg PO q 12h to q 8h) for 4 weeks or combination of trimethoprim/sulfadiazine (TMS; 15 mg/kg PO q 12h) and pyrimethamine (1 mg/kg PO q 24h).
- Metronidazole toxicity: discontinue metronidazole. In dogs, diazepam administration (0.5 mg/kg IV once, followed by 0.5 mg/kg PO q 8h until resolution of signs) appears to shorten the duration of clinical signs. Oral diazepam should be used with extreme caution in cats due to the reported incidence of idiosyncratic hepatic necrosis.

POSSIBLE COMPLICATIONS

A permanent mild head tilt may persist after resolution of other clinical signs

RECOMMENDED MONITORING

- Serial neurologic exam every 4 weeks
- Serial infectious disease titers if indicated

PROGNOSIS AND OUTCOME

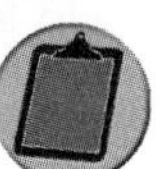

- Prognosis for most peripheral vestibular diseases is good with specific treatment, with the exception of neoplasia, which carries a guarded-to-poor prognosis.
- CDV and FIP encephalomyelitis: poor even with treatment.
- Rickettsial and protozoal encephalitis: good with early and specific treatment.
- Fungal encephalitis: fair to guarded. Long-term treatment may be required to control clinical signs.
- GME: fair to guarded. Many dogs respond initially to treatment; however, relapse is common. In some dogs, corticosteroids eventually can be discontinued.
- Neoplasia: generally poor long-term prognosis.
- Metronidazole toxicity: excellent.

PEARLS & CONSIDERATIONS

COMMENTS

- Compensation for vestibular diseases will occur in many animals, regardless of lesion location, and clinical signs may improve slightly if the lesion is slow growing.
- In general, animals with PVD carry a good prognosis for recovery following specific therapy.
- The long-term prognosis for animals with CVD is variable depending upon the specific cause; however, treatment should be attempted to alleviate clinical signs.

PREVENTION

- Thyroid supplementation in dogs with hypothyroidism.
- Avoidance of high doses and/or prolonged courses of metronidazole treatment. A common error is to prescribe a high dose of the drug (e.g., 30–65 mg/kg PO q 12h). The recommendation is to limit the maximum daily dose to 30 mg/kg/day, or else divide it into two daily doses.

CLIENT EDUCATION

Head tilt may be persistent

SUGGESTED READING

LeCouteur RA, Vernau KM: Feline vestibular disorders. Part I: Anatomy and clinical signs. *J Fel Med Surg* 1:71, 1999.

LeCouteur RA, Vernau KM: Feline vestibular disorders. Part II: Diagnostics approach and differential diagnosis. *J Fel Med Surg* 1:81, 1999.

Thomas WB: Vestibular dysfunction. *Vet Clin North Amer Small Anim Pract* 30(1):227, 2000.

AUTHOR: **MARK T. TROXEL**
EDITOR: **CURTIS W. DEWEY**

Vitamin A Toxicosis

BASIC INFORMATION

DEFINITION

Usually a chronic toxicosis seen in dogs and cats after repeated ingestion of high doses of vitamin A; characterized by lethargy, anorexia, weight loss, cervical neck pain, skin conditions, and possibly reproductive problems. Acute intoxication may present as vomiting, diarrhea, abdominal pain, and rarely hepatitis.

SYNONYM(S)

Retinoids are vitamin A derivatives.

EPIDEMIOLOGY

SPECIES, AGE, SEX

- All mammals are susceptible, but vitamin A intoxication clinically occurs mainly in the cat.
- Intoxication is more likely with repeated exposures than with a single acute exposure.
- Toxicity can occur in cats 2 to 9 years of age that are fed a diet high in raw liver (e.g., 4 days per week).
- Experimentally, dogs fed a daily diet containing 10,000 IU vitamin A/kg diet (dry matter) for several months developed hypervitaminosis A.

CLINICAL PRESENTATION

DISEASE FORMS/SUBTYPES

- Acute: very rare
- Chronic: after months of high levels of vitamin A ingestion

HISTORY, CHIEF COMPLAINT

- History of chronic exposure to excesses of a high vitamin A-containing product (capsules) or diet (mainly or exclusively raw liver diet: most common)
- Acute (rare): self-limiting mild vomiting, diarrhea, anorexia, depression
- Chronic: lethargy, anorexia, weight loss, gingivitis, matted haircoat, irritability, may resent handling; signs typically develop over several months
- Pregnant animals: deformed fetus (cleft palate, hydrocephalus, microencephaly), reproductive failure

PHYSICAL EXAM FINDINGS

- Neck and limb rigidity due to exostosis (proliferation from bone)
- Tense musculature
- Neck ventroflexion possible:
    - In contrast to neck ventroflexion from hypokalemia or thiamine deficiency, characterized by a flaccid neck, in patients with vitamin A intoxication the ventroflexion is stiff (caused by bony exostoses).
    - Exfoliation, matted coat.

ETIOLOGY AND PATHOPHYSIOLOGY

Source:

- Vitamin A and its congeners are not produced endogenously and must be supplied exogenously through different sources (dietary or oral supplementation); β-carotene is a plant pigment found in a number of foods. It is converted to retinal in the intestine and is further oxidized to retinoic acid and retinol.
- Acidic forms of vitamin A (*cis*- or *trans*-retinoic acid), vitamin A derivatives (retinol, *trans*-retinyl palmitate, retinyl stearate), synthetic retinoids (tretinoin, isotretinoin, etretinate), and vitamin A

capsules, tablets, and injections all represent potential pharmaceutical sources of vitamin A.
- Liver (typically from chicken, beef, seal, or fish) is a common nutritional source of vitamin A.

Disease:
- Vitamin A plays an essential role in normal night vision, reproductive processes, maintenance of epithelial and membrane structure, normal cellular growth, and immune functions.
- Hypervitaminosis A can inhibit keratinization of epithelial cells, which can lead to skin problems.
- High concentrations of vitamin A induce chondrocytes to produce more extracellular matrix, which forms a framework for mineralization (exostoses: abnormal bone growth, cervical spondylosis).
- In humans, neurologic toxicity is due to increased intracranial pressure.

DIAGNOSIS

Clinical diagnosis is based almost entirely on unusual nutritional/dietary supplement history and characteristic exostotic bony changes on radiographs (especially cervicothoracic vertebrae)

DIFFERENTIAL DIAGNOSIS

Other causes of acute gastrointestinal (GI) signs (vomiting, diarrhea) or liver damage (rare because acute vitamin A toxicosis is very uncommon)

INITIAL DATABASE

- Complete blood count (CBC): nonspecific changes or no significant changes expected
- Serum chemistry profile: liver enzymes elevated with acute intoxication
- Urinalysis: generally unremarkable
- Cervical radiograph: may show bone-density cervical mass ventral to C1-C2 intervertebral space

ADVANCED OR CONFIRMATORY TESTING

- Cats: serum retinol more than 3145 μg/L is considered toxic (normal 200-1600)
- Toxic levels in feline liver (postmortem) 8590-39,570 μg/g
- In dogs, serum retinol > 20,000 μg/L is considered toxic

TREATMENT

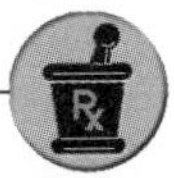

THERAPEUTIC GOAL(S)

- Decontaminate the GI tract (acute exposure)
- Remove source (chronic use)
- Provide supportive care as needed

ACUTE GENERAL TREATMENT

- Decontamination of patient:
  - Emesis: 3% hydrogen peroxide at 2 ml/kg PO (maximum of 45 ml) if recent large ingestion (within few hours); repeated once in 10-15 minutes if no emesis first time
  - Activated charcoal: 1-2 g/kg PO if recent large ingestion (within few hours)
- Remove source (excess vitamin A)
- Supportive care:
  - IV fluids
  - Vomiting may be controlled with metoclopramide at 0.1-0.4 mg/kg bodyweight PO, SC, or IM
  - Management of liver damage (rare) as needed (see Hepatic Injury, Acute, p 491)

DRUG INTERACTIONS

Hypervitaminosis A can interfere with the action of other fat-soluble vitamins.

POSSIBLE COMPLICATIONS

Liver damage (rare)

RECOMMENDED MONITORING

- Serum biochemistry profile
- Body weight

PROGNOSIS AND OUTCOME

- Excellent in acute cases
- Chronic: guarded prognosis; bony changes are permanent; some cats that were fed only liver may refuse to eat anything else

PEARLS & CONSIDERATIONS

COMMENTS

- Deficiency far more common than intoxication.
- Dogs can convert β-carotene into vitamin A but cats cannot.
- The amount of vitamin A needed to cause toxic effects is usually 10-1000 times the dietary requirements for most species.
- The vitamin A requirement for cats is 10,000 IU/kg of diet fed, with levels up to 100,000 IU/kg of diet tolerated.
- For dogs, the requirement is 3333 IU/kg of diet fed, with up to 33,330 IU/kg of diet tolerated.
- Vitamin A is fat soluble; 90% is stored in the liver and 10% in adipose tissue.

PREVENTION

Do not overfeed raw beef liver to cats

CLIENT EDUCATION

Teach owners the value of a balanced diet

SUGGESTED READING

Doireau V, et al: Vitamin A poisoning revealed by hypercalcemia in a child with kidney failure. *Arch Pediatr* 3(9):888-890, 1996.

Puls R: Vitamin A in dogs, vitamin A in cats. In *Vitamin Levels in Animal Health.* Clearbrook, British Columbia, Sherpa International, 1994, pp 14, 20.

Rader JD: Vitamin A. In Plumlee K (ed): *Clinical Veterinary Toxicology*. St. Louis, Mosby, 2003, p 330.

AUTHOR: **MARY M. SCHELL**
EDITOR: **SAFDAR A. KHAN**

Voice Change

BASIC INFORMATION

DEFINITION

Condition characterized by reduced vocalization and/or change in pitch of vocalization

EPIDEMIOLOGY

SPECIES, AGE, SEX

- Canine and feline
- Apparent male predisposition (3:1) for idiopathic laryngeal paralysis

GENETICS AND BREED PREDISPOSITION

- Hereditary laryngeal paralysis (Bouvier des Flandres, Siberian husky, pit bull terrier)
- Generalized polyneuropathy (dalmatian)

- Acquired laryngeal paralysis (giant and large breeds have been reported to be overrepresented)
- Laryngeal edema/eversion of laryngeal saccules (brachycephalic breeds)

CONTAGION AND ZOONOSIS: If secondary to infectious diseases (e.g., infectious tracheobronchitis [kennel cough]); potential but rare zoonosis (e.g., immunocompromised persons) with *Bordetella bronchiseptica*.

ASSOCIATED CONDITIONS AND DISORDERS

- In dogs:
  - Infectious tracheobronchitis (kennel cough)
  - Laryngeal paralysis
  - Brachycephalic airway syndrome
- In cats:
  - Lymphosarcoma
  - Squamous cell carcinoma (SCC)
  - Secondary to thyroidectomy

CLINICAL PRESENTATION

HISTORY, CHIEF COMPLAINT: Voice change may be described as a change in pitch of bark or meow (dog/cat, respectively) or a persistent hoarseness.

- Variable voice change depending on condition:
  - Peracute if traumatic
  - Acute if infectious
  - Subclinical and subtle if associated with neoplasia or with laryngeal paralysis
- May be associated with:
  - Exercise intolerance if mild upper airway obstruction (structural or functional)
  - Inspiratory stridor and respiratory distress (dyspnea, cyanosis, syncope) if substantial upper airway obstruction (structural or functional)

PHYSICAL EXAM FINDINGS: Variable: dependent on primary cause.

ETIOLOGY AND PATHOPHYSIOLOGY

- Anatomic cause: structure of the larynx affected
- Functional cause: innervation of the larynx affected

DIAGNOSIS

DIFFERENTIAL DIAGNOSIS

- Anatomic cause:
  - Laryngeal distortion:
    - Blunt trauma (e.g., choke chain, hit by car, kicked by horse)
    - Penetrating trauma (e.g., stick, gunshot, dog/snake bite)
  - Laryngeal edema (elongated soft palate, insect bite, chronic barking)
  - Eversion of the laryngeal saccules
  - Laryngeal/pharyngeal foreign body
  - Laryngeal inflammation (polyp, traumatic, infectious [viral, bacterial], granulomatous, immune mediated)
  - Laryngeal neoplasia (mast cell tumor, SCC, leiomyoma/sarcoma, rhabdomyoma/sarcoma, fibroma/fibrosarcoma, lymphosarcoma)
- Functional cause:
  - Dysfunction of the recurrent laryngeal nerve:
    - Congenital/idiopathic laryngeal paralysis
    - Trauma to the nerve (direct or indirect)
      - Occurs after thyroidectomy in cats
    - Nerve compression (hematoma, abscess, tumor [thyroid carcinoma, lymphosarcoma])
    - Neuropathy, polyneuritis
  - Myopathy (including cricoarytenoid dorsalis muscle)
  - Neuromuscular disease (myasthenia gravis)

INITIAL DATABASE

- Complete blood count (CBC), serum biochemistry panel, and urinalysis
- Cervical/thoracic imaging:
  - Radiographs: The normal larynx, especially if mineralized, should not be mistaken for a foreign body
  - Ultrasound (mass lesions, laryngeal paralysis)
- Oral/laryngeal/pharyngeal examination (visual ± endoscopy); may require sedation depending on whether severe inspiratory dyspnea is present (with severe dyspnea, the laryngeal exam often may be performed while the patient is awake because the patient is breathing with mouth and oropharynx maximally opened)

ADVANCED OR CONFIRMATORY TESTING

- CT scan or MRI of larynx
- Serum acetylcholine receptor antibodies titer (myasthenia gravis)
- Electromyography (myopathies)
- Exploratory surgery ± biopsy and histopathologic examination

TREATMENT

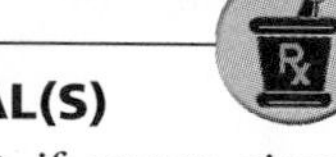

THERAPEUTIC GOAL(S)

- Stabilize the patient if upper airway obstruction/dyspnea
- Determine cause of voice change
- Address primary cause of the condition

ACUTE GENERAL TREATMENT

- Stabilization of the patient:
  - If associated with mild inspiratory stridor:
    - Sedation of the patient, oxygen supplementation
  - If associated with severe inspiratory stridor and dyspnea:
    - Sedation of the patient, oxygen supplementation, intubation/ventilation if necessary, emergency tracheostomy if indicated
- Addressing the primary cause:
  - If secondary to anatomic cause:
    - See Tracheobronchitis (Infectious): Dogs, p 1096
    - Local trauma/inflammation: foreign body removal, anti-inflammatory drugs (e.g., carprofen 2 mg/kg PO q 12h, or meloxicam 0.1 mg/kg PO q 24h); antibiotics if indicated (penetrating wound; consider amoxicillin-clavulanate 12.5 mg/kg PO q 12h and then base the decision on aerobic and anaerobic culture and sensitivity [C&S]); soft palate resection
    - Eversion of laryngeal saccules: resection
    - Laryngeal mass: resection (ventriculocordectomy/partial laryngectomy), radiation therapy, or chemotherapy
    - If mass resection impossible: total laryngectomy with permanent tracheostomy
  - If secondary to functional cause:
    - Laryngeal paralysis: unilateral cricoarytenoid lateralization
    - Surgical decompression of recurrent laryngeal nerve (hematoma, abscess drainage, mass excision)
    - Acquired neuropathy/neuromuscular disease: treat according to primary cause

CHRONIC TREATMENT

Variable: dependent on primary cause

POSSIBLE COMPLICATIONS

Variable, dependent on primary cause:

- Laryngeal paralysis: aspiration pneumonia
- Tumor, recurrence, progression of disease (local, regional, systemic)
- Inflammation, infection, or foreign body: recurrence possible
- Trauma: potential irreversible nerve damage

RECOMMENDED MONITORING

Variable: dependent on primary cause

PROGNOSIS AND OUTCOME

Variable, depending on condition:

- Infectious tracheobronchitis: excellent
- Trauma, inflammation, or foreign body: good to guarded
- Laryngeal paralysis: good to guarded with surgery
- Resectable laryngeal mass: good if benign and clean resection; poor if malignant, nonresectable, and/or not responsive to chemotherapy or radiation therapy

PEARLS & CONSIDERATIONS

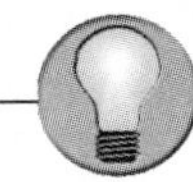

COMMENTS

A very common underlying cause in dogs is laryngeal paralysis

CLIENT EDUCATION

If the cause is infectious tracheobronchitis, the affected dog should avoid contact with other dogs, especially those that are unvaccinated.

SUGGESTED READING

Monnet E: Laryngeal paralysis and devocalization. In Slatter D: *Textbook of Small Animal Surgery*, ed 3. Philadelphia, WB Saunders, 2003, pp 837–845.

Nelson AW: Laryngeal trauma and stenosis. In Slatter D: *Textbook of Small Animal Surgery*, ed 3. Philadelphia, WB Saunders, 2003, pp 845–857.

Venker-van Hagen AJ: Diseases of the throat. In Ettinger SJ, Feldman EC (eds): *Textbook of Veterinary Internal Medicine*, ed 5. Philadelphia, WB Saunders, 2000, pp 1025–1031.

AUTHOR: **BERTRAND LUSSIER**

EDITOR: **ETIENNE CÔTÉ**

Vomiting, Acute

BASIC INFORMATION

DEFINITION

Active expulsion of stomach and sometimes duodenal contents preceded by nausea and retching; duration is less than 7 days

SYNONYM(S)

Acute emesis

EPIDEMIOLOGY

SPECIES, AGE, SEX: Any animal can be affected; epidemiology depends on the underlying cause.

Young animals are more likely to ingest foreign bodies or acquire infectious diseases (viral and parasitic).

RISK FACTORS: Use of drugs, such as nonsteroidal anti-inflammatory drugs (NSAIDs) and glucocorticoids; chemotherapy.

GEOGRAPHY AND SEASONALITY: Infectious causes often are more prevalent in specific geographic regions.

ASSOCIATED CONDITIONS AND DISORDERS: The most common cause of acute vomiting is dietary indiscretion; however, numerous gastrointestinal (GI) or systemic diseases can also cause vomiting.

CLINICAL PRESENTATION

DISEASE FORMS/SUBTYPES

- Patients can be presented looking healthy with no concurrent signs of systemic involvement. These are classified as "nonserious cases."
- Patients can be presented with concurrent systemic clinical signs (e.g., lethargy, dehydration, icterus, fever). These are classified as "serious cases."

HISTORY, CHIEF COMPLAINT: It is important to differentiate vomiting (active expulsion of GI contents) from dysphagia (difficulty swallowing) and regurgitation (passive movement of ingesta from the esophagus out the mouth).

Important components of the history:

- Vaccination status (parvoviral enteritis and canine distemper are more likely in unvaccinated than vaccinated dogs)
- Administration or ingestion of potentially ulcerogenic drugs, such as NSAIDs or glucocorticoids
- Possibility of ingestion of a foreign body (e.g., exposure to objects that could be ingested; individual propensity to such ingestions)
- Dietary history (e.g., recent changes; content and volume of recent and typical meals)
- Description of the vomitus (e.g., hematemesis) and productiveness (e.g., nonproductive with gastric dilatation-volvulus)
- Time relation of vomiting to food intake (if vomiting of undigested or partially digested food occurs >7–10 hours after ingestion, a gastric outflow obstruction or gastric hypomotility is likely)

PHYSICAL EXAM FINDINGS: A thorough physical examination is mandatory. Specific points requiring extra attention include:

- Hydration status
- Mouth inspection (e.g., linear foreign body in cats, ulcerations suggesting intoxication or uremia)
- Abdominal palpation (e.g., abdominal pain, abdominal distention, foreign body, mass, organomegaly)
- Rectal examination (e.g., presence of melena, foreign material)

ETIOLOGY AND PATHOPHYSIOLOGY

- Stimulation of humoral (blood-borne substances) or neural (especially via receptors located throughout the GI tract) pathways can lead to activation of the vomiting center located in the medulla oblongata.
- Certain drugs (e.g., apomorphine [dogs], xylazine [cats]), uremic toxins, and electrolyte, osmolar, or acid-base disorders can also activate the chemoreceptor trigger zone (CRTZ), which in turn triggers the vomiting center, causing vomiting.

DIAGNOSIS

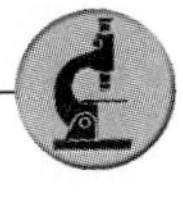

DIFFERENTIAL DIAGNOSIS

- GI causes:
  - Adverse food reactions (dietary indiscretion, intolerance)
  - Gastritis: viral (parvovirus, coronavirus, distemper), bacterial
  - Foreign body
  - Parasites (*Physaloptera* spp., *Ollulanus tricuspis*)
  - Motility disorders
  - Gastric dilatation/volvulus
- Extra-GI causes
  - Extra-abdominal disorders:
    - Azotemia/uremia
    - Hypoadrenocorticism
    - Diabetic ketoacidosis
    - Intoxications
    - Drugs (NSAIDs, chemotherapy, glucocorticoids)
    - Neurologic disorders (especially vestibular)
  - Intra-abdominal disorders:
    - Hepatic failure
    - Pancreatitis
    - Peritonitis
    - Pyometra

INITIAL DATABASE

- If the animal is classified as a nonserious case: history and thorough physical examination are most important; further work-up is determined by status and response to treatment
- If the animal is classified as a serious case and/or if vomiting was nonproductive: further diagnostic work-up is always warranted:
  - Complete bood count (CBC), serum chemistry profile (including sodium and potassium)
  - Urinalysis

- Fecal examination
- Medical imaging:
  - Abdominal radiographs: radio-opaque foreign bodies, signs of intestinal obstruction, ileus, gastric dilation/volvulus, or loss of abdominal detail, suggesting pancreatitis or peritonitis
  - Abdominal ultrasound: changes associated with organomegaly; identification of origin and extent of masses and other such findings
- With hematemesis: review medication/drug exposure history, coagulation profile, adrenocorticotropic hormone (ACTH) stimulation, gastroduodenoscopy

ADVANCED OR CONFIRMATORY TESTING

- If clinically relevant: liver function tests, ACTH stimulation test to rule out hypoadrenocorticism, toxicologic testing, neurologic examination, canine or feline pancreatic lipase immunoreactivity.
- In some cases, especially to evaluate motility disorders or gastric outflow obstruction, GI contrast studies can be performed.
- If vomiting persists (for more than 3 to 4 days) or worsens, approach the animal as a chronic vomiting case (see Vomiting, Chronic, p 1158); endoscopy is warranted if previous tests fail to identify the cause.

TREATMENT

THERAPEUTIC GOAL(S)

- Rehydrate the animal if needed.
- Allow the GI tract to "rest" by giving nothing per os (NPO).

ACUTE GENERAL TREATMENT

Nonserious cases: These animals are generally treated as outpatients:

- NPO for 12-24 hours. If vomiting resolves, initiate a small amount of water or ice cubes. Thereafter, initiate feeding with small quantities of a highly digestible, low-fat diet for several days. Gradually transition to using the regular food

Serious cases: hospitalize the animal and perform further diagnostic steps as described above (Initial Database and Advanced or Confirmatory Testing).

- NPO; water; and food identical as for the nonserious cases
- IV fluid therapy (crystalloids)
- Antiemetics:
  - Indications: when vomiting is severe and animal is at risk for dehydration or for developing electrolyte/acid-base imbalances or reflux esophagitis
  - Should only be used if the possibility of GI obstruction has been ruled out
  - Metoclopramide 0.2-0.5 mg/kg IM or SC q 8h (dopamine antagonist; central and peripheral antiemetic agent), or
  - Chlorpromazine 0.1-0.5 mg/kg IM or SC q 8-24h, based on response (phenothiazine derivate with central antiemetic activity, α-antagonist, can cause hypotension especially in dehydrated animals). Avoid chlorpromazine in epileptic animals (may lower seizure threshold)

POSSIBLE COMPLICATIONS

- Dehydration
- Reflux esophagitis
- Aspiration pneumonia
- Electrolyte and acid-base imbalances (especially hypokalemia and sometimes metabolic acidosis)

RECOMMENDED MONITORING

- Signs of dehydration
- Abdominal pain
- Frequency of the vomiting

PROGNOSIS AND OUTCOME

Very good with dietary indiscretion; otherwise, depends on underlying etiology

PEARLS & CONSIDERATIONS

COMMENTS

- Most cases of acute vomiting are self-limiting and do not require further diagnostics. However, it is important not to miss the more seriously sick animals and also to recommend further work-up and treatment if the vomiting does not subside within a few days.
- Use antiemetics carefully because they can mask progressive disease and reponse to primary therapy.

CLIENT EDUCATION

Avoid dietary indiscretion (whenever possible)

SUGGESTED READING

Tams TR: Gastrointestinal symptoms. In Tams TR (ed): *Handbook of Small Animal Gastroenterology*. Philadelphia, WB Saunders, 2003, pp 1-50.

Tilley LP, Smith FWK Jr. (eds): *The 5-Minute Veterinary Consult, Canine and Feline*. Baltimore, Lippincott, Williams & Wilkins, 2000.

AUTHOR: **SYLVIE DAMINET**

EDITOR: **ETIENNE CÔTÉ**

Vomiting, Chronic

BASIC INFORMATION

DEFINITION

- Active expulsion of stomach and sometimes duodenal content preceded by nausea and retching.
- Either intermittent course or persistent vomiting for more than 7 days.
- Chronic vomiting is a very common clinical sign and can be associated with a variety of disorders.

SYNONYM(S)

Chronic emesis

EPIDEMIOLOGY

SPECIES, AGE, SEX

- Any animal can be affected; epidemiology depends on the underlying cause.
- Young animals are more likely to ingest foreign bodies.

GENETICS AND BREED PREDISPOSITION

- Brachycephalic breeds: pyloric stenosis
- Airedale terriers: pancreatic carcinoma
- Shar-pei, rottweiler, German shepherd: inflammatory bowel disease (IBD)

RISK FACTORS

- Use of drugs, such as nonsteroidal anti-inflammatory drugs (NSAIDs) and glucocorticoids; chemotherapy.
- Numerous nongastrointestinal (GI) systemic diseases can cause vomiting.

CONTAGION AND ZOONOSIS: Zoonotic potential of *Helicobacter heilmanii* and *H. felis* unclear.

ASSOCIATED CONDITIONS AND DISORDERS: Hypochloremic metabolic alkalosis initially; progression leads to dehydration and hypovolemia, and metabolic acidosis may emerge.

CLINICAL PRESENTATION

DISEASE FORMS/SUBTYPES

- Owners may present animals that look healthy with no obvious signs of systemic disease.
- Owners may present animals that have signs of systemic disease (e.g., dehydration, icterus).

HISTORY, CHIEF COMPLAINT

- It is important to differentiate vomiting from dysphagia and regurgitation.
    - Vomiting involves forceful retching and abdominal contraction and may produce bile-stained contents.
- Administration of potentially ulcerogenic drugs, such as NSAIDs or glucocorticoids.
- The possibility of ingestion of a foreign body.
- Dietary history, a description of the vomitus (e.g., possible hematemesis), and its time relation to food intake.
- If vomiting of undigested or partially digested food occurs >7-10 hours after ingestion, a gastric outflow obstruction or gastric hypomotility is likely.

PHYSICAL EXAM FINDINGS

- A thorough physical examination is mandatory.
- Extra attention is warranted regarding:
    - Hydration status
    - Mouth inspection (sublingual linear foreign body in cats, ulcerations)
    - Abdominal palpation (abdominal mass, thickened bowel loops)
    - Rectal examination (presence of melena or hematochezia)
- In cats older than 6 years, palpation of the neck region for thyroid nodules is essential.

ETIOLOGY AND PATHOPHYSIOLOGY

- Stimulation of humoral (blood-borne substances) or neural (especially via receptors located throughout the GI tract) pathways can lead to activation of the vomiting center located in the brain (medulla oblongata).
- Certain drugs (e.g., apomorphine, xylazine), uremic toxins, and electrolyte, osmolar, or acid-base disorders can activate the chemoreceptor trigger zone (CRTZ), which is also in the medulla oblongata, and cause vomiting.

DIAGNOSIS

DIFFERENTIAL DIAGNOSIS

Extra-GI causes:

- Extra-abdominal disorders:
    - Azotemia/uremia
    - Hypoadrenocorticism
    - Especially in cats: hyperthyroidism, heartworm disease
    - Intoxications
    - Drugs
    - Neurologic disorders (especially vestibular)
- Intra-abdominal disorders:
    - Hepatic disease
    - Pancreatitis
    - Peritonitis

GI causes:

- Gastritis (lymphocytic-plasmacytic, eosinophilic)
- Food intolerance/food allergy
- Foreign body
- Parasites (*Physaloptera* spp., *Ollulanus tricuspis*)
- Neoplasia
- Inflammatory bowel disease
- Bilious vomiting syndrome
- Motility disorders
- Colitis (up to 30% of dogs with colitis may vomit)
- Hiatal hernia

INITIAL DATABASE

- Complete blood count (CBC), serum biochemistry profile (including sodium and potassium)
- Urinalysis
- Fecal examination
- Total thyroxine (older cats)
- Medical imaging: abdominal radiographs and/or abdominal ultrasound
- With hematemesis: check drug history, platelet count, coagulation profile, adrenocorticotropic hormone (ACTH) stimulation, and possibly serum gastrin concentration (gastrinoma); gastroduodenoscopy may be indicated

ADVANCED OR CONFIRMATORY TESTING

- If clinically relevant, based on history, exam, and minimum database: liver function tests, ACTH stimulation test to rule out hypoadrenocorticism, toxicologic testing, neurologic examination, canine or feline pancreatic lipase immunoreactivity, feline heartworm antibody testing.
- In some cases, especially to evaluate motility disorders or gastric outflow obstruction, GI contrast studies may be indicated.
- If all previous tests fail to identify a non-GI cause for chronic vomiting, gastroduodenoscopy or an exploratory laparotomy with GI and hepatic biopsies is indicated.

TREATMENT

THERAPEUTIC GOAL(S)

- Supportive treatment if needed
- Elimination of the underlying cause and/or specific treatment is warranted

CHRONIC TREATMENT

- Causative treatment is warranted especially if the patient shows systemic clinical signs. If the patient seems otherwise healthy, dietary therapy alone can be tried if the initial database fails to identify abnormalities. If the response to this treatment is insufficient, further diagnostics are necessary, followed by specific treatment based on results.
- Antiemetics (e.g., metoclopramide 0.2-0.4 mg/kg SC q 8h) can be used empirically after the presence of a foreign body is ruled out. Metoclopramide can cause lethargy and restlessness, especially in cats
- Dietary manipulations (often low-fat, hypoallergenic diets containing a single and novel source of protein)
- Specific treatments (see specific information for individual disorders):
    - Foreign body removal
    - Inflammatory bowel disease: diet, glucocorticoids, azathioprine
    - Antiparasitic treatments
    - Hypoadrenocorticism: mineralocorticoid and glucocorticoid replacement

DRUG INTERACTIONS

Cimetidine and ranitidine can interfere with hepatic metabolism of other drugs

POSSIBLE COMPLICATIONS

- Weight loss due to malnutrition
- Dehydration
- Hypokalemia
- Sometimes metabolic alkalosis with hypochloremia if a pyloric (sub) obstruction is present

PROGNOSIS AND OUTCOME

Dependent on etiology

PEARLS & CONSIDERATIONS

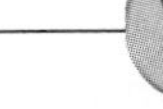

COMMENTS

- Numerous causes of chronic vomiting exist. A first step is to rule out extra-GI causes with initial (imaging and laboratory-based) work-up. If these results are not significantly abnormal, gastroduodenoscopy or exploratory laparotomy with hepatic and GI biopsies is recommended for animals that chronically vomit.
- Caution is warranted: often, concentrating only on the GI tract too early can lead to misdiagnosis and erroneous treatment.
- Some dogs or cats with vomiting due to IBD show no abnormalities on gastric endoscopy and biopsies. Therefore, endoscopy of the small intestine is important even with a history of chronic vomiting without diarrhea.
- The area under the tongue must be examined in every cat that has a chronic vomiting condition; this area is most easily visualized by pressing dor-

sally on the skin of the underside (ventral surface) of the mandible, between the bodies of the mandible, while the mouth is open. This pressure elevates the sublingual tissues and tongue, exposing the region of interest.

SUGGESTED READING

Tams TR: Gastrointestinal symptoms. In Tams TR (ed): *Handbook of Small Animal Gastroenterology*. Philadelphia, WB Saunders, 2003, pp 1-50.

Tilley LP, FWK Smith Jr (eds): *The 5-Minute Veterinary Consult, Canine and Feline*. Baltimore, Lippincott, Williams & Wilkins, 2000.

AUTHOR: **SYLVIE DAMINET**
EDITOR: **ETIENNE CÔTÉ**

von Willebrand Disease

BASIC INFORMATION

DEFINITION

Hereditary primary hemostatic defect caused by a quantitative or functional deficiency of von Willebrand factor (vWF). vWF is an adhesive protein required for normal platelet-collagen binding at sites of small vessel injury. Clinical expression varies in severity from a mild bleeding tendency manifesting primarily after injury to more severe forms characterized by recurrent mucosal hemorrhage and prolonged bleeding from normal processes, such as deciduous tooth loss

SYNONYM(S)

Factor-VIII related antigen (old terminology; protein is now referred to as vWF)
vWD

EPIDEMIOLOGY

SPECIES, AGE, SEX

- von Willebrand disease (vWD) is the most common hereditary bleeding disorder of dogs. It is a rare hemostatic defect of cats.
- Severe forms typically manifest by 1 year of age, and milder forms may be inapparent unless the patient undergoes surgery or trauma.

GENETICS AND BREED PREDISPOSITION

- Autosomal trait with three type classifications:
  - Severe (types 2 and 3 vWD): recessive inheritance
  - Mild to moderate (type 1 vWD): recessive or incomplete dominant inheritance
- Males and females express and transmit vWD with equal frequency
- In recessive forms, affected pups inherit a vWF mutation from both dam and sire
- Affected breeds:
  - Type 1 vWD: Airedale, Akita, Bernese mountain dog, dachshund, Doberman pinscher, German shepherd, golden retriever, greyhound, Irish wolfhound, Manchester terrier, miniature pinscher, Pembroke Welsh corgi, poodle, schnauzer, and sporadic cases in any breed
  - Type 2 vWD: German short-haired pointer, German wirehaired pointer
  - Type 3 vWD: Chesapeake Bay retriever, Dutch kooiker, Scottish terrier, Shetland sheepdog, and sporadic cases (recent cases in Australian shepherd, Border collie, cocker spaniel, Labrador retriever, Maltese)

CLINICAL PRESENTATION

DISEASE FORMS/SUBTYPES

- Type 1 vWD: quantitative protein deficiency. Low plasma concentration of vWF (von Willebrand factor antigen [vWF:Ag]) with proportionate reduction in vWF function; the vWF protein has a full distribution of multimeric forms
- Type 2 vWD: both quantitative and functional protein deficiency; low plasma vWF:Ag has a disproportionate decrease in vWF function measured by collagen binding or support of platelet agglutination. vWF protein lacks the high molecular weight multimers
- Type 3 vWD: severe vWF deficiency, no detectable plasma vWF

HISTORY, CHIEF COMPLAINT

- Severe forms: recurrent mucosal bleeds, prolonged bleeding from loss of deciduous teeth or minor wounds, blood loss anemia after surgery or trauma
- Mild forms: few spontaneous or severe bleeds; abnormal bleeding typically observed after surgical or traumatic injury

PHYSICAL EXAM FINDINGS

- Abnormal hemorrhage:
  - Mucosal bleeding
  - Abnormal bleeding from traumatic/surgical wounds
- Pallor due to blood loss anemia

ETIOLOGY AND PATHOPHYSIOLOGY

- Distinct vWF mutations causative for type 3 vWD have been described in Scottish terriers and Dutch kooiker dogs.
- Homozygosity for a mutation located at a splice site of the vWF gene has been associated with low vWF protein in type 1 vWD.
- Types 2 and 3 vWD cause a moderate to severe bleeding tendency.
- The clinical severity of type 1 vWD generally correlates with decrease in vWF concentration.
- vWF is an adhesive protein required for normal platelet-collagen binding at sites of small vessel injury under high shear.
- A lack of vWF impairs platelet plug formation and causes bleeding despite normal in vitro platelet numbers, normal platelet aggregation, and normal coagulation cascade parameters (normal coagulation profile).

DIAGNOSIS

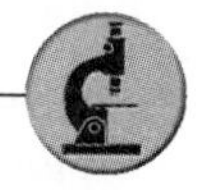

DIFFERENTIAL DIAGNOSIS

- Primary hemostatic defects:
  - Thrombocytopenia
  - Acquired or hereditary platelet dysfunction (thrombocytopathias; e.g., animal taking aspirin)
- Coagulation factor deficiency
- Vasculopathy or erosive/infiltrative vessel defect causing mucosal hemorrhage

INITIAL DATABASE

- Thorough physical exam to define single versus multiple sites of hemorrhage
- Baseline hematocrit and plasma protein: normal or decreased if bleeding is severe and chronic
- Platelet count or platelet estimate from blood smear: usually normal
- Point-of-care coagulation screening tests: usually normal:
  - Activated clotting time (ACT)
  - Activated partial thromboplastin time (aPTT)
  - Prothrombin time (PT)
- Bleeding time (buccal mucosal bleeding time): increased (see Buccal Mucosal Bleeding Time, p 1201)

ADVANCED OR CONFIRMATORY TESTING

Clinical diagnosis is based on specific measurement of plasma vWF concentration:

- vWF concentration (vWF:Ag):
  - vWF:Ag <50% is evidence of vWF deficiency, but clinical bleeding tendency is usually seen in animals having more severe deficiency (<25%).

- Types 1 and 2 vWD in dogs are characterized by the presence of low protein concentration, whereas type 3 vWD is characterized by a complete absence of vWF (vWF:Ag <0.1%).
- Differentiation of types 1 and 2 vWD is based on the presence of dysfunctional and structurally abnormal protein in the type 2 form. Abnormal protein is identified based on the following tests:
  - vWF:CBA = vWF collagen binding activity (functional assay).
  - vWF multimer analyses = Western blot to visualize vWF subunit structure.
- Hereditary type 2 vWD has been identified only in two breeds: German wire-haired and short-haired pointers.
- An acquired type 2 vWD occurs in human beings with aortic stenosis. A recent study of mitral valve disease in Cavalier King Charles spaniels revealed abnormal vWF multimer distribution, compatible with classification of type 2 vWD.

TREATMENT

THERAPEUTIC GOAL(S)

- Control active bleeding with transfusion therapy and local wound care
- Minimize frequency of induced bleeds by avoiding surgery, trauma, and any drug therapy that inhibits platelet function or coagulation factor activity
- Correct any underlying medical conditions that might impair hemostasis

ACUTE GENERAL TREATMENT

A patient that had a normal preoperative platelet count but that bleeds persistently during a surgical procedure, that shows no physical evidence of severe systemic illness (vasculitis), and that is not known to have been exposed to anticoagulant (e.g., rodenticide) or antiplatelet (e.g., aspirin) substances, should be suspected of having vWD and may be treated as follows pending the results of confirmatory tests (see Advanced or Confirmatory Testing above):

- Transfusion to supply hemostatic levels of vWF is the best strategy to control active hemorrhage refractory to local wound care. Patients with severe vWD (typically types 2 and 3 vWD) may require a second or third transfusion within the first 24 hours of presentation to sustain hemostasis after an initial response.
- Transfusion of plasma components reduces risk of volume overload or red cell sensitization while maximizing vWF replacement.
- Fresh frozen plasma (10–12 ml/kg IV):
  - Transfuse at the high end of dosage range for the initial transfusion.
  - Severely deficient patients may require repeated transfusions at q 8–12h intervals.
- Cryoprecipitate (unit dosage varies for different suppliers):
  - Cryoprecipitate is prepared from fresh frozen plasma and contains a fivefold to tenfold concentration of vWF in approximately one-tenth the volume of the starting plasma.
  - Cryoprecipitate's low volume eliminates the risk of volume overload if repeated transfusion is needed for high-dose vWF replacement.
- Fresh whole blood (12–20 ml/kg) can be used as a source of vWF replacement if plasma components are unavailable or if replacement of red blood cells (RBCs) and vWF is desired to treat ongoing blood-loss anemia.
  - Risk of volume overload generally limits whole blood transfusion to q 24h intervals.
  - See Transfusion Therapy and Collection Techniques for Blood Banking, p 1312.
- Packed RBC transfusion (6–12 ml/kg) is indicated to treat severe blood-loss anemia.
- Use local wound care (suture, pressure wrap, tissue glue) to help control bleeding from cutaneous or superficial sites.

CHRONIC TREATMENT

- Intermittent transfusion may be needed to control hemorrhagic events in patients with severe (types 2 and 3) vWD.
- Preoperative transfusion to patients with type 2 or 3 vWD or severe expression of type 1 vWD to replace vWF before surgical procedures.
  - Fresh frozen plasma and cryoprecipitate are the best products for preoperative prophylaxis: same dose as described previously.
  - Transfusion is administered just before the surgical procedure. Peak vWF is obtained immediately post-transfusion, and values fall to baseline by 24 hours.
  - Close monitoring is required during the first 24 hours after the operation. Repeat tranfusion (at q 8–12h) may be required during this period for severe vWD.
- Desmopressin acetate (DDAVP; deamino 8 D-arginine vasopressin) is a synthetic vasopressin analog that can be used preoperatively to enhance surgical hemostasis in patients with mild to moderate vWD (type 1 vWD); dosage is 1 μg/kg SQ, given 30 minutes preoperatively.
  - The response to DDAVP varies, and transfusion should be available if hemorrhage develops in spite of DDAVP therapy.
- The development of endocrinopathy (e.g., hypothyroidism, hypoadrenocorticism) or thrombocytopenia may exacerbate the bleeding tendency of vWF-deficient patients. Identification and correction of these disorders are indicated to help reduce risk of clinical signs.

DRUG INTERACTIONS

Avoid drugs with anticoagulant or antiplatelet effects in animals with vWD:

- Nonsteroidal anti-inflammatory drugs (NSAIDs)
- Sulfonamide antibiotics
- Heparin, coumadin
- Plasma expanders
- Estrogens
- Cytotoxic drugs

POSSIBLE COMPLICATIONS

RBC sensitization causing transfusion reactions:

- Transfuse plasma components when possible
- Dogs with severe vWD should be blood-typed because repeated transfusion may be required. Choose type-matched donors for RBC or whole blood transfusions
- Canine transfusion: after a first RBC transfusion, perform a cross-match before subsequent transfusions

RECOMMENDED MONITORING

Adequate vWF replacement is demonstrated by:

- Cessation of active bleeding
- Stabilization of hematocrit/plasma protein

PROGNOSIS AND OUTCOME

- Most dogs clinically affected with vWD have a good quality of life and only require transfusions intermittently or rarely.
  - Animals with severe vWD (types 2 and 3 vWD) are most likely to develop spontaneous bleeds or require repeated transfusion.All dogs affected with types 2 and 3 vWD should receive a preoperative transfusion before surgical procedures.
  - Many dogs with type 1 vWD have mild disease expression. Clinical signs of abnormal bleeding are most likely to develop in dogs with vWF:Ag <25%.
- Acute bleeding crises may require aggressive transfusion support to rapidly provide hemostatic levels of vWF protein. High-dose component therapy (fresh frozen plasma or cryoprecipitate) may be needed to control severe bleeds.

PEARLS & CONSIDERATIONS

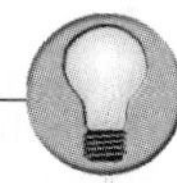

COMMENTS

- Specific diagnosis of vWD requires measurement of plasma vWF concentration (vWF:Ag):
  - The findings of normal coagulation panel and platelet count do not rule out vWD
- Signs of mucosal hemorrhage (rather than petechiae) are typical manifestations of vWD.

PREVENTION

- Screen animals preoperatively to determine baseline vWF:Ag for breeds or lines with a high prevalence of vWD. The risk of abnormal bleeding is greatest for dogs with vWF:Ag that is <25%.
- Clinically affected dogs should not be used for breeding. Carriers of the vWD trait can be identified based on vWF:Ag that is <50% or based on detection of specific mutations in DNA analyses. Protein analyses are relatively fast and inexpensive and do not require knowledge of mutation type; however, values for carrier and clear dogs may overlap at the low end of the normal range (50–70% vWF:Ag). A commercial company (Vetgen) offers vWF mutation detection for several breed-variants of vWD, using cheek swabs for isolation of DNA. Dogs that are heterozygous for a specific mutation type are considered vWD "carriers," whereas homozygotes are considered vWD "affected."
- Selective breeding practices can reduce the prevalence or eliminate vWD from an affected pedigree. Breeding two clear parents is ideal and is expected to produce entire litters of clear pups. Breeding one carrier parent to a clear mate may be acceptable, and the clear pups produced from these matings can be used for subsequent generations. Carrier to carrier matings may produce affected pups and therefore should be avoided.

CLIENT EDUCATION

Owners and breeders should be aware of vWD and be advised to screen their pets to prevent propagation of the trait.

SUGGESTED READING

Brooks MB, Catalfamo JL: Platelet disorders and von Willebrand disease. In Ettinger S, Feldman E (eds): *Textbook of Veterinary Internal Medicine*, ed 6. St. Louis, Elsevier, 2004, pp 1918–1929.

Johnson GS, Turrentine MA, Kraus KH: Canine von Willebrand disease. *Vet Clin North Am Small An Pract* 18:195–229, 1988.

Venta PJ, Li J, Yuzbasiyan-Gurkan V, Brewer GJ, Schall W: Mutation causing vWD in Scottish terriers. *J Vet Int Med* 14:10–19, 2000.

AUTHOR: **MARJORY B. BROOKS**

EDITOR: **SUSAN M. COTTER**

Weight Loss

BASIC INFORMATION

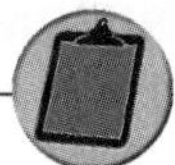

DEFINITION

Spontaneous decrease in body mass, not resulting from a deliberate intervention for obesity control

SYNONYM(S)

Cachexia
Emaciation

EPIDEMIOLOGY

SPECIES, AGE, SEX: Dogs and cats of any age and either sex.

GENETICS AND BREED PREDISPOSITION: Dependent on the underlying cause.

RISK FACTORS: Dependent on the underlying cause.

CLINICAL PRESENTATION

DISEASE FORMS/SUBTYPES

- Weight loss with localizing gastrointestinal (GI) signs (e.g., dysphagia, regurgitation, vomiting, diarrhea)
- Weight loss without localizing GI signs:
  - Associated with polyphagia and increased appetite
  - Associated with anorexia and decreased food intake

HISTORY, CHIEF COMPLAINT

- Thin appearance, lethargy, decreased appetite
- It is essential to determine (1) quantity, quality, and appropriateness of the diet being fed; (2) appetite (increased or decreased); (3) daily activity; (4) presence of conditions increasing energy requirements (e.g., growth, pregnancy/lactation); and (5) presence of localizing GI signs (dysphagia, regurgitation, vomiting, and diarrhea)

PHYSICAL EXAM FINDINGS

- Poor body condition (or decrease in weight in comparison to historic body weight) with poor haircoat and muscle atrophy (temporal muscle atrophy often is the most noticeable)
- Physical examination should be aimed at detecting clues for the underlying disease (e.g., abdominal masses on palpation, fever)

ETIOLOGY AND PATHOPHYSIOLOGY

- Body weight is determined by caloric intake, absorptive capacity, metabolic rate, and energy losses.
- Weight loss may result from (1) decreased caloric intake usually due to anorexia but also from inadequate feeding or inability to eat; (2) inability to digest or absorb ingested nutrients caused by GI disorders or lack of pancreatic enzymes; (3) inability to utilize absorbed nutrients due to a metabolic problem (e.g., diabetes mellitus); (4) increased metabolic rate (e.g., hyperthyroidism); (5) increased catabolic rate in diseases associated with insulin resistance or increased inflammatory cytokines; and (6) loss of nutrients through the GI or urinary tract or because of extensive skin lesions.
- Weight loss is regarded as clinically important when it exceeds 5% or more of the body weight over a 2 to 4 week period, is not deliberate (e.g., obesity reduction), and is not associated with fluid loss.
- Physical causes are usually obvious during physical examination.
- Neoplasia and chronic infections can be indicated by weight loss as the sole clinical sign.

DIAGNOSIS

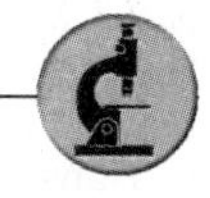

DIFFERENTIAL DIAGNOSIS

- Weight loss with localizing GI signs:
  - Inability to prehend, masticate, or chew food
  - Dysphagia
  - Regurgitation
    - Esophageal disorders
  - Vomiting
    - GI diseases
    - Systemic diseases associated with vomiting
  - Small bowel diarrhea
    - Inflammatory bowel disease
    - Intestinal lymphoma
    - Lymphangiectasia
    - Exocrine pancreatic insufficiency
    - Intestinal parasites

- Pure large bowel diarrhea not associated with weight loss
- Weight loss without localizing GI signs:
  - Polyphagia/increased appetite
    - Related to diet:
      - Inadequate feeding
      - Poor quality diet
    - Increased energy demand:
      - Pregnancy
      - Lactation
      - Increased physical activity
      - Growth
    - Increased metabolic rate:
      - Hyperthyroidism (cats)
    - Inability to utilize nutrients:
      - Diabetes mellitus
  - Anorexia/decreased appetite
    - Related to diet:
      - Poor-tasting diet
      - Inability to eat (e.g., neurologic disorders)
    - Systemic diseases leading to anorexia or increased catabolic rate:
      - Neoplasia (anywhere)
      - Chronic infections:
        - Viral:
          - Feline leukemia virus (FeLV) infection
          - Feline immunodeficiency virus (FIV) infection
          - Feline infectious peritonitis (FIP)
        - Systemic mycoses:
          - Blastomycosis
          - Histoplasmosis
          - Cryptococcosis
          - Coccidioidomycosis
        - Bacterial:
          - Bacterial endocarditis
          - Chronic bacterial pneumonia
          - Rickettsial infections (e.g., chronic ehrlichiosis)
          - Mycobacterial infections
        - Protozoal infections:
          - Leishmaniasis
          - Hepatozoonosis
      - Chronic inflammation:
        - Immune-mediated diseases (e.g., polyarthritis)
        - Chronic pancreatitis
      - Organ failure:
        - Renal failure
        - Liver failure
        - Congestive heart failure (CHF)
      - GI disorders (without vomiting or diarrhea):
        - Gastric ulcers
        - Inflammatory bowel disease
        - Lymphangiectasia
        - GI tumors
    - Diseases associated with loss of nutrients:
      - Glomerular diseases
      - Renal tubular loss (e.g., Fanconi syndrome)
      - Protein-losing enteropathy

INITIAL DATABASE

- Complete blood count (CBC), serum biochemistry panel, urinalysis
- FeLV/FIV serologic examination: all cats
- Serum T4 (cats >5 years old)
- Fecal flotation and direct smears

ADVANCED OR CONFIRMATORY TESTING

In animals with localizing GI signs:

- Trypsin-like immunoreactivity (TLI) if small bowel diarrhea: exocrine pancreatic insufficiency
- Fecal α-1 protease inhibitor activity: protein-losing enteropathy
- Abdominal ultrasound: GI tract thickness, hidden tumors
- Upper GI endoscopy
- GI biopsies by endoscopy or exploratory laparotomy
- Bile acids to rule out liver failure (particularly in young dogs with a portosystemic shunt)

In all other animals, specific tests to "rule out" or "rule in" a particular disease or group of diseases:

- Thoracic radiographs: left-sided CHF, metastatic disease, and bacterial and fungal pneumonia
- Abdominal ultrasonography: pancreatitis, hidden tumors or infections
- Urine protein:creatinine (UPC) ratio: protein-losing nephropathy
- Appropriate tests for suspected infectious agents

TREATMENT

THERAPEUTIC GOAL(S)

- Treat underlying disease
- Provide nutritional support

ACUTE GENERAL TREATMENT

- Improve appetite:
  - Diet change.
  - Antacids (H_2 blockers [famotidine, ranitidine] or proton pump inhibitors [omeprazole]).
  - Antinausea medications (metoclopramide, ondansetron).
  - Appetite stimulant (cyproheptadine may be helpful in some animals).
- Increase caloric intake:
  - Feeding plan should be individualized. Enteral nutrition is preferred in animals that have a functioning GI tract and are not vomiting. Assisted feeding through a nasoesophageal, esophagostomy, gastrostomy, or jejunostomy tube may be required in some animals. Parenteral nutrition may be necessary in animals that cannot tolerate enteral feeding.
  - Caloric requirements are estimated by calculating resting energy requirements (RER in kilocalories = 70 × body weight in kilograms$^{0.75}$) and illness energy requirements (IER).
    - RER can be estimated clinically as:
      - Animals that are <2 kg:
        - RER (kilocalories) = 50 × body weight in kilograms + 18
      - Animals that are 2-45 kg:
        - RER (kilocalories) = 30 × body weight in kilograms + 70
      - Animals that are >45 kg:
        - RER (kilocalories) = 18 × body weight in kilograms + 400
    - IER is calculated by multiplying RER by an illness factor (1.2 to 1.4 for dogs; 1.1 to 1.2 for cats).

CHRONIC TREATMENT

- Treat underlying disease
- Maintain adequate caloric intake

POSSIBLE COMPLICATIONS

Dependent on underlying disease

RECOMMENDED MONITORING

- Body weight
- Other parameters based on underlying cause

PROGNOSIS AND OUTCOME

Weight stabilization occurs in the majority of surviving patients through treatment of the underlying disease and caloric supplementation.

PEARLS & CONSIDERATIONS

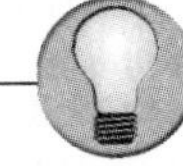

COMMENTS

- If the patient has other clinical signs, the diagnostic approach should not focus on the weight loss alone.
- Weight loss and decreased appetite are often caused by a systemic disease.
- Weight loss and increased appetite are commonly associated with increased energetic demands (pregnancy and lactation), increased metabolic rate (hyperthyroidism in cats), and diabetes mellitus.
- Presence of fever is consistent with infectious or inflammatory causes of weight loss although paraneoplastic fever and weight loss are also possible.
- In the initial stages of therapy, changes in body weight often reflect changes in fluid dynamics.

PREVENTION

Dependent on the underlying cause

CLIENT EDUCATION

Dependent on the underlying cause

SUGGESTED READING

Remillard RL, Armstrong PJ, Davenport DJ: Assisted feeding in hospitalized animals. In Hand MS, Thatcher CD, Remillard RL, Roudebush R (eds): *Small Animal Clinical Nutrition*, ed 4. Topeka, KS, Mark Morris Institute, 2000, pp 351–399.

Sanderson S, Bartges JW: Management of anorexia. In Bonagura JD (ed): *Current Veterinary Therapy XIII*, ed 13. Philadelphia, WB Saunders, 2000, pp 69–74.

AUTHORS: **BRADLEY A. GREEN, HELIO AUTRAN DE MORAIS**
EDITOR: **ETIENNE CÔTÉ**

West Nile Virus Infection

BASIC INFORMATION

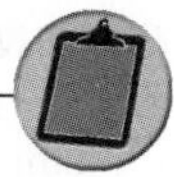

DEFINITION

Mosquito-borne virus that affects humans and animals

EPIDEMIOLOGY

SPECIES, AGE, SEX: Wild birds are the principal hosts of West Nile virus. More than 14 species of birds have been infected. Horses and humans may also develop clinical signs of infection. Dogs and cats are considered resistant to infection, with rare single-case reports describing natural infection in dogs. Although the few rare reported dogs were older adults, no sex or age predilection is apparent.
RISK FACTORS: Age and immunosuppression are considered risk factors for people but have not been objectively documented as such in animals.
CONTAGION AND ZOONOSIS: Domestic animals are not considered a risk factor for amplification of West Nile virus.
GEOGRAPHY AND SEASONALITY: Infections are more common during warm seasons in wetland ecosystems where there are greater numbers of mosquitoes.

CLINICAL PRESENTATION

DISEASE FORMS/SUBTYPES: Most infections with West Nile virus in domestic species are subclinical.
HISTORY, CHIEF COMPLAINT: The location and extent of renal, central nervous system (CNS), and myocardial lesions in dogs suggest that signs of renal failure, central neurologic deficits, and either syncope or signs of congestive heart failure (CHF), respectively, could be presenting chief complaints.
PHYSICAL EXAM FINDINGS: Histopathologic findings suggest that nonspecific malaise (lethargy, anorexia, weight loss) and mentation changes (e.g., depression) as well as signs of renal failure (e.g., halitosis, oral mucosal ulcers), neurologic involvement (central neurologic deficits), and myocarditis (e.g., cardiac arrhythmia on auscultation, pulse deficits) may be expected in advanced cases. The physical exam is likely often normal, and the infection is not suspected (nor necessarily of clinical concern).

ETIOLOGY AND PATHOPHYSIOLOGY

- West Nile virus is a mosquito-borne disease. The natural hosts are wild birds of the Corvidae family (crows, blue jays) and other passerines (e.g., finches, blackbirds, warblers), which serve as a reservoir for infection. Mosquitoes (*Culex* spp.) feed on infected birds and are vectors, transmitting disease to other animals and to people.
- Dogs and cats may become viremic after experimental exposure to West Nile virus, but they do not commonly develop clinical signs.

DIAGNOSIS

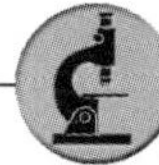

INITIAL DATABASE

- Complete blood count (CBC), serum chemistry profile, urinalysis: too few cases in small animals to identify common abnormalities. Histopathologic lesions suggest that results consistent with renal failure (e.g., azotemia and isosthenuria; pathologic proteinuria) could be expected in some cases.
- Neurologic examination may localize a lesion. Other differential diagnoses (other encephalitides; neoplasia; metabolic disease) should be considered more likely.
- Electrocardiogram (ECG): arrhythmias are more likely to be due to causes other than West Nile virus infection, and such causes should be ruled out first.

ADVANCED OR CONFIRMATORY TESTING

- Cerebrospinal fluid (CSF) tap: mononuclear pleocytosis is typically identified in other species
- Serologic titers are the test of choice for confirmation of infection in other species but have not been clinically validated for dogs or cats

TREATMENT

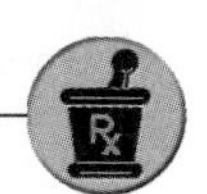

THERAPEUTIC GOAL(S)

Supportive care; no specific treatment has been identified as effective in small animal medicine due to the rarity of cases

ACUTE GENERAL TREATMENT

- As determined by clinical manifestations of disease
- Neurologic manifestations: see Seizures, p 990; Disorientation/Confusion, p 312
- Renal failure: see Chronic Renal Failure, Overt ("Symptomatic"), p 205; Chronic Renal Failure, Occult ("Asymptomatic"), p 204
- Myocarditis: treatment of arrhythmias if negatively affecting perfusion; see Ventricular Arrhythmias, p 1148; Atrial Premature Complexes and Supraventricular Tachycardia, p 100

PROGNOSIS AND OUTCOME

Too few cases are documented to formulate a reliable prognosis.

PEARLS & CONSIDERATIONS

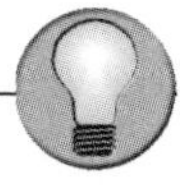

COMMENTS

- The epidemics of West Nile virus in horses and humans in the United States between 2000 and 2002 were the largest reported epidemics to this date.
- Domestic species do not contribute to the incidence of human disease because the reservoir is in wild birds.
- Dogs and cats have not routinely been diagnosed with West Nile virus but may become viremic after experimental exposure to infected mosquitoes.

PREVENTION

- Control of West Nile virus is best accomplished by control of mosquito populations.
- Dogs and cats appear to be sufficiently resistant to infection that the role of pre-

vention (e.g., use of insecticides) remains poorly defined, and there is no proven benefit to implementing preventive measures in small animal medicine.

CLIENT EDUCATION

- Prevention of mosquito breeding grounds and mosquito exposure is the most effective method of preventing human infection.
- Domestic species are not a risk to people.

SUGGESTED READING

Austgen LE, et al: Experimental infection of cats and dogs with West Nile virus. *Emerg Infect Dis* 10(1):82-86, 2004.

Buckweitz S, et al: Serological, reverse transcriptase-polymerase chain reaction, and immunohistochemical detection of West Nile virus in a clinically affected dog. *J Vet Diagn Invest* 15:324-329, 2004.

Lichtensteiger CA, et al: West Nile virus encephalitis and myocarditis in wolf and dog. *Emerg Infect Dis* 9:1303-1306, 2003.

Solomon T: Flavivirus encephalitis. *N Engl J Med* 351:370-387, 2004.

Wilkins PA, Del Piero F: West Nile virus: Lessons from the 21st century. *J Vet Emerg Crit Care* 14(1):2-14, 2004.

AUTHOR: **KATHRYN TAYLOR**

EDITOR: **DOUGLASS K. MACINTIRE**

Whipworm Infection

BASIC INFORMATION

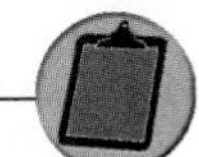

DEFINITION

Infection of the cecum (and possibly ileum and colon) with *Trichuris vulpis* (canine); rare in cats: *T. campanula* or *T. serrata*

SYNONYM(S)

Trichuriasis

EPIDEMIOLOGY

SPECIES, AGE, SEX: Primarily in dogs; rarely a problem in cats.

RISK FACTORS

- Roaming
- Exposure to feces or a contaminated environment

CONTAGION AND ZOONOSIS: Humans are rare aberrant hosts.

GEOGRAPHY AND SEASONALITY

- Common in the eastern and southern United States
- Ova are extremely resistant in the environment, surviving 4 to 5 years, and demonstrating no seasonality

CLINICAL PRESENTATION

DISEASE FORMS/SUBTYPES

- Large bowel diarrhea (mucoid stool, hematochezia, tenesmus) of variable degrees of severity
- Hypoadrenocorticism-like syndrome: hyponatremia, hyperkalemia, azotemia, metabolic acidosis
- Rarely, typhlitis or cecocolic intussusception may occur

HISTORY, CHIEF COMPLAINT

- None (incidental finding on fecal flotation)
- Clinical signs of large bowel diarrhea: frequent, urgent defecation of loose or watery feces, possibly containing mucus or fresh blood (hematochezia). Tenesmus, flatulence possible
- Occasionally associated with weight loss and protein-losing enteropathy
- In dogs with hypoadrenal-like illness, lethargy, vomiting, or severe diarrhea may be present

PHYSICAL EXAM FINDINGS

- Commonly, animals with mild whipworm infections have a normal physical examination.
- Vague signs of midabdominal pain/tenderness, often characterized by flank licking, have been associated with granulomatous typhlitis.
- Rarely, physical signs of systemic disease are present (weight loss/cachexia) with hypoadrenal-like illness related to whipworm infection.

ETIOLOGY AND PATHOPHYSIOLOGY

- Direct life cycle begins with ingestion of embryonated eggs.
- Ova hatch in small intestine and larvae burrow into mucosa for a 1-week period not causing clinical signs.
- Young adults emerge, relocate to the cecum/colon, and deeply embed the thread-like head (the "whip") into the mucosa to feed on blood and tissue fluids.
- Three month prepatent period precedes the appearance of ova in feces.
- Host response varies from mild, localized inflammation to mucosal hyperplasia to granulomatous inflammation, resulting in variable degrees of gastrointestinal (GI) clinical signs.
- Affected animals can develop large bowel diarrhea that ranges in severity from intermittent soft stool to severe, copious mucoid or hemorrhagic diarrhea with tenesmus.
- Whipworm-related enteritis may produce biochemical changes falsely suggesting hypoadrenocorticism.
    - Hyponatremia: due to concurrent diarrhea-associated sodium loss, water consumption, and anorexia.
    - Hyperkalemia: due to metabolic acidosis, decreased kaliuresis from reduced flow in the distal renal tubules, and/or laboratory artifact (normal platelet K^+ release when clotting).
    - Primary enteritis-associated hyponatremia and hyperkalemia are not caused by aldosterone deficiency (hypoadrenocorticism), as confirmed by normal adrenocorticotropic hormone (ACTH) stimulation test results.
- Whipworm infection has been suggested as a cause for cecocolic intussusception.

DIAGNOSIS

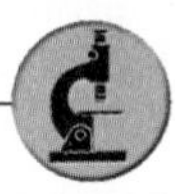

DIFFERENTIAL DIAGNOSIS

- *Capillaria* spp. infection (ova appear similar, but *Capillaria* spp. do not cause enteritis)
- Dietary-responsive large bowel diarrhea
- *Clostridium perfringens* enterotoxicosis
- Inflammatory bowel disease (large intestine)
- Chronic colitis (e.g., histiocytic ulcerative colitis)
- Eosinophilic colitis
- Histoplasmosis (large bowel)
- Neoplasia (carcinoma, lymphoma)
- Hypoadrenocorticisim
- Protein-losing enteropathy
- Intussusception

INITIAL DATABASE

- Serial fecal flotations to identify characteristic golden-brown bioperculated smooth ova: they are dense, and intermittently shed—often in low numbers—making multiple examinations necessary with adequately dense flotation solution (specific gravity >1.200; e.g., sugar or zinc sulfate).
- Empiric anthelmintic treatment with fenbendazole is rational in mild cases.
- Complete blood count: occasional eosinophilia and mild to moderate anemia.
- Serum biochemistry profile: hyponatremia, hyperkalemia, azotemia, hypoalbuminemia, metabolic acidosis are occasionally seen.
- Rectal cytology: insensitive for ova, but may demonstrate clostridial spores, inflammatory cells, neoplastic cells.
- ACTH response testing is recommended to rule out hypoadrenocorti-

cism in dogs with hyponatremia and hyperkalemia.

ADVANCED OR CONFIRMATORY TESTING

Colonoscopy is an expensive way to detect the presence of adult worms in the cecum and proximal colon.

TREATMENT

THERAPEUTIC GOAL(S)

Eliminate parasites from the GI tract

ACUTE GENERAL TREATMENT

- Anthelmintic therapy:
  - Fenbendazole 50 mg/kg PO q 24h × 3 days is the preferred treatment.
  - Febantel 10 mg/kg PO q 24h × 3 days is an acceptable alternative.
  - Drontal Plus (contains febantel) is also an appropriate therapy.
- Re-treat monthly for 3 months due to the long prepatent period
- Supportive care (e.g., intravenous fluids) for electrolyte abnormalities and azotemia in severe cases
- Typhlectomy for granulomatous typhlitis or cecocolic intussusception (rare)

CHRONIC TREATMENT

Milbemycin oxime is an effective preventative for chronic, recurrent trichuriasis.

DRUG INTERACTIONS

Dogs should be evaluated for presence of heartworm infection before instituting milbemycin oxime

POSSIBLE COMPLICATIONS

Possible adverse reaction with milbemycin oxime in heartworm positive dogs

RECOMMENDED MONITORING

Frequent fecal examinations for chronic infections

PROGNOSIS AND OUTCOME

- Excellent with appropriate therapy
- Reinfection likely due to environmental contamination with resistant ova

PEARLS & CONSIDERATIONS

COMMENTS

- *T. vulpis* is a common cause of large bowel diarrhea in dogs in the eastern and southern United States.
- Empiric treatment is recommended in uncomplicated cases before pursuing a lengthy, expensive diagnostic work-up.
- The potential for hypoadrenocorticism-like findings with trichuriasis must be recognized when hypoadrenocorticism is suspected in any dog based on history, clinical signs, and serum biochemistry/electrolyte results.
- Seizures have been reported in dogs with trichuriasis, most likely associated with profound hyponatremia.

PREVENTION

Milbemycin oxime in endemic areas or with chronic infections is an excellent preventative against *T. vulpis* and *D. immitis* infection.

CLIENT EDUCATION

Environmental contamination is the source for reinfection and is difficult to eliminate; monthly prophylaxis is recommended after treatment.

SUGGESTED READING

Graves TK, et al: Basal and ACTH-stimulated plasma aldosterone concentrations are normal or increased in dogs with trichuriasis-associated pseudohypoadrenocorticism. *J Vet Intern Med* 8:287–289, 1994.

Jergens AE, Willard MD: Diseases of the large intestine. In Ettinger SJ, Feldman ED (eds): *Textbook of Veterinary Internal Medicine*. Philadelphia, WB Saunders, 2000, pp 1238–1256.

Nelson RW, Couto CG: Disorder of the intestinal tract. In Nelson RW, Cuoto CG (eds): *Small Animal Internal Medicine*. St. Louis, Mosby, 1998, pp 433–467.

Reinemeyer CR: Canine gastrointestinal parasites. In Bonagura JD, Kirk RW (eds): *Current Veterinary Therapy XII*. Philadelphia, WB Saunders, 1995, pp 711–716.

Sherding RG, Burrows CF: Diarrhea. In Anderson NV (ed): *Veterinary Gastroenterology*, ed 2. Malvern, PA, Lea & Febiger, 1992, pp 399–477.

AUTHOR: **E. KELLY NITSCHE**
EDITOR: **DEBRA L. ZORAN**

Wolff-Parkinson-White Syndrome

BASIC INFORMATION

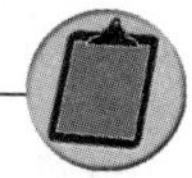

DEFINITION

The underlying defect is an accessory pathway or additional conductive fiber connection between atria and ventricles, separate and parallel to the normal atrioventricular (AV) node-bundle of His connection. The accessory pathway can participate as one limb of a rapid, re-entrant tachycardia.

SYNONYM(S)

WPW
General:
- Accessory atrioventricular pathway
- AV reciprocating tachycardia
- Ventricular pre-excitation

EPIDEMIOLOGY

SPECIES, AGE, SEX: Any; most commonly identified in dogs <6 years old.

GENETICS AND BREED PREDISPOSITION: Labrador retrievers and brachycephalic breeds appear to be predisposed.

ASSOCIATED CONDITIONS AND DISORDERS: In dogs, there is a possible association between tricuspid valve dysplasia and accessory AV pathways.

CLINICAL PRESENTATION

DISEASE FORMS/SUBTYPES
- Manifest accessory AV pathway: capable of antegrade (atrioventricular) conduction, bypassing the AV node. The result is ventricular pre-excitation during normal sinus rhythm. Manifest accessory pathways can also participate as the antegrade or retrograde limb of a tachyarrhythmia.
- Concealed accessory AV pathway: capable of retrograde conduction (ventricle to atrium) only. Therefore, there is no ventricular pre-excitation. Concealed AV pathways can participate as the retrograde limb of a tachyarrhythmia.

HISTORY, CHIEF COMPLAINT: Related to resultant tachyarrhythmias:
- Decreased exercise tolerance/weakness
- Vomiting, inappetence
- Racing heart/pulsing ears or head
- Dyspnea/coughing
- Abdominal distention
- Acute collapse
- Sudden death

PHYSICAL EXAM FINDINGS: Patient may be normal at the time of exam or may show the following signs:
- Tachyarrhythmia
- Decreased femoral pulse quality
- Tachypnea/dyspnea
- Peritoneal fluid wave
- Mucous membrane pallor

ETIOLOGY AND PATHOPHYSIOLOGY

- The accessory AV pathway is composed of working myocardial fibers that exist outside the confines of the normal conduction system and connect atrial and ventricular myocardium.
- The antegrade (atria to ventricles) conduction of an atrial impulse over the accessory AV pathway activates a portion of the ventricular myocardium early and then spreads in a cell-to-cell fashion. The result is a short PR interval and a wide, abnormal QRS complex (i.e., ventricular pre-excitation).
- Retrograde (ventricles to atria) conduction of a ventricular impulse over the accessory AV pathway activates a portion of the atrium and then spreads in a cell-to-cell fashion, eventually reaching the AV node. If the AV node conducts the impulse to the ventricles, this cycle can be repeated in a self-perpetuating loop and result in a narrow complex tachyarrhythmia.
- If a tachyarrhythmia is frequent or sustained, it can lead to tachycardia-induced cardiomyopathy, a dilated poorly contractile heart that is indistinguishable from idiopathic dilated cardiomyopathy, except that it is reversible with control of the tachyarrhythmia.
- Pathways capable of rapid antegrade conduction can conduct atrial tachyarrhythmias rapidly to the ventricles, bypassing the normal delay imposed by the AV node.

DIAGNOSIS

DIFFERENTIAL DIAGNOSIS

- Electrocardiographic (ECG):
  - Narrow complex, regular tachyarrhythmias: automatic or re-entrant atrial tachycardias, AV re-entrant tachycardia, junctional tachycardias
  - Pre-excited tachyarrhythmias: ventricular tachycardias
- Radiographic/echocardiographic (in cases progressing to tachycardia-induced cardiomyopathy):
  - Idiopathic dilated cardiomyopathy

INITIAL DATABASE

- ECG:
  - Ventricular pre-excitation may be present during sinus rhythm: short PR interval (usually <0.06 seconds); initial portion of the QRS slurred (i.e., slowly rises or descends); QRS duration prolonged (>0.06 seconds); QRS axis may be abnormal ("delta wave")
  - Tachyarrhythmias: tend to be narrow complex (QRS <0.06 seconds), 250–400+ bpm; when patients are not on antiarrhythmic drugs, the ECG may have a visible deflection in ST segment (retrograde P wave); tachyarrhythmias are often intermittent or may be intermittent, so they are not necessarily captured on a baseline ECG
- Echocardiogram:
  - May be normal
  - May mimic dilated cardiomyopathy
  - Assess for congenital heart defects; examine tricuspid valve
- Thoracic radiographs:
  - Assess cardiac silhouette (normal to severely enlarged)
  - Assess pulmonary vasculature and lung fields (for congestion and edema)
- Physical tests:
  - Vagal maneuver: may terminate a tachyarrhythmia by inducing AV nodal blockade but generally unsuccessful (see Vagal Maneuver, p 1323)

ADVANCED OR CONFIRMATORY TESTS

- Holter monitoring: can be helpful in capturing intermittent pre-excitation or tachyarrhythmias.
- Drug administration: IV diltiazem can terminate AV reciprocating tachycardia by inducing AV block; however, it can terminate certain other tachyarrhythmias as well. Blood pressure (BP) monitoring and resuscitation equipment should be available.
- Electrophysiologic testing: definitively establishes the presence or absence of an accessory pathway and its location along the AV groove.

TREATMENT

THERAPEUTIC GOAL(S)

Terminate any tachyarrhythmia present and control its reoccurrence

ACUTE GENERAL TREATMENT

- Incessant narrow complex tachyarrhythmias: aimed at slowing AV nodal conduction or blocking the accessory pathway: diltiazem (0.125–0.35 mg/kg, slow IV over 3 to 4 minutes) or procainamide (6–20 mg/kg slow IV over 30 minutes) most commonly used.
- Synchronized direct current (DC) cardioversion can be used once the patient is anesthetized or unconscious if drugs are unsuccessful.

CHRONIC TREATMENT

- Antiarrhythmic drug therapy to control tachyarrhythmias.
- Radiofrequency catheter ablation of the accessory pathway is a curative procedure.

DRUG INTERACTIONS

Potential interactions between digoxin and several antiarrhythmic and commonly used drugs

POSSIBLE COMPLICATIONS

- Tachycardia-induced cardiomyopathy
- Congestive heart failure (CHF)
- Sudden death
- Side effects of antiarrhythmic drugs

RECOMMENDED MONITORING

- Follow-up exam, ECG, and Holter monitoring: frequency dependent on the severity of the tachyarrhythmias documented
- Radiographic and echocardiographic monitoring for dogs with tachycardia-induced cardiomyopathy: with adequate control of tachyarrhythmias, myocardial function should improve within 3 months

PROGNOSIS AND OUTCOME

- Excellent with radiofrequency catheter ablation.
- Fair long term with antiarrhythmic drug administration.
- Poor if tachyarrhythmias are not controlled: progressive cardiomyopathic changes (eventually not completely reversible) and recurrent CHF result. Sudden death becomes more common.

PEARLS & CONSIDERATIONS

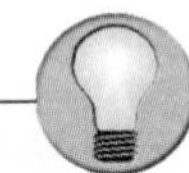

COMMENTS

- Should be a differential diagnosis in a young (<6 years old) dog presenting with dilated cardiomyopathy (DCM)-like signs.
- May require Holter monitoring for documentation.
- Even dogs with tachycardiomyopathy and CHF can be cured with successful ablation of the accessory pathway.

CLIENT EDUCATION

- Monitor heart rate carefully at home.
- Sustained tachyarrhythmias are life threatening.
- Curative procedures are available.

SUGGESTED READING

Atkins CE, Wright KN: Supraventricular tachycardia associated with accessory atrioventricular pathways in dogs. In Bonagura JD (ed): *Kirk's Current Veterinary Therapy XII*. Philadelphia, WB Saunders, 1995, pp 807–813.

Wright KN, et al: Radiofrequency catheter ablation of atrioventricular accessory pathways in 3 dogs with subsequent resolution of tachycardia-induced cardiomyopathy. *J Vet Intern Med* 13:361-371, 1999.

Wright KN: Assessment and treatment of supraventricular tachyarrhythmias. In Bonagura JD (ed): *Kirk's Current Veterinary Therapy XIII*. Philadelphia, WB Saunders, 2000, pp 726-730.

Wright KN: Interventional catheterization for tachyarrhythmias. In Abbott J (ed): *Veterinary Clinics of North America: Small Animal Practice*. Philadelphia, Elsevier, 2004, pp 1171-1185.

AUTHOR: **KATHY WRIGHT**

EDITOR: **ETIENNE CÔTÉ**

Yew Toxicosis

BASIC INFORMATION

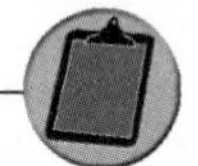

DEFINITION

Systemic adverse effects due to accidental ingestion, typically by dogs, of dried or fresh yew plant material. Characteristic signs are often severe and can include vomiting, muscle weakness, seizures, cardiac arrhythmias, coma, and death.

SYNONYM(S)

Taxines (*Taxus* alkaloids) are the toxic components of the yew plant.

EPIDEMIOLOGY

SPECIES, AGE, SEX: Dogs are more likely to be involved than cats; all breeds, sexes, and ages are susceptible.

RISK FACTORS

- Yews are toxic both as green and as dried plant material.
- All parts of the yew are toxic except for the red, fleshy fruit surrounding the hard seed. The hard seed coat is resistant to digestive enzymes. Clinical signs are unlikely if the seed is swallowed whole, but absorption from a cracked or partly chewed seed is possible.

GEOGRAPHY AND SEASONALITY

- The most common ornamental yews are *T. baccata* (English yew) and *T. cuspidata* (Japanese yew).
- In the eastern United States, *T. canadensis* (American yew) is the most common native yew; in Florida, *T. floridana* is the most common native species, and in the western United States, *T. brevifolia* (Western or Pacific yew) is most frequently seen.
- Taxine content is often higher in the winter than in the summer.

CLINICAL PRESENTATION

HISTORY, CHIEF COMPLAINT

- History of exposure to dried or fresh plant material.
- Recent history of vomiting, with the presence of plant material noted in the vomitus.
- The onset of systemic clinical signs is extremely rapid (within 30 minutes to 3 hours postingestion), and progression to death may happen within a few hours.
- In increasing degree of severity over time, the spectrum of clinical complaints includes vomiting, muscle weakness, seizures, coma, and death.

PHYSICAL EXAM FINDINGS

- Signs of abdominal pain
- Mydriasis
- Tachycardia or bradycardia (both occur fairly commonly with yew toxicosis)
- Hypotension
- Respiratory distress or arrest

ETIOLOGY AND PATHOPHYSIOLOGY

- *Taxus* spp. (yew) are commonly used as ornamental evergreen shrubs.
- Yew alkaloids (taxines) are calcium and sodium ion channel blockers that gradually induce bradycardia and, ultimately, cardiac arrest.

DIAGNOSIS

Generally based on known or possible ingestion of yew; confirmation is via identification of plant parts in vomitus

DIFFERENTIAL DIAGNOSIS

- Cardiac glycoside-containing plants (e.g., oleander, foxglove)
- Ca channel blockers (diltiazem, verapamil) toxicosis
- Caffeine toxicosis (methylxanthines)

INITIAL DATABASE

Complete blood count (CBC), serum biochemistry profile, urinalysis: hypokalemia possible

- Electrocardiogram (ECG): A wide variety of arrhythmias is possible and fairly common, most commonly atrioventricular (AV) block, ventricular tachycardia, and (ultimately with severe intoxications) ventricular fibrillation/cardiac arrest

ADVANCED OR CONFIRMATORY TESTING

- Taxines (or metabolites) can be identified in vomitus and stomach contents by gas chromatography, mass spectrometry, and silica gel thin layer chromatography although the lengthy turnaround time of such advanced testing usually precludes its use clinically.
- Necropsy: The diagnosis of yew poisoning is generally based on the presence of yew plant in the gut. Taxine depresses the conduction system of the heart; therefore, no significant lesions are typically found on necropsy.
- Histopathologic examination: no characteristic lesions; fatty degeneration of the kidney, congestion of lungs, and inflammation of the gastrointestinal (GI) tract are possible.

TREATMENT

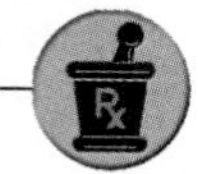

THERAPEUTIC GOAL(S)

- Stop absorption and increase excretion of taxines
- Correct cardiac arrhythmias associated with yew ingestion

ACUTE GENERAL TREATMENT

- Emesis: in animals not showing clinical signs:
  - Apomorphine: 0.03-0.04 mg/kg IV or IM, or crush tablet portion with water and instill into conjunctival sac and rinse following emesis.
  - Hydrogen peroxide 3%: 2 ml/kg PO (max 45 ml [in large dogs]), repeat in 10 to 15 minutes if no vomiting.
  - Emesis may not remove all plant material from the GI tract.
  - Gastric lavage (plant material not easily removed through tube).
  - Endoscopic removal of plant parts.
  - Activated charcoal (1-2 g/kg PO) with a cathartic, such as sorbitol (70%) 1-3 ml/kg; mix with charcoal; use labeled dose for commercial products.
- Treat cardiac arrhythmias as needed:
  - Ventricular tachyarrhythmias: correct hypokalemia if present and consider lidocaine (dogs: 2 mg/kg IV; cats: use with caution), amiodarone (dogs: 10-25 mg/kg PO q 12h), procainamide (dogs: 6-8 mg/kg IV; cats: 1-2 mg/kg IV) or sotalol (dogs/cats: 2 mg/kg PO q 12h). See Ventricular Arrhythmias, p 1148.
  - Bradycardia: atropine 0.04 mg/kg IV.

- Control seizures: diazepam (dogs/cats: 0.25–0.5 mg/kg IV) or phenobarbital (dogs/cats: 2–5 mg/kg IV, higher doses often used in dogs [see Epilepsy, Idiopathic, p 351; Seizures, p 990])
- IV fluids and oxygen as needed
- Correct electrolyte abnormalities as needed

DRUG INTERACTIONS

- Na channel blockers (proarrhythmia)
- Ca channel blockers

RECOMMENDED MONITORING

- ECG
- Serum electrolytes
- Central nervous system (CNS) signs
- Respiratory effort

PROGNOSIS AND OUTCOME

- Good if treated early and aggressively (prior to onset of clinical signs)
- Poor if systemic effects are present, especially cardiac arrhythmias

PEARLS & CONSIDERATIONS

COMMENTS

- All species of yews should be considered toxic, but there is great variability in taxine content.
- Tetanic epileptiform seizures are reported clinically in dogs but not reproduced experimentally.
- Toxic dose for dogs is 30 g (approximately 2 tbsp) of plant material.

PREVENTION

Keep pets away from yew bushes and clippings

CLIENT EDUCATION

Dried shrubbery and trimmings are still toxic.

SUGGESTED READING

Burrows GE, Tyrl RJ: Taxaceae. In Burrows GE, Tyrl RJ (eds): *Toxic Plants of North America*. Ames, IA, Iowa State Press, 2001, pp 1149–1157.

AUTHOR: **TINA WISMER**
EDITOR: **SAFDAR A. KHAN**

Zinc Oxide Toxicosis

BASIC INFORMATION

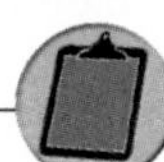

DEFINITION

Generally acute self-limiting nausea, vomiting, lethargy, and anorexia occurring after ingestion of concentrated (10–40%) zinc oxide-containing products, such as diaper rash ointments, creams, hemorrhoid preparations, calamine lotion, and some sun blocks

SYNONYM(S)

Chinese white
Zinc white
ZnO

EPIDEMIOLOGY

SPECIES, AGE, SEX: All animals susceptible; cases commonly involve dogs.
RISK FACTORS: Younger, unsupervised pets are most likely to ingest products containing zinc oxide.

CLINICAL PRESENTATION

HISTORY, CHIEF COMPLAINT
- Acute onset of vomiting.
- White color material present in the vomitus (looks like product ingested) within hours of the ingestion.
- Animals usually remain bright, alert, and responsive.

PHYSICAL EXAM FINDINGS: Unremarkable, aside from nausea, vomiting, and mild lethargy.

ETIOLOGY AND PATHOPHYSIOLOGY

- Zinc oxide-containing ointments or creams are used as topical skin protectants, astringents, and bactericidal agents.
- Most zinc oxide ointments or creams contain 10–40% zinc oxide.
- Some commercial zinc ointment preparations may also contain varying concentrations of vitamin A or D or local anesthetics (benzocaine), cod liver oil, beeswax, petrolatum, or mineral oil.
- Zinc salts are usually irritating to gastrointestinal (GI) mucosa.
- Mild to moderate vomiting occurs due to acute gastric irritation.
- Vomiting is self-limiting but exacerbated if unlimited water ingestion is allowed before resolution.
- Some dogs will occasionally show an allergic-type reaction (urticaria, angioedema).

DIAGNOSIS

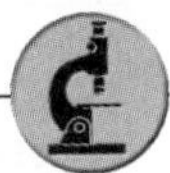

DIFFERENTIAL DIAGNOSIS

- Dietary indiscretion/indigestion.
- Pancreatitis.
- Parvoviral enteritis.
- Zinc oxide characteristically gives stools/vomit a white color.

INITIAL DATABASE

Not generally required; no systemic signs are expected, and diagnostic testing is rarely indicated (self-resolving problem)

TREATMENT

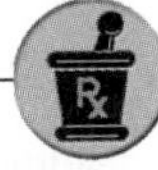

THERAPEUTIC GOAL(S)

- Control vomiting
- Provide supportive care (e.g., with IV fluids) if needed; rarely necessary
- Treat allergic-type reaction with antihistamines as needed

ACUTE GENERAL TREATMENT

- Nothing by mouth (NPO) until 2 hours after last episode of vomiting.
- Most cases do not require IV fluids because clinical signs resolve within 12 hours. Allergic reactions may persist longer (24 hours).
- For allergic reaction: diphenhydramine 2–4 mg/kg PO q 8–12h, or 1 mg/kg IM or SC q 8–12h for dogs; 0.5 mg/kg PO q 12h or 2 mg/kg IM q 12h for cats.

POSSIBLE COMPLICATIONS

GI foreign body if the container was ingested

PROGNOSIS AND OUTCOME

- Expect rapid and complete recovery within 24 hours
- Ingestion is not expected to result in zinc toxicosis (hemolytic anemia, renal damage) because most dogs vomit. Unlike a solid zinc-containing object, which tends to remain in the GI tract long enough to allow absorption of zinc, ointment/cream is readily removed from stomach—minimal risk for zinc intoxication with single ingestion of a zinc oxide topical product

PEARLS & CONSIDERATIONS

COMMENTS

- Single acute ingestion of zinc oxide-containing ointments or creams is not likely to result in zinc toxicosis.
- Repeated use of concentrated zinc oxide-containing products can result in zinc toxicosis, however. Zinc toxicosis has been reported in a dog when 40% zinc oxide ointment was applied dermally for 4 days and dog licked most of the ointment after application.
- Cod liver oil in products containing zinc oxide makes them attractive to dogs.
- Zinc metal toxicosis (see Zinc Toxicosis, p 1171) can cause systemic signs, whereas zinc oxide toxicosis generally does not.
- There has been one case report in which repeated use and subsequent licking of zinc oxide ointment in a dog resulted in typical signs of zinc toxicosis (hemolytic anemia, hemoglobinuria); however, generally acute single ingestion of zinc oxide-containing products is not likely to result in typical signs of zinc toxicosis.

PREVENTION

Keep diaper rash products out of pet's reach

SUGGESTED READING

National Library of Medicine, Medline Plus http://www.nlm.nih.gov/medlineplus/ency/article/002571.htm.

Welch SL: Oral toxicity of topical preparations. *Vet Clin North Am Small Anim Pract* 32(2):443–453, 2002.

AUTHOR: **MARY M. SCHELL**

EDITOR: **SAFDAR A. KHAN**

Zinc Phosphide Intoxication

BASIC INFORMATION

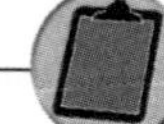

DEFINITION

Zinc phosphide is a metallophosphide rodenticide available as 0.5–10% bait. Acute toxicosis occurs from ingestion of bait and is characterized by progressive bloody vomiting, agitation, discomfort, constant movement or running, vocalization, bruxism (teeth grinding), respiratory distress, muscle tremors, seizures, and death

SYNONYM(S)

Gopher or mole killer

Zn_3P_2, trizinc diphosphide

EPIDEMIOLOGY

SPECIES, AGE, SEX: All species are susceptible; dogs are more frequently involved.

GENETICS AND BREED PREDISPOSITION: Animals unable to vomit are at greater risk.

GEOGRAPHY AND SEASONALITY: Increased incidence during greater rodent activity and mobility following harvest.

CONTAGION AND ZOONOSIS: Public health significance to veterinary personnel: Human inhalation of phosphine off-gas during decontamination procedures can occur (risk of pulmonary and other effects in humans). Typical garlic odor of phosphine may not be detectable at low yet hazardous concentrations to humans. If handling a phosphine-intoxicated animal, ensure good ventilation and contact regional hazardous materials authority for safest procedure guidelines and refer to acute treatment guidelines as described in this entry

CLINICAL PRESENTATION

HISTORY, CHIEF COMPLAINT

- History of exposure
- Vomiting often with blood
- Agitation, discomfort, constant movement or running
- Vocalization, teeth grinding
- Muscle tremors, seizure

PHYSICAL EXAM FINDINGS

- Agitation, vocalization
- Retching, hematemesis
- Dyspnea, harsh lung sounds (due to pulmonary edema)
- Signs of cranial abdominal pain
- Cardiac arrhythmia
- Shock
- Slight garlic or rotten fish odor

ETIOLOGY AND PATHOPHYSIOLOGY

The toxin:

- Baits are available as commercial grain-based pellet, tracking powder, or paste.
- Fumigants aluminum phosphide and magnesium phosphide are similar to zinc phosphide in toxicity.
- Some commercial names are Sweeneys Poison Peanuts Mole and Gopher Bait, Dragon Gopher and Mole Killer Pellets, and Dexol Gopher Killing Pellets 2.

Pathophysiology:

- Onset of clinical signs in most cases is 15 minutes to 4 hours after ingestion; occasionally delayed up to 18 hours.
- Corrosive effects of zinc phosphide can cause signs of cranial abdominal (gastric) pain and bloody vomiting.
- Gastric acid hydrolysis of zinc phosphide liberates highly toxic phosphine gas, which is rapidly absorbed by passive diffusion.
- Phosphine disrupts cellular respiration by interfering with electron transport (cytochrome C) in the mitochondrion, leading to cellular hypoxia, generation of reactive oxygen species, and lipid peroxidation, especially in tissues of high oxygen demand.
- Death is from cardiac arrest most commonly resulting from hypotensive shock, seizures, and pulmonary compromise.

DIAGNOSIS

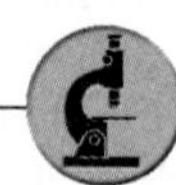

DIFFERENTIAL DIAGNOSIS

- Strychnine intoxication
- Metaldehyde intoxication
- Organophosphate or carbamate insecticides intoxication
- Arsenic intoxication
- Primary central nervous system (CNS) disease (neoplasia, encephalitis, other)
- Hepatic encephalopathy

INITIAL DATABASE

- Chest radiographs (pulmonary edema)
- Acid-base status (respiratory and metabolic acidosis)
- Electrocardiogram (ECG) (arrhythmias, nonspecific evidence of myocardial ischemia [e.g., ST segment elevation or depression])
- Baseline complete blood count (CBC) and serum chemistries (unremarkable)
  - Baseline electrolytes (possibly decreased Mg^{++}, Ca^{++})
- Coagulation profile (increased)

ADVANCED OR CONFIRMATORY TESTING

- Freeze gastric contents, vomitus, liver, and kidney in airtight containers for zinc phosphide analysis.
- Silver nitrate paper qualitative screen of gastric fluid may help detect presence of phosphine gas. Phosphine reacts with silver nitrate, changing the test paper color

to black and indicating a positive reaction (follow label directions).

TREATMENT

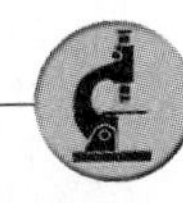

THERAPEUTIC GOAL(S)

- Decontamination of patient (remove remaining toxin)
- Reduce liberation of phosphine gas (public health concerns)
- Control seizures
- Support pulmonary, cardiovascular, acid-base, and neuromuscular systems
- Correction of acid-base, electrolyte, and chemical abnormalities
- Use exogenous scavenging precursors (prevent ongoing organ damage)

ACUTE GENERAL TREATMENT

- Decontamination of patient:
  - Emesis (see Vomiting, Induction of, p 1328).
  - Animal not showing clinical signs: 1-2 ml/kg 3% hydrogen peroxide PO, maximum dose 45 ml for largest dogs or apomorphine 0.04 mg/kg IM or IV, or instill into conjunctival sac part of a crushed tablet dissolved in water.
  - Activated charcoal 1-3 g/kg PO (caution: aspiration risk in vomiting animal) (see Gastric Intubation, Gavage, Lavage, p 1258).
- Reduce liberation of phosphine gas:
  - 1-3 tbsp (15-45 ml) margarine or olive/corn/vegetable oil (high in unsaturated lipids) fed on a piece of bread to an affected, conscious animal PO may help quench reactive oxygen species from phosphine in the stomach. Useful prior to presentation and decontamination of patient.
  - Magnesium hydroxide 10-60 ml PO/animal prior to presentation and decontamination to increase gastric pH. A common preparation of magnesium hydroxide is Milk of Magnesia.
- Control seizures. One of the following may be used:
  - Diazepam 0.5-2 mg/kg IV; repeat as needed.
  - Pentobarbital 10-30 mg/kg IV to effect, repeat as needed.
  - Propofol up to 5-6 mg/kg slow IV to effect, then constant rate IV infusion 0.1-0.6 mg/kg/min titrated to effect.
- Stabilize respiratory, cardiovascular, and neuromuscular systems:
  - Place endotracheal tube if needed with proper gas evacuation.
  - Supplemental oxygen.
  - Treat shock with crystalloids or colloids; crystalloid dose 80-90 ml/kg/hr for dogs; 40-60 ml/kg/hr for cats. Synthetic colloid dose approximately 20 ml/kg per day for dogs; 10-20 ml/kg per day for cats (adjust based on case parameters).
  - Corticosteroids (dexamethasone 0.1-0.2 mg/kg IV) if needed.
  - Monitor acid-base status and correct it with sodium bicarbonate as needed.
  - Monitor electrolytes; correct any deficiency (Ca^{++}, Mg^{++}, and K^{+}).
  - Control pain with narcotic analgesics (e.g., fentanyl transdermal patches 25-100 µg/hr; injectable opiates first if acute pain).
  - Monitor serum biochemistry profiles for 72 hours for delayed hepatic and renal injury.
- Exogenous scavengers:
  - *N*-acetylcysteine reduced myocardial injury in laboratory animals exposed to aluminum phosphide: loading dose 140-280 mg/kg PO or slow IV, then 70 mg/kg PO q 6h for six treatments.

POSSIBLE COMPLICATIONS

Renal, cardiac, and/or hepatic compromise

RECOMMENDED MONITORING

Respiratory, cardiac, hepatic, and renal functions for 72 hours after exposure

PROGNOSIS AND OUTCOME

- Good for animals not showing clinical signs 8 to 16 hours after exposure
- Guarded to poor if cardiac arrhythmias, shock, or pulmonary edema develop; death usually within 6 hours
- Fair to good for cases surviving 24 hours

PEARLS & CONSIDERATIONS

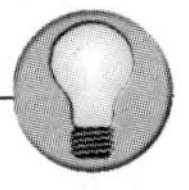

COMMENTS

- Early vomiting may reduce risk of serious toxicity in dogs.
- Human inhalation of phosphine off-gas during decontamination procedures can occur and is hazardous. Typical garlic odor of phosphine may not be detectable at low yet hazardous concentrations to humans.
- Baits may retain potency for 3 years in a dry environment.
- Toxic dose in dogs and cats is 20-40 mg/kg.
- Only 1 tbsp of 2% pellet bait contains approximately 180 mg zinc phosphide, a significant risk for a 10-kg dog.
- Delayed hepatic or renal injury is possible 48 to 72 hours following exposure.

CLIENT EDUCATION

- Keep all baits away from dogs
- Dogs can dig mole/gopher holes and retrieve the bait in the yard/garden

SUGGESTED READING

Knight MW: Zinc phosphide. In Peterson ME, Talcott PA (eds): *Small Animal Toxicology*. Philadelphia, WB Saunders, 2001, pp 748-755.

Phosphine and selected metal phosphides. *International Programme on Chemical Safety, Environmental Health Criteria* 73: www.inchem.org.

AUTHOR: **MICHAEL W. KNIGHT**

EDITOR: **SAFDAR A. KHAN**

Zinc Toxicosis

BASIC INFORMATION

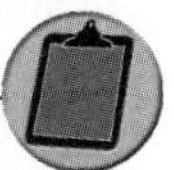

DEFINITION

Occurs after ingestion of zinc-containing objects such as pennies, scrap metal pieces, and hardware. Clinical signs arise due to acute gastrointestinal (GI) irritation or hemolysis (zinc-mediated red blood cell [RBC] injury).

SYNONYM(S)

Elemental zinc

Zn

EPIDEMIOLOGY

SPECIES, AGE, SEX: Toxicity is reported mostly in dogs (all breeds, sexes, ages) from ingesting zinc-containing objects (pennies, hardware nuts, wires); cats are less likely cases.

CLINICAL PRESENTATION

HISTORY, CHIEF COMPLAINT

- Inappetence, lethargy, protracted vomiting, diarrhea
- Red-colored urine
- Animal occasionally may vomit up pennies or other metallic objects or pass pennies in the feces

- Animal owners often are unaware of ingestion of any foreign metallic object by their pets
    - In these cases, zinc toxicosis becomes suspected based on hemolytic anemia and/or presence of metallic object in the GI tract on radiographs

PHYSICAL EXAM FINDINGS

- As already described
- Signs of abdominal discomfort or pain on palpation
- Pale mucous membranes
- Icterus
- Discolored urine (hemoglobinuria)

ETIOLOGY AND PATHOPHYSIOLOGY

The toxin:

- Metallic zinc is used in galvanizing, welding, and soldering. Zinc salts are used as astringents, antiseptics, deodorants; in galvanized nuts and cage wires; and in smoke generators, wood preservatives, pigments, and insecticides. Zinc gluconate is about 14% elemental zinc.
- U.S. pennies minted after 1982 weigh 2.5 g and are 97.6% zinc and 2.4% copper. Canadian pennies prior to 1997 were approximately 98% copper and 1.75% zinc. From 1997 to 2001, Canadian pennies were made with 96% zinc and 4% copper. Since 2001, Canadian pennies have been made of copper-plated steel (94% steel, 1.5% nickel, 4.5% copper).

Pathophysiology:

- Zinc has an antagonistic effect on copper and iron. It can interfere with iron absorption, making RBCs susceptible to hemolysis. Zinc also causes direct, severe GI mucosal irritation.
- Zinc leaches from metallic objects due to an acidic gastric pH, providing continuous GI absorption. Toxicosis occurs when zinc-containing objects are retained or embedded in the GI tract.

DIAGNOSIS

Tentative diagnosis is based on presence of radiopaque material in the GI tract (pennies, wires, nuts) and clinical signs; hemolytic anemia provides further support

DIFFERENTIAL DIAGNOSIS

- Other toxicoses: onions/garlic, acetaminophen, mothballs, local anesthetics
- Immune-mediated hemolytic anemia
- Tick-borne diseases

INITIAL DATABASE

- Complete blood count (CBC): regenerative anemia, hemoglobinemia, reticulocytosis, spherocytosis; neutrophilic leukocytosis
- Serum biochemistry profile: azotemia; elevation in serum bilirubin, liver enzymes, amylase, lipase
- Urinalysis: hemoglobinuria, proteinuria

ADVANCED OR CONFIRMATORY TESTING

Definitive diagnosis: blood or tissue zinc levels

- For blood collection, use special tubes (royal blue top) and syringes that contain no rubber grommets. Do not use traditional syringes, rubber grommets, and Vacutainer tubes because these contain some amount of zinc and may give erroneous results.
- Toxic levels in dogs:
    - Serum: 10–54 ppm (adequate levels 0.7–2 ppm)
    - Whole blood: 45 ppm (note: this dog ended up dying)
    - Liver: 130–436 ppm (adequate levels 30–70 ppm)
    - Kidney: 175–295 ppm (adequate levels 16–30 ppm)
    - Urine: 10–25 ppm (adequate levels 2–5 ppm)

TREATMENT

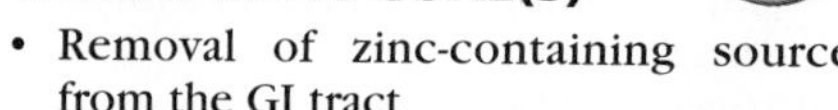

THERAPEUTIC GOAL(S)

- Removal of zinc-containing source from the GI tract
- Chelation therapy with calcium EDTA or dimercaprol or d-penicillamine
- Supportive care

ACUTE GENERAL TREATMENT

- Removal of zinc source from GI tract:
    - Emesis (see Vomiting, Induction of, p 1328): do not induce if animal is already vomiting; always feed the animal first (avoid unproductive vomiting)
    - Removal through an endoscope: this may be possible if the metallic object is small and present in the stomach. However, difficult/impossible if there is food in the stomach or with smooth, slippery objects
    - Surgical removal (gastrostomy/enterotomy): last resort; weigh all the risks and benefits before performing surgery; stabilize the animal first (fluids, blood transfusion as needed)
    - Activated charcoal: does not adsorb zinc well; not indicated
- Chelation therapy: Note that most cases of zinc poisoning do not require chelation therapy. Animals with zinc toxicosis usually respond well to fluid therapy and other supportive measures once the source of zinc has been removed. Options for chelation therapy include one of the following treatments:
    - Calcium EDTA (6.6% solution) in dogs: 100 mg/kg 2–5 days; divide dose into four portions and dilute to 10 mg CaEDTA/ml of 5% dextrose; administer SC at different sites. Do not exceed 2 g per day and do not treat for more than 5 consecutive days. In cats: 27.5 mg/kg in 15 ml of 5% dextrose SC q 6h for 5 days. Use with extreme caution due to risk of nephrotoxicity
    - Dimercaprol 2–4 mg/kg SC or IM q 8–12h for 2 days
    - D-penicillamine: 110 mg/kg per day PO divided into 3–4 doses, 7 to 14 days
    - Efficacy of dimercaprol and d-penicillamine has not been validated for zinc toxicosis
- Supportive care:
    - Fluid diuresis with a balanced cystalloid solution to promote zinc excretion and prevent hemoglobinuric nephrosis
    - Blood transfusion as needed
    - Control severe vomiting with metoclopramide (0.2–0.5 mg/kg SC q 8h) if needed, provided GI obstruction is ruled out

POSSIBLE COMPLICATIONS

Liver and renal compromise

RECOMMENDED MONITORING

- Complete blood count (CBC)
- Serum biochemistry profile (serum bilirubin, renal, and liver values for 1 to 3 days or until resolution of signs; pancreatic enzymes)
- Hematocrit
- Urinalysis

PROGNOSIS AND OUTCOME

- Good with aggressive supportive care after removing the source
- Poor if there is overt clinical evidence of multiple organ system damage or failure (liver, kidney, and/or pancreas)

PEARLS & CONSIDERATIONS

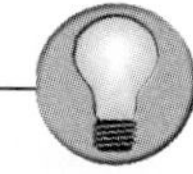

COMMENTS

- Toxicosis not likely to occur if zinc-containing objects move out of the GI tract quickly.
- The hematologic and clinical findings in animals with zinc toxicosis are similar to those found for immune-mediated hemolytic anemia (IMHA).
- Zinc toxicosis can cause a positive direct antiglobulin test (Coombs' test) result. Therefore, Coombs' test is not a reliable method of differentiating between IMHA and zinc toxicosis.
- The LD_{50} of zinc chloride is approximately 100 mg/kg PO.

- The greatest amounts of zinc are present in blood, liver, kidney, skin, lung, brain, heart, and pancreas. Excretion of zinc occurs through the bile and kidneys.

SUGGESTED READING

Breitschwerdt EB, et al: Three cases of acute zinc toxicosis in dogs. *Vet Hum Toxicol* 28(2):109–117, 1986.

Ogden L: Zinc toxicosis. In Kirk RW, Bonagura JD (eds): *Current Veterinary Therapy XI: Small Animal Practice*. Philadelphia, WB Saunders, 1992, pp 197–200.

AUTHOR & EDITOR: **SAFDAR A. KHAN**

Zinc-Responsive Dermatosis

BASIC INFORMATION

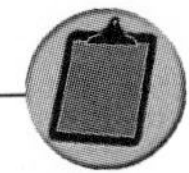

DEFINITION

Uncommon zinc-responsive scaling disorder of the skin that can be hereditary or secondary to a dietary imbalance

EPIDEMIOLOGY

SPECIES, AGE, SEX

- No sex predilection
- Syndrome I: age of onset is typically 1 to 3 years; range: 2 months to 11 years
- Syndrome II: most common in young, rapidly growing dogs

GENETICS AND BREED PREDISPOSITION

- Syndrome I: northern breeds, such as Alaskan malamute, Siberian husky, and Samoyed; also reported in Doberman pinschers and Great Danes
- Syndrome II: any breed; Great Dane, Doberman pinscher, beagle, German shepherd, German short-haired pointer, Labrador retriever, Rhodesian Ridgeback, and standard poodle may be predisposed

RISK FACTORS: Rapidly growing puppies fed diets deficient in zinc or high in phytates (high plant/grain content) or calcium.

CLINICAL PRESENTATION

DISEASE FORMS/SUBTYPES

- Syndrome I: hereditary
- Syndrome II: dietary

HISTORY, CHIEF COMPLAINT

- Owner may note scaling and crusting dermatosis.
- Pruritus may precede development of other clinical signs and is present in nearly half of animals.
- Some puppies with syndrome II present with depression, anorexia, delayed growth, fever, and lymphadenopathy.

PHYSICAL EXAM FINDINGS

- Focal erythema and alopecia progress to scaly and crusted lesions.
- Dull, dry coat.
- Secondary microbial (bacterial and yeast) dermatitis.
- Predilection sites: periocular, ears, nose, perioral, footpads, pressure points on limbs.
- Scrotum, prepuce, perianal region, and vulva may also be affected.

ETIOLOGY AND PATHOPHYSIOLOGY

- Genetic defect involving zinc absorption reported in Alaskan malamutes.
- Diets high in calcium or phytates (plant/grain products) bind to zinc and decrease absorption.
- Zinc absorption is also negatively affected by essential fatty acid deficiency, high levels of iron in water, or prolonged diarrhea.
- It is suspected that low zinc levels cause poor lytic enzyme function (thus affecting skin maturation) or increased epidermal turnover rate (leading to hyperkeratosis).

DIAGNOSIS

The diagnosis is essentially based on identification of lesions both clinically and histopathologically in an animal of a breed that is at risk, an animal that has a current history of nutritional inadequacy (high in phytates, high iron-content drinking water), or an animal with chronic diarrhea.

DIFFERENTIAL DIAGNOSIS

- Hepatocutaneous syndrome
- Dermatophytosis
- Generic dog food disease (nutritionally deficient diets)
- Demodicosis
- Pemphigus foliaceus

INITIAL DATABASE

- Skin scrapings: generally negative
- Fungal culture: expect negative result
- If diarrhea is noted, perform fecal flotation and any additional appropriate testing

ADVANCED OR CONFIRMATORY TESTING

Skin biopsy: epidermal hyperkeratosis; parakeratotic hyperkeratosis is the most common finding, and follicular parakeratosis is highly suggestive

TREATMENT

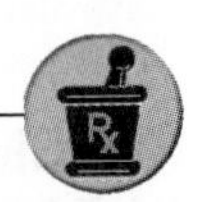

THERAPEUTIC GOAL(S)

- Eliminate scaling
- Eliminate secondary microbial dermatitis

ACUTE GENERAL TREATMENT

- Assess and correct dietary deficiencies.
- Treat secondary bacterial or yeast dermatitis (see Pyoderma, p 930; *Malassezia* Dermatitis, p 664).
- Antiseborrheic shampoos to remove scales and crusts.
- Syndrome I: Supplementation is recommended at 1–3 mg/kg of elemental zinc daily. Zinc gluconate (generic) 5 mg/kg PO q 24h, or zinc sulfate 10 mg/kg PO q 24h. Response to treatment is usually noted within 6 weeks. Lifelong treatment is required.
- Syndrome II: Correct diet. Lesions improve within 2 to 6 weeks in most cases. Some animals require zinc supplementation.
- Essential fatty acid supplementation (omega-3 and omega-6) may aid zinc absorption.

CHRONIC TREATMENT

- It has been suggested that low (0.15 mg/kg PO q 24h) doses of prednisone or prednisolone can be added to the regimen to aid gastrointestinal (GI) absorption if response is inadequate. Improved response may also be due to an anti-inflammatory effect on the skin.
- Different forms of zinc may be tried if there is poor response to therapy. It has been suggested that IV sterile zinc sulfate administration (10–15 mg/kg diluted 1:1 with saline) may help animals that do not respond to oral supplementation (due to poor intestinal absorption). Treat weekly for at least 4 weeks (monitor with electrocardiogram [ECG] when administering), then every 1 to 6 months as maintenance.

DRUG INTERACTIONS

- Zinc salts may reduce the absorption of some fluoroquinolones and chelate oral tetracycline, reducing the absorption of zinc.

- Penicillamine and ursodiol may inhibit zinc absorption.

POSSIBLE COMPLICATIONS

- Emesis: zinc in the form of methionine or acetate may be less likely to cause stomach irritation. If vomiting occurs, lower the dose or give with food.
- Large doses of zinc can inhibit copper absorption in the intestine. Carefully consider the use of zinc in copper deficient animals.
- IV zinc sulfate treatment may result in cardiac arrhythmias.

PROGNOSIS AND OUTCOME

- Syndrome I: fair to good prognosis in most animals
- Syndrome II: excellent prognosis if cause is of dietary origin

PEARLS & CONSIDERATIONS

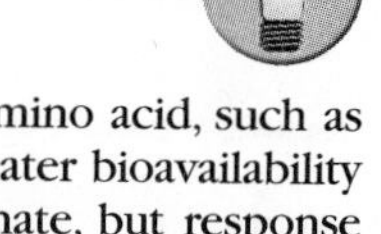

COMMENTS

- Zinc chelated as an amino acid, such as methionine, offers greater bioavailability than sulfate or gluconate, but response has been noted using all forms. If one form is not working, try another.
- Zinc plus linoleic acid (e.g., safflower oil) has been shown to improve skin and coat condition in normal dogs eating a properly balanced diet.

CLIENT EDUCATION

- Syndrome I: animals should not be used for breeding purposes
- Syndrome II: nutritional counseling on benefits of feeding good quality diets

SUGGESTED READING

Columbini S: Canine zinc responsive dermatosis. *Vet Clin North Am Small Anim Pract* 29(6):1373–1383, 1999.

White SD, et al: Zinc-responsive dermatosis in dogs: 41 cases and literature review. *Vet Dermatol* 12:101–109, 2001.

AUTHOR: **STEPHEN WAISGLASS**
EDITOR: **JAN A. HALL**

SECTION II

Procedures and Techniques

EDITOR

Etienne Côté, DVM, DACVIM (Cardiology, SAIM)

Abdominal Drainage

BASIC INFORMATION

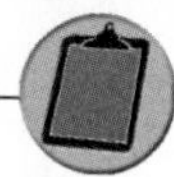

SYNONYM(S)

Large-volume abdominal paracentesis
Peritoneal drainage

OVERVIEW AND GOAL(S)

To evacuate large-volume ascites via percutaneous placement of a sterile tube into the abdomen

INDICATIONS

- Tense ascites caused by chronic passive congestion (right heart failure, chronic hepatopathies)
- Abdominal compartment syndrome

CONTRAINDICATIONS

- Hemoabdomen: voids autotransfusion; delays control of cause of hemoabdomen
- Coagulopathy: risk of hemorrhage if laceration of abdominal organ occurs with needle tip

EQUIPMENT, ANESTHESIA

- Local anesthesia.
- Manual restraint; sedation needed only rarely. NOTE: Animals often are restless during restraint due to pressure of ascites on diaphragm; in such cases, the procedure may be preceded by large-volume needle centesis or may need to be performed with the animal in standing position.
- Hair clippers.
- Surgical scrub solution, rubbing alcohol, and gauze/sponge for prepping skin.
- Use 0.5–15 ml 2% lidocaine for local anesthesia. The volume is based on body weight, 1–70 kg. Discomfort from lidocaine infusion can be reduced by adding 0.05–0.2 ml sodium bicarbonate for injection (8.4% = 84 mg/ml = 1 mEq/L) and by warming solution to body temperature (armpit method).
- Alligator forceps (preferable) or mosquito hemostats, 1 pair (Fig. II-1B).
- Red rubber feeding tube: sterile 5–16 Fr tube, based on body size (Fig. II-1C).
- Sterile surgical gloves.
- Suture material (e.g., nylon 2-0) and needle (Fig. II-1D),
- A #11 sterile scalpel blade (Fig. II-1E).
- Sterile needle holders (Fig. II-1F).
- Sterile suture scissors.
- Elizabethan collar.
- Sterile gauze squares (postprocedure).
- Tissue glue (postprocedure).

ANTICIPATED TIME

15 to 40 minutes, plus drainage time

PREPARATION: IMPORTANT CHECKPOINTS

- Weigh animal immediately before procedure (to quantify volume of fluid lost)
- Advise owner of possible drawbacks:
  - Hair clipping required
  - Procedure generally palliative; underlying problem not corrected
  - Low risk of infection or other complications
- Have Elizabethan collar ready to place on the animal as soon as procedure is complete

POSSIBLE COMPLICATIONS AND COMMON ERRORS TO AVOID

- Overall, complications very uncommon; approximately 5–10% incidence of irritation or dehiscence of incision, responding to topical treatment. Major complications are <1%.
- Concerns for hypovolemia, hypotension, hypoalbuminemia, and ascending bacterial peritonitis appear unjustified given lack of occurrence in large case series (unpublished data).
- Elizabethan collar must be on the animal at all times during drainage to avoid self-induced damage to the tube.
- Once in place in the standing animal, the tube ± stopcock may be caught in the grate flooring of the cage when the animal lies down. Covering the grate on the floor of the cage with towels helps prevent this complication.

PROCEDURE

- Clip hair widely (ventral abdomen), with umbilicus approximately at center of clipped area. Since the procedure does not require surgical draping, long hair must be trimmed back extensively.
- Restrain in lateral recumbency.
- Wide surgical scrub and prep, centered on ventral abdominal midline and just cranial to the umbilicus.
- Lidocaine infusion at planned point of entry; on abdominal midline, generally just cranial to the umbilicus. Use multiple (e.g., six to eight) small subcutaneous boluses.
- NOTE: More cranial is better in most males (greater distance from prepuce, so less risk of contamination), but it is important to avoid too cranial in animals with hepatomegaly (right-sided heart failure, some liver diseases).
- NOTE: Lidocaine infusion must be wide (cranial-caudal, left-right) and deep (reaching all layers, including peritoneum) and involves injecting many small pockets of lidocaine throughout the region of the planned incision.
- CAUTION: Avoid subcutaneous tissue laceration with the needle tip. After each infiltration of a small pocket of lidocaine, partially withdraw the needle, redirect it, and then readvance it for the next infiltration. The multiple infiltrations can all be accomplished via a single point of needle entry (i.e., radial redirection of the needle).
- After opening the sterile gloves, keep the paper wrapper flat and use as a

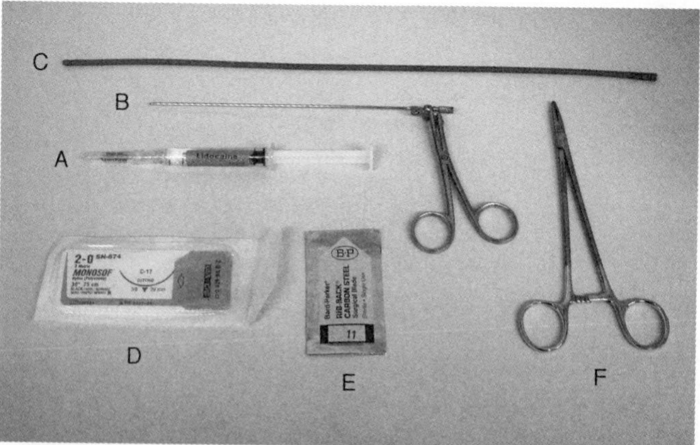

FIGURE II-1 Equipment and materials used for abdominal drainage. **A,** 0.5–15 ml 2% lidocaine for local anesthesia. **B,** Alligator forceps. **C,** Sterile red rubber feeding tube 5–16 Fr gauge. **D,** Suture material (e.g., nylon 2-0) and needle. **E,** #11 sterile scalpel blade. **F,** Sterile needle holders.

sterile surface. Wear the sterile gloves from this point onward. Use the suture scissors for making three to five additional drainage holes in the red rubber feeding tube to avoid omental plugging during drainage.

- NOTE: To make extra holes prior to inserting the tube into the abdomen, kink the red rubber feeding tube with thumb and forefinger and snip off the corner of the folded edge; unfolded edge reveals a small oval hole (needs to be <50% of tube's circumference to prevent weakening it). Repeat to make several holes along the distal half of the tube. The suture scissors are kept sterile for later in the procedure.
- Using the #11 scalpel blade, make a stab incision cranial to the umbilicus on the ventral abdominal midline, at the center of the lidocaine-infiltrated area.
- NOTE: To avoid an excessively large incision, hold the #11 scalpel blade between the thumb and forefinger. The point at which the blade is held between the thumb and forefinger leaves a maximal width of the exposed blade that is the same as, or just slightly greater than, the diameter of the red rubber feeding tube to be inserted; that is, the fingertips act as a guard to prevent excessive insertion of the blade. For example, if a 10 Fr red rubber feeding tube will be used (approximate outer diameter of tube is 6 mm), then the scalpel blade should be held such that the maximum exposed width of the blade (at the fingertips) is 6 or 7 mm.
- The blade is set aside but kept sterile in case enlargement of the incision is necessary.
- The tube is inserted into the abdomen. Tube insertion is facilitated by grasping the tip in the lower jaw of an alligator forceps, closing the forceps, and advancing tube and forceps through the hole. Mosquito forceps are an acceptable alternative. Often, the hole in the skin and the hole in the body wall are not exactly aligned due to imperceptible shifting of the tissue planes. Blunt probing with the tube and forceps may be necessary to find the hole in the abdominal wall. If excessive pressure is required, the incision may need to be enlarged using the #11 scalpel blade.
- Any sign of discomfort on the animal's part is an indication for additional lidocaine infiltration at and around the insertion site.
- Once the tube is inserted appropriately (a release of pressure may be apparent as the tube pierces the peritoneum and then experience voluminous flow of ascites), it is advanced until it protrudes from the abdominal wall by only 1–2 inches (several cm).
- The tube is sutured in place, using 2-0 or 3-0 nylon, with both a circumferential purse string and a transfixation (suture through the tube) ligature.
- If a rapid flow of fluid occurs, a clamp or partially closed three-way stopcock (usually requiring a "Christmas tree" type of adapter to fit most red rubber feeding tubes) can be used for moderating the rate of flow.
- Complete drainage is possible in minutes (often 15–20 minutes) or 2–6 hours (animal is placed in a cage with a grated floor to allow drainage and if towels are placed on top of the grate to prevent a clamp/stopcock from becoming caught in the grate).
- CAUTION: An Elizabethan collar is essential for preventing the animal from chewing at, and transecting, the tube.
- The system may be closed (drainage bag) or open; if open, as is done most commonly, the animal must be monitored for ongoing drainage, and the tube needs to be removed immediately when flow ceases, to reduce the risk of ascending infection.
- When drainage has ended, the animal is again restrained in lateral recumbency, and the nylon ligatures are cut. The tube is removed, taking care not to withdraw omentum. The skin incision may be dried with a sterile gauze, and tissue glue may be applied to close it. If the incision is >5 mm, a skin suture or staple may be placed.

POSTPROCEDURE

- Weigh the animal; record weight of lost fluid (for future reference and also to know accurate lean body weight for medication dosages).
- Dripping of ascitic fluid from incision is common despite tissue glue and generally resolves in minutes to hours. If it is persistent, a skin suture or staple may be necessary.
- Dripping and any subcutaneous pooling of ascetic fluid are minimized by allowing complete rather than partial drainage during procedure.

ALTERNATIVES AND THEIR RELATIVE MERITS

Abdominocentesis with needle and syringe:

- Less invasive
- Very time-consuming for large volumes (e.g., 1 L or more)
- Generally ineffective at removing most or all of ascites

AUTHOR: **ETIENNE CÔTÉ**

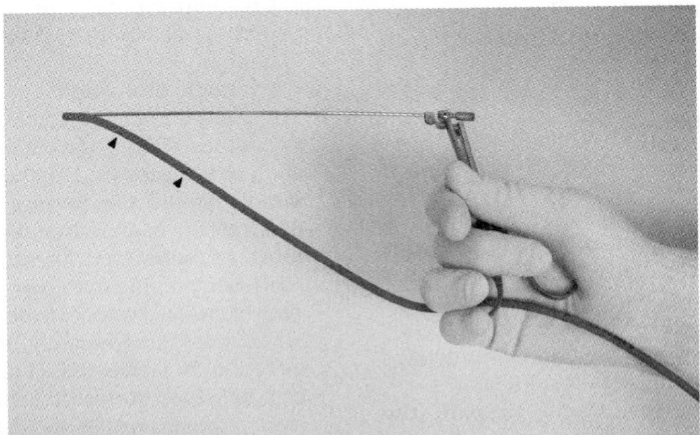

FIGURE II-2 A sterile red rubber feeding tube with additional holes in its distal part (*arrowheads*). This tube is grasped in the jaws of the alligator forceps, which allows the tube to be passed into the abdominal cavity through a small incision on the ventral abdominal midline.

Abdominocentesis

BASIC INFORMATION

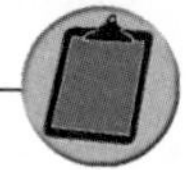

SYNONYM(S)

Abdominal paracentesis
Abdominal tap
Belly tap

OVERVIEW AND GOAL(S)

To use a needle and syringe to obtain a sample of abdominal fluid

INDICATIONS

- Visible abdominal distention with palpable fluid wave
- Ultrasound-detected ascites
- Generally diagnostic, not therapeutic (versus abdominal drainage as already described, p 1176)

CONTRAINDICATIONS

- Abdominal enlargement due to mass or organomegaly, without ascites, because of risk of organ damage without benefit of fluid retrieval for analysis
- Bleeding disorders

EQUIPMENT, ANESTHESIA

- Procedure is done with manual restraint only and without anesthesia (local or general), except in fractious or excited animals.
- NOTE: Animals may be distressed during restraint due to pressure of large-volume ascites on the diaphragm; in such cases, sedation should not be administered, but rather the procedure may be performed with the animal in lateral recumbency or in standing position.
- Hair clippers.
- Surgical scrub solution, rubbing alcohol, and gauze/sponge for prepping skin.
- Six to ten 4 × 4 inch gauze pads.
- Needles (one to five; 2 inches long; 20, 22, or 25 gauge based on animal size and body wall thickness). A 22-gauge needle is generally preferred.
- Syringes (one to three; 6 cc or greater).
- Sterile tubes for cytologic examination and fluid analysis (red and lavender tops).
- Ultrasound guidance optional.

ANTICIPATED TIME

About 1 to 10 minutes

PREPARATION: IMPORTANT CHECKPOINTS

- Assess for risk of coagulopathy if indicated overtly (e.g., epistaxis, hematuria, melena, petechiae/ecchymoses) or suspected via primary diagnosis (e.g., hepatopathy)
- Use ultrasound guidance if necessary for small volumes of ascites
- Advise owner of possible complications, as listed in the following paragraphs

POSSIBLE COMPLICATIONS AND COMMON ERRORS TO AVOID

- "Dry tap," no fluid withdrawn: insufficient abdominal fluid (check with ultrasound); fluid is too viscous or particulate (change needle and syringe because clot may be in needle; check fluid appearance with ultrasound); wrong area was sampled (change animal's posture or site of centesis).
- Centesis nonrepresentative of underlying process: assess for extra-abdominal causes of ascites, such as cardiovascular, hypoalbuminemia, and vasculitis as indicated, and pursue primary intra-abdominal causes further, beginning with abdominal ultrasound. If negative, consider nonexfoliating intra-abdominal disease.
- Laceration of organ with needle tip. Decrease risk with:
  - Good animal restraint (sedation if animal is fractious or excited)
  - Ultrasound guidance if volume of ascites is small
  - Single-dimensional, in-out motion of needle with minimal or no redirecting
- Pooling of ascitic fluid subcutaneously postprocedure; usually resolves on its own

PROCEDURE

- Place animal in dorsal recumbency or lateral recumbency. If dyspnea is present, lateral recumbency is preferable. Very small, dyspneic animals (cats, toy breed dogs) that are cooperative may be restrained in an upright sitting position ("begging" posture) in a technician's arms; muzzling is recommended due to proximity to technician.
- Aseptically scrub and prepare the clipped area, which typically will be on the midline just cranial or just caudal to the umbilicus. Position adjusted according to any known risk (e.g., cavitated abdominal mass in that location).
- Advance needle through skin and body wall, directing the needle cranially and dorsally into the abdomen. The needle is meant to pass through the linea alba/body wall slightly obliquely, such that the tract left when the needle is removed can close on itself. The obliquity comes from the dorsocranial orientation of the needle on the midline instead of direct dorsal orientation.
- Once tip of needle is just under the skin, pull back on plunger intermittently or continuously and observe for fluid "flashback" into syringe.
- Depth of penetration (2-3 mm to 3 cm) is relative to the animal's size and amount of body fat.
- Once fluid flow is established, the desired amount of fluid can be aspirated, and then the needle is withdrawn from the abdomen smoothly and quickly.
- Immediate tests that can be performed include:
  - Visual inspection for turbidity and color. NOTE: Hemorrhagic samples that have any hematocrit >5% appear equally red.
  - Odor; foul smell commonly associated with anaerobic infections. NOTE: Be aware of the possibility of airborne zoonoses if applicable (e.g., systemic fungal, other), and avoid assessing odor in such cases.
  - Hematocrit: compare to peripheral blood to rule out hemorrhage.
  - Total protein: compare to peripheral blood to rule out hemorrhage, exudative process.
  - Creatinine, potassium: compare to peripheral blood to rule out uroabdomen.
  - Cytologic evaluation.
- The fluid should be fractionated into two tubes (EDTA [lavender-top tube] and sterile glass [red-top tube]), and a sample should also be saved on a sterile swab for bacterial culture. The two tubes are submitted for standard fluid analysis including cytologic evaluation. The bacterial swab can be submitted for culture immediately if bacterial infection is suspected clinically, or it can be saved for later submission in case cytologic results indicate the possibility of bacterial infection.

POSTPROCEDURE

Subcutaneous pooling of ascitic fluid is common with partial drainage of large volume ascites; may resolve spontaneously or require abdominal wrap (barring dyspnea)

ALTERNATIVES AND THEIR RELATIVE MERITS

- Repeat centesis under ultrasound guidance
  - Better ability to reach small pockets of ascites
- Diagnostic peritoneal lavage
  - Increases ability to sample small volumes of ascites
  - Often poorly diagnostic, somewhat cumbersome
  - Generally replaced by ultrasound-guided centesis
- Laparoscopy or exploratory laparotomy for nonexfoliating, primary intra-abdominal disorders causing ascites
  - Definitive diagnosis for abdominal masses, mesothelioma/carcinomatosis, and other such conditions

AUTHOR: **ETIENNE CÔTÉ**

PROCEDURES AND TECHNIQUES

Angiogram, Nonselective

BASIC INFORMATION

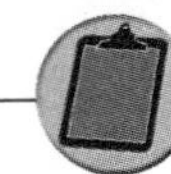

SYNONYM(S)

Nonselective radiographic contrast study of the heart

OVERVIEW AND GOAL(S)

To perform an IV contrast study that highlights the venous return to the heart and the right-sided cardiac structures

INDICATIONS

- Suspected venous obstruction (see Cranial Vena Cava Syndrome, p 256)
- Ill-defined abnormalities of the right side of the heart when echocardiography is equivocal or unavailable
- Pulmonary thromboembolism: rarely diagnostic as a nonselective procedure (often requires power-injected contrast through large-bore catheter in pulmonary artery)

CONTRAINDICATIONS

- Lesions that are equally or better defined without the administration of contrast (i.e., via echocardiography).
- Hypersensitivity to contrast material.
- Acute renal failure (decreased ability to excrete contrast material and/or risk of contrast-induced renal failure).
- Arteriovenous (AV) fistulae are not an indication for this procedure. AV fistulae shunt from artery to vein and require selective arteriography.

EQUIPMENT, ANESTHESIA

- Can be done with or without anesthesia; sedation in most patients (see end pages inside text cover).
- Hair clippers.
- Surgical scrub solution, rubbing alcohol, and gauze/sponge for prepping skin.
- IV catheter (jugular or peripheral).
  - A 19- or 20-gauge catheter for cats or small dogs; a 16- or 18-gauge catheter for medium or large dogs.
- The catheter cap or T-port should be a screw tip to avoid detachment under high pressure of contrast injection.
- ± Sterile surgical gloves if using a non-sheathed jugular catheter.
- ± Lidocaine for local anesthesia if large jugular catheter (e.g., 18 gauge or larger).
- Routine tape and bandage material for catheter fixation to skin.
- ± Suture material (e.g., 3-0 nylon), needle holders, and suture scissors if anchoring jugular catheter to skin of neck.
- Syringe for IV contrast material. A syringe with a screw tip is recommended to avoid pressure-induced separation of the syringe from the T-port or catheter cap during high-pressure injection of contrast.
- Transparent, aqueous IV contrast material (iodinated, ionic; e.g., Renograffin 76, Renovist 69%, Hypaque M 75, Conray 60%); maximal total cumulative dose given during procedure, assuming maintenance IV fluid administration to promote diuresis: 3 ml/kg.
- Radiographic facility, including radiographic machine, films and cassette, and developer and/or fluoroscopic unit.

ANTICIPATED TIME

About 15 to 30 minutes after catheter placement

PREPARATION: IMPORTANT CHECKPOINTS

- Thoracic radiographs: must precede contrast study, because a diagnosis may be apparent from these alone.
- Congestive heart failure must be controlled prior to procedure.
- Clipping of hair over vein to be catheterized (typically jugular or cephalic; jugular may be preferable in small animals (<10 kg) because the cephalic can be too small to allow easy flow of viscous contrast solution through catheter.
- A 12-hour fast if sedating animal.
- Placement of IV catheter.
- Discuss possible complications with owner. As indicated in the following paragraphs (see Jugular Catheter Placement and Management, p 1270).

POSSIBLE COMPICATIONS AND COMMON ERRORS TO AVOID

Nondiagnostic study; improve likelihood of diagnostic result by:

- Using large-diameter catheter
- Using fluoroscopy instead of serial radiographs
- Injecting contrast rapidly
- Injecting adequate volume of contrast

PROCEDURE

- Catheter patency is checked.
- Animal is placed on radiographic table, usually in lateral recumbency.
- Position of radiographic beam is set over area of interest (usually thorax, neck, or limb).
- Contrast is injected IV by hand as quickly as possible (maximal manual pressure). Recommended single dose is 1–2 ml/kg (440 mg iodine/kg).
- Radiographic views are obtained at the appropriate times (Table II-1), or the flow of contrast is observed in real-time with fluoroscopy.

POSTPROCEDURE

IV fluid diuresis is provided if appropriate. The goal is to increase excretion of contrast medium, but excessive volume load must be avoided if heart disease exists.

ALTERNATIVES AND THEIR RELATIVE MERITS

- An echocardiogram and thoracic radiographs should be performed prior to angiography:
  - Noninvasive, excellent diagnostic yield
- Vascular ultrasound:

TABLE II-1*

Site enhanced by contrast	Dog Time (sec) from start of injection	Cat Time (sec) from start of injection
Cranial vena cava	1-2.5	0.5-1.5
Right ventricle	2-3	1.5-2.5
Pulmonary arteries	2-3	1.5-2.5
Left atrium	4-5.5	4.5-7
Left ventricle	4.5-6	5-7
Aorta	4.5-6.5	5-7

*Adapted from Wise M: Nonselective angiocardiography in the normal dog and cat. *Vet Radiol* 23:144-151, 1982.

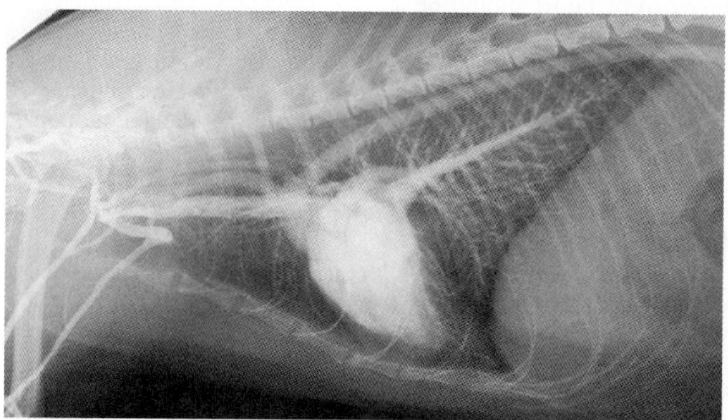

FIGURE II-3 Lateral nonselective angiogram in a normal cat. The contrast was injected in a cephalic vein; the right side of the heart and pulmonary circulation are opacified, and early opacification of the left side of the heart and aorta is also seen. Courtesy of Dr. Brett Kantrowitz.

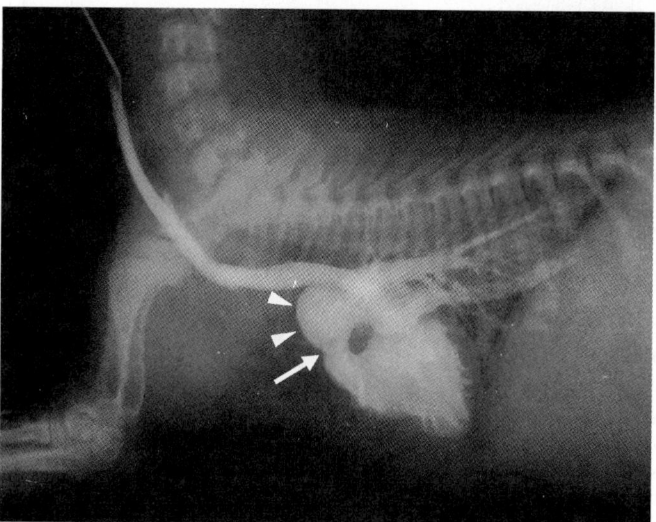

FIGURE II-4 Lateral nonselective angiogram in a dog with valvular pulmonic stenosis. The contrast was injected in a jugular vein. Narrowing (stenosis) is seen at the level of the pulmonic valve (*arrow*). Marked poststenotic dilatation of the pulmonary trunk is apparent (*arrowheads*). Courtesy of Dr. Brett Kantrowitz.

- ◦ Noninvasive but limited by lungs: poor visualization of intrathoracic vessels
- Arterial blood gas (ABG) analysis:
  - ◦ If pulmonary vascular disease
- Selective angiography/cardiac catheterization:
  - ◦ If cardiac or pulmonary vascular lesion still unclear

AUTHORS: **ETIENNE CÔTÉ, BRETT KANTROWITZ**

Arterial Blood Sampling and Arterial Catheterization

BASIC INFORMATION

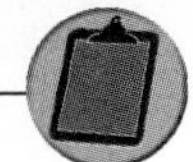

SYNONYM(S)

Arterial phlebotomy
Arterial puncture

OVERVIEW AND GOAL(S)

To access the peripheral artery with a needle or catheter, typically for arterial blood gas (ABG) analysis or for arterial blood pressure (BP) monitoring, respectively

INDICATIONS

- Assessment of ABG and acid-base status, usually in animals with systemic illness or a respiratory problem
- Placement of an arterial catheter for BP measurement, usually in critically ill or anesthetized animals

CONTRAINDICATIONS

Bleeding disorder: assess for overt signs of bleeding or historic evidence of bleeding

EQUIPMENT, ANESTHESIA

Sedation or general anesthesia not usually required; manual restraint only. One or two assistants may be needed.

- Hair clippers
- Sterile scrub material
- Six to ten 3 × 3 inch gauze squares

Arterial catheter:

- Standard over-the-needle IV-type catheter
  - Cats, dogs <10 kg: 24 or 25 gauge.
  - Dogs 10–25 kg: 22 gauge.
  - Dogs >25 kg: 20 gauge.
- White tape, 2 cm (1 inch) width
- Heparinized sterile saline flush
- Pressure transducer and monitor (if continuously monitoring direct arterial pressure)

Arterial blood sample (one time):

- 1-ml heparinized syringe
- Needles (guidelines for size: same as for arterial catheters as already described)

ANTICIPATED TIME

- About 5 minutes (arterial blood sample)
- About 10 to 15 minutes (arterial catheter)

PREPARATION: IMPORTANT CHECKPOINTS

- Thoracic radiographs are indicated prior to, or concurrently with, ABG sampling when the purpose of arterial sampling is to assess arterial oxygen or CO_2 levels.
- Samples for venous blood gas measurement generally are easier to obtain and may be useful for measuring certain parameters in arterial blood (e.g., pH, pCO_2, HCO_3^-).
- Confirmation of normal platelet count.
- Confirmation of absence of overt signs of bleeding disorders or historic evidence of bleeding.

POSSIBLE COMPLICATIONS AND COMMON ERRORS TO AVOID

- Pressing excessively firmly on the artery when palpating for the pulse to locate the proper site for puncture; excessive pressure abolishes the pulse and makes accurate puncture virtually impossible.
- Inserting the needle or catheter without having convincingly identified the course of the artery (by repeated palpation of the arterial pulse).
- Crossing both artery and vein with the needle, resulting in venous contamination of arterial sample (artifactual low pO_2 result).
- Mistakenly advancing the needle or catheter with the bevel up rather than down.
- Inadequate manual pressure on the site after the procedure.
  - Hematoma possible if inadequate direct pressure is applied after the procedure or if animal has a bleeding disorder or vasculitis.
- Artery may not be patent after arterial catheterization, but the effect of this loss of patency on the animal typically is minimal (limits the source of access for arterial blood samples in the immediate future, but rarely causes ischemia distal to the site of puncture).

PROCEDURE

See Figs. II-5 and II-6

- Clip hair over the area of interest (dorsal metatarsus: dorsal surface of distal hind limb, from hock to beginning of phalanges; inguinal area: femoral triangle, from inguinal crease [medial side of proximal hind limb, where thigh meets caudal abdomen] toward stifle).
- Restrain animal in lateral recumbency (e.g., left lateral).
  - Dorsal metatarsal arterial approach:
    - Right-handed clinician: fully extend animal's hock by drawing paw of upper hind limb (right paw, if animal is in left lateral recumbency) toward self using the left hand.
    - While keeping leg extended using traction on the right hind paw with the left hand, palpate the dorsal metatarsal pulse with the tips

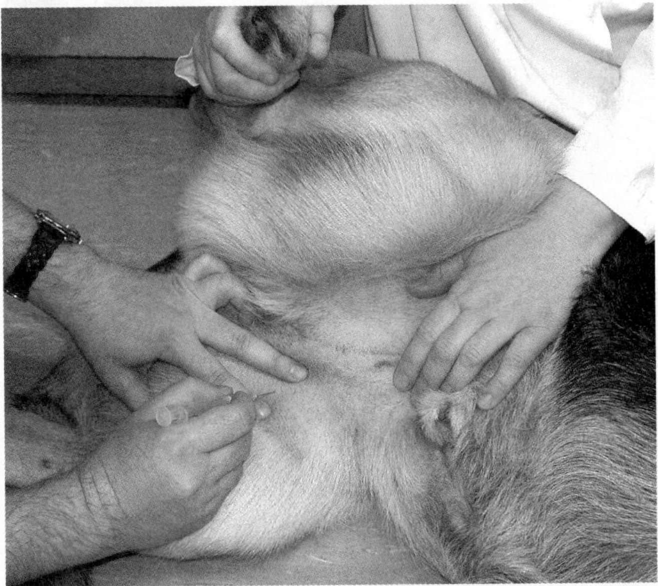

FIGURE II-5 Blood sample from the femoral artery, dog in left lateral recumbency. Cranial is to the lower right. While an assistant holds the right hind limb elevated and the prepuce retracted, the phlebotomist identifies the course of the left femoral artery between the middle and index fingers by palpation of the femoral pulse with both fingers and prepares to enter the artery with the needle, bevel down.

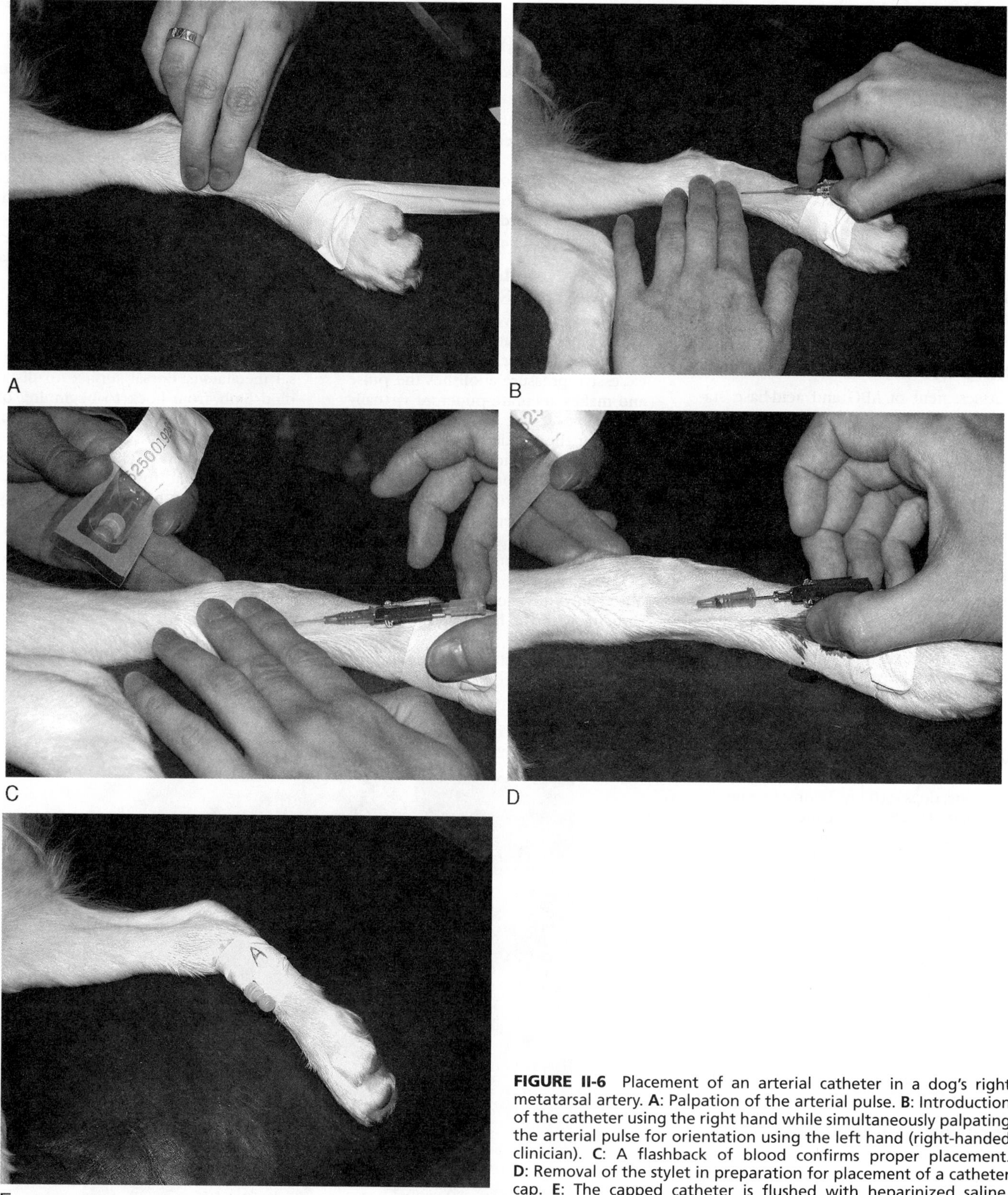

FIGURE II-6 Placement of an arterial catheter in a dog's right metatarsal artery. **A**: Palpation of the arterial pulse. **B**: Introduction of the catheter using the right hand while simultaneously palpating the arterial pulse for orientation using the left hand (right-handed clinician). **C**: A flashback of blood confirms proper placement. **D**: Removal of the stylet in preparation for placement of a catheter cap. **E**: The capped catheter is flushed with heparinized saline, wrapped, and clearly marked as arterial.

of the index and middle fingers of the right hand on the dorsal surface of the right metatarsus. The pulse lies between the third and fourth metatarsal bones (see Fig. II-6).

- Palpating the dorsal metatarsal pulse simultaneously with two fingers reveals the course of the dorsal metatarsal artery.
- CAUTION: The course of the metatarsal artery must be identified convincingly by repeated palpation of the dorsal metatarsal pulse before beginning to insert the needle or catheter.
  - Both dorsal metatarsal and femoral approach.

- Continue as described for both dorsal metatarsal and femoral arterial approaches in the upcoming step: Repeat brief aseptic scrubbing procedure.
  - Femoral arterial approach:
    - Right-handed clinician: Fully extend the animal's dependent hind limb (e.g., left hind leg, if in left lateral recumbency) to expose the medial inguinal area of that leg. In cooperative (or anesthetized) cats and dogs, the leg may be restrained minimally or not at all. In recalcitrant animals, a second restrainer is needed to hold the leg in an extended, stable position.
    - Palpate the femoral pulse at its dorsal-most location, near the inguinal crease. It should be palpated with the tips of the index and middle fingers of the right hand (for a right-handed clinician). The femoral artery lies midway between the cranial-most and caudal-most aspects of the thigh, at the usual location for palpation during physical examination.
    - Palpating the pulse of a femoral artery simultaneously with two fingers 1–2 cm apart reveals the course of the femoral artery, namely a straight line between the two points on the artery where the pulse is palpated (i.e., between the two fingers).
    - CAUTION: This line (the artery) must be identified convincingly by repeated palpation of the femoral pulse before beginning to insert the needle or catheter.
  - Both dorsal metatarsal and femoral approach.
    - Repeat brief aseptic scrubbing procedure once pulse has been palpated satisfactorily.
    - There is no need for the assistant to "hold off" or "raise" the vessel as is done for venous samples because of the normal arterial pressure.
    - The syringe (with needle) is held in the right hand in the same way a pen is held (see Figs. II-5 and II-6). It enters the skin obliquely at 45 degrees. If placing an arterial catheter, the 45-degree angle between skin and catheter is also necessary, but the catheter is held the same way an IV catheter is normally held (see Fig. II-6).
    - The bevel of the needle/catheter points down, not up (contrary to venous blood samples and IV catheters).
    - The needle is introduced under the skin and into the artery, again advancing while maintaining a 45-degree angle between the syringe and the vessel.
    - A flashback of blood indicates successful entry into the artery. Pulsatile flow is visible when an uncapped catheter is used. With a needle and syringe, arterial pressure will slowly but steadily "self-fill" the syringe, and negative pressure (as with a venous blood sample) is not necessary.
    - Typically, a sample for ABG analysis requires approximately 0.5 ml of blood, which should be placed in an ice bath if analysis in the following 10 minutes is not possible.
    - An arterial catheter should be fixed in place and either capped and flushed, or it should be connected to a pressure transducer for pressure measurement. It should be identified clearly with a label as being arterial.

POSTPROCEDURE

Successful outcome:

- Successful arterial puncture for blood gas measurement improves animal care via treatment adjustments.
- Successful arterial catheter placement improves animal care via minute-by-minute adjustments of factors that influence arterial BP (e.g., IV fluids, pressor drugs, anesthetic agents) in anesthetized or critically ill animals.

ALTERNATIVES AND THEIR RELATIVE MERITS

- Repeat thoracic radiographs:
  - Noninvasive; provides information on lesions of respiratory system only. Minimal usefulness for assessing subtle, moment-by-moment changes
- Venous blood gas analysis:
  - Sampling is easier
  - Few other advantages over arterial blood, unhelpful regarding pO_2
- Arterial cutdown for arterial blood sampling:
  - Easier access to vessel
  - More invasive

AUTHOR: **ETIENNE CÔTÉ**

PROCEDURES AND TECHNIQUES

Arthrocentesis

BASIC INFORMATION

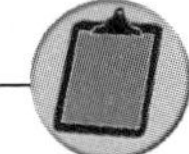

SYNONYM(S)

Joint tap
Joint aspirate
Synovial tap

OVERVIEW AND GOAL(S)

To use a needle and syringe and obtain a sample of fluid from a synovial (joint) space for analysis

INDICATIONS

- Joint pain (arthralgia)
- Joint swelling, joint effusion
- Radiographic evidence of joint disease
- As part of evaluation of nonspecific systemic signs

CONTRAINDICATIONS

Severe coagulopathy (risk of hemarthrosis)

EQUIPMENT, ANESTHESIA

- Generally performed with mild sedation but not local or general anesthesia.
- Skilled clinicians sometimes use no sedation or anesthesia unless the animal shows signs of resentment or discomfort.
- The procedure may be performed during general anesthesia if the animal is anesthetized for another reason.
- Hair clippers.
- Surgical scrub solution, rubbing alcohol, and gauze/sponge for prepping skin.
- Six to ten 4 × 4 inch gauze pads.
- Microscope slides (at least 10), cleaned and spread out on a table or tray.
- Five to ten sterile needles (20, 22, or 23 gauge, depending on the animal's size).
- Three or four sterile syringes (1, 3, or 6 cc).
- Red-top test tube.
- Lavender-top test tube.
- Sterile culture swab.
- Sterile gloves.

ANTICIPATED TIME

About 10 to 30 minutes

PREPARATION: IMPORTANT CHECKPOINTS

- The joints to be aspirated should be clearly identified in the medical record.

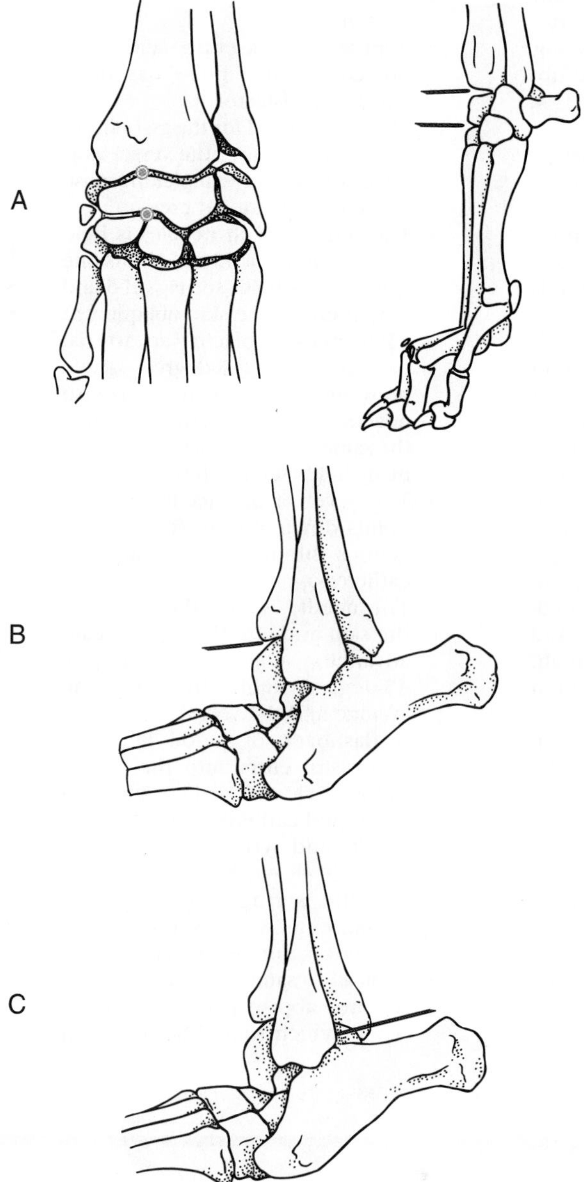

FIGURE II-7 Schematic representation of recommended sites for arthrocentesis in the dog and cat. **A,** Carpus: partially flex joint. Palpate and enter anteromedial aspect of carpometacarpal or radiocarpal space. **B,** Hock: cranial approach. Palpate space between tibia and tibiotarsal bone on anterolateral surface of hock; insert needle in shallow, palpable space. **C,** Hock: lateral approach. Partially flex joint and insert needle under lateral malleolus of fibula. Reprinted with permission from Nelson RW, Couto CG: *Small Animal Internal Medicine,* ed 3. Mosby, Inc., St. Louis, 2003, pp 1074, 1075.

- As a general rule, the carpi, tarsi, and stifles are the most easily accessed joints.

POSSIBLE COMPLICATIONS AND COMMON ERRORS TO AVOID

- Blood contamination of sample: very common and detrimental to obtaining accurate diagnosis. Be sure to release negative pressure on syringe before withdrawing needle from joint.
- Iatrogenic hemarthrosis: very uncommon unless underlying coagulopathy.
- Lameness induced by procedure: very rare.

PROCEDURE

- The skin is clipped and aseptically prepped over the relevant joint(s).
- Bony landmarks are palpated to have the most direct access to the joint space.
- NOTE: An important rule of thumb is to first palpate a joint in a gentle and superficial manner to find areas of gross joint swelling. When they occur, joint swellings can often be felt as soft, flocculent, "puffy" subcutaneous pockets of synovial fluid and are the easiest source of access to a joint. This is especially true for the carpi, tarsi, and stifles.

CARPUS

- On the cranial-most surface of the flexed carpus, a space is delineated by the distal radius proximally, the carpal bones distally, and the tendons of the extensor carpi radialis and common digital extensor on either side.
- The space is 2-3 mm in diameter in a medium-size dog.
- It is a natural depression that is best felt when the carpus is flexed (Fig. II-7A).
- An assistant maintains the carpus in a gently but fully flexed position to open the radiocarpal angle and increase access to the joint space during the procedure.

TARSUS

- The tarsal joint is not excessively flexed or extended.
- The caudal aspect of the tarsus presents both medial and lateral access to the tarsal joint.
- The lateral and medial malleoli of the distal tibia are palpated; immediately medial and caudal to each one is a depression in which the joint space can be accessed (Fig. II-7B).

STIFLE

- The stifle joint is not excessively flexed or extended.
- From a cranial approach, the needle is passed laterally or medially to the patellar tendon and is directed caudally and toward the center of the tibial plateau.

Once the landmarks have been established for the chosen joint(s):

- Aseptically scrub the site once more.
- Open sterile syringes onto sterile field (e.g., onto opened paper wrapper for sterile gloves).
- Put on both sterile gloves.
- With the help of an assistant, attach sterile needle to sterile syringe.
- Have assistant hold joint in the desired position to maximize access with needle.
- Palpate landmarks once more.
- Advance needle and syringe, applying gentle negative pressure with syringe once the needle tip is below the skin until synovial fluid is seen in the needle hub and syringe.
- Often, the needle tip will strike bone. If so, the pressure should be released from the syringe, and the needle tip "walked" off the bone and further into the joint space. "Walking" refers to gentle probing using the needle tip, seeking out a path of lesser resistance within a few millimeters of the site where bone was encountered. The needle is partially withdrawn—but remains below the skin surface—and is redirected and readvanced during "walking."
- When the needle tip advances without striking bone, negative pressure may be reapplied with the syringe until synovial fluid enters the hub of the needle and the syringe.
- If blood is encountered, the procedure should be stopped and then restarted with a new needle and syringe.
- At least 1 ml should be sought if possible, but many successful arthrocentesis procedures will only produce <0.5 ml of joint fluid.
- It is essential to release the negative pressure from the syringe prior to withdrawing the needle to avoid blood contamination.

POSTPROCEDURE

- Immediate assessment of the synovial fluid includes:
  - Turbidity; the fluid should be clear and pale tan or pale yellow.
  - Viscosity test; a drop of fluid placed between two slides, which are then separated, should appear somewhat viscous or gummy. Synovial fluid that has little viscosity, like water, is abnormal.
  - Odor; none is expected in normal synovial fluid. NOTE: If an airborne zoonotic organism is part of the differential diagnosis, assessing the odor may be hazardous and should be avoided.
- Laboratory samples to be submitted include (in general order of priority because volume of fluid retrieved may be small):
  - Fresh smears on microscope slides.
  - Whole fluid, in red-top tube.
  - Whole fluid, in lavender-top tube.
  - Culture swab.
- Routine sedation/anesthetic recovery as needed.

ALTERNATIVES AND THEIR RELATIVE MERITS

- Radiographs:
  - Useful for detecting subchondral bone lesions.
  - Do not replace synovial fluid analysis.
- Bone scan:
  - Identifies multiple joint involvement.
  - Identifies relative degree of severity between joints.
  - Does not give etiologic diagnosis.
- Synovial biopsy:
  - Appropriate if joint capsule is thickened or deformed (grossly, radiographically) and synovial fluid analysis is unrewarding.

AUTHOR: **ETIENNE CÔTÉ**

PROCEDURES AND TECHNIQUES

Barium Enema

SYNONYM(S)

Large bowel/rectal contrast study

OVERVIEW AND GOAL(S)

To perform a radiographic contrast procedure that provides information on the gross structure of the colon and rectum. This information generally is not available by other routine imaging means: abdominal ultrasound is limited by the presence of gas in the colon, and plain radiography cannot evaluate the mucosal surface of the colon and cannot evaluate colonic distensibility.

INDICATIONS

- Persistent tenesmus
- Pelvic canal/rectal mass effect on rectal palpation and/or on plain radiographs
- Severe constipation/obstipation not responsive to simple medical management

CONTRAINDICATIONS

NOTE: Organic iodine contrast material (e.g., sodium iothalamate, sodium diatrizoate, diluted 1:1 with water) should be used instead of barium if rectal or colonic perforation is suspected.

EQUIPMENT

- General anesthesia is usually required; otherwise, barium is often expelled from the rectum by the animal's straining.
- Enema bag/set; for smaller animals, large syringes may be used instead.
- Barium sulfate suspension with concentration 15–20% weight per volume.
- Foley urinary catheter (e.g., 10–18 Fr tube for body range of cats to large dogs, respectively) or Bardex catheter.
- Sterile, water-soluble lubricant.

ANTICIPATED TIME

Approximately 40 to 60 minutes

PREPARATION: IMPORTANT CHECKPOINTS

- Fecal occult blood testing is highly specific using o-Tolidine-based test kits and may be performed to further increase an index of suspicion for a colonic abnormality.
- Prepare an adequate volume of barium. Using too low of a barium dose is a very common problem, causing pseudolesions or missing lesions altogether.
- Barring excessive anal pain, any dog weighing 6 kg or more needs to have a simple but complete rectal palpation prior to barium enema to better localize any focal lesions.
- Animal fasted 24 hours.
- A maximum amount of feces is evacuated from the colon prior to the administration of the barium enema.
- Metastasis imaging (three-view thoracic radiographs; abdominal ultrasound to assess liver, lymph nodes, etc.) is indicated if malignancy is part of the differential diagnosis.

PROCEDURE

- Obtain preliminary abdominal radiographs to confirm adequate animal preparation (colon is as empty as possible) and to set radiographic technique. The barium contrast dose of 10 ml/kg is placed into enema reservoir.
- Lubricate catheter and insert sufficiently such that Foley balloon is well beyond the anus and within the rectum.
- Inflate Foley balloon to reduce or prevent outflow of contrast from the anus, and gently tug on catheter to bring Foley balloon to seal caudally and prevent contrast leakage from anus.
- Slowly administer barium with the animal in right lateral recumbency, using gravity for colonic filling (raise the reservoir above the animal)
- Once the colon has been distended, clamp the infusion tubing to prevent backflow of the contrast material.
- Obtain both lateral views and oblique views (45 degrees), and a ventrodorsal view (Fig. II-8).

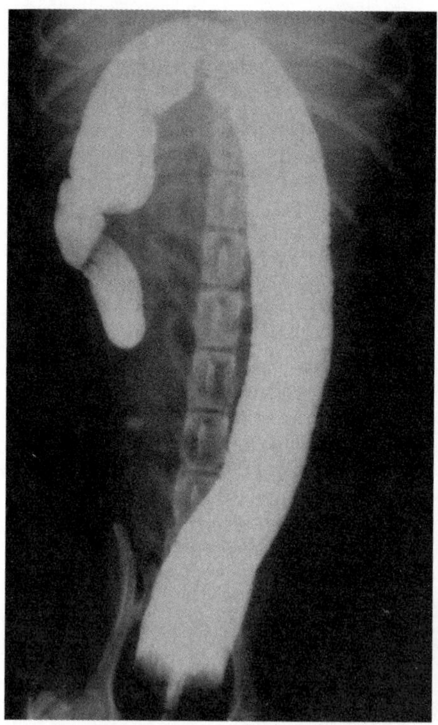

A

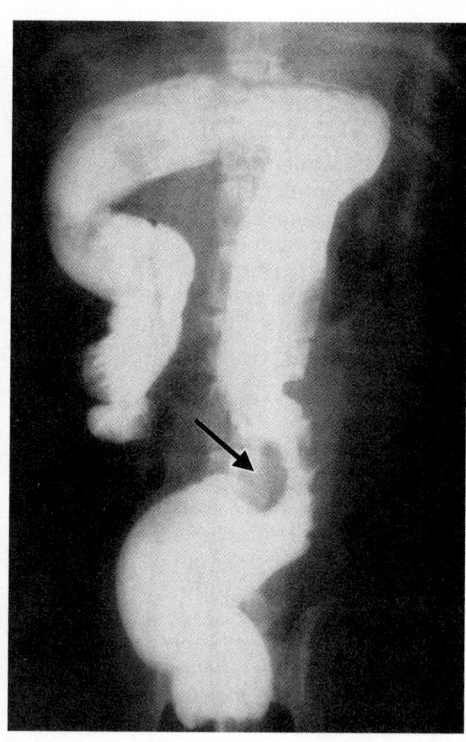

B

FIGURE II-8 **A**, Ventrodorsal projection, normal study. **B**, Ventrodorsal projection, abnormal study. A large filling defect in the distal colon (*arrow*) causes marked narrowing of the lumen, suggesting a mass lesion.

POSTPROCEDURE

- Routine anesthetic recovery.
- The clinician should tell the client that it is normal for the stools to be loose and grey or pale brown in color for several defecations after the procedure.

POSSIBLE COMPLICATIONS AND COMMON ERRORS TO AVOID

Perianal trauma and iatrogenic colonic perforation are very rare; use Foley catheter instead of rigid enema tube.

ALTERNATIVES AND THEIR RELATIVE MERITS

- Endoscopy has largely replaced barium enemas.
- Abdominal ultrasound: the potential for visualizing the structure of the colonic wall is often severely restricted by the pelvis and by presence of air in the colon.
- Plain radiographs: diagnostic test of choice for bony obstruction of the pelvic canal (fracture, malformation, mass); poor sensitivity for soft-tissue lesions of the colon.
- Colonic biopsy: diagnostic test of choice once a focal or diffuse mucosal lesion is suspected or identified.

AUTHORS: **LEEANN PACK, ETIENNE CÔTÉ**

Barium Esophagram, Dynamic

BASIC INFORMATION

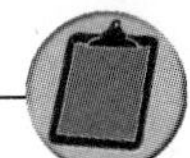

SYNONYM(S)

Barium swallow
Fluoroscopic esophagram

OVERVIEW AND GOAL(S)

To administer a contrast agent *per os* and observe the oral and pharyngeal phases of swallowing and esophageal transit using fluoroscopy. The goal of the study is to define abnormalities of swallowing and/or esophageal transit.

INDICATIONS

Functional abnormalities of swallowing (dysphagia, abnormal esophageal motility); can be used for evaluating mechanical abnormalities (mass, foreign body, extrinsic compression), but a static esophagram is usually sufficient for this purpose.

CONTRAINDICATIONS

- Evidence or risk of esophageal perforation
- Megaesophagus (not an absolute contraindication, but the study is not needed for diagnosis)

EQUIPMENT, ANESTHESIA

- Contrast agent.
  - Liquid barium (30% weight/volume and higher density)
  - Iodinated contrast agent:
    - Nonionic (iohexol, iopamidol, ioxaglate compounds)
    - Diluted 1:1 with water
- Highly palatable canned food
- Syringes for barium administration
- Bowl and utensil for mixing barium and food
- X-ray unit:
  - Fluoroscopic capability
  - Spot-film capability
  - Video recording capability
- Protective clothing (lead aprons, gloves, thyroid shields) for personnel
- Paper towels or similar for cleanup of barium on animal and x-ray table

ANTICIPATED TIME

15 to 20 minutes

PREPARATION: IMPORTANT CHECKPOINTS

- Survey films of thorax and cervical region.
  - If contraindications are present (as previously mentioned), then study should not be performed.
  - If plain films are diagnostic (i.e., megaesophagus), the study is unnecessary.
- Prepare contrast agents.
  - Barium:
    - Liquid barium in appropriately sized syringe.
    - Liquid barium mixed with canned food. Only a small amount of barium (~5 ml) is needed, which also will keep the solid consistency of the food.
  - Nonionic iodinated contrast agent:
    - Iohexol, iopamidol, ioxaglate compounds.
    - Liquid diluted 1:1.
    - Diluted liquid is mixed with canned food.
- Personnel needed for procedure (restraint and administration of contrast). This may require two to three people, depending on animal's size and temperament.
- All personnel should have appropriate lead protective apparel (aprons, thyroid shield, gloves).
- Paper towels or other barrier drapes to limit excess contrast agent on table and animal.

POSSIBLE COMPLICATIONS AND COMMON ERRORS TO AVOID

- Aspiration of contrast agent: The study is always begun with a liquid contrast agent and no food. Animals with disorders requiring these evaluations may be prone to dysphagia and aspiration of contrast. If a small amount of liquid contrast agent is aspirated, it can be coughed up. If the animal aspirates a substantial amount of liquid contrast agent, the study should be aborted.
- Ionic iodinated contrast agents: These agents should not be used because clinically significant (potentially fatal) pulmonary edema can occur if these agents are aspirated. Ionic agents include diatrizoate, iothalamate, and iodamide compounds: All must be avoided.
- Nonionic iodinated contrast agents: These agents can be used if esophageal perforation is suspected.
- Leakage of contrast agent: Evidence or risk of esophageal perforation is considered a contraindication for this study: If contrast agent leakage is suspected at any time, the study should be aborted.

Assuming that the procedure is not stopped due to aspiration of contrast agent or evidence of leakage of contrast agent, it is important to perform the study with both liquid contrast agent and liquid contrast agent mixed with food to give as full an assessment of esophageal function as possible.

Fluoroscopic procedures involve a substantial radiation dose to the animal and to personnel. Radiation safety (e.g., proper protective clothing, collimation so that personnel are not included in the primary beam) is paramount.

PROCEDURE

Dynamic esophagram: barium:

- Survey films of thorax and cervical region (already described in preparation).
- Position animal in right lateral recumbency (if a C-arm fluoroscopy unit is used, it may be possible to place the animal in sternal recumbency) with appropriate restraint.
- Activate fluoroscopy unit briefly to determine correct positioning and collimation.
- Activate the video recorder.
- Administer liquid barium *per os* (~5 ml for a cat and 5-10 ml depending on the size of the dog), and activate fluoroscopic unit; image the oral and pharyngeal phases of swallowing (progression of barium from mouth to esophagus). Repeat two to three times even if no abnormality is defined.
- Spot film any areas of abnormality; lateral views are generally sufficient.
- Repeat above procedure with barium paste (OPTIONAL).
- Administer barium and canned food mixture *per os*. Appropriately sized food balls (1-3 cm in diameter) may be fed to the animal or placed in the mouth. Activate fluoroscopic unit and image the oral and pharyngeal phases of swallowing (progression of barium and food from mouth to esophagus). Repeat two to three times even if no abnormality is defined.
- Spot film any areas of abnormality; lateral views are generally sufficient.

Dynamic esophagram: iodinated contrast agent:

- This study may be performed if esophageal rupture is suspected or if endoscopy is to be performed immediately following the esophagram. If an esophageal perforation is suspected, a static esophagram is usually performed instead, using a nonionic iodinated compound.
- The dynamic esophagram using an iodinated contrast agent follows the same procedure as the barium esophagram.

POSTPROCEDURE

No information on the oral and pharyngeal phases of swallowing

ALTERNATIVES AND THEIR RELATIVE MERITS

Static esophagram: A static esophagram (administration of barium and routine films) can be used in place of a dynamic study for certain indications. A static study does not require the use of a fluoroscopy unit and is generally sufficient for most suspected mechanical abnormalities of the esophagus (e.g., megaesophagus, esophageal foreign body, esophageal mass, esophageal stricture). However, subtle abnormalities of swallowing and esophageal transit are rarely identified in this study, and it provides no information on the pharyngeal phase of swallowing.

AUTHOR: **PATRICIA L. ROSE**

Behavioral Assessment

BASIC INFORMATION

SYNONYM(S)

Behavioral problems: misbehavior, aggression, house soiling, destructiveness, barking

OVERVIEW AND GOAL(S)

- To reestablish the owner-animal bond
- To protect the owner and the public from injury or loss of property

INDICATIONS

- Owner requests information on behavior.
- Better yet, practitioner asks the client how satisfied he or she is with the animal.
- It is often too late if the owners are already contemplating getting rid of the pet.

CONTRAINDICATIONS

If the dog or cat is very aggressive, the animal should probably be euthanized. Finding a new home for this animal is not an option. If the original owner cannot live with the animal, no one should have to.

EQUIPMENT, ANESTHESIA

- Assess-a-Hand
- Child-sized doll
- Closed-circuit television (camera and time-lapse video recorder)

ANTICIPATED TIME

About 1 hour for cats or 2 hours for dogs, including diagnosis and treatment.

PREPARATION: IMPORTANT CHECKPOINTS

- Have a history form, preferably one for each species.
- Pictures of dogs and cat in various moods are very helpful.
- Have the most commonly used tools available, as appropriate:
  - Basket muzzle
  - Gentle Leader
  - Kong dog toy
  - Catalogs or websites of less commonly recommended products

POSSIBLE COMPLICATIONS AND COMMON ERRORS TO AVOID

Dealing with aggressive animals is a hazard, so liability is great; however, it is also essential to address an owner's problems correctly or a life will be lost when the animal is euthanized.

PROCEDURE

The overall goal specifically is to determine the exact nature of the problem, resulting in appropriate intervention and prognosis when possible. With the increased use of facsimile machines and electronic mail, sending and receiving histories before the consultation is a convenient as well as time-saving strategy. A sample set of history forms can be found at www.vet.cornell.edu/abc.

1. Rule out medical disorders (e.g., urinary tract infection, feline lower urinary tract signs/disease, or ectopic ureters for soiling an area the house; metabolic, central neurologic, endocrine, or pain-producing conditions for aggression) and treat appropriately if present.
2. Clarify the nature of the environment surrounding the behavioral problem:
   - Number of people and animals in the household.
   - Amount of space at the animal's disposal, both with owners at home and when absent.
   - For cats, the location, type, and contents of litter boxes.
   - Change in the people or pets in the household or their schedules.
   - If the presenting problem is destructive behavior, soiling an area in the house, or barking, an important step is to determine whether these events occur when the owners are at home or only when they are gone.
3. Clarify the reaction of the owners and others to the animal's misbehavior. Do they punish or soothe the animal?
4. Help the owner to avoid misdirected intervention, such as punishing after the fact, rewarding the dog for aggressive behavior, or rewarding jumping up.
5. The owner should be given a reasonable treatment plan that does not involve risk to the owner or the public.
6. A detailed history should be taken carefully. A destructive dog can be used as an example.
   - When is the animal destructive?
   - Where is the animal destructive?
   - With what methods have the owners tried to address the problem?

NOTE: It is always important to maintain a neutral attitude when taking a history, because any criticism of the owners' methods at this time will probably inhibit owners from volunteering any additional information as the interview continues.

The dog's early history often gives clues regarding the cause of misbehavior:

- If the dog was obtained from a kennel at 6 months of age, it may never have been properly socialized to people during the socialization period of 7 to 14 weeks of age.
- If the dog was obtained as a 3-week-old puppy or was hand raised, it may be too dependent on people and not properly socialized with dogs.

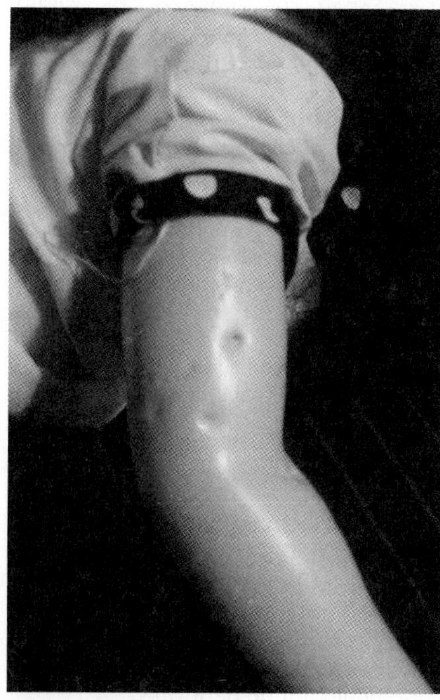

FIGURE II-9 Bite marks on a doll's arm inflicted by an aggressive dog during a behavioral assessment.

- If the dog was obtained from a pound or an animal shelter, it may have been placed there because it was destructive or aggressive in the original home.

The owners should be able to supply this information and to indicate why they obtained the animal. Hand-raised kittens are frequently presented for aggression as adults, and feral or free-ranging cats may be reluctant to remain indoors and may vocalize, claw, or spray when confined.

7. NOTE: Canine aggression is much more complicated. The victim, time, place, and circumstances of the aggressive episode must be known. The owner should be asked to describe the dog's posture: the position of its ears and tail as well as its vocalization and mouth position. Pupillary dilation and raised hackles indicate sympathetic stimulation. A temperament test should be performed. A toddler-sized doll can be walked toward the dog. Although some dogs are frightened, aggressive ones will bark and even bite the doll (Fig. II-9). An artificial hand (Assess-a-Hand) can be used for determining how responsive the dog is to touching of its head, abdomen, paws, and tail. The artificial hand can also be used for pulling food from the dog in a safe manner.

Behavior history forms for cats can be shorter than those for dogs because cats rarely are trained and do not require the attention that dogs do. Because cats are much less likely to demonstrate their misbehavior during an interview, a video recording of the cat when it is aggressive is very helpful. If the problem is soiling an area the house, time lapse videorecording can elucidate which cat in a multicat household is soiling and what its pre-elimination and postelimination behaviors are. Many cats visit the litter box but eliminate elsewhere, indicating an aversion to the litter or to the box.

POSTPROCEDURE

Recheck the animal at 3 and 6 weeks to determine the success of the treatment and compliance of the owner.

ALTERNATIVES AND THEIR RELATIVE MERITS

Behavioral problems can be referred to trainers, but there is no quality assurance. Herbal remedies also lack quality control or controlled studies of their efficacy.

AUTHOR: **KATHERINE ALBRO HOUPT**

Biopsy: Ultrasound-Guided, Percutaneous

BASIC INFORMATION

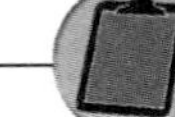

SYNONYM(S)

Tissue core biopsy
Tru-Cut biopsy

OVERVIEW AND GOAL(S)

Procedure to obtain tissue core sample using ultrasound guidance and real-time monitoring of needle instrument placement

INDICATIONS

- Ultrasonographic detection of focal mass lesion
- Ultrasonographic detection of diffuse or focal parenchymal organ abnormalities

CONTRAINDICATIONS

- Cavitated mass or coagulopathy: risk of hemorrhage
- If abscess possible: risk of leakage/sepsis
- Intrathoracic masses not in contact with the chest wall: poor visualization
- Diffuse lung disease: risk of pneumothorax

EQUIPMENT, ANESTHESIA

- Biopsy instrument:
  - Automatic:
    - Manually advanced to a point 1.5–2.0 cm superficial to lesion
    - When triggered, cutting needle and external shaft automatically advance a specific distance
  - Semiautomatic:
    - Inner cutting needle manually advanced to desired depth
    - When triggered, external shaft automatically advances over cutting needle
  - Manual:
    - Operator controls depth of needle and length of tissue sampled
    - Requires two hands to operate device
- Formalin container
- A #11 scalpel blade to incise skin
- A set of 25-gauge standard injection needles
- Hair clippers
- Surgical scrub, rubbing alcohol, gauze
- Sector or linear-array ultrasound transducer:
  - Sector transducers allow sampling of deep structures.
  - Linear-array transducers provide better resolution of superficial structures.
- ± Biopsy guide: easiest method but angle of needle insertion fixed
- Anesthesia: IV or gas anesthesia required

ANTICIPATED TIME

The procedure time is 10 to 15 minutes, plus anesthesia preparation/recovery time

PREPARATION: IMPORTANT CHECKPOINTS

- Perform coagulation profile, platelet count, and blood pressure (BP) measurement
- Place IV catheter
- Ensure proper function of biopsy instrument

POSSIBLE COMPLICATIONS AND COMMON ERRORS TO AVOID

- Avoid overly rapid advancement and activation of the instrument.
  - A common, serious error of inexperienced veterinarians is to both advance and activate the instrument in one motion, which is contraindicated (poor placement/control of instrument tip).
  - The full extent of the instrument must be observed and monitored carefully and advanced with caution to the area to be sampled.
- Identify and avoid large vessels in the organ being sampled or in those adjacent to the structure to minimize hemorrhage.
- Avoid penetrating bowel lumen, especially with larger gauge instruments, due to risk of peritonitis.
- Ensure that the ultrasound beam captures the full length and orientation of the instrument in the animal (see Fine-Needle Aspirate: Ultrasound Guided, p 1252).
- Sample the left aspect of the liver when possible to avoid the gallbladder and hilar vessels on the right. If the liver is small or cranially located, consider a caudal intercostal approach.
- In cases of bilateral renal abnormalities, the left kidney should be sampled due to its more caudal location.
- Sample the caudal cortex of the kidney to avoid the medulla and arcuate and hilar vessels.

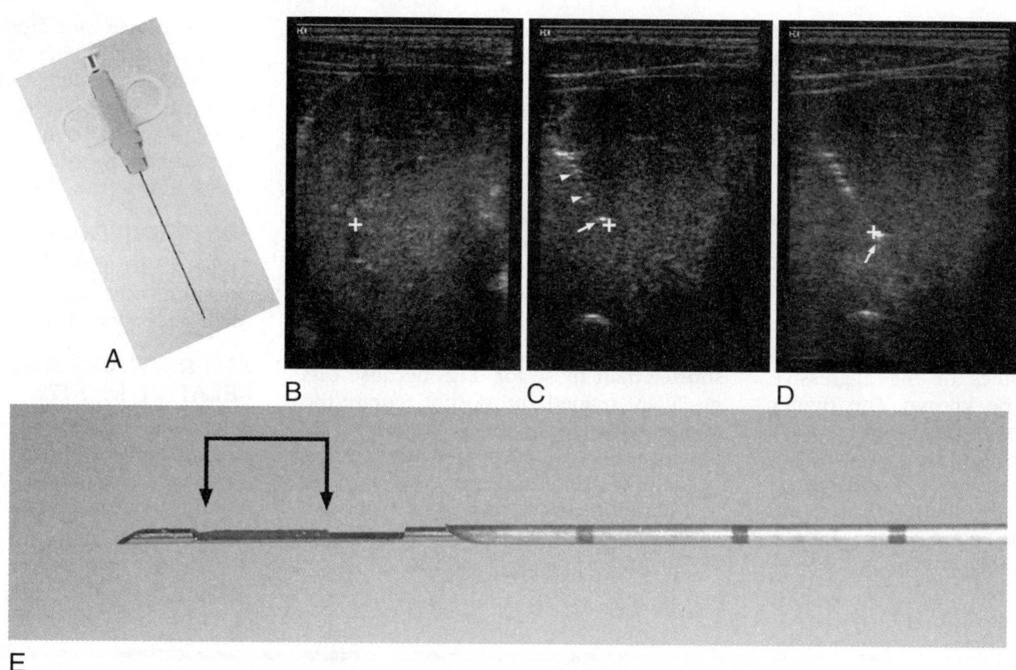

FIGURE II-10 **A**, A semiautomatic-type instrument used for ultrasound-guided core biopsy. **B**, Ultrasound of a dog's liver in preparation for core biopsy. The targeted area chosen for biopsy is marked (+). **C**, Ultrasound of the same dog's liver, biopsy underway. The semiautomatic instrument shown in panel A has been advanced (*arrowheads*) until its tip (*arrow*) is immediately above the target. **D**, Internal stylet advancing with instrument held immobile. With the instrument held immobile, the internal stylet is slowly advanced, crossing through the targeted area or lesion. Once the stylet is in the fully deployed position shown here, the instrument can be triggered, which obtains the sample. **E**, Core of liver tissue (*between arrows*) is shown within the chamber of the stylet.

- Do not pass through an organ other than the one being aspirated.
- Avoid using preanesthetic drugs that cause splenomegaly or panting.

PROCEDURE

- Restrain the animal in dorsal or lateral recumbency. A padded V-trough can be used.
- Clip hair from the ventral abdomen.
- Thoroughly evaluate area of interest sonographically, characterize lesion, identify adjacent or internal vessels to be avoided, and determine least traumatic location and direction of needle placement.
- Prepare skin with surgical scrub.
- Obtain ultrasound image of area to be sampled.
- Ensure that probe marker location on screen corresponds with desired needle course.
- Prepare biopsy instrument.
- Make a small skin incision with a scalpel blade at the site needle will be introduced.
- Introduce needle parallel to plane of ultrasound beam, visualizing it as it is advanced.
- Slowly fan transducer side to side to identify needle as necessary.
- Automatic:
    - Determine throw length of biopsy device before triggering the device. This is the additional distance the instrument advances when triggered.
    - Manually advance the needle, stopping at this distance superficial to desired biopsy site. CAUTION: When triggered, needle will advance predetermined throw length to obtain biopsy.
    - Trigger needle: cutting needle and external shaft will advance the predetermined throw length to obtain sample.
- Semiautomatic:
    - Manually advance the inner cutting needle to desired biopsy depth.
    - Trigger needle: External shaft will automatically advance over cutting needle to obtain sample.
- Manual:
    - Manually advance the inner cutting needle to desired biopsy depth.
    - Manually advance the external shaft over the cutting needle to obtain sample.
    - Requires two hands to operate, so two people are required for biopsy procedure.
- Withdraw needle from animal.
- Use a 25-gauge needle to gently lift sample from biopsy needle.
- Place sample in formalin container.
- Two to three samples of each organ or lesion are obtained.

POSTPROCEDURE

- Scan to evaluate for hemorrhage. A very small amount of hemorrhage is not uncommon.
- If small amount of hemorrhage is noted, reevaluate after several additional minutes.
- Hematuria is common following renal biopsy.

ALTERNATIVES AND THEIR RELATIVE MERITS

Laparoscopic and surgical biopsies are more invasive but have higher diagnostic quality in some cases.

SUGGESTED READING

Nyland TG, et al: Ultrasound-guided biopsy. In Nyland TG, Mattoon JS (eds): *Small Animal Diagnostic Ultrasound*, ed 2. Philadelphia, WB Saunders, 2002, pp 30–48.

Penninck DG, Finn-Bodner ST: Updates in interventional ultrasonography. *Vet Clin North Am Small Anim Pract* 28: 1017–1040, 1998.

AUTHOR: **WENDY D. FIFE**

Blood Pressure Measurement

BASIC INFORMATION

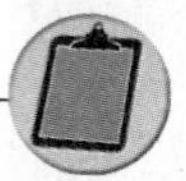

OVERVIEW AND GOAL(S)

- The goal of noninvasive blood pressure (BP) assessment in animals in a veterinary setting is to accurately measure arterial BP and detect abnormal BP, particularly systemic hypertension.
- Doppler sphygomanometric methods or automated oscillometric methods may be used.
- Doppler methods deliver systolic BP values.
- Oscillometric methods deliver systolic, diastolic, and mean BP values.
- Systolic BP is the value of interest in most clinical cases of systemic hypertension (see Systemic Hypertension, p 1058).

INDICATIONS

- Presence of clinical signs of systemic hypertension (see Systemic Hypertension, p 1058).
- Presence of systemic disease known to be associated with systemic hypertension (e.g., renal disease, hyperthyroidism, hyperadrenocorticism, diabetes mellitus, pheochromocytoma).
- Random BP screening in young healthy animals is not recommended.

EQUIPMENT, ANESTHESIA

Doppler method (used in dogs and cats; the preferred method for cats):

- Commercial Doppler amplifier with attached piezoelectric crystal for detection of blood flow
- Sphygmomanometer previously calibrated for accuracy
- A variety of cuff sizes based on animal limb circumference
- Pliable measuring tape to measure animal limb circumference
- Ultrasound coupling gel
- Hair clippers and isopropyl alcohol, if desired, for preparation of site of piezoelectric crystal application

Oscillometric method (automated system; used in dogs, less reliable in cats):

- Commercial automated oscillometric BP monitor, with either print or data storage capability
- A variety of cuff sizes based on animal limb circumference
- Pliable measuring tape to measure animal limb circumference

ANTICIPATED TIME

- Doppler method: approximately 10 minutes.
- Oscillometric method: approximately 20 minutes.

PREPARATION: IMPORTANT CHECKPOINTS

- Be sure that the animal has acclimated to the clinic's environment and is calm and comfortable in lateral or sternal recumbency or sitting. BP values may be obtained in standing animals only if a tail cuff is used. Owner presence and assurance may help to calm the animal.
- Be sure that the cuff size used is appropriate and is noted in the record for future reference. The width of the cuff should be ~40% of the circumference of the limb or tail at the cuff site.
- During measurements with either method, the cuff should be at the level of the right atrium. This may involve elevating a forelimb during measurement if the animal is sitting.
- BP should be measured by well-trained individuals in the practice to maximize consistency. This is especially important when Doppler methods are used.

POSSIBLE COMPLICATIONS AND COMMON ERRORS TO AVOID

- Erratic oscillometric readings may be obtained if an arrhythmia or very high heart rate is present.
- For maximal accuracy in Doppler readings, be sure that the audible signal is strong before beginning cuff occlusions.

PROCEDURE

Doppler method (Fig. II-11):

- Restrain the animal in a comfortable position and allow time and reassurance for acclimatization. The position of the animal is dependent on the animal's temperament and mobility and on the planned position of the cuff.
  - Cuff on forelimb at level of radius: sternal or lateral recumbency or sitting position.
  - Cuff on hind limb proximal to hock (tibial level): lateral recumbency preferred; sternal recumbency may be used if leg is in gentle extension during measurement.
- Measure the circumference of the limb or tail at the intended cuff site and select an appropriately sized cuff (as already described when preparing the animal).
- Wrap the cuff snugly around the limb and attach to sphygmomanometer.
- Clip or dampen hair as needed at site of Doppler crystal application distal to the cuff (palmar or plantar arterial

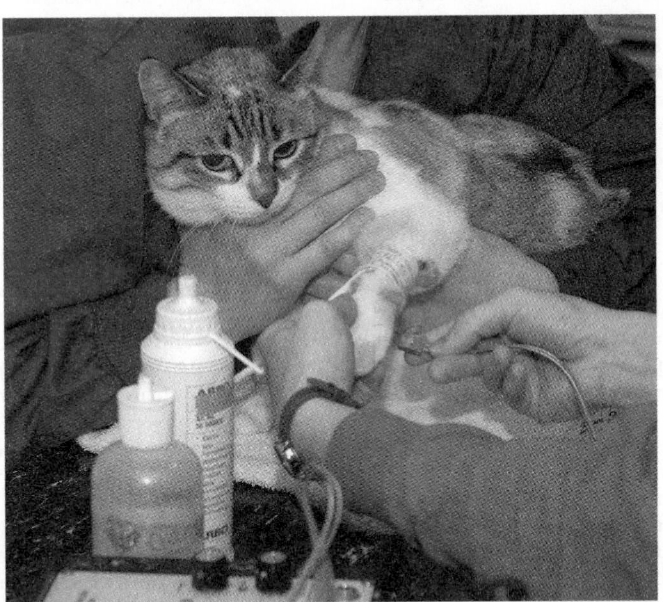

FIGURE II-11 Doppler method is used for estimating BP in a cat. Note that the animal is restrained in a calm, comfortable position. The cuff is applied to a distal forelimb, and the limb is elevated such that the cuff is at the level of the right atrium during readings. Coupling gel is applied to the Doppler crystal (shown). After the Doppler crystal is positioned over the palmar arterial arch and a strong audible signal is obtained, a bulb sphygmomanometer is used for inflating the cuff and occluding the arterial flow and then slowly deflated. The pressure at which arterial flow is again audible is recorded as the systolic BP.

arch, proximal to the metatcarpal/metatarsal pad and slightly medial); apply coupling gel and hold or tape crystal in position (see Fig. II-11).
- The crystal is placed against the skin concave side down; the flat aspect of the crystal faces out.
- Verify correct position by listening for clear pulsatile sounds of flow in the artery beneath the crystal. Adjust the crystal position or angle as necessary to improve signal strength if sounds are soft, distant, or muffled.
- Gently position limb so that the cuff is at the level of the right atrium during readings.
  - Sternum level if animal is in lateral position.
  - Thoracic inlet level if animal is sternal or sitting.
- While listening to sound of flow, inflate the cuff using the bulb manometer to approximately 20 mmHg greater than the pressure needed to cut off flow sounds.
- Slowly deflate the cuff (1-3 mmHg per second) and note the pressure at which pulsatile sounds of flow recur. This pressure is recorded as the systolic pressure.
- Completely deflate the cuff and count the heart rate in the approximately 30 seconds between pressure readings. A contemporary heart rate can be recorded with each BP reading.
- Record at least six measurements in succession, allowing approximately 30 seconds to 1 minute between measurements to allow for limb reperfusion.
- Discard the first reading and average the results of the remaining readings to obtain a representative number of systolic pressure and heart rate. High heart rate may indicate that increased levels of stress have affected readings.

Oscillometric method (Fig. II-12):
- Restrain the animal in a comfortable position and allow time and reassurance for acclimatization. The position of the animal is dependent on animal's temperament and mobility and on the planned position of the cuff.
  - Cuff on forelimb at level of radius: sternal or lateral recumbency or sitting position.
  - Cuff on proximal forelimb at level of humerus (cats): sternal recumbency.
  - Cuff on distal hind limb at level of metatarsus (median artery): lateral recumbency preferred; sternal recumbency may be used if leg is in gentle extension during measurement.
  - Cuff on proximal tailhead: sternal or lateral recumbency or standing if animal is relatively immobile during readings.
  - Limb cuffs should not be used in standing animals.
- Measure the circumference of the limb or tail at the intended cuff site and choose an appropriately sized cuff (as already noted when preparing the animal).
- Wrap the cuff snugly around the limb, with the center of the inflatable bladder of the cuff positioned over the artery, and attach to the BP monitor.
- Gently position limb so that the cuff is at the level of the right atrium during readings (no repositioning required if tail cuff is used) (see Fig. II-12).
  - Sternum level if animal is in lateral position.
  - Thoracic inlet level if animal is sternal or sitting.
- Record at least six measurements in succession, allowing approximately 30 seconds to 1 minute between measurements to allow for limb reperfusion.
- Discard the first reading and any readings with clearly spurious results, and average the results of the remaining readings to obtain a representative number for systolic, diastolic, and mean pressures, respectively.
- Note the heart rate readings associated with the BP readings. If heart rate is clearly incorrect, BP values may be spurious. In addition, high heart rate during recording may indicate high animal stress levels and possible elevated BP due to stress of procedure.

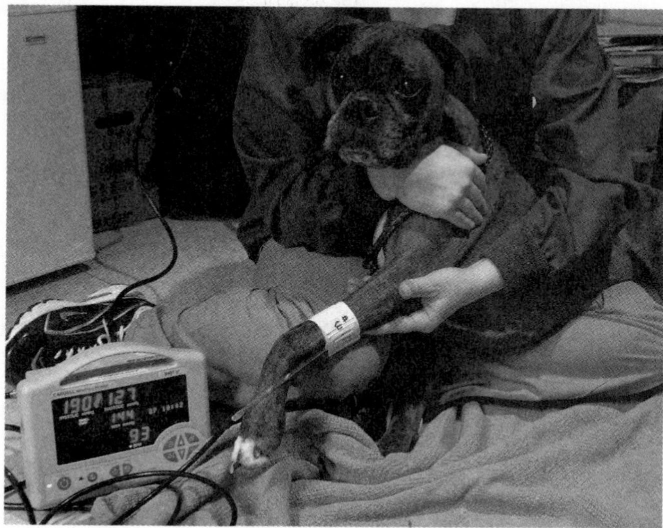

FIGURE II-12 An automated oscillometric method used with a forelimb cuff to obtain systolic, diastolic, and mean BP in a dog. The dog is restrained in a comfortable position with the intended cuff-site limb gently extended. The cuff is positioned at the midradius level, and the limb is positioned such that the cuff is at the level of the right atrium during readings.

POSTPROCEDURE

- Record the average values in animal's record with notation of method, cuff size, and cuff site used.
- Evaluate BP values in light of clinical findings and level of anxiety or excitement during BP measurement.

ALTERNATIVES AND THEIR RELATIVE MERITS

Invasive BP measurement involves acute arterial puncture (typically femoral artery) with a small gauge needle attached to a pressure transducer or the placement of a catheter in a distal artery (typically dorsal pedal) that is attached to pressure tubing and a pressure transducer. A BP tracing is printed out, and systolic and diastolic pressure can be determined from the pressure tracing.
- Highly accurate information since direct measure is used.
- Local anesthesia is used for minimizing discomfort.
- Arterial puncture or arterial catheter placement requires more technical skill than noninvasive methods.
- Bleeding may occur at site of femoral puncture if care is not taken to apply pressure for at least 5 minutes after the needle is withdrawn.
- Invasive methods are rarely used in conscious clinical patients, but indwelling arterial catheters are frequently used for continuous BP assessment in anesthetized or critically ill patients.

AUTHOR: **REBECCA L. STEPIEN**

Bone Biopsy

BASIC INFORMATION

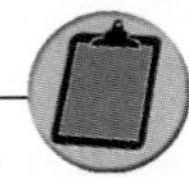

OVERVIEW AND GOAL(S)

Percutaneous sampling procedure using a minimally invasive approach to obtain cortical and cancellous bone for histologic analysis

INDICATIONS

Investigation of primary bone lesions, most commonly suspected neoplasms or bony infections:

- Focal, palpable, hard bone swellings
- Radiographic evidence of lytic and/or productive focal bone lesions
- Pathologic fractures

CONTRAINDICATIONS

- Bleeding disorders
- If iatrogenic/pathologic fracture appears likely as a result of the procedure (radiographic appearance of severe osteolysis)

EQUIPMENT AND ANESTHESIA

- General anesthesia
- Clippers for hair
- Routine antiseptic surgical scrub material and isopropyl alcohol
- A 22-gauge needle
- A #11 scalpel blade
- Sterile surgical gloves
- Bone biopsy needle, either a purpose-made Jamshidi-type needle or a routine bone marrow aspiration needle and stylet

ANTICIPATED TIME

About 20 to 30 minutes plus anesthesia induction and recovery

PREPARATION: IMPORTANT CHECKPOINTS

- Radiographs of the region to be biopsied always are indicated first to confirm bony nature of enlargement.
- Thoracic radiographs (three views, metastasis check) if bony mass is cause for biopsy.
- Platelet count; severe thrombocytopenia (10,000 platelets/μl and/or overt clinical signs of hemorrhage) is a contraindication for the procedure.
- Discuss risks with owner, including possible need for amputation if iatrogenic pathologic fracture occurs.

POSSIBLE COMPLICATIONS AND COMMON ERRORS TO AVOID

- Bone biopsy tends to be unrewarding in cases of diffuse osteopenia. These animals benefit more from review of signalment and history and assessments of serum ionized calcium, phosphorus, parathyroid hormone (PTH), and vitamin D levels.
- Iatrogenic pathologic fracture: This complication is best avoided by ensuring that if serial samples are taken, they are taken at multiple different angles and positions on the bone to avoid circumferential or linear sets of biopsy punch holes.
- Iatrogenic nerve damage, vessel trauma: The course of regional nerves, veins, and arteries needs to be known and properly identified before proceeding. Doing so may require a "mini-cutdown" or keyhole (1-cm) skin incision and blunt dissection through the soft tissues to reach bone.

PROCEDURE

- The area of greatest bony abnormality is identified on the radiographs, and the hair over that area is clipped widely (usually at least 3 × 3 inches).
- An approximate measurement of the thickness of the lesion should be made from the radiographs (distance from skin to marrow cavity) to anticipate the desired depth of needle penetration.
- General anesthesia is induced.
- The skin overlying the area of greatest radiographic abnormality is aseptically scrubbed. Surgical draping often can be avoided, provided a sufficiently wide area of hair has been clipped.
- The clinician puts on surgical gloves and pinch-elevates the skin to make a small (2–3 mm) stab incision using the scalpel blade. CAUTION: Be sure that nerves and vessels do not course in the chosen area.
- The biopsy needle is advanced into the lesion using gentle, consistent forward pressure and a rotatory, clockwise-counterclockwise twisting motion. CAUTION: The resistance of the abnormal tissue may be variable, and a sudden push could damage the bone or deeper structures on the other side of the lesion; the biopsy needle should therefore be "palmed" (butt of the needle in palm, needle shaft held firmly between index finger and thumb) so that the fingertips of the thumb and index act as a buttress.
- The stylet is generally removed from the biopsy needle and set aside after the soft tissues have been passed and the needle is in bone.
- The biopsy needle has been sufficiently advanced when the cortex and marrow of one side of a bone (and its lesion) have been traversed (i.e., when the marrow cavity is reached, as estimated from the radiographs).
- Before withdrawing the needle, a gentle rocking of the needle (a few millimeters) side to side will break off any attachments of the biopsy core to deeper bone. Not doing this could cause the core biopsy to be retained in the bone rather than coming out with the needle.
- The needle is withdrawn, again with a rotatory clockwise-counterclockwise motion to decrease friction.
- The sample is expelled from the shaft of the needle. The stylet is inserted normograde (usual direction) if using a bone marrow aspirate-type needle; however, the stylet is inserted retrograde (up the tip of the needle) if using a Jamshidi-type needle because these usually are tapered at the tip.
- Multiple (two or three) samples often are obtained during one procedure to increase diagnostic yield. The samples are drawn away from each other to reduce the risk of weakening/fracturing the bone.
- If a very small skin incision was made, then direct pressure alone (or possibly tissue glue) usually is sufficient for clo-

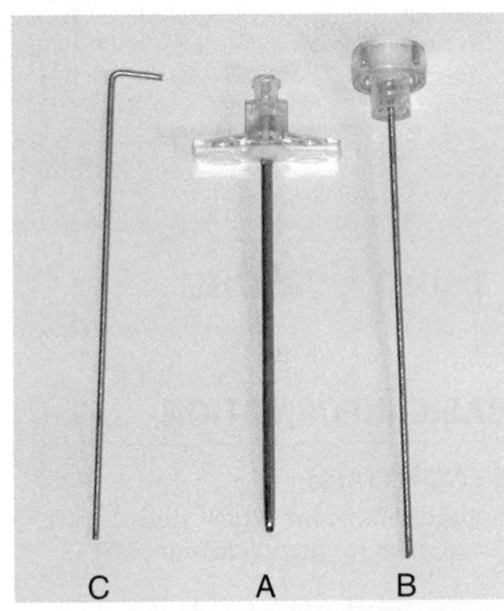

FIGURE II-13 Jamshidi-type needles for bone biopsies. **A,** Needle. **B,** Stylet that remains inside the needle while crossing the soft tissues but is removed before entering bone. **C,** A second stylet that is inserted retrograde into the needle after the procedure is finished to expel the biopsy specimen from the needle shaft.

sure; larger incisions (rare) may require skin sutures or staples.

POSTPROCEDURE

- Sedation/prolongation of recovery if animal flails its biopsied limb (to reduce risk of self-induced pathologic fracture).
- Radiograph biopsied limb if the animal experiences markedly worse lameness after the procedure (rule out pathologic fracture).
- Evaluate site several minutes later. If a hematoma is present, direct pressure is indicated.

ALTERNATIVES AND THEIR RELATIVE MERITS

- Open biopsy; more invasive, but specimen is larger.
- Amputation (if area being biopsied is on a limb); indicated if pathologic fracture is present.

AUTHOR: **ETIENNE CÔTÉ**

Bone Grafting

BASIC INFORMATION

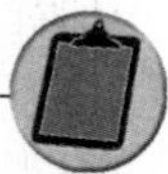

SYNONYM(S)

Autogenous cancellous bone grafting (used most frequently in animals)

OVERVIEW AND GOAL(S)

- Adjunct to surgical bone repair
- Enhances bone healing by osteogenesis, osteoconduction, and osteoinduction:
  - About 10% of donor cells survive and contain osteoblastic potential.
  - Grafted cells serve as a trellis for ingrowing recipient vascular and cellular elements.
  - Bone morphogenic proteins in graft stimulate recipient mesenchymal cells to form bone.
- Provides structural support with cortical graft placed in bone defect

INDICATIONS

- Fractures
- Delayed unions or nonunions
- Osteomyelitis:
  - Infection of the recipient site is not a contraindication to bone grafting.
  - The selected site from which the graft is harvested (donor site), however, must be aseptic.
- Arthrodesis
- Corrective osteotomies
- Ablation of bone cysts
- Limb-sparing surgery

CONTRAINDICATIONS

Prolonged anesthesia/operative time in compromised animal

EQUIPMENT, ANESTHESIA

Standard orthopedic equipment and anesthesia are used during fracture repair, osteotomy, or arthrodesis.

ANTICIPATED TIME

An additional 15 to 30 minutes of operative time (autogenous cancellous bone grafting)

PREPARATION: IMPORTANT CHECKPOINTS

Donor graft site:

- In the same animal (autogenous)
- Common locations: proximal lateral humerus, proximal lateral femur, proximal medial tibia, or dorsolateral ilial wing
- Needs to be aseptically prepared preoperatively

POSSIBLE COMPLICATIONS AND COMMON ERRORS TO AVOID

- Hematoma formation
- Loss of graft by inadvertent discard of graft-laden sponge
- Contamination of donor site by infection or neoplasia from recipient site
- Inadequate graft harvest
- Iatrogenic fracture at donor site
- Iatrogenic physeal damage at donor site

PROCEDURE

For autogenous cancellous bone graft:

- Primary orthopedic procedure is performed, and then fresh graft is obtained from a separate (donor) site in the animal.
- Skin incision carried through subcutaneous tissues directly to bone at donor site.
- Near cortex penetrated by pin or drill bit.
- Curette used for collecting intramedullary contents: cancellous bone graft.
- Material collected in sterile container or gauze sponge and soaked with blood to prevent dessication.
- Graft transferred to, and placed in, recipient site around implants and fracture(s).
- Routine closure of primary operative site and then donor site.

For commercially available (allograft) cancellous bone graft:

- The graft is placed in sterile container and covered with the animal's blood to congeal while the primary orthopedic procedure is performed. The graft is placed at the operative site, as already described, prior to closure.

For autogenous corticocancellous graft from ilium:

- Rongeurs or bone cutters are used for resecting ilium and collecting cortical and cancellous bone.

ALTERNATIVES AND THEIR RELATIVE MERITS

Autogenous cancellous graft is the "gold" standard; commercial preparations lack osteogenic potential but are technically easier to obtain.

SUGGESTED READING

Johnson AL, Hulse DA: Fundamentals of orthopaedic surgery and fracture management. In Fossum TW (ed): *Small Animal Surgery*, ed 2. St. Louis, Mosby, 2002, pp 821–900.

Millis DL, Martinez SM: Bone grafts. In Slatter D (ed): *Textbook of Small Animal Surgery*, ed 3. Philadelphia, WB Saunders, 2002, pp 1875–1891.

AUTHOR: **JOSEPH C. GLENNON**

Bone Marrow Aspiration/Core Biopsy

BASIC INFORMATION

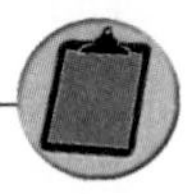

OVERVIEW AND GOAL(S)

To obtain a sample of bone marrow cells for cytologic (aspiration) or histologic (core biopsy) analysis

INDICATIONS

- Cytopenias without identifiable underlying cause
- Unusual blood cell morphologic abnormalities on blood smear
- Staging of neoplasia (especially lymphoma and mast cell tumor)

CONTRAINDICATIONS

- Contraindications to sedation or anesthesia
- Infection of overlying soft tissues
- Not a contraindication: thrombocytopenia

EQUIPMENT, ANESTHESIA

- Either sedation plus analgesia and local anesthesia may be used, or general anesthesia can be used.
- Typical protocol: butorphanol 0.2 mg/kg IV, plus lidocaine 2% local infiltration (1-8 ml SC for cats to large dogs, respectively) and propofol 3-6 mg/kg IV to effect. Propofol and local anesthesia are inadequate without an analgesic such as butorphanol because neither propofol nor lidocaine provides systemic analgesia, and aspiration is painful.
- Clippers for hair.
- Antiseptic scrub solution, isopropyl alcohol, and gauze squares for preparing the skin.
- Sterile surgical gloves.
- A #11 scalpel blade.
- Bone marrow aspiration/biopsy needle, typically 18 gauge.
- Microscope slides and/or laboratory container with anticoagulant and/or sterile test tube. The preferred method of submission varies from laboratory to laboratory.
- Tissue glue.
- A 10% formalin and biopsy jar (if core biopsy).

ANTICIPATED TIME

About 20 minutes

PREPARATION: IMPORTANT CHECKPOINTS

- For larger patients (large-breed dogs, obese animals), the needle guard should be removed (Fig. II-14); otherwise, the exposed amount of needle shaft may not reach the marrow cavity.
- A whole blood sample for complete blood count (CBC) should be drawn before the procedure and submitted at the same time as the cytologic examination slides/biopsy specimen.
- The laboratory to which the sample is being submitted should be consulted beforehand. Some clinical pathologists require fresh smears, others require anticoagulated samples, and still others require clotted samples. Depending on the desired sample submission, anticoagulant may be placed in the aspirating syringe.

POSSIBLE COMPLICATIONS AND COMMON ERRORS TO AVOID

Aspirate:

- Inadvertent clotting of sample; preventable by reducing the time between aspiration and smearing to a few seconds.
- Sliding off the bone on initial approach, causing soft tissue trauma; prevented with good anatomic landmarking, firm but not excessive pressure when advancing the needle, perpendicular positioning of the needle tip against the bone surface, and keeping one's hand close to one's body for greater control when advancing the needle into bone.
- Submitting all slides for routine staining; it is worthwhile to keep one or two slides, unstained because there may be additional indications (e.g., feline leukemia immunofluorescence, antimegakaryocyte antibody testing) that emerge later in the case and for which additional slides would be useful.

Core biopsy:

- Assumption that a core biopsy is superior to a marrow aspirate/cytologic examination. In most cases, a cytologic examination is more informative.
- Sliding off the bone on initial approach, causing soft tissue trauma: as already described.
- For core biopsies, failing to slightly rock the biopsy needle when it is fully embedded before withdrawing. This rocking motion breaks off attachments to the core and prevents the biopsy sample from remaining attached to bone and sliding out of the needle on withdrawal.

PROCEDURE

An ilial or humeral approach may be used.

Aspirate: humerus:

- Sedation or general anesthesia is induced.
- For a right-handed clinician, the animal's left humerus is easiest. The animal is placed in right lateral recumbency on a table, and the clinician stands behind (dorsal to) the animal (Fig. II-15).
- The area over the animal's left shoulder is clipped of hair and aseptically scrubbed. Generally, a hairless, disinfected surface of skin that is a minimum of 3 × 3 inches is necessary, centered on the point of the shoulder.
- Unless the animal is under general anesthesia, a local anesthetic is infiltrated (SC and through the soft tissues to the level of the periosteum) according to the following landmarks:
  - The site of entry into the marrow cavity is the craniolateral, proximal humerus, just distal to the joint space of the shoulder.
  - On palpation of the cranial aspect of the shoulder, a depression is felt (shoulder joint), and the site of entry with the needle is 3-10 mm (cat to large dog) distal and lateral to this point.
  - A broad surface of bone with little overlying muscle—the lateral, distal aspect of the greater tubercle—is the target. The needle should not enter the joint space.
- A brief aseptic scrub of the site is repeated after local anesthesia injection.
- The clinician puts on sterile gloves.
- Using his or her left hand, the clinician takes the animal's proximal left humerus firmly, holding the limb just distal to the aseptically scrubbed area. In this way, the left hand is no longer sterile but the right hand is still sterile.
- The landmarks just described are palpated again with the right hand; using the scalpel blade, the clinician makes a 2-3 mm skin incision over the lateral, distal greater tubercle.
- Using the right hand, the clinician places the bone marrow needle in the skin incision, exactly perpendicular to the bone surface, and advances it using a clockwise-counterclockwise rotatory motion and firm forward pressure. The bone marrow biopsy needle must be held firmly in the right hand, with the butt of the needle seated in the palm of the hand.
- If properly directed, the bone marrow needle should be difficult to advance and should feel firmly seated in bone.

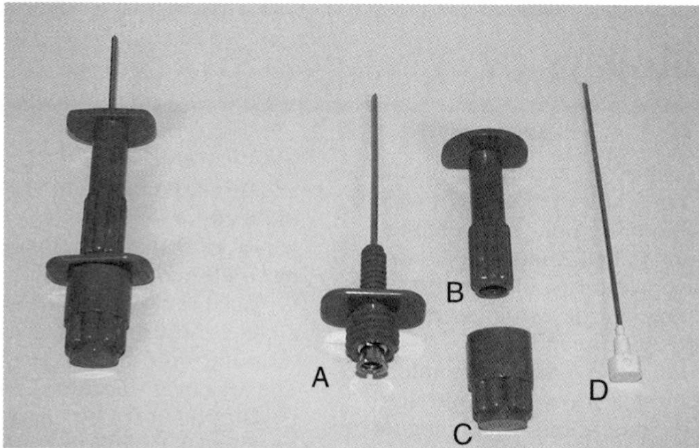

FIGURE II-14 Assembled (*left*) and disassembled (*right*) bone marrow needles. **A**, Needle. **B**, Needle guard. **C**, Cap. **D**, Stylet.

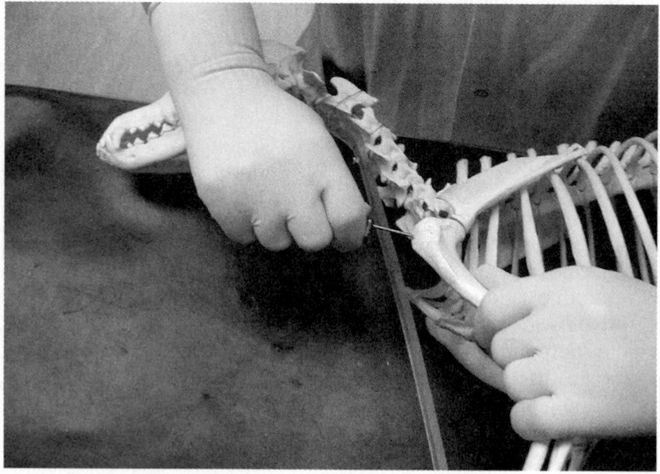

FIGURE II-15 Position for bone marrow aspiration from the proximal humerus using a skeleton for demonstration. The clinician is standing dorsal to the recumbent animal and is holding the humerus firmly. The needle tip is on the distal, lateral surface of the greater tubercle, ready to be advanced.

- The needle is advanced 0.5–2 cm (cat to small dog/big dog) to reach the marrow cavity.
- The needle cap and stylet are then removed, a syringe is attached to the needle, and negative pressure is created by drawing back on the syringe plunger.
- Marrow (looks like blood) enters the syringe; 1–2 ml should be harvested if possible.
- As soon as marrow is in the syringe, the syringe and needle are withdrawn together, and the sample is instantly prepared for submission according to the laboratory's specifications.
  - Fresh smears: with the needle and syringe still connected to each other, a sample of marrow is expelled such that it partially floods the microscope slide. The sample is then reaspirated into the needle and syringe. This process leaves behind marrow spicules (1–2 mm specks) on the slide, and spicules contain the greatest concentration of marrow cells.
  - Anticoagulated samples: The marrow is placed in a purpose-made dish with anticoagulant or in a lavender-top tube.
- The skin incision is closed with tissue glue, and mild direct pressure is applied for hemostasis.

Aspirate: ilium:

- Sedation or general anesthesia is induced.
- The animal is placed in ventral recumbency.
- The skin over the dorsal-most aspect of the right or left ilial wing is clipped of hair and aseptically scrubbed. Generally, a hairless, disinfected surface of skin that is a minimum of 3 × 3 inches is necessary, centered on the palpable dorsal-most aspect of the wing of the ilium.
- Unless the animal is under general anesthesia, local anesthetic is infiltrated SC and through the soft tissues to the level of the periosteum. The site of entry, and therefore the site requiring local anesthesia, is the dorsal-most/slightly medial aspect of the ilial wing.
- A brief aseptic scrub of the site is repeated after local anesthesia injection.
- The clinician puts on sterile gloves.
- Standing over the animal, the clinician palpates the dorsal wing of the ilium and makes a small (2–3 mm) skin incision using the scalpel blade.
- Using the right hand, the clinician places the bone marrow needle in the skin incision until it touches ilial bone and then advances it using a clockwise-counterclockwise rotatory motion and a moderate amount of forward (downward) pressure. The bone marrow biopsy needle must be held firmly in the right hand, with the butt of the needle seated in the palm of the hand.
- If properly directed, the bone marrow needle should be difficult to advance and should feel firmly seated in bone.
- The needle is advanced 0.5–2 cm (cat to small or big dog) to reach the marrow cavity.
- The needle cap and stylet are then removed, a syringe is attached to the needle, and negative pressure is created by drawing back on the syringe plunger.
- Marrow (looks like blood) enters the syringe; 1–2 ml should be harvested if possible.
- As soon as marrow is in the syringe, the syringe and needle are withdrawn together, and the sample is instantly prepared for submission according to the laboratory's specifications.
  - Fresh smears: With the needle and syringe still connected to each other, a sample of marrow is expelled such that it partially floods the microscope slide. The sample is then reaspirated into the needle and syringe. This process leaves behind marrow spicules (1–2 mm specks) on the slide, and spicules contain the greatest concentration of marrow cells.
  - Anticoagulated samples: The marrow is placed in a purpose-made dish with anticoagulant or in a lavender-top tube.
- The skin incision is closed with tissue glue, and mild direct pressure is applied for hemostasis.

Core biopsy: humerus or ilium:

- The same procedure as for bone marrow aspiration is followed, up to the point of advancing the needle into bone.
- When the needle is initially in bone (first few rotations, but before having advanced the full 0.5–2 cm), the procedure is stopped, the needle cap is unscrewed, and the stylet is removed.
- In this way, the cortex is not included in the sample (in contrast to bone biopsy, p 1193).
- The cap is then replaced on the needle, and the procedure is continued, advancing the needle into the marrow cavity.

- No aspiration is involved. Rather, when the needle has been advanced a total of 0.5–2 cm (cat to small or big dog, respectively) without a stylet, a core of marrow should be in the shaft of the needle. The twisting and advancing motion is stopped, and the needle is gently tilted or rocked very slightly (perhaps 10 degrees side to side), to break the core of marrow free from its attachments.
- The needle is then withdrawn and examined; a white plug of marrow should be obstructing the tip of the needle. This plug is expelled into 10% formalin using the stylet inserted in the normal (normograde) direction.

POSTPROCEDURE

Routine recovery from sedation/anesthesia and submission of samples for analysis

ALTERNATIVES AND THEIR RELATIVE MERITS

- Repeated CBC: assesses trends in cytopenias and morphologic blood cell abnormalities but does not show precursors and maturation sequence of blood cells.
- Buffy coat examination: unreliable for malignant mast cell disease (poor sensitivity, poor specificity compared to bone marrow evaluation).

AUTHOR: **ETIENNE CÔTÉ**

Brainstem Auditory Evoked Response

BASIC INFORMATION

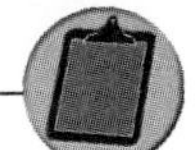

SYNONYM(S)

Auditory brainstem response (ABR)
Hearing test

OVERVIEW AND GOAL(S)

- The brainstem auditory evoked response (BAER) test is done to evaluate and record the electrical response in the brainstem to an auditory stimulus.
- Between 1000 and 1500 auditory stimuli (usually a click sound) are delivered to each ear, and the brainstem electrical responses are averaged together and recorded. This results in a characteristic waveform with about five discernable peaks.
- The BAER test does not actually assess conscious perception of hearing; however, because there are very few diseases that would interrupt the hearing pathways after they have left the brainstem, it is accepted as a tacit test of hearing.
- BAER waveforms can be altered (absent, decreased amplitude [height]; increased latency [delayed appearance]) by abnormalities within the ear (e.g., middle ear infection) or brainstem (e.g., neoplasia).
- Conductive (obstruction to sound in the ear canal or middle ear) and sensorineural (abnormality with the nerves or receptors in the inner ear) deafness both result in an abnormal BAER test.
- Although BAER testing is commonly used to diagnose congenital deafness (an absolute yes/no assessment) (Figs. II-16, II-17, and II-18), it can also be used to assess the level of hearing function by performing threshold analyses. Most dogs can hear sounds at a level of sound intensity of 0–5 dB. By gradual reduction of the sound intensity during testing (from an initial level of 80 dB), the examiner can establish whether the threshold is abnormally increased.

INDICATIONS

- Suspected deafness or hearing loss (unilateral or bilateral). Screening for congenital deafness is the most common reason for BAER testing. It is frequently done in puppies of those breeds commonly affected with congenital deafness (e.g., dalmatian, bull terrier, English setter). Puppies should be at least 6 weeks of age when tested.
- Suspected brainstem disease (neoplasia, infarction).
- Confirmation of brain death (complete loss of brainstem function).

EQUIPMENT, ANESTHESIA

- A computer with a signal averager and software capable of labeling and analysis of waveforms.
- Subdermal electrodes.
- Headphones, foam insert microphones, or a bone conductor.
- Otoscope.

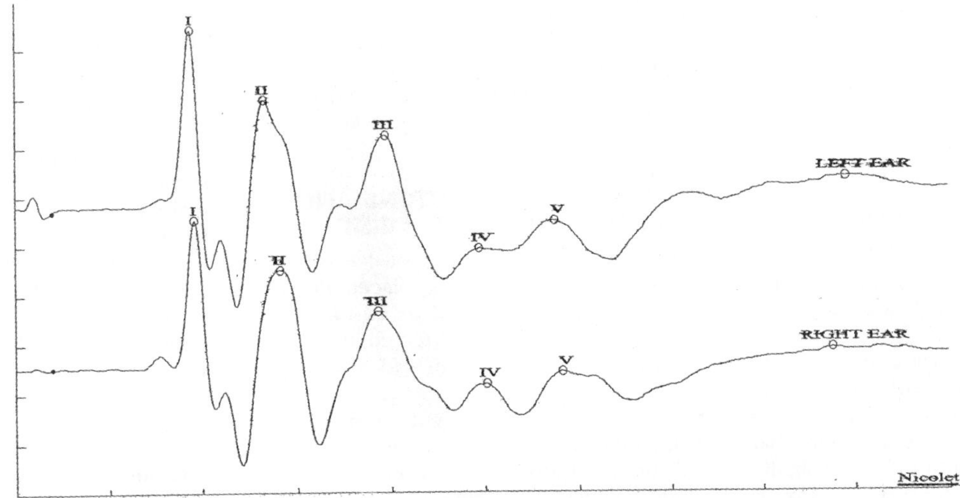

FIGURE II-16 Normal study. Courtesy of Dr. Peter Foley.

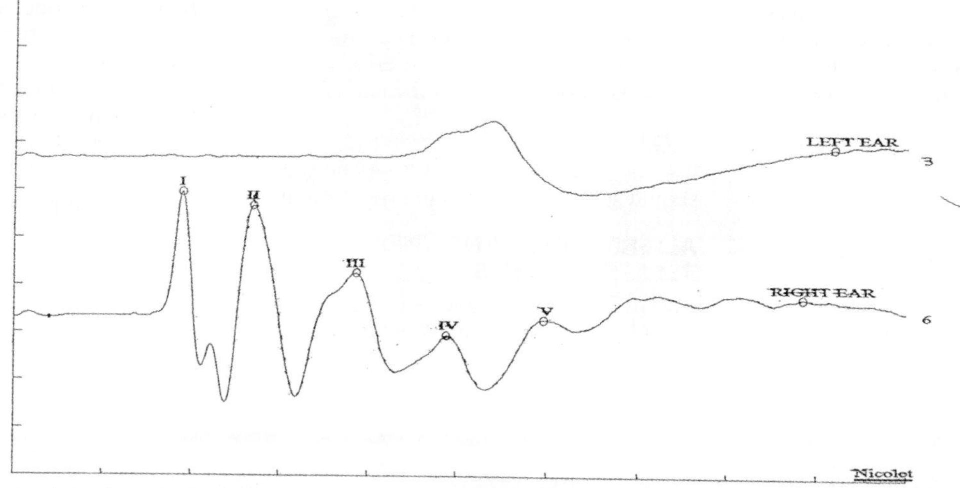

FIGURE II-17 Unilateral deafness in the left ear. Courtesy of Dr. Peter Foley.

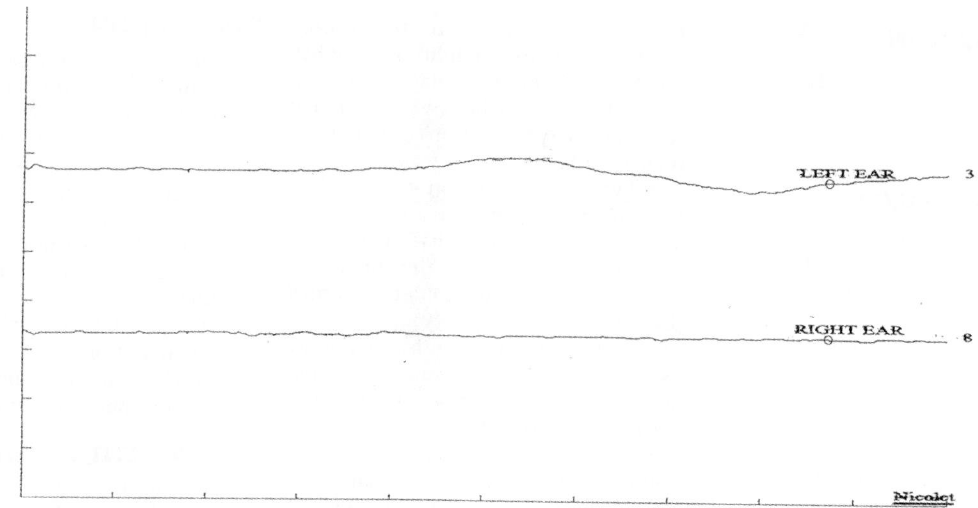

FIGURE II-18 Bilateral deafness. Courtesy of Dr. Peter Foley.

- Sedation may or may not be required depending on how quiet the animal is and if it will lie still for 10 to 15 minutes. If sedation is required, light sedation is usually sufficient, and it will not significantly alter the characteristics of the recorded waveforms.

ANTICIPATED TIME

Usually 15 to 30 minutes depending on how quiet the animal is being

PREPARATION: IMPORTANT CHECKPOINTS

- Computer check to see that established protocols have been loaded appropriately and settings are correct.
- Impedence check (via computer software program) to ensure that all the electrodes are operating effectively.
- Otoscopic examination: to ensure that ear canal is open and free from significant amounts of debris or wax. A stenotic or occluded ear canal will not transmit sound to the tympanum and will result in subnormal waveform amplitudes and prolonged latencies. Ear canals may need to be cleaned thoroughly prior to the BAER test. Clinicians should visually assess the integrity of the tympanic membrane.
- Ensure that right and left ear electrodes are appropriately placed and noted correctly on the computer.

POSSIBLE COMPLICATIONS AND COMMON ERRORS TO AVOID

- Ear canals filled with wax or debris.
- Insert microphones not placed deep enough in the ear canal or positioned such that the sound is directed into the wall of the ear canal instead of down the lumen.
- Subdermal electrodes become dislodged.
- If flatline or grossly abnormal recording is obtained, always do a thorough technical check (e.g., computer working, sound is actually generated in the microphones, subdermal electrodes in place and not dislodged, inserted microphones placed appropriately in the ear canal) to ensure that the result is real.

PROCEDURE

- Place animal in sternal recumbency on a well-padded table (or floor) in a quiet and dimly lit room.
- Turn on computer, load appropriate software and protocols, and set up animal record.
- Insert subdermal electrodes:
  - Right and left ears: Place electrode subcutaneously adjacent to where the horizontal ear canal begins (usually at the caudal end of the zygomatic arch).
  - Reference electrode: Place the electrode midline, halfway between the occipital crest and orbits.
  - Ground electrode: Place the electrode midline over the second and fourth cervical vertebra.

- Check electrode impedence (usually in the computer software) to ensure that electrodes are working appropriately.
- Perform an otoscopic examination and clean ears if necessary.
- Place foam insert microphones in right and left ear canals: Place them so that they are well seated in the upper (distal) third of the vertical ear canal. If using headphones, ensure that the pinnae are not obstructing the headphones and a snug seal is established over the ear canal.
- Set sound intensity at 80 dB. There is no established appropriate sound intensity to do initial screening, but this level has been determined to be comfortable for the animal and effective at identifying potential hearing deficits.
- Set signal averager to average 1000 signals, and select right or left ear to begin recording.
- Each ear should be recorded twice, and the recorded waveforms should be compared. They should be very similar. If not, do a technical check and repeat the test.
- Once good quality recordings have been recorded for both ears, the waveforms should be labeled and amplitudes and latencies calculated.
- Subdermal electrodes and inserted microphones are then removed, and the animal can be discharged.

POSTPROCEDURE

If the animal has been sedated, allow it to recover sufficiently before discharge.

ALTERNATIVES AND THEIR RELATIVE MERITS

There are no practical and accurate alternatives to establishing unilateral or bilateral deafness in dogs and cats. Bilateral deafness can usually be suspected but not confirmed by subjective assessment of the animal's response to loud noises.

AUTHOR: **DARCY H. SHAW**

Bronchoscopy

BASIC INFORMATION

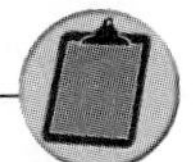

OVERVIEW AND GOAL(S)

To view and assess both the anatomy (mucosal, structural) and function (dynamic collapse) of the airways from larynx to distal bronchi and to obtain samples from the distal airways for analysis

INDICATIONS

- Diagnostic: evaluation of lower airway and parenchymal disease (culture/cytologic examination, biopsy) and documentation of airway caliber disorders (malacia, collapse, compression, bronchiectasis)
- Therapeutic: foreign body/secretion removal

CONTRAINDICATIONS

- Major: severe hypoxemia, unstable cardiac arrhythmias, heart failure
- Minor: significant resting expiratory effort, bronchomalacia, inexperience

EQUIPMENT, ANESTHESIA

- Equipment:
  - Flexible endoscope: 3-5 mm in diameter, 55-85 cm in length.
  - Mouth gag, sterile gauze, suction capabilities.
  - Sterile saline:
    - Preloaded in three to four 10-20 ml syringes for bronchoalveolar lavage (BAL).
    - For rinsing and cleaning.
  - Sterile, water-soluble lubricant.
  - Forceps: if foreign body removal or mucosal biopsy is required.
- Anesthesia:
  - Pretreatment with a bronchodilator is recommended, especially in cats; use injectable terbutaline, 0.01 mg/kg SQ at least 15 minutes prior to the procedure.
  - IV catheter for administration of a short-acting injectable anesthetic protocol: either atropine 0.02-0.04 mg/kg IM or glycopyrrolate 0.01-0.02 mg/kg IM; in addition, butorphanol 0.05-0.1 mg/kg IM and diazepam 0.1 mg/kg IV followed by propofol 3-6 mg/kg, slow IV titrated to effect, with repeated miniboluses of propofol (1 mg/kg) as needed over the duration of the procedure to maintain anesthetized state.
  - Intubation is rarely used for the procedure; an anesthesia "T" piece is required if the scope will be passed through the tube; jet ventilation can be used if available.
  - Provide oxygen before, during, and after the procedure; insufflate oxygen through the endoscope channel or via a 3-8 Fr urinary catheter passed alongside the scope during the procedure; use an endotracheal tube or a face mask for oxygen administration before and after.
  - Topical 2% lidocaine if needed to decrease pharyngeal/laryngeal sensation and movement.
  - Doxapram HCl 2.2 mg/kg IV once to assist with laryngeal evaluation.
  - Electrocardiogram (ECG), blood pressure (BP) cuff, and other monitoring equipment.

ANTICIPATED TIME

A complete bronchoscopy and bronchoalveolar lavage can be completed within 10 to 20 minutes by an experienced endoscopist; animal recovery time is additional and varies with the type of anesthetic used.

PREPARATION: IMPORTANT CHECKPOINTS

- The bronchoscopist must have a good understanding of normal bronchial mucosa and lung anatomy (Fig. II-19) to diagnose subtle airway abnormalities.
- The bronchoscope should be cleaned and ready for use.
- All supplies and equipment should be available before starting the procedure; anesthetic monitoring and image capture equipment should be turned on and ready to use.
- Antibiotics should be discontinued at least 72 hours prior to the procedure for accurate culture results.
- Chest radiographs are useful to help select specific lung regions for examination and for BAL.

POSSIBLE COMPLICATIONS AND COMMON ERRORS TO AVOID

- Contamination of the BAL sample is possible if care is not taken to avoid touching the upper airways during insertion of the scope. Guarded catheters may be used for decreasing the potential for BAL contamination, although catheter cost limits their use.
- Pulmonary barotrauma (tracheobronchial or lung rupture) is possible if the oxygen insufflation rate exceeds the ability of the gas to exit the lungs; this is of concern in smaller animals when the bronchoscope diameter is close to the tracheal size and pressure builds up in the lungs as active insufflation continues.
- Airway collapse during recovery can result in severe hypoxemia; anticipate when active expiratory effort is noted prior to anesthesia; slow recovery from anesthesia helps minimize this concern.

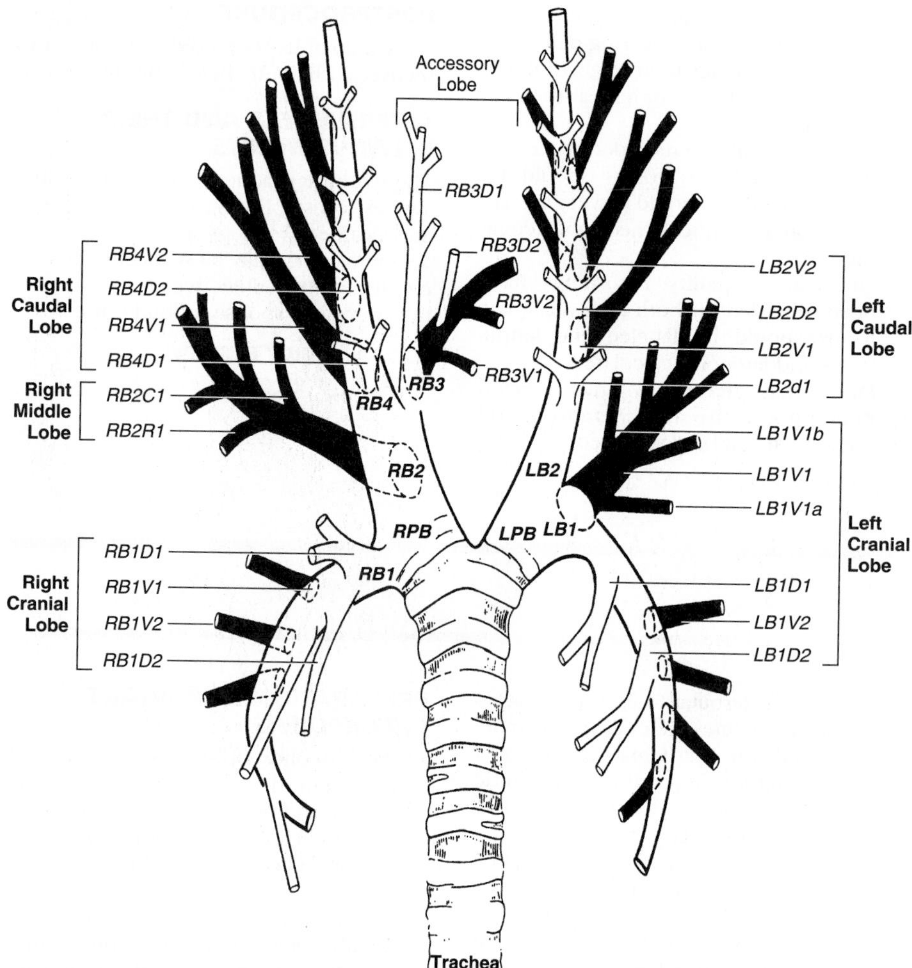

FIGURE II-19 Diagrammatic representation of the normal canine tracheobronchial tree. Reprinted with permission from Amis T, McKiernan BC: Systematic identification of endobronchial anatomy during bronchoscopy in the dog. *Am J Vet Res* 47:2649–2657, 1986.

PROCEDURE

- Sternal recumbency is the recommended position in cats and dogs.
- Topical anesthesia (1–2% lidocaine) may be applied to the pharyngeal/laryngeal mucosa to minimize laryngospasm or excessive coughing.
- Provide oxygen as already outlined.
- Evaluate the oropharyngeal/laryngeal region; use IV doxapram HCl (2.2 mg/kg once) to stimulate intrinsic laryngeal function motion.
- Insert the bronchoscope into the airways, noting changes in shape (hypoplasia, stricture), dynamic caliber (malacia, collapse), and mucosa (secretions, erythema, edema, masses).
- In the normal animal, the dorsal tracheal membrane is taut so that there is little if any redundancy (no visible protrusion or collapse into the airway).
- The healthy tracheobronchial mucosa is a smooth, light pink surface with a rich supply of submucosal capillaries; if these capillaries are not visible, mucosal edema or cellular infiltration is likely present.
- Healthy mucosa has a slightly glistening appearance; mucosal edema is readily apparent because it imparts a gelatinous appearance to the epithelial surface.
- The clinician should examine the carina for abnormalities (widening, compression, mucosal infiltration) before evaluating each lobar and as many segmental and/or subsegmental bronchi as possible (as both the animal and endoscope size will allow).
- Airway bifurcations beyond the carina are referred to simply as a spur. Like the carina, these should also form a sharp V, but they become widened and appear U shaped with chronic airway inflammation and/or mucosal edema.
- Small polypoid mucosal nodules are commonly encountered in the bronchi of dogs with chronic bronchitis.
- Small amounts of white or slightly opaque mucus may be noted in a healthy animal, but larger accumulations or secretions of unusual color are abnormal.
- The normal monopodial branching system results in a gentle, smooth tapering of the airways. Changes may be focal or generalized and include those of shape and size of the airway lumen, such as an intraluminal stricture/tumor, external compression (tumor or lymphadenopathy), bronchiectasis or dynamic collapse (malacia).
- Whether or not abnormalities are noted, samples should be obtained for culture and cytologic examination. Following the initial airway evaluation, the endoscope is removed from the animal and cleaned by alternatively suctioning the channel with sterile saline and air immediately prior to reinsertion.
- The BAL site (lobe and bronchus) is chosen based on both radiographic and gross bronchoscopic findings. If no site is clearly abnormal, BALs from both "middle" lung lobes should be collected.
- To perform a BAL, the bronchoscope is first gently wedged into a segmental or smaller bronchus. Aliquots of 10–20 ml sterile saline (depending on the size of the animal) are instilled into the airway (via the suction channel or a washing pipette) and then immediately aspirated using slow, gentle hand suction.
- Ideally at least two different sites (lung lobes) should be lavaged, with two aliquots per site.
- A 40–90% return of the volume instilled is expected. Difficulty in fluid recovery results when a proportionately large endoscope is used (prevents wedging into a small bronchus) or when malacic airways collapse when suction is applied.
- If there is enough time and anesthetic depth is appropriate, the nasopharynx should also be examined.

POSTPROCEDURE

- Provide supplemental oxygen until fully recovered.
- Crackles are commonly noted on auscultation for a short time following a BAL procedure.
- Process samples immediately.
  - Quantitated aerobic cultures should be made if possible.
  - *Mycoplasma* and anaerobic cultures are processed using Amies transport swabs.
  - Cytology:
    - Total white blood cell (WBC) and differential cell counts should be done.
    - The predominant cell in all species should be the alveolar macrophage (70+%), with usually less than 3–8% of all other cell types (except the cat, which may have up to 20+% eosinophils and still be normal).
- Handling the scope:
  - Immediately rinse/wipe the scope down when finished to prevent secretions from drying.
  - Clean and sterilize the scope as outlined in the manufacturer's manual.
  - Store the scope hanging up (to fully dry it) in a protected space/closet.

ALTERNATIVES AND THEIR RELATIVE MERITS

- Tracheal wash procedures are less expensive and easier to perform; however, they lack the ability to direct sampling into specific sites; they provide no information regarding anatomic, structural, or functional airway abnormalities; and have no therapeutic capability.
- Fine-needle lung aspiration biopsy has been used successfully to sample consolidated lung lobes and larger masses.

AUTHOR: **BRENDAN C. MCKIERNAN**

Buccal Mucosal Bleeding Time

BASIC INFORMATION

SYNONYM(S)

Bleeding time
BMBT

OVERVIEW AND GOAL(S)

To quickly and easily assess primary hemostasis and evaluate formation of a platelet plug

INDICATIONS

Presence of mucosal hemorrhage (petechiae/ecchymoses, gingival bleeding, epistaxis, melena, hematuria) in animals with a normal platelet count. May also be used for assessing primary hemostasis in preoperative animals

CONTRAINDICATIONS

Thrombocytopenia

EQUIPMENT, ANESTHESIA

- Anesthesia is generally not required in dogs.
- Sedation or general anesthesia necessary in cats.
- Template bleeding device (device with a spring-loaded blade that creates a standard incision in the buccal mucosa).
- Filter paper or gauze for blotting blood.
- Muzzle gauze (or equivalent).
- Stopwatch.

ANTICIPATED TIME

A total of 5 to 10 minutes

PREPARATION: IMPORTANT CHECKPOINTS

Evaluate platelet count prior to evaluating buccal mucosal bleeding time (BMBT).

POSSIBLE COMPLICATIONS AND COMMON ERRORS TO AVOID

- Animal may become agitated; use sedation as needed to keep animal still for entire test.
- Do not manually disrupt clot while assessing clotting time.

PROCEDURE

- Place animal in lateral recumbency.
- Evert upper lip and secure in everted position with muzzle gauze. This allows exposure of the buccal mucosa and causes the vessels to become slightly engorged.
- Place template firmly on mucosa, and activate the blade (Fig. II-20).
- Begin timing when the incision is made.
- Hold filter paper beneath the incision to absorb blood (Fig. II-21).
- Continue timing until a clot has formed and bleeding has ceased.
- Normal BMBT is about 3 minutes in cats and about 4 minutes in dogs.

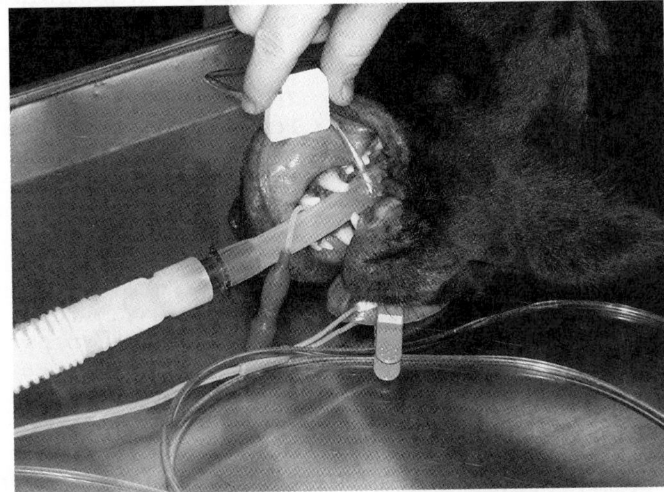

FIGURE II-20 Template bleeding device placed against buccal mucosa.

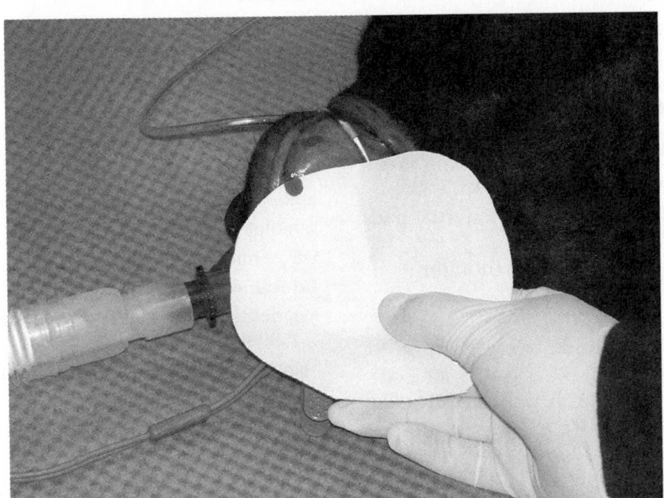

FIGURE II-21 Blotting blood below the incision.

POSTPROCEDURE

After the clot has formed and the test is completed, it may be necessary to apply pressure as needed if the clot becomes disrupted and bleeding resumes.

ALTERNATIVES AND THEIR RELATIVE MERITS

Cuticle ("toenail") bleeding time; less reliable as a measure of primary hemostasis and more painful to the animal.

AUTHOR: **ERIKA DE PAPP**

Cardiopulmonary Cerebral Resuscitation

BASIC INFORMATION

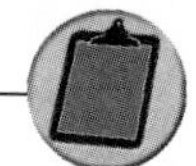

SYNONYM(S)

Cardiopulmonary resuscitation
CPCR
CPR

OVERVIEW AND GOAL(S)

Cardiopulmonary cerebral resuscitation (CPCR) is instituted for cardiorespiratory arrest or near arrest. The goal is return of spontaneous and effective circulation and, ultimately, unassisted ventilation and appropriate cerebral function.

INDICATIONS

Cardiopulmonary arrest or near arrest; signs of impending arrest may include bradycardia, hypoventilation, hypothermia, hypotension, and progressive obtundation. These indicate action should be taken to ensure continued effective circulation and ventilation. There are four cardiac rhythms that enter the definition of cardiac arrest: asystole, ventricular fibrillation, pulseless ventricular tachycardia or ventricular flutter, and electromechanical dissociation.

EQUIPMENT

- Endotracheal tube and laryngoscope
- Ambu-Bag, Bain Circuit, or mechanical ventilator
- Blood pressure (BP) measuring device (Doppler preferable)
- Electrocardiogram (ECG) (monitor preferable to printer)
- Defibrillator; internal and external paddles
- End Tidal carbon dioxide monitor
- Pulse oximetry
- Oxygen source
- Fluids: crystalloids (e.g., lactated Ringer's solution, 0.9% NaCl) and colloids (e.g., hetastarch, pentastarch)
- Blood products (e.g., whole blood, packed red blood cells, polymerized bovine hemoglobin)
- Lubricant for eyes
- Point of care testing for blood glucose, electrolytes, packed cell volume, total solids, lactate, blood gases
- Other items that should be nearby: lidocaine jelly, suction tubing and means of generating suction, IV and urethral catheters, thoracotomy tubes, laceration packs
- Items for doing open thoracic cardiac massage and vascular cut-down procedures, self retaining retractors
- Sterile gloves, means of warming fluids

The data collection sheet for record keeping should include:

- Date and time of arrest and institution of CPCR.
- Animal medical record number, body weight, signalment and underlying disease, as well as assumed cause of the arrest.
- A table or another quick and clear way to list which drugs are given, at what time they are given and at what dosage, and their effects.
- Listing of fluid type and volume administered.
- Time and energy of any defibrillation.
- Pertinent laboratory results as tests are run during the procedure.
- Personnel present during the event.
- Time of return to spontaneous circulation or ending CPCR efforts.
- Outcome.
- Data that should be noted as well include size of endotracheal tube, time and settings if mechanical ventilation is instituted, changes in status of mentation, presence or absence of urine output, and BP measurement results.

PREPARATION: IMPORTANT CHECKPOINTS

- The owners of any critically ill animal must be consulted at the time of the animal's admission regarding their resuscitation wishes for the pet. In many cases of advanced disease, advanced age, and even financial limitations of the family, CPCR may not be appropriate, and the pet should be allowed to pass away peacefully.
- Successful CPCR is a team effort. The team consists of the clinician leading the arrest and individuals who are keeping a record of the event, acquiring the requested drugs or materials, administering the drugs and therapies, providing the chest compressions, and communicating with the animal's family. The team may contain any number of people, from one or two to many, with some having multiple roles.
- A senior knowledgeable individual must take charge in fostering a calm

TABLE II-2 **Emergency Drugs**

Aminophylline: 25 mg/ml
Atropine*[1]: 0.54 mg/ml
Bretylium tosylate: 50 mg/ml
Calcium gluconate*: (10% = 100 mg/ml [calcium: 27.2 mg/ml or 1.36 mEq/ml])
Dextrose*: 5% (50 mg/ml) or 50% (500 mg/ml)
Dobutamine*: 12.5 mg/ml
Dopamine*: 40, 80, 160 mg/ml
Doxapram: 20 mg/ml
Epinephrine*[1]: 1:1000 (1 mg/ml) or 1:10,000 (0.1 mg/ml)
Esmolol: 10 mg/ml
Furosemide*: 5% (50 mg/ml)
Lidocaine*: 2% (20 mg/ml)
Magnesium sulphate*: 10% (100 mg/ml, 0.8 mEq/ml), 12.5% (125 mg/ml, 1 mEq/ml), 50% (500 mg/ml, 4 mEq/ml)
Mannitol*: 5% (50 mg/ml, 275 mOsm/L), 10% (100 mg/ml, 550 mOsm/L)
Norepinephrine*[1]: 1 mg/ml
Phenylephrine: 10 mg/ml
Procainamide*: 100 mg/ml
Sodium bicarbonate*: 8.4% (1 mEq/ml)

Glucocorticoids:
Dexamethasone: SP (4 mg/ml)
Prednisolone sodium succinate: (10 or 50 mg/ml)
Methylprednisolone sodium succinate: (62.5 mg/ml)

Reversal agents*:
Flumazenil: 0.1 mg/ml
Naloxone: 0.4 or 1 mg/ml
Atipamezole: 5 mg/ml
Yohimbine: 2 mg/ml

Sample concentrations are listed; it is essential to check the actual concentration of available product.
*Indicates drugs that should be in all basic emergency kits. The others may be beneficial, and their use is dependent on clinician knowledge and familiarity.
[1]Indicates that the drug can be administered intratracheally using a long catheter, generally at double the dose and followed by several deep breaths.

environment during CPCR, directing the other team members in their tasks, and keeping the team informed of progress. One responsible team member should be in communication with the owners to keep them apprised of progress and inform the team of changes in the family's wishes.

- Team members must be fully trained and prepared ahead of time concerning their responsibilities.
- All of the equipment that was previously listed (e.g., endotracheal tubes, breathing circuits, IV catheters, defibrillation paddles, sterile gloves, etc.) should be available in sizes appropriate for a wide variety of animals.
- Drug boxes should be checked weekly at least to ensure all drugs are available and have not reached their expiration dates.
- Equipment should be checked regularly for malfunctions and cleaned immediately after each use so that each piece is ready to be used again without notice.
- Data sheets need to be kept nearby so that events, drug administration, animal information, and responses to treatments can be recorded in a timely and accurate fashion.
- After every CPCR event, the team should review the process to assess whether changes in plan, arrangement, or protocols are necessary for improvement of efforts in the future.

POSSIBLE COMPLICATIONS AND COMMON ERRORS TO AVOID

- Inaccurate drug dosage administration.
- Hyperventilation .
- Inadequate fluid resuscitation.
- Incorrect assessment of ECG, especially false interpretation of bad contact between ECG machine and animal as "ventricular fibrillation."
- Inadequately trained personnel.
- Delayed defibrillation. The success of defibrillation approaches 100% when instituted within 1 minute of onset of fibrillation and falls precipitously to virtually 0% after 15 minutes.
- Monitoring electrolytes, blood glucose, and physiologic parameters too infrequently.
- Malfunctioning or unavailable equipment.
- Not opening the chest early enough. The decision should be made by no later than 10 minutes into an arrest to do open-chest CPR.
- Acute renal failure, diarrhea, liver dysfunction, and altered mentation and reflexes are common sequelae to inadequate oxygen delivery and tissue perfusion. Organ function must be closely monitored to take preemptive action should parameters deteriorate.

Prognosis overall is guarded to grave, depending on the underlying disease process, age, and overall state of debilitation of the animal. The number of successful resuscitations (i.e., survive to discharge) approaches 5%; however, the fact that they occur with good critical care management means that every effort should be made to resuscitate animals when appropriate.

PROCEDURE

Most of the initial tasks listed here should be occurring simultaneously.

- Identify lack of effective spontaneous circulation and ventilation.
- Initiate chest compressions.
- Intubate the airway and place ECG.
- Begin assisted ventilation with 100% inspired oxygen.
- Identify cardiac rhythm if any.
- Establish vascular access (IV catheter) if not already established.
- If anesthetized, turn off inhalant anesthetics, and reverse any injectable drugs that have reversal agents.
- If thoracic compromise exists (e.g., pleural effusion, pneumothorax) or arrest is due to pericardial effusion, open-chest CPR must be instituted immediately. With pericardial effusion, open the pericardium ventral to the phrenic nerve to improve diastolic function of the heart and remove effusion.
- Fluid administration: IV (or intraosseous [IO], especially in pediatric animals). Shock rate (e.g., one blood volume over the first hour, with constant monitoring and adjustments as needed; approximate blood volume = 90 cc/lb [200 cc/kg] in dogs, 65 cc/lb [150 cc/kg] in cats) is usually appropriate; use caution with cardiac or renal disease.
- Administer epinephrine (low dose: 0.02 mg/kg IV; high dose: 0.2 mg/kg) for pulseless electrical activity (i.e., rapid, pulseless ventricular tachycardia or flutter; electromechanical dissociation) or for asystole.
- Defibrillate electrically (e.g., starting with 2–4 J/kg if closed chest) or medically (e.g., bretylium tosylate 5 mg/kg IV) if ventricular fibrillation.
- Treat arrhythmias: atropine (0.04 mg/kg IV) followed by epinephrine again if asystole unresponsive to initial epinephrine; repeat defibrillation if ventricular fibrillation persists; lidocaine (2–3 mg/kg IV) for ventricular tachycardia or flutter; atropine for persistent bradycardia.
- Start vasopressors if BP not adequate once appropriate fluid resuscitation is administered.
- Assess metabolic condition with repeated blood gas analysis and electrolyte and blood glucose monitoring: treat abnormalities accordingly.
- Monitor body temperature, cranial nerve reflexes.

POSTPROCEDURE

MONITOR, MONITOR, MONITOR: ideally continuously; if not, then very frequent intermittent monitoring is required. A majority of critically ill animals that have been resuscitated will arrest again within a few hours.

Clinicians should monitor the following:

- BP
- Ventilation
- Oxygenation
- Cranial nerve reflexes
- Mentation
- Blood gases
- Organ-specific chemistries
- Urine output
- Electrolytes
- Blood glucose
- Central venous pressure
- Lactate
- Packed cell volume (PCV)

Clinicians should also note the following during the monitoring period:

- Administration of mannitol, at 1–2 g/kg IV over 30 minutes, is useful to reduce cerebral edema secondary to hypoxic brain injury as well as to support renal perfusion and improve circulation to tissues.
- Maintain adequate vascular volume with crystalloid, colloid, and blood product administration as indicated by perfusion status (temperature of extremities, mucous membrane color, pulse quality, hydration).
- Until the animal is conscious and mobile, recumbent animal care protocols must be used. Frequently turning the animal, lubricating its eyes, keeping it clean of eliminations, and keeping the oropharynx clean and/or suctioning the endotracheal tube are imperative. Monitor for pressure-induced sores and blood flow impairment.
- If postarrest recumbency lasts hours or more, passive range-of-motion exercises may help with improving ultimate recovery as well as helping to assess the progress of the animal's muscle strength.

ALTERNATIVES AND THEIR RELATIVE MERITS

There are many approaches to and controversies associated with CPCR. Many books and/or articles list different drug dosages and indications or contraindications. The reader is advised to be prepared by reading multiple sources and generating a customized flow chart that takes into consideration the personnel, drugs, and equipment available at a particular practice. If the animal is stable to move, postresuscitation management should ideally be handled in a well-staffed 24-hour facility.

SUGGESTED READING

Hackett TB: Cardiopulmonary cerebral resuscitation. *Vet Clin North Am Small Animal Prac* 31:6, pp 1253–1264, 2001.

AUTHOR: **SHARON DRELLICH**

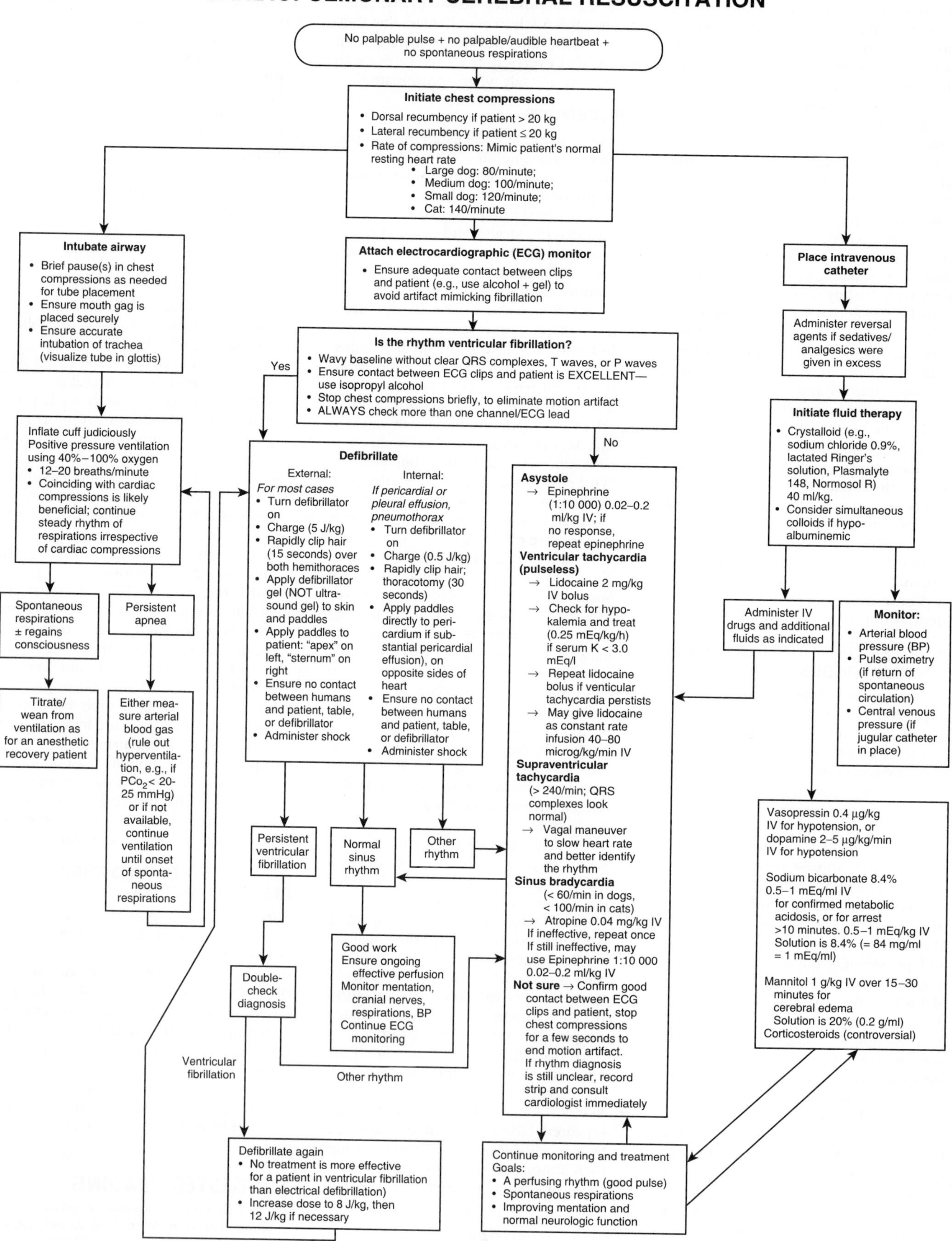

Author: Etienne Côté

Catheterization, Urethral

BASIC INFORMATION

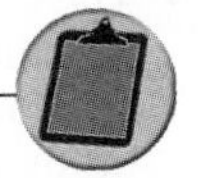

SYNONYM(S)

Urinary catheterization (see Urethral Obstruction [Feline]: Medical Management, p 1319 for catheterization of cats)

OVERVIEW AND GOAL(S)

To pass a sterile catheter from the urethral orifice into the urinary bladder to obtain a urine sample or to evacuate the bladder

INDICATIONS

- Urine sample for urinalysis/urine culture
- Temporary management of urinary retention syndromes

CONTRAINDICATIONS

- Urethral pain.
- Preputial/vulvar mass.
- An animal that might otherwise be eligible for renal transplantation can be eliminated from the transplant list on the basis of prior urethral catheterization.

EQUIPMENT, ANESTHESIA

- Sterile polypropylene or red rubber-type catheter (or Foley catheter if indwelling); size ranges from 5–14 Fr, depending on the animal's size.
- Sterile lubricant.
- Sterile syringe (3–20 ml).
- Sterile gloves.
- ± Sterile tubing and urine collection bag (if indwelling catheter).

ANTICIPATED TIME

About 10 minutes

PREPARATION: IMPORTANT CHECKPOINTS

Rectal palpation is indicated as part of the physical examination of any adult dog, particularly prior to passing a urethral catheter (identify masses, sources of pain, or other factors that would affect passage of the catheter).

POSSIBLE COMPLICATIONS AND COMMON ERRORS TO AVOID

- Incorrect orientation (female): Upon entry into the vulva, the directing (index) finger must be oriented dorsally in the vulva and vestibule, not cranially (Fig. II-22).
- Incorrect catheter position (female): The clitoral fossa externally and vagina internally, must be avoided in catheterizing female dog.
- Forceful advancement of the catheter: The catheter should pass with no resistance and no discomfort. Otherwise,-consider free catch, cystocentesis, or sedation/anesthesia (if indwelling catheter).
- Excessive advancement of the catheter: Risks include bladder perforation and catheter looping/knot formation (requiring laparotomy).

PROCEDURE

Female (see Fig. II-22):

- The dog stands on an exam table or on the ground (giant-breed dogs). The procedure is also easily performed on the laterally recumbent (e.g., anesthetized) dog.
- While an assistant holds the dog's head, the examiner opens the sterile catheter wrapper, applies sterile lubricant to the catheter tip, and ensures that the catheter remains in a sterile field (e.g., the opened catheter wrapper).
- The right-handed examiner puts on sterile gloves, lubricates the right index finger, and takes the urinary catheter under his or her right index finger (palmar surface of finger), catheter tip at fingertip.
- The examiner lifts the dog's tail with the left hand and places the index finger on the vulva, pointing dorsally, and then enters the vulva by gently everting the vulvar lips and pressing cranially.
- The examiner advances the index finger and catheter directly dorsally (i.e., toward the ceiling in the standing dog) to a narrowing, which is the vestibulovaginal junction. The ischial arch also is palpable cranially.
- The urethral opening is on the cranial/ventral surface in this region, immediately adjacent to the ischial arch. Therefore, the catheter is advanced under the index finger, such that the index finger blocks off the vestibulovaginal route and directs the catheter ventrally into the urethra (see Fig. II-22). There should be no palpable resistance when advancing the catheter.
- Once urine flows from the catheter, it is advanced 2–3 cm (small dog) to 10–15 cm (large dog) into its final position.

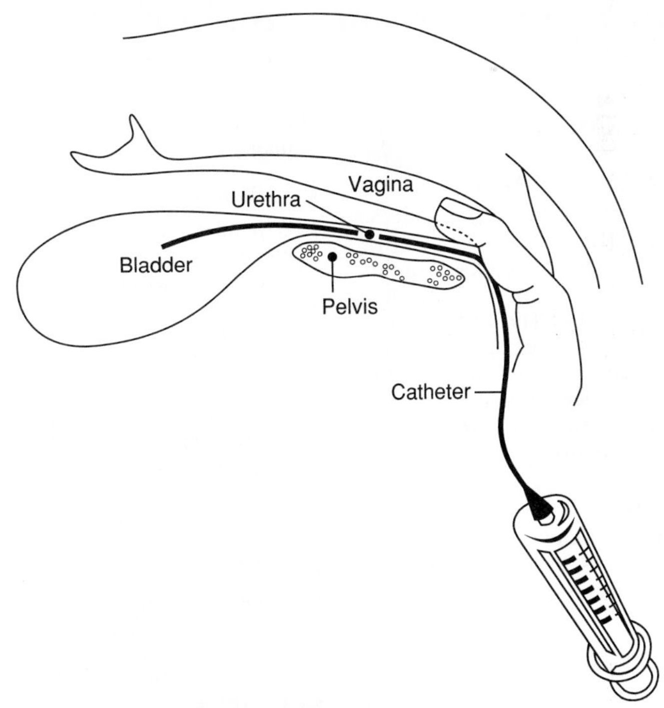

FIGURE II-22 Cross-sectional anatomy of the female urogenital tract, demonstrating the proper position of catheter and index finger.

Male (Fig. II-23):

- An assistant positions himself or herself dorsal to the laterally recumbent dog, elevates the dog's nondependent leg, and retracts the prepuce to expose the penis (see Fig. 23). A second assistant is usually needed to restrain the dog's head.
- The sterile catheter is kept within its sterile wrapper except for the distal end of the wrapper, which is cut off (see Fig. II-23A).
- The next 3–5 cm of sterile wrapper is then cut and left overlying the catheter (see Fig. II-23B); it will serve as a sliding sterile cuff for advancing the catheter out of the wrapper and up the urethra without touching the catheter directly with the fingers. This approach minimizes contamination without requiring sterile gloves.
- The catheter is placed into the urethral opening and is advanced until urine is obtained. Minor resistance may be felt at the ischium or prostate, but the procedure should be aborted if force seems necessary or if the animal seems uncomfortable.

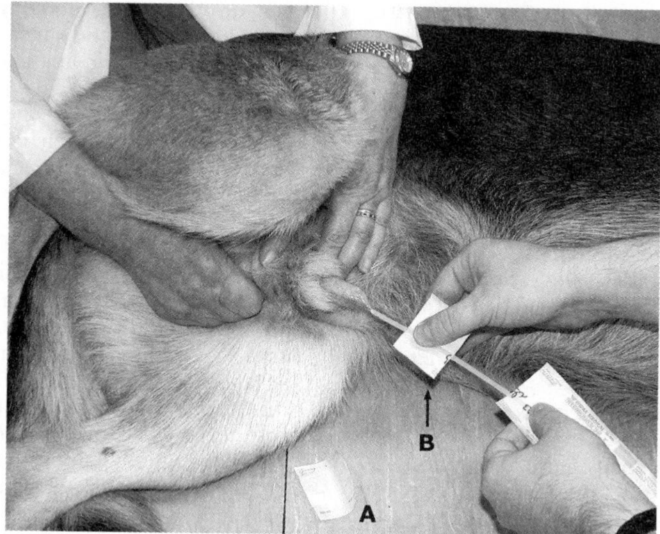

FIGURE II-23 Urethral catheterization of the male dog. **A,** Distal end of wrapper cut off. **B,** Segment of sterile wrapper functioning as a sliding cuff for advancing the catheter.

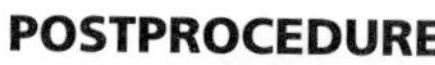

POSTPROCEDURE

If an indwelling system is used, the catheter is fixed in place, and the extension tubing and collection bag are connected to the catheter.

ALTERNATIVES AND THEIR RELATIVE MERITS

- Free-catch urine sample: simple and noninvasive but contaminates sample with urethral and genital bacteria and cells
- Cystocentesis: more invasive but may be less uncomfortable than catheterization; avoids urethral contamination

AUTHOR: **ETIENNE CÔTÉ**

Central Venous Pressure Monitoring

BASIC INFORMATION

OVERVIEW AND GOAL(S)

Central venous pressure (CVP) is a measurement that reflects the ability of the heart, and specifically the right side of the heart, to accept and pump blood through the circulatory system. The CVP reflects the interaction of the heart, vascular tone, and blood volume. Monitoring of CVP allows a better understanding of the circulatory status of the body and of the impact of fluid therapy.

INDICATIONS

- Monitoring the administration of large volumes of fluids in animals that are in shock or have impaired urine production
- Diagnostic help in difficult-to-diagnose right heart failure cases (e.g., constrictive pericarditis)

CONTRAINDICATIONS

Only those of jugular catheter placement (e.g., hypercoagulable or hypocoagulable states, skin infection over jugular site); see Jugular Catheter Placement and Management, p 1270

EQUIPMENT, ANESTHESIA

- IV jugular catheter (Mila or Arrow double-lumen catheters).
- Sterile 500-ml saline bag with IV drip set.
- CVP set (Universal CVP set, Abbott Laboratories). Alternatively, if a purpose-made kit is not available, use the following: a sterile three-way stopcock, sterile IV fluid-type tubing, and a ruler (centimeter grading and at least 30-cm long). The sterile tubing is taped to the ruler, and it is held vertically, creating a simple pressure manometer.

ANTICIPATED TIME

- About 15 minutes to install the set
- About 2 minutes for each CVP reading

PREPARATION: IMPORTANT CHECKPOINTS

- The prerequisite is the placement of an IV jugular catheter (see Jugular Catheter Placement and Management, p 1270).
  - The distal tip of this catheter should be in the cranial vena cava, just cranial to the right atrium, which allows accurate measurement of CVP without inducing premature atrial contractions. Confirm position radiographically.
  - Mila or Arrow catheters are the most commonly used because their double lumen allows simultaneous sampling and fluid delivery.

PROCEDURE

- One end (female end) of the CVP set goes to a suspended IV fluid bag (Fig. II-24). The line on that end should be closed using a clamp.
- A second end connects to tubing that is fixed to a scale (e.g., manometer scale or ruler) (see Fig. II-24). This line also should be closed using a clamp.
- The manometer tubing is pressed into the scale groove.
  - If using individual materials, tape the sterile IV fluid-type plastic tubing to the ruler.
- Using adhesive strips, fix the manometer on a vertical surface, such as the wall of a cage or a vertical stand, next to the animal and at a height such that

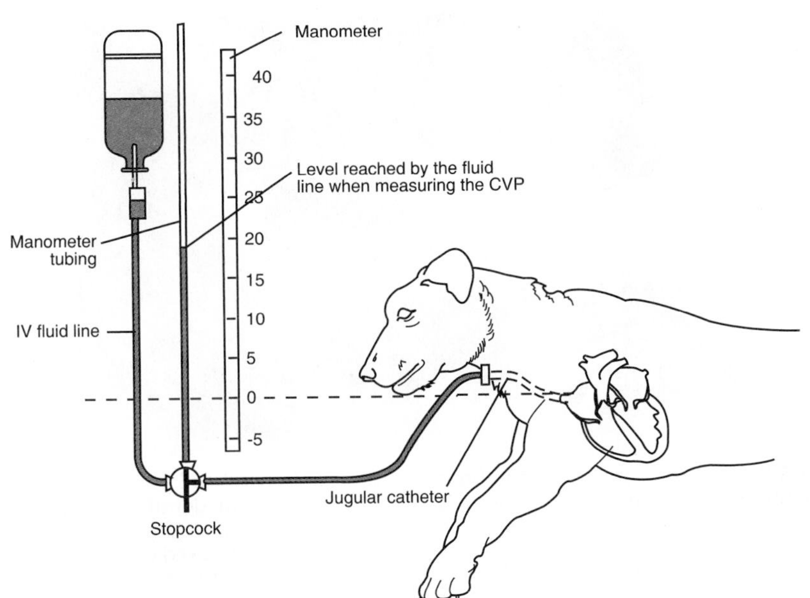

FIGURE II-24 CVP monitoring. The dashed line represents the level of the right atrium, and therefore the zero point for setting the manometer. Reprinted with permission from Sattler FP: Shock. In Kirk RW (ed): *Current Veterinary Therapy III*. Philadelphia, WB Saunders, 1968.

the 0 on the scale of the manometer/ruler is at the level of the animal's heart (right atrium).
- Unclamp the fluid line coming from the fluid bag (see Fig. II-24).
  - Fluid should run through the line until the line contains only fluid and no air.
- Then unclamp the manometer tubing and turn the three-way stopcock such that flow exists between the fluid line from the fluid bag (see Fig. II-24) and the fluid line of the manometer (see Fig. II-24).
- Fill the manometer line (see Fig. II-24) with fluid, to within 3 cm of its extremity.
- Next, connect the remaining end (male end) of the CVP set to the jugular catheter. The stopcock is usually integral to the set.
  - If using individual materials rather than a purpose-made set, connect the male end of the three-way stopcock directly to the jugular catheter.
- Finally, turn the stopcock so that a column of fluid exists between the jugular catheter and the manometer.
- The fluid in the manometer will fall until it reflects the CVP (measured in centimeters of water).

POSSIBLE COMPLICATIONS AND COMMON ERRORS TO AVOID

- One must allow fluid to flow frequently through the IV line to avoid plugging of the catheter by a blood clot. Periodic flushing with heparinized saline is desirable.
- Cardiac function needs to be factored in when interpreting results. For example, animals with tricuspid regurgitation may have elevated CVP irrespective of intravascular volume loads.
- The CVP level represents mostly loading conditions of the heart (preload), not afterload.

INTERPRETATION

- Normal CVP: variable; oscillates between −1 and +5 cm H_2O.
- Values between +5 and +10 cm H_2O are borderline.
- Values above +10 cm H_2O may indicate too much blood volume expansion. IV fluids should no longer be administered.
- Values above +15 cm H_2O may indicate right-sided congestive heart failure.

ALTERNATIVES AND THEIR RELATIVE MERITS

- Blood pressure (BP) monitoring: easier to use and represents another way to monitor the cardiovascular status and the impact of IV fluids. This is the best alternative to CVP monitoring. It does not require an IV jugular catheter.
- Weight: can be used for documenting rehydration; excessive weight gain could be a signal to slow/stop IV fluids.
- Packed cell volume/total solids (PCV/TS): A drop in the PCV/TS may indicate hemodilution.
- Urine specific gravity: A drop in the specific gravity could document successful restoration of plasma volume but is very dependent on kidney function.
- Pulmonary capillary wedge pressure/Swan-Ganz catheterization: accurately measures left-sided heart pressures, which CVP does not; however, this technique is much more technically demanding.

AUTHOR: **ERIC DE MADRON**

PROCEDURES AND TECHNIQUES

Cerebrospinal Fluid Collection

BASIC INFORMATION

SYNONYM(S)

Spinal tap
CSF tap

OVERVIEW AND GOAL(S)

- To safely collect an uncontaminated sample of cerebrospinal fluid (CSF) from an animal with suspected central nervous system (CNS) disease.
- CSF analysis is the single most valuable diagnostic test for evaluating inflammatory CNS disorders and aids in the diagnosis of other encephalopathies and myelopathies.

INDICATIONS

- Clinical signs consistent with CNS or nerve root dysfunction
- Monitoring treatment efficacy of confirmed inflammatory CNS disease
- Intrathecal administration of contrast material (myelography)

CONTRAINDICATIONS

Absolute:
- Increased intracranial pressure (depressed mental status, bradycardia, hypertension, miosis, anisocoria)
- Any condition in which general anesthesia is contraindicated

Relative:
- Advanced imaging results identifying a noninflammatory disease process, which explains the animal's clinical signs

EQUIPMENT, ANESTHESIA

- General anesthesia and endotracheal intubation
- A few 20- or 22-gauge, 1.5-inch spinal needles (2.5- or 3.5-inch needle may be needed for large dogs or for lumbar approach)
- Hair clippers
- Surgical scrub solution, isopropyl alcohol, and gauze
- Sterile surgical gloves
- Sterile collection tubes (do not use tubes containing EDTA [lavender-top tubes])
- An assistant to position the animal and stabilize the animal's head and neck
- Level stationary or locked table

ANTICIPATED TIME

About 30 minutes of anesthesia

PREPARATION: IMPORTANT CHECKPOINTS

- Performed preferably after advanced imaging has ruled out both noninflammatory processes (neoplasia, malformation, vascular) and obvious increased intracranial pressure (coning and caudal displacement of the cerebellum, flattening of gyri, loss of sulci).
- Make arrangements for laboratory transport within 30 minutes of collection, or have in-house analysis equipment prepared and calibrated.
- If immediate analysis of the CSF is not possible, special preservation techniques may be required (prior laboratory consultation is recommended).
- Warn owners of hair clipping and low risk of complications. Complications associated with the procedure, although rare, can be fatal.

PROCEDURE

- General anesthesia and intubation
- Preparation and positioning for centesis from the cerebellomedullary cistern (preferred due to ease and lower risk of blood contamination):
  - Shave and surgically scrub the skin from the occipital protuberance rostrally to the dorsal spine of C3 caudally and to the base of each pinna laterally.
  - Sterile gloves are worn, but the field is not usually draped.
  - Lateral recumbency: right lateral for the right-handed clinician and left lateral for the left-handed clinician.
  - An assistant holds the head at a 90-degree angle to the neck and parallel to the table. Care must be taken not to overflex the neck, which could result in obstruction of the endotracheal tube or compress the jugular veins and would increase the intracranial pressure. For the head to be parallel to the table, the assistant must hold the nose slightly elevated from the table.
  - The assistant positions the dorsal aspect of the neck at the edge or slightly over the edge of the table.
  - The clinician should sit on a stool or kneel to be at eye level with the animal's head.
- Landmarking and puncture:
  - The right-handed clinician places the left thumb on the right wing of the atlas and the left ring or middle finger on the left wing of the atlas (Figs. II-25 and II-26).
  - The left index finger is used for identifying the midline by palpating the occipital protuberance and the dorsal spine of C2, drawing an invisible line between these points.
  - Many cats and toy-breed dogs do not have a well-defined occipital protuberance. In these cases, the dorsal spine of C2 should be used as the sole landmark for identifying the midline.
  - The orientation of the needle's path will be parallel to the table's surface and toward the angle of the animal's mandible.
  - For dogs, using the right hand, the needle with stylette in place is inserted through the skin along the midline just cranial to the wings of the atlas.
  - In cats, the skin is tough, and the distance between the skin and subarachnoid space is very small. Therefore, although the same point of insertion is identified, the skin should be tented prior to inserting the needle through the skin into the subcutaneous tissues.
  - The needle is directed through subcutaneous fat and muscle toward the subarachnoid space, taking care to avoid lateral, caudal, or cranial deviation of the spinal needle.
  - Occasionally, a loss of resistance to the needle insertion is felt as the needle passes through the fascial planes of the muscle and, eventually, the dorsal atlantooccipital membrane; this so-called pop is not reliable and should not be used as an indicator of appropriate depth of the needle.
  - While maintaining a grip on the hub of the needle with the right hand, the left hand now grasps the needle near its insertion into the skin.
  - The stylette is withdrawn with the right hand, and the hub of the needle is examined for the presence of CSF.
  - If no CSF is present, the needle is first withdrawn a few millimeters while watching for the appearance of CSF to ensure the needle has not been inserted too deep (into nervous tissue), and then the needle is advanced. The stylette need not be replaced at this point. (Although advancing the needle without the stylette creates a slight risk of creating a tissue plug in the needle, it decreases the risk of advancing the needle too deeply as CSF will appear as soon as the subarachnoid space is entered).
  - As the needle is advanced one of three things will happen:
    - CSF appears in the hub of the needle and will begin to drip out. The needle should then be advanced 1 mm to place the entire bevel in the cerebellomedullary cistern, and the needle is grasped firmly against the skin. The slight advancement and firm hold on the needle reduce the risk of blood contamination from meningeal vessels.
    - The needle hits bone. This is usually the occipital bone, and the needle should be redirected caudally to enter the cerebellomedullary

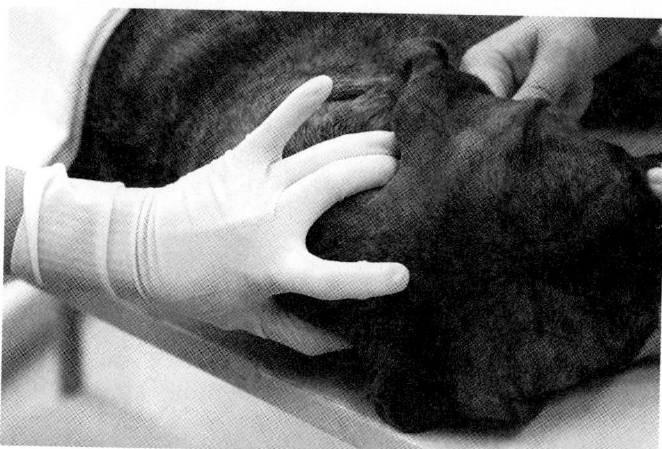

FIGURE II-25 Landmarks. Dog is in right lateral recumbency, head pointing to the right of the photo. This right-handed clinician is using the left hand to identify the occipital protuberance (index finger) and wings of the atlas (right wing of the atlas: thumb; left wing of the atlas: middle and ring fingers). The neck is appropriately flexed (≈90°) and the nose is elevated by an assistant so that the muzzle is parallel to the table surface.

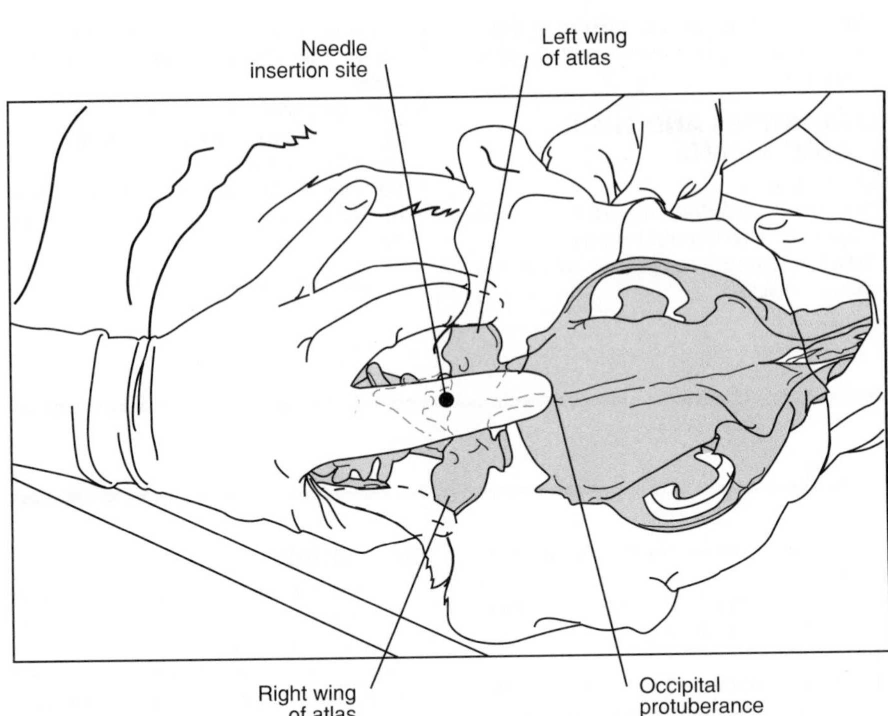

FIGURE II-26 Diagram of the same image as in Fig. II-25, showing the bony landmarks and site of needle insertion.

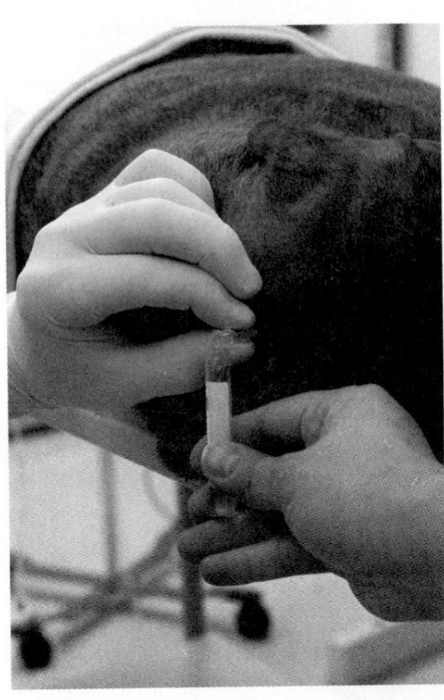

FIGURE II-27 Same animal as in Figs. II-25 and II-26. While the clinician holds the needle, an assistant collects the CSF.

cistern; if it strikes the atlas, the needle needs to be redirected cranially. The needle may be walked along the bone to find the cistern, bearing in mind that it will be only millimeters deeper, but this may result in blood contamination from trauma to the periosteum.

- Frank blood appears in the hub. This most likely indicates that the needle is off midline and has punctured a venous sinus. In this case, the needle is removed and discarded, gloves are changed, the surgical prep is repeated, and the procedure is started again. NOTE: If blood is encountered, it is typically from a location outside the subarachnoid space and does not limit the ability to obtain an uncontaminated sample when the procedure is repeated.

- Once CSF begins to drip from the hub, it is collected into two plain, sterile red-top tubes. Ideally, an assistant collects the sample, and the examiner does not release the needle during collection (Fig. II-27).
- In general, 1 ml of CSF is required for assessment of the white blood cell (WBC) count, protein determination, and cytologic examination (1 ml/5 kg of body weight can be obtained safely).
- If the animal weighs more than 5 kg, additional CSF can and should be collected for possible culture or ancillary diagnostics, such as infectious titers or immunoglobulin indices.
- Once the appropriate amount of CSF has been collected, the needle is removed.
- NOTE: If during the procedure the heart rate acutely decreases or if fluid streams rather than drips from the hub when the subarachnoid space is entered, the needle should be removed and the procedure aborted.

- Preparation and positioning (for centesis from the lumbar subarachnoid space) is technically more difficult, yields less fluid, and is more likely to involve blood contamination but is more sensitive for focal thoracolumbar lesions:
  - The skin is shaved and surgically scrubbed over the dorsal midline from L3 cranially to the midsacrum caudally and the wings of the ilium laterally.
  - Sterile gloves are worn, but the field is not usually draped.
  - The animal is positioned in lateral recumbency with the lumbar spine flexed ("tucked" posture).
- Landmarking and puncture:
  - The needle enters the L5–L6 or L6–L7 interspace in dogs, or the L7–S1 interspace in cats.
  - Except in very small or thin animals, the L6 dorsal spine is typically the most caudal and can be palpated just cranial to the wings of the ilium.
  - If the L7 dorsal spine is palpable, it is usually much smaller than that of L6 and lies between the wings of the ilium.
  - Radiographs can demonstrate individual differences in anatomy.
  - The needle is inserted into the skin just caudolaterally to the caudal dorsal spine of the space to be entered (i.e., caudolaterally to L6 for puncture between L5 and L6).
  - The needle is directed craniomedially to puncture the interarcuate space between the vertebrae.
  - If bone is encountered, the needle is redirected (usually cranially) until the space is identified.
  - If the needle is inserted to the hub and no bone is encountered, the needle is either too short or directed too far laterally.
  - Fluid can be collected from the dorsal subarachnoid space, but more often the needle is passed through the nervous tissue to the floor of the vertebral canal.
  - The stylette is removed, and if CSF is not recovered, the needle is withdrawn slightly to enter the ventral subarachnoid space while the exam-

iner watches for the appearance of fluid in the hub of the needle.
  - The CSF typically flows much more slowly from this site when compared with the cerebellomedullary cistern.

POSTPROCEDURE

- Routine postanesthetic monitoring.
- Monitor for neurologic deficits due to iatrogenic trauma (respiratory difficulty or vestibular ataxia with puncture from the cerebellomedullary cistern; paresis and proprioceptive ataxia with lumbar puncture).

ALTERNATIVES AND THEIR RELATIVE MERITS

MRI or CT scan:
- Advanced imaging superior for the diagnosis of structural lesions.
- May be strongly suggestive of inflammatory disease.
- Typically used in addition to CSF analysis to fully evaluate disorders of the CNS.

Serum infectious titers:
- Systemic disease not necessarily reflective of CNS disease.
- For most inflammatory nervous system diseases, no infectious agent is identified.

AUTHOR: **GREG KILBURN**

Chest Tube Placement

BASIC INFORMATION

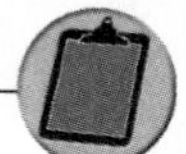

SYNONYM(S)

Thoracostomy tube placement

OVERVIEW AND GOAL(S)

To provide means for frequent or continuous drainage of fluid or air from the pleural cavity

INDICATIONS

- Pyothorax
- Rapidly forming pleural effusion
- Recurring pneumothorax requiring repeated thoracocentesis
- Tension pneumothorax
- Postoperative thoracotomy management

CONTRAINDICATIONS

Severe coagulopathy

EQUIPMENT, ANESTHESIA

- General anesthesia with intubation (ideally) or sedation
- Clippers
- Surgical scrub
- A #11 scalpel blade
- Local anesthetic (e.g., 2% lidocaine 0.2–0.5 ml/kg, SC; maximum of 7 ml)
- Small surgical pack
- Suture material (e.g., 2-0 to 4-0 nylon)
- An assistant (if possible)
- Thoracostomy tube
- Catheter adapter
- A three-way stopcock
- Injection caps
- ± Continuous drainage device
- 20-gauge orthopedic wire
- Wire twister and cutter

ANTICIPATED TIME

About 15 to 45 minutes

PREPARATION: IMPORTANT CHECKPOINTS

- Make extra drainage holes in chest tube with scalpel blade if fluid is present in pleural space (<50% of the diameter of tube).
- Monitor animal's oxygenation with pulse oximetry during anesthesia and placement.
- If tension pneumothorax is present, continuous evacuation of pleural space by thoracocentesis until chest wall is opened will help stabilize animal.

POSSIBLE COMPLICATIONS AND COMMON ERRORS TO AVOID

- Improper (SC) placement of tube
- Impaling the heart or lungs with the tube's stylet/trochar
- Pulmonary contusions
- Placement of the tube into the abdominal cavity with abdominal organ trauma
- Aforementioned complications are more common with the trochar method
- Tube migration or premature removal of tube by animal
- Development of life-threatening pneumothorax if tube becomes open to atmosphere

PROCEDURE

- General anesthesia (preferable). Can be done with sedation for an emergency case.
- Lateral recumbency.
- Clip hair from lateral thorax, extending from axilla cranially to the last rib caudally, and from dorsal spine to ventral midline (Fig. II-28).
- Aseptically prep and drape area.
- Using scalpel blade, make a small stab incision in the skin over the highest point of the thorax at the ninth through tenth intercostal spaces (ICS).
- The assistant then pulls the skin cranially several centimeters, and the assistant holds the skin in that position. The chest tube will be placed into the thorax via seventh or eighth ICS. Later, when the skin is released, the result will be a SC tunnel, from which the tube should emerge through the skin around the ninth or tenth ICS.
- Lidocaine is injected into intercostal muscle at the tube insertion site, or an

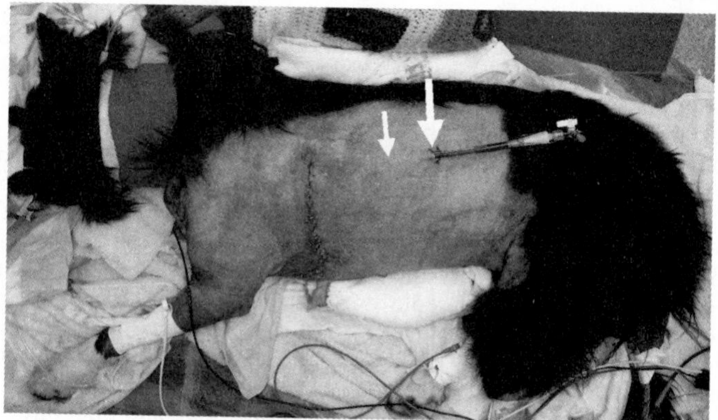

FIGURE II-28 Chest tube in place after lateral thoracotomy for a penetrating wound. The tube enters the skin at approximately the tenth ICS (*large arrow*), tunnels under the skin for three rib spaces, and enters the thorax (*small arrow*) through the seventh ICS. Note the Chinese finger-trap suture pattern to secure the tube and the use of wire to secure the tube-to-adapter and adapter-to-stopcock connections.

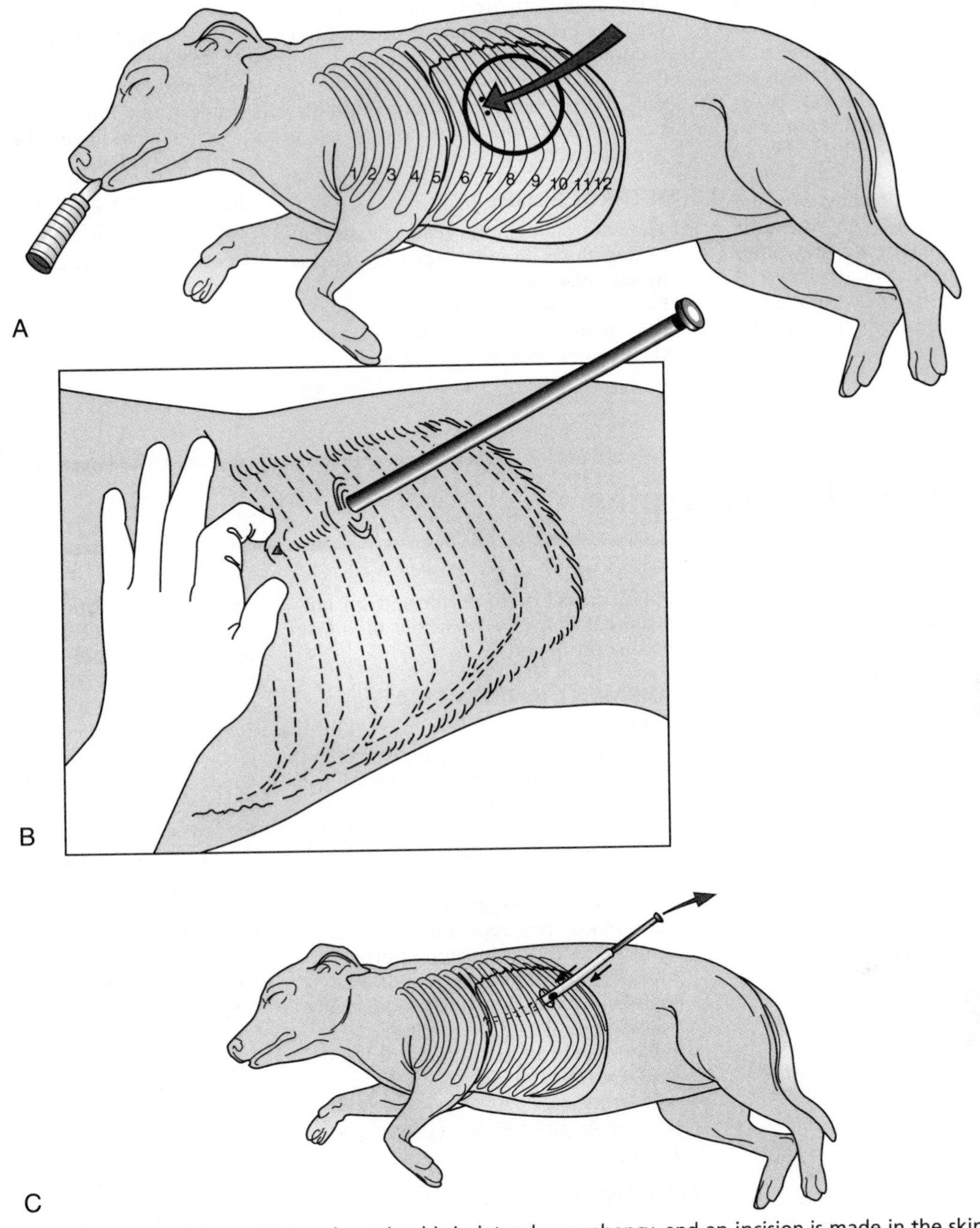

FIGURE II-29 **A**, For placement of a chest tube, the animal is in lateral recumbency, and an incision is made in the skin at least two ICS caudal to the planned site of entry into the thorax. **B**, The chest tube and the trocar within it are tunneled together SC to the appropriate ICS, and the chest is entered with the tube. **C**, The tube is then advanced off the trocar (*small arrows*), such that all side holes of the chest tube are within the pleural space and the trocar has not advanced farther into the chest. The trocar is then withdrawn (*larger arrow*), and the chest tube is capped and secured as shown in Fig. II-28.

intercostal block can be performed, injecting lidocaine just ventral and caudal to the transverse processes of the thoracic vertebrae/head of ribs one space cranial and caudal and at the site of insertion. Before injecting, aspirate back to determine that needle is not in the intercostal artery or vein.

- Stop manual ventilation while inserting tube to deflate lungs and decrease risk of trauma to lungs.
- With the skin still drawn cranially, hemostats are used for bluntly dissecting vertically into the pleural space, spreading the jaws wide enough for the tube to snugly fit through the opening. The tube is inserted and advanced, making sure that all side holes in the tube are well within the thorax.
- Connect tube to a three-way stopcock and injection caps or a pleural drainage system (see Fig. II-28).
- Secure to skin with a purse-string suture around the tube at the entry site and a "Chinese finger trap" suture pattern to reduce sliding of the tube.
- Place sterile dressing and light bandage.
- Tube connection sites can be secured with orthopedic wire in figure-eight patterns.

Alternate method, trochar technique (Fig. II-29):

- Sedation or anesthesia should be provided if possible.
- Initial prep as previously described.
- Tube and trochar/stylet within it are tunneled SC by two to three rib spaces and then positioned perpendicular to the chest wall and grasped tightly 1–2 inches from distal tip.
- Top of the tube is hit bluntly with the palm of other hand, popping the tube through into pleural space; the other hand grasping tube and trochar 1–2 inches from the distal tip acts as a guard to prevent the tube from entering the thorax excessively.
- Tube is slid off the trochar/stylet, cranially and ventrally, then connected and secured as described previously.
- This very rapid placement technique is only recommended in emergency situations, due to increased risk of iatrogenic trauma.

POSTPROCEDURE

- Thoracic radiographs (lateral and ventrodorsal or dorsoventral) to check tube(s) placement.
- Bandage to secure tube(s).
- Pain management: injectable opioids versus intrathoracic bupivacaine.
    - Bupivacaine can be given at a dose of 1.5 mg/kg through tube every 6–8 hours.
- Continuous monitoring as long as the chest tube is in place due to the risk of disconnection and the development of pneumothorax.

ALTERNATIVES AND THEIR RELATIVE MERITS

Repeat thoracocentesis: may become difficult to manage animal if pleural evacuation is needed frequently.

AUTHOR: **LORI S. WADDELL**

Cross-Match and Blood Typing

BASIC INFORMATION

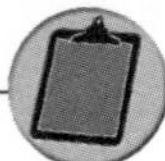

SYNONYM(S)

Blood typing: determines if the primary red blood cell (RBC) antigens of the donor and the primary RBC antigens of the recipient are identical

Major cross-match: evaluates incompatibilities between the donor's RBCs and recipient's plasma

Minor cross-match: evaluates incompatibilities between recipient's RBCs and donor's plasma

OVERVIEW AND GOAL(S)

- Minimize transfusion reactions and maximize longevity of post-transfusion RBCs.
- Cross-matching and/or blood typing eliminates most transfusion reactions.

INDICATIONS

- Blood typing: performed prior to administering a blood transfusion to allow selection of blood that will minimize sensitization; should be performed on all donor animals.
- Major cross-match: performed on animals receiving whole blood or packed RBCs.
    - First-time transfusions to dogs are usually safe without prior cross-matching (blood typing is generally sufficient).
    - Strongly recommended in dogs that have whelped or that received a transfusion more than 4 days previously (even if blood typed).
    - Strongly recommended in all cats, even with first transfusion. Transfusing cats without prior blood typing and/or cross-matching is dangerous.
- Minor cross-match: performed on animals that will receive whole blood or plasma products.

EQUIPMENT, ANESTHESIA

Blood typing:

- Commercially available canine or feline blood-typing cards (DMS Laboratories, 2 Darts Mill Road, Flemington, NJ 08822)
- Approximatley ≥0.4 ml EDTA anticoagulated (purple-top tube) whole blood

Cross-match:

- 1 ml EDTA-anticoagulated (purple-top tube) blood from recipient
- 1 ml EDTA-anticoagulated (purple-top tube) blood from donor or cross-match segments from units of blood being considered
- Tabletop centrifuge
- 3-ml test tubes
- 0.9% saline
- Disposable pipettes or 1-cc syringes
- Test tube rack

ANTICIPATED TIME

- Blood typing: 2 minutes.
- Major and minor cross-match: 40 minutes.

PREPARATION: IMPORTANT CHECKPOINTS

- In-house canine blood-typing cards only detect dog erythrocyte antigen (DEA) 1.1 antigen.
- The stability and expiration of components of blood typing kits vary: Ensure proper storage and check expiration dates.

POSSIBLE COMPLICATIONS AND COMMON ERRORS TO AVOID

Dogs or cats that are autoagglutinating due to underlying disease (e.g., immune-mediated hemolytic anemia [IMHA]) or that have had a recent incompatible blood transfusion cannot be accurately blood typed and will have false-positive cross-match and blood typing card results.

Severely anemic cats or dogs (<10% hematocrit) may not show agglutination when reagent is added to blood-typing cards (prozone effect): Remove some of the plasma to concentrate the RBCs before adding a drop to the test cards.

PROCEDURE

BLOOD TYPING: commercially available blood-typing cards (see package inserts).

CROSS-MATCH (MAJOR AND MINOR)

Step 1

- Collect 1–2 ml of donor blood in an EDTA (purple-top) tube, or use an equivalent 1–2 ml of cross-match segments from stored whole blood or PRBCs.
- Collect 1–2 ml of recipient blood in an EDTA tube.
- Place donor blood in one red-top tube and recipient blood in a different red-top tube.
- Centrifuge the two red-top tubes for 10 minutes (1000 × g).
- Separate donor plasma from donor RBCs using a pipette and save the plasma in a labeled red-top tube for later use.
- Separate recipient plasma from recipient RBCs using a new pipette and save the recipient plasma in a labeled red-top tube for later use.
- Wash the remaining packed RBCs three times by filling tubes with 0.9% saline, gently resuspending, centrifuging (1000 × g) for 5 minutes, and decanting off the saline (discard the saline).
- After a third wash, add 0.2 ml of remaining PRBCs from the donor red-top tube to 4.8 ml of 0.9% saline (in a

separate red-top tube) and gently mix (makes a 4% RBC solution).

- Add 0.2 ml of remaining PRBCs from the recipient red-top tube to 4.8 ml of 0.9% saline and gently mix.

Step 2A

On a glass slide:

- Mix 2 drops of recipient plasma and 1 drop of donor RBC suspension (major cross-match).
- Mix 2 drops of donor plasma and 1 drop of recipient RBC suspension (minor cross-match).
- For recipient control, mix 2 drops of recipient plasma and 1 drop of recipient RBC suspension.
- Gently rock slides back and forth, and note presence of macroagglutination within 2 minutes.
- Add coverslip, and examine microscopically for microagglutination within 5 minutes.

Step 2B

In a red-top tube:

- Mix 2 drops of recipient plasma and 1 drop of donor RBC suspension (major cross-match).
- Mix 2 drops of donor plasma and 1 drop of recipient RBC suspension (minor cross-match).
- Incubate at room temperature for 15 minutes.
- Centrifuge for 1 minute.
- Observe the plasma for hemolysis or agglutination.
- Hemolysis or agglutination indicates incompatibility.

POSTPROCEDURE

DEA 1.1^+ dogs can receive DEA 1.1^+ or DEA 1.1^- blood. DEA 1.1^- dogs should only receive DEA 1.1^- blood. The following should be noted if autoagglutination occurs:

- When the recipient control shows hemolysis or agglutination (common in IMHA cases), the cross-match cannot be interpreted. In such cases, use "universal blood" (determined by complete blood typing) if no prior transfusion has been given or use hemoglobin-based oxygen carriers (i.e., Oxyglobin).
- If all available units are incompatible, the least reactive unit may need to be administered.
- Cats that show a positive result in both wells of blood-typing cards should be retested in a reference laboratory for the rare AB blood type.

ALTERNATIVES AND THEIR RELATIVE MERITS

An EDTA-collected blood sample can be sent to commercial laboratories for complete blood typing of dogs and cats: advised for all blood donors. In dogs, "universal donors" (DEA 1.1^-, DEA 1.2^-, and DEA 7^-) can also be identified through laboratory blood typing. Consultation with the laboratory is advised because different labs test for different canine erythrocyte antigens.

AUTHOR: **SØREN R. BOYSEN**

Cystocentesis

BASIC INFORMATION

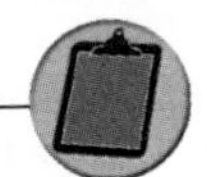

OVERVIEW AND GOAL(S)

To obtain a sample of urine from the bladder

INDICATIONS

- Urinalysis
- Urine culture and sensitivity (C&S)
- Diagnostic evaluation of vaginal or preputial discharge or of discolored urine

CONTRAINDICATIONS

- Bleeding disorder
- Ascites
- Peritonitis
- Dyspnea, back/hip pain, or other conditions causing distress during dorsal recumbency

EQUIPMENT, ANESTHESIA

The procedure is generally performed awake, but sedation or general anesthesia does not preclude it. The following equipment should be available:

- A 22-gauge, 1.5-inch needle
- A 12-cc syringe
- Cotton balls or gauze squares (e.g., 3 × 3 inches)
- Isopropyl alcohol

ANTICIPATED TIME

About 5 minutes

PREPARATION: IMPORTANT CHECKPOINTS

Identify contraindications on physical examination, and perform any diagnostic tests, including (as applicable) abdominal radiographs, abdominal ultrasound, complete blood count (CBC) with platelet count, coagulation profile.

POSSIBLE COMPLICATOINS AND COMMON ERRORS TO AVOID

The bladder is variable in its exact location from one individual to the next as well as in its degree of fullness in every individual. Therefore, it should be identified by palpation prior to cystocentesis.

PROCEDURE

- The animal is placed in dorsal recumbency (Fig. II-30). The help of one or more assistants may be necessary to keep the animal in this position. In addition, a U-shaped trough may be used for keeping the animal comfortably recumbent (Fig. II-31). The examiner stands or kneels beside the animal (either side).
- The right-handed examiner palpates the animal's caudal abdomen with the left hand and holds the syringe—with needle attached—in the right hand.
- Landmarks:
  - General guidelines: cranial to the brim of the pelvis, caudal to the umbilicus.
  - A commonly used landmark in female dogs, especially obese dogs, is the natural depression that forms on the caudal abdominal surface just cranial to the inguinal mammary glands on the ventral midline (see Fig. II-30). Cystocentesis is performed with the needle entering perpendicularly at this point is generally successful if the bladder is moderately or markedly full of urine.
  - In general, the urinary bladder is more easily palpated in cats than dogs and in thinner animals.
- With cystocentesis in male dogs, an assistant can retract the prepuce laterally. Alternatively, the prepuce may be drawn to one side by the examiner in the palm of the palpating hand.
- With the bladder encircled with the fingers of the left hand, the examiner cleans the overlying skin on the ventral midline with isopropyl alcohol-soaked gauze or cotton.
- The examiner then introduces the needle through the overlying skin on the ventral midline, directed perpendicular

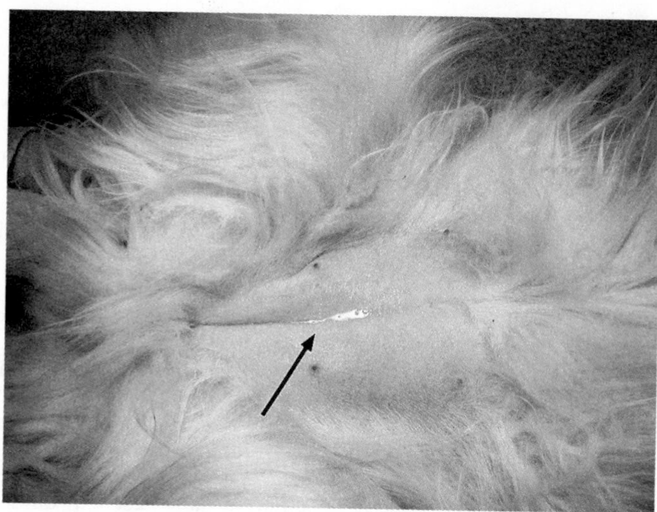

FIGURE II-30 Ventral abdomen of a female dog in dorsal recumbency; cranial is to the right. A natural depression occurs on the ventral midline of the caudal abdomen of female dogs (*arrow*), where isopropyl alcohol pools.

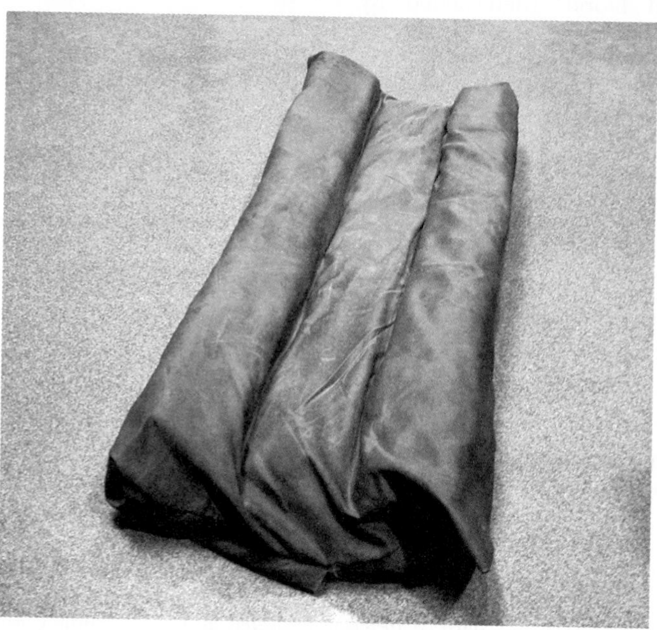

FIGURE II-31 U-shaped foam trough used for maintaining an animal comfortably in dorsal recumbency.

to the skin (i.e., vertically downward when the dog is in dorsal recumbency). The examiner pulls back on the syringe plunger, creating negative pressure from the moment the needle is through the skin. Doing so helps identify penetration of the bladder as soon as it occurs.

- If no urine is obtained, it is important to NOT redirect the needle while it is in the abdomen; doing so could cause laceration of abdominal structures with the needle tip. When no urine is obtained, the needle may be withdrawn until it is just within the abdominal wall, redirected to a new angle, and then readvanced.
- Once urine flows into the syringe, the examiner withdraws the desired amount of urine and then withdraws the needle and submits the sample for analysis.

POSTPROCEDURE

No discomfort, gross hematuria, or other abnormality is expected after a properly performed cystocentesis.

ALTERNATIVES AND THEIR RELATIVE MERITS

- Free-catch: atraumatic, but the sample is contaminated with urethral, preputial/vulvar, and cutaneous bacteria.
- Urethral catheterization: minimally invasive; may be more uncomfortable than cystocentesis in many animals and is not practical for urine sampling in cats.
- Ultrasound-guided cystocentesis: useful when the bladder is small, when the animal is very obese, or when there is ascites or any mass lesion in the caudal abdomen.

AUTHOR: **ETIENNE CÔTÉ**

Cystogram

BASIC INFORMATION

OVERVIEW AND GOAL(S)

On survey radiographs, the urinary bladder is often visualized. However, if further evaluation of the urinary bladder is needed or if the urinary bladder is not adequately seen on survey films, a cystogram may be needed.

A cystogram is a radiographic study of the urinary bladder following intraluminal administration of a positive contrast medium, negative contrast medium, or both. Evaluation of the urinary bladder with ultrasound has largely replaced many functions of the cystogram.

INDICATIONS

- Dysuria, pollakiuria, hematuria, stranguria
- Evaluation of caudal abdominal masses
- Increased or decreased opacity associated with the bladder
- Nonvisualization of the bladder after abdominal or pelvic trauma; suspected bladder rupture
- Abnormally shaped or located bladder
- Congenital abnormalities
- Recurrent or nonresponsive urinary tract infection (UTI)
- Suspected neoplasia
- Suspected polyp(s)
- Suspected radiolucent calculi
- Posturethral/cystic surgical evaluation

SPECIFIC STUDY FOR SUSPECTED DISEASE

- Negative-contrast cystogram: bladder position
- Positive-contrast cystogram: bladder rupture, bladder position
- Double-contrast cystogram: mucosal thickness (cystitis), mucosal margination, luminal contents (calculi), neoplasia

EQUIPMENT, ANESTHESIA

- General anesthesia or heavy sedation
- Agents:
  - Negative-contrast cystogram: room air, carbon dioxide, nitrous oxide.
  - Positive-contrast cystogram: iodinated contrast medium (sodium iothalamate, sodium diatrizoate) or nonionidinated contrast medium (iohexol, iopamidol) if clinically warranted.
- Urinary catheter with inflatable bulb (Foley catheter) appropriately sized for the animal
- Tomcat catheter used for male cats
- Sterile lubricating jelly
- Surgical gloves
- Sterile syringe for contrast
- Sterile syringe for withdrawing urine from bladder
- Sterile syringe to inflate Foley balloon
- Mild surgical scrub solution and gauze/sponges for prepping the penis/vulva
- Sterile three-way stopcock
- Sterile catheter adapter (Christmas tree)
- Enema bag/set
- Sterile saline

ANTICIPATED TIME

Approximately 30 minutes

PREPARATION

- Animal fasted 24 hours.
- Water *ad libitum*.
- Enema given at least 2 hours prior to study to remove a maximum of fecal material from the colon to allow visualization of the urinary bladder.
- Sterile gloves should be worn from this point forward.
- Positive-contrast cystogram:
  - Dilute positive contrast agent to 15–30% with sterile saline.
  - Dose of diluted contrast is 10 ml/kg.
  - Draw appropriate dose into a syringe.
- Negative-contrast cystogram:
  - Use 10 ml/kg of chosen negative agent (cats: 4–50 ml generally adequate).
  - Draw appropriate dose into a syringe.
- Double-contrast cystogram:
  - Use 10 ml of undiluted positive-contrast agent (cats: 2–4 ml).
  - Use 10 ml/kg of chosen negative-contrast agent (cats: 40–50 ml generally adequate).
  - Draw appropriate doses into syringes.
- Remove Foley catheter from packaging using aseptic technique.
- Attach catheter adapter (Christmas tree) to Foley catheter.
- Attach three-way stopcock to catheter adapter.
- Draw appropriate amount of air into a syringe to inflate the Foley bulb.
- Attach syringe containing air to the three-way stopcock.
- Open three-way stopcock to allow air flow into the catheter bulb to ensure that the bulb is intact. Fill the bulb to the recommended level, and close the three-way stopcock.
- Once it is clear that the bulb will hold air, release the air from the bulb, leaving the air in the syringe.
- Attach the syringe filled with selected contrast onto the three-way stopcock (and fill the catheter with positive contrast if performing a positive contrast study).
- Close the stopcock to the contrast material, and open to the syringe filled with air for bulb inflation.
- In male cats, a sterile tomcat catheter is used. Contrast material is drawn into the syringe, and the syringe is attached directly to the catheter.

POSSIBLE COMPLICATIONS AND COMMON ERRORS TO AVOID

- Urinary bladder rupture
- Cystitis: hemorrhagic, emphysematous
- Bacterial contamination: iatrogenic UTI
- Bladder or urethral trauma
- Catheter kinking or knotting
- Positive-contrast media reaction (rare)
- Negative-contrast: possibility of air embolism with severe mucosal disease (rare)

PROCEDURE

- Preliminary abdominal radiographs are made to determine adequate animal preparation and to set radiographic technique.
- The kilovoltage peak (kVp) should be set between 65 and 75 to maximize contrast due to the photoelectric effect (K edge of iodine).
- Milliampere seconds (mAs) may need to be increased 25–50% over surveys.
- The animal should be placed in left lateral recumbency.
- An assistant should extrude the penis in the male.
- The penis/vulva should be prepped with mild surgical scrub solution.
- Sterile lubricating jelly is placed onto the top of the Foley catheter.
- The catheter is then gently advanced into the urinary bladder (a stylet can be used with the Foley if necessary) (see Catheterization, Urethral, p 1205).
- Inflate the catheter bulb with air, and then close the stopcock to maintain inflation.
- Attach a syringe onto the stopcock, and open the stopcock to this syringe.
- Remove as much urine as possible from the bladder (repeat as necessary to allow total emptying).
- Close stopcock to this syringe and discard syringe
- Turn stopcock open to the contrast medium, and inject the dose of chosen agent.
- Palpate the bladder periodically to ensure that the bladder is not overdistended.
- Stop if back pressure is felt, if reflux is seen around the catheter, or if the bladder feels full.
  - Positive: Once the contrast is in the bladder, images can be obtained (Figs. II-32 and II-33).
  - Negative: Once the contrast is in the bladder, images can be obtained.
  - Double: Inject the positive contrast, and then roll the animal to ensure good mucosal coating; follow this with injection of the negative contrast, and then images can be made (Fig. II-34).
  - NOTE: If a double-contrast study is desired after a positive-contrast study, the majority of the positive contrast is removed from the bladder, leaving only a small puddle; then negative contrast is injected.
- Ventrodorsal and lateral radiographs are made immediately after injection.

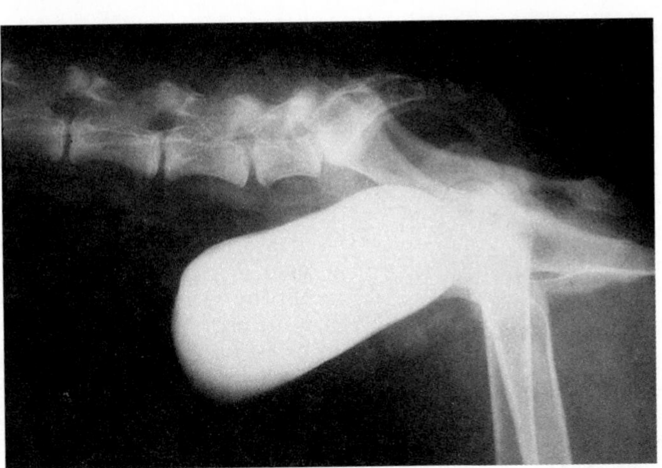

FIGURE II-32 Positive-contrast cystogram, lateral projection. Normal study.

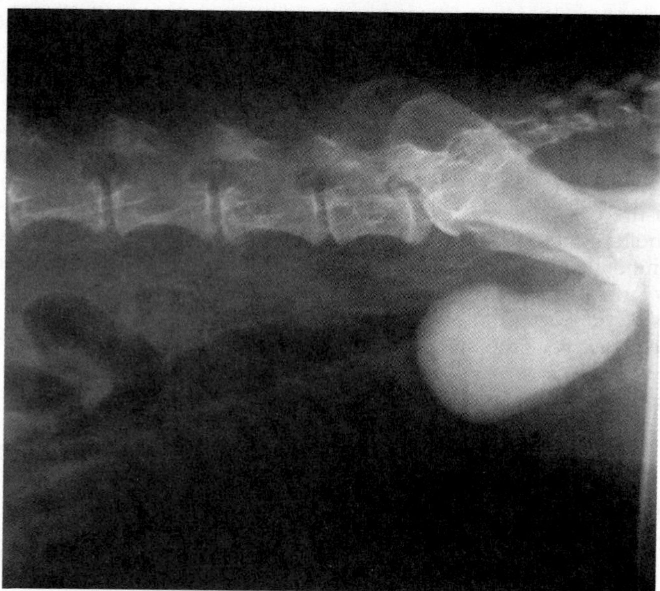

FIGURE II-33 Positive-contrast cystogram, lateral projection. A large filling defect is seen along the caudodorsal aspect of the urinary bladder. This was later diagnosed as transitional cell carcinoma.

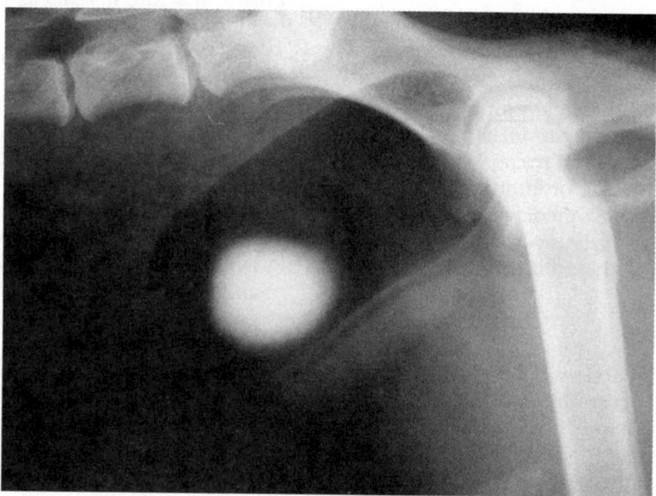

FIGURE II-34 Double-contrast cystogram, lateral projection. Normal study.

POSTPROCEDURE

- Once the study is complete, the recoverable volume (majority) of contrast is withdrawn from the urinary bladder.
- Air should be removed from the catheter bulb before the catheter is withdrawn.
- If anesthesia used, expect a routine anesthetic recovery.

ALTERNATIVES AND THEIR RELATIVE MERITS

- Plain abdominal radiographs: inexpensive means to survey the abdomen. Radiopaque cystic calculi can be visualized. Size and shape of the bladder often obvious.
- Abdominal ultrasound: excellent for visualization of bladder, especially the wall thickness, luminal contents, and trigone region. Urinary bladder rupture not definitive with ultrasound; noninvasive and readily available.
- CT scan and MRI: provide excellent study of the bladder; however, these are costly and rarely performed for this indication.

AUTHOR: **LEEANN PACK**

Cystoscopy

BASIC INFORMATION

SYNONYM(S)

Transurethral cystoscopy
Urethrocystoscopy
Uroendoscopy

OVERVIEW AND GOAL(S)

Transurethral cystoscopy (TUC) involves the use of rigid or flexible endoscopes for examination of the urinary bladder via passage through the urethra. Most anatomic structures of the lower urinary tract can be visualized: vulvar vestibule, vagina, urethral orifice, urethra, urinary bladder, and ureteral orifices.

INDICATIONS

Transurethral cystoscopy is most often used in chronic conditions, but it may also be beneficial in cases with severe acute presentations. A differential diagnosis list for any of the following disorders or clinical signs could be an indication for transurethral cystoscopy.

- Anatomic abnormalities: vaginal strictures, persistent vaginal membranes, ectopic ureters.
- Cystitis: chronic infectious, idiopathic, interstitial.
- Post-traumatic or postsurgical assessment: pelvic fractures, abdominal trauma, prior surgery.
- Hematuria: examination to identify origin of bleeding and observation of ureteral orifices (unilateral versus bilateral hematuria of renal origin).
- Urethritis: infectious, inflammatory, granulomatous.
- Stranguria.
- Urinary incontinence: identification of possible causes; therapeutic periurethral

submucosal injections of glutaraldehyde cross-linked collagen.
- Pollakiuria.
- Calculi: urethral or cystic calculi retrieval and identification (Figs. II-35 and II-36).
- Tumor: urethral, urinary bladder, prostatic, vaginal.
- Obstruction: tumor, stricture, calculi, hyperplasia (vaginal).
- Urethral stricture: diagnosis and dilations.
- Removal of small polyps and tumors.
- Ureteroscopy: for advanced endoscopists; generally requires concurrent fluoroscopy.
- Holmium: YAG (Ho:YAG) laser: used for laser lithotripsy; this is of growing interest and of proven benefit for the fragmentation of urinary calculi. As of 2005, the cost and advanced training involved have left the use of this laser largely as a procedure available at just a few veterinary teaching hospitals or larger referral centers.

CONTRAINDICATIONS

- Animal size and sex are the most common limiting factors; the exact limitations depend on endoscope size (external diameter), as described in the following paragraphs.
- Known severe bacterial urinary tract infection is a relative risk factor.
- Known perforation or rupture of bladder or urethra.

EQUIPMENT, ANESTHESIA

There is a wide array of possible equipment to use for transurethral cystoscopy. The marked differences between the male anatomy and female anatomy and between dogs and cats lead to the common veterinary statement of "You can never have enough scopes." To be prepared for *any* size and sex of animal may require a mix of six to seven flexible and rigid scopes.

- Review of the normal anatomy of the lower urinary tract.
- Preparation of the preputial or perineal area by clipping interfering hair and gentle cleansing.
- General anesthesia with tracheal intubation is required.
- Between 1 to 2 L of body temperature sterile saline for flush and infusion during procedure via IV infusion set.
- Water-soluble sterile lubricant with or without lidocaine jelly.
- Bacterial culture tubes.
- Biopsy jars with 10% buffered formalin.
- Flexible-tipped ureteral guide wires can be helpful for bypassing obstructions, strictures, and tears (serving a stylet-type function), then allowing catheters to be passed over them; human ureteral dilation catheters can be used with the guide wires if urethral stricture is present.
- Accessory implements include sterile brushes, guide wires, biopsy forceps, balloon catheters, sterile catheters, stone retrieval baskets, and polypectomy snares (with or without electrocautery).
- Appropriate light source and light cables.
- Documentation equipment (videocassette, digital video, prints).
- Flexible endoscopes:
  - Size of scopes varies by both anticipated length of the urinary tract segment to be assessed (cranial tip of filled bladder extending to perineum or preputial opening) and diameter of the urethra.
  - As examples: A larger female dog may be examined cystoscopically using a 5-mm, two-way deflecting fiberendoscope (e.g., bronchoscope), while a small male cat may allow passage of a 1.2-mm pediatric ureterocystoscope.
  - Ancillary catheters, brushes, stone retrieval baskets, and biopsy forceps.
  - Flexible endoscopes may require more positioning and manipulation of the animal because they tend to be deflected easily by external pressures.
- Rigid endoscopes:
  - A wide array of rigid endoscopes from human medicine can be used for transurethral cystoscopy, including purpose-designed cystoscopes, small laparoscopes, and adapted arthroscopes.
  - Rigid telescope sizes can range from 2.7–5 mm in diameter, with respective cannula diameters ranging from 3.8–6 mm; length of the scopes ranges from 7–30 cm.
  - A 0-degree viewing angle may be better for viewing the urethra, and a 30-degree viewing angle may be preferred for viewing the bladder.
  - A "bridge" is used for connecting some scopes with their cannulas (cannula-bridge-scope) and to provide additional access ports (generally one or two) for flushing or infusion of saline and passage of other instruments.
  - The Albarran lever is a "deflecting bridge" that forces flexible biopsy instruments to exit the bridge at an angle; this facilitates biopsy and grasping of structures that are almost parallel to the scope.
  - The Ellik evacuator allows for rapid saline lavage to provide for collection of small calculi when attached to a rigid cystoscope cannula.
  - Rigid scopes tend to provide superior images.

ANTICIPATED TIME

- About 30 to 75 minutes depending on ease of passage, extent of lesion(s), and whether the procedure is diagnostic or also therapeutic (e.g., stone retrieval).

PREPARATION: IMPORTANT CHECKPOINTS

- Have clear goals for the procedure based on case assessment.
- Know the appearance of normal structures in the lower urinary tract via textbooks or continuing education/training.
- Plan ahead for staff involvement with setup, procedural assistance, and cleaning the equipment.
- Discuss with owner that repeated procedures can be required (e.g., stone retrievals, stricture dilation, reassessments, etc.).
- Make alternative plans for surgery if goals are not achieved.

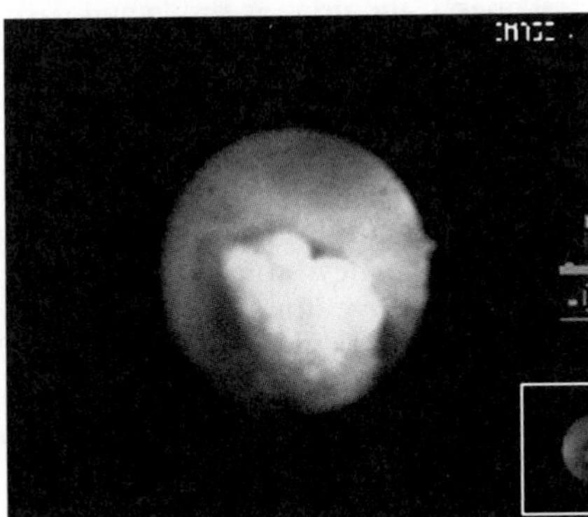

FIGURE II-35 Endoscopic view of the urethra of a dog with severe stanguria and hematuria. A large urolith is occluding most of the lumen. Courtesy of Dr. Etienne Côté.

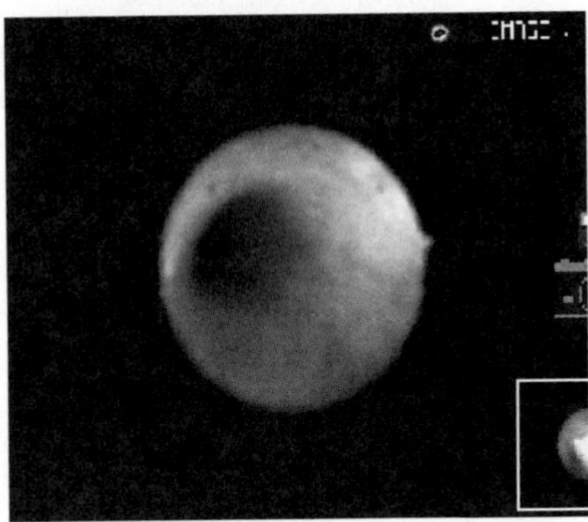

FIGURE II-36 Endoscopic view of the same site in the same dog as in Fig. II-34. Using an older set of dull biopsy forceps, the urolith was fragmented into several pieces within the urethral lumen, and the fragments passed easily through the urethra during the procedure. Moderate mucosal erythema remains (bottom half of the image), but the dog's recovery was uneventful and complete. Courtesy of Dr. Etienne Côté.

POSSIBLE COMPLICATIONS AND COMMON ERRORS TO AVOID

- Mistaking the fossa clitoridis in female dogs for the urethral orifice.
- Prior digital- or catheter-induced trauma to the urethral tubercle (papilla), thereby hindering entry of the endoscope into the urethra.
- Iatrogenic urinary tract infections (UTIs).
- Rupture of the urinary bladder or urethra due to inappropriate technique or existing disease.
- Urethral mucosal edema due to inherent trauma from endoscopy can be a limiting factor in uroendoscopy, particularly in the urethra of male dogs.
- Operator reliance on visual impressions rather than histopathologic or cytologic evaluation of samples.

PROCEDURE

- If using small-diameter flexible endoscopes, if the urine is turbid and dark, or if there is gross hematuria, it may be best to empty the bladder prior to the procedure via urethral catheterization (see Catheterization, Urethral, p 1205).
- Transurethral cystoscopy can be done with the animal in either ventral or dorsal recumbency; some veterinarians prefer to have the animal in dorsal recumbency for most procedures, but in some cases, it is necessary to reverse the position.
- The perineum and the prepuce or vulva are cleansed; it is preferable that an aseptic technique be the goal and that any procedure-related materials be kept sterile (away from surrounding hospital-related contamination). However, it is expected that contamination from the animal will occur via the urethra, vulva, or prepuce.
- For female dogs and cats, the fiberendoscope or cannula with a rigid scope assembly is placed in the vulva, and the vulvar skin is gently pinched externally (by an assistant) to create a seal; then a saline infusion is started until the vault is distended. When the vulvovaginal area has been examined and the urethral orifice identified, the urethra is cannulated with the scope and distended with saline as the scope is passed to the bladder. The bladder is then emptied via the biopsy channel of the fiberscope or the cannula (remember that the rigid scope slides through the cannula) and then refilled with saline; it is important to visualize the appearance of mucosa both when the bladder is empty and when it is filled.
- For male dogs and cats, the technique is similar except that the prepuce is held to form a seal around a flexible fiberendoscope.
- The bladder is examined in a methodical pattern inclusive of the apex of the bladder.
- The ureteral orifices are identified, and in many cases, pulsatile flow of urine can be observed. Then the trigonal area is examined. Biopsies are taken for histopathologic evaluation and culture, and stones may be examined and samples taken for analysis.
- The endoscope is then withdrawn slowly while the clinician observes for abnormalities.
- Visualization of the urethral mucosa is often superior during withdrawal of the endoscope.
- Biopsies, brush cytologies, and other procedures are done as warranted.
- Ectopic ureteral openings can be identified in most cases with more accuracy than with the use of contrast radiography when the urethra is examined with care; multiple sites of ectopic openings might be identified, and the trigonal region should be examined for normal orifice appearances.
- Colliculus seminalis can be seen more prominently in intact male dogs as well as in the prostatic openings and deferent duct openings into the proximal urethra.
- Vaginal and cervical os can be visualized in female dogs.
- The goals of the procedure should be reviewed prior to final withdrawal.

POSTPROCEDURE

- Consider antibiotic use when it is appropriate for the case.
- Use appropriate pain management for the animal.

ALTERNATIVES AND THEIR RELATIVE MERITS

Suprapubic (prepubic) percutaneous cystoscopy: more involved with equipment and invasiveness; may be used when larger tumors obstruct the trigonal region or when placing retrograde guide wire to facilitate antegrade catheterization.

AUTHOR: **MARK E. HITT**

Defibrillation, Electrical

BASIC INFORMATION

OVERVIEW AND GOAL(S)

Electrical defibrillation is the treatment of choice for cardiac arrest characterized by ventricular fibrillation. It consists of application of an electric shock to the heart, causing massive depolarization; when defibrillation is successful, this massive depolarization is immediately followed by spontaneous resumption of sinus rhythm.

INDICATIONS

Ventricular fibrillation

CONTRAINDICATIONS

- Conscious animal
- Normal cardiac rhythm but electrocardiographic (ECG) artifact mimics ventricular fibrillation
- Poor or inappropriate contact between defibrillation paddles and animal
- Inability to electrically isolate animal from surrounding animals or humans (e.g., in contact with same pool of water/urine/other conductive medium)
- Ventricular fibrillation > 10 minutes' duration

EQUIPMENT, ANESTHESIA

- Clippers for hair
- Defibrillator; ideally, combined defibrillator-electrocardiograph to avoid risk of electrical damage to stand-alone ECG machine (Fig. II-37)
- Defibrillation coupling gel (Fig. II-38)

ANTICIPATED TIME

About 1 to 10 minutes

PREPARATION: IMPORTANT CHECKPOINTS

- Is it ventricular fibrillation?
  - ECG shows coarse or fine patternless electrical activity with no synchronized activity (no QRS complexes) when ventricular fibrillation is present.

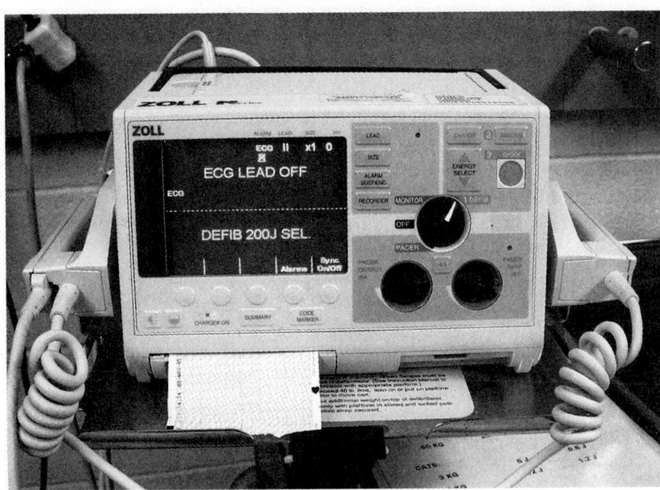

FIGURE II-37 Typical defibrillator. The paddles are clipped to the side of the unit, and the screen displays both ECG information and defibrillation charge (at 200 J in image). The controls for energy selection, for charging, and for shock administration on the front panel are also present as finger controls directly on the paddles (not shown).

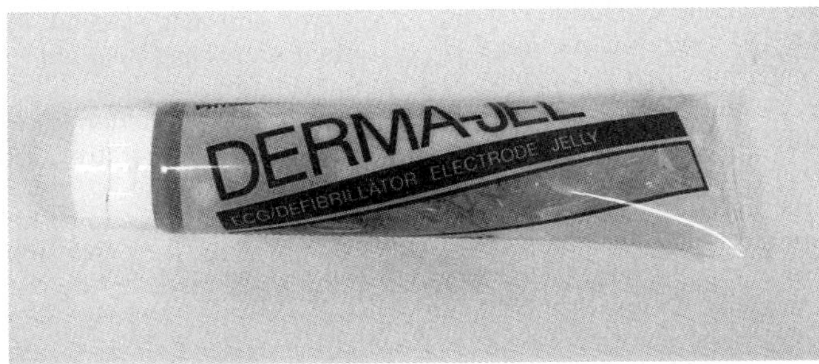

FIGURE II-38 Tube of defibrillator gel.

- If the animal is conscious, the rhythm is not ventricular fibrillation.
- If a pulse is palpable, the rhythm is not ventricular fibrillation.
- Is the animal prepared correctly?
  - Dorsal or lateral recumbency, on a dry, insulated surface (e.g., foam mat or linoleum floor).
  - Hair clipped from both hemithoraces over heart (fourth through sixth intercostal spaces [ICS], right and left).

NOTE: The limbs of the animal will flail when the shock is administered, and any objects (e.g., monitoring instruments, drug bottles, etc.) in their trajectory must be removed prior to shock delivery.

POSSIBLE COMPLICATIONS AND COMMON ERRORS TO AVOID

- Electric shock can be transmitted to bystanders: NOTE: This complication can cause cardiac arrest in human or animal onlookers. This result is best avoided by ensuring that no one is in contact with the animal or anything the animal is touching before delivering a shock. It is also important to ensure that no indirect contact from urine, saline, or any other fluids that may be trickling from the animal is occurring between the animal and the shoes of surrounding individuals. Shouting "clear" is not enough since most people do not know what to do in response.
- Defibrillation is too late: The success of defibrillation approaches 100% when it is performed within the first minute of ventricular fibrillation, then decreases by 10–15% per minute. Defibrillation is the most important treatment when there is ventricular fibrillation, and some have suggested revising the "ABCs" of resuscitation to the "DABCs" with D for defibrillation.
- Poor application of paddles on animal.
  - Paddles must be set widely apart (i.e., one on each side of the thorax); if too close, an electrical arc between them can cause severe skin burns and operator injury.
  - Defibrillator gel must be applied between the defibrillator paddles and the animal's skin. NOTE: Any facility that owns a defibrillator must also own a tube of defibrillator gel because alternatives are inadequate: Ultrasound gel is contraindicated, alcohol is flammable, and bare skin without a coupling agent can be burned by electrical arcs.

PROCEDURE

- The animal is placed in lateral or dorsal recumbency.
- Rapid clip of hair over the left and right precordia (area of chest overlying the heart): 20 seconds.
- The ECG diagnosis of ventricular fibrillation is confirmed.
  - Animals with ventricular fibrillation are always unconscious (nonperfusing rhythm) and pulseless.
  - Alcohol or gel must be present at all points of contact between the ECG wires/clips and the animal (to rule out poor connection artifact/"pseudofibrillation").
  - Click from leads I to II and then to III on the ECG monitor to check for organized electrical cardiac activity in any lead. If present, defibrillation is contraindicated.
- The defibrillator is charged: 5 J/kg.
- Defibrillator gel is smeared on the surface of both paddles.
- The paddles are applied to the thorax: paddle marked "Left" or "Apex" is on left hemithorax, and paddle marked "Right" or "Sternum" is on the right.
- All onlookers and assistants must stand back and be neither in direct nor indirect contact with the animal. The only contact point between the animal and the person administering the shock is the paddles.
- The shock is delivered.
- The ensuing ECG rhythm is assessed immediately.

POSTPROCEDURE

If the rhythm still appears to be ventricular fibrillation, it should be quickly confirmed (check other ECG leads on the monitor, and ensure ECG connection between animal and machine is good); if confirmed, defibrillation is immediately warranted once again at 8 J/kg. Up to 12 J/kg may be administered. When the rhythm is any other than defibrillation, standard cardiopulmonary resuscitation procedures are followed (see Cardiopulmonary Cerebral Resuscitation, p 1202).

ALTERNATIVES AND THEIR RELATIVE MERITS

- Precordial thump (physical blow to the chest); theory: delivers physical "equivalent" of electrical shock; unproven value, many potential drawbacks, and never preferred over electrical defibrillation.
- Pharmacologic defibrillation (bretylium, potassium chloride/calcium chloride, etc.). Unproven and not known to be widely successful in the clinical setting.

AUTHOR: **ETIENNE CÔTÉ**

Dental Extraction

BASIC INFORMATION

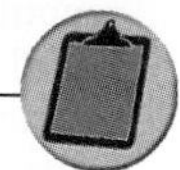

SYNONYM(S)

Exodontics

OVERVIEW AND GOAL(S)

- Removal of a tooth in a way that ensures complete removal of the root(s) and rapid healing of the dental alveolus and oral soft tissue.
- Simple extraction is indicated for simple rooted teeth except canine teeth or indicated for teeth that have already lost most of their attachment. Canines and multirooted teeth usually require surgical extraction.

INDICATIONS

- Nonvital (dead) tooth; tooth with exposure or contamination of the endodontic system.
- Moderate to severe periodontal disease.
- Nonrestorable dental lesions: dental resorptions, dental fractures.
- Persistent primary teeth; retained roots or impacted teeth. Some teeth involved in jaw fracture.
- Dental malocclusions.
- Oral surgery, removal of oral tumors, oral cysts.

CONTRAINDICATIONS

- When general anesthesia is contraindicated because of severe uncontrolled metabolic disease
- Animals with a bleeding disorder
- Animals undergoing chemotherapy or radiotherapy

EQUIPMENT, ANESTHESIA

- General anesthesia, preemptive pain control, and regional or local anesthesia are utilized as needed.
- Simple extraction:
  - Dental radiograph
  - A #11 or #15 scalpel blade
  - Dental elevator(s)
  - Dental forceps
- Surgical extraction: as above, plus:
  - Periosteal elevator
  - Dental unit with high-speed handpiece and FG dental burs (no. 699-701, regular, long shank, and surgical lengths)
  - Bone rongeurs or bone rasp
  - Bone curette
  - Sterile saline with syringe and atraumatic needle
  - Soft-tissue scissors (LaGrange)
  - Tissue forceps
  - Needle holder, 4-0 resorbable suture material with swaged on needle

ANTICIPATED TIME

About 5 minutes for most simple extractions and 20 minutes for most surgical extractions

PREPARATION: IMPORTANT CHECKPOINTS

Dental radiographs: check for the number of roots, their shape, and their structural integrity (root resorption); the condition of the surrounding bone; and the presence or absence of a periodontal ligament with possible root ankylosis.

POSSIBLE COMPLICATIONS AND COMMON ERRORS TO AVOID

- Oronasal fistula: if occurs, should be closed with a mucoperiosteal flap, either at the time the extraction is done or as a delayed surgery if the gingival tissue is so inflamed that its capacity to hold sutures is questionable.
- Root fracture:
  - Most easily prevented by examination of the preoperative radiographs and proper treatment planning. If the root is in advanced stage of resorption, is ankylosed, and has no evidence of periodontal or endodontic infection, it could be left in place for continued resorption.
  - Although the clinician should try to remove as much root material as possible in an animal with root fracture, the risk of damaging surrounding tissue should be weighed against the benefit of finding the last piece of root material.
  - When a root fragment is left *in situ*, the owner should be informed of that aspect of the surgery, and follow-up radiographs should be included in the treatment plan. The risk of causing an abscess is higher when the root fragment has been mobilized and its blood supply severed during its attempted extraction.
- Jaw fracture: usually the result of a blind attempt at extracting a tooth on the mandible without preoperative dental radiographs and appropriate treatment planning. Small breed dogs with severe periodontal disease of the first lower molars are the most likely to be at risk for jaw fracture during dental extraction.
- Root fragments in the nasal cavity or the mandibular canal need to be retrieved.

PROCEDURE

Simple extraction:

- Incision of the gingival attachment around the tooth with a scalpel blade.
- Mobilization of the tooth with dental elevators using a first-class lever, wheel-and-axle, or wedge types of forces.
  - The tip of the elevator is used circumferentially as a wedge between the root and the bone to stretch the periodontal ligament or as a wheel and axle with the side of the blade engaged under the enamel bulge, mesial or distal to the tooth, to elevate the tooth out of the alveolus.
  - Use light forces over a longer period (at least 10 seconds each time) to break the attachment without fracturing the root.
  - Extend the index finger (of the hand holding the elevator) along the shaft of the elevator to protect deeper sturctures in case of slippage.
- Extraction with dental forceps once the tooth is mobile. Light rotation force may help.
- Check that extraction is complete; perform a postoperative radiograph if needed.
- Brief digital pressure to help hemostasis, to reduce the expansion of the alveolar wall caused by the extraction, and to approximate the gingival margins.
- Suture if needed.

Surgical extraction:

- Incision of the gingival attachment around the tooth with a scalpel blade.
- Elevation of a mucoperiosteal flap with a periosteal elevator.
- With a dental bur, buccal cortical bone and alveolar bone is removed to expose the root surface up to half its length.
- On a multirooted tooth, the crown is sectioned between the roots.
- Each individual root with its attached piece of crown is elevated.
- Check that the extraction is complete.
- Smooth the edge of the alveolar bone with a bone rongeur or rasp; curette and flush debris out of the alveolus.
- Trim the border of the soft tissue if needed.
- Suture with a simple suture pattern.
  - After a surgical extraction, the gingiva is sutured back in place, even in the case of an abscess.
  - It is important to cover the bone exposed during the elevation of the soft tissue.

POSTPROCEDURE

- Surgical extractions: pain medication for 4 days, soft food for 10 days.
- Antibiotics are used if the animal shows systemic clinical signs (fever, loss of appetite, etc.) or if the condition has progressed to osteomyelitis.
- Recheck in 10 to 14 days.

ALTERNATIVES AND THEIR RELATIVE MERITS

Endodontics, periodontics, and orthodontics are other alternative treatments. They have the advantage of preserving the teeth. They are often a better option when the owner is interested in doing the necessary aftercare and home dental care.

AUTHOR: **YVAN DUMAIS**

Dental Preventative (Home) Care

BASIC INFORMATION

OVERVIEW AND GOAL(S)

A regimen of home dental care is designed to help keep the periodontium healthy in between professional oral prophylactic or therapeutic treatments.

INDICATIONS

- Accumulation of bacterial plaque (soft) or dental calculus (hard) on the dental surface
- Prevention of gingivitis and periodontal disease
- Part of the maintenance phase in the treatment of periodontitis

CONTRAINDICATIONS

- When the animal needs professional dental prophylactic treatment (gingivitis, calculus, or plaque buildup) or periodontal treatment (periodontitis, loss of dentogingival attachment)
- Oral hygiene complements and does not replace professional dental care

EQUIPMENT, MATERIAL

- Soft-bristle toothbrush; pet toothpaste
- Food that is specially designed to reduce dental plaque or calculus formation
- Oral rinses to help reduce dental plaque formation
- Chew toys

ANTICIPATED TIME

The home dental care regimen is discussed during regular visits or as part of a comprehensive oral prophylactic treatment or periodontal treatment. Once the regimen is well accepted by the pet and the owner, it is a daily routine that takes only 1 or 2 minutes.

PREPARATION: IMPORTANT CHECKPOINTS

The home dental care regimen should be selected after considering the animal's needs; the will, availability, and dexterity of the owner; and the compliance of the animal.

The implementation may require some form of training or behavior positive reinforcement before the pet associates home dental care with something fun.

POSSIBLE COMPLICATIONS AND COMMON ERRORS TO AVOID

- The desire to achieve thorough oral hygiene right at the beginning is often a deterrent for the owner and the animal. Most pets will not tolerate more than 20 seconds of toothbrushing and will not allow brushing the aspect of the teeth facing the palate or the tongue.
- In pets that have minimal calculus buildup, an annual thorough dental examination/cleaning under anesthesia often is not recommended. As a result, these animals may end up having severe dental or periodontal problems for an extended period of time before the problem gets noticed. It is sad that after investing a lot of effort in home dental care for prevention, these owners are not getting the success they were expecting because the recommendation for professional dental care was never made until it was clinically obvious that a problem was present. Pets, just as humans, need both: home dental care and professional dental care.
- Many chew toys have a round cross-sectional shape and are so hard that the carnassial teeth are prone to break when the pet bites down on them.
- There are so many products on the market and so many claims, most unsupported by credible independent research, that it is difficult to choose what to recommend to clients. A credible and independent source of information on the efficacy of dental products is the Veterinary Oral Health Council website (www.vohc.org), and products bearing the council's seal are recommended.

PROCEDURE

Training for toothbrushing; instructions for the owner:

- Start with a bare finger and apply pet toothpaste on the rostral (front) teeth.
- Massage the gingiva for a few seconds. Repeat many times a day.
- As the pet gets used to it, go farther caudally in the mouth until the pet tolerates the procedure being done up to and including the molars.
- Once the pet is comfortable with the procedure, start using a toothbrush with soft bristles and apply the toothpaste again on the rostral teeth, brushing for a few seconds.
- Go farther caudally as the pet tolerates the procedure. Give praise and rewards immediately after. Brush daily.
- Movement: For the incisors, brush from the gingiva toward the tip of the teeth. For the other teeth, brush with a circulatory movement with the bristles slightly oriented toward the gingiva of the upper jaw, then lower jaw, so that the action is focused on the area next to the gingival border. With the mouth closed, the last teeth of the lower jaw are hidden behind the teeth of the upper jaw; however, the area next to the gingiva can still be brushed.

Other alternatives:

- Food specially designed to prevent calculus or plaque formation either mechanically (fibers) or chemically. Fibers help clean the caudal teeth.
- Rinses: Chlorhexidine 0.12% for treatment and prevention of gingivitis (not for periodontitis because it is ineffective in organic material, cannot reach bottom of periodontal pockets); zinc and ascorbic acid, mainly for their action on epithelium and connective tissue post-treatment.
- Products containing enzymes that enhance the antimicrobial action of the saliva and leukocytes.
- Products that stimulate oral exercise, the production of saliva, and the removal of plaque and calculus.

POSTPROCEDURE

Professional dental care once a year to allow complete oral examination, removal of plaque and calculus in areas where they still build up despite home dental care, and tooth polishing.

ALTERNATIVES AND THEIR RELATIVE MERITS

In absence or ineffectiveness of home dental care, the frequency of professional dental care is adjusted to prevent or control periodontal disease.

AUTHOR: **YVAN DUMAIS**

Dental Prophylactic Treatment

BASIC INFORMATION

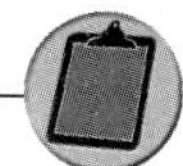

SYNONYM(S)

Dental cleaning and polishing
Dental prophylaxis

OVERVIEW AND GOAL(S)

- Complete oral examination
- Removal of calculus and plaque buildup on teeth to create a healthier dentogingival environment
- Polishing of the teeth surface to make it less prone to calculus accumulation

INDICATIONS

- Accumulation of bacterial plaque (soft) or dental calculus (hard) on the dental surface
- Treatment of gingivitis
- Prevention of periodontal disease
- Annual dental examination
- Part of the maintenance phase in the treatment of periodontitis

CONTRAINDICATIONS

- Established periodontitis: The animal should receive more involved diagnostic and treatment procedures rather than prophylactic treatment. Diagnosis (including dental examination, periodontal probing, and full-mouth intraoral radiographic examination) and treatment (dental cleaning and polishing, root planing, dental extractions, antimicrobials, periodontal surgery—therapies aimed at removing the cause of the disease) may be performed in stages, with a period of maintenance and reevaluation between them.
- When general anesthesia is contraindicated because of systemic illness.
- Old age is not a contraindication.
- NOTE: Dogs with mitral valve endocardiosis have not been shown to have a greater risk of dental procedure-associated bacterial endocarditis than dogs with normal heart valves.

EQUIPMENT, ANESTHESIA

- General anesthesia and tracheal intubation.
- Hand instruments:
  - Scalers (H 6-7).
  - Curettes (Gracey 3/4, Gracey 13/14, Mini-five 1/2).
  - Dental explorer and periodontal probe (XP-17/0W).
  - Dental mirror.
  - Instrument tray.
  - Ceramic sharpening stone.
- Power instruments:
  - Ultrasonic (magnetostrictive with metal stack, magnetostrictive with ferrite rods, or piezoelectric) or sonic scaler.
  - One tip for removal of gross and moderate calculus buildup.
  - One perio (or universal) tip for removal of subgingival calculus and debris. The energized water spray at the end of the tip also kills the bacteria with what is referred to as the *cavitation effect*.
  - Dental unit, either air or electric powered, with low-speed handpiece and straight attachment. Since the speed of the prophy cup should be around 4000 rpm, a straight attachment 4:1 gear ratio is usually necessary with air-driven units.
  - Prophy head for straight attachment, multi-use or single-use.
  - Rubber prophy cups; prophy paste (jars or uni-dose cups) or flour pumice medium grit.
- Dental fluoride (APF 1.23% or NaF 2%), mainly for cats if fluoride is not included in the prophy paste.
- Chlorhexidine solution 0.12%.
- Good lighting conditions, magnifying glasses.
- Dental chart.

ANTICIPATED TIME

About 20 minutes for a cat and 45 minutes for a dog

PREPARATION: IMPORTANT CHECKPOINTS

Operator protection:

- Surgical mask, gloves, eye protection, scrub top or gown.
- Instill 0.12 % chlorhexidine solution in the animal's mouth before starting the procedure to reduce bacterial counts in the aerosols generated during power scaling.

Animal protection:

- Keep the animal warm because of the cooling effect of the water-spray during power scaling; protect the eyes (lubrication, towel) and sterilize the instruments. Appropriately inflate the cuff of the endotracheal tube.
- Administer antibiotics only if animal is immunosuppressed, has internal prosthesis, or has a severe infection: 20 mg/kg ampicillin IV 1-hour prior to the procedure or clindamycin 5 mg/kg or clavulanic acid-amoxicilin 13.5 mg/kg PO 12 hours prior to the procedure.
- Place cotton gauze in the oropharynx to catch pieces of calculus that could otherwise enter the trachea after extubation.

POSSIBLE COMPLICATIONS AND COMMON ERRORS TO AVOID

- Forgetting to remove the cotton gauze in the oropharynx before extubation.
- Causing thermal damage to the dental pulp by staying too long over a tooth during power scaling or polishing or inadequate water spray during power scaling.
- Damaging the tooth surface by being heavy-handed during scaling and polishing or by using burs (Rotosonics) to remove calculus.
- Dental cusp (tip) fracture caused when using extraction forceps to chip away the calculus (not recommended).
- Power instrumentation: Use the lowest effective intensity setting; use a light touch; work with the last 3 mm at the end of the tip; keep the tip moving with adequate water spray. Use a gauge to check tip wear and replace when 2 mm has been lost (50% loss of efficacy).

PROCEDURE

- The anesthetized, intubated animal is placed in lateral recumbency, and all stages of the procedure described here are performed on the lingual side of the teeth on the recumbent side and the labial side of the teeth on the nonrecumbent side. Then the animal is turned over, and the procedure can be repeated (avoids turning the animal multiple times).
- Removal of very heavy calculus deposits with a dental scaler or hoe.
- Removal of the gross and moderate supragingival calculus using hand instrumentation (dental curette, scaler) or power intrumentation (sonic or ultrasonic with a heavier tip at moderate- to high-intensity setting).
- The working surface of the power scaler should be held parallel not perpendicular to the tooth surface.
- Removal of light supragingival (finition) and subgingival calculus with hand instrumentation (dental curette) or power instrumentation (sonic or ultrasonic with slim perio or universal tip at low-to-moderate intensity setting).
- A disclosing solution can be used for checking for the presence of dental plaque or an air syringe for the presence of calculus.
- The teeth are polished with prophy paste or flour pumice.
- Dental examination with dental explorer; periodontal examination with periodontal probe. Chart all the findings.

- Flush the gingival sulcus with an atraumatic needle and saline to remove the prophy paste or flour pumice, calculus debris, and bacteria.
- Dry the teeth, apply fluoride for 4 minutes, wipe it off.
- Perform final rinse with 0.12% chlorhexidine.

POSTPROCEDURE

- Discuss home oral care with owners and find appropriate regimen.
- Provide the owner with information about the postoperative treatment plan, including the date of the next dental appointment.

ALTERNATIVES AND THEIR RELATIVE MERITS

- The wrong alternative to the prevention of periodontal disease with dental prophylactic treatment and home dental care is to wait until periodontal disease has progressed and periodontal treatment is necessary to help control the progression of the disease. This is obviously not an option that benefits the animal or the owner.
- Brushing the teeth will not remove existing calculus.
- Dental prophylactic treatment performed without general anesthesia provides some cosmetic improvement but no long-term benefit.

AUTHOR: **YVAN DUMAIS**

Dermatologic Diagnostic Procedures

BASIC INFORMATION

SYNONYM(S)

Diagnostic techniques in dermatology
Diagnostic testing in dermatology

OVERVIEW AND GOAL(S)

- Tests that are performed to confirm a diagnosis and/or to rule out differential diagnoses for skin lesions.
- The most common diagnostic procedures in dermatology are examination of the haircoat and skin with a good light source and magnifying lens, flea combing, acetate tape preparation, skin scrapings, skin cytology, Wood's lamp examination, fungal culture for dermatophytes, and skin biopsies.

INDICATIONS

- Skin scrapings: used primarily to find mites and occasionally nematode infestation.
- Skin cytologic examination: extremely useful diagnostic procedure indicated in almost every dermatology case. It can rapidly and inexpensively detect the presence of inflammation, infection, (bacteria, fungi), autoimmune disease (acantholytic keratinocytes in pemphigus), or neoplasia.
- Wood's lamp examination: useful screening tool when dermatophytosis caused by *Microsporum canis* is suspected.
- Dermatophyte culture: indicated when a dermatophytosis is suspected. In fact, it is indicated in virtually any cat with undiagnosed skin disease.
- Skin biopsies: performed to confirm a diagnosis or to provide direction (without always receiving a definitive diagnosis). Skin biopsies are recommended with any neoplastic or suspected neoplastic lesion, any persistent or unusual lesion, any vesicular dermatosis, and any undiagnosed alopecia.

CONTRAINDICATIONS

Virtually none

EQUIPMENT, ANESTHESIA

Simple equipment is required to perform veterinary dermatologic tests. Standard equipment and materials consist of:

- Biopsy kit, including biopsy punches (Fig. II-39A)
- One or two #10 scalpel blades (Fig. II-39B)
- Glass microscope slides (Fig. II-39C) and coverslips (20 × 40 or 22 × 50 mm)
- Mineral oil (Fig. II-39D)
- Cotton-tip applicators (Fig. II-39E)
- Acetate tape (clear adhesive tape) (Fig. II-39F)
- Microscope
- Hemostat
- Handheld magnifying lens
- Flea combs
- Cytologic examination stain
- Wood's lamp
- Dermatophyte test media
- Sterile toothbrushes
- Syringes
- A few 22-, 23-, and 25-gauge needles
- Biopsy kit
- Local anesthetic (e.g., lidocaine 2%)
- Biopsy jars containing 10% neutral buffered formalin

ANTICIPATED TIME

The procedure takes a few minutes.

POSSIBLE COMPLICATIONS AND COMMON ERRORS TO AVOID

- Skin scrapings: It is important to clip hair before performing skin scrapings to avoid false-negative results. However, it is preferable to use scissors when surface mites, such as *Cheyletiella*, are

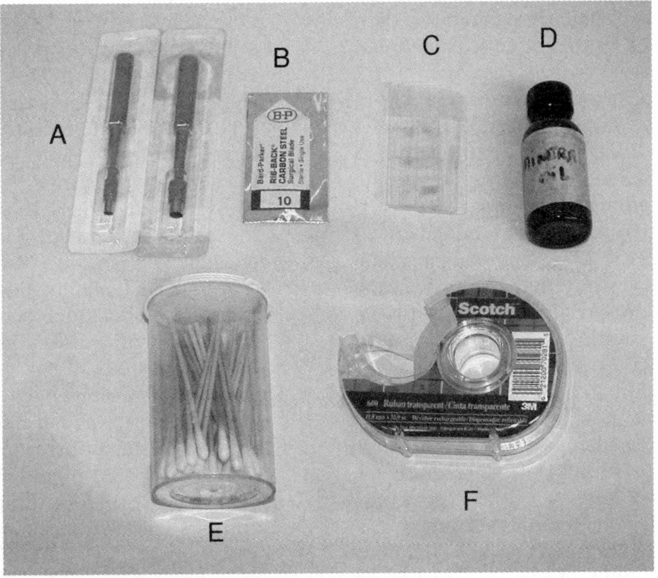

FIGURE II-39 Materials used for performing dermatologic diagnostic tests. **A,** Biopsy punches. **B,** #10 scalpel blades. **C,** Glass microscope slides. **D,** Mineral oil. **E,** Cotton tip applicators. **F,** Acetate tape (clear adhesive tape).

suspected because they can be lost if electric clippers are used.
- NOTE: A positive scraping allows the clinician to find and identify a parasitic infestation, but its sensitivity in ruling out a diagnosis depends on the parasitic disease and the aggressiveness of sampling.
- Skin biopsies: Do not scrub—or wipe or rub with alcohol or antiseptic—the surface of a biopsy site prior to performing punch biopsies because pathologic changes on the skin surface, which often are critical in making a diagnosis, may be altered or removed. For the same reason, do not shave the area of interest; gently clip the hair with scissors if necessary.

PROCEDURE

- Skin scrapings:
  - Apply a few drops of mineral oil to the area of skin selected for scraping or coat the scalpel blade that is used for performing the scraping with mineral oil. Broad superficial scrapings that collect scales and crusts should be performed when looking for mites living on the surface (*Cheyletiella*) or in the superficial layers of the skin (*Sarcoptes, Notoedres*). Deeper skin scrapings must be performed when suspecting the presence of deep dwelling mites (*Demodex*). In the latter case, the skin must be squeezed to help extrude the mites from the hair follicles first, and the scrapings should be deep enough to create capillary oozing.
  - The skin scraping material that is collected on the scalpel blade is then smeared on a glass slide; additional mineral oil is added, and a cover slip is applied. The specimen is then examined with 40X (*Cheyletiella, Sarcoptes, Notoedres*) or 100X (*Demodex*) magnification.
  - *Demodex* mites are part of the skin's normal flora, but it is extremely rare to find them on skin scrapings. If one or few mites are found, more deep skin scrapings should be taken to confirm the diagnosis of demodicosis. Conversely, numerous negative skin scrapings from appropriate areas should reliably eliminate demodicosis and notoedric mange. In addition, in areas that are difficult to scrape, hair can be plucked, and the proximal ends examined under a microscope for the presence of *Demodex* mites.
  - Negative skin scrapings (even if several are performed) do not eliminate the possibility of sarcoptic mange or cheyletiellosis.
- Skin cytologic examination:
  - Allows microscopic examination of fluid or material collected from nodules, tumors, cysts, plaques, draining tracts, ulcers, pustules, vesicles, papules, and surface of the skin or ears. Several techniques may be used for obtaining samples. Specimens may be collected by
    (1) impression smears made from the surface of intact lesions or from cut surfaces of surgically excised lesions, such as nodules or tumors;
    (2) impression smears made after lancing pustules or papules;
    (3) fine-needle aspiration (FNA) of cells or material from lesions;
    (4) smears made by rolling the cotton-tipped applicator across a glass slide (particularly useful for ear specimens); and
    (5) scrapings of superficial epithelial cells with a dry, dull scalpel blade. This cellular material is then pressed firmly onto a glass slide.
  - After the specimen has dried, the slide is stained with a modified Wright's stain (e.g., Diff Quik) and examined microscopically. When a drop of mineral oil is put on the stained dried specimen and then covered with a large coverslip (22 × 40 or 22 × 50 mm), visualization of cells and most microorganisms at 400X is enhanced; thus, there is no need to perform an examination under oil immersion (1000X) in most cases.
- Wood's lamp examination:
  - This ultraviolet light's wavelength of 253.7 nm is temperature dependent, and the lamp should be turned on for 5-10 minutes before use. Certain dermatophytes (mainly *Microsporum canis* in veterinary medicine) may cause infected hairs (not scales or crusts) to fluoresce an apple-green color. This occurs in about 50% of cases with *M. canis*.
  - It is a fast and inexpensive screening tool for dermatophytosis. False positives are unfortunately frequent. Glowing hair should be plucked and the proximal end further examined with the Wood's lamp or used for culture or direct examination for fungal elements under microscope. A negative examination does not rule out dermatophytosis.
- Dermatophyte culture:
  - Generally performed in clinics on commercial dermatophyte test medium (DTM), available in either glass jars or flat plates. The culture medium consists of Sabouraud's dextrose agar, antibacterial and antifungal agents to inhibit growth of contaminants, and phenol red (pH indicator).
  - Select hairs and scales for culture along the edge of newly developing lesions. Broken or frayed hairs and those that fluoresce with Wood's lamp are the best specimens. The plucked hairs should be firmly pressed onto the surface of the medium. Alternatively, vigorous brushing of the animal's haircoat with a sterile toothbrush or a small piece of sterile carpet can be used for collecting hairs and scales (more useful to identify carriers not showing obvious lesions). This material can be removed from the toothbrush with a sterile hemostat and placed into the culture medium. Alternately, if plates are used, the DTM is inoculated by gently embedding or repeatedly dabbing the toothbrush into the medium.
  - Ideally, the culture medium should be incubated in the dark at 22-30°C (72-86°F) and at about 30% of relative humidity for 10 to 14 days, and it should be checked daily for fungal growth. Dessication and exposure to ultraviolet light hinder growth.
  - A red color change with visible mycelial growth (typically cream color) is seen with dermatophytes on DTM. Contaminants (environmental molds) will eventually turn the media red; however, colony growth is usually well established before any color change appears in the medium. In addition, most saprophyte colonies are pigmented. Nonetheless, identification of the fungi is essential if a suspected dermatophyte is grown on culture.
  - Macroconidia must be collected from the mycelial surface by gently applying the sticky side of clear acetate tape to the aerial surface. The tape with sample is then pressed onto a glass slide over a drop of methylene blue or lactophenol cotton blue stain and examined under microscope for characteristic macroconidia.
- Skin biopsies:
  - The biopsy technique selected (punch biopsy, wedge biopsy, excisional biopsy) varies according to the type of lesions.
  - Site selection is crucial. Choose several representative lesions that may represent various stages of the same pathologic process or multiple problems, with emphasis on primary lesions if possible (e.g., pustules, vesicles).
  - Punch biopsy specimens (usually 6 mm) can be obtained under local anesthesia (1 ml of 2% lidocaine per site, injected subcutaneously beneath the specimen; do not exceed 1 ml per 5 kg of body weight). If a papule, pustule, vesicle, or any small lesion is selected, the lesion should be centered in the

biopsy specimen. The biopsy punch should be rotated in only one direction to minimize shearing artifact. Handle the specimen carefully. The forceps should grasp either the hairs of the biopsy sample or its deepest surface (e.g., subcutis), never the core of the biopsy sample itself. The specimen must be put rapidly in 10% neutral buffered formalin. Skin biopsy punch sites can be sutured with one or two interrupted sutures.
- Skin biopsies, along with a detailed history and animal description, should be submitted to a veterinary dermatopathologist.

ALTERNATIVES AND THEIR RELATIVE MERITS

Therapeutic trials (e.g., antiparasitic, antimicrobial) are frequently performed in veterinary dermatology and represent very useful diagnostic tools. For example, therapeutic trials with acaricidal agents, such as the avermectins, are often required when sarcoptic acariosis or cheyletiellosis is suspected but skin scrapings are negative.

AUTHOR: **MANON PARADIS**

Diagnostic Peritoneal Lavage

BASIC INFORMATION

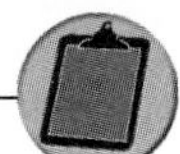

SYNONYM(S)

Abdominal lavage
DPL

OVERVIEW AND GOAL(S)

Instillation and subsequent evacuation of lavage fluid to evaluate suspected intra-abdominal disease

INDICATIONS

Animals with suspected abdominal disorders for which other noninvasive/less invasive testing has been inconclusive or unavailable. Animals that might benefit from diagnostic peritoneal lavage (DPL) include those with:
- Abdominal trauma
- Acute abdomen
- Sepsis with no source identified
- Shock with no source identified

CONTRAINDICATIONS

- Cardiovascular/respiratory compromise that may be exacerbated by lavage fluid administration
- Coagulopathy
- Recent abdominal surgery
- Diaphragmatic hernia

EQUIPMENT, ANESTHESIA

- Minimum of two assistants.
- Sedation may be necessary; local anesthesia and manual restraint may be sufficient for some animals.
- Hair clippers.
- Surgical scrub solution.
- Isopropyl alcohol.
- Sterile gauze for scrubbing skin.
- Local anesthesia (2% lidocaine).
- Sterile drape.
- Sterile surgical gloves.
- Sterile needle holders.
- Sterile scissors.
- A #11 blade for stab incision of skin.
- Sterile drainage catheter—various devices can be used, including:
  - Peritoneal dialysis catheter (recommended).
  - Over-the-needle large gauge IV catheter: may be prone to kinking.
  - Abdominal drainage catheter.
  - Red rubber feeding tube.
- Sterile collection system consisting of "Christmas tree" adapter, three-way stopcock, IV drip set, and collection bag.
- 2-0 or 3-0 nylon suture to anchor the catheter to the skin.
- Bandage material:
  - Nonadhesive, absorbent, sterile pad.
  - Cast padding.
  - Kling-type bandage roll.
  - Protective outer layer (Vet-wrap, etc.).
- Elizabethan collar.
- Lavage fluid (typically lukewarm saline) and administration supplies that depend on the volume of lavage infused (syringe/needle versus fluid bag with drip set).

ANTICIPATED TIME

About 15 to 40 minutes for placement. Additional time required for drainage depends on type of catheter selected, degree of flow obstruction encountered, and variation between animals.

PREPARATION: IMPORTANT CHECKPOINTS

- Ensure adequate manual or chemical restraint. Excessive struggling by the animal may result in contamination of the sterile field or increased risk of abdominal trauma during catheter placement.
- Maximize cardiovascular stability prior to the procedure.
- Receive owner approval for invasive procedure.
- Perform all abdominal imaging prior to the procedure because the lavage fluid instillation will affect future imaging interpretation.

POSSIBLE COMPLICATIONS AND COMMON ERRORS TO AVOID

- Care must be taken during placement to avoid internal organ damage. Possible traumatic injury includes:
  - Vessel or organ laceration leading to hemoabdomen.
  - GI tract perforation leading to septic peritonitis.
  - Urinary tract laceration leading to uroabdomen.
- Obstruction of catheter drainage holes with omentum is a frequent occurrence and can limit complete retrieval of lavage fluid. Repositioning the animal and flushing the catheter may help to relieve the obstruction. Use of commercially available peritoneal dialysis catheters with numerous (50–100) small diameter side holes may minimize complete omental plugging. Cutting additional side holes (never more than one-third the circumference because tube breakage may occur) into a nonperitoneal dialysis-specific catheter can be performed to decrease plugging of a single distal opening.
  - If sufficient lavage fluid cannot be retrieved, complications such as animal discomfort, cardiovascular or respiratory compromise, or overhydration may ensue.
- Subcutaneous or external leakage of lavage fluid may occur, especially if the body wall incision is large. Tunneling the catheter at least 2 cm through the subcutaneous space will help minimize external leakage. Keep the body wall and skin incisions small; the tube should be inserted with a snug fit through the incisions.
- Ascending infection into the peritoneal cavity is infrequent but possible. Sterile technique must be maintained during placement and when manipulating the lavage materials. A bandage should be maintained over the catheter site, and

the catheter should be removed when the procedure has been completed.

PROCEDURE

PREPARATION OF ANIMAL

- Sedate the animal if it is fractious or likely to struggle or if the clinician's ability to maintain a sterile technique throughout the procedure is questionable.
- Empty urinary bladder through catheterization or manual expression (decreases potential for bladder trauma or laceration during catheter placement).
- Place in dorsal recumbency. (Left lateral recumbency is also possible but not preferred.)
- Clip hair from abdomen, from xiphoid to pubis.
- Surgical scrub.
- Determine catheter insertion sites for the skin and body wall.
  - Recommended skin insertion site is 1–2 cm to the right of the umbilicus.
  - Recommended body wall insertion site is 1.5–3 cm caudal to the skin insertion site.
- Administer lidocaine injection at skin and body wall insertion sites, penetrating all tissue layers to be incised. NOTE: Pain with lidocaine injection can be minimized by mixing lidocaine with one-tenth the volume of 8.4 mEq/L sodium bicarbonate (adjusts to a more neutral pH) and by warming to body temperature (e.g., once filled, keep syringe tucked in clinician's axilla).
- Repeat surgical scrub.
- Wear sterile gloves.
- Drape sterile field.

PLACEMENT: The technique will vary depending on the chosen catheter device.

- Trochar-type peritoneal dialysis catheter:
  - Incise skin using a #11 blade: incision should be no larger than the catheter diameter.
  - Tunnel the catheter through the subcutaneous space to the desired body wall entry site.
  - Insert trochar and catheter through the body wall at a 45-degree angle, directed caudally.
    - A turgid abdomen allows easier placement.
    - With a flaccid abdomen, insertion may be facilitated by grasping and "tenting" the abdomen with one free hand while advancing the catheter with another hand.
  - After passage through the body wall, advance the catheter off the trochar to minimize the potential for trauma with the sharp trochar.
  - Final catheter placement should be within the abdominal cavity, along the ventral midline, adjacent to the urinary bladder.
- Seldinger-type peritoneal dialysis/abdominal drainage catheter:
  - Insert using the same anatomic markers.
  - Use the Seldinger technique of initial guide wire placement, dilation, and subsequent catheter insertion along the guide wire.
- Over-the-needle IV catheter:
  - Make two to four additional side holes <30% of the diameter of the catheter using a #10 blade.
  - Insert using the same anatomic markers, and advance the catheter off the stylet once the body wall has been fully penetrated.
- Red rubber feeding tube: see Abdominal Drainage, p 1176

ANCHORING

- Anchor the catheter in place using 3-0 or 2-0 nylon. A purse-string suture should be placed in the skin, followed by a Roman sandal/Chinese finger-trap suture.
- Attach the sterile collection system to the catheter port.
- Apply a sterile dressing at the insertion site followed by a bandage.
- CAUTION: An Elizabethan collar should be used if the animal is left unsupervised at any time with the tube in place.

LAVAGE

- Instill 22 ml/kg of warm saline into the abdominal cavity through the three-way stopcock. Closely monitor the cardiovascular and respiratory status of the animal during infusion for early detection of deterioration, warranting termination of the procedure. Place a sterile male adapter into the port when completed to maintain a closed system.
- Gently rock the animal from side to side and massage the abdomen to promote fluid dispersion.
- Attach a 6–20 ml syringe (dependent on body size and fluid volume instilled), and slowly (to avoid omental plugging) aspirate to obtain the fluid sample for analysis. Replace male adapter when completed.
- Open stopcock to the collection system and allow gravity to drain the remaining lavage fluid. Incomplete retrieval is likely due to partial absorption and ineffective retrieval. Maximum retrieval should be attempted.

REMOVAL

- Cut the purse-string suture and remove the catheter.
- Place a skin suture if the incision >5 mm.
- Maintain a sterile dressing and bandage over the incision site for 12 to 24 hours.

ANALYSIS

- Evaluate color: Clear fluid is not expected when peritonitis exists. Flocculent fluid indicates possible peritonitis. Red fluid indicates hemoabdomen. Green fluid likely contains bile.
- Perform packed cell volume (PCV) count: >5% indicates significant hemoabdomen.
- Perform white blood cell (WBC) count: normal is approximately 1000 cells/mm^3.
- Perform cytologic examination of fluid for degenerative neutrophils, toxic change, intracellular bacteria, bilirubin crystals, neoplastic cells, and other such abnormalities.
- Consider aerobic/anaerobic culture if septic peritonitis is suspected.
- Consider chemistry evaluation of lavage fluid with comparison to peripheral blood:
  - Elevated creatinine in lavage fluid indicates ruptured urinary tract.
  - Elevated bilirubin indicates ruptured biliary tree.
  - Elevated amylase indicates pancreatitis.

POSTPROCEDURE

- Monitor recovery from sedation/anesthesia.
- Supportive care as indicated for condition.

ALTERNATIVES AND THEIR RELATIVE MERITS

- Percutaneous needle abdominocentesis:
  - Technically easier to perform.
  - Requires less equipment.
  - Higher probability of a negative tap with small fluid volumes or pocketed areas of disease.
- Abdominal ultrasonography:
  - Noninvasive.
  - Allows visualization of the entire abdomen and detection of small or pocketed areas of fluid accumulation.
  - Ultrasound-guided aspiration allows fluid collection without risk of side effects secondary to instillation of lavage fluid.
  - Diagnostic accuracy is operator dependent.
  - Not available at all veterinary facilities.
- Abdominal CT scan or MRI:
  - High diagnostic accuracy rate.
  - Typically requires anesthesia.
  - Limited to referral institutions.
  - Expensive.
- Laparoscopy:
  - High diagnostic accuracy rate.
  - Requires anesthesia.
  - Not available at many veterinary facilities.
- Exploratory laparotomy:
  - High diagnostic accuracy rate.
  - Requires anesthesia.
  - Highly invasive.

AUTHOR: **LILLIAN I. GOOD**

Echocardiography

BASIC INFORMATION

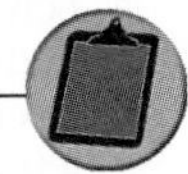

SYNONYM(S)

Cardiac ultrasound
Echo
Transthoracic echocardiography

OVERVIEW AND GOAL(S)

A complete echocardiographic study should:

(1) reveal the pertinent acquired or congenital lesions;
(2) evaluate valvular function;
(3) quantify ventricular systolic and diastolic function; and
(4) estimate the hemodynamic burden through quantification of chamber size (dilatation, hypertrophy).

INDICATIONS

- Congenital or acquired cardiac disease (valvular, myocardial, pericardial), cardiac neoplasia, pulmonary hypertension, systemic hypertension, and pleural effusion or respiratory distress of uncertain etiology.
- Limited echo studies can be useful in selected emergency situations (e.g., pericardial effusion, estimation of atrial size, or ventricle ejection fraction during initial stabilization if other initial diagnostic modalities are hazardous or nondiagnostic).

CONTRAINDICATIONS

- Animal should be stable enough to handle restraint.
- Animals with life-threatening problems (e.g., pleural effusion, pulmonary edema, and other causes of respiratory distress) need to be stabilized (limited echo study might be warranted or postponed).

EQUIPMENT, ANESTHESIA

- Scanning table with holes cut out (examination from beneath the animal improves image quality).
- Ultrasonic transmission gel.
- Isopropyl alcohol.
- Hair clippers might be needed.
- Ultrasound equipment: sector scanning transducers are preferred.
    - Cats and small dogs (usually 7.0-8.0-MHz transducer), medium-sized dogs (5.0-MHz transducer), large dogs (2.5-3.5-MHz transducer).
    - It may be necessary to use two different probes during one examination.
- The echocardiography machine should have M-mode, two-dimensional (2-D), Doppler (pulsed-wave, continuous-wave, and color-coded), and electrocardiogram (ECG) capabilities.
- Sedation/anesthesia is neither required nor desired except in very uncooperative animals.

ANTICIPATED TIME

Variable due to experience and case complexity (5-40 minutes).

PREPARATION: IMPORTANT CHECKPOINTS

- Dogs and cats usually require little preparation for echocardiographic examination.
- Fasting is not needed.
- Hair might be clipped over the right third to the sixth intercostal spaces (ICS) and left at the fourth to the seventh ICS (precordial transducer locations); however, in most dogs and cats, satisfactory images can be obtained by parting the haircoat, applying isopropyl alcohol liberally over area of interest, and finally applying transmission gel.

POSSIBLE COMPLICATIONS AND COMMON ERRORS TO AVOID

- Although the technique has no known physical hazard, there are risks associated with the improper interpretation or use of the results of the test.
- Use high-frequency transducers to obtain quality images of near field structures.
- Use low-frequency transducers for quality Doppler (color, pulse wave, continuous wave) signals.
- Adjust depth of the real-time image to fill the field of view (reduce amount of lung field).
- Adjust gain to avoid producing a white distorted image due to a high setting; too low of a setting will produce a weak signal.
- Remember the concept of blue/away and red/toward (BART) for color-flow Doppler studies.

PROCEDURE

- Image quality is improved in lateral recumbency; however, dogs and cats may be examined in a standing, sitting, or sternal position.
- The ultrasound machine's ECG clips are attached to the legs as recommended by the manufacturer (ECG is used for measurements and timing within the cardiac cycle).
- Starting in right lateral recumbency (animal's legs toward the examiner), the right parasternal location (window) is between the right third and sixth ICS, between the sternum and costochondral junctions (landmark: palpate right precordial heartbeat and place transducer at this location to start). Attention is paid to having the assistant restrain the animal with the forelegs drawn cranially to open the axilla/acoustic window.
- Long-axis views: The beam plane is oriented slightly clockwise from perpendicular to long axis of the body, parallel to the long axis of the heart, and with the transducer index mark pointing toward the heart base (craniodorsal, approximately toward the animal's shoulder); the following two views are obtained. First, a four-chamber view with the ventricles displayed to the left and the atria to the right (Fig. II-40).

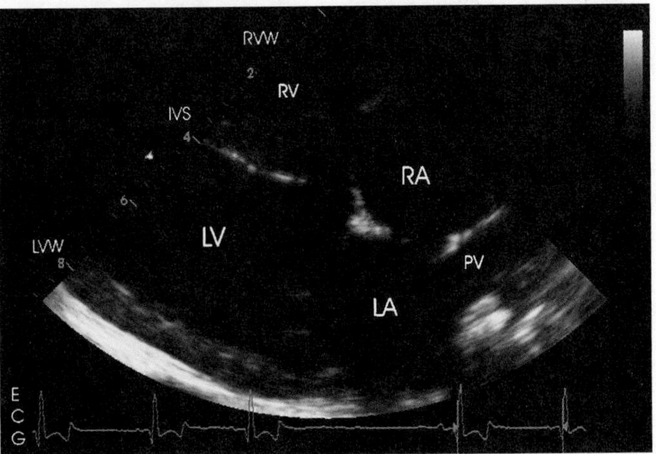

FIGURE II-40 Right parasternal four-chamber long-axis view in a normal dog (obtained without shaving). IVS, interventricular septum; LA, left atrium; LV, left ventricle; LVW, left ventricular wall; PV, pulmonary vein; RA, right atrium; RV, right ventricle; RVW, right ventricular wall.

The second view is obtained by slight clockwise rotation of the transducer from the four-chamber view into a slightly more craniodorsal orientation revealing the left ventricular outflow tract, aortic valve, and aortic root.

- Short-axis views: Rotate the transducer about 90 degrees toward the sternum from the four-chamber view (keep probe in same position except for the rotation) such that the beam plane is oriented perpendicular to the long axis of the heart with the transducer index mark now pointing cranially toward the animal's elbow (proper orientation identified by circular symmetry of the left ventricle or aortic root). There are five standard transverse images (left ventricle with papillary muscles [Fig. II-41], left ventricle at mitral chordae tendineae level, left ventricle at mitral valve level, heart base-aorta/left atrium level [Fig. II-42], and heart base-pulmonary artery) obtained from this position by pivoting the transducer from the apex to the base of the heart (caudal/ventral to cranial/dorsal).
- Turn animal over into left lateral recumbency, with the animal's legs still toward the sonographer.
- Left caudal (apical) parasternal location: The location is between the left fifth and seventh ICS, as close to the sternum as possible (landmark: palpable left apical heartbeat):
  - Left apical two-chamber views: The transducer index mark is pointing toward the heart base (dorsal), and the beam plane parallel to the long axis of the heart, the left side of the heart, is visualized (left atrium, left ventricle, and mitral valve). Slight rotation of the transducer into a craniodorsal to caudoventral orientation reveals left ventricle, outflow tract, aortic valve, and aortic root in a long-axis view.
  - Left apical four-chamber views: This is the only view in which the transducer index mark is pointing to the left and caudally, opposite of all other views. NOTE: The transducer should be as far back toward the apex of the heart as possible, often around the seventh ICS, and tilted to point cranially. The beam plane is in a left caudal to right cranial orientation and then directed dorsally toward the heart base, revealing the ventricles in the near field closest to the transducer and the atria in the far field (heart is oriented vertically; left ventricle, mitral valve, and left atrium should appear to the right). Modest cranial tilting of the beam from the above view will bring the left ventricular outflow region into view (five-chamber view) (Fig. II-43).
- Left cranial parasternal location: The location is between the left third and fourth ICS, between the sternum and costochondral junctions.
  - Long-axis views: With the transducer index mark pointing cranially and the beam plane oriented parallel to the long axis of the body and heart, a view of the left ventricular outflow tract, aortic valve, and ascending aorta is obtained (left ventricle will be displayed to the left and aorta to the right). From this position, angling of the beam ventral (toward the sternum) to the aorta brings out the right atrium/right auricle, tricuspid valve, and inflow region of the right ventricle (displayed to the right, while the left ventricle will be noted to the left). Finally, angling the transducer dorsally (transducer will almost be horizontal and parallel with the table) in relation to the ascending aorta produces a view of the main pulmonary artery, pulmonary valve, and right ventricular outflow tract.
  - Short-axis views: Remain in the same location as for the cranial long axis, and rotate the transducer until the transducer's index mark is toward the thoracic spine (dorsally, about 90 degrees from the location of long-axis view; aorta should appear circular in the center of the image). The right ventricular inflow tract should be to the left, and outflow tract and pulmonary artery to the right.

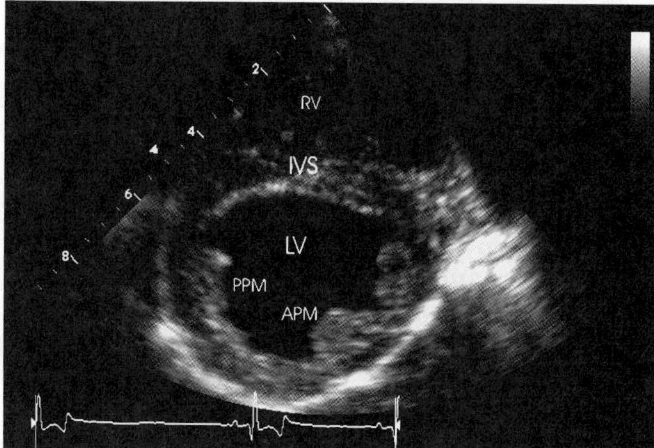

FIGURE II-41 Right parasternal short-axis view at the left ventricular papillary muscle level in the same dog. From this view, gentle pivoting motion (caudal/ventral to cranial/dorsal) of the transducer beam toward the base will reveal the other four standard views obtained from this location. APM, anterior papillary muscle; IVS, interventricular septum; LV, left ventricle; PPM, posterior papillary muscle; RV, right ventricle.

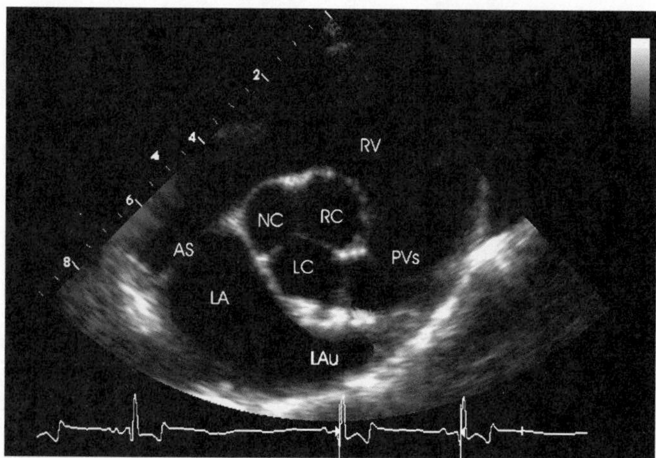

FIGURE II-42 Remaining in the same right parasternal window as the two previous views in Figs. II-40 and II-41, gentle pivoting toward the heart base, the right parasternal short-axis view at the left atrium/aorta level was obtained in the same dog. AS, atrial septum; LA, left atrium; LAu, left auricle; LC, left coronary cusp; NC, noncoronary cusp; PV, pulmonary vein; PVs, pulmonic valve; RC, right coronary cusp; RV, right ventricle.

POSTPROCEDURE

- Remove ECG clips.
- Wipe gel and alcohol from animal.

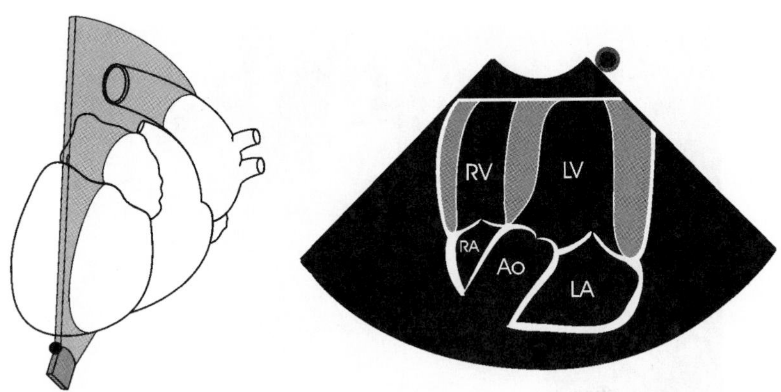

FIGURE II-43 The five-chamber view is obtained at the left apical parasternal location. The left apical parasternal location is the only time during the echocardiographic examination when the index mark on the head of the transducer is directed caudally. Ao, aorta; LA, left atrium; LV, left ventricle; RA, right atrium; RV, right ventricle.

ALTERNATIVES AND THEIR RELATIVE MERITS

Transesophageal echocardiography:
- Semi-invasive procedure.
- Requires general anesthesia in animals.
- Provides superb clarity and resolution.

SUGGESTED READING

Bonagura JD: Echocardiography. *J Am Vet Med Assoc* 204:516–522, 1994.
Oyama MA: Advances in echocardiography. *Vet Clin North Am Small Anim Pract* 34(5):1083–1104, 2001.
Thomas WP, Gaber CE, Jacobs GJ, et al: Recommendations for standards in transthoracic two-dimesional echocardiography in the dog and cat. *J Vet Int Med* 7:247–252, 1993.

AUTHOR: **ROBERT PROŠEK**

Electrocardiography

BASIC INFORMATION

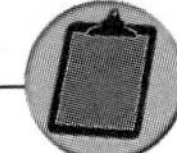

SYNONYM(S)

Electrocardiogram: ECG, EKG
Electrocardiograph: ECG machine

OVERVIEW AND GOAL(S)

- To obtain a tracing that represents the rhythm of the heartbeat.
- Electrocardiography is the diagnostic test of choice for evaluating cardiac arrhythmias.
- Electrocardiography may also provide some limited information regarding cardiac structure (sizes and proportions of waves and complexes sometimes indicate chamber enlargement) and systemic disturbances (e.g., hyperkalemia, hypoxemia).

INDICATIONS

- Evaluation of a cardiac arrhythmia noted during physical examination.
- Part of routine cardiovascular monitoring during general anesthesia or intensive care.
- Monitoring of a cardiac arrhythmia noted during anesthesia or hospitalization.
- Evaluation of an animal with clinical signs suggesting syncope.
- Evaluation of an animal with suspected or confirmed hyperkalemia.

CONTRAINDICATIONS

Severe dyspnea contraindicates restraint in lateral recumbency for ECG.

EQUIPMENT, ANESTHESIA

- Electrocardiograph (ECG machine). Each ECG wire should end in an atraumatic clip that connects the machine to the animal's skin.
- A table with a waterproof, foam core pad on which the animal can lie comfortably (to reduce electrical interference emerging through the table).
- Isopropyl alcohol for improving contact between ECG clips and skin.

ANTICIPATED TIME

- Basic tracing: 5 minutes.
- Ongoing monitoring: any duration.
- For prolonged monitoring, see Holter/Cardiac Event Monitoring, p 1264.

PREPARATION: IMPORTANT CHECKPOINTS

Check that the electrocardiograph has sufficient paper supply and is functioning. There is no ink in most electrocardiographs (heat-sensitive paper and thermal stylus).

POSSIBLE COMPLICATIONS AND COMMON ERRORS TO AVOID

- Animals that are in respiratory distress should not be restrained for electrocardiography; these animals should be assessed while they are standing (or in any other position in which they are not distressed), or the ECG should be postponed until dyspnea has improved or resolved.
- Artifact can be minimized by:
  - Using enough isopropyl alcohol at the point of contact between the skin clips and skin.
  - Avoiding metal-on-metal contact between clips; often, with smaller dogs and cats, the wires need to be held apart by the person performing the ECG to avoid wire-to-wire or clip-to-clip contact during the procedure.
  - Choosing a quiet, comfortable environment to perform the tracing; a cold or stressful environment may trigger shivering (and motion artifact), whereas an excessively warm or stressful environment can induce panting in dogs (and motion artifact).
  - Replacing the ECG wire set every 5 years under all circumstances or annually with heavy use (e.g., used multiple times weekly) because the wires tend to fracture internally with age.
  - Evaluating multiple ECG leads rather than just one lead; each lead provides a different perspective on the electrical activity of the heartbeat, and lead II is not necessarily the lead in which the clearest P waves, QRS complexes, T waves, and minimal artifact are seen.
- Overinterpretation of the dimensions of P waves and T waves as indicating cardiac chamber enlargement is a common pitfall; echocardiography is much more sensitive and specific than electrocardiography for assessing cardiac structure.

- Motion artifact may mimic abnormal cardiac activity and cause misdiagnosis.
- In-hospital monitoring that lasts for hours or more should involve the use of atraumatic or minimally traumatic skin clips: either (1) a small patch of skin can be shaved on each side of the thorax and stick-on, human ECG patches can be used or (2) loops of small-gauge steel suture may be passed through the skin in the usual locations on the four limbs (Table II-3), and the ECG wires are clamped to these loops instead of directly to the skin.

PROCEDURE

- The procedure is the same for cats and dogs.
- Performing an ECG requires two people (clinician and assistant), unless animal restraint is not necessary (anesthetized or unconscious animal).
- The assistant restrains the animal in right lateral recumbency (Fig. II-44). Sitting, sternal, and dorsal positions are equally acceptable; determination of the mean electrical axis from these other positions is inaccurate, but this has no effect on assessing the cardiac rhythm.
- The assistant stands or sits behind (dorsal to) the right-laterally recumbent animal and holds the animal's limbs perpendicular to the long axis of the animal's body. NOTE: For the humeri and femurs to be truly perpendicular to the long axis of the body, the assistant

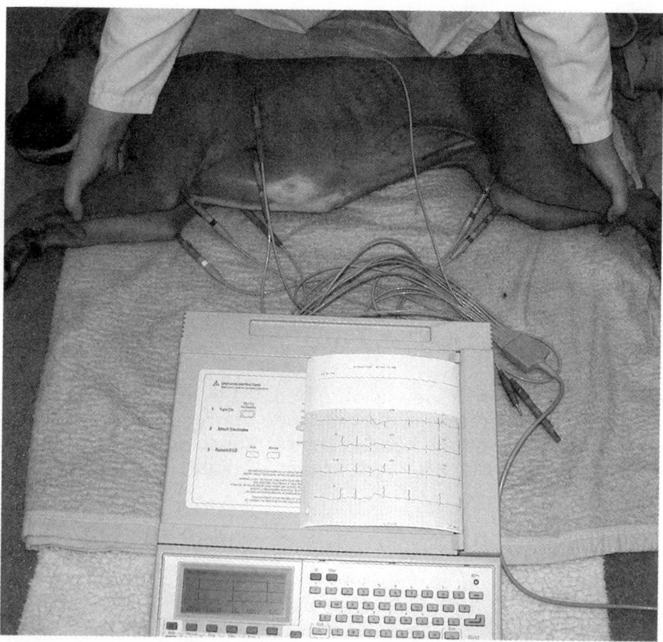

FIGURE II-44 The patient is comfortably restrained in right lateral recumbency, with the limbs perpendicular to the long axis of the body. An insulating (waterproof, foam core) pad is under the patient to reduce the influence of electrical interference.

TABLE II-3 ECG Clip/Electrode Placement for Standard Limb Leads (I, II, III, aVR, aVL, aVF):

RA, white	Right forelimb; clip to skin just proximal to the olecranon (caudal triceps region).
LA, black	Left forelimb; clip to skin just proximal to the olecranon (caudal triceps region).
RL, green	Right hind limb; clip to skin just proximal to the stifle (cranial thigh); ground wire.
LL, red	Left hind limb; clip to skin just proximal to the stifle (cranial thigh).

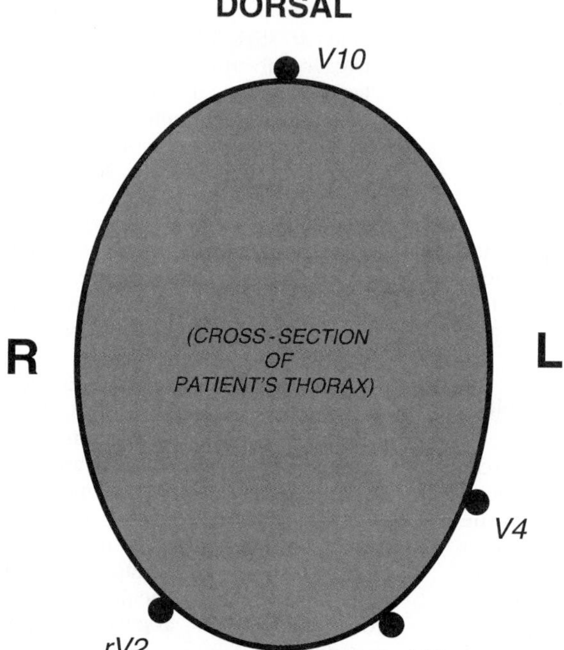

AS WRITTEN ON CABLES (=HUMAN*)	VETERINARY TERMS (and previous vet nomenclature)	LOCATION ON THE PATIENT'S CHEST
V1	rV2 (CV5RL)	RIGHT 5TH INTERCOSTAL SPACE, JUST TO RIGHT OF STERNUM
V2	V2 (CV6LL)	LEFT 6TH INTERCOSTAL SPACE, JUST TO LEFT OF STERNUM
V3	V4 (CV6LU)	LEFT 6TH INTERCOSTAL SPACE, AT THE COSTOCHONDRAL JUNCTION
V4	V10	DORSAL MIDLINE, DIRECTLY DORSAL TO V4 (APPROXIMATELY @ 7TH THORACIC VERTEBRA)

*V5 and V6 are not used in veterinary medicine.

FIGURE II-45 The placement and utility of precordial leads.

needs to extend the limbs sometimes quite substantially. Forelimbs (at the level of the carpi) are held in the assistant's right hand and hind limbs (at the level of the tarsi) in the left.

- The clinician attaches the ECG clips (electrodes) to the appropriate points on the animal for the limb leads (see Table II-3) as well as the precordial leads (Fig. II-45).
- A standard ECG includes representative recordings from all six limb leads, usually 5-15 seconds each for I, II, III, aVR, aVL, and aVF, and will provide further information if precordial leads are also recorded (see Fig. II-45).
- A standard ECG also includes a "rhythm strip," which is a continuous tracing of the same lead for 30 seconds to 1 minute or more.
    - The most commonly used lead for the rhythm strip is lead II, but the lead that is chosen should be the one that shows the clearest P waves, QRS complexes, and T waves.
    - The duration of the rhythm strip depends on the reason for performing the ECG and can be as long as is needed (several minutes) when an intermittent arrhythmia is being sought.
- Generally, if an abnormality has not been detected over a period of 3-4 minutes of ECG recoding on paper, then the procedure is terminated. The tracing obtained thus far is reviewed meticulously, and if further ECG evaluation is needed, ongoing ECG monitoring either with an in-hospital display monitor (e.g., oscilloscope) or portable telemetry (e.g., see Holter/Cardiac Event Monitoring, p 1264) can be used.

POSTPROCEDURE

The clips are carefully detached from the skin prior to releasing the animal's restraint.

ALTERNATIVES AND THEIR RELATIVE MERITS

- Thoracic radiographs: provide some information on cardiac structure (e.g., chamber enlargement), but this information is limited by substantial overlap between normal and mild to moderate abnormalities. Also indicated when ST segment elevation or depression is present (assess for pulmonary or airway lesions).
- Echocardiography: the clinical gold standard for assessing cardiac chamber size; indicated if cardiac enlargement is suspected based on ECG and/or radiographs.
- Pulse oximetry/arterial blood gas measurement: If ST segment elevation or depression is noted in the absence of structural heart disease (e.g., cardiomyopathy, advanced valvular disease, congenital heart disease).
- Serum potassium measurement: if lack of P waves is noted, especially in an animal with a history and/or physical findings suggesting a reason for hyperkalemia (urgent).

AUTHOR: **ETIENNE CÔTÉ**

PROCEDURES AND TECHNIQUES

Electromyography (EMG) and Nerve Conduction Velocity (NCV)

BASIC INFORMATION

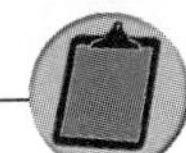

SYNONYM(S)

Electrodiagnostics
EMG and NCV

OVERVIEW AND GOAL(S)

- Noninvasive method of evaluating animals that are showing clinical signs consistent with neuromuscular disease.
- May confirm the presence of nerve, neuromuscular junction, or muscle disease in these animals.

INDICATIONS

- Animals with clinical signs and neurologic examination suggestive of neuromuscular disease (diffuse or focal).
- Animals with peripheral nerve injuries.
- May help confirm the presence of endocrine disease (hyperadrenocorticism-pseudomyotonia).

CONTRAINDICATIONS

Animals with megaesophagus ± severe diffuse neuromuscular signs are poor anesthetic candidates due to risk of regurgitation, aspiration pneumonia, and hypoventilation.

EQUIPMENT, ANESTHESIA

- General anesthesia and tracheal intubation are required. For some more advanced electrodiagnostic testing, animals must be paralyzed with atracurium, and therefore manual or mechanical ventilation may be required.
- Should ideally be performed in electrically shielded room to minimize background noise.
- Differential amplifier, needle electrodes for stimulating and recording impulses (concentric needle electrode preferred for electromyography [EMG]), isopropyl alcohol, and measuring tape.
- Surgical pack: often, muscle and nerve biopsies (see Muscle and Nerve Biopsy, p 1279) are done following electrodiagnostics.
- In some cases, percutaneous endoscopic gastric (PEG) tube placement (see Feeding Tube Placement: Percutaneous Endoscopic Gastrostomy [PEG], p 1247) is beneficial while animal is anesthetized (providing nutritional support, administering medications, etc.).

ANTICIPATED TIME

- EMG: 10-20 minutes
- EMG + nerve conduction velocity (NCV): 40-60 minutes

PREPARATION: IMPORTANT CHECKPOINTS

Monitor body temperature because hypothermia can prolong nerve conduction times

POSSIBLE COMPLICATIONS AND COMMON ERRORS TO AVOID

- Complications related to anesthesia
- Regurgitation and aspiration pneumonia in animals with megaesophagus/esophageal dysfunction or dysphagia

PROCEDURE

- Animal is premedicated, anesthetized, intubated, and then maintained with inhalational anesthetic (isoflurane, sevoflurane).
- Placed in lateral recumbancy.
- EMG:
    - Noninvasive method of evaluating animals with myopathy or denervation.
    - Needle electrodes are used for recording electrical activity in major muscle groups in appendicular muscles and in epaxial and masticatory muscles; rarely esophageal, laryngeal muscles, and tongue.
    - Normal healthy muscle is electrically silent at rest, aside from normal background end-plate activity due to random release of small vesicles (quanta) of acetylcholine at neuromuscular junction.
    - Short bursts of electrical activity during needle placement are also normal and are due to temporary disruption of muscle fibers (insertional activity).
    - Other spontaneous electrical discharges or in resting muscle (i.e., anesthetized animal) are abnormal and indicate neuromuscular disease.

- Abnormal EMG activity confirms the presence of neuromuscular disease and helps localize which muscle groups affected; however, abnormal EMG activity cannot differentiate between myopathic or neuropathic disease.
- Abnormal EMG activity includes fibrillation potentials, positive sharp waves, complex repetitive discharges, or myotonic discharges. In general, the type of waveform is not specific for neuroanatomic location (nerve versus muscle) or pathophysiologic mechanism of disease.
- EMG changes due to denervation may not be detected for 5 to 10 days after initial injury.
- Severity of clinical signs does not always correlate with severity of EMG changes.

• Motor NCV:
- Using stimulating needle electrodes, a nerve is stimulated at various accessible points along its anatomic pathway.
- Recording needle electrodes used for recording compound muscle action potential in myofibers innervated by that nerve.
- Nerve conduction velocity along various segments of axon may be determined by measuring distance between points of stimulation and difference in latency of waveforms (velocity [meters per second] = Δ distance/Δ time).
- Nerves are composed of multiple fiber types of varying diameter and amounts of myelination, thus will conduct at different velocities.
- The compound muscle action potential (CMAP) waveform represents electrical activity of different myofibers as action potentials travel down axons at different speeds and reach the neuromuscular junction, stimulating myofiber contraction at different times. Thus, the CMAP waveform represents the summation of action potentials of a group of myofibers over time.
- The amplitude of the waveform is proportional to the number of available axons. Axonal disease results in a decreased number of axons and a decreased CMAP amplitude and may also cause secondary EMG changes due to denervation.
- Nerve conduction velocity measures the speed at which action potentials travel down the axon. Decreases in NCV may be due to demyelination or due to loss of the large, fastest conducting fibers.
- Demyelinating diseases slow conduction along the axon and result in a longer onset latency of the waveform, a widening and distortion of the CMAP waveform, and physiologic dispersion or distortion of the waveform over the time axis.
- Many peripheral nerve diseases result in both axonal loss and demyelination, causing decreased amplitude, physiologic dispersion, and abnormal EMG activity due to denervation.
- Nerves commonly tested in domestic animals include the sciatic, peroneal, cranial tibial, radial, musculocutaneous, and median.
- The recurrent laryngeal, facial nerve, and trigeminal nerves are rarely tested.
- Measuring nerve conduction velocity is helpful in determining whether disease is demyelinating, axonal, or both, as well as whether the nerves are more affected proximally or distally. It is also helpful in determining which nerves are affected.

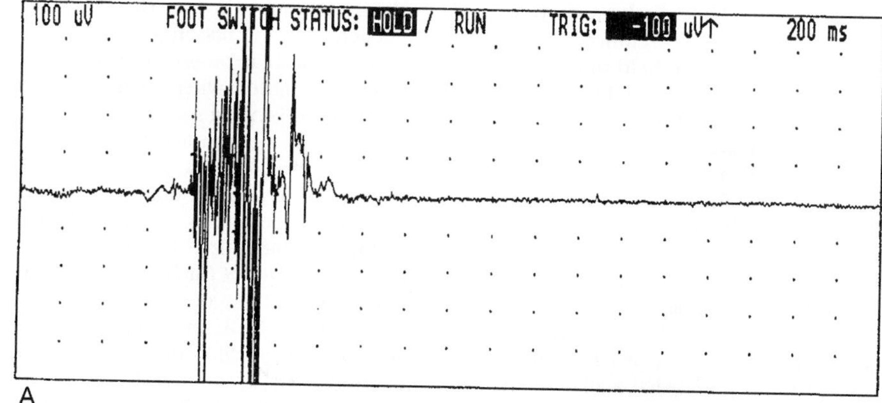

A

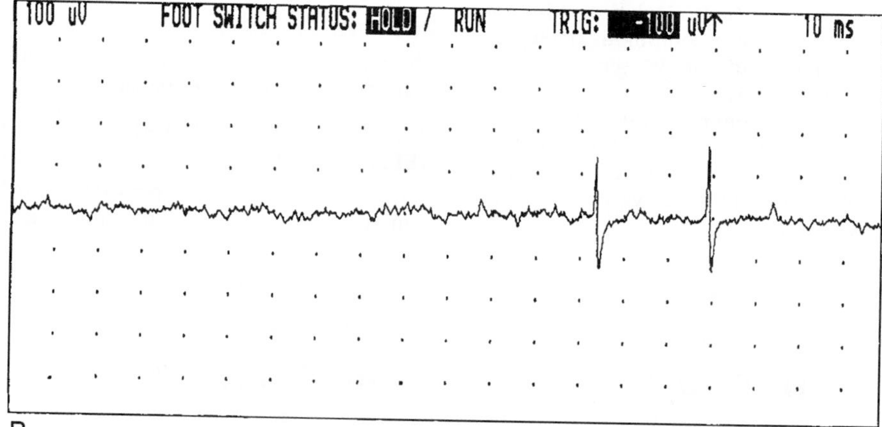

B

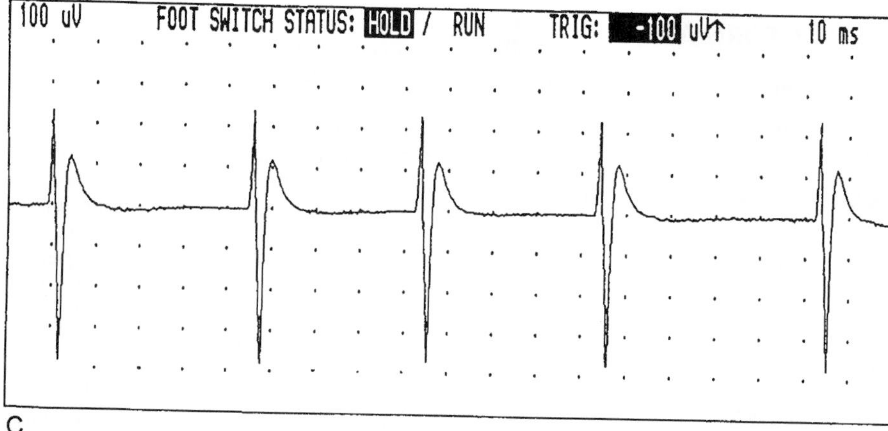

C

FIGURE II-46 Types of electrical activity seen in normal muscle during EMG evaluation. **A**, Insertional activity. Note the abrupt onset and termination of activity associated with needle placement (100 μV/div; 200 msec/div). **B**, Miniature end-plate potentials with two end-plate spikes indicating close proximity of the needle to an end-place (100 μV/div; 10 msec/div). **C**, Motor unit action potentials seen during voluntary muscle activity in an awake animal (100 μV/div; 10 msec/div). Reprinted with permission from Cuddon PA: Electrophysiology in neuromuscular disease. *Vet Clin N Am Small An Prac* 32:31–62, 2002.

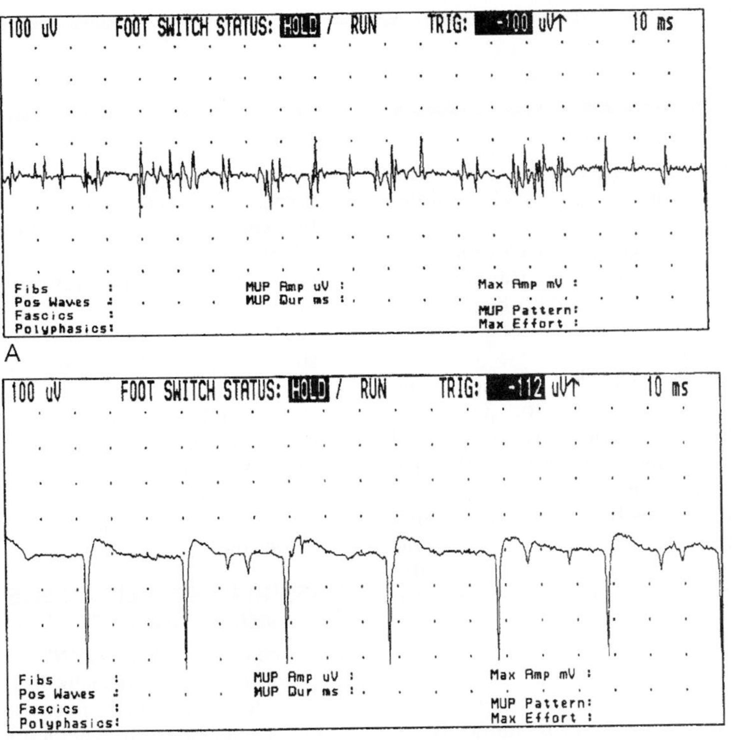

FIGURE II-47 Electromyography: abnormal spontaneous electrical activity. **A,** Fibrillation potentials, moderate density (100 μV/div, 10 msec/div). Fibrillation potentials may be associated either with denervation secondary to axonopathy or with primary myopathy. The density and consistency of observed fibrillation potentials is an accurate reflection on the severity of muscle involvement. **B,** Spontaneous electrical activity in the form of positive sharp waves (100 μV/div; 10 msec/div). Reprinted with permission from Cuddon PA: Electrophysiology in neuromuscular disease. *Vet Clin N Am Sm An Prac* 32:31–62, 2002.

- Pathophysiologic mechanism of disease cannot be determined using NCV.
- Nerve and muscle biopsies are often necessary to determine the etiology of disease, although EMG and nerve conduction velocity help determine the nature of disease (demyelinating versus axonal versus myopathy) and optimal biopsy sample site.

POSTPROCEDURE

- Monitor recovery from anesthesia.
- Nerve and muscle biopsies are often indicated after electrodiagnostic testing to determine the pathophysiology of disease (e.g., inflammatory, infectious, neoplastic, degenerative, toxic, endocrine).
  - See Muscle and Nerve Biopsy, p 1279.
  - For additional details, consult recommended methods for submission of samples in Shelton and Engvall, 2002.
- In some cases, PEG tube placement is indicated while the animal is anesthetized.

ALTERNATIVES AND THEIR RELATIVE MERITS

Muscle and nerve biopsies as already described

SUGGESTED READING

Shelton GD, Engvall E: Muscular dystrophies and other inherited myopathies. *Vet Clin North Am Small An Pract* 32(1):103–124, 2002.

AUTHOR: **MICHELLE MURRAY SCIBELLI**

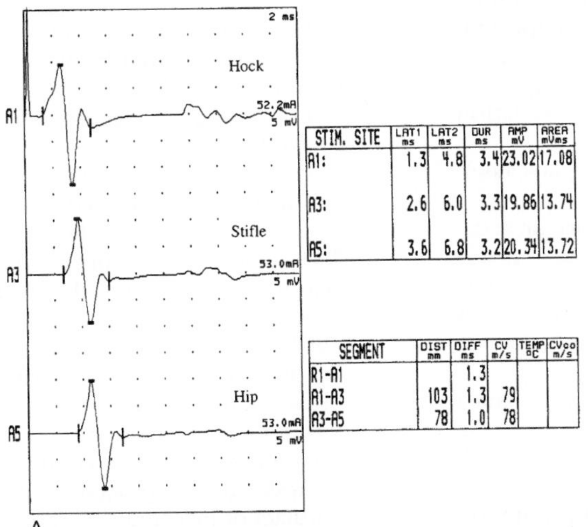

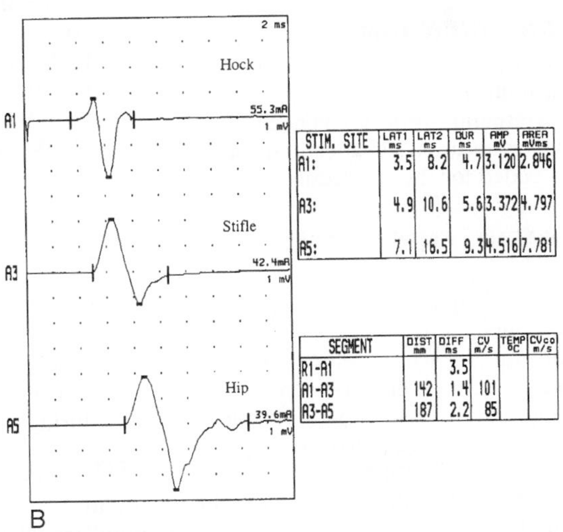

FIGURE II-48 Motor nerve conduction studies recorded from the plantar interosseous muscles following stimulation of the sciatic-tibial nerve at the hock, stifle, and hip in a normal dog (*A*) and in a dog with generalized muscle disease (*B*) (mitochondrial myopathy). Note the marked generalized decrease in CMAP amplitudes (3.12, 3.37, and 4.51 mV) from all sites of stimulation in the myopathic dog when compared with the normal dog (23.02, 19.86, and 20.34 mV). Despite CMAP amplitude reduction, the dog with myopathy has normal MNCVs (101 and 85 m/sec). Generalized CMAP amplitude decrease can also be observed in prejunctional neuromuscular diseases, such as botulism, as well as in primary axonopathies. Recording parameters: *A*, 5 mV/div and 2 msec/div and *B*, 1 mV/div and 2 msec/div. Reprinted with permission from Cuddon PA: Electrophysiology in neuromuscular disease. *Vet Clin N Am Sm An Prac* 32:31–62, 2002.

Electroretinogram

BASIC INFORMATION

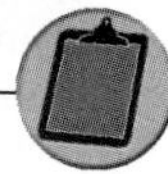

SYNONYM(S)

ERG

OVERVIEW AND GOAL(S)

- Evaluation of retinal function (quantitative or qualitative) through measurement of the electrical response generated after the photoreceptors receive a light stimulus.
- An electroretinogram (ERG) by itself does not determine whether an animal can see; the retina is only one part of the visual system.

INDICATIONS

- Differentiation of causes of sudden blindness (i.e., sudden acquired retinal degeneration syndrome [SARDS]) and optic neuritis
- Evaluation of retinal function to determine cataract surgery suitability
- Identifying inherited retinal disease (i.e., progressive retinal atrophy [progressive rod-cone degeneration] or progressive rod-cone dysplasias) at an early age well before clinical signs and gross retinal changes occur
- Evaluation of damage incurred by glaucoma or toxic effects of drugs
- Evaluation of the effects of optic nerve hypoplasia on retinal function

CONTRAINDICATIONS

- Panuveitis
- Corneal ulcer
- Any contraindication for general anesthesia or sedation (if anesthesia/sedation needed for the procedure)

EQUIPMENT, ANESTHESIA

- Equipment:
  - ERG recording unit (Retinographics, LKC, Nicolet).
  - Gold-foil contact lens electrode or an atraumatic wire electrode (placed in conjunctival cul-de-sac). Contact lens electrodes are used most often.
  - Reference and ground electrodes.
  - Standardized light source for light stimulus.
  - "Safe" light, red light, or small red penlight.
  - Timer for dark adaptation.
  - Conducting agent to facilitate electrical contact between the contact lens electrode and the eye; methylcellulose (Gonak) or GenTeal Tear Gel.
  - Table; if stainless steel, cover with nonconducting material (rubber padding).
  - Optional: head rest for elevation and positioning of head; this may be made of foam, rolled-up blankets, or sandbags.
- Anesthesia:
  - General anesthesia or sedation; some animals will tolerate the procedure with topical anesthesia only (and contact lens electrode), but the risk of artifact is increased.
  - General anesthesia prevents animal movement (artifact source) and allows more precise direction of the light stimulus into the eye via fixation of the eye.
  - Sedation. One of these three protocols can be considered:
    - Acepromazine (0.03 mg/kg IV) and butorphanol (0.3 mg/kg IV).
      - Observe precautions/contraindications, especially with acepromazine.
      - Butorphanol can be partially reversed with naloxone (0.02 mg/kg IM).
    - Propofol 4-6 mg/kg IV to effect (low doses will be sufficient in most cases).
    - Medetomidine (0.005-0.01 mg/kg [dogs, cats] IM) combined with butorphanol (0.2-0.4 mg/kg [dogs, cats] IM).
  - Other anesthetic or sedation protocols may be employed; it is important to be consistent to aid in correct interpretation of the recordings.
  - General anesthesia and sedation depress the ERG response.
  - Topical anesthetic (i.e., proparacaine).
- Personnel (two people):
  - One to monitor anesthesia or sedation, position the animal's head, ensure that light stimulus is directed into the eye during the flash, and check to see that all electrodes are in position during test.
  - One to run the computer program during the test.

ANTICIPATED TIME

About 1 to 1.5 hours, including time for pupillary dilation

PREPARATION: IMPORTANT CHECKPOINTS

- Knowledge of retinal physiology.
- Familiarity with ERG equipment.
- Control of inflammation; especially important in a precataract surgery evaluation.
- Dilation of pupils.
- Bleaching of retinal pigments in rods by exposure to bright light before dark adaptation.
- Dark adaptation (4 minutes minimum, 20 minutes desirable).
- Lock room to avoid inadvertent exposure to light and necessity of starting procedure again.
- Use grounded outlet to decrease/eliminate 60-cycle interference.
- Take off wristwatch to decrease 60-cycle interference.
- Set up computer, supplies, equipment before dark adaptation.

POSSIBLE COMPLICATIONS AND COMMON ERRORS TO AVOID

POSSIBLE COMPLICATIONS

- Corneal ulcers, especially in diabetics with decreased corneal sensitivity and increased risk of corneal ulceration.
- Hypoxemia or death due to failure to monitor animal during general anesthesia.

COMMON ERRORS

- Preparation errors:
  - Failure to dilate pupils fully.
- Procedural errors:
  - Failure to direct light stimulus directly into eye.
  - Error in labeling which eye is which on recordings.
  - Lack of standardized protocol for specific model of equipment on premises.
  - Lack of standardized anesthesia/sedation, leading to difficulty in interpretation of results.
  - Excess noise due to failure to use signal averaging and filters.
  - Excess muscle fasciculations in eyelids due to inadequate sedation, leading to excess noise in the readings. The use of an eyelid speculum exacerbates muscle activity due to muscle stretching.
  - Dull electrode needles.
  - Gap in gold-foil electrode ring on contact lens electrode, leading to inaccurate reading or artifact.
  - Expulsion of contact lens or reference electrodes during procedure, leading to artifact or inaccurate reading.
  - 60-cycle interference caused by lights, appliances in same room, using a noninsulated table.
  - "Stray" light stimulus from computer monitor during procedure, leading to lower amplitude readings.
- Animal-derived errors:
  - Eyes are closed, leading to very low amplitude readings.

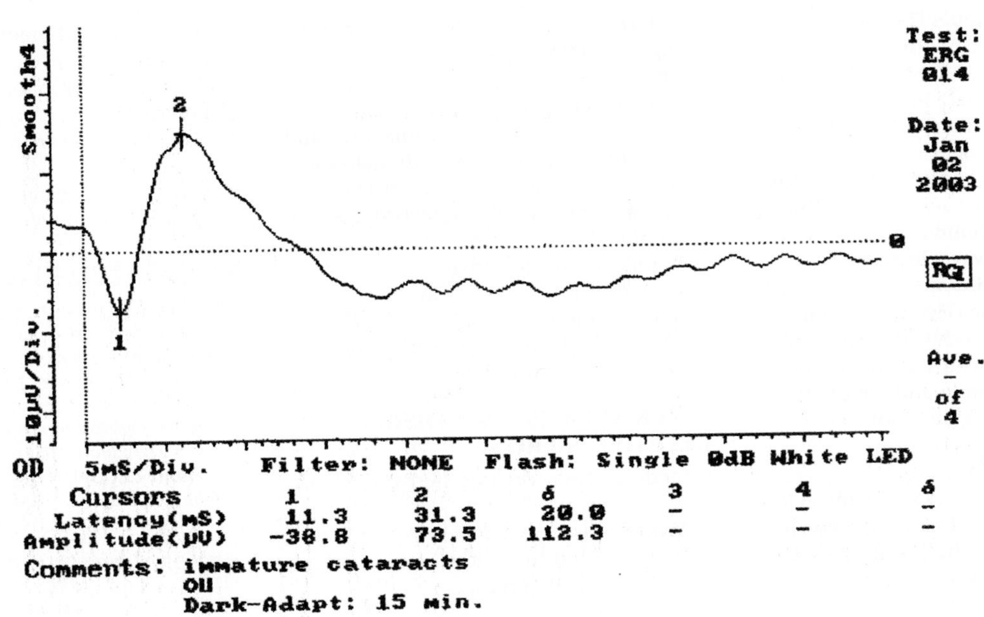

FIGURE II-49 Normal ERG. The number 1 marks the nadir of the a-wave, and the number 2 marks the peak of the b-wave.

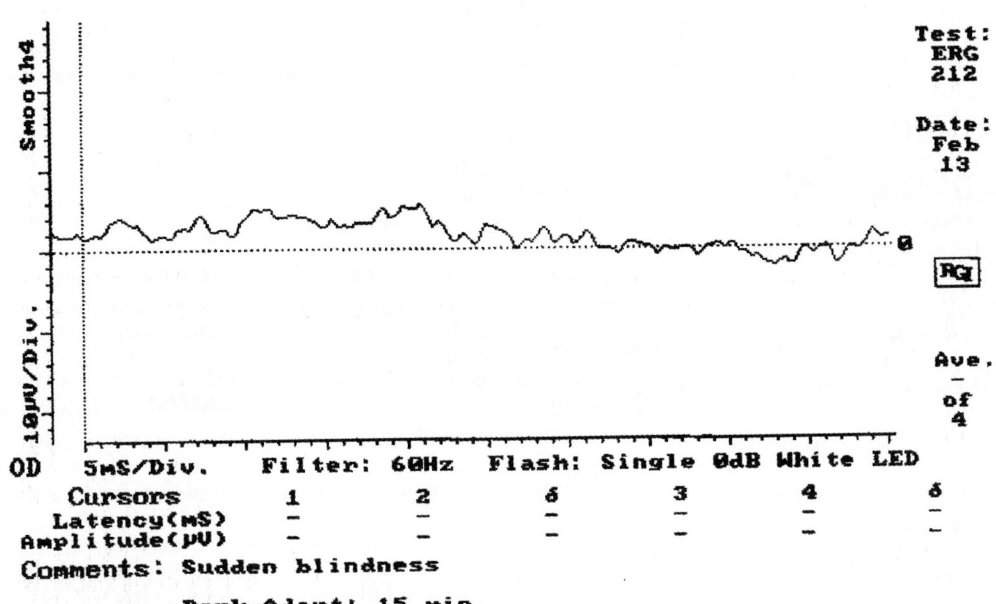

FIGURE II-50 ERG from dog with SARDS. No normal waves are detectable.

- ◦ Blinking during light stimulation, leading to low amplitude readings.
- ◦ Third eyelid is prolapsed, expelling the contact lens or leading to very low amplitude readings due to the failure of light to reach retina.

Interpretation errors:

- Misinterpretation of findings due to lack of knowledge of retinal physiology and basis of the test.
- Believing, in error, that cataracts will depress or eliminate the passage of light to the retina. Cataracts can amplify the ERG response due to increased scattered light.

PROCEDURE

- Dilate pupils with short-acting mydriatic (i.e. tropicamide) 30 minutes before sedation.
- Sedate or induce general anesthesia as necessary.
- Place reference electrode in skin over ipsilateral zygomatic arch, halfway between the eye and ear.
- Place ground electrode in skin over top of muzzle. If dog must be muzzled, place ground electrode in skin on forehead. If electrode needles do not go into skin easily, discard and use new electrodes to avoid discomfort to animal and to increase accuracy of reading.
- Place topical anesthetic in eye.
- Place conducting gel on concave surface of contact lens.
- Place contact lens in eye, ensuring that the lens is centered on the cornea and not on top of the nictitating membrane.
- Perform standardized protocol. Protocols are available in ERG units' software. To determine rod function, important in progressive rod-cone degeneration, a blue filter under scotopic conditions must be used.

- Use signal averaging. This produces an averaged response after a predetermined number of flashes (5–10) and enhances the signal-to-noise ratio.
- Use band-pass filters to screen out unwanted frequencies.
- A normal ERG consists of a low-amplitude negative a-wave 10–12 msec after the light stimulus, followed by a large positive b-wave. In some tracings, the c-wave (a third wave) is seen as a positive deflection (Figs. II-49 and II-50).
- The a-wave is produced by the photoreceptors and the b-wave by movement of potassium in and out of Müller cells and indirectly by bipolar cells.

POSTPROCEDURE

- Remove electrodes from eye and skin.
- Soak contact lens electrode in distilled water; do not rub the inside surface of the lens to clean it because this action will remove the gold-foil circle, rendering it useless.
- Flush eye with sterile eye wash and stain for corneal ulcer.
- Partially reverse acepromazine and butorphanol sedation with naloxone, or recover from general anesthesia.
- Measure amplitude of recordings, the amplitude from the nadir (lowest point) of the negative a-wave to the peak of the positive b-wave.
- Record findings on a separate disc or CD for a backup copy, and print hard copy for animal's record.

ALTERNATIVES AND THEIR RELATIVE MERITS

Genetic testing for inherited retinal disease:

- Many tests are available for specific dog breed-related inherited retinopathies but not for all breeds.
- Only requires blood test, so simpler than ERG.

Maze test under photopic and scotopic conditions:

- May be gross screening test for retinal atrophy.
- Unable to determine anatomic source of defect in sudden blindness cases.

SUGGESTED READING

Aguirre G: Electroretinography—Are we misusing an excellent diagnostic tool? *Vet Comp Ophthalmol* 5(1):2-3, 1995.

Komaromy AM, Brooks DE, Dawson WW, et al: Technical issues in electrodiagnostic recording. *Vet Ophthalmol* 5(2):85-91, 2002.

Sims MH: Electrodiagnostic evaluation of vision. In Gelatt KN (ed): *Veterinary Ophthalmology*. Baltimore, Lippincott, Williams & Wilkins, 1999, pp 484-504.

AUTHOR: **NANCY B. COTTRILL**

Enema (Evacuation, Retention)

BASIC INFORMATION

OVERVIEW AND GOAL(S)

Emptying of colonic content (evacuation) and/or administration of substrates through enema (retention)

INDICATIONS

Evacuation enema:

- Treatment of colonic impaction/constipation
- Preparation of the animal for colonoscopy

Retention enema:

- Treatment of severe hepatic encephalopathy

CONTRAINDICATIONS

Painful anus, rectal mass

EQUIPMENT, ANESTHESIA

- Enema solutions:
  - Warm tap water or isotonic saline (5–10 ml/kg).
  - Docusate (emollient enema promoting water penetration within the feces).
  - Mineral oil (lubricant enema; 5–10 ml for small dogs and cats, 10–20 ml for medium-size dogs, 20–30 ml for larger dogs).
  - Lactulose (hyperosmotic laxative; 5–10 ml for cats).
- Preparation of the animal for flexible colonoscopy: To perform a successful colonic examination, thorough preparation of the animal is mandatory. Enema administration alone is often not enough to obtain a fully clean colon. Therefore, the following should also be performed in those animals to ensure a successful colonoscopy:
  - The animal should have fasted for 24 to 36 hours.
  - The use of an oral gastrointestinal (GI) isosmotic lavage solution, such as Golytely, Colopeg, or Colyte, is recommended two times, a few hours apart, in the afternoon preceding the colonoscopy.
    - Dogs: 30 ml/kg through an orogastric tube.
    - Cats: 30 ml/kg through a nasoesophageal tube.
  - One or two enemas are administered the afternoon before and the morning of the colonoscopy until the animal is evacuating watery fluid. Often "larger" quantities of water are necessary to obtain an adequately cleaned colon (dogs >20 kg: 1 L; dogs >40 kg: 2 L). Use a funnel and a large tube.
- Treatment of severe acute hepatic encephalopathy:
  - First perform a cleansing enema to evacuate all remaining colonic content.
  - Retention enema (total amount of 15 ml/kg): allows the delivery of fermentable substrates or colonic pH modification.
    - Lactulose (1:2 dilution with water).
    - Neomycin in water (10–20 mg/kg).
    - An alternative is to use diluted Betadine (1:10, rinse thoroughly after 15 minutes).
  - See also Hepatic Encephalopathy, p 489.

ANTICIPATED TIME

About 15 minutes

PREPARATION: IMPORTANT CHECKPOINTS

- Fluid therapy is an essential part of the management of colon impaction.
- Animals should be well hydrated.

POSSIBLE COMPLICATIONS AND COMMON ERRORS TO AVOID

- Some enemas, such as docusate, can promote GI water loss. Therefore, they should be used with caution if the animal is dehydrated.
- If enemas are administered too quickly, they can lead to discomfort and vomiting.
- Enemas should be administered after they are warmed to body temperature.
- Do not administer mineral oil with docusate.
- Do not administer sodium phosphate enemas to small dogs or cats because such enemas can induce dehydration, neurologic signs, and severe hyperphosphatemia, hypernatremia, and hypocalcemia.
- If the animal has much anal or rectal pain, enemas should be replaced by an extra administration of an oral GI lavage solution.
- If the animal is not cooperative, sedation or general anesthesia can be necessary.

PROCEDURE

- Slowly insert a very well-lubricated catheter or feeding tube through the anus (10–14 Fr) (Fig. II-51). In cats, a

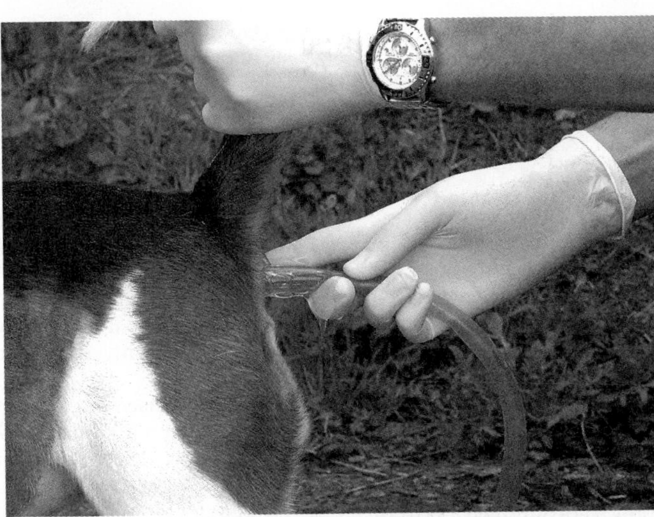

FIGURE II-51 An enema tube that is well lubricated before going into the anus. The distal end of the tube must be smooth and rounded and not have sharp edges. It is generously lubricated and passed into the anus and then advanced to a maximum point that corresponds to the distance from the anus to the last rib.

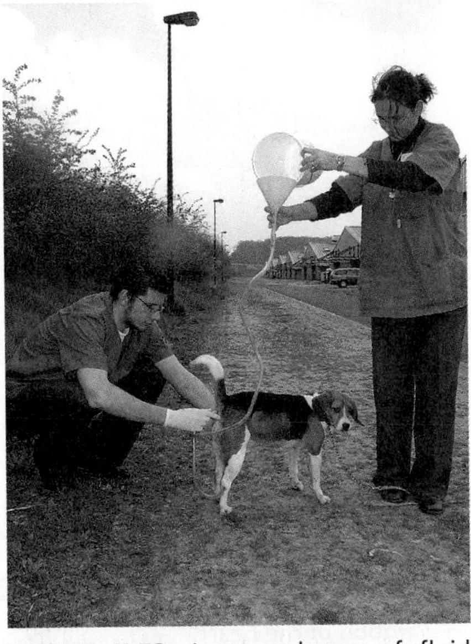

FIGURE II-52 Large volumes of fluid instilled using gravity, a funnel, and tube. This procedure is performed either for preparation for colonoscopy or as a treatment for constipation.

60-ml syringe and a urinary catheter can be used.
- Enema solution should be warmed and administered slowly. It may be administered by syringe, or larger volumes may be instilled more easily using a funnel and gravitational flow (Fig. II-52).
- When there is no resistance, the tube is inserted for a total length equal to that from the anus to the last rib (premeasure the tube).

POSTPROCEDURE

- Animals can have diarrhea.
- If enema administration was unsuccessful, animals with colon impaction may require manual extraction of impacted feces (under anesthesia).
- After the administration of an oral GI lavage solution, the animal should be kept quiet in a cage to avoid the potential risk of developing gastric dilation/volvulus.
- Dogs should be regularly walked on a leash to allow defecation.

ALTERNATIVES AND THEIR RELATIVE MERITS

Pediatric suppositories (dosage is 1 to 3), such as glycerol, docusate (Colace), or bisacodyl (Dulcolax), can be used as an alternative to enemas. These are safer than the use of phosphate enemas, especially for cats or smaller dogs.

AUTHOR: **SYLVIE DAMINET**

Enema: Scintigraphic (Radionuclide)

BASIC INFORMATION

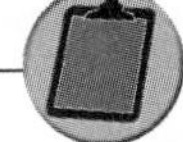

SYNONYM(S)

Nuclear portogram
Per rectum portal scintigraphy
Transcolonic portal scintigraphy

OVERVIEW AND GOAL(S)

Portosystemic shunts (PSS) are a relatively common congenital disorder in dogs and cats. Scintigraphy provides a rapid, noninvasive screening test for this disorder.

INDICATIONS

- Confirm the presence of a macroscopic portosystemic shunt.
- Evaluate the effectiveness of previous surgical shunt vessel attenuation.
- Provide limited information regarding the number (single versus multiple) and location (intrahepatic versus extrahepatic) of the portosystemic shunt vessel(s).

CONTRAINDICATIONS

Critical animal condition precluding relative isolation necessary to comply with regulatory requirements.

EQUIPMENT, ANESTHESIA

Gamma camera and either an analog recorder (microdot) or preferably a nuclear medicine computer are necessary for calculation of shunt fraction.

ANTICIPATED TIME

- Procedure time of 5 minutes
- Isolation time (varies by local regulatory agency) of 6 to 60 hours

PREPARATION: IMPORTANT CHECKPOINTS

Animal:
- No animal preparation is required.
- Ideally, animals are fed the morning of the procedure.
- Evacuation enemas are encouraged as a form of preparation by some clinicians but may not be routinely used by other clinicians.

Radionuclide setup:
- Prepare a dose of sodium ^{99m}T-pertechnetate (37–74 MBq/kg) in a small volume (<1.0 cc) in a shielded syringe case.

POSSIBLE COMPLICATIONS AND COMMON ERRORS TO AVOID

- Delivery of isotope into transverse colon
- Poor positioning of animal on camera relative to location of radionuclide delivery in colon
- Inadequate radionuclide uptake

PROCEDURE

Technique: initial:
- Position the animal in right lateral recumbancy on a Plexiglas table positioned over the gamma camera.

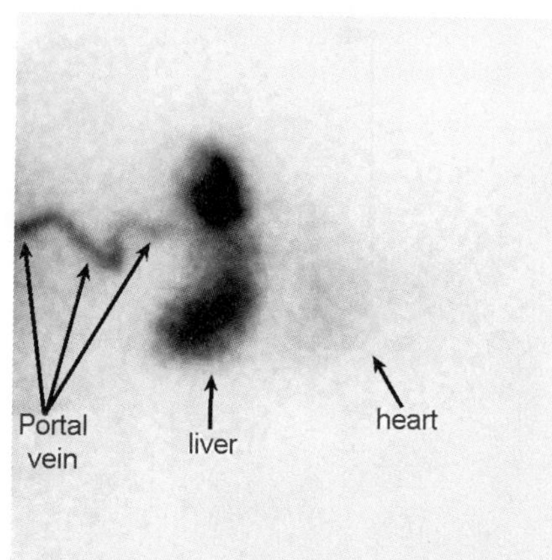

FIGURE II-53 Composite image of the early phase of a scintigraphic enema in a normal dog. Lateral projection; cranial is to the right. Note the clear visualization of the portal vein and liver with incomplete visualization of the heart.

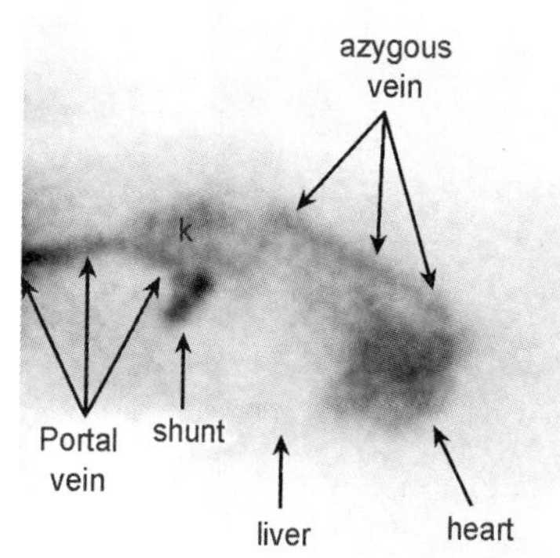

FIGURE II-54 Composite image of the early phase of a scintigraphic enema in a dog with a surgically confirmed portoazygous shunt. Same orientation as in Fig. II-52. Note the visualization of the portal vein, shunt vessel at the level of the right kidney (*k*) as well as the visualization of the azygous vein. Minimal visualization of the liver is due to reduced portal blood flow.

- Place the lubricated end of a pediatric feeding tube or IV extension set into the rectum.
- Connect a three-way stopcock to the end of the delivery tubing.
- Connect a syringe containing 5–10 ml of air to the three-way stopcock.
- Connect the shielded syringe containing the sodium ^{99m}T-pertechnetate dose.

Technique: main:
- Introduce dose into feeding tube.
- Begin dynamic image acquisition.
- Flush dose into colon using room air flush.

Dynamic image acquisition parameters:
- Analog (microdot): 16 dynamic images of 5-second duration.
- Digital (computer): 100 dynamic images of 2-second duration using 128 × 128 matrix.

POSTPROCEDURE

Isolation of animal in a radiation safety area until animal monitoring consistent with local release criteria. Collection of animal waste produced during isolation; the waste is treated as radioactive and typically held for decay before disposal.

ALTERNATIVES AND THEIR RELATIVE MERITS

- Ultrasound:
  - More readily available.
  - Very operator dependent.
  - Good success for diagnosis of intrahepatic shunts, limited by overlying ribs and lungs.
  - Limited success for diagnosis of extrahepatic shunts due to interference by adjacent gas-filled intestines.
  - Contrast harmonic ultrasonography may reduce operator dependence.
- Helical CT scan contrast portography:
  - Requires anesthesia.
  - More expensive.
  - Provides global perspective of entire abdomen with excellent anatomic detail.
  - Generally used in cases of confirmed PSS when additional anatomic information is desired prior to surgical intervention.
- MRI angiography:
  - Least available.
  - Requires anesthesia.
  - More expensive.
  - Provides global perspective of entire abdomen with excellent anatomic detail.
  - Generally used in cases of confirmed PSS when additional anatomic information is desired prior to surgical intervention.
- Intraoperative mesenteric portography:
  - Generally considered the gold standard for diagnosis of PSS.
  - Requires anesthesia.
  - Invasive.
  - Expensive.
- Liver biopsy:
  - Requires anesthesia.
  - Invasive.
  - Unable to confidently distinguish between macroscopic shunt and intrahepatic microvascular dysplasia.

AUTHOR: **MICHAEL R. BROOME**

Epidural Analgesia/Anesthesia

BASIC INFORMATION

SYNONYM(S)

Extradural blockade

OVERVIEW AND GOAL(S)

Administration of drugs into the epidural space to provide decreased sensory and sympathetic pain transmission, modulation (analgesia), and/or complete motor blockade (anesthesia). Drugs can be administered in one dose (single shot), repetitively, or by continuous infusion.
- Epidural analgesia: injection of an opioid, a phencyclidine, an α-agonist, or a nonsteroidal anti-inflammatory drug (NSAID)
- Epidural anesthesia: injection of a local anesthetic

INDICATIONS

Caesarean section, thoracostomy, pelvic or hind limb orthopedic manipulations, amputations (forelimb and hind limb), abdominal procedures, tail or perineal procedures, diaphragmatic repair, pancreatitis, peritonitis, intervertebral disk disease (IVDD).

Advantages:
- Lengthy, quick-onset analgesia
- Few systemic side effects for acute/chronic medical surgical pain
- Reduced requirements for parenteral and inhalant drugs
- Alternative to general anesthesia for animals that are at high risk (American Society of Anesthesiologists III, IV, V, E categories) (see American Society of Anesthesiologists Classification System, p 1334)
- Adjunct to balanced anesthesia regimes

CONTRAINDICATIONS

Absolute contraindications:
- Coagulopathies
- Localized infection/inflammation over entry to epidural space

- Increased intracranial pressure (head trauma, space-occupying mass)
- Risk of or present severe respiratory depression (phrenic nerve injury, tentorial herniation)

Relative contraindications (requires alteration of dose, frequency, drugs, or placement site):

- Urinary retention
- Meningitis, encephalitis, diskospondylitis
- Severe anatomical/neurologic disturbance or obesity at landmarks
- Inexperienced administration

Contraindications for use of local anesthetics in epidurals:

- Uncorrected hypovolemia
- Vasodilatory shock
- Severe clinical cardiac or liver impairment (third-spaced fluid disease, ascites)
- Acute renal failure
- Sympathetic disturbance (e.g., autonomic disease, dysautonomia)
- Use of potent systemic vasodilators

EQUIPMENT, ANESTHESIA

Most animals that receive an epidural are heavily sedated or under general anesthesia at the time of administration. Premedication with both anxiolytic and analgesic drugs (opioid, α-agonist) is recommended even if continued progression into general anesthesia is not anticipated due to the pain of positioning, approach, and administration of epidural agents.

Equipment:

- Hair clippers.
- Surgical scrub solution, isopropyl alcohol or saline, gauze/sponge.
- Epidural or spinal needle (Quincke, Husted, or Tuohy needles); 22-20 gauge, 1.5- to 3.5-inch small hypodermic needles (22 gauge, 0.5-1.5 inch) can also be used for tiny animals.
- Sterile gloves.
- Sterile saline.
- "Test syringe" for saline and air mix.
- Syringe for administration of combination of local and/or opioid.
- A few 20-gauge needles.
- Local anesthetics for epidural injection: 0.5% bupivacaine or 2% lidocaine (preservative- and epinephrine-free).
- Opioids for epidural injection: morphine, preferably preservative free (Duramorph, Astramorph, preservative-free morph), but parenteral morphine has been used for single-dose injection without complications anecdotally; buprenorphine, oxymorphone, and hydromorphone may also be utilized.
- A second operator (assistant) to allow strict attention to aseptic technique.

For epidural catheterization, the following will also be required:

- Blunt-tipped, lateral-faced opening needle with curved bevel (Tuohy needle).
- Continuous or indwelling epidural catheter.
- Injection port with screw or lock fitting to avoid inadvertent disconnection.
- Sterile scissors.
- Microfilter.
- Sterile covering for site and/or part/total catheter (Tegaderm).
- Suture material (3-0 nylon or other monofilament, nonabsorbable suture).
- Needle holders.
- Suture scissors.

ANTICIPATED TIME

- Experienced operator: 5-10 minutes.
- Inexperienced operator, anatomic/animal positioning issues, dermatologic uncleanliness: 20 minutes.

PREPARATION: IMPORTANT CHECKPOINTS

- Base doses on lean body weight.
- Review anatomy and placement of drugs: Most epidurals are performed at the lumbosacral junction because the cord terminates cranial to this area in dogs and near this area in cats; however, epidurals can be administered at any intervertebral space if lumbosacral (LS) access is limited.
- Consider use of local and narcotic drugs, and if used, determine the ratio of each. Narcotics are almost always utilized; locals are questionable.
- Positioning of animal: sternal with hind legs pulled fully cranially under body or else flexed and stable under pelvis ("frog-legged"). Aged, debilitated, or traumatized animals may be uncomfortable in either position, so lateral positioning is also used (Fig. II-55). Obese animals are best placed in sternal not only because of ease in identifying LS space but also because oxygenation and ventilation may be optimal.
- Premedication:
    - Medetomidine 0.005-0.01 mg/kg (5-10 μg/kg) IM or IV.
    - Can also instead use a combination of anxiolytic plus analgesic: anxiolytic (acepromazine 0.02-0.05 mg/kg IM or IV or midazolam 0.2-0.5 mg/kg IM or IV), plus analgesic (hydromorphone 0.1 mg/kg IM or morphine 0.5-2 mg/kg IM).

POSSIBLE COMPLICATIONS AND COMMON ERRORS TO AVOID

- Infection.
- Hemorrhage.
- Spinal or nerve root trauma.
- Respiratory depression.
- Urinary retention.
- Pruritus.
- Nausea and vomiting.
- Systemic vasodilatation secondary to sympathetic blockade if local anesthetic is used.
- Motor paralysis if lidocaine or concentrated bupivacaine is used.
- Subarachnoid injection—respiratory and cardiac arrest possible with cranial advancement of drugs; seizures possible.

PROCEDURE

- The animal is positioned appropriately (as previously described).
- The lumbosacral space is identified by palpating the most cranial dorsal aspects of each ilial wing, drawing an imaginary line between wings, and palpating the spinous process of L7 caudal to this line. The spinous process of L7 is smaller and shorter than that of L6 and, as such, is often more difficult to find. Staying directly on midline, the site of entry (LS space) is identified by placing a fingertip on the spinous process of L7 and gently rocking the finger caudally into the depression behind the process. The

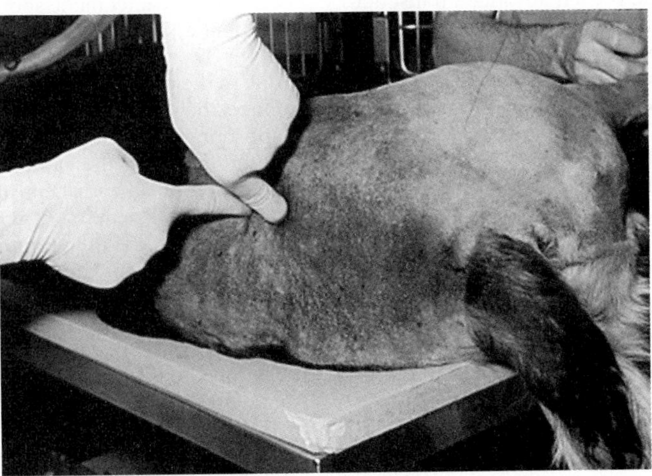

FIGURE II-55 Lumbosacral region of dog in left lateral recumbency. On the dorsal midline, the caudal-most dorsal spinous process, L7, is palpated (clinician's left hand). This process, shorter and smaller than that of L6 (clinician's right hand), is located caudal to an imaginary line that joins the most cranial dorsal aspects of both iliac crests. The point of epidural entry is the lumbosacral space, which is directly caudal to the dorsal spinous process of L7.

needle entry site is within this depression. (See Fig. II-55.)

- Once the entry site has been identified, the LS area should be clipped and aseptically prepped three times using alternating chlorhexidine scrub and alcohol/saline.
- Sterile gloves are opened, and the sleeve is used as a sterile field; syringes, needles, and instruments are opened on the sleeve around the gloves.
- Epidural drugs are aseptically drawn into a syringe; dosages: some clinicians prefer combined local anesthetic bupivacaine 0.1–0.3 mg/kg (motor sparing at 0.5%) with morphine 0.1 mg/kg for canine patients. This combination can be diluted to a total volume of 0.1–0.15 ml/kg with saline if advancement of the solution into the thoracic area is needed (thoracotomy, forelimb amputation, diaphragmatic repair, etc.). Total volume rarely exceeds 6 ml of saline, local, and opioid combined for canine patients. This calculation is appropriate for an injection made from the lumbosacral space. Injections made more cranially are reduced in volume by 25% per four to five vertebral bodies.
- For cats, 0.1 mg/kg morphine is diluted with saline to a total volume of 0.1–0.2 ml/kg. Local anesthetic is rarely used because of the propensity to administer this into the subarachnoid space and the increased toxicity potential in this species.
- Both species: 0.5–2 ml saline with 0.5–2 ml of air are drawn into another syringe, which will act as an epidural space "tester" or identifier.

TECHNIQUE OF EPIDURAL INJECTION

- Brace the hand holding the needle on the animal's back. Use the other hand to identify the LS space as already outlined.
- The needle is then advanced transcutaneously at a 90-degree angle to the skin surface over the LS site.
- The primary source of resistance is the dorsal spinous ligament (ligamentum flavum). This is the hardest layer to penetrate, and 1-mm depth pushes are required to realize entry into the ligament and the classic loss of resistance, or "pop" as the epidural space is entered ventral to the ligament.
- At that time, the stylet is removed, and the hub of the needle is inspected for presence of blood or cerebrospinal fluid (CSF).
    - If blood is seen, the needle tip is partially redrawn and redirected.
    - If CSF is encountered, the needle is probably in the subarachnoid space and should be withdrawn slightly.
    - If no blood or CSF is seen, assurance of presence in the epidural space is made by:
        - "Loss of resistance" technique: The syringe containing the saline and air is attached onto the hub of the needle. The syringe plunger is then depressed slightly (0.05–0.2 ml). If there is no increase in resistance to pushing the plunger, then the needle is correctly positioned in the epidural space. If the air bubble in the syringe is compressed or pushed against the saline as the plunger is depressed, then the needle tip lies in the paraspinal tissue, which indicates incorrect placement.
        - "Hanging drop" technique: When the ligamentum flavum is encountered (i.e., first sign of resistance), the stylet is withdrawn, and the hub of the epidural/spinal needle is filled with one to two drops of saline so that the liquid forms a meniscus in the hub. As the epidural space is entered, the normally negative pressure will cause aspiration down the needle shaft, and the saline will disappear.
- Once the correct positioning is confirmed, the injection proceeds over a 30- to 60-second time frame. Often, respiratory and cardiac rate increase during injection.

TECHNIQUE OF EPIDURAL CATHETERIZATION

- Once the needle enters the space, the bevel of the needle must face cranially.
- The catheter is then threaded down the needle.
- Catheter advancement should proceed without resistance. The catheter should never be withdrawn into the needle due to the possibility of shear/breakage.
- Once the catheter is advanced to the appropriate space, the needle is then withdrawn over the catheter.
- A section of skin adjacent to the site of entry is then penetrated with the needle. The needle is then tunneled parallel to the surface of skin for 1.5–2 cm and then exits the skin.
- The catheter's free end is then fed retrograde up the needle.
- The needle is then withdrawn, and the catheter is effectively "tunneled" away from the epidural site. This provides for decreased chances of bacteremia/infection in the epidural space.
- Excess catheter length is cut from the catheter using sterile scissors.
- The filter and injection port are secured.
- The epidural medications are then administered through the catheter, with the amount reduced to accommodate for placement of catheter tip.
- The catheter cap and filter are secured with suture. A protective sterile covering is placed over the catheter and LS space.

POSTPROCEDURE

- Onset of analgesia varies from immediate for lidocaine epidurals, 30–60 minutes for bupivacaine epidurals, to 2–4 hours for morphine and oxymorphone epidurals.
- Duration of analgesia varies from 1 hour for lidocaine epidurals, 3–6 hours for bupivacaine epidurals, to 12–15 hours for morphine epidurals.
- Pain of injection is severe with local anesthetics and ketamine. Some clinicians strongly suggest utilizing each as diluted solutions only and administering bupivacaine only if the animal is under the influence of heavy sedation/analgesia or is anesthetized.
- Vomition, nausea, and drooling are common when catheters are placed in the thoracic spinal canal, when heavy volumes or concentrated morphine is used, or when pain/sudden hypotension is sensed during an injection ("awake bupivacaine epidurals").
- The injection cap, filter, and dressing should be replaced every 72–96 hours using aseptic technique in catheters that are routinely used (q 12h to q 8h treatments).
- Swelling or pain over the tunneled site or, more importantly, over the catheter entry site warrants removal of the catheter. Replacement should then be questioned; alternative analgesic methods are suggested instead.

ALTERNATIVES AND THEIR RELATIVE MERITS

- General inhalant anesthesia: cardiorespiratory depression; expense.
- Systemic narcotic administration: side effects of gastrointestinal (GI) stasis, respiratory depression, and mild anxiety; expense.
- Local nerve blocks: probably the best option for analgesia if an epidural cannot be performed.

AUTHOR: **ANDREA L. LOONEY**

Excretory Urogram

BASIC INFORMATION

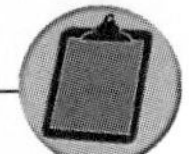

SYNONYM(S)

IVP
IV pyelogram
IV urogram

OVERVIEW AND GOAL(S)

When the kidneys are difficult to assess by plain film radiography or when qualitative functional information is needed, an excretory urogram could be performed. On survey abdominal radiographs, the renal silhouette may not be visualized in animals that have decreased abdominal detail (young, thin, peritoneal fluid).

INDICATIONS

- Identify kidneys (if poor abdominal detail) (Fig. II-56)
- Mass lesions of kidneys (or mass in region of kidney)
- Qualitative assessment of renal function
- Patency, continuity of urinary tract
- Prior to nephrectomy
- Abnormal renal size, shape
- Persistent hematuria
- Suspected renal or ureteral calculi
- Suspected hydronephrosis (Fig. II-59)
- Suspected ureteral ectopia, ureterocele (Fig. II-57)
- Suspected ureteral rupture
- To evaluate the urinary bladder when it cannot be catheterized
- Postoperative assessment of urinary tract (patency, strictures, leakage)

CONTRAINDICATIONS

- Dehydration
- Previous reaction to iodinated contrast medium (a nonionic medium should be used)
- Caution should be used in animals with the following conditions:
  - Diabetes mellitus
  - Multiple myeloma
  - Congestive heart failure
  - Hypertension
  - Concurrent drug administration (cardiac glycosides)
  - Severe debilitation

EQUIPMENT, ANESTHESIA

- Many recommend the use of general anesthesia or heavy sedation; however, an excretory urogram can be performed in an unanesthetized animal.
- IV catheter.
- Hair clippers.
- Surgical scrub solution, rubbing alcohol, and gauze/sponges for prepping skin where catheter is placed.

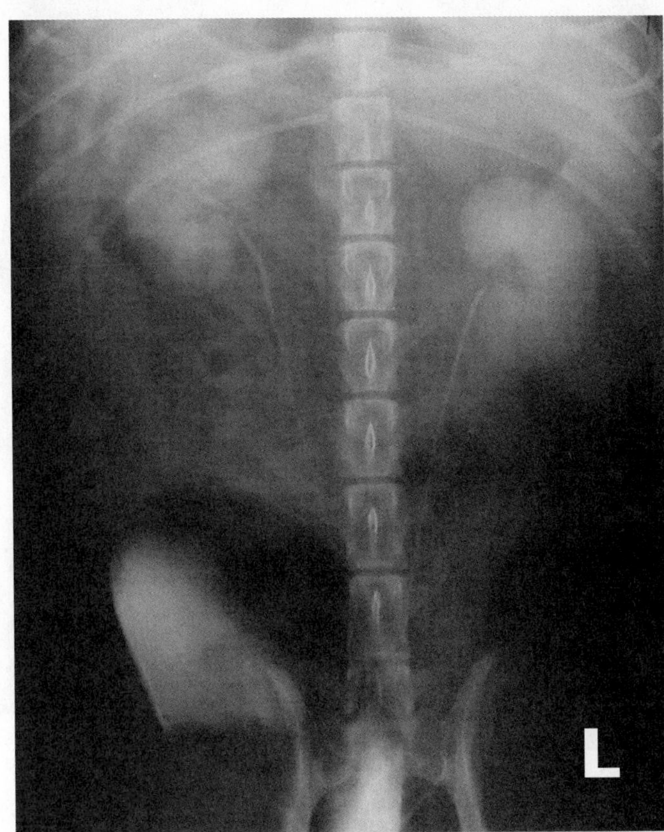

FIGURE II-56 Excretory urogram, ventrodorsal view; normal study. Both kidneys and both ureters are clearly seen; contrast material is also seen in the urinary bladder (to the right of midline). L, left.

- Tape/releasing elastic (Vetrap-type) bandage.
- Iodinated contrast medium (sodium iothalamate, sodium diatrizoate).
- Nonionic contrast medium (iohexol, iopamidol) if clinically warranted.
- Syringe.
- Heparin/saline for flush.
- Enema set.
- Antianaphylactic agents (e.g., diphenhydramine 2-4 mg/kg for IM injection).
- Oxygen and a drug cart to reverse any possible complication during the procedure (see complications in following paragraphs).

ANTICIPATED TIME

Approximately 1 hour

PREPARATION: IMPORTANT CHECKPOINTS

- The owner should be advised that hair will be removed from the site of IV catheter placement.
- Animal should have fasted 24 hours.
- Water given *ad libitum*.
- Enema given at least 2 hours prior to study to remove a maximum of the fecal material from the colon to allow visualization of kidneys and ureters.
- Assess hydration: proceed only if normal.
- Clip the hair where the IV catheter is to be placed.
- The site for the catheter placement should be prepped with surgical scrub solution, rubbing alcohol, and gauze/sponges.
- Place an IV catheter in a cephalic or jugular vein; it is imperative that the catheter be properly placed.
- Secure the catheter in place with tape or releasing elastic (VetRap-type) bandage.
- Add 900-mg iodine/kg body weight contrast material into syringe.
- Add an appropriate amount of heparin/saline flush into syringe.

POSSIBLE COMPLICATIONS AND COMMON ERRORS TO AVOID

- Vomiting: this often occurs immediately after injection of the contrast medium. If the animal is muzzled, the

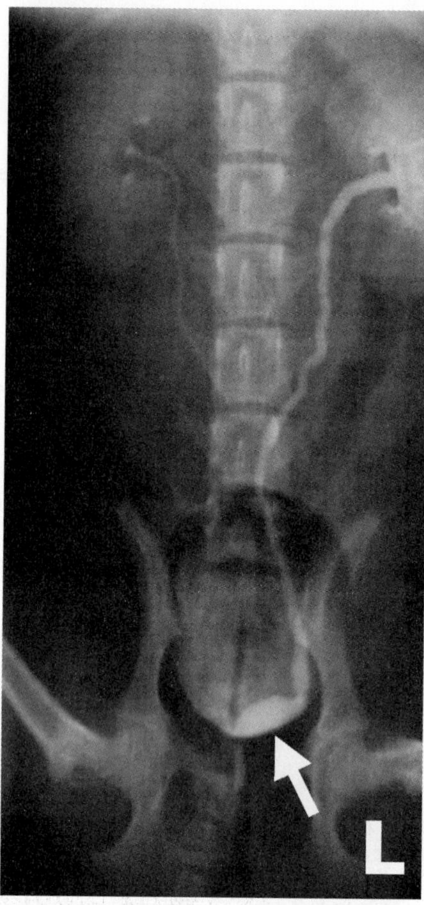

FIGURE II-57 Excretory urogram, ventrodorsal view; ectopic ureter (left side), normal ureter (right side). The ectopic ureter is diffusely enlarged (hydroureter), especially distally where it inserts in an ectopic location (*arrow*). L, left.

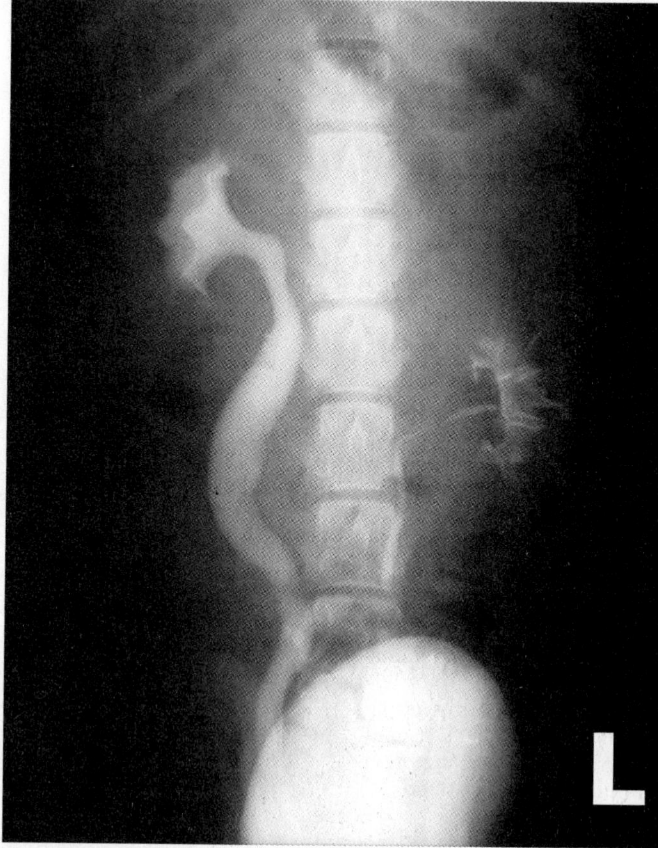

FIGURE II-58 Excretory urogram, ventrodorsal view; pyelonephritis (right side). Right-sided hydronephrosis and severe hydroureter are apparent. L, left.

muzzle should be removed immediately to avoid aspiration.
- Systemic hypotension, bradycardia.
- Anaphylaxis (airway edema, vascular collapse, bronchospasm).
- Perivascular injection may result in sloughing of surrounding tissue.
- Contrast media-induced renal failure.
- The administration of iodinated contrast media may affect urine specific gravity, urine sediment, and urine culture results for 24 hours following administration.
- Blood values (blood urea nitrogen [BUN], creatinine, prothrombin time [PT], partial thromboplastin time [PTT], activated partial thromboplastin time [APTT], thromboplastin time [TT], and hematocrit) might also be affected for up to 24 hours after contrast administration.

PROCEDURE

- Preliminary abdominal radiographs are made to determine adequate animal preparation and to set radiographic technique.
- The kilovoltage peak (kVp) should be set between 65 and 75 to maximize contrast due to the photoelectric effect (K edge of iodine).
- Flush the catheter to again ensure patency.
- Inject contrast material rapidly as a bolus.
- Flush the catheter of residual contrast material.
- A ventrodorsal view is obtained at 20 seconds.
- Ventrodorsal and right lateral views are obtained at 5 minutes, 20 minutes, and 40 minutes (Figs. II-58 and II-59).
- Oblique views are obtained at 5 minutes to visualize ureteral termination at the urinary bladder.

POSTPROCEDURE

- If anesthesia is used: routine anesthetic recovery.
- Maintain adequate hydration.
- The IV catheter should remain in place for at least 15 to 20 minutes after the study is completed. The port for venous access might be necessary should a contrast media adverse reaction occur.
- Remove the catheter >20 minutes after the procedure.

ALTERNATIVES AND THEIR RELATIVE MERITS

- Plain abdominal radiographs: inexpensive means to survey the abdomen. Radiopaque renal or ureteral calculi can be visualized. Size and shape of the kidneys can be assessed if abdominal detail is adequate and fecal material is not obscuring their visualization.
- Abdominal ultrasound: excellent potential for visualization of kidneys, especially in animals that show poor radiographic abdominal detail. Renal size, shape, position, and relative echogenicity to the liver and spleen can be assessed. The size of the renal pelvis can also be evaluated. The internal architecture of the kidneys can be assessed. Ultrasound can determine if masses are solid or cystic in nature. Resistive index can be calculated.
- CT scan: provides excellent detail of the size, shape, and margination of the kidneys. IV contrast media can also be used to enhance findings in the kidneys and or ureters. This imaging modality can also be used for assessing renal vas-

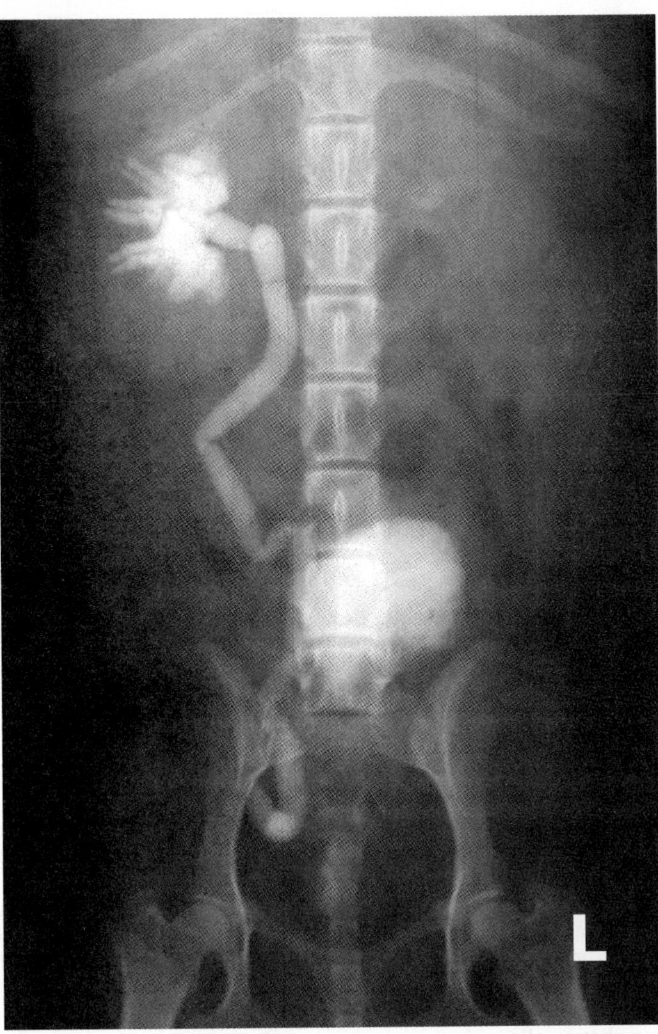

FIGURE II-59 Excretory urogram, ventrodorsal view; hydronephrosis and hydroureter, right side. L, left.

cular anatomy when screening feline renal transplant donors. CT scans, however, are more costly to perform than other studies already listed and require general anesthesia.
- Nuclear scintigraphy:
  - Diethylenetriaminepentaacetate (DTPA): to determine global and individual kidney glomerular filtration rates (GFRs); to evaluate the animal's response to treatment; to evaluate function of contralateral kidney prior to surgery and possible removal of diseased kidney; to identify and determine the severity of subclinical renal disease in an animal receiving nephrotoxic agents; and to examine renal perfusion by obtaining rapid serial images during first pass circulation.
  - Mercaptoacetyltriglycine (MAG_3): to determine global and individual kidney effective renal plasma flow (ERPF).

AUTHOR: **LEEANN PACK**

Feeding Tube Placement: Esophagostomy Tube

BASIC INFORMATION

SYNONYM(S)

Esophageal feeding tube
E-tube

OVERVIEW AND GOAL(S)

A simple method to place a large-bore feeding tube into an animal without hindering the animal's normal ability to eat and drink

INDICATIONS

- Anorexia with a functional lower gastrointestinal (GI) tract
- Disorders of the oral cavity or pharynx

CONTRAINDICATIONS

- Poor anesthetic candidate
- Prolonged vomiting
- Esophageal disease:
  - Stricture
  - Foreign body
  - Megaesophagus

EQUIPMENT, ANESTHESIA

- General anesthesia required.
- Tracheal intubation required.
- Mouth gag (speculum).
- Sterile gloves.
- Curved forceps (e.g., curved Carmalt forceps).
- A #15 scalpel blade.
- Feeding tube (sterile; 10 Fr, minimum size): red rubber or polypropylene.
- Long polypropylene catheter (optional). If used, it should be as long as, or longer than, the feeding tube.
- Needle holders.
- Suture: nonabsorbable (e.g., 0 to 4-0 nylon for large dogs to cats, respectively).
- Bandage material: sterile dressing, roll gauze, dry adherent wrap (e.g., Vetrap or Elastikon-type).
- Radiology equipment (optional).

ANTICIPATED TIME

- Between 20 and 30 minutes anesthesia time
- Between 5 and 10 minutes of procedure

PREPARATION: IMPORTANT CHECKPOINTS

Familiarization with the locations of the great vessels (Fig. II-60):
- The left external jugular vein is adjacent to the esophagus and may overlie it.

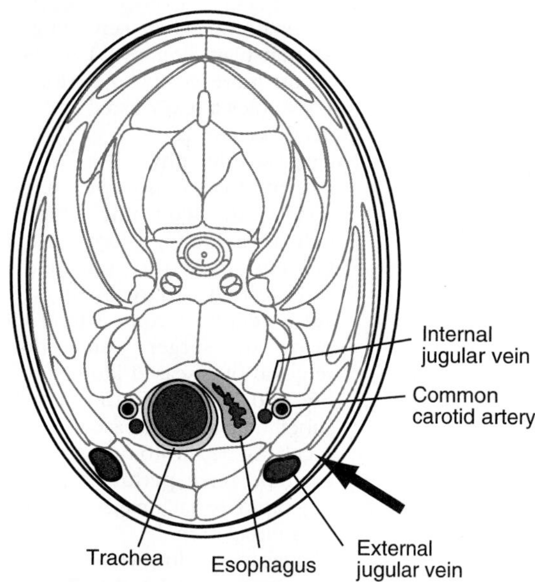

FIGURE II-60 Cross-section of the midcervical region, cranial view (animal's left is on the right of the image). The external jugular vein and, to a lesser extent, the common carotid artery and internal jugular vein may lie between the esophagus and the skin insertion site (*arrow*).

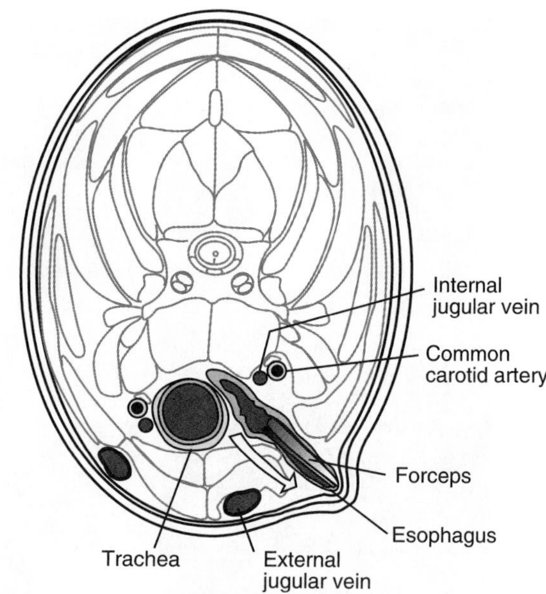

FIGURE II-61 Tips of curved forceps placing pressure in the esophagus so that the esophagus is brought toward the skin (*curved arrow at bottom of figure*). This process helps to move vessels aside and reduces the risk of vascular complications during tube placement.

- When preparing the site of esophageal tube placement, it is essential to distend the jugular vein periodically by occluding it manually at the thoracic inlet. This allows the location of the jugular vein to be clearer so that it can be avoided during tube placement.
- The common carotid arteries are located immediately dorsolateral to the trachea and are not at risk with this procedure when it is performed correctly.

POSSIBLE COMPLICATIONS AND COMMON ERRORS TO AVOID

- Procedural:
  - Severing of a great vessel
  - Excessively cranial placement (in the pharynx, instead of the esophagus)
- Postprocedural:
  - Excessively tight neck bandage
  - Reflux esophagitis
  - Vomiting/regurgitation, including expulsion of the distal part of the tube during vomiting
  - Aspiration pneumonia
  - Occlusion of the tube:
    - Can be prevented by ensuring that foods and medications administered through the tube are pulverized to a fine consistency.
    - If occlusion occurs, it may be possible to relieve it by repeatedly instilling a few milliliters of carbonated water (seltzer or club soda) to help dissolve the obstruction.

PROCEDURE

- Induce anesthesia and intubate the animal.
- Place the animal in right lateral recumbency.
- Clip and aseptically prep the midcervical region: most or all of the left side of the neck is prepared. In smaller patients (cats, small dogs), the area extends from the angle of the mandible to the thoracic inlet and covers the entire left side of the neck from dorsal to ventral midlines; however, in larger dogs, a somewhat smaller relative area (e.g., 15-cm square) is sufficient.
- Trim the tube to the correct length:
  - Determine the proper length of the feeding tube by measuring the distance from the midcervical region (midpoint between angle of mandible and thoracic inlet) to the seventh or eighth intercostal space (ICS) using the tube itself as a measuring stick. In addition to this measured length, add approximately 6 cm of extra length to the measurement to account for the segment of tube that will remain outside the animal.
  - Trim the distal aspect of the tube to leave the correct length, including the 6-cm exterior segment.
  - Create two lateral openings in the distal part of the tube: a few millimeters in size but no greater than 30% of the circumference of the tube to avoid kinking or breakage. These holes will allow food to flow even if the end hole is obstructed.
- Place the mouth gag to keep the patient's mouth open.
- Introduce curved forceps into the oral cavity with the tips of the forceps pointing up (left lateral direction).
  - The forceps will be pointed caudally (into the esophagus), with the handles oriented ventrodorsally in the animal's mouth so that the forcep tips in the esophagus point up/laterally, toward the animal's skin.
  - Advance the forceps maximally into the animal's mouth such that the forcep tips enter the esophagus and can be felt through the skin.
  - Palpate the desired region (the left hand orients the forceps deep into the animal's mouth, and the right hand palpates the forcep tips through the esophagus and skin) until forcep tips are in the proper location (Fig. II-61):
    - Avoid placement that is too cranial (pharynx, large veins), which is a common and serious problem caused by incomplete insertion of the forceps.The tips of the forceps should be caudal to the point at which the maxillary and sublingual veins converge into the external jugular vein and must be caudal to the entire larynx.
    - Avoid placement that overlies the jugular vein. Raising the jugular vein by applying pressure at the thoracic inlet allows it to be more clearly visualized. This should be done repeatedly when identifying the site of tube insertion and preparing to make the incision (see Figure II-61).
    - Placement that is too distal is not a common problem, provided the point of placement remains in the midcervical region.

- Elevate (lateral pressure, upward away from the table) the distal part of the forceps, and again confirm a proper location.
- Force the forcep tips through the esophageal wall and skin by incising over the instrument tips with a scalpel. The distal-most tips of the forceps should now have emerged through a snug, very small (a few millimeters) incision in the skin and lateral esophagus.
- Open the forceps tips slightly, just enough to grasp the distal tip of the feeding tube. Close the forceps on the feeding tube tip, and draw the feeding tube out with the forceps (cranially) through the opening and most of the way out the oral cavity, leaving only about 6 cm of tube protruding through the skin.
- Use the polypropylene catheter as a guide to feed the tube back into the esophagus.
- Place a purse-string suture around the stoma (skin opening), and secure the tube with a Chinese finger-trap suture.

POSTPROCEDURE

- Place a light bandage for several days as the wound heals.
- Postprocedure radiographs will ensure proper placement prior to anesthetic recovery. The tube should extend to the distal esophagus but should not enter the stomach.
- Most animals tolerate these feeding tubes well, but some may need an Elizabethan collar to prevent damaging the tube.
- Feedings may be started as soon as the animal recovers from anesthesia, and the tube may be removed at any time. Removal generally does not require anesthesia or sedation, and the stoma heals by second intention.
- Blended watery diets will pass through the tube, but the tube should be flushed after each feeding to help ensure that it does not become obstructed.

ALTERNATIVES AND THEIR RELATIVE MERITS

- Nasoesophagostomy tube: typically only liquid diets (much smaller in diameter); however, the tube can be placed without general anesthesia. Animals generally do not tolerate this type of tube as well as other tubes.
- Percutaneous endoscopic gastrostomy (PEG) tube: can place a larger diameter tube and provide bolus feedings. Appropriate in cases of esophageal disease, whereas esophagostomy tubes are not; well tolerated, but unlike esophagostomy tube, gastrostomy tubes cannot be used for 24 hours postplacement during healing of the stoma and should not be removed before several days or 1 week postplacement.

AUTHOR: **ANDREW CRUIKSHANK**

Feeding Tube Placement: Nasoesophageal and Nasogastric

BASIC INFORMATION

OVERVIEW AND GOAL(S)

Nourishment via enteral feeding helps prevent bacterial translocation from the intestine, absorption of endotoxins, and development of sepsis in critically ill animals that are unable or unwilling to maintain adequate caloric intake. Enteral nutrition plays a very important role in enterocyte health. Placement of a nasogastric tube or nasoesophageal tube facilitates administration of correct nutrition to satisfy nutritional requirements.

INDICATIONS

- Nasoesophageal and nasogastric tubes:
  - Short-term enteral feeding (usually less than 7 days)
  - Administration of oral liquid medication
- Nasogastric tube:
  - Suctioning of gastric fluid, gastric decompression, and prevention of gastric distention

CONTRAINDICATIONS

- Animals with severe facial trauma involving the nares and nasal turbinates
- Animals with severe pharyngeal, laryngeal, or esophageal physical or functional abnormalities (e.g., severe megaesophagus, esophageal surgery, or perforation)
- Animals with repeated, uncontrolled vomition or regurgitation
- Semiconscious and unconscious animals
- Severe coagulopathies

EQUIPMENT, ANESTHESIA

- Usually placed without sedation, but in very fractious animals, sedation might be indicated.
- Topical local anesthetic (2% lidocaine can be used).
- Syringe and needle.
- Permanent marker or tape to mark length of tube required.
- Lubricating jelly.
- Flexible feeding tube (polyvinyl, polyurethane, or silicone).
- Suture material or quick-drying glue.
- Elizabethan collar.
- Radiography.

ANTICIPATED TIME

About 5 minutes

PREPARATION: IMPORTANT CHECKPOINTS

- Select the largest tube that will be able to pass through the nares. Approximate guidelines: puppies and kittens, 3 Fr gauge; cats and small dogs, 5 Fr gauge; larger cats and dogs, 8 Fr gauge or bigger; giant dog breeds, typically 12–18 Fr gauge. If the tube diameter is too small, even the most dilute solutions will not be able to pass through the tube.
- Premeasure and mark the length of the tube that should be passed. For nasogastric intubations, the tube is measured from the nostril to the ninth intercostal space (ICS); for nasoesophageal feeding, the tube is measured up to the sixth ICS.
- The author prefers making use of nasoesophageal placement in cases requiring nutritional support (rather than nasogastric) because this method does not interfere with the lower esophageal sphincter and therefore potentially lowers the risk of esophageal reflux.

POSSIBLE COMPLICATIONS AND COMMON ERRORS TO AVOID

- Excessive lidocaine administration in cats and possibly smaller dogs (toxic dose 4 mg/kg)
- Tracheal intubation
- Epistaxis
- Tube blockage with food particles, mucus, or esophageal or gastric mucosa
- Rhinitis
- Esophageal reflux, especially with nasogastric tubes
- Vomition or regurgitation with expulsion of the tube
- Aspiration of esophageal contents and aspiration pneumonia

PROCEDURE

- Manual restraint of animal with or without sedation.
- Elevate the nose so the animal is looking at the ceiling, and, with the animal's mouth closed, instill approximately 0.25–0.5 ml lidocaine in each nostril, depending on the size of the animal. NOTE: Remember toxic dose in cats. It is helpful to time the instillation when the animal is inhaling, so as to minimize the amount of anesthetic blown or sneezed out of the nares. Both nostrils are anesthetized at this time to avoid delay if it becomes necessary to use the other nostril. The head and restraint are released while allowing lidocaine to take effect: typically 1–2 minutes.
- The premeasured tube is well lubricated with lubricating jelly.
- The tube is directed ventromedially into the nostril and passed via the ventral meatus. In dogs, the nostril can be pushed dorsally to assist easy passing of the tube (Fig. II-62).
- The tube is advanced up to the premeasured mark. Avoid extending the neck because this will increase the risk of tracheal intubation. Slight flexion of the neck will help the animal to swallow the distal end of the tube and facilitate proper placement.
- Check correct placement of tube in the esophagus or stomach:
    - Attempts to aspirate air from the tube with a syringe will create negative pressure if the tube ends appropriately in the esophagus. If air is easily withdrawn during aspiration from the tube, it is likely in the pharynx or trachea.
    - Injecting air through the tube should create gurgling sounds on auscultation of the stomach if the tube was successfully placed into the stomach.
    - Radiographs may be taken of the cervical and thoracic esophagus to visually confirm location of the tube.
    - NOTE: Do not check tube placement by injecting water into the tube. Theoretically, an animal will cough if the tube is placed in the trachea, but some animals may be too weak to cough; in cats in particular, coughing is a very poor indicator of tube placement because the majority of cats will not cough.
- The tube can either be sutured or glued into place (Fig. II-63). The first point of attachment to the skin is as close to the nares as possible. Additional sutures or glue should be placed on the dorsum of the muzzle or on the cheek. Make sure to avoid the whiskers in cats to prevent irritation.

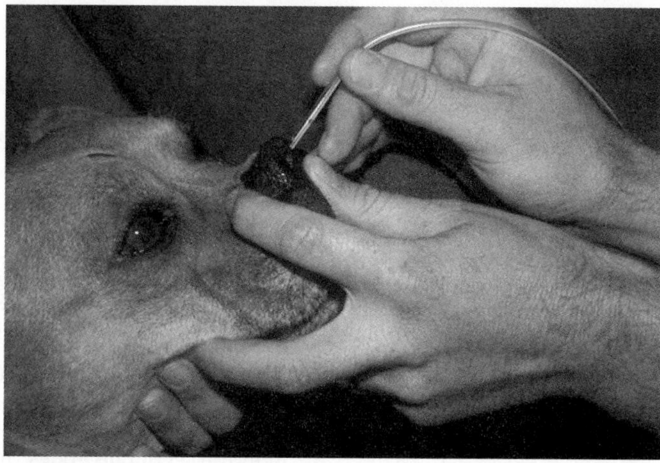

FIGURE II-62 The nostril of a dog being pushed dorsally to facilitate tube placement.

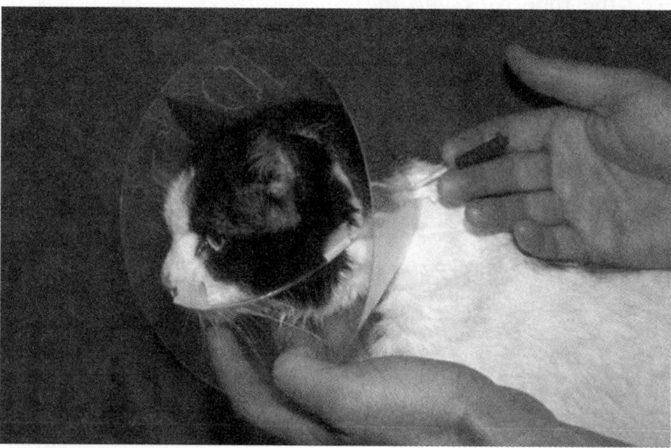

FIGURE II-63 Cat after placement of nasoesophageal tube and Elizabethan collar.

- Some animals do not tolerate the tubes due to irritation, and the use of an Elizabethan collar can be indicated depending on the temperament of the animal.

POSTPROCEDURE

- Ensure that the tube does not migrate out.
- Regularly flush the tube with a volume of water equivalent to or greater than the volume of the tube itself. Doing so helps to avoid blockage and is indicated especially prior to and immediately after administering food.
- Food should be administered slowly to avoid rapid distention of the esophagus or stomach.
- Keep the tube opening closed between feedings to avoid air buildup in the stomach.
- A prokinetic (e.g., metoclopramide) could be used to assist with the functioning of the lower esophageal sphincter to minimize the risk of esophageal reflux.
- If obstruction of the tube with food or medication occurs, one or more instillations of a few milliliters of carbonated water (seltzer/mineral water/club soda) may dissolve the obstruction.

ALTERNATIVES AND THEIR RELATIVE MERITS

- Alternative feeding tubes could be placed with minor surgery and short general anesthesia (e.g., a percutaneous endoscopic gastrostomy [PEG] tube or esophagostomy tube) or major surgical procedures requiring long general anesthetics (e.g., gastrostomy and jejunostomy tubes).
- These tubes are often indicated for animals in which nasoesophageal and nasogastric tubes are contraindicated (see Contraindications above).

AUTHOR: **MIRINDA NEL (VAN SCHOOR)**

Feeding Tube Placement: Percutaneous Endoscopic Gastrostomy (PEG)

BASIC INFORMATION

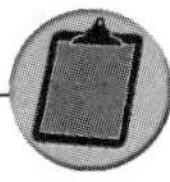

OVERVIEW AND GOAL(S)

Placement of a tube (using minimally invasive techniques) that provides a portal of entry into the stomach for administration of food and medications. These tubes typically can be left in place for days to several weeks.

INDICATIONS

To enable enteral nutrition and/or medication delivery in an animal that is unable or unwilling to eat on its own for an extended period of time (e.g., cat with hepatic lipidosis, animal with a jaw fracture)

CONTRAINDICATIONS

- Intestinal obstruction
- Pancreatitis

EQUIPMENT, ANESTHESIA

- Endoscope with a biopsy forceps
- Rusch-Pezzer tube (16–20 Fr in diameter, according to animal size) (Fig. II-64, number 1)
- A sterile #11 scalpel blade (see Fig. II-64, number 2)
- Tomcat catheter (see Fig. II-64, number 3)
- A 16-gauge sterile needle (see Fig. II-64, number 4)
- Sturdy suture material (e.g., polyamide, nonabsorbable, 0 or larger gauge), at least 1-m/3-ft long for most animals and up to 1.5 m (5 ft) for large dogs (see Fig. II-67, number 5)
- Over-the-needle IV catheter (18-gauge, 2-inch Terumo) (see Fig. II-64, number 6)
- Suture material for the skin (e.g., 2-0, 3-0 nylon) (see Fig. II-64, number 7)
- Suture scissors and needle holder (see Fig. II-64, number 8)
- Female Luerlock Connector (Argyle)
- BD prn adaptor

ANTICIPATED TIME

About 15 to 20 minutes of procedure and 30 minutes of anesthesia time

PREPARATION: IMPORTANT CHECKPOINTS

- Preparation of the animal: the left side of the abdomen is shaved and aseptically scrubbed. The animal is anesthetized and placed in right lateral recumbency.
- Preparation of the Pezzer tube:
  - The 3-mm blunted protuberance ("nipple") at the extremity of the ampulla ("mushroom head") of the Pezzer tube should be cut off with scissors to facilitate the passage of food (see Fig. II-64, number 1a). NOTE: The ampulla/ mushroom head itself is not cut; only the small protuberance on it is cut, creating an additional end hole in the ampulla. It is important also not to cut into the adjacent end holes in the ampulla, which would weaken the ampulla's structure.
  - The proximal, flared end of the Pezzer tube should then be cut, just prior to the wider cylindrical extremity (i.e., cutting off the most proximal 3–4 cm of tube) (see Fig. II-64, number 1b). The cut segment is important and must not be discarded.
  - Next, the clinician trims the proximal extremity (the nonmushroom end, Fig. II-65A) of the Pezzer tube into an arrow shape to allow the fitting of this end inside the wide extremity of a tomcat catheter (Fig. II-65B). The 16-gauge needle should then be passed through the walls of this end (see Fig. II-65C).
  - The 3–4 cm cut segment is kept to create a flange, which will ultimately stabilize the tube (Fig. II-68, number 1b). To create a flange, the clinician takes the 3–4 cm segment of tube and, using a #11 scalpel blade, makes a 5-mm stab incision in the midbody of the tube segment. The clinician then repeats the stab incision on the opposite side of the tube segment, such that two parallel and longitudinal 5-mm incisions are created in alignment to each other in the middle of the segment. These transverse incisions will allow the passage of the Pezzer tube through them, such that the flange prevents inward migration of the tube when the animal is awake and mobile.
  - Preparation of the Pezzer tube is now complete.

POSSIBLE COMPLICATIONS AND COMMON ERRORS TO AVOID

- The thread needs to be sturdy because otherwise it may break during the pulling of the Pezzar tube through the gastric and abdominal wall.
- The ampulla of the Pezzer tube may be blocked at the level of the gastroesophageal sphincter. A firmer pull will allow the ampulla to pass this obstacle. NOTE: It is essential to brace this traction on the tube with counterpressure at the level of the body wall. If pulling the Pezzar tube into place with the right hand, the clinician's left thumb and forefinger are on the body wall, adjacent to the tube, and are exerting counterpressure to make sure the ampulla stops at the stomach wall and does not come out entirely.
- The Pezzer tube needs to be left in place for at least 2 weeks to allow fibrous tissue to surround the portion of the tube between the stomach and

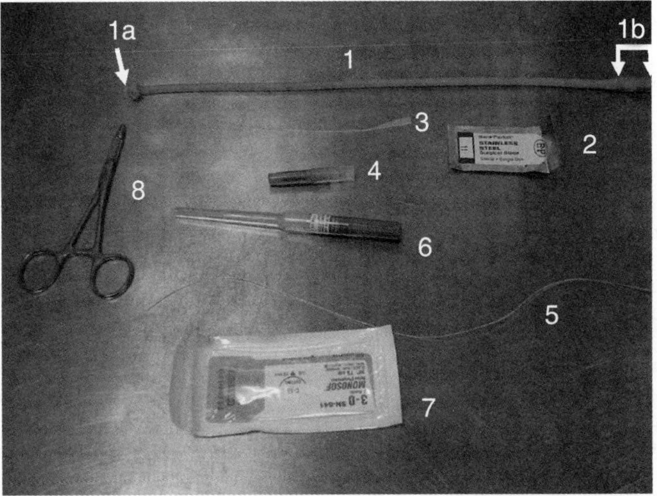

FIGURE II-64 Equipment necessary for PEG tube placement: **1**, Pezzer tube (**1a**, blunted protuberance/"nipple"; **1b**, segment to be cut; will become the flange). **2**, #11 scalpel blade. **3**, Tomcat catheter. **4**, 16-gauge needle; **5**, Thread; **6**, IV-type catheter; **7**, Suture material; **8**, Needle holder/scissors.

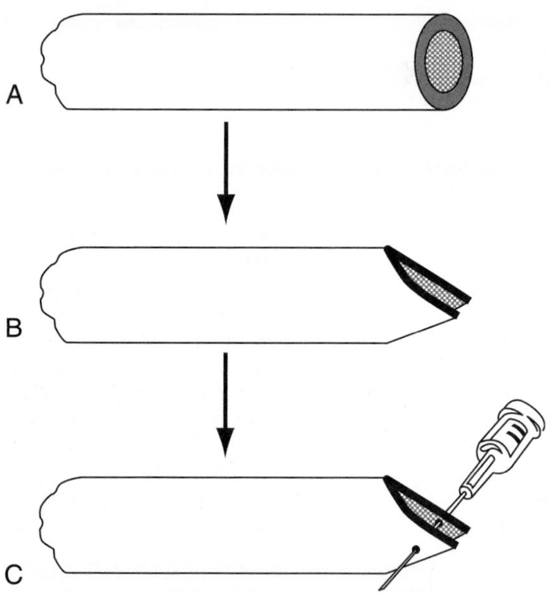

FIGURE II-65 Preparation prior to anesthetizing the animal. **A**, The cut segment (as in Fig. II-63B) of the proximal (nonampulla) end of the Pezzer tube. **B**, The proximal end trimmed into an arrowhead shape. **C**, The end pierced side-to-side with the needle. The location of the needle insertion should be at the base of the arrowhead (i.e., just before the trimmed sections, where the diameter of the tube is still complete).

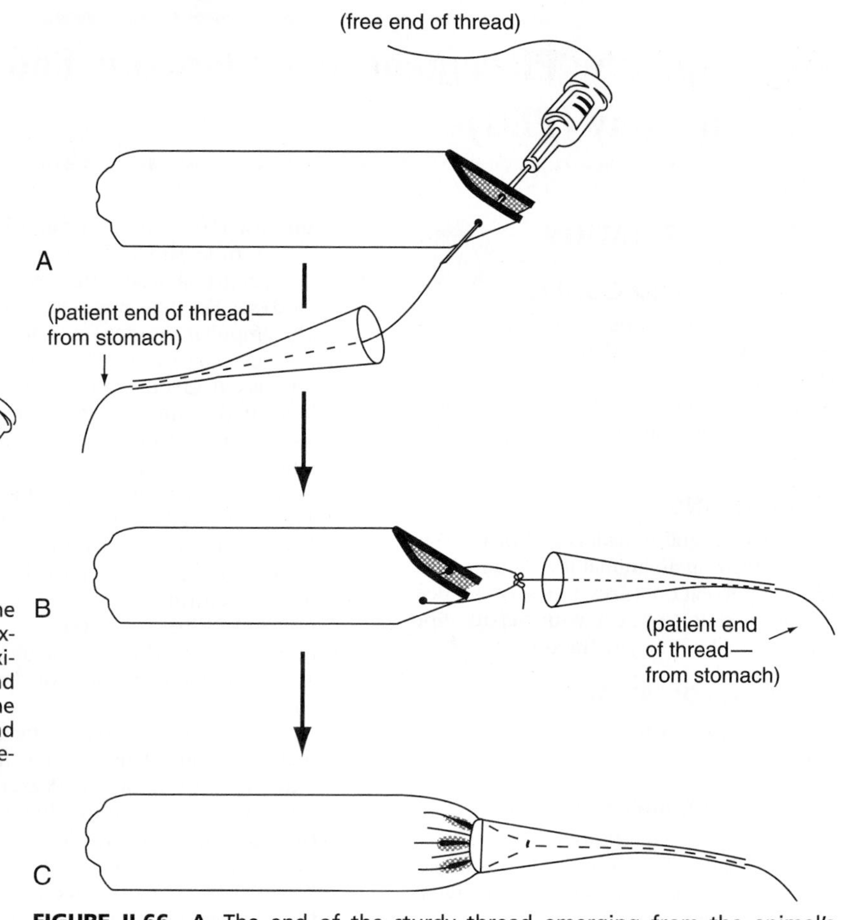

FIGURE II-66 **A**, The end of the sturdy thread emerging from the animal's mouth passed into the narrow end of the tomcat catheter and then into the tip of the needle (i.e., retrograde up the needle). The needle is removed, leaving the thread through the tip of the Pezzer tube. The thread is tied to itself with several surgeon's knots. **B**, Free end of the thread trimmed off. **C**, The tomcat catheter wedged over the Pezzer tube and knots.

the abdominal wall, therefore sealing it off from the abdominal cavity. This is important for the safe removal of the Pezzer tube and minimizes the risk of peritonitis.

- The incisions in the flange need to be long enough to avoid creating a stricture of the Pezzer tube.
- Blockage of the Pezzer tube by dried food should be avoided by careful rinsing of the tube after use. If blockage occurs, it can be addressed by repeatedly administering a few milliliters of carbonated water (seltzer/club soda/mineral water) into the tube until the obstruction dissolves.

PROCEDURE

- The endoscope is introduced into the stomach, and the extremity of the endoscope should be pointing toward the left side of the antrum. The light at the endoscope tip should be visible through the skin.
- The stomach is then inflated with air until the skin becomes tense.
- The extremity of the over-the-needle IV catheter is then introduced into the gastric cavity through the skin, aiming for the light of the endoscope.
- Once the catheter is introduced into the stomach, the stylet is removed. The thread can then be introduced through the catheter into the stomach.
- With the endoscope, the extremity of the thread inside the stomach is grabbed using the biopsy forceps of the endoscope; thread, biopsy forceps, and endoscope are pulled outside all together through the esophagus and the mouth. NOTE: Ensure that the proximal end of the thread is kept outside to avoid the whole length of the thread being pulled through.
- The extremity of the thread that is emerging from the animal's mouth is then passed through the narrow end (tip) of the tomcat catheter.
- Then this thread is passed though the 16-gauge needle that is already going through the extremity of the Pezzer tube (see Fig. II-66A). The needle is then removed, leaving the thread embedded through the tip of the Pezzer tube. The extremities of the thread are tied to the Pezzer tube using several surgeon's knots (Fig. II-66B).
- By pulling on the "abdominal" extremity of the thread, the clinician fits the extremity of the Pezzer tube inside the wide part of the tomcat catheter (see Fig. II-66C). It is a very snug fit, and as much of the Pezzer tube tip is crammed into the broad end of the tomcat catheter as possible. Once this is done, the clinician can start to pull the tomcat catheter connected to its Pezzer tube into the stomach.
- By continuing to pull on the "abdominal" (proximal) extremity of the thread, the clinician will see the tomcat catheter soon appear through the skin. Here again, bracing with digital counterpressure at the abdominal wall is essential. To also allow the bigger Pezzer tube to pass through the skin, the clinician often has to widen the skin incision using a scalpel blade. Caution is warranted to avoid cutting the thread.
- The Pezzer tube will have to be pulled all the way until the ampulla lies against the gastric wall (this can be checked by endoscopy; see Fig. II-67).
- The extremity of the Pezzer tube is cut again and inserted through the flange. The flange is then pushed all the way against the abdominal skin (see Fig. II-68).
- A Chinese finger-trap suture can be placed to prevent accidental removal of the tube.
- The Luerlock adaptor and the PRN adaptor are then fitted to the extremity of the Pezzer tube.

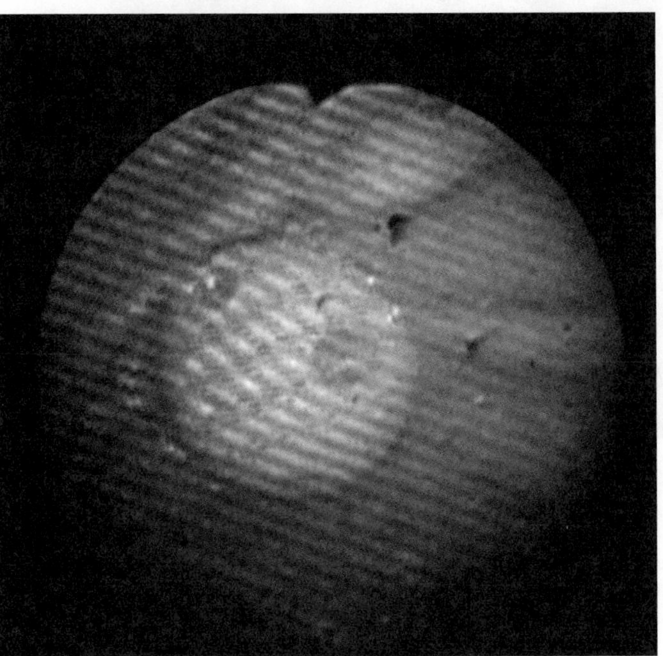

FIGURE II-67 Ampulla of the Pezzer tube seen from the inside of the stomach.

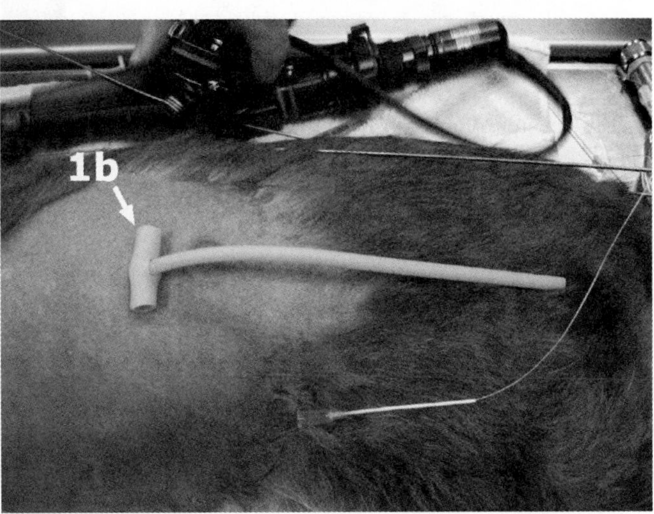

FIGURE II-68 Anesthetized cat in right lateral recumbency, cranial to the left. The PEG tube is in place, and the procedure is complete (the number 1b indicates the flange).

POSTPROCEDURE

- An Elizabethan collar may be necessary to prevent removal of the percutaneous endoscopic gastrostomy (PEG) tube by the animal.
- Removal of the Pezzer tube: This should be done no sooner than 2 weeks after the placement (as already described) to avoid possible leakage of food from the stomach into the abdominal cavity.

ALTERNATIVES AND THEIR RELATIVE MERITS

- Pharyngostomy/esophageal tubes: These tubes do not require an endoscope for placement and therefore can be cheaper alternatives. They work well but can be associated with local infection (uncommon). They are usually good for a few weeks. Their use requires normal esophageal function.
- Nasoesophageal tubes: These tubes provide a short-term solution (a few days). They are easy to place and also easily removed by the animal. They are smaller in diameter, and this may limit the rate of delivery of food.
- Jejunostomy tube: These tubes require surgical or endoscopic placement. They are used for bypassing the stomach and thus providing enteric feedings in animals with pancreatitis, for example.
- Parenteral nutrition: not as complete as enteral nutrition; requires a jugular catheter.

AUTHOR: **ERIC DE MADRON**

Feeding Tube Placement: Percutaneous Endoscopic Jejunostomy (PEJ)

BASIC INFORMATION

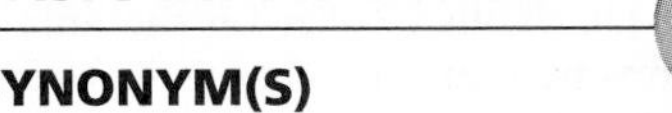

SYNONYM(S)

Percutaneous endoscopic-assisted placement of jejunostomy feeding tube
Percutaneous gastrojejunostomy feeding tube

OVERVIEW AND GOAL(S)

Placement of a jejunal feeding tube using endoscopic assistance, rather than laparotomy or laparoscopy, to provide postgastric enteral feeding to nutritionally deficient or debilitated animals. Enteral feeding provides the advantage of improved overall metabolism and health of the intestinal tract. Enteral feeding reduces intestinal bacterial translocation, maintains glutamine synthesis, and improves and maintains gut immunologic barrier functions.

INDICATIONS

- Postgastric feeding is advised for animals with uncontrolled vomiting from any cause.
- Following gastric or biliary surgery.
- Pancreatitis.
- Disorders causing persistent gastroparesis (e.g., following intestinal surgery).
- Animals at increased risk of active or passive gastroesophageal reflux and aspiration (e.g., prolonged recumbency, laryngeal paralysis, altered mentation).

CONTRAINDICATIONS

- Unresolved peritonitis
- Anesthetic risks
- Large-volume peritoneal effusion

EQUIPMENT, ANESTHESIA

- General anesthesia is required with endotracheal intubation.
- Postprocedural analgesia.
- Mouth gag.
- Sterile water-soluble lubricant for endoscope passage.
- Supplies as needed to place percutaneous endoscopic gastrostomy (PEG) tube (see Feeding Tube Placement: Percutaneous Endoscopic Gastrostomy [PEG], p 1247).
- 2-0 monofilament suture material.
- Iohexol as water-soluble radiographic contrast agent.
- Flexible video or fiberoptic endoscope and ancillary equipment appropriate to size of animal (generally 7.9 mm diameter with 100 cm length is acceptable for most cases).
- Endoscopic snare or grasping forceps.
- Vacuum source for endoscopic suction.
- PEG tube that is 18–24 Fr as a kit with percutaneous endoscopic jejunostomy (PEJ) or as a separate item (e.g., Pezzer mushroom-tip catheter).
- PEJ tube that is 8–12 Fr in diameter (e.g., Wilson-Cook Medical, Global Veterinary Products, Compat brand by Novartis [Fig. II-69]) and 35–150 cm in length; PEJ kits with gastrostomy tubes are also available; variable diameters and lengths based on supplier and animal size; internally coated catheters have an internal lubricant that activates when flushed with sterile water; 1 mm = 3 Fr.
- Weighted PEJ tubes are less commonly used; they have a tungsten bulb at the tip that adds weight to help prevent migration of the tube back to the stomach; these are preferred by some endoscopists and not by others.
- A 0.021–0.037 mm (50–150 cm) flexible guide wire matched to selected PEJ feeding tube.
- Fluoroscopy is preferred to be available, especially while staff is learning the technique.
- Elizabethan collar or other restraint to prevent patient's removal of PEJ or PEG tubes.
- Orthopedic stockinette appropriate to size of animal to create a "sweater-like effect."

ANTICIPATED TIME

About 40 to 80 minutes (including placement of PEG tube)

PREPARATION: IMPORTANT CHECKPOINTS

- Test or check integration of guide wire, PEG tube, and PEJ tube for compatibility of diameters and lengths.
- Plan for coordination of staff regarding anesthesia, endoscopy, and fluoroscopy.

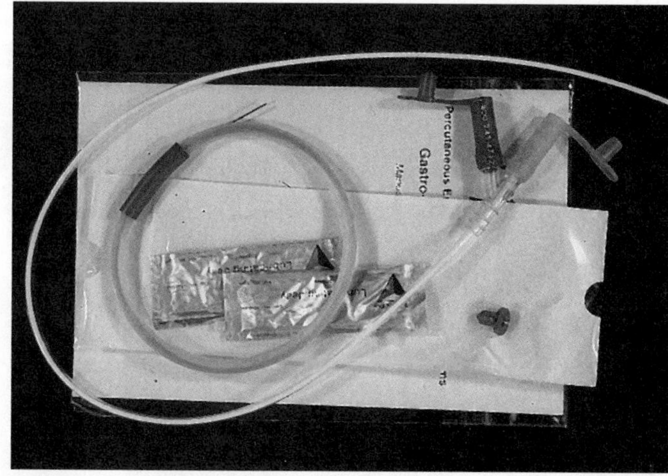

FIGURE II-69 Gastrojejunostomy combined kit from Wilson-Cook. Courtesy of Dr. Al Jergens.

- Discuss with client the potential that the PEJ tube may become occluded or may migrate back to stomach despite best efforts and cost of catheters.
- Check or estimate the fill volume of catheter prior to placement.

POSSIBLE COMPLICATIONS AND COMMON ERRORS TO AVOID

- Stoma site infection
- Premature removal by animal of tube (teeth, rubbing on objects in environment)
- Peritonitis if adhesion of body wall to stomach breaks down
- Diarrhea induced by feeding enteral formula
- Reflux of enteral feeding product aborally
- PEJ tube migration back to the stomach and possible vomition of the tube aborally

PROCEDURE

- Clip and prep left side of animal from approximately the eighth intercostal space (ICS) to just cranial to the stifle and from dorsal spinous process to ventral midline.
- General anesthesia with endotracheal intubation.
- Animal is positioned in right lateral recumbency.
- A PEG tube is placed (see Feeding Tube Placement: Percutaneous Endoscopic Gastrostomy [PEG], p 1247).
- Endoscope is passed to stomach from oral cavity.
- A snare or retrieval basket is passed via the gastrostomy (PEG) tube to the stomach.
- Endoscope is then maneuvered through the snare or basket.
- Pylorus is then visualized, and the endoscope is passed through to the mid-duodenum.
- Guide wire is passed via the operating channel of endoscope and continued forward blindly along the lumen of the small intestine until it is estimated that the tip is located in the proximal third of the jejunum.
- Guide wire is held stable as the scope is slowly withdrawn from the body.
- Guide wire should then be in the center of the snare or basket. This is tightened and withdrawn via the gastrostomy tube to the exterior so as to pull guide wire through the gastrostomy tube (proximal tip is in jejunum, and distal end extends out the gastrostomy tube).
- Location of proximal tip of guide wire is checked with fluoroscopy and may be adjusted in position.
- PEJ tube is flushed with copious amounts of water to activate lubricant.
- PEJ tube is passed over the guide wire until it extends a length adequate for the proximal tip to be in the proximal third of the jejunum (Fig. II-70).
- PEJ tube location is assessed with fluoroscopy or radiography with test infusion of a few milliliters of water-soluble contrast agent (iohexol); the PEJ tube may be repositioned as needed.
- Guide wire is removed slowly while the PEJ is held stable (Fig. II-71).
- PEJ tube is secured to animal's body or to the PEG tube as it exits the left side of the abdomen.

POSTPROCEDURE

- Place Elizabethan collar on the animal to prevent removal of both PEG and PEJ tubes.
- Place and adjust orthopedic stockinette "sweater" over animal's body, including two holes cut for the forelegs, to protect tubes; this should be "comfortable" to reduce stimulus for premature removal by animal.
- Monitor recovery from anesthesia.
- Instill the volume of sterile water needed to fill tube every 2 hours to keep tube patent.

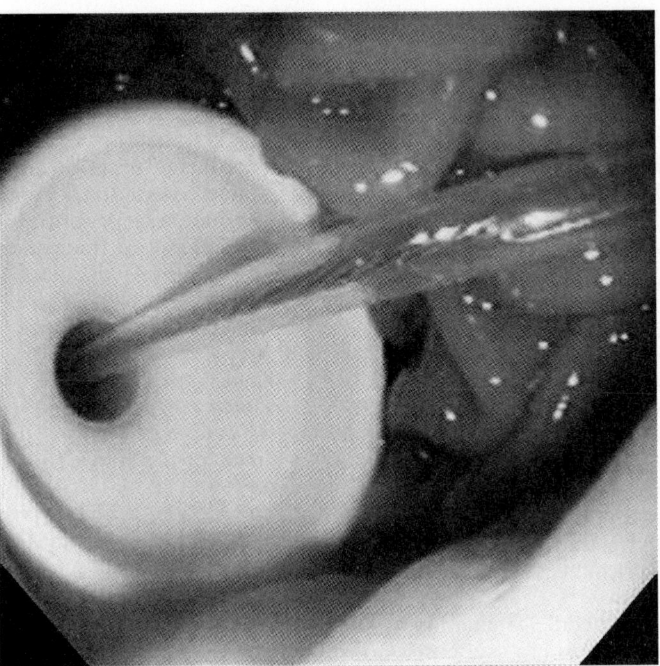

FIGURE II-70 Endoscopic image. Luminal view of the stomach, showing the gastrostomy/PEG tube with jejunostomy/PEJ tube inserted. Courtesy of Dr. Al Jergens.

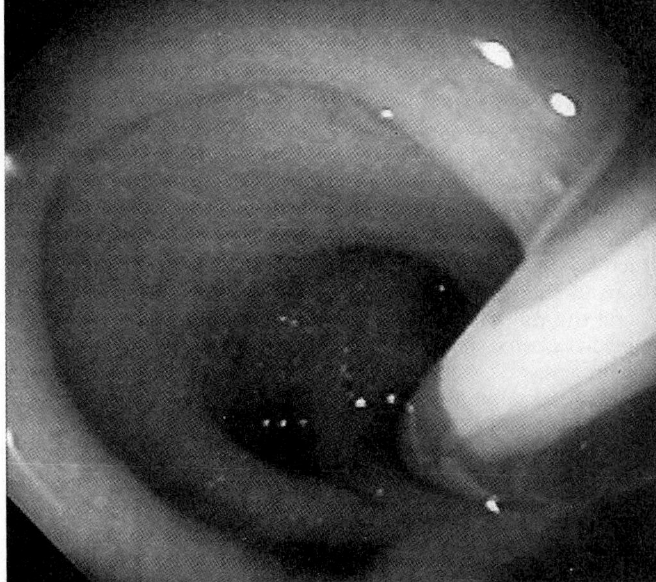

FIGURE II-71 Endoscopic image. Luminal view of the duodenum, showing the jejunostomy/PEJ tube over the guide wire (not seen). Courtesy of Dr. Al Jergens.

- Begin enteral nutrition 12 hours following tube placement.
- Monitor stoma site; expect mild inflammation and swelling; discharge from stoma may appear serous or mildly purulent, but cytologic analysis should reveal no bacteria; cleanse stoma gently with sterile saline and gauze squares as needed; surgical scrub can be used if needed but should be rinsed off completely.
- PEJ tube may be used as long as it remains functional and needed; often used for days to many weeks.
- Enteral feedings, either as boluses or constant drip infusion, are started with goal of one-third of daily caloric requirements being given the first day, two-thirds the second day, and full feedings by the third day.
- After removal of the PEJ tube, the remaining gastrostomy (PEG) tube may be used for nutrition if appropriate.
- The gastrostomy tube is generally left in place a minimum of 10 days to ensure adequate adhesion of stomach to the abdominal wall.
- The gastrostomy tube is removed by gentle progressive traction in a caudal direction that is also directed slightly away from the body; the remaining stoma will often close over within 4 to 8 hours after tube is removed.

ALTERNATIVES AND THEIR RELATIVE MERITS

- Nasojejunostomy tubes are placed with endoscopic or fluoroscopic assistance. These have the advantage of not requiring a gastrostomy tube. However, they have problems with nasal irritation, short duration of use (often a few days), difficulty in placing the tip distally enough in the jejunum, and problems with postprocedural retrograde migration (flex orally instead of aborally) back to the stomach or being vomited orally.
- Laparoscopic-assisted jejunostomy tubes can be placed at the end of a diagnostic or therapeutic laparoscopy. This technique allows for exteriorizing a loop of jejunum, which then is held with four stay sutures while a purse-string suture is placed in the antimesenteric side. The jejunostomy tube is placed through an incision in the center of the purse-string suture. This suture is tightened when the tube has been placed successfully (using fluoroscopy to confirm location and aboral direction). A box suture technique is used for creating an adhesion of the intestine to the body wall that secures the safe position of the jejunostomy tube. Problems can involve aboral migration or confusion in the direction for placement of the tube. Other complications include those that would be possible with surgically placed jejunostomy tubes.

AUTHOR: **MARK E. HITT**

Fine-Needle Aspirate, Ultrasound Guided

BASIC INFORMATION

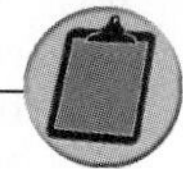

SYNONYM(S)

Needle biopsy

OVERVIEW AND GOAL(S)

Procedure to obtain small tissue or fluid samples using ultrasound guidance and real-time monitoring of needle placement

INDICATIONS

- Ultrasonographic evaluation of focal mass lesion or nodule
- Ultrasonographic evaluation of diffuse or focal parenchymal organ abnormalities
- Drainage of cysts, abscesses, or fluid

CONTRAINDICATIONS

- Cavitated mass: risk of hemorrhage
- Coagulopathy: risk of hemorrhage
- Suspected transitional cell carcinoma: possibility of seeding tumor along needle tract

EQUIPMENT, ANESTHESIA

- A few 22- or 25-gauge standard sterile injection needles, 1.5 inches in length
  - Longer needle (3.5 inch) required if using biopsy guide
- A few 6-ml syringes
- Glass microscope slides
- Hair clippers
- Surgical scrub, rubbing alcohol, gauze
- Sector or linear-array ultrasound transducer
  - Sector transducers allow sampling of deep structures
  - Linear-array transducers provide better resolution of superficial structures
  - ± Biopsy guide: easiest method but angle of needle insertion is fixed
  - Sedation often not needed for fine-needle aspirate (FNA)
  - Occasionally, IV or gas anesthesia required (e.g., anxious animal, small structure in close proximity to large vessel)

ANTICIPATED TIME

About 5 to 10 minutes

PREPARATION: IMPORTANT CHECKPOINTS

- Perform coagulation profile, platelet count, and arterial blood pressure (BP) measurement if animal is at an increased risk of bleeding.
- Determine if sedation is required; place IV catheter if needed.
- Ensure proper animal restraint.

POSSIBLE COMPLICATIONS AND COMMON ERRORS TO AVOID

- Avoid the suction method in sampling vascular organs (e.g., spleen) to decrease hemodilution.
- Identify and avoid large vessels within the organ being sampled or those adjacent to the structure (e.g., aorta adjacent to lymph node).
- Hemorrhage is uncommon if 22- or 25-gauge needle is used and the movement of the needle through the entire procedure is one-dimensional (in and out only, with no side-to-side motion).
- Do not move the needle side to side within an organ because this will cause tissue trauma.
- If redirecting needle orientation, withdraw needle tip to subcutis and then reinsert. Redirecting with needle fully advanced is ineffective (position changes little or not at all) and dangerous (shearing of tissue with needle tip).
- Cells may dry and clot in the needle very quickly. Therefore, when the needle is withdrawn, the expulsion of needle contents onto a microscope slide and the slide smearing technique should all be completed within seconds.
- Avoid penetrating bowel lumen, especially with larger gauge needles, due to risk of peritonitis.
- Sample the left aspect of the liver when possible to avoid the gallbladder and hilar vessels on the right. If the liver is small or cranially located, consider an intercostal approach.
- With renal aspirates, sample the caudal cortex of the kidney to avoid the medulla and hilar vessels.
- In cases of bilateral renal abnormalities, the left kidney should be sampled due to its more caudal location.
- Do not pass through an organ other than the one being aspirated.
- Avoid administering drugs that cause splenomegaly or panting (e.g., phenothiazines, some opiates).
- If aspirating an adrenal gland mass, be aware of possible BP alterations and severe hemorrhage in the case of pheochromocytoma.

PROCEDURE

- Restrain the animal in dorsal or lateral recumbency. A padded V-trough can be used for the animal so that it is more comfortable when lying down. (See Fig. II-31.)
- Clip hair from the ventral abdomen.
- Thoroughly evaluate area of interest, characterize lesion, identify adjacent or internal vessels to be avoided, and determine least traumatic location and direction of needle placement.
- Prepare skin with surgical scrub.
- Obtain ultrasound image of area to be sampled.
- Ensure probe marker location on screen corresponds with desired needle course.
- Freehand technique: Hold transducer in one hand and insert needle with other.
- The suction technique is useful in aspirates of less vascular structures (e.g., lymph node) but often results in hemodilution when aspirating vascular organs like the spleen.
  - Without syringe suction:
    - Introduce a 22- or 25-gauge needle parallel to plane of ultrasound beam, visualizing needle as it is advanced.
    - Slowly fan transducer side to side to identify entire needle length to tip (Figs. II-72 and II-73).
    - Advance and retract needle three to four times to fill needle shaft with tissue cells. If using a spinal needle, remove the stylet before beginning the advancing and retracting of the needle.
    - Withdraw needle from animal and quickly attach a 6-ml syringe prefilled with 5 cc room air.
    - Expel contents onto microscopic slide(s) immediately, and lightly smear using standard blood smear technique.
  - With syringe suction:
    - Attach 6-ml syringe to 22- or 25-gauge needle.
    - Introduce needle parallel to plane of ultrasound beam, as already described.
    - Apply suction to syringe three to four times while gently advancing and retracting needle.
    - Withdraw needle from animal and disconnect syringe.
    - Retract plunger to fill syringe with air and reconnect syringe to needle.
    - Expel contents onto microscopic slide(s) immediately, and lightly smear using standard blood smear technique.
    - Multiple samples of each organ or lesion should be obtained.

POSTPROCEDURE

Scan to evaluate for hemorrhage (very uncommon with this procedure).

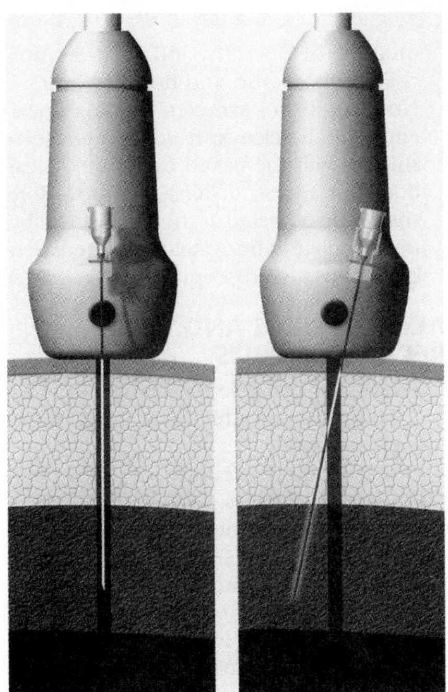

FIGURE II-72 Importance of correct alignment between needle and ultrasound probe. Left panel: Correct alignment is present, and the full extent of the needle is seen. Right panel: The needle is not aligned with the ultrasound beam, and only the proximal portion of the needle is seen. Here, trauma to deeper tissues is possible because the location of the tip of the needle is unknown. Reprinted from Fife WD: Abdominal ultrasound: Aspirations and biopsies. In Ettinger SJ, Feldman EC (eds): *Textbook of Veterinary Internal Medicine*, ed 6. St. Louis, Elsevier Saunders, 2005, pp 271–275.

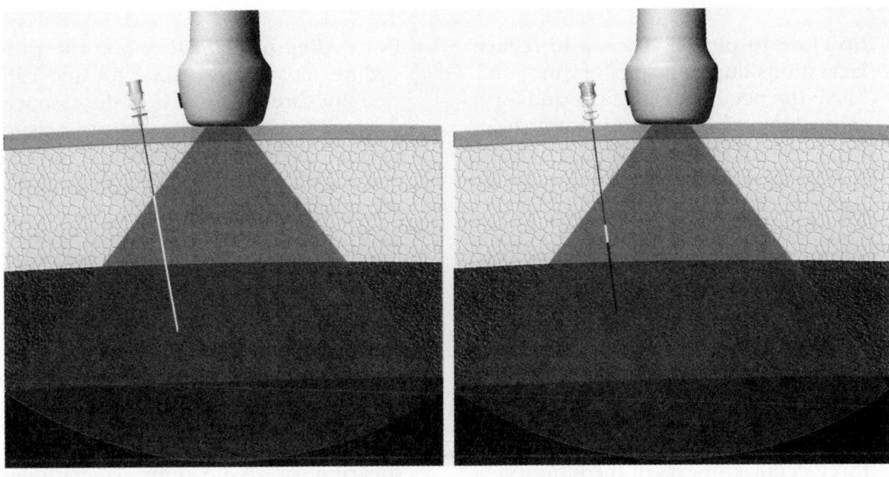

FIGURE II-73 Views as seen on monitor of the ultrasound machine, perpendicular to Fig. II-72. Left panel: Correct alignment produces complete visualization of needle. Right panel: Probe-needle malalignment underrepresents the depth of the needle.

ALTERNATIVES AND THEIR RELATIVE MERITS

Tissue-core and surgical biopsy are more invasive but of greater diagnostic quality due to the ability to collect larger tissue samples.

SUGGESTED READING

Nyland TG, et al: Ultrasound-guided biopsy. In Nyland TG, Mattoon JS (eds): *Small Animal Diagnostic Ultrasound*, ed 2. Philadelphia, WB Saunders, 2002, pp 30–48.

Penninck DG, Finn-Bodner ST: Updates in interventional ultrasonography. *Vet Clin North Am Small Anim Pract* 28:1017–1040, 1998.

AUTHOR: **WENDY D. FIFE**

Fine-Needle Sampling for Cytologic Analysis: Lung

BASIC INFORMATION

OVERVIEW AND GOAL(S)

Minimally invasive diagnostic tool with a good diagnostic yield for focal lesions. Good technique increases the diagnostic yield and reduces complications.

INDICATIONS

- Pulmonary masses and nodules
- Areas of pulmonary consolidation
- Lower diagnostic yield and greater risk to animal for diffuse (interstitial) pulmonary diseases

CONTRAINDICATIONS

Bleeding disorders (coagulopathy, thrombocytopenia, thrombocytopathia)

EQUIPMENT, ANESTHESIA

- A few sterile 22-gauge needles (2.5–8.9 cm)
- A 12-ml syringe
- An 84-cm flexible extension set for IV lines
- Glass slides
- Blow dryer
- Image guidance if possible (ultrasound, CT scan, fluoroscopy, radiology)
- General anesthesia is recommended to reduce risks of pulmonary lacerations and pneumothorax

ANTICIPATED TIME

About 30 minutes

PREPARATION: IMPORTANT CHECKPOINTS

- Warn owners that hemorrhage and pneumothorax are possible complications, warranting intensive care and sometimes presenting a life-threatening situation.
- Rule out bleeding disorders.

PROCEDURE

- Induce general anesthesia, including endotracheal intubation.
- Clip the hair from the biopsy site(s), and clean the site with surgical soap.
- Connect extension set between syringe and needle.
- Fill syringe with 5–10 ml of air.
- The clinician hangs the syringe and extension tubing around his or her neck and holds the needle like a pen to allow precise manipulations.
- Localize lesion with diagnostic imaging. Fine-needle procedures guided only by radiographs can be performed on large masses or when large areas of the lungs are affected. NOTE: Sonographic guidance works only if the mass, nodule, or consolidated lobe is in contact with the thoracic wall.
- Rapidly position the needle tip within the lesion. Avoid keeping the needle

tip close to pleural surfaces to reduce lacerations during respiratory motion.
- Move the needle rapidly back and forth using long needle passes (away from major blood vessels) and try staying within the lesion. Do not use negative pressure.
- Rapidly withdraw the needle.
- Immediately expel the sample on glass slides using the air-filled syringe.
- Make smear using the standard blood smear technique or a gentle squash technique.
- Immediately air-dry the smear with a blow dryer.
- Repeat the procedure to obtain two to three cellular smears of the lesion(s).

POSTPROCEDURE

Risks of pneumothorax are significantly reduced (5% versus 40–50%) if the animal is kept in lateral recumbency (biopsy side down) for 30 to 60 minutes following the procedure. If the animal is stable, keep under anesthesia 15 to 20 minutes after the procedure. This simple precaution takes advantage of recumbency atelectasis to rapidly seal any lung perforations or lacerations.

POSSIBLE COMPLICATIONS AND COMMON ERRORS TO AVOID

- Hemorrhage (pulmonary, pleural, airways).
- Pneumothorax.
- Proceeding too slowly: While the procedure must be prepared for and carried out carefully, time is of the essence during fine-needle sampling. Tissue trauma activates coagulation, which can rapidly plug the needle or degrade the quality of the sample.
- Short- and slow-needle passes: A slow or timid back-and-forth motion does not detach a sufficient number of cells. The needle tip, however, must remain within the target tissue during this part of the procedure to avoid contamination by, or damage to, surrounding tissues.
- Changing directions while the needle is deep in the lesion: doing so causes shearing of tissue, lung lacerations, bleeding, and pain. The needle should always be withdrawn to the skin's surface (almost out but not quite) before being redirected.
- Aspiration: When aspiration is used in the lungs, air is aspirated as soon as the bevel enters an air-filled space, and the sample is lost in the syringe or extension set. A vigorous back-and-forth motion without aspiration is sufficient to detach cells, create mild bleeding, and fill the needle with a diagnostic sample.
- Multiple sites: An important point is to obtain three to five cellular biopsies of different areas of large lesions because masses or large lesions may contain a mixture of necrotic, inflamed, hemorrhagic, neoplastic, and normal tissues.
- Nondiagnostic samples: With experience, a clinician can identify cellular smears with the naked eye. If the smear does not appear cellular, the procedure should be repeated. If there is any doubt, the sample can be evaluated immediately by in-house microscopic examination.

ALTERNATIVES AND THEIR RELATIVE MERITS

- Tru-Cut or core biopsy:
  - May be associated with more complications.
  - May be more accurate for diffuse pulmonary diseases.
- Bronchoscopy/bronchoalveolar lavage:
  - Minimally invasive: lowest risk of iatrogenic pneumothorax.
  - Requires disease process that is exfoliating cells into the alveoli or airways (e.g., useful for lung consolidation due to pneumonia). Therefore, false negatives are possible.
- Surgical biopsy:
  - More costly.
  - More invasive.
  - Most definitive diagnostic sampling technique for diffuse (interstitial) pulmonary diseases.

AUTHORS: **MARC PAPAGEORGES, MICHÈLE MENARD**

Fine-Needle Sampling for Cytologic Analysis: Subcutaneous Mass

BASIC INFORMATION

OVERVIEW AND GOAL(S)

Minimally invasive diagnostic tool; good technique increases diagnostic yield. The use of a nonaspiration technique produces superior results due to decreased hemodilution.

INDICATIONS

All cutaneous and subcutaneous masses

CONTRAINDICATIONS

Hematoma in an animal with systemic evidence of bleeding tendency

EQUIPMENT, ANESTHESIA

- A few sterile 22-gauge needles of various lengths (2.5–8.9 cm), without stylet (Fig. II-74A)
- A 12-ml syringe (Fig. II-74D)
- An 84-cm flexible extension set for IV lines (optional) (Fig. II-74C)

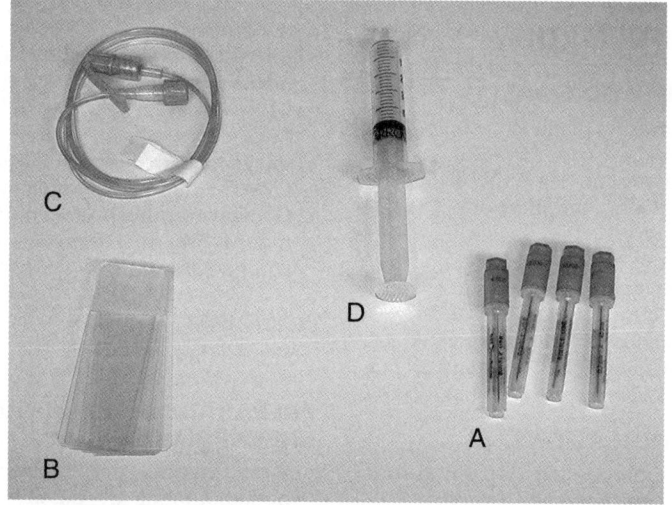

FIGURE II-74 Materials used for fine-needle sampling. **A,** Four 22-gauge, 1.5-inch needle(s). **B,** Microscope slides. **C,** Extension tubing. **D,** A syringe filled with air.

- Glass slides
- Blow dryer
- Sedation or general anesthesia required only with fractious animals

ANTICIPATED TIME

About 5 to 10 minutes

PROCEDURE

- Clip the hair from the site and clean the site with surgical soap.
- Connect needle directly to syringe or use extension set (easier manipulations).
- Fill syringe with 5-10 ml of air before proceeding further.
- If extension set is used, hang the syringe and extension tubing around the neck and hold the needle like a pen to allow precise manipulations. If the extension set is not used, the air-filled syringe is attached to the needle.
- Immobilize lesion with one hand.
- With the other hand, rapidly position the needle tip within the lesion.
- Rapidly move the needle tip back and forth 8 to 10 times without changing its path. CAUTION: Depth and orientation must be sufficiently controlled to avoid reaching tissues outside the lesion, including the risk of needlestick injury to the clinician.
- Long-needle passes are better, but the needle tip must remain within the lesion.
- At no time does the volume of air in the syringe change. NOTE: The purpose of the syringe will be to eject the contents of the needle onto a slide, and the syringe is not involved in suction.
- Rapidly withdraw the needle.
- Immediately expel the sample on glass slides using the air-filled syringe.
- Make smear using the standard blood smear technique or a gentle squash preparation.
- Immediately air-dry the smear with a blow dryer.
- Repeat the procedure to obtain three to five cellular smears of each mass.

NOTE: The use of an extension set for IV lines serves several purposes. The procedure is less cumbersome because the needle is separated from the syringe. Thus, by being able to manipulate the needle more precisely, the clinician can obtain more accurate samples. By prefilling the syringe with air, the transfer of the sample onto glass slides is expedited, which reduces sample clotting. Clinicians should not use negative pressure during fine-needle sampling. Rather, the vigorous back-and-forth motion and the capillary pressure in the needle appear to be sufficient to detach cells, create mild bleeding, and fill the lumen of the needle with a cellular sample. The sample volume is reduced, but representative cellularity is increased.

POSSIBLE COMPLICATIONS AND COMMON ERRORS TO AVOID

- Hemorrhage (rare and usually easy to control).
- Proceeding too slowly: Time is of the essence during fine-needle sampling. Tissue trauma activates coagulation, which can rapidly plug the needle or degrade the quality of the sample.
- Short- and slow-needle passes: A slow or timid back-and-forth motion does not detach a sufficient number of cells. The needle tip, however, must remain within the target tissue during this part of the procedure to avoid contamination by surrounding tissues. This becomes more of a challenge with very small masses.
- Changing directions: doing so while the needle is deep in the lesion causes shearing of tissue, bleeding, and pain. The needle should always be withdrawn to the skin surface (almost out but not quite) before being redirected.
- Only one sample: An important point is to obtain three to five cellular samples of different areas of large lesions because masses or large lesions may contain a mixture of necrotic, inflamed, hemorrhagic, neoplastic, and normal tissues.
- Nondiagnostic samples: With experience, a clinician can identify cellular smears with the naked eye. If the smear does not appear cellular, the procedure should be repeated. The sample quality can also be evaluated immediately by in-house microscopic examination.
- Not sending all smears when an expert opinion is desired: Sometimes the answer is found only on one or two smears. Send all smears when consulting a cytopathologist.

ALTERNATIVES AND THEIR RELATIVE MERITS

- Tru-Cut or core biopsy:
  - More expensive
  - Requires local anesthesia
  - May be useful for more precise identification of some tumors
- Surgical biopsy:
  - More expensive
  - Requires local or general anesthesia
  - May be useful for more precise identification of some tumors
  - May be curative if entire lesion is removed

AUTHORS: **MICHÈLE MENARD, MARC PAPAGEORGES**

Fistulogram

BASIC INFORMATION

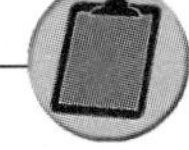

SYNONYM(S)

Positive-contrast fistulogram

OVERVIEW AND GOAL(S)

Fistulograms are radiographic contrast procedures that may be utilized in the evaluation of a cutaneous draining tract.

INDICATIONS

- Identify soft-tissue foreign bodies (e.g., splinters, plant awns, glass)
- Locate potential source of a draining tract (e.g., orthopedic implants, sutures)
- Identify communication of tract with body cavity or organ

CONTRAINDICATIONS

Known sensitivity to contrast media

EQUIPMENT, ANESTHESIA

- Contrast media:
  - Ionic or nonionic organic iodinated contrast agents
- Catheters:
  - Variable length and size depending on extent of lesion
  - Preferably semirigid without balloon tip, such as a tomcat catheter; no stylets
- Sedation/anesthesia may be required for fractious animals.

ANTICIPATED TIME

About 5 to 20 minutes

PREPARATION: IMPORTANT CHECKPOINTS

- Sedation/anesthesia if required
- Hair clipped and area scrubbed/disinfected
- Survey radiograph of region

POSSIBLE COMPLICATIONS AND COMMON ERRORS TO AVOID

- Systemic reaction to contrast agents (rare)

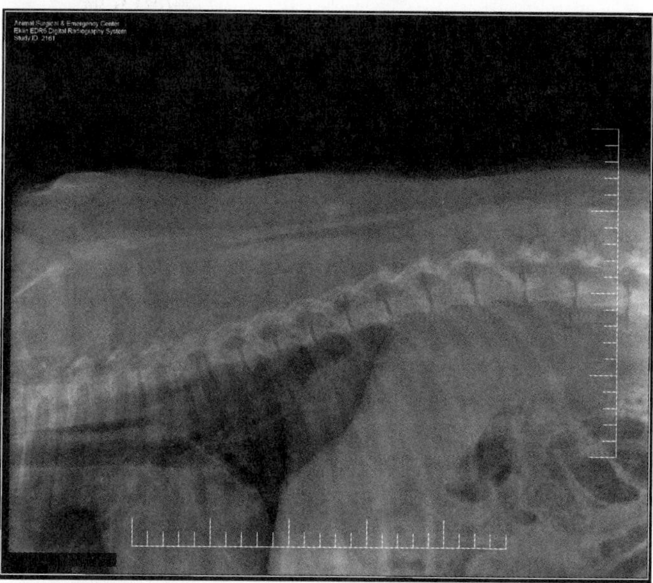

FIGURE II-75 Lateral radiographic projection of the torso of a dog prior to contrast injection. There is a suggestion of minor radiopacity in dorsal body wall dorsal to location of a draining tract. Courtesy of Dr. Phil Gill.

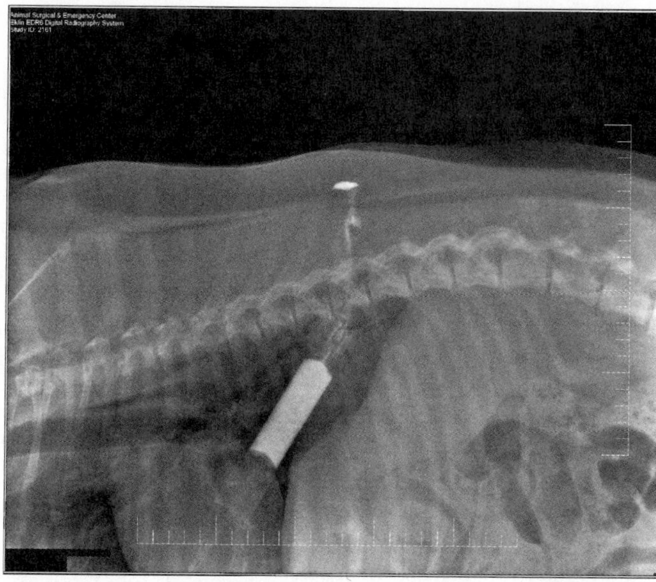

FIGURE II-76 Lateral radiographic projection of the same dog after contrast injection into a cutaneous raining tract on the lateral thorax. The study shows the extent of the draining tract, with pooling of contrast media in the dorsal body wall. Filling defect in contrast-filled tract created by catheter. Courtesy of Dr. Phil Gill.

- Local irritation from hypertonic contrast agents (rare; can dilute with saline or sterile water for prevention)
- Leakage of contrast into fascial planes leading to nondiagnostic study (common)
- Inability to follow full extent of draining tract (common)
- Masking of small foreign bodies by opacity of contrast agent (common)

PROCEDURE

- Catheter is placed retrograde into draining tract as far as possible.
- Injection (usually 1–2 cc) while catheter in place or while drawing it back out.
- Appropriate radiographic projections; two views at right angles are usually sufficient.

ALTERNATIVES AND THEIR RELATIVE MERITS

- Ultrasound:
  - Easy to perform.
  - Variable information obtained; may detect foreign bodies.
  - Difficult to follow extent of tract.
- CT scan and MRI:
  - Expensive.
  - Variable information obtained.

AUTHOR: **BRETT KANTROWITZ**

Foreign Body Removal, Esophageal (Endoscopic)

BASIC INFORMATION

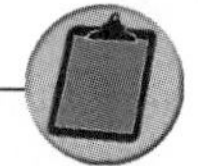

SYNONYM(S)

Minimally invasive removal of esophageal foreign bodies

OVERVIEW AND GOAL(S)

- Objects causing esophageal obstruction are most commonly located in one of three locations: at the thoracic inlet, at the level of the base of the heart, or immediately cranial to the gastroesophageal sphincter.
- About 90% of foreign bodies obstructing the esophagus can be removed without performing a thoracotomy. Removal of these objects is achieved by making use of rigid or flexible endoscopes.
- If a foreign object cannot be removed via the oral route, an attempt can be made to pass the object through into the stomach using a large-bore stomach tube and copious lubrication, provided complications such as esophageal perforation (from a sharp-edged foreign body, esophageal wall devitalization, or overly aggressive forward pressure) are avoided. Objects passed from the esophagus into the stomach may then be removed via a gastrostomy or left to be digested (in the case of bones and other digestible objects).

INDICATIONS

Presence of foreign objects lodged in the esophagus (e.g., bones, fishhooks, needles, toys)

CONTRAINDICATIONS

Esophageal perforation is an absolute contraindication to minimally invasive approaches; thoracotomy is indicated in these cases.

EQUIPMENT, ANESTHESIA

- General anesthesia.
- Cuffed endotracheal tube.
- Mouth gag/speculum.
- Rigid tube for esophageal dilation (optional); typical external diameters are

2 cm (cat, small dog), 3 cm (medium-size dog), and 4 cm (large dog). The end of the tube should have smooth edges (may heat with flame, then trim edges when cool before using).
- Rigid proctoscope or flexible fiberoptic endoscope.
- Endoscopic basket or grasping forceps (recommended) or endoscopic biopsy forceps (second choice).
- Water-soluble lubricating jelly.
- Polyethylene catheter or feeding tube (optional).
- Suctioning apparatus.

ANTICIPATED TIME

Approximately 20-90 minutes, depending on size of object and ease with which it can be grasped, atraumatically dislodged, and retrieved

PREPARATION: IMPORTANT CHECKPOINTS

- Assess for location of foreign body, presence of signs of aspiration pneumonia, and evidence of esophageal perforation by performing survey and contrast radiography using low osmolality, nonionic contrast medium. Radiographs should be performed or repeated immediately prior to induction of general anesthesia to avoid anesthetizing an animal in which a foreign body has spontaneously passed into the stomach.
- Endoscopic evaluation of location of foreign body and state of esophageal mucosa.
- Ensure adequate hydration and perfusion.
- Antibiotic therapy, if indicated by complications (described in following paragraphs); often empirically at first (e.g., ampicillin 22 mg/kg IV q 8h and enrofloxacin 5 mg/kg diluted 1:1 in 0.9% saline and given slowly IV, q 24h [cats] or q 12h [dogs]) and then guided by results of culture and sensitivity (C&S).
- Advise the owner of possible complications.
  - There may be a need for emergency thoracotomy if perforation occurs or if removal via the oral route is impossible; possible gastrostomy may result if the foreign body has to be pushed through into the stomach and is unlikely to be digested.

POSSIBLE COMPLICATIONS AND COMMON ERRORS TO AVOID

- Esophageal mucosal trauma (erosion, ulceration)
- Esophageal perforation, pyothorax, pleuritis, mediastinitis
- Aspiration of esophageal contents and aspiration pneumonia
- Tension pneumothorax (associated with esophageal insufflation when using flexible fiberoptic endoscope)
- Bradycardia due to vagal stimulation
- Sepsis (due to aspiration or to esophageal rupture)
- Esophageal stricture (first clinical manifestations: usually >2 weeks postoperatively)
- Bronchoesophageal fistulation (rare)
- Failure to radiograph immediately prior to induction (foreign body may have passed spontaneously)

PROCEDURE

- General anesthesia.
- Place endotracheal tube and inflate cuff to prevent aspiration of esophageal contents.
- Animal in sternal or left lateral recumbency (allows the esophagus to lie over the aorta).
- Examine the mouth (especially the sublingual region) for the presence of objects, such as thread, needles, or fishhooks.
- Suction esophagus to remove any liquid contents and contrast medium.
- Insert mouth gag/speculum.
- Rigid proctoscope technique:
  - Lubricate proctoscope.
  - Pass the proctoscope orally and into the esophagus to the level of the foreign body, visualizing the foreign body and any evidence of perforation that would contraindicate further endoscopic manipulations.
  - Lubrication can be placed at the site of the foreign body using a polyethylene catheter with the tip placed at the level of the foreign body, between the foreign body and esophageal mucosa.
  - Using grasping forceps, bring the foreign body close to the end of the proctoscope.
  - If the foreign body is small enough, it can be partially pulled into the lumen of the proctoscope.
  - The foreign body, proctoscope, and grasping forceps are pulled out together via the mouth by gentle manipulation and with adequate lubrication. Continuous visualization and gentleness of traction are essential through this process. This is to ensure that complications such as esophageal laceration or perforation are noticed immediately if they occur, that the retrieval can be stopped immediately, and that the foreign body be reposi-

PROCEDURES AND TECHNIQUES

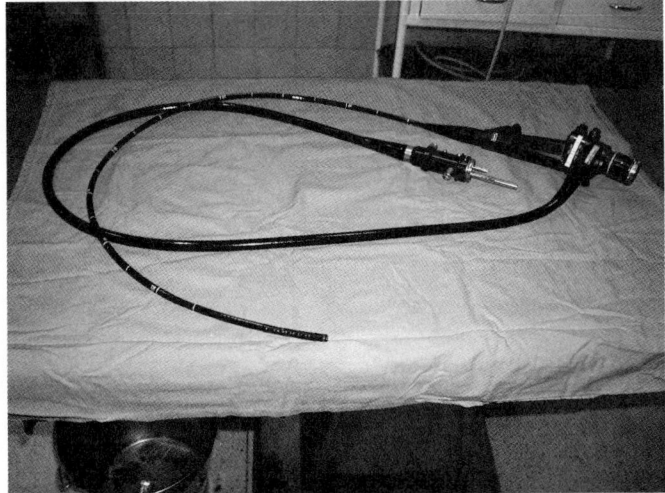

FIGURE II-77 A 1-m flexible fiberoptic endoscope. This endoscope is adequate for esophageal procedures in dogs and cats of all body sizes.

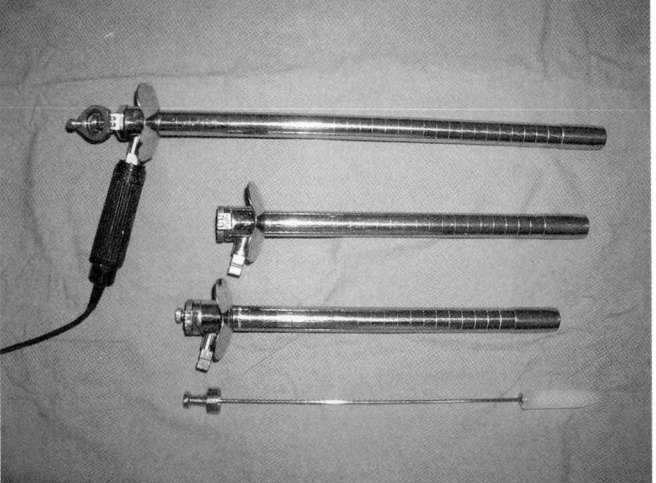

FIGURE II-78 A large (top) and two small (below) rigid proctoscopes used for retrieving esophageal foreign bodies and a small proctoscopic stylet (bottom). The stylet is placed into the proctoscope for advancing into the esophagus. Once the desired degree of insertion is achieved, the stylet is withdrawn, and the glass port (seen in the open position in the large proctoscope, top) may be closed for the most effective visualization.

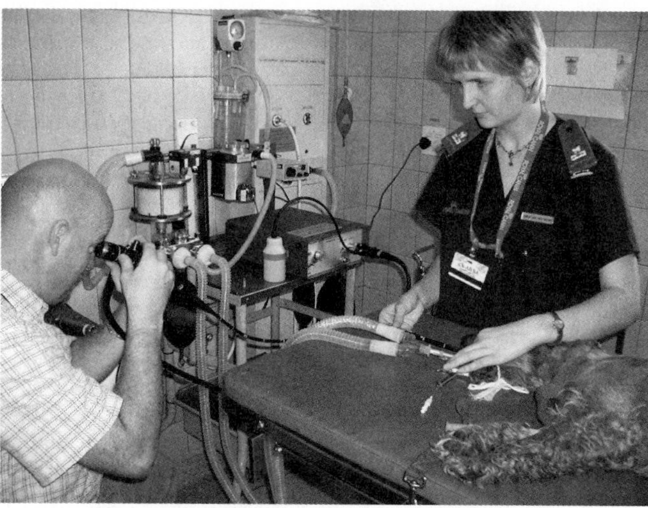

FIGURE II-79 The operator (left) examines the esophagus of an animal using a flexible fiberoptic endoscope, while an assistant adjusts the endoscope's insertion and rotation according to the operator's instructions.

tioned or the procedure be aborted in favor of thoracotomy if serious complications are noted.
 - If retrieval is not possible, an attempt should be made to gently push the foreign body through to the stomach using a well-lubricated stomach tube, provided no evidence of esophageal devitalization (e.g., deep mucosal lacerations and discolorations or other signs of possibly imminent perforation) are seen.
 - Careful examination of the esophageal wall after foreign body removal; any suspicion of possible esophageal perforation warrants close radiographic and clinical monitoring.
- Flexible fiberoptic endoscope technique:
 - For medium-size or larger dogs, a rigid tube can first be placed to assist in dilating the esophagus. The endoscope can then be passed through this tube.
 - Lubricate the endoscope.
 - Pass the endoscope to the level of the foreign body, visualizing the foreign body and assessing the integrity of the adjacent esophagus.
 - Insufflation of air will allow dilation of the esophagus around the foreign body.
 - Lubrication can also be placed at the site of the foreign body, using a catheter or feeding tube, as already described.
 - Grasping forceps or biopsy forceps can be passed through the endoscope biopsy channel. The use of biopsy forceps is a last resort because dulling and damage to the instrument are possible.
 - Grasp the foreign body and pull it close to the endoscope.
 - The endoscope, forceps, and foreign body are gently pulled out together via the mouth while ensuring adequate esophageal dilation and lubrication.
 - If retrieval is not possible, an attempt should be made to push the foreign body through to the stomach.
 - The esophageal mucosa is carefully examined endoscopically after removal of the foreign body.

POSTPROCEDURE

- If esophageal mucosa is damaged (e.g., suspected on endoscopic observation of darkened/discolored esophageal mucosa, deep mucosal lacerations, or after prolonged, difficult procedure; confirmation comes from intraprocedure or postprocedure radiographs):
 - Clean lacerations that do not extend through the full thickness of the esophageal wall can be left to heal by epithelialization.
 - Full-thickness tears and areas of esophageal necrosis require immediate surgical resection or repair.
- Withhold food and water for 24 hours.
- Maintain hydration and electrolyte balance.
- Pain management: antibiotics (as already described), prokinetic agents, corticosteroids, and/or gastric antacids may be indicated (see Foreign Body Removal, Esophageal [Endoscopic], p 1256; Esophagitis, p 366; Esophageal Stricture, p 363).
- Gastrostomy feeding tube placed distal to the site of the foreign body if prolonged withholding of food is indicated (such as in cases of esophageal mucosal damage).
- Once the animal has recovered, first introduce liquids, followed by gruel if no adverse reactions are noted once liquids have been introduced.

ALTERNATIVES AND THEIR RELATIVE MERITS

- Advancement of foreign body into stomach followed by gastrostomy:
 - If a foreign body is too large or awkward to grasp, an attempt could be made to gently push it through into the stomach. Digestible objects, such as bones, could be left in the stomach to digest, but sharp objects and objects such as toys should not be pushed into the stomach (risk of esophageal perforation). Follow-up radiography is advised to ensure that foreign bodies were either digested or passed through the digestive tract.
- For cases in which esophageal perforation and its complications have already developed, surgical removal of the foreign body via thoracotomy is the only alternative.

AUTHOR: **MIRINDA NEL (VAN SCHOOR)**

Gastric Intubation, Gavage, Lavage

BASIC INFORMATION

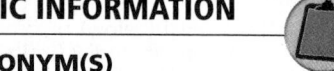

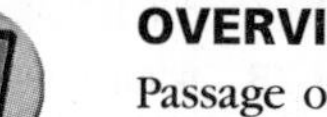

SYNONYM(S)

Gastric decompression
Orogastric feeding
Orogastric intubation

OVERVIEW AND GOAL(S)

Passage of a hollow tube into the mouth and through the oropharynx into the stomach to facilitate decompression of gas, removal of stomach contents (lavage), or administration of large volumes of liquid, food, or medication (gavage).

INDICATIONS

- Gastric intubation:
 - Preoperative stabilization of gastric dilatation volvulus (GDV); allows evacuation of gas and fluid, resulting in an improved hemodynamic state.

- Relief of discomfort associated with gaseous dilatation (without torsion) of the stomach.
- Gavage:
  - Administration of large volumes of liquid medication, including:
    - Activated charcoal after toxin ingestion.
    - Barium for gastrointestinal (GI)-contrast radiography.
    - Hyperosmotic laxative agent prior to colonoscopy.
  - Administration of formula to neonatal animals that are not nursing on their own.
- Lavage:
  - Preoperative stabilization of GDV. Removal of stomach contents may help decrease the speed of gas reaccumulation while the animal is being prepared for surgery, thus slowing or preventing cardiovascular deterioration.
  - Removal of stomach contents with suspected intoxications.

NOTE: Gastric lavage may not be indicated in all cases of toxin ingestion. Substance ingested, consistency, time since ingestion, and animal status will influence whether gastric lavage is appropriate.

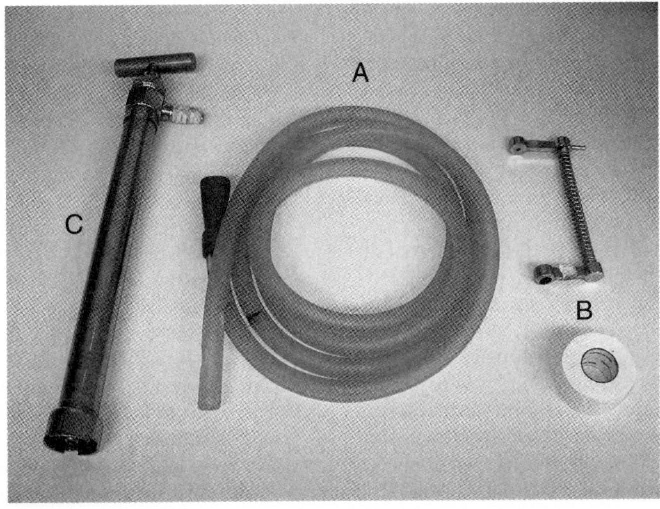

FIGURE II-80 Materials and equipment used for gastric intubation and lavage. **A,** Orogastric tube. **B,** Metal speculum or roll of tape to be used as a mouth gag. **C,** Stomach pump for lavage.

CONTRAINDICATIONS

- Esophageal disease that could lead to tube-induced trauma or perforation. Conditions of concern include esophageal stricture, neoplasia, ulceration, megaesophagus, and recent esophageal surgery.
- Gastric disease that could lead to tube-induced trauma or perforation. Conditions of concern include neoplasia, ulceration, and recent gastric surgery.
- Any swallowing disorder (megaesophagus, esophageal motility disorder, etc.), pharyngeal disorder, or laryngeal disorder (paralysis, previous tie-back surgery, etc.) that could predispose a nonendotracheally intubated animal to aspiration.
- If even one of these conditions is present, the risk of the procedure versus its benefits must be considered (and will vary from case to case) before deciding whether to perform the procedure.

EQUIPMENT, ANESTHESIA

- Gastric intubation:
  - Two assistants (minimum).
  - Flexible plastic tubing of various length and diameter (Fig. II-80A). The distal end must be smooth and atraumatic; smoothing may be achieved by brief heating of the end of the tube over a flame, cooling, and trimming edges with a scalpel blade. One to three side holes may facilitate evacuation of stomach contents by minimizing obstruction of a single distal hole with gastric mucosa or ingesta.
  - A roll of clinic-type white cloth tape (Fig. II-80B).
  - Water-soluble lubrication jelly.
  - Mouth gag/speculum (see Fig. II-80B).
- If gastric lavage, all of the above, plus:
  - Funnel or stomach pump (Fig. II-80C).
  - Container (e.g., bucket) to collect stomach contents and lavage fluid.
  - Lavage fluid: usually warm (body temperature) water.

ANTICIPATED TIME

Dependent on cooperation of animal; additional time may be needed for sedation or general anesthesia:

- Gastric intubation: 2–5 minutes.
- Gavage: 3–10 minutes.
- Lavage: 10–60 minutes.

PREPARATION: IMPORTANT CHECKPOINTS

- Ensure that adequate manual or chemical restraint for the procedure is planned. Personal preference and animal stability may dictate the degree of sedation or anesthesia chosen. NOTE: Some clinicians prefer to ensure a patent and protected airway through the use of general anesthesia and a cuffed endotracheal (ET) tube when gastric lavage is performed to minimize the potential for aspiration pneumonia.
- Maximize cardiovascular stability prior to the procedure.

POSSIBLE COMPLICATIONS AND COMMON ERRORS TO AVOID

- Inadvertent passage of the orogastric tube into the trachea can result in mild to severe complications.
  - Tracheal irritation leading to transient coughing or mucosal bleeding is possible.
  - Tracheal or bronchial placement of the gastric tube can result in airway obstruction until the tube is repositioned.
  - Tracheal or bronchial tearing can result in pneumomediastinum, pneumothorax, and death.
  - Tracheal or bronchial administration of gavage or lavage fluids can result in severe aspiration pneumonia and death.
  - See procedure (as explained in following paragraphs) for avoidance of this complication.
- Oral, pharyngeal, laryngeal, esophageal, or gastric trauma can result if excessive force is used for passing the gastric tube. Full-thickness tearing is possible, especially with a preexisting underlying disease.
- Inability to pass the tube into the stomach may be due to the choice of a tube with a diameter that is too large, esophageal obstruction (foreign body, stricture, neoplasia), torsion of the stomach, or excessive lower esophageal sphincter (LES) tone. Discontinuation of metoclopramide prior to elective gastric intubation is recommended to minimize LES tone.
- Inadequate sedation of an uncooperative animal will lead to longer procedure times and increased risk of injury to the animal and veterinary staff.
- Inability to effectively remove gastric contents through lavage may be related to excessive size or adhesive nature of gastric contents, gastric compartmentalization, or other factors.
- Regurgitation during lavage, gastric overfilling, or esophageal administration of large volumes of lavage fluid can result in aspiration if a cuffed ET tube is not in place.
- Excessive tube advancement can cause occlusion of the distal end of the tube

against stomach mucosa. Palpation of the tube pressing against the stomach wall may indicate a need for partial retraction.

PROCEDURE

Manual restraint, sedation, or general anesthesia as indicated.

- Position animal in sternal recumbency. If animal is uncomfortable, alternate positions may be better tolerated (sitting, standing, lateral, etc.).
    - Placement of the animal on an elevated surface will allow gravity-assisted efflux of stomach contents and lavage fluid.
- Choose appropriate tube diameter for esophageal size and procedure planned. Example: A tube with an outer diameter of 1.5 inches (3.5 cm) is appropriate for most medium-sized dogs (45 lb [20 kg]). A larger tube size may be necessary for effective lavage versus gas decompression.
- Measure the length of tube necessary to pass from the nose to the xiphoid. Mark this distance on the tube with a piece of tape or nontoxic marker.
- Place a mouth gag (speculum) to prevent the animal from chewing on the tube.
    - A roll of 2-inch clinic-type white cloth tape works well in many animals. The tube will pass through the hole in the tape roll. Place tape roll on top of the tongue and behind the canine teeth.
    - Have an assistant hold the mouth closed around the mouth gag.
    - Avoid using a gag that will damage the teeth.
- Generously lubricate the distal portion of the stomach tube.
- Pass the tube into the mouth through the mouth gag.
- Advance the tube through the oropharynx and into the esophagus. Steps to promote and confirm esophageal and subsequent gastric intubation include the following:
    - Choice of a larger gastric tube size than appropriate ET tube size will lessen the possibility of tracheal intubation.
    - A neutral or very slightly ventroflexed position of the head (i.e., avoiding extension of the neck) will reduce the opportunity for the tube to pass into the trachea.
    - In the awake animal, allow the swallowing reflex to facilitate tube passage through the pharynx.
    - If substantial coughing occurs, reassess placement because the orogastric tube may be in the trachea.
    - Palpate the tube in the esophagus (separate from the tracheal rings).
    - Direct visualization of tube passage through the esophagus along the left side of the neck (lean, short-haired patients).
    - Small amounts of air infused into the stomach tube result in a gurgling sound when the stomach is ausculted.
    - Mild suction applied to the tube should reveal negative pressure, stomach contents, or odorous gastric gas with proper gastric intubation, whereas air flow and absence of negative pressure suggest that the tube is in the airways.
- Pass the tube up to the marked point that indicates where the tube should have entered the stomach. Relief of gas pressure can be assessed through auditory, tactile, and olfactory observations.
    - Certain conditions such as GDV may inhibit tube passage into the stomach. Choice of a smaller tube, gentle rotational pressure on the tube, repositioning of the animal, or percutaneous needle gastric decompression may facilitate passage.

DECOMPRESSION

- Place the external portion of the stomach tube lower than the animal's head and body to allow gravity-assisted evacuation of stomach contents.
- Gentle massage of the stomach through the body wall may help to increase efflux.

GAVAGE

- Using syringe, funnel, or stomach pump, instill the desired medication through the tube into the stomach.
- With administration of viscous materials, dilution with water may facilitate passage through the tube.
- Coughing, dysnea, or cyanosis at any point suggests the tube may be in the respiratory tree. The procedure is terminated immediately, with kinking of the proximal tube (to avoid leakage of tube contents during withdrawal), tube removal, and animal care (physical examination, thoracic radiography as warranted, etc.).

LAVAGE

- Using a funnel or stomach pump, instill approximately 5–10 ml/kg of lukewarm (body temperature) water into the tube.
- Acute onset of coughing, dyspnea, or cyanosis warrants immediate termination, as already described.
- Hold the tube higher than the animal's head to prevent efflux of the lavage fluid until desired.
- Gently massage the stomach to facilitate mixing of the stomach contents with the lavage.
- Lower the stomach tube below the level of the head to allow the lavage fluid to efflux. Gentle manipulation of the tube forward or backward 1–3 cm may improve efflux.
- If the tube obstructs with stomach contents, flushing or manual breakdown may relieve the obstruction. If this is unsuccessful, the tube should be removed and the entire process repeated.
- Repeat lavage administration and efflux until the efflux is clear and the stomach contents have been removed.

REMOVAL

- Kink the tube during removal to prevent laryngeal/pharyngeal contamination with liquid remaining in the tube lumen.
- Remove the mouth gag.

POSTPROCEDURE

- Monitor recovery from sedation/anesthesia.
- Supportive care as indicated for the condition.

ALTERNATIVES AND THEIR RELATIVE MERITS

- Nasoesophageal/nasogastric intubation:
    - May be less stressful to the animal than orogastric intubation.
    - Tube can be left in place for repeated aspirations/instillations.
    - Small tube diameter prevents administration of viscous substances and effective lavage. Withdrawal of large volumes of gastric contents is not possible.
- Percutaneous needle decompression/gastrocentesis:
    - May be easier to perform in a fractious animal.
    - Allows gastric gas decompression when degree of torsion or another esophageal obstruction prevents tube passage.
    - Potential for splenic puncture/laceration, gastric vessel or wall laceration, or other abdominal trauma.
    - Ineffective for removing ingesta or large volumes of gastric contents.
- Manual oral administration of medications or formula (pediatric animals):
    - Decreased chance of complications associated with orogastric intubation and gavage.
    - Administration of large volumes to an uncooperative animal is labor intensive.
    - Risk of aspiration with force-feeding.
- Induced emesis to clear gastric contents:
    - Often more effective at removing stomach contents than lavage.
    - Risk of aspiration, especially with decreased mentation or laryngeal/pharyngeal dysfunction.
    - Not indicated with caustic ingestions.
    - Not effective in all animals.

AUTHOR: **LILLIAN I. GOOD**

Gastroscopy/Duodenoscopy

BASIC INFORMATION

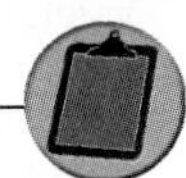

SYNONYM(S)

Upper gastrointestinal (GI) endoscopy

OVERVIEW AND GOAL(S)

Minimally invasive, endoscopic method of visualizing the mucosal surface of the stomach and proximal duodenum. This procedure offers the possibility of retrieving foreign bodies, performing mucosal biopsies, and placing a gastrostomy or jejunostomy tube.

INDICATIONS

- Chronic or acute vomiting
- Gastric foreign body
- Suspicion of gastric or duodenal ulcer
- Suspicion of gastric or duodenal neoplasia
- Suspicion of inflammatory bowel disease or gastric/duodenal neoplasia
- Placement of percutaneous endoscopic gastrostomy (PEG) tube for enteral feeding

CONTRAINDICATIONS

- Food in stomach
- Large and/or sharp foreign body

EQUIPMENT, ANESTHESIA

- General anesthesia required.
- Endotracheal intubation required.
- Mouth gag/speculum.
- Flexible fiberoptic endoscope with monocular or video display:
  - Diameter of 9-10 mm and length of 1000-1250 mm are sufficient for both gastroscopy and duodenoscopy of most medium- to large-sized dogs and for only gastroscopy of cats and small dogs.
  - A diameter of 5.5 mm or less is usually necessary to enter the duodenum of cats or small dogs. A length of 900-1000 mm is usually sufficient for cats and small dogs.
- Vacuum source for endoscopic suction.
- Endoscopic biopsy forceps.
- Endoscopic foreign body retrieval forceps, snares, or baskets.
- Biopsy jar with 10% buffered formalin.

ANTICIPATED TIME

- Usually 60-90 minutes anesthesia time (30-60 minutes endoscopy time).
- Complex foreign body retrieval may take >60 minutes.

PREPARATION: IMPORTANT CHECKPOINTS

- Animal should have fasted for 12 hours prior to the procedure if possible.
- Simpler, less invasive diagnostic procedures are performed prior to endoscopy (e.g., complete blood count [CBC], serum biochemistry profile, urinalysis, abdominal radiographs in all cases, abdominal ultrasound, fecal flotation, adrenocorticotropic hormone [ACTH] stimulation test, and others as indicated by the specific features of each case).

POSSIBLE COMPLICATIONS AND COMMON ERRORS TO AVOID

- Narcotic analgesics (e.g., morphine, meperidine, and butorphanol) increase motility of the pyloric antrum and may make passage of the endoscope into the duodenum difficult.
- Gastric or duodenal rupture:
  - Usually only occurs when the wall is compromised by a deep ulcer or neoplasia.
- Overinsufflation, usually of the stomach, may cause potentially severe bradycardia due to abdominal compartment syndrome (see Abdominal Compartment Syndrome, p 2) and creates the risk of gastric rupture.
- Prior administration of barium may make visualization difficult, and aspirating it with suction through the endoscope may be damaging to the suction channel of the endoscope.
- Failure to recognize the major duodenal papilla as a normal structure (major and minor duodenal papillae in cats) could lead to inadvertent biopsy, which in turn presents the potential for fibrosis and obstruction of the pancreatic and common bile ducts.

PROCEDURE

- Induce general anesthesia.
- Position the animal in left lateral recumbency. This is the position in which the pylorus is most easily entered.
- Place a mouth gag to keep the jaws open.
- Lubricate the endoscope with water-based lubricating jelly.
- Introduce the endoscope into the mouth, and feed it gently through the upper esophageal sphincter.
- Examine the esophageal mucosa as the scope is advanced down to the lower esophageal sphincter.
- Insufflate the esophagus with enough air to prevent the walls from collapsing on the scope and reducing visibility. An assistant may be required to gently occlude the upper esophagus by gently squeezing the cervical region externally, immediately cranial to the larynx, to prevent insufflated air from escaping out of the mouth. This will not be necessary once the tip of the endoscope is in the stomach.
- Whenever the scope is traveling down a tubular structure, such as the esophagus or duodenum, it is important to keep repositioning the scope so that the lumen of the tube is kept in the center of the screen. This maximizes visibility and minimizes trauma to the gut wall.
- Thread the scope through the lower esophageal sphincter by keeping the opening to the stomach in the center of the screen/view piece while gently advancing the scope.
- Once the distal end of the endoscope is in the stomach, insufflate the stomach with air to separate the walls and improve visibility. Insufflate until the rugal folds of the stomach are less prominent but still present. If the rugal folds are completely flattened, the stomach is so inflated that there is risk of compromising respiration or rupturing the stomach.
- If duodenoscopy is to be performed, it is best to proceed directly to the pylorus while it still may be relaxed. Prolonged insufflation or other activity in the stomach stimulates pyloric tone and motility, making threading the scope through the pylorus more difficult.
- Advancing the scope through the pylorus is usually the most difficult part of this procedure. The tone and degree of patency of the pylorus can be quite variable.
- If it is difficult to advance the scope to the opening of the pylorus (i.e., the scope is fed into the animal but advances no closer to the pylorus), suction some air out of the stomach—it may have been overinflated. This is common in large-breed dogs.
- If the pylorus is open, immediately advance the scope into the duodenum. If the pylorus is closed, maintain the opening to the pylorus in the middle of the screen while gently advancing the scope. If resistance is encountered, do not force the scope. Sometimes insufflating some air at the

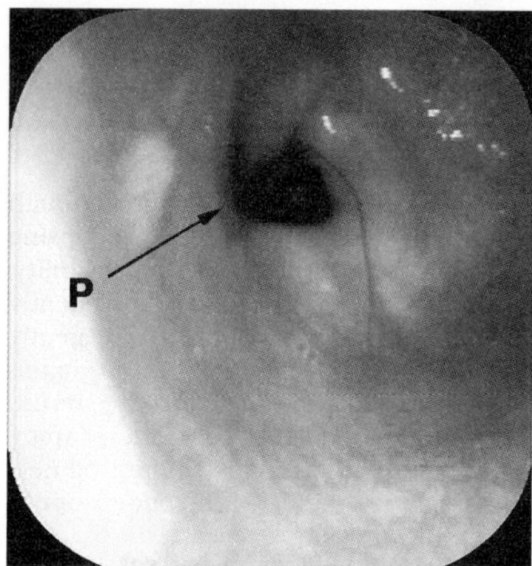

FIGURE II-81 Endoscopic view of the normal pylorus (P).

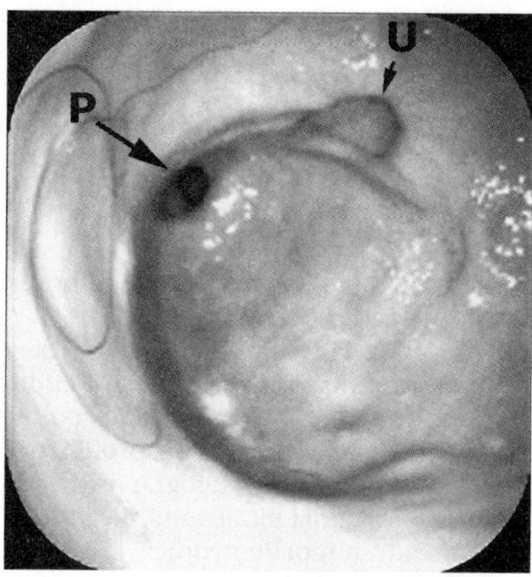

FIGURE II-82 Endoscopic view of the pylorus (P) and a large, crater-like gastric ulcer (U).

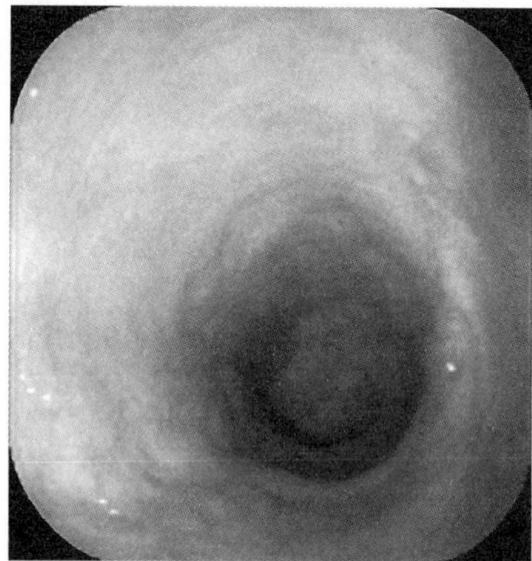

FIGURE II-83 Endoscopic view of the normal duodenum.

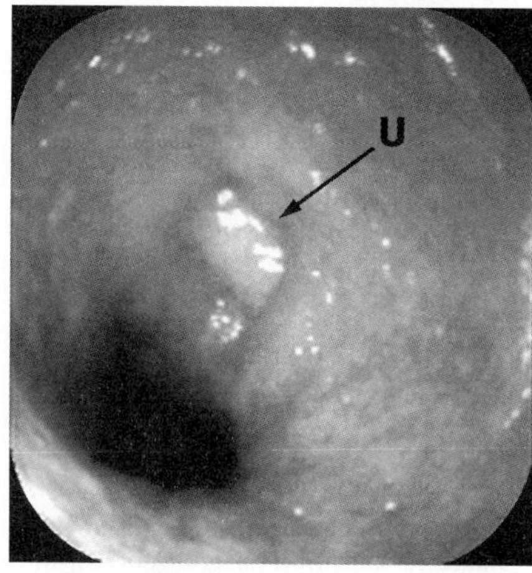

FIGURE II-84 Endoscopic view of a duodenal ulcer (U).

opening of the pylorus will stimulate it to open.

- If the pylorus is impossible to thread, try feeding a closed pair of endoscopic biopsy forceps through the pylorus. Use the threaded forceps as a stylet to feed the scope into the duodenum. If the scope still will not pass through the pylorus, consider using a smaller scope.
- Once the distal end of the endoscope is in the duodenum, advance the scope down to the limit of its length.
- Identify, if possible, the major duodenal papilla where the pancreatic duct and the common bile duct empty into the duodenum. Do not biopsy this structure accidentally.
- Examine and identify any irregularities to the duodenal mucosa and any foreign bodies.
- Obtain multiple (6–12) mucosal biopsies using biopsy forceps. Store these biopsies in 10% formalin. Any brushings or fluid samples for cytologic analysis or culture may be obtained now as well.
- Slowly withdraw the endoscope from the duodenum while obtaining mucosal biopsies and deflating the duodenum.
- Once back in the stomach, examine the entire stomach, including obtaining a retroflexed view to visualize the gastric cardia. This maneuver requires maximal flexion of the endoscope tip, such that the endoscope itself is seen emerging through the cardia. Identify any mucosal irregularities, masses, ulcers, or foreign bodies.
- Obtain multiple (6–12) biopsies of any irregular structures and normal mucosa. Be cautious about taking a biopsy of deep gastric ulcers because this could cause perforation of the stomach wall.
- Deflate the stomach before withdrawing the endoscope into the esophagus.
- Deflate the esophagus while slowly continuing to withdraw the endoscope from the esophagus. Suction any fluid in the esophagus because it may be refluxed gastric acid that may ulcerate the esophagus if left behind.
- Take the scope out of the animal, remove the mouth gag, and recover the animal from anesthesia.

POSTPROCEDURE

- This procedure is minimally invasive, and the animal rarely requires analgesics after the endoscopy.
- Anesthetic recovery is usually routine.
- Clean the endoscope (internal and external surfaces) immediately before secretions and fluid have dried and are difficult to remove.

ALTERNATIVES AND THEIR RELATIVE MERITS

Exploratory laparotomy:

- Large, full-thickness biopsies may be taken from anywhere in the GI tract.
- All the abdominal organs may be visualized and biopsied if needed.
- Virtually any foreign body may be retrieved anywhere in the stomach or intestine.
- Serosal surfaces and wall thickness can be evaluated.
- Gastrostomy tube or jejunostomy tube may be placed.
- Tumors or abnormal tissue may be surgically excised.
- More invasive.
- May be more costly.
- May be more time consuming.
- More painful for the animal/longer recovery time.
- Greater risk of peritonitis and incisional dehiscence.
- Unable to visualize the esophagus.
- Unable to visualize the mucosal surface of stomach or intestines unless a gastrostomy or an enterotomy is performed.

AUTHOR: **PETER FOLEY**

Hemodialysis

BASIC INFORMATION

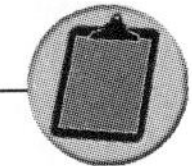

SYNONYM(S)

Blood purification
Renal replacement therapy

OVERVIEW AND GOAL(S)

Hemodialysis is a blood purification procedure used for correcting the azotemia and for normalizing the fluid, electrolyte, and acid-base imbalances resulting from renal failure. In this procedure, the animal's anticoagulated blood circulates through an artificial kidney (hemodialyzer) and is exposed to an electrolyte solution (dialysate) across a semipermeable membrane. Metabolic waste products, exogenous toxins, and excess water are removed from the bloodstream by diffusion (concentration gradient) and convection (hydrostatic gradient) through the dialysis membrane.

In acute uremia, hemodialysis restores metabolic stability and is provided for a finite period of time to allow animals to use their potential of recovery from acute renal injury. Hemodialysis itself has no direct effect on renal recovery. Hemodialysis can be used further for indefinite renal replacement in end-stage chronic renal failure.

INDICATIONS

- Acute uremia: worsening azotemia and clinical signs of uremia despite adequate conventional therapy, anuria, fluid overload, severe azotemia (blood urea nitrogen [BUN] >100 mg/dl, creatinine >10 mg/dl); severe refractory hyperkalemia.
- Chronic renal failure: acute decompensation, preanesthetic stabilization, pretransplant conditioning, chronic renal replacement therapy.
- Miscellaneous: fluid overload; acute poisoning; drug overdose (removal of small-molecular-weight toxins or drugs that have minimal protein binding capacity).

CONTRAINDICATIONS

- Small animal size (<2 kg) (relative contraindication)
- Severe pulmonary or cerebral hemorrhage (due to required anticoagulation)

EQUIPMENT, ANESTHESIA

Sedation/anesthesia: required for the placement of a large-bore double-lumen catheter (vascular access) but not for the hemodialysis procedure itself once vascular access is established.

- Vascular access: short-term, temporary double-lumen catheter (minimum of 7 Fr for cats and small dogs; 11.5 Fr for larger dogs); long-term, permanent double-lumen or twin-lumen catheter with subcutaneous tunneling; typically placed in the external jugular vein.
- Hemodialysis delivery system (hemodialysis machine).
- Disposable extracorporeal circuit.
- Disposable dialyzer (artificial kidney).
- Water purification system: particulate filter, carbon sorbent, water softener, deionization bed, and reverse osmosis.
- Dialysate concentrates: acid concentrate, bicarbonate.
- Monitoring equipment: blood pressure (BP) monitor, coagulation timer (e.g., activated clotting time [ACT]), in-line blood volume and oxygen saturation monitor (e.g., Critline), electrocardiogram (ECG).
- Emergency cart: cardiopulmonary resuscitation drugs, oxygen, endotracheal tube.
- Protamine (for excessive heparinization and active hemorrhage).
- Physical restraint (i.e., harness and table straps).

ANTICIPATED TIME

- Chronic treatments: 4-5 hours, three times a week.
- Acute treatments: depending on the degree of azotemia and the selected therapeutic schedule, initial treatments can be shorter (3-4 hours) or longer (extended slow therapy); they are provided daily until normalization of azotemia is achieved; a three times a week schedule is then maintained until recovery of renal function.
- Every treatment necessitates 2 additional hours for setup, animal preparation, and completion.

PREPARATION: IMPORTANT CHECKPOINTS

- Initial database for animal evaluation and formulation of the dialysis prescription: body weight, physical exam, body temperature, heart rate, BP, hematocrit/total solids, serum chemistry profile (especially BUN, creatinine, electrolytes, TCO_2 [HCO_3^-]), coagulation time (e.g., ACT).
- Adequacy of vascular access: should deliver between 15-50 ml/min in cats and very small dogs and 200-500 ml/min in large-breed dogs.
- Preparation of the dialysis system: priming and recirculation of the extracorporeal circuit, alarm testing, refreshing of the extracorporeal circuit.
- Dialysis prescription: type and size of dialyzer and extracorporeal circuit; total volume of blood to be processed; duration of the treatment; ultrafiltration (fluid removal); dialysate composition and modeling (Na^+, K^+, bicarbonate, additives); dialysate flow rate, direction, and temperature; anticoagulation (type, prime, constant infusion rate); type of fluid used to prime the extracorporeal circuit (crystalloid, colloid, blood); and special procedures (e.g., single-needle operation, bypass time).

POSSIBLE COMPLICATIONS AND COMMON ERRORS TO AVOID

- Intradialytic complications: hemorrhage, hypotension, vomiting (hypovolemia, dialyzer reaction), dialysis disequilibrium (osmotic fluid shift into the intracellular compartment due to rapid correction of the azotemia; cellular edema; can progress to cerebral edema and death), malfunction of vascular access, clotting of the extracorporeal circulation.
- Interdialytic complications: hemorrhage, delayed dialysis disequilibrium, catheter complications (thrombosis, vascular stenosis, infection, chylothorax).
- Other complications: related to severe uremia (i.e., uremic pneumonitis, encephalopathy, ulcers), its treatment (i.e., fluid overload, drug toxicity), or to the underlying etiology precipitating the renal failure (i.e., sepsis, hypovolemic shock).

PROCEDURE

Establishment of vascular access:

- A temporary or permanent dialysis catheter is placed aseptically in the external jugular vein, with the tip reaching in the cranial vena cava or the right atrium. Permanent catheters require placement with the animal under general anesthesia because they involve venotomy and subcutaneous tunneling. Proper placement is confirmed by adequate blood flow and thoracic radiographs/fluoroscopy. The dialysis catheter is dedicated to dialysis therapy, and it is never used for other indications. It is prepared and handled aseptically for each use.

Initiation of dialysis therapy:

- The dialysis machine is equipped with appropriate disposables (extracorporeal circuit, hemodialyzer), and its function is tested according to the manufacturer's protocols. Animals are equipped with a harness and strapped to the table to loosely restrain their activity.

- The catheter is connected to the extracorporeal circuit using aseptic techniques, and the extension lines are secured to the animal's body to avoid accidental catheter removal. The extracorporeal circulation is established under close monitoring of cardiovascular and respiratory status, and it is progressively increased to reach the prescribed blood flow.

Monitoring:

- Cardiovascular parameters (heart rate, BP, venous oxygen saturation, relative blood volume change), general condition (mentation, pupillary light reflexes), anticoagulation (i.e., ACT), and machine function (extracorporeal blood flow, dialyzer clearance) are monitored and recorded every 15-30 minutes for the duration of the treatment.
- Initial dialysis treatments commonly necessitate additional monitoring, including ECG and pulse oximetry.

End of therapy:

- The blood circulating in the extracorporeal circuit is returned to the animal, and the disposables are discarded.
- The dialysis catheter is locked with a solution of concentrated heparin (100-500 U/ml in cats; 1000-5000 U/ml in dogs) and protected with a neck bandage until the next treatment.

POSTPROCEDURE

- Monitor for hemorrhage and dialysis disequilibrium (neurologic changes).
- Because of the persisting effect of systemic heparinization: no needle stick (IV, IM, SQ), no placement or removal of IV or arterial catheters, and no procedure that could potentially cause mucosal or internal hemorrhages for 6-8 hours following discontinuation of dialysis.
- Assessment of dialysis adequacy: treatment adequacy implies global control of all the individual problems of renal failure, of which dialysis only addresses a few. Nutrition; pain control; treatment of renal hyperparathyroidism, anemia, and metabolic acidosis; and further supportive care are critical for successful therapy and are not corrected by hemodialysis. Predialysis and postdialysis serum biochemistry profiles are routinely performed to assess the adequacy of the dialysis treatment. Blood volume processed, time on dialysis, convective fluid removal (ultrafiltration), normalization of chemistry parameters, and reduction ratios of urea and creatinine are commonly used for describing treatments. However, dialytic adequacy is better assessed and more accurately described using kinetic modeling of dialytic removal and interdialytic generation of urea. Because urea kinetic modeling provides additional insight into the nutritional adequacy of animals undergoing dialysis, it should be considered as part of the global assessment for animals treated with this form of renal replacement therapy.
- Maintenance of the dialysis equipment is critical for adequate operation and safety of the procedure: Before each treatment, dialysate is controlled for traces of residual chlorine; at the end of each treatment, the machine is rinsed with acid and bleach to remove bicarbonate and protein deposits, respectively. At the end of every dialysis day, the machine is disinfected with a chemical or heat cycle. Once a week, the machine is disinfected with a dwell cycle, and once a month, a quantitative bacteriologic culture of the dialysate water is performed. A chemical water analysis for trace elements is scheduled once a year.

ALTERNATIVES AND THEIR RELATIVE MERITS

- Continuous renal replacement therapy (CRRT): a slower but extended form of dialysis therapy with more gradual correction of hydration and metabolic imbalances; lower blood and dialysate flow rates imply fewer treatment interruptions and alarms and, potentially, a technically less demanding form of therapy. Therapeutic decisions and design of adequate and safe treatment plans still require a thorough understanding of renal pathophysiology and of dialysis technology, especially when used for treating severely uremic animals that are a very small size. After initial correction of the azotemia, maintenance of uremic animals with CRRT is hampered by the low efficiency of the treatments and the need for continuous therapy.
- Renal transplantation: offers the potential of long-term replacement of all renal functions when recovery can no longer be expected; requires surgical expertise and experience with the management of the long-term immunosuppression required to avoid graft rejection.

AUTHOR: **THIERRY FRANCEY**

Holter/Cardiac Event Monitoring

BASIC INFORMATION

SYNONYM(S)

Cardiac telemetry

OVERVIEW AND GOAL(S)

To assess the cardiac rhythm during a period of hours or more. The monitor may record the rhythm continuously for 24 to 48 hours (Holter monitor) or intermittently over a period of days to weeks, during which time the owner observes clinical signs (event monitor).

INDICATIONS

- Syncope
- Episodic clinical signs of uncertain type but that might represent syncope
- Screening of animals for latent arrhythmia (arrhythmia not causing overt clinical signs)
- Monitoring of antiarrhythmic drug effects (Holter monitor only)

CONTRAINDICATIONS

- Animal thought to be likely to damage a portable monitor
- Animal that will be bathed or will be swimming
- Animal too small to carry monitor (monitoring may still take place, but animal stays mainly in pet carrier or cage for recording period)

EQUIPMENT, ANESTHESIA

- Clippers for hair.
- Isopropyl alcohol.
- Gauze squares or cotton balls.
- Cardiac electrode adhesive patches (cutaneous).

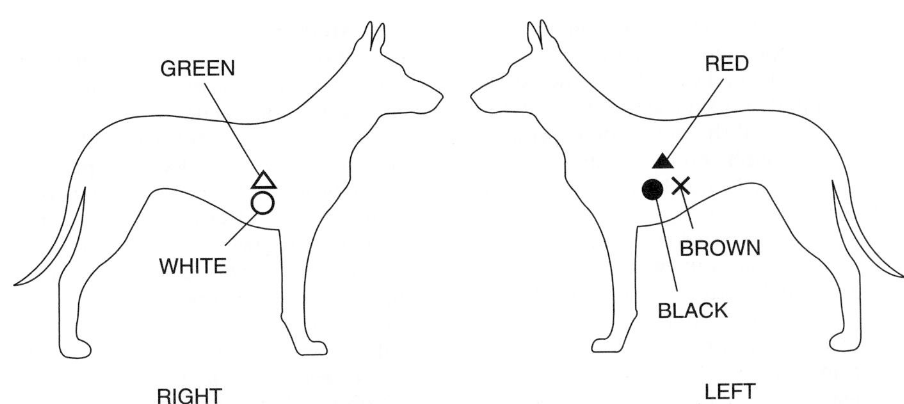

FIGURE II-85 Electrode patch placement for Holter monitor. Colors correspond to the colors of the connecting tips on the ends of the Holter monitor wires. Reprinted with permission from Côté E, Ettinger SJ: Electrocardiography and cardiac arrhythmias. In Ettinger SJ, Feldman EC (eds): *Textbook of Veterinary Internal Medicine*, ed 6. St. Louis, WB Saunders, 2005.

- Tissue glue.
- Ultrasound gel.
- Bandage material: roll gauze, Esmarch-type bandage material (e.g., Vetrap), stretch adhesive-type cotton bandage (e.g., Elastikon, Elastoplast), white medical tape.
- Holter or event monitor, including wires to connect to animal, new batteries, and a blank audio cassette tape (Holter only).
- Interpretation system and printer or access to such a system.

NOTE: Monitors are expensive systems not routinely owned by general practices. They are available for rental from many sources, including www.labcorp.com, www.vetheart.com, www.idexx.com, and www. pdsheart.com. The monitor itself is sent by courier to the hospital for placement on the animal. When the monitoring period is over, the supplier receives the tape (Holter) or transtelephonic signal (event monitor) and reports the findings and interpretations.

ANTICIPATED TIME

- Installation: 10 minutes (event monitor) or 20 minutes (Holter).
- Monitoring period: 24 or 48 hours (Holter); 7-18 days (event monitor; weeks to many months for surgically implanted event monitors).

PREPARATION: IMPORTANT CHECKPOINTS

If the reason for using cardiac monitoring is the occurrence of sporadic clinical signs, a complete medical evaluation is usually indicated first:

- Complete blood count (CBC), serum biochemistry panel, urinalysis; all cases, hypoglycemia, hypocalcemia.
- Serum preprandial and postprandial bile acids (if consistent with case): hepatic encephalopathy.
- Electrocardiogram (ECG; standard, in-hospital): all cases; the diagnosis may be apparent without the need for Holter or cardiac event monitoring.
- Thoracic radiographs, echocardiogram: all cases; assessment of cardiac structure, presence or absence of signs of congestive heart failure.

The monitor itself is checked for proper function before preparing to install it on the animal. For the Holter monitor, the audiotape should be seen to advance; event monitor: digital display of remaining episodes available in memory (large number) and days of battery life remaining (small number).

Discussion of care of the monitor with the owner: The monitor must stay dry, clean, intact, and undamaged. It is customary to have the owner leave a deposit in the sum of the replacement cost of the monitor before leaving the hospital with the machine.

POSSIBLE COMPLICATIONS AND COMMON ERRORS TO AVOID

- Wet monitor: no swimming or bathing during the recording period; in the rain: a plastic bag needs to be placed over the monitor by the owner.
- Damaged/chewed monitor or wires: If the owner observes the animal damaging the monitor, an immediate recheck is warranted. The equipment can be examined and, subsequently, the monitor may simply be more heavily wrapped to prevent damage, or the monitoring period may be terminated and the monitor removed.
- Unstuck electrode patches: prevented by cleaning and preparing the skin with isopropyl alcohol prior to patch placement and by using an extremely small

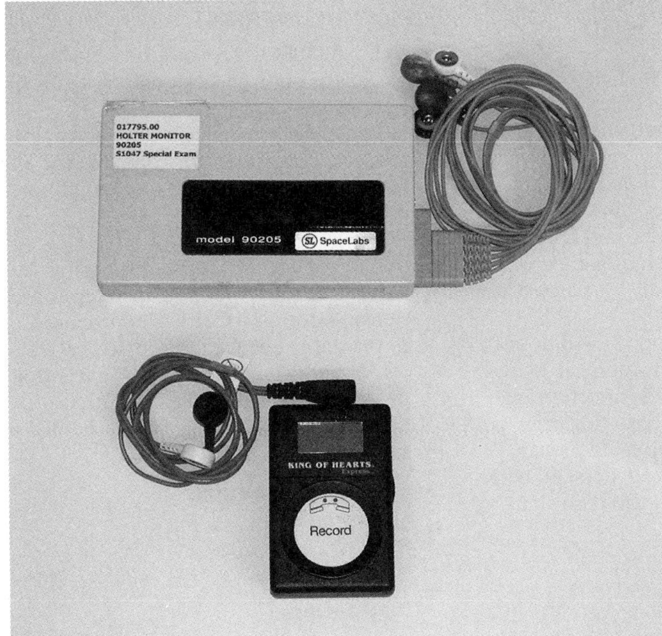

FIGURE II-86 Holter monitor (above) and event monitor (below), with wires and connecting electrodes at the ends of the wires (five wires for the Holter; two wires for the event monitor).

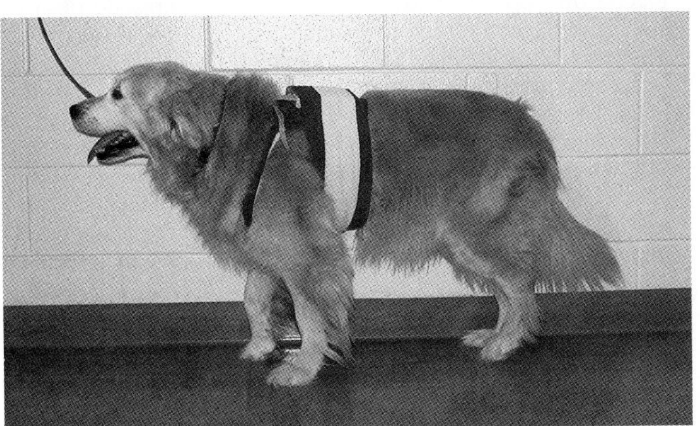

FIGURE II-87 Final appearance of a properly placed Holter monitor on a medium-sized dog.

amount of tissue glue to attach the patches to the skin, as described below.
- Poor electrode patch contact with skin: prevented by cleaning and preparing the skin with isopropyl alcohol prior to patch placement and by adding a small amount of ultrasound gel to the center of the patch before applying it to the skin (see following paragraphs).
- Monitoring period is inexplicably shorter than expected: prevented by using new batteries every time. In addition, for Holter monitors, it is important to be sure that the audiotape is not put into the monitor backwards.
- Poor triggering of event button (Holter) or record button (event monitor): prevented by carefully showing the owners how to trigger the event and record buttons on the monitor at the time of installation.
- Letting batteries run out, causing the captured events to be deleted (event monitor): Clients need to return 1 day prior to expected end of battery life.

PROCEDURE

HOLTER MONITOR

- The animal's apex beat (heartbeat on the thorax) is palpated on both the right and left side of the chest. These will be the sites of electrode patch placement.
- The hair is clipped over these areas bilaterally, ensuring a generous clip: There must be room for the electrode patches and a few centimeters of space separating them.
- The hairless skin is wiped clean with isopropyl alcohol–soaked gauze or cotton and allowed to dry.
- Some cardiologists prefer to attach the patches to the wires of the monitor prior to placing the patches on the animal, which is acceptable. The following method will describe the alternative approach.
- Patch preparation: A very small dollop of ultrasound gel is placed on the center of each electrode patch, and a tiny amount of tissue glue (<1 full drop) is placed on opposite ends of the adhesive band of each electrode patch.
- The patches are attached to the animal's skin: three patches on the left in a triangular conformation and two patches (one ventral to the other) on the right.
- The wires are attached to the patches according to the color scheme shown in Fig. II-85. Pressing the wire attachments directly onto the patches on the thorax can be painful to the animal and is not recommended. Rather, after the patch is attached to the skin, the patch and underlying skin are elevated with the finger, and the electrode is pressed in using thumb and forefinger.
- The monitor is attached to the animal as follows:
  - The monitor is held in a dorsal midline location but not wrapped at first; rather, roll gauze is wrapped around the chest, incorporating the wires such that they emerge at the dorsal midline.
  - Esmarch-type (e.g., Vetrap) bandage material is wrapped over the gauze, around the thorax, as well as cranial to the shoulders in a figure-eight pattern, creating a "vest" of bandage material. The monitor is not included in this layer.
  - Finally, the monitor is attached over the dorsal midline using elastic cotton adhesive (Elastikon-type) bandage material that encircles the chest. It is often useful to place a roll of gauze under each side of the monitor to stabilize it directly on the midline when it is wrapped.
  - This last step can be replaced with the use of a dog backpack (available in stores that sell equipment for outdoor activities) or a purpose-made Holter vest for dogs.
  - The monitor's event button should still be visible and accessible to the owner, but connections onto the thorax, loops of wire, and the rest of the monitor itself should be protected.
- If a clock setting can be adjusted on the monitor, it is set to the current time. If not, the times at which the battery was installed and the recording began are noted as time zero in the medical record.
- The owner needs to be instructed to keep a diary of the dog's activities, including the time of the observed activity. This includes both normal activities and events thought to be of clinical relevance. They also may press the event button on the monitor if an episode of apparent significance (e.g., collapse) occurs; it will be flagged on the Holter recording.

After the recording period (24–48 hours):
- The bandage material, monitor, wires, and electrode patches are removed. Removal of the skin patches may be facilitated with isopropyl alcohol.
- The cassette is analyzed or sent back for analysis along with the recorder.

EVENT MONITOR

- Animal preparation and patch preparation are the same as for Holter monitors (as already described).
- There are only two wires/electrodes and, therefore, only two electrode patches. The right-sided electrode (white) is connected to the electrode patch on the right hemithorax, and the left-sided electrode is connected to the patch on the left, as described previously.
- The monitor is wrapped onto the animal also as described above. It is essential to leave the large white record button visible and accessible.
- When the animal has an episode, the owner must press the record button. Doing so captures the ECG preceding and following the time the button was pressed. Typically, the monitors are set to store the preceding 45-second time period of ECG and the subsequent 15 seconds, for a total of 1 minute of ECG spanning the clinical episode.
- Immediately after pressing the record button, the owner will recognize that the monitor has been successfully activated because it emits a whistling sound for several seconds while it is recording.
- Event monitors typically have a total memory of 5 minutes (i.e., five 1-minute episodes), though newer models can store 18 minutes or more.

After the recording period (usually 6 days):
- The bandaging, wires, and monitor are removed, and the stored information is immediately transmitted transtelephonically to the receiving station. Otherwise, the batteries continue to be drained, and the information eventually will be lost.

ALTERNATIVES AND THEIR RELATIVE MERITS

- In-hospital ECG: less motion artifact but generally shorter and under artificial conditions.
- Holter monitor instead of event monitor: for screening for occurrence of latent arrhythmia; for antiarrhythmic drug monitoring.
- Event monitor instead of Holter monitor: for long-term (days) monitoring; for smaller animals; for transtelephonic transmission of recorded information.
- Implantable event monitor (Reveal Plus [Medtronics]): Allows an extended period of monitoring (months) but implantation is invasive and monitors are costly.

AUTHOR: **ETIENNE CÔTÉ**

Intraosseous Catheter Placement

BASIC INFORMATION

OVERVIEW AND GOAL(S)

- Insertion and maintenance of a patent catheter in the marrow cavity of a long bone for purposes of administering parenteral fluids, drugs, blood, or virtually any other agent that is routinely given IV.
- The technique is most commonly used in debilitated neonatal and pediatric animals, in which peripheral veins may be very small and difficult to access but also in which the bone is soft and entered fairly easily.

INDICATIONS

- Urgent fluid replacement in a severely dehydrated/hypovolemic kitten or puppy (most common indication)
- Plasma or blood transfusion in an animal that has poor peripheral or jugular venous access
- Administration of drugs when IV access is not available

CONTRAINDICATIONS

- Osteopenia (nutritional or metabolic bone disease) or fracture affecting the target bone.
- Infection of the overlying soft tissues.
- Sepsis is a relative contraindication. The benefit of fluid administration must be felt to outweigh the risk of osteomyelitis.

EQUIPMENT, ANESTHESIA

Sedation or general anesthesia is necessary for animals that are otherwise well. However, intraosseous catheters are often placed in severely debilitated animals; local anesthesia with 2% lidocaine (typical kitten/puppy dose: 0.25 ml) is sufficient for these animals.

- Clippers for hair.
- Isopropyl alcohol, surgical scrub supplies, and sterile gauze squares.
- Spinal needle: typically 20 gauge, 1.5 or 2.5 inches long.
- T-port-type injection cap with side connector.
- Sterile gloves.
- Tissue glue.
- Heparinized saline flushes.
- Bandage material: roll gauze, cast padding, Esmarch-type bandage (e.g., Vetrap), white medical tape.
- Suture scissors and bandage scissors.
- ± Splint material (e.g., wooden tongue depressor in pediatric patients) to protect the spinal needle after placement.

ANTICIPATED TIME

About 20 minutes

PREPARATION: IMPORTANT CHECKPOINTS

- Review anatomic landmarks.
- Consider alternatives (e.g., IV catheter).

POSSIBLE COMPLICATIONS AND COMMON ERRORS TO AVOID

- Damage to nerves (especially sciatic) or vessels. Risk is minimized by manipulating the limbs as described in the following paragraphs.
- Spinal needle kinking, causing obstruction; common: minimized by using a needle that is not excessively long, that is not overly thin (a 22-gauge needle should probably be the smallest used in even the smallest animals), and by bandaging the proximal/protruding part of the needle in a way that reduces the lateral forces applied to it when the animal bumps against the cage wall, lies down, or rolls over.
- Using a regular 18-gauge needle (hypodermic/injection-type) instead of a spinal needle has been described, but this approach is not recommended. The procedure involves "coring out" a path by placing an 18-gauge needle in the appropriate place, immediately removing it (since, without a stylet, it will be plugged with bone), and placing a second, new 18-gauge needle in the tract just created by the previous needle. Complications, including replugging with bone in the second needle, inability to find the hole when placing the second needle, and leakage of fluid around the needle are extremely common. Therefore, only spinal needles (with stylets) should be used, not regular hypodermic needles.

PROCEDURE

FEMORAL APPROACH

- Sedation/general anesthesia is administered if deemed necessary based on animal parameters (e.g., mentation, extent of illness, vital signs).
- The animal is placed in lateral recumbency, and the nondependent leg is used.
- The clinician palpates the hip; the greater trochanter of the femur is the outer/lateral landmark, and the trochanteric fossa medial to the greater trochanter is the target.
- The overlying skin is clipped of hair and aseptically prepped.
- If no sedation or general anesthetic has been administered, local anesthetic is infiltrated into the trochanteric fossa at this time.
- A 2-mm stab incision is made in the skin overlying the trochanteric fossa.
- The femur is rotated internally and adducted and is held in this position during needle placement to reduce the risk of traumatizing the sciatic nerve.
- The sciatic nerve courses medial to the trochanteric fossa, dorsal to the acetabulum. Therefore, entering the trochanteric fossa from its lateral-most aspect minimizes the risk of sciatic nerve damage.
- The spinal needle is placed through the stab incision in the skin and onto the greater trochanter (lateral to target). It is then moved gradually in a medial direction until it enters the trochanteric fossa.
- Once in the trochanteric fossa, the needle is advanced parallel to the long axis of the bone, with the hub of the needle held firmly to allow a burrowing, clockwise-counterclockwise rotating motion to facilitate advancement of the needle. A mild loss of resistance is usually felt when the needle reaches the marrow cavity. NOTE: It is important not to advance the needle the length of the entire bone and into the distal cortex because this could block flow through the needle.
- When the needle is sufficiently advanced, the stylet is withdrawn. The T-port is filled with heparinized saline, fitted onto the spinal needle hub, and flushed with heparinized saline.
- The spinal needle is sutured in place (to prevent migration outward) using a Chinese finger-trap suture pattern. This may be further solidified by applying tissue glue to the suture as it courses over the hub of the spinal needle and the T-port.
- Cast padding, roll gauze, and bandage material are rolled around and over the needle hub and T-port in a way that protects the needle from becoming kinked or damaged with the animal's movements. Wooden tongue depressors or other splint materials can be useful for protecting the part of the needle that protrudes from the femur.
- The T-port can be connected to an IV fluid set, a blood transfusion set, or other, based on the animal's needs.
- There should be no outward signs of discomfort; if there are, nerve damage or other complications should be sus-

PROCEDURES AND TECHNIQUES

pected, and the spinal needle may need to be withdrawn.

TIBIAL APPROACH

- The preparation is as described for the femoral approach, but the target area is the medial, proximal tibia (Fig. II-89B).
- The spinal needle enters the tibia on the medial surface of the tibial tuberosity and is directed laterodistally, as shown.
- The protocol is otherwise the same from the removal of the stylet to the end of the procedure.

POSTPROCEDURE

- Catheter care includes flushing with 0.2–0.4 ml sterile saline every 6–8 hours if an infusion is not being administered through the needle. It is important not to overflush the system in small animals, causing systemic heparinization.
- Catheter obstruction is a common problem. Most cases are prevented by proper placement (not too deep in the bone, causing blockage from the distal cortex), and proper securing and protection of the spinal needle so the animal does not bend it; prevention

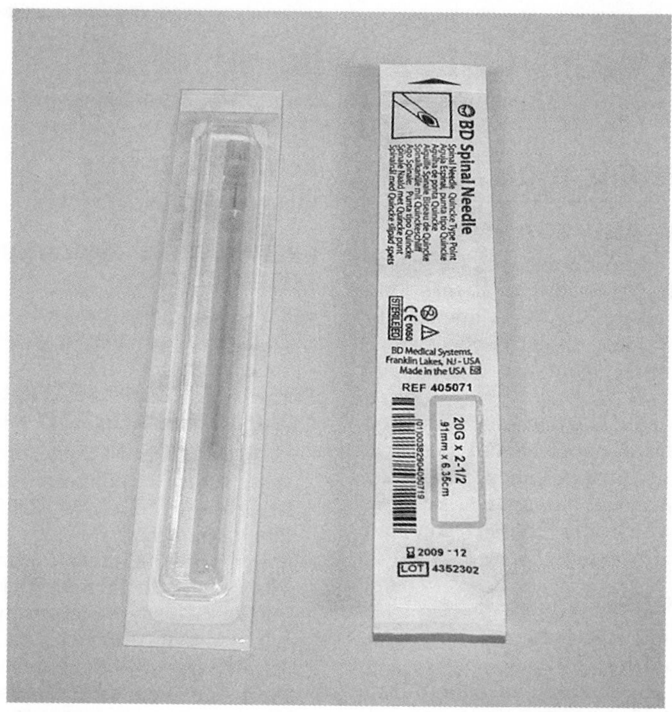

FIGURE II-88 Different views of two 20-gauge, 2.5-inch spinal needles used for intraosseous catheterization.

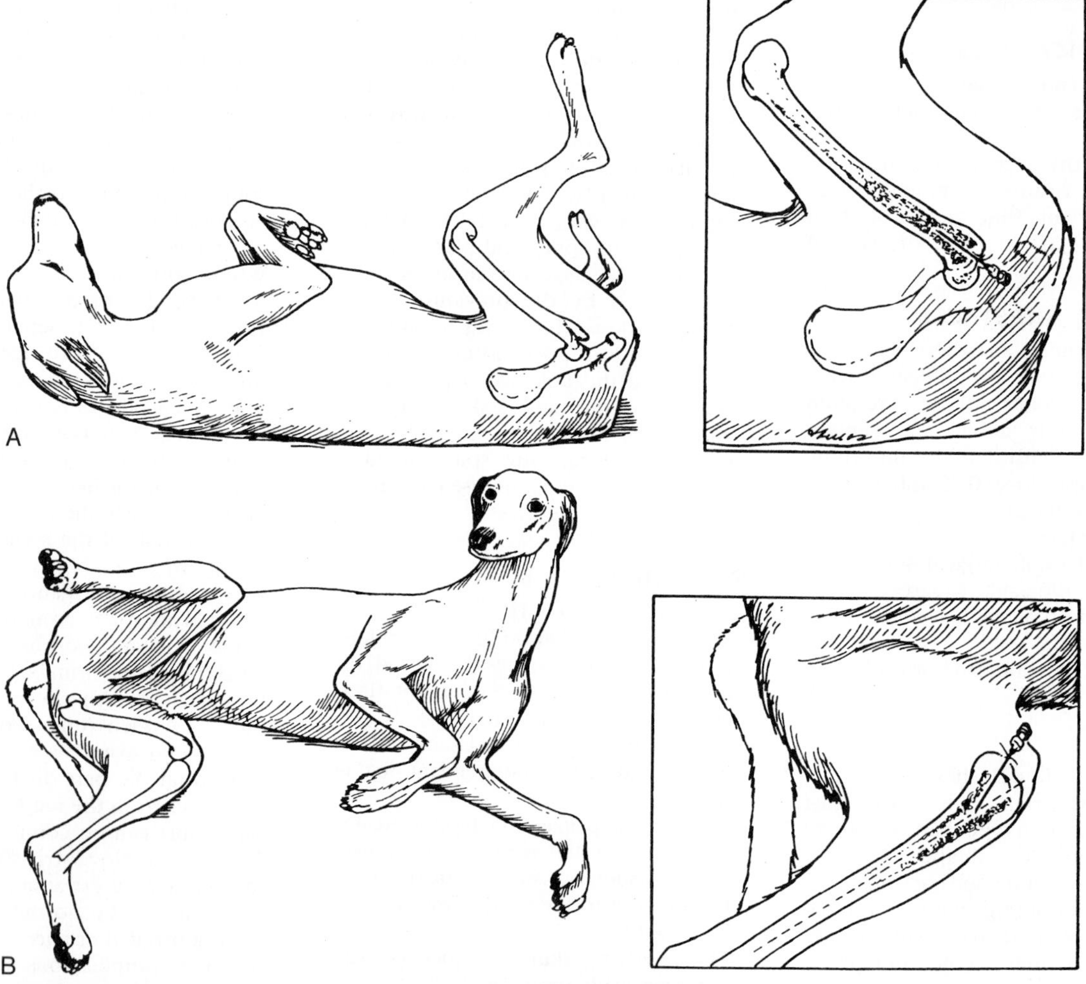

FIGURE II-89 Intraosseous catheter placement. **A**, Femoral approach. **B**, Tibial approach. Reprinted with permission from Otto CM, Crowe DT Jr. Intraosseous resuscitation techniques and applications. In Kirk RW, Bonagura JD (eds): *Kirk's Current Veterinary Therapy XI.* Philadelphia, WB Saunders, 1992.

also is possible by regular flushing or infusion to keep the catheter patent.
- If the spinal needle becomes obstructed or bent and needs to be replaced, a different bone should be chosen for intraosseous catheter placement because a minimum of 24 to 48 hours are needed for the bone to heal. Otherwise, leakage from the original needle site of entry and subcutaneous pooling of the administered fluid/blood/drug commonly occur.
- The spinal needle can usually be removed without sedation or general or local anesthesia and without eliciting signs of pain from the animal.

ALTERNATIVES AND THEIR RELATIVE MERITS

- Venous cutdown for peripheral or jugular catheter: acceptable alternative but more invasive, possibly with a greater risk of local infection.
- Intraperitoneal administration: acceptable in mildly/moderately ill pediatric animals, including for blood transfusion. Lack of direct access to the circulation is a substantial drawback compared to intraosseous catheterization.

AUTHOR: **ETIENNE CÔTÉ**

Intubation, Endotracheal

BASIC INFORMATION

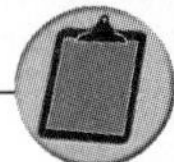

SYNONYM(S)

Placement of a tube into the tracheal lumen via an oral approach

OVERVIEW AND GOAL(S)

Endotracheal intubation is performed routinely in dogs and cats undergoing general anesthesia and is also a fundamental technique in emergency/critical care situations.

INDICATION

- To establish and maintain airway patency in animals under general anesthesia
- To protect respiratory tract from aspiration of foreign material during anesthesia
- To facilitate delivery of supplemental oxygen and volatile inhalant anesthetic agents
- To minimize exposure of hospital personnel to waste anesthetic gases
- To minimize anatomic dead space and optimize respiratory efficiency
- To facilitate delivery of positive-pressure ventilation

CONTRAINDICATIONS

Oral approach may not be possible with mandibular/maxillary trauma, temporomandibular disorders, oropharyngeal lesions, or oropharyngeal surgery where endotracheal tube placement would interfere with the surgical field.

EQUIPMENT, ANESTHESIA

Primary equipment:
- Appropriate endotracheal tube
- Adequate lighting
- Roll gauze to secure tube

Supplemental equipment:
- Laryngoscope
- Local anesthetic
- Stylet or guide tube
- Sterile, water-soluble lubricant
- Mouth speculum

ANTICIPATED TIME

- Routine: <30 seconds in an adequately anesthetized animal
- Difficult airway: <3-4 minutes

PREPARATION: IMPORTANT CHECKPOINTS

- Adequate anesthetic depth required to provide good muscle relaxation and inhibit airway reflexes.
- Preoxygenation indicated in select animals.
- Measurement of tube length and trimming if necessary (see Procedure below).

POSSIBLE COMPLICATIONS AND COMMON ERRORS TO AVOID

- Laryngospasm
- Trauma to larynx/trachea
- Vagal reflex activity
- Unrecognized esophageal intubation
- Bronchial intubation
- Postextubation upper airway obstruction

PROCEDURE

- Place anesthetized/unconscious animal in sternal recumbency.
- An assistant opens the animal's mouth by placing one finger and thumb behind the maxillary canine teeth. Lips are pulled upward and out of oral cavity. The animal's head and neck are extended to form a straight line (Fig. II-90).
- Do *not* support or put pressure under animal's neck.
- Grasp the animal's tongue, and use gentle pressure to extend it rostrally and ventrally. Excessive traction on the tongue should be avoided.
- With laryngoscope: Place tip of blade at base of tongue underneath epiglottis, and exert downward (ventral) pressure. This disengages the epiglottis from the soft palate and directs it rostrally, allowing the laryngeal opening to be visualized. NOTE: Do not place laryngoscope blade on top of epiglottis.
- Without a laryngoscope: Use the endotracheal tube to disengage the epiglottis from the soft palate and expose laryngeal opening.
- If local anesthetic is used for desensitizing the larynx, apply it to vocal folds using spray dispenser, cotton swab, or hypodermic needle and syringe for topical application.
- Advance endotracheal tube between the vocal folds into trachea. In cats, wait until the folds separate during inspiration before attempting to advance tube.
- Do not force tube. If resistance is encountered, back out slightly, maneuver tip of tube's bevel between the vocal folds, and gently rotate tube while advancing.
- Ensure that distal portion of tube lies at level of thoracic inlet and that proximal end terminates at level of animal's incisors. Tubes may need to be shortened to appropriate length before placement.
- Tie piece of roll gauze tightly around tube, without constricting lumen, at a point caudal to animal's incisor teeth. Secure gauze around maxilla or back of animal's head.
- Connect endotracheal tube to breathing system and begin delivery of oxygen.
- Close pop-off valve and gently squeeze reservoir bag until a pressure of 20 cm of H_2O is reached in breathing system while listening for sound of leaking air exiting oral cavity around tube. Incrementally inflate cuff on tube using an "air syringe" until sound of leak is terminated. Avoid cuff overinflation, and remember to open pop-off valve once cuff is inflated.
- Correct tube placement may be confirmed by:
  - Palpation of single tubular structure in cervical region (as opposed to two tubes, representing an intubated

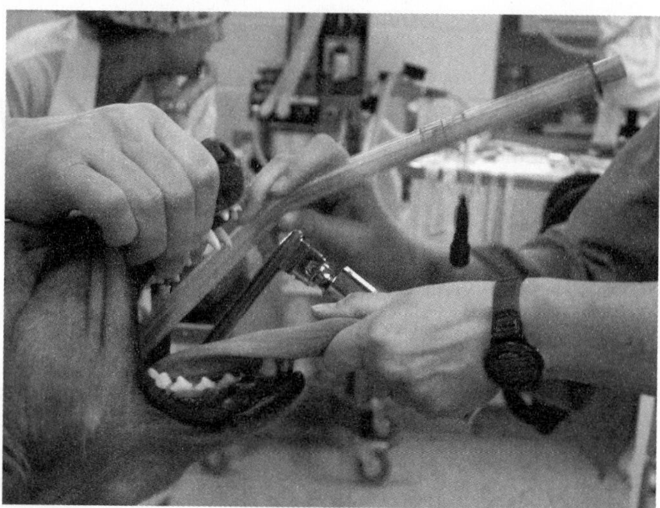

FIGURE II-90 Intubation of an anesthetized dog. An assistant extends the dog's neck and retracts the lips. The right-handed clinician is holding both a laryngoscope and the dog's tongue in the left hand and is placing the endotracheal tube using the right hand.

esophagus alongside a trachea that is not intubated).
  - Movement of reservoir bag corresponding to thoracic wall movements associated with animal inspiration/expiration.
  - Auscultation of good breath sounds bilaterally during positive-pressure ventilation.
  - Detection of carbon dioxide in animal's exhaled gases and evidence of normal capnographic tracing.

POSTPROCEDURE

- Extubate when animal's oral/pharyngeal reflexes have returned.
- In brachycephalic animals, endotracheal tube should be left in place as long as possible during recovery.
- In animals undergoing procedures associated with accumulation of blood/fluid in oral cavity, cuff may be left partially inflated during extubation.

ALTERNATIVES AND THEIR RELATIVE MERITS

Tracheostomy or pharyngostomy: Oral approach is preferred in routine cases (no tissue trauma and technically simple to perform).

AUTHOR: **LEIGH A. LAMONT**

Jugular Catheter Placement and Management

BASIC INFORMATION

OVERVIEW AND GOAL(S)

Jugular venous access is essential in small animal critical care and general medicine for a variety of therapeutic and diagnostic reasons.

- The duration of catheter patency and function tends to be longer with jugular catheters compared to peripheral catheters.
- Higher osmolar solutions (parenteral nutritional solutions, glucose solutions) may be administered more safely through these catheters compared to peripheral venous catheters.
- Jugular venous catheters allow for easier through-the-catheter blood sampling and are necessary for measuring central venous pressure.
- Finally, jugular catheter sites are less likely to be contaminated from vomit and diarrhea in animals with those problems.

INDICATIONS

- When multiple/serial blood samples are required (e.g., diabetic ketoacidotic animals)
- Measuring central venous pressure (CVP)
- Constant rate infusions of hyperosmolar solutions (e.g., dextrose solutions >5%)
- Total/partial parenteral nutrition (T/PPN) administration
- In animals with severe vomiting and diarrhea that require IV access

CONTRAINDICATIONS

- Hypercoagulable states (e.g., protein-losing nephropathy)
- Increased intracranial pressure (holding off jugular vein may increase intracranial pressure)
- Hypocoagulable states (e.g., liver failure, rodenticide anticoagulant toxicity)
- Thrombocytopenia
- Thrombocytopathia
- Skin infection over site of jugular catheter placement

EQUIPMENT, ANESTHESIA

- Sedation generally not necessary in critically ill animals but may be needed in fractious animals.
- Clippers.
- Sterile surgical gloves.
- Surgical scrub soap.
- Gauze squares for surgical prep of site.
- Heparinized saline flushes.
- Suture material.
- White cloth-type tape.
- Bandaging material (e.g., roll gauze, cast padding, and Elastikon/Elastoplast-type adhesive roll bandage).
- Injection cap.
- Triple antibiotic ointment.
- Guide-wire technique: the following four items are available in kits manufactured by Cook, Mila, and Arrow:
  - Hypodermic needle
  - Guide wire
  - Dilator
  - Polyurethane IV catheter
- Other materials:
  - A #11 scalpel blade
  - Suture material (e.g., 2-0 to 4-0 nylon)

ANTICIPATED TIME

About 20 minutes

PREPARATION: IMPORTANT CHECKPOINTS

Check coagulation profile (prothrombin time [PT], partial thromboplastin time [PTT], platelet count, platelet function)

POSSIBLE COMPLICATIONS AND COMMON ERRORS TO AVOID

- Do not use leashes that go around the neck (neck leads) when a jugular catheter is in place.

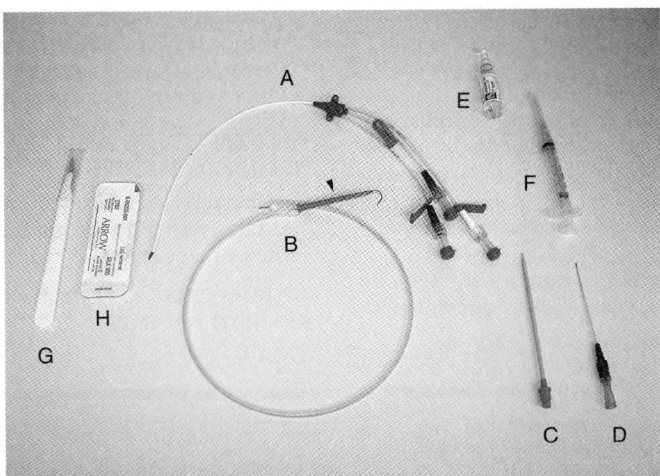

FIGURE II-91 Guide wire-type jugular catheter kit. **A**, Triple-lumen jugular catheter. **B**, Flexible, Teflon-coated stylet with J-tip straightening sleeve (*arrowhead*). **C**, Vessel dilator. **D**, Peripheral IV catheter (a large-bore needle may be used instead, but the guide wire must fit through it). **E**, Local anesthetic. **F**, Syringe with which to inject the anesthetic. **G**, Disposable scalpel for making a skin incision. **H**, Suture material.

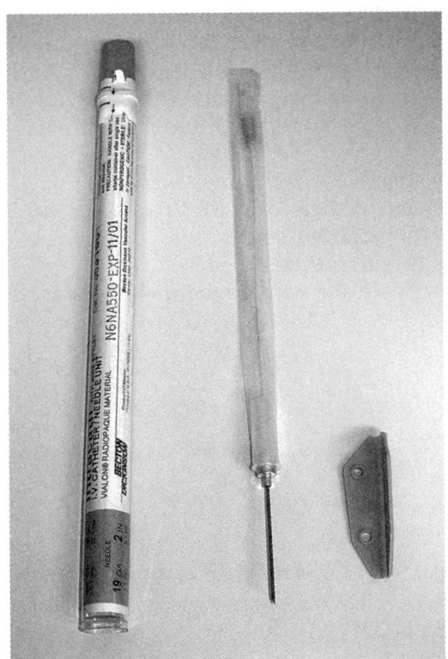

FIGURE II-92 Through-the-needle type jugular catheter. Inside the kit (left) are the catheter (center) and the needle guard (right). Note the plastic sheath of the catheter, which allows the catheter to be advanced through the needle into the animal without wearing sterile gloves; also note the large needle that remains with the animal and must be covered with the needle guard.

- Place needle guard when using through-the-needle catheters before removing the stylet. Otherwise, the needle can lacerate or transect the catheter.
- Avoid excessively tight neck bandaging.

PROCEDURE

- Catheter placement should always be done aseptically.
- Animal should be in lateral recumbency, with the nonrecumbent side being the side with the jugular to be catheterized.
- Clip hair from site. Centered over the jugular furrow, the clip and aseptic prep extend approximately as follows:
  - From slightly beyond the ventral midline of the neck ventrally to halfway between the ventral and dorsal midlines dorsally
  - From the thoracic inlet caudally to the angle of the mandible cranially
- Prepare site aseptically with complete surgical scrub.

GUIDE-WIRE TECHNIQUE

- Use sterile surgical gloves when placing the catheter.
- Drape site with sterile drape.
- Check that catheter or needle about to be used for venipuncture can accept guide wire (compatible diameters).
- Insert needle in vessel (jugular venipuncture):
  - Catheter (generally needs to be larger than 20 gauge) may used in place of needle.
  - In thick-skinned animals, a two-step approach may be better:
    (1) raise the jugular vein;
    (2) lift (tent) the skin overlying the jugular vein;
    (3) enter only the skin with the needle/catheter, or make a small stab incision in the skin with a sterile scalpel blade;
    (4) gently return the skin to a normal position (keeping the needle in place in the skin); and
    (5) advance the needle into the raised jugular vein.
- Place guide wire into vessel through needle or catheter, J-tip (not straight tip) first. To do so, the guide wire is retracted into the J-tip straightening device (a small, tapered sleeve), and the device with the straightened J-tip is placed into the catheter. The guide wire may then be advanced easily through the catheter and into the jugular vein, with the J-shape emerging from the peripheral catheter in the jugular vein to avoid trauma from a straight guide wire tip.
- After advancing the guide wire a few cm into the jugular vein (4–10 cm, depending on the patient's size), do not move the guide wire for the rest of the procedure, until the catheter is in place.
- While holding the guide wire firmly with one hand (guide wires are Teflon-coated and slippery), remove needle or catheter from vessel and off the wire while ensuring the guide wire stays in the vessel.
- Maintain digital pressure over the catheter placement site to minimize hemorrhage.
- Measure length of guide wire protruding from skin; it should be a few cm greater than the length of the dilator (withdraw guide wire slightly as needed).
- Place dilator over the wire into the vessel (this dilates the vessel insertion site so the catheter can be placed more easily into the vessel). Expect some bleeding around the site, which should be controlled with direct pressure. Some jugular catheter kits have a combined catheter-dilator configuration (Fig. II-91), which allows the dilation step and the catheter placement step to occur simultaneously.
- While holding the guide wire firmly in place, remove the dilator back over the wire, making sure that wire stays in the vessel. Apply pressure over the site to minimize hemorrhage.
- Thread IV catheter over the wire, and advance catheter into the vessel.
- Remove wire, making sure the catheter stays in place.
- Remove air in the catheter line with the use of a 3-cc syringe that contains heparinized saline.
- Flush catheter with heparinized saline without administering air to animal.
- Suture catheter to skin.
- Cover site with nonadhesive bandage.
- Bandage catheter in a stable position (neck wrap).

THROUGH-THE-NEEDLE CATHETER TECHNIQUE

- Insert needle into vessel. The two-step technique may help (as just described).
- Advance catheter through the needle into the vessel.

- Lock catheter into needle hub.
- Withdraw needle from vessel and skin (i.e., withdraw needle by 3–4 cm, ensuring that the catheter remains well in the jugular vein), and place the needle guard over needle.
- Remove stylet from catheter.
- Cap catheter and flush catheter with heparinized saline.
- Suture catheter to skin.
- Cover site with nonadhesive bandage.
- Bandage catheter in a stable position (neck wrap).

POSTPROCEDURE

- Assess tightness of bandage around animal's neck after each layer is placed. A finger should easily pass between skin and bandage.
- Leashes should be placed around shoulders, or use a harness.
- If using multiple lumen catheters, be sure animal cannot chew lumen lines.
- When using multiple lumens, designate one for TPN (usually the most distal).
- Flush line(s) with heparinized saline every 6 hours to maintain patency.

ALTERNATIVES AND THEIR RELATIVE MERITS

Peripheral catheter: technically simpler and cheaper but does not allow jugular catheter functions as already described.

AUTHORS: **ELISA A. PETROLLINI, KENNETH DROBATZ**

Laryngeal, Pharyngeal, or Oral Examination

BASIC INFORMATION

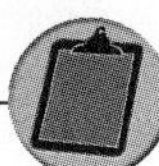

SYNONYM(S)

Laryngoscopy
Pharyngoscopy

OVERVIEW AND GOAL(S)

Complete examination of oral cavity, oropharynx, larynx, and part of the nasopharynx

INDICATIONS

- Anorexia (secondary to oral discomfort)
- Oronasal fistula evaluation
- Mandibular/maxillary fracture assessment
- Precise occlusion evaluation
- Ptyalism/hypersalivation
- Gagging
- Halitosis
- Facial deformity
- Voice change
- Dysphagia
- Noisy respiration, especially inspiratory stridor with a radiographically normal trachea
- Respiratory distress, especially inspiratory

CONTRAINDICATIONS

Severe respiratory distress necessitating oxygen supplementation, endotracheal intubation, or emergency tracheostomy

EQUIPMENT, ANESTHESIA

VENOUS ACCESS

- Hair clippers with a #40 blade
- Surgical skin scrub preparation materials
- IV over-the-needle catheter of appropriate size for the animal (18–24 gauge)
- T-port or prn to cap catheter
- White cloth tape, 1.5 inches and 1 inch, for catheter fixation
- 5-ml heparinized saline

ANESTHETIC AGENTS

- Premedication:
  - It may be preferrable to avoid premedication when evaluating laryngeal function. The use of thiopental without premedication significantly increases arytenoid motion before recovery, which is optimal, when compared to other protocols (propofol, ketamine, and diazepam; acepromazine and thiopental; acepromazine and propofol). This is the recommended protocol for evaluating laryngeal function (Tobias, et al, 2004).
  - If the lack of premedication when potentially evaluating laryngeal function is unacceptable to the clinician, an alternative is glycopyrrolate (0.01 mg/kg IV, IM, or SC) and butorphanol (0.1 mg/kg IV, IM, or SC).
  - If no evaluation of laryngeal function is judged necessary, then a standard sedation or premedication protocol is acceptable if the animal is stable. Examples:
    - Glycopyrrolate (0.01 mg/kg IV, IM, or SC) + acepromazine (0.05 mg/kg IM or SC) + butorphanol (0.1 mg/kg IM or SC); or
    - Glycopyrrolate (0.01 mg/kg IV, IM, or SC) + hydromorphone (0.1 mg/kg IM) ± acepromazine (0.05 mg/kg IM or SC).
- Induction:
  - For evaluation of laryngeal function, thiopental (20 mg/kg IV, give half the volume as a bolus and then "to effect") or propofol (2 mg/kg with premedication, or 6 mg/kg if no premedication) are preferred over ketamine-diazepam (Gross, et al., 2002).
  - If no evaluation of laryngeal function is judged necessary, routine agents are appropriate. Examples in stable animals include:
    - Thiopental (20 mg/kg IV, give half the volume as a bolus and then "to effect"); or
    - Propofol (2 mg/kg with premedication; 6 mg/kg if no premedication); or
    - Ketamine (10 mg/kg) + diazepam (0.5 mg/kg) IV.
- Stimulation of respiration:
  - The use of doxapram HCl helps differentiate normal dogs from dogs with laryngeal paralysis. In these dogs, administration of doxapram seems to enhance paradoxical arytenoid motion (Tobias, Jackson, Harvey, 2004).
    - Doxapram HCl 5–10 mg/kg IV.

POSITIONING

- To maintain head in the upright position:
  - Conformable roll gauze (e.g., 2-inch Kling)
  - Two poles (of the type used for IV fluid administration, optional)

ORAL EXAMINATION

- Oral speculum (mouth gag)
- Light source/transilluminator
- Laryngoscope
- Dry gauze sponges:
  - For manipulating the tongue
  - To dry up secretions

LARYNGEAL EXAMINATION

- Oral speculum
- Light source/transilluminator
- Laryngoscope
- One or two tongue depressors taped end to end for dorsal retraction/elevation of the soft palate

OROPHARYNGEAL AND NASOPHARYNGEAL EXAMINATION

- As for oral and laryngeal examination (above) + spay hook for cranial retraction of soft palate
- Small mirror used in dentistry with antifogging agent or immersed in warm (38°C) water/saline

FINE-NEEDLE ASPIRATION/BIOPSIES

- A set of 10-ml syringes, 22-gauge needles, and microscope slides for fine-needle aspiration and cytologic examination
- Biopsy kit:
  - A #15 scalpel bladder
  - Adson forceps
  - Needle holder
  - Small scissors

- Suture scissors
- Appropriate size suture that can be resorbed (surgeon's preference)

ENDOTRACHEAL INTUBATION

- Appropriate size tube (see Intubation, Endotracheal, p 1269)
- Conformable 1- or 2-inch tape or gauze for tube fixation
- A 5–10 ml empty syringe for cuff inflation
- Anesthesia machine verified with appropriate circuit for the animal (semiopened or semiclosed):
  - Functional
  - Oxygen
  - Inhalant anesthetic agent

ANTICIPATED TIME

About 15 to 30 minutes

PREPARATION: IMPORTANT CHECKPOINTS

- Use preoxygenation with a mask if possible.
- Always perform this examination on animals that have been fasted, because the airway is not always protected during the exam. There is the possibility of regurgitation of gastric contents and subsequent aspiration pneumonia.
- Always be prepared for orotracheal intubation of animal and possible ventilation with oxygen through an anesthetic circuit.
- In animals in respiratory distress, always be prepared to perform an emergency tracheostomy.
- In animals with moderate or marked inspiratory stridor or any degree of upper airway distress, owners must hear and understand options to consider (surgical intervention if problem correctable, euthanasia on the table if nonresectable disorder) if severe laryngeal infiltration, a nonresectable mass, or other equally serious problem is identified.

POSSIBLE COMPLICATIONS AND COMMON ERRORS TO AVOID

- Incomplete examination.
- May give a false-positive diagnosis of laryngeal paralysis because animal is too heavily sedated or not enough time is given for animal to come out of light anesthesia. To avoid this situation, prepare doxapram HCl and administer if needed.

PROCEDURE

- When dogs are extremely dyspneic due to laryngeal paralysis, the diagnosis often can be made on the awake animal.
  - A bright light source (e.g., Finnoff transilluminator) is directed into the oral cavity during the severe dyspnea, and failure of the arytemoid cartilages to abduct is clearly apparent in the conscious animal.
- Otherwise, proceed as follows.
- Venous access:
  - Prepare site for IV catheter insertion (clip, clean, and prep skin).
  - Insert IV catheter.
  - Close catheter with a T tube or a prn.
  - Fixation of catheter to skin.
  - Flush catheter with heparinized saline.
- Premedication:
  - Administer premedication if judged necessary.
- Preoxygenation:
  - Animal in sternal recumbency.
  - If possible, use a mask to preoxygenate animal for 5 minutes.
- Induction of anesthesia:
  - IV administration of predetermined anesthetic agent.
    - Very light anesthetic plane is used for evaluation of laryngeal function.
      - If anesthetic plane is too deep, give time (5–10 minutes) for animal to partially recover from anesthesia, and then continue to evaluate.
    - Deeper anesthetic plane is used for evaluation of oral cavity and pharynx and anatomic evaluation of the larynx.
- Positioning of the head:
  - Assistant holds head upright using a piece of conformable roll gauze (Kling) passed behind the upper canine teeth.
  - Alternatively, two IV poles, one on each side of the table, can be used; the conformable gauze is passed behind the upper canine teeth, and the gauze is attached to each IV pole, thus supporting the head in the upright position.
  - Place oral speculum of appropriate size.
- Oral examination:
  - All structures of the oral cavity should be evaluated.
    - Lips, cheeks, teeth (abscess, fracture, occlusion), gingiva, tongue (under and at the base), hard palate, soft palate (mass, elongation), tonsillar crypts/tonsils.
- Oropharyngeal examination:
  - Soft palate should be palpated for thickness, mobility.
  - Elevate soft palate dorsally with a tongue depressor or two depressors taped end to end in a large dog.
  - Depress base of the tongue ventrally with a laryngoscope. This permits the evaluation of the upper esophageal sphincter.
- Laryngeal examination:
  - After the evaluation of the oropharynx, it is appropriate to evaluate the anatomy of the larynx (Fig. II-93): epiglottis, aryepiglottic folds, arytenoid cartilages (cuneiform and corniculate processes) vocal cords, laryngeal ventricles (Monnet, 2003).
  - Then evaluate the function of the larynx.
    - Normal:
      - Observe active abduction of the arytenoid cartilages synchronized with inspiration.
      - Observe passive adduction of the arytenoid cartilages synchronized with expiration.
    - Abnormal:
      - Observe no movement of cartilages.
        - Is it significant? Animal is usually too deeply anesthetized; wait until motion returns or administer doxapram HCl (see Laryngeal Paralysis, p 619).
      - Observe paradoxical movement of arytenoid cartilages, indicating laryngeal paralysis:
        - Adduction at inspiration.
        - Abduction at expiration.
- Nasopharyngeal examination:
  - Palpate the soft palate, and then press firmly to detect masses that could be in the nasopharynx (e.g., a nasopharyngeal polyp could deform the soft palate and could be palpated).
  - Use a spay hook to retract the caudal edge of the soft palate cranially, permitting the visualization of part of the nasopharynx.
  - Use a small, dental-type mirror to "look back" into the nasopharynx.

POSTPROCEDURE

- Airway protection:
  - When the examination is completed, perform orotracheal intubation, inflate cuff, and secure tube to avoid complications secondary to regurgitation/aspiration pneumonia.
- Administer oxygen via anesthesia circuit.
- Monitor recovery from anesthesia.
- Extubation of animal when reflexes are reestablished, especially the deglutition reflex.

ALTERNATIVES AND THEIR RELATIVE MERITS

NASOPHARYNGEAL ENDOSCOPY

- The use of a small flexible endoscope can permit a more precise evaluation of the nasopharynx because it can be retroflexed 180 degrees and advanced in the nasopharynx, permitting visualization of the nasal choanae.
- Involves a substantial investment (endoscope, monitor, camera, image processor, light source).

TRANSNASAL ENDOSCOPY

- The use of transnasal endoscopy has been reported in large dogs (over 20 kg) for the evaluation of the nasopharynx and of laryngeal structure and function. General anesthesia was not required, which might be an advantage. Dogs were heavily sedated, and topical anesthesia was used in the left nasal

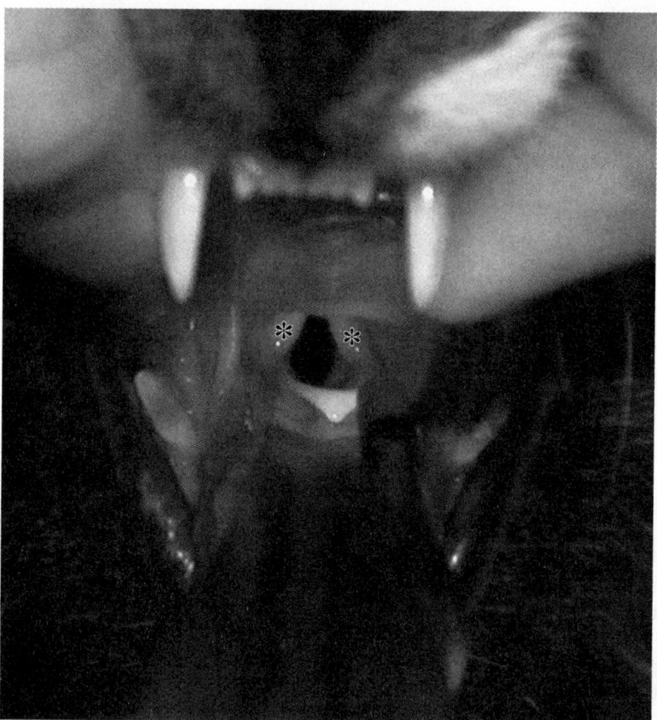

FIGURE II-93 Typical appearance of the glottis of a healthy, anesthetized cat. The tongue is depressed with a laryngoscope, revealing the epiglottis ventrally (tip appears as a white triangle in the center of the image), the soft palate dorsally, and the arytenoid cartilages laterally (*asterisks*). Slightly deeper and ventral to the arytenoid cartilages, the vocal cords are seen (slight obliquity; animal's left vocal cord is seen more clearly here than the right one).

passage. The procedure was successful (Radlinsky, Mason, Hodgson 2004).

- This technique does not permit the evaluation of the oral cavity and of the oropharynx, so it is of limited use for a complete evaluation as described here.
- Involves a substantial investment (endoscope, monitor, camera, image processor, light source).

ULTRASOUND

- Sonographic evaluation of laryngeal paralysis has been evaluated in 40 dogs (30 with laryngeal paralysis and 10 normal).
- The results showed a high degree of sensitivity and specificity with this technique (Rudorf, Barr, Lane 2001).

SUGGESTED READING

Gross ME, et al: A comparison of thiopental, propofol, and diazepam-ketamine anesthesia for evaluation of laryngeal function in dogs premedicated with butorphanol-glycopyrrolate. *J Am Anim Hosp Assoc* 38:503, 2002.

Monnet E: Laryngeal paralysis and devocalization. In Slatter D (ed): *Textbook of Small Animal Surgery*, ed 3. Philadelphia, WB Saunders, 2003, pp 837–845.

Radlinsky MG, Mason DE, Hodgson D: Transnasal laryngoscopy for the diagnosis of laryngeal paralysis in dogs. *J Am Anim Hosp Assoc* 40:211, 2004.

Rudorf H, Barr FJ, Lane GJ: The role of ultrasound in the assessment of laryngeal paralysis in the dog. *Vet Radiol Ultrasound* 42(4):338–343, 2001.

Tobias KM, et al: Effects of various anesthetic agents on laryngeal motion during laryngoscopy in normal dogs. *Vet Surg* 33(2):102, 2004.

Tobias KM, Jackson AM, Harvey RC: Effects of doxapram HCl on laryngeal function of normal dogs and dogs with naturally occurring laryngeal paralysis. *Vet Anesth Anal* 31(4):258, 2004

AUTHOR: **BERTRAND LUSSIER**

Local Anesthesia and Regional Anesthesia

BASIC INFORMATION

SYNONYM(S)

Local blocks

OVERVIEW AND GOAL(S)

- Local anesthesia and regional anesthesia refer to a broad range of techniques that utilize local anesthetic agents delivered to a discrete anatomic area (as opposed to systemic delivery).
- With these techniques, the local anesthetic agent inhibits pain by blocking transmission of noxious input (and other types of sensory input) before it ever reaches the brain. The animal's level of consciousness is not affected.
- This contrasts with general anesthesia, during which nociceptive processing continues to occur but the animal is not able to perceive pain due to the unconscious state.

INDICATION

- Infiltrative anesthesia:
  - Incisional block: supplemental analgesia for a variety of surgical procedures (e.g., abdominal wall incisions, total ear canal ablation incisions).
- Peripheral nerve blocks:
  - Dental nerve block: supplemental analgesia for tooth extractions, maxillary/mandibular surgeries.
  - Brachial plexus block: supplemental analgesia for surgical procedures involving the forelimb distal to shoulder.
  - Distal radial, ulnar, and median nerve blocks: supplemental analgesia for feline onychectomy or any surgical procedure involving the distal forepaw.
  - Intercostal nerve blocks: supplemental analgesia after lateral thoracotomy or desensitizing area around isolated rib fractures.
- Epidural anesthesia/analgesia:
  - Lumbosacral injection of local anesthetic: indicated for caudal procedures/injuries only (e.g., involving hind limb, tail, perineum, caudal abdomen).
  - Lumbosacral injection of opioid: hydrophilic opioids (i.e., morphine) indicated to supplement analgesia for a variety of procedures (e.g., hind limb, tail, abdominal, forelimb, thoracic, cervical procedures).
- Other regional techniques:

- Intra-articular anesthesia/analgesia supplemental analgesia for intra-articular procedures (stifle most common).
- Interpleural anesthesia supplemental analgesia for thoracic and cranial abdominal pain (especially pancreatitis).
- IV regional anesthesia desensitization of a distal limb to facilitate surgery.

CONTRAINDICATIONS

- Infiltrative anesthesia, peripheral nerve blocks, others:
  - Injection into infected tissue
- Epidural anesthesia/analgesia (see Epidural Analgesia/Anesthesia, p 1238):
  - Injection into infected tissue (at lumbosacral junction)
  - Coagulopathy
  - Septicemia
  - Uncorrected hypotension (especially with local anesthetics)
  - Significant trauma/lesion at lumbosacral junction

EQUIPMENT, ANESTHESIA

- Infiltrative anesthesia:
  - Incisional block:
    - Hypodermic needle (22, 25 gauge), syringe, sterile gloves, local anesthetic.
    - Dosages (total per animal): lidocaine ≤5 mg/kg (dog); ≤3 mg/kg (cat). Bupivacaine: ≤2 mg/kg (dog); ≤1 mg/kg (cat).
    - Animal is usually under general anesthesia, and block is done either before incision is made or at the end of the surgery prior to complete closure.
- Peripheral nerve blocks:
  - Dental nerve block:
    - Hypodermic needle (22, 25 gauge), syringe, local anesthetic.
    - Dosages (total per animal): lidocaine ≤5 mg/kg (dog); ≤3 mg/kg (cat). Bupivacaine: ≤2 mg/kg (dog); ≤1 mg/kg (cat).
    - Animal is usually under general anesthesia.
  - Brachial plexus block:
    - Hypodermic needle (22 gauge) or spinal needle (22 gauge, 2–3 inches), syringe, local anesthetic.
    - Dosages (total per animal): lidocaine ≤5 mg/kg (dog); ≤3 mg/kg (cat). Bupivacaine: ≤2 mg/kg (dog); ≤1 mg/kg (cat).
    - Specialized insulated needle (22 gauge, 3 inches) required if a nerve locator is to be used.
    - Animal is usually sedated or under general anesthesia.
  - Distal radial, ulnar, median nerve blocks:
    - Hypodermic needle (22, 25 gauge), syringe, local anesthetic.
    - Dosages (total per animal): lidocaine ≤5 mg/kg (dog); ≤3 mg/kg (cat). Bupivacaine: ≤2 mg/kg (dog); ≤1 mg/kg (cat).
    - Animal is usually under general anesthesia, and block is done prior to surgical procedure.
  - Intercostal nerve block:
    - Hypodermic needle (22, 25 gauge), syringe, local anesthetic.
    - Dosages (total per animal): lidocaine ≤5 mg/kg (dog); ≤3 mg/kg (cat). Bupivacaine: ≤2 mg/kg (dog); ≤1 mg/kg (cat).
    - Animal is usually sedated or under general anesthesia.
- Epidural anesthesia/analgesia (see Epidural Analgesia/Anesthesia, p 1238).
  - Spinal needle (18, 20, 22 gauge; Quincke or Huber point, 1.5–3.5 inches), syringe, sterile gloves, local anesthetic (preservative-free lidocaine, bupivacaine), ± opioid (preservative-free morphine).
- Other regional techniques
  - Intra-articular anesthesia/analgesia:
    - Hypodermic needle (22 gauge), syringe, sterile gloves, local anesthetic (lidocaine, bupivacaine) ± opioid (morphine).
    - Dosages (total per animal): lidocaine ≤5 mg/kg (dog); ≤3 mg/kg (cat). Bupivacaine: ≤2 mg/kg (dog); ≤1 mg/kg (cat).
    - Animal is usually sedated or under general anesthesia.
  - Interpleural anesthesia:
    - Butterfly catheter (22 gauge) or through-the-needle catheter (20 gauge, 2 inches); preplaced chest tube or commercial interpleural anesthesia tray, syringe, sterile gloves, local anesthetic.
    - Dosages: lidocaine ≤5 mg/kg (dog), q 2–4h; ≤3 mg/kg (cat), q 4h. Bupivacaine: ≤2 mg/kg (dog) initially, then ≤1 mg/kg q 6h; ≤1 mg/kg (cat) initially, then ≤0.5 mg/kg q 6h.
    - Animals are usually sedated or under general anesthesia
  - IV regional anesthesia:
    - Esmarch bandage material (e.g., Vetrap), IV catheter (22 gauge), tourniquet, hypodermic needle (22 gauge), syringe, local anesthetic (lidocaine).
    - Dose: lidocaine, 2.5–5 mg/kg (dog only).
    - Animal is usually sedated.

ANTICIPATED TIME

This time period does not include clip and preparation of the site where indicated.

- Infiltrative anesthesia:
  - Incisional block: <1 to 2 minutes.
- Peripheral nerve blocks:
  - Dental nerve blocks: <1 to 2 minutes.
  - Brachial plexus block: <5 to 10 minutes.
  - Distal radial, ulnar, median nerve blocks: <1 to 2 minutes.
  - Intercostal nerve blocks: <1 to 2 minutes.
- Epidural anesthesia/analgesia: <5 to 10 minutes.
- Other regional techniques:
  - Intra-articular anesthesia/analgesia: <1 to 2 minutes.
  - Interpleural anesthesia: <5 to 10 minutes.
  - IV regional anesthesia: <5 to 10 minutes.

PREPARATION: IMPORTANT CHECKPOINTS

- Ensure that injection site(s) is clipped (if applicable) and aseptically prepared.
- Adhere to strict aseptic technique during all procedures—doing this is mandatory.
- Ensure that drug solutions are free from contamination (especially for epidural and intra-articular techniques).

POSSIBLE COMPLICATIONS AND COMMON ERRORS TO AVOID

- Systemic local anesthetic toxicity is possible with any technique and is usually associated with inadvertent IV injection/excessive drug doses.
- Infiltrative anesthesia:
  - Incisional block: inadvertent IV or intra-arterial injection, penetration of body cavities/organs.
- Peripheral nerve blocks:
  - Dental nerve block: self-mutilation following sensory loss to tongue and lips (rare).
  - Brachial plexus block: inadvertent IV or intra-arterial injection or injection into the thoracic cavity with possible pneumothorax/pulmonary laceration.
  - Distal radial, ulnar, median nerve blocks: self-mutilation following sensory loss to distal paws (very rare).
  - Intercostal nerve block: inadvertent intrathoracic injection with possible pneumothorax/pulmonary laceration.
- Epidural anesthesia/analgesia: inadequate block, hypotension, urinary retention, transient neurologic deficits (rare).
- Other regional techniques:
  - Intra-articular anesthesia/analgesia: articular cartilage damage.
  - Interpleural anesthesia: pneumothorax, pulmonary laceration.
  - IV regional anesthesia: ischemic limb damage; systemic local anesthetic toxicity due to tourniquet failure.

PROCEDURE

For selected techniques only.

- Peripheral nerve blocks:
  - Dental nerve blocks:
    - Infraorbital: Palpate infraorbital foramen rostral and ventral to medial canthus of eye; insert needle into foramen and aspirate. If there is negative pressure (no blood), inject local anesthetic.
    - Mandibular: Palpate mandibular foramen intraorally on the medial surface of the ramus of the mandible, and insert needle percutaneously from the ventromedial aspect of the mandible toward the foramen and aspirate; if there is negative pressure (no blood), inject local anesthetic.
  - Brachial plexus block (Fig. II-94):
    - From a cranial approach, insert the needle medial to the scapula just ventral to the body of the sixth cervical vertebra; advance until the tip of the needle is just beyond the first rib and aspirate; if negative pressure (no blood), inject one-fourth dose of a local anesthetic; withdraw needle partially and aspirate; if there is negative pressure (no blood), inject another one-fourth dose of anesthetic; repeat until needle is completely withdrawn and all drug has been injected.
  - Distal radial, ulnar, median nerve blocks; three injections required per paw:
    - On dorsal aspect, insert needle just proximal to the first phalanx and aspirate; if there is negative pressure (no blood), inject local anesthetic.
    - On palmar aspect, insert needle just medial to accessory carpal pad and aspirate; if negative pressure (no blood), inject local anesthetic.
    - Remove needle and insert just lateral and proximal to accessory carpal pad and aspirate; if there is negative pressure (no blood), inject local anesthetic.
- Epidural anesthesia/analgesia (see also Epidural Analgesia/Anesthesia, p 1238).
  - Place the animal in lateral or sternal recumbency, and locate the lumbosacral space as follows: Palpate the cranial edges of the ilial wings (this is at the level of the sixth lumbar vertebra), palpate the dorsal process of the seventh lumbar vertebra caudal to this area, and then palpate a large depression corresponding to the lumbosacral space farther caudally.
  - Insert spinal needle directly over the lumbosacral space at an angle perpendicular to the skin, and advance needle slowly through the ligamentum flavum until a loss of resistance and characteristic "pop" is appreciated, indicating that the epidural space has been penetrated.
  - Remove stylet and ensure that blood or cerebrospinal fluid (CSF) is not evident in needle hub.
  - Inject 1 ml of air using a glass syringe to confirm lack of resistance and correct needle placement; inject local anesthetic, opioid, or other analgesic.
- Other regional techniques.
  - Interpleural anesthesia:
    - Insert catheter in the ninth intercostal space on the midlateral aspect of thorax.
    - Aspirate to remove air/blood.
    - Inject local anesthetic (lidocaine should be injected first in conscious animals to minimize discomfort and can be followed by bupivacaine if a long duration block is desired).

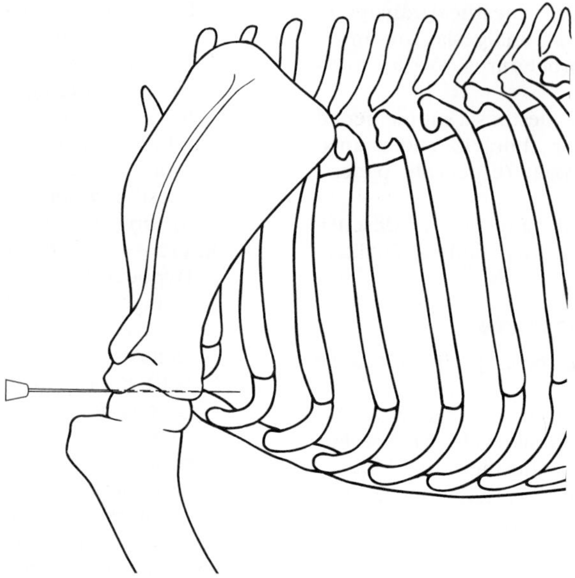

FIGURE II-94 Brachial plexus nerve block. Place the needle medial to the scapulohumeral joint, lateral to the thoracic wall, toward the costochondral junction, and parallel to the vertebral column. From Fossum TW, et al: *Small Animal Surgery*, ed 2. St. Louis, Mosby, 2002.

POSTPROCEDURE

- If local/regional anesthesia is being used for supplementing analgesia in conjunction with general anesthesia, injectable and inhalant anesthetic requirements may be markedly reduced.
- Animals must be monitored for adequacy of analgesia and treated accordingly.

ALTERNATIVES AND THEIR RELATIVE MERITS

Pain associated with surgery, trauma, and a variety of medical conditions can usually be managed using systemic analgesics (e.g., opioids, nonsteroidal anti-inflammatory drugs [NSAIDs]); however, these agents are not able to block peripheral nociceptive input. The inclusion of a local or regional technique constitutes a multimodal approach to anesthesia and pain management and is simply good medical practice.

AUTHOR: **LEIGH A. LAMONT**

Luxation Reduction (Closed): Shoulder, Elbow, or Hip

BASIC INFORMATION

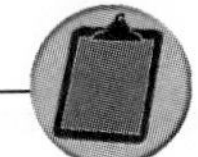

SYNONYM(S)

Coxofemoral luxation (hip)
Dislocated shoulder, elbow, hip
Scapulohumeral luxation (shoulder)

OVERVIEW AND GOAL(S)

- Severe joint trauma can cause ligament/ joint capsule damage, resulting in displacement of the bones of the joint.
- Closed reduction aims to restore the normal alignment of the joint, without surgical intervention, and to maintain stability until these soft tissues heal.

INDICATIONS

- Traumatic luxation of normal shoulder, elbow, hip joints
- Acute luxation (<5 days)

CONTRAINDICATIONS

- Luxation associated with severe ligament damage or avulsion fractures that impede normal joint function and/or leave the joint unstable after closed reduction.
- Failure of closed reduction due to interposed soft tissue, hematoma, or recurrent luxation necessitates open (surgical) reduction.
- Chronic luxation (>5 to 7 days).
- Dysplastic joint:
  - Glenoid dysplasia.
  - Total hip replacement may be a better option in cases of severe hip dysplasia.
- Femoral head and neck ostectomy (FHO) may be an acceptable alternative to closed/open hip reduction in a small dog or cat.

EQUIPMENT, ANESTHESIA

- General anesthesia
- Rope or leash to provide counter pressure (hip luxation)
- Assistant
- Bandage material

ANTICIPATED TIME

About 10 to 30 minutes

PREPARATION: IMPORTANT CHECKPOINTS

- Advise owner of aftercare and possible drawbacks:
  - Recurrence
  - Degenerative joint disease
  - Decreased range of motion
  - Possible need for open reduction
  - Postreduction bandage care
  - Postreduction exercise restriction

After anesthetic induction:

- Minimum of two views of the joint to confirm luxation versus fracture
- Animal in lateral recumbency affected limb up (affected limb on the nonrecumbent side)
- Hanging the affected limb can be useful (elbow luxation) for 5 to 10 minutes: secure the carpus and hoist the limb vertically with traction

POSSIBLE COMPLICATIONS AND COMMON ERRORS TO AVOID

- If there is excessive instability following closed reduction, open reduction should be performed.
- Failure to critically evaluate plain radiographs to assess joint anatomy or damage, avulsion fragments, and intra-articular debris.
- Trying to reduce a luxation with sedation alone.
- Failure to appropriately bandage the luxation.
- Removal of bandage too soon.
- Inadequate patient exercise restriction.

PROCEDURE

All luxation reductions are performed with the animal under general anesthesia.

- Shoulder:
  - Forelimb held in extension (in a ventral direction perpendicular to the long axis of the body, as in the standing animal).
  - For lateral luxation of the humeral head, apply medial pressure to the head at the same time as lateral pressure on the scapula.
  - Check range of motion and stability.
  - Place leg in a Spica splint.
  - For medial luxation of the humeral head, apply lateral pressure to the head at the same time as medial pressure on the scapula.
  - Check range of motion and stability.
  - Place the leg in a Velpeau sling.
  - Splint or sling can be removed after 2 weeks.
  - Passive range of motion exercises can begin after bandage removal, but restricted exercise is essential for another 2 to 4 weeks.
- Elbow:
  - Radius and ulna are usually luxated laterally relative to the distal humerus.
  - With the elbow in flexion, inwardly rotate the antebrachium.
  - Combined with elbow flexion, this movement enables the anconeal process of the ulna (caudal-most extent of the trochlear notch in the ulna) to hook into the olecranon fossa of the humerus. This maneuver is followed by careful extension of the elbow.
  - Hook the anconeal process of the ulna between the humeral condyles and carefully extend the elbow. With this part of the maneuver, the joint should now be reduced.
  - Passive range-of-motion exercises can begin after bandage removal, but restricted exercise is essential for 4 to 6 weeks, followed by 2 weeks of leash exercise only.
- Hip:
  - Assistant stands on opposite side of animal holding the ends of a rope or leash placed in the animal's groin to provide counterpressure.
  - Craniodorsal hip luxation:
    - The tarsus is grasped and externally rotated while the femur is pulled caudally.
    - The head of the femur rides up and over the dorsal acetabular rim.
    - Internal rotation while maintaining the pull on the femur together with direct pressure on the greater trochanter will seat the head in the acetabulum.
    - Place hip in an Ehmer or modified Ehmer sling for 2 weeks.
  - Caudoventral luxation:
    - The femur should be abducted and externally rotated to seat the femoral head in the acetabulum.
    - Hobbles may be applied for 10 to 14 days.
  - Lateral pressure can be applied to the reduced proximal femur as the hip is passively flexed and extended in an attempt to drive debris from the acetabulum.

POSTPROCEDURE

- Radiograph to evaluate the reduction.
- Toes should be accessible or visible to monitor for heat, cold, swelling, or pain.
- Bandage needs to be protected from moisture and kept clean and dry.

ALTERNATIVES AND THEIR RELATIVE MERITS

- Open reduction:
  - Requires surgical intervention
  - Greater cost
  - Carries a higher rate of success than closed reduction for the shoulder, elbow, and hip
- FHO may be worth considering for cats and small dogs as the possibility of hip re-luxation is elminated.
- Arthrodesis can provide pain relief for a chronically unstable joint. Aside from cost, complications include nonunion,

stress fractures, implant failure and infection.

- Excision glenoid arthroplasty for the shoulder joint. There are few reports of glenoid arthroplasty, but an abnormal gait is to be expected.
- Amputation.

AUTHOR: **NICHOLAS J. TROUT**

Medication Administration by Inhalation

BASIC INFORMATION

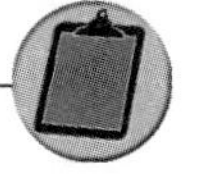

OVERVIEW AND GOAL(S)

To deliver medication to the respiratory tract with maximal efficacy and minimal side effects

INDICATIONS

Virtually any disease of the respiratory tract for which oral or injectable corticosteroids are indicated:

- Lymphocytic-plasmacytic rhinitis
- Allergic rhinitis
- Laryngeal edema secondary to laryngeal paresis/paralysis or mass
- Reverse sneeze
- Chronic bronchitis
- Asthma
- Eosinophilic pneumonia

Any disease of the respiratory tract for which oral or injectable bronchodilators are indicated:

- Asthma
- Chronic bronchitis (occasional)
- Bronchial compression secondary to left heart enlargement (occasional)

CONTRAINDICATIONS

Prior known sensitivity to inhaled medications

EQUIPMENT, ANESTHESIA

- Face mask: specific to species and size of animal's muzzle
- Spacer: specific to size of animal
- Metered dose inhaler (MDI)

ANTICIPATED TIME

- Inhalation time is usually 7-10 seconds, q 24h to q 12h or as needed (bronchodilator).
- Preparation time for animal may be a matter of seconds if animal is trained and comfortable with the device or may last weeks if training is required.

PREPARATION: IMPORTANT CHECKPOINTS

- Approximately 90% of dogs and 65% of all cats will tolerate the placement of the mask and spacer apparatus the very first time.
- Animals that will not tolerate this device initially still can be trained to acceptance. This usually takes a few days to a few weeks.
- Approximately 5% of dogs and 20% of cats will not accept this form of medication delivery even after weeks of training.

POSSIBLE COMPLICATIONS AND COMMON ERRORS TO AVOID

- Some animals cough immediately after inhaling the medications. No treatment for this is required.
- Mild conjunctivitis occasionally occurs if the top of the mask is in contact with the lower conjunctival lid margins.
- Contact dermatitis of the muzzle occasionally occurs.
- "Thrush," a yeast infection within the posterior pharynx, is a frequent complication in humans. This has not been reported in dogs or cats using inhaled corticosteroids.
- Growth retardation is a potential concern in children using inhaled corticosteroids. This has not been reported in dogs and cats.
- Cats with respiratory distress due to bronchoconstriction will very quickly benefit from inhalation of bronchodilator drugs. The temporary restraint required to administer these drugs has not been reported to result in clinically significant complications in this setting.
- Some cats will hold their breath. If this occurs, it is essential to wait until the animal begins breathing for 7 to 10 breaths.

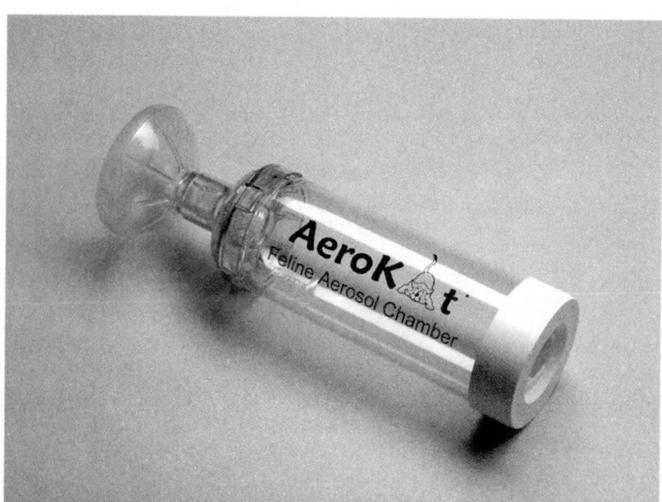

FIGURE II-95 The spacer device connected to a face mask.

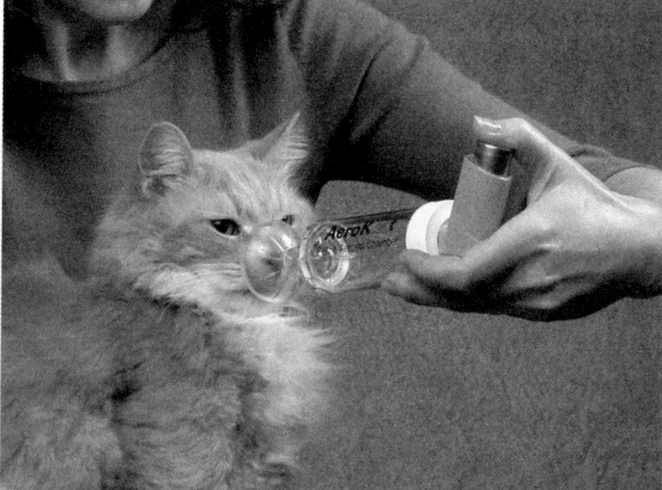

FIGURE II-96 The spacer connected to an MDI and a self-sealing mask of the type commonly used for induction of anesthesia. The spacer acts as a reservoir for the inhaled medication, so the animal breathes the drug into its airways whenever it breathes through the face mask.

- Some dogs and cats have nasal congestion that prevents inhalation by this method. In these cases, it is useful to instill a drop of a topical nasal decongestant (e.g., phenylephrine drops [Neosynephrine]) into either or both nostrils and wait 10 to 15 minutes before using the inhaled medications.

PROCEDURE

Technique, initial:

- Shake MDI three to five times vigorously.
- Attach MDI to spacer.
- Position the animal to restrain it and prevent side-to-side movement.

Technique, main:

- Place the mask over the animal's nose (cats) or muzzle (dog). If right-handed, use left hand to place mask.
- Use right hand to actuate (spray) medication, one puff into spacer.
- MDI for albuterol comes as one dose only.
- MDI for fluticasone comes as 44, 110, and 220 μg/actuation.
- Watch animal breathe for 7 to 10 breaths by watching the rib cage/abdomen.
- Alternatively, count 7 to 10 condensations of breath within the plastic mask.
- If an animal is resistant and in respiratory distress, it is usually safe to administer the medication with two people involved to temporarily restrain the animal. This is true even in the case of respiratory distress due to asthma.

POSTPROCEDURE

- Wipe patient's face/muzzle with washcloth
- Maintain cleanliness of spacer according to manufacturer's recommendations

ALTERNATIVES AND THEIR RELATIVE MERITS

- Nebulization does not offer superior drug-delivery results compared to the simple mask/spacer combination.
- Long-acting corticosteroids cannot be administered by inhalation.
- Oral prednisone should be considered when the animal requires immediate anti-inflammatory treatment. Inhaled corticosteroids may take 7 to 10 days to reach full effect. In these cases, prednisone/prednisolone should be administered for the first week concomitantly with the inhaled corticosteroid.
- Parenteral bronchodilators can be used (e.g., terbutaline, subcutaneously [SC]) if an animal is fractious and cannot be easily restrained.
- Topical medications: There are no current or prior objective data that document the effectiveness of topical corticosteroids or bronchodilators in the treatment of respiratory disorders in dogs or cats.
- Alternative therapies: There are many unproven alternative, evolving, and experimental approaches to treating respiratory disease in the canine and feline species.

AUTHOR: **PHILIP PADRID**

PROCEDURES AND TECHNIQUES

Muscle and Nerve Biopsy

BASIC INFORMATION

OVERVIEW AND GOAL(S)

Minimally invasive procedure for collection of muscle specimens for histologic, histochemical, immunohistochemical, and ultrastructural analyses. Nerve biopsy should only be performed by persons trained in the procedure.

INDICATIONS

- Chronic muscle atrophy, hypertrophy
- Weakness, hypotonia
- Exercise intolerance
- Nonorthopedic gait abnormalities
- Contractures
- Chronically elevated creatine kinase, myoglobinuria
- Myalgia, cramping
- Clinical evidence of muscle or peripheral nerve disease

CONTRAINDICATIONS

- Coagulopathy
- Poor anesthetic risk

EQUIPMENT, ANESTHESIA

- General anesthesia usually required; muscle biopsies can be taken under heavy sedation and local anesthetic if indicated.
- General surgical pack including self-retaining retractors.
- Containers for biopsy specimens:
  - Plain red-top tubes (5-10 ml) for unfixed biopsy specimens.
  - Biopsy jars containing fixatives: 10% formalin for routine histopathology, 2.5% glutaraldehyde in phosphate buffer, or Karnovsky's fixative for electron microscopy.
- Tongue depressors or wooden sticks and suture material or pins: for maintaining length of nerve specimens.
- Method of refrigeration prior to shipping specimens.
- Styrofoam containers for shipping refrigerated specimens to a specialized laboratory.

ANTICIPATED TIME

- About 60 to 90 minutes if the biopsy is combined with electrophysiologic examinations (see Electromyography [EMG] and Nerve Conduction Velocity [NCV], p 1231)
- About 30 to 45 minutes if nerve and muscle biopsy only

PREPARATION: IMPORTANT CHECKPOINTS

- It is essential that details of fixation and transportation be obtained from the laboratory that processes the tissues prior to taking biopsies.
- Determine if problem is generalized or localized to specific muscle groups: this will help in the selection of which muscle and nerve should be biopsied.
- Knowledge of anatomic localization of specific muscle groups.
- It is critical that unfixed biopsy specimens are kept refrigerated and shipped by courier for processing within 24 to 36 hours. Do not ship biopsy specimens on a Friday.

POSSIBLE COMPLICATIONS AND COMMON ERRORS TO AVOID

- Complications (hematoma, swelling) are rare following muscle biopsy.
- Transient neurologic dysfunction (knuckling, proprioceptive deficits) possible on the side of a nerve biopsy. The owner should be warned of the expected short-term deficits before the procedure.
- Artifacts in histologic specimens due to poor fixation or traumatic collection; handle tissue carefully.
- Biopsy of wrong muscle (e.g., frontalis instead of temporalis for masticatory muscle myositis).

PROCEDURE

For biopsy of muscle (biceps femoris) and nerve (common peroneal) through the same incision, an open biopsy procedure is necessary:

- Palpate the location of the common peroneal nerve on the lateral aspect of the distal femur just caudal to the proximal tibia.
- Clip hair, aseptic scrub/prep.

- Incise skin and overlying fascia to expose muscle.
- Establish orientation of the muscle fibers.
- Make parallel incisions along the longitudinal direction of the muscle fibers.
- Collect biopsy specimens 0.5 cm (width) × 0.5 cm (depth) × 1 cm (length).
- Transect the ends of the biopsy, handling carefully to minimize artifact.
- Wrap tissue in a saline-moistened gauze sponge (only moistened, not dripping wet).
- Place in dry, watertight container and keep chilled (not frozen).
- Collect a second smaller piece of muscle from same site and place freely in 10% buffered formalin.
- Locate the nerve as it passes over the lateral head of the gastrocnemius muscle.
- Isolate the nerve carefully by blunt dissection.
- A 5-0 or 6-0 silk suture is placed through the caudal one-third to one-half of the nerve at the proximal end of the biopsy site, allowing minimal gentle traction.
- A 3–4 cm fascicular biopsy is excised using fine iris scissors.
- Lay nerve specimen on a tongue depressor or stick, and either pin or tie ends with suture to maintain length. Do not stretch.
- Immerse nerve biopsy into either 10% buffered formalin or Karnovsky's fixative.
- The fascial layer is closed with absorbable suture (e.g., polydioxanone).
- Skin closure with monofilament nylon or staples.

Open muscle biopsy procedures are also recommended if a peripheral nerve biopsy is not collected at the same time. For collection of temporalis muscle, make sure that the frontalis muscle is not collected by mistake (Fig. II-97).

Percutaneous biopsy is not recommended for routine muscle biopsy collection in dogs and cats:

- Inadequate sample size.
- Difficult to orient tissue.
- Artifact.

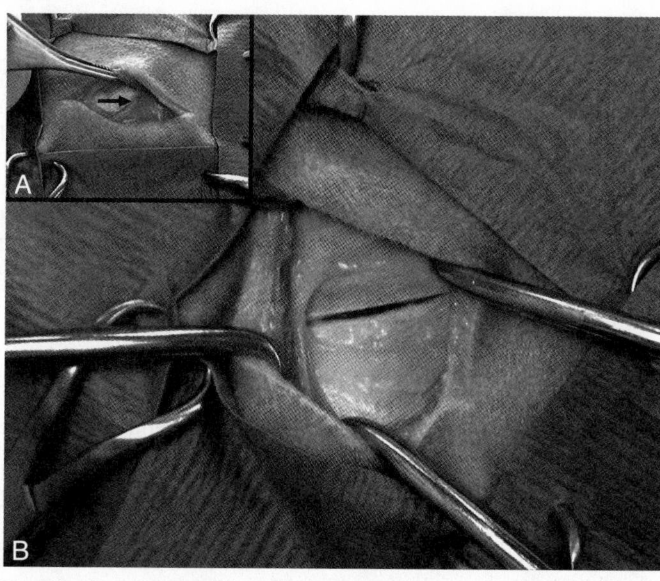

FIGURE II-97 Biopsies obtained from the temporalis muscle for a diagnosis of masticatory muscle myositis. **A,** Frontalis muscle (first muscle encountered, *arrow*) after making a skin incision. This muscle should be incised and retracted, allowing visualization of the thick fascia that overlies the temporalis muscle. **B,** Fascia has been incised and retracted, allowing access to the temporalis muscle. For a more complete description of anatomy of the masticatory muscles, refer to Melmed, et al, 2004.

Needle biopsies may be beneficial in research situations where sequential biopsy samples may be required over time; may be guided by ultrasonographic localization of specific lesions.

POSTPROCEDURE

- Treatment of hemorrhage, swelling, or hematoma if these occur (rare).
- External dressings are not normally required.
- Animals should be monitored to prevent interference with the sutures.
- Proprioceptive deficits as already described; usually self-resolving in 3 to 4 days; long-term deficits are extremely uncommon.

ALTERNATIVES AND THEIR RELATIVE MERIT

- For muscle diseases, there is no alternative to the muscle biopsy for determining the specific diagnosis and therapeutic options.
- MRI studies may help localize focal lesions and allow for guided muscle biopsies.
- Electrophysiologic examinations can provide important information on peripheral nerve diseases, but a peripheral nerve biopsy should still be collected for histologic evaluation.

SUGGESTED READING

Dickinson PJ, LeCouteur RA: Muscle and nerve biopsy. *Vet Clin North Am Small An Pract* 32:63–102, 2002.

Melmed C, Shelton GD, Bergman R, Barton C: Masticatory muscle myositis: Pathogenesis, diagnosis, and treatment. *Comp Contin Ed Pract Vet* 26:590–605, 2004.

AUTHOR: **G. DIANE SHELTON**

Myelography

BASIC INFORMATION

OVERVIEW AND GOAL(S)

Myelography is the introduction of positive-contrast media into the subarachnoid space. Myelography is used for demonstrating lesions in the spinal cord or lesions extrinsic to the spinal cord that may be causing cord compression. This procedure is used for supplementing or confirming information obtained with plain film radiography.

INDICATIONS

- Clinical signs of spinal cord disease (± spinal trauma).
- Spinal pain or neurologic deficits without diagnosis on plain films or laboratory tests.
- Confirmation of suspected lesion on plain films.
- Aid in surgical planning (define exact location of lesion).
- Determine amount of spinal cord swelling.

- Exclude compressive lesions of the spinal cord; by process of elimination, make presumptive diagnosis of noncompressive spinal disorder.
- Rule out intraspinal lesion.
- Disparity between clinical signs and plain radiographs.
- Recurrence of clinical signs after decompressive surgery.

CONTRAINDICATIONS

- Cerebrospinal fluid (CSF) analysis indicates inflammation or infection: condition aggravated by irritation from contrast medium.
- Increased CSF pressure: possible herniation of cerebellum through foramen magnum.
- Known hypersensitivity to contrast medium.

EQUIPMENT, ANESTHESIA

- General anesthesia.
- Intrathecal contrast material: low osmolar, nonionic, water-soluble iodines, such as iohexol or iopamidol (180–300 mg iodine/ml most commonly used).
  - Full spine dose is 0.45 ml/kg; regional dose is 0.30 ml/kg.
- A 20–22-gauge spinal needle with stylet and short bevel, 1.5–3.5 inches (depending on size of animal).
- Appropriate size syringe.
- Flexible extension tubing or T-port (catheter cap with side line and port).
- Hair clippers.
- Surgical scrub solution, rubbing alcohol, and gauze/sponge for prepping skin.
- Sterile surgical gloves.

ANTICIPATED TIME

About 45 to 60 minutes, not including preprocedural anesthesia time

PREPARATION: IMPORTANT CHECKPOINTS

- Perform CSF analysis to ensure no evidence of infection or inflammation.
- Ensure adequate hydration status to decrease risk of neurotoxicity. Administer IV fluids as appropriate.
- Metastasis imaging (3-view thoracic radiographs are also indicated if malignancy is part of the differential diagnosis for the spinal problem).
- Advise owner the hair will be clipped in a large area near the injection site.

POSSIBLE COMPLICATIONS AND COMMON ERRORS TO AVOID

- The most common complication of myelography is postprocedure seizures. Recover the animal with head elevated to minimize risk. If directly induced by contrast, seizures are expected to occur during anesthetic recovery. Seizures occurring thereafter are virtually never caused by the contrast injection.
- Bradycardia is sometimes seen in animals during injection of the contrast material.
- Epidural injection may occur with lumbar puncture: wavy pattern is apparent radiographically both dorsally and ventrally.
- Subdural injection.
  - Central canal filling: thin line in center of cord
- Administration of air bubbles.
- Use of the incorrect type of contrast agent can be fatal. Ionic contrast agents (e.g., diatriazoate or any other product) should never be used in any amount in myelography; only low osmolar, nonionic, water-soluble iodines are indicated.
- Lumbar puncture: Inability to enter the space is commonly due to a nonmidline location of the needle (needle is inadvertently located parallel to, and lateral to, dorsal midline).
- Extension of the neck for neck-extended views can cause permanent cord injury, especially in animals with neck pain prior to the procedure and animals with severe cervical intervertebral disk disease (IVDD). These views should be preceded by nonextended views (diagnosis may be apparent without extension) or avoided altogether.

PROCEDURE

- Obtain survey radiographs of the area of interest (ventrodorsal and lateral views).
- Clip a large area of hair near the injection site (depending on cisternal or lumbar puncture).
- Sterile surgical gloves should be worn from this point on, and a sterile technique should be used (nonsterile materials will need to be handled by an assistant).
- Aseptically prepare the site for injection with surgical scrub solution, isopropyl alcohol, and gauze/sponges.
- Draw correct contrast dose into syringe.
- Attach flexible extension tubing to the syringe, and fill with contrast so no air bubbles are present.
- Cisternal puncture (see Cerebrospinal Fluid Collection, p 1207):
  - Commonly used for evaluating suspected cervical spinal cord lesions.
  - Animal is placed in lateral recumbency with neck fully flexed at atlanto-occipital joint.
  - Insert needle on midline, with bevel directed caudally, at the center of the triangle formed by the external occipital protuberance and the wings of the atlas.
  - Advance needle slowly until ligamentum flavum and dorsal dura are punctured. Since the puncturing may not be apparent, a good approach is to advance 1–2 mm at a time, removing the stylet and checking for CSF in the hub of the needle each time before replacing the stylet and advancing further.
  - Once the subarachnoid space is entered and CSF flows, obtain a CSF sample for immediate analysis.
  - If CSF analysis does not provide a diagnosis, the procedure may be continued.
  - Attach tubing to the needle and inject contrast material slowly.
  - Once contrast material is injected completely, the needle is removed.
  - Elevate head prior to obtaining radiographs to allow contrast material to flow caudally from the atlanto-occipital site of injection.
  - Standard radiographic views (lateral, ventrodorsal, 45-degree obliques) are then obtained.
  - Optional views (lateral, neck flexed, neck extended, and traction views). Caution with neck-extended views, which may cause permanent damage to the spinal cord in some animals, particularly those with severe cervical IVDD.
- Lumbar puncture:
  - Commonly used for evaluating suspected thoracolumbar lesions.
  - More technically difficult—fluoroscopy beneficial (see Cerebrospinal Fluid Collection, p 1207).
  - Animal in lateral recumbency.
  - Sixth lumbar spinous process is palpated. For anatomic localization of this spinous process, see Epidural Analgesia/Anesthesia, p 1238.
  - With bevel directed cranially, introduce needle at 30–60-degree angle at this site just to the side of the spinous process.

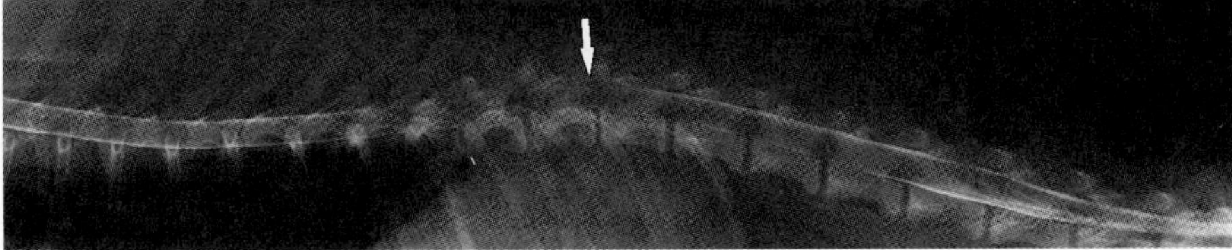

FIGURE II-98 Myelogram of a dog, lateral projection. Mild dorsal deviation of the ventral subarachnoid contrast column and attenuation of the dorsal contrast column, most pronounced at T12–T13 (*arrow*) are seen, identifying the lesion as extradural. Mineralization of the T11–T12 intervertebral disk is an incidental finding.

PROCEDURES AND TECHNIQUES

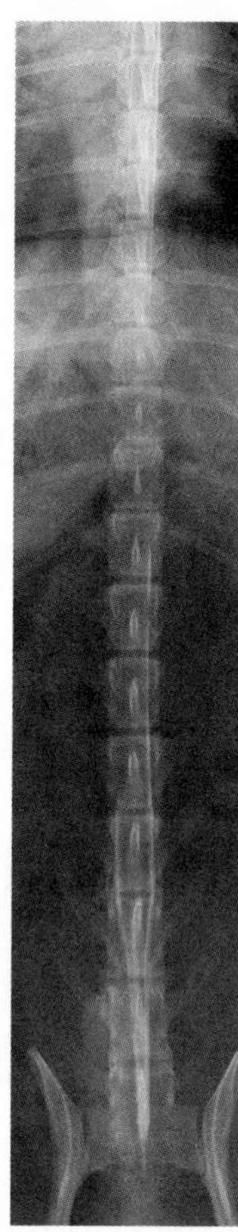

FIGURE II-99 Myelogram, ventrodorsal projection; same animal as in Fig. II-98. The contrast column is similarly attenuated over the caudal thoracic vertebral segments. The T12–T13 focus is less clearly seen.

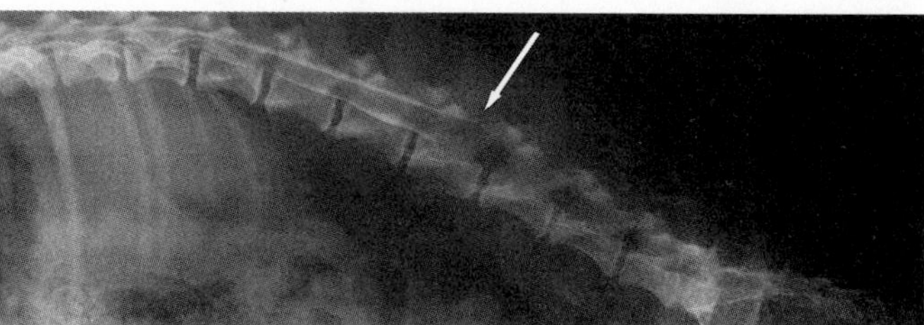

FIGURE II-100 Myelogram of a dog. Attenuation of both the dorsal and ventral contrast columns over L4 on this lateral projection is consistent with either an intramedullary lesion or a lateralizing extramedullary lesion (*arrow*).

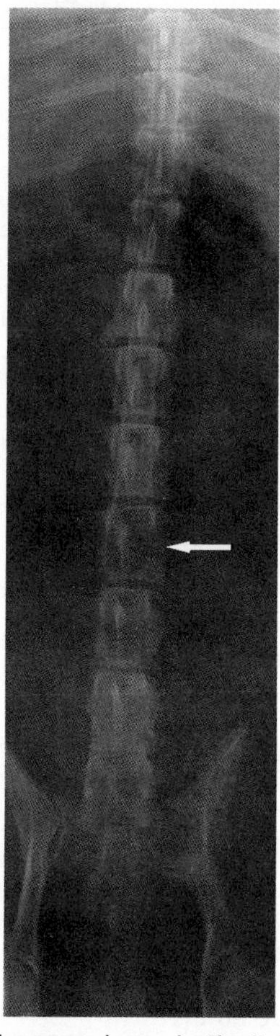

FIGURE II-101 Myelogram of the same dog as in Fig. II-100, ventrodorsal projection. The attenuation of both lateral contrast columns with a widened appearance of the spinal cord seen on this projection (*arrow*), together with Fig. II-100, identifies this lesion as intramedullary. The principal differential diagnosis is neoplasia.

- Reposition needle until tip enters interarcuate space between L5 and L6. It may be necessary to flex the spine—especially in older animals with degenerative bony changes.
- The tail or hind limbs may twitch as the needle enters the spinal cord.
- Advance needle to canal floor.
- Remove stylet and check for CSF; if no CSF is visualized, withdraw needle slowly until flow is obtained.
- Compressing the jugular veins may increase CSF pressure, allowing CSF to flow more readily.
- Once CSF is obtained and no contraindications have been identified on analysis, attach tubing to the needle and inject contrast material slowly into subarachnoid space.
- Once contrast material is injected, the needle is removed.
- Standard radiographic views (lateral, ventrodorsal, 45-degree obliques) are then obtained (Figs. II-98 to II-103).

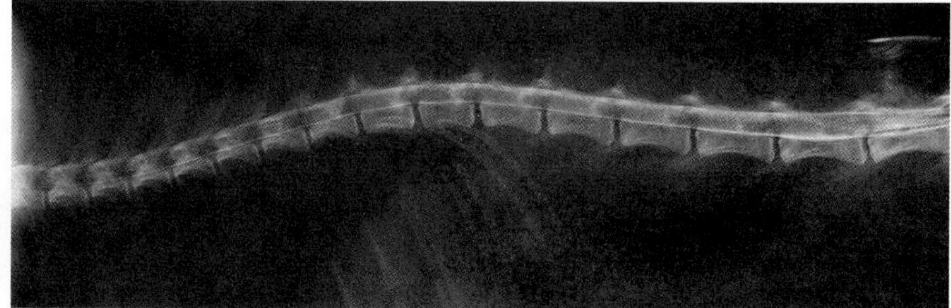

FIGURE II-102 Myelogram of a cat, lateral projection. Lumbar and caudal thoracic portion. Normal study. An incidental finding is a small amount of intramuscular and subcutaneous accumulation of contrast material at the site of the lumbar injection.

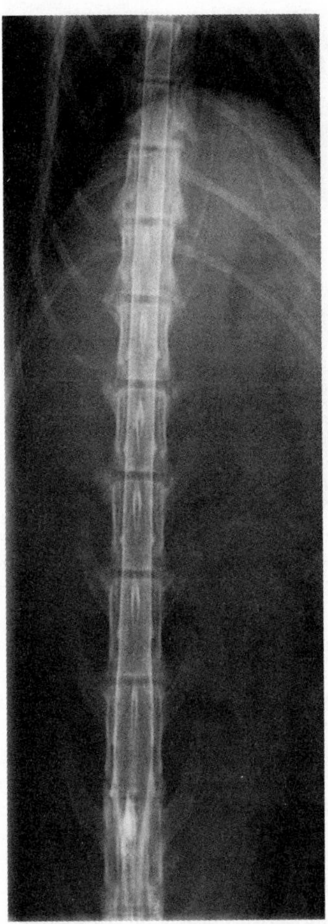

FIGURE II-103 Myelogram of a cat, ventrodorsal projection; same cat as in Fig. II-102. Lumbar and caudal thoracic portion. Normal study. An incidental finding is a small amount of intramuscular and subcutaneous accumulation of contrast material at the site of the lumbar injection.

POSTPROCEDURE

- The animal's head should be elevated so contrast material does not accumulate around the brain.
- The animal should be monitored for seizure activity.
- If seizures are encountered, diazepam (0.5–1 mg/kg IV) can be administered.
- Many clinicians recommend keeping the animal under general anesthesia for 30 minutes to 1 hour after myelography to decrease the incidence of seizures.
- Myelographic effect on CSF: increased cell count (pleocytosis), increased percentage of neutrophils, increased protein, false-positive Pandy score, and high specific gravity. These effects are transient, and the normal state usually returns in 24 to 48 hours.
- Maintain adequate hydration status: IV fluids ± fluid diuresis.

ALTERNATIVES AND THEIR RELATIVE MERITS

- CT scan:
  - Requires general anesthesia and knowledge of cross-sectional anatomy.
  - Provides axial images without superimposition of other structures, more detailed than standard radiography, ability to postprocess.
  - Equipment and CT scan examination more costly than myelography and CT often requires intrathecal injection of contrast prior to the scan.
- MRI:
  - Requires general anesthesia and knowledge of cross-sectional anatomy.
  - Provides axial images without superimposition of other structures; more detailed than standard radiography.
  - Sensitive, accurate, noninvasive, and does not involve the use of ionizing radiation.
  - Equipment and MRI examination more costly than myelography or CT scan.

AUTHOR: **LEEANN PACK**

Nasal Flush

BASIC INFORMATION

SYNONYM(S)

Nasal lavage

OVERVIEW AND GOAL(S)

- To obtain cells and/or tissue for diagnostic sampling of intranasal inflammation, infection, or neoplasia.
- To remove small nasal foreign bodies.

INDICATIONS

- Chronic nasal discharge (unilateral or bilateral)
- Intranasal obstruction
- Chronic sneezing
- Nasal foreign body
- Epistaxis with normal coagulation profile and blood pressure (BP)
- Maxillary mass/deformity

CONTRAINDICATIONS

- High-risk anesthetic animals (i.e., severely compromised metabolic, cardiac, or neurologic disease)
- Coagulopathy/bleeding disorder

EQUIPMENT, ANESTHESIA

- General anesthesia
- Endotracheal intubation
- Bowl of lukewarm tap water
- Rolls of gauze to pack the pharynx (one to three rolls, depending on size of animal)
- A 60-ml feeding-tip syringe; the larger the diameter of the syringe tip, the more forceful the water jet can be generated by pushing on the plunger
- Sterile saline solution for flush (1 L bag)
- Two bath towels
- Sterile, water-soluble lubricant

ANTICIPATED TIME

- Time for general anesthesia.
- Actual procedure takes <10 minutes per nostril.

PREPARATION: IMPORTANT CHECKPOINTS

- Thoroughly soak the rolled gauze in tap water, and then wring it out just before using it.
- Fill the 60-ml syringe to capacity with sterile saline solution.

POSSIBLE COMPLICATIONS AND COMMON ERRORS TO AVOID

- Improper placement or insufflation of the cuffed endotracheal tube, thus allowing water to enter the trachea of the anesthetized animal.

- Unevenly distributed or insufficient gauze, allowing the diagnosis (cells and tissue) to be flushed back into the esophagus.
- Forgetting to remove the gauze from the pharynx once the flush is finished.
- Using loose 4 × 4-inch gauze sponges—some may be forgotten after the procedure is finished and may occlude the larynx or trachea.
- In case of severe nasal destruction, epistaxis may develop.

PROCEDURE

- General anesthesia induction and maintenance; endotracheal intubation.
  - Verification of appropriate endotracheal tube cuff inflation.
- Sternal recumbency, head and neck extended.
- Unwind gauze and soak in water, and then retrieve and wring out excess water.
- Place damp gauze dorsal to and on both sides of the endotracheal tube as far caudally as possible, past the caudal edge of the soft palate.
- Gently insert lubricated end of syringe into the ventral meatus of the nose as far as it will go. This is most easily achieved by pushing the philtrum of the nose dorsally while aiming the tip of the syringe toward the septum. Slide into the nasal passage without using force.
- Place towel over the head and nose of the dog to avoid a spray of back flush onto the operator.

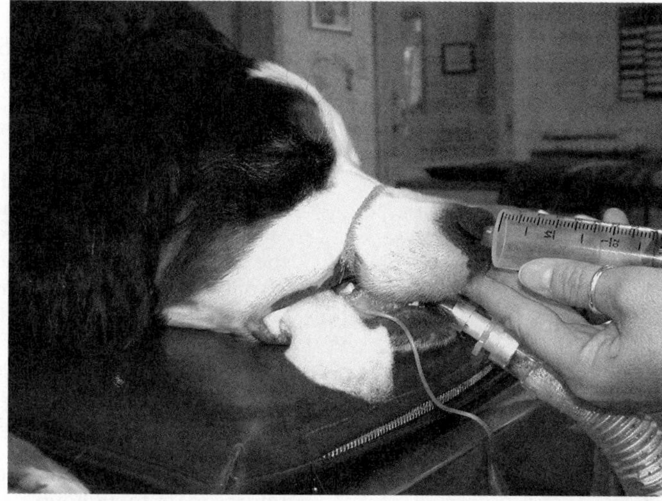

FIGURE II-104 A large-bore syringe is inserted into the nostril of this anesthetized patient to perform the nasal flush procedure. End of gauze roll can be seen protruding from the mouth.

- While holding the syringe firmly in place, forcefully empty the 60 cc of saline into the nasal passage.
- A powerful stream of fluid is required to dislodge foreign bodies or pieces of abnormal tissue.
- Repeat several times for each nostril; other towel may be used to control spillage if saline flows from mouth.
- When finished, gently pull gauze from the pharynx and examine carefully for foreign bodies or tissue clumps.

POSTPROCEDURE

- Remove the gauze from the caudal pharynx.
- Once the gauze is removed, examine the animal's mouth and pharynx for any material that was flushed out of the nose but not trapped into the gauze.
- Observe the animal for sneezing and bleeding after termination of general anesthesia.

ALTERNATIVES AND THEIR RELATIVE MERITS

- Rhinoscopy normally precedes nasal flush.
- CT scans and MRIs provide specific information on intranasal structure that is not obtained with nasal flush.

AUTHOR: **HANS GELENS**

Nasal Infusion of Clotrimazole

BASIC INFORMATION

OVERVIEW AND GOAL(S)

Intranasal infusion of clotrimazole is a minimally invasive technique for treating confirmed nasal aspergillosis in dogs. Treatment is performed for more than 1 hour. Resolution of clinical signs is achieved in two-thirds of dogs with fungal rhinitis after a single treatment.

INDICATIONS

Dogs with confirmed nasal aspergillosis; confirmation requires either histopathologic confirmation of fungal hyphae in nasal tissues or at least two of the following: positive *Aspergillus fumigatus* titer, positive *Aspergillus* culture, and radiographic/CT scan findings suggestive of fungal rhinitis (turbinate loss, fungal granulomas) (see Aspergillosis, p 87).

CONTRAINDICATIONS

- Cribriform plate erosion/damage secondary to fungal rhinitis. If advanced imaging (CT scan or MRI) of the cribriform plate is not available, owners should be warned that cribriform integrity has not been assessed. Topical therapy in animals with known cribriform damage has not been reported.
- Bulky fungal granulomas within the frontal sinus. Massive fungal disease within the frontal sinuses often recurs following topical therapy. It is assumed that the treatment does not adequately penetrate the center of these granulomas. Sinusotomy, surgical removal of bulky disease, followed by topical clotrimazole applied through the surgical incision should be considered.

EQUIPMENT, ANESTHESIA

- General anesthesia is required
- A cuffed endotracheal tube (mandatory)
- Two 12-Fr Foley catheters, one 24-Fr Foley catheter, and two 10-Fr polypropylene or red-rubber catheters
- Laparotomy sponges
- Two 60-ml syringes, one 12-ml syringe
- One pack of 3-0 nylon suture
- Suction canister and tubing
- Three hemostats
- One pair operating scissors
- One long-handled needle holder
- Four 30-ml vials of 1% clotrimazole

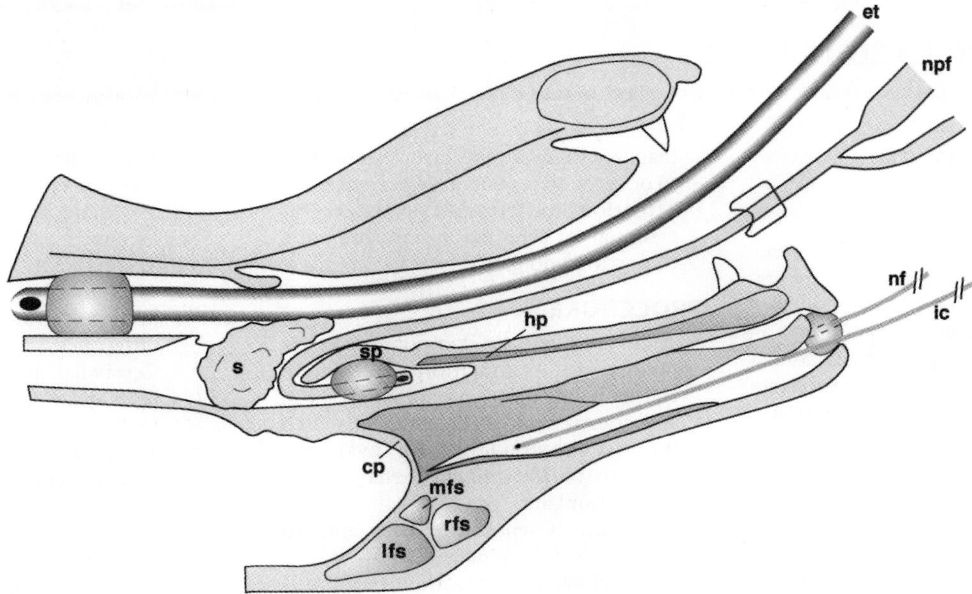

FIGURE II-105 Sagittal section of an anesthetized dog in dorsal recumbency. The image shows the position of the endotracheal tube (et), nasopharyngeal Foley catheter (npf), pharyngeal sponges (s), infusion catheter (ic), and rostral nasal Foley catheter (nf) in relation to the hard palate (hp), soft palate (sp), cribriform plate (cp), rostral frontal sinus (rfs), medial frontal sinus (mfs), and lateral frontal sinus (lfs). Reprinted with permission from Mathews KG, Koblik PD, Richardson EF, et al: Computed tomographic assessment of noninvasive intranasal infusion in dogs with fungal rhinitis. *Vet Surg* 25:309–319, 1996.

ANTICIPATED TIME

About 2 hours total: 30 minutes for setup and induction, 1 hour for treatment, and 30 minutes for recovery.

PREPARATION: IMPORTANT CHECKPOINTS

Imaging studies are followed by rhinoscopic evaluation and then clotrimazole infusion during the same anesthetic episode if diagnostic results are highly suggestive of fungal rhinitis.

POSSIBLE COMPLICATIONS AND COMMON ERRORS TO AVOID

The inflated balloon of the nasopharyngeal Foley catheter must be palpated through the soft palate, just caudal to the hard palate. The balloon is initially held in place with a finger, which is then replaced with laparotomy sponges. Failure to fully inflate the balloon or ensure proper positioning will result in leakage of clotrimazole into the oropharynx.

PROCEDURE

- Place animal into lateral recumbency.
- Pass a 24-Fr Foley catheter orally and then into the nasopharynx with the aid of a long needle holder. Bend the Foley catheter tip 180 degrees so that the tip flips and comes to be seated dorsal to the soft palate. While palpating through the soft palate, fill the Foley balloon with air. Withdraw the balloon if necessary until it is just caudal to the hard palate. Place laparotomy sponges in the oropharynx to prevent caudal migration of the balloon.
- Pass a 10-Fr polypropylene or red-rubber infusion catheter through each nostril and into each dorsal meatus (premeasure to the medial canthus).
- Place a 12-Fr Foley catheter into each nostril to prevent solution from leaking out the nostrils. Place a single nylon suture in each nostril to prevent rostral balloon migration. Fill balloons with air until obstruction occurs.
- Roll animal into dorsal recumbency.
- Fill two 60-ml syringes with the 1% clotrimazole solution (Lotrimin solution, Schering Corporation, Kenilworth, NJ). Administer 60 ml/side each hour via the infusion catheters.
- Place hemostats across any Foley if fluid is present within the catheter.
- Position the animal's head during infusion: 15 minutes, dorsal; 15 minutes, left lateral; 15 minutes, right lateral; and 15 minutes, dorsal again. The animal's body should remain in dorsal recumbency.

POSTPROCEDURE

Following treatment, the animal is placed in sternal recumbency. All catheters and sponges are removed and counted. Clotrimazole is allowed to drain out of the nares by tilting the animal's nose downward at the edge of the treatment table. Suction and dry sponges are used for ensuring that the pharynx is dry prior to recovery from anesthesia. Retreat the animal if nasal discharge does not cease by 2 weeks after treatment.

ALTERNATIVES AND THEIR RELATIVE MERITS

- Oral antifungals may be used in place of intranasal infusion of clotrimazole or as an adjunct to topical therapy. Itraconazole (5 mg/kg, q 12h PO for at least 2 months) has been associated with the greatest response rate (60–70%) and requires intermittent monitoring of liver enzymes. A single 1-hour infusion of clotrimazole is equally effective if the medication is injected via catheters placed in dorsal sinusotomies.
- Enilconazole can also be applied topically via dorsal sinusotomy catheters but requires daily administration of small volumes (5 to 10 ml/side) for 10 to 14 days.

AUTHOR: **KYLE G. MATHEWS**

Neurologic Examination

BASIC INFORMATION

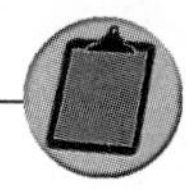

OVERVIEW AND GOAL(S)

To evaluate a patient's neurologic function through clinical assessment of mentation, gait, posture, facial and body symmetry, and responses (voluntary and involuntary). Specifically, the goal in an animal with a nervous system lesion is to establish the anatomic location of that lesion.

INDICATIONS

- Clinical signs suggesting either an intracranial lesion or a systemic disorder with intracranial effects (e.g., seizures, altered mentation/behavior, propulsive circling, whole-body tremor)
- Cranial nerve deficits (e.g., blindness without ophthalmic cause, strabismus, inability to close eyelids, head tilt, resting nystagmus, dysphagia)
- Horner's syndrome
- Gait abnormalities without an apparent orthopedic/soft tissue cause (weakness, spasticity, ataxia, lameness)
- Massive trauma with uncertain neurologic effects
- Clinical signs suggesting dysautonomia

CONTRAINDICATIONS

- Situations posing danger to the examiner (aggression; zoonosis [rabies])
- Disorders with which manipulation may worsen the lesion (relative contraindication; for example, for an animal with spinal trauma, much or all of the exam may need to be performed when the animal is in a recumbent position)

EQUIPMENT, ANESTHESIA

- Quiet, enclosed room to allow uninterrupted observation
- Floor with nonskid surface
- Pleximeter
- Light source/transilluminator
- Mosquito forceps

ANTICIPATED TIME

About 10 to 20 minutes

PREPARATION: IMPORTANT CHECKPOINTS

- Assess for contraindications (as already noted).
- Note: Review existing diagnostic test results (lab tests, radiographs, etc.) after performing the neurologic examination to avoid introducing bias.

POSSIBLE COMPLICATIONS AND COMMON ERRORS AVOID

- Inaccurate diagnosis (clinicians may think the condition is more or less severe than it actually is); this error is less likely to occur with repetition/experience.
- Attention to left-right symmetry is essential for avoiding misinterpretation of posture and gait.

PROCEDURE

- There are five main components to the neurologic examination: sensorium, gait, postural reactions, spinal reflexes, and cranial nerves. The order in which the five components are evaluated depends on the animal's behavior and chief complaint.
- Sensorium: Owners are best able to evaluate subtle changes in their animal's behavior or sensorium. In increasing severity, sensorium changes are depression, lethargy, obtundation, semicoma (stupor), and coma.
- Gait: Diagnosis of gait disorders is based on pattern recognition for specific anatomic sites in the nervous system (and musculoskeletal system). These are best evaluated with the animal moving on grass or a rug where slipping is not a problem. As a rule, changes are best seen with the animal walking slowly and taking numerous slow turns. There are two qualities of paresis and three qualities of ataxia that are considered in gait analysis.
  - Paresis (neurogenic abnormality of muscle tone/strength):
    - Lower motor neuron (LMN) paresis causes a loss of ability to support weight, reflected in rapid short strides with collapsing on the affected limb. The animal walks with a "lame" gait.
    - Upper motor neuron (UMN) paresis interferes with gait generation, delaying the protraction of the affected limb and lengthening the stride. This form of paresis cannot be separated from general proprioceptive (GP) ataxia because of the close association of the descending upper motor neuron tracts and ascending general proprioceptive tracts in any transverse section of the spinal cord.
  - Ataxia ("incoordination"):
    - General proprioceptive (GP) ataxia creates the appearance of the animal not knowing where its limb(s) is/are located in space. This also results in a delay in protraction of the limb, and the animal may show an excessive medial (adduction) or lateral (abduction) excursion of the limb as it is protracted. The stride may also be prolonged. Both UMN and GP deficits can cause the animal to occasionally stand on the dorsal aspect of its paw.
    - Vestibular ataxia is evident when the animal has a head tilt and drifts or stumbles to the side from loss of balance.
    - Cerebellar ataxia is characterized by a delay in protraction and an excessive response, a dysmetric abrupt gait generation that usually is associated with some balance loss.
- Postural reactions: Normal postural reactions require that most components of the peripheral and central nervous systems be intact. The most reliable of the postural reactions is the hopping response.
  - Hopping response: Each limb is tested by holding the animal so that most of the weight is borne on the limb to be tested and the animal is moved laterally on that limb.
    - First, straddle the animal so that both you and the animal are facing in the same direction.
    - Palpate the thoracic limbs to determine if any denervation or disuse atrophy is present.
    - Flex and extend the limbs to determine range of motion and muscle tone.
    - Place the paw on its dorsal surface—the paw replacement test—and observe how quickly it is replaced. NOTE: This is not just a test of conscious proprioception (CP), because disorders of the UMN, LMN, and/or general somatic afferent cutaneous receptors all can result in a delay in this response. A sole CP deficit cannot be determined, and that term should be discarded from the neurologic examination. Be aware that many normal animals may delay in replacing their paw to its supporting position.
    - Brace elbow on knee and support the abdomen so that most of the animal's weight is on its thoracic limbs.
    - With a free arm, pick up the animal's thoracic limb on that side and push the animal laterally away from that limb. This will force the animal to hop on the opposite thoracic limb.
    - After three or four hops, do not move, but just reverse both arms so that you can pick up the opposite forelimb and hop the animal back on the contralateral thoracic limb.

- Compare one forelimb with the other only when it is being hopped laterally.
- Move back to the pelvic limbs and repeat the muscle palpation, range of motion, and paw replacement.
- At that time, check the tail and anus for tone and reflex response.
- Stand beside the animal, and with one arm placed under the sternum, pick the animal up so it is standing on its pelvic limbs.
- Pick up the closest pelvic limb, and push the animal away so that it hops laterally on the opposite pelvic limb.
- Repeat this maneuver on the opposite side.
- Always compare the thoracic limbs with each other and then the pelvic limbs with each other because the pelvic limbs normally tend to be slower than the thoracic limbs.
- For very large dogs, it is easier to make the same observations while the dog is "hemiwalked."
- For hemi-walking stand beside the dog and pick up both limbs so that they are located at your side; then push the animal gently away.
- These hopping responses are much more reliable than the paw replacement test.

- Spinal reflexes: For spinal reflex testing, the animal should be placed in lateral recumbency.
  - Manipulate the limbs to assess muscle tone.
  - With the animal relaxed and the stifle slighty flexed, elicit the patellar reflex by tapping on the patellar tendon. If it is not present in one or both limbs, always place the dog in the opposite recumbency, and repeat the patellar reflex before concluding that it is absent. Some old dogs with no neurologic complaints lack the patellar reflex. This may be the only reliable tendon reflex because the other myotactic reflexes (triceps, biceps, extensor carpi radialis, etc.) may not be present in some normal animals.
  - The withdrawal-flexor reflex is routinely tested by gently compressing the base of the claw in each paw with forceps and observing the strength of the limb flexion and the animal's response (e.g., abrupt turning, vocalization) to the noxious stimulus. NOTE: The sensory modality that is tested is not pain. It is a noxious stimulus that is used, and what is observed is the animal's reaction to this conscious perception (nociception). Pain is the animal's response to a noxious stimulus. It is difficult to determine an animal's response to a minimal noxious stimulus, and there is no practical value to differentiating light and deep pain.
- Cranial nerves: sitting down on the floor with your back against the wall and knees flexed is the best position from which to evaluate small dogs and cats. Place the animal between your thighs and hold its head while testing the function of the cranial nerves. You can perform this cranial nerve exam on larger dogs by straddling them so that you and the dog are both looking in the same direction. Proper evaluation requires a relaxed, nearly motionless animal. Use a regional approach, starting with the eyes.
  - Menace response:
    - The menace response assesses vision and facial nerve function as long as the stimulus of the hand thrust at the animal's face does not touch the face or create excessive air movement.
    - If there is no response, be sure the eyelids are able to close (i.e., there is no facial paralysis).
    - If there is a normal palpebral reflex or spontaneous eyelid closure but still no menace response, then tap the eyelids or face gently to get the animal's attention, and then repeat the menace gesture.
    - Failure to close the eyelids to a menace in an animal >10 weeks old with normal facial nerve function or the lack of eyeball or head retraction in a patient with facial paralysis indicates a lesion in some part of the visual pathway from the eyeball to the occipital lobe.
    - Animals with significant cerebellar disorders that have no menace response are still visual.
    - Assessing the menace response prior to shining a light in the animal's eyes avoids falsely compromising the menace response with the glare of the light.
  - Pupil size and pupillary light reflex:
    - With a strong light source, assess the size and symmetry of the pupils from a distance.
    - Bring the light to about 1-2 cm from the eye, and swing it from one eye to the other and back again.
    - Repeat this to be sure that with the light in one eye, the pupils of both eyes are constricting.
    - Deficits in this light reflex implicate a lesion in the eye/optic nerve (optic chiasm or tracts) and/or the general visceral efferent component of the oculomotor nerve.
  - Ocular position and movement:
    - Observe the position of the eyeballs for strabismus, and test abduction (abducent, VI) and adduction (oculomotor, III) nerve function by moving the head side to side while observing the eyes.
    - Look for a resting nystagmus. If not present, then look for a positional nystagmus with the head held flexed laterally to either side and then extended dorsally. Occasionally, it is worthwhile to look for this sign with the animal placed in dorsal recumbency.
  - Trigeminal nerve (V):
    - Palpate the muscles of mastication (motor V) for denervation atrophy.
    - Recheck the palpebral reflex by stimulating the lateral and medial canthi with blunt forceps (sensory V).
    - Place the blunt forceps against the nasal septum on each side to assess ophthalmic V and the nociceptive pathway to the opposite somesthetic cortex.
    - Recheck the palpebral reflex by stimulating the lateral and medial canthi with a touch from the tip of blunt forceps (sensory V; VII [facial]). Observe for ear movement and lip symmetry and tone (VII).
    - Open the jaw to assess muscle tone (motor V) and range of motion.
  - Glossopharyngeal (IX), vagus (X), and hypoglossal (XII):
    - Observe the tongue for its size and movements (XII).
    - Place one finger in the oropharynx to determine the muscle tone and the animal's response to the presence of the finger—the gag reflex (IX and X).

POSTPROCEDURE

By establishing the anatomic diagnosis (the location of the lesion in the nervous system), the results of the neurologic exam will allow a differential diagnosis to be established and a diagnostic plan to be created.

AUTHOR: **ALEXANDER DELAHUNTA**

Ophthalmic Examination

BASIC INFORMATION

OVERVIEW AND GOAL(S)

Basic examination of the structure and function of the eyes and adnexa (surrounding structures) to establish an ophthalmic diagnosis, prognosis, and treatment plan, and to evaluate the need for additional diagnostic testing or referral.

INDICATIONS

- An abnormal appearance to the eye(s) or adnexa
- Ocular discomfort or trauma
- Vision impairment/loss
- Systemic disease that may have ocular manifestations

EQUIPMENT, ANESTHESIA

- An exam table in a quiet room that can be darkened.
- A bright focal light source (Finnoff transilluminator or otoscope without a cone) (Fig. II-106).
- Schirmer tear test (STT) strips—optional.
- Fluorescein dye-impregnated strips.
- Sterile saline/irrigating solution.
- Topical anesthetic (e.g., proparacaine).
- Tonometer (Schiøtz, Tonopen).
- 1% tropicamide—optional.
- Condensing/fundic or magnifying lens (lens strength of 20–28D is best for general use).
- Direct ophthalmoscope—optional.
- Muzzle for aggressive dogs.
- Sedation and/or anesthesia are generally not necessary and may in fact hinder a good examination due to globe position, reduced alertness, and anesthetic drug effects.

ANTICIPATED TIME

About 10 to 20 minutes

PREPARATION: IMPORTANT CHECKPOINTS

- Adequate restraint will greatly aid examination and is generally best performed by an assistant, not the owner.
- Examine the animal at eye level (on exam table); large dogs may be examined on the floor, sitting up, and, if cooperative, backed into a corner.

POSSIBLE COMPLICATIONS AND COMMON ERRORS TO AVOID

- Fragile eyes (ruptured eyes, descemetoceles) should be handled extremely gently if at all. NOTE: Do not palpate, retropulse, or measure intraocular pressure.
- Perform STT before any solutions are applied (solutions alter fluid content of tears); assess fluorescein staining before tonometry (tonometer may give false appearance of corneal lesion); assess pupillary motion before pharmacologic mydriasis (mydriatic drugs block miotic response).

PROCEDURE

- Grossly assess functional vision as the animal walks to the exam room: Does the animal show signs of adequate vision, such as successfully avoiding objects? Or conversely, does it walk cautiously with head down, using its whiskers and other senses to navigate? Is it easily frightened by obstacles? Does vision appear to be worse on one side than the other?
- Looking at the face head-on in normal room light, assess the overall appearance and symmetry of the head, orbits, and globe size and position. Note any ocular discharge or tear staining.
    - Evaluate the eyelid shape and conformation before manipulating the head and eyes.
    - Palpate the muscles of mastication, and assess the degree of globe retropulsion through the closed lids. Palpate both eyes simultaneously to best assess symmetry.
    - Retropulsing each eye individually also elevates the nictitans, which can then be evaluated for presence, shape, coloration, and abnormalities.
- Assess the cranial nerves bilaterally:
    - Menace response (II in, VII out): Covering one eye, perform a menacing gesture to the open eye to elicit a blink, without stimulating the face. Hold the hand flat and vertical with its lateral aspect toward the animal's eye to allow testing of different areas of the visual field while minimizing air motion.
        - Note that diffuse cerebellar disease may cause absence of the menace response without loss of vision.
        - Note that very young puppies and kittens normally do not menace.
    - Palpebral reflex (sensory V in, VII out): Lightly touch the lateral and medial canthi to stimulate blinking.
        - Note that facial paralysis disables blinking, in which case globe retraction and nictitans elevation (VI, ± III, IV out) or head withdrawal may be seen instead.
    - Dazzle reflex (II in, VII out): Rapidly apply a very bright focal light to one eye. This should cause a blink response. This subcortical response does not alone signify vision so much as some degree of retinal and optic nerve function.

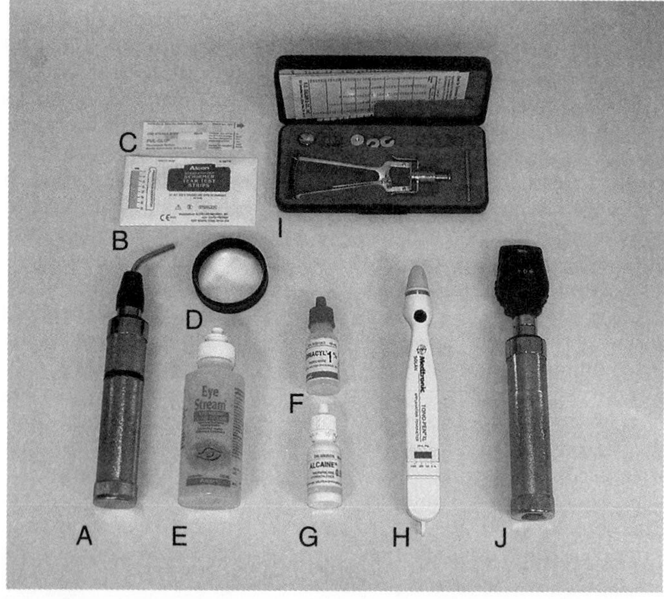

FIGURE II-106 Equipment and materials that may be used during an ophthalmic examination. **A,** Finnoff transilluminator. **B,** STT strips. **C,** Fluorescein dye-impregnated strip. **D,** Lens. **E,** Sterile irrigating solution. **F,** 1% tropicamide solution. **G,** 0.5% proparacaine solution. **H,** Tonometer—Tonopen. **I,** Tonometer—Schiøtz. **J,** Direct ophthalmoscope.

- Pupillary light reflex (PLR) (II in, III out): Apply a bright light to one eye and observe ipsilateral (direct PLR) and contralateral (indirect or consensual PLR) pupillary closure.
- Test vision by tossing cotton balls or gauze into the visual field.
  - Functional vision can also be tested utilizing an obstacle course in an enclosed area. The best obstacles are relatively large, safe to bump into, and free of odor. Vary the course during the test. Do not provide excessive nonvisual guidance (sound, food). Repeat in dim light if indicated.
- If significant mucoid ocular discharge is present, measure tear production.
  - Gently wipe away very large clumps of discharge without touching the lid margins or ocular surface.
  - Keeping the proximal end of the STT strip in the package, fold at the notch. Place the folded tip between the lower lid and globe. Close lids if necessary; keep strip in for 60 seconds, and immediately replace if blinked out.
  - Borderline result is 10–15 mm; normal is >15 mm wetting per minute in dogs and cats (even lower for many normal cats).
- If corneal ulceration is suspected, apply fluorescein. Place a drop of sterile saline on a fluorescein strip, and lightly touch the strip to the bulbar conjunctiva. Allow the lids to blink. Flush excess fluorescein with saline to prevent false-positive results. Examine in a darkened room, ideally with cobalt light/Wood's lamp.
  - In 1–5 minutes, fluorescein may appear at the nostril(s) or mouth, indicating nasolacrimal patency (positive Jones test). Note that a negative Jones test does not necessarily indicate nasolacrimal obstruction.
- Retroilluminate the eyes to identify opacities in the visual axis.
  - Hold the transilluminator above your ear and shine it into the animal's eyes. Adjust your position (usually to below the level of the animal) until you see the fundic reflection, and then scan from side to side to visualize opacities, which will appear silhouetted.
- Carefully examine the surface and anterior segments of the eyes in dim light with the transilluminator. Note the lid margins, nasolacrimal puncta, bulbar and palpebral conjunctiva, cornea and anterior chamber, iris surface, pupil, and anterior lens.
  - Holding the light from the side will aid greatly in accentuating the three-dimensionality of anterior chamber structures.
- Examine the fundus, noting the optic nerve, retinal vessels, tapetum, and nontapetum.
  - A drop of 1% tropicamide may be given for mydriasis if there is no suspicion of glaucoma. Wait 20 to 30 minutes after applying; the effects will last for 2 to 4 hours.
  - Indirect ophthalmoscopy: the preferred method, as it provides a wider view that is easier to interpret, allows three-dimensional visualization, and is safer for the examiner.
    - Using a fundic lens and transilluminator, position yourself as for performing retroillumination (as already described) an arm's length away from the animal. The assistant should hold the lids open. If using an aspheric lens, hold the lens' flatter side (white rim) toward the animal. Place the lens 1–2 inches from the animal's eye, and then move it toward you slightly until the fundic view appears (inverted and backwards) in the lens. Examine the whole fundus, adjusting as if the "fulcrum" of the line of sight is at the animal's lens (e.g., moving laterally for a more medial view).
  - Direct ophthalmoscopy: provides a highly magnified view of very small areas of the fundus.
    - To allow the widest area to be examined, use your right eye to examine the animal's right eye, and use your left eye to examine the animal's left eye.
    - With the largest white circle setting and the diopter dial set on 0, focus on the fundus by viewing the eye from 2–6 inches from the animal. View as many areas as possible, adjusting the focus if needed by changing diopter settings. These lenses allow for focusing at different depths (for a fixed distance from the animal) and also can adjust for any correction required by your eyes. The view through the direct ophthalmoscope is a direct image (not reversed).
    - If the light causes blepharospasm or resistance on the part of the animal, dim the light, apply the polarizing filter, or use a smaller circle size.
    - The slit beam (rectangle) setting may help in detecting three-dimensionality in anterior segment or fundic lesions.
    - The crosshairs in the fixation aperture may be used for measuring very small retinal lesions.
    - The red-free (green) filter allows differentiation between fundic blood, which appears black, and melanin, which appears brown.
    - An optional cobalt filter may be used for detecting fluorescein-positive corneal lesions.
- If the eye is red or cloudy or there is vision loss, perform tonometry. Note that "digital tonometry" (mere globe palpation) is inadequate to measure intraocular pressure. Apply a drop of topical anesthetic.
  - Schiøtz: Assemble the tonometer and clean the footplate. Test the tonometer by placing it on the included test block (gives a scale reading of 0). Position the animal with iris plane parallel to floor (dorsal recumbency or sitting up, nose pointed to the ceiling). Holding the tonometer by the handles and keeping it vertical, gently rest the footplate on the central cornea (not the third eyelid or sclera) until a single reading is produced. Repeat two to three times, and use included chart to get actual intraocular pressure (IOP). If IOP is >25 mmHg, repeat with next additional weight. Record IOP in millimeters of mercury (not as scale readings).
  - Tonopen: Properly fit a clean tip cover, turn on, and calibrate if necessary. Gently touch the instrument tip to the cornea, keeping it perpendicular to the eye; it does not need to be horizontal. Repeat several times until a long beep is heard. A bar over the 5% reading at the bottom indicates a statistically significant reading (mean given in millimeters of mercury).
  - Normal IOP in dogs and cats is 15–25 mmHg.

AUTHOR: **JANE O. CHO**

Orthopedic Examination

BASIC INFORMATION

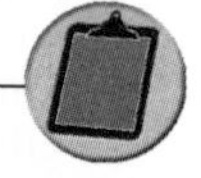

OVERVIEW AND GOAL(S)

To identify and localize an orthopedic disorder by performing a thorough and reproducible examination of the axial and appendicular skeleton, joints, and musculature

INDICATIONS

Any animal with abnormal musculoskeletal function due to injury, joint, muscle, or bone related disease

CONTRAINDICATIONS

In trauma cases, life-threatening problems should be addressed and animal stabilization ensured before performing a detailed orthopedic evaluation.

EQUIPMENT, ANESTHESIA

- Specialized equipment is usually not required.
- Goniometer to measure joint angles is optional.
- Sedation/general anesthesia is rarely necessary.

ANTICIPATED TIME

About 20-30 minutes

PREPARATION: IMPORTANT CHECKPOINTS

Detailed history, tailored to the individual case, including:

- Signalment:
  - Breed-specific orthopedic disorders
- Owner assessment of problem
- Duration of problem
- Speed of onset
- Relationship to trauma, exercise, or time of day
- Course of problem
- Influence of rest or medications
- Associated or independent systemic disease
- Previous orthopedic problems and associated treatments and outcomes
- "Family" history
- Diet and exercise regimen
- Observation in the examination room noting how the animal sits, stands, and moves around
- Observation of different gaits in an open area

POSSIBLE COMPLICATIONS AND COMMON ERRORS TO AVOID

- Do not overinterpret breed-specific disorders.
- Beware of misinterpretation of neurologic disorders for orthopedic problems and vice versa.
  - Postural reactions, such as proprioceptive testing and tactile placement responses, together with spinal cord reflexes can help differentiate between orthopedic and neurologic disorders.
- Perform neurologic examination after orthopedic examination (see Neurologic Examination, p 1286).

PROCEDURE

- Strive to palpate entire musculoskeletal system.
- Palpate all joints for swelling, thickening, crepitus, pain, and instability.
- Palpate all muscles for swelling, atrophy, pain, and asymmetry.
- Palpate bones for irregularity, pain, and instability.
- Palpate entire spine (including flexion, extension, and lateral deviation of the head and neck; tail head flexion and flexion and extension of the lumbosacral joint) for pain and sensitivity.
- Place all joints through a full range of motion.
- Know normal range of motion for all joints.
- When appropriate, use opposite limb as "normal" for comparison, best achieved in a standing position.
- Specific orthopedic tests include an Ortolani maneuver for hip joint laxity and a cranial drawer/sign test or a tibial thrust test for stifle joint instability.
- Ortolani maneuver:
  - The femur is forced dorsally and perpendicular to the spine in an attempt to subluxate the hip joint.
  - Slow abduction of the limb allows the femoral head to return to the acetabulum.
  - An audible or palpable "clunk" is a positive sign, suggesting hip laxity.
- Cranial drawer/sign test (see Cranial Cruciate Ligament Injury, p 253):
  - The examiner places a finger and thumb of one hand on the patella and lateral fabella proximal to the joint; he or she also places the finger and thumb of the other hand on the fibular head and tibial crest distal to the joint.
  - Cranial translation of the tibia can be applied to the joint in stifle flexion and extension. A torn cranial cruciate ligament will produce cranial subluxation (cranial movement) of the tibia relative to the femur.
- Tibial thrust test (see Cranial Cruciate Ligament Injury, p 253):
  - Evaluates the same instability as a cranial drawer test (i.e., tests mainly for cranial cruciate ligament integrity).
  - Dorsoflexion of the hock while the stifle is in slight flexion.
  - Positive result consists of a tibial thrust motion (cranial movement of the tibial plateau relative to the rest of the stifle), appreciated by placement of an index finger on the tibial crest.
  - Animal cooperation will determine whether the examination requires sedation or even general anesthesia.
- Perform a rectal examination in cases of pelvic trauma.

POSTPROCEDURE

- Inform owner that some animals may be sore or painful after an orthopedic examination.
- Use nonsteroidal anti-inflammatory drugs (NSAIDs) if the animal appears sore after manipulation.

ALTERNATIVES AND THEIR RELATIVE MERITS

Plain radiographs:

- May require sedation.
- Minimum of two views of the localized region.
- Normal opposite limb can be useful as a control for comparison.
- In trauma patients, thoracic radiographs should precede orthopedic radiographs as part of a minimum database.
- Initial radiographic assessment of spinal injuries should ideally be performed without sedation.
- Radiographic information and clinical/physical examination are complementary; one cannot entirely replace the other because some animals with radiographically severe lesions are clinically mildly affected and vice-versa.

Specific radiographic studies may be indicated (e.g., PennHIP, dorsal acetabular rim [DAR] view of pelvis, hyperflexed or hyperextended view of joint).

ARTHROCENTESIS: Where joint swelling is palpated, arthrocentesis may be indicated for cytologic evaluation of synovial fluid.

CT SCAN AND MRI: Imaging techniques can be extremely useful in specific cases:

- Rule in or rule out diagnosis that is unclear from examination and routine testing.
- CT scan is usually preferred for bone analysis, and MRI is usually preferred for soft tissue analysis, including ligament and articular cartilage damage.
- Requires general anesthesia.
- Cost or availability may be prohibitive.

BONE SCAN AND NUCLEAR SCINTIGRAPHY

- Helpful to localize an occult orthopedic lameness.

- Highly sensitive yet nonspecific.
- Requires sedation and hospitalization of "hot" animal, and cost or availability may be prohibitive.

DIAGNOSTIC ULTRASOUND

- Limited uses in identifying orthopedic disorders.
- In skilled hands, can identify biceps, triceps, infraspinatus, and Achilles and iliopsoas tendon lesions.

ARTHROSCOPY

- Allows minimally invasive visualization and diagnosis ± surgical repair of a joint disorder.
- Requires general anesthesia, and cost or availability may be prohibitive.

AUTHOR: **NICHOLAS J. TROUT**

Otoscopy (Video)

BASIC INFORMATION

OVERVIEW AND GOAL(S)

- Minimally invasive examination technique for the external ear canal, tympanic membrane, and middle ear.
- Allows excellent visualization, sampling, and documentation during ear flushing, myringotomy (deliberate perforation of the tympanum), and biopsy procedures.

INDICATIONS

- When clinical signs of ear disease are present: otic discomfort, pruritus, discharge, swelling or erythema, headshaking, Horner's syndrome, vestibular signs, deafness.
- Ear flushing using video otoscopy is indicated in unresponsive or recurrent otitis or if otitis media is suspected.

CONTRAINDICATIONS

- Very painful ears (in conscious animal)
- Severely stenotic ear canals

EQUIPMENT, ANESTHESIA

The main piece of equipment for the procedure is a video otoscope.

- Ear examination:
  - The examination can be performed in a conscious animal if the ear is not too painful.
  - Manual restraint is required.
  - A small amount of isopropyl alcohol is needed for cleaning the otoscope tip.
- Ear flushing:
  - Many techniques have been described.
  - Ear flushing, myringotomy, and biopsy procedures require general anesthesia and endotracheal intubation.
  - Ceruminolytic agent (dogs only).
  - Bulb syringe.
  - Sterile physiologic saline solution, approximately 1 L in bowl (may be warmed to body temperature).
  - A 5 Fr, 22-inch polypropylene urinary catheter, tip dulled by heating briefly over a flame.
  - Two 35-ml syringes.
  - Culturette tubes.
  - Video otoscope: compatible biopsy and grasping instruments and ear curettes are available.
  - Optional: suction unit and flushing and suction apparatus.

ANTICIPATED TIME

- Ear examination: <5 minutes in conscious animal.
- Ear flushing: 10–30 minutes per ear, 30–60 minutes for anesthesia.

PREPARATION: IMPORTANT CHECKPOINTS

Ear examination:

- Avoid having topical medication or cleaning solution instilled in the ears for 12 hours prior to procedure.
- Use adequate restraint to prevent harm to pet and handler.

Ear flushing:

- Collect cytologic analysis and culture samples before instilling fluids or cleaning solutions in the ear.

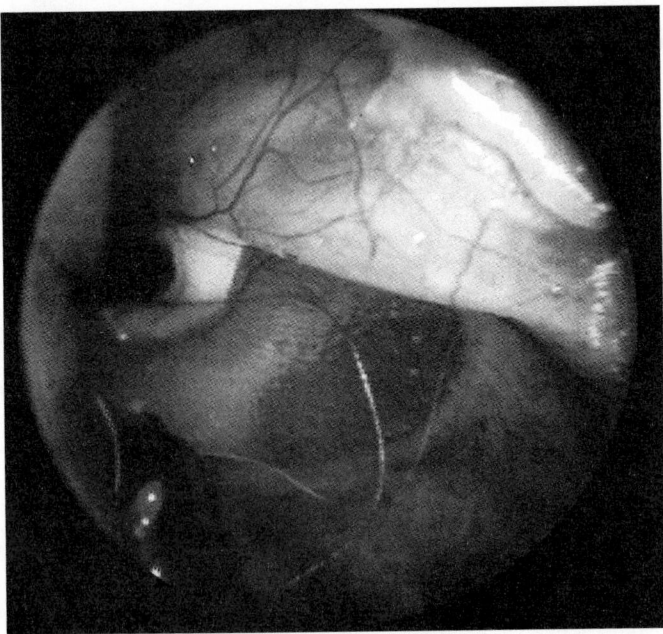

FIGURE II-107 Otoscopic view of a normal ear canal and tympanum.

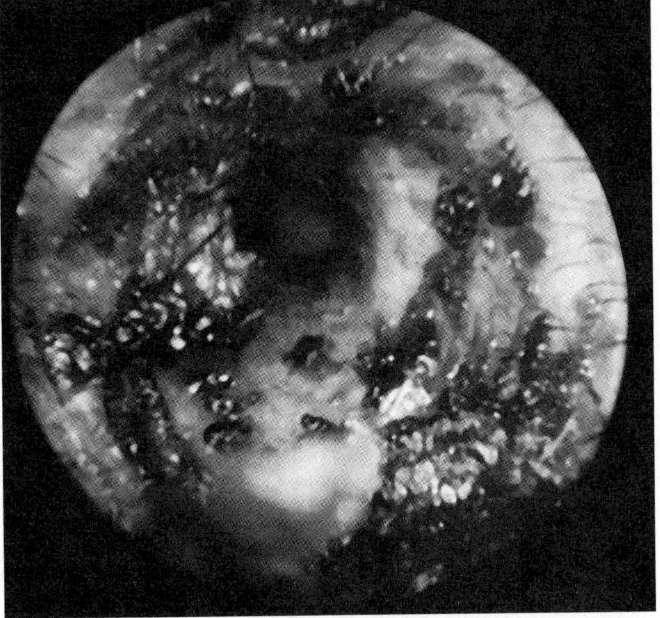

FIGURE II-108 Otoscopic view of an external ear canal with erythema and copious cerumen.

POSSIBLE COMPLICATIONS AND COMMON ERRORS TO AVOID

Ear examination:
- Discomfort, trauma to ear canal.

Ear flushing:
- Vestibular signs, deafness, Horner's syndrome, facial nerve injury, pain, tympanic membrane rupture.
- Usually temporary but may persist.
- More common in cats; therefore, the use of strong ceruminolytic agents should be avoided in this species.
- Flushing very inflamed ears may increase discomfort and induce a rapid return of debris to the ear canal.
- Should not be attempted in extremely stenotic ear.
- Use oral ± topical corticosteroids in inflamed or stenotic ears before and after flushing.

PROCEDURE

Ear examination:
- Wipe otoscope tip with isopropyl alcohol.
- Pull pinna gently away from skull.
- Slowly introduce otoscope into ear canal, using video image for guidance (Figs. II-107 and II-108).
- If thorough examination is not possible, the procedure may be attempted after 1 to 2 weeks of topical therapy, cleaning, ± oral corticosteroids (no topical medication on day of recheck).

Ear flushing:
- Sternal recumbency, head may be tilted to each side slightly as needed.
- Inflate endotracheal tube cuff.
- Tilt head down so that solutions exit from the nose if the tympanic membrane is ruptured.
- Collect cytologic analysis and culture samples.
- For tenacious or waxy debris, instill ceruminolytic agent, massage, and remove using saline and bulb syringe (dogs only).
- Introduce catheter through otoscope so that tip is visible, and attach 35-ml saline-filled syringe.
- Assistant flushes saline solution using small pulses.
- Direct catheter tip as needed to dislodge debris.
- Removal of debris reveals area of tympanic membrane at end of ear canal.
- If tympanic membrane is ruptured, the catheter can be advanced a short distance ventrally into the middle ear cavity.
- If the cavity is intact but otitis media is suspected, myringotomy may be performed by introducing a fine instrument (catheter cut to create a beveled edge, or a small culture swab) through the otoscope and directing it through the caudoventral portion of the pars tensa.
- May collect samples for cultures and cytologic analysis from middle ear.
- Gently flush middle ear with saline solution at body temperature.
- Suction excess saline solution from the ear canal, and instill topical medication if appropriate.

POSTPROCEDURE

- Oral ± topical corticosteroids reduce the inflammation induced by otoscopy and flushing.
- Ear medications should be started immediately after flushing; start cleaning ear the following day.

ALTERNATIVES AND THEIR RELATIVE MERITS

Handheld otoscopes are adequate for cursory examination of the ear canal but much less useful for ear flushing procedures. Advantages of hand-held otoscope:
- Less expensive.
- Convenient and portable.
- Less prone to condensation.
- Smaller plastic tip may be better tolerated.

Advantages of video otoscope:
- Greatly improved optics and magnification.
- Allows documentation.
- Vastly superior for ear flush procedures because the ear canal can be visualized very well through saline solution during the flush procedure, allowing for a very thorough cleaning with minimal trauma.
- Allows for much more precise and thus safe placement of instruments for biopsy, myringotomy, and foreign body removal.

AUTHOR: **KINGA GORTEL**

Oxygen Supplementation

BASIC INFORMATION

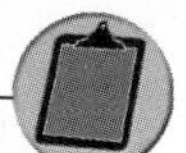

SYNONYM(S)

Oxygen therapy

OVERVIEW AND GOAL(S)

Oxygen is easily administered, readily available, and, if used correctly, safe. There are very few contraindications to oxygen supplementation. Oxygen therapy is often used in emergency and critical care medicine because hypoxic cellular metabolism is less efficient and may lead to organ dysfunction and death. The critical care supplier must understand the physiology of oxygen delivery and recognize cases that will benefit from oxygen therapy. A worthwhile rule of thumb is if there is uncertainty about whether to supplement oxygen, supplementation should be initiated pending clarification.

INDICATIONS

- Clinical situations in which oxygen therapy may be of benefit include: respiratory distress, sepsis, pyometra, severe bite wounds, hyperthermia, pleural space disease, congestive heart failure, anemia, all forms of shock, pulmonary contusions, pulmonary hypertension, seizures, and head trauma.
- Clinical signs caused by hypoxemia include an anxious expression, extended head and neck, open mouth breathing, abducted elbows, tachypnea, tachycardia, cyanosis, cardiac arrhythmias, and syncope.
- The hallmark clinical sign of diminished arterial oxygen content is cyanosis. For cyanosis to be detected, there must be >5 g/dl of unoxygenated hemoglobin in the peripheral capillaries (corresponds to SpO_2 75–80%); therefore, cyanosis indicates severe hypoxemia, and anemic animals may have critical hypoxemia without cyanosis.

CONTRAINDICATIONS

Causing distress to an already compromised animal is a contraindication. Several methods of oxygen delivery are available. Selection of the optimal technique depends on the animal's respiratory status, desired inspired O_2 content, anticipated duration of therapy, equipment available and its size, and conformation and temperament of the animal.

EQUIPMENT, ANESTHESIA

See description for placement of devices

ANTICIPATED TIME

Less than 10 minutes for any of the procedures

PREPARATION: IMPORTANT CHECKPOINTS

Pretreat animal with an anxiolytic that is not hypotensive and that does not decrease respiratory effort. Most of these cases are in respiratory distress, so the less anxiety the better. Low-dose benzodiazepines or morphine, buprenorphine, or fentanyl are feasible choices.

POSSIBLE COMPLICATIONS AND COMMON ERRORS TO AVOID

Excessive oxygen supplementation: Administration of 100% oxygen for 12 hours or 80–90% for 18 hours can lead to alterations in pulmonary function and signs of oxygen toxicity. Oxygen toxicity is often difficult to recognize because the clinical signs can be similar to those seen with hypoxemia. However, oxygen toxicity is relatively uncommon, it takes at least 12 hours to occur, it is preventable, and it is reversible in the early stages if oxygen is discontinued. Supplementation with 50% oxygen appears safe in the dog.

PROCEDURE

Emergency oxygen supply: Holding an oxygen delivery tube so that a high flow occurs directly into the animal's mouth is an option that can be used in an emergency situation until more optimal oxygen delivery methods are instituted.

MASK: The mask is perhaps the easiest and least invasive technique for oxygen supplementation. Purpose-made veterinary masks are preferable (better fit). These masks come in an assortment of sizes that range from pediatric size to large dog size and are designed to fit over the muzzle. It is often awkward to administer oxygen via mask to brachycephalic dogs and some cats. The mask can be connected via tubing to a 100% oxygen source, and if used for long periods of time, the oxygen should be humidified. With a well-fitted mask, flow rates of 8–12 L per minute achieve a fraction of inspired oxygen (FIO_2) of 0.4 to 0.5 (room air 0.2). The advantages of a mask are related to ease and speed of administration, and no specialized equipment is required. In addition, during oxygen administration, the animal can be closely monitored. Disadvantages of this technique include lack of tolerance by some animals and the requirement of constant manual application of the mask unless the animal is moribund or otherwise immobile.

INTRANASAL CANNULA: (Fig. II-109) There are various types of tubes available for nasal catheterization, including feeding tubes and urinary catheters. Some clinics use flexible feeding tubes or Foley catheters with multiple fenestrations to avoid mucosal jet lesions. The largest tube size possible should be passed. These tubes are placed in the conscious animal, but local anesthesia is recommended. Topical 2% lidocaine is used. The toxic lidocaine dose is 4 mg/kg in the cat, and one-fourth to one-half this dose is usually sufficient therapeutically.

- The tube is premeasured to the medial canthus of the eye, and the level of the external nares is marked on the tube to indicate the maximal distance of insertion.
- The animal's head is tilted with the muzzle pointing upwards. A few drops of lidocaine are applied to the external nares to desensitize the nasal mucosa.
- The tube is advanced until the tip is at the level of the medial canthus of the eye (until mark on tube is at nares). Insertion is usually easier if the nostril is pushed dorsally and the tube is directed medially.
- Once placed, the tube can be secured as close to the nostril as possible with suture or methacrylate glue (superglue).
- The tube should also be attached on the muzzle, below the eye and on the neck.
- These animals should also be fitted with an Elizabethan collar to prevent self-directed removal of the tube.

The advantages of this technique include ease of application, no special equipment required, versatility in animals that are different sizes, and the lack of interference with animal monitoring. Disadvantages include lack of animal tolerance, variable flow rates required to provide oxygen, nasal mucosal irritation, and gastric distention at high flow rates (rare). Recommended flow rates to achieve a specific FIO_2 are listed in Table II-4.

TRANSTRACHEAL: Oxygen may be administered transtracheally via a nasal catheter, which is advanced through the nasopharynx to the proximal trachea or through a catheter placed percutaneously through the cervical trachea. A long, flexible IV (jugular-type) catheter can be placed percutaneously into the trachea through the cricothyroid membrane or between tracheal rings. These catheters can be over-the-needle types or through-the-needle types. The entry area should be infiltrated with a local anesthetic prior to catheter introduction. In an emergency situation (e.g., cat with critical laryngeal spasm), a hypodermic needle or an over-the-needle catheter attached to a fluid extension set can be used for administering oxygen intratracheally. Oxygen lines used with this technique should be humidified. The disadvantages of this technique include difficulty with tube placement and poor animal tolerance when it awakens or is more alert.

OXYGEN CAGE: Oxygen cage equipment usually involves a chamber that can be flooded with oxygen to provide an oxygen-enriched environment. The advantage of this equipment is a controlled environment. The disadvantages include poor access to animal, difficulty in monitoring the animal, and inadvertent uncontrolled environmental conditions (especially overheating). Alternative oxygen-enriched environments include oxygen tents (Fig. II-110) or a cage with a "fitted door" into which O_2 is pumped. These systems are

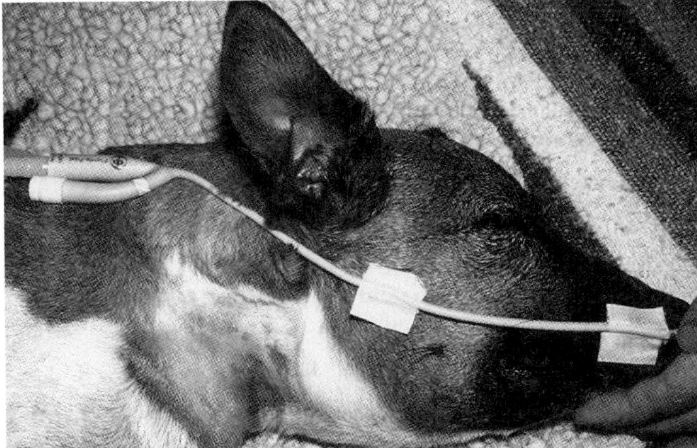

FIGURE II-109 Animal receiving oxygen supplementation via an intranasal Foley catheter.

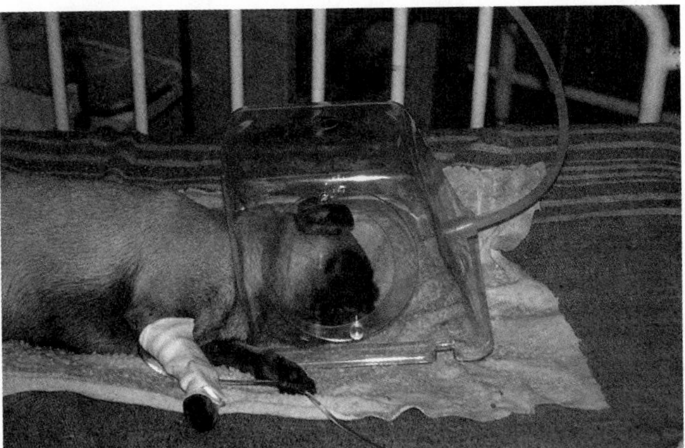

FIGURE II-110 Animal receiving oxygen supplementation via a tent.

TABLE II-4 **Approximate Oxygen Flow Rates for Supplementation Administration with a Nasal Catheter***

Oxygen Flow Rates (L/min) Required to Deliver an FIO_2 of:			
Weight (kg)	30–50%	30–75%	75–100%
0–10	0.5–1	1–2	3–5
10–20	1–2	3–5	>5
20–40	3–5	>5	?

*Reproduced with permission from Drobatz KJ, Hackner S, Powell S: Oxygen supplementation. In Bonagura JD (ed): *Kirk's Current Veterinary Therapy XII, Small Animal Practice*. Philadelphia, WB Saunders, 1995, pp 175–179.

Intranasal flow rates of >3l per minute often are not tolerated by animals; these rates may cause the animal to close its oropharynx in response to rapid air/O_2 flow. If a hissing sound is heard because oxygen is mostly or entirely refluxing from the nostrils, common sense dictates that the tube and apparatus be checked; if no defects are found, the clinician should try a lower flow rate.

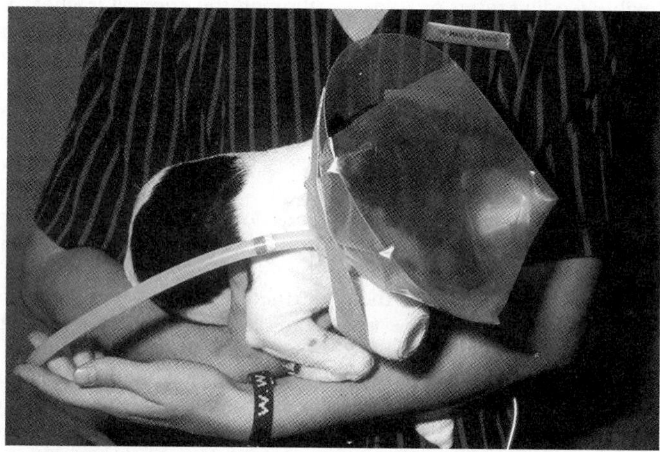

FIGURE II-111 Animal receiving oxygen supplementation via an Elizabethan collar partly covered with cellophane, creating an oxygen canopy. Note the oxygen tube entering through the caudal edge of the collar.

inefficient and generally have no way to remove or scavenge CO_2. This works well for cats that present in acute left heart failure because the clinician can supplement oxygen for a period of time without the stress of nasal oxygen. Human neonatal incubators have also been used for supplementing oxygen in small animals, and kits to modify normal clinic cages into oxygen cages are available. Covering some of the carrier holes with cellophane and providing a humidified oxygen source can convert pet carriers into emergency oxygen cages. Elevated temperatures and carbon dioxide levels may be a problem with this technique, however.

MISCELLANEOUS: With an Elizabethan collar, cellophane, and a humidified oxygen line, it is possible to easily create an oxygen canopy (Fig. II-111).

- The animal is fitted with an Elizabethan collar (E-collar), and the lower 50-75% of the collar diameter is covered with cellophane.
- The oxygen line is run inside the E-collar and provides oxygen into the cellophane-covered area.
- In this way, the animal's head is essentially within an oxygen tent.
- In areas with high ambient temperatures, this device is poorly tolerated.
- The advantages of this technique include ease of application and no special equipment requirements.
- The major disadvantage is animal intolerance.

NOTE: Oxygen can also be administered in acute situations via a transparent plastic bag placed over the animal's head.

POSTPROCEDURE

- Most animals requiring oxygen supplementation will be hospitalized in an intensive care unit and observed closely due to the nature of the underlying disease. In addition, it is important to closely monitor the typical vital parameters, including temperature, pulse, and respiratory rate. Specific evaluation for animals on oxygen supplementation includes thoracic auscultation, observation of respiratory effort, evaluation of mucous membrane color, capillary refill time, blood gas analysis, and/or pulse oximetry.
- Knowing when and how to discontinue oxygen therapy can present the clinician with a dilemma. Generally, it is worthwhile to slowly wean animals off oxygen supplementation. The rate of tapering should be based on the animal's condition and response but is generally done over a 24-48 hour period. It is also important to remember that oxygen is often an adjunctive therapy, and treatment directed toward the underlying disease process is paramount.

AUTHOR: **DAVID MILLER**

Pacemaker: Transthoracic Cardiac Pacing

BASIC INFORMATION

SYNONYM(S)

Temporary cardiac pacing

OVERVIEW AND GOAL(S)

Noninvasive, rapidly implemented temporary cardiac pacing system used for support of heart rate and blood pressure (BP) in animals that are under anesthesia and that have medically refractory bradyarrhythmias. Typical applications are stabilization for permanent pacemaker implantation and emergency treatment of life-threatening bradyarrhythmias.

INDICATIONS

- Support of heart rate and BP during general anesthesia for dogs with medically refractory bradyarrhythmias undergoing permanent pacemaker implantation or another surgery unrelated to pacemaker implantation
- Emergency treatment of hemodynamically unstable, medically refractory, complete atrioventricular block until more definitive therapy can be instituted
- Bradyasystolic arrests (e.g., digoxin overdose)

EQUIPMENT, ANESTHESIA

- General anesthesia and tracheal intubation required.
- Continuous electrocardiogram (ECG) and transthoracic pacing system

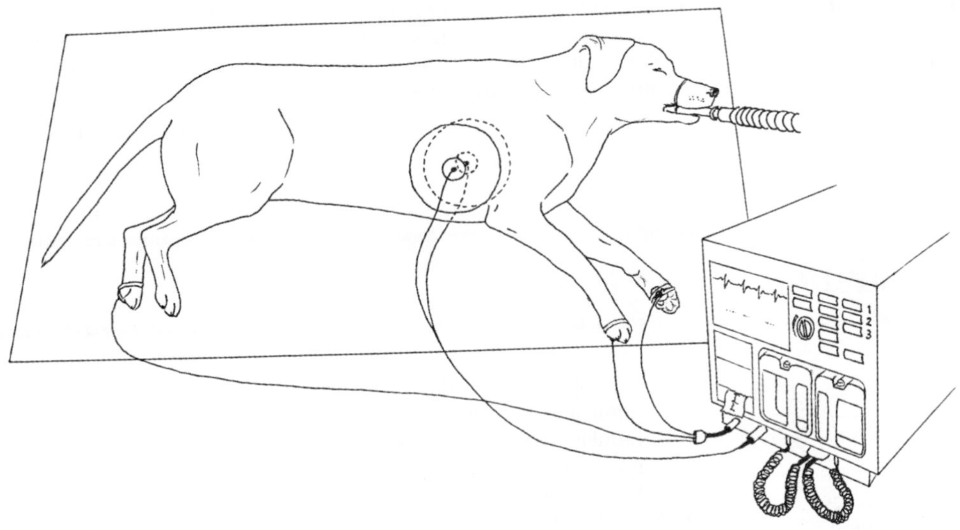

FIGURE II-112 Illustration of anesthetized, laterally recumbent dog with properly placed electrode patches and connection to pacing system. Courtesy of DeFrancesco TC, et al: Noninvasive transthoracic temporary cardiac pacing in dogs. *J Vet Internal Med* 17:663–667, 2003.

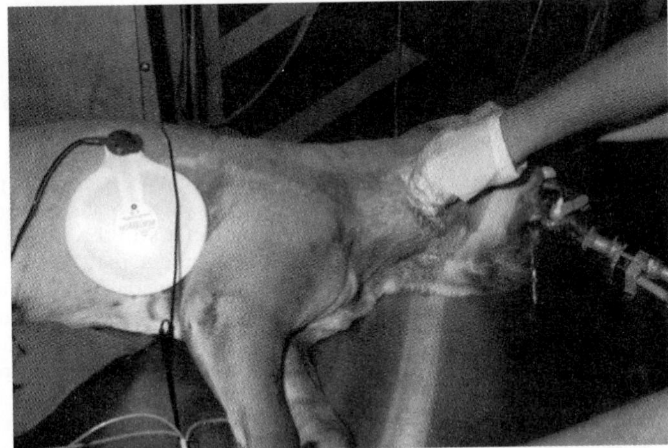

FIGURE II-113 Animal undergoing transthoracic pacing while the neck is aseptically prepared for permanent transvenous pacemaker implantation.

required, including disposable adhesive transthoracic patch electrodes.
- A #10 clipper blade (to shave the hair from the left and right precordia (area of the thorax overlying the heart).
- Occasionally, a neuromuscular blocker (and hence mechanical ventilation) may be desirable to limit jerking of skeletal muscles during surgical procedure.

ANTICIPATED TIME

Pacing system can be attached and pacing implemented in just a few minutes, especially in urgent situations.

PREPARATION: IMPORTANT CHECKPOINTS

- Have pacing system prepared (patch electrodes on chest and ECG monitoring ongoing) at induction of general anesthesia in dogs undergoing permanent pacemaker implantation or other dogs at risk for bradyarrhythmic complications with general anesthesia. This is a precaution in the event of bradyasystole during induction.
- Ensure clear ECG tracing to allow accurate sensing of dog's intrinsic heartbeat before starting transthoracic pacing.

POSSIBLE COMPLICATIONS AND COMMON ERRORS TO AVOID

- Most common complications are skeletal muscle twitching and pain associated with pacing stimulus.
- Pain or distress experienced in awake dogs requires rapid induction of general anesthesia for continued use of the temporary pacemaker. Analgesia (opiate or nonsteroidal anti-inflammatory drug [NSAID]) is also recommended.
- Skeletal muscle twitching, more pronounced in smaller dogs, may require neuromuscular blockade to lessen the jerking of forelimbs and chest during surgical procedure.
- Most common error is suboptimal placement of patch electrodes causing inconsistent pacing. Ensure placement directly over the palpable cardiac impulse beats. Readjustment of patch electrodes may be necessary.
- Obese dogs or dogs with pleural space disease may require higher than expected pacing threshold.

PROCEDURE

The procedure is typically performed in dogs undergoing anesthesia for permanent pacemaker implantation. ECG and pacing patch electrodes are in place prior to induction. The pacing system is usually turned on shortly after induction of anesthesia.

- ECG leads are connected to the dog, and a good quality ECG tracing is obtained.
- Patch electrodes are placed directly over cardiac impulse on left and right hemithorax. The fur on the chest is shaved, and a small dollop of ECG paste is placed on the surface of the patch electrode facing the skin. Dogs ideally should be placed in lateral recumbency (Figs. II-112 and II-113).
- Ensure accurate ECG sensing of dog's intrinsic cardiac rhythm by adjusting ECG gain and lead selection. A sensing marker will appear on the animal's QRS complex, signaling accurate sensing.
- After setting the pacing rate (range 40–170 beats per minute), the pacing current (range 0–200 mA) is gradually increased until ventricular capture is confirmed on the ECG monitor and by palpation of a corresponding arterial pulse. Ventricular capture is recognized by a wide QRST complex following a pacing spike on the ECG. The pacing current is maintained just above the capture threshold.
- Pacing rate and current usually ranges between 60–80 beats per minute and from 50–110 mA, respectively.

POSTPROCEDURE

Pacing patch electrodes are removed from skin. Adhesive remover can be used.

ALTERNATIVES AND THEIR RELATIVE MERITS

Transvenous transthoracic pacing:

- Specialized transthoracic pacing system not required (very expensive).
- No skeletal muscle twitching or pain associated with pacing stimulus.
- Procedure is more invasive, and implementation requires more time and expertise.
- Can be associated with infection, bleeding, lead wire displacement, lead wire-induced arrhythmia, cardiac perforation, and thromboembolism.

AUTHOR: **TERESA DEFRANCESCO**

Parenteral Nutrition

BASIC INFORMATION

SYNONYM(S)

PN

Partial parenteral nutrition (PPN)

Total parenteral nutrition (TPN)

OVERVIEW AND GOAL(S)

- Parenteral nutrition (PN) is nutrition delivered by the IV route.
- It can be life saving in animals that cannot tolerate enteral feeding.
- Used when no other feeding option exists and the need for nourishment is a critical factor in clinical outcome.

INDICATIONS

Animals in need of nutritional support when:

- Enteral nutrition is contraindicated (e.g., gastrointestinal [GI] dysfunction or risk of pulmonary aspiration)
- Sufficient nutrition cannot be provided by the enteral route alone (e.g., severe malabsorptive disease)

CONTRAINDICATIONS

- Animals that can be fed safely and effectively by the enteral route
- Animals that are at risk with catheter placement:
  - Central venous catheters in animals at high risk of thromboembolic disease (e.g., protein-losing nephropathy or enteropathy, hyperadrenocorticism, disseminated intravascular coagulopathy)
  - Jugular catheters in animals with increased cerebral pressure (e.g., head trauma)
- Animals experiencing fluid overload (e.g., animals with heart failure, oliguria, or severe hypoproteinemia)

EQUIPMENT, ANESTHESIA

- Venous access:
  - A dedicated catheter is required for delivery of the nutrient solution to avoid septic complications and drug-nutrient interactions.
  - Treat catheter placement as a surgical procedure (surgical prep, draping, and the use of sterile gloves) (see Jugular Catheter Placement and Management, p 1270).
  - Place a central venous catheter to deliver TPN because the nutrient solution is hyperosmolar. Solutions that are more dilute can be prepared, but the resulting large volume that must be infused can become a limiting factor.
  - Catheters made of nonthrombogenic materials (polyurethane or silicone) are preferred, particularly for peripheral infusion.
  - Multilumen central or peripherally placed central catheters (PICC lines) can be used if one of the ports is dedicated for PN.
- Nutrient admixture:
  - Amino acid solutions (3–10%) are used for providing protein. These solutions come with and without added electrolytes (Fig. II-114).
  - Nonprotein calories can be provided by a combination of lipid emulsions (10% or 20%) and dextrose (10–50%) or dextrose alone (see Fig. II-114).
  - Electrolytes can be added to the nutrient solution as needed or provided separately in the animal's crystalloid fluid therapy. The latter allows greater flexibility. Alternatively, a combination amino acid and electrolyte solution can be used.
  - Special parenteral vitamin and mineral preparations are available. However, because most companion animals receive PN for relatively short periods of time (<2 weeks), only certain vitamins and minerals are commonly added to the nutrient admixture (B complex, ± potassium phosphate, magnesium sulfate, and trace elements [zinc, copper, manganese, and chromium]) (Fig. II-115).

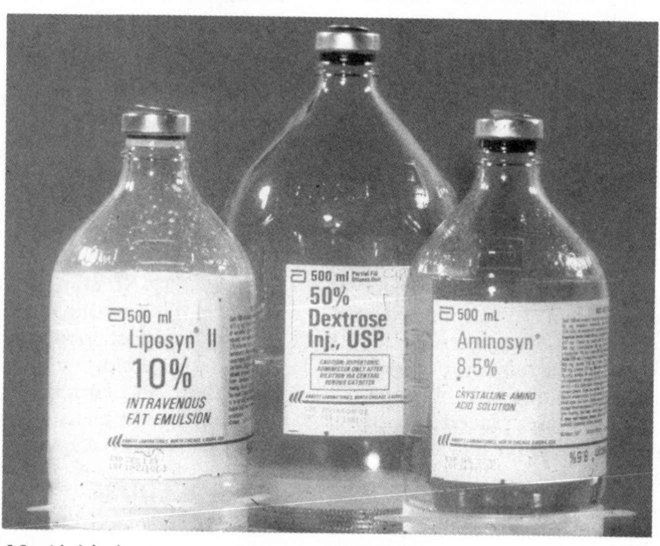

FIGURE II-114 Lipid, dextrose, and amino acid solutions.

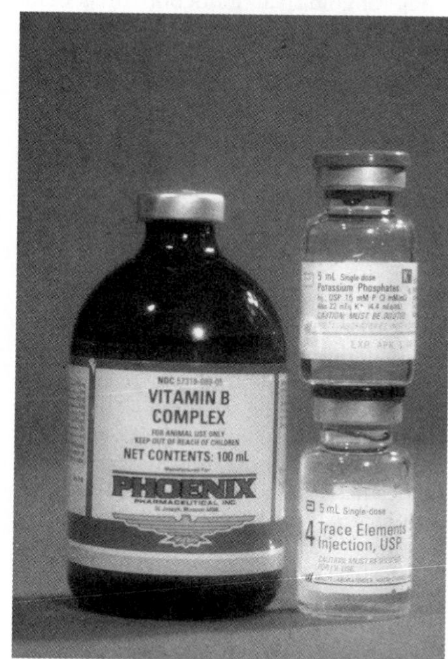

FIGURE II-115 Vitamin, electrolyte, and mineral solutions.

- Monitoring and nursing care:
  - PN is best delivered continuously (although this is not absolutely necessary), so 24-hour nursing care is desirable both for administration and for catheter vigilance/catheter care.
  - Many of the complications of PN can be life threatening, so careful monitoring of the animal is mandated. This includes frequent checking of serum glucose and electrolyte concentrations; hence, the ability to do some in-house serum chemistry analyses is necessary.

PREPARATION: IMPORTANT CHECKPOINTS

- Venous access:
  - Reserve a dedicated venous catheter (or port of a multilumen catheter) for PN. Insert the catheter under aseptic conditions, and do not use for any other purpose.
- Nutrient admixture:
  - Prepare PN solutions under aseptic conditions. In addition, solutions must be compounded in a specific sequence and carefully mixed.
  - Use the services of a home infusion service or a human hospital pharmacy to compound PN solutions when the veterinary practice lacks the facilities and expertise.

POSSIBLE COMPLICATIONS AND COMMON ERRORS TO AVOID

- Common metabolic complications:
  - NOTE: When addressing electrolyte abnormalities, delivering supplements in the IV fluids rather than in the PN solution allows greater flexibility. Later, when the amount of supplementation for maintenance is established, it can be included in the PN formulation.
  - Hyperglycemia: If present, reduce the percentage of nonprotein calories from dextrose, or give regular insulin.
  - Hypokalemia: If present, supplement IV fluids with potassium chloride. Monitor for hypomagnesemia (see Refeeding Syndrome, p 948).
  - Hypophosphatemia: If present, supplement IV fluids with potassium phosphate, or add potassium phosphate to PN formulation.
  - Hypomagnesemia: If present, supplement IV fluids with magnesium sulfate or add magnesium sulfate to PN formulations.
  - Hyperlipidemia: If present, reduce or omit the lipid emulsion.
- Catheter complications:
  - Loss of venous access secondary to catheter malposition or thrombosis: If occurs, replace catheter.
  - Thrombophlebitis: If occurs, replace catheter. Select peripheral catheters that are long and made of nonthrombogenic materials.

TABLE II-5 Sample PN Worksheet for a 17-kg Dog: Centrally Administered PN Calculation

CANINE HIGH-PROTEIN REGIMEN

Weight: 17.5 kg	RER = 600 kcal/day
Day 1 Goal:	50% RER = 0.5(600) = 300 kcal
Day 2 Goal:	100% RER = 600 kcal
% Protein calories:	25%
Nonprotein calories:	50% from lipid
	50% from dextrose

Solutions:

- 8.5% amino acids (without electrolytes)
- 50% dextrose
- 20% lipid emulsion
- MTE-4 trace element solution containing 0.8 mg zinc/ml
- Potassium phosphate (3 mM/ml)
- Injectable B complex

Day 1 Calculations

Amino Acids

- (0.25)(300 kcal) = 75 kcal from protein.
- There are 4 kcal/g protein; therefore, the animal needs 18.75 grams of protein: (75 kcal ÷ 4 kcal/g = 18.75 g).
- 8.5% amino acid solution = 0.085 g protein/ml; therefore, the animal needs 220 ml 8.5% amino acid solution: (220 ml = 18.75 g ÷ 0.085 g/ml).

Nonprotein Calories

- (0.75)(300 kcal) = 225 kcal.
  - 50% dextrose to provide 50% nonprotein calories = 112.5 kcal.
    - 50% dextrose solution = 1.7 kcal/ml; therefore, the animal needs 66 ml 50% dextrose solution: (66 ml = 112.5 kcal ÷ 1.7 kcal/ml).
  - 20% lipid emulsion to provide 50% nonprotein calories = 112.5 kcal.
    - 20% lipid emulsion = 2 kcal/ml; therefore, the animal needs 56 ml 20% lipid emulsion: (56 ml = 112.5 kcal ÷ 2 kcal/ml).

Trace Elements

- Dosed at 1 μg zinc/kcal delivered MTE-4; contains 0.8 mg zinc/ml.
- Therefore, the animal needs 0.37 ml: (0.37 ml = 300 kcal ÷ [0.8 mg/ml × 1000]).

Potassium Phosphate

- Dosed at 8 mM/1000 kcal delivered.
  - Therefore, the animal needs 2.4 mM potassium phosphate: (2.4 mM = [8 mM × 300 kcal] ÷ 1000 kcal).
  - Potassium phosphate solution = 3 mM/ml.
  - Therefore, the animal needs 0.8 ml potassium phosphate: (0.8 ml = 2.4 mM ÷ 3 mM/ml).

Vitamin B Complex

- Dosed at approximately 2 ml/L infused.
- Total infusate for day 1 = 343 ml.
- Therefore, 1.0 ml B complex should be sufficient.

Infusion Rate

343 ml ÷ 24 hr = 14 ml/hr.

Day 2 Calculations

Same calculations as those for day 1, but substitute 600 kcal for 300 kcal

  - Infection: If occurs, remove catheter and culture the tip. Replace with a new catheter in a new location.

PROCEDURE

PN PRESCRIPTION FORMULATION

- Choose between central or peripheral venous administration.
  - Central venous administration is preferred because smaller volumes of PN solution are required, and thrombophlebitis is less likely to occur.
  - Peripheral venous administration is possible when central venous access is not available, but the animal must be fluid tolerant.
  - NOTE: For peripheral venous infusion, long catheters made of nonthrombogenic materials reduce the likelihood of thrombophlebitis.
- Calculating the caloric goal:
  - Calculate the resting energy requirement (RER) using the animal's current body weight (or the animal's estimated ideal weight if overweight).
  - Formula: RER = 70 + 30 × (body weight in kilograms) for animals weighing 2-30 kg; use 70 × (body

weight in kilograms)$^{0.75}$ for animals that weigh outside this range.
  - Start with a caloric goal of RER, and adjust based on animal response.
- Decide what percentage of calories will be delivered as protein depending on the animal's level of protein tolerance or deficiency.
  - Dogs: Provide 15–25% of goal calories as protein.
  - Cats: Provide 25–30% of goal calories as protein.
  - Amino acid solutions: provide 4 kcal/g.
  - To calculate the volume of amino acid solution required:
    1. Divide the protein calories by 4 kcal/g = grams of amino acids required.
    2. Divide the grams of amino acids required by the grams of amino acids per milliliter in the solution = volume of amino acid solution.
  - NOTE: For peripheral infusion, use ≤6% amino acid solutions due to high osmolarity.
- Decide what percentage of nonprotein calories will be delivered as dextrose with the remainder to be delivered as lipid:
  - 100% of the nonprotein calories can be delivered as dextrose, but hyperglycemia is a common sequela. 50% dextrose provides 1.7 kcal/ml.
  - Alternatively, lipid emulsions can be used for delivering 50–70% of the nonprotein calories; 20% lipid emulsions provide 2 kcal/ml.
  - NOTE: For peripheral venous infusion, a high percentage of nonprotein calories from lipid is preferred because the lipid emulsions are isoosmolar. They are also more calorically dense than the dextrose solutions that can be safely infused peripherally (≤20% dextrose).
- Add 0.2 ml/100 kcal vitamin B complex.
- Decide whether electrolytes and minerals will be added.
  - Supplementation may not be necessary if amino acid solutions containing additional electrolytes are used.
  - CAUTION: Supplementation is contraindicated in animals with renal failure.
  - Potassium phosphate: 8 mEq/1000 kcal.
  - Magnesium sulfate: 0.8 mEq/100 kcal.
  - Zinc: 1 μg/kcal.
- Calculate the hourly infusion rate by dividing the total volume by 24.

POSTPROCEDURE

- Delivery:
  - Deliver the solution at a constant rate using an infusion pump if possible (Fig. I-116).
  - Administer 50% of the goal infusion, and monitor for metabolic complications the first day, advancing to the goal rate the next day if no problems occur that cannot be addressed.
  - Do not discontinue PN abruptly, especially in animals that are not eating. If an animal cannot be weaned, monitor for hypoglycemia.
- Catheter care:
  - Examine the catheter site at least daily for signs of phlebitis or infection, changing the dressing as needed.
  - Change the drip set at least every other day.
  - Never use the catheter for any purpose other than the delivery of PN (no blood sampling, administering medications, fluid therapy, or measuring central venous pressure).
- Monitoring:
  - In addition to the routine monitoring appropriate for any animal on IV fluid therapy, animals receiving PN should be monitored for metabolic complications.
  - Animals should have blood glucose monitored at least every 12 hours and serum electrolytes at least once daily depending on circumstances and whether any PN supplementation is required.
  - When a packed cell volume (PCV) is performed, the serum should be examined for evidence of lipemia.
  - A complete serum chemistry profile and blood count should be performed as indicated but at least once weekly.

ALTERNATIVES AND THEIR RELATIVE MERITS

Enteral nutrition:

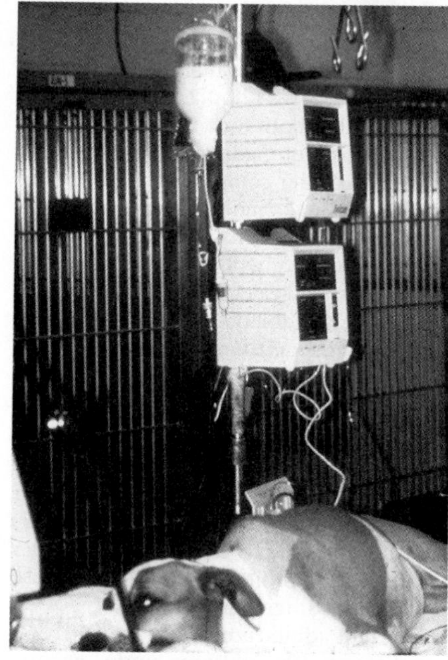

FIGURE II-116 Animal receiving PN.

- In general, nutrient delivery by the enteral route is safer and less costly than PN.
- Enteral nutrition has trophic effects on the GI tract and supports both the structure and function of the mucosa and the barrier function of the gut.
- Preferred over PN whenever feasible.

SUGGESTED READING

Chan DL: Parenteral nutritional support. In Ettinger SJ, Feldman EC (eds): *Textbook of Veterinary Internal Medicine*, ed 6. Philadelphia, Elsevier, 2005, pp 586–591.

Chan DL, Freeman LM, Labato MA, Rush JE: Retrospective evaluation of partial parenteral nutrition in dogs and cats. *J Vet Intern Med* 16(4):440–445, 2002.

Pyle SC, Marks SL, Kass PH: Evaluation of complications and prognostic factors associated with administration of total parenteral nutrition in cats: 75 cases (1994–2001). *J Am Vet Med Assoc* 225(2):242–250, 2004.

AUTHOR: **KATHRYN E. MICHEL**
EDITOR: **C. A. TONY BUFFINGTON**

Pericardiocentesis

BASIC INFORMATION

SYNONYM(S)

Pericardial drainage
Pericardial tap

OVERVIEW AND GOAL(S)

A catheter is used for removing a volume of pericardial effusion for diagnostic and/or therapeutic purposes.

INDICATIONS

- Pericardial effusion causing cardiac tamponade
- Pericardial effusion of unknown etiology

CONTRAINDICATIONS

Small volume of pericardial effusion (difficult to safely enter the pericardial space)

EQUIPMENT, ANESTHESIA

- Local anesthesia (2% lidocaine).

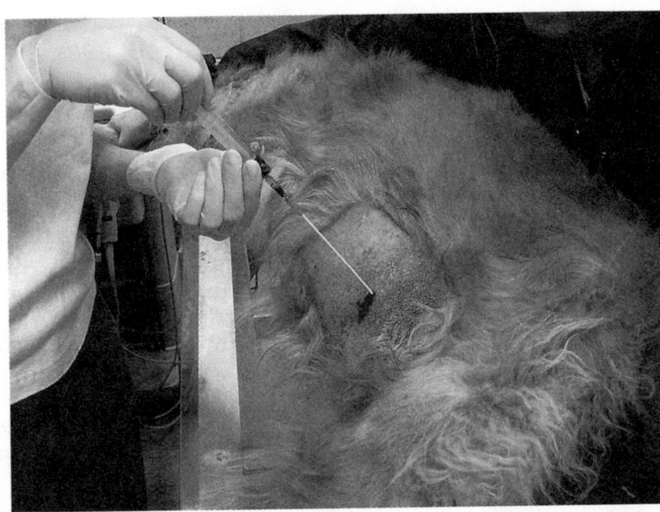

FIGURE II-117 Pericardiocentesis in a dog with severe cardiac tamponade and hemorrhagic pericardial effusion. Left lateral recumbency; head is beyond the lower right corner of the image. The syringe-catheter-stylet combination has been advanced to the point of entering the pericardium, and effusion is seen in the hub of the stylet and the syringe. Next, the catheter will be advanced off the stylet.

- Manual restraint; sedation needed only rarely.
- Hair clippers.
- Surgical scrub solution, rubbing alcohol, and gauze/sponge for prepping skin.
- 0.5–12 ml 2% lidocaine for local anesthesia; volume based on body weight, 1–70 kg. NOTE: Discomfort of lidocaine infusion can be reduced by adding 0.05–0.2 ml 8.4% sodium bicarbonate and warming to body temperature (armpit method).
- Sterile surgical gloves.
- A #11 scalpel blade.
- A 14-gauge over-the-needle catheter (e.g., equine IV catheter).
- A 6-cc syringe.
- Two 35- or 60-ml syringes.
- Kidney bowl for effusion.
- Lavender- and red-top tubes for sample.
- Tissue glue.

ANTICIPATED TIME

About 15 to 40 minutes

PREPARATION: IMPORTANT CHECKPOINTS

- Ultrasound guidance: not usually used during the procedure. Immediately prior to the procedure, however, ultrasound-based localization of an area with maximal pericardial effusion and minimal lung is extremely useful.
- ECG may be used during the procedure; appearance of premature ventricular complexes (PVCs) suggests catheter/stylet is touching heart and should not be advanced farther. However, such contact with the heart is generally palpable (heartbeat hitting catheter tip), and PVCs may occur independently of the catheter in animals with pericardial effusion.
- Clinicians should tell clients that the procedure is often palliative and that effusion can recur, with the likelihood and speed of recurrence depending on the underlying cause. Rapid re-effusion or even hemodynamic collapse postcentesis is possible with atrial tear and with malignancies such as hemangiosarcomas.

POSSIBLE COMPLICATIONS AND COMMON ERRORS TO AVOID

- Inability to obtain pericardial fluid. Ultrasound guidance is useful before reattempting.
- Effusion that clots in the syringe, either due to excessive advancement (catheter tip is in the heart) or to a rapidly bleeding pericardial effusion. Differentiation: disconnect syringe from catheter/stylet. If catheter is intracardiac, flow should be pulsatile ± vigorous.
- Coronary artery laceration; unlikely with right-sided approach.

PROCEDURE

- The animal is restrained in left lateral recumbency for the whole procedure. The approach will be via the right side of the thorax to minimize the risk of catheter-induced coronary artery laceration.
- Ultrasound is used for confirming that pericardial effusion is present in sufficient volume to allow safe centesis (width of effusion on echocardiogram >1 cm). In the absence of ultrasound guidance, the site of entry is at the level of the costochondral junction, right fifth intercostal space.
- The area is widely clipped of hair and aseptically prepared. The wide clipping of hair should allow the procedure to be done without a sterile drape.
- The designated site of centesis is again confirmed with ultrasound.
- Lidocaine is infused subcutaneously, intramuscularly (intercostal muscle), and subpleurally. Doing so requires that the needle be repeatedly withdrawn until almost out of the skin and then redirected and reinserted until a region at least 2 cm square, and spanning the entire thickness of the chest wall, has been infiltrated.
- The clinician puts on sterile gloves and makes a 3-mm skin incision in the center of the site using the scalpel blade.
- The catheter, which covers a metal stylet, is attached to the 6-ml syringe, and the tip of the catheter-stylet combination is inserted into the skin incision.
- The clinician advances the syringe-catheter-stylet combination (which is grasped in the palm as a handle to advance the catheter and stylet) while drawing back on the syringe plunger to create negative pressure. The orientation is perpendicular to the chest wall and is neither cranially nor caudally directed.
- When a flashback of effusion is seen to enter the syringe, the syringe-stylet-catheter apparatus is advanced only 2–3 mm farther into the chest.
- With continuing negative pressure on the syringe (effusion flowing into syringe), the syringe and stylet are kept in the same position, while the catheter is advanced several centimeters farther. In this way, the catheter is seated well within the pericardial space.
- Using a large-volume syringe (35 or 60 ml), the effusion is withdrawn. Ideally, an assistant helps by emptying one syringe while the clinician is filling the other with pericardial effusion; thus, two syringes can aseptically be traded back and forth until the pericardium is empty.
- When the effusion has partially or completely been removed, the catheter is withdrawn, and the skin incision is closed with tissue glue.

POSTPROCEDURE

- Ascites caused by cardiac tamponade should resolve spontaneously over the 12- to 36-hour period following pericardiocentesis.
- A recheck echocardiogram immediately postcentesis and another echocardiogram 12–24 hours later are recommended (assess remaining volume and note in record). Rapid reaccumulation of effusion suggests malignancy, atrial rupture from stretch, or coagulopathy.

ALTERNATIVES AND THEIR RELATIVE MERITS

- Pericardiectomy: long-term palliation.
- Diuretic: contraindicated in acute treatment (does not mobilize effusion but does deplete circulating blood volume, worsening cardiac filling); advocated by some for delay of recurrence of idiopathic or malignant effusions.

AUTHOR: **ETIENNE CÔTÉ**

Physical Rehabilitation

BASIC INFORMATION

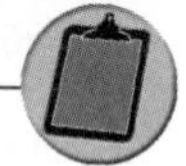

SYNONYM(S)

Physical therapy
Physiotherapy

NOTE: In some U.S. states, the term physical therapy (and possibly physiotherapy) is a protected term reserved only for human physical therapists. Therefore, claiming to practice such therapy without being a licensed physical therapist is potentially misleading and illegal. The term physical rehabilitation is safe and is recommended for veterinary medicine.

OVERVIEW AND GOAL(S)

Using modalities, manual therapies, and therapeutic exercises to increase function by strengthening an animal's muscles, accelerating the healing of damaged tissues, increasing flexibility and ranges of motion, and decreasing pain.

INDICATIONS

- Postoperative orthopedic/joint surgery (e.g., fractures, cranial cruciate ligament tears, total hip replacements, femoral head and neck ostectomy)
- Postoperative laminectomy/hemilaminectomy or other spinal surgery
- Acute neurologic diseases (fibrocartilaginous embolism/stroke, trauma, intervertebral disk disease [IVDD])
- Osteoarthritis/spondylosis
- Vestibular disease and other balance/proprioceptive problems
- Postoperative amputation
- Soft-tissue injuries (e.g., sprains and strains, tendon repairs, muscle tears)
- Obesity/conditioning

CONTRAINDICATIONS

- Unstable fractures and joints.
- Therapeutic ultrasound is contraindicated over metal implants, tumors, growth plates, eyes, heart, and pregnant uteruses.
- Neuromuscular electrical stimulation may be contraindicated in animals with seizure disorders.
- Heat is contraindicated over acutely inflamed tissues.
- Swimming and underwater treadmill exercise are contraindicated in animals with diarrhea.

EQUIPMENT, ANESTHESIA

Physical rehabilitation can be successfully performed with a minimal amount of equipment. The practitioner's hands are the greatest asset. The following are, however, recommended for optimal results, depending on the case:

- Manual restraint at times
- Goniometer to measure angles of joints
- Gulick II tape measure (to measure limb circumference/muscle mass)
- Heat packs
- Cold/ice packs
- Inflatable exercise/yoga balls and/or rolls
- Therapeutic ultrasound unit (with ultrasound gel)
- Neuromuscular electrical stimulation (NMES) unit (www.fernovetsystems.com)
- Treadmills (underwater or land) (www.fernovetsystems.com)
- Swimming area (pools for larger animals, tubs for smaller animals)
- Canine life vests
- Various slings and carts
- Cavaletti rails (horizontal bars or poles at varying heights for the animal to walk over; a ladder lying flat works well)
- Stairs
- Balance boards ("wobble" and "rocker" boards)
- Elastic resistance bands
- Leg weights
- Extracorporeal shockwave therapy unit (usually requires sedation) (www.hmt-usa.com)
- Cold lasers
- Various splints and orthotics

ANTICIPATED TIME

- About 20 to 60 minutes
- Usually performed several times a week

PREPARATION: IMPORTANT CHECKPOINTS

- Be sure that any surgical repair is stable.
- Watch for any swelling or signs of infected tissues, which could contraindicate treatment.
- Be sure that the animal's condition is not deteriorating with rehabilitation.
- Exercise animals on an empty stomach (subjectively may decrease risk of gastric dilation-volvulus).
- Take joint range-of-motion measurements (goniometry) in flexion and extension using a goniometer:
  - Normal values are published for some breeds.
  - The measurements should be rechecked every 2 to 4 weeks to monitor progress.
- Measure thigh or forearm circumference as a rough measure of muscle mass.
  - The measurement of this circumference is done with a tape measure, preferably the Gulick II to decrease margin of error.
  - This measurement also should be monitored every few weeks for progress.

POSSIBLE COMPLICATIONS AND COMMON ERRORS TO AVOID

- Do not institute hydrotherapy (e.g., swimming, underwater treadmill) until skin incisions have successfully sealed (at least 5 days).
- It is easy to overwork the animal, especially in the initial treatments. Be sure the animal can easily handle the work regimen in the beginning. As a general rule, exercise can be increased about 20% per week if the animal is improving.
- Do not stress the tissues too much (remember time frames for tissue healing).
  - For example, bone healing (fracture, surgical osteotomy) takes 8 to 12 weeks to be complete under ideal conditions. A classic pitfall would be applying too much force too early or allowing the dog to apply too much via inappropriate exercise. Signs of pain and palpable instability could be warning signs. Consultation with the surgeon on the stability of the repair is recommended.
- In the immediate postoperative period, therapeutic exercise may be contraindicated. These animals may still benefit from cryotherapy and gentle passive range-of-motion exercises three to four times daily.

PROCEDURE

- Thermal treatments (cryotherapy, heat therapy) are applied to the affected area and should not create discomfort.
- If acute inflammation is present (e.g., first few days after surgery, flare-up of chronic conditions), initiate cryotherapy with an ice pack or cold pack first. Apply for 10 to 15 minutes over the site of the inflammation. Cryotherapy aims to decrease edema, inflammation, and pain.
- For chronic situations, heat therapy is indicated. This is accomplished by massage, warm packs for superficial areas, or therapeutic ultrasound for deeper tissues (2-5 cm under the skin). Heat will increase blood flow to the tissues, increasing flexibility and decreasing the chance of injury with exercise. It can also reduce pain.
- After the warm-up period, stretching can be instituted if the procedure does not contribute to tissue injury. Tissue injury is avoided through precautions, including heeding the normal time frame of bone healing if relevant (as already described) and using an appropriately limited degree of force during healing, such as avoiding excessive force (animal vocalizes or resists).

- If the animal is vocalizing, then the practitioner is going too far. Of course, some animals will squirm or vocalize without even being touched, so individual personalities are taken into consideration.
- The individual joints are brought to a comfortable end range in flexion and then extension for 10 to 15 seconds each. This is repeated 6 to 15 times.
- Passive range-of-motion (PROM) exercises are also instituted at this point. The entire limb is cycled through its ranges of motion, being sure to incorporate all desired joints. This will increase flexibility and minimize adhesions and contractures.
- Neuromuscular electrical stimulation (NMES) can be used for artificially eliciting a muscle contraction:
  - Electrical current is delivered by pads through the skin to the motor end plate, thereby causing the muscle belly to contract.
  - NMES is primarily used for strengthening muscles and increasing endurance as well as to attenuate atrophy.
  - This modality is most helpful in animals that are paralyzed and paretic.
- The animal (depending on the individual case) may now be ready for therapeutic exercises. These are designed to increase strength, balance, and proprioception as well as encourage weight bearing on affected limbs as indicated. Therapeutic exercise is also helpful in improving active range-of-motion (AROM) in joints, flexibility, and overall function. Therapeutic exercises include the following:
  - Assisted-standing exercises, using slings or exercise balls and rolls, are used in the early stages, especially for patients that are paralyzed or paretic.
  - These exercises are designed to encourage the patient to bear as much of his/her own weight as possible.
  - The patient is supported in a standing position with the assistance of either slings or yoga balls under the trunk.
  - The patient can be rocked side to side or front to back. If the patient begins to collapse, he/she is then lifted back up to the original position and the exercise begins anew.
  - Weight-shifting exercises are designed to shift the patient's weight onto the affected limb(s) to encourage weight bearing. This is achieved with balls and rolls, balance boards, wheelbarrowing and dancing exercises, or simply discouraging use of the contralateral limb in a normal standing position.
  - Sit-to-stand exercises are used for increasing ranges of motion and strength in the hind limbs. The dog is commanded to sit squarely on its rear end and then to stand up. Small treats can be used. To get the dog to flex the hind limb squarely, the affected limb can be positioned against a wall to prevent "cheating."
  - Stair climbing is used for improving strength, coordination, and flexibility.
  - Underwater treadmills (Fig. II-118) are valuable tools that can be used in most cases:
    - Water height can be adjusted to different levels to change the animal's buoyancy and, thereby, the amount of weight the limbs are bearing.
    - Changing water heights also changes the active ranges of motion for all the joints of the limbs, depending on which ones are breaking the plane of the water.
    - Most units will also allow variations in speed, time, and incline.
    - Resistance jets can be installed.
    - Life vests and slings for assistance should be used as needed.
  - Land treadmills can also be used.
  - Cavaletti rails are used for increasing AROM, strength, balance, and coordination:
    - These are typically created with traffic cones with holes drilled through at different heights.
    - PVC pipes can then be inserted at the desired heights to create an obstacle course for the dog to negotiate.
    - The dog must lift its limbs to walk over these rails, thus encouraging active range of motion.
    - The cones and poles can be arranged to also force the dog to weave in and out of the cones, further strengthening the patient's balance and coordination skills.
  - Elastic resistance bands and leg weights can be used to further challenge the dog with many activities. Be careful where these are placed—do not put undue stress or torque on susceptible tissues; usually reserved for advanced cases, when a patient has progressed from simpler exercises:
    - Can be used for a postoperative patient with cranial cruciate ligament repair toward the end of its treatments or a patient with osteoarthritis that has successfully progressed to a point that it needs to be further challenged.
  - Balance boards are used for increasing proprioceptive awareness and balance as well as strength:
    - These are typically flat wooden boards, with a fulcrum underneath, on which the dog stands and tries to balance itself.
    - Indications in some animals with vestibular disease, ataxia of various causes, amputees.

POSTPROCEDURE

- Stretching after exercise is usually indicated.
- Cryotherapy (10–15 minutes) is also frequently indicated after the treatment to reduce muscle spasms, pain, and swelling.
- Any progression of lameness or signs of pain must be noted. If observed, reduce the next treatment by about 50%. NOTE: Be careful to differentiate orthopedic pain from muscle soreness. Muscle soreness is expected after the first few treatments.
  - Palpate the muscle bellies and move the joints to identify the source of pain.
- Anti-inflammatory medications can be used as needed:
  - Carprofen: 2.2 mg/kg PO q 24h to q 12h.
  - Deracoxib: 1–2 mg/kg PO q 24h.

ALTERNATIVES AND THEIR RELATIVE MERITS

- Acupuncture may also be helpful with pain control and neurologic diseases.

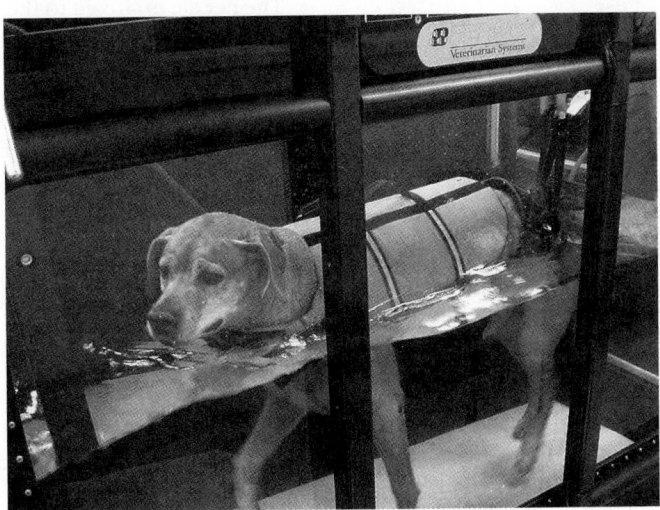

FIGURE II-118 Dog on underwater treadmill. The treadmill speed and depth of water can be adjusted to optimize the level of activity.

- Chiropractic therapy may be helpful in some cases.

SUGGESTED READING

Bockstahler B, Levine D, Millis D: *Essential Facts of Physiotherapy in Dogs and Cats*. Guelph, Lifelearn, 2004.

Gross DM: *Canine Physical Therapy: Orthopedic Physical Therapy*. East Lyme, CT, Wizard of Paws, 2002.

Marsolais GS, Dvorak G, Conzemius MG: Effects of postoperative rehabilitation on limb function after cranial cruciate ligament repair in dogs. *J Am Vet Med Assoc* 220:1325–1330, 2002.

Millis DL, Levine D, Taylor RA: *Canine Rehabilitation and Physical Therapy*. St. Louis, WB Saunders, 2004.

AUTHOR: **TIMOTHY V. HATT**

Prostatic Diagnostic Sampling: Biopsy, Fine-Needle Aspiration

BASIC INFORMATION

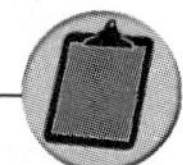

SYNONYM(S)

Needle aspiration biopsy
Guided needle aspiration biopsy
Nonguided needle aspiration biopsy
Tru-Cut needle biopsy

OVERVIEW AND GOAL(S)

Nonsurgical technique for obtaining prostate tissue samples for cytologic and histopathologic analysis. These techniques can also be performed when prostatic wash samples have provided inconclusive or inadequate results.

INDICATIONS

- Pyuria
- Hematuria
- Penile/urethral discharge
- Prostate enlargement
- Asymmetric, irregular, or nodular prostate

CONTRAINDICATIONS

- Inadequate restraint
- Bleeding disorder
- Acute prostatitis

EQUIPMENT, ANESTHESIA

- A 22-gauge sterile needle.
- A 2-cc or 3-cc sterile syringe.
- Ultrasound machine.
- Sterile Tru-Cut-type core biopsy needle.
- General anesthesia for core biopsy; needle aspiration usually does not require sedation or general anesthesia.

ANTICIPATED TIME

Abdominal ultrasound time takes 10 to 40 minutes depending on operator expertise. Fine-needle aspiration typically then takes about 1 to 3 minutes. Core biopsy with general anesthesia takes about 20 to 30 minutes.

PREPARATION: IMPORTANT CHECKPOINTS

The patient can be standing or in lateral or dorsal recumbency for needle aspiration.

These procedures usually require two people: the veterinarian and one assistant. Needle aspiration can be performed on a fully awake animal provided the animal is adequately restrained. Core biopsies require heavy sedation or general anesthesia.

POSSIBLE COMPLICATIONS AND COMMON ERRORS TO AVOID

This procedure requires the placement of a needle or biopsy instrument directly into the prostate. If an abscess or cyst is present, rupture of the cyst or abscess is possible secondary to this procedure. These procedures should not be performed on animals with inadequate coagulation systems/bleeding tendencies.

PROCEDURE

Needle aspirations can be performed as either ultrasound guided or nonguided.

NONGUIDED NEEDLE ASPIRATION: If the prostate is sufficiently enlarged that it can be palpated externally (abdominally) and stabilized by caudal abdominal palpation, then the procedure can be performed nonguided (without the use of ultrasound).

- The external surface of the skin over the prostate is clipped of hair and aseptically prepared as would be done for a surgical procedure.
- The needle is affixed to the syringe, the needle tip is placed through the prepared skin, and the tip is advanced into the prostate gland.
- Material is aspirated into the needle by drawing on the syringe plunger to create negative pressure in the syringe.
- Negative pressure is released before withdrawing the needle.
- The needle and syringe are then withdrawn quickly, the syringe is detached from the needle and filled with air, and then the syringe is reattached to the needle; the contents are vigorously expelled onto a microscope slide to make fresh smears for cytologic analysis.
- A portion of the material can be placed in appropriate media for culture and sensitivity (C&S) instead of being smeared, or else the procedure can be repeated to obtain more material for this purpose.

GUIDED NEEDLE ASPIRATION: If the prostate gland cannot be palpated externally or if a needle aspirate needs to be directed into a portion of the gland that cannot be identified by external palpation, an ultrasound guided aspiration can be obtained.

- The animal should undergo a full abdominal ultrasound evaluation, and an appropriate area for aspiration should be identified.
- The skin is prepared as for a nonguided aspiration (as already described).
- The needle with a syringe attached is then advanced through the skin into the prostate.
- Using ultrasound, the needle is visualized advancing to the appropriate area of the prostate.
- The prostate gland is aspirated, and the sample is handled for evaluation (as already described).

CORE BIOPSIES: GUIDED OR NONGUIDED: Core biopsies are obtained either guided or nonguided as already described for needle aspiration.

- Because a core biopsy is a more invasive and painful procedure, general anesthesia is necessary.
- Care must be taken not to transect the urethra with this full-thickness biopsy procedure. With this guideline in mind, the clinician should take the biopsy in an orientation parallel to the urethra (i.e., parallel to the long axis of the animal's body) and not perpendicular or oblique.
- A portion of the biopsy is taken for bacterial culture.
- The remaining portion of the biopsy is then rolled on a slide for cytologic examination. The sample is then placed in formalin and processed for histopathologic evaluation.
- The region of the biopsy is examined ultrasonographically for evidence of bleeding.

POSTPROCEDURE

These are outpatient procedures. The patient may be sent home the same day provided that its clinical condition is stable and that any anesthetic/sedation recovery is complete. The patient should be sent home with a course of antibiotics for 5 days or a longer course if the culture results are positive (see Prostatitis, p 897).

ALTERNATIVES AND THEIR RELATIVE MERITS

A technique of performing a needle aspiration biopsy of the prostate per-rectum using a guarded needle has been described. This technique has the problem of injecting bacteria directly into the prostate because the colon cannot be sterilized. The advent of ultrasound-guided techniques has made this procedure obsolete.

AUTHOR: **DONALD R. KRAWIEC**

Prostatic Massage

BASIC INFORMATION

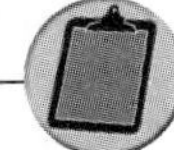

SYNONYM(S)

Expressed prostatic fluid sampling by urethral catheter
Prostatic wash or washing
Traumatic catheter biopsy

OVERVIEW AND GOAL(S)

Nonsurgical technique for obtaining prostate tissue samples for practices without ultrasound capabilities. This technique can also be performed when needle aspiration of the prostate has provided inconclusive or inadequate results.

INDICATIONS

- Pyuria
- Hematuria
- Penile/urethral discharge
- Prostate enlargement
- Asymmetric, irregular, or nodular prostate

CONTRAINDICATIONS

- Inadequate restraint
- Bleeding disorder
- Acute prostatitis

EQUIPMENT, ANESTHESIA

- Urinary catheter of sufficient length to reach the urinary bladder. A soft, red, rubber (Sovereign-type) feeding tube is preferable because it is less traumatic than a polypropylene catheter.
- Two 5-ml syringes.
- Two 5-ml aliquots of sterile saline solution.
- Two sterile sample containers capable of holding at least 5 ml of fluid.
- Routine surgical scrub soap and gauze squares for disinfecting the distal penis.
- Manual restraint to general anesthesia, depending on the demeanor of the animal.

ANTICIPATED TIME

Approximately 20 to 30 minutes

PREPARATION: IMPORTANT CHECKPOINTS

- The patient can be standing or in lateral recumbency.
- The procedure usually requires three people: the veterinarian and two assistants.
- The procedure requires both digital rectal palpation and urethral catheterization. If the animal resists these procedures, sedation is advised.

POSSIBLE COMPLICATIONS AND COMMON ERRORS TO AVOID

- This procedure requires digital massage of the prostate. If acute bacterial prostatitis is present, the prostatic massage could result in release of bacteria into the bloodstream and septicemia.
- If an abscess or cyst is present, rupture is possible secondary to this procedure.
- The urinary bladder must be completely empty before starting the procedure, or the prostate sample will be diluted by the excess urine.
- Premeasuring the catheter makes it possible to place the catheter into the urinary bladder without causing catheter-induced bladder trauma or allowing it to loop back on itself to form a knot.
- Bladder infections will make the prostate wash difficult to interpret. Animals with bacterial cystitis should be treated with an appropriate antibiotic before undergoing a prostatic wash.

PROCEDURE

- While one assistant restrains the animal, the other assistant retracts the prepuce to expose the penis and cleans the distal penis with a mild surgical disinfectant.
- The veterinarian passes a urinary catheter into the urethra until the tip is in the bladder and completely removes the urine.
- The veterinarian instills 5 ml of sterile saline via the catheter into the bladder.
- This fluid is then aspirated back with a syringe and placed in a sterile tube labeled *tube #1*.
- The veterinarian then places an index finger in the animal's rectum and palpates both the prostate and the catheter.
- The catheter is retracted until the tip can be felt to be distal (caudal) to the prostate.
- The prostate is then gently massaged for 1 minute.
- The palpating finger is retracted until it is distal/caudal to the holes in the catheter, and gentle pressure is applied to the catheter rectally so that fluid injected into the catheter will not leak out of the penis but will move cranially into the bladder.
- A total of 5 ml of sterile saline is then injected into the catheter so the fluid flows across the prostatic urethra into the bladder.
- The catheter is then advanced into the bladder, and the fluid is aspirated into a syringe and placed into a sterile tube labeled *tube #2*.
- Both tubes are presented for fluid analysis and culture.

If the above procedure yields either inadequate sample size or equivocal results, a traumatic catheter biopsy can be performed. General anesthesia or sedation with systemic analgesia is indicated.

- The urinary catheter in placed into the urethra as already described.The tip of the catheter should be in the prostatic urethra. Correct catheter placement can be verified by digital rectal examination or by radiograph.
- A 12-cc syringe is attached to the catheter, and negative pressure is applied so that prostatic tissue is aspirated into the holes of the catheter.
- While maintaining negative pressure on the syringe, the catheter is withdrawn from the urethra. Doing so will tear tissue from the prostate that is aspirated into the catheter. This prostatic tissue can be used for cytologic evaluation, and sometimes a sufficiently large piece is obtained to allow histopathologic examination.

POSTPROCEDURE

- The animal should be discharged with an antibiotic for 5 days to reduce the risk of inducing a bladder infection.
- Sample #1 will have only bladder material, whereas sample #2 will have both

prostate and bladder material. Comparing the two samples allows the clinician to localize the disease process to the prostate and/or the urinary bladder.

ALTERNATIVES AND THEIR RELATIVE MERITS

Prostatic washings are done infrequently due to the advent of ultrasound-guided prostate biopsy procedures; however, washings do provide a representative prostate tissue sample.

AUTHOR: **DONALD R. KRAWIEC**

Rectal Palpation

BASIC INFORMATION

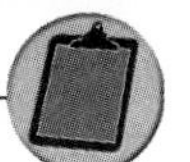

SYNONYM(S)

Digital palpation
Rectal exam
Transrectal palpation

OVERVIEW AND GOAL(S)

Tactile assessment of the urethra, caudal aspect of the trigone of the urinary bladder, bony pelvic canal, aortic trifurcation, pelvic diaphragm, anal sacs, rectal mucosa, and either the prostate gland (males) or caudal vagina (females)

INDICATIONS

Part of any complete routine physical exam in adult dogs; generally not feasible in puppies or cats.

CONTRAINDICATIONS

- Animals weighing <5 kg
- Relative contraindication: anal/rectal pain. Requires that the rectal exam be performed under sedation or general anesthesia

EQUIPMENT, ANESTHESIA

- Sedation or anesthesia only if required for patient comfort.
- Latex or other clean, nonsterile exam glove
- Lubricant (e.g., K-Y Jelly or Vaseline)
- Cotton wool or other absorbent material to receive contents expressed from anal sacs
- Microscope slide with drop of saline

ANTICIPATED TIME

About 10 to 60 seconds

PREPARATION: IMPORTANT CHECKPOINTS

Review elements of animal's history (dysuria, hematuria, tenesmus, hind limb lameness, etc.), remainder of physical exam, and any diagnostic findings (e.g., hypercalcemia) that could be pertinent to rectal examination findings.

POSSIBLE COMPLICATIONS AND COMMON ERRORS TO AVOID

- Rectal perforation: extremely uncommon when gentle technique is used.
- Anal sac rupture: also uncommon; however, impacted, infected/abscessed sacs may be more fragile. If anal sacs are large and/or painful, and gentle pressure is unrewarding or distressing to the patient, anesthesia is recommended and anal sac cannulation may then be performed.
- Perianal fistulae may make it difficult to assess the exact location of the anal opening; time and caution are warranted to avoid exacerbating a fistula through blunt probing.
- Rectal peristalsis may be confused with perineal hernia or rectal stricture. If uncertainty exists, the rectal exam can be prolonged by 1 to 2 minutes because a wave of peristalsis will pass but a stricture will not.

PROCEDURE

- Animal is restrained in a standing position by technician holding the head and neck.
- The right-handed examiner puts a glove on his or her right hand; the right index finger is lubricated.
- The examiner stands behind the animal and lifts its tail with the left hand to expose the anus.
- The right index finger is placed on the anus, and then after a few seconds, the finger is gently introduced through the external anal sphincter.
- The tail may be released; most dogs will hold the tail elevated during the rectal exam.
- The left hand, no longer holding the tail, reaches under to the animal's caudal abdomen and cups the ventrocaudal abdomen.
- In addition to this cupping motion, the examiner draws the hand caudally toward his or her body to elevate the viscera of the caudal abdomen toward the right index (palpating) finger. With sufficient upward pressure, and without discomfort to the animal, it is possible to palpate the prostate of even giant breed dogs this way.
- The palpation reaches to the maximal depth allowed by the examiner's finger and the animal's comfort; the examiner can also turn the finger circumferentially to assess both left and right walls of the pelvic canal and the roof of the pelvic canal.
- Once the exam is completed, the examiner withdraws the index finger, ensuring to first palpate the integrity of the pelvic diaphragm (assess for perineal hernia) and, if necessary, to express the anal sacs located at the 4 and 8 o'clock positions if the anus is pictured as a clockface.
- Finally, the feces coating the glove are examined grossly for blood or other abnormalities and smeared on a microscope slide for cytologic examination.

ALTERNATIVES AND THEIR RELATIVE MERITS

- Fecal flotation and fecal occult blood test: identifies microscopic abnormalities (parasites, blood) but is of little use regarding structural malformations of the rectum and perirectal area.
- Abdominal ultrasound: excellent visualization of many organs of caudal abdomen and cranial pelvic canal; however, the bony pelvis and colon severely narrow the acoustic window and compromise ultrasound assessment of urethra, distal colon, and much of pelvic canal, which is the area that a rectal examination accesses best.

AUTHOR: **ETIENNE CÔTÉ**

Rhinoscopy

BASIC INFORMATION

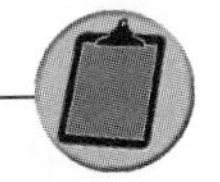

OVERVIEW AND GOAL(S)

Minimally invasive, endoscopic approach to the nasal cavity for visual evaluation and swab, flush, and biopsy procedures

INDICATIONS

- Chronic nasal discharge
- Intranasal obstruction
- Chronic sneezing
- Nasal foreign body
- Epistaxis with normal coagulation profile and blood pressure (BP)
- Maxillary mass/deformity

CONTRAINDICATIONS

Coagulopathy/bleeding disorder

EQUIPMENT, ANESTHESIA

General anesthesia and endotracheal intubation are required. The following equipment is recommended:

- Mouth gag (speculum)
- Sterile, water-soluble lubricant
- Sterile saline solution for flush
- Gauze squares for packing off pharynx
- Flexible, fiber-optic endoscope (small; 3 mm diameter maximum for patients <20 lb)
- Vacuum source for endoscopic suction
- Microbial culture swab
- Biopsy forceps (intraendoscopic or separate, such as Jackson mare 2-, 4-, or 6-Fr endometrial biopsy forceps)
- Biopsy jar with 10% buffered formalin
- Phenylephrine (e.g., Neosynephrine drops) for postoperative epistaxis

ANTICIPATED TIME

- Usually 60 to 90 minutes anesthesia time (about 30 to 60 minutes endoscopy time)
- Up to 3 to 4 hours possible with complex foreign bodies

PREPARATION: IMPORTANT CHECKPOINTS

- Warn owners that epistaxis is common for at least 1 to 3 days after the procedure.
- Check that current coagulation profile (prothrombin [PT], activated partial thromboplastin time [APTT], platelets) and BP are normal.

POSSIBLE COMPLICATIONS AND COMMON ERRORS TO AVOID

- Biopsy sample not representative of entire process (very common with small through-the-endoscope pinch forceps, especially if dull)
- Inability to see beyond first few millimeters of nasal passages (common, especially in cats and small dogs; an endoscope that is too big can be a contributing factor)
- Hemorrhage after biopsy (rarely before biopsy although blood from scraping mucosa with scope can obscure view)
- Inability to see choanae during retroflexed view of nasopharynx (common in large dogs)
- Anesthetic complications

PROCEDURE

TECHNIQUE: INITIAL

- General anesthesia.
- Endotracheal intubation; check good seal on cuff (but not excessive inflation pressure).
- Ventral recumbency.
- Animal facing endoscopist; head at edge of table elevated on folded towels.
- Fill caudal pharynx with gauze (one to two 3 × 3-inch squares for cats, several for dogs; count number to ensure complete retrieval after procedure).
- Swab with sterile culture swab for microbial culture (usually aerobic bacterial).
- Measure length from tip of nostril to medial canthus of eye:
  - This is the maximal length of insertion of the endoscope.
  - Going farther than this measurement can perforate cribriform plate if diseased and enter the brain.

TECHNIQUE: MAIN

- Advance endoscope into one nostril.
- Easiest route is medial and very dorsal.
  - Push dorsal edge of nostril caudally and dorsally with thumb.
  - Enter just alongside nasal septum for easiest access.
- Begin saline infusion through endoscope for better visualization.
  - Catch outpouring of saline in waste bucket or on towels on floor.
- Examine dorsal, middle, and ventral nasal meatus systematically.
- If lesion noted, biopsy after completing visualization (otherwise, blood obscures field).
- Repeat process for contralateral nostril.
- When finished with both nostrils, prop mouth open with speculum.
- Enter oral cavity with endoscope.
- Curve endoscope tip to about 160 degrees so that it reaches behind edge of soft palate.
- Examine choanae.
- Pull body of endoscope gently forward (cranially) to better observe choanae.
- Biopsy lesions if applicable.
- Withdraw endoscope.

TECHNIQUE: COMPLETION

- Suction caudal pharynx as necessary.
- Remove gauze sponges in caudal pharynx. Count number to confirm all removed.
- Instill phenylephrine (few drops in each nostril) if voluminous epistaxis.
- Anesthetic recovery:
  - Neck elevated/nose down to reduce inhalation of blood.
  - Extubation as late as safely possible to avoid inhalation of blood.

POSTPROCEDURE

- Epistaxis common. Treatment options:
  - Instill two to five drops of phenylephrine in bleeding nostril (best time is prior to complete anesthetic recovery—deeper instillation).
  - Tranquilization (butorphanol IV and/or low-dose acepromazine IM).
  - Very rarely, large-volume arterial epistaxis requires carotid ligation (bilateral carotid ligation can safely be done without risking hypoperfusion).
  - Phenylephrine nasal drops may be tried at home.
- Sneezing is common (often decreases to the same intensity as sneezing prior to procedure—if any—within 48 hours after the procedure).

ALTERNATIVES AND THEIR RELATIVE MERITS

- Nasal swab:
  - No anesthesia.
  - Possibly acceptable for culture and sensitivity (C&S) of nasal discharge but commonly contaminated with normal flora.
  - Poor cytologic yield because animal is awake.
- Nasal flush:
  - Minimal tissue disruption means less epistaxis but also fewer cells for diagnosis.
  - Can flush out foreign material/foreign body.
- Blind nasal biopsy:
  - Quick.
  - Location nonspecific.
  - May provide good yield if large sample (e.g., with Jackson forceps) and if oriented based on imaging results (radiographs, CT scan, MRI).
- Open-mouth transpalatal biopsy:

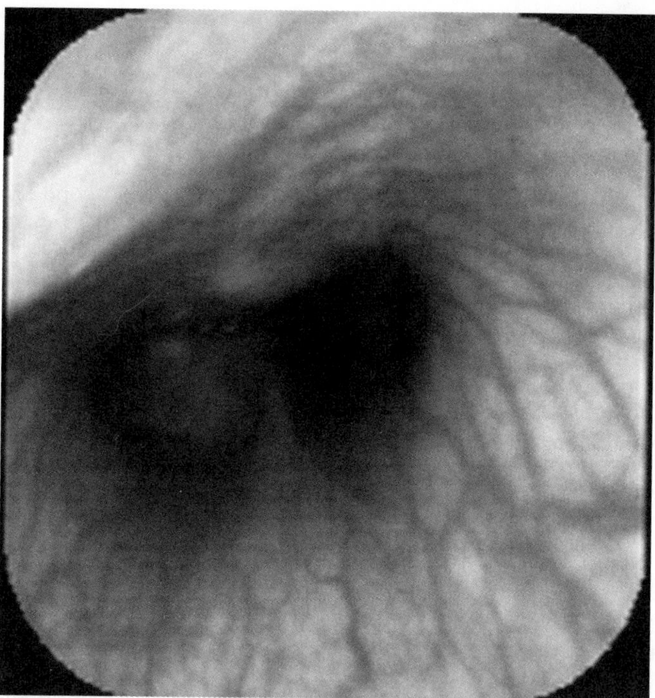

FIGURE II-119 Endoscopic view, retroflexed behind the soft palate to show the choanae. Dog's right is on the left side of the image. A fleshy mass is present in the right choana.

- Caudal nasal biopsy possible without rhinotomy.
- Nasopharyngeal biopsy possible.
- Palatine artery must be avoided.

• Rhinotomy:
  - Most likely to give definitive diagnosis of nasal disease.
  - Most invasive: incision through maxillary bones, disruption of large amounts of nasal mucosa.
  - Often delayed until lesser invasive means have failed.

• CT scan or MRI:
  - Imaging techniques: no therapeutic value by themselves.
  - More specific localization of lesion (CT scan usually preferred because of bone).

AUTHOR: **ETIENNE CÔTÉ**

Slings, Casts, and Other Forms of Immobilization

BASIC INFORMATION

SYNONYM(S)

External coaptation

OVERVIEW AND GOAL(S)

To provide appropriate temporary support and allow healing of musculoskeletal injuries, either alone or as augmentation of surgical repairs.

INDICATIONS

- Robert Jones bandage: temporary immobilization of unstable fractures; control of edema and swelling. Appropriate for open fractures following wound dressing.
- Splints: temporary immobilization of fractures or peripheral joint luxations; also used following surgery for joint injuries, arthrodeses, or tendon injuries.
- Casts: immobilization of distal limb fractures when mechanically stable; also appropriate following surgical repair—similar to splints.
- Slings: partial immobilization of all joints of the limb and prevention of weight bearing. Ehmer sling is used primarily following reduction of hip luxation to prevent recurrence.

CONTRAINDICATIONS

Excessive duration of immobilization may lead to muscle and joint contracture and permanent loss of mobility. Use with caution, especially in pediatric animals.

EQUIPMENT, ANESTHESIA

Sedation may be required for appropriate placement of splints and bandages if animal is in pain or uncooperative. General anesthesia is required for reduction of fractures or joint luxations prior to immobilization.

Materials required (amounts and material widths depend on animal size):

- Appropriate wound dressing, if needed
- A 0.5- or 1-inch roll of tape
- Rolls of cast padding, 2-6 inches (in width)
- Rolls of conforming gauze, 2-6 inches (in width)
- Rolls of self-adherent stretch tape

Additional materials:

- Roll of cotton, 12-inch width (for Robert Jones bandage)
- Fiberglass resin or plaster-impregnated casting tape, 2-4 inches (in width) for casts
- Stretch stockinette (for casts, optional)
- Rigid Mason metasplint, lateral plastic limb splint, fiberglass or thermoplastic splint (for splints)

ANTICIPATED TIME

About 10 to 30 minutes for application of most casts, splints, and slings

PREPARATION: IMPORTANT CHECKPOINTS

Wounds should be treated, and an appropriate dressing should be applied before splinting or bandaging.

POSSIBLE COMPLICATIONS AND COMMON ERRORS TO AVOID

- Toes of the third and fourth digits should be left visible whenever possible to allow monitoring for coolness, swelling, cyanosis, or discharge, any of which warrants removal of the splint, cast, or bandage for closer evaluation of the soft tissues.
- All bandages, splints, slings, and casts should be checked frequently for limb swelling or discoloration, skin abrasions, loosening or slippage, moisture, or odor.
- Severe ischemia can result from poor application or management.

PROCEDURE

ROBERT JONES BANDAGE

- Divide bulky roll cotton lengthwise and in thickness; reroll to create several smaller, narrower rolls.
- Apply adhesive tape stirrups directly to the skin of the medial and lateral or cranial and caudal surfaces of the distal limb, extending from the carpus or tarsus distally 4–6 inches beyond the toes.
- Apply cotton, winding it around the leg from distal to proximal, as far as possible into the axillary or inguinal space.
- Each turn of the cotton should overlap the last layer by 50%.
- Wrap the cotton as evenly as possible.
- Apply conforming gauze around the cotton, as tightly as possible, working from distal to proximal.
- Cotton should be evenly compressed until the bandage is firm to the touch.
- Pull the tape stirrups proximally, and apply them onto the bandage. Their purpose is to prevent the bandage from slipping off the limb.
- Cover with a tertiary layer of conforming tape.
- Goal of this bandage is even compression and firm support over the entire limb.
- Properly applied, the finished bandage should make a thumping sound like a ripe melon when it is percussed.
- Tips of toes must be visible for monitoring. Due to the high compression, this bandage can cause severe ischemic injury if applied poorly.

SPLINTS

- Apply tape stirrups as for the Robert Jones bandage.
- Apply cast padding, starting distally and winding around the limb as far proximally as needed.
- Apply a layer of conforming gauze from distal to proximal area.
- Place rigid splint material, usually on the caudal or lateral side of the limb.
- Repeat another one to two layers of conforming gauze.
- Cover with an outer layer of conforming tape.

CASTS

- Apply adhesive tape stirrups.
- Roll stockinette over the limb, allowing extra length proximally and distally. Stockinette is optional but does give the cast a more finished appearance.
- Apply a light layer of cast padding over stockinette.
- Apply roll gauze with light and even compression.
- Apply casting tape over the gauze in distal to proximal direction, overlapping by 50% and avoiding digital pressure and wrinkles during application. Layer as needed for appropriate strength.
- Support the limb at multiple points while hardening to avoid dents or incorrect alignment.
- Roll stockinette ends over the cast ends.
- Apply the stirrups to the cast. Their purpose is to prevent the cast from slipping off the limb.
- Cover with an outer tertiary layer of elastic conforming tape.

SLINGS

- *Velpeau sling (forelimb)* (Fig. II-120):
  - Lightly pad the foot and carpus with cast padding to prevent excessive flexion.
  - Wrap conforming gauze around the foot from medial to lateral (see Fig. II-120A).
  - Hold the limb adducted against the body wall with the carpus, elbow, and shoulder in flexion (see Fig. II-120B).
  - Roll the conforming roll gauze around the limb and thorax, passing

PROCEDURES AND TECHNIQUES

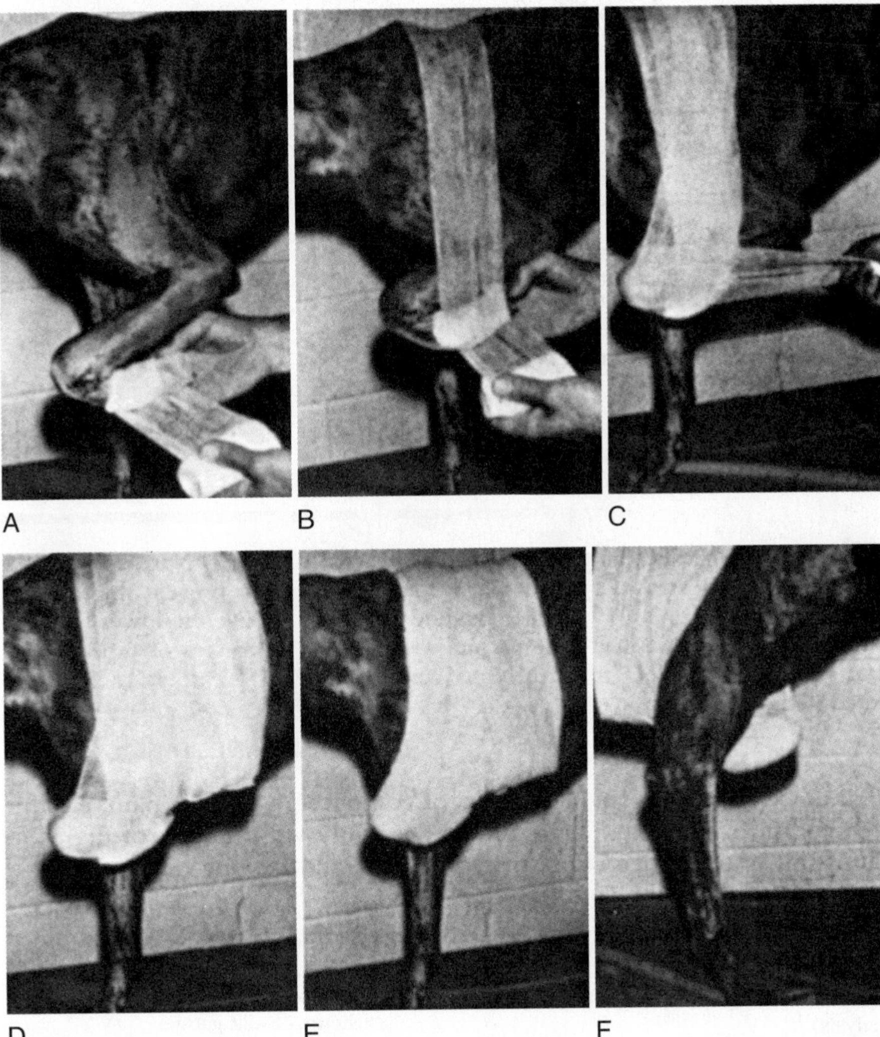

FIGURE II-120 Velpeau sling. **A**, Conforming gauze bandage material is wrapped loosely around the paw, with the direction of wrapping causing the gauze to pass from medial to lateral on the dorsal surface of the paw, as shown. **B**, With the carpus, elbow, and shoulder all flexed, the gauze is brought from the paw over the lateral aspect of the limb and shoulder, over the chest and back, and caudal to the opposite axilla. It then continues across the ventral chest, back to the starting point. **C**, Several more layers of gauze are applied in a similar manner, and a few layers are brought around the flexed carpus to prevent extension of the elbow. Such extension could force the distal limb out of the bandage. **D**, Gauze bandaging is completed. **E**, Wide elastic tape is used for covering the gauze in a pattern similar to that used for the gauze application, which completes the application of the splint. **F**, View of the opposite side of the patient, showing that both gauze and adhesive are caudal to the opposite axilla. Reprinted with permission from Piermattei DL, Flo GL, DeCamp CE: *Brinker, Piermattei and Flo's: Handbook of Small Animal Orthopedics and Fracture Treatment*, ed 2. Philadelphia, WB Saunders, 1990.

caudally to the opposite forelimb to prevent slipping (see Fig. II-120C).
  - Continue on the same pattern for two to three layers, incorporating the entire carpus and foot (see Fig. II-120D–F).
  - Apply a light tertiary layer of conforming tape over the gauze in the same pattern (see Figs. II-120E and II-120F).
  - The easiest way to perform these steps is with the patient awake and standing.
  - The sling should not be used for more than 2 weeks in order to avoid joint contracture.
- *Ehmer sling (hind limb)* (Fig. II-121):
  - Lightly pad the metatarsal region with cast padding.
  - Hold the stifle and tarsus in flexion.
  - Pass adhesive tape around the padded metatarsal region, coming up the lateral side.
  - Twist tape 180 degrees to keep the adhesive side against the skin and pass medially to the stifle.
  - Pass the tape over the lateral thigh, as far proximally into the inguinal region as possible.
  - Again twist the tape to keep the adhesive against the skin and pass distally medial to the hock.
  - Continue tape back up to the starting point at the lateral side of the metatarsal region.
  - Repeat the pattern two to three times to layer the tape.
  - If maintaining hip reduction, following the last pattern, pass the tape over the lateral side of the flexed leg over the back and around the abdomen as a belly band; stick the tape to itself on the abdominal wall, taking care to exclude the prepuce in males. NOTE: Adhesive tape must be stuck directly to haired skin to avoid slippage.
  - The sling should not be used for more than 2 weeks, in order to avoid joint contracture.
  - The limb must be monitored frequently for swelling or skin abrasion.

POSTPROCEDURE

- Check toes and distal limb at least twice daily for any signs of ischemic injury.
- Monitor contact points of bandage materials, especially around bony prominences and joints.

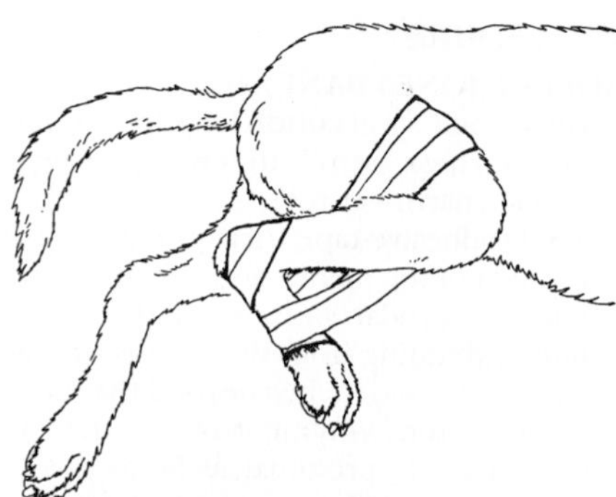

FIGURE II-121 Ehmer sling. Reprinted with permission from Piermattei DL, Flo GL, DeCamp CE: *Brinker, Piermattei and Flo's: Handbook of Small Animal Orthopedics and Fracture Treatment*, ed 2. Philadelphia, WB Saunders, 1990.

SUGGESTED READING

Simpson AM, Beale BS, Radlinsky MA: Bandaging in dogs and cats: External coaptation. *Comp Cont Educ Pract Vet* 23(2):157–164, 2001.

Bandage techniques. In Bojrab MJ, Ellison GW, Slocum B (eds): *Current Techniques in Small Animal Surgery*. Baltimore, Williams & Wilkens, 1998, pp 1295–1318.

AUTHOR: **PETER MOAK**

Thoracocentesis

BASIC INFORMATION

SYNONYM(S)

Chest tap
Pleural tap
Thoracentesis (human medicine)

OVERVIEW AND GOAL(S)

Rapid and technically easy procedure that is both therapeutic (removing air or fluid from the pleural space) and diagnostic (confirming the presence of air or fluid and obtaining samples of fluid for further analysis)

INDICATIONS

- Animals with respiratory distress (increased respiratory rate and effort) and dull lung sounds on auscultation
- Animals that present after trauma (hit by car, bite wounds, falling from height) and those that have undergone positive-pressure ventilation have increased risk for pneumothorax and may require thoracocentesis
- May also be used in the evaluation of smaller volume pleural effusions that are not causing significant clinical signs (diagnostic only; generally more challenging and greater risk of iatrogenic lung laceration)

CONTRAINDICATIONS

Severe coagulopathy; fractious behavior

EQUIPMENT, ANESTHESIA

- Clippers.
- Antiseptic scrub (e.g., chlorhexidine).
- Sterile gloves.
- Large syringe (10–60 ml, depending on size of animal).
- Three-way stopcock.
- Sterile extension tubing and a sterile needle, catheter, or butterfly catheter:
  - Large dogs: 1.5-inch needle or longer catheter, 18–22 gauge.
  - Medium dogs, large cats: 1-inch needle or catheter, 20–22 gauge.
  - Cats, small dogs: 3/4 to 7/8-inch butterfly needle, 22–23 gauge; 25-gauge needle possible for diagnostic centesis.
- Bowl (for fluid).
- Red- and purple-top tubes for sample submission.
- Sedation may be needed depending on animal's disposition and stability.

ANTICIPATED TIME

Procedure is relatively fast (<5 minutes) although can be prolonged (45–60 minutes) if a large amount of fluid or air (i.e., several liters) needs to be removed or if effusion is viscous, contains fibrin clumps or blood clots, or is compartmentalized.

PREPARATION: IMPORTANT CHECKPOINTS

- If the patient is in severe respiratory distress and has dull lung sounds on auscultation, thoracocentesis should be performed prior to thoracic radiographs.
- In cases where respiratory signs are less severe, thoracic radiographs can be used for confirming the presence of fluid or air in the pleural space prior to thoracocentesis.
- Discuss possible complications with owners.
- Rule out coagulopathy as likely cause of respiratory signs first (from history, physical examination, ± coagulation screening).
- Prepare equipment and supplies (Fig. II-122).
- Be able to keep animal relatively still, either with restraint or sedation, to minimize risk of iatrogenic pneumothorax or hemothorax.

POSSIBLE COMPLICATIONS AND COMMON ERRORS TO AVOID

- Iatrogenic pneumothorax

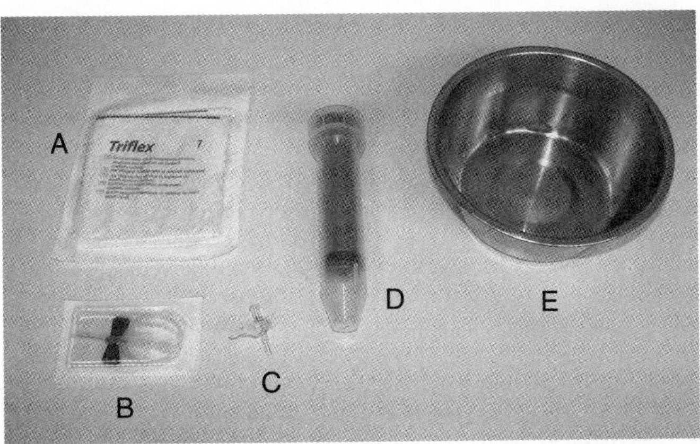

FIGURE II-122 Materials used for thoracocentesis. **A,** Sterile gloves. **B,** Butterfly-type catheter. **C,** Three-way stopcock. **D,** Large syringe. **E,** Bowl.

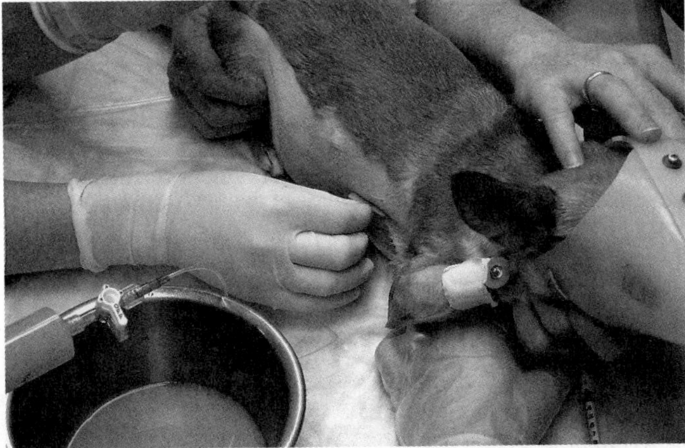

FIGURE II-123 Thoracocentesis for removal of septic pleural effusion from a Chihuahua. A butterfly catheter with three-way stopcock and a 60-ml syringe are in use. The entry site is at the right seventh or eighth ICS, approximately at the level of the costochondral junction. An open muzzle is placed loosely for protection of staff without compromising the animal's respirations.

- Intrathoracic hemorrhage
- Reexpansion pulmonary edema in situations of chronic pleural space disease
- Acute death from stress of restraint in animals with severe respiratory compromise

PROCEDURE

- Position animal, preferably in sternal recumbency or standing, but lateral recumbency is also acceptable for pneumothorax.
- Have assistant available to restrain animal or give sedation as needed.
  - Consider brief, quiet rest in oxygen cage if extreme dyspnea (any restraint or sedation appears hazardous).
  - With mild or no dyspnea, butorphanol 0.05-0.1 mg/kg IV may be used for light sedation; protocols for heavy sedation or anesthesia (e.g., propofol) will likely require intubation in the pleural effusion/pneumothorax animal.
- Clip and aseptically prepare appropriate rib space:
  - If expecting fluid, or if unsure (fluid versus air), clip at the seventh or eighth intercostal space (ICS), about at the level of the costochondral junction.
  - If expecting air, clip at the eighth or ninth ICS space, approximately one-third of the way down the chest.
- Wear sterile gloves for the insertion of the appropriate-size needle or butterfly catheter.
- Attach needle to syringe.
- Insert needle slowly just cranial to the rib to avoid intercostal blood vessels (Fig. II-123). When through skin (beveled edge of needle is no longer visible), begin aspirating with a few tenths of 1 ml to 1-2 ml of negative pressure for small to large animals, respectively.
- Observe hub of needle for signs of fluid ("flashback"):
  - If a small amount of frank blood is aspirated or if lungs can be felt rubbing against needle, needle should be moved to a different location.
  - If large amount of blood is obtained, place 1-2 ml in a red-top tube to see if it clots.
  - Blood from hemothorax should not clot, whereas blood from the heart or a blood vessel should clot normally if the animal does not have significant coagulopathy.
- For any other fluid, aspiration should continue until no more fluid can be removed.
- Directing the needle ventrally, rolling the animal slightly to the side on which thoracocentesis is being performed and reaspirating from a more ventral location can facilitate removal of as much fluid as possible.
- Fluid is submitted for fluid analysis and cytologic examination and is saved for future bacterial culture and sensitivity (C&S) (aerobic, anaerobic) if cytologic examination suggests septic exudate.
- Aspiration of air will turn the tubing a slightly foggy white color as the warm air from the thoracic cavity encounters the room temperature tubing.
  - Aspirate until negative pressure is reached.
  - If negative pressure is never obtained, a tension pneumothorax may be present, and chest tubes with continuous suction are needed (see Chest Tube Placement, p 1210).

POSTPROCEDURE

Monitor for returning signs of respiratory distress: could represent return of underlying pleural disease or iatrogenic pneumothorax or hemothorax.

ALTERNATIVES AND THEIR RELATIVE MERITS

- Chest tube placement: continuous removal of fluid and air but is more invasive and is associated with a greater risk of iatrogenic complications.
- Diuretics: slow mobilization of modified transudates (e.g., heart failure) compared to thoracocentesis and ineffective with other causes (e.g., exudates, hemorrhage).

AUTHOR: **LORI S. WADDELL**

Tracheostomy

BASIC INFORMATION

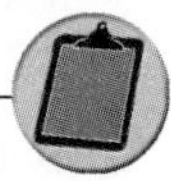

OVERVIEW AND GOAL(S)

The creation of a temporary hole through which a tube or a permanent stoma in the trachea can be placed. Tracheostomy facilitates airflow into the trachea distal to the nose, mouth, nasopharynx, and larynx.

INDICATIONS

- Temporary tube tracheostomy:
  - Emergency procedure to establish airflow in situations of acute upper respiratory distress or upper respiratory obstruction that does not allow stabilization with supplemental oxygen or oral intubation; occurs with trauma, neoplasia, laryngeal edema/collapse, certain foreign bodies.
  - Elective procedure to provide alternative airflow for surgical procedures of the oropharynx.
  - Long-term ventilatory support.
- Permanent tracheostoma:
  - Salvage or palliative procedure.
  - Upper respiratory obstructions causing respiratory distress that cannot be treated otherwise; occurs in neoplasia, hemorrhage, laryngeal collapse.

CONTRAINDICATIONS

Respiratory distress due to intrathoracic disease

EQUIPMENT, ANESTHESIA

- Anesthesia:
  - General anesthesia if elective procedure.
  - Local anesthesia if too unstable for general anesthesia ± analgesia/sedative.
  - If the animal is unconscious due to upper airway obstruction, tracheostomy is generally indicated in the absence of general or local anesthesia. Anesthesia is then administered/titrated if necessary after the tracheostomy has been performed but prior to the return of consciousness.
- Aseptic surgical preparation if elective procedure (and if time allows in cases of emergency tracheostomy):
  - Hair clippers.
  - Surgical scrub solution, alcohol, gauze sponges.
- Instruments:
  - Sterile gloves.
  - A #11 sterile scalpel blade.
  - Scalpel handle.
  - 2-0 to 4-0 polydioxanone/polypropylene suture on a taper needle.
  - Needle holders.
  - Brown-Adson forceps.
  - Kelly hemostat forceps.
- Tracheostomy tubes:
  - Diameter: Tubes should be no larger than one-half the size of the trachea. Intratracheal length: The tube should extend six to seven tracheal rings. Composition: Tubes should be made of autoclavable, nonreactive material (silver, silicone, nylon).
  - Single lumen tubes must be removed and replaced for cleaning (Fig. II-124).
  - Double lumen tubes have a removable inner cannula for cleaning, which is more convenient and is comfortable for the animal, but they may be too large for smaller animals and mucus can still accumulate distal to the inner cannula.
  - Cuffed tubes are used for ventilator support: High-volume, high-compliance cuffs that are able to inflate with low pressures and less blood-flow compromise are indicated.
  - The Shiley tracheostomy tube is the most common, and the company offers many varieties for treating veterinary patients.

ANTICIPATED TIME

- Temporary 10 minutes
- Permanent 30 minutes

PREPARATION: IMPORTANT CHECKPOINTS

- Have all supplies at hand before beginning procedure.
- Label stay sutures to aid in replacement of tube.
- Inform owner of potential complications of procedure and long-term prognosis of condition.

POSSIBLE COMPLICATIONS AND COMMON ERRORS TO AVOID

- Tracheostomy emergencies: obstruction, extubation, and cuff leakage.
- Tube "cleaning" cannot involve pushing secretions and debris back into the trachea. Proper suctioning and, if double-lumen tube, removal of the inner cannula are essential.
- Infection.
- Hemorrhage.
- Subcutaneous emphysema, pneumomediastinum, pneumothorax.
- Tracheal malacia.
- Tube tracheostomy:
  - Gagging, vomiting, and coughing, especially during suctioning
  - Tube obstruction
  - Tube dislodgement
  - Tracheal irritation causing tracheocutaneous or tracheoesophageal fistulas
  - Vascular erosions
  - Stricture or stenosis from pressure necrosis and mucosal erosions
- Permanent tracheostomy:
  - Stomal occlusion by mucus, skin folds, stenosis
  - Mucus accumulation
  - Coughing and gagging from tracheal irritation

PROCEDURE

TEMPORARY TRACHEOSTOMY

- Place animal in dorsal recumbency, and clip hair of ventral and lateral neck.
- Surgically prep the skin if time permits (all elective procedures and as much as possible with emergency cases).
- Make a ventral, cervical midline skin incision extending caudally from the distal aspect of the larynx. A typical length for the incision is 2–3 cm in a medium-sized dog.
- Expose the trachea by bluntly dissecting on the midline between the paired sternohyoid muscles and retracting the muscles and skin laterally.
- Either a horizontal (transverse) or a vertical (midline) incision can be made into the trachea.

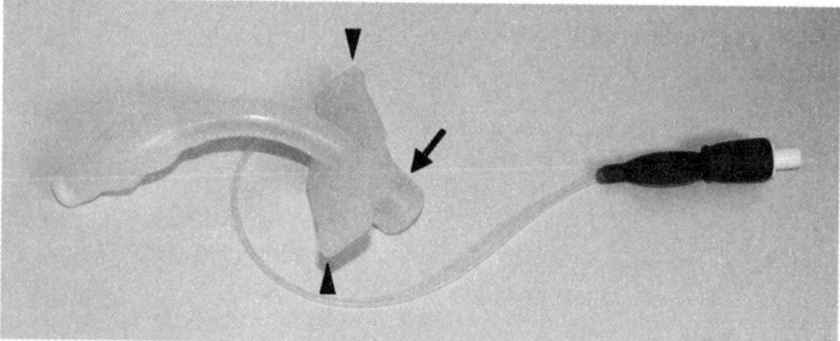

FIGURE II-124 A single-lumen, cuffed tracheostomy tube. The curved and cuffed portions are inside the patient. The external plate (*arrowheads*) is sutured to the skin of the ventral neck or is tied around the neck with umbilical tape; the proximal extremity of the tube (*arrow*) either is left open or is attached to a ventilator.

- Prior to incising the tracheal cartilages/rings, stay sutures should be placed encircling cartilages proximally and distally (horizontal tracheostomy) or laterally (vertical tracheostomy) to the proposed tracheal incision.
- A horizontal tracheostomy can be made by incising through the annular ligament between the third and fourth tracheal cartilages, with the incision not extending more than half the circumference of the trachea.
- A vertical tracheostomy can be made by incising through the ventral midline of the third through the fifth tracheal cartilages.
- Insert a tracheostomy tube by placing tension on the sutures to temporarily enlarge the tracheal opening and using a hemostat to manipulate the tube through the incision.
- Alternatively, a tracheal flap tracheostomy can be performed by making a U-shaped incision into the cartilage based at the second tracheal ring and extending distally two to three rings. The cartilage flap is raised, and the endotracheal or tracheostomy tube is inserted. This technique is best for long-term intubation or ventilation because it decreases pressure on the tissue and granulation tissue formation.
- Secure the tube by suturing it to the skin or tying it with gauze around the neck.
- If necessary, skin cranial and caudal to the tube can be sutured together.
- Leave stay sutures in place while tracheostomy tube is present to aid in tube replacement should it become dislodged or obstructed.

PERMANENT TRACHEOSTOMY

- Place animal in dorsal recumbency, and clip hair of the ventral and lateral neck.
- Surgically prep the skin.
- Make a ventral cervical midline skin incision extending caudally from the distal aspect of the larynx. A typical length for the incision is 6–8 cm in a medium-size dog.
- Expose the trachea by bluntly dissecting between the paired sternohyoid muscles and retracting laterally.
- Identify the third through sixth tracheal cartilages/rings.
- Create a tunnel dorsal to the trachea in this region through gentle blunt dissection and, using this tunnel, place several horizontal mattress sutures with 2-0 or 3-0 polydioxanone/polypropylene through the tunnel and sternohyoid muscles to deviate the trachea ventrally and decrease tension.
- Make an incision through the ventral aspect of the third to sixth tracheal cartilages to the mucosal level, and remove a rectangular segment with a length of three to four cartilages and a width one-third of the tracheal circumference. The size of the segment removed should be approximately 50% larger than the size of the desired stoma.
- Using thumb forceps and the blunt edge of the scalpel blade, dissect free the edges of the incised cartilage from the underlying mucosa.
- Resect a rectangular segment of skin from the edges adjacent to the tracheostomy site similar to the size and shape of the tracheostoma. Excise excess skin or fat if present.
- Using interrupted intradermal sutures of 3-0 polydioxanone/polypropylene, suture the skin around the tracheostoma to the peritracheal tissues laterally and the annular ligaments proximally and distally. These sutures will promote skin adhesion to the trachea and decrease seroma formation and suture tension.
- Make an I- or H-shaped incision into the tracheal mucosa.
- Fold the mucosa over the cartilage edges, and suture it to the skin edges using simple interrupted sutures at the corners and a simple continuous pattern of 4-0 polypropylene for the remainder of the area.

POSTPROCEDURE

TEMPORARY TRACHEOSTOMY TUBE CARE

- Proper care is necessary to prevent airway infection and occlusion.
- Inner cannulas are removed and cleaned or replaced at least every 24 hours or as needed. The inner cannula is soaked in 2% chlorhexidine solution and rinsed before replacement.
- Aseptic technique and sterile equipment should always be used when clearing the airways.
- Preoxygenation is performed for 2 to 5 minutes prior to suctioning to minimize hypoxemia.
- A sterile suction catheter no larger than one-half the size of the tracheostomy tube with a blunt end and side suction holes should be used. The catheter should be inserted without vacuum until obstruction is encountered, and then intermittent suction is performed while rotating the catheter as it is removed.The catheter should not remain in the airway for more than 15 seconds.
- Frequency of suctioning is determined by the amount of secretions produced by the animal and may range from every 15 minutes to 6 to 8 hours.
- Humidification or instillation of 0.1 ml/kg (minimum 1 ml and maximum 5 ml) sterile saline every 1 to 2 hours as well as coupage to aid in clearing secretions.

CUFFED TUBES

- Cuffs are inflated for airway sealing to prevent air leakage during ventilatory support.
- A stethoscope is placed over the trachea adjacent to the cuff to auscultate leaks.
- Air is removed in 0.25-ml increments until a small leak is detected at maximal airway pressure, which is considered minimal occluding volume.
- Cuff deflation is not recommended unless there is evidence of difficulty achieving positive-pressure ventilation or airway pressure.

PERMANENT TRACHEOSTOMY CARE

- Frequent cleaning of the opening (often every few hours for an indefinite period of time) is necessary to remove mucus, hair, and foreign material.
- Application of ointment, such as petroleum jelly, decreases mucosal drying and aids in removal of debris.
- Monthly clipping of the hair around the stoma to prevent matting.
- No swimming; avoidance of environments that may allow aspiration of particulate debris.

TEMPORARY TRACHEOSTOMY: TUBE REMOVAL

- The tube should be removed as soon as upper airway airflow has been reestablished. The original tube is removed and replaced with a smaller tube, and respirations are observed for 10 minutes for appropriate ventilation through and around the smaller tube. If respiratory effort is satisfactory, the tube is then occluded, and the animal is observed for appropriate ventilation via oral-nasal respirations. If the animal continues to breathe comfortably, then the tube is removed.
- The surgical site should be allowed to heal by second intention.
- For flap tracheostomy, the site should be debrided of granulation tissue and the flap sutured back into its original area using interrupted sutures of absorbable suture to align the cartilages.

ALTERNATIVES AND THEIR RELATIVE MERITS

- Oral/endotracheal intubation: always attempted first in patients with acute onset, severe upper airway obstruction. Advantages over tracheostomy are speed of mobilization of the airway, technical simplicity, and minimal invasiveness. When such intubation is not possible (e.g., upper airway obstruction cannot be relieved and patient is suffocating), tracheostomy is the procedure of choice.
- Oxygen supplementation: sufficient as initial management in patients with mild upper airway obstruction but often inadequate as sole therapy in cases of moderate or severe obstruction.

AUTHORS: **SARAH ALLEN, ANN MARIE MANNING**

Transfusion Therapy and Collection Techniques for Blood Banking

BASIC INFORMATION

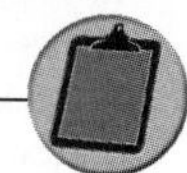

SYNONYM(S)

Blood transfusion
Component therapy

OVERVIEW AND GOAL(S)

Safely collect and administer blood products.

INDICATIONS

FRESH WHOLE BLOOD

- Improve oxygen delivery:
  - Hemolysis
  - Blood loss
  - Nonregenerative anemia
- Provide clotting factors:
  - Anticoagulant rodenticide toxicity
  - Liver disease
  - von Willebrand disease (vWD)
  - Disseminated intravascular coagulation (DIC)
  - Hemophilia A
  - Other factor deficiencies
- Support oncotic pressure:
  - Protein-losing disease (enteropathy, nephropathy, massive skin wounds or burns, serosal inflammation)
- Fresh whole blood is not recommended for treatment of thrombocytopenia unless significant active hemorrhage and anemia exist.

STORED WHOLE BLOOD: Same as for fresh whole blood except for vWD, liver disease, hemophilia A, and DIC: After 6 hours of storage, platelets, factors V and VIII, and von Willebrand factor all decrease.

PACKED RED BLOOD CELLS (PRBCs)

- Improve oxygen delivery:
  - When oncotic support and clotting factors are not required
  - When volume overload is a concern (cardiac disease, renal failure, chronic anemia)

FRESH FROZEN PLASMA

- Provide clotting factors (same as fresh whole blood)
- Support oncotic pressure (same as fresh whole blood)
- Pancreatitis (controversial) or colostrum replacement
- Must be separated and frozen within 6 hours of collection

FROZEN PLASMA: Plasma frozen more than 6 hours after collection or fresh frozen plasma stored more than 1 year:

- Anticoagulant rodenticide toxicity and hemophilia B (factors II, VII, IX, and X preserved).
- Support oncotic pressure.
- Pancreatitis (controversial) or colostrum replacement.

OTHERS: Platelet-rich plasma and platelet concentrate are rarely used in private practice (labor intensive, 2 to 3 day storage times, special storage conditions).

CONTRAINDICATIONS

- Animals with normal to increased packed cell volume (PCV).
- Administer cautiously in patients with volume overload, heart disease, or renal failure.
- Incompatible recipients:
  - Cross-match dogs that have whelped or have received a transfusion more than 4 days previously.
  - Cats: all require blood typing and/or cross-matching prior to transfusion.
- First-time transfusions to dogs are usually safe without prior blood typing and/or cross-matching.

EQUIPMENT, ANESTHESIA

BLOOD COLLECTION: Need clippers and material for sterile prep.

- Dogs:
  - Donor dogs should be healthy adults, weigh >30 kg, and have a normal physical exam and negative heartworm and rickettsial serologies.
  - Butorphanol 0.1–0.2 mg/kg for IV use.
  - Sterile 450-ml collection bag with tubing, needle, and anticoagulant (commercially available) (Fig. II-126).
  - Digital gram scale.
  - Hemostat forceps.
  - Scissors.
  - Hemoclips and stripper sealer (optional).
- Cats:
  - Donor cats should be healthy adults, weigh >4 kg, have a normal physical exam and normal blood smear, and be negative for feline leukemia and feline immunodeficiency virus serologies.
  - Ketamine HCl: 1–2 mg/kg for IV use.
  - Two 35-ml syringes (a 60-ml syringe may collapse the vein).
  - Anticoagulant (citrate-phosphate-dextrose-adenine-1 or adenine-citrate-dextrose).
  - A 19-gauge butterfly needle.
  - NOTE: Heparin (300 units per 50 ml blood collected) can be used as an anticoagulant in an emergency.
    - Dilute heparin in 3 ml of saline to facilitate mixing.
    - Heparin contains no preservatives: administer blood within 24 hours.
    - Heparin activates platelets: avoid in thrombocytopenic animals.

BLOOD ADMINISTRATION (Fig. II-125)

- IV or intraosseous (IO) catheter
- Transfusion set with filter (dogs)
- A 170-μm syringe filter and an IV extension set (cats)

ANTICIPATED TIME

- Whole blood collection: 20 to 40 minutes.
- Administration: minutes to maximum of 4 hours depending on animal's condition.

PREPARATION: IMPORTANT CHECKPOINTS

- Check PCV of recipient and donor prior to transfusion.
- Save hematocrit tube containing recipient plasma for future comparison if hemolytic reactions occur.
- Aseptic technique is essential.
- See Cross-Match and Blood Typing, p 1212.

POSSIBLE COMPLICATIONS AND COMMON ERRORS TO AVOID

TRANSFUSION REACTIONS (see also Transfusion Reactions, p 1098)

- Monitor temperature, heart rate, and respiratory rate every 10 minutes for 30 minutes, then every 60 minutes until transfusion completed.
- Uncommon (3%) and rarely fatal (<1%) if cross-matched.
- Stop transfusion.
- Evaluate signs: If mild without evidence of hemolysis or bacterial contamination, restart transfusion at a slower rate and monitor closely.
- Risk of reactions is reduced by:
  - Using donor dogs negative for DEA 1.1 and preferably negative for DEA 1.2 and DEA 7
  - Cross-matching all donors with recipients
  - Using proper collection, administration, and storage techniques
  - Not adding anything other than 0.9% saline to blood products

Hemolytic transfusion reaction: may be acute or delayed:

- Acute:
  - Can see signs within 20 minutes.
  - Restlessness, fever, tachycardia, vomiting, hemoglobinuria, hemoglobinemia.

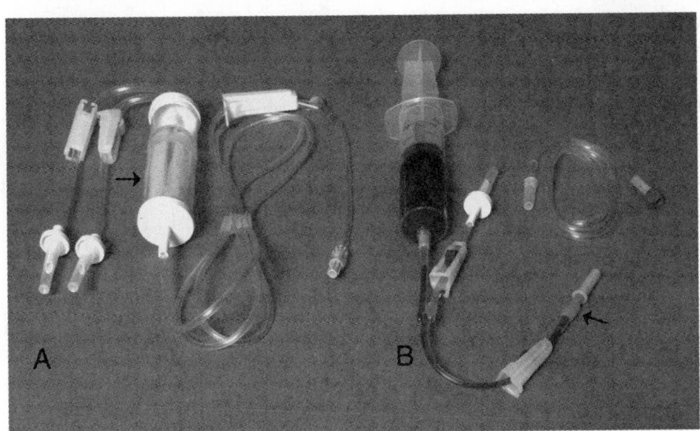

FIGURE II-125 Two blood transfusion systems. Arrows indicate filters. A, A transfusion set with filter chamber typically used for larger volumes (medium- and large-breed dogs). B, A 170-μm syringe filter and IV extension set typically used for cats and toy breed dogs.

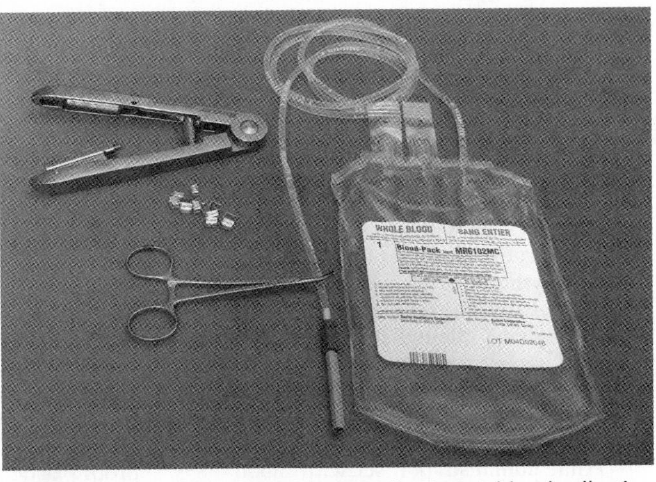

FIGURE II-126 Materials for blood collection. A blood collection bag, tubing, and needle (right) are shown, with a hemostatic clamp placed on the tubing to prevent leakage of the anticoagulant. Hemoclips and a stripper sealer (left) are also shown.

- Very rarely: renal failure, collapse, shock, and death.
- Stop transfusion.
- Look for hemolysis: check plasma color of a spun hematocrit tube (compare to pretransfusion plasma color).
- Check blood pressure (BP) and urine output.
- Administer fluids (address shock, prevent DIC).
- Corticosteroids and antihistamines will not prevent acute hemolytic reactions.

- Delayed:
  - Can occur 3–14 days after transfusion.
  - Decrease transfusion efficacy but usually produces no clinical signs.

Anaphylactic reactions:
- Usually mild.
- Fever, urticaria, erythema, pruritus.
- Stop transfusion.
- Administer antihistamines (e.g., diphenhydramine 1–2 mg/kg IM) and glucocorticoids (e.g., dexamethasone SP 0.1–0.2 mg/kg IV).
- Can usually restart transfusion at a slower rate.

Volume overload:
- Cough, dyspnea, jugular distention.
- Stop transfusion.
- Administer furosemide (e.g., 2 mg/kg IV) ± oxygen supplementation.

Bacterial contamination: Examine blood for discoloration, and submit blood for culture and Gram stain if animal is febrile.

OTHER CONCERNS
- Microembolism
- Hypothermia
- Acidosis
- Citrate toxicity

PROCEDURE

BLOOD COLLECTION FOR BANKING
- Blood donor dogs:
  - Administer butorphanol 0.2 mg/kg IV.
  - Place in lateral recumbency on an elevated surface.
  - Clip ventral neck (center over jugular furrow).
  - Perform sterile scrub.
  - Place collection bag on the scale at a level below the animal (blood collects via gravity).
  - Zero the scale (collection bag + anticoagulant ≈ 85 g).
  - NOTE: If less than 450 ml of blood is to be collected, anticoagulant must be expressed from the collection bag to maintain the 1:7 anticoagulant to blood ratio (e.g., to collect 225 ml blood, discard half the anticoagulant [32 g]).
  - Clamp tubing with hemostat (near needle).
  - Hold off jugular vein for visualization.
  - Remove needle cap and insert needle (16–17 gauge) into jugular vein.
  - Remove hemostat; collection begins.
  - During collection, gently rock the bag intermittently to mix blood with the anticoagulant.
  - Rotate/adjust needle delicately if flow stops.
  - Continue collection until scale reads 450 g (± 45 g).
  - Release jugular vein pressure.
  - Reclamp tubing near needle.
  - Remove needle from jugular vein.
  - Recap needle.
  - Strip blood from tubing into bag to mix with anticoagulant.
  - Allow tubing to refill.
  - Tie/hemoclip tubing at 6- to 10-cm intervals for storage and cross-match.
  - Remove hemostat.
  - If collection technique is questionable, blood should be used within 24 hours.
- Blood donor cats:
  - Sedate (1–2 mg/kg ketamine IV; may add diazepam 0.1 mg/kg IV if necessary).
  - Clip ventral neck (center over jugular furrow).
  - Perform sterile scrub.
  - Use a separate needle to put 4 ml ACD or CPDA-1 into each sterile 35-ml syringe.
  - Connect one 35-ml syringe to a butterfly needle.
  - Hold off jugular vein to visualize.
  - Remove needle guard.
  - Insert butterfly needle into jugular vein.
  - Gently aspirate 27 ml of blood while slowly rocking the syringe to mix anticoagulant and blood.
  - Disconnect syringe from butterfly catheter.
  - Cap syringe with a sterile needle.
  - Attach second anticoagulant-filled syringe, and gently aspirate 27 ml of blood as already described.
  - Release jugular pressure.
  - Remove needle from jugular vein.
  - NOTE: A similar technique can be used in dogs (60-ml syringe with 7 ml ACD or CPDA-1) if collection bags are unavailable; refrigerate and use within 24 hours.

ADMINISTRATION
- For all blood products:
  - Always use a filter.
  - Start slowly (0.5 ml/kg/hr) for 15–20 minutes.
  - Monitor for reactions.
  - Increase rate if no reactions occur.
  - Complete transfusion by 4 hours (decreases bacterial contamination).
  - Normal rate is 5–10 ml/kg/hr.
  - Can increase to 20 ml/kg/hr in unstable hypovolemic animals.
  - Can administer as rapidly as possible in a severe crisis.
  - For heart disease, renal failure, or potential volume overload, administer at 1–4 ml/kg/hr and monitor for volume overload (as already described).

- Can divide dosage into smaller aliquots and refrigerate up to 24 hours (allows slower administration with minimal risk of bacterial contamination).
- From a syringe (see Fig. II-125B):
  - Attach syringe filter to syringe.
  - Attach IV extension set to filter.
  - Prime system with blood product.
  - Connect extension set to IV catheter.
  - Use syringe pump or intermittent administration (i.e., healthy cats: 5 ml over 5 minutes then wait 6–12 minutes and repeat).
- From a collection bag (see Fig. II-125A):
  - Use blood administration set with filter (see manufacturer instructions).
  - Prime administration set with blood product.
  - Attach to IV catheter.
  - Set drip rate.
  - Some infusion pumps can be used; check manufacturer specifications.
- Dosages:
  - Whole blood: 10–20 ml/kg.
    - Generally: 2 ml/kg increases PCV ≈1%.
  - PRBCs: 5–10 ml/kg.
    - Generally: 1 ml/kg increases PCV 1%.
    - Can dilute with 50–125 ml of 0.9% saline to decrease viscosity.
  - Alternatively: PRBCs or whole blood (milliliters) dose = BW (kilograms) × 90 × (PCV desired – PCV recipient)/PCV of donor blood; substitute 90 with 60 for cats.
- Warming whole blood or PRBCs is not essential; indications to warm:
  - Multiple transfusions.
  - Hypothermic animals.
  - Neonates.
  - Warm by room air or water bath.
  - Do not exceed 37°C (hemolysis).
- Fresh frozen/frozen plasma: 10–20 ml/kg.
  - Plastic is fragile when frozen; handle frozen units delicately.
  - Thaw in 37°C water bath in a waterproof plastic bag.
  - Give within 4 hours for clotting factors.
  - Can store 24 hours in refrigerator after thawing if clotting factors not required.
  - Repeat dosage if coagulopathy persists.

POSTPROCEDURE

- Blood donors: Administer fluids if hypovolemic (tachycardia, pale mucous membranes, prolonged capillary refill time) or if the fluid equivalent of more than 2% of the body weight in kilograms is collected.
- Patients/recipients: Check PCV 2 hours after the transfusion is complete, and check coagulation profile after administering plasma for coagulopathies.

ALTERNATIVES AND THEIR RELATIVE MERITS

- Polymerized hemoglobin (Oxyglobin):
  - Improves oxygen delivery.
  - Provides colloidal support but no other plasma benefits.
  - Dogs: 10–30 ml/kg at a maximum of 10 ml/kg/hr.
  - Cats: 5–10 ml/kg at a maximum of 5 ml/kg/hr.
  - Monitor closely for signs of volume overload, especially in cats.
- Synthetic colloids:
  - Hypoalbuminemia requires large volumes of whole blood or plasma to correct.
  - Synthetic colloids should be considered instead to support colloidal pressure (bolus 5–20 ml/kg then 10–20 ml/kg/day; use lower doses for cats).
  - Human albumin: Role is controversial; further studies are required before recommendations can be made (suggested guidelines: dogs, 2–7 ml/kg of 25% or 10–35 ml/kg of 5% over 4–6 hours).

AUTHOR: **SØREN R. BOYSEN**

Transtracheal Wash

BASIC INFORMATION

SYNONYM(S)

Tracheal lavage
Tracheal wash
Tracheal wash via endotracheal tube

OVERVIEW AND GOAL(S)

Minimally invasive method of obtaining specimens from the trachea for cytologic examination and culture

INDICATIONS

- Chronic cough
- Alveolar and bronchial radiographic lung patterns

CONTRAINDICATIONS

Compromise of unstable animal with respiratory disease via stress, sedation, anesthesia, or restraint.

EQUIPMENT, ANESTHESIA

- May only need restraint in depressed animal, or use minimal sedation/anesthesia, to avoid suppressing the cough reflex and to minimally depress respiration.
- Administration of supplemental oxygen is possible through a catheter placed in trachea via oral cavity or endotracheal tube. Ensure that the patient cannot bite/sever the catheter or tube.
- Both the transtracheal wash and the tracheal wash via endotracheal tube require:
  - Sterile saline 0.5–2.0 ml/kg (often separated into two syringes to allow repetition).
  - Additional sterile syringe (empty) for aspiration.
    - Should be larger than infusion syringe for better aspiration.
  - Sterile tube designated for aerobic and fungal cultures.
  - Microscope slides (for fresh smears/cytologic analysis).
  - EDTA (purple top) tube for aliquot for cytologic analysis (may improve cell preservation) or cell counts.

TRANSTRACHEAL WASH

- Clipper for hair
- Sterile scrub supplies and isopropyl alcohol
- Sterile paper/cloth drape if desired
- 2% lidocaine for local subcutaneous injection (0.5–1.0 ml)
- A sterile #11 scalpel blade for small nick in skin (<1 mm)
- A sterile 18- to 22-gauge through-the-needle (introducer) jugular catheter of appropriate length
- Roll cast padding and Vetrap-type releasing elastic bandaging for cervical wrap

TRACHEAL WASH WITH USE OF STERILE ENDOTRACHEAL TUBE

- Topical 2% lidocaine solution applied by spray or swab as needed to laryngeal and pharyngeal regions (notably in cats)
- Sterile endotracheal tube
- Sterile red rubber catheter 5 Fr, preferably long enough to reach fourth through sixth intercostal space (ICS)

ANTICIPATED TIME

About 15 to 20 minutes

PREPARATION: IMPORTANT CHECKPOINTS

- Recent thoracic radiographs.
- Supplemental oxygen available.

- Advise owner of risks of techniques, including possible nondiagnostic findings.

POSSIBLE COMPLICATIONS AND COMMON ERRORS TO AVOID

- Contamination of specimens via oral cavity if using endotracheal tube technique.
- Subcutaneous emphysema or pneumomediastinum with transtracheal approach.
- Being too hesitant in volume of saline instilled.
- Withdrawal of catheter against the insertion needle can cut catheter off in the tracheal lumen.
- Cyanosis/hypoxemia in animals with borderline hypoxemia prior to procedure.

PROCEDURE

Decide between techniques based on value of sample purity versus patient risk factors; transtracheal approach lessens contamination but slightly increases risk of complications.

TRANSTRACHEAL WASH

- Patient in sitting or sternal position, ideally at the front end of a table to have the site of entry into the trachea at eye level.
- Head and neck elevated to horizontal or further vertical (45 degrees toward ceiling); if one side of the lungs is of greater interest, then have this be the dependent (down) side using lateral recumbency.
- Palpate the small cricothyroid membrane at the caudal aspect of the ventral larynx (Fig. II-127).

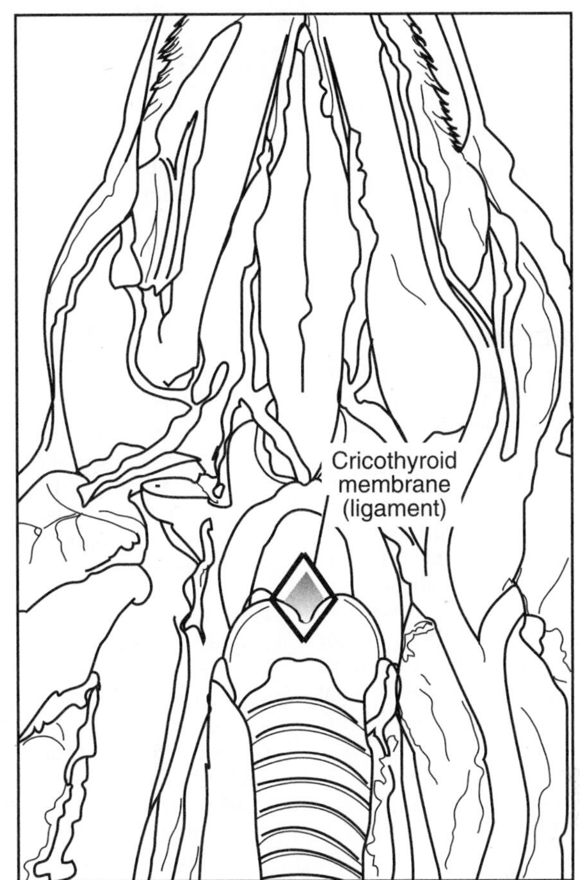

FIGURE II-127 Anatomic diagram of the ventral neck of a dog; dissected specimen. Cranial is toward the top of the image. A diamond-shaped outline identifies the cricothyroid membrane, through which a catheter is introduced for performing a transtracheal wash.

- Clip and prepare the area using sterile technique.
- Infiltrate 0.5–1.0 ml lidocaine in SC tissue overlying the cricothyroid membrane.
- Make a small (<1 mm) incision with the #11 scalpel blade.
- Prepare jugular catheter.
- Insert jugular catheter needle at oblique angle caudodorsally through the small incision in the skin, then through the cricothyroid membrane.
- When the needle is in the tracheal lumen, a slight cough upon entry is common. Take care to avoid lacerating the dorsal wall of the trachea with the needle tip.
- Slide the catheter down into the tracheal lumen; remove the stylet partially.
- Back out the insertion needle so it is outside the trachea and skin, hold catheter steady (catheter position stays unchanged), and apply the needle guard.
- Remove stylet and flush initial volume. It is important to aspirate immediately after flushing and to not aspirate against negative pressure (catheter tip lodged against respiratory mucosa; release negative pressure and reposition). May switch to larger syringe to aspirate as much fluid sample as possible; if no specimen is obtained, then the second volume is flushed and aspirated again. Saline that passes down the trachea is expectorated or coughed back toward the catheter; mucus and turbidity are seen in the fluid; often, only 1–2 ml will be retrieved out of every 10 ml infused.
- Withdraw catheter.
- Gently wrap neck over insertion site with cast padding, roll gauze, and VetWrap to reduce risk of SC emphysema; keep the neck wrap in place preferably 12 hours, ensuring that it is not too tight.

TRACHEAL WASH VIA ENDOTRACHEAL TUBE

- Sedate or anesthetize animal, and place oral speculum to hold mouth open.
- Pass sterile endotracheal tube to an appropriate level; use topical lidocaine on larynx if needed.
- Pass sterile red rubber catheter through the endotracheal tube to level of thoracic inlet or bronchial bifurcation; lavage with same technique as already described.
- Can follow flush procedure with covered endoscopic cytology brush if desired.

POSTPROCEDURE

- Provide supplemental oxygen if needed.
- Divide specimen into aliquots for cytologic analysis and cultures, and fresh slides for cytologic analysis; can request routine staining and Gram stain.
- If respiratory distress occurs, tilt the animal's body (head down, allowing fluid to flow cranially), perform coupage, consider reintubation and oxygen supplementation/positive-pressure ventilation.
- Radiographs to assess for pneumomediastinum if needed.

ALTERNATIVES AND THEIR RELATIVE MERITS

Tracheobronchoscopy:

- Visualization of airways to bronchi.
- Catheter lavage and brush cytologic analysis can be performed.
- Requires longer time.
- Tracheobronchoscopy is more accurate than tracheal wash if both options are available.

AUTHOR: **MARK E. HITT**

Upper Gastrointestinal Radiographic Contrast Series

BASIC INFORMATION

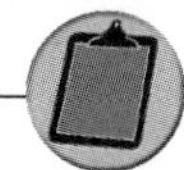

SYNONYM(S)

Barium series
UGI

OVERVIEW AND GOAL(S)

- To identify abnormalities of the stomach and/or small intestinal tract. Morphologic and/or functional abnormalities may be identified.
- The upper gastrointestinal (UGI) radiographic contrast series is most commonly performed using barium, which gives the best mucosal detail and therefore the best evaluation of morphology. The study may be performed with an iodinated contrast agent; these do not give good mucosal detail and are most useful for evaluating gastrointestinal (GI) integrity and patency (Fig. II-128).

INDICATIONS

- Severe or protracted vomiting
- Hematemesis or melena
- Abdominal pain
- Abnormalities of survey radiographs requiring further investigation
- Determine location of GI structures (i.e., herniation)

CONTRAINDICATIONS

- Survey radiographic evidence of perforation:
  - If perforation is suspected, the study may be performed with an iodinated contrast agent; however, because of their relatively poor opacity, iodinated contrast agents may fail to demonstrate GI leakage.
- Survey radiographic evidence of obstruction:
  - Not an absolute contraindication but the study is not needed for diagnosis.
- Projectile vomiting:
  - Not an absolute contraindication but the risks involved in performing the study may outweigh the potential benefits.

EQUIPMENT, ANESTHESIA

- Contrast agent:
  - Liquid barium (30% weight/volume):
    - 10 ml/kg PO.
    - In very obese patients, it may be preferable to dose for desired/lean body weight, not actual weight.
  - Ionic iodinated contrast agent:
    - Gastrografin/Renografin: 2–7 ml/kg PO; total dose not to exceed 50 ml.
    - Gastrografin is a contrast agent that was marketed for oral use only; this product is no longer available. Renografin is a contrast agent used for IV injection and may be given orally instead of Gastrografin.
  - Nonionic iodinated contrast agent:
    - Iohexol (Omnipaque).
      - 10 ml/kg PO of diluted iohexol (240–875 mg I/ml, diluted 1:1 to 1:3 with tap water).
      - The greater the iodine concentration of the iohexol, the better the mucosal detail.
      - Administration of undiluted iohexol causes vomiting.
- Syringes for contrast administration.
- Orogastric tube of the appropriate size.
- X-ray unit.
- Protective clothing (lead aprons, gloves, thyroid shields) for personnel.
- Paper towels or similar material for cleanup of barium on animal and x-ray table.
- Drugs for restraint (used only if absolutely necessary): The following agents have the least effect on motility and should be used if a motility disorder is suspected:
  - Dogs: acepromazine 0.055–0.1 mg/kg IV; avoid if animal is elderly or systemically ill.
  - Cats: diazepam 0.44 mg/kg; ketamine 13.2 mg/kg.
  - These drugs are given in separate syringes IM approximately 20 minutes prior to the procedure. If a motility abnormality is not of concern (i.e., determining if obstruction is present), the following combination is recommended for cats. This will give better and more consistent restraint than the diazepam/ketamine combination; the following drugs are also given IM approximately 20 minutes prior to the procedure and should be avoided if animal is elderly or systemically ill:
    - Acepromazine: 0.22 mg/kg.
    - Ketamine: 13.2 mg/kg.

ANTICIPATED TIME

- About 6 hours to complete the study (barium); actual time spent performing the study is approximately 1.5 hours.
- About 2 to 3 hours to complete the study (iodinated contrast agents); actual time spent performing the study is approximately 1 hour.
- ± Additional film at 24 hours postcontrast administration.

PREPARATION: IMPORTANT CHECKPOINTS

- Empty GI tract:
  - Fasting to empty the stomach
  - Remove excess fluid from stomach via tube if present
  - Enema: only if colon is very full

POSSIBLE COMPLICATIONS AND COMMON ERRORS TO AVOID

- Complications:
  - Vomiting and aspiration of barium: If the animal has projectile vomiting and/or radiographic evidence of severe gastric fluid retention, the risks involved in performing the UGI radiographic contrast series may outweigh the potential benefits.
  - Aspiration of iodinated contrast agents: Ionic iodinated contrast agents can cause severe (and fatal) pulmonary edema if aspirated. These agents should be administered only via orogastric intubation.
- Common errors:
  - Administration of too low a volume of barium.
  - Administration of barium prior to abdominal ultrasound or endoscopy (may interfere with visualization; however, sequence of testing may make this unavoidable).

PROCEDURE

- Obtain survey (plain) right lateral and dorsoventral radiographs of the abdomen.
  - Dorsoventral views provide better evaluation of the body and pyloric region of the stomach and are preferred for the UGI radiographic contrast series.
- Administer contrast:
  - Barium dosage: 10 ml/kg PO. If too low a volume of barium is used, artifactual delayed gastric emptying can occur. Administration via orogastric tube is preferred, but barium may be administered per os.
  - Iodinated contrast agents Gastrografin/Renografin: 2–7 ml/kg PO, with total dose not to exceed 50 ml; iohexol: 10 ml/kg PO of diluted iohexol (240–875 mg I/ml diluted 1:1 to 1:3). Administration via orogastric tube is preferred.
- Obtain films:
  - Film sequence and views for barium: This sequence is a routine timetable. The timing of films can be altered as the study progresses, based on what is found in the study.
    - Immediate: right and left lateral, ventrodorsal and dorsoventral.
    - 30 minutes: right lateral and dorsoventral.
    - 60 minutes: right lateral and dorsoventral.

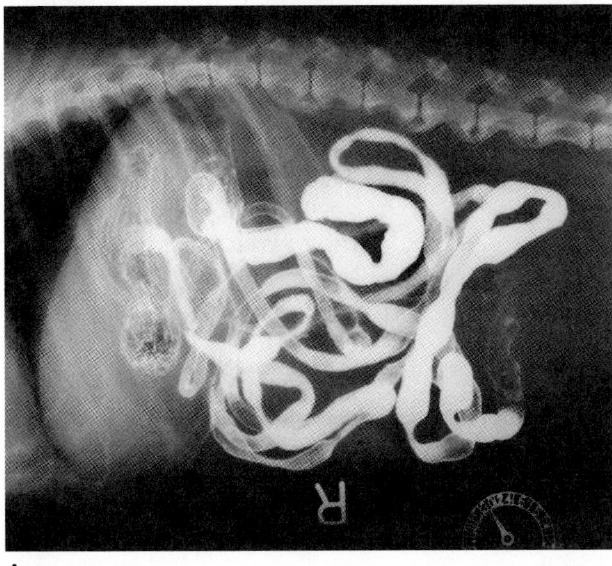

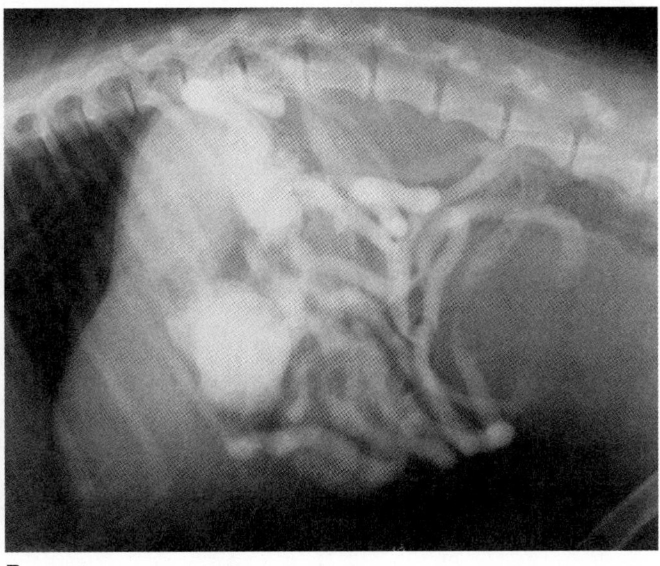

A B

FIGURE II-128 **A,** Right lateral radiograph obtained 30 minutes after administration of liquid barium. Note the high opacity of the contrast agent and the good mucosal detail. **B,** Right lateral radiograph obtained 30 minutes after administration of iohexol. The contrast agent is much less opaque, and the mucosal surface is poorly defined.

- 90 minutes: right lateral and dorsoventral.
- 3 hours: right lateral and dorsoventral.
- 5 hours: right lateral and dorsoventral.
- ± 24 hours: right lateral and dorsoventral.

◦ Film sequence and views for iodinated contrast agents: This sequence is a routine timetable. The timing of films can be altered as the study progresses, based on what is found in the study.
- Immediate: right and left lateral, ventrodorsal and dorsoventral.
- 15 minutes: right lateral and dorsoventral.
- 30 minutes: right lateral and dorsoventral.
- 60 minutes: right lateral and dorsoventral.
- 2 hours: right lateral and dorsoventral.

- By definition, the UGI radiographic contrast series is considered to be complete when contrast has both emptied from the stomach and has entered the large intestine (Fig. II-129).
- Films may be taken beyond this point if an abnormality has been noted during the examination; for example, in an animal with retention of barium in the stomach, the UGI radiographic contrast series should be continued until the stomach empties or an abnormality to account for the barium retention is noted.
- If an abnormality (i.e., obstruction) is identified, the study is considered to be complete even if barium is still present in the stomach and/or has not entered the large intestine.

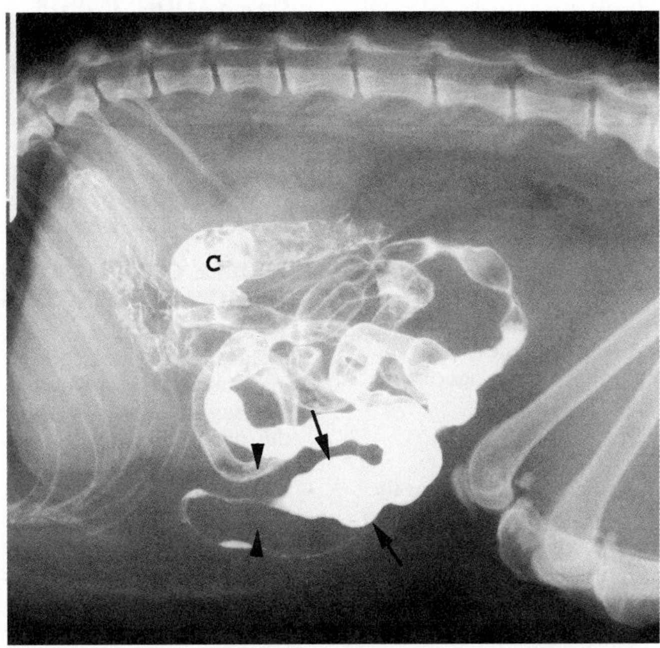

FIGURE II-129 Right lateral radiograph obtained 2 hours after administration of liquid barium. A distended segment of small intestine (*arrows*) suddenly narrows at an area of intramural thickening (*arrowheads*) caused by a circumferential soft-tissue mass in this dog. Barium is present in the cecum (C), indicating that the bowel is patent.

POSTPROCEDURE

- There are no postprocedure considerations for a routine UGI radiographic contrast series other than informing the client that stools may have a paler color for several defecations after the procedure.
- The findings of the UGI radiographic contrast series may lead to an additional diagnostic test, such as exploratory laparotomy or endoscopy.

ALTERNATIVES AND THEIR RELATIVE MERITS

- Endoscopy:
  - Endoscopy allows visualization of the mucosal surface of the stomach

and duodenum and allows tissue biopsies to be performed.
  - However, endoscopy does not evaluate the entire small intestinal tract and requires the use of general anesthesia.
- Abdominal ultrasonography:
  - Ultrasonography is rapid and noninvasive and does not involve ionizing radiation.
  - However, ultrasonographic evaluation of the GI tract can be severely limited by gas in the tract. Interpretation of ultrasound images of the GI tract requires an experienced sonographer, and many GI disease processes do not cause significant changes in the ultrasonographic appearance of the intestine.
- Exploratory laparotomy:
  - Allows assessment of the entire length of the GI tract and full-thickness gastric and intestinal biopsies. However, general anesthesia, invasiveness, and recovery/incision healing time make laparotomy a second-order diagnostic modality after lesser invasive evaluations, such as plain radiography, UGI radiographic contrast series, ultrasonography, and/or endoscopy.

AUTHOR: **PATRICIA L. ROSE**

Urethral Obstruction (Canine): Medical Management

BASIC INFORMATION

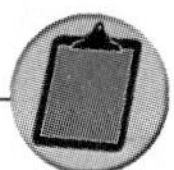

OVERVIEW AND GOAL(S)

Compete urethral obstruction is a potentially life-threatening event, culminating in death from uremia within 2 to 5 days if untreated. Although most causes for urethral obstruction are intraluminal (e.g., urethroliths, foreign material, urethral plugs), mural (e.g., tumors, urethral strictures) and extramural causes (e.g., pelvic fractures, iatrogenic urethral ligation), and functional disorders (e.g., detrusor-sphincter dyssynergia) result in identical clinical consequences.

INDICATIONS

- Urethroliths (common)
- Blood clots
- Intraurethral foreign bodies
- Matrix-crystalline urethral plugs (uncommon)

EQUIPMENT, ANESTHESIA

The type and degree of sedation/anesthesia varies depending on patient status and veterinarian's preference.

- Cardiovascular stabilization:
  - Heating pad
  - IV catheter
  - Warm IV replacement fluids
  - Sodium bicarbonate
- Decompressive cystocentesis:
  - A sterile 1.5-inch, 22-gauge needle
  - IV extension tubing
  - Three-way stopcock
  - Large syringe (20–60 ml)
- Retrograde urethral flushing:
  - Sterile isotonic nonirritating solutions (e.g., normal saline, lactated Ringer's solution)
  - Long, flexible large-bore sterile catheter (e.g., 8-Fr, 22-inch red rubber feeding tubes)
  - Large sterile syringe (20–60 ml)
  - Moistened gauze sponges
- Indwelling catheter placement:
  - Nonabsorbable suture and needle holders
  - Soft, flexible, inert sterile urinary catheter

ANTICIPATED TIME

About 20 minutes to 1 hour

PREPARATION: IMPORTANT CHECKPOINTS

- Inform owners of the possibility of urinary bladder rupture and guarded short-term prognosis with and without therapy.
- Inform owners that in many cases, surgery or lithotripsy will be needed to correct an underlying problem.

POSSIBLE COMPLICATIONS AND COMMON ERRORS TO AVOID

- Survey radiography is essential to verify, localize, and search for the underlying cause of obstruction. Therefore, radiographs should be obtained early in the diagnostic process prior to initiation of therapy.
- Unsuccessful transurethral insertion and passage of urinary catheters is an unreliable and sometimes unsafe (i.e., urethral tear, rupture, and subsequent stricture) method of confirming and localizing urethral obstruction.

PROCEDURE

- Sedate or anesthetize animal.
- Decompressive cystocentesis:
  - Attach a 1.5-inch, 22-gauge needle; IV extension tubing; and three-way stopcock; then use a large-volume syringe (20–60 ml) to remove urine from bladder.
  - By using the IV extension tubing and three-way stopcock between the needle and syringe, the urinary bladder will not have to be repunctured to empty a syringe full of urine.
  - Excessive digital pressure should not be applied to the bladder wall while the needle is in the lumen to prevent urine from being forced around the needle into the peritoneal cavity.
  - Attempting complete evacuation of the bladder lumen is undesirable because the sharp point of the needle may then damage the bladder wall. We recommend that 10–15 ml of urine remain in the bladder.
  - Cystocentesis should not contribute to bladder rupture. Excessive manipulation of a devitalized, overdistended bladder is usually the cause of bladder rupture.
  - Advantages:
    - Obtaining urine sample for analysis and culture.
    - Temporarily halting the adverse metabolic consequences of obstruction.
    - Reducing intraluminal bladder pressure to facilitate retropulsion.
    - Reducing pain associated with bladder overdistention.
  - Disadvantages:
    - Potential extravasation of urine into peritoneal cavity.
    - Bladder wall trauma.
- Retrograde urethral flushing:
  - Lubricate around the urethroliths.
    - Fill one 12-ml syringe with 5 ml of saline and another 12-ml syringe with 5 ml of sterile water-soluble lubricant.
    - Attach these two syringes with a three-way stopcock.
    - Mix the contents of both syringes by emptying one syringe into the other several times.
    - After inserting a urethral catheter, inject 3–8 ml of mixture to lubricate around uroliths.
    - This step is not always necessary.
  - Insert a lubricated large-bore flexible catheter into the distal urethra. The tip of the catheter should remain distal to urethroliths.
  - Occlude pelvic urethra: Insert a gloved index finger into the rectum, and occlude the urethral lumen by compressing the urethra against the floor of the bony pelvis.

- Occlude distal urethra: With a moistened gauze sponge, occlude the distal urethra by compressing the distal tip of penis around the catheter.
- Forcefully flush fluid through catheter:
  - Fill a large syringe (20-35 ml) with sterile isotonic solution (e.g., saline, lactated Ringer's solution, etc.). The normal bladder holds approximately 7-11 ml/kg of the patient's weight.
  - With the syringe attached to the catheter, turn it upside down, and place the top of the plunger against the tabletop.
  - Hold the syringe by the barrel, and forcefully push it down over the plunger with the goal of dilating the urethral lumen with saline.
- Relieve occlusion of pelvic urethra: once the urethra becomes dilated, digital pressure applied to the pelvic urethra (but not the penile urethra) should be rapidly released.
- Continue flushing:
  - Continue flushing fluid through the catheter and urethral lumen to propel urethroliths into the urinary bladder. Use caution not to overdistend the bladder lumen with saline.
  - If the technique is repeated, accumulation of saline in the bladder lumen necessitates repeating decompressive cystocentesis.
- To perform this technique in female dogs, insert the index finger into the vagina, and apply digital pressure and occlude the distal urethra over the catheter at the urethral papilla. Inserting the index finger in the rectum and applying digital pressure over the catheter in the pelvic urethra can also achieve distal urethral occlusion.

POSTPROCEDURE

- Medical imaging:
  - Radiography provides an appropriate method of assessing whether all of the uroliths have been flushed into the bladder lumen.
  - Transurethral catheterization is not a reliable method of verifying that all uroliths have been flushed out of the urethra.
- Pain medication (i.e., butorphanol, hydromorphone, etc.) is indicated for a short duration (1-2 days). Nonsteroidal anti-inflammatory drugs (NSAIDs) are contraindicated in animals with compromised renal function or dehydration.
- Prevent negative fluid balance associated with postobstructive diuresis by administering parenteral fluids.

ALTERNATIVES AND THEIR RELATIVE MERITS

To minimize surgical disfigurement of the urethra (e.g., urethrotomy, urethrostomy) consider lithotripsy to shatter obstructing urethroliths if retrograde urohydropropulsion is not successful.

AUTHORS: **JODY P. LULICH, CARL A. OSBORNE**

Urethral Obstruction (Feline): Medical Management

BASIC INFORMATION

OVERVIEW AND GOAL(S)

Compete urethral obstruction is a potentially life-threatening event, culminating in death from uremia within 2 to 5 days if untreated. Although most causes for urethral obstruction are intraluminal (e.g., urethral plugs, urethroliths, foreign material), mural (e.g., tumors, urethral strictures) and extramural causes (e.g., pelvic fractures, iatrogenic urethral ligation) result in identical clinical consequences.

INDICATIONS

- Matrix-crystalline urethral plugs (common)
- Urethroliths (common)
- Blood clots
- Intraurethral foreign bodies (i.e., buckshot)

EQUIPMENT, ANESTHESIA

The type and degree of sedation/anesthesia vary depending on patient status and veterinarian's preference.

- Cardiovascular stabilization:
  - Heating pad
  - IV catheter
  - Warm IV replacement fluids
  - Sodium bicarbonate
  - Insulin and glucose to manage hyperkalemia (rare)
  - Calcium gluconate to manage hyperkalemia (rare); see Hyperkalemia, p 546
- Decompressive cystocentesis:
  - Sterile 1.5-inch, 22-gauge needle
  - IV extension tubing
  - Three-way stopcock
  - Several syringes (size: 3-20 ml)
- Retrograde urethral flushing:
  - Sterile isotonic nonirritating solutions (e.g., normal saline, lactated Ringer's solution)
  - Sterile open-ended catheter (e.g., Minnesota olive tip catheter)
  - IV extension tubing
  - Large syringe (12-35 ml)
  - Moistened gauze sponges
- Indwelling urinary catheter placement:
  - Nonabsorbable suture and needle holders
  - Soft, flexible, inert sterile urinary catheter
  - Elizabethan collar

ANTICIPATED TIME

About 20 minutes to 1 hour

PREPARATION: IMPORTANT CHECKPOINTS

- Ensure cardiovascular stabilization prior to general anesthesia or urethral flushing.
- Prevalence of potentially life-threatening abnormalities in cats with urethral obstruction:
  - Hypothermia (<100° F) = 39%
  - Acidemia (pH <7.2) = 16%
  - Bradycardia (<149 bpm) = 12%
  - Hyperkalemia (>8 mEq/l) = 12%
  - Hypocalcemia (<0.8 mmol/l) = 6%
- Inform owners of the possibility of urinary bladder rupture and guarded short-term prognosis with and without therapy.

POSSIBLE COMPLICATIONS AND COMMON ERRORS TO AVOID

- Cats with urethral obstruction and cardiovascular collapse rarely present with signs referable to the urinary system. Therefore, assessment of urinary bladder size (i.e., palpation or medical imaging) is essential to avoid overlooking urethral obstruction as the primary cause for cardiovascular or respiratory distress.
- Survey radiography is essential to verify, localize, and search for the underlying cause of obstruction. Therefore, radiographs should be performed early in the diagnostic process prior to initiation of therapy. Nonobstructed dysuric cats usually do not have obstructed urethras.
- Unsuccessful transurethral insertion of urinary catheters is an unreliable and sometimes unsafe (i.e., urethral tear, rupture, and subsequent stricture) method of confirming and localizing urethral obstruction.
- Caustic, strongly acidic flushing solutions are contraindicated.

PROCEDURE

- Sedate or anesthetize the patient.
- To fragment urethral plugs, gently massage the distal urethra and cautiously compress the urinary bladder with the goal of promoting expulsion of plugs. This is easy to perform but not commonly effective.
- Decompressive cystocentesis:
  - Attach a 1.5-inch, 22-gauge needle; IV extension tubing; and a three-way stopcock; then use a large-volume syringe (20–60 ml) to remove urine from bladder.
  - By using the IV extension tubing and three-way stopcock between the needle and syringe, the urinary bladder will not have to be repunctured to empty a syringe full of urine.
  - Excessive digital pressure should not be applied to the bladder wall while the needle is in the lumen to prevent urine from being forced around the needle into the peritoneal cavity.
  - Attempting complete evacuation of the bladder lumen is undesirable because the sharp point of the needle may then damage the bladder wall; the authors recommend that 10–15 ml of urine remain in the bladder.
  - Properly performed cystocentesis should not contribute to bladder rupture. Any excessive manipulation of a devitalized, overdistended bladder wall may promote rupture.
- Advantages of decompressive cystocentesis:
  - Obtaining urine sample for analysis and culture.
  - Temporarily halting the adverse effects of obstruction.
  - Reducing intraluminal bladder pressure to facilitate retropulsion.
  - Reducing pain associated with bladder overdistention.
- Disadvantages of decompressive cystocentesis:
  - Potential extravasation of urine into peritoneal cavity.
  - Bladder wall trauma.
- Flushing plug contents out the external urethral orifice:
  - Attach open-ended catheter, IV extension tubing, and large (35-ml) fluid-filled syringe in that order (Fig. II-130). Displace air in the tubing by filling tubing and catheter with fluid from the syringe prior to insertion in the urethra.
  - Insert tip of catheter into distal urethral opening.
  - Flush a large quantity of sterile isotonic solution into the urethral lumen, allowing it to reflux out the external urethral orifice.
  - Subsequent application of steady but gentle digital pressure to the bladder wall may result in expulsion of a urethral plug.
- Retrograde urethral flushing (to propel intraluminal contents into urinary bladder):
  - Attach open-ended catheter, IV extension tubing, and fluid-filled syringe (12–20 ml) in that order (see Fig. II-130). Displace air in the tubing by filling tubing and catheter with fluid from the syringe prior to insertion in the urethra.
  - Insert tip of catheter into distal urethral opening.
  - With a moistened gauze sponge, occlude the distal urethra around the catheter.
  - Pull the penile urethra caudally to extending it parallel to the vertebral column (Fig. II-131).
  - Flush fluid vigorously by emptying syringe.
  - Repeat urethral flushing if needed while also remembering to repeat decompressive cystocentesis if bladder lumen becomes distended with flushing solution.
  - The greatest pressure to retrograde hydropropulse is achieved with the smallest syringe.

POSTPROCEDURE

In some cases, radiographs are indicated to verify return of uroliths into urinary bladder.

INDWELLING TRANSURETHRAL CATHETERS

- To minimize urethral trauma, avoid open-end catheters with sharp stylets.
- Not always indicated.
- When indicated, 3-Fr or 5-Fr flexible feeding tubes composed of material that minimizes foreign body inflammatory response are preferred.
- Indications:
  - Inadequate/poor urine stream following urethral flushing:
    - Urethral spasm/swelling (~1–3 days)
    - Excessive urinary precipitates (~1–2 days)
  - Assist correction of postrenal azotemia (~1–2 days).
  - Promote recovery of detrusor contractility (~1–5 days).

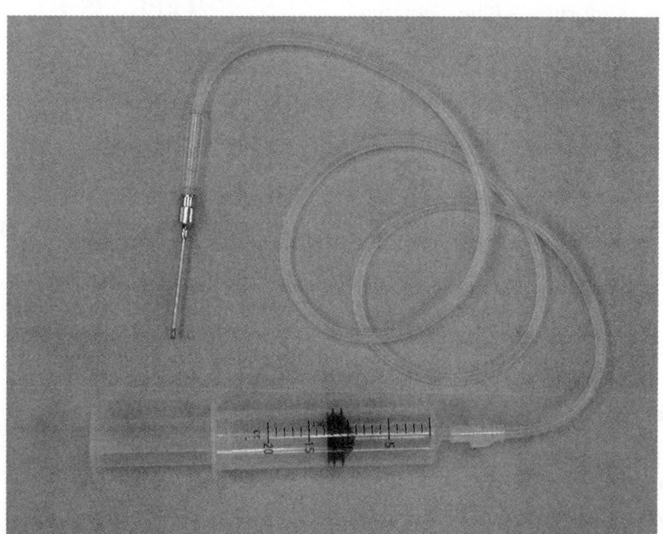

FIGURE II-130 Assembled catheter, IV extension tubing, and syringe to facilitate removing the obstruction in the urethra of cats.

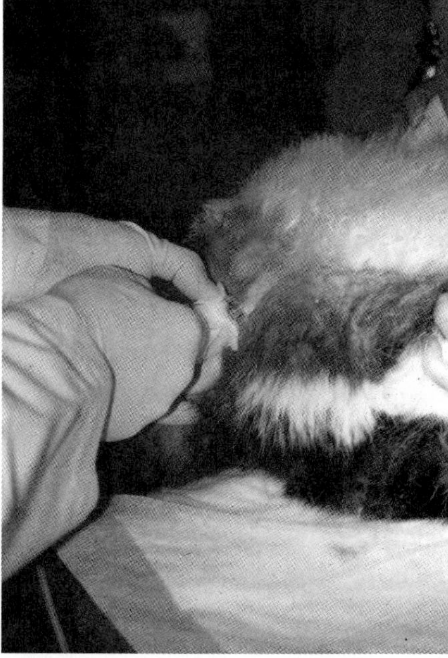

FIGURE II-131 Perineum of an anesthetized cat undergoing medical management of urethral obstruction. Cat is in dorsal recumbency; cranial is to the right of the photo. Occluding the distal urethra around the catheter and pulling the urethra caudally and dorsally to displace urethral kinking will facilitate retrograde flushing of plugs and stones into the urinary bladder.

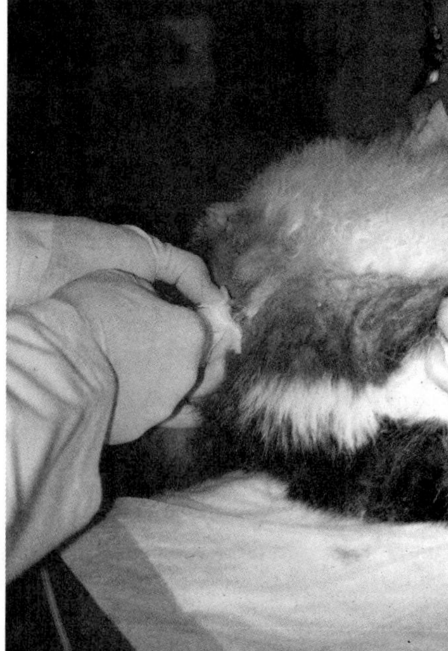

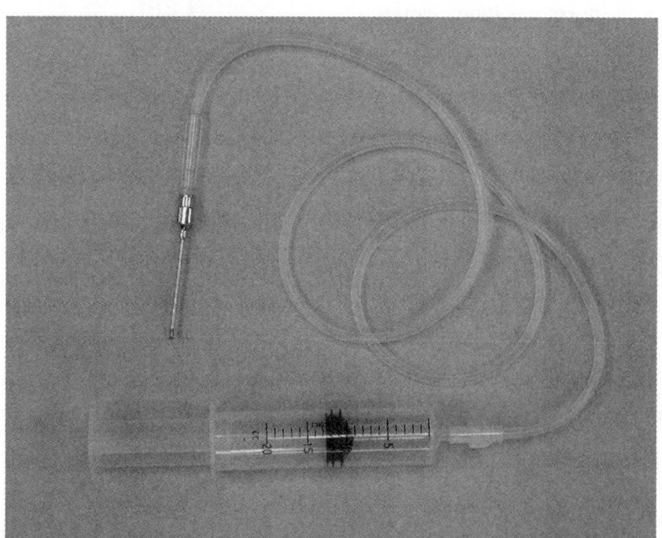

- Promote repair of urothelial urethral tear (~3-10 days).
- Care and management:
  - Place as atraumatically and cleanly as possible.
  - Maintain a closed collection system.
  - Remove indwelling catheters as soon as possible.
  - If urine is initially sterile, avoid antimicrobial therapy until catheter is removed.
  - If urine is initially infected, treat the infection (see Cystitis, Bacterial, p 270).
  - Treat potentially life-threatening infections.
  - Do not give the cat corticosteroids.
- Pain medication (buprenorphine, butorphanol, etc.) is indicated for a short duration (1 to 4 days). Nonsteroidal anti-inflammatory drugs (NSAIDs) are contraindicated in cats with compromised renal function or dehydration.
- Prevent negative fluid balance associated with postobstructive diuresis by giving parenteral fluids.
- Not recommended: routine use of urethral smooth muscle relaxants (e.g., phenoxybenzamine, prazosin), urethral antispasmodics (e.g., propantheline, oxybutynin), and parasympathomimetics (e.g., bethanechol) following urethral manipulation; the efficacy of these agents has not been established by properly controlled clinical trials.

ALTERNATIVES AND THEIR RELATIVE MERITS

Urethrostomy may be indicated if obstruction cannot be corrected. Contrast urethrography is indicated to localize the site(s) of obstruction and to select the location of surgery.

AUTHORS: **JODY P. LULICH, CARL A. OSBORNE**

Urethrogram

BASIC INFORMATION

SYNONYM(S)

Retrograde urethrogram

OVERVIEW AND GOAL(S)

- The urethra cannot be seen on survey radiographs; therefore, a positive-contrast examination is necessary for radiographic evaluation.
- Ultrasound can be used for seeing small portions of the urethra in the male; however, adequate diagnostic imaging of the entire urethra requires radiographic assessment with the injection of water-soluble organic iodide contrast material.
- A simple urethrogram is quick and easy to perform.
- A vaginocystourethrogram is usually performed in the female due to the difficulty of catheterizing the female urethra.

INDICATIONS

- Clinical signs:
  - Dysuria, stranguria
  - Difficulty catheterizing, urethral obstruction
  - Trauma to pelvis or os penis
  - Hematuria in a voided or catheterized urine sample but normal urine on cystocentesis
  - Hemorrhagic preputial discharge with a normal penile/preputial physical exam
- Differential diagnosis:
  - Urethral calculi
  - Urethral tear/rupture
  - Urethral stricture
  - Iatrogenic urethral trauma
  - Urethral neoplasia
  - Urethral fistula
  - Other urethral mucosal abnormalities
  - Penile or extrapelvic urethral disease
  - Congenital anomalies
  - Postoperative evaluation of urethra to assess patency and completeness of healing (prostatic disease with communication with urethra)
  - Evaluation of perineal or caudal abdominal masses

EQUIPMENT, ANESTHESIA

- Heavy sedation is often all that is needed to perform the study in male dogs. General anesthesia can be used if necessary. The male cat should be under general anesthesia for the study.
- Mild surgical scrub solution and gauze/sponges for disinfecting the penis prior to catheterization.
- Urinary catheter (preferably with inflatable bulb), such as a Foley catheter.
- Iodinated contrast medium (sodium iothalamate, sodium diatrizoate).
- Sterile lubricating jelly.
- Sterile syringe for contrast (e.g., 12 ml).
- Sterile syringe for inflating the catheter bulb.
- Sterile catheter adapter (Christmas-tree type).
- Sterile three-way stopcock.
- Sterile saline.
- Sterile gloves.
- Enema bag/set.
- Open-ended tomcat catheter (e.g., 3.5 Fr) used for male cats.

ANTICIPATED TIME

Approximately 20 to 30 minutes

PREPARATION: IMPORTANT CHECKPOINTS

- An enema is given approximately 2 hours prior to the study to ensure the removal of fecal material from the colon. Fecal material may compromise visualization of the urethra.
- Dilute organic iodinated contrast media to 50% solution with sterile saline.
- Sterile gloves should be worn from this point forward in the preparation.
- Draw 12 ml of diluted contrast material into the 12-ml syringe.
- Remove Foley catheter from packaging in a sterile manner, and remove guide wire.
- Attach catheter adapter (Christmas tree) to Foley catheter.
- Attach three-way stopcock to catheter adapter.
- Load syringe with air for inflating cuff later by drawing appropriate amount of air into the syringe (based on recommendation of Foley bulb size).
- Attach syringe containing air to the three-way stopcock.
- Open three-way stopcock to allow airflow into the catheter bulb to ensure that the bulb is intact. Fill the bulb to recommended level, and close the three-way stopcock.
- Once it is clear the bulb will hold air, withdraw the air from the bulb back into the syringe.
- Attach syringe filled with contrast material onto the three-way stopcock, and fill the Foley catheter with contrast material. If this step is bypassed, air bubbles will be injected, resulting in a suboptimal study.
- Close the stopcock to the contrast material, and open to the syringe filled with air.
- In male cats, a sterile tomcat catheter is used. Diluted contrast material is drawn into the syringe, and the syringe is attached directly to the catheter.

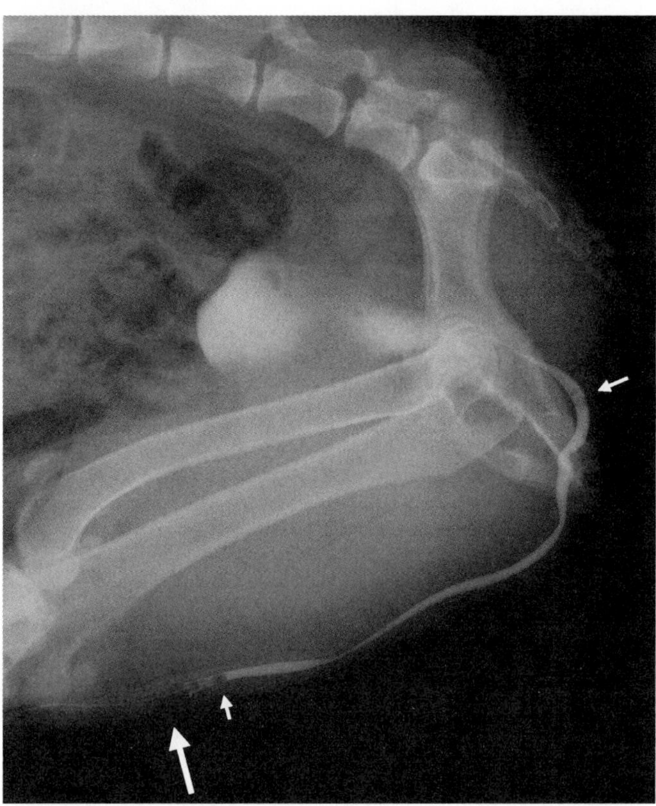

FIGURE II-132 Normal male urethrogram (lateral view, cranial to the left). Small air bubbles are seen in the pelvic urethra and distal urethra (*small arrow*), and the inflated bulb of the Foley catheter is also seen (*large arrow*).

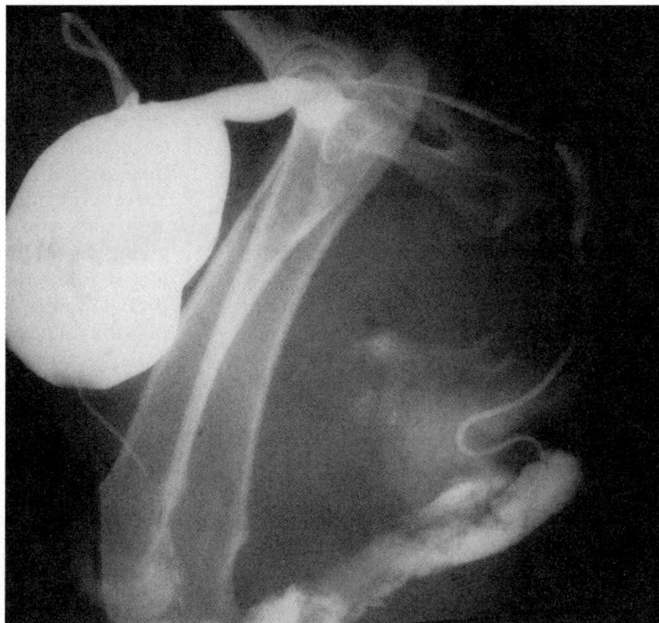

FIGURE II-133 Male dog with urethral rupture (lateral view, cranial to the left). Contrast material has leaked widely throughout the soft tissues of the prepuce as a result of the ruptured urethra (bottom right of image).

POSSIBLE COMPLICATIONS AND COMMON ERRORS TO AVOID

- Trauma due to overdistention of the cuff; risk is minimized by advancing the catheter.
- Rupture of the urethra; forceful injection when the urethra is obstructed can lead to urethral rupture (see Fig. II-133).
- Mild transient submucosal hemorrhage secondary to balloon (try not to leave urethral catheter in place longer than 15 minutes [urethral trauma caused by local ischemia and mechanical trauma]).
- Urinary bladder-associated complications (hemorrhagic cystitis, catheter kinking or knotting in the bladder lumen, pulmonary air embolism, bladder rupture secondary to overdistention of the bladder) are extremely rare because the catheter remains in distal urethra.
- Bacterial contamination.
- False results: catheter in too far (past lesion site), too little contrast, air bubbles.
- Contrast media reactions (absorbed systemically though mucosa).
- Anaphylactic reactions: very rare.

PROCEDURE

- Preliminary caudal abdominal radiographs (lateral and oblique ventrodorsal) are made to set radiographic technique and ensure adequate preparation of the animal.
- The kilovoltage peak should be set between 65 and 75 to maximize contrast due to the photoelectric effect (K edge of iodine).
- The animal should be placed in left lateral recumbency (to reduce the risk of air embolism going to the lungs).
- An assistant should then extrude the penis from the prepuce.
- The penis should be prepped with a mild surgical scrub solution.
- Sterile lubricating jelly is placed onto the tip of the Foley catheter.
- Insert Foley catheter into the distal urethra until the bulb can no longer be seen, but no farther; the procedure is conducted with the catheter inserted into the urethra a very short distance to avoid passing beyond the site of the lesion.
- Inject air into bulb to inflate bulb, and then close the stopcock to maintain inflation. A suitable volume of air should meet little resistance and yet should provide enough of a seal to prevent backflow of contrast out the urethra during injection.
- Tug very lightly on the catheter to ensure the bulb seal is tight, and adjust bulb inflation (increase or decrease) accordingly.
- With the animal's hind limbs pulled forward to allow an unobstructed radiographic projection of the urethra, inject 12 ml of contrast material rapidly into the urethral catheter. NOTE: The contrast material should flow smoothly and with no resistance; if resistance is met, stop the injection and make the radiographic exposure.
- Make radiographic exposure just before the end of injection (Figs. II-132 to II-135).
- Close the stopcock to the syringe that contained the contrast material, and remove syringe.
- Refill syringe with diluted contrast material in preparation for second injection, and reattach syringe to stopcock; open stopcock to allow contrast flow.
- Place animal in an oblique ventrodorsal position and inject 12 cc of contrast rapidly. NOTE: Here again, the contrast material should flow smoothly and with no resistance; if resistance is met, stop the injection, and make the radiographic exposure.
- Make radiographic exposure just before the end of injection.
- For male cats, the animal preparation and survey radiographs are the same as the dog. The penis is extruded and prepped, a lubricated tomcat catheter

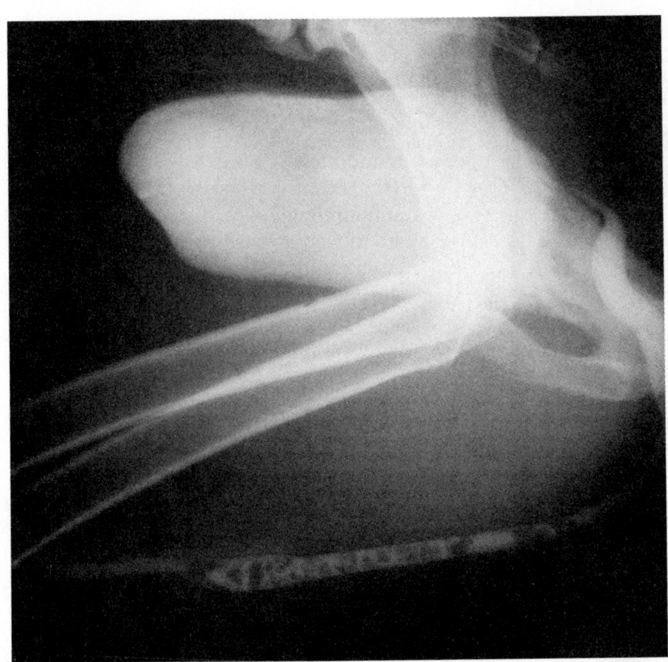
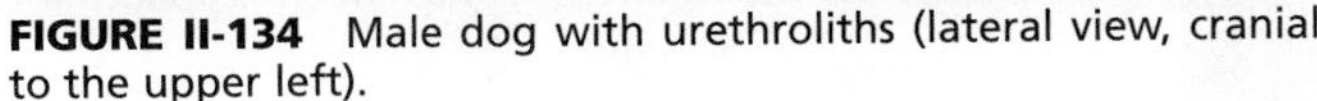

FIGURE II-134 Male dog with urethroliths (lateral view, cranial to the upper left).

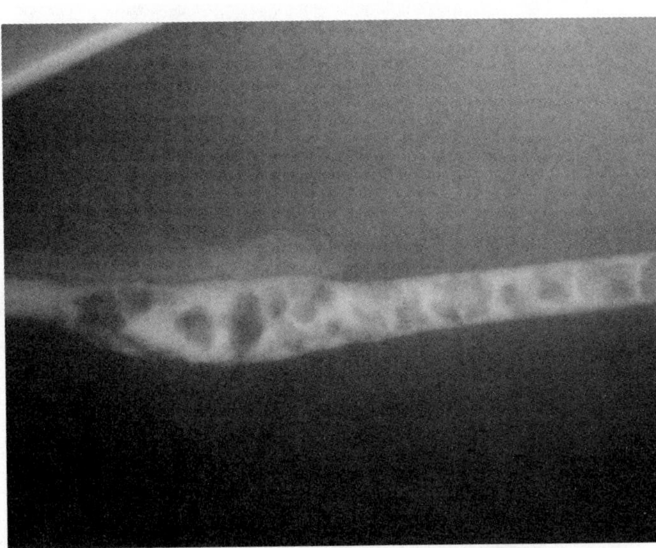

FIGURE II-135 Zoomed view of Fig. II-134, showing multiple urethroliths.

is placed just inside the distal urethra, and contrast material is injected.

POSTPROCEDURE

- Once the study is complete, the air should be removed from the Foley bulb before the catheter is withdrawn from the penis.
- If general anesthesia was used: routine anesthetic recovery.

ALTERNATIVES AND THEIR RELATIVE MERITS

- Plain abdominal radiographs: inexpensive means to survey the urethra for radiopaque urethral calculi. Otherwise, contrast medium is needed to visualize the urethra and most of its associated lesions.
- Abdominal ultrasound: can be used for assessing a portion of the urethra; however, ultrasound should only be used in certain instances (e.g., proximal urethral disorders).

AUTHOR: **LEEANN PACK**

Vagal Maneuver

BASIC INFORMATION

SYNONYM(S)

- Carotid sinus massage
- Ocular pressure
- Valsalva maneuver

OVERVIEW AND GOAL(S)

A physical manipulation that temporarily increases parasympathetic tone, mainly for diagnostic—and occasionally therapeutic—cardiac rhythm effects

INDICATIONS

Tachycardia in which the rate is so rapid that it is unclear whether the rhythm is ventricular or supraventricular (e.g., heart rate is >260 bpm)

CONTRAINDICATIONS

- Ocular disease (for ocular pressure)
- Disorders of the ventral neck (for carotid sinus massage)
- Bradycardia, including the bradycardia-tachycardia syndrome (sick sinus syndrome)

EQUIPMENT, ANESTHESIA

No anesthetic requirement; procedure is performed when the animal is awake. Procedure requires electrocardiogram (ECG) machine with printer to assess and record initial cardiac rhythm and to record effect of vagal maneuver.

ANTICIPATED TIME

About <1 minute

PREPARATION: IMPORTANT CHECKPOINTS

A printed ECG tracing of the rhythm prior to the vagal maneuver is necessary.

POSSIBLE COMPLICATIONS AND COMMON ERRORS TO AVOID

- Inadequate vagal response: Subjectively, carotid sinus massage appears to be more effective than ocular pressure in some patients and vice-versa in others, but some supraventricular tachycardias (and essentially all cases of ventricular tachycardia) are resistant to both.
- Concerns regarding vagal maneuver: Related harm due to carotid artery atherosclerosis is based on human cardiology but is not expected to be relevant to small animal medicine.

PROCEDURE

- Patient may be standing or recumbent.
- ECG leads are connected, and a good ECG signal should be seen.
- The prevagal-maneuver ECG is traced/printed; about 20 to 30 seconds of tracing should be recorded.

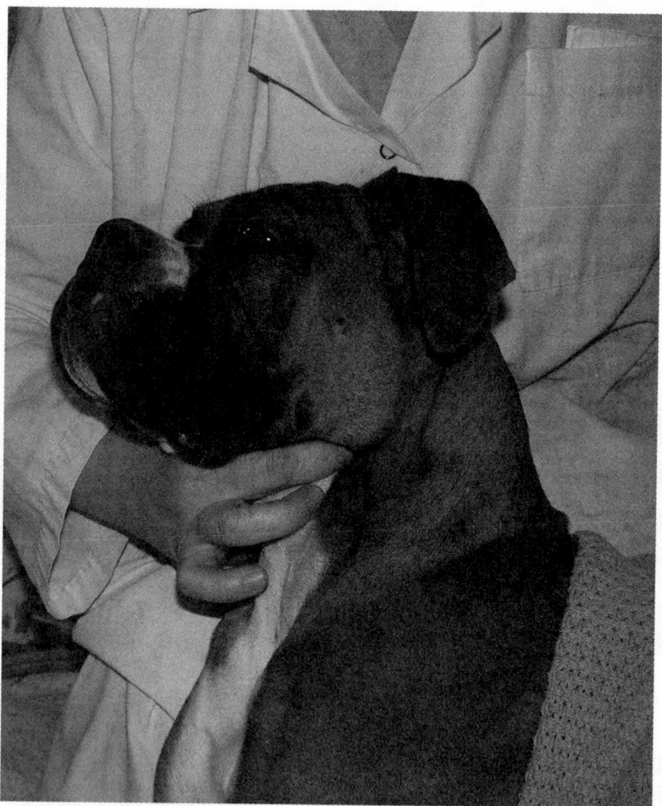

FIGURE II-136 Placement of fingers for performing carotid sinus massage in a dog.

- The vagal maneuver is applied, with the ECG printing continuously. The ECG paper should be marked at the time of onset of the vagal maneuver. Usually, only one maneuver is performed. The ECG should be allowed to continue to run (printing) throughout the duration of the vagal maneuver and for at least 15 seconds after its termination.

OCULAR PRESSURE

- The patient's eyelids are closed, and using the thumb and middle finger of the same hand, both globes are depressed caudally into the orbit.
- A small, smooth massaging motion may be applied to the eyes along with the direct pressure.
- The degree of pressure should be sufficient that the eyes are substantially retracted caudally without, however, provoking any sign of discomfort or resentment. The exact extent of retraction will vary depending on orbit shape and size.
- Pressure is maintained until a substantial decrease in heart rate is noted and the rhythm can be identified or until the maneuver has been applied for 15 seconds.

CAROTID SINUS MASSAGE

- The target area is the base of the internal carotid artery, which is not palpable as such but is located dorsocranially to the larynx, medial to the angle of the mandible.
- The larynx is palpated using the thumb and forefinger. The thumb and forefinger are moved dorsally and cranially from the larynx until resting in the natural depression medial to the angle of the mandible and ventral to the occipital bone.
- Gentle, pincer-like pressure is applied in this area with the thumb and forefinger.
- Pressure is maintained, and a small, smooth, circular massaging motion may be performed.
- The pressure exerted is often sufficient to elicit a gag reflex but should not be so great as to cause discomfort or resentment.
- Pressure is maintained until a substantial decrease in heart rate is noted and the rhythm can be identified or until the maneuver has been applied for 15 seconds.

POSTPROCEDURE

- A vagal maneuver can routinely be terminated abruptly.
- Failure to slow tachycardia with a vagal maneuver should prompt a search for the tachycardia's possible causes, including anxiety/stress of hospitalization, respiratory compromise, structural cardiac disease, and systemic illness.

ALTERNATIVES AND THEIR RELATIVE MERITS

Pharmacologic slowing of tachycardias, such as with injectable propranolol, verapamil, or adenosine, should only be considered once the aforementioned possible inciting factors have been ruled out or addressed.

AUTHOR: **ETIENNE CÔTÉ**

Vaginal Examination in the Bitch

BASIC INFORMATION

SYNONYM(S)

Digital vaginal examination

OVERVIEW AND GOAL(S)

- Minimally invasive, digital examination of the vagina to evaluate the vaginal anatomy
- Possible lesions in bitches include:
  - Vaginal strictures
  - Vaginal tumors
  - Trauma during breeding
  - Congenital anatomic anomalies

INDICATIONS

- Vaginal discharge
- Poor breeding experience
- Urinary incontinence (urine pooling)
- Dystocia

CONTRAINDICATIONS

- There are relatively few contraindications to this procedure.
- If infection of the reproductive tract is a consideration:
  - Vaginal culture should be taken first.
  - Culture is followed by vaginal cytologic analysis before a digital examination is performed.

EQUIPMENT, ANESTHESIA

- Minimal restraint usually required
- Antiseptic cleanser
- Sterile exam glove
- Sterile, water-soluble lubricant

ANTICIPATED TIME

With a cooperative bitch, the procedure should take less than 5 minutes, from gentle cleansing of the vulvar lips to finishing the exam.

POSSIBLE COMPLICATIONS AND COMMON ERRORS TO AVOID

- Urethral opening lies on the ventral surface of the vestibule and should be avoided (Fig. II-137).
  - This is not difficult if the finger is passed up to the vestibulovaginal junction perpendicularly to the ground in the standing bitch.
- Vestibulovaginal junction is one barrier to the entrance of the uterus and should not be mistaken for the cervix or a stricture (see Fig. II-137).
  - The canine vagina is very long (up to 12 inches [29 cm] in giant-breed dogs), and thus the cervix is unlikely to be palpated on digital examination of the vagina.
  - The junction acts a barrier to pathogens and will be narrower than the vestibule or vagina. If the examiner proceeds slowly, he or she should be able to pass the finger beyond the junction in most bitches (depending on the size of the bitch and the size of the finger).

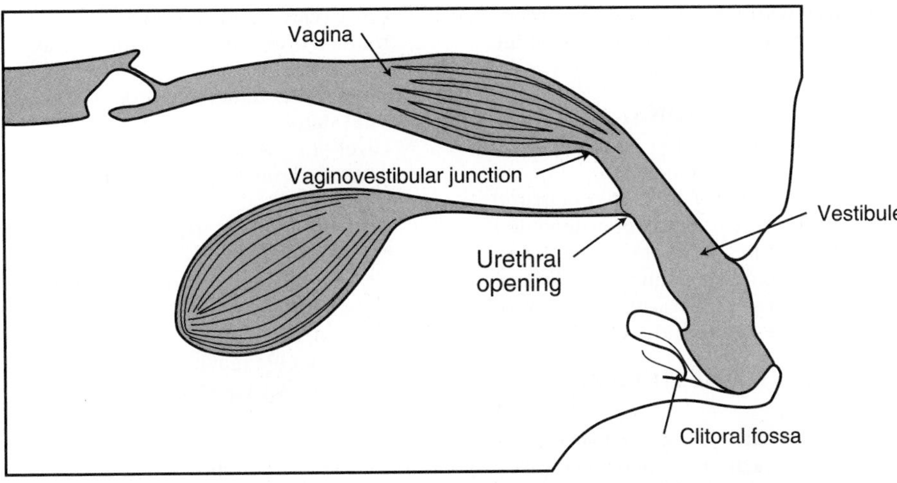

FIGURE II-137 Anatomic relationship of the vestibule and the vagina in the bitch. Dorsal is toward the top of the image, cranial to the left.

PROCEDURE

- Animal should be restrained in standing position.
- Vulvar lips should be gently wiped with a mild antibacterial cleanser.
- Examiner should wear sterile gloves.
- After coating the gloved index finger with the sterile lubricant, the finger is passed into the vulva and turned directly upward (90-degree angle to the floor in the standing animal). The upward direction is important so the urethral opening is avoided (see Fig. II-137).
- When the finger cannot go any farther dorsally, it is turned directly cranially (parallel to the floor) and advanced over the ischium and into the vaginal vault.
  - As the finger passes over the ischium into the vagina, there may be a slight tightening at the vestibulovaginal junction. Depending on the size of the bitch and the size of the hand, most fingers should pass through this junction.
  - If the finger is well lubricated and it does not pass this point, a vaginal stricture should be considered.

ALTERNATIVES AND THEIR RELATIVE MERITS

- Speculum examination (vaginoscopy) may be performed for the visualization of the vaginal walls and vault:
  - Inflamed walls in vaginitis cases
  - Urine on the floor of the vagina in urine pooling disorders
  - Evidence of trauma in difficult breeding
  - Evaluation of vaginal folds and mucosa for timing of estrus
- Vaginoscopy with an endoscope to visualize vagina and potentially the cervix

AUTHOR: **CAROL A. MCCLURE**

Ventilation, Positive Pressure

BASIC INFORMATION

SYNONYM(S)

Artificial ventilation
Assisted ventilation
Mechanical ventilation

OVERVIEW AND GOAL(S)

- Positive-pressure ventilation (PPV) requires intensive 24-hour monitoring and nursing care but can be lifesaving.
- Owner communication and highly trained staff are essential.
- Manual PPV requires a person to manually deliver a breath to the animal.
- Mechanical PPV involves a machine that takes the place of the person to deliver a breath.
- Manual PPV is only practical for short-term use (up to several hours), while mechanical PPV is required for long-term cases (>6–12 hours).
- The objective of PPV is to maintain normal arterial oxygen (PaO_2) and carbon dioxide pressure ($PaCO_2$) until an underlying disease can be identified and treated.
- Therapeutic goal:
  - PaO_2 is >60 mmHg (minimum, >80 mmHg preferred).
  - $PaCO_2$ is <50 mmHg.
  - End-tidal CO_2 is <50 mmHg.
  - Arterial oxygen saturation (SaO_2) is >90% (minimum, >96% preferred)
  - Measure PaO_2 and $PaCO_2$ with arterial blood gases (ABGs); measure end-tidal CO_2 with capnometry (inserted between endotracheal tube and breathing device) and oxygen saturation (SaO_2) with pulse oximetry (attached to the tongue).
- Prognosis varies with underlying disease:
  - A reasonable goal is to discharge 25–40% of mechanically ventilated cases.
  - Animals with ventilatory failure and normal lung function (i.e., opioid or barbituate overdose, certain toxins, tick paralysis, botulism) have the best prognosis.

INDICATIONS

- Early intervention has the greatest chance of success.
- Ventilatory failure: $PaCO_2$ is >50 mmHg and pH is <7.3.
- Some can be managed with short-term PPV (e.g., reversible opioid overdose).
- Respiratory failure: PaO_2 is <50 mmHg, or SaO_2 is <88% despite supplemental oxygen.
- Often requires >12 hours of PPV.

- Animals with sustained extreme respiratory distress: increased work of breathing.
- Often requires >12 hours of PPV.

CONTRAINDICATIONS

- Irreversible underlying disease
- Lack of trained personnel
- If >6–12 hours of PPV is anticipated, initiating manual PPV is questionable if mechanical PPV is not available.
- There should be a trained technician with the animal and a veterinarian on the premises around the clock.

EQUIPMENT, ANESTHESIA

- Intubation:
  - Animals can be ventilated via inflated endotracheal or tracheostomy tubes.
  - Low-pressure, high-volume cuffs are preferred.
  - Endotracheal intubation is more common due to familiarity, ease of procedure, and minimal risk of tissue damage.
  - If PPV exceeds 24 hours or when heavy sedation is not desired, a tracheostomy may be preferred (allows some dogs to eat and drink).
- Sedation (as needed; more common with endotracheal intubation):
  - Pentobarbital: 2 mg/kg boluses to effect (up to 12 mg/kg) q 4-6h or as needed to maintain sedation.
  - Fentanyl: 5 μg/kg boluses to effect up to 50 μg/kg, then 5–7 μg/kg/hr constant-rate infusion (CRI) (can add diazepam).
  - Propofol: 2–8 mg/kg bolus to effect, then 0.1–0.3 mg/kg/min CRI.
  - Close cardiovascular monitoring is required in animals under heavy sedation.
- Minimum recommended monitoring:
  - Vital signs.
  - Level of consciousness.
  - ABGs or pulse oximetry and end-tidal CO_2.
  - Arterial blood pressure (BP).
  - Continuous ECG.
  - Volume of fluids in and out (urinary catheter).
  - Hematocrit, total solids, glucose, and urine specific gravity.
  - Ventilator setting should be recorded every hour.

MANUAL

- Ambubag and attached oxygen:
  - Inexpensive.
  - Readily available.
  - Pediatric-size bag most common (typically 450–950 ml volume).
  - Can be used without supplemental oxygen (not ideal).
  - Excellent for short-term use (i.e., during cardiopulmonary resuscitation [CPR]).
  - Can add positive-end expiratory valves, which create positive-end expiratory pressure (PEEP) to recruit collapsed alveoli and improve oxygen exchange (typically in 0–10 cm or 0–20 cm H_2O sizes).
  - Some Ambu bags have a removable safety valve that will open when a specific airway pressure is exceeded (typically 40 cm H_2O).
  - Difficult to determine tidal volume and airway pressures delivered (vary with size and degree of manual pressure applied to the bag).
- Anesthesia machine with manual ventilation:
  - Readily available.
  - Estimate tidal volume delivered with the size of the reservoir bag.
  - Can monitor airway pressure with attached pressure gauge.
  - Can apply adjustable PEEP valves (typically range from 0–40 cm H_2O).

MECHANICAL

- Anesthesia ventilators:
  - Limited choice of ventilator modes.
  - Typically deliver only 100% inspired oxygen concentrations (FiO_2).
  - Increased risk of oxygen toxicity if ventilating >12 hours.
- Mechanical ventilators (Figs. II-138 and II-139):
  - Allow greatest control over type of breath delivered (pressure, volume, flow rate, FiO_2, respiratory rate, sensitivity to trigger a breath, and PEEP).
  - Supply humidified oxygen.
  - Can be used for long-term care (days to weeks).
  - Relatively expensive.

ANTICIPATED TIME

- It can take several minutes to set up mechanical ventilators.
- Initiate manual PPV (takes seconds to initiate) while mechanical ventilators are being set up.
- The overall duration of ventilation time varies with the underlying disease and animal's response.

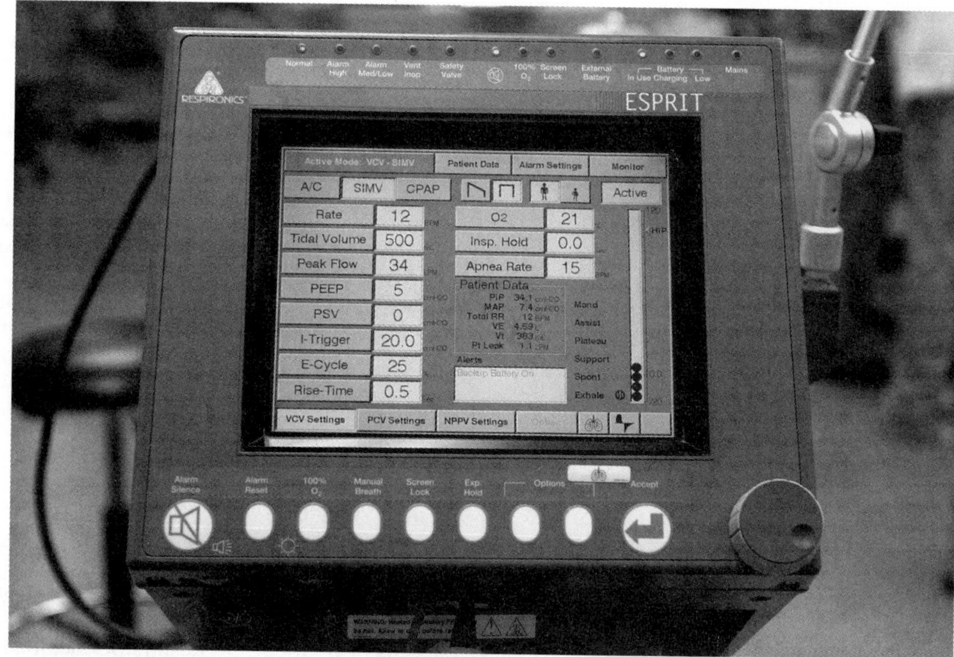

FIGURE II-138 Potential ventilator settings for a 40- to 60-kg animal. Volume control ventilation (VCV) with synchronized intermittent mandatory ventilation (SIMV) is shown. The inspired oxygen content is 21% (room air). The peak inspiratory pressure (PIP) is high (34 cm H_2O), and efforts should be made to decrease this value by decreasing the tidal volume, increasing peak flow rate, or decreasing the PEEP.

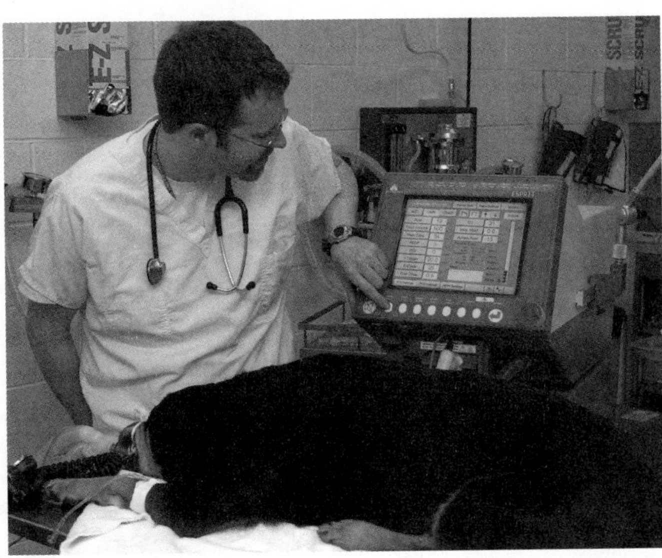

FIGURE II-139 Ventilator in use.

PREPARATION: IMPORTANT CHECKPOINTS

- Ensure oxygen source, monitoring equipment, and suction devices are available.
- Nutritional support should be available for long-term cases.
- Pleural space disease (pneumothorax, pleural effusion) should be identified and treated prior to ventilation.
- Perform thoracocentesis in suspected cases; untreated pleural space disease is associated with higher incidence of ventilatory complications.
- Check that valves on Ambu bag are functioning properly (not sticking) between uses.
- Check anesthetic machine and anesthesia ventilator, and check that mechanical ventilator tubing is correctly connected, valves are functioning, humidifiers are full, and there are no leaks in the system.

POSSIBLE COMPLICATIONS AND COMMON ERRORS TO AVOID

- Barotrauma: Avoid exceeding 30 cm of H_2O airway pressure.
- Cardiovascular effects: PPV increases intrathoracic pressures, which may impede venous return to the heart and can subsequently decrease cardiac output; at a minimum, monitor heart rate and BP closely.
- Oxygen toxicity: significant risk after 12 hours if FiO_2 remains above 60%.
- Ventilator-associated pneumonia: Monitor for deterioration of respiratory function or unexplained fever.
- Confirm diagnosis with radiographs and endotracheal wash.
- Pneumothorax: more common with high airway pressures (>30 cm H_2O).
  - Can cause acute deterioration in ventilatory parameters.
  - Auscultation usually reveals dull breath sounds in upper parts of thorax (i.e., dorsally when animal is in sternal recumbency).
  - Perform thoracocentesis in suspected cases.
  - Tension pneumothorax is associated with a severe decrease in cardiac output and hypotension; check for tension pneumothorax in ventilated animals that suddenly develop shock.
- Oral and ocular ulcers: usually avoided with good nursing care.
  - Lubricate eyes with sterile eye lubricant and cleanse mouth with 0.1% chlorhexidine solution-soaked gauze sponges every 4 hours.

PROCEDURE

NOTE: Step-by-step guidelines to initiate PPV are beyond the scope of this text, and clinicians should consult more extensive reviews to become familiar with different ventilator modes and their indications. The following are suggested guidelines for starting PPV. Most cases do better in sternal recumbency.

- Ambu bag:
  - Bag size (in milliliters) should be at least 15 × BW (kilograms) to be able to deliver adequate tidal volumes.
  - Set oxygen flow rates at 10–15 L/min (delivers 50–90% oxygen levels).
  - Attach adjustable PEEP valve to exhaust limb if PEEP desired (requires compatible attachment site). Adjust PEEP by turning valve to the desired level (start with 5 cm H_2O).
  - If an oxygen reservoir bag is used, higher (90–100%) inspired oxygen levels can be achieved.
  - Animals can breathe spontaneously while connected to Ambu bags although airway resistance is higher.
- Anesthetic machine with manual ventilation:
  - Insert adjustable PEEP valve in the expiratory limb of tubing (bidirectional valves eliminate the risk of occlusion associated with backward insertion of unidirectional valves) if PEEP is desired.

SUGGESTED INITIAL PPV SETTING GUIDELINES (see Fig. II-138)

- Inspired oxygen concentration (FiO_2):
  - Start with 100% FiO_2.
  - For long-term (many hours) use, decrease to the lowest FiO_2 that maintains desired PaO_2/SaO_2 to reduce the risk of oxygen toxicity.
  - Respiratory rate (RR):
    - 8–20 breaths per minute (bpm).
    - Increase the RR to decrease the $PaCO_2$ if >50 mmHg.
    - New RR = RR × $PaCO_2$/desired $PaCO_2$.
    - RR: Often >20 breaths/minute if underlying pulmonary disease is present.
- Oxygen flow rates:
  - Start with 0.5–1.0 L/kg/min.
  - Often need to increase if underlying pulmonary disease is present.
- Tidal volume:
  - Amount of air delivered with each breath.
  - Normal values: 10–15 ml/kg.
  - Values of 4–6 ml/kg are associated with fewer lung injuries in people.
  - Volumes in excess of 20 ml/kg are likely to cause lung injury (barotrauma and volutrauma).
  - May need to increase tidal volume if $PaCO_2$ does not respond to increased RR.
  - General rule: Use lowest volume possible to achieve oxygen and carbon dioxide goals.
- Airway pressure:
  - If pressure gauge available.
  - Normal airway pressures reach 15–20 cm H_2O.
  - Values that are >30 cm H_2O are to be avoided (likely to result in lung injury).
- Inspiratory time:
  - Inspiratory time is normally between 1.5–2.5 seconds.
- Inspiratory to expiratory (I:E) ratio:
  - Start with values of 1:2–1:4.
  - Try to stay >1:2 to prevent the next breath being delivered before exhalation is complete.
  - Increasing RR or tidal volume will decrease I:E ratio.
  - Increasing oxygen flow rates will increase I:E ratio.
  - Changing one parameter may require a change in another to maintain desired I:E ratio.
- PEEP:
  - Healthy lungs do not require PEEP.
  - Adding PEEP to diseased lungs often improves oxygenation.
  - A common starting value is 3 cm H_2O.
  - If 3 cm H_2O does not achieve desired results (based on PaO_2/SaO_2), increase the PEEP by 2–4 cm H_2O until desired values are achieved.

- Exceeding 15 cm H_2O of PEEP increases the risk of lung injury and may decrease cardiac output.

POSTPROCEDURE

- Supplemental oxygen is often required after weaning from ventilation.
- Oxygen supplementation should be set up prior to extubation (nasal oxygen is frequently used).

ALTERNATIVES AND THEIR RELATIVE MERITS

Liquid ventilation using perfluorocarbons shows promise in managing some forms of respiratory failure in people but is cost prohibitive to most veterinary practices and clients.

SUGGESTED READING

Campbell VL, King LG: Pulmonary function, ventilator management, and outcome of dogs with thoracic trauma and pulmonary contusions: 10 cases (1994–1998). *J Am Vet Med Assoc* 217(10):1505–1509, 2000.

Drellich S: Principles of mechanical ventilation. *Vet Clin North Am Sm Anim Pract* 32(5):1087–1100, 2002.

Mueller ER: Suggested strategies for ventilatory management of veterinary patients with acute respiratory distress. *J Vet Emerg Crit Care* 11(3)191–198, 2001.

AUTHOR: **SØREN R. BOYSEN**

Vomiting, Induction of

BASIC INFORMATION

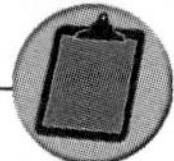

SYNONYM(S)

Emesis, induction of

OVERVIEW AND GOAL(S)

Deliberate induction of vomiting for elimination of ingested noxious materials

INDICATIONS

Confirmed or suspected ingestion of toxic substance

CONTRAINDICATIONS

- Ingestion of alkaline toxic substances: risk of reflux esophagitis
- Ingestion of oily substances: risk of aspiration pneumonia
- Ingestion of sharp or pointed foreign bodies: risk of gastrointestinal (GI) tract perforation
- Ingestions having occurred too long in the past to be effectively offset by vomiting (time is dependent on substance ingested)
- Sedated, mentally depressed, or comatose animal: risk of aspiration pneumonia

EQUIPMENT, ANESTHESIA

- No anesthesia; the procedure is performed awake
- 3% hydrogen peroxide (NOTE: not 30% hydrogen peroxide used for hair bleaching)
- Sterile or nonsterile syringe
- Gastric gavage tube and oral speculum/ mouth gag (rarely necessary)
- Alternative for dogs or cats: syrup of ipecac
- Alternative for cats: xylazine 0.44 mg/kg IV, IM, or SC single dose

ANTICIPATED TIME

About 5 minutes

PREPARATION: IMPORTANT CHECKPOINTS

- Identification of the ingested substance is essential. NOTE: Vomiting should not be induced unless a known substance was ingested or exam findings are indicative of such an ingestion (e.g., antifreeze on muzzle, lead pellets in stomach on radiograph).
- If the animal has not eaten recently, canned food corresponding to approximately half a meal can be fed prior to induction of emesis to avoid nonproductive vomiting/dry heaving. If no appetite, simply proceed with emesis.

POSSIBLE COMPLICATIONS AND COMMON ERRORS TO AVOID

- Aspiration pneumonia: Monitor for dyspnea, coughing, fever, and lethargy postemesis. If present, proceed to thoracic radiographs.
- Gastric irritation: common and usually benign.
- Esophagitis: usually benign and self-resolving if secondary to vomiting induction alone; may be more serious (e.g., esophageal perforation or stricture) if caused by ingestion of corrosive substance or lacerating foreign body.

PROCEDURE

- Calculate appropriate dose of emetic (choose one):
  - Hydrogen peroxide 3%: 0.25–0.5 ml/kg PO once.
  - Syrup of ipecac: 2–6 ml total dose PO once.
  - Xylazine: 0.44 mg/kg IV, IM, or SC once (cats only).
- NOTE: 1 teaspoon = 5 ml; 1 tablespoon = 15 ml; 1 fluid ounce = 28 ml.
- Administer once. For orals (hydrogen peroxide or ipecac), it is best to administer via cheek pouch:
  - With animal in sitting position, elevate animal's chin (mouth closed) so neck is extended.
  - Insert tip of syringe into canthus of lips on one side (corner of mouth), with mouth still closed.
  - Infuse peroxide or ipecac over several seconds, watching for swallowing motions.
  - If not swallowed (e.g., if entirely spit up), may redose once immediately.
  - If a syringe is not available, alternatives include plastic human dosing cups, turkey basters (large volumes of peroxide for big dogs), or teaspoons/ tablespoons.
- Vomiting should occur within 5 to 10 minutes; if not, repeat.
- The patient must not have his/her head raised and should not be wearing a muzzle when vomiting is expected; either of these factors would greatly increase the risk of aspiration pneumonia.

POSTPROCEDURE

- Oral emetics: may administer a total of three doses.
- Persistent vomiting usually subsides in 15 to 30 minutes; otherwise, an antiemetic may be given (very uncommon).
- Treatment for ulcerative gastritis (e.g., H_2 blocker) may be instituted prophylactically.

ALTERNATIVES AND THEIR RELATIVE MERITS

- Table salt for emesis: not recommended due to risk of critical hypernatremia if emesis does not occur.
- Activated charcoal:
  - Reduces bioavailability of many overdosed drugs and toxic substances.
  - Often coadministered 30 minutes after induction of emesis or instead of induction of emesis if vomiting is contraindicated.
  - Minimal or no efficacy with corrosive alkalis, mineral acids, or petroleum distillates.
- Gastric lavage:
  - Best approach if animal is unconscious (emesis is contraindicated).
  - No proven benefit over induction of emesis in terms of efficacy of purging gastric ingesta.

AUTHOR: **ETIENNE CÔTÉ**

SECTION III

Differential Diagnosis

EDITOR

Etienne Côté, DVM, DACVIM (Cardiology, SAIM)

Abortion, Canine

Differential diagnosis list available on the companion online site at www.cote.clinicalvetadvisor.com.

Acidosis, Lactic

Causes*

Type A: Hypoxic

I. Increased oxygen demand
   A. Severe exercise
   B. Convulsions
II. Decreased oxygen availability
   A. Reduced tissue perfusion
      1. Cardiac arrest, cardiopulmonary resuscitation
      2. Shock
      3. Hypovolemia
      4. Left ventricular failure
      5. Low cardiac output
      6. Acute pulmonary edema
   B. Reduced arterial oxygen content
      1. Hypoxemia ($PO_2 \leq 30$ mmHg)
      2. Extremely severe anemia (packed cell volume [PCV] <10%)

Type B: Nonhypoxic

I. Drugs and toxins
   A. Phenformin
   B. Salicylates
   C. Ethylene glycol
   D. Many others
II. Diabetes mellitus
III. Liver failure
IV. Neoplasia (e.g., lymphosarcoma)
V. Sepsis
VI. Renal failure
VII. Hypoglycemia
VIII. Hereditary defects
   A. Mitochondrial myopathies
   B. Defects in gluconeogenesis

From Dibartola S: *Fluid, Electrolyte, and Acid-Base Disorders in Small Animal Practice.* St. Louis, WB Saunders, 2006.

*D-Lactic acidosis occurs with short bowel syndrome in human beings and has been observed in cats fed propylene glycol.

Acidosis, Metabolic

Causes

Increased Anion Gap (Normochloremic)

Ethylene glycol intoxication
Salicylate intoxication
Other rare intoxications (e.g., paraldehyde, methanol)
Diabetic ketoacidosis*
Uremic acidosis†
Lactic acidosis

Normal Anion Gap (Hyperchloremic)

Diarrhea
Renal tubular acidosis
Carbonic anhydrase inhibitors (e.g., acetazolamide)
Ammonium chloride
Cationic amino acids (e.g., lysine, arginine, histidine)
Posthypocapnic metabolic acidosis
Dilutional acidosis (e.g., rapid administration of 0.9% saline)
Hypoadrenocorticism‡

From Dibartola S: *Fluid, Electrolyte, and Acid-Base Disorders in Small Animal Practice.* St. Louis, WB Saunders, 2006.

*Patients with diabetic ketoacidosis may have some component of hyperchloremic metabolic acidosis in conjunction with increased anion gap acidosis.

†The metabolic acidosis early in renal failure may be hyperchloremic and later convert to typical increased anion gap acidosis.

‡Patients with hypoadrenocorticism typically present with hypochloremia due to impaired water excretion, absence of aldosterone, impaired renal function, and lactic acidosis. These factors prevent manifestation of hyperchloremia.

Acidosis, Respiratory

Causes	
Airway Obstruction Aspiration (e.g., foreign body, vomitus) **Respiratory Center Depression** Neurologic disease (e.g., brainstem, high cervical spinal cord lesion) Drugs (e.g., narcotics, sedatives, barbiturates, inhalation anesthetics) **Cardiopulmonary Arrest** **Neuromuscular Defects** Myasthenia gravis Tetanus Botulism Polyradiculoneuritis Polymyositis Tick paralysis Hypokalemic myopathy in cats Hypokalemic periodic paralysis in Burmese cats Drug-induced (succinylcholine, pancuronium, aminoglycosides with anesthetics, organophosphates)	**Restrictive Defects** Diaphragmatic hernia Pneumothorax Pleural effusion Hemothorax Chest wall trauma Pulmonary fibrosis Pyothorax **Pulmonary Disease** Respiratory distress syndrome Pneumonia Severe pulmonary edema Diffuse metastatic disease Smoke inhalation Pulmonary thromboembolism Chronic obstructive pulmonary disease Pulmonary fibrosis **Inadequate Mechanical Ventilation**

From Dibartola S: *Fluid, Electrolyte, and Acid-Base Disorders in Small Animal Practice*. St. Louis, WB Saunders, 2006.

DIFFERENTIAL DIAGNOSIS

Acute Abdomen

Differential diagnosis list available on the companion online site at www.cote.clinicalvetadvisor.com.

Acute Renal Failure

Causes

Prerenal
- Anesthesia
- Congestive heart failure (CHF)
- Dehydration
- Heatstroke
- Hemorrhagic shock
- Hypoadrenocorticism
- Hypoalbuminemia
- Hypotensive shock
- Hypovolemic shock
- Septic shock
- Surgery
- Trauma

Intrinsic Renal

Nephrotoxins
- Aminoglycosides
- Amphotericin B
- Cisplatin
- Ethylene glycol
- Heavy metals
- Hemoglobinuria
- Myoglobinuria
- Nonsteroidal anti-inflammatory drugs (NSAIDs)
- Radiocontrast agents
- Snake venom

Hemodynamic
- Anesthesia
- Cardiovascular shock
- Hemorrhagic shock
- Hypotensive shock
- Hypovolemic shock
- Septic shock
- Surgery

Other Conditions
- Cardiovascular failure
- Glomerulonephritis
- Hypercalcemia
- Leptospirosis
- Lymphoma
- Pyelonephritis
- Renal arterial thromboembolism
- Rickettsial infections
- Trauma

Postrenal
- Bilateral renal calculi
- Bilateral ureteral calculi
- Extraluminal obstruction
- Prostatic disease
- Rupture of outflow tracts
- Urethral calculi
- Urethral neoplasia

*Modified from Bonagura J: *Kirk's Current Veterinary Therapy XIII*, ed 13. St. Louis, WB Saunders, 2000.

Acute Respiratory Distress Syndrome (ARDS)

Causes, Predispositions, and Risk Factors*

- Electrocution
- Near drowning
- Neurologic insult (e.g., brain injury)
- Noxious gas inhalation (e.g., phosphine toxicosis)
- Oxygen toxicity
- Pneumonia (aspiration, other)
- Pulmonary contusions
- Pulmonary embolism
- Sepsis (e.g., secondary to parvoviral enteritis or other processes)
- Smoke inhalation
- Strangulation
- Trauma (massive)
- Upper airway obstruction (laryngeal paralysis, elongated soft palate, foreign body, mass)
- Vasculitis/systemic inflammatory response syndrome (SIRS) (e.g., secondary to necrotizing pancreatitis or other generalized inflammatory states)

*Risk factors may apply to veterinary patients, human patients, or both.

Adrenal Mass/Nodule

List of Possibilities in the Differential Diagnosis of an Incidentally Discovered Mass in the Adrenal Region

Adrenal Cortex
- Nodular hyperplasia
- Adenoma
- Carcinoma

Adrenal Medulla
- Pheochromocytoma
- Ganglioneuroma

Extra-adrenal Masses
- Extra-adrenal pheochromocytoma (paraganglioma)

Other Adrenal Masses
- Myelolipoma
- Granulomatous disease (fungal, feline infectious peritonitis [FIP])
- Teratoma
- Adrenal cyst
- Hematoma

Metastasis
- Mammary gland tumors
- Lymphoma
- Leukemia
- Pulmonary adenocarcinoma
- Other carcinomas (prostate, bladder, gastric)

Pseudoadrenal Masses
- Arising from kidney, pancreas, lymph nodes, and blood vessels

Technical Artifacts

From Bonagura J: *Kirk's Current Veterinary Therapy XIII*, ed 13. St. Louis, WB Saunders, 2000.

Alkalosis, Metabolic

Causes
Chloride Responsive
Vomiting of stomach contents
Diuretic therapy
Posthypercapnia
Chloride Resistant
Primary hyperaldosteronism
Hyperadrenocorticism
Alkali Administration
Oral administration of sodium bicarbonate or other organic anions (e.g., lactate, citrate, gluconate, acetate)
Oral administration of cation-exchange resin with nonabsorbable alkali (e.g., phosphorus binder)
Miscellaneous
Refeeding after fasting
High-dose penicillin
Severe potassium or magnesium deficiency

From Dibartola S: *Fluid, Electrolyte, and Acid-Base Disorders in Small Animal Practice*. St. Louis, WB Saunders, 2006.

Alkalosis, Respiratory

Causes
Hypoxemia (stimulation of peripheral chemoreceptors by decreased oxygen delivery)
Right-to-left shunting
Decreased P_iO_2 (e.g., residence at high altitude)
Congestive heart failure (CHF)
Severe anemia
Hypotension
Pulmonary diseases (causing ventilation-perfusion inequality)
Pneumonia
Pulmonary embolism
Pulmonary fibrosis
Pulmonary edema
Acute pulmonary distress syndrome (ARDS)
Pulmonary Disease (stimulation of nociceptive receptors independent of hypoxemia)
Pneumonia
Pulmonary embolism
Interstitial lung disease
Pulmonary edema
ARDS
Central Nervous System (CNS)–Mediated Hypocapnia (direct stimulation of medullary respiratory center)
Liver disease
Gram-negative sepsis
Drugs: salicylate intoxication, progesterone, xanthines (e.g., aminophylline)
Recovery from metabolic acidosis
Central neurologic disease
Trauma
Tumor
Infection
Inflammation (e.g., granulomatous meningoencephalitis)
Cerebrovascular accident
Exercise
Heatstroke
Mechanical Ventilation

From DiBartola S: *Fluid, Electrolyte, and Acid-Base Disorders in Small Animal Practice*. St. Louis, WB Saunders, 2006.

Alopecia (Endocrine)

Differential diagnosis list available on the companion online site at www.cote.clinicalvetadvisor.com.

Alopecia, Periocular

Differential diagnosis list available on the companion online site at www.cote.clinicalvetadvisor.com.

American Society of Anesthesiologists Classification System

American Society of Anesthesiologists: Classification System for Physical Status and Recommended Tests for Each Class

Physical Status	Definition	Examples	Recommended Laboratory Tests: Minor*	Recommended Laboratory Tests: Major†	Prognosis
I	Healthy with no organic disease	Elective procedures not necessary for health (ovariohysterectomy)	PCV, TP, urine specific gravity	CBC, U/A, surgical panel‡	Excellent
II	Local disease with no systemic signs	Healthy nonelective surgery (skin laceration, simple fracture)	PCV, TP, urine specific gravity	CBC, U/A, surgical panel‡	Good
III	Disease causes moderate systemic signs that limit function	Heart murmur, anemia, pneumonia, mild chest trauma, moderate dehydration	CBC, U/A, surgical panel‡	CBC, U/A, biochemical§ panel	Fair
IV	Disease causes severe systemic signs that threatens life	Gastric torsion, diaphragmatic hernia, severe chest trauma, severe anemia or dehydration	CBC, U/A, biochemical panel§	CBC, U/A, biochemical§ panel	Guarded
V	Moribund, not expected to live for more than 24 hours with or without surgery	Endotoxic shock, severe trauma, multiorgan failure	CBC, U/A, biochemical panel§	CBC, U/A, biochemical§ panel	Grave
E	Emergency	Qualifier of above classes	PCV, TP, urine specific gravity	Depends on facilities available	Variable

From Slatter D: *Textbook of Small Animal Surgery*, St. Louis, Elsevier, 2003.
*Minor is duration less than 60 minutes.
†Major is duration longer than 60 minutes or concerns patients older than 7 years.
‡Surgical panel: urea, creatinine, alkaline phosphatase, alanine aminotransferase, glucose, sodium, potassium chloride, total protein.
§Biochemical panel: the full panel includes surgical panel tests plus bicarbonate, anion gap, calcium, phosphorus, cholesterol, total bilirubin, γ-glutamyltransferase, and albumin.
CBC, complete blood cell count; PCV, packed cell volume; TP, total protein; U/A, urinalysis.

Amyloidosis

Diseases Reported in Association with Amyloidosis in Dogs

SYSTEMIC DISEASE (Glomerular Disease)

Infectious

Bacterial
Pyelonephritis (A)
Pyometra (A,G)
Pyoderma (A,G)
Other chronic bacterial infections (A,G)

Protozoal
Leishmaniasis (A, MN, P-E, and M)

Rickettsial

Viral
Canine adenovirus type 1 (P-M)

Fungal
Blastomycosis (A)
Coccidioidomycosis (A,G)

Inflammatory
Chronic dermatitis (A,G)
Pancreatitis (A,G)
Periodontal disease (A,G)
Polyarthritis (A,G)
Systemic lupus erythematosus (A, MN, P-E, and M)

Neoplastic
Lymphosarcoma (A,G)
Primary erythrocytosis (MCD?)
Other neoplasms (A,G, MN)

Miscellaneous
Hyperlipidemia (?)
Chronic insulin infusion (A)
Cyclic hematopoiesis in gray collies (A)

Familial

Idiopathic (A, G, MN, MCD, P-E, or M)

Modified from Ettinger S, Feldman E: *Textbook of Veterinary Internal Medicine*, ed 6. St. Louis, WB Saunders, 2005.
A, amyloidosis; G, glomerulonephritis–uncharacterized; MN, membranous nephropathy; MCD, minimal change disease; P, proliferative; E, endocapillary; M, mesangial.

Anaphylaxis

Causes

Venoms
Insects of the *Hymenoptera* order: bees, wasps, ants
Spiders: black widow, brown recluse
Lizards: gila monster, Mexican beaded lizard
Snakes: pit vipers (rattlesnakes, copperheads, water moccasins), coral snakes

Hormones
Insulin
Corticotropin
Vasopressin
Parathyroid hormone
Betamethasone
Triamcinolone

Antibiotics
Pencillins-amoxicillin, ampicillin, procaine penicillin
Chloramphenicol
Lincomycin
Gentamicin
Tetracycline
Sulfonamides
Cephalosporins
Polymyxin B
Doxorubicin

Nonsteroidal Anti-inflammatory Drugs (NSAIDs)
Aspirin
Ibuprofen

Anesthetics and Sedatives
Acepromazine
Ketamine
Barbiturates
Lidocaine and other local anesthetics
Narcotics
Diazepam

Parasiticides
Dichlorophen
Levamisole
Piperazine
Dichlorvos
Diethylcarbamazine
Thiacetarsemide

Miscellaneous
Blood products
Aminophylline
Asparaginase
Calcium disodium edetate
Iodinated contrast media
Neostigmine
Amphotericin B
Vaccines
Allergen extracts: pollens, molds, foods
Enzymes: chymotrypsin and trypsin
Vitamins: vitamin K, thiamine, and folic acid
Dextrans and gelatins
Sulfonamides

Foods
Milk
Egg white
Shellfish
Legumes
Fruits: citrus
Chocolate
Grains

Physical Factors
Cold
Heat
Exercise

Modified from Ettinger S, Feldman E: Textbook of Veterinary Internal Medicine, ed 6. St. Louis, WB Saunders, 2005.

Anemia (Aplastic)

Differential diagnosis list available on the companion online site at www.cote.clinicalvetadvisor.com.

Anemia: Causes

Causes

Hemorrhage
- ***Surgery/trauma***
- ***Coagulopathy:***
  - von Willebrand disease/thrombopathia
  - Thrombocytopenia
  - Hemophilia A, B/decreases in other factors
  - DIC
- ***Ectoparasiticism (fleas, ticks, lice)***
- ***GI (hookworms, neoplasia, ulceration)***
- ***Neoplasia (hemangiosarcoma)***

Hemolysis
- ***Antibody-mediated***
  - Warm-reactive IgG IHA
  - Cold-reactive IgM IHA
  - Transfusion reaction
- ***Congenital***
  - Phosphofructokinase deficiency (English springer spaniels, American cocker spaniel)
  - Familial nonspherocytic, hemolytic anemia (poodles)
  - Elliptocytosis (one crossbred dog)
  - NADH methomoglobin reductase deficiency (several breeds of dogs)
  - Hemolytic anemia secondary to RBC membrane defect (beagles)
  - Pyruvate kinase deficiency (beagles, Basenjis,
  - West Highland white terriers, giant schnauzers, Abyssinians)
  - Vitamin B_{12} deficiency (giant schnauzers)
  - Predisposition to oxidant injury, high erythrocyte potassium and low glutathione levels (Akitas, Shiba Inus)
- ***Toxin/Drug-Induced***
  - Propylthiouracil
  - Lead
  - DL-methionine
  - Cephalosporins
  - Fenbendazole
  - Dapsone
  - Gold salts
  - MLV vaccines
  - Oxidants
  - Onions
  - Acetaminophen
  - Methylene blue
  - Phenacetin
  - Propylene glycol
  - Phenol compounds (mothballs)
  - Benzocaine
  - Hydroxyurea
  - Vitamin K_3
- ***Parasites***
  - Hemobartonellosis (*Haemobartonella canis, M. haemofelis* and *M. haemominutum*)
  - *Cytauxzoon felis*
  - Babesiosis (*Babesia canis, B. gibsoni*)
  - Ehrlichiosis (*Ehrlichia canis*)
- ***Microangiopathic***
  - Splenic torsion
  - Cranial vena cava syndrome
  - Hemangiosarcoma

Decreased Production
- ***Bone marrow disorder***
  - Hematopoietic malignancy
  - Myelofibrosis
  - Idiopathic aplastic anemia
  - Irradiation
  - Myelodysplasia
- ***Systemic disease***
  - Anemia of chronic disease/inflammation
  - FeLV
  - Parvovirus
  - Renal failure
  - Liver disease
  - Endocrine disease (hypothyroidism, hypoadrenocorticism)
  - Neoplasia
- ***Toxin/Drug***
  - Estrogen
  - Chemotherapy
  - Phenylbutazone
  - TMS
  - Griseofulvin
  - Quinidine
  - Thiacetarsemide
  - NSAIDs
- ***Nutritional***
  - Mineral deficiency (iron)
  - Vitamin deficiency (B complex)
  - Inadequate protein intake

Modified with permission from Bonagura J: *Kirk's Current Veterinary Therapy XII: Small Animal Practice*. St. Louis, WB Saunders, 1995, p 448.
DIC, disseminated intravascular coagulation; FeLV, feline leukemia virus; GI, gastrointestinal; IHA, immune-mediated hemolytic anemia; MLV, modified live virus; NSAIDs, nonsteroidal anti-inflammatory drugs; TMS, trimethoprim/sulfadiazine.

Anemia (Hemolytic)

Differential diagnosis list available on the companion online site at www.cote.clinicalvetadvisor.com.

Anemia, Immune-Mediated

Examples of Underlying Disorders and Triggers

Infectious
Viral: FeLV, FIV, FIP infection, transient or chronic persistent upper respiratory or GI viral diseases
Bacterial: leptospirosis, hemobartonellosis, various acute and chronic infections (e.g., abscess, pyometra, diskospondylitis)
Parasitic: babesiosis, leishmaniasis, dirofilariasis, ehrlichiosis, *Ancylostoma caninum*
Other emerging infectious diseases (e.g., bartonellosis), bee stings

Drugs
Sulfonamides
Cephalosporins
Penicillins
Vaccines
Propylthiouracil (cats)
Methimazole (cats)
Procainamide

Neoplasia
Hemolymphatic: leukemias, lymphoma, multiple myeloma
Solid tumors

Immune Disorders
SLE
Hypothyroidism
Primary and secondary immunodeficiencies

Genetic Predisposition
American cocker spaniel (one-third of all cases)
English springer spaniel
Old English sheepdog
Irish setter
Poodle
Dachshund

From Ettinger S, Feldman E: *Textbook of Veterinary Internal Medicine*, ed 6. St. Louis, WB Saunders, 2005.
FeLV, feline leukemia virus; FIP, feline infectious peritonitis; FIV, feline immunodeficiency virus; GI, gastrointestinal; SLE, systemic lupus erythematosus.

Anemias: Characteristics

Differential diagnosis list available on the companion online site at www.cote.clinicalvetadvisor.com.

Anemias: Evaluation

Approach to Anemia Diagnosis

I. Determine Severity of the Anemia
   A. *Mild anemia (PCV >30% dog, >20% cat).*
      1. Consider age, breed, and statistical chance of normality.
      2. Check for laboratory or sample error; repeat venipuncture.
      3. For a secondary problem, go to step IV.
   B. *For moderate -to-severe anemia, go to step II.*

II. Determine Bone Marrow Responsiveness
   A. *No reticulocytosis or polychromasia expected during first 2 to 3 days or in mild anemia (PCV >30% dog, >20% cat).*
   B. *Reticulocytosis and polychromasia peak 4 to 5 days if bone marrow function normal.*
      1. Marked canine reticulocytosis >500,000.
      2. Marked feline aggregate reticulocytosis >200,000.
   C. *Later-stage responsiveness at 7 to 14 days:*
      1. Feline punctate reticulocytosis, marked >1,500,000.
      2. Dogs: increase in macrocytic hypochromic RBCs.
   D. *Classification by RBC indices and hematology instrument graphics.*
      1. Macrocytic hypochromic: regenerative anemia.
      2. Normocytic normochromic: nonregenerative or preregenerative anemia.
      3. Microcytic hypochromic: iron deficiency anemia.
      4. Macrocytic normochromic.
   E. *If adequately regenerative, go to step III; if inadequately regenerative, go to step IV.*

III. Regenerative Anemia Diagnosis
   A. *Blood smear analysis critical in hemolytic anemia diagnosis.*
      1. Spherocytes, autoagglutination, Heinz bodies, polychromasia, blood parasites, eccentrocytes, RBC fragmentation.
   B. *Hemoglobinuria is best proof of intravascular hemolytic anemia.*
   C. *Internal blood loss resembles hemolytic anemia.*
      1. Document hemorrhage with cytologic examination and other such tests.
   D. *External blood loss.*
      1. Often in history.
      2. Tendency toward hypoproteinemia, hypoalbuminemia, or both.
      3. Check for thrombocytopenia or bleeding tendency.

IV. Nonregenerative Anemia Diagnosis
   A. *Way to a diagnosis varies with case presentation.*
   B. *Use history and severity of anemia to reevaluate reticulocyte numbers to see if anemia is truly nonregenerative; duration exceeding 3 to 4 days excludes preregenerative anemia; reticulocyte response is weak or absent 2 weeks after the cause of an anemia ceases; mild anemia will not stimulate much reticulocytosis.*
   C. *Evaluate rest of the hematology report*
      1. Microcytic hypochromic RBCs usually indicate iron deficiency anemia
         a. RBC *cytograms* and histograms more sensitive than MCV and MCHC
         b. Half of iron deficiency anemia cases regenerative
      2. Normocytic normochromic anemia most common but nonspecific
      3. Macrocytic normochromic feline RBCs without reticulocytosis, suggests FeLV-induced myelodysplasia (see text)

(*Continued*)

Approach to Anemia Diagnosis—(*Continued*)

4. Evidence of inflammation (see Chapter 4); anemia of inflammatory diseases is very common (i.e., mild, normocytic normochromic anemia)
5. Evidence of leukemia or dysplastic hematopoiesis (see Chapter 4) usually indicates bone marrow evaluation; go to H
6. Thrombocytopenia (see Chapter 5); consider *Ehrlichia* or other infections (see Chapter 15)
7. Pancytopenia or bicytopenia indicates bone marrow disease and bone marrow evaluation; go to H

D. Clinical chemistry profile

1. Renal or hepatic failure causes secondary anemia (see Chapters 7 and 9)
2. Systemic diseases have variable causes of anemia

E. Virology, serology if infection is likely (e.g., fever, lymphadenopathy)

F. Endocrinologic examination for hypothyroidism or other dysfunction (see Chapter 8) (e.g., mild, normocytic normochromic anemia)

G. Toxicity

1. Check for testicular neoplasm or access to estrogen
2. Withhold any current drug therapy and monitor for recovery
3. Check for toxicants in environment

H. Bone marrow examination reveals many diagnoses (see text and Chapter 2)

1. Myelofibrosis, aplastic pancytopenia, dyserythropoiesis, leukemia, myelodysplasia, refractory anemia with excessive blasts, etc.

From Willard M, Tvedten H: *Small Animal Clinical Diagnosis by Laboratory Methods*, ed 4. St. Louis, WB Saunders, 2004.

PCV, packed cell volume; RBC, red blood cell; MCV, mean corpuscular volume; MCHC, mean corpuscular hemoglobin concentration; FeLV, feline leukemia virus.

Anisocoria

Differential diagnosis list available on the companion online site at www.cote.clinicalvetadvisor.com.

Anorexia

I. Psychologic (especially cats)

II. Inability to Smell Food

III. Dysphagia (especially when it causes pain)

IV. Inflammation
- Because of an infectious agent
- Because of immune-mediated disease
- Because of neoplasia
- Because of necrosis
- Because of drugs

V. Alimentary and Abdominal Diseases (especially those causing nausea or abdominal pain)

VI. Neoplasia
- Because of the neoplasm itself
- Because of secondary bacterial infection when neoplasia impairs natural defense mechanisms

VII. Toxins
- Exogenous (various ones)
- Endogenous (e.g., renal failure, hepatic encephalopathy)

VIII. Endocrine Disease
- Hypoadrenocorticism
- Hyperthyroidism

IX. Central Nervous System (CNS) Disease
- Primary
- Secondary

From Willard M, Tvedten H: *Small Animal Clinical Diagnosis by Laboratory Methods*, ed 4. St. Louis, WB Saunders, 2004.

Anticoagulant Rodenticides: Brand Names and Corresponding Active Ingredients

Differential diagnosis list available on the companion online site at www.cote.clinicalvetadvisor.com.

Antidotes to Common Poisons

Differential diagnosis list available on the companion online site at www.cote.clinicalvetadvisor.com.

Arrhythmias

Causes of or Predisposing Factors for Ventricular Arrhythmias (Premature Ventricular Complexes, Ventricular Tachycardia)
Hypokalemia
Hypoxemia (e.g., from pulmonary edema, other causes)
Anemia
Structural heart disease (valvular heart disease, cardiomyopathy, congenital heart disease, others)
Blunt chest trauma (e.g., hit by car)
Gastric dilatation and volvulus
Abdominal mass (splenic, hepatic, others)
Sepsis
Acidosis
Systemic inflammatory response syndrome (SIRS)
Intoxications (digitalis, pseudoephedrine, many other pharmaceuticals; oleander, yew, many other plants)
Excess catecholamines
Myocarditis (diagnosis of exclusion)

Arrhythmias: ECG Characteristics

Differential diagnosis list available on the companion online site at www.cote.clinicalvetadvisor.com.

Arrhythmias: Ventricular Versus Supraventricular

Differential diagnosis list available on the companion online site at www.cote.clinicalvetadvisor.com.

Azoospermia

Differential diagnosis list available on the companion online site at www.cote.clinicalvetadvisor.com.

Azotemia

Differential diagnosis list available on the companion online site at www.cote.clinicalvetadvisor.com.

Azotemia: Blood Urea Nitrogen/Creatinine Mismatch

Differential diagnosis list available on the companion online site at www.cote.clinicalvetadvisor.com.

Bacteria Isolated from Sites of Infection

Bacteria Commonly Isolated from Various Sites in Infectious Disorders in Dogs and Cats

Integument
Pyoderma
Staphylococcus aureus/intermedius
Proteus spp.
Pseudomonas spp.
Escherichia coli (usually secondary to staphylococci)
Ear
Pseudomonas spp.
S. aureus/intermedius
Proteus spp.

Respiratory System
Pneumonia
Pseudomonas spp.
E. coli
Klebsiella spp.
Pasteurella spp.
Bordetella spp.
Staphylococcus spp.
Streptococcus spp.
Mycoplasma spp.
Pleural Cavity
Nocardia spp.
Actinomyces spp.
Pasteurella spp.
Anaerobes

GI Tract
Intestine
Salmonella spp.
Campylobacter spp.
Clostridium perfringens
E. coli
Genitourinary Tract
E. coli
Proteus spp.
Klebsiella spp.
S. aureus/intermedius
Eye (conjunctiva and cornea)
S. aureus (coagulase positive and negative)
Streptococcus spp.
S. epidermidis
E. coli
Proteus spp.
Bacillus spp.

Cardiovascular System
Aerobes
S. aureus
ß-hemolytic streptococci
E. coli
Klebsiella spp.
Pseudomonas spp.
Proteus spp.
Salmonella spp.
Anaerobes
Bacteroides spp.
Fusobacterium spp.
Clostridium spp.

Data compiled from Greene CE (ed): *Clinical Microbiology and Infectious Diseases of the Dog and Cat.* Philadelphia, WB Saunders, 1998.
GI, gastrointestinal.

Behavioral Change: Primary Behavioral Versus Neurologic

Differential diagnosis list available on the companion online site at www.cote.clinicalvetadvisor.com.

Bleeding Disorders

Expected Hemostatic Test Results in Selected Diseases

Disease	Hemostatic Profile				
	BMBT	Platelet Count	APTT	PT	FDP
Thrombocytopenia (e.g., ehrlichiosis)	I	D	N	N	N
Platelet dysfunction (e.g., aspirin treatment)	I	N	I	N	N
Intrinsic pathway defect (e.g., hemophilia A or B)	N*	N	I	N	N
Factor VII deficiency	N	N	N	I	N
Multiple factor defects (e.g., vitamin K antagonism)	N*	N	I	I	N
Common pathway defect (e.g., factor X deficiency)	N*	N	I	I	N
DIC	I	D	I	I	I
von Willebrand disease	I	N†	N‡	N	N

Modified from Willard M, Tvedten H: *Small Animal Clinical Diagnosis by Laboratory Methods*, ed 4. St. Louis, WB Saunders, 2004.
*Initially stops in normal time period but may start bleeding again.
†Mild thrombocytopenia may occur if patient is concurrently hypothyroid.
‡Usually normal but may be increased.
BMBT, buccal mucosal bleeding time; APTT, activated partial thromboplastin time; PT, prothrombin time; FDP, fibrin degradation products; I, increased; D, decreased; N, normal; DIC, disseminated intravascular coagulation. DIC can have widely variable results.

Bleeding Disorders: Primary Versus Secondary

Differential diagnosis list available on the companion online site at www.cote.clinicalvetadvisor.com.

Blindness

Differential diagnosis list available on the companion online site at www.cote.clinicalvetadvisor.com.

Blood Type Frequencies, Cats

Differential diagnosis list available on the companion online site at www.cote.clinicalvetadvisor.com.

Blood Type Frequencies, Dogs

Differential diagnosis list available on the companion online site at www.cote.clinicalvetadvisor.com.

Bone Diseases, Congenital

Congenital Skeletal Disorders of Small Animals

Osteochondrodysplasias: Abnormalities of Cartilage, Bone Growth, and Development

A. Defects of Growth of Tubular Bone or Spine
1. Multiple epiphyseal dysplasia: beagle
2. Pseudoachondrodysplasia: miniature poodle, Scottish deerhound
3. Chondrodysplasia: Alaskan malamute, cocker spaniel, English pointer, Great Pyrenees, Norwegian elkhound
4. Ocular-skeletal dysplasia: Labrador retriever, Samoyed
5. Pelger-Huet anomaly: cats
6. Scottish fold osteochondrodysplasia: cats

B. Disorganized Development of Cartilage and Fibrous Components
1. Multiple cartilaginous exostoses (osteochondromatosis)
2. Enchondroma
3. Fibrous dysplasia

C. Abnormalities of Density, Cortical Diaphyseal Structure, or Metaphyseal Molding
1. Osteogenesis imperfecta
2. Osteopetrosis

Primary Metabolic Abnormalities
- Vitamin D–dependent rickets
- Mucopolysaccharidosis (MPS)
- Fucosidosis
- GM gangliosidosis
- Gaucher's disease

Dysostoses with Malformation of Individual Bones, Singly or in Combination
- Hemimelia
- Phocomelia
- Amelia
- Syndactyly
- Polydactyly
- Ectrodactyly
- Segmental hemiatrophy

Adapted from Sharrard WJW: *Pediatric Orthopaedics and Fractures*, ed 3. London, Blackwell Scientific Publications, 1993.

Bone Marrow Disorders

Differential diagnosis list available on the companion online site at www.cote.clinicalvetadvisor.com.

Bone Neoplasia

Differential diagnosis list available on the companion online site at www.cote.clinicalvetadvisor.com.

Bradycardia

Causes of Bradycardia in Dogs and Cats

A. Arrhythmias
1. Second-degree AV block
2. Third-degree AV block
3. SSS/sinus node dysfunction
4. Atrial standstill (hyperkalemia, atrial myopathy)

B. Hypothermia

C. Hypothyroidism

D. Organophosphate toxicosis

E. Pharmacologic (e.g., due to β-blockers, calcium channel blockers, digitalis, opiates, α_2 blocking drugs)

F. Vagal tone high: normal
1. Brachycephalic breed
2. Athletic animal at rest
3. Sleep

G. Vagal tone high: abnormal
1. GI disturbances
2. Upper respiratory obstruction (e.g., foreign body, laryngeal paralysis, elongated soft palate, mass, anesthetic circuit problem)
3. Neurologic lesions (central and severe: usually coma)

Notes: First-degree AV block does not affect the heart rate.

In critically ill or anesthetized animals, an acute transition from tachycardia to bradycardia may indicate an upcoming cardiac arrest.

Definition of bradycardia in the clinical setting: heart rate <60 bpm (large-breed dogs), <70 bpm (medium-breed dogs), <90 bpm (small-breed dogs), <130 bpm (cats). AV, atrioventricular; GI, gastrointestinal; SSS, sick sinus syndrome.

Bronchial Disease: Chronic

Possible Causes of Chronic Bronchitis in Dogs

Atmospheric pollution

Passive smoking
- Chronic exposure to smoke in poorly ventilated confined spaces

Respiratory tract infections
- Chronic fungal infection
- Chronic bacterial infection: *Bordetella bronchiseptica*, *Mycoplasma* spp.
- Viral infection: canine distemper virus, adenovirus (types 1 and 2), herpesvirus
- Parasites: *Filaroides milksi*, *F. hirthi*, *Crenosoma vulpis*, *Capillaria aerophila*, *Dirofilaria immitis*

Genetic or acquired defects
- α_1-Antitrypsin deficiency
- Mucociliary defects
- Immunodeficiency

Hypersensitivity (allergic) lung disease

Modified with permission from King L: In *Textbook of Respiratory Disease in Dogs and Cats*. WB Saunders, 2004, p 381.

Central Nervous System Disorders: Multifocal

Diseases That Commonly Result in Multifocal CNS Signs

Degenerative
- Storage disease
- Multineuronal degeneration

Anomalous
- Hydrocephalus/syringomyelia/hydromyelia complex

Metabolic
- Hepatic
- Renal
- Hypoglycemia
- Hyperthyroidism
- Hypothyroidism
- Hyperadrenocorticism
- Hyperosmolar syndromes
  - Adipsia

Neoplastic
- Lymphoma
- Leukemias
- Metastatic tumors

Nutritional
- Thiamine

Inflammatory
- ***Infectious***
  - Viral
    - Distemper
    - Herpes
    - Parvovirus
    - Parainfluenza
    - FIP
    - FIV
  - Bacterial
    - Bacterial encephalitis
    - Tetanus
  - Fungal
    - Cryptococcosis
    - Blastomycosis
    - Coccidioidomycosis
    - Candidiasis
    - Aspergillosis
  - Protozoal
    - Toxoplasmosis
    - Neosporosis
  - Parasitic
    - *Toxocara*
    - *Cuterebra*
  - Rickettsial
    - RMSF
    - *Ehrlichia*
  - Unclassified
    - Protothecosis
- ***Noninfectious***
  - GME
  - Breed-associated CNS inflammation (necrotizing encephalitis): pug encephalitis, Maltese encephalitis, Yorkshire terrier encephalitis
  - Spinal cord vasculitis
  - Nonclassified
    - Steroid-responsive meningitis

Idiopathic
- Dysautonomia

Toxins

Vascular disease
- Intracranial hemorrhage
- Thromboembolism
- Hypertension
- Spinal hemorrhage

Modified from Ettinger S, Feldman E: *Textbook of Veterinary Internal Medicine*, ed 6. St. Louis, WB Saunders, 2005.
CNS, central nervous system; FIV, feline immunodeficiency virus; FIP, feline infectious peritonitis virus; GME, granulomatous meningoencephalitis; RMSF, Rocky Mountain spotted fever.

Cerebrospinal Fluid Abnormalities

CSF Determinations and Diseases of the Nervous System

	Disease	
Determination	**Meningitis** Bacterial disease: suppurative inflammation	**Parenchymal Disease** Tissue necrosis: neoplasia, degenerations Viral disease: nonsuppurative inflammation
Physical	Turbid, clot	Clear, colorless
Cytologic (WBC)		
Quantitative	Large increase: >100/cmm	Small increase: <100/cmm
Differential	Mostly neutrophils	Mostly mononuclear cells
Chemical		
Protein		
Quantitative (total)	Large increase: >100 mg/dl	Small increase: <100 mg/dl
Glucose: normally about 80% of blood level	Normal or decreased to below 50% of the blood level	Normal

Modified from de Lahunta A: *Veterinary Neuroanatomy and Clinical Neurology*. St. Louis, WB Saunders, 1983.
CSF, cerebrospinal fluid; WBC, white blood cell; cmm, cubic millimeter.

Chronic Renal Failure: Causes

Causes

Familial or Congenital

I. Dogs
  A. Amyloidosis in shar-pei and beagle dogs
  B. Cystadenocarcinoma in German shepherd dogs
  C. Renal dysplasia in shih tzus, Lhasa apso, golden retrievers, Norwegian Elkhounds, Chow Chows, and others
  D. Glomerulopathy in English cocker spaniels, Doberman pinschers, bull terriers, soft-coated Wheaten terriers, Samoyeds
  E. Fanconi syndrome in Basenjis
  F. Polycystic kidney disease in Cairn terriers
II. Cats
  A. Amyloidosis in Abyssinian cats and oriental short-haired cats
  B. Polycystic kidney disease in Persians and Himalayans

Acquired

I. Infectious
  A. Bacterial
  B. Mycotic-blastomycosis
  C. Leptospirosis
  D. Leishmaniasis
  E. Feline infectious peritonitis (FIP)
II. Immune complex glomerulopathy
  A. Amyloidosis
  B. Neoplasia
    1. Lymphosarcoma
    2. Renal cell carcinoma
    3. Nephroblastoma
    4. Others
  C. Sequela of acute renal failure
  D. Bilateral hydronephrosis
    1. Spay granulomas
    2. Transitional cell carcinoma: bladder trigone location
    3. Nephrolithiasis
  E. Polycystic kidney disease
  F. Hypercalcemia
    1. Malignancy
    2. Primary hyperparathyroidism
  G. Idiopathic

From Ettinger S, Feldman E: *Textbook of Veterinary Internal Medicine*, ed 6. St. Louis, WB Saunders, 2005.

Chronic Renal Failure: Complications

Complications and Comorbid Conditions in Animals with Chronic Kidney Disease

Complications of Chronic Kidney Disease

- Anemia
- Systemic hypertension
- Dehydration
- Hyperparathyroidism
- Hyperphosphatemia
- Hypocalcemia and hypercalcemia
- Hypokalemia
- Malnutrition
- Metabolic acidosis
- Uremic signs

Comorbid Conditions

- Cardiac disease
- Degenerative joint disease
- Dental and oral diseases
- Hyperthyroidism (cats)
- Nephroliths and ureteroliths
- Urinary tract infections

From Ettinger S, Feldman E: *Textbook of Veterinary Internal Medicine*, ed 6. St. Louis, WB Saunders, 2005.

Coma, Stupor

Causes of Stupor and Coma

Congenital or Familial Disorders
Hydrocephalus
Lysosomal storage disorders
Lissencephaly

Metabolic Disorders
Hepatic encephalopathy
Hypoadrenocorticism
Diabetes mellitus
Hypoglycemia
Hypothyroidism
Uremia
Hypoxia
Acid-base imbalance
Osmolality imbalance
Heatstroke
Hyperlipidemia

Nutritional Disorders
Thiamine deficiency (end-stage)

Neoplasia
Primary lesions
Metastatic lesions

Inflammation
Canine distemper
Rabies
Rocky Mountain spotted fever
Ehrlichia infection
Feline infectious peritonitis
Fungal, protozoal, and bacterial infections
Granulomatous meningoencephalitis

Toxins/Drugs
Ethylene glycol
Lead
Barbiturates
Mushroom poisoning
Alcohol
Cannabinoids
Hallucinogens

Trauma
Cranial trauma

Vascular
Coagulopathies
Hypertension
Cardiomyopathy
Bacterial emboli
Feline ischemic encephalopathy
Ischemia

Other
Status epilepticus

From Ettinger S, Feldman E: *Textbook of Veterinary Internal Medicine*, ed 5. St. Louis, WB Saunders, 2000.

Congenital Heart Disease: Breed Predilections

Breed Predilections in Dogs with CHD

Breed	Condition
Airedale terrier	Pulmonic stenosis (PS)-2
Beagle	PS*
Bichon frise	Patent ductus arteriosus (PDA)-2
Boxer	Aortic stenosis (AS)-3
Boykin spaniel	PS*
Bull terrier	Mitral dysplasia (MD)*
Chihuahua	PS,* PDA*
Cocker spaniel	PDA-1, PS-1
Collie	PDA-1
Doberman pinscher	Atrial septal defect (ASD)*
English bulldog	PS-3, ventricular septal defect (VSD)-3, AS-1, tetralogy of Fallot (TF)*
English springer spaniel	PDA-2
German shepherd	Tricuspid dysplasia (TD)-3, AS-1, persistent right aortic arch (PRAA)-2, MD,* PDA*
German shorthaired pointer	AS*
Golden retriever	AS-3, TD*
Great Dane	AS-1, PRAA-3, MD,* TD*
Irish setter	PRAA*
Keeshond	PDA-2, TF*
Kerry blue terrier	PDA-3
Labrador retriever	TD-3
Maltese	PDA-3
Mastiff	PS-3
Miniature schnauzer	PS-2
Newfoundland	AS-3
Pomeranian	PDA-3
Poodles	PDA-2
Rottweiler	AS-3
Samoyed	PS-3, AS-1, ASD*
Scottish terrier	PS-2
Shetland sheepdog	PDA-3
West Highland white terrier	PS-3
Weimaraner	TD,* peritoneopericardial hernia*
Yorkshire terrier	PDA-1

With permission from Kirk R and Bonagura J, eds: ***Kirk's** Current Veterinary Therapy XI: Small Animal Practice*. St. Louis, WB Saunders, 1993, p 650. Data from Veterinary Medical Data Base (VMDB) at Purdue University, 1987–1989: 1320 dogs with congenital heart disease (CHD) out of 154,233 dogs. Numbers 1, 2, and 3 identify predisposed breeds represented by four or more affected dogs in which relative risk for the indicated abnormality was significantly elevated in this series (P 0.05 to P 0.0001):
1: Mildly increased risk (odds ratio 1.5–2.9 times all other dogs).
2: Moderate risk (odds ratio 3–4.9 times others).
3: Marked risk (odds ratio 5 times others).
*Breed-associated diseases were not confirmed in this study but suggested or confirmed by others.
Sex predominance: PDA (females 3:1), PS in English bulldogs (males 4:1), mitral and tricuspid dysplasia (males 2:1).

DIFFERENTIAL DIAGNOSIS

Congestive Heart Failure: Causes

Causes

Valvular Heart Disease
Congenital malformations: aortic or subaortic stenosis, mitral valve malformation, pulmonic stenosis, tricuspid valve malformation
Acquired diseases: myxomatous atrioventricular valvular disease, ruptured chordae tendineae, bacterial endocarditis

Myocardial Diseases
Malformations: defects of the atrial and ventricular septum
Dilated cardiomyopathy
Hypertrophic cardiomyopathy
Restrictive cardiomyopathy (endomyocardial fibrosis)
Undefined feline cardiomyopathies
Atrial muscle degeneration
Right ventricular cardiomyopathy
Myocarditis
Secondary myocardial diseases: hyperthyroidism, acromegaly, hypertension

Pericardial Diseases
Idiopathic pericardial hemorrhage/pericarditis
Cardiac neoplasia leading to pericardial effusion
Infectious

Vascular Diseases
Malformation: patent ductus arteriosus, arteriovenous fistula
Heartworm disease

High-Output States
Anemia
Thyrotoxicosis

Cardiac Arrhythmia
Chronic bradyarrhythmia
Chronic tachyarrhythmia

From DiBartola S: *Fluid, Electrolyte, and Acid-Base Disorders in Small Animal Practice*. St. Louis, WB Saunders, 2000.

Congestive Heart Failure: Classification

Functional Classification of CHF

New York Heart Association Classification*

I. Normal activity does not produce undue fatigue, dypsnea, or coughing.
II. The dog or cat is comfortable at rest, but ordinary physical activity causes fatigue, dyspnea, or coughing.
III. The dog or cat is comfortable at rest, but minimal exercise may produce fatigue, dyspnea, or coughing. Signs may also develop while the animal is in a recumbent position (orthopnea).
IV. CHF, dyspnea, and coughing are present even when the dog or cat is at rest. Signs are exaggerated by any physical activity.

International Small Animal Cardiac Health Council†

I. Asymptomatic patient.
   A. Signs of heart disease but no cardiomegaly.
   B. Signs of heart disease and evidence of compensation (cardiomegaly).
II. Mild to moderate CHF.
   A. Clinical signs of CHF are evident at rest or with mild exercise and adversely affect the quality of life.
III. Advanced CHF
   A. Clinical signs of CHF are immediately obvious.
      1. Home care is possible.
      2. Hospitalization is recommended (cardiogenic shock, life-threatening edema, large pleural effusion, refractory ascites).

*Adapted from the New York Heart Association Classification in Ettinger SJ, Suter PF: The recognition of cardiac disease and congestive heart failure. In Ettinger SJ, Suter PF (eds): *Canine Cardiology*. Philadelphia, WB Saunders, 1970, p 215.
†Adapted from International Small Animal Cardiac Health Council: Recommendations for the diagnosis of heart disease and the treatment of heart failure in small animals. In Miller MS, Tilley LP (eds): *Manual of Canine and Feline Cardiology*. Philadelphia, WB Saunders, 1995, p 473.
CHF, congestive heart failure.

Congestive Heart Failure: Physical Signs

Physical Signs Associated with CHF

Pulmonary Signs (Left-Sided CHF)
Rales (alveolar edema)
Frothy, pink sputum
Shortness of breath, tachypnea
Dyspnea during recumbency (orthopnea)
Cough

Signs Attributable to Either Left or Right CHF
Weakness and fatigue (general exercise intolerance)
Exertional dyspnea
Gallop sound/"gallop rhythm" (accentuated third heart sound)
Poor peripheral perfusion: pale mucous membranes, slow capillary refill time, mild cyanosis, cool extremities
Tachycardia
Weight loss (cachexia)

Systemic Signs (Right-Sided CHF)
Generalized venous engorgement
Hepatomegaly
Body cavity effusions (modified transudate): ascites, pleural effusion, pericardial effusion
Dependent peripheral edema
Weight gain (retained fluid)

Modified from Ettinger S, Feldman E: *Textbook of Veterinary Internal Medicine*, ed 4. St. Louis, WB Saunders, 1994.
CHF, congestive heart failure.

Conjunctivitis, Canine (Chronic)

Differential diagnosis list available on the companion online site at www.cote.clinicalvetadvisor.com.

Conjunctivitis, Feline

Differential diagnosis list available on the companion online site at www.cote.clinicalvetadvisor.com.

Constipation

Differential Diagnosis of Constipation in the Cat

Neuromuscular Dysfunction
Colonic smooth muscle: idiopathic megacolon, aging
Spinal cord disease: lumbosacral disease, cauda equina syndrome, sacral spinal cord deformity (Manx cat)
Hypogastric or pelvic nerve disorders: traumatic injury, malignant disease, dysautonomia
Submucosal or myenteric plexus neuropathy: dysautonomia, aging

Mechanical Obstruction
Intraluminal: foreign material (bones, plant material, hair), neoplasia, rectal diverticulum, perineal hernia, anorectal stricture
Intramural: neoplasia
Extraluminal: pelvic fracture, neoplasia, prostatic disease

Inflammation
Perianal fistula, proctitis, anal sac abscess, anorectal foreign body, perianal bite wound

Metabolic and Endocrine
Metabolic: dehydration, hypokalemia, hypocalcemia, and hypercalcemia
Endocrine: hypothyroidism, obesity, nutritional secondary hyperparathyroidism

Pharmacologic
Opioid agonists, cholinergic antagonists, diuretics, barium sulfate, phenothiazines

Environmental and Behavioral
Soiled litter box, inactivity, hospitalization, change in environment

Adapted from Washabau RJ, Hasler AH: Constipation, obstipation, and megacolon. In August JR (ed): *Consultations in Feline Internal Medicine*, ed 3. Philadelphia, WB Saunders, 1997, p 106.

Corneal Ulcer

Underlying Causes of Corneal Ulceration in Dogs and Cats

Entropion
Other lid defects
Distichiasis
Ectopic cilia
Lagophthalmos
Exophthalmos
Foreign body
KCS
Severe debilitation
Neural defects; CN V and/or VII

Modified with permission from Kirk R: *Kirk's Current Veterinary Therapy XI: Small Animal Practice*. Philadelphia, WB Saunders, 1993, p 1103.
CN, cranial nerve; KCS, keratoconjunctivitis sicca.

Coughing

Causes of Cough in Small Animals

Allergic/Inflammatory
Feline asthma
Chronic bronchitis
COPD
PIE
Eosinophilic pneumonitis

Cardiovascular
Pulmonary edema
Left atrial enlargement
Pulmonary thromboembolism

Infectious
Tracheobronchitis
Pneumonia
- Bacterial
- Viral
- Fungal
- Protozoal

Neoplastic
Primary
- Lung
- Trachea
- Larynx

Metastatic
- Heart-base tumor
- Compression due to enlarged lymph nodes

Parasites
Filaroides
Aelurostrongylus
Paragonimus
Capillaria
Dirofilaria, especially postadulticide treatment
Larval migration (*Toxocara* spp., *Ancylostoma caninum*, *Strongyloides stercoralis*)
Other

Trauma and Physical Abnormalities
Foreign body
Collapsing trachea
Tracheal hypoplasia
Tracheal stenosis
Smoke inhalation
Pulmonary hemorrhage

Modified with permission from King L: In *Textbook of Respiratory Disease in Dogs and Cats*. Philadelphia, WB Saunders, 2004, p 44.
COPD, chronic obstructive pulmonary disease; PIE, pulmonary infiltrates with eosinophils.

Cranial Nerve Deficits

Cranial Nerve Dysfunction

Nerve	Clinical Signs	Clinical Tests	Normal Response	Abnormal Response
I. Olfactory	Hyposmia or anosmia	Smell of food or nonirritating, volatile substance	Interest in food; sniff, recoil, or nose lick with volatile substance	No reaction
II. Optic	Visual impairment and hesitancy in moving	1. Obstacle test 2. Visual placing reaction 3. Menace reaction 4. Following movement test	1. Avoidance of obstacle 2. Visual placement of limbs 3. Eye blink 4. Eyes following objects	1. Bumping objects 2–4. No reaction
III. Oculomotor	Ventrolateral strabismus	1. Ocular movement in horizontal and vertical planes	1. Normal ocular excursion	1. Impaired movements of affected eye
	Paralysis of upper eyelid (ptosis), mydriasis	2. Point source of light in each eye	2. Direct and consensual pupillary light reflexes	2. On affected side, direct pupillary reflex absent, consensual reflex present; on normal side, direct pupillary reflex present, consensual reflex absent
Sympathetic control of pupillary function	Constricted pupil (miosis), enophthalmos, prolapse of third eyelid, ptosis of upper lid			
IV. Trochlear	Usually not noted			
V. Trigeminal (motor and sensory)	Atrophy of masticatory muscles Inability to close mouth	1. Jaw tone 2. Palpate and observe masticatory muscles 3. Palpebral reflex 4. Corneal reflex 5. Probe nasal mucosa 6. Touch face	1. Resistance to opening jaws 2. Normal muscle contour and resilience 3. Eye blink 4. Eye blink and globe retraction 5. Recoil 6. No reaction	1. Lack of resistance 2. Atrophy, hypotonia 3–5. No reaction 6. Intense discomfort
VI. Abducent	Medial strabismus	Ocular movements in horizontal plane	Normal ocular excursion	Impaired lateral movement of affected eye
VII. Facial	Asymmetry of facial expression Inability to close eyelids Lip commissure paralysis Ear paralysis	1. Palpebral reflex 2. Corneal reflex 3. Menace reaction 4. Tickle ear	1–3. Eye blink 4. Ear flick	1–4. No reaction
VIII. Vestibulocochlear Vestibular	Nystagmus, head tilt, circling Falling and rolling	1. Ocular movements in horizontal and vertical planes 2. Caloric and rotatory test 3. Righting reactions	1–2. Normal physiologic nystagmus 3. Normal righting	1–3. No reaction, ventrolateral strabismus on dorsal extension of head
Cochlear	Deafness	Hand clap	Startle reaction, blink ear contraction	No reaction
IX. Glossopharyngeal	Dysphagia	Gag reflex	Swallowing response	No reaction
X. Vagus	Dysphagia Abnormal vocalizing Inspiratory dyspnea Megaesophagus	1. Gag reflex 2. Laryngeal reflex 3. Oculocardiac reflex	1. Swallow 2. Cough 3. Bradycardia	1–3. No reaction
XI. Spinal accessory	Usually not noted			
XII. Hypoglossal	Deviation of tongue	1. Tongue stretch 2. Nose rub	1. Retraction 2. Lick response	1–2. No reaction

With permission from Braund KG: In *Clinical Syndromes in Veterinary Neurology*. St. Louis, Mosby, 1994,

Cyanosis: Causes

Causes of Central and Peripheral Cyanosis

Central Cyanosis
- ***Cardiac (Right-to-Left Shunting)***
  - Intracardiac:
    - Tetralogy of Fallot
    - Atrial or ventricular septal defect with pulmonic stenosis or pulmonary hypertension
  - Extracardiac:
    - Reversed patent ductus arteriosus (PDA) (differential cyanosis)
    - Pulmonary arteriovenous fistulas
- ***Pulmonary***
  - Hypoventilation:
    - Pleural effusion, pneumothorax
    - Respiratory muscle failure (e.g., fatigue, myopathy, or neurologic abnormalities)
    - Toxicity (e.g., sedative or anesthetic overdose)
    - Primary neurologic disease (e.g., neoplasia, inflammatory)
  - Obstruction:
    - Laryngeal paralysis
    - Foreign body (e.g., laryngeal, tracheal)
    - Mass lesion of large airways (e.g., neoplasia, parasitic, inflammatory)
    - Inadequate oxygen concentration of inspired gas (e.g., high-altitude, anesthetic complication)
- ***Ventilation-Perfusion Mismatch***
  - Pulmonary thromboembolism
  - Pulmonary infiltration
    - Edema
    - Inflammation
    - Neoplasia
    - Acute respiratory distress syndrome (ARDS)
  - Chronic obstructive pulmonary disease or pulmonary fibrosis
- ***Nonoxygen-Carrying Hemoglobin (Hg) (e.g., methemoglobinemia)***

Peripheral Cyanosis
- Central cyanosis (e.g., congestive heart failure)
- Decreased arterial supply (e.g., surgical ligation of artery)
- Peripheral vasoconstriction (e.g., hypothermia, shock)
- Arterial thromboembolism
- Low cardiac output
- Obstruction of venous drainage: tourniquet or foreign object (i.e., rubber band), venous thrombosis, right-sided heart failure

Modified from Ettinger S, Feldman E: *Textbook of Veterinary Internal Medicine*, ed 6. St. Louis, WB Saunders, 2005.

Cyanosis: Differentiation

Differential diagnosis list available on the companion online site at www.cote.clinicalvetadvisor.com.

Dermatoses

Differential diagnosis list available on the companion online site at www.cote.clinicalvetadvisor.com.

Dermatoses, Scaling and Crusting

Differential diagnosis list available on the companion online site at www.cote.clinicalvetadvisor.com.

Diabetes Insipidus, Nephrogenic

Causes

Congenital (primary)

Acquired (secondary)
- Functional
  - Drugs
    - Glucocorticoids
    - Lithium
    - Demeclocycline
    - Methoxyflurane
    - *Escherichia coli* endotoxin (e.g., pyelonephritis, pyometra)
    - Diuretics
  - Electrolyte disturbances
    - Hypokalemia
    - Hypercalcemia
  - Altered medullary hypertonicity
    - Hypoadrenocorticism
  - Multifactorial or unknown mechanism
    - Hepatic insufficiency
    - Hyperthyroidism
    - Hyperadrenocorticism
    - Postobstructive diuresis
    - Acromegaly
- Structural
  - Medullary interstitial amyloidosis (e.g., in cats, shar-pei dogs)
  - Polycystic kidney disease
  - Chronic pyelonephritis
  - Chronic interstitial nephritis

From DiBartola S: *Fluid, Electrolyte, and Acid-Base Disorders in Small Animal Practice*. St. Louis, WB Saunders, 2000.

Diabetes Ketoacidosis

Triggers and Predisposing Conditions

- Acromegaly
- Congestive heart failure
- Epinephrine release
- Glucagonoma
- Glucocorticoid treatment
- Hepatitis/cholangiohepatitis
- Hyperadrenocorticism
- Infection
  - Abscess (subcutaneous, other)
  - Periodontal/oral
  - Pneumonia
  - Pyoderma
  - Pyometra
  - Urinary tract infection
- Pancreatitis
- Pulmonary thromboembolism
- Progesterone (diestrus; progestogen treatment)
- Renal failure

Diabetes Mellitus

Complications in Dogs and Cats

Common
- Iatrogenic hypoglycemia
- Persistent polyuria and polydipsia (PU/PD)
- Weight loss
- Cataracts (dogs)
- Bacterial infections, especially in the urinary tract
- Pancreatitis
- Ketoacidosis
- Hepatic lipidosis
- Peripheral neuropathy (cat)

Uncommon
- Peripheral neuropathy (dog)
- Glomerulonephropathy, glomerulosclerosis
- Retinopathy
- Exocrine pancreatic insufficiency
- Gastric paresis
- Diabetic diarrhea
- Diabetic dermatopathy (dog) (i.e., superficial necrolytic dermatitis/hepatocutaneous syndrome)

From Feldman E, Nelson R: *Canine and Feline Endocrinology and Reproduction*, ed 3. St. Louis, WB Saunders, 2004.

Diarrhea

Major Categories and Causes for Acute Diarrhea in Dogs and Cats

Intestinal Parasites
- Hookworms
- Roundworms
- Whipworms
- Coccidia
- *Giardia lamblia* (sometimes difficult to diagnose)
- *Strongyloides*
- *Tritrichomonas*

Dietary Problems
- Poor-quality food or food poisoning
- Sudden dietary change (especially in young animals)
- Food intolerance or allergy

Acute Viral or Bacterial Enteritis
- Parvovirus (canine and feline)
- Coronavirus (canine and feline)
- *Clostridium perfringens*–associated enteritis
- Campylobacteriosis
- Salmonellosis
- *Escherichia coli*–associated enteritis (verotoxin-producing strains)

Intussusception

Intoxication
- Garbage
- Food poisoning
- Heavy metal
- Organophosphate

Hemorrhagic Gastroenteritis

From Willard M, Tvedten H: *Small Animal Clinical Diagnosis by Laboratory Methods*, ed 4. St. Louis, WB Saunders, 2004.

Diarrhea, Chronic Large Intestinal: Causes

Differential diagnosis list available on the companion online site at www.cote.clinicalvetadvisor.com.

Diarrhea, Neonatal

Differential diagnosis list available on the companion online site at www.cote.clinicalvetadvisor.com.

Diarrhea, Small Versus Large Intestine

Differential diagnosis list available on the companion online site at www.cote.clinicalvetadvisor.com.

Dilated Cardiomyopathy Differential Diagnosis: Myocardial Failure

Differential diagnosis list available on the companion online site at www.cote.clinicalvetadvisor.com.

Discolored Urine

Differential diagnosis list available on the companion online site at www.cote.clinicalvetadvisor.com.

Diskospondylitis: Microorganisms

Infectious Agents Associated with Diskospondylitis in Dogs and Cats

Dogs

Bacterial

Staphylococcus intermedius
Brucella canis
Nocardia
Actinomyces
Streptococcus canis
Escherichia coli
Alcaligenes
Micrococcus
Proteus
Mycobacterium
Corynebacterium

Fungal

Aspergillus terreus
Paecilomyces varioti
Fusarium
Mucor

Cats

S. canis
Actinomyces
E. coli

Modified from Greene C: *Infectious Diseases of the Dog and Cat*, ed 2. St. Louis, WB Saunders, 1999.

Disseminated Intravascular Coagulation

Conditions

Intravascular Hemolysis
Hemolytic transfusion reaction
Hemolytic anemia

Septicemia
Gram-negative bacteria (endotoxin)
Gram-positive bacteria (bacterial coat mucopolysaccharide)

Viremia

Parasitic Infections
Protozoal infection
Metazoal infection

Obstetric Complications

Miscellaneous
Gastric dilatation-volvulus
Diabetes mellitus

Neoplasia

Massive Tissue Injury
Burns
Trauma
Surgical procedures
Heatstroke

Venoms and Toxins
Snakebites
Insect stings
Aflatoxin

Hepatic Disease

Pancreatitis

From Bonagura J: *Kirk's Current Veterinary Therapy XIII*, ed 13. St. Louis, WB Saunders, 2000.

Dysphagia

Causes

Anatomic or Mechanical Lesions
Pharyngeal inflammation (e.g., abscess, inflammatory polyps, oral eosinophilic granulomas)
Foreign body obstruction (oral, pharyngeal, nasopharyngeal, proximal esophagus)
Neoplasia
Retropharyngeal lymphadenomegaly
Sialocele
Mandibular fracture
Lingual frenulum disorder
Cricopharyngeal achalasia or asynchrony
TMJ disorder (e.g., luxation, fracture)
Cleft palate
Pharyngeal trauma

Pain
Stomatitis/glossitis/pharyngitis (FIV, FeLV, immune-mediated disease, uremic glossitis, ingestion of a caustic substance)
Tooth-related problems (tooth root abscess, fracture, periodontitis)
Trauma
Electric cord burns
Retrobulbar abscess

Neuromuscular Disorders
Myasthenia gravis (focalized or generalized)
Acute polyradiculoneuritis
Masticatory myositis
Tick paralysis
Botulism
Polymyositis
TMJ disease

Neurologic Disorders
Rabies
Trigeminal paralysis or neuritis
Neuropathies of CN VII, IX, X, or XII
CNS disease (brainstem lesion)

From Ettinger S, Feldman E: *Textbook of Veterinary Internal Medicine*, ed 6. St. Louis, WB Saunders, 2005.
CN, cranial nerve; CNS, central nervous system; FIV, feline immunodeficiency virus; FeLV, feline leukemia virus; TMJ, temporomandibular joint.

DIFFERENTIAL DIAGNOSIS

Dyspnea

Causes

Upper Airway Disorders
Nasal cavity*
- Stenotic nares
- Obstruction (infection, inflammation, neoplasia, trauma, bleeding disorders)

Pharynx, larynx
- Elongated or edematous soft palate
- Pharyngeal polyp (cat)
- Laryngeal edema, collapse, foreign body, inflammation, trauma, paralysis, spasm, neoplasia, vocal fold webbing
- Everted laryngeal saccules

Cervical trachea
- Collapse, stenosis
- Trauma, foreign body
- Neoplasia, osteochondral dysplasia
- Parasites (*Oslerus osleri*)

Lower Airway Disorders
Thoracic trachea (see Cervical Trachea, above)
- Extraluminal compression (lymphadenopathy, heart-based tumors, enlarged left atrium)

Bronchial disease (allergic, infectious, parasitic, chronic obstructive pulmonary disease)

Pulmonary Parenchymal Disorders
Edema (cardiogenic, noncardiogenic)
Pneumonia (infectious, parasitic, inhalation)
Neoplasia
Allergy (allergic pneumonitis, including heartworm; eosinophilic granuloma; pulmonary infiltrates with eosinophils)
Embolism (dirofilariasis, hyperadrenocorticism, disseminated intravascular coagulation)
Trauma, bleeding disorders

Pleural/Body Wall Disorders
Pneumothorax
Pleural effusion
Congenital body wall disorders (pectus excavatum)
Thoracic wall trauma
Thoracic wall neoplasia
Thoracic wall paralysis
Diaphragmatic hernia (congenital, acquired)

Mediastinal Disorders
Infection
Trauma, including pneumomediastinum
Neoplasia

Peritoneal Cavity Disorders
Organomegaly, obesity
Effusion
Gastric torsion/dilatation-volvulus

Hemoglobin Disorders
Anemia
Methemoglobinemia
Cyanosis

Miscellaneous
Central nervous system (brain, spinal cord)
Peripheral nerve, neuromuscular, muscular
Metabolic (acidemia; severe hypokalemia in cats)
Anxiety
- Fear
- Pain

From Ettinger S, Feldman E: *Textbook of Veterinary Internal Medicine*, ed 5. St. Louis, WB Saunders, 2000.
*Only if the animal does not mouth-breathe.

Dystocia: Causes

Differential diagnosis list available on the companion online site at www.cote.clinicalvetadvisor.com.

Dystocia Versus Other Periparturient Phenomena

Differential diagnosis list available on the companion online site at www.cote.clinicalvetadvisor.com.

Edema

Differential diagnosis list available on the companion online site at www.cote.clinicalvetadvisor.com.

Effusions

Differential diagnosis list available on the companion online site at www.cote.clinicalvetadvisor.com.

Effusions, Bicavitary

Conditions Associated with Bicavitary Effusions

Cardiovascular conditions
  Pericardial effusion of any cause (neoplastic, idiopathic, toxic [anticoagulant], other) causing cardiac tamponade
  Constrictive pericardial disease
  Right-sided congestive failure: dilated cardiomyopathy, tricuspid regurgitation of any cause (tricuspid dysplasia, myxomatous tricuspid valve disease/endocardiosis, other), severe pulmonic stenosis, or pulmonale or any cause (heartworm disease/caval syndrome, idiopathic pulmonary hypertension, other)
  Right ventricular thromboembolism
  Caudal vena cava thromboembolism
Congenital obstruction: caudal vena cava
Hypoalbuminemia: protein-losing nephropathy, protein-losing enteropathy, advanced hepatic disease, pancreatitis, extensive burns
Bile peritonitis
Vasculitis (e.g., FIP)
Neoplastic conditions
  Right atrial fibroma
  Metastatic adenocarcinoma
  Lymphoma
  Hemangiosarcoma
  Mesothelioma
  Cholangiocellular carcinoma
  Chemodectoma
  Prostatic adenocarcinoma
  Diffuse carcinomatosis

Modified from Willard M, Tvedten H: *Small Animal Clinical Diagnosis by Laboratory Methods*, ed 4. St. Louis, WB Saunders, 2004.
"Bicavitary" is defined here as concurrent pleural effusion and ascites.
FIP, feline infectious peritonitis.

Electrocardiogram (ECG) Abnormalities

COMMON ASSOCIATIONS

Baseline

1. Sawtooth: atrial flutter versus artifact (panting, purring, electrical interference).

P waves

1. Tall (>0.4 mV [dog], >0.2 mV [cat]): *P pulmonale*. Rule out right atrial enlargement. Tall P waves are normal if R-R interval is short (i.e., normal during sinus tachycardia), but P wave height should normalize when heart rate slows.
2. Wide (>0.05 sec [dog], >0.04 sec [cat]): *P mitrale*. Rule out left atrial enlargement.
3. Cyclical increase and decrease in P wave amplitude: wandering pacemaker.
4. Absent: isoelectric to that lead (P waves are present but visible only in other leads), atrial standstill due to hyperkalemia, atrial standstill due to atrial myocardial disorder (rare), atrial fibrillation (fine, wavy baseline and irregularly irregular R-R interval must be present also).

PR Association

1. Long PR interval (>0.13 sec [dog], >0.09 sec [cat]): first-degree atrioventricular (AV) block.
2. Progressive lengthening of PR interval until longest one is followed by P wave without QRS complex: second-degree AV block, Mobitz type I.
3. Two or more consecutive P waves without QRS complexes, then a P wave triggers a QRS complex: second-degree AV block, Mobitz type II.
4. P waves and QRS complexes occur independently: third-degree AV block (normal or high atrial [P wave] rate, ventricular escape rhythm [wide, bizarre QRS complexes] slower than atrial rate) or ventricular tachycardia (wide, bizarre QRS complexes occur at a faster rate than P waves, which are often buried within the QRS complexes).
5. Short PR interval (<0.06 sec [dog[, <0.05 sec [cat]): preexcitation/Wolff-Parkinson-White syndrome (PR interval is short at any heart rate) or sinus tachycardia (PR interval normally shortens as heart rate increases).

QRS Complexes

1. Wide (>0.06 sec [dogs], >0.04 sec [cats]): diagnostic of left bundle branch block. Strongly suggests left ventricular enlargement; also occurs with severe hyperkalemia, quinidine toxicity.
2. Small (short): rule out hypothyroidism, pericardial effusion, pleural effusion, ascites, obesity, pneumothorax, intrathoracic mass, hypothermia (dogs); rule out normal (cats).

(*Continued*)

Q Waves (Lead II)
1. Deep: generally normal, especially in young, large breed dogs; has been loosely associated with interventricular septal hypertrophy in dogs.

R Waves (Lead II)
1. Tall (>2.5 mV [dogs that are small or medium breeds], >3.0 mV [dogs that are large breeds], >0.9 mV [cats]): left ventricular enlargement.

S Waves (Lead II)
1. Deep: rule out right ventricular enlargement.
2. $S_1S_2S_3$ (S wave present in leads I, II, and III): strongly suggests right ventricular enlargement.

ST Segment
1. Elevation (>0.15 mV [dog], any [cat]) or depression (>0.2 mV [dog], any [cat]): myocardial hypoxia, electrolyte disturbances.
2. Slurring/coving: myocardial hypoxia.

T Waves
1. Tall (>1 mV or >1/4 of height of R wave [dog]; >0.3 mV [cats]): commonly normal. If onset of tall T waves is noted during ECG monitoring over time: rule out hyperkalemia, myocardial hypoxia, movement artifact (change in limb position).
2. Different from rest of T waves: indicates abnormal repolarization, which in turn suggests abnormal ventricular depolarization of that heartbeat (e.g., premature ventricular complex).

Widespread availability of echocardiography has demonstrated that ECG is of limited accuracy for inferring cardiac structure. Indications of abnormal cardiac chamber size based on ECG features should be considered tentative and are best assessed using echocardiography.

Endocarditis

Differential diagnosis list available on the companion online site at www.cote.clinicalvetadvisor.com.

Enteropathies: Breed-Related

Differential diagnosis list available on the companion online site at www.cote.clinicalvetadvisor.com.

Eosinophilia

Potential Causes of Eosinophilia in Dogs and Cats
Parasitism
Heartworm disease
GI
Dermatologic
Other
Asthma
Nonparasitic dermatologic disease
Mast cell tumor
Hypoadrenocorticism (Addison's disease)
Uterine disease
Eosinophilic myositis
Eosinophilic pneumonitis/rhinitis/conjunctivitis
Eosinophilic enterocolitis (allergic colitis)
Eosinophilic leukemia
Eosinophilic granuloma complex
Eosinophilic vasculitis
Drug reaction

From Feldman E, Nelson R: Canine and Feline Endocrinology and Reproduction, ed 3. St. Louis, WB Saunders, 2004.GI, gastrointestinal.

Feline Leukemia Virus and Feline Immunodeficiency Virus

Associated Diseases
Immunosuppression with opportunistic infections
Gingivitis/stomatitis (FIV>FeLV)
Myeloproliferative disease/erythroleukemia (FeLV>>FIV)
Lymphosarcoma/lymphoid leukemias (FeLV>>FIV)
Diarrhea/panleukopenia-like syndrome
Weight loss/cachexia
Chronic fever
Glomerulonephritis
Anterior uveitis/pars planitis/glaucoma (FIV>>FeLV)
Behavioral changes/dementia/peripheral neuropathies
Hypergammaglobulinemia (FIV>FeLV)
Hemolytic anemias/aplastic anemias (FeLV>>FIV)
Lymphopenia/neutropenia
Thrombocytopenia (FeLV>>FIV)
Abortion/fetal resorptions/thymic atrophy (FeLV>>FIV)
Chronic progressive polyarthritis

From Ettinger S, Feldman E: *Textbook of Veterinary Internal Medicine*, ed 5. St. Louis, WB Saunders, 2000.
FeLV, feline leukemia virus; FIV, feline immunodeficiency virus.

Fever of Unknown Origin

Associated Conditions

Systemic Infections

Dogs

Bacterial endocarditis, bacteremias from an inapparent focus (e.g., secondary to persistent neutropenia or a congenital/acquired immunodeficiency syndrome); Lyme borreliosis (acute); leptospirosis; brucellosis infection; mycobacterial infections; rickettsial disease (e.g., ehrlichiosis, RMSF, haemobartonellosis); protozoal infections (e.g., babesiosis, leishmaniasis, disseminated toxoplasmosis, neosporosis); disseminated mycotic infections (e.g., histoplasmosis, blastomycosis, cryptococcosis, coccidioidomycosis, aspergillosis)

Cats

FIV infection; FeLV infection; feline infectious anemia (*Haemobartonella felis*); feline infectious peritonitis; bacteremias from an inapparent focus; systemic mycoses (e.g., histoplasmosis, cryptococcosis); mycobacterial infections (often atypical); atypical calicivirus infection

Localized Infections

Dogs

Bacterial endocarditis; urogenital infections (e.g., pyelonephritis, chronic prostatitis/prostatic abscess, stump pyometra); pyothorax and lung infections (e.g., inhaled pulmonary foreign bodies/pulmonary abscess, bronchopneumonia); occult hepatic abscess or cholangitis; localized peritonitis; diskospondylitis; juvenile metaphyseal osteomyelitis; retrobulbar or tooth root abscess; oropharyngeal stick injuries, septic thrombi

Cats

Pyothorax and lung infections (e.g., pulmonary abscess, bronchopneumonia), upper respiratory infections; occult hepatic abscess or cholangiohepatitis; urogenital infections (e.g., pyelonephritis); localized peritonitis; osteomyelitis; cat bite abscess/cellulitis

Immune-Mediated Diseases

Dogs

SLE; immune-mediated polyarthropathies: rheumatoid arthritis (erosive); nonerosive, nonseptic polyarthritis; idiopathic diseases; polyarthritis-meningitis complex (weimaraner, Newfoundland, German shorthaired pointer, boxer, beagle); polyarthritis-polymyositis complex (spaniel breeds); polyarthritis of Akitas; polyarthritis and amyloidosis of the Chinese shar-pei (shar-pei hock); polyarteritis nodosa; autoimmune hemolytic anemia and immune-mediated thrombocytopenia; steroid-responsive meningitis; immunodeficiency syndromes

Cats

SLE (rare in cats); chronic progressive polyarthropathy, including the ankylosing (periosteal proliferative) and luxating (erosive) forms; autoimmune hemolytic anemia (rare; may be FeLV associated); immune-mediated thrombocytopenia (rare; may be FeLV associated)

Neoplasia

Dogs

Solid neoplasms (especially those that are necrotic, elicit an inflammatory response, or have widespread metastases); lymphoproliferative or myeloproliferative disease

Cats

FeLV-related lymphoproliferative and myeloproliferative disorders

Miscellaneous

Dogs

Metaphyseal osteopathy, panosteitis; inflammatory-granulomatous bowel disease; liver disease (e.g., hepatic necrosis, cirrhosis, portosystemic shunts); pulmonary emboli; nodular panniculitis; drug reactions (tetracyclines, penicillin, sulfonamides, amphotericin B, quinidine)

Cats

Pansteatitis (cats on fish-rich diets); hypervitaminosis A; drug reactions (e.g., tetracycline, levamisole)

With permission from Greene C: Table 96–3: Conditions associated with fevers of unknown origin. In Greene C (ed): *Infectious Diseases of the Dog and Cat*, ed 2. St. Louis, WB Saunders, 1999, p 696.

FIV, feline immunodeficiency virus; FeLV, feline leukemia virus; SLE, systemic lupus erythematosus; RMSF, Rocky Mountain spotted fever.

DIFFERENTIAL DIAGNOSIS

Gastric Outflow Obstruction

Differential diagnosis list available on the companion online site at www.cote.clinicalvetadvisor.com.

Gastrointestinal Endocrine Diseases

Differential diagnosis list available on the companion online site at www.cote.clinicalvetadvisor.com.

Gastrointestinal Ulceration

Conditions and Drugs Associated with GI Ulceration in Small Animals

Impaired Mucosal Defense
- Drugs
  - NSAIDs*
  - Corticosteroids
- Stress
  - Shock
  - Sepsis
  - Trauma
  - Major surgery
- Neurologic disease
  - Head trauma
  - Intervertebral disk disease†
- Metabolic disorders
  - Liver disease
  - Renal disease
  - Pancreatitis
- Inflammatory bowel disease
- GI neoplasia
- Mastocytosis
- Gastric motility disorders

Hyperacidity
- Gastrinoma
- Mastocytosis

From Bonagura J: *Kirk's Current Veterinary Therapy XII: Small Animal Practice*, ed 12. St. Louis, WB Saunders, 1995.

*NSAIDs that have been associated with GI ulcers in small animals include aspirin, indomethacin, phenylbutazone, flunixin, ibuprofen, meloxicam, naproxen, and piroxicam.

†Treated with corticosteroids.

NSAIDs, nonsteroidal anti-inflammatory drugs; GI, gastrointestinal.

Glomerular Diseases, Cats

Associated Diseases Reported in Cats

Systemic Disease (Glomerular Disease)
- Infectious
  - Bacterial
    - Chronic bacterial infections (G)
    - Mycoplasmal polyarthritis (G)
  - Viral
    - FIV (G)
    - FIP (MN)
    - FeLV (G, MN)
- Inflammatory
  - Pancreatitis (G)
  - Cholangiohepatitis (G)
  - Chronic progressive polyarthritis (G)
  - SLE (MN)
  - Other immune-mediated diseases (G)
- Neoplastic
  - Leukemia (MN)
  - Lymphosarcoma (MN)
  - Mastocytosis (G)
  - Other neoplasms (G)
- Miscellaneous
  - Acromegaly (?)
  - Mercury toxicity (MN)
- Familial (MN)
- Idiopathic (MN)

From Ettinger S, Feldman E: *Textbook of Veterinary Internal Medicine*, ed 6. St. Louis, WB Saunders, 2005.

FeLV, feline leukemia virus; FIP, feline infectious peritonitis; FIV, feline immunodeficiency virus; G, glomerulonephritis, uncharacterized; MN, membranous nephropathy; SLE, systemic lupus erythematosus; ?, uncertain association.

Glomerulonephritis, Dogs

Associated Diseases Reported in Dogs

Systemic Disease (Glomerular Disease)
- Infectious
  - Bacterial
    - Bartonellosis (G)
    - Brucellosis (G)
    - Endocarditis (G)
    - Pyometra (A,G)
    - Pyoderma (A,G)
    - Other chronic bacterial infections (A,G)
  - Protozoal
    - Babesiosis (MPGN)
    - Hepatozoonosis (G)
    - Leishmaniasis (A, MN, P-E and P-M)
    - Trypanosomiasis (G)
  - Rickettsial
    - Ehrlichiosis (G)
  - Viral
    - Canine adenovirus type 1 (P-M)
  - Parasitic
    - Dirofilariasis (A, MN)
  - Fungal
    - Coccidioidomycosis (A,G)
- Inflammatory
  - Chronic dermatitis (A,G)
  - Inflammatory bowel disease (G)
  - Pancreatitis (A,G)
  - Periodontal disease (A,G)
  - Polyarthritis (A,G)
  - SLE (A, MN, P-E and P-M)
  - Other immune-mediated diseases (G)
- Neoplastic
  - Leukemia (G)
  - Lymphosarcoma (A,G)
  - Mastocytosis (G)
  - Primary erythrocytosis (MCD?)
  - Systemic histiocytosis (G)
  - Other neoplasms (A, G, MN)
- Miscellaneous
  - Corticosteroid excess (G)
  - Trimethoprim-sulfatherapy (G)
  - Hyperlipidemia (?)
  - Congenital C3 deficiency
- Familial
- Idiopathic (A, G, MN, MCD, P-E or M)

Modified from Ettinger S, Feldman E: *Textbook of Veterinary Internal Medicine*, ed 6. St. Louis, WB Saunders, 2005.

A, amyloidosis; G, glomerulonephritis, uncharacterized; MN, membranous nephropathy; MCD, minimal change disease; P, proliferative (E, endocapillary; M, mesangial); SLE, systemic lupus erythematosus; MPGN, membranoproliferative (mesangiocapillary) glomerulonephritis; ?, association uncertain.

Glucosuria

Causes in Dogs and Cats

Blood glucose concentration exceeding renal threshold	Diabetes mellitus Stress (especially in cats) Infusion of dextrose-containing fluids Hyperadrenocorticism (rarely causes glucose >180 mg/dl) Pheochromocytoma (rare)
Abnormal proximal renal tubular function	Aminoglycoside toxicity Acute renal failure Fanconi syndrome Primary renal glucosuria
Contamination	Urinary hemorrhage in an animal with mild hyperglycemia

From Willard M, Tvedten H: Small Animal Clinical Diagnosis by Laboratory Methods, ed 4. St. Louis, WB Saunders, 2004.

Halitosis

Causes

Oral Diseases
Periodontal disease (gingivitis, periodontitis, abscessation)
Neoplasia (melanoma, fibrosarcoma, SCC)
Foreign body or trauma (fractures, electrical cord injury)
Pharyngitis
Stomatitis, lymphocytic-plasmacytic feline stomatitis

Respiratory Diseases
Rhinitis and/or sinusitis
Neoplasia
Pneumonia or pulmonary abscess

Dermatologic Diseases
Lip fold pyoderma
Ulcerative mucocutaneous pyoderma
Feline or canine eosinophilic granulomas
Pemphigus complex, bullous pemphigoid, systemic lupus erythematosus
Drug eruptions
Cutaneous lymphoma
Exposure to DMSO

Metabolic Diseases
Renal failure/uremia
Diabetic ketoacidosis

GI Diseases
Megaesophagus
Inflammatory bowel disease
Exocrine pancreatic insufficiency
Neoplasia
Constipation

Dietary
Aromatic foods (onions, garlic)
Fetid foodstuffs (e.g., ingestion of carrion)
Coprophagy

Grooming Behavior
Anal sacculitis
Vaginitis/balanoposthitis
Lower UTI

Adapted from *Veterinary Guide to Odor and Disease: The Oral Cavity and Dermatology*. Veterinary Learning Systems, 1997.
DMSO, dimethyl sulfoxide; GI, gastrointestinal; SCC, squamous cell carcinoma; UTI, urinary tract infection.

Heart Murmurs

Characteristics and Clinical Signs Associated with "Innocent" Murmurs Versus Murmurs Associated with CHD

Innocent Murmur
Grade usually <III/VI
Systolic
PMI: usually left base
Murmur characteristics may change with animal position
Murmur intensity may increase or decrease with increasing heart rate
Decreased intensity with age
Inaudible after ~16 weeks of age
Animal clinically normal

Congenital Heart Disease
Grade ≥III/VI
Any timing possible
PMI: any possible
Similar murmur characteristics in all body positions
Murmur intensity increases with increase in heart rate
Same or increasing intensity up to and beyond 16 weeks of age
Persists after ~16 weeks of age
Stunting, unthriftiness, cyanosis, or signs of heart failure may be present

Modified from Bonagura J: *Kirk's Current Veterinary Therapy XIII*, ed 13. St. Louis, WB Saunders, 2000.
CHD, congenital heart disease; PMI, point of maximal murmur intensity.

Heart Murmurs: Congenital Heart Defect-Associated

Differential diagnosis list available on the companion online site at www.cote.clinicalvetadvisor.com.

Heartworm: Clinical Severity

Differential diagnosis list available on the companion online site at www.cote.clinicalvetadvisor.com.

Heartworm: *Dirofilaria* Versus *Dipetalonema*

Differential diagnosis list available on the companion online site at www.cote.clinicalvetadvisor.com.

Heartworm Disease: Complications

Complications

Untreated
Eosinophilic granulomatosis
Eosinophilic pneumonitis
Right-sided congestive heart failure*
Hemoglobinuria, "pigment nephropathy"*
Hemolytic anemia*
Pulmonary thromboembolism

During or Shortly after Treatment Period
Acute (surgical removal):
Anaphylaxis
Hypotension
Cardiac arrest
Subacute (medical treatment):
Eosinophilic pneumonitis
Pain at injection site (melarsomine)
Pulmonary thromboembolism (possibly massive, especially if inadequate exercise restriction)
Sudden death (especially if inadequate exercise restriction)

*Together, comprise the "caval syndrome" of heartworm disease.

Hematochezia

Causes

Anal Disease
Perianal fistulas
Anal sacculitis or abscess
Stricture
Neoplasia (e.g., anal sac tumor)
Trauma (e.g., bite wound)
Perianal hernia
Foreign body

Rectum and Colon
Proctitis (inflammation of the rectal mucosa)
Colitis
- Idiopathic
- Inflammatory bowel disease
- Stress
- Infectious
  - *Campylobacter* spp.
  - *Clostridium perfringens*

Parvovirus
Parasitism
- Hookworms
- Whipworms
- Coccidia
- Roundworms

Neoplasia
- Rectal polyp
- Adenocarcinoma
- Lymphoma

Rectal prolapse
Mucosal trauma
- Movement of foreign material (e.g., hairballs)
- Iatrogenic (e.g., thermometers, enemas, fecal loops)

Automobile trauma
Ileocecocolic area: intussusception

Modified from Tams TR: Gastrointestinal symptoms. In *Handbook of Small Animal Gastroenterology*. Philadelphia, WB Saunders, 1996.
Constipation often can cause excessive straining, which can result in formed stools with blood on the surface.

Hematemesis

Bleeding Disorders
Disseminated intravascular coagulation
Anticoagulant rodenticide toxicity
Thrombocytopenia
Congenital or acquired coagulation factor deficiencies/defects

Heavy Metal Toxicity
Arsenic
Lead
Zinc

Infectious Disorders
GI parasitism
Viral gastroenteritis
Bacterial gastroenteritis

Perioperative Hemorrhage
Gastric-dilatation volvulus
Gastrectomy
Gastrostomy

Gastric/Duodenal Erosions/Ulcerations
Infiltrative disease
- Neoplasia
- Inflammatory bowel disease
- Phycomycosis

Metabolic disorders
- Renal disease
- Liver disease
- Hypoadrenocorticism

Stress erosions/ulcerations
- Burns (Curling's ulcer)
- Neurologic disorders
  - Head trauma (Cushing's ulcer)
  - Spinal cord disorders
- Sepsis/septic shock
- Hypovolemic shock
- Multiple trauma

Drug Administration
- Glucocorticoids
- NSAIDs
  - Aspirin
  - Indomethacin
  - Phenylbutazone
  - Naproxen
  - Sulindac
  - Ibuprofen
  - Flunixin meglumine
  - Meclofenamic acid
  - Piroxicam

Gastric/Duodenal Foreign Bodies

Neoplasia
- Mast cell tumor
- Gastrinoma (Zollinger-Ellison syndrome)
- Pancreatic polypeptide secreting tumor
- Basophilic leukemia

Hemorrhagic Gastroenteritis

Esophageal Disorders
Esophagitis
Esophageal neoplasia
Esophageal foreign bodies

With permission from Kirk RW, Bonagura JD, eds: *Kirk's Current Veterinary Therapy XI: Small Animal Practice*. St. Louis, WB Saunders, 1992, p 133.
GI, gastrointestinal; NSAIDs, nonsteroidal anti-inflammatory drugs.

Hematuria

Causes
Urinary Tract Origin (Kidneys, Ureters, Bladder, Urethra)
Trauma
Traumatic collection (e.g., catheter, cystocentesis)
Renal biopsy
Blunt trauma (e.g., automobile accident)
Urolithiasis
Neoplasia
Inflammatory disease
Urinary tract infection
Feline urologic syndrome (idiopathic feline lower urinary tract disease)
Chemically induced inflammation (e.g., cyclophosphamide-induced cystitis)
Parasites
Dioctophyma renale
Capillaria plica
Bleeding disorder
Warfarin intoxication
Disseminated intravascular coagulation
Thrombocytopenia
Renal infarction
Renal pelvic hematoma
Vascular malformation
Renal telangiectasia (Welsh corgi)
Idiopathic renal hematuria
Genital Tract Contamination (Prostate, Prepuce, Vagina)
Estrus
Inflammatory, neoplastic, and traumatic lesions of the genital tract

From Ettinger S, Feldman E: *Textbook of Veterinary Internal Medicine*, ed 6. St. Louis, WB Saunders, 2005.

Hemolytic Anemia: Suspected or Documented Causes

Selected Substances Documented or Suspected to Cause Hemolytic Anemia
Acetaminophen (especially cats)
Benzocaine (especially cats)
Cephalosporins
Dapsone
Methylene blue (especially cats)
Nitrofurantoin
Onions
Penicillins
Phenacetin (especially cats)
Phenazopyridine
Phenylbutazone
Sulfonamides
Vaccinations
Vitamin K_3 (cats)
Zinc

From Willard M, Tvedten H: *Small Animal Clinical Diagnosis by Laboratory Methods*, ed 4. St. Louis, WB Saunders, 2004.

These substances do not always cause anemia, but they have the potential and should be withdrawn, if possible, in animals with hemolytic anemia.

Hemoptysis

Causes
Pulmonary
Pulmonary thromboembolism: secondary to neoplastic, endocrine, cardiac, metabolic disease
Pulmonary hypertension: secondary to heartworm disease; congenital or acquired cardiac defects that result in shunting of blood
Chronic bronchitis/bronchiectasis
Bacterial pneumonia
Nocardiosis
Pulmonary abscess
Kennel cough (rare)
Fungal pneumonia: blastomycosis, histoplasmosis, coccidioidomycosis
Parasites: *Paragonimus kellicotti*, *Capillaria aerophila*, *Aelurostrongylus abstrusus*
Pulmonary infiltrate with eosinophils
Neoplasia, lung: primary adenocarcinoma, undifferentiated carcinoma, SCC, chondrosarcoma; metastatic; primary tracheal tumors
Lung lobe torsion
Cardiovascular
Heartworm disease
Cardiogenic pulmonary edema
Arteriovenous fistula
Bacterial endocarditis
Systemic
Coagulopathies: primary (quantitative or qualitative platelet defects) or secondary hemostatic (factor deficiencies, anticoagulant rodenticide toxicity, DIC) abnormalities
Trauma: pulmonary contusion, tracheal rupture, FB
Iatrogenic: endotracheal intubation; complication of lung biopsy/aspirate, transtracheal wash, or bronchoscopy

From Ettinger S, Feldman E: *Textbook of Veterinary Internal Medicine*, ed 6. St. Louis, WB Saunders, 2005.

FB, foreign body; DIC, disseminated intravascular coagulopathy; SCC, squamous cell carcinoma.

Hemothorax

Causes of Hemothorax and Sanguineous Effusions

- Trauma
- Malignancy
- Coagulopathy
- Diaphragmatic hernia
- Lung lobe torsion
- Pulmonary infarction
- Pulmonary abscessation
- Recent surgery
- Aortic aneurysm
- Swan-Ganz catheter placement*
- Tube thoracostomy*
- Hemopneumothorax*
- Costal exostosis*
- Endometriosis*
- Foreign body
- Heartworm disease
- Central venous catheter placement

Modified with permission from King L: *Textbook of Respiratory Disease in Dogs and Cats*. St. Louis, WB Saunders, 2004, p 611.

*Reported only in human literature.

Hepatic Failure, Acute

Clinically Relevant Causes

Category of Injury	Examples
Trauma	Automobile accident High-rise syndrome
Toxin	**Environmental Agents:** Aflatoxin *Amanita pantherina, phalloides* Cycadaceae Heavy metals **Therapeutic Agents:** Thiacetarsemide Mebendazole Diethylcarbamazine-oxibendazole Acetaminophen Methoxyflurane, halothane Diethylcarbamazine Tetracycline Trimethoprim-sulfadiazine Griseofulvin Diazepam (cats)
Infectious agents	Infectious canine hepatitis Leptospirosis Toxoplasmosis Vena cava syndrome Bacterial sepsis
Thermal	Heatstroke
Extension of abdominal inflammation	Pancreatitis Peritonitis Inflammatory bowel disease
Metabolic disorder	Lipidosis (cats)

From Ettinger S, Feldman E: *Textbook of Veterinary Internal Medicine*, ed 4. St. Louis, WB Saunders, 1994.

Hepatic Fibrosis

Causes in Dogs

Chronic hepatitis
- Hepatic copper accumulation
  - Primary (Bedlington terriers, West Highland white terriers)
  - Secondary (Doberman pinschers, Skye terriers)
- Infectious
- Drug-induced
  - Primidone
- Metabolic
  - α-Antitrypsin deficiency
- Others
  - Lobular dissecting hepatitis
  - Idiopathic chronic hepatitis

Toxins, chemicals
- Pyrrolizidine alkaloids, CCl_4

Postnecrotic fibrosis
Chronic congestive heart failure
Chronic cholangiohepatitis
Chronic biliary obstruction
Idiopathic hepatic fibrosis
- Perivenous
- Diffuse pericellular
- Periportal

From Bonagura J: *Kirk's Current Veterinary Therapy XIII*, ed 13. St. Louis, WB Saunders, 2000.

Hepatic Infections and Abscesses

Bacteria Isolated from Hepatobiliary Suppurative Inflammation and Abscesses

Aerobic Cultures (Positive Cultures: *n* = 54)

***n* ≥3 each**
Escherichia coli
Staphylococcus intermedius
S. aureus
S. epidermidis
Streptococcus group D *enterococci*
Streptococcus β-hemolytic
Enterococcus
Enterobacter aerogenes
E. agglomerans
Pseudomonas aeruginosa

***n* = 1 each**
Pseudomonas fluorescens
Klebsiella pneumoniae
Bacillus spp.
Acinetobacter calcoacetics
Citrobacter freundii
Moraxella phenylpyruvica
Pasteurella multocida
Bordetella bronchiseptica
Nocardia
Salmonella
Campylobacter jejuni

Anaerobic Cultures (Positive Cultures: *n* = 26)
Propionibacterium acnes
Clostridium perfringens
Clostridium
Bacteroides melaninogenicus
Corynebacterium spp.
Actinomyces
Peptostreptococcus
Fusobacterium
Anaerobic streptococci

Additional Microbes Reported Elsewhere
Bacillus piliformis
Corynebacterium spp.
Proteus spp.
Francisella tularensis
Listeria monocytogenes
Eugenic fermenter-4 bacilli

With permission from Greene C: *Infectious Diseases of the Dog and Cat*, ed 2. St. Louis, WB Saunders, 1999, p 616.
In order from most to least common. Data acquired from case records, Companion Animal Hospital, College of Veterinary Medicine, Cornell University, Ithaca, NY, 1985–1996.

Hepatic Neoplasia

Dogs
***Primary Hepatic Tumors (26%)**
Hepatocellular carcinoma
Hepatocellular adenoma
Hepatic hemangiosarcoma
Biliary carcinoma
Other
Leiomyosarcoma
Liposarcoma
Myxosarcoma
Fibrosarcoma
Biliary adenoma
Hepatic carcinoid
Hemolymphatic Neoplasia (28%)
Lymphosarcoma
MCT
Plasma cell tumor
Metastatic Neoplasia (46%)

Cats
***Primary Hepatic Tumors (20%)**
Biliary carcinoma
Hepatocellular carcinoma
Hepatic hemangiosarcoma
Other
Biliary cystadenoma
Myelolipoma
Hepatic carcinoid
Hemolymphatic Neoplasia (60%)
Lymphosarcoma
MCT
Plasma cell tumor
Metastatic Neoplasia (20%)

From Ettinger S, Feldman E: *Textbook of Veterinary Internal Medicine*, ed 6. St. Louis, WB Saunders, 2005.
*Primary tumors: in order of prevalence.
MCT, mast cell tumor.

Hepatopathy, Vacuolar

Differential Diagnoses for Canine Vacuolar Hepatopathy

Hyperadrenocorticism
Spontaneous disease
Pituitary or adrenal origin
Iatrogenic, glucocorticoids therapy:
PO, IM, SQ, topical (skin, eye, ear)

Adrenal Hyperplasia Syndrome
Abnormal sex hormone production (aberrant adrenocortical disease)

Hepatocutaneous Syndrome

Chronic Stress
Illness > 4 weeks

Severe Dental Disease
Infection

Chronic Infections or Inflammation
Pyelonephritis, chronic dermatitis (examples)

Inflammatory Bowel Disease (IBD)
Lymphoplasmacytic
Eosinophilic

Neoplasia
Lymphoma, other

Disorders Influencing Lipid Metabolism
Diabetes mellitus
Idiopathic hyperlipidemia (e.g., schnauzer, sheltie, other)

Pancreatitis, Chronic

Hypothyroidism, Severe

Congestive Heart Failure (CHF)

From Ettinger S, Feldman E: *Textbook of Veterinary Internal Medicine*, ed 6. St. Louis, WB Saunders, 2005.

Hepatotoxins

Differential diagnosis list available on the companion online site at www.cote.clinicalvetadvisor.com.

Horner's Syndrome

Summary of Lesions

Location	Lesion	Associated Neurologic Deficit
Cervical spinal cord	External injury	Tetraplegia-spastic, dyspnea
	Focal leukomyelomalacia, embolic infarct, disk compression	Hemiplegia-ipsilateral, spastic
T1–T3 spinal cord	External injury	Pelvic and thoracic limb
	Neoplasm	Paresis or paralysis with lower motor neuron deficit in thoracic limbs and upper motor neuron deficit in pelvic limbs
	Focal poliomyelomalacia (embolic infarct)	
	Diffuse myelomalacia (ascending and descending)	Lower motor neuron deficit; analgesia of tail, anus, pelvic limbs, abdomen, and thorax with paretic thoracic limbs
T1–T3 ventral roots	Avulsion of roots of brachial plexus	Brachial plexus paresis or paralysis of the thoracic limb on the same side
Proximal spinal nerves	Lymphosarcoma	None if confined to the trunk
Cranial thoracic sympathetic trunk	Neurofibroma	
Cervical sympathetic trunk	Injury from surgical intervention in the area or from dog bites	None if unilateral; bilateral lesions interfere with laryngeal and esophageal function because of vagal involvement
Middle ear cavity (small animals)	Otitis media Neoplasia	Signs of peripheral vestibular disturbance; ipsilateral ataxia, head tilt, nystagmus, and sometimes facial palsy or hemifacial spasm
Retrobulbar	Contusion Neoplasia	Varies with degree of contusion to the optic and oculomotor nerves, which also influence pupillary size

From Delahunta A: *Veterinary Neuroanatomy and Clinical Neurology*. St. Louis, WB Saunders, 1983.

Hypercalcemia: Causes

Causes

Nonpathologic
- Nonfasting (minimal increase)
- Physiologic growth of young
- Laboratory error
- Spurious
  - Lipemia
  - Detergent contamination of sample or tube

Transient or Inconsequential
- Hemoconcentration
- Hyperproteinemia
- Hypoadrenocorticism
- Severe environmental hypothermia

Pathologic or Consequential—Persistent
- Associated with malignancy
  - Humoral hypercalcemia of malignancy
    - Lymphoma (common)
    - Anal sac apocrine gland adenocarcinoma (common)
    - Carcinoma (sporadic): lung, pancreas, skin, nasal cavity, thyroid, mammary gland, adrenal medulla
    - Thymoma (rare)
  - Hematologic malignancies (bone marrow osteolysis)
    - Lymphoma
    - Multiple myeloma
    - Myeloproliferative disease (rare)
    - Leukemia (rare)
  - Metastatic or primary bone neoplasia (very uncommon)
- Chronic renal failure
- Hypervitaminosis D
  - Iatrogenic
  - Plants (calcitriol glycosides)
  - Vitamin D_3 ointments
  - Rodenticide
- Granulomatous disease
  - Blastomycosis
  - Schistosomiasis
  - Dermatitis
- Primary hyperparathyroidism
  - Adenoma (common)
  - Adenocarcinoma (rare)
  - Hyperplasia (uncommon)
- Acute renal failure
- Skeletal lesions (nonmalignant, uncommon)
  - Osteomyelitis (bacterial or mycotic)
  - Hypertrophic osteodystrophy
  - Disuse osteoporosis (immobilization)
- Excessive calcium-containing intestinal phosphate binders
- Excessive calcium supplementation (calcium carbonate)
- Hypervitaminosis A
- Hypercalcemic conditions in human medicine
  - Milk-alkali syndrome (rare in dogs)
  - Thiazide diuretics
  - Acromegaly
  - Thyrotoxicosis
  - Postrenal transplantation
  - Aluminum exposure (dogs?)

From Dibartola S: *Fluid, Electrolyte, and Acid-Base Disorders in Small Animal Practice*. St. Louis, WB Saunders, 2006.

Hypercalcemia: Lab

Differential diagnosis list available on the companion online site at www.cote.clinicalvetadvisor.com.

Hypercapnia

Causes

Hypoventilation
- Neuromuscular disorder
- Medullary dysfunction (excessive depth of anesthesia; intracranial disease)
- Cervical disease or neuromuscular disease

Airway Obstruction
- Large airway obstruction (laryngeal paralysis; tracheal collapse)
- Small airway obstruction (chronic airway disease; bronchoconstriction)

Thoracic Wall Problems
- Open pneumothorax
- Flail chest
- Anterior displacement of the diaphragm by abdominal space filling disorders
- Pleural space filling disorder (air; fluid; diaphragmatic hernia)
- Pleural fibrosis

Pulmonary Parenchymal Disease (Late)

Inappropriate ventilator settings

Dead space rebreathing

Recent bicarbonate therapy (in ventilatory compromised animals)

Compensation for metabolic acidosis

Malignant hyperthermia

With permission from King L: *Textbook of Respiratory Disease in Dogs and Cats*. St. Louis, WB Saunders, 2004, p 184.

Definition of hypercapnia (synonym: hypercarbia): abnormally increased arterial carbon dioxide tension (e.g., in dogs: pCO_2 50 mmHg [venous], 44 mmHG [arterial]; in cats: pCO_2 45 mmHg [venous], 32 mmHg [arterial]).

Hyperchloremia

Causes of Corrected Hyperchloremia

Pseudohyperchloremia
- Lipemic samples (colorimetric methods)
- Potassium bromide therapy

Excessive Loss of Sodium Relative to Chloride
- Diarrhea

Excessive Gain of Chloride Relative to Sodium
- Therapy with chloride salts (NH_4Cl, KCl)
- Total parenteral nutrition
- Fluid therapy (e.g., 0.9% NaCl, hypertonic saline, KCl-supplemented fluids)
- Salt poisoning

Renal Chloride Retention
- Renal failure
- Renal tubular acidosis
- Hypoadrenocorticism*
- Diabetes mellitus*
- Chronic respiratory alkalosis
- Drug-induced: acetazolamide, spironolactone

Adapted from de Morais: Chloride ion in small animal practice: The forgotten ion. *J Vet Emerg Crit Care* 2:11–24, 1992.

*May be associated with corrected hypochloremia in cats.

Hyperglobulinemia

Causes

Polyclonal
- Infections
  - Bacterial*†
    - Brucellosis
    - Pyoderma
    - Bacterial endocarditis
  - Viral
    - FIP‡
    - FIV
    - FeLV
  - Fungal*†
    - Systemic fungal infections (e.g., blastomycosis, histoplasmosis, coccidioidomycosis)
  - Rickettsial†‡
    - Ehrlichiosis
  - Parasitic
    - Dirofilariasis*†
    - Demodicosis
    - Scabies
  - Immune-mediated disease
    - Infections (immune complex)
      - Dirofilariasis*†
      - Feline cholangitis/cholangiohepatitis
      - Pyometra
    - SLE, including glomerulonephritis, IMHA, IMT, and polyarthritis*
    - IMHA, IMT (not because of SLE)*
    - Pemphigus complex, bullous pemphigoid*
    - Rheumatoid arthritis*
  - Neoplasia†‡

Monoclonal
- Infection
  - Ehrlichiosis†‡
  - Leishmaniasis†‡
  - FIP (rare)
  - Idiopathic†‡
  - Benign monoclonal gammopathy
- Neoplasia†‡
  - Multiple myeloma‡
  - Macroglobulinemia
  - Lymphosarcoma
  - Extramedullary plasmacytoma (rare)
- Miscellaneous
  - Cutaneous amyloidosis
  - Plasmacytic gastroenterocolitis*

From Willard M, Tvedten H: *Small Animal Clinical Diagnosis by Laboratory Methods* (4th ed). St. Louis, WB Saunders, 2004.
*Mild (4–5 g/dl).
† Moderate (5–6 g/dl).
‡ Severe (>6 g/dl).
Effect of age should be considered when assessing globulin value. FeLV, feline leukemia virus; FIP, feline infectious peritonitis; FIV, feline immunodeficiency virus; IMHA, immune-mediated hemolytic anemia; IMT, immune-mediated thrombocytopenia; SLE, systemic lupus erythematosus.

Hyperglycemia

Causes of Altered Blood Glucose in Dogs and Cats*

Hyperglycemia
- Diabetes mellitus*
- "Stress" (cat)*
- Postprandial
- Hyperadrenocorticism*
- Acromegaly (cat)
- Diestrus (bitch)
- Pheochromocytoma (dog)
- Pancreatitis
- Exocrine pancreatic neoplasia
- Renal insufficiency
- Drug therapy*
  - Glucocorticoids
  - Progestogens
  - Megestrol acetate
  - Thiazide diuretics
- Parenteral nutrition

*Modified from Willard M, Tvedten H: *Small Animal Clinical Diagnosis by Laboratory Methods*, ed 4. St. Louis, WB Saunders, 2004.

Hyperkalemia

Causes

Pseudohyperkalemia
Thrombocytosis
Hemolysis

Increased Intake
Unlikely to cause hyperkalemia in presence of normal renal function unless iatrogenic (e.g., continuous infusion of excessive amounts of potassium)

Translocation (ICF→ECF)
Acute mineral acidosis (e.g., HCl, NH_4Cl)
Insulin deficiency (e.g., diabetic ketoacidosis)
Acute tumor lysis syndrome
Reperfusion of extremities after aortic thromboembolism in cats with cardiomyopathy
Hyperkalemic periodic paralysis (one case report in a pit bull)
Drugs: nonspecific β-blockers (e.g., propranolol)*

Decreased Urinary Excretion
Urethral obstruction
Ruptured bladder
Anuric or oliguric renal failure
Hypoadrenocorticism
Selected GI disease (e.g., trichuriasis, salmonellosis, perforated duodenal ulcer)
Chylothorax with repeated pleural fluid drainage
Hyporeninemic hypoaldosteronism

Drugs
Angiotensin-converting enzyme inhibitors (e.g., captopril, enalapril)*
Potassium-sparing diuretics (e.g., spironolactone, amiloride, triamterene)*
Prostaglandin inhibitors (e.g., indomethacin)*
Heparin*
Other

Normal platelet clotting (need heparinized/green top tube sample to avoid artifactual hyperkalemia)

Modified from Dibartola S: *Fluid, Electrolyte and Acid-Base Disorders in Small Animal Practice*. St. Louis, Saunders, 2006.

*Likely to cause hyperkalemia only in conjunction with other contributing factors (e.g., decreased renal function, concurrent administration of potassium supplements); not well documented in veterinary medicine.

ECF, extracellular fluid; GI, gastrointestinal; ICF, intracellular fluid.

Hyperlipidemia

Diseases and Conditions That Cause Hypertriglyceridemia and Hypercholesterolemia*

Causes of Hypertriglyceridemia
Increased Triglyceride Production
By hepatocytes
By enterocytes:
Postprandial hyperlipidemia
Decreased Lipolysis or Intravascular Processing of Lipoproteins
Hypothyroidism
Nephrotic syndrome
Lipoprotein lipase deficiency (rare in cats, very rare in dogs)
Other, Unknown, or Multiple Mechanisms
Acute pancreatitis
Diabetes mellitus
High-lipid diet
Hyperadrenocorticism or excess glucocorticoids
Hyperlipidemia in a Brittany spaniel
Idiopathic hyperlipidemia of miniature schnauzers

Causes of Hypercholesterolemia
Increased Cholesterol Production
By hepatocytes:
Nephrotic syndrome or protein-losing nephropathy
By enterocytes:
Postprandial hyperlipidemia
Decreased Lipolysis or Intravascular Processing of Lipoproteins
Hypothyroidism
Nephrotic syndrome or protein-losing nephropathy
Lipoprotein lipase deficiency (very rare in dogs)
Other, Unknown, or Multiple Mechanisms
Acute pancreatitis
Cholestasis (obstructive)
Diabetes mellitus
Hyperadrenocorticism
Hypercholesterolemia in briards
Idiopathic hyperlipidemia of miniature schnauzers

*Data from Stockham FL, Scott MA: Lipids. In *Fundamentals of Veterinary Clinical Pathology*. Ames, IA, Iowa State Press, 2002, pp 521–537.

Hypernatremia

Causes

Pure Water Deficit
Primary hypodipsia (e.g., in miniature schnauzers)
Diabetes insipidus
- Central
- Nephrogenic

High environmental temperature
Fever
Inadequate access to water

Hypotonic Fluid Loss
Extrarenal
- GI
  - Vomiting
  - Diarrhea
  - Small intestinal obstruction
- Third-space loss
  - Peritonitis
  - Pancreatitis
- Cutaneous
  - Burns

Renal
- Osmotic diuresis
  - Diabetes mellitus
  - Mannitol infusion
- Chemical diuretics
- Chronic renal failure
- Nonoliguric acute renal failure
- Postobstructive diuresis

Impermeable Solute Gain
Salt poisoning
Hypertonic fluid administration
- Hypertonic saline
- Sodium bicarbonate
- Parenteral nutrition
- Sodium phosphate enema

Hyperaldosteronism
Hyperadrenocorticism

From DiBartola S: *Fluid, Electrolyte, and Acid-Base Disorders in Small Animal Practice.* St. Louis, WB Saunders, 2000.
GI, gastrointestinal.

Hyperphosphatemia

Causes

Maldistribution (Translocation)
- Tumor cell lysis
- Tissue trauma or rhabdomyolysis
- Hemolysis
- Metabolic acidosis

Increased Intake
- GI
  - Phosphate enemas
  - Vitamin D intoxication
- Parenteral
  - IV phosphate

Decreased Loss
- Acute or chronic renal failure
- Uroabdomen or urethral obstruction
- Hypoparathyroidism
- Acromegaly (?)*
- Hyperthyroidism

Physiologic: Young Growing Animal

Laboratory Error (e.g., lipemia, hyperproteinemia, depending on methodology)

From DiBartola S: *Fluid, Electrolyte, and Acid-Base Disorders in Small Animal Practice.* St. Louis, WB Saunders, 2000.
*(?) Importance in veterinary medicine uncertain.
GI, gastrointestinal.

Hypersensitivity

Types and Examples

Features: Type and Mechanism	Examples	Pathophysiology	Signs
Type I Immediate (anaphylactic)	Food allergy Atopy Insect bite hypersensitivity Adverse vaccine reaction Adverse drug reaction	Acute, systemic inflammation is triggered by IgE-mediated degranulation of mast cells and basophils; degranulation releases histamine, leukotrienes, interleukins, and other vasodilatory and inflammatory substances.	Urticaria (plaques of skin swelling) Angioedema (regional or diffuse cutaneous or visceral swelling) Pruritus If severe: hypotension and shock (dogs) or dyspnea (cats)
Type II Cytotoxic	Immune-mediated hemolytic anemia Immune-mediated thrombocytopenia Hypothyroidism (lymphocytic thyroiditis) Hemolytic reaction (incompatible transfusion donor-recipient match; neonatal isoerythrolysis) Pemphigus Adverse drug reaction	Antibody (IgM or IgG) binds to surface molecules (rightly or wrongly perceived as antigenic) on cells of body tissues. The antibody-tagged cells are destroyed by the mononuclear-phagocytic (reticuloendothelial) system.	Signs depend on body tissue cells involved. Examples include hemolysis and cutaneous lesions.
Type III Immune-complex mediated	Systemic lupus erythematosus Rheumatoid arthritis Feline infectious peritonitis	Complexing of antibody with soluble antigen (slight excess of antigen causes the most intense reactions). Deposition of antigen-antibody complexes in tissues elicits neutrophil release of enzymes and free radicals, causing tissue damage. Common sites of tissue damage include glomeruli, synovium, and vascular endothelium.	Signs of protein-losing nephropathy, polyarthritis, polyarteritis
Type IV Delayed cell mediated	Contact hypersensitivity Transplanted organ rejection	T lymphocyte-mediated (rather than primarily antibody-mediated) interaction with antigen. "Delay" refers to late onset of reaction (>12 hours after beginning of exposure) due to mobilization and infiltration of T lymphocytes, usually "memory T cells" from prior or ongoing exposure to antigen. These T lymphocytes secrete inflammatory substances and attract macrophages and more lymphocytes, leading to tissue destruction.	Signs depend on body tissue involved. Examples include cutaneous lesions (contact hypersensitivity) and organ dysfunction (transplant rejection).

Hypertension, Systemic

Diseases/Clinical Findings Commonly Associated with Systemic Hypertension
Dogs
Ocular findings consistent with hypertensive choroidopathy, hypertensive retinopathy, or intraocular hemorrhage
Chronic or acute renal failure
Hyperadrenocorticism
Diabetes mellitus
Neurologic signs unexplained by other causes
Pheochromocytoma
Unexplained left ventricular hypertrophy (uniform/symmetrical)
Cats
Ocular findings consistent with hypertensive choroidopathy, hypertensive retinopathy, or intraocular hemorrhage
Chronic or acute renal failure
Hyperthyroidism
Diabetes mellitus
Any neurologic signs
Age >10 years
Heart murmur caused by uniform/symmetrical left ventricular hypertrophy (reversible with long-term control of hypertension)

From Ettinger S, Feldman E: *Textbook of Veterinary Internal Medicine*, ed 6. St. Louis, WB Saunders, 2005.

A complete funduscopic examination and BP measurement are indicated in animals known to have or suspected of having these disease conditions. Conditions that are rare in the species (e.g., hyperthyroidism in dogs) are not included. BP measurement is often included in routine cardiac evaluations. Idiopathic hypertrophic cardiomyopathy cannot be diagnosed without excluding hypertension unless the left ventricular hypertrophy is asymmetrical or regional (always idiopathic hypertrophic cardiomyopathy) rather than diffuse.

Hyperthermia

Causes
Impaired Heat Loss
Exposure to high ambient temperatures in a closed, poorly ventilated environment (heatstroke)
Strenuous exercise, especially if concurrent respiratory embarrassment (e.g., if animal is brachycephalic or has laryngeal paralysis)
Hypermetabolic Disorders
Malignant hyperthermia
Hyperthyroidism
Pheochromocytoma
Increased Muscle Activity
Tetanus
Seizure activity
Metaldehyde intoxication
Hypocalcemia
Miscellaneous Causes
Hypothalamic tumor
Certain drugs (phenothiazines, cholinergics)

Modified with permission from Greene C: *Infectious Diseases of the Dog and Cat*, ed 2. St. Louis, WB Saunders, 1999, p 694.

Hyperthyroid Therapy

Differential diagnosis list available on the companion online site at www.cote.clinicalvetadvisor.com.

Hypoalbuminemia

Causes
Decreased Production
Chronic hepatic insuffiency*
Inadequate protein intake†‡
Maldigestion†
Malabsorption†
Hypergammaglobulinemia
Sequestration
Body cavity effusion
Vasculopathy
Increased Loss
PLN because of glomerular disease*
GI: PLE*
Cutaneous
Whole blood loss
Dilution

From Willard M, Tvedten H: *Small Animal Clinical Diagnosis by Laboratory Methods*, ed 4. St. Louis, WB Saunders, 2004.

*Most common and important causes of serum albumin ≤2.0 g/dl. Other causes rarely, if ever, cause serum albumin ≤2.0 g/dl.

†Of very doubtful importance as a sole cause of serum albumin ≤2.0g/dl. Probably more important as a contributing factor when there is another problem that results in hypoalbuminemia.

‡Can be important in very young animals or animals fed diets that are extremely restricted in protein for prolonged periods.

GI, gastrointestinal; PLE, protein-losing enteropathy; PLN, protein-losing nephropathy.

Hypocalcemia

Conditions Associated with Hypocalcemia
Common
Hypoalbuminemia
Chronic renal failure
Puerperal tetany (eclampsia)
Acute renal failure
Acute pancreatitis
Undefined cause (mild hypocalcemia)
Occasional
Soft-tissue trauma or rhabdomyolysis
Hypoparathyroidism
Primary
Idiopathic or spontaneous
Postoperative bilateral thyroidectomy
After sudden reversal of chronic hypercalcemia
Ethylene glycol intoxication
Phosphate enema
After $NaHCO_3$ administration
Uncommon
Laboratory error
Improper sample anticoagulant (EDTA)
Infarction of parathyroid gland adenoma
Rapid IV infusion of phosphates
Acute calcium-free IV infusion (dilutional)
Intestinal malabsorption or severe starvation
Hypovitaminosis D
Blood transfusion (citrated anticoagulant)
Hypomagnesemia
Nutritional secondary hyperparathyroidism
Acute tumor lysis syndrome
Human
Pseudohypoparathyroidism
Drug-induced
Hypercalcitoninism
Osteoblastic bone neoplasia (prostate cancer)

From DiBartola S: *Fluid, Electrolyte, and Acid-Base Disorders in Small Animal Practice*. St. Louis, WB Saunders, 2000.
EDTA, ethylenediamine tetraacetic acid.

Hypocapnia

Causes
Hypotension
Fever
Sepsis
Excitement
Exercise
Pain
Pulmonary thromboembolism
Early pulmonary parenchymal disease
Cytokine release in the systemic inflammatory response syndrome
Inappropriate ventilator settings
Compensation for metabolic acidosis

Modified with permission from King L: *Textbook of Respiratory Disease in Dogs and Cats*. St. Louis, WB Saunders, 2004, p 183.
Definition of hypocapnia: abnormally decreased arterial carbon dioxide tension (e.g., in dogs: pCO_2 <33 mmHg [venous], <36 mmHg [arterial]; in cats: pCO_2 <33 mmHg [venous], <28 mmHg [arterial]).

Hypochloremia

Causes
Pseudohypochloremia
Lipemic samples (titrimetric methods)
Excessive loss of chloride relative to sodium
Vomiting of stomach contents*
Therapy with thiazides or loop diuretics*
Chronic respiratory acidosis
Hyperadrenocorticism
Exercise
Therapy with solutions containing high sodium concentration relative to chloride
Sodium bicarbonate
Sodium penicillin (extremely high doses)

Adapted from de Morais: Chloride ion in small animal practice: The forgotten ion. *J Vet Emerg Crit Care* 2:11–24, 1992.
*Most important causes in small animal practice.

Hypoglycemia

Causes
β-Cell tumor (insulinoma)
Extrapancreatic neoplasia
Hepatocellular carcinoma, hepatoma
Leiomyosarcoma, leiomyoma
Hemangiosarcoma
Hepatic insufficiency*
Portal caval shunts
Chronic fibrosis, cirrhosis
Sepsis*
Hypoadrenocorticism
Hypopituitarism
Idiopathic hypoglycemia*
Neonatal hypoglycemia
Juvenile hypoglycemia (esp. toy breeds)
Hunting dog hypoglycemia
Renal failure
Exocrine pancreatic neoplasia
Hepatic enzyme deficiencies
von Gierke's disease (type 1 glycogen storage disease)
Cori's disease (type 3 glycogen storage disease)
Severe polycythemia
Prolonged starvation
Prolonged sample storage*
Iatrogenic*
Insulin therapy
Sulfonylurea therapy
Ethanol
Ethylene glycol
Artifact
Glucometers
Laboratory error

Modified from Willard M, Tvedten H: *Small Animal Clinical Diagnosis by Laboratory Methods*, ed 4. St. Louis, WB Saunders, 2004.
*Common cause.

Hypokalemia: Associated Disorders (Cats)

Conditions Associated with Hypokalemia in Cats

Thyrotoxicosis
Chronic renal failure
Metabolic acidosis
Dietary
- Potassium deficient
- Acidified diets

Insulin overdose
Diuretic therapy (furosemide)
Metabolic alkalosis
Chronic vomiting/diarrhea
Fluid administration (plasma dilution and volume-induced diuresis)
Idiopathic (Burmese breed)
Systemic diseases
- Hepatic disease
- Infectious disease

Hyperaldosteronism (Conn's syndrome) caused by an adrenocortical tumor
Renal tubular acidosis

From Bonagura J: *Kirk's Current Veterinary Therapy XIII*, ed 13. St. Louis, WB Saunders, 2000.

Hypokalemia: Causes

Causes

Decreased intake
- Alone unlikely to cause hypokalemia unless diet is aberrant
- Administration of potassium-free fluids (e.g., 0.9% NaCl, 5% dextrose in water)

Translocation (ECF→ICF)
- Alkalemia
- Insulin/glucose-containing fluids
- Catecholamines
- Hypothermia?
- Hypokalemic periodic paralysis (Burmese cats)

Increased loss
- GI (FE_k < 4–6%)
  - Vomiting of stomach contents
  - Diarrhea
- Urinary (FE_k > 4–6%)
  - Chronic renal failure in cats
  - Diet-induced hypokalemic nephropathy in cats
  - Distal (type I) RTA
  - Proximal (type II) RTA after $NaHCO_3$ treatment
  - Postobstructive diuresis
  - Dialysis
  - Mineralocorticoid excess
    - Hyperadrenocorticism
    - Primary hyperaldosteronism (adenoma, hyperplasia)
  - Drugs
    - Loop diuretics (e.g., furosemide, ethacrynic acid)
    - Thiazide diuretics (e.g., chlorothiazide, hydrochlorothiazide)
    - Amphotericin B
    - Penicillins
    - Albuterol overdosage

From DiBartola S: *Fluid, Electrolyte, and Acid-Base Disorders in Small Animal Practice.* St. Louis, WB Saunders, 2000.
ECF, extracellular fluid; FE_k, fractional excretion of potassium; GI, gastrointestinal; ICF, intracellular fluid; RTA, renal tubular acidosis.

Hypomagnesemia

Causes of Magnesium Depletion in Humans

Inadequate Dietary Intake
Protein-calorie malnutrition
Magnesium-free fluids and total parenteral nutrition

GI Disorders
Prolonged nasogastric suction
Chronic diarrhea
Malabsorption syndromes
Extensive bowel resection
Intestinal and biliary fistulas
Primary infantile hypomagnesemia

Renal Loss
Chronic parenteral fluid therapy with magnesium-free fluids
Intrinsic tubular disorders
- Chronic interstitial nephritis, pyelonephritis, glomerulonephritis
- Acute tubular necrosis (diuretic phase)
- Postobstructive diuresis
- Renal tubular acidosis
- Congenital magnesium wasting
- Drug injury
  - Aminoglycosides
  - Amphotericin B
  - Cisplatin
  - Cyclosporine

Loop diuretics
Osmotic diuretics: glucose, mannitol, urea
Hypercalcemia
Hypokalemia
Alcohol

Metabolic
Hypercalcemia
Hypophosphatemia

Endocrine
Diabetes mellitus
Hyperthyroidism
Primary hyperparathyroidism
Hyperadrenocorticism
Inappropriate secretion of antidiuretic hormone

Redistribution
Pancreatitis
Hyperadrenergic states
Massive blood transfusion
Insulin therapy
Refeeding syndrome
Hypothermia
Acute respiratory alkalosis
Sepsis
Cardiopulmonary bypass

Miscellaneous
Severe burns
Excessive lactation
Excessive sweating

From DiBartola S: *Fluid, Electrolyte, and Acid-Base Disorders in Small Animal Practice.* St. Louis, WB Saunders, 2000.
GI, gastrointestinal.

Hyponatremia

Causes

With Normal Plasma Osmolality
Hyperlipidemia
Hyperproteinemia

With High Plasma Osmolality
Hyperglycemia
Mannitol infusion

With Low Plasma Osmolality
- Including hypervolemia
  - Severe liver disease
  - CHF
  - Nephrotic syndrome
  - Advanced renal failure
- Including normovolemia
  - Psychogenic polydipsia
  - Syndrome of inappropriate antidiuretic hormone secretion
  - Antidiuretic drugs
  - Myxedema coma of hypothyroidism
  - Hypotonic fluid infusion
- Including hypovolemia
  - GI loss
    - Vomiting
    - Diarrhea
  - Third-space loss
    - Pancreatitis
    - Peritonitis
    - Uroabdomen
    - Pleural effusion (e.g., chylothorax)
    - Peritoneal effusion
  - Cutaneous loss
    - Burns
  - Hypoadrenocorticism
  - Diuretic administration

From DiBartola S: *Fluid, Electrolyte, and Acid-Base Disorders in Small Animal Practice*. St. Louis, WB Saunders, 2000.
CHF, congestive heart failure; GI, gastrointestinal.

Hypophosphatemia

Causes

Maldistribution (Translocation)
Treatment of diabetic ketoacidosis
Carbohydrate load or insulin administration
Respiratory alkalosis or hyperventilation
Total parenteral nutrition or nutritional recovery
Hypothermia

Increased Loss (Reduced Renal Resorption)
Primary hyperparathyroidism
Renal tubular disorders (e.g., Fanconi's syndrome)
Proximally acting diuretics (e.g., carbonic anhydrase inhibitors) (?)*
Eclampsia
Hyperadrenocorticism (?)

Decreased Intake (Reduced Intestinal Absorption)
Dietary deficiency (?)
Vomiting (?)
Malabsorption (?)
Phosphate binders
Vitamin D deficiency

Laboratory Error
Example: mannitol administration

From DiBartola S: *Fluid, Electrolyte, and Acid-Base Disorders in Small Animal Practice*. St. Louis, WB Saunders, 2000.
*(?) Importance in veterinary medicine uncertain.

Hypotension, Systemic

Causes

Decreased Preload
Hypovolemia
Hemorrhage
Trauma
GI losses
Polyuria
Hypoadrenocorticism
Effusions or third spacing of fluid
Burns
Heatstroke
Decreased Venous Return
Pericardial effusion/cardiac tamponade
Restrictive pericarditis
Severe pneumothorax
Positive-pressure ventilation
Gastric dilatation and volvulus
Heartworm disease (caval syndrome)

Decreased Cardiac Function
Cardiomyopathy
Valvular disease
Bradyarrhythmias
Tachyarrhythmias
Electrolyte abnormalities
Acid-base disturbances
Severe hypoxia

Decreased Vascular Tone
SIRS
Anaphylaxis
Neurogenic
Drug induced (anesthetic agent, vasodilators [e.g., β-blockers, Ca channel blockers])
Electrolyte abnormalities
Acid-base disturbances
Severe hypoxia

From Ettinger S, Feldman E: *Textbook of Veterinary Internal Medicine*, ed 6. St. Louis, WB Saunders, 2005.
GI, gastrointestinal; SIRS, sepsis/systemic inflammatory response syndrome.

Hypothermia

Causes

Iatrogenic
Surgery
Anesthesia
Overzealous treatment of hyperthermia

Systemic Disease
Cardiac
Hypothyroidism
Sepsis
Chronic renal failure
Hypoadrenocorticism
Malnutrition
Hypoglycemia
Neurologic
  Head trauma
  Neoplasia
  Cerebrovascular accident

Environmental
Exposure
Trauma

Modified with permission from Bonagura J: *Kirk's Current Veterinary Therapy XII: Small Animal Practice*. St. Louis, WB Saunders, 1995, p 159.

Hypothyroidism

Neurologic Associations (Confirmed or Suspected)

Neuromuscular weakness (slowly progressive)
Muscle atrophy (scapular, masticatory muscle)
Facial nerve paralysis
Vestibular signs (peripheral)
Laryngeal paralysis
Megaesophagus

Hypoxemia

Causes

Hypoventilation*
Acute barbiturate toxicosis, CNS lesion, neuromuscular disease (e.g., botulism, polyradiculoneuritis), pneumothorax, flail chest, pleural effusion, upper airway obstruction (e.g., laryngeal paralysis, foreign body, large airway trauma, large airway mass), anesthetic circuit problems

Diffusion/Gas Exchange Disorder*
Pneumonia, pulmonary edema, pulmonary hemorrhage

Ventilation-Perfusion Mismatch*
Pulmonary thromboembolism, prolonged recumbency

Right-to-Left Cardiovascular Shunt
Tetralogy of Fallot, right-to-left shunting patent ductus arteriosus, other forms of Eisenmenger's physiology

*Possibility of positive response to supplemental oxygen.
CNS, central nervous system.

Icterus

Differential diagnosis list available on the companion online site at www.cote.clinicalvetadvisor.com.

Ileus

Causes

Physical
Intestinal obstruction
Overdistention by aerophagia

Neuromuscular
Anticholinergic drugs
Dysautonomia
Spinal cord injury
Visceral myopathies

Metabolic
Hypokalemia
Uremia
Endotoxemia

Functional
Abdominal surgery
Ischemia
Inflammatory causes
Peritonitis
Pancreatitis
Parvovirus

From Ettinger S, Feldman E: *Textbook of Veterinary Internal Medicine*, ed 6. St. Louis, WB Saunders, 2005.

Immunodeficiency Syndromes: Acquired

Common Acquired Causes of Compromised Immune System Function

Drugs
Antineoplastics
Corticosteroids
Other immunosuppressive agents (e.g., azathioprine, gold salts)

Malnutrition
Intestinal parasitism
Inflammatory bowel disease
Protein-calorie deficiency
Obesity

Infections
Viral infection (FeLV, FIV, FIP, CDV, parvovirus)
Ehrlichia canis

Endocrine Disease
Hyperadrenocorticism
Diabetes mellitus

Neoplasia

Miscellaneous
Neonatal animals
Colostrum deprivation

From Bonagura J: *Kirk's Current Veterinary Therapy XIII*, ed 13. St. Louis, WB Saunders, 2000.
CDV, canine distemper virus; FeLV, feline leukemia virus; FIP, feline infectious peritonitis; FIV, feline immunodeficiency virus.

Immunodeficiency Syndromes: Congenital

Differential diagnosis list available on the companion online site at www.cote.clinicalvetadvisor.com.

Immunodeficiency-Related Complications

Organisms and Medical Problems Commonly Implicated in Immunocompromised Hosts

Opportunistic Organisms
Viruses: feline herpesvirus, FIP, feline calicivirus, canine papillomavirus, canine herpesvirus
Rickettsia: *Haemobartonella*
Bacteria: *Citrobacter* sp., *Escherichia coli, Enterobacter, Klebsiella pneumoniae, Mycobacterium* spp., *Nocardia asteroids, Proteus, Pseudomonas aeruginosa, Serratia marcescens, Staphyloccoccus intermedius*
Fungi: *Aspergillus* sp., *Candida* sp., *Cryptococcus, Histoplasma, Mucor*
Protozoa: *Pneumocystis carinii, Toxoplasma gondii, Cryptosporidium*
Metazoa: *Demodex canis, Otodectes notoedres*

Medical Problems
Recurrent skin infections
Recurrent mucosal infections
Neonatal sepsis and mortality
Reactive amyloidosis
Vasculitis, arteritis, polyarthritis
Recurrent bacteremia
Granulomatous infections
Chronic hypersensitivity reactions
Autoimmune diseases
Persistent intracellular rickettsial or bacterial infections
Disproportional leukocytosis
Persistent lymphopenia

With permission from Greene C: *Infectious Diseases of the Dog and Cat*, ed 2. St. Louis, WB Saunders, 1999, p 684.

Incontinence, Fecal

Causes

Neurologic Disease
Sacral spinal cord
Congenital vertebral malformation
Meningomyelocele
Sacrococcygeal hypoplasia of Manx cats
Sacral fracture
Sacrococcygeal subluxation
Lumbosacral instability
Viral meningomyelitis
Diskospondylitis
Degenerative myelopathy
Neoplasia
Peripheral neuropathy
Trauma
Repair of perineal hernia
Perineal urethrostomy
Penetrating wounds
Dysautonomia
Hypothyroidism
Diabetes mellitus

Non-neurologic Disease
Colorectal causes
Inflammatory bowel disease
Neoplasia
Constipation
Anorectal causes
Trauma
Surgery (anal sac, perineal hernia, rectal resection)
Perianal fistula
Neoplasia
Miscellaneous causes
Severe diarrhea
Irritable bowel syndrome
Decreased mentation
Old age

From Ettinger S, Feldman E: *Textbook of Veterinary Internal Medicine*, ed 6. St. Louis, WB Saunders, 2005.

Incontinence, Urinary

Causes

Urethral incompetence
Ectopic ureters
Neurologic disorders
Urge incontinence (secondary to urinary tract infection [UTI] or uroliths)
Idiopathic detrusor instability
Paradoxic (overflow) incontinence
Ureterocele
Pelvic bladder
Ureterovaginal or urethrorectal fistula
Patent urachus

From Ettinger S, Feldman E: *Textbook of Veterinary Internal Medicine*, ed 6. St. Louis, WB Saunders, 2005.

Infertility, Male

Based on Inability to Sire a Litter

Congenital Infertility
- Hormonal
  - Hypopituitarism
  - Hypothyroidism
- Chromosomal aberration
- Developmental
  - Cryptorchidism
  - Penis, prepuce, os penis anomaly
  - Testicular hypoplasia
  - Duct aplasia
- Motility defect
  - Kartagener's syndrome
- Retrograde ejaculation

Acquired Infertility
- Hormonal
  - Hypopituitarism
  - Hypothyroidism
  - Hyperadrenocorticism
- Metabolic
  - Uremia
  - Hepatic
- Neoplasia
  - Compression
  - Hormonal secretion
- Stress
- Infection
- Fever
- Duct obstruction
- Immune-mediated orchitis
- Drugs, exogenous hormone therapy
- Retrograde ejaculation
- Idiopathic testicular degeneration
- Sexual overuse?
- Psychological?

Modified from Feldman E, Nelson R: Canine and Feline Endocrinology and Reproduction, ed 3. St. Louis, WB Saunders, 2004.

Infertility with Preserved Libido

Drugs and Exogenous Hormones That Affect Fertility in Humans and Possibly Dogs

Chemotherapeutic Drugs
- Busulfan
- Chlorambucil
- Cisplatin
- Cyclophosphamide
- Methotrexate
- Vinblastine
- Vincristine

Miscellaneous Drugs
- Amphotericin B*
- Alloxan
- Cimetidine*
- Clomipramine
- Ketoconazole*
- Spironolactone
- Sulfasalazine

Hormones

Anabolic steroids
- Methyltestosterone*
- Testosterone esters*

Estrogens
- Estradiol 17B*
- Diethylstilbestrol*
- KABI 1774*

Progestogens
- Medroxyprogesterone acetate*
- Megestrol acetate*
- Delmadinone acetate*

Glucocorticoids*

Tamoxifen citrate*

Gossypol*

GnRH antagonists*

GnRH agonists*

From Feldman E, Nelson R: Canine and Feline Endocrinology and Reproduction, ed 3. St. Louis, WB Saunders, 2004.

*Documented in the dog.

Inflammatory Bowel Diseases

Causes of Chronic Small Bowel Inflammation

Chronic Infection
Giardia sp.
Histoplasma sp.
Toxoplasma sp.
Mycobacteria sp.
Protothecosis
Pythiosis
Pathogenic bacteria (*Campylobacter*, *Salmonella* spp., pathogenic *Escherichia coli*)

Food Allergy

Small Bowel Inflammation Associated with Other Primary Gastrointestinal Diseases
Lymphoma
Lymphangiectasia

Idiopathic Causes
Lymphocytic-plasmacytic enteritis (LPE)
Eosinophilic gastroenterocolitis (EGE)
Granulomatous enteritis (same as regional enteritis?)

From Ettinger S, Feldman E: *Textbook of Veterinary Internal Medicine*, ed 6. St. Louis, WB Saunders, 2005.

Insulin Resistance

Recognized Causes of Insulin Ineffectiveness or Insulin Resistance in Diabetic Dogs and Cats

Caused by Insulin Therapy
Inactive insulin
Diluted insulin
Improper administration technique
Inadequate dose
Somogyi effect
Inadequate frequency of insulin administration
Impaired insulin absorption, especially ultralente insulin
Anti-insulin antibody excess

Caused by Concurrent Disorder
Diabetogenic drugs
Hyperadrenocorticism
Diestrus (bitch)
Acromegaly (cat)
Infection, especially of oral cavity and urinary tract
Hypothyroidism (dog)
Hyperthyroidism (cat)
Renal insufficiency
Liver insufficiency
Cardiac insufficiency
Glucagonoma (dog)
Pheochromocytoma
Chronic inflammation, especially pancreatitis
Pancreatic exocrine insufficiency
Severe obesity
Hyperlipidemia
Neoplasia

From Feldman E, Nelson R: *Canine and Feline Endocrinology and Reproduction*, ed 3. St. Louis, WB Saunders, 2004.

Iron Abnormalities

Differential diagnosis list available on the companion online site at www.cote.clinicalvetadvisor.com.

Joint Effusion

Differential diagnosis list available on the companion online site at www.cote.clinicalvetadvisor.com.

Keratoconjunctivitis Sicca

Causes

Breed predisposition
Congenital anomaly
Drug-induced toxicity
Iatrogenic
  Surgical or drug related
Idiopathic
Immune-mediated condition
Infectious agents
  Canine distemper virus
  Feline herpesvirus
Neurogenic
Radiation therapy for nasal or intracranial neoplasms
Trauma to orbit or eye

With permission from Bonagura J: *Kirk's Current Veterinary Therapy XII: Small Animal Practice*. St. Louis, WB Saunders, 1995, p. 1232.
KCS, keratoconjunctivitis sicca.

Ketonuria

Causes

Diabetes mellitus/diabetic ketoacidosis
Starvation
Lactation
Pregnancy
Fever
Renal glucosuria
Severely carbohydrate-restricted diet
Glycogen storage disease

Lacrimation/Epiphora, Chronic

Differential diagnosis list available on the companion online site at www.cote.clinicalvetadvisor.com.

Lactate: Elevated Serum Levels

Major Causes
Type A: Clinical Evidence of Absolute or Relative Tissue Hypoxia
Shock (systemic hypoperfusion)
Hypovolemic
Cardiogenic
Septic
Local hypoperfusion
Gastric necrosis and other causes of splanchnic ischemia
Aortic thromboembolism
Severe hypoxemia (PaO_2 <30–40 mmHg)
Severe anemia (packed cell volume <15%)
Carbon monoxide toxicity
Excessive muscular activity
Exercise
Trembling
Seizures
Type B: No Clinical Evidence of Tissue Hypoxia
Type B_1 (in association with an underlying disease)
Diabetes mellitus
Severe liver disease
Malignancy
Sepsis
Pheochromocytoma
Thiamine deficiency
Type B_2 (due to drugs and toxins)
Acetaminophen
Cyanide
Epinephrine
Ethanol
Ethylene glycol
Insulin
Methanol
Morphine
Nitroprusside
Propylene glycol
Salicylates
Terbutaline
Type B_3 (due to inborn metabolic defects)
Mitochondrial myopathy
Miscellaneous
Alkalosis: hyperventilation
Hypoglycemia

From Bonagura J: *Kirk's Current Veterinary Therapy XIII*, ed 13. St. Louis, WB Saunders, 2000.

Laryngeal Neoplasia

Malignant Tumors of the Canine and Feline Larynx
Lymphoma
Squamous cell carcinoma
Mast cell tumor
Osteosarcoma
Melanoma
Adenocarcinoma
Chondrosarcoma
Granular cell myoblastoma
Fibrosarcoma
Anaplastic carcinoma
Leiomyoma

Modified from Bonagura J: *Kirk's Current Veterinary Therapy XIII*, ed 13. St. Louis, WB Saunders, 2000.

Liver Enzyme Elevations

Conditions That Cause Liver Enzyme Elevations in the Absence of Primary Liver Disease

Drug Induction
Corticosteroids (dogs): ↑↑↑ ALP, ↑↑ GGT, ↑ ALT, ↑ AST
Anticonvulsants (phenobarbital, phenytoin, primidone): ↑ ALT, ↑ ALP, ↑ AST, ↑ GGT

Endocrinopathies
Hyperthyroidism (cats): ↑ ALP, ↑ ALT
Hypothyroidism (dogs): ↑ ALP
Diabetes mellitus: ↑ ALP
Hyperadrenocorticism (dogs): ↑↑↑ ALP, ↑ ALT, ↑ GGT, ↑ AST

Hypoxia/Hypotension: ↑↑ ALT, ↑ ALP, ↑ GGT, ↑ AST
Congestive heart failure
Severe acute blood loss
Status epilepticus
Hypotensive crisis
Surgery
Septic shock
Hypoadrenocorticism
Hypovolemic shock

Muscle Injury: ↑ ALT, ↑ AST
Acute muscle necrosis/trauma
Malignant hyperthermia
Myopathies

Neoplasia
Adenocarcinomas: pancreatic, intestinal, adrenocortical, mammary
Sarcomas: hemangiosarcoma, leiomyosarcoma
Hepatic metastasis: ↑ AST, ↑ ALT, ↑ ALP
Unique enzyme induction: ↑↑ ALP, ↑↑ GGT

Miscellaneous
Systemic infections
Pregnancy (cats): ↑ placental ALP
Colostrum-fed neonates (dogs): ↑ GGT

Bone Disorders: ↑ ALP
Young animals (up to 7 months)
Osteosarcoma
Osteomyelitis

From Ettinger S, Feldman E: *Textbook of Veterinary Internal Medicine*, ed 5. St. Louis, WB Saunders, 2000.
ALP, alkaline phosphatase; ALT, alanine aminotransferase; AST, aspartate aminotransferase; GGT, gamma-glutamyl transpeptidase.

Lymphatic Disorders

Causes

Lymphangitis, Lymphedema, Lymphadenitis, Lymphadenopathy
Infection
Neoplasia
Reactive hyperplasia
Granuloma

Lymphedema
Primary developmental abnormality of lymphatics
Hypoplasia
Aplasia
Lymphangiectasia
Hyperplasia
Secondary acquired abnormalities of lymphatics
Surgical excision of lymphatics or lymph nodes
Post-traumatic lymphangiopathy
Neoplastic invasion
Extrinsic compression of lymph vessels or tissue
Acute obstructive lymphadenitis
Chronic sclerosing lymphadenitis/lymphangitis
Lymphatic atrophy with interstitial fibrosis
Radiation therapy

Lymphocysts
Cystic hygroma, lymphoceles, pseudocyst

Lymphangiomas

From Ettinger S, Feldman E: *Textbook of Veterinary Internal Medicine*, ed 6. St. Louis, WB Saunders, 2005.

Lymphatic Drainage

Normally Palpable Lymph Nodes and Body Regions That Nodes Drain

Lymph Node	Area Drained
Mandibular	All parts of the head not drained by the parotid node (parotid node drains the cutaneous area of the caudal half of dorsum of muzzle, and the lateral cranium, parotid gland, and muscles of mastication)
Superficial cervical (prescapular)	Skin on caudal part of head, including pharynx, part of pinna, lateral surface of neck and the thoracic limb except the shoulder, and medial side of the brachium and antebrachium
Axillary and accessory axillary	Mammary glands, thoracic wall, and deep structures of the thoracic limb
Superficial inguinal	Ventral half of the abdominal wall, including the abdominal and inguinal mammary glands as well as efferent vessels from the popliteal lymph nodes, penis, prepuce, and scrotum in the male
Popliteal	All parts of the pelvic limb distal to the node

From Slatter D: *Textbook of Small Animal Surgery*. St. Louis, Elsevier, 2003.

Lymphoma and Lymphoid Neoplasia

Anatomical Classification of Lymphoid Neoplasms

Name	Incidence in Dogs	Incidence in Cats (FeLV status)	Selected Clinicopathologic Characteristics
Lymphoma			
Multicentric	80–85%	20–40% (80% FeLV+)	In cats, spleen and liver are virtually always affected; feline lymphoid hyperplasia is a common cause of generalized lymphadenopathy; in dogs, diffuse pulmonary infiltrates are in 25–35% of cases.
Alimentary	<7%	15–45% (30% FeLV+)	Regional lymph nodes are commonly affected; late-stage disease affects kidneys; in some cats, the condition may be associated with FIV.
Mediastinal (thymic)	<5%	20–50% (80% FeLV+)	Sternal lymph nodes are affected in dogs, and nodes and thymus are affected in cats; pleural effusion and hypercalcemia are common (40%).
Extranodal sites Cutaneous	7%	5–10%	B-cell tumors are termed *cutaneous lymphoma*; T-cell tumors are termed *mycosis fungoides*.
Nervous system		(80% FeLV+)	This is the most common cause of posterior paresis in cats; the bone marrow is often affected; in dogs, the condition usually reflects late-stage multicentric disease.
Renal			Late-stage disease affects CNS and is often present in renal failure.
Plasma Cell Tumors			
Multiple myeloma	Uncommon	Rare (no association with FeLV)	75% of dogs have immunoglobulin or monoclonal gammopathy, and 10% have circulating plasmacytes; immunoglobulin M-producing tumor termed *macroglobulinemia* (Waldenstrom's).
Cutaneous	Infrequent	Extremely rare	Rarely metastasize (<5%)
GI	Infrequent	Unreported	Uncommonly metastasize
Osseous	Rare	Unreported	Often progress to systemic myeloma within 6 months

From Slatter D: *Textbook of Small Animal Surgery*. St. Louis, Elsevier, 2003.
FeLV, feline leukemia virus; FIV, feline immunodeficiency virus; GI, gastrointestinal.

Lymphoma Staging Classification

The World Health Organization (WHO) Clinical Staging System for Lymphoma

Stage I	Single lymph node involved
Stage II	Multiple lymph nodes involved on one side of the diaphragm
Stage III	Generalized peripheral lymph node involvement
Stage IV	Stages I–III with liver and/or splenic involvement
Stage V	Stages I–IV with blood and/or bone marrow involvement

Substage A: no signs of systemic illness
Substage B: signs of systemic illness
E: designation used for extranodal tumors

From Slatter D: *Textbook of Small Animal Surgery*. St. Louis, Elsevier, 2003.

Lymphoproliferative and Myeloproliferative Disorders

Lymphoproliferative Disorders
Preneoplastic:
Persistent lymphocytosis
Leukemia/Disseminated Forms:
Lymphoblastic leukemia (B-, T-, null-cell types)
Lymphocytic leukemia (B-, T-cell types)
Granular lymphocyte leukemia (T-, NK-cell types)
Plasma cell myeloma
Mycosis fungoides/Sézary syndrome
Neoplastic Solid Tissue Forms:
Lymphoma (B- and T-cell types of nodal and extranodal sites)
Plasmacytoma (extramedullary sites)

Myeloproliferative Disorders*
Preneoplastic:
Myelodysplastic syndrome (primary)
Leukemic/Disseminated Forms:
Acute myeloid leukemia (types M1–M7)
Chronic Myeloproliferative Disease†
Chronic myelogenous leukemia (neutrophils)
Eosinophilic leukemia
Basophilic leukemia
Chronic myelomonocytic leukemia
Polycythemia vera
Essential thrombocythemia
Myeloid metaplasia/myelofibrosis or idiopathic myelofibrosis
Mast Cell Leukemia/Mastocythemia
Malignant Histiocytosis or Disseminated Histiocytic Sarcoma (Dendritic Cells)
Neoplastic Solid Tissue Forms:
Cutaneous histiocytoma (dendritic cells)
Localized histiocytic sarcoma (dendritic cells)

From Willard M, Tvedten H: *Small Animal Clinical Diagnosis by Laboratory Methods*, ed 4. St. Louis, WB Saunders, 2004.
*The term *myeloproliferative* is used in its broadest sense to include nonlymphoid dysplastic and neoplastic conditions.
†Uncommon disease states.

Mediastinal Enlargement

Differential diagnosis list available on the companion online site at www.cote.clinicalvetadvisor.com.

Megaesophagus

Associated Diseases and Causes in Dogs

Central Nervous System
Distemper
Cervical vertebral instability with leukomalacia
Brainstem lesions
Neoplasia
Trauma

Peripheral Neuropathies
Polyneuritis
Polyradiculoneuritis
Ganglioradiculitis
Dysautonomia
Giant cell axonal neuropathy
Spinal muscular atrophy
Toxicity
- Lead
- Thallium
- Acrylamide

Bilateral vagal damage

Neuromuscular Junction
Myasthenia gravis
Botulism
Tetanus
Anticholinesterase toxicity

Esophageal Musculature
Esophagitis
Systemic lupus erythematosus
Glycogen storage disease
Polymyositis
Dermatomyositis
Cachexia
Trypanosomiasis
Hypoadrenocorticism
Hypothyroidism?

Miscellaneous
Pyloric stenosis
Gastric dilatation volvulus
Pituitary dwarfism
Thymoma
Mediastinitis

From Bonagura J: *Kirk's Current Veterinary Therapy XIII*, ed 13. St. Louis, WB Saunders, 2000.
?, cause-and-effect relationship not established.

Melena

Causes

Ingested Blood
Oral lesions
Nasopharyngeal lesions
Pulmonary lesions
Diet

Parasitism
Hookworms

Neoplasia
Adenocarcinoma
Lymphoma
Leiomyoma or leiomyosarcoma
Mast cell tumor
Gastrinoma

Coagulopathies
DIC
Rodenticide intoxication

Drug Administration
NSAIDs
Glucocorticoids

Miscellaneous
Liver failure
Pancreatitis
Renal failure
Inflammation (e.g., foreign body, acute gastritis, hemorrhagic gastroenteritis, inflammatory bowel disease)
Hypoadrenocorticism
GI ischemia (e.g., shock, volvulus, intussusception)
Foreign bodies
GI blood vessel malformations (e.g., arteriovenous fistula)
Polyps

From Ettinger S, Feldman E: *Textbook of Veterinary Internal Medicine*, ed 6. St. Louis, WB Saunders, 2005.

DIC, disseminated intravascular coagulation; GI, gastrointestinal; NSAIDs, nonsteroidal anti-inflammatory drugs.

Monoclonal Gammopathy

Associated Conditions

Multiple myeloma
Waldenstrom's macroglobulinemia
Plasma cell leukemia
Nonsecretory myeloma
Extramedullary plasmacytoma
Monoclonal gammopathy of undetermined significance
Chronic lymphocytic leukemia
Lymphoma
Feline infectious peritonitis
Ehrlichiosis
Amyloidosis
Lymphocytic enteritis

With permission from Bonagura J: *Kirk's Current Veterinary Therapy XII: Small Animal Practice*. St. Louis, WB Saunders, 1995, p 525.

Myocardial Diseases (Feline)

Causes

Idiopathic
Hypertrophic cardiomyopathy
Restrictive cardiomyopathy
Dilated cardiomyopathy
Arrhythmogenic right ventricular cardiomyopathy

Secondary (Including Specific Cardiomyopathies)
Inflammatory
Viral (panleukopenia?)
Bacterial
Protozoal
Fungal
Algal
Parasitic
Metabolic
Nutritional
  Taurine deficiency
Endocrine
  Thyrotoxicosis
  Acromegaly
  Diabetes mellitus
Toxic
  Anthracyclines (doxorubicin)
Vascular
Systemic hypertension
Infiltrative
Neoplastic
Glycogen storage disorders
Mucopolysaccharidosis
Fibroplastic
Endomyocardial fibrosis
Endocardial fibroelastosis
Genetic
Hypertrophic cardiomyopathy
Physical agents
Heatstroke

Unclassified Cardiomyopathies
Idiopathic unclassified cardiomyopathy
Persistent atrial standstill

Miscellaneous
Ischemia
Excessive left ventricular moderator bands

From Ettinger S, Feldman E: *Textbook of Veterinary Internal Medicine*, ed 5. St. Louis, WB Saunders, 2000.

Myocarditis

Causes

Viral
Canine distemper virus (neonate)
Canine parvovirus (prenatal, neonate)

Rickettsial
Rickettsia rickettsii

Bacterial
Numerous genera
Borrelia burgdorferi

Algal
Prototheca spp.

Fungal
Cryptococcus neoformans
Coccidioides immitis
Aspergillus terreus
Paecilomyces varioti

Protozoal
Trypanosoma cruzi
Toxoplasma gondii
Hepatozoon canis
Neospora caninum

Traumatic
Automobile trauma
Injury from falling
Penetrating trauma
Cardiac catheterization

Immune-Mediated Conditions
Rarely reported in veterinary medicine

Unknown
Transmissible myocarditis-diaphragmitis of cats

Modified with permission from Greene C: *Infectious Disease of the Dog and Cat*, ed 2. St. Louis, WB Saunders, 1999, p 580.

Myopathies

Classification

Inflammatory
Infectious
  Bacterial: leptospirosis
  Protozoal: toxoplasmosis/neosporosis
  Parasitic: *Toxocara,* others

Immune Mediated
Masticatory muscle myositis
Polymyositis
Dermatomyositis

Degenerative
Acquired
Endocrine
  Hyperadrenocorticism
  Hypothyroidism
  Hypokalemic polymyopathy (cats)
Fibrotic/ossifying myopathies
Ischemic
Nutritional
Neoplastic
Toxic
Inherited
Muscular dystrophy
  X-linked muscular dystrophy (dystrophin deficient)
  Other muscular dystrophies (dystrophin positive)
Myotonia
Metabolic
  Glycogen storage disease
  Mitochondrial myopathy
  Lipidic myopathy
  Malignant hyperthermia
Centronuclear myopathy (Labrador retriever)

From Ettinger S, Feldman E: *Textbook of Veterinary Internal Medicine*, ed 6. St. Louis, WB Saunders, 2005.

Myopathies, Congenital

Differential diagnosis list available on the companion online site at www.cote.clinicalvetadvisor.com.

Myositis

Microorganisms Associated with Musculoskeletal Infections

Causes of Myositis Infection
Hepatozoon
Toxoplasma gondii
Neospora caninum
Leptospira
Borrelia
Numerous bacteria
Toxigenic *Streptococcus canis*

Modified with permission from Greene C: *Infectious Diseases of the Dog and Cat*, ed 2. St. Louis, WB Saunders, 1999, p 555.

Nasal Discharge, Sneezing

Causes

Structural Anomalies
Cleft palate
Oronasal fistula
Cricopharyngeal achalasia
Megaesophagus

Allergic/Immunologic
Allergic rhinitis
Lymphoplasmacytic rhinitis

Bleeding Disorder
Factor deficiency (congenital and acquired)
Thrombocytopenia (infectious and immune mediated)
Vessel wall (trauma and vasculitis)
Foreign bodies/trauma

Infections
Viral: distemper, parainfluenza, adenovirus type 2 (dogs); herpesvirus, calicivirus (cats)
Bacterial: including dental disease, chronic feline rhinosinusitis
Fungal: *Aspergillus* spp., *Penicillium* spp., *Cryptococcus neoformans*, Rhinosporidium seeberi; other opportunistic fungi are rare (e.g., *Trichosporon*)
Rickettsial (*Ehrlichia canis*, Rocky Mountain spotted fever)
Parasitic (*Pneumonyssoides caninum*, *Linguatula serrata*, *Capillaria aerophila*, *Syngamus ierei*, *Cuterebra* spp.)
Other (*Chlamydia* spp.)

Neoplasia/Polyps
Carcinomas, sarcomas, transmissible venereal tumor
Polyp (nasopharyngeal in cats)

From Willard M, Tvedten H: *Small Animal Clinical Diagnosis by Laboratory Methods*, ed 4. St. Louis, WB Saunders, 2004.

Nasal Neoplasia

Malignant Tumors of the Canine and Feline Nasal and Paranasal Sinuses

Canine
Adenocarcinoma
- Differentiated
- Undifferentiated

Squamous cell carcinoma
Chondrosarcoma
Fibrosarcoma
Lymphosarcoma

Feline
Adenocarcinoma
Lymphoma

Infrequently Reported
Osteosarcoma
Hemangiosarcoma
Rhabdomyosarcoma
Leiomyosarcoma
Nerve sheath tumors
Neuroblastoma

Modified from Bonagura J: *Kirk's Current Veterinary Therapy XIII*, ed 13. St. Louis, WB Saunders, 2000.

Nasal Obstruction/Discharge in Cats, Chronic

Causes

Viral rhinitis with or without secondary bacterial infection
- Herpesvirus (feline viral rhinotracheitis)
- Calicivirus

Nasopharyngeal stenosis
Esophageal motility dysfunction
Foreign body (typically blade of grass)
Allergic rhinitis
Nasopharyngeal polyp
Neoplasia (nasal lymphoma, other)
Cryptococcal rhinitis
Cleft palate (congenital) (uncommon)

Nephrotic Drugs and Substances*

Aminoglycoside antibiotics, such as neomycin, kanamycin, gentamicin, amikacin, and tobramycin (important)
Amphotericin B (important)
Arsenic
Cephalothin (uncommon)
Cisplatin (important)
Cyclophosphamide (nephrotoxicity is uncommon; sterile cystitis is more common)
Dextran (low molecular weight)
Ethylene glycol (important)
Furosemide (uncommon)
Heavy metals (i.e., gold, lead, mercury)
Nonsteroidal anti-inflammatory drugs (NSAIDs), such as aspirin or ibuprofen (important when there is preexisting renal disease or hypotension)
Polymyxin B (important)
Radiographic contrast media (important when there is preexisting azotemia and dehydration)
Sulfonamides (uncommon if more soluble sulfonamides are used)
Tetracyclines (uncommon)
Thallium
Thiazides (uncommon)
Vancomycin (uncommon)
Zinc

Modified from Willard M, Tvedten H: *Small Animal Clinical Diagnosis by Laboratory Methods*, ed 4. St. Louis, WB Saunders, 2004.

*Not all these drugs reliably produce nephrotoxicity. Those drugs recognized as the most dangerous are denoted important.

Nerves of the Forelimb: Cutaneous Distribution

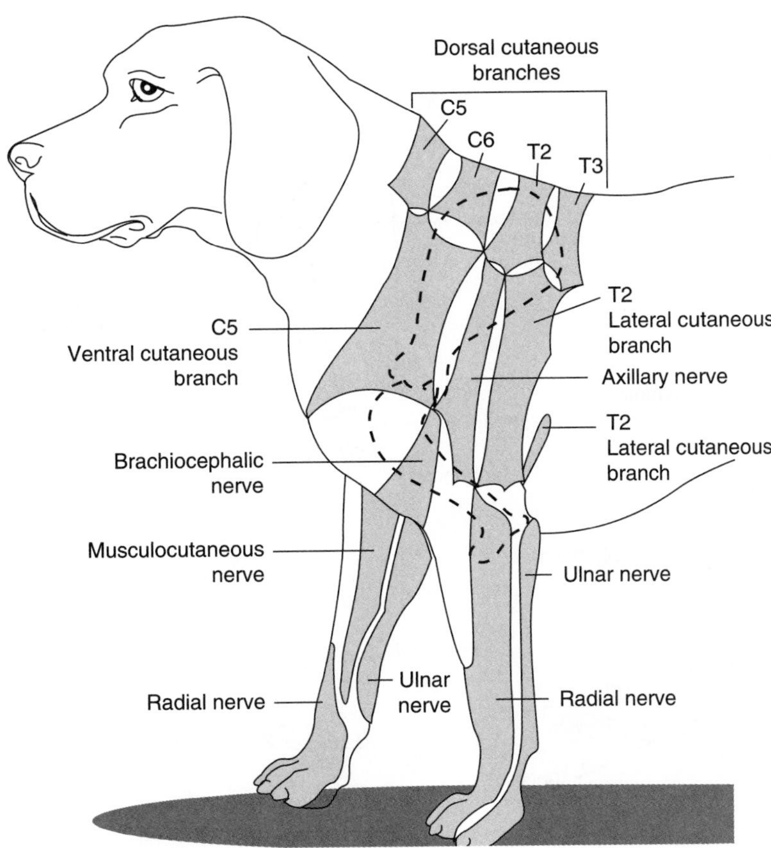

Nerves of the Forelimb: Localization of Contributing Spinal Cord Segments

Nerves of the Forelimb

Nerve	Spinal Cord Segments
Phrenic	$C_{5,6,7}$
Cranial pectoral	$C_{6,7,8}$
Suprascapular	$C_{6,7}$
Subscapular	$C_{6,7}$
Musculocutaneous	$C_{6,7,8}$
Axillary	$C_{7,8}$
Thoracodorsal	C_{8}
Lateral thoracic	C_{8}, T_{1}
Radial	$C_{7,8}$, $T_{1,2}$
Median and ulnar	C_{8}, $T_{1,2}$
Caudal pectoral	C_{8}, $T_{1,2}$
Sympathetics (Horner's)	$T_{1,2,3}$

From Evans H, de Lahunta A: *Guide to the Dissection of the Dog*, ed 6. St. Louis, WB Saunders, 2004.

Nerves of the Hind Limb: Cutaneous Distribution

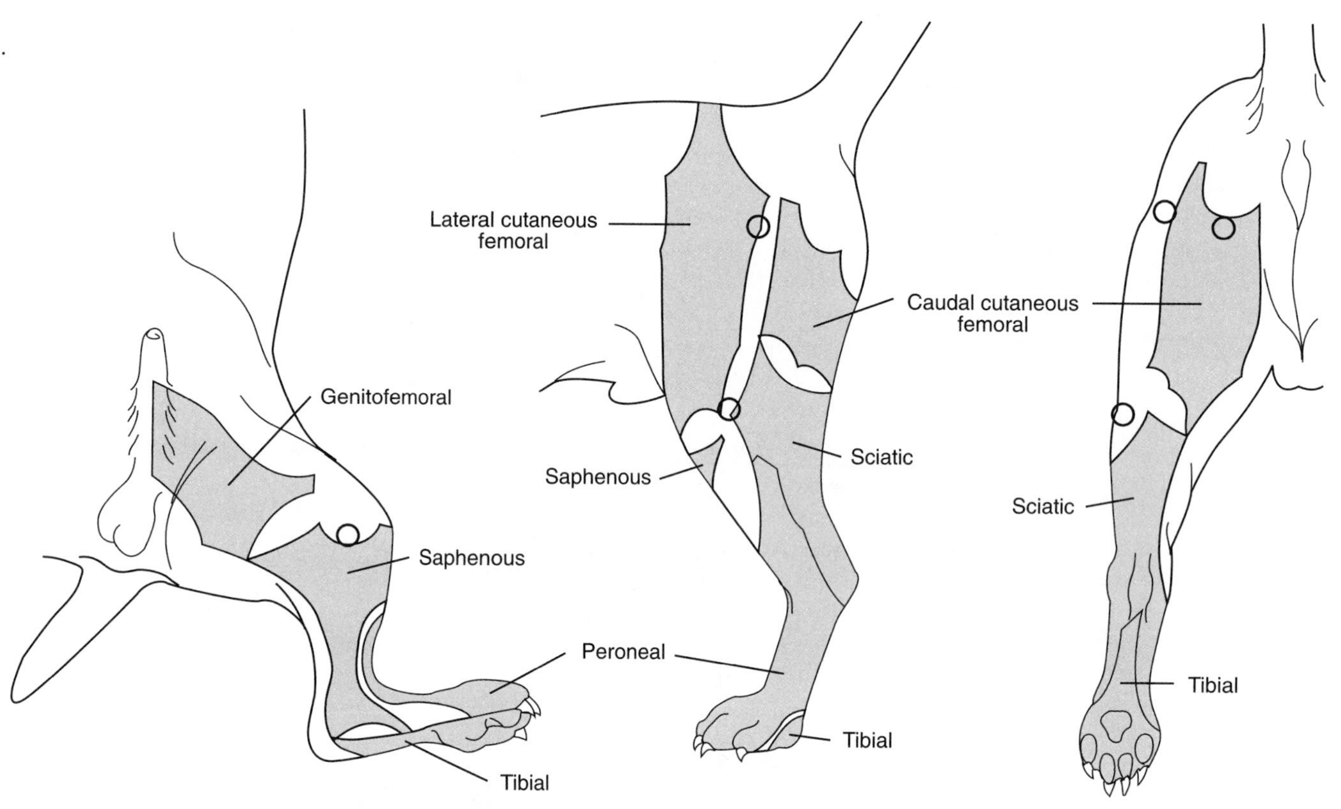

Nerves of the Hind Limb: Localization of Contributing Spinal Cord Segments

Nerves of the Hind Limb

Nerve	Spinal Cord Segments
Femoral	$L_{4,5,6}$
Obturator	$L_{(4),5,6}$
Cranial gluteal	$L_{6,7}, S_1$
Caudal gluteal	$L_7, S_{1,2}$
Sciatic	$L_{6,7}, S_{1,2}$
Pudendal	$S_{1,2,3}$

From Evans H, de Lahunta A: *Guide to the Dissection of the Dog*, ed 6. St. Louis, WB Saunders, 2004.

Neurologic Signs and Underlying Causes

Relationship of Clinical Signs to Anatomic Site of Lesion

Clinical Signs	Functional System	Anatomic Location
Inability to prehend	Masticatory and tongue muscles	CN V, XII, pons-medulla
Dysphagia	Tongue, palatal, pharyngeal, and esophageal muscles	CN IX, X, XI, XII, medulla
Drooling	Facial paralysis, dysphagia	CN VII, middle ear, medulla
		CN IX, X, medulla
Head tilt, nystagmus, loss of balance, rolling	Vestibular system	CN VIII: inner ear, medulla, cerebellum
Strabismus	CN to extraocular muscles, vestibular system	CN III, IV, VI, midbrain-medulla
		Inner ear-medulla-cerebellum
Circling		
With loss of balance	Vestibular system	Inner ear, medulla, cerebellum
Without loss of balance	Limbic system (?)	Frontal lobe, rostral thalamus
Head and eye deviation-turning to one side	Limbic system (?)	Frontal lobe, rostral thalamus
Pacing, head pressing	Limbic system	Frontal lobe, rostral thalamus
Opisthotonos	Upper motor neuron	Rostral cerebellum, midbrain
Blindness	Visual system	
	Dilated unresponsive pupils	Eyeball, optic nerves
	Normal pupils	Visual cortex-cerebrum, (midbrain)
Depression, semicoma, coma	Ascending reticular activating system	Pons to thalamus-cerebral cortex
Seizures		Cerebrum, thalamus-hypothalamus
Hyperesthesia, hyperactivity to external stimuli	Ascending reticular activating system	Thalamus, cerebrum
Aggressive behavior, mania-hysteria, odontoprisis	Limbic system	Thalamus, cerebrum
Tremor		
Associated with movements, head, and neck	Cerebellar system	Cerebellum
Associated with movements, head, trunk, limbs	Multiple systems	Diffuse CNS
Episodic, not associated with movements, head, trunk, limbs		Thalamus, cerebrum
Bradycardia, hypothermia, hyperthermia	UMN for general visceral efferent system	Hypothalamus
Irregular-ataxic respirations	UMN for respiratory muscle LMN	Pons-medulla

From de Lahunta A: *Veterinary Neuroanatomy and Clinical Neurology*. St. Louis, WB Saunders, 1983.
CN, cranial nerve; CNS, central nervous system; LMN, lower motor neuron; UMN, upper motor neuron; ?, may occur with lesion in this location.

Neuromuscular Diseases

Diseases of the Lower Motor Neuron
- ***Neuromuscular Junction***
  - Botulism
  - Tick paralysis
  - Myasthenia gravis
  - Organophosphate intoxication
- ***Peripheral Nerve***
  - Trauma
  - Neoplasia
  - Ischemia—caudal aortic thrombosis-embolism
- ***Spinal Roots and Nerves***
  - Trauma—root avulsion
  - Lumbosacral stenosis—cauda equina syndrome
  - Neoplasia—neurofibroma
  - Inflammation
- ***Spinal Roots and/or Nerves and Peripheral Nerves***
  - Inflammation
    - *Acute polyneuritis: polyneuropathy*
      - Dog: idiopathic polyradiculoneuritis/coonhound paralysis
        - Acute idiopathic polyneuropathy
        - Postrabies vaccination
        - Distal denervating disease
        - Brachial plexus neuritis
    - *Chronic polyneuritis: polyneuropathy*
      - Dog: chronic polyneuritis
        - Inherited hypertrophic neuropathy
        - Giant axonal neuropathy
        - Distal symmetric polyneuropathy
        - Metabolic neuropathy

Spinal Cord
- Focal myelopathy from compression
- Acute ischemic myelopathy: fibrocartilaginous emboli
- Diffuse myelomalacia
- Inflammations: viral, protozoal
- Hereditary neuronal abiotrophy in Swedish Lapland dogs
- Hereditary spinal muscular atrophy in Brittany spaniels
- Stockard's paralysis

Muscle Disease
- *Myositis*
  - Infectious
  - Idiopathic—immune mediated
    - Masticatory
    - Polymyositis
- *Myotonia*
  - Hereditary myopathic myotonia of young animals
  - Acquired myopathic myotonia of old dogs
- *Other myopathies*

From de Lahunta A: *Veterinary Neuroanatomy and Clinical Neurology*. St. Louis, WB Saunders, 1983.

Neutropenia

Differential diagnosis list available on the companion online site at www.cote.clinicalvetadvisor.com.

Neutrophil Dysfunction

Causes of Congenital and Acquired Neutrophil Dysfunction

Dysfunction	Species
Chemotactic Factor Generation	
Congenital	
C3 deficiency (Brittany spaniel)	Dog
Adherence	
Congenital	
CD11-CD18 adhesion protein deficiency (Irish setter)	Dog
Acquired	
Diabetes mellitus (poorly regulated)	Dog
Chemotaxis	
Congenital	
C3 deficiency (Brittany spaniel)	Dog
CD11-CD18 adhesion protein deficiency (Irish setter)	Dog
Chédiak-Higashi syndrome (Persian)	Cat
Pelger-Huët anomaly? (foxhound)	Dog*
Primary ciliary dyskinesia (pointer)	Dog
Recurrent infections (weimaraner)	Dog
Acquired	
Bacterial pyoderma	Dog
Demodicosis (serum inhibitor?)	Dog
FeLV infection	Cat
FIP	Cat
Hyperalimentation-induced hypophosphatemia	Dog
Protothecosis (serum inhibitor?)	Dog
Phagocytosis	
Congenital	
C3 deficiency (Brittany spaniel)	Dog
CD11-CD18 adhesion protein deficiency (Irish setter)	Dog
Recurrent and persistent infections (weimaraner)	Dog
Acquired	
Continuous-flow centrifugation and filtration-leukapheresis	
Collected neutrophils	Dog
Hyperalimentation-induced hypophosphatemia	Dog
Bacterial Killing	
Congenital	
CD11-CD18 adhesion protein deficiency (Irish setter)	Dog
Cyclic neutropenia (Gray collies)	Dog
Recurrent and persistent infections (weimaraner)	Dog
Rhinitis-pneumonia syndrome (Doberman pinscher)	Dog
Acquired	
FeLV infection	Cat
Hyperalimentation-induced hypophosphatemia	Dog
Lead toxicosis	Dog
Turpentine-induced inflammation	Dog

From Bonagura J: *Kirk's Current Veterinary Therapy XIII*, ed 13. St. Louis, WB Saunders, 2000.

*Neutrophil chemotaxis was tested in only one of four English-American (Walker) foxhounds with Pelger-Huët anomaly; defective chemotaxis has not been found in other dogs, including foxhounds, with the anomaly.

FeLV, feline leukemia virus; FIP, feline infectious peritonitis.

Optic Nerve Disorders

Differential diagnosis list available on the companion online site at www.cote.clinicalvetadvisor.com.

Oral Ulcers

Differential diagnosis list available on the companion online site at www.cote.clinicalvetadvisor.com.

Orbital Diseases

Differential diagnosis list available on the companion online site at www.cote.clinicalvetadvisor.com.

Osteomyelitis

Causes in Dogs

Bacterial
Aerobes
Escherichia coli
Klebsiella spp.
Pasteurella spp.
Proteus spp.
Pseudomonas spp.
Staphylococcus spp. (most common of the bacteria that cause osteomyelitis)
S. intermedius
Streptococcus spp.
Anaerobes
Actinomyces spp.
Bacteroides spp.
Clostridium spp.
Fusobacterium spp.
Nocardia spp.
Peptostreptococcus spp.

Viral
Canine distemper virus

Fungal
Aspergillus spp.
Blastomyces dermatitidis
Candida spp.
Coccidioides immitis
Cryptococcus neoformans
Histoplasma capsulatum

Ototoxic Drugs

Aminoglycoside Antibiotics
Neomycin
Dihydrostreptomycin
Gentamicin
Streptomycin
Kanamycin
Tobramycin
Amikacin

Other Antibiotics
Polymyxin B&E
Minocycline
Erythromycin
Chloramphenicol
Vancomycin

Loop Diuretics
Furosemide
Bumetanide
Ethacrynic acid

Antiseptics
Chlorhexidine
Iodine and iodophores
Ethanol
Benzalkonium chloride
Benzethonium chloride
Cantrimide

Antineoplastic Agents
Cisplatin
Nitrogen mustard

Miscellaneous
Quinine
Salicylates
Propylene glycol
Detergents
Arsenic
Lead
Mercury

From Ettinger S, Feldman E: *Textbook of Veterinary Internal Medicine*, ed 6. St. Louis, WB Saunders, 2005.

Panting

Causes

Elevated ambient temperature
Fever, hyperthermia
Anxiety, nervousness
Pain
Hyperadrenocorticism
Glucocorticosteroid therapy
Pheochromocytoma
Hyperthyroidism
Hypocalcemia
Narcotic administration
Cardiac disease/tachyarrhythmias
Brain disease

With permission from King L: *Textbook of Respiratory Disease in Dogs and Cats*. St. Louis, WB Saunders, 2004, p 47.

Paraneoplastic Syndromes

Paraneoplastic Disorder	Clinical Features	Associated Neoplasms in Companion Animals
Malignancy-associated hypercalcemia	Dehydration, depression, muscular weakness, anorexia, polyuria and polydipsia, vomiting, arrhythmias	Lymphoma (thymic, multicentric, extranodal leukemia), carcinomas (nasal, pulmonary, mammary, squamous cell, thyroid, apocrine gland of anal sac, gastric, pancreatic, testicular, parathyroid gland), thymomas, multiple myeloma, epidermoid carcinoma of the lung
Extrapancreatic hypoglycemia	Weakness, seizures	Hepatocellular carcinoma, hepatoma, hemangiosarcoma, leiomyosarcoma, splenic hemangiosarcoma, salivary gland adenocarcinoma, metastatic oral melanoma, mammary carcinoma, pulmonary carcinoma, plasma cell tumor, lymphocytic leukemia, renal carcinoma
Hyperhistaminemia, mast cell degranulation	Gastrointestinal ulceration with melena and hematemesis, urticaria, erythema, pruritus, poor wound healing, anaphylactoid reaction, hypotension/arrhythmias, altered coagulation	Mast cell tumor
Cancer anorexia/cachexia syndrome	Weight loss >5–10% BW kg, anorexia >2–3 days' duration, early satiety	Any tumors
Syndrome of inappropriate antidiuretic hormone secretion	Hyponatremia, polyuria and polydipsia, edema	Pulmonary carcinoma (dog)
Fever	Persistent pyrexia >39.7°C (103°F) without infection	Lymphoproliferative and myeloproliferative neoplasms; mast cell, hepatic, and brain tumors
Polycythemia	Exercise intolerance, seizures, red mucous membranes, PCV >60	Renal tumors, lymphoma, polycythemia vera, hepatic tumors
Hypertrophic osteopathy	Painful, hard, swollen distal limbs, reluctance to walk	Primary lung tumors, rhabdomyosarcoma (bladder), esophageal sarcomas, pulmonary metastatis, carcinoma, renal carcinomas, hepatic adenocarcinoma, pulmonary carcinoma, and renal papillary adenoma (cat)
Dermatologic disorders	Nodular, dermatofibrosis, erythema, flushing, necrolytic migratory erythema	Renal cystadenocarcinoma, mast cell tumor, pheochromocytoma, pancreatic adenocarcinoma
Renal disorders	Amyloid deposition, glomerulonephritis, concentrating defects, proteinuria, nephrotic syndrome	Many tumors, including lymphoma, plasma cell tumors, mast cell tumors
Central nervous system	Hyperviscosity syndrome (seizures, dementia)	Lymphoma, plasma cell tumors
Peripheral nervous system		
Neuromuscular junction	Myasthenia gravis (weakness with exercise that improves with rest)	Thymoma, hepatocellular carcinoma, osteosarcoma, mammary adenocarcinoma, pheochromocytoma, pulmonary adenocarcinoma
Neuropathy	Weakness, cranial nerve abnormalities	Lymphoma, bronchogenic carcinoma, insulinoma, leiomyosarcoma, hemangiosarcoma, and undifferentiated sarcomas
Neuromyopathy	Weakness, muscle pain, proprioception deficits	Pulmonary carcinoma
Myopathy	Myositis	Thymoma

With permission from Bonagura J: *Kirk's Current Veterinary Therapy XII: Small Animal Practice*. St. Louis, WB Saunders, 1995, p 531.

Paronychia and Other Claw Fold Disorders

Differential diagnosis list available on the companion online site at www.cote.clinicalvetadvisor.com.

Pericardial Diseases

Congenital Disorders
Pericardial defects*
Peritoneopericardial diaphragmatic hernia*
Pericardial cyst

Acquired Disorders
Pericardial effusion
Hydropericardium (transudate)*
  Congestive heart failure
  Hypoalbuminemia
  Peritoneopericardial diaphragmatic hernia
Pericarditis (exudates)
  Infectious (bacterial, fungal)
  Sterile (idiopathic, metabolic, viral)
Hemopericardium (hemorrhage)
  Neoplastic
  Traumatic
  Cardiac rupture (especially left atrial)
  Idiopathic
Pericardial Mass Lesions (± effusion)
Neoplastic
Granulomatous (actinomycosis, coccidioidomycosis)
Pericardial abscess
Constrictive Pericardial Disease
Idiopathic
Infectious
Pericardial foreign body
Neoplastic

With permission from Kittleson M: *Small Animal Cardiovascular Medicine*. St. Louis, Mosby, 1998, p 417.
*Conditions that rarely compromise cardiac function.

Pericardial Effusion in the Dog

Differential diagnosis list available on the companion online site at www.cote.clinicalvetadvisor.com.

Peritonitis

Causes of Peritonitis

Aseptic Peritonitis
Chemical peritonitis
  Bile peritonitis
  Uroperitoneum
Peritoneal foreign body
Starch granulomatous peritonitis
Sclerosing encapsulating peritonitis
Mechanical peritonitis

Septic Peritonitis
Leakage of gastrointestinal contents
  Perforating intestinal foreign body
  Gastric rupture in gastric dilation-volvulus
  Perforating gastric or intestinal ulcers
  Colonic perforation (steroidal or nonsteroidal anti-inflammatory drug induced)
  Dehiscence of intestinal surgical wound
Iatrogenic perforation
  Intraperitoneal alimentation
Penetrating abdominal wounds
Blunt abdominal trauma
Ischemic intestinal injury
Pancreatitis
Ruptured pyometra
Uterine torsion
Ruptured prostatic abscess
Liver abscess or hepatitis
Splenic abscess or splenitis
Splenic torsion
Mesenteric lymph node abscess
Ruptured gallbladder or bile duct with bacterobilia
Ruptured bladder with cystitis
Umbilical abscess
Surgical peritoneal contamination
Peritoneal dialysis

From Slatter D: *Textbook of Small Animal Surgery*. St. Louis, Elsevier, 2003.

Petechiae, Ecchymoses

Causes

Thrombocytopenia
Decreased platelet production
Drug
- Albendazole (D)
- Azathioprine (D,C)
- Chemotherapeutic agents (D,C)
- Chloramphenicol (D,C)
- Estrogen (D)
- Griseofulvin (C)
- Meclofenamic acid (D)
- Phenobarbital (D)
- Phenylbutazone (D)
- Trimethoprim-sulfadiazine (D)

Infection
- *Ehrlichia* spp.
- FeLV
- FIV
- Disseminated histoplasmosis

Myelophthisis
Myelofibrosis
Immune-mediated disorder (antimegakaryocytic)
Increased platelet destruction
IMT
- Primary IMT
  - ITP
  - SLE
- Secondary IMT
  - Infection
  - Neoplasia
  - Vaccine
  - Drug
    - Sulfonamides (D)
    - Cephalosporins (D)
    - Gold salts (D)
    - Methimazole (C)
    - Propylthiouracil (C)
    - Dextrans (D)

Ehrlichia spp. infection
Increased platelet consumption
Disseminated intravascular coagulation
Vasculitis
- Infection
- *Rickettsia rickettsii*
- *Leptospira* spp.
- *Ehrlichia* spp.
- FIP

Neoplasia
Inflammation
Immune-mediated disorder
Drug reaction

Thrombopathia
Inherited
Chédiak-Higashi syndrome of Persian cat
Thrombasthenia of otterhound
Delta-storage pool disease of American cocker spaniel
Other thrombopathias
- Basset hound
- Spitz
- Grey collies with cyclic hematopoiesis
- Domestic shorthair

Acquired
Drug
- Aspirin
- Cephalothin
- Acepromazine

Systemic disease
- Uremia
- Liver disease

Hematologic disorders
- IMT
- Myelo-/lymphoproliferative disorders
- Dysproteinemia (e.g., multiple myeloma)

Vascular Disorders
Vasculitis (see increased platelet consumption)
Hyperadrenocorticism
Dysproteinemia

From Ettinger S, Feldman E: *Textbook of Veterinary Internal Medicine*, ed 5. St. Louis, WB Saunders, 2000.
C, cats; D, dogs; IMT, immune-mediated thrombocytopenia; FeLV, feline leukemia virus; FIP, feline infectious peritonitis; FIV, feline immunodeficiency virus; ITP, idiopathic thrombocytopenic purpura; SLE, systemic lupus erythematosus.

Pleural Effusion

Cause, Appearance, Total Protein, and Cytologic Examination Findings of Pleural Effusions

Cause	Appearance	Total Protein	Cytologic Examination	Other Tests
Pyothorax (*septic exudate*)	Cloudy, tomato soup, malodor	>4 g/dl	Degenerative neutrophils, intracellular and extracellular bacteria, macrophages, RBCs	Aerobic C&S
Idiopathic chylothorax (*modified transudate*)	Milky white	≤3 g/dl	Mature lymphocytes, few RBCs, few macrophages, few neutrophils	Effusion and serum triglyceride levels
Right-sided (± left-sided in cats) heart failure (*modified transudate*)	Clear	≤2 g/dl	Very few cells: RBCs, lymphocytes	Echocardiogram
Lymphosarcoma (*modified transudate or nonseptic exudate*)	Clear, milky, serosanguineous	2–4 g/dl	Immature lymphoblasts, few mature lymphocytes, few RBCs	Thoracic radiographs, thoracic ultrasound, aspirate/cytologic examination of mass
Thymoma (*modified transudate or nonseptic exudate*)	Clear, milky, serosanguineous	2–4 g/dl	Mesothelial cells, mature lymphocytes, few RBCs, few macrophages	Thoracic radiographs, thoracic ultrasound, aspirate/cytologic examination of mass
Neoplasia (e.g., carcinoma) (*modified transudate or nonseptic exudate*)	Clear, cloudy, serosanguineous, bloody	2–4 g/dl	Clumps of neoplastic cells	Thoracic radiographs, thoracic ultrasound
Hypoalbuminemia (*pure transudate*)	Clear, watery	<2.5 g/dl	Mononuclear cells (mesothelial cells, lymphocytes, macrophages)	Serum albumin, urine protein: creatinine ratio, bile acids
FIP (cats) (*nonseptic exudate*)	Straw-colored, cloudy	>4 g/dl	Macrophages, lymphocytes, RBCs, fibrin	FIP PCR on fluid serum FIP titer

Modified with permission from King L: *Textbook of Respiratory Disease in Dogs and Cats*. St. Louis, WB Saunders, 2004, p 16.
C&S, culture and sensitivity; FIP, feline infectious peritonitis; PCR, polymerase chain reaction; RBCs, red blood cells.

Pneumonia, Aspiration

Conditions Predisposing an Animal to Aspiration of Stomach Contents

Impairment of Protective Airway Reflexes
Coma
Head trauma
Metabolic derangements
Central depressant medications (sedation, general anesthesia)
Muscle relaxants
Seizures
Airway trauma
Laryngeal/pharyngeal dysfunction

Large Volumes of Intragastric Food/Fluid
Delayed gastric emptying
- Ileus
- Bowel obstruction
- Pain
- Anxiety
- Opioid medication
- Peristaltic abnormalities
- Pregnancy
- Obesity

Overfeeding by enteral tube
Recent meal (before emergency anesthesia/surgery)

Impaired Function of Gastroesophageal Sphincter
Presence of a nasogastric feeding tube
Achalasia
Esophageal obstruction
Abnormalities of esophageal function
- Megaesophagus
- Reflux esophagitis
- Myasthenia gravis

With permission from King L: *Textbook of Respiratory Disease in Dogs and Cats*. St. Louis, WB Saunders, 2004, p 423.

Pneumonia, Bacteria Isolated In

Differential diagnosis list available on the companion online site at www.cote.clinicalvetadvisor.com.

Polyarthritis

Classification of Immune-Based Arthritis

Erosive
Rheumatoid arthritis
Periosteal proliferative polyarthritis
Polyarthritis of greyhounds

Nonerosive
Systemic lupus erythematosus
Polyarthritis/polymyositis
Polyarthritis/meningitis
Arthritis of Akita
Amyloidosis of shar-pei
Polyarteritis nodosa
Idiopathic
- Type I (uncomplicated)
- Type II (reactive)
- Type III (enteropathic)
- Type IV (malignancy)

Miscellaneous
Vaccination "reactions"
Plasmacytic/lymphocytic synovitis
Drug-induced

With permission from Bonagura J: *Kirk's Current Veterinary Therapy XII: Small Animal Practice*. St. Louis, WB Saunders, 1995, p 1189.

Polycythemia

Relative
Dehydration
Splenic contraction

Absolute
Hypoxemia (respiratory disease, obesity, high altitude)
Renal neoplasm
Pyelonephritis
Renal cyst
Hydronephrosis
Hepatoma
Right-to-left shunting cardiovascular malformation (Eisenmenger's physiology)
- Tetralogy of Fallot
- Right-to-left patent ductus arteriosus
- Septal defect with concurrent severe pulmonic stenosis or pulmonary hypertension
- Double outlet right ventricle
- Transposition of the great arteries

Polycythemia vera

Polyphagia

Primary Polyphagia
Destruction of satiety center
Trauma
Mass lesion (e.g., neoplasia)
Infection
Psychogenic causes
Stress
Introduction of a more palatable diet
Gluttony

Drug-Induced Polyphagia
Glucocorticoids
Anticonvulsants
Antihistamines
Progestins
Benzodiazepines
Amitraz
Cyproheptadine

Reported Specific Disorders Associated with Polyphagia
FIP
Lymphocytic cholangitis (feline)
Spongiform encephalopathy (feline)
Foreign body encephalitis (feline)

Secondary Polyphagia
Physiologic increase in metabolic rate
Cold temperature
Lactation
Pregnancy
Growth
Increased exercise
Pathologic increase in metabolic rate
Hyperthyroidism
Acromegaly
Decreased energy supply
Diabetes mellitus
Malassimilation syndromes
- Pancreatic exocrine insufficiency
- Infiltrative bowel disease
- Parasites
- Lymphangiectasia

Decreased intake
Megaesophagus (congenital)
Low-calorie diet
Hypoglycemia
Unknown
Hyperadrenocorticism
Portosystemic shunt/hepatoencephalopathy
SARDS

Modified from Ettinger S, Feldman E: *Textbook of Veterinary Internal Medicine*, ed 6. St. Louis, WB Saunders, 2005.
FIP, feline infectious peritonitis; SARDS, sudden acquired retinal degeneration.

Polyuria and Polydipsia: Differential Diagnosis

Differential diagnosis list available on the companion online site at www.cote.clinicalvetadvisor.com.

Polyuria and Polydipsia: Drug-Induced

Differential diagnosis list available on the companion online site at www.cote.clinicalvetadvisor.com.

Portosystemic Shunts

Breeds
More commonly single, intrahepatic in large breed dogs
More commonly single, extrahepatic in small breed dogs and cats

Multiple Shunts
Multiple shunts are extrahepatic and are most commonly acquired rather than congenital. They occur secondary to portal hypertension induced by chronic hepatopathies or surgical intervention in an animal with hepatic microvascular dysplasia.

Location on Portogram
If shunt is cranial to T 13, more likely intrahepatic
If any part of the shunt is caudal to T 13, more likely extrahepatic

Preputial Discharge

Urine
PU/PD
Ectopic ureters
Urethral sphincter dysfunction
UTI
Urolithiasis

Hemorrhagic
Bleeding disorder (thrombocytopenia, coagulopathy)
Neoplasia (bladder, urethra, prostate, testicle)
Inflammation/infection (bladder, urethra, prostate, testicle, penis/prepuce [balanoposthitis])
Foreign body (bladder, urethra, prepuce)
Trauma
Urolithiasis

Mucopurulent
Penile and preputial inflammation/infection (balanoposthitis)
Neoplasia
Foreign body (preputial, urethral)
Phimosis

PU/PD, polyuria/polydipsia; UTI, urinary tract infection.

Prostatomegaly

Abscess (asymmetric, often painful)
Benign prostatic hyperplasia (symmetric, nonpainful; uncommon in castrated dogs)
Cyst (prostatic, paraprostatic; asymmetric, nonpainful)
Neoplasia (adenocarcinoma, others; asymmetric, usually nonpainful)
Prostatitis (asymmetric; painful [acute prostatitis] or nonpainful [chronic])

Protein-Losing Enteropathies

Differential diagnosis list available on the companion online site at www.cote.clinicalvetadvisor.com.

Proteinuria

Preglomerular
Physiologic
Stress
Extreme temperatures
Strenuous exercise
Renal venous congestion
Overload
Hyperproteinemia (total protein >9 g/dl)
Hemoglobinemia
Myoglobinemia
Paraproteinemia

Glomerular
Glomerulonephritis
Infectious
- Dirofilariasis
- *Ehrlichia canis*
- Chronic bacterial infections
- Bacterial endocarditis
- Brucellosis
- Leishmaniasis
- Borreliosis
- Septicemia

Inflammatory
- SLE

Neoplastic
Familial
Idiopathic
Amyloidosis
Familial
Inflammatory
- SLE

Neoplastic
Idiopathic
Glomerulosclerosis
Diabetes mellitus
Hyperfiltration
Hypertension

Postglomerular
Tubular dysfunction
Fanconi's syndrome
Acute tubular necrosis
Hemorrhage
UTI
Urolithiasis
Trauma
Neoplasia

With permission from Bonagura J: *Kirk's Current Veterinary Therapy XII: Small Animal Practice*. St. Louis, WB Saunders, 1995, p 938.
SLE, systemic lupus erythematosus; UTI, urinary tract infection.

Pruritus, Cats

Differential diagnosis list available on the companion online site at www.cote.clinicalvetadvisor.com.

Pruritus, Dogs

Differential diagnosis list available on the companion online site at www.cote.clinicalvetadvisor.com.

Pulmonary Hypertension

Causes

Airway or pulmonary parenchymal disease (chronic)
Branch pulmonary artery stenosis (congenital)
Congestive heart failure (chronic left-sided)
Heartworm disease
Hypoxia (chronic): high altitude, chronic airway obstruction
Idiopathic/"primary"
Left-to-right shunting congenital malformations
Persistently underdeveloped/"fetal" pulmonary circulation
Pulmonary thromboembolism

Pulmonary Markings

Differential Diagnoses for the Various Lung Patterns on Thoracic Radiographs

Bronchial Pattern
Chronic bronchitis (irritant, allergic, parasitic)
Calcification
Peribronchial cuffing (edema, bronchopneumonia, pulmonary infiltrates with eosinophilia)

Interstitial Pattern
Nodular
Neoplasia
Granuloma (eosinophilic, fungal, parasitic or heartworm-associated, foreign body)
Bulla with fluid
Hematoma, abscess, cyst
Mucus-filled bronchus
Bronchiectasis
Hazy and unstructured
Diffuse
- Artifact (underexposure, obesity, end-expiratory film)
- Degenerative changes ("old dog lung")
- Neoplasia (lymphosarcoma, metastasis)
- Pneumonitis (toxic, inhalant, metabolic, viral, parasitic)
- ARDS
- Transitional stages of diseases, such as edema, hemorrhage, bronchopneumonia

Localized
- Hemorrhage
- PTE
- Foreign body
- Partial atelectasis
- Transitional stages of disease, such as edema, bronchopneumonia, hemorrhage, or parasites

Alveolar Pattern
Diffuse
Edema (cardiogenic or noncardiogenic)
Bronchopneumonia
Hemorrhage
Smoke inhalation
Near-drowning incident
Acute respiratory distress syndrome
Localized
Edema
Bronchopneumonia
Hemorrhage
Primary lung tumor or metastasis
Lobar collapse or atelectasis
Heartworm disease
Infarct

From Ettinger S, Feldman E: *Textbook of Veterinary Internal Medicine*, ed 6. St. Louis, WB Saunders, 2005.
ARDS, acute respiratory distress syndrome; PTE, pulmonary embolism.

DIFFERENTIAL DIAGNOSIS

Pupil Size Abnormalities, Neurogenic

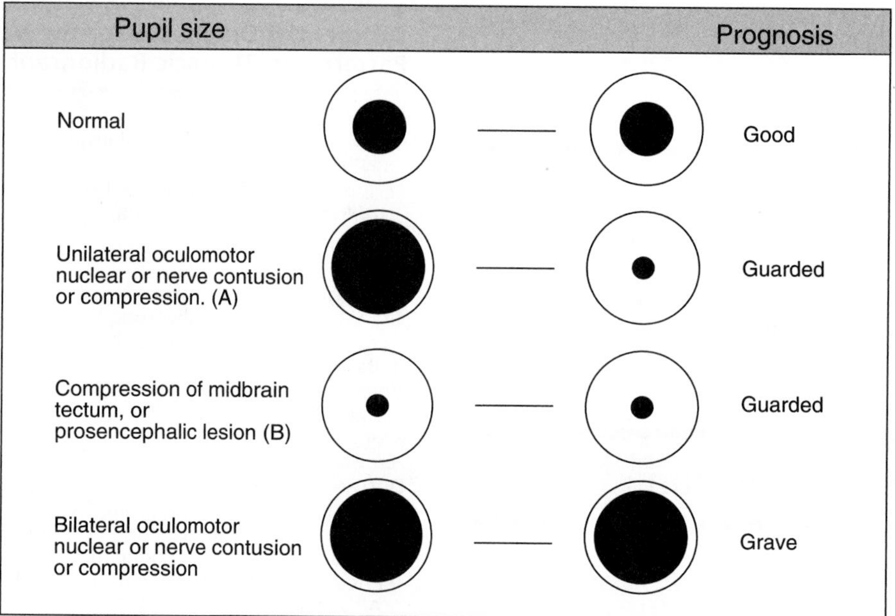

FIGURE III-1 **A**, Asymmetric interference with cerebral control of oculomotor neurons and/or the sympathetic upper motor neuron system. **B**, Bilateral sympathetic upper motor neuron deficiency or loss of facilitation; bilateral release of oculomotor general visceral efferent neurons from cerebral inhibition.

Pyoderma

Differential Diagnosis of Canine Pyoderma

Surface

Pyotraumatic dermatitis (acute moist dermatitis, hot spots): pyotraumatic folliculitis, demodicosis, neoplasia (especially sweat gland adenocarcinoma), cutaneous metastasis, fixed drug eruption, early necrotizing form of idiopathic nodular panniculitis, early localized vasculitis, focal *Malassezia* dermatitis, candidiasis

Intertrigo (skinfold pyoderma)

- Lip-fold intertrigo: localized demodicosis, fixed drug eruption, superficial necrolytic dermatitis, *Malassezia* dermatitis or candidiasis, zinc-responsive dermatosis, muzzle folliculitis and furunculosis (canine acne), localized pemphigus foliaceus, early pemphigus vulgaris, early bullous pemphigoid
- Facial-fold intertrigo: localized demodicosis, *Malassezia* dermatitis, dermatophytosis
- Vulvar-fold intertrigo: urinary tract infection with self-trauma, ulcerative dermatosis of the Shetland sheepdog and collie, drug eruption, canine familial dermatomyositis, pemphigus vulgaris, bullous pemphigoid
- Tail-fold intertrigo: flea allergy dermatitis
- Obesity-fold intertrigo: *Malassezia* dermatitis

Mucocutaneous pyoderma: lip-fold intertrigo, localized demodicosis, early discoid lupus erythematosus, zinc-responsive dermatosis, generic dog food skin disease, muzzle folliculitis and furunculosis (canine acne)

Superficial

Impetigo (puppy pyoderma): early flea allergy dermatitis, superficial folliculitis

Superficial bacterial folliculitis: superficial spreading pyoderma, flea allergy dermatitis, demodicosis, pemphigus foliaceus, sarcoptic acariasis, severe impetigo, drug eruption, erythema multiforme, seborrheic dermatitis, sterile eosinophilic pustulosis

Deep

Deep folliculitis and furunculosis: demodicosis, subcutaneous and deep mycoses, severe maladapted dermatophytosis, sterile granuloma-pyogranuloma, histiocytosis, idiopathic nodular panniculitis, juvenile sterile granulomatous dermatitis and lymphadenitis, vasculitis

Pyotraumatic folliculitis: pyotraumatic dermatitis, demodicosis, neoplasia (especially sweat gland adenocarcinoma), cutaneous metastasis, fixed drug eruption, early necrotizing form of idiopathic nodular panniculitis, early localized vasculitis, focal *Malassezia* dermatitis, candidiasis

Muzzle folliculitis and furunculosis (canine acne): localized demodicosis, early juvenile sterile granulomatous dermatitis and lymphadenitis

Pedal folliculitis and furunculosis: demodicosis, dermatophytosis, subcutaneous and deep mycoses, opportunistic fungal diseases, *Pelodera* dermatitis

Callus pyoderma (pressure-point pyoderma): acral lick dermatitis, generic dog food skin disease, focal actinic comedones

German shepherd dog pyoderma: demodicosis with secondary deep pyoderma, subcutaneous and deep mycoses, opportunistic fungal diseases

Cellulitis (+ demodicosis): juvenile sterile granulomatous dermatitis and lymphadenitis (juvenile cellulites), subcutaneous and deep mycoses, German shepherd dog pyoderma, sterile granuloma-pyogranuloma, idiopathic liquefying panniculitis

Reprinted with permission from Ihrke PJ: *Bacterial Skin Disease in the Dog: A Guide to Canine Pyoderma*. Princeton, NJ, Veterinary Learning Systems, 1996. With permission from Greene C: *Infectious Diseases of the Dog and Cat*, ed 2. St. Louis, WB Saunders, 1999, p 544.

Red Eye

Parameter	Anterior Uveitis	Conjunctivitis	Superficial Keratitis	Glaucoma
Conjunctiva	Not thickened, vessels easily seen	Thick, folded and hyperemic, vessels concealed	Not thickened	Not thickened
Conjunctival vessels	Circumcorneal and straight, not movable with conjunctiva	Superficial, diffuse, and tortuous	Diffuse, vessels form fine network in vicinity of cornea	Diffuse, superficial and prominent
Secretion or discharge	None	Moderate to copious	Serous to purulent	None
Pain	Moderate	None to slight	Moderate to severe	Severe to acute
Photophobia	Moderate	None	Severe	Slight
Cornea	Clear to steamy	Clear	Clouded to opaque	Steamy
Pupil size	Small, sluggish, irregular, or fixed	Normal	Normal	Dilated, moderate to complete, and fixed
Pupillary light response	Poor	Normal	Normal	Absent
Intraocular pressure	Variable; may be normal, slightly elevated, or diminished	Normal	Normal	Elevated

With permission from Lavignette AM: Differential diagnosis and treatment of anterior uveitis. *Vet Clin North Am* 3:504, 1973. Modified from Slatter D: *Fundamentals of Veterinary Ophthalmology*. St. Louis, WB Saunders, 2001.

Regurgitation

Causes

Esophageal Disease
Megaesophagus (primary or secondary)
Esophagitis
Mechanical obstruction (foreign body, stricture, vascular ring anomaly)

Alimentary Disorders
Pyloric outflow obstruction
Gastric dilatation volvulus
Hiatal hernia

Neuropathies
Peripheral (polyradiculitis, giant cell axonal neuropathy, polyneuritis, lead poisoning)
Central (distemper, brainstem lesion, neoplasia, trauma)

Neuromuscular Junction Abnormalities
Myasthenia gravis (focalized or generalized)
Botulism
Tetanus
AChE toxicity

Immune-Mediated Causes
SLE
Polymyositis
Dermatomyositis

Endocrine
Hypothyroidism
Hypoadrenocorticism

From Ettinger S, Feldman E: *Textbook of Veterinary Internal Medicine*, ed 6. St. Louis, WB Saunders, 2005.
AChE, acetylcholinesterase; SLE, systemic lupus erythematosus.

Renal Failure, Acute

Causes of Intrinsic Acute Renal Failure

Renal Ischemia
Progression of prerenal azotemia
Renal vascular disease (avulsion, thrombosis, stenosis)

Nephrotoxicity
Exogenous toxins
Endogenous toxins
Drugs

Primary Renal Diseases
Infections: pyelonephritis, leptospirosis, infectious canine hepatitis
Immune-mediated desease: acute glomerulonephritis, SLE, renal transplant rejection
Neoplasia: lymphoma
Miscellaneous: "Alabama rot"

Systemic Diseases with Renal Manifestations
Infections: FIP, borreliosis, babesiosis, leishmaniasis, bacterial endocarditis
Pancreatitis
SIRS, sepsis, mutiple organ failure, DIC
Heart failure
SLE
Hepatorenal syndrome
Malignant hypertension
Hyperviscosity syndrome: polycythemia, multiple myeloma

From Ettinger S, Feldman E: *Textbook of Veterinary Internal Medicine*, ed 6. St. Louis, WB Saunders, 2005.
DIC, disseminated intravascular coagulopathy; FIP, feline infectious peritonitis; SIRS, systemic inflammatory response syndrome; SLE, systemic lupus erythematosus.

Renal Failure, Acute Versus Chronic

Differential diagnosis list available on the companion online site at www.cote.clinicalvetadvisor.com.

Respiratory Parasites

Parasite (host)	Comment
Aelurostrongylus abstrusus (cats)	Coughing, sneezing, lethargy possible but usually no signs
Capillaria aerophila (dogs, cats)	Chronic cough or no clinical signs
Crenosoma vulpis (wild canids; rarely dogs)	Chronic cough clinically mimicking chronic sterile bronchitis
Eucoleus boehmi (dogs, cats)	Chronic sneezing, nasal discharge, facial rubbing
Filaroides hirthi (dogs only)	Breeding kennels; zinc sulfate flotation is best (not Baermann)
Oslerus osleri (wild canids; rarely dogs)	Nodules in large airway mucosa; treatment difficult
Paragonimus kellicotti (dogs, cats)	Chronic cough ± pneumothorax; rust-colored pharyngeal phlegm
Pneumonyssoides caninum (dogs)	Nasal mite; sensitive to parenteral (and presumably oral) ivermectin

Retinopathies

Common Systemic Disorders Affecting the Retina

Dog
Blastomycosis
Coccidioidomycosis
Cryptococcosis
Distemper
Ehrlichiosis
Histoplasmosis
Hypertension
Larva migrans (*Toxocara* spp.)
Leishmaniasis
Lymphosarcoma
Multiple myeloma
Toxoplasmosis

Cat
Blastomycosis
Cryptococcosis
FIP
Histoplasmosis
Hypertension
Lymphosarcoma (both FeLV positive and negative)
Toxoplasmosis
Tuberculosis

Modified from Slatter D: *Fundamentals of Veterinary Ophthalmology*. St. Louis, WB Saunders, 2001.
FeLV, feline leukemia virus; FIP, feline infectious peritonitis.

Salter-Harris Fracture Classification

Salter-Harris Classification of Separations or Fracture-Separations Involving a Growth Plate and the Adjacent Metaphysis and Epiphysis

Type of Fracture	Radiographic Findings	Principal Anatomic Region Involved
Type 1	Physeal separation, displacement of the epiphysis from the metaphysis at the growth plate	Proximal humerus and femur, distal femur
Type 2	Small corner of the metaphyseal bone fractured, with displacement of the epiphysis from the metaphysis at the growth plate	Distal femur and humerus, proximal humerus, proximal tibia
Type 3	Fracture through the epiphysis and part of the growth plate, with the metaphysis unaffected	Distal humerus
Type 4	Fracture through the epiphysis, growth plate, and metaphysis; several fracture lines possible	Distal femur, distal humerus
Type 5	Compression of the growth plate. Soft tissue swelling, but no bony abnormalities seen following the injury	Distal ulna, distal radius, distal femur

Modified from Piermattei D, Flo G: *Brinker, Piermattei, and Flo's Handbook of Small Animal Orthopedics and Fracture Repair*, ed 3. St. Louis, WB Saunders, 1997.

Seizures

Causes

Extracranial
Hypoglycemia
- Glycogen storage diseases
- β-Cell neoplasm of pancreas
- Youth and malnutrition (especially small or toy breeds)
- Youth and GI disease (especially small or toy breeds)
- Insulin excess during treatment for diabetes mellitus
- Intestinal leiomyosarcoma

Hypoxia
- Cardiorespiratory disease (e.g., severe bradycardia or severe tachycardia, disorders producing polycythemia)
- Hepatoencephalopathy
- Renal disease
- Hypocalcemia
- Hyperkalemia
- Hyperlipoproteinemia
- GI disease
  - Parasitism
  - "Garbage" toxicity
- Polycythemia
  - Right-to-left shunt (e.g., reversed patent ductus arteriosus, tetralogy of Fallot, atrial or ventricular septal defect with concurrent pulmonic stenosis or pulmonary hypertension)
  - Renal neoplasm (erythropoietin-producing)
  - Chronic lung disease
  - Polycythemia vera

Intracranial
Inflammations
- Canine distemper encephalitis, toxoplasmosis, cryptococcosis, neosporosis
- Other viral encephalitides: rabies
- FIP meningoencephalitis in cats

Neoplasia
- Primary or metastatic

Malformations
- Hydrocephalus, lissencephaly-pachygyria

Injury
Degenerations
- Thiamine deficiency in cats
- Cerebral infarction in cats
- Intoxications: lead, mercury, arsenic, chlorinated hydrocarbons, organophosphates, hexachlorophene, ethylene glycol; radiopaque media for myelography, metaldehyde, tremorgenic mycotoxins (penitrem A, roquefortine), blue-green algae, chocolate, marijuana, ethanol/methanol/ fermented materials (e.g., bread dough), prescription human medications

Idiopathic Epilepsy

Modified from de Lahunta A: *Veterinary Neuroanatomy and Clinical Neurology*. St. Louis, WB Saunders, 1983.
FIP, feline infectious peritonitis; GI, gastrointestinal.

Seizures: Causes Grouped According to Age

Prevalence of Common Seizure Disorders in Relation to Patient's Age at the Time of Onset of the First Seizure

Age of the Seizure Disorder Onset: Before 8 Months
Rare: idiopathic epilepsy
Mainly:
Developmental disorders (e.g., malformations, hydrocephalus)
Encephalitis or meningitis
Trauma
Extracranial causes
- Hepatic encephalopathy (e.g., portocaval shunt)
- Hypoglycemia
- Intoxications
- Intestinal parasitism

Age of Onset: 8 Months to 4 Years
Mainly: idiopathic epilepsy
Seldom:
Developmental disorders (e.g., malformations, hydrocephalus)
Trauma
Encephalitis or meningitis
Acquired hydrocephalus
Neoplasia
Extracranial causes
- Hepatic encephalopathy (e.g., portacaval shunt, liver disease)
- Hypocalcemia
- Electrolyte disturbances
- Hypothyroidism
- Intoxications

Age of Onset: More Than 4 Years
Seldom:
Idiopathic epilepsy
Trauma
Encephalitis or meningitis
Acquired hydrocephalus
Extracranial causes
- Hepatic encephalopathy (e.g., serious liver disease)
- Hypocalcemia
- Electrolyte disturbances
- Hypothyroidism

Increasing:
Neoplasia
Degenerative disorders
Vascular disorders
Extracranial causes
- Hypoxia
- Hypoglycemia

Modified with permission from Braund KB: *Clinical Syndromes in Veterinary Neurology*. St. Louis, Mosby, 1994, p 242.

Seizures: Characteristics and Differentiation

Seizures, Differentiation from Other Events

	Seizure (Grand Mal)	Seizure (Partial)	Syncope	Episodic Weakness	Narcolepsy/ Cataplexy
Precipitating event			Exertion, pain, micturition, defecation, cough, stressful event	Exertion or none	Excitement, feeding
Prodrome	Minutes to days; atypical behavior (e.g., anxious, more withdrawn, attention-seeking) ± vomiting		Seconds; acute weakness, staggering, vocalization, autonomic stimulation	None (disorder is neuromuscular)	None
Aura	None	Marks onset of partial seizure	None	None	None
Event features	Chomping, hypersalivation, tonic-clonic limb motion; duration often 1–2 minutes; duration >5 minutes consistent with seizure, highly inconsistent with syncope.	Localized signs	Motionlessness; flaccid or rigid extension of limbs; opisthotonus possible; no tonic-clonic activity; duration generally transient (<1 minute)	Gradual or sudden loss of muscle tone, causing recumbency; mentation and consciousness remain normal; no tonic-clonic activity	Instantaneous loss of muscle tone; animal is immobile (sleeping) but appears to be aware of its surroundings
Recovery	Slowness returning to consciousness; disorientation (commonly 10 minutes or longer); blindness, circling, and other signs of central nervous system dysfunction common	Varies	Rapid recovery of normal mentation; often able to walk (and considered back to normal by owner) within minutes	Highly variable; generally reflective of course of onset (gradual onset associated with slow recovery); in some cases, rapid onset disorders may have a protracted course	Fairly rapid (several seconds to 1 minute), with appearance of waking from sleep

Modified from Ettinger SJ, Feldman EC: *Textbook of Veterinary Internal Medicine*, ed 6. St. Louis, Elsevier, 2005, p 27.

Convulsive syncope ("Stokes-Adams seizures" or "Stokes-Adams attacks") are syncopal events generally caused by cardiac arrhythmias that produce profound syncope, causing temporary cerebral hypoxia and seizures. Therefore, clarification of the type of event observed by the owner (syncope versus seizure) may be difficult and generally rests on the observation of an episode, the presence of heart disease, and the documentation of a severe bradycardia or tachycardia during the event. Videotaping of an episode by the owner and cardiac event monitoring (pager-size portable electrocardiographic [ECG] unit that is triggered by the owner when an event occurs) can be invaluable in clarifying whether an animal is experiencing seizures versus syncope.

Seizures, Refractory or Poorly Controlled

Factors Responsible for Inadequate Control of Seizures

Medication and Dosage
- Improper choice of drug
- Insufficient drug dosage
- Delayed increase in dosage
- Inadequate increase in dosage
- Too rapid change of medication
- Too rapid reduction of dosage
- Excessive fluctuations in serum concentrations
- Inappropriately combined drugs
- Failure to monitor serum levels.

Noncompliance

Drug-drug interactions

Other precipitating factors
- Additional medications
- Additional diseases
- Physical or psychologic stress

Diagnostic failures
- Extracerebral causes of seizures
- Progressive brain lesions
- Misidentification of episodes
- Syncope
- Myasthenia gravis
- Narcolepsy/cataplexy

Modified with permission from Kirk RW, Bonagura JD (eds): *Kirk's Current Veterinary Therapy XI: Small Animal Practice*. St. Louis, WB Saunders, 1993, p 986.

Shock

Differential diagnosis list available on the companion online site at www.cote.clinicalvetadvisor.com.

Skin Tumors

Epithelial Tumors

Epidermal tumors
- Papilloma
- Squamous cell carcinoma
- Basal cell tumors
- Intracutaneous cornifying epithelioma

Follicular tumors
- Trichoepithelioma
- Pilomatricoma

Sebaceous gland tumors

Sweat gland tumors

Perianal gland tumors

Anal sac apocrine gland tumors

Ceruminous gland tumors

Spindle Cell Tumors

Soft-tissue sarcoma

Round Cell Tumors

Canine cutaneous histiocytoma

Mast cell tumor

Plasmacytoma

Lymphoma

Transmissible venereal tumor

Neuroendocrine Tumors

Melanocytic tumors

From Ettinger S, Feldman E: *Textbook of Veterinary Internal Medicine*, ed 5. St. Louis, WB Saunders, 2000.

Spinal Reflexes

Differential diagnosis list available on the companion online site at www.cote.clinicalvetadvisor.com.

Splenic Diseases: Infectious

Infectious Causes of Splenomegaly/Splenitis*

Viral Diseases
FIP (C)
FeLV (C)
FIV (C)
Infectious canine hepatitis (D)

Rickettsial and mycoplasmal diseases
Ehrlichiosis (*canine and feline*)
RMSF (*Rickettsia rickettsii*)
Q fever (*Coxiella burnetii*)
Hemotropic mycoplasmosis (*Mycoplasma haemofelis*, formerly *Haemobartonella felis* Ohio)

Bacterial Infections
Canine brucellosis
Mycoplasmosis
Florida borreliosis
Plague
Tularemia
Streptococcosis
Staphylococcosis
Salmonellosis
Francisella infection
Endotoxemia

Fungal Diseases
Cryptococcosis
Histoplasmosis
Blastomycosis

Protozoal Diseases
Toxoplasmosis
Cytauxzoonosis (C)
Babesiosis (*Babesia canis* and *B. gibsoni*)
Leishmaniasis (D)

From Ettinger S, Feldman E: *Textbook of Veterinary Internal Medicine*, ed 6. St. Louis, WB Saunders, 2005.

*Infectious disease may affect the spleen directly or may indirectly cause splenomegaly by causing chronic anemia, chronic antigen stimulation, or disturbances in blood flow (e.g., endotoxmia).

C, cats; D, dogs; FeLV, feline leukemia virus; FIP, feline infectious peritonitis; FIV, feline immunodeficiency virus; RMSF, Rocky Mountain spotted fever.

Splenomegaly

Causes of Splenomegaly

Causes of Generalized Splenomegaly
Inflammation
- Infectious
- Granulomatous condition

Neoplasia
- Primary
  - Lymphoma
  - Mastocytosis
  - Histiocytosis
- Metastatic

Hyperplasia
- Extramedullary hematopoiesis

Amyloidosis

Congestion
- *Pharmacologic*
  - Phenothiazine tranquilizer
  - Barbiturates
- *Torsion of splenic pedicle*
  - Isolated
  - With gastric dilatation-volvulus
- *Portal vein/caudal vena cava hypertension*
  - Vascular anomaly
  - Cardiac failure
  - Hepatic cirrhosis
  - Neoplasia

Causes of Localized Splenomegaly
Neoplasia
- Hemangiosarcoma
- Hemangioma
- Lymphosarcoma
- Leiomyosarcoma
- Fibrosarcoma

Non-neoplasia
- Hematoma
- Nodular hyperplasia
- Abscess

Modified from Bonagura J: *Kirk's Current Veterinary Therapy XIII*, ed 13. St. Louis, WB Saunders, 2000.

Stomatitis

Stomatitis	
Conditions associated with immune system depression or dysfunction	Necrotizing ulcerative gingivostomatitis
	Mycotic infections (commonly candidiasis)
	Neutrophil dysfunction; gray collie syndrome, drug therapy, viral infection (e.g., FeLV)
Autoimmune disorders	Vesiculobullous skin diseases (e.g., pemphigus and pemphigoid)
	Systemic or discoid lupus erythematosus
	Sjögren-like syndrome
Hypersensitivity	Drug eruptions
	Insect stings
Viral infections	FeLV
	FIV
	Calicivirus
Miscellaneous conditions	Eosinophilic granuloma complex
	Feline chronic gingivostomatitis

Modified from Slatter D: *Textbook of Small Animal Surgery*. St. Louis, Elsevier, 2003.
FeLV, feline leukemia virus; FIV, feline immunodeficiency virus.

Storage Disorders

Differential diagnosis list available on the companion online site at www.cote.clinicalvetadvisor.com.

Stunted Growth

Potential Causes of Small Stature in Dogs and Cats

Endocrine
Hyposomatotropism
Hypothyroidism
Hyperadrenocorticism
Hypoadrenocorticism
Diabetes mellitus

Nonendocrine
Malnutrition
Gastrointestinal
- Maldigestion
- Pancreatic exocrine insufficiency
- Malabsorption
- Heavy intestinal parasitism

Hepatic
- Portosystemic vascular shunt
- Glycogen storage disease

Renal disease
Cardiovascular disease (especially congenital heart defects)
Skeletal dysplasia; chondrodystrophy
Mucopolysaccharidosis
Hydrocephalus

From Feldman E, Nelson R: *Canine and Feline Endocrinology and Reproduction*, ed 3. St. Louis, WB Saunders, 2004.

Subcutaneous and Skin Masses

Common Skin and Subcutaneous Tumors

Epithelial Tumors
Papilloma
Intracutaneous cornifying epithelioma
Squamous cell carcinoma
Basal cell tumors
Trichoepithelioma
Pilomatricoma
Trichoblastoma
Sebaceous gland tumors
Hepatoid gland tumors (perianal gland tumors)
Sweat gland tumors (apocrine gland tumors)
Ceruminous gland tumors
Anal sac apocrine gland tumors

Mesenchymal Tumors
Soft-tissue sarcomas

Round Cell Tumors
Plasmacytoma
Mast cell tumor
Lymphoma
Histiocytoma
Transmissible venereal tumor

Melanocytic Tumors
Melanoma

From Ettinger S, Feldman E: *Textbook of Veterinary Internal Medicine*, ed 6. St. Louis, WB Saunders, 2005.

Syncope

Differential Diagnoses for Syncope and Episodic Weakness

Primary Cardiac Causes
Arrhythmias
Obstruction to cardiac filling
Obstruction of ventricular ejection

Hypotension
Inadequate cardiac output (e.g., dilated cardiomyopathy)
Inadequate vascular tone (e.g., vasodilators, β-blockers)
Inadequate blood volume
- Blood loss
  - Internal (e.g., splenic hemangiosarcoma, GI blood loss)
  - External (e.g., trauma)
- Diuresis (e.g., furosemide)
- Hypoadrenocorticism
- Fluid loss (e.g., emesis, diarrhea)

Hypoxemia
Respiratory failure
Pulmonary thromboembolism

Abnormalities of Blood Constituents
Hypoglycemia
Hypokalemia
Anemia
Hepatoencephalopathy

Neurologic and Neuromuscular Disorders
Epilepsy
Structural CNS disorders
- Neoplasia
- Cerebral arterial disease
- Thromboembolism

Narcolepsy
Myasthenia gravis

From Fox P: *Textbook of Canine and Feline Cardiology: Principles and Practice*. St. Louis, WB Saunders, 2000, p 447.

Syncope, Disease Associations

Differential diagnosis list available on the companion online site at www.cote.clinicalvetadvisor.com.

Systemic Inflammatory Response and Multiple Organ Dysfunction

Differential diagnosis list available on the companion online site at www.cote.clinicalvetadvisor.com.

Tachycardia

Differential Diagnosis for a Rapid Heart Rate

Sinus tachycardia
- Excitement
- Pain
- Toxicosis (e.g., chocolate; digitalis; aminophylline/theophylline; pseudoephedrine, phenylpropanolamine, and related compounds)
- Sepsis
- Hypotension
- Congestive heart failure
- Systemic illness (e.g., hyperthyroidism, fever, anemia)

Atrial flutter
Atrial fibrillation
Atrial/junctional tachycardias
Preexcitation (Wolff-Parkinson-White syndrome, others)
Ventricular tachycardia
Ventricular flutter
Torsade de pointes

Tenesmus/Dyschezia

Causes

Colorectal Disease
Constipation
Colitis-proctitis
- Inflammatory bowel disease
- *Histoplasma capsulatum* (histoplasmosis)
- *Clostridium perfringens* (enterotoxicosis)
- *Prototheca zopfii* (protothecosis)

Rectal stricture
Neoplasia: polyps
Foreign material
Irritable bowel syndrome

Perineal-Perianal Disease
Anal sacculitis, impaction, or abscess
Anal sac neoplasia
Perianal fistula
Perineal hernia

Urogenital Disease
Cystitis-urethritis-vaginitis
Obstructive material—urethral calculi, foreign body
Prostatitis-prostatic abscess
Parturition
Neoplasia of the urethra, bladder, prostate, or vagina

Miscellaneous Causes
Caudal abdominal cavity mass
Pelvic fracture: neoplasia

From Ettinger S, Feldman E: *Textbook of Veterinary Internal Medicine*, ed 6. St. Louis, WB Saunders, 2005.

Testicular Dimension Abnormalities

Diseases That Cause Change in Testicular Size

Large Testes
Neoplasia
Acute infection
Testicular torsion
Inguinoscrotal hernia
Sperm granuloma

Small Testes
Hypoplasia
Chronic inflammation
Cryptorchidism
Degeneration
Intersex

From Bonagura J: *Kirk's Current Veterinary Therapy XIII*, ed 13. St. Louis, WB Saunders, 2000.

Third Eyelid Disorders

Differential Diagnosis of Prominent Third Eyelid/Third Eyelid Protrusion, and Treatment Approaches

Prominent Third Eyelid with Focal Abnormality
- Curled or scrolled leading edge: excise abnormal cartilage
- Pink, fleshy mass protruding between the globe and the third eyelid in a young dog ("cherry eye"): surgically reposition the gland
- Pink, fleshy mass protruding between the globe and the third eyelid in an old dog: possible neoplasia; biopsy or complete excision of third eyelid
- Mass within or on anterior surface of third eyelid: biopsy or local excision with or without adjunctive therapy; larger masses may require complete excision of third eyelid

Generalized Enlargement of the Third Eyelid
- Thickened and depgimented; may have corneal involvement ("pannus"): conjunctival scraping or biopsy; treat with topical steroids, cyclosporine
- Thickened and inflamed with firm, fibrous nodules; cornea, episclera, and bulbar conjunctiva are also often involved; biopsy: collie-nodular granulomatous episclerokeratitis, other breeds: ocular nodular fasciitis; treat on basis of breed and biopsy results
- Diffuse, generalized enlargement of third eyelid or gland of the third eyelid: aspiration or biopsy; lymphosarcoma or other systemic neoplasia

Prominent Third Eyelid Only
- Nonpigmented leading edge: appears prominent but needs no therapy
- Secondary to pain: check for corneal ulcer, foreign body, or other source of ocular or intraocular pain
- Horner's syndrome: look for other signs of miosis, ptosis, and enophthalmos; attempt to localize lesion and treat if needed
- Secondary to orbital disease: enophthalmos may lead to passive protrusion or orbital mass; cellulitis or myositis may displace third eyelid, causing protrusion
- Systemic disease, such as tetanus

From Slatter D: *Textbook of Small Animal Surgery*. St. Louis, Elsevier, 2003.

Thromboembolism

Causes and Predisposing Factors of Thrombosis and Thromboembolism

Vascular Endothelial Damage
Arteriosclerosis
Atherosclerosis
Vasculitis
Heartworm disease
Catheterization
Injection of irritating substances
Neoplasia
Vascular incarceration/compression
Hyperhomocysteinemia
FIE
Fibrocartilaginous embolism

Hypercoagulability
Infection/sepsis/abscess
Neoplasia
Hyperadrenocorticism
PLN
PLE
DIC
Thrombocytosis
Platelet hyperreactivity
IHA
Parvovirus infection

Abnormal Blood Flow
Neoplasia
Cardiomyopathy
CHF
Endocarditis
Hypovolemia
Shock
Anemia
Polycythemia
Dehydration
Hyperviscosity

From Ettinger S, Feldman E: *Textbook of Veterinary Internal Medicine*, ed 6. St. Louis, WB Saunders, 2005.
CHF, congestive heart failure; DIC, disseminated intravascular coagulation; FIE, feline ischemic encephalopathy; IHA, immune-mediated hemolytic anemia; PLE, protein-losing enteropathy; PLN, protein-losing nephropathy.

Thyroid Hormone Alterations

Differential diagnosis list available on the companion online site at www.cote.clinicalvetadvisor.com.

Total Protein Elevation (Serum)

Inflammation
Infectious
Bacterial (e.g., deep pyoderma)
Viral (e.g., feline infectious peritonitis)
Protozoal (e.g., leishmaniasis)
Fungal (e.g., blastomycosis)
Rickettsial (e.g., ehrlichiosis)
Noninfectious
Neoplasia (especially if necrotic areas are present)
Foreign body granuloma
Antigenic response (e.g., inflammatory bowel disease)
Paraneoplastic protein synthesis
Multiple myeloma
Lymphoma
Dehydration
Hemoconcentration can elevate both albumin and globulin fractions.
Dehydration/hemoconcentration is the only differential diagnosis to explain hyperalbuminemia.

Modified from Cowell R: *Veterinary Clinical Pathology Secrets*. St. Louis, Elsevier, 2004, p 56.

Toxins, Radiopaque

Potentially Toxic Substances That May Be Detected Radiographically

Ammonium chloride
Antivert (meclizine, an antiemetic)
Aspirin (enteric-coated)
Bethanechol
Calcium carbonate
Chloral hydrate
Compazine (prochlorperazine)
Copper (coins)
Crack vials
Drug packets
Elavil (amitriptyline)
Iron
Lead (fishing sinkers)
Mothballs
  Paradichlorobenzene (highly opaque)
  Naphthalene (faintly opaque)
Multivitamins with iron
Placidyl
Potassium chloride
Sustained-release products
Thorazine (chlorpromazine)
Zinc (pennies)

With permission from Peterson ME, Talcott PA: *Small Animal Toxicology*. St. Louis, WB Saunders, 2006.

Tracheal Neoplasia

Malignant Tumors of the Canine and Feline Trachea
Tracheal Tumors
Lymphoma
Squamous cell carcinoma
Mast cell tumor
Chondrosarcoma
Adenocarcinoma
Osteosarcoma
Anaplastic carcinoma
Leiomyoma

Modified from Bonagura JD: *Kirk's Current Veterinary Therapy XIII*, ed 13. WB Saunders, 1999, p 503.

Ulcerative/Erosive Skin Lesions

Differential diagnosis list available on the companion online site at www.cote.clinicalvetadvisor.com.

Ulcers and Erosions (Cutaneous), Distribution

Differential diagnosis list available on the companion online site at www.cote.clinicalvetadvisor.com.

Upper Respiratory Infection, Feline

Essential Clinical Features of Respiratory Disease Related to Pathogen Involved

Feature	FVR	FCV*	FCh	Bb
Lethargy	+++	+	+	+
Sneezing	+++	+	+	++
Conjunctivitis	++	++	+++**	–
Hypersalivation	++	–†	–	–
Ocular discharge	+++	++	+++	(+)
Nasal discharge	+++	++	+	++
Oral ulceration	+	+++	–	–
Keratitis	+	–	–	–
Coughing	(+)	–	–	++
Pneumonia	(+)	+	±	+
Lameness	–	++	–	–

Based on a table previously published in Gaskell RM, Bennett M: *Feline and Canine Infectious Diseases*. Blackwell Science, 1996, p 8.

* Strain variation.

** Often persistent.

† Slight wetness may be seen around the mouth if ulcers present.

FVR, feline viral rhinotracheitis (feline herpesvirus infection; FCV, feline calcivirus infection; FCh, *Chlamydophila felis* (formerly *Chlamydia psittaci)* infection; Bb, *Bordetella bronchiseptica* infection; (+), uncommon but may occur; ±, lesions may be present but are not usually seen clinically.

Urinary Crystals

Name	Description	Significance
Struvite (magnesium ammonium phosphate)	Colorless prisms with three to six sides (coffin lid)	Common in mildly acidic to alkaline urine in normal dogs and cats; may be associated with struvite calculi and infection with urease-producing bacteria
Calcium oxalate (monohydrate)	Dumbbells or small spindles	May be normal (especially if delay in analysis after urine collection), or due to ethylene glycol intoxication; may be associated with oxalate calculi
Calcium oxalate (dihydrate)	Colorless envelopes or small stars	May be normal (especially if delay in analysis after urine collection), or due to ethylene glycol intoxication; may be associated with oxalate calculi
Calcium phosphate	Prisms (long) or amorphous	May be normal or associated with calculi
Ammonium urate	Yellow-brown "thorn apples"	Normal in dalmatians and English bulldogs; associated with hepatic insufficiency and portosystemic shunts; may be associated with urate calculi
Uric acid	Yellow to yellow-brown prisms, diamonds, or rosettes	Same as ammonium urate
Bilirubin	Golden-yellow to brown needles or granules	May be present in normal dogs with concentrated urine or may be due to bilirubinuria
Cystine	Colorless, flat hexagonal plates	Due to cystinuria; may be associated with calculi
Cholesterol	Colorless, flat, notched plates	May be found in normal dogs and cats
Hippuric acid	Prisms (four to six) sides with rounded corners	Uncertain; have been confused with calcium oxalate monohydrate crystals
Sulfonamide	Clear to brown eccentrically bound needles in sheaves	Associated with sulfonamide administration

Modified from Willard M, Tvedten H: *Small Animal Clinical Diagnosis by Laboratory Methods*, ed 4. St. Louis, WB Saunders, 2004.

Urinary Tract Infections, Recurrent and Persistent

Underlying Causes of a Recurrent or Persistent Urinary Tract Infection

Cause	Means of Diagnosis
Lack of owner compliance in drug administration	History (check for leftover medications)
Upper UTI	Excretory urogram showing dilated pelvis, culture urine from renal pelvis, urinalysis demonstrating WBC casts, ultrasonography
Calculi	Survey and/or contrast radiographs, ultrasonography, cystoscopy
Prostatitis	Rectal palpation, ejaculate cytologic examination and culture, prostatic aspirate, prostatic biopsy, ultrasonography
Neoplasm	Rectal palpation, vaginal palpation, cytologic examination of urine sediment, contrast radiographs, biopsy, ultrasonography, urethrocystoscopy
Diverticulum	Positive-contrast radiographs
Granuloma	Contrast radiographs, urethrocystoscopy, biopsy
Urinary incontinence or urine retention due to any cause	History, physical examination, determination of residual urine volume
Decreased resistance to infection	History, physical exam, medical evaluation to detect hyperadrenocorticism, diabetes mellitus, retroviral infection in cats, or other causes of immune compromise
Urinary catheterization	History, physical examination
Antibiotic resistance	Urine C&S
Foreign body	Ultrasound, cystoscopy
PU/PD (severe): antibiotic fails to attain adequate concentration in urine	Measure water intake; urinalysis
Vaginal or preputial conformational abnormalities	Physical exam

Modified from Willard M, Tvedten H: *Small Animal Clinical Diagnosis by Laboratory Methods*, ed 4. St. Louis, WB Saunders, 2004.
C&S, culture and sensitivity; PU/PD, polyuria and polydipsia; UTI, urinary tract infection; WBC, white blood cell.

Uroliths

Radiographic Characteristics of Common Uroliths

Mineral Type	Degree of Radiopacity	Shape
Cystine	+ to ++	Smooth; usually small; round to oval
Calcium oxalate dihydrate	++++	Often rough; round to oval (occasionally jackstone)
Calcium oxalate monohydrate	+++	Often smooth, round (occasionally jackstone)
Struvite	+ to ++++	Smooth; round or faceted; sometimes assumes shape of renal pelvis, ureter, bladder, or urethra; sometimes laminated
Calcium phosphate	++++	Smooth; round or faceted
Ammonium urate and uric acid	0 to ++	Smooth but occasionally irregular; round or oval
Silica*	++ to ++++	Typically jackstone
Mixed and compound	+ to ++++	Varies with composition; may have detectable nucleus and shell
Matrix	0 to +	Usually round but may be influenced by location

From Slatter D: *Textbook of Small Animal Surgery*. St. Louis, Elsevier, 2003.
*Not observed as a primary mineral in cats.

DIFFERENTIAL DIAGNOSIS

Uveitis

Systemic Etiologies of Anterior and Posterior Uveitis

Infectious
Mycotic: blastomycosis, cryptococcosis, histoplasmosis, coccidioidomycosis, aspergillosis, other
Rickettsia: *Ehrlichia canis*, *E. platys*, RMSF
Toxoplasmosis
FIV, FeLV, FIP
Lyme disease (borreliosis)
Bacteremia/septicemia
Brucella canis
Aberrant parasitic migration: heartworm, *Toxocara*, hookworm, others
Infectious canine hepatitis
Protothecosis
Mycobacteria
Leptospirosis
Leishmaniasis
Distemper
Other

Noninfectious
Neoplasia: lymphosarcoma, adenocarcinoma, reticulosis, other
Autoimmune: uveodermatologic syndrome (Vogt-Koyanagi-Harada-like syndrome)
Other

With permission from Kirk RW, Bonagura JD (eds): *Kirk's Current Veterinary Therapy XI: Small Animal Practice*. St. Louis, WB Saunders, 1993, p 1114.
FeLV, feline leukemia virus infection; FIP, feline infectious peritonitis; FIV, feline immunodeficiency virus; RMSF, Rocky Mountain spotted fever.

Vaccine Failure

Causes

Host Factors
Primary immunodeficiencies
Maternal antibody interference
Age: very young or very old
Pregnancy
Stress, concurrent illness
Pyrexia, hypothermia
Incubating disease at time of vaccination
Drugs: cytotoxic, glucocorticoids
Anesthesia?
Hormonal fluctuations
General debilitation, malnutrition

Vaccine Factors
Rendered noninfectious during handling
Improper storage
Vaccines not protecting 100% of population (biologic variation)
Disinfectant used on needles and syringes
Wrong strain
Excessive attenuation
Overwhelming exposure

Human Error
Improper mixing of products
Exposed at time of vaccination
Concurrent use of antimicrobials or immunosuppressive drugs
Simultaneous use of antisera
Too frequent administration (<2-week interval)
Disinfection of skin?
Wrong route of administration
Delay between vaccines in initial series
Omission of booster vaccination

From Greene C: *Infectious Diseases of the Dog and Cat*, ed 2. St. Louis, WB Saunders, 1999.
?, uncertain.

Vascular Disorders

Peripheral Vascular Diseases

Diseases of Arteries and Arterioles
Occlusive diseases
Arterial embolism
Arterial thrombosis
Angiitis, vasculitis
Vasospasm, traumatic, toxic
Diabetic arteriopathy
Nonocclusive diseases
Arteriovenous (AV) fistula
Arterial aneurysm
Arterial calcification
Arteriosclerosis, hyalinosis, amyloidosis
Atherosclerosis
Vasculitis

Diseases of Veins
Phlebectasia
Varicosis
Phlebitis and thrombophlebitis
Venous thrombosis
Venous malformations

Diseases of Lymphatics
Lymphangitis
Lymphedema
Lymphangiectasia
Lymphatic hypoplasia, aplasia, hyperplasia
Lymphangioma, lymphocysts
Lymphangiosarcoma

Tumors of Peripheral Blood Vessels
Angioma, hemangioma, hemangiosarcoma

From Ettinger S, Feldman E: *Textbook of Veterinary Internal Medicine*, ed 6. St. Louis, WB Saunders, 2005.

DIFFERENTIAL DIAGNOSIS

Vestibular Disease: Central Versus Peripheral

	Central Vestibular Disease	Peripheral Vestibular Disease
Loss of balance	Yes	Yes
Head tilt	Yes	Yes
Falling/rolling	Yes (greater tendency to roll)	Yes
Nystagmus	Yes	Yes
Horizontal	Yes	Yes
Rotatory	Yes	Yes
Vertical	Yes	No
Positional	Yes	No
Strabismus (ventrolateral)	Yes	Yes
Cranial nerve deficits	Possible I–XII, especially V, VI, VII	Possible VII
Horner's syndrome	No	Possible
Cerebellar signs	Possible	No
Mental depression	Possible	No
Hemiparesis with ipsilateral postural reaction deficits	Possible	No

Modified with permission from Braund KG: *Clinical Syndromes in Veterinary Neurology*. St. Louis, Mosby, 1994, p 65.

Vomiting

Common Causes

Metabolic/Endocrine Disorders
Uremia
Hypoadrenocorticism
Diabetes mellitus
Hyperthyroidism
Hepatic disease
Endotoxemia/septicemia
Electrolyte disorders
Acid-base disorders

Intoxicants
Lead
Ethylene glycol
Zinc
Strychnine

Drugs
Cardiac glycosides
Erythromycin
Chemotherapy agents
Apomorphine
Xylazine
Medetomidine
Penicillamine
Tetracycline
NSAIDs

Abdominal Disorders
Pancreatitis
Peritonitis
Neoplasia

Dietary Causes
Indiscretions
Intolerances
Allergy

Gastric Disorders
Gastritis
Helicobacter infection
Parasites
Ulceration
Neoplasia
Foreign bodies
Dilatation-volvulus
Hiatal hernia
Obstruction
Motility disorders

Disorders of the Small Intestine
Inflammatory bowel disease
Neoplasia
Foreign body
Intussusception
Parasites
Parvovirus
Bacterial overgrowth

Disorders of the Large Intestine
Colitis
Obstipation
Parasites

From Ettinger S, Feldman E: *Textbook of Veterinary Internal Medicine*, ed 6. St. Louis, WB Saunders, 2005.
NSAIDs, nonsteroidal anti-inflammatory drugs.

Vomiting, Acute

Differential diagnosis list available on the companion online site at www.cote.clinicalvetadvisor.com.

Vomiting, Chronic

Differential diagnosis list available on the companion online site at www.cote.clinicalvetadvisor.com.

Vulvar Discharge

Hemorrhagic
With Mainly Superficial (Mature) Epithelial Cells
Normal proestrus, estrus, or early diestrus
Ovarian remnant
Ovarian pathologic condition (i.e., cystic follicles, functional ovarian tumor)
Exogenous estrogen
Without Superficial (Mature) Epithelial Cells
Normal lochia
Subinvoluted placental sites
Vaginal laceration
Neoplasia of vagina or uterus
Uterine torsion
Bleeding disorder

Mucoid
Normal
- Lochia
- Late pregnancy
- Luteal phase (diestrus)

Androgenic stimulation
- Endogenous (intersex)
- Exogenous (mibolerone, testosterone)

Cervicitis
Mucometra
Idiopathic (?)

Modified from Willard M, Tvedten H: *Small Animal Clinical Diagnosis by Laboratory Methods*, ed 4. St. Louis, WB Saunders, 2004.

Weakness

Major Causes

Anemia
Abdominal effusions
Cardiovascular
Chronic inflammation/infections
Chronic wasting diseases
Drug related
Electrolyte disorders
Endocrine disorders
Fever
Metabolic dysfunction states
Neoplasia
Neurologic disorders
Neuromuscular/polyneuropathies
Nutritional disorders
Overactivity
Psychological disorders
Pulmonary diseases
Skeletal diseases

Modified from Ettinger S, Feldman E: *Textbook of Veterinary Internal Medicine*, ed 5. St. Louis, WB Saunders, 2000.

Weight Loss

Diagnostic Considerations for Animals with Marked Weight Loss

Dietary History: Inadequate Diet
Starvation
Underfeeding
Poor-quality food

Dietary History: Adequate Diet
Environmental/housing factors
- Competition for food from other pets
- Limited access to food

Oral and dental disease
Impaired use of nutrients
- Specific nutrient deficiency
- Maldigestion of any cause
- Malabsorption of any cause
- Diabetes mellitus
- Protein-losing disease
  - Nephropathy
  - Gastroenteropathy
- Cardiac disease*

Elevated metabolism
- Hyperthyroidism
- Chronic fever of any cause*

End-stage renal disease*
Neoplasia*
Chronic infection*
Chronic inflammation of any cause (e.g., immunologic disease*)

From Ettinger S, Feldman E: *Textbook of Veterinary Internal Medicine*, ed 6. St. Louis, WB Saunders, 2005.
*Diseases typically associated with cachexia in humans and animals. Note: Animals may present with or without a loss of appetite.

Zoonotic Diseases

Zoonoses: Diseases for Which Immunocompromised People Are at Increased Risk, and Means of Disease Transmission

Direct Zoonoses from Pets*
Bite, saliva: rabies, pasteurellosis, capnocytophagiosis, helicobacteriosis
Scratch, contact: dermatophytosis, bartonellosis
Inhaled, aerosols: plague (cat), tularemia, bordetellosis
Feces: toxoplasmosis, cryptosporidiosis, campylobacteriosis, helicobacteriosis, salmonellosis, giardiasis, ancylostomiasis, toxocariasis
Urine: brucellosis (dog), leptospirosis (dog)
Transport of insect vector: bartonellosis, tularemia, plague, RMSF, dipylidiasis
Other animal hosts: *Rhodococcus equi* infection (horse), *Mycobacterium marinum* infection (fish), psittacosis (birds), salmonellosis (reptiles and amphibians)

Environmentally Acquired Zoonoses
Saprophytic: pneumocystosis, microsporidiosis, *Mycobacterium avium*-complex infection, cryptococcosis, coccidioidomycosis, histoplasmosis, blastomycosis, aspergillosis
Vector acquired: ehrlichiosis, borreliosis, babesiosis, plague, RMSF, tularemia, bartonellosis

With permission from Greene C: *Infectious Diseases of the Dog and Cat*, ed 2. St. Louis, WB Saunders, 1999, p 711.
*Predominantly dogs and cats, except where otherwise indicated.
RMSF, Rocky Mountain spotted fever.

SECTION IV

Laboratory Tests

EDITOR
Lois Roth-Johnson, DVM, PhD, DACVP

Acanthocyte

BASIC INFORMATION

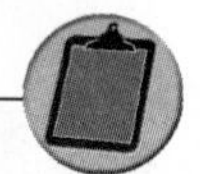

DEFINITION

Erythrocyte morphologic abnormality characterized by irregular, usually blunt, projections from the normally smooth round cell membrane (from the Greek *akantha,* meaning "thorn").

SYNONYM(S)

Burr cell
Echinoacanthocyte
Spur cell

TYPICAL NORMAL RANGE

Normally none to rare. Not reported unless seen on blood film.

PHYSIOLOGY

Mechanism for membrane shape abnormality is not known. Associated with abnormalities in red blood cell membrane lipids.

CAUSES OF ABNORMALLY HIGH LEVELS: Hemangiosarcoma; liver, splenic or renal disease; artifact of blood film preparation

NEXT DIAGNOSTIC STEP TO CONSIDER IF LEVELS HIGH: Repeat complete blood count to confirm; if consistent finding, evaluate for liver, splenic, or renal disease and metabolic abnormalities as suggested by clinical signs.

LAB ARTIFACTS THAT MAY INTERFERE WITH READINGS OF LEVELS OF THIS SUBSTANCE: Specimen age artifact (delay in preparing blood film, sample not refrigerated); artifact of blood film preparation

SAMPLE FOR COLLECTION AND ANY SPECIAL SPECIMEN HANDLING NOTES: Whole blood in ethylenediamine tetraacetic acid (lavender top tube) or heparin (green top tube); include a blood film prepared when specimen is collected to help rule out specimen age artifact.

PEARLS: Considered nonspecific and a common artifact; should be evaluated in a second, fresh specimen prior to drawing diagnostic conclusions.

AUTHOR: **ETIENNE CÔTÉ**

Acetylcholine Receptor Antibody Test

BASIC INFORMATION

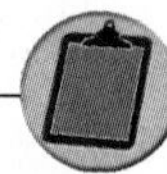

DEFINITION

Test for detection of antiacetylcholine-receptor (AChR) antibodies, which cause acquired myasthenia gravis.

SYNONYM(S)

ARAT
Myasthenia gravis titer

TYPICAL NORMAL RANGE

Normally 0 to 0.6 nmol/L (dogs), 0 to 0.3 nmol/L (cats)

PHYSIOLOGY

Acetylcholine is released from a neuron's presynaptic membrane at the neuromuscular junction. In myasthenia gravis patients, the acetylcholine fails to adequately bind to muscle-based receptors in the postsynaptic membrane (sarcolemma) because the receptors are inactivated by autoantibodies. This test is for detection of these autoantibodies in the serum.

CAUSES OF ABNORMALLY HIGH LEVELS: Myasthenia gravis

NEXT DIAGNOSTIC STEP TO CONSIDER IF LEVELS HIGH: Assess response to immunosuppressive and/or oral pyridostigmine treatment or intravenous edrophonium (Tensilon). Both should alleviate clinical signs. However, response to treatment is considered less diagnostically reliable (lower sensitivity) than the acetylcholine receptor antibody test.

DRUG EFFECTS ON LEVELS: False negative: corticosteroid or other immunosuppressive therapy. If clinically feasible, treatment should be stopped at least 4 weeks prior to testing.

LAB ARTIFACTS THAT MAY INTERFERE WITH READINGS OF LEVELS OF THIS SUBSTANCE: False negative: failure to keep specimen chilled.

SAMPLE FOR COLLECTION AND ANY SPECIAL SPECIMEN HANDLING NOTES: Serum (2 ml minimum): separate from clot as soon as possible. Should be frozen and sent on dry ice (preferable) or cold pack to reference lab overnight.

PEARLS: Some dogs with myasthenia gravis are negative for AChR antibodies, but have immune complexes associated with other antigens at the neuromuscular junction that interfere with neurotransmission. Nerve stimulation studies may be needed in these patients.

AUTHOR: **ETIENNE CÔTÉ**

Acetylcholinesterase Level

BASIC INFORMATION

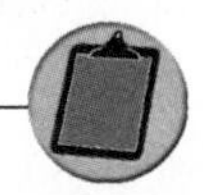

DEFINITION

Blood level of the enzyme that catabolizes acetylcholine.

SYNONYM(S)

Cholinesterase level

TYPICAL NORMAL RANGE

About 500 to 1500 U/L for dogs, but specific ranges vary with the reference laboratory. A positive diagnosis of low level means that the animal's level is at least 25% less than the lower limit of normal range.

PHYSIOLOGY

Acetylcholine is the main neurotransmitter at the neuromuscular junction and the enzyme responsible for catabolism of acetylcholine is acetylcholinesterase. When acetylcholinesterase levels are low, there is decreased catabolism of acetylcholine, resulting in poorly controlled or uncontrolled neuromuscular activation. Muscle tremors and smooth muscle activation (gastrointestinal signs and other autonomic signs) occur. Organophosphates antagonize acetylcholinesterase, leading to these clinical signs. Organophosphate toxicity is the most common cause of low blood levels of this enzyme. Measurement of red blood cell acetylcholinesterase concentration helps to diagnose toxicity with organophosphate containing insecticides.

CAUSES OF ABNORMALLY LOW LEVELS: Organophosphate toxicity, carbamate toxicity

NEXT DIAGNOSTIC STEP TO CONSIDER IF LEVELS LOW: Response to treatment

IMPORTANT INTERSPECIES DIFFERENCES: Cats naturally have lower cholinesterase levels, making tests less reliable in this species.

SAMPLE FOR COLLECTION AND ANY SPECIAL SPECIMEN HANDLING NOTES: Whole blood in ethylenediamine tetraacetic acid (lavender top tube) or heparin (green top); 20 grams of brain tissue may be used for postmortem diagnosis.

PEARLS: Turnaround time is usually longer than clinical condition allows; therefore, the test is often confirmatory (retrospective) because the decision to treat must be made on the basis of clinical information, before results are available.

AUTHOR: **ETIENNE CÔTÉ**

ACTH (Adrenocorticotropic Hormone), Endogenous/Baseline

BASIC INFORMATION

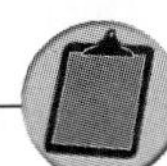

DEFINITION

Hormone secreted by anterior pituitary in response to corticotropin releasing hormone (CRH) secreted by hypothalamus.

SYNONYM(S)

Corticotropin

TYPICAL NORMAL RANGE

For dogs: 10 to 110 pg/ml; for cats: 0 to 110 pg/ml. To convert pg/ml to pmol/L, multiply pg/ml by 0.22.

PHYSIOLOGY

Stress causes hypothalamic release of CRH. CRH stimulates anterior pituitary release of ACTH. Proteolytic fragmentation of large precursor hormone, proopiomelanocortin (POMC), is the source of ACTH and other hormones. ACTH stimulates cortisol and aldosterone release from the adrenal cortex. High circulating levels of cortisol inhibit release of CRH (feedback inhibition). High baseline ACTH concentrations help differentiate between pituitary-dependent hyperadrenocorticism and a functional adrenal cortical tumor, which produces low ACTH concentrations.

CAUSES OF ABNORMALLY HIGH LEVELS: Hypocortisolism, either natural (primary Addison's disease) or iatrogenic (sudden cessation of chronic glucocorticoid administration); pituitary dependent hyperadrenocorticism due to pituitary neoplasia

NEXT DIAGNOSTIC STEP TO CONSIDER IF LEVELS HIGH

- Determine treatment (glucocorticoid, including topical medications) history.
- ACTH stimulation test if no history of steroid administration.

CAUSES OF ABNORMALLY LOW LEVELS: High endogenous cortisol levels, either spontaneously (hyperadrenocorticism/Cushing's disease) or iatrogenic (administration of glucocorticoids); panhypopituitarism

NEXT DIAGNOSTIC STEP TO CONSIDER IF LEVELS LOW: Rule out sampling error; see specimen collection/special handling. Evaluate for hyperadrenocorticism. If history, physical examination, and diagnostic tests support hyperadrenocorticism and ACTH level is abnormally low, a diagnosis of adrenal cortical neoplasia is suspected and further testing (e.g., abdominal ultrasonography) is warranted.

IMPORTANT INTERSPECIES DIFFERENCES: Adrenal disease is uncommon in cats; test is infrequently done.

DRUG EFFECTS ON LEVELS

- Increase: insulin.
- Decrease: glucocorticoid administration.

LAB ARTIFACTS THAT MAY INTERFERE WITH READINGS OF LEVELS OF THIS SUBSTANCE: Decrease: thawing of specimen; collection or storage in glass tubes.

SAMPLE FOR COLLECTION AND ANY SPECIAL SPECIMEN HANDLING NOTES: Morning sample preferred. Collect in cold, heparinized plastic syringe; centrifuge; collect plasma immediately; freeze in plastic tubes. Samples must be shipped frozen and remain frozen until analysis.

PEARLS: Useful test for differentiating pituitary-dependent Cushing's disease from adrenal cortical tumor. The hormone is very labile, however; inappropriate specimen handling yields false-negative results.

AUTHOR: **ETIENNE CÔTÉ**

Activated Coagulation Time (ACT)

BASIC INFORMATION

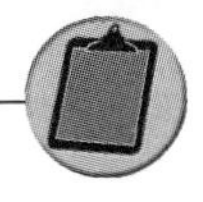

DEFINITION

The time interval from contact of blood with diatomaceous earth pellets to formation of a clot.

SYNONYM(S)

Activated clotting time

TYPICAL NORMAL RANGE

Less than 140 seconds

PHYSIOLOGY

Contact activation of the coagulation cascade occurs when whole blood is drawn into a warmed (37°C) tube containing diatomaceous earth pellets. The intrinsic and common coagulation pathways are activated. After multiple inversions for mixing, the tube is kept in a heating block or tucked in the clinician's axilla and checked for clot formation every 5 to 10 seconds.

CAUSES OF ABNORMALLY HIGH LEVELS: Decreased concentration of any of coagulation factors of the intrinsic or common coagulation pathways (all factors

except VII) to less than 5% of normal; severe thrombocytopenia (<10,000 platelets/μL); uremia
NEXT DIAGNOSTIC STEP TO CONSIDER IF LEVELS HIGH: Confirm with more sensitive tests (activated partial thromboplastin time); platelet count
DRUG EFFECTS ON LEVELS: Prolonged by heparin or aspirin therapy
LAB ARTIFACTS THAT MAY INTERFERE WITH READINGS OF LEVELS OF THIS SUBSTANCE: Considered an in-office test. Any variation in test protocol may alter results. End point (visual clot detection) is subject to observer variability.
SAMPLE FOR COLLECTION AND ANY SPECIAL SPECIMEN HANDLING NOTES: Whole blood into siliceous (gray top, with large granules) tube, prewarmed to 37°C. Mix by inversion, incubate at 37°C (purpose-made heating block or human axilla), and check for clot formation every 5 to 10 seconds.
PEARLS: Considered an insensitive test. Carriers of hemophilia (coagulation factors are 40–60% of normal) would not be detected by this test.

AUTHOR: **ETIENNE CÔTÉ**

Activated Partial Thromboplastin Time (aPTT)

BASIC INFORMATION

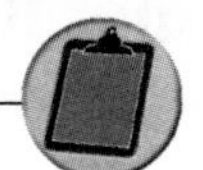

DEFINITION

Screening test for intrinsic and common coagulation pathways.

SYNONYM(S)

aPTT
Partial thromboplastin time (PTT)

TYPICAL NORMAL RANGE

Reported in seconds. Laboratory, instrument, and species specific reference ranges must be used. Prolonged when at least one coagulation factor is <70% of normal.

PHYSIOLOGY

Citrated plasma is incubated at 37° C with excess procoagulant phospholipid. Contact activator is added to activate the intrinsic pathway via Factors XII and XI. Citrate in the specimen chelates Ca^{2+}, limiting activation beyond Factor XIa. After additional incubation, $CaCl_2$ is added to saturate the citrate and allow the reaction to continue to clot fomation. The aPTT is the time from addition of $CaCl_2$ to clot formation.
CAUSES OF ABNORMALLY HIGH LEVELS: Liver disease (decreased factor production), vitamin K inactivation (anticoagulant rodenticides, coumarin therapy), decreased vitamin K absorption (biliary obstruction), increased factor inactivation or consumption (disseminated intravascular coagulation [DIC]), factor dilution (massive blood loss with colloid or crystalloid fluid replacement), hereditary factor defects, heparin therapy.
NEXT DIAGNOSTIC STEP TO CONSIDER IF LEVELS HIGH: Assess history for exposure to toxic substances or treatment. Measurement of individual factors if hereditary disease is suspected.
IMPORTANT INTERSPECIES DIFFERENCES: Prolonged aPTT is reported in cats without evidence of clinical hemostatic disease.
DRUG EFFECTS ON LEVELS: Increased: heparin, aspirin. Polymerized bovine hemoglobin (Oxyglobin) administration interferes with ability to detect clot.
LAB ARTIFACTS THAT MAY INTERFERE WITH READINGS OF LEVELS OF THIS SUBSTANCE
- Decrease: contamination with tissue factor when specimen obtained, overfilling citrate tube.
- Increase: incomplete filling of citrate tube dilutes specimen, old specimen.

SAMPLE FOR COLLECTION AND ANY SPECIAL SPECIMEN HANDLING NOTES: "Clean stick" (minimally traumatic phlebotomy) required; otherwise, tissue factor from traumatized subcutaneous tissue can falsely lower the result. Ideally, collect a sufficient volume of blood to place first aliquot in red top tube and discard (or use for serology). Collect specimen in citrate (blue top) tube. Fill completely. Refrigerate and submit to reference lab. If time interval for testing is >6 hours, mix thoroughly, centrifuge, collect plasma, freeze.
PEARLS: aPTT increases before PT with heparin therapy, but not with warfarin/anticoagulant rodenticide toxicosis or coagulopathy of liver disease.

AUTHOR: **ETIENNE CÔTÉ**

Alanine Aminotransferase (ALT)

BASIC INFORMATION

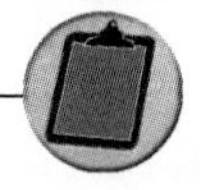

DEFINITION

Enzyme located in hepatocyte cytoplasm.

SYNONYM(S)

Serum glutamic pyruvate transaminase (SGPT)

TYPICAL NORMAL RANGE

Dogs: 0 to 30 U/L; cats: 10 to 25 U/L. Specific values vary among laboratories.

PHYSIOLOGY

Enzyme primarily found in hepatocyte cytoplasm that "leaks" into blood when hepatocyte cell membrane injury occurs. Low concentrations in erythrocytes or skeletal muscle may cause minor (insignificant) increases in hemolytic diseases or with muscle injury, respectively.
CAUSES OF ABNORMALLY HIGH LEVELS: Hepatocellular injury from any cause. Liver injury may be primary or secondary. Dystrophin deficient muscular dystrophy causes slight to moderate increases in dogs and slight to marked increases in cats.
NEXT DIAGNOSTIC STEP TO CONSIDER IF LEVELS HIGH: If elevations >2 times the upper limit of reference range persist, assess history for exposure to hepatotoxins (including medications). If none, begin assessing hepatic structure (e.g., abdominal radiographs, ultrasound) and function (preprandial and postprandial serum bile acids; alkaline phosphatase, bilirubin). Consider biopsy if values remain elevated or increase.

DRUG EFFECTS ON LEVELS: Many drugs induce hepatocellular injury. Drugs commonly implicated include glucocorticoids and phenobarbital.
LAB ARTIFACTS THAT MAY INTERFERE WITH READINGS OF LEVELS OF THIS SUBSTANCE: Increase: lipemia, hemolysis (*in vivo* or artifactual).
SAMPLE FOR COLLECTION AND ANY SPECIAL SPECIMEN HANDLING NOTES: Serum (red top tube); allow to clot, centrifuge, separate serum from clot.
PEARLS: Mild elevations in ALT may just as likely be due to serious disease processes as benign fluctuation; correlating the finding to the remainder of the case, and monitoring trends if necessary, are essential for properly interpreting high ALT values. ALT elevation indicates hepatocyte damage, but does not necessarily reflect on overall hepatic function.

AUTHOR: **ETIENNE CÔTÉ**

Albumin

BASIC INFORMATION

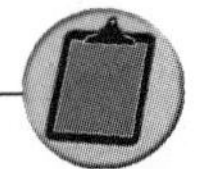

DEFINITION

Small protein comprising the highest proportion of protein in blood. Serum albumin is measured.

TYPICAL NORMAL RANGE

Dogs and cats: 2.5 to 4.0 g/dl (25 to 40 mg/ml); neonates and young animals often have slightly lower concentrations.

PHYSIOLOGY

Synthesized in liver. Functions to maintain oncotic pressure and as a transport protein for ions, bilirubin, thyroxine, and other compounds. Spectrophotometric method is usually used for measuring serum albumin.
CAUSES OF ABNORMALLY HIGH LEVELS: Dehydration, laboratory error
NEXT DIAGNOSTIC STEP TO CONSIDER IF LEVELS HIGH: Assess hydration status; if normal, recheck results.

CAUSES OF ABNORMALLY LOW LEVELS

- Loss: enteropathy, nephropathy/glomerular disease, severe exudative skin lesions (burn), massive hemorrhage (total protein and globulin are also low).
- Decreased production: severe chronic liver disease.

NEXT DIAGNOSTIC STEP TO CONSIDER IF LEVELS LOW: Review history and physical exam with respect to intestinal, renal, and liver function. Assess in conjunction with hematocrit, total protein, serum globulin, liver enzymes, and renal function. If a cause is not determined, additional testing to be considered includes preprandial and postprandial bile acids, urine protein-to-creatinine ratio, fecal flotation, fecal occult blood. Additional tests (radiographs, ultrasound, biopsy) should be dictated by history, physical examination, and previous test results.

DRUG EFFECTS ON LEVELS: Long-term therapy with hepatotoxic drugs (e.g., anticonvulsants) may cause low levels secondary to liver injury.
LAB ARTIFACTS THAT MAY INTERFERE WITH READINGS OF LEVELS OF THIS SUBSTANCE

- Decrease: use of reagents for human testing (BCP dye binding reaction).
- Increase: BCG dye may bind to globulin.

SAMPLE FOR COLLECTION AND ANY SPECIAL SPECIMEN HANDLING NOTES: Serum (red top); allow specimen to clot, centrifuge, collect serum, refrigerate, ship on ice.
PEARLS: Concentration may be slightly lower in very young and very old patients.

AUTHOR: **ETIENNE CÔTÉ**

Albuminuria and Proteinuria

BASIC INFORMATION

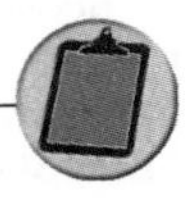

DEFINITION

The presence of excess protein and/or albumin in urine.

TYPICAL NORMAL RANGE

About 4 to 95 mg/dl protein (wet chemistry instrument methods) negative, trace, +1 on dipstick methods (with no evidence of urinary tract disease).

PHYSIOLOGY

- Proteins <68,000 daltons readily pass the glomerular filter, but most are resorbed in the proximal tubules. Alhough it is a relatively small protein, albumin is too large to filter through the normal glomerulus and thus stays in the circulation of healthy animals.
- Tamm-Horsfall protein—a mucoprotein secreted by tubular and collecting duct cells—and albumin make up most of the protein found in the urine of healthy animals.

CAUSES OF ABNORMALLY HIGH LEVELS

- Overflow proteinuria: caused by increased plasma levels of protein such as hemoglobinuria, hyperglobulinemia, and myoglobinuria.
- Tubular proteinuria: caused by decreased protein resorption.
- Glomerular proteinuria: caused by increased glomeular permeability.
- Hemorrhage in urinary system.
- Inflammation in urinary system, causing increased vascular permeability.

NEXT DIAGNOSTIC STEP TO CONSIDER IF LEVELS HIGH

- Examine urine sediment for evidence of inflammation or hemorrhage.
- Examine serum for evidence of hemolysis.
- Measure serum protein (hyperproteinemia, hyperglobulinemia, or hypoalbuminemia).
- Urine protein-to-creatinine ratio.

LAB ARTIFACTS THAT MAY INTERFERE WITH READINGS OF LEVELS OF THIS SUBSTANCE

- False increase (with dipstick method): prolonged contact with alkaline urine.
- False decrease (with dipstick method): if protein is other than albumin (e.g., Bence Jones proteinuria).
- False decrease (acid precipitation method): if urine is highly alkaline.

- False increase (sulfosalicyclic acid method): after administration of iodine-based contrast media, sulfisoxazole, very large doses of penicillin, and precipitation of crystals owing to low pH.

SAMPLE FOR COLLECTION AND ANY SPECIAL SPECIMEN HANDLING NOTES: Urine in clean container

AUTHOR: **ELIZABETH G. WELLES**

Aldosterone, Endogenous

BASIC INFORMATION

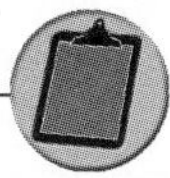

DEFINITION

Mineralocorticoid secreted by adrenal cortex. Endogenous aldosterone is a test of aldosterone concentration in circulation.

TYPICAL NORMAL RANGE

Dog: 2–96 pg/ml. To convert pg/ml to ng/dl, divide pg/ml result by 10. To convert pg/ml to pmol/L, multiply pg/ml result by 2.775.

PHYSIOLOGY

Synthesized by adrenal cortex in response to angiotensin II. Acts on receptors throughout the body, but primarily distal renal tubules to enhance retention of sodium and water and promote excretion of potassium, effectively maintaining or increasing blood pressure.

CAUSES OF ABNORMALLY HIGH LEVELS: Adrenal neoplasia or hyperplasia, low sodium intake.

NEXT DIAGNOSTIC STEP TO CONSIDER IF LEVELS HIGH: If associated with hypokalemia/hyperkaluria, hypernatremia with decreased urine excretion, and/or hypertension, then evaluation for adrenal neoplasia is warranted.

CAUSES OF ABNORMALLY LOW LEVELS: Adrenal atrophy (idiopathic, secondary to medication, pituitary disease), high sodium intake.

NEXT DIAGNOSTIC STEP TO CONSIDER IF LEVELS LOW: Review treatment/medication history; adrenocorticotropic hormone stimulation test to evaluate hypothalamic, pituitary, adrenal axis.

DRUG EFFECTS ON LEVELS

- Decrease: angiotensin-converting enzyme inhibitors, nonsteroidal anti-inflammatory drugs, propanolol.
- Increase: lithium, spironolactone.

LAB ARTIFACTS THAT MAY INTERFERE WITH READINGS OF LEVELS OF THIS SUBSTANCE

- Artifactual decrease: storage at 22°C for ≥3 days or at 37° C for 1 day.

SAMPLE FOR COLLECTION AND ANY SPECIAL SPECIMEN HANDLING NOTES: Plasma collected in ethylenediamine tetraacetic acid (lavender top) or heparin (green top). Centrifuge, collect plasma as soon as possible. Freeze, ship on ice.

PEARLS: Test is rarely indicated.

AUTHOR: **ETIENNE CÔTÉ**

Alkaline Phosphatase

BASIC INFORMATION

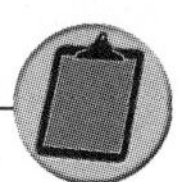

DEFINITION

Alkaline phosphatase (ALP) is a membrane-associated enzyme found in liver, bone, colostrum, and many other tissues. Its physiologic function is not known.

SYNONYM(S)

Alk phos
ALP
sALP

TYPICAL NORMAL RANGE

Dogs: 0 to 90 U/L; cats 4 to 80 U/L. Specific values vary among reference laboratories.

PHYSIOLOGY

Domestic mammals have two genes responsible for ALP production. I-ALP is not associated with measured serum increases. Tissue-nonspecific ALP is modified to form to isoforms, L-ALP (liver associated) and B-ALP (bone associated). C-ALP appears unique to dogs. Increased C-ALP is stimulated by corticosteroids. Most routine assays measure total serum ALP.

CAUSES OF ABNORMALLY HIGH LEVELS: Cholestasis, hormone (corticosteroids) or drug (prednisone, phenobarbital) induction, osteoblast activity (normal growth in young dogs, fracture repair, osteosarcoma)

NEXT DIAGNOSTIC STEP TO CONSIDER IF LEVELS HIGH: Disregard in young animals (if no other abnormalities found); evaluate hepatobiliary structure and function; review medication history; assess for Cushing's disease only if consistent history and physical examination.

IMPORTANT INTERSPECIES DIFFERENCES

- Dogs: Corticosteroid induction seems unique to dogs; can specifically measure for this form. Does not differentiate source of corticosteroid, however (e.g., endogenous—stress, adrenal hyperplasia, hyperadrenocorticism—versus exogenous/iatrogenic all are measured as corticosteroid isoenzyme).
- Cats: ALP has poor sensitivity for cholestasis, except in hepatic lipidosis. Short serum half-life (8 hours in cats versus 24 hours in dogs) makes even low-magnitude ALP elevations generally more clinically significant in the cat than in the dog.

DRUG EFFECTS ON LEVELS: Increase: corticosteroid, phenobarbital, primidone, prednisone, thyroxine.

LAB ARTIFACTS THAT MAY INTERFERE WITH READINGS OF LEVELS OF THIS SUBSTANCE: Increase: marked hemolysis.

SAMPLE FOR COLLECTION AND ANY SPECIAL SPECIMEN HANDLING NOTES: Serum (red top tube), allow to clot, centrifuge, collect serum, refrigerate, and ship on ice

PEARLS: The vast majority of dogs with increased ALP do not have hyperadrenocorticism (Cushing's disease). Therefore, an elevated serum alkaline phosphatase level warrants a detailed review of history and physical examination before determining whether testing for Cushing's disease is warranted.

AUTHOR: **ETIENNE CÔTÉ**

Ammonia

BASIC INFORMATION

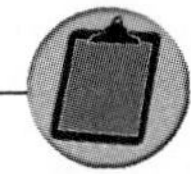

DEFINITION

Measurement of ammonium (NH_4^+) concentration in plasma. NH_4^+ is the predominant form of the analyte in blood. Routine assays require plasma, not whole blood.

SYNONYM(S)

Ammonia: NH_3
Ammonium
Ammonium: NH_4^+
Blood ammonia
Plasma ammonium

TYPICAL NORMAL RANGE

- Dogs: 45 to 120 μg/dl; cats: 30 to 100 μg/dl.

PHYSIOLOGY

Ammonium is produced in the gastrointestinal tract and carried via the portal circulation to the liver. Hepatic transformation of two ammonium molecules into one urea molecule requires adequate hepatic function. High circulating ammonium concentrations have been treated as a marker of hepatic dysfunction.

CAUSES OF ABNORMALLY HIGH LEVELS: Decreased clearance from blood: decreased functional liver mass, decreased portal blood flow, urea cycle abnormalities. Increased production: post race (greyhounds, other racing dogs).

NEXT DIAGNOSTIC STEP TO CONSIDER IF LEVELS HIGH: Review history, examination, complete blood count, serum chemistry panel, and abdominal imaging results to assess for signs of hepatobiliary disease and portal circulation abnormalities; serum preprandial and postprandial bile acids.

DRUG EFFECTS ON LEVELS: Decrease: antibiotics that affect gastrointestinal flora (aminoglycosides), lactulose, *Lactobacillus acidophilus* culture, enema. Increase: asparaginase, narcotics, diuretics causing hypokalemia, high-protein diet.

LAB ARTIFACTS THAT MAY INTERFERE WITH READINGS OF LEVELS OF THIS SUBSTANCE: Increase: delay in harvesting plasma, specimen processing; hemolysis (if assay depends on light transmittance).

SAMPLE FOR COLLECTION AND ANY SPECIAL SPECIMEN HANDLING NOTES: Twelve-hour fasting specimen preferred. Collect blood into ammonia-free heparin (green) tube; separate plasma from cells immediately; store on ice and test within 1 hour or freeze (−20°C) and test within 49 hours.

PEARLS: Because of difficulty in proper specimen handling, measurement of preprandial and postprandial serum bile acids and urine bile acid-to-creatitine ratio has replaced ammonium measurement.

AUTHOR: **ETIENNE CÔTÉ**

Amylase

BASIC INFORMATION

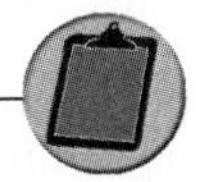

DEFINITION

Enzyme principally involved in hydrolysis of complex carbohydrates (starches); concentrations measured in serum. Spectrophotometric methods are most often used; "dry reagents" are used less frequently.

SYNONYM(S)

AMS

TYPICAL NORMAL RANGE

Dogs: 371 to 1,503 U/L. Cats: 530 to 1660 U/L. Specific values vary among laboratories.

PHYSIOLOGY

Amylase is a cytoplasmic enzyme found in high concentration in the pancreas, intestine, and liver. It functions to catabolize complex starches. Ca^{2+} is a required cofactor. Amylase is eliminated via the urinary tract.

CAUSES OF ABNORMALLY HIGH LEVELS: Pancreatitis (may be normal to markedly increased) in dogs; vomiting; decreased glomerular filtration (increase is usually less than three times upper reference range value)

NEXT DIAGNOSTIC STEP TO CONSIDER IF LEVELS HIGH: Correlate to history, examination, complete blood count, and remainder of serum chemistry panel. If consistent with pancreatitis, consider abdominal ultrasonography to assess further.

IMPORTANT INTERSPECIES DIFFERENCES

- Cats with pancreatitis often do not have elevated serum amylase concentration.
- The diagnostic value of amylase levels in cats is minimal.

SAMPLE FOR COLLECTION AND ANY SPECIAL SPECIMEN HANDLING NOTES: Serum (red top tube), allow to clot, centrifuge, separate serum, refrigerate, and ship on ice. Amylase is fairly stable compared to other analytes measured in routine chemistry panels.

PEARLS: One-time measurement of amylase level in a dog is of very little significance with respect to pancreatitis (neither normal nor elevated levels rule out or rule in pancreatitis); trends in amylase levels over time (e.g., daily) may be more informative in terms of disease progression in patients with acute pancreatitis. A nonseptic abdominal effusion with an amylase concentration greater than serum amylase is supportive of a diagnosis of pancreatitis.

AUTHOR: **ETIENNE CÔTÉ**

Anemia, Nonregenerative

BASIC INFORMATION

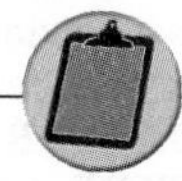

DEFINITION

Anemia characterized by a lack of or inadequate polychromasia or reticulocytosis.

SYNONYM(S)

Nonresponsive anemia

PHYSIOLOGY

Primary cause is decreased erythrocyte (red blood cell [RBC]) production. If decreased production is the sole cause, it may take weeks to months for anemia to be clinically evident, depending on the RBC lifespan.

CAUSES: Nutritional deficiency (iron, copper, folate, or vitamin B_{12}), chronic disease (renal disease, endocrinopathies, neoplasia, many others) or inflammation, primary bone marrow disease, therapeutic agents (hydroxyurea, phenylbutazone, sulfa containing antibiotics, estrogen). Long-term treatment with erythropoietin.

NEXT DIAGNOSTIC STEP TO CONSIDER IF PRESENT: Identification of underlying cause: serum biochemical profile, urinalysis, diagnostic imaging if systemic illness is present and anemia of chronic disease is suspected. Advanced diagnostic testing may then include bone marrow evaluation, serologic tests for infectious disease (e.g., feline leukemia virus, ehrlichiosis), thyroid function tests, serum ferritin.

SAMPLE FOR COLLECTION AND ANY SPECIAL SPECIMEN HANDLING NOTES: Ethylenediamine tetraacetic acid anticoagulated blood (lavender top) for complete blood count (CBC) and reticulocyte count; freshly made direct blood smear for morphologic evaluation; serum (red top) for chemistry panel.

PEARLS: Anemia due to early or acute hemolysis and blood loss may initially appear nonregenerative when the bone marrow has not had time to respond. It takes about 2 to 3 days after acute hemolysis or blood loss for reticulocytosis to be evident, and 7 days for optimum response. Thus, in cases of nonregenerative anemia where a very recent onset of the anemia is possible, serial CBC, blood smear evaluation, and reticulocyte counts are recommended to assess eventual bone marrow response. Once lack of regeneration has been determined, bone marrow assessment may be considered to help determine cause.

AUTHOR: **FIDELIA R. FERNANDEZ**

Anemia, Regenerative

BASIC INFORMATION

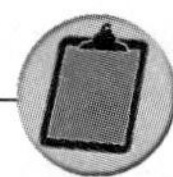

DEFINITION

Anemia characterized by reticulocytosis, indicating bone marrow response. Polychromasia occurs and may be accompanied by basophilic stippling, Howell-Jolly bodies, and nucleated red blood cells (normoblastemia).

SYNONYM(S)

Responsive anemia

TYPICAL NORMAL RANGE

Anemias with absolute reticulocyte count (percent reticulocyte × red blood cell count/μL) of >50,000/μL (cats) and >60,000/μL (dogs) indicate regeneration.

PHYSIOLOGY

Hypoxia induced by decreased red cell mass stimulates erythropoietin production and, subsequently, erythropoiesis.

CAUSES: Blood loss and/or hemolysis.

NEXT DIAGNOSTIC STEP TO CONSIDER IF PRESENT: Blood smear evaluation of red cell morphology for evidence of size and shape changes and parasitic inclusions; physical examination for evidence of blood loss via gastrointestinal tract or elsewhere, ectoparasites, neoplasia; biochemical profile; fecal analysis, urinalysis; serology for infectious agents.

IMPORTANT INTERSPECIES DIFFERENCES: Dogs can mount a greater regenerative response than cats. Both aggregate and punctuate reticulocytes are enumerated in cats to assess reticulocyte response.

LAB ARTIFACTS THAT MAY INTERFERE WITH READINGS OF LEVELS OF THIS SUBSTANCE: Presence of *Mycoplasma hemofelis* (formerly *Haemobartonella felis*) inclusions may falsely increase flow cytometric reticulocyte counts.

SAMPLE FOR COLLECTION AND ANY SPECIAL SPECIMEN HANDLING NOTES: Ethylenediamine tetraacetic acid anticoagulated blood (lavender top) for complete blood cell and reticulocyte count; fresh direct blood smear for morphologic evaluation of red cells.

PEARLS: A reticulocyte count is the most reliable assessment of red blood cell regeneration. On peripheral blood smears, polychromasia is considered characteristic but not diagnostic of orderly regeneration. Presence of nucleated red blood cells, Howell-Jolly bodies, and basophilic stippling without polychromasia may indicate bone marrow injury or toxicity (such as lead poisoning) interfering with red blood cell maturation.

AUTHOR: **FIDELIA R. FERNANDEZ**

Anion Gap

BASIC INFORMATION

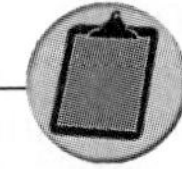

DEFINITION

Calculated value using the formula $[(Na^+ + K^+) - (Cl^- + HCO_3^-)]$. Represents the negatively charged atoms and molecules in the bloodstream that are not measured by the analysis of these four electrolytes.

TYPICAL NORMAL RANGE

Dogs, cats: approximately 5 to 15 mEq/L (mEq/L = mmol/L).

PHYSIOLOGY

The total of positive and negative charges in the blood must be equal. Routine chemistry profile measures only some cations (positively charged particles) and anions (negatively charged particles). "Unmeasured anions" (e.g., lactate, charges on proteins) and "unmeasured cations" (e.g., magnesium, calcium) exist. Unmeasured refers to anything other than the four ions included in the anion gap formula. Measured cations (Na^+, K^+) normally exceed measured anions (Cl^-, HCO_3^-) by about 5 to 15 mEq/L. Because total positive and negative charges must be equal, unmeasured anions must outnumber unmeasured cations by that same amount. In health, excess unmeasured anions are mostly charges on proteins. An increased anion gap indicates an increase in unmeasured anions, usually resulting from organic acid (e.g., lactic acid) accumulation.

CAUSES OF ABNORMALLY HIGH LEVELS: Lactic acidosis, uremia, ketoacidosis, ethylene glycol toxicity

NEXT DIAGNOSTIC STEP TO CONSIDER IF LEVELS HIGH: Evaluate chemistry profile for azotemia, diabetes mellitus. Collect urine for ketone measurement. Review history for ethylene glycol exposure. Examine urine sediment for calcium oxalate monohydrate crystals.

CAUSES OF ABNORMALLY LOW LEVELS: Decreases are not clinically relevant.

DRUG EFFECTS ON LEVELS: Potassium bromide may falsely increased serum chloride measurement, decreasing the anion gap, often producing a negative number.

LAB ARTIFACTS THAT MAY INTERFERE WITH READINGS OF LEVELS OF THIS SUBSTANCE: Anything interfering with the measurement of the electrolytes included in the anion gap calculation will alter the anion gap value (e.g., lipemia, hemolysis).

SAMPLE FOR COLLECTION AND ANY SPECIAL SPECIMEN HANDLING NOTES: Serum (red top) for routine chemistry/electrolyte profile.

PEARLS

- The anion gap is usually used for differentiating between bicarbonate loss (normal anion gap) and organic acid accumulation (high anion gap) in patients with metabolic acidosis.
- In mixed acid-base disorders, an animal may have metabolic acidosis, but the pH may be in the normal or alkaline range because of competing factors. In this situation, a high anion gap helps identify "occult" acidosis.

AUTHOR: **JAMES H. MEINKOTH**

Antinuclear Antibody (ANA)

BASIC INFORMATION

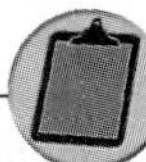

DEFINITION

Indirect immunofluorescent antibody (IFA) test to detect antibodies specific for DNA, RNA, and nucleoprotein.

TYPICAL NORMAL RANGE

Reported as negative or positive; positive results will have a titer and a pattern associated with it (homogeneous nuclear, speckled nuclear, nuclear rim, or nucleolar).

PHYSIOLOGY

Antinuclear antibodies are associated with autoimmune disorders, most prominently systemic lupus erythematosus (SLE).

CAUSES OF ABNORMALLY HIGH LEVELS: SLE, some bacterial and protozoal infections

NEXT DIAGNOSTIC STEP TO CONSIDER IF LEVELS HIGH: Assess for other systemic signs consistent with SLE, rule out other infections.

IMPORTANT INTERSPECIES DIFFERENCES: Requires use of species specific fluorescent antibody

DRUG EFFECTS ON LEVELS: Decreased or false negative titers: cytotoxic drugs, high doses of corticosteroids. False positive tests: sulfonamides, tetracycline, hydralazine, procainamide, griseofulvin. False positive tests are reported in cats treated with propylthiouracil, methimazole.

SAMPLE FOR COLLECTION AND ANY SPECIAL SPECIMEN HANDLING NOTES: Serum (red top tube). Store at 2-8°C (refrigeration).

PEARLS

- Significance of pattern in domestic animals is unclear.
- Positive ANA titers support a clinical diagnosis of SLE in dogs, but are not specific.
- Low positive titers can be seen with various diseases and in older animals.
- ANA titer is much more sensitive (better screening test) for SLE than is the LE prep.

AUTHOR: **FONZIE QUANCE-FITCH**

Antithrombin III (ATIII)

BASIC INFORMATION

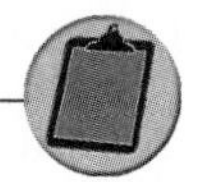

DEFINITION

Endogenous anticoagulant. Major plasma inhibitor of serine protease factors of the coagulation cascade (factors XII, XI, X, and IX; thrombin and plasmin).

SYNONYM(S)

Antithrombin
Heparin cofactor

TYPICAL NORMAL RANGE

Dogs: 75–120%. Cats: 75–110%. Measured as a percentage of species-specific pooled samples.

PHYSIOLOGY

Synthesized in liver and endothelial cells; ATIII (with the help of heparin) binds to thrombin, preventing conversion of fibrinogen to fibrin; ATIII forms a 1:1 complex with thrombin (and other serine proteases). Heparin functions as an anticoagulant by accelerating the reaction that alters the configuration of ATIII (potentiates ATIII), increasing the rate of complex formation. Complex is cleared by hepatocytes.

CAUSES OF ABNORMALLY HIGH LEVELS: Exogenous cortisol administration, inflammation (as part of positive acute phase response)

NEXT DIAGNOSTIC STEP TO CONSIDER IF LEVELS HIGH: Increased ATIII is not clinically significant.

CAUSES OF ABNORMALLY LOW LEVELS: Decreased production (liver disease, portosystemic shunts), increased loss (protein losing nephropathy, glomerular nephritis, renal amyloidosis, protein-losing enteropathy), increased hepatic clearance of ATIII-enzyme complexes (disseminated intravascular coagulation [DIC], heparin therapy)

NEXT DIAGNOSTIC STEP TO CONSIDER IF LEVELS LOW: Assess other aspects of the coagulation cascade (activated partial thromboplastin time or activated coagulation time and prothrombin time), platelet count, fibrinogen level, D-dimers and fibrin degradation products. A procoagulant state may exist due to low ATIII levels alone or in conjunction with other disorders (e.g., DIC).

DRUG EFFECTS ON LEVELS: Exogenous cortisol administration has been associated with mild to moderate increases in ATIII in dogs (dogs with hyperadrenocorticism have decreased levels, perhaps secondary to the associated changes in the liver, which may explain the association of hyperadrenocorticism with thromboembolic disease).

LAB ARTIFACTS THAT MAY INTERFERE WITH READINGS OF LEVELS OF THIS SUBSTANCE: Age: Lower levels of ATIII have been reported in young animals. Assay differences: ATIII may be overestimated in certain thrombin chromogenic assays (heparin cofactor II activity in addition to ATIII is detected).

SAMPLE FOR COLLECTION AND ANY SPECIAL SPECIMEN HANDLING NOTES: Blue top (citrated tube), separate plasma into a plastic tube; freeze (store at 0–4° C).

PEARLS: If the ATIII activity is <70% of the control, the animal will be unresponsive to heparin treatment; ATIII replacement therapy is required for heparin to be effective in such cases.

AUTHOR: **DEBORAH G. DAVIS**

Aspergillus spp. Serology

BASIC INFORMATION

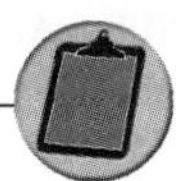

DEFINITION

Specific tests may detect either antibodies to *Aspergillus* spp. (by enzyme-linked immunosorbent assay [ELISA], agarose gel immunodiffusion, or counterimmunoelectrophoresis) or the presence of *Aspergillus* antigen (ELISA) in the blood.

PHYSIOLOGY

Aspergillus spp. are common environmental fungi (saprophytes) and opportunistic pathogens. Nasal aspergillosis—characterized by nasal discharge, ulceration of nares, and facial pain—is the most common manifestation of disease. Infection is more common in dogs than cats. Disseminated aspergillosis also occurs in dogs (most commonly German shepherd dogs).

CAUSES OF ABNORMALLY HIGH LEVELS: Antibody tests: The presence of antibodies indicates exposure, but not necessarily active infection. Antigen: The presence of serum antigen indicates systemic infection or, at the very least, colonization of skin or mucosal surfaces.

NEXT DIAGNOSTIC STEP TO CONSIDER IF LEVELS HIGH: False positive and false negative tests results can occur with all tests for aspergillosis (including culture, cytology, histopathology). No single test is diagnostic. Nasal radiography or computed tomography (turbinate destruction and increased areas of radiolucency) and rhinoscopy (for direct visualization and for cytologic, histopathologic, or culture specimens) are the most informative tests.

IMPORTANT INTERSPECIES DIFFERENCES: Serologic tests often use species specific antibodies. Confirm with the lab that the specific test being used is valid for the species in question.

SAMPLE FOR COLLECTION AND ANY SPECIAL SPECIMEN HANDLING NOTES: Serum, refrigerated

PEARLS: *Penicillium* spp. is another genus of fungus that can cause nasal disease in dogs. The organisms appear similar and can only be differentiated via culture or serology, not cytologic appearance alone. Antibody serologic tests that detect antibody to either antigen are preferred.

Both *Penicillium* spp. and *Aspergillus* spp. are ubiquitous in the environment and common contaminants. Positive blind culture of nasal discharge without cytologic/histologic evidence of inflammation and tissue invasion may represent only contamination. Conversely, the fungal plaques are localized and blind biopsy/cytology collection often shows only nonspecific inflammation if the fungal plaques are missed. Rhinoscopy guided collection of tissue samples is most likely to yield a positive diagnosis.

AUTHOR: **JAMES H. MEINKOTH**

Baermann Fecal Flotation

BASIC INFORMATION

DEFINITION

A method used for examination of fecal specimens for parasite larvae. Rather than being drawn to the surface, as with a fecal flotation, parasites are detected after being drawn to the bottom of the Baermann apparatus. The Baermann apparatus is a funnel with a rubber tube attached to the stem, usually supported by a ring stand. Feces are put on cheesecloth in a strainer, which is placed in the funnel. Water is added to cover the specimen, which is then macerated. An aliquot of fluid collected after a few hours is examined microscopically for parasitic larvae.

SYNONYM(S)

Baermann's funnel apparatus

TYPICAL NORMAL RANGE

Reported as negative or positive with species identification

PHYSIOLOGY

The Baermann apparatus uses the larvae's tendency to migrate from fecal matter to warm water.

CAUSES OF ABNORMALLY HIGH LEVELS: Filarid parasite (*Filaroides osleri, F. milksi, F. hirthi, Crenosoma vulpis*, and *Aelurostrongylus abstrusus*) infections are most likely to be detected by this method of fecal examination.

NEXT DIAGNOSTIC STEP TO CONSIDER IF LEVELS HIGH: Positive fecal with parasite identification is considered diagnostic.

DRUG EFFECTS ON LEVELS: Antihelmintics may decrease larval shedding.

LAB ARTIFACTS THAT MAY INTERFERE WITH READINGS OF LEVELS OF THIS SUBSTANCE: Test is not sensitive. A negative test does not rule out infection because fecal shedding of larvae is intermittent.

SAMPLE FOR COLLECTION AND ANY SPECIAL SPECIMEN HANDLING NOTES: Fresh (24 hours old) fecal specimen submitted in dry container.

PEARLS: Bronchoscopy is preferred for detection of *F. osleri,* but the procedure is time consuming, more costly, and requires general anesthesia. Baermann fecal flotation is considered to have a slight advantage over usual fecal flotation for detection of larvae in feces. No advantage for detection of ova.

AUTHOR: **LOIS ROTH-JOHNSON**

Bartonellosis Serology

BASIC INFORMATION

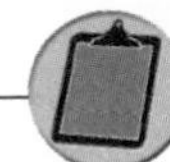

DEFINITION

Bartonella spp. are a group of vector-transmitted, intraerythrocytic bacterial organisms that can induce persistent infections in dogs, cats, and humans.

Formerly *Rochalimaea* (*quintana, henselae, elizabethae, vinsonii*).

SYNONYM(S)

Cat scratch fever
Oroya fever (humans)
Trench fever

TYPICAL NORMAL RANGE

Consult the laboratory conducting the test for information regarding reference ranges. Some general guidelines include:

- Immunofluorescence antibody (IFA) test for *B. vinsonii* and *B. henselae*. Negative titer is <1:64.
- Western immunoblot (FeBart) for multiple *Bartonella* spp. in dogs and cats. Results available as negative or +1 to +4, with +3 and +4 considered to be positive and +2 considered to be possibly affected.

PHYSIOLOGY

Following vector transmission, chronic intravascular infections may produce no clinical signs or cause acute, life-threatening disease, or chronic debilitating illness. Cats may exhibit fever, lymphadenopathy, or central nervous system (CNS) signs. Seropositive dogs may exhibit polyarthritis, endocarditis, myocarditis, CNS signs, granulomatous disease, cutaneous vasculitis, uveitis, immune-mediated hemolytic anemia, or immune-mediated thrombocytopenia.

CAUSES OF ABNORMALLY HIGH LEVELS: Seropositivity indicates exposure to *Bartonella* spp.

NEXT DIAGNOSTIC STEP TO CONSIDER IF LEVELS HIGH: If seropositive, consider submitting whole blood for culture or polymerase chain reaction (PCR), or tissue biopsy for histopathology, Warthin-Starry stain, and PCR. Speciation for *B. henselae, B. clarridgeae, B. quintona*, and *B. vinsonii* is possible with PCR testing. Diagnosis may be difficult to confirm.

IMPORTANT INTERSPECIES DIFFERENCES: Although blood culture is currently the gold standard for confirming a diagnosis in cats, culture appears to be insensitive for isolation of *Bartonella* spp. from dogs. In both species, cyclic bacteremia can result in false negatives for both blood culture and PCR.

DRUG EFFECTS ON LEVELS: Effective treatment with macrolide antibiotics may decrease serology titers.

LAB ARTIFACTS THAT MAY INTERFERE WITH READINGS OF LEVELS OF THIS SUBSTANCE: PCR: false-positive results via contamination of samples; false-negative results due to degradation of nucleic acids via improperly sample handling and storage.

SAMPLE FOR COLLECTION AND ANY SPECIAL SPECIMEN HANDLING NOTES: Contact laboratory for specific instructions. IFA: submit 1 ml serum (red top tube). Western immunoblot (FeBart): submit whole blood, serum (red top), or plasma (green or purple top). PCR: submit whole blood collected into an EDTA (purple top) tube.

AUTHOR: **PATTY J. EWING**

Basophils

BASIC INFORMATION

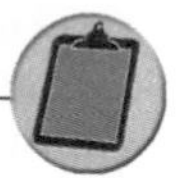

DEFINITION

White blood cell (granulocytic leukocyte) that has a segmented nucleus and metachromatic or purple ("basophilic") granules in cytoplasm. Basophils are rarely encountered in the blood of healthy animals.

TYPICAL NORMAL RANGE

Dogs and cats: 0 to 0.1×10^3 basophils/μL.

PHYSIOLOGY

Basophilic precursors undergo differentiation in the bone marrow, enter peripheral blood circulation for a few hours, and then enter tissue. Basophils produce leukotrienes and release histamine, heparin, and other mediators from their granules. Basophils participate in immunoglobulin E-mediated hypersensitivity reactions. They are similar in morphology to mast cells, but mast cells have a mononuclear nucleus and primarily reside in tissue.

CAUSES OF ABNORMALLY HIGH LEVELS: Allergic reactions (e.g., food, insect sting); parasitism (e.g., dirofilariasis/heartworm disease, flea infestation); mast cell neoplasm; basophilic leukemia; myeloproliferative diseases (e.g., polycythemia vera)

NEXT DIAGNOSTIC STEP TO CONSIDER IF LEVELS HIGH: Additional tests directed by clinical signs to rule out causes of high values listed above.

IMPORTANT INTERSPECIES DIFFERENCES: The granules in feline basophils stain lavender or light violet. The metachromatic staining of granules in feline basophilic myelocytes diminishes as the basophils undergo maturation in the marrow. Canine basophils have very low numbers of metachromatic granules. Because canine basophils are large and have grey basophilic cytoplasm, they can be misidentified as monocytes on blood smear.

SAMPLE FOR COLLECTION AND ANY SPECIAL SPECIMEN HANDLING NOTES: Ethylenediamine tetraacetic acid (purple tube) blood sample and freshly prepared blood smear

PEARLS: Basophilia often accompanies eosinophilia, a further indication of allergic or parastic dissease. Careful examination is necessary to identify basophils; when stained with the rapid Romanowsky stains (e.g., Diff Quik), the cytoplasmic granules of canine basophils may be even less apparent.

AUTHOR: **STEPHEN D. GAUNT**

Bence Jones Urinary Proteins

BASIC INFORMATION

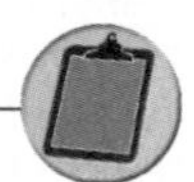

DEFINITION

Unassociated immunoglobulin light chains produced in excess by abnormal plasma cells as occurring with malignant plasma cell neoplasia (multiple myeloma).

SYNONYM(S)

Free immunoglobulin light chains
M-proteins
Myeloma proteins
Paraproteinuria

TYPICAL NORMAL RANGE

Reported as negative or positive

PHYSIOLOGY

Light chains are a component of immunoglobulins. Increased production occurs with increased immunoglobulin production or catabolism, as with multiple myeloma or (rarely) plasma cell tumors, the benign counterpart. Bence Jones proteins precipitate when heated, followed by redissolving when boiled and precipitation again when cooled.

CAUSES OF ABNORMALLY HIGH LEVELS: Multiple myeloma; less often associated with extramedullary plasmacytoma or chronic lymphocytic leukemia; rarely associated with chronic infectious diseases.

NEXT DIAGNOSTIC STEP TO CONSIDER IF LEVELS HIGH: Confirm monoclonal gammopathy with plasma immunoelectrophoresis. Assess for osteolytic bone lesions (radiographs); bone marrow plasmacytosis or plasma cell neoplasia (cytology or biopsy); urine protein electrophoresis (monoclonal spike in β or δ regions).

LAB ARTIFACTS THAT MAY INTERFERE WITH READINGS OF LEVELS OF THIS SUBSTANCE: False positives can occur with marked proteinuria.

SAMPLE FOR COLLECTION AND ANY SPECIAL SPECIMEN HANDLING NOTES: Urine: Store at 2–8° C (refrigeration).

PEARLS: Heat precipitation method is not highly sensitive. Urine protein dipstick tests do not detect Bence Jones protein. The presence of Bence Jones proteins in the urine does not indicate glomerular disease (the molecules are sufficiently small to pass through normal glomerular fenestrations).

AUTHOR: **FONZIE QUANCE-FITCH**

Bicarbonate

BASIC INFORMATION

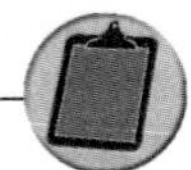

DEFINITION

An anion that is the major extracellular buffer in blood.

SYNONYM(S)

HCO_3^-

TYPICAL NORMAL RANGE

Dogs and cats: 17 to 24 mEq/L (mEq/L = mmol/L).

PHYSIOLOGY

Bicarbonate is formed from the conversion of carbon dioxide and water to carbonic acid by carbonic anhydrase. Carbonic acid dissociates into bicarbonate and hydrogen ion. During metabolic acidosis, bicarbonate minimizes pH changes by binding to excess H^+. Binding excess H^+ decreases measurable HCO_3^-.

CAUSES OF ABNORMALLY HIGH LEVELS: Metabolic alkalosis (causes: vomiting, diuretics, overadministration of bicarbonate) or respiratory acidosis (causes: pulmonary parenchymal disease [pneumonia, pulmonary edema], pulmonary restrictive disease [pleural effusion, pneumothorax, diaphragmatic hernia], central nervous system depression [anesthesia, narcotics, brain stem disease], airway obstruction)

NEXT DIAGNOSTIC STEP TO CONSIDER IF LEVELS HIGH: Evaluate arterial blood gas profile (particularly pH and PCO_2) to differentiate between metabolic alkalosis (high pH, high HCO_3^-, high PCO_2) and metabolic compensation for respiratory acidosis (low pH, high PCO_2, high HCO_3^-). Evaluate for causes (listed above) of underlying process.

CAUSES OF ABNORMALLY LOW LEVELS: Metabolic acidosis (causes: bicarbonate loss due to diarrhea, lactic acidosis, ketoacidosis, uremia and ingestion of ethylene glycol) or compensation for respiratory alkalosis (causes: pulmonary disease [pneumonia, pulmonary edema], direct stimulation of central nervous system [pain, anxiety], septicemia).

NEXT DIAGNOSTIC STEP TO CONSIDER IF LEVELS LOW: Evaluate arterial blood gas profile to differentiate between metabolic acidosis (low pH, low HCO_3^-, low PCO_2) and metabolic compensation for respiratory alkalosis (high pH, low PCO_2, low HCO_3^-). Evaluate for causes (listed above) of underlying process.

LAB ARTIFACTS THAT MAY INTERFERE WITH READINGS OF LEVELS OF THIS SUBSTANCE: Decrease: processing delay. Specimens analyzed within 15 minutes of collections are preferred. Storage in a capped syringe on ice at 4° C for up to 2 hours is acceptable.

SAMPLE FOR COLLECTION AND ANY SPECIAL SPECIMEN HANDLING NOTES: Bicarbonate is a calculated value provided as part of a blood gas analysis. Whole blood in a heparinized syringe, avoiding exposure to room air, is used as described for blood gas analysis.

PEARLS: Total carbon dioxide (TCO_2) estimates plasma bicarbonate, which is part of most serum chemistry profiles. TCO_2 is the total amount of CO_2 gas that can be released from serum. At physiologic pH (7.4), about 95% of the potential gas is CO_2 and 5% is HCO_3^-. Therefore, although TCO_2 is usually slightly higher (1 to 2 mEq/L) than the bicarbonate on a blood gas profile, it is considered a clinically accurate assessment of bicarbonate.

AUTHOR: **JAMES H. MEINKOTH**

LABORATORY TESTS

Bile Acids (Blood, Urinary)

BASIC INFORMATION

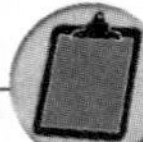

DEFINITION

Family of detergent-like compounds (predominately cholic acid and chenodeoxycholic acid in animals) synthesized in the liver from cholesterol and secreted in bile to aid in digestion and absorption of fat and fat-soluble vitamins.

TYPICAL NORMAL RANGE

- Fasting bile acids normally <5 μmol/L.
- Fasting bile acids >20 μmol/L, postprandial samples >25 μmol/L, and urine bile acid/creatinine >7.1 indicate liver disease.

PHYSIOLOGY

Stored in the gallbladder. Released as a bolus into the small intestines upon feeding. An efficient enterohepatic circulation exists when up to 95% of bile acids are recycled. Serum bile acids are evaluated in paired samples (fasting, postprandial). Urinary bile acid: creatinine ratios reflect an average serum bile acid concentration and only a single sample is required.

CAUSES OF ABNORMALLY HIGH LEVELS: Cholestasis, liver disease, portosystemic shunt

NEXT DIAGNOSTIC STEP TO CONSIDER IF LEVELS HIGH: Assess for cholestasis (bilirubin, alkaline phosphatase), portosystemic shunt (imaging), other liver diseases (alanine aminotransferase, imaging, liver biopsy).

LAB ARTIFACTS THAT MAY INTERFERE WITH READINGS OF LEVELS OF THIS SUBSTANCE

- Decrease: hemolysis, lipemia (spectrophotometric method), no effect on radioimmunoassay.
- Increase: hypertriglyceridemia (spectrophotometric method), no effect on radioimmunoassay.

SAMPLE FOR COLLECTION AND ANY SPECIAL SPECIMEN HANDLING NOTES

- Serum: 12-hour fasting sample and 2-hour postprandial sample recommended. Separate serum from red blood cells as soon as possible. Store at 2–8° C (refrigeration).
- Urine: fresh urine, avoid blood contamination.

PEARLS

- If cholestasis is present (e.g., patient is icteric without evidence of hemolysis), bile acids do not provide any additional information on hepatic function. Bile acids are a good indicator of hepatobiliary function, but are not specific for the type of underlying disease. Extrahepatic diseases can elevate bile acid concentrations. Urine bile acids are more specific for canine liver dysfunction than serum bile acids.
- Occasional preprandial values that exceed postprandial values are attributed to spontaneous gallbladder contraction.

AUTHOR: **FONZIE QUANCE-FITCH**

Bilirubin

BASIC INFORMATION

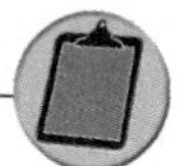

DEFINITION

A pigment produced by the degradation of the heme portion of hemoglobin (and, to a lesser extent, other porphyrin-containing compounds).

TYPICAL NORMAL RANGE

- Dogs: approximately 0-0.3 mg/dl.
- Cats: approximately 0-0.1 mg/dl. Specific values vary among laboratories. For mmol/L, multiply mg/dl × 17.1.

PHYSIOLOGY

During the breakdown of red blood cells (either senescent or pathologic hemolysis), heme is split to iron and protoporphyrin; protoporphyrin is converted to biliverdin then to unconjugated bilirubin predominately in macrophages of spleen, bone marrow, and liver. Unconjugated bilirubin is released into circulation, where it is bound to carrier proteins (albumin, globulins) and transported to the liver for uptake, conjugation, and secretion into bile. Conjugation renders bilirubin water-soluble. Laboratory assays include total serum bilirubin, direct (conjugated) bilirubin, and indirect (unconjugated) bilirubin, which is a calculated value.

CAUSES OF ABNORMALLY HIGH LEVELS: Hemolysis, decreased hepatic uptake, decreased functional liver mass, decreased bile excretion (intrahepatic or extrahepatic)

NEXT DIAGNOSTIC STEP TO CONSIDER IF LEVELS HIGH: Assess for hemolytic disease (complete blood count, Coomb's test), bile obstruction (alkaline phosphatase [ALP], imaging), hepatic disease (alanine aminotransferase, ALP, liver biopsy).

LAB ARTIFACTS THAT MAY INTERFERE WITH READINGS OF LEVELS OF THIS SUBSTANCE

- Hemolysis interferes with (either increases or decreases, depending on the method) measurement.
- Lipemia falsely increases bilirubin.
- Light degrades bilirubin (up to 50% in 1 hour in direct sunlight or fluorescent light).

SAMPLE FOR COLLECTION AND ANY SPECIAL SPECIMEN HANDLING NOTES: Nonhemolyzed serum (red-top tube). Separate serum from red blood cells as soon as possible. Store at 2-8°C (refrigeration). Protect from light.

PEARLS: Determination of conjugated and unconjugated forms of bilirubin is not usually useful in differentiating hemolytic from hepatic/biliary causes of icterus in dogs and cats.

AUTHOR: **FONZIE QUANCE-FITCH**

Bilirubinuria

BASIC INFORMATION

DEFINITION

The presence of bilirubin in urine. Most common is conjugated bilirubin, which is water soluble; some unconjugated bilirubin is bound to albumin if albuminuria or proteinuria is present.

TYPICAL NORMAL RANGE

- Negative in healthy cats; rarely trace or +1 in normal cats with extremely concentrated urine (>1.055 specific gravity).
- Negative in healthy dogs, trace or +1 in normal dogs with moderately or highly concentrated urine.

PHYSIOLOGY

Bilirubin is a byproduct of erythrocyte hemoglobin metabolism. Increased bilirubin production/release is caused by hemolytic states and abnormalities in hepatobiliary excretion of bilirubin. Water soluble conjugated bilirubin is readily filtered through the glomerulus; dogs have especially low renal thresholds with minimal tubular resorption of bilirubin, such that bilirubinuria precedes hyperbilirubinemia (icterus). Also, canine renal tubular epithelial cells are capable of bilirubin production from hemoglobin resorbed from urine. Cats have higher thresholds and greater tubular resorption of conjugated bilirubin; therefore, bilirubinuria is more clinically significant compared with dogs and usually indicates hepatobiliary disease. Albumin bound unconjugated bilirubin does not pass the glomerulus readily. However, animals with albuminuria/proteinuria may have enough albumin/protein in urine to get measurable amounts of unconjugated bilirubin in urine.

CAUSES OF ABNORMALLY HIGH LEVELS: Hemolytic diseases and decreased hepatobiliary excretion of bilirubin

NEXT DIAGNOSTIC STEP TO CONSIDER IF LEVELS HIGH: Assess urine specific gravity, hematocrit, and liver enzymes (alanine aminotransferase, alkaline phosphatase, ± γ-glutamyl transferase).

IMPORTANT INTERSPECIES DIFFERENCES: In health, only dogs are expected to have bilirubinuria; however, cats with extremely concentrated urine may have trace or +1 reaction.

DRUG EFFECTS ON LEVELS

- Indican (a substance that may occur in the urine of normal animals) and etodolac metabolites may cause spurious increase.
- Ascorbic acid may cause spurious decrease.

LAB ARTIFACTS THAT MAY INTERFERE WITH READINGS OF LEVELS OF THIS SUBSTANCE: Ultraviolet light causes bilirubin degradation. It is best if the urine sample has less than 30 minutes of direct ultraviolet light exposure prior to analysis.

SAMPLE FOR COLLECTION AND ANY SPECIAL SPECIMEN HANDLING NOTES: Minimum of 5 ml of urine in clean/sterile container collected by free catch, catheterization, or cystocentesis

AUTHOR: **ELIZABETH G. WELLES**

Blastomyces Serology

BASIC INFORMATION

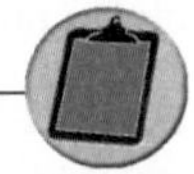

DEFINITION

Blastomycosis is a systemic fungal infection caused by the dimorphic fungus *Blastomyces dermatitidis*.

SYNONYM(S)

Agar-gel immunodiffusion (AGID) test

PHYSIOLOGY

Following inhalation of *Blastomyces* spores, a primary lung infection develops with subsequent spread via blood and lymphatics to multiple tissues, most notably skin, eye, bone, lymph nodes, and brain.

CAUSES OF ABNORMALLY HIGH LEVELS: A positive AGID test indicates exposure to *Blastomyces*.

NEXT DIAGNOSTIC STEP TO CONSIDER IF TEST IS POSITIVE: Correlate serology results with clinical signs and radiographic findings. Demonstration of the organism in cytologic or tissue biopsy samples is required for definitive diagnosis. PCR testing is also available.

CAUSES OF NEGATIVE RESULT: Negative test result indicates lack of exposure, early infection, or inadequate immune response to exposure.

NEXT DIAGNOSTIC STEP TO CONSIDER IF LEVELS LOW: If high clinical suspicion of *Blastomyces* spp. exists but antibody test is negative, consider collection of relevant cytologic samples or biopsy samples to demonstrate organisms. PCR testing may detect early infections.

IMPORTANT INTERSPECIES DIFFERENCES: Blastomycosis is more common in dogs living in endemic areas, such as the Mississippi, Ohio, and the Missouri river valleys. Infection rarely occurs in cats.

SAMPLE FOR COLLECTION AND ANY SPECIAL SPECIMEN HANDLING NOTES: Submit 1 ml of serum (red-top tube) for AGID serology test. For PCR testing, submit 3 ml of blood in EDTA tube, throat swabs or lung aspirates in sterile container, and/or tissue. Samples for PCR should be stored at 4°C until shipped.

PEARLS: In dogs, the blastomyces AGID has a sensitivity of 91% and a specificity of 96%.

AUTHOR: **PATTY J. EWING**

Blood Gas Analysis

BASIC INFORMATION

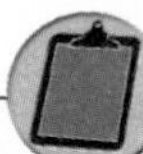

DEFINITION

- Evaluation of blood pH, pCO_2, pO_2, and bicarbonate. Other calculated parameters may be included.
- A blood pH lower than normal indicates *acidosis*, whereas a blood pH higher than normal indicates *alkalosis*. The acidosis or alkalosis is considered *metabolic* if a low HCO_3^- is a predominant coabnormality, or conversely is considered *respiratory* if high pCO_2 is a predominant coabnormality.

SYNONYM(S)

Acid-base analysis

TYPICAL NORMAL RANGE

- Arterial pH: dog = 7.35 to 7.45, cat = 7.30 to 7.42
- PCO_2 (mmHg): dog = 31 to 42, cat = 25 to 37
- PO_2 (mmHg): dog = 90 to 100, cat = 90 to 100
- HCO_3^- (mEq/L): dog = 19 to 26, cat = 14 to 21

PHYSIOLOGY

- Blood pH is maintained within narrow limits by a variety of buffers acting in concert. pCO_2 and bicarbonate (HCO_3) are the main parameters used for detecting respiratory and metabolic (respectively) derangements altering pH. Arterial pO_2 is used for evaluating pulmonary function. Normal respiration maintains high pO_2 and relatively low pCO_2 concentration.
- General interpretive steps are to determine if the pH has changed significantly and then evaluate the HCO_3^- and pCO_2 to determine if the change is due to metabolic or respiratory abnormalities, respectively.

CAUSES OF ABNORMALLY HIGH LEVELS: See individual tests, particularly pH.

CAUSES OF ABNORMALLY LOW LEVELS: See individual tests, particularly pH.

DRUG EFFECTS ON LEVELS: Diuretics such as furosemide can cause metabolic alkalosis.

LAB ARTIFACTS THAT MAY INTERFERE WITH READINGS OF LEVELS OF THIS SUBSTANCE: Exposure to room air will result in falsely increased pO_2 and decreased pCO_2. Failure to analyze samples promptly can result in decreases in pH and PO_2.

SAMPLE FOR COLLECTION AND ANY SPECIAL SPECIMEN HANDLING NOTES: Whole blood collected and maintained in heparinized syringe (0.05 to 0.1 ml of heparin [1000 units/ml] per ml blood). Cap end of needle to limit exposure to room air. Specimens analyzed within 15 minutes of collections are preferred. Storage in a capped syringe on ice at 4°C for up to 2 hours is acceptable.

PEARLS

- Alterations in pH can be life threatening. Handheld point-of-care analyzers are available for use in clinics.
- Venous blood samples are sufficient for routine evaluation of pH, pCO_2, and HCO_3^-. Arterial samples are more difficult to obtain, but are needed for meaningful interpretation of pO_2 levels.

AUTHOR: **JAMES H. MEINKOTH**

Blood pH

BASIC INFORMATION

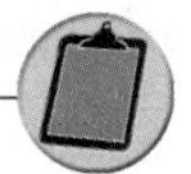

DEFINITION

Measure of the hydrogen ion (H^+) concentration (acidity) of the blood.

TYPICAL NORMAL RANGE

Dogs: 7.31 to 7.42; cats: 7.24 to 7.40.

PHYSIOLOGY

pH is inversely related to H^+ concentration; increased $[H^+]$ = decreased pH. Hydrogen ions are continuously produced by metabolic processes and excreted via the kidneys or bound to buffers.

CAUSES OF ABNORMALLY HIGH LEVELS: Increased pH indicates alkalosis, either respiratory (decreased pCO_2) or metabolic (increased bicarbonate). Metabolic causes: vomiting, diuretics, overadministration of bicarbonate. Respiratory alkalosis is caused by hyperventilation due to pulmonary disease, direct stimulation of central nervous system (pain, anxiety), septicemia.

NEXT DIAGNOSTIC STEP TO CONSIDER IF LEVELS HIGH: Respiratory: thoracic radiography/ultrasound, evaluate mentation, blood cultures. Metabolic: evaluate for vomiting, review treatment history.

CAUSES OF ABNORMALLY LOW LEVELS: Decreased pH indicates acidosis, either metabolic (low bicarbonate) or respiratory (increased pCO_2). Metabolic causes: bicarbonate loss (and/or production of endogenous acids) due to diarrhea, lactic acidosis, ketoacidosis, uremia, ingestion of exogenous toxins (ethylene glycol). Respiratory causes: pulmonary parenchymal disease, pulmonary restrictive disease (pleural effusion, pneumothorax, diaphragmatic hernia), central nervous system depression (anesthesia, narcotics, brainstem disease), airway obstruction.

NEXT DIAGNOSTIC STEP TO CONSIDER IF LEVELS LOW: Metabolic: calculate anion gap to determine if due to loss of bicarbonate (anion gap normal) or accumulation of organic acid (high anion gap). Evaluate serum biochemistry profile for renal disease, diabetes mellitus. Respiratory: ensure patent airway, thoracic radiography/ultrasound, evaluate mentation.

DRUG EFFECTS ON LEVELS: Decrease: sedative, narcotic, general anesthetics causing respiratory depression. Increase: bicarbonate or diuretic administration.

LAB ARTIFACTS THAT MAY INTERFERE WITH READINGS OF LEVELS OF THIS SUBSTANCE: Decrease: delayed analysis of sample, excessive heparin in syringe. Increase: sample exposure to room air.

SAMPLE FOR COLLECTION AND ANY SPECIAL SPECIMEN HANDLING NOTES: Whole blood collected and maintained in heparinized syringe, 0.05–0.1 ml of heparin/ml blood. Cap syringe end to limit exposure to room air. Specimens analyzed within 15 minutes of collections are preferred. Storage in a capped syringe on ice at 4° C for up to 2 hours is acceptable.

PEARLS: Disturbances of pH can be life threatening. Periodic monitoring during prolonged anesthesia and in patients with severe metabolic illness (vomiting, diarrhea, shock) is critical.

AUTHOR: **JAMES H. MEINKOTH**

Blood Typing

BASIC INFORMATION

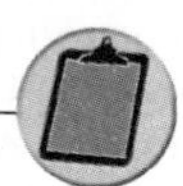

DEFINITION

Identification of specific inherited characteristic cell surface antigens on erythrocyte membrane.

TYPICAL NORMAL RANGE

- Canine: dog erythrocyte antigen (DEA) 1.1, 1.2, 1.3 ("A" system). Other systems exist, but the "A" system is most important for transfusion purposes. DEA 7 can cause antibody response in dogs that lack it.
- Feline: type A (most common), type B (less common), type AB (rare).

PHYSIOLOGY

- Canine: DEA 1.1 antigen is capable of producing acute hemolytic reactions in sensitized dogs; identified by monoclonal antibodies on blood typing cards.
- Feline: type A (>95%), type B (<5%); defined by preexisting, naturally occurring isoantibodies against the antigen they lack; type AB lacks antibodies; isoantibodies responsible for transfusion reactions and neonatal isoerythrolysis.

CAUSES OF ABNORMALLY HIGH LEVELS: Reported result is individual animal's blood type.

IMPORTANT INTERSPECIES DIFFERENCES

- Dogs do not have naturally occurring antibodies; first transfusion will not cause hemolytic reaction (typing unnecessary for first transfusion).
- All type B cats >3 months of age have high titers of naturally occurring type A antibodies that act as strong hemagglutinins and hemolysins. Type A or AB kittens born to type B queens are at risk of developing neonatal isoerythrolysis. Higher incidence of type B blood: British shorthair, Devon Rex, Cornish Rex breeds, DSH and DLH on U.S. west coast, Europe, Japan, and Australia.

SAMPLE FOR COLLECTION AND ANY SPECIAL SPECIMEN HANDLING NOTES

- Ethylenediamine tetraacetic acid (purple top) tube.
- Typing cards are species specific. Dog blood typing cards are for DEA 1.1 antigen and cards for cats can be used to determine type A, B, or AB.

PEARLS

- Dog: blood from dogs positive for DEA 1.1 should never be given to DEA 1.1 negative dogs.
- Cats: blood from type B cats should never be given to type A cats.

AUTHOR: **DEBORAH G. DAVIS**

Blood Urea Nitrogen (BUN)

BASIC INFORMATION

DEFINITION

Concentration of urea in serum, plasma, or whole blood (usually measured in serum).

SYNONYM(S)

Increased BUN/SUN is azotemia (with or without increased creatinine)
Serum urea nitrogen (SUN)
Urea nitrogen

TYPICAL NORMAL RANGE

- Dogs: 10–25 mg/dl.
- Cats: 5–30 mg/dl.

PHYSIOLOGY

Most of serum urea is synthesized via hepatic urea cycle, which converts ammonia derived from bacterial metabolism of dietary protein to urea. A small amount of ammonia is derived from deamination of amino acids. The kidneys excrete urea. Urea is freely filtered by glomeruli: some is resorbed by tubular epithelial cells to establish (with sodium) the medullary concentration gradient. Serum urea concentration often parallels creatinine concentration.

CAUSES OF ABNORMALLY HIGH LEVELS

- Mild to moderate increases can result from prerenal causes such as dehydration, decreased cardiac output, or shock (increased concentration of BUN exceeds creatinine).
- Renal disease of virtually any etiology (inflammatory, degenerative, neoplastic, congenital, toxic, or other) can cause azotemia (concentrations of BUN and creatinine often parallel).
- Urinary outflow obstruction results in postrenal azotemia (increased BUN and creatinine).
- Gastrointestinal hemorrhage results in increased urea production (less effect on creatinine concentration).

NEXT DIAGNOSTIC STEP TO CONSIDER IF LEVELS HIGH: Urine specific gravity, measurement of amount of urine production.

CAUSES OF ABNORMALLY LOW LEVELS

- Lack of hepatic urea production owing to decreased dietary protein (low protein diet, anorexia), hepatic failure, decreased functional hepatic mass, portosystemic shunt, congenital deficiency of urea cycle enzymes (rare).
- Increased urea excretion is due to crystalloid or osmotic diuresis or marked polydipsia/polyuria, such as iatrogenic water drinkers (rare) or renal or central diabetes insipidus.

NEXT DIAGNOSTIC STEP TO CONSIDER IF LEVELS LOW: Assess urine specific gravity, quantity of urine output, quantity of water intake, concentrations of electrolytes and calcium.

SAMPLE FOR COLLECTION AND ANY SPECIAL SPECIMEN HANDLING NOTES: Serum (red-top tube) preferred. Heparinized plasma (green-top tube) acceptable.

Some instruments can use ethylenediamine tetraacetic acid plasma (lavender-top tube) or whole blood.

PEARLS: High doses of gastroduodenal ulcerogenic drugs (corticosteroids, nonsteroidal anti-inflammatories) may cause intestinal hemorrhage, increasing BUN.

AUTHOR: **ELIZABETH G. WELLES**

Bone Marrow Cytology

BASIC INFORMATION

DEFINITION

Cytologic evaluation allows assessment of blood precursor cell production and morphology.

TYPICAL NORMAL RANGE

Marrow particles should contain 25–75% hematopoietic cells, with all cell lines exhibiting orderly, complete maturation and normal shape, size, and features (morphology).

PHYSIOLOGY

Bone marrow contains trabecular bone with marrow spaces containing capillaries, hematopoietic cells, and adipocytes. Hematopoietic activity occurs in response to peripheral demand. Bone marrow aspiration is indicated when there are unexplained cytopenias (nonregenerative anemia, neutropenia, and/or thrombocytopenia), hyperglobulinemia, or suspicion for neoplasia.

CAUSES OF ABNORMALLY HIGH LEVELS: Hyperplasia indicates increased peripheral demand for cells due to cell destruction, increased utilization, or loss. Lymphocytes and plasma cells may be increased due to antigenic stimulation neoplasia. Iron stores may be increased with anemia of chronic disease and hemolytic anemia.

NEXT DIAGNOSTIC STEP TO CONSIDER IF LEVELS HIGH: Dependent on clinical signs, laboratory results

CAUSES OF ABNORMALLY LOW LEVELS

- Hypoplasia indicates decreased cell production. Causes: anemia of chronic disease, chronic renal disease, feline leukemia virus (FeLV), ehrlichiosis (dogs), estrogen toxicity depress red blood cell production. Drug induced or immune mediated destruction of precursor cells in the marrow, viral infection (i.e., parvovirus, canine distemper) may affect either erythroid series or myeloid series or both.
- Maturation arrest and dysplastic changes of red blood cells occur with FeLV infection, iron deficiency; myelodysplastic syndrome or toxic injury may affect erythroid or myeloid series.
- Iron stores are decreased with blood loss and iron deficiency.

NEXT DIAGNOSTIC STEP TO CONSIDER IF LEVELS LOW: Dependent on clinical signs and laboratory findings. For example, nonregenerative anemia with erythroid hypoplasia of the marrow warrants measurement of serum erythropoietin levels.

IMPORTANT INTERSPECIES DIFFERENCES: Iron stores are not usually visible in cat bone marrow and cannot be evaluated cytologically.

SAMPLE FOR COLLECTION AND ANY SPECIAL SPECIMEN HANDLING NOTES: Aspirated marrow should immediately be made into fresh smears and also be placed in a lavender-top tube. Proper collection and preparation of slides are essential for accurate interpretation. Hematopoietic cells degenerate rapidly after collection. Slides must be prepared immediately (before a clot forms) or within 30 minutes after collection if anticoagulant is used. A good bone marrow aspirate has several marrow particles for evaluation with spreading of the cells in a monolayer for evaluation of morphology.

PEARLS: Bone marrow aspirates must be interpreted concurrently with complete blood count results. An accompanying bone marrow core may help interpret the overall cellularity of the bone marrow. A fresh smear should be stained and examined for the presence of marrow spicules/cells while the animal is still sedated/anesthetized; if spicules are not adequate, the procedure may be repeated immediately.

AUTHOR: **RUANNA GOSSETT**

Borreliosis (Lyme Disease) Serology

BASIC INFORMATION

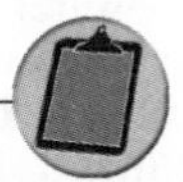

DEFINITION

Lyme borreliosis is a tick-borne disease of dogs, cats, and humans that is caused by the spirochete *Borrelia burgdorferi*.

SYNONYM(S)

Borrelia burgdorferi infection
Lyme disease

TYPICAL NORMAL RANGE

Consult laboratory conducting the test. Some guidelines include: qualitative enzyme-linked immunosorbent assay (ELISA) for antibody to the C_6 peptide of *B. burgdorferi* antigen, positive or negative result; quantitative C_6 antibody test negative result: <30 units/ml; immunofluorescent antibody (IFA) negative result: <1:64.

PHYSIOLOGY

Borrelia spp. organisms are inoculated into the skin via *Ixodes* tick bite where they proliferate and spread to many tissues, including joints and the central nervous system. Persistent infections are common and they may produce no clinical sings, or may result in chronic debilitating disease such as arthritis, meningitis, or protein-losing nephropathy. Host's own inflammatory response likely plays a role in development of disease.

CAUSES OF ABNORMALLY HIGH LEVELS: Qualitative or quantitative C_6 ELISA assay: positive test indicates natural exposure to *B. burgdorferi*. Whole-cell ELISA or IFA: seropositivity indicates natural exposure to pathogenic or nonpathogenic *Borrelia* organisms, or vaccination with borreliosis vaccine.

NEXT DIAGNOSTIC STEP TO CONSIDER IF LEVELS HIGH: If the qualitative C_6 ELISA test is positive, consider the quantitative C_6 antibody test to establish a baseline titer for monitoring treatment in dogs. If IFA is positive, consider Western blot, ELISA testing for specific outer surface proteins, or C_6 ELISA assay. Polymerase chain reaction and blood culture have been used for confirming a diagnosis; however, these tests have low sensitivity (difficult to find organisms).

CAUSES OF NEGATIVE TEST/TITER: Early infection or noninfected.

NEXT DIAGNOSTIC STEP TO CONSIDER IF LEVELS LOW: Consider repeating C_6 antibody test or IFA in 3 to 5 weeks if clinically appropriate.

DRUG EFFECTS ON LEVELS: C_6 titer may decrease within 4 to 5 months following successful treatment with doxycycline or amoxicillin.

SAMPLE FOR COLLECTION AND ANY SPECIAL SPECIMEN HANDLING NOTES: C_6 qualitative ELISA test requires 1 ml of serum or plasma (red-top or purple-top tube). IFA and Western blot: 1 ml of serum (red-top tube). Samples are stable for up to 4 days at refrigerator temperature.

PEARLS: A large proportion of dogs exposed to *Borrelia* (and therefore, a positive test result) do not develop clinical signs of Lyme disease; the decision to treat should always be based on clinical characteristics in addition to serology results.

AUTHOR: **PATTY J. EWING**

Bromide

BASIC INFORMATION

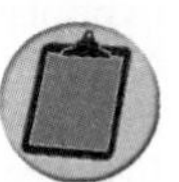

DEFINITION

Active ingredient in potassium or sodium bromide, drugs used for treating seizure disorders.

TYPICAL NORMAL RANGE

Target therapeutic range: 200–300 mg/dl.

PHYSIOLOGY

- As a seizure-controlling drug, bromide competes with chloride transport across cell membranes, resulting in neuronal hyperpolarization and increased seizure threshold. Neuron excitability is depressed.
- The standard method for measuring serum concentration is spectrophotometrically using the gold chloride method. Measurement by ion selective electrode is considered inaccurate.

CAUSES OF ABNORMALLY HIGH LEVELS: Excessive therapeutic dose.

NEXT DIAGNOSTIC STEP TO CONSIDER IF LEVELS HIGH: Lower dose

IMPORTANT INTERSPECIES DIFFERENCES: Used primarily in dogs; cats are more prone to exhibiting toxic side effects (lethargy, vomiting, polydipsia, polyuria, constipation, pancreatitis).

DRUG EFFECTS ON LEVELS: High chloride diets and diuretics enhance bromide elimination, increasing the bromide dose required for therapeutic effect. Conversely, low chloride diets and concurrent use of central nervous system depressents can enhance bromide effects/toxicity.

LAB ARTIFACTS THAT MAY INTERFERE WITH READINGS OF LEVELS OF THIS SUBSTANCE: Increase: ion-selective electrode method of measurement (chloride interference).

SAMPLE FOR COLLECTION AND ANY SPECIAL SPECIMEN HANDLING NOTES: Serum (red top), refrigerate. First sample should be submitted within 1 week of loading dose; second specimen at 1 month; monitor every 3 to 6 months.

PEARLS: Higher incidence of adverse reaction in older patients and patients with renal dysfunction. KBr is not approved by the U.S. Food and Drug Administration for use in animals.

AUTHOR: **SHERRY J. MORGAN**

Brucella Slide Agglutination

BASIC INFORMATION

DEFINITION

Enzyme-linked immunosorbent assay (ELISA) test for detection of *Brucella canis* antibody in patient serum.

SYNONYM(S)

Rapid slide agglutination test (RSAT)

TYPICAL NORMAL RANGE

Agglutination indicates positive test; serum from noninfected dogs fails to agglutinate.

PHYSIOLOGY

Highly sensitive screening test used for detecting active *B. canis* infection. Patient serum is mixed with heat-killed *B. ovis* on slide. Specimens from patients with antibodies to *B. canis* have positive agglutination.

CAUSES OF ABNORMALLY HIGH LEVELS: *B. canis* infection; false-positive test may occur in patients with antibodies to *Bordetella bronchiseptica*, *Pseudomonas* spp., *Moraxella* spp., or other gram-negative bacteria. Overall, approximately 40% of positive tests are associated with true *B. canis* infection.

NEXT DIAGNOSTIC STEP TO CONSIDER IF LEVELS HIGH: Confirm positive test results with 2-mercaptoethanol tube agglutination, agar gel immunodiffusion, or culture. Appropriate culture specimens (vaginal exudate, aborted pups, semen) depend on clinical signs.

SAMPLE FOR COLLECTION AND ANY SPECIAL SPECIMEN HANDLING NOTES: Serum (red-top tube); separate serum from clot, refrigerate sample.

PEARLS: Humans are susceptible (zoonosis), but infections are rare.

AUTHOR: **LOIS ROTH-JOHNSON**

Buffy Coat

BASIC INFORMATION

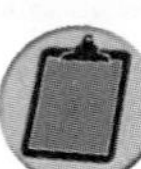

DEFINITION

The thin white layer of packed leukocytes and platelets found atop the packed erythrocytes following high-speed centrifugation of anticoagulated blood in tube.

TYPICAL NORMAL RANGE

Typically not measured. The height of this layer in a spun blood specimen was previously used as a crude index of the total leukocyte count.

PHYSIOLOGY

Leukocytes and platelets are less dense than erythrocytes, so deposit above the packed erythrocytes following centrifugation. A special instrument (IDEXX QBC) can expand and differentiate the layers of buffy coat, and thereby generate useful leukocyte and platelet data.

CAUSES OF ABNORMALLY HIGH LEVELS: Any condition causing leukocytosis or thrombocytosis will increase the thickness of buffy coat layer.

NEXT DIAGNOSTIC STEP TO CONSIDER IF LEVELS HIGH: Complete blood count (CBC) with blood smear examination

CAUSES OF ABNORMALLY LOW LEVELS: Leukopenia

NEXT DIAGNOSTIC STEP TO CONSIDER IF LEVELS LOW: CBC with blood smear examination

SAMPLE FOR COLLECTION AND ANY SPECIAL SPECIMEN HANDLING NOTES: Ethylenediamine tetraacetic acid (purple tube) blood

PEARLS

- Smears of buffy coat can be an important tool for concentrating abnormal leukocytes that occur in very low number. Examples: detection of mastocytemia as a staging tool in dogs with mast cell neoplasm, detection of infectious agents in neutrophils or monocytes (e.g., *Histoplasma* in cats, *Hepatozoon* in dogs).
- Circulating mast cells occur more often as an incidental finding in dogs with various inflammatory diseases, compared to dogs with systemic mast cell neoplasms. Buffy coat detection of mast cells should be restricted to potential staging tool for dogs with confirmed mast cell neoplasms, rather than a means to diagnose mast cell neoplasms.

AUTHOR: **STEPHEN D. GAUNT**

Calcium, Serum

BASIC INFORMATION

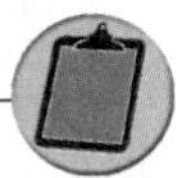

DEFINITION

Essential mineral with regulatory functions (cell signaling). Serum total calcium includes protein-bound (35%), anion complexed (10%), and ionized (55%) fractions.

SYNONYM(S)

Ca

Ca^{2+}

TYPICAL NORMAL RANGE

- Total Ca: 8 to 11.5 mg/dl; 2 to 3.8 mmol/L.
- Ionized Ca: 4.5 to 6 mg/dl; 1.1 to 1.5 mmol/L.
- Unit conversion: mg/dl × 0.2495 = mEq/L × 0.5 = mmol/L.

PHYSIOLOGY

Regulated by parathyroid hormone (PTH), calcitriol (vitamin D metabolite) affecting intestine, kidney, and bone. Dietary absorption depends on calcitriol. Glomeruli filter nonprotein-bound Ca; 98% reabsorbed by tubules. Low ionized Ca stimulates PTH production, mobilizing Ca from bone, increasing renal tubular resorption, stimulating calcitriol synthesis.

CAUSES OF ABNORMALLY HIGH LEVELS: Hypercalcemia of malignancy; hypoadrenocorticism, primary hyperparathyroidism, osteolysis, granulomatous conditions, hypervitaminosis D, renal failure, excess supplementation

NEXT DIAGNOSTIC STEP TO CONSIDER IF LEVELS HIGH: Measure ionized Ca. Evaluate for neoplasia, exposure to oral vitamin D (rodenticides, supplements, ointments). Measure serum phosphorus, parathormone-related peptide, PTH.

CAUSES OF ABNORMALLY LOW LEVELS: Hypoalbuminemia, renal failure, pancreatitis, eclampsia, hypoparathyroidism, severe tissue trauma, ethylene glycol intoxication, exocrine pancreatic insufficiency, malabsorption syndromes, hypomagnesemia, phosphate enema, acute tumor lysis syndrome

NEXT DIAGNOSTIC STEP TO CONSIDER IF LEVELS LOW
- Measure serum albumin. Correct Ca for a low serum albumin (dogs). Evaluate for renal failure, gastrointestinal diseases.
- Measure PTH, magnesium.

DRUG EFFECTS ON LEVELS
- Increase: thiazide diuretics, supplements containing vitamin D, rodenticides, excess oral phosphate binders.
- Decrease: furosemide, glucocorticoids, phosphate enemas, Ca-binding anticoagulants.

LAB ARTIFACTS THAT MAY INTERFERE WITH READINGS OF LEVELS OF THIS SUBSTANCE
- Decreased: Ca-binding anticoagulants (artifacts: ethylenediamine tetraacetic acid, citrate, oxalate).
- Increased: lipemia, hemolysis.
- Decreased ionized Ca: aerobic sample handling, overheparinization. Increased ionized Ca: prolonged exposure to erythrocytes, serum separator tubes.

SAMPLE FOR COLLECTION AND ANY SPECIAL SPECIMEN HANDLING NOTES
- Serum preferred, heparinized plasma may be used.
- Ionized Ca: anaerobic handling necessary. Harvest serum, plasma within 1 hour. Stable in heparinized blood for 9 hours (4°C), serum or plasma for 1 week (4°C). Do not use serum separator tubes. Heparin concentration should not exceed 15 U/ml of blood.

PEARLS
- Acidosis increases ionized serum Ca concentration; alkalosis decreases it.
- Acid-base status affects signs associated with hypocalcemia.

AUTHOR: **ROBIN W. ALLISON**

Canine Distemper Testing

BASIC INFORMATION

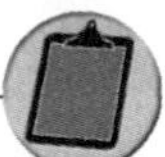

DEFINITION

Canine distemper is a multisystemic disease caused by a *Morbillivirus*.

TYPICAL NORMAL RANGE

Refer to laboratory conducting the tests. Available tests include serum immunofluorescent antibody test (IFA) titer, direct IFA, and viral neutralization assay.

PHYSIOLOGY

Distemper is spread via inhalation. Virus attaches to upper respiratory tract epithelium and replicates in macrophages. It spreads to regional lymph nodes and subsequently to bone marrow, thymus, spleen, mesenteric lymph nodes, and gastrointestinal tract. Then 8 to 14 days later, it spreads to epithelial tissue and central nervous system. Young dogs may develop fever, leukopenia, respiratory signs, and demyelinating encephalomyelitis. Chronic encephalitis is associated with viral persistence.

CAUSES OF ABNORMALLY HIGH LEVELS
- Positive IFA immunoglobulin (Ig) M titer indicates recent exposure to vaccine or acute natural infection. IgM is detectable from 1 to 4 weeks postexposure. Positive IFA IgG titer indicates exposure to vaccine, presence of maternal antibody, or chronic natural infection. Serum viral neutralization assay is preferred for determining protective antibody response to vaccination.
- Positive direct IFA on cytologic or histopathologic sample is diagnostic of infection.

NEXT DIAGNOSTIC STEP TO CONSIDER IF LEVELS HIGH
- Direct immunofluorescence is used for detecting antigen in cytologic smears of conjunctival, tonsillar, genital, or urinary bladder epithelium, or in white blood cells (buffy coat or bone marrow).
- Cerebrospinal fluid (CSF): increased protein and lymphocytic pleocytosis.
- Distemper IgG titer in CSF is a sensitive and specific indicator of distemper encephalitis. Histopathologic lesions and positive immunohistochemistry for CDV antigen are diagnostic.
- Routine cytologic evaluation of conjunctival smears for inclusions (routine staining, with or without IFA) is generally unrewarding.

CAUSES OF ABNORMALLY LOW LEVELS: Lack of protective vaccine antibody titer. Early infection with natural exposure.

NEXT DIAGNOSTIC STEP TO CONSIDER IF LEVELS LOW: If clinically indicated, evaluate IgM titer or repeat IgG titer in 2 to 3 weeks (expect increase if original low/absent level was due to early infection).

SAMPLE FOR COLLECTION AND ANY SPECIAL SPECIMEN HANDLING NOTES: Serology: 1 ml of serum (red-top tube). May store 4 days (refrigerated) or longer (frozen). IFA: conjunctival, urinary sediment, buffy coat smears air dried and preferably fixed in acetone for 5 minutes. Whole blood in EDTA (purple-top tube) stored for no more than 48 hours (refrigerated) may be used in place of buffy coat smear.

PEARLS
- Serologic testing is the most sensitive and specific test in the live patient.
- Although studies suggest that currently available commercial vaccinations offer protection from disease for 3 years, determination of protective serum titer values has not been done. Immunologically competent dogs that have been vaccinated should be able to mount an amnestic response that would prevent viral exposure leading to disease.

AUTHOR: **PATTY J. EWING**

Canine Parvovirus Tests

BASIC INFORMATION

DEFINITION

Canine parvoviral enteritis is a highly infectious, often fatal disease of Canidae caused by a small, nonenveloped DNA virus, CPV-2, that requires rapidly dividing cells for replication.

SYNONYM(S)

CPV-2
Parvo

TYPICAL NORMAL RANGE

Negative or positive with titer. Available tests: serum immunoglobulin (Ig) M and IgG immunofluorescent antibody (IFA); serum antibody by hemagglutination inhibition; and fecal antigen enzyme-linked immunosorbent assay (ELISA).

PHYSIOLOGY

Following oronasal exposure to contaminated feces, CPV-2 replicates in oropharyngeal lymphoid tissue, mesenteric lymph nodes, and thymus. Viremia develops 1 to 5 days postexposure. Virus infects intestinal crypt epithelium causing necrosis and clinical signs of anorexia, vomiting, and bloody diarrhea. Virus spreads to lymphoid tissue and bone marrow causing necrosis, subsequent leukopenia, and immunosuppression. Without treatment, secondary infection, gram-negative sepsis, disseminated intravascular coagulation, and death may ensue.

CAUSES OF ABNORMALLY HIGH LEVELS

- Positive fecal ELISA test indicates viral antigen shedding due to natural infection or recent (5 to 12 days) vaccination with modified live vaccine.
- Positive serum IgM by IFA indicates recent exposure (natural or vaccination); usually positive by time clinical signs are present.
- Positive IgG titer by IFA indicates exposure (natural or vaccination); can demonstrate rising titer in acute and 10- to 14-day convalescent serum samples, although urgency of initial diagnosis and treatment usually minimizes utility of this approach.
- Serum antibody titer by hemagglutination inhibition (HI) of ≥1:64 indicates previous exposure (natural or vaccination) and protective antibody.

NEXT DIAGNOSTIC STEP TO CONSIDER IF LEVELS HIGH: Positive fecal ELISA with appropriate clinical signs is generally diagnostic.

CAUSES OF ABNORMALLY LOW LEVELS

- Negative fecal ELISA indicates uninfected, very early postexposure, or end of viral shedding (virus seldom detectable 10 to 12 days after natural infection; 5 to 7 days of clinical signs).
- False-negative fecal ELISA may occur if the sample is obtained ex vivo (e.g., defecated stool) rather than being swabbed from the rectum.
- Negative serology indicates lack of exposure to virus and inadequate vaccine protection.

NEXT DIAGNOSTIC STEP TO CONSIDER IF LEVELS LOW: If clinical signs and laboratory findings are consistent but ELISA and IFA are negative, electron microscopic exam of feces can be performed. Additional tests—such as histopathologic evaluation of necropsy or biopsy tissue, or tissue culture—are possible, but are invasive and potentially hazardous to the patient.

LAB ARTIFACTS THAT MAY INTERFERE WITH READINGS OF LEVELS OF THIS SUBSTANCE: Severe hemolysis and lipemia interferes with IFA.

SAMPLE FOR COLLECTION AND ANY SPECIAL SPECIMEN HANDLING NOTES: ELISA: fresh feces, store for 48 hours (2-8° C). HI, IFA: serum (red-top tube) can store at 2-8° C up to 4 days.

PEARLS: Some (but not all) ELISA tests for canine parvovirus also will detect feline parvovirus (panleukopenia) in the feces of cats that are shedding virus. False-negative results occur in early stages (prior to fecal shedding) or late stages (virus has become bound to specific antibody). False-positive results are attributed to vaccination.

AUTHOR: **PATTY J. EWING**

Casts in Urine Sediment

BASIC INFORMATION

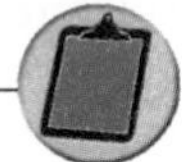

DEFINITION

Coagulum of protein, cells, and/or cell debris forming in renal tubules and observed during microscopic examination of urine sediment.

SYNONYM(S)

Cylindruria

TYPICAL NORMAL RANGE

- Reported as negative or average number of casts per low-power microscope field with cast identification.
- Zero, one, or two hyaline casts in moderately concentrated urine is considered normal.

PHYSIOLOGY

Tamm Horsfall mucoprotein, secreted by renal tubular epithelium, combines with cells in renal tubules, forming cylindrical structures (casts) that are passed in urine. This type of cast is occasionally referred to as a hyaline cast. Some casts (granular, cellular, fatty) are composed of renal tubular epithelial cells or material that reflects their degeneration. Waxy casts are uncommon and indicative of chronic disease. They form from granular casts that have degenerated. Others are composed of leukocytes or red blood cells, indicating inflammation or hemorrhage.

CAUSES OF ABNORMALLY HIGH LEVELS: Toxic renal tubular injury, pyelonephritis

NEXT DIAGNOSTIC STEP TO CONSIDER IF LEVELS HIGH: Evaluate history for exposure to renal toxins; kidney biopsy if otherwise clinically indicated.

DRUG EFFECTS ON LEVELS: Gentamicin, amikacin, or other renal tubular toxins may cause granular, cellular, or fatty casts.

LAB ARTIFACTS THAT MAY INTERFERE WITH READINGS OF LEVELS OF THIS SUBSTANCE: Delay in examination, excessive specimen mixing, and alkaline urine promote disintegration of casts and false-negative results.

SAMPLE FOR COLLECTION AND ANY SPECIAL SPECIMEN HANDLING NOTES: Fresh urine (at least 10 ml) in clean, sterile container for urinalysis

PEARLS: Failure to see casts does not rule out renal tubular disease.

AUTHOR: **LOIS ROTH-JOHNSON**

Cerebrospinal Fluid (CSF) Analysis

BASIC INFORMATION

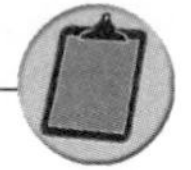

DEFINITION

Cerebrospinal fluid (CSF) is the aqueous fluid that surrounds the brain and spinal cord. *Pleocytosis* refers to an increased cellularity of the CSF sample. *Xanthochromia* refers to a yellow discoloration of the sample, typically from blood that has been present in the CSF for days or longer. *Albuminocytologic dissociation* refers to a disproportionate elevation of CSF protein compared to minimally elevated, or normal, CSF cell count.

TYPICAL NORMAL RANGE

Dogs: red blood cell (RBC), <30/μL; white blood cell (WBC), 0–4/μL; protein, <35 mg/dl. Cats: RBC, <30/μL; WBC, 0–4/μL; protein, <36 mg/dl.

PHYSIOLOGY

Cerebrospinal fluid provides support and protection for neural structures, serves as a transport medium for metabolic products to and from the brain, and provides a barrier to control the microenvironment of the nervous system. It is normally colorless, clear, and almost acellular. Cytocentrifugation is required for cytologic evaluation of cells to assess for inflammation, hemorrhage, and infectious agents. Protein (primarily albumin) concentration is normally very low and requires microprotein assays for accurate assessment.

CAUSES OF ABNORMALLY HIGH LEVELS

- Increased protein: hemorrhage, increased permeability of the blood-CSF barrier, or localized production of immunoglobulins.
- Increased protein with normal cellularity: degenerative disease, intervertebral disc disease, trauma, fibrocartilaginous embolism, cervical spondylomyelopathy, neoplasia, and viral infections.
- Increased protein and cell counts: inflammation, infection (viral, fungal, bacterial, rickettsial, parasitic), granulomatous meningoencephalitis, neoplasia, immune mediated disease, vasculitis, and necrotizing meningoencephalitis. Neoplastic cells are rare in CSF.

NEXT DIAGNOSTIC STEP TO CONSIDER IF LEVELS HIGH: Correlate CSF findings with history, clinical, neurologic, and radiographic findings.

DRUG EFFECTS ON LEVELS: Glucocorticoids may reduce inflammatory cell counts.

SAMPLE FOR COLLECTION AND ANY SPECIAL SPECIMEN HANDLING NOTES: Fluid in lavender-top or red-top tube; refrigerate. Analysis should be performed as soon as possible because cells deteriorate and lyse rapidly due to the low protein concentration. Addition of autologous serum to CSF (1:1) helps preserve cells for cytologic evaluation. However, a separate aliquot of CSF must be submitted for protein determination and cell counts.

AUTHOR: **RUANNA GOSSETT**

Chloride

BASIC INFORMATION

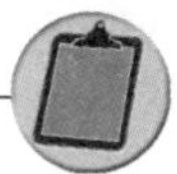

DEFINITION

Major extracellular fluid (ECF) anion. Serum Cl essentially equals ECF Cl: Na, HCO_3 influence concentrations.

SYNONYM(S)

Cl

Cl^-

TYPICAL NORMAL RANGE

Canine: 105 to 115 mEq/L; feline: 115 to 125 mEq/L; mEq/L = mmol/L.

PHYSIOLOGY

Major component of gastric juices; intestinal resorption coupled to Na resorption, HCO_3 secretion. Kidneys play major regulatory role: filtered by glomeruli, reabsorbed in renal tubules following Na and water. Acid-base balance helps regulate serum levels: inverse relationship between Cl and HCO_3 concentrations. Na and Cl concentrations change proportionally, but if Na concentration remains the same, increased Cl causes hyperchloremic acidosis; decrease causes hypochloremic alkalosis.

CAUSES OF ABNORMALLY HIGH LEVELS

- With proportional Na increase: same as hypernatremia.
- Without proportional increase in Na: hyperchloremic acidosis caused by gastrointestinal (GI) or renal loss of HCO_3, compensation for chronic respiratory alkalosis.

NEXT DIAGNOSTIC STEP TO CONSIDER IF LEVELS HIGH

- Evaluate in relation to Na, acid-base balance.
- Calculate corrected Cl to determine if proportional change relative to Na: Cl (corrected) = Cl (measured) × [Na (mean normal)/Na (measured)]. Reference interval for corrected Cl is the same as for Cl.

CAUSES OF ABNORMALLY LOW LEVELS

- With proportional decrease in Na: same as hyponatremia.
- Without proportional decrease in Na: hypochloremic alkalosis caused by loss/sequestration of HCl (gastric vomiting, upper GI obstruction), compensation for chronic respiratory acidosis.

NEXT DIAGNOSTIC STEP TO CONSIDER IF LEVELS LOW

- Evaluate in relation to Na, acid-base balance.
- Calculate corrected Cl to determine if proportional change.

DRUG EFFECTS ON LEVELS

- Decreased: thiazide or loop diuretics, furosemide, $NaHCO_3$, Na penicillin (high doses).
- Increased: NH_4Cl, KCl, parenteral saline administration, acetazolamide, spironolactone.

LAB ARTIFACTS THAT MAY INTERFERE WITH READINGS OF LEVELS OF THIS SUBSTANCE

- Marked hyperlipidemia or hyperproteinemia: decreased measurement (method dependent). Serum osmolality is normal.
- False increase: halides (bromide, iodide) are measured as Cl.

SAMPLE FOR COLLECTION AND ANY SPECIAL SPECIMEN HANDLING NOTES: Serum (red-top tube) preferred; heparinized plasma (green-top tube) may be used.

PEARLS: Changes independent of Na should be interpreted in conjuntion with the anion gap. They suggest mixed acid-base disorders (hypochloremic alkalosis, if the anion gap is not increased or high anion-gap acidosis) because simple hyperchloremic metabolic acidosis typically does not have an increased anion gap.

AUTHOR: **ROBIN W. ALLISON**

Cholesterol

BASIC INFORMATION

DEFINITION

- A lipid that is found only in animal tissues. The test measures circulating blood (serum) levels.
- Hyperlipidemia is a term that groups hypercholesterolemia and hypertriglyceridemia.

TYPICAL NORMAL RANGE

Dogs: 112 to 328 mg/dl.
Cats: 82 to 218 mg/dl.

PHYSIOLOGY

Synthesized by the liver or absorbed in intestines from dietary sources. Cholesterol is essential to life, as a major component of cell membranes and a precursor for the synthesis of steroid hormones and bile acids. Cholesterol and other lipids are insoluble in water. They are transported in the blood attached to apoproteins. Lipid-apoprotein complexes are called lipoproteins. They contain variable proportions of triglycerides, cholesterol, cholesterol esters, and phospholipid. In laboratory analysis, lipoproteins can be separated by ultracentrifugation into chylomicrons, high-density lipoproteins (HDL), intermediate density lipoproteins, low-density lipoproteins (LDL), and very low-density lipoproteins (VLDL), but the clinical importance of lipoprotein profiling in small animal medicine is minimal, compared to human medicine.

CAUSES OF ABNORMALLY HIGH LEVELS

- Primary hyperlipidemia: idiopathic in schnauzer dogs and rarely in other breeds; hypercholesterolemia of Briard dogs, Doberman pinschers, and Rottweilers; familial hyperchylomicronemia of cats.
- Secondary hyperlipidemia: postprandial (most common), hypothyroidism, diabetes mellitus, liver disease, hyperadrenocorticism, pancreatitis in dogs and cats, nephrotic syndrome, high fat diet.

NEXT DIAGNOSTIC STEP TO CONSIDER IF LEVELS HIGH

- Ensure that blood sample was drawn after ≥12-hour fast.
- Assess for causes of secondary hyperlipidemia (endocrine or metabolic disease). If no cause is identified, consider primary hyperlipidemia.

CAUSES OF ABNORMALLY LOW LEVELS: Chronic liver disease, starvation.

NEXT DIAGNOSTIC STEP TO CONSIDER IF LEVELS LOW: Evaluate for chronic liver disease. Rule out starvation.

IMPORTANT INTERSPECIES DIFFERENCES: Dogs and cats are resistant to atherosclerosis partly due to the low concentration of very low density lipoproteins in these species. High density lipoproteins are the major lipoproteins in dogs and cats.

DRUG EFFECTS ON LEVELS

- Increase: exogenous corticosteroids.
- Decrease: lipid lowering diets, bile acid sequestrants, and hepatic hydroxymethylglutaryl coenzyme A reductase inhibitors (statins) lower cholesterol levels.

LAB ARTIFACTS THAT MAY INTERFERE WITH READINGS OF LEVELS OF THIS SUBSTANCE: Increase: hemolysis.

SAMPLE FOR COLLECTION AND ANY SPECIAL SPECIMEN HANDLING NOTES

- A 10- to 12-hour fast is required. Postprandial hypercholesterolemia is usually mild, however (<twofold elevation).
- Serum (red top), heparinized plasma (green top), or ethylenediamine tetraacetic acid plasma (lavender top). Stable for 1 week at 2-8°C and 4 weeks at −20°C.

PEARLS: The most common cause for hypercholesterolemia and no other complete blood count/serum biochemistry abnormalities in an adult, fasted dog is hypothyroidism.

AUTHOR: **RUANNA GOSSETT**

Coagulation Profile

BASIC INFORMATION

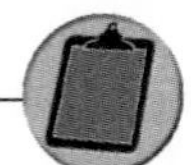

DEFINITION

Series of tests designed to assess the coagulation pathway and localize specific hemostatic defects causing coagulopathies. Consists of partial thromboplastin time (PT), activated partial thromboplastin time (aPTT), and activated clotting time (ACT).

SYNONYM(S)

Activated partial thromboplastin time (aPTT) and partial thromboplastin time (PTT) are synonymous.

TYPICAL NORMAL RANGE

- ACT: 60 to 100 seconds (canine) and <65 seconds (feline).
- aPTT: 8.6 to 12.9 seconds (canine) and 13.7 to 30.2 seconds (feline).
- PT: 5.1 to 7.9 seconds (canine) and 8.4 to 10.8 seconds (feline).
- Reference values are laboratory- and instrument-specific.
- Neonates (<24 hours old) may have greater values than adults.

PHYSIOLOGY

Coagulation factors are a cascade of enzymes that require sequential activation. They stabilize the platelet plug through the conversion of fibrinogen to fibrin, forming a fibrin platelet plug that resists plasmin degradation. The coagulation cascade is divided into intrinsic, extrinsic, and common pathways. Pathways of activation are through tissue thromboplastin (extrinsic; released from cell surface membranes of injured tissues) and by contact activation of basement membranes and negatively charged surfaces of collagen or platelets (intrinsic; e.g., contact with a vessel denuded of endothelium). The division is somewhat artificial, because the tissue factor/factor VIIa complex is a potent activator of both factors IX and X.

CAUSES OF ABNORMALLY HIGH LEVELS

- Prolonged PT: extrinsic (factor VII) or common coagulation (X, V, II, thrombin, and fibrinogen) pathway defect; most sensitive test of warfarin-type toxicity; increased with a decrease/absence of factors of extrinsic or common pathway, disseminated intravascular coagulation (DIC), acquired vitamin K deficiency, biliary obstruction, liver failure.
- Prolonged aPTT: defects in intrinsic pathway (factors XII, XI, IX, VIII); hemophilia, von Willebrand's disease, DIC, acquired vitamin K deficiency, bile insufficiency or liver failure.
- Prolonged ACT: any disorder that sufficiently increases PT, aPTT, or both (common pathway) can cause increased ACT.

NEXT DIAGNOSTIC STEP TO CONSIDER IF LEVELS HIGH: Platelet count, buccal mucosal bleeding time, fibrin degradation products, specific factor analysis

CAUSES OF ABNORMALLY LOW LEVELS: Clotting times shorter than reference range are uncommon and unlikely associated with clinical disease.

DRUG EFFECTS ON LEVELS: Increased: warfarin, heparin therapy.

LAB ARTIFACTS THAT MAY INTERFERE WITH READINGS OF LEVELS OF THIS SUBSTANCE: Increase: inadequately filled tubes because of specimen dilution by anticoagulant.

SAMPLE FOR COLLECTION AND ANY SPECIAL SPECIMEN HANDLING NOTES: Citrated plasma (blue top) for most tests. Diatomaceous earth (gray top) for ACT. Fill tubes completely. Refrigerate, send to lab on ice.

PEARLS: ACT is insensitive except in cases of severe coagulopathy (e.g., severe warfarin intoxication); it should always be followed up with PT and aPTT assessments. Low PT, aPTT, ACT values do *not* indicate a procoagulant or thrombogenic state.

AUTHOR: **DEBORAH G. DAVIS**

Cobalamin

BASIC INFORMATION

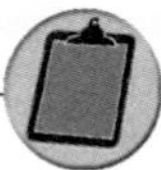

DEFINITION

Water soluble vitamin with a porphyrin ring; side chains bound to cobalt.

SYNONYM(S)

Cyanocobalamin
Vitamin B_{12}

TYPICAL NORMAL RANGE

- Dogs: 238–733 ng/dl.
- Cats: 290–1500 ng/dl.
- Conversion:
  - 1 pg/ml = 0.1 ng/dl
  - 1 pg/ml × 0.7378 = pmol/L

PHYSIOLOGY

Source is dietary. Released from food during gastric digestion and bound to R-proteins (nonspecific binding proteins) found in salivary and gastric secretions. Transferred to intrinsic factor (IF) in the alkaline pH of the intestine. IF enhances the absorption of cobalamin in the ileum. Cobalamin is stored in the liver.

CAUSES OF ABNORMALLY HIGH LEVELS: Uncommon; dietary supplementation and hepatocellular necrosis (theoretical).

NEXT DIAGNOSTIC STEP TO CONSIDER IF LEVELS HIGH: Review oral or parenteral supplements.

CAUSES OF ABNORMALLY LOW LEVELS: Decreased ileal absorption due to inflammation, villus atrophy or other mucosal disease; decreased IF production due to gastric disease in dogs and exocrine pancreatic insufficiency in dogs and cats; congenital insufficiency of IF in giant schnauzers, border collies; malabsorption; bacterial overgrowth in proximal small intestine (enteric bacteria bind cobalamin).

NEXT DIAGNOSTIC STEP TO CONSIDER IF LEVELS LOW: Assess for inflammatory bowel disease (IBD; history, physical exam, serial fecal flotations, and possibly empiric parasiticide treatment and/or abdominal ultrasonography to rule out other causes; biopsy of small intestine ultimately needed for diagnosis of IBD). Assess for pancreatic insufficiency (serum trypsin like immunoreactivity)

DRUG EFFECTS ON LEVELS: Oral or parenteral supplements increase concentration.

LAB ARTIFACTS THAT MAY INTERFERE WITH READINGS OF LEVELS OF THIS SUBSTANCE

- Falsely increased by hemolysis or heparin.
- Falsely decreased by excessive light exposure.

SAMPLE FOR COLLECTION AND ANY SPECIAL SPECIMEN HANDLING NOTES: Serum; separate as soon as possible; store at 8° C.

PEARLS

- Assays for human specimens are unreliable in dogs and cats because of species specific carrier.
- Assessment of cobalamin (and folate) levels is no longer considered reliable for the diagnosis of antibiotic responsive enteritis/small intestinal bacterial overgrowth.

AUTHOR: **LOIS ROTH-JOHNSON**

Coccidioides immitis Serology

BASIC INFORMATION

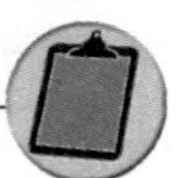

DEFINITION

Coccidioides immitis is a soil-borne dimorphic fungus restricted to certain geographic regions, specifically the Lower Sonoran life zone within the southwestern United States, Mexico, and Central and South America. Serology measures the anti-coccidioides antibodies that may be present in serum by one of several methods.

SYNONYM(S)

Valley fever serology

PHYSIOLOGY

Infection is typically acquired by inhalation, initially causing pulmonary infection that may disseminate to lymph nodes, bones, eyes, heart, testicles, brain, spinal cord, and other visceral organs.

CAUSES OF ABNORMALLY HIGH LEVELS: Interpretation of positive titers varies substantially depending upon the type of test performed. Consult with individual laboratory.

- Tube precipitin (TP) antibody: detects immunoglobulin (Ig) M, positive early in infection only.
- Complement fixation (CF) antibody: detects IgG, positive with past exposure or active infection; titers ≥1:64 usually indicate severe or disseminated disease.
- Latex agglutination: detects IgM, positive early, some false-positive results in dogs.
- Agar gel immunodiffusion (AGID) with TP antigen: more sensitive than TP antibody in early infection.
- AGID with CF antigen: detects IgG, more sensitive than CF antibody.
- Enzyme-linked immunosorbent assay (ELISA) for IgM: ~15% false positives, may cross react with blastomycosis.
- ELISA for IgG: similar to CF and AGID/CF, may cross react with blastomycosis.

NEXT DIAGNOSTIC STEP TO CONSIDER IF LEVELS HIGH: Confirm diagnosis with cytology or histopathology if appropriate samples can be obtained.

IMPORTANT INTERSPECIES DIFFERENCES: Both CF and TP antibodies may persist in cats for long periods of time, even with therapy.

LAB ARTIFACTS THAT MAY INTERFERE WITH READINGS OF LEVELS OF THIS SUBSTANCE

- False-negative CF antibody test in dogs may be due to interference from anticomplement factors in 15–25% of normal dog sera.
- Cross reactivity with blastomycosis possible in ELISA tests.

SAMPLE FOR COLLECTION AND ANY SPECIAL SPECIMEN HANDLING NOTES: Serum, single sample or paired 4 to 6 weeks apart. Refrigerate.

PEARLS: Should not be cultured without biosafety precautions; mycelial phase is highly infectious to humans.

AUTHOR: **ROBIN W. ALLISON**

Colloid Osmotic Pressure

BASIC INFORMATION

DEFINITION

The portion of serum osmotic pressure generated by colloids (typically proteins) and other molecules that are too large to freely cross the vasculature.

SYNONYM(S)

Oncotic pressure

TYPICAL NORMAL RANGE

Dogs: 14–27 mmHg.
Cats: 21–34 mmHg.

PHYSIOLOGY

Colloid osmotic pressure (COP) and hydrostatic pressure control fluid movement between the intravascular and interstitial spaces. In health, COP is generated largely by albumin (~80%) with the remainder being mostly fibrinogen and globulins. Therapeutic administration of colloidal solutions (plasma, polymerized bovine hemoglobin [Oxyglobin], hetastarch) can be used for compensating for pathologic decreases in COP.

CAUSES OF ABNORMALLY HIGH LEVELS: Marked hyperglobulinemia (e.g., plasma cell myeloma, feline infectious peritonitis), overadministration of therapeutic colloids (i.e., Oxyglobin)

NEXT DIAGNOSTIC STEP TO CONSIDER IF LEVELS HIGH: Evaluate serum proteins; review drug history for administration of colloids.

CAUSES OF ABNORMALLY LOW LEVELS: As for hypoalbuminemia (hemorrhage, gastrointestinal or renal protein loss, hepatic failure). Acidosis lowers COP independently of protein concentration.

NEXT DIAGNOSTIC STEP TO CONSIDER IF LEVELS LOW: Evaluate serum proteins, screen for blood/plasma loss, urine protein, liver function.

DRUG EFFECTS ON LEVELS: Increase: therapeutic administration of colloids (intended affect).

LAB ARTIFACTS THAT MAY INTERFERE WITH READINGS OF LEVELS OF THIS SUBSTANCE: Marked hemolysis may increase COP.

SAMPLE FOR COLLECTION AND ANY SPECIAL SPECIMEN HANDLING NOTES: Plasma collected in heparin (green top) or EDTA (lavender top), spun and separated from cells. A specific instrument (colloid osmometer) is required for measurement; COP is not reported routinely on small animal blood profiles.

PEARLS

- COP is superior to albumin measurement (and therefore is most useful) when evaluating and monitoring the oncotic pressure of an animal receiving treatment with nonalbumin-type colloids such as synthetic colloids (hetastarch, pentastarch).
- COP must be interpreted in context of clinical situation.
  - Decreased COP due to acute changes in protein concentration (hemorrhage) is more likely to result in clinical abnormalities than chronic hypoalbuminemia.
  - Trends in COP change may be more significant than a single value.
  - COP may be useful in differentiating causes of edema (decreased COP vs. increased hydrostatic pressure vs. vasculitis [COP normal for the latter]).
- Equations to estimate COP using serum/plasma protein concentration are not reliable in critically ill animals. Direct measurement using a colloid osmometer is needed.

AUTHOR: **JAMES H. MEINKOTH**

Complete Blood Count

BASIC INFORMATION

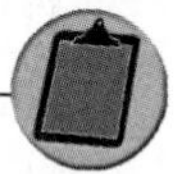

DEFINITION

A group of routine tests for measuring several parameters of erythrocytes, leukocytes, and platelets. Tests include blood cell concentrations, measurement of cell sizes and hemoglobin concentration, differential leukocyte count, and morphology of blood cells on a stained blood smear. Plasma protein concentration is also included by many labs.

SYNONYM(S)

CBC
Hemogram

TYPICAL NORMAL RANGE

See hematocrit, leukocytes, and other specific parameters.

PHYSIOLOGY

See hematocrit, leukocytes, and other specific parameters.

SAMPLE FOR COLLECTION AND ANY SPECIAL SPECIMEN HANDLING NOTES: Ethylenediamine tetraacetic acid (purple tube) blood sample and freshly prepared blood smear for lab to stain.

AUTHOR: **STEPHEN D. GAUNT**

Cell Name	Appearance	Clinical Relevance
Acanthocyte (burr cell)	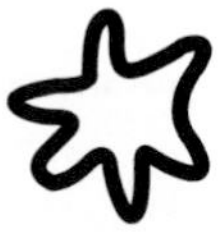	Associated with vascular, liver, or renal disease
Codocyte (target cell)	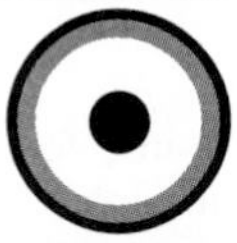	Regenerative anemia; liver or renal disease; abnormal lipid metabolism
Eccentrocyte (burr cell)	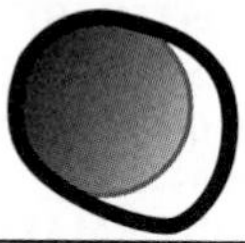	Oxidative injury
Keratocyte	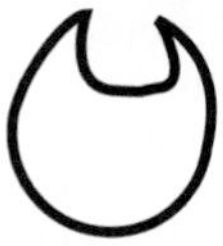	Vascular disease including hemangiosarcoma, disseminated intravascular coagulation
Heinz body	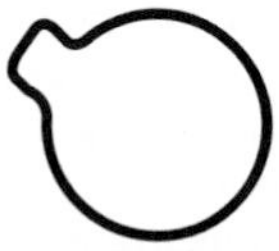	Oxidative injury
Leptocyte	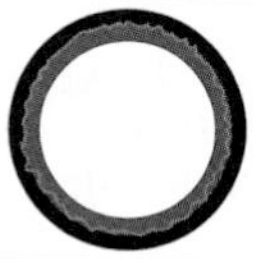	Iron deficiency
Schistocyte	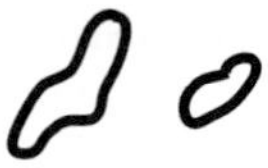	Vascular disease including hemangiosarcoma, disseminated intravascular coagulation
Spherocyte	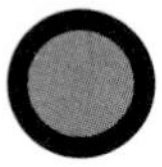	Immune-mediated hemolysis or partial phagocytosis. Unlike small red blood cells (microcytosis), spherocytes have no central pallor

FIGURE IV-1 Red cell abnormalities.

Coombs' Test

BASIC INFORMATION

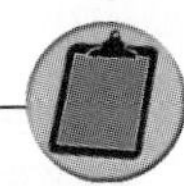

DEFINITION

Demonstrates the presence of erythrocyte-bound immunoglobulin (Ig) or complement.

SYNONYM(S)

Direct antiglobulin test (DAT)

TYPICAL NORMAL RANGE

Reported as negative or positive

PHYSIOLOGY

Coomb's reagent (polyvalent, species-specific anti-IgG, anti-IgM, and anti-complement antibodies) is added to animal's washed red blood cells. If Ig or complement is present on the animal's red blood cells, crosslinking will occur, resulting in agglutination (positive result).

CAUSES OF ABNORMALLY HIGH LEVELS: Immune-mediated hemolytic anemia (IMHA)

NEXT DIAGNOSTIC STEP TO CONSIDER IF LEVELS HIGH: Examine blood smear for spherocytes, assess for anemia, rule out infectious or neoplastic conditions that may cause positive test.

IMPORTANT INTERSPECIES DIFFERENCES: Species-specific Coomb's reagent is required.

DRUG EFFECTS ON LEVELS: Treatment with glucocorticosteroids may cause false-negative results.

LAB ARTIFACTS THAT MAY INTERFERE WITH READINGS OF LEVELS OF THIS SUBSTANCE

- Positive result not associated with IMHA may be seen: posttransfusion (>3 to 7 days after transfusion), with nonspecific coating of erythrocytes, or with in vitro complement binding during storage.
- False-negative result may be seen if: antibody is present in too low a titer to be detected by test, weakly bound antibody elutes during washing, or antibody or complement detaches from RBCs due to sample aging.

SAMPLE FOR COLLECTION AND ANY SPECIAL SPECIMEN HANDLING NOTES: Whole blood (ethylenediamine tetraacetic acid, purple-top tube), store at 8° C, test as soon as possible after collection to avoid erroneous results.

PEARLS: Test is supportive of but not specific for IMHA. Positive results can occur in patients with infectious or neoplastic disease. Coombs' test is unnecessary (already "positive") in patients with spontaneous autoagglutination.

AUTHOR: **FONZIE QUANCE-FITCH**

Cortisol

BASIC INFORMATION

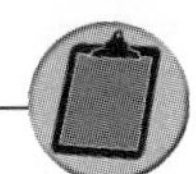

DEFINITION

Cortisol is a product of the adrenal gland cortex that initiates synthesis of proteins and receptors for hormones and cytokines involved in gluconeogenesis, protein catabolism, lipolysis, immune responses, and water balance.

TYPICAL NORMAL RANGE

Baseline cortisol concentration is 10–160 nmol/L in dogs and 10–110 nmol/L in cats

PHYSIOLOGY

Causes of hypercortisolemia include hyperadrenocorticism (Cushing's disease), either functional adrenocortical adenoma/adenocarcinoma or pituitary dependent hyperadrenocorticism; stress induced hypercortisolemia; Sertoli cell tumor; or exogenous administration of ACTH (adrenocorticotropic hormone). ACTH released from pituitary adenomas/adenocarcinomas stimulates adrenal cortical release of cortisol. Adrenocortical adenoma/adenocarcinoma in dogs and most cats overproduce cortisol. In ferrets and some cats, adrenocortical tumors produce other steroid hormones such as estrogen or progesterone and result in clinical signs of hyperadrenocorticism. Ovarian/Sertoli cell tumors in dogs can produce cortisol-like compounds. Stress of disease causes increased release of ACTH from the pituitary gland with subsequent increased release of cortisol from adrenal glands. Administration of exogenous ACTH for use in the diagnosis of Cushing's disease causes increased adrenal gland production and release of cortisol. Administration of exogenous corticosteroids (specifically dexamethasone) is used for suppressing production/release of ACTH with subsequent decrease in adrenal release of cortisol. (Dexamethasone is used for this test because it cross-reacts with cortisol minimally (<0.1%), which is considerably less than most of the other available corticosteroids.)

With the lack of appropriate ACTH secretion from pituitary gland or atrophy or destruction/necrosis of adrenal cortex, cortisol concentration can be low. Sudden withdrawal of administration of exogenous glucocorticoids, which has caused adrenal gland atrophy, can precipitate iatrogenic hypoadrenocorticism.

CAUSES OF ABNORMALLY HIGH LEVELS

- Identifying a naturally-occurring, abnormally high concentration of cortisol may be helpful because increases may be intermittent
- Increased concentrations may need to be provoked or suppressed for diagnostic purposes
- Pituitary tumor production of excess ACTH—pituitary dependent hyperadrenocorticism (Cushing's disease)
- Adrenal tumor production of excess cortisol—functional adrenal adenoma or adenocarcinoma
- Stress of disease (endogenous production of increased ACTH)
- Ovarian/Sertoli tumor production of cortisol-like compounds
- Administration of exogenous ACTH

NEXT DIAGNOSTIC STEP TO CONSIDER IF LEVELS HIGH: Low-dose dexamethasone suppression test.

CAUSES OF ABNORMALLY LOW LEVELS

- Primary hypoadrenocorticism (Addison's disease) caused by immune-mediated atrophy or destruction of the adrenal cortex can result in low concentrations of cortisol, cortisol and aldosterone, or only aldosterone.
- Secondary hypoadrenocorticism (ACTH deficiency) is caused by destruction, necrosis, or removal of the pituitary gland.
- Iatrogenic hypoadrenocorticism occurs secondary to sudden withdrawal of exogenously administered corticos-

teroids, which have caused atrophy of the adrenal glands.
- Ketoconazole inhibits steroid biosynthesis, which can cause low concentrations of cortisol.

NEXT DIAGNOSTIC STEP TO CONSIDER IF LEVELS LOW: ACTH stimulation test.

IMPORTANT INTERSPECIES DIFFERENCES
- Cat adrenal tumors may produce hormones (progesterone) other than cortisol.
- Ferret adrenal tumors usually produce hormones (estrogen and progesterone) other than cortisol.

DRUG EFFECTS ON LEVELS
- Immunoassays for cortisol measurement have significant cross-reactivity with other glucocorticoids: cortisol (100%), prednisolone (69%), prednisone (6.4%), 11-deoxycortisol (7.5%), cortisone (4.2%), corticosterone (3.5%), spironolactone (<0.2%), and dexamethasone (<0.1%).
- Ketoconazole can cause low cortisol concentration because of steroid biosynthesis inhibition.

SAMPLE FOR COLLECTION AND ANY SPECIAL SPECIMEN HANDLING NOTES
- Serum (red top tube) or EDTA plasma (lavender top tube).
- Cortisol in EDTA plasma is more stable than in serum and more stable in cooled samples compared with warm samples. Cortisol is equally distributed between red cells and plasma; therefore, rapid separation of plasma from cells (previously reported) is of no added benefit.

AUTHOR: **ELIZABETH G. WELLES**

Creatine Kinase (CK)

BASIC INFORMATION

DEFINITION

Cytosolic enzyme has the highest activity in skeletal muscle, cardiac muscle, smooth muscle, brain, and nerves. Skeletal muscle is responsible for clinically signifcant elevations in dogs and cats.

SYNONYM(S)

Creatine phosphokinase (CPK)

TYPICAL NORMAL RANGE

Dogs: 10–200 U/L.
Cat: 64–440 U/L.

PHYSIOLOGY

- CK is critical for energy production in muscle tissue for contraction.
- CK catalyzes the formation of adenosine triphosphate (ATP) by transfer of high energy phosphate from creatine phosphate to adenosine diphosphate (ADP). It also catalyses the reverse reaction when muscles are at rest.
- Serum CK activity is primarily of muscle origin. It is a sensitive indicator of skeletal or cardiac muscle damage.
- Increased serum concentration occurs 4 to 6 hours after injury. Values return to normal within 24 to 48 hours.
- Persisting elevation of CK indicates ongoing muscle damage.
- CK isoenzymes may be measured to more specifically localize muscle damage to cardiac or skeletal muscle.

CAUSES OF ABNORMALLY HIGH LEVELS: Trauma, exertion, intramuscular injections, degenerative muscle disease, infectious and noninfectious myopathies, ischemia, metabolic disease, toxic insult, nutritional, anorexia in cats

NEXT DIAGNOSTIC STEP TO CONSIDER IF LEVELS HIGH: Evaluate for muscle disease or injury or muscle catabolism. In dogs, as in people, serum cardiac troponin-I levels are probably more sensitive and specific for myocardial damage than CK myocardial isoenzyme.

IMPORTANT INTERSPECIES DIFFERENCES: CK elevation is commonly seen in anorexic cats.

LAB ARTIFACTS THAT MAY INTERFERE WITH READINGS OF LEVELS OF THIS SUBSTANCE
- Increase: hemolysis, lipemia, contamination of blood with muscle fluid during difficult venipuncture; dilution of samples (attributed to dilution of CK inhibitors in serum).
- Decrease: collection in citrate or flouride tubes.

SAMPLE FOR COLLECTION AND ANY SPECIAL SPECIMEN HANDLING NOTES: Serum (red top), heparinized plasma (green top), or ethylenediamine tetraacetic acid (lavender top) plasma. Refrigerated samples are stable for 8 to 12 hours; samples stored at –20° C are stable for 2 to 3 days.

PEARLS: Persistent, exceedingly high CK levels (e.g., >200,000 U/L) are strongly suggestive of muscular dystrophy.

AUTHOR: **RUANNA GOSSETT**

Creatinine

BASIC INFORMATION

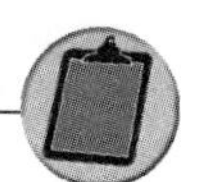

DEFINITION

Creatinine is a waste product that results from degradation of muscle creatine or creatine phosphate.

TYPICAL NORMAL RANGE

Dogs and cats: approximately 0–1.5 mg/dl (0–133 umol/L)

PHYSIOLOGY

Creatinine is continuously produced from slow daily degradation of muscle creatine and is excreted in urine. It is freely filtered by the glomerulus and is not resorbed by renal tubular epithelial cells.

CAUSES OF ABNORMALLY HIGH LEVELS
- Decreased glomerular filtration rate (GFR) causes increased creatinine concentration.
- Animals with greater muscle mass, such as greyhounds, have higher creatinine concentrations than less well muscled animals. Greyhounds often have creatinine concentration of 1.5–2.5 mg/dl.

NEXT DIAGNOSTIC STEP TO CONSIDER IF LEVELS HIGH: Check serum urea (BUN) concentration and urine specific gravity. Urea and creatinine concentrations increase in parallel in many urinary tract disorders dogs and cats.

CAUSES OF ABNORMALLY LOW LEVELS: Thin body condition/muscle loss may result in low creatinine concentration.
NEXT DIAGNOSTIC STEP TO CONSIDER IF LEVELS LOW: Evaluate for causes of muscle loss/pathological weight loss.
SAMPLE FOR COLLECTION AND ANY SPECIAL SPECIMEN HANDLING NOTES: Serum (red top tube) or heparinized plasma (green top tube).

AUTHOR: **ELIZABETH G. WELLES**

Cross-Matching

BASIC INFORMATION

DEFINITION

A laboratory procedure to detect antibodies between an animal and potential blood donor. Major cross-match involves animal serum and donor cells; the minor uses donor serum and animal cells.

TYPICAL NORMAL RANGE

Lack of agglutination

PHYSIOLOGY

Major cross-match determines if there are agglutinating and/or hemolytic antibodies in the animal against the donor antigens. Incompatible reactions occur when blood is transfused to an animal having antibodies (whether naturally occurring antibodies, as occurs in all cats, or antibodies induced by a previous mismatched transfusion, which can occur in any species) or isosensitization from transplacental immunization (the placenta is impermeable to immunoglobulins, such that a developing fetus's blood type may be different from its dam's, even if the dam has circulating antibodies against the fetal erythrocytes; ingestion of immunoglobulin-rich colostrum by the neonate in the first day postpartum allows maternal antibodies to lyse neonatal erythrocytes because of neonatal gastrointestinal permeability). Incompatible minor cross-match is not associated with severe transfusion reactions.
CAUSES OF ABNORMALLY HIGH LEVELS: Agglutination (either macroscopic or microscopic) or significant hemolysis in the cross-match tubes, but not in control indicates an incompatible donor.
IMPORTANT INTERSPECIES DIFFERENCES: Cross-matching should always be performed prior to transfusion in cats, regardless of previous transfusion history, due to the presence of naturally occurring antibodies. Transfusion of type A blood into type B cats causes rapid hemolysis (in minutes to two days, instead of the typical, 29- to 39-day transfused erythrocyte lifespan in cats) and severe anaphylaxis.
DRUG EFFECTS ON LEVELS: Glucocorticoids and other immunosuppressants may reduce the incidence of incompatibility (reduce negative cross-matches).
LAB ARTIFACTS THAT MAY INTERFERE WITH READINGS OF LEVELS OF THIS SUBSTANCE: Agglutination in the control tubes (patient serum added to patient red blood cells [RBCs] or donor serum added to donor RBCs) indicates reagent contamination or autoagglutination.
SAMPLE FOR COLLECTION AND ANY SPECIAL SPECIMEN HANDLING NOTES: Two tubes are preferred, one ethylenediamine tetraacetic acid (purple-top tube) and one tube without anticoagulant (red-top tube or serum separator tube).
PEARLS: A compatible cross-match does not indicate that the animal and the donor have the same blood type, merely that erythrocyte antibodies were not detected.

AUTHOR: **DEBORAH G. DAVIS**

LABORATORY TESTS

Cryptococcus Antigen Test

BASIC INFORMATION

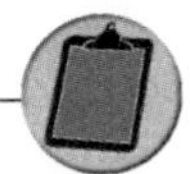

DEFINITION

Cryptococcus is a saprophytic dimorphic fungus with a worldwide distribution. *C. neoformans* is the most common species to cause disease in animals. The antigen test detects capsular antigen present in the animal's serum.

PHYSIOLOGY

- Pigeon droppings are considered the main reservoir. Inhalation is presumed mode of infection. Nasal or pulmonary infection occurs; potential dissemination to central nervous system, eyes, skin, bones, lymph nodes.
- Colonization of nasal passages can occur without producing overt clinical signs.

CAUSES OF ABNORMALLY HIGH LEVELS: Methods include latex agglutination and enzyme-linked immunosorbent assay. Positive titer confirms active infection. Ability to detect antigen is high (sensitivity ~97%) but false-negative results do occur, possibly due to localized disease or a prozone effect. False-positive results are very uncommon (specificity approaches 100%). Higher titers are seen with disseminated disease. Monitoring titers is useful to evaluate therapeutic success; declining titers are considered a good prognostic sign.
NEXT DIAGNOSTIC STEP TO CONSIDER IF LEVELS HIGH: Cytology, histopathology, and culture may be useful to confirm but generally are unnecessary when a positive antigen test result occurs in a patient with compatible clinical signs.
SAMPLE FOR COLLECTION AND ANY SPECIAL SPECIMEN HANDLING NOTES

- Serum (most common), urine, or cerebrospinal fluid (CSF); check with individual laboratory.
- CSF is preferred if central nervous system signs are present, may be more sensitive.

PEARLS: Titers from different laboratories using different methods can vary considerably; use the same method if performing repeated titers to monitor treatment.

AUTHOR: **ROBIN W. ALLISON**

Crystals in Urine Sediment

BASIC INFORMATION

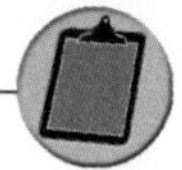

DEFINITION

Precipitation of salts of metabolic products forming crystals observed in urine sediment.

SYNONYM(S)

Crystalluria

TYPICAL NORMAL RANGE

- Reported as negative or number of crystals per high power field with specific identification.
- Normal dogs and cats may have low numbers of crystals.

PHYSIOLOGY

Metabolic products that are normal, abnormal, or related to medication may precipitate, forming crystals that may be seen in urine sediment. Crystal formation depends on urine pH, temperature, and compound concentration.

CAUSES OF ABNORMALLY HIGH LEVELS: Abnormal or increased metabolic products, changes in urine pH enhancing formation of specific crystals.

NEXT DIAGNOSTIC STEP TO CONSIDER IF LEVELS HIGH

- Assess diet, medication history, or evaluate for metabolic abnormalities suggested by specific crystals.
- Urine culture and sensitivity in all dogs with struvite crystalluria because infection with urease-producing bacteria is the most common cause.

IMPORTANT INTERSPECIES DIFFERENCES: Dalmatian dogs normally have ammonium urate crystals; in other breeds, this may indicate hepatic dysfunction.

DRUG EFFECTS ON LEVELS: Sulfonamides, radiopaque injectable contrast are associated with crystalluria.

LAB ARTIFACTS THAT MAY INTERFERE WITH READINGS OF LEVELS OF THIS SUBSTANCE: Crystals may dissolve as urine pH changes following voiding. Refrigeration of specimens may result in *in vitro* formation of both struvite (ammonium magnesium phosphate, triple phosphate) and oxalate crystals which remain when specimens are returned to room temperature. Retesting of fresh specimens is suggested if numbers are high and the possibility of clinical significance exists.

SAMPLE FOR COLLECTION AND ANY SPECIAL SPECIMEN HANDLING NOTES: Fresh specimen in sterile container for urinalysis

PEARLS: Crystalluria may be indicative of urolithiasis. Absence of crystals does not rule out disease. If clinically significant (calcium oxalate) crystalluria is suspected, a fresh specimen should be analyzed.

AUTHOR: **LOIS ROTH-JOHNSON**

Cell Name	Appearance	Clinical Relevance
Ammonium magnesium phosphate (triple phosphate, struvite)	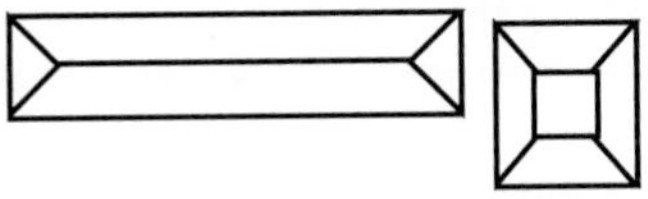	Common in dogs (infection) and cats (nutrition), especially with alkaline urine or as artifact
Ammonium biurate	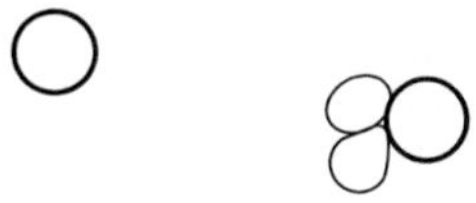	Infrequent in healthy patients except Dalmatians and English bulldogs; if numerous, suggests liver dysfunction or shunt in dogs and cats
Bilirubin		Associated with bilirubinuria
Calcium oxalate monohydrate	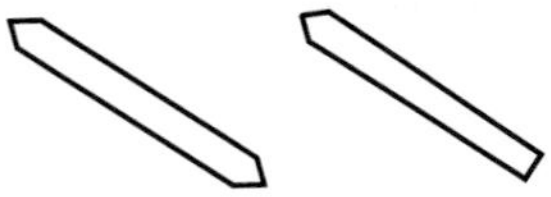	Suggests ethylene glycol toxicity
Calcium oxalate dihydrate	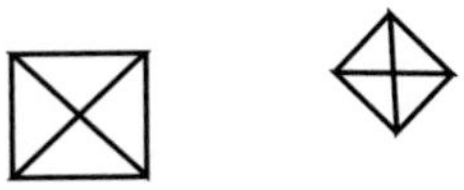	Seen in healthy patients; suggests ethylene glycol toxicity
Calcium phosphate	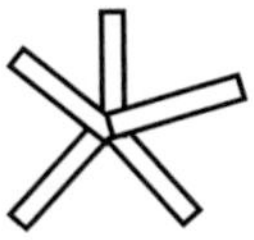	Seen in healthy dogs
Cyst(e)ine		Rare; suggests liver disease or primary cyst(e)inuria (e.g., breed-related)
Cholesterol	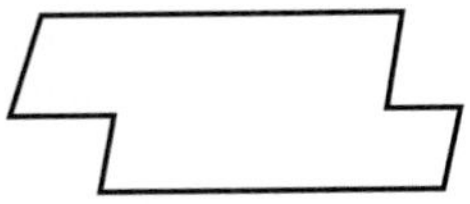	Uncommon in healthy dogs; may occur with hypercholesterolemia or renal disease
Drug crystals	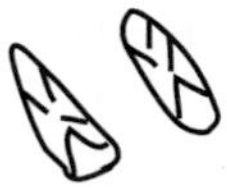	Sulfa, contrast media; renal elimination of material
Hippuric acid	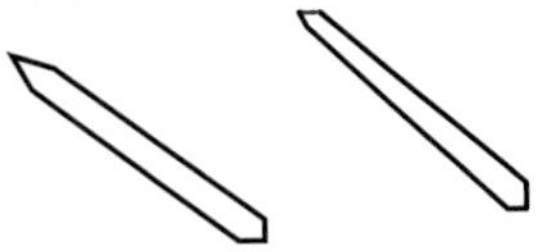	Rare; should be distinguished from calcium oxalate monohydrate (history, physical exam)

FIGURE IV-2 Urine crystals.

Culture and Sensitivity, Bacterial

BASIC INFORMATION

DEFINITION

Submission of infected tissue for enhanced growth and isolation of pathogens and their evaluation of the antibiotics that would kill or inactivate them.

TYPICAL NORMAL RANGE

- Bacterial isolates are reported by genus and species.
- Antibiotic sensitivity, which is determined either by disk diffusion method (Kirby-Bauer) or determination of minimum inhibitory concentration (MIC) method, is reported as sensitive, intermediate (or indeterminant), or resistant.

PHYSIOLOGY

Small quantities of suspect tissues are aseptically plated on media that enhance the growth of bacteria. Individual colonies are isolated and identified by morphologic features (texture, color) and specific chemical reactions. Isolated colonies are exposed to known concentrations of antibiotics and evaluated for growth inhibition.

CAUSES OF ABNORMALLY HIGH LEVELS: Bacterial infection or contamination

NEXT DIAGNOSTIC STEP TO CONSIDER IF LEVELS HIGH: Select an appropriate antibiotic based on sensitivity, appropriate method of delivery (e.g., injection, oral, topical), and site of infection.

IMPORTANT INTERSPECIES DIFFERENCES

- Some organisms are normal flora in some species but pathogens in others.
- Some antibiotics are appropriate for one species of patient but toxic in another.

DRUG EFFECTS ON LEVELS: Previous or concurrent antibiotic therapy, even if not the drug of choice, may inhibit culture growth.

LAB ARTIFACTS THAT MAY INTERFERE WITH READINGS OF LEVELS OF THIS SUBSTANCE

- Contamination (during collection by use of nonsterile containers, prolonged storage at room temperature, or delays in shipment) may result in overgrowth.
- Contaminant organisms may inhibit growth of more fastidious organisms.

SAMPLE FOR COLLECTION (TYPE OF SPECIMEN, COLOR TUBE) AND ANY SPECIAL SPECIMEN HANDLING NOTES: Fresh tissue in sterile container; culture swab is acceptable for both aerobic and anerobic culture.

PEARLS: Monitor potential antibiotic toxicity by appropriate clinical monitoring and laboratory tests.

AUTHOR: **LOIS ROTH-JOHNSON**

Cyclosporine Serum Levels

BASIC INFORMATION

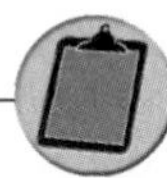

DEFINITION

Cyclosporine is an immunosuppressant drug that has a selective inhibitory effect on T lymphocytes, suppressing the early cellular response to antigenic and regulatory stimuli.

SYNONYM(S)

Cyclosporine A (CsA)

TYPICAL NORMAL RANGE

400-600 ng/dl

PHYSIOLOGY

Peak plasma levels usually occur 1.3 to 4 hours after oral administration. Ingestion of a fatty meal significantly delays absorption of cyclosporine in the gelatin capsule formulation (Sandimmune) but not in the microemulsion formulation (Neoral, Atopica). In whole blood, 50-60% of cyclosporine accumulates within erythrocytes, 10-20% accumulates within leukocytes, and the remainder of drug in circulation is associated with plasma lipoproteins. Half-life is approximately 6 hours. Extensive metabolism in the liver to >30 metabolites. Elimination primarily via bile. In the presence of hepatic dysfunction, dosage adjustments may be necessary. Major toxic effect is renal but other potential toxicities include hypertension, hepatotoxicity, neurotoxicity, gingival hyperplasia, gastrointestinal toxicity.

CAUSES OF ABNORMALLY HIGH LEVELS: Overdosage, hepatic impairment, interaction with drugs (see below).

CAUSES OF ABNORMALLY LOW LEVELS: Interaction with drugs (see below).

DRUG EFFECTS ON LEVELS: Interacts with a variety of commonly used drugs. Clearance is accelerated with coadministration of phenobarbital, phenytoin, trimethoprime-sulfamethoxazole and rifampin (induction of hepatic P-450). Clearance is decreased when coadministered with amphotericin B, erythromycin, or ketoconazole.

SAMPLE FOR COLLECTION AND ANY SPECIAL SPECIMEN HANDLING NOTES: A blood cyclosporine level is typically checked 1 to 2 days after initiating therapy and then at 2- to 4-week intervals. Trough levels (24 hour): either whole blood or plasma is satisfactory but due to binding to red/white blood cells values will vary depending upon sample submitted; check with laboratory prior to submission.

PEARLS: The decrease in cyclosporine excretion caused by ketoconazole can be used advantageously. Cyclosporine is a costly medication, whereas ketoconazole is inexpensive. Therefore, ketoconazole 5 mg/kg by mouth every 24 hours may be coadministered with cyclosporine microemulsion (e.g., Neoral) 5 mg/kg by mouth every 24 hours, which halves the required cyclosporine dose (every 12 hours to every 24 hours) while maintaining the same serum cyclosporine concentration.

AUTHOR: **SHERRY J. MORGAN**

D-Dimer

BASIC INFORMATION

DEFINITION

Protein fragments that are formed from the degradation of cross-linked fibrin. They are specific for fibrin degradation products (fibrinolysis). This is a specific method of detecting active coagulation and fibrinolysis.

TYPICAL NORMAL RANGE

0.02–0.28 μg/ml

PHYSIOLOGY

D-dimers form when plasmin digests cross-linked fibrin; the test is more specific than fibrin[ogen] degradation products (FDPs) because only the fibrin-derived products are detected.

CAUSES OF ABNORMALLY HIGH LEVELS: Increased fibrinolysis or decreased clearance of fibrin degradation products by the liver or mononuclear phagocytic system; specific causes include local and disseminated intravascular coagulation, internal hemorrhage, liver disease, chronic renal failure.

NEXT DIAGNOSTIC STEP TO CONSIDER IF LEVELS HIGH: Evaluation of the coagulation system: platelet count, antithrombin III, activated coagulation time (ACT) or activated partial thromboplastin time (PTT), prothrombin time (PT), thrombin time (TT), fibrinogen. If clinical suspicion of pulmonary thromboembolism exists, further evaluation (ultrasound, angiography; thoracic radiography and arterial blood gas measurement) may be indicated.

SAMPLE FOR COLLECTION AND ANY SPECIAL SPECIMEN HANDLING NOTES: Citrate (blue top) tubes are used; it is important that traumatic venipuncture be avoided to prevent activation of platelets and the coagulation systems; blood and anticoagulant should be mixed thoroughly immediately after collection.

PEARLS: Assays for D-dimers are still being evaluated for their usefulness in veterinary medicine. Semiquantitative (latex agglutination) and quantitative (immunoturbimetric) methods have been evaluated in dogs.

AUTHOR: **DEBORAH G. DAVIS**

Digoxin, Serum Level

BASIC INFORMATION

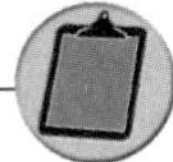

DEFINITION

Digoxin is a drug in the cardiac glycoside class that has complex cardiovascular actions. It is used in the management of supraventricular arrhythmias (e.g., atrial fibrillation) and certain cases of congestive heart failure.

SYNONYM(S)

Digitalis

TYPICAL RANGE

In humans, serum level >2 ng/ml is suggestive of toxicity; therapeutic levels range from 0.5–1.5 ng/dl or 0.8–2.0 ng/ml (see below). In veterinary medicine, the same values are used, but no clinical trial has ever proven that "therapeutic levels" are beneficial over empiric dosing.

PHYSIOLOGY

Digoxin is rapidly absorbed as an oral elixir (serum levels detectable in 45 minutes; bioavailability 100%) and slightly less so in the tablet form (hours; bioavailability 80%). Intravenous administration is no loner recommended. Regardless of administration route, excretion is renal. The linear dose-response curve of digoxin suggests that "subtherapeutic" serum levels, which are associated with fewer side effects, may provide beneficial effects, and revised therapeutic serum levels of 0.5–1.5 ng/ml have been suggested in human cardiology. The primary mechanism of action of the cardioglycosides is interference with Na/K-ATP-ase with resultant increase in intracellular calcium. Adverse effects including severe lethargy and anorexia, and arrythmias such as atrioventricular block due to progressive interference with electrical conduction and increase in vagal tone, may occur.

CAUSES OF ABNORMALLY HIGH LEVELS: Large body size, obesity (digoxin is not distributed in fat), and renal failure warrant lowering digoxin dose; otherwise, high serum levels and toxicity may occur. Dosing based on surface area has been recommended. The half-life of cardiac glycosides is highly variable among patients.

NEXT DIAGNOSTIC STEP TO CONSIDER IF LEVELS HIGH: Adjust dose, depending on suspected cause.

CAUSES OF ABNORMALLY LOW LEVELS: Hypokalemia potentiates digitalis-induced arrhythmias. If toxicity is evident but the serum concentration is not excessive, serum potassium should be evaluated.

NEXT DIAGNOSTIC STEP TO CONSIDER IF LEVELS LOW: Measure serum potassium.

IMPORTANT INTERSPECIES DIFFERENCES: Enterohepatic recycling of cardiac glycosides is very important in humans, less so in dogs.

DRUG EFFECTS ON LEVEL: Drugs inducing hepatic metabolism (phenytoin, rifampin) accelerate digoxin metabolism resulting in higher than expected serum levels. Quinidine elevates serum concentrations by decreasing clearance and volume of distribution. Other drugs that may increase serum digoxin concentrations include verapamil, diltiazem, amiodarone, flecainide, and spironolactone.

SAMPLE FOR COLLECTION AND ANY SPECIAL SPECIMEN HANDLING NOTES: Serum (red top); store at 2–8°C.

PEARLS: Serum digoxin levels may be used to confirm ingestion of plants (milkweed, foxglove, oleander, dogbane) that contain cardiac glycosides.

AUTHOR: **SHERRY J. MORGAN**

Eccentrocyte

BASIC INFORMATION

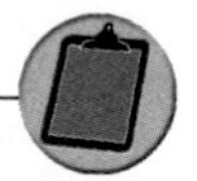

DEFINITION

Erythrocyte damaged by oxidants. Characterized by focal area of fused membranes and eccentric displacement of hemoglobinized cytosol. The fused membranes appear as a clear area at periphery of erythrocyte and outlined by membrane, with shifting of the cytoplasm and loss of any central pallor.

SYNONYM(S)

Bite cell
Hemighost

TYPICAL NORMAL RANGE

Absent in health

PHYSIOLOGY

During oxidative damage, hemichromes (oxidized forms of hemoglobin) bind to the band 3 protein of the membrane cytoskeleton. This creates cross-linking and fusion of the erythrocyte cytoskeleton, and alters the membrane with externalization of antigenic proteins and attachment of autoantibodies. Hemichromes can also precipitate to form Heinz bodies.

CAUSES OF ABNORMALLY HIGH LEVELS

- Oxidative damage to erythrocyte from toxins such as acetaminophen, onions, and benzocaine in dogs and cats, zinc and garlic in dogs. Heinz bodies may also be seen in conjunction with eccentrocytes.
- Decreased antioxidant activity of erythrocytes: congenital deficiency of glucose-6-phosphate dehydrogenase with decreased production of reduced nicotinamide adenine dinucleotide phosphate (NADPH) in erythrocytes.

NEXT DIAGNOSTIC STEP TO CONSIDER IF LEVELS HIGH: Evaluate history for source of oxidative damage to erythrocytes.

SAMPLE FOR COLLECTION AND ANY SPECIAL SPECIMEN HANDLING NOTES: Ethylenediamine tetraacetic acid blood and freshly prepared blood smear for lab to stain.

AUTHOR: **STEPHEN D. GAUNT**

Ehrlichia Serology

BASIC INFORMATION

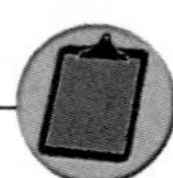

DEFINITION

Detection of serum antibodies directed against *Ehrlichia* spp. (most commonly *E. canis*).

SYNONYM(S)

Ehrlichia titer

PHYSIOLOGY

Ehrlichia spp. are rickettsial agents that infect a wide range of host species. Numerous species of *Ehrlichia* have been shown to infect dogs. *E. canis* produces an acute disease from which animals recover, but typically remain subclinical and may later present with more severe disease.

CAUSES OF ABNORMALLY HIGH LEVELS

- The presence of antibodies directed against *E. canis* indicates exposure to *E. canis* or related organisms. Some antigens of *E. canis*, *E. ewingii*, and *E. chaffeensis* are cross reactive, whereas others are not.
- A positive titer indicates only exposure and does not prove that the current clinical signs are due to active infection.
- *E. canis* can cause a persistent subclinical infection, so a dog with a positive titer is likely to still be infected unless treated with appropriate antimicrobial therapy.

NEXT DIAGNOSTIC STEP TO CONSIDER IF LEVELS HIGH: Treatment with appropriate antimicrobial therapy. Evaluate whether the patient's current signs are consistent with ehrlichiosis. A positive test for ehrlichial DNA via the polymerase chain reaction (PCR) supports active infection and can determine the specific species of *Ehrlichia* involved.

CAUSES OF ABNORMALLY LOW LEVELS: Infection with different *Ehrlichia* spp.

NEXT DIAGNOSTIC STEP TO CONSIDER IF LEVELS LOW: If a clinical suspicion for ehrlichiosis persists despite a negative titer to *E. canis*, then titers to other ehrlichial species (e.g., *E. equi*) should be performed because cross-reactivity does not occur reliably.

IMPORTANT INTERSPECIES DIFFERENCES: Serology often uses species specific reagents. *Ehrlichia* serology is most often performed on dogs. Check with lab as to appropriateness if testing cats.

SAMPLE FOR COLLECTION AND ANY SPECIAL SPECIMEN HANDLING NOTES: Serum (red top)

PEARLS

- Some dogs maintain persistent titers for years despite appropriate therapy and apparent resolution of disease.
- An in-clinic, enzyme-linked immunosorbent assay (ELISA)-based serology test (SNAP3Dx, IDEXX Labs) for detecting *E. canis* antibody appears to have high specificity when compared with immunofluorescent assay, but may not detect low titers.
- Dogs infected with one species of ehrlichial organism may have negative titers if early in infection or if infected with other species of ehrlichia.
- Ehrlichia serology is much more sensitive (i.e., better screening test) that evaluating a blood smear for the presence of ehrlichial inclusions in leukocytes.

AUTHOR: **JAMES H. MEINKOTH**

Eosinophils

BASIC INFORMATION

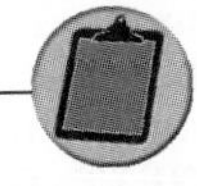

DEFINITION

Granulocytic leukocyte with eosinophilic granules in cytoplasm and a segmented nucleus.

TYPICAL NORMAL RANGE

- Dogs: 0.1–1.3 × 10^3 eosinophils/μL.
- Cats: 0–1.5 × 10^3 eosinophils/μL.

PHYSIOLOGY

Eosinophilic precursors develop in the marrow under influence of interleukin-5. Mature eosinophils are released into blood to circulate for a few hours and then enter tissue. Eosinophils contain major basic protein, which is important in attacking helminthic parasites. Eosinophils can both promote and inhibit hypersensitivity reactions. Eosinophilic inflammation occurs more often in cutaneous, respiratory, and intestinal tissues.

CAUSES OF ABNORMALLY HIGH LEVELS: Parasitism (e.g., dirofilariasis, larval migration in tissues); allergic reactions (e.g., flea bite hypersensitivity); idiopathic eosinophilic inflammation (e.g., hypereosinophilic syndrome in cats); hypoadrenocorticism ("relaxed" leukogram, which is the unexpected absence of stress leukogram and eosinopenia in ill patient); mast cell neoplasm; eosinophilic leukemia (rare).

NEXT DIAGNOSTIC STEP TO CONSIDER IF LEVELS HIGH: Use clinical history/signs to assess for causes listed.

CAUSES OF ABNORMALLY LOW LEVELS: Stress leukogram, from enodogenous or exogenous glucocorticoids; acute inflammation.

NEXT DIAGNOSTIC STEP TO CONSIDER IF LEVELS LOW: Low values are rarely of clinical signficance.

IMPORTANT INTERSPECIES DIFFERENCES

- In canine eosinophils, the granules are round and can vary considerably in size and number. In some dogs (especially greyhounds), clear vacuoles appear instead of eosinophilic granules.
- Feline eosinophils have distinctive rod-shaped granules.

DRUG EFFECTS ON LEVELS: Glucocorticoids cause increased sequestration of eosinophils in tissues, with development of eosinopenia.

SAMPLE FOR COLLECTION AND ANY SPECIAL SPECIMEN HANDLING NOTES: Ethylenediamine tetraacetic acid blood and freshly prepared blood smear for lab to stain.

AUTHOR: **STEPHEN D. GAUNT**

Erythropoietin

BASIC INFORMATION

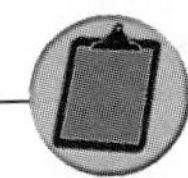

DEFINITION

Renal hormone that stimulates erythropoiesis in the presence of tissue hypoxia.

SYNONYM(S)

EPO

TYPICAL NORMAL RANGE

Radioimmunoassay method: dogs, 8.4–28 mU/ml; cats, 10–30 mU/ml.

PHYSIOLOGY

Erythropoietin (EPO) is produced primarily by the kidney (sole source in dogs) with small amounts produced by the liver. Tissue hypoxia stimulates EPO production. EPO induces differentiation of erythroid progenitor cells to rubriblasts; stimulates mitosis of erythroid cells; reduces maturation time; and accelerates release of reticulocytes from the bone marrow into circulation.

CAUSES OF ABNORMALLY HIGH LEVELS: Hypoxemia inducing cardiovascular or pulmonary disease; hypoxemia due to high altitude; inappropriate EPO production due to EPO-producing neoplasia, renal cyst, or hydronephrosis; hyperthyroidism; EPO therapy. Regardless of cause, secondary polycythemia is the result.

NEXT DIAGNOSTIC STEP TO CONSIDER IF LEVELS HIGH

- Confirm polycythemia. If polycythemia is absent, EPO result may be spurious, or may represent early disease. Serial monitoring of hematocrit is warranted in these cases.
- Identify cause of any hypoxemia inducing condition: thoracic radiographs, arterial blood gas measurement, possibly echocardiography.
- Evaluate for neoplasia, renal disease, and endocrinopathy.

CAUSES OF ABNORMALLY LOW LEVELS: Decreased EPO in the presence of polycythemia and normal PO_2 suggests polycythemia vera; chronic renal failure.

NEXT DIAGNOSTIC STEP TO CONSIDER IF LEVELS LOW: Assess renal function.

LAB ARTIFACTS THAT MAY INTERFERE WITH READINGS OF LEVELS OF THIS SUBSTANCE: Increased: hemolyzed or lipemic specimens.

SAMPLE FOR COLLECTION (TYPE OF SPECIMEN, COLOR TUBE) AND ANY SPECIAL SPECIMEN HANDLING NOTES: Serum (red top) or heparinized plasma (green top); separate serum or plasma from erythrocytes, freeze, and transport frozen.

PEARLS: Measurement of serum EPO levels is an appropriate test in patients with repeatable absolute polycythemia. It generally precedes bone marrow evaluation in these cases.

AUTHOR: **FIDELIA R. FERNANDEZ**

Estradiol/Estrogen

BASIC INFORMATION

DEFINITION

Hormone synthesized and secreted by developing ovarian follicles.

TYPICAL NORMAL RANGE

Baseline estradiol/estrogen in canine anestrus is 5-15 pg/ml

PHYSIOLOGY

- Dogs: Proestrus is under the influence of progressively increasing circulating concentrations of estradiol, which is produced by the developing ovarian follicles. A rising estradiol level correlates with marked development changes in the vaginal mucosa, vulva, and uterus. Serum estradiol concentrations start to increase just before proestrus becomes clinically detectable. Estradiol concentrations above 25 pg/ml are typical of early proestrus and concentrations greater than 60–70 pg/dl are typical of late proestrus. Peak estradiol serum concentrations are reached 24 to 48 hours prior to the end of proestrus before standing heat (estrus).
- Cats: Anestrus and interestrous periods typically have estradiol serum concentrations less than 12–15 pg/ml. Estradiol concentrations greater than 20 pg/ml typically accompany follicular activity (follicular phase of the feline cycle averages 7.0 to 7.7 days, depending on whether coitus is experienced and whether ovulation is induced. Day 1 of the follicular phase of estrus typically is associated with an estradiol concentration ≈25 pg/ml; at day 3 it is ≈45 pg/ml, at day 5 it is ≈50 pg/ml or above, at day 5 it is ≈20–25 pg/ml, and by day 8 it has returned to ≈10 pg/ml.

CAUSES OF ABNORMALLY HIGH LEVELS: In intact female dogs, high levels indicate mid- to late proestrus. In intact female cats, high levels indicate the mid follicular phase of the cycle. In ovariectomized female cats, high levels (above baseline) suggest incomplete excision of ovarian tissue.

NEXT DIAGNOSTIC STEP TO CONSIDER IF LEVELS HIGH: In ovariectomized cats: administer HCG to cause luteolysis of follicles, check for increasing progesterone. If progesterone increases above 2.5 ng/ml 5-7 days later, exploratory surgery is recommended (persistent ovarian tissue).

This test is not used in dogs.

CAUSES OF ABNORMALLY LOW LEVELS

- Ovariectomy
- Basal (low) concentrations of estradiol occur in anestrus and diestrus

IMPORTANT INTERSPECIES DIFFERENCES: Cats are induced ovulators and are seasonally polyestrous.

SAMPLE FOR COLLECTION AND ANY SPECIAL SPECIMEN HANDLING NOTES: Serum (red top tube).

AUTHOR: **ELIZABETH G. WELLES**

Ethylene Glycol Bench Test

BASIC INFORMATION

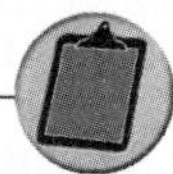

DEFINITION

Test kit for diagnosing ethylene glycol (antifreeze) poisoning.

SYNONYM(S)

EGT kit (manufactured by PRN Pharmacal)

TYPICAL NORMAL RANGE

Qualitative test reported as positive or negative.

PHYSIOLOGY

Poisoning occurs from consumption of antifreeze or "snow globe" liquid. Following ingestion, ethylene glycol is metabolized to toxic metabolites via the action of alcohol dehydrogenase. The glycolic acid metabolite causes severe, high anion gap metabolic acidosis. The oxalic acid metabolite combines with serum calcium, forming calcium oxalate crystals that deposit in renal tubules. Severe renal tubular damage can lead to anuric or oliguric renal failure. The test kit detects only ethylene glycol, not the metabolites.

CAUSES OF ABNORMALLY HIGH LEVELS: Positive result indicates recent consumption (usually within 12 hours) of ethylene glycol.

NEXT DIAGNOSTIC STEP TO CONSIDER IF LEVELS HIGH: Determination of anion and osmolal gap (increased in ethylene glycol poisoning). Electrolyte panel and blood gas determination to evaluate for metabolic acidosis and electrolyte abnormalities (hypochloridemia/hyperkalemia). Renal profile and urinalysis to evaluate for renal failure and presence of calcium oxalate monohydrate crystals.

CAUSES OF ABNORMALLY LOW LEVELS: Ethylene glycol rapidly metabolized and excreted. Test results are negative if >12 to 18 hours since consumption.

NEXT DIAGNOSTIC STEP TO CONSIDER IF LEVELS LOW: If historic evidence suggests toxicity is suspected, evaluate renal function, electrolyte status. Determine serum levels of metabolite (glycolic acid).

IMPORTANT INTERSPECIES DIFFERENCES: The bench test is approved for use in dogs only.

DRUG EFFECTS ON LEVELS: Positive: propylene glycol or glycerol.

SAMPLE FOR COLLECTION AND ANY SPECIAL SPECIMEN HANDLING NOTES: One milliliter of anticoagulated whole blood (lavender-top tube). Even though sample is stable for 48 hours at 0–4° C, sample should be brought to laboratory and run as a stat test because of clinical urgency.

PEARLS

- If antifreeze toxicity is suspected but it has been >48 hours since ingestion, blood urea nitrogen and creatinine are increased and patients are acidotic with an increased anion gap.
- Local human hospitals may also be able to perform the test. Because the test evaluates only the concentration of ethylene glycol, a human assay can be used for animals.

AUTHOR: **SHERRY J. MORGAN**

Fecal Culture

BASIC INFORMATION

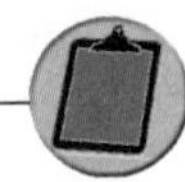

DEFINITION

Analysis of feces for enteric bacterial pathogens.

TYPICAL NORMAL RANGE

Reported as negative or degree (slight, moderate, heavy) of growth of specific pathogens.

PHYSIOLOGY

Chronic diarrhea, especially in patients with signs of systemic disease (intermittent or persistent fever, leukocytosis or leukopenia) or melena, may be due to bacterial infection. Laboratory conditions enhance growth of pathogens, allowing isolation of bacterial colonies and their identification by morphologic features and chemical tests.

CAUSES OF ABNORMALLY HIGH LEVELS: Enteric infection. Common enteric pathogens include *Salmonella* spp., *Clostridium* spp., *Shigella* spp., *Yersinia* spp., *Escherichia coli* and *Campylobacter* spp.

NEXT DIAGNOSTIC STEP TO CONSIDER IF LEVELS HIGH: Request specific antibiotic sensitivity.

IMPORTANT INTERSPECIES DIFFERENCES: Bacterial enteritis is an uncommon but serious disease in dogs. Bacterial enteritis is very rare in cats.

DRUG EFFECTS ON LEVELS: Low level antibiotic therapy may inhibit culture growth.

LAB ARTIFACTS THAT MAY INTERFERE WITH READINGS OF LEVELS OF THIS SUBSTANCE: False negative results: delay in setting up culture; contamination or overgrowth of normal flora; failure to notify lab of suspected fastidious pathogens requiring special handling; exposure of anaerobes to oxygen.

SAMPLE FOR COLLECTION AND ANY SPECIAL SPECIMEN HANDLING NOTES: Fresh feces in sterile container. If shigellosis, campylobacterisosis, or clostridium infection is suspected, special transport media may be needed, depending on transport time to reference laboratory. Contact laboratory to obtain appropriate transport media.

PEARLS

- Most enteric pathogens cause disease in humans; specimen handling precautions are necessary to reduce risk of zoonosis.
- Much overlap exists between bacterial flora of dogs with enteritis and normal dogs. Identification of certain fecal bacteria does not necessarily indicate a cause and effect relationship.

AUTHOR: **LOIS ROTH-JOHNSON**

Fecal Flotation

BASIC INFORMATION

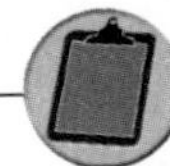

DEFINITION

Screening test for detection of ova and larvae in feces.

TYPICAL NORMAL RANGE

Reported as negative or positive with species identification

PHYSIOLOGY

Flotation of parasitic ova and cysts is promoted in solutions with a greater osmolarity than water. Fecal specimens are mixed with saturated sugar or zinc sulfate solution in a small cylinder topped with a cover slip. After allowing time for ova or cysts to rise to the surface, the coverslip is examined microscopically.

CAUSES OF ABNORMALLY HIGH LEVELS: Gastrointestinal, or less commonly respiratory, parasitic infection. Ova of ascarids, hookworms, and flukes. Coccidia, tapeworm segments, and protozoa may be identified.

NEXT DIAGNOSTIC STEP TO CONSIDER IF LEVELS HIGH: Positive test is definitive.

CAUSES OF ABNORMALLY LOW LEVELS: Intermittent shedding of ova.

NEXT DIAGNOSTIC STEP TO CONSIDER IF LEVELS LOW: Serial fecal analyses; empiric anthelmintic treatment; further diagnostic testing of gastrointestinal system.

DRUG EFFECTS ON LEVELS: Anthelmintic treatment may decrease parasite burden.

LAB ARTIFACTS THAT MAY INTERFERE WITH READINGS OF LEVELS OF THIS SUBSTANCE: Freezing or delayed specimen processing distorts or destroys ova, decreasing detection.

SAMPLE FOR COLLECTION AND ANY SPECIAL SPECIMEN HANDLING NOTES: Fresh feces (≤24 hours, room temperature or refrigerated) in dry container. If a delay in processing is anticipated, a solution of feces (one part) and sodium acetate-acetic acid formalin (three parts) may be submitted. To prepare solution, combine 1.5 g sodium acetate, 2 ml glacial acetic acid, 4 ml 40% formaldehyde, and 92.5 ml water. Indicate that specimen has been diluted.

PEARLS

- Diarrhea may decrease ova concentration.
- Ova shedding is intermittent. Therefore, a single negative test does not rule out infection. Serial testing (at least three) should be done if parasitic disease is suspected.

AUTHOR: **LOIS ROTH-JOHNSON**

Feline Coronavirus Serology

BASIC INFORMATION

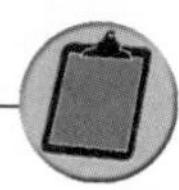

DEFINITION

Feline coronavirus infection refers to two distinct entities: feline infectious *peritonitis* (FIP) and feline enteric coronaviral (FECV) enteritis. FIP is a systemic, viral disease of high mortality characterized by insidious onset, *fever*, disseminated pyogranulomatous inflammation, and in some cases, proteinaceous exudative effusions in body cavities ("wet form"). FECV causes mild transient diarrhea and/or vomiting and, less commonly, chronic or severe diarrhea.

SYNONYM(S)

Feline enteric coronavirus
Feline infectious peritonitis (FIP)

TYPICAL NORMAL RANGE

Consult with laboratory conducting the test.

PHYSIOLOGY

Following ingestion, FIP virus replicates in intestinal epithelial cells and probably tonsils and oropharynx. The virus infects macrophages with subsequent extension to multiple tissues. Antiviral antibodies are produced. Immune complexes form and are deposited in blood vessels of serosal surfaces, uvea, kidney, liver, and other tissues. A pyogranulomatous response develops. Proteinaceous abdominal or thoracic effusion results from increased vascular permeability. FIP-type coronavirus is thought to represent a spontaneous mutation of feline enteric coronavirus that occurs *in vivo* in certain individual cats.

CAUSES OF ABNORMALLY HIGH LEVELS: Positive FECV titer indicates nonspecific exposure to FIP coronavirus, feline enteric coronavirus, other coronaviruses, or FIP vaccine. Serology is relatively nonspecific.

NEXT DIAGNOSTIC STEP TO CONSIDER IF LEVELS HIGH: Correlate with clinical signs/laboratory data. Consider cytologic evaluation, A:G ratio, polymerase chain reaction (PCR), or immunofluorescent antibody on effusion fluid, all of which are supportive but not definitive (none of these tests differentiates between FIP-coronavirus and enteric coronavirus). Histopathology of biopsy or necropsy tissue is required for definitive diagnosis.

CAUSES OF ABNORMALLY LOW LEVELS: False-negative serology tests result from peracute infection, low antibody level, lack of antibody production, or antibody bound within immune complexes.

NEXT DIAGNOSTIC STEP TO CONSIDER IF LEVELS LOW: If FIP is still suspected, consider same diagnostic steps as if test is positive.

SAMPLE FOR COLLECTION AND ANY SPECIAL SPECIMEN HANDLING NOTES: One ml serum (red-top tube) for serology. One ml effusion fluid collected into purple-top tube for PCR. Samples for serology can be stored for up to 4 days at refrigerator temperature or for longer periods at −20° C without loss of antibody.

PEARLS: A negative titer alone does not rule out FIP, nor does a positive titer alone indicate FIP.

AUTHOR: **PATTY J. EWING**

Feline Immunodeficiency Virus Tests

BASIC INFORMATION

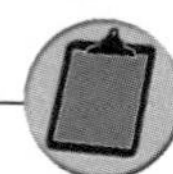

DEFINITION

Feline immunodeficiency virus (FIV) is a retrovirus (lentivirus) that attacks the immune system of cats and results in progressive immunosuppressive disease.

SYNONYM(S)

Enzyme-linked immunosorbent assay (ELISA)
Immunofluorescent antibody (IFA)

TYPICAL NORMAL RANGE

Reported as positive or negative

PHYSIOLOGY

FIV is inoculated via saliva or blood from bite wounds. There are three stages of infections. Acute phase: FIV initially infects T-lymphocytes and salivary glands with subsequently spread to other mononuclear cells; cats may have fever, leukopenia and lymphadenopathy. Subclinical phase: cats may be without clinical signs for years. Chronic phase: progressive immunosuppression with development of wide variety of clinical disorders including stomatitis/gingivitis, anemia and leukopenia, neurologic signs, enteritis, weight loss, and opportunistic infections. A cat may have no clinical signs for years due to a prolonged subclinical phase that follows acute infection. Available tests measure circulating FIV antibody levels, not viral antigen. The natural history of lentiviruses makes the presence of antibody essentially equivalent to infection (exceptions: maternal antibody, vaccination).

CAUSES OF ABNORMALLY HIGH LEVELS: Screening test: ELISA or rapid immunomigration assay—positive indicates possible exposure to FIV or FIV vaccine; positive or equivocal result requires confirmatory testing. Due to maternally transferred antibody, FIV testing of kittens ≤6 months of age is unreliable (false positives) and is not recommended.

NEXT DIAGNOSTIC STEP TO CONSIDER IF LEVELS HIGH: Confirmatory tests: Western blot or IFA. Positive Western blot or IFA indicates maternal antibody (kittens <6 months old) or exposure to FIV or the vaccine. Polymerase chain reaction (PCR) test may be a useful test in the future for differentiating vaccine exposure from true infection; however, currently available tests vary significantly in their diagnostic accuracy and should be interpreted with caution.

CAUSES OF ABNORMALLY LOW LEVELS: Negative ELISA indicates lack of exposure or acute infection.

NEXT DIAGNOSTIC STEP TO CONSIDER IF LEVELS LOW: If clinical signs suggest FIV infection, retest in 4 to 12 weeks.

SAMPLE FOR COLLECTION AND ANY SPECIAL SPECIMEN HANDLING NOTES

- ELISA: 0.5 ml serum (red-top tube) or plasma (purple- or green-top tube).
- Western blot or IFA: 1 ml of serum (red-top tube).

AUTHOR: **PATTY J. EWING**

Feline Leukemia Virus Enzyme-Linked Immunosorbent Assay (ELISA)

BASIC INFORMATION

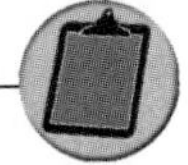

DEFINITION

Feline leukemia virus (FeLV) is a retrovirus of cats that causes hematopoietic neoplasia, immunosuppression, and/or anemia.

SYNONYMS

ELISA: enzyme-linked immunosorbent assay
FeLV

TYPICAL NORMAL RANGE

Reported as positive or negative

PHYSIOLOGY

Following exposure to FeLV via the oronasal route, the virus replicates in oropharyngeal lymphoid tissue. The virus may be cleared with an effective immune response. An ineffective immune response results in viremia and replication in marrow and lymphoid cells. Affected cats may be transiently viremic with latent virus residing in the marrow, may become persistently viremic, or may be overtly healthy carriers. Persistent viremia may result in immunosuppression, myelosuppression, hematopoietic neoplasia, immune complex diseases, or reproductive disorders.

CAUSES OF ABNORMALLY HIGH LEVELS: ELISA detects the free soluble FeLV core antigen, p27; therefore, a positive ELISA indicates that the cat is viremic (infected with FeLV). False-positive results due to technical error can occur, but this occurs infrequently.

NEXT DIAGNOSTIC STEP TO CONSIDER IF LEVELS HIGH: Confirm with FeLV IFA test.

CAUSES OF ABNORMALLY LOW LEVELS: A negative ELISA indicates that either the cat is not infected or has an early infection.

NEXT DIAGNOSTIC STEP TO CONSIDER IF LEVELS LOW: If the cat was recently exposed to an FeLV positive cat but the ELISA is negative, retesting in 30 to 90 days is recommended.

LAB ARTIFACTS THAT MAY INTERFERE WITH READINGS OF LEVELS OF THIS SUBSTANCE: Hemolysis may cause a false-positive or false-negative result.

SAMPLE FOR COLLECTION AND ANY SPECIAL SPECIMEN HANDLING NOTES: One ml serum (red-top tube) or plasma (purple-top tube).

PEARLS

- Vaccination for FeLV involves a different component of the virus (gp70 protein) than the one detected by ELISA. Therefore, prior vaccination does not affect test results.
- The FeLV ELISA test is more sensitive (more likely to "catch" all FeLV positive cases) but less specific (may also erroneously identify a few FeLV negative cases as positive) compared to the FeLV IFA. Therefore, FeLV ELISA is a good initial screening test, but positive results may or may not be true positives and need to be confirmed with IFA.

AUTHOR: **PATTY J. EWING**

Feline Leukemia Virus Immunofluorescent Antibody (IFA)

BASIC INFORMATION

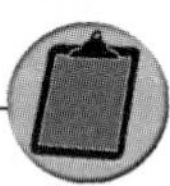

DEFINITION

Feline leukemia virus (FeLV) is a retrovirus of cats that causes hematopoietic neoplasia, immunosuppression, and/or anemia.

SYNONYM(S)

FeLV
IFA: immunofluorescent antibody

TYPICAL NORMAL RANGE

Reported as positive or negative

PHYSIOLOGY

Following exposure to FeLV via the oronasal route, the virus replicates in oropharyngeal lymphoid tissue. The virus may be cleared with an effective immune response. An ineffective immune response results in viremia and replication in bone marrow and lymphoid cells. Affected cats may be transiently viremic with latent virus residing in the marrow, may become persistently viremic, or may be overtly healthy carriers. Persistent viremia may result in immunosuppression, myelosuppression, hematopoietic neoplasia, immune complex diseases, or reproductive disorders.

CAUSES OF ABNORMALLY HIGH LEVELS: IFA detects the cell-associated FeLV core antigen, p27, in cells; therefore, a positive IFA indicates infection with FeLV and probable bone marrow infection. A positive IFA with a negative enzyme-linked immunosorbent assay (ELISA) is always a false result and testing should be repeated.

NEXT DIAGNOSTIC STEP TO CONSIDER IF LEVELS HIGH: Correlate with history, clinical findings, and laboratory data.

CAUSES OF ABNORMALLY LOW LEVELS: A negative IFA with a positive ELISA indicates either uninfected (false positive ELISA) or early infection.

NEXT DIAGNOSTIC STEP TO CONSIDER IF LEVELS LOW: If positive ELISA and negative IFA, repeat assay in 6 to 8 weeks.

LAB ARTIFACTS THAT MAY INTERFERE WITH READINGS OF LEVELS OF THIS SUBSTANCE: Marked thrombocytopenia, marked leukopenia, eosinophilia, or poor quality buffy coat or bone marrow smear may cause false-negative or false-positive results.

SAMPLE FOR COLLECTION AND ANY SPECIAL SPECIMEN HANDLING NOTES

- One ml of whole blood (EDTA: purple-top tube): stable at 4°C for 4 days.
- Air-dried buffy coat smears or bone marrow smears: store at room temperature.

PEARLS

- Vaccination for FeLV involves a different component of the virus (gp70 protein) than the one detected by IFA. Therefore, prior vaccination does not affect test results.
- The FeLV IFA test is less sensitive (does not "catch" all FeLV positive cases) but more specific (positive result is reliably positive) compared to the FeLV ELISA. Therefore, FeLV IFA is not a good initial screening test, but is an excellent confirmatory test.

AUTHOR: **PATTY J. EWING**

Fibrin or Fibrinogen Degradation Products

BASIC INFORMATION

DEFINITION

Fibrin or fibrinogen degradation products (FDPs) are protein fragments of fibrin or fibrinogen that have been cleaved by plasmin as part of fibrinolysis. Assays to detect FDPs are used for identifying increased fibrin or fibrinogen breakdown that is seen with excessive coagulation (disseminated intravascular coagulation [DIC]). Plasmin can act on both fibrinogen and fibrin, and assays for FDPs do not differentiate between fibrinolysis and fibrinogenolysis.

SYNONYM(S)

FDPs

TYPICAL NORMAL RANGE

Semiquantitative normal values: dogs, 0–10 μg/ml; cats, 0–8 μg/ml. Abnormal values are reported as moderately increased or markedly increased. Exact values are laboratory dependent.

PHYSIOLOGY

- FDPs are formed by plasmin breakdown of noncross-linked fibrin and fibrinogen. FDPs are potent inhibitors of coagulation; they compete with fibrinogen for the active sites on thrombin and interfere with the conversion of fibrinogen to fibrin.
- FDPs interfere with platelet aggregation; they bind to the fibrinogen-binding site on platelets.
- FDPs are eliminated by the liver and the kidney, so patients with hepatic or renal disease can have elevated FDPs.

CAUSES OF ABNORMALLY HIGH LEVELS

- Increased fibrinolysis: internal hemorrhage, local or disseminated intravascular coagulation.
- Decreased FDP clearance: hepatic disease, renal failure.

NEXT DIAGNOSTIC STEP TO CONSIDER IF LEVELS HIGH

- Complete blood count with platelet count/serum chemistry profile/urinalysis.
- Coagulation profile: activated partial thromboplastin time, prothrombin time, thrombin time, angiotensin III, D-dimer.

LAB ARTIFACTS THAT MAY INTERFERE WITH READINGS OF LEVELS OF THIS SUBSTANCE: False increases can be seen when FDP generation occurs during collection (traumatic venipuncture).

SAMPLE FOR COLLECTION AND ANY SPECIAL SPECIMEN HANDLING NOTES: Serum assay: use tubes filled with thrombin, or reptilase (snake venom) with soybean trypsin inhibitor or aprotinin (light-blue tubes with yellow label). Plasma assays: citrated tube (light-blue top).

PEARLS: Serum specimens cannot be used because clot formation consumes FDPs, lowering measurement.

AUTHOR: **DEBORAH G. DAVIS**

Fibrinogen

BASIC INFORMATION

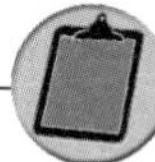

DEFINITION

A glycoprotein important in hemostasis; a positive acute-phase protein that increases due to inflammation or tissue injury; important in tissue repair.

TYPICAL NORMAL RANGE

Dogs: 150–300 mg/dl; cats: 150–300 mg/dl.

PHYSIOLOGY

Made in the liver; production is upregulated with inflammation or tissue damage (due to cytokines interleukin [IL]-1, IL-6, and tumor necrosis factor [TNF]). It is a nonenzymatic coagulation factor (factor I), cleaved (activated) by thrombin to form fibrin and promote stable clot formation.

CAUSES OF ABNORMALLY HIGH LEVELS: Two major causes include dehydration (hemoconcentration) and increased production by the liver (positive acute phase protein) in response to cytokines IL-1, IL-6, and TNF due to inflammation or tissue damage. Can also increase with physiologic stress (pregnancy).

NEXT DIAGNOSTIC STEP TO CONSIDER IF LEVELS HIGH: Look for source of inflammation/tissue injury: complete blood count (determine if inflammatory leukogram is present), serum chemistry profile; if hyperglobulinemia, serum protein electrophoresis is warranted to document a polyclonal gammopathy supportive of an inflammatory process.

CAUSES OF ABNORMALLY LOW LEVELS: Increased consumption in disseminated intravascular coagulation or increased fibrinogenolysis, decreased hepatic fibrinogen synthesis, inherited/congenital disorders (documented in bichon frise, Bernese mountain dogs, Lhasa apso, vizsla, and collie).

NEXT DIAGNOSTIC STEP TO CONSIDER IF LEVELS LOW: Full coagulation profile (activated partial thromboplastin time, prothrombin time, thrombin time, platelet count, and fibrinogen degradation products) to assess for disseminated intravascular coagulation. Serum chemistry profile to evaluate hepatic parameters. Serum bile acids to evaluate hepatobiliary function.

SAMPLE FOR COLLECTION AND ANY SPECIAL SPECIMEN HANDLING NOTES: Citrated plasma (blue-top tube), recommended to centrifuge and remove plasma within 1 hour of collection and test as soon as possible.

AUTHOR: **DEBORAH G. DAVIS**

Folate

BASIC INFORMATION

DEFINITION

The anionic form of folic acid. Part of B-vitamin complex.

SYNONYM(S)

Folic acid

TYPICAL NORMAL RANGE

Dogs: 6.5 to 11.5 µg/L.
Cats: 9.7 to 21.6 µg/L.
Check with individual laboratories.

PHYSIOLOGY

Primary source is diet; also produced by enteric bacteria. Ingested folate is released from food and hydrolyzed in proximal small intestine. Dietary and bacteria produced folate are taken up by intestinal epithelium, metabolized, and systemically absorbed (blood).

CAUSES OF ABNORMALLY HIGH LEVELS: Intestinal bacterial overgrowth, exocrine pancreatic insufficiency (EPI), excessive gastric acid production, oversupplementation

NEXT DIAGNOSTIC STEP TO CONSIDER IF LEVELS HIGH: Test for bacterial overgrowth, EPI. Evaluate diet.

CAUSES OF ABNORMALLY LOW LEVELS: Small intestinal mucosal disease, dietary deficiency, medication (sulfasalazine, phenytoin, antibiotics that deplete gastrointestinal flora causing decreased folate production), extensive intestinal neoplasia.

NEXT DIAGNOSTIC STEP TO CONSIDER IF LEVELS LOW: Evaluate diet, medication history. Assess for intestinal mucosal disease (endoscopy or surgery).

IMPORTANT INTERSPECIES DIFFERENCES: Different reference ranges for dogs and cats. High serum concentration in cats is of no known clinical signficance. Increased serum folate (due to bacterial overgrowth) associated with low immunoglobulin A in German shepherd dogs

DRUG EFFECTS ON LEVELS: Decrease: associated with sulfasalazine, phenytoin, and antibiotics that disturb intestinal flora.

LAB ARTIFACTS THAT MAY INTERFERE WITH READINGS OF LEVELS OF THIS SUBSTANCE: False increase: hemolyzed specimens (released from red blood cells).

SAMPLE FOR COLLECTION AND ANY SPECIAL SPECIMEN HANDLING NOTES: Nonhemolyzed serum (red-top tube; separate serum from clot immediately and place in fresh red top tube for submission). Stable at 4°C for 1 day, −20°C for 6 to 8 weeks. Avoid repeated freezing, thawing.

PEARLS

- Folate should be evaluated in conjunction with cobalamin, trypsin-like immunoreactivity for best interpretation.
- Maternal folate deficiency is associated with congenital malformations (neural tube and conotruncal cardiac defects) in humans but there is no evidence of a similar problem in dogs and cats

AUTHOR: **LOIS ROTH-JOHNSON**

Fructosamine

BASIC INFORMATION

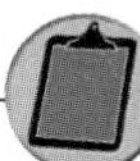

DEFINITION

Fructosamine is an amino sugar formed by the reduction of osazone glucosamine. It is dependent on the concentration of glucose-bound serum proteins. The test is used for assessing the average serum glucose concentration over the preceding 2 to 3 weeks.

SYNONYM(S)

Glycated proteins
Glycosylated proteins

TYPICAL NORMAL RANGE

Range varies with instrument (personal experience with Heska SpotChem, fructosamine is usually <200 µmol/L in healthy animals).

PHYSIOLOGY

Persistent hyperglycemia results in irreversible binding of glucose to reactive molecules, such as serum proteins, erythrocyte membranes, and other cell membranes. Transient hyperglycemia may result in noncovalent, reversible binding of glucose to reactive molecules. Therefore, this test may help differentiate transient stress-induced hyperglycemia from diabetes mellitus in cats.

CAUSES OF ABNORMALLY HIGH LEVELS: Persistent hyperglycemia.

NEXT DIAGNOSTIC STEP TO CONSIDER IF LEVELS HIGH: Review history and physical exam for findings indicative of diabetes mellitus. Check serum glucose and for the presence of urine glucose and urine ketones.

CAUSES OF ABNORMALLY LOW LEVELS

- Animals with hypoproteinemia and hypoalbuminemia may have lowered fructosamine. If hypoalbuminemia is concurrent with diabetes mellitus, the fructosamine level may appear falsely low.
- Hyperthyroid cats have lower fructosamine than healthy cats owing to accelerated protein (albumin) turnover.

NEXT DIAGNOSTIC STEP TO CONSIDER IF LEVELS LOW: In cats, test for hyperthyroidism. Check serum/plasma proteins/albumin concentrations.

IMPORTANT INTERSPECIES DIFFERENCES: Glucose has a higher for albumin in dogs and globulins in cats.

SAMPLE FOR COLLECTION AND ANY SPECIAL SPECIMEN HANDLING NOTES: Serum (red-top tube) or heparinized plasma (green-top tube).

PEARLS: Fructosamine is not typically used to assess persistent hypoglycemia as would occur in patients with insulinoma.

AUTHOR: **ELIZABETH G. WELLES**

Fungal Culture

BASIC INFORMATION

DEFINITION

Analysis of tissue or exudate for fungal organisms.

TYPICAL NORMAL RANGE

Reported as negative or degree (slight, moderate, heavy) of growth of specific pathogens

PHYSIOLOGY

Laboratory conditions enhance growth of pathogens and allow isolation of fungal colonies and their identification by morphologic features and chemical tests.

CAUSES OF ABNORMALLY HIGH LEVELS: Fungal infection. Common fungal infections include dermatophytosis, aspergillosis, cryptococcosis, blastomycosis, histoplasmosis, and coccidioimycosis. Saprophytes may cause skin lesions or systemic disease in immune compromised patients.

NEXT DIAGNOSTIC STEP TO CONSIDER IF LEVELS HIGH: Culture is definitive. Used as a confirmatory test for dermatophytes; *Aspergillus* spp. may be cultured for specific identification if organisms seen in cytologic or histologic specimens. Dimorphic fungi are typically not cultured due to health risk for laboratory personnel; instead, serologic tests and/or cytologic demonstration of organisms are confirmatory.

IMPORTANT INTERSPECIES DIFFERENCES: Dermatophytes may cause pseudomycetoma (deep granulomatous or pyogranulomatous lesions) in Persian cats.

DRUG EFFECTS ON LEVELS: Corticosteroid therapy decreases patient resistance, enhancing organism growth.

LAB ARTIFACTS THAT MAY INTERFERE WITH READINGS OF LEVELS OF THIS SUBSTANCE: False negative: improper media or growth conditions.

SAMPLE FOR COLLECTION AND ANY SPECIAL SPECIMEN HANDLING NOTES

- Dermatophytes: hair plucked from affected areas should be submitted in dermatophyte test media or sterile dry containers.
- Tissue or exudate: sterile, dry container.

PEARLS: Do not submit specimens for culture if cryptococcosis, blastomycosis, histoplasmosis, or coccidioimycosis is suspected. In culture, these organisms are health hazards to laboratory personnel (zoonosis via inhalation or accidental inoculation). Serologic tests coupled with cytologic or histologic lesions are appropriate for diagnosis.

AUTHOR: **LOIS ROTH-JOHNSON**

Gamma-glutamyltransferase

BASIC INFORMATION

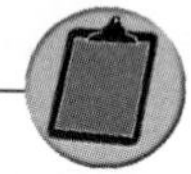

DEFINITION

Serum enzyme used as marker for liver disease associated with cholestasis.

SYNONYM(S)

GGT

TYPICAL NORMAL RANGE

Dogs: ~0–6 U/L; cats: ~0–4 U/L.
Specific values vary among laboratories.

PHYSIOLOGY

Membrane-bound enzymes present in many cells with biliary epithelium, renal tubular epithelial cells, pancreatic cells, and mammary epithelial cells (especially during lactation) having the greatest activity. Significant increases in serum activity associated primarily with liver disease. Renal urinary GGT may be measured as evidence for renal tubular damage. Colostrum of some species contains high levels of GGT.

CAUSES OF ABNORMALLY HIGH LEVELS: Cholestasis; biliary hyperplasia; ingestion of colostrum in neonates; may be induced by corticosteroid administration in dogs.

NEXT DIAGNOSTIC STEP TO CONSIDER IF LEVELS HIGH

- Evaluate recent drug administration in the dog.
- Alkaline phosphatase (ALP), bilirubin, bile acids, liver biopsy.

CAUSES OF ABNORMALLY LOW LEVELS: Low end of reference intervals are usually very low. Low levels are not clinically significant.

IMPORTANT INTERSPECIES DIFFERENCES: Colostrum in most species contains high GGT concentrations. Increases in GGT occurs within 24 hours of suckling: sensitive indicator of passive transfer. In pups, levels fall to within reference intervals by 10 days of age.

DRUG EFFECTS ON LEVELS: Increases secondary to therapeutic drugs causing cholestasis. Increases also seen with anticonvulsant and corticosteroid therapy.

LAB ARTIFACTS THAT MAY INTERFERE WITH READINGS OF LEVELS OF THIS SUBSTANCE: Increase: heparin (therapy or use as anticoagulant for collection).

SAMPLE FOR COLLECTION AND ANY SPECIAL SPECIMEN HANDLING NOTES: Serum; separate as soon as possible; store at 8° C.

PEARLS: GGT is more sensitive but less specific than ALP in the cat (for all diseases except hepatic lipidosis) and more specific but less sensitive in the dog.

AUTHOR: **FONZIE QUANCE-FITCH**

Gastrin

BASIC INFORMATION

DEFINITION

Group of peptide hormones secreted by G-cells of gastric antrum and duodenum in response to protein meal. Functions to stimulate parietal cell secretion of gastric acid and histamine release by enterochromaffin cells. Also stimulates pancreatic acinar cells when bound to cholecystokinin.

SYNONYM(S)

G-34 (big gastrin)
G-17
g-14 (mini gastrin)

TYPICAL NORMAL RANGE

0–100 pg/ml

PHYSIOLOGY

Ingestion of protein meal stimulates release. Binds to receptors (parietal, enterochromaffin cells), regulating gastric acid release for protein digestion. Enhances digestion by stimulating gastric blood flow, antral motility, and pancreatic secretion. Stimulates DNA, RNA production, and proliferation of parietal cells and gastric mucosa.

CAUSES OF ABNORMALLY HIGH LEVELS: Excess secretion (gastrinoma/ Zollinger-Ellison syndrome) associated with gastric mucosa hypertrophy, gastric, duodenal ulceration. The underlying cause is typically a neoplasm of pancreatic islet δ cells; when these cells undergo neoplastic transformation, they regain the ability to produce gastrin (normally only occurs in the fetus).

NEXT DIAGNOSTIC STEP TO CONSIDER IF LEVELS HIGH: Evaluate gastric mucosa (endoscopy) for hypertrophy, ulceration; assess for pancreatic islet (δ cell) tumor (abdominal ultrasound and, if a pancreatic mass is seen, laparotomy).

SAMPLE FOR COLLECTION AND ANY SPECIAL SPECIMEN HANDLING NOTES: Frozen serum; fasting specimen suggested.

AUTHOR: **LOIS ROTH-JOHNSON**

Giardiasis Testing: Fecal Flotation and Enzyme-Linked Immunosorbent Assay (ELISA)

BASIC INFORMATION

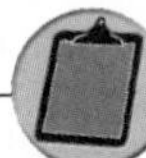

DEFINITION

Giardia lamblia is a protozoan causing chronic, severe diarrhea in pets and humans. Contaminated water is the usual source of infection. Fecal flotation using zinc sulfate and fecal ELISA tests are used for detection of the organism.

SYNONYM(S)

Lamblia intestinalis

TYPICAL NORMAL RANGE

Reported as negative for trophozoites or fecal antigen, or positive.

PHYSIOLOGY

- Zinc sulfate fecal flotation depends on accurate identification of trophozoites in fecal specimens combined with zinc sulfate solution. Trophozoites float to the surface and an aliquot of fluid is examined microscopically.
- ELISA test detects specific antigens in feces.

CAUSES OF ABNORMALLY HIGH LEVELS: Intestinal infection

NEXT DIAGNOSTIC STEP TO CONSIDER IF LEVELS HIGH: Identification of organisms in fecal flotation or by ELISA is considered diagnostic.

DRUG EFFECTS ON LEVELS: Anthelmintic drug treatment may lower fecal shedding of organisms.

LAB ARTIFACTS THAT MAY INTERFERE WITH READINGS OF LEVELS OF THIS SUBSTANCE: Feces for flotation must be fresh. Fecal flotation has low sensitivity (50%) and specificity (76%). Specimens should be examined within 15 minutes of flotation set-up to minimize cyst rupture or distortion. At least three negative results should be obtained before giardiasis is ruled out. ELISA test is more sensitive (92%) and specific (99%). In-office testing devices are available.

SAMPLE FOR COLLECTION AND ANY SPECIAL SPECIMEN HANDLING NOTES: Fresh (≤24 hours) fecal specimen in clean dry container. ELISA test kits are available for in-office testing.

PEARLS: Affects humans. The disease is especially severe in immunocompromised humans, dogs, and cats. Thorough washing of hands with soap should be done following cleaning up pet waste. Babies should be kept away from pets with diarrhea.

AUTHOR: **LOIS ROTH-JOHNSON**

Globulins

BASIC INFORMATION

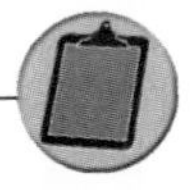

DEFINITION

In routine chemistry profiles, globulin concentration is calculated from subtraction of measured albumin from measured total serum protein. Globulins are typically classified as α, β, or γ depending on electophoretic mobility.

TYPICAL NORMAL RANGE

Dogs: ~2–4 g/dl.
Cats: ~2.5–5 g/dl.
Specific values vary among laboratories.
Conversion: g/dl × 10 = g/L.

PHYSIOLOGY

Globulins are a heterogeneous group of large serum proteins including immunoglobulins, clotting proteins, complement, and many acute phase proteins and lipoproteins, with a wide variety of physiologic functions.

CAUSES OF ABNORMALLY HIGH LEVELS

- Polyclonal gammopathy: chronic inflammation, hepatic disease, feline infectious peritonitis, immune-mediated disease.
- Monoclonal gammopathy: multiple myeloma, lymphosarcoma, canine ehrlichiosis, leishmaniasis.
- If concurrent hyperalbuminemia: dehydration.

NEXT DIAGNOSTIC STEP TO CONSIDER IF LEVELS HIGH

- Evaluate albumin:globulin (A:G) ratio. Decreased A:G ratio when albumin within reference interval and increased globulin indicates increased globulin production. If the A:G ratio is close to 1, consider dehydration as a cause for a relative increase in globulin.
- Protein electrophoresis and/or immunoelectrophoresis.

CAUSES OF ABNORMALLY LOW LEVELS

- If concurrent with normal albumin level: failure of passive transfer (neonates), immunodeficiencies, hepatic insufficiency.
- If concurrent with hypoalbuminemia: hemorrhage, gastrointestinal or renal protein loss, severe malnutrition/ maldigestion/malabsorption, hepatic insufficiency.

NEXT DIAGNOSTIC STEP TO CONSIDER IF LEVELS LOW

- Evaluate albumin:globulin ratio.
- Evaluate for possible hemorrhage.
- Assess for renal or gastrointestinal protein loss, hepatic failure, malnutrition, maldigestion, or malabsorption.

LAB ARTIFACTS THAT MAY INTERFERE WITH READINGS OF LEVELS OF THIS SUBSTANCE: As a calculated value, anything affecting accuracy of total protein or albumin measurements will be reflected in globulin concentration.

PEARLS: Magnitude of increase of α and β globulins are usually insufficient to cause an increase in globulin values. An electrophoresis is needed to identify increased peaks.

AUTHOR: **FONZIE QUANCE-FITCH**

Glucose, Blood

BASIC INFORMATION

DEFINITION

Blood concentration of the sugar that is utilized for energy production.

SYNONYM(S)

Blood sugar

TYPICAL NORMAL RANGE

Dogs: 60–125 mg/dl (3.3–6.9 mmol/L).
Cats: 70–150 mg/dl (3.9–8.3 mmol/L).

PHYSIOLOGY

Carbohydrates in the diet are catabolized to glucose for absorption and transport to the liver and other tissues. The liver produces glucose via gluconeogenesis and glycogenolysis, and stores glucose in the form of glycogen or converts glucose to amino acids and lipids. Blood glucose levels are regulated by dietary intake, hormones such as insulin and glucagon, and tissue utilization. Glucose metabolism and blood glucose concentration are affected by many disorders.

CAUSES OF ABNORMALLY HIGH LEVELS: Diabetes mellitus, hyperadrenocorticism, stress, hyperthyroidism, hyperpituitarism, acute pancreatitis, excitement induced epinephrine release (primarily cats), postprandial (minor elevations).

NEXT DIAGNOSTIC STEP TO CONSIDER IF LEVELS HIGH: Assess for persistent hyperglycemia, glucosuria and ketonuria, serum fructosamine.

CAUSES OF ABNORMALLY LOW LEVELS: Long-term starvation or malabsorption, insulin overdose, paraneoplastic (insulinoma, leimyosarcoma), chronic liver disease, extreme exertion, sepsis, neonatal or juvenile hypoglycemia, hypoadrenocorticism, glycogen storage diseases, artifact (delay in processing, or centrifuging and separating red blood cells from whole blood sample).

NEXT DIAGNOSTIC STEP TO CONSIDER IF LEVELS LOW: Resample to verify persistent hypoglycemia. Correlate with other clinical and laboratory findings. Serum insulin levels to assess for hyperinsulinism due to insulinoma.

IMPORTANT INTERSPECIES DIFFERENCE: Hyperglycemia due to excitement induced epinephrine release is common in cats.

DRUG EFFECTS ON LEVELS

- Increase: glucocorticoids; adrenocorticotropic hormone; intravenous fluids containing dextrose, growth hormone, megestrol acetate, thiazide diuretics, xylazine, ketamine in cats, morphine, and phenothiazine.
- Decrease: insulin injection, ethanol, salicylates, sulfonylurea, and o,p'-DDD.

LAB ARTIFACTS THAT MAY INTERFERE WITH READINGS OF LEVELS OF THIS SUBSTANCE

- Decrease: Delayed separation of serum or plasma from red blood cells results in artificial depression due to utilization of glucose by blood cells.
- Increase: lipemia.

SAMPLE FOR COLLECTION AND ANY SPECIAL SPECIMEN HANDLING NOTES: Serum (red top) or heparinized plasma (green top). Separate from cells within 30 minutes after sample collection. Stable at 2–8° C for 4 days.

AUTHOR: **RUANNA GOSSETT**

Glucosuria

BASIC INFORMATION

DEFINITION

Glucose in urine.

SYNONYM(S)

Glycosuria

TYPICAL NORMAL RANGE (US UNITS; SI UNITS)

Negative in healthy dogs and cats

PHYSIOLOGY

Glucose is a small molecule and is freely filtered by glomeruli. Renal tubular epithelium normally resorbs all glucose. Serum glucose concentrations above which tubular cells are unable to fully resorb glucose from urine filtrate (renal threshold) are 180–220 mg/dl (dogs) and 250–300 mg/dl (cats).

CAUSES OF ABNORMALLY HIGH LEVELS

- Persistent (several hours to days) hyperglycemia caused by diabetes mellitus or administration of glucose containing fluids.
- Transient hyperglycemia if the renal threshold is exceeded for sufficient time and bladder has minimal glucose-free urine to result in dilution (e.g., stress hyperglycemia in cats).
- Defective renal tubular resorption due to acute tubular disease, acute renal failure, or Fanconi syndrome (an inherited disorder of basenjis, Norwegian elkhounds, and Shetland sheepdogs).

NEXT DIAGNOSTIC STEP TO CONSIDER IF LEVELS HIGH: Check serum glucose concentration. May need to measure serum fructosamine to differentiate diabetes mellitus from transient hyperglycemia, especially in cats, owing to transient hyperglycemia caused by excitement, fear, or stress.

IMPORTANT INTERSPECIES DIFFERENCES: Cats have a higher renal threshold for hyperglycemia before glucosuria occurs, but are also prone to much greater levels of hyperglycemia caused by stress.

DRUG EFFECTS ON LEVELS: With most urine dipsticks (glucose oxidase method), vitamin C/ascorbic acid causes a false decreased reaction. With the Clinitest (copper reduction method), ascorbic acid and cephalosporin antibiotics can cause false-positive reactions.

LAB ARTIFACTS THAT MAY INTERFERE WITH READINGS OF LEVELS OF THIS SUBSTANCE: False positive/increase: hydrogen peroxide and sodium hypochlorite (bleach). False negative/decrease: ketones, very concentrated samples, and cold urine.

SAMPLE FOR COLLECTION AND ANY SPECIAL SPECIMEN HANDLING NOTES: Clean urine collected as free catch, catheterization, or cystocentesis and of sufficient quantity into which to dip the urine dipstick. Alternatively, a large drop can be placed on the specific reagent pad on the dipstick.

PEARLS: Urine should be at least room temperature or warmer (>20° C or 70° F) for enzymes in reagent pad of dipstick to have appropriate activity.

AUTHOR: **ELIZABETH G. WELLES**

Glycated Hemoglobin

BASIC INFORMATION

DEFINITION

The concentration of glucose bound to hemoglobin. The test is used for assessing the average serum glucose concentration over the preceding 2 to 3 months.

SYNONYM(S)

Glycosylated hemoglobin
Hemoglobin A1c

TYPICAL NORMAL RANGE

Interval varies with laboratory.

PHYSIOLOGY

Persistent hyperglycemia results in irreversible binding of glucose to reactive molecules, such as hemoglobin. The time frame over which glycated hemoglobin indicates glucose levels (2 to 3 months) is a reflection of the average blood glucose concentration and red blood cell lifespan.

CAUSES OF ABNORMALLY HIGH LEVELS: Persistent hyperglycemia, uncontrolled diabetes mellitus

NEXT DIAGNOSTIC STEP TO CONSIDER IF LEVELS HIGH: Review history and physical exam for findings indicative of diabetes mellitus. Check serum glucose and check for the presence of urine glucose and urine ketones. If the animal is diabetic and is being treated with insulin: check the insulin; check how the owners are storing, preparing and administering the insulin; reassess the dosage (may be too low or too high); and investigate insulin antagonistic disorders if relevant.

SAMPLE FOR COLLECTION AND ANY SPECIAL SPECIMEN HANDLING NOTES: Whole anticoagulated blood (ethylenediamine tetraacetic acid [purple top] or heparin [green top])

PEARLS: Glycated hemoglobin is used less often than fructosamine values to assess hyperglycemic conditions. Increased glycated hemoglobin values take longer to develop and are dependent upon hematocrit and red blood cell life span.

AUTHOR: **ELIZABETH G. WELLES**

Heartworm Antigen and Antibody Tests

BASIC INFORMATION

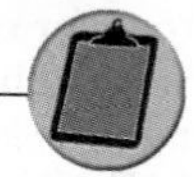

DEFINITION

Antigen test kits detect adult heartworm (*Dirofilaria immitis*) antigen. Antibody tests detect circulating antibody to either microfilarial cuticular antigen or adult heartworm antigen.

SYNONYM(S)

Occult heartworm test

TYPICAL NORMAL RANGE

Results are reported as negative or positive. Some tests are semiquantitative, reported as weakly positive. This is not necessarily indicative of worm burden (see causes of abnormally low levels).

PHYSIOLOGY

- Antigen tests detect an antigen primarily derived from adult female heartworm reproductive tract in the circulating blood of the host.
- Antibody tests detect species-specific circulating antibodies against either adult heartworms or larvae.

CAUSES OF ABNORMALLY HIGH LEVELS

- Antigen: infection with adult heartworms.
- Antibody: indicates exposure to *D. immitis,* but not all larval-infected animals will develop adult heartworms.

NEXT DIAGNOSTIC STEP TO CONSIDER IF LEVELS HIGH: Thoracic radiographs, electrocardiogram, cardiac ultrasound, complete blood count, chemistry panel.

CAUSES OF ABNORMALLY LOW LEVELS

- Antigen test: false low levels may be seen with very low worm burden (one or two female worms), single sex (male) infection, immature worms (<5 months old).
- Antibody test: false negatives may occur <30 days postinfection or if animal fails to produce detectable antibodies.

NEXT DIAGNOSTIC STEP TO CONSIDER IF LEVELS LOW: Retest in 1 to 2 months, assess for clinical signs of heartworm disease.

IMPORTANT INTERSPECIES DIFFERENCES: Antigen tests are less sensitive in the cat (low worm burden, single sex infections). Antibody tests can be useful in cats with clinical signs. Combination of an antigen and antibody test may improve overall sensitivity compared to the use of individual antibody tests alone.

DRUG EFFECTS ON LEVELS: Antigen test may remain positive up to 16 weeks postadulticide treatment.

LAB ARTIFACTS THAT MAY INTERFERE WITH READINGS OF LEVELS OF THIS SUBSTANCE: Severe hemolysis or lipemia may interfere with test. Antigen may degrade if sample not properly handled or stored.

SAMPLE FOR COLLECTION AND ANY SPECIAL SPECIMEN HANDLING NOTES: Serum (red-top tube). Store at 2–8° C. Some assays may also allow whole blood or plasma.

PEARLS: Echocardiography (cardiac ultrasound) rivals the heartworm antibody test for sensitivity of detection of adult heartworms in cats.

AUTHOR: **FONZIE QUANCE-FITCH**

Heartworm Filter Test

BASIC INFORMATION

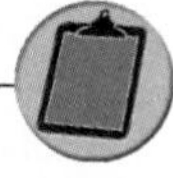

DEFINITION

Concentration method for the detection of circulating microfilariae of *Dirofilaria immitis*.

SYNONYM(S)

Difil test
Filaria filter test
Knott's test

TYPICAL NORMAL RANGE

Reported as negative or positive

PHYSIOLOGY

Circulating microfilariae are the larval (L1) stage of adult heartworms (*D. immitis*). Must be distinguished from circulating larval form of *Dipetalonema reconditum*.

CAUSES OF ABNORMALLY HIGH LEVELS: Circulating microfilaria of *D. immitis* or *D. reconditum*

NEXT DIAGNOSTIC STEP TO CONSIDER IF LEVELS HIGH: Confirm with heartworm antigen test; thoracic radiographs or ultrasound may be useful to stage the disease.

CAUSES OF ABNORMALLY LOW LEVELS: Occult infections (adult heartworms are present but ciculating microfilariae are absent) may be present due to single sex infection, immature worms, immune mediated destruction of microfilaria, prophylactic administration without initial testing.

NEXT DIAGNOSTIC STEP TO CONSIDER IF LEVELS LOW: Heartworm antigen tests, thoracic radiographs, ultrasound

IMPORTANT INTERSPECIES DIFFERENCES: Cats with heartworm disease are frequently microfilaria negative.

DRUG EFFECTS ON LEVELS: Animals on monthly preventative may be microfilaremia negative despite having heartworm disease.

SAMPLE FOR COLLECTION AND ANY SPECIAL SPECIMEN HANDLING NOTES: Whole blood (ethylenediamine tetraacetic acid, citrated or heparin)

PEARLS: As a screening test, the heartworm microfilaria test is less sensitive than the heartworm antigen test.

AUTHOR: **FONZIE QUANCE-FITCH**

Heinz Bodies

BASIC INFORMATION

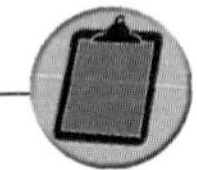

DEFINITION

Single or multiple precipitated denatured hemoglobin on the red cell (erythrocyte) membrane often associated with oxidative damage.

SYNONYM(S)

Erythrocyte refractile body
HB
Schmauch body

TYPICAL NORMAL RANGE

Low proportion seen in red blood cells of normal cats.

PHYSIOLOGY

Oxidants may cause irreversible denaturation of hemoglobin molecule and Heinz body formation. Heinz bodies have affinity for membrane protein band 3, forming a complex with it, resulting in clustering of membrane protein band 3 on both the internal and external red blood cell membrane. External clustering of protein band 3 creates a recognition site for auto-antibodies. Heinz bodies also make red blood cells rigid and less deformable (via cross-linking of spectrin and hemoglobin). These mechanisms make red blood cells prone to lysis (intravascular hemolysis) or phagocytosis by macrophages in the spleen (extravascular hemolysis).

CAUSES OF ABNORMALLY HIGH LEVELS: Drugs (see drug effects) and chemicals from food (onions, garlic, chives) or other substances (zinc); deficiency of enzymes that protect against oxidants.

NEXT DIAGNOSTIC STEP TO CONSIDER IF LEVELS HIGH

- Review patient history (diet, drug exposure).
- Check complete blood count, urinalysis, chemistry profile for anemia, hemolysis.

IMPORTANT INTERSPECIES DIFFERENCES: Normal in feline red blood cells (5-96% may have HBs) due to innately unstable hemoglobin structure, predisposition to form methemoglobin (low methemoglobin reductase activity), and inefficient removal by spleen. Normal HBs not associated with anemia. Increased HB formation may also occur without significant anemia in diabetes mellitus, hyperthyroidism, and lymphoma. In other species, increased numbers of HBs may be seen postsplenectomy.

DRUG EFFECTS ON LEVELS: Acetaminophen, benzocaine containing products, DL methionine, methylene blue, phenacetin, phenazopyridine, phenothiazine, and vitamin K_3 cause HB formation and hemolytic anemia.

SAMPLE FOR COLLECTION AND ANY SPECIAL SPECIMEN HANDLING NOTES: Purple top (ethylenediamine tetraacetic acid) tube for complete blood count and new methylene blue stained smears.

PEARLS: Free HBs may falsely increase instrument platelet counts and hemoglobin measurement.

AUTHOR: **FIDELIA R. FERNANDEZ**

Hematocrit

BASIC INFORMATION

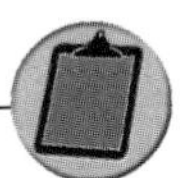

DEFINITION

The percentage of blood composed of red cells. Electronic cell counters calculate hematocrit using the formula: (MCV × RBC)/10 = HCT, where HCT is hematocrit, MCV is mean corpuscular volume (in femtoliters, fl), and RBC is erythrocyte count (× 10^6/fl).

SYNONYM(S)

Centrifugal microhematocrit
HCT
Packed cell volume

TYPICAL NORMAL RANGE

Dogs: 36–60%; cats: 29–48%.
Specific values vary among laboratories.

PHYSIOLOGY

- HCT values are slightly less than packed cell volume (PCV) because there is no trapped plasma in an automated hematocrit calculation as can occur with spun, packed cell values.
- Sources of variation:
  - Due to the variable MCV of domestic animals, values for HCT may be erroneous if the instrument is not calibrated for specific species.
  - Abnormal plasma osmolality and electrolyte balance may also result in a difference between HCT and PCV.
  - Although PCV measures change in red cell volume as they occur *in vivo*, dilution of red cells with normal saline and standing in hematology instruments may cause red cells to return to their normal volume.

CAUSES OF ABNORMALLY HIGH LEVELS: Polycythemia due to breed (sight hounds), dehydration, or splenic contraction ("relative polycythemia"), or due to hypoxemia, independent erythropoietin production (renal lesions), or polycythemia vera (myeloproliferative disease of erythrocytes) ("absolute polycythemia").

NEXT DIAGNOSTIC STEP TO CONSIDER IF LEVELS HIGH: Assess hydration status, review clinical history; evaluate for causes of polycythemia.

CAUSES OF ABNORMALLY LOW LEVELS: Anemia, overhydration.

NEXT DIAGNOSTIC STEP TO CONSIDER IF LEVELS LOW: Blood smear evaluation for type of anemia and evidence of polychromasia; reticulocyte count; bone marrow evaluation if anemia is nonregenerative; serology for parasites and infectious disease; Coombs' test.

IMPORTANT INTERSPECIES DIFFERENCES: Greyhounds and whippets have slightly higher normal values (up to 65% is considered normal, with some individuals exceeding even this level).

DRUG EFFECTS ON LEVELS: Erythropoietin injections increase HCT; drugs toxic to bone marrow (hydroxyurea, methimazole, many others) and drugs that cause hemolysis (e.g., zinc, methylene blue, benzocaine) can decrease HCT.

LAB ARTIFACTS THAT MAY INTERFERE WITH READINGS OF LEVELS OF THIS SUBSTANCE

- Hemolysis and specimen clotting prevent accurate reading.

- Decrease: insufficient filling of ethylenediamine tetraacetic acid (EDTA) tube dilutes specimen.

SAMPLE FOR COLLECTION (TYPE OF SPECIMEN, COLOR TUBE) AND ANY SPECIAL SPECIMEN HANDLING NOTES: EDTA-anticoagulated blood (lavender top); two capillary tubes for PCV; transport at room temperature or refrigerate if sample is held in the clinic. Follow proper filling of Vacutainer tubes.

PEARLS: The differences between HCT and PCV values are not clinically significant, except at very high values (PCV/HCT >65%), where plasma trapping becomes substantial.

AUTHOR: **FIDELIA R. FERNANDEZ**

Hemoglobinuria and Hematuria

BASIC INFORMATION

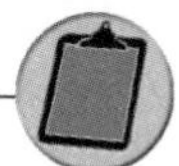

DEFINITION

Hemoglobinuria is the presence of hemoglobin in urine and is associated with red to brown urine that persists even with centrifugation. Hematuria is the presence of red cells in urine and is associated with red cloudy urine that clears with centrifugation.

TYPICAL NORMAL RANGE

Hemoglobin is not found in normal urine. Less than five red blood cells (RBCs) per high-power microscope field is considered normal in urine sediment.

PHYSIOLOGY

- Free hemoglobin in the plasma binds haptoglobin. Complex is cleared in the liver. When haptoglobin becomes saturated, the free hemoglobin splits into dimers which are excreted by the kidneys. Hemoglobin in glomerular filtrate is absorbed by proximal tubules and metabolized to bilirubin, iron, and globin. Unabsorbed hemoglobin appears in urine (hemoglobinuria).
- Erythrocytes may appear in the urine from upper urinary (renal, rarely ureteral), lower urinary (bladder, urethra), urogenital (prostate, testes, prepuce, uterus, vagina, vulva), or artifactual (traumatic sampling) sources.

CAUSES OF ABNORMALLY HIGH LEVELS

- Hemoglobinuria: severe intravascular hemolysis. Free hemoglobin may appear in urine in cases of hematuria where large numbers of red cells lyse in very dilute (specific gravity ≤1.008) or alkaline urine.
- Hematuria may be associated with hemorrhage, trauma, inflammation/necrosis, or neoplasia in the urinary tract.

NEXT DIAGNOSTIC STEP TO CONSIDER IF LEVELS HIGH

- Hemoglobinuria: identify cause of hemolysis by blood smear evaluation for hemic parasites, Heinz bodies, spherocytes, and red blood cell membrane defect. Systemic evaluation (complete blood count, serum chemistry profile, abdominal and thoracic imaging) may be indicated for identifying triggers of hemolytic anemia.
- Hematuria: determine when hematuria occurs during micturition. Hematuria at the beginning of urination suggests lower urinary or genital origin; at the end of urination, bladder origin (calculi, polyps); throughout urination, renal disease, diffuse bladder disease, prostatic disease. Radiography and ultrasonography are helpful in localizing the lesion.

DRUG EFFECTS ON LEVELS: Drugs causing intravascular hemolysis can also result in hemoglobinuria.

PEARLS: Cystocentesis and catherization are frequently associated with microscopic hematuria. These collection methods are not recommended for monitoring remission or progression of hematuria.

Free-catch urine from bitches in heat (proestrus) may be contaminated with blood.

AUTHOR: **FIDELIA R. FERNANDEZ**

Hemolysis

BASIC INFORMATION

DEFINITION

Hemolysis is lysis of erythrocytes releasing hemoglobin. It results in red discoloration of serum or plasma.

PHYSIOLOGY

Hemolysis is most commonly an *in vitro* artifact from traumatic venipuncture or improper sample handling. It may also occur *in vivo* due to pathologic intravascular or extravascular hemolysis. Hemolysis may interfere with certain laboratory assays by: discoloration of sample altering spectrophotometric assay results, dilution of normal substances in serum, or leakage of analytes from red blood cells resulting in false increase in these substances the in the serum or plasma.

CAUSES OF ABNORMALLY HIGH LEVELS: Hemolysis causes artifactual increase in hemoglobin, mean corpuscular hemoglobin concentration, alanine aminotransferase, aspartate aminotransferase, creatine kinase, lactate dehydrogenase, triglycerides, and total protein.

CAUSES OF ABNORMALLY LOW LEVELS: Hemolysis causes artifactual decrease in total bilirubin, direct bilirubin, alkaline phosphatase, γ-glutamyltransferase, and lipase.

LAB ARTIFACTS THAT MAY INTERFERE WITH READINGS OF LEVELS OF THIS SUBSTANCE: Ways to prevent *in vitro* hemolysis include: avoid traumatic venipuncture and excess negative pressure when drawing blood into syringe; prompt separation of serum from the clot; proper storage of samples (refrigeration); and avoid delay in sample analysis or delayed transport of samples to the laboratory for analysis.

AUTHOR: **RUANNA GOSSETT**

High-Dose Dexamethasone Suppression Test

BASIC INFORMATION

DEFINITION

Administration of dexamethasone suppresses production/release of hypothalamic corticosteroid releasing hormone (CRH) and pituitary adrenocorticotrophic hormone (ACTH), with subsequent reduction in production/release of cortisol from adrenal glands.

SYNONYM(S)

HDDST
High dose dex

TYPICAL NORMAL RANGE

- Baseline cortisol: 10–160 nmol/L (dogs); 10–110 nmol/L (cats).
- Postdexamethasone cortisol concentration: <40 nmol/L or <1.4 μg/dl (dogs); <35 nmol/L (cats). A 50% reduction in cortisol concentration from baseline has been interpreted as adequate suppression.

PHYSIOLOGY

- The high-dose dexamethasone suppression test (HDDST) is used for helping to differentiate pituitary-dependent hyperadrenocorticism from functional adrenal adenoma/adenocarcinoma. Dexamethasone is administered intravenously at 0.1 mg/kg. Serum cortisol level is measured at 4 and 8 hours postadministration.
- HDDST typically results in adequately decreased cortisol concentration in hyperadrenocorticism caused by pituitary tumors, whereas hyperadrenocorticism caused by adrenal tumors does not result in adequately decreased cortisol concentration with HDDST. Dogs with nonadrenal illness and healthy dogs should have adequately decreased cortisol concentration (same response as dogs with pituitary dependent hyperadrenocorticism).

CAUSES OF ABNORMALLY HIGH LEVELS: Adrenal neoplasia.

NEXT DIAGNOSTIC STEP TO CONSIDER IF LEVELS HIGH: Abdominal ultrasound to assess for adrenal neoplasia.

CAUSES OF ABNORMALLY LOW LEVELS: If cortisol concentration is adequately decreased after HDDST, patient has either pituitary-dependent hyperadrenocorticism or nonadrenal illness.

NEXT DIAGNOSTIC STEP TO CONSIDER IF LEVELS LOW

- Evaluate for nonadrenal disease.
- Magnetic resonance imaging of brain to assess for pituitary lesion.

DRUG EFFECTS ON LEVELS

- Immunoassays for cortisol measurement have significant cross-reactivity with other glucocorticoids: prednisolone (69%), prednisone (6.4%), 11-deoxycortisol (7.5%), cortisone (4.2%), corticosterone (3.5%), spironolactone (<0.2%), and dexamethasone (<0.1%).
- Ketoconazole inhibits steroid biosynthesis causing low cortisol concentration.

SAMPLE FOR COLLECTION AND ANY SPECIAL SPECIMEN HANDLING NOTES

- Serum (red-top tube) or ethylenediamine tetraacetic acid (EDTA) plasma (lavender-top tube).
- Cortisol in EDTA plasma is more stable than in serum and more stable in cooled samples compared with warm samples. Cortisol is equally distributed between red cells and plasma; therefore, rapid separation of plasma from cells (previously reported) is of no added benefit.

PEARLS

- Careful measurement of dexamethasone dose is important for accuracy. For small dogs, an insulin syringe may be used (no dead space in hub of needle and syringe); if diluting for accuracy, dexamethasone should be added to diluent and not vice versa.
- When a highly skilled ultrasonogapher and high-resolution ultrasound machine are available, imaging often supersedes HDDST testing.

AUTHOR: **ELIZABETH G. WELLES**

Insulin and Insulin:Glucose Ratio

BASIC INFORMATION

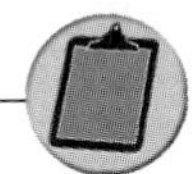

DEFINITION

Insulin is a hormone produced and secreted by the β-cells of the pancreatic islets of Langerhans. It promotes uptake of glucose by all tissues. It promotes anabolic metabolism of carbohydrates, proteins, lipids, and nucleic acids. The main targets of insulin are fat, skeletal muscle, and liver. Some tissues are not dependent on insulin for glucose uptake, including neurons, erythrocytes, renal tubular epithelial cells, enterocytes, pancreatic β-cells, ocular lens, exercising muscle, and basal metabolism in hepatocytes. The amended insulin:glucose ratio is calculated according to the following formula: serum insulin (μU/ml) × 100/serum glucose (mg/dl) − 30. This formula compares the insulin concentration in relationship with serum glucose concentration, but is generally considered inaccurate and should not be used.

TYPICAL NORMAL RANGE

Serum insulin interval varies with laboratory. Reference interval should be established for each laboratory. Insulin: glucose ratio <30 is considered normal, ratio >30 is suggestive of hyperinsulinism (it is not 100% diagnostic).

PHYSIOLOGY

Under normal conditions, high blood glucose levels trigger insulin release, and high insulin levels decrease blood glucose levels. This feedback mechanism ensures glucose homeostasis and is the reason that the insulin:glucose ratio is <30 in health. Persistent and/or excessive hyperinsulinism (e.g., paraneoplastic) may cause rapid, excessive cellular uptake of glucose, which results in hypoglycemia and varied clinical signs such as weakness, muscle tremors, collapse, seizures, and coma. Decreased concentrations of insulin are absolute with type I diabetes mellitus and often relative with type II and type III diabetes mellitus.

CAUSES OF ABNORMALLY HIGH LEVELS: Pancreatic β-cell neoplasia (insulinoma), leiomyosarcoma; insulin therapy; artifact (see below).

NEXT DIAGNOSTIC STEP TO CONSIDER IF LEVELS HIGH: Measure serum glucose concentration simultaneously.

Assess pancreas and small intestine by ultrasonographic examination.
CAUSES OF ABNORMALLY LOW LEVELS: Diabetes mellitus.
NEXT DIAGNOSTIC STEP TO CONSIDER IF LEVELS LOW: Check serum glucose concentration, urine glucose, and urine ketones. In diabetes mellitus, the serum glucose is increased; if untreated, there is often glucosuria ± ketonuria.
LAB ARTIFACTS THAT MAY INTERFERE WITH READINGS OF LEVELS OF THIS SUBSTANCE: Anti-insulin antibodies (contributors to diabetes mellitus) interfere with insulin assays and cause false, markedly elevated insulin concentration results.
SAMPLE FOR COLLECTION AND ANY SPECIAL SPECIMEN HANDLING NOTES: Serum (red-top tube).
PEARLS: Insulin should always be assessed concurrently with serum glucose. Insulin levels are almost always measured when investigating hypoglycemia and are virtually never indicated for assessment of hyperglycemia.

AUTHOR: **ELIZABETH G. WELLES**

Ketonuria

BASIC INFORMATION

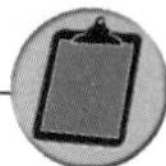

DEFINITION

Ketones (acetoacetate, β-hydroxybutyrate, acetone) in urine.

TYPICAL NORMAL RANGE

Reported as negative or slight (1+), moderate (2+), marked (+3).

PHYSIOLOGY

Urine is normally negative for ketones. Their presence in urine is the result of increased fat/lipid metabolism and decreased utilization of carbohydrates as an energy source. The standard laboratory (dipstick) test only detects acetoacetate and acetone.
CAUSES OF ABNORMALLY HIGH LEVELS: Diabetes mellitus, hypoglycemia, starvation.
NEXT DIAGNOSTIC STEP TO CONSIDER IF LEVELS HIGH: Assess nutritional condition; evaluate for diabetes mellitus (serum glucose, ± insulin concentration); evaluate for disorders of glucose metabolism (especially in young patients).
DRUG EFFECTS ON LEVELS: False increases: streptozotocin, aspirin.
LAB ARTIFACTS THAT MAY INTERFERE WITH READINGS OF LEVELS OF THIS SUBSTANCE: Standard test does not detect β-hydroxybutyrate, considered the ketone excreted in the earliest cases. Acetate tablet method (Bayer) is considered a more sensitive method and is recommended if ketonuria is suspected.
SAMPLE FOR COLLECTION AND ANY SPECIAL SPECIMEN HANDLING NOTES: Fresh urine specimen in sterile container for standard urinalysis.
PEARLS: If ketonuria coexists with glucosuria and hyperglycemia, diabetes mellitus ± diabetic ketoacidosis is likely. Serum Na, K, P, and blood gas determinations are recommended. Ketonuria without glucosuria is suggestive of starvation, fasting.

AUTHOR: **LOIS ROTH-JOHNSON**

Lactate

BASIC INFORMATION

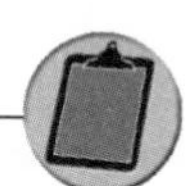

DEFINITION

Metabolic end product of anaerobic glycolysis.

SYNONYM(S)

Lactic acid

TYPICAL NORMAL RANGE

- Range: 1.8–22.5 mg/dl; <2 mEq/L (experimental studies, primarily in dogs).
- Unit conversion: mg/dl × 0.111 = mEq/L; 1 mmol/L = 1 mEq/L.

PHYSIOLOGY

Normally produced in small quantities in skin, erythrocytes, brain, skeletal muscle, gut. Increased production occurs when tissues (primarily skeletal muscle and gut) must maintain energy production under anaerobic conditions (tissue hypoxia). Abnormal carbohydrate metabolism associated with some diseases may also increase production. Liver and kidney are the primary consumers of lactate. Lactic acidosis occurs when production exceeds utilization.

CAUSES OF ABNORMALLY HIGH LEVELS
- Hypoxia: severe exercise, seizures, any cause of decreased oxygen availability (shock, hypovolemia, cardiac disease, pulmonary edema).
- Nonhypoxia: gastric dilatation/volvulus, diabetes mellitus, liver failure, neoplasia, sepsis, renal failure, hypoglycemia, babesiosis, rare hereditary defects (mitochondrial myopathy, pyruvate dehydrogenase deficiency).

NEXT DIAGNOSTIC STEP TO CONSIDER IF LEVELS HIGH
- Not measured as part of routine biochemical profile, but cageside use becoming increasingly common in emergency/critical care setting.
- Lactic acidosis should be suspected when there is an unexplained increase in the anion gap. Evaluate underlying causes.

DRUG EFFECTS ON LEVELS: Increases associated with salicylates, ethylene glycol, epinephrine, and phenobarbital
LAB ARTIFACTS THAT MAY INTERFERE WITH READINGS OF LEVELS OF THIS SUBSTANCE: Increased: delayed plasma harvest, venous stasis (prolonged holding off of the vein), struggling during venipuncture.
SAMPLE FOR COLLECTION AND ANY SPECIAL SPECIMEN HANDLING NOTES: Plasma (lithium heparin or sodium fluoride); must be centrifuged immediately and removed from erythrocytes. Refrigerate immediately or freeze.
PEARLS: Markedly elevated lactate concentrations have been associated with a poor prognosis in critical care settings. For example, dogs with gastric dilation/volvulus have a 99% survival rate if plasma lactate <6 mmol/L but a 58% survival rate if plasma lactate >6 mmol/L.

AUTHOR: **ROBIN W. ALLISON**

Lactate Dehydrogenase

BASIC INFORMATION

DEFINITION

Cytosolic enzyme found in most cells in the body.

TYPICAL NORMAL RANGE

Dogs: 50–380 U/L; cats: 46–350 U/L.

PHYSIOLOGY

Lactate dehydrogenase (LDH) catalyzes the oxidation of L-lactate to pyruvate and the reverse reaction. LDH is nonspecific because it is present in many tissues. It is concentrated in heart, skeletal muscle, liver, kidney, and erythrocytes. There are five LDH isoenzymes that can be separated electrophoretically. One is found primarily in cardiac muscle and another one is found primarily in skeletal muscle. Isoenzyme determination allows more specificity in identifying cardiac or skeletal muscle injury. LDH isoenzyme measurement is rarely performed because there are other more sensitive and specific markers of muscle and hepatic injury.

CAUSES OF ABNORMALLY HIGH LEVELS: Cardiac disease, skeletal muscle disease, renal damage, liver disease, and hemolysis.

NEXT DIAGNOSTIC STEP TO CONSIDER IF LEVELS HIGH: Evaluate for muscle injury, hepatic disease, or hemolytic anemia.

LAB ARTIFACTS THAT MAY INTERFERE WITH READINGS OF LEVELS OF THIS SUBSTANCE: Hemolysis results in false elevation because red blood cells contain LDH.

SAMPLE FOR COLLECTION AND ANY SPECIAL SPECIMEN HANDLING NOTES: Serum (red top). Store at 4°C.

AUTHOR: **RUANNA GOSSETT**

Lead, Blood Level

BASIC INFORMATION

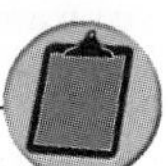

DEFINITION

Lead toxicity is relatively common. Exposure is usually by ingestion. Inhalation, dermal, subcutaneous/intramuscular exposure occur uncommonly.

TYPICAL TOXIC RANGE

- 0.6 ppm or greater is diagnostic.
- 0.35 ppm or greater with signs and confirmatory tests (δ-aminolevulinic acid [ALA] or fecal lead) is also diagnostic.

PHYSIOLOGY

- Although lead is poorly absorbed from the digestive tract, once absorbed, it is retained by tissues (kidney, bone). Blood levels may be elevated for 1 to 2 months after a single exposure. Levels decline slowly. Blood concentration indicates exposure but does not reflect exposure duration or total body concentration. Lead crosses the placental barrier and is excreted in the milk. Young animals are more susceptible to toxicity.
- Lead exposure results in increased urinary excretion of ALA and inhibits the conversion of coproporphyrinogen III to protoporphyrin and heme synthetase.
- The interference with hemoglobin synthesis, hemogram abnormalities such as basophilic stippling, and increased number of nucleated red blood cells in nonanemic patients are suggestive, but not diagnostic, of lead poisoning.

CAUSES OF ABNORMALLY HIGH LEVELS: Exposure to lead.

NEXT DIAGNOSTIC STEP TO CONSIDER IF LEVELS HIGH: Serum ALA dehydratase inhibition and erythrocyte protoporphyrin assays are highly sensitive tests for exposure and an indication of possible effect of lead. They are not a substitute for blood lead assay, which confirms the presence of lead. Fecal lead may be of benefit; a value of 35 ppm is suspect.

IMPORTANT INTERSPECIES DIFFERENCES: Less common in cats.

SAMPLE FOR COLLECTION AND ANY SPECIAL SPECIMEN HANDLING NOTES: Heparinized (green top) or ethylenediamine tetraacetic acid (lavender) whole blood. Ninety percent of circulating lead is bound to erythrocytes. Serum lead is *not* routinely used and is not readily interpretable.

PEARLS

- Kidney and liver tissue may be submitted if blood is not available. Kidney is considered preferable (≥10 ppm is diagnostic). Formalin fixed samples may be used for retrospective analyses.
- Chronic exposure is more likely than acute exposure.
- Blood levels and clinical signs do not always correlate. Blood levels are the best indicator of lead exposure, but may not indicate duration or dose of exposure.
- Ingested items containing lead may be seen radiographically.

AUTHOR: **SHERRY J. MORGAN**

Left Shift

BASIC INFORMATION

DEFINITION

The presence of band neutrophils (or earlier neutrophilic precursors such as metamyelocytes or myelocytes) in peripheral blood. This finding nearly always indicates active inflammation. When segmented neutrophils are also increased, the left shift can be described as "regenerative," suggesting appropriate marrow response to increased tissue demands for neutrophils. Alternately, when the segmented neutrophil count is unchanged or decreased, a left shift would be described as "degenerative," suggesting that the granulopoietic response of marrow is outweighed by tissue demand. That said, the use of these specific terms is not universally accepted.

TYPICAL NORMAL RANGE

- Dogs: 0–0.3 × 10^3 band neutrophils/μL.
- Cats: 0–0.2 × 10^3 band neutrophils/μL.

PHYSIOLOGY

Band neutrophils, metamyelocytes, and myelocytes are late precursors that normally remain in the marrow storage pool to differentiate into segmented neutrophils. If intense tissue demand for neutrophils during inflammation depletes the segmented neutrophils from the marrow storage pool, band neutrophils (and earlier precursors) can be prematurely released from the marrow into blood.

CAUSES OF ABNORMALLY HIGH LEVELS: Acute inflammation, granulocytic leukemia

NEXT DIAGNOSTIC STEP TO CONSIDER IF LEVELS HIGH: Identify source of inflammation.

SAMPLE FOR COLLECTION AND ANY SPECIAL SPECIMEN HANDLING NOTES: Ethylenediamine tetraacetic acid blood tube and freshly prepared blood smear for laboratory to stain

PEARLS

- Always examine stained blood smear for band neutrophils, because the neutrophil counts generated by automated hematology analyzers do not distinguish between segmented and band neutrophils. The presence of toxic changes in neutrophils is another indicator of intense inflammation.
- The hyposegmentation of Pelger Huët syndrome is not considered a left shift.

AUTHOR: **STEPHEN D. GAUNT**

Leptospira Serology, Canine

BASIC INFORMATION

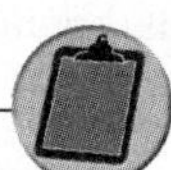

DEFINITION

Leptospirosis is a zoonotic disease caused by pathogenic serovars of *Leptospira interrogans*, a motile, spiral-shaped bacterium (spirochete). Serovars of importance include canicola, icterohaemorrhagiae, grippotyphosa, pomona, hardjo, bratislava, autumnalis.

TYPICAL NORMAL RANGE

Reported as titer values; panel of serovars varies among laboratories.

PHYSIOLOGY

- Organisms penetrate abraded skin and/or mucous membranes, replicate within bloodstream; rapid dissemination to multiple organs, most importantly liver and kidney (allows shedding in urine). Organisms replicate in the renal tubular epithelium, causing chronic tubulointerstitial nephritis and persistent carrier state if untreated.
- Vaccines elicit immunity against canicola and icterohaemorrhagiae serovars; newer vaccine (Fort Dodge Duramune) elicits immunity against these plus grippotyphosa and pomona.

CAUSES OF ABNORMALLY HIGH LEVELS: Microscopic agglutination test (MAT): a titer of ≥ 1:800 or fourfold rise in titer (paired serum 3 weeks apart) to a serovar against which the dog has not previously been vaccinated suggests active disease. Vaccine-induced titers are generally low (<1:800), but may be as high as 1:3200; these higher titers generally do not persist longer than 3 months.

NEXT DIAGNOSTIC STEP TO CONSIDER IF LEVELS HIGH: Polymerase chain reaction (PCR) using urine, blood, cerebrospinal fluid, aqueous humor, or tissue is possible, as is direct fluorescent antibody testing on tissue (kidney, liver). Darkfield microscopy or culture (blood, urine) prior to antibiotic therapy can be performed, but is technically difficult and not widely available.

CAUSES OF ABNORMALLY LOW LEVELS: Early infection, antibiotic treatment.

NEXT DIAGNOSTIC STEP TO CONSIDER IF LEVELS LOW: Enzyme-linked immunosorbent assay for immunoglobulin (Ig) G and IgM antileptospiral antibodies. IgM may be detected 1 week after infection. May be useful in detecting acute leptospirosis prior to IgG increase.

DRUG EFFECTS ON LEVELS: Antibiotic therapy may cause a decreased MAT titer, prevent a rising titer in paired sample, and cause negative PCR results and negative culture results.

SAMPLE FOR COLLECTION AND ANY SPECIAL SPECIMEN HANDLING NOTES: Collect 2 ml of serum (red-top tube). Stable for 4 days at 4°C or longer at 0°C.

PEARLS: The diagnosis can be missed if relevant serovars are excluded from serologic testing, because there is no consistent serologic cross-reactivity from one serovar to another. Serovars currently recommended for testing: canicola, pomona, grippotyphosa, bratislava, icterohaemorrhagiae, hardjo and autumnalis.

AUTHOR: **PATTY J. EWING**

Leukocyte Function Test

BASIC INFORMATION

DEFINITION

Tests of the *in vitro* ability of leukocytes to perform specific functions unique to that cell type (e.g., neutrophils, lymphocytes). These tests are not routine because the specific leukocyte may have to be isolated from blood. The tests are only available at research laboratories.

PHYSIOLOGY

Neutrophil function tests include measuring response to chemotatic stimuli, respiratory burst and release of oxidative metabolites, phagocytosis and killing of bacteria, and expression of activation cell markers (e.g., CD18). Monocytes are tested for ability to phagocytose particles. Lymphocyte tests include proliferative response to specific mitogens (e.g., concanavalin A, pokeweed mitogen), expression of B- and T-cell receptors and other markers using flow cytometry or polymerase chain reaction (PCR), and immunoelectrophoresis and quantitation of serum antibodies.

CAUSES OF ABNORMALLY LOW LEVELS

- Abnormal function of neutrophils: congenital disorders such as canine leukocyte adhesion defect, cyclic hematopoiesis of grey collies.
- Abnormal function of lymphocytes: congenital disorders such as severe combined immunodeficiency.

NEXT DIAGNOSTIC STEP TO CONSIDER IF LEVELS LOW: Tests are diagnostic of cell function abnormalities.

SAMPLE FOR COLLECTION AND ANY SPECIAL SPECIMEN HANDLING NOTES: The laboratory performing tests should be contacted for specific sample collection and shipment handling, although heparinized blood is typically used for leukocyte isolation and function testing.

AUTHOR: **STEPHEN D. GAUNT**

Leukocytes (Leukocytosis/Leukopenia)

BASIC INFORMATION

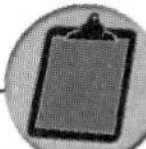

DEFINITION

Leukocyte is the term for blood cells that can be categorized as either granulocytic (neutrophils, eosinophils, and basophils) or mononuclear (lymphocytes and monocytes). Leukocytosis indicates an increase above the normal range; leukopenia indicates a decrease below the normal range.

SYNONYM(S)

White blood cells (WBC)

TYPICAL NORMAL RANGE

- Dogs: 6–17 × $10^3/\mu L$.
- Cats: 6–19 × 10^3 leukocytes/μL.

PHYSIOLOGY

Encompasses several different types of cells with different functions and kinetics. More specific analysis of neutrophils, lymphocytes, monocytes, eosinophils, and basophils is indicated. Changes in the number and morphology of each different leukocyte should be investigated.

CAUSES OF ABNORMALLY HIGH LEVELS: Increased numbers of neutrophils (neutrophilia) and lymphocytes (lymphocytosis) are the most common contributor to leukocytosis. Leukocytosis does not equal inflammation. Leukocytosis caused by inflammation can be accompanied by band neutrophils/left shift, toxic neutrophilic changes, or both. Leukocytosis should be interpreted with physical exam findings and other laboratory test results.

NEXT DIAGNOSTIC STEP TO CONSIDER IF LEVELS HIGH: Evaluate the absolute concentrations of each leukocyte type to determine the specific cause of leukocytosis.

CAUSES OF ABNORMALLY LOW LEVELS

- Leukopenia is most often attributed to neutropenia or lymphopenia.
- The most common next diagnostic step indicated in patients with persistent leukopenia attributed to neutropenia without an identifiable systemic cause is bone marrow aspiration for cytology, although in cats, retroviral testing (feline leukemia virus, feline immunodeficiency virus) should be performed first.

NEXT DIAGNOSTIC STEP TO CONSIDER IF LEVELS LOW: Evaluate the absolute concentration of each leukocyte type to determine the specific cause of leukopenia.

LAB ARTIFACTS THAT MAY INTERFERE WITH READINGS OF LEVELS OF THIS SUBSTANCE: Nucleated erythrocytes (NRBC) cannot be accurately differentiated from leukocytes by leukocyte counting instruments, so any NRBC present would add to the total leukocyte concentration. A formula must be used to calculate the number of total leukocytes: correct WBC/μL = counted WBC/μL × 100/100 + number of NRBC. Be aware that not all laboratories necessarily make this correction on the final complete blood count report.

SAMPLE FOR COLLECTION AND ANY SPECIAL SPECIMEN HANDLING NOTES: Ethylenediamine tetraacetic acid and freshly prepared blood smear for laboratory to stain

PEARLS

- Rather than the total leukocyte count (even if it is within the reference interval), the absolute concentrations of the individual leukocytes should be evaluated: neutrophil, lymphocyte, monocyte, eosinophil, and basophil.
- Severe leukocytosis (>50,000), regardless of cause, is associated with a guarded to poor prognosis.

AUTHOR: **STEPHEN D. GAUNT**

Lipase

BASIC INFORMATION

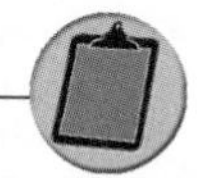

DEFINITION

Enzyme that hydrolyzes triglycerides to fatty acids and glycerol.

TYPICAL NORMAL RANGE

- Serum lipase activity based on enzymatic activity:
  - Dogs: 100–750 IU/L.
  - Cats: 10–195 IU/L.
- Pancreatic lipase immunoreactivity:
  - Dogs: 2.2–102.1 μg/L.
  - Cats: 2.0–6.8 μl/L.

PHYSIOLOGY

Lipase is present in pancreas, adipose tissue, gastric mucosa, and duodenal mucosa. Pancreatic lipase catabolizes triglycerides into fatty acids and glycerol, monoglycerides, and diglycerides in the proximal small intestine. Bile salts and colipase enhance the efficiency of lipase activity. The pancreas is considered the primary source of serum lipase concentration, although other tissues may contribute.

CAUSES OF ABNORMALLY HIGH LEVELS: Pancreatitis, renal failure, azotemia, hepatic disease, gastrointestinal disease (gastroenteritis, duodenal obstruction, peritonitis), neoplasia.

NEXT DIAGNOSTIC STEP TO CONSIDER IF LEVELS HIGH: Evaluate for pancreatitis (pancreatic lipase immunoreactivity, abdominal ultrasound) and renal disease.

CAUSES OF ABNORMALLY LOW LEVELS: Exocrine pancreatic insufficiency

NEXT DIAGNOSTIC STEP TO CONSIDER IF LEVELS LOW: Assess for pancreatic insufficiency (serum trypsin-like immunoreactivity).

IMPORTANT INTERSPECIES DIFFERENCES: Lipase measured by enzymatic activity is not a reliable indicator of pancreatitis in cats. Pancreatic lipase immunoreactivity is a more sensitive and specific test for diagnosis of pancreatitis in cats.

DRUG EFFECTS ON LEVELS: Dexamethasone and prednisone therapy increase lipase activity without concurrent increase in amylase.

LAB ARTIFACTS THAT MAY INTERFERE WITH READINGS OF LEVELS OF THIS SUBSTANCE: Decrease: lipemia, hemolysis, icterus.

SAMPLE FOR COLLECTION AND ANY SPECIAL SPECIMEN HANDLING NOTES: Serum (red top), heparinized plasma (green top) or ethylenediamine tetraacetic acid plasma (lavender top). Stable at 2–8° C for 3 weeks. Avoid freeze/thaw.

PEARLS: Degree of elevation in serum does not correlate with severity of pancreatitis; rather than using individual values, continued elevations, decreases, or plateau of levels are likely to provide more diagnostic information.

AUTHOR: **RUANNA GOSSETT**

Lipemia

BASIC INFORMATION

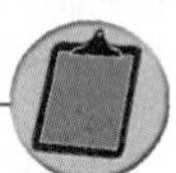

DEFINITION

Lipemia is the cloudy appearance of serum or plasma due to the presence of increased concentration of triglyceride rich lipoproteins (chylomicrons and very low density lipoproteins).

TYPICAL NORMAL RANGE

Normally absent from a fasting blood sample

PHYSIOLOGY

Lipemia may interfere with certain laboratory assays by causing dilution of substances in serum, or turbidity of the sample which affects the results of spectrophotometric assays. Lipemia causes hemolysis that contributes to interference with laboratory assays. Lipemia occurs in postprandial samples, primary hyperlipidemia, and secondary hyperlipidemia.

CAUSES OF ABNORMALLY HIGH LEVELS: Postprandial specimens, primary hyperlipidemia, secondary hyperlipidemia.

NEXT DIAGNOSTIC STEP TO CONSIDER IF LEVELS HIGH

- Determine if specimen is postprandial. Lipemia may be avoided by fasting for 12 to 24 hours prior to sample collection. Ultracentrifugation may clear lipemic serum. If lipemia in dogs persists with fasting, it may be cleared (for purposes of eliminating lipemia related artifacts) by injection of 100 U/kg of sodium heparin intravenously and collection of the blood sample 15 minutes later.
- Evaluation for causes of secondary hyperlipidemia (hypothyroidism, diabetes mellitus, acute pancreatitis, hyperadrenocorticism, nephrotic syndrome, and high fat diet) is indicated if lipemia is present in a fasted blood sample. If no evidence of these conditions is found, consider primary hyperlipidemia.

PEARLS

- Examples of analytes artifactually increased by lipemia include: hemoglobin, mean corpuscular hemoglobin concentration, triglycerides, plasma protein measured by refractometer, and spectrophotometric assays for glucose, calcium, phosphorus, and total bilirubin.
- Examples of analytes artifactually decreased by lipemia include: lipase, sodium, potassium, and aspartate aminotransferase.
- Hypercholesterolemia does *not* cause lipemia.

AUTHOR: **RUANNA GOSSETT**

Low-Dose Dexamethasone Suppression Test

BASIC INFORMATION

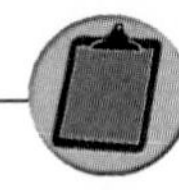

DEFINITION

Administration of dexamethasone suppresses production/release of hypothalamic corticosteroid releasing hormone (CRH) and pituitary adrenocorticotrophic hormone (ACTH), with subsequent reduction in production/release of cortisol from adrenal glands.

SYNONYM(S)

LDDST
Low-dose dex

TYPICAL NORMAL RANGE

Baseline cortisol: 10–160 nmol/L (dogs); 10–110 nmol/L (cats). After dexamethasone administration: expect cortisol concentration <40 nmol/L or <1.4 μg/dl (healthy dogs); <35 nmol/L (healthy cats). Reduction in cortisol concentration of 50% or more from baseline has also been interpreted as adequate suppression. Failure to suppress is strongly suggestive of hyperadrenocorticism (either pituitary based or primary adrenal based).

PHYSIOLOGY

Low-dose dexamethasone suppression test (LDDST) is a screening test for hyperadrenocorticism. Serum or plasma cortisol concentration is determined before administration (0.01 mg/kg intravenously) of dexamethasone. In health, hypothalamic CRH and pituitary ACTH production/release are suppressed for several hours with subsequent reduction in adrenal cortisol production/release. Cortisol half-life is 2 hours; at 4 and 8 hours postdexamethasone administration, cortisol concentration should be markedly decreased. LDDST virtually never causes adequately decreased cortisol in dogs with hyperadrenocorticism, but nonadrenal illness also may cause failure of LDDST to suppress cortisol levels (false positive).

CAUSES OF ABNORMALLY HIGH LEVELS (FAILURE TO SUPPRESS)

- Hyperadrenocorticism: pituitary dependent or adrenal neoplasia.
- Nonadrenal illness.

NEXT DIAGNOSTIC STEP TO CONSIDER IF LEVELS HIGH

- Abdominal ultrasound for adrenal enlargement.
- Repeat LDDST when other (nonadrenal) problems are controlled.

CAUSES OF ABNORMALLY LOW LEVELS (ADEQUATE SUPPRESSION): Patients with adequate cortisol suppression are either healthy (vast majority) or have pituitary dependent hyperadrenocorticism (rare exception).

NEXT DIAGNOSTIC STEP TO CONSIDER IF LEVELS LOW: Reassess history, physical exam, complete blood count, serum chemistry profile, urinalysis, blood pressure measurement, and abdominal ultrasound for other causes of clinical signs. If hyperadrenocorticism remains possible, LDDST may be repeated 1 to 3 months later.

IMPORTANT INTERSPECIES DIFFERENCES: Hyperadrenocorticism is extremely rare in cats.

DRUG EFFECTS ON LEVELS

- Immunoassays for cortisol measurement have significant cross reactivity with other glucocorticoids: prednisolone (69%), prednisone (6.4%), 11-deoxycortisol (7.5%), cortisone (4.2%), corticosterone (3.5%), spironolactone (<0.2%), and dexamethasone (<0.1%).
- Ketoconazole inhibits steroid biosynthesis causing low cortisol concentration.

SAMPLE FOR COLLECTION AND ANY SPECIAL SPECIMEN HANDLING NOTES

- Serum (red-top tube) or ethylenediamine tetraacetic acid (EDTA) plasma (lavender-top tube).
- Cortisol in EDTA plasma is more stable than in serum. Cool specimens are more stable than warm samples. Cortisol is equally distributed between red cells and plasma; therefore, rapid separation of plasma from cells (previously reported) is of no benefit.

PEARLS: Very small volumes of dexamethasone are used (0.01 mg/kg using dexamethasone 4 mg/ml equals 0.01 ml for a 4 kg [9 lb] dog, for example). Therefore, dead space in a regular syringe and needle hub should be considered. Either dilution (add dexamethasone to diluent, not the other way around) or use of an insulin syringe (no dead space in hub) should be considered for accurate dosing.

AUTHOR: **ELIZABETH G. WELLES**

LABORATORY TESTS

Lupus Erythematosus Preparation (LE Prep)

BASIC INFORMATION

DEFINITION

Preparation of incubated clotted blood crushed through a wire sieve. Fluid is collected and centrifuged; buffy coat is mixed with equal amounts of serum, smeared, and stained with Wright's stain or new methylene blue. Lupus erythematosus (LE) positive preparations show rosetting of neutrophils around nuclear material and LE cells (neutrophils with phagocytized smooth, homogeneous nuclear material).

SYNONYM(S)

LE clot test
LE prep
LE preparation

TYPICAL NORMAL RANGE

Reported as negative or positive. Positive test indicates active disease (systemic lupus erythematosus [SLE]).

PHYSIOLOGY

LE cell formation occurs in the presence of sufficient immunoglobulin G antibody to deoxyribonucleoprotein along with complement. This antinuclear antibody binds the nuclei of traumatized or nonviable leukocytes. Viable neutrophils then phagocytize the opsonized nuclear material, forming the LE cell.

CAUSES OF ABNORMALLY HIGH LEVELS: Active systemic lupus erythematosus

NEXT DIAGNOSTIC STEP TO CONSIDER IF LEVELS HIGH: Assess presence of antinuclear antibodies by indirect immunofluorescence (ANA test).

LAB ARTIFACTS THAT MAY INTERFERE WITH READINGS OF LEVELS OF THIS SUBSTANCE: Mere phagocytosis of nuclear material with intact chromatin

pattern (tart cell) does not constitute an LE cell.
SAMPLE FOR COLLECTION AND ANY SPECIAL SPECIMEN HANDLING NOTES: Five to 10 ml of blood in a glass test tube; heparinized blood (green-top tube) may also be used.

PEARLS

- LE cells may occur in skin lesions and joint fluid of patients with active SLE.
- Absence of LE cells does not rule out SLE: the test is specific (positive is true positive) but is a very poor screening test (positives are seen very uncommonly in patients with SLE).
- ANA testing and correlation with clinical signs are needed for diagnosis of SLE.

AUTHOR: **FIDELIA R. FERNANDEZ**

Lymphocyte (Lymphocytosis, Lymphopenia)

BASIC INFORMATION

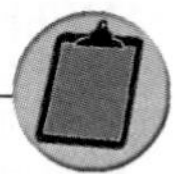

DEFINITION

The mononuclear leukocytes that mediate immune responses. Most lymphocytes are small with scant basophilic cytoplasm, although very low numbers have fine magenta granules clustered near nucleus (granular lymphocytes).

TYPICAL NORMAL RANGE

- Dogs: 1.0–5.0 × 10^3 lymphocytes/μL.
- Cats: 1.5–7.0 × 10^3 lymphocytes/μL.

PHYSIOLOGY

Most lymphocytes are produced in lymphoid tissues such as lymph nodes, spleen, and thymus. Lymphocytes are long-lived cells. They emigrate from blood into lymphoid tissues, but then circulate in the lymphatic system to re-enter venous circulation via the thoracic duct. Using surface receptors as markers, lymphocytes can be classified as T-lymphocytes (e.g., CD3 positive) that mediate cell-mediated responses, B-lymphocytes (e.g., CD79a positive) that mediate humoral responses, or null cells that mediate cytotoxicity. Most of the circulating lymphocytes in blood are T-cells.
CAUSES OF ABNORMALLY HIGH LEVELS

- Inflammatory diseases with antigenic stimulation
- Excitement with epinephrine release (especially young cats)
- Lymphoid neoplasms (e.g., leukemia, lymphoma)
- Hypoadrenocorticism ("relaxed" leukogram: lymphocytosis without neutrophilia in an obviously stressed animal)

NEXT DIAGNOSTIC STEP TO CONSIDER IF LEVELS HIGH: Evaluate for causes listed, depending on clinical signs.
CAUSES OF ABNORMALLY LOW LEVELS

- Endogenous or exogenous glucocorticoids (stress leukogram)
- Acute inflammation (especially viral infections)
- Disruption of lymphatic flow (e.g., chylothorax, lymphadenopathy, lymphangiectasia)
- Immunodeficiency (e.g., severe combined immunodeficiency)

NEXT DIAGNOSTIC STEP TO CONSIDER IF LEVELS LOW: Evaluate for causes listed, depending on clinical signs.
DRUG EFFECTS ON LEVELS: Glucocorticoids cause lymphopenia by causing sequestration of lymphocytes in lymphoid tissue and lympholysis.
SAMPLE FOR COLLECTION AND ANY SPECIAL SPECIMEN HANDLING NOTES: Ethylenediamine tetraacetic acid tube and freshly prepared blood smear for laboratory to stain.
PEARLS: In evaluating lymphocytosis, cell morphology is important. Significantly increased numbers of large or atypical lymphocytes indicate lymphoblastic leukemia, whereas a marked increase in small, well-differentiated lymphocytes occurs with chronic lymphocytic leukemia.

AUTHOR: **STEPHEN D. GAUNT**

Magnesium

BASIC INFORMATION

DEFINITION

Essential nutrient, major divalent cation. Serum total magnesium includes protein bound (30%), anion complexed (15%), and ionized (55%) fractions.

SYNONYM(S)

Mg
Mg^{2+}

TYPICAL NORMAL RANGE

- Range: 1.5–2.7 mg/dl
- Unit conversion: mg/dl × 0.4114 = mEq/L; mEq/L × 0.5 = mmol/L

PHYSIOLOGY

Sources: dietary; commercial foods are fortified. Absorbed in small intestine; vitamin D may enhance absorption. Excreted in urine, feces, milk. Extracellular fluids contain <2% of total, bone contains 50–60%, remainder is intracellular. Shifts from extracellular to intracellular compartments. Ionized Mg is the biologically active form.
CAUSES OF ABNORMALLY HIGH LEVELS

- Decreased urinary excretion (decreased glomerular filtration rate, renal failure).
- Uncommon: excess oral administration (antacids, laxatives), intravenous Mg.

NEXT DIAGNOSTIC STEP TO CONSIDER IF LEVELS HIGH

- Evaluate renal function.
- Review oral and parenteral supplements.

CAUSES OF ABNORMALLY LOW LEVELS

- Hypoproteinemia: decreases protein-bound Mg; no effect on ionized Mg.
- Excess urinary excretion: diuresis; renal tubular disease.
- Inadequate gastrointestinal absorption: chronic diarrhea, malabsorption syndromes, binding to other nutrients (excess fatty acids, oxalate, phosphate, fiber).

- Shifts from extracellular to intracellular compartments: treatment for diabetic ketoacidosis (insulin, bicarbonate infusions).
- Diabetes mellitus, hyperparathyroidism, hyperthyroidism, pancreatitis, trauma, sepsis may predispose.

NEXT DIAGNOSTIC STEP TO CONSIDER IF LEVELS LOW

- Measure serum albumin; measure serum ionized magnesium.
- Evaluate for renal, gastrointestinal disease as a primary or contributing cause.

DRUG EFFECTS ON LEVELS

- Renal excretion increased by loop and osmotic diuretics, and drug-induced renal tubular injury (e.g., aminoglycosides, cisplatin, amphotericin B).
- Insulin, glucose, or bicarbonate infusions promote intracellular shifting, decreasing serum Mg.
- Administration of Mg-containing laxatives, antacids causes increases.

LAB ARTIFACTS THAT MAY INTERFERE WITH READINGS OF LEVELS OF THIS SUBSTANCE

- Falsely increased by hemolysis or delayed removal of serum from clot.
- Falsely decreased if anticoagulants that bind Mg are used (ethylenediamine tetraacetic acid [purple-top tube], citrate [blue-top tube], oxalate).

SAMPLE FOR COLLECTION AND ANY SPECIAL SPECIMEN HANDLING NOTES: Serum preferred (red-top tube); heparinized plasma (green-top tube) may be used. Remove serum from erythrocytes promptly after centrifugation.

PEARLS: Concurrent hypocalcemia, hypokalemia may be refractory to therapy until hypomagnesemia is corrected.

AUTHOR: **ROBIN W. ALLISON**

Methemoglobinemia, Methemoglobinuria

BASIC INFORMATION

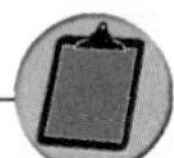

DEFINITION

Methemoglobinemia: accumulation of methemoglobin in blood. Methemoglobinuria: presence of methemoglobin in urine. Methemoglobin has an iron moiety that has been oxidized to the ferric (Fe^{3+}) state.

SYNONYM(S)

MetHb

TYPICAL NORMAL RANGE

- Methemoglobin spot test: drop of venous blood on a white paper towel normally is bright red; if methemoglobin concentration is >10%, spot remains dark with a brown tinge.
- Blood/urine levels: methemoglobin normally represents <1% of total hemoglobin.

PHYSIOLOGY

Increased production of methemoglobin results from exposure to oxidant chemicals, drugs, plants, or decreased reduction of methemoglobin due to a hereditary deficiency of erythrocyte methemoglobin reductase. Methemoglobin cannot bind and carry oxygen to tissue. If sufficient amounts of methemoglobin are present, low blood oxygen tension (hypoxia) results.

CAUSES OF ABNORMALLY HIGH LEVELS: Hereditary deficiency of methemoglobin reductase, or exposure to oxidant chemicals (nitrite, copper), drugs (e.g., acetaminophen, benzocaine, phenazopyridine, zinc), or plants.

NEXT DIAGNOSTIC STEP TO CONSIDER IF LEVELS HIGH

- If spot test is positive, consider arterial blood gas, pulse oximetry and co-oximetry analysis, if available.
- Complete blood count to determine if hemolytic anemia is present, because it is a common sequela to oxidant injury of erythrocytes.
- Evaluation of red blood cell morphology for Heinz bodies and eccentrocytes (hallmarks of oxidant injury).
- Methemoglobin reductase level determination if hereditary deficiency is suspected.

SAMPLE FOR COLLECTION AND ANY SPECIAL SPECIMEN HANDLING NOTES

- Collect 0.5 ml of anticoagulated blood (ethylenediamine tetraacetic acid tube [EDTA]) for spot test.
- Methemoglobin reductase level determination: Prior arrangements must be made with a laboratory before submitting samples. One milliliter anticoagulated blood (EDTA tube) should be refrigerated and sent chilled (not frozen) to a laboratory allowing assay to be done the same day the specimen is collected. One or more samples collected from normal animals should be submitted with the patient samples for use as controls.

PEARLS

- Severe methemoglobinemia produces chocolate brown discoloration of the blood.
- Most chemicals producing methemoglobinemia also produce Heinz body hemolytic anemia.

AUTHOR: **SHERRY J. MORGAN**

Monocyte (Monocytosis, Monocytopenia)

BASIC INFORMATION

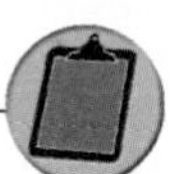

DEFINITION

Largest leukocyte on blood smear. It has an oval to lobulated nucleus and gray-basophilic cytoplasm with fine azurophilic granules and occasionally clear vacuoles. Monocytes become macrophages in tissues and fluids.

SYNONYM(S)

Leukocyte
White blood cell

TYPICAL NORMAL RANGE

- Dogs: $0.1–1.5 \times 10^3$ monocytes/μL.
- Cats: $0–1.0 \times 10^3$ monocytes/μL.

PHYSIOLOGY

Monocytes are produced in the marrow with a short transit time from monoblast to monocyte, which quickly enters blood. Monocytes and macrophages are involved in several different functions that include killing bacteria and fungi, presenting antigens to lymphocytes, removal of necrotic and apoptotic cell debris, and erythrocyte destruction.

CAUSES OF ABNORMALLY HIGH LEVELS

- Inflammation, acute or chronic
- Stress leukogram, from endogenous or exogenous glucocorticoids
- Monocytic leukemia, myelomonocytic leukemia

NEXT DIAGNOSTIC STEP TO CONSIDER IF LEVELS HIGH: Evaluate for given causes, depending on clinical signs.

CAUSES OF ABNORMALLY LOW LEVELS: Monocytopenia is not considered a clinically significant abnormality because monocytes can normally occur in very low numbers.

SAMPLE FOR COLLECTION AND ANY SPECIAL SPECIMEN HANDLING NOTES: Blood in ethylenediamine tetraacetic acid (lavender top) and freshly prepared blood smear for laboratory to stain

PEARLS: After acute onset of neutropenia caused by transient suppression of hematopoiesis (e.g., chemotherapy), monocytes return to high levels in blood sooner than neutrophils. Therefore, in neutropenic patients, monocytosis can signal return of hematopoietic function and impending resolution of neutropenia.

AUTHOR: **STEPHEN D. GAUNT**

Mycobacterial Culture

BASIC INFORMATION

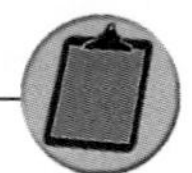

DEFINITION

Growth, isolation, and identification of *Mycobacterium* spp.

TYPICAL NORMAL RANGE

Reported as growth or no growth, with identification of organisms.

PHYSIOLOGY

Organisms may be intermittent in respiratory specimens (tracheal exudate) but should be constant in solid tissue specimens (skin, lymph node). The organism must be isolated from other flora and grown in media specific for *Mycobacteria* spp. Growth and identification of these fastidious organisms may take 2 to 4 months.

CAUSES OF ABNORMALLY HIGH LEVELS: Infection with *Mycobacterium* spp. Common sites of infection include skin and respiratory tract. Infections may become systemic, involving lymphatics system and bone marrow.

NEXT DIAGNOSTIC STEP TO CONSIDER IF LEVELS HIGH: Determine appropriate antibiotic for treatment.

IMPORTANT INTERSPECIES DIFFERENCES

- Feline leprosy (*M. lepraemurium*) and atypical mycobacteriosis (*M. avium, M. fortuitum, M. thermoresistibile, M. xenopi, M. phlei and M. smegmatis*) are considered unique to the cat.
- Dogs, especially basset hounds, are susceptible to systemic disease caused by *M. avium*.
- Humans can transmit *M. bovis* to dogs.

DRUG EFFECTS ON LEVELS: Concurrent or recent antibiotic therapy may inhibit growth.

LAB ARTIFACTS THAT MAY INTERFERE WITH READINGS OF LEVELS OF THIS SUBSTANCE: Contamination or overgrowth by commensal organisms may mask growth.

SAMPLE FOR COLLECTION AND ANY SPECIAL SPECIMEN HANDLING NOTES: Tissue or exudate from lesion in a sterile container. If zoonotic *Mycobacterium* spp. is suspected, the container should have a screw top and a double outer container should be used; label as biohazard. Submit to laboratory as soon as possible.

PEARLS

- Cutaneous or localized infections are more likely to become systemic in immunocompromised hosts. Immunocompromised owners may be susceptible to infection.
- Fine needle aspirates of solid tissue lesions are characterized by macrophages containing rod-shaped organisms that appear as negative images with Wright-Giemsa or Diff-Quik stains.
- Organisms will stain with acid-fast stains.

AUTHOR: **LOIS ROTH-JOHNSON**

Mycoplasma spp. Culture

BASIC INFORMATION

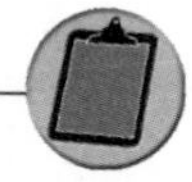

DEFINITION

Laboratory growth of infectious *Mycoplasma* spp. agents to allow isolation and identification.

TYPICAL NORMAL RANGE

Reported as no growth or growth with identification of pathogens

PHYSIOLOGY

Mycoplasma spp. are the smallest, simplest self-replicating bacteria. Infection is uncommon but is associated with arthritis, respiratory disease, and conjunctivitis, especially in immunocompromised patients. The organism is fastidious and grows slowly in culture.

CAUSES OF ABNORMALLY HIGH LEVELS: Infection is associated with arthritis, respiratory disease, and conjunctivitis.

NEXT DIAGNOSTIC STEP TO CONSIDER IF LEVELS HIGH: Assess immune function because clinical disease is more likely in immunocompromised patients.

IMPORTANT INTERSPECIES DIFFERENCE: Diseases caused by *Mycoplasma* spp. are uncommon in cats and dogs. Mycoplasmal conjunctivitis and respiratory disease are more likely to occur in cats; arthritis is more likely to occur in dogs.

DRUG EFFECTS ON LEVELS: Glucocorticoid or other immunosuppressive therapies may enhance growth.

LAB ARTIFACTS THAT MAY INTERFERE WITH READINGS OF LEVELS OF THIS SUBSTANCE: Contamination with commensals may mask growth. Organism takes a long time to grow in culture and cultures may be discarded inadvertently if laboratory personnel are not informed that *Mycoplasma* spp. infection is suspected.

SAMPLE FOR COLLECTION AND ANY SPECIAL SPECIMEN HANDLING NOTES: Swabs, exudate, or tissue should be submitted in specific transport media to enhance growth. Laboratory should be contacted to obtain media for sample submission.

PEARLS: Growth in culture may take up to two weeks: serologic tests or polymerase chain reaction should be used for confirming infection.

AUTHOR: **LOIS ROTH-JOHNSON**

Myoglobinemia, Myoglobinuria

BASIC INFORMATION

DEFINITION

Myoglobin is a low molecular weight heme protein found in muscle tissue.

TYPICAL NORMAL RANGE

- Serum myoglobin in dogs: <10.0–136.0 ng/ml; cats <10.0–13.8 ng/ml.
- Not present in urine of healthy animals.

PHYSIOLOGY

Myoglobin stores and transports oxygen in muscle fibers. It is released from muscle when there is severe disruption of the muscle membrane or necrosis. Myoglobin is detected in the serum within 2 to 4 hours after injury. Myoglobin does not significantly bind serum proteins. It passes quickly through the glomerulus and is excreted in urine. Red to brown urine discoloration due to myoglobinuria occurs before plasma appears discolored (observable hemoglobinemia). Myoglobin causes a positive occult blood test on urine dipstick and must be distinguished from blood or hemoglobin in the urine.

CAUSES OF ABNORMALLY HIGH LEVELS: Trauma, ischemia, toxic injury, or necrosis of muscle tissue

NEXT DIAGNOSTIC STEP TO CONSIDER IF LEVELS HIGH: Evaluate for muscle injury or necrosis (e.g., serum creatine kinase level) versus laboratory evidence of hemolysis.

LAB ARTIFACTS THAT MAY INTERFERE WITH READINGS OF LEVELS OF THIS SUBSTANCE: False positive reaction for blood on urine dipstick is due to high bilirubin concentration, contamination of urine with oxidizing agents in disinfectants, leukocytes, bacteria, peroxidase, or iodine.

SAMPLE FOR COLLECTION AND ANY SPECIAL SPECIMEN HANDLING NOTES

- Myoglobinemia: serum (red top), heparinized plasma (green top), or ethylenediamine tetraacetic acid plasma (lavender top). Refrigerate at 2–8°C.
- Myoglobinuria: 1 ml urine.

PEARLS: To distinguish myoglobinuria from hemoglobinuria and hematuria, examine serum and urine sediment. To distinguish myoglobinuria from hemoglobinuria and hematuria, examine serum and urine sediment. In a patient with a positive blood result on urine dipstick, evaluate color of serum (e.g., in microhematocrit tube); pink discoloration indicates hemolysis and suggests hemoglobinuria as cause for positive urine blood result. If no evidence of hemolysis, evaluate urine sediment for presence of red blood cells, which indicates hematuria as cause for positive urine blood result. If no hematuria and no hemolysis, positive blood result on urine dipstick is due to myoglobinuria by process of elimination and it may be confirmed with an ammonium sulphate precipitation test on urine.

AUTHOR: **RUANNA GOSSETT**

Neospora caninum Serology

BASIC INFORMATION

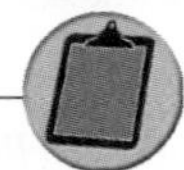

DEFINITION

Detection of serum antibody to *Neospora caninum* by immunofluorescent assay (IFA) or enzyme-linked immunosorbent assay (ELISA).

PHYSIOLOGY

N. caninum is a coccidian parasite whose morphology is identical to *Toxoplasma gondii* under light microscopy. Clinical manifestations of *N. caninum* in dogs are primarily neurologic and musculoskeletal. Transplacental transmission occurs.

CAUSES OF ABNORMALLY HIGH LEVELS

- Infection with, or prior exposure to, *N. caninum*. Rising titer (>fourfold) confirms active infection. Positive cerebrospinal fluid titers are considered suggestive of disease.
- IFA tests have little cross reactivity with other parasites, including *T. gondii*. However, cross reactivity depends on the antigen source used for the assay (among other things) and may vary.
- Most dogs with confirmed neosporosis have titers ≥200. High titers have been found in clinically normal dogs suggesting subclinical disease.

NEXT DIAGNOSTIC STEP TO CONSIDER IF LEVELS HIGH: Treatment for neosporosis, if clinical signs are compatible with this disease.

IMPORTANT INTERSPECIES DIFFERENCES: Serologic tests use species specific reagents and must be adapted for the species of interest. Cats have been experimentally infected, but clinically neosporosis in cats is unknown; natural disease in small animals is mainly seen in dogs. *N. caninum* is an important cause of abortion in ruminants.

SAMPLE FOR COLLECTION AND ANY SPECIAL SPECIMEN HANDLING NOTES: Serum, refrigerated.

PEARLS

- Diagnosis is sometimes made via observation of tachyzoites of *N. caninum* in biopsy/necropsy tissue or in cytologic preparations. The morphology of the tachyzoites of *N. caninum* and *T. gondii* is identical, but differentiation can be made via direct fluorescent antibody or immunohistochemistry of tissue samples using species specific antibodies. Alternatively, molecular techniques (PCR) have been used for differentiating the two organisms.
- Almost all commercially available laboratory tests for antibody are for immunoglobulin G.

AUTHOR: **JAMES H. MEINKOTH**

Neutrophil (Neutrophilia, Neutropenia)

BASIC INFORMATION

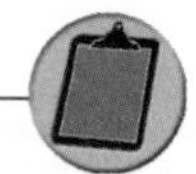

DEFINITION

Blood leukocyte with segmented nucleus and inconspicuous cytoplasmic granules. Its primary functions during inflammation are phagocytosis and killing bacteria.

SYNONYM(S)

Polymorphonuclear neutrophil (PMN)
Segmented neutrophil

TYPICAL NORMAL RANGE

- Dogs: 3.0–11.5 × 10^3 neutrophils/µL.
- Cats: 2.5–12.5 × 10^3 neutrophils/µL.

PHYSIOLOGY

Precursors in bone marrow respond to colony-stimulating factors produced during inflammatory and immune responses. Mature neutrophils are initially retained in marrow as part of *storage pool*. In blood, neutrophils occur either in the *circulating pool* or are associated with endothelial cells as *marginal pool*, and then emigrate into tissue. Neutrophils circulate for only a few hours. In blood samples collected for complete blood count, only neutrophils in circulating pool are counted.

CAUSES OF ABNORMALLY HIGH LEVELS (NEUTROPHILIA)

- Inflammation, whether acute or chronic, infectious or noninfectious. If acute inflammation, left shift and/or toxic changes may be present.
- Stress leukogram (glucocorticoids shift neutrophils from marrow storage pool and from marginal pool into circulating pool).
- Excitement leukocytosis (increased blood flow shifts neutrophils from marginal to circulating pool).
- Paraneoplastic production of colony-stimulating factor.
- Granulocytic leukemia.
- Canine leukocyte adhesion deficiency.

NEXT DIAGNOSTIC STEP TO CONSIDER IF LEVELS HIGH: Assess for cause depending on clinical signs.

CAUSES OF ABNORMALLY LOW LEVELS (NEUTROPENIA)

- Intense inflammation (increased tissue demand)
- Endotoxemia (shift from circulating to marginal pool)
- Acute parvoviral infection (decreased marrow production and endotoxemia)
- Decreased granulopoiesis (e.g., feline leukemia virus [FeLV] infection, feline immunodeficiency virus [FIV] infection, drugs [see below], myelophthisis)
- Destruction of mature neutrophils (e.g., immune-mediated)
- Previous use of recombinant human colony stimulating factor.

NEXT DIAGNOSTIC STEP TO CONSIDER IF LEVELS LOW: Bone marrow aspirate or core biopsy

IMPORTANT INTERSPECIES DIFFERENCES

- Neutrophilia from excitement is more likely in young cats, whereas neutrophilia from glucocorticoids (stress leukogram) is more likely in dogs.
- Dogs typically have higher degrees of neutrophilia than cats.
- Belgian Tervuren dogs have benign, familial neutropenia.
- Cats may have benign, idiopathic neutropenia (diagnosis of exclusion).

DRUG EFFECTS ON LEVELS

- Increase: glucocorticoids.
- Decrease: albendazole, methimazole, trimethoprim-sulfa, many chemotherapeutic anticancer agents, many others.

SAMPLE FOR COLLECTION AND ANY SPECIAL SPECIMEN HANDLING NOTES: Ethylenediamine tetraacetic acid tube of blood and freshly prepared blood smear for laboratory to stain

PEARLS: Inflammation is not the only cause of neutrophilia; other causes are stress leukogram and excitement leukocytosis.

AUTHOR: **STEPHEN D. GAUNT**

Parathyroid Hormone

BASIC INFORMATION

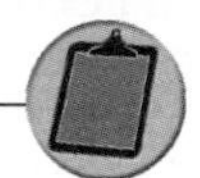

DEFINITION

Hormone produced by parathyroid glands in response to low blood calcium levels; important in the rapid and precise regulation of calcium.

SYNONYM(S)

Parathormone
PTH

TYPICAL NORMAL RANGE

- Canine and feline: 2–13 pmol/L.
- Results may vary among laboratories and the established reference ranges for the laboratory should be used for exact interpretation of results.

PHYSIOLOGY

Parathyroid hormone (PTH) acts directly on the bone and kidney and indirectly on the intestine to increase serum calcium levels. PTH acts on the kidney to increase renal excretion of phosphate, increase tubular resorption of calcium and convert vitamin D precursors to active vitamin D (which, along with PTH, increases calcium absorption from the gastrointestinal tract). PTH acts on the bone to mobilize calcium and phosphate. Ultimately, these actions result in elevation of blood calcium and hypophosphatemia.

CAUSES OF ABNORMALLY HIGH LEVELS: Hyperparathyroidism: primary hyperparathyroidism (parathyroid adenoma/hyperplasia), multiple endocrine neoplasia, chronic renal disease (renal secondary hyperparathyroidism), pseudohyperparathyroidism (decreased PTH receptor receptiveness). Rare: nutritional secondary hyperparathyroidism.

NEXT DIAGNOSTIC STEP TO CONSIDER IF LEVELS HIGH: Serum ionized calcium, complete blood count, serum chemistry profile, urinalysis, thoracic and abdominal imaging of other endocrine organs.

CAUSES OF ABNORMALLY LOW LEVELS: Parathyroid inflammation and degeneration (lymphocytic parathyroiditis) and inadvertent surgical removal of parathyroid (thyroidectomy in cats), decreased PTH production due to inhibition (hypervitaminosis D, hypercalcemic disorders except primary hyperparathyroidism).

NEXT DIAGNOSTIC STEP TO CONSIDER IF LEVELS LOW: Same as for elevated PTH

LAB ARTIFACTS THAT MAY INTERFERE WITH READINGS OF LEVELS OF THIS SUBSTANCE: Prolonged storage or thawing of sample may cause artificial results, either increased or decreased.

SAMPLE FOR COLLECTION (TYPE OF SPECIMEN, COLOR TUBE) AND ANY SPECIAL SPECIMEN HANDLING NOTES: Serum is used for the assay. The samples should be centrifuged immediately after clotting, frozen, and shipped frozen for analysis as soon as possible.

PEARLS: It is important to know both the serum ionized calcium and the PTH levels in order to correctly correlate the laboratory results. For example, ionized hypercalcemia should cause PTH levels to be low or undetectable; PTH levels in the mid- or high-normal range (or higher) with concurrently elevated ionized calcium suggest primary hyperparathyroidism.

AUTHOR: **DEBORAH G. DAVIS**

Parathyroid Hormone Related Protein

BASIC INFORMATION

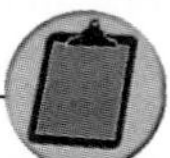

DEFINITION

Humoral factor with a molecular structure similar to parathyroid hormone (PTH); can bind to PTH receptors. It plays an important role in humoral hypercalcemia of malignancy.

SYNONYM(S)

Parathormone
Parathyroid hormone
PTHrP

TYPICAL NORMAL RANGE

Not normally found circulating in the blood. Canine: <2 pmol/L.

PHYSIOLOGY

Produced in minimal amounts in tissues of normal adults and functions in a paracrine manner. In humoral hypercalcemia of malignancy, neoplastic cells secrete excess amounts of PTH related protein (PTHrP) and other cytokines. PTHrP binds to the PTH receptors in the bone and kidney and mimics the effects of PTH. It results in osteoclastic bone resorption, increased renal resorption of calcium and decreased renal resorption of phosphate. Malignancies associated with increased levels of PTHrP are T-cell lymphoma, thymoma, and apocrine gland adenocarcinoma of the anal sac. Sporadic cases of humoral hypercalcemia of malignancy have been seen with other carcinomas as well.

CAUSES OF ABNORMALLY HIGH LEVELS: Humoral hypercalcemia of malignancy.

NEXT DIAGNOSTIC STEP TO CONSIDER IF LEVELS HIGH: Review physical exam, including rectal palpation in all dogs (apocrine gland adenocarcinoma, sublumbar lymphadenopathy). Serum ionized calcium, serum phosphorus, serum PTH. Humoral hypercalcemia of malignancy usually causes elevated ionized calcium level, low-normal or low PTH level, and low phosphorus level. Complete blood count, serum chemistry profile, urinalysis, and diagnostic imaging to identify and define extent of neoplastic disease.

LAB ARTIFACTS THAT MAY INTERFERE WITH READINGS OF LEVELS OF THIS SUBSTANCE: Thawing causes degradation of the protein and interferes with validity of results (either falsely increasing or decreasing).

SAMPLE FOR COLLECTION AND ANY SPECIAL SPECIMEN HANDLING NOTES: See laboratory for specifics. If serum is sent, immediately spin the sample after it clots, separate serum, and freeze. Ship frozen. If plasma is used, ethylenediamine tetraacetic acid (purple top) with a protease inhibitor (apoprotinin or leupeptin) should be added. Plasma should be separated from the erythrocytes and shipped frozen.

PEARLS: Three mechanisms can cause cancer-associated hypercalcemia: humoral hypercalcemia of malignancy, local bone resorption induced by hematologic neoplasms growing into the bone marrow (multiple myeloma), and local bone resorption induced by metastatic bone lesions.

AUTHOR: **DEBORAH G. DAVIS**

Pelger Huët

BASIC INFORMATION

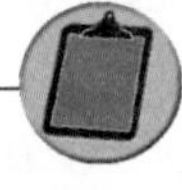

DEFINITION

A congenital defect in nuclear lobulation of leukocytes that is rarely reported in dogs and cats. The characteristic appearance of a hyposegmented nucleus is most evident in neutrophils, but also occurs in eosinophils, basophils, monocytes, and megakaryocytes. The nuclear shape of affected neutrophils can be bilobed ("pince nez" cell), band, round, or oval, similar to neutrophilic precursors, but the nuclear chromatin of affected neutrophils is coarsely condensed, similar to mature neutrophils.

SYNONYM(S)

Pelger Huët anomaly
Pelger Huët syndrome
Pseudo Pelger-Huët

PHYSIOLOGY

Segmented neutrophils in dogs and cats typically have three to five nuclear lobes. In the congenital form of Pelger-Huët, heterozygotes are most common and exhibit hyposegmented neutrophils, many of which resemble band neutrophils. The heterozygous condition is considered benign because affected animals have no ill effects and neutrophil function tests are not significantly altered. The low incidence of homozygotes is attributed to embryonic death. Rarely, during the course of severe inflammatory disease in unaffected animals, hyposegmentation of neutrophils will occur as a transient, reversible condition ("pseudo" Pelger Huët).

SAMPLE FOR COLLECTION AND ANY SPECIAL SPECIMEN HANDLING NOTES: Ethylenediamine tetraacetic acid blood and freshly prepared blood smear for laboratory to stain.

PEARLS

- When an otherwise unremarkable complete blood count report has a significant left shift in an apparently healthy dog or cat, consider the likelihood of Pelger Huët anomaly.
- Pelger Huët is essentially an incidental finding with no clinical adverse effect.

AUTHOR: **STEPHEN D. GAUNT**

Phenobarbital Serum Level

BASIC INFORMATION

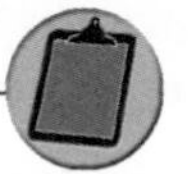

DEFINITION

Used for monitoring patients receiving phenobarbital for treating seizures, and for determining if therapeutic or potentially toxic levels have been reached.

SYNONYM(S)

PB
PhB
Pheno

TYPICAL NORMAL RANGE

Therapeutic range: 15–40 μg/ml.

PHYSIOLOGY

The elimination half-life of orally administered phenobarbital in dogs ranges widely, from 12 to 125 hours (average approximately 48 hours). Peak levels occur 4 to 8 hours after administration. Pharmacokinetics can be altered by chronic administration, concurrent disease (especially liver disease), age, and concurrent administration of other drugs. For this reason, monitoring of serum drug levels at steady state (14 to 16 days after starting treatment) is recommended. Peak and trough levels, which were previously recommended, are not considered necessary for making therapeutic decisions.

CAUSES OF ABNORMALLY HIGH LEVELS: Greater than 45 μg/ml: considered toxic.

NEXT DIAGNOSTIC STEP TO CONSIDER IF LEVELS HIGH: Correlate levels with clinical signs (i.e., presence or absence of seizures). Consider effect that concurrently administered drugs or concurrent disease may be having on pharmacokinetics. Evaluate a liver profile. Whether liver disease, other disease, or drugs are present, high levels should prompt the consideration of dose reduction, with institution of a second antiseizure drug if needed.

CAUSES OF ABNORMALLY LOW LEVELS: Serum levels <10 μg/ml are subtherapeutic.

NEXT DIAGNOSTIC STEP TO CONSIDER IF LEVELS LOW: Correlate drug levels with clinical signs (seizures).

DRUG EFFECTS ON LEVELS: Concurrent administration of many other drugs, such as certain antibiotics (e.g., doxycycline, chloramphenicol, metronidazole), anticoagulants (warfarin), cardiopulmonary drugs (e.g., aminophylline/theophylline, certain β-blockers, quinidine), glucocorticoids (prednisone, others) and many others, may increase or decrease levels of phenobarbital. Consult a pharmacology textbook or pharmacist for information regarding specific drug interactions.

LAB ARTIFACTS THAT MAY INTERFERE WITH READINGS OF LEVELS OF THIS SUBSTANCE: Collection of blood in a serum separator tube can falsely decrease levels. Moderate to marked lipemia or icterus may also interfere with determination of drug levels.

SAMPLE FOR COLLECTION AND ANY SPECIAL SPECIMEN HANDLING NOTES: One milliliter of serum (not in serum separator tube).

PEARLS

- Measurement of peak and/or trough levels, which were previously recommended, are not considered necessary for making therapeutic decisions.
- Phenobarbital is involved in many drug interactions; consult a pharmacology textbook or pharmacist if multiple medications.

AUTHOR: **SHERRY J. MORGAN**

Phosphorus

BASIC INFORMATION

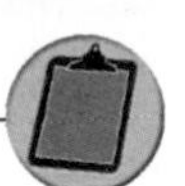

DEFINITION

Inorganic form of phosphate; the major intracellular anion; primarily located in bone (as hydroxyapatite) with the remainder in soft tissues and in the circulation.

SYNONYM(S)

Phosphate

TYPICAL NORMAL RANGE

- Canine: 3.2–8.1 mg/dl (1.03 to 2.61 mmol/L).
- Feline: 3.2–6.5 mg/dl (1.03 to 2.09 mmol/L).

PHYSIOLOGY

Clinical assays measure only the total inorganic phosphorus, although both organic and inorganic phosphorus are present. Form depends on pH. Blood levels are affected by intestinal absorption, shifting between intracellular and extracellular compartments, renal clearance, and animal age. Parathyroid hormone (PTH) triggers phosphaturia.

CAUSES OF ABNORMALLY HIGH LEVELS: Decreased glomerular filtration rate (decreased renal excretion due to renal failure, prerenal or postrenal azotemia), hypoparathyroidism, acromegaly, increased intestinal absorption (phosphate enema, increased vitamin D, ischemic intestinal lesions), myopathies, hyperthyroidism in cats, osteolytic bone lesions, normal bone growth.

NEXT DIAGNOSTIC STEP TO CONSIDER IF LEVELS HIGH

- Rule out artifact (repeat test).
- Evaluate kidney function, rule out urinary obstruction or rupture; determine PTH levels, thyroid hormone level (cats), ionized calcium; survey skeletal radiographs.

CAUSES OF ABNORMALLY LOW LEVELS: Increased renal excretion (Fanconi syndrome in dogs, prolonged diuresis), prolonged anorexia, intestinal malabsorption, hypovitaminosis D, humoral hypercalcemia of malignancy, primary hyperparathyroidism, hyperinsulinism (endogenous or treatment for diabetic ketoacidosis)

NEXT DIAGNOSTIC STEP TO CONSIDER IF LEVELS LOW: Complete blood count/chemistry profile/urinalysis, rule out artifact, iatrogenic, ionized calcium

DRUG EFFECTS ON LEVELS

- Decrease: phosphate binding antacids, anesthetics, diuretics, insulin, anticonvulsants, bicarbonate, mithramycin, salicylates.
- Increase: phosphate enemas, intravenous supplementation, furosemide, vitamin D, hydrochlorothiazide, minocycline.

LAB ARTIFACTS THAT MAY INTERFERE WITH READINGS OF LEVELS OF THIS SUBSTANCE

- Increase: hemolysis (in vivo or in vitro), delayed removal of serum from clot, hyperlipidemia, hyperproteinemia, thrombocytosis.
- Decrease: postprandial carbohydrates (mild).

SAMPLE FOR COLLECTION AND ANY SPECIAL SPECIMEN HANDLING NOTES: Serum (red-top tube) preferred; can also be measured in heparinized plasma and urine.

PEARLS

- Healthy animals less than 1 year of age may normally have elevated serum phosphorus levels.
- Acute hypophosphatemia (e.g., during initial management of diabetic ketoacidosis) carries the risk of severe hemolysis.

AUTHOR: **DEBORAH G. DAVIS**

Platelets

BASIC INFORMATION

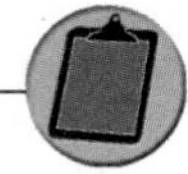

DEFINITION

- Thrombocytopenia: decreased platelet count.
- Thrombocytosis: increased platelet count.
- Thrombopathia: abnormal platelet function.

TYPICAL NORMAL RANGE

- Canine: 150,000–500,000/μL.
- Feline: 150,000–400,000/μL.
- Seven to 15 platelets per 100× field (blood film) is associated with adequate platelet numbers.

PHYSIOLOGY

Platelets form from megakaryocytes in bone marrow, spleen, lung. Platelets are discoid, anucleate 5- to 7-μm cytoplasmic fragments; important in primary hemostasis. They adhere to subendothelium by the binding of von Willebrand factor (vWF) to platelet GPIb. Aggregation occurs through binding of platelet membrane $\alpha_{IIb}\beta_3$ with fibrinogen or vWF. Activated platelets release granule contents (fibrinogen, factor V, ADP, ATP, plasminogen), thromboxane A2, arachidonic acid. Mediator release and reactions with leukocytes are important in inflammation and wound healing.

CAUSES OF ABNORMALLY HIGH LEVELS: Redistribution (exercise, epinephrine release), neoplasia (essential thrombocythemia, acute megakaryocytic leukemia), increased production (inflammation, iron deficiency, rebound from thrombocytopenia). Associated with hyperadrenocorticism and administration of glucocorticoid, although the mechanism is not known.

NEXT DIAGNOSTIC STEP TO CONSIDER IF LEVELS HIGH: Examine blood film to confirm increase; serum iron profile, complete blood count/serum chemistry profile for evidence of inflammation (neutrophilia with left shift, elevated globulins); bone marrow aspirate.

CAUSES OF ABNORMALLY LOW LEVELS: Thrombocytopenia: acute, severe blood loss; drugs (myelotoxic); immune-mediated destruction; bone marrow replacement (myelofibrosis, neoplasia); megakaryocytic neoplasia; localized or disseminated intravascular coagulation (DIC); infectious diseases (canine distemper, canine parvovirus, cytauxzoonosis, endotoxemia, feline leukemia virus [FeLV], feline infectious peritonitis [FIP], ehrlichiosis, babesiosis, histoplasmosis, leptospirosis, Rocky Mountain spotted fever, leishmaniasis).

NEXT DIAGNOSTIC STEP TO CONSIDER IF LEVELS LOW: Review history and physical exam for signs of underlying disorder/trigger; evaluation of blood film for hemotropic infectious agents, clumping; coagulation profile to rule out bleeding, DIC; bone marrow aspirate; serologic titers for infectious diseases.

DRUG EFFECTS ON LEVELS

- Thrombocytosis: vincristine, vinblastine exogenous corticosteroids.
- Thrombocytopenia: chemotherapeutic agents, estrogens, phenylbutazone, certain diuretics, certain antibiotics, antimicrobials.

LAB ARTIFACTS THAT MAY INTERFERE WITH READINGS OF LEVELS OF THIS SUBSTANCE: Clumping, large platelets (macroplatelets) falsely decrease analyzer count. Heparinized samples often have excessive platelet clumping; macroplatelets (and resultant undercounting by automated analyzers, "pseudothrombocytopenia") are an incidental finding in Cavalier King Charles spaniels.

SAMPLE FOR COLLECTION AND ANY SPECIAL SPECIMEN HANDLING NOTES: Ethylenediamine tetraacetic acid (purple top) preferred; citrated blood (blue top) can be used.

PEARLS: Suspect thrombopathia if platelet count, hematocrit, coagulation parameters (prothrombin time, activated partial thromboplastin time), and vWF are normal but buccal mucosal bleeding time is prolonged. Causes include hereditary, drug associated (barbiturate anesthetics, nonsteroidal anti-inflammatory drugs, antihistamines, penicillin), fibrin degradation products, hepatic disease, hyperglobulinemia (with multiple myeloma, ehrlichiosis), FeLV, uremia. Document with specific platelet function tests.

AUTHOR: **DEBORAH G. DAVIS**

Poikilocyte

BASIC INFORMATION

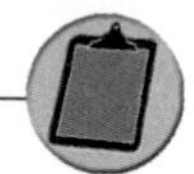

DEFINITION

General term for presence of abnormally shaped mature erythrocytes in blood. This shape change can be artifactual (e.g., crenation) or pathologic (e.g., spherocytes, schistocytes).

SYNONYM(S)

Poikilocytosis

TYPICAL NORMAL RANGE

Only artifactually induced poikilocytes (e.g., crenation) would be observed in the blood of healthy animals.

PHYSIOLOGY

Normal shape of mature erythrocyte is discocyte (biconcave disk). With damage to cell membrane (e.g., antibodies, toxins, or lipid accumulation) or damage to hemoglobin (e.g., oxidation), the plasma membrane and/or protein cytoskeleton of the erythrocyte is altered and an abnormal erythrocyte shape results.

CAUSES OF ABNORMALLY HIGH LEVELS: Immune-mediated hemolytic anemias (spherocytes), erythrocyte fragmentation (schistocytes, acanthocytes), oxidative damage (Heinz bodies, eccentrocytes), hepatic diseases (acanthocytes), venomous snake bite (echinocytes, spherocytes), bee sting (spherocytes).

NEXT DIAGNOSTIC STEP TO CONSIDER IF LEVELS HIGH: Definitive determination of the specific type of poikilocytes present.

IMPORTANT INTERSPECIES DIFFERENCES: Crenation (artifact) occurs more commonly in feline erythrocytes. Spherocytes are more easily detected in the erythrocytes of dogs because normal canine erythrocytes have a prominent central pallor.

LAB ARTIFACTS THAT MAY INTERFERE WITH READINGS OF LEVELS OF THIS SUBSTANCE

- Poorly prepared blood smear will distort canine erythrocytes so that central pallor is lost and cells may resemble spherocytes.
- Erythrocytes on blood smears allowed to slowly air dry during preparation could have refractile markings and distortion; best to rapidly dry smears by waving or use heat block.
- Lipemia will cause lysis and distortion of erythrocyte morphology.
- Crenation often occurs from effects of smear preparation on erythrocytes.

SAMPLE FOR COLLECTION AND ANY SPECIAL SPECIMEN HANDLING NOTES: Ethylenediamine tetraacetic acid blood and freshly prepared blood smear for laboratory to stain.

AUTHOR: **STEPHEN D. GAUNT**

Polycythemia

BASIC INFORMATION

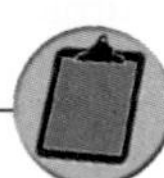

DEFINITION

Increased circulating erythrocyte mass, with increased hematocrit (or packed cell volume [PCV]), hemoglobin concentration, and/or erythrocyte count of blood. Occurs from increase in the circulating erythrocytes only (*relative* polychythemia) or an increase in both circulating erythrocytes and erythropoietic cells (*absolute* polycythemia).

SYNONYM(S)

Erythrocytosis

PHYSIOLOGY

Relative polycythemia occurs most commonly, with the increase in circulating erthrocytes from decreased plasma volume (e.g., dehydration) or the release of sequestered erythrocytes following epinephrine-induced splenic contraction. *Absolute* polycythemia indicates an increase in circulating and erythropoietic cells, the result of increased erythropoietin concentration or heightened response to erythropoietin. *Appropriate* increase in erythropoietin occurs secondary to systemic hypoxia. *Inappropriate* production of erythropoietin occurs uncommonly, from hypoxia restricted to kidneys (e.g., right to left shunting patent ductus arteriosus) or paraneoplastc expression of erythropoietin from neoplasm (usually renal). *Polycythemia vera* is a myeloproliferative disease resulting from clonal proliferation of well-differentiated erythrocytes without any increase in basal levels of erythropoietin. The resultant erythrocytosis, especially in cases of absolute polycythemia, can cause increased viscosity of blood, sludging of blood flow, and resultant hypoxia and thrombosis.

CAUSES OF ABNORMALLY HIGH LEVELS: Dehydration (relative polycythemia); splenic contraction (relative polycythemia); high altitude, right-to-left cardiac shunts, or chronic pulmonary diseases (appropriate absolute polycythemia); renal hypoxia, renal carcinoma with erythropoietin secretion (inappropriate absolute polycythemia); polycythemia vera.

NEXT DIAGNOSTIC STEP TO CONSIDER IF LEVELS HIGH: Verify instrument PCV with manual test (spun hematocrit). After ruling out the more common causes of relative polycythemia (e.g., physical exam and evaluation of serum albumin concentration for dehydration), urinalysis and abdominal ultrasound (evaluate kidneys), echocardiography, arterial pO_2 measurement, and erythropoietin assay are needed.

IMPORTANT INTERSPECIES DIFFERENCES

- Polycythemia caused by epinephrine-induced splenic contraction is more likely in cats, although it may be appreciated in breeds of dogs (e.g., dachshunds, greyhounds) with normally higher hematocrits.
- Sight hounds (e.g., greyhounds, deerhounds, wolfhounds, Afghan hounds) have a higher normal hematocrit/PCV (may exceed 55%).

SAMPLE FOR COLLECTION AND ANY SPECIAL SPECIMEN HANDLING NOTES: Ethylenediamine tetraacetic acid blood

PEARLS: Hypovolemia/dehydration is the most common cause of polycythemia in dogs and cats.

AUTHOR: **STEPHEN D. GAUNT**

Potassium

BASIC INFORMATION

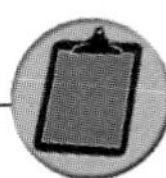

DEFINITION

Major intracellular cation continually pumped into cell by energy-dependent sodium-potassium pump at cell membrane; important in cardiac and neuromuscular membrane potentials/excitability.

SYNONYM(S)

K+

TYPICAL NORMAL RANGE

Typically 3.5–5.5 mEq/L (mmol/L)

PHYSIOLOGY

Influenced by acid-base status. Inorganic or mineral acidosis (e.g., with renal failure) causes extracellular shift and hyperkalemia. Under normal conditions, renal regulation of plasma K+ shifts K+ from extracellular fluid to intracellular fluid. Hyperkalemia is uncommon if renal function is normal (exceptions: postrenal lesions, hypoadrenocorticism, iatrogenic). Potassium is released during normal platelet coagulation, potentially causing artifactual hyperkalemia.

CAUSES OF ABNORMALLY HIGH LEVELS: Decreased renal excretion (renal failure, urinary tract obstruction or rupture), hypoadrenocorticism, artifact (as a result of normal platelet clumping, or else in Asian dog breeds [e.g., Akita]), gastrointestinal disease (salmonellosis, trichuriasis), chylothorax with repeated drainage, diabetic ketoacidosis, metabolic acidosis (due to inorganic acids), rhabdomyolysis.

NEXT DIAGNOSTIC STEP TO CONSIDER IF LEVELS HIGH: Repeat measurement using green-top tube to collect blood sample (heparin), complete blood count/profile, evaluate for drugs that can cause hyperkalemia, abdominal ultrasound/radiographs (check integrity of urinary tract), adrenocorticotropic hormone stimulation, blood gas to assess acid-base status.

CAUSES OF ABNORMALLY LOW LEVELS: Increased loss (vomiting, diarrhea), chronic renal failure (cats), postobstructive diuresis, inappropriate fluid therapy, diuresis associated with diabetes mellitus/ketoacidosis, hyperaldosteronism, alkalemia and hypokalemic periodic paralysis of Burmese cats.

NEXT DIAGNOSTIC STEP TO CONSIDER IF LEVELS LOW: Complete blood count/profile/urinalysis/blood gas.

DRUG EFFECTS ON LEVELS

- Hyperkalemia: angiotensin-converting enzyme-inhibitors, potassium-sparing diuretics (e.g., spironolactone), K+ penicillin G, oversupplementation of fluids with K+, o,p'-DDD (iatrogenic hypoadrenocorticism).
- Hypokalemia: loop diuretics (furosemide), thiazide diuretics, amphotericin B, penicillin, administration of K+ free fluids.

LAB ARTIFACTS THAT MAY INTERFERE WITH READINGS OF LEVELS OF THIS SUBSTANCE: Serum K+ is higher than plasma K+, especially if a thrombocytosis is present; marked hemolysis in dogs (Akitas, English Springer spaniels) with high K+ red blood cell concentration, marked leukocytosis. Avoid by prompt separation of plasma from cells. Drawing blood through an intravenous catheter may dilute sample resulting in false decrease.

SAMPLE FOR COLLECTION AND ANY SPECIAL SPECIMEN HANDLING NOTES: Serum (red-top tube); K+ will remain stable for extended periods of time. K+ ethylenediamine tetraacetic acid (purple-top tube) should not be used as an anticoagulant.

PEARLS

- It is important to measure the acid-base status of hypokalemic/hyperkalemic animals.
- Normal K+ levels in the presence of an inorganic acidemia suggest low K+ stores. Normal K+ in an alkalotic animal suggests the total body K+ is high.

AUTHOR: **DEBORAH G. DAVIS**

Progesterone

BASIC INFORMATION

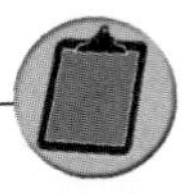

DEFINITION

Steroid hormone secreted by corpora lutea of the ovaries and by the placenta.

TYPICAL NORMAL RANGE

Depends on stage of estrous cycle; concentrations exceeding 2 ng/ml indicate luteal function.

PHYSIOLOGY

Progesterone is secreted by the cells of developing corpus luteum, the presence of which indicates pregnancy, diestrus, or an ovarian lesion (e.g., cyst or neoplasm). Concentrations greater than those of anestrus (i.e., greater than 2 ng/ml) are used for predicting time of ovulation in bitches. Proestrus is characterized by increased estrogen concentration, vulvar swelling, and vaginal discharge; decreasing estrogen concentration and increasing progesterone concentration, resulting from increased luteinizing hormone (LH) indicates estrus. Behavioral changes (receptivity to breeding) are also important features to be observed. Ovulation occurs approximately 48 hours after the LH surge. Progesterone is needed to maintain pregnancy and is secreted by the placenta. Decreasing progesterone concentrations (<2 ng/ml) indicate the onset of parturition within 24 hours in most bitches.

CAUSES OF ABNORMALLY HIGH LEVELS: Developing corpora lutea followed by pregnancy; residual ovarian tissue in a patient thought to have been spayed; luteal cysts; granulosa cell tumor.

NEXT DIAGNOSTIC STEP TO CONSIDER IF LEVELS HIGH: Confirm the presence of ovarian abnormalities (e.g., with abdominal ultrasound) if not evaluating a breeding bitch.

CAUSES OF ABNORMALLY LOW LEVELS: Depends on stage of cycle; may indicate normal anestrus, failure to ovulate, become pregnant, or maintain pregnancy; parturition.

IMPORTANT INTERSPECIES DIFFERENCES: Used primarily in dogs; not used in cats because they are induced ovulators.

DRUG EFFECTS ON LEVELS: Minimal interference by deoxycortisol, deoxycortisone, and dihydroprogesterone

LAB ARTIFACTS THAT MAY INTERFERE WITH READINGS OF LEVELS OF THIS SUBSTANCE: Falsely decreased with storage at room temperature or delay in separation of serum or plasma from red blood cells; lipemia interference if measured by chemiluminescence; use of serum separator tubes (SST) falsely decreases values.

SAMPLE FOR COLLECTION AND ANY SPECIAL SPECIMEN HANDLING NOTES: Depends on the laboratory; both serum (red top) or heparinized or ethylenediamine tetraacetic acid plasma may be used. Do not use SST. Separate serum or plasma from red blood cells as soon as possible. Store at 2–8°C.

AUTHOR: **LOIS ROTH-JOHNSON**

Protein Electrophoresis

BASIC INFORMATION

DEFINITION

Qualitative and quantitative determination of proteins, typically measured in serum, but may also be performed on cerebrospinal fluid and urine. Proteins separate into groups (fractions) based on their rate of migration in an electric field. Protein charge and size determine migration rate.

TYPICAL NORMAL RANGE

	Dogs:	*Cats:*
α-1	0.2–0.5 g/dl	0.2–1.1 g/dl
α-2	0.3–1.1 g/dl	0.4–0.9 g/dl
β-1	0.6–1.2 g/dl	0.3–0.9 g/dl
β-2	0.6–1.4 g/dl	0.6–1.0 g/dl
γ-1	0.5–1.3 g/dl	0.6–1.0 g/dl
γ-2	0.4–0.9 g/dl	1.4–1.9 g/dl

PHYSIOLOGY

The five major fractions of soluble body proteins are albumin and the four globulin fractions: α-1, α-2, β, and γ. β and γ globulins each have two fractions. Albumin is the largest fraction in healthy animals. The α-1 globulin fraction primarily contains acute phase proteins. The α-2 globulin and β globulin fractions contain acute phase proteins, lipoproteins, and some immunoglobulins. The γ globulin fraction contains immunoglobulin (Ig) A, IgG, and IgM. Elevation of γ globulins may be seen on the electrophoresis tracing as a broad based peak (*polyclonal*) or a single narrow peak (*monoclonal*).

CAUSES OF ABNORMALLY HIGH LEVELS

- Increased α globulin: acute inflammation, nephrotic syndrome, corticosteroid administration.
- Increased β globulin: acute inflammation, nephrotic syndrome, liver disease, immune responses.
- Increased γ globulins: immune stimulation, neoplasia.

NEXT DIAGNOSTIC STEP TO CONSIDER IF LEVELS HIGH

- Polyclonal gammopathy: assess for inflammation, infection, immune mediated disease, liver disease, neoplasia.
- Monoclonal gammopathy: assess for plasma cell myeloma, B-cell lymphoma, lymphocytic leukemia; infectious disease (ehrlichiosis, feline infectious peritonitis, leishmaniasis, plasmacytic stomatitis, lymphoplasmacytic enterocolitis).

CAUSES OF ABNORMALLY LOW LEVELS

- Albumin: acute phase response, glomerular disease, liver disease, gastrointestinal disease, blood loss, sequestration in body cavity effusion.
- Globulins: inherited or acquired immunodeficiency.

NEXT DIAGNOSTIC STEP TO CONSIDER IF LEVELS LOW: Investigate for albumin loss or decreased synthesis.

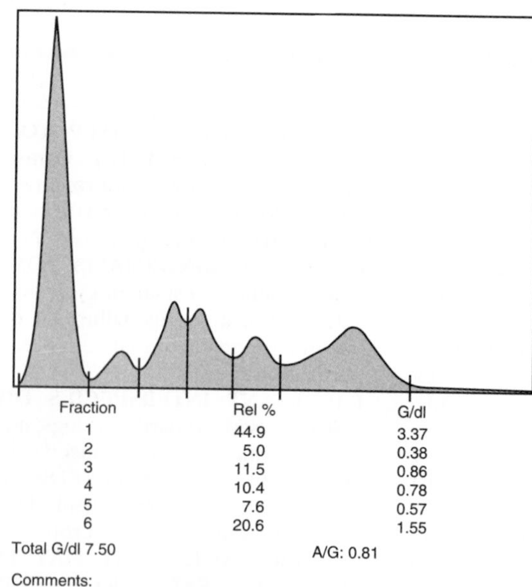

Fraction	Rel %	G/dl
1	44.9	3.37
2	5.0	0.38
3	11.5	0.86
4	10.4	0.78
5	7.6	0.57
6	20.6	1.55

Total G/dl 7.50 A/G: 0.81

Comments:

FIGURE IV-3 Serum protein electrophoresis tracing demonstrating a normal distribution of serum proteins.

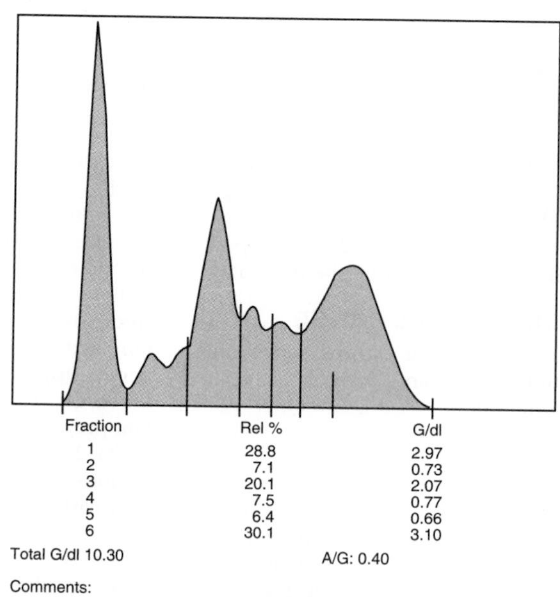

Fraction	Rel %	G/dl
1	28.8	2.97
2	7.1	0.73
3	20.1	2.07
4	7.5	0.77
5	6.4	0.66
6	30.1	3.10

Total G/dl 10.30 A/G: 0.40

Comments:

FIGURE IV-4 Serum protein electrophoresis tracing demonstrating hyperglobuinemia that is polyclonal in distribution, as is typical of inflammation.

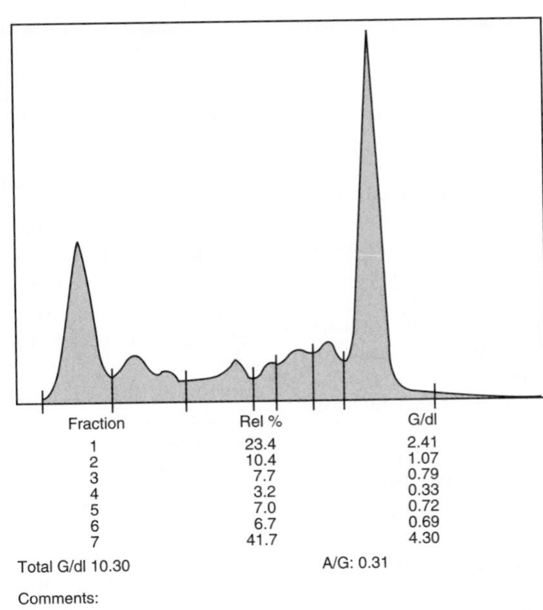

Fraction
1
2
3
4
5
6
7
Rel %
23.4
10.4
7.7
3.2
7.0
6.7
41.7
G/dl
2.41
1.07
0.79
0.33
0.72
0.69
4.30
Total G/dl 10.30
A/G: 0.31
Comments:

FIGURE IV-5 Serum protein electrophoresis tracing demonstrating hyperglobulinemia that is monoclonal in distribution (single peak). This patient had multiple myeloma.

LAB ARTIFACTS THAT MAY INTERFERE WITH READINGS OF LEVELS OF THIS SUBSTANCE: Hemolysis artificially elevates β globulins because hemoglobin migrates in this region; lipemia promotes hemolysis.
SAMPLE FOR COLLECTION AND ANY SPECIAL SPECIMEN HANDLING NOTES: Serum (red top), refrigerate. Heparinized plasma (green top) is acceptable.

AUTHOR: **RUANNA GOSSETT**

Proteins Induced by Vitamin K Absence or Antagonism (PIVKA)

BASIC INFORMATION

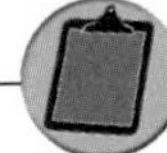

DEFINITION

Proteins induced by vitamin K absence or antagonism (PIVKA) are precursor coagulation proteins that accumulate in the peripheral blood when vitamin K is absent or inhibited.

SYNONYM(S)

PIVKA
Thrombotest

TYPICAL NORMAL RANGE

Canine: 12 to 20 seconds. Feline: 20 to 30 seconds.

PHYSIOLOGY

Factors II, VII, IX, and X, factor C, and factor S are all vitamin-K dependent coagulation factors. They are proteins synthesized in inactive precursor form in the liver. They require carboxylation of their glutamyl residues by vitamin K prior to activation. The enzyme vitamin K epoxide reductase is critical for carboxylation. In the absence of vitamin K or if vitamin K epoxide reductase is inhibited (by anticoagulant rodenticides), the inactive coagulation precursors (PIVKAs) and vitamin K epoxide accumulate in the blood, where they can be measured. The PIVKA test is a sensitive indicator of anticoagulant intoxication.
CAUSES OF ABNORMALLY HIGH LEVELS: Decreased vitamin K: neonate born to malnourished mother, sterilization of gastrointestinal tract (due to antibiotic therapy), prolonged anorexia/abnormal diet, malabsorption of vitamin K (cholestasis, exocrine pancreatic insufficiency, infiltrative bowel disease). Vitamin K antagonism: anticoagulant rodenticides, cephalosporins, and sulfonamides.
NEXT DIAGNOSTIC STEP TO CONSIDER IF LEVELS HIGH: Complete blood count/profile, urinalysis, full coagulation profile, determine if recent exposure to drugs or anticoagulant rodenticides. Urinalysis should not be obtained by cystocentesis and blood sampling should be drawn from a compressible vein (e.g., limb, not jugular) in patients with elevated PIVKA concentrations and therefore with a bleeding tendency.
DRUG EFFECTS ON LEVELS: Numerous drugs can worsen the effects of anticoagulant rodenticide toxicity through platelet inhibition (nonsteroidal anti-inflammatory drugs, steroids), decreased protein binding (phenylbutazone, corticosteroids and sulfonamides), and increased hepatic metabolism (antibiotics, rifampin, chloramphenicol, barbiturates).
SAMPLE FOR COLLECTION AND ANY SPECIAL SPECIMEN HANDLING NOTES: Plasma in citrated tube (blue top). Spin and separate plasma. May refrigerate specimens that will be analyzed within 3 hours; freeze >3 hours.
PEARLS: Alhough helpful in confirming a diagnosis of rodenticide toxicity, in most cases treatment decisions must be made before test results are available.

AUTHOR: **DEBORAH G. DAVIS**

Prothrombin Time

BASIC INFORMATION

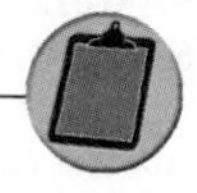

DEFINITION

Screening coagulation test of the extrinsic and common coagulation pathways.

SYNONYM(S)

One-stage prothrombin time (OSPT)
PT

TYPICAL NORMAL RANGE

Values are approximate (normals are laboratory and instrument specific).

- Canine: 5 to 8 seconds.
- Feline: 7 to 11 seconds.

PHYSIOLOGY

Plasma to be tested and the reagent (Ca^{2+}-thromboplastin reagent) are warmed and mixed together to allow tissue factor in the reagent to activate factor VII in the plasma, initiating the extrinsic pathway and then the common pathway. A fibrin clot is formed that is detected by the instrument. The prothrombin time (PT) is the time from the plasma and reagent mixing to the formation of the clot.

CAUSES OF ABNORMALLY HIGH LEVELS: Prolonged PT: hepatic disease, vitamin K deficiency, disseminated intravascular coagulation (DIC), anticoagulant intoxication, hereditary defects in extrinsic or common pathway (factors VII, X, V, II and I), heparin, presence of fibrin degradation products (FDPs), antibodies to phospholipids or coagulation factors.

NEXT DIAGNOSTIC STEP TO CONSIDER IF LEVELS HIGH: Rule out acquired causes and DIC; specific coagulation factor assays (rare).

CAUSES OF ABNORMALLY LOW LEVELS: Shortened PT is not a reliable measure of hypercoagulability.

DRUG EFFECTS ON LEVELS: Heparin can cause a prolonged PT. PT is often the first coagulation test affected by heparin administration.

LAB ARTIFACTS THAT MAY INTERFERE WITH READINGS OF LEVELS OF THIS SUBSTANCE: Different thromboplastin reagents can produce different results; improper blood-to-citrate ratios falsify results (too little blood can prolong results and too much blood can shorten coagulation times).

SAMPLE FOR COLLECTION AND ANY SPECIAL SPECIMEN HANDLING NOTES: Citrated plasma (blue-top tube). Care should be taken to avoid traumatic venipuncture which can cause in vitro activation of tissue factor, artifactually shortening the PT. Immediately mix the blood and anticoagulant.

PEARLS: Antagonism or absence of vitamin K-dependent coagulation factors, as occurs in anticoagulant rodenticide intoxication or liver disease, tends to increase PT before activated partial thromboplastic time. This is due to the short half life of factor VII.

A patient with overt clinical signs of hemorrhage due to anticoagulant rodenticide intoxication will invariably have an elevated PT (usually markedly elevated).

Decreased PT does not indicate hypercoagulability; rather, it is usually a result of suboptimal phlebotomy (sample collection artifact).

AUTHOR: **DEBORAH G. DAVIS**

Pyuria

BASIC INFORMATION

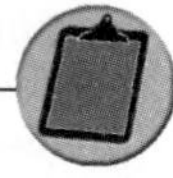

DEFINITION

The presence of increased leukocytes in urine sediment.

TYPICAL NORMAL RANGE

Less than 5 leukocytes/high power field (HPF = 40× objective)

PHYSIOLOGY

In health, few leukocytes from the kidneys, urinary bladder, reproductive tract, or urethra enter the urine (free catch or catheterization).

CAUSES OF ABNORMALLY HIGH LEVELS: Inflammation of genital or urinary tract.

NEXT DIAGNOSTIC STEP TO CONSIDER IF LEVELS HIGH

- Assess method of urine collection: free catch, catheterization, cystocentesis.
  - If free catch, obtain fresh sample (for further evaluation) via cystocentesis if possible, or via urethral catheter or midstream catch if not possible.
  - Similarly, if catheter sample, obtain fresh sample by cystocentesis if possible.
- Assess other findings in urinalysis, such as pH, numbers of red cells, and presence of bacteria.
- Bacterial culture and sensitivity of urine.

CAUSES OF ABNORMALLY LOW LEVELS

- Diseases that hamper neutrophil function (e.g., diabetes mellitus, hyperadrenocorticism) may falsely reduce the number of leukocytes observed in a patient with urinary tract infection.
- Diseases that cause urine to be dilute (endocrinopathies, liver disease, renal failure, others) may give the misleading appearance of a low concentration of leukocytes (or their absence) in the urine of patients with urinary tract infections.

SAMPLE FOR COLLECTION AND ANY SPECIAL SPECIMEN HANDLING NOTES: Urine in clean/sterile container.

PEARLS

- Should be detected during sediment examination, a part of urinalysis.
- For negative bacterial urine culture with concurrent pyuria, consider:
  - Antibiotic effect
  - Fungal or algal urinary tract infection
- A urine culture and sensitivity is indicated even when pyuria is absent if the differential diagnosis includes diseases that reduce neutrophil function and/or cause dilute urine.
- Patients with chronic renal failure, in particular, may not show pyuria despite having low-grade pyelonephritis, and identifying such an infection through culture and sensitivity offers the possibility of reversing renal tubular damage with appropriate antibiotic treatment.

AUTHOR: **ELIZABETH G. WELLES**

Rabies Diagnostic Testing

BASIC INFORMATION

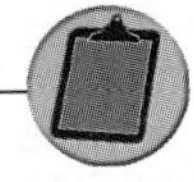

DEFINITION

Evaluation of presence or absence of rabies virus infection.

TYPICAL NORMAL RANGE

Results are reported as positive or negative.

PHYSIOLOGY

Rabies is an acute encephalitis caused by an RNA virus of the rhabdovirus family. Infection almost always results in death. Disease transmission is most often through bites with inoculation of virus-containing saliva into the wound. Inhalation and mucous membrane contamination are other, very rare, routes of infection. Virus localizes to central nervous system. Direct immunofluorescent antibody (IFA) testing of brain tissue is the method used for definitive diagnosis. Submission of appropriate specimens requires necropsy examination. The test detects viral antigen in the neural tissue of infected animals.

CAUSES OF ABNORMALLY HIGH LEVELS: Viral infection

NEXT DIAGNOSTIC STEP TO CONSIDER IF LEVELS HIGH: Exposed personnel should consult their physicians immediately. Exposed animals should be quarantined and observed for development of clinical signs.

SAMPLE FOR COLLECTION AND ANY SPECIAL SPECIMEN HANDLING NOTES: Fresh brain tissue. Note: aerosolization of rabies virus is possible during craniotomy portion of necropsy or during removal of head (exposure of spinal cord). Therefore, removal of head or of brain should be reserved for qualified personnel (e.g., pathologist or state veterinarian). Body of rabies suspect should be chilled (refrigerated), not frozen. Cut brain in sagittal (longitudinal) section. Submit half in clean, dry double bag for IFA test. Clearly label as rabies suspect.

PEARLS

- Most testing is done at state diagnostic laboratories.
- Half of the brain should be submitted in formalin to assess for other diseases if rabies tests are negative.
- Brain tissue is the only suitable specimen; other tissue such as whiskers or peripheral nerve are not.
- Dogs and cats that have an implanted microchip, are vaccinated for rabies, and have a protective titer certified by the FVNA Laboratory at Kansas State University or the Veterinary Command Food and Diagnostic Laboratory, Fort Sam Houston, Texas may avoid quarantine when traveling to Hawaii or the United Kingdom if they meet other criteria. Refer to http://www.aphis.usda.gov/NCIE/pdf/vet-fs-usa_canada.pdf for more details regarding pet travel to the United Kingdom or Hawaii without a quarantine period.

AUTHOR: **LOIS ROTH-JOHNSON**

Reticulocytes

BASIC INFORMATION

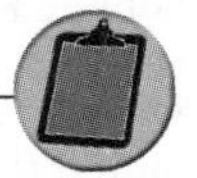

DEFINITION

Erythroid precursor that have expelled their nuclei, with larger volume, more ribosomes, and less hemoglobin than mature erythrocytes. Name derived from *reticulum* that forms after ribosomes are precipitated by supravital dyes (e.g., new methylene blue).

SYNONYM(S)

Polychromatophilic erythrocyte

TYPICAL NORMAL RANGE

Dogs (nonanemic): <80 × 10^3 reticulocytes/μL (or × 10^9/L). Cats (nonanemic): <60 × 10^3 reticulocytes/μL (or × 10^9/L).

PHYSIOLOGY

With increased erythropoietin and proliferation of erythroid precursors, increased numbers of reticulocytes are released into blood. Two forms of maturating reticulocytes are identified in cats. *Aggregate* reticulocytes have many ribosomes forming prominent reticulum with supravital staining appear as polychromatophilic erythrocytes on Romanowsky-stained smears. *Punctate* reticulocytes have fewer ribosomes that form pin-point inclusions on supravital stain. They are not apparent on Romanowsky-stained smears.

CAUSES OF ABNORMALLY HIGH LEVELS: Regenerative anemias from blood loss or hemolysis (e.g., immune-mediated hemolytic anemia, mycoplasmosis, oxidative anemias, fragmentation anemia).

NEXT DIAGNOSTIC STEP TO CONSIDER IF LEVELS HIGH: Determine specific cause of blood loss or hemolysis.

CAUSES OF ABNORMALLY LOW LEVELS: Decreased erythropoietin (e.g., chronic renal failure), inflammation-induced suppression, iron deficiency, decreased erythroid percursors in marrow (e.g., immune-mediated attack on erythroid precursors, feline leukemia virus or feline immunodeficiency virus infection, myelophthisis).

NEXT DIAGNOSTIC STEP TO CONSIDER IF LEVELS LOW: Bone marrow aspirate or core biopsy.

IMPORTANT INTERSPECIES DIFFERENCES

- In cats, punctate reticulocytes circulate for 10 to 14 days, so they occur after erythropoietic response and increase in aggregate reticulocytes have abated. Only aggregate reticulocytes should be counted in cats.
- In dogs, punctate reticulocytes do not persist significantly longer than aggregate reticulocytes.
- Dogs mount a higher reticulocyte response than cats during regenerative anemias.

LAB ARTIFACTS THAT MAY INTERFERE WITH READINGS OF LEVELS OF THIS SUBSTANCE: Autoagglutination decreases the number of detectable reticulocytes.

SAMPLE FOR COLLECTION AND ANY SPECIAL SPECIMEN HANDLING NOTES: Ethylenediamine tetraacetic acid blood for flow-cytometric counting by analyzers (preferred) or manual counting of supravital stained smears.

PEARLS

- An increase in *absolute concentration* of reticulocytes is the gold standard for determining whether anemia is regenerative or nonregenerative.
- Reticulocyte counts may not be included in routine complete blood count; be sure it is included for anemic patients.

AUTHOR: **STEPHEN D. GAUNT**

Rheumatoid Factor

BASIC INFORMATION

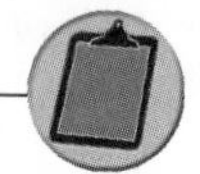

DEFINITION

Autoantibodies to the Fc portion of autologous immunoglobulin (Ig) G.

TYPICAL NORMAL RANGE

Reported as negative or positive; positive results will have an associated titer specific for reference laboratory.

PHYSIOLOGY

Predominately IgM antibodies that form immune complexes in sera, synovial fluid, and synovial membranes. Immune complexes localized within inflamed cartilage activating complement and contributing to synovial inflammation.

CAUSES OF ABNORMALLY HIGH LEVELS: Rheumatoid arthritis. False-positive results are common and seen in healthy dogs or animals with other causes of polyarthritis, heartworm disease, pyometra, leishmaniasis, and systemic lupus erythematosus.

NEXT DIAGNOSTIC STEP TO CONSIDER IF LEVELS HIGH: Synovial fluid analysis, synovial biopsy, serologic testing for infectious diseases (fungal, heartworm disease, rickettsial, borreliosis), radiography of affected joint(s).

LAB ARTIFACTS THAT MAY INTERFERE WITH READINGS OF LEVELS OF THIS SUBSTANCE

- Decrease/false negative: freezing of specimen destroys antibodies.
- Increase/false positive: animals with antibodies to sheep red blood cells.

SAMPLE FOR COLLECTION AND ANY SPECIAL SPECIMEN HANDLING NOTES: Serum (red-top tube).

PEARLS: Not a good test in dogs, neither sensitive nor specific for routine diagnostic use. Rheumatoid factors are only present in about one-fourth of dogs with rheumatoid arthritis. Also can be present in animals with other polyarthritis, heartworm disease, pyometra, leishmaniasis, and systemic lupus erythematosus.

AUTHOR: **FONZIE QUANCE-FITCH**

Rocky Mountain Spotted Fever Serology

BASIC INFORMATION

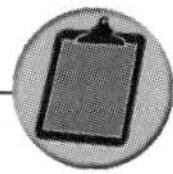

DEFINITION

Rocky Mountain spotted fever (RMSF) is a tick-borne, acute systemic disease caused by *Rickettsia rickettsii*. It is characterized by fever, anorexia, thrombocytopenia, uveitis, and necrotizing vasculitis in dogs.

TYPICAL NORMAL RANGE

Consult the laboratory conducting the test for information regarding reference ranges. General guideline: immunofluorescent antibody negative titer is <1:64.

PHYSIOLOGY

R. rickettsii is inoculated via a tick bite (*Dermacentor* spp.; possibly *Amblyomma* sp. or *Rhipicephalus* sp.), enters the circulatory system and infects and replicates within endothelial cells of small blood vessels, where it induces a vasculitis. Vasculitis leads to increased vascular permeability, microvascular hemorrhage, thrombocytopenia, disseminated intravascular coagulation (DIC), edema, and ultimately hypotensive shock with multiple organ damage.

CAUSES OF ABNORMALLY HIGH LEVELS: A positive titer indicates exposure to the RMSF organism. A very high single IgG titer (≥1:1024), fourfold increase in paired IgG titers (2 to 4 weeks apart), or a positive IgM titer with characteristic signs is consistent with active infection.

NEXT DIAGNOSTIC STEP TO CONSIDER IF LEVELS HIGH: A polymerase chain reaction (PCR) test is available, but may not be necessary if clinical signs are compatible with RMSF and the titer(s) are positive.

CAUSES OF ABNORMALLY LOW LEVELS: A negative titer indicates lack of exposure or early/acute infection.

NEXT DIAGNOSTIC STEP TO CONSIDER IF LEVELS LOW: If clinical signs of RMSF are present and initial titer is negative, submit a convalescent titer in 2 to 4 weeks.

SAMPLE FOR COLLECTION AND ANY SPECIAL SPECIMEN HANDLING NOTES: Submit 1 ml of serum (red-top tube). Can store for 4 days at 4°C or at 0°C for several weeks. Paired IgG titers should be submitted to the same laboratory for testing at the same time.

PEARLS: Because of the rapid progression of clinical RMSF, the diagnosis often is made on suggestive physical and general clinicopathologic findings in order to institute treatment rapidly; the turnaround time of RMSF serology may make the result confirmatory in retrospect (i.e., the decision to treat cannot always wait for the test result).

AUTHOR: **PATTY J. EWING**

Schistocytes

BASIC INFORMATION

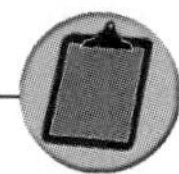

DEFINITION

Red cell fragments are considered to be the hallmark of microangiopathic hemolysis.

SYNONYM(S)

Schizocyte

PHYSIOLOGY

Schistocytes result from shredding of red cells as they pass through the microvasculature containing fibrin thrombi or altered endothelium. Any traumatic or physical injury to red cells can lead to schistocyte formation.

CAUSES OF ABNORMALLY HIGH LEVELS: Disseminated intravascular coagula-

tion (DIC), vasculitis, hemangiosarcoma, dirofilariasis, intravenous catheters, burns, heart valve disease, myelofibrosis, glomerulonephritis. May be seen in severe iron deficiency anemia (increased red blood cell fragility causes fragmentation).
NEXT DIAGNOSTIC STEP TO CONSIDER IF LEVELS HIGH: Evaluate patient's clinical history, heartworm status, coagulation profile, tick titers.

IMPORTANT INTERSPECIES DIFFERENCES: Schistocytes are not typically seen in cats with DIC, possibly because their smaller red blood cells are less likely to be damaged by fibrin in vascular spaces.
SAMPLE FOR COLLECTION AND ANY SPECIAL SPECIMEN HANDLING NOTES: Ethylene diamine tetraacetic acid (purple top) for complete blood count.

PEARLS: Even small numbers of schistocytes are significant, indicating underlying microangiopathy; unlikely to be induced artifactually by smear preparation technique.

AUTHOR: **FIDELIA R. FERNANDEZ**

Semen Analysis

BASIC INFORMATION

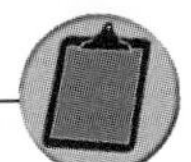

DEFINITION

Assessment of male ejaculate for volume, sperm number and morphology, percent of live sperm, presence of other cells, bacteria, and, occasionally, alkaline phosphatase and carnitine concentration; used as part of assessment of male fertility.

TYPICAL NORMAL RANGE

Normal total sperm is 400×10^6 with 52–90% classified as live and normal in most dogs. Motility, which is often considered an indicator of viability, should be approximately 80%; motility patterns are random. Sperm should have single heads of uniform shape and size; free heads should be rare; tails are normally straight to slightly curved; hooked, kinked or multiple tails are considered abnormal. It is common to see few urethral, prostatic, or squamous epithelial cells; low numbers of bacteria are also common. Alkaline phosphatase >10,000 U/L.

PHYSIOLOGY

Ejaculate is divided into three fractions. First and third fractions are mostly prostatic secretion; the second sperm-rich fraction should be used for evaluation.
CAUSES OF ABNORMALLY LOW LEVELS: Decreased numbers of normal, viable sperm suggest testicular injury, neoplasia, or atrophy. Decreased concentration of seminal alkaline phosphatase and/or carnitine indicates obstruction of genital tubular structures.
NEXT DIAGNOSTIC STEP TO CONSIDER IF LEVELS LOW: Examination of testicle and epididymis on physical examination and using ultrasound; measurement of resting plasma testosterone
SAMPLE FOR COLLECTION AND ANY SPECIAL SPECIMEN HANDLING NOTES: Motility must be evaluated immediately; it cannot be assessed in specimens transported to a reference laboratory.
PEARLS: History is an important aspect of fertility assessment. Do not rely on a single test.

AUTHOR: **LOIS ROTH-JOHNSON**

Sodium

BASIC INFORMATION

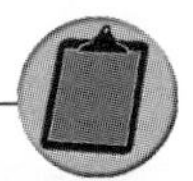

DEFINITION

Electrolyte, major extracellular cation. Concentration is relative to hydration status and extracellular fluid (ECF) volume. Does not indicate total body content. Serum Na concentration essentially equals ECF Na concentration.

SYNONYM(S)

Na
Na^+

TYPICAL NORMAL RANGE

Canine: 140–150 mEq/L; feline: 150–160 mEq/L. Conversion: mEq/L = mmol/L.

PHYSIOLOGY

Serum concentration is net of oral intake, excretion, water shifts between ECF and ICF (intracellular fluid). Na (and water) lost via kidneys, intestine, skin, respiratory tract. Concentration is regulated via balance of blood volume and plasma osmolality by glomerular filtration and renal tubular resorption. With hypovolemia, aldosterone promotes Na resorption, antidiuretic hormone (ADH) promotes water resorption. Hypoosmolality causes decreased water intake, increased urinary water excretion. Hypervolemia reduces Na resorption. Hyperosmolality promotes water intake, ADH-mediated water resorption. Water shifting from ICF to ECF dilutes serum Na.

CAUSES OF ABNORMALLY HIGH LEVELS
- Hypovolemia; hypotonic fluid loss: vomiting, diarrhea, pancreatitis, peritonitis, osmotic diuresis, renal failure, postobstructive diuresis.
- Normovolemia; pure water loss: diabetes insipidus, water deprivation, high temperature, brainstem disease.
- Hypervolemia; Na gain (uncommon): salt poisoning, hypertonic fluid administration, hyperaldosteronism.

NEXT DIAGNOSTIC STEP TO CONSIDER IF LEVELS HIGH: Evaluate hydration status; test for listed diseases.
CAUSES OF ABNORMALLY LOW LEVELS
- High measured osmolality: hyperglycemia, mannitol administration.

- Low measured osmolality:
  - Hypovolemia: vomiting, diarrhea, pancreatitis, peritonitis, pleural effusion, uroabdomen, hypoadrenocorticism, prolonged diuretic administration, ketonuria, Na-wasting nephropathy.
  - Hypervolemia: heart failure, severe hepatopathy, nephrotic syndrome, advanced renal disease (oliguric/anuric).
  - Normovolemia: hypotonic fluid therapy, psychogenic polydipsia, syndrome of inappropriate antidiuretic hormone secretion (SIADH; rare).

NEXT DIAGNOSTIC STEP TO CONSIDER IF LEVELS LOW

- Evaluate hydration status; test for listed diseases.
- Measure plasma osmolality.
- Measure urinary fractional Na excretion.

DRUG EFFECTS ON LEVELS

- Increase: osmotic diuretics, phosphate enema, furosemide, corticosteroids.
- Decrease: furosemide, prolonged diuresis (osmotic, thiazides).

LAB ARTIFACTS THAT MAY INTERFERE WITH READINGS OF LEVELS OF THIS SUBSTANCE: Marked hyperlipidemia, hyperproteinemia may decrease measured Na (method dependent). Serum osmolality is normal.

SAMPLE FOR COLLECTION AND ANY SPECIAL SPECIMEN HANDLING NOTES: Serum preferred. Heparinized plasma may be used (lithium or ammonium heparin, green-top tube).

PEARLS: Sampling from an improperly cleared intravenous catheter commonly causes inaccurate values.

AUTHOR: **ROBIN W. ALLISON**

Spherocytes

BASIC INFORMATION

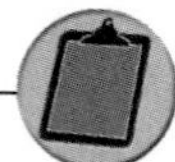

DEFINITION

Small, dense staining red cells with no central pallor, considered the hallmark of immune mediated hemolytic anemia (IMHA) or a normal finding post transfusion.

PHYSIOLOGY

Partial phagocytosis of antibody coated red cells by macrophages results in loss of surface membrane without loss of volume, resulting in spherocyte formation. Pitting (excision) of Heinz bodies in the spleen also leads to spherocyte formation. May also be seen in cases of canine babesiosis and hemotropic mycoplasmosis (previously haemobartonellosis) in cats and dogs.

CAUSES OF ABNORMALLY HIGH LEVELS: Immune mediated hemolysis or erythrocyte fragmentation associated with snake bite, bee sting, hemoparasitism, zinc toxicosis, neoplasia, or idiopathic; normal phenomenon beginning 2 to 3 days after transfusion of red cells (even if properly cross-matched).

NEXT DIAGNOSTIC STEP TO CONSIDER IF LEVELS HIGH: Evaluate history for causes of anemia; Coombs' test and slide autoagglutination test if IMHA suspected.

IMPORTANT INTERSPECIES DIFFERENCES: Spherocytes are easily detected in dogs due to normally prominent central pallor; difficult to identify in other domestic animals (cats) that normally have no central pallor in their red cells. Some breeds of dogs (Shiba Inu and Akita) normally have microcytic red cells that should not be confused with spherocytes.

SAMPLE FOR COLLECTION AND ANY SPECIAL SPECIMEN HANDLING NOTES: Ethylenediamine tetraacetic acid (purple top) for evaluation of gross agglutination, blood smear evaluation.

PEARLS

- Microcytic red blood cells of severe iron deficiency anemia differ from spherocytes in that microcytic red cells are hypochromic and truly microcytic (their mean corpuscular volume is decreased); spherocytes have normal red cell volume.
- In anemic patients, a complete blood count and/or fresh blood smears should always be obtained *before* transfusion, to screen for spherocytes (suggesting IMHA); spherocytosis *after* transfusion does not discriminate between IMHA and normal post transfusion phenomenon.

AUTHOR: **FIDELIA R. FERNANDEZ**

Synovial Fluid Analysis

BASIC INFORMATION

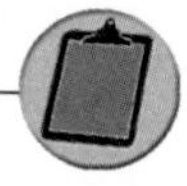

DEFINITION

Analysis of the viscous fluid secreted by synoviocytes that lubricates joints and transports nutrients to articular cartilage.

SYNONYM(S)

Joint fluid analysis

TYPICAL NORMAL RANGE

Normal synovial fluid is colorless to pale yellow, viscous, has high mucin (hyaluronic acid) content, and does not clot. Red blood cells are absent. Nucleated cell counts vary among species and the joint sampled, but are usually ≤500/μL (up to 3000 cells/μL occasionally reported in normal joints). Synoviocytes and macrophages predominate. Protein concentration ranges from 1.8–4.8 g/dL (refractometer).

PHYSIOLOGY

Analysis includes assessment of viscosity, mucin clot test, cell counts, protein concentration, and cytologic evaluation. Microscopic examination assesses cell population distribution and may detect infectious agents.

CAUSES OF ABNORMALLY HIGH LEVELS

- Increased erythrocytes indicate iatrogenic blood contamination or hemarthrosis.
- Increased nucleated cells occur with degenerative and inflammatory arthropathies.
  - Mononuclear cells predominate in degenerative arthropathy or joint instability. Causes include trauma, osteoarthrosis, osteochondritis disse-

cans, or avascular necrosis of the femoral head.

- Neutrophils predominate in inflammatory arthropathies (infectious, noninfectious, immune mediated). Bacterial infection is usually monoarticular and due to penetrating trauma. Polyarticular infection may be due to systemic bacterial infection, tick borne disease, fungal infection, and, rarely, mycoplasmosis infection. Noninfectious inflammatory arthropathies are polyarticular or have shifting leg lameness (immune mediated diseases; chronic progressive polyarthritis in cats).

NEXT DIAGNOSTIC STEP TO CONSIDER IF LEVELS HIGH

- Hemorrhage: distinguish iatrogenic versus pathologic. Erythrocytophagia suggests hemarthrosis.
- Degenerative arthropathy: joint radiographs, assess for joint instability or ligament tear.
- Inflammatory arthropathy: culture synovial fluid, *Borrelia* spp. and *Ehrlichia* spp. serology, serum antinuclear antibody test, assess for systemic disease, and joint radiographs.

SAMPLE FOR COLLECTION AND ANY SPECIAL SPECIMEN HANDLING NOTES: Ethylene diamine tetraacetic acid (lavender top) (cell counts, cytologic evaluation); red top tube (culture); refrigerate.

PEARLS: Some samples are very viscous, and the addition of a drop of crystalline hyaluronidase allows more accurate assessment of cell counts. Addition of hyaluronidase should be done at the reference laboratory after viscosity and protein concentration are measured and after the mucin clot test is done and slides for cytologic evaluation are prepared.

AUTHOR: **RUANNA GOSSETT**

Taurine Blood Levels

BASIC INFORMATION

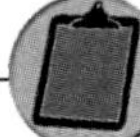

DEFINITION

Amino acid with a poorly understood role in cardiac metabolism.

TYPICAL NORMAL RANGE

- Consult with laboratory conducting the test.
- Cats: <20 nmol/ml (plasma) is considered diagnostic of cardiomyopathy; cats with <60 nmol/ml should receive supplementation.

PHYSIOLOGY

Low blood levels of taurine have been associated with dilated cardiomyopathy in cats and certain breeds of dogs, such as cocker spaniels, retrievers, and many other breeds. Determination of plasma and/or whole blood levels of taurine may be useful in determining role in dilated cardiomyopathy and need for supplementation.

CAUSES OF ABNORMALLY LOW LEVELS: Dietary deficiency or familial predisposition.

NEXT DIAGNOSTIC STEP TO CONSIDER IF LEVELS LOW: Correlate with cardiac and/or ophthalmologic evaluation findings.

IMPORTANT INTERSPECIES DIFFERENCES: Fasting may decrease plasma levels of taurine in feline samples; therefore, whole blood is the preferred sample for cats. Ideally, both whole blood and plasma taurine levels should be determined for dogs.

LAB ARTIFACTS THAT MAY INTERFERE WITH READINGS OF LEVELS OF THIS SUBSTANCE: Bacterial contamination may falsely decrease blood taurine levels. Delay in separating and chilling plasma or poor blood collection technique may result in falsely increased levels of plasma taurine because taurine is released from leukocytes and activated platelets.

SAMPLE FOR COLLECTION AND ANY SPECIAL SPECIMEN HANDLING NOTES: Collect 2 ml frozen heparinized whole blood. Collect whole blood in green top tube and freeze. Alternatively, collect 1 ml of frozen heparinized plasma. Chill sodium heparin collection tube (green-top tube) and separate plasma immediately after collection in a refrigerated centrifuge. After centrifugation, transfer plasma to plain red-top tube for submission.

PEARLS

- Dogs do not need to be eating a taurine-deficient diet to develop taurine-deficient dilated cardiomyopathy; poor bioavailability of nutritional taurine (e.g., binding by rice husks) and excess urinary excretion of taurine precursors (e.g., cystine) have been proposed as mechanisms.
- Oral taurine supplementation is inexpensive and safe.
- Low taurine levels may be used to confirm a diagnosis of cardiomyopathy, but are generally not used as a screening test.

AUTHOR: **SHERRY J. MORGAN**

Testosterone

BASIC INFORMATION

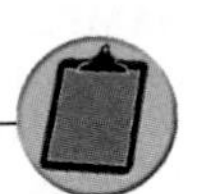

DEFINITION

Hormone responsible for development of male characteristics.

TYPICAL NORMAL RANGE

Usually >1 ng/ml indicates an intact male.

PHYSIOLOGY

Derived from cholesterol; primarily produced by the interstitial cells of the testes; ovarian theca cells, zona reticularis of the adrenal cortex, and placenta produce lesser amounts; hematogenous distribution to target tissue; affects bone growth and muscle mass, development of spermiogenic tissue in testes, and behavior. Extratesticular production accounts for sexual behavior in castrated males or animals with ovarian or adrenal tumors.

CAUSES OF ABNORMALLY HIGH LEVELS: Cryptorchid or intersex patients may have concentrations consistent with intact male.

NEXT DIAGNOSTIC STEP TO CONSIDER IF LEVELS HIGH: Investigate for

presence of abdominal testicle(s) or abnormal gonadal tissue.
CAUSES OF ABNORMALLY LOW LEVELS: Infertility.
NEXT DIAGNOSTIC STEP TO CONSIDER IF LEVELS LOW: Resample because cyclic low levels may occur in fertile patients; pulses of testosterone may occur throughout the day; increased concentration over basal levels following administration of human chorionic gonadotropin (HCG) or gonadotropin-releasing hormone (GnRH) indicates functional testicular tissue.
IMPORTANT INTERSPECIES DIFFERENCES: Cats (intact males, castrated males, and females) tend to have higher basal levels than other species; should assess by increase of basal concentration 60 minutes following HCG or GnRH injection at doses of 2 μg/kg up to 50 μg/kg.
DRUG EFFECTS ON LEVELS: False increases due to administration of androgenic drugs, such as methyltestosterone; administration of radioisotopes falsely increases values measured by radioimmunoassay; chronic administration of androgenic drugs suppresses natural production.
LAB ARTIFACTS THAT MAY INTERFERE WITH READINGS OF LEVELS OF THIS SUBSTANCE: Delayed separation from red blood cells, collection in ethylenediamine tetraacetic acid, and storage at room temperature falsely decrease values.
SAMPLE FOR COLLECTION AND ANY SPECIAL SPECIMEN HANDLING NOTES: Heparinized (green top) plasma or serum; separate plasma or serum from red blood cells as soon as possible; store specimen at 2–8°C.
PEARLS: Main indications are the assessment of infertile male patients, and to help determine whether a male without external testicles is cryptorchid or has been neutered.

AUTHOR: **LOIS ROTH-JOHNSON**

Thyroglobulin Antibody

BASIC INFORMATION

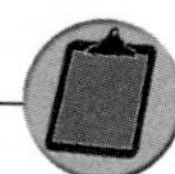

DEFINITION

Autoantibodies against thyroglobulin, the major storage form for thyroxine and triiodothyronine in the thyroid follicle.

SYNONYM(S)

TgAA

TYPICAL NORMAL RANGE

Results reported as negative or positive or inconclusive.

PHYSIOLOGY

The presence of thyroglobulin antibody (TgAA) is an indicator of immune-mediated thyroiditis and homozygous carriers for the disease.
CAUSES OF ABNORMALLY HIGH LEVELS: Immune-mediated thyroiditis; low-grade false-positive results may occur if vaccinated in the previous 30 to 40 days.
NEXT DIAGNOSTIC STEP TO CONSIDER IF LEVELS HIGH: Free T4 (equilibrium dialysis). Repeat test in 2 to 4 months.
DRUG EFFECTS ON LEVELS: Thyroid supplement associated with false-negative test. Treatment should be discontinued for at least 90 days prior to testing.
SAMPLE FOR COLLECTION AND ANY SPECIAL SPECIMEN HANDLING NOTES: Serum (red-top tube) or ethylenediamine tetraacetic acid plasma (purple-top tube). Separate serum or plasma from red blood cells as soon as possible. Store at 2–8°C (refrigeration).
PEARLS: Positive dogs not recommended for breeding due to hereditary nature of disease. Many dogs may develop TgAA prior to clinically evident immune-mediated thyroiditis and hypothyroidism. Carriers (heterozygotes) are negative. Dogs with chronic disease, with thyroid destruction may have negative results.

AUTHOR: **FONZIE QUANCE-FITCH**

Thyroid-Stimulating Hormone

BASIC INFORMATION

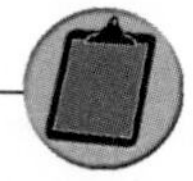

DEFINITION

Pituitary-derived hormone that acts on the thyroid gland to produce and secrete thyroid hormones.

SYNONYM(S)

Canine TSH (cTSH)
Thyrotropin
TSH

TYPICAL NORMAL RANGE

Dogs: 0.1–0.5 ng/ml (ug/dl × 10 = ng/ml). Values vary with laboratory; be sure test method has been validated for dogs.

PHYSIOLOGY

TSH is released from the pituitary from stimulation by thyrotropin-releasing hormone (TRH), acts on the thyroid gland to stimulate synthesis and release of thyroxine (T4) and triiodothyronine (T3). T3 and T4 act as negative feedback to reduce TSH and TRH secretion.
CAUSES OF ABNORMALLY HIGH LEVELS: Hypothyroidism
NEXT DIAGNOSTIC STEP TO CONSIDER IF LEVELS HIGH: Free T4 by equilibrium dialysis (free T4 ED) and total T4.
CAUSES OF ABNORMALLY LOW LEVELS: Sensitivity of the test is not sufficient to differentiate normal from low concentrations.
IMPORTANT INTERSPECIES DIFFERENCES: Species-specific immunoassay required. No valid measurement of feline TSH available. May be some crossreactivity with the canine TSH assay.
SAMPLE FOR COLLECTION AND ANY SPECIAL SPECIMEN HANDLING NOTES: Serum (red-top tube) or ethylenediamine tetraacetic acid plasma (purple-top tube). Separate serum or plasma from red blood cells as soon as possible. Store at 2–8°C (refrigeration).
PEARLS
- Canine patients having low free T4 (ED) and increased cTSH concentra-

tions are extremely likely to have hypothyroidism.
- May increase ability to assess thyroid function when evaluated in conjunction with thyroid hormone concentrations.

AUTHOR: **FONZIE QUANCE-FITCH**

Thyroxine, fT4ed

BASIC INFORMATION

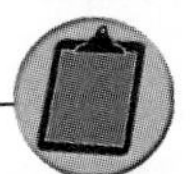

DEFINITION

- Thyroxine (T4) is the major storage form of iodine-containing thyroid hormone. Chief function is to increase rate of cell metabolism.
- Free T4 (fT4) is the biologically available, non-protein-bound form of the hormone able to enter cells.

SYNONYM(S)

Tetraiodothyronine

TYPICAL NORMAL RANGE

- fT4 averages approximately 2.0 ng/dl; specific values vary among laboratories.
- To convert μg/dl × 10 = ng/ml; μg/dl × 12.87 = nmol/L; ng/ml × 1.287 = nmol/L (SI unit nearest 1 nmol/L).

PHYSIOLOGY

Up to 99.9% protein bound in circulation and therefore not biologically active. Thyroxine is deiodinated to active form of the hormone (T3) in cells. Binds to receptor proteins in cells, inducing DNA translation and production of proteins associated with cell growth, oxidative phosphorylation, and membrane transport of electrolytes resulting in an increase in metabolic rate and growth stimulation.

CAUSES OF ABNORMALLY HIGH LEVELS: Hyperthyroidism; presence of autoantibodies; exogenous T4, TSH, or TRH; administration of iodine (or compounds containing iodine)

NEXT DIAGNOSTIC STEP TO CONSIDER IF LEVELS HIGH

- If hyperthyroidism is suspected: other thyroid tests (fT4, TSH), imaging.
- If autoantibodies: run thyroglobulin autoantibodies (TGAA).
- Evaluate diet, supplements for iodine content.

CAUSES OF ABNORMALLY LOW LEVELS: Hypothyroidism, euthyroid sick syndrome

NEXT DIAGNOSTIC STEP TO CONSIDER IF LEVELS LOW: TSH, evaluate for nonthyroidal diseases.

DRUG EFFECTS ON LEVELS: Glucocorticoids, sulfonamides, phenobarbital, nonsteroidal anti-inflammatory drugs may decrease concentration.

LAB ARTIFACTS THAT MAY INTERFERE WITH READINGS OF LEVELS OF THIS SUBSTANCE

- Artifactual increase of free T4 if sample is not kept cold.
- Artifactual increase of free and total T4 if stored in glass tubes at 37°C.

SAMPLE FOR COLLECTION AND ANY SPECIAL SPECIMEN HANDLING NOTES: Serum (red-top tube) or ethylenediamine tetraacetic acid plasma (purple-top tube). Separate serum or plasma from red blood cells as soon as possible. Store at 2–8°C.

PEARLS

- Breed differences occur: T4 and free T4 can be markedly lower in sight-hounds; small breeds tend to have higher reference intervals.
- Total T4 is a good screening test because of its sensitivity to disease but a poor confirmatory test due to its lower specificity.
- Free T4 is not as likely to be affected by nonthyroidal illness or drugs.
- Diurnal fluctuations occur in dogs but are not predictable, up to 20% below normal reference interval.
- Free T4 is also measured by radioimmunoassay, which is cheaper but of no apparent benefit over total T4 and less accurate than free T4 by equilibrium dialysis.

AUTHOR: **FONZIE QUANCE-FITCH**

Total Protein (Serum)

BASIC INFORMATION

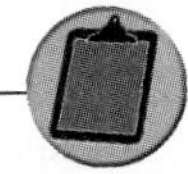

DEFINITION

Serum proteins consist of albumin, antibodies, complement, enzymes, coagulation factors, and transport proteins. Albumin and globulin make up the majority of serum total proteins. Fibrinogen, factor V, and factor VIII are present in plasma but not in serum because they are utilized in clot formation.

SYNONYM(S)

Total solids

TYPICAL NORMAL RANGE

- Dogs: 5.1–7.8 g/dl.
- Cats: 5.9–8.5 g/dl.

PHYSIOLOGY

The proteins in serum are important for maintaining colloid osmotic pressure, hemostasis, transport of molecules, and immune response. Most of these proteins are synthesized in the liver and immune system.

CAUSES OF ABNORMALLY HIGH LEVELS: Increased globulin: inflammation, neoplasia (myeloma, lymphoma). Increased albumin occurs with dehydration and is "relative"; increased production does not occur.

NEXT DIAGNOSTIC STEP TO CONSIDER IF LEVELS HIGH: Measure serum albumin and globulin levels; assess hydration status; serum protein electrophoresis.

CAUSES OF ABNORMALLY LOW LEVELS: Protein losing nephropathy: typically, albumin is lost but globulins are not, resulting in hypoalbuminemia only. Similarly, with chronic hepatopathies, albumin is not synthesized, leading to hypoalbuminemia. With protein losing enteropathy, whole blood loss (gastroin-

testinal, lacerations/trauma, other hemorrhage), or massive burns, all serum proteins can be decreased, leading to hypoalbuminemia and hypoglobulinemia.
NEXT DIAGNOSTIC STEP TO CONSIDER IF LEVELS LOW: Measure serum albumin and globulin levels. Evaluate for gastrointestinal disease. Assess renal, liver function.

DRUG EFFECTS ON LEVELS

- Increase: testosterone, estrogens, growth hormone.
- Decrease: thyroxine, cortisol.

LAB ARTIFACTS THAT MAY INTERFERE WITH READINGS OF LEVELS OF THIS SUBSTANCE: Increase: lipemia, hemolysis.

SAMPLE FOR COLLECTION AND ANY SPECIAL SPECIMEN HANDLING NOTES: Serum (red top). Can be evaluated using heparinized plasma (green top) or ethylenediamine tetraacetic acid plasma (lavender top). Stable for 1 month at 2–8°C .

AUTHOR: **RUANNA GOSSETT**

Toxoplasma gondii Serology

BASIC INFORMATION

DEFINITION

Toxoplasmosis is a protozoan disease caused by *Toxoplasma gondii*, an intracellular parasite that infects many tissues of birds and mammals, including humans.

TYPICAL NORMAL RANGE

Reported as titer values; consult with reference laboratory.

PHYSIOLOGY

The enteroepithelial life cycle with sexual and asexual phases is completed only in the definitive host (cats). Transmission is by congenital infection, ingestion of cysts in tissue, or ingestion of oocyst-contaminated water or food. Infected animals may show no clinical signs or may develop a variety of clinical signs such as neurologic, ocular, respiratory, cardiac, muscular, or stillbirths, depending on tissues infected.
CAUSES OF ABNORMALLY HIGH LEVELS: Enzyme-linked immunosorbent assay (ELISA) positive immunoglobulin (Ig) G with negative IgM titer most consistent with chronic exposure to *T. gondii*, although some IgM titers decrease rapidly in acute infections, as seen in 20–85% of the cat population (geographically variable). Positive IgM with negative IgG titer most consistent with recent exposure or active infection with *T. gondii*. Positive IgG with positive IgM titer consistent with recent exposure or active infection.
NEXT DIAGNOSTIC STEP TO CONSIDER IF LEVELS HIGH: If IgG titer is positive, evaluate IgM titer or paired IgG titers (at least 2 weeks apart). Greater than fourfold increase in paired IgG titers indicates recent exposure. Polymerase chain reaction (PCR) test on cerebrospinal fluid, aqueous humor, or fresh tissue to demonstrate presence of *Toxoplasma* DNA. Definitive diagnosis requires demonstration of organisms in tissue via histopathology, immunohistochemistry, and/or PCR, or via animal or cell culture inoculation. Some infectious disease specialists recommend response to treatment (e.g., with clindamycin) as a diagnostic test in patients with compatible clinical signs and a positive IgM or rising IgG titer.
CAUSES OF ABNORMALLY LOW LEVELS: Negative IgG and IgM titers indicate absence of exposure or peracute infection.
NEXT DIAGNOSTIC STEP TO CONSIDER IF LEVELS LOW: If clinical signs are suggestive of acute toxoplasmosis, reevaluate IgM and IgG titers in 3 weeks.
LAB ARTIFACTS THAT MAY INTERFERE WITH READINGS OF LEVELS OF THIS SUBSTANCE: Lipemia and hemolysis interfere with the ELISA.
SAMPLE FOR COLLECTION AND ANY SPECIAL SPECIMEN HANDLING NOTES: Submit 1 ml of serum (red-top tube). Stable for 4 days at 4°C or 0°C for several weeks.
PEARLS: Value of a single IgG measurement in cats is highly limited because a large proportion of healthy cats (20–85% of the population) has a positive result.

AUTHOR: **PATTY J. EWING**

Triglycerides

BASIC INFORMATION

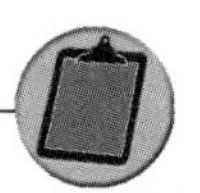

DEFINITION

Main storage form of long chain fatty acids.

SYNONYM(S)

Triacylglycerol

TYPICAL NORMAL RANGE

Dogs: 20–150 mg/dL. Cats: 20–90 mg/dL.

PHYSIOLOGY

Three fatty acid molecules are bound (esterified) to a glycerol backbone to form a triglyceride molecule, the main lipid in adipose tissue and primary form of body fat. Primary sites of triglyceride synthesis are liver, small intestine, adipose tissue and mammary gland, but synthesis occurs in most cells. Triglycerides are transported in the blood bound to apoproteins, forming complexes called lipoproteins. Circulating triglyceride levels reflect a balance of absorption and synthesis by the small intestine, synthesis and secretion by hepatocytes, and uptake by adipose tissue. These processes are affected by dietary fat intake and hormones (insulin, glucagon).
CAUSES OF ABNORMALLY HIGH LEVELS

- Primary hyperlipidemia: idiopathic hyperlipidemia (schnauzer, beagles, and rarely in Brittany spaniels, mixed breed dogs and cats); familial hyperchylomicronemia in cats.

- Secondary hyperlipidemia: postprandial, hypothyroidism (dogs), diabetes mellitus, pancreatitis, hepatic disease, nephrotic syndrome, hyperadrenocorticism, high fat diet, acromegaly (cats).

NEXT DIAGNOSTIC STEP TO CONSIDER IF LEVELS HIGH: Measure fasting levels (minimum 12-hour fast). If persistent, assess for causes of secondary hyperlipidemia. If secondary hyperlipidemia is ruled out, primary hyperlipidemia is diagnosis of exclusion.

CAUSES OF ABNORMALLY LOW LEVELS: Malabsorption/maldigestion; hepatic synthetic failure (chronic hepatopathies).

NEXT DIAGNOSTIC STEP TO CONSIDER IF LEVELS LOW: Trypsin-like immunoreactivity (TLI), cobalamin (vitamin B_{12}) and folate, assess for panhypoproteinemia; serum bile acids (preprandial and postprandial).

IMPORTANT INTERSPECIES DIFFERENCES: Hyperlipidemia may occur in cholestatic liver disease. Cats with hepatic lipidosis do not have hyperlipidemia.

DRUG EFFECTS ON LEVELS

- Increased: doxorubicin therapy, exogenous corticosteroids.
- Decreased: lipid-lowering diets, supplementation with fish oils, nicotinic acid and fibric acid derivatives such as gemfibrozil.

LAB ARTIFACTS THAT MAY INTERFERE WITH READINGS OF LEVELS OF THIS SUBSTANCE: Hemolysis, lipemia, increased fluid viscosity and glycerol artificially elevate triglyceride levels.

SAMPLE FOR COLLECTION AND ANY SPECIAL SPECIMEN HANDLING NOTES: Serum (red top), heparinized plasma (green top), or ethylenediamine tetraacetic plasma (lavender top). Stable at 2–8°C for 1 week, 3 months frozen at −20°C.

PEARLS: Triglyceride levels may be measured in suspected chylous effusions. Triglyceride levels in the fluid that are greater than serum triglyceride levels in effusion indicates chylous effusion, even if the effusion is not grossly milky in appearance.

AUTHOR: **RUANNA GOSSETT**

Tri-Iodothyronine (T3)

BASIC INFORMATION

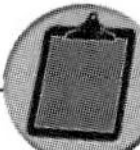

DEFINITION

Active form of iodine-containing thyroid hormone. Chief function is to increase rate of cell metabolism.

SYNONYM(S)

3,5,3′ tri-iodothyroinine

TYPICAL NORMAL RANGE

- Dogs: 0.5–1.8 ng/ml; cats: 0.4–1.6 ng/ml.
- Values vary with laboratory.
- Conversion: ng/dl × 10 = pg/ml; ng/dl × 0.01536 = nmol/L; pg/dl × 15.4 = nmol/L = SI unit.
- Specific values vary among laboratories and assay types.

PHYSIOLOGY

Approximately 20% of T3 produced from thyroid gland; the rest is from conversion of T4 to T3 in cells. More biologically active than thyroxine (T4). In circulation, 99% is protein bound. Dissociates to free T3 to enter cells. Binds to receptor proteins in cells, which induces DNA translation and production of proteins associated with cell growth, oxidative phosphorylation, and membrane transport of electrolytes resulting in an increase in metabolic rate and growth stimulation.

CAUSES OF ABNORMALLY HIGH LEVELS: Hyperthyroidism; presence of autoantibodies; exogenous T3, TSH or TRH; administration of iodine (or compounds containing iodine).

NEXT DIAGNOSTIC STEP TO CONSIDER IF LEVELS HIGH

- If hyperthyroidism suspected: other thyroid tests, clinical signs, imaging.
- If autoantibodies: run thyroglobulin autoantibody test (TGAA).
- Evaluate diet and supplements for iodine content.

CAUSES OF ABNORMALLY LOW LEVELS: Hypothyroidism, euthyroid sick syndrome.

NEXT DIAGNOSTIC STEP TO CONSIDER IF LEVELS LOW: T4, free T4, evaluate for nonthyroidal diseases.

LAB ARTIFACTS THAT MAY INTERFERE WITH READINGS OF LEVELS OF THIS SUBSTANCE: Decrease: moderate to marked hemolysis.

SAMPLE FOR COLLECTION AND ANY SPECIAL SPECIMEN HANDLING NOTES: Serum (red-top tube) or ethylenediamine tetraacetic acid plasma (purple-top tube). Separate serum or plasma from red blood cells as soon as possible. Store at 2–8°C (refrigeration).

PEARLS: Test is of little diagnostic value. Broad overlap in T3 serum levels within euthyroid, hypothyroid, and euthyroid sick dogs. Total T3 is relatively insensitive and often nonspecific in assessment of hypothyroidism. Total and free T3 provide little additional information over total and free T4 by equilibrium dialysis. Serum T3 correlates poorly with thyroid disease.

AUTHOR: **FONZIE QUANCE-FITCH**

Troponins, Cardiac

BASIC INFORMATION

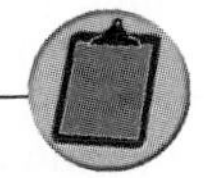

DEFINITION

Troponins are intracellular myofibrillar proteins expressed in cardiac and skeletal muscle. Cardiac troponin I (Tn-I) is the most diagnostically accurate.

TYPICAL NORMAL RANGE

- Dogs: 0.03–0.07 ng/ml (Tn-I), 0.01–0.15 ng/ml (troponin T), 0.05–0.21 ng/ml (troponin C).
- Cats: 0.03–0.16 ng/ml (Tn-I), 0.05–0.22 ng/ml (troponin T).

PHYSIOLOGY

- Troponins regulate the contractility of striated muscle. They mediate the interaction between the sarcomeric proteins actin and myosin. The troponin complex is composed of three proteins. Troponin I is the inhibitory com-

ponent that prevents interaction between actin and myosin until intracellular calcium is bound by troponin C. Troponin T is the tropomyosin binding element that binds troponin I to the actin filament.
- The cardiac isoforms of troponins I and T are specific markers for myocardial injury because they are antigenically distinct from skeletal muscle troponins. They are found in high concentration only in cardiac myocytes.
- Cardiac troponins are released into the circulation when there is cardiac ischemia and necrosis. Troponins increase in the circulation within 4 to 6 hours after myocyte injury and may persist up to 1 or 2 weeks. They appear to be earlier, more specific markers of cardiac injury than traditional methods (echocardiography, electrocardiography) for many veterinary cardiac disorders.

CAUSES OF ABNORMALLY HIGH LEVELS: Pericardial effusion caused by hemangiosarcoma or idiopathic pericarditis in dogs (elevations greater with hemangiosarcoma), cardiomyopathy, myocardial contusion, gastric dilatation—volvulus, myocarditis, structural heart disease associated with congestive heart failure in dogs and cats, high-dose doxorubicin toxicity in dogs, and canine babesiosis.

SAMPLE FOR COLLECTION AND ANY SPECIAL SPECIMEN HANDLING NOTES: Serum (red top), heparinized plasma (green top), or ethylenediamine tetraacetic acid plasma (lavender top); refrigerate or freeze to −20° C.

PEARLS: Cardiac troponin concentrations are diagnostically superior to other enzyme assessments (e.g., myocardial isoenzyme of creatine kinase) in human beings and appear to be promising, valuable detection and monitoring tools in veterinary cardiology.

AUTHOR: **RUANNA GOSSETT**

Trypsin-Like Immunoreactivity

BASIC INFORMATION

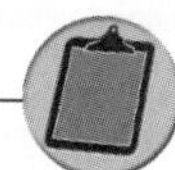

DEFINITION

Immunologic assay that detects trypsinogen, trypsin, and trypsin bound to protease inhibitors. Most detected activity due to trypsinogen.

SYNONYM(S)

TLI

TYPICAL NORMAL RANGE

- Canine: 5.0–35.0 μg/L.
- Feline:12.0–82.0 μg/L.

PHYSIOLOGY

Trypsinogen, the inactive (zymogen) form of trypsin, is produced by pancreatic acinar epithelial cells and is present in low concentration in the blood of normal patients. The assay also detects the active enzyme, trypsin, which may be increased in concentration in the blood of patients with pancreatitis.

CAUSES OF ABNORMALLY HIGH LEVELS: Pancreatitis.

NEXT DIAGNOSTIC STEP TO CONSIDER IF LEVELS HIGH: Not usually used for diagnosis of pancreatitis; clinical signs, diagnostic imaging results, and possibly increased serum amylase, lipase usually adequate. TLI >50 μg/L (dogs), >100 μg/L (cats) are consistent with pancreatitis.

CAUSES OF ABNORMALLY LOW LEVELS: Exocrine pancreatic insufficiency (EPI); severe, chronic, persistent pancreatitis or lymphocytic pancreatitis associated with parenchymal destruction.

NEXT DIAGNOSTIC STEP TO CONSIDER IF LEVELS LOW: Less than 2.5 μg/L (dogs) and <8.0 μg/L (cats) are diagnostic for EPI. Values between these and reference range are equivocal. If EPI is suspected, repeat test in 4 weeks. May also indicate chronic, persistent pancreatitis.

IMPORTANT INTERSPECIES DIFFERENCES
- Cats: age-related increases, associated with acinar adenomas.
- Dogs: increased values associated with malnutrition.

SAMPLE FOR COLLECTION AND ANY SPECIAL SPECIMEN HANDLING NOTES: Serum (red-top tube), nonhemolyzed, fasting (12 to 18 hours) sample.

PEARLS: Assays are species specific. Check with reference laboratory to be sure that species specific assays are being run.

AUTHOR: **LOIS ROTH-JOHNSON**

Urinalysis

BASIC INFORMATION

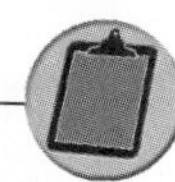

DEFINITION

Panel of screening tests done on urine to evaluate for inflammation, degenerative lesions, protein loss, and neoplasia in the urinary tract and systemic metabolic disease.

TYPICAL NORMAL RANGE

- Color: yellow; appearance: clear; pH: 6.0 to 7.5; specific gravity: >1.012; protein, glucose, ketones, bilirubin, blood, bacteria: negative; red blood cells, leukocytes, epithelial cells: 0 to 5 per high-power field; casts: 0 to 2 per low-power field.
- Some values depend on collection method.

PHYSIOLOGY

Urine constituents and composition reflect lesions of the urinary tract and may provide an indication of metabolic abnormalities.

LAB ARTIFACTS THAT MAY INTERFERE WITH READINGS OF LEVELS OF THIS SUBSTANCE: Delay in specimen processing may decrease some values and increase others. See specific tests. Generally, 10 ml of urine is recommended because reference range quantitation of urine sediment is usually based on this volume.

SAMPLE FOR COLLECTION AND ANY SPECIAL SPECIMEN HANDLING NOTES: Collect 10 ml of fresh urine in sterile container. Indicate method of collection (cystocentesis, catheterization, or free catch).

PEARLS: Collection method may influence interpretation. Blood and epithelial cells in catheterized specimens or bacteria in free-catch specimens may not indicate disease.

AUTHOR: **LOIS ROTH-JOHNSON**

Urine Cortisol:Creatinine Ratio

BASIC INFORMATION

DEFINITION

Screening test for hyperadrenocorticism that measures the ratio of urinary cortisol to creatinine excretion.

TYPICAL NORMAL RANGE

- Ratios less than approximately 10×10^{-6} rule out hyperadrenocorticism.
- Ratios greater than approximately 10×10^{-6} indicate elevated serum cortisol (adrenal or nonadrenal disease). Specific values vary among laboratories.

PHYSIOLOGY

Because urine excretion of creatinine is fairly constant, its ratio to urine cortisol excretion provides a measurement of average serum cortisol levels.

CAUSES OF ABNORMALLY HIGH LEVELS: Hyperadrenocorticism, many nonadrenal diseases, and physiologic conditions.

NEXT DIAGNOSTIC STEP TO CONSIDER IF LEVELS HIGH: Adrenocorticotropic hormone (ACTH) stimulation, low-dose dexamethasone suppression test (LDDS).

IMPORTANT INTERSPECIES DIFFERENCES: Ratio may be abnormally high in cats with hyperthyroidism.

DRUG EFFECTS ON LEVELS: Corticosteroid administration increases levels; ketoconazole therapy decreases levels.

LAB ARTIFACTS THAT MAY INTERFERE WITH READINGS OF LEVELS OF THIS SUBSTANCE: Increase: anticoagulants, bilirubin.

SAMPLE FOR COLLECTION AND ANY SPECIAL SPECIMEN HANDLING NOTES: Fresh urine, morning collection preferred.

PEARLS

- Increased ratio is a sensitive but nonspecific test for hyperadrenocorticism. High ratios are associated with stress, nonadrenal disease, as well as hyperadrenocorticism.
- Values within reference range strongly indicate patient does not have hyperadrenocorticism.
- Increased urinary cortisol excretion may be physiologic or pathologic.

AUTHOR: **FONZIE QUANCE-FITCH**

Urine pH Abnormalities

BASIC INFORMATION

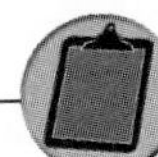

DEFINITION

Urine pH higher or lower than reference range; the negative logarithm of hydrogen ion concentration in urine.

SYNONYM(S)

Aciduria (low urine pH)
Alkaliuria (high urine pH)

TYPICAL NORMAL RANGE

Dogs and cats: 6.0–7.5.

PHYSIOLOGY

Dietary constituents influence urine pH in health.

CAUSES OF ABNORMALLY HIGH LEVELS: Alkaliuria:

- Expected postprandially in monogastric mammals.
- Infections (usually cystitis) in dogs/cats caused by bacteria that contain/produce urease (urea is degraded to ammonia, which is a weak base and removes free hydrogen ion from urine).
- Excess base is excreted or increased acid (free hydrogen ions) is retained (renal proximal and distal tubules) in some cases of metabolic alkalosis and occasionally in cases of chronic respiratory alkalosis.
- Distal renal tubular acidosis (decreased hydrogen ion excretion in distal nephron) may result in alkaline urine or a disproportionately high urine pH (>6) compared with the blood pH (acidemia).
- Proximal renal tubular acidosis (inability to conserve bicarbonate in proximal tubules) may result in high urine pH early in the disorder.

NEXT DIAGNOSTIC STEP TO CONSIDER IF LEVELS HIGH: Urine sediment examination and/or culture for bacteria.

CAUSES OF ABNORMALLY LOW LEVELS: Aciduria:

- Severe cases of metabolic alkalosis with hypochloridemia ± hypokalemia
- Hypokalemia (H+ excretion in exchange for K+ resorption in intercalated cells of distal tubules)
- Loop diuretic treatment (e.g., furosemide)
- Excretion of excess acid (H+) in metabolic or respiratory acidosis

NEXT DIAGNOSTIC STEP TO CONSIDER IF LEVELS LOW: Determine serum electrolyte status (Na+, K+, Cl–, HCO_3^-).

IMPORTANT INTERSPECIES DIFFERENCES: Dogs and cats typically have more acid urine than other species.

DRUG EFFECTS ON LEVELS: Potassium wasting diuretics may result in renal K+ conservation and excess H+ excretion (aciduria).

LAB ARTIFACTS THAT MAY INTERFERE WITH READINGS OF LEVELS OF THIS SUBSTANCE

- Marked delay in analysis may result in urine alkalinization (urea converts to ammonia spontaneously or via urease containing bacteria).
- High pH (≥9) may cause a false positive urine dipstick protein reading.

SAMPLE FOR COLLECTION AND ANY SPECIAL SPECIMEN HANDLING NOTES: Minimum of 5 ml of urine in clean/sterile container collected by free catch, catheterization, or cystocentesis (if culture also needed).

AUTHOR: **ELIZABETH G. WELLES**

Urine Protein:Creatinine Ratio

BASIC INFORMATION

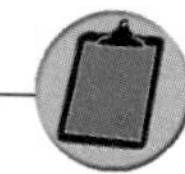

DEFINITION

Amount of protein excreted in urine compared with (ratio) the concentration of urine, as determined in a single sample collection (spot check).

SYNONYM(S)

UP:C ratio

TYPICAL NORMAL RANGE

Urine protein:creatinine (UP:C) ratio in healthy individuals is <0.6 (cats) or <1 (dogs).

PHYSIOLOGY

- Increased urinary protein loss can be assessed for significance when compared to the concentration of creatinine in the urine.
- Glomeruli normally allow the passage of only trace amounts of protein (if any) into the urine. Glomerular damage, renal tubular damage, or inflammation in the urinary tract can cause proteinuria and an elevated UP:C.
- UP:C has traditionally been used in the diagnosis of protein losing nephropathies (glomerulonephritis, amyloidosis), for which it remains the initial diagnostic test of choice.
- More recently, renal tubular protein loss and associated UP:C elevation have also emerged as early markers of chronic renal failure, with important treatment and prognostic implications in dogs and cats.
- An inactive urine sediment exam and negative bacterial urine culture (to exclude urinary tract infection as a source of urine protein) are necessary before a diagnosis of renal protein loss can be made from an elevated UP:C.

CAUSES OF ABNORMALLY HIGH LEVELS

- Urinary tract inflammation may result in modest UP:C ratio elevations (e.g., 1-3), although very high values (e.g., 40) have been reported in patients with bacterial cystitis.
- Tubular loss of protein may result in a UP:C ratio of 1-5.
- Glomerular loss of protein usually results in UP:C >1, usually >3, and renal amyloidosis usually has UP:C ratio >15.

NEXT DIAGNOSTIC STEP TO CONSIDER IF LEVELS HIGH: Full urinalysis, serum protein concentration, serum urea and creatinine, urine bacterial culture, and sensitivity.

SAMPLE FOR COLLECTION AND ANY SPECIAL SPECIMEN HANDLING NOTES: Urine in clean container.

PEARLS: Albumin is a major component of the urinary protein excreted in protein losing nephropathy. Because it is of a similar molecular size as antithrombin III, a markedly elevated UP:C with a sterile urine sample may indicate a hypercoagulable state.

AUTHOR: **ELIZABETH G. WELLES**

Urine Specific Gravity

BASIC INFORMATION

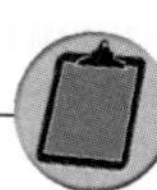

DEFINITION

Urine specific gravity (USG) is an estimate of urine osmolality.

SYNONYM(S)

Concentrated urine: USG >1.030 (dog), >1.035 (cat)
Isosthenuria: USG = 1.008-1.012
Hyposthenuria: USG <1.008

TYPICAL NORMAL RANGE

Normally 1.001-1.060, depending on hydration status.

PHYSIOLOGY

Assessment of ability to concentrate urine. Depends upon hydration status as well as renal function.

CAUSES OF ABNORMALLY HIGH LEVELS

- Dehydration, proteinuria, and glucosuria may cause falsely high estimates of value, though values are rarely greater than reference range:
- 2% glucosuria (4+ on urine dipsticks) increases USG by 0.008-0.010.

CAUSES OF ABNORMALLY LOW LEVELS

- If low USG (1.008-1.012) is concurrent with normal serum blood urea nitrogen (BUN) and creatinine levels, the most likely explanation is normal formation of dilute urine to preserve euvolemia (e.g., after drinking water).
- No conclusion can be drawn concerning renal function, except that at least 25% of renal tubules must be functioning for BUN and creatinine levels to be normal.

If low USG (1.008-1.012) plus azotemia, glucosuria, dehydration, polyuria, or oliguria, then renal tubular concentrating ability is impaired. Underlying causes include:

- Decreased numbers of functional nephrons (>75% nonfunctioning tubules); chronic renal failure
- Osmotic diuresis (iatrogenic, other)
- Diabetes insipidus (central, nephrogenic)
- Aldosterone deficit (hypoadrenocorticism) or resistance (spironolactone)

NEXT DIAGNOSTIC STEP TO CONSIDER IF LEVELS LOW: Determine hydration status, evaluate serum chemistry values, especially urea, creatinine, inorganic phosphate, glucose, calcium, sodium, and potassium.

IMPORTANT INTERSPECIES DIFFERENCES

- Concentrating abilities vary among species: cat > dog > horse/cow.
- Adults have greater concentrating ability than neonates.

DRUG EFFECTS ON LEVELS: Diuretics cause USG to decrease (sodium and water excretion).

SAMPLE FOR COLLECTION AND ANY SPECIAL SPECIMEN HANDLING NOTES: Urine in clean container.

PEARLS

- A low USG is meaningless with respect to renal function unless it is accompanied by BUN and creatinine levels measured on a blood sample drawn at the same time as the urine sample.
- Acute anuric renal failure may be associated with a normal USG (residual urine).
- USG in untreated diabetics is usually 1.025-1.035; isosthenuria suggests concomitant renal disease or hyperadrenocorticism.

AUTHOR: **ELIZABETH G. WELLES**

von Willebrand Factor Assay

BASIC INFORMATION

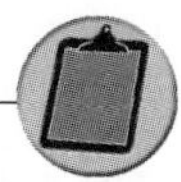

DEFINITION

von Willebrand disease (vWD) results from decreased functional von Willebrand factor (vWF), causing prolonged bleeding time and abnormal primary hemostasis.

TYPICAL NORMAL RANGE

Canine: 60–172% of normal pooled plasma.

PHYSIOLOGY

- vWF is produced by endothelial cells and megakaryocytes. vWF circulates with factor VIII, which prolongs its stability. Stored in endothelial cells and platelet α-granules. vWF acts as a bridge between exposed subendothelial collagen and platelets, and among platelets. Platelet binding of vWF triggers a cascade of hemostatic and thrombotic events. Low levels of vWF result in lack of platelet activation.
- Measured by quantitative enzyme-linked immunosorbent assay (ELISA) with species-specific antibodies to vWF. Multimeric analysis (separates the different vWF multimers) can distinguish between type 1 and 2 vWD.

CAUSES OF ABNORMALLY HIGH LEVELS: Azotemia, liver disease

NEXT DIAGNOSTIC STEP TO CONSIDER IF LEVELS HIGH: No clinical importance

CAUSES OF ABNORMALLY LOW LEVELS: vWD (type 1, 2, or 3) is the most common hereditary bleeding disorder in dogs. ELISA is typically <35% in vWD. No detectable vWF indicates type 3 vWD. vWF 30–70% indicates a carrier.

NEXT DIAGNOSTIC STEP TO CONSIDER IF LEVELS LOW: Genetic tests to identify gene mutations to detect carriers in certain dog breeds. Any dog with factor levels <70% is considered a carrier and not appropriate for breeding.

IMPORTANT INTERSPECIES DIFFERENCES: Feline platelets contain vWF; canine platelets do not contain significant levels. Thrombocytopenia does not affect vWF values in dogs.

DRUG EFFECTS ON LEVELS: Epinephrine, endotoxin, and 1-deamino-8-D-arginine vasopressin (DDAVP) can increase vWF. DDAVP will increase vWF both in dogs with type 1 vWD and in normal dogs.

LAB ARTIFACTS THAT MAY INTERFERE WITH READINGS OF LEVELS OF THIS SUBSTANCE: Decrease: hemolysis, clotting.

SAMPLE FOR COLLECTION AND ANY SPECIAL SPECIMEN HANDLING NOTES: Sodium citrate (blue top) or ethylenediamine tetraacetic acid (purple top) tube. After centrifugation, plasma should be promptly collected, frozen, and shipped overnight.

PEARLS: If the platelet counts and coagulation times are within normal limits, buccal mucosal bleeding time may help diagnose vWD. Affected patients will have prolonged buccal mucosal bleeding times.

AUTHOR: **DEBORAH G. DAVIS**

Warfarin

BASIC INFORMATION

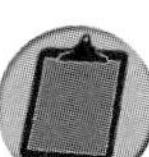

DEFINITION

- Commonly used rodenticide; testing is typically for retrospective confirmation (e.g., identification and prevention of future reintoxication, or for legal purposes).
- Note: animals suspected of active hemorrhage due to ingestion of warfarin or other anticoagulant toxicosis should be evaluated with prothrombin time (PT) or assessment of proteins inhibited by vitamin K absence/antagonism (PIVKA), because turnaround time to warfarin assay results is typically long and it is less widely available.

SYNONYM(S)

First-generation compounds: warfarin, indanedione-containing rodenticides.

Second-generation compounds: coumarin-based generics (brodifacoum, difenacoum, bromadiolone) and the indanedione diphacinone.

TYPICAL TOXIC RANGE

Consult laboratory for reference range and for inclusion of both first- and second-generation compounds in test panel.

PHYSIOLOGY

Well, but slowly, absorbed following oral administration. Peak plasma levels in 6 to 12 hours. Most is plasma protein-bound but high concentrations in liver, spleen, kidney. Metabolism occurs in the liver. Elimination rate depends on compound, amount ingested; may accumulate if small amounts ingested over several days. Warfarin half-life in dog plasma is 14.5 hours; the half-life of diphacinone is suspected to be days. Brodifacoum is assumed to be similar or longer than that of diphacinone. The differences in residual half-lives have important therapeutic implications. Compounds interfere with coagulation by decreasing clotting factors II, VII, IX and X (competitive inhibition of vitamin K epoxide-reductase).

CAUSES OF ABNORMALLY HIGH LEVELS: Ingestion of compounds or of animals who have consumed compounds. Relay toxicosis (incurred from consumption of prey [e.g., rodents] that have eaten warfarin) rarely occurs with second-generation anticoagulants, other than diphacinone.

NEXT DIAGNOSTIC STEP TO CONSIDER IF LEVELS HIGH: Remove source; administer vitamin K; whole blood transfusion.

DRUG EFFECTS ON LEVELS: Oxyphenbutazone, phenylbutazone, diphenylhydantoin, sulfonamides, and adrenocorticosteroids increase toxicity.

SAMPLE FOR COLLECTION AND ANY SPECIAL SPECIMEN HANDLING NOTES: Chemical detection of specific anticoagulants in vomitus or baits. Liver tissue (frozen) for postmortem diagnosis. Unclotted blood, stomach contents, intestinal content, feces, spleen, and kidney should also be submitted.

PEARLS: Conditions enhancing susceptibility are: high dietary fat as fatty acids displace the plasma protein bound anticoagulant, prolonged oral antibiotic therapy, biliary obstruction, liver disease, hypoalbuminemia (warfarin is highly plasma protein bound), renal disease.

AUTHOR: **SHERRY J. MORGAN**

Zinc, Serum Level

BASIC INFORMATION

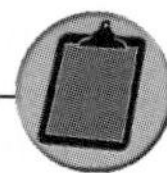

DEFINITION

Zinc is an essential trace mineral that serves as a cofactor for enzymes in many tissues. It is important in regulation of the immune response, modulation of keratogenesis, wound healing, maintenance of normal reproductive function, and acuity of taste and smell.

TYPICAL TOXIC RANGE

Dogs, cats: <2.0 mg/ml (serum); <30-70 ppm, wet weight (liver). Check with laboratory for values considered diagnostic of toxicity.

PHYSIOLOGY

Source is dietary. Zinc is absorbed via the intestine, metabolized in the liver, and exported to peripheral tissues.

CAUSES OF ABNORMALLY HIGH LEVELS: Ingestion of excessive levels of zinc phosphide (either as powder, bait). Toxicity may also result from relay toxicosis associated with eating tissues of zinc phosphide poisoned animals or ingestion of pennies minted after 1983.

NEXT DIAGNOSTIC STEP TO CONSIDER IF LEVELS HIGH: Vomitus/gastric lavage (phosphine gas) is actually the preferred method of diagnosis in case of toxicity. *Caution*: phosphine gas (faint garlic or rotten fish odor; gas is liberated in the breath of animals with zinc phospide intoxication such as during gastric lavage) is a public health hazard and may cause severe/permanent respiratory injury to veterinary personnel or bystanders.

CAUSES OF ABNORMALLY LOW LEVELS: Malnutrition, malabsorption, animals on total parenteral nutrition.

NEXT DIAGNOSTIC STEP TO CONSIDER IF LEVELS LOW: Skin biopsy if zinc-deficient dermatosis is suspected.

IMPORTANT INTERSPECIES DIFFERENCES: Zinc-responsive dermatosis occurs in dogs. Familial form (Alaskan malamutes, Siberian huskies) and from affecting puppies fed zinc-deficient or oversupplemented diets. Lethal acrodermatitis is a rare inherited disorder of bull terriers that does not respond to zinc supplementation and is invariably fatal.

SAMPLE FOR COLLECTION AND ANY SPECIAL SPECIMEN HANDLING NOTES

- Serum: Because of the use of zinc stearate to coat rubber, serum samples must be drawn in all glass or all plastic syringes and all glass or all plastic vials must be used for transport.
- Toxicity: test for toxic metabolite, phosphine gas. Submit frozen vomitus or gastric lavage in airtight containers.

PEARLS

- In zinc phosphide toxicity, there may be a characteristic acetylene odor to the gastric contents and may be bloody.
- Zinc phosphide causes emesis in dogs and cats so fatal intoxication is not frequent. Ingestion with a meal enhances toxicity, by promoting conversion to zinc phosphine gas.
- Ingested pennies may be detected radiographically.

AUTHOR: **SHERRY J. MORGAN**

SECTION V

Clinical Algorithms

EDITORS

Leah A. Cohn, DVM, PhD, DACVIM (SAIM)
Urology

Etienne Côté, DVM, DACVIM (Cardiology, SAIM) Cardiology

Cheryl L. Cullen, DVM, MVetSc, DACVO
Ophthalmology

Jan A. Hall, BVM&S, MS, MRCVS, DACVD
Dermatology

Joseph Harari, DVM, MS, DACVS
Orthopedics

Sherri Ihle, DVM, MSc, DACVIM (SAIM)
Endocrinology

Safdar A. Khan, DVM, MS, PhD, DABVT
Toxicology

Michelle A. Kutzler, DVM, PhD, DACT
Theriogenology

Karen L. Overall, MA, VMD, PhD, DACVB
Behavior

Kenneth M. Rassnick, DVM, DACVIM (Oncology) Oncology

Elizabeth Rozanski, DVM, DACVECC, DACVIM (SAIM) Emergency and Critical Care

Rance K. Sellon, DVM, PhD, DACVIM (SAIM) Respiratory Diseases

ABORTION:

Diagnostic Approach to Abortion in the Dog

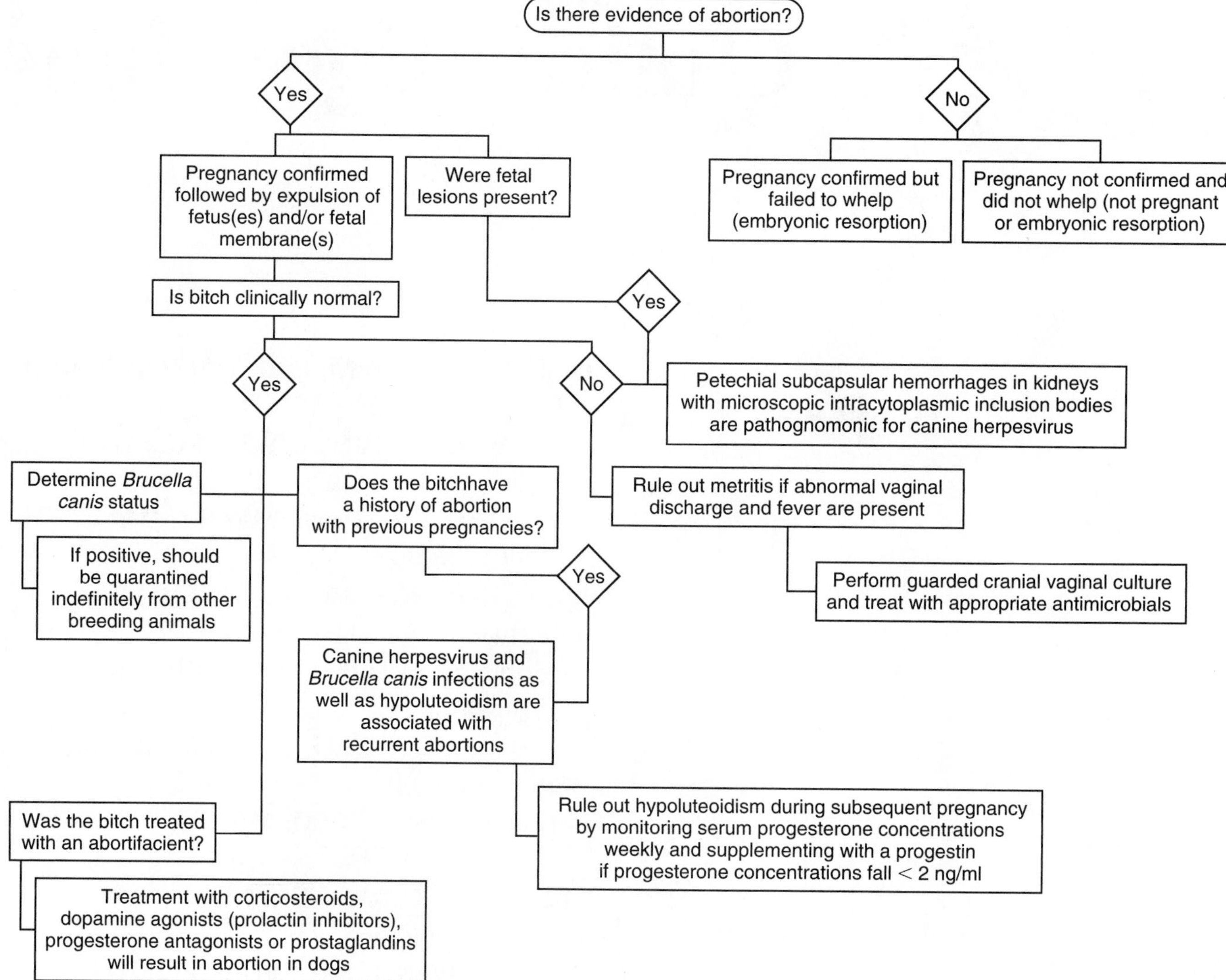

Author: Wenche Farstad
Editor: Michelle A. Kutzler

ACID-BASE DISORDERS

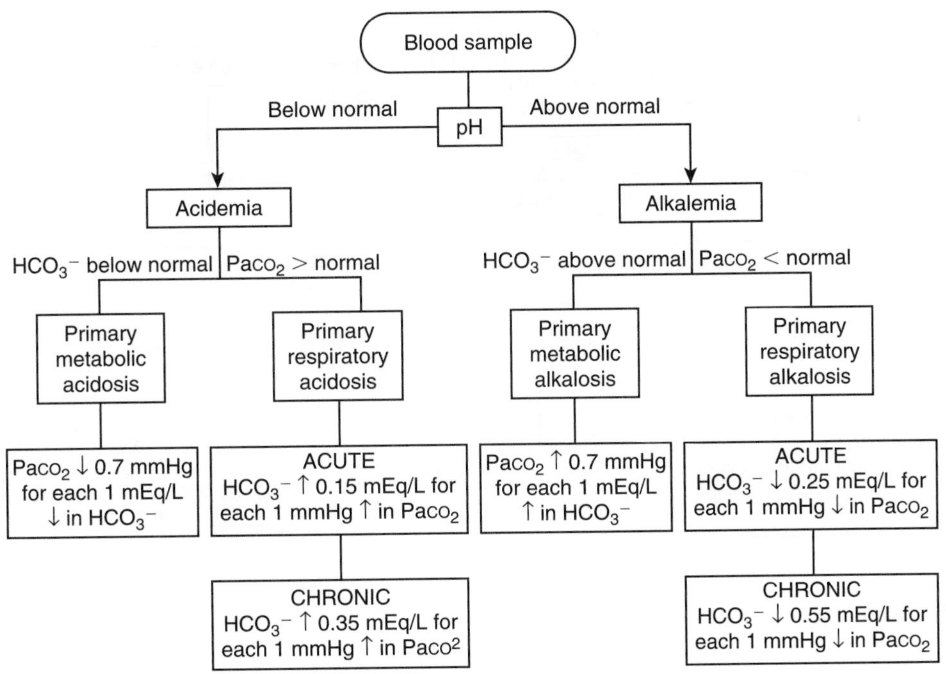

From Slatter DH: *Textbook of Small Animal Surgery,* ed 3. St. Louis, WB Saunders, 2003.

ACUTE ABDOMEN

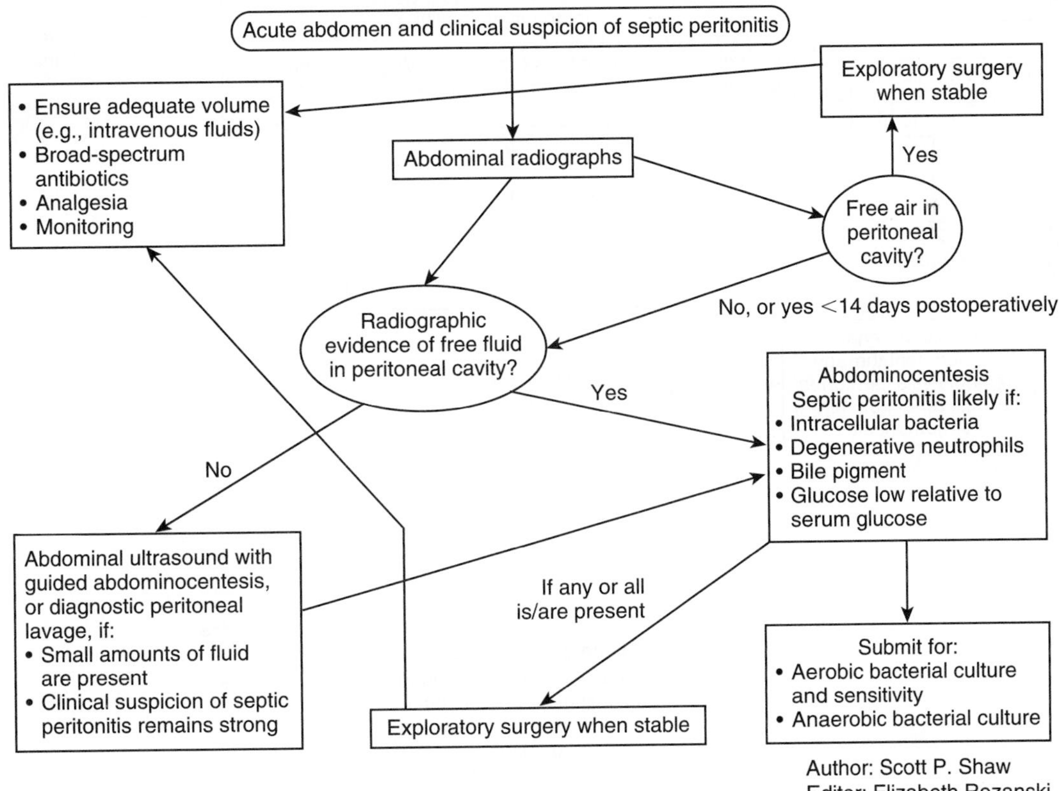

Author: Scott P. Shaw
Editor: Elizabeth Rozanski

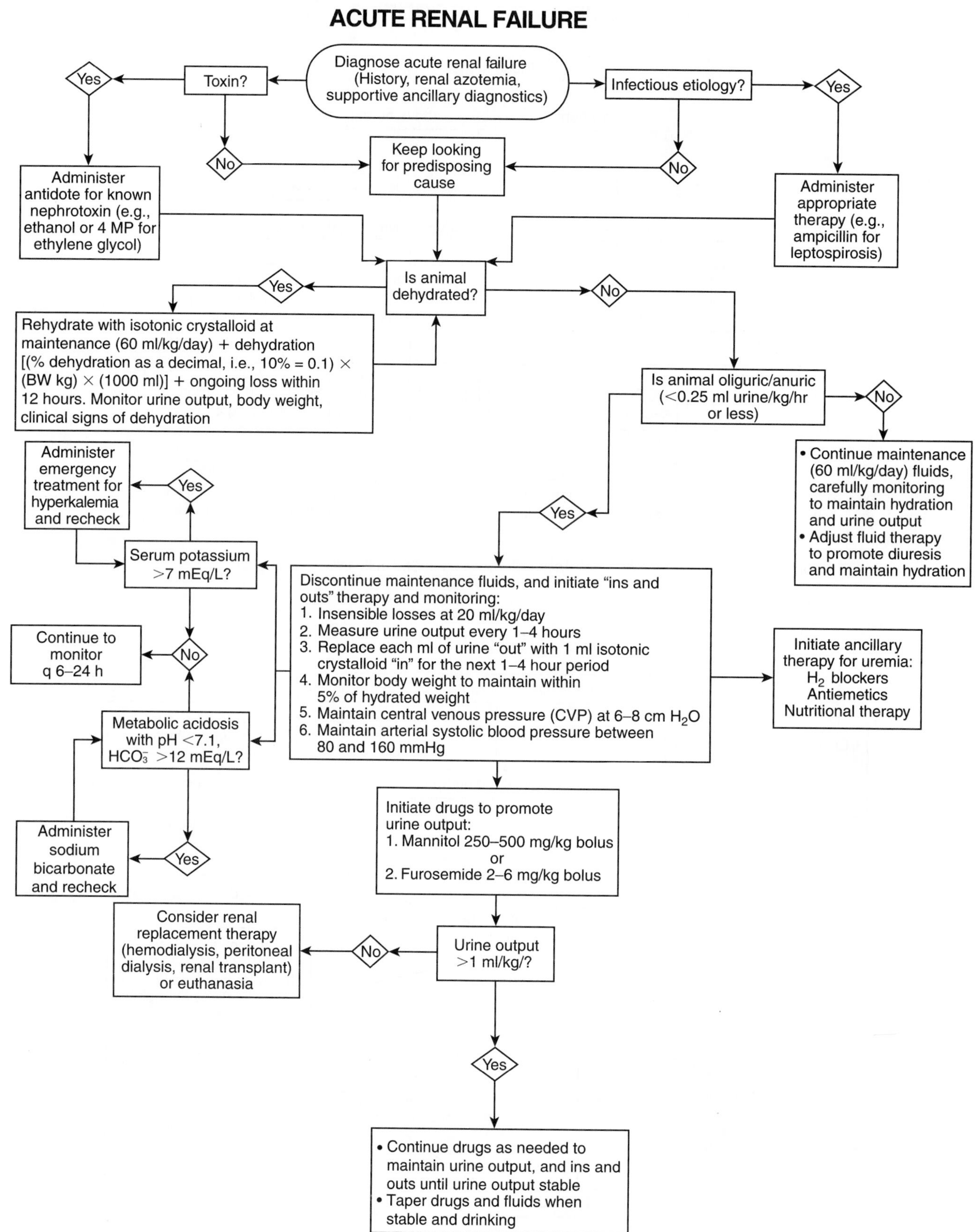

Author: Marie E. Kerl
Editor: Leah A. Cohn

ADENOCARCINOMA OF THE ANAL SACS

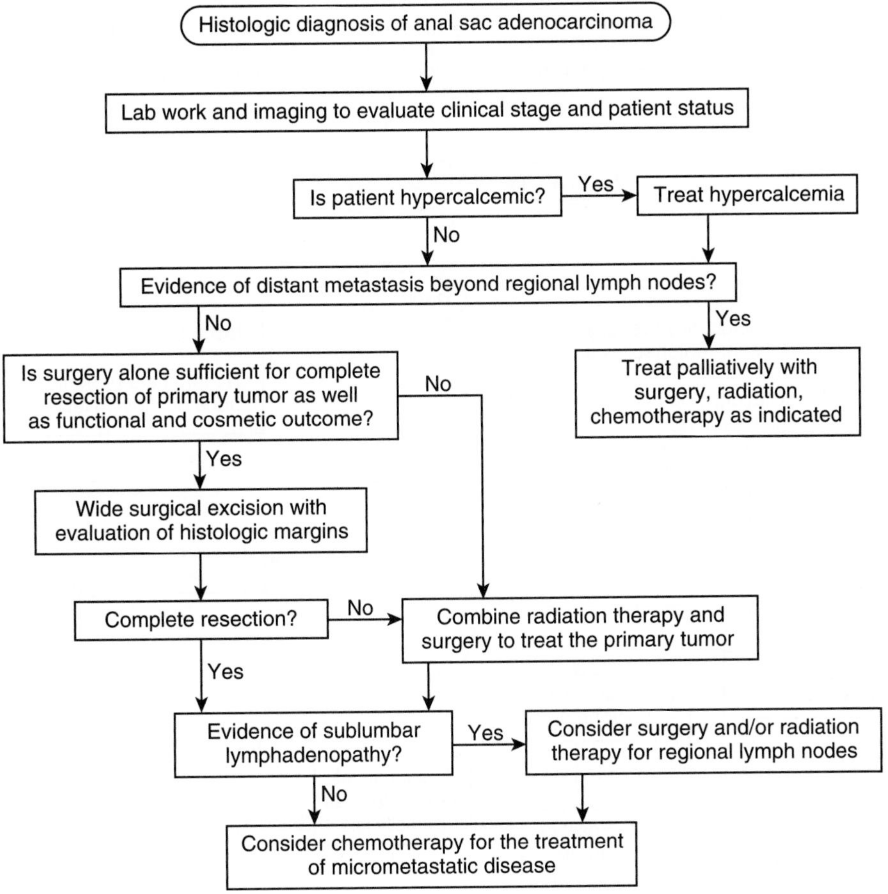

Author: Elizabeth A. McNiel
Editor: Kenneth M. Rassnick

ANESTHETIC COMPLICATIONS

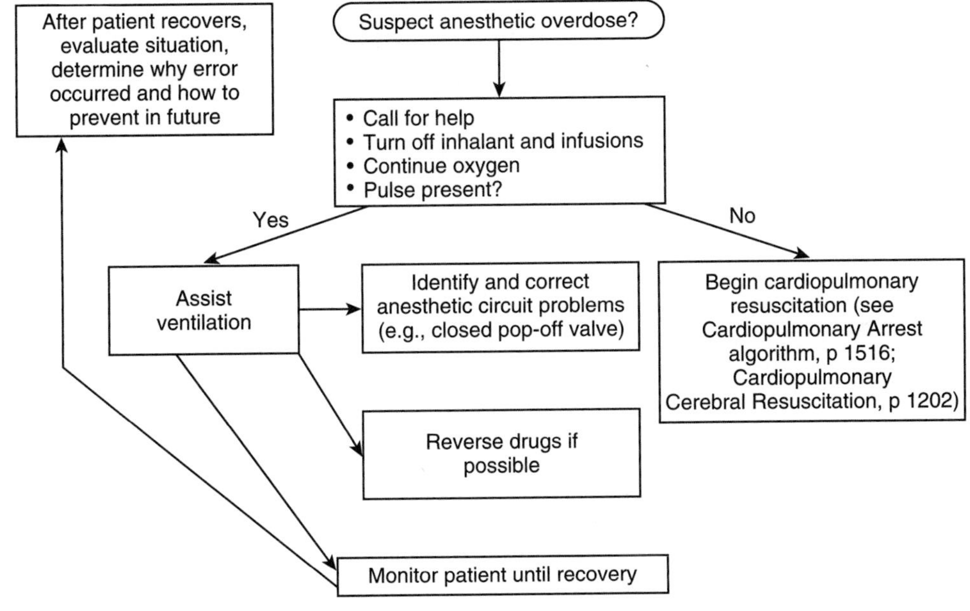

Author: Scott P. Shaw
Editor: Elizabeth Rozanski

CLINICAL ALGORITHMS

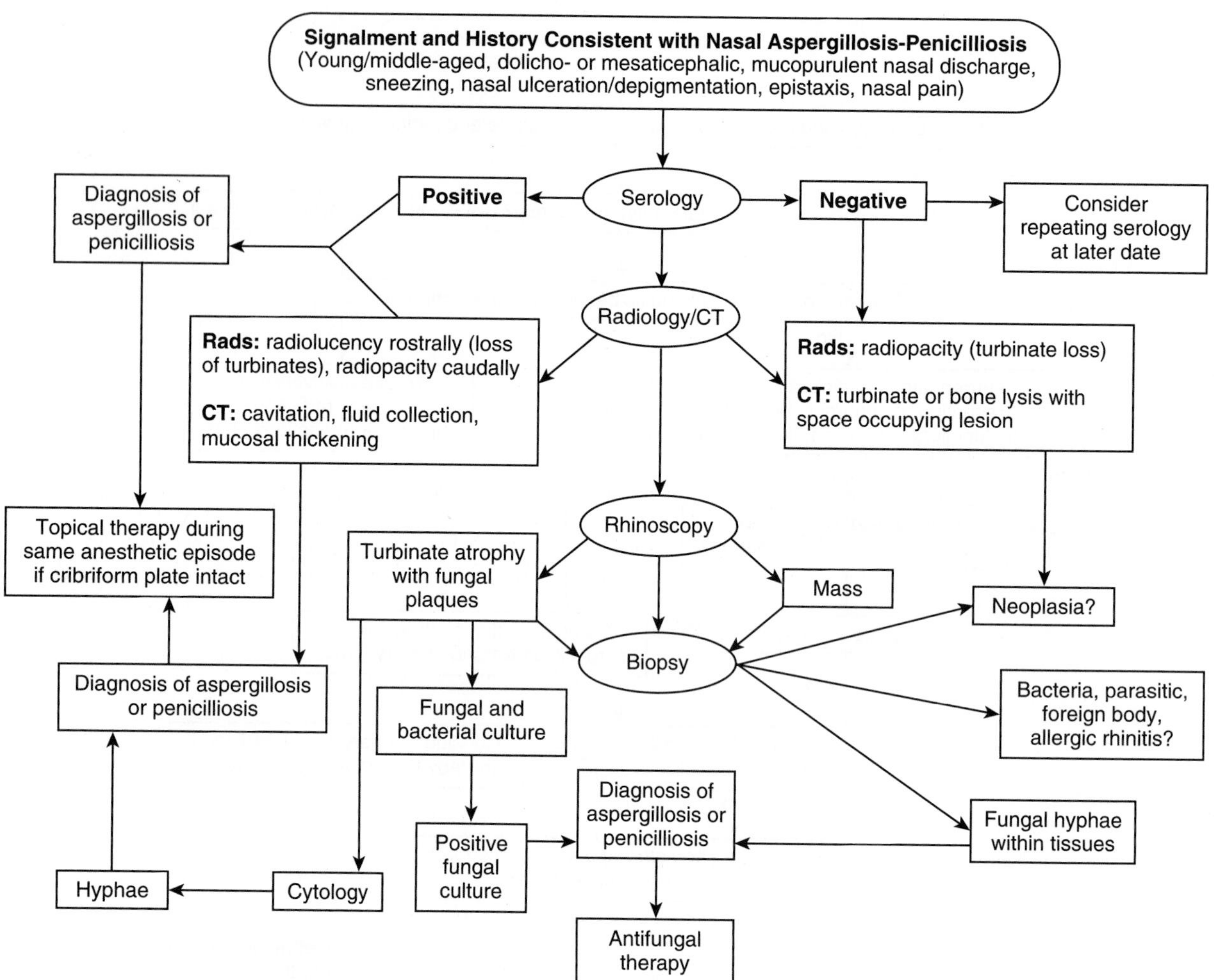

From Greene CE: *Infectious Diseases of the Dog and Cat* (revised reprint), ed 3. St. Louis, WB Saunders, 2006.

ASTHMA

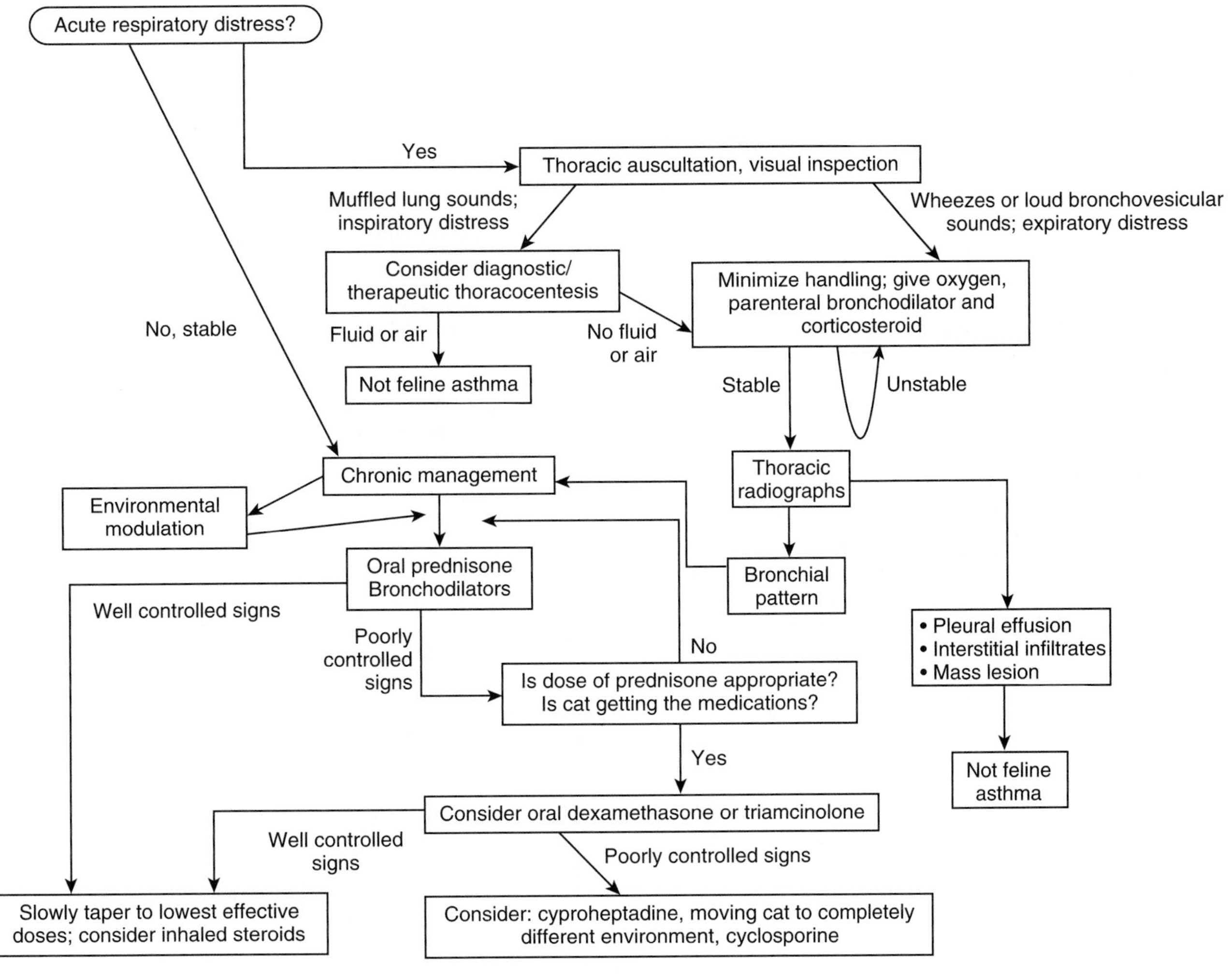

Author: Carol Reinero
Editor: Rance K. Sellon

ATRIAL FIBRILLATION

Atrial fibrillation (AF)

Do the patient's electrocardiograms (ECGs) show that the AF began in the preceding 72 hours?

Yes → Are the atria structurally normal (radiographs, echocardiogram)?

- **Yes** → Consider conversion (atrial defibrillation) or watchful waiting
  - Electrical (with short-acting intravenous [IV] general anesthesia) at 100 to 200 joules
  - Amiodarone
  - Sotalol
  - Quinidine
- **No** → Treatment for chronic AF
  - Watchful waiting if rate is not excessive
  - Triggering event gone?
    - Gastric dilation-volvulus (GDV)
    - Other gastrointestinal (GI) or vagal event
    - Addison's disease
    - Hit by car (HBC)
    - Postpericardiocentesis
    - Hypothyroidism
    - Volume load
    - General anesthesia

No, or not sure → Treatment for chronic AF → Does the patient have cardiogenic pulmonary edema?

- **No** → Is the ventricular rate rapid?
  - >140 bpm (big dog)
  - >180 bpm (small dog)
  - >240 bpm (cat)
  - **No** → No antiarrhythmic treatment
  - **Yes** → Treat with negative dromotropic drug(s) (AV nodal–delaying agents) based on underlying heart structure
    - Dilated cardiomyopathy (DCM)
      - Digoxin
      - ± β-blocker
    - Hypertrophic cardiomyopathy (HCM) or left ventricular hypertrophy (LVH)
      - β-Blocker *or*
      - Calcium channel blocker (CCB) *or*
      - Both
    - Normal heart
      - β-Blocker *or*
      - Digoxin *or*
      - CCB *or*
      - Combination
- **Yes** → Treat with furosemide → Has pulmonary edema resolved?
  - **Yes** → Is the ventricular rate rapid?
    - >140 bpm (big dog)
    - >180 bpm (small dog)
    - >240 bpm (cat)
    - **No** → No antiarrhythmic treatment
    - **Yes** → Treatment with negative dromotropic drug(s) (AV nodal–delaying agents) based on underlying heart structure:
      - Dilated cardiomyopathy (DCM)
        - Digoxin
        - ± β-blocker
      - HCM or LVH
        - β-Blocker *or*
        - CCB *or*
        - Both
      - Normal heart
        - β-Blocker *or*
        - Digoxin *or*
        - CCB *or*
        - Combination
  - **No** → Is the ventricular rate excessive at rest?
    - >180 bpm (big dog)
    - >200 bpm (small dog)
    - >300 bpm (cat)
    - **Yes** → Tachycardia may be contributing to congestive heart failure (CHF). Consider combination or solo-negative dromotropes:
      - Digoxin
      - β-Blockers (low, incremental doses)
      - CCBs

      Goal is to decrease heart rate slightly (10% to 20%)

      → Has pulmonary edema resolved?
      - **Yes** → Is the ventricular rate rapid? (above)
      - **No** → Is the ventricular rate excessive at rest? (above)
    - **No** →
      - Increase diuretic dose until signs of edema have improved or resolved or until maximum diuretic dose is reached
      - Add diuretic (Thiazide)
      - Give diuretic IV or intramuscularly (IM) or constant rate infusion (CRI) to improve efficacy

From Ettinger SJ, Feldman EC: *Textbook of Veterinary Internal Medicine,* ed 6. St. Louis, WB Saunders, 2005.

BLEEDING DISORDER

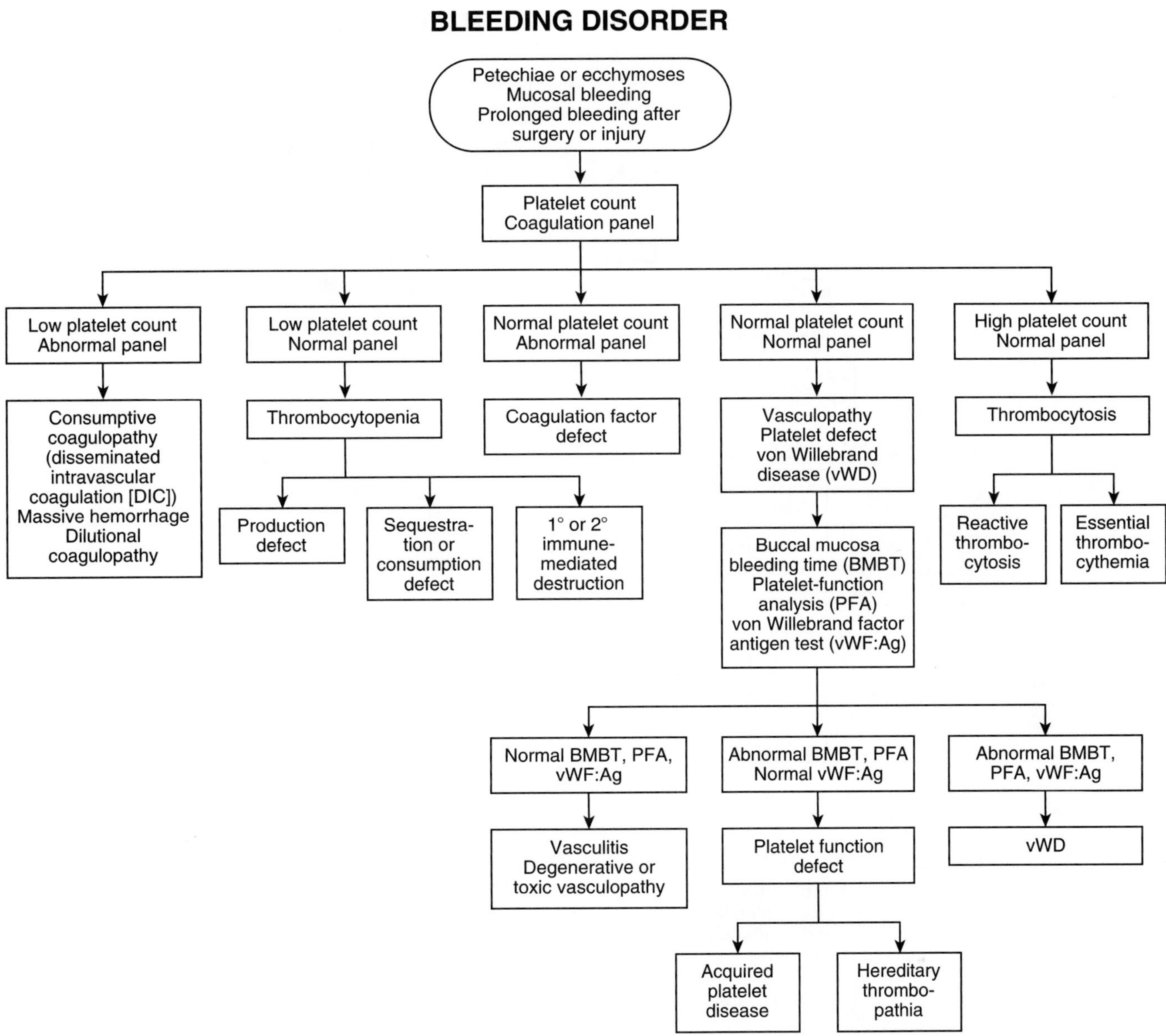

From Ettinger SJ, Feldman EC: *Textbook of Veterinary Internal Medicine,* ed 6. St. Louis, WB Saunders, 2005.

BLEEDING PATIENT: INITIAL APPROACH

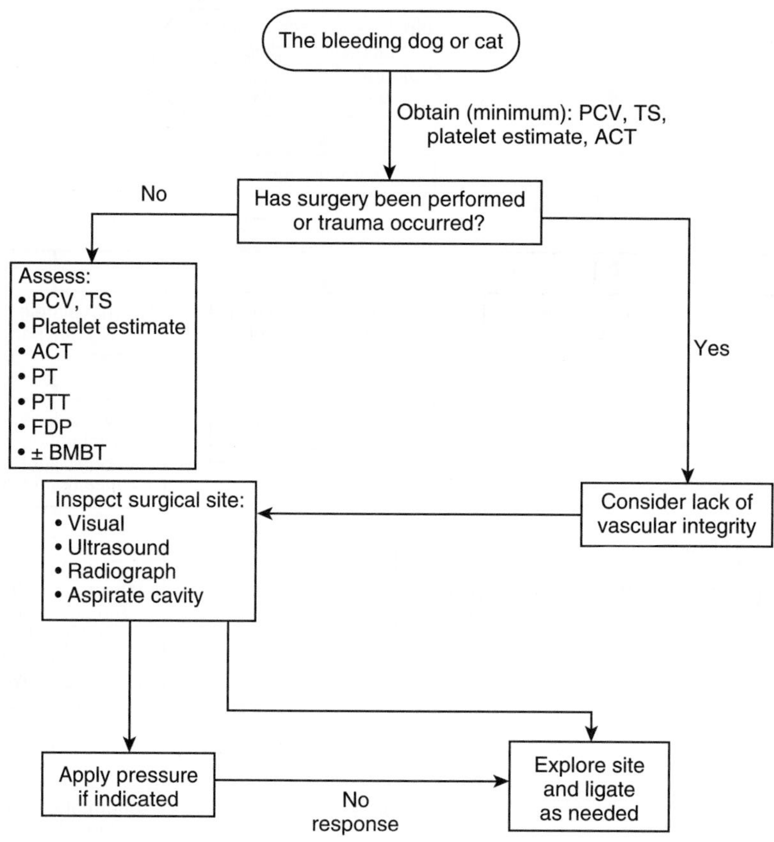

Modified from Slatter DH: *Textbook of Small Animal Surgery,* ed 3. St. Louis, WB Saunders, 2003.

- ACT: activated clotting time
- BMBT: buccal mucosal bleeding time
- FDP: fibrin(ogen) degradation products
- PCV: packed cell volume
- PT: prothrombin time
- PTT: partial thromboplastin time
- TS: total solids

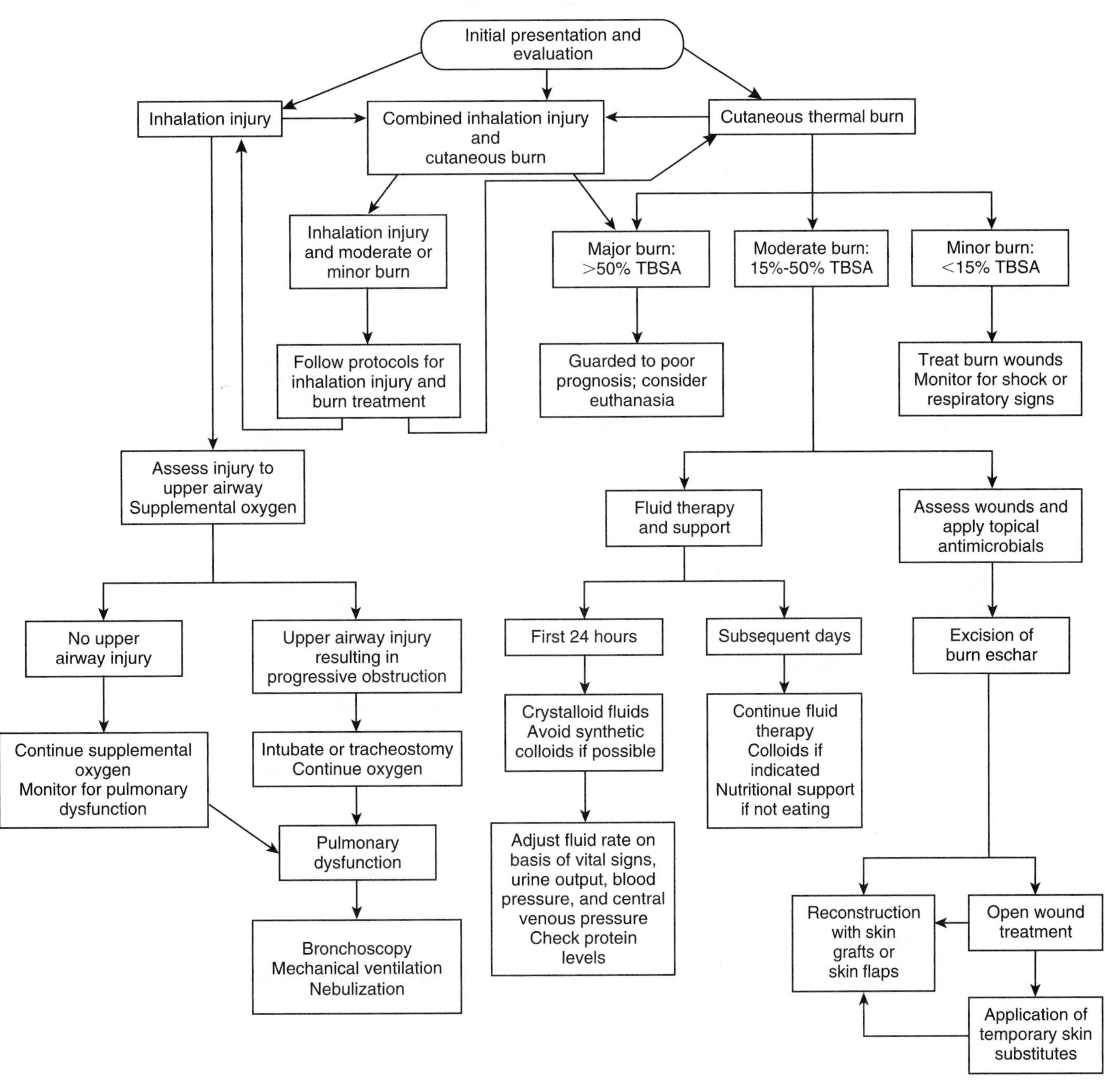

Modified from Slatter DH: *Textbook of Small Animal Surgery,* ed 3. St. Louis, WB Saunders, 2003.

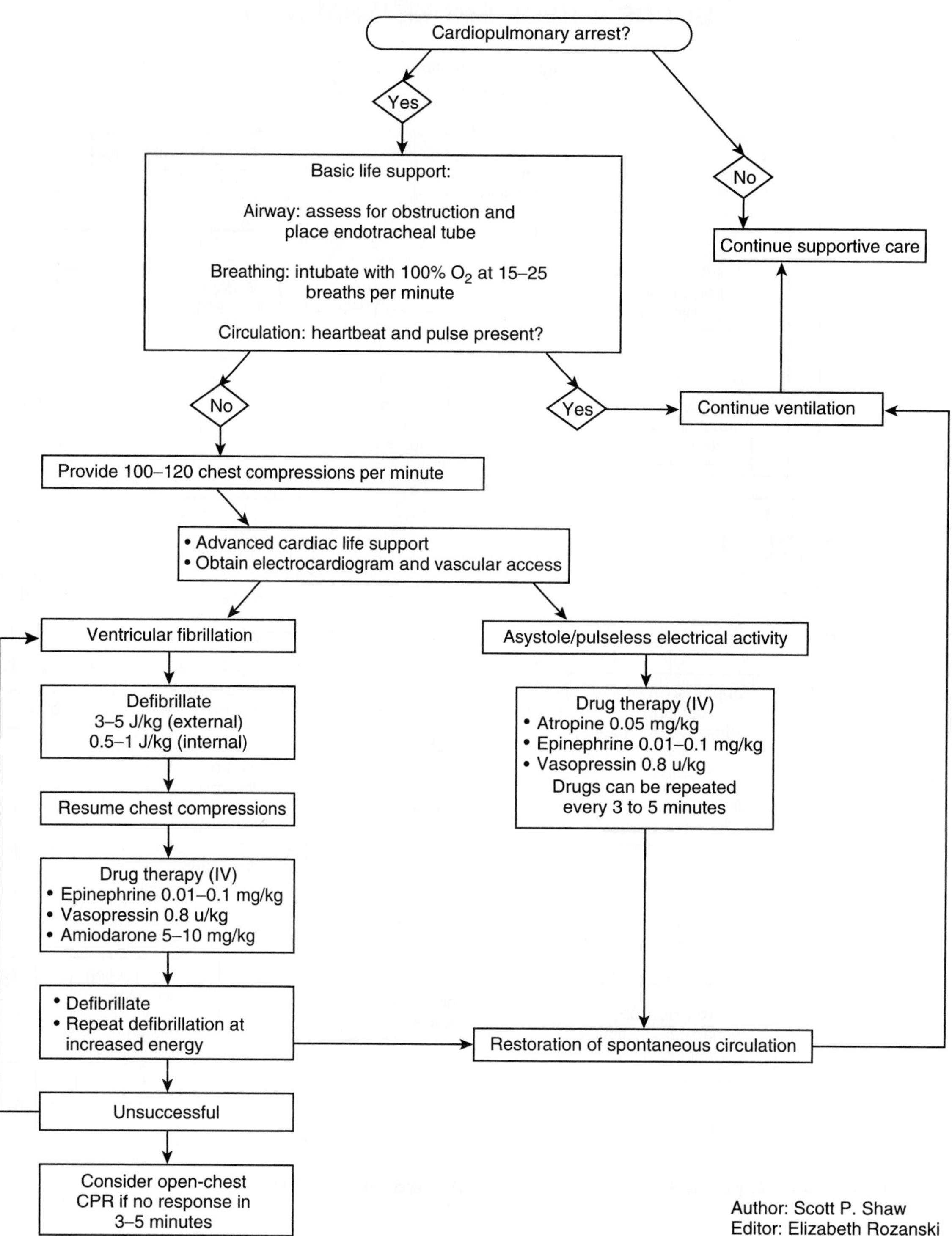

Author: Scott P. Shaw
Editor: Elizabeth Rozanski

CHRONIC RENAL FAILURE: MANAGEMENT

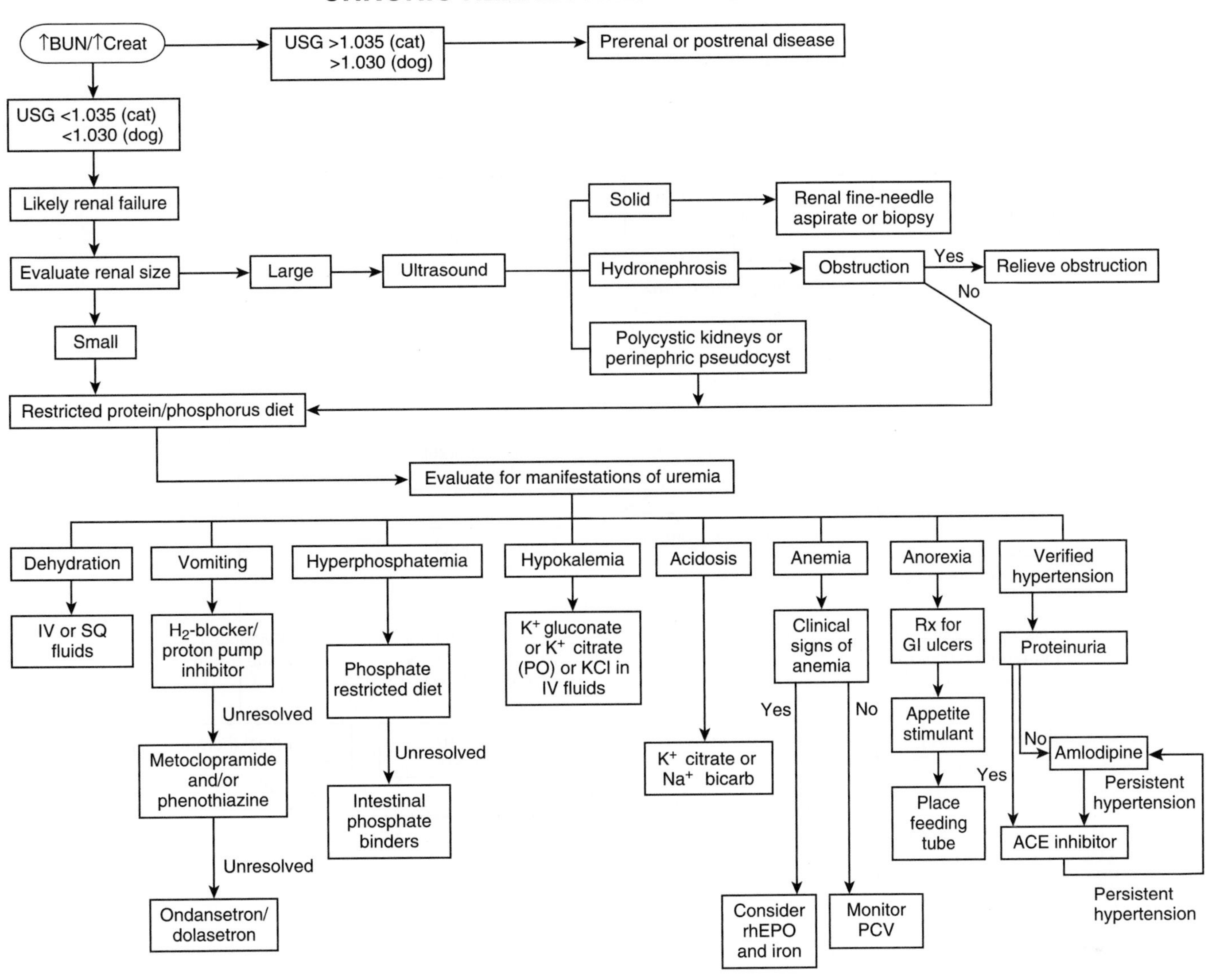

Author: Cathy Langston
Editor: Leah A. Cohn

ACE: angiotensin-converting enzyme
Bicarb: bicarbonate
BUN: blood urea nitrogen
Creat: creatinine
GI: gastrointestinal
IV: intravenous
PCV: packed cell volume
PO: per os
rhEPO: recombinant human erythropoietin
Rx: treatment
SQ: subcutaneous
USG: urine specific gravity

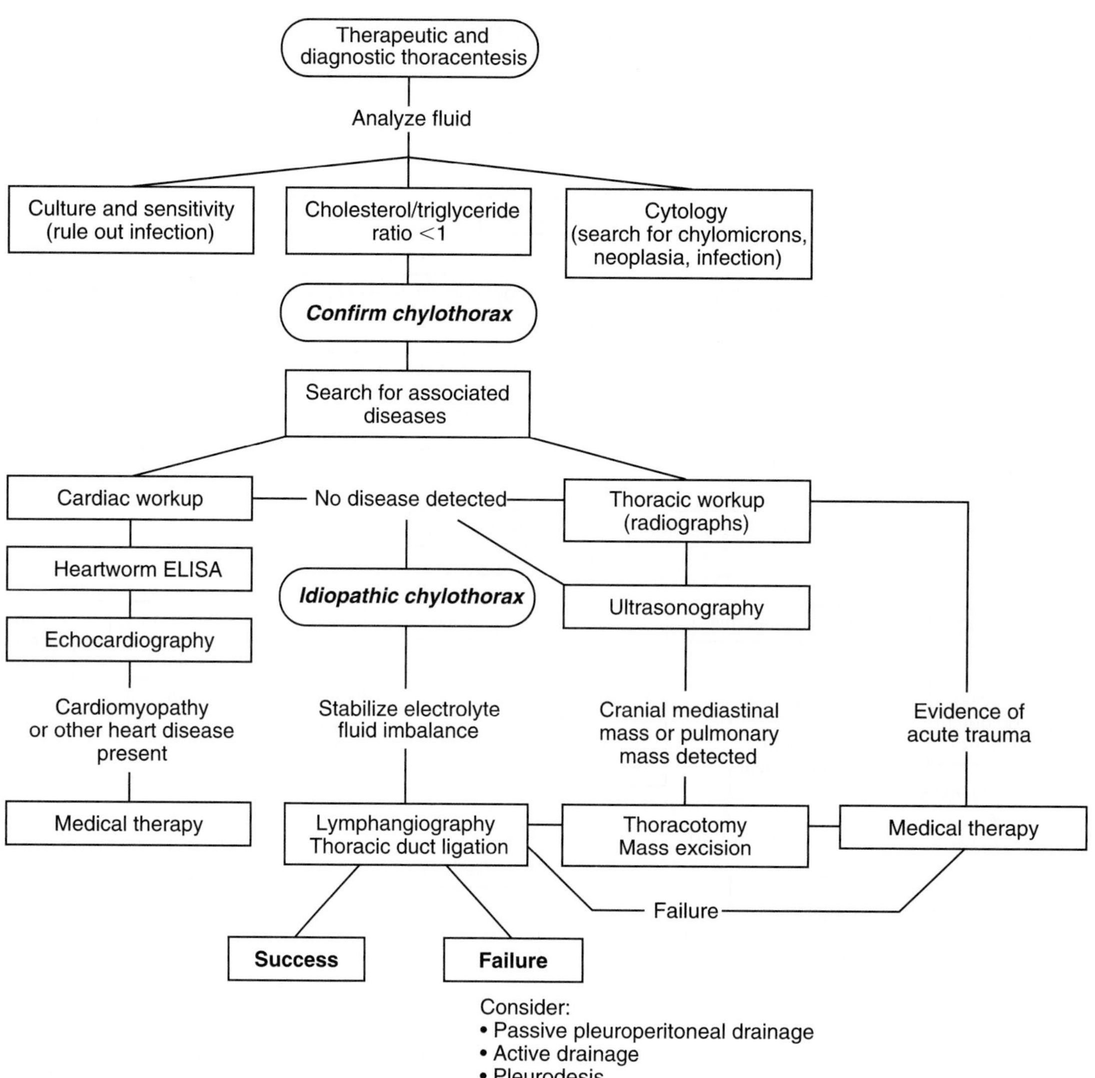

From Bonagura JD: *Kirk's Current Veterinary Therapy XII*, ed 12. St. Louis, WB Saunders, 1995.

CONSTIPATION, OBSTIPATION, AND MEGACOLON

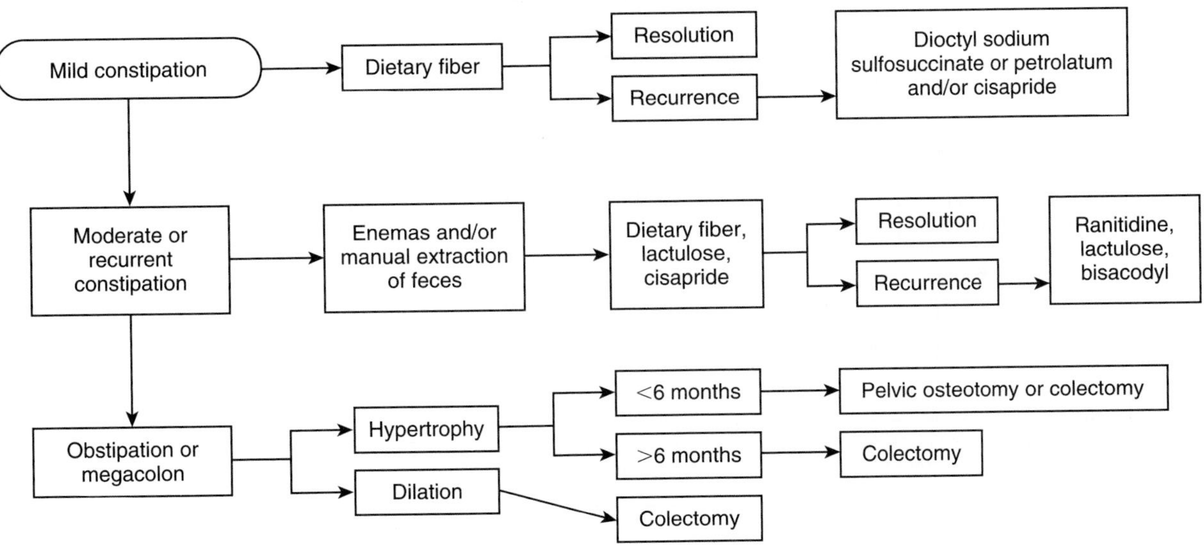

From Slatter DH: *Textbook of Small Animal Surgery,* ed 3. St. Louis, WB Saunders, 2003.

CRANIAL CRUCIATE LIGAMENT INJURY

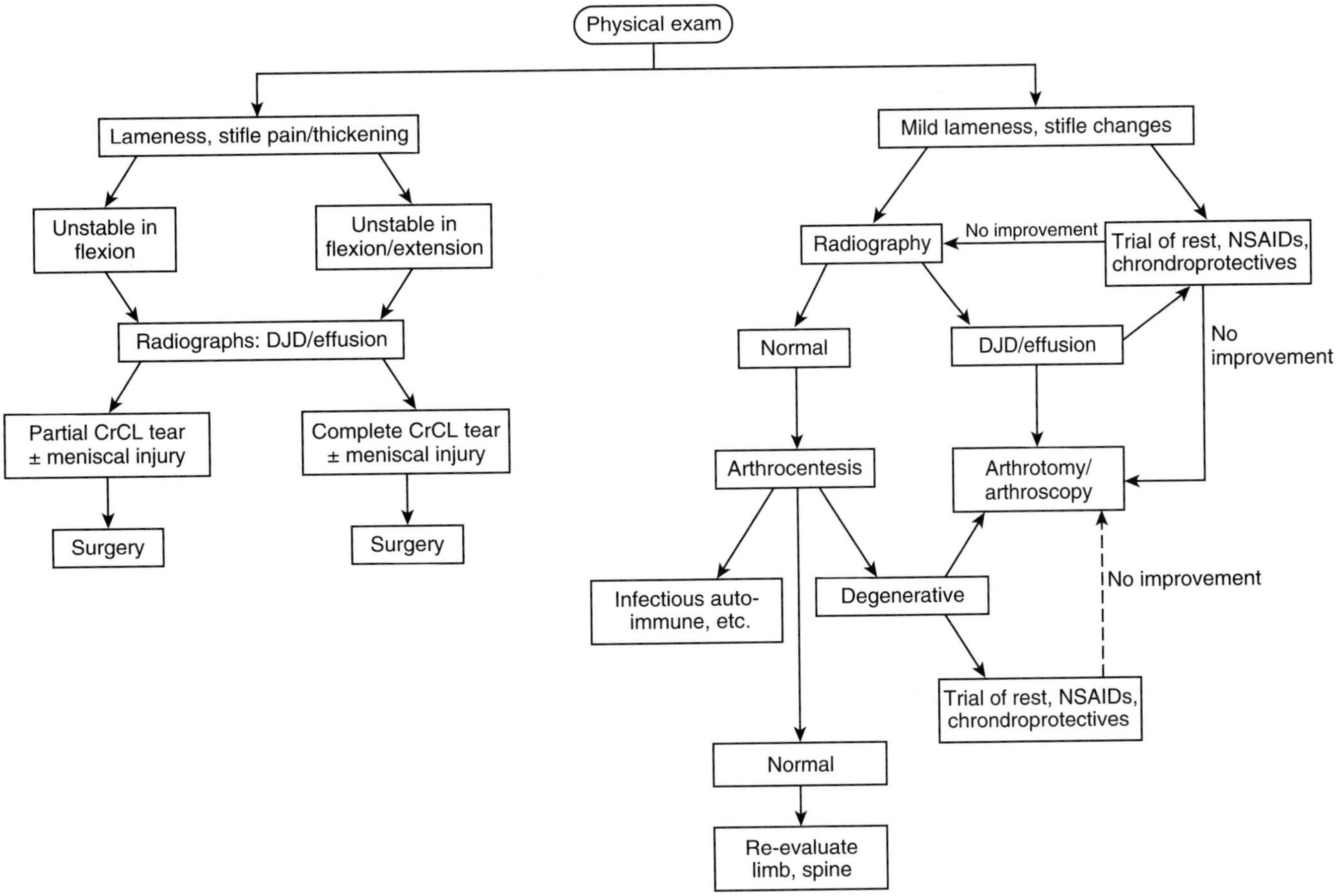

Physical exam

Lameness, stifle pain/thickening

Unstable in flexion

Unstable in flexion/extension

Radiographs: DJD/effusion

Partial CrCL tear ± meniscal injury

Surgery

Complete CrCL tear ± meniscal injury

Surgery

Mild lameness, stifle changes

Radiography

No improvement

Trial of rest, NSAIDs, chrondroprotectives

No improvement

Normal

DJD/effusion

Arthrocentesis

Arthrotomy/ arthroscopy

Infectious auto-immune, etc.

Degenerative

No improvement

Trial of rest, NSAIDs, chrondroprotectives

Normal

Re-evaluate limb, spine

NSAIDs, nonsteroidal anti-inflammatory drugs; DJD, degenerative joint disease.

Author & Editor: Joseph Harari

CLINICAL ALGORITHMS

CYANOSIS

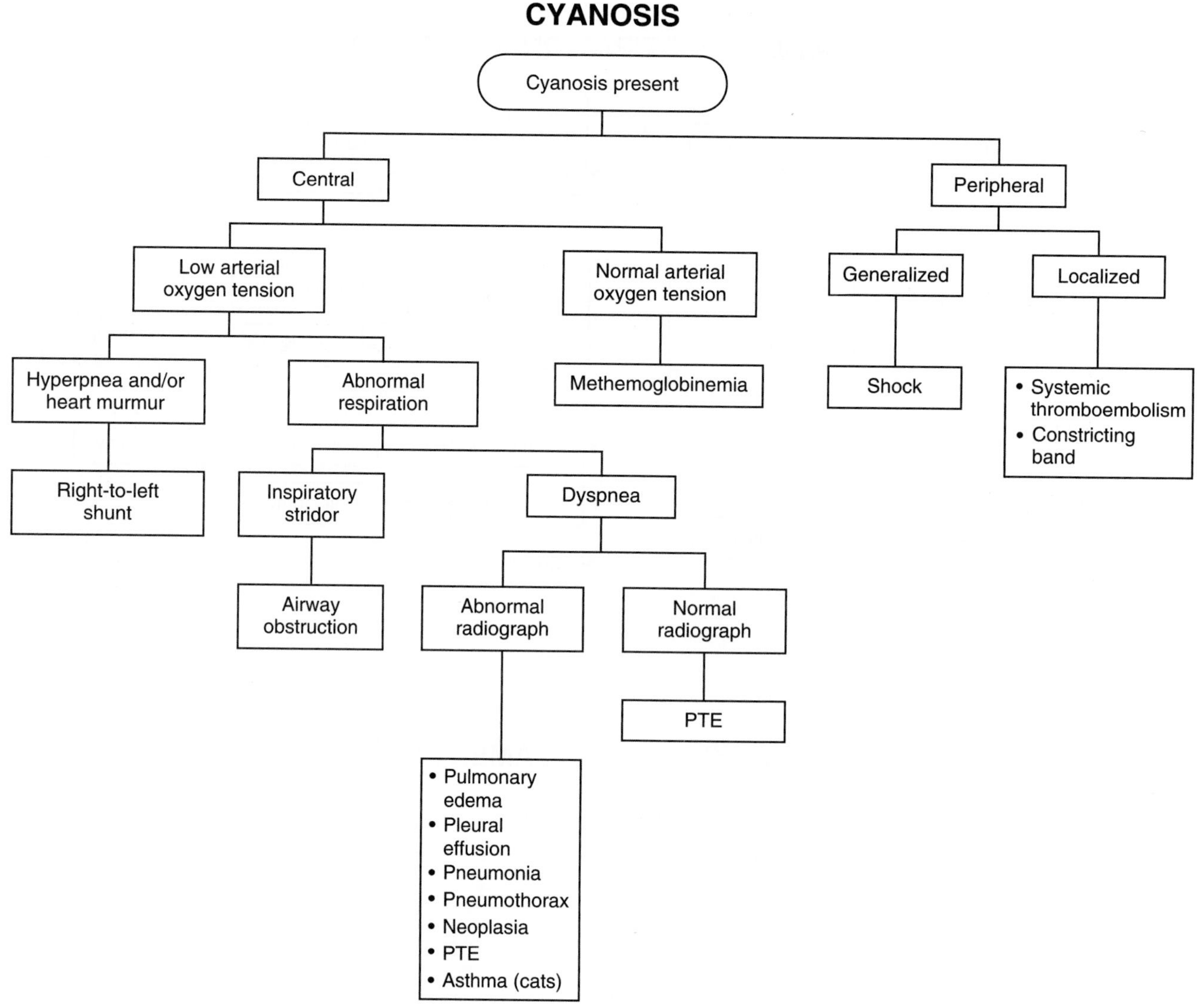

Modified from Kittleson MD, Kienle RD: *Small Animal Cardiovascular Medicine*. St. Louis, Mosby, 1999.
PTE: pulmonary thromboembolism

DIABETES INSIPIDUS

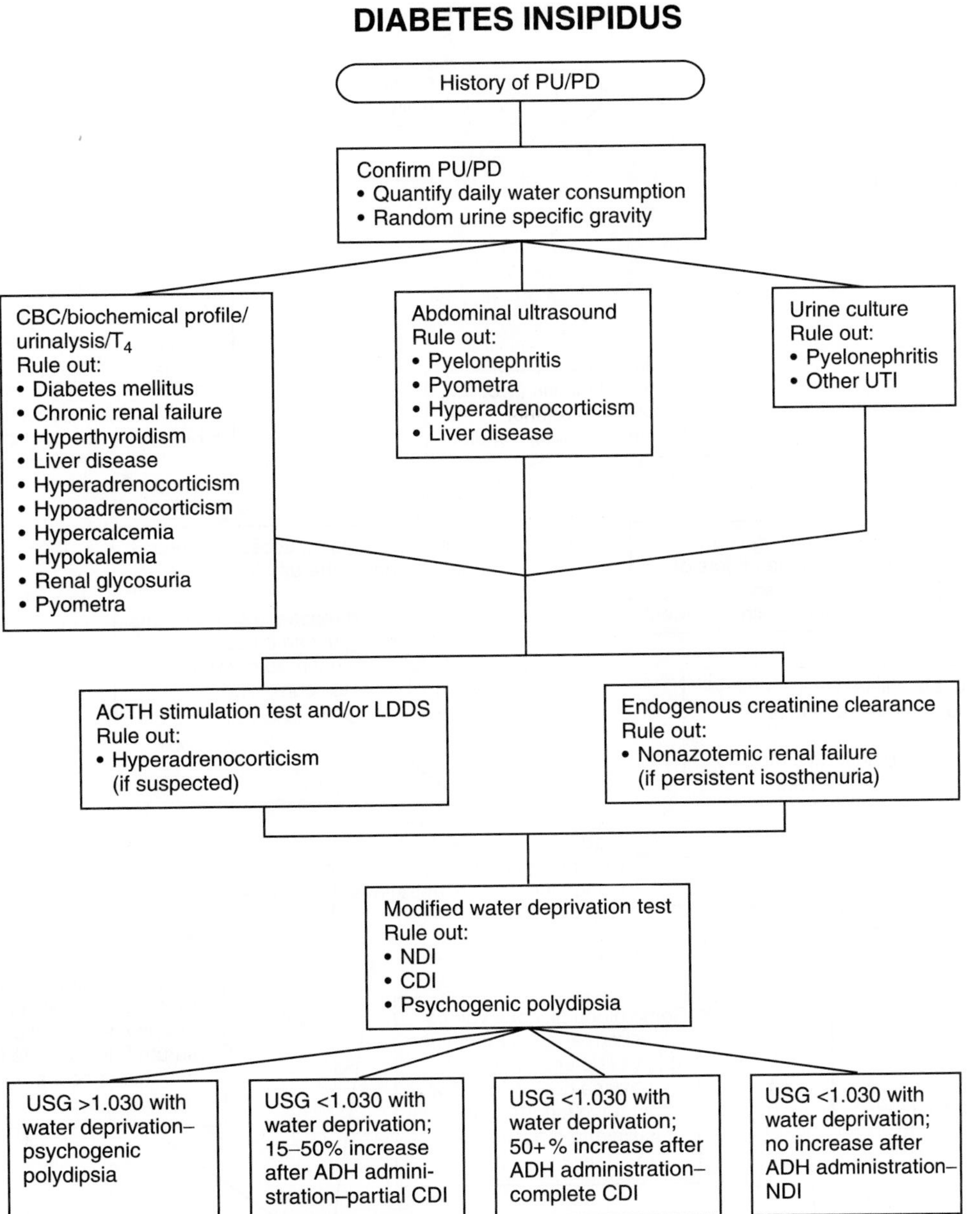

ACTH, adrenocorticotropic hormone; ADH, antidiuretic hormone; CBC, complete blood count; CDI, central diabetes insipidus; LDDS, low-dose dexamethasone suppression test; NDI, nephrogenic diabetes insipidus; PU/PD, polyuria/polydipsia; USG, urine specific gravity; UTI, urinary tract infection.

Author: Sarah L. Naidoo
Editor: Sherri Ihle

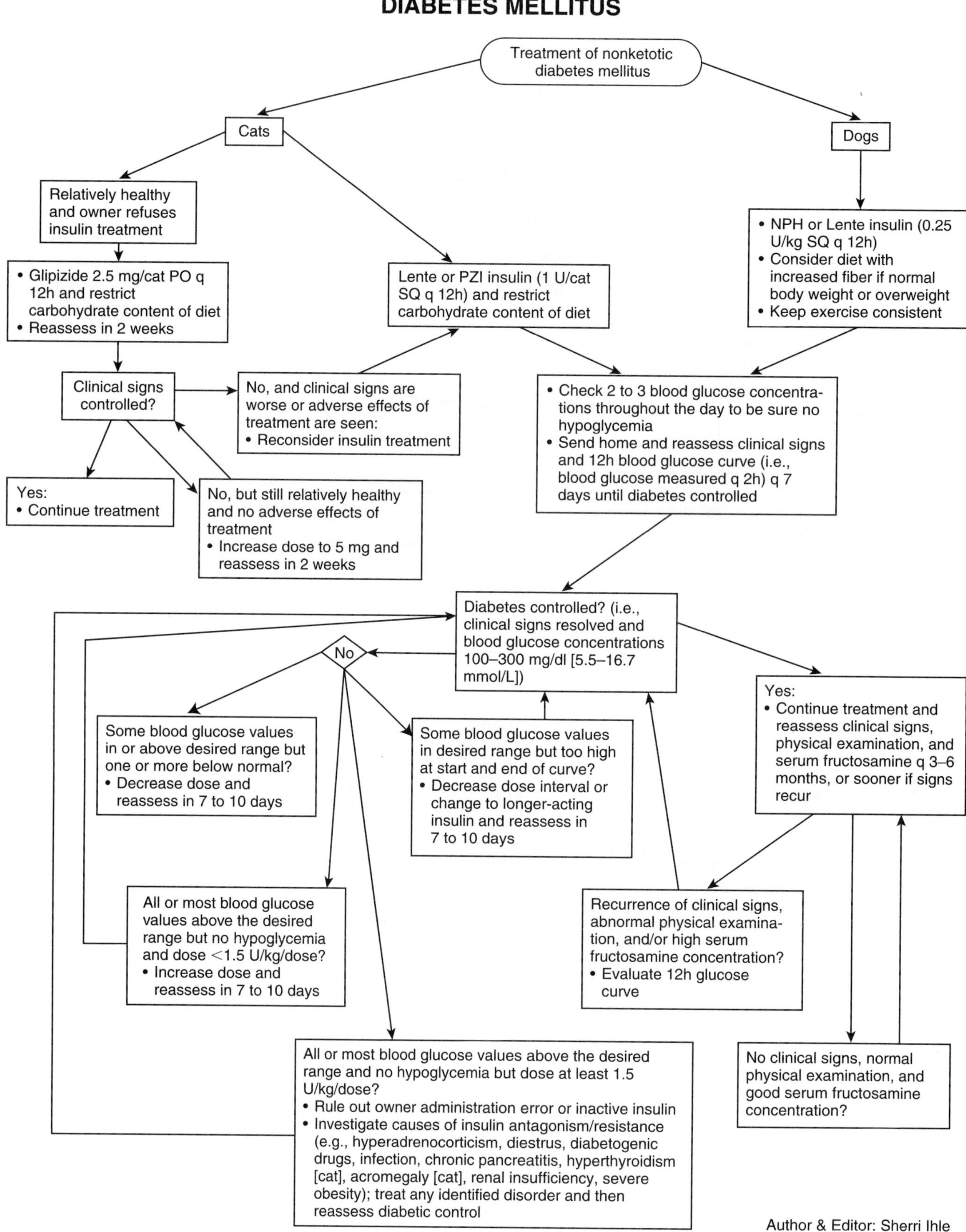

Author & Editor: Sherri Ihle

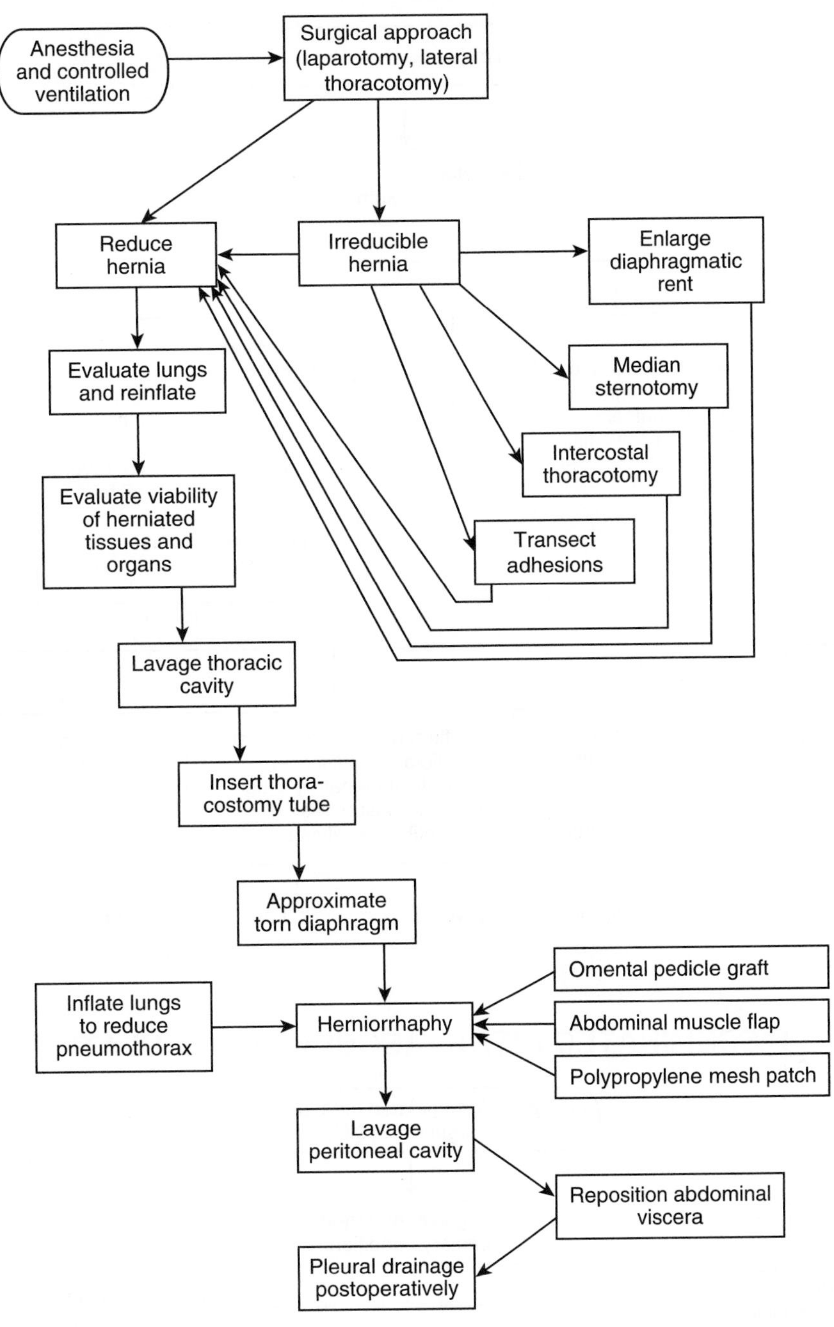

Modified from Slatter DH: *Textbook of Small Animal Surgery,* ed 3. St. Louis, WB Saunders, 2003.

DIARRHEA, LARGE BOWEL

Large bowel diarrhea

- History
- Physical examination

First episode:
- Rehydration if needed
- Fecal examination
- Empiric anthelmintics
- Dietary modifications

No improvement or recurrence:
- Complete blood count (CBC), serum chemistry, urinalysis
- Fecal culture, polymerase chain reaction (PCR), reverse transcriptase PCR (RT-PCR)
- Exfoliative cytology
- Abdominal imaging
- Colonoscopy

Irritable bowel syndrome:
- Fiber supplementation
- Loperamide
- Propantheline

Dietary sensitivity:
- Novel protein diets
- Hydrolyzed diets
- Antioxidant diets
- Fiber supplementation

Inflammatory bowel disease:
- Dietary modification
- Antiinflammatory drugs
- Immunosuppressive drugs
- Motility-modifying drugs

Infection:
- Antibiotics
- Anthelmintics
- Antiprotozoals
- Antifungals

Lymphoma:
- Chemotherapy

From Ettinger SJ, Feldman EC: *Textbook of Veterinary Internal Medicine*, ed 6. St. Louis, WB Saunders, 2006.

DISSEMINATED INTRAVASCULAR COAGULATION

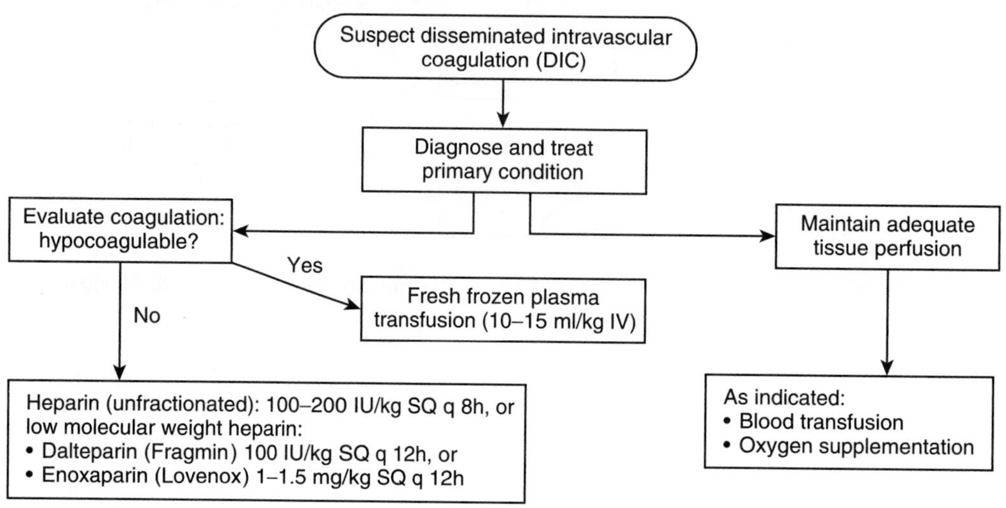
Suspect disseminated intravascular coagulation (DIC)
Diagnose and treat primary condition
Evaluate coagulation: hypocoagulable?
Yes
Fresh frozen plasma transfusion (10–15 ml/kg IV)
No
Heparin (unfractionated): 100–200 IU/kg SQ q 8h, or low molecular weight heparin:
• Dalteparin (Fragmin) 100 IU/kg SQ q 12h, or
• Enoxaparin (Lovenox) 1–1.5 mg/kg SQ q 12h
Maintain adequate tissue perfusion
As indicated:
• Blood transfusion
• Oxygen supplementation

Author: Scott P. Shaw
Editor: Elizabeth Rozanski

DRAINING TRACTS, CUTANEOUS

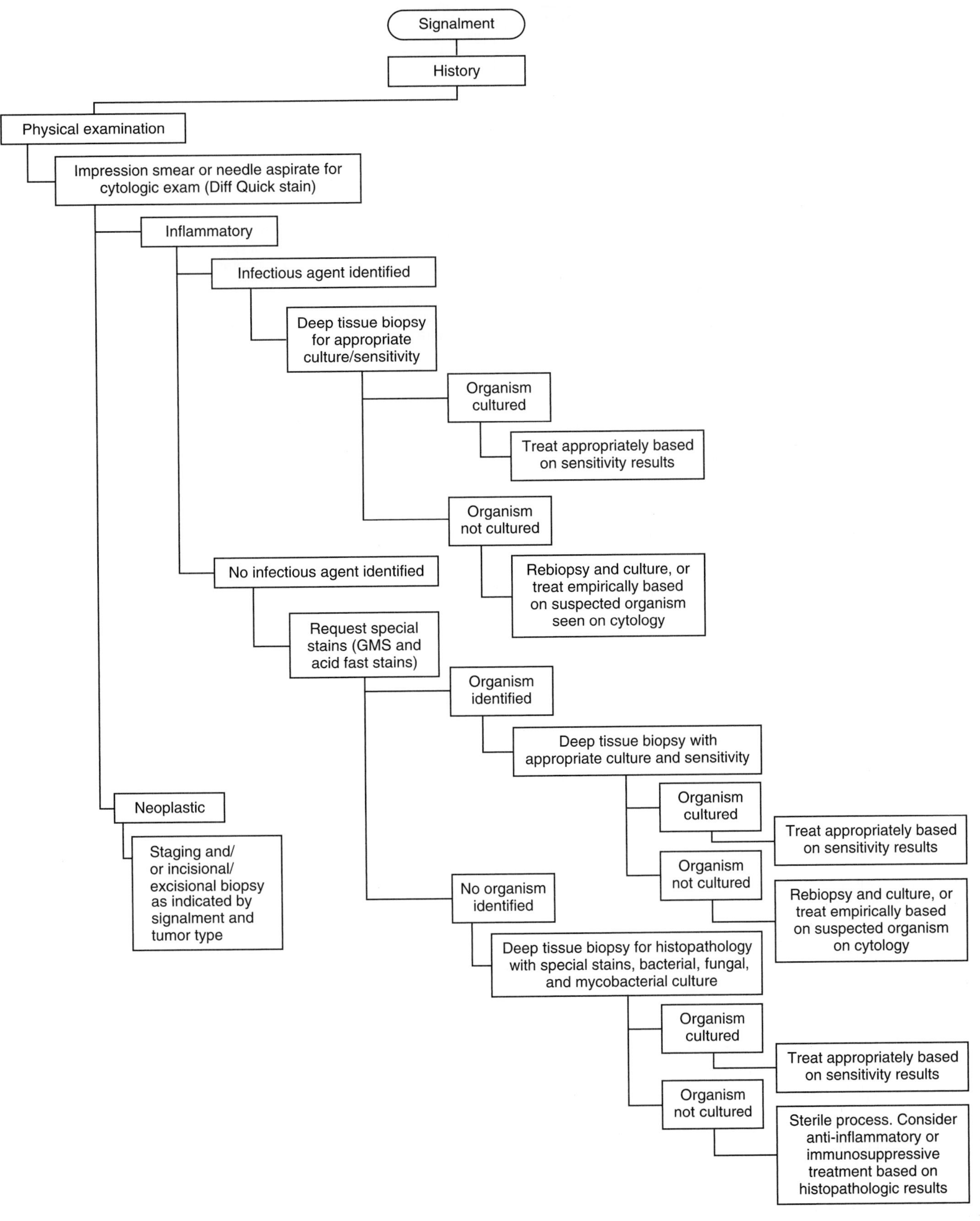

Author: Andrew Lowe
Editor: Jan A. Hall

DYSPNEA AND RESPIRATORY DISTRESS: HOSPITAL-ACQUIRED

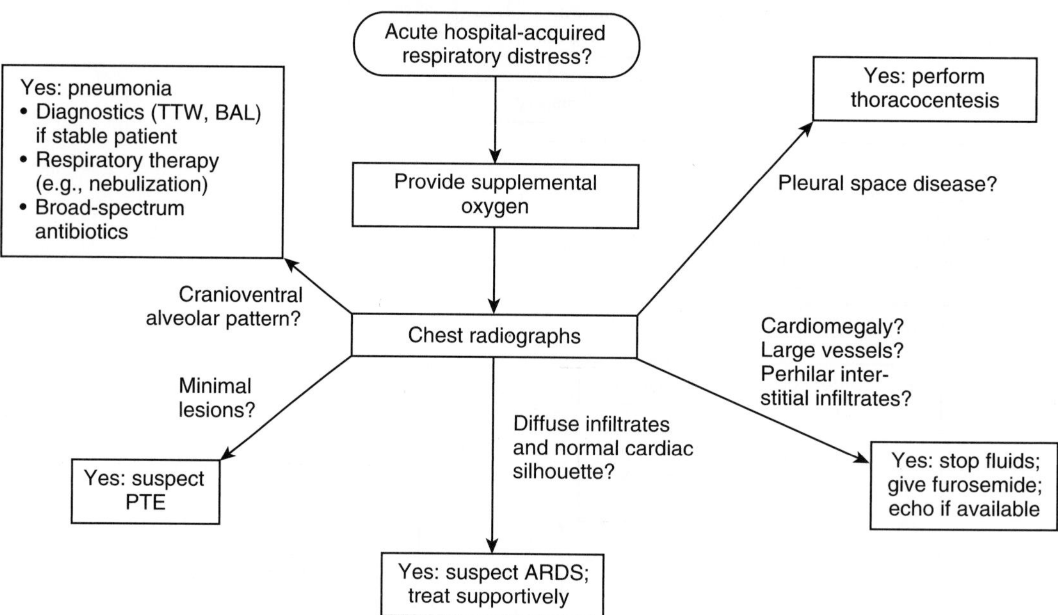
Acute hospital-acquired respiratory distress?
Provide supplemental oxygen
Chest radiographs
Craniovental alveolar pattern?
Yes: pneumonia
• Diagnostics (TTW, BAL) if stable patient
• Respiratory therapy (e.g., nebulization)
• Broad-spectrum antibiotics
Pleural space disease?
Yes: perform thoracocentesis
Minimal lesions?
Yes: suspect PTE
Diffuse infiltrates and normal cardiac silhouette?
Yes: suspect ARDS; treat supportively
Cardiomegaly? Large vessels? Perhilar interstitial infiltrates?
Yes: stop fluids; give furosemide; echo if available

ARDS, adult respiratory distress syndrome; PTE, pulmonary thromboembolism.

Author: Scott P. Shaw
Editor: Elizabeth Rozanski

DYSTOCIA

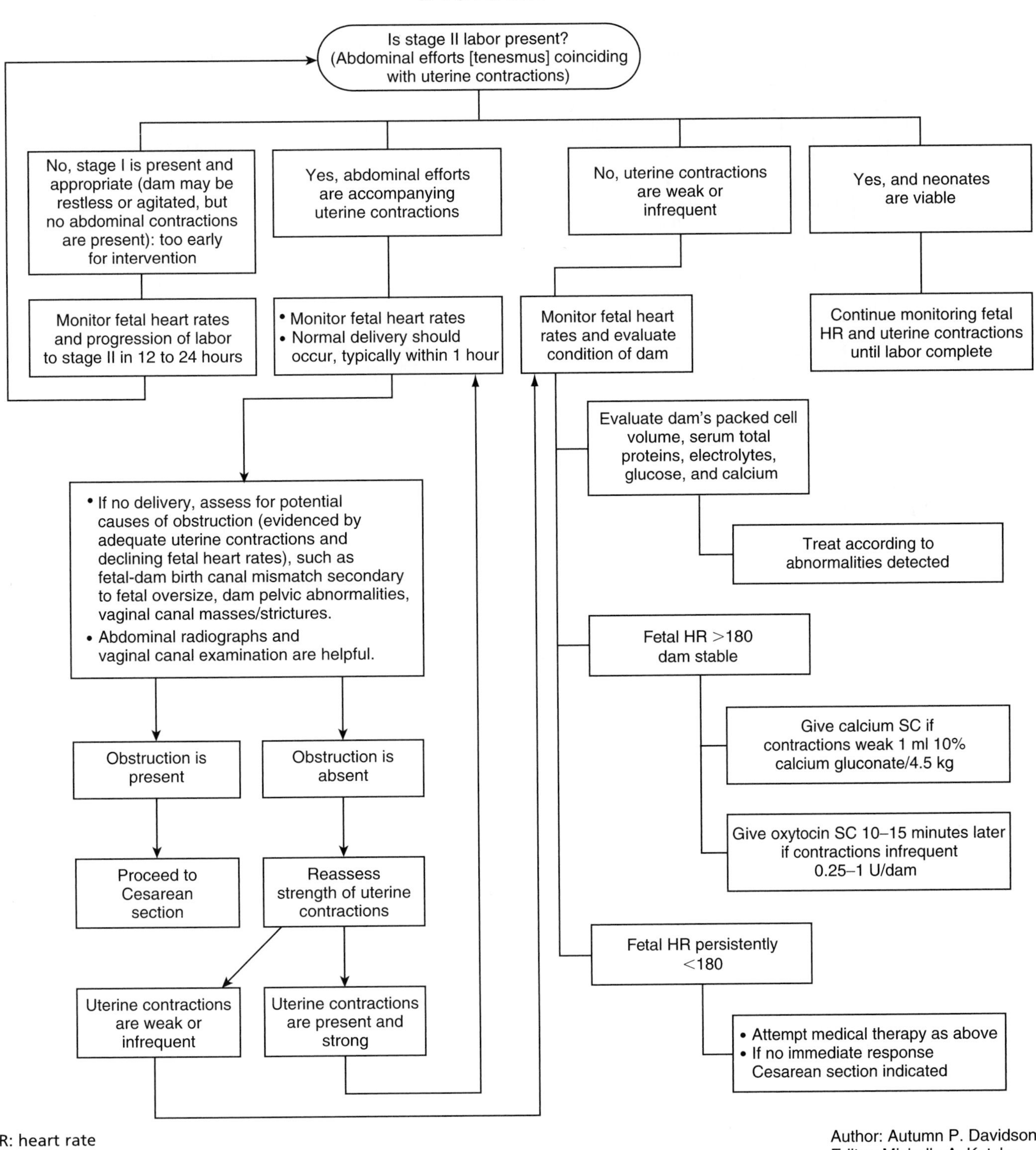
Is stage II labor present? (Abdominal efforts [tenesmus] coinciding with uterine contractions)
No, stage I is present and appropriate (dam may be restless or agitated, but no abdominal contractions are present): too early for intervention
Yes, abdominal efforts are accompanying uterine contractions
No, uterine contractions are weak or infrequent
Yes, and neonates are viable
Monitor fetal heart rates and progression of labor to stage II in 12 to 24 hours
• Monitor fetal heart rates
• Normal delivery should occur, typically within 1 hour
Monitor fetal heart rates and evaluate condition of dam
Continue monitoring fetal HR and uterine contractions until labor complete
Evaluate dam's packed cell volume, serum total proteins, electrolytes, glucose, and calcium
Treat according to abnormalities detected
• If no delivery, assess for potential causes of obstruction (evidenced by adequate uterine contractions and declining fetal heart rates), such as fetal-dam birth canal mismatch secondary to fetal oversize, dam pelvic abnormalities, vaginal canal masses/strictures.
• Abdominal radiographs and vaginal canal examination are helpful.
Fetal HR >180 dam stable
Give calcium SC if contractions weak 1 ml 10% calcium gluconate/4.5 kg
Give oxytocin SC 10–15 minutes later if contractions infrequent 0.25–1 U/dam
Obstruction is present
Obstruction is absent
Proceed to Cesarean section
Reassess strength of uterine contractions
Fetal HR persistently <180
Uterine contractions are weak or infrequent
Uterine contractions are present and strong
• Attempt medical therapy as above
• If no immediate response Cesarean section indicated

HR: heart rate
SC: subcutaneous

Author: Autumn P. Davidson
Editor: Michelle A. Kutzler

ESOPHAGEAL MOTILITY DISORDER: TREATMENT

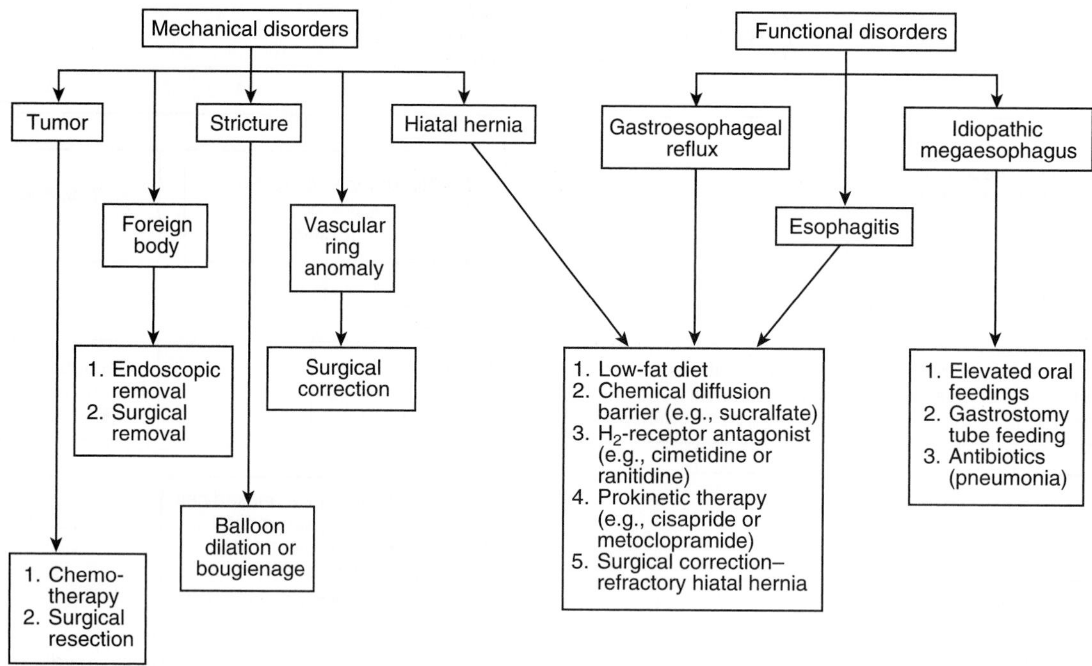

Modified from Slatter DH: *Textbook of Small Animal Surgery*, ed 3. St. Louis, WB Saunders, 2003.

ETHYLENE GLYCOL TOXICITY

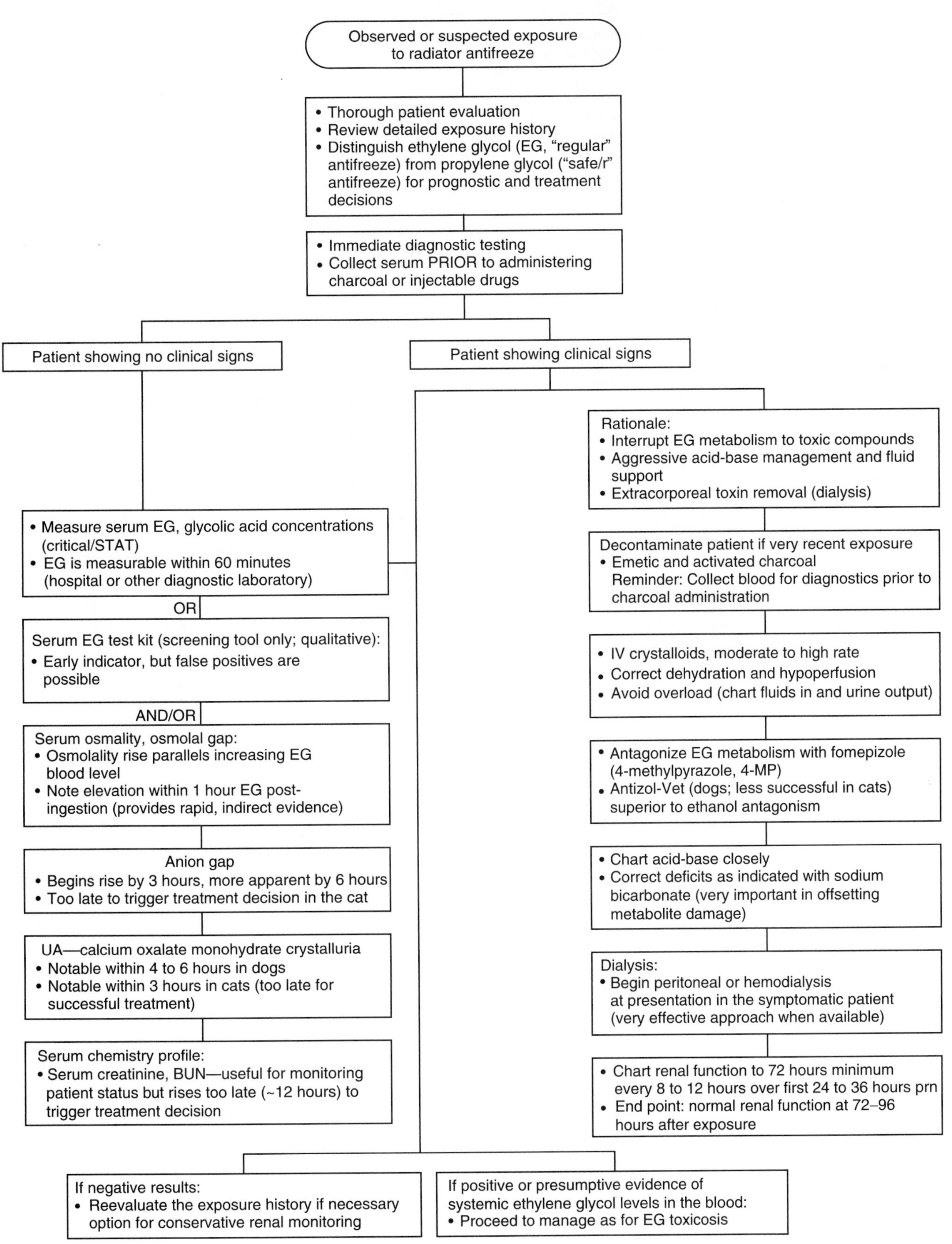

Observed or suspected exposure to radiator antifreeze
• Thorough patient evaluation
• Review detailed exposure history
• Distinguish ethylene glycol (EG, "regular" antifreeze) from propylene glycol ("safe/r" antifreeze) for prognostic and treatment decisions
• Immediate diagnostic testing
• Collect serum PRIOR to administering charcoal or injectable drugs
Patient showing no clinical signs
Patient showing clinical signs
Rationale:
• Interrupt EG metabolism to toxic compounds
• Aggressive acid-base management and fluid support
• Extracorporeal toxin removal (dialysis)
• Measure serum EG, glycolic acid concentrations (critical/STAT)
• EG is measurable within 60 minutes (hospital or other diagnostic laboratory)
OR
Serum EG test kit (screening tool only; qualitative):
• Early indicator, but false positives are possible
AND/OR
Serum osmality, osmolal gap:
• Osmolality rise parallels increasing EG blood level
• Note elevation within 1 hour EG post-ingestion (provides rapid, indirect evidence)
Anion gap
• Begins rise by 3 hours, more apparent by 6 hours
• Too late to trigger treatment decision in the cat
UA—calcium oxalate monohydrate crystalluria
• Notable within 4 to 6 hours in dogs
• Notable within 3 hours in cats (too late for successful treatment)
Serum chemistry profile:
• Serum creatinine, BUN—useful for monitoring patient status but rises too late (~12 hours) to trigger treatment decision
Decontaminate patient if very recent exposure
• Emetic and activated charcoal
Reminder: Collect blood for diagnostics prior to charcoal administration
• IV crystalloids, moderate to high rate
• Correct dehydration and hypoperfusion
• Avoid overload (chart fluids in and urine output)
• Antagonize EG metabolism with fomepizole (4-methylpyrazole, 4-MP)
• Antizol-Vet (dogs; less successful in cats) superior to ethanol antagonism
• Chart acid-base closely
• Correct deficits as indicated with sodium bicarbonate (very important in offsetting metabolite damage)
Dialysis:
• Begin peritoneal or hemodialysis at presentation in the symptomatic patient (very effective approach when available)
• Chart renal function to 72 hours minimum every 8 to 12 hours over first 24 to 36 hours prn
• End point: normal renal function at 72–96 hours after exposure
If negative results:
• Reevaluate the exposure history if necessary option for conservative renal monitoring
If positive or presumptive evidence of systemic ethylene glycol levels in the blood:
• Proceed to manage as for EG toxicosis

Author: Michael W. Knight
Editor: Safdar A. Khan

FELINE IMMUNODEFICIENCY VIRUS INFECTION

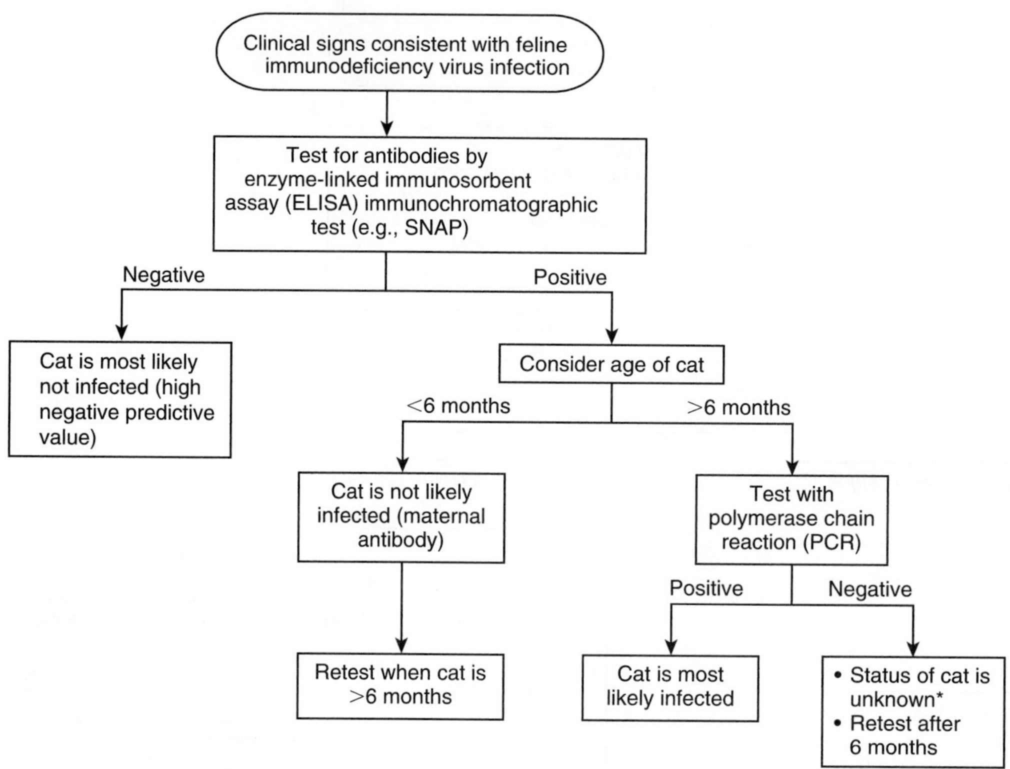

*Cats can be vaccinated; PCR can be false-negative.

Modified from Ettinger SJ, Feldman EC: *Textbook of Veterinary Internal Medicine*, ed 6. St. Louis, WB Saunders, 2005.

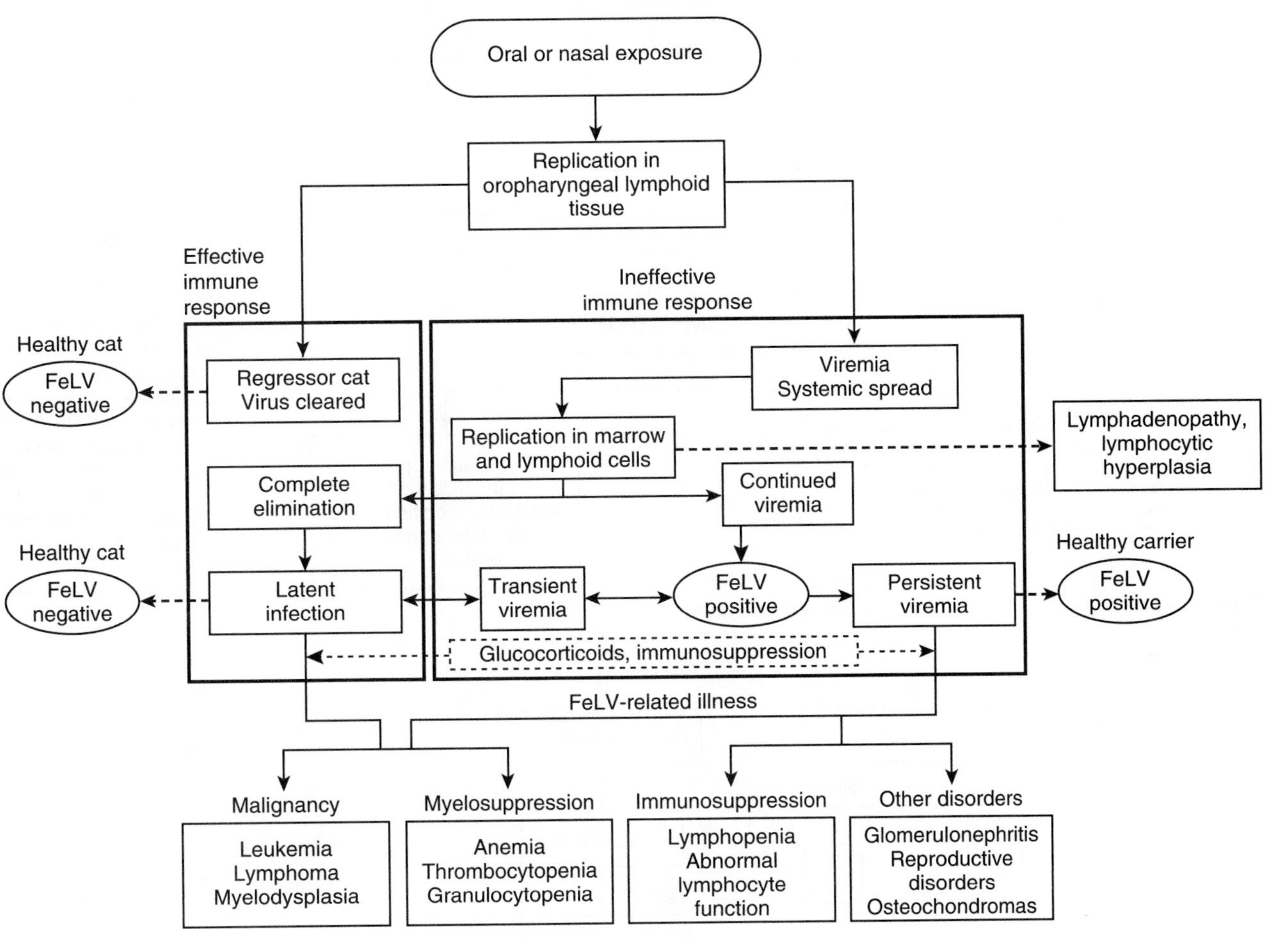

From Greene CE: *Infectious Diseases of the Dog and Cat* (revised reprint), ed 3. St. Louis, WB Saunders, 2006.

FELINE LOWER URINARY TRACT SIGNS

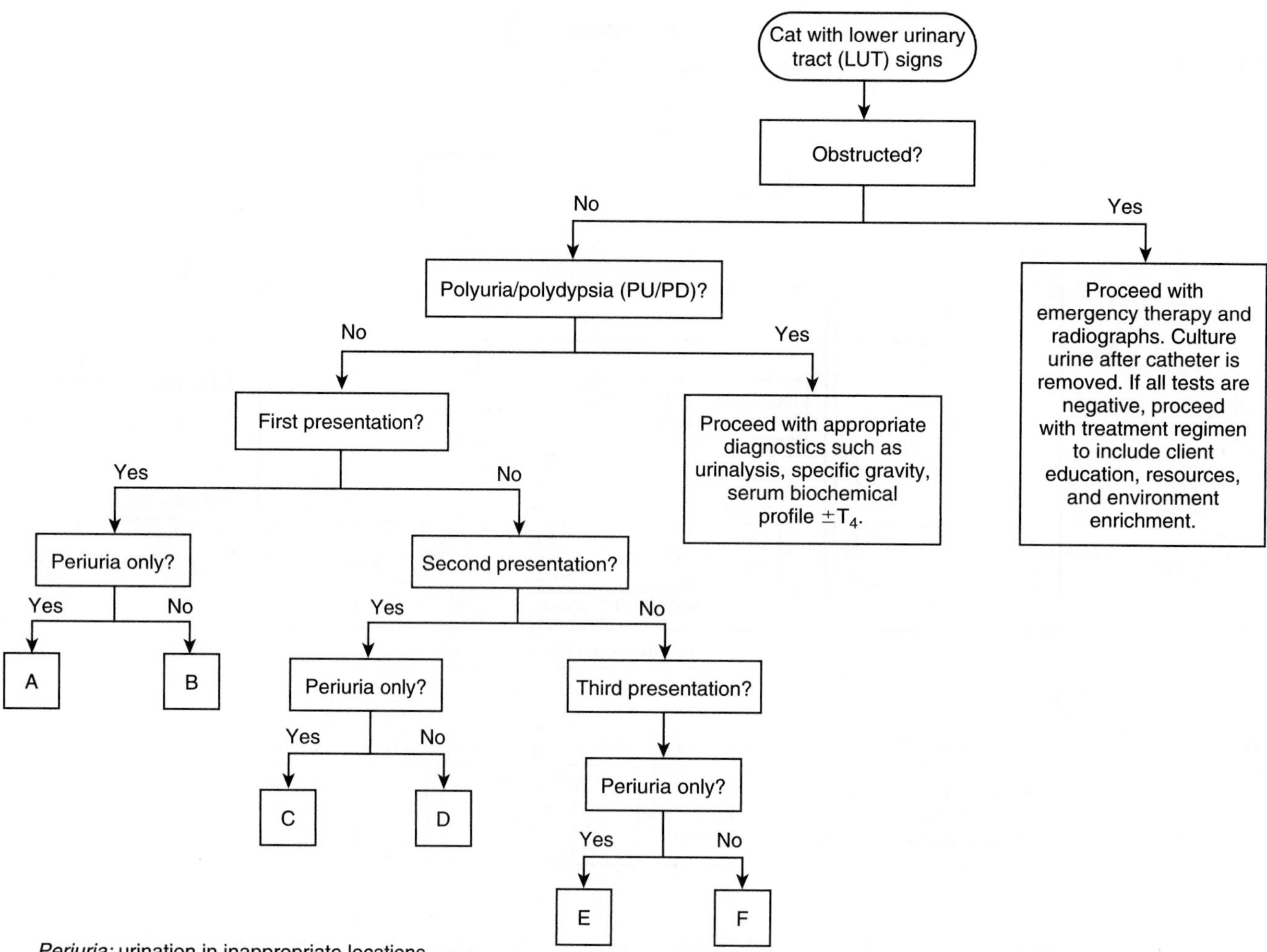

Periuria: urination in inappropriate locations.

A Diagnostic: None is usually necessary.
Treatment: Litter box management and cleaning of soiled areas should be addressed.
Medications: No medications are recommended.

B Diagnostic: A radiograph should be considered, especially if hematuria is present.
Treatment: If the radiograph is negative, therapy should include analgesia for 2 to 3 days during the acute episode. Litter box management and cleaning of soiled areas should be addressed.
Medications: No medications are recommended.

C Diagnostic: A urinalysis is recommended. If submaximal urine specific gravity is present, then appropriate diagnostics are needed.
Treatment: If diagnostic tests are negative, then the resource checklist should be reviewed and additional areas that were not previously addressed should be incorporated.
Medications: Phermonotherapy is recommended.

D Diagnostic: A radiograph, urinalysis, and urine culture are recommended.
Treatment: If all tests are negative, analgesia should be provided for 2 to 3 days during acute episode. Canned food is encouraged for the cat in addition to litter box management and cleaning of soiled areas. The cat's urine specity gravity is monitored for 3 to 4 weeks to assess the cat's water intake.
Medications: Phermonotherapy is recommended.

E Diagnostic: A urinalysis should be performed if it has not already been done. Radiographs, urine culture, and biochemical profile are also recommended.
Treatment: If all tests are negative, then the resource checklist is formally reviewed and those areas that have not already been addressed should be incorporated. Further information for cleaning soiled areas should be provided. Additional resources (web sites, books) on how to provide an enhanced indoor environment for cats should be provided to clients. Intercat conflict issues should also be addressed.
Medications: Phermonotherapy should be used in conjunction with behavior-altering medications such as tricyclic antidepressants (TCAs) or buspirone. The medication should be taken for 4 weeks; if no improvement is seen, a referral for further diagnostics and consultation should be considered.

F Diagnostic: A radiograph, a urinalysis, and a urine culture should be performed. A complete blood count (CBC) and biochemical profile should also be submitted. If all tests are negative, a contrast study or abdominal ultrasound of the bladder and urethra should be considered to rule out radiolucent calculi and other mass lesions.
Treatment: If all diagnostics are negative, analgesia should be provided for 2 to 3 days during acute episode. In addition to canned food, the sheet on "Increasing your cat's water intake" should be reviewed. Water should be viewed as a "drug," and the cat's urine specific gravity should be monitored to evaluate water intake. The resource checklist should be formally reviewed, and those areas that have not already been addressed should be incorporated. Additional resources (web sites, books) on how to provide an enhanced indoor environment for cats should be provided to clients. Intercat conflict issues should also be addressed. Follow up and support for clients are essential.
Medications: Phermonotherapy should be used in conjunction with behavior-altering medications such as TCAs or anxiolytics. Medication should be taken for 4 weeks; if no improvement is seen, a referral for further diagnostics such as a cystoscopy should be considered.

From Ettinger SJ, Feldman EC: *Textbook of Veterinary Internal Medicine*, ed 6. St. Louis, WB Saunders, 2005.

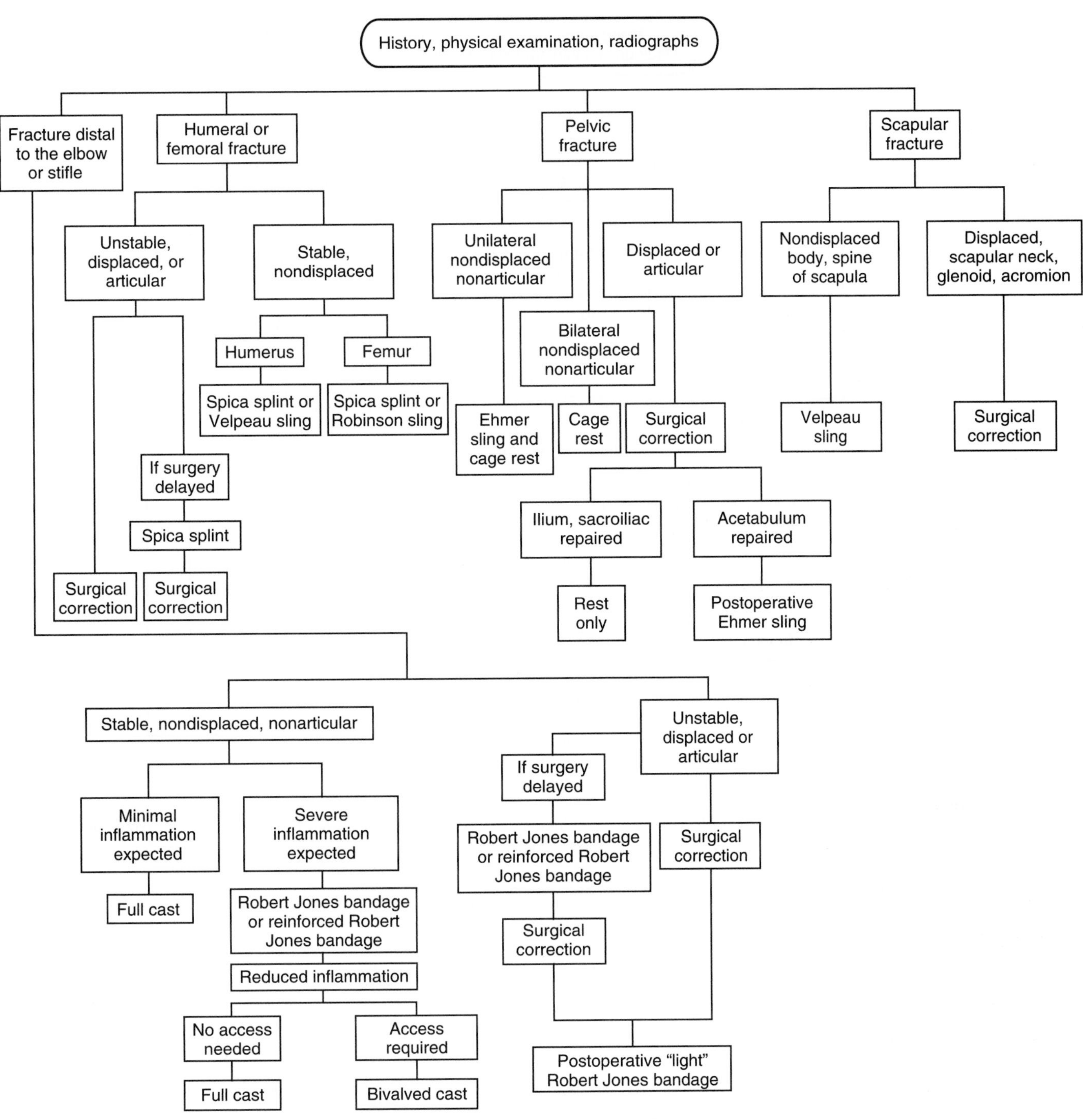

From Slatter DH: *Textbook of Small Animal Surgery*, ed 3. St. Louis, WB Saunders, 2003.

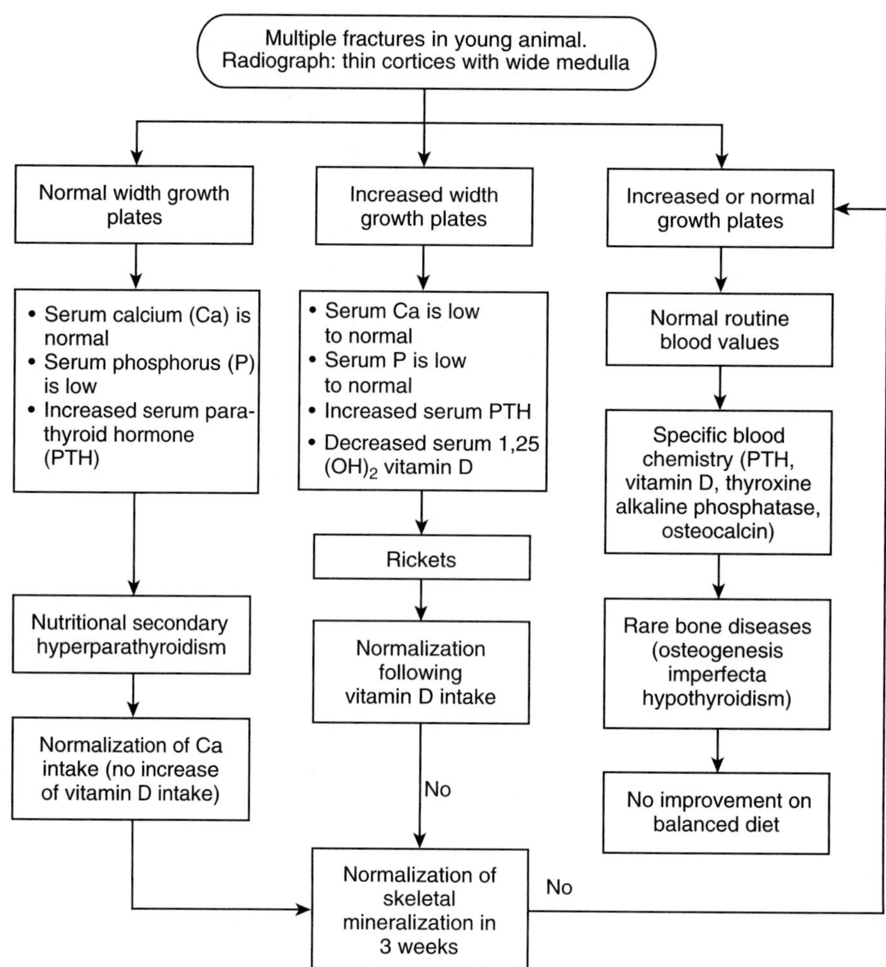

Modified from Ettinger SJ, Feldman EC: *Textbook of Veterinary Internal Medicine*, ed 6. St. Louis, WB Saunders, 2005.

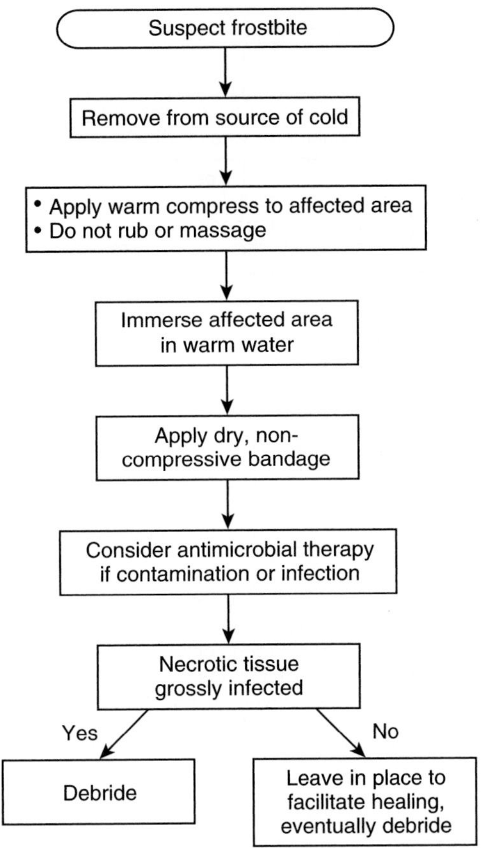
FROSTBITE
Suspect frostbite
Remove from source of cold
• Apply warm compress to affected area
• Do not rub or massage
Immerse affected area in warm water
Apply dry, non-compressive bandage
Consider antimicrobial therapy if contamination or infection
Necrotic tissue grossly infected
Yes
No
Debride
Leave in place to facilitate healing, eventually debride

Author: Scott P. Shaw
Editor: Elizabeth Rozanski

GLAUCOMA

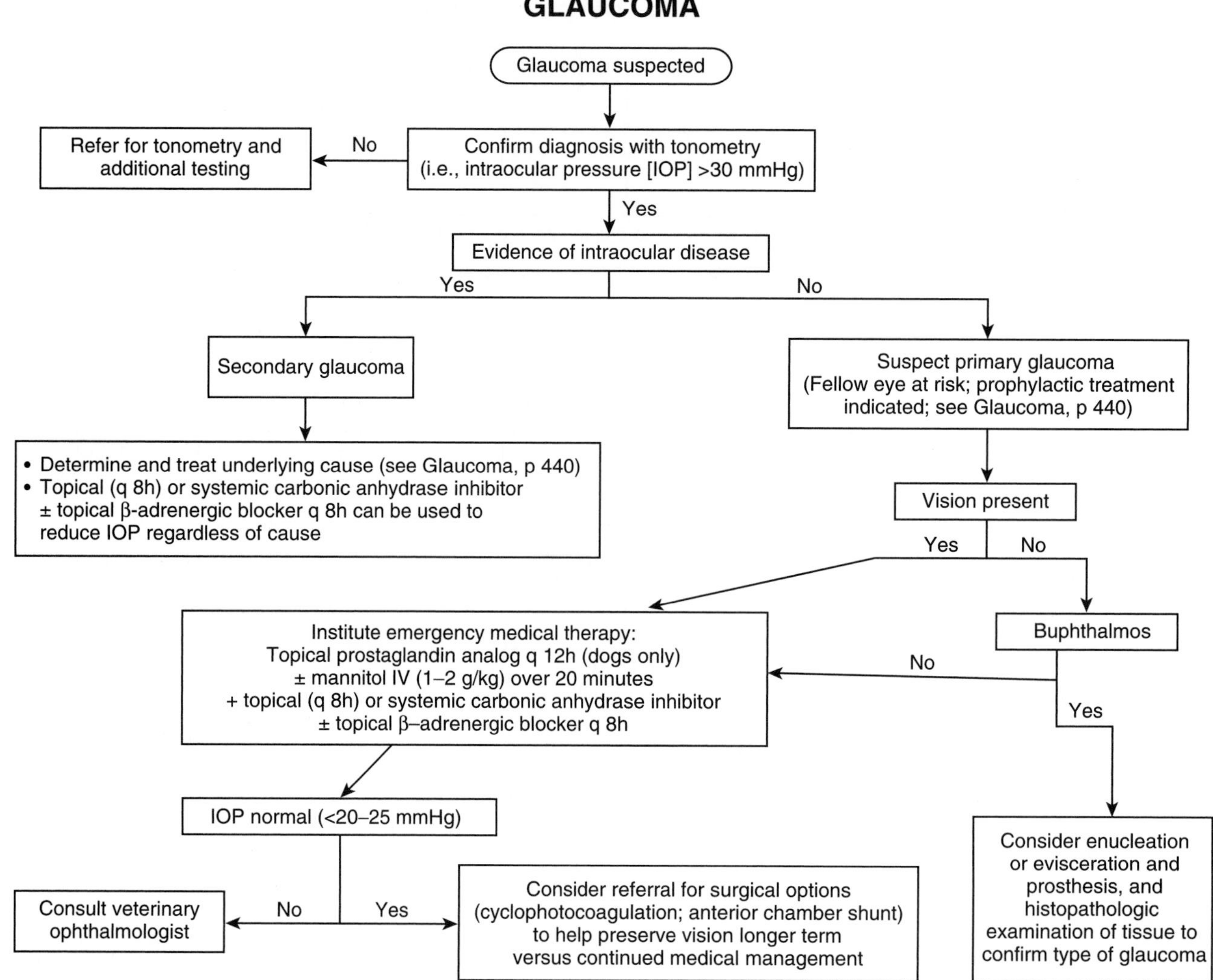
Glaucoma suspected
Confirm diagnosis with tonometry (i.e., intraocular pressure [IOP] >30 mmHg)
No
Refer for tonometry and additional testing
Yes
Evidence of intraocular disease
Yes
No
Secondary glaucoma
• Determine and treat underlying cause (see Glaucoma, p 440)
• Topical (q 8h) or systemic carbonic anhydrase inhibitor ± topical β-adrenergic blocker q 8h can be used to reduce IOP regardless of cause
Suspect primary glaucoma (Fellow eye at risk; prophylactic treatment indicated; see Glaucoma, p 440)
Vision present
Yes
No
Buphthalmos
No
Yes
Institute emergency medical therapy: Topical prostaglandin analog q 12h (dogs only) ± mannitol IV (1–2 g/kg) over 20 minutes + topical (q 8h) or systemic carbonic anhydrase inhibitor ± topical β–adrenergic blocker q 8h
IOP normal (<20–25 mmHg)
No
Yes
Consult veterinary ophthalmologist
Consider referral for surgical options (cyclophotocoagulation; anterior chamber shunt) to help preserve vision longer term versus continued medical management
Consider enucleation or evisceration and prosthesis, and histopathologic examination of tissue to confirm type of glaucoma

Author & Editor: Cheryl L. Cullen

GLOMERULONEPHRITIS: MANAGEMENT

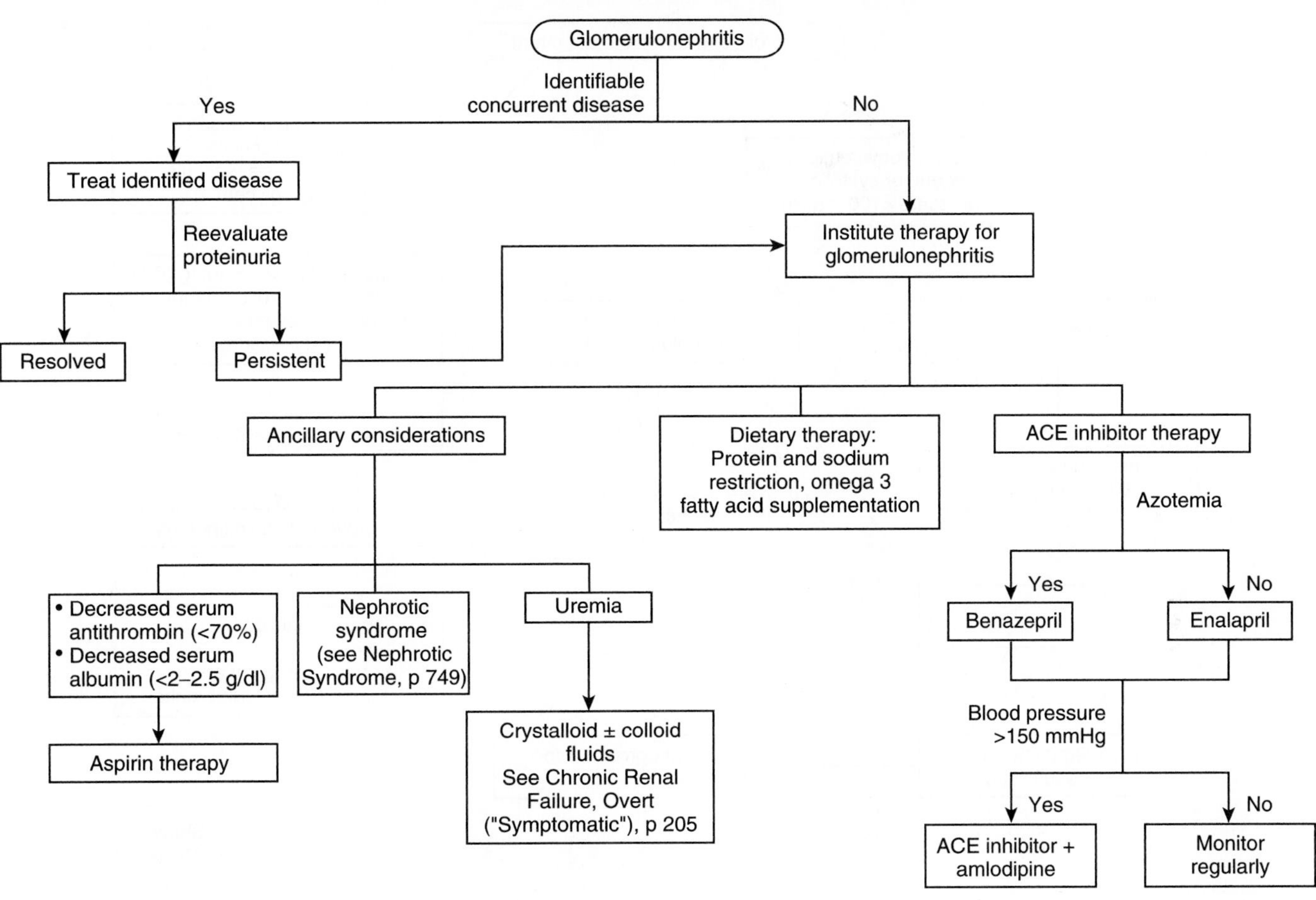

Author: Anne M. Dalby
Editor: Leah A. Cohn

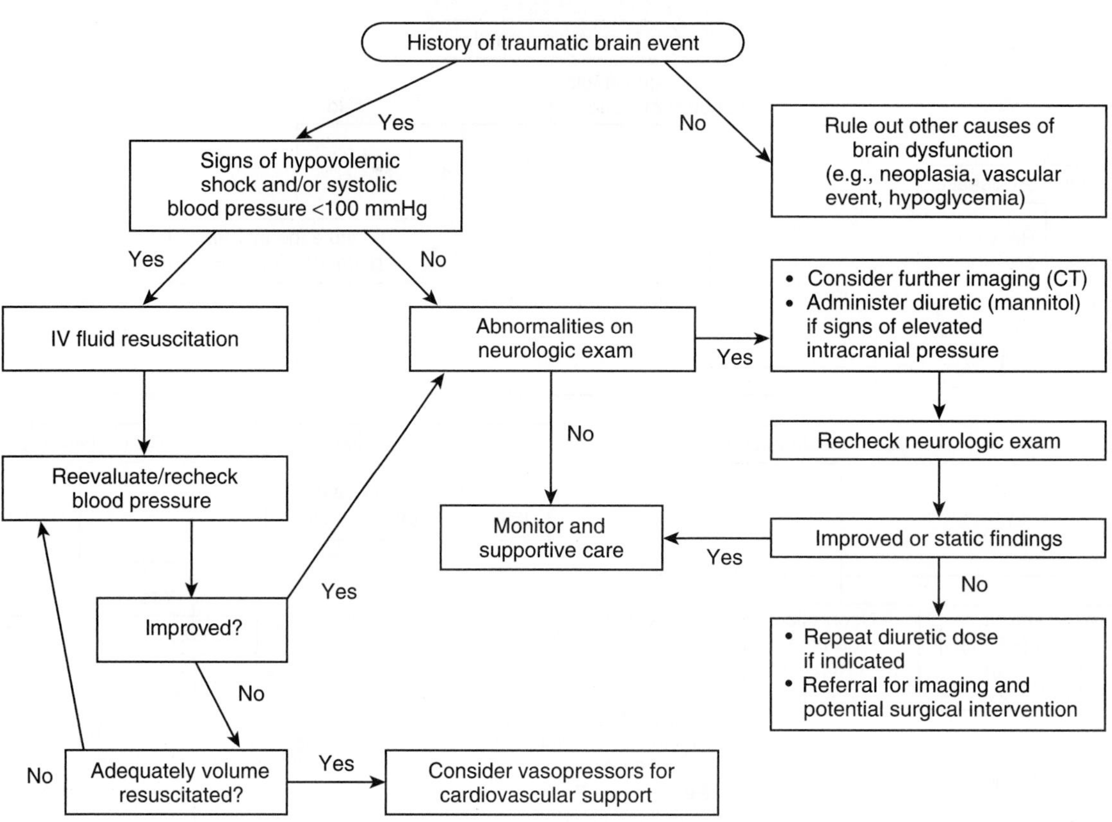

Author: Scott P. Shaw
Editor: Elizabeth Rozanski

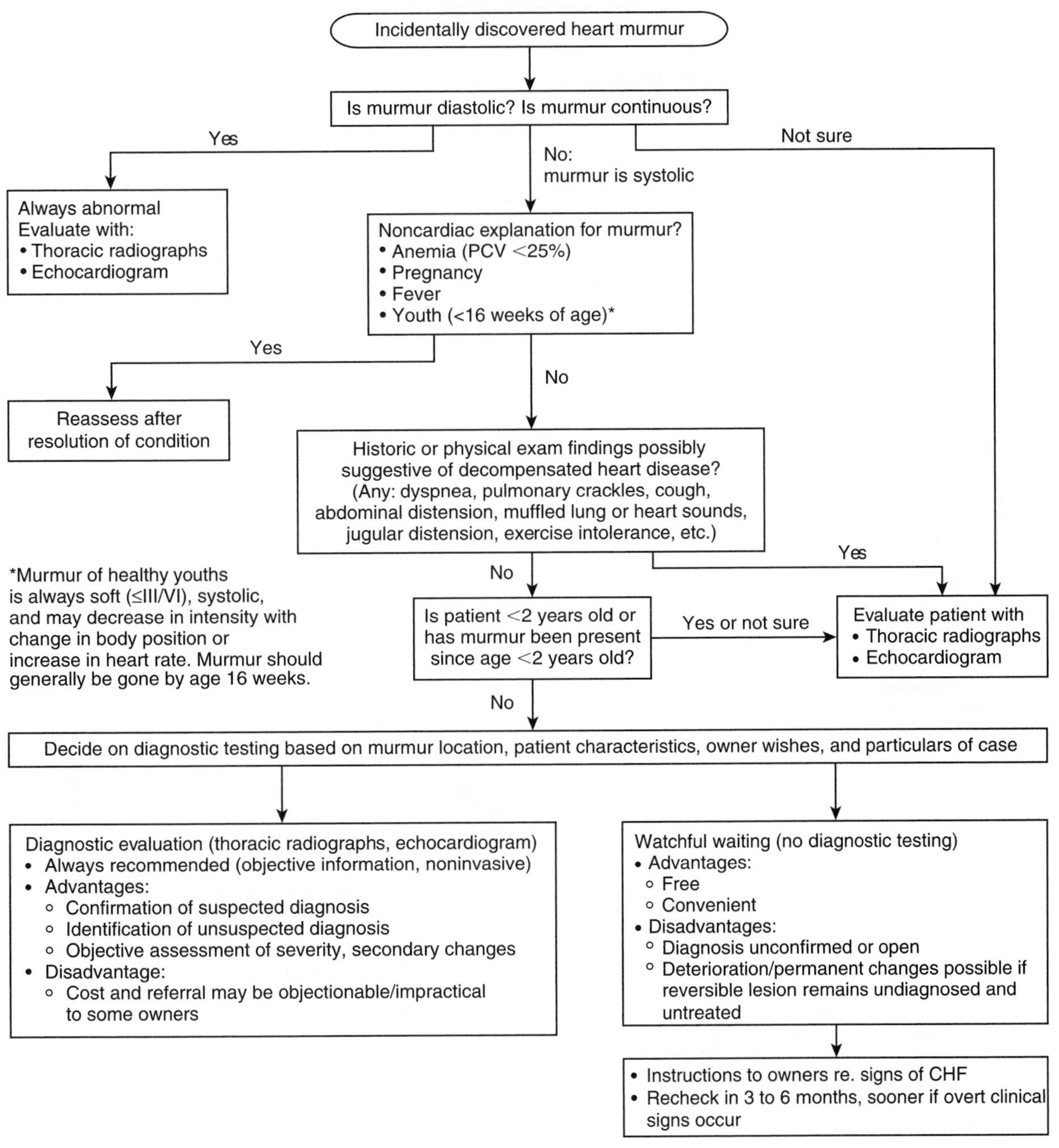

PCV, packed cell volume; CHF, congestive heart failure.

Author & Editor: Etienne Côté

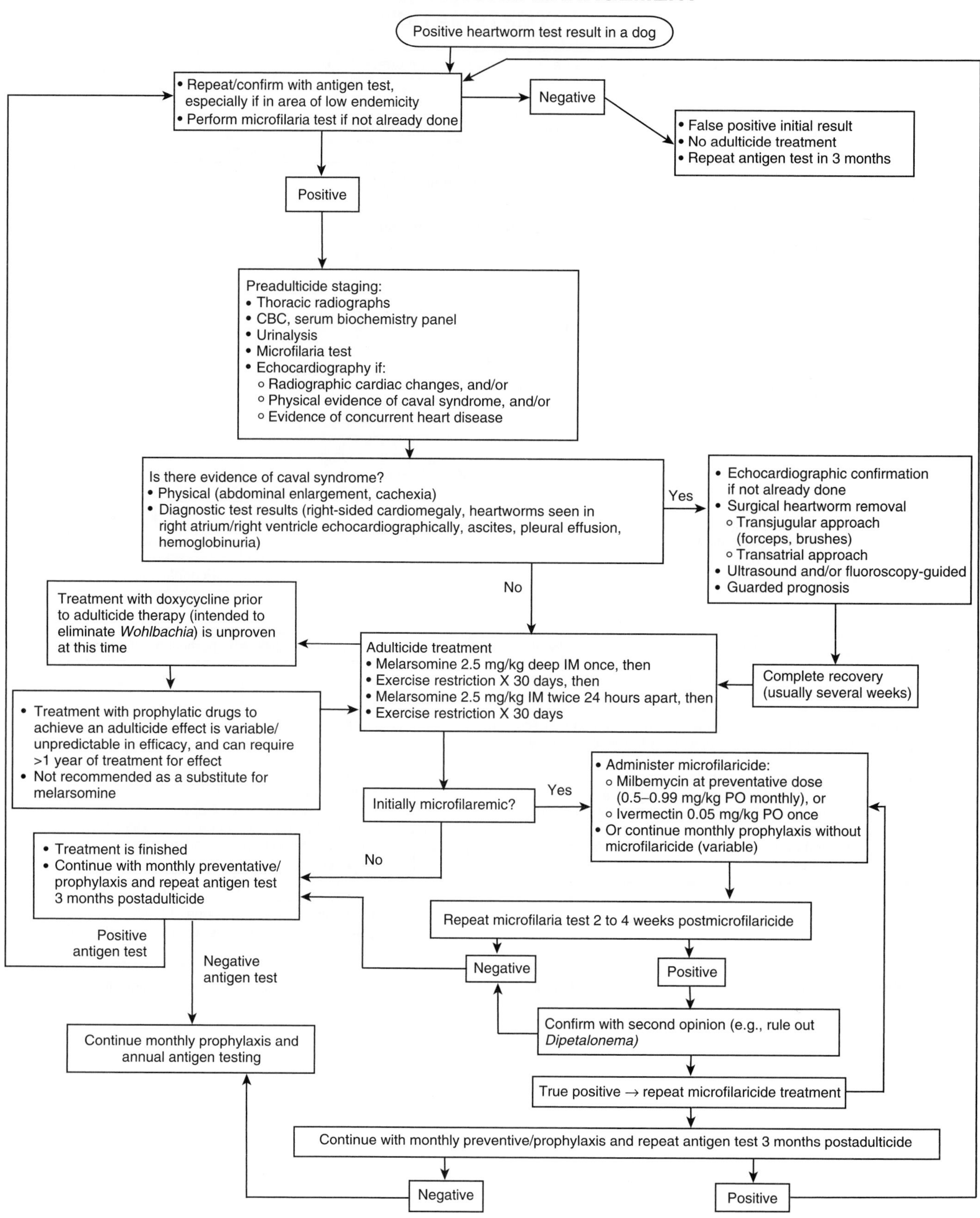
HEARTWORM MANAGEMENT
Positive heartworm test result in a dog
• Repeat/confirm with antigen test, especially if in area of low endemicity
• Perform microfilaria test if not already done
Negative
• False positive initial result
• No adulticide treatment
• Repeat antigen test in 3 months
Positive
Preadulticide staging:
• Thoracic radiographs
• CBC, serum biochemistry panel
• Urinalysis
• Microfilaria test
• Echocardiography if:
○ Radiographic cardiac changes, and/or
○ Physical evidence of caval syndrome, and/or
○ Evidence of concurrent heart disease
Is there evidence of caval syndrome?
• Physical (abdominal enlargement, cachexia)
• Diagnostic test results (right-sided cardiomegaly, heartworms seen in right atrium/right ventricle echocardiographically, ascites, pleural effusion, hemoglobinuria)
Yes
• Echocardiographic confirmation if not already done
• Surgical heartworm removal
○ Transjugular approach (forceps, brushes)
○ Transatrial approach
• Ultrasound and/or fluoroscopy-guided
• Guarded prognosis
No
Treatment with doxycycline prior to adulticide therapy (intended to eliminate Wohlbachia) is unproven at this time
Adulticide treatment
• Melarsomine 2.5 mg/kg deep IM once, then
• Exercise restriction X 30 days, then
• Melarsomine 2.5 mg/kg IM twice 24 hours apart, then
• Exercise restriction X 30 days
Complete recovery (usually several weeks)
• Treatment with prophylatic drugs to achieve an adulticide effect is variable/unpredictable in efficacy, and can require >1 year of treatment for effect
• Not recommended as a substitute for melarsomine
Initially microfilaremic?
Yes
• Administer microfilaricide:
○ Milbemycin at preventative dose (0.5–0.99 mg/kg PO monthly), or
○ Ivermectin 0.05 mg/kg PO once
• Or continue monthly prophylaxis without microfilaricide (variable)
No
• Treatment is finished
• Continue with monthly preventative/prophylaxis and repeat antigen test 3 months postadulticide
Repeat microfilaria test 2 to 4 weeks postmicrofilaricide
Positive antigen test
Negative antigen test
Negative
Positive
Confirm with second opinion (e.g., rule out Dipetalonema)
Continue monthly prophylaxis and annual antigen testing
True positive → repeat microfilaricide treatment
Continue with monthly preventive/prophylaxis and repeat antigen test 3 months postadulticide
Negative
Positive

Author & Editor: Etienne Côté

Additional information available on the American Heartworm Society website: www.heartwormsociety.com.

HEAT STROKE—HYPERTHERMIA

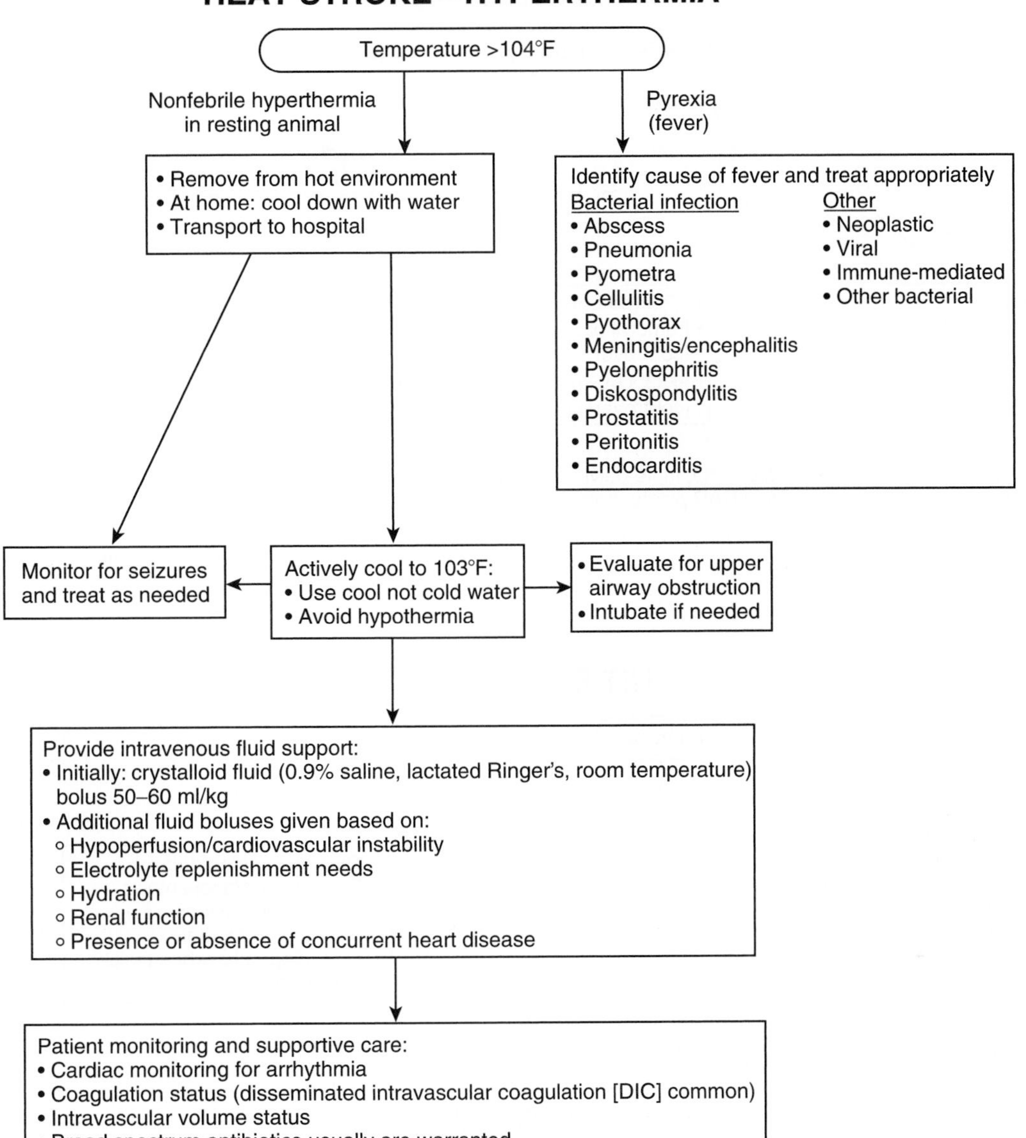

Temperature >104°F
Nonfebrile hyperthermia in resting animal
Pyrexia (fever)
• Remove from hot environment
• At home: cool down with water
• Transport to hospital
Identify cause of fever and treat appropriately
Bacterial infection
• Abscess
• Pneumonia
• Pyometra
• Cellulitis
• Pyothorax
• Meningitis/encephalitis
• Pyelonephritis
• Diskospondylitis
• Prostatitis
• Peritonitis
• Endocarditis
Other
• Neoplastic
• Viral
• Immune-mediated
• Other bacterial
Monitor for seizures and treat as needed
Actively cool to 103°F:
• Use cool not cold water
• Avoid hypothermia
• Evaluate for upper airway obstruction
• Intubate if needed
Provide intravenous fluid support:
• Initially: crystalloid fluid (0.9% saline, lactated Ringer's, room temperature) bolus 50–60 ml/kg
• Additional fluid boluses given based on:
○ Hypoperfusion/cardiovascular instability
○ Electrolyte replenishment needs
○ Hydration
○ Renal function
○ Presence or absence of concurrent heart disease
Patient monitoring and supportive care:
• Cardiac monitoring for arrhythmia
• Coagulation status (disseminated intravascular coagulation [DIC] common)
• Intravascular volume status
• Broad spectrum antibiotics usually are warranted

Author: Scott P. Shaw
Editor: Elizabeth Rozanski

HIP DYSPLASIA

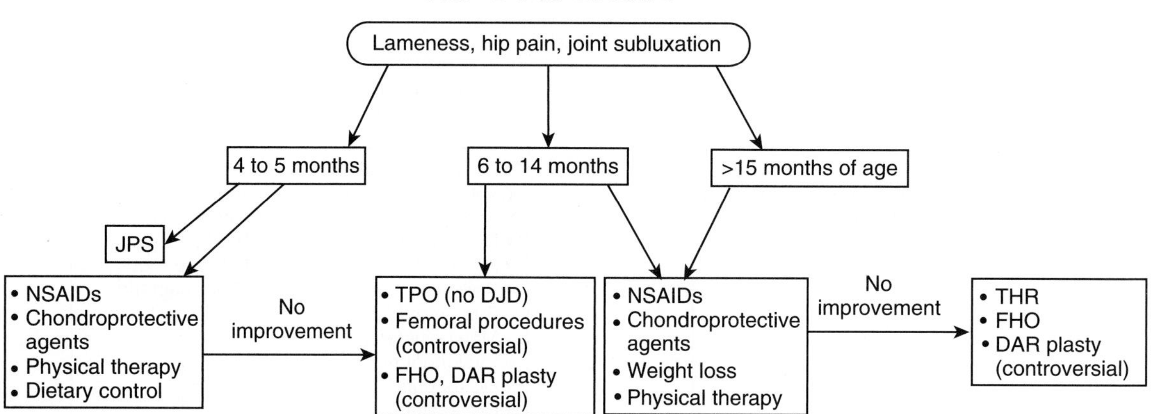

JPS, juvenile pubic symphysiodesis; TPO, triple pelvic osteotomy; THR, total hip replacement; FHO, femoral head/neck ostectomy; DAR plasty, dorsal acetabular rim arthroplasty.

Author & Editor: Joseph Harari

HIT BY CAR

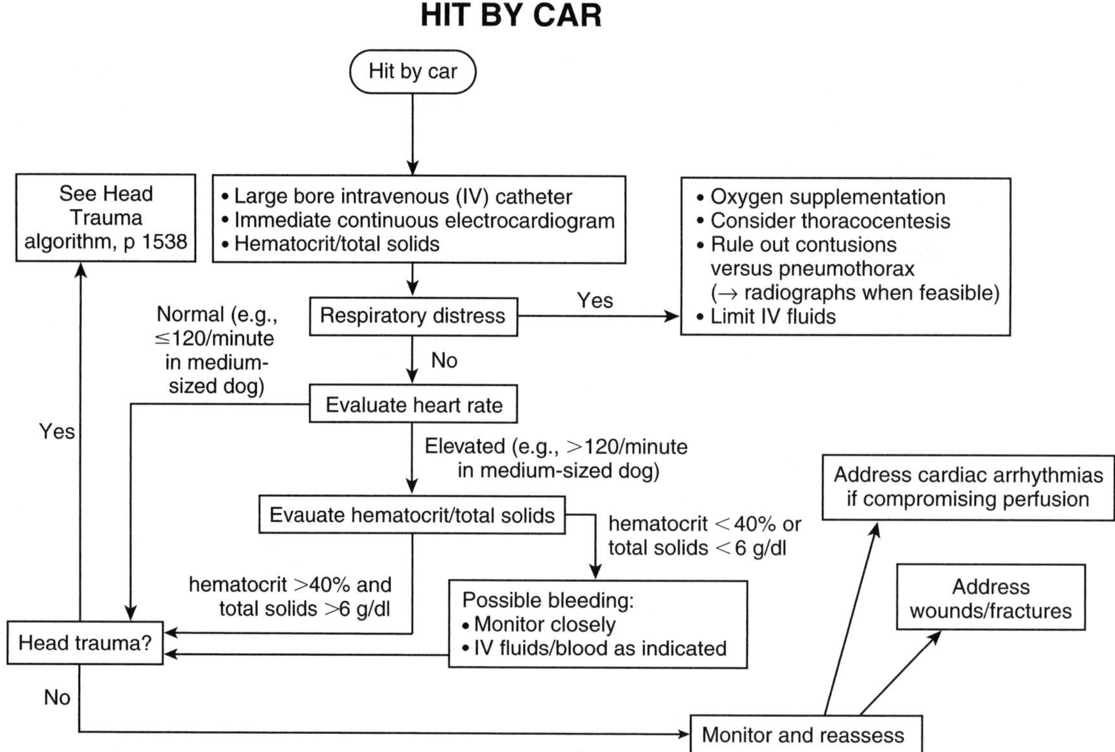

Author: Scott P. Shaw
Editor: Elizabeth Rozanski

HYPERADRENOCORTICISM: TREATMENT

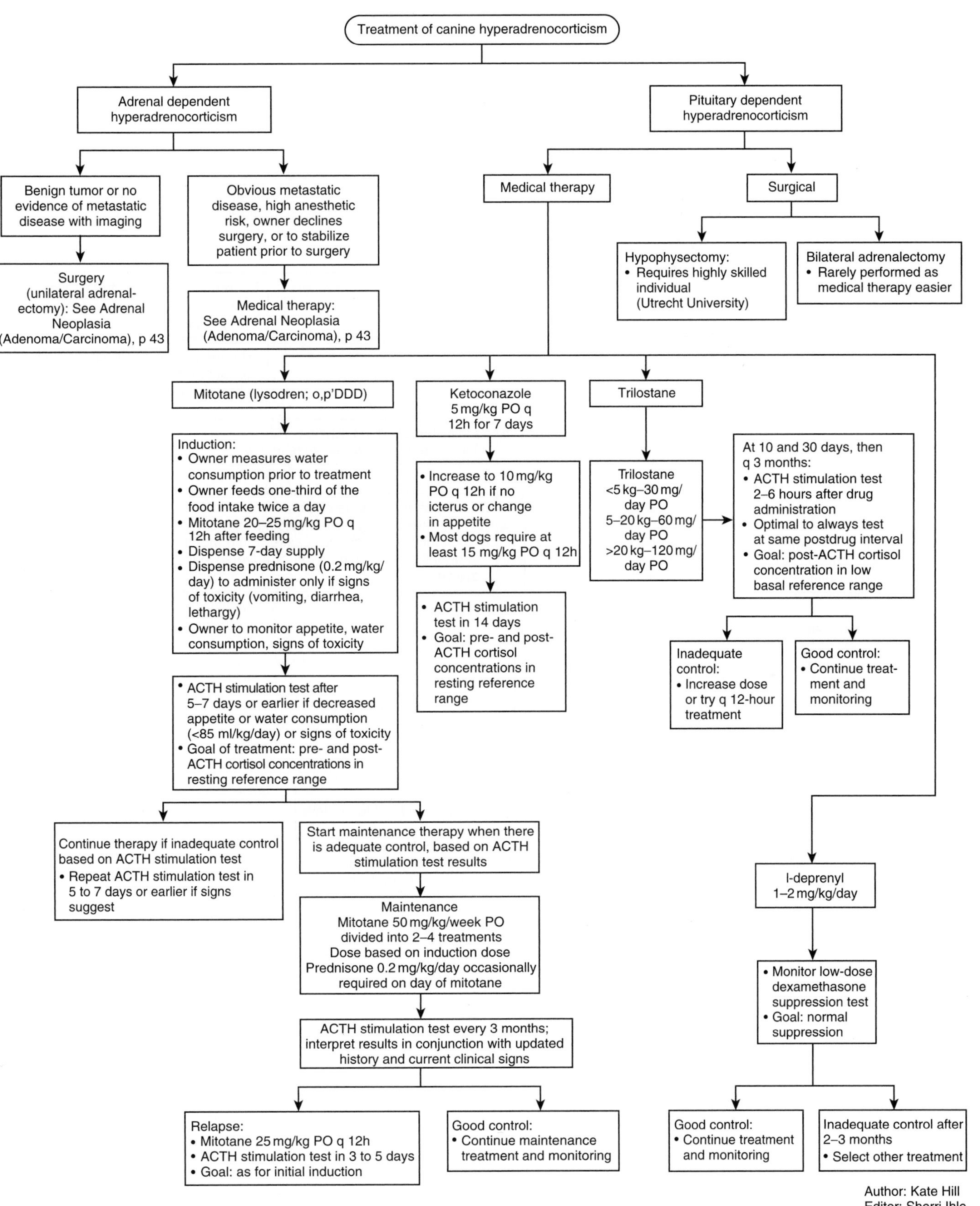
Treatment of canine hyperadrenocorticism
Adrenal dependent hyperadrenocorticism
Pituitary dependent hyperadrenocorticism
Benign tumor or no evidence of metastatic disease with imaging
Obvious metastatic disease, high anesthetic risk, owner declines surgery, or to stabilize patient prior to surgery
Medical therapy
Surgical
Surgery (unilateral adrenal-ectomy): See Adrenal Neoplasia (Adenoma/Carcinoma), p 43
Medical therapy: See Adrenal Neoplasia (Adenoma/Carcinoma), p 43
Hypophysectomy: • Requires highly skilled individual (Utrecht University)
Bilateral adrenalectomy • Rarely performed as medical therapy easier
Mitotane (lysodren; o,p'DDD)
Ketoconazole 5 mg/kg PO q 12h for 7 days
Trilostane
Induction: • Owner measures water consumption prior to treatment • Owner feeds one-third of the food intake twice a day • Mitotane 20–25 mg/kg PO q 12h after feeding • Dispense 7-day supply • Dispense prednisone (0.2 mg/kg/day) to administer only if signs of toxicity (vomiting, diarrhea, lethargy) • Owner to monitor appetite, water consumption, signs of toxicity
• Increase to 10 mg/kg PO q 12h if no icterus or change in appetite • Most dogs require at least 15 mg/kg PO q 12h
Trilostane <5 kg–30 mg/day PO 5–20 kg–60 mg/day PO >20 kg–120 mg/day PO
At 10 and 30 days, then q 3 months: • ACTH stimulation test 2–6 hours after drug administration • Optimal to always test at same postdrug interval • Goal: post-ACTH cortisol concentration in low basal reference range
• ACTH stimulation test in 14 days • Goal: pre- and post-ACTH cortisol concentrations in resting reference range
Inadequate control: • Increase dose or try q 12-hour treatment
Good control: • Continue treatment and monitoring
• ACTH stimulation test after 5–7 days or earlier if decreased appetite or water consumption (<85 ml/kg/day) or signs of toxicity • Goal of treatment: pre- and post-ACTH cortisol concentrations in resting reference range
Continue therapy if inadequate control based on ACTH stimulation test • Repeat ACTH stimulation test in 5 to 7 days or earlier if signs suggest
Start maintenance therapy when there is adequate control, based on ACTH stimulation test results
Maintenance Mitotane 50 mg/kg/week PO divided into 2–4 treatments Dose based on induction dose Prednisone 0.2 mg/kg/day occasionally required on day of mitotane
ACTH stimulation test every 3 months; interpret results in conjunction with updated history and current clinical signs
Relapse: • Mitotane 25 mg/kg PO q 12h • ACTH stimulation test in 3 to 5 days • Goal: as for initial induction
Good control: • Continue maintenance treatment and monitoring
l-deprenyl 1–2 mg/kg/day
• Monitor low-dose dexamethasone suppression test • Goal: normal suppression
Good control: • Continue treatment and monitoring
Inadequate control after 2–3 months • Select other treatment

Author: Kate Hill
Editor: Sherri Ihle

HYPERTHYROIDISM

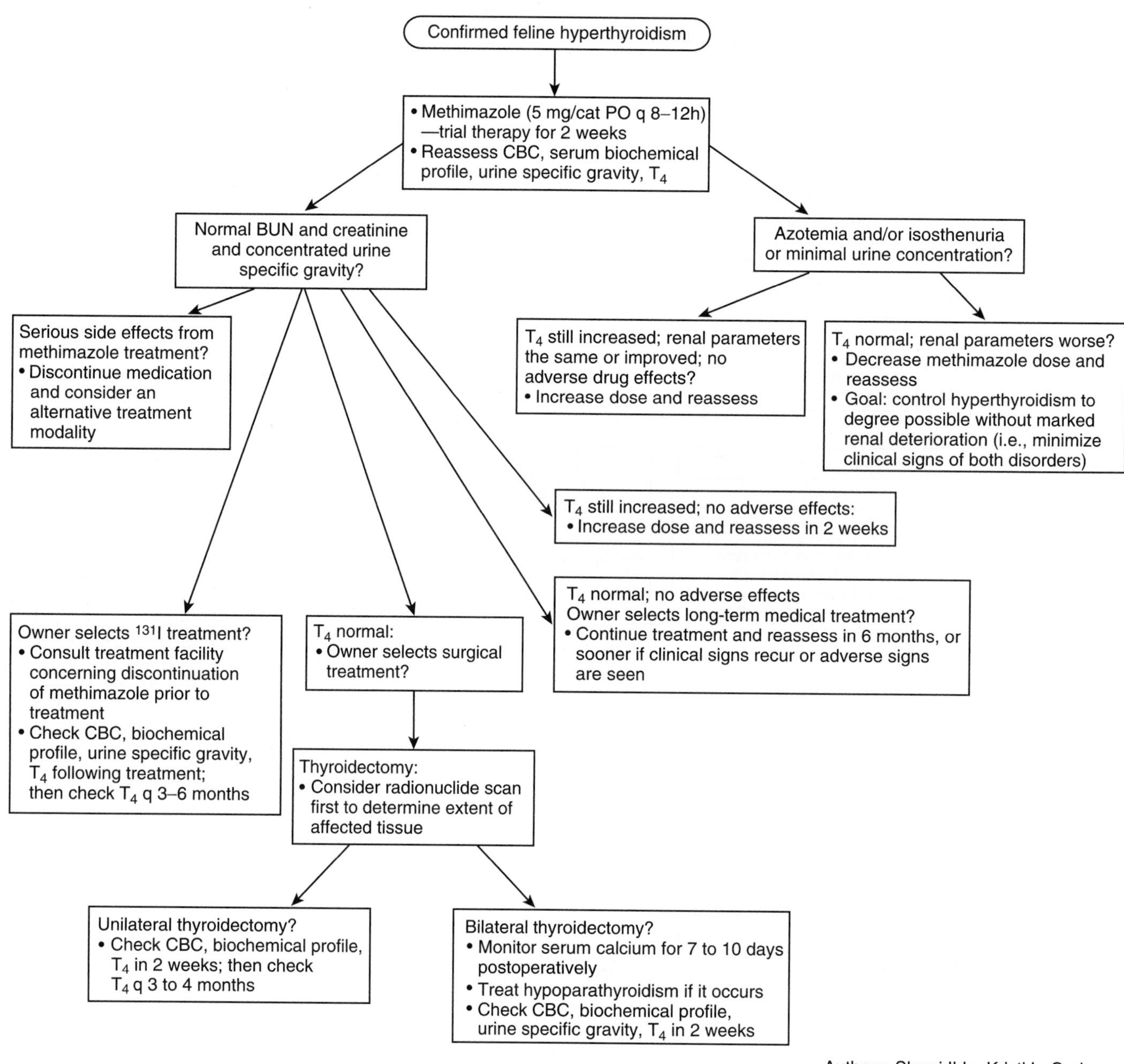

Confirmed feline hyperthyroidism
• Methimazole (5 mg/cat PO q 8–12h) —trial therapy for 2 weeks
• Reassess CBC, serum biochemical profile, urine specific gravity, T_4
Normal BUN and creatinine and concentrated urine specific gravity?
Azotemia and/or isosthenuria or minimal urine concentration?
Serious side effects from methimazole treatment?
• Discontinue medication and consider an alternative treatment modality
T_4 still increased; renal parameters the same or improved; no adverse drug effects?
• Increase dose and reassess
T_4 normal; renal parameters worse?
• Decrease methimazole dose and reassess
• Goal: control hyperthyroidism to degree possible without marked renal deterioration (i.e., minimize clinical signs of both disorders)
T_4 still increased; no adverse effects:
• Increase dose and reassess in 2 weeks
T_4 normal; no adverse effects
Owner selects long-term medical treatment?
• Continue treatment and reassess in 6 months, or sooner if clinical signs recur or adverse signs are seen
Owner selects ^{131}I treatment?
• Consult treatment facility concerning discontinuation of methimazole prior to treatment
• Check CBC, biochemical profile, urine specific gravity, T_4 following treatment; then check T_4 q 3–6 months
T_4 normal:
• Owner selects surgical treatment?
Thyroidectomy:
• Consider radionuclide scan first to determine extent of affected tissue
Unilateral thyroidectomy?
• Check CBC, biochemical profile, T_4 in 2 weeks; then check T_4 q 3 to 4 months
Bilateral thyroidectomy?
• Monitor serum calcium for 7 to 10 days postoperatively
• Treat hypoparathyroidism if it occurs
• Check CBC, biochemical profile, urine specific gravity, T_4 in 2 weeks

Authors: Sherri Ihle, Kristi L. Graham
Editor: Sherri Ihle

HYPOADRENOCORTICISM

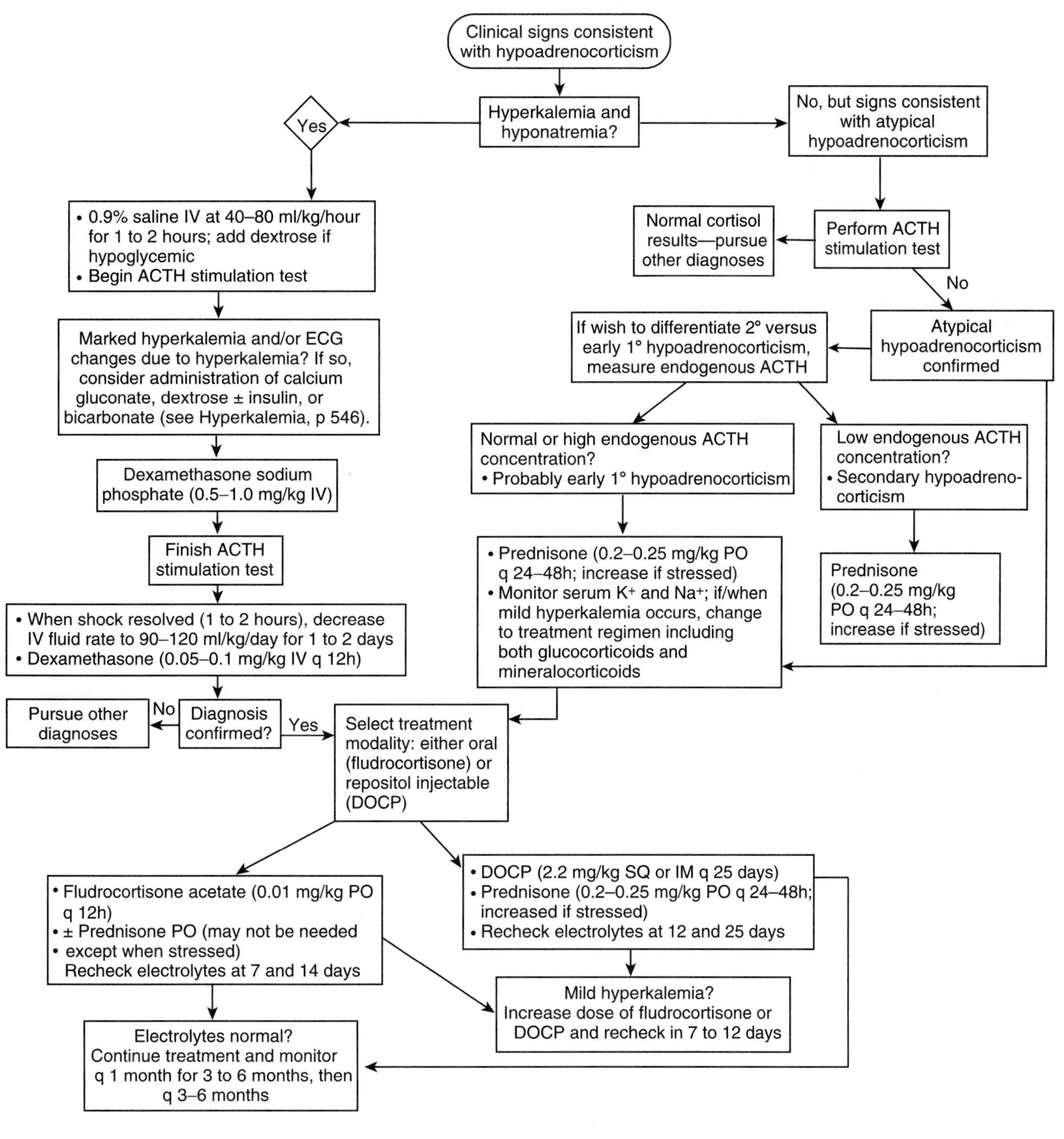

Author: Cary L. M. Bassett
Editor: Sherri Ihle

HYPOPARATHYROIDISM: MANAGEMENT

Confirmed hypocalcemia and hyperphosphatemia

→ Decreased serum albumin and/or increased BUN and serum creatinine
→ • Investigate other causes of hypocalcemia
• Measure serum ionized calcium level

→ Normal serum albumin concentration and normal BUN and serum creatinine levels
→ Normal or increased PTH? — Yes → • Investigate other causes of hypocalcemia • Measure serum ionized calcium level
→ Decreased or low-normal serum parathyroid hormone (PTH) level?
Yes → Initiate treatment for hypoparathyroidism

Patient is stable, and showing no overt clinical signs referable to hypocalcemia
→ • Dihydrotachysterol 0.02–0.03 mg/kg PO q 24h
• Calcium carbonate 1–4 g PO q 24h
→ Recheck serum calcium

Patient is showing mild clinical signs (e.g., intermittent muscle fasciculations) but is otherwise well
→ Administer calcium gluconate 10% SC

Patient is showing severe clinical signs referable to hypocalcemia (e.g., tetany, hyperthermia)
→ Connect ECG monitor and administer calcium gluconate 10% injectable solution: 1–1.5 ml/kg IV to effect, while monitoring for efficacy (visible reduction in clinical signs) and/or signs of excess (e.g., bradycardia or QT interval shortening on ECG)
→ • Administer calcium gluconate 10% injectable solution: 0.5–1.5 ml/kg SC diluted in 0.5–1.5 ml/kg sterile saline and with dosage adjusted according to serum calcium
• Dosage interval = q 6–12h
• Duration of treatment: typically 1–4 days, depending on severity of signs and time of onset of efficacy of dihydrotachysterol
→ Recheck serum calcium once weekly until in mid-normal range; adjust dihydrotachysterol dose accordingly (typical long-term dose = 0.01–0.02 mg/kg PO q 24h)

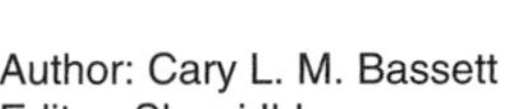
Author: Cary L. M. Bassett
Editor: Sherri Ihle

HYPOTHYROIDISM: TREATMENT

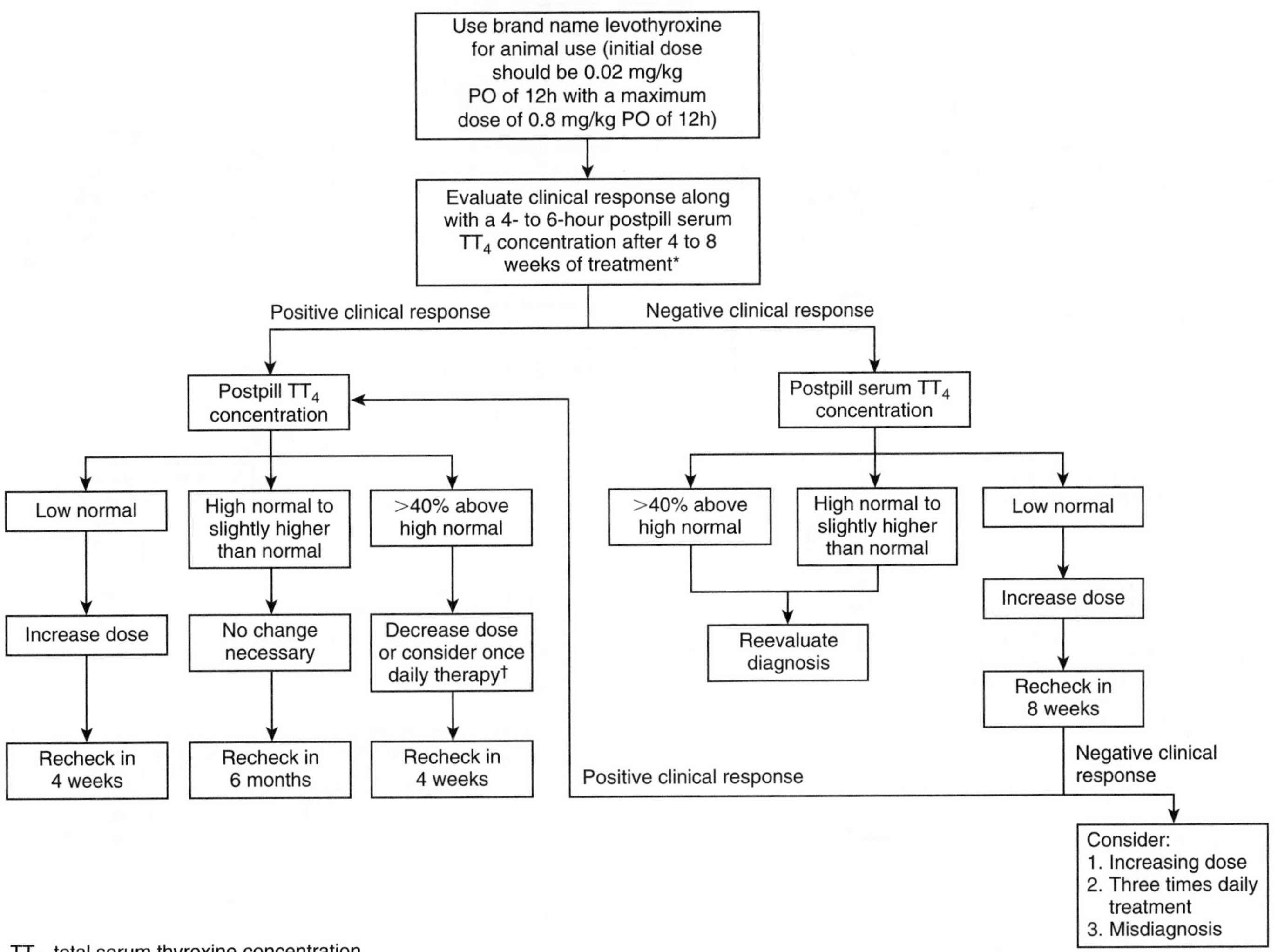

TT_4, total serum thyroxine concentration.
*Serum free T_4 by equilibrium dialysis can also be measured.
†Prepill serum T_4 also recommended if once daily therapy is administered.

Modified from Ettinger SJ, Feldman EC: *Textbook of Veterinary Internal Medicine*, ed 6. St. Louis, WB Saunders, 2005.

ICTERUS: MANAGEMENT

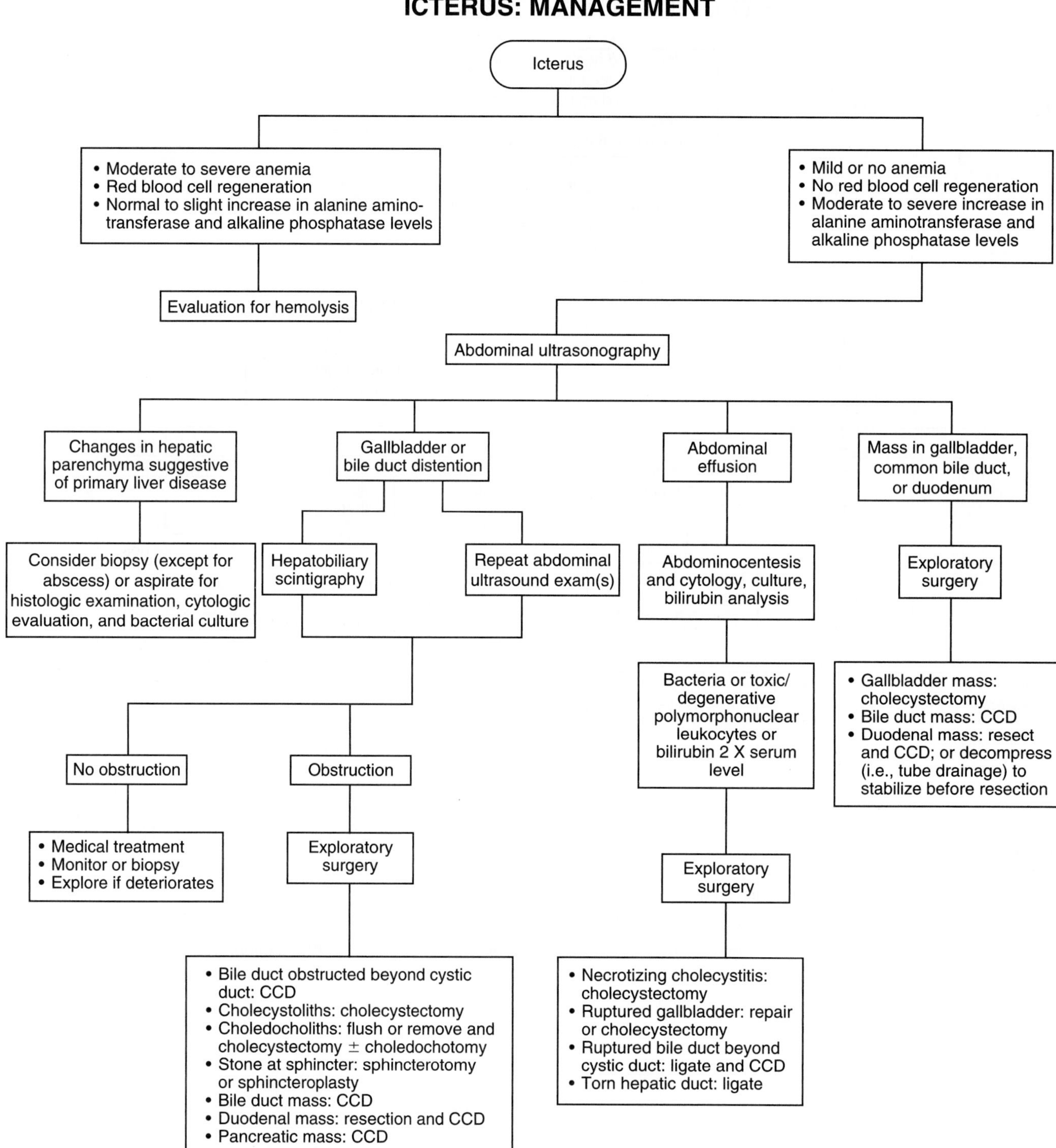

Modified from Slatter DH: *Textbook of Small Animal Surgery*, ed 3. St. Louis, WB Saunders, 2003.

CCD, cholecystoduodenostomy.

INAPPROPRIATE ELIMINATION, CAT

Diagnostic tree for feline elimination disorders

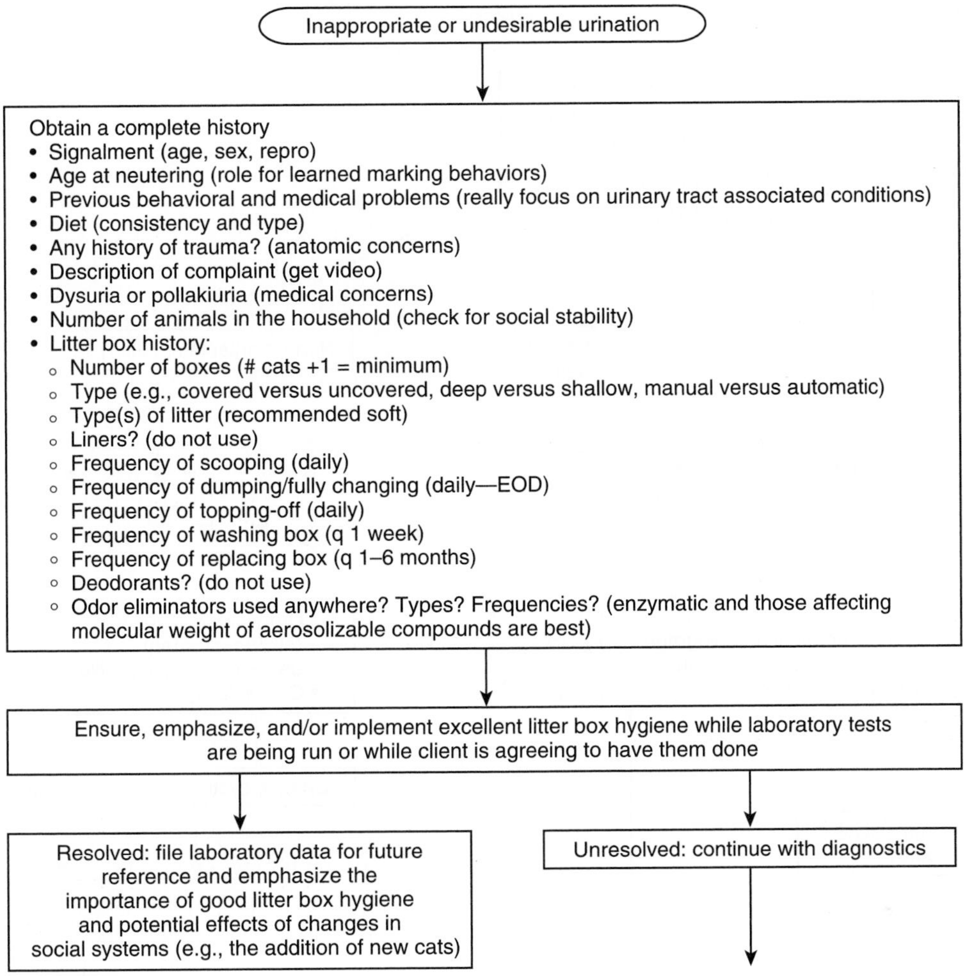

Inappropriate or undesirable urination

↓

Obtain a complete history
- Signalment (age, sex, repro)
- Age at neutering (role for learned marking behaviors)
- Previous behavioral and medical problems (really focus on urinary tract associated conditions)
- Diet (consistency and type)
- Any history of trauma? (anatomic concerns)
- Description of complaint (get video)
- Dysuria or pollakiuria (medical concerns)
- Number of animals in the household (check for social stability)
- Litter box history:
  - Number of boxes (# cats +1 = minimum)
  - Type (e.g., covered versus uncovered, deep versus shallow, manual versus automatic)
  - Type(s) of litter (recommended soft)
  - Liners? (do not use)
  - Frequency of scooping (daily)
  - Frequency of dumping/fully changing (daily—EOD)
  - Frequency of topping-off (daily)
  - Frequency of washing box (q 1 week)
  - Frequency of replacing box (q 1–6 months)
  - Deodorants? (do not use)
  - Odor eliminators used anywhere? Types? Frequencies? (enzymatic and those affecting molecular weight of aerosolizable compounds are best)

↓

Ensure, emphasize, and/or implement excellent litter box hygiene while laboratory tests are being run or while client is agreeing to have them done

↓ (left)

Resolved: file laboratory data for future reference and emphasize the importance of good litter box hygiene and potential effects of changes in social systems (e.g., the addition of new cats)

↓ (right)

Unresolved: continue with diagnostics

↓

Overall K: *Manual of Clinical Behavior Medicine.* St. Louis, Elsevier, 2007 (in press).
Some parts adapted from Overall KL, Labato M, 2006 (unpublished).

(Continued)

INAPPROPRIATE ELIMINATION, CAT—*(Continued)*

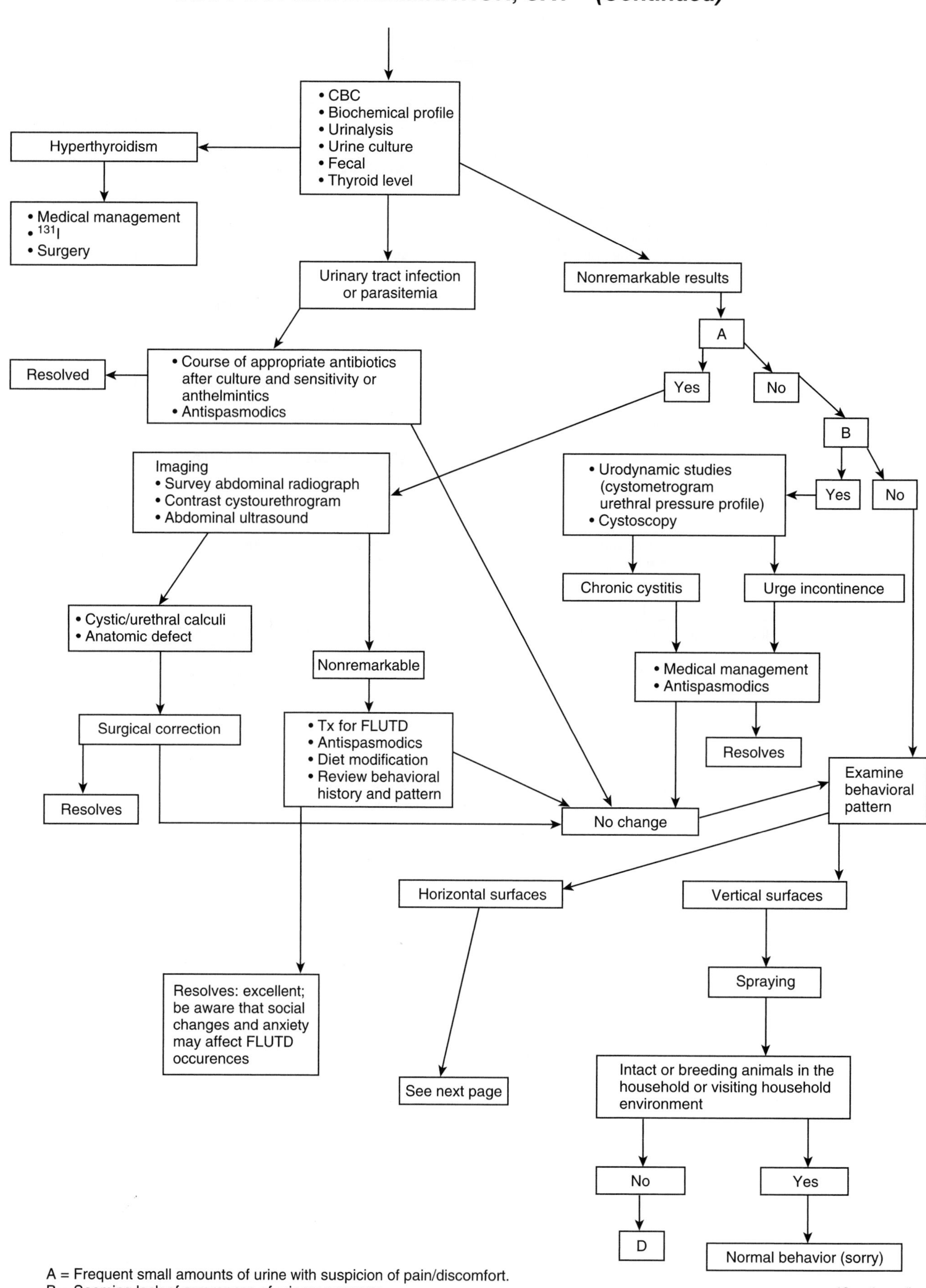

(Continued)

INAPPROPRIATE ELIMINATION, CAT—*(Continued)*

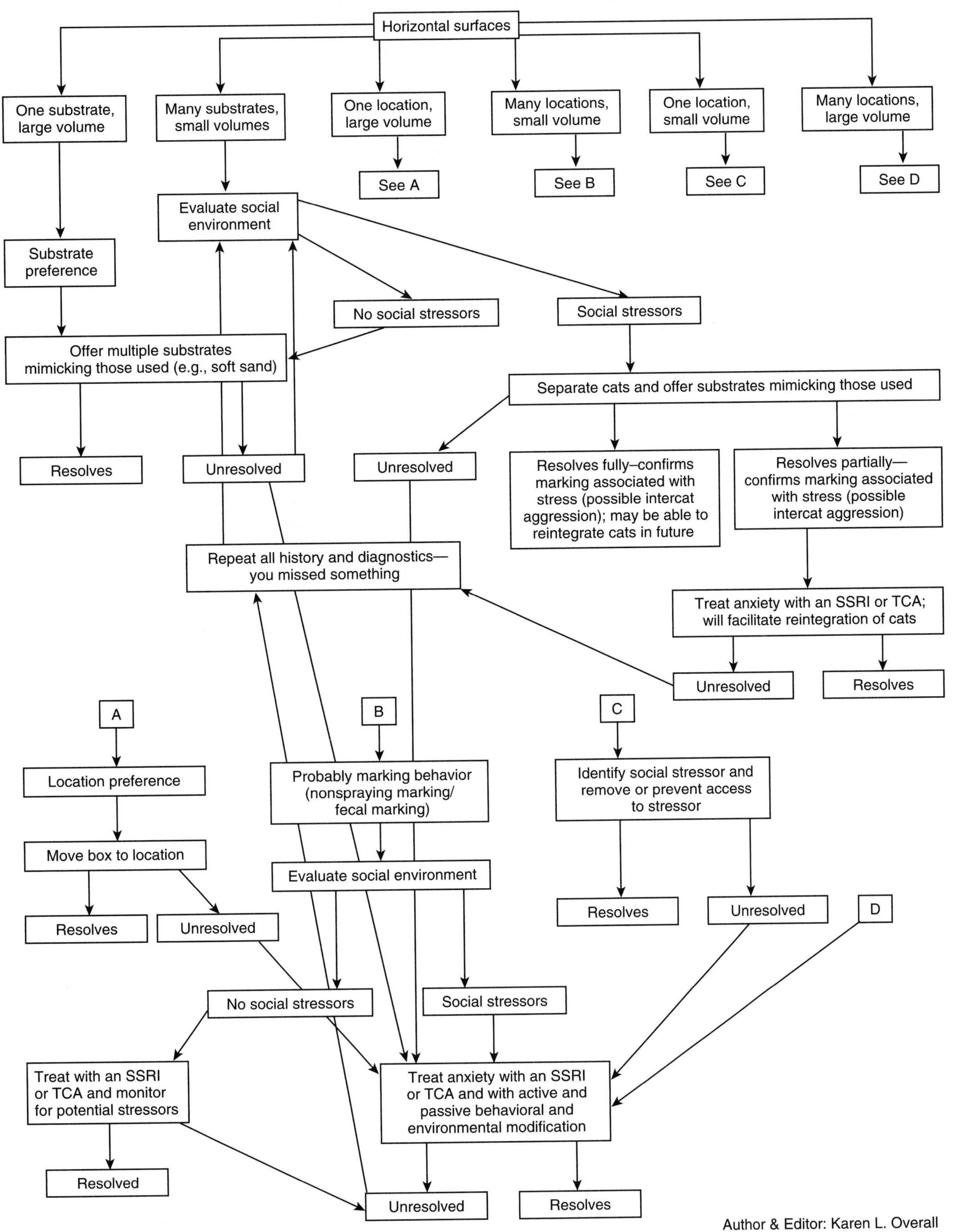

Author & Editor: Karen L. Overall

INFERTILITY IN THE CANINE FEMALE:

Keys to Solving Infertility Problems

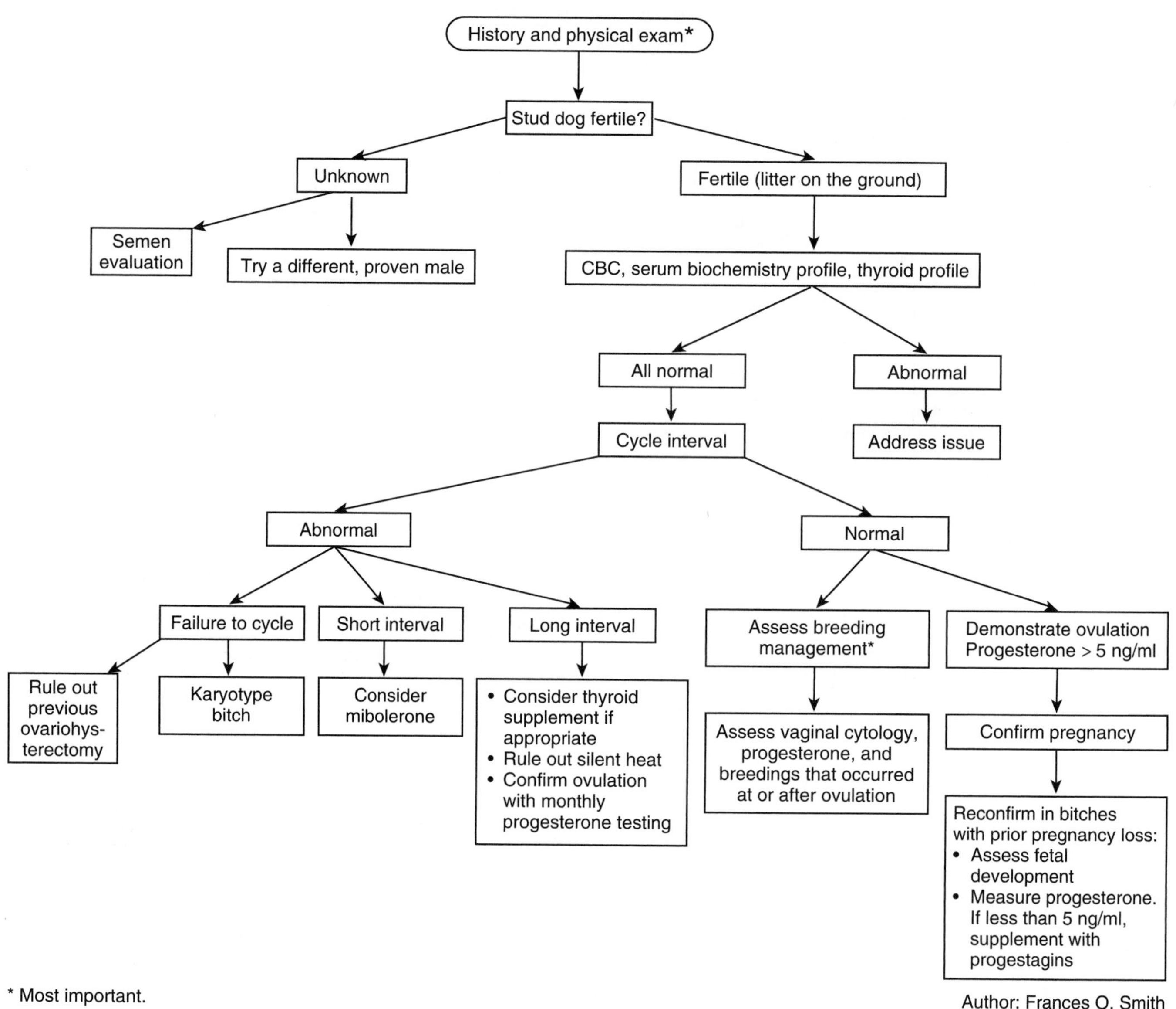

* Most important.

Author: Frances O. Smith
Editor: Michelle A. Kutzler

INSULINOMA

Clinical signs of insulinoma → CBC, serum biochemical profile, UA

CBC, serum biochemical profile, UA → Normal?; Normal except for hypoglycemia?; Abnormalities other than hypoglycemia

Normal? → Fast the animal, checking blood glucose q 1–2h or if clinical signs seen

Fast the animal, checking blood glucose q 1–2h or if clinical signs seen → No hypoglycemia and normal serum fructosamine; Hypoglycemia

No hypoglycemia and normal serum fructosamine → Pursue other diagnoses

Hypoglycemia → Submit concurrent sample for serum insulin assay

Normal except for hypoglycemia? → Yes → Submit concurrent sample for serum insulin assay

Normal except for hypoglycemia? → No → Pursue other diagnoses

Abnormalities other than hypoglycemia → Pursue other diagnoses

Submit concurrent sample for serum insulin assay → Low serum insulin; Increased serum insulin or serum insulin in the normal range despite hypoglycemia

Low serum insulin → Pursue other diagnoses

Increased serum insulin or serum insulin in the normal range despite hypoglycemia → Insulinoma

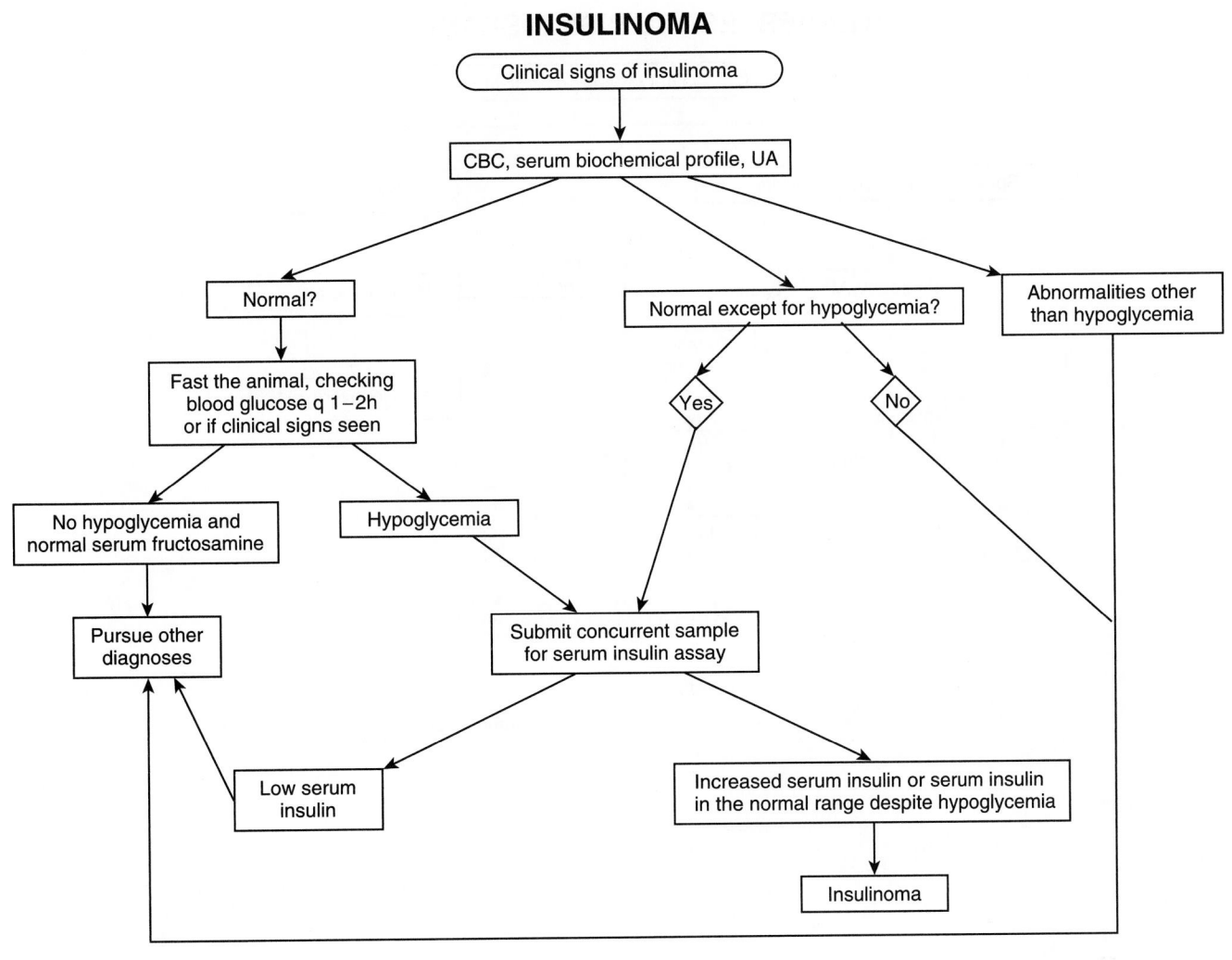

Author: Ninette Keller
Editor: Sherri Ihle

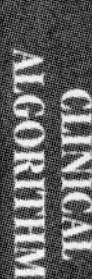

INTERVERTEBRAL DISK DISEASE

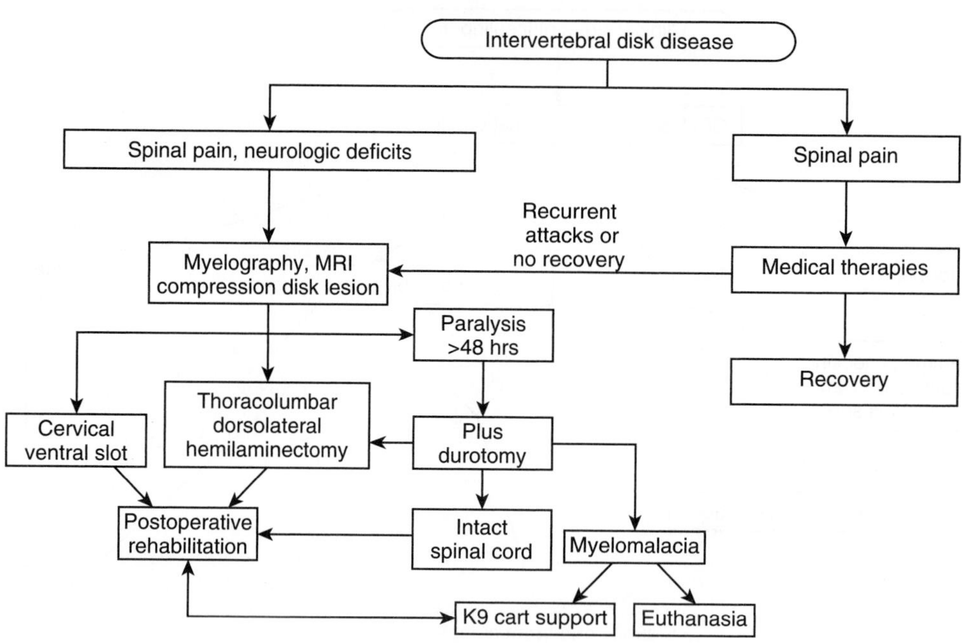

Author & Editor: Joseph Harari

LEUKEMIAS: CLASSIFICATION AND TREATMENT

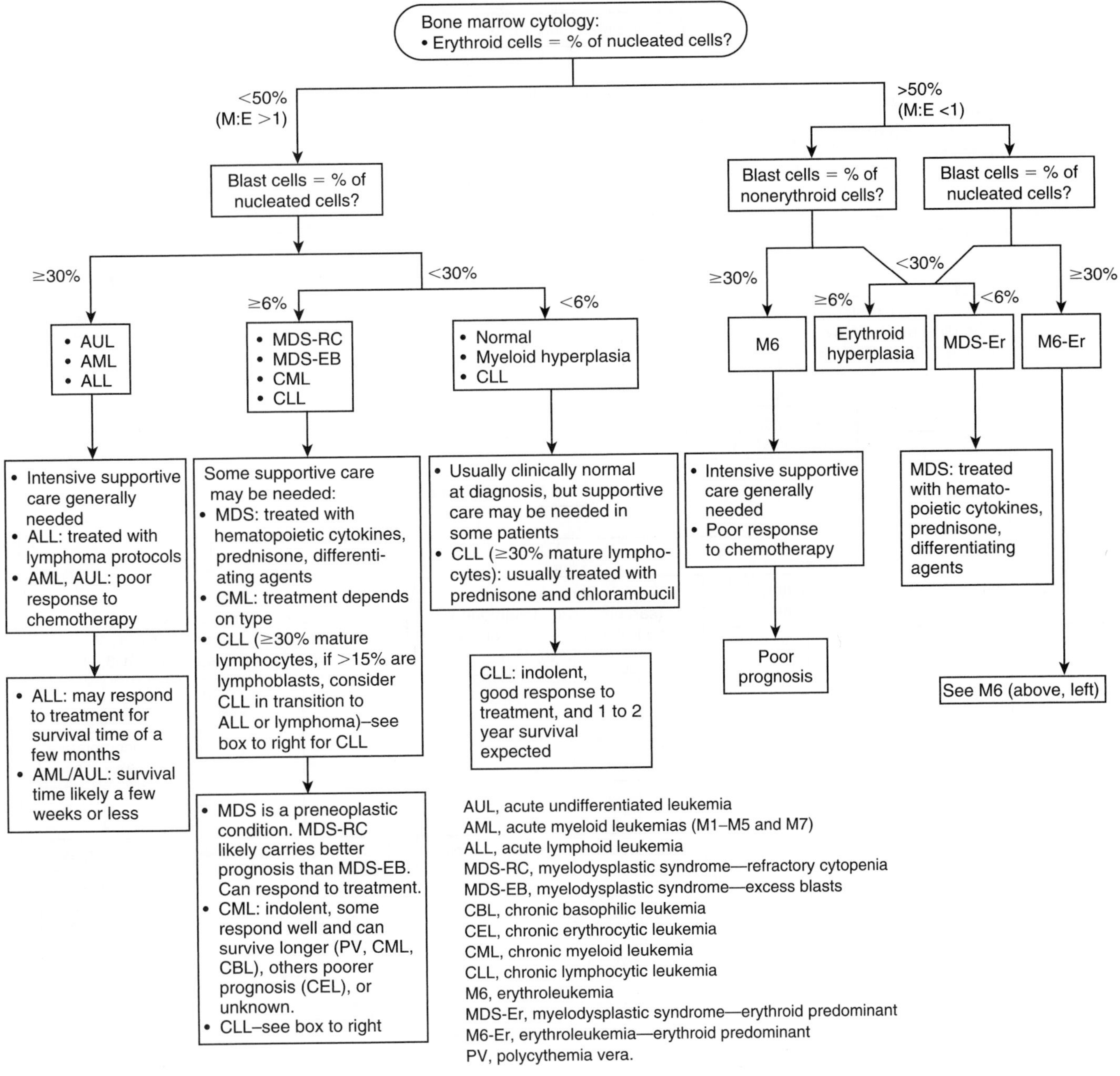

AUL, acute undifferentiated leukemia
AML, acute myeloid leukemias (M1–M5 and M7)
ALL, acute lymphoid leukemia
MDS-RC, myelodysplastic syndrome—refractory cytopenia
MDS-EB, myelodysplastic syndrome—excess blasts
CBL, chronic basophilic leukemia
CEL, chronic erythrocytic leukemia
CML, chronic myeloid leukemia
CLL, chronic lymphocytic leukemia
M6, erythroleukemia
MDS-Er, myelodysplastic syndrome—erythroid predominant
M6-Er, erythroleukemia—erythroid predominant
PV, polycythemia vera.

Author: Nicole C. Northrup
Editor: Kenneth M. Rassnick

Based on the Animal Leukemia Study Group criteria for classification of acute myeloid leukemias in dogs and cats, and modified from Jacobs RM, Messick JB, Valli VE: Tumors of the hemolymphatic system. In Meuten DJ (ed): *Tumors in Domestic Animals*, ed 4. Ames, IA, Iowa State Press, 2002, pp 119–198.

MAMMARY GLAND TUMORS, CAT

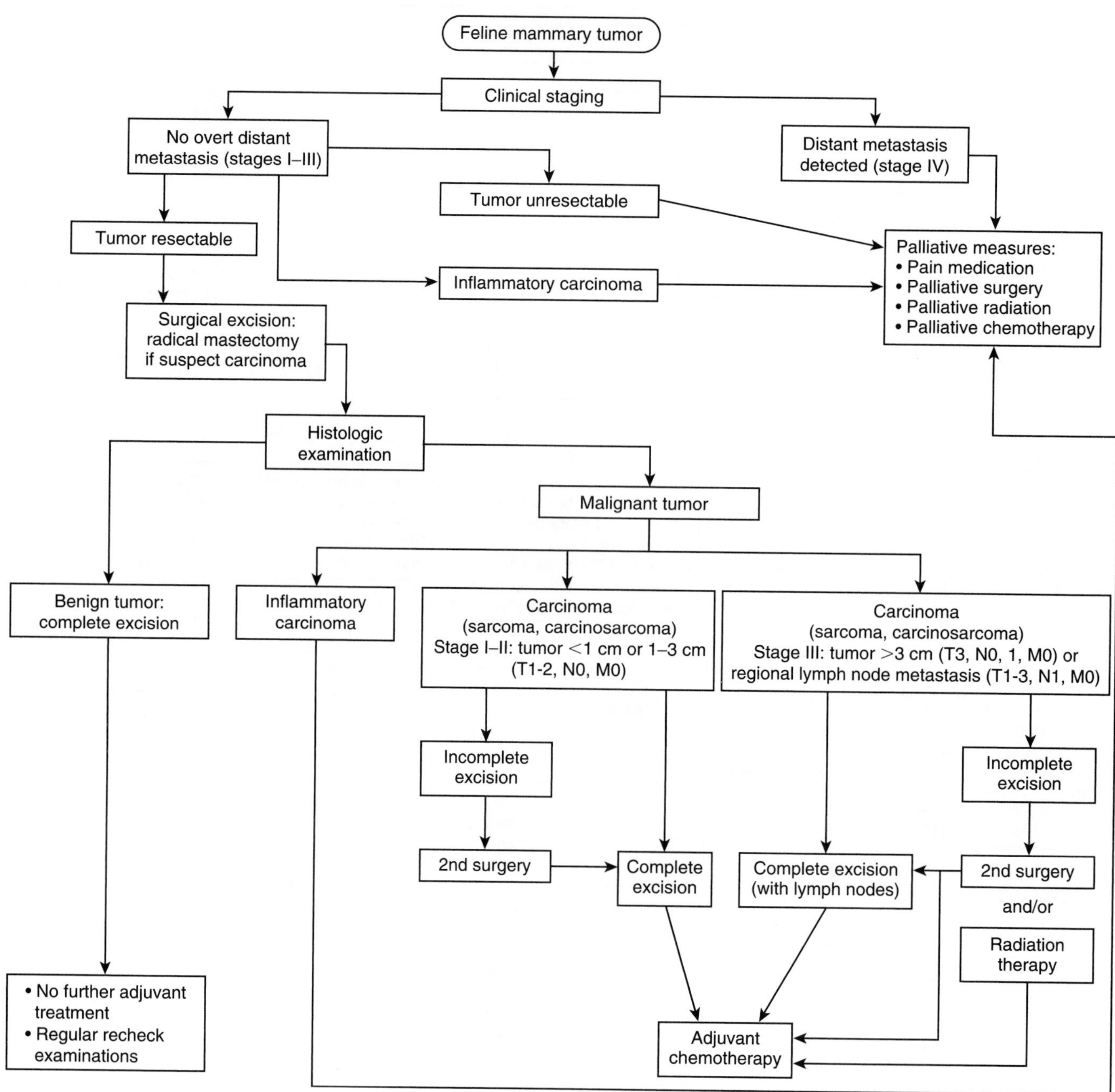
Feline mammary tumor
Clinical staging
No overt distant metastasis (stages I–III)
Distant metastasis detected (stage IV)
Tumor unresectable
Tumor resectable
Inflammatory carcinoma
Palliative measures:
• Pain medication
• Palliative surgery
• Palliative radiation
• Palliative chemotherapy
Surgical excision: radical mastectomy if suspect carcinoma
Histologic examination
Malignant tumor
Benign tumor: complete excision
Inflammatory carcinoma
Carcinoma (sarcoma, carcinosarcoma) Stage I–II: tumor <1 cm or 1–3 cm (T1-2, N0, M0)
Carcinoma (sarcoma, carcinosarcoma) Stage III: tumor >3 cm (T3, N0, 1, M0) or regional lymph node metastasis (T1-3, N1, M0)
Incomplete excision
Incomplete excision
2nd surgery
Complete excision
Complete excision (with lymph nodes)
2nd surgery
and/or
Radiation therapy
• No further adjuvant treatment
• Regular recheck examinations
Adjuvant chemotherapy

Author: Daniela Simon
Editor: Kenneth M. Rassnick

MAMMARY GLAND TUMORS, DOG

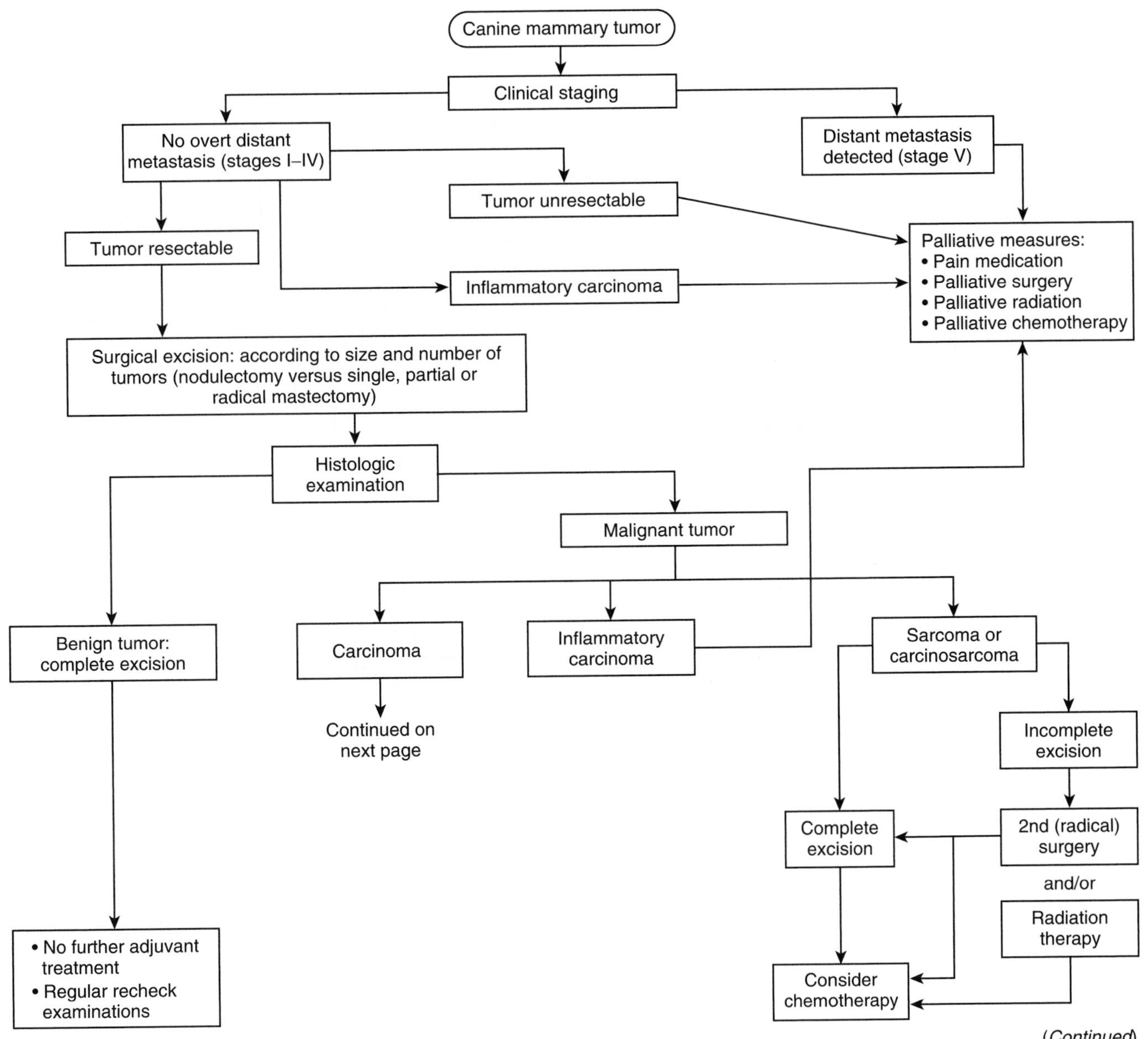

(*Continued*)

MAMMARY GLAND TUMORS, DOG—*(Continued)*

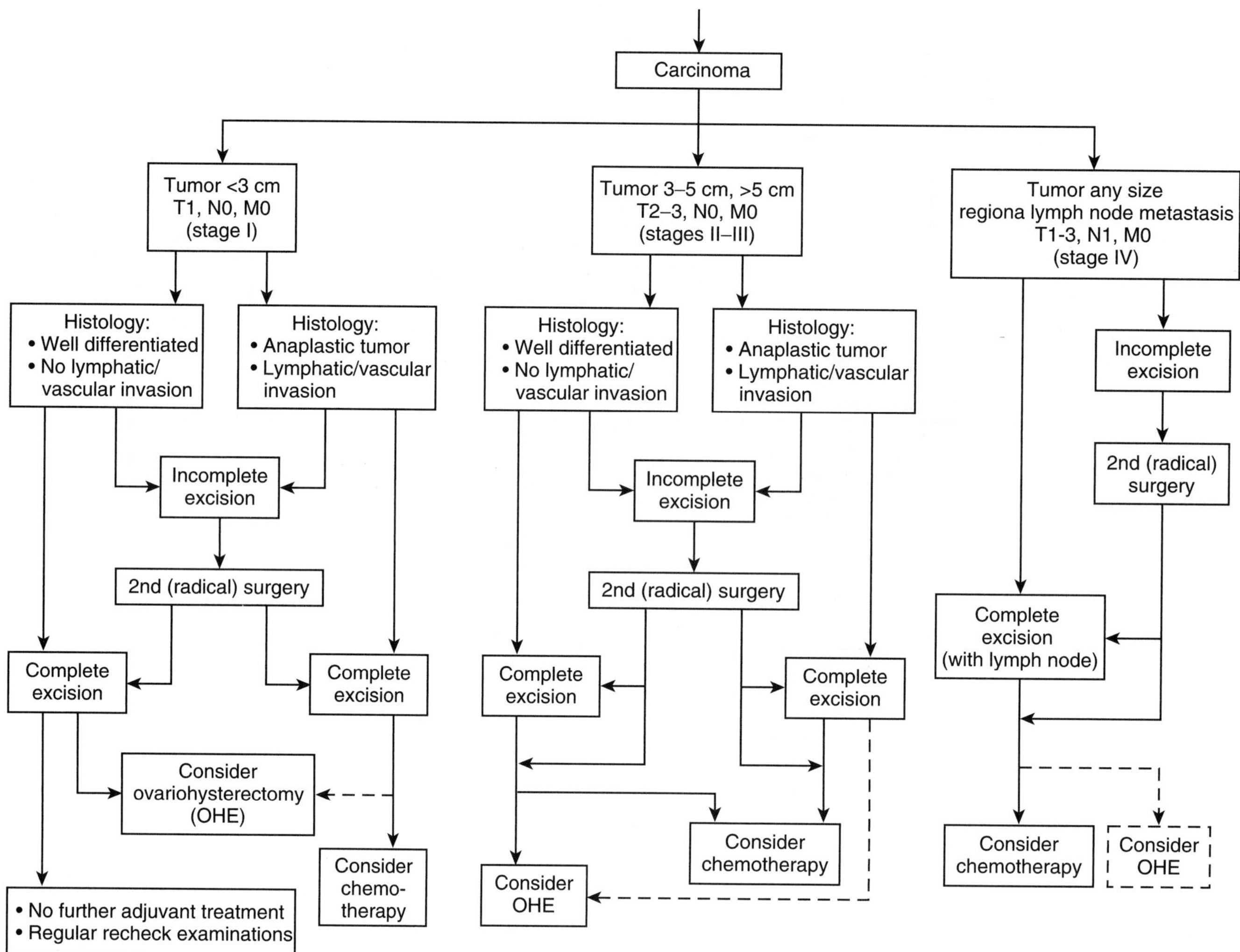

Author: Daniela Simon
Editor: Kenneth M. Rassnick

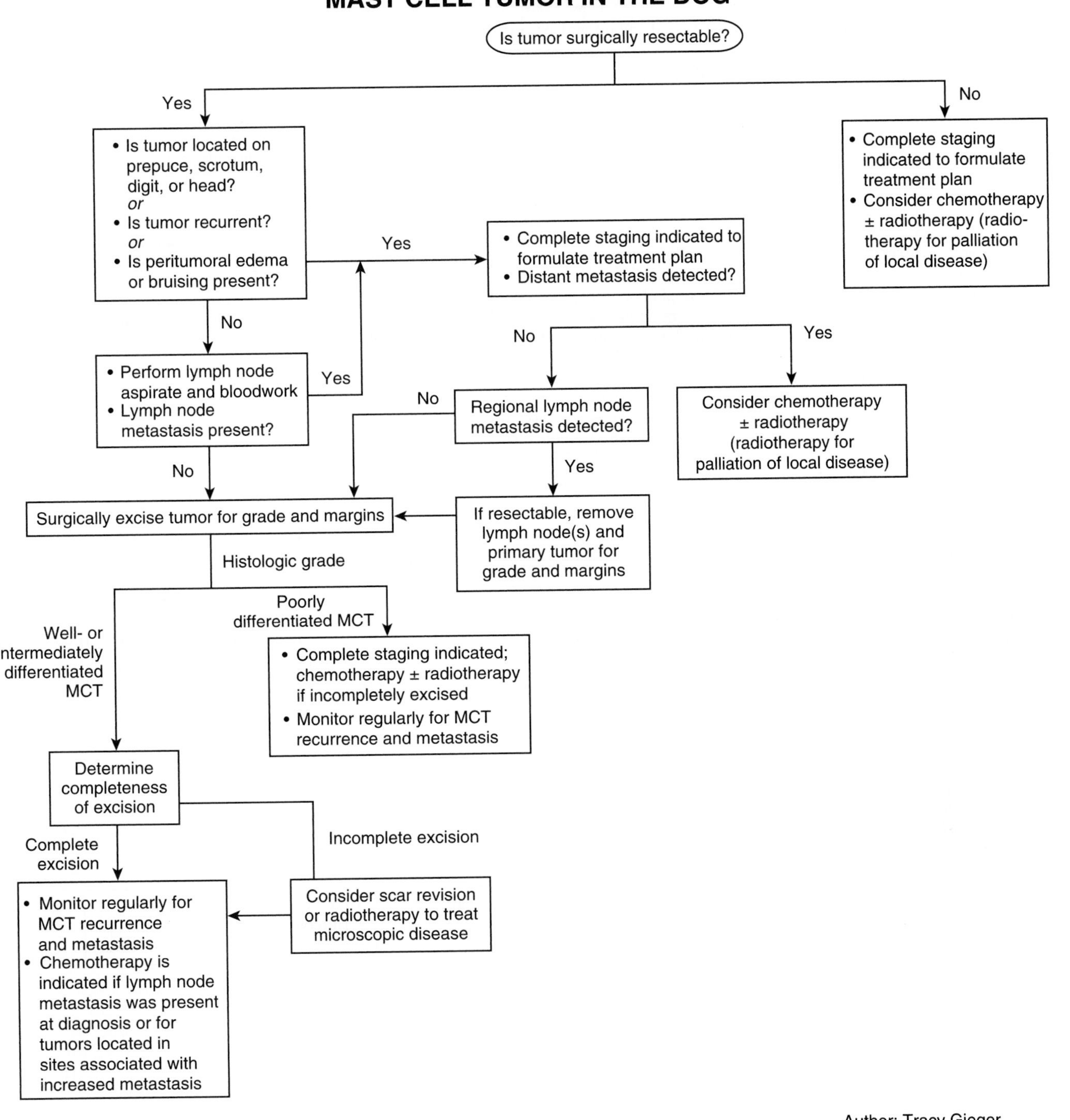
MAST CELL TUMOR IN THE DOG
Is tumor surgically resectable?
Yes
No
• Is tumor located on prepuce, scrotum, digit, or head? or • Is tumor recurrent? or • Is peritumoral edema or bruising present?
• Complete staging indicated to formulate treatment plan • Consider chemotherapy ± radiotherapy (radiotherapy for palliation of local disease)
Yes
• Complete staging indicated to formulate treatment plan • Distant metastasis detected?
No
• Perform lymph node aspirate and bloodwork • Lymph node metastasis present?
Yes
No
Yes
No
Regional lymph node metastasis detected?
Consider chemotherapy ± radiotherapy (radiotherapy for palliation of local disease)
No
Yes
Surgically excise tumor for grade and margins
If resectable, remove lymph node(s) and primary tumor for grade and margins
Histologic grade
Poorly differentiated MCT
Well- or intermediately differentiated MCT
• Complete staging indicated; chemotherapy ± radiotherapy if incompletely excised • Monitor regularly for MCT recurrence and metastasis
Determine completeness of excision
Incomplete excision
Complete excision
• Monitor regularly for MCT recurrence and metastasis • Chemotherapy is indicated if lymph node metastasis was present at diagnosis or for tumors located in sites associated with increased metastasis
Consider scar revision or radiotherapy to treat microscopic disease

Author: Tracy Gieger
Editor: Kenneth M. Rassnick

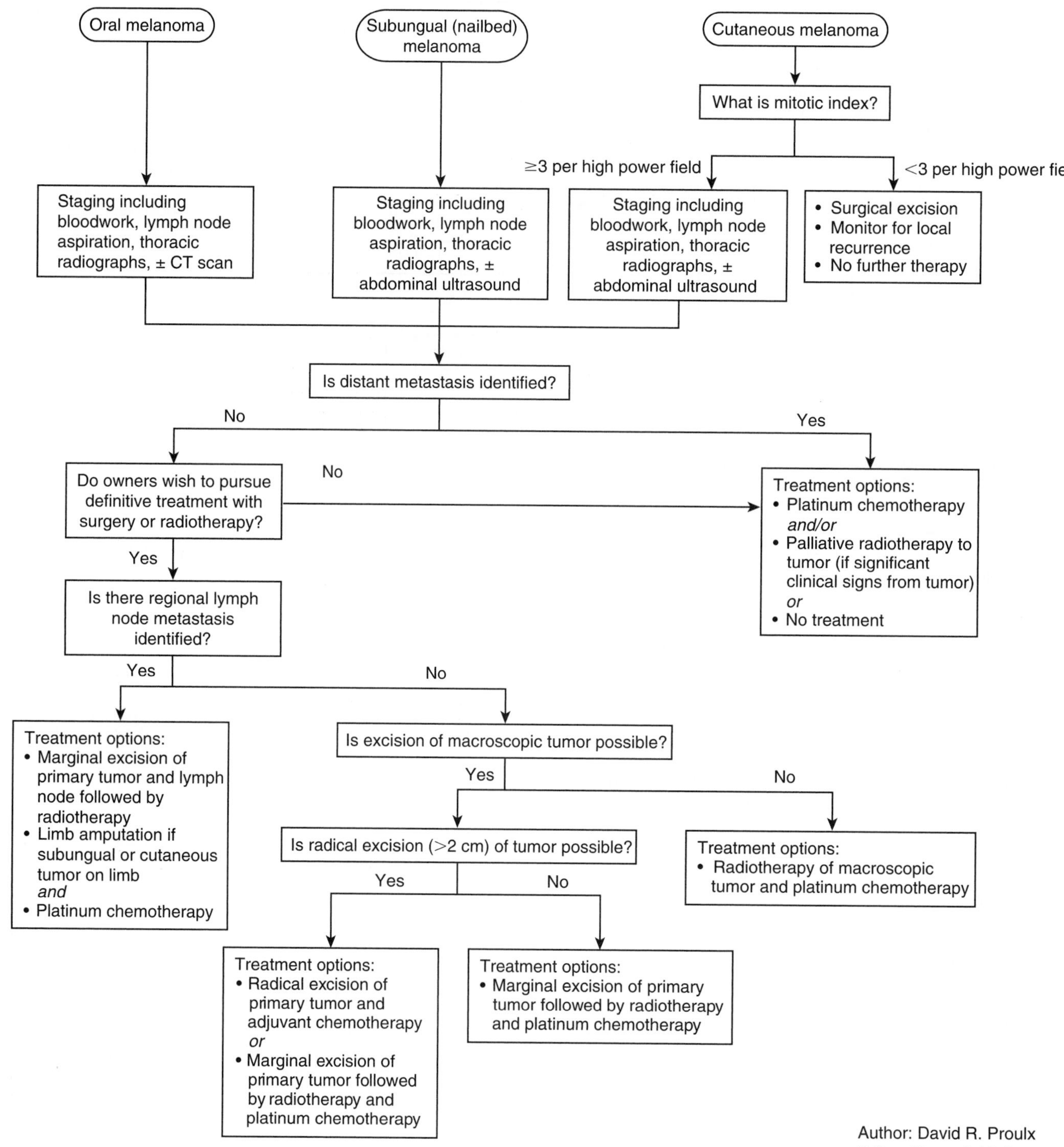

Author: David R. Proulx
Editor: Kenneth M. Rassnick

MUCOCELE, SALIVARY

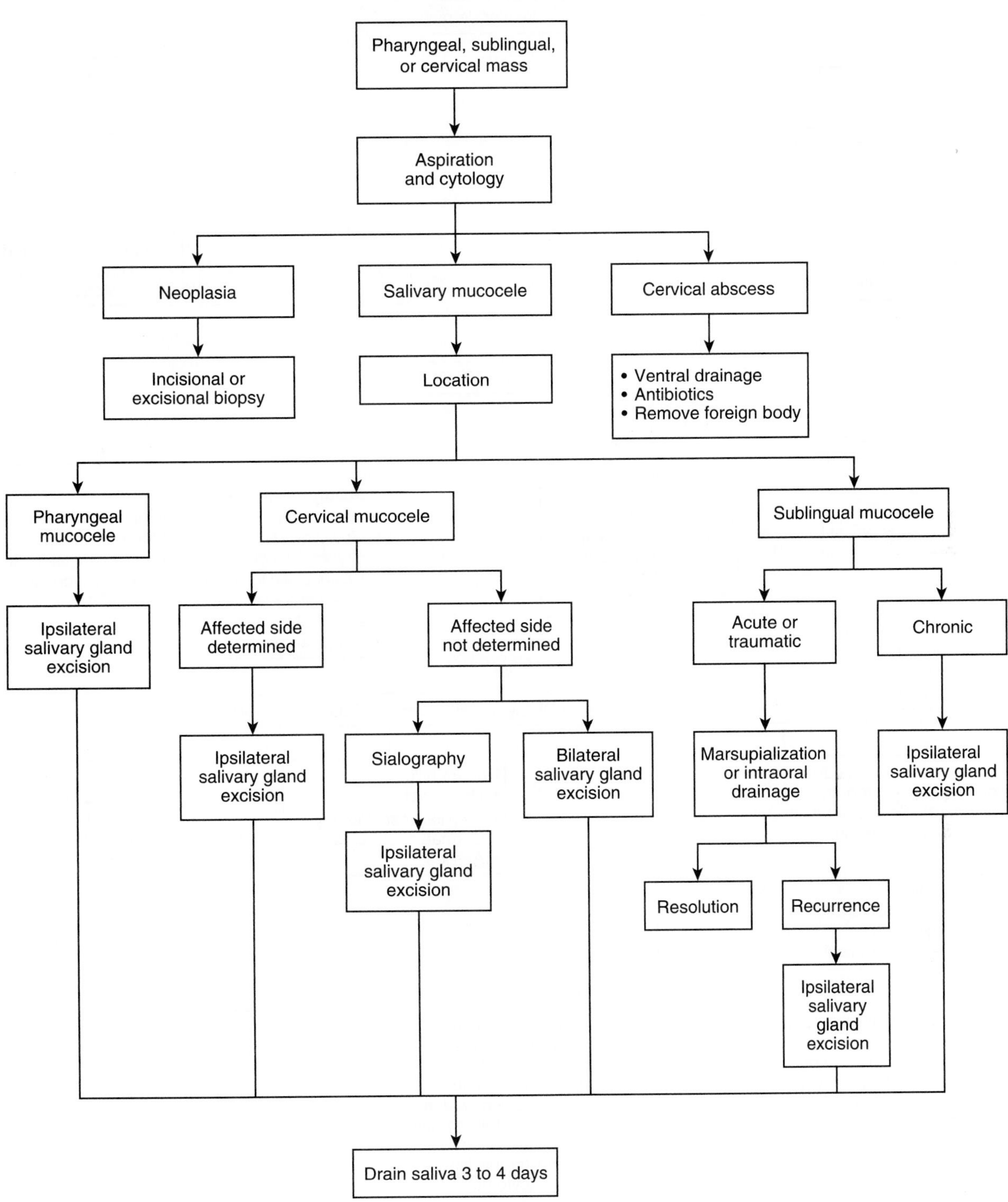

Modified from Ettinger SJ, Feldman EC: *Textbook of Veterinary Internal Medicine*, ed 6. St. Louis, WB Saunders, 2005.

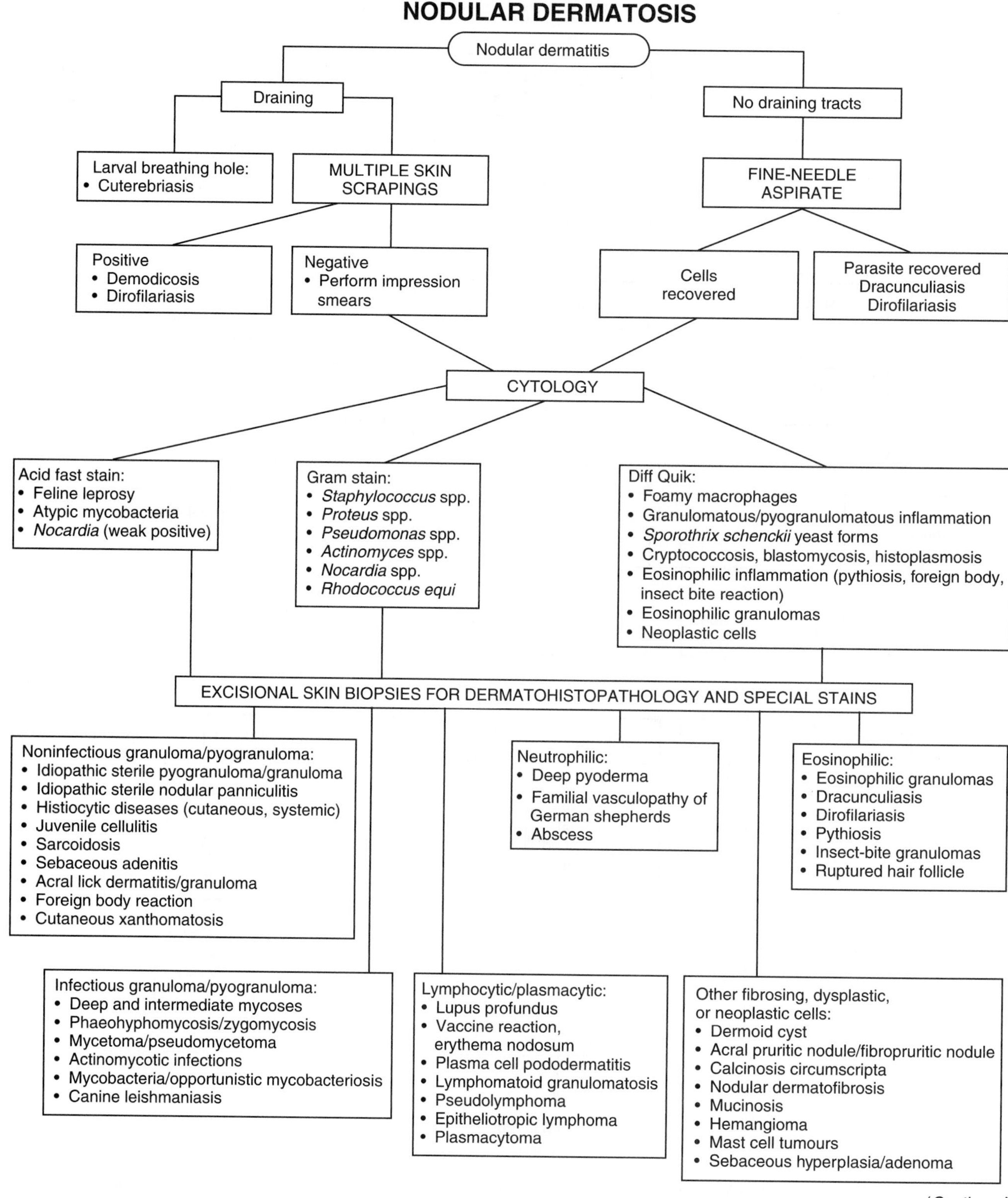
NODULAR DERMATOSIS
Nodular dermatitis
Draining
No draining tracts
Larval breathing hole:
• Cuterebriasis
MULTIPLE SKIN SCRAPINGS
FINE-NEEDLE ASPIRATE
Positive
• Demodicosis
• Dirofilariasis
Negative
• Perform impression smears
Cells recovered
Parasite recovered
Dracunculiasis
Dirofilariasis
CYTOLOGY
Acid fast stain:
• Feline leprosy
• Atypic mycobacteria
• Nocardia (weak positive)
Gram stain:
• Staphylococcus spp.
• Proteus spp.
• Pseudomonas spp.
• Actinomyces spp.
• Nocardia spp.
• Rhodococcus equi
Diff Quik:
• Foamy macrophages
• Granulomatous/pyogranulomatous inflammation
• Sporothrix schenckii yeast forms
• Cryptococcosis, blastomycosis, histoplasmosis
• Eosinophilic inflammation (pythiosis, foreign body, insect bite reaction)
• Eosinophilic granulomas
• Neoplastic cells
EXCISIONAL SKIN BIOPSIES FOR DERMATOHISTOPATHOLOGY AND SPECIAL STAINS
Noninfectious granuloma/pyogranuloma:
• Idiopathic sterile pyogranuloma/granuloma
• Idiopathic sterile nodular panniculitis
• Histiocytic diseases (cutaneous, systemic)
• Juvenile cellulitis
• Sarcoidosis
• Sebaceous adenitis
• Acral lick dermatitis/granuloma
• Foreign body reaction
• Cutaneous xanthomatosis
Neutrophilic:
• Deep pyoderma
• Familial vasculopathy of German shepherds
• Abscess
Eosinophilic:
• Eosinophilic granulomas
• Dracunculiasis
• Dirofilariasis
• Pythiosis
• Insect-bite granulomas
• Ruptured hair follicle
Infectious granuloma/pyogranuloma:
• Deep and intermediate mycoses
• Phaeohyphomycosis/zygomycosis
• Mycetoma/pseudomycetoma
• Actinomycotic infections
• Mycobacteria/opportunistic mycobacteriosis
• Canine leishmaniasis
Lymphocytic/plasmacytic:
• Lupus profundus
• Vaccine reaction, erythema nodosum
• Plasma cell pododermatitis
• Lymphomatoid granulomatosis
• Pseudolymphoma
• Epitheliotropic lymphoma
• Plasmacytoma
Other fibrosing, dysplastic, or neoplastic cells:
• Dermoid cyst
• Acral pruritic nodule/fibropruritic nodule
• Calcinosis circumscripta
• Nodular dermatofibrosis
• Mucinosis
• Hemangioma
• Mast cell tumours
• Sebaceous hyperplasia/adenoma

(*Continued*)

NODULAR DERMATOSIS—*(Continued)*

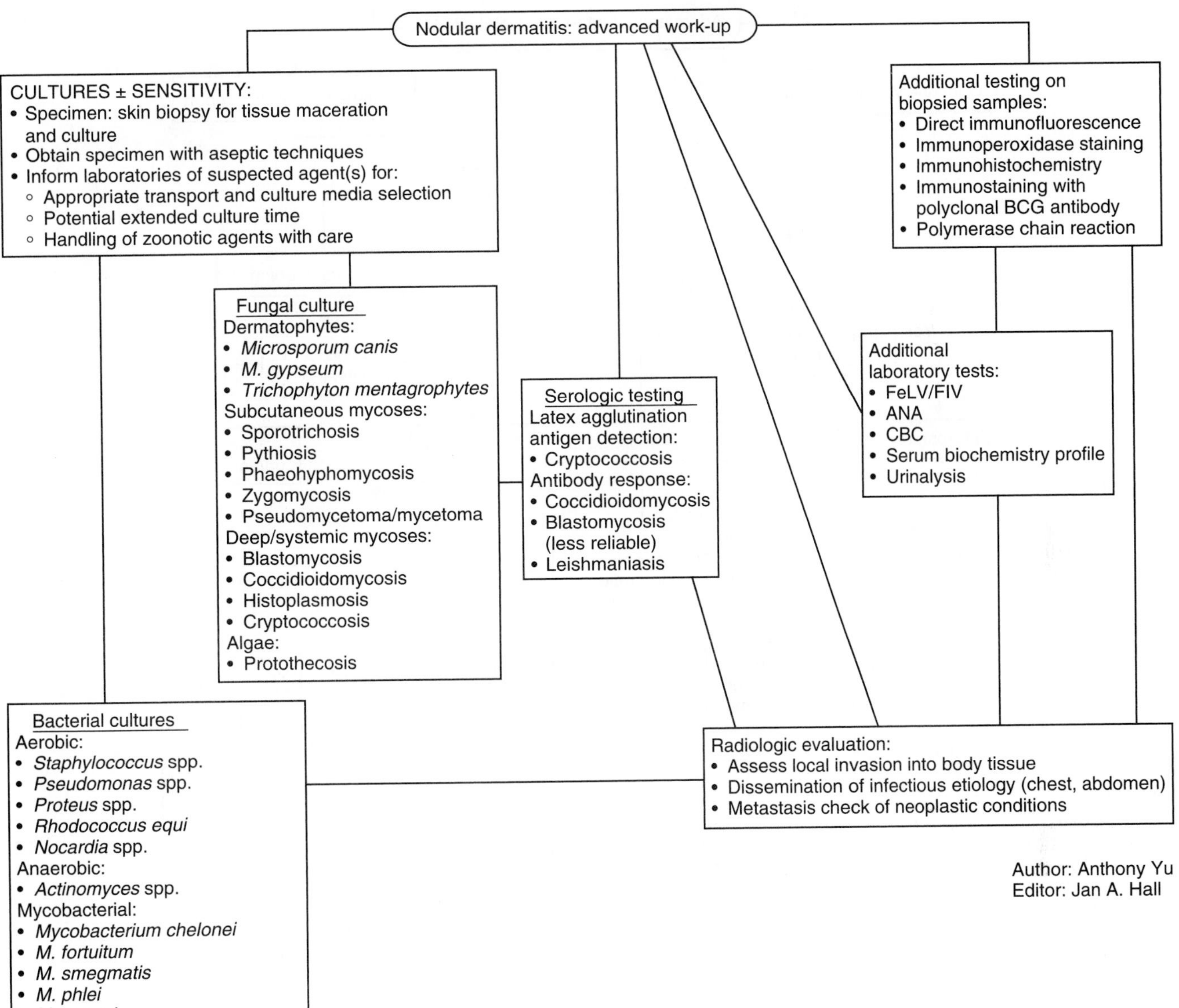

Nodular dermatitis: advanced work-up
CULTURES ± SENSITIVITY:
• Specimen: skin biopsy for tissue maceration and culture
• Obtain specimen with aseptic techniques
• Inform laboratories of suspected agent(s) for:
◦ Appropriate transport and culture media selection
◦ Potential extended culture time
◦ Handling of zoonotic agents with care
Additional testing on biopsied samples:
• Direct immunofluorescence
• Immunoperoxidase staining
• Immunohistochemistry
• Immunostaining with polyclonal BCG antibody
• Polymerase chain reaction
Fungal culture
Dermatophytes:
• *Microsporum canis*
• *M. gypseum*
• *Trichophyton mentagrophytes*
Subcutaneous mycoses:
• Sporotrichosis
• Pythiosis
• Phaeohyphomycosis
• Zygomycosis
• Pseudomycetoma/mycetoma
Deep/systemic mycoses:
• Blastomycosis
• Coccidioidomycosis
• Histoplasmosis
• Cryptococcosis
Algae:
• Protothecosis
Serologic testing
Latex agglutination antigen detection:
• Cryptococcosis
Antibody response:
• Coccidioidomycosis
• Blastomycosis (less reliable)
• Leishmaniasis
Additional laboratory tests:
• FeLV/FIV
• ANA
• CBC
• Serum biochemistry profile
• Urinalysis
Bacterial cultures
Aerobic:
• *Staphylococcus* spp.
• *Pseudomonas* spp.
• *Proteus* spp.
• *Rhodococcus equi*
• *Nocardia* spp.
Anaerobic:
• *Actinomyces* spp.
Mycobacterial:
• *Mycobacterium chelonei*
• *M. fortuitum*
• *M. smegmatis*
• *M. phlei*
• *M. xenopi*
• *M. thermoresistible*
Radiologic evaluation:
• Assess local invasion into body tissue
• Dissemination of infectious etiology (chest, abdomen)
• Metastasis check of neoplastic conditions

Author: Anthony Yu
Editor: Jan A. Hall

NUTRITIONAL SUPPORT, DECISION-MAKING

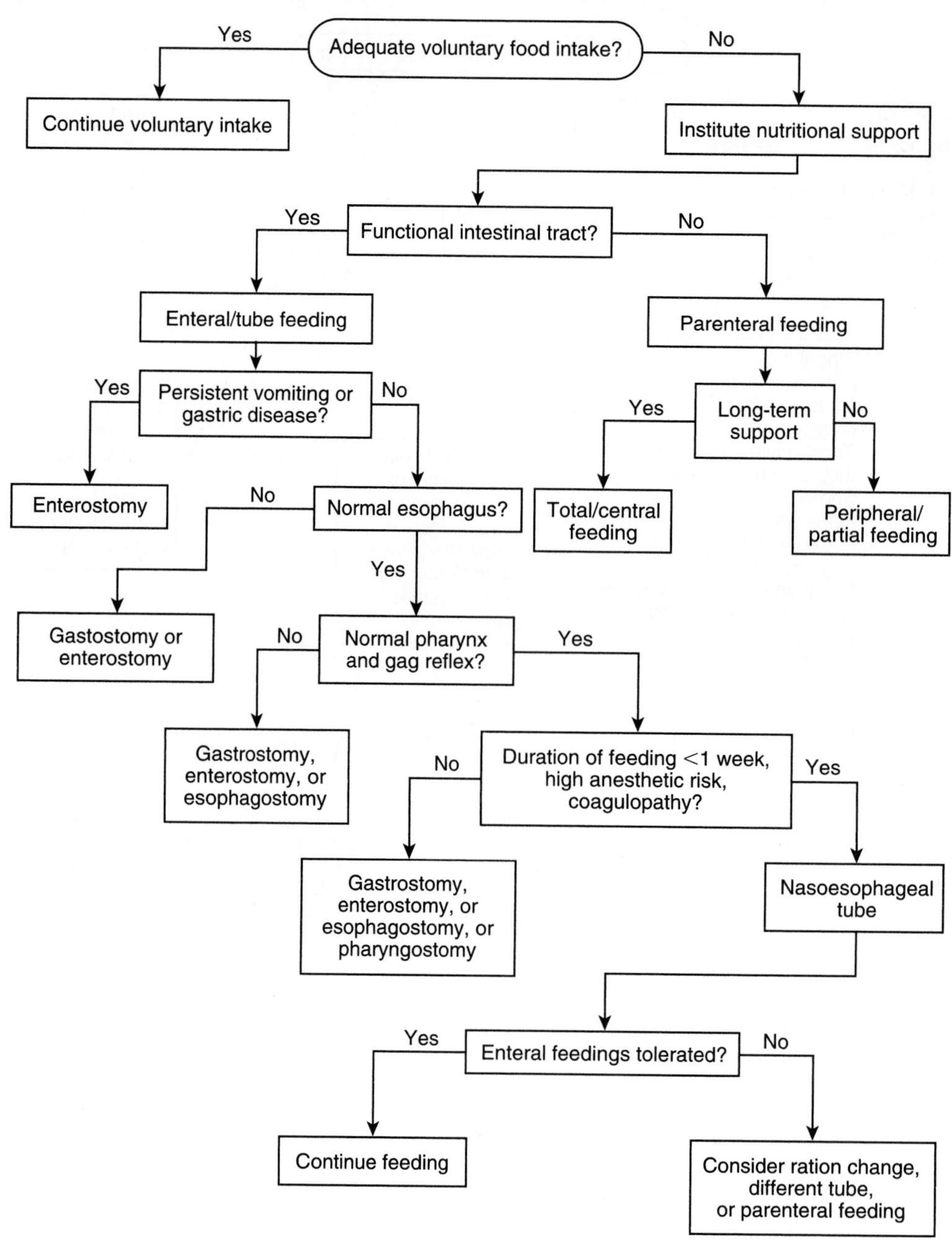

From Slatter DH: *Textbook of Small Animal Surgery*, ed 3. St. Louis, WB Saunders, 2003.

ORGANOPHOSPHATE AND CARBAMATE TOXICITY

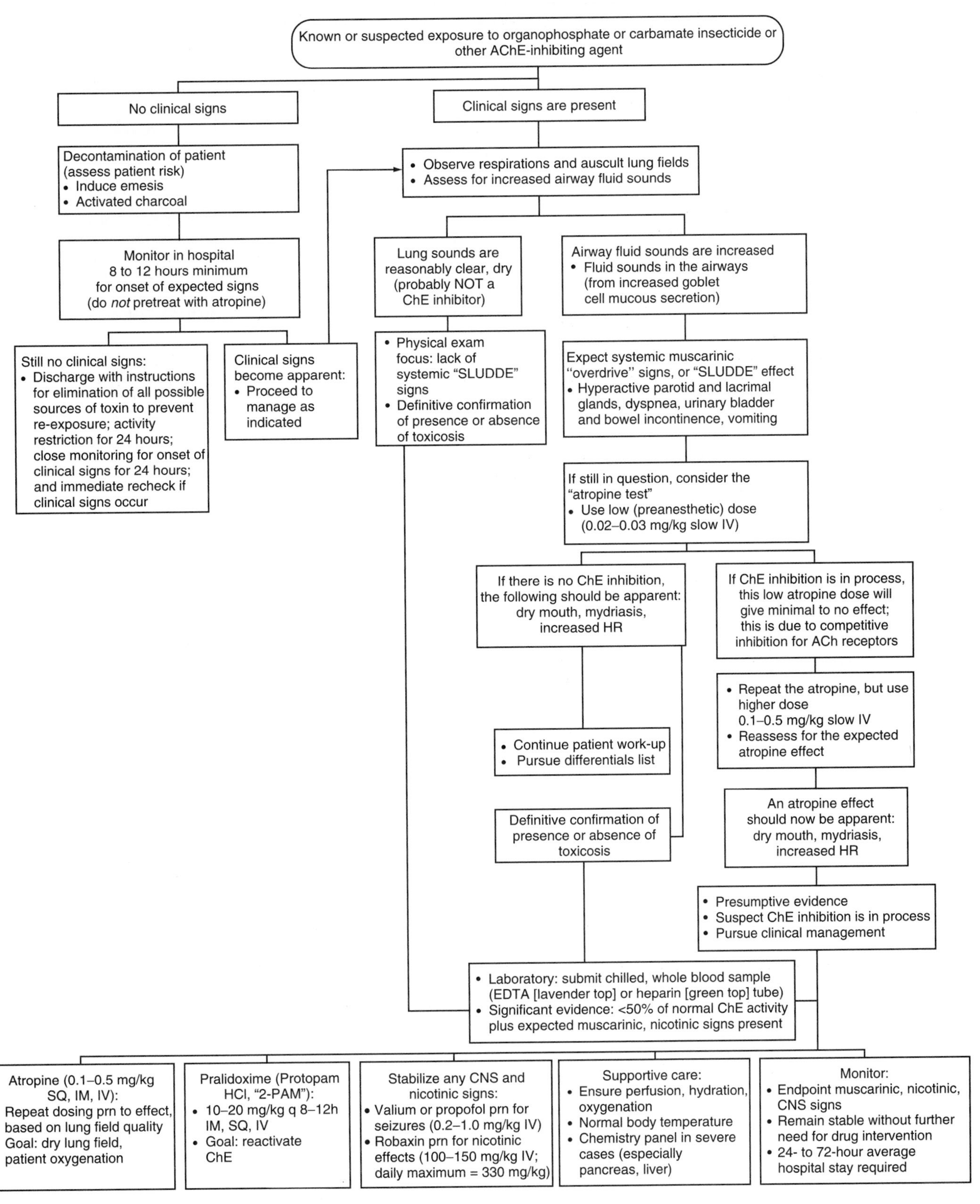

ACh: acetylcholine
AChE: acetylcholinesterase, cholinesterase
HR: heart rate
SLUDDE: salivation, lacrimation, urination, diarrhea, dyspnea, emesis

Author: Michael W. Knight
Editor: Safdar A. Khan

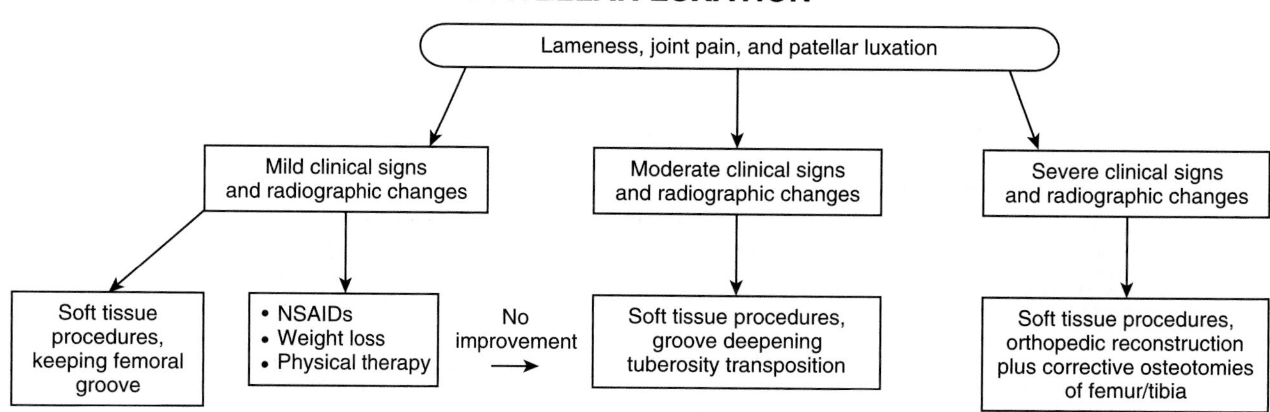

Author & Editor: Joseph Harari

PERINEAL HERNIA

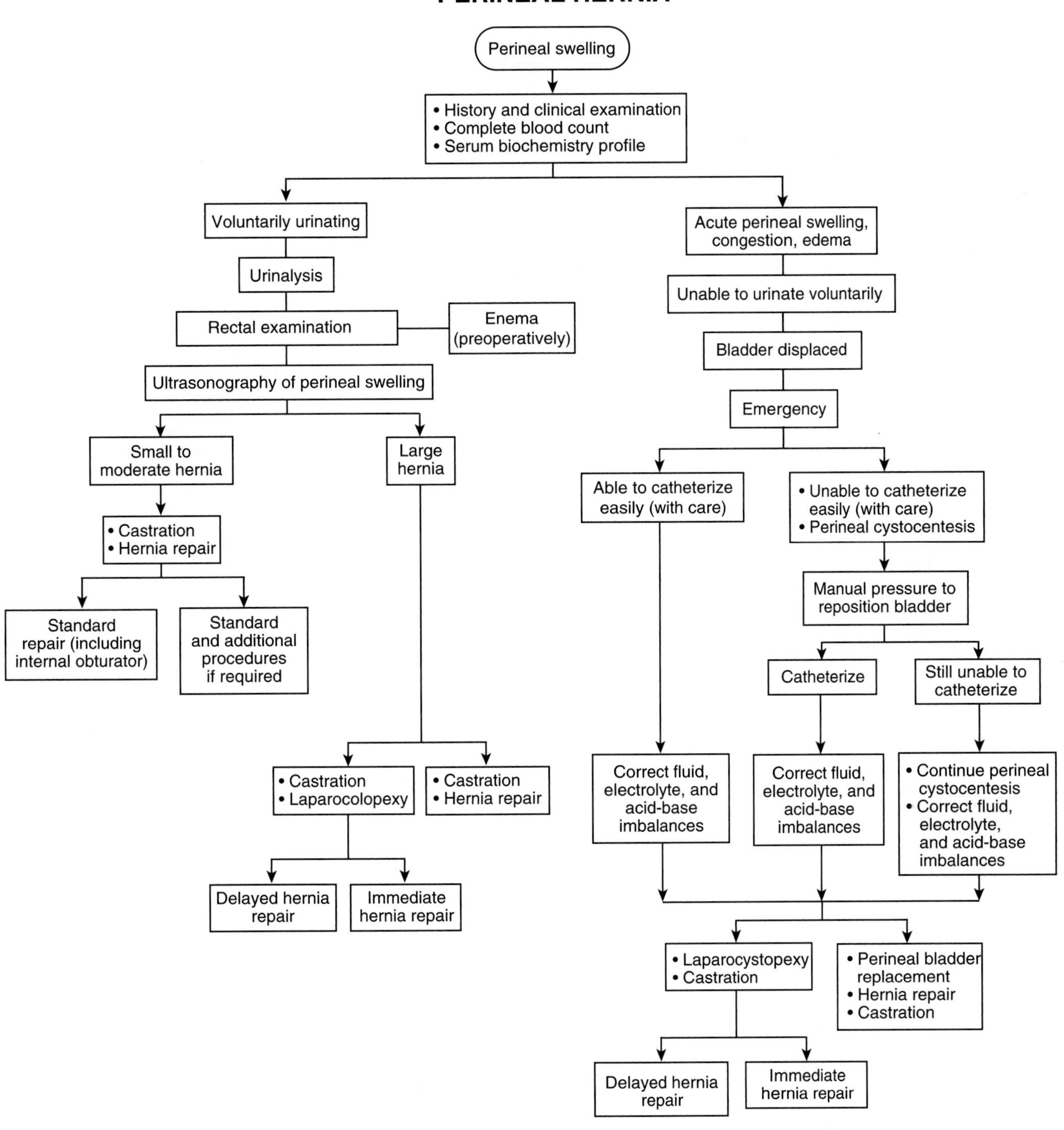

Modified from Slatter DH: *Textbook of Small Animal Surgery*, ed 3. St. Louis, WB Saunders, 2003.

PERITONITIS, SEPTIC

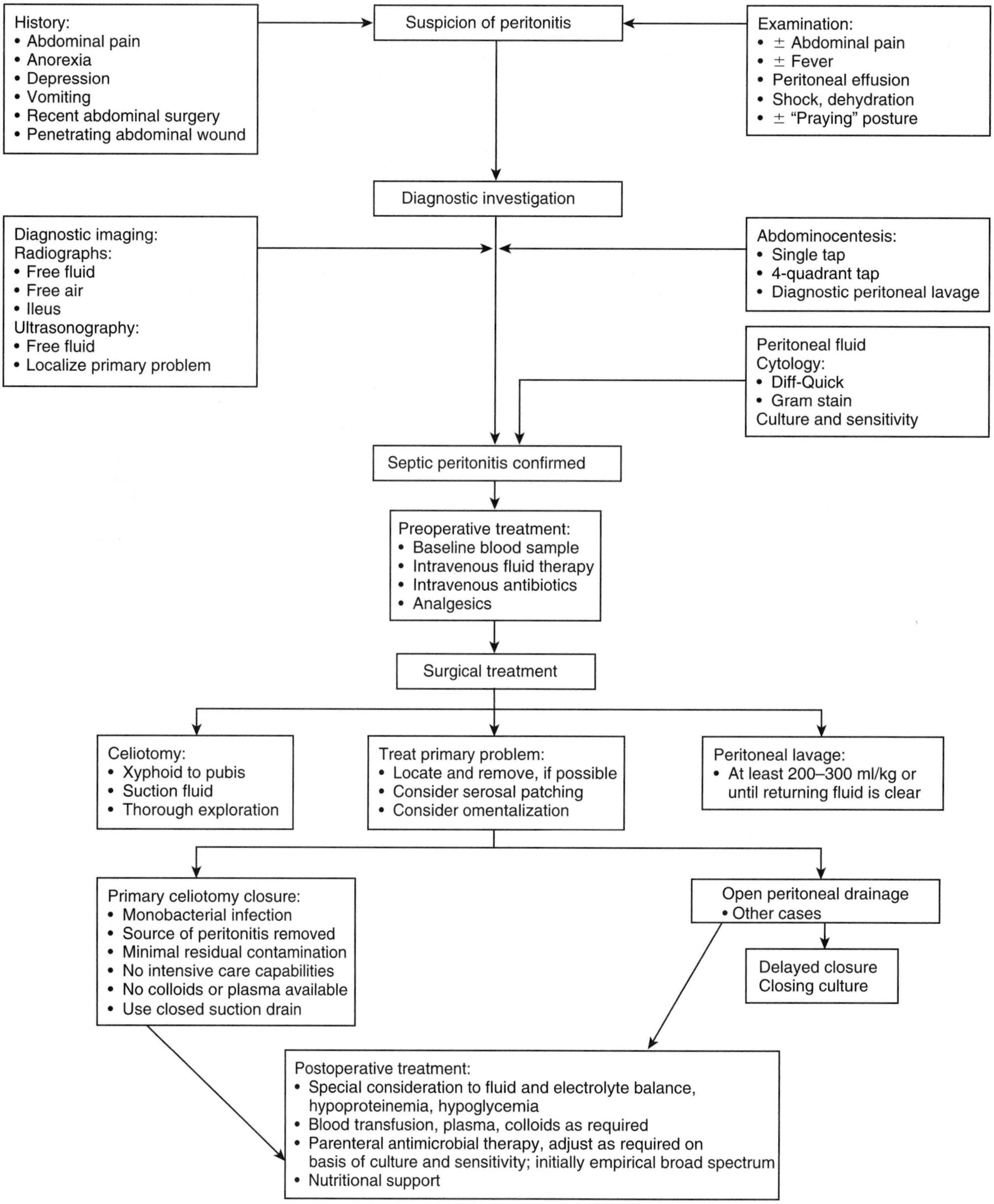

History:
- Abdominal pain
- Anorexia
- Depression
- Vomiting
- Recent abdominal surgery
- Penetrating abdominal wound

Suspicion of peritonitis

Examination:
- ± Abdominal pain
- ± Fever
- Peritoneal effusion
- Shock, dehydration
- ± "Praying" posture

Diagnostic investigation

Diagnostic imaging:
Radiographs:
- Free fluid
- Free air
- Ileus

Ultrasonography:
- Free fluid
- Localize primary problem

Abdominocentesis:
- Single tap
- 4-quadrant tap
- Diagnostic peritoneal lavage

Peritoneal fluid
Cytology:
- Diff-Quick
- Gram stain

Culture and sensitivity

Septic peritonitis confirmed

Preoperative treatment:
- Baseline blood sample
- Intravenous fluid therapy
- Intravenous antibiotics
- Analgesics

Surgical treatment

Celiotomy:
- Xyphoid to pubis
- Suction fluid
- Thorough exploration

Treat primary problem:
- Locate and remove, if possible
- Consider serosal patching
- Consider omentalization

Peritoneal lavage:
- At least 200–300 ml/kg or until returning fluid is clear

Primary celiotomy closure:
- Monobacterial infection
- Source of peritonitis removed
- Minimal residual contamination
- No intensive care capabilities
- No colloids or plasma available
- Use closed suction drain

Open peritoneal drainage
- Other cases

Delayed closure
Closing culture

Postoperative treatment:
- Special consideration to fluid and electrolyte balance, hypoproteinemia, hypoglycemia
- Blood transfusion, plasma, colloids as required
- Parenteral antimicrobial therapy, adjust as required on basis of culture and sensitivity; initially empirical broad spectrum
- Nutritional support

Modified from Slatter DH: *Textbook of Small Animal Surgery*, ed 3. St. Louis, WB Saunders, 2003.

PHEOCHROMOCYTOMA

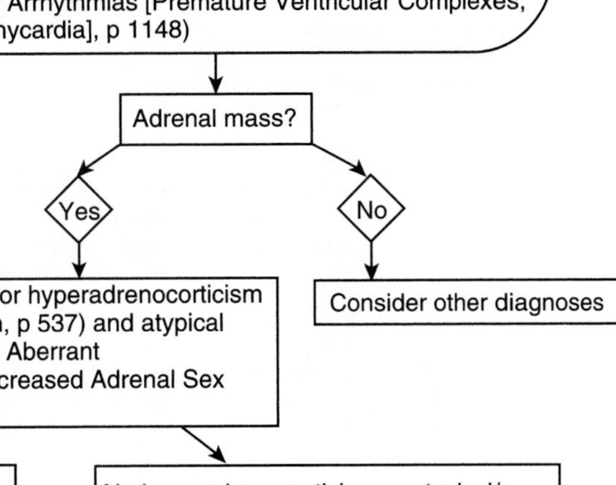
• Unexplained hypertension (see Systemic Hypertension, p 1058)
or
• Unexplained paroxysmal ventricular arrhythmia (see Ventricular Arrhythmias [Premature Ventricular Complexes, Ventricular Tachycardia], p 1148)
Adrenal mass?
Yes
No
Perform screening test(s) for hyperadrenocorticism (see Hyperadrenocorticism, p 537) and atypical hyperadrenocorticism (see Aberrant Adrenocortical Disease [Increased Adrenal Sex Hormone Production], p 5)
Consider other diagnoses
Hyperadrenocorticism: treat appropriately (see algorithm for Hyperadrenocorticism: Treatment, p 539)
No hyperadrenocorticism or atypical/ aberrant adrenocortical disease: consider surgical excision (if possible) or biopsy with immunohistochemical staining of excised tissue

Author: Elisabeth Snead
Editor: Sherri Ihle

PNEUMONIA, ASPIRATION

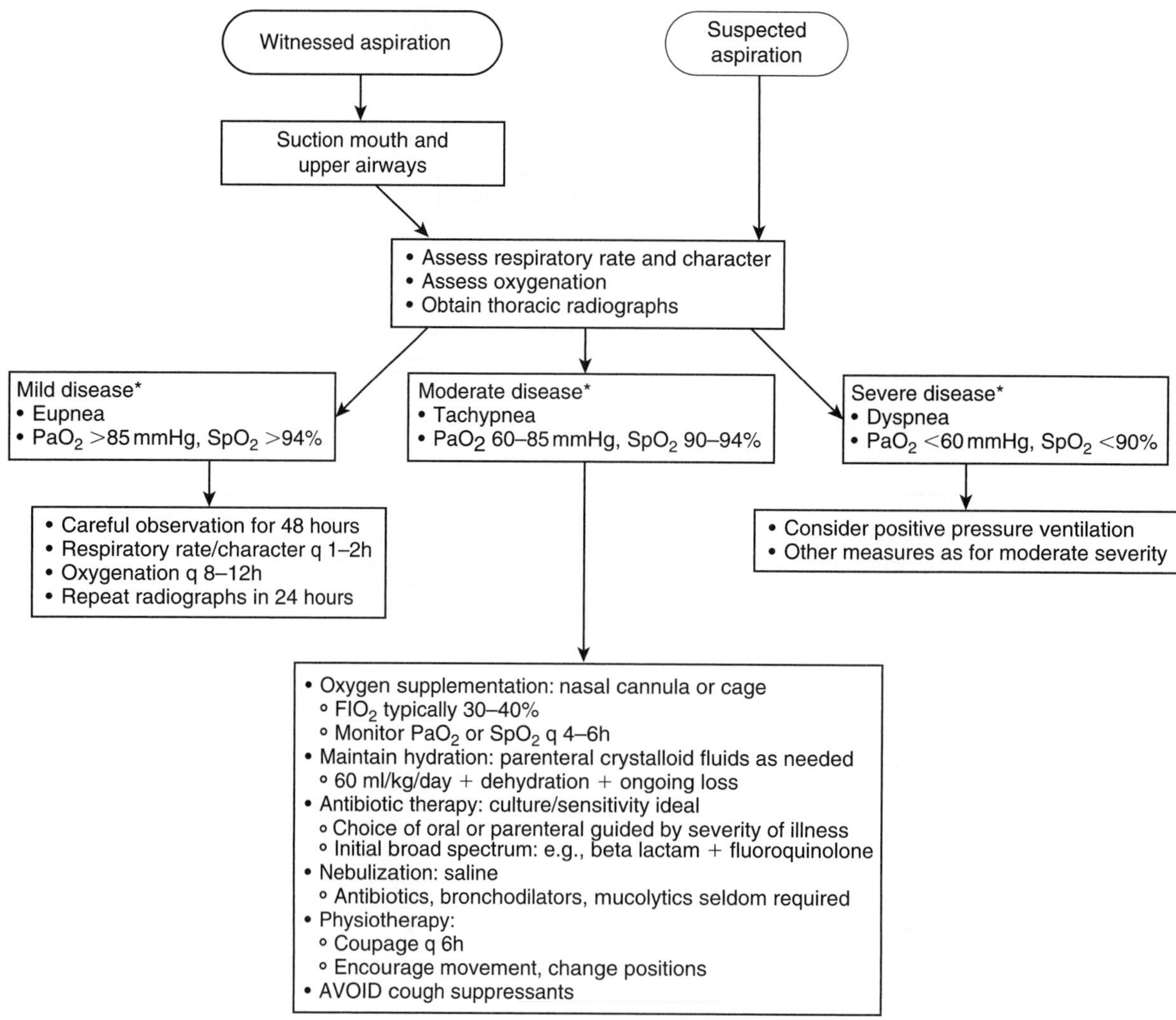

Witnessed aspiration
Suspected aspiration
Suction mouth and upper airways
• Assess respiratory rate and character
• Assess oxygenation
• Obtain thoracic radiographs
Mild disease*
• Eupnea
• PaO_2 >85 mmHg, SpO_2 >94%
Moderate disease*
• Tachypnea
• PaO_2 60–85 mmHg, SpO_2 90–94%
Severe disease*
• Dyspnea
• PaO_2 <60 mmHg, SpO_2 <90%
• Careful observation for 48 hours
• Respiratory rate/character q 1–2h
• Oxygenation q 8–12h
• Repeat radiographs in 24 hours
• Consider positive pressure ventilation
• Other measures as for moderate severity
• Oxygen supplementation: nasal cannula or cage
◦ FIO_2 typically 30–40%
◦ Monitor PaO_2 or SpO_2 q 4–6h
• Maintain hydration: parenteral crystalloid fluids as needed
◦ 60 ml/kg/day + dehydration + ongoing loss
• Antibiotic therapy: culture/sensitivity ideal
◦ Choice of oral or parenteral guided by severity of illness
◦ Initial broad spectrum: e.g., beta lactam + fluoroquinolone
• Nebulization: saline
◦ Antibiotics, bronchodilators, mucolytics seldom required
• Physiotherapy:
◦ Coupage q 6h
◦ Encourage movement, change positions
• AVOID cough suppressants

*For all, minimize risk of further aspiration or damage from aspiration.

Author: Leah A. Cohn
Editor: Rance K. Sellon

POLYARTHRITIS

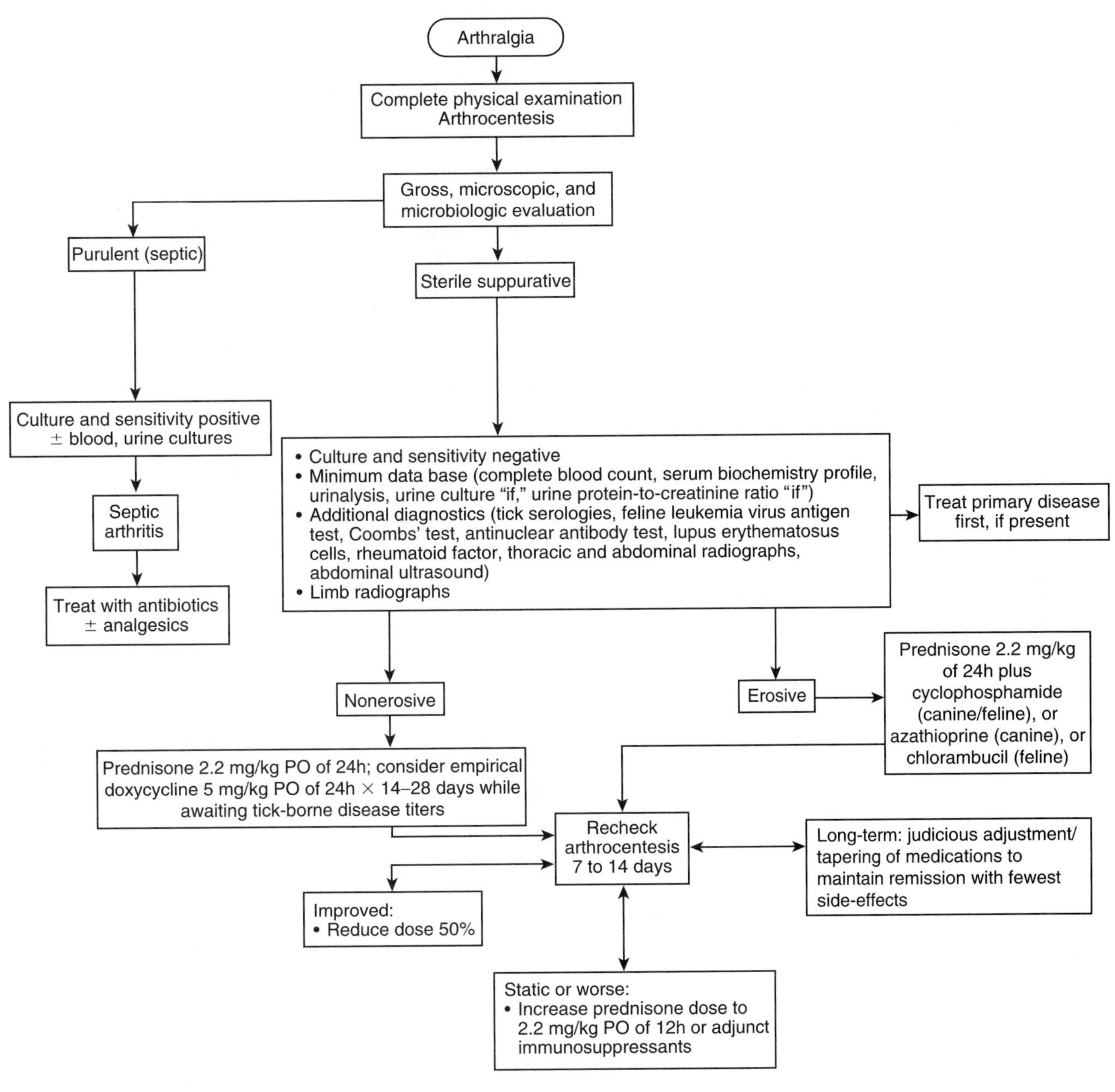
Arthralgia
Complete physical examination
Arthrocentesis
Gross, microscopic, and microbiologic evaluation
Purulent (septic)
Sterile suppurative
Culture and sensitivity positive ± blood, urine cultures
Septic arthritis
Treat with antibiotics ± analgesics
• Culture and sensitivity negative
• Minimum data base (complete blood count, serum biochemistry profile, urinalysis, urine culture "if," urine protein-to-creatinine ratio "if")
• Additional diagnostics (tick serologies, feline leukemia virus antigen test, Coombs' test, antinuclear antibody test, lupus erythematosus cells, rheumatoid factor, thoracic and abdominal radiographs, abdominal ultrasound)
• Limb radiographs
Treat primary disease first, if present
Nonerosive
Erosive
Prednisone 2.2 mg/kg of 24h plus cyclophosphamide (canine/feline), or azathioprine (canine), or chlorambucil (feline)
Prednisone 2.2 mg/kg PO of 24h; consider empirical doxycycline 5 mg/kg PO of 24h × 14–28 days while awaiting tick-borne disease titers
Recheck arthrocentesis 7 to 14 days
Long-term: judicious adjustment/ tapering of medications to maintain remission with fewest side-effects
Improved:
• Reduce dose 50%
Static or worse:
• Increase prednisone dose to 2.2 mg/kg PO of 12h or adjunct immunosuppressants

Modified from Slatter DH: *Textbook of Small Animal Surgery*, ed 3. St. Louis, WB Saunders, 2003.

POLYURIA AND POLYDIPSIA

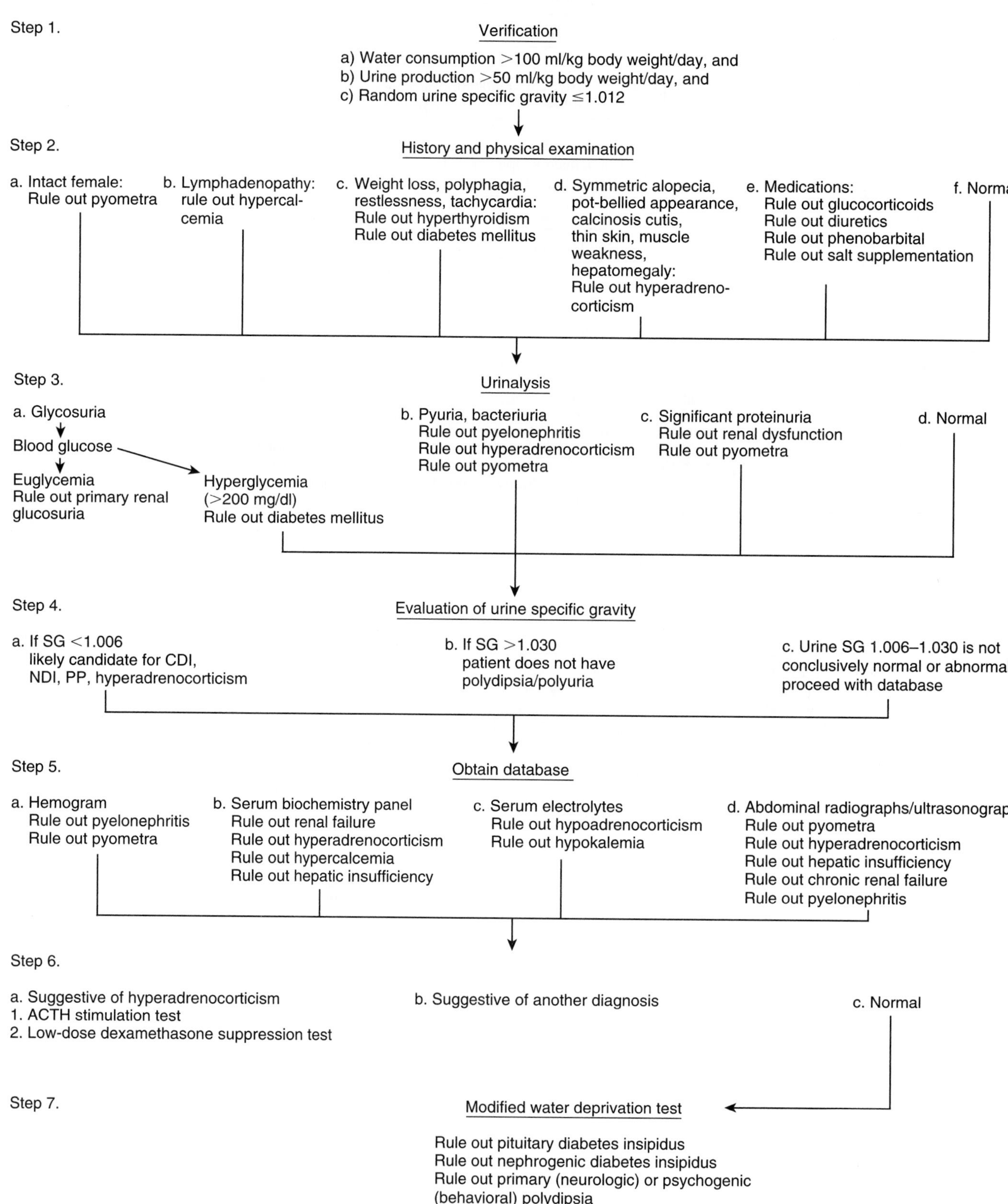
Step 1.
Verification
a) Water consumption >100 ml/kg body weight/day, and
b) Urine production >50 ml/kg body weight/day, and
c) Random urine specific gravity ≤1.012
Step 2.
History and physical examination
a. Intact female: Rule out pyometra
b. Lymphadenopathy: rule out hypercalcemia
c. Weight loss, polyphagia, restlessness, tachycardia: Rule out hyperthyroidism Rule out diabetes mellitus
d. Symmetric alopecia, pot-bellied appearance, calcinosis cutis, thin skin, muscle weakness, hepatomegaly: Rule out hyperadrenocorticism
e. Medications: Rule out glucocorticoids Rule out diuretics Rule out phenobarbital Rule out salt supplementation
f. Normal
Step 3.
Urinalysis
a. Glycosuria
Blood glucose
Euglycemia Rule out primary renal glucosuria
Hyperglycemia (>200 mg/dl) Rule out diabetes mellitus
b. Pyuria, bacteriuria Rule out pyelonephritis Rule out hyperadrenocorticism Rule out pyometra
c. Significant proteinuria Rule out renal dysfunction Rule out pyometra
d. Normal
Step 4.
Evaluation of urine specific gravity
a. If SG <1.006 likely candidate for CDI, NDI, PP, hyperadrenocorticism
b. If SG >1.030 patient does not have polydipsia/polyuria
c. Urine SG 1.006–1.030 is not conclusively normal or abnormal; proceed with database
Step 5.
Obtain database
a. Hemogram Rule out pyelonephritis Rule out pyometra
b. Serum biochemistry panel Rule out renal failure Rule out hyperadrenocorticism Rule out hypercalcemia Rule out hepatic insufficiency
c. Serum electrolytes Rule out hypoadrenocorticism Rule out hypokalemia
d. Abdominal radiographs/ultrasonograpl Rule out pyometra Rule out hyperadrenocorticism Rule out hepatic insufficiency Rule out chronic renal failure Rule out pyelonephritis
Step 6.
a. Suggestive of hyperadrenocorticism
1. ACTH stimulation test
2. Low-dose dexamethasone suppression test
b. Suggestive of another diagnosis
c. Normal
Step 7.
Modified water deprivation test
Rule out pituitary diabetes insipidus
Rule out nephrogenic diabetes insipidus
Rule out primary (neurologic) or psychogenic (behavioral) polydipsia

CDI, central diabetes insipidus; NDI, nephrogenic diabetes insipidus; PP, primary or psychogenic polydipsia; SG, specific gravity.
Modified from Feldman EC, Nelson RW: *Canine and Feline Endocrinology and Reproduction*, ed 3. St. Louis, WB Saunders, 2004.

PROSTATITIS

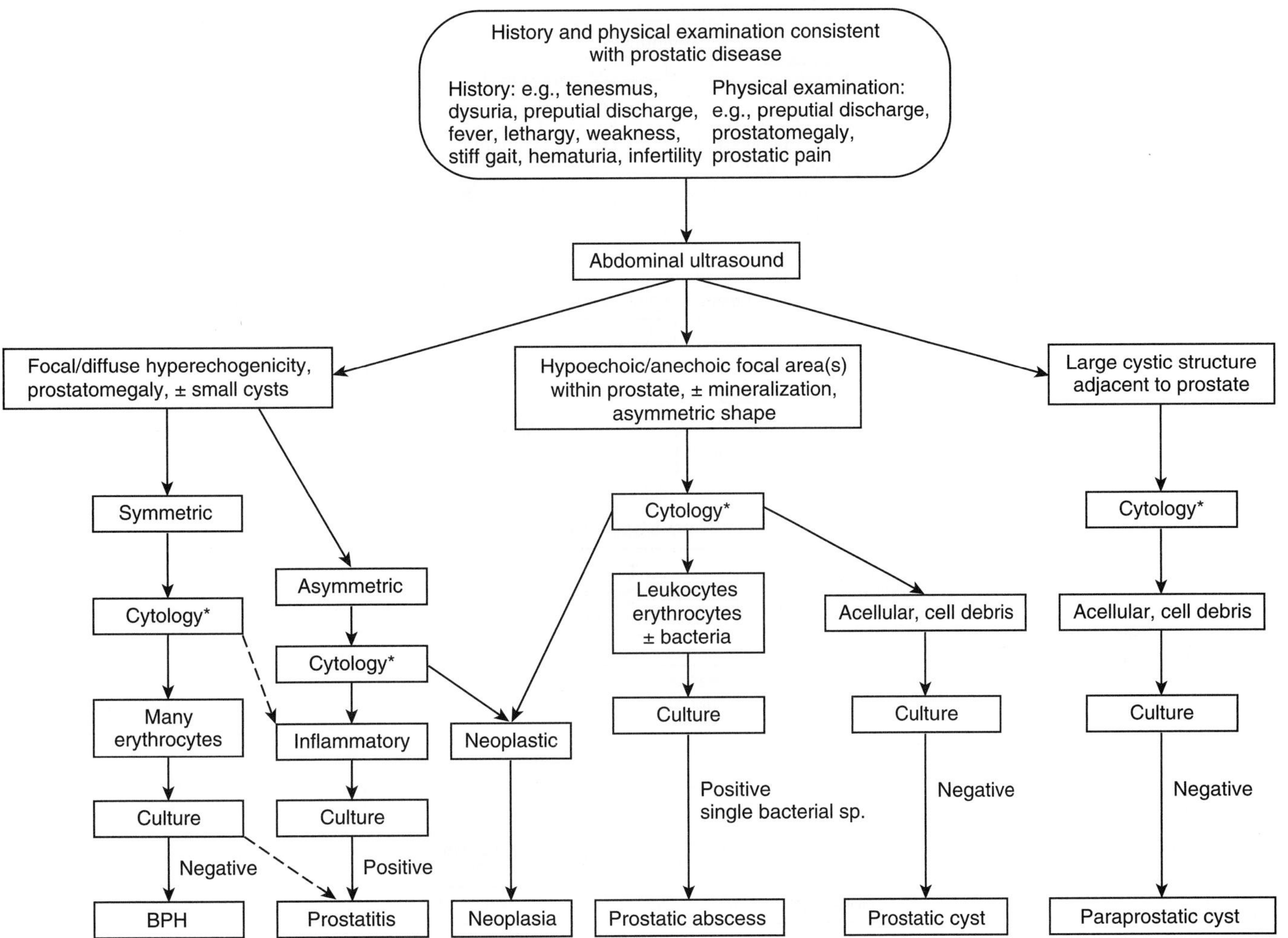

*Cytology can be obtained from a fine-needle aspirate, a prostatic massage, or an ejaculate depending on circumstances.

Author: Lisa Brownlee
Editor: Leah A. Cohn

PROTEIN-LOSING NEPHROPATHY

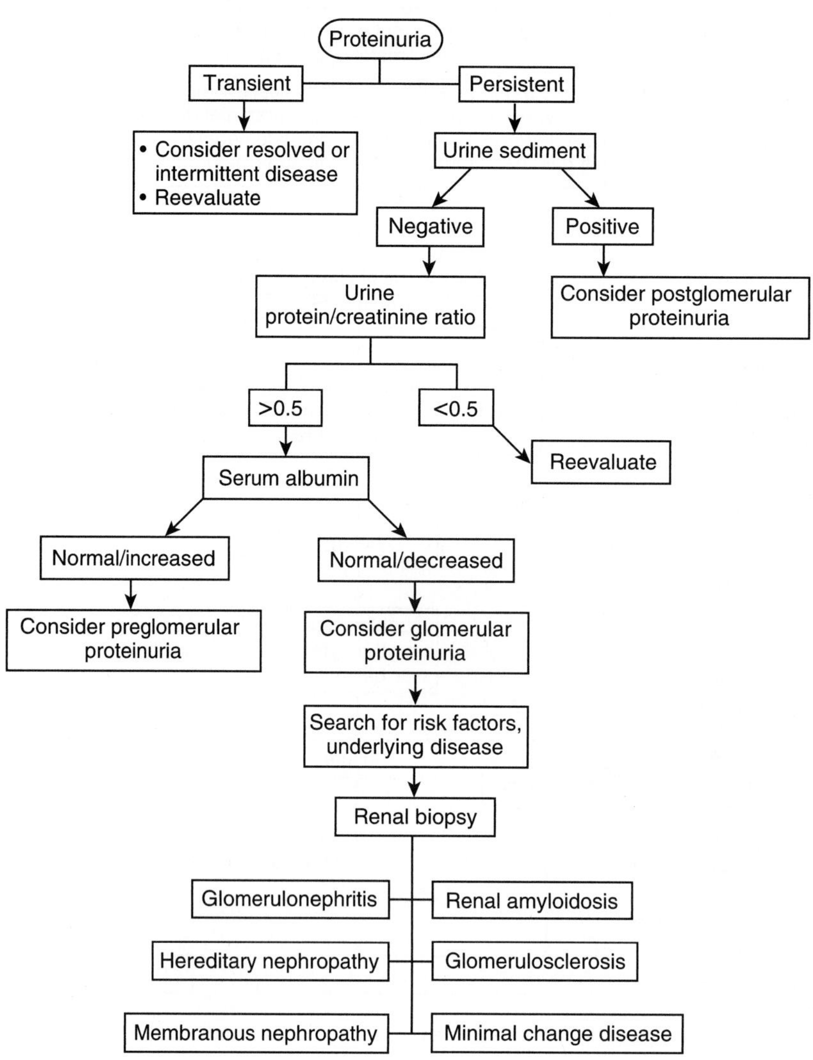

Author: Anne M. Dalby
Editor: Leah A. Cohn

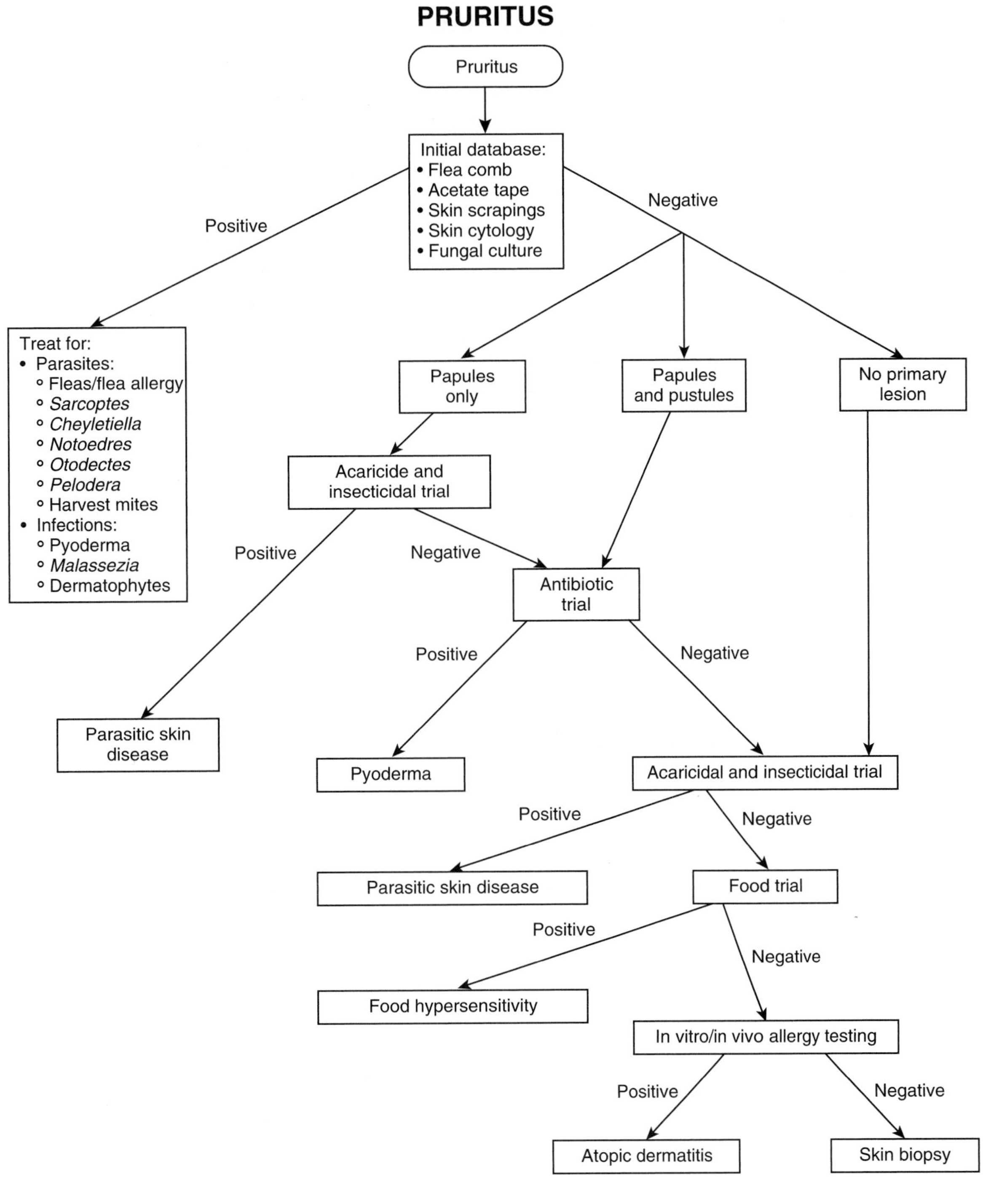
PRURITUS
Pruritus
Initial database:
• Flea comb
• Acetate tape
• Skin scrapings
• Skin cytology
• Fungal culture
Positive
Negative
Treat for:
• Parasites:
◦ Fleas/flea allergy
◦ Sarcoptes
◦ Cheyletiella
◦ Notoedres
◦ Otodectes
◦ Pelodera
◦ Harvest mites
• Infections:
◦ Pyoderma
◦ Malassezia
◦ Dermatophytes
Papules only
Papules and pustules
No primary lesion
Acaricide and insecticidal trial
Positive
Negative
Antibiotic trial
Positive
Negative
Parasitic skin disease
Pyoderma
Acaricidal and insecticidal trial
Positive
Negative
Parasitic skin disease
Food trial
Positive
Negative
Food hypersensitivity
In vitro/in vivo allergy testing
Positive
Negative
Atopic dermatitis
Skin biopsy

Author: Manon Paradis
Editor: Jan A. Hall

PUSTULAR AND CRUSTING SKIN DISORDERS

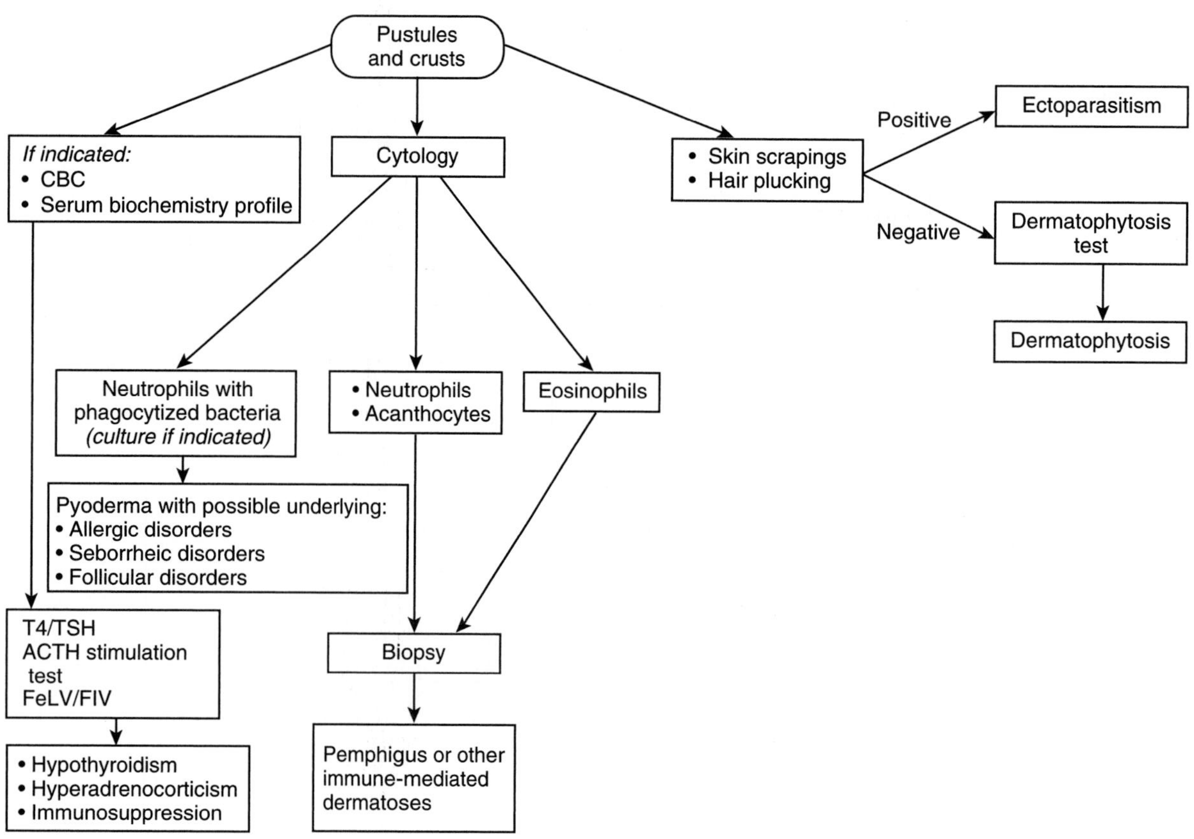

Author: Caroline de Jaham
Editor: Jan A. Hall

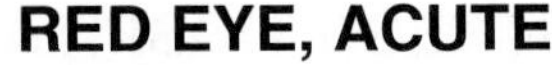

- Acute red eye
  - Exophthalmos
    - Yes → Orbital disease → Schirmer tear test (STT)
    - No → Schirmer tear test (STT)
  - Schirmer tear test (STT)
    - Decreased (< 10 mm wetting/min) → Keratoconjunctivitis sicca (KCS) → Fluorescein stain
    - Normal or increased (≥ 15 mm/min) → Fluorescein stain
  - Fluorescein stain
    - Positive → Corneal ulceration
    - Negative → Intraocular pressure (IOP)
  - Intraocular pressure (IOP)
    - Decreased <10 mmHg → Uveitis
    - Normal 15–25 mmHg → Corneal discoloration
    - Increased >30 mmHg → Glaucoma
  - Corneal discoloration
    - Yes → Nonulcerative keratitis
      See:
      - Corneal vascularization, p 249
      - Corneal pigmentation, p 242
      - Corneal lipid infiltrates, p 241
      - Episcleritis/scleritis, p 353
    - No → Conjunctivitis, Blepharitis

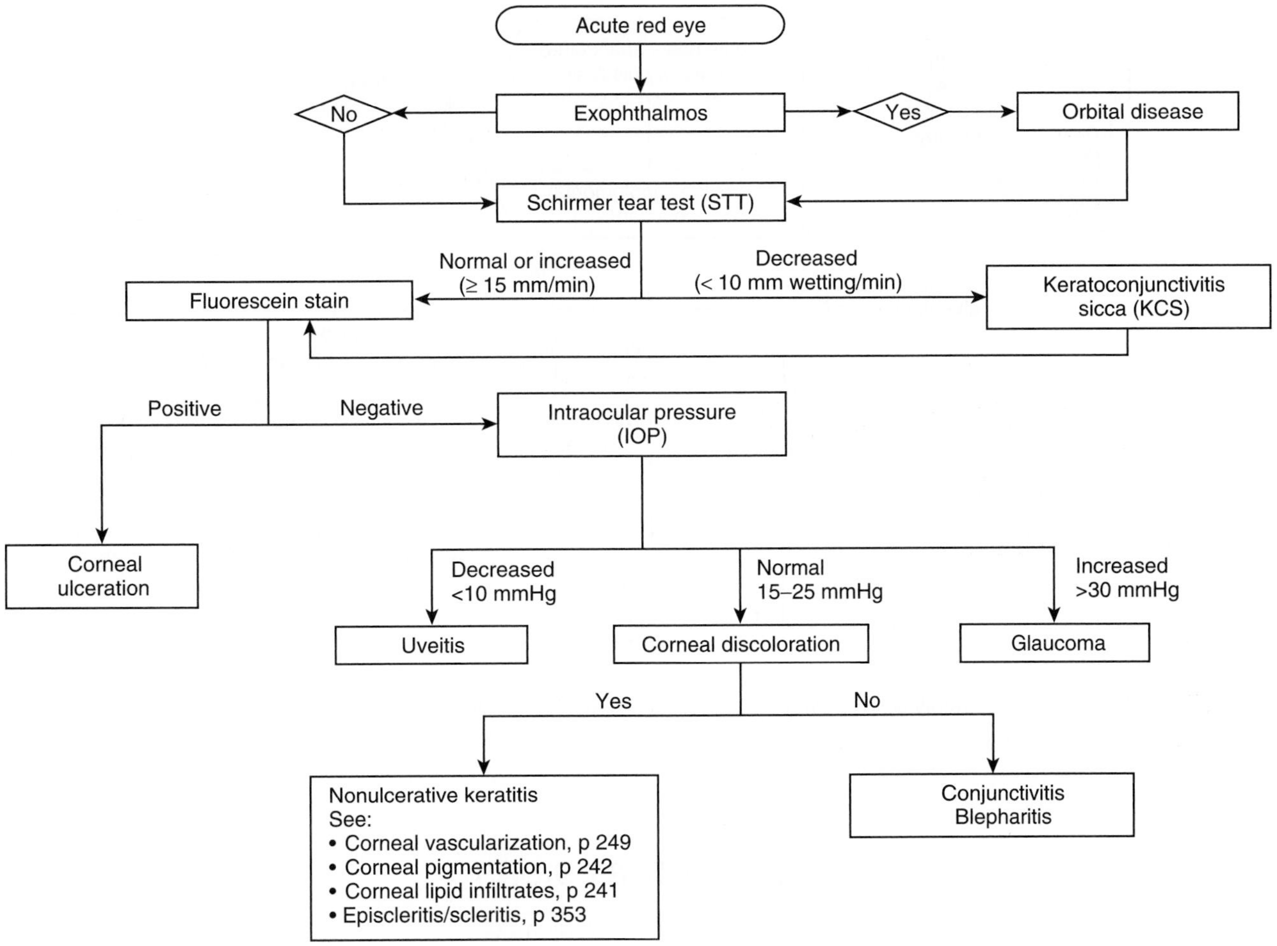

Author & Editor: Cheryl L. Cullen

Note: STT values ≥10 but <15 mm wetting/minute may be normal or indicative of early KCS; IOPs between 10–15 and 25–30 mmHg may be normal for some animals (interpret STT values and IOPs in light of other ophthalmic findings).

RESPIRATORY DISTRESS, HOSPITAL-ACQUIRED

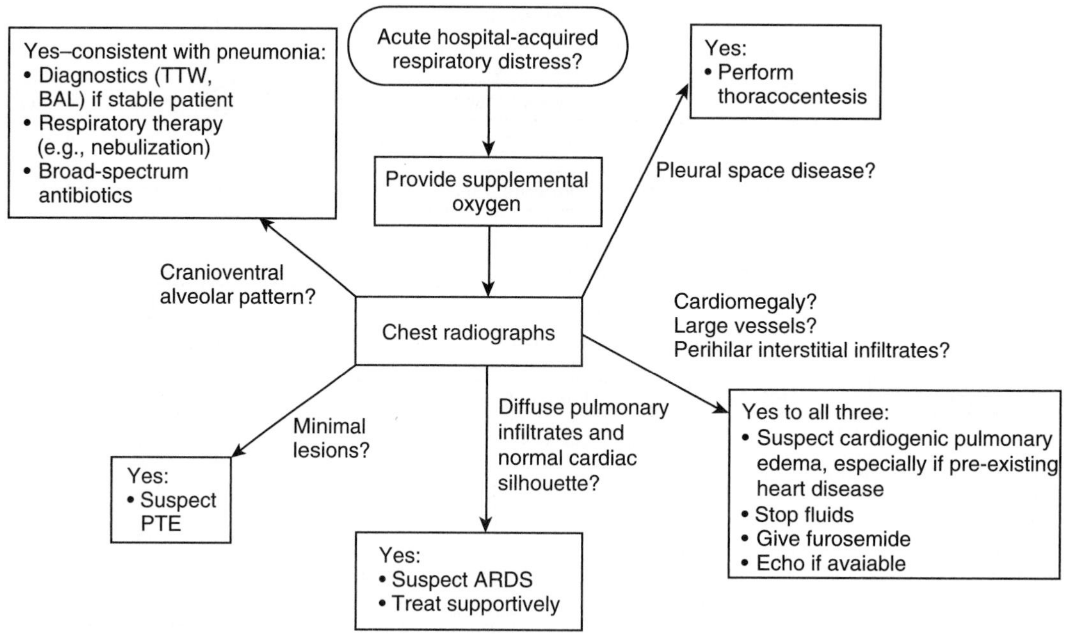

ARDS, adult respiratory distress syndrome; PTE, pulmonary thromboembolism.

Author: Scott P. Shaw
Editor: Elizabeth Rozanski

RESPIRATORY SIGNS

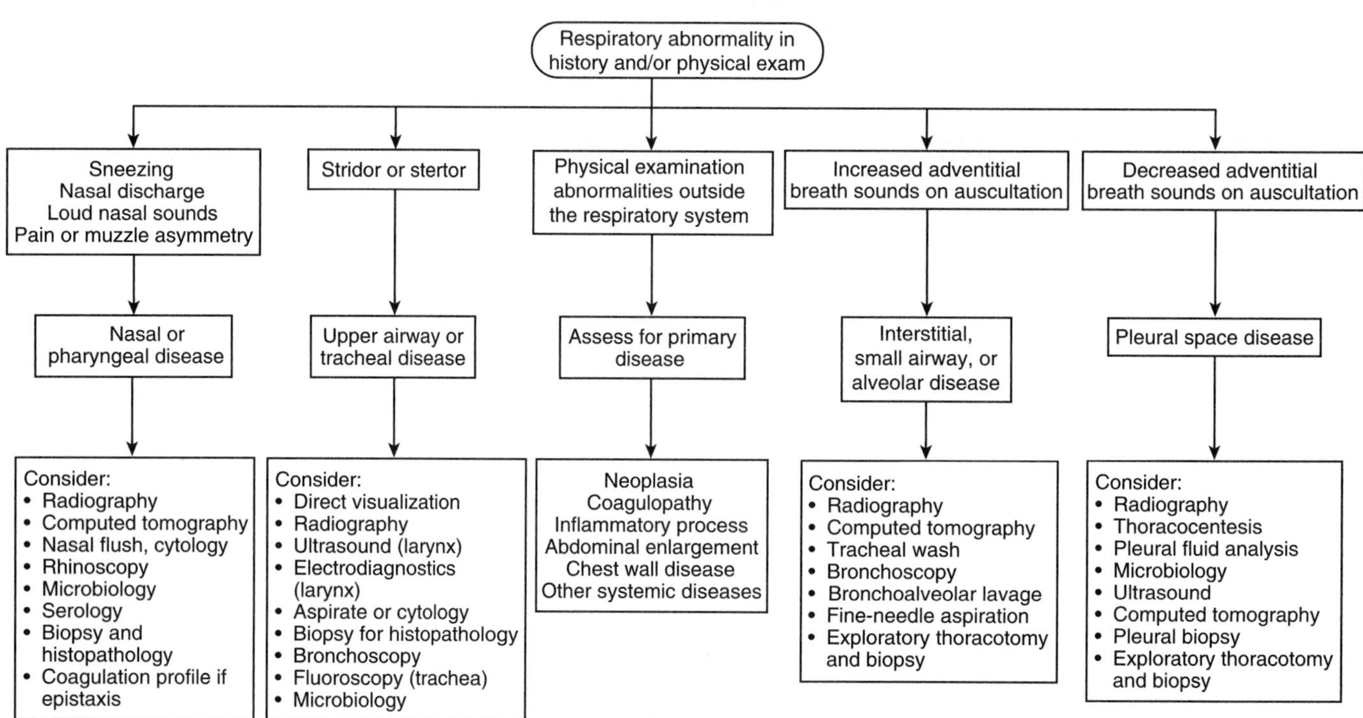

Modified from Ettinger SJ, Feldman EC: *Textbook of Veterinary Internal Medicine*, ed 6. St. Louis, WB Saunders, 2005.

SEPSIS AND SEPTIC SHOCK

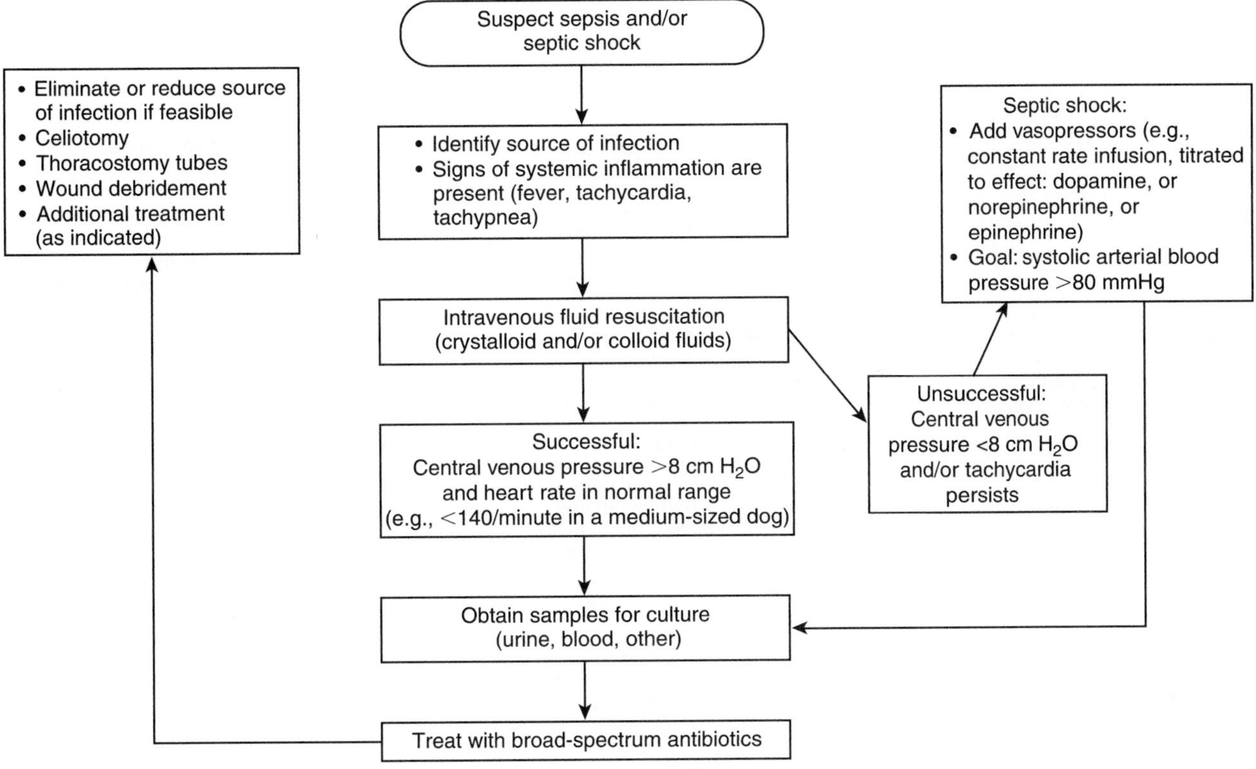

Author: Scott P. Shaw
Editor: Elizabeth Rozanski

SHOCK, HYPOVOLEMIC

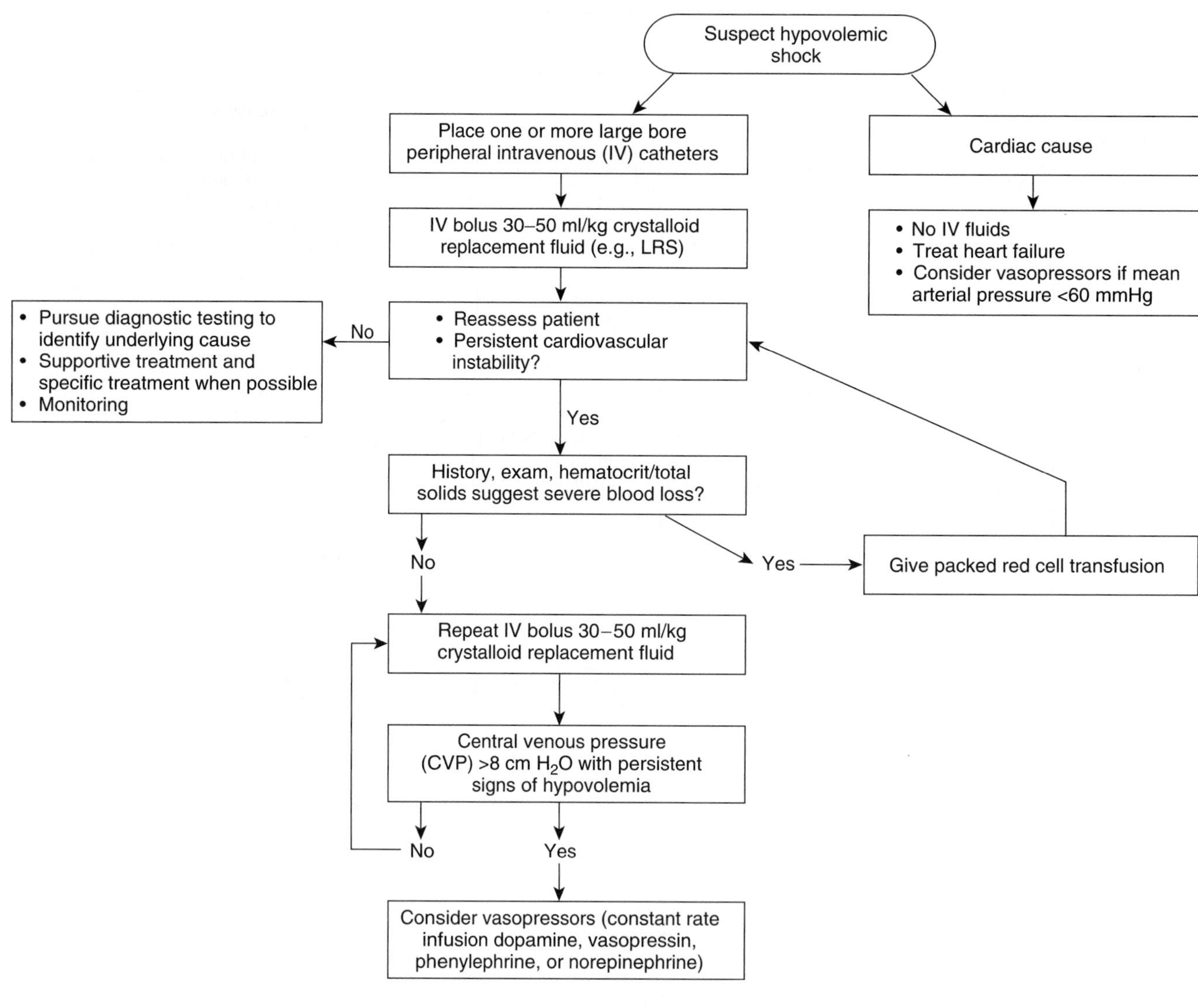

Resuscitation goals/endpoints:
- Normalization of heart rate
- Normalization of blood pressure
- CVP between 8 and 12 cm H_2O
- Adequate urine production

Author: Scott P. Shaw
Editor: Elizabeth Rozanski

SMOKE INHALATION

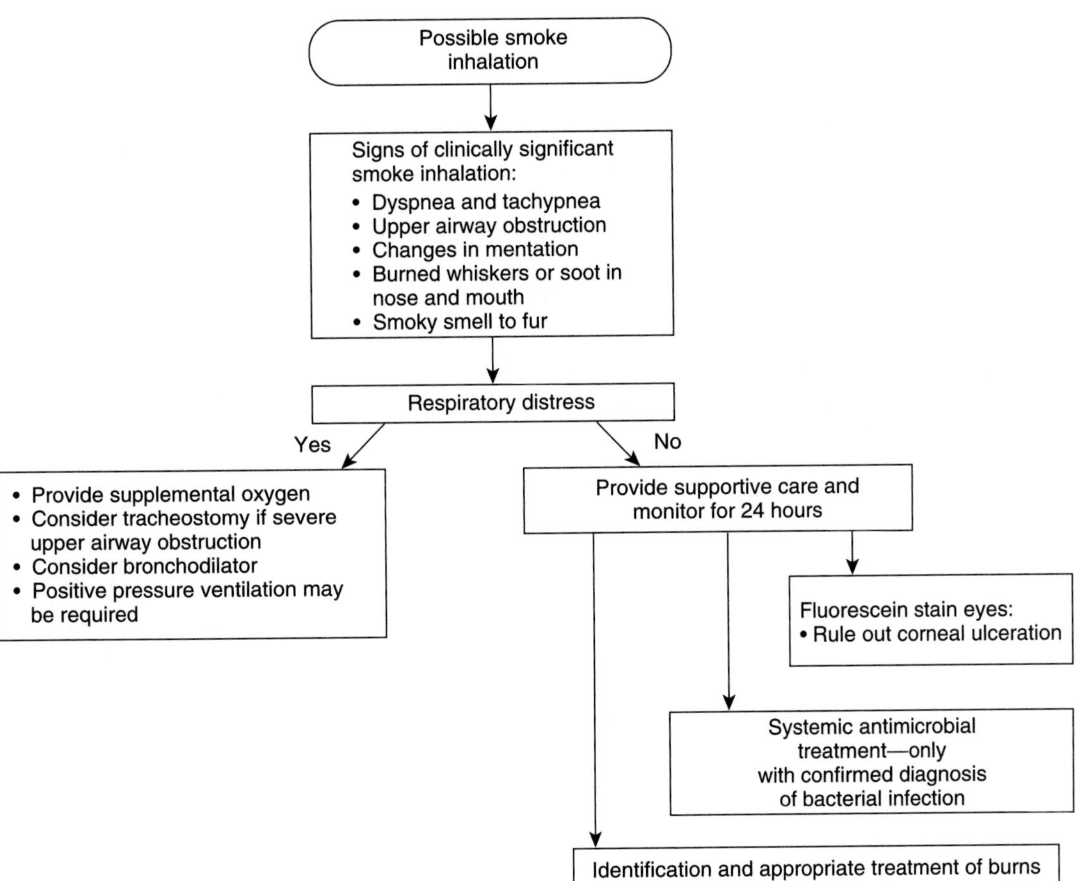
Possible smoke inhalation
Signs of clinically significant smoke inhalation:
• Dyspnea and tachypnea
• Upper airway obstruction
• Changes in mentation
• Burned whiskers or soot in nose and mouth
• Smoky smell to fur
Respiratory distress
Yes
No
• Provide supplemental oxygen
• Consider tracheostomy if severe upper airway obstruction
• Consider bronchodilator
• Positive pressure ventilation may be required
Provide supportive care and monitor for 24 hours
Fluorescein stain eyes:
• Rule out corneal ulceration
Systemic antimicrobial treatment—only with confirmed diagnosis of bacterial infection
Identification and appropriate treatment of burns

Important considerations:

- It can take up to 24 hours after exposure for signs of respiratory distress to develop
- Animals with neurologic signs have a poor prognosis

Author: Scott P. Shaw
Editor: Elizabeth Rozanski

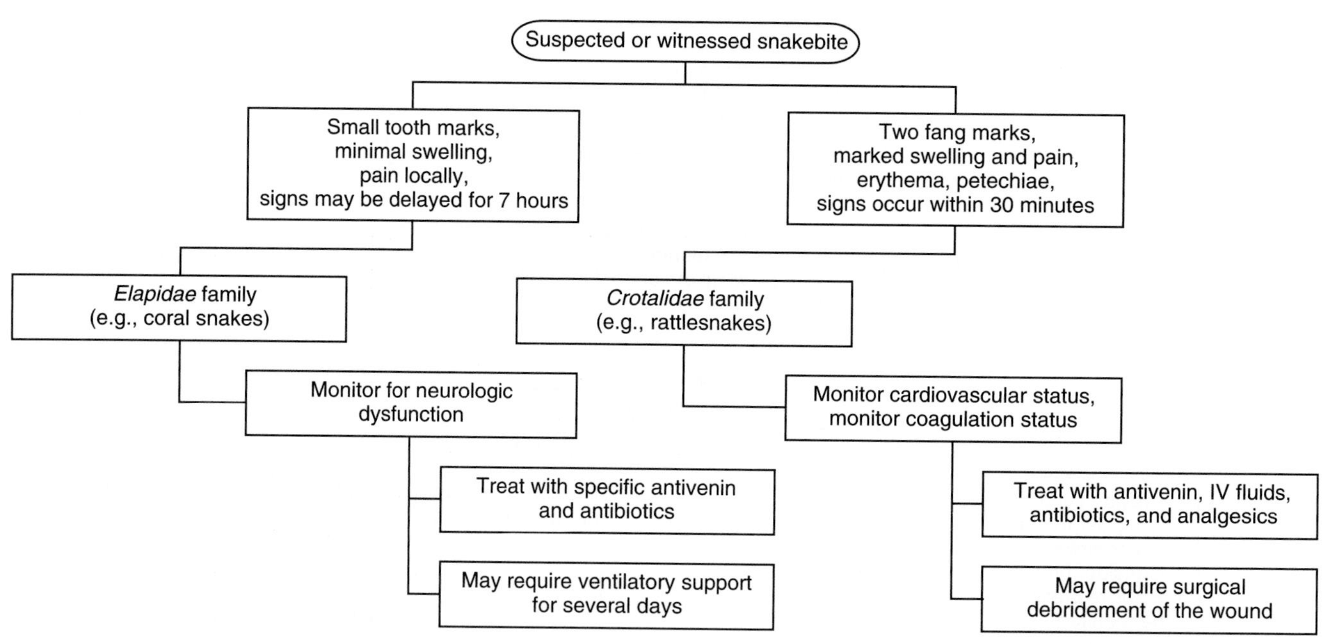
SNAKEBITE
Suspected or witnessed snakebite
Small tooth marks, minimal swelling, pain locally, signs may be delayed for 7 hours
Two fang marks, marked swelling and pain, erythema, petechiae, signs occur within 30 minutes
Elapidae family (e.g., coral snakes)
Crotalidae family (e.g., rattlesnakes)
Monitor for neurologic dysfunction
Monitor cardiovascular status, monitor coagulation status
Treat with specific antivenin and antibiotics
May require ventilatory support for several days
Treat with antivenin, IV fluids, antibiotics, and analgesics
May require surgical debridement of the wound

Author: April Paul
Editor: Elizabeth Rozanski

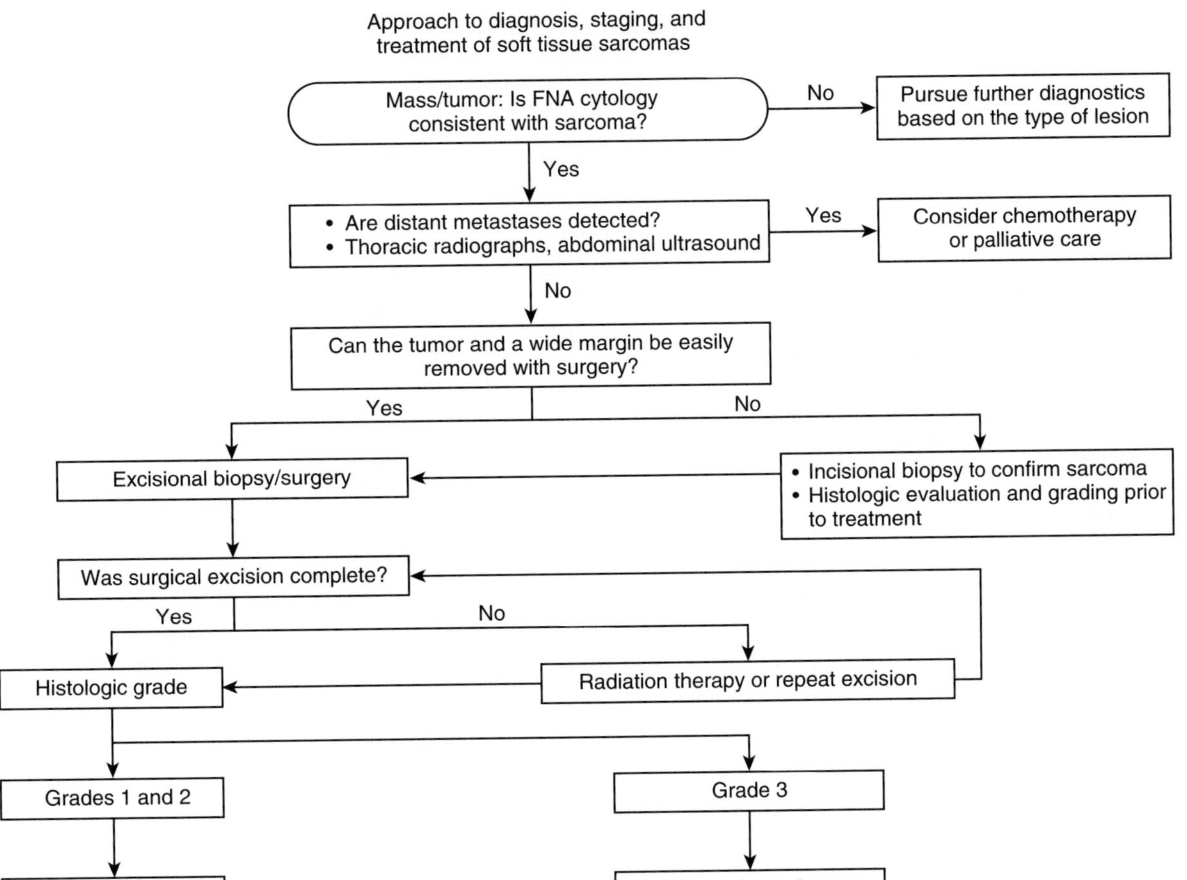

Author: John Farrelly
Editor: Kenneth M. Rassnick

CLINICAL ALGORITHMS

SYNCOPE

- Patient presented for evaluation of syncope
  - Cardiac disease
    - Period of cessation of heartbeat not responsive to atropine
      - Sick sinus syndrome
      - High-grade second-degree atrioventricular block
      - Third-degree atrioventricular block
      - Atrial standstill
    - Increased heart rate
      - Ventricular tachycardia/flutter
      - Supraventricular tachycardia
    - Obstructive lesion
      - Subaortic stenosis
      - Pulmonic stenosis
      - Pulmonary hypertension including heartworm disease
      - Hypertrophic cardiomyopathy
      - Intracardiac neoplasia or thrombus
  - No cardiac disease
    - Obstruction to cerebral blood flow
      - Cough syncope
    - Decreased blood pressure
      - Decreased cardiac output
        - Sinus arrest or atrioventricular block responsive to atropine (vagally induced)
          - Idiopathic
          - Mechanoreceptor stimulation
          - Respiratory or abdominal disease
          - Carotid sinus hypersensitivity
        - Decreased stroke volume
          - No common causes in dogs or cats
      - Decreased peripheral vascular resistance → Drug-induced
        - Increased vagal tone
          - Mechanoreceptor stimulation
          - Idiopathic
    - Metabolic
      - Hypoglycemia

Modified from Kittleson MD, Kienle RD: *Small Animal Cardiovascular Medicine.* St. Louis, Mosby, 1999.

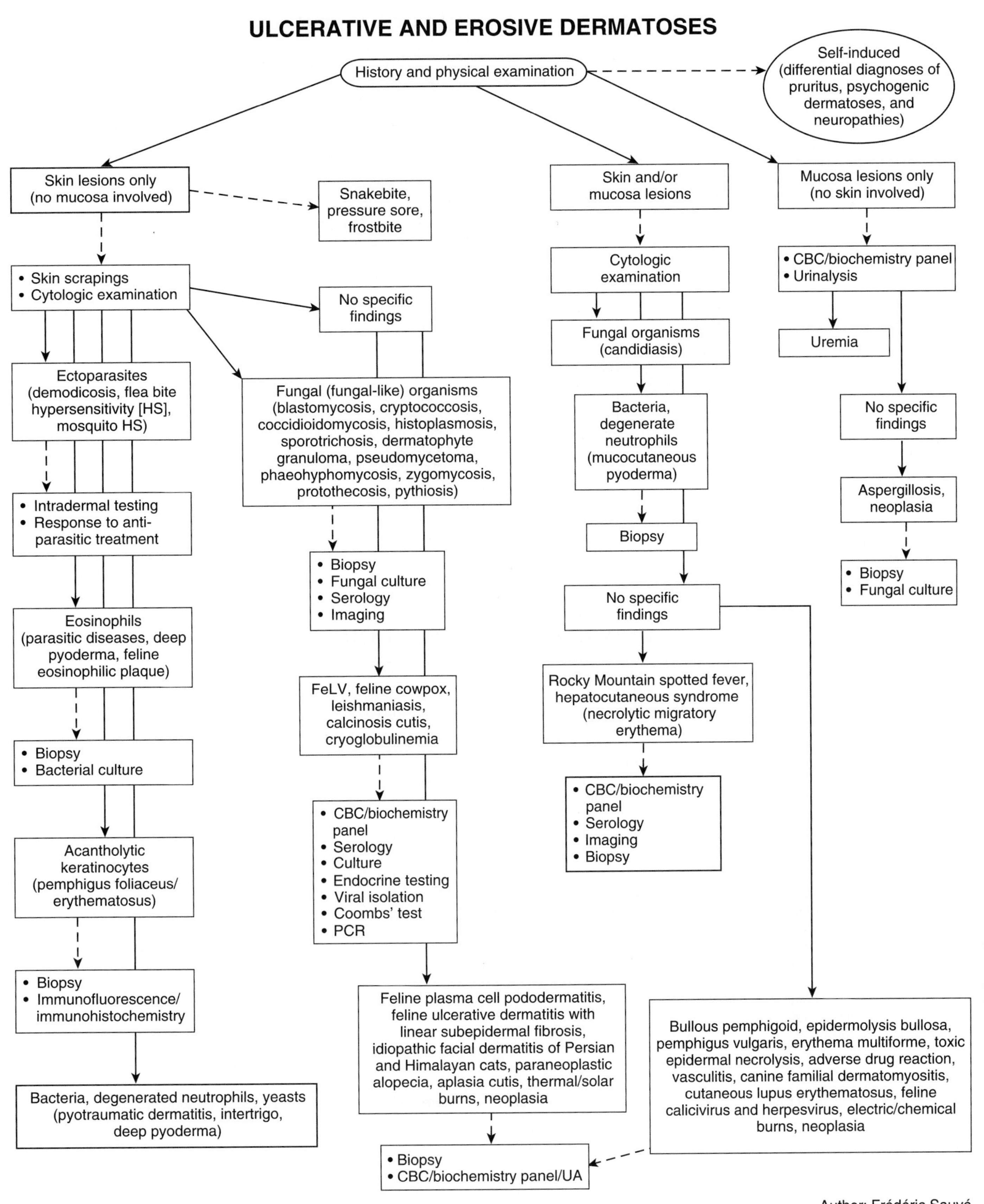

Author: Frédéric Sauvé
Editor: Jan A. Hall

UPPER AIRWAY OBSTRUCTION/CHOKING

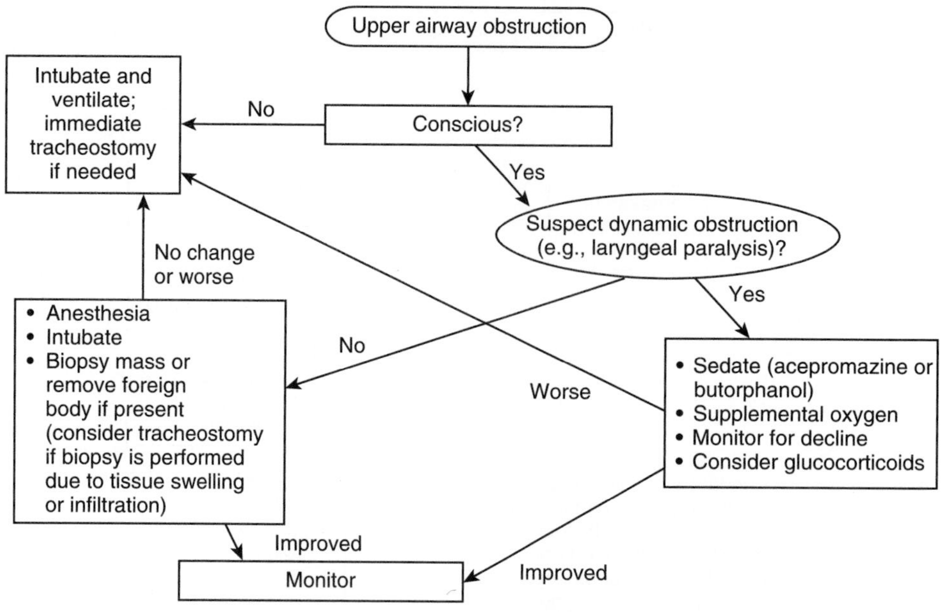

Author: Scott P. Shaw
Editor: Elizabeth Rozanski

URINARY TRACT INFECTION

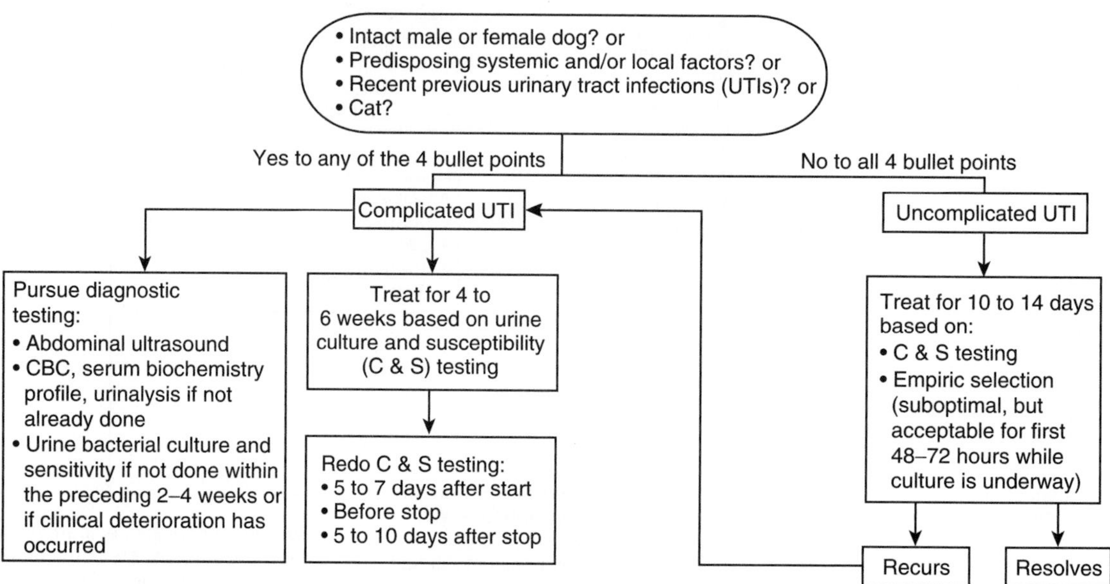

Modified from Ettiinger SJ, Feldman EC: *Textbook of Verterinary Internal Medicine*, ed 6. St. Louis, WB Saunders, 2005.

UROABDOMEN

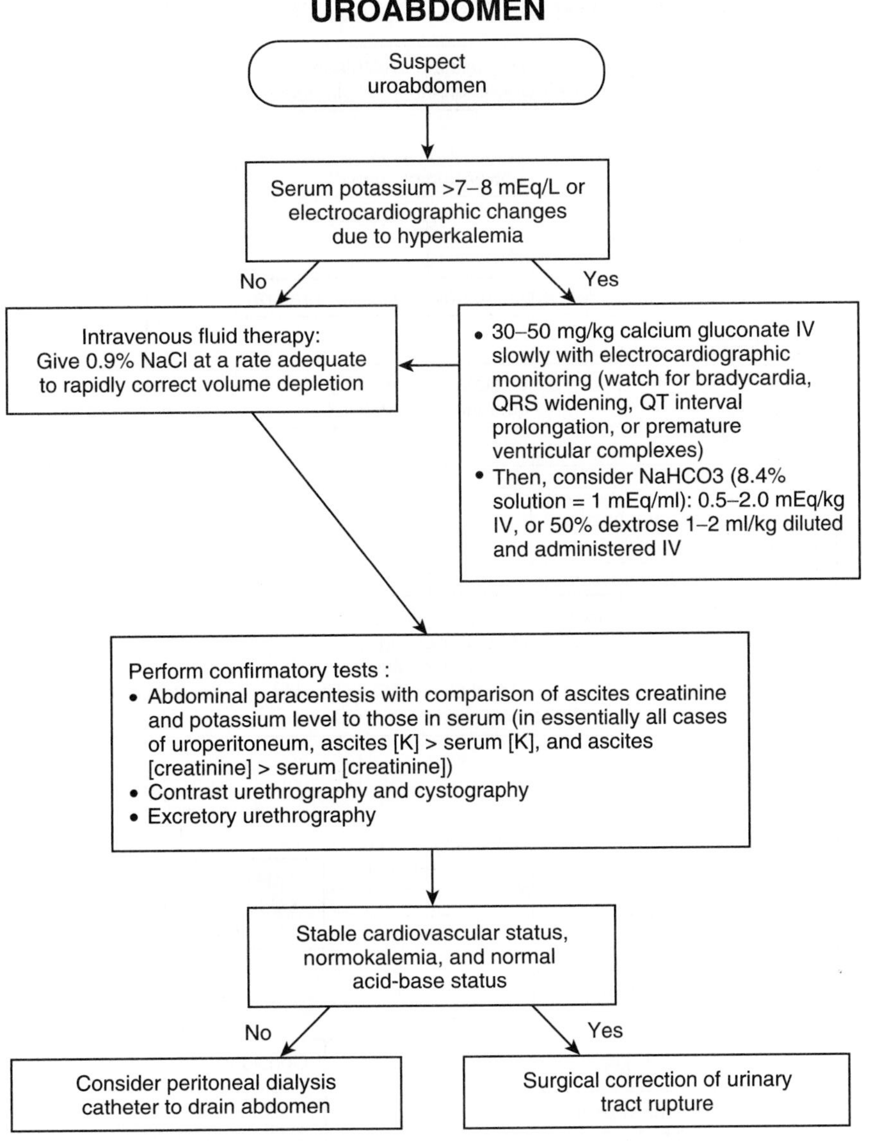

Author: Scott P. Shaw
Editor: Elizabeth Rozanski

UROLITHS, OXALATE

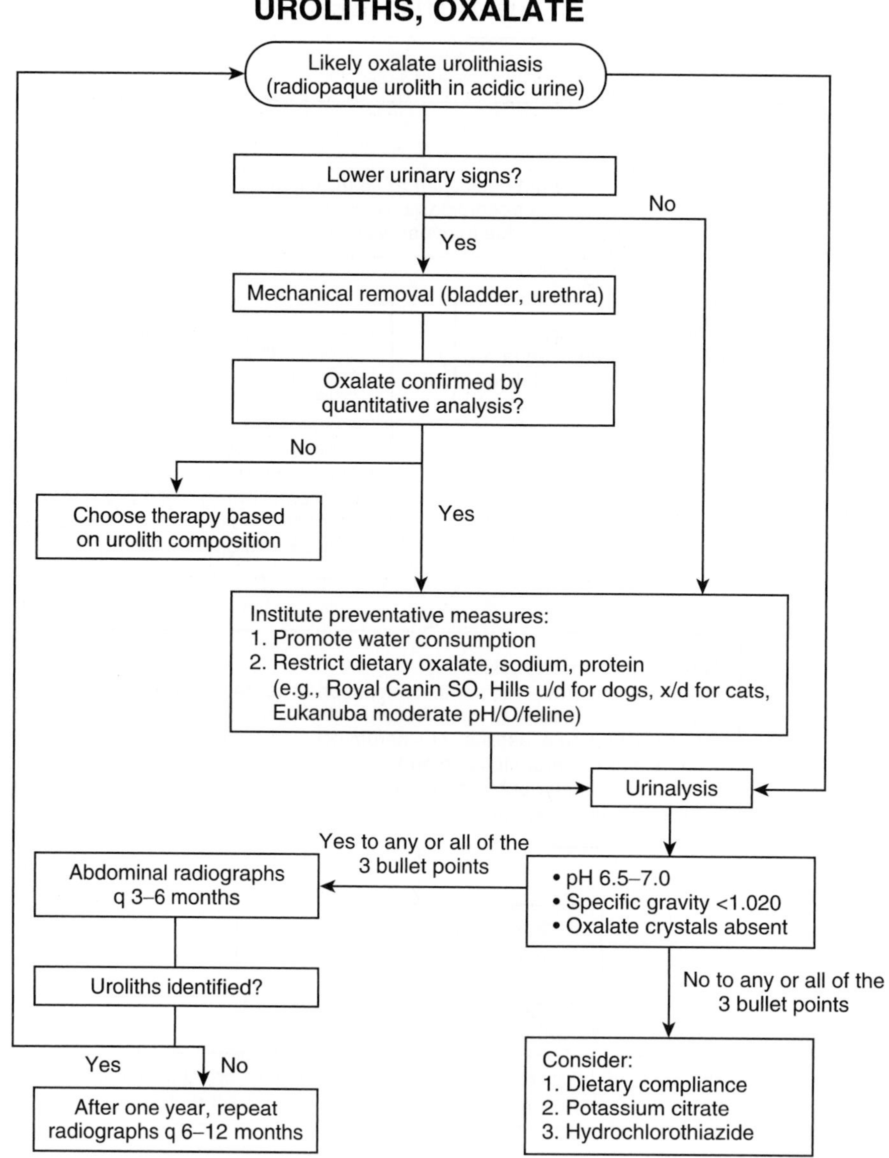

Author: Karen K. Faunt
Editor: Leah A. Cohn

UROLITHS, STRUVITE

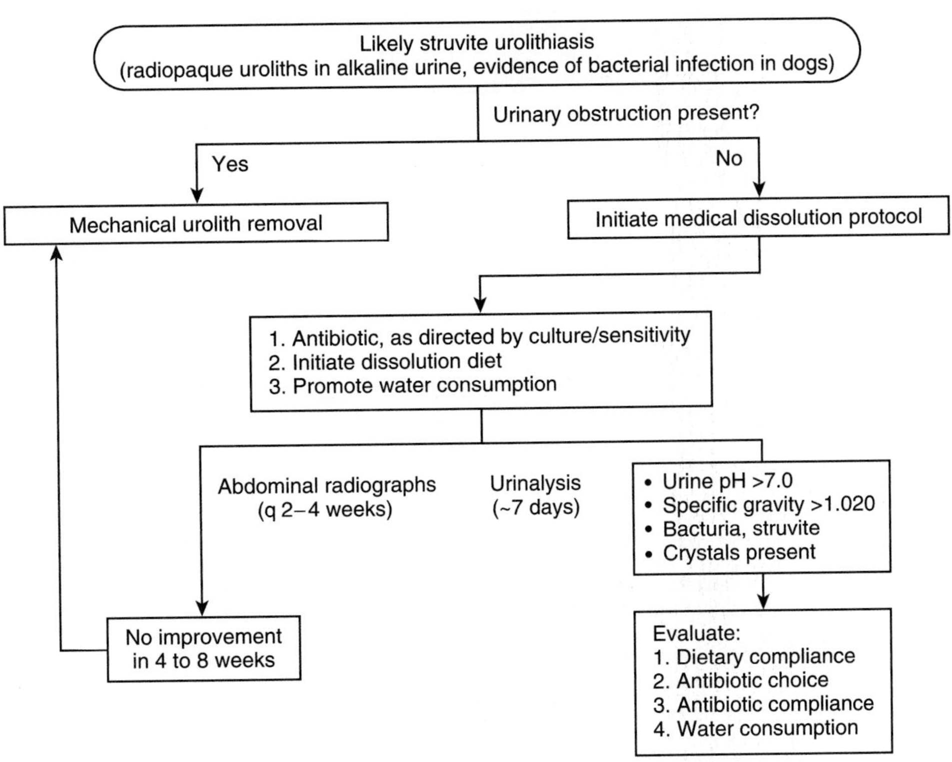

Author: Karen K. Faunt
Editor: Leah A. Cohn

VENTRICULAR TACHYCARDIA: MANAGEMENT

Electrocardiographic (ECG) rhythm consists only of wide, bizarre QRS complexes

↓

Is the rate high?
- >160 bpm for giant-breed dog
- >180 bpm for small-breed dog
- > 240 bpm for cat

No → This is not ventricular tachycardia (VT):
- Ventricular escape rhythm
- Accelerated idioventricular rhythm
- Motion artifact
- Conduction defect such as right bundle branch block

→ Do not treat with antiarrhythmics

Yes → Is there a P wave for every QRS and is the PR interval constant?

- **No to either or both** → VT
- **No to either or both** → • Atrial flutter • Atrial fibrillation (AF) plus right bundle branch block (rare) → Treat accordingly
- **Yes to both** → This is not VT. Consider:
  - Right bundle branch block
  - Another conduction defect

VT → Are there clinical signs directly attributable to the arrhythmia?
- Syncope
- Other (present when arrhythmia is present; gone when it is gone)

Yes → Treatment is indicated. Options include:
- Intravenous (IV)
  - Lidocaine
- Oral (PO)
  - Solatol
  - Mexiletine plus β-blocker
  - Tocainide plus β-blocker
  - Amiodarone

No → Is there an underlying problem that may be triggering the VT and that must be dealt with first?*
- Hypoxemia (congestive heart failureem [CHF], other)†
- Anemia (packed cell volume <25%)†
- Hypokalemia†
- Hypomagnesemia
- Sepsis
- Acidosis
- Abdominal mass†
- Blunt trauma†
- Intoxication
- Excess catecholamines
- Structural heart disease†
- Myocarditis (diagnosis by exclusion)
- Gastric dilation-volvulus (GDV)†

Yes → Address the underlying problem first (→ return to "Are there clinical signs directly attributable to the arrhythmia?")

No (or is being corrected) → Is rate sustained at greater than parameters above? Is pulse (or arterial blood pressure measurement) suboptimal?

- **Yes to either or both** → Treatment is indicated. Options include:
  - Intravenous (IV)
    - Lidocaine
  - Oral (PO)
    - Sotalol
    - Mexiletine plus β-blocker
    - Tocainide plus β-blocker
    - Amiodarone
- **No to both** → Reassess but no antiarrhythmic treatment for now (→ return to "Is the rate high?")

*Virtually any medical problem, if severe enough, can cause ventricular arrhythmias.
†Most common.

Modified from Ettinger SJ, Feldman EC: *Textbook of Veterinary Internal Medicine*, ed 6. St. Louis, WB Saunders, 2005.

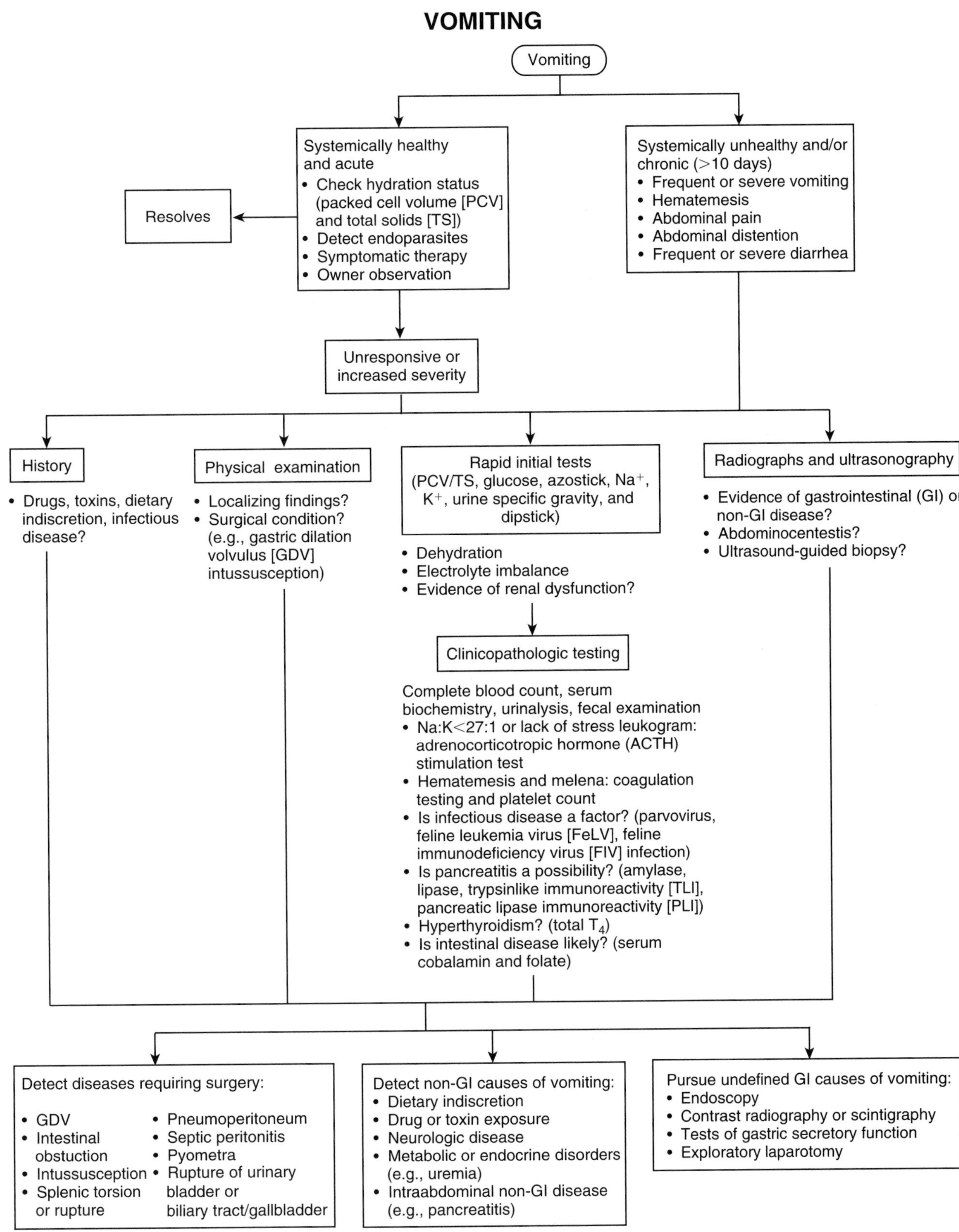

VOMITING
Vomiting
Systemically healthy and acute
• Check hydration status (packed cell volume [PCV] and total solids [TS])
• Detect endoparasites
• Symptomatic therapy
• Owner observation
Resolves
Systemically unhealthy and/or chronic (>10 days)
• Frequent or severe vomiting
• Hematemesis
• Abdominal pain
• Abdominal distention
• Frequent or severe diarrhea
Unresponsive or increased severity
History
• Drugs, toxins, dietary indiscretion, infectious disease?
Physical examination
• Localizing findings?
• Surgical condition? (e.g., gastric dilation volvulus [GDV] intussusception)
Rapid initial tests (PCV/TS, glucose, azostick, Na+, K+, urine specific gravity, and dipstick)
• Dehydration
• Electrolyte imbalance
• Evidence of renal dysfunction?
Radiographs and ultrasonography
• Evidence of gastrointestinal (GI) or non-GI disease?
• Abdominocentestis?
• Ultrasound-guided biopsy?
Clinicopathologic testing
Complete blood count, serum biochemistry, urinalysis, fecal examination
• Na:K<27:1 or lack of stress leukogram: adrenocorticotropic hormone (ACTH) stimulation test
• Hematemesis and melena: coagulation testing and platelet count
• Is infectious disease a factor? (parvovirus, feline leukemia virus [FeLV], feline immunodeficiency virus [FIV] infection)
• Is pancreatitis a possibility? (amylase, lipase, trypsinlike immunoreactivity [TLI], pancreatic lipase immunoreactivity [PLI])
• Hyperthyroidism? (total T_4)
• Is intestinal disease likely? (serum cobalamin and folate)
Detect diseases requiring surgery:
• GDV
• Intestinal obstuction
• Intussusception
• Splenic torsion or rupture
• Pneumoperitoneum
• Septic peritonitis
• Pyometra
• Rupture of urinary bladder or biliary tract/gallbladder
Detect non-GI causes of vomiting:
• Dietary indiscretion
• Drug or toxin exposure
• Neurologic disease
• Metabolic or endocrine disorders (e.g., uremia)
• Intraabdominal non-GI disease (e.g., pancreatitis)
Pursue undefined GI causes of vomiting:
• Endoscopy
• Contrast radiography or scintigraphy
• Tests of gastric secretory function
• Exploratory laparotomy

Modified from Ettinger SJ, Feldman EC: *Textbook of Veterinary Internal Medicine*, ed 6. St. Louis, WB Saunders, 2005.

SECTION VI

Drug Formulary

REDACTORS

Stephen J. Ettinger, DVM, DACVIM (Cardiology, SAIM), FACC, FAHA

Etienne Côté, DVM, DACVIM (Cardiology, SAIM)

Wayne S. Schwark, DVM, MSc, PhD

The drugs listed in this formulary represent a compilation of the more commonly used therapeutic agents in small animal practice, without implying endorsement (or lack thereof) of specific medications. Not all drugs used in veterinary practice are included, and clinicians may infrequently or never use some of those listed.

Drugs are organized in alphabetical order by generic names, with trade names in parentheses under the generic title, and the drugs also are listed alphabetically by brand name, with a cross-reference. A brief description of the drug's actions or indications is also provided. Canine and feline dosage levels are given individually. Note that *total dose* is the amount given to an animal in each single dose (in contrast to *dose per kilogram body weight*) and not the total amount of drug given for the full course of treatment (dosage). The fifth column, entitled Comments, describes commonly seen side effects, specific important observations, or other characteristics that are particularly important to the clinician. A sixth column, entitled How the Drug Is Supplied, includes commonly available sizes and formulations. Abbreviations used in the formulary are first defined on this page for the reader's reference.

Entries that are preceded by letters or modifiers are listed according to the principal word in the name of the drug. For example, L-asparaginase is listed under the letter *A*, DL-methionine is listed under the letter *M*, and s-adenosyl methionine is also listed under the letter *M*. Entries that are preceded by numbers (e.g., 4-methylpyrazole) are listed together at the very beginning of the formulary.

While every effort has been made to include clinically useful, important, and accurate information, a comprehensive review of the details of individual drugs is too voluminous to be listed in this format. Therefore, it remains the prescriber's and clinician's responsibility to ensure that the particulars of any drug are appropriate for the intended application. The clinician should recheck drug dosages for accuracy as well as for specific indications, contraindications, and warnings. Drugs are listed not only by their licensed uses but also by commonly practiced uses. Again, the clinician needs to identify the specific and recommended indications for each drug by reviewing relevant information (e.g., product insert, primary sources) before prescribing, recommending, or using a drug.

Drugs dosages, comments, and side effects are taken from several sources:

1. The clinical experience of the redactors of this formulary.
2. Drug-related information from the other sections of this textbook.
3. Ettinger SJ, Feldman, EC: *Textbook of Veterinary Internal Medicine*, ed 6. St. Louis, WB Saunders, 2005.
4. Allen D, et al (eds): *Handbook of Veterinary Drugs*. Philadelphia, Lippincott, Williams & Wilkins, 2004.
5. Plumb DC: *Veterinary Drug Handbook*, ed 4. Ames, IA, Blackwell, 2005.
6. Kirk RW, Bonagura JD: *Current Veterinary Therapy* IX, X, XI, XII, and XIII. Philadelphia, WB Saunders, 1986–1999.
7. Greene CE (ed): *Infectious Diseases of the Dog and Cat,* ed 2. St. Louis, WB Saunders, 1999.

ABBREVIATIONS

AA: amino acid
ACE: angiotensin-converting enzyme
ACS: American Chemical Society
ACT: activated coagulation time
ACTH: adrenocorticotropic hormone
AV: atrioventricular
BM: bone marrow
BP: blood pressure
BUN: blood urea nitrogen
BW: body weight
C: capsules
C-II: class 2 controlled drug
C-III: class 3 controlled drug
C-IV: class 4 controlled drug
CA: carbonic anhydrase
CBC: complete blood count
CDI: central diabetes insipidus
CHF: congestive heart failure
CLL: chronic lymphocytic leukemia
CNS: central nervous system
COX: cyclooxygenase
CRI: constant rate infusion
D5W: sterile 5% dextrose in water
DCM: dilated cardiomyopathy
DIC: disseminated intravascular coagulation
DJD: degenerative joint disease
DOCA: deoxycorticosterone acetate
ECG: electrocardiogram
EDTA: ethylenediamine tetraacetic acid
ER: extended release
ES: extra strength
FAIDS: feline immunodeficiency virus-induced acquired immunodeficiency syndrome
FDA: Food and Drug Administration
FeLV: feline leukemia virus
FIP: feline infectious peritonitis
G–: gram negative
G+: gram positive
GABA: γ-aminobutyric acid
GI: gastrointestinal
GM: Gram
HDDST: high-dose dexamethasone suppression test
HM: human medicine
HPA: hypothalamic-pituitary-adrenal
HR: heart rate
HW: heartworm
I: injectable
IBD: inflammatory bowel disease
IC: intracardiac
ICU: intensive care unit
IHA: immune-mediated hemolytic anemia
IM: intramuscular
IP: intraperitoneal
ITP: immune-mediated thrombocytopenia
IU: international unit(s)
IV: intravenous
KCS: keratoconjunctivitis sicca
LDDST: low-dose dexamethasone suppression test
LES: lower esophageal (gastroesophageal) sphincter
LRS: lactated Ringer's solution
MAO: monoamine oxidase
MVO_2: myocardial oxygen consumption
NDI: nephrogenic diabetes insipidus
NPH: isophane
NSAID: nonsteroidal anti-inflammatory drug
O: topical ointment
OO: ophthalmic ointment
OS: ophthalmic solution
OTC: over-the-counter, nonprescription item
P: powder
PCV: packed cell volume
PDH: pituitary-dependent hyperadrenocorticism
PO: per os; oral
PP: polyphagia
PRN: as needed
PSS: physiologic saline solution
PTE: pulmonary thromboembolism
PTT: activated partial thromboplastin time
PU/PD: polyuria and polydipsia
q: every
RA: rheumatoid arthritis
RBC: red blood cell
RS: regular strength
S: oral solution
SC: subcutaneous
SIBO: small intestinal bacterial overgrowth/antibiotic-responsive enteritis
SLE: systemic lupus erythematosus
SQ: subcutaneous
SVT: supraventricular tachycardia
T: tablet
T1/2: serum half-life
T3: triiodothyronine
T4: thyroxine
TCC: transitional cell carcinoma
tbsp: tablespoon (= 15 ml)
tsp: teaspoon (= 5 ml)
TVT: transmissible venereal tumor
Tx: treatment
U: unit(s)
USP: United States Phamacopeia
UTI: urinary tract infection
V/D: vomiting/diarrhea
VM: veterinary medicine
vWF: von Willebrand factor
WBC: white blood cell

TABLE VI-1 **Drug Formulary**

Generic Name (Trade Name)	Indications/ Drug Type	Canine Dose	Feline Dose	Comments	How the Drug Is Supplied
2-PAM	*(see pralidoxime)*				
4-methylpyrazole, 4-MP	*(see fomepizole)*				
5-ASA	*(see mesalamine)*				
5-FU	*(see fluorouracil)*				
Abelcet	*(see amphotericin B, liposomal encapsulated)*				
Acarbose (Precose)	Oral hypoglycemic drug used for treating diabetes mellitus; α-glucosidase inhibitor	12.5–25 mg per dog PO for initial dose; if ineffective, may increase to 50–100 mg per dog if no adverse effects	Not recommended	Adverse effects (diarrhea, weight loss) common: 35% of dogs	25, 50, 100 mg T HM
Accolate	*(see zafirlukast)*				
Accutane	*(see isotretinoin)*				
Acepromazine (acetylpromazine, PromAce, AtraVet, "ace")	Sedation, preanesthetic, central antiemetic	Premedication or as part of sedative protocol: 0.03–0.15 mg/kg SQ, IM, IV; as oral sedative (e.g., prior to travel): 0.5–1 mg/kg PO	Same	Oversedation causes CNS depression; in old or systemically ill animals, use at fraction of low dose (e.g., one-fourth) or not at all; do not use in animals with seizures or hypotension; breed sensitivities; has no anxiolytic or analgesic properties on its own (travel); hypotensive agent	5, 10, 25 mg T; 10 mg/ml I VM
Acetaminophen (Tylenol, Excedrin, Feverall, Liquiprin, Midol, Pamprin, Panadol, Percogesic, Tempra, Bromo-Seltzer, paracetamol, and most "aspirin-free" preparations)	Antipyretic, analgesic	10–20 mg/kg PO q 12h	Do not use	Toxic to cats (methemoglobinemia); gastric irritation; hepatotoxicity if overdose; analgesic, not anti-inflammatory	Many sizes T OTC
Acetazolamide (Diamox)	Glaucoma, CA inhibitor	2–10 mg/kg PO q 8h	2–10 mg/kg PO q 8h	Hypokalemia, panting, acidosis	125, 250 mg T,C HM
Acetylcysteine (Mucomyst)	1. Acetaminophen toxicosis in cats 2. Decrease bronchial secretion viscosity 3. Collagenase-complicated corneal ulcers	1. Same as for cats 2. Nebulize as 2% solution q 12h 3. One drop 10% solution q 2–4h in eye	First dose 140 mg/kg, then 70 mg/kg PO q 6h for three to seven treatments; may be given as slow bolus IV	Tastes bad, bronchospasm possible, conjunctivitis if prolonged topical use	100, 200 mg/ml, I HM
Acetylsalicylic acid (ASA, aspirin)	Analgesia, antiinflammatory, antipyretic, DIC, antithrombotic via decreased platelet aggregation	10–25 mg/kg PO q 8–24h; 0.5 mg/kg PO q 12h as antithrombotic	Per cat: 40.5–81 mg (10–20 mg/kg) PO q 48–72h; minidose: 5 mg (1 mg/kg) PO q 72h	Anorexia—nausea, GI irritation, gastric ulcer—bleeding, platelet dysfunction, anemia, doses higher than minidose are *less* anticoagulant in dogs	81, 300, 600 mg, T OTC
Acitretin (Soriatane)	Synthetic retinoid for keratinization disorders in specific breeds (e.g., cocker spaniels)	0.5–1.32 mg/kg PO q 24h	—	Teratogenic; excreted in milk; adverse effects similar to etretinate?	10, 25 mg T HM
ACTH gel	Provocative agent for diagnosis of hyperadrenocorticism or hypoadrenocorticism	2 IU/kg IM, obtain blood preinjection and at 2 hours postinjection for cortisol levels	Per cat (IM): 10 IU, obtain blood preinjection and 1–2 hours postinjection	Rare allergic reaction, do not give IV	40, 80 IU/ml I HM

(Continued)

TABLE VI-1 **Drug Formulary—(*Continued*)**

Generic Name (Trade Name)	Indications/ Drug Type	Canine Dose	Feline Dose	Comments	How the Drug Is Supplied
ACTH-like solution, aqueous (tetracosactrin, cosyntropin, Cortrosyn)	Provocative agent for diagnosis of hyperadrenocorticism or hypoadreno-corticism; appears superior to ACTH gel but more costly	Standard dose: 250 µg/dog (0.25 mg/dog) once, IV or IM. Low dose: 5 µg/kg (0.005 mg/kg) IV once; with either protocol, obtain blood preinjection and at 1 hour postinjection for cortisol levels	Per cat: 0.125 mg IM or IV total dose; obtain blood preinjection and at 30 and 60 minutes postinjection	Costly; however, low dose and standard dose are equally effective when used IV; also remains effective if diluted, fractionated, and frozen for use at low dose (dogs) (Peterson ME: *J Am Vet Med Assoc* 224: 198–199, 2004)	250 µg (0.25 mg) per ampule I HM
Actigall	*(see ursodeoxycholic acid)*				
Activated charcoal (Requa)	GI adsorbent	1 g/5 ml water: give 10 ml of slurry/ kilogram; best administered via stomach tube	1 g/5 ml water: give 10 ml of slurry/kilo-gram; best administered via stomach tube	Do not induce vomiting; Inhalation pneumonia may occur; Follow with cathartic.	VM HM (various)
Adenosyl methionine, s-	*(see methionine, s-adenosyl)*				
Adequan	*(see glycosamino-glycan—polysulfated)*				
Adrenalin	*(see epinephrine)*				
Adriamycin	*(see doxorubicin)*				
Adrucil	*(see fluorouracil)*				
Advantage	*(see imidacloprid)*				
Advil	*(see ibuprofen)*				
Aglepristone (Alizine, RU-46534)	Progesterone receptor antagonist	10 mg/kg SQ twice, 24h apart	—	Not licensed or widely used in the United States, abortifacient	300 mg/ml I VM
Albendazole (Valbazen)	*Giardia*; other endoparasites	25–50 mg/kg PO q 12h for maximum 5 days	15–25 mg/kg PO q 12h for 5 days	May cause bone marrow suppression at recorded dosages; 4 doses total (2-day course) recommended for giardiasis; up to 10–21 days for *Paragonimus*	300 mg/g (paste) S VM
Albeta	*(see methionine, DL-)*				
Albon	*(see sulfadimetho-xine)*				
Albuterol (Ventolin, Proventil, Volmax, salbutamol)	Immediate but short-acting β-2 adrenergic agonist bronchodilator	0.02–0.05 mg/kg (20–50 µg/kg) PO q 8–12h Inhalant: one puff PRN, up to q 12h	One puff PRN	Beneficial effect lasts <4 hours; restlessness, muscle tremors; use with caution in patients where sympathetic drive could be harmful (e.g., heart disease, hypertension, hyperthyroidism, seizure disorders)	2, 4, 5 mg T, 2.5 mg/ml S, 6.8, 17 g inhalation canisters (0.1 mg [100 µg] per puff) HM
Aldactazide	*(see hydrochlorothia-zide/spironolactone)*				
Aldactone	*(see spironolactone)*				
Aleve	*(see naproxen)*				
Alkeran	*(see melphalan)*				
Allopurinol (Zyloprim)	Urate urolithiasis Leishmaniasis	10 mg/kg PO q 8h, then reduce to 10 mg/kg PO q 24h after 1 month	None	q 8h Tx for 30 days then q 24h	100, 300 mg T HM

TABLE VI-1 **Drug Formulary—(*Continued*)**

Generic Name (Trade Name)	Indications/ Drug Type	Canine Dose	Feline Dose	Comments	How the Drug Is Supplied
Alprazolam (Xanax)	Benzodiazepine Separation anxiety		0.0125–0.025 mg/kg PO q 12–24h	Feline dose range of 0.125–0.25 mg/kg published in other sources represents a 10-fold excess and should not be used	0.25, 0.5, 1, 2 mg T HM
Altace	*(see ramipril)*				
AlternaGEL	*(see aluminum hydroxide)*				
Aluminum hydroxide (Amphojel, AlternaGEL)	Phosphate binder, antacid	Initially, 10–30 mg/kg PO q 8–12h; titrate based on PO_4 to 10–90 mg/kg PO q 6–12h; 5–10 ml/dog	Same dose; per cat: approx. 1–3 ml q 8–12h	May cause metabolic alkalosis; Amphojel = 64 mg $Al(OH)_3$/ml; AlternaGEL = 120 mg $Al(OH)_3$/ml; decreases absorption of concurrent drugs (e.g., tetracyclines, ketoconazole)	OTC, S HM
Amantadine (Symmetrel)	NDMA antagonist analgesic drug	2 mg/kg PO q 24h	3–5 mg/kg PO q 24h	New agent with little published clinical use; safety and efficacy profiles undetermined	100 mg C, 10 mg/ml S HM
AmBisome	*(see amphotericin B, liposomal encapsulated)*				
Amicar	*(see aminocaproic acid)*				
Amiglyde-V	*(see amikacin)*				
Amikacin (Amikin, Amiglyde-V)	Aminoglycoside, GM + and – agent	10–20 mg/kg q 24h or 5–10 mg/kg q 12h IV, IM, SQ	Same	Nephrotoxic, ototoxic, neuromuscular blockade, poor GI absorption	50 mg/ml I VM
Amikin	*(see amikacin)*				
Amino acids 3% and glycerin injection with electrolytes (ProcalAmine)	Partial parenteral nutrition	Maintenance rate	Maintenance rate	Essential and nonessential amino acids, carbohydrates, and electrolytes for IV infusion; see Parenteral Nutrition, p 1296	IV solution bags, S
Aminocaproic acid (Amicar)	Antiprotease activity for degenerative myelopathy	15 mg/kg PO q 8h	—	Limited information on side effects or benefits	200 mg T, 250 mg/ml S, 250 mg/ml I HM
Aminopentamide (Centrine)	Antispasmodic, cholinergic blocking agent, similar to atropine	0.01–0.03 mg/kg PO, IM, SQ, q 8–12h	0.01–0.03 mg/kg PO, IM, SQ, q 8–12h	Dryness of the mouth, atropine-like side effects; contraindicated in GI obstruction, GI infection/toxin, glaucoma, heart disease, tachycardia	0.2 mg T, 0.5 mg/ml I VM
Aminophylline	Bronchodilator, diuretic (very mild)	5–10 mg/kg PO, IV, q 8–24h	2–6 mg/kg PO, q 12–24h	Hyperexcitability, tachycardia, gastric irritation, PU/PD, anorexia; therapeutic serum level = 10–20 µg/ml, administer IV slowly	100, 200 mg T, 25 mg/ml I VM
Aminopropazine (Jenotone)	Used in urethral obstructions, smooth muscle relaxant	2.2–4.4 mg/kg IM, q 12–24h	Per cat: 6.25–12.5 mg IM, q 12–24h for 48 hours	Do not use with cystic atony; contraindicated in hypotension	25 mg T, 25 mg/ml I VM
Amiodarone (Cordarone)	Type III antiarrhythmic agent for serious/life-threatening ventricular tachyarrhythmias	10 mg/kg PO q 12h for 1 week (loading), then 8 mg/kg PO q 24h	—	Photosensitivity, liver necrosis, keratopathy, positive Coombs' test; may be proarrhythmic	200 mg T HM

(*Continued*)

TABLE VI-1 **Drug Formulary—(*Continued*)**

Generic Name (Trade Name)	Indications/ Drug Type	Canine Dose	Feline Dose	Comments	How the Drug Is Supplied
Amitraz (Mitaban)	Demodicosis, mites, ticks	5–10 ml/gallon H_2O, dip dog; air dry; = 0.025 to 0.05% solution; use three times per week on feet with a fresh solution of 0.5 ml in 30 ml propylene glycol or mineral oil	—	CNS depression; wear gloves when applying; requires multiple dips; transient pruritus noted; small breeds more susceptible; use in ventilated areas and in accordance with relevant regulations (e.g., EPA)	19.9% solution for dilution and topical skin application VM
Amitriptyline HCl (Elavil)	Separation anxiety-related disorders, destructive disorders, feline inappropriate elimination; tricyclic antidepressant; long onset to clinical benefit	1.1–4.4 mg/kg PO q 12–24h	Per cat: 2.5–5 mg total dose (0.5–1 mg/kg) PO q 12–24h	Sedation, psychosis, anticholinergic side effects; caution if seizure history, glaucoma, dysuria	10, 25, 50, 75, 100, 150 mg T HM
Amlodipine (Norvasc)	Long-acting Ca channel blocking agent for hypertension	0.0625–0.25 mg/kg PO q 24h	0.125–0.25 mg/kg PO q 24h	Somnolence, hypotension	2.5, 5, 10 mg T HM
Ammonium chloride (Uroeze)	Urinary acidifier	100 mg/kg PO q 12h	20–40 mg/kg PO q 12h	Poor palatability, GI signs; contraindicated in liver disease and in renal failure; granules = 200 or 400 mg in 1/4 tsp	500 mg T, HM; 400 mg T; 200, 400 mg per 1/4 tsp P VM
Amoxicillin (Amoxi-tabs, Amoxi-drops, Robamox-V)	Penicillin class antibiotic, GM + (not GM–) and anaerobic antibacterial agent,	10–20 mg/kg PO, SQ, IM, IV, q 8–12h	Same	Penicillin contraindications	50, 100, 150, 200, 400 mg T, 25, 50 mg/ml S VM, HM
Amoxicillin/ clavulanic acid (Clavamox, Augmentin)	*(see amoxicillin);* no penicillinase inactivation	10–20 mg/kg PO q 12h	Same	Penicillin sensitivity, vomiting in cats; tablets must remain in foil until used	62.5, 125, 250, 375 mg T; 50 mg/ml S VM, HM
Amoxitabs	*(see amoxicillin)*				
Amphojel	*(see aluminum hydroxide)*				
Amphotericin B (Fungizone)	Systemic mycoses	Test dose (monitor for acute febrile reaction) = 0.25 mg/kg IV; if okay, then 0.5 mg/kg in D5W given IV CRI three times weekly for 2–4 months; do not exceed 5–10 mg/kg	Test dose (monitor for acute febrile reaction) = 0.1 mg/kg IV; if okay, then 0.1–0.25 mg/kg in 5–20 ml of 5% dextrose in water given slowly IV three times weekly for up to 6 weeks	Nephrotoxic; monitor BUN; pretreat with antiemetics; extravasation injury; anaphylaxis possible; may administer at lower dosage SQ in 0.45% saline plus 2.5% dextrose; combination with oral azoles to decrease dose/ toxicity	50 mg/vial (or 100 mg/vial [*Abelcet*]) I HM
Amphotericin B, liposomal encapsulated (AmBisome, Abelcet)	Blastomycosis, histoplasmosis, cryptococcosis, coccidioidomycosis	0.5 mg/kg IV test dose; then 1–2.5 mg/kg IV, q 48h; recommended cumulative dose = 12 mg/kg	—	Anaphylaxis possible; less nephrotoxic than aqueous amphotericin B (as already described)	50 mg/vial I HM
Ampicillin	Penicillin class antibiotic; routine G+ and anaerobic infections, some G–	10–20 mg/kg PO, SQ, IM, IV, q 8h	Same	Penicillin contra-indications, phlebitis	125, 250, 500 mg C; 125 mg/5 ml S; 1, 3, 6 g vials I VM, HM

TABLE VI-1 **Drug Formulary—(*Continued*)**

Generic Name (Trade Name)	Indications/ Drug Type	Canine Dose	Feline Dose	Comments	How the Drug Is Supplied
Amprolium (Corid)	Enteric coccidiostat	Per pup: 100 mg total dose q 24h in food or water (not both) for 10 days; per adult dog: 300 mg total dose q 24h in food or water (not both) for 10 days	—	Overdosage causes CNS disturbances; thiamine is antidote	9.6% S VM
Amrinone (Inocor)	Low-output systolic myocardial failure; phosphodiesterase inhibitor	1–3 mg bolus IV, then 0.01–0.1 mg/kg/min (10–100 μg/kg/min) IV CRI	—	Tachycardia, anxiety; monitor pulse and BP	5 mg/ml I HM
Anafranil	*(see clomipramine)*				
Ancef	*(see cephalosporin antibiotics)*				
Ancobon	*(see flucytosine)*				
Ancotil	*(see flucytosine)*				
Anipryl	*(see selegiline)*				
Antirobe	*(see clindamycin)*				
Antisedan	*(see atipamezole)*				
Antivert	*(see meclizine)*				
Antizol-Vet	*(see fomepizole)*				
Anzemet	*(see dolasetron)*				
Apomorphine	Induction of vomiting	0.03 mg/kg IV or 1/4–1/2 tab in conjunctival sac (flush out after onset of emesis)	Same	Do not use if decreased consciousness; do not use in cases of corrosive poisoning; periocular irritation	6 mg T HM
Apresoline	*(see hydralazine)*				
Aqua-Mephyton	*(see vitamin K_1)*				
ARA-C	*(see cytosine arabinoside)*				
Arava	*(see leflunomide)*				
Aredia	*(see pamidronate)*				
Artificial tears ointment (Adapt, Lacrilube)	Used for insufficient tear production or with decreased blinking	One drop in affected eye PRN	Same	Hypersensitivity	OTC HM
ASA	*(see acetylsalicylic acid)*				
Asacol	*(see mesalamine)*				
Ascorbic acid (vitamin C)	Acetominophen-induced methemoglobin toxicity, copper hepatotoxicity	Per dog: 100–500 mg PO, total dose q 8h	30 mg/kg PO, SQ, IM, IV, q 6h, for acetaminophen toxicity	Caution in urolithiasis	500 mg/ml I; 50, 100, 250, 500 mg, 1 g T HM, OTC
Ascriptin	*(see acetylsalicylic acid)*				
L-asparaginase (Elspar)	Induction therapy for lymphoreticular neoplasms, ITP	400 IU/kg IM, IP once or as part of a protocol; or 10,000–20,000 IU/m^2 IM, IP, SQ	Same	Allergic reactions; anaphylaxis; pretreat with antihistamines; pancreatitis; coagulopathies	10,000 IU/vial I HM
Aspirin	*(see acetylsalicylic acid)*				
Atabrine	*(see quinacrine)*				
Atarax	*(see hydroxyzine)*				

(Continued)

TABLE VI-1 **Drug Formulary—(*Continued*)**

Generic Name (Trade Name)	Indications/ Drug Type	Canine Dose	Feline Dose	Comments	How the Drug Is Supplied
Atenolol (Tenormin)	β-1 adrenergic blockade; supraventricular tachyarrhythmias, systemic hypertension, hypertrophic cardiomyopathy	0.25–1 mg/kg PO q 24h to q 12h	Per cat: 1/8–1/4 of 25 mg tab PO total dose, q 24h to q 12h	Hypotension, depression, β-blockade induced CHF, inappetence, bradycardia; generally start at low dose and titrate up as necessary	25, 50, 100 mg T HM
Atipamezole (Antisedan)	Synthetic α-2 adrenergic antagonist; used for reversing analgesic-sedative effects of medetomidine	Administer a volume of atipamezole equal to the volume of medetomidine used (meaning the atipamezole dose equals five times the medetomidine dose [in mg] because the atipamezole concentration is five times higher); use IV or IM; give less if >1 hour since medetomidine	Same	The return to normal state may not be immediate	5 mg/ml I VM
Atopica	*(see cyclosporine)*				
Atravet	*(see acepromazine)*				
Atropine SO_4	Parasympatholytic, anticholinergic; preanesthetic agent, organophosphate toxicity; supraventricular bradyarrhythmia; atropine response test	0.02–0.044 mg/kg IM, SQ, IV. Atropine response test: give IV only, and recheck ECG after 2–15 minutes. For organophosphate poisoning, give 0.2–2 mg/kg IV, IM, or SQ (give ¼ dose IV and the remainder IM or SQ)	Same	Tachycardia, mydriasis, ileus, photophobia, dysuria; do not use in CHF unless bradycardia is present	0.54 mg/ml I VM various HM
Atropine sulfate ophthalmic solution or ointment	Used when pupillary dilation is desired (e.g., uveitis)	One drop in affected eye q 12–24h	Same: one drop in affected eye q 12–24h	Atropine side effects; contraindicated in the presence of glaucoma; cats may salivate	0.5, 1% OO; 0.5, 1, 2, and 3% OS HM
Augmentin	*(see amoxicillin/ clavulanic acid)*				
Aurothioglucose (Solganal)	Pemphigus complex, autoimmune diseases, rheumatoid arthritis	Week 1: 0.1 mg/kg IM single dose; week 2: 0.2 mg/kg single dose; then 1 mg/kg once a week IM, decreasing to once a month for maintenance immunosuppression	Per cat: week 1: 1 mg IM; week 2: 2 mg IM; then 1 mg/kg once a week IM, decreasing to once a month	Blood dyscrasias, renal and hepatotoxicity, neuritis-encephalitis, cutaneous toxicity, pain at injection site, many others	50 mg/ml I HM
Avlosulfon	*(see dapsone)*				
Axid	*(see nizatidine)*				
Azathioprine (Imuran)	Immunosuppressive agent (SLE, RA, immune-mediated hepatopathies, pemphigus, polymyositis, ITP, IHA, etc.)	1–2 mg/kg PO q 24–48h	Do not use: toxic	Monitor CBC; bone marrow suppression (leukopenia, thrombocytopenia); rarely hepatotoxic; use chemo precautions when handling or administering	50 mg T HM
Azidothymidine (AZT, zidovudine, Retrovir)	Antiretroviral agent	—	5–15 mg/kg PO q 12h for 21 days	Monitor for anemia	100 mg C; 300 mg T; 10 mg/ml S HM

TABLE VI-1 **Drug Formulary—*(Continued)***

Generic Name (Trade Name)	Indications/ Drug Type	Canine Dose	Feline Dose	Comments	How the Drug Is Supplied
Azithromycin (Zithromax)	Broad-spectrum static macrolide antibiotic; refractory respiratory infections, other infections	5–10 mg/kg PO q 24h for 1–5 days	5 mg/kg PO q 24h for 1–5 days; pulse therapy or long-term treatment possible (weeks)	Resistant infections, GI effects, perishable (oral solution expires after 1 week despite refrigeration)	250, 600 mg T; 20, 40 mg/ml S HM
Azium	*(see dexamethasone)*				
AZT	*(see azidothymidine)*				
Azulfidine	*(see sulfasalazine)*				
Bactrim	*(see trimethoprim/ sulfamethoxazole)*				
Bactrovet	*(see sulfadimethoxine)*				
BAL	*(see dimercaprol)*				
Banamine	*(see flunixin meglumine)*				
Baytril	*(see enrofloxacin)*				
Benadryl	*(see diphenhydramine)*				
Benazepril (Fortekor, Lotensin)	ACE inhibitor, vasodilator. CHF therapy; glomerulopathy; systemic hypertension (usually in conjuction with other Tx; ineffective as antihypertensive monotherapy)	0.25–0.33 mg/kg PO q 24h	0.25 mg/kg PO q 24h	Dual renal-hepatic elimination; sedation, anorexia (both very rare); monitor potassium, renal, and liver values; veterinary formulation not available nor approved in United States	5, 20 mg VM (Canada, Europe, others); 5, 10, 20, 40 mg T HM
Bentyl	*(see dicyclomine)*				
Benzapen	*(see penicillin-benzathine)*				
Benzoyl peroxide (Oxydex, Pyoben)	Acne, seborrhea, pyoderma, pruritus	Shampoo PRN; leave on skin for 10 minutes and rinse. Gel: apply topically q 8–12h	Shampoo PRN; leave on skin for 10 minutes and rinse. Gel: apply topically q 8–12h	Bleaches fabric; may be skin irritant	OTC, VM, HM
Betamethasone (Betasone)	Injectable or topical long-acting steroid	0.1–0.4 mg/kg IM; apply ointment topically PRN up to q 8h	Apply ointment topically PRN up to q 8h	Glucocorticoid, adverse effects; 7–10 times the potency of prednisone	2, 5 mg/ml I, VM; 0.6 mg T; 3 mg/ml I HM
Betapace	*(see sotalol)*				
Betasone	*(see betamethasone)*				
Bethanechol (Urecholine)	Bladder atony (nonobstructive), cholinergic agent	Per dog: 5–25 mg PO total dose, q 8h, or 2.5–15 mg SQ, q 8h	Per cat: 2.5–5.0 mg PO, total dose q 12h	Do not use with obstruction or areflexic bladder; GI adverse effects possible	5, 10, 25, 50 mg T HM
Biaxin	*(see clarithromycin)*				
Biosol	*(see neomycin)*				
Bisacodyl (Dulcolax)	Laxative (stimulant and cathartic)	5–20 mg/dog PO q 24h	5 mg/cat PO q 24h	Short-term use only; may cause cramping, diarrhea	5 mg T OTC, HM
Bismuth subsalicylate (Pepto-Bismol)	GI tract protectant, antidiarrheic, *Helicobacter* protocols	1 ml per 4 kg BW PO up to q 6h	Same with caution due to salicylate composition	Side effect (uncommon): vomiting; causes stool to develop dark grey or black discoloration	17, 35 mg/ml S; 262 mg T OTC, HM

(Continued)

TABLE VI-1 **Drug Formulary—(*Continued*)**

Generic Name (Trade Name)	Indications/ Drug Type	Canine Dose	Feline Dose	Comments	How the Drug Is Supplied
Blood products	From typed donors: 1. Whole, if fresh: RBC, WBCs, platelets, plasma proteins, and coagulation factors; if >8 hours, RBCs and plasma proteins only; packed RBCs for anemia 2. Fresh frozen plasma. 2a. Standard dose, then titrated based on need. 2b. Dose necessary to increase plasma albumin by 1 g/dl. 3. For coagulation factors 4. Cryoprecipitate for vWF, hemophilia A, and fibrinogen deficiencies	1. 5–22 ml/kg slowly IV; rapid if active hemorrhage is present 2. a. 6–10 ml/kg IV b. 45 ml/kg IV 3. 6–10 ml/kg IV 4. 1 unit (225 ml)/ 10 kg BW IV	Same	Precautions are detailed in respective chapters (see Transfusion Reactions, p 1098; Transfusion Therapy and Collection Techniques for Blood Banking, p 1312)	VM, I
Bonine	*(see meclizine)*				
Bovine polymerized hemoglobin	*(see hemoglobin glutamer)*				
Brethine	*(see terbutaline)*				
Breviblock	*(see esmolol)*				
British anti-Lewisite	*(see dimercaprol)*				
Bromide (KBr-generic)	Anticonvulsant	20–35 mg/kg PO q 24h or divided q 12h (if GI signs are a problem); may require an initial loading dose of 400–600 mg/kg given in divided doses with food over a 24-hour period; dose in conjunction with phenobarbital may be lower; adjust based on serum bromide levels and clinical response	Do not use; may trigger severe airway disease (asthma-like) in cats	Used with phenobarbital or alone; may potentiate side effects of sedation, ataxia, and pelvic limb weakness; effective serum range 500–1000 μg/ml in some labs, 1000–2500 μg/ml in others; use ACS grade; some labs use 14-oz KBr powder + 1 L NaCl; 60 ml of this mixture in 8 oz Karo syrup = 400 mg KBr/ml; also available as Na+ salt; may be administered per rectum to achieve more rapid blood levels; dietary chloride intake should be constant: can affect rate of elimination; pancreatitis reported sporadically	400 mg/ml S VM

TABLE VI-1 **Drug Formulary—(*Continued*)**

Generic Name (Trade Name)	Indications/ Drug Type	Canine Dose	Feline Dose	Comments	How the Drug Is Supplied
Bromocriptine (Parlodel)	Dopamine agonist prolactin inhibitor; causes luteolysis	Pyometra: 0.03 mg/kg PO q 8h for 10 days; pregnancy termination: 0.01 mg/kg PO q 8h for 3–4 days		Used in conjunction with prostaglandin F2α inhibitor; adverse side effects include nausea, neurologic signs; mainly seen at higher dose; abortifacient	2.5, 5 mg T HM
Bromo-Seltzer	*(see acetaminophen)*				
Budesonide (Entocort)	Glucocorticoid with minimal systemic effects due to topical GI distribution and rapid first-pass hepatic metabolism; inflammatory bowel disease	Per dog: 1–6 mg PO total dose, q 24–48h; for noninfectious colitis: 1/2 to 1 enema (based on body size) per rectum q 24h after defecation		Dosing limited by formulation (one-size unbreakable capsule); capsule dissolution designed for human ileum, unproven in VM	1, 3 mg C; 2 mg enema HM
Bufferin	*(see acetylsalicylic acid)*				
Bunamidine (Scolaban)	*Taenia, Dipylidium, Echinococcus*	25–50 mg/kg PO once; fast 3 hours before and after administration	Same	V/D rarely observed	100, 200, 400 mg T VM
Buprenex	*(see buprenorphine)*				
Buprenorphine HCl (Buprenex)	Opiate agonist: 1. Analgesia 2. Sedative for medical procedures	1. 0.01–0.02 mg/kg (10–20 μg/kg) IV, IM 2. 0.0075–0.01 mg/kg (7.5–10 μ/kg) IV, IM	0.005–0.01 mg/kg (5–10 μg/kg) IV, IM	Respiratory depression; use cautiously in aged or debilitated patients; neuroleptanalgesia when used with diazepam or acepromazine	0.324 mg/ml I HM
BuSpar	*(see buspirone)*				
Busiprone (BuSpar)	Anxiolytic agent; urine spraying, aggression, repetitive behaviors	Per dog: 2.5–10 mg PO total dose, q 8–12h	Per cat: 2.5–5 mg PO total dose, q 12–24h	Caution when used with hepatic or renal disease; may induce CNS stimulation or depression	5, 10, 15 mg T HM
Butazolidin	*(see phenylbutazone)*				
Butorphanol tartrate (Torbutrol, Torbugesic, Stadol)	Cough suppressant, narcotic agonist/ antagonist, analgesia, sedative	Analgesia, sedation: 0.2–1 mg/kg PO, IM, SQ, q 12h to q 6h; 0.1–0.2 mg/kg IV; antitussive: 0.5–1 mg/kg PO q 6–12h	Analgesia, sedation: 0.1–0.4 mg/kg, SQ, IM, IV, q 6–12h	Vomiting, sedation; possible overexcitement in cats	1, 5, 10 mg T; 1 mg/ml, 10 mg/ml I VM, HM
B vitamins	*(see thiamine, cobalamin)*				
Cabergoline (Dostinex)	Dopamine agonist prolactin inhibitor; causes luteolysis	Pyometra: 0.005 mg/kg PO q 24h for 10 days; pregnancy termination: 0.005 mg/kg PO q 8h for 3–4 days	—	Abortifacient	0.5 mg T HM
Calan	*(see verapamil)*				
Calcet	*(see calcium gluconate)*				
Calcimar	*(see calcitonin)*				
Calcitonin (Calcimar, Miacalcin)	Reduces serum calcium in hypercalcemic states, especially cholecalciferol toxicity	4–8 IU/kg IV, IM, SQ, q 12h	4–8 IU/kg IV, IM, SQ, q 12h	Injections are irritating; GI upset possible	200 IU/ml I HM

(*Continued*)

TABLE VI-1 **Drug Formulary—(*Continued*)**

Generic Name (Trade Name)	Indications/ Drug Type	Canine Dose	Feline Dose	Comments	How the Drug Is Supplied
Calcitriol	Vitamin D analog; hypocalcemia	0.02 μg/kg PO q 24h (hypoparathyroidism) or 0.002–0.004 μg/kg PO q 24h (adjunct treatment of chronic renal failure/renal secondary hyperpara-thyroidism) titrate according to response	Per cat: 0.01–0.04 μg/kg PO q 24h; titrate according to response	Rapid onset of action and short activity (days), versus other drugs (e.g., DHT)	0.25, 0.5 μg C; 1 μg/ml S
Calcium carbonate (Titralac, Tums)	Hypocalcemia, adjunct treatment	1–4 g/day PO	Same	Could cause alkalosis	OTC, HM
Calcium chloride (10% solution)	Ventricular asystole	0.1 ml/kg IV slowly, or IC	Same		100 mg/ml I HM
Calcium EDTA (Versenate, Edetate, Havidote)	Lead, zinc, and other metal poisoning	25 mg/kg SC q 6h for 5 days maximum; dilute in 5% D5W or 0.9% saline	Same	Empty gut of lead prior to use; injection may be painful despite dilution; potentially nephrotoxic	200 mg/ml I HM
Calcium gluconate (Calcet)	Critical hypocalcemia, ventricular asystole	10% infusion: 50–200 mg/kg IV slowly over 15–30 minutes, up to q 6h; 50–150 mg Ca++/kg per day in continuous IV infusion; oral: 150–250 mg/kg PO q 8h	Same	Arrhythmias; monitor ECG and overt response to treatment during infusion; V/D; dystrophic calcification	100 mg/ml I HM
Caninsulin	*(see insulin)*				
Caparsolate	*(see thiacetarsemide)*				
Capoten	*(see captopril)*				
Capstar	*(see nitenpyram)*				
Captan powder 50% (Orthocide)	Dermatomycoses	Mix 2 tbsp per gallon of water, and apply topically every 3–7 days; do not rinse after applying	Same	May induce contact sensitization in humans	VM
Captopril (Capoten)	Vasodilator, CHF, hypertension, ACE inhibitor	0.5–1.5 mg/kg PO q 8–12h	Per cat: 3.125–6.25 mg PO, q 12h total dose	Hypotension-depression, anorexia, V/D; could exacerbate renal failure; less effective and shorter duration of action than most other ACE inhibitors	12.5, 25, 50, 100 mg T HM
Carafate	*(see sucralfate)*				
Carbaryl	Cholinesterase inhibitor for fleas, ticks, cheyletiellic mange	Use as a dip every 7–14 days; do not rinse off; spray q 48h	Same	Do not use on animals under 4 weeks old; cholinesterase toxicity—treat with atropine and bathing; may stain hair yellow	0.5–2% topical solution VM
Carbenicillin (Geocillin, Geopen, Pyopen)	Bacterial infections, broad-spectrum penicillin derivative	40–100 mg/kg IV, IM, SQ q 6–8h (carbenicillin sodium; systemic infections); 10–33 mg/kg PO q 8h (carbenicillin indanyl disodium; UTI)	Same, but do not exceed 55 mg/kg with parenteral formulation	*(see penicillin)*	382 mg T; 1, 2, 5, 10, 20, 30 g I HM
Carbazole	*(see carbimazole)*				

TABLE VI-1 **Drug Formulary—(*Continued*)**

Generic Name (Trade Name)	Indications/ Drug Type	Canine Dose	Feline Dose	Comments	How the Drug Is Supplied
Carbimazole (Carbazole)	Hyperthyroidism; is metabolized to methimazole		Per cat: 5 mg PO total dose, q 8–12h; titrate after 1–3 weeks based on response	Adverse effects similar to methimazole; not available nor approved in United States	5, 20 mg T HM
Carboplatin (Paraplatin)	Antineoplastic for many carcinoma and sarcoma therapies	300 mg/m² IV in D5W over 15 minutes every 3 weeks for 4 treatments	200 mg/m² IV in D5W over 15 minutes every 4 weeks	Myelosuppression; expensive; advantageous to *cis*-platinum (renal); use chemo precautions when handling or administering	50, 150, 450 mg I HM
Cardioxane	*(see dexrazoxane)*				
Cardizem	*(see diltiazem)*				
Cardoxin	*(see digoxin)*				
Caricide	*(see diethylcarbamazine)*				
L-carnitine	AA transports fatty acids into mitochondria for energy metabolism; some dilated cardiomyopathy cases; feline hepatic lipidosis	50–100 mg/kg PO q 8h	50–100 mg/kg PO q 24h for hepatic lipidosis	Expensive in big dogs; to be used with other Tx; effects uncertain	250, 500 mg T/C; 100 mg/ml S HM
Carprofen (Rimadyl)	NSAID with analgesic and antipyretic effects	2 mg/kg PO q 12h	—	Hepatotoxicity: do not use with bleeding disorders, inflammatory bowel disease, or GI ulcers; monitor liver values; do not use with corticosteroids or ASA; may decrease ACE inhibition	25, 75, 100 mg T VM
Carvedilol (Coreg)	α_1-blocking agent with nonselective β-blockade; used in CHF and primary tachycardias	0.1–0.2 mg/kg PO q 24h starting dose; may increase to 0.4 mg/kg PO q 24h	Unknown	Lethargy; GI signs; iatrogenic relapse of CHF; if prior CHF, begin at low dose and increase slowly over several weeks; possible danger in asthmatics	3.125, 6.25, 12.5, 25 mg T HM
Castor oil	Irritant cathartic	8–30 ml PO	4–10 ml PO	Gripping catharsis may develop; do not use if obstructed or atonic	OTC, HM
CCNU	*(see lomustine)*				
CeeNu	*(see lomustine)*				
Cefa-Drops	*(see cefadroxil)*				
Cefadroxil (Cefa-Tabs, Cefa-Drops, Duricef)	First-generation cephalosporin antibiotic	22 mg/kg PO q 8h	Same	First-generation cephalosporin; mainly active against G+	50, 100, 200 mg, 1 g T; 50 mg/ml S, VM; 1 g T; 500 mg C; 25, 50, 100 mg/ml S HM
Cefa-Tabs	*(see cefadroxil)*				
Cefotaxime (Claforan)	Third-generation cephalosporin; G+ and G– organisms and many anaerobes	20–40 mg/kg slow IV, q 8h for 7 days	Same	Pain if injected IM; BM toxicity uncommon	500 mg, 1, 2, 10 g I HM
Cefoxitin (Mefoxin)	Cephamycin grouped with second-generation cephalosporins; some G+, G–, and anaerobic bactericidal activity	10–30 mg/kg IV, q 6–8h	Same	Pain if injected IM; BM toxicity uncommon	1, 2, 10 g vials I HM

(*Continued*)

TABLE VI-1 **Drug Formulary—(*Continued*)**

Generic Name (Trade Name)	Indications/ Drug Type	Canine Dose	Feline Dose	Comments	How the Drug Is Supplied
Cefpodoxime (Simplicef, Vantin)	Third-generation cephalosporin antibiotic	5 mg/kg PO q 12h, or 10 mg/kg PO q 24h	Same	New agent; efficacy against G– organisms and *Staphylococcal* spp.	100, 200 mg T; 10, 20 mg/ml S HM
Ceftiofur (Naxcel)	Third-generation cephalosporin	2.2–4.4 mg/kg SQ, q 12–24h	Same	—	1, 4 g vials I VM
CellCept	*(see mycophenolate mofetil)*				
Centrine	*(see aminopentamide)*				
Cephalosporin antibiotics	Broad-spectrum bactericidal β-lactamase inactivation although second- and third-generation more resistant	10–30 mg/kg PO, SQ, IM, IV, q 12h to q 6h; review each product for specific dosage, handling, and administration	Same	GI side effects, penicillin contra-indications; possibly nephrotoxic at high dosages or if used with aminoglycoside antibiotics	250, 500 mg C; 25, 50, 100 mg/ml S; 1, 2, 20 g vials I VM, HM
Cephulac	*(see lactulose)*				
Cestex	*(see epsiprantel)*				
Charcoal	*(see activated charcoal)*				
Chemet	*(see succimer)*				
Cheque	*(see mibolerone)*				
Chlorambucil (Leukeran)	Lymphoreticular neoplasia, chronic lymphocytic leukemia, macro-globulinemia, feline IBD	2 mg/m^2 PO q 24h for 3 weeks beyond remission; then 1.5 mg/m^2 PO q 24h for 15 days and then every third day; or 0.1–0.2 mg/kg PO q 24–72h	1.5 mg/m^2 PO q 24h as for dog, or 0.1 mg/kg PO q 48–72h; or total dose per cat 2 mg/cat PO q 48h	Bone marrow suppression; usually a second line agent often used with prednisone and/or other agents; use chemo precautions when handling or administering; do not break or crush tablets	2 mg T HM
Chloramphenicol (Chloromycetin)	1. Broad-spectrum bacteriostatic agent; *Mycoplasma, Rickettsia, Chlamydia*, and anaerobic bacteria; excellent lipid solubility (intracellular access)	1. 30–50 mg/kg PO, IV, IM, SQ, q 8h	1. 15–50 mg/kg PO, IV, IM, SQ, q 12h	Hepatic microsomal enzyme inhibitor; may potentiate some Rx-use caution; do not use with "cidal" agents; monitor CBC and chemistries; caution in pregnancy/neonates; avoid human exposure: risk of irreversible human bone marrow suppression	100 mg/ml I; 100, 250, 500 mg; 1 g T VM, HM
	2. 1% ophthalmic ointment: corneal ulcers and infections; 0.5% ophthalmic solution: corneal ulcers and infections	2. Apply to eye q 6h	2. Apply to eye q 4–8h		1% OO, 0.5% OS VM, HM
Chlorhexidine 0.5% (Nolvasan)	1. Topical antiseptic shampoo 2. Topical antiseptic solution	1. Shampoo every 3–7 days 2. Dilute the solution 1:10 with water and apply to lesions, q 8–24h	Same	—	OTC, HM, VM
Chloromycetin	*(see chloramphenicol)*				
Chlorothiazide (Diuril)	Diuretic/hypotensive, nonhormonal Tx for CDI and NDI, urolithiasis—decreased calcium elimination	20–40 mg/kg PO q 12h	Same	Hyponatremia, hypokalemia; use cautiously with digitalis	250, 500 mg T; 50 mg/ml S HM

TABLE VI-1 **Drug Formulary—(*Continued*)**

Generic Name (Trade Name)	Indications/ Drug Type	Canine Dose	Feline Dose	Comments	How the Drug Is Supplied
Chlorpheniramine (Chlor-Trimeton, ChlorTripolon)	Decongestant, antihistamine, antipruritic	Per dog: 2–8 mg PO total dose, q 8–12h	Per cat: 1–2 mg PO total dose, q 8–12h	May cause drowsiness or restlessness; anticholinergic side effects	10 mg/ml I; 0.4 mg/ml S; 2, 4, 8, 12 mg T OTC, HM
Chlorpromazine (Thorazine)	Tranquilization, antiemetic	Oral tranquilization: 1–3 mg/kg PO up to q 6h Sedation: 0.1–1 mg/kg SQ, IM Antiemetic: 0.5 mg/kg IM or IV, up to q 6h	Same	Severe CNS depression with overdosage; may potentiate seizures; use sparingly or not at all in older or systemically ill patients; hypotension	10, 25, 50, 100, 200 mg T; 2 mg/ml S; 25 mg suppository; 25 mg/ml I HM
Chlor-Trimeton	*(see chlorpheniramine)*				
ChlorTripolon	*(see chlorpheniramine)*				
Choledyl	*(see oxtriphylline)*				
Chronulac	*(see lactulose)*				
Ciloxan	*(see ciprofloxacin)*				
Cimetidine (Tagamet)	H_2 receptor antagonist, esophagitis, gastric reflux, chronic gastritis, GI tract ulceration, hypergastrinemia, effects of mast cell tumors	5–10 mg/kg PO q 6–12h; 5 mg/kg IV, q 8h	2.5–5 mg/kg PO q 8–12h	Hepatic microsomal enzyme inhibitor; administer slowly IV	200, 300, 400, 800 mg T; 60 mg/ml S; 150 mg/ml I HM
Ciprofloxacin (Cipro, Ciloxan)	Fluoroquinolone antibacterial agent, broad-spectrum "cidal"; *Mycoplasma*	5–15 mg/kg PO q 12h	—	Incompletely bioavailable in dogs; see other fluoroquinolone comments under *Enrofloxacin*	100, 250, 500, 750 mg T HM
Cisapride (Propulsid, Prepulsid)	Prokinetic serotonergic for feline megacolon; gastroesophageal reflux; first- and second-degree GI motility disorders	0.1–0.5 mg/kg PO q 8–12h	Per cat: 2.5–5 mg total dose PO q 8–12h	Requires adjunctive Rx as stool softener; does not increase gastric secretions; increases esophageal peristalsis; reported to be associated with ventricular arrhythmias in HM and no longer available on the human market; toxic interaction with ketoconazole, cimetidine, macrolide antibiotics	10, 20 mg T; 1 mg/ml S HM
Cisplatin (Platinol)	Solid carcinomas, osteosarcoma	50–70 mg/m² IV every 3–5 weeks; pretreat with IV fluids 12 hours before and after Rx Intracavitary: same protocol, using 50 mg/m² dose diluted into 250 ml 0.9% sterile NaCl and administered into the peritoneal or pleural space immediately after effusion evacuation	None: do not use	Use antiemetic agent; BM suppression; renal toxicity; fatal pulmonary edema in cats; anaphylaxis; use chemo precautions when handling or administering	10 and 50 mg vials I HM
Citrate	*(see potassium citrate)*				

(*Continued*)

TABLE VI-1 **Drug Formulary—*(Continued)***

Generic Name (Trade Name)	Indications/ Drug Type	Canine Dose	Feline Dose	Comments	How the Drug Is Supplied
Claforan	*(see cefotaxime)*				
Clarithromycin (Biaxin)	Broad-spectrum macrolide antibacterial; resistant respiratory or skin infections	5–10 mg/kg PO q 12h	Same	GI, liver disturbances; bone marrow toxicity rarely	250, 500 mg T; 25, 50 mg/ml S HM
Clavamox	*(see amoxicillin/ clavulanic acid)*				
Clemastine fumarate (Tavist products, Contac products, many others)	Antihistamine; allergic skin disease, other allergies, mast cell tumor	0.05–0.1 mg/kg PO q 12h	0.3–0.6 mg/cat PO q 12h	Lethargy/drowsiness or restlessness; caution: other active ingredients in OTC combo formulations	1.34, 2.68 mg T HM OTC
Cleocin	*(see clindamycin)*				
Clindamycin (Cleocin, Antirobe)	Lincosamide antibiotic, G+, *Streptococcus, Staphylococcus*, anaerobes, *Bacteroides*, toxoplasmosis, neosporosis, babesiosis, osteomyelitis	5–10 mg/kg PO q 12h; toxoplasmosis: 5–20 mg/kg PO q 12h	Same; toxoplasmosis: 12.5–25 mg/kg PO q 12h	May cause V/D and very rarely hepatotoxicity; do not use with erythromycin or chloramphenicol Oral solution has unpleasant taste	150 mg/ml I; 25, 75, 150 mg C; 25 mg/ml S VM, HM
Clomicalm	*(see clomipramine)*				
Clomipramine (Anafranil, Clomicalm)	Separation anxiety in the dog, acral lick dermatitis in cats; tricyclic antidepressant agent	1–2 mg/kg PO q 12h	0.5–1 mg/kg PO q 24h	Do not use in breeding dogs or if dog is receiving or has received MAO inhibitors (e.g., anipryl, amitraz, etc); vomiting, lethargy, diarrhea, and polydipsia are adverse reactions most often noted; caution in animals with GI motility or seizure disorders	5, 20, 40, 80 mg T VM
Clonazepam (Klonopin)	Seizure disorders, panic disorders, sedation	0.5 mg/kg PO q 8–12h; titrate as required to effect	—	Second-line seizure Rx; sedation; duration of action in dogs may be short (few hours)	0.5, 1, 2 mg T HM
Clopidogrel (Plavix)	Antiplatelet drug (glycoprotein IIb/IIIa inhibitor)	—	18.75 mg/cat PO q 24h	Emerging application in cats at risk of thromboembolism. Clinical efficacy/safety promising but unproven	75 mg T HM
Cloprostenol	Abortifacient for mismating (early, prior to ossification of fetal bones)	1–2.5 μg/kg SQ, q 24–48h for 5 days	Same	Dilute 1:10 with sterile 0.9% NaCl for accurate dosing	250 μg/ml I VM
Clorazepate (Tranxene)	Second- or third-line antiepileptic drug; benzodiazepine	0.5–1 mg/kg PO q 8h	0.5–1 mg/kg PO q 8h	0.5–1 mg/kg PO q 8h New agent; safety and efficacy profile poorly defined at this time	3.75, 7.5, 15 mg T HM
Clotrimazole (Veltrim, Lotrimin, Mycelex)	Used topically for nasal aspergillosis; also externally for *Malassezia* and other fungi	PRN to fill nasal cavity for nasal aspergillosis (follow precautions and protocol)	—	Intranasal administration requires preplacing catheters surgically or via endoscope; use propylene glycol preparation for this indication	10 mg/ml topical solution OTC, HM

TABLE VI-1 **Drug Formulary—(*Continued*)**

Generic Name (Trade Name)	Indications/ Drug Type	Canine Dose	Feline Dose	Comments	How the Drug Is Supplied
Coal tar (0.5% to 8%)	Shampoo; seborrhea, dermatitis, eczema, keratolytic	Bathe every 3–14 days; leave in contact with skin for 10 minutes and rinse thoroughly	Same	May irritate skin	VM
Cobalamin (vitamin B_{12}, cyanocobalamin)	Used for treating vitamin B_{12} deficiency from exocrine pancreatic disease, SIBO, and in giant schnauzers	Total dose: 250–500 µg (0.25–0.5 mg) per dog IM, SQ once weekly or less, based on serum levels	Total dose: 125–250 µg (0.125–0.25 mg) per cat IM, SQ		1000 µg/ml (= 1 mg/ml) I HM, VM
Codeine	Opiate antitussive	1–2 mg/kg PO PRN, up to q 6h		May cause sedation at higher doses; schedule C-II	15, 30, 60 T HM
Colace	*(see dioctyl sodium sulfosuccinate)*				
Colchicine	Hepatic fibrosis	0.03 mg/kg/day PO q 24h	No reported use	Not well described; GI effects, bone marrow toxicity, teratogenicity possible	0.5, 0.6 mg T HM
Compazine	*(see prochlorperazine)*				
Conofite	*(see miconazole)*				
Cordarone	*(see amiodarone)*				
Coreg	*(see carvedilol)*				
Corid	*(see amprolium)*				
Cortrosyn	*(see ACTH-like solution, aqueous)*				
Cosequin	*(see glucosamine—chondroitin sulfate)*				
Cosyntropin	*(see ACTH-like solution, aqueous)*				
Coumadin	*(see warfarin)*				
Covera	*(see verapamil)*				
Cuprimine	*(see penicillamine)*				
Cyanocobalamin	*(see cobalamin)*				
Cyclophosphamide (Cytoxan, Neosar)	Lymphoreticular tumors, solid carcinomas, immune-mediated disease	50 mg/m² (or 2 mg/kg) PO, 4 days on, 3 days off, or use q 48h; or 200–300 mg/m² IV q 3 weeks	Same	GI signs; BM suppression; hemorrhagic cystitis, especially with higher (weekly) dose; alopecia; use with caution; use chemo precautions when handling or administering (see Chemotherapy: Adverse Reactions, p 189); do not crush or break tablets; caution: cyclosporine brand names almost identical (Neosar versus Neoral)	25, 50 mg T; 100, 200, 500 mg and 1 and 2 g vials I HM
Cyclosporine—ophthalmic (Optimmune)	T-lymphocyte inhibitor; KCS in dogs	0.2% ophthalmic ointment or solution in oil base; use one drop/short (1/4-in) strip q 12h in affected eye(s) until improvement occurs, then q 24h	Do not use	May be ophthalmic irritant; monitor for infections	HM, VM, OO, OS; 4 ml olive oil and 1 ml cyclosporine

(*Continued*)

TABLE VI-1 **Drug Formulary—(*Continued*)**

Generic Name (Trade Name)	Indications/ Drug Type	Canine Dose	Feline Dose	Comments	How the Drug Is Supplied
Cyclosporine—systemic (Sandimmune, Atopica, Neoral)	IHA, ITP, perianal fistula, atopic dermatitis, feline necrotizing gingivitis, renal transplantation, other immunosuppressive purposes	1. Emulsion forms: (Neoral, Atopica): 2-5 mg/kg PO q 12h (2-5 mg/kg PO q 24h if concurrent ketoconazole administration) 2. Nonemulsion form: (Sandimmune, very rarely available now): 5-10 mg/kg PO q 12h (5-10 mg/kg PO q 24h if concurrent ketoconazole administration) 3. 2-3 mg/kg slow IV over 4 hours q 12h; dilute to 1 mg/ml in D5W or 0.9% NaCl before administration	Same	Adjust dose to attain good clinical response and 200-500 ng/ml blood level (for autoimmune diseases; 300-800 ng/ml for renal transplant patients). Oral doses based on greater absorption of emulsion forms versus nonemulsion forms; can cause nephrotoxicity (protein-losing nephropathy), gingival hyperplasia; anaphylaxis possible with IV; little clinical experience with IV to date. Caution: cyclophosphamide brand name is almost identical (Neoral versus Neosar)	25, 50, 100 mg C; 100 mg/ml S; 50 mg/ml I, HM; 10, 25, 50, 100 mg C VM
Cypip	*(see diethylcarbamazine)*				
Cyproheptadine (Periactin)	Serotonin and H_1 antagonist: 1. Appetite stimulant via hypothalamic action 2. Feline pica 3. Antihistamine 4. Urine spraying 5. Add-on for feline asthma	3. 1 mg/kg PO q 8-12h	1-5. Total dose = 1-4 mg/cat PO q 12-24h	Can cause excitability or depression, especially at higher doses; vomiting, aggressiveness	4 mg T; 0.4 mg/ml S HM
Cytarabine	*(see cytosine arabinoside)*				
Cytobin	*(see triiodothyronine)*				
Cytomel	*(see triiodothyronine)*				
Cytosar	*(see cytosine arabinoside)*				
Cytosine arabinoside (cytarabine, Cytosar, ARA-C)	Antineoplastic, lymphoma protocol	100 mg/m² SQ or slow IV, q 24h for 2-4 days	Same	Leukopenia-BM suppression, GI toxicity, reconstituted vial good for 48 hours; use along with cancer protocol; use chemo precautions when handling or administering	100, 500 mg; 1 and 2 g vials I HM
Cytotec	*(see misoprostol)*				
Cytoxan	*(see cyclophosphamide)*				
Dacarbazine (DTIC)	Melanoma, sarcoma	800-1000 mg/m² IV, CRI (8 hours) every 3-4 weeks	Not recommended	GI toxicity, BM suppression, extravasation injury	100, 200 mg vials, I HM

TABLE VI-1 **Drug Formulary—(*Continued*)**

Generic Name (Trade Name)	Indications/ Drug Type	Canine Dose	Feline Dose	Comments	How the Drug Is Supplied
Dalteparin	*(see heparin—low molecular weight)*				
Danazol (Danocrine)	Modified androgen; used for ITP, IHA; anabolic; used for prostatic hypertrophy or androgen-dependent neoplasia	5–10 mg/kg PO q 12h	5 mg/kg PO q 12h	Adjunctive Rx for ITP and IHA; hepatotoxicity; bone marrow toxicity possible; immunosuppressive response may take weeks or months; androgen effects faster	50, 100, 200 mg, C HM
Danocrine	*(see danazol)*				
Dapsone (Avlosulfon)	1. Antibacterial-anti-inflammatory agent used for some skin disorders 2. Antiprotozoal/antimycobacterial effects	1. 1 mg/kg PO q 8h 2. 1 mg/kg PO q 8h initially until remission, then 0.3 mg/kg maintenance	Total dose: 25–50 mg per cat PO q 12h	Hepatotoxicity and BM suppression may occur early in therapy; hemolysis, GI signs, skin eruptions possible	25 and 100 mg T HM
Daranide	*(see dichlorphenamide)*				
Daraprim	*(see pyrimethamine)*				
DDAVP	*(see desmopressin acetate)*				
DDVP	*(see dichlorvos)*				
DEC	*(see diethylcarbamazine)*				
Decadron	*(see dexamethasone)*				
Deca-Durabolin	*(see nandrolone decanoate)*				
Decholin	*(see dehydrocholic acid)*				
Deferoxamine (Desferal, DFO)	Iron chelator; treatment of iron toxicity	10–15 mg/kg/hr IV CRI, then titrate based on serum iron levels; alternatively, if CRI not possible, give 10–40 mg/kg IM q 8h for 24–72 hours, based on serum iron levels	—	Arrhythmia, hypotension, wheezing if CRI too rapid; hypocalcemia, thrombocytopenia possible; do not use in cases of renal failure; potential teratogen	500 mg vials I HM
Dehydrocholic acid (Decholin)	Used to stimulate bile flow	10–15 mg/kg PO q 8h for 7–10 days	Same	Do not use with biliary obstruction	HM
Demerol	*(see meperidine HCl)*				
Denosyl	*(see methionine, s-adenosyl)*				
Depakene	*(see valproic acid)*				
Depakote	*(see valproic acid)*				
Depen	*(see penicillamine)*				
Depo-Medrol	*(see methylprednisolone acetate)*				
Depo-Provera	*(see medroxyprogesterone acetate)*				
Deprenyl	*(see selegiline)*				
Deracoxib (Deramaxx)	COX-2-inhibiting NSAID drug; for treatment of osteoarthritis, perioperative pain management	1–2 mg/kg PO q 24h (long-term use); 3–4 mg/kg PO q 24h (max. 7 days)	—	GI signs (vomiting, anorexia)	25, 100 mg chewable T VM
Deramaxx	*(see deracoxib)*				

(Continued)

TABLE VI-1 **Drug Formulary—(*Continued*)**

Generic Name (Trade Name)	Indications/ Drug Type	Canine Dose	Feline Dose	Comments	How the Drug Is Supplied
Dermathycin	*(see thyrotropin)*				
Derm Caps	*(see fatty acid nutritional supplement)*				
DES	*(see diethylstilbestrol)*				
Desferal	*(see deferoxamine)*				
Desitin	*(see zinc oxide)*				
Desmopressin acetate (DDAVP)	1. Vasopressin analog (1-desamino-8-D-arginine-vasopressin) to manage central diabetes insipidus 2. von Willebrand disease	One to four drops intranasally or in subconjunctival sac, q 6–24h (diabetes insipidus) or 1–2 µg/kg SQ, q 24h to q 12h; oral dose not yet determined	Same (intranasal or subconjunctival)	Rhinorrhea, hypersensitivity reactions, water retention; use nasal spray form topically (1.5–4 µg/drop); 40 times stronger than parenteral (4 µg/ml)	10 µg/spray (= 0.1 ml) in 2.5- or 5-ml bottles; 4 µg/ml I; 0.1 and 0.2 mg, T HM
Desoxycorticosterone pivalate (DOCP) (Percorten-V)	Replacement therapy for mineralocorticoid deficiency (hypoadreno-corticism); each 25 mg releases 1 mg DOCA/day for 21–26 days	1 ml/12 kg, q 25 days (i.e., 2 mg/kg) IM or SQ	—	Titrate dosage to effect; monitor serum electrolytes; no glucocorticoid activity; may require oral prednisolone 0.2–0.4 mg/kg per day as adjunctive therapy	25 mg/ml I VM
Dexamethasone (Azium, Dexate, Decadron); Dexamethasone sodium phosphate (SP)	Potent glucocorticoid for anti-inflammatory, immune suppression, hypoadrenocorticism, shock, pituitary-adrenal axis testing	Anti-inflammatory: 0.1–0.2 mg/kg per day PO, SC, or IV; immunosuppressive: 0.2–0.4 mg/kg per day PO, SC, or IV; long-term oral: q 48h best Hypoadrenocorticism: 0.1–0.8 mg/kg IV (initial treatment; e.g., hypovolemic shock) but maintenance = <0.1 mg/kg PO PRN up to q 24h. LDDST = 0.01 mg/kg IV; HDDST = 0.1 mg/kg IV	Same	HPA axis suppression, multiorgan steroid effects; very high CNS doses (e.g., 4–8 mg/kg) of unproven clinical benefit and almost always associated with short-term adverse effects (e.g., severe GI bleeding); if more than several consecutive days of treatment, taper dose gradually before stopping	0.25, 0.5, 0.75, 1, 1.5, 2, 4, 6 mg T; 2, 8, 16 mg/ml I (dexamethasone); 4, 10, 20, 24 mg/ml I (dexamethasone SP) VM, HM
Dexasporin ophthalmic solution or ointment (Maxitrol)	Neomycin, polymyxin, and dexamethasone combination used for steroid-responsive ophthalmic inflammation where a combined antibiotic is desirable	One drop in affected eye q 6–12h	One drop in affected eye q 6–12h	Steroids are contraindicated in some specific eye diseases (e.g., corneal ulcers, feline herpetic keratitis); systemic corticosteroid side effects are possible	0.05% ointment, 0.1% solution HM
Dexadrine	*(see dextroamphetamine)*				
Dexate	*(see dexamethasone)*				
Dexrazoxane (Zinecard, Cardioxane)	EDTA derivative that protects against doxorubicin-induced cardiomyopathy; may also be used for doxorubicin extravasation lesions	10:1 ratio to doxorubicin dose (i.e., administer 10 times more dexrazoxane than doxorubicin); IV CRI over 30 minutes, begun 45 minutes prior to doxorubicin		Myelosuppression possible	250 and 500 mg vials I HM
Dextran (Rheomacrodex)	Hypovolemia, plasma volume expander	Approximately 20 ml/kg IV, titrated to effect	Same	Platelet dysfunction—hemorrhage, circulatory overload	10% dextran in PSS or D5W I HM

TABLE VI-1 **Drug Formulary—(*Continued*)**

Generic Name (Trade Name)	Indications/ Drug Type	Canine Dose	Feline Dose	Comments	How the Drug Is Supplied
Dextroamphetamine (Dexedrine)	Amphetamine; narcolepsy, hyperkinesis	5–10 mg total dose per dog PO q 8h; 0.2–1.3 mg/kg PO PRN	—	—	5 mg T; 5, 10, 15 mg; ER HM
Dextromethorphan	Antitussive	0.5–2 mg/kg PO q 8h	Same	Usually in association with other drugs (i.e., OTC cough syrup viz. Robitussin); efficacy questioned; avoid with moist/ productive coughs; avoid aspirin-containing or acetaminophen-containing combination in cats (OTC)	Many OTC, HM
Dextrose 50%	Hypoglycemia	Administer 1–5 ml IV for hypoglycemic crisis; dilute with sterile water or 0.9% NaCl (three to five times the volume) before administering	1 ml IV for hypoglycemic crisis; dilute as for dogs	Dilution decreases viscosity and reduces risk of perivascular injury if extravasation; repeated dosing in insulinoma may worsen insulin secretion	50% dextrose = 500 mg/ml VM
DFO	*(see deferoxamine)*				
DHT	*(see dihydrotachysterol)*				
Diamox	*(see acetazolamide)*				
Diastat	*(see diazepam)*				
Diazepam (Valium, Diastat)	1. Tranquilizer, component of anesthetic induction protocol 2. Anticonvulsant 3. Muscle relaxant 4. Appetite stimulant (cats) 5. Urine marking/ spraying (cats) 6. Sedative/ anxiolytic	1. With ketamine for sedation/ anesthetic induction: 0.5 mg/kg IV or to effect, maximum 20 mg/dose 2. 0.5–1 mg/kg IV to effect; enema: 1–2 mg/kg made up as 4 mg/ml enema solution; or IV CRI: 0.5 mg/kg/hr, titrated PRN 3. 0.25–1 mg/kg PO q 12h to q 8h 6. 0.05–0.2 mg/kg IV or 0.25–1 mg/kg PO, PRN up to q 12h	1, 2. Total dose: 0.25–2 mg IV per cat, to effect 3, 5. Total dose: 1–2 mg per cat PO q 12h 4. 0.2 mg/kg IV prior to feeding 6. Same as for dog	Sedation; ataxia; paradoxical excitement/ aggression; hepato-pathy in some cats within days or weeks of starting PO; CRI: diazepam is inactivated by light and adsorbs onto plastic; use glass syringe and short tubing if possible; class IV	2, 5, 10 mg T; 5 mg/ml I; 2.5, 5, 10, 15, 20 mg (rectal gel) HM
Diazoxide (Proglycem)	Hypoglycemia associated with insulinoma	5–20 mg/kg PO q 12h	None	Vomiting, anorexia	50 mg C; 50 mg/ml S HM
Dibenzyline	*(see phenoxybenzamine HCl)*				
Dichlorphenamide (Daranide)	Glaucoma; carbonic anhydrase inhibitor	2–4 mg/kg PO q 8h	Same	Weakness, lethargy, diarrhea, hypokalemia, hyperchloremic metabolic acidosis	50 mg T HM

(Continued)

TABLE VI-1 **Drug Formulary—(*Continued*)**

Generic Name (Trade Name)	Indications/ Drug Type	Canine Dose	Feline Dose	Comments	How the Drug Is Supplied
Dichlorvos (Task, Vapona, DDVP)	Hookworms, whipworms, roundworms; flea collars and tags	27–33 mg/kg PO once; 11 mg/kg PO once (puppies); change collar every 4 months	11 mg/kg PO once; change collar every 4 months	Organophosphate toxicity; do not use with constipation, intestinal obstruction, or hepatic, cardiac, or heartworm disease; no effect on larval form of whipworms	10, 20 mg T; 68, 136, 204 mg C; 136, 204, 544 mg paste VM
Dicural	*(see difloxacin)*				
Dicyclomine (Bentyl)	Irritable bowel syndrome, detrusor hyperspasticity causing urge incontinence	0.15 mg/kg PO q 8–12h	—	—	10 mg C; 20 mg T HM
Diethylcarbamazine (DEC, Caricide, Cypip, Filaribits)	1. Heartworm (HW) prophylaxis 2. *Crenosoma* lungworm treatment 3. Ascarid infections	1. 6–7 mg/kg PO q 24h, from start of HW season to 2 months after end of HW season 2. 70 mg/kg PO q 12h, for 3 days 3. 55–100 mg/kg PO; repeat in 10–20 days	55–110 mg/kg PO once for ascarids	Vomiting; may decrease sperm count; anaphylaxis if microfilaria positive dog	50, 60, 100, 120, 180, 200, 300, 400 mg T; 60 mg/ml S; other sizes VM, HM
Diethylstilbestrol (DES)	1. Estrogen-responsive incontinence 2. Perianal gland adenoma, benign prostatic hyperplasia	1. Total dose: 0.1–1 mg per dog PO q 24h for 4–7 days, then once weekly 2. Total dose: 0.25–1 mg per dog PO, q 24–48h for 2–7 days	0.05–0.1 mg/day PO	May induce signs of estrus—decrease to lowest effective dosage; high dosages may cause anemia, leukopenia, thrombocytopenia; ineffective for pregnancy termination; limited availability in U.S. market	1, 5 mg T; 50 mg/ml I; other sizes HM
Difloxacin (Dicural)	Fluoroquinolone antibacterial	5–10 mg/kg PO q 24h; maximum = 30 days		GI effects, cartilage damage possible in pups; avoid in seizure animals	11, 45, 136 mg T VM
Diflucan	*(see fluconazole)*				
Digoxin (Cardoxin, Lanoxin)	Supraventricular tachyarrhythmias, systolic dysfunction; positive inotrope, negative chronotrope, negative dromotrope, baroreceptor upregulator	0.005 mg/kg PO q 12h; maximum dose for largest dog = 0.25 mg PO q 12h; can double dose for first 24 hours only	Total dose: 1/4 of a 0.125 mg tablet per cat PO q 48h	Injectable form not recommended; see also Digoxin Toxicity, p 301	0.125, 0.25 mg T; 0.05 mg/ml S HM
Dihydrotachysterol (DHT, Hytakerol)	Hypocalcemia	0.03–0.06 mg/kg PO, q 24h initially for 2–3 days; then 0.01–0.02 mg/kg PO q 24–48h, titrated to response	Same	Hypercalcemia; monitor serum calcium and patient until well stabilized; when stable, monitor long-term use	0.125, 0.2, 0.4 mg T; 0.125 mg C; 0.2 mg/ml S HM
Dilacor-XL	*(see diltiazem)*				
Dilantin	*(see phenytoin)*				
Dilaudid	*(see hydromorphone)*				
Diltiazem hydrochloride (Cardizem) (sustained release forms: Dilacor-XL, Cardizem CD)	Ca channel blocking agent; hypertrophic cardiomyopathy (in felines), acute SVT	0.5–1.5 mg/kg PO q 8h; for acute SVT: 0.01–0.02 mg/kg IV initial dose; repeat PRN; maximum cumulative IV dose = 1 mg/kg; may start at 0.1–0.2 mg/kg IV if heart is structurally normal	0.8–2.5 mg/kg PO q 12h to q 8h; 10 mg/kg PO q 24h, in sustained release form	Bradycardia, hypotension, anorexia; sustained release form often causes adverse reactions (hepatic, GI) in cats; dose-dependent AV block	30, 60, 90, 120 mg T; 120, 180, 240, 320 mg C; 60, 90, 120, 240, 360, 420 mg; ER HM

TABLE VI-1 **Drug Formulary—(*Continued*)**

Generic Name (Trade Name)	Indications/ Drug Type	Canine Dose	Feline Dose	Comments	How the Drug Is Supplied
Dimenhydrinate (Dramamine, Gravol)	Motion sickness	4-8 mg/kg PO, up to q 8h	Total dose: 12.5 mg per cat PO, up to q 8h	Lethargy, drowsiness; administer 1 hour prior to travel for best antinausea effect	80 mg T; 12.5 mg/ 4 ml S; 50 mg/ml I HM, OTC
Dimercaprol (BAL, British anti-Lewisite)	Chelating agent; heavy metal toxicosis, such as mercury, lead, and arsenic	2.5-5 mg/kg IM (dose of 5 mg/kg used only in acute cases and only on first day) q 4h on days 1 and 2; q 8h on day 3; q 12h for next 10 days	Same	Injections sting; caution: renal insufficiency; sulfurous odor of breath	100 mg/ml I HM
Dimercaptosuccinic acid	*(see succimer)*				
Dimethyl sulfoxide (DoMoSo, DMSO)	1. Topical anti-inflammatory 2. Renal amyloidosis 3. CNS trauma	1. Apply solution topically q 12h to q 8h; use 60% otic solution, q 12h 2. 80 mg/kg SQ, q 48h (dilute solution 1:4 with sterile water) 3. 1 g/kg of 10% solution over 45 minutes IV	None	Erythema, pruritus; investigational except as otic solution; wear gloves; readily absorbed; sulfurous odor of breath; teratogen: not for breeding animals	90% gel; 90% solution; topical VM, HM
Dinoprost	*(see Prostaglandin)*				
Dioctyl sodium sulfosuccinate (docusate, DSS, Colace, Surfak)	Stool softener	One or two 50-mg capsules PO q 12-24h; per rectum: 60-90 ml (8 mg docusate/ml)	One 50-mg capsule PO q 12-24h	Also available as enema preparation for cats and small dogs	25, 50, 100 mg hard caplets OTC, HM, VM
Dipentum	*(see olsalazine)*				
Diphenhydramine HCl (Benadryl Allergy)	H_1 receptor antihistamine	2-4 mg/kg PO q 12h to q 8h; 1-2 mg/kg IM, SC, q 12h	Same	Sedative, anticholinergic, antiemetic; use with caution in seizure animals; avoid IV use (seizures)	25, 50 mg C, T; 2.5 mg/ml S; 10 mg/ml I HM
Diphenoxylate HCl with atropine (Lomotil)	Antidiarrheal, nonanalgesic opiate	0.1-0.2 mg/kg PO up to q 8h; total dose: 0.625-2.5 mg PO per dog, up to q 8h	0.6-1.2 mg total dose per cat PO q 12h	Sedation, constipation, ileus; use with caution in cats (opiate adverse effects) and in patients with respiratory or cardiovascular compromise	2.5 mg T; 0.5 mg/ml S HM
Diprivan	*(see propofol)*				
Dipyrone (Novin)	Antipyretic Injectable NSAID	25 mg/kg SQ, IM, IV, up to q 8h	Same	Hypothermia, BM suppression; do not use if hyperthermia is not true fever (contraindicated if elevated temperature is due to heat stroke, seizures, brachycephalic crisis, etc.)	300 mg T; 500 mg/ml I HM
Disopyramide (Norpace)	Ventricular dysrhythmias, type IA agent	6-22 mg/kg PO q 8h	None	Rarely used; may be used with quinidine or procainamide	100, 150 mg C; 100, 150 mg; ER HM
Dithiazanine iodide (Dizan)	Microfilaricide	6.6-11 mg/kg PO, q 24h for 7-10 days	None	Stains stool purple, V/D, anorexia	10, 50, 100, 200 mg T VM
Ditrim	*(see trimethoprim/ sulfadiazine)*				
Diuril	*(see chlorothiazide)*				

(Continued)

TABLE VI-1 **Drug Formulary—(*Continued*)**

Generic Name (Trade Name)	Indications/ Drug Type	Canine Dose	Feline Dose	Comments	How the Drug Is Supplied
Dizan	*(see dithiazanine iodide)*				
DMSO	*(see dimethyl sulfoxide)*				
DMSO with flucinolone (Synotic)	*(see flucinolone)*				
Dobutamine HCl (Dobutrex)	Inotropic agent for very severe dilated cardiomyopathy; short-term usage, only in ICU setting; β-1 agonist	0.0025–0.02 mg/kg/min (2.5–20 μg/kg/min) IV CRI in sterile LRS, 0.9% NaCl, or D5W	0.004–0.005 mg/kg/min (4–5 μg/kg/min) IV CRI	Use 48 hours maximum; may increase HR; monitor for arrhythmias; continue usual cardiac therapy; cats are very sensitive to Rx and may have seizures; doses above 0.01 mg/kg/min (10 μg/kg/min) in dogs are more likely to be arrhythmogenic	12.5 mg/ml I HM
Dobutrex	*(see dobutamine)*				
DOCP	*(see desoxycorticosterone pivalate)*				
Docusate	*(see dioctyl sodium sulfosuccinate)*				
Dolasetron (Anzemet)	Serotonin-inhibiting central antiemetic	0.3–0.6 mg/kg IV or SC q 12–24h	Same	Dose extrapolated from human medicine; little supportive evidence, negative effects poorly established at this time	20 mg/ml I; 50, 100 mg T HM
Domitor	*(see medetomidine)*				
DoMoSo	*(see dimethyl sulfoxide)*				
Dopamine HCl (Inotropin)	α-1, β-1, and dopaminergic agent; inotropic agent for heart failure; pressor agent—hypotension	0.002–0.008 mg/kg/min (2–8 μg/kg/min) IV CRI in LRS, 0.9% saline, or D5W	Same	Tachycardia, vasoconstriction; requires ICU monitoring; acute renal failure application no longer considered valid; 1. 1–3 μg/kg/min = dopamine receptor stimulation = visceral vasodilation 2. 3–10 μg/kg/min = β-1 cardiac receptor stimulation = positive inotrope 3. >10 μg/kg/min = positive chronotrope = increased cardiac output but also α-1 stimulation, which leads to vasoconstriction, possible reflex bradycardia	40, 80, 160 mg/ml, I HM
Dopram	*(see doxapram)*				

TABLE VI-1 **Drug Formulary—(*Continued*)**

Generic Name (Trade Name)	Indications/ Drug Type	Canine Dose	Feline Dose	Comments	How the Drug Is Supplied
Doramectin (Dectomax)	Avermectin antiparasitic; spirocercosis	0.2 mg/kg SQ q 2 weeks for 3 treatments; if lesions persist, additional treatment with 0.5 mg/kg PO q 24h for 6 weeks has been successful	—	Currently the treatment of choice for canine spirocercosis; caution with avermectin-susceptible individuals and breeds	10 mg/ml I VM
Dorzolamide (Trusopt)	Carbonic anhydrase inhibitor, glaucoma	One drop per eye q 8h, adjusted PRN	Same	Monitor for hypokalemia	2% OS; 5, 10, 15 ml HM
Doxapram (Dopram)	1. Respiratory stimulant 2. Diagnostic aid for laryngeal paralysis suspects	1. 1.5–10 mg/kg once IV; repeat if needed 2. 2.2 mg/kg IV	Same	For puppy/kitten respiratory stimulation, use one to five drops under tongue or via umbilical vein	20 mg/ml I HM
Doxepin (Sinequan)	Tricyclic antidepressant; pruritic dermatoses in dogs, especially if there is a behavioral component	0.5–5 mg/kg PO q 12h		Some antihistamine effects; contraindicated if concurrent MAO inhibitors (e.g., anipryl, amitraz)	10, 25, 50, 75, 100, 150 mg C; 10 mg/ml S HM
Doxorubicin (Adriamycin)	Lymphomas, carcinomas, solid tumors	According to chemo protocol; either 30 mg/m² IV CRI once every 3 weeks (for dogs >10 kg) or 1 mg/kg IV once every 3 weeks (for dogs ≤10 kg); not to exceed total cumulative dose of 250 mg/m²	According to chemo protocol; 20–25 mg/m² once every 3 weeks IV CRI to maximum total dose of 90 mg/m²	Anaphylaxis, BM suppression, GI toxicity, cardiotoxic, severe vesicant (extravasation injury); use chemo precautions when handling or administering drug and with patient's urine and feces; reddish discoloration to urine due to drug pigment	2 mg/ml I HM
Doxycycline (Vibramycin)	Tetracycline antibiotic; *Rickettsia*, *Ehrlichia*, *Haemobartonella*/*Anaplasma*, and *Chlamydia* infections; brucellosis; intracellular penetration	5 mg/kg PO q 24h; 2–5 mg/kg IV CRI q 12h	Same	Do not use in puppies, kittens, or animals that are pregnant; may cause anorexia, vomiting, depression; hyperthermia in cats; photosensitization; administer water post-pilling to reduce esophagitis risk	20, 50, 100 mg T/C; 5, 10 mg/ml S HM
Dramamine	*(see dimenhydrinate)*				
Dramamine II	*(see meclizine)*				
Droncit	*(see praziquantel)*				
DTIC	*(see dacarbazine)*				
Dulcolax	*(see bisacodyl)*				
Duragesic	*(see fentanyl)*				
Duricef	*(see cefadroxil)*				
Ecotrin	*(see acetylsalicylic acid)*				
ECP	*(see estradiol cypionate)*				
Edrophonium Cl (Tensilon)	Diagnostic agent for cholinergic stimulation; myasthenia gravis; may slow some supraventricular tachycardias	0.1–0.2 mg/kg IV; max = 5 mg total dose	Total dose = 0.25–1 mg IV per cat	Muscarinic signs	10 mg/ml I HM
EDTA	*(see calcium EDTA)*				

(Continued)

TABLE VI-1 **Drug Formulary—*(Continued)***

Generic Name (Trade Name)	Indications/ Drug Type	Canine Dose	Feline Dose	Comments	How the Drug Is Supplied
Elavil	*(see amitriptyline)*				
Eldepryl	*(see selegiline)*				
Elixophyllin	*(see theophylline elixir)*				
Ellence	*(see epirubicin)*				
Elmiron	*(see pentosan polysulfate)*				
Elspar	*(see asparaginase, L-)*				
Enacard	*(see enalapril maleate)*				
Enalapril maleate (Vasotec, Enacard)	ACE inhibitor, vasodilator; CHF, systemic hypertension, glomerulopathy	0.5 mg/kg PO, q 24h initially, then to q 12h if necessary	0.25 mg/kg PO q 24h	Hypotension, weakness, anorexia; avoid increasing furosemide dosage when initiating or increasing enalapril dosage; human adverse effects (renal effects, cough, hyperkalemia); very uncommon in the dog	1, 2.5, 5, 10, 20 mg T; 1.25 mg/ml I VM, HM
Enilconazole (Imaverol)	Nasal aspergillosis	10 mg/kg diluted with equal amount sterile water and administered intranasally via tubes placed in frontal sinuses	—	Not approved; possible allergic reactions	Use poultry-grade product; 10% emulsion
Enoxaparin	*(see heparin—low molecular weight)*				
Enrofloxacin (Baytril)	Broad-spectrum fluoroquinolone class antibacterial	2.5–10 mg/kg PO, IM q 12h; double dosage single adminstration per day may be equally effective	2.5–5 mg/kg PO q 24h (this dose is the maximum in cats)	Do not use in puppies or kittens (causes cartilage lesions); cats: avoid doses >5 mg/kg per day and/or long courses of treatment (risk of irreversible retinopathy); caution in seizure patients (as with all fluoro-quinolones); drug interactions (e.g., inhibits theophylline metabolism)	5.7, 22.7, 68 mg T; 22.7 mg/ml I VM
Entocort	*(see budesonide)*				
Ephedrine	Bronchodilator Urinary incontinence	1–2 mg/kg PO q 8–12h	2–5 mg per cat PO q 8–12h	For bronchospasm: usually used in combination with sedatives and/or bronchodilators; use with caution if sympathetic drive could be harmful (heart disease, hypertension, hyperthyroidism, etc.); narrow therapeutic-toxic range; CNS stimulation, restlessness, irritability	25, 50 mg C; 50 mg/ml I HM

TABLE VI-1 **Drug Formulary—(*Continued*)**

Generic Name (Trade Name)	Indications/ Drug Type	Canine Dose	Feline Dose	Comments	How the Drug Is Supplied
Epinephrine (Adrenalin)	α-adrenergic agent and β-adrenergic agent used for inotropic and chronotropic support: 1. Cardiac arrest 2. Bronchodilation 3. Anaphylaxis 4. Hemostasis (topical)	1. 0.0025 mg/kg IV, repeated to effect (= 1 ml of 1:10,000 per 40 kg BW); triple if administering intratracheally 2, 3. 0.025 mg/kg IV, IM, SC 4. Topical use: place 1 or 2 drops after applying pressure to, and dabbing blood from, a persistently bleeding wound	Same	Arrhythmogenic: increases MVO_2; avoid high doses (tachycardia); vasoconstriction; avoid direct sunlight exposure; note: 1:1000 and 1:10,000 solution both commonly available, caution (10-fold difference)	1:1000 (1 mg/ml) I; 1:10,000 (0.1 mg/ml) I Epipen: 0.15 mg (0.15 ml) or 0.3 mg (0.3 ml),one-time dose HM
Epirubicin (Ellence, Pharmorubicin, 4'-epi-doxorubicin)	Anthracycline antineoplastic	Same as for doxorubicin according to chemo protocol (e.g., 30 mg/m², IV CRI, q 21 days)	—	Same as for doxorubicin but with generally fewer adverse effects (especially lesser incidence and extent of cardiotoxicity)	10, 50, 200 mg I (2 mg/ml) HM
EPO	*(see erythropoietin)*				
Epoetin-α	*(see erythropoietin)*				
Epogen	*(see erythropoietin)*				
Epsiprantel (Cestex)	Tapeworms (cesticide)	5.5 mg/kg PO once	2.75 mg/kg PO once	GI signs possible	12.5, 25, 50, 100 mg, T VM
Erythromycin	1. Macrolide antibiotic, GM+ drug, *Campylobacter, Mycoplasma, Rickettsia, Chlamydia* 2. GI prokinetic	1. 10–20 mg/kg PO q 8h 2. 0.5–1 mg/kg PO q 8h	Same	Hypersensitivity; GI upsets	200, 250, 333, 400, 500 mg T; 100 mg/ml I HM
Erythropoietin (EPO, Epoetin, Epogen, r-Hu EPO, Procrit)	Recombinant human erythropoietin	100 U/kg three times per week SQ until RBC levels increase; then 1 time per week thereafter, titrated based on response	Same	Anaphylaxis, hypertension, GI signs; autoantibodies may develop	2000, 3000, 4000, 10,000, 20,000 I HM
Eskalith	*(see lithium carbonate)*				
Esmolol (Brevibloc)	β-blocker with very rapid onset and offset	0.05–0.1 mg/kg/min (50–100 μg/kg/min) IV CRI, titrated to effect	Same	Contraindicated with pre-existing bradycardia, CHF	10 mg/ml HM
Estradiol cyclopentane-propionate (ECP)	Estradiol to terminate pregnancy	—	—	Repeatably shown to be toxic to bone marrow; unpredictable abortefacient; not recommended	—
Estrogen—conjugated (Premarin)	Estrogen derived from pregnant mare serum; used for treating post-ovariohysterectomy estrogen insufficiency causing urinary incontinence	0.625 mg = 1.0 mg DES; use PO for urinary incontinence (see diethylstilbestrol)	—	May induce signs of estrus	0.3, 0.625, 0.9, 1.25, 2.5 mg T HM
Ethanol 20%	Ethylene glycol toxicosis	Dilute to 20% ethanol in saline; administer 5.5 ml/kg IV q 4h for 5 Rx, then q 6h for 4 Rx	Dilute to 20% ethanol in saline; administer 5 ml/kg IV q 6h for 5 Rx, then q 8h for 4 Rx	May cause or exacerbate CNS depression; monitor hydration, electrolytes, acid-base status, perivascular (*continued*)	—

(*Continued*)

TABLE VI-1 **Drug Formulary—(*Continued*)**

Generic Name (Trade Name)	Indications/ Drug Type	Canine Dose	Feline Dose	Comments	How the Drug Is Supplied
				damage. If alternatives are lacking, an 80 proof alcoholic beverage (40% ethanol) such as vodka may be diluted 1:1 in sterile 0.9% NaCl to create a 20% ethanol solution	
Etodolac (EtoGesic, Lodine)	NSAID; selective COX-2 inhibitor for DJD in dogs	10–15 mg/kg PO q 24h		GI and renal toxicity; if long-term, use low dose; do not administer with ASA or corticosteroids	150, 300 mg T VM; 200, 300 mg C; 400, 500 mg T HM
EtoGesic	*(see etodolac)*				
Etretinate (Tegison)	Synthetic retinoid used to treat disorders of keratinization in specific breeds (primarily cocker spaniels)	1 mg/kg PO q 24h	Total dose: 10 mg per cat PO q 24h	Vomiting, anemia KCS, increased liver enzymes, expensive	10, 25 mg C HM
Excedrin	*(see acetaminophen)*				
Famotidine (Pepcid)	H_2 receptor antagonist	0.5–1 mg/kg PO, IV, q 12–24h	0.5 mg/kg PO, IV, q 24h	Advantages over other similar agents: once-a-day dosage, minimal p450 inhibition	10, 20, 40 mg T; 8 mg/ml S; 10 mg/ml I HM, OTC
Fatty acid nutritional supplement (Derm Caps)	Dietary supplement, allergic skin disease, dry skin	One regular capsule PO, q 24h, per 9 kg BW; one ES capsule PO, q 24h, per 25–30 kg BW; one "100s" capsule PO, q 24h, per 45 kg BW	—	GI upset, increased bleeding times, "fishy" breath	Regular, ES, 100s, C VM
Febantel (Rintal)	Acaricidal, phenylguanidine, antiparasitic	10–15 mg/kg PO q 24h for 3 days	Same	Is metabolized to fenbendazole and oxfendazole	27.2, 163.3 mg T VM
Felbamate (Felbatol)	Antiseizure drug used when seizures are refractory to pheno-barbital and bromide	15 mg/kg PO q 8h; can increase to 60 mg/kg PRN		Monitor for BM suppression; hepatotoxic; expensive	400, 600 mg T; 600 mg/tsp S HM
Felbatol	*(see felbamate)*				
Feldene	*(see piroxicam)*				
Feline synthetic pheromones	*(see pheromones, feline synthetic)*				
Feliway	*(see pheromones, feline synthetic)*				
Fenbendazole (Panacur)	Hookworm, whipworm, roundworm, *Taenia, Paragonimus, Filaroides, Giardia, Capillaria*, lungworm *(Aelurostrongylus)*	50 mg/kg PO q 24h for 3 days; repeat in 3 weeks; whipworms, also repeat in 3 months; lung-worms: 50 mg/kg PO, q 24h, for 10 days	Same; not FDA approved	Vomiting (rare); safe in dogs with heart-worms	222 mg/g granules; 100 mg/ml S VM
Fentanyl (Duragesic)	Transdermal opioid patch—usually lasts at least 72 hours; requires 12 hours to be effective; injectable is ultrashort acting	Patches: 5–10 kg = 25 µg/hr; 10–20 kg = 50 µg/hr; 20–30 kg = 75 µg/hr; >30 kg = 100 µg/hr Injectable: 0.01–0.04 mg/kg SC, IM, IV; CRI: 0.003–0.006 mg/kg/hr (3–6 µg/kg/hr) IV	2.5-mg patch	Apply patch to a small clipped area on thorax; never cut patch; prevent human contact with gel surface of patches; avoid heat exposure (e.g., heat-ing pad)—increases absorption; respira-tory depression and hypoventilation	2.5 mg (25 µg/h), 5 mg (50 µg/h), 7.5 mg (75 µg/h), 10 mg (100 µg/h) patches; 0.05 mg/ml (50 µg/ml) I, HM; former VM injectable (Innovar) was eight times more concentrated than human injectable; do not confuse.

TABLE VI-1 **Drug Formulary—*(Continued)***

Generic Name (Trade Name)	Indications/ Drug Type	Canine Dose	Feline Dose	Comments	How the Drug Is Supplied
Fenthion (Prospot, Spot-on)	Organophosphate insecticide	4–8 mg/kg topically to unbroken skin; follow instructions; do not apply more than once every 2 weeks	None	Do not use with other cholinesterase inhibiting agents; do not use in puppies or sick or debilitated dogs	5.6 and 13.8% solution VM
Ferric cyanoferrate (Prussian blue, Radiogardase)	Thallium poisoning	100–200 mg/kg PO q 8h	None	Administer as capsule or in a glucose solution orally; constipation, vomiting	500 mg C HM
Ferrous sulfate	Iron supplementation	Total dose: 100–300 mg per dog PO q 24h	Total dose: 50–100 mg per cat PO q 24h	Common side effect: minor GI upset; overdose: severe GI signs, hypotension, collapse; delayed toxicity = pulmonary edema, liver failure (*see deferoxamine*)	325 mg (65 mg Fe) T; 18, 44 mg Fe/5 ml S HM, OTC
Feverall	*(see acetaminophen)*				
Fiber (soluble dietary)	*(see psyllium mucilloid)*				
Filaribits	*(see diethylcarbamazine)*				
Filgrastim (Neupogen, r-Hu G-CSF)	Recombinant human granulocyte colony-stimulating factor; used for chemotherapy-induced neutropenia	1–5 μg/kg per day SQ for 3–5 days maximum	1–5 μg/kg per day SQ for 3–5 days maximum	Antibodies develop after several days of therapy	300 μg/ml I HM
Finasteride (Proscar)	Used for treating benign prostatic hyperplasia by inhibiting enzyme that changes testosterone to active dihydroxy-testosterone	Total dose: 5 mg per dog (BW 10–40 kg) PO q 24h	—	Little published objective information about use, efficacy, or side effects in canine medicine	1, 5 mg T HM
Fipronil (Frontline)	Topical parasiticide for fleas and ticks	9.7% solution; apply topically by weight once monthly	Same	Keep away from children, food, water; avoid contact with pet if fipronil is still wet on skin; use on puppies only if >10 weeks old, kittens if >12 weeks old	9.7% solution, 0.29% spray VM
Flagyl	*(see metronidazole)*				
Fleet	*(see phosphate enemas)*				
Florinef	*(see fludrocortisone)*				
Flovent	*(see fluticasone)*				
Fluconazole (Diflucan)	Imidazole antifungal compound: especially useful for cryptococcosis or CNS/ocular mycoses	2.5–5 mg/kg PO q 24h or divided q 12h	Same; up to 50 mg PO total dose per cat q 12h	Historically was expensive, though generic form now available (cheaper)	50, 100, 200 mg T; 2 mg/ml I HM
Flucort	*(see flumethasone)*				
Flucytosine (Ancobon, Ancotil)	Aspergillosis, cryptococcosis, candidiasis	100 mg/kg PO q 12h, or 25–50 mg/kg PO q 6h	Same	Renal, bone marrow, and hepatotoxicity; may cause GI upset; do not administer to pregnant animals; neurologic side effects in cats	250, 500 mg C; 75 mg/ml S HM

(Continued)

TABLE VI-1 **Drug Formulary—(*Continued*)**

Generic Name (Trade Name)	Indications/ Drug Type	Canine Dose	Feline Dose	Comments	How the Drug Is Supplied
Fludrocortisone (Florinef)	Hypoadrenocorticism, mineralocorticoid replacement therapy	0.1 mg/5 kg PO q 24h or q 12h; adjust dosage by need and laboratory testing	0.1 mg/5 kg per day PO; adjust dosage by need and laboratory testing	Systemic hypertension, PU/PD, weight gain, Cushing's-like side effects possible (some glucocorticoid activity)	0.1 mg T HM
Flumazenil (Romazicon)	Benzodiazepine antagonist, possibly management of hepatic encephalopathy	0.01–0.02 mg/kg IV (titrate depending on benzodiazepine dose)	Same	—	0.1 mg/ml I HM
Flumethasone (Flucort)	Anti-inflammatory, corticosteroid	Total dose: 0.06–0.25 mg PO, IV, IM, SQ, q 24h, per dog; intralesional, intra-articular	Total dose: 0.03–0.125 mg PO, IV, IM, SQ, q 24h, per cat	Glucocorticoid-related side effects	0.0625 mg T; 0.5 mg/ml I VM
Flunixin meglumine (Banamine)	NSAID analgesic agent	0.25–1.0 mg/kg IV, IM, SQ, q 24h; maximum 3–5 days dosage	0.25 mg/kg IV, IM, q 24h; maximum 3–5 days dosage	Platelet dysfunction; ulcerative gastritis; kidney damage; risk often outweighs benefit of use; use with extreme caution; multiple safer alternatives	50 mg/ml I VM
Fluocinolone 0.01% with 60% DMSO (Synotic)	Topical corticosteroid plus DMSO for severe otic inflammation	2–12 drops applied topically to ear, q 12h	Two to four drops applied topically to ear, q 12h	Systemic corticosteroid effects; wear gloves (to avoid transcutaneous absorption by owner/tech/vet)	0.1% otic solution VM
Fluorouracil	Chemotherapy agent for carcinomas	150 mg/m^2 IV weekly or 2–10 mg/kg IV weekly	Do not use	Part of a chemotherapy protocol; bone marrow toxicity, GI toxicity, and neurotoxicity possible	50 mg/ml I HM
Fluoxetine (Prozac)	Serotonin reuptake inhibitor	0.5–2 mg/kg PO q 24h	0.5 mg/kg PO q 24h	Used for treating behavioral disorders; acral lick dermatitis; efficacy uncertain	10 mg T; 10, 20, 40 mg C; 4 mg/ml S HM
Flurbiprofen 0.03% solution (Ocufen)	Topical ocular NSAID	One drop instilled in eye q 12h, adjusted PRN	—	Caution with corneal ulcers; contraindicated in infected corneal ulcers	2.5, 5, 10 ml OS HM
Fluticasone (Flovent)	Inhaled glucocorticoid	One puff PRN, up to q 12–24h	Same	Need inhaler apparatus; some patients are reluctant to accept placement of a mask at first; maximum effect only after 7–14 days of use; see Medication Administration by Inhalation, p 1278	7.9 g and 13 g inhalation canisters (0.044, 0.11, or 0.22 mg [44, 110, or 220 μg] per puff) HM
Folate	B vitamin	Total dose: 2.5–5 mg PO per dog q 24h	Total dose: 2.5 mg PO per cat q 24h	—	5 mg/ml I; 5 mg T HM
Fomepizole (Antizol-Vet, 4-methylpyrazole, 4-MP)	Treatment of known or suspected ethylene glycol toxicity	22 mg/kg IV; then 15, 15, and 5 mg/kg IV at 12, 24, and 36 hours following initial dose; then 3–5 mg/kg IV, q 12h, until recovery	—	Dilute drug properly; monitor renal, electrolyte, and hydration status	1.5-g kit I VM, HM
Fortekor	*(see benazepril)*				
Fragmin	*(see heparin—low molecular weight)*				
Frontline	*(see fipronil)*				

TABLE VI-1 **Drug Formulary—*(Continued)***

Generic Name (Trade Name)	Indications/ Drug Type	Canine Dose	Feline Dose	Comments	How the Drug Is Supplied
Fulvicin	*(see griseofulvin)*				
Fungizone	*(see amphotericin B)*				
Furadantin	*(see nitrofurantoin)*				
Furazolidone (Furoxone)	1. Amebiasis 2. Enteric coccidiosis 3. Giardiasis	1. 2.2 mg/kg PO q 8h for 7 days 2. 8–20 mg/kg PO for 7 days 3. 4 mg/kg PO q 12h for 7 days	Same	—	100 mg T; 3.3 mg/ml S HM
Furosemide (Lasix, Salix)	Potent loop duretic agent; used in acute renal failure; hypercalcemia; hypertension, CHF (especially pulmonary edema), ascites, and fluid retention	0.5–6 mg/kg PO, SQ, IM, IV, q 8–12h	0.5–4 mg/kg PO, SQ, IM, IV, q 8–12h	Use lowest effective dosage; high doses reserved for IV use in acute severe pulmonary edema; monitor for hypokalemia, hyponatremia, and hypochloremic alkalosis; caution: azotemia and dehydration	12.5, 20, 40, 50, 80 mg T; 10 mg/ml S; 50 mg/ml I VM, HM
Furoxone	*(see furazolidone)*				
Gammagard S/D	*(see immunoglobulin)*				
Garamycin	*(see gentamicin)*				
Gemcitabine (Gemzar)	Various forms of neoplasia	10 mg/kg IV CRI over 30 minutes; 275 mg/m^2 IV CRI	25 mg/m^2 diluted and given IV slowly twice weekly, according to chemo protocol	Very new drug in veterinary oncology at time of this writing, with dosage, efficacy, and side effects poorly characterized	200 mg, 1g vials I VM, HM
Gemfibrozil (Lopid)	Lipid-lowering agent	7.5 mg/kg PO q 12h	—	—	300, 600 mg T HM
Gemzar	*(see gemcitabine)*				
Genoptic	*(see gentamicin, ophthalmic)*				
Gentamicin (Garamycin, Gentocin)	Broad-spectrum aminoglycoside antibiotic most effective against G– bacteria	6 mg/kg IV, q 24h, or 2–4 mg/kg IM, SQ, IV, q 8h, maximum 7 days	Same	Higher dosage given q 24h is preferred (less nephrotoxic); not effective orally; do not use in renal failure or dehydrated/hypovolemic patients; reserved for serious identified infections only; not for anaerobic infections; nephrotoxic-ototoxic	50 mg/ml I VM, HM
Gentamicin, otic (Gentocin otic)	Ear infections, especially *Pseudomonas* or *Proteus*	Apply q 8h	Apply q 8h	Includes betamethasone 1 mg/ml, which can have topical and/or systemic corticosteroid effects; ototoxic risk (aminoglycoside)	3 mg/ml otic solution VM, HM
Gentamicin, ophthalmic (Gentocin, Genoptic)	Conjunctival/corneal infections, especially *Pseudomonas*	Apply q 4–8h	Apply q 4–8h	Rarely irritating; a preparation that contains corticosteroids also exists in nearly identical packaging; use caution when selecting product	3 mg/g OO; 3 mg/ml OS VM, HM
Gentocin	*(see gentamicin)*				
Geopen	*(see carbenicillin)*				
Glargine	*(see Insulin)*				

(Continued)

TABLE VI-1 **Drug Formulary—(*Continued*)**

Generic Name (Trade Name)	Indications/ Drug Type	Canine Dose	Feline Dose	Comments	How the Drug Is Supplied
Glipizide (Glucotrol)	Oral hyperglycemic agent; useful in some type II diabetes mellitus in cats	0.25–0.5 mg/kg PO q 12h; generally not recommended	0.25–0.5 mg/kg PO q 12h	Hypoglycemia, GI effects, hepatopathy; eventual loss of efficacy (very common); no objective information available on extended-release formulation in veterinary diabetic patients	5, 10 mg T HM
Glucagon	Provocative testing agent for insulinoma, diabetes mellitus, and hyperadrenocorticism	0.03 mg/kg IV	None	May induce hypoglycemia; 1 unit = 1 mg	1 mg/ml I HM
Glucosamine—chondroitin sulfate (Cosequin)	Chondroprotective agent for osteoarthritis	Small and medium-size dogs: one to two RS capsules PO q 24h; big dogs: 1 to 2 DS capsules PO q 24h, or 2 to 4 RS capsules PO q 24h	One RS capsule PO q 24h	—	RS and DS, C VM
Glucotrol	*(see glipizide)*				
Glycerin 50% solution (oral) (Osmoglyn)	Glaucoma	1–2 ml/kg PO once	Same	50% solution = 500 mg/ml; do not use if anuria, CHF, severe dehydration	220 ml S HM
Glycerin suppositories	Constipation	One suppository per rectum	Same or 3 ml liquid per rectum	—	OTC, HM
Glycopyrrolate (Robinul)	Anticholinergic preanesthetic agent	0.01 mg/kg SQ, IM, IV	Same	Tachycardia, arrhythmias, intestinal ileus, mydriasis, and photophobia; avoid in narrow-angle glaucoma	0.2 mg/ml I VM, HM
Glycosaminoglycan—polysulfated (Adequan)	Chondroprotective agent; slows ± helps heal noninfectious, degenerative, and traumatic arthritis	2–4 mg/kg IM twice weekly for 4 weeks; then once every 2–4 weeks	2 mg/kg IM q 4 days for 6 doses; then PRN	Occasional pain at injection site; possibly inhibits coagulation	100 mg/ml I VM
GoLYTELY (polyethylene glycol-electrolyte solution)	Large bowel evacuant/cathartic	22–33 ml/kg via stomach tube	20–30 ml/kg via stomach tube	Withhold food; administer twice q 2h apart prior to GI endoscopic procedure	Powder or concentrate for dilution HM
Goodwinol	Demodecosis (localized)	Apply topically q 24h	Same	Rotenone, orthophenyl phenol, and benzocaine mixture; efficacy not demonstrated	1.25% Rotenone O VM
Gravol	*(see dimenhydrinate)*				
Griseofulvin (Fulvicin)	Dermatophytoses	50–150 mg/kg PO q 24h to q 12h; 25–50 mg/kg q 24h if using microsize product (U/F); 5–15 mg/kg PO q 12h, if using ultramicrosize product (P/G)	Same	U/F prep better absorbed than regular: therefore, dosage is 50% lower for this formulation; P/G even more so: therefore, dosage is a further 30% lower for this formulation; GI signs, teratogen, granulocytopenia, anemia, hepatopathy	125, 250 500 mg T; 250, 500 mg microsize formulation T; 125, 165, 250, 330 mg ultramicrosize formulation T; 125 mg/5 ml S VM/HM
Havidote	*(see Calcium EDTA)*				
Heartgard-30	*(see ivermectin)*				

TABLE VI-1 **Drug Formulary—(*Continued*)**

Generic Name (Trade Name)	Indications/ Drug Type	Canine Dose	Feline Dose	Comments	How the Drug Is Supplied
Hemoglobin glutamer (Oxyglobin)	Bovine hemoglobin-based oxygen-carrying fluid; used to treat hemolytic, blood loss, or ineffective erythropoietic anemias	10–30 ml/kg IV at 10 ml/kg/hr in a one-time single infusion; some administer partial dosages daily instead	Not licensed; used IV by some at 15 ml/kg IV in a slow single dose or daily split doses	Overdosage may cause cardiopulmonary signs; hemoglobinuria; has no clotting factors; interferes with clinical pathologic testing; half-life *in vivo* = 18–43 hours	125 ml I; single-use bags VM
Heparin	1. Anticoagulation 2. DIC therapy	1. 200–300 IU/kg SQ or IV, q 8h to q 6h, for thromboembolism; increase PTT to 1.5–2.5 times normal or ACT to 1.2–1.4 times normal; 10 IU/kg SQ, q 8h, (minidose therapy for ITP) 2. 50–100 IU/kg SQ, q 6–8h	75–150 IU/kg q 6–8h SQ	Prolongs bleeding time; not thrombolytic; ineffective in the absence of antithrombin III (e.g., protein-losing diseases); "regular" heparin is unfractionated heparin (versus low-molecular-weight heparin)	1000, 2000, 5000, 10,000, 20,000, 40,000 mg/ml I HM
Heparin—low molecular weight (Dalteparin [Lovenox], Enoxaparin [Fragmin])	Anticoagulant	Dalteparin (Fragmin): 100–150 IU/kg SQ, q 12h	Dalteparin (Fragmin): 100–150 IU/kg SQ, q 12h Enoxaparin (Lovenox): 1 mg/kg SQ, q 12h	Outpatient (owner-administered) SQ anticoagulant; main differences versus unfractionated heparin: low-molecular-weight heparin is longer-lasting, more predictable in its activity, apparently more effective, less antigenic (not important in VM), and much more expensive; clinical efficacy and advantages not yet proven in VM	Enoxaparin: 100 mg/ml I; 30, 40, 60, 80, 100, 120, 150 mg I (prefilled syringes) Dalteparin: 10,000 or 25,000 IU/ml I; 2500, 5000, 10,000 IU I (prefilled syringes) HM
Herplex	*(see idoxuridine)*				
Hespan	*(see hetastarch)*				
Hetacillin (Hetacin)	Similar to penicillin	10–20 mg/kg PO q 8h	Same	Penicillin reactions	50, 100, 200 mg T VM
Hetacin	*(see hetacillin)*				
Hetastarch 6% (Hespan)	Colloid and plasma volume expansion, shock, sepsis, head trauma	10–20 ml/kg per day IV	10–15 ml/kg per day IV	Rapid IV bolus initially over 5–10 minutes; titrate crystalloids slowly; volume overload possible	500 ml package of 6% hetastarch in 0.9% NaCl I HM
Hu G-CSF	*(see filgrastim)*				
Humulin	*(see insulin)*				
Hycodan	*(see hydrocodone)*				
Hydralazine (Apresoline)	Arteriolar vasodilator, CHF	0.5–3 mg/kg PO q 8–12h	2.5–5 mg/cat total dose PO q 12h	Hypotension, tachycardia malaise, depression, anorexia	10, 25, 50, 100 mg T; 20 mg/ml S HM
Hydrea	*(see hydroxyurea)*				
Hydrochlorothiazide (HydroDIURIL)	Diuretic, nonhormonal therapy for CDI and NDI, urolithiasis (calcium containing)	2–4 mg/kg PO q 12h, initially; then decrease by 50% or to q 24h	1–2 mg/kg PO q 12h, initially; then decrease by 50% or to q 24h	Hypokalemia; exacerbates digitalis toxicity; dehydration	25, 50, 100 mg T HM

(Continued)

TABLE VI-1 **Drug Formulary—(*Continued*)**

Generic Name (Trade Name)	Indications/ Drug Type	Canine Dose	Feline Dose	Comments	How the Drug Is Supplied
Hydrochlorothiazide/ spironolactone (Aldactazide)	Diuretic plus aldosterone blocker	Use on basis of 1 mg/kg of spironolactone PO q 12–24h	Rarely used	Often used in conjunction with furosemide in chronic, recurrent CHF	25/25 mg T; 50/ 50 mg T HM
Hydrocodone bitartrate (Hycodan)	Narcotic antitussive	0.22 mg/kg PO q 6–24h	Rarely used	Sedation; C-III substance; Hycodan contains hydrocodone 5 mg/tab and homatropine 1.5 mg/tab; constipation (rare)	5 mg T; 1 mg/ml S HM
Hydrocortisone acetate 1% cream	Topical corticosteroid for focal dermatitis	Apply topically q 6–12h	Same	Prolonged usage may result in iatrogenic Cushing's syndrome	1% O HM
HydroDIURIL	*(see hydrochlorothiazide)*				
Hydrogen peroxide 3%	Emetic	0.25–0.5 ml/kg PO (3% solution); repeat once in 5–15 minutes PO if emesis does not occur	Same	Do not use if a caustic agent was ingested, if level of consciousness is decreased, or if the patient is unable to swallow; see Vomiting, Induction of, p 1328	3% topical solution HM OTC
Hydromorphone (Dilaudid)	Analgesia, preanesthetic	0.1–0.2 mg/kg SQ, IM, or IV once or PRN up to q 2–4h	Same	Vomiting common immediately postinjection, bradycardia, second-degree AV block, dysphoria in some cats	1, 2, 4, 10 mg/ml I HM
Hydroxyurea (Hydrea)	Chemotherapeutic compound; disorders of RBC excess, especially polycythemia vera and right-to-left cardiac shunts	20–25 mg/kg PO q 12–24h; when PCV decreases, then 25–50 mg/kg PO q 48h and adjust based on PCV	10–15 mg/kg PO q 24h; then q 48h based on PCV	Anorexia, vomiting, BM suppression possible; monitor CBC regularly	500 mg C HM
Hydroxyzine (Atarax)	H_1 receptor antihistamine for allergic skin disorders	1–2 mg/kg PO q 8–12h	0.5–1 mg/kg PO q 12h to q 8h	Sedative, anticholinergic side effects	10, 25, 50, 100 mg T; 10 mg/5 ml S; 25, 50 mg/ml I HM
Hyoscyamine (Levsin)	Antimuscarinic, inhibits propulsive GI motility	0.003–0.006 mg/kg PO q 8h	Same: infrequently used	Useful in irritable bowel syndrome and functional intestinal disorders; dry mouth; urinary retention; tachycardia	0.125 mg T; 0.125 mg/5 ml S; 0.375 mg ER; 0.5 mg/ml I HM
Hytakerol	*(see dihydrotachysterol)*				
Ibuprofen (Advil, Motrin, Nuprin)	Nonsalicylate, NSAID	Not recommended	Not recommended	Frequently causes GI bleeding and irritation; many safer alternatives	OTC, HM
Idoxuridine (Herplex, Stoxil)	Used for treating feline herpesviral keratitis, KCS		One drop q 4h initially, then q 6–8h	Occasional ophthalmic irritation	0.1% OS HM
Ifex	*(see ifosfamide)*				
Ifosfamide (Ifex)	Various neoplasms	350–375 mg/m² IV once every 3 weeks for three treatments maximum	—	Efficacy under investigation; dosing interval according to chemo protocol; pretreat with mesna and IV diuresis to reduce risk of hemorrhagic cystitis; neutropenia possible	50 mg/ml I

TABLE VI-1 **Drug Formulary—(*Continued*)**

Generic Name (Trade Name)	Indications/ Drug Type	Canine Dose	Feline Dose	Comments	How the Drug Is Supplied
Imaverol	*(see enilconazole)*				
Imferon	*(see iron dextran injection)*				
Imidacloprid (Advantage)	Topical treatment for adult and larval stage of fleas	Apply topically to intact skin; dose monthly by BW from prepackaged cards	Same	Avoid contact with skin, food, or water; avoid eye exposure.	9.1% topical solution VM
Imidocarb (Imizole)	*Babesia gibsoni, Ehrlichia canis;* hepatozoonosis	5–7.5 mg/kg IM or SQ once; repeat in 2–3 weeks	—	Painful injection: give IM; cholinergic side effects	120 mg/ml I VM
Imipenem-cilastatin (Primaxin)	Broad-spectrum bactericidal carbapenem antibacterial	2–10 mg/kg slow IV (over 30 minutes), q 6–8h for 3–5 days	Same	Adverse effects possible: GI, CNS, hypersensitivity; reduce dose if renal compromise	250, 500 mg vials I HM
Imipramine (Tofranil)	Tricyclic antidepressant; behavioral changes, narcolepsy, cataplexy, inappropriate elimination	0.5–2 mg/kg PO q 8–12h	0.5 mg/kg PO q 12–24h, or total dose 2.5–5 mg per cat PO q 12h	Prolonged onset of action, drowsiness, behavioral changes	10, 25, 50 mg T; 125 mg/ml I HM
Imizole	*(see imidocarb)*				
Immiticide	*(see melarsomine)*				
Immunoglobulin (Gammagard S/D, human intravenous immunoglobulin G, IVIG)	Treatment of primary immunodeficient states; also IHA, ITP, and CLL	0.5–1.5 g/kg slow IV infusion	—	Must be given IV; very expensive; hypersensitivity; not reported as first-line therapy	2.5, 5, 10 g single-dose vials I HM
ImmunoRegulin	*(see Propionibacterium acnes)*				
Imodium	*(see loperamide)*				
Imuran	*(see azathioprine)*				
Inocor	*(see amrinone)*				
Inderal	*(see propranolol)*				
Inotropin	*(see dopamine)*				
Insulin (Humulin R, N, U, PZI, Vetsulin, Caninsulin, Glargine)	Diabetes mellitus, diabetic ketoacidosis, severe hyperkalemia	REGULAR: 0.5–1.0 U/kg initially IM or SQ; then q 4–6h. NPH: 0.5–1.0 U/kg q 12–24h SQ. All insulins may be diluted with diluents provided by drug company for more precise administration of small doses	NPH: total dose (starting): 1–2 U per cat SQ, q 24h to q 12h. LENTE, ULTRALENTE, PZI, GLARGINE: total dose 1–3 U per cat SQ, q 12–24h	Dosage variable: adjust and monitor accordingly; these are average approximate dosages; maintain hydration; avoid hypoglycemia and hypokalemia	100 U/ml I HM, VM
Interceptor	*(see milbemycin)*				
Interferon (Roferon)	Immune modulator with antiviral and antiproliferative effects; used for FeLV and FAIDS, leukemia, lymphoma, FIP	1 IU/5 kg BW, PO every 2 weeks to stimulate appetite	Total dose: 30 IU per cat PO: 7 days on, then 7 days off	Studies uncontrolled; used mostly in FeLV+ cats	3, 18, 36 million IU per vial I HM
Iodides	*(see sodium iodide 20%)*				
Ipecac syrup	Induce vomiting	0.25–0.5 ml/kg PO; can repeat once after 5–15 minutes if no vomiting	Not recommended in cats; use 3% hydrogen peroxide PO instead	Do not use with activated charcoal (ineffective)	70 mg/ml S; OTC, HM; many oral OTC; 50 mg/ml I HM
Ipodate (Oragrafin)	Oral radiographic contrast agent with antithyroid effects; used for hyperthyroidism	—	Total dose: 15–100 mg per cat PO q 12h; titrated based on clinical response and T3	Blocks T4 conversion to T3; therefore, blood monitoring = serum T3 levels	500 mg C HM
Iron-dextran injection (Imferon)	Iron-deficiency anemia	10 mg/kg in divided doses IM or total dose 100–300 mg PO per day for one dog	Same: IM or total dose 50–100 mg PO per day for one cat	Irritating IM	Many oral OTC; 50 mg/ml I HM

DRUG FORMULARY

(Continued)

TABLE VI-1 **Drug Formulary—(*Continued*)**

Generic Name (Trade Name)	Indications/ Drug Type	Canine Dose	Feline Dose	Comments	How the Drug Is Supplied
Isoproterenol (Isuprel)	β-adrenergic agonist	0.2 mg in 250 ml 5% dextrose, IV CRI at a rate of 0.05–0.1 μg/kg/min; titrate to effect, adequate HR	0.2 mg in 250 ml 5% dextrose, IV to effect, adequate HR	Increased HR, increased or decreased BP, CNS stimulation, arrhythmogenic	0.2 mg/ml (=200 μg/ml) I HM
Isoptin	*(see verapamil)*				
Isosorbide dinitrate	Orally administered vasodilator	—	—	No recognized therapeutic efficacy in small animals	—
Isotretinoin (Accutane)	Sebaceous adenitis, keratinization disorders, mycosis fungoides, feline acne	1–2 mg/kg PO q 12h; reduce dosage after 1 month if improving	Total dose: 5–10 mg PO q 24h, per cat	GI and CNS effects may occur; if so, reduce dosage by 50% or stop; teratogen; KCS in dogs; other muco-cutaneous side effects	10, 20, 40 mg C HM
Isuprel	*(see isoproterenol)*				
Itraconazole (Sporanox)	Antimycotic fungistatic imidazole compound for blastomycosis, coccidioidomycosis, cryptococcosis; histoplasmosis *M. canis*, dermato-phytosis, candidiasis	5–10 mg/kg PO q 12–24h	5–10 mg/kg PO q 24h; 1.5–3.0 mg/kg PO q 24h	Long-term therapy (months or more) often required; must be taken with food; open capsules and place pellets in food if necessary; antiacid GI drugs will reduce efficacy (decrease absorption); monitor liver status	100 mg C; 10 mg/ml S HM
Ivermectin (Heartgard-30, Ivomec)	GABA agonist, anti-parasiticide 1. Heartworm prophylaxis, microfilaricide 2. Endoparasites 3. Sarcoptic mange 4. Demodectic mange 5. Otodectic mange 6. Cheyletiellosis	1. Prophylaxis: 0.006 mg/kg (6 μg/kg) PO, once monthly; microfilaricide: 0.05 mg/kg (50 μg/kg) once PO, 2–4 weeks after adulticide Rx 2. 0.2 mg/kg (200 μg/kg) PO 3. 0.3 mg/kg (300 μg/kg) PO or 0.2 mg/kg (200 μg/kg) SQ two times, 14 days apart 4. 0.05 mg/kg (50 μg/kg) PO; increase to 0.3 mg/kg (300 μg/kg) by day 5; increase to 0.6 mg/kg (600 μg/kg) once daily PO after 30 days if necessary 5. 0.3 mg/kg (300 μg/kg) PO, SQ, two times at 14 days apart 6. 0.3 mg/kg (300 μg/kg) SQ two times at 21 days apart	1. Prophylaxis: 0.024 mg/kg (24 μg/kg) SQ; repeat in 3–4 wks (usually under 0.1 cc) Same (2) Same (4) Same (5) Same (6)	Do not use in collies or other dogs sensitive to drug (exception: collies and similar breeds usually tolerate low [HW prophylaxis] dose); CNS, vomiting, anaphylaxis; can give injectable solution PO; of questionable value in treating feline heartworm disease; consider testing individual patients prior to treatment for the MDR-1 gene mutation if ivermectin is the treatment of choice in patients where susceptibility to toxicosis is possible (see Ivermectin Toxicosis, p 610)	68, 136, 272 μg T or chewables; 10 mg/ml (=10,000 μg/ml) I VM
Ivomec	*(see ivermectin)*				

TABLE VI-1 **Drug Formulary—(*Continued*)**

Generic Name (Trade Name)	Indications/ Drug Type	Canine Dose	Feline Dose	Comments	How the Drug Is Supplied
Jenotone	*(see aminopropazine)*				
Kaolin/pectin	GI tract protectant	1–2 ml/kg PO q 2–6h	Same	May limit absorption of other Rx; may constipate; products that historically contained kaolin/pectin (e.g., Kaopectate) now often have bismuth subsalicylate or attapulgite instead—check ingredients	Many OTC preparations; T/S VM, HM
Kabikinase	*(see streptokinase)*				
Kaon	*(see potassium salts oral supplement)*				
KBr	*(see bromide)*				
Keflex	*(see cephalosporin antibiotics)*				
Kenalog	*(see triamcinolone)*				
Keppra	*(see levetiracetam)*				
Ketamine HCl (Ketaset, Vetalar)	Dissociative anesthetic agent; short-action when given IV in healthy dogs/cats: 10–20 minutes	When diazepam (at dose of 0.5 mg/kg) given IV first: immediately follow with ketamine 5–7 mg/kg IV bolus for sedation and minor procedures (diazepam [5 mg/ml]: ketamine combination in ratio of 1:1 → use 0.5 ml/10 kg of each [in separate syringes] IV)	Restraint: 11 mg/kg IM; anesthesia (but does not provide deep analgesia): 22–33 mg/kg IM or 2.2–4.4 mg/kg IV	Eyes remain open: use ophthalmic ointment; salivation, seizures, respiratory depression, laryngospasm, hypothermia; do not use with renal failure or glaucoma; reduce dose by 50–75% if stable but systemically ill; avoid if hypertrophic cardiomyopathy; controlled drug	100 mg/ml I VM, HM
Ketaset	*(see ketamine)*				
Ketoconazole (Nizoral)	Antifungal agent; protothecosis; inhibits glucocorticoid synthesis	10–15 mg/kg PO q 12h; long-term 10 mg/kg PO q 24h; Cushing's syndrome Rx: 15 mg/kg PO q 12h	5–10 mg/kg q 12h PO or q 24h; long term: 10 mg/kg q 48h PO	Anorexia, nausea, vomiting, constipation, hepatotoxicity; monitor liver status; begin lower and titrate upwards to reduce risk of side effects; must be given with food (for good absorption); drug interaction potential: DMSO inhibitor; antacids decrease absorption	200 mg T HM
Ketofen	*(see ketoprofen)*				
Ketoprofen (Orudis KT; Ketofen)	NSAID	0.5–1 mg/kg PO q 12h; 1–2 mg/kg SQ, IM, or IV once or q 24h up to 3 days maximum	Same	GI ulceration, renal effects possible	25, 50, 75 mg C; 12.5 mg T, HM, OTC; 5, 10, 20 mg T; 10, 100 mg/ml I, VM (not approved in United States)
Kitten Milk Replacer (KMR)	Milk replacement	—	30 ml per 1/4 lb BW PO daily, divided into three to six meals	—	OTC, VM
Klonopin	*(see clonazepam)*				
KMR	*(see kitten milk replacer)*				

(*Continued*)

TABLE VI-1 **Drug Formulary—(*Continued*)**

Generic Name (Trade Name)	Indications/ Drug Type	Canine Dose	Feline Dose	Comments	How the Drug Is Supplied
Lactulose (Cephulac, Chronulac)	Hepatic encephalopathy is treated by acidifying colon contents, trapping NH_4 that is then expelled; the drug is also a stool softener	0.25–0.5 ml/kg PO q 8–12h. As a retention enema: Total volume = 10–20 ml/kg (consisting of 3 parts lactulose plus 7 parts water) per rectum	Total dose: 1–5 ml PO q 8h, per cat. Enema: same as for dog	Loose stools/ diarrhea; flatulence; cramping; may use per rectum in patients with hepatic coma	666 mg/ml S HM
Lacrilube	*(see artificial tears ointment)*				
Lanoxin	*(see digoxin)*				
Lasix	*(see furosemide)*				
Latanoprost (Xalatan)	Topical prostaglandin analog used in the treatment of glaucoma	One drop to affected eye, q 12–24h	—	Generally effective and potent; may combine with oral carbonic anhydrase inhibitor; one drop equals approximately 0.0015 mg	0.05 mg/ml OS HM
Laxative paste (Laxatone, Cat-a-Lax, etc.)	Oral laxative, hairball Tx	1/2–2 inches PO daily until nonconstipated, then weekly or PRN	Same	Large amounts daily could result in malabsorption (e.g., fat-soluble vitamins)	OTC, S, VM
Leflunomide (Arava)	Autoimmune disorders (IHA, ITP, sterile meningitis, systemic histiocytosis)	1.5–4 mg/kg PO q 24h	—	New agent; beneficial and adverse effects sparsely documented to date; GI and bone marrow effects possible; seek trough serum level of 20 μg/ml	10, 20, 100 mg T HM
Leukeran	*(see chlorambucil)*				
Levamisole (Levasole, Ripercol, Tramisol)	Heartworm microfilaricide, immune stimulant, feline lungworms	10 mg/kg PO, q 24h, 7–14 days as a microfilaricide; 2.5–5 mg/kg PO, q 48h, for immune modulation	2.5–5 mg/kg PO, q 48h, for immune modulation; 10–20 mg/kg PO, q 48h, for *Aelurostrongylus* and *Capillaria*	Salivation, vomiting, shock-like syndrome with excessive microfilaricide death, neurotoxic, sudden death; not FDA approved for small animal medicine	184 mg T; 136 mg/ml S; 11.5% gel VM 50 mg T HM
Levarterenol	*(see norepinephrine)*				
Levasol	*(see levamisole)*				
Levetiracetam (Keppra)	Third-line anticonvulsant for refractory seizures	20 mg/kg PO q 8h, in addition to KBr and phenobarbital	—	Clinical VM use very new as of this writing, few adverse effects reported; can uptitrate if starting dose ineffective; expensive	500 mg T HM
Levophed	*(see norepinephrine)*				
Levothyroxine sodium (Soloxine, Synthroid)	Synthetic thyroid hormone replacement therapy	0.04 mg/kg PO q 12h Myxedema coma: 0.005 mg/kg slow IV q 12h	Total dose: 0.05–0.1 mg PO, q 24h, per cat	Thyrotoxicosis; do not give only on basis of low T4 (assess clinical signs and other lab results); adjust dose based on response and blood levels; concurrent antiepiletics (e.g., phenobarbital) may affect levels; maximum dose for largest dog: 0.8 mg PO q 12h	0.025, 0.05, 0.075, 0.125, 0.15 mg T HM 0.1, 0.2, 0.3, 0.4, 0.5, 0.6, 0.8 mg T VM
Levsin	*(see hyoscyamine)*				

TABLE VI-1 **Drug Formulary—(*Continued*)**

Generic Name (Trade Name)	Indications/ Drug Type	Canine Dose	Feline Dose	Comments	How the Drug Is Supplied
Lidocaine (Xylocaine)	Ventricular arrhythmias, local anesthesia	2–4 mg/kg IV over 1–2 minutes, then 0.5–2 mg/kg every 20–60 minutes, or 0.04–0.08 mg/kg/min (40–80 µg/kg/min) CRI IV; inject up to 4 mg/kg SQ for local anesthesia	0.25–1.0 mg/kg slowly over 5 minutes; give 1–4 mg bolus maximum over 5 minutes; use diluted solution as CRI 0.01–0.04 mg/kg/min (10–40 µg/kg/min)	Give initial bolus slowly; seizures, hypotension; use lidocaine preparations *without* epinephrine for cardiac arrhythmia therapy; use only for life-threatening arrhythmias	20 mg/ml I HM
Lime sulfur solution (LymDyp, Sulfodip)	Bacterial and fungal dermatosis, sarcoptic mange	Dip once to twice weekly; let air dry; use 4–6 weeks (ideally until two to three fungal cultures are negative)	Same	Offensive odor; stains furniture; wear gloves to avoid hypersensitivity	2% dip VM
Lincocin	*(see lincomycin)*				
Lincomycin (Lincocin)	Staphylococcal and anaerobic infections, some *Mycoplasma* infections	15–25 mg/kg PO, IV, IM, q 8–12h	Same	Vomiting, hepatotoxicity; do not use in combination with chloramphenicol or erythromycin	250, 500 mg T, HM; 100, 200, 500 mg T; 50 mg/ml S; 100 mg/ml I VM
Liothyronine, T3 (Cytobin, Cytomel)	T3 suppression testing; treatment of hypothyroidism in dogs that do not absorb levothyroxine	0.004–0.006 mg/kg (4–6 µg/kg) PO q 8h	0.0044 mg/kg (4.4 µg/kg) PO q 12h to q 8h; 0.025 mg (25 µg) PO q 8h, per cat for eight dosages as testing agent for T3 suppression	Thyrotoxicosis	5, 25, 50 µg T HM
Liquiprin	*(see acetaminophen)*				
Lisinopril (Zestril, Prinivil)	ACE inhibitor; CHF, protein-losing nephropathy	0.5–0.75 mg/kg PO q 24h	0.25 mg/kg PO q 24h	Monitor BUN, creatinine; lethargy, anorexia	2.5, 5, 10, 20, 40 mg T HM
Lithane	*(see lithium carbonate)*				
Lithium carbonate (Eskalith, Lithane, Lithotabs)	Increased production of all cell lines by bone marrow	21–26 mg/kg per day PO	Unknown	Nausea, diarrhea, vertigo	300 mg C; 450 mg ER HM
Lithotabs	*(see lithium carbonate)*				
Lodine	*(see etodolac)*				
Lomotil	*(see diphenoxylate with atropine)*				
Lomustine (CCNU, CeeNu)	Nitrosourea alkylating agent for brain tumors, mast cell tumors, relapse or failure to respond to lymphoma therapy	60–90 mg/m^2 PO, once every 3 weeks	—	Neutropenia may develop after 7 days; GI adverse effects, anemia; its active metabolites reach the CNS	10, 40, 100 mg C HM
Loperamide (Imodium)	Opiate antidiarrheal, acute colitis	0.1–0.2 mg/kg PO q 8h	0.1–0.15 mg/kg PO q 12h	Discontinue if not effective within 48 hours; collie sensitivity; CNS adverse effects possible in dogs and cats	2 mg C; 1 mg/5 ml S HM, OTC
Lopid	*(see gemfibrozil)*				
Lopressor	*(see metoprolol)*				
Losec	*(see omeprazole)*				
Lotensin	*(see benazepril)*				
Lotrimin	*(see clotrimazole)*				
Lovenox	*(see heparin—low molecular weight)*				

(*Continued*)

TABLE VI-1 **Drug Formulary—(*Continued*)**

Generic Name (Trade Name)	Indications/ Drug Type	Canine Dose	Feline Dose	Comments	How the Drug Is Supplied
Lufenuron (Program)	Insect development inhibitor; inhibits chitin synthesis: 1. Prevents flea eggs from developing into adults 2. Coccidioidomycosis 3. Dermatophytosis	Administer PO in conjunction with food. 1. 10 mg/kg PO, once every 30 days 2. 5–10 mg/kg PO q 24h 3. 54–100 mg/kg PO once q 2–4 weeks	1. 30 mg/kg PO, one time per month or 10 mg/kg once every 6 months by SQ injection 3. 51–266 mg/kg PO, once	Expensive as long-term daily Rx for fungal disease; efficacy in dermatophytosis questionable; may be combined with milbemycin for control of fleas, heartworms, roundworms, and whipworms	Sold in packets for varying BW by T, S, solution, or 10 mg/ml T or I
Lutalyse	*(see prostaglandin F2-α)*				
Lym-DYP	*(see lime sulfur solution)*				
Lysodren	*(see o,p'-DDD)*				
Macrobid	*(see nitrofurantoin)*				
Macrodantin	*(see nitrofurantoin)*				
Magnesium hydroxide (Milk of Magnesia)	Antacid, laxative	Total dose: 5–10 ml PO, q 4–6h, per dog	—	Cathartic agent at three to five times the antacid dosage; rarely used because high dosing frequency and rebound acid secretion	77.5 mg/g S OTC, HM
Magnesium sulfate	Hypomagnesemia	0.75–1 mEq/kg/day as IV CRI; for hypomagnesemia-associated life-threatening ventricular arrhythmias: 0.15–0.3 mEq/kg slow IV (15–30 minutes) while monitoring for adverse effects	Same	Monitor for acute toxicosis: increased QT interval on ECG; lethargy, hypotension, weakness, collapse	100 mg/ml (0.8 mEq/ml), 125 mg/ml (1 mEq/ml), 500 mg/ml (4 mEq/ml) I HM
Mannitol 20%	Osmotic diuretic used for treating acute glaucoma, cerebral edema, and oliguria/ anuria; aids in elimination of certain toxins (e.g., ethylene glycol)	0.5–1 g/kg IV slowly over 15–20 minutes for anuria; double dosage for acute glaucoma or cerebral edema	Same	Rehydrate patient prior to use; can repeat twice if renal output is not increased; resolubilize (by warming) if crystallized, ensuring to cool to body temperature before administering; overzealous use: circulatory overload/ pulmonary edema	100 mg/ml (10%); 200 mg/ml (20%) I HM
Marbofloxicin (Zeniquin)	Fluoroquinolone class antibiotic	2–4 mg/kg PO q 24h	Not licensed	Anorexia and vomiting; not recommended for rapidly growing dogs due to possible arthropathy; caution in seizure patients (as with all fluoroquinolones)	25, 50, 100, 200 mg T VM
Maxitrol	*(see dexasporin)*				
MCT oil	*(see medium chain triglycerides)*				
Mebendazole (Telmintic)	Hookworm, whipworm, and roundworm	22 mg/kg with food once daily for 3 days	—	Repeat as indicated; V/D may develop; hepatopathies have been incriminated in a small number of cases	VM

TABLE VI-1 **Drug Formulary—(*Continued*)**

Generic Name (Trade Name)	Indications/ Drug Type	Canine Dose	Feline Dose	Comments	How the Drug Is Supplied
Meclizine (Bonine, Dramamine II, Antivert)	Antiemetic, motion sickness	1.25 mg/kg PO q 24h	12.5 mg per cat PO q 24h	Lethargy, CNS depression possible	12.5, 25, 50 mg T OTC HM
Medetomidine (Domitor)	Synthetic α-2 adrenoreceptor agonist; provides sedation-analgesia as chemical restraint for healthy exercise tolerant dogs; useful for sedation of cats that have compensated ("asymptomatic") hypertrophic cardiomyopathy	0.005–0.02 mg/kg (5–20 μg/kg) IM as a single agent; used by some at half or quarter dose in combination with butorphanol, ketamine, morphine, or oxymorphone	0.02 mg (20 μg/kg) IM	Do not use if hypertensive; allow dog or cat to rest quietly after administration; do not use in older, younger (<12 weeks old), sick, or debilitated dogs or cats; reversed with equal volume of atipamezole; reflex bradycardia is result of drug-induced hypertension; do not attempt to "correct" bradycardia with atropine or other antibradycardiac drugs; nonopiate/not controlled; sedation outlasts analgesia	1 mg/ml I VM
Medium chain triglycerides (MCT oil)	Nutritional supplement used in protein-losing diseases (lymphangiectasia) and when long-term triglyceride intake should be reduced, such as in chylothorax	1–2 ml/kg daily in food	Same	May be unpalatable; efficacy not demonstrated; GI upset (V/D)	OTC, HM
Medroxy-progesterone acetate (Depo-Provera, Provera)	Long-acting progesterone compound used for decreasing male dog libido and aggression, rarely as a contraceptive; in cats, used for psychogenic and miliary dermatitis and inappropriate elimination	2–20 mg/kg IM, SQ, every 4–6 months	Total dose: 10–100 mg IM, SQ, every 4 months, per cat	Overdosage may cause cystic endometritis, diabetes mellitus, hypoadrenocorticism, and mammary hyperplasia/ adenocarcinoma; local alopecia may occur; carefully weigh risks versus benefits	2.5, 5, 10 mg T; 150, 400 mg/ml I HM
Mefoxin	*(see cefoxitin)*				
Megace	*(see megesterol acetate)*				
Megestrol acetate (Ovaban, Megace)	Oral progestogen used for delaying estrus and treating canine pseudopregnancy; canine and feline behavioral modification; eosinophilic granuloma and some chronic feline skin disorders	Anestrus Rx: 0.5 mg/kg PO for 32 days; proestrus Rx: 2.0 mg/kg PO for 8 days; behavior modification: 2–4 mg/kg PO, q 24h, for 14 days, then decrease and stop after 6 weeks	Estrus suppression total dose: 5–10 mg PO, q 24h, per cat for 7 days, then twice weekly; same dose as for dog for behavior modification	See specific diseases; do not use in pregnant pets or pets with uterine problems; avoid use with mammary tumors or hyperplasia; may cause PU/PD, polyphagia, diabetes mellitus	5, 20 mg T, VM; 20, 40 mg T HM
Melarsomine (Immiticide)	Organic arsenical for treatment of adult heartworms	2.5 mg/kg IM, q 24h, for two doses at 24 hours apart, or split protocol (preferred): one dose, then 30 days later, two dosages IM at 24 hours apart	None	Painful after few days: give in epaxial muscles; cellulitis or salivation may occur; PTE occurs when worms die; absolute cage rest for 4 weeks post-Tx; not for class IV HW disease	50 mg/vial I VM

(Continued)

TABLE VI-1 **Drug Formulary—*(Continued)***

Generic Name (Trade Name)	Indications/ Drug Type	Canine Dose	Feline Dose	Comments	How the Drug Is Supplied
Meloxicam (Metacam, Mobic)	COX-2-inhibiting NSAID; for treatment of osteoarthritis; perioperative pain management	0.1 mg/kg PO, SC, q 24h (may be preceded by single 0.2 mg/kg loading dose, PO, SC, IV)	Chronic use: 0.025 mg/kg PO q 24h (can be preceded by perioperative dose below as loading dose); perioperative pain control: 0.1–0.2 mg/kg PO, SC, IV once only	GI signs (vomiting, anorexia), GI ulceration, perforation	1.5 mg/ml S; 5 mg/ml I, VM; 7.5, 15 mg T HM
Melphalan (Alkeran)	Multiple myeloma; lymphoreticular and other neoplasms; alkylating agent	0.1 mg/kg PO q 24h for 10 days, then 0.05 mg/kg PO q 24h; or 1.5 mg/m^2 PO q 24h for 7–10 days; or 7 mg/m^2, q 24h, for 5 days every 3 weeks	Same	Anorexia, nausea, vomiting, leukopenia, thrombocytopenia, anemia	2 mg T HM
Meperidine HCl (Demerol)	Narcotic analgesic with short-term (1–4 hours) effect	3–10 mg/kg IM or slow IV PRN	1–4 mg/kg IM PRN	Watch for signs of narcotic overdosage (i.e., sedation, depression, seizures, hypotension, [especially in cats]); can reverse with naloxone	50, 100 mg/ml I; 50, 100 mg T; 10 mg/ml S HM
Mephyton	*(see vitamin K_1)*				
Meropenem (Merrem IV)	Carbapenem antibiotic, especially for G– bacteria (alternative to aminoglycosides)	12 mg/kg SQ, q 12h, or 24 mg/kg IV, q 24h, for UTI	—	Clinical VM use very new at time of this writing; efficacy and side effects sparsely reported	500, 1000 g vial I HM
Merrem IV	*(see meropenem)*				
Mesalamine (5-ASA, Asacol, Pentasa)	Inhibits prostaglandin production in the colon; irritable bowel syndrome, ulcerative colitis	10–20 mg/kg PO q 8h	—	Clinical VM use very new at time of this writing; efficacy unproven; may be infused rectally (enema formulations)	400 mg T; 250 mg C; 4 g/60 ml enema HM
Mesna (Mesnex)	Urothelial protection preceding ifosfamide chemotherapy	Dose is 20% of ifosfamide dose	—	Administered as pretreatment before ifosfamide: reconstitute as 20 mg/ml and give calculated dose as IV bolus, followed by 9 ml/kg 0.9% NaCl IV over 30 minutes, then ifosfamide	100 mg/ml I HM
Mesnex	*(see mesna)*				
Mestinon	*(see pyridostigmine bromide)*				
Metacam	*(see meloxicam)*				
Metamucil	*(see psyllium mucilloid)*				
Methazolamide (Neptazane)	Oral carbonic anhydrase inhibitor, glaucoma	5 mg/kg PO q 8–12h		Induces mild metabolic acidosis (bicarbonaturia); GI and CNS adverse effects possible	25, 50 mg T, HM
Methigel	*(see methionine, DL-)*				

TABLE VI-1 **Drug Formulary—(*Continued*)**

Generic Name (Trade Name)	Indications/ Drug Type	Canine Dose	Feline Dose	Comments	How the Drug Is Supplied
Methimazole (Tapazole)	Feline hyperthyroidism, palliative Rx for canine functional thyroid neoplasia	Total dose 2.5–5 mg PO q 12h, per dog	Total dose 2.5–5 mg PO q 8–12h, per cat	Possible side effects: anorexia, vomiting, and blood dyscrasias; intense facial pruritus; monitor CBC and T4; start at 1/2 dosage, then increase after 7–10 days based on clinical response and T4 level; monitor renal function	5, 10 mg T HM
DL-methionine (Methigel, Albeta)	Urinary acidifier	0.2–1 g PO q 8h, per dog	0.2–1 g PO q 24h, per cat	Contraindicated for renal failure, acidosis, pancreatic disease, hepatic insufficiency/encephalopathy; GI irritability; blood dyscrasias, in cats especially	15 mg/ml S; 200, 200, 500 mg T, C OTC, VM, HM
S-adenosyl methionine (SAMe, Denosyl)	Adjunctive treatment for certain liver diseases, steroid hepatopathy, acetaminophen toxicity	Total dose per dog: 90 mg PO q 24h (small dog), or 225 mg or more PO q 24h (large dog)	Total dose per cat: 90 mg PO q 24h	—	90, 225 mg T VM
Methocarbamol (Robaxin)	Muscle relaxant	20–45 mg/kg PO q 12h to q 8h; 44–220 mg/kg slow IV (few minutes); use high end of dose range if strychnine, metaldehyde, tetanus; maximum = 330 mg/kg per day	20–45 mg/kg PO q 8–12h	Ataxia, sedation, ptyalism, emesis	100 mg/ml I; 500 mg T, VM; 100 mg/ml I; 500, 750 mg T HM
Methotrexate	Antimetabolite, antineoplastic agent that inhibits dihydrofolate reductase; used to treat some cancers or for immunosuppression; sclerosing cholangiohepatitis	0.06 mg/kg PO q 24–48h; or 2.5 mg/m^2 PO q 24–48h	2.5 mg/m^2 PO q 2–3 days	Leukopenia, GI bleeding, hepatotoxicity; see specific cancer or disease state	2.5 mg T; 2.5 mg/ml I HM
Methylene blue (new methylene blue)	1. For treatment of methemoglobinemia in dogs 2. As intraop insulinoma Dx test	1. 1–2 mg/kg slowly IV, once 2. Dilute 3 mg/kg in sterile saline, and administer as CRI	—	Use once only; can induce Heinz body anemia; islet cell tumors = purple (versus pale blue background); best contrast 30 minutes after onset of CRI	10 mg/ml I HM
Methylprednisolone acetate (Depo-Medrol)	Repositol corticosteroid; feline asthma, eosinophilic granuloma complex; for intralesional skin injections	1–2 mg/kg IM, SQ	Same; total dose: 10–20 mg per cat	Glucocorticoid contraindications and side effects	20, 40, 80 mg/ml I VM, HM
Methylprednisolone sodium succinate (Solu-Medrol)	See prednisolone sodium succinate	30 mg/kg slow IV once, then 15 mg/kg IV in 2–6 hours	Same	GI ulcers very common; assess need for this Tx based on acuity (time frame) and severity	40, 125, 500, 1000, 2000 mg/vial I HM
Methyltestosterone	Anabolic drug, androgenic steroid; used in testosterone-responsive incontinence	0.5 mg/kg PO	Same	May increase creatinine and glucose levels	10 mg C HM

(*Continued*)

TABLE VI-1 **Drug Formulary—*(Continued)***

Generic Name (Trade Name)	Indications/ Drug Type	Canine Dose	Feline Dose	Comments	How the Drug Is Supplied
Metoclopramide (Reglan)	Antiemetic with both central (chemoreceptor trigger zone) and peripheral (GI prokinetic) effects; increases LES pressure; promotes gastric emptying	0.2–0.5 mg/kg PO, SQ, q 6–12h, or 1–2 mg/kg per day given as IV infusion over 24 hours	Same	Do not use with GI obstruction, with phenothiazines, or with narcotic analgesics; atropine blocks effect; may increase seizure activity; extrapyramidal effects, avoid in epileptics	5, 10 mg T; 1 mg/ml S; 5 mg/ml I HM
Metoprolol (Lopressor, Toprol XL)	Antiarrhythmic, β-1 selective blockade; may provide support for CHF animals on traditional therapy	0.4–1 mg/kg PO q 8–12h; q 24h for extended release	Total dose: 2–10 mg PO, q 12–24h, per cat	Lethargy, depression; decreased HR; β-blockade-induced CHF; always begin low and titrate up	50, 100 mg T; 50, 100, 200 mg ER; 1 mg/ml I HM
Metronidazole (Flagyl)	Anaerobic infections; antiprotozoal (*Giardia, Entamoeba, Balantidium, Pentatrichomonas*); IBD, SIBO; *Helicobacter* therapy, colitis therapy	10–20 mg/kg PO q 12h; for sepsis: 15 mg/kg slow IV (30-minute infusion) q 12h	Same	Anorexia and vomiting; neurotoxicity and hepatotoxicity may develop at high and/or prolonged dosages; hepatic metabolism; use 7.5 mg/kg PO q 12h if liver disease	250, 500 mg T; 500 mg/100 ml I HM
Mexiletine (Mexitil)	Type 1B antiarrhythmic drug used for treating ventricular arrhythmias; lidocaine-like oral agent	4–10 mg/kg PO q 8–12h	—	Anorexia, depression; CNS stimulatory signs; side effects rare	150, 200, 250 mg C HM
Mexitil	*(see mexiletine)*				
Miacalcin	*(see calcitonin)*				
Mibolerone (Cheque)	Prevents estrus (dogs only); pseudocyesis; synthetic androgenic anabolic steroid	Total dose per dog for estrus suppression (initiate Tx 30 days prior to proestrus): 1. 1–11 kg: 30 μ PO per day, per dog 2. 12–22 kg: 60 μg PO per day, per dog 3. 23–45 kg: 120 μg PO per day, per dog 4. >45 kg, or German shepherd dog (mix), 180 μg PO per day, per dog Pseudocyesis: 10 times above dosage for 5 days PO	—	Do not use in pregnant dogs or in those with renal or hepatic disease	100 μg/ml S VM
Miconazole (Conofite)	Topical antifungal	Apply q 12h to lesion; continue after resolution of lesions for 2 weeks	Same	Contact hypersensitivity; caution: re. zoonosis if dermatophytosis (wear gloves)	OTC, topical cream, and solution HM
Micro-K extencaps	*(see potassium salts)*				
Midazolam (Versed)	Benzodiazepine tranquilizer; three to four times more potent than diazepam	Preanesthetic dose: 0.1–0.3 mg/kg IV, IM, SQ (lower end of range if IV)	0.05–0.3 mg/kg IV, IM, SQ (mid- to lower end of range if IV and/or if combined with ketamine)	Caution if liver disease, avoid if glaucoma	1 mg/ml, 5 mg/ml I HM
Midol	*(see acetaminophen)*				
Mifepristone (Mifeprex, RU-486)	Progesterone receptor antagonist	2.5 mg/kg PO, q 12–24h, for 5 days	—	Abortifacient	200 mg T HM

TABLE VI-1 **Drug Formulary—(*Continued*)**

Generic Name (Trade Name)	Indications/ Drug Type	Canine Dose	Feline Dose	Comments	How the Drug Is Supplied
Milbemycin (Interceptor)	Anthelmintic action in HW prevention, HW microfilaricide, hookworm, and roundworm control; demodicosis; *Pneumonyssoides caninum*	0.5–1.0 mg/kg orally once monthly; 0.5–2.3 mg/kg PO, q 12–24h, 2–4 weeks for demodicosis, longer if skin scrapings fail to clear mites; may use low dose for 30 days, two times after if necessary; 0.5–1.0 mg/kg per week for 3 weeks	—	Test for heartworms prior to initial administration	2.3, 5.75, 11.5, 23 mg T VM
Milk of Magnesia	*(see magnesium hydroxide)*				
Minipress	*(see prazosin)*				
Mintezol	*(see thiabendazole)*				
Misoprostol (Cytotec)	Prostaglandin E-1 analog; used for gastric ulcers (especially those associated with NSAID use)	2–8 μg/kg PO q 8–12h	—	Secretory diarrhea, vomiting, anorexia; may induce abortion in pregnant mammals (also avoid client exposure); side effects are dose dependent	100, 200 μg T HM
Mitaban	*(see amitraz)*				
Mitotane	*(see o,p'-DDD)*				
Mitoxantrone (Novantrone)	Chemotherapeutic agent closely related to doxorubicin but no cumulative cardiotoxicity	5 mg/m² once every 3 weeks IV	6.25 mg/m² once every 3 weeks IV	Depression, GI signs, leukopenia, hepatotoxicity, extravasation injury	2 mg/ml I HM
Mobic	*(see meloxicam)*				
Morphine sulfate	Narcotic analgesic; acute CHF as adjunctive therapeutic agent to relieve anxiety	0.1–1 mg/kg q 2–6h IM, SQ, IV, epidural; or sustained release 1.5–3.0 mg/kg PO q 12h (ER)	0.05–0.2 mg/kg IM, SQ, q 2–6h	Hyperexcitability in cats; vomiting, respiratory, and CNS depression; hypotension, especially if given IV; constipation	30 mg ER; 5, 10, 20 mg suppository; 10, 20 mg/5 ml S; 15, 30 mg T; 2, 4, 5, 8, 10, 15 mg/ml I HM
Motrin	*(see ibuprofen)*				
Moxidectin (Proheart)	1. Avermectin antiparasitic 2. Heartworm prophylaxis, demodicosis	1. HW prevention: 3 μg/kg PO once monthly 2. Demodicosis: 0.2–0.4 mg/kg PO q 24h	—	Not FDA approved; sustained-release injection (Proheart) removed from market due to adverse effects; demodicosis dose: monitor for adverse effects *(see ivermectin)*	30, 68, 136 μg T; large animal product available as 1.3-g tube VM
Mucomyst	*(see acetylcysteine)*				
Mycelex	*(see clotrimazole)*				
Mycophenolate mofetil (CellCept)	Immunosuppression via inhibition of T- and B-cell proliferation; steroid-responsive meningitis-arteritis, necrotizing encephalitis, other immune-mediated disorders	20 mg/kg PO q 12h; reduce to 10 mg/kg PO q 12h after 3–4 weeks if ongoing treatment	—	Clinical use in veterinary medicine still new as of this writing; reported adverse effects include hemorrhagic diarrhea, vomiting, and myelosuppression	250 mg C, 500 mg T, 250 mg/ml S HM
Mycostatin	*(see nystatin)*				
Mydriacyl	*(see tropicamide)*				
Mylepsin	*(see primidone)*				

(Continued)

TABLE VI-1 **Drug Formulary—(*Continued*)**

Generic Name (Trade Name)	Indications/ Drug Type	Canine Dose	Feline Dose	Comments	How the Drug Is Supplied
Naloxone (Narcan)	Narcotic antagonist	0.004–0.04 mg/kg IV, IM, SC	Same	The effect of the narcotic may last longer than the naloxone, requiring redosing; this is particularly true in end-stage liver disease, portosystemic shunts, or with drugs that are P-450 blockers	0.02, 0.4, 1 mg/ml I HM
Naltrexone (ReVia)	Partial opiate antagonist; certain behavioral disorders	1–2.2 mg/kg PO q 12–24h	25–50 mg PO, q 24h, per cat	Contraindicated in hepatopathies; antagonizes opiate drugs (e.g., certain antitussives, antidiarrheals)	50 mg T HM
Nandrolone decanoate (Deca-Durabolin)	Anabolic steroid and bone marrow stimulant (erythropoiesis only)	1 mg/kg/week IM	0.5–1.0 mg/kg per week IM	Give deep IM; do not administer to pregnant or hepato-insufficient animals or animals with hormone-sensitive tumors. C-III drug	100 and 200 mg/ml I HM
Naprosyn	*(see naproxen)*				
Naproxen (Naprosyn, Aleve)	NSAID	1.2–2.8 mg/kg PO, once daily or every other day	Do not use	Severe GI ulceration/ perforation very common; renal, CNS; not a preferred drug; serum half-life is 32–92 hours in dogs; many safer alternatives	200, 250, 375, 500 mg T; 125 mg/ 5 ml S HM
Narcan	*(see naloxone)*				
Naxcel	*(see ceftiofur)*				
Nembutal	*(see pentobarbital)*				
Nemex	*(see pyrantel pamoate)*				
Neomycin (Biosol)	Aminoglycoside used orally for SIBO, hepatic encephalopathy	10–20 mg/kg PO q 8–12h	Same	Ototoxicity and nephrotoxicity are rare with oral dosage; in severe intestinal disease, toxicity may be more likely (systemic absorption)	200 mg/ml S; 100, 500 mg, T VM, HM
Neoral	*(see cyclosporine—systemic)*				
Neosar	*(see cyclophosphamide)*				
Neostigmine (Prostigmin)	Anticholinesterase agent for myasthenia gravis	0.01–0.05 mg/kg IM, SQ, PRN	Same	Muscarinic effects: vomiting, diarrhea, bradycardia are reversed by atropine	0.25, 0.5, 1, 2 mg/ml I; 15 mg T HM
Neo-Synephrine	*(see phenylephrine)*				
Neptazane	*(see methazolamide)*				
Neupogen	*(see filgrastim)*				
Niacinamide (nicotinamide)	Usually used in combination with a tetracycline for immune-mediated dermatopathies	<5 kg: 100 mg PO q 8h; 5–10 kg: 250 mg PO q 8h; >10 kg: 500 mg PO q 8h	—	GI adverse effects possible	50, 100, 125, 250, 500 mg T HM
Niclosamide (Yomesan)	Tapeworm anthelmintic	154 mg/kg PO; fast 24 hours before; repeat in 2–3 weeks	Same	Occasionally soft stools; generally replaced by praziquantel	VM
Nicotinamide	*(see niacinamide)*				
Nilstat	*(see nystatin)*				
Nipride	*(see nitroprusside)*				

TABLE VI-1 **Drug Formulary—(*Continued*)**

Generic Name (Trade Name)	Indications/ Drug Type	Canine Dose	Feline Dose	Comments	How the Drug Is Supplied
Nitenpyram (Capstar)	Flea adulticide; inhibits insect specific nicotinic receptors	Dogs up to 11 kg: total dose 11.4 mg PO per dog, maximum q 24h; dogs >11 kg: total dose 57 mg PO per dog, maximum q 24h	Total dose: 11.4 mg PO per cat, max. q 24h	Onset of action: rapid (minutes to hours), but duration of activity limited (day[s])	11.4, 57 mg T VM
Nitrofurantoin (Furadantin, Macrobid, Macrodantin)	UTIs	4 mg/kg PO q 8h	Same	Oral form used only for UTIs; GI, hepatotoxicity	50, 100 mg T; 5 mg/ml S; 25, 50, 100 mg macrocrystals C HM
Nitroglycerin 2% ointment (Nitrol ointment)	Transdermal venodilator for reducing cardiac preload in acute CHF	Apply 1/4–2 inch strip q 6–8h topically to skin	Apply 1/8–1/4 inch strip q 8h topically to skin	May cause hypotension; apply with glove to hairless region (i.e., pinna or inguinal area); clinical efficacy questionable; nitrate tolerance/loss of efficacy in 48 hours	2% O HM
Nitrol ointment	*(see nitroglycerin)*				
Nitroprusside (Nipride)	Arterial dilator, venodilator; reduces preload and afterload in CHF	1–7 μg/kg/min IV CRI	1–2 μg/kg/min IV CRI	Hypotension; use 2–3 days IV maximum; avoid extravasation	50 mg/vial I HM
Nizatidine (Axid)	H_2 receptor antagonist	5 mg/kg PO q 24h	2.5–5 mg/kg PO q 24h (for colonic motility effects)	Has GI prokinetic effects (via anti-cholinesterase activity)	75, 150, 300 mg T HM
Nizoral	*(see ketoconazole)*				
Nolvasan	*(see chlorhexidine)*				
Norepinephrine (Levophed, Levarterenol)	β-1 and α-agonist; used for treating shock	1–2 ml in 250 ml of 0.9% NaCl, IV CRI to effect	None	Hypertension, tachycardia	1 mg/ml I HM
Norpace	*(see disopyramide)*				
Norvasc	*(see amlodipine)*				
Novantrone	*(see mitoxantrone)*				
Novin	*(see dipyrone)*				
Numorphan	*(see oxymorphone)*				
Nuprin	*(see ibuprofen)*				
Nystatin (Nilstat, Mycostatin, Nystex)	Topical antifungal, oral candidiasis	50,000–150,000 IU PO q 6–8h	100,000 IU PO q 6h	Fungicidal; not appreciably absorbed in GI tract, so useful for topical oral application	100,000 IU/ml S HM
Nystex	*(see nystatin)*				
Octreotide (Sandostatin)	Somatostatin analog with primary inhibitory effect on intestinal and pancreatic secretions; insulinoma, glucagonoma	Total dose: 10–40 μg (0.01–0.04 mg) SQ, q 8h, per dog		Nausea, vomiting, abdominal discomfort	50, 100, 200, 500 μg/ml I HM
Ocufen	*(see flurbiprofen)*				
Ofloxacin (Ocuflox)	Topical fluoroquinolone antibiotic for ophthalmic use	One drop topically in affected eye q 12h; adjust as necessary	Same	Bactericidal G– and G+	3 mg/ml OS HM
Olsalazine (Dipentum)	Salicylate; anti-inflammatory activity in ulcerative colitis (5-ASA)	5–20 mg/kg PO q 8h	Unknown	See sulfasalazine	250 mg C HM
Omeprazole (Prilosec, Losec)	Proton pump acid blocker; used in reflux esophagitis and hyperacidity syndromes	0.7 mg/kg PO q 24h	Total dose: 5 mg per cat PO q 24h	Few side effects noted	10, 20 mg C HM

(Continued)

TABLE VI-1 **Drug Formulary—(*Continued*)**

Generic Name (Trade Name)	Indications/ Drug Type	Canine Dose	Feline Dose	Comments	How the Drug Is Supplied
Oncovin	*(see vincristine)*				
Ondansetron (Zofran)	5-HT3 receptor antagonist (serotonin inhibitor); used in conjunction with emetogenic cancer chemotherapy; used in protracted vomiting unresponsive to other treatments	0.1-0.2 mg/kg IV bolus, q 12h	—	Used before and for 48 hours following specific IV; cancer Rx; efficacy and safety in cats still under investigation; collies could be more sensitive	4, 8 mg T; 2 mg/ml I; 1.25 mg/ml S HM
o,p'-DDD (Lysodren, Mitotane)	Hyperadrenocorticism; selective necrosis of the zonae fasciculata and reticularis of the adrenal gland	25 mg/kg PO q 12h with food to effect (approximately 5-10 days); then 25-50 mg/kg once every 7-14 days to effect (based on monitoring adrenocortical function); give with food	None	Vomiting, diarrhea, weakness, glucocorticoid ± mineralocorticoid deficiency; hepatotoxicity; best if given in divided doses; insulin dose in diabetics may need to be altered	500 mg T VM
Optimmune	*(see cyclosporine—ophthalmic)*				
Oragrafin	*(see ipodate)*				
Oral rehydration solution (ORS; Pedialyte)	Oral electrolyte and glucose replacement	Up to maintenance (60 ml/kg per day PO) and replacement (based on physical exam); PO divided into several doses as low-cost rehydration/ volume expansion	Same	—	Many HM, OTC
Orbax	*(see orbifloxacin)*				
Orbifloxacin (Orbax)	Fluoroquinolone antibacterial	2.5-7.5 mg/kg PO q 24h	Same	May cause arthropathy in immature dogs; caution in seizure patients (as with all fluoroquinolones)	5.7, 22.7, 68 mg T VM
Ormetoprim-sulfadimethoxine	*(see sulfadimethoxine/ ormetoprim)*				
ORS	*(see oral rehydration solution)*				
Orthocide	*(see captan powder 50%)*				
Orudis KT	*(see ketoprofen)*				
Osmoglyn	*(see glycerin 50% solution [oral])*				
Ovaban	*(see megesterol acetate)*				
Oxacillin (Prostaphlin)	Penicillin derivative used for staphylococcal skin infections	22-40 mg/kg PO q 8h; 5-20 mg/kg IV q 6-8h	Same	Best if not given with food; GI upset possible	250 mg/5 ml S; 250, 500 mg C; 250, 500 mg, 1, 2 g I HM
Oxazepam (Serax)	Appetite stimulant (oral benzodiazepine agent)	—	Total dose: 2.5 mg per cat PO once; do not use long term because it can lead to hepatotoxicity	Overdosage results in sedation and incoordination	10, 15, 30 mg C; 15 mg T HM
Oxtriphylline (Choledyl)	Bronchodilator (theophylline derivative)	4-10 mg/kg PO q 8h	4-10 mg/kg PO q 8h	Vomiting, diarrhea, hyperexcitability	100, 200 mg T; 400, 600 mg ER HM
Oxydex	*(see benzoyl peroxide)*				
Oxyglobin	*(see hemoglobin glutamer)*				

TABLE VI-1 **Drug Formulary—(*Continued*)**

Generic Name (Trade Name)	Indications/ Drug Type	Canine Dose	Feline Dose	Comments	How the Drug Is Supplied
Oxymorphone (Numorphan)	Narcotic agonist for analgesia, anesthetic induction, and minor procedures	Preanesthesia: 0.1–0.2 mg/kg IM, SQ; 0.02–0.05 mg/kg IV; analgesia: 0.03–0.2 mg/kg IV, IM, SQ, PRN	0.01–0.1 mg/kg IV, IM, SQ, PRN	Respiratory and CNS depression; hypotension, sedation, bradycardia, feline hyperexcitability; panting (dogs); reverse with naloxone	1, 1.5 mg/ml I HM
Oxytetracycline (Terramycin)	Broad-spectrum bacteriostatic agent; also used for rickettsiae, *Mycoplasma* spp., spirochetes, and chlamydiae; used for treating SIBO	10–20 mg/kg PO q 8h to q 6h; as OO, apply q 12h to q 6h	Same	Do not use in pregnancy (last trimester) or in first month of life (dental staining); GI side effects; photosensitivity; caution with liver and kidney disease; do not administer with antacids, dairy products, or intestinal adsorbents	50, 125 mg/ml I; 250 mg C HM
Oxytocin (Pitocin, Syntocinon)	Pituitary hormone used for uterine inertia; to stimulate milk flow; vasopressive effects and as an antidiuretic	Obstetrics (uterine inertia): 5–25 U IM total dose, every 30 minutes, or 1–2 U/kg; milk production: 2–10 U IM or via intranasal spray	Obstetrics: 2 U/kg IM, every 30 minutes; milk production: 1 U IM	Do not use if birth canal obstructed; refrigerate vial and warm syringe before injection	10 U/ml I; 40 U/ml nasal spray HM
Pamidronate (Aredia)	Bisphosphonate compound; hypercalcemia (e.g., due to cholecalciferol intoxication)	0.65–2 mg/kg diluted in 0.9% NaCl and given as IV CRI	—	Clinical VM use very new at time of this writing; efficacy and adverse effects sparsely reported	30, 60, 90 mg vials I HM
Pamprin	*(see acetaminophen)*				
Panacur	*(see fenbendazole)*				
Panadol	*(see acetaminophen)*				
Pancreatic enzymes (Pancrelipase, Viokase)	Pancreatic exocrine insufficiency	½–2 tsp powder in 1 lb (500 g) of canned food or 2 cups of moistened dry food; allow to stand 15–30 minutes, then feed	Same proportional to size of feeding	Avoid inhaling powder dust; Viokase brand has superior efficacy; gingival bleeding possible	VM, HM
Pancrelipase	*(see pancreatic enzymes)*				
Paracetamol	*(see acetaminophen)*				
Paramite	*(see phosmet dip)*				
Paraplatin	*(see carboplatin)*				
Paregoric	Opiate antidiarrheal	0.05–0.06 mg/kg PO q 12h to q 8h	None	May cause constipation; controlled drug	HM, S
Paroxetine (Paxil)	Selective serotonin reuptake inhibitor	Total dose: 2.5–5 mg PO, q 24h, per dog	Total dose: 1.25–2.5 mg PO, q 24h, per cat	Behavioral changes, anorexia possible; avoid combining with MAO inhibitors (anipryl, amitraz, etc.)	10, 20, 30, 40 mg T; 12.5, 25 mg ER (Paxil CR) T HM
Paxil	*(see paroxetine)*				
Pedialyte	*(see oral rehydration solution)*				
D-penicillamine (Cuprimine, Depen)	Orally active chelating agent for lead and copper; used for aiding in the prevention of cysteine urolithiasis, copper storage disease	10–15 mg/kg PO q 12h	—	Administer on empty stomach if tolerable; may cause vomiting, skin eruptions, and vascular lesions; monitor CBC	250 mg (Depen) T; 125, 250 mg (Cuprimine) C HM

(*Continued*)

TABLE VI-1 **Drug Formulary—(*Continued*)**

Generic Name (Trade Name)	Indications/ Drug Type	Canine Dose	Feline Dose	Comments	How the Drug Is Supplied
Penicillin, benzathine (Benzapen)	G+ infections; some activity against anaerobes; bactericidal	20,000–40,000 U/kg IM, SQ, q 48–72h	Same	Long-acting formulation; do not use with penicillin hypersensitivity; do not use if serious infection is suspected; IM or SQ injection only	150,000 U/ml I VM
Penicillin G procaine (Wycillin, many others)	G+ infections; some activity against anaerobes; bactericidal	20,000–40,000 units/ kg IM, SQ, q 12–24h	Same	Solution for injection is opaque = for IM/ SQ injection only; penicillin hypersensitivity contraindicates	300,000 U/ml I VM
Penicillin G potassium or sodium	G+ infections; some activity against anaerobes; bactericidal	20,000–40,000 U/kg IV, IM, SQ, q 4–6h	Same	Penicillin hypersensitivity contraindicates; may contain high levels K+ (administer judiciously and monitor); solution for injection should be completely transparent; not effective orally	1 million, 5 million, 10 million, and 20 million U vials I HM
Penicillin-V	G+ infections; bactericidal; effective orally	5.5–11 mg/kg PO q 6–8h	Same	250 mg = 400,000 U; avoid if penicillin hypersensitivity; GI upset possible	250, 500 mg T; 125, 250 mg/5 ml S; many other sizes HM
Pentasa	*(see mesalamine)*				
Pentazocine (Talwin)	Narcotic agonist/ antagonist used for short-term analgesia	1–3 mg/kg IM, 2–6 mg/kg PO	2–3 mg/kg SQ, IM, IV	May cause salivation and/or sedation; reverse with naloxone; may cause dysphoria in cats	30 mg/ml I, HM; often combined with other Rx VM, HM
Pentobarbital (Nembutal, pentobarbitone)	Status epilepticus, general anesthesia	Anesthesia: 10–30 mg/kg IV slowly to effect; seizures: 3–15 mg/kg IV slowly to effect	Anesthesia: 10–30 mg/kg IV slowly to effect; seizures: 3–15 mg/kg IV slowly to effect	Respiratory depression and hypotension may develop if used alone or especially with or after diazepam	50 mg/ml I; available as tablets, elixir, suppositories VM, HM
Pentosan polysulfate (Elmiron)	Glycosaminoglycan-like agent; osteoarthritis (dogs); idiopathic cystitis (cats)	10 mg/kg PO or 3 mg/kg IM; given once weekly for 4 weeks	8 mg/kg PO q 12h	Rare adverse effects (e.g., vomiting) in dogs; experimental drug with minimal clinical data in cats; efficacy and safety unproven	100 mg C HM
Pentostam	*(see sodium stibogluconate)*				
Pentothal	*(see thiopental)*				
Pentoxifylline (Trental)	Increases plasticity of RBC membranes; used in many dermatoses, including dermatomyositis	10–25 mg/kg PO q 12h	—	Clinical VM use still new at time of this writing; few adverse effects reported	400 mg T HM
Pepcid	*(see famotidine)*				
Pepto-Bismol	*(see bismuth subsalicylate)*				
Percogesic	*(see acetaminophen)*				
Percorten-V	*(see desoxycorticosterone pivalate)*				
Periactin	*(see cyproheptadine)*				
PGF2-alpha	*(see Prostaglandin)*				
Pharmorubicin	*(see epirubicin)*				

TABLE VI-1 **Drug Formulary—(*Continued*)**

Generic Name (Trade Name)	Indications/ Drug Type	Canine Dose	Feline Dose	Comments	How the Drug Is Supplied
Phenobarbital	Long-acting barbiturate used for seizure control; occasionally used as a sedative	1–2 mg/kg PO q 8–12h; okay to titrate slowly up to 16 mg/kg per day in divided doses; may be given IV as a bolus of 2–15 mg/kg slowly for status epilepticus followed by 2–6 mg/hr CRI if necessary; maintain trough serum levels at 15–45 μg/ml	Same	Ataxia, sedation, PU/PD; long-term (especially if >35 μg/ml serum levels) hepatotoxicity occurs; initial adjustment period is required (liver enzyme inducer); if using higher dose IV, monitor respirations; controlled substance; see also Phenobarbital: Adverse Effects/ Toxicosis, p 844	8, 16, 32, 65, 100 mg T; 15, 20 mg/5 ml S; 30, 60, 65, 130 mg/ml I HM
Phenoxybenzamine HCl (Dibenzyline)	Adrenergic, α-receptor blocking agent; urinary incontinence due to detrusor sphincter dyssynergia	0.25–1 mg/kg PO q 12h	Total dose: 2.5–5 mg PO, q 12–24h, per cat	May result in vomiting, hypotension/ hypertension, rapid HR, miosis; long (4–7 days) onset of action; no effect on postprostatic urethra of cats	10 mg C HM
Phenylbutazone (Butazolidin)	NSAID	10–15 mg/kg PO q 8–12h	Not recommended	Use lowest effective dosage; do not exceed 800 mg per day; may cause vomiting, GI ulceration, BM suppression, nephrotoxicity; incidence of toxicosis is high; not generally recommended	100, 400, 1000 mg T VM, HM
Phenylephrine (Neo-Synephrine)	Postsynaptic α-adrenergic stimulant used as the following: 1. As nasal drops for rhinitis 2. As IV infusion for treatment of hypotension	1. One to two drops intranasal pediatric solution, q 8–24h 2. 1–3 μg/kg per minute as IV CRI, adjusted to effect	Same	May cause nasal irritation if used chronically; vasoconstriction (systemic hypertension) and pupillary dilation if given parenterally (constant BP monitoring necessary); arrhythmogenic in combination with halothane	10 mg/ml I; OS and intranasal OTC products HM
Phenylpropanolamine HCl	α-adrenergic agonist used for treating hormone-responsive urinary sphincter hypotonus (incontinence) by increasing urethral smooth muscle activity	1 mg/kg PO q 8h	1–2 mg/kg PO q 8–12h	Anxiety, dizziness, hypertension, tachycardia, urinary retention; no longer available as human OTC product	50 mg T VM
Phenytoin (Dilantin)	Anticonvulsant agent	—	—	No longer recommended	—
Pheromones, feline synthetic facial (Feliway)	Behavioral disorders, acclimation to new environment	—	Topical application to surroundings	Spray may be applied to objects, or diffuser disseminates product in room	Spray pump or diffuser VM

(*Continued*)

TABLE VI-1 **Drug Formulary—(*Continued*)**

Generic Name (Trade Name)	Indications/ Drug Type	Canine Dose	Feline Dose	Comments	How the Drug Is Supplied
Phosmet dip (Paramite)	Organophosphate dip for fleas, ticks, and canine sarcoptic mange	2 tbsp (1 oz) per gallon H_2O; sponge on and let air dry	Do not use	Wear gloves to use; use once weekly maximum; do not use in puppies if under 8 weeks old; avoid eye exposures; fever, salivation, seizures, and CNS signs suggest organophosphate toxicity (if such signs occur, use atropine injection and wash off dog)	11.6% dip VM
Phosphate (IV supplementation)	*(see potassium phosphate)*				
Phosphate enemas (Fleet)	Treatment of constipation, bowel evacuation	For large dogs, use one adult bottle; for medium dogs, use 1/2 bottle or a pediatric enema; not recommended for use in small dogs (toxicity: hyperphosphatemia/ hypocalcemia)	Not recommended	May cause severe hyperphosphatemia and hypocalcemia in patients weighing <10 kg; do not use if patient is dehydrated, with renal or cardiac failure, or in very sick patients	OTC, HM
Phytonadione	*(see vitamin K_1)*				
Pilocarpine ophthalmic solution	Miotic (muscarinic) agent useful in glaucoma, KCS	1. One drop in affected eye, q 6–12h 2. For KCS: two to five drops of 1% or 2% solution in food, q 24h	Same	Ciliary spasms; systemic signs rare when used topically; adjust dose according to time and response; V/D and better alternatives (cyclosporine) have meant less use for KCS	0.25, 0.5, 1, 2, 3, 4, 6, 8% OS HM
Pimobendan (Vetmedin)	Oral positive inotrope and vasodilator; effective adjunct Tx in CHF caused by DCM in Dobermans but not cocker spaniels	0.25 mg/kg PO q 12h	None	Not approved for VM or human use in United States	1.25, 2.5, 5 mg C VM
Piperacillin (Pipracil)	Broad-spectrum parenteral penicillin	25–50 mg/kg IM or slow IV (20–30 minute infusion), q 8–12h	—	Penetrates blood-brain barrier; CSF: serum concentration ratio = 0.06 (non-inflamed) to 0.3 (inflammatory diseases)	2, 3, 4, 40 g I HM
Piperacillin + tazobactam (Zosyn)	Broad-spectrum parenteral penicillin with β-lactamase inhibitor	3.4 g per dog slow IV (30-minute infusion), q 6h	—	Not compatible with LRS	2, 3, 4 g (with 0.25, 0.375, 0.5 g tazobactam, respectively) I HM
Piperazine	Ascarid infection	50–100 mg/kg PO	Same	Repeat in 3 weeks; vomiting and diarrhea may occur at higher dosages	250 mg T; 100 mg/ml S VM, HM
Pipracil	*(see piperacillin)*				
Piroxicam (Feldene)	NSAID: as primary or secondary Rx for bladder TCC due to immunomodulatory effect; for chronic sterile rhinitis in cats	0.3 mg/kg PO q 48h or q 24h	Chronic sterile rhinitis: same, plus doxycycline, for 2–6 weeks	GI irritation, renal damage possible; must open capsules and put in food for most animals; often coadministered with misoprostol	10, 20 mg C HM
Pitocin	*(see oxytocin)*				

TABLE VI-1 **Drug Formulary—(*Continued*)**

Generic Name (Trade Name)	Indications/ Drug Type	Canine Dose	Feline Dose	Comments	How the Drug Is Supplied
Pitressin	*(see vasopressin)*				
Platinol	*(see cisplatin)*				
Plavix	*(see clopidogrel)*				
Polysulfated glycosaminoglycan	*(see glycosaminogly-can—polysulfated)*				
Potassium bromide (KBr)	*(see bromide)*				
Potassium chloride injection	Treatment and prevention of hypokalemia	Add to IV fluid per liter based on serum K+ level; serum K: 3.5–5 mEq/L = add 20 mEq KCl/L; 3–3.4 mEq/L = add 30 mEq KCl/L; 2.5–2.9 mEq/L = add 40 mEq KCl/L; 2–2.4 mEq/L = add 60 mEq KCl/L; <2 mEq/L = add 80 mEq KCl/L	Same	Never infuse rapidly; rate of infusion must never exceed 0.5 mEq K+/kg/hr; monitor serum K+ regularly	2, 10, 20, 30, 40, 60, 90 mEq/ml I HM
Potassium chloride, oral	*(see potassium salts)*				
Potassium citrate (Urocit-K)	Inhibits Ca oxalate crystal formation in urine; alkalinizing agent for urine	75 mg/kg PO q 12h; 1–2 mEq/kg PO per day		GI irritation; 5 mEq = 540 mg	5, 10 mEq T HM
Potassium gluconate	*(see potassium salts)*				
Potassium phosphate	Hypophosphatemia	0.01–0.03 mM/kg/hr IV	Same	Hyperphosphatemia; recheck serum levels after 6 hours and adjust or stop; for potassium phosphate, 1 mM phosphate = 33 mg/dl phosphate; avoid calcium-containing fluids	5, 10, 15, 30, 50 ml vials (3 mM PO4 and 4.4 mEq K per ml for all) I HM
Potassium salts (Kaon Elixir, Micro-K Extencaps, Tumil-K)	Potassium supplements in various oral formulations	1/4–1 tbsp (or oral paste or caps) PO q 8–12h	1/8–1/4 tbsp (or oral paste or caps) PO q 8–12h	Dose according to deficit; monitor serum K; may cause gastric irritation	Many OTC preparations, different sizes VM, HM
Pralidoxime chloride (2-PAM, Protopam)	Reactivates cholinesterase inactivated by organophosphate	20–50 mg/kg IM or SQ; then q 8–12h, PRN	20 mg/kg IM or SQ, q 6–8h, PRN	Monitor patient continuously; avoid IV administration (may cause acute laryngospasm); do not use for carbamate toxicity	1 g vial I HM
Praziquantel (Droncit)	*Taenia, Dipylidium, Echinococcus, Heterobilharzia*	Use according to instructions on product according to weight; PO or SQ, IM	Same	Fasting not required; do not use in puppies under 4 weeks old or kittens under 6 weeks of age	23, 34 mg T; 56.8 mg/ml VM; 600 mg T HM
Prazosin (Minipress)	α-adrenergic antagonist; balanced vasodilator; decreases urethral smooth muscle tone	Total dose: 0.5–2 mg PO, q 12h or q 8h, per dog	Total dose: 0.5–1 mg PO, q 12h to q 8h, per cat	Hypotension, depression, malaise	1, 2, 5 mg C
Precose	*(see acarbose)*				
Pred Forte	*(see prednisolone, ophthalmic suspension)*				

(*Continued*)

TABLE VI-1 **Drug Formulary—(*Continued*)**

Generic Name (Trade Name)	Indications/ Drug Type	Canine Dose	Feline Dose	Comments	How the Drug Is Supplied
Prednisolone, prednisone	1. Replacement therapy (hypoadrenocorticism) 2. Anti-inflammatory: antipruritic immune system suppression 3. Antineoplastic chemotherapy	1. Anti-inflammatory: 0.5–1 mg/kg PO, IM, SQ, per day 2. Immune suppression: 2–4.4 mg/kg, usually PO, per day 3. 40 mg/m² PO, per day for 7 days; then 20 mg/m² PO, q 48h	Same	PU/PD; polyphagia; suppression of HPA axis: Cushing's syndrome; hepatopathy; opportunistic infections; muscle wasting; connective tissue and skin fragility; taper dosage if used long term	1, 2.5, 5, 10, 20, 25, 50 mg T; 1 mg/ml S; 10, 25 mg/ml I HM, VM
Prednisolone, ophthalmic suspension (Pred Forte)	Steroid responsive inflammation of the lids, conjunctiva, sclera, cornea, and anterior segment of the eye	One drop in affected eye, q 6–12h	Same	Variable strength products (0.12–1%) used as required; do not use with purulent, viral, or fungal infection or with corneal ulcers; systemic side effects are possible but rare	0.12, 0.125, 1% OS HM
Prednisolone sodium succinate (Solu-Delta-Cortef)	Soluble corticosteroid used IV for shock of multiple causes	5–33 mg/kg IV slow bolus; repeat up to q 6h; spinal injury: 30 mg/kg IV	Same	Causes vomiting if administered too rapidly	100, 500 mg vials I VM
Premarin	*(see estrogen—conjugated)*				
Prilosec	*(see omeprazole)*				
Primaxin	*(see imipenem)*				
Primidone (Mylepsin)	Anticonvulsant medication hepatically converted to phenobarbital	3–8 mg/kg PO q 8h; initially up to 16 mg/kg PO q 8h (adjust based on serum phenobarbital levels)		Causes PU/PD/PP, sedation, and ataxia. Often hepatotoxic with prolonged use. No benefit over phenobarbital; no longer recommended	50, 250 mg T; 50 mg/ml S HM
Primor	*(see sulfadimethoxine/ormetoprim)*				
Prinivil	*(see lisinopril)*				
Pro-Banthine	*(see propantheline)*				
Procainamide (Pronestyl SR, Procan-SR)	Ventricular arrhythmias	6–20 mg/kg IV slowly over 30 minutes, then IV CRI 0.02–0.04 mg/kg/min (20–40 µg/kg/min) if life threatening; 6–20 mg/kg IM, q 4h, or 6–20 mg/kg PO, q 6h	1–2 mg/kg bolus IV; then 0.01–0.02 mg/kg/min (10–20 µg/kg/min) IV CRI	Available as sustained release tablet for q 8h administration (absorption questionable); this is a negative inotrope; use serum levels for long-term dosing adjustments (optimum: 3–20 µg/ml); may cause hypotension, tachycardia, and ECG changes; dermatologic side effects	100, 500 mg/ml I; 250, 375, 500 mg C, T; 250, 500, 750, 1000 mg ER C, T HM
ProcalAmine	*(see amino acid solution 3% and glycerin injection with electrolytes)*				
Procan-SR	*(see procainamide)*				
Prochlorperazine (Compazine)	Antiemetic	0.11–0.44 mg/kg SQ, IM, q 6–12h	Same	Sedation, hypotension, anticholinergic side effects (dry mouth, GI hypomotility); do not use in epileptic patients; available also in suppository formulation	5 mg/ml I; 1 mg/ml S; 5, 10, 25 mg T; 10, 15, 30 mg ER HM

TABLE VI-1 **Drug Formulary—(*Continued*)**

Generic Name (Trade Name)	Indications/ Drug Type	Canine Dose	Feline Dose	Comments	How the Drug Is Supplied
Procrit	*(see erythropoietin)*				
Proglycem	*(see diazoxide)*				
Prograf	*(see tacrolimus)*				
Program	*(see lufenuron)*				
ProHeart	*(see moxidectin)*				
PromAce	*(see acepromazine)*				
Pronestyl	*(see procainamide)*				
Propantheline (Pro-Banthine)	Anticholinergic agent used for treating diarrhea, bradycardia syndromes, and detrusor hyperreflexia	0.2–0.5 mg/kg PO, q 8–24h; increase to effect for bradycardia syndromes	Same	Tachycardia, dry mouth, constipation, mydriasis, ileus, urinary retention	7.5, 15 mg T HM
Propionibacterium acnes (Immuno-regulin)	Immune modulator/ potentiator	0.03–0.07 mg/kg IV at 2–3 day intervals	Total dose: 0.2 mg per cat IV, 1–2 times a week	No controlled studies	0.4 mg/ml I VM
Propofol (Diprivan, Rapinovet)	Ultrashort (5–7 minutes) acting anesthetic; no cumulative effect with repeated administration	3–6 mg/kg IV	Same	Give slowly over 1–2 mintues in equal dosages to effect; agent provides no analgesia: consider opiate premed and/ or inhalant anesthetic if minor (or other) surgical procedures	10 mg/ml I HM, VM
Propranolol (Inderal)	β-adrenergic blocking agent used for treating supraventricular arrhythmias, some ventricular arrhythmias, and feline hypertrophic cardiomyopathy	For acute tachycardias: 0.1–0.5 mg IV total dose per bolus; no more frequently than 1 bolus q 1–3 minutes to 5 mg maximum (largest dog); administer until the rate slows; chronic use: 0.2–1 mg/kg q 8–12h PO, usually start low and titrate dosage upward to effect	0.1–0.5 mg IV bolus slowly; 2.5–5.0 mg PO q 8–12h, begin low and titrate dosage	Anorexia, apnea, depression, ataxia; bradycardia, negative inotropic effect: potentiates AV nodal depression of digoxin and Ca channel blockers; underlying cause of tachycardia (e.g., heart failure, hypovolemia) must be addressed before IV propranolol	10, 20, 40, 60, 80, 90 mg T; 60, 80, 120, 160 mg ER; 4, 8, 80 mg/ml S; 1 mg/ml I HM
Propylthiouracil (PTU)	Feline hyper-thyroidism	Not used	10 mg/kg PO q 8–12h	Immune-mediated hemolytic anemia and thrombo-cytopenia; anorexia, vomiting, and lethargy; risk of adverse effects frequently outweighs potential benefit	50 mg T HM
Proscar	*(see finasteride)*				
Prostaglandin (PGF2-α, Lutalyse, Dinoprost)	1. Open-cervix pyometra 2. Abortive agent at 31–35 days	1. Day 1: 0.1 mg/kg SQ once; day 2: 0.2 mg/kg SQ once; days 3–7: 0.25 mg/kg SQ, q 24h 2. 0.1 mg/kg SQ, q 8h for 2 days, then 0.2 mg/kg SQ, q 8h for 3–7 days (or until fetuses are expelled)	1. 0.1 mg/kg SQ, q 12h for 5 days 2. 0.5–1 mg/kg SQ for 2 days	Panting, salivation, vomiting, diarrhea, colic, and tachycardia lasting about 30 minutes; should be given under hospital supervision	5 mg/ml I VM
Prostaphlin	*(see oxacillin)*				
Prostigmin	*(see neostigmine)*				
Protopam	*(see pralidoxime)*				
Protopic	*(see tacrolimus)*				

(Continued)

TABLE VI-1 **Drug Formulary—(*Continued*)**

Generic Name (Trade Name)	Indications/ Drug Type	Canine Dose	Feline Dose	Comments	How the Drug Is Supplied
Proventil	*(see albuterol)*				
Provera	*(see medroxyprogesterone acetate)*				
Prozac	*(see fluoxetine)*				
Prussian blue	*(see ferric cyanoferrate)*				
Pseudoephedrine (Sudafed, others)	Hormone-deficient urinary incontinence of bitches	0.2–0.4 mg/kg PO q 8–12h	—	Narrow window between therapeutic and toxic doses; use with caution if sympathetic drive could be harmful (heart disease, hypertension, hyperthyroidism, etc.) or if CNS abnormalities	30, 60, 120 mg T HM, OTC
Psyllium mucilloid (Metamucil)	Bulk laxative, stool softener	2–10 g PO, q 12–24h, in moistened food	2–4 g PO, q 12–24h, in moistened food	Titrate dose based on stool consistency; may also be used for treating fiber-responsive diarrhea	OTC, HM
PTU	*(see propylthiouracil)*				
Pyoben	*(see benzoyl peroxide)*				
Pyopen	*(see carbenicillin)*				
Pyrantel pamoate (Nemex, Pyr-A-Pam, Strongid-T)	Roundworm and hookworm anthelmintic	5–10 mg/kg PO	10 mg/kg PO	Repeat in 3 weeks; safe at recommended dosages including in dogs with heartworms	22.7, 113.5 mg T; 2.27, 4.54, 50 mg/ml S VM
Pyr-A-Pam	*(see pyrantel pamoate)*				
Pyridostigmine bromide (Mestinon)	Anticholinesterase agent used for treating myasthenia gravis	0.2–2 mg/kg PO q 8–12h	0.25 mg/kg PO maximum of once daily	Available as soft tablet and syrup (60 mg/5 ml); vomiting, diarrhea, salivation, and weakness may develop	60 mg T; 180 mg ER; 12 mg/ml S; 5 mg/ml I HM
Pyrimethamine (Daraprim)	Folic acid antagonist, toxoplasmosis, neosporosis	0.5–1 mg/kg PO, q 24h, for 48 hours; then 0.25 mg/kg PO, q 24h, for 14 days	Same	Often used with sulfonamides to treat toxoplasmosis; bone marrow suppression due to folate deficiency; may need to supplement with folic or folinic acid; teratogenic	25 mg T HM
PZI	*(see insulin)*				
Quibron	Bronchodilator-expectorant; combination of theophylline and guaifenesin	One capsule PO, q 8–12h, in large breeds only	Not recommended	Hyperexcitability, vomiting	150, 300 mg C; 300 mg T; 300 mg ER HM
Quinacrine (Atabrine)	Giardiasis, enteric coccidiosis	10 mg/kg PO q 24h for 5–12 days	11 mg/kg PO q 24h, for 5 days	May cause enteric signs; considered second line agent	100 mg T HM
Quinaglute	*(see quinidine)*				
Quinidex	*(see quinidine)*				
Quinidine (Quinaglute, Quinidex)	Type Ia antiarrhythmic agent; used mostly for ventricular dysrhythmias; conversion of acute-onset atrial fibrillation	6–20 mg/kg PO, IM, q 6–8h	Not recommended	Do not give IV or use with Digitalis; negative inotropic agent; available in long-acting tablet forms	100, 200, 300 mg T; 275, 300, 330 mg ER; 80 mg/ml I HM

TABLE VI-1 **Drug Formulary—(*Continued*)**

Generic Name (Trade Name)	Indications/ Drug Type	Canine Dose	Feline Dose	Comments	How the Drug Is Supplied
Radiogardase	*(see ferric cyanoferrate)*				
Ramipril (Altace)	ACE inhibitor	0.125 mg/kg PO q 12h	—	Clinical VM use still new at time of this writing; efficacy and adverse effects sparsely reported	1.25, 2.5, 5, 10 mg C HM
Ranitidine HCl (Zantac)	H_2 histamine receptor antagonist; promotility agent (e.g., cats with constipation)	1–2 mg/kg PO, SQ, IM, slow IV, q 8–12h	Same	GI prokinetic effects due to anti-cholinesterase activity; slow IV (bolus may cause immediate vomiting)	75, 150, 300 mg T; 15 mg/ml S; 25 mg/ml I HM
Rapinovet	*(see propofol)*				
Reglan	*(see metoclopramide)*				
Requa	*(see activated charcoal)*				
Retrovir	*(see azidothymidine)*				
ReVia	*(see naltrexone)*				
Revolution	*(see selamectin)*				
Rheomacrodex	*(see dextran)*				
r-Hu-EPO	*(see erythropoietin)*				
Rifadin	*(see rifampin)*				
Rifampin (Rifadin)	Antimycobacterial antibacterial agent	5–10 mg/kg PO, IV q 12–24h	5–10 mg/kg PO, IV q 24h	A part of protocols with other anti-infectives for better efficacy, less resistance	150, 300 mg T; 600 mg I HM
Rimadyl	*(see carprofen)*				
Rintal	*(see febantel)*				
Ripercol	*(see levamisole)*				
Robamox-V	*(see amoxicillin)*				
Robaxin	*(see methocarbamol)*				
Robinul	*(see glycopyrrolate)*				
Roferon	*(see interferon)*				
Romazicon	*(see flumazenil)*				
Rompun	*(see xylazine)*				
Rotenone (topical ointment)	*(see Goodwinol)*				
RU-486	*(see mifepristone)*				
Rutin	Chylothorax; benzopyrone recommended for treatment of chylous pleural effusion; reportedly potentiates macrophage function	—	50 mg/kg PO q 8h; total dose 250 mg PO q 8h, per cat or 500 mg PO q 12h, per cat	Generally purchased in health food stores	500 mg T OTC
s-adenosyl methionine	*(see methionine, s-adenosyl)*				
Salix	*(see furosemide)*				
Salbutamol	*(see albuterol)*				
Salmeterol (Serevent)	Inhaled long-acting β-2 agonist bronchodilator	One puff PRN, q 12–24h	Same	Takes >1 hour to take effect	6.5, 13 g inhalation canisters (0.025 mg [25 μg] per puff) HM
SAMe	*(see methionine, s-adenosyl)*				
Sandimmune	*(see cyclosporine—systemic)*				
Sandostatin	*(see octreotide)*				
Scolaban	*(see bunamidine)*				

(*Continued*)

TABLE VI-1 **Drug Formulary—(*Continued*)**

Generic Name (Trade Name)	Indications/ Drug Type	Canine Dose	Feline Dose	Comments	How the Drug Is Supplied
Selamectin (Revolution)	Endectocide: topical for fleas, ticks, ear mites, heartworm prevention, sarcoptic mange, intestinal hookworms, and roundworms	Approximately 6 mg/kg topically according to dosage on packaging; one application per month	Same	Use in dogs or cats over 6 weeks old; for heartworm prevention: give within 1 month of first exposure to mosquitos and continue until within 1 month of last exposure	Prepackaged doses (topical liquid in plastic ampules) VM
Selegiline (deprenyl, Anipryl, Eldepryl)	Restores central dopamine levels: MAO inhibitor; used for treating cognitive dysfunction syndrome; may be helpful in selected PDH canine Cushing's cases	PDH: 1 mg/kg PO per day for 30 days, then may increase dosage to 2 mg/kg per day if no response; CDS: 0.5 mg/kg daily; may double dose after 1 month if ineffective	Not recommended	Low level of effectiveness reported; not to be used with other MAO inhibitors (e.g., antidepressants, amitraz)	2, 5, 10, 15, 30 mg T, VM; 5 mg C,T HM
Septra	*(see trimethoprim/ sulfamethoxazole)*				
Serax	*(see oxazepam)*				
Serevent	*(see salmeterol)*				
Sildenafil (Viagra)	Pulmonary hypertension	0.5–1 mg/kg PO q 8h	—	Dosage extrapolated from human pulmonary hypetension use; efficacy, correct dosing, adverse effects, and other factors unproven for dogs	25, 50, 100 mg T HM
Silvadene cream	*(see silver sulfadiazine)*				
Silver sulfadiazine (Silvadene cream)	Topical anti-infective preparation for complications of burns	Apply to burn area q 12h as necessary	Same	Hypersensitivity to sulfonamides; KCS; Dobermans	10 mg/g O HM
Simplicef	*(see cefpodoxime)*				
Sinequan	*(see doxepin)*				
Slo-Bid	*(see theophylline, sustained action)*				
Sodium bicarbonate	Metabolic acidosis, urine alkalinization (e.g., intoxication)	mEq/day = (desired serum [HCO_3] − present serum [HCO_3]) × 0.3 × BW (kilograms); administer 50% over 15 minutes and recheck serum levels; then give the balance over 24 hours	Same	Alkalosis, hypernatremia, CHF, hypokalemia; correct inciting factors concurrently (or prior to HCO_3 Tx); 84 mg $NaHCO_3$ contains 1 mEq HCO_3	0.6, 1 mEq/ml I; 5, 10 grain T HM
Sodium iodide 10%	Sporotrichosis	15 mg/kg PO q 8h; some higher doses reported	Same	Monitor for iodinism: fever, ptyalism, GI signs; contains 0.1 mg iodine/ml	10% I VM
Sodium stibolgluconate (Pentostam)	Leishmaniasis	30–50 mg/kg SQ, IV, q 24h, or 10–20 mg/kg IM, q 24h, for 20–28 days	—	Not available in United States except through the Centers for Disease Control and Prevention	100 ml vials (100 mg/ml) I HM
Solganal	*(see aurothioglucose)*				
Soloxine	*(see levothyroxine sodium)*				

TABLE VI-1 **Drug Formulary—(*Continued*)**

Generic Name (Trade Name)	Indications/ Drug Type	Canine Dose	Feline Dose	Comments	How the Drug Is Supplied
Solu-Delta-Cortef	*(see prednisolone sodium succinate)*				
Solu-Medrol	*(see methylprednisolone sodium succinate)*				
Soriatane	*(see acitretin)*				
Sotalol (Betapace)	Classes II and III antiarrhythmic agent; used primarily for treating ventricular tachyarrhythmias	1–6.6 mg/kg PO q 12h	Total dose: 10–40 mg PO, q 12h, per cat; very little published experience with drug in cats	β-blocking effects seen at low dosages; type III effects at higher levels; begin low and titrate upwards to effect	80, 120, 160, 240 mg T HM
Spironolactone (Aldactone)	Potassium-sparing diuretic; inhibits aldosterone	1–4 mg/kg PO q 12–24h	Same	Usually used with other diuretic agents; monitor potassium (hyperkalemia); used with ACEI agents usually once per day and at low dose Spironolactone with hydrochlorothiazide is a 1:1 combination of the two drugs (brand names for the combined product include Aldactazide and Spirozide)	25, 50, 100 mg T HM
Sporanox	*(see itraconazole)*				
Spot-On	*(see fenthion)*				
Stadol	*(see butorphanol)*				
Stanozolol (Winstrol)	Anabolic steroid used for treating anorexia, debilitation, and anemia	0.1–0.2 mg/kg PO q 12–24h; total dose: 25–50 mg IM weekly per dog	0.1–0.2 mg/kg PO q 24h to q 12h; total dose: 12.5–25 mg IM weekly per cat	Contraindicated in pregnancy; hepatotoxicity in cats; controlled drug	2 mg T; 50 mg/ml I VM, HM
Stilbogluconate	*(see sodium stilbogluconate)*				
Stoxil	*(see idoxuridine)*				
Streptase	*(see streptokinase)*				
Streptokinase (Kabikinase, Streptase)	Thrombolytic drug; arterial or pulmonary thromboembolism	90,000 IU/kg IV over 30 minutes, then 45,000 IU/kg per hour for 7–12 hours based on response	Same	Bleeding diathesis; hyperkalemia from reperfusion; intracardiac thrombus is an absolute contraindication; complications cancel benefits in feline aortic thromboemboli	250,000, 600,000, 750,000, 1.5 million U vials I HM
Streptozotocin (streptozocin, Zanosar)	Insulinoma chemotherapy	500 mg/m^2 infusion preceded and followed by extensive IV fluid diuresis	—	Nephrotoxicity, hepatotoxicity, BM suppression	1g I HM
Strongid-T	*(see pyrantel pamoate)*				
Succimer (*meso*-2,3 dimercaptosuccinic acid, Chemet)	Lead toxicity chelating agent	10 mg/kg PO, q 8h, for 10–17 days	Same	May need second course of therapy; accesses intracellular sites, including CNS vomiting, sulfurous odor of breath	100 mg C HM
Sucralfate (Carafate)	Complexes with proteinaceous materials in stomach, thereby preventing undesirable effects of acids on the gastric mucosa	Total dose: 1/4–1 tab PO, q 6–8h, per dog	Total dose: 1/4 tab PO, q 6–12h, per cat	May constipate; interferes with absorption of many drugs administered concurrently	1 g T, 100 mg/ml S HM
Sudafed	*(see pseudoephedrine)*				

(*Continued*)

TABLE VI-1 **Drug Formulary—(*Continued*)**

Generic Name (Trade Name)	Indications/ Drug Type	Canine Dose	Feline Dose	Comments	How the Drug Is Supplied
Sulfadiazine (Sulfadyne)	Bacteriostatic agent used for treating the following: 1. Toxoplasmosis and nocardiosis 2. Soft tissue/UTIs	1. 80 mg/kg PO q 8h 2. 30 mg/kg PO q 24h	Same	Sulfonamide precautions, KCS, idiosyncratic toxicities, Dobermans	500 mg T VM, HM
Sulfadiazine/ trimethoprim	*(see trimethoprim/ sulfadiazine)*				
Sulfadimethoxine (Bactrovet, Albon)	Bacteriostatic agent used for treating toxoplasmosis, nocardiosis, and coccidiosis	50 mg/kg PO day 1; then 25 mg/kg PO q 24h	Same	KCS, nephrotoxicity, and hypersensitivity	400 mg/ml I; 125, 250, 500 mg T; 50, 125 mg/ml S VM, HM
Sulfadimethoxine/ ormetroprim (Primor)	Potentiated sulfonamide	27–55 mg/kg PO q 24h on day 1; then 13.5–27.5 mg/kg q 24h thereafter for a maximum of 21 days	None	Sulfonamide contraindications	120, 240, 600, 1200 mg T VM
Sulfadyne	*(see sulfadiazine)*				
Sulfamethoxazole/ trimethoprim	*(see trimethoprim/ sulfamethoxazole)*				
Sulfasalazine (Azulfidine)	Anti-inflammatory effect on the colon; ulcerative and idiopathic colitis	22–55 mg/kg PO q 8h	10–20 mg/kg PO, q 12h, 3–5 days	Avoid prolonged treatment; KCS; blood dyscrasias, vomiting; caution in cats: salicylate component could be toxic	500 mg T HM
Sulfodip	*(see lime sulfur solution)*				
Surfak	*(see dioctyl sodium sulfosuccinate)*				
Surital	*(see thiamylal Na)*				
Symmetrel	*(see amantadine)*				
Synotic	*(see fluocinolone 0.01% with 60% DMSO)*				
Synthroid	*(see levothyroxine sodium)*				
Syntocinon	*(see oxytocin)*				
Syprine	*(see trientene)*				
Tacrolimus (Prograf, Protopic)	Immune-mediated hemolytic anemia and other autoimmune disorders; topical: atopy, perianal fistula	0.16 mg/kg IM, q 24h; 1 mg/kg PO q 24h	—	Sparsely reported use at the time of this writing; narrow therapeutic-toxic range, with frequent negative side effects; these doses are associated with adverse effects, so titrate to keep trough serum level 0.1–0.4 ng/ml (dogs); vasculitis, anorexia, intussusception; wear gloves when applying topical formulation	1 mg, 5 mg T; 5 mg/ml, I; 0.3% lotion HM
Tadalafil (Cialis)	Longer-acting phosphodiesterase inhibitor; pulmonary hypertension	1 mg/kg PO q 48h	—	Very new drug; investigational and unsupported use in veterinary medicine at this time; case report and anecdotal descriptions of benefit, but side-effects poorly documented	5, 10, 20 mg T HM

TABLE VI-1 **Drug Formulary—*(Continued)***

Generic Name (Trade Name)	Indications/ Drug Type	Canine Dose	Feline Dose	Comments	How the Drug Is Supplied
Tagamet	*(see cimetidine)*				
Talwin	*(see pentazocine)*				
Tapazole	*(see methimazole)*				
Task	*(see dichlorvos)*				
Taurine	Feline DCM; canine DCM in American cocker spaniels, retriever breeds, many others; retinopathy	50 mg/kg PO q 8h, or total dose 500–1000 mg PO, q 12h, per dog	Total dose: 125–250 mg PO, q 12h, per cat	Switch to taurine-enriched diet if relevant (many are already on balanced diet)	250 mg T OTC, HM
Tavist	*(see clemastine fumarate)*				
Tegison	*(see etretinate)*				
Telazol	*(see tiletamine—zolazepam)*				
Telmintic	*(see mebendazole)*				
Temaril-P	*(see trimeprazine)*				
Tempra	*(see acetaminophen)*				
Tenormin	*(see atenolol)*				
Tensilon	*(see edrophonium Cl)*				
Tepoxalin (Zubrin)	NSAID (broad-spectrum COX and leukotrienes)	10 mg/kg PO q 24h	—	Gastritis, diarrhea, hepatopathy, renal effects	30, 50, 100, 200 mg T VM
Terbutaline (Brethine)	Bronchodilator via specific β-2 stimulation	Total dose: 0.625–5 mg PO, q 8–12h, per dog	Total dose: 0.625–1.25 mg PO, q 12h, per cat	Excitability, vomiting, tachycardia	2.5, 5 mg T; 1 mg/ml I HM
Terramycin	*(see oxytetracycline)*				
Testosterone	Testosterone responsive incontinence in male dogs and cats	2.2 mg/kg IM, monthly	Total dose: 5–10 mg IM, per cat	Hepatopathy; behavioral changes; controlled drug	25, 50, 100, 200 mg/ml I HM
Tetracycline	Broad-spectrum antibiotic; bacteriostatic; used especially for *Brucella*, *Chlamydia*, *Leptospira*, *Mycoplasma*, and *Rickettsia*; used for pleurodesis; used with niacinamide for autoimmune dermatopathies; used as an ophthalmic ointment	10–22 mg/kg q 8h PO for 3 weeks; pleurodesis: 20 mg/kg in 4 ml saline/kg intrapleural; ophthalmic ointment: apply q 6–8h	Same	Fever, vomiting, diarrhea, photosensitivity; do not administer with dairy products, antacids, intestinal adsorbents; do not give in last 3 weeks of pregnancy or to newborns/pediatric animals; cats more sensitive to adverse effects	100, 250, 500 mg T/C; 25 mg/ml S; 250, 500 mg/vial I; 10 mg/g OO; 10 mg/ml OS HM, VM
Theo-Dur	*(see theophylline, sustained action)*				
Theophylline elixir (Elixophyllin)	Bronchodilator	6–11 mg/kg PO q 8h	Rarely used: 8 mg/kg PO q 12h	*(see aminophylline)*; restlessness, vomiting	16 mg/ml S HM
Theophylline, sustained action (Slo-Bid, Theo-Dur)	Long-acting bronchodilator	5–15 mg/kg PO q 12–24h	Same but infrequently utilized (adverse effects)	Hyperexcitability common; nausea or vomiting: stop drug	100, 200, 300 mg ER HM
Thiabendazole (Mintezol)	Aspergillosis, penicilliosis, *Filaroides* (*Oslerus*), and feline eosinophilic granuloma complex; topical: ear mites, dermatophytes	50 mg/kg PO, q 24h, for 3 days, repeat in 1 month	5–10 mg/kg PO, q 24h, three times weekly	Not licensed for feline use; dachshunds uniquely sensitive	500 mg T; 100 mg/ml S VM

(Continued)

TABLE VI-1 **Drug Formulary—(*Continued*)**

Generic Name (Trade Name)	Indications/ Drug Type	Canine Dose	Feline Dose	Comments	How the Drug Is Supplied
Thiacetarsamide (Caparsolate)	Heartworm adulticide; hemobartonellosis (*Mycoplasma felis*)	2.2 mg/kg q 12h, slow IV for four doses	1.1–2.2 mg/kg q 12h, slow IV for four doses; often not recommended	Largely replaced by melarsomine; vomiting, depression, hepatotoxicity (icterus), nephrotoxicity; thromboembolic phenomena 7–28 days post-Rx; perivenous injection causes sloughing; acute pulmonary edema in cats	10 mg/ml I VM
Thiamine (vitamin B_1)	Thiamine deficiency; lead poisoning	Total dose: 10–100 mg IM, IV, PO, q 12h, per dog	Total dose: 50 mg IM, IV, PO, q 12h, per cat	Stings IM	100, 200 mg/ml I; 5, 10, 25, 50, 100, 250, 500 mg T; HM
Thiamylal Na (Surital)	Ultrashort-acting barbiturate anesthetic	11–17.5 mg/kg IV titrated to induction of anesthesia	Same	(*see thiopental*)	Not available currently; may return to the market; 1, 5, 10 g vials I
Thioguanine	Antineoplastic, acute leukemias	40 mg/m² PO, q 24h, for 4–5 days, then every 3 days	25 mg/m² PO, q 24h, for 1–5 days, then every 30 days	Bone marrow, GI, hepatic adverse effects possible	40 mg T HM
Thiopental sodium (Pentothal)	Ultrashort-acting anesthetic (similar to thiamylal Na)	13–26 mg/kg IV titrated to induction of anesthesia	Same	Respiratory and cardiac depression; avoid perivenous administration; ventricular bigeminy common; sight hounds more sensitive	1, 2.5, 5 g vials I HM
Thorazine	(*see chlorpromazine*)				
Thytropar	(*see thyrotropin TSH*)				
Thyrotropin TSH (thyroid-stimulating hormone, Dermathycin, Thytropar)	Hormone used for diagnosis of hypothyroidism	Total doses: 5 U per dog to 10 kg IV, IM, SQ; 10 U per dog over 10 kg IV, IM, SQ	Total dose: 2.5 U per cat IM or IV	Follow protocol for testing: preinjection and 6 hours post-IM or post-IV injection	5, 10 U/vial I VM, HM
Thyroxine	(*see levothyroxine sodium*)				
Ticarcillin—clavulanate (Timentin)	Broad-spectrum penicillin-clavulanic acid combination	50–100 mg/kg slow IV, q 8h	40–50 mg/kg IM or slow IV, q 6–8h	GI upset	3 g vials I HM
Tiletamine—zolazepam (Telazol)	Tranquilizer, dissociative anesthetic combination agent; used for chemical restraint or minor surgical procedures	5–12 mg/kg IM	Same	Rapid onset; respiratory depression may occur quickly (be prepared for intubation); controlled drug	100 mg/ml combined (50 mg each per ml) I VM
Tigan	(*see trimethobenzamide*)				
Timentin	(*see ticarcillin-clavulanate*)				
Timolol solution (Timoptic)	β-blocking topical agent used for decreasing intraocular pressures due to glaucoma	One drop in eye, q 12h	Same	Potentiation of β-blocking effects possible (asthmatics, cardiac patients); avoid 0.25% solution (ineffective); often used in combination with other glaucoma drugs (weak action)	0.25, 0.5% OS HM
Timoptic	(*see timolol solution*)				
Titralac	(*see calcium carbonate*)				

TABLE VI-1 **Drug Formulary—(*Continued*)**

Generic Name (Trade Name)	Indications/ Drug Type	Canine Dose	Feline Dose	Comments	How the Drug Is Supplied
Tocainide (Tonocard)	Class Ib antiarrhythmic agent for ventricular tachyarrhythmias	15–20 mg/kg q 8–12h PO	—	Anorexia, GI signs, weakness, head bobbing, other CNS effects possible (lidocaine-like), corneal dystrophy; possibly adverse renal effects; may need to use with other class Ia drugs for maximum effect	400, 600 mg T HM
Tocopherol	*(see vitamin E)*				
Tofranil	*(see imipramine)*				
Tolfedine	*(see tolfenamic acid)*				
Tolfenamic acid (Tolfedine)	Oral/injectable NSAID	4 mg/kg SC or IM once, then PO, q 24h, for 2–4 days; may continue oral regimen 3–5 consecutive days per week	4 mg/kg SC or IM once, then PO, q 24h, for 2–4 days	Approved for veterinary use in Canada and Europe but not in the United States	6, 30, 60 mg T; 40 mg/ml I VM
Tonocard	*(see tocainide)*				
Toprol-XL	*(see metoprolol)*				
Torbugesic	*(see butorphanol)*				
Torbutrol	*(see butorphanol)*				
Tramadol (Ultram)	Analgesia; orally active opiate (mu-receptor agonist)	1–4 mg/kg PO q 8–12h	1–2 mg/kg PO q 12h	New agent; clinical efficacy and safety profile still incomplete; Tramacet, Ultracet are tramadol + acetaminophen (do not use in cats); partial antagonism possible with naloxone	50 mg T HM
Tramisol	*(see levamisole)*				
Tranxene	*(see clorazepate)*				
Trental	*(see pentoxifylline)*				
Tresaderm	Otitis externa with allergic/bacterial/ fungal component(s)	2–12 drops per ear; (proportional to size of ear), q 12h	Two drops per ear, q 12h	Combination neomycin + thiabendazole + triamcinolone; corticosteroid is absorbed systemically; avoid prolonged daily use	Neomycin 0.25% + thiabendazole 4% + triamcinolone 0.1% otic VM
Triamcinolone (Vetalog, Kenalog)	Intermediate-acting corticosteroid used PO; by injection IM, SQ, or intralesional	0.1–0.22 mg/kg IM, SQ, PO	Same	Corticosteroid effects	0.5, 1.5 mg T; 2, 6 mg/ml I HM, VM
Tribrissen	*(see trimethoprim/ sulfadiazine)*				
Trientine (Syprine)	Alternative to penicillamine to chelate copper	10–15 mg/kg PO q 12h	—	See penicillamine	250 mg C HM
Trifluridine (Viroptic)	Antiherpetic viral agent	—	At least two to four times daily in eyes	—	1% OS
Triiodothyronine (T3, Cytomel, Cytobin, Liothyronine)	Hypothyroidism; used when patient is unable to convert thyroxine to triiodothyroxine; also diagnostically as T3 suppression test	0.004–0.006 mg/kg (4–6 µg/kg) PO q 8h	0.0044 mg/kg (4.4 µg/kg) PO q 8–12h; T3 suppression: 0.025 mg (25 µg) total per cat dose PO, q 8h for seven doses, then blood for T4 and T3 (control)	Thyrotoxicosis, PU/PD, polyphagia, nervousness, panting, tachycardia	5, 25, 50 µg T

(Continued)

TABLE VI-1 **Drug Formulary—(*Continued*)**

Generic Name (Trade Name)	Indications/ Drug Type	Canine Dose	Feline Dose	Comments	How the Drug Is Supplied
Trilostane (Vetoryl)	Steroid analog (competitive inhibitor of 3β-hydroxysteroid dehydrogenase); treatment for pituitary-dependent hyperadrenocorticism	Dogs <5 kg: 30 mg PO q 24h. Dogs ≥5 kg: 60 mg PO q 24h	—	Not approved for VM or human use in United States; adrenal necrosis possible; with long-term treatment, make adjustments in 20- or 30-mg increments as dictated by clinical response and ACTH stimulation testing	60, 120 mg T,C VM
Trimeprazine (Termaril-P, Vanectyl-P)	Anti-inflammatory antipruritic antitussive antihistamine agent; usually combined with prednisolone	Total dose: 1/2–2 tablets PO, q 12h, per dog to effect	Total dose: 1/4–1/2 tablet PO, q 12–24h, per cat to effect	Steroid effect; drowsiness; Temaril-P contains 5 mg trimeprazine 2 mg prednisolone per tablet	5 + 2 mg T; 3.7 mg + 1 mg C; 7.5 mg + 2 mg C VM
Trimethobenzamide (Tigan)	Antiemetic	3 mg/kg IM, PO q 8–12h	None	CNS reactions; hypersensitivity	100, 250 mg C; 100, 200 mg suppositories; 100 mg/ml I HM
Trimethoprim/ sulfadiazine (Tribrissen, Ditrim)	Potentiated sulfonamide; bactericidal broad-spectrum combination agent against G+ and G– bacteria, *Toxoplasma, Nocardia, Pneumocystis*	Routine infections: 15 mg/kg PO, SQ, IM, q 12h; toxoplasmosis: 30 mg/kg PO q 12h	Routine infections: 15 mg/kg PO, SQ, IM, q 12h; toxoplasmosis: 30 mg/kg PO q 12h	Cats: salivation; dogs: KCS syndrome; Dobermans: polyarthropathy; ITP; hepatotoxicity and blood dyscrasias have been reported	30, 120, 480, 960 mg T; 60 mg/ml S; 24, 48% I VM, HM
Trimethoprim/ sulfamethoxazole (Bactrim, Septra)	Same as for trimethoprim/ sulfadiazine	Same as for trimethoprim/ sulfadiazine	Same as for trimethoprim/ sulfadiazine	Same as for trimethoprim/ sulfadiazine	Same as for trimethoprim/ sulfadiazine
Tropicamide ophthalmic solution (Mydriacyl)	Anticholinergic mydriatic agent for eye examination	One drop 15 minutes prior to ophthalmic examination	Same	Causes mydriasis and photophobia; do not use in suspected cases of glaucoma	0.5, 1% OS HM
Trusopt	*(see dorzolamide)*				
Tumil-K	*(see potassium salts)*				
Tums	*(see calcium carbonate)*				
Tylan	*(see tylosin)*				
Tylenol	*(see acetaminophen)*				
Tylosin (Tylan)	Macrolide antibiotic used for treating colitis and small bowel bacterial overgrowth syndrome	5–10 mg/kg PO q 12h; may increase slowly to 40 mg/kg PO q 12h	5–10 mg/kg PO q 12h	Usually used as powder sprinkled on food; bitter taste	50, 200 mg/ml I; 3000 mg/5 ml P VM
Ultram	*(see tramadol)*				
Unique E	*(see vitamin E)*				
Urecholine	*(see bethanechol)*				
Urocit-K	*(see potassium citrate)*				
Uroeze	*(see ammonium chloride)*				
Ursodeoxycholic acid (ursodiol, Actigall)	Synthetic hydrophilic bile acid; suppresses hepatic secretion and synthesis of cholesterol; choleretic agent via solubilizing cholesterol (sludged bile) and increase in gallbladder contractions	10–15 mg/kg PO q 12–24h	7.5–15 mg/kg PO q 12–24h	Anecdotal reports of beneficial effects in sclerosing cholangitis and biliary cirrhosis; may induce diarrhea; contraindicated if gallbladder obstruction; minimal contribution (<10%) to endogenous measured serum bile acids level	300 mg C HM

TABLE VI-1 **Drug Formulary—(*Continued*)**

Generic Name (Trade Name)	Indications/ Drug Type	Canine Dose	Feline Dose	Comments	How the Drug Is Supplied
Ursodiol	*(see ursodeoxycholic acid)*				
Valacyclovir	Antiviral	—	Do not use	Severe bone marrow, renal, and hepatic toxicities common even at subtherapeutic doses	—
Valbazen	*(see albendazole)*				
Valium	*(see diazepam)*				
Valproic acid (Depakene, Depakote)	Seizures	60–100 mg/kg PO q 8h	Unknown	CNS depression, GI disturbances initially; hepatotoxicity with chronic use; considered third-line therapeutic drug	125, 250, 500 mg T; 250 mg C; 50 mg/ml S HM
Vancomycin (Vancocin)	Bactericidal glycopeptide antibacterial	10–20 mg/kg slow IV (30–60 minutes) q 6–12h for 7–10 days	—	Reserved for resistant *Staphylococcus, Enterococcus, Clostridium difficile,* especially when sepsis possible or present and when resistance to other agents is documented	500 mg, 1g, 5g I HM
Vanectyl-P	*(see trimeprazine)*				
Vantin	*(see cefpodoxime)*				
Vapona	*(see dichlorvos)*				
Vasopressin (vasopressin aqueous, Pitressin)	Diagnostic agent for central or nephrogenic diabetes insipidus; emerging application in cardiopulmonary cerebral resuscitation is not yet validated in clinical veterinary medicine	Diagnostic: 0.5 U/kg IM to maximum 5 U after 5% weight loss from water deprivation	Same	Not available as tannate in oil	20 U/ml I HM
Vasotec	*(see enalapril)*				
Velban	*(see vinblastine)*				
Veltrim	*(see clotrimazole)*				
Ventolin	*(see albuterol)*				
Verapamil (Calan, Covera, Isoptin, Verelan)	Ca channel-blocking agent used principally to treat supraventricular tachyarrhythmias	1–4.4 mg/kg PO q 8–12h; 0.05 mg/kg slowly IV; may repeat twice, 5–30 minutes between doses	Not recommended as oral Ca channel blocker for cardiomyopathy; *(see diltiazem instead)*	Not suggested for IV use clinically if structural heart disease or systemic illness (e.g., hypovolemia) present; negative inotropic agent; usually do not use with β-blockers; may cause heart block	40, 80, 120 mg T; 120, 180, 240, 360 mg ER; 2.5 mg/ml I HM
Verelan	*(see verapamil)*				
Versed	*(see midazolam)*				
Versenate	*(see calcium EDTA)*				
Veta-K1	*(see vitamin K_1)*				
Vetalar	*(see ketamine HCl)*				
Vetalog	*(see triamcinolone)*				
Vetmedin	*(see pimobendan)*				
Vetoryl	*(see trilostane)*				
Vetsulin	*(see insulin)*				

(*Continued*)

TABLE VI-1 **Drug Formulary—(*Continued*)**

Generic Name (Trade Name)	Indications/ Drug Type	Canine Dose	Feline Dose	Comments	How the Drug Is Supplied
Viagra	*(see sildenafil)*				
Vibramycin	*(see doxycycline)*				
Vidarabine (Vira-A)	Antiherpetic antiviral agent	—	Apply four to six times daily in eyes	—	3% OO HM
Vinblastine (Velban)	Vinca alkaloid used in cancer chemotherapy, esp. lymphoreticular and mast cell cancers; also ITP	2 mg/m^2 IV q 1-2 weeks, or 0.05-0.1 mg/kg IV weekly	Same	*(see vincristine)*	1 mg/ml I HM
Vincristine (Oncovin)	Vinca alkaloid (see vinblastine, above); used also for TVT	0.5 mg/m^2 IV weekly; TVT: 0.025 mg/kg IV weekly, maximum 1 mg per dose	Same	Perivascular irritant, leukopenia, constipation, local neuropathy (especially in cats)	1 mg/ml I HM
Viokase	*(see pancreatic enzymes)*				
Vira-A	*(see vidarabine)*				
Viroptic	*(see trifluridine)*				
Vitamin B_1	*(see thiamine)*				
Vitamin B_{12}	*(see cobalamin)*				
Vitamin E (tocopherol, Unique E)	Antioxidant; steatitis, discoid lupus, dermatitis	Total dose: 100–400 IU PO, q 24h, per dog	Total dose: 30 IU PO, q 24h, per cat	May use serum tocopherol levels to adjust dose	700 mg C HM
Vitamin K_1 (Phytonadione, Aqua-MEPHYTON, Mephyton, Veta-K1)	Coumarin, indanedione, diphacinone, brodifacoum, and other anticoagulant rodenticide intoxications and coagulopathy due to decreased levels of vitamin K-dependent clotting factors	Load with 2.5–3.3 mg/kg SQ multiple sites, then 1.1–3.3 mg/kg q 12h PO; do not give IV; for replacement therapy in chronic hepatopathies: 2.5 mg SQ, IM, or PO, q 12h, for 3–5 days, then once weekly	Same	Anaphylaxis risk if given IV; second generation anticoagulants usually require 3–4 weeks of therapy; use parenteral form if inhibited absorption (small gauge needle to minimize hematoma risk in rodenticide patients); hepatotoxicity risk with chronic use	5 mg T; 25 mg C; 2, 10 mg/ml I VM, HM
Volmax	*(see albuterol)*				
Warfarin (Coumadin)	Anticoagulant; inhibits vitamin K epoxide reductase, blocking activation of vitamin K-dependent factors	0.1–0.2 mg/kg PO q 24h, to maintain PT at 1.5–2 times the baseline	Total dose: 0.2–0.5 mg PO, q 24h, per cat for most cats	Fatal or nonfatal hemorrhage; widely variable interindividual effects requiring close monitoring	1, 2, 2.5, 3, 4, 5, 6, 7.5, 10 mg T; 2 mg/ml I HM
Winstrol	*(see stanozolol)*				
Wycillin	*(see penicillin G procaine)*				
Xalatan	*(see latanoprost)*				
Xanax	*(see alprazolam)*				
Xylazine (Rompun)	α-adrenergic agonist agent with sedation and analgesia of 15–30 minutes; emetic effect in cats	0.66–2.0 mg/kg IM; 0.66–1.1 mg/kg IV	Emetic agent: 0.44–1.1 mg/kg IM or IV	Many side effects include arrhythmias, transient second-degree AV block, hypotension, increased sensitization to catecholamines in halothane anesthesia; reversal with yohimbine	20 mg/ml I VM
Xylocaine	*(see lidocaine)*				
Yobine	*(see yohimbine)*				
Yohimbine (Yobine)	α-2 (xylazine) antagonist	0.1–0.25 mg/kg slow IV; 0.2–0.5 mg/kg IM, SQ	Same	Apprehension, salivation, tremors, excitability	2 mg/ml I VM
Yomesan	*(see niclosamide)*				

TABLE VI-1 **Drug Formulary—(*Continued*)**

Generic Name (Trade Name)	Indications/ Drug Type	Canine Dose	Feline Dose	Comments	How the Drug Is Supplied
Zafirlukast (Accolate)	Leukotriene receptor antagonist; feline asthma: not for acute attacks	—	Total dose: 5 mg per cat PO q 24h	New drug at time of this writing; very limited use in VM	10, 20 mg T HM
Zanosar	*(see streptozocin)*				
Zantac	*(see ranitidine)*				
Zeniquin	*(see marbofloxacin)*				
Zestril	*(see lisinopril)*				
Zidovudine	*(see azidothymidine)*				
Zinc oxide (Desitin)	Promotes healing of irritated or abraded skin	Apply a thin film q 12h	Same	GI effects and hemolytic anemia if chronically ingested	OTC, HM, O
Zinc sulfate, acetate, gluconate, or methionine	Zn responsive dermatoses; copper storage disease	5–10 mg/kg elemental Zn PO q 12h	7–10 mg/kg PO q 24h, for hepatic lipidosis	GI irritability: administer with food; Zn-induced hemolysis if plasma levels exceed 1000 mg/dl; blood Zn levels require special blood tubes (normal rubber caps contain Zn)	66, 100, 200, 220 mg T; 1 mg/ml I HM
Zinecard	*(see dexrazoxane)*				
Zithromax	*(see azithromycin)*				
Zofran	*(see ondansetron)*				
Zonisamide (Zonegran)	Sulfonamide-based compound; second- or third-line antiepileptic drug	10 mg/kg PO q 24h	—	Sulfa precautions; new agent with incompletely defined, evolving safety and efficacy profiles	100 mg C HM
Zosyn	*(see piperacillin + tazobactam)*				
Zubrin	*(see tepoxalin)*				
Zyloprim	*(see allopurinol)*				

Index

Bolded page numbers indicate principal textual treatment. Page numbers followed by (a), indicate algorithms; (b), boxes; (f), figures; (t), tables.

Sedation and Chemical Restraint in Small Animal Practice

Etienne Côté, DVM, DACVIM
Leigh Lamont, DVM, MS, DACVA

Disclaimer: The following drugs and applications are recommended based on published reports and clinical experience. Specific use must be guided by appropriate and reasonable precautions, preparation, and information on the part of the veterinarian using or advocating the use of these products. Descriptions of drug effects and parameters of usage are likely to vary from one patient to the next and the description of the drug characteristics listed here applies to patients that are otherwise healthy.

Acepromazine

Expected observable effect: tranquilization, ± hypotension. With encouragement, the animal should still be able to rise and walk but with obvious mental depression.

Dose and route (dog or cat): 0.025–0.05 mg/kg IV or 0.05–0.15 mg/kg IM or SQ (oral tablet dose is 5–10 times higher).

Pain control: none.

Time to desired effect of sedation: 2–3 minutes (IV), 5–15 minutes (IM or SQ), 10–20 minutes (oral).

Indications: tranquilization of otherwise healthy, young- to middle-aged dogs and cats.

Contraindications (relative): old age; hypotension; most heart diseases; most liver diseases; most renal diseases and other disorders in which arterial hypoperfusion could be deleterious.

Advantages: substantial, effective sedation/mental depression, effect is often prolonged.

Drawbacks: no analgesia, no antianxiety effects; highly variable/unpredictable duration and intensity of effect, especially in older or systemically ill patients. Rare manic/hyperaggressive reactions.

Expected duration of effect/recovery: 30 minutes to several hours.

Alternative: for milder sedation: butorphanol + either diazepam or midazolam (e.g., healthy but older dog or cat)—see below.

Notes and comments: seizure threshold-lowering effects are unproven.

Butorphanol

Expected observable effect: mild to moderate sedation. Does not cause immobilization, but prolongs the duration and degree of tolerance to restraint.

Dose and route (dog or cat): butorphanol 0.1–0.4 mg/kg IV or IM + acepromazine 0.025–0.05 mg/kg IV or IM. Butorphanol and acepromazine can be mixed in the same syringe for immediate use.

Pain control: mild.

Time to desired effect of sedation: <1 minute (IV), 10–15 minutes (IM).

Indications: sedation and immobilization for minimally painful procedures. Useful for very active or agitated young animals.

Contraindications: older animals (relative contraindication to acepromazine); hypovolemia, dehydration, hypotension, most heart diseases, marked acid-base imbalance, or other instances of systemic illness.

Advantages: prolonged sustained sedation; flexibility of IM or IV route.

Drawbacks: prolonged recovery period and interindividual variability of effect, especially with acepromazine.

Expected duration of effect/recovery: 20–30 minutes (IV use), variable up to hours (IM route).

Alternatives: for slightly greater sedation: butorphanol + diazepam/midazolam (e.g., healthy but older dog or cat)—see below. For greater sedation: add acepromazine 0.025–0.05 mg/kg IV or 0.05–0.15 mg/kg IM (e.g., healthy young dog or cat).

Notes and comments: acepromazine 0.05 mg/kg and glycopyrrolate 0.01 mg/kg are commonly added to create a preanesthetic combination ("B-A-G") for healthy dogs and cats.

Buprenorphine

Expected observable effect: prolonged mild to moderate sedation.

Dose and route (dog or cat): 0.005–0.02 mg/kg IV or IM. Alternatively, 0.01 mg/kg sublingually (transmucosal absorption) is possible in cats only.

Pain control: mild to moderate.

Time to desired effect of sedation: 15–30 minutes (longer to achieve peak analgesic effects). Clinical sedation may be apparent sooner when buprenorphine is combined with other sedatives/tranquilizers.

Indications: sedation and immobilization for minimally painful procedures. Useful for very active or agitated young animals.

Contraindications: older animals (relative contraindication to acepromazine); hypovolemia, dehydration, hypotension, most heart diseases, marked acid-base imbalance, or other instances of systemic illness.

Expected duration of effect/recovery: up to 6–8 hours.

Alternatives: for greater sedation (e.g., diagnostic imaging in a very agitated but stable puppy), add acepromazine 0.02–0.05 mg/kg (IM or IV).

Notes and comments: This is a long acting opioid and its effects are not easily reversed with naloxone. Buprenorphine is used frequently for postoperative analgesia due to the prolonged dosing interval that is required.

Butorphanol + diazepam (or butorphanol + midazolam)

Expected observable effect: The animal becomes quieter but remains responsive, and is less likely to feel mildly noxious stimuli or to struggle during manual restraint.

Dose and route (dog or cat): butorphanol 0.1–0.4 mg/kg IV or IM + either diazepam 0.1–0.2 mg/kg IV or midazolam 0.1–0.2 mg/mg IV or IM. Butorphanol can be combined in the same syringe with either diazepam or midazolam for immediate use.

Pain control: mild.

Time to desired effect of sedation: <1 minute (IV) or 5–15 minutes (IM).

Indications: mild sedation and analgesia. Examples: ultrasound exam or radiographs of very restless young animal or of mildly fractious cat.

Contraindications: liver disease (diazepam, midazolam); hypovolemia, dehydration, marked acid-base imbalance, or other instances of severe systemic illness.

Advantages: provides light sedation.

Drawbacks: IV administration (only diazepam); short duration of action.

Expected duration of effect/recovery: animals that are otherwise healthy generally remain able to ambulate with this protocol or regain the ability to do so within 15–20 minutes of administration (IV use).

Alternatives: for greater sedation: omit diazepam/midazolam and replace with medetomidine 0.01 mg/kg IM or IV, or omit butorphanol and replace with hydromorphone 0.1–0.2 mg/kg IM or IV, or add acepromazine 0.025–0.05 mg/kg IM or IV.

Notes and comments: midazolam historically was expensive but is now available as generic (cost is similar to diazepam).